**The authorized list of established names
for drugs in the United States of America**

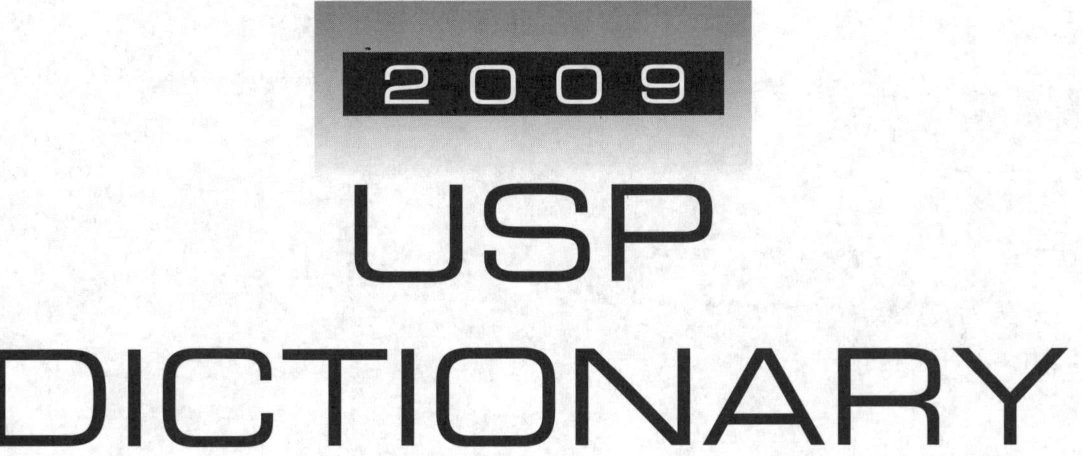

USP DICTIONARY

Of USAN and International Drug Names

**Published in accordance with the directions of the Expert Committee
on Nomenclature of the USP Council of Experts, with the cooperation of the
United States Adopted Names Council**

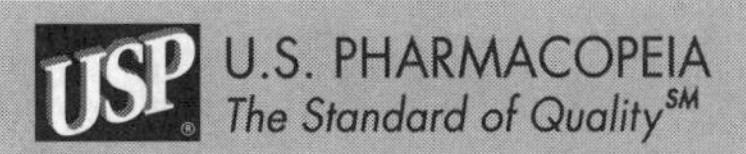

12601 Twinbrook Parkway
Rockville, MD 20852

"Interested persons, in the absence of the designation by the Food and Drug Administration of an official name, may rely on as the established name for any drug the current compendial name or the USAN adopted name listed in the *USAN and the USP Dictionary of Drug Names.*" [21 CFR299.4]

A compilation of the United States Adopted Names (USAN) selected and released from June 15, 1961, through January 31, 2009, current USP and NF names for drugs, and other nonproprietary drug names, the *USP Dictionary* incorporates the text previously published under the title *USAN and the USP Dictionary of Drug Names*.

Executive Vice President / Roger L. Williams

Library of Congress Catalog Card Number: sn 94001224
ISSN 1076-4275
ISBN 978-1-889788-78-4

Contents

For the most effective use of this book, the reader is urged to read the Preface and to consult the list of Abbreviations as needed. In addition, the following notes and examples are provided as pointers on how to use the book.

Each U.S. Adopted Name is shown in **boldface** type. The USAN entry typically includes:

1 U.S. Adopted Name (USAN)

2 Year of publication as a USAN, in brackets and italicized

3 Pronunciation guide

4 Designation of official compendium in which title occurs; e.g., boldface **USP** or **NF** if current, or specific edition in lightface type if not current

5 Molecular formula and weight

6 International nonproprietary name (INN)

7 Chemical name(s)

8 CAS registry number(s)

9 Other nonproprietary name(s)

10 Pharmacologic and/or therapeutic activity (italicized), based largely on representations from the sponsor of the USAN and subject to possible change as additional information becomes available

11 Brand name(s)

12 Name(s) of manufacturer(s) [a † symbol appears if the firm is no longer associated with the product]

13 Code designation(s) (italicized), preceded by the symbol ✧

14 Graphic formula

15 UNII Code

ILLUSTRATIVE USAN ENTRY

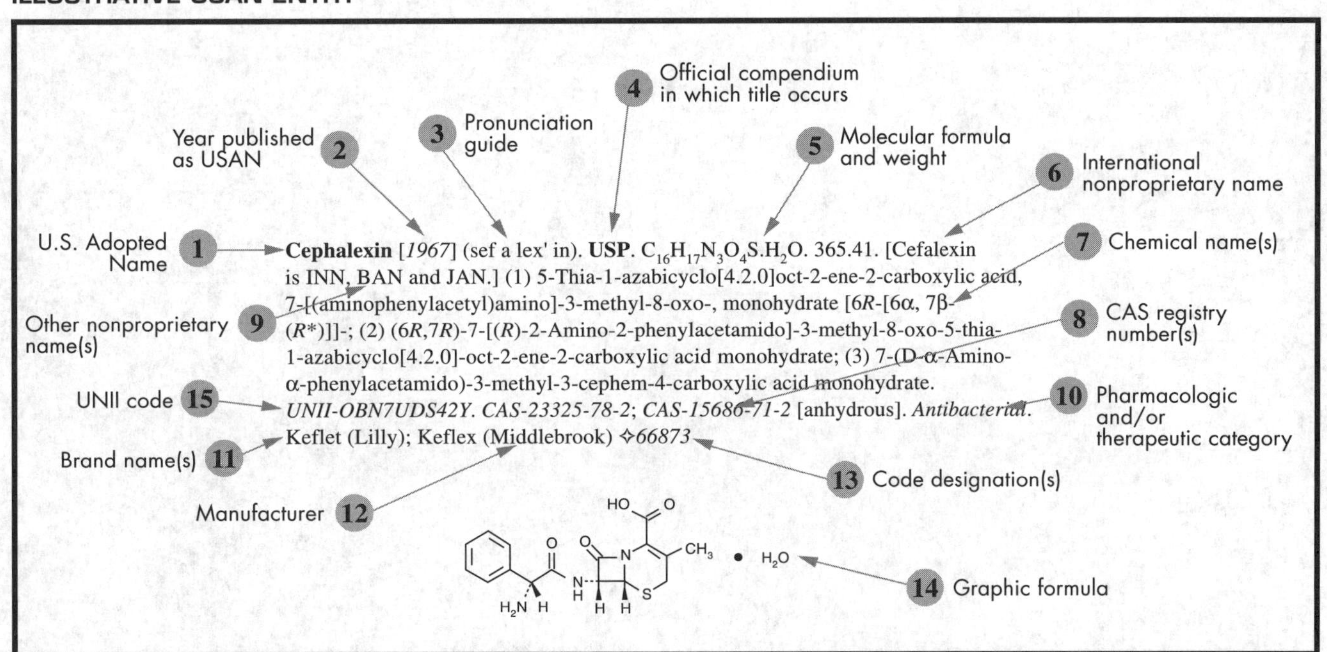

TYPES OF ENTRIES IN THE BOOK

USAN (in **boldface** type and accompanied by [date])

Current USP and NF titles followed by USP or NF (in **boldface** type)

International and other nonproprietary names

Brand names

Code designations

Cross-references

USAN APPENDICES

I Brand Names for USAN and Other Nonproprietary Names
II USAN and USP and NF Names Listed by Categories
III Molecular Formulas
IV Code Designations for USAN and Other Nonproprietary Names
V UNII Codes for USAN and Other Nonproprietary Names
VI CAS Registry Numbers and NSC Numbers
VII Guiding Principles for Coining U.S. Adopted Names for Drugs
VIII Guiding Principles for Coining U.S. Adopted Names for Contact Lens Materials
IX USAN Submission Forms

Preface

The text of this dictionary of nonproprietary names, brand names, code designations, and Chemical Abstracts Service registry numbers for drugs has been published continually since 1963 by the United States Pharmacopeial Convention, Inc. (USP), as a public service and particularly to support the United States Adopted Names (USAN) program which began in 1961. It is prepared under the aegis of the USP Nomenclature Expert Committee.

45th Edition

This Dictionary, now in its forty-fifth edition, is the annual compilation of United States Adopted Names (for which the abbreviation, USAN, generally is used). It is cumulative from June 15, 1961, when the U.S. Adopted Names program began. It incorporates the text of the publication previously known as *USAN and the USP Dictionary of Drug Names* and supersedes the 2008 edition and all earlier editions of the dictionary.

Supplements to the Dictionary are published bimonthly in the *Nomenclature* section of *Pharmacopeial Forum* (*PF*), USP's Journal of Standards Development and Official Compendia Revision. The new names and revisions of existing names in supplements are cumulatively included in the next published edition of the Dictionary.

The Federal Food and Drug Administration (FDA) has stated that interested persons may, in the absence of the designation of an official name, rely on *USAN and the USP Dictionary of Drug Names* (now known as the *USP Dictionary of USAN and International Drug Names*) for the established name for any drug in the U.S.A. (see *FDA Established Names*). The FDA has indicated also that it will not routinely designate official names and will do so only under certain specific conditions.

The USAN and the current compendial—*United States Pharmacopeia* (*USP*) and *National Formulary* (*NF*)—names are printed in **boldface** type. The International Nonproprietary Names (INN), British Approved Names (BAN) and Japanese Accepted Names (JAN), along with other miscellaneous names, appear in regular lightface type.

Included herein are 131 new U.S. Adopted Names released since publication of the previous edition of this book, as well as additions of other names for drugs. This edition reflects also hundreds of changes affecting information given in previously published entries.

The need for such compilations grows ever greater as the lists lengthen. The body of compounds in active use as drugs does not increase greatly, because new and better drugs tend to displace older drugs intended for the same purposes. On the other hand, new brand names may appear long after a drug is first marketed. The number of nonproprietary names increases steadily because, once assigned, a name remains on record and may not be reassigned even though the compound that it designates has been abandoned.

Although rarely done, a brand name may be recycled and applied to another drug. Notable, too, are changes in the ingredients of combination drug products, while retaining the same brand name.

This book lists 10,351 nonproprietary drug name entries. These entries contain more than 3,393 brand names; 4,846 code designations (including 399 NSC numbers); and more than 11,303 CAS registry numbers. There are 8,163 graphics depicted. The total number of USAN herein is 4,549.

All International Nonproprietary Names (INN) published by the World Health Organization from the start of the INN program in 1953 through 2008 are included in this book. Where an INN or other international name (BAN, JAN) exists for a drug that is covered by a **boldface** entry, the entry designates whether the INN, BAN, or JAN is the same as the corresponding USAN or *USP* or *NF* name or differs, in which case the difference is shown.

As is stated in this preface under *USAN Procedure*, there is increasing emphasis on the worldwide adoption of the same name for each therapeutic substance in view of the manifest advantages it offers to better communication and world trade. Thus the policy of including *all* INN in this Dictionary lends added perspective and serves to reinforce the aim for more uniformity.

Appendixes, which follow the main alphabetic list, are included on (I) brand names for USAN and other nonproprietary names; (II) USAN and USP and NF names listed by categories; (III) molecular formulas; (IV) code designations for USAN and other nonproprietary names; (V) UNII codes for USAN and other nonproprietary names; (VI) CAS registry numbers and NSC numbers; (VII) guiding principles for coining U.S. Adopted Names for drugs; (VIII) guiding principles for coining U.S. Adopted Names for contact lens materials; and (IX) USAN submission forms.

With respect to the legal status of trademarks cited as brand names herein, inquiries should be directed to the U.S. Patent Office.

The database of this Dictionary is maintained on a computer with storage and retrieval capabilities designed to facilitate future revisions and additions to the text as needed. Completeness and accuracy are of course paramount objectives in a compilation such as this. Suggestions of corrections or additions to the text will be welcomed for future consideration.

USP Nomenclature Expert Committee

A USP Drug Nomenclature Committee was established in 1985. The designation was changed subsequently to the USP Nomenclature Committee, the term Drug being removed when it became necessary for the Committee to address the nomenclature of articles other than drugs (e.g., dietary supplements and devices) that were introduced into the official compendia. The designation was changed again to the Expert Committee on Nomenclature and Labeling. The responsibility for labeling was added to reflect the close interdependence of nomenclature and labeling that had become evident. Requiring certain information via labeling can afford an opportunity to leave it out of an article's name itself. However, since nomenclature is the essence of the Expert Committee's work, the name was simplified to the Nomenclature Expert Committee for the 2005–2010 revision cycle.

In accordance with the Rules and Procedures of the 2005–2010 Council of Experts as adopted pursuant to the USP Bylaws, this Dictionary is prepared under the aegis of the USP Nomenclature Expert Committee for 2005–2010, which currently comprises:

Loyd V. Allen, Jr., Ph.D.
Mary B. Baker, Pharm.D.
Dawn M. Boothe, DVM, Ph.D.
Herbert S. Carlin, D.Sc.
Mrunal S. Chapekar, Ph.D.
Edward M. Cohen, Ph.D.
Stephanie Y. Crawford, Ph.D.
Everett Flanigan, Ph.D.
Thomas S. Foster, Pharm.D.
Michael J. Groves, Ph.D.
William M. Heller, Ph.D.
David F. Long, Ph.D.
Joan C. May, Ph.D.
Ginette A. Pepper, Ph.D., R.N.
Jerry Phillips, B.S., R.Ph.
Thomas P. Reinders, Pharm.D., *Chair*
Harold N. Rode, Ph.D.
Philip D. Walson, M.D.
Darin J. Weber, Ph.D.
Chao-Mei Yu, Ph.D.

The Nomenclature Expert Committee is responsible for promoting uniformity and consistency among official titles in the *USP* and the *NF*, coining suitable titles where such are needed because of the lack of public (nonproprietary) names or to improve the names already in use. The titles are designed to be in harmony with convenience in prescribing and with accepted tenets of general usage and are intended to be simple, useful, and clearly distinguishing and differentiating. The Nomenclature Expert Committee also determines the parameters of content, format, and style of the information contained in the Dictionary, and receives and rules upon all questions and appeals for reconsideration of text prepared by USP staff and appearing in the Dictionary. These responsibilities of the Nomenclature Expert Committee represent no change from the responsibilities relative to drug nomenclature that have resided with the Pharmacopeia since its founding in 1820. The appointment of the Nomenclature Expert Committee in no way alters the way in which the USP organization as a co-sponsor of the USAN Program, or the USP Council of Experts, works closely and cordially with the USAN Council. Indeed, the Nomenclature Expert Committee is concerned with several areas not within the scope of the USAN Council, e.g., nomenclature for dosage form monographs, applying the established policy of using the same terminology in both the monograph title and the strength expression for the article. The Expert Committee likewise deals with other aspects of the language used in the prescription, dispensing, sale, or manufacture of drugs.

The Nomenclature Expert Committee is supported by the U.S. Pharmacopeia. Andrzej Wilk, Ph.D., is the USP Department of Healthcare Quality and Information's liaison to the Nomenclature Expert Committee.

USAN Council

The three organizations that sponsor the USAN Program, i.e., the American Medical Association, the American Pharmacists Association, and the U.S. Pharmacopeia, do so through representation on the USAN Council. Members are appointed by their sponsors, subject to acceptance by the other sponsors. In addition, the three organizations jointly select a member-at-large. Members are appointed for one-year terms and may serve no more than ten consecutive terms.

In 1967, negotiations were completed to provide for participation by the U.S. Food and Drug Administration in the program as a means of consolidating the work of selecting suitable nonproprietary names for drugs on the part of the federal government and the existing Council. Thus, a liaison representative of the FDA sits on the Council. The roster of the Council for 2008, with member appointment or designation shown parenthetically, includes:

John Bergen, Ph.D. (Member-at-Large)
David Lewis, Ph.D., (FDA)
Anthony Palmieri III, Ph.D. (APhA), *Chair*
Peter Rheinstein, M.D., J.D. (AMA)
Darin J. Weber, Ph.D. (USP)

The USAN Council was formed January 2, 1964, to succeed the AMA–USP Nomenclature Committee. It works mainly by correspondence and e-mail, although Council meetings are held twice a year.

The USAN Council Secretariat is located at the American Medical Association, and is housed in the AMA headquarters. Inquiries and communications pertaining to USAN should be addressed to the USAN Council Secretary.[1]

USAN Review Board

The six-member USAN Review Board was established to provide an effective means of settling controversy stemming from irreconcilable differences of opinion regarding drug name selection. Two members are appointed by each sponsoring organization for one-year terms, subject to indefinite renewal.

Recourse to the Review Board in settling disputes over selection of the names has been relatively rare; in fact, its services have been employed in only five cases to date. Participants agree at the outset that the determination of the USAN Review Board is final and beyond appeal.

The USAN Review Board for 2009 comprises:

Donald R. Bennett, M.D., Ph.D. (AMA)
John E. Kasik, M.D., Ph.D. (AMA)
Stuart Feldman, Ph.D. (APhA)
Alice J. Matuszak, Ph.D. (APhA)
Jordan L. Cohen, Ph.D. (USP)
Gary L. Yingling, J.D., M.S. (USP)

The USAN Review Board secretariat is supported by the U.S. Pharmacopeia. Susan S. de Mars, J.D., serves the Board as Secretary.

USAN Program

The USAN Program is the specifically organized effort in the United States directed to producing simple and useful nonproprietary names for drugs and certain other related agents (e.g., small molecule drugs; biotechnology drugs; gene therapies; cellular therapies; contact lens materials; active ingredients in sunscreens; veterinary products; the base, salt, solvate, hydrate, or ester or other chemical derivative of a substance that has recevied a USAN). The name-selection process should be initiated when the drug enters the clinical investigation stage. Indeed, USAN are often created for compounds that never come to be marketed as drugs.

The adoption of a name is independent of clinical evaluation or acceptance by the medical profession of the article to which the name applies. Nevertheless, the USAN Council chooses each U.S. Adopted Name with the expectation that it will be suitable

---

[1] Secretary, USAN Council, c/o American Medical Association, 515 North State Street, Chicago, Illinois 60610 [Telephone: (312) 464-4046].

for prescribing and dispensing purposes and for designation as the title of the monograph, should the article be recognized in the official *United States Pharmacopeia* or *National Formulary*.

The USAN Program has earned a measure of prestige and world-wide recognition as an undertaking in the public interest. In addition to long-standing prejudices that work against instituting an orderly and effectual system of name selection, there also is widespread misunderstanding with respect to what constitutes good nonproprietary names and what purposes they serve. The USAN Council is committed to following established principles for coining nonproprietary names (see Appendixes VII and VIII) and to enlisting the cooperation of the pharmaceutical industry in this country and of nomenclature groups abroad with a view to selecting a single, good nonproprietary name for each promising new drug. The most up-to-date copy of these principles, and specific nomenclature schemes for gene therapies, monoclonal antibodies, and cell therapies, are maintained at the USAN Program web site, www.ama-assn.org/go/usan.

The Purpose of USAN—A nonproprietary name of a drug serves numerous and varied purposes. Its principal functions are to identify the substance to which it applies and to serve as a designation that may be used without restriction by the public at large, both lay and professional. The importance of the latter function is enhanced by the restrictions necessarily imposed upon the nature and use of a trademark, particularly in the pharmaceutical field. Teaching in pharmacy and medicine requires a common designation, especially for a drug that is available from several sources or in a combination of two or more drugs. Nonproprietary names greatly facilitate communication between health professionals, and most journals demand their use. State formularies and hospital and managed care organization formularies generally use nonproprietary names as the titles of the articles recognized. A nonproprietary name is essential to the pharmaceutical manufacturer as a means of preserving trade mark rights to a brand name for the article concerned. Finally, federal law obliges the manufacturer to use the "established" nonproprietary name in advertising, labels, and brochures.

It is this wide variety of functions that makes difficult the task of expressing very exactly the criteria for judging simplicity and usefulness in drug names, attributes generally conceded to be desirable.

The Philosophy of the USAN Program—An examination of nonproprietary names for drugs currently in use is likely to result in an inaccurate evaluation of present nomenclature practices. Many of those names were coined prior to the adoption of current nomenclature procedures and principles. Indeed, many of those older names demonstrated the obvious need for an organized effort in the U.S. directed toward producing useful, simple and appropriate nonproprietary names for drugs. Existing names, then, reflect a mixture of old and new nomenclature practices and philosophy.

In many instances poor naming of drugs was due to the earlier practice of condensing the full chemical name into a chemically oriented nonproprietary name. At the time this practice came into being, the chemistry of most drugs was not too complex. With advancing chemical complexity of drug entities, however, nonproprietary names so derived became increasingly long and difficult to spell, pronounce, and remember.

In addition to the problems caused by the complexity of the word itself, chemically derived names have been criticized because they fail to provide useful information to anyone but a scientist involved in drug development. (Although the scientist's need is recognized, there exists more scientific and accurate chemical nomenclature to serve the purpose.)

Nonproprietary nomenclature is intended primarily for physicians, pharmacists, and those in related health professions concerned with the understanding of the drug's pharmacological and therapeutic properties. Therefore, it must be emphasized again that nonproprietary names should be coined in such a way as to be most useful to, and usable by, their primary users, i.e., those in the health professions.

USAN Procedure

A submission[2] for a USAN originates usually from a firm or an individual who has developed a substance of potential therapeutic utility to the point where there is a distinct possibility of its being marketed in the United States of America.

In the case of a substance that is regarded as an "Investigational New Drug" (IND) within the terms of the Federal Food, Drug, and Cosmetic Act of 1938, the process of selecting a USAN should be initiated preferably during the period of investigation when the substance is under clinical study so that the adoption of the USAN will be complete by the time the relevant New Drug Application is filed. The USAN Program requires submission of the IND number as part of the application.

A submission for a USAN is expected to conform to the established Guiding Principles (see Appendixes VII and VIII) and to be reasonably free from conflict with other names, including both trademarks and nonproprietary names. USAN and INN stems are building blocks of nonproprietary names. Nonproprietary names, by their very nature, are in the public domain. These USAN and INN stems will be utilized in creating USAN and INN for compounds manufactured by several pharmaceutical companies and are not available for ownership by an individual company or person. For these reasons, the USAN Council makes an effort to discourage the occasional, undesirable practice of incorporating in trademarks the syllables used in an established nonproprietary name, or syllables recommended for USAN. Such trademarks might act as a bar to the subsequent adoption of appropriate nonproprietary names for closely related drugs. Failure to recognize this is an impediment to the work of the USAN Council in establishing new USAN in a class of drugs and the freedom of both the USAN and INN programs in selecting further nonproprietary names in the same series of substances is seriously diminished. Where the initial screening of the application suggests that the name fails to conform, or that it appears to conflict with an existing name, the USAN Council Secretary may offer suggestions with a view to expediting the selection process.

A user's fee for each U.S. Adopted Name is to be submitted with the form, "Request for a United States Adopted Name (USAN)," copies of which are included in this Dictionary (see Appendix IX). An editable version of the USAN application form is available as a MS-Word document at the USAN Program web site, www.ama-assn.org/go/usan. Additional information about the application process is also available at that web site.

Each application should be accompanied by the appropriate form. This information, supplemented by the results of searches conducted by the Secretary, is referred to the Council members, whose views then are exchanged until a tentative decision can be submitted to the sponsor for comment. It should be emphasized that while the Council can ascertain the preferred chemical nomenclature for a structure claimed for any compound of definite composition, the Council is not in a position to confirm the structure or the claims for pharmacologic activity. The information given under the category Therapeutic Claim is based on the manufacturer's claims as submitted to FDA for investigational new drug approval or as approved by the firm for publication when the name is

---

† Brand name formerly used, and/or firm no longer concerned with this product.

[2] Inquiries and submissions for USAN should be addressed to the Secretary, USAN Council, c/o American Medical Association, 515 North State Street, Chicago, Illinois 60610.

adopted. Adoption of a USAN does not imply endorsement of the claims or products by the USAN Council or its sponsoring organizations—the American Medical Association, the American Pharmacists Association, and the United States Pharmacopeia.

Suggested USAN are published on the USAN Program web site and are also sent to the World Health Organization (WHO) nomenclature secretariat. These publications and reviews serve as invitations for comments or protests. No disclosure of the name of the applicant or of the chemical nature of the substance appears in these statements.

Once the USAN Council and the applicant have agreed on a name, the tentatively adopted USAN is ordinarily submitted for consideration to the World Health Organization. If no objections are raised, adoption is considered final and newly approved USAN (updated monthly) are published electronically on the web site, www.ama-assn.org/go/usan. Soon thereafter the USAN is published in the USP bi-monthly publication *Pharmacopeial Forum*[3] as a Supplement to this Dictionary.

Despite the efforts to give notice of the proposed adoption of a USAN in the early stages and to exercise care in avoiding conflicts with established names, valid objections sometimes arise rather late. All such objections receive conscientious attention from the Council.

Occasionally, a USAN will be found unsuitable for adoption elsewhere, either internationally by the WHO or by one or more national bodies. Sometimes a closely similar name proves acceptable to one or more of these agencies, as in the case of the British Approved Name (BAN) "Cyclobarbitone" and its U.S. counterpart "Cyclobarbital." There is increasing emphasis, however, on the worldwide adoption of the same name for each therapeutic substance in view of the manifest advantages it offers to better communication and world trade.

Among the Guiding Principles for Coining U.S. Adopted Names for Drugs (see Appendix VII) is the principle that for most organic compounds, the designation for the pharmacologically active portion should appear first in the name; e.g., oxacillin sodium. This principle is applied generally in the entries herein.

Pronunciation

Responding to the continual introduction of new drug classes, the USAN Council develops common stems for which chemical and/or pharmacologic parameters are established (Appendix VII). In using such common stems for coining new nonproprietary names for drugs that belong to a series of related agents, the Council intends that they be pronounced consistently, thus bringing attention both orally and in writing to the presence of the stem and the prefixes or suffixes that distinguish one from another in the series.

Over the four decades of the USAN Program, inconsistencies in the Council's own suggested pronunciations became all too apparent. At its 10 June 2002 meeting, the Council adopted the Pronunciation Guide that follows (see page 17). The pronunciation of USANs adopted subsequently are to follow this Guide.

For over 3 years, culminating with 2,979 changes in the *2006 Dictionary*, the USP Expert Committees (Nomenclature and Labeling, 2000–2005, and Labeling, 2005–2010) reviewed the suggested pronunciations: first, to conform to the Pronunciation Guide in expressing the way the pronunciation is presented in the Dictionary; second, to standardize the pronunciations—"if it's spelled the same, it should be pronounced the same," applying particularly to the stems and to the first syllables; and third, to modify that standardization where a particular name had become pronounced differently in the popular culture.

Many of the changes involved adding a secondary accent, a feature which was rare in the original pronunciations. The stem syllable is generally the primary accent, and the secondary accent helps to differentiate the names within the class. In a few cases, suggested alternate pronunciations were provided. The Nomenclature Expert Committee continued to fine tune its review for the 2007 USP Dictionary. Revisions were made in 4,032 names.

For 2007, as a convenience to the reader, the pronunciation of each word within a bold-faced name was provided in every entry. This is in contrast to the usual dictionary style of providing the pronunciation of a word only on its first appearance. In addition, the pronunciations of those "Other Words"—secondary words—that are part of a name but do not appear alphabetically in the main entries, are provided in a list following the Pronunciation Guide. To save space, pronunciations have been deleted from names that were never USAN and are no longer USP or NF (exception: co-names created by USP for selected combination products, but never made official).

FDA Established Names

Under the terms of the Drug Amendments of 1962 to the Federal Food, Drug, and Cosmetic Act, which became law October 10, 1962, the Secretary of Health and Human Services is authorized to designate an official name for any drug wherever deemed "necessary or desirable in the interest of usefulness and simplicity."[4]

The Commissioner of Food and Drugs and the Secretary of Health and Human Services published in the *Federal Register* regulations effective November 26, 1984, and elucidated February 16, 1988, which state, in part:

Sec.299.4 Established names of drugs.

(d) "...the Food and Drug Administration agrees with 'Guiding Principles for Coining U.S. Adopted Names for Drugs,' published in *USAN and the USP Dictionary of Drug Names*...."

(e) "The Food and Drug Administration will not routinely designate official names under subsection 508 of the act. As a result, the established name under subsection 502(e) of the act will ordinarily be either the compendial name of the drug or, if there is no compendial name, the common and usual name of the drug. Interested persons, in the absence of the designation by the Food and Drug Administration of an official name, may rely on as the established name for any drug the current compendial name or the USAN adopted name listed in *USAN and the USP Dictionary of Drug Names*...."[5]

This Dictionary incorporates the text previously published under the title, *USAN and the USP Dictionary of Drug Names*. It is to make absolutely clear which names are compendial (*USP* or *NF*) or common or usual (USAN) that this Dictionary sets off the entries on these by showing them in **boldface** type.

International Nonproprietary Names

Under its charter, the World Health Organization (WHO) is empowered simply to *recommend* specific actions or procedures to its Member States. This limitation is incorporated into the WHO program concerned with the selection of international nonproprietary

[3] Published by the United States Pharmacopeia, 12601 Twinbrook Parkway, Rockville, Maryland 20852.

[4] F.D. & C. Act, Sec. 508 [358].

[5] 49 Fed. Reg. 37575 (1984) as amended by 53 Fed. Reg. 5369 (1988), amending 21 CFR 299.4.

names for pharmaceutical substances, in that the WHO first publishes the selected names as proposals (PINN; i.e., "Proposed International Nonproprietary Names"). A period of four months from the date of publication in *WHO Drug Information* is allowed for entering comments on, or objections to, any proposal on the part of Member States or other interested parties. In general, an objection reflects a belief that the proposal concerned is confusingly close to (i.e., conflicts with) a name already in use, perhaps in only a restricted area in which the party has a proprietary interest in the form of trademark rights. In the event that no objection is received, the WHO proceeds with listing and publishing the PINN as a RINN ("Recommended International Nonproprietary Name"), which almost all Member States then recognize as the sole or preferred nonproprietary name for use within their respective territories.

International nonproprietary names selected during 1953–2007 are included herein. Some are identical to, and identified with, USAN, *USP*, or *NF* entries; others are independent entries designated as INN. Where an INN is given in this volume as an independent entry, the chemical name and any graphic formula shown are generally those provided by the WHO.

International Cooperation

The USAN Council functions primarily to serve the health professions in the U.S. However, in an age when drug manufacturers market their products in many countries, when international travel is increasing steadily, and medical and pharmaceutical literature is translated and read widely around the world, the need for cooperation regarding nomenclature activities among the major drug-producing countries clearly is evident.

In addition to the USAN Council, active nomenclature agencies exist for example in Great Britain, Japan, France, Spain, and Russia. These agencies operate at varying levels of authority and cooperate with pharmaceutical manufacturers within areas of jurisdiction in the selection of appropriate nonproprietary names.

The agencies maintain liaison with one another in an effort to secure the wide adoption of the most appropriate and universally acceptable designation for each drug. The natural concern of each of the groups is with the drugs that are being synthesized, isolated, investigated, produced, or marketed in its own national area.

To prevent the confusion that arises when several nonproprietary names are used for a single drug, either in the same country or in several different countries, the WHO has assumed the responsibility of coordinating existing nomenclature at the international level.

Through its Expert Group on International Nonproprietary Names, whose members are drawn primarily from representatives of the national nomenclature agencies, the WHO has developed a procedure and formulated guiding principles for the selection of International Nonproprietary Names (INN). Where national nomenclature agencies exist, they usually act as agents for manufacturers by referring mutually selected designations (usually prior to national adoption) to the WHO with the request that these be considered for selection as INNs.

A manufacturer located in a country without a nomenclature agency can make a direct request for a nonproprietary name to the WHO or, in some instances, to an existing agency in another country, preferably one in which the pharmaceutical preparation is likely to be marketed.

After the selection of INNs, the WHO proposes and, unless an objection is raised, recommends to all its member states that such names be adopted at the local level. Formal adoption in accordance with national practice is necessary to provide a review of the suitability of the INN for national use.

Pharmacy Equivalent Names

A Pharmacy Equivalent (PEN) name was a short and simple name offered by USP as a standardized and useful term that may be used for convenience by practitioners where it may be impractical to use the complete official monograph title of a compendial article.

The PEN name for a dosage form containing two or more therapeutic drug substances was devised by combining portions of the official names of the component drug substances. A "Co-" prefix, not used elsewhere in compendial terminology, indicated that the article was a combination dosage form. For example, the PEN name Co-triamterzide is a representation of the *Co*mbination of *triamter*ene and hydrochlorothia*zide*.

PEN names were intended to be informative and to discourage the proliferation of trivial names and undefined abbreviations. Because a PEN name is not an official *USP* or *NF* title, it is not necessary that it appear on the label or in the labeling of a drug product. The USP Nomenclature Expert Committee no longer creates PEN names.

FDA Orphan Drugs

Under the terms of the Orphan Drug Act[6] of 1983, the development and marketing of drug products expected to be of limited commercial appeal but potentially useful in relatively rare disease conditions are encouraged. When the FDA makes an orphan product designation, if the product has not already been approved for marketing for some other use, the name designated may not be the established or proper name approved by the FDA for the product if eventually approved or licensed for marketing.

The ultimate selection of a U.S. Adopted Name for an orphan drug may be based on special considerations that pertain to this rather select group of drugs. Therefore, where a USAN for an orphan drug appears to follow a more chemically oriented terminology than is customary for drug nomenclature generally, such instance is not to be regarded as a basis or a precedent for a future selection of a U.S. Adopted Name.

Chemical Nomenclature

A nonproprietary name (often referred to as a *generic* name) and a proprietary name (often referred to as a *brand name* or a *trademark*) serve different useful purposes, but neither is designed to provide precise information concerning the chemical structure of the drug substance. To describe the chemical structure, a third type of name, i.e., a *chemical name*, is needed.

Chemical names tend to be complex and cumbersome; thus, although they may provide, for scientific and technical personnel, a complete, precise, and unambiguous description of the substance, they fail to constitute a concise, convenient designation that meets the day-to-day needs of the pharmacist, the physician, the patient, the jurist, and others functioning in related activities that involve pharmaceuticals. These latter needs are more appropriately served by nonproprietary names, of which USAN are primary examples.

For USAN entries pertaining to drugs that are strictly definable chemical substances (and the vast majority of single-entity drugs are of this type), two *chemical names* are usually included in each entry to provide such definition. Of the many chemical names that

---

† Brand name formerly used, and/or firm no longer concerned with this product.

6 Pub.L. 97-414.

could be used, the ones selected for this compilation are those that have been used as the American Chemical Society's *Chemical Abstracts* (CA) index names; thus, fundamentally and advantageously, they all stem from the same basic system of chemical nomenclature, and they function, through CA, as keys to the world's chemical literature.

The first of these two names usually is the inverted form of the systematic chemical name developed by Chemical Abstracts Service (CAS), in general accordance with the recommendations of the International Union of Pure and Applied Chemistry (IUPAC) and the International Union of Biochemistry and Molecular Biology (IUBMB), and employed in the current issues of CA. The second name, generated in accordance with the recommendations of these scientific unions, is included in view of the general recognition that it is neither practical nor desirable to rely solely on the CA index names for all purposes of identification and reference. The inverted form of the first name is provided because it guides the user *directly* to the CA literature—since that is the style in which chemical substances are indexed in that literature. Conversion to the uninverted form of the name is readily accomplished. Thus:

Hydrazinecarboximidamide, 2-[-(2,6-dichlorophenoxy)ethyl]-, sulfate, (2:1)

becomes

2-[2-(2,6-Dichlorophenoxy)ethyl]hydrazinecarboximidamide sulfate (2:1).

Benzeneacetic acid, α-(hydroxymethyl)-8-methyl-8-azabicyclo[3.2.1]oct-3-yl ester, 8-oxide, hydrochloride, *endo*-($\pm$)-

becomes

($\pm$)-*endo*-α-(Hydroxymethyl)-8-methyl-8-azabicyclo[3.2.1]oct-3-yl benzeneacetate 8-oxide hydrochloride.

This second name is given in uninverted form and is of a systematic type formerly used in CA; it is identical with, or closely resembles, the chemical name sanctioned and employed by the IUPAC and by the WHO.

These two types of chemical names differ primarily in that while the IUPAC names make generous use of nonsystematic and semisystematic (often referred to as *trivial*) names and qualifying terms, all of which impede electro-mechanical manipulation, the CAS names are more systematic for most substances. It is primarily by virtue of this stricter adherence to systematic nomenclature that the CAS chemical names are more readily amenable to the ever-increasing demand for electronic processing by various means, thus greatly facilitating literature searches and the processing of other queries based on chemical composition described in terms of nomenclature.

A third chemical name is occasionally supplied in an entry herein, especially in instances where that name is of a type that has become firmly established through long-continued use, e.g., see bolasterone; calcium glubionate; panthenol; and taleranol. Also, a CAS chemical synonym is occasionally supplied as an additional name in the relatively rare instances where the CA index name for a chemical substance is not a chemical name, e.g., see cosyntropin; pepstatin.

[NOTE—The foregoing does not apply to chemical names shown for entries other than USAN and current compendial names established before the USAN Program began. In those other entries, any chemical name shown, whether conforming to CAS nomenclature or otherwise, is given only for descriptive purposes to help identify the substance. The chemical name shown in an independent INN entry is usually that provided by the WHO.]

Identification of Names by Number

To meet the need for rapid handling of data on drugs for many purposes, compounds and preparations are being identified by number. This trend in no way minimizes the importance of adopting the best possible nonproprietary names for drugs; indeed, its success is related to the soundness of the names program, to the end that taken together the nonproprietary name and the number(s) assigned to it provide increasingly effective control of data and information on drugs.

In the system developed and being used by the CAS, registry numbers are assigned to compounds at random, and although unique, the numbers convey no compositional or other kinds of information. The FDA maintains the National Drug Code Directory, in which a three-part number is assigned to identify the manufacturer or distributor or repackager, the drug product, and the package. Other numerical classifications exist for literature searching.

In this book USAN entries and other entries, such as from current or former revisions of the *USP* and the *NF*, carry CAS registry numbers. A given entry usually carries only one such number, but because of (a) variations in the way in which information is reported in the literature, and therefore stored in automated files, and (b) the variety of searches expected to be conducted on such files, sometimes two, or occasionally more, CAS numbers are pertinent to a single entry. For example, information on the pharmacology of ampicillin may be stored in a file under either ampicillin anhydrous or ampicillin trihydrate, depending on how it was reported in the literature, and each of these substances carries its own CAS registry number. Similarly, information on the synthesis of doxorubicin hydrochloride may be stored under that entry or under the parent substance, doxorubicin.

With entries carrying multiple CAS registry numbers, the one carrying no annotation enclosed within brackets (usually the first one) is the registry number assigned to that entry. Each additional number is followed by a bracketed term which, as is apparent from the following examples, discloses its relationship to the assigned number. Prominent categories of entries carrying more than one CAS registry number are exemplified in the following:

Hydrated substances carry one registry number for the hydrate and another one for the anhydrous substance. Examples:
  Theophylline 5967-84-0; 58-55-9 [anhydrous]
  Ampicillin 69-53-4; 7177-48-2 [trihydrate]

Addition salts of organic bases carry one registry number for the salt and another one for the organic base. Examples:
  Promethazine Hydrochloride 58-33-3; 60-87-7 [promethazine]
  Acetophenazine Maleate 5714-00-1; 2751-68-0 [acetophenazine]

Quaternary salts carry one registry number for the salt and another one for the quaternary radical, if that radical has had a number assigned to it by CAS. Examples:
  Bretylium Tosylate 61-75-6; 59-41-6 [bretylium]
  Choline Chloride 67-48-1; 62-49-7 [choline]

Metal salts of uncommon organic acids and all salt-like substances carry one registry number for the salt and another one for the acid or acidic substance. Examples:
  Edetate Sodium 64-02-8; 60-00-4 [edetic acid]
  Hexobarbital Sodium 50-09-9; 56-29-1 [hexobarbital]

Entries for which CAS has replaced a registry number with another one carry both numbers, as recommended by CAS since the replaced number was in use prior to its replacement. Examples:
  Aspartocin 4117-65-1; 1402-89-7 [replaced]
  Phendimetrazine Tartrate 50-58-8; 21102-82-9 [replaced]; 634-03-7 [phendimetrazine]

In general, when using CAS registry numbers as search terms, all numbers *deemed pertinent* to the search at hand should be used. To omit one or more of such numbers is to risk failing to retrieve all of the stored information pertinent to the search. This does not mean that all of the registry numbers associated with a substance in this book must always be used in searches involving that substance. According to the nature of the query that has prompted the search, one can decide whether one or more of the registry numbers are not pertinent and can therefore be omitted.

Appendix VI provides a tabulation of entries in the order of increasing CAS registry number. This is followed by a similar tabulation in the order of increasing NSC (National Service Center of the National Cancer Institute, National Institutes of Health) number; the corresponding NSC numbers are also in the respective individual entries.

UNII Description

Unique ingredient identifiers (UNIIs) are non-proprietary, permanent, unique, unambiguous identifiers based on molecular structure and/or descriptive information. UNIIs are generated by the joint FDA/USP Substance Registration System (SRS) and are used to support health information technology initiatives for substances in drugs, biologics, foods, and devices. The UNII is one of the core components of the United States Federal Medication Terminology, has been adopted by the United States Consolidated Health Informatics initiative, and is part of the FDA's Structured Product Labeling. The UNII consists of ten alphanumeric characters. The first nine are randomly generated and the tenth character is determined through a mathematical algorithm and is appended to the first nine. Substances that are registered in the SRS follow detailed business rules for that registration which were developed by the SRS Project Management Team. In addition, substances that are registered in the SRS follow a detailed and robust set of data rules that were developed by the SRS Board for drawing molecular structures and representing descriptive information. The SRS Board consists of experts from both the USP and FDA, and it works very closely with drug regulators from other nations in the development of these rules.

Graphic Formulas

Consonant with the employment of Chemical Abstracts nomenclature, and also in the interest of uniformity of style, the orientation of ring systems and the depiction of stereoisomeric features in graphic formulas are generally consistent with CAS practices. Either alternating double bonds or a circle within a hexagon is used in graphic formulas to represent the bonding in benzene rings and all others that contain six atoms of any kind that are connected in conjugate (Kekulé) style in one or more of the individual resonant structures that contribute to the hybrid structure actually present in the molecule.

Many structures depicted in the Dictionary were drawn by hand. All the USP and NF graphic formulas contained herein were drawn electronically to achieve a consistent style and uniform format. The existing hand-drawn structures were converted to bit-mapped images in the Tagged Image File Format (TIFF) that were then converted with commercial structure-recognition software to display the structure.

Molecular Weights

The standard atomic weights of the elements that are used in the tabulation of molecular weights are those recommended in 2005 by the IUPAC Commission on Atomic Weights and Isotopic Abundances. The exact atomic weights are used in the computations. The molecular weights derived from these atomic weights are systematically rounded off to two decimal places using the method adopted by the Executive Committee of the USP Division of General Policies, Requirements, Nomenclature. That is, retain only the number to include the digits in the first three decimal places of the sum of the atomic weights: discard the last digit if it is smaller than 5 to obtain the molecular weight or discard the last digit if it is 5 or larger and increase the digit in the second decimal place by one to obtain the molecular weight.

Radioactive Pharmaceuticals

Since the radioactive pharmaceuticals are specially packaged in distinctive containers, labeled with the internationally recognized symbols for radioactivity, and available only to specially trained personnel, the USAN Council has agreed on the general principle that for these drugs the nonproprietary name should include the name of the basic compound serving as the carrier for the radioactivity, the symbol for the radioactive isotope, and the atomic weight (inasmuch as several radioactive isotopes of a given element may be in use).

Brand Names

The *2007 USP Dictionary* showed the beginnings of a change in philosophy on the inclusion of brand names. Emphasizing that this is a dictionary of drug substance names, not a list of drug products, references to combination drug products and their brand names were dropped. References to manufacturers of drug products marketed only under their nonproprietary names were dropped. Brand names no longer used in the USA, as determined primarily by reference to FDA s Orange Book, and occasionally to the National Drug Code Directory and various other sources, have been dropped.

Brand names still being used are sometimes difficult to attribute ownership thereof. The sale of a drug name from one company to another, the many company mergers on the one hand and spinoffs on the other and the consequent name changes of companies, plus the trend for two companies to co-market the same drug under one brand name are challenging to keep up with. In general, only one player in a co-marketing arrangement is listed.

Current labelers (marketers) of a drug may have had nothing to do with its original research. However, that connection is not necessarily lost, as the researcher's code for the drug, where available, is included in the main entry and cross-referenced to Appendix IV.

The formulator and labeler of a drug product are not necessarily the same firm. Moreover, sometimes a single formulator produces a drug product for several labelers and sometimes a single labeler purchases a drug product from more than one formulator. There is no general effort to make in this book a distinction between the formulator and the labeler of a product.

It should be noted that the pharmacologic and/or therapeutic category stated in an entry may not necessarily apply to every brand name listed in that entry; e.g., the category may pertain to one or more dosage forms whereas a particular brand name may represent such dosage form(s) or perhaps some other dosage form not contemplated by the stated category.

---

† Brand name formerly used, and/or firm no longer concerned with this product.

Code Designations

Alphanumeric combinations frequently are used during the investigational phase required to demonstrate the utility of new, potentially therapeutic substances. The alphabetic portion of a code designation usually is identifiable with the institution or firm that assigns the code designation to the agent under test. For example, among the code designations commonly encountered are some that include the initials "NSC." Code designations find their way into the scientific literature because it is customary to use them in identifying the compounds in early publications prior to adoption of a USAN.

Summary of Types of Information Provided

The individual entries in this volume comprise, in general, the following: (1) USAN (in **boldface** type), with year of its adoption in brackets; (2) official names (usually of the drug substances as distinct from the dosage forms) from the current revisions of the *United States Pharmacopeia* and the *National Formulary* (in **boldface** type), with some exceptions, e.g., combinations; (3) names that were official in previous revisions of the *USP* and the *NF*; (4) international and other nonproprietary names; (5) miscellaneous older names that had been in general use at various times in the past; (6) brand names; and (7) code designations.

The statement of a category or categories of pharmacologic and/or therapeutic activity is italicized in USAN entries and in entries for current *USP* and *NF* names. In the case of many new entries, the sponsors of the USAN may not have complete information insofar as all of the categories of activity are concerned. Comments aimed toward the attainment of greater uniformity and usefulness in the pharmacologic classification system used herein will be welcomed, particularly if they are supported by authoritative information.

Literature references (e.g., "MI" for Merck Index) are given in some entries solely as sources of possible further information about the compound and do not imply any connection with the program for selection of nonproprietary names.

The names of the manufacturers currently or formerly concerned with the respective compounds are mentioned. Mergers and name changes of manufacturers and sales of brand names from one manufacturer to another are common. Where known, the name of the current owner of the brand name is given, but no special attempt is made to be up to date in all entries. Information that a manufacturer is no longer concerned with a compound will be gratefully received.

Further analysis of the content of this edition is given on page 7 under *How to Use This Book*.

Acknowledgments

Stephanie Shubat, M.S., Gail Karet, Ph.D., Helene Biernacki, and Julie Murphy of the USAN Council Secretariat, and Dr. Raffaella Balocco-Mattavelli and Sophie Lasseur, Quality Assurance-INN, World Health Organization (WHO), rendered invaluable assistance during the preparation of this book. Dr. Raymond Boudet-Dalbin, Université René Descartes, and Dr. Sabine Kuhn, Chemical Abstracts Service, made significant contributions with their help on the graphic formulas and CAS registry numbers, and in providing chemical names consistent with the *Chemical Abstracts* conventions. Don L. Barker, Spectrum Computer Services, Inc., provided skillful database analyses and programming. Also assisting commendably in the production of this edition were USP staff Andrzej Wilk, Ph.D., Scientist, Healthcare Quality and Information; Shawn C. Becker, R.N., M.S., Healthcare Quality and Information; Amy Strasser, Production Coordinator; Irena Smith, Publishing Specialist III; Deborah R. Miller, Manager, Publications Production.

Each of these individuals contributed significantly to this book. They all generously provided their expert knowledge, expeditious cooperation, and patience. Their contributions are sincerely appreciated.

Much of the work on the USAN Program is hidden from view. The results, however, are shared by many, all of whom thus benefit from the labors of the few who give freely of time and effort and of others whose cooperation makes success possible. The continued willing cooperation from all segments of the pharmaceutical industry, which contributes immeasurably to the success of the USAN Program as well as provides helpful information on the various entries throughout this book, is gratefully recorded.

Andrzej Wilk, Ph.D., *Senior Scientist,*
   USP Nomenclature Expert Committee

PRONUNCIATION GUIDE FOR DRUG NAMES
Adopted by the USAN Council, 10 June 2002
(Revised 14 July 2006)

This pronunciation guide has been developed and approved by the USAN Council, and was revised at the USAN Countil meeting, July 14, 2006, to facilitate pronunciation of USAN and will be used on all future Statements of Adoption.

SYLLABLES: Syllable designations are based upon phonetic considerations. They are meant to show pronunciation without ambiguity, even though word breaks may not follow those that are normally considered correct American English language word breaks.

A prime mark (′) follows the primary accent syllable; a double prime mark (″) follows any secondary accent syllable. All syllables are separated by a blank space. No diacritical marks are used.

SOUNDS AND SPELLING: Vowels, long—spelling designations in all syllables **except the last syllable**, unless indicated otherwise:

a	ay	(may)
e	ee	(lee) (same in last syllable also)
i	eye	(when by itself as a syllable)
	ye	(when in conjunction with a consonant: lye)
o	oh	(when by itself as a syllable)
	oe	(when in conjunction with a consonant: toe)
u	ue	(cue; cure) (same in last syllable also)
y	ee	(oxytocin, ox ee toe′ sin)
	i	(thrombolytic, throm boe lit′ ik)
	eye	(kanamycin, kan a mye′ sin)

Spelling designation **in the last syllable**:   The vowels a, i and o assume long vowel sounds by the addition of an e at the end of the syllable.

    rate
    bite
    toe

Short vowel sounds receive no special designations in any syllable.

Digraphs:

ah	father	oo	food
aw	paw	ou	ought
ch	child	ow	out
ng	sing	oy	oil
oi	oil	wh	when

Consonant sounds and examples:

b	bed	q	queen (**kween**)
c	citrate (**si′ trate**)	r	rot
	carbon (**kar′ bon**)	s	sing
d	door		osmotic (**oz mot′ ik**)
f	floor		aspirin (**as′ pir in**)
g	gore		vision (**vi′ zhun**)
	digital (**di′ ji tal**)	t	taught
h	hat	v	vote
j	jar	w	wing
k	king	x	ox
l	low		xanthines (**zan′ theens**)
m	my	y	yes
n	no	z	zinc (**zink**)
p	pot		

PRONUNCIATION OF OTHER WORDS (SECONDARY WORDS)

Acedoben	a″ se doe′ ben	Camsylate	kam′ si late
Acefurate	a″ se fue′ rate	Caproate	kap′ roe ate
Acesulfame	a″ se sul′ fame	Caprylate	kap′ ri late
Acetate	as′ e tate	Carbonate	kar′ bo nate
Acetonide	a seet′ oh nide	Carboxymaltose	kar box″ ee mawl′ tose
Acetophenide	a seet″ oh fen′ ide	Carnauba	kar noe′ ba
Aceturate	a set′ ue rate	Carotene	kar′ oh teen
Acid	as′ id	Celmoleukin	sel″ moe loo′ kin
Acistrate	a sis′ trate	Chloride	klor′ ide
Activated	ak′ ti vay″ ted	Chlorohydrate	klor″ oh hychlorohydrex e′ drate
Aggregated	ag′ re gay″ ted	Chlorohydrex	klor″ oh hye′ drex
Alaninate	al″ a nin′ ate	Chorionic	kor″ ee on′ ok
Alfa	al′ fa	Chromate	kroe′ mate
Alfacon	al′ fa kon	Chromated	kroe′ may ted
Alginate	al′ ji nate	Cilexetil	sye lex′ e til
Aliplasmid	al″ i plas′ mid	Cinnamate	sin′ a mate
Altumomab	al toom′ oh mab	Citrate	sit′ rate
Aluminate	a loo′ mi nate	Cituxetan	sye tux′ e tan
Aluminometasilicate	a loo″ mi noe met″ a sil′ i kate	Clathrate	klath′ rate
Aluminosilicate	a loo″ mi noe sil′ i kate	Closylate	kloe′ si late
Amide	a′ mide	Colloid	kol′ oid
Aminoacetate	a mee″ noe as′ e tate	Colloidal	koe loid′ al
Aminolevulinate	a mee″ noe lev″ ue lin′ ate	Conjugated	kon′ joo gay″ ted
Ammoniated	a moe′ nee ay″ ted	Copolymer	koe pol′ i mer
Amylase	am′ i lase	Cresyl	kres′ il
Amylosulfate	am″ i loe sul′ fate	Crosfumaril	kros fue′ ma ril
Anhydrous	an hye′ drus	Crotalidae	kroe tal′ i dee
Anisatil	a ni′ sa til	Cyclamate	sye′ kla mate
Antitoxin	an″ tee tox′ in	Cyclotate	sye′ kloe tate
Apcitide	ap′ si tide	Cypionate	sip′ ee oh nate
Aritox	ar′ i tox	Dalanated	dal′ a nay″ ted
Arsenate	ar′ se nate	Decanoate	dek″ a noe′ ate
Ascorbate	a skor′ bate	Dehydroacetate	dee hye″ droe as′ e tate
Aspart	as′ part	Delta	del′ ta
Aspartate	a spar′ tate	Detemir	de′ te mir
Axetil	ax′ e til	Diacetate	dye as′ e tate
Balsam	bawl′ sam	Dibasic	dye bat′ sik
Behenate	be hen′ ate	Dibunate	dye′ bue nate
Beloxil	bel ox′ il	Dibutyrate	dye bue′ ti rate
Bengal	ben′ gal	Dichloroacetate	dye klor″ oh as′ e tate
Benzathine	ben′ za theen	Dichlorohydrate	dye klor″ oh hye′ drate
Benzenesulfonate	ben″ zeen sul′ foe nate	Dichlorohydrex	dye klor″ oh hye′ drex
Benzoate	ben′ zoe ate	Dicholine	dye koe′ leen
Bepiplasmid	bep″ i plas′ mid	Dicitrate	dye sit′ rate
Besudotox	be soo′ doe tox	Dicloacetate	dye″ kloe as′ e tate
Besylate	bes′ i late	Diethylamine	dye eth′ il a meen
Bicarbonate	bye kar′ bo nate	Diftitox	dif′ ti tox
Bicisate	bye sis′ ate	Difumarate	dye fue′ ma rate
Bisulfate	bye sul′ fate	Dihydrate	dye hye′ drate
Bisulfite	bye sul′ fite	Dihydrochloride	dye hye″ droe klor′ ide
Bitartrate	bye tar′ trate	Dilaurate	dye lawr′ ate
Borate	bore′ ate	Dimaleate	dye mal′ ee ate
Bovine	boe′ vine	Dimeglumine	dye meg′ loo meen
Bromide	broe′ mide	Dimesylate	dye mes′ i late
Butyrate	bue′ ti rate	Dinitrate	dye nye′ trate
Caltespen	kal tes′ pen	Diolamine	dye ole′ a meen
Camphorated	kam′ for ay″ ted	Dioxide	dye ox′ ide
		Diphosphate	dye fos′ fate

Dipivoxil — dye″ piv ox′ il
Dipotassium — dye″ poe tas′ ee um
Dipropionate — dye proe′ pee oh nate
Disalicylate — dye″ sa lis′ i late
Disodium — dye soe′ dee um
Disoproxil — dye″ soe prox′ il
Distearate — dye steer′ ate
Ditartrate — dye tar′ trate
Ditosylate — dye tos′ i late
Ditriflutate — dye trye floo′ tate
Edamine — ed′ a meen
Edisylate — e dis′ i late
Elaidate — el″ a id′ ate
Emulsifying — ee mul″ si fye′ ing
Enanthate — e nan′ thate
Enzymatic — en″ zi mat′ ik
Erbumine — er′ bue meen
Esterified — es ter′ i fide
Esters — es′ ters
Estolate — es′ toe late
Esylate — es′ i late
Etabonate — et′ a boe′ nate
Etexilate — e tex′ i late
Ethasulfate — eth″ a sul′ fate
Ethyl — eth′ il
Ethylsuccinate — eth″ il sux′ i nate
Ethylsulfate — eth″ il sul′ fate
Excipient — ex sip′ ee ent
Fanolesomab — fan″ oh les′ oh mab
Ferpentetate — fer pen′ te tate
Fever — fee′ ver
Fluoride — floor′ ide
Fosamil — fos′ a mil
Fosfatex — fos′ fa tex
Fulvius — ful′ vi us
Fumarate — fue′ ma rate
Furifosmin — fure″ i fos′ min
Furoate — fure′ oh ate
Gadolinium — gad″ oh lin′ ee um
Galactarate — gal ak′ tar ate
Gallate — gal′ ate
Glacial — glay′ shil
Glargine — glar′ jeen
Glubionate — gloo bye′ oh nate
Glucaldrate — gloo kal′ drate
Gluconate — gloo′ koe nate
Glucuronate — gloo″ kure on′ ate
Glucuronide — gloo″ kure on′ ide
Glulisine — gloo′ lis een
Glutamate — gloo′ ta mate
Glutamer — gloo′ ta mer
Gly — glye
Glycerate — glis′ er ate
Glycinate — glye′ sin ate
Glycolate — glye′ koe late
Guaiacolsulfonate — gwye″ a kol sul′ foe nate
Hazel — hay′ zel
Hemicellulose — hem″ ee sel′ ue lose
Hemifumarate — hem″ ee fue′ ma rate
Hemisuccinate — hem″ ee sux′ i nate
Hexacetonide — hex″ a seet′ oh nide
Hexafluoride — hex″ a floor′ ide
Hexasodium — hex″ a soe′ dee um
Hippurate — hip′ ure ate
Homopolymer — hoe″ moe pol′ i mer
Hormone — hor′ mone
Hyclate — hye′ klate

Hydrabamine — hye″ dra bam′ een
Hydrate — hye′ drate
Hydrobromide — hye″ droe broe′ mide
Hydrochloride — hye″ droe klor′ ide
Hydrogenated — hye droj′ en ay″ ted
Hydrolysate — hye drol′ i sate
Hydrophilic — hye″ droe fil′ ik
Hydroxide — hye drox′ ide
Hydroxyanisole — hye drox″ ee an′ i sole
Hydroxytoluene — hye drox″ ee tol′ ue een
Hypochlorite — hye″ poe klor′ ite
Iberfilcon — eye″ ber fil′ kon
Immune — i mune′
Inactivated — in ak′ ti vay″ ted
Indanyl — in′ da nil
Interpolymer — in″ ter pol′ i mer
Iodide — eye′ oh dide
Iodinated — eye′ oh di nay″ ted
Isethionate — eye″ se thye′ oh nate
Isobutyl — eye″ soe bue′ til
Isophane — eye′ soe fane
Isoquinolinium — eye″ soe kwin″ oh lin′ i um
Isothiocyanate — eye″ soe thye″ oh sye′ a nate
Kamedoxomil — kay″ me dox′ oh mil
Ketolaurate — kee″ toe lawr′ ate
Ketone — kee′ tone
Lactate — lak′ tate
Lactobionate — lak″ toe bye′ oh nate
Ladenovec — la den′ oh vek
Latrodectus — lat′ roe dek′ tus
Levulinate — lev″ ue lin′ ate
Lexidronam — lex id′ roe nam
Lispro — lis′ pro
Lutetium — loo tee′ shee um
Mactans — mak′ tans
Magsulfex — mag sul′ fex
Malate — mal′ ate
Maleate — mal′ ee ate
Mandelate — man′ de late
Mebutate — meb′ ue tate
Medocaril — me dok′ a ril
Medoxil — me dox′ il
Medoxomil — me dox′ oh mil
Medronate — me′ droe nate
Mepesuccinate — mep″ e sux′ i nate
Merpentan — mer pen′ tan
Mertansine — mer tan′ seen
Mertiatide — mer tye′ a tide
Mesylate — mes′ i late
Mesylates — mes′ i lates
Metabisulfite — met″ a bye sul′ fite
Metaphosphate — met″ a fos′ fate
Methacrylate — meth ak′ ri late
Methylbromide — meth″ il broe′ mide
Methylsulfate — meth″ il sul′ fate
Microaggregated — mye″ kroe ag′ re gay″ ted
Microcrystalline — mye″ kroe kris′ ta lin
Microspheres — mye′ froe sfeerz″
Micrurus — mye kroo′ rus
Mofetil — moe′ fe til
Molybdate — moe lib′ date
Monoacetate — mon″ oh as′ e tate
Monobasic — mon″ oh bay′ sik
Monoethyl — mon″ oh eth″ il
Monofluorophosphate — mon″ oh floor″ oh fos′ fate
Monoglycerides — mon″ oh glis′ er idze
Monohydrate — mon″ oh hye′ drate

Monolaurate	mon″ oh lawr′ ate	Polylysine	pol″ ee lye′ seen
Monolinoleate	mon″ oh lin oh′ lee ate	Polyoxylglycerides	pol″ ee ox″ il glis′ er ides
Monomethyl	mon″ oh meth′ il	Polyphosphate	pol″ ee fos′ fate
Mononitrate	mon″ oh nye′ trate	Polystyrene	pol″ ee stye′ reen
Monooleate	mon″ oh oh′ lee ate	Polysulfate	pol″ ee sul′ fate
Monopalmitate	mon″ oh pal′ mi tate	Polyvalent	pol″ ee vay′ lent
Monopotassium	mon″ oh poe tas′ ee um	Porcine	por′ sine
Monostearate	mon″ oh steer′ ate	Povacrylex	poe″ va krye′ lex
Monosulfate	mon″ oh sul′ fate	Precipitated	pre sip′ i tay″ ted
Monoxide	mon ox′ ide	Pregelatinized	pree jel at′ i nized
Mucate	mue′ kate	Probenate	proe′ be nate
Mustard	mus′ tard	Probutate	proe bue′ tate
Myristate	mir′ is tate	Propionate	proe′ pee oh nate
Nafate	naf′ ate	Proxetil	prox′ e til
Napsylate	nap′ si late	Pullus	pool′ us
Niacinate	nye′ a sin ate	Purified	
Nicotinate	nik″ oh tin′ ate	Pyro-	pye″ roe
Nitrate	nye′ trate	Pyrophosphate	pye″ roe fos′ fate
Nitridocade	nye trid′ oh kade	Racemic	ray see′ mik
Nitrite	nye′ trite	Raffimer	raf′ fi mer
Nitroprusside	nye″ troe prus′ ide	Recombinant	ree kom′ bi nant
Nofetumomab	noe″ fe toom′ oh mab	Resin	rez′ in
Octaacetate	ok″ ta as′ e tate	Rinfabate	rin′ fa bate
Octachlorohydrate	ok″ ta klor″ oh hye′ drate	Saccharate	sak′ a rate
Octachlorohydrex	ok″ ta klor″ oh hye′ drex	Sagrada	sa gra′ da
Olamine	ole′ a meen	Salnacedin	sal na′ se din
Oleate	oh′ lee ate	Satumomab	sa toom′ oh mab
Oleoresin	oh″ lee oh rez′ in	Sebacate	seb′ a kate
Ovine	oh′ vine	Serpentina	ser″ pen teen′ a
Oxalate	ox′ a late	Sesquichlorohydrate	ses″ kwi klor″ oh hye′ drate
Oxide	ox′ ide	Sesquichlorohydrex	ses″ kwi klor″ oh hye′ drex
Oxidized	ox′ i dized	Sesquifumarate	ses″ kwi fue′ ma rate
Oxidronate	ox″ i droe′ nate	Sesquioleate	ses″ kwi oh′ lee ate
Oxybate	ox′ i bate	Sestamibi	ses″ ta mib′ ee
Ozogamicin	oh″ zoe ga mye′ sin	Siboroxime	sye″ boe rox′ eem
Palmitate	pal′ mi tate	Silicate	sil′ i kate
Pamoate	pam′ oh ate	Sorbate	sor′ bate
Pantothenate	pan toe′ then ate	Sorbitex	sor′ bi tex
Pegol	peg′ ol	Stearate	steer′ ate
Pendetide	pen′ de tide	Stearates	steer′ ates
Pentachlorohydrate	pen″ ta klor″ oh hye′ drate	Subacetate	sub as′ e tate
Pentachlorohydrex	pen″ ta klor″ oh hye′ drex	Subcarbonate	sub kar′ bo nate
Pentahydrochloride	pen″ ta hye″ droe klor′ ide	Subcitrate	sub cit′ rate
Pentasodium	pen″ ta soe′ dee um	Subgallate	sub gal′ ate
Pentetreotide	pen″ te tree′ oh tide	Sublimed	sub lymed
Perborate	per bore′ ate	Subnitrate	sub nye′ trate
Percha	per′ cha	Subsalicylate	sub″ sa lis′ i late
Perchlorate	per klor′ ate	Subsulfate	sub sul′ fate
Permanganate	per man′ ga nate	Succinate	sux′ i nate
Peroxide	per ox′ ide	Sudotox	soo′ doe tox
Persodium	per soe′ dee um	Suleptanate	sul ep′ ta nate
Pertechnetate	per tek′ ne tate	Sulfa	sul′ fa
Phenpropionate	fen proe′ pee oh nate	Sulfate	sul′ fate
Phenylacetate	fen″ il as′ e tate	Sulfide	sul′ fide
Phenylbutyrate	fen″ il bue′ ti rate	Sulfite	sul′ fite
Phosphanilate	fos fan′ i late	Sulfonate	sul′ foe nate
Phosphate	fos′ fate	Sulfosalicylate	sul″ foe sa lis′ i late
Phthalate	thal′ ate	Sulfoxide	sul fox′ ide
Piconol	pik′ o nol	Sulfoxylate	sul fox′ il ate
Picrate	pik′ rate	Sulfurated	sul′ fur ay″ ted
Pivalate	piv′ a late	Tacatuzumab	tak″ a tooz′ oo mab
Pivoxetil	piv ox′ e til	Tadenovec	ta den′ oh vek
Pivoxil	piv ox′ il	Tannate	tan′ ate
Placarbil	pla kar′ bil	Tannex	tan′ ex
Polacrilex	pol″ a kril′ ex	Tartrate	tar′ trate
Poliglumex	pol″ ee gloo′ mex	Teboroxime	te″ boe rox′ eem
Polistirex	pol″ ee stye′ rex	Tebutate	teb′ ue tate

Terephthalate	ter″ e thal′ ate	Trimetaphosphate	trye met″ a fos′ fate
Tetrachlorohydrate	tet″ ra klor″ oh hye′ drate	Trioleate	trye oh′ lee ate
Tetrachlorohydrex	tet″ ra klor″ oh hye′ drex	Trioxide	trye ox′ ide
Tetranitrate	tet″ ra nye′ trate	Trisilicate	trye sil′ i kate
Tetrasodium	tet″ ra soe′ dee um	Trisodium	trye soe′ dee um
Thiomalate	thye″ oh mal′ ate	Tristearate	trye steer′ ate
Thiosulfate	thye″ oh sul′ fate	Trisulfide	trye sul′ fide
Tiuxetan	tye ux′ e tan	Tritiated	trit′ ee ay″ ted
Tosylate	tos′ i late	Undecanoate	un dek″ a noe′ ate
Tribasic	trye bay′ sik	Undecylate	un de′ sil ate
Trichlorohydrate	trye″ klor oh hye′ drate	Undecylenate	un de′ sil en ate
Trichlorohydrex	trye″ klor oh hye′ drex	Vaccine	vax′ een
Trichloromonofluoromethane	trye klor″ oh mon″ oh floor″ oh meth′ ane	Vaccinia	vax in′ ee a
		Valerate	val′ er ate
Triethiodide	trye″ eth eye′ oh dide	Vanillin	va nil′ in
Triflutate	trye′ floo tate	Xinafoate	zye naf′ oh ate
Trihydrochloride	trye hye″ droe klor′ ide	Zirconium	zir koe′ nee um
Trimeta-	trye met″ a	Zoster	zos′ ter

ABBREVIATIONS

AMA-DE	*AMA Drug Evaluations,* former publication of the American Medical Association
BAN	British Approved Name
BVC	British Veterinary Codex
CA	*Chemical Abstracts,* published by the American Chemical Society
CAS	Chemical Abstracts Service
CID	*CTFA Cosmetic Ingredient Dictionary,* published by The Cosmetic, Toiletry and Fragrance Association, Inc.
DCF	Dénomination Commune Française (French approved nonproprietary name)
INN	International Nonproprietary Name
JAN	Japanese Accepted Name
MI	*Merck Index,* published by Merck & Company, Inc.
ND	*New Drugs,* former publication of the American Medical Association
NF	National Formulary
NND	*New and Nonofficial Drugs,* former publication of the American Medical Association
NNR	*New and Nonofficial Remedies,* former publication of the American Medical Association
NSC	National Service Center, National Cancer Institute, National Institutes of Health
PEN	Pharmacy Equivalent Name
PHS	Public Health Service [United States]
SRS	Substance Registration System
UNII	Unique Ingredient Identifier
USAN	United States Adopted Names
USP	United States Pharmacopeia
USP DI	Vol. I—*Drug Information for the HealthCare Professional*

Revisions to the 2008 Dictionary

The following is a list of new nonproprietary names appearing in the *2009 USP Dictionary*. Names shown in **boldface type** are USAN and/or *USP* or *NF* monograph titles.

Aderbasib
Adoprazine
Afutuzumab
Alacizumab Pegol
Aleplasinin
Alipogene Tiparvovec
Almorexant
Amsilarotene
Apricoxib
Ataluren
Bafetinib
Bederocin
Befiradol
Bentamapimod
Blinatumomab
Bupropion Hydrobromide
Cabazitaxel
Caraway Oil
Cardamon Oil
Cardamon Seed
Cariprazine
Carlecortemcel-L
Carmegliptin
Carmegliptin Dihydrochloride
Catridecacog
Citatuzumab Bogatox
Cixutumumab
Coleneuramide
Conatumumab
Conestat Alfa
Cositecan
Custirsen Sodium
Dabigatran Etexilate Mesylate
Danusertib
Daporinad
Darotropium Bromide
Davunetide
Degarelix Acetate
Delafloxacin
Delafloxacin Meglumine
Demiditraz
Denenicokin
Derquantel
Dexnebivolol
Dirucotide
Dirucotide Acetate
Disitertide
Drinabant
Dulanermin
Dutogliptin
Dutogliptin Tartrate
Edoxaban
Elagolix
Elagolix Sodium
Elotuzumab
Entinostat

Eprotirome
Esomeprazole Potassium
Esreboxetine
Esreboxetine Succinate
Etaracizumab
Farletuzumab
Fasobegron
Favipiravir
Fermagate
Fidaxomicin
Figitumumab
Flopristin
Foravirumab
Fosbretabulin Disodium
Fostamatinib
Fostamatinib Disodium
Hydroxyethyl Starch 130/0.4
Ibipinabant
Ibodutant
Iclaprim
Imeglimin
Indacaterol Maleate
Indeglitazar
Ingenol Mebutate
Inolitazone
Lancovutide
Larazotide
Larazotide Acetate
Lensiprazine
Levomefolate Calcium
Levomefolic Acid
Levomilnacipran
Levonebivolol
Linaclotide
Linagliptin
Linopristin
Liprotamase
Lixisenatide
Macitentan
Melogliptin
Mimopezil
Mirabegron
Mocetinostat Dihydrobromide
Monepantel
Nabiximols
Naluzotan
Naluzotan Hydrochloride
Nelivaptan
Obeticholic Acid
Olesoxime
Oleyl Oleate
Ombrabulin
Orange Peel Tincture, Sweet
Otenabant
Otenabant Hydrochloride
Palifosfamide

Palovarotene
Pardoprunox Hydrochloride
Pozanicline
Pozanicline Tartrate
Radezolid
Radezolid Hydrochloride
Radiprodil
Rafivirumab
Ramucirumab
Ranagengliotucel-T
Rapeseed Oil, Fully Hydrogenated
Rapeseed Oil, Fully Hydrogenated Superglycerinated
Remogliflozin Etabonate
Retaspimycin
Retaspimycin Hydrochloride
Riociguat
Saracatinib
Semagacestat
Semuloparin Sodium
Serlopitant
Sifilcon A
Sivifene
Sobetirome
Sofinicline
Sofinicline Benzenesulfonate
Spinosad
Talarozole
Talmapimod
Tanezumab

Tasimelteon
Tasisulam Sodium
Taspoglutide
Tecovirimat
Telcagepant
Telcagepant Potassium
Tenatumomab
Teneligliptin
Tertomotide
Tigatuzumab
Tildipirosin
Tiprolisant
Toceranib
Toceranib Phosphate
Tosedostat
Tozasertib
Tozasertib Lactate
Troplasminogen Alfa
Turofexorate Isopropyl
Tylvalosin Tartrate
Ustekinumab
Vadimezan
Varespladib
Varespladib Methyl
Vedolizumab
Velneperit
Viquidacin
Voreloxin

United States Adopted Names
(USAN)

AND INTERNATIONAL DRUG NAMES

A/16686 — *See* Ramoplanin.

A-16686 — *See* Ramoplanin.

Abacavir Succinate [*1996*] (a bak′ a vir sux′ i nate). $C_{14}H_{18}N_6O.C_4H_6O_4$. 404.42. [Abacavir is INN and BAN.] (1) 2-Cyclopentene-1-methanol, 4-[2-amino-6-(cyclopropylamino)-9*H*-purin-9-yl]-, (1*S-cis*)-, butanedioate (1:1) (salt); (2) (1*S*,4*R*)-4-[2-Amino-6-(cyclopropylamino)-9*H*-purin-9-yl]-2-cyclopentene-1-methanol succinate (1:1) (salt). *UNII-40FH6D8CHK; UNII-WR2TIP26VS* [abacavir]. *CAS-168146-84-7; CAS-136470-78-5* [abacavir]. *Antiviral.* ◇*1592U89*

Abacavir Sulfate [*1997*] (a bak′ a vir sul′ fate). $(C_{14}H_{18}N_6O)_2.H_2SO_4$. 670.74. (1*S*,4*R*)-4-[2-Amino-6-(cyclopropylamino)-9*H*-purin-9-yl]-2-cyclopentene-1-methanol sulfate (salt) (2:1). *UNII-J220T4J9Q2. CAS-188062-50-2. Antiviral.* Ziagen (GlaxoSmithKline) ◇*1592U89*

Abafilcon A [*1996*] (a″ ba fil′ kon). $(C_5H_9NO)_w(C_{16}H_{38}O_5\text{-}Si_4)_x(C_{11}H_{14})_y(C_{10}H_{14}O_4)_z$. (1) 2-Propenamide, *N,N*-dimethyl-, polymer with 3-[3,3,3-trimethyl-1,1-bis[(trimethylsilyl)oxy]disiloxanyl]propyl 2-methyl-2-propenoate, 2-ethenyl-1,3,5-trimethylbenzene, and 1,2-ethanediyl bis(2-methyl-2-propenoate); (2) *N,N*-Dimethylacrylamide polymer with 3-[3,3,3-trimethyl-1,1-bis(trimethylsiloxy)disiloxanyl]propyl methacrylate, 2,4,6-trimethylstyrene and ethylene dimethacrylate. *CAS-165253-33-8. Contact lens material (hydrophilic).* [*Note—The water content of the contact lens material is 27.0±0.6% at ambient temperature (23±2°C), and the oxygen permeability is 69 ± 1.1 × 10⁻¹¹(cm²/sec)(ml O₂/ml × mm Hg) at 35°C (Dk value).*]

Abafungin. $C_{21}H_{22}N_4OS$. 378.49. Hexahydro-2-[[4-[*o*-(2,4-xylyloxy)phenyl]-2-thiazolyl]imino]pyrimidine. *UNII-11DI31LWXF. CAS-129639-79-8.* INN; BAN. ◇*Bay w 6341*

Abagovomab. Immunoglobulin G1, anti-idiotype anti-[anti-(*Homo sapiens* cancer antigen 125, CA 125, MUC-16) *Mus musculus* monoclonal antibody OC125] *Mus musculus* monoclonal antibody ACA125, clone 3D5 gamma1 heavy chain disulfide with clone 3D5 kappa light chain; (223-223″:226-226″:228-228″) trisdisulfide dimer. *CAS-792921-10-9.* INN.

Abamectin [*1988*] (a″ ba mek′ tin). A mixture consisting of 80% or more of Abamectin Component B_{1a} and 20% or less of Abamectin Component B_{1b}. *CAS-65195-55-3* [Component B_{1a}]; *CAS-65195-56-4* [Component B_{1b}]. INN. *Antiparasitic.* Avomec [Veterinary] (Merial); Bovitin [Veterinary] (Merial); Doratect [Veterinary] (Merial); Duomectin [Veterinary] (Merial); Duotin [Veterinary] (Merial); Endecto (Merck); Enzec (Merck); Enzek (Merck); Parafoil (Merck); Vertimil (Merck); Zectin (Merck) ◇*MK-0936*

Abamectin Component B_{1a}. $C_{48}H_{72}O_{14}$. 873.08. Component of Abamectin. (1) Avermectin A_{1a}, 5-*O*-demethyl-; (2) (2a*E*,4*E*,8*E*)-(5′*S*,6*S*,6′*R*,7*S*,11*R*,13*S*,15*S*,17a*R*,20*R*,20a*R*,20b*S*)-6′-[(*S*)-*sec*-Butyl]-5′,6,6′,7,10,11,14,15,17a,20,20a,20b-dodecahydro-20,20b-dihydroxy-5′,6,8,19-tetramethyl-17-oxospiro[11,15-methano-2*H*,13*H*,17*H*-furo[4,3,2-*pq*][2,6]benzodioxacyclooctadecin-13,2′-[2*H*]pyran]-7-yl 2,6-dideoxy-4-*O*-(2,6-dideoxy-3-*O*-methyl-α-L-*arabino*-hexopyranosyl)-3-*O*-methyl-α-L-*arabino*-hexopyranoside. *CAS-65195-55-3.*

Abamectin Component B_{1b}. $C_{47}H_{70}O_{14}$. 859.05. Component of Abamectin. (1)Avermectin A_{1a}, 5-*O*-demethyl-25-de(1-methylpropyl)-25-(1-methylethyl)-; (2) (2a*E*,4*E*,8*E*)-(5′*S*,6*S*,6′*R*,7*S*,11*R*,13*S*,15*S*,17a*R*,20*R*,20a*R*,20b*S*)-5′,6,6′,7,10,11,14,15,17a,20,20a,20b-Dodecahydro-20,20b-dihydroxy-6′-isopropyl-5′,6,8,19-tetramethyl-17-oxospiro[11,15-methano-2*H*,13*H*,17*H*-furo[4,3,2-*pq*][2,6]benzodioxacyclooctadecin-13,2′-[2*H*]pyran]-7-yl

2,6-dideoxy-4-*O*-(2,6-dideoxy-3-*O*-methyl-α-L-*arabino*-hexopyranosyl)-3-*O*-methyl-α-L-*arabino*-hexopyranoside. *CAS-65195-56-4.*

Abanoquil. $C_{22}H_{25}N_3O_4$. 395.45. 4-Amino-2-(3,4-dihydro-6,7-dimethoxy-2(1*H*)-isoquinolyl)-6,7-dimethoxyquinoline. *UNII-F738MWY53L. CAS-90402-40-7.* INN; BAN.

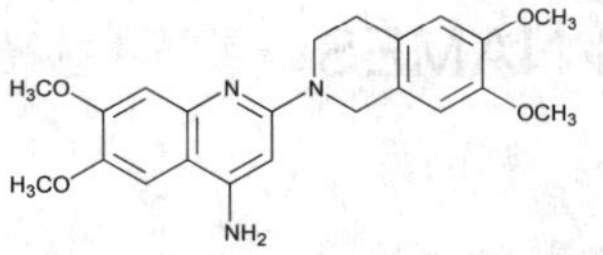

Abaperidone. $C_{25}H_{25}FN_2O_5$. 452.47. 7-[3-[4-(6-Fluoro-1,2-benzisoxazol-3-yl)piperidino]propoxy]-3-(hydroxymethyl)-4*H*-1-benzopyran-4-one. *UNII-40755Z8956. CAS-183849-43-6.* INN.

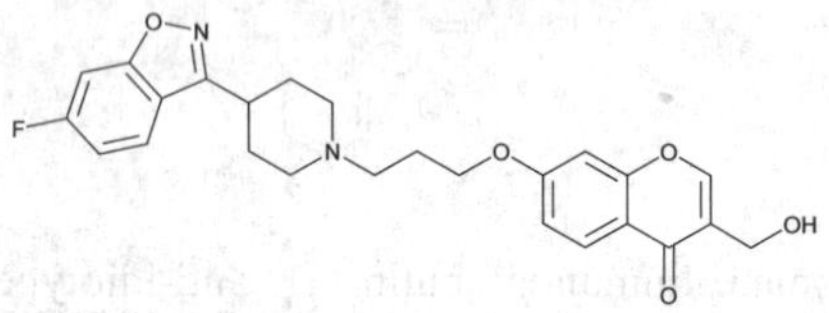

Abarelix [*1997*] (a″ ba rel′ ix). $C_{72}H_{95}ClN_{14}O_{14}$. 1416.06. *N*-Acetyl-3-(2-naphthyl)-D-alanyl-4-chloro-D-phenylalanyl-3-(3-pyridyl)-D-alanyl-L-seryl-*N*-methyl-L-tyrosyl-D-asparaginyl-L-leucyl-*N*^6^-isopropyl-L-lysyl-L-prolyl-D-alaninamide. *UNII-W486SJ5824. CAS-183552-38-7.* INN. *Gonad-stimulating principle; antagonist (LHRH).* Plenaxis (Praecis) ◇*PPI-149; R3827*

Abatacept [*2004*] (a bat′ a sept). $(C_{1965}H_{3080}N_{479}O_{695}S_{16})$. 1-25-Oncostatin M (human precursor) fusion protein with CTLA-4 (antigen) (human) fusion protein with immunoglobulin G1 (human heavy chain fragment). Molecular weight is approximately 92,000 daltons (46,000 daltons per chain). *UNII-7D0YB67S97. CAS-332348-12-6.* INN; BAN; JAN. *Treatment of autoimmune diseases such as rheumatoid arthritis (selective co-stimulation modulator; binds to the B7 family of molecules expressed on antigen-presenting cells (APC)).* ◇*BMS-188667*

```
MGVLLTQRTL LSLVLALLFP SMASMAMHVA QPAVVLASSR GIASFVCEYA
SPGKATEVRV TVLRQADSQV TEVCAATYMM GNELTFLDDS ICTGTSSGNQ
VNLTIQGLRA MDTGLYICKV ELMYPPPYYL GIGNGTQIYV IDPEPCPDSD
QEPKSSDKTH TSPPSPAPEL LGGSSVFLFP PKPKDTLMIS RTPEVTCVVV
DVSHEDPEVK FNWYVDGVEV HNAKTKPREE QYNSTYRVVS VLTVLHQDWL
NGKEYKCKVS NKALPAPIEK TISKAKGQPR EPQVYTLPPS RDELTKNQVS
LTCLVKGFYP SDIAVEWESN GQPENNYKTT PPVLDSDGSF FLYSKLTVDK
SRWQQGNVFS CSVMHEALHN HYTQKSLSLS PG**K*
```

** - C-terminus (predominant species)
  * - C-terminus (cDNA)
 <u>underline</u> - N-glycosylation

Abciximab [*1994*] (ab six′ i mab). (1) Immunoglobulin G1, (human-mouse monoclonal c7E3 clone p7E3V$_H$hC$_{γ1}$ Fab fragment anti-human glycoprotein IIb/IIIa receptor), disulfide with human-mouse monoclonal c7E3 clone p7E3V$_κ$hC$_κ$ light chain; (2) Immunoglobulin G1 (human-mouse monoclonal c7E3 clone p7E3V$_H$hC$_{γ1}$ Fab fragment anti-human glycoprotein IIb/IIIa receptor), disulfide with human-mouse monoclonal c7E3 clone p7E3V$_κ$hC$_κ$ light chain. Molecular weight is approximately 47,600 daltons. *UNII-X85G7936GV. CAS-143653-53-6.* INN; BAN. *Monoclonal antibody (antithrombotic).* ReoPro (Lilly) ◇*c7E3*

Abecarnil. $C_{24}H_{24}N_2O_4$. 404.46. Isopropyl 6-(benzyloxy)-4-(methoxymethyl)-9*H*-pyrido[3,4-*b*]indole-3-carboxylate. *UNII-IZM1PNJ3JL. CAS-111841-85-1.* INN.

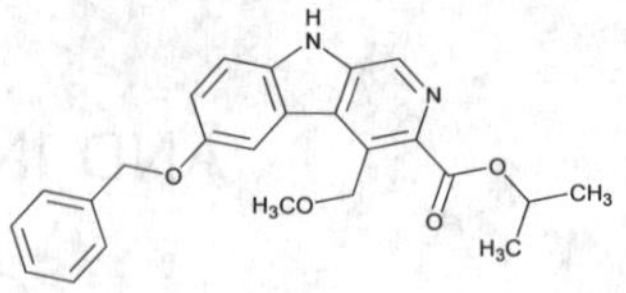

Abetimus. $C_{1632}H_{2100}N_{610}O_{970}P_{156}S_4$. 50,741.84. d(C-A-C-A-C-A-C-A-C-A-C-A-C-A-C-A-C-A-C-A-C-A)-*P*,5′,5‴,5‴′,5‴″″″-Tetraester with ethylenebis(oxyethylene)bis[bis[2-[6-[2-[(6-hydroxyhexyl)thio]acetamido]hexanamido]ethyl]carbamate], complex with d(T-G-T-G-T-G-T-G-T-G-T-G-T-G-T-G) (1:4). *CAS-167362-48-3.* INN.

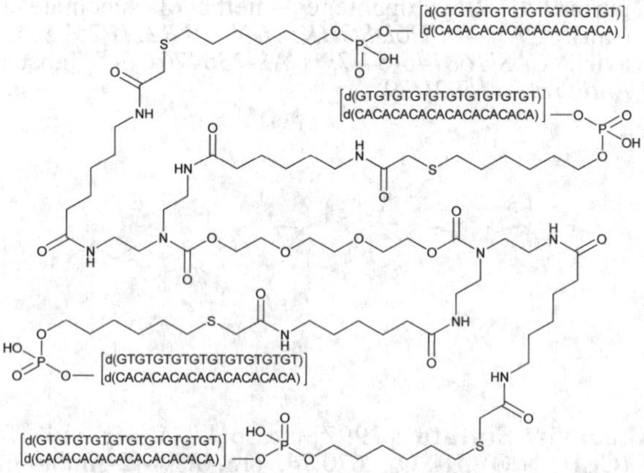

Abetimus Sodium [*1998*] (a bet′ i mus soe′ dee um). $C_{1632}H_{1944}N_{610}Na_{156}O_{970}P_{156}S_4$. 54,172 daltons. Deoxyribonucleic acid d(C-A-C-A-C-A-C-A-C-A-C-A-C-A-C-A-C-A), 5′-ester with 1,2-ethanediylbis(oxy-2,1-ethanediyl)bis[2-(21,21-dihydroxy-4,11-dioxo-20-oxa-13-thia-3,10-diaza-21-phosphaheneicos-1-yl)-23,23-dihydroxy-6,13-dioxo-22-oxa-15-thia-2,5,12-triaza-23-phosphatricosanoate] (4:1), *P*,*P*′,23,23′-tetraoxide, complex with deoxyribonucleic acid d(T-G-T-G-T-G-T-G-T-G-T-G-T-G-T-G-T-G) (1:1), hexapentacontahectasodium salt. *CAS-169147-32-4.* *Treatment of systemic lupus erythematosus and diseases-associated nephritis (immunosuppressant).* ◇*LJP 394*

Abiraterone. $C_{24}H_{31}NO$. 349.51. 17-(3-Pyridyl)androsta-5,16-dien-3β-ol. *UNII-G819A456D0. CAS-154229-19-3.* INN; BAN. ◇*CB 7598; CB 7630 [as acetate]*

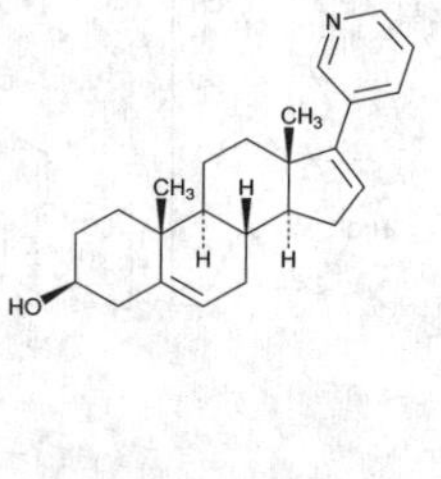

Abitesartan. $C_{26}H_{31}N_5O_3$. 461.56. 1-[[*N*-[*p*-(*o*-1*H*-Tetrazol-5-ylphenyl)benzyl]valeramido]methyl-1-cyclopentane carboxylic acid. *UNII-3YY13B9G25. CAS-137882-98-5.* INN. *[Name previously used: Tisartan.]*

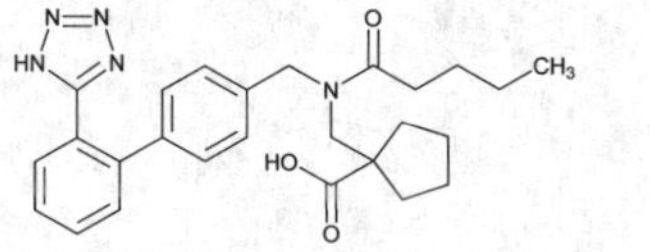

Ablukast [*1989*] (ab loo′ kast). $C_{28}H_{34}O_8$. 498.56. (1) 2*H*-1-Benzopyran-2-carboxylic acid, 6-acetyl-7-[[5-(4-acetyl-3-hydroxy-2-propylphenoxy)pentyl]oxy]-3,4-dihydro-, (±)-; (2) (±)-6-Acetyl-7-[[5-(4-acetyl-3-hydroxy-2-propylphenoxy)pentyl]oxy]-2-chromancarboxylic acid. *UNII-000TKM5BBQ. CAS-96566-25-5.* INN. *Anti-asthmatic (leukotriene antagonist).* ◇*Ro 23-3544/000*

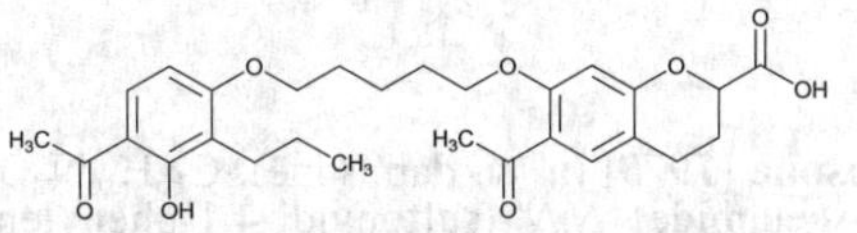

Ablukast Sodium [*1989*] (ab loo′ kast soe′ dee um). $C_{28}H_{33}NaO_8$. 520.55. (1) 2*H*-1-Benzopyran-2-carboxylic acid, 6-acetyl-7-[[5-(4-acetyl-3-hydroxy-2-propylphenoxy)pentyl]oxy]-3,4-dihydro-, monosodium salt, (±)-; (2) Sodium (±)-6-acetyl-7-[[5-(4-acetyl-3-hydroxy-2-propylphenoxy)pentyl]oxy]-2-chromancarboxylate. *CAS-96565-55-8. Anti-asthmatic (leukotriene antagonist).* Ulpax (Hoffmann-LaRoche†) ◇*Ro 23-3544/001*

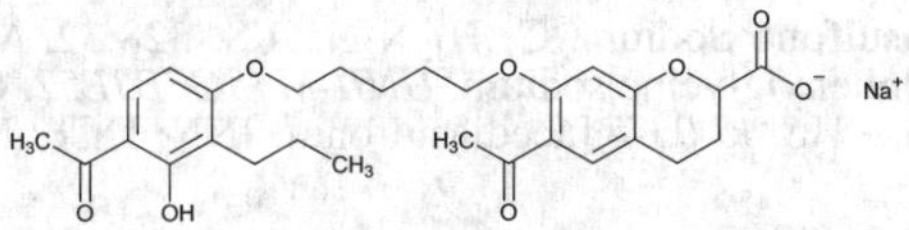

Abrineurin [*2000*] (a″ bri noor′ in). $C_{587}H_{947}N_{177}S_{10}$. (1) *N*-L-Methionylneurotrophic factor (human brain-derived) cyclic (14→81), (59→110), (69→112)-tris(disulfide) dimer; (2) *N*-L-Methionylneurotrophic factor (human brain-derived) cyclic (13→80), (58→109), (68→111)-tris(disulfide), dimer. Molecular weight is approximately 27,200 daltons for the dimer. *CAS-178535-92-7; CAS-178535-93-8* [monomer]. INN. *Treatment of amyotrophic lateral sclerosis (ALS).*[*Name previously used: Brineurin.*]

```
                                              M
HSDPARRGEL SVCDSISEWV TAADKKTAVD MSGGTVTVLE KVPVSKGQLK
QYFYETKCNP MGYTKEGCRG IDKRHWNSQC RTTQSYVRAL TMDSKKRIGW
RFIRIDTSCV CTLTIKRGR
```

Abunidazole. $C_{15}H_{19}N_3O_4$. 305.33. α-(5-*tert*-Butyl-2-hydroxyphenyl)-1-methyl-5-nitroimidazole-2-methanol. *UNII-6EH821150I. CAS-91017-58-2.* INN.

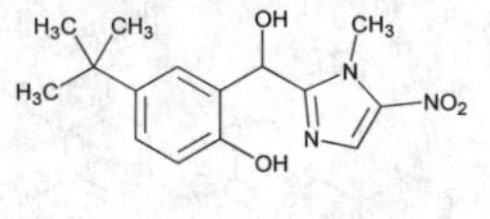

Acacia (a kay′ sha). **NF**. The dried gummy exudate from the stems and branches of *Acacia senegal* (Linné) Willdenow or of other related African species of *Acacia* (Fam. Leguminosae). *UNII-5C5403N26O. CAS-9000-01-5.* JAN. *Pharmaceutic aid (suspending and/or viscosity agent).*

Acadesine [*1992*] (a ka′ de seen). $C_9H_{14}N_4O_5$. 258.23. (1) 1*H*-Imidazole-4-carboxamide, 5-amino-1-β-D-ribofuranosyl-; (2) 5-Amino-1-β-D-ribofuranosylimidazole-4-carboxamide. *UNII-531EF47846. CAS-2627-69-2.* INN; BAN. *Platelet aggregation inhibitor.* ◇*GP-1-110*

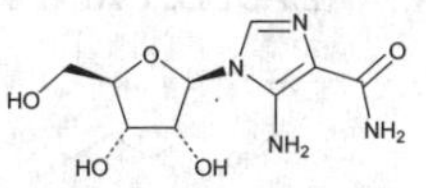

Acamprosate Calcium [*2002*] (a kam′ proe sate kal′ see um). $C_{10}H_{20}CaN_2O_8S_2$. 400.48. [Acamprosate is INN and BAN.] (1) 1-Propanesulfonic acid, 3-(acetylamino)-, calcium salt (2:1); (2) Calcium 3-(acetylamino)propane-1-sulfonate. *UNII-59375N1D0U. CAS-77337-73-6; CAS-77337-76-9* [acamprosate]. *Treatment of alcohol dependency.* Campral (Forest)

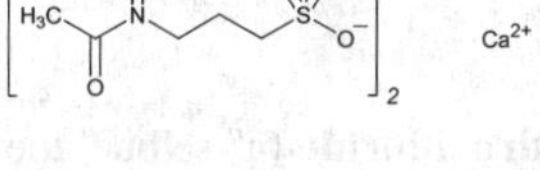

Acamylophenine — *See* Camylofin.

Acamylophenine Hydrochloride (JAN) — *See* Camylofin.

Acaprazine. $C_{15}H_{21}Cl_2N_3O$. 330.25. *N*-[3-[4-(2,5-Dichlorophenyl)-1-piperazinyl]propyl]acetamide. *UNII-F2S6Z4SB8T. CAS-55485-20-6.* INN.

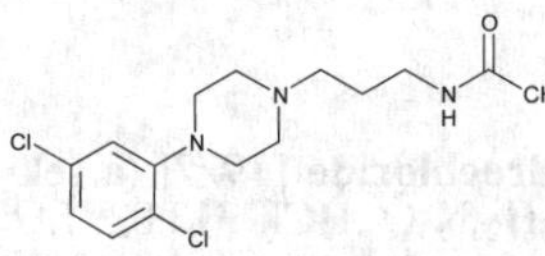

Acarbose [*1983*] (ay′ kar bose). $C_{25}H_{43}NO_{18}$. 645.60. (1) D-Glucose, *O*-4,6-dideoxy-4-[[[1*S*-(1α,4α,5β,6α)]-4,5,6-trihydroxy-3-(hydroxymethyl)-2-cyclohexen-1-yl]amino]-α-D-glucopyranosyl-(1→4)-*O*-α-D-glucopyranosyl-(1→4)-; (2) *O*-4,6-Dideoxy-4-[[(1*S*,4*R*,5*S*,6*S*)-4,5,6-trihydroxy-3-(hydroxymethyl)-2-cyclohexen-1-yl]amino]-α-D-glucopyranosyl-(1→4)-*O*-α-D-glucopyranosyl-(1→4)-D-glucose. *UNII-T58MSI464G. CAS-56180-94-0.* INN; BAN; JAN. *Inhibitor (α-glucosidase).* Precose (Bayer) ◇*Bay g 5421*

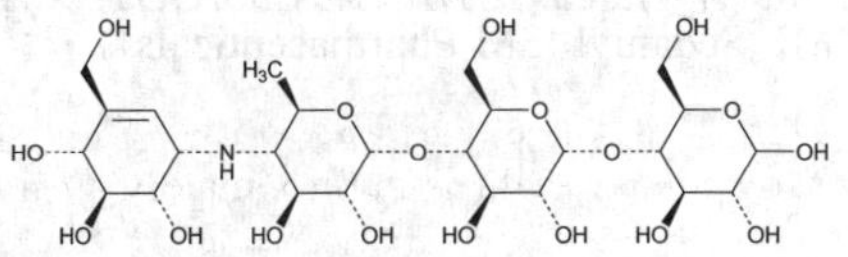

---

† Brand name formerly used, and/or firm no longer concerned with this product.

Acebrochol. $C_{29}H_{48}Br_2O_2$. 588.50. 5,6-β-Dibromo-5α-cholestan-3β-ol acetate. *UNII-7XZB016MY5. CAS-514-50-1.* INN; DCF.

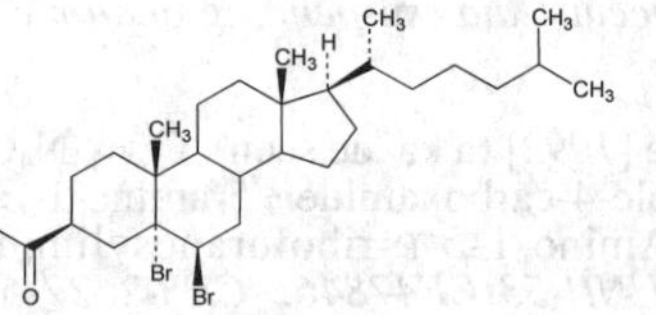

Aceburic Acid. $C_6H_{10}O_4$. 146.14. 4-Hydroxybutyric acid acetate. *UNII-F777XEP0LL. CAS-26976-72-7.* INN; DCF.

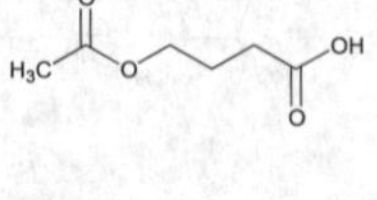

Acebutolol [*1973*] (a″ se bue′ toe lol). $C_{18}H_{28}N_2O_4$. 336.43. (1) Butanamide, *N*-[3-acetyl-4-[2-hydroxy-3-[(1-methylethyl)amino]propoxy]phenyl]-, ($\pm$)-; (2) ($\pm$)-3′-Acetyl-4′-[2-hydroxy-3-(isopropylamino)propoxy]butyranilide. *UNII-67P356D8GH. CAS-37517-30-9.* INN; BAN. *Antiadrenergic (β-receptor).*

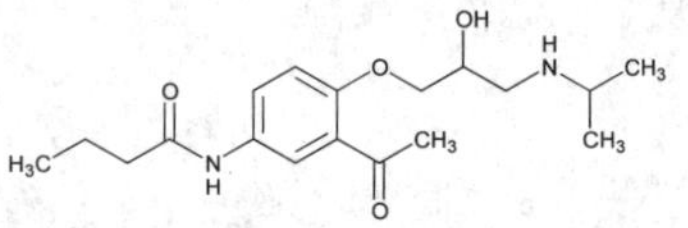

Acebutolol Hydrochloride (a″ se bue′ toe lol hye″ droe klor′ ide). USP. $C_{18}H_{28}N_2O_4$·HCl. 372.89. (1) Butanamide, *N*-[3-acetyl-4-[2-hydroxy-3-[(1-methylethyl)amino]propoxy]phenyl]-, monohydrochloride, ($\pm$)-; (2) ($\pm$)-3′-Acetyl-4′-[2-hydroxy-3-(isopropylamino)propoxy]butyranilide monohydrochloride. *UNII-B025Y34C54; UNII-67P356D8GH* [acebutolol]. *CAS-34381-68-5; CAS-37517-30-9* [acebutolol]. JAN. *Anti-adrenergic (β-receptor).* Sectral (Dr. Reddy's) ◇*M&B 17803A; IL-17803A*

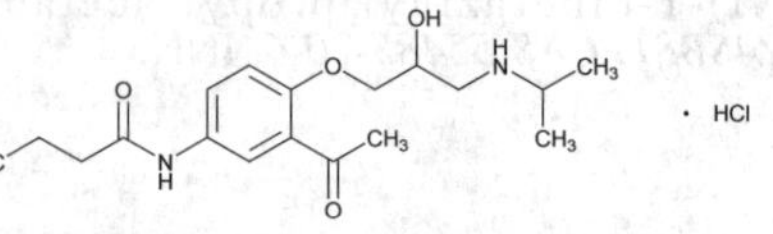

Acecainide Hydrochloride [*1977*] (a sek′ a nide hye″ droe klor′ ide). $C_{15}H_{23}N_3O_2$·HCl. 313.82. [Acecainide is INN.] (1) Benzamide, 4-(acetylamino)-*N*-[2-(diethylamino)ethyl]-, monohydrochloride; (2) 4′-[[2-(Diethylamino)ethyl]carbamoyl]acetanilide monohydrochloride. *UNII-B9K738KX14; UNII-910Q707V6F* [acecainide]. *CAS-34118-92-8; CAS-32795-44-1* [acecainide]. *Cardiac depressant (anti-arrhythmic).* ◇*ASL-601*

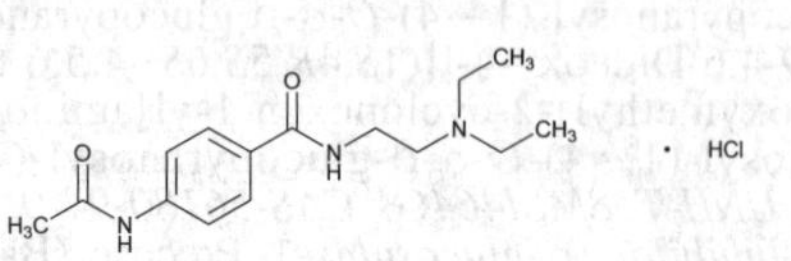

Acecarbromal. $C_9H_{15}BrN_2O_3$. 279.13. 1-Acetyl-3-(α-bromo-α-ethylbutyryl)urea. *UNII-E47C56IGOY. CAS-77-66-7.* INN; MI. Sedamyl (3M Pharmaceuticals†)

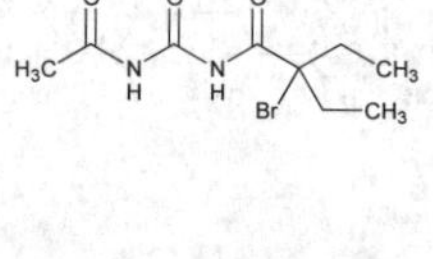

Aceclidine [*1967*] (a sek′ li deen). $C_9H_{15}NO_2$. 169.22. (1) 1-Azabicyclo[2.2.2]octan-3-ol, acetate (ester); (2) 3-Quinuclidinol acetate (ester); (3) 3-Acetoxyquinuclidine. *UNII-0578K3ELIO. CAS-827-61-2.* INN. *Cholinergic.* Glaucostat (Kingshill Pharmaceuticals, Inc., Switzerland)

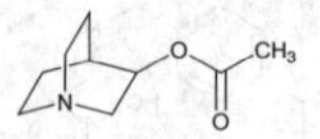

Aceclofenac. $C_{16}H_{13}Cl_2NO_4$. 354.18. Glycolic acid, [*o*-(2,6-dichloroanilino)phenyl]acetate (ester). *CAS-89796-99-6.* INN; BAN.

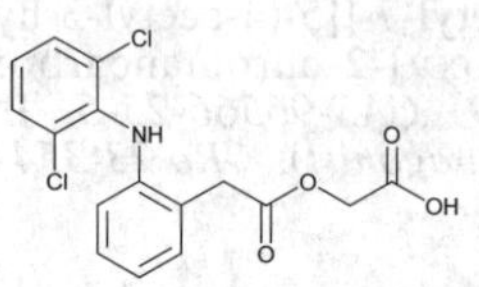

Acedapsone [*1970*] (a″ se dap′ sone). $C_{16}H_{16}N_2O_4S$. 332.37. (1) Acetamide, *N,N′*-(sulfonyldi-4,1-phenylene)bis-; (2) 4′,4‴-Sulfonylbis[acetanilidec]. *UNII-0GZ72U84TN. CAS-77-46-3.* INN; BAN. *Antimalarial; antibacterial (leprostatic).* Hansolar (Parke-Davis†) ◇*CI 556; CN-1883; DADDS; PAM-MR-1165*

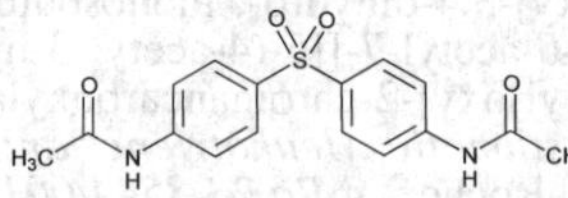

Acediasulfone Sodium. $C_{14}H_{13}N_2NaO_4S$. 328.32. *N*-*p*-Sulfanilylphenylglycine sodium. *UNII-M45G7BJL52. CAS-127-60-6; CAS-80-03-5* [acediasulfone]. INN; DCF; MI.

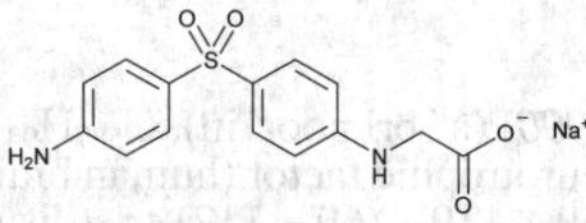

Acedoben. $C_9H_9NO_3$. 179.17. *p*-Acetamidobenzoic acid. *UNII-04Z20NMK31. CAS-556-08-1.* INN.

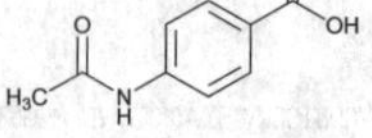

Acefluranol. $C_{25}H_{26}F_2O_8$. 492.47. 4,4′-[(1*RS*,2*SR*)-1-Ethyl-2-methylethylene]bis[6-fluoropyrocatechol] tetraacetate. *UNII-3K0BN50QXD. CAS-80595-73-9.* INN; BAN. ◇*BX 591*

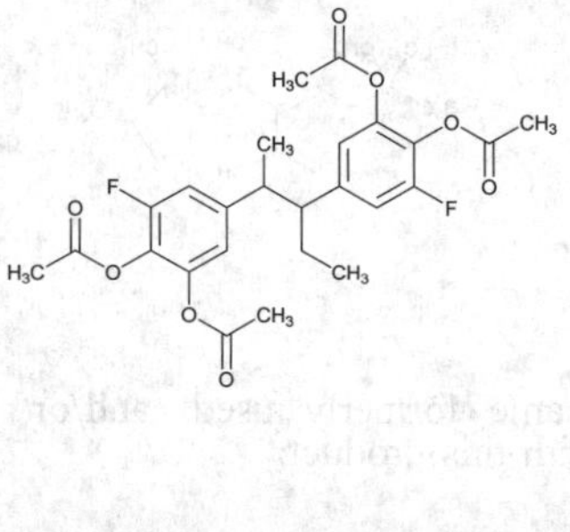

Acefurtiamine. $C_{21}H_{24}N_4O_7S$. 476.50. *S*-Ester of thio-2-furoic acid with *N*-[(4-amino-2-methyl-5-pyrimidinyl)methyl]-*N*-(4-hydroxy-2-mercapto-1-methyl-1-butenyl)formamide *O*-glycolate acetate. *UNII-6APJ3D1308. CAS-10072-48-7.* INN.

Acefylline Clofibrol. $C_{19}H_{21}ClN_4O_5$. 420.85. 2-(*p*-Chlorophenoxy)-2-methylpropyl 1,2,3,6-tetrahydro-1,3-dimethyl-2,6-dioxopurine-7-acetate. *UNII-WY672D78VW. CAS-70788-27-1.* INN.

Acefylline Piperazine. $(C_9H_{10}N_4O_4)_2 \cdot C_4H_{10}N_2$. 562.54. Piperazine 7-theophyllineacetate. *UNII-12I91IOS6Z. CAS-18833-13-1; CAS-15302-00-8* [replaced]. INN; BAN; DCF; MI. *[Name previously used: Acepifylline.]*

Aceglatone. $C_{10}H_{10}O_8$. 258.18. D-Glucaric acid 1,4:6,3-dilactone diacetate. *UNII-347Q3OOJ13. CAS-642-83-1.* INN; JAN; MI.

Aceglutamide Aluminum [*1984*] (a″ se gloo′ ta mide a loo′ mi num). $C_{35}H_{59}Al_3N_{10}O_{24}$. 1084.84. [Aceglutamide is INN.] (1) Aluminum, pentakis(*N*²-acetyl-L-glutaminato)tetrahydroxytri-; (2) Pentakis (*N*²-acetyl-L-glutaminato)tetrahydroxytrialuminum. *UNII-R7QTG0PMPX; UNII-01J18G9G97* [aceglutamide]. *CAS-12607-92-0; CAS-2490-97-3* [aceglutamide]. JAN. *Anti-ulcerative*. Glumal (Kyowa Hakko Kogyo Co., Ltd., Japan) ◇*KW-110*

Acemannan [*1990*] (a″ se man′ nan). Acemannan is a highly acetylated, polydispersed, linear mannan obtained from the mucilage of *Aloe barbadensis*, Miller (aloe vera). Molecular weight is 1–2 million daltons. *CAS-110042-95-0.* INN. *Antiviral; immunomodulator*. Carraklenz Wound & Skin Cleanser (Carrington); Carrisyn (Carrington); Snow & Sun Sports Gel (Carrington) *[Name previously used: Polymanoacetate.]*

Acemetacin. $C_{21}H_{18}ClNO_6$. 415.82. 1-(*p*-Chlorobenzoyl)-5-methoxy-2-methylindole-3-acetic acid ester with glycolic acid. *UNII-5V141XK28X. CAS-53164-05-9.* INN; BAN; JAN; MI.

Acemethadone — *See* Methadyl Acetate.

Aceneuramic Acid. $C_{11}H_{19}NO_9$. 309.27. (-)-5-Acetamido-3,5-dideoxy-D-*glycero*-D-*galacto*-nonulosonic acid. *CAS-131-48-6.* INN.

Acenocoumarin — *See* Acenocoumarol.

Acenocoumarol. $C_{19}H_{15}NO_6$. 353.33. (1) 2*H*-1-Benzopyran-2-one, 4-hydroxy-3-[1-(4-nitrophenyl)-3-oxobutyl]-; (2) 3-(α-Acetonyl-*p*-nitrobenzyl)-4-hydroxycoumarin. *UNII-I6WP63U32H. CAS-152-72-7.* NF XIV; INN; BAN; MI.

Aceperone. $C_{24}H_{29}FN_2O_2$. 396.50. 4-[4-(Acetamidomethyl)-4-phenylpiperidino]-4′-fluorobutyrophenone. *UNII-S69KXZ59AB. CAS-807-31-8.* INN; MI. ◇*R 3248*

Acephenazine Dimaleate — *See* Acetophenazine Maleate.

Acepifylline (previously used name) — *See* Acefylline Piperazine.

---

† Brand name formerly used, and/or firm no longer concerned with this product.

Acepromazine Maleate [*1973*] (a″ se proe′ ma zeen mal′ ee ate). **USP.** $C_{19}H_{22}N_2OS.C_4H_4O_4$. 442.53. [Acepromazine is INN and BAN.] (1) Ethanone, 1-[10-[3-(dimethylamino)propyl]-10*H*-phenothiazin-2-yl]-, (*Z*)-2-butenedioate (1:1); (2) 10-[3-(Dimethylamino)propyl]phenothiazin-2-yl methyl ketone maleate (1:1). *UNII-37862HP2OM. CAS-3598-37-6; CAS-61-00-7* [acepromazine]. *Sedative (veterinary).*

Aceprometazine. $C_{19}H_{22}N_2OS$. 326.46. 10-[2-(Dimethylamino)propyl]phenothiazin-2-yl methyl ketone. *UNII-984N9YTM4Y. CAS-13461-01-3.* INN; DCF. ◇*CB 1664*

Acequinoline. $C_{14}H_{15}NO_2$. 229.27. 7-Methoxy-2,4-dimethyl-3-quinolyl methyl ketone. *UNII-FKJ64U4XOB. CAS-42465-20-3.* INN; DCF. ◇*CB 4985*

Acesulfame. $C_4H_5NO_4S$. 163.15. 6-Methyl-1,2,3-oxathiazin-4(3*H*)-one 2,2-dioxide. *UNII-MA3UYZ6K1H. CAS-33665-90-6.* INN; BAN; MI.

Acesulfame Potassium. NF. $C_4H_4NO_4SK$. 201.24. (1) 6-Methyl-1,2,3-oxathiazine-4(3*H*)-one-2,2-dioxide potassium salt; (2) 3,4-Dihydro-6-methyl-1,2,3-oxathiazine-4-one-2,2-dioxide potassium salt. *UNII-23OV73Q5G9. CAS-55589-62-3.*

Acetaminocaproic Acid — *See* Acexamic Acid.

Acetaminophen (a seet″ a min′ oh fen). **USP.** $C_8H_9NO_2$. 151.16. [Paracetamol is INN and BAN.] (1) Acetamide, *N*-(4-hydroxyphenyl)-; (2) 4′-Hydroxyacetanilide. *UNII-362O9ITL9D. CAS-103-90-2.* JAN. *Analgesic; antipyretic.* Acephen (G & W); Infants' Feverall (Actavis); Injectapap (Ortho-McNeil); Neopap (Polymedica); Tylenol (McNeil)

Acetaminosalol. $C_{15}H_{13}NO_4$. 271.27. 4′-Hydroxyacetanilide salicylate. *UNII-O3J7H54KMD. CAS-118-57-0.* INN; DCF; MI.

Acetanilide. *UNII-SP86R356CC. CAS-103-84-4.* NF X [Acetanilid]; MI.

Acetannin — *See* Acetyltannic Acid.

Acetarsol (INN, BAN, DCF) — *See* Acetarsone.

Acetarsone. $C_8H_{10}AsNO_5$. 275.09. [Acetarsol is INN and BAN.] *N*-Acetyl-4-hydroxy-*m*-arsanilic acid. *UNII-806529YU1N. CAS-97-44-9.* NF XI; MI. Stovarsol (Abbott†)

Acetazolamide (a seet″ a zole′ a mide). **USP.** $C_4H_6N_4O_3S_2$. 222.25. (1) Acetamide, *N*-[5-(aminosulfonyl)-1,3,4-thiadiazol-2-yl]-; (2) *N*-(5-Sulfamoyl-1,3,4-thiadiazol-2-yl)acetamide. *UNII-O3FX965V0I. CAS-59-66-5.* INN; BAN; JAN. *Carbonic anhydrase inhibitor.* Diamox (Duramed)

Acetazolamide Sodium. $C_4H_5N_4NaO_3S_2$. 244.23. (1) Acetamide, *N*-[5-(aminosulfonyl)-1,3,4-thiadiazol-2-yl]-, monosodium salt; (2) *N*-(5-Sulfamoyl-1,3,4-thiadiazol-2-yl)acetamide monosodium salt. *UNII-429ZT169UH. CAS-1424-27-7.* JAN. Diamox (Duramed)

Acetergamine. $C_{18}H_{23}N_3O$. 297.39. (+)-*N*-Acetyl-9,10-dihydrolysergamine. *UNII-O60O0JB93O. CAS-3031-48-9.* INN.

Acetiamine. $C_{16}H_{22}N_4O_4S$. 366.44. *N*-[(4-Amino-2-methyl-5-pyrimidinyl)methyl]-*N*-(4-hydroxy-2-mercapto-1-methyl-1-butenyl)formamide *O,S*-diacetate. *CAS-299-89-8.* INN; MI. ◇*D.A.T.*

Acetic Acid (a see′ tik as′ id). **NF.** (1) Acetic acid; (2) Acetic acid. *UNII-Q40Q9N063P. CAS-64-19-7.* JAN. *Pharmaceutic aid (acidifying agent).* Vosol (Carter-Wallace)

Acetic Acid, Glacial (a see′ tik as′ id glay′ shil). **USP.** $C_2H_4O_2$. 60.05. (1) Acetic acid; (2) Acetic acid. *UNII-Q40Q9N063P. CAS-64-19-7.* JAN. *Pharmaceutic aid (acidifying agent).* Acetasol (Actavis); Orlex (Procter & Gamble)

Acetiromate. $C_{15}H_9I_3O_5$. 649.94. 4-(4-Hydroxy-3-iodophenoxy)-3,5-diiodobenzoic acid acetate. *UNII-8Q5153W1NW. CAS-2260-08-4.* INN.

Acetohexamide [*1962*] (a seet″ oh hex′ a mide). **USP.** $C_{15}H_{20}N_2O_4S$. 324.40. (1) Benzenesulfonamide, 4-acetyl-*N*-[[cyclohexylamino]carbonyl]-; (2) 1-[(*p*-Acetylphenyl)-sulfonyl]-3-cyclohexylurea. *UNII-QGC8W08I6I. CAS-968-81-0.* INN; BAN; JAN. *Antidiabetic.* Dymelor (Lilly) ◇33006

Acetohydroxamic Acid [*1984*] (a seet″ oh hye″ drox am′ ik as′ id). **USP.** $C_2H_5NO_2$. 75.07. (1) *N*-Acetyl hydroxyacetamide; (2) Acetohydroxamic acid. *UNII-4RZ82L2GY5. CAS-546-88-3.* INN. *Enzyme inhibitor (urease).* Lithostat (Mission)

Acetomenaphthone. [Acetomenaphtone is JAN.] 2-Methyl-1,4-naphthylene diacetate. *UNII-DWG8UZD9HT. CAS-573-20-6.* BAN.

Acetomenaphtone (JAN) — *See* Acetomenaphthone.

Acetomeroctol. *UNII-W8OY9Y1132. CAS-584-18-9.* MI.

Acetone (as′ e tone). **NF.** C_3H_6O. 58.08. (1) 2-Propanone; (2) Acetone. *UNII-1364PS73AF. CAS-67-64-1. Pharmaceutic aid (solvent).*

Acetophenazine Maleate [*1963*] (a seet″ oh fen′ a zeen mal′ ee ate). $C_{23}H_{29}N_3O_2S \cdot 2C_4H_4O_4$. 643.70. [Acetophenazine is INN.] (1) Ethanone, 1-[10-[3-[4-(2-hydroxyethyl)-1-piperazinyl]propyl]-10*H*-phenothiazin-2-yl]-, (*Z*) 2-butenedioate (1:2) (salt); (2) 10-[3-[4-(2-Hydroxyethyl)-1-piperazinyl]propyl]phenothiazin-2-yl methyl ketone mal-

---

eate (1:2) (salt). *UNII-3P5HNU5JTC. CAS-5714-00-1; CAS-2751-68-0* [acetophenazine]. USP XXII. *Antipsychotic.* Tindal (Schering) ◇*Sch 6673; NSC-70600*

Acetophenetidin (previously used name) — *See* Phenacetin.

Acetorphine. $C_{27}H_{35}NO_5$. 453.57. 6,7,8,14-Tetrahydro-7α-(1-hydroxy-1-methylbutyl)-6,14-*endo*-ethenooripavine 3-acetate. *UNII-2OGQ81529L. CAS-25333-77-1.* INN; BAN.

Acetosulfone Sodium [*1964*] (a seet″ oh sul′ fone soe′ dee um). $C_{14}H_{14}N_3NaO_5S_2$. 391.40. [Sulfadiasulfone is INN.] (1) Acetamide, *N*-[[5-amino-2-[(4-aminophenyl)sulfonyl]-phenyl]sulfonyl]-, monosodium salt; (2) *N*-(6-Sulfanilylmetanilyl)acetamide monosodium salt. *UNII-FQ3M2Y4BU3. CAS-128-12-1; CAS-80-80-8* [acetosulfone]. *Antibacterial (leprostatic).* Promacetin (Parke-Davis†) ◇*CI-100; IA-307; NSC-107528*

Acetoxythymoxamine — *See* Moxisylyte.

Acetphenetidin (previously used name) — *See* Phenacetin.

Acetphenolisatin — *See* Oxyphenisatin Acetate.

Acetrizoate Sodium. $C_9H_5I_3NNaO_3$. 578.84. [Sodium Acetrizoate is INN and BAN.] Sodium 3-acetamido-2,4,6-triiodobenzoate. *UNII-5GF4B2I1DD. CAS-129-63-5; CAS-85-36-9* [acetrizoic acid]. USP XVI; MI. Salpix (Ortho-McNeil)

Acetrizoic Acid. *CAS-85-36-9.* USP XV.

Acetryptine. $C_{12}H_{14}N_2O$. 202.25. 3-(2-Aminoethyl)indol-5-yl methyl ketone. *UNII-N9VWZ34G5E. CAS-3551-18-6.* INN. ◇*W 2965 A*

Acetsalicylamide — *See* Salacetamide.

Acetylcarbromal — *See* Acecarbromal.

Acetylcholine Chloride (a seet″ il koe′ leen klor′ ide). **USP**. $C_7H_{16}ClNO_2$. 181.66. [Acetylcholine Chloride for Injection is JAN.] (1) Ethanaminium, 2-(acetyloxy)-*N,N,N*-trimethyl-, chloride; (2) Choline acetate (ester) chloride. *UNII-AF73293C2R. CAS-60-31-1; CAS-51-84-3* [acetylcholine]. INN; BAN; JAN. *Cardiac depressant; cholinergic; miotic; vasodilator (peripheral).* Miochol (Novartis)

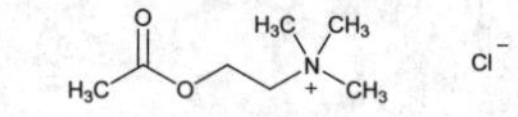

Acetylcysteine [*1963*] (a seet″ il sis′ teen). **USP**. $C_5H_9NO_3S$. 163.19. (1) L-Cysteine, *N*-acetyl-; (2) *N*-Acetyl-L-cysteine. *UNII-WYQ7N0BPYC. CAS-616-91-1.* INN; BAN; JAN. *Mucolytic.* Acetadote (Cumberland); Mucomyst (Apothecon); Mucosil (Dey) ◇*5052; NSC-111180*

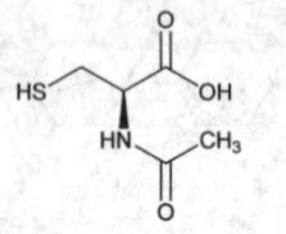

N-Acetyl-L-Cysteine (JAN) — *See* Acetylcysteine.

Acetyldigitoxin. $C_{43}H_{66}O_{14}$. 806.98. (3β,5β)-3-[(*O*-3-*O*-Acetyl-2,6-dideoxy-β-D-*ribo*-hexopyranosyl-(1→4)-*O*-2,6-dideoxy-β-D-*ribo*-hexopyranosyl-(1→4)-2,6-dideoxy-β-D-*ribo*-hexopyranosyl)oxy]-14-hydroxycard-20(22)-enolide. *UNII-0ZV4Q4L2FU. CAS-1111-39-3.* NF XIV; INN; MI. Acylanid (Novartis)

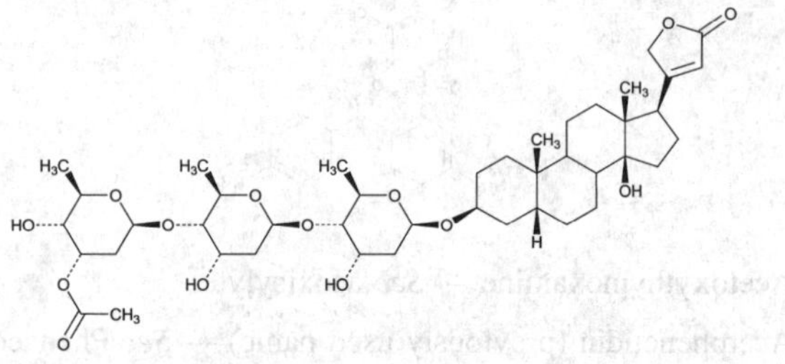

Acetylkitasamycin (JAN) — *See* Kitasamycin.

Acetylleucine. $C_8H_{15}NO_3$. 173.21. *N*-Acetyl-DL-leucine. *UNII-K76S41V71X. CAS-99-15-0.* INN.

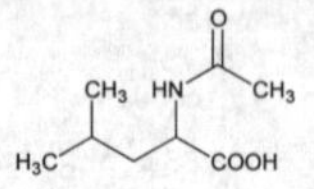

Acetylmethadol (INN, BAN, DCF) — *See* Methadyl Acetate.

Acetyloleandomycin — *See* Troleandomycin.

Acetylpheneturide (JAN) — *See* Pheneturide.

Acetylpropylorvinol — *See* Acetorphine.

Acetylsalicylate Aluminum — *See* Aspirin Aluminum.

Acetylsalicylic Acid (previously used name) — *See* Aspirin.

Acetylspiramycin (JAN) — *See* Spiramycin.

Acetylsulfamethoxazole (JAN) — *See* Sulfamethoxazole.

Acetylsulfisoxazole (JAN) — *See* Sulfisoxazole Acetyl.

Acetyltannic Acid. *CAS-1397-74-6.* USP XI; MI.

Acetyltributyl Citrate (a seet″ il trye bue′ til sit′ rate). **NF**. $C_{20}H_{34}O_8$. 402.48. (1) Citric acid, *O*-acetyltributyl ester; (2) Tributyl 2-acetoxypropane-1,2,3-tricarboxylate. *CAS-77-90-7.*

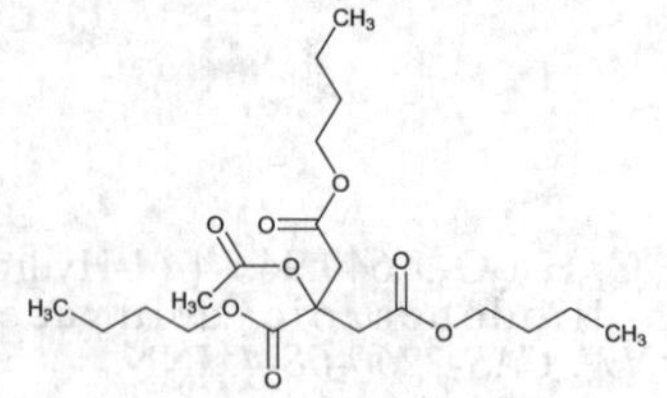

Acetyltriethyl Citrate (a seet″ il trye eth′ il sit′ rate). **NF**. $C_{14}H_{22}O_8$. 318.32. (1) Citric acid, *O*-acetyltriethyl ester; (2) Triethyl 2-acetoxypropane-1,2,3-tricarboxylate. *CAS-77-89-4.*

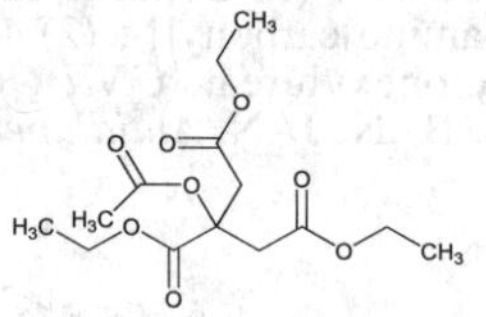

Acevaltrate. $C_{24}H_{32}O_{10}$. 480.50. 1,7a-Dihydro-1,6-dihydroxyspiro[cyclopenta[*c*]pyran-7(6*H*), 2′-oxirane]-4-methanol 4-acetate 1(or 6)-isovalerate 6(or 1)-(3-hydroxy-3-methylbutyrate, acetate). *UNII-S9MFK45GY9. CAS-25161-41-5.* INN.

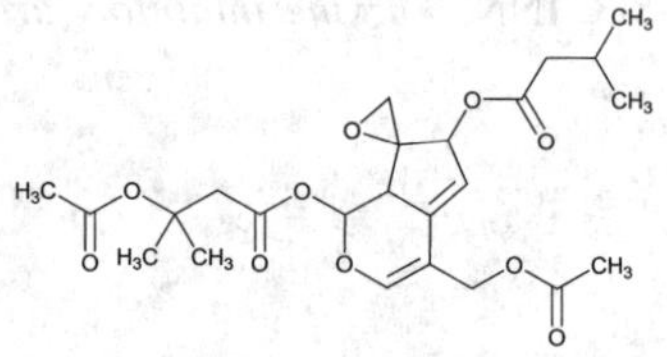

Acexamic Acid. $C_8H_{15}NO_3$. 173.21. 6-Acetamidohexanoic acid. *CAS-57-08-9.* INN; BAN; DCF. ◇*CY 153*

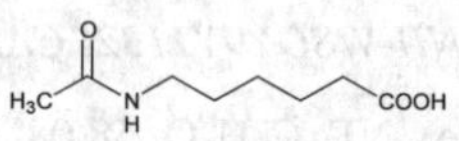

Aciclovir (INN, BAN, JAN) — *See* Acyclovir.

Acifran [*1984*] (a′ si fran). $C_{12}H_{10}O_4$. 218.21. (1) 2-Furancarboxylic acid, 4,5-dihydro-5-methyl-4-oxo-5-phenyl-, (±)-; (2) (±)-4,5-Dihydro-5-methyl-4-oxo-5-phenyl-2-furoic acid. *UNII-B1X701S0MV. CAS-72420-38-3.* INN. *Antihyperlipoproteinemic.* Reductol (Wyeth-Ayerst†) ◇*AY-25,712*

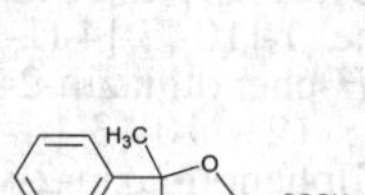

Acinitrazole (previously used name) — *See* Nithiamide.

Acipimox. $C_6H_6N_2O_3$. 154.12. 5-Methylpyrazinecarboxylic acid 4-oxide. *UNII-K9AY9IR2SD. CAS-51037-30-0.* INN; BAN; MI.

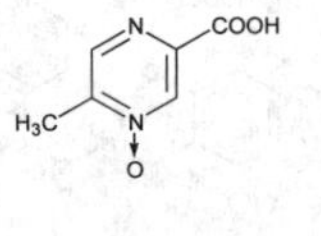

Acitazanolast. $C_9H_7N_5O_3$. 233.18. 3′-(1*H*-Tetrazol-5-yl)oxanilic acid. *UNII-99Y8VJ356G. CAS-114607-46-4.* INN.

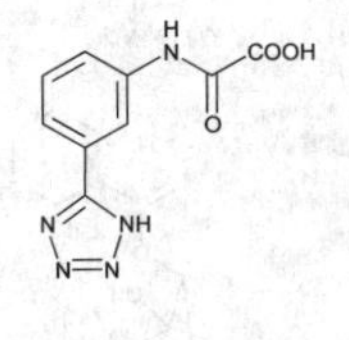

Acitemate. $C_{14}H_{18}N_2O_5$. 294.30. (±)-*cis*-3-Carboxy-6,7,8,9-tetrahydro-6-methyl-4-oxo-4*H*-pyrido[1,2-*a*]pyrimidine-9-acetic acid, 3-ethyl ester. *UNII-HM4L00P85U. CAS-101197-99-3.* INN.

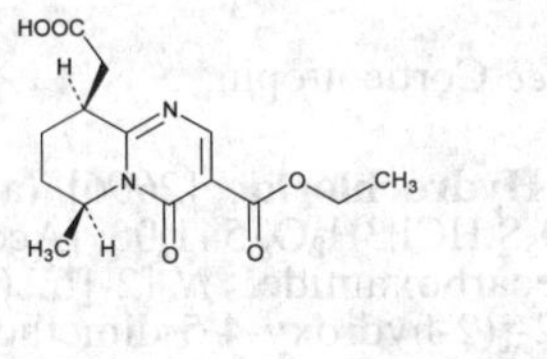

Acitretin [*1987*] (a″ si tre′ tin). $C_{21}H_{26}O_3$. 326.43. (1) 2,4,6,8-Nonatetraenoic acid, 9-(4-methoxy-2,3,6-trimethylphenyl)-3,7-dimethyl-, (*all-E*)-; (2) (*all-E*)-9-(4-Methoxy-2,3,6-trimethylphenyl)-3,7-dimethyl-2,4,6,8-nonatetraenoic acid. *UNII-LCH760E9T7. CAS-55079-83-9.* INN; BAN. *Antipsoriatic.* Soriatane (Connetics) ◇*Ro 10-1670/000*

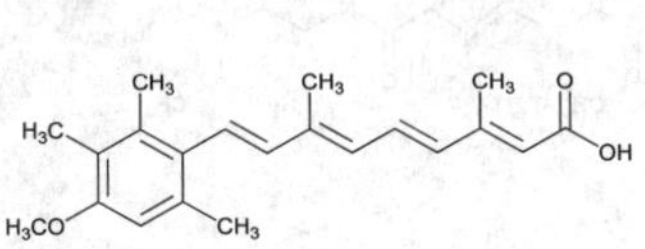

Acivicin [*1980*] (a″ si vye′ sin). $C_5H_7ClN_2O_3$. 178.57. (1) 5-Isoxazoleacetic acid, α-amino-3-chloro-4,5-dihydro-, [*S*-(*R**,*R**)]-; (2) (α*S*,5*S*)-α-Amino-3-chloro-2-isoxazoline-5-acetic acid. *UNII-O0X60K76I6. CAS-42228-92-2.* INN. *Antineoplastic.* ◇*U-42,126; AT-125*

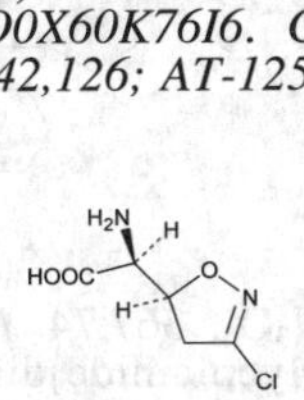

Aclacinomycin A (previously used name) — *See* Aclarubicin.

Aclantate. $C_{15}H_{14}ClNO_4S$. 339.79. 4-(2-Chloro-*m*-toluidino)-3-thiophenecarboxylic acid, hydroxymethyl ester, acetate (ester). *UNII-281Y036E0W. CAS-39633-62-0.* INN. ◇*Hoe 473*

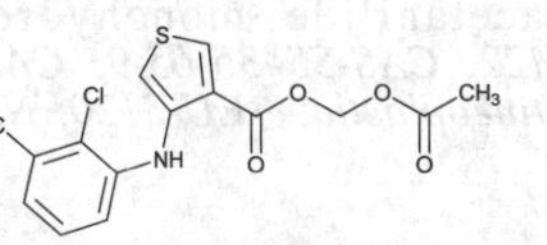

Aclarubicin [*1981*] (a″ kla roo′ bi sin). $C_{42}H_{53}NO_{15}$. 811.87. [Aclarubicin Hydrochloride is JAN.] (1) 1-Naphthacenecarboxylic acid, 2-ethyl-1,2,3,4,6,11-hexahydro-2,5,7-trihydroxy-6,11-dioxo-4-[[2,3,6-trideoxy-4-*O*-[2,6-dideoxy-4-*O*-[(2*R*-*trans*)-tetrahydro-6-methyl-5-oxo-2*H*-pyran-2-yl]-α-L-*lyxo*-hexopyranosyl]-3-(dimethylamino)-α-L-*lyxo*-hexopyranosyl]oxy]-, methyl ester, [1*R*-(1α,2β,4β)]-; (2) Methyl (1*R*,2*R*,4*S*)-2-ethyl-1,2,3,4,6,11-hexahydro-2,5,7-trihydroxy-6,11-dioxo-4-[[2,3,6-trideoxy-4-*O*-[2,6-dideoxy-4-*O*-[(2*R*,6*S*)-tetrahydro-6-methyl-5-oxo-2*H*-pyran-2-yl]-α-L-*lyxo*-hexopyranosyl]-3-(dimethylamino)-α-L-*lyxo*-hexopyranosyl]oxy]-1-naphthacenecarboxylate. *UNII-74KXF8I502. CAS-57576-44-0.* INN; BAN. *Antineoplastic. [Name previously used: Aclacinomycin A.]* ◇*NSC-208734*

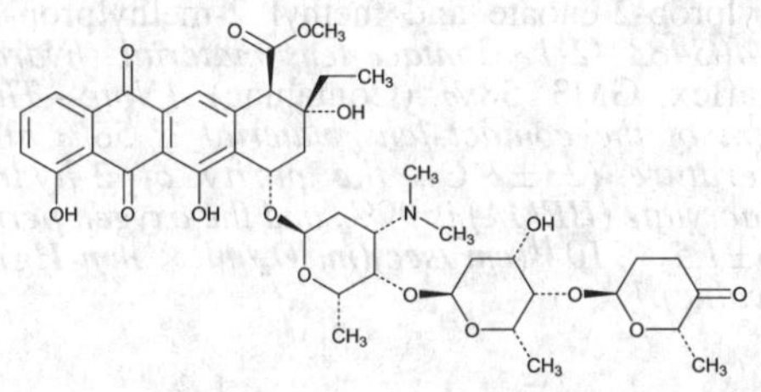

Aclatonium Napadisilate. $C_{30}H_{46}N_2O_{14}S_2$. 722.82. Choline 1,5-naphthalenedisulfonate (2:1), dilactate, diacetate. *CAS-55077-30-0.* INN; BAN; JAN; MI.

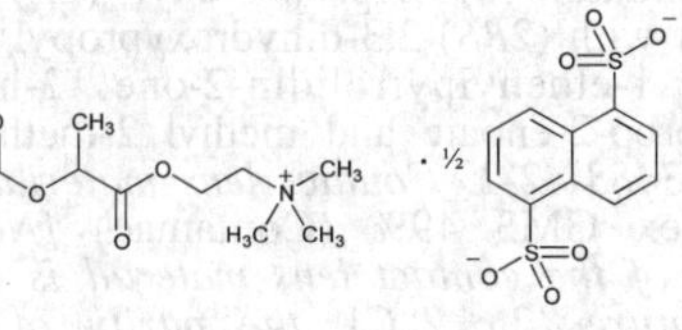

Aclatonium Napadisylate (former BAN) — *See* Aclatonium Napadisilate.

Aclidinium Bromide [*2007*] (a″ kli din′ ee um broe′ mide). $C_{26}H_{30}BrNO_4S_2$. 564.55. (1) 1-Azoniabicyclo[2.2.2]octane, 3-[(hydroxydi-2-thienylacetyl)oxy]-1-(3-phenoxypropyl)-, bromide, (3*R*)-; (2) (3*R*)-3-{[Hydroxydi(thiophen-2-yl)acetyl]oxy}-1-(3-phenoxypropyl)-1-azoniabicyclo[2.2.2]octane bromide. *UNII-UQW7UF9N91. CAS-320345-99-1.* INN. *Treatment of symptoms related to chronic obstructive pulmonary disease.* ◇*LAS 34273; LAS 34273 micronized; 14115700; LAS W-330*

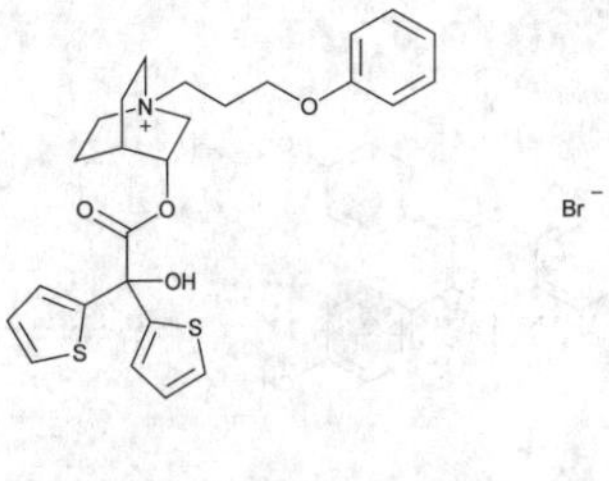

---

† Brand name formerly used, and/or firm no longer concerned with this product.

Acodazole Hydrochloride [*1982*] (a koe′ da zole hye″ droe klor′ ide). C$_{20}$H$_{19}$N$_5$O.HCl. 381.86. [Acodazole is INN.] (1) Acetamide, *N*-methyl-*N*-[4-[(7-methyl-1*H*-imidazo[4,5-*f*]quinolin-9-yl)amino]phenyl]-, monohydrochloride; (2) *N*-Methyl-4′-[(7-methyl-1*H*-imidazo[4,5-*f*]quinolin-9-yl)amino]acetanilide monohydrochloride. *UNII-6D7W9EAH22. CAS-55435-65-9; CAS-79152-85-5* [acodazole]. *Antineoplastic.* ◇*EU-3120; NSC-305884*

Acofilcon A [*2002*] (a″ koe fil′ kon). (C$_{10}$H$_{12}$O$_4$)$_v$ (C$_7$H$_{12}$O$_4$)$_w$ (C$_6$H$_{10}$O$_3$)$_x$ (C$_6$H$_9$NO)$_y$ (C$_5$H$_8$O$_2$).yz. (1) 2-Butenedioic acid (2*Z*)-, di-2-propenyl ester, polymer with 2,3-dihydroxypropyl 2-methyl-2-propenoate, 1-ethenyl-2-pyrrolidinone, 2-hydroxyethyl 2-methyl-2-propenoate and methyl 2-methyl-2-propenoate; (2) Diprop-2-enyl (2*Z*)-but-2-enedioate polymer with (2*RS*)-2,3-dihydroxypropyl 2-methylprop-2-enoate, 1-ethenylpyrrolidin-2-one, 2-hydroxyethyl 2-methylprop-2-enoate and methyl 2-methylprop-2-enoate. *CAS-403483-42-1. Contact lens material (hydrophobic).* Contaflex GM3 58% (Contamac) *[Note—The water content of the contact lens material is 58% at ambient temperature (23±2°C), the purity of 2-hydroxyethyl methacrylate (HEMA) is 99%, and the oxygen permeability is 26±1.5 × 10^{-11}(cm^2/sec)(ml O$_2$/ml × mm Hg) at 35°C (Dk value).]*

Acofilcon B [*2002*] (a″ koe fil′ kon). (C$_{10}$H$_{12}$O$_4$)$_v$ (C$_7$H$_{12}$O$_4$)$_w$ (C$_6$H$_{10}$O$_3$)$_x$ (C$_6$H$_9$NO)$_y$ (C$_5$H$_8$O$_2$).yz. (1) 2-Butenedioic acid (2*Z*)-, di-2-propenyl ester, polymer with 2,3-dihydroxypropyl 2-methyl-2-propenoate, 1-ethenyl-2-pyrrolidinone, 2-hydroxyethyl 2-methyl-2-propenoate and methyl 2-methyl-2-propenoate; (2) Diprop-2-enyl (2*Z*)-but-2-enedioate polymer with (2*RS*)-2,3-dihydroxypropyl 2-methylprop-2-enoate, 1-ethenylpyrrolidin-2-one, 2-hydroxyethyl 2-methylprop-2-enoate and methyl 2-methylprop-2-enoate. *CAS-403483-42-1. Contact lens material (hydrophobic).* Contaflex GM3 49% (Contamac) *[Note—The water content of the contact lens material is 49% at ambient temperature (23±2°C), the purity of 2-hydroxyethyl methacrylate (HEMA) is 99%, and the oxygen permeability is 13±1.5 × 10^{-11}(cm^2/sec)(ml O$_2$/ml × mm Hg) at 35°C (Dk value).]*

Acolbifene Hydrochloride [*2002*] (a kol′ bi feen hye″ droe klor′ ide). C$_{29}$H$_{31}$NO$_4$.HCl. 494.02. [Acolbifene is INN and BAN.] (1) 2*H*-1-Benzopyran-7-ol, 3-(4-hydroxyphenyl)-4-methyl-2-[4-[2-(1-piperidinyl)ethoxy]phenyl]-, hydrochloride, (2*S*)-; (2) (2*S*)-3-(4-Hydroxyphenyl)-4-methyl-2-[4-(2-piperidin-1-yl-ethoxy)phenyl]-2*H*-chromen-7-ol. *UNII-KXC7811DBY. CAS-252555-01-4; CAS-182167-02-8* [acolbifene]. *Prevention or treatment of breast and uterine proliferation or cancer.* ◇*SCH57068·HCl*

Aconiazide. C$_{15}$H$_{13}$N$_3$O$_4$. 299.28. Isonicotinic acid [*o*-(carboxymethoxy)benzylidene]hydrazide. *UNII-8OKQ9NS8-MO. CAS-13410-86-1.* INN.

Aconitine. C$_{34}$H$_{47}$NO$_{11}$. 645.74. (1α,3α,6α,14α,15α,16β)-20-Ethyl-1,6,16-trimethoxy-4-(methoxymethyl)aconitane-3,8,13,14,15-pentol 8-acetate 14-benzoate. *CAS-302-27-2.* USP X; MI.

Acortan — *See* Corticotropin.

Acotiamide Hydrochloride [*2006*] (a″ koe tye′ a mide). C$_{21}$H$_{30}$N$_4$O$_5$S.HCl.3H$_2$O. 541.06. [Acotiamide is INN.] (1) 4-Thiazolecarboxamide, *N*-[2-[bis(1-methylethyl)amino]ethyl]-2-[(2-hydroxy-4,5-dimethoxybenzoyl)amino]-, monohydrochloride, trihydrate; (2) *N*-[2-[Bis(1-methylethyl)amino]ethyl]-2-[(2-hydroxy-4,5-dimethoxybenzoyl)amino]thiazole-4-carboxamide monohydrochloride trihydrate. *UNII-NMW7447A9A; UNII-D42OWK5383* [acotiamide]. *CAS-773092-05-0; CAS-185106-16-5* [acotiamide]. *Functional dyspepsia.* ◇*Z-338; YM443*

Acoxatrine. C$_{23}$H$_{28}$N$_2$O$_3$. 380.48. (±)-*N*-[[1-(1,4-Benzodioxan-2-ylmethyl)-4-phenyl-4-piperidyl]methyl]acetamide. *UNII-7IGS0KX75Q. CAS-748-44-7.* INN. ◇*R 5385*

Acreozast. C$_{15}$H$_{14}$ClN$_3$O$_6$. 367.74. *N,N′*-(2-Chloro-5-cyano-*m*-phenylene)bis[glycolamide]diacetate (ester). *UNII-84DZ9RW4WK. CAS-123548-56-1.* INN.

Acridorex. $C_{24}H_{24}N_2$. 340.46. 9-{2-[(α-Methylphenethyl)amino]ethyl}acridine. *UNII-7SGV5HQH8B. CAS-47487-22-9.* INN. ◇*B.S. 7573-a*

Acriflavine. *UNII-1T3A50395T.* NF X; MI.

Acriflavine Hydrochloride. [Acriflavinium Chloride is INN.] A mixture of the hydrochlorides of 3,6-diamino-10-methylacridinium chloride and 3,6-diaminoacridine. NF X; MI.

Acriflavinium Chloride (INN) — *See* Acriflavine Hydrochloride.

Acrihellin. $C_{29}H_{38}O_7$. 498.61. 3β,5,14-Trihydroxy-19-oxo-5β-bufa-20,22-dienolide 3-(3-methylcrotonate). *CAS-67696-82-6.* INN.

Acrinol (JAN) — *See* Ethacridine Lactate.

Acrisorcin [*1962*] (a″ kri sor′ sin). $C_{12}H_{18}O_2 \cdot C_{13}H_{10}N_2$. 388.50. (1) 1,3-Benzenediol, 4-hexyl-, compd. with 9-acridinamine (1:1); (2) 4-Hexylresorcinol compound with 9-aminoacridine (1:1). *UNII-2U918O4BEV. CAS-7527-91-5.* USP XXII; INN. *Antifungal.* Akrinol (Schering) ◇*Sch 7056*

Acrivastine [*1985*] (ak″ ri vas′ teen). $C_{22}H_{24}N_2O_2$. 348.44. (1) 2-Propenoic acid, 3-[6-[1-(4-methylphenyl)-3-(1-pyrrolidinyl)-1-propenyl]-2-pyridinyl]-, (*E,E*)-; (2) (*E*)-6-[(*E*)-3-(1-Pyrrolidinyl)-1-*p*-tolylpropenyl]-2-pyridineacrylic acid. *UNII-A20F9XAI7W. CAS-87848-99-5.* INN; BAN. *Antihistaminic.* ◇*BW 825C*

Acrocinonide. $C_{24}H_{29}FO_6$. 432.48. 9-Fluoro-11β,16α,17,21-tetrahydroxypregna-1,4-diene-3,20-dione cyclic 16,17-acetal with acrolein. *UNII-67N58AU0IZ. CAS-28971-58-6.* INN; DCF. ◇*SD 2102-18*

Acronine [*1969*] (a′ kroe neen). $C_{20}H_{19}NO_3$. 321.37. (1) 7*H*-Pyrano[2,3-*c*]acridin-7-one, 3,12-dihydro-6-methoxy-3,3,12-trimethyl-; (2) 3,12-Dihydro-6-methoxy-3,3,12-trimethyl-7*H*-pyrano[2,3-*c*]acridin-7-one. *UNII-QE0G097358. CAS-7008-42-6.* INN. *Antineoplastic.* ◇*Compound 42339; NSC-403169*

Acrosoxacin (BAN) — *See* Rosoxacin.

Actagardin. A polypeptide antibiotic obtained from cultures of *Actinoplanes garbadinensis* or *Actinoplanes liguriae*, or the same substance produced by any other means. INN.

Actaplanin [*1975*] (ak″ ta plan′ in). A complex of glycopeptide-type antibiotics derived from a new species of the genus *Actinoplanes*, strain ATCC 23342. It contains three aromatic amino acids, a cyclic peptide, glucose, mannose, rhamnose, and ristosamine. (1) Actaplanin; (2) Actaplanin. *CAS-37305-75-2.* INN; BAN. *Growth stimulant (veterinary).* Kamoran (Lilly†) ◇*A-4696*

Actarit. $C_{10}H_{11}NO_3$. 193.20. (*p*-Acetamidophenyl)acetic acid. *UNII-HW5B6351RZ. CAS-18699-02-0.* INN; JAN.

Actinomycin C (BAN and previously used name) — *See* Cactinomycin.

Actinomycin D (JAN) — *See* Dactinomycin.

Actinoquinol Sodium [*1965*] (ak tin″ oh kwin′ ol soe′ dee um). $C_{11}H_{10}NNaO_4S$. 275.26. [Actinoquinol is INN.] (1) 5-Quinolinesulfonic acid, 8-ethoxy-, sodium salt; (2) 8-

---

Ethoxy-5-quinolinesulfonic acid sodium salt. *UNII-8PW272ITDS. CAS-7246-07-3; CAS-15301-40-3* [actinoquinol]. *Ultraviolet screen.*

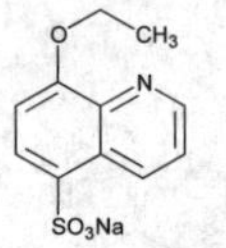

Actisomide [*1989*] (ak tis'pr oh mide). $C_{23}H_{35}N_3O$. 369.54. (1) 3*H*-Pyrido[1,2-*c*]pyrimidin-3-one, 4-[2-[bis(1-methylethyl)amino]ethyl]-4,4a,5,6,7,8-hexahydro-1-methyl-4-phenyl-, *cis*-(±)-; (2) (±)-*cis*-4-[2-(Diisopropylamino)ethyl]-4,4a,5,6,7,8-hexahydro-1-methyl-4-phenyl-3*H*-pyrido[1,2-*c*]pyrimidin-3-one. *CAS-96914-39-5.* INN. *Cardiac depressant (anti-arrhythmic).* ◇*SC-36602*

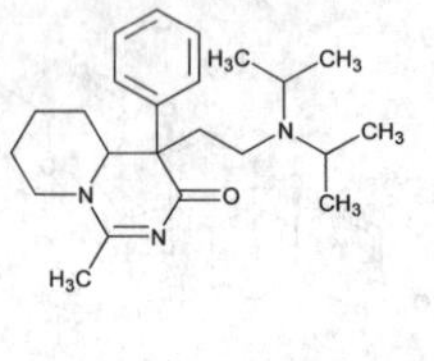

Actodigin [*1974*] (ak″ toe di' jin). $C_{29}H_{44}O_9$. 536.65. (1) 24-Nor-5,14-chol-20(22)-en-21-oic acid, 3-(β-D-glucopyranosyloxy)-14,23-dihydroxy-, γ-lactone, (3β,5β,14β)-; (2) 3β-(β-D-Glucopyranosyloxy)-14,23-dihydroxy-24-nor-5β,14β-chol-20(22)-en-21-oic acid γ-lactone. *CAS-36983-69-4.* INN. *Cardiotonic.* ◇*AY-22,241*

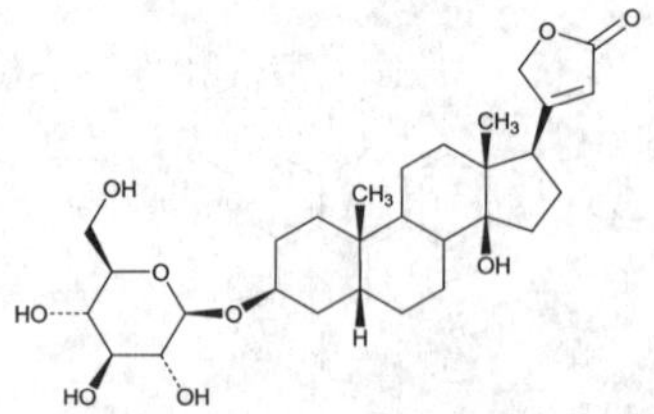

Actovegin. An extract from hemolysed blood of young oxen. JAN.

Acyclovir [*1979*] (ay sye' kloe vir). **USP.** $C_8H_{11}N_5O_3$. 225.20. [Aciclovir is INN, BAN, and JAN.] (1) 6*H*-Purin-6-one, 2-amino-1,9-dihydro-9-[(2-hydroxyethoxy)methyl]-; (2) 9-[(2-Hydroxyethoxy)methyl]guanine. *UNII-X4HES1O11F. CAS-59277-89-3. Antiviral.* Zovirax (GlaxoSmithKline)

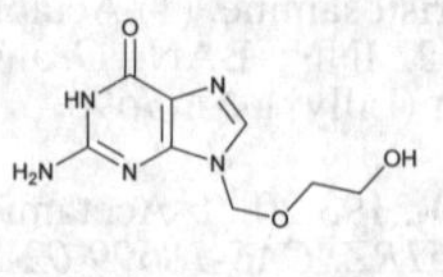

Acyclovir Sodium [*1984*] (ay sye' kloe vir soe' dee um). $C_8H_{10}N_5NaO_3$. 247.19. (1) 6*H*-Purin-6-one, 2-amino-1,9-dihydro-9-[(2-hydroxyethoxy)methyl]-, monosodium salt; (2) 9-[(2-Hydroxyethoxy)methyl]guanine monosodium salt. *UNII-927L42J563. CAS-69657-51-8. Antiviral.* Zovirax (GlaxoSmithKline) ◇*BW 248U sodium*

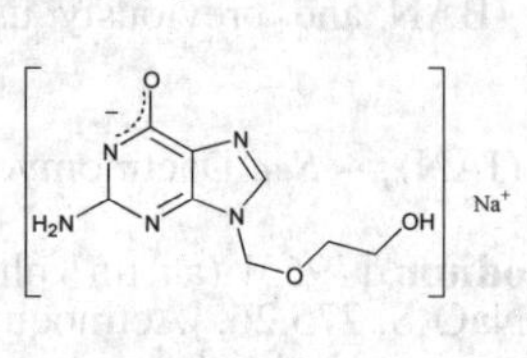

Adafenoxate. $C_{20}H_{26}ClNO_3$. 363.88. 2-(1-Adamantylamino)ethyl (*p*-chlorophenoxy)acetate. *UNII-B8VQU4C05J. CAS-82168-26-1.* INN.

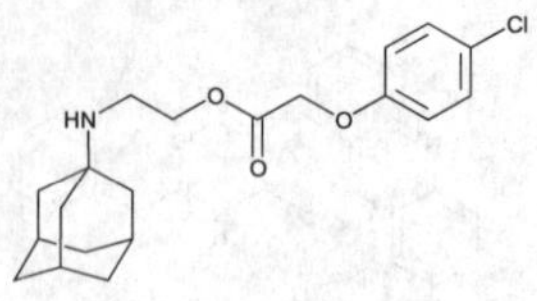

Adalimumab [*2002*] (a″ da lim' ue mab). Immunoglobulin G1, anti-(human tumor necrosis factor) (human monoclonal D2E7 heavy chain), disulfide with human monoclonal D2E7 light chain, dimer. Molecular weight is approximately 148,000 daltons. *UNII-FYS6T7F842. CAS-331731-18-1.* INN; BAN. *Treatment of rheumatoid arthritis and other chronic inflammatory diseases (monoclonal antibody).* ◇*D2E7; LU200134*

Adamantanamine Hydrochloride — *See* Amantadine Hydrochloride.

Adamexine. $C_{20}H_{26}Br_2N_2O$. 470.24. α-(1-Adamantylmethylamino)-4',6'-dibromo-*o*-acetotoluidide. *UNII-6LPU49W75V. CAS-54785-02-3.* INN.

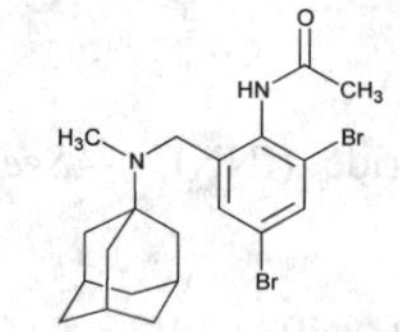

Adapalene [*1991*] (a dap' a leen). $C_{28}H_{28}O_3$. 412.52. (1) 2-Naphthalenecarboxylic acid, 6-(4-methoxy-3-tricyclo[3.3.1.1^{3,7}]dec-1-ylphenyl)-; (2) 6-[3-(1-Adamantyl)-4-methoxyphenyl]-2-naphthoic acid. *UNII-1L4806J2QF. CAS-106685-40-9.* INN; BAN. *Anti-acne.* Differin (Galderma) ◇*CD 271*

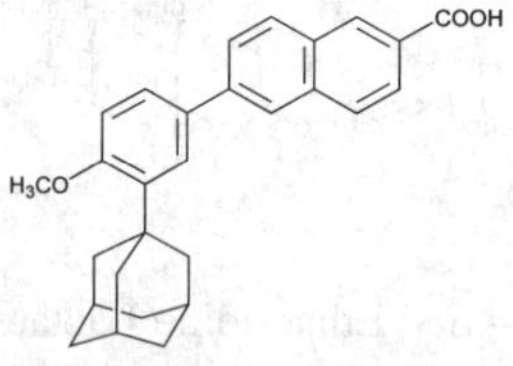

Adaprolol Maleate [*1990*] (a da' proe lol mal' ee ate). $C_{26}H_{39}NO_4 \cdot C_4H_4O_4$. 545.66. [Adaprolol is INN.] (1) Benzeneacetic acid, 4-[2-hydroxy-3-[(1-methylethyl)amino]propoxy]-, 2-tricyclo[3.3.1.1^{3,7}]dec-1-ylethyl ester, (±)-, (*Z*)-2-butenedioate (1:1) (salt); (2) (±)-2-(1-Adamantyl)ethyl [*p*-[2-hydroxy-3-(isopropylamino)propoxy]phenyl]acetate, maleate (1:1) (salt). *UNII-2I8RV6WL9A; UNII-XP991I11WL* [adaprolol]. *CAS-121009-31-2; CAS-101479-70-3* [adaprolol]. *Antihypertensive (β-blocker, ophthalmic).* ◇*HGP-2; CDDD 2803*

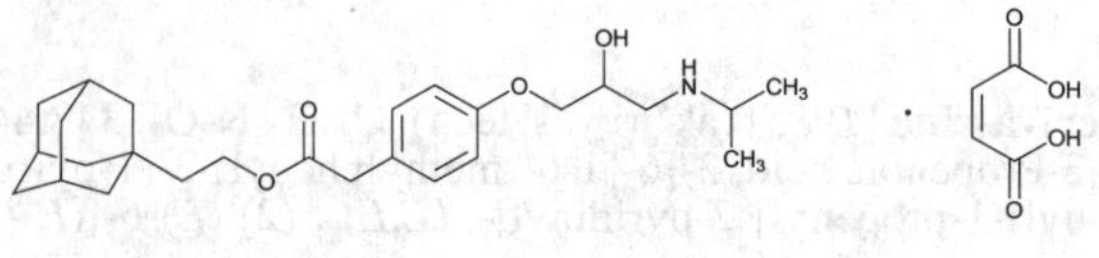

Adargileukin Alfa. $C_{695}H_{1124}N_{180}O_{202}S_7$ (peptide). [88-Arginine]interleukin 2 (human clone pTIL2-21a) (partly glycosylated). *CAS-250710-65-7.* INN.

Adatanserin Hydrochloride [*1993*] (a″ da tan′ ser in hye″ droe klor′ ide). $C_{21}H_{31}N_5O.HCl$. 405.96. [Adatanserin is INN.] (1) Tricyclo[3.3.1.1^{3,7}]decane-1-carboxamide, *N*-[2-[4-(2-pyrimidinyl)-1-piperazinyl]ethyl]-, monohydrochloride; (2) *N*-[2-[4-(2-Pyrimidinyl)-1-piperazinyl]ethyl]-1-adamantanecarboxamide monohydrochloride. *UNII-48BX75B06D. CAS-144966-96-1; CAS-127266-56-2* [adatanserin]. *Anti-anxiety agent; antidepressant.* ◇*WY-50324 HCl*

Adecatumumab. $C_{6552}H_{10080}N_{1740}O_{2052}S_{46}$. Immunoglobulin G1, anti-(human antigen 17-1A) (human monoclonal MT201 γ1-chain), disulfide with human monoclonal MT201 κ-chain, dimer. *CAS-503605-66-1.* INN.

Adefovir [*1994*] (a def′ oh vir). $C_8H_{12}N_5O_4P$. 273.19. (1) Phosphonic acid, [[2-(6-amino-9*H*-purin-9-yl)ethoxy]methyl]-; (2) [[2-(6-Amino-9*H*-purin-9-yl)ethoxy]methyl]phosphonic acid; (3) 9-[2-(Phosphonomethoxy)ethyl]adenine. *UNII-6GQP90I798. CAS-106941-25-7.* INN; BAN. *Antiviral.* ◇*GS-0393*

Adefovir Dipivoxil [*1996*] (a def′ oh vir dye piv ox′ il). $C_{20}H_{32}N_5O_8P$. 501.47. (1) Propanoic acid, 2,2-dimethyl-, [[[2-(6-amino-9*H*-purin-9-yl)ethoxy]methyl]phosphinylidene]bis(oxymethylene) ester; (2) [[2-(6-Amino-9*H*-purin-9-yl)ethoxy]methyl]phosphonic acid, diester with hydroxymethyl pivalate; (3) 9-[2-[[Bis[(pivaloyloxy)methoxy]phosphinyl]methoxy]ethyl]adenine. *UNII-U6Q8Z01514. CAS-142340-99-6. Antiviral.* Hepsera (Gilead Sciences) ◇*GS-0840*

Adekalant. $C_{22}H_{31}N_3O_4$. 401.50. *tert*-Butyl 7-[(*S*)-3-(*p*-cyanophenoxy)-2-hydroxypropyl]-3,7-diazabicyclo [3.3.1] nonane-3-carboxylate. *UNII-62R1A43O49. CAS-227940-00-3.* INN.

Adelavin. A mixture of flavin adenin dinucleotide and liver extract. JAN.

---

† Brand name formerly used, and/or firm no longer concerned with this product.

Adelmidrol. $C_{13}H_{26}N_2O_4$. 274.36. *N,N′*-bis(2-Hydroxyethyl)-nonanediamide. *UNII-1BUC3685QU. CAS-1675-66-7.* INN.

Ademetionine. $C_{15}H_{22}N_6O_5S$. 398.44. (±)-5′-[(*R**)-[(*R**)-3-Amino-3-carboxypropyl]methylsulfonio]-5′-deoxyadenosine hydroxide, inner salt. *CAS-17176-17-9.* INN.

Adenazole (previously used name) — *See* Tocladesine.

Adenine (ad′ e neen). USP. $C_5H_5N_5$. 135.13. (1) 1*H*-Purin-6-amine; (2) 1,6-Dihydro-6-iminopurine. *CAS-73-24-5.* JAN. *Vitamin.*

Adenosine [*1988*] (a den′ oh seen). USP. $C_{10}H_{13}N_5O_4$. 267.24. (1) Adenosine; (2) 6-Amino-9-β-D-ribofuranosyl-9*H*-purine; (3) 9-β-D-Ribofuranosyladenine. *UNII-K72T3FS567. CAS-58-61-7.* BAN. *Cardiac depressant (anti-arrhythmic).* Adenocard (Astellas); Adenoscan (Astellas) ◇*SR 96225*

Adenosine Phosphate [*1963*] (a den′ oh seen fos′ fate). $C_{10}H_{14}N_5O_7P$. 347.22. (1) 5′-Adenylic acid; (2) 5′-Adenylic acid; (3) Adenosine 5′-(dihydrogen phosphate). *CAS-61-19-8.* INN; BAN. *Nutrient.* Adenyl (Wyeth-Ayerst); My-B-Den (Bayer†) ◇*A 5MP; NSC-20264*

Adenosine Triphosphate Disodium. $C_{10}H_{14}N_5Na_2O_{13}P_3$. 551.14. Adenosine 5′-(disodium triphosphate). *CAS-987-65-5.* JAN. ATP (Medco Research)

Aderbasib [*2007*] (a der′ ba sib). $C_{21}H_{28}N_4O_5$. 416.47. (1) 5-Azaspiro[2.5]octane-5-carboxylic acid, 7-[(hydroxyamino)carbonyl]-6-[(4-phenyl-1-piperazinyl)carbonyl]-, methyl ester, (6*S*,7*S*)-; (2) Methyl (6*S*,7*S*)-7-[(hydroxyamino)carbonyl]-6-[(4-phenylpiperazin-1-yl)carbonyl]-5-azaspiro[2.5]octane-5-carboxylate. *UNII-V9YL6NEJ3G. CAS-791828-58-5.* INN. *Antineoplastic; ErbB Sheddase (ADAM) Inhibitor.* ◇*INCB 007839*

Adibendan. $C_{16}H_{14}N_4O$. 278.31. 5,7-Dihydro-7,7-dimethyl-2-(4-pyridyl)pyrrolo[2,3-*f*]benzimidazol-6(3*H*)-one. *UNII-E87N3L27KX. CAS-100510-33-6.* INN.

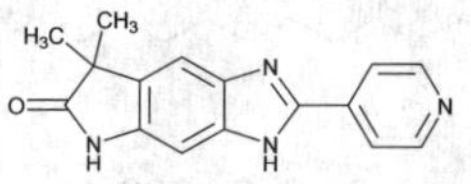

Adicillin. $C_{14}H_{21}N_3O_6S$. 359.40. (1) (4-Amino-4-carboxybutyl)penicillin; (2) 6-(5-Amino-5-carboxyvaleramido)-3,3-dimethyl-7-oxo-4-thia-1-azabicyclo[3.2.0]heptane-2-carboxylic acid. *UNII-NOF9U9EYQ4. CAS-525-94-0.* INN; BAN.

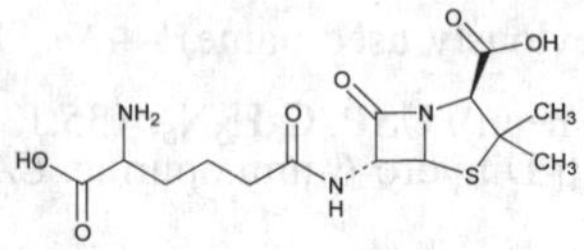

Adimolol. $C_{25}H_{29}N_3O_3$. 419.52. (±)-1-[3-[[2-Hydroxy-3-(1-naphthyloxy)propyl]amino]-3-methylbutyl]-2-benzimidazolinone. *UNII-B6CJY5K2ST. CAS-78459-19-5.* INN.

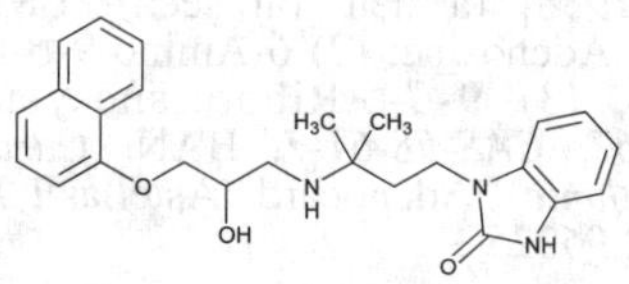

Adinazolam [*1980*] (a″ din az′ oh lam). $C_{19}H_{18}ClN_5$. 351.83. (1) 4*H*-[1,2,4]Triazolo[4,3-*a*][1,4]benzodiazepine-1-methanamine, 8-chloro-*N*-*N*-dimethyl-6-phenyl-; (2) 8-Chloro-1-[(dimethylamino)methyl]-6-phenyl-4*H*-*s*-triazolo[4,3-*a*][1,4]benzodiazepine. *UNII-KN08449444. CAS-37115-32-5.* INN; BAN. *Antidepressant; sedative-hypnotic.* ◇*U-41,123*

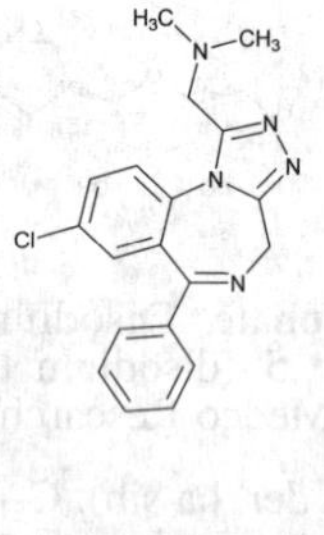

Adinazolam Mesylate [*1984*] (a″ din az′ oh lam mes′ i late). $C_{20}H_{22}ClN_5O_3S$. 447.94. (1) 4*H*-[1,2,4]Triazolo[4,3-*a*][1,4]benzodiazepine-1-methanamine, 8-chloro-*N*,*N*-dimethyl-6-phenyl-, monomethanesulfonate; (2) 8-Chloro-1-[(dimethylamino)methyl]-6-phenyl-4*H*-*s*-triazolo[4,3-*a*][1,4]benzodiazepine monomethanesulfonate. *UNII-NT8S62A727; UNII-KN08449444* [adinazolam]. *CAS-57938-82-6; CAS-37115-32-5* [adinazolam]. *Antidepressant.* ◇*U-41,123F*

Adiphenine Hydrochloride [*1969*] (a dif′ e neen hye″ droe klor′ ide). $C_{20}H_{25}NO_2$·HCl. 347.88. [Adiphenine is INN.] (1) Benzeneacetic acid, α-phenyl-2-(diethylamino)ethyl ester hydrochloride; (2) 2-(Diethylamino)ethyl diphenyl-

acetate hydrochloride. *UNII-42B4PDY0AV. CAS-50-42-0; CAS-64-95-9* [adiphenine]. *Relaxant (smooth muscle).* ◇*NSC-129224*

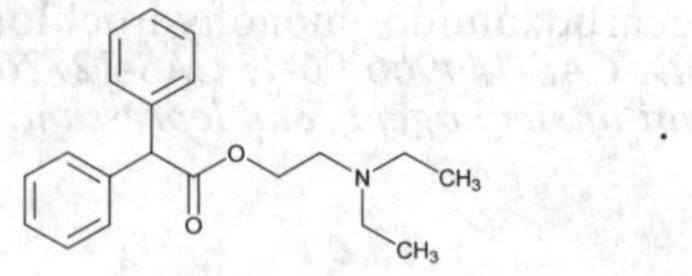

Adipic Acid. NF. $C_6H_{10}O_4$. 146.14. (1) Hexanedioic acid; (2) 1,4-Butanedicarboxylic acid. *UNII-76A0JE0FKJ. CAS-124-04-9.*

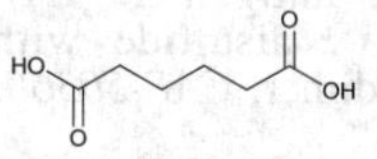

Adipiodone (INN, BAN, JAN) — *See* Iodipamide.

Adipiodone Meglumine Injection (JAN) — *See* Iodipamide Meglumine.

Adipiplon [*2007*] (a dip′ i plon). $C_{18}H_{18}FN_7$. 351.38. (1) [1,2,4]Triazolo[1,5-*c*]pyrimidine, 7-[[2-(3-fluoro-2-pyridinyl)-1*H*-imidazol-1-yl]methyl]-2-methyl-8-propyl-; (2) 7-[[2-(3-Fluoropyridin-2-yl)-1*H*-imidazol-1-yl]methyl]-2-methyl-8-propyl-[1,2,4]triazolo[1,5-*c*]pyrimidine. *UNII-OPL214POJ1. CAS-840486-93-3.* INN. *Sedative/hypnotic.[Name previously used: Apiplon.]* ◇*NG2-73*

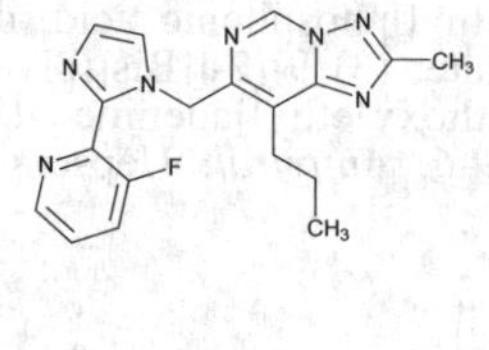

Aditeren. $C_{13}H_{17}N_5O_2$. 275.31. 2,4-Diamino-5-(4-amino-3,5-dimethoxybenzyl)pyrimidine. *UNII-L4F80M873G. CAS-56066-19-4.* INN.

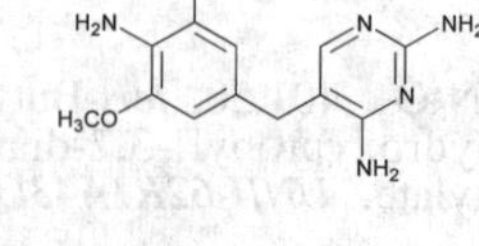

Aditoprim. $C_{15}H_{21}N_5O_2$. 303.36. 2,4-Diamino-5-[4-(dimethylamino)-3,5-dimethoxybenzyl]pyrimidine. *UNII-2Z81WDX2ZH. CAS-56066-63-8.* INN.

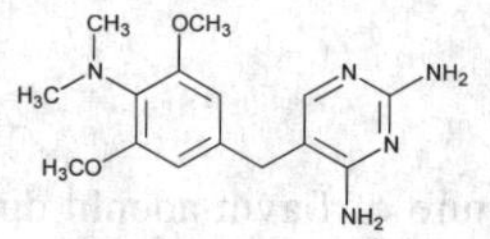

Adoprazine. $C_{24}H_{24}FN_3O_2$. 405.46. 1-(2,3-Dihydro-1,4-benzodioxin-5-yl)-4-{[5-(4-fluorophenyl)pyridin-3-yl]methyl}piperazine. *CAS-222551-17-9.* INN.

Adosopine. $C_{17}H_{14}N_2O_3$. 294.30. *N*-(5,6-Dihydro-5-methyl-6,11-dioxo-10-morphanthridinyl)acetamide. *UNII-OKB1O47Q6F. CAS-88124-26-9*. INN.

Adozelesin [*1990*] (a″ doe zel′ e sin). $C_{30}H_{22}N_4O_4$. 502.52. (1) 2-Benzofurancarboxamide, *N*-[2-[(4,5,8,8a-tetrahydro-7-methyl-4-oxocyclopropa[*c*]pyrrolo[3,2-*e*]indol-2(1*H*)-yl)-carbonyl]-1*H*-indol-5-yl]-, (7b*R*)-; (2) (7b*R*,8a*S*)-*N*-[2-[(4,5,8,8a-Tetrahydro-7-methyl-4-oxocyclopropa[*c*]-pyrrolo[3,2-*e*]indol-2(1*H*)-yl)carbonyl]indol-5-yl]-2-benzofurancarboxamide. *CAS-110314-48-2*. INN. *Antineoplastic*. ◇U-73,975

Adrafinil. $C_{15}H_{15}NO_3S$. 289.35. 2-[(Diphenyl-methyl)sulfinyl]acetohydroxamic acid. *UNII-BI81Z4542G. CAS-63547-13-7*. INN; MI.

Adrenaline (BAN) — *See* Epinephrine.

Adrenaline Bitartrate — *See* Epinephrine Bitartrate.

Adrenalone [*1971*] (a dren′ a lone). $C_9H_{11}NO_3$. 181.19. (1) Ethanone, 1-(3,4-dihydroxyphenyl)-2-(methylamino)-; (2) 3′,4′-Dihydroxy-2-(methylamino)acetophenone. *CAS-99-45-6*. INN. *Adrenergic (ophthalmic)*.

Adrenochrome Monoaminoguanidine Mesilate. $C_{10}H_{13}N_5O_2 \cdot CH_4O_3S \cdot H_2O$. 349.36. *CAS-4009-68-1* [Adrenochrome Guanylhydrazone Mesilate, anhydrous]. JAN.

Adrenochrome Monosemicarbazone Sodium Salicylate Complex — *See* Carbazochrome Salicylate.

Adrenocorticotrophic Hormone — *See* Corticotropin.

Adrenocorticotrophin — *See* Corticotropin.

Adrenone — *See* Adrenalone.

---

† Brand name formerly used, and/or firm no longer concerned with this product.

Adrogolide. $C_{22}H_{25}NO_4S$. 399.50. (5a*R*,11b*S*)-4,5,5a,6,7,11b-Hexahydro-2-propylbenzo[*f*]thienol[2,3-*c*]quinoline-9,10-diol diacetate (ester). *UNII-YC3281G42A. CAS-171752-56-0*. INN.

Adrogolide Hydrochloride [*1999*] (a droe′ goe lide hye″ droe klor′ ide). $C_{22}H_{25}NO_4S \cdot HCl$. 435.96. (1) Benzo[*f*]thieno[2,3-*c*]quinoline-9,10-diol, 4,5,5a,6,7,11b-hexahydro-2-propyl-, diacetate (ester), hydrochloride, (5a*R-trans*)-; (2) (5a*R*,11b*S*)-4,5,5a,6,7,11b-Hexahydro-2-propylbenzo[*f*]thieno[2,3-*c*]quinoline-9,10-diol diacetate (ester), hydrochloride. *UNII-69MG3OZA0H. CAS-166591-11-3*. *Treatment of the symptoms of Parkinson's disease (dopamine D_1 receptor agonist)*. ◇ABT-431; A-93431.1

ADS — *See* Olsalazine Sodium.

Afalanine. $C_{11}H_{13}NO_3$. 207.23. *N*-Acetyl-3-phenyl-DL-alanine. *UNII-FFW2NGO18S. CAS-2901-75-9*. INN.

Afeletecan. $C_{45}H_{49}N_7O_{11}S$. 895.98. Camptothecin, ester with *N*-[[*p*-[(3-*O*-methyl-β-L-fucopyranosyl)oxy]phenyl]thiocarbamoyl]-L-histidyl-L-valine. *UNII-IX0QAD6RD2. CAS-215604-75-4*. INN.

Afelimomab. Immunoglobulin G3, anti-(human tumor necrosis factor α) F(ab′)2 fragment (mouse monoclonal LU54107 γ3-chain), disulfide with mouse monoclonal LU54107 κ-chain, dimer. *CAS-156227-98-4*. INN.

Afimoxifene [*2006*] (a″ fi mox′ i feen). $C_{26}H_{29}NO_2$. 387.51. (1) Phenol, 4-[1-[4-[2-(dimethylamino)ethoxy]phenyl]-2-phenyl-1-butenyl]-; (2) 4-[1-[4-[2-(Dimethylamino)ethoxy]phenyl]-2-phenylbut-1-enyl]phenol. *UNII-*

17197F0KYM. CAS-68392-35-8. INN. *Local treatment of estrogen dependent conditions of the breast.* TamoGel (Ascend Therapeutics) ◇4-OHT

Aflibercept [*2008*] (a flib′ er sept). $C_{4318}H_{6788}N_{1164}O_{1304}S_{32}$. (1) Vascular endothelial growth factor receptor type VEGFR1 (synthetic human immunoglobulin domain 2 fragment) fusion protein with vascular endothelial growth factor receptor type VEGFR2 (synthetic human immunoglobulin domain 3 fragment) fusion protein with immunoglobulin G1 (synthetic Fc fragment), dimer, (2) Des-432-lysine-[human vascular endothelial growth factor receptor 1-(103-204)-peptide (containing Ig-like C2-type 2 domain) fusion protein with human vascular endothelial growth factor receptor 2-(207-308)-peptide (containing Ig-like C2-type 3 domain fragment) fusion protein with human immunoglobulin G1-(227 *C*-terminal residues)-peptide (Fc fragment)], (211-211′:214-214′)-bisdisulfide dimer. Molecular weight is approximately 96,900 daltons. *UNII-15C2VL427D. CAS-862111-32-8.* INN. *Inhibitor of aberrant angiogenesis-vascular leak and inflammation; angiogenesis inhibitor for treatment of cancer.* ◇AVE0005; VEGF Trap

```
SDTGRPFVEM YSEIPEIIHM TEGRELVIPC RVTSPNITVT LKKFPLDTLI
PDGKRIIWDS RKGFIISNAT YKEIGLLTCE ATVNGHLYKT NYLTHRQTNT
IIDVVLSPSH GIELSVGEKL VLNCTARTEL NVGIDFNWEY PSSKHQHKKL
VNRDLKTQSG SEMKKFLSTL TIDGVTRSDQ GLYTCAASSG LMTKKNSTFV
RVHEKDKTHT CPPCPAPELL GGPSVFLFPP KPKDTLMISR TPEVTCVVVD
VSHEDPEVKF NWYVDGVEVH NAKTKPREEQ YNSTYRVVSV LTVLHQDWLN
GKEYKCKVSN KALPAPIEKT ISKAKGQPRE PQVYTLPPSR DELTKNQVSL
TCLVKGFYPS DIAVEWESNG QPENNYKTTP PVLDSDGSFF LYSKLTVDKS
RWQQGNVFSC SVMHEALHNH YTQKSLSLSP G
```

Afloqualone. $C_{16}H_{14}FN_3O$. 283.30. 6-Amino-2-(fluoromethyl)-3-*o*-tolyl-4(3*H*)-quinazolinone. *CAS-56287-74-2.* INN; JAN; MI.

Afovirsen Sodium [*1997*] (a″ foe vir′ sen soe′ dee um). $C_{192}H_{231}N_{57}Na_{19}O_{107}P_{19}S_{19}$. 6683.75. [Afovirsen is INN.] 2′-Deoxy-*P*-thiocytidylyl-(5′→3′)-*P*-thiothymidylyl-(5′→3′)-2′-deoxy-*P*-thioguanylyl-(5′→3′)-2′-deoxy-*P*-thiocytidylyl-(5′→3′)-*P*-thiothymidylyl-(5′→3′)-2′-deoxy-*P*-thiocytidylyl-(5′→3′)-2′-deoxy-*P*-thiocytidylyl-(5′→3′)-*P*-thiothymidylyl-(5′→3′)-*P*-thiothymidylyl-(5′→3′)-2′-deoxy-*P*-thiocytidylyl-(5′→3′)-2′-deoxy-*P*-thioadenylyl-(5′→3′)-2′-deoxy-*P*-thiocytidylyl-(5′→3′)-2′-deoxy-*P*-thiocytidylyl-(5′→3′)-*P*-thiothymidylyl-(5′→3′)-*P*-thiothymidylyl-(5′→3′)-2′-deoxy-*P*-thiocytidylyl-(5′→3′)-2′-deoxy-*P*-thioguanylyl-(5′→3′)-*P*-thiothymidylyl-(5′→3′)-thymidine, nonadecasodium salt. *CAS-138330-98-0; CAS-151356-08-0* [afovirsen]. *Antiviral.* ◇ISIS-2105; I-2105; IP-2105

Afurolol. $C_{15}H_{21}NO_4$. 279.33. 7-[3-(*tert*-Butylamino)-2-hydroxypropoxy]phthalide. *UNII-WQ1WRV49R9. CAS-65776-67-2.* INN.

Afutuzumab [*2008*] (a″ fue tooz′ oo mab). $C_{6512}H_{10060}N_{1712}O_{2020}S_{44}$. (1) Immunoglobulin G1, anti-(human CD20 (antigen)) (human-mouse monoclonal GA101 heavy chain), disulfide with human-mouse monoclonal GA101 κ-chain, dimer; (2) Immunoglobulin G1, anti-(human B-lymphocyte antigen CD20 (membrane-spanning 4-domains subfamily A member 1, B-lymphocyte surface antigen B1, Leu-16 or Bp35)), humanized mouse monoclonal GA101 des-CH3[107]-K-γ1 heavy chain (222-219′)-disulfide with humanized mouse monoclonal GA101 κ light chain dimer (228-228″:231-231″)-bisdisulfide. Molecular weight is approximately 146,100 daltons. *CAS-949142-50-1.* INN. *Oncology, treatment of lymphoma.* ◇RO 5072759; huMABCD20; GA101

Agalsidase Alfa [*2000*] (ay gal′ si dase al′ fa). $C_{2029}H_{3080}N_{544}O_{587}S_{27}$ (subunit protein moiety reduced). (1) Galactosidase, α- (human clone λAG18 isoenzyme A subunit protein moiety reduced); (2) α-Galactosidase (human-clone λAG[18] isoenzyme A subunit protein moiety reduced). Molecular weight is approximately 45,351 daltons. *UNII-2HLC17MX9G. CAS-104138-64-9.* INN; BAN. *Treatment of Fabry Disease.* Replagal (Transkaryotic Therapies) ◇EC 3.2.1.22

```
LDNGLARTPT MGWLHWERFM CNLDCQEEPD SCISEKLFME MAELMVSEGW
KDAGYEYLCI DDCWMAPQRD SEGRLQADPQ RFPHGIRQLA NYVHSKGLKL
GIYADVGNKT CAGFPGSFGY YDIDAQTFAD WGVDLLKFDG CYCDSLENLA
DGYKHMSLAL NRTGRSIVYS CEWPLYMWPF QKPNYTEIRQ YCNHWRNFAD
IDDSWKSIKS ILDWTSFNQE RIVDVAGPGG WNDPDMLVIG NFGLSWNQQV
TQMALWAIMA APLFMSNDLR HISPQAKALL QDKDVIAINQ DPLGKQGYQL
RQGDNFEVWE RPLSGLAWAV AMINRQEIGG PRSYTIAVAS LGKGVACNPA
CFITQLLPVK RKLGFYEWTS RLRSHINPTG TVLLQLENTM QMSLKDLL
```

* glycosylation site

Agalsidase Beta. $C_{2029}H_{3080}N_{544}O_{587}S_{27}$ (subunit protein moiety reduced). α-Galactosidase (human clone λAG[18] isoenzyme A subunit protein moiety reduced), glycoform β. *UNII-RZD65TSM9U. CAS-104138-64-9.* INN.

```
LDNGLARTPT MGWLHWERFM CNLDCQEEPD SCISEKLFME MAELMVSEGW
KDAGYEYLCI DDCWMAPQRD SEGRLQADPQ RFPHGIRQLA NYVHSKGLKL
GIYADVGNKT CAGFPGSFGY YDIDAQTFAD WGVDLLKFDG CYCDSLENLA
DGYKHMSLAL NRTGRSIVYS CEWPLYMWPF QKPNYTEIRQ YCNHWRNFAD
IDDSWKSIKS ILDWTSFNQE RIVDVAGPGG WNDPDMLVIG NFGLSWNQQV
TQMALWAIMA APLFMSNDLR HISPQAKALL QDKDVIAINQ DPLGKQGYQL
RQGDNFEVWE RPLSGLAWAV AMINRQEIGG PRSYTIAVAS LGKGVACNPA
CFITQLLPVK RKLGFYEWTS RLRSHINPTG TVLLQLENTM QMSLKDLL
```

Aganodine. $C_9H_{10}Cl_2N_4$. 245.11. (4,7-Dichloro-2-isoindolinyl)guanidine. *UNII-670P9AQR46. CAS-86696-87-9.* INN.

Agar (a′ gar). **NF.** The dried, hydrophilic, colloidal substance extracted from *Gelidium cartilagineum* (Linné) Gaillon (Fam. Gelidiaceae), *Gracilaria Confervoides* (Linné)

Greville (Fam. Sphaerococcaceae), and related red algae (Class Rhodophyceae). JAN. *Pharmaceutic aid (suspending agent).*

Agatolimod [*2007*] (a″ ga tol′ i mod). $C_{236}H_{303}N_{70}O_{133}P_{23}S_{23}$. 7698.21. (1) DNA, d(*P*-thio)(T-C-G-T-C-G-T-T-T-T-G-T-C-G-T-T-T-T-G-T-C-G-T-T); (2) *P*-Thiothymidylyl-(3′→5′)-2′-deoxy-*P*-thiocytidylyl-(3′→5′)-2′-deoxy-*P*-thioguanylyl-(3′→5′)-*P*-thiothymidylyl-(3′→5′)-2′-deoxy-*P*-thiocytidylyl-(3′→5′)-2′-deoxy-*P*-thioguanylyl-(3′→5′)-*P*-thiothymidylyl-(3′→5′)-*P*-thiothymidylyl-(3′→5′)-*P*-thiothymidylyl-(3′→5′)-2′-deoxy-*P*-thioguanylyl-(3′→5′)-*P*-thiothymidylyl-(3′→5′)-2′-deoxy-*P*-thiocytidylyl-(3′→5′)-2′-deoxy-*P*-thioguanylyl-(3′→5′)-*P*-thiothymidylyl-(3′→5′)-*P*-thiothymidylyl-(3′→5′)-*P*-thiothymidylyl-(3′→5′)-*P*-thiothymidylyl-(3′→5′)-2′-deoxy-*P*-thioguanylyl-(3′→5′)-*P*-thiothymidylyl-(3′→5′)-2′-deoxy-*P*-thiocytidylyl-(3′→5′)-2′-deoxy-*P*-thioguanylyl-(3′→5′)-*P*-thiothymidylyl-(3′→5′)-thymidine, triacosasodium salt. *CAS-207623-20-9.* INN. *Treatment of cancer; oligonucleotide.* ◇*PF-3512676*

Agatolimod Sodium [*2007*] (a″ ga tol′ i mod soe′ dee um). $C_{236}H_{303}N_{70}O_{133}P_{23}S_{23}Na_{23}$. (1) DNA, d(*P*-thio)(T-C-G-T-C-G-T-T-T-T-G-T-C-G-T-T-T-T-G-T-C-G-T-T) tricosasodium salt; (2) *P*-Thiothymidylyl-(3′→5′)-2′-deoxy-*P*-thiocytidylyl-(3′→5′)-2′-deoxy-*P*-thioguanylyl-(3′→5′)-*P*-thiothymidylyl-(3′→5′)-2′-deoxy-*P*-thiocytidylyl-(3′→5′)-2′-deoxy-*P*-thioguanylyl-(3′→5′)-*P*-thiothymidylyl-(3′→5′)-*P*-thiothymidylyl-(3′→5′)-*P*-thiothymidylyl-(3′→5′)-2′-deoxy-*P*-thioguanylyl-(3′→5′)-*P*-thiothymidylyl-(3′→5′)-2′-deoxy-*P*-thiocytidylyl-(3′→5′)-2′-deoxy-*P*-thioguanylyl-(3′→5′)-*P*-thiothymidylyl-(3′→5′)-*P*-thiothymidylyl-(3′→5′)-*P*-thiothymidylyl-(3′→5′)-*P*-thiothymidylyl-(3′→5′)-2′-deoxy-*P*-thioguanylyl-(3′→5′)-*P*-thiothymidylyl-(3′→5′)-2′-deoxy-*P*-thiocytidylyl-(3′→5′)-2′-deoxy-*P*-thioguanylyl-(3′→5′)-*P*-thiothymidylyl-(3′→5′)-thymidine tricosasodium salt. Molecular weight is approximately 8,204 daltons. *CAS-541547-35-7. Treatment of cancer; oligonucleotide.* ◇*PF-3512676*

Aglepristone. $C_{29}H_{37}NO_2$. 431.61. 11β-[*p*-(Dimethylamino)phenyl]-17β-hydroxy-17-[(*Z*)-propenyl]estra-4,9-dien-3-one. *UNII-0UT4JLE1CM. CAS-124478-60-0.* INN.

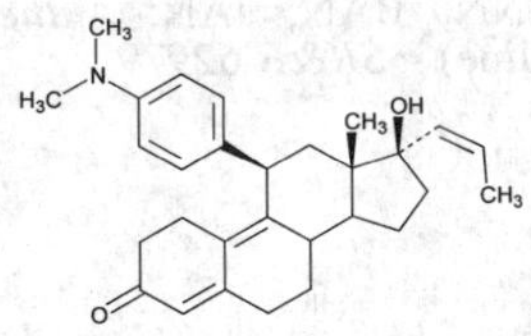

Agofollin — *See* Estradiol.

Agomelatine. $C_{15}H_{17}NO_2$. 243.30. *N*-[2-(7-Methoxy-1-naphthyl)ethyl]acetamide. *UNII-137R1N49AD. CAS-138112-76-2.* INN.

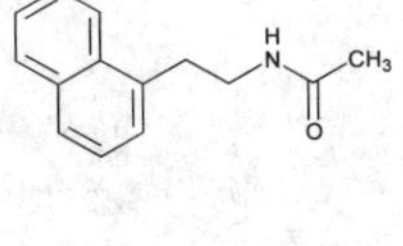

Air, Compressed — *See* Air, Medical.

Air, Medical (air, med′ i kal). **USP.** A natural or synthetic mixture of gases consisting largely of nitrogen and 21.5 ± 2.0% oxygen by volume. *Gas, medicinal.*

Ajmaline. $C_{20}H_{26}N_2O_2$. 326.43. Ajmalan-17,21-diol. *CAS-4360-12-7.* JAN.

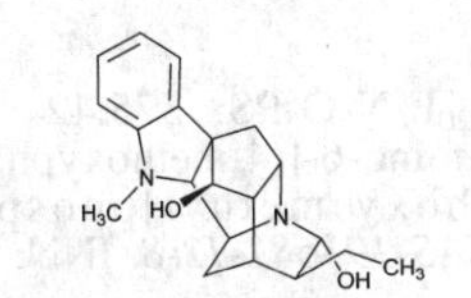

Aklomide [*1964*] (ak′ loe mide). $C_7H_5ClN_2O_3$. 200.58. (1) Benzamide, 2-chloro-4-nitro-; (2) 2-Chloro-4-nitrobenzamide. *UNII-B0E341RA20. CAS-3011-89-0.* INN; BAN. *Coccidiostat (for poultry).*

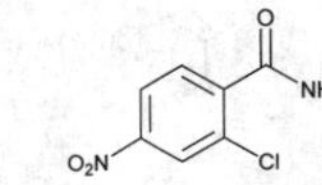

5 ALA HCl (trivial name) — *See* Aminolevulinic Acid Hydrochloride.

Alacepril. $C_{20}H_{26}N_2O_5S$. 406.50. *N*-[1-[(*S*)-3-Mercapto-2-methylpropionyl]-L-prolyl]-3-phenyl-L-alanine acetate (ester). *UNII-X39TL7JDPF. CAS-74258-86-9.* INN; JAN; MI.

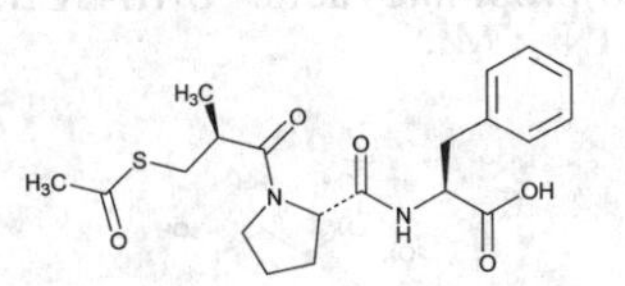

Alacizumab Pegol. Immunoglobulin di-Fab′ fragment, anti-[*Homo sapiens* VEGFR2 (vascular endothelial growth factor receptor 2, KDR, kinase insert domain receptor, FLK1, CD309)] pegylated humanized monoclonal antibody di-Fab′ CDP791 (or g165 DFM-PEG); VH-gamma1CH1 [humanized VH (*Homo sapiens* FR/*Mus musculus* CDR) [8.8.10] - *Homo sapiens* IGHG1*01 CH1-hinge (hinge PPCP12-15>AA)] (220-214′)-disulfide with kappa light chain [humanized V-KAPPA (*Homo sapiens* FR/*Mus musculus* CDR) [6.3.9] -*Homo sapiens* IGKC*01]; (226-bis-[maleimide-PEG (polyethylene glycol) 20 kDa]-226″)-dimer. *CAS-934216-54-3.* INN.

Alafosfalin. $C_5H_{13}N_2O_4P$. 196.14. [(1*R*)-1-[(2*S*)-2-Aminopropionamido]ethyl]phosphonic acid. *UNII-0M8OM373BS. CAS-60668-24-8.* INN; BAN; MI.

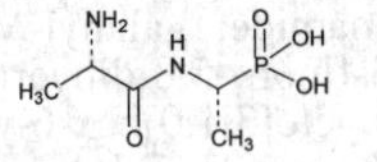

Alagebrium Chloride [*2004*] (al a″ je bree′ um klor′ ide). $C_{13}H_{14}ClNOS$. 267.77. (1) Thiazolium, 4,5-dimethyl-3-(2-oxo-2-phenylethyl)-, chloride; (2) 4,5-Dimethyl-3-(2-oxo-2-phenylethyl)thiazolium chloride. *UNII-79QS8K2877. CAS-341028-37-3.* INN. *Prevention and treatment of cardiovascular complications of aging, diabetes, and end stage renal disease; diabetic multisymptom pathology (other than cardiovascular) including retinopathy, neuphropathy, neuropathy, and ulcers (advanced glycosylation endproduct (AGE) crosslink inhibitor).* ◇*ALT-711*

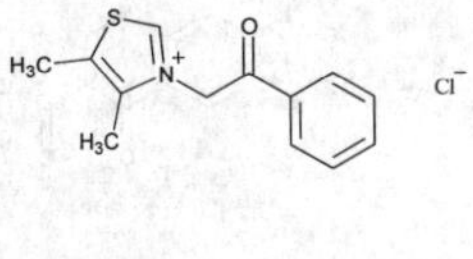

---

† Brand name formerly used, and/or firm no longer concerned with this product.

Alamecin [*1971*] (al″ a mee′ sin). Antibiotic produced by *Trichoderma viride Pers. ex fries.* Alamecin. *CAS-11096-79-0. Antibacterial.*

Alamifovir. $C_{19}H_{20}F_6N_5O_5PS$. 575.42. Bis(2,2,2-trifluoroethyl) [(2-{2-amino-6-[(4-methoxyphenyl)sulfanyl]-9*H*-purin-9-yl}ethoxy)methyl]phosphonate. *UNII-0N739K2A8A. CAS-193681-12-8.* INN.

Alanine [*1979*] (al′ a neen). **USP.** $C_3H_7NO_2$. 89.09. [L-Alanine is JAN.] (1) L-Alanine; (2) L-Alanine. *UNII-OF5P57N2ZX. CAS-56-41-7* [L]. INN. *Amino acid.*

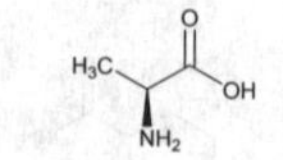

L-Alanine (JAN) — *See* Alanine.

Alanine Nitrogen Mustard — *See* Melphalan.

Alanosine. $C_3H_7N_3O_4$. 149.11. (-)-(*S*)-2-Amino-3-(hydroxynitrosamino)propionic acid. *UNII-2CNI71214Y. CAS-5854-93-3.* INN; MI.

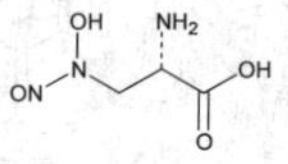

Alaproclate [*1981*] (al″ a proe′ klate). $C_{13}H_{18}ClNO_2$. 255.74. (1) DL-Alanine, 2-(4-chlorophenyl)-1,1-dimethylethyl ester; (2) DL-Alanine *p*-chloro-α,α-dimethylphenethyl ester. *UNII-C4R42570ZO. CAS-60719-82-6.* INN. *Antidepressant.* ◇*GEA 654*

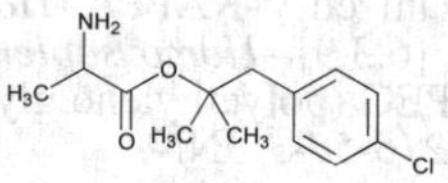

Alatrofloxacin Mesylate [*1996*] (al at″ roe flox′ a sin mes′ i late). $C_{26}H_{25}F_3N_6O_5 \cdot CH_4O_3S$. 654.61. [Alatrofloxacin is INN.] (1) L-Alaninamide, L-alanyl-*N*-[3-[6-carboxy-8-(2,4-difluorophenyl)-3-fluoro-5,8-dihydro-5-oxo-1,8-naphthyridin-2-yl]-3-azabicyclo[3.1.0]hex-6-yl]-, monomethanesulfonate, (1α,5α,6α); (2) 7-[(1*R*,5*S*,6*s*)-6-[(*S*)-2-[(*S*)-2-Aminopropionamido]propionamido]-3-azabicyclo[3.1.0]hex-3-yl]-1-(2,4-difluorophenyl)-6-fluoro-1,4-dihydro-4-oxo-1,8-naphthyridine-3-carboxylic acid, monomethanesulfonate. *UNII-2IXX802851. CAS-157605-25-9; CAS-157182-32-6* [alatrofloxacin]. *Antibacterial.* Trovan (Pfizer) ◇*CP-116,517-27*

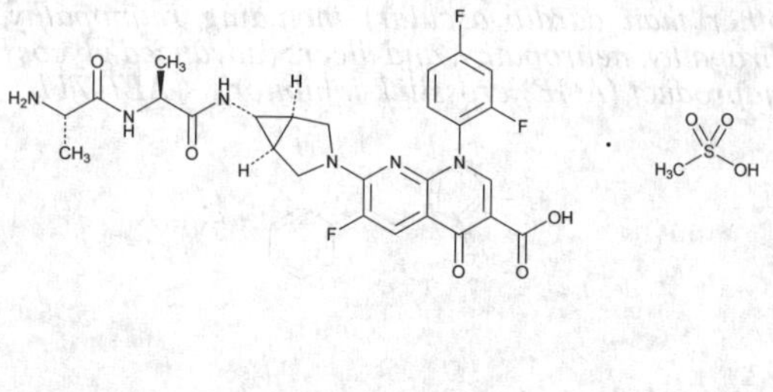

Alazanine Triclofenate. $C_{27}H_{23}Cl_3N_2OS_2 \cdot (C_6H_3Cl_3O)_2$. 956.87. A mixture of one molecule of 3-ethyl-2-[3-(3-ethyl-2-benzothiazolinylidene)propenyl]benzothiazolium 2,4,5-trichlorophenate and two molecules of 2,4,5-trichlorophenol. *CAS-5779-59-9.* INN.

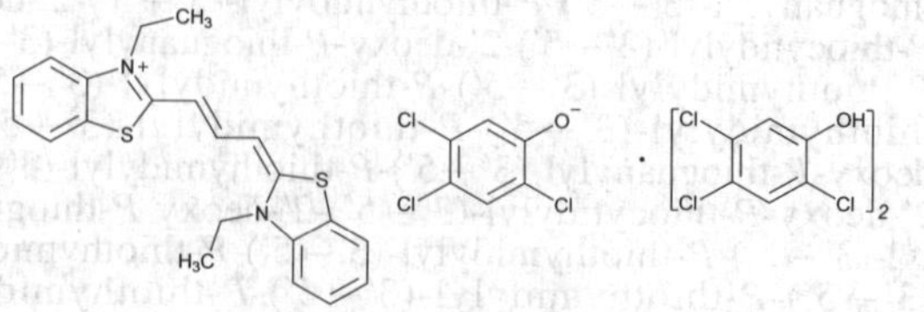

Albaconazole [*2008*] (al″ ba kon′ a zole). $C_{20}H_{16}ClF_2N_5O_2$. 431.82. (1) 4(3*H*)-Quinazolinone, 7-chloro-3-[(1*R*,2*R*)-2-(2,4-difluorophenyl)-2-hydroxy-1-methyl-3-(1*H*-1,2,4-triazol-1-yl)propyl]-; (2) 7-Chloro-3-[(1*R*,2*R*)-2-(2,4-difluorophenyl)-2-hydroxy-1-methyl-3-(1*H*-1,2,4-triazol-1-yl)propyl]quinazolin-4(3*H*)-one. *UNII-YDW24Y8IAB. CAS-187949-02-6.* INN. *Treatment of fungal infections.* ◇*UR-9825*

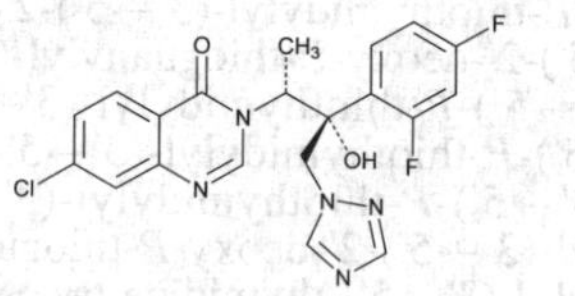

Albendazole [*1976*] (al ben′ da zole). **USP.** $C_{12}H_{15}N_3O_2S$. 265.33. (1) Carbamic acid, [5-(propylthio)-1*H*-benzimidazol-2-yl]-, methyl ester; (2) Methyl 5-(propylthio)-2-benzimidazolecarbamate. *UNII-F4216019LN. CAS-54965-21-8.* INN; BAN; JAN. *Anthelmintic.* Albenza (GlaxoSmithKline) ◇*SK&F 62979*

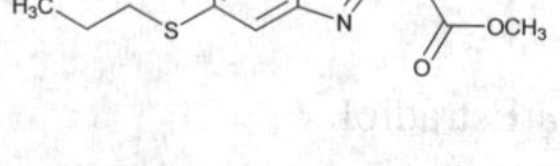

Albendazole Oxide. $C_{12}H_{15}N_3O_3S$. 281.33. Methyl 5-(propylsulfinyl)-2-benzimidazolecarbamate. *UNII-J39B52TV34. CAS-54029-12-8.* INN; BAN.

Albiglutide [*2007*] (al″ bi gloo′ tide). $C_{3232}H_{5032}N_{864}O_{979}S_{41}$. 72,971.40. (1) Albugon, a recombinant human glucagon-like peptide 1-albumin protein; (2) ([8-Glycine]human glucagon-like peptide 1-(7-36)-peptidyl)([8-glycine]human glucagon-like peptide 1-(7-36)-peptidyl)(human serum albumin (585 residues)). *UNII-5E7U48495E. CAS-782500-75-8.* INN. *Treatment of type 2 diabetes.* ◇*GSK716155*

```
HGEGTFTSDV SSYLEGQAAK EFIAWLVKGR HGEGTFTSDV SSYLEGQAAK
EFIAWLVKGR DAHKSEVAHR FKDLGEENFK ALVLIAFAQY LQQCPFEDHV
KLVNEVTEFA KTCVADESAE NCDKSLHTLF GDKLCTVATL RETYGEMADC
CAKQEPERNE CFLQHKDDNP NLPRLVRPEV DVMCTAFHDN EETFLKKYLY
EIARRHPYFY APELLFFAKR YKAAFTECCQ AADKAACLLP KLDELRDEGK
ASSAKQRLKC ASLQKFGERA FKAWAVARLS QRFPKAEFAE VSKLVTDLTK
VHTECCHGDL LECADDRADL AKYICENQDS ISSKLKECCE KPLLEKSHCI
AEVENDEMPA DLPSLAADFV ESKDVCKNYA EAKDVFLGMF LYEYARRHPD
YSVVLLLRLA KTYETTLEKC CAAADPHECY AKVFDEFKPL VEEPQNLIKQ
NCELFEQLGE YKFQNALLVR YTKKVPQVST PTLVEVSRNL GKVGSKCCKH
PEAKRMPCAE DYLSVVLNQL CVLHEKTPVS DRVTKCCTES LVNRRPCFSA
LEVDETYVPK EFNAETFTFH ADICTLSEKE RQIKKQTALV ELVKHKPKAT
KEQLKAVMDD FAAFVEKCCK ADDKETCFAE EGKKLVAASQ AALGL
```

Albinterferon Alfa-2b [*2007*] (al bin″ ter feer′ on al′ fa). $C_{3796}H_{5937}N_{1015}O_{1143}S_{50}$. (1) 1-585-Serum albumin (human) fusion protein with interferon α-2b (human); (2) Human serum albumin (585 residues) fusion protein with human interferon alpha-2 (165 residues). Molecular weight is approximately 85,700 daltons. *CAS-472960-22-8.* INN. *Treatment of chronic hepatitis C.* Albuferon (Human Genome Sciences)

```
DAHKSEVAHR FKDLGEENFK ALVLIAFAQY LQQCPFEDHV KLVNEVTEFA
KTCVADESAE NCDKSLHTLF GDKLCTVATL RETYGEMADC CAKQEPERNE
CFLQHKDDNP NLPRLVRPEV DVMCTAFHDN EETFLKKYLY EIARRHPYFY
APELLFFAKR YKAAFTECCQ AADKAACLLP KLDELRDEGK ASSAKQRLKC
ASLQKFGERA FKAWAVARLS QRFPKAEFAE VSKLVTDLTK VHTECCHGDL
LECADDRADL AKYICENQDS ISSKLKECCE KPLLEKSHCI AEVENDEMPA
DLPSLAADFV ESKDVCKNYA EAKDVFLGMF LYEYARRHPD YSVVLLLRLA
KTYETTLEKC CAAADPHECY AKVFDEFKPL VEEPQNLIKQ NCELFEQLGE
YKFQNALLVR YTKKVPQVST PTLVEVSRNL GKVGSKCCKH PEAKRMPCAE
DYLSVVLNQL CVLHEKTPVS DRVTKCCTES LVNRRPCFSA LEVDETYVPK
EFNAETFTFH ADICTLSEKE RQIKKQTALV ELVKHKPKAT KEQLKAVMDD
FAAFVEKCCK ADDKETCFAE EGKKLVAASQ AALGLCDLPQ THSLGSRRTL
MLLAQMRRIS LFSCLKDRHD FGFPQEEFGN QFQKAETIPV LHEMIQQIFN
LFSTKDSSAA WDETLLDKFY TELYQQLNDL EACVIQGVGV TETPLMKEDS
ILAVRKYFQR ITLYLKEKKY SPCAWEVVRA EIMRSFSLST NLQESLRSKE
```

Albumin, Aggregated [*1974*] (al bue′ min ag′ re gay″ ted). *Diagnostic aid (lung imaging)* [when combined with technetium Tc 99m]. ◇*MP 4006*

Albumin, Aggregated Iodinated I 131 Serum [*1966*] (al bue′ min ag′ re gay″ ted eye′ oh di nay″ ted). (1) Albumin, blood serum, aggregates of, labeled with iodine-131; (2) Albumin, blood serum, aggregates of, labeled with iodine-131. *Radioactive agent.* Albumotope-LS (Bristol-Myers Squibb†); MAA I 131 (Mallinckrodt†); Macroscan-131 (Abbott†)

Albumin, Chromated Cr 51 Serum [*1966*] (al bue′ min kroe′ may ted). (1) Albumin, blood serum, labeled with chromium-51; (2) Albumin, blood serum, labeled with chromium-51. *Radioactive agent.* Chromalbin (Bristol-Myers Squibb†)

Albumin Human (al bue′ min hue′ man). **USP.** A sterile, nonpyrogenic preparation of serum albumin obtained by fractionating material (source blood, plasma, serum, or placentas) from healthy human donors, the source material being tested for the absence of hepatitis B surface antigen. *UNII-ZIF514RVZR. Blood volume supporter.* Optison (GE Healthcare) [*Name previously used: Albumin, Normal Human Serum.*]

---

† Brand name formerly used, and/or firm no longer concerned with this product.

Albumin, Iodinated (^{131}I) Human Serum (INN) — *See* Albumin, Iodinated I 131 Serum.

Albumin, Iodinated (^{131}I) Human Serum, Injection (JAN) — *See* Albumin, Iodinated I 131 Serum.

Albumin, Iodinated I 125 Serum [*1966*] (al bue′ min eye′ oh di nay″ ted). [Iodinated (^{125}I) Human Serum Albumin is INN.] (1) Albumin, blood serum, labeled with iodine-125; (2) Albumin, blood serum, labeled with iodine-125. *CAS-9048-49-1.* USP XIX. *Diagnostic aid (blood volume determination); radioactive agent.* Albumotope I-125 (Bristol-Myers Squibb†); IHSA I-125 (Mallinckrodt); RISA-125 (Abbott†)

Albumin, Iodinated I 131 Serum [*1966*] (al bue′ min eye′ oh di nay″ ted). [Iodinated (^{131}I) Human Serum Albumin is INN; Iodinated (^{131}I) Human Serum Albumin Injection is JAN.] (1) Albumin, blood serum, labeled with iodine-131; (2) Albumin, blood serum, labeled with iodine-131. *CAS-9048-49-1.* USP XIX. *Diagnostic aid (blood volume determination); diagnostic aid (intrathecal imaging); radioactive agent.* Albumotope I-131 (Bristol-Myers Squibb†); IHSA I-131 (Mallinckrodt†); RISA-131 (Abbott†)

Albumin, Normal Human Serum (previously used name) — *See* Albumin Human.

Albumin Tannate. Compound of albumin with tannic acid. *CAS-9006-52-4.* JAN.

Albuterol [*1971*] (al bue′ ter ol). **USP.** $C_{13}H_{21}NO_3$. 239.31. [Salbutamol is INN and BAN.] (1) 1,3-Benzenedimethanol, α^1-[[(1,1-dimethylethyl)amino]methyl]-4-hydroxy-; (2) α^1-[(*tert*-Butylamino)methyl]-4-hydroxy-*m*-xylene-α,α'-diol. *UNII-QF8SVZ843E. CAS-18559-94-9. Bronchodilator.* Proventil (Schering); Ventolin (GlaxoSmithKline)

Albuterol Sulfate [*1974*] (al bue′ ter ol sul′ fate). **USP.** $(C_{13}H_{21}NO_3)_2 \cdot H_2SO_4$. 576.70. [Salbutamol Sulfate is JAN.] (1) 1,3-Benzenedimethanol, α^1-[[(1,1-dimethylethyl)amino]methyl]-4-hydroxy-, sulfate (2:1) (salt); (2) α^1-[(*tert*-Butylamino)methyl]-4-hydroxy-*m*-xylene-α,α'-diol sulfate (2:1) (salt). *UNII-021SEF373I; UNII-QF8SVZ843E* [albuterol]. *CAS-51022-70-9; CAS-18559-94-9* [albuterol]. *Bronchodilator.* Accuneb (Dey); Proair (Teva); Proventil (Schering); Ventolin (GlaxoSmithKline); Volmax (Muro) ◇*Sch 13949W Sulfate*

Albutoin [*1964*] (al bue′ toin; al bue′ toe in). $C_{10}H_{16}N_2OS$. 212.31. (1) 4-Imidazolidinone, 5-(2-methylpropyl)-3-(2-propenyl)-2-thioxo-; (2) 3-Allyl-5-isobutyl-2-thiohydantoin. *CAS-830-89-7.* INN. *Anticonvulsant.* ◇*BAX 422Z*

Alcaftadine [*2006*] (al kaf′ ta deen). $C_{19}H_{21}N_3O$. 307.39. (1) 5*H*-Imidazo[2,1-*b*][3]benzazepine-3-carboxaldehyde, 6,11-dihydro-11-(1-methyl-4-piperidinylidene)-; (2) 11-(1-Methylpiperidin-4-ylidene)-6,11-dihydro-5*H*-imidazolo[2,1-*b*][3]benzazepine-3-carbaldehyde; (3) 4-(1-Methyl-piperidin-4-ylidene)-9,10-dihydro-4H-3,10a-diaza-benzo[f]azulene-1-carbaldehyde. *UNII-7Z8O94ECSX. CAS-147084-10-4.* INN. *Antiallergic, histaminic H-1 receptor antagonist, anti-inflammatory.* ◇*R 89674*

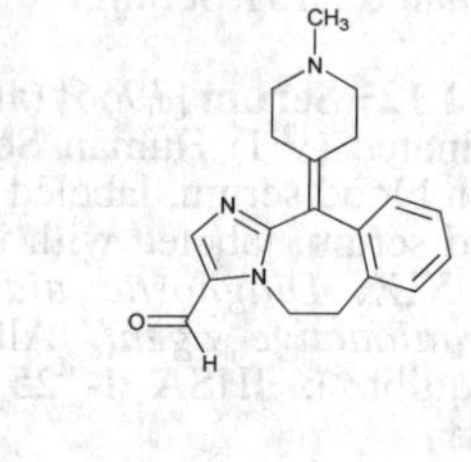

Alclofenac [*1971*] (al kloe′ fen ak). $C_{11}H_{11}ClO_3$. 226.66. (1) Benzeneacetic acid, 3-chloro-4-(2-propenyloxy)-; (2) [4-(Allyloxy)-3-chlorophenyl]acetic acid. *CAS-22131-79-9.* INN; BAN; JAN. *Anti-inflammatory.* Mervan (Continental Pharma, Belgium) ◇*W 7320*

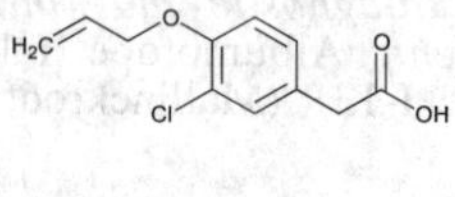

Alclometasone Dipropionate [*1979*] (al″ kloe met′ a sone dye proe′ pee oh nate). **USP.** $C_{28}H_{37}ClO_7$. 521.04. [Alclometasone is INN and BAN.] (1) Pregna-1,4-diene-3,20-dione, 7-chloro-11-hydroxy-16-methyl-17,21-bis(1-oxopropoxy)-, (7α,11β,16α)-; (2) 7α-Chloro-11β,17,21-trihydroxy-16α-methylpregna-1,4-diene-3,20-dione 17,21-dipropionate. *UNII-S56PQL4N1V; UNII-136H45TB7B* [alclometasone]. *CAS-66734-13-2; CAS-67452-97-5* [alclometasone]. JAN. *Anti-inflammatory (topical).* Aclovate (GlaxoSmithKline) ◇*Sch 22219*

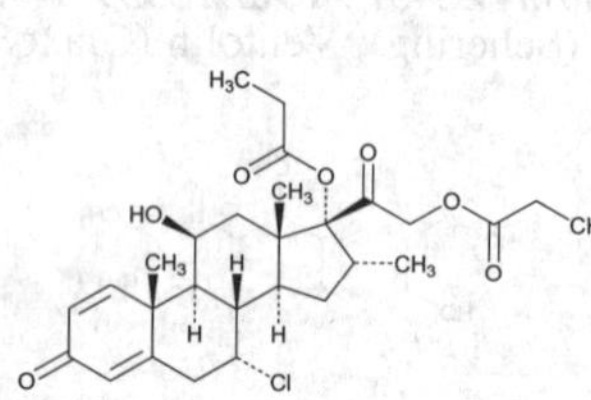

Alcloxa [*1963*] (al klox′ a). $C_4H_9Al_2ClN_4O_7$. 314.55. [Aluminum Chlorohydroxy Allantoinate is JAN.] (1) Aluminum, chlorotetrahydroxy[(4,5-dihydro-2-hydroxy-5-oxo-1*H*-imidazol-4-yl)ureato]di-; (2) Chlorotetrahydroxy[(2-hydroxy-5-oxo-2-imidazolin-4-yl)ureato]dialuminum; (3) Aluminum chlorhydroxy allantoinate. *UNII-18B8O9DQA2. CAS-1317-25-5.* INN. *Astringent; keratolytic.* ◇*ALCA; RC-173*

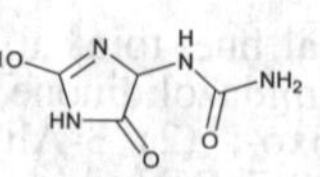

Alcohol (al′ ka hol). **USP.** C_2H_6O. 46.07. [Ethanol is JAN.] (1) Ethanol; (2) Ethyl alcohol. *UNII-3K9958V90M. CAS-64-17-5. Anti-infective, topical; pharmaceutic aid (solvent).*

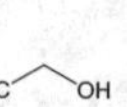

Alcuronium Chloride [*1967*] (al kure oh′ nee um klor′ ide). $C_{44}H_{50}Cl_2N_4O_2$. 737.80. (1) Toxiferine I, 4,4′-didemethyl-4,4′-di-2-propenyl-, dichloride; (2) *N,N*′-Diallylnortoxifer-

inium dichloride. *UNII-490DW6501Y. CAS-15180-03-7.* INN; BAN; JAN. *Relaxant (skeletal muscle).* Alloferin (Hoffmann-LaRoche-International) ◇*RO 4-3816*

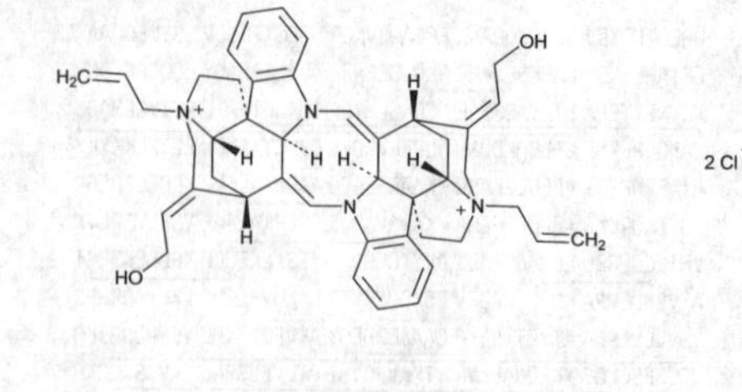

Aldesleukin [*1990*] (al″ des loo′ kin). $C_{690}H_{1115}N_{177}O_{203}S_6$. 15,600 daltons. (1) 2-133-Interleukin 2 (human reduced), 125-L-serine-; (2) 125-L-Serine-2-133-interleukin 2 (human reduced). *CAS-110942-02-4.* INN; BAN. *Antineoplastic; biological response modifier; immunostimulant.* Proleukin (Chiron)

```
PTSSSTKKT   QLQLEHLLLD   LQMILNGINN   YKNPKLTRML   TFKFYMPKKA
TELKHLQCLE  EELKPLEEVL   NLAQSKNFHL   RPRDLISNIN   VIVLELKGSE
TTFMCEYADE  TATIVEFLNR   WITFSQSIIS   TLT
```

Aldesulfone Sodium (INN, DCF) — *See* Sulfoxone Sodium.

Aldioxa [*1963*] (al dye ox′ a). $C_4H_7AlN_4O_5$. 218.10. (1) Aluminum, dihydroxy[(4,5-dihydro-2-hydroxy-5-oxo-1*H*-imidazol-4-yl)ureato]-; (2) Dihydroxy[2-hydroxy-5-oxo-2-imidazolin-4-yl)ureato]aluminum; (3) Aluminum dihydroxy allantoinate. *UNII-8T66I31YNK. CAS-5579-81-7.* INN; JAN. *Astringent; keratolytic.* ◇*ALDA; RC-172*

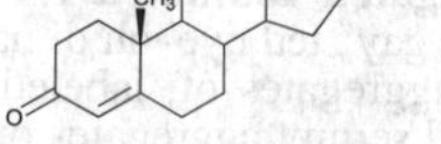

Aldosterone. $C_{21}H_{28}O_5$. 360.44. 11β,21-Dihydroxypregn-4-ene-3,18,20-trione. *UNII-4964P6T9RB. CAS-52-39-1.* INN; BAN; DCF; MI.

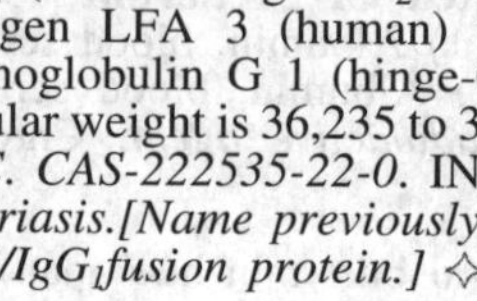

Alefacept [*2000*] (a lef′ a sept). $C_{3264}H_{5002}N_{840}O_{988}S_{20}$. (1) 1-92-LFA-3 (Antigen) (human) fusion protein with immunoglobulin G_1 (human hinge-CH_2-CH_3 γ1-chain), dimer; (2) 1-92-Antigen LFA 3 (human) fusion protein with human immunoglobulin G 1 (hinge-CH_2-CH_3 γ1-chain), dimer. Molecular weight is 36,235 to 36,837 daltons. *UNII-ELK3V90G6C. CAS-222535-22-0.* INN; BAN. *Treatment of plaque psoriasis.[Name previously used: Recombinant human LFA-3/IgG₁fusion protein.]* ◇*BG9712; LFA3TIP; BG9273*

```
FSQQIYGVVY GNVTFHVPSN VPLKEVLWKK QKDKVAELEN SEFRAFSSFK
NRVYLDTVSG SLTIYNLTSS DEDEYEMESP NITDTMKFFL YVDKTHTCPP
CPAPELLGGP SVFLFPPKPK DTLMISRTPE VTCVVVDVSH EDPEVKFNWY
VDGVEVHNAK TKPREEQYNS TYRVVSVLTV LHQDWLNGKE YKCKVSNKAL
PAPIEKTISK AKGQPREPQV YTLPPSRDEL TKNQVSLTCL VKGFYPSDIA
VEWESNGQPE NNYKTTPPVL DSDGSFFLYS KLTVDKSRWQ QGNVFSCSVM
HEALHNHYTQ KSLSLSPGK
```

Aleglitazar [*2007*] (al″ e gli′ ta zar). $C_{24}H_{23}NO_5S$. 437.51. (1) Benzo[*b*]thiophene-7-propanoic acid, α-methoxy-4-[2-(5-methyl-2-phenyl-4-oxazolyl)ethoxy]-, (α*S*)-; (2) (2*S*)-2-Methoxy-3-{4-[2-(5-methyl-2-phenyl-1,3-oxazol-4-yl)ethoxy]-benzothiophen-7-yl}propionic acid; (3) (*S*)-2-Methoxy-3-[4-[2-(5-methyl-2-phenyloxazol-4-yl-ethoxy]-benzo[*b*]thiophen-7-yl]propionic acid. *UNII-41T4OAG59U. CAS-475479-34-6.* INN. *Treatment of type II diabetes.* ◇*RO0728804; R1439*

Alemcinal [*1999*] (a lem′ si nal). $C_{38}H_{67}NO_{10}$. 697.94. 8,9-Didehydro-*N*-demethyl-9-deoxo-4″,6,12-trideoxy-6,9-epoxy-*N*-ethylerythromycin. *UNII-5DS173ODI4. CAS-150785-53-8.* INN. *Gastrointestinal prokinetic (motilin agonist).* ◇*Abbott-81229.0; ABT-229; A-81229*

Alemtuzumab [*1999*] (al″ em tooz′ oo mab). (1) Immunoglobulin G1, anti-(human CD52 (antigen)) (human-rat monoclonal CAMPATH-1H, γ1-chain), disulfide with human-rat monoclonal CAMPATH-1H light chain, dimer; (2) Immunoglobulin G 1 (human-rat monoclonal CAMPATH-1H γ1-chain anti-human antigen CD52), disulfide with human-rat monoclonal CAMPATH-1H light chain, dimer. Molecular weight is approximately 150,000 daltons. *UNII-3A189DH42V. CAS-216503-57-0.* INN; BAN. *Antineoplastic (monoclonal antibody).* Campath (Boehringer Ingelheim KG, Germany) ◇*LDP-03*

Alendronate Sodium [*1990*] (a len′ droe nate soe′ dee um). **USP**. $C_4H_{12}NNaO_7P_2.3H_2O$. 325.12. (1) Phosphonic acid, (4-amino-1-hydroxybutylidene)bis-, monosodium salt, trihydrate; (2) Sodium trihydrogen (4-amino-1-hydroxybutylidene)diphosphonate, trihydrate. *UNII-2UY4M2U3RA. CAS-121268-17-5.* *Bone resorption inhibitor.* Fosamax (Merck) ◇*MK-217; G-704,650*

Alendronic Acid. **USP**. $C_4H_{13}NO_7P_2$. 249.10. (4-Amino-1-hydroxybutylidene)diphosphonic acid. *UNII-X1J18R4W8P. CAS-66376-36-1.* INN; BAN.

Alentemol Hydrobromide [*1990*] (a len′ te mol hye″ droe broe′ mide). $C_{19}H_{25}NO.HBr$. 364.32. [Alentemol is INN.] (1) 1*H*-Phenalen-5-ol, 2-(dipropylamino)-2,3-dihydro-, hydrobromide, (+)-; (2) (+)-2-(Dipropylamino)-2,3-dihydrophenalen-5-ol hydrobromide. *UNII-Y67FY3RWN1; UNII-F6S91MHL3E* [alentemol]. *CAS-112892-81-6; CAS-112891-97-1* [alentemol]. *Antipsychotic; dopamine agonist.* ◇*U-68,553B*

Aleplasinin [*2007*] (al″ e plas′ in in). $C_{28}H_{27}NO_3$. 425.52. (1) 1*H*-Indol-3-acetic acid, 1-[[4-(1,1-dimethylethyl)phenyl]methyl]-5-(3-methylphenyl)-α-oxo-; (2) [1-[4-(1,1-Dimethylethyl)benzyl]-5-(3-methylphenyl)-1*H*-indol-3-yl]oxoacetic acid. *UNII-LL56J87F3X. CAS-481629-87-2.* INN. *Treatment of Alzheimer's disease.* ◇*PAZ-417*

Alepride. $C_{22}H_{30}ClN_3O_2$. 403.95. 2-(Allyloxy)-4-amino-5-chloro-*N*-[1-(3-cyclohexen-1-ylmethyl)-4-piperidyl]benzamide. *UNII-R6G1M06TPO. CAS-66564-15-6.* INN.

Alestramustine. $C_{26}H_{36}Cl_2N_2O_4$. 511.48. Estradiol 3-[bis(2-chloroethyl)carbamate], 17-ester with L-alanine. *UNII-81U8A51CHK. CAS-139402-18-9.* INN.

Aletamine Hydrochloride [*1965*] (a let′ a meen hye″ droe klor′ ide). $C_{11}H_{15}N \cdot HCl$. 197.70. [Alfetamine is INN.] (1) Benzeneethanamine, α-2-propenyl-, hydrochloride; (2) α-Allylphenethylamine hydrochloride. *CAS-4255-24-7; CAS-4255-23-6* [aletamine]. *Antidepressant.* ◇*NDR-5061A*

Alexidine [*1969*] (a lex′ i deen). $C_{26}H_{56}N_{10}$. 508.79. (1) 2,4,11,13-Tetraazatetradecanediimidamide, *N,N‴*-bis(2-ethylhexyl)-3,12-diimino-; (2) 1,1′-Hexamethylenebis[5-(2-ethylhexyl)biguanide]. *UNII-GVN71CAL3G. CAS-22573-93-9; CAS-22782-69-0* [replaced]. INN. *Antibacterial.* ◇*Win 21,904; Compound 904*

Alexitol Sodium. Sodium polyhydroxyaluminium monocarbonate hexitol complex where *n* = 0 or an integer, controlled by the preparative conditions. *CAS-66813-51-2.* INN; BAN; MI.

Alexomycin [*1996*] (a lex″ oh mye′ sin). A mixture composed mainly of isolate 10381b which contains several cyclic sulfur peptides produced by *Streptomyces arginensis* and purified by solvent extraction. The purified material has been shown to contain several related cyclic sulfur peptide structures. (1) Alexomycin; (2) Alexomycin. *CAS-165101-50-8. Growth stimulant (veterinary).* ◇*U-82127*

Alfacalcidol. $C_{27}H_{44}O_2$. 400.64. (5Z,7E)-9,10-Secocholesta-5,7,10(19)-triene-1α,3β-diol. *CAS-41294-56-8.* INN; BAN; JAN.

Alfadex. NF. $C_{36}H_{60}O_{30}$. 972.84. α-Cyclodextrin. *UNII-Z1LH97KTRM. CAS-10016-20-3.* INN; BAN.

Alfadolone. $C_{21}H_{32}O_4$. 348.48. 3α,21-Dihydroxy-5α-pregnane-11,20-dione. *UNII-OE1C96974E. CAS-14107-37-0.* INN; BAN; DCF. [*Name previously used: Alphadolone.*] ◇*GR 2/1574*

Alfaprostol [*1982*] (al″ fa prost′ ol). $C_{24}H_{38}O_5$. 406.56. (1) 5-Heptenoic acid, 7-[2-(5-cyclohexyl-3-hydroxy-1-pentynyl)-3,5-dihydroxycyclopentyl]-, methyl ester, [1*R*-[1α(Z),2β(*S**),3α,5α]]-; (2) Methyl (Z)-7-[(1*R*,2*S*,3*R*,5*S*)-2-[(3*S*)-5-cyclohexyl-3-hydroxy-1-pentynyl]-3,5-dihydroxycyclopentyl]-5-heptenoate. *UNII-4XKL2JJ08I. CAS-74176-31-1.* INN; BAN. *Prostaglandin (veterinary).* ◇*Ro 22-9000; K 11941*

Alfatradiol. $C_{18}H_{24}O_2$. 272.38. Estra-1,3,5(10)-triene-3,17α-diol. *CAS-57-91-0.* INN.

Alfaxalone. $C_{21}H_{32}O_3$. 332.48. 3α-Hydroxy-5α-pregnane-11,20-dione. *UNII-BD07M97B2A. CAS-23930-19-0.* INN; BAN; JAN; MI; DCF. [*Name previously used: Alphaxalone.*] ◇*GR 2/234*

Alfentanil Hydrochloride [*1980*] (al fen′ ta nil hye″ droe klor′ ide). **USP.** $C_{21}H_{32}N_6O_3 \cdot HCl \cdot H_2O$. 470.99. [Alfentanil is INN and BAN.] (1) Propanamide, *N*-[1-[2-(4-ethyl-4,5-dihydro-5-oxo-1*H*-tetrazol-1-yl)ethyl]-4-(methoxymethyl)-4-piperidinyl]-*N*-phenyl, monohydrochloride, monohydrate; (2) *N*-[1-[2-(4-Ethyl-5-oxo-2-tetrazolin-1-yl)-ethyl]-4-(methoxymethyl)-4-piperidyl]propionanilide monohydrochloride monohydrate. *UNII-11S92G0TIW; UNII-1N74HM2BS7* [alfentanil]. *CAS-70879-28-6; CAS-69049-06-5* [anhydrous]; *CAS-71195-58-9* [alfentanil]. *Analgesic (narcotic).* Alfenta (Akorn) ◇*R 39,209*

Alferminogene Tadenovec [*2007*] (al″ fer min′ oh jeen ta den′ oh vek). (1) DNA (synthetic human adenovirus 5 human fibroblast growth factor 4 gene-containing 35506-nucleotide fragment ZK 205368; (2) Recombinant human adenovirus 5 (replication-deficient, E1-deleted) containing a human fibroblast growth factor-4 cDNA sequence driven by a cytomegalovirus promoter. *CAS-473553-86-5.* INN. *Gene therapy product; promotes angiogenesis.* Generx (Cardium Therapeutics)

Alfetamine (INN) Hydrochloride — *See* Aletamine Hydrochloride.

Alfimeprase [*2000*] (al fim′ e prase). $C_{985}H_{1541}N_{285}O_{301}S_{12}$. 3-203-Fibrolase [3-serine] [Agkistrodon contortrix contortrix recombinant]. Molecular weight is approximately 22,576 daltons. *UNII-GPN9HBH1HS. CAS-259074-76-5.* INN; BAN. *Thrombolytic.* (Amgen)

```
SFPQRYVQ LVIVADHRMN TKYNGDSDKI RQWVHQIVNT INEIYRPLNI
QFTLVGLEIW SNQDLITVTS VSHDTLASFG NWRETDLLRR QRHDNAQLLT
AIDFDGDTVG LAYVGGMCQL KHSTGVIQDH SAINLLVALT MAHELGHNLG
MNHDGNQCHC GANSCVMAAM LSDQPSKLFS DCSKKDYQTF LTVNNPQCIL
NKP
```

Alfuzosin Hydrochloride [*1984*] (al fue′ zoe sin hye″ droe klor′ ide). $C_{19}H_{27}N_5O_4.HCl$. 425.91. [Alfuzosin is INN and BAN.] (1) 2-Furancarboxamide, (±)-*N*-[3-[(4-amino-6,7-dimethoxy-2-quinazolinyl)methylamino]propyl]tetrahydro-, monohydrochloride; (2) (±)-*N*-[3-[(4-Amino-6,7-dimethoxy-2-quinazolinyl)methylamino]propyl]tetrahydro-2-furamide monohydrochloride. *UNII-75046A1XTN; UNII-90347YTW5F* [alfuzosin]. *CAS-81403-68-1; CAS-81403-80-7* [alfuzosin]. *Antihypertensive (α-blocker).* Uroxatral (Sanofi Aventis) ◇*SL 77 499-10*

Algeldrate [*1967*] (al jel′ drate). $AlH_3O_3.xH_2O$. 78.00 (anhydrous). A non-reactive, powdered, aluminum hydroxide hydrate. (1) Aluminum hydroxide, hydrate; (2) Aluminum hydroxide hydrate. *UNII-03J11K103C. CAS-1330-44-5.* INN. *Antacid.* ◇*W 4600*

Algestone Acetonide [*1966*] (al jes′ tone a seet′ oh nide). $C_{24}H_{34}O_4$. 386.52. [Algestone is INN.] (1) Pregn-4-ene-3,20-dione, 16,17-[(1-methylethylidene)bis(oxy)], (16α)-; (2) 16α,17-Dihydroxypregn-4-ene-3,20-dione cyclic acetal with acetone. *CAS-4968-09-6; CAS-595-77-7* [algestone]. BAN. *Anti-inflammatory.* ◇*W3395*

Algestone Acetophenide [*1969*] (al jes′ tone a seet″ oh fen′ ide). $C_{29}H_{36}O_4$. 448.59. (1) Pregn-4-ene-3,20-dione, 16,17-[(1-phenylethylidene)bis(oxy)]-, [16α(*R*)]-; (2) (*R*)-16α,17-Dihydroxypregn-4-ene-3,20-dione cyclic acetal

with acetophenone. *CAS-24356-94-3. Progestin.* Deladroxone (Bristol-Myers Squibb†); Droxone (Bristol-Myers Squibb†) ◇*SQ 15,101*

Algin — *See* Sodium Alginate.

Alginic Acid (al jin′ ik as′ id). **NF.** $(C_6H_8O_6)_n$. Alginic acid, Poly. *UNII-8C3Z4148WZ. CAS-9005-32-7.* BAN. *Pharmaceutic aid (tablet binder and emulsifying agent).*

Alglucerase [*1992*] (al gloo′ ser ase). $C_{2532}H_{3854}N_{672}O_{711}S_{16}$ (protein moiety). 59,300 (SDS-PAGE determined). A modified form of human placental tissue β-glucocerebrosidase (β-D-glucosyl-*N*-acylsphingosine glucohydrolase). It is a monomeric glycoprotein of 497 amino acids; approximately 12% of the glycoprotein consists of *N*-linked carbohydrate chains of the complex and high mannose type. (1) Glucosylceramidase (human placenta isoenzyme protein moiety reduced); (2) Glucosylceramidase (human placenta isoenzyme protein moiety reduced). *UNII-27T56C7KK0. CAS-143003-46-7.* INN; BAN. *Enzyme replenisher (glucocerebrosidase).* Ceredase (Genzyme) [*Name previously used: Macrophage-targeted β-glucocerebrosidase.*]

```
ARPCIPKSFG  YSSVVCVCNA  TYCDSFDPPT  FPALGTFSRY  ESTRSGRRME
LSMGPIQANH  TGTGLLLTLQ  PEQKFQKVKG  FGGAMTDAAA  LNILALSPPA
QNLLLKSYFS  EEGIGYNIIR  VPMASCDFSI  RTYTYADTPD  DFQLHNFSLP
EEDTKLKIPL  IHRALQLAQR  PVSLLASPWT  SPTWLKTNGA  VNGKGSLKGQ
PGDIYHQTWA  RYFVKFLDAY  AEHKLQFWAV  TAENEPSAGL  LSGYPFQCLG
FTPEHQRDFI  ARDLGPTLAN  STHHNVRLLM  LDDQRLLLPH  WAKVVLTDPE
AAKYVHGIAV  HWYLDFLAPA  KATLGETHRL  FPNTMLFASE  ACVGSKFWEQ
SVRLGSWDRG  MQYSHSIITN  LLYHVVGWTD  WNLALNPEGG  PNWVRNFVDS
PIIVDITKDT  FYKQPMFYHL  GHFSKFIPEG  SQRVGLVASQ  KNDLDAVALM
HPDGSAVVVV  LNRSSKDVPP  TIKDPAVGFL  ETISPGYSIH  TYLWHRQ
```

Alglucosidase Alfa [*2004*] (al″ gloo koe′ si dase al′ fa). $C_{4758}H_{7262}N_{1274}O_{1369}S_{35}$. 105,338. [Alglucosidase Alfa (genetical recombination) is JAN.] (1) Glucosidase, pre-pro-α-[199-arginine,223-histidine] (human); (2) [199-Ar-

---

† Brand name formerly used, and/or firm no longer concerned with this product.

ginine,223-histidine]prepro-α-glucosidase (human). *UNII-DTI67O9503*. *CAS-420794-05-0*. INN. *Treatment of Pompe's disease (enzyme replacement therapy).* ◇*rhGAA*

```
MGVRHPPCSH RLLAVCALVS LATAALLGHI LLHDFLLVPR ELSGSSPVLE
ETHPAHQQGA SRPGPRDAQA HPGRPRAVPT QCDVPPNSRF DCAPDKAITQ
EQCEARGCCY IPAKQGLQGA QMGQPWCFFP PSYPSYKLEN LSSSEMGYTA
TLTRTTPTFF PKDILTLRLD VMMETENRLH FTIKDPANRR YEVPLETPRV
HSRAPSPLYS VEFSEEPFGV IVHRQLDGRV LLNTTVAPLF FADQFLQLST
SLPSQYITGL AEHLSPLMLS TSWTRITLWN RDLAPTPGAN LYGSHPFYLA
LEDGGSAHGV FLLNSNAMDV VLQPSPALSW RSTGGILDVY IFLGPEPKSV
VQQYLDVVGY PFMPPYWGLG FHLCRWGYSS TAITRQVVEN MTRAHFPLDV
QWNDLDYMDS RRDFTFNKDG FRDFPAMVQE LHQGGRRYMM IVDPAISSSG
PAGSYRPYDE GLRRGVFITN ETGQPLIGKV WPGSTAFPDF TNPTALAWWE
DMVAEFHDQV PFDGMWIDMN EPSNFIRGSE DGCPNNELEN PPYVPGVVGG
TLQAATICAS SHQFLSTHYN LHNLYGLTEA IASHRALVKA RGTRPFVISR
STFAGHGRYA GHWTGDVWSS WEQLASSVPE ILQFNLLGVP LVGADVCGFL
GNTSEELCVR WTQLGAFYPF MRNHNSLLSL PQEPYSFSEP AQQAMRKALT
LRYALLPHLY TLFHQAHVAG ETVARPLFLE FPKDSSTWTV DHQLLWGEAL
LITPVLQAGK AEVTGYFPLG TWYDLQTVPI EALGSLPPPP AAPREPAIHS
EGQWVTLPAP LDTINVHLRA GYIIPLQGPG LTTTESRQQP MALAVALTKG
GEARGELFWD DGESLEVLER GAYTQVIFLA RNNTIVNELV RVTSEGAGLQ
LQKVTVLGVA TAPQQVLSNG VPVSNFTYSP DTKVLDICVS LLMGEQFLVS
WC
```

* - glycosylation sites

Alibendol. $C_{13}H_{17}NO_4$. 251.28. 5-Allyl-*N*-(2-hydroxyethyl)-3-methoxysalicylamide. *UNII-A8CO1VZK2Z*. *CAS-26750-81-2*. INN; DCF; MI. ◇*H 3774*

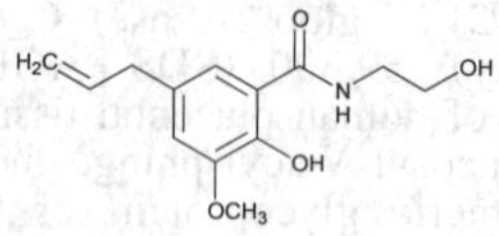

Alicaforsen Sodium [*2002*] (a lik″ a for′ sen soe′ dee um). $C_{192}H_{225}N_{75}Na_{19}O_{98}P_{19}S_{19}$. 6785.83. [Alicaforsen is INN.] (1) DNA, *d*[(*R*)-*P-thio*](G-C-C-C-A-A-G-C-T-G-G-C-A-T-C-C-G-T-C-A) nonadecasodium salt; (2) 2′-Deoxy-*P*-thioguanylyl-(3′→5′)-2′-deoxy-*P*-thiocytidylyl-(3′→5′)-2′-deoxy-*P*-thiocytidylyl-(3′→5′)-2′-deoxy-*P*-thiocytidylyl-(3′→5′)-2′-deoxy-*P*-thioadenylyl-(3′→5′)-2′-deoxy-*P*-thioadenylyl-(3′→5′)-2′-deoxy-*P*-thioguanylyl-(3′→5′)-2′-deoxy-*P*-thiocytidylyl-(3′→5′)-*P*-thiothymidylyl-(3′→5′)-2′-deoxy-*P*-thioguanylyl-(3′→5′)-2′-deoxy-*P*-thioguanylyl-(3′→5′)-2′-deoxy-*P*-thiocytidylyl-(3′→5′)-2′-deoxy-*P*-thioadenylyl-(3′→5′)-2′-*P*-thiothymidylyl-(3′→5′)-2′-deoxy-*P*-thiocytidylyl-(3′→5′)-2′-deoxy-*P*-thiocytidylyl-(3′→5′)-2′-deoxy-*P*-thioguanylyl-(3′→5′)-2′-*P*-thiothymidylyl-(3′→5′)-2′-deoxy-*P*-thiocytidylyl (3′→5′)-2′-deoxyadenosine, nonadecasodium salt. *CAS-331257-52-4; CAS-185229-68-9* [alicaforsen]. INN. *Anti-inflammatory used in the treatment of steroid dependent Crohn's disease, ulcerative colitis, psoriasis, rheumatoid arthritis, and renal transplant (anti-ICAM-1 antisense).* ◇*ISIS 2302*

PS-d(GCCCAAGCTGGCATCCGTCA)

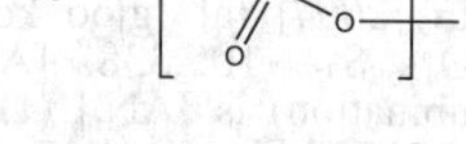

Aliconazole. $C_{18}H_{13}Cl_3N_2$. 363.67. (Z)-1-[2,4-Dichloro-β-(*p*-chlorophenyl)cinnamyl]imidazole. *UNII-51HX72H34H*. *CAS-63824-12-4*. INN.

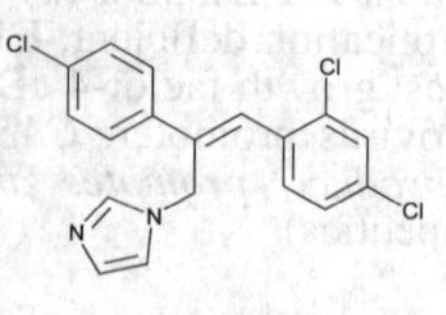

Alifedrine. $C_{18}H_{27}NO_2$. 289.41. 1-Cyclohexyl-3-[[(α*S*,β*R*)-β-hydroxy-α-methylphenethyl]amino]-1-propanone. *UNII-K2PM66M0VQ*. *CAS-78756-61-3*. INN.

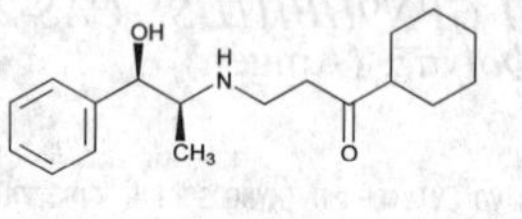

Aliflurane [*1976*] (a″ li flur′ ane). $C_4H_3ClF_4O$. 178.51. (1) Cyclopropane, 1-chloro-1,2,2,3-tetrafluoro-3-methoxy-; (2) 2-Chloro-1,2,3,3-tetrafluorocyclopropyl methyl ether. *UNII-Q1069WKM8G*. *CAS-56689-41-9*. INN. *Anesthetic (inhalation).* ◇*26P*

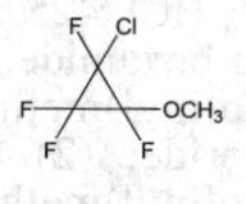

Alilusem. $C_{17}H_{15}ClN_2O_5S$. 394.83. 7-Chloro-1-(2-methylbenzoyl)-2,3-dihydroquinolin-4(1*H*)-one (*E*)-*O*-sulfooxime. *UNII-37376U135T*. *CAS-144506-11-6*. INN.

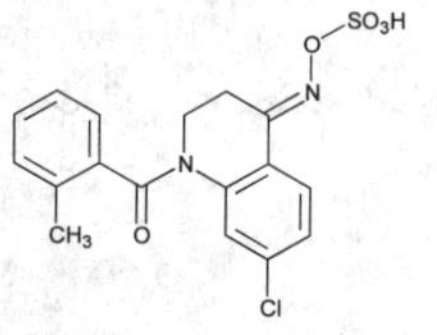

Alimadol. $C_{19}H_{23}NO$. 281.39. *N*-(3-Methoxy-3,3-diphenylpropyl)allylamine. *UNII-8ET970D66K*. *CAS-52742-40-2*. INN.

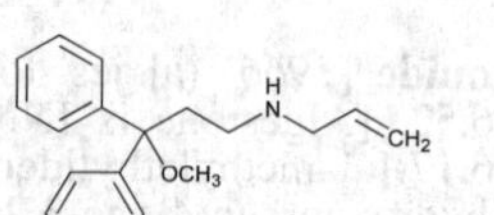

Alimemazine (INN, BAN) — *See* Trimeprazine Tartrate.

Alimemazine Tartrate (JAN) — *See* Trimeprazine Tartrate.

Alinastine. $C_{28}H_{39}N_3O$. 433.63. 2-[1-(*p-tert*-Butylphenethyl)-4-piperidyl]-1-(2-ethoxyethyl)benzimidazole. *UNII-FDP9A2F6YL*. *CAS-154541-72-7*. INN.

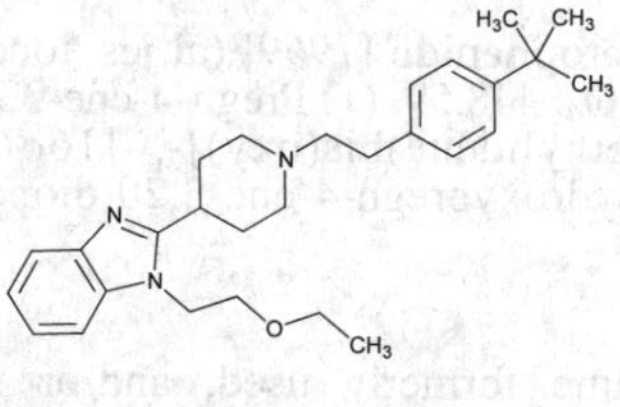

Alinidine. $C_{12}H_{13}Cl_2N_3$. 270.16. 2-(*N*-Allyl-2,6-dichloroanilino)-2-imidazoline. *UNII-E7IDJ8DS1D. CAS-33178-86-8.* INN; BAN; MI. ⬦*St 567-BR [as hydrobromide]*

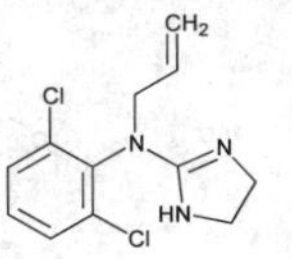

Alipamide [*1969*] (a li′ pa mide). $C_9H_{12}ClN_3O_3S$. 277.73. (1) Benzoic acid, 3-(aminosulfonyl)-4-chloro-2,2-dimethylhydrazide; (2) 4-Chloro-3-sulfamoylbenzoic acid 2,2-dimethylhydrazide. *UNII-PE8925K9EY. CAS-3184-59-6.* INN; BAN. *Diuretic; antihypertensive.* ⬦*CI-546; CN-38,474; D-1721*

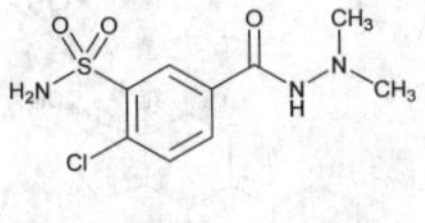

Alipogene Tiparvovec. Recombinant adeno-associated virus serotype 1 (AAV1) vector expressing the S447X variant of the human lipoprotein lipase (LPL) gene. *CAS-929881-05-0.* INN.

Alisactide — *See* Alsactide.

Aliskiren [*2005*] (a lis kye′ ren). $C_{30}H_{53}N_3O_6$. 551.76. (1) Benzeneoctanamide, δ-amino-*N*-(3-amino-2,2-dimethyl-3-oxopropyl)-γ-hydroxy-4-methoxy-3-(3-methoxypropoxy)-α,ζ-bis(1-methylethyl)-, (α*S*, γ*S*, δ*S*, ζ*S*)-; (2) (2*S*,4*S*,5*S*,7*S*)-5-Amino-*N*-(2-carbamoyl-2-methylpropyl)-4-hydroxy-2-isopropyl-7-[4-methoxy-3-(3-methoxypropoxy)benzyl]-8-methylnonamide. *UNII-502FWN4Q32. CAS-173334-57-1.* INN. *Treatment of essential hypertension (renin inhibitor).* ⬦*SPP100*

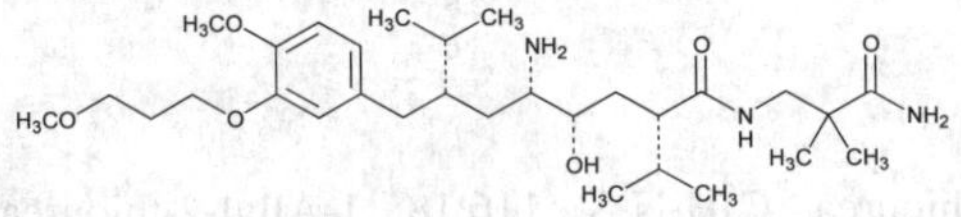

Aliskiren Fumarate [*2006*] (a lis kye′ ren fue′ ma rate). $(C_{30}H_{53}N_3O_6)_2.C_4H_4O_4$. 1219.59. (1) Benzeneoctanamide, δ-amino-*N*-(3-amino-2,2-dimethyl-3-oxopropyl)-γ-hydroxy-4-methoxy-3-(3-methoxypropoxy)-α,ζ-bis(1-methylethyl)-, (α*S*, γ*S*, δ*S*, ζ*S*)-, (2*E*)-2-butenedioate (2:1) (salt); (2) Bis(2*S*,4*S*,5*S*,7*S*)-5-amino-*N*-(3-amino-2,2-dimethyl-3-oxopropyl)-4-hydroxy-7-[4-methoxy-3-(3-methoxypropoxy)benzyl]-8-methyl-2-(1-methylethyl)nonanamide] (2*E*)-but-2-enedioate. *UNII-C8A0P8G029. CAS-173334-58-2.* JAN. *Treatment of essential hypertension (renin inhibitor).* ⬦*SPP100*

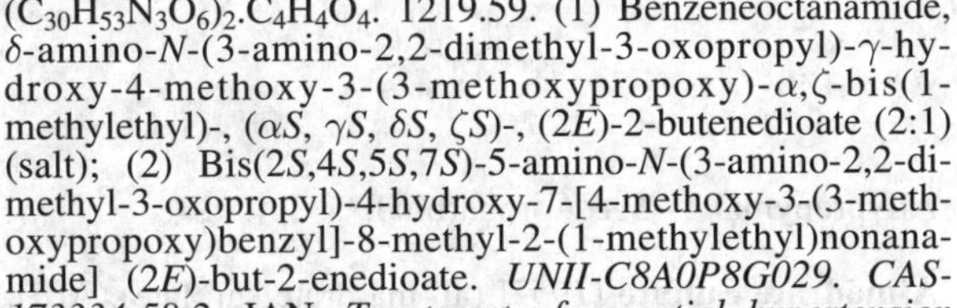

Alisobumal — *See* Butalbital.

Alitame [*1988*] (a′ li tame). $C_{14}H_{25}N_3O_4S.2½H_2O$. 376.47. (1) D-Alaninamide, L-α-aspartyl-*N*-(2,2,4,4-tetramethyl-3-thietanyl)-, hydrate (2:5); (2) (3*S*)-Amino-*N*-[(1*R*)-1-[(2,2,4,4-tetramethyl-3-thietanyl)carbamoyl]ethyl]succinamic acid hydrate (2:5). *UNII-6KI9M51JOG. CAS-99016-42-9; CAS-80863-62-3* [anhydrous]. *Sweetener.* ⬦*CP-54,802*

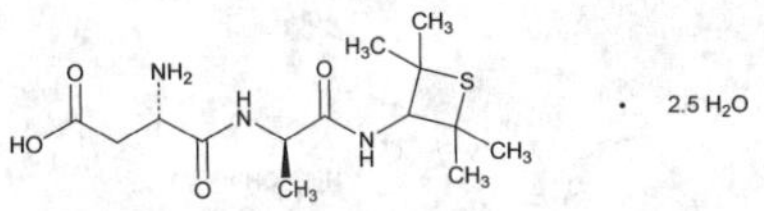

Alitretinoin [*1998*] (a″ li tret′ i noin). $C_{20}H_{28}O_2$. 300.44. (1) 9-*cis*-Retinoic acid; (2) (2*E*,4*E*,6*Z*,8*E*)-3,7-Dimethyl-9-(2,6,6-trimethyl-1-cyclohexen-1-yl)-2,4,6,8-nonatetraenoic acid. *UNII-1UA8E65KDZ. CAS-5300-03-8.* INN; BAN. *Antineoplastic used in the treatment of AIDS-related Kaposi's sarcoma and in the treatment of acute promyelocytic leukemia.* Panretin (Eisai Medical Research) ⬦*LG100057; LGD1057; ALRT1057; AGN 192013; NSC-659772*

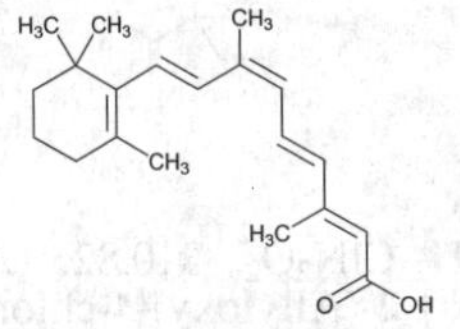

Alizapride. $C_{16}H_{21}N_5O_2$. 315.37. *N*-[(1-Allyl-2-pyrrolidinyl)methyl]-6-methoxy-1*H*-benzotriazole-5-carboxamide. *CAS-59338-93-1.* INN; MI.

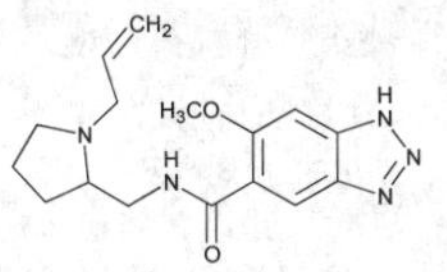

Alkavervir. *Veratrum viride* alkaloids. MI. Veriloid (3M Pharmaceuticals)

Alkyl (C12-15) Benzoate (al′ kil ben′ zoe ate). **NF.** $C_{20}H_{32}O_2$. 304.47 (average). Benzoic acid, C12-15 alkyl ester. *CAS-68411-27-8. Pharmaceutic aid (vehicle, oleaginous); pharmaceutic aid (emollient).*

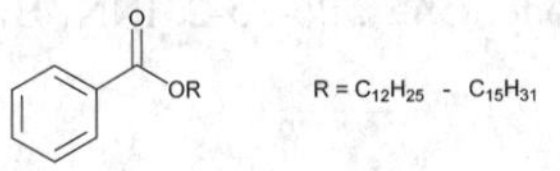

Alkylpolyaminoethylglycine. JAN.

Alkylpolyaminoethylglycine Hydrochloride. JAN.

Allantoin [*1981*] (a lan′ toin; a lan′ toe in). **USP.** $C_4H_6N_4O_3$. 158.12. (1) Urea, (2,5-dioxo-4-imidazolidinyl)-; (2) Allantoin. *UNII-344S277G0Z. CAS-97-59-6.* BAN; JAN. *Vulnerary (topical).*

---

† Brand name formerly used, and/or firm no longer concerned with this product.

Alletorphine. $C_{27}H_{35}NO_4$. 437.57. 17-Allyl-17-demethyl-7α-((R)-1-hydroxy-1-methylbutyl)-6,14-*endo*-ethenotetrahydrooripavine. *UNII-4UWR086NOA. CAS-23758-80-7.* INN; BAN. ◇*R&S 218-M*

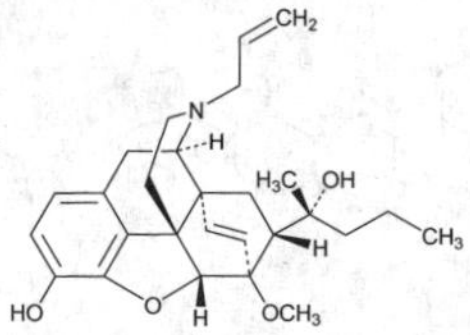

Allobarbital [*1966*] (al″ oh bar′ bi tal). $C_{10}H_{12}N_2O_3$. 208.21. (1) 2,4,6(1H,3H,5H)-Pyrimidinetrione, 5,5-di-2-propenyl-; (2) 5,5-Diallylbarbituric acid. *UNII-8NT43GG2HA. CAS-52-43-7.* INN. *Sedative-hypnotic. [Name previously used: Diallylbarbituric Acid.]* ◇*NSC-9324*

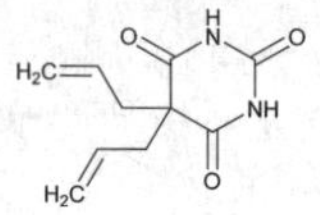

Alloclamide. $C_{16}H_{23}ClN_2O_2$. 310.82. [Alloclamide Hydrochloride is JAN.] 2-(Allyloxy)-4-chloro-N-[2-(diethylamino)ethyl]benzamide. *UNII-H7B263Z7AQ. CAS-5486-77-1.* INN; DCF; MI.

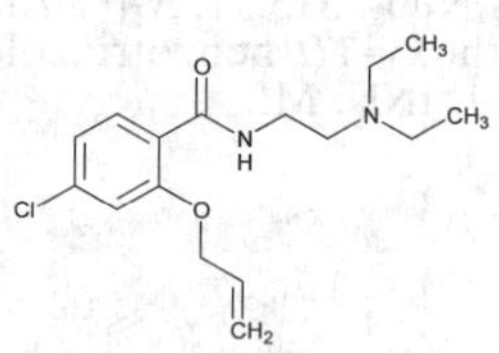

Allocupreide Sodium. $C_{11}H_{10}CuN_2NaO_2S$. 320.81. Sodium 3-(3-allyl-S-cupropseudothioureido)benzoate. *CAS-5965-40-2.* INN; DCF; MI. Ebesal (Hoechst-Roussel†)

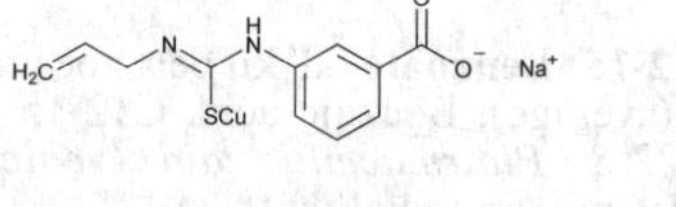

Allomethadione. $C_7H_9NO_3$. 155.15. 3-Allyl-5-methyloxazolidine-2,4-dione. *CAS-526-35-2.* INN; BAN; DCF.

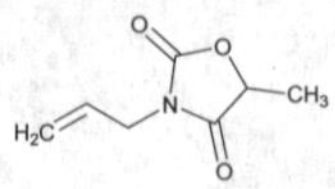

Allopurinol [*1964*] (al″ oh pure′ i nol). USP. $C_5H_4N_4O$. 136.11. (1) 4H-Pyrazolo[3,4-d]pyrimidin-4-one, 1,5-dihydro-; (2) 1,5-Dihydro-4H-pyrazolo[3,4-d]pyrimidin-4-one; (3) 1H-Pyrazolo[3,4-d]pyrimidin-4-ol. *UNII-63CZ7GJN5I. CAS-315-30-0.* INN; BAN; JAN. *Xanthine oxidase inhibitor.* Zyloprim (Promethus) ◇*BW 56-158; NSC-1390*

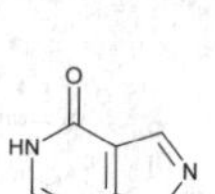

Allyl Isothiocyanate [*1988*] (al′ il eye″ soe thye″ oh sye′ a nate). USP. C_4H_5NS. 99.15. (1) 3-Isothiocyanato-1-propene; (2) Isothiocyanic acid allyl ester. *UNII-BN34FX42G3. CAS-57-06-7.*

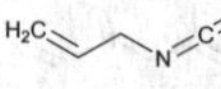

Allylbarbituric Acid (previously used name) — *See* Butalbital.

Allylestrenol. $C_{21}H_{32}O$. 300.48. 17α-Allylestr-4-en-17β-ol. *CAS-432-60-0.* INN; BAN; JAN; MI. *[Name previously used: Allyloestrenol.]*

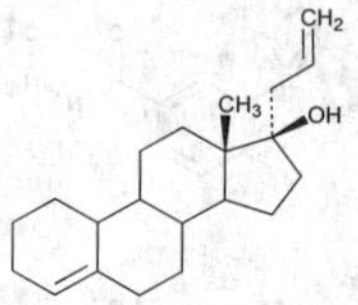

N-Allylnoretorphine — *See* Alletorphine.

Allyloestrenol (previously used name) — *See* Allylestrenol.

Allylprodine. $C_{18}H_{25}NO_2$. 287.40. 3-Allyl-1-methyl-4-phenyl-4-propionyloxypiperidine. *UNII-4343OEZ18O. CAS-25384-17-2.* INN; BAN; DCF; MI.

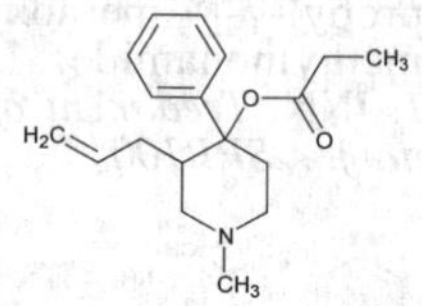

Allylthiourea. $C_4H_8N_2S$. 116.18. 1-Allyl-2-thiourea. *CAS-109-57-9.* INN.

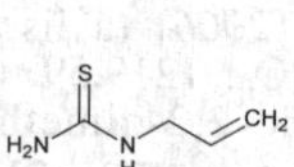

Allypropymal — *See* Aprobarbital.

Almadrate Sulfate [*1967*] (al′ ma drate sul′ fate). $Al_4H_6Mg_2O_{14}S.xH_2O$. 418.64 (anhydrous). (1) Aluminum magnesium hydroxide oxide sulfate; (2) Aluminum magnesium hydroxide oxide sulfate hydrate. *CAS-12125-11-0.* INN. *Antacid.* ◇*W 4425*

Almagate [*1987*] (al′ ma gate). $CH_7AlMg_3O_{10}.2H_2O$. 314.99. (1) Magnesium, [carbonato(2-)]heptahydroxy(aluminum)-tri-, dihydrate; (2) Aluminum magnesium carbonate hydroxide $(AlMg_3(CO_3)(OH)_7)$ dihydrate. *CAS-66827-12-1; CAS-72526-11-5* [anhydrous]. INN; BAN. *Antacid.* ◇*LAS 3876*

Almagodrate. $Al_{10}H_{26}Mg_5O_{39}S_2.nH_2O$. 1105.65 (anhydrous). Decaaluminum pentamagnesium hexacosahydroxide pentaoxide bis(sulfate) hydrate. INN.

Almasilate. $Al_2MgO_8Si_2.xH_2O$. 262.43 (anhydrous). Magnesium aluminosilicate $(MgAl_2Si_2O_8)$ hydrate. *CAS-71205-22-6.* INN; BAN.

Almecillin. $C_{13}H_{18}N_2O_4S_2$. 330.42. 3,3-Dimethyl-7-oxo-6-[[(2-propenylthio)acetyl]amino]-4-thia-1-azabicyclo[3.2.0]heptane-2-carboxylic acid. *CAS-87-09-2.* INN.

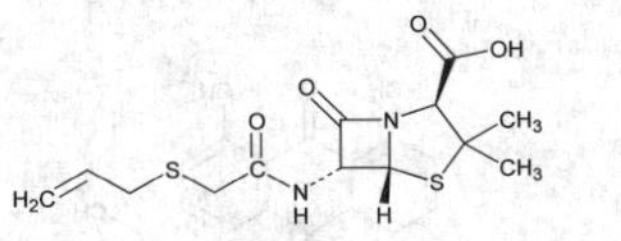

Almestrone. $C_{19}H_{24}O_2$. 284.39. 3-Hydroxy-7α-methylestra-1,3,5(10)-trien-17-one. *UNII-N18A31MTB0. CAS-10448-96-1.* INN.

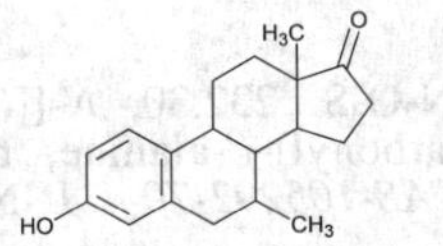

Alminoprofen. $C_{13}H_{17}NO_2$. 219.28. *p*-[(2-Methylallyl)amino]hydratropic acid. *UNII-0255AHR9GJ. CAS-39718-89-3.* INN; JAN; MI.

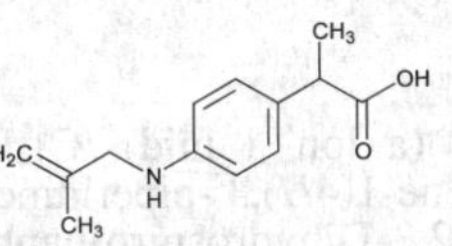

Almitrine Mesylate [*1984*] (al' mi treen mes' i late). $C_{26}H_{29}F_2N_7.2CH_4O_3S$. 669.76. [Almitrine is INN and BAN.] (1) 6-[4-[Bis(4-fluorophenyl)methyl]-1-piperazinyl]-*N*,*N'*-di-2-propenyl-1,3,5-triazine-2,4-diamine dimethanesulfonate; (2) 2,4-Bis(allylamino)-6-[4-[bis(*p*-fluorophenyl)methyl]-1-piperazinyl]-*s*-triazine dimethanesulfonate. *UNII-6RY6V6XM8T; UNII-9A1222NBG4* [almitrine]. *CAS-29608-49-9; CAS-27469-53-0* [almitrine]. *Respiratory stimulant.* Vectarion (Oril S.A., France) ◇*S-2620*

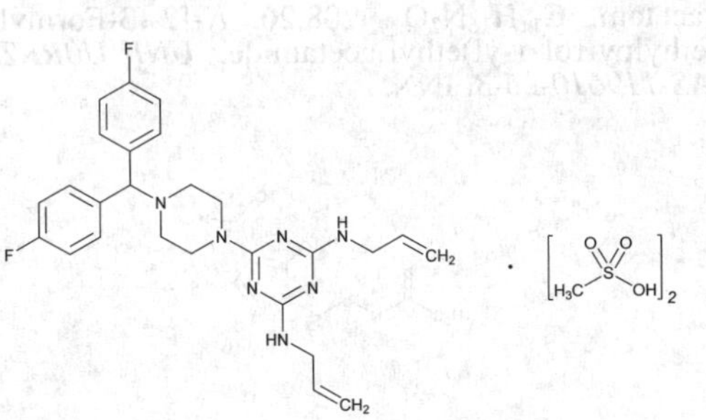

Almokalant. $C_{18}H_{28}N_2O_3S$. 352.49. ($\pm$)-*p*-[3-[Ethyl[3-(propylsulfinyl)propyl]amino]-2-hydroxypropoxy]benzonitrile. *UNII-I9NG89L275. CAS-123955-10-2.* INN.

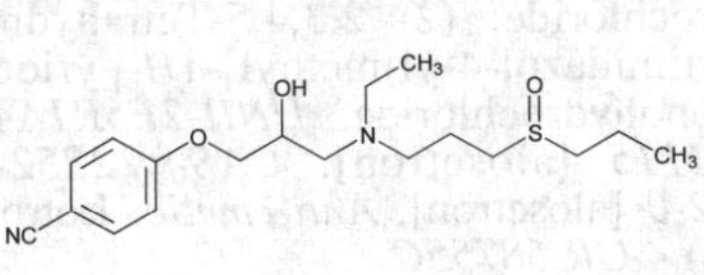

Almond Oil (ah' mund). **NF.** (1) Almond Oil; (2) Almond Oil. *CAS-8007-69-0. Pharmaceutic aid (emollient and perfume); pharmaceutic aid (vehicle, oleaginous).*

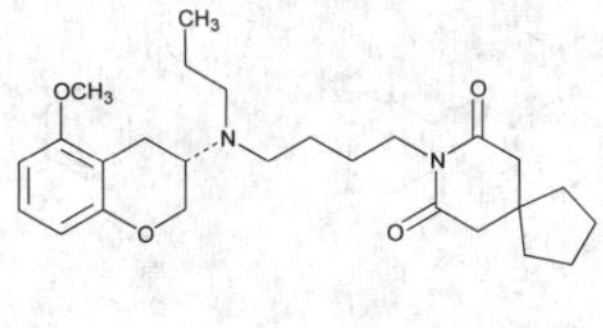

† Brand name formerly used, and/or firm no longer concerned with this product.

Almorexant. $C_{29}H_{31}F_3N_2O_3$. 512.56. (2*R*)-2-[(1*S*)-6,7-Dimethoxy-1-{2-[4-(trifluoromethyl)phenyl]ethyl}-3,4-dihydroisoquinolin-2(1*H*)-yl]-*N*-methyl-2-phenylacetamide. *CAS-871224-64-5.* INN.

Almotriptan [*1997*] (al″ moe trip′ tan). $C_{17}H_{25}N_3O_2S$. 335.46. (1) Pyrrolidine, 1-[[[3-[2-(dimethylamino)ethyl]-1*H*-indol-5-yl]methyl]sulfonyl]-; (2) 1-[[[3-[2-(Dimethylamino)ethyl]indol-5-yl]methyl]sulfonyl]pyrrolidine. *UNII-1O4XL5SN61. CAS-154323-57-6.* INN; BAN. *Antimigraine.* ◇*LAS 31416*

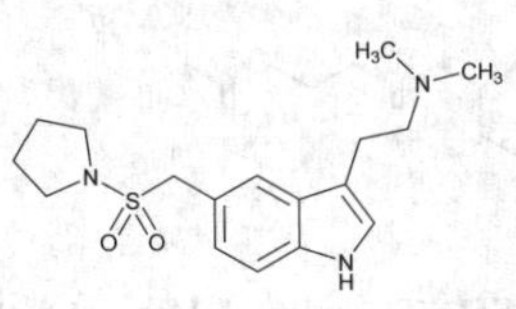

Almotriptan Malate [*1998*] (al″ moe trip′ tan mal′ ate). $C_{17}H_{25}N_3O_2S.C_4H_6O_5$. 469.55. (1) 1-[[[3-[2-(Dimethylamino)ethyl]-1*H*-indol-5-yl]methyl]sulfonyl]pyrrolidine, hydroxybutanedioate (1:1); (2) 1-[[[3-[2-(Dimethylamino)ethyl]indol-5-yl]methyl]sulfonyl]pyrrolidine malate (1:1). *UNII-PJP3I2605E. CAS-181183-52-8. Antimigraine (5HT$_{1D}$agonist).* Axert (Ortho-McNeil) ◇*PNU-180638E; LAS 31416 D,L-malate acid*

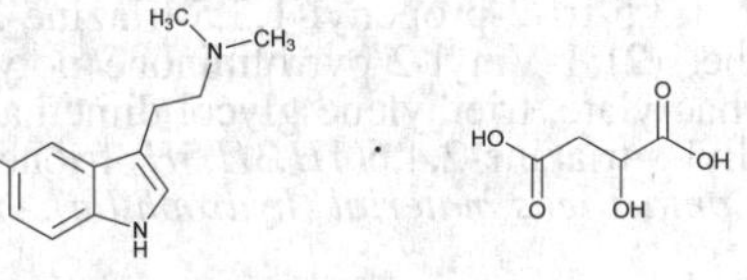

Almoxatone. $C_{18}H_{19}ClN_2O_3$. 346.81. (+)-(*R*)-3-[*p*-[(*m*-Chlorobenzyl)oxy]phenyl]-5-[(methylamino)methyl]-2-oxazolidinone. *UNII-85V47MCE4Z. CAS-84145-89-1.* INN.

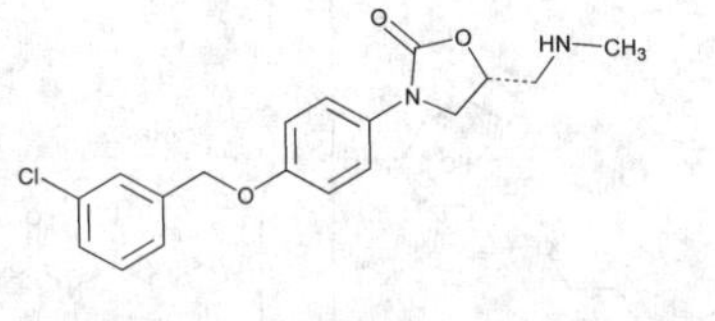

Almurtide. $C_{18}H_{30}N_4O_{11}$. 478.45. 2-Acetamido-3-*O*-[[[(1*S*)-1-[[(1*R*)-1-carbamoyl-3-carboxypropyl]carbamoyl]ethyl]carbamoyl]methyl]-2-deoxy-D-glucopyranose. *UNII-1DCO35D4OR. CAS-61136-12-7.* INN; BAN. ◇*NorMDP*

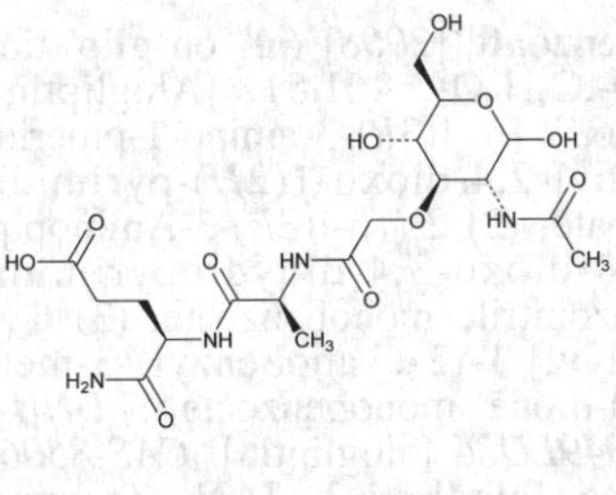

Alnespirone. $C_{26}H_{38}N_2O_4$. 442.59. (+)-(*S*)-*N*-[4-[(5-Methoxy-3-chromanyl)propylamino]butyl]-1,1-cyclopentanediacetimide. *UNII-34E28BM822. CAS-138298-79-0.* INN.

Alniditan Dihydrochloride [*1997*] (al ni′ di tan dye hye″ droe klor′ ide). $C_{17}H_{26}N_4O\cdot2HCl$. 375.34. [Alniditan is INN and BAN.] (1) 1,3-Propanediamine, *N*-[(3,4-dihydro-2*H*-1-benzopyran-2-yl)methyl]-*N′*-(1,4,5,6-tetrahydro-2-pyrimidinyl)-, dihydrochloride, (*R*)-; (2) (-)-2-[[3-[[(*R*)-2-Chromanylmethyl]amino]propyl]amino]-1,4,5,6-tetrahydropyrimidine dihydrochloride. *UNII-B57Z82EOGE* [alniditan]. *CAS-155428-00-5; CAS-152317-89-0* [alniditan]. *Antimigraine.* ◇*R-91274*

Aloe (al′ oh). **USP.** The dried latex of the leaves of *Aloe barbadensis* Miller (*Aloe vera* Linné), known in commerce as Curaçao Aloe, or of *Aloe ferox* Miller and hybrids of this species with *Aloe africana* Miller and *Aloe spicata* Baker, known in commerce as Cape Aloe (Fam. Liliaceae). *UNII-V5VD430YW9.* JAN.

Alofilcon A [*1979*] (al″ oh fil′ kon). $(C_6H_9NO)_w(C_5H_8O_2)_x$ $(C_{14}H_{22}O_6)_y(C_{12}H_{15}N_3O_3)_z$. (1) 2-Pyrrolidinone, 1-ethenyl-, polymer with methyl 2-methyl-2-propenoate, 1,2-ethanediylbis(oxy-2,1-ethanediyl) bis(2-methyl 2-propenoate) and 1,3,5-tri-2-propenyl-1,3,5-triazine-2,4,6(1*H*,3*H*,5*H*)-trione; (2) 1-Vinyl-2-pyrrolidinone polymer with methyl methacrylate, triethylene glycol dimethacrylate and 1,3,5-triallyl-*s*-triazine-2,4,6(1*H*,3*H*,5*H*)-trione. *CAS-67101-27-3. Contact lens material (hydrophilic).* ◇*WX 14812; SCL-70*

Alogliptin Benzoate [*2008*] (al″ oh glip′ tin ben′ zoe ate). $C_{18}H_{21}N_5O_2\cdot C_7H_6O_2$. 461.51. [Alogliptin is INN.] (1) Benzonitrile, 2-[[6-[(3*R*)-3-amino-1-piperidinyl]-3,4-dihydro-3-methyl-2,4-dioxo-1(2*H*)-pyrimidinyl]methyl]-, monobenzoate; (2) 2-({6-[(3*R*)-3-Aminopiperidin-1-yl]-3-methyl-2,4-dioxo-3,4-dihydropyrimidin-1(2*H*)-yl}-methyl)benzonitrile monobenzoate; (3) 6-[(3*R*)-3-Aminopiperidin-1-yl]-1-(2-cyanobenzyl)-3-methylpyrimidin-2,4(1*H*,3*H*)-dione monobenzoate . *UNII-EEN99869SC; UNII-JHC049LO86* [alogliptin]. *CAS-850649-62-6; CAS-850649-61-5* [alogliptin]. JAN. *Treatment of type 2 diabetes.* ◇*SYR-322*

Aloin. $C_{20}H_{14}O_4$. 318.32. 10-*β*-D-Glucopyranosyl-1,8-dihydroxy-3-hydroxymethyl-9(10*H*)-anthrone. *UNII-W41H6S09F4. CAS-5133-19-7.* BAN.

Alonacic. $C_9H_{16}N_2O_3S$. 232.30. *N*-[[(2*RS*,4*R*)-2-Methyl-4-thiazolidinyl]carbonyl]-*β*-alanine, methyl ester. *UNII-J7RT0951E3. CAS-105292-70-4.* INN.

Alonimid [*1971*] (a lon′ i mid). $C_{14}H_{13}NO_3$. 243.26. (1) Spiro[naphthalene-1(4*H*),3′-piperidine]-2′,4,6′-trione, 2,3-dihydro-; (2) 2,3-Dihydrospiro[naphthalene-1(4*H*),3′-piperidine]-2′,4,6′-trione. *CAS-2897-83-8.* INN. *Sedative-hypnotic.*

Aloracetam. $C_{11}H_{16}N_2O_2$. 208.26. *N*-[2-(3-Formyl-2,5-dimethylpyrrol-1-yl)ethyl]acetamide. *UNII-U0RKZ75D0T. CAS-119610-26-3.* INN.

Alosetron Hydrochloride [*1992*] (a loe′ se tron hye″ droe klor′ ide). $C_{17}H_{18}N_4O\cdot HCl$. 330.81. [Alosetron is INN and BAN.] (1) 1*H*-Pyrido[4,3-*b*]indol-1-one, 2,3,4,5-tetrahydro-5-methyl-2-[(5-methyl-1*H*-imidazol-4-yl)methyl]-, monohydrochloride; (2) 2,3,4,5-Tetrahydro-5-methyl-2-[(5-methylimidazol-4-yl)methyl]-1*H*-pyrido[4,3-*b*]indol-1-one monohydrochloride. *UNII-2F5R1A46YW; UNII-13Z9HTH115* [alosetron]. *CAS-122852-69-1; CAS-122852-42-0* [alosetron]. *Anti-emetic.* Lotronex (GlaxoSmithKline) ◇*GR 68755C*

Alovudine [*1992*] (a loe′ vue deen). $C_{10}H_{13}FN_2O_4$. 244.22. (1) Thymidine, 3′-deoxy-3′-fluoro-; (2) 3′-Deoxy-3′-fluorothymidine. *UNII-PG53R0DWDQ. CAS-25526-93-6.* INN. *Antiviral.* ◇*CL 184,824*

Aloxidone (former BAN) — *See* Allomethadione.

Aloxiprin. Polymeric condensation product of aluminum oxide and *o*-acetylsalicylic acid. *CAS-9014-67-9.* INN; BAN; DCF; MI.

Aloxistatin. $C_{17}H_{30}N_2O_5$. 342.43. Ethyl (+)-(2*S*,3*S*)-2,3-epoxy-*N*-[(*S*)-1-(isopentylcarbamoyl)-3-methylbutyl]succinamate. *UNII-L5W337AOUR. CAS-88321-09-9.* INN.

Alozafone. $C_{21}H_{21}ClFN_3O_2$. 401.86. 4′-Chloro-2-[(2-cyano-1-methylethyl)methylamino]-2′-(*o*-fluorobenzoyl)-*N*-methylacetanilide. *UNII-PF3UC3747Y. CAS-65899-72-1.* INN.

Alpertine [*1976*] (al per′ teen). $C_{25}H_{31}N_3O_4$. 437.53. (1) 1*H*-Indole-2-carboxylic acid, 5,6-dimethoxy-3-[2-(4-phenyl-1-piperazinyl)ethyl]-, ethyl ester; (2) Ethyl 5,6-dimethoxy-3-[2-(4-phenyl-1-piperazinyl)ethyl]indole-2-carboxylate. *UNII-KYT38QTB4K. CAS-27076-46-6.* INN. *Antipsychotic.* ◇*Win 31,665*

Alpha Amylase [*1962*] (al′ fa am′ i lase). A concentrate of amylolytic enzyme of bacterial or animal origin. (1) α-Amylase; (2) Amylase, α-. *CAS-9000-90-2. Anti-inflammatory.* Fortizyme (Sterling Winthrop†)

Alphacemethadone — *See* Alphacetylmethadol.

Alphacetylmethadol. $C_{23}H_{31}NO_2$. 353.50. (3*R*,6*R*)-3-Acetoxy-6-dimethylamino-4,4-diphenylheptane. *UNII-BXF83S0HEL. CAS-17199-58-5.* INN; BAN; DCF.

Alpha-Cypermethrin. $C_{22}H_{19}Cl_2NO_3$. 416.30. (*SR*)-α-Cyano-3-phenoxybenzyl (1*RS*,3*RS*)-3-(2,2-dichlorovinyl)-2,2-dimethylcyclopropanecarboxylate. *UNII-99W8X078CA. CAS-67375-30-8.* BAN.

Alphadolone (previously used name) — *See* Alfadolone.

Alphafilcon A [*1997*] (al fa fil′ kon). $(C_6H_{10}O_3)_v(C_6H_9NO)_w(C_{14}H_{24}O_3)_x(C_{10}H_{14}O_4)_y(C_9H_{12}O_5)_z$. (1) 2-Propenoic acid, 2-methyl-, 2-hydroxyethyl ester, polymer with 1-ethenyl-2-pyrrolidinone, 4-(1,1-dimethylethyl)-2-hydroxycyclohexyl 2-methyl-2-propenoate, 1,2-ethanediyl bis(2-methyl-2-propenoate) and 2-[[(ethenyloxy)carbonyl]oxy]ethyl 2-methyl-2-propenoate; (2) 2-Hydroxyethyl methacrylate polymer with 1-vinyl-2-pyrrolidinone, 4-*tert*-butyl-2-hydroxycyclohexyl methacrylate, ethylene dimethacrylate and 2-(methacryloyloxy)ethyl vinyl carbonate. *CAS-145497-36-5. Contact lens material (hydrophilic).* SofLens66 (Bausch & Lomb) *[Note—The water content of the contact lens material is 66±2% at ambient temperature (23±2°C), and the oxygen permeability is 32 × 10⁻¹¹(cm²/sec)(ml O₂/ml × mmHg) at 35°C (Dk value).]*

Alphameprodine. $C_{17}H_{25}NO_2$. 275.39. *cis*-3-Ethyl-1-methyl-4-phenyl-4-propionyloxypiperidine. *UNII-11771648L1. CAS-468-51-9.* INN; BAN; DCF.

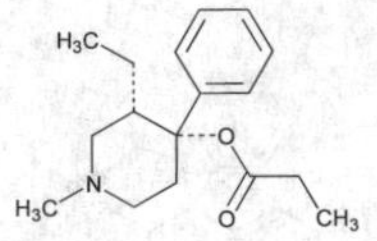

Alphamethadol. $C_{21}H_{29}NO$. 311.46. (3R,6R)-6-Dimethylamino-4,4-diphenyl-3-heptanol. *UNII-XBD99QNI42. CAS-17199-54-1.* INN; BAN; DCF.

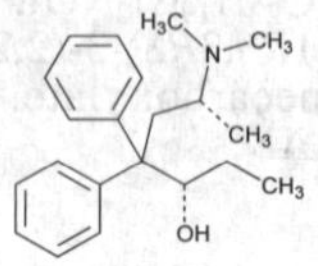

Alpha-Methyldopa (previously used name) — *See* Methyldopa.

Alphaprodine Hydrochloride. $C_{16}H_{23}NO_2 \cdot HCl$. 297.82. [Alphaprodine is INN and BAN.] (1) 4-Piperidinol, 1,3-dimethyl-4-phenyl-, propanoate (ester), hydrochloride, *cis*-(±)-; (2) (±)-1,3-Dimethyl-4-phenyl-4-piperidinol propionate (ester) hydrochloride. *UNII-CO51Q2EI5Z. CAS-561-78-4; CAS-14405-05-1* [stereononspecific]; *CAS-77-20-3* [alphaprodine]. USP XXI; MI. Nisentil (Hoffmann-LaRoche†)

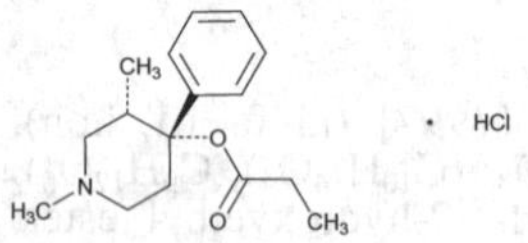

Alphaxalone (previously used name) — *See* Alfaxalone.

Alpidem [*1987*] (al' pi dem). $C_{21}H_{23}Cl_2N_3O$. 404.33. (1) Imidazo[1,2-*a*]pyridine-3-acetamide, 6-chloro-2-(4-chlorophenyl)-*N,N*-dipropyl-; (2) 6-Chloro-2-(*p*-chlorophenyl)-*N,N*-dipropylimidazo[1,2-*a*]pyridine-3-acetamide. *CAS-82626-01-5.* INN; BAN. *Anti-anxiety agent.* ◇*SL 80.0342-00*

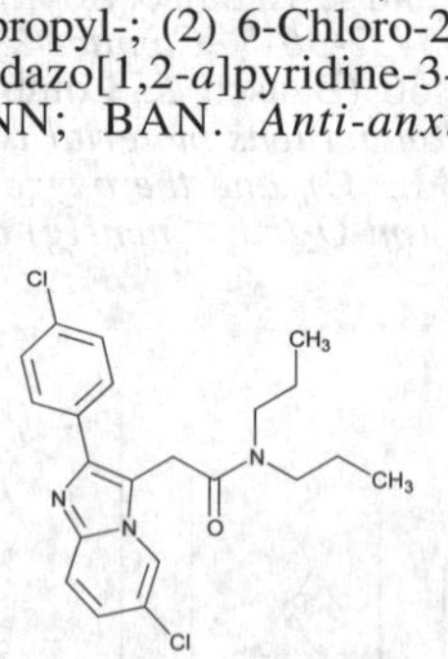

Alpiropride. $C_{17}H_{26}N_4O_4S$. 382.48. (±)-*N*-[(1-Allyl-2-pyrrolidinyl)methyl]-4-amino-5-(methylsulfamoyl)-*o*-anisamide. *UNII-1768UW0XS1. CAS-81982-32-3.* INN; MI.

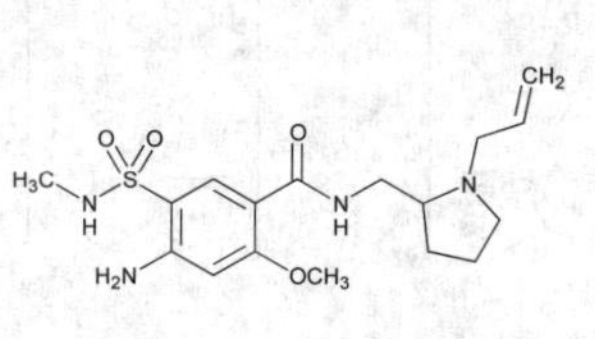

Alprafenone. $C_{25}H_{35}NO_4$. 413.55. (±)-3-[3-[2-Hydroxy-3-(*tert*-pentylamino)propoxy]-4-methoxyphenyl]-4'-methyl-propiophenone. *UNII-D5H25D039V. CAS-124316-02-5.* INN.

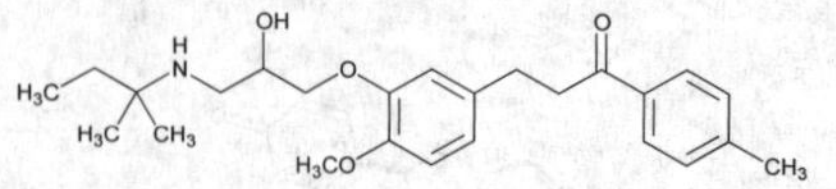

Alprazolam [*1973*] (al pra' zoe lam). **USP.** $C_{17}H_{13}ClN_4$. 308.76. (1) 4*H*-[1,2,4]Triazolo[4,3-*α*][1,4]benzodiazepine, 8-chloro-1-methyl-6-phenyl-; (2) 8-Chloro-1-methyl-6-phenyl-4*H*-*s*-triazolo[4,3-*α*][1,4]benzodiazepine. *UNII-YU55MQ3IZY. CAS-28981-97-7.* INN; BAN; JAN. *Sedative-hypnotic.* Niravam (Schwarz Pharma); Xanax (Pfizer) ◇*U-31,889*

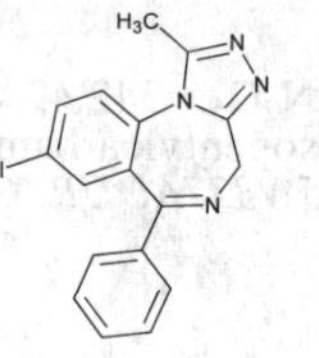

Alprenolol Hydrochloride [*1968*] (al pren' oh lol hye″ droe klor' ide). $C_{15}H_{23}NO_2 \cdot HCl$. 285.81. [Alprenolol is INN and BAN.] (1) 2-Propanol, 1-[(1-methylethyl)amino]-3-[2-(2-propenyl)phenoxy]-, hydrochloride; (2) 1-(*o*-Allylphenoxy)-3-(isopropylamino)-2-propanol hydrochloride. *CAS-13707-88-5; CAS-13655-52-2* [alprenolol]. JAN. *Antiadrenergic* (*β-receptor*). ◇*H 56/28*

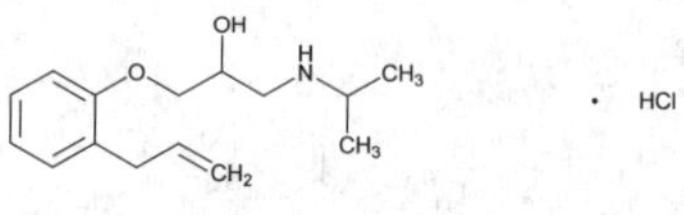

Alprenoxime Hydrochloride [*1990*] (al pren' ox eem hye″ droe klor' ide). $C_{15}H_{22}N_2O_2 \cdot HCl$. 298.81. (1) 2-Propanone, 1-[(1-methylethyl)amino]-3-[2-(2-propenyl)phenoxy]-, oxime, monohydrochloride; (2) 1-(*o*-Allylphenoxy)-3-(isopropylamino)-2-propanone oxime, monohydrochloride. *CAS-121009-30-1. Antiglaucoma agent.* ◇*HGP-5; CDDD 1815*

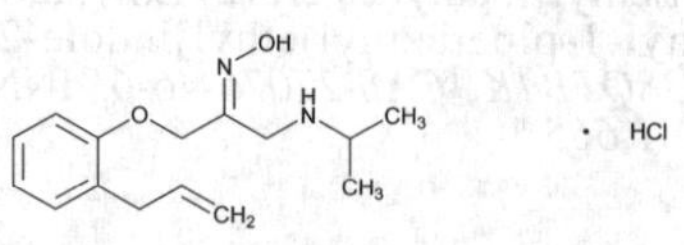

Alprostadil [*1977*] (al pros' ta dil). **USP.** $C_{20}H_{34}O_5$. 354.48. (1) Prost-13-en-1-oic acid, 11,15-dihydroxy-9-oxo-, (11*α*,13*E*,15*S*)-; (2) (1*R*,2*R*,3*R*)-3-Hydroxy-2-[(*E*)-(3*S*)-3-hydroxy-1-octenyl]-5-oxocyclopentaneheptanoic acid. *UNII-F5TD010360. CAS-745-65-3.* INN; BAN; JAN. *Vasodilator.* Caverject (Pfizer); Edex (Schwarz Pharma); Muse (Vivus); Prostin (Pfizer) [*Names previously used: Prostaglandin E₁; PGE₁.*] ◇*U-10,136*

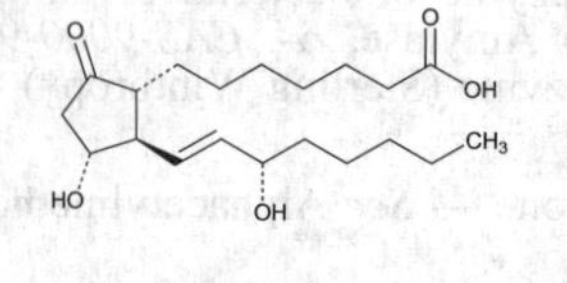

Alprostadil Alfadex. $C_{20}H_{34}O_5 \cdot x(C_{36}H_{60}O_{30})$. *α*-Cyclodextrin—7-{(1*R*,2*R*,3*R*)-3-hydroxy-2-[(*E*)-(3*S*)-3-hydroxyoct-1-enyl]-5-oxo-cyclopentyl}heptanoic acid. BAN; JAN.

Alrestatin Sodium [*1976*] (al″ re stat′ in soe′ dee um). $C_{14}H_8NNaO_4$. 277.21. [Alrestatin is INN.] (1) 1*H*-Benz[*de*]isoquinoline-2(3*H*)acetic acid, 1,3-dioxo-, sodium salt; (2) Sodium 1,3-dioxo-1*H*-benz[*de*]isoquinoline-2(3*H*)-acetate. *UNII-018XNU6812; UNII-515DHK15LG* [alrestatin]. *CAS-51876-97-2; CAS-51411-04-2* [alrestatin]. *Enzyme inhibitor (aldose reductase).* ◇*AY-22,284A*

Alsactide. $C_{99}H_{155}N_{29}O_{21}S$. 2119.54. 1-β-Alanine-17-[L-2,6-diamino-*N*-(4-aminobutyl)hexanamide]-α$^{1-17}$-corticotropin. *CAS-34765-96-3.* INN; MI.

Alseroxylon. *CAS-8001-95-4.* JAN. Rautensin (Novartis); Rauwiloid (3M Pharmaceuticals)

Altanserin Tartrate [*1984*] (al tan′ ser in tar′ trate). $C_{26}H_{28}FN_3O_8S$. 561.58. [Altanserin is INN.] (1) 4(1*H*)-Quinazolinone, 3-[2-[4-(4-fluorobenzoyl)-1-piperidinyl]ethyl]-2,3-dihydro-2-thioxo-, [*R*-(*R**,*R**)]-2,3-dihydroxybutanedioate; (2) 3-[2-[4-(*p*-Fluorobenzoyl)piperidino]ethyl]-2-thio-2,4(1*H*,3*H*)-quinazolinedione L-(+)-tartrate (1:1). *UNII-9P204CHE8J; UNII-5015H744JQ* [altanserin]. *CAS-79449-96-0; CAS-76330-71-7* [altanserin]. *Serotonin antagonist.* ◇*R-53,200*

Altapizone. $C_{24}H_{28}N_4O_2$. 404.50. 4-Phenyl-4′-(1,4,5,6-tetrahydro-6-oxo-3-pyridazinyl)-1-piperidinepropionanilide. *UNII-SW3OJS6TOD. CAS-93277-96-4.* INN.

Alteconazole. $C_{17}H_{12}Cl_3N_3O$. 380.66. *cis*-1-[2-(*p*-Chlorophenyl)-3-(2,4-dichlorophenyl)-2,3-epoxypropyl]-1*H*-1,2,4-triazole. *UNII-EA590X615B. CAS-93479-96-0.* INN.

Alteplase [*1989*] (al′ te plase). **USP.** $C_{2569}H_{3894}N_{746}O_{781}S_{40}$. 59,007.61. A serine protease with a primary sequence composed of 527 amino acids. The sequence is identical to the naturally occurring protease produced by endothelial cells of vessel walls. Plasminogen activator (human tissue-type protein moiety). *CAS-105857-23-6.* INN; BAN; JAN. *Plasminogen activator.* Activase (Genentech) ◇*rt-PA*

```
SYQVICRDEK   TQMIYQQHQS   WLRPVLRSNR   VEYCWCNSGR
AQCHSVPVKS   CSEPRCFNGG   TCQQALYFSD   FVCQCPEGFA
GKCCEIDTRA   TCYEDQGISY   RGTWSTAESG   AECTNWNSSA
LAQKPYSGRR   PDAIRLGLGN   HNYCRNPDRD   SKPWCYVFKA
GKYSSEFCST   PACSEGNSDC   YFGNGSAYRG   THSLTESGAS
CLPWNSMILI   GKVYTAQNPS   AQALGLGKHN   YCRNPDGDAK
PWCHVLKNRR   LTWEYCDVPS   CSTCGLRQYS   QPQFR

IKGGLFADIA   SHPWQAAIFA   KHRRSPGERF   LCGGILISSC
WILSAAHCFQ   ERFPPHHLTV   ILGRTYRVVP   GEEEQKFEVE
KYIVHKEFDD   DTYDNDIALL   QLKSDSSRCA   QESSVVRTVC
LPPADLQLPD   WTECELSGYG   KHEALSPFYS   ERLKEAHVRL
YPSSRCTSQH   LLNRTVTDNM   LCAGDTRSGG   PQANLHDACQ
GDSGGPLVCL   NDGRMTLVGI   ISWGLGCGQK   DVPGVYTKVT
NYLDWIRDNM   RP
```

Althiazide [*1962*] (al thye′ a zide). $C_{11}H_{14}ClN_3O_4S_3$. 383.89. [Altizide is INN.] (1) 2*H*-1,2,4-Benzothiadiazine-7-sulfonamide, 6-chloro-3,4-dihydro-3-[(2-propenylthio)methyl]-, 1,1-dioxide; (2) 3-[(Allylthio)methyl]-6-chloro-3,4-dihydro-2*H*-1,2,4-benzothiadiazine-7-sulfonamide 1,1-dioxide. *CAS-5588-16-9. Antihypertensive.* ◇*P-1779*

Altinicline Maleate [*1999*] (al tin′ i kleen mal′ ee ate). $C_{12}H_{14}N_2.C_4H_4O_4$. 302.33. [Altinicline is INN.] (1) (*S*)-3-Ethynyl-5-(1-methyl-2-pyrrolidinyl)pyridine (*Z*)-2-butenedioate (1:1); (2) (-)-5-Ethynylnicotine maleate (1:1); (3) (-)-3-Ethynyl-5-[(*S*)-1-methyl-2-pyrrolidinyl]pyridine maleate (1:1). *UNII-RJ9V9V09VM* [altinicline]. *CAS-192231-16-6; CAS-179120-92-4* [altinicline]. *Antiparkinsonian (nicotinic acetylcholine receptor subtype selective agonist).* ◇*SIB-1508Y*

Altizide (INN, DCF) — *See* Althiazide.

---

† Brand name formerly used, and/or firm no longer concerned with this product.

Altoqualine. $C_{27}H_{36}N_2O_8$. 516.58. (3*S*)-7-Amino-4,5,6-triethoxy-3-[(1*R*)-1,2,3,4-tetrahydro-6,7,8-trimethoxy-2-methyl-1-isoquinolyl]phthalide. *UNII-56G228IW9Q. CAS-121029-11-6.* INN.

Altrenogest [*1981*] (al tren′ oh jest). $C_{21}H_{26}O_2$. 310.43. (1) Estra-4,9,11-trien-3-one, 17β-hydroxy-17-(2-propenyl)-; (2) 17α-Allyl-17-hydroxyestra-4,9,11-trien-3-one. *CAS-850-52-2.* INN; BAN. *Progestin (veterinary).* REGU-MATE (Roussel-UCLAF, France) ◇*RU-2267; A-35957*

Altretamine [*1990*] (al tret′ a meen). **USP.** $C_9H_{18}N_6$. 210.28. (1) 1,3,5-Triazine-2,4,6-triamine, *N,N,N′,N′,N″,N″*-hexamethyl-; (2) Hexamethylmelamine. *UNII-Q8BIH59O7H. CAS-645-05-6.* INN; BAN. *Antineoplastic.* Hexalen (MGI Pharma) ◇*NSC-13875*

Altumomab (INN) — *See* Indium In 111 Altumomab Pentetate.

Altumomab Pentetate — *See* Indium In 111 Altumomab Pentetate.

Alum, Ammonium (al′ um a moe′ nee um). **USP.** $AlNH_4(SO_4)_2.12H_2O$. 453.33. (1) Sulfuric acid, aluminum ammonium salt (2:1:1), dodecahydrate; (2) Aluminum ammonium sulfate (1:1:2) dodecahydrate. *CAS-7784-26-1; CAS-7784-25-0* [anhydrous]. *Astringent (topical).*

Alum, Potassium (al′ um poe tas′ ee um). **USP.** $AlK(SO_4)_2.12H_2O$. 474.39. [Aluminum Potassium Sulfate is JAN.] (1) Sulfuric acid, aluminum potassium salt (2:1:1), dodecahydrate; (2) Aluminum potassium sulfate (1:1:2) dodecahydrate. *CAS-7784-24-9; CAS-10043-67-1* [anhydrous]. *Astringent (topical).*

Aluminoparaaminosalicylate Calcium. $C_{14}H_{13}AlCaN_2O_8.5H_2O$. 494.40. Alumino *p*-aminosalicylate calcium. *CAS-14641-21-5* [anhydrous]. JAN.

Aluminum Acetate (a loo′ mi num as′ e tate). **USP** [Topical Solution]. $C_6H_9AlO_6$. 204.11. (1) Acetic acid, aluminum salt; (2) Aluminum acetate. *UNII-80EHD8I43D. CAS-139-12-8. Astringent.* Buro-Sol Concentrate (Doak); Domeboro (Bayer)

Aluminum Aminoacetate — *See* Dihydroxyaluminum Aminoacetate.

Aluminum Carbonate, Basic [*1988*] (a loo′ mi num kar′ bo nate). Basic Aluminum Carbonate. Ingredient of an aluminum hydroxide–aluminum carbonate gel. USP XXII. *Antacid.* Basaljel (Wyeth-Ayerst)

Aluminum Chlorhydroxide (previously used name) — *See* Aluminum Chlorohydrate.

Aluminum Chlorhydroxide Alcohol Soluble Complex (previously used name) — *See* Aluminum Chlorohydrex.

Aluminum Chloride (a loo′ mi num klor′ ide). **USP.** $AlCl_3.6H_2O$. 241.43. (1) Aluminum chloride, hexahydrate; (2) Aluminum chloride hexahydrate. *CAS-7784-13-6; CAS-7446-70-0* [anhydrous]. *Astringent (topical).*

Aluminum Chlorohydrate [*1979*] (a loo′ mi num klor″ oh hye′ drate). **USP.** $Al_y(OH)_{3y-z}Cl_z.H_2O$. (1) Aluminum chlorohydroxide; (2) Aluminum hydroxychloride. *CAS-12042-91-0* [dihydrate]; *CAS-1327-41-9* [anhydrous]. *Anhidrotic. [Names previously used: Aluminum Chlorhydroxide; Aluminum Hydroxychloride.]*

Aluminum Chlorohydrex [*1978*] (a loo′ mi num klor″ oh hye′ drex). Derivative of aluminum chlorohydrate. It is reported to be a coordination complex of basic aluminum chloride and propylene glycol or polyethylene glycol in which the water molecules normally coordinated to the aluminum in aluminum chlorohydrate have been displaced by the glycol, resulting in a relatively less-polar complex of low water content. (1) Aluminum chlorohydrex. *CAS-53026-85-0. Astringent (topical). [Names previously used: Aluminum Chlorhydroxide Alcohol Soluble Complex; Aluminum Chlorohydrol Propylene Glycol Complex.]*

Aluminum Chlorohydrex Polyethylene Glycol (a loo′ mi num klor″ oh hye′ drex pol″ ee eth′ i leen glye′ kol). **USP.** $Al_y(OH)_{3y-z}Cl_z.nH_2O.mH(OCH_2CH_2)_nOH$. (1) Aluminum chlorohydroxide polyethylene glycol complex; (2) Aluminum hydroxychloride polyethylene glycol complex. *Anhidrotic.*

Aluminum Chlorohydrex Propylene Glycol (a loo′ mi num klor″ oh hye′ drex proe′ pi leen glye′ kol). **USP.** $Al_y(OH)_{3y-z}Cl_z.nH_2O.mC_3H_8O_2$. (1) Aluminum chlorohydroxide, hydrate: propylene glycol complex (1:1); (2) Aluminum hydroxychloride, hydrate: propylene glycol complex (1:1). *CAS-53026-85-0. Anhidrotic.*

Aluminum Chlorohydrol Propylene Glycol Complex (previously used name) — *See* Aluminum Chlorohydrex.

Aluminum Chlorohydroxy Allantoinate (JAN) — *See* Alcloxa.

Aluminum Clofibrate. $C_{20}H_{21}AlCl_2O_7$. 471.26. Bis[2-(*p*-chlorophenoxy)-2-methylpropionato]hydroxyaluminum. *UNII-56203T2K2X. CAS-14613-01-5; CAS-882-09-7* [clofibric acid]. INN; BAN; JAN.

Aluminum Dichlorohydrate (a loo′ mi num dye klor″ oh hye′ drate). **USP.** $Al_y(OH)_{3y-z}Cl_z.nH_2O$. (1) Aluminum chlorohydroxide; (2) Aluminum hydroxychloride. *Anhidrotic.*

Aluminum Dichlorohydrex Polyethylene Glycol (a loo′ mi num dye klor″ oh hye′ drex pol″ ee eth′ i leen glye′ kol). **USP.** $Al_y(OH)_{3y-z}Cl_z.nH_2O.mH(OCH_2CH_2)_nOH$. (1) Aluminum chlorohydroxide polyethylene glycol complex; (2) Aluminum hydroxychloride polyethylene glycol complex. *Anhidrotic.*

Aluminum Dichlorohydrex Propylene Glycol (a loo' mi num dye klor" oh hye' drex proe' pi leen glye' kol). **USP**. $Al_y(OH)_{3-z}Cl_z.nH_2O.mC_3H_8O_2$. (1) Aluminum chlorohydroxide propylene glycol complex; (2) Aluminum hydroxychloride propylene glycol complex. *Anhidrotic.*

Aluminum Flufenamate. $(C_{14}H_9F_3NO_2)_3Al$. 867.65. Aluminum *N*-(3'-trifluoromethylpheny)anthranilate. *UNII-9NZ7H8YAHG. CAS-16449-54-0.* JAN.

Aluminum Glycinate, Basic — *See* Dihydroxyaluminum Aminoacetate.

Aluminum Hydroxide (a loo' mi num hye drox' ide). **USP** [Gel]. $Al(OH)_3$. 78.00. (1) Aluminum hydroxide; (2) Aluminum hydroxide. *UNII-5QB0T2IUN0. CAS-21645-51-2. Antacid.* Amphojel (Wyeth-Ayerst); Dialume (Rhone-Poulenc Rorer†)

Aluminum Hydroxide, Dried (a loo' mi num hye drox' ide). **USP**. $Al(OH)_3$. 78.00. Aluminum hydroxide. *CAS-21645-51-2.* JAN. *Antacid.* ALternaGEL (Johnson & Johnson-Merck Consumer); Alu-Cap (3M Pharmaceuticals)

Aluminum Hydroxychloride (previously used name) — *See* Aluminum Chlorohydrate.

Aluminum Lactate. $C_9H_{15}AlO_9$. 294.19. *UNII-V797H4GG0Z. CAS-18917-91-4.* JAN.

Aluminum Monostearate (a loo' mi num mon" oh steer' ate). **NF**. (1) Aluminum, dihydroxy(octadecanoato-*O*-)-; (2) Dihydroxy(stearato)aluminum. *UNII-P9BC99461E. CAS-7047-84-9.* JAN. Component of Penicillin G Procaine with Aluminum Stearate Suspension.

Aluminum Phosphate (a loo' mi num fos' fate). **USP** [Gel]. (1) Phosphoric acid, aluminum salt (1:1); (2) Aluminum phosphate (1:1). *CAS-7784-30-7. Antacid.* Phosphaljel (Wyeth-Ayerst)

Aluminum Potassium Sulfate (JAN) — *See* Alum, Potassium.

Aluminum Sesquichlorohydrate [*1980*] (a loo' mi num ses" kwi klor" oh hye' drate). **USP**. $Al_y(OH)_{3-z}Cl_z.nH_2O$. A polymeric, loosely hydrated complex encompassing a range of aluminum to chloride atomic ratios between 1.26:1 and 1.90:1. (1) Aluminum chlorohydroxide; (2) Aluminum hydroxychloride. *CAS-11097-68-0. Anhidrotic.*

Aluminum Sesquichlorohydrex Polyethylene Glycol (a loo' mi num ses" kwi klor" oh hye' drex pol" ee eth' i leen glye' kol). **USP**. $Al_y(OH)_{3-z}Cl_z.nH_2O.mH(OCH_2CH_2)_nOH$. (1) Aluminum chlorohydroxide polyethylene glycol complex; (2) Aluminum hydroxychloride polyethylene glycol complex. *Anhidrotic.*

Aluminum Sesquichlorohydrex Propylene Glycol (a loo' mi num ses" kwi klor" oh hye' drex proe' pi leen glye' kol). **USP**. $Al_y(OH)_{3-z}Cl_z.nH_2O.mC_3H_8O_2$. (1) Aluminum chlorohydroxide propylene glycol complex; (2) Aluminum hydroxychloride propylene glycol complex. *Anhidrotic.*

Aluminum Silicate, Natural. *CAS-12141-46-7.* JAN.

Aluminum Silicate, Synthetic. *CAS-12141-46-7.* JAN.

Aluminum Subacetate (a loo' mi num sub as' e tate). **USP** [Topical Solution]. $C_4H_7AlO_5$. 162.08. (1) Aluminum, bis(acetato-*O*)hydroxy-; (2) Bis(acetato)hydroxyaluminum; (3) Basic aluminum acetate. *CAS-142-03-0; CAS-8000-61-1. Astringent.*

Aluminum Sulfate (a loo' mi num sul' fate). **USP**. $Al_2(SO_4)_3.xH_2O$. 342.15 (anhydrous). (1) Sulfuric acid, aluminum salt (3:2), hydrate; (2) Aluminum sulfate (2:3) hydrate. *CAS-17927-65-0; CAS-10043-01-3* [anhydrous]. Component of Aluminum Subacetate Solution.

Aluminum Zirconium Octachlorohydrate (a loo' mi num zir koe' nee um ok" ta klor" oh hye' drate). **USP**. $Al_yZr(OH)_{3y+4-x}Cl_x.nH_2O$. A polymeric, loosely hydrated complex of basic aluminum zirconium chloride that encompasses a range of aluminum-to-zirconium atomic ratios between 6.0:1 and 10.0:1, and a range of (aluminum plus zirconium)-to-chloride atomic ratios between 1.5:1 and 0.9:1. *Anhidrotic.*

Aluminum Zirconium Octachlorohydrex Gly (a loo' mi num zir koe' nee um ok" ta klor" oh hye' drex glye). **USP**. A derivative of Aluminum Zirconium Octachlorohydrate in which some of the water molecules have been displaced by glycine. *Anhidrotic.*

Aluminum Zirconium Pentachlorohydrate (a loo' mi num zir koe' nee um pen" ta klor" oh hye' drate). **USP**. $Al_yZr(OH)_{3y+4-x}Cl_x.nH_2O$. A polymeric, loosely hydrated complex of basic aluminum zirconium chloride that encompasses a range of aluminum-to-zirconium atomic ratios between 6.0:1 and 10.0:1, and a range of (aluminum plus zirconium)-to-chloride atomic ratios between 2.1:1 and 1.51:1. *Anhidrotic.*

Aluminum Zirconium Pentachlorohydrex Gly (a loo' mi num zir koe' nee um pen" ta klor" oh hye' drex glye). **USP**. A derivative of Aluminum Zirconium Pentachlorohydrate in which some of the water molecules have been displaced by glycine. *Anhidrotic.*

Aluminum Zirconium Tetrachlorohydrate (a loo' mi num zir koe' nee um tet" ra klor" oh hye' drate). **USP**. $Al_yZr(OH)_{3y+4-x}Cl_x.nH_2O$. A polymeric, loosely hydrated complex of basic aluminum zirconium chloride that encompasses a range of aluminum-to-zirconium atomic ratios between 2.0:1 and 5.99:1 and a range of (aluminum plus zirconium)-to-chloride atomic ratios between 1.5:1 and 0.9:1. *Anhidrotic.*

Aluminum Zirconium Tetrachlorohydrex Gly [*1980*] (a loo' mi num zir koe' nee um tet" ra klor" oh hye' drex glye). **USP**. A coordination complex of aluminum zirconium tetrachlorohydrate $[Al_yZr(OH)_{3y+4-x}Cl_x.nH_2O]$ and glycine in which some of the water molecules normally coordinated to the metals have been displaced by the glycine. (1) Glycine aluminum-zirconium complex; (2) Aluminum zirconium glycine tetrachloro hydrate complex. *Anhidrotic.*

Aluminum Zirconium Trichlorohydrate (a loo' mi num zir koe' nee um trye klor" oh hye' drate). **USP**. $Al_yZr(OH)_{3y+4-x}Cl_x.nH_2O$. A polymeric, loosely hydrated complex of basic aluminum zirconium chloride that encompasses a range of aluminum-to-zirconium atomic ratios between 2.0:1 and 5.99:1 and a range of (aluminum plus zirconium)-to-chloride atomic ratios between 2.1:1 and 1.51:1. *Anhidrotic.*

Aluminum Zirconium Trichlorohydrex Gly [*1980*] (a loo' mi num zir koe' nee um trye klor" oh hye' drex glye). **USP**. A coordination complex of aluminum zirconium trichlorohydrate $[Al_yZr(OH)_{3y+4-x}Cl_x.nH_2O]$ and glycine in which some of the water molecules normally coordinated to the

---

† Brand name formerly used, and/or firm no longer concerned with this product.

metals have been displaced by the glycine. (1) Glycine aluminum-zirconium complex; (2) Aluminum zirconium glycine trichloro hydrate complex. *Anhidrotic.*

Alusulf. $Al_7H_{17}O_{25}S_2 \cdot xH_2O$. 670.12 (anhydrous). Heptaaluminum heptadecahydroxide bis(sulfate) hydrate. *CAS-61115-28-4.* INN.

Alvameline Maleate [*2002*] (al va′ me leen mal′ ee ate). $C_9H_{15}N_5 \cdot C_4H_4O_4$. 309.32. [Alvameline is INN.] Pyridine, 3-(2-ethyl-2*H*-tetrazol-5-yl)-1,2,5,6-tetrahydro-1-methyl-, (2Z)-2-butenedioate (1:1). *UNII-76732QSQ30. CAS-219581-36-9; CAS-120241-31-8* [alvameline]. *A partial M_1agonist and M_2/M_3antagonist.* ◇*Lu 25-109-M*

Alverine Citrate [*1965*] (al′ ve reen sit′ rate). $C_{20}H_{27}N \cdot C_6H_8O_7$. 473.56. [Alverine is INN and BAN.] *N*-Ethyl-3,3′-diphenyldipropylamine citrate (1:1). *UNII-9JFB58YK1E. CAS-5560-59-8; CAS-150-59-4* [alverine]. NF XIII. *Anticholinergic.*

Alvespimycin Hydrochloride [*2006*] (al ves″ pi mye′ sin hye″ droe klor′ ide). $C_{32}H_{48}N_4O_8 \cdot HCl$. 653.21. [Alvespimycin is INN.] (1) Geldanamycin,17-demethoxy-17-[[2-(dimethylamino)ethyl]amino]-, monohydrochloride; (2) Hydrochloride of (4*E*,6*Z*,8*S*,9*S*,10*E*,12*S*,13*R*,14*S*,16*R*)-19-[[2-(dimethylamino)ethyl]amino]-13-hydroxy-8,14-dimethoxy-4,10,12,16-tetramethyl-3,20,22-trioxo-2-azabicyclo[16.3.1]docosa-1(21),4,6,10,18-pentaen-9-yl carbamate. *UNII-612K359T69; UNII-001L2FE0M3* [alvespimycin]. *CAS-467214-21-7; CAS-467214-20-6* [alvespimycin]. *Treatment of solid and hematological tumors.* ◇*KOS-1022; 17-DMAG.HCl*

Alvimopan [*2002*] (al″ vi moe′ pan). $C_{25}H_{32}N_2O_4 \cdot 2H_2O$. 460.56. (1) Glycine, *N*-[2-[[4-(3-hydroxyphenyl)-3,4-dimethyl-1-piperidinyl]methyl]-1-oxo-3-phenylpropyl]-, dihydrate, [3*R*-[1(*S**),3α,4α]]-; (2) [[(2*S*)-2-[[(3*R*,4*R*)-4-(3-Hydroxyphenyl)-3,4-dimethylpiperidin-1-yl]methyl]-3-phenylpropanoyl]amino]acetic acid dihydrate. *UNII-677C126AET. CAS-170098-38-1; CAS-156053-89-3* [anhydrous]. INN; BAN. *Treatment of opioid-induced bowel dysfunction, opioid-induced nausea and vomiting, post-operative ileus, idiopathic constipation, and irritable bowel syndrome (peripherally restricted mu opioid receptor antagonist).* ◇*ADL 8-2698; LY246736*

Alvircept Sudotox [*1993*] (al′ vir sept soo′ doe tox). $C_{2600}H_{4130}N_{748}O_{812}S_{10}$ (protein moiety). 59,187 daltons. Biotechnologically-derived chimeric protein engineered to link the first 178 amino acids of the extracellular domain of CD_4 via two linker residues to amino acids 1-3 and 253-613 of *Pseudomonas* exotoxin A. (1) 1-178-Antigen CD 4 (human clone pT4B protein moiety reduced), N^2-L-methionyl-, (178→248′)-protein with 248-L-histidine-249-L-methionine-250-L-alanine-251-L-glutamic acid-248-613-exotoxin A (Pseudomonas aeruginosa reduced); (2) N^2-L-Methionyl-1-178-antigen CD 4 (human clone pT4B protein moiety reduced)(178→248′)-protein with 248-L-histidine-249-L-methionine-250-L-alanine-251-L-glutamic acid-248-613-exotoxin A (*Pseudomonas aeruginosa* reduced). *CAS-137487-62-8.* INN. *Antiviral.* ◇*U-85,855*

MKKVVLGKKG	DTVELTCTAS	QKKSIQFHWK	NSNQIKILGN	QGSFLTKGPS
KLNDRADSRR	SLWDQGNFPL	IIKNLKIEDS	DTYICEVEDQ	KEEVQLLVFG
LTANSDTHLL	QGQSLTLTLE	SPPGSSPSVQ	CRSPRGKNIQ	GGKTLSVSQL
ELQDSGTWTC	TVLQNQKKVE	FKIDIVVLAH	MAEEGGSLAA	LTAHQACHLP
LETFTRHRQP	RGWEQLEQCG	YPVQRLVALY	LAARLSWNQV	DQVIRNALAS
PGSGGDLGEA	IREQPEQARL	ALTLAAAESE	RFVRQGTGND	EAGAANADVV
SLTCPVAAGE	CAGPADSGDA	LLERNYPTGA	EFLGDGGDVS	FSTRGTQNWT
VERLLQAHRQ	LEERGYVFVG	YHGTFLEAAQ	SIVFGGVRAR	SQDLDAIWRG
FYIAGDPALA	YGYAQDQEPD	ARGRIRNGAL	LRVYVPRSSL	PGFYRTSLTL
AAPEAAGEVE	RLIGHPLPLR	LDAITGPEEE	GGRLETILGW	PLAERTVVIP
SAIPTDPRNV	GGDLDPSSIP	DKEQAISALP	DYASQPGKPP	REDLK

Alvocidib [*2002*] (al voe′ si dib). $C_{21}H_{20}ClNO_5 \cdot HCl$. 438.30. (1) 4*H*-1-Benzopyran-4-one, 2-(2-chlorophenyl)-5,7-dihydroxy-8-[(3*R*,4*S*)-3-hydroxy-1-methyl-4-piperidinyl]-, hydrochloride, *rel*-(-)-; (2) (-)-*cis*-2-(2-Chlorophenyl)-5,7-dihydroxy-8-(3-hydroxy-1-methylpiperidin-4-yl)-4*H*-1-benzopyran-4-one hydrochloride. *UNII-D48MS3A6N9. CAS-131740-09-5; CAS-146426-40-6.* INN. *Antineoplastic (cyclin-dependent kinase inhibitor).[Note—The trivial name, flavopiridol, has appeared in literature.]* ◇*HMR 1275; MDL 107,826A; L 86 8275; HL 275; NSC-649890*

Amacetam Hydrochloride (previously used name) — *See* Pramiracetam Hydrochloride.

Amacetam Sulfate (previously used name) — *See* Pramiracetam Sulfate.

Amadinone Acetate [*1970*] (a ma′ di none as′ e tate). $C_{22}H_{27}ClO_4$. 390.90. [Amadinone is INN.] (1) 19-Norpregna-4,6-diene-3,20-dione, 17-(acetyloxy)-6-chloro-; (2) 6-

Chloro-17-hydroxy-19-norpregna-4,6-diene-3,20-dione acetate. *UNII-6MB06022N0* [amadinone]. *CAS-22304-34-3; CAS-30781-27-2* [amadinone]. *Progestin.* ◇*RS-2208*

Amafolone. $C_{19}H_{31}NO_2$. 305.45. 3α-Amino-2β-hydroxy-5α-androstan-17-one. *UNII-N8Y78OKP8D. CAS-50588-47-1.* INN; BAN.

Amalgucin. NNR 1955.

Amanozine. $C_9H_9N_5$. 187.20. 2-Amino-4-anilino-*s*-triazine. *UNII-X43W7JDA8L. CAS-537-17-7.* INN; MI.

Amantadine Hydrochloride [*1964*] (a man′ ta deen hye″ droe klor′ ide). **USP.** $C_{10}H_{17}N \cdot HCl$. 187.71. [Amantadine is INN and BAN.] (1) Tricyclo[3.3.1.1^{3,7}]decan-1-amine, hydrochloride; (2) 1-Adamantanamine hydrochloride. *UNII-M6Q1EO9TD0; UNII-BF4C9Z1J53* [amantadine]. *CAS-665-66-7; CAS-768-94-5* [amantadine]. JAN. *Antiviral.* Symadine (Solvay Pharmaceuticals); Symmetrel (Endo) ◇*EXP-105-1; NSC-83653*

Amantanium Bromide. $C_{25}H_{46}BrNO_2$. 472.54. Decyl(2-hydroxyethyl)dimethylammonium bromide 1-adamantanecarboxylate. *UNII-K0435HZQ57. CAS-58158-77-3.* INN; MI.

Amantocillin. $C_{19}H_{27}N_3O_4S$. 393.50. (1) (3-Amino-1-adamantyl)penicillin; (2) 6-(3-Amino-1-adamantanecarboxamido)-3,3-dimethyl-7-oxo-4-thia-1-azabicyclo[3.2.0]heptane-2-carboxylic acid. *UNII-GV5ZHU20H9. CAS-10004-67-8.* INN.

Amaranth. *CAS-915-67-3.* USP XIX; MI.

Ambamustine. $C_{29}H_{39}Cl_2FN_4O_4S$. 629.61. *N*-[3-[*m*-[Bis(2-chloroethyl)amino]phenyl]-*N*-[3-(*p*-fluorophenyl)-L-alanyl]-L-alanyl]-L-methionine, ethyl ester. *UNII-IB1H345F24. CAS-85754-59-2.* INN.

Ambasilide. $C_{21}H_{25}N_3O$. 335.44. 3-(*p*-Aminobenzoyl)-7-benzyl-3,7-diazabicyclo[3.3.1]nonane. *UNII-012LYD6KXM. CAS-83991-25-7.* INN.

Ambazone. $C_8H_{11}N_7S$. 237.28. *p*-Benzoquinone amidinohydrazone thiosemicarbazone hydrate. *UNII-BYK4592A3Q. CAS-6011-12-7.* INN; BAN; DCF; MI.

Ambenonium Chloride. $C_{28}H_{42}Cl_4N_4O_2$. 608.47. (1) Benzenemethanaminium, *N,N*′-[(1,2-dioxo-1,2-ethanediyl)bis(imino-2,1-ethanediyl)]bis[2-chloro-*N,N*-diethyl-, dichloride; (2) [Oxalylbis(iminoethylene)]bis[(*o*-chlorobenzyl)diethylammonium] dichloride. *UNII-51FOB87G3I. CAS-115-79-7; CAS-52022-31-8* [tetrahydrate]; *CAS-7648-98-8* [ambenonium]. USP XX; INN; BAN; JAN; MI. Mytelase (Sanofi Aventis)

---

† Brand name formerly used, and/or firm no longer concerned with this product.

Ambenoxan. $C_{14}H_{21}NO_4$. 267.32. *N*-[2-(2-Methoxy-ethoxy)ethyl]-1,4-benzodioxan-2-methylamine. *UNII-YBP650462L. CAS-2455-84-7.* INN; BAN.

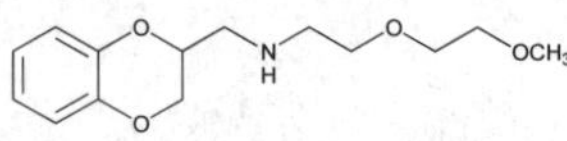

Ambicromil (INN, BAN) — *See* Probicromil Calcium.

Ambomycin [*1962*] (am″ boe mye′ sin). Antibiotic produced by *Streptomyces ambofaciens.* Ambomycin. *CAS-1402-81-9.* INN. *Antineoplastic.* ◇*NSC-53397*

Ambrisentan. $C_{22}H_{22}N_2O_4$. 378.42. (+)-(2*S*)-2-[(4,6-Dimethylpyrimidin-2-yl)oxy]-3-methoxy-3,3-diphenylpropanoic acid. *UNII-HW6NV07QEC. CAS-177036-94-1.* INN; BAN; JAN. Letairis (Gilead Sciences)

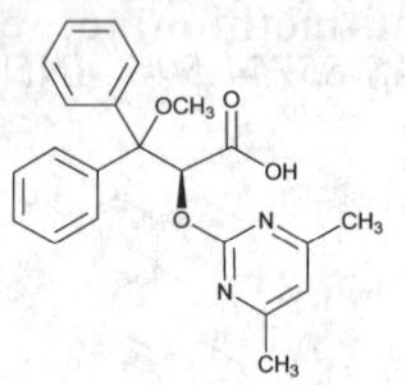

Ambroxol. $C_{13}H_{18}Br_2N_2O$. 378.10. [Ambroxol Hydrochloride is JAN.] *trans*-4-[(2-Amino-3,5-dibromobenzyl)amino]cyclohexanol. *UNII-200168S0CL; UNII-CC995ZMV90* [ambroxol hydrochloride]. *CAS-18683-91-5; CAS-23828-92-4* [hydrochloride]. INN; BAN; MI.

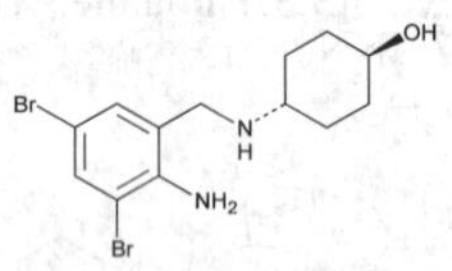

Ambruticin [*1978*] (am″ broo tye′ sin). $C_{28}H_{42}O_6$. 474.63. Antibiotic derived from *Polyangium cellulosum* subsp. *fulvum.* (1) 2*H*-Pyran-2-acetic acid, 6-[2-[2-[5-(6-ethyl-3,6-dihydro-5-methyl-2*H*-pyran-2-yl)-3-methyl-1,4-hexadienyl]-3-methylcyclopropyl]ethenyl]tetrahydro-4,5-dihydroxy-; (2) 6-[2-[2-[5-(6-Ethyl-3,6-dihydro-5-methyl-2*H*-pyran-2-yl)-3-methyl-1,4-hexadienyl]-3-methylcyclopropyl]vinyl]tetrahydro-4,5-dihydroxy-2*H*-pyran-2-acetic acid. *UNII-X794618736. CAS-58857-02-6.* INN. *Antifungal.* ◇*W7783; SMP-78 Acid S*

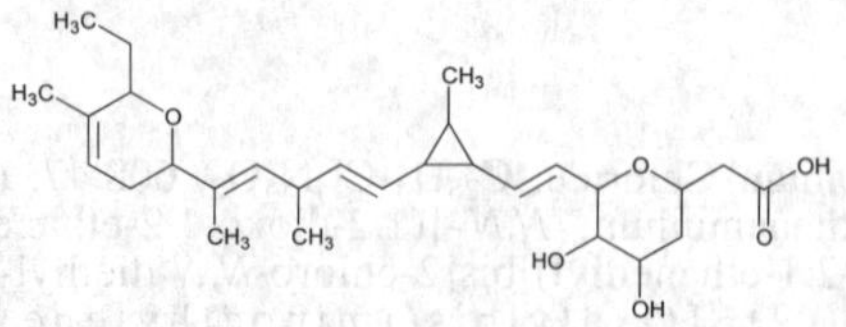

Ambucaine. $C_{17}H_{28}N_2O_3$. 308.42. 2-Diethylaminoethyl 4-amino-2-butoxybenzoate. *UNII-M7G4B57ZCB. CAS-119-29-9.* INN; DCF; MI.

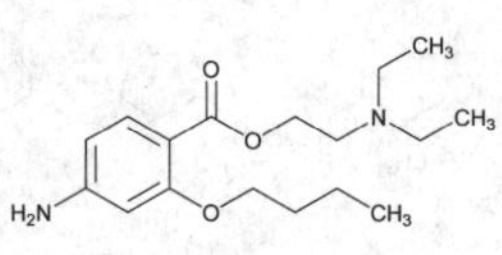

Ambucetamide. $C_{17}H_{28}N_2O_2$. 292.42. 2-(Dibutylamino)-2-(*p*-methoxyphenyl)acetamide. *CAS-519-88-0.* INN; BAN; MI.

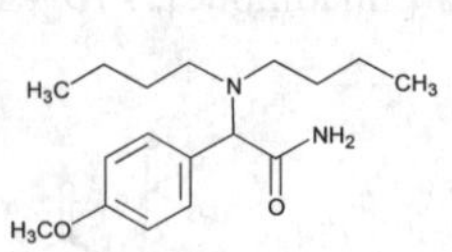

Ambuphylline [*1964*] (am bue′ fi lin). $C_7H_8N_4O_2.C_4H_{11}NO$. 269.30. [Bufylline is BAN.] (1) 1*H*-Purine-2,6-dione, 3,7-dihydro-1,3-dimethyl-, compd. with 2-amino-2-methyl-1-propanol (1:1); (2) Theophylline compound with 2-amino-2-methyl-1-propanol (1:1). *UNII-VOU5V0B772. CAS-5634-34-4. Diuretic; relaxant (smooth muscle).* Butaphyllamine (Marion Merrell Dow†) *[Name previously used: Bufylline.]*

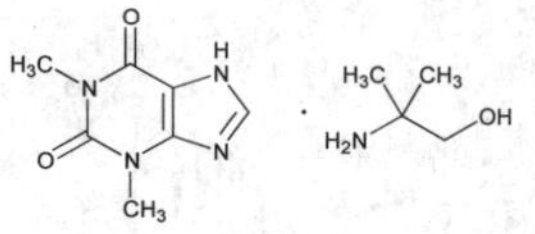

Ambuside [*1968*] (am′ bue side). $C_{13}H_{16}ClN_3O_5S_2$. 393.87. (1) 1,3-Benzenedisulfonamide, 4-chloro-6-[(3-hydroxy-2-butenylidene)amino]-*N*^{1}-2-propenyl-; (2) *N*^{1}-Allyl-4-chloro-6-[(3-hydroxy-2-butenylidene)amino]-*m*-benzenedisulfonamide. *CAS-3754-19-6.* INN; BAN. *Diuretic.* ◇*EX 4810; RMI 83,047*

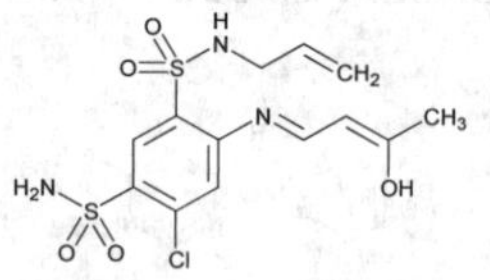

Ambuterol — *See* Mabuterol.

Ambutonium Bromide. (3-Carbamoyl-3,3-diphenylpropyl)ethyldimethylammonium bromide. *UNII-9J8YA3ZT14. CAS-115-51-5; CAS-14007-49-9* [ambutonium]. BAN; MI.

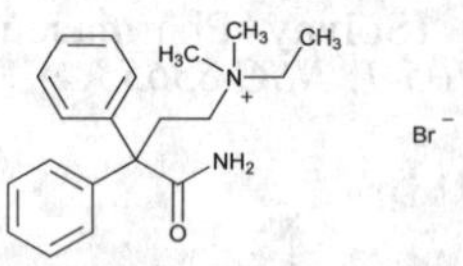

Ambutoxate — *See* Ambucaine.

Amcinafal [*1970*] (am sin′ a fal). $C_{26}H_{35}FO_6$. 462.55. (1) Pregna-1,4-diene-3,20-dione, 9-fluoro-11,21-dihydroxy-16,17-[(1-ethylpropylidene)bis(oxy)]-, (11β,16α)-; (2) 9-Fluoro-11β,16α,17,21-tetrahydroxypregna-1,4-diene-3,20-dione cyclic 16,17-acetal with 3-pentanone. *CAS-3924-70-7.* INN. *Anti-inflammatory.* ◇*SQ 15,102*

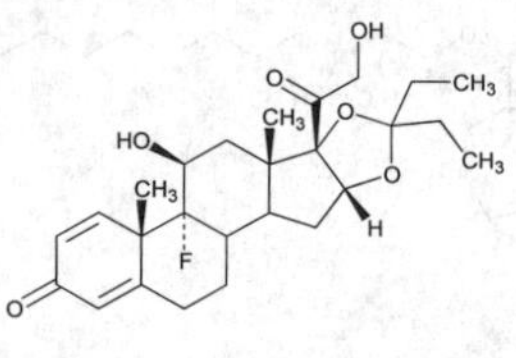

Amcinafide [*1970*] (am sin′ a fide). $C_{29}H_{33}FO_6$. 496.57. (1) Pregna-1,4-diene-3,20-dione, 9-fluoro-11,21-dihydroxy-16,17-[(1-phenylethylidene)bis(oxy)]-, [11β,16α(*R*)]-; (2)

(*R*)-9-Fluoro-11β,16α,17,21-tetrahydroxypregna-1,4-diene-3,20-dione cyclic 16,17-acetal with acetophenone. *CAS-7332-27-6*. INN. *Anti-inflammatory.* ◇*SQ 15,112*

Amcinonide [*1975*] (am sin′ oh nide). **USP.** $C_{28}H_{35}FO_7$. 502.57. (1) Pregna-1,4-diene-3,20-dione, 21-(acetyloxy)-16,17-[cyclopentylidenebis(oxy)]-9-fluoro-11-hydroxy-, (11β,16α)-; (2) 9-Fluoro-11β,16α,17,21-tetrahydroxy-pregna-1,4-diene-3,20-dione cyclic 16,17-acetal with cyclopentanone, 21-acetate. *UNII-423W026MA9*. *CAS-51022-69-6*. INN; BAN; JAN. *Glucocorticoid.* Cyclocort (Astellas) ◇*CL 34699*

Amdinocillin [*1981*] (am dee″ noe sil′ in). $C_{15}H_{23}N_3O_3S$. 325.43. [Mecillinam is INN and BAN.] (1) 4-Thia-1-azabicyclo[3.2.0]heptane-2-carboxylic acid, 6-[[(hexahydro-1*H*-azepin-1-yl)methylene]amino]-3,3-dimethyl-7-oxo-, [2*S*-(2α,5α,6β)]-; (2) (2*S*,5*R*,6*R*)-6-[[(Hexahydro-1*H*-azepin-1-yl)methylene]amino]-3,3-dimethyl-7-oxo-4-thia-1-azabicyclo[3.2.0]heptane-2-carboxylic acid. *UNII-V10579P3QZ*. *CAS-32887-01-7*. USP XXIII. *Antibacterial.* Coactin (Roche) ◇*Ro 10-9070*

Amdinocillin Pivoxil [*1981*] (am dee″ noe sil′ in piv ox′ il). $C_{21}H_{33}N_3O_5S$. 439.57. [Pivmecillinam is INN and BAN; Pivmecillinam Hydrochloride is JAN.] (1) 4-Thia-1-azabicyclo[3.2.0]heptane-2-carboxylic acid, 6-[[(hexahydro-1*H*-azepin-1-yl)methylene]amino]-3,3-dimethyl-7-oxo-, (2,2-dimethyl-1-oxopropoxy)methyl ester, [2*S*-(2α,5α,6β)]-; (2) Hydroxymethyl (2*S*,5*R*,6*R*)-6-[[(hexahydro-1*H*-azepin-1-yl)methylene]amino]-3,3-dimethyl-7-oxo-4-thia-1-azabicyclo[3.2.0]heptane-2-carboxylate pivalate (ester). *UNII-1WAM1OQ30B*. *CAS-32886-97-8*. *Antibacterial.* Coactabs (Hoffmann-LaRoche†) ◇*Ro 10-9071*

Amdoxovir [*2001*] (am dox′ oh vir). $C_9H_{12}N_6O_3$. 252.23. (1) 1,3-Dioxolane-2-methanol, 4-(2,6-diamino-9*H*-purin-9-yl)-, (2*R*,4*R*)-; (2) (2*R*,4*R*)-4-(2,6-Diamino-9*H*-purin-9-yl)-1,3-dioxolane-2-methanol. *UNII-54I81H0M9C*. *CAS-*

145514-04-1. INN. *Antiviral used in the treatment of HIV-1 and hepatitis B infections (reverse transcriptase inhibitor).* ◇◇*(-)-DAPD; DAPD*

Ameban — *See* Carbarsone.

Amebarsone — *See* Carbarsone.

Amebucort. $C_{28}H_{40}O_7$. 488.61. 11β,17,21-Trihydroxy-6α-methylpregn-4-ene-3,20-dione 21-acetate 17-butyrate. *UNII-7YRF8G0G0F*. *CAS-83625-35-8*. INN.

Amedalin Hydrochloride [*1970*] (a med′ a lin hye″ droe klor′ ide). $C_{19}H_{22}N_2O \cdot HCl$. 330.85. [Amedalin is INN.] (1) 2*H*-Indol-2-one, 1,3-dihydro-3-methyl-3-[3-(methylamino)propyl]-1-phenyl-, monohydrochloride; (2) 3-Methyl-3-[3-(methylamino)propyl]-1-phenyl-2-indolinone monohydrochloride. *UNII-0EMF539HN0*. *CAS-22232-73-1; CAS-22136-26-1* [amedalin]. *Antidepressant.* ◇*UK-3540-1*

Amediplase. 173-L-Serine-174-L-tyrosine-175-L-glutamine-173-275-plasminogen activator (human tissue-type reduced), fusion protein with urokinase (human urine β-chain reduced). *CAS-151912-11-7*. INN.

```
SYQGNSDCYF  GNGSAYRGTH  SLTESGASCL  PWNSMILIGK  VYTAQNPSAQ
ALGLGKHNYC  RNPDGDAKPW  CHVLKNRRLT  WEYCDVPSCS  TCGLRQYSQP
QFRIIGGEFT  TIENQPWFAA  IYRRHRGGSV  TYVCGGSLMS  PCWVISATHC
FIDYPKKEDY  IVYLGRSRLN  SNTQGEMKFE  VENLILHKDY  SADTLAHHND
IALLKIRSKE  GRCAQPSRTI  QTICLPSMYN  DPQFGTSCEI  TGFGKENSTD
YLYPEQLKMT  VVKLISHREC  QQPHYYGSEV  TTKMLCAADP  QWKTDSCQGD
SGGPLVCSLQ  GRMTLTGIVS  WGRGCALKDK  PGVYTRVSHF  LPWIRSHTKE
ENGLAL
```

Amelometasone. $C_{26}H_{35}FO_6$. 462.55. (+)-9-Fluoro-11β,17-dihydroxy-21-methoxy-16β-methylpregna-1,4-diene-3,20-dione 17-propionate. *UNII-T01B0RCE7T*. *CAS-123013-22-9*. INN.

---

† Brand name formerly used, and/or firm no longer concerned with this product.

Ameltolide [*1990*] (a mel′ toe lide). $C_{15}H_{16}N_2O$. 240.30. (1) Benzamide, 4-amino-*N*-(2,6-dimethylphenyl)-; (2) 4-Amino-2′,6′-benzoxylidide. *CAS-787-93-9*. INN; BAN. *Anticonvulsant*. ◇*LY 201116*

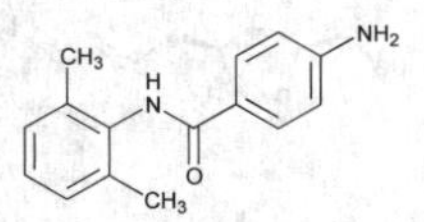

Amelubant. $C_{33}H_{34}N_2O_5$. 538.63. Ethyl [[4-[[3-[[4-[1-(4-hydroxyphenyl)-1-methylethyl]phenoxy]methyl]benzyl]oxy]phenyl](imino)methyl]carbamate. *UNII-E0018IF0K4*. *CAS-346735-24-8*. INN.

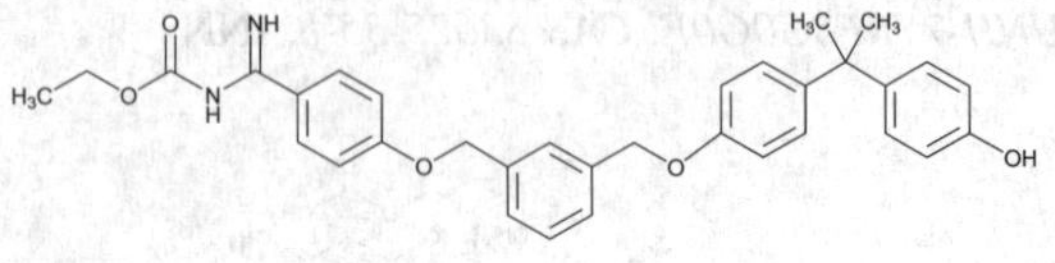

Amenozine — *See* Amanozine.

Amesergide [*1992*] (am e ser′ jide). $C_{25}H_{35}N_3O$. 393.56. (1) Ergoline-8-carboxamide, *N*-cyclohexyl-6-methyl-1-(1-methylethyl)-, (8β)-; (2) *N*-Cyclohexyl-1-isopropyl-6-methylergoline-8β-carboxamide. *CAS-121588-75-8*. INN. *Serotonin antagonist*. ◇*LY237733*

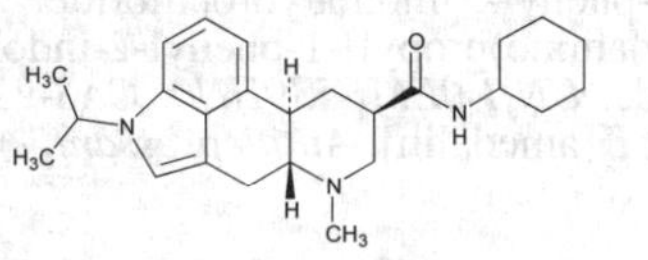

Ametantrone Acetate [*1981*] (a met′ an trone as′ e tate). $C_{22}H_{28}N_4O_4.2C_2H_4O_2$. 532.59. [Ametantrone is INN.] (1) 9,10-Anthracenedione, 1,4-bis[[2-[(2-hydroxyethyl)amino]ethyl]amino]-, diacetate (salt); (2) 1,4-Bis[[2-[(2-hydroxyethyl)amino]ethyl]amino]anthraquinone diacetate (salt). *UNII-6FH145297U*. *CAS-70711-40-9*. *Antineoplastic*. ◇*CI-881*

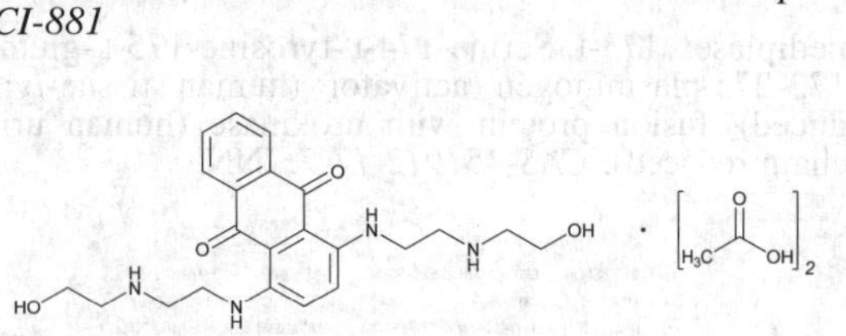

Ametazole (BAN) — *See* Betazole Hydrochloride.

Amethocaine (former BAN) — *See* Tetracaine.

Amethopterin (previously used name) — *See* Methotrexate.

Amezepine. $C_{18}H_{20}N_2$. 264.36. 5-Methyl-10-[2-(methylamino)ethyl]-5*H*-dibenz[*b,f*]azepine. *UNII-RZ5COP6XI5*. *CAS-60575-32-8*. INN.

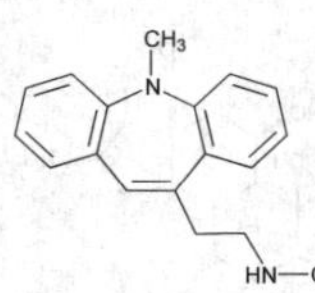

Amezinium Metilsulfate. $C_{12}H_{15}N_3O_5S$. 313.33. 4-Amino-6-methoxy-1-phenylpyridazinium methyl sulfate. *UNII-03NR868ICX*. *CAS-30578-37-1*. INN; JAN; MI.

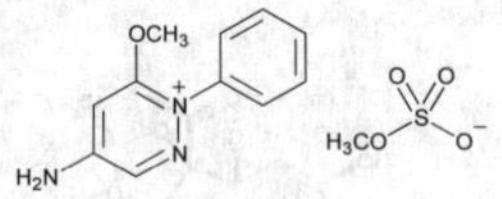

Amfebutamone Hydrochloride (previously used name) — *See* Bupropion Hydrochloride.

Amfecloral (INN, BAN) — *See* Amphecloral.

Amfenac Sodium [*1977*] (am′ fen ak soe′ dee um). $C_{15}H_{12}NNaO_3.H_2O$. 295.27. [Amfenac is INN and BAN.] (1) Benzeneacetic acid, 2-amino-3-benzoyl-, sodium salt, monohydrate; (2) Sodium (2-amino-3-benzoylphenyl)acetate monohydrate. *UNII-28O5C1J38A* [amfenac]. *CAS-61618-27-7*; *CAS-51579-82-9* [amfenac]. JAN. *Anti-inflammatory*. ◇*AHR-5850D*

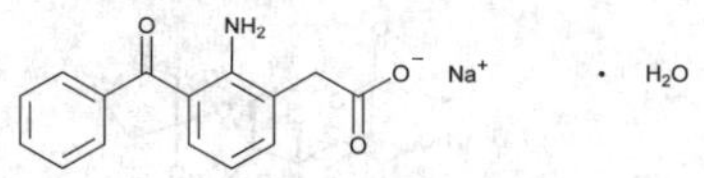

Amfepentorex. $C_{15}H_{25}N$. 219.37. *N,α*-Dimethyl-*p*-pentylphenethylamine. *UNII-OPE7BD4AAA*. *CAS-15686-27-8*. INN; DCF. ◇*CB 2201*

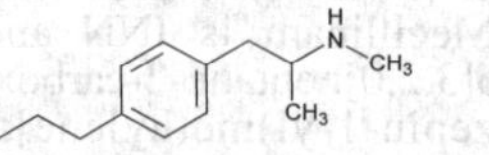

Amfepramone (INN, DCF) **Hydrochloride** — *See* Diethylpropion Hydrochloride.

Amfetamine (INN, BAN) — *See* Amphetamine Sulfate.

Amfetaminil. $C_{17}H_{18}N_2$. 250.34. [(*α*-Methylphenethyl)amino]phenylacetonitrile. *UNII-0XU0V77JVE*. *CAS-17590-01-1*. INN.

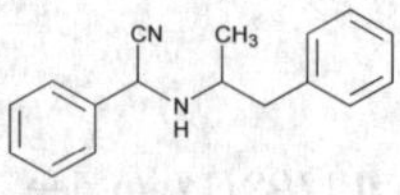

Amfilcon A [*1985*] (am fil′ kon). $(C_6H_{10}O_3)_x(C_4H_6O_2)_y(C_{10}H_{14}O_4)_z$. (1) 2-Propenoic acid, 2-methyl-, 2-hydroxyethyl ester, polymer with 2-methyl-2-propenoic acid and 1,2-ethanediyl bis(2-methyl-2-propenoate); (2) 2-Hydroxyethyl methacrylate polymer with methacrylic acid and ethylene dimethacrylate. *CAS-33410-59-2*. *Contact lens material (hydrophilic)*.

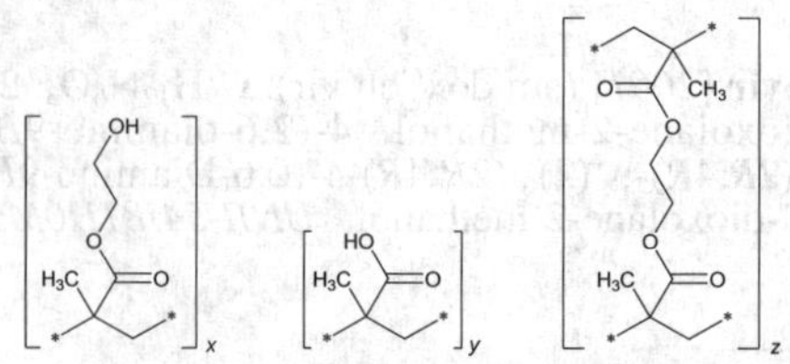

Amflutizole [*1983*] (am floo′ ti zole). $C_{11}H_7F_3N_2O_2S$. 288.25. (1) 5-Isothiazolecarboxylic acid, 4-amino-3-[3-(trifluoromethyl)phenyl]-; (2) 4-Amino-3-(α,α,α-trifluoro-*m*-tolyl)-5-isothiazolecarboxylic acid. *CAS-82114-19-0*. INN. *Suppressant (gout).* ◇*LY 141894*

Amfomycin (INN, DCF) — *See* Amphomycin.

Amfonelic Acid [*1967*] (am″ foe nee′ lik as′ id). $C_{18}H_{16}N_2O_3$. 308.33. (1) 1,8-Naphthyridine-3-carboxylic acid, 1-ethyl-1,4-dihydro-4-oxo-7-(phenylmethyl)-; (2) 7-Benzyl-1-ethyl-1,4-dihydro-4-oxo-1,8-naphthyridine-3-carboxylic acid. *CAS-15180-02-6*. INN; BAN. *Stimulant (central).* ◇*Win 25,978; NSC-100638*

Amibegron [*2007*] (a″ mi beg′ ron). $C_{22}H_{26}ClNO_4$. 403.90. (1) Acetic acid, [[(7*S*)-7-[[(2*R*)-2-(3-chlorophenyl)-2-hydroxyethyl]amino]-5,6,7,8-tetrahydro-2-naphthalenyl]oxy]-, ethyl ester; (2) Ethyl {[(7*S*)-7-{[(2*R*)-2-(3-chlorophenyl)-2-hydroxyethyl]amino}-5,6,7,8-tetrahydronaphthalen-2-yl]oxy}acetate. *UNII-PDQ3ME68U3*. *CAS-121524-08-1*. INN. *Antidepressant.* ◇*SR58611*

Amibegron Hydrochloride [*2007*] (a″ mi beg′ ron hye″ droe klor′ ide). $C_{22}H_{26}ClNO_4 \cdot HCl$. 440.36. (1) Acetic acid, [[(7*S*)-7-[[(2*R*)-2-(3-chlorophenyl)-2-hydroxyethyl]amino]-5,6,7,8-tetrahydro-2-naphthalenyl]oxy]-, ethyl ester, hydrochloride; (2) Ethyl {[(7*S*)-7-{[(2*R*)-2-(3-chlorophenyl)-2-hydroxyethyl]amino}-5,6,7,8-tetrahydronaphthalen-2-yl]oxy}acetate hydrochloride. *CAS-121524-09-2*. *Antidepressant.* ◇*SR58611A*

Amibiarson — *See* Carbarsone.

Amicarbalide. $C_{15}H_{16}N_6O$. 296.33. 3,3′-Diamidinocarbanilide. *UNII-D7CJB20DJO*. *CAS-3459-96-9*. INN; BAN; MI. ◇*M&B 5062 A*

Amicibone. $C_{22}H_{31}NO_3$. 357.49. Benzyl-1-[2-(hexahydro-1*H*-azepin-1-yl)ethyl]-2-oxocyclohexanecarboxylate. *CAS-23271-63-8*. INN; MI.

Amicloral [*1972*] (a″ mi klor′ al). $(C_8H_{11}Cl_3O_6)_x(C_6H_{10}O_5)_y$. (1) α-D-Glucopyranose, 6-*O*-(2,2,2-trichloro-1-hydroxyethyl)-, polymer with α-D-glucopyranose; (2) 6-*O*-(2,2,2-Trichloro-1-hydroxyethyl)-α-D-glucopyranose 1→4 polymer with α-D-glucopyranose. *CAS-34398-83-9*. *Food additive (veterinary).* ◇*SK&F 39186*

Amicycline [*1964*] (a″ mi sye′ kleen). $C_{21}H_{23}N_3O_7$. 429.42. (1) 2-Naphthacenecarboxamide, 9-amino-4-(dimethylamino)-1,4,4a,5,5a,6,11,12a-octahydro-3,10,12,12a-tetrahydroxy-1,11-dioxo-, [4*S*-(4α,4aα,5aα,12aα)]-; (2) 9-Amino-4-(dimethylamino)-1,4,4a,5,5a,6,11,12a-octahydro-3,10,12,12a-tetrahydroxy-1,11-dioxo-2-naphthacenecarboxamide. *CAS-5874-95-3*. INN. *Antibacterial.*

Amidantel. $C_{13}H_{19}N_3O_2$. 249.31. 4′-[[1-(Dimethylamino)ethylidene]amino]-2-methoxyacetanilide. *UNII-C67IS11N0O*. *CAS-49745-00-8*. INN; BAN. ◇*BAY d 8815 [hydrochloride]*

Amidapsone [*1972*] (a″ mi dap′ sone). $C_{13}H_{13}N_3O_3S$. 291.33. (1) Urea, [4-[(4-aminophenyl)sulfonyl]phenyl]-; (2) (*p*-Sulfanilylphenyl)urea. *UNII-8N5BE1142E*. *CAS-3569-77-5*. INN. *Antiviral (for poultry).* ◇*NSC-28120*

Amidefrine (BAN) — *See* Amidephrine Mesylate.

Amidefrine Mesilate (INN) — *See* Amidephrine Mesylate.

Amidephrine Mesylate [*1965*] (a″ mi def′ rin mes′ i late). $C_{10}H_{16}N_2O_3S \cdot CH_4O_3S$. 340.42. [Amidefrine Mesilate is INN; Amidefrine is BAN.] (1) Methanesulfonamide, *N*-[3-[1-hydroxy-2-(methylamino)ethyl]phenyl]-, monomethanesulfonate (salt); (2) 3′-[1-Hydroxy-2-(methylami-

---

† Brand name formerly used, and/or firm no longer concerned with this product.

no)ethyl]methanesulfonanilide monomethanesulfonate (salt). *UNII-S3IG39T94B. CAS-1421-68-7; CAS-3354-67-4* [replaced]; *CAS-37571-84-9* [amidephrine]. *Adrenergic.* ◇*5190*

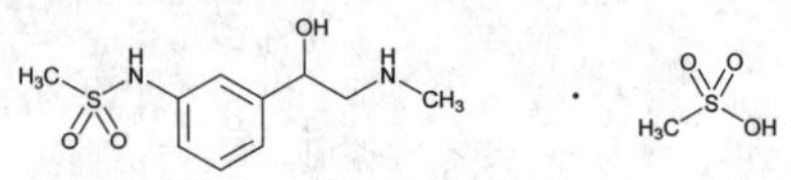

Amidol — *See* Dimepheptanol.

Amidopyrine (previously used name) — *See* Aminopyrine.

Amidotrizoic Acid (BAN, JAN) — *See* Diatrizoic Acid.

Amifampridine. $C_5H_7N_3$. 109.13. Pyridine-3,4-diamine. *CAS-54-96-6*. INN.

Amiflamine. $C_{12}H_{20}N_2$. 192.30. (+)-4-(Dimethylamino)-α-2-dimethylphenethylamine. *UNII-NE25WV9C8S. CAS-77518-07-1*. INN.

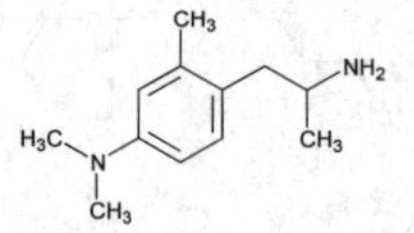

Amifloverine. $C_{16}H_{27}NO_3$. 281.39. 2-(3,5-Diethoxyphenoxy)triethylamine. *UNII-X154DLC3EY. CAS-54063-24-0*. INN; DCF.

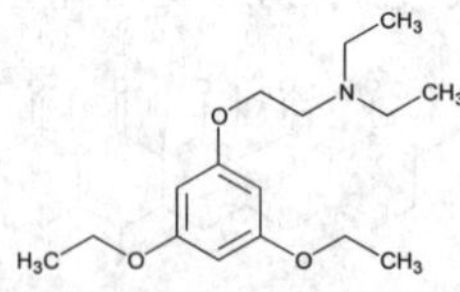

Amifloxacin [*1984*] (a″ mi flox′ a sin). $C_{16}H_{19}FN_4O_3$. 334.35. (1) 3-Quinolinecarboxylic acid, 6-fluoro-1,4-dihydro-1-(methylamino)-7-(4-methyl-1-piperazinyl)-4-oxo-; (2) 6-Fluoro-1,4-dihydro-1-(methylamino)-7-(4-methyl-1-piperazinyl)-4-oxo-3-quinolinecarboxylic acid. *UNII-5TU5227-KYQ. CAS-86393-37-5*. INN; BAN. *Antibacterial.* ◇*Win 49,375*

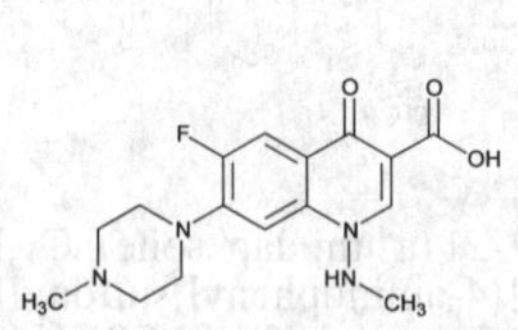

Amifloxacin Mesylate [*1984*] (a″ mi flox′ a sin mes′ i late). $C_{16}H_{19}FN_4O_3 \cdot CH_4O_3S$. 430.45. [Amifloxacin is BAN.] (1) 3-Quinolinecarboxylic acid, 6-fluoro-1,4-dihydro-1-(methylamino)-7-(4-methyl-1-piperazinyl)-4-oxo-, monomethanesulfonate; (2) 6-Fluoro-1,4-dihydro-1-(methylamino)-7-(4-methyl-1-piperazinyl)-4-oxo-3-quinolinecarboxylic acid monomethanesulfonate. *UNII-2C21AN130I; UNII-5TU5227KYQ* [amifloxacin]. *CAS-88036-80-0; CAS-86393-37-5* [amifloxacin]. *Antibacterial.* ◇*Win 49,375-3*

Amifostine [*1991*] (a″ mi fos′ teen). **USP**. $C_5H_{15}N_2O_3P \cdot S \cdot 3H_2O$. 268.27. (1) Ethanethiol, 2-[(3-aminopropyl)amino]-, dihydrogen phosphate (ester), trihydrate; (2) *S*-[2-[(3-Aminopropyl)amino]ethyl] dihydrogen phosphorothioate, trihydrate. *UNII-M487QF2F4V. CAS-112901-68-5; CAS-*

20537-88-6 [anhydrous]. INN; BAN. *Protectant (topical); radioprotector.* Ethyol (MedImmune) *[USAN previously used: Ethiofos.]* ◇*WR-2721; NSC-296961*

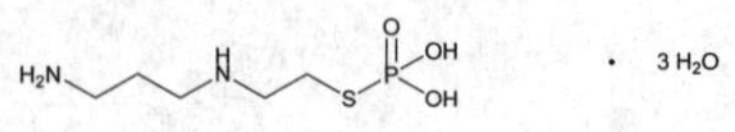

Amiglumide. $C_{26}H_{36}N_2O_4$. 440.58. (*R*)-4-(2-Naphthamido)-*N,N*-dipentylglutaramic acid. *UNII-H48W1A97VB. CAS-119363-62-1*. INN.

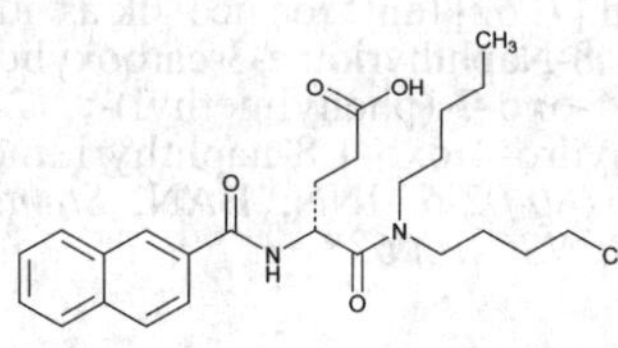

Amikacin (a″ mi kay′ sin). **USP**. $C_{22}H_{43}N_5O_{13}$. 585.60. (1) D-Streptamine, *O*-3-amino-3-deoxy-α-D-glucopyranosyl-(1→6)-*O*-[6-amino-6-deoxy-α-D-glucopyranosyl-(1→4)]-N^1-(4-amino-2-hydroxy-1-oxobutyl)-2-deoxy-, (*S*)-; (2) *O*-3-Amino-3-deoxy-α-D-glucopyranosyl-(1→4)-*O*-[6-amino-6-deoxy-α-D-glucopyranosyl-(1→6)]-N^3-(4-amino-L-2-hydroxybutyryl)-2-deoxy-L-streptamine. *UNII-84319SGC3C. CAS-37517-28-5*. INN; BAN. *Antibacterial.*

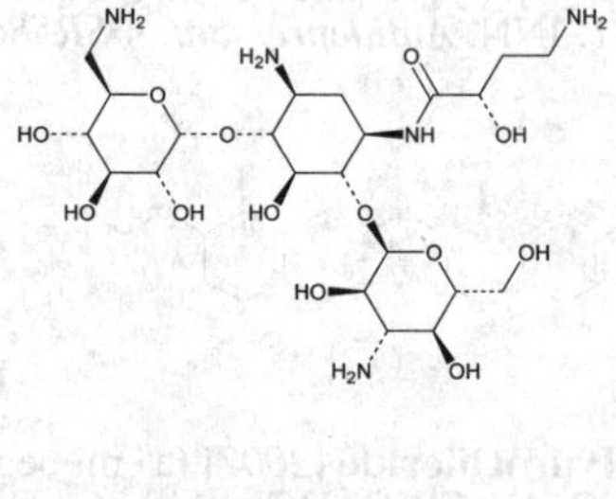

Amikacin Sulfate [*1973*] (a″ mi kay′ sin sul′ fate). **USP**. $C_{22}H_{43}N_5O_{13} \cdot 2H_2SO_4$. 781.76. (1) D-Streptamine, *O*-3-amino-3-deoxy-α-D-glucopyranosyl-(1→6)-*O*-[6-amino-6-deoxy-α-D-glucopyranosyl-(1→4)]-N^1-(4-amino-2-hydroxy-1-oxobutyl)-2-deoxy-, (*S*)-, sulfate (1:2) (salt); (2) *O*-3-Amino-3-deoxy-α-D-glucopyranosyl-(1→4)-*O*-[6-amino-6-deoxy-α-D-glucopyranosyl-(1→6)]-N^3-(4-amino-L-2-hydroxybutyryl)-2-deoxy-L-streptamine sulfate (1:2). *UNII-N6M33094FD; UNII-84319SGC3C* [amikacin]. *CAS-39831-55-5; CAS-37517-28-5* [amikacin]. JAN. *Antibacterial.* Amikin (Apothecon) ◇*BB-K8*

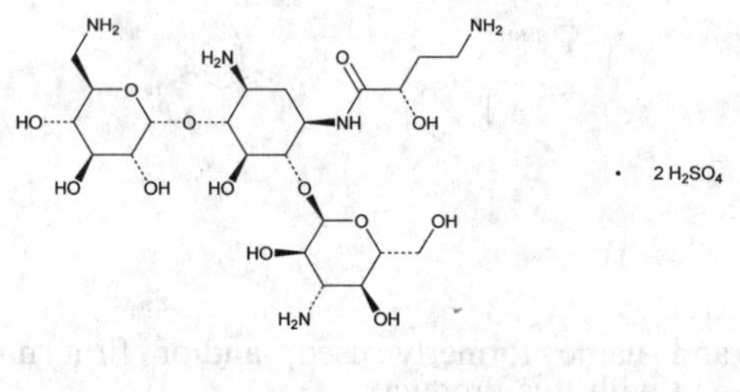

Amikhelline. $C_{18}H_{21}NO_5$. 331.36. 9[2-(Diethylamino)ethoxy]-4-hydroxy-7-methyl-5*H*-furo[3,2-*g*][1]benzopyran-5-one. *UNII-BD9T227F6M. CAS-4439-67-2.* INN.

Amilomer. Microspheres produced by reaction of partially hydrolysed starch with epichlorohydrin, quickly degradable by amylase (with a half-life of less than 120 minutes). *CAS-42615-49-6.* INN.

Amiloride Hydrochloride [*1967*] (a mil′ oh ride hye″ droe klor′ ide). **USP**. $C_6H_8ClN_7O.HCl.2H_2O$. 302.12. [Amiloride is INN and BAN.] (1) Pyrazinecarboxamide, 3,5-diamino-*N*-(aminoiminomethyl)-6-chloro-, monohydrochloride dihydrate; (2) *N*-Amidino-3,5-diamino-6-chloropyrazinecarboxamide monohydrochloride dihydrate. *UNII-FZJ37245UC; UNII-7DZO8EB0Z3* [amiloride]. *CAS-17440-83-4; CAS-2016-88-8* [anhydrous]; *CAS-2609-46-3* [amiloride]. *Diuretic.* Midamor (Merck)

Amiloxate [*1999*] (a″ mil ox′ ate). **USP**. $C_{15}H_{20}O_3$. 248.32. (1) 4-Methoxycinnamic acid, isoamyl ester; (2) 2-Benzoic acid, 2-propenoic acid, 3-(4-methoxyphenyl)-3-methylbutyl ester. *CAS-71617-10-2.* INN. *Sunscreen (ultraviolet B absorber).* Neo Heliopan (H & R Florasynth) *[Name previously used: Isoamyl Methoxycinnamate.] [Note—The International Cosmetic Ingredient (INCI) name for amiloxate is isoamyl p-methoxycinnamate.]* ◇*E-1000*

Aminacrine Hydrochloride [*1964*] (am in ak′ rin hye″ droe klor′ ide). $C_{13}H_{10}N_2.HCl$. 230.69. [Aminoacridine is INN and BAN.] (1) 9-Acridinamine monohydrochloride; (2) 9-Aminoacridine monohydrochloride. *UNII-OR5RM3Q5QL;*

UNII-78OY3Z0P7Z [aminacrine]. *CAS-134-50-9; CAS-90-45-9* [aminacrine]. *Anti-infective, topical.* Monacrin (Sterling Winthrop†) ◇*NSC-7571*

Aminarsone — *See* Carbarsone.

Amindocate. $C_{19}H_{29}N_3O_2$. 331.45. 2-(Dimethylamino)ethyl 1-[2-(dimethylamino)ethyl]-2,3-dimethylindole-5-carboxylate. *UNII-5C193VF4V3. CAS-31386-24-0.* INN.

Amineptine. $C_{22}H_{27}NO_2$. 337.46. 7-[(10,11-Dihydro-5*H*-dibenzo[*a,d*]cyclohepten-5-yl)amino]heptanoic acid. *UNII-27T1I13L6G. CAS-57574-09-1.* INN; MI.

Aminitrozole (INN, BAN) — *See* Nithiamide.

Amino Methacrylate Copolymer. **NF**. A fully polymerized copolymer of (2-dimethylaminoethyl) methacrylate, butyl methacrylate, and methyl methacrylate.

Aminoacetic Acid (JAN and previously used name) — *See* Glycine.

Aminoacridine (INN, BAN) — *See* Aminacrine Hydrochloride.

Aminobenzoate Potassium (a mee″ noe ben′ zoe ate poe tas′ ee um). **USP**. $C_7H_6KNO_2$. 175.23. (1) Benzoic acid, 4-amino-, potassium salt; (2) Potassium 4-aminobenzoate. *UNII-41KZS5432U. CAS-138-84-1; CAS-150-13-0* [*p*-aminobenzoic acid]. *Analgesic.* Potaba (Glenwood)

Aminobenzoate Sodium (a mee″ noe ben′ zoe ate soe′ dee um). **USP**. $C_7H_6NNaO_2$. 159.12. (1) Benzoic acid, 4-amino-, sodium salt; (2) Sodium 4-aminobenzoate. *Analgesic.*

Aminobenzoic Acid (a mee″ noe ben zoe′ ik as′ id). **USP**. $C_7H_7NO_2$. 137.14. (1) Benzoic acid, 4-amino; (2) *p*-Aminobenzoic acid. *UNII-TL2TJE8QTX. CAS-150-13-0. Ultraviolet screen.* RVPaba Lipstick (ICN†) *[Name previously used: Para-Aminobenzoic Acid.]*

Aminobenzylpenicillin — *See* Ampicillin.

γ-Aminobutyric Acid. $C_4H_9NO_2$. 103.12. γ-Aminobutyric acid. *UNII-2ACZ6IPC6I. CAS-56-12-2.* JAN.

---

† Brand name formerly used, and/or firm no longer concerned with this product.

Aminocaproic Acid [*1963*] (a mee″ noe ka proe′ ik as′ id). **USP.** C₆H₁₃NO₂. 131.17. [ε-Aminocaproic Acid is JAN.] (1) Hexanoic acid, 6-amino-; (2) 6-Aminohexanoic acid. *UNII-U6F3787206. CAS-60-32-2.* INN; BAN. *Hemostatic.* Amicar (Xanodyne) ◇*CL 10304; CY-116; EACA; 177 J.D.; NSC-26154*

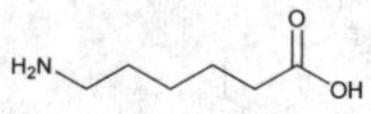

Aminodeoxykanamycin — *See* Bekanamycin.

Aminoethyl Nitrate. C₂H₆N₂O₃. 106.08. 2-Aminoethyl nitrate. *UNII-S1IA7R2J48. CAS-646-02-6.* INN; DCF.

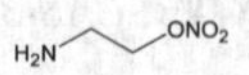

Aminoethylsulfonic Acid (JAN) — *See* Taurine.

Aminoglutethimide (a mee″ noe gloo teth′ i mide). **USP.** C₁₃H₁₆N₂O₂. 232.28. (1) 2,6-Piperidinedione, 3-(4-aminophenyl)-3-ethyl-; (2) 2-(*p*-Aminophenyl)-2-ethylglutarimide. *UNII-0O54ZQ14I9. CAS-125-84-8.* INN; BAN. *Adrenocortical suppressant; antineoplastic.* Cytadren (Novartis)

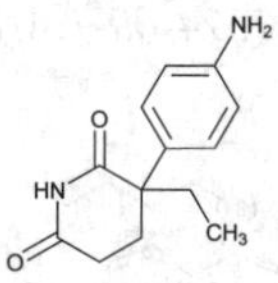

Aminohippurate Sodium (a mee″ noe hip′ ure ate soe′ dee um). **USP** [Injection]. C₉H₉N₂NaO₃. 216.17. [*p*-Aminohippurate Sodium is JAN.] (1) Glycine, *N*-(4-aminobenzoyl)-, monosodium salt; (2) Monosodium *p*-aminohippurate. *UNII-SUO3KVS1O9. CAS-94-16-6; CAS-61-78-9* [aminohippuric acid]. *Diagnostic aid (renal function determination).*

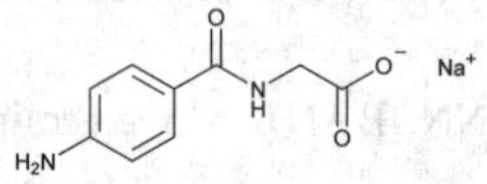

Aminohippuric Acid (a mee″ noe hi pure′ ik as′ id). **USP.** C₉H₁₀N₂O₃. 194.19. (1) Glycine, *N*-(4-aminobenzoyl)-; (2) *p*-Aminohippuric acid. *CAS-61-78-9.* Component of Aminohippurate Sodium [Injection].

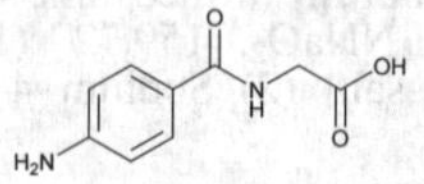

γ-Amino-β-hydroxybutyric acid. C₄H₉NO₃. 119.12. γ-Amino-β-hydroxybutyric acid. *CAS-352-21-6.* JAN.

Aminolevulinic Acid Hydrochloride [*1997*] (a mee″ noe lev″ ue lin′ ik as′ id hye″ droe klor′ ide). C₅H₉NO₃.HCl. 167.59. 5-Aminolevulinic acid hydrochloride. *UNII-V35KBM8JGR. CAS-5451-09-2. Antineoplastic.* Levulan (Dusa)

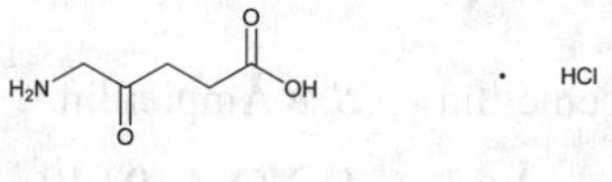

Aminometradine. C₉H₁₃N₃O₂. 195.22. 1-Allyl-6-amino-3-ethyluracil. *UNII-PPM8SX5Q3V. CAS-642-44-4.* INN; BAN; MI.

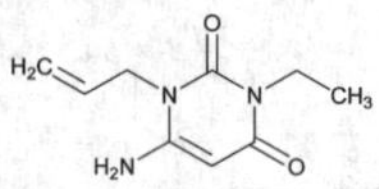

Aminopentamide Sulfate (a mee″ noe pen′ ta mide sul′ fate). **USP.** C₁₉H₂₄N₂O.H₂SO₄. 394.49. [Dimevamide is INN.] α-[2-(Dimethylamino)propyl]-α-phenylbenzeneacetamide sulfate. *UNII-20P9NI883O. CAS-60-46-8.* NND 1962.

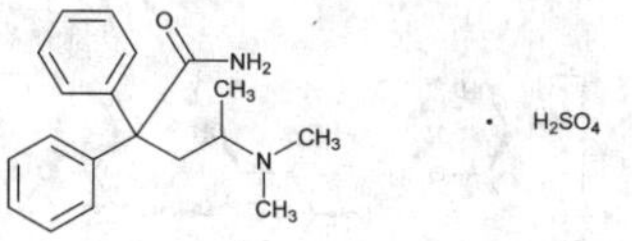

Aminophenazone (INN) — *See* Aminopyrine.

Aminophenazone Cyclamate. C₁₃H₁₇N₃O.C₆H₁₃NO₃S. 410.53. 4-Dimethylamino-2,3-dimethyl-1-phenyl-3-pyrazolin-5-one cyclohexylsulfamate. *UNII-RM5BP192F9. CAS-747-30-8.* INN.

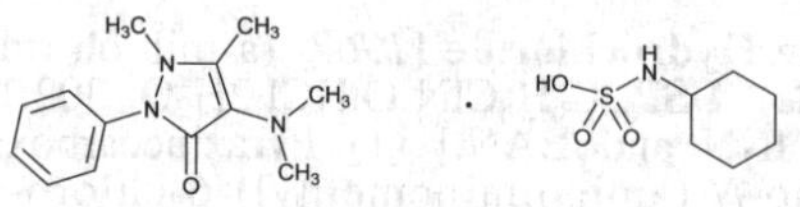

Aminophylline (am″ i nof′ i lin). **USP.** C₁₆H₂₄N₁₀O₄. 420.43. (1) 1*H*-Purine-2,6-dione, 3,7-dihydro-1,3-dimethyl-, compd. with 1,2-ethanediamine (2:1); (2) Theophylline compound with ethylenediamine (2:1). *UNII-27Y3KJK423; UNII-C229N9DX94* [aminophylline dihydrate]. *CAS-317-34-0; CAS-5897-66-5* [dihydrate]; *CAS-49746-06-7* [replaced]. INN; BAN; JAN. *Relaxant (smooth muscle).* Somophyllin (Fisons); Truphylline (G & W) [*Name previously used: Theophylline Ethylenediamine.*]

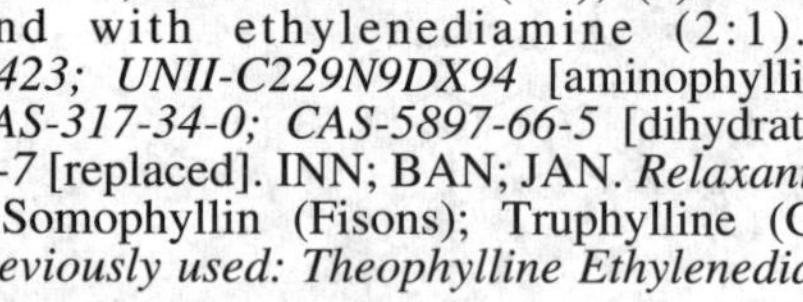

Aminopromazine. C₁₉H₂₅N₃S. 327.49. 10-[2,3-Bis(dimethylamino)propyl]phenothiazine. *UNII-S9SDD93U5U. CAS-58-37-7.* INN; BAN; DCF; MI. [*Name previously used: Proquamezine.*]

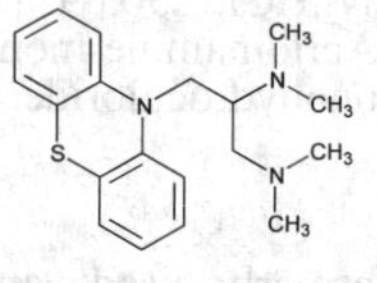

Aminopterin Sodium. $C_{19}H_{18}N_8Na_2O_5$. 484.38. Sodium salt of N-[p-[[(2,4-diamino-6-pteridinyl)methyl]amino]benzoyl]glutamic acid. *UNII-FZU1QI13O9. CAS-58602-66-7; CAS-54-62-6 [aminopterin].* INN; BAN; DCF. ◇*NSC-739 [as the base]*

Aminopyrine. $C_{13}H_{17}N_3O$. 231.29. [Aminophenazone is INN.] 4-Dimethylamino-2,3-dimethyl-1-phenyl-3-pyrazolin-5-one. *UNII-01704YP3MO. CAS-58-15-1.* NF X; JAN; MI. *[Name previously used: Amidopyrine.]*

Aminoquin Naphthoate — *See* Pamaquine Naphthoate.

Aminoquinol. $C_{26}H_{31}Cl_2N_3$. 456.45. 7-Chloro-2-(o-chlorostyryl)-4-[[4-(diethylamino)-1-methylbutyl]amino]quinoline. *UNII-CH1Y88E2AY. CAS-10023-54-8.* INN.

Aminoquinoline — *See* Aminoquinol.

Aminoquinuride. $C_{21}H_{20}N_6O$. 372.42. 1,3-Bis(4-amino-2-methyl-6-quinolyl)urea. *UNII-08T7936572. CAS-3811-56-1.* INN; MI.

Aminorex [*1963*] (a min′ oh rex). $C_9H_{10}N_2O$. 162.19. (1) 2-Oxazolamine, 4,5-dihydro-5-phenyl-; (2) 2-Amino-5-phenyl-2-oxazoline. *UNII-2SH16612I9. CAS-2207-50-3.* INN; BAN. *Anorexic.* Apiquel (Ortho-McNeil†) ◇*McN-742; NSC-66952*

Aminosalicylate Calcium. $C_{14}H_{12}CaN_2O_6.3H_2O$. 398.38. [Calcium Para-aminosalicylate is JAN.] (1) Benzoic acid, 4-amino-2-hydroxy-, calcium salt (2:1), trihydrate; (2) Calcium 4-aminosalicylate (1:2) trihydrate. *UNII-*

9VF16M7FWU. CAS-133-15-3 [anhydrous]; CAS-6059-16-1 [calcium 4-aminosalicylate]; CAS-65-49-6 [4-aminosalicylic acid]. USP XXI.

Aminosalicylate Potassium. $C_7H_6KNO_3$. 191.23. (1) Benzoic acid, 4-amino-2-hydroxy-, potassium salt (1:1); (2) Monopotassium 4-aminosalicylate. *UNII-7N21461LKD. CAS-133-09-5 [potassium 4-aminosalicylate]; CAS-65-49-6 [4-aminosalicylic acid].* USP XX.

Aminosalicylate Sodium (a mee″ noe sa lis′ i late soe′ dee um). **USP.** $C_7H_6NNaO_3.2H_2O$. 211.15. (1) Benzoic acid, 4-amino-2-hydroxy-, monosodium salt, dihydrate; (2) Monosodium 4-aminosalicylate dihydrate. *UNII-S38B9W6AXW. CAS-6018-19-5; CAS-133-10-8 [anhydrous]; CAS-65-49-6 [4-aminosalicylic acid]. Antibacterial (tuberculostatic).* Parasal Sodium (Panray); Teebacin (Consolidated Midland)

Aminosalicylic Acid (a mee″ noe sal i sil′ ik as′ id). **USP.** $C_7H_7NO_3$. 153.14. (1) Benzoic acid, 4-amino-2-hydroxy-; (2) 4-Aminosalicylic acid. *UNII-5B2658E0N2. CAS-65-49-6. Antibacterial (tuberculostatic).* Parasal (Panray); Paser (Jacobus)

Aminosalyle Sodium — *See* Aminosalicylate Sodium.

Aminosidine Sulfate — *See* Paromomycin Sulfate.

Aminothiazole. $C_3H_4N_2S$. 100.14. 2-Aminothiazole. *UNII-5K8WKN668K. CAS-96-50-4.* INN; MI. ◇*RP 2921*

Aminotrate Phosphate — *See* Trolnitrate Phosphate.

Aminoxaphen — *See* Aminorex.

Aminoxytriphene (INN) — *See* Amotriphene.

Aminoxytropine Tropate Hydrochloride — *See* Atropine Oxide Hydrochloride.

Amiodarone [*1987*] (a″ mi oh′ da rone). $C_{25}H_{29}I_2NO_3$. 645.31. [Amiodarone Hydrochloride is JAN.] (1) Methanone, (2-butyl-3-benzofuranyl)[4-[2-(diethylamino)ethoxy]-3,5-diiodophenyl]-; (2) 2-Butyl-3-benzofuranyl 4-[2-(diethylamino)ethoxy]-3,5-diiodophenyl ketone. *UNII-N3RQ532IUT. CAS-1951-25-3.* INN; BAN. *Cardiac depressant (anti-arrhythmic, ventricular).* Cordarone (Wyeth-Ayerst) ◇*L-3428; SKF 33134-A*

---

† Brand name formerly used, and/or firm no longer concerned with this product.

Amiperone. $C_{24}H_{28}ClFN_2O_2$. 430.94. 4-(*p*-Chlorophenyl)-1-[3-(*p*-fluorobenzoyl)propyl]-*N,N*-dimethylisonipecotamide. *UNII-FTX5V7543O. CAS-1580-71-8.* INN. ◇*R 2962*

Amiphenazole. $C_9H_9N_3S$. 191.25. 2,4-Diamino-5-phenylthiazole. *UNII-7ZJ8PWY0XD. CAS-490-55-1.* INN; BAN; MI.

Amipizone. $C_{14}H_{16}ClN_3O_2$. 293.75. 2-Chloro-4′-(1,4,5,6-tetrahydro-4-methyl-6-oxo-3-pyridazinyl)propionanilide. *UNII-7OT95Q2G4E. CAS-69635-63-8.* INN.

Amipramidine — *See* Amiloride Hydrochloride.

Amiprilose Hydrochloride [*1987*] (a″ mi pril′ ose hye″ droe klor′ ide). $C_{14}H_{27}NO_6$.HCl. 341.83. [Amiprilose is INN.] (1) α-D-Glucofuranose, 3-*O*-[3-(dimethylamino)propyl]-1,2-*O*-(1-methylethylidene)-, hydrochloride; (2) 3-*O*-[3-(Dimethylamino)propyl]-1,2-*O*-isopropylidene-α-D-glucofuranose hydrochloride. *UNII-546994B3VA; UNII-S0FG5X68QT* [amiprilose]. *CAS-60414-06-4; CAS-56824-20-5* [amiprilose]. *Anti-inflammatory.* Therafectin (Greenwich) ◇*SM-1213 (free base)*

Amiquinsin Hydrochloride [*1966*] (a″ mi kwin′ sin hye″ droe klor′ ide). $C_{11}H_{12}N_2O_2$.HCl.H₂O. 258.70. [Amiquinsin is INN.] (1) 4-Quinolinamine, 6,7-dimethoxy-, monohydrochloride, monohydrate; (2) 4-Amino-6,7-dimethoxyquinoline hydrochloride monohydrate. *UNII-EZ270U8Z9W. CAS-7125-70-4; CAS-1696-79-3* [anhydrous]; *CAS-13425-92-8* [amiquinsin]. *Antihypertensive.* ◇*U-935*

Amisometradine. $C_9H_{13}N_3O_2$. 195.22. 6-Amino-3-methyl-1-(2-methylallyl)-2,4(1*H*,3*H*)-pyrimidinedione. *UNII-30973N61ZF. CAS-550-28-7.* NF XI; INN; BAN; MI.

Amisulpride. $C_{17}H_{27}N_3O_4S$. 369.48. 4-Amino-*N*-[(1-ethyl-2-pyrrolidinyl)methyl]-5-(ethylsulfonyl)-*o*-anisamide. *CAS-71675-85-9.* INN; BAN; MI.

Amiterol. $C_{12}H_{20}N_2O$. 208.30. DL-*p*-Amino-α-[(*sec*-butylamino)methyl]benzyl alcohol. *UNII-W09SX84JTI. CAS-54063-25-1.* INN.

Amithiozone. $C_{10}H_{12}N_4OS$. 236.29. [Thioacetazone is INN and BAN.] 4′-Formylacetanilide thiosemicarbazone. *CAS-104-06-3.* MI. [*Name previously used: Thiacetazone.*]

Amitivir [*1991*] (a mit′ i vir). $C_3H_2N_4S$. 126.14. 1,3,4-Thiadiazole-2-carbamonitrile. *UNII-R4KR9A9165. CAS-111393-84-1.* INN.

Amitraz [*1981*] (a′ mi traz). **USP.** $C_{19}H_{23}N_3$. 293.41. (1) Methanimidamide, *N*′-(2,4-dimethylphenyl)-*N*-[[(2,4-dimethylphenyl)imino]methyl]-*N*-methyl-; (2) *N*-Methyl-*N*′-2,4-xylyl-*N*-(*N*-2,4-xylylformimidoyl)formamidine; (3) *N*-Methylbis(2,4-xylyliminomethyl)amine. *UNII-33IAH5017S. CAS-33089-61-1.* INN; BAN. *Scabicide.* ◇*U-36,059*

Amitriptyline Hydrochloride (am″ i trip′ ti leen hye″ droe klor′ ide). **USP.** $C_{20}H_{23}N$.HCl. 313.86. [Amitriptyline is INN and BAN.] (1) 1-Propanamine, 3-(10,11-dihydro-5*H*-dibenzo[*a,d*]cyclohepten-5-ylidene)-*N,N*-dimethyl-, hydrochloride; (2) 10,11-Dihydro-*N,N*-dimethyl-5*H*-dibenzo[*a,d*]cycloheptene-$\Delta^{5,\gamma}$-propylamine hydrochloride. *UNII-26LUD4JO9K; UNII-1806D8D52K* [amitriptyline].

CAS-549-18-8; CAS-50-48-6 [amitriptyline]. JAN. *Antidepressant*. Amitril (Warner Chilcott); Elavil (AstraZeneca); Endep (Roche)

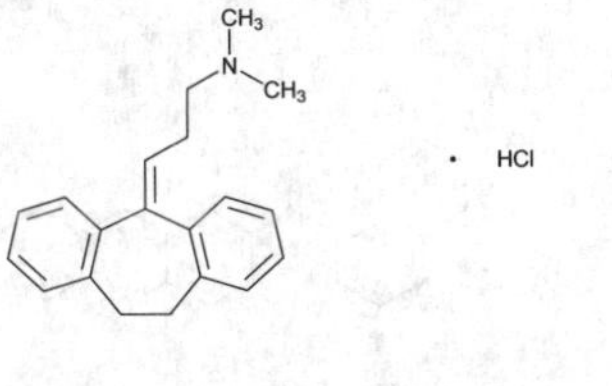

Amitriptylinoxide. $C_{20}H_{23}NO$. 293.40. 10,11-Dihydro-*N*,*N*-dimethyl-5*H*-dibenzo[*a*,*d*]cycloheptene-$\Delta^{5,\gamma}$-propylamine *N*-oxide. *UNII-TYR2U59WMA. CAS-4317-14-0*. INN; MI.

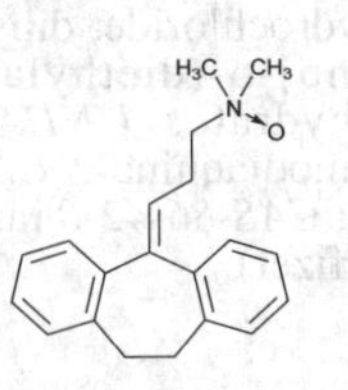

Amixetrine. $C_{17}H_{27}NO$. 261.40. 1-[β-(Isopentyloxy)phenethyl]pyrrolidine. *UNII-7UL287YTPJ. CAS-24622-72-8*. INN; DCF; MI.

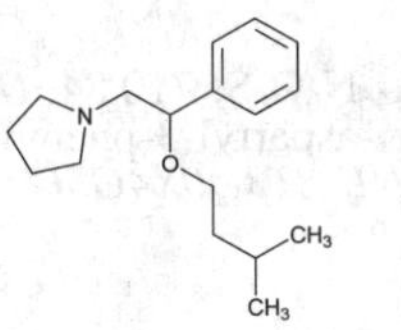

Amlexanox [*1995*] (am lex′ a nox). $C_{16}H_{14}N_2O_4$. 298.29. (1) 5*H*-[1]Benzopyrano[2,3-*b*]pyridine-3-carboxylic acid, 2-amino-7-(1-methylethyl)-5-oxo-; (2) 2-Amino-7-isopropyl-5-oxo-5*H*-[1]benzopyrano[2,3-*b*]pyridine-3-carboxylic acid. *UNII-BRL1C2459K. CAS-68302-57-8*. INN; BAN; JAN; MI. *Anti-allergic*. Aphthasol (Uluru) ◇*AA-673; CHX 3673*

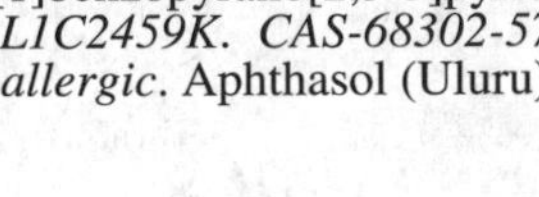

Amlintide [*1996*] (am′ lin tide). $C_{165}H_{261}N_{51}O_{55}S_2$. 3903.28. (1) L-Tyrosinamide, L-lysyl-L-cysteinyl-L-asparaginyl-L-threonyl-L-alanyl-L-threonyl-L-cysteinyl-L-alanyl-L-threonyl-L-glutaminyl-L-arginyl-L-leucyl-L-alanyl-L-asparaginyl-L-phenylalanyl-L-leucyl-L-valyl-L-histidyl-L-seryl-L-seryl-L-asparaginyl-L-asparaginyl-L-phenylalanylglycyl-L-alanyl-L-isoleucyl-L-leucyl-L-seryl-L-seryl-L-threonyl-L-asparaginyl-L-valylglycyl-L-seryl-L-asparaginyl-L-threonyl-, cyclic (2→7)-disulfide; (2) L-Lysyl-L-cysteinyl-L-asparaginyl-L-threonyl-L-alanyl-L-threonyl-L-cysteinyl-L-alanyl-L-threonyl-L-glutaminyl-L-arginyl-L-leucyl-L-alanyl-L-asparaginyl-L-phenylalanyl-L-leucyl-L-valyl-L-histidyl-L-seryl-L-seryl-L-asparaginyl-L-asparaginyl-L-phenylalanylglycyl-L-alanyl-L-isoleucyl-L-leucyl-L-seryl-L-seryl-

L-threonyl-L-asparaginyl-L-valylglycyl-L-seryl-L-asparaginyl-L-threonyl-L-tyrosinamide, cyclic (2→7)-disulfide. *CAS-122384-88-7*. INN. *Antidiabetic*. ◇*AC001*

KCNTATCATQ RLANFLVHSS NNFGAILSST NVGSNTY —NH₂

Amlodipine Besylate [*1988*] (am loe′ di peen bes′ i late). **USP.** $C_{20}H_{25}ClN_2O_5 \cdot C_6H_6O_3S$. 567.05. [Amlodipine is INN and BAN; Amlodipine Besilate is JAN.] (1) 3,5-Pyridinedicarboxylic acid, 2-[(2-aminoethoxy)methyl]-4-(2-chlorophenyl)-1,4-dihydro-6-methyl-, 3-ethyl 5-methyl ester, (±)-, monobenzenesulfonate; (2) 3-Ethyl 5-methyl (±)-2-[(2-aminoethoxy)methyl]-4-(*o*-chlorophenyl)-1,4-dihydro-6-methyl-3,5-pyridinedicarboxylate, monobenzenesulfonate. *UNII-864V2Q084H; UNII-1J444QC288* [amlodipine]. *CAS-111470-99-6; CAS-88150-42-9* [amlodipine]. *Anti-anginal; antihypertensive*. Norvasc (Pfizer) ◇*UK-48,340-26*

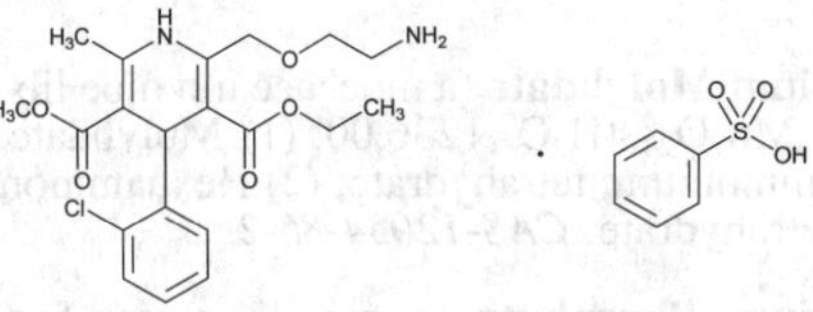

Amlodipine Maleate [*1986*] (am loe′ di peen mal′ ee ate). $C_{20}H_{25}ClN_2O_5 \cdot C_4H_4O_4$. 524.95. (1) 3,5-Pyridinedicarboxylic acid, 2-[(2-aminoethoxy)methyl]-4-(2-chlorophenyl)-1,4-dihydro-6-methyl-, 3-ethyl 5-methyl ester, (±)-, (*Z*)-2-butenedioate (1:1); (2) 3-Ethyl 5-methyl (±)-2-[(2-aminoethoxy)methyl]-4-(*o*-chlorophenyl)-1,4-dihydro-6-methyl-3,5-pyridinedicarboxylate, maleate (1:1). *UNII-CQ27G2BZJM. CAS-88150-47-4. Anti-anginal; antihypertensive*. Amvaz (Dr. Reddy's) ◇*UK-48,340-11*

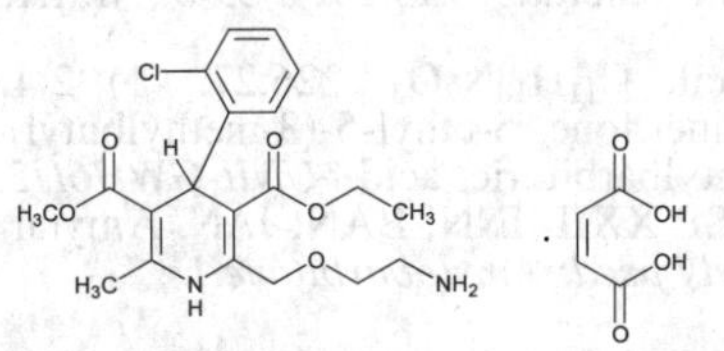

Ammonia N 13 [*1990*] (a mone′ ya). **USP** [Injection]. $H_3{}^{13}N$. (1) Ammonia-^{13}N; (2) [^{13}N]Ammonia. *UNII-9OQO0E343Z. CAS-34819-78-8. Diagnostic aid (cardiac imaging); diagnostic aid (liver imaging); radioactive agent. [Note—This radiopharmaceutical, labeled with a cyclotron-generated radionuclide, is prepared in individual nuclear medical centers.]*

Ammonia Solution, Strong (a mone′ ya). **NF.** NH_3. 17.03. [Ammonia Water is JAN.] A solution containing 29.0 ± 2.0% NH_3 by weight. *CAS-7664-41-7. Pharmaceutic aid (solvent and source of ammonia)*.

Ammonia Water (JAN) — *See* Ammonia Solution, Strong.

Ammonio Methacrylate Copolymer (a moe′ nee oh meth ak′ ri late koe pol′ i mer). **NF.** A fully polymerized copolymer of acrylic and methacrylic acid esters with a low content of quaternary ammonium groups having two types, A and B. *Pharmaceutic aid (coating agent)*.

Ammonium Benzoate. *UNII-AC80WD7GPF. CAS-1863-63-4*. USP XI; MI.

Ammonium Carbonate (a moe′ nee um kar′ bo nate). **NF.** (1) Carbonic acid, monoammonium salt, mixt. with ammonium carbamate; (2) Monoammonium carbonate mixture with ammonium carbamate. *CAS-8000-73-5. Pharmaceutic aid (source of ammonia)*.

---

† Brand name formerly used, and/or firm no longer concerned with this product.

Ammonium Chloride (a moe′ nee um klor′ ide). **USP.** NH₄Cl. 53.49. (1) Ammonium chloride; (2) Ammonium chloride. *UNII-01Q9PC255D. CAS-12125-02-9.* JAN. *Acidifier; diuretic.*

Ammonium Ichthosulfonate — *See* Ichthammol.

Ammonium Lactate [*1994*] (a moe′ nee um lak′ tate). C₃H₉NO₃. 107.11. (1) Propanoic acid, 2-hydroxy-, mono-ammonium salt, (±)-; (2) Ammonium (±)-lactate. *UNII-67M901L9NQ. CAS-52003-58-4. Antipruritic (topical).* ◇*BMS-186091*

Ammonium Mandelate. *UNII-NH496X0UJX* [mandelic acid]. *CAS-530-31-4; CAS-90-64-2* [mandelic acid]. USP XIV; MI.

Ammonium Molybdate (a moe′ nee um moe lib′ date). **USP.** (NH₄)₆Mo₇O₂₄.4H₂O. 1236.00. (1) Molybdate (Mo₇O₂₄⁶⁻), hexaammonium, tetrahydrate; (2) Hexaammonium molybdate tetrahydrate. *CAS-12054-85-2.*

Ammonium Phosphate (a moe′ nee um fos′ fate). **NF.** (NH₄)₂HPO₄. 132.06. (1) Phosphoric acid, diammonium salt; (2) Diammonium phosphate. *UNII-10LGE70FSU. CAS-7783-28-0. Pharmaceutic aid.*

Ammonium Salicylate. *UNII-0T3Q181657. CAS-528-94-9.* NF X; MI.

Ammonium Sulfate (a moe′ nee um sul′ fate). **NF.** (NH₄)₂SO₄. 132.14. Ammonium sulfate. *UNII-SU46B-AM238. CAS-7783-20-2.*

Ammonium Valerate. *CAS-5972-85-0.* NF IX; MI.

Amobarbital. C₁₁H₁₈N₂O₃. 226.27. (1) 2,4,6(1*H*,3*H*,5*H*)-Pyrimidinetrione, 5-ethyl-5-(3-methylbutyl)-; (2) 5-Ethyl-5-isopentylbarbituric acid. *UNII-GWH6IJ239E. CAS-57-43-2.* USP XXII; INN; BAN; JAN. Amytal (Lilly) [*Name previously used: Amylobarbitone.*]

Amobarbital Sodium (am″ oh bar′ bi tal soe′ dee um). **USP.** C₁₁H₁₇N₂NaO₃. 248.25. [Amobarbital Sodium for Injection is JAN.] (1) 2,4,6(1*H*,3*H*,5*H*)-Pyrimidinetrione, 5-ethyl-5-(3-methylbutyl)-, monosodium salt; (2) Sodium 5-ethyl-5-isopentylbarbiturate. *UNII-G0313KNC7D; UNII-GWH6IJ239E* [amobarbital]. *CAS-64-43-7; CAS-57-43-2* [amobarbital]. *Sedative-hypnotic.* Amytal Sodium (Lilly); Talamo (Marion Merrell Dow†)

Amocaine Chloride — *See* Amolanone Hydrochloride.

Amocarzine. C₁₈H₂₁N₅O₂S. 371.46. 4-Methyl-4′-(*p*-nitroanilino)thio-1-piperazinecarboxanilide. *UNII-99807U412Y. CAS-36590-19-9.* INN.

Amodiaquine (am″ oh dye′ a kwin). **USP.** C₂₀H₂₂ClN₃O. 355.86. (1) Phenol, 4-[(7-chloro-4-quinolinyl)amino]-2-[(diethylamino)methyl]-; (2) 4-[(7-Chloro-4-quinolyl)amino]-α-(diethylamino)-*o*-cresol. *UNII-220236ED28. CAS-86-42-0.* INN; BAN. *Antiprotozoal.*

Amodiaquine Hydrochloride (am″ oh dye′ a kwin hye″ droe klor′ ide). **USP.** C₂₀H₂₂ClN₃O.2HCl.2H₂O. 464.81. (1) Phenol, 4-[(7-chloro-4-quinolinyl)amino]-2-[(diethylamino)methyl]-, dihydrochloride, dihydrate; (2) 4-[(7-Chloro-4-quinolyl)amino]-α-(diethylamino)-*o*-cresol dihydrochloride dihydrate. *UNII-K6PW2S574L; UNII-220236ED28* [amodiaquine]. *CAS-6398-98-7; CAS-69-44-3* [anhydrous]; *CAS-86-42-0* [amodiaquine]. *Antimalarial.* Camoquin (Pfizer)

Amogastrin. C₃₅H₄₆N₆O₈S. 710.84. *N*-Carboxy-L-tryptophyl-L-methionyl-L-α-aspartyl-3-phenyl-L-alaninamide *N-tert*-pentyl ester. *UNII-8T3Q0X4G5G. CAS-16870-37-4.* INN; JAN.

Amolanone Hydrochloride. C₂₀H₂₃NO₂.HCl. 345.86. [Amolanone is INN.] 3-[2-(Diethylamino)ethyl]-3-phenyl-2(3*H*)-benzofuranone hydrochloride. *UNII-M36927R46E; UNII-1ALL724WB1* [amolanone]. *CAS-6009-67-2; CAS-76-65-3* [amolanone]. NND 1964; MI. Amethone Hydrochloride (Abbott†)

Amolimogene Bepiplasmid [*2006*] (am″ oh lim′ oh jeen bep″ i plas′ mid). (1) DNA (synthetic plasmid p3kDRαHPV16-18); (2) Bacterially derived DNA and microparticles made of poly(D,L-lactide-co-glydolide). *CAS-870524-46-2.* INN. *Treatment of HPV-mediated disease.* ◇*ZYC101a*

Amonafide. $C_{16}H_{17}N_3O_2$. 283.33. 3-Amino-*N*-[2-(dimethylamino)ethyl]naphthalimide. *UNII-1Q8D39N37L.* *CAS-69408-81-7.* INN.

Amoproxan. $C_{22}H_{35}NO_7$. 425.52. α-(Isopentyloxymethyl)-4-morpholineethanol 3,4,5-trimethoxybenzoate (ester). *UNII-27RL57FCYM.* *CAS-22661-76-3.* INN; DCF; MI. ◇*CERM 730*

Amopyroquine. $C_{20}H_{20}ClN_5$. 365.86. 4-[(7-Chloro-4-quinolyl)amino]-α-1-pyrrolidinyl-*o*-cresol. *UNII-SV6L22Y9QF.* *CAS-550-81-2.* INN.

Amorolfine [*1990*] (a moe′ role feen). $C_{21}H_{35}NO$. 317.51. [Amorolfine Hydrochloride is JAN.] (1) Morpholine, 4-[3-[4-(1,1-dimethylpropyl)phenyl]-2-methylpropyl]-2,6-dimethyl-, *cis*-, (±)-; (2) (±)-*cis*-2,6-Dimethyl-4-[2-methyl-3-(*p-tert*-pentylphenyl)propyl]morpholine. *CAS-78613-35-1; CAS-78613-38-4* [hydrochloride]. INN; BAN. *Antimycotic.* Loceryl (Hoffmann-LaRoche) ◇*Ro 14-4767/000*

Amoscanate. $C_{13}H_9N_3O_2S$. 271.29. *p*-(*p*-Nitroanilino)phenyl isothiocyanate. *CAS-26328-53-0.* INN; MI.

Amosulalol. $C_{18}H_{24}N_2O_5S$. 380.46. [Amosulalol Hydrochloride is JAN.] (±)-5-[1-Hydroxy-2-[[2-(*o*-methoxyphenoxy)ethyl]amino]ethyl]-*o*-toluenesulfonamide. *UNII-C69JI1BAU8.* *CAS-85320-68-9.* INN; MI.

Amotosalen Hydrochloride [*2001*] (a″ moe toe′ sa len hye″ droe klor′ ide). $C_{17}H_{19}NO_4.HCl$. 337.80. [Amotosalen is INN.] (1) 7*H*-Furo[3,2-*g*][1]benzopyran-7-one, 3-[(2-aminoethoxy)methyl]-2,5,9-trimethyl-, hydrochloride; (2) 3-[(2-Aminoethoxy)methyl]-2,5,9-trimethyl-7*H*-furo[3,2-*g*][1]benzopyran-7-one hydrochloride. *UNII-67B255SI5F; UNII-K1LDZ0VBC0* [amotosalen]. *CAS-161262-29-9; CAS-161262-29-9* [amotosalen]. INN. *Photochemical treatment (light-activated psoralen derivative intended for use in the inactivation of viruses, bacteria, and leukocytes in platelet concentrates and fresh frozen plasma in blood bank settings).* ◇*S-59*

Amotriphene. $C_{26}H_{29}NO_3$. 403.51. [Aminoxytriphene is INN.] 2,3,3-Tris(*p*-methoxyphenyl)-*N,N*-dimethylallylamine. *CAS-5585-64-8.* MI. Myordil (Sterling Winthrop†)

Amoxapine [*1971*] (a mox′ a peen). **USP.** $C_{17}H_{16}ClN_3O$. 313.78. (1) Dibenz[*b,f*][1,4]oxazepine, 2-chloro-11-(1-piperazinyl)-; (2) 2-Chloro-11-(1-piperazinyl)dibenz[*b,-f*][1,4]oxazepine. *UNII-R63VQ857OT.* *CAS-14028-44-5.* INN; BAN; JAN. *Antidepressant.* Asendin (Lederle) ◇*CL 67,772*

Amoxecaine. $C_{17}H_{29}N_3O_2$. 307.43. 2-[(2-Diethylaminoethyl)ethylamino]ethyl *p*-aminobenzoate. *UNII-4N3QA02VE5.* *CAS-553-65-1.* INN; DCF.

Amoxicillin [*1972*] (a mox″ i sil′ in). **USP.** $C_{16}H_{19}N_3O_5S.3H_2O$. 419.45. [Amoxicilline is INN.] (1) 4-Thia-1-azabicyclo[3.2.0]heptane-2-carboxylic acid, 6-[[amino(4-hydroxyphenyl)acetyl]amino]-3,3-dimethyl-7-oxo-, trihydrate[2*S*-[2α,5α,6β(*S**)]]-; (2) (2*S*,5*R*,6*R*)-6-[(*R*)-(-)-2-Amino-2-(*p*-hydroxyphenyl)acetamido]-3,3-dimethyl-7-oxo-4-thia-1-azabicyclo[3.2.0]heptane-2-carboxylic acid trihydrate. *UNII-804826J2HU.* *CAS-61336-70-7; CAS-26787-78-0* [anhydrous]. BAN; JAN. *Antibac-*

terial. Amoxil (GlaxoSmithKline); Dispermox (Ranbaxy); Larotid (GlaxoSmithKline); Trimox (Apothecon) *[Name previously used: Amoxycillin.]* ◇BRL 2333

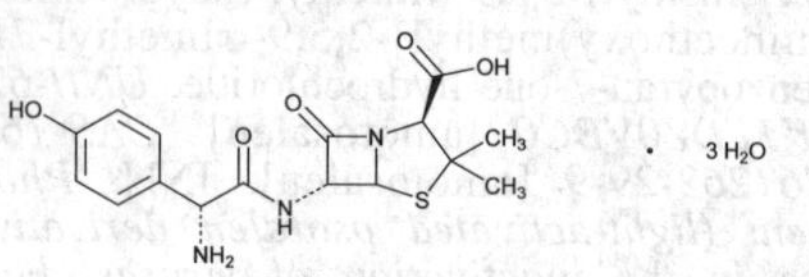

Amoxicillin Sodium *[1998]* (a mox″ i sil′ in soe′ dee um). $C_{16}H_{18}N_3NaO_5S$. 387.39. (1) [2S-[2α,5α.6β(S*)]]-6-[[Amino(4-hydroxyphenyl)acetyl]amino]-3,3-dimethyl-7-oxo-4-thia-1-azabicyclo[3.2.0]heptane-2-carboxylic acid monosodium salt; (2) Monosodium (-)-(2S,5R,6R)-6-[(R)-2-amino-2-(p-hydroxyphenyl)acetamido]-3,3-dimethyl-7-oxo-4-thia-1-azabicyclo[3.2.0]heptane-2-carboxylate. *UNII-544Y3D6MYH. CAS-34642-77-8. Antibiotic.[Note— Amoxicillin sodium will be used in combination with clavulanate potassium and marketed as "Augmentin for intravenous administration."]* ◇BRL-2333AB-B

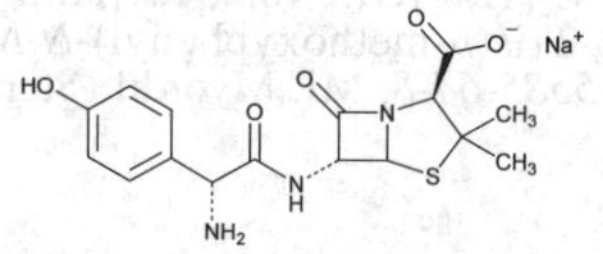

Amoxicilline (INN) — *See* Amoxicillin.

Amoxycillin (previously used name) — *See* Amoxicillin.

Amoxydramine Camsilate. $C_{27}H_{37}NO_6S$. 503.65. 2-(Diphenylmethoxy)-*N,N*-dimethylethylamine-*N*-oxide 2-oxo-10-bornanesulfonate. *UNII-3L1FU2EO79. CAS-15350-99-9.* INN.

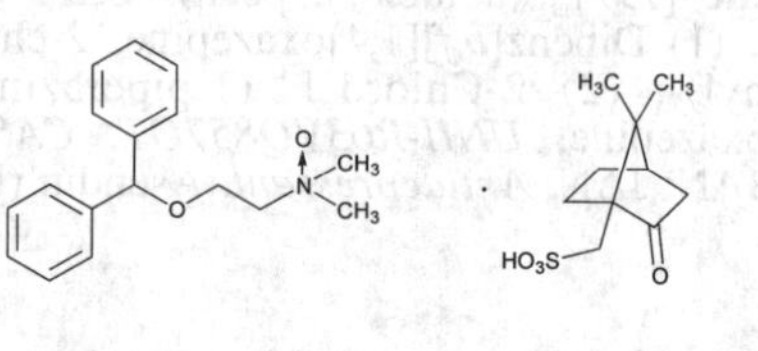

Amoxydramine Camsylate (DCF) — *See* Amoxydramine Camsilate.

Amperozide. $C_{23}H_{29}F_2N_3O$. 401.49. 4-[4,4-Bis(p-fluorophenyl)butyl]-*N*-ethyl-1-piperazinecarboxamide. *UNII-0M2W3TAG39; UNII-8V2171U69N* [amperozide hydrochloride]. *CAS-75558-90-6; CAS-75529-73-6* [hydrochloride]. INN; BAN; MI.

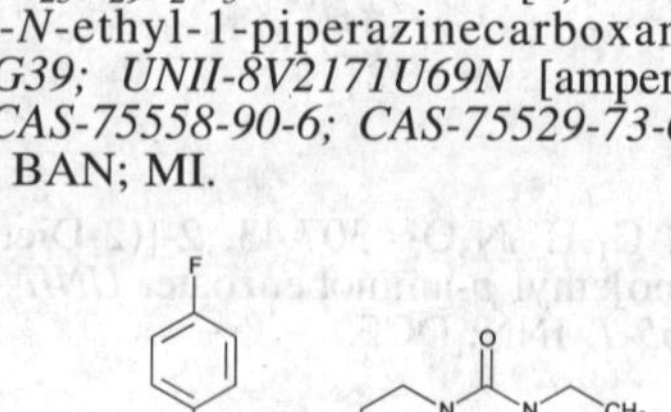

Amphecloral *[1961]* (am fe klor′ al). $C_{11}H_{12}Cl_3N$. 264.58. [Amfecloral is INN and BAN.] (1) Benzeneethanamine, α-methyl-*N*-(2,2,2-trichloroethylidene)-; (2) α-Methyl-*N*-(2,2,2-trichloroethylidene)phenethylamine. *CAS-5581-35-1. Anorexic.*

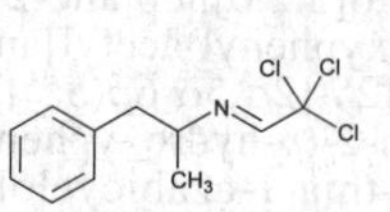

Amphenidone. $C_{11}H_{10}N_2O$. 186.21. 1-(*m*-Aminophenyl)-2[1*H*]-pyridone. *UNII-M61FM2VCSV. CAS-134-37-2.* INN; MI.

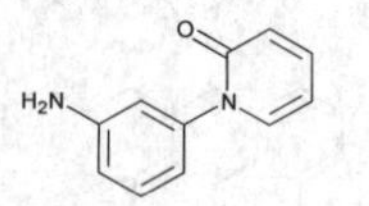

Amphetamine Sulfate (am fet′ a meen sul′ fate). **USP**. $(C_9H_{13}N)_2.H_2SO_4$. 368.49. [Amfetamine is INN and BAN.] (1) Benzeneethanamine, α-methyl-, sulfate (2:1), (±)-; (2) (±)-α-Methylphenethylamine sulfate (2:1). *UNII-6DPV8NK46S; UNII-CK833KGX7E* [amphetamine]. *CAS-60-13-9; CAS-300-62-9* [amphetamine]. *Stimulant (central)*. Benzadrine (GlaxoSmithKline)

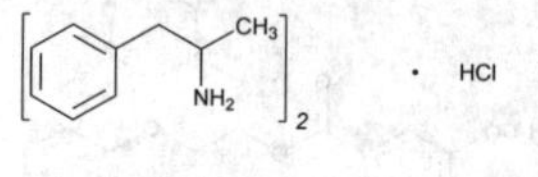

Amphetamine Sulfate, Dextro — *See* Dextroamphetamine Sulfate.

Amphomycin *[1964]* (am″ foe mye′ sin). [Amfomycin is INN.] A substance produced by *Streptomyces canus*. (1) Amphomycin; (2) Amphomycin. *UNII-4P63B997RT. CAS-1402-82-0.* BAN. *Antibacterial.*

Amphotalide. $C_{19}H_{20}N_2O_3$. 324.37. *N*-[5-(*p*-Aminophenoxy)-pentyl]phthalimide. *UNII-95818EH730. CAS-1673-06-9.* INN; DCF; MI.

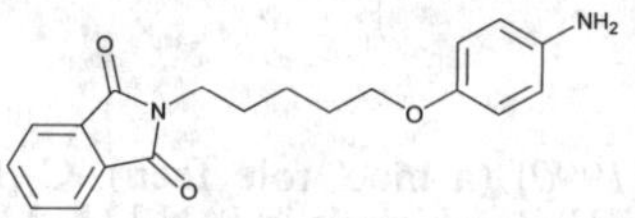

Amphotericin B (am″ foe ter′ i sin). **USP**. $C_{47}H_{73}NO_{17}$. 924.08. [Amphotericin is BAN.] (1) Amphotericin B; (2) Amphotericin B; (3) [1*R*-(1*R*,3*S*,5*R*,6*R*,9*R*,11*R*,15*S*,16*R*,17*R*,18*S*,19-*,3*S*,5*R*,6*R*,9*R*,11*R*,15*S*,16*R*,17*R*,18*S*,19*E*,21-*E*,23*E*,25*E*,27*E*,29*E*,31*E*,33*R*,35*S*,36*R*,37*S*)]]-33-[(3-Amino-3,6-dideoxy-β-D-mannopyranosyl)oxy]-1,3,5,6,9,11,17,37-octahydroxy-15,16,18-trimethyl-13-oxo-14,39-dioxabicyclo[33.3.1]nonatriaconta-19,21,23,25,27,29,31-heptaene-36-carboxylic acid. *UNII-7XU7A7DROE. CAS-1397-89-3.* INN; JAN. *Antifungal.* Abelcet (Enzon); Ambisome (Astellas); Amphotec (Three Rivers); Fungizone (Apothecon)

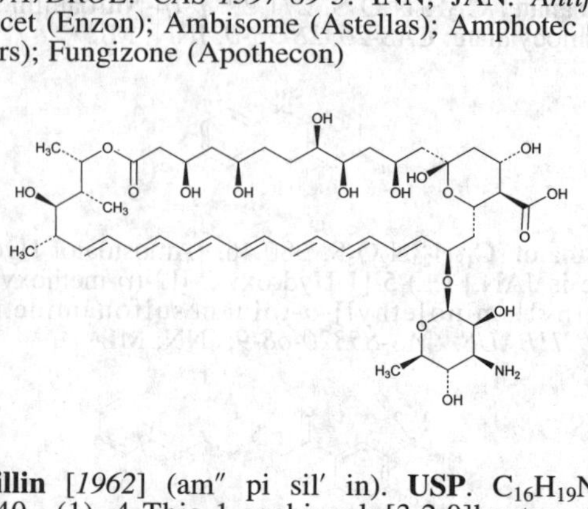

Ampicillin *[1962]* (am″ pi sil′ in). **USP**. $C_{16}H_{19}N_3O_4S$. 349.40. (1) 4-Thia-1-azabicyclo[3.2.0]heptane-2-carboxylic acid, 6-[(aminophenylacetyl)amino]-3,3-dimethyl-7-oxo-, [2S-[2α,5α,6β(S*)]]-; (2) (2S,5R,6R)-6-[(R)-2-Amino-2-phenylacetamido]-3,3-dimethyl-7-oxo-4-thia-1-azabicyclo[3.2.0]heptane-2-carboxylic acid. *UNII-7C782967RD. CAS-69-53-4; CAS-7177-48-2* [trihydrate]. INN; BAN; JAN. *Antibacterial.* Amcill (Parke-Davis†);

Omnipen (Wyeth-Ayerst); Polycillin (Apothecon†); Principen (Apothecon) ◇*BRL-1341; P-50; AY-6108; NSC-528986*

Ampicillin Sodium [*1966*] (am″ pi sil′ in soe′ dee um). **USP.** $C_{16}H_{18}N_3NaO_4S$. 371.39. (1) 4-Thia-1-azabicyclo[3.2.0]-heptane-2-carboxylic acid, 6-[(aminophenylacetyl)amino]-3,3-dimethyl-7-oxo-, monosodium salt, [2*S*-[2α,5α,6β(*S**)]]-; (2) Monosodium D-(-)-6-(2-amino-2-phenylacetamido)-3,3-dimethyl-7-oxo-4-thia-1-azabicyclo[3.2.0]heptane-2-carboxylate. *UNII-JFN36L5S8K. CAS-69-52-3.* JAN. *Antibacterial.* Omnipen (Wyeth); Penbritin (Wyeth); Polycillin (Bristol-Myers Squibb); Totacillin (GlaxoSmithKline); Principen (Apothecon)

Ampiroxicam. $C_{20}H_{21}N_3O_7S$. 447.46. (±)-4-(1-Hydroxyethoxy)-2-methyl-*N*-2-pyridyl-2*H*-1,2-benzothiazine-3-carboxamide ethyl carbonate (ester), 1,1-dioxide. *UNII-0PV32JZB1J. CAS-99464-64-9.* INN; BAN; JAN. ◇*CP-65703*

Amprenavir [*1997*] (am pren′ a vir). $C_{25}H_{35}N_3O_6S$. 505.63. (1) [3*S*-[3*R**(1*R**,2*S**)]]-[3-[[(4-Aminophenyl)sulfonyl](2-methylpropyl)amino]-2-hydroxy-1-(phenylmethyl)propyl] tetrahydro-3-furanyl carbamate; (2) (3*S*)-Tetrahydro-3-furyl [(α*S*)-α-[(1*R*-1-hydroxy-2-(*N*¹-isobutylsulfanilamido)ethyl]phenethyl]carbamate. *UNII-5S0W860XNR. CAS-161814-49-9.* INN; BAN. *Antiviral (HIV protease inhibitor).* Agenerase (GlaxoSmithKline) ◇*VX-478; 141W94; KVX-478*

Amprocidum — *See* Amprolium.

Amprolium (am proe′ lee um). **USP.** $C_{14}H_{19}ClN_4 \cdot HCl$. 315.24. (1) 1-[(4-Amino-2-propyl-5-pyrimidinyl)methyl]-2-methylpyridinium chloride monohydrochloride; (2) 1-[(4-Amino-2-propyl-5-pyrimidinyl)methyl]-2-picolinium chloride monohydrochloride. *UNII-95CO6N199Q. CAS-*

---

† Brand name formerly used, and/or firm no longer concerned with this product.

121-25-5. INN; BAN. *Coccidiostat (for poultry).* Amprol [Veterinary] (Merial); Amprovine [Veterinary] (Merial); Corid [Veterinary] (Merial)

Amprotropine Phosphate. *UNII-6831EK981Y. CAS-134-53-2; CAS-148-32-3* [amprotropine]. MI.

Ampyrimine. $C_{12}H_{11}N_7$. 253.26. 2,4,7-Triamino-5-phenylpyrimido[4,5-*d*]pyrimidine. *CAS-5587-93-9.* INN. ◇*SKF 13338*

Ampyzine Sulfate [*1966*] (am′ pi zeen sul′ fate). $C_6H_9N_3 \cdot H_2SO_4$. 221.23. [Ampyzine is INN.] (1) Pyrazinamine, *N,N*-dimethyl-, sulfate (1:1); (2) (Dimethylamino)pyrazine sulfate (1:1). *UNII-B8L03Q9MME. CAS-7082-29-3; CAS-5214-29-9* [ampyzine]. *Stimulant (central).* ◇*W 3580B*

Amquinate [*1968*] (am kwin′ ate). $C_{18}H_{24}N_2O_3$. 316.39. (1) 3-Quinolinecarboxylic acid 7-(diethylamino)-4-hydroxy-6-propyl-, methyl ester; (2) Methyl 7-(diethylamino)-4-hydroxy-6-propyl-3-quinolinecarboxylate. *CAS-17230-85-2.* INN. *Antimalarial.*

Amrinone (previously used name) — *See* Inamrinone.

Amrubicin [*2007*] (am roo′ bi sin). $C_{25}H_{25}NO_9$. 483.47. (1) 5,12-Naphthacenedione, 9-acetyl-9-amino-7-[(2-deoxy-β-D-*erythro*-pentopyranosyl)oxy]-7,8,9,10-tetrahydro-6,11-dihydroxy-, (7*S*,9*S*)-; (2) (+)-(7*S*,9*S*)-9-Acetyl-9-amino-7-[(2-deoxy-β-D-*erythro*-pentopyranosyl)oxy]-6,11-dihydroxy-7,8,9,10-tetrahydrotetracene-5,12-dione. *UNII-93N13LB4Z2. CAS-110267-81-7.* INN. *Antineoplastic.*

Amrubicin Hydrochloride [*2007*] (am roo′ bi sin hye″ droe klor′ ide). $C_{25}H_{25}NO_9 \cdot HCl$. 519.93. (1) 5,12-Naphthacenedione, 9-acetyl-9-amino-7-[(2-deoxy-β-D-*erythro*-pentopyranosyl)oxy]-7,8,9,10-tetrahydro-6,11-dihydroxy-, hydrochloride, (7*S*,9*S*)-; (2) (+)-(7*S*,9*S*)-9-Acetyl-9-amino-7-

[(2-deoxy-β-D-*erythro*-pentopyranosyl)oxy]-6,11-dihydroxy-7,8,9,10-tetrahydrotetracene-5,12-dione hydrochloride. *CAS-110311-30-3. Antineoplastic.* Calsed (Pharmion) ◇*SM-5887*

Amsacrine [*1980*] (am′ sa kreen). $C_{21}H_{19}N_3O_3S$. 393.46. (1) Methanesulfonamide, *N*-[4-(9-acridinylamino)-3-methoxyphenyl]-; (2) 4′-(9-Acridinylamino)methanesulfon-*m*-anisidide. *UNII-00DPD30SOY. CAS-51264-14-3.* INN; BAN. *Antineoplastic.* Amsidyl (Parke-Davis†) ◇*CI-880; m-AMSA; NSC-249992*

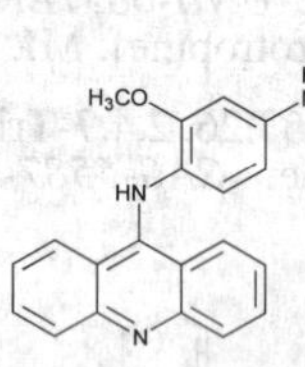

Amsilarotene. $C_{20}H_{27}NO_3Si_2$. 385.60. 4-[3,5-Bis(trimethylsilyl)benzamido]benzoic acid. *CAS-125973-56-0.* INN.

Amtolmetin Guacil. $C_{24}H_{24}N_2O_5$. 420.46. *N*-[(1-Methyl-5-*p*-toluoylpyrrol-2-yl)acetyl]glycine *o*-methoxyphenyl ester. *UNII-323A00CRO9. CAS-87344-06-7.* INN.

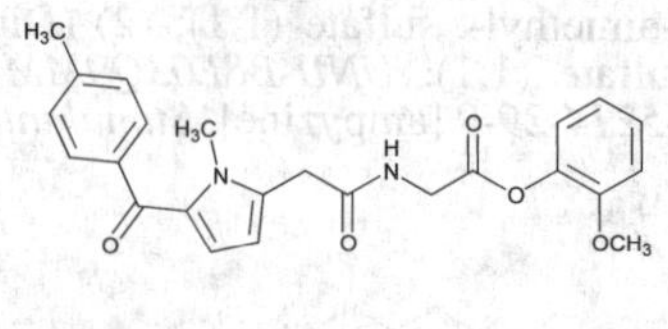

Amustaline Dihydrochloride [*2004*] (ay mus′ ta leen dye hye″ droe klor′ ide). $C_{22}H_{25}Cl_2N_3O_2 \cdot 2HCl$. 507.28. (1) β-Alanine, *N*-9-acridinyl-, 2-[bis(2-chloroethyl)amino]ethyl ester, dihydrochloride; (2) 2-[Bis(2-chloroethyl)amino]ethyl 3-(acridin-9-ylamino)propanoate dihydrochloride. *UNII-C5MKX7XOYA. CAS-210584-54-6. Ex-vivo blood bank process for inactivation of viruses, bacteria, parasites, and leukocytes in red blood cells (nucleic acid alkylator).* ◇*S-303.2HCl*

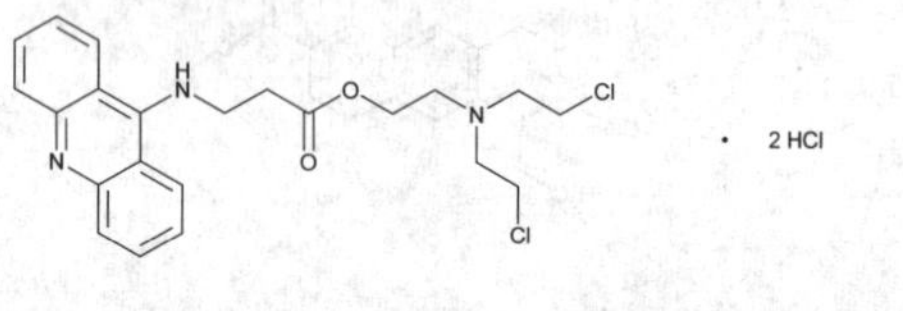

Amyl Nitrite (a′ mil nye′ trite). **USP.** $C_5H_{11}NO_2$. 117.15. A mixture of nitrous acid, 2-methylbutyl ester, and nitrous acid, 3-methylbutyl ester. *CAS-110-46-3; CAS-8017-89-8* [mixture]. JAN. *Vasodilator.*

Amylene Hydrate (am′ i leen hye′ drate). **NF.** $C_5H_{12}O$. 88.15. (1) 2-Butanol, 2-methyl-; (2) *tert*-Pentyl alcohol. *CAS-75-85-4. Pharmaceutic aid (solvent).*

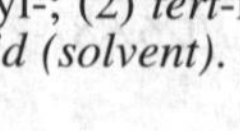

Amylin — *See* Amlintide.

Amylmetacresol. $C_{12}H_{18}O$. 178.27. 6-Pentyl-*m*-cresol. *CAS-1300-94-3.* INN; BAN.

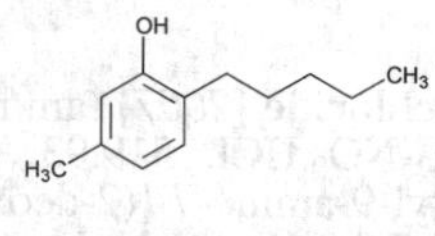

Amylobarbitone (previously used name) — *See* Amobarbital.

Amylocaine. 1-(Dimethylaminomethyl)-1-methylpropyl benzoate. *UNII-QRW683O56T. CAS-644-26-8.* BAN.

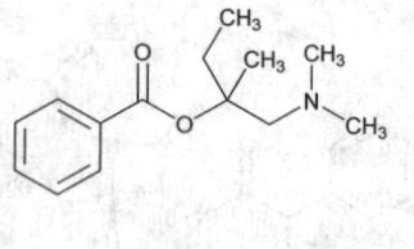

Anacetrapib [*2007*] (a″ na set′ ra pib). $C_{30}H_{25}F_{10}NO_3$. 637.51. (1) 2-Oxazolidinone, 5-[3,5-bis(trifluoromethyl)phenyl]-3-[[4′-fluoro-2′-methoxy-5′-(1-methylethyl)-4-(trifluoromethyl)[1,1′-biphenyl]-2-yl]methyl]-4-methyl-, (4*S*,5*R*)-; (2) (4*S*,5*R*)-5-[3,5-Bis(trifluoromethyl)phenyl]-3-{[4′-fluoro-2′-methoxy-5′-(propan-2-yl)-4-(trifluoromethyl)[1,1′-biphenyl]-2-yl]methyl}-4-methyl-1,3-oxazolidin-2-one. *UNII-P7T269PR6S. CAS-875446-37-0.* INN. *Treatment of atherosclerosis.*

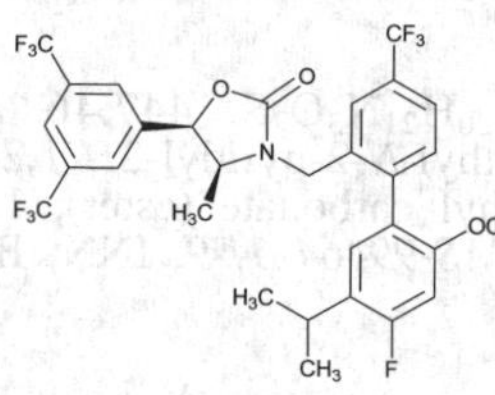

Anagestone Acetate [*1965*] (an a jes′ tone as′ e tate). $C_{24}H_{36}O_3$. 372.54. [Anagestone is INN.] (1) Pregn-4-en-20-one, 17-(acetyloxy)-6-methyl-, (6α)-; (2) 17-Hydroxy-6α-methylpregn-4-en-20-one acetate. *UNII-GNT396G9QT. CAS-3137-73-3; CAS-2740-52-5* [anagestone]. *Progestin.* Anatropin (Ortho Pharmaceutical†)

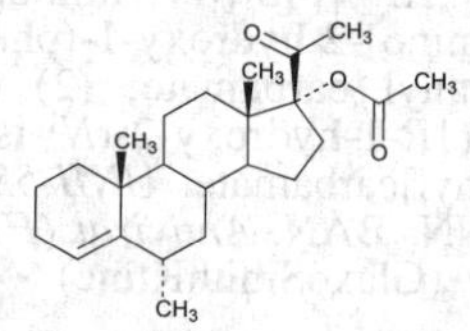

Anagrelide Hydrochloride [*1979*] (an ag′ re lide hye″ droe klor′ ide). $C_{10}H_7Cl_2N_3O \cdot HCl$. 292.55. [Anagrelide is INN and BAN.] (1) Imidazo[2,1-*b*]quinazolin-2(3*H*)-one, 6,7-dichloro-1,5-dihydro-, monohydrochloride; (2) 6,7-Dichloro-1,5-dihydroimidazo[2,1-*b*]-quinazolin-2(3*H*)-one monohydrochloride. *UNII-VNS4435G39; UNII-K9X45X0051* [anagrelide]. *CAS-58579-51-4; CAS-68475-42-3* [anagrelide]. *Antithrombotic.* Agrylin (Shire) ◇*BL-4162a*

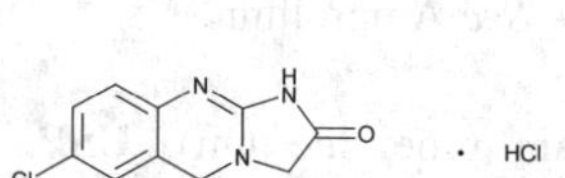

Anakinra [*1994*] (an a kin′ ra). $C_{759}H_{1186}N_{208}O_{232}S_{10}$. 17,258 daltons. (1) Interleukin 1 receptor antagonist (human isoform x reduced), N^2-L-methionyl-; (2) N^2-L-Methionylinterleukin 1 receptor antagonist (human isoform x reduced). *UNII-9013DUQ28K. CAS-143090-92-0.* INN; BAN. *Anti-inflammatory (nonsteroidal); suppressant (inflammatory bowel disease).* Antril (Synergen)

```
                                                              M
RPSGRKSSKM   QAFRIWDVNQ   KTFYLRNNQL   VAGYLQGPNV   NLEEKIDVVP
IEPHALFLGI   HGGKMCLSCV   KSGDETRLQL   EAVNITDLSE   NRKQDKRFAF
IRSDSGPTTS   FESAACPGWF   LCTAMEADQP   VSLTNMPDEG   VMVTKFYFQE
DE
```

Anamorelin Hydrochloride [*2006*] (an″ a moe rel′ in hye″ droe klor′ ide). $C_{31}H_{42}N_6O_3 \cdot HCl$. 583.16. [Anamorelin is INN.] (1) 3-Piperidinecarboxylic acid, 1-(2-methylalanyl-D-tryptophyl)-3-(phenylmethyl)-, trimethylhydrazide, monohydrochloride, (3R)-; (2) (3R)-1-{(2R)-2-[(2-Amino-2-methylpropanoyl)amino]-3-(indol-3-yl)propanoyl}-3-benzyl-*N,N′,N′*-trimethylpiperidine-3-carbohydrazide hydrochloride. *UNII-55F75LJQ0V. CAS-861998-00-7. Treatment of cancer anorexia and cancer cachexia.* ◇*RC-1291 HCl*

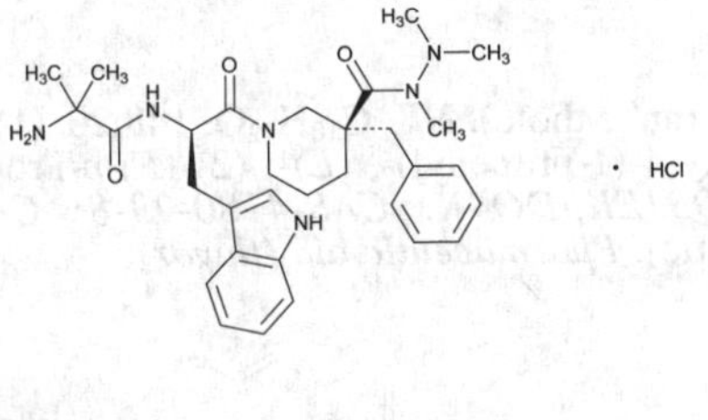

Anaritide Acetate [*1987*] (an ar′ i tide as′ e tate). $C_{112}H_{175}N_{39}O_{35}S_3 \cdot xC_2H_4O_2$. [Anaritide is INN and BAN.] (1) Atriopeptin-21 (rat), *N*-L-arginyl-8-L-methionine-21a-L-phenylalanine-21b-L-arginine-21c-L-tyrosine-, acetate (salt); (2) L-Arginyl-L-seryl-L-seryl-L-cysteinyl-L-phenylalanylglycylglycyl-L-arginyl-L-methionyl-L-aspartyl-L-arginyl-L-isoleucylglycyl-L-alanyl-L-glutaminyl-L-serylglycyl-L-leucylglycyl-L-cysteinyl-L-asparaginyl-L-seryl-L-phenylalanyl-L-arginyl-L-tyrosine cyclic (4→20)-disulfide, acetate (salt). *UNII-EGV6V52K6N. CAS-104595-79-1; CAS-95896-08-5* [anaritide]. *Antihypertensive; diuretic.* ◇*WY-47,663 acetate*

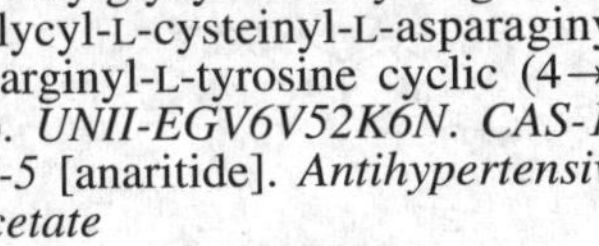

```
RSSCFGGRMDR IGAQSGLGCN SFRY
```

Anastrozole [*1995*] (an as′ troe zole). $C_{17}H_{19}N_5$. 293.37. (1) 1,3-Benzenediacetonitrile, α,α,α′,α′-tetramethyl-5-(1*H*-1,2,4-triazol-1-ylmethyl)-; (2) α,α,α′,α′-Tetramethyl-5-(1*H*-1,2,4-triazol-1-ylmethyl)-*m*-benzenediacetonitrile. *UNII-2Z07MYW1AZ. CAS-120511-73-1.* INN; BAN. *Antineoplastic.* Arimidex (AstraZeneca) ◇*ICI D1033; ZD1033*

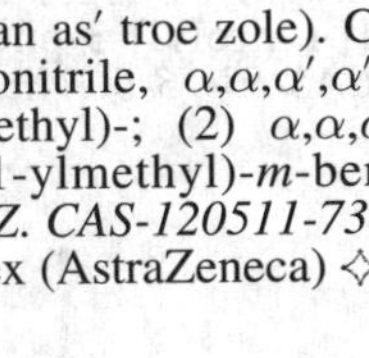

Anatibant. $C_{34}H_{36}Cl_2N_6O_5S$. 711.66. (2*S*)-*N*-[3-(4-Carbamimidoylbenzamido)propyl]-1-{2,4-dichloro-3-[(2,4-dimethyl-8-quinolyloxy)methyl]phenylsulfonyl}pyrrolidine-2-carboxamide. *UNII-CLO4JRD21F. CAS-209733-45-9.* INN.

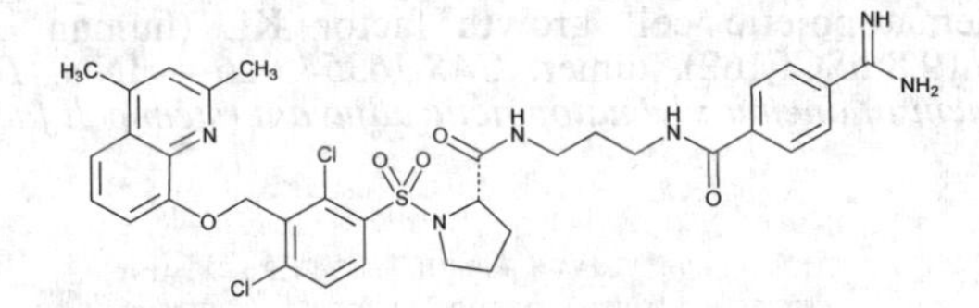

Anatumomab Mafenatox. Immunoglobulin G 1, anti-(human tumor-associated glycoprotein 72) (human-mouse clone pMB125 Fab fragment γ1-chain) fusion protein with enterotoxin A (227-alanine) (*Staphylococcus aureus*) complex with mouse clone pMB 125 κ-chain). INN.

Anaxirone. $C_{11}H_{15}N_3O_5$. 269.25. Tris(2,3-epoxypropyl)bicarbamimide. *UNII-36R61Y789T. CAS-77658-97-0.* INN.

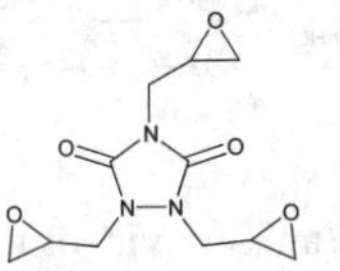

Anazocine. $C_{16}H_{23}NO$. 245.36. 9-*syn*-Methoxy-3-methyl-9-phenyl-3-azabicyclo[3.3.1]nonane. *UNII-K2S5VMM2SG. CAS-15378-99-1.* INN.

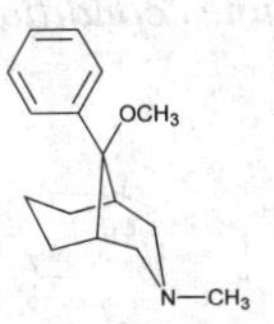

Anazolene Sodium [*1962*] (an az′ oh leen soe′ dee um). $C_{26}H_{16}N_3Na_3O_{10}S_3$. 695.58. [Sodium Anoxynaphthonate is BAN.] (1) 2,7-Naphthalenedisulfonic acid, 4-hydroxy-5-[[4-(phenylamino)-5-sulfo-1-naphthalenyl]azo], trisodium salt; (2) 4-[(4-Anilino-5-sulfo-1-naphthyl)azo]-5-hydroxy-2,7-naphthalenedisulfonic acid trisodium salt; (3) C.I. acid blue 92 trisodium salt. *UNII-F6G1K9WJU4. CAS-3861-73-2; CAS-7488-76-8* [anazolene, acid]. INN. *Diagnostic aid (blood volume and cardiac output determination).*

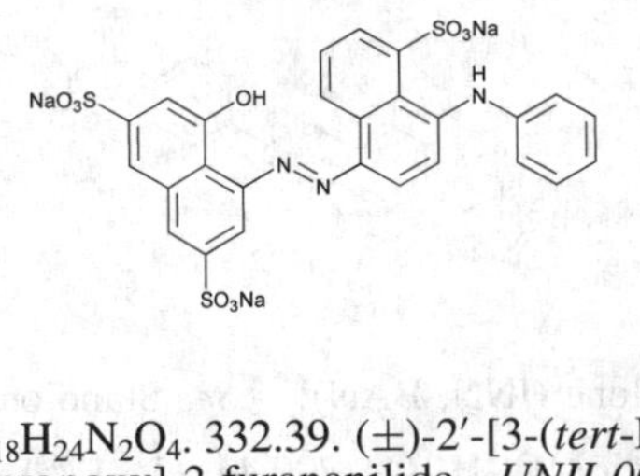

Ancarolol. $C_{18}H_{24}N_2O_4$. 332.39. (±)-2′-[3-(*tert*-Butylamino)-2-hydroxypropoxy]-2-furananilide. *UNII-00EED65INL. CAS-75748-50-4.* INN.

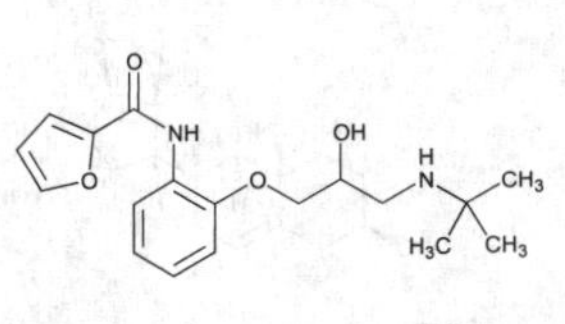

---

† Brand name formerly used, and/or firm no longer concerned with this product.

Ancer-20. A mixture containing polysaccharides (mainly composed of arabinose, mannose and glucose) and nucleic acid obtained from hot water extracts of *Mycobacterium tuberculosis* strain Aoyama B. JAN.

Ancestim [*1997*] (an′ se stim). $C_{1662}H_{2650}N_{422}O_{512}S_{18}$. 18,600 ± 100 daltons (for the monomer). *N*-L-Methionyl-1-165-hematopoietic cell growth factor KL (human clone V19.8:hSCF162), dimer. *CAS-163545-26-4*. INN. *Treatment of anemia; hematopoietic adjuvant (stem cell factor).*

```
            M
EGICRCTVTN NVKDVTKLVA NLPKDYMITL KYVPGMDVLP SHCWISEMVV
QLSDSLTDLL DKFSNISEGL SNYSIIDKLV NIVDDLVECV KENSSKDLKK
SFKSPEPRLF TPEEFFRIFN RSIDAFKDFV VASETSDCVV SSTLSPEKDS
RVSVTKPFML PPVAA
```

Ancitabine. $C_9H_{11}N_3O_4$. 225.20. [Ancitabine Hydrochloride is JAN.] (2*R*,3*R*,3a*S*,9a*R*)-2,3,3a,9a-Tetrahydro-3-hydroxy-6-imino-6*H*-furo[2′,3′;4,5]oxazolo[3,2-*a*]pyrimidine-2-methanol. *UNII-DO2D32W0VC*. *CAS-31698-14-3*. INN; MI.

Ancriviroc [*2005*] (an″ kri vir′ ok). $C_{28}H_{37}BrN_4O_3$. 557.52. (1) [1,4′-Bipiperidine]-4-methanimine, α-(4-bromophenyl)-1′-[(2,4-dimethyl-1-oxido-3-pyridinyl)carbonyl]-*N*-ethoxy-4′-methyl-, (α*Z*)-; (2) 4-[(*Z*)-(4-Bromophenyl)(ethoxyimino)methyl]-1′-[(2,4-dimethyl-1-oxidopyridin-3-yl)carbonyl]-4′-methyl[1,4′-bipiperidinyl]. *UNII-322WXU4AU2*. *CAS-370893-06-4*. INN. *Antiviral; treatment of autoimmune conditions (CCR5 antagonist).* ◇*SCH351125*

Ancrod [*1975*] (an′ krod). Proteinase obtained from the venom of the Malayan pit-viper *Agkistrodon rhodostoma*, acting specifically on fibrinogen. *CAS-9046-56-4*. INN; BAN. *Anticoagulant.* Venacil (Abbott†)

Andolast. $C_{15}H_{11}N_9O$. 333.31. 4,4′-Di-1*H*-tetrazol-5-ylbenzanilide. *UNII-6513M33209*. *CAS-132640-22-3*. INN.

Androstanolone (INN, BAN) — *See* Stanolone.

Androstenediol. $C_{19}H_{30}O_2$. 290.44. (3β,17β)-Androst-5-ene-3,17-diol. *CAS-521-17-5*. JAN.

Androstenedione. $C_{19}H_{26}O_2$. 286.41. 4-Androstene-3,17-dione. *CAS-63-05-8*. JAN.

Anecortave Acetate [*1998*] (an e kor′ tave as′ e tate). $C_{23}H_{30}O_5$. 386.48. [Anecortave is INN.] (1) 21-(Acetyloxy)-17-hydroxypregna-4,9(11)-diene-3,20-dione; (2) 17,21-Dihydroxypregna-4,9(11)-diene-3,20-dione 21-acetate. *CAS-7753-60-8*. *Treatment of diseases involving neovascularization of the eye (angiostatic steroid).* ◇*AL-3789*

Anethole (an′ e thole). **NF**. $C_{10}H_{12}O$. 148.20. (1) Benzene, 1-methoxy-4-(1-propenyl)-, (*E*)-; (2) (*E*)-*p*-Propenylanisole. *UNII-Q3JEK5DO4K*. *CAS-4180-23-8; CAS-104-46-1* [synthetic]. *Pharmaceutic aid (flavor).*

Anetholtrithion. $C_{10}H_7OS_2$. 207.29. 5-(*p*-Methoxyphenyl)-3*H*-1,2-dithiole-3-thione. *CAS-532-11-6*. JAN.

Aneurine Hydrochloride — *See* Thiamine Hydrochloride.

Angiotensin Amide [*1962*] (an″ jee oh ten′ sin a′ mide). $C_{49}H_{70}N_{14}O_{11}$. 1031.17. [Angiotensinamide is INN and BAN.] (1) Angiotensin II, 1-L-asparagine-5-L-valine-; (2) 1-L-Asparagine-5-L-valineangiotensin II; (3) *N*-[1-[*N*-[*N*-[*N*-(*N*²-L-Asparaginyl)-L-arginyl)-L-valyl]-L-tyrosyl]-L-valyl]-L-histidyl]-L-prolyl]-3-phenyl-L-alanine. *UNII-7WAL1X78KV*. *CAS-53-73-6*. NF XIII. *Vasoconstrictor.* ◇*NSC-107678*

```
NRVYVHPF —NH₂
```

Angiotensin II. $C_{50}H_{71}N_{13}O_{12}$. 1046.18. 5-L-Isoleucineangiotensin II. *CAS-4474-91-3*. INN; JAN.

```
NRVYIHPF —NH₂
```

Anhydrohydroxyprogesterone (previously used name) — *See* Ethisterone.

Anidoxime [*1973*] (an i dox′ eem). $C_{21}H_{27}N_3O_3$. 369.46. (1) 1-Propanone, 3-(diethylamino)-1-phenyl-, *O*-[[(4-methoxyphenyl)amino]carbonyl]oxime; (2) 3-(Diethylamino)propiophenone *O*-[(*p*-methoxyphenyl)carbamoyl]oxime. *UNII-88ETS2Q7LZ. CAS-34297-34-2.* INN; BAN. *Analgesic.*

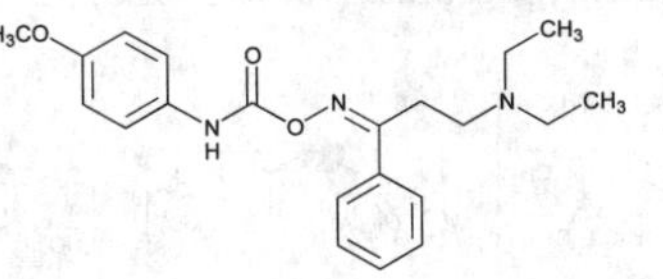

Anidulafungin [*1998*] (ay nid″ ue la fun′ jin). $C_{58}H_{73}N_7O_{17}$. 1140.24. (1) Echinocandin B, 1-[(4*R*,5*R*)-4,5-dihydroxy-N^2-[[4″-(pentyloxy)[1,1′:4′,1″-terphenyl]-4-yl]carbonyl]-L-ornithine]-; (2) (4*R*,5*R*)-4,5-Dihydroxy-N^2-[[4″-(pentyloxy)-*p*-terphenyl-4-yl]carbonyl]-L-ornithyl-L-threonyl-*trans*-4-hydroxy-L-prolyl-(*S*)-4-hydroxy-4-(*p*-hydroxyphenyl)-L-threonyl-L-threonyl-(3*S*,4*S*)-3-hydroxy-4-methyl-L-proline cyclic (6→1)-peptide. *UNII-9HLM53094I. CAS-166663-25-8.* INN. *Antifungal used in the treatment of infections caused by Candida (all species), Aspergillus, and Pneumocystis.* Eraxis (Pfizer) ◇*LY303366*

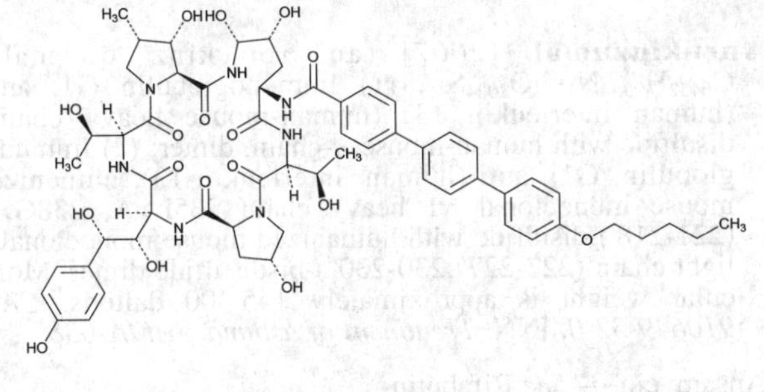

Anilamate. $C_{15}H_{14}N_2O_3$. 270.28. Methylcarbamate of salicylanilide. *CAS-5591-49-1.* INN.

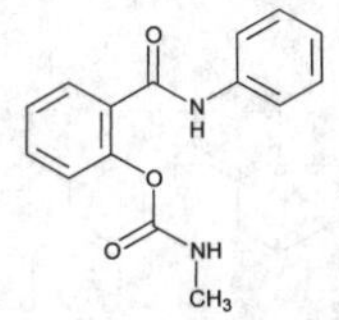

Anileridine (an″ i ler′ i deen). **USP.** $C_{22}H_{28}N_2O_2$. 352.47. (1) 4-Piperidinecarboxylic acid, 1-[2-(4-aminophenyl)ethyl]-4-phenyl-, ethyl ester; (2) Ethyl 1-(*p*-aminophenethyl)-4-phenylisonipecotate. *UNII-71Q1A3O279. CAS-144-14-9.* INN; BAN. *Analgesic (narcotic).*

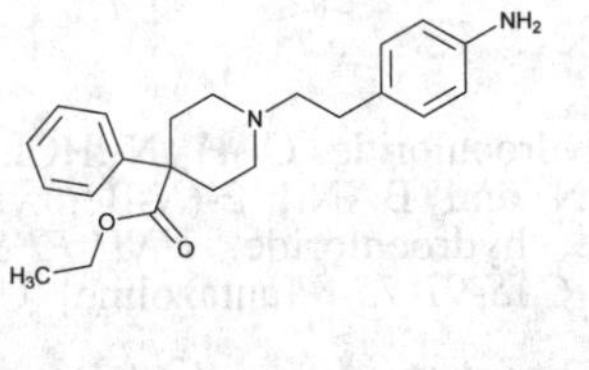

Anileridine Hydrochloride (an″ i ler′ i deen hye″ droe klor′ ide). **USP.** $C_{22}H_{28}N_2O_2 \cdot 2HCl$. 425.39. (1) 4-Piperidinecarboxylic acid, 1-[2-(4-aminophenyl)ethyl]-4-phenyl-, ethyl ester, dihydrochloride; (2) Ethyl 1-(*p*-aminophenethyl)-4-phenylisonipecotate dihydrochloride. *UNII-915Q054DLC; UNII-71Q1A3O279* [anileridine]. *CAS-126-12-5; CAS-144-14-9* [anileridine]. *Analgesic (narcotic).* Leritine (Merck)

---

† Brand name formerly used, and/or firm no longer concerned with this product.

Anilopam Hydrochloride [*1976*] (an il′ oh pam hye″ droe klor′ ide). $C_{20}H_{26}N_2O \cdot 2HCl$. 383.36. [Anilopam is INN.] (1) Benzenamine, 4-[2-(1,2,4,5-tetrahydro-8-methoxy-2-methyl-3*H*-3-benzazepin-3-yl)ethyl]-, dihydrochloride, (-)-; (2) (-)-3-(*p*-Aminophenethyl)-2,3,4,5-tetrahydro-8-methoxy-2-methyl-1*H*-3-benzazepine dihydrochloride. *UNII-JOT47SVI4K; UNII-34E9Q468RT* [anilopam]. *CAS-53716-45-3; CAS-53716-46-4* [anilopam]. *Analgesic.* ◇*786-723*

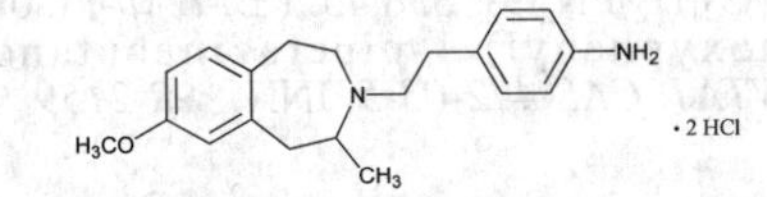

Anipamil. $C_{34}H_{52}N_2O_2$. 520.79. 2-[3-[(*m*-Methoxyphenethyl)methylamino]propyl]-2-(*m*-methoxyphenyl)tetradecanenitrile. *UNII-9Y54WZV1CJ. CAS-83200-10-6.* INN.

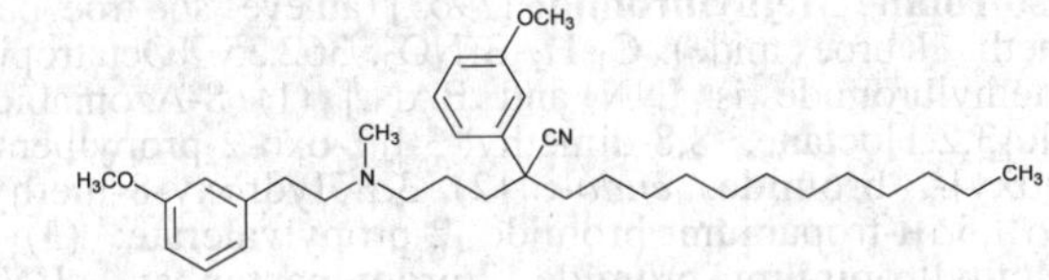

Aniracetam [*1981*] (an″ i ra′ se tam). $C_{12}H_{13}NO_3$. 219.24. (1) 2-Pyrrolidinone, 1-(4-methoxybenzoyl)-; (2) 1-*p*-Anisoyl-2-pyrrolidinone. *UNII-5L16LKN964. CAS-72432-10-1.* INN; JAN. *Mental performance enhancer.* ◇*Ro 13-5057*

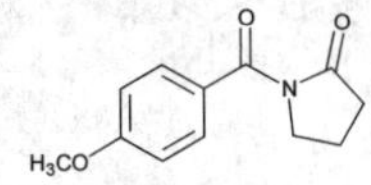

Anirolac [*1985*] (a nye′ role ak). $C_{16}H_{15}NO_4$. 285.29. (1) 1*H*-Pyrrolizine-1-carboxylic acid, 2,3-dihydro-5-(4-methoxybenzoyl)-, (±)-; (2) (±)-5-*p*-Anisoyl-2,3-dihydro-1*H*-pyrrolizine-1-carboxylic acid. *UNII-S9B9E35WUX. CAS-66635-85-6.* INN. *Anti-inflammatory; analgesic.* ◇*RS-37326*

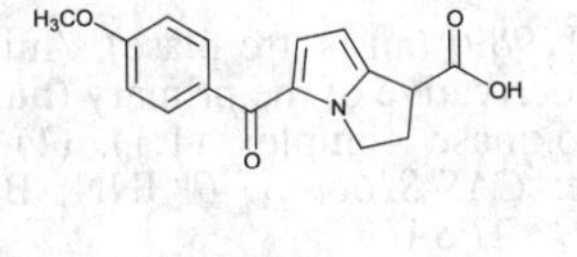

Anisacril. $C_{22}H_{18}O_3$. 330.38. 2-(*o*-Methoxyphenyl)-3,3-diphenyl acrylic acid. *CAS-5129-14-6.* INN. ◇*SKF 16046*

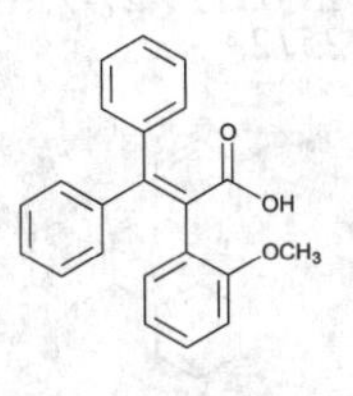

Anise Oil (an′ is). **NF.** The volatile oil distilled with steam from the dried, ripe fruit of *Pimpinella ansium* L. (Fam. Apiaceae) or from the dried ripe fruit of *Illicium verum* Hook. f. (Fam. Illiciaceae). *CAS-8007-70-3. Pharmaceutic aid (flavor).*

Anisindione. $C_{16}H_{12}O_3$. 252.26. 2-(*p*-Methoxyphenyl)indane-1,3-dione. *UNII-S747T1ERAJ. CAS-117-37-3.* NF XIII; INN; BAN; MI. Miradon (Schering)

Anisopirol. $C_{21}H_{27}FN_2O_2$. 358.45. (±)-α-(*p*-Fluorophenyl-4-(*o*-methoxyphenyl)-1-piperazinebutanol. *UNII-162A01WTAJ. CAS-442-03-5.* INN. ◇*R 2159*

Anisotropine Methylbromide [*1963*] (an eye″ soe troe′ peen meth″ il broe′ mide). $C_{17}H_{32}BrNO_2$. 362.35. [Octatropine Methylbromide is INN and BAN.] (1) 8-Azoniabicyclo[3.2.1]octane, 8,8-dimethyl-3-[(1-oxo-2-propylpentyl)oxy]-, bromide, *endo*-; (2) 3α-Hydroxy-8-methyl-1αH,5αH-tropanium bromide 2-propylvalerate; (3) 8-Methyltropinium bromide 2-propylpentanoate. *UNII-62M960DHIL. CAS-80-50-2.* JAN. *Anticholinergic.* Valpin (Endo)

Anisperimus. $C_{18}H_{39}N_7O_3$. 401.55. [(6-Guanidinohexyl)carbamomoyl]methyl[4-[[(*R*)-3-aminobutyl]amino]butyl]carbamate. *UNII-D0514P112G. CAS-170368-04-4.* INN.

Anistreplase [*1989*] (an is′ tre plase). Anistreplase is the *p*-anisoylated derivative of the primary (human) lys-plasminogen streptokinase complex (1:1). (1) Anistreplase; (2) Anistreplase. *CAS-81669-57-0.* INN; BAN. *Fibrinolytic.* ◇*BRL 26921; APSAC*

Anitrazafen [*1980*] (an″ i traz′ a fen). $C_{18}H_{17}N_3O_2$. 307.35. (1) 1,2,4-Triazine, 5,6-bis(4-methoxyphenyl)-3-methyl-; (2) 5,6-Bis(*p*-methoxyphenyl)-3-methyl-*as*-triazine. *UNII-2Y065P7MYR. CAS-63119-27-7.* INN. *Anti-inflammatory (topical).* ◇*LY 122512*

Anoxomer [*1980*] (an ox′ oh mer). $(C_{10}H_{14}O_2)_u(C_{10}H_{10})_v(C_{10}H_{14}O)_w(C_7H_8O_2)_x(C_{16}H_{16}O_2)_y(C_7H_8O)_z$. (1) 1,4-Benzenediol, 2-(1,1-dimethylethyl)-, polymer with diethenylbenzene, 4-(1,1-dimethylethyl)phenol, 4-methoxyphenol, 4,4′-(1-methylethylidene)bis[phenol] and 4-methylphenol; (2)

tert-Butylhydroquinone polymer with divinylbenzene, *p*-*tert*-butylphenol, *p*-methoxyphenol, 4,4′-isopropylidenediphenol and *p*-cresol. *CAS-60837-57-2. Pharmaceutic aid (antioxidant); food additive.* ◇*D 00079*

Anpirtoline. $C_{10}H_{13}ClN_2S$. 228.74. 4-[(6-Chloro-2-pyridyl)thio]piperidine. *UNII-32K9S228IK. CAS-98330-05-3.* INN.

Anrukinzumab [*2007*] (an″ roo kinz′ oo mab). $C_{6452}H_{9954}N_{1714}O_{2024}S_{46}$. (1) Immunoglobulin G1, anti-(human interleukin 13) (human-mouse heavy chain), disulfide with human-mouse κ-chain, dimer; (2) Immunoglobulin G1, anti-(human interleukin-13) humanized mouse monoclonal γ1 heavy chain 235L>A, 238G>A (221-218′)-disulfide with humanized mouse monoclonal κ light chain (227-227″:230-230″)-bisdisulfide dimer. Molecular weight is approximately 145,400 daltons. *CAS-910649-32-0.* INN. *Treatment of asthma.* ◇*IMA-638*

Ansamycin — *See* Rifabutin.

Ansoxetine. $C_{26}H_{25}NO_3$. 399.48. (±)-6-[[α-[2-(Dimethylamino)ethyl]benzyl]oxy]flavone. *UNII-3LY71185IQ. CAS-79130-64-6.* INN.

Antafenite. $C_{11}H_{10}N_2S$. 202.28. (±)-5,6-Dihydro-6-phenylimidazo[2,1-*b*]thiazole. *UNII-89846MU42L. CAS-15301-45-8.* INN. ◇*R-8193*

Antazoline Hydrochloride. $C_{17}H_{19}N_3$·HCl. 301.81. [Antazoline is INN and BAN.] 2-(*N*-Benzylanilino)methyl-2-imidazoline, hydrochloride. *UNII-FP8Q8F72JH. CAS-2508-72-7; CAS-91-75-8* [antazoline]. USP XV; MI.

Antazoline Phosphate (an taz′ oh leen fos′ fate). **USP.** $C_{17}H_{19}N_3$·H_3PO_4. 363.35. (1) 1*H*-Imidazole-2-methanamine, 4,5-dihydro-*N*-phenyl-*N*-(phenylmethyl)-, phosphate (1:1); (2) 2-[(*N*-Benzylanilino)methyl]-2-imidazoline phosphate (1:1). *UNII-VPR5FPH326. CAS-154-68-7; CAS-91-75-8* [antazoline]. *Antihistaminic.*

Antazonite. $C_{11}H_{12}N_2O_2S_2$. 268.36. (±)-*N*-[3-[2-Hydroxy-2-(2-thienyl)ethyl]-4-thiazolin-2-ylidene]acetamide. *UNII-K9RLQ5L66X. CAS-25422-75-7.* INN. ◇*R 6438*

Antelmycin (INN) — *See* Anthelmycin.

Anthelmycin [*1964*] (an″ thel mye′ sin). Antibiotic substance produced by *Streptomyces longissimus*. [Antelmycin is INN.] (1) Anthelmycin; (2) Anthelmycin. *CAS-1402-84-2. Anthelmintic.* ◇*33876*

Anthiolimine. $C_{12}H_9Li_6O_{12}S_3Sb$. 604.79. Mercaptosuccinic acid triester with thioantimonic acid (H_3SbS_3), hexalithium salt. *UNII-TX973XBY8N. CAS-305-97-5.* INN; MI.

Anthralin (an′ thra lin). **USP**. $C_{14}H_{10}O_3$. 226.23. [Dithranol is INN and BAN.] (1) 9(10*H*)-Anthracenone, 1,8-dihydroxy-; (2) 1,8-Dihydroxy-9-anthrone. *UNII-U8CJK0JH5M. CAS-480-22-8; CAS-1143-38-0. Antipsoriatic.* Anthra-Derm (Dermik); DrithoCreme (Dermik); Drithoscalp (Dermik); Lasan (Stiefel†)

Anthramycin [*1966*] (an″ thra mye′ sin). $C_{16}H_{17}N_3O_4$. 315.32. [Antramycin is INN.] (1) 2-Propenamide, 3-(5,10,11,11a-tetrahydro-9,11-dihydroxy-8-methyl-5-oxo-1*H*-pyrrolo[2,1-*c*][1,4]benzodiazepin-2-yl)-, (*E*)-; (2) (*E*)-5,10,11,11a-Tetrahydro-9,11-dihydroxy-8-methyl-5-oxo-1*H*-pyrrolo[2,1-*c*][1,4]-benzodiazepine-2-acrylamide. *CAS-4803-27-4. Antineoplastic.*

Anthrax Vaccine Adsorbed (an′ thrax vax′ een). **USP**. A sterile, milky-white suspension made from cell-free filtrates of microaerophilic cultures of an avirulent, nonencapsulated strain of *Bacillus anthracis*.

Antibiotic 273a₁ — *See* Paldimycin.

Anti-CD3 — *See* Muromonab-CD3.

Anticoagulant Citrate Dextrose (an″ tee koe ag′ ue lant sit′ rate dex′ trose). **USP** [Solution]. A sterile solution of Citric Acid, Sodium Citrate, and Dextrose in Water for Injection. *Anticoagulant (for storage of whole blood).*

Anticoagulant Citrate Phosphate Dextrose (an″ tee koe ag′ ue lant sit′ rate fos′ fate dex′ trose). **USP** [Solution]. A sterile solution of Citric Acid, Sodium Citrate, Monobasic Sodium Phosphate, and Dextrose in Water for Injection. *Anticoagulant (for storage of whole blood).*

Anticoagulant Citrate Phosphate Dextrose Adenine (an″ tee koe ag′ ue lant sit′ rate fos′ fate dex′ trose ad″ e neen). **USP** [Solution]. A sterile solution of Citric Acid, Sodium Citrate, Monobasic Sodium Phosphate, Dextrose, and Adenine in Water for Injection. *Anticoagulant (for storage of whole blood).*

Anticoagulant Heparin (an″ tee koe ag′ ue lant hep′ a rin). **USP** [Solution]. A sterile solution of Heparin Sodium in Sodium Chloride Injection. *Anticoagulant (for storage of whole blood).*

Anticoagulant Sodium Citrate (an″ tee koe ag′ ue lant soe′ dee um sit′ rate). **USP** [Solution]. A sterile solution of Sodium Citrate in Water for Injection. *Anticoagulant (for plasma and for blood for fractionation).*

Antienite. $C_9H_8N_2S_2$. 208.30. (±)-5,6-Dihydro-6-(2-thienyl)imidazo[2,1-*b*]thiazole. *UNII-50Z1JVP72H. CAS-5029-05-0.* INN. ◇*R 8025; R 8141*

Antiepilepsirine (previously used name) — *See* Ilepcimide.

Antifebrin — *See* Acetanilide.

Antiformin, Dental (JAN) — *See* Sodium Hypochlorite [Solution, Diluted].

Antihemophilic Factor (an″ tee hee″ moe fil′ ik fak′ tor). **USP**. A sterile, freeze-dried powder containing the Factor VIII fraction prepared from units of human venous plasma that have been tested for the absence of hepatitis B surface antigen, obtained from whole-blood donors and pooled. *Antihemophilic.* Alphanate (Alpha Therapeutic); Bioclate (Centeon); Haemate-P (Hoechst-Roussel); Helixate (Centeon); Hemofil M (Hyland); Humafac (Parke-Davis†); Humate-P (Centeon); Koate-HP (Bayer); KOGENATE (Bayer); Monoclate-P (Centeon); Profilate Heat-Treated (Alpha Therapeutic†); Profilate HP (Alpha Therapeutic†); Profilate OSD (Alpha Therapeutic); Profilate SD (Alpha Therapeutic†) *[Name previously used: Antihemophilic Factor, Human.]*

Antihemophilic Factor, Human (previously used name) — *See* Antihemophilic Factor.

Antilymphocyte Immunoglobulin (Horse). A preparation of horse immunoglobulins containing antibodies to human lymphocytes. BAN.

Antimony Potassium Tartrate (an′ ti moe″ nee poe tas′ ee um tar′ trate). **USP**. $C_8H_4K_2O_{12}Sb_2.3H_2O$. 667.87. (1) Antimonate(2-), bis[μ-[2,3-dihydroxybutanedioato(4-)-$O^1,O^2:O^3,O^4$]]-di-, dipotassium, trihydrate, stereoisomer; (2) Dipotassium bis[μ-[L-(+)-tartrato(4-)]]diantimonate (2-) trihydrate. *CAS-28300-74-5; CAS-11071-15-1* [anhydrous]. *Antischistosomal.*

Antimony Sodium Tartrate (an′ ti moe″ nee soe′ dee um tar′ trate). **USP**. $C_8H_4Na_2O_{12}Sb_2$. 581.61. (1) Antimonate(2-), bis[μ-[2,3-dihydroxybutanedioato(4-)-$O^1,O^2:O^3,O^4$]]di-,

disodium, stereoisomer; (2) Disodium bis[μ-[L-(+)-tartrato(4-)]]diantimonate(2-). *CAS-34521-09-0*. JAN. *Antischistosomal.*

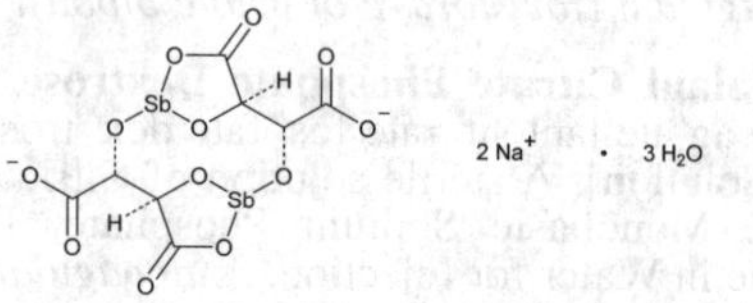

Antimony Sodium Thioglycollate. *CAS-539-54-8*. USP XIV; MI.

Antimony Trisulfide Colloid [*1978*] (an′ ti moe″ nee trye sul′ fide kol′ oid). Sb₂S₃. 339.72. (1) Antimony sulfide (Sb₂S₃); (2) Antimony sulfide (Sb₂S₃). *CAS-1345-04-6*. *Pharmaceutic aid.*

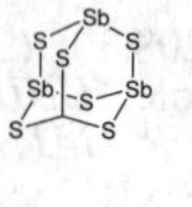

Antipyrine (an″ tee pye′ reen). **USP**. C₁₁H₁₂N₂O. 188.23. [Phenazone is INN and BAN.] (1) 1,2-Dihydro-1,5-dimethyl-2-phenyl-3*H*-pyrazol-3-one; (2) 2,3-Dimethyl-1-phenyl-3-pyrazolin-5-one. *UNII-T3CHA1B51H*. *CAS-60-80-0*. JAN; MI. *Analgesic.*

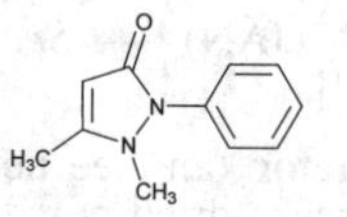

Antirabies Serum. USP XXVI. *Immunizing agent (passive).*

Anti-Rh Typing Serums (previously used name) — *See* Blood Grouping Serums Anti-D, Anti-C, Anti-E, Anti-c, Anti-e.

Antithrombin Alfa [*2007*] (an″ tee throm′ bin al′ fa). C₂₁₉₁H₃₄₅₁N₅₈₃O₆₅₆S₁₈. (1) Antithrombin (human reduced); (2) Human antithrombin-III (ATIII). Molecular weight is approximately 49,000 daltons. *CAS-84720-88-7*. INN. *Anticlotting agent.* Atryn (GTC Biotherapeutics)

```
HGSPVDICTA KPRDIPMNPM CIYRSPEKKA TEDEGSEQKI PEATNRRVWE
LSKANSRFAT TFYQHLADSK NDNDNIFLSP LSISTAFAMT KLGACNDTLQ
QLMEVFKFDT ISEKTSDQIH FFFAKLNCRL YRKANKSSKL VSANRLFGDK
SLTFNETYQD ISELVYGAKL QPLDFKENAE QSRAAINKWV SNKTEGRITD
VIPSEAINEL TVLVLVNTIY FKGLWKSKFS PENTRKELFY KADGESCSAS
MMYQEGKFRY RRVAEGTQVL ELPFKGDDIT MVLILPKPEK SLAKVEKELT
PEVLQEWLDE LEEMMLVVHM PRFRIEDGFS LKEQLQDMGL VDLFSPEKSK
LPGIVAEGRD DLYVSDAFHK AFLEVNEEGS EAAASTAVVI AGRSLNPNRV
TFKANRPFLV FIREVPLNTI IFMGRVANPC VK
```

• glycosylation sites

Antithrombin III Human. **USP**. [Antithrombin III is INN and BAN.] The glycoprotein antithrombin obtained from human plasma. *CAS-52014-67-2*. Kybernin (Hoechst-Roussel); THROMBATE III (Bayer)

Antivenin (Latrodectus mactans) (an″ tee ven′ in lat″ roe dek′ tus mak′ tans). **USP**. A sterile, non-pyrogenic preparation derived by drying a frozen solution of specific venom-neutralizing globulins obtained from the serum of healthy horses immunized against venom of black widow spiders (*Latrodectus mactans*). *Immunizing agent (passive).* Antivenin (Merck) [*Name previously used: Widow Spider Species Antivenin (Latrodectus mactans).*]

Antivenin (Micrurus Fulvius) (an″ tee ven′ in mye kroo′ rus ful′ vi us). **USP**. A sterile, non-pyrogenic preparation derived by drying a frozen solution of specific venom-neutralizing globulins obtained from the serum of healthy horses immunized against venom of the Eastern Coral snake (*Micrurus fulvius*). *Immunizing agent (passive).*

Antivenin (Crotalidae) Polyvalent (an″ tee ven′ in kroe tal′ i dee pol″ ee vay′ lent). **USP**. A sterile, non-pyrogenic preparation derived by drying a frozen solution of specific venom-neutralizing globulins obtained from the serum of healthy horses immunized against venoms of four species of pit vipers, *Crotalus atrox*, *Crotalus adamanteus*, *Crotalus durissus terrificus*, and *Bothrops atrox* (Fam. Crotalidae). *Immunizing agent (passive).*

Antrafenine. C₃₀H₂₆F₆N₄O₂. 588.54. 2-[4-(α,α,α-Trifluoro-*m*-tolyl)-1-piperazinyl]ethyl *N*-[7-(trifluoromethyl)-4-quinolyl]anthranilate. *UNII-21FS93Y6OE*. *CAS-55300-29-3*. INN; MI.

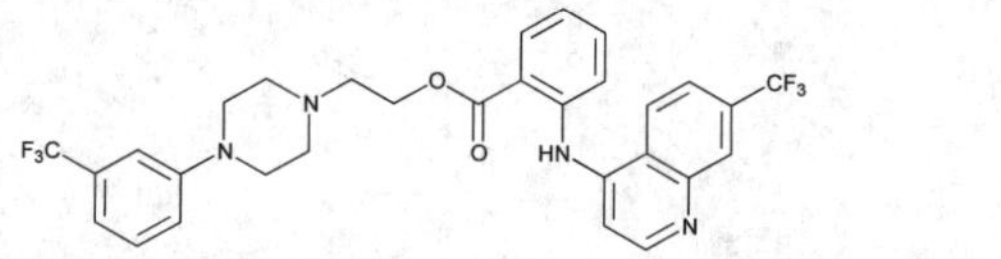

Antramycin (INN) — *See* Anthramycin.

Apadenoson [*2005*] (a″ pa den′ oh son). C₂₃H₃₀N₆O₆. 486.52. (1) Cyclohexanecarboxylic acid, 4-[3-[6-amino-9-(*N*-ethyl-β-D-ribofuranuronamidosyl)-9*H*-purin-2-yl]-2-propynyl]-, methyl ester, *trans*-; (2) Methyl *trans*-4-[3-[6-amino-9-(*N*-ethyl-β-D-ribofuranosyluronamide)-9*H*-purin-2-yl]prop-2-ynyl]cyclohexanecarboxylate. *UNII-BTS1Y6777M*. *CAS-250386-15-3*. INN. *Adjunct to nuclear myocardial perfusion imaging in patients unable to exercise adequately.* ◇BMS068645

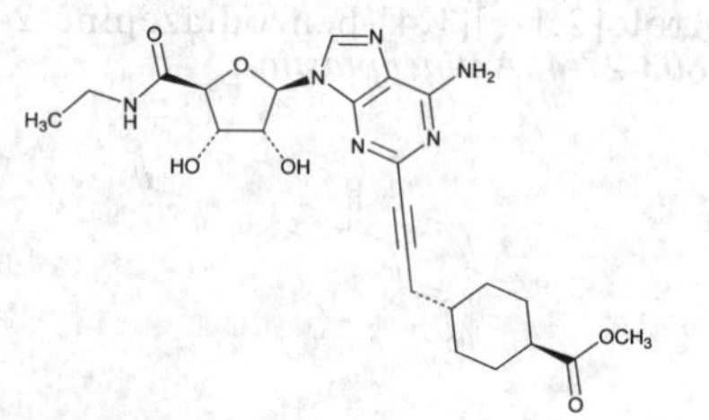

Apadoline. C₂₃H₂₉N₃OS. 395.56. (+)-10-[(1*R*)-Methyl-2-(1-pyrrolidinyl)ethyl]-*N*-propylphenothiazine-2-carboxamide. *UNII-5Q36UVB8YA*. *CAS-135003-30-4*. INN.

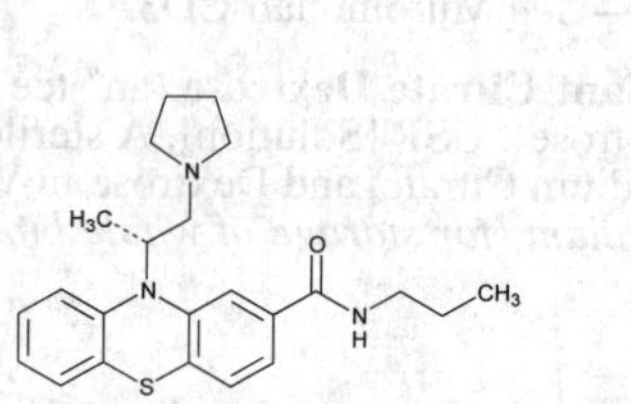

Apafant [*1997*] (a′ pa fant). $C_{22}H_{22}ClN_5O_2S$. 455.96. 4-[3-[4-(*o*-Chlorophenyl)-9-methyl-6*H*-thieno[3,2-*f*]-*s*-triazolo[4,3-*a*][1,4]diazepin-2-yl]propionyl]morpholine. *UNII-J613NI05SV. CAS-105219-56-5*. INN. *Platelet activating factor antagonist.* ◇*WEB 2086 BS*

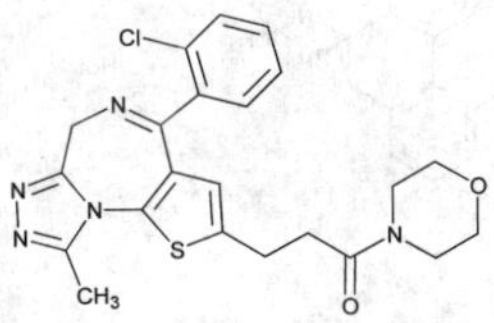

Apaflurane. C_3HF_7. 170.03. 1,1,1,2,3,3,3-Heptafluoropropane. *UNII-R40P36GDK6. CAS-431-89-0*. INN; BAN.

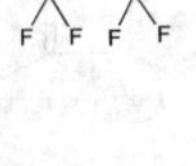

Apalcillin Sodium [*1986*] (ay″ pal sil′ in soe′ dee um). $C_{25}H_{22}N_5NaO_6S$. 543.53. (1) 4-Thia-1-azabicyclo[3.2.0]-heptane-2-carboxylic acid, 6-[[[[(4-hydroxy-1,5-naphthyridin-3-yl)carbonyl]amino]phenylacetyl]amino]-3,3-dimethyl-7-oxo-, monosodium salt, [2*S*-[2α,5α,6β(*S**)]]-; (2) Sodium (2*S*,5*R*,6*R*)-6-[(*R*)-2-(4-hydroxy-1,5-naphthyridine-3-carboxamido)-2-phenylacetamido]-3,3-dimethyl-7-oxo-4-thia-1-azabicyclo[3.2.0]heptane-2-carboxylate. *UNII-3XQ12NYC0Q. CAS-58795-03-2; CAS-63469-19-2* [apalcillin]. INN. *Antibacterial.* ◇*WY-44,417 sodium*

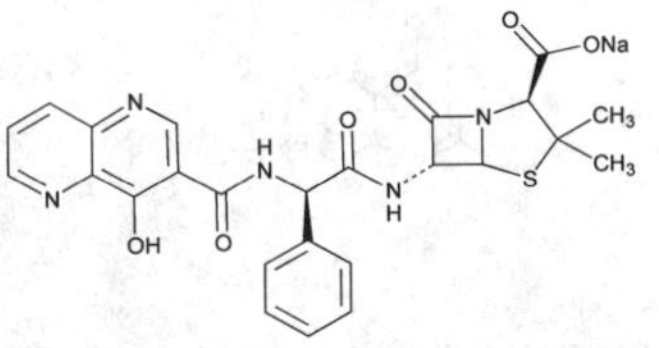

APAP — *See* Acetaminophen.

Apaxifylline [*1995*] (ay″ pax if′ i lin). $C_{16}H_{22}N_4O_3$. 318.37. (1) 1*H*-Purine-2,6-dione, 3,7-dihydro-8-(3-oxocyclopentyl)-1,3-dipropyl-, (*S*)-; (2) (-)-(*S*)-8-(3-Oxocyclopentyl)-1,3-dipropylxanthine. *UNII-OG8HSX6N6H. CAS-151581-23-6*. INN. *Selective adenosine A₁ antagonist.* ◇*BIIP 20 XX*

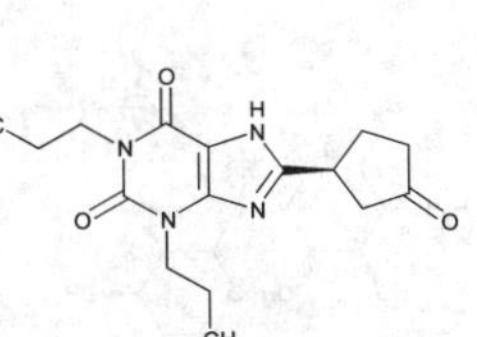

Apaziquone [*2002*] (ay paz′ i kwone). $C_{15}H_{16}N_2O_4$. 288.30. (1) 1*H*-Indole-4,7-dione, 5-(1-aziridinyl)-3-(hydroxymethyl)-2-[(1*E*)-3-hydroxy-1-propenyl]-1-methyl-; (2) 5-(Azridin-1-yl)-3-(hydroxymethyl)-2-[(1*E*)-3-hydroxyprop-1-enyl]-methyl-1*H*-indole-4,7-dione. *UNII-H464ZO600O. CAS-114560-48-4*. INN. *Antineoplastic.* ◇*EO9; NOR-701*

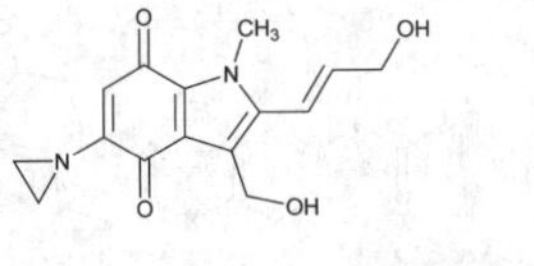

Apazone [*1969*] (ap′ a zone). $C_{16}H_{20}N_4O_2$. 300.36. [Azapropazone is INN and BAN.] (1) 1*H*-Pyrazolo[1,2-*a*][1,2,4]benzotriazine-1,3(2*H*)-dione, 5-(dimethylamino)-9-methyl-2-propyl-; (2) 5-(Dimethylamino)-9-methyl-2-propyl-1*H*-pyrazolo[1,2-*a*][1,2,4]benzotriazine-1,3(2*H*)-dione. *UNII-K2VOT966ZI. CAS-13539-59-8. Anti-inflammatory.* ◇*AHR-3018; Mi-85; NSC-102824*

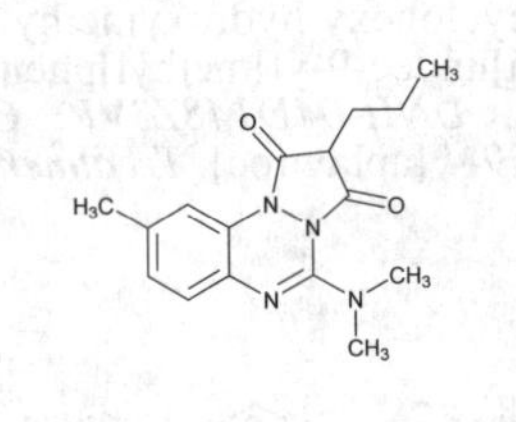

Apicycline. $C_{30}H_{38}N_4O_{11}$. 630.64. α-[4-(Dimethylamino)-1,4,4a,5,5a,6,11,12a-octahydro-3,6,10,12,12a-pentahydroxy-6-methyl-1,11-dioxo-2-naphthacenecarboxamido]-4-(2-hydroxyethyl)-1-piperazineacetic acid. *UNII-T1Y573BS7H. CAS-15599-51-6*. INN; MI. ◇*RIT 1140*

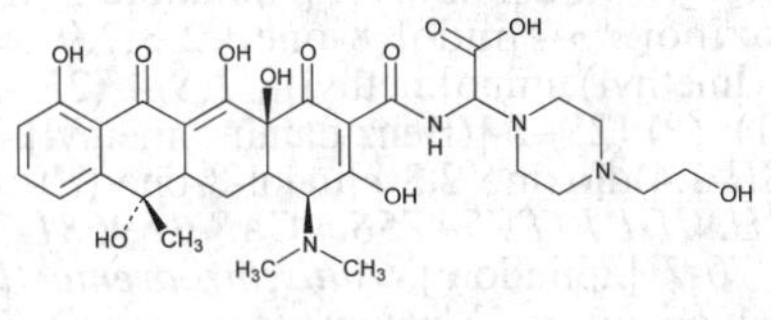

Apilimod Mesylate [*2006*] (a pil′ i mod mes′ i late). $C_{23}H_{26}N_6O_2$. 418.49. [Apilimod is INN.] (1) Benzaldehyde, 3-methyl-, [6-(4-morpholinyl)-2-[2-(2-pyridinyl)ethoxy]-4-pyrimidinyl]hydrazone mesylate; (2) N-(3-Methylbensylidene) N-[6-morpholin-4-yl-2(2-pyridin-2-yl-ethoxy)-pyrimidin-4-yl]-hydrazine bismesylate. *CAS-870087-36-8; CAS-541550-19-0* [apilimod]. *Treatment of inflammatory diseases (inhibits production of IL-12).* ◇*STA-5326 mesylate*

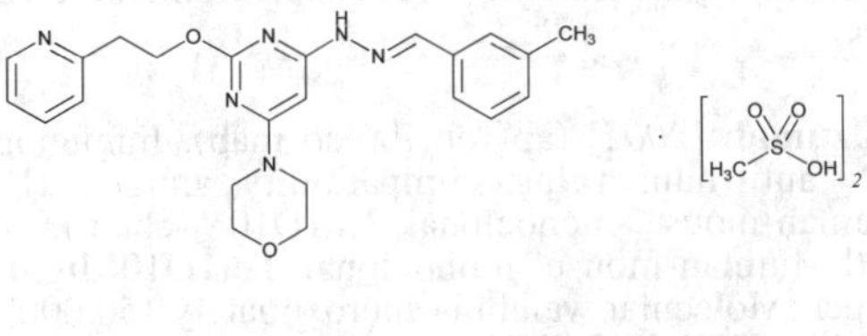

Apiplon (previously used name) — *See* Adipiplon.

Apixaban [*2005*] (a pix′ a ban). $C_{25}H_{25}N_5O_4$. 459.50. (1) 1*H*-Pyrazolo[3,4-*c*]pyridine-3-carboxamide,4,5,6,7-tetrahydro-1-(4-methoxyphenyl)-7-oxo-6-[4-(2-oxo-1-piperidinyl)phenyl]-; (2) 1-(4-Methoxyphenyl)-7-oxo-6-[4-(2-oxopiperidin-1-yl)phenyl]-4,5,6,7-tetrahydro-1*H*-pyrazo-

---

† Brand name formerly used, and/or firm no longer concerned with this product.

lo[3,4-*c*]pyridine-3-carboxamide. *UNII-3Z9Y7UWC1J. CAS-503612-47-3.* INN; JAN. *Anticoagulant, antithrombotic.* ◇*BMS-562247-01*

Aplaviroc Hydrochloride [*2005*] (ap″ la vir′ ok hye″ droe klor′ ide). C$_{33}$H$_{43}$N$_3$O$_6$.HCl. 614.17. [Aplaviroc is INN.] (1) Benzoic acid, 4-[4-[[(3*R*)-1-butyl-3-[(*R*)-cyclohexylhydroxymethyl]-2,5-dioxo-1,4,9-triazaspiro[5.5]undec-9-yl]-methyl]phenoxy]-, monohydrochloride; (2) 4-[4-[[(3*R*)-1-Butyl-3-[(*R*)-cyclohexylhydroxymethyl]-2,5-dioxo-1,4,9-triazaspiro[5.5]undec-9-yl]methyl]phenoxy]benzoic acid hydrochloride. *UNII-04D148Z3VR. CAS-461023-63-2; CAS-461443-59-4* [aplaviroc]. *Treatment of HIV infection.* ◇*GW873140A*

Aplindore Fumarate [*2004*] (ap′ lin dor fue′ ma rate). C$_{18}$H$_{18}$N$_2$O$_3$.C$_4$H$_4$O$_4$. 426.42. [Aplindore is INN.] (1) 8*H*-1,4-Dioxino[2,3-*e*]indol-8-one, 2,3,7,9-tetrahydro-2-[[(phenylmethyl)amino]methyl]-, 2(*S*)-, (2*E*)-2-butenedioate (1:1); (2) (2*S*)-2-[(Benzylamino)methyl]-2,3,7,9-tetrahydro-8*H*-1,4-dioxino[2,3-*e*]indol-8-one (*E*)- butenedioate (1:1). *UNII-P13TV5A758. CAS-189681-71-8; CAS-189681-70-7* [aplindore]. *Antischizoprenic (low intrinsic activity modulator of human dopamine D$_2$/D$_3$receptors). [Name previously used: Palindore Fumarate.]* ◇*DAB-452*

Aplonidine Hydrochloride — *See* Apraclonidine Hydrochloride.

Apolizumab [*2002*] (ap″ oh liz′ oo mab). Immunoglobulin G1, anti-(human histocompatibility antigen HLA-DR) (human-mouse monoclonal Hu1D10γ$_1$-chain), disulfide with human-mouse monoclonal Hu1D10 light chain, dimer. Molecular weight is approximately 150,000 daltons. *CAS-267227-08-7.* INN; BAN. *Anti-cancer agent against 1D10 antigen positive B-cell malignancies.* ◇*HU1D10*

Apomorphine Hydrochloride (a poe mor′ feen hye″ droe klor′ ide). **USP.** C$_{17}$H$_{17}$NO$_2$.HCl.½H$_2$O. 312.79. [Apomorphine is BAN.] (1) 4*H*-Dibenzo[*de,g*]quinoline-10,11-diol, 5,6,6a,7-tetrahydro-6-methyl-, hydrochloride, hemihydrate, (*R*)-; (2) 6a*β*-Aporphine-10,11-diol hydrochloride hemihydrate. *UNII-F39049Y068; UNII-N21FAR7B4S*

[apomorphine]. *CAS-41372-20-7; CAS-314-19-2* [anhydrous]; *CAS-58-00-4* [apomorphine]. *Emetic.* Apokyn (Vernalis)

Apovincamine. C$_{21}$H$_{24}$N$_2$O$_2$. 336.43. Methyl(3*α*,16*α*)-eburnamenine-14-carboxylate. *UNII-504R182ZX7. CAS-4880-92-6.* INN.

Apraclonidine Hydrochloride [*1988*] (a pra klon′ i deen hye″ droe klor′ ide). **USP.** C$_9$H$_{10}$Cl$_2$N$_4$.HCl. 281.57. [Apraclonidine is INN and BAN.] (1) 1,4-Benzenediamine, 2,6-dichloro-*N*^{1}-2-imidazolidinylidene-, monohydrochloride; (2) 2-[(4-Amino-2,6-dichlorophenyl)imino]imidazolidine monohydrochloride. *UNII-D2VW67N38H; UNII-843CEN85DI* [apraclonidine]. *CAS-73218-79-8; CAS-66711-21-5* [apraclonidine]. *Adrenergic (α$_2$-agonist).* Iopidine (Alcon) ◇*AL02145*

Apramycin [*1972*] (a″ pra mye′ sin). C$_{21}$H$_{41}$N$_5$O$_{11}$. 539.58. Antibiotic produced by *Streptomyces tenebrarius.* (1) D-Streptamine, 4-*O*-[(8*R*)-2-amino-8-*O*-(4-amino-4-deoxy-α-D-glucopyranosyl)-2,3,7-trideoxy-7-(methylamino)-D-*glycero*-α-D-*allo*-octodialdo-1,5:8,4-dipyranos-1-yl]-2-deoxy-; (2) 4-*O*-[(8*R*)-2-Amino-8-*O*-(4-amino-4-deoxy-α-D-glucopyranosyl)-2,3,7-trideoxy-7-(methylamino)-D-*gly-cero*-α-D-*allo*-octodialdo-1,5:8,4-dipyranos-1-yl]-2-deoxy-D-streptamine. *UNII-388K3TR36Z. CAS-37321-09-8; CAS-41194-16-5* [replaced]. INN; BAN. *Antibacterial.* ◇*EL-857; 47657*

Apratastat [*2004*] (a pra′ ta stat). C$_{17}$H$_{22}$N$_2$O$_6$S$_2$. 414.50. (1) 3-Thiomorpholinecarboxamide, *N*-hydroxy-4-[[4-[(4-hydroxy-2-butynyl)oxy]phenyl]sulfonyl]-2,2-dimethyl-, (3*S*)-; (2) (3*S*)-*N*-Hydroxy-4-[[4-[(4-hydroxybut-2-ynyl)oxy]phenyl]sulfonyl]-2,2-dimethylthiomorpholine-3-car-boxamide. *UNII-C6BZ5263BJ. CAS-287405-51-0.* INN. *Treatment of rheumatoid arthritis.* (Wyeth) ✧*TMI-005*

Apremilast [*2006*] (a pre′ mi last). $C_{22}H_{24}N_2O_7S$. 460.50. (1) Acetamide, *N*-[2-[(1*S*)-1-(3-ethoxy-4-methoxyphenyl)-2-(methylsulfonyl)ethyl]-2,3-dihydro-1,3-dioxo-1*H*-isoindol-4-yl]-; (2) (+)-*N*-[2-[(1*S*)-1-(3-Ethoxy-4-methoxyphenyl)-2-(methylsulfonyl)ethyl]-1,3-dioxo-2,3-dihydro-1*H*-isoindol-4-yl]acetamide. *UNII-UP7QBP99PN. CAS-608141-41-9.* INN. *Treatment of chronic inflammatory conditions including psoriasis, arthritis, asthma and cutaneous lupus erythematosus (CLE).* ✧*CC-10004*

Aprepitant [*2000*] (a pre′ pi tant). $C_{23}H_{21}F_7N_4O_3$. 534.43. (1) 3*H*-1,2,4-Triazol-3-one, 5-[[(2*R*,3*S*)-2-[(1*R*)-1-[3,5-bis(trifluoromethyl)phenyl]ethoxy]-3-(4-fluorophenyl)-4-morpholinyl]methyl]-1,2-dihydro-; (2) 3-[[(2*R*,3*S*)-3-(*p*-Fluorophenyl)-2-[[(α*R*)-α-methyl-3,5-bis(trifluoromethyl)benzyl]oxy]morpholino]methyl]-Δ²-1,2,4-triazolin-5-one. *UNII-1NF15YR6UY. CAS-170729-80-3.* INN; JAN. *Antiemetic in chemotherapy-induced emesis; antidepressant; treatment of psychiatric conditions [substance P antagonist (neurokinin NK₁antagonist)].* Emend (Merck) ✧*MK-0869*

Apricitabine. $C_8H_{11}N_3O_3S$. 229.26. 4-Amino-1-[(2*R*,4*R*)-2-(hydroxymethyl)-1,3-oxathiolan-4-yl]pyrimidin-2(1*H*)-one. *UNII-K1YX059ML1. CAS-160707-69-7.* INN.

Apricot Kernel Water. JAN.

Apricoxib [*2008*] (a″ pri kox′ ib). $C_{19}H_{20}N_2O_3S$. 356.44. (1) Benzenesulfonamide, 4-[2-(4-ethoxyphenyl)-4-methyl-1*H*-pyrrol-1-yl]-; (2) 4-[2-(4-Ethoxyphenyl)-4-methyl-1*H*-pyr-rol-1-yl]benzenesulfonamide. *UNII-5X5HB3VZ3Z. CAS-197904-84-0.* INN. *Treatment of pain and inflammation, oncology.* ✧*TG01; R-109339; CS-706*

Aprikalim. $C_{12}H_{16}N_2OS_2$. 268.40. (-)-(1*R*,2*R*)-Tetrahydro-*N*-methyl-2-(3-pyridyl)thio-2*H*-thiopyran-2-carboxamide 1-oxide. *UNII-374BH4KVRG. CAS-92569-65-8.* INN.

Aprindine [*1973*] (a prin′ deen). $C_{22}H_{30}N_2$. 322.49. (1) 1,3-Propanediamine, *N*-(2,3-dihydro-1*H*-inden-2-yl)-*N*′,*N*′-diethyl-*N*-phenyl-; (2) *N*,*N*-Diethyl-*N*′-2-indanyl-*N*′-phenyl-1,3-propanediamine. *UNII-5Y48085P9Q. CAS-37640-71-4.* INN; BAN. *Cardiac depressant (anti-arrhythmic).* ✧*Compound 99170*

Aprindine Hydrochloride [*1975*] (a prin′ deen hye″ droe klor′ ide). $C_{22}H_{30}N_2$·HCl. 358.95. (1) 1,3-Propanediamine, *N*-(2,3-dihydro-1*H*-inden-2-yl)-*N*′,*N*′-diethyl-*N*-phenyl-, monohydrochloride; (2) *N*,*N*-Diethyl-*N*′-2-indanyl-*N*′-phenyl-1,3-propanediamine monohydrochloride. *UNII-PB5EKT7Q2V; UNII-5Y48085P9Q* [aprindine]. *CAS-33237-74-0; CAS-37640-71-4* [aprindine]. JAN. *Cardiac depressant (anti-arrhythmic).* Fibocil (Lilly†) ✧*Compound 83846*

Aprinocarsen Sodium [*2003*] (a prin″ oh kar′ sen soe′ dee um). $C_{196}H_{230}N_{68}Na_{19}O_{105}P_{19}S_{19}$. 6852.86. [Aprinocarsen is INN.] (1) DNA, d(P-thio)(G-T-T-C-T-C-G-C-T-G-G-T-G-A-G-T-T-T-C-A) nonadecasodium salt; (2) 2′-Deoxy-*P*-thioadenylyl-(5′→3′)-2′-deoxy-*P*-thiocytidylyl-(5′→3′)-*P*-thiothymidylyl-(5′→3′)-*P*-thiothymidylyl-(5′→3′)-*P*-thiothymidylyl-(5′→3′)-2′-deoxy-*P*-thioguanylyl-(5′→3)-2′-deoxy-*P*-thioadenylyl-(5′→3′)-2′-deoxy-*P*-thioguany-lyl-(5′→3′)-*P*-thiothymidylyl-(5′→3′)-2′-deoxy-*P*-thioguanylyl-(5′→3′)-2′-deoxy-*P*-thioguanylyl-(5′→3′)-*P*-thiothy-midylyl-(5′→3′)-2′-deoxy-*P* thiocyticylyl-(5′→3′)-2′-deoxy-*P*-thioguanylyl-(5′→3′)-2′-deoxy-*P*-thiocytidylyl-(5′→3′)-*P*-thiothymidylyl-(5′→3′)-2′-deoxy-*P*-thiocytidylyl-(5′→3′)-*P*-thiothymidylyl-(5′→3′)-*P*-thiothymidylyl-(5′→3′)-2′-deoxyguanosine nonadecasodium salt. *CAS-151879-73-1* [for base substance]. *Treatment of non-small cell lung cancer (antisense oligonucleotide; protein kinase C-alpha inhibitor).* Affinitak (Isis) ✧*ISIS 5321*

---

† Brand name formerly used, and/or firm no longer concerned with this product.

Aprobarbital. $C_{10}H_{14}N_2O_3$. 210.23. 5-Allyl-5-isopropylbarbituric acid. *UNII-Q0YKG9L6RF. CAS-77-02-1.* NF XIII; INN; DCF; MI. Alurate (Hoffmann-LaRoche)

Aprofene. $C_{21}H_{27}NO_2$. 325.44. 2-Diethylaminoethyl 2,2-diphenylpropionate. *UNII-PL791XXJ7B. CAS-3563-01-7.* INN.

Aprosulate Sodium. $C_{27}H_{34}N_2Na_{16}O_{70}S_{16}$. 2387.41. N,N'-Trimethylenebis[actobionamide] hexadecakis(sodium sulfate) (ester). *UNII-311154J4LN. CAS-123072-45-7.* INN.

Aprotinin [*1968*] (a″ proe tye′ nin). **USP.** $C_{284}H_{432}N_{84}O_{79}S_7$. 6511.44. [Aprotinin Solution is JAN.] (1) Trypsin inhibitor, pancreatic basic; (2) L-Arginyl-L-prolyl-L-aspartyl-L-phenylalanyl-L-cysteinyl-L-leucyl-L-glutamyl-L-prolyl-L-prolyl-L-tyrosyl-L-threonylglycyl-L-prolyl-L-cysteinyl-L-lysyl-L-alanyl-L-arginyl-L-isoleucyl-L-isoleucyl-L-arginyl-L-tyrosyl-L-phenylalanyl-L-tyrosyl-L-asparaginyl-L-alanyl-L-lysyl-L-alanylglycyl-L-leucyl-L-cysteinyl-L-glutaminyl-L-threonyl-L-phenylalanyl-L-valyl-L-tyrosylglycylglycyl-L-cysteinyl-L-arginyl-L-alanyl-L-lysyl-L-arginyl-L-asparaginyl-L-asparaginyl-L-phenylalanyl-L-lysyl-L-seryl-L-alanyl-L-glutamyl-L-aspartyl-L-cysteinyl-L-methionyl-L-arginyl-L-threonyl-L-cysteinylglycylglycyl-L-alanine cyclic (5→55), (14→38), (30→51) tris(disulfide). *UNII-04XPW8C0FL. CAS-9087-70-1; CAS-12407-79-3* [ox pancreas basic]; *CAS-11061-94-2* [ox pancreas basic reduced]. INN; BAN. *Enzyme inhibitor (proteinase).* Trasylol (Bayer) ◇*RP 9921; Riker 52G; Bayer A 128*

```
RPDFCLEPPY  TGPCKARIIR  YFYNAKAGLC  QTFVYGGCRA  KRNNFKSAED
CMRTCGGA
```

Aptazapine Maleate [*1984*] (ap taz′ a peen mal′ ee ate). $C_{16}H_{19}N_3 \cdot C_4H_4O_4$. 369.41. [Aptazapine is INN.] (1) $2H,10H$-Pyrazino[1,2-*a*]pyrrolo[2,1-*c*][1,4]benzodiazepine, 1,3,4,14b-tetrahydro-2-methyl-, (±)-, (*Z*)-2-butenedioate (1:1); (2) (±)-1,3,4,14b-Tetrahydro-2-methyl-$2H,10H$-pyrazino[1,2-*a*]pyrrolo[2,1-*c*][1,4]benzodiazepine maleate (1:1). *UNII-7X768418RT. CAS-71576-41-5; CAS-71576-40-4* [aptazapine]. *Antidepressant.* ◇*CGS 7525A*

Aptiganel Hydrochloride [*1996*] (ap ti ga′ nel hye″ droe klor′ ide). $C_{20}H_{21}N_3 \cdot HCl$. 339.86. [Aptiganel is INN.] (1) Guanidine, N-(3-ethylphenyl)-N-methyl-N'-1-naphthalenyl, monohydrochloride; (2) 1-(*m*-Ethylphenyl)-1-methyl-3-(1-naphthyl)guanidine monohydrochloride. *UNII-46475LV84I* [aptiganel]. *CAS-137160-11-3; CAS-137159-92-3* [aptiganel]. *Stroke and traumatic brain injury treatment (NMDA ion channel blocker).* Cerestat (Cambridge) ◇*CNS 1102*

Aptocaine. $C_{14}H_{20}N_2O$. 232.32. 2-Methyl-1-pyrrolidineaceto-*o*-toluidide. *UNII-08K838NNTE. CAS-19281-29-9.* INN; BAN; DCF.

Arabinosyl Cytosine — *See* Cytarabine.

Arachis Oil — *See* Peanut Oil.

Ara-Cytidine — *See* Cytarabine.

Aranidipine. $C_{19}H_{20}N_2O_7$. 388.37. (±)-Acetonyl methyl 1,4-dihydro-2,6-dimethyl-4-(*o*-nitrophenyl)-3,5-pyridinedicarboxylate. *UNII-4Y7UR6X2PO. CAS-86780-90-7.* INN.

Aranotin [*1968*] (ar″ a noe′ tin). $C_{20}H_{18}N_2O_7S_2$. 462.50. (1) $8H,16H$-7a,15a-Epidithio-$7H,15H$-bisoxepino[3′,4′:4,5]pyrrolo[1,2-*a*:1′,2′-*d*]pyrazine-7,15-dione, 5-(acetyloxy)-5,5a,13,13a-tetrahydro-13-hydroxy-; (2) 5,5a,13,13a-Tetrahydro-5,13-dihydroxy-$8H,16H$-7a,15a-epidithio-$7H,15H$-bisoxepino[3′,4′:4,5]pyrrolo[1,2-a:1′,2′-*d*]pyrazine-7,15-dione 5-acetate. *UNII-H56CKB2FFV. CAS-19885-51-9.* INN. *Antiviral.* ◇*53183*

Araprofen. $C_{16}H_{15}NO_4$. 285.29. ($\pm$)-*p*-(*o*-Carboxyanilino)hydratropic acid. *UNII-BIQ52YQ7VG. CAS-15250-13-2.* INN.

Arasertaconazole. $C_{20}H_{15}Cl_3N_2OS$. 437.77. 1-{(2*R*)-2-[(7-Chloro-1-benzothiophen-3-yl)methoxy]-2-(2,4-dichlorophenyl)ethyl}-1*H*-imidazole. *UNII-PR82C5R514. CAS-583057-48-1.* INN.

Arbaclofen Placarbil [*2006*] (ar bak′ loe fen pla kar′ bil). $C_{19}H_{26}ClNO_6$. 399.87. (1) Benzenepropanoic acid, 4-chloro-*β*-[[[[(1*S*)-2-methyl-1-(2-methyl-1-oxopropoxy)-propoxy]carbonyl]amino]methyl]-, (*βR*)-; (2) (3*R*)-3-(4-Chlorophenyl)-4-[[[(1*S*)-2-methyl-1-[(2-methylpropanoyl)oxy]propoxy]carbonyl]amino]butanoic acid. *UNII-W89H91R7VX. CAS-847353-30-4.* INN. *Treatment of gastro-esophageal reflux disease (GERD) and spasticity.* ◇*XP19986*

Arbaprostil [*1976*] (ar″ ba prost′ il). $C_{21}H_{34}O_5$. 366.49. (1) Prosta-5,13-dien-1-oic acid, 11,15-dihydroxy-15-methyl-9-oxo-, (5*Z*,11*α*,13*E*,15*R*)-; (2) (*E,Z*)-(1*R*,2*R*,3*R*)-7-[3-Hydroxy-2-[(3*R*)-(3-hydroxy-3-methyl-1-octenyl)]-5-oxo-cyclopentyl]-5-heptenoic acid; (3) (15*R*)-15-Methylprostaglandin E_2. *UNII-M6B59S6MEF. CAS-55028-70-1.* INN. *Antisecretory (gastric).* ◇*U 42,842*

Arbekacin. $C_{22}H_{44}N_6O_{10}$. 552.62. [Arbekacin Sulfate is JAN.] *O*-3-Amino-3-deoxy-*α*-D-glucopyranosyl-(1→4)-*O*-[2,6-diamino-2,3,4,6-tetradeoxy-*α*-D-*erythro*-hexopyranosyl-(1→6)]-*N′*-[(2*S*)-4-amino-2-hydroxybutyryl]-2-deoxy-L-streptamine. *UNII-G7V6SLI20L. CAS-51025-85-5.* INN; MI.

Arbutamine Hydrochloride [*1992*] (ar bue′ ta meen hye″ droe klor′ ide). $C_{18}H_{23}NO_4 \cdot HCl$. 353.84. [Arbutamine is INN and BAN.] (1) 1,2-Benzenediol, 4-[1-hydroxy-2-[[4-(4-hydroxyphenyl)butyl]amino]ethyl]-, (*R*)-hydrochloride; (2) (*R*)-3,4-Dihydroxy-*α*-[[[4-(*p*-hydroxyphenyl)butyl]amino]methyl]benzyl alcohol hydrochloride. *UNII-K0NF2CPJ7F; UNII-B07L15YAEV* [arbutamine]. *CAS-125251-66-3; CAS-128470-16-6* [arbutamine]. *Stimulant (cardiac).* Genesa (Gensia) ◇*GP-2-121-3*

Arcitumomab [*1995*] (ar″ si toom′ oh mab). (1) Immunoglobulin G 1 (mouse monoclonal IMMU-4 Fab′ fragment *γ*-chain anti-human antigen CEA), disulfide with mouse monoclonal IMMU-4 light chain; (2) Immunoglobulin G 1 (mouse monoclonal IMMU-4 Fab′ fragment *γ*-chain anti-human antigen CEA), disulfide with mouse monoclonal IMMU-4 light chain. Molecular weight is approximately 54,000 daltons. *CAS-154361-48-5; CAS-154361-49-6* [technetium Tc 99m arcitumomab]. INN. *Monoclonal antibody.* CEA-Scan (Immunomedics) *[Note—The clinically administered preparation is the monoclonal antibody (arcitumomab) labeled with technetium Tc 99m, or technetium Tc 99m arcitumomab. The CAS name for this preparation is Immunoglobulin G 1 (mouse monoclonal IMMU-4 Fab′ fragment γ-chain anti-human antigen CEA), disulfide with mouse monoclonal IMMU-4 light chain, technetium-^{99m}Tc salt.]* ◇*IMMU-4*

Arclofenin [*1984*] (ar″ kloe fen′ in). $C_{19}H_{17}ClN_2O_6$. 404.80. (1) Glycine, *N*-[2-[(2-benzoyl-4-chlorophenyl)amino]-2-oxoethyl]-*N*-(carboxymethyl)-; (2) [[[(2-Benzoyl-4-chlorophenyl)carbamoyl]methyl]imino]diacetic acid. *UNII-RN145A0SVL. CAS-87071-16-7.* INN. *Diagnostic aid (hepatic function determination).*

Ardacin. $C_{81}H_{82}Cl_4N_8O_{30}$ (aridicin A). 1789.37; $C_{82}H_{84}Cl_4N_8O_{30}$ (aridicin B). 1803.39; $C_{83}H_{86}Cl_4N_8O_{30}$ (aridicin C). 1817.42; $C_{83}H_{86}Cl_4N_8O_{30}$ (aridicin C_2). 1817.42. A mixture of aridicin A, aridicin B, aridicin C and aridicin C_2; the latter are glucopeptide antibiotics derived from a new species of the genus *Kibdelosporangium aridum*, strain ATCC 39323. They contain a

---

† Brand name formerly used, and/or firm no longer concerned with this product.

mannose and a glycolipid group attached at as yet undetermined sites. *CAS-117742-13-9*. INN; BAN. ◇*AAD AAD 216; SK&F 100814*

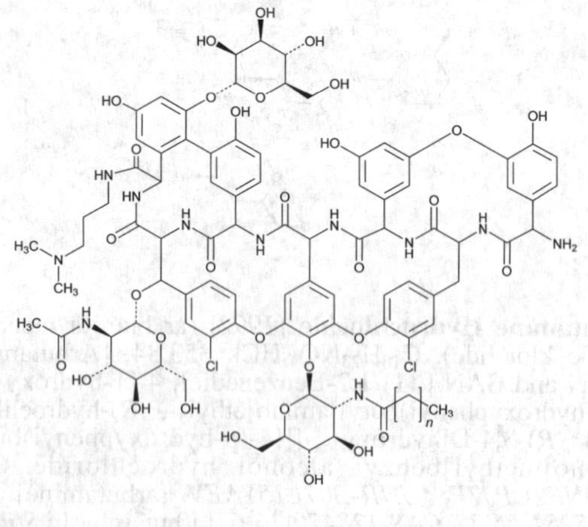

Ardenermin [*2002*] (ar″ de ner′ min). $C_{770}H_{1207}N_{193}O_{232}S_5$ (reduced protein). 134-285-Neutrokine α (human clone HNEDU15 precursor). *CAS-305391-49-5*. INN. *B cell survival factor that affects B cell representation and serum immunoglobulins in patients with congenital or acquired immunodeficiencies (tumor necrosis factor).* BLyS (Human Genome Sciences) ◇*BLyS; TNFSF20; BAFF; TALL-1; zTNF4; THANK; TL7; TNFSBF13B*

```
AVQGPEETVT   QDCLQLIADS   ETPTIQKGSY   TFVPWLLSFK   RGSALEEKEN
KILVKETGYF   FIYGQVLYTD   KTYAMGHLIQ   RKKVHVFGDE   LSLVTLFRCI
QNMPETLPNN   SCYSAGIAKL   EEGDELQLAI   PRENAQISLD   GDVTFFGALK
LL
```

Ardeparin Sodium [*1993*] (ar dep′ a rin soe′ dee um; ar″ de par′ in soe′ dee um). Depolymerized heparin obtained by peroxide fragmentation of heparin sodium (USP). The end chain structure appears to be the same as the starting material with no unusual sugar residues present. The low molecular weight heparin produced differs from the starting material in molecular weight only. The average relative molecular mass range is 5,500 to 6,500 daltons, with not less than 98%, by weight, of the compounds between 2,000 and 15,000 daltons. The degree of sulfation is approximately 2.7 sulfate residues per disaccharide unit. The substance is the sodium salt. *CAS-9041-08-1*. INN. *Anticoagulant.* Normiflo (Pfizer) ◇*WY-90493 RD*

Arecoline Hydrobromide. *UNII-24S79B9CX7; UNII-4ALN5933BH* [arecoline]. *CAS-300-08-3; CAS-63-75-2* [arecoline]. NF XII; MI.

Arfalasin. $C_{48}H_{67}N_{13}O_{11}$. 1002.13. 1-Succinamic acid-5-L-valine-8-(L-2-phenylglycine)angiotensin II. *CAS-60173-73-1*. INN.

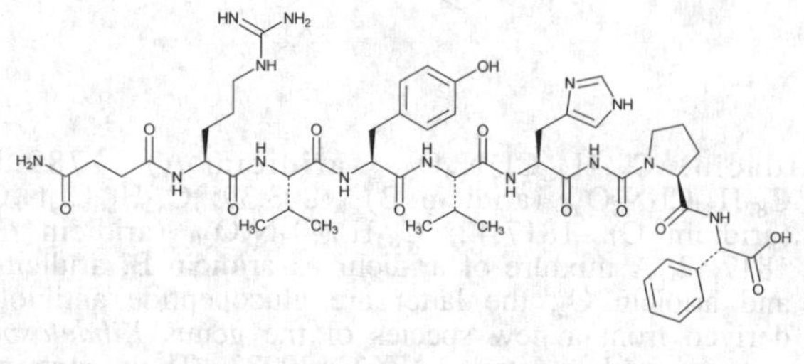

Arfendazam. $C_{18}H_{17}ClN_2O_3$. 344.79. Ethyl 7-chloro-2,3,4,5-tetrahydro-4-oxo-5-phenyl-1*H*-1,5-benzodiazepine-1-carboxylate. *UNII-P37G7BTX8V. CAS-37669-57-1*. INN.

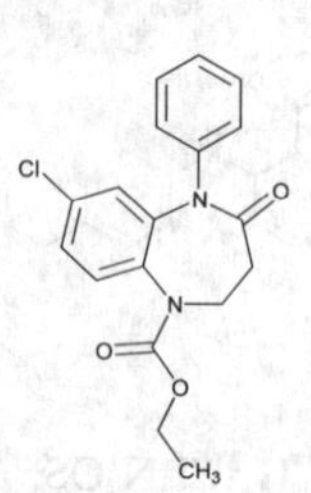

Arformoterol Tartrate [*2003*] (ar″ for moe′ ter ol tar′ trate). $C_{19}H_{24}N_2O_4.C_4H_6O_6$. 494.49. [Arformoterol is INN.] (1) Formamide, *N*-[2-hydroxy-5-[(1*R*)-1-hydroxy-2-[[(1*R*)-2-(4-methoxyphenyl)-1-methylethyl]amino]ethyl]phenyl]-, (2*R*,3*R*)-2,3-dihydroxybutanedioate (1:1) (salt); (2) (-)-*N*-[2-Hydroxy-5-[(1*R*)-1-hydroxy-2-[[(1*R*)-2-(4-methoxyphenyl)-1-methylethyl]amino]ethyl]phenyl]formamide hydrogen (2*R*,3*R*)-2,3-dihydroxybutanedioate (salt). *UNII-5P8VJ2I235; UNII-F91H02EBWT* [arformoterol]. *CAS-200815-49-2; CAS-67346-49-0* [arformoterol]. *Anti-asthmatic and bronchodilator.* Brovana (Sepracor)

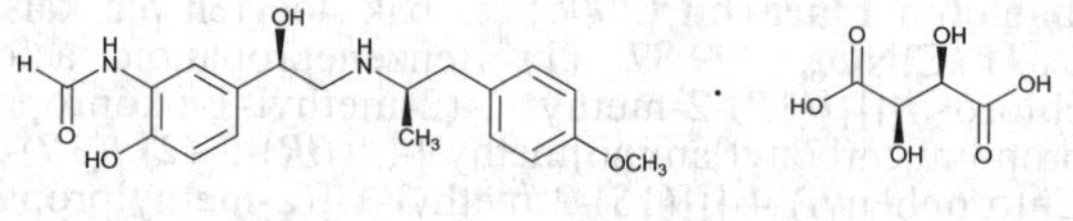

Argatroban [*1997*] (ar gat′ roe ban). $C_{23}H_{36}N_6O_5S.H_2O$. 526.65. (1) 2-Piperidinecarboxylic acid, 1-[5-[(aminoiminomethyl)amino]-1-oxo-2-[[(1,2,3,4-tetrahydro-3-methyl-8-quinolinyl)sulfonyl]amino]pentyl]-4-methyl-, monohydrate; (2) (2*R*,4*R*)-4-Methyl-1-[*N*²-[(1,2,3,4-tetrahydro-3-methyl-8-quinolyl)sulfonyl]-L-arginyl]pipecolic acid, monohydrate. *UNII-IY90U61Z3S; UNII-OCY3U280Y3* [argatroban anhydrous]. *CAS-141396-28-3; CAS-74863-84-6* [anhydrous]. INN; BAN; JAN. *Anticoagulant.* ◇*MCI-9038; MD-805; DK-7419; GN1600*

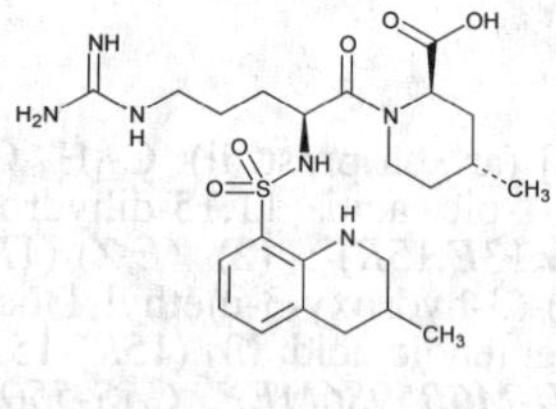

Argimesna. $C_8H_{20}N_4O_5S_2$. 316.40. L-Arginine mono(2-mercaptoethanesulfonate). *UNII-62V6QH821R. CAS-106854-46-0*. INN.

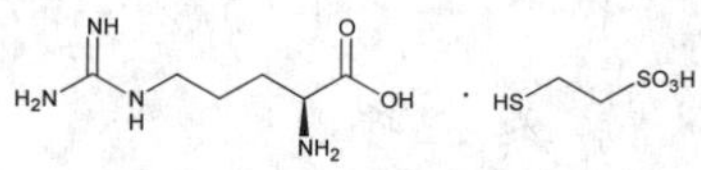

Arginine (ar′ ji neen). **USP.** $C_6H_{14}N_4O_2$. 174.20. (1) L-Arginine; (2) L-Arginine. *UNII-94ZLA3W45F. CAS-74-79-3*. INN. *Ammonia detoxicant; diagnostic aid (pituitary function determination).*

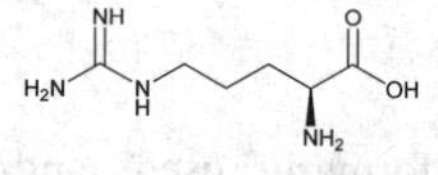

Arginine Glutamate [*1963*] (ar′ ji neen gloo′ ta mate). $C_6H_{14}N_4O_2 \cdot C_5H_9NO_4$. 321.33. (1) L-Arginine L-glutamate (1:1); (2) L-Arginine L-glutamate (1:1). *UNII-TU1X77K34Q*. *CAS-4320-30-3*. BAN; JAN. *Ammonia detoxicant*. Modumate (Abbott†)

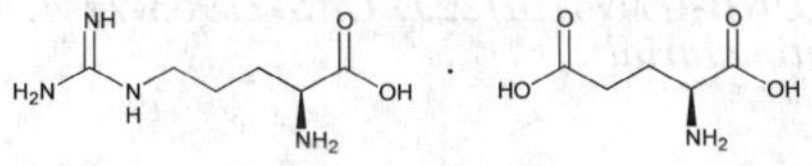

Arginine Hydrochloride [*1970*] (ar′ ji neen hye″ droe klor′ ide). **USP**. $C_6H_{14}N_4O_2 \cdot HCl$. 210.66. (1) L-Arginine monohydrochloride; (2) L-(+)-Arginine monohydrochloride. *UNII-F7LTH1E20Y; UNII-94ZLA3W45F* [arginine]. *CAS-1119-34-2* [L]; *CAS-74-79-3* [L-arginine]. JAN. *Ammonia detoxicant*. R-gene 10 (Pfizer)

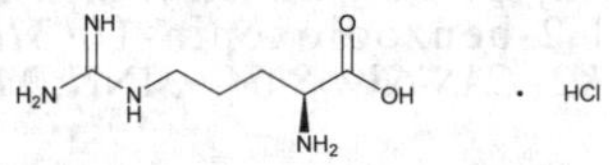

Argipressin Tannate [*1977*] (ar″ ji pres′ in tan′ ate). [Argipressin is INN and BAN.] (1) Vasopressin, 8-L-arginine-, tannate; (2) 8-L-Argininevasopressin tannate; (3) Tannins, compound with 8-L-argininevasopressin. *CAS-113-79-1* [argipressin]. *Antidiuretic*. Pitressin Tannate (Synthetic) (Parke-Davis†) ◇*CI-107*

Argiprestocin. $C_{43}H_{67}N_{15}O_{12}S_2$. 1050.22. 8-Arginineoxytocin. *CAS-113-80-4*. INN.

Arildone [*1977*] (ar′ il done). $C_{20}H_{29}ClO_4$. 368.89. (1) 3,5-Heptanedione, 4-[6-(2-chloro-4-methoxyphenoxy)hexyl]-; (2) 4-[6-(2-Chloro-4-methoxyphenoxy)hexyl]-3,5-heptanedione. *UNII-69MBN7JF59*. *CAS-56219-57-9*. INN. *Antiviral*. ◇*Win 38020*

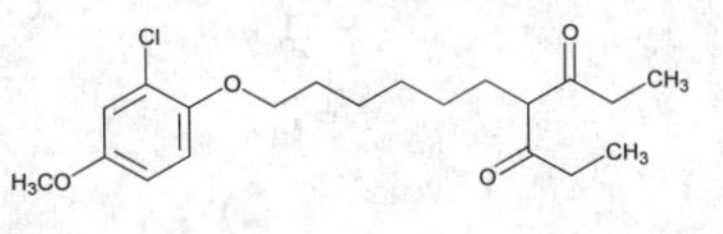

Arimoclomol. $C_{14}H_{20}ClN_3O_3$. 313.78. *N*-[(2*R*)-2-Hydroxy-3-(1-piperidyl)propoxy]pyridine-3-carboximidoyl chloride, 1-oxide. *UNII-EUT3557RT5*. *CAS-289893-25-0*. INN.

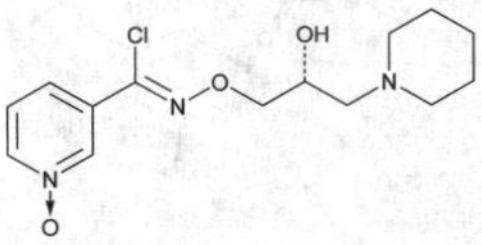

Aripiprazole [*1997*] (ar″ i pip′ ra zole). $C_{23}H_{27}Cl_2N_3O_2$. 448.39. (1) 2(1*H*)-Quinolinone, 7-[4-[4-(2,3-dichlorophenyl)-1-piperazinyl]butoxy]-3,4-dihydro-; (2) 7-[4-[4-(2,3-Dichlorophenyl)-1-piperazinyl]butoxy]-3,4-dihydrocar

bostyril. *UNII-82VFR53I78*. *CAS-129722-12-9*. INN; BAN. *Antipsychotic; antischizophrenic*. Abilify (Otsuka) ◇*OPC-14597; OPC-31*

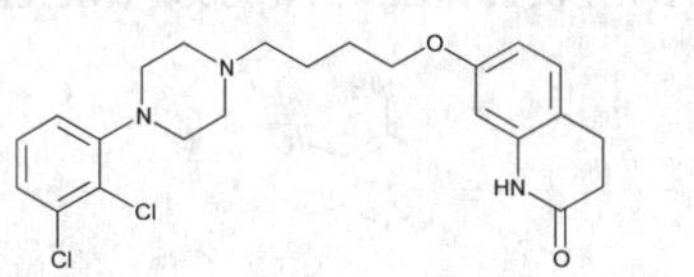

Armodafinil [*2004*] (ar moe daf′ i nil). $C_{15}H_{15}NO_2S$. 273.35. (1) Acetamide, 2-[(diphenylmethyl)sulfinyl]-, (-)-; (2) (-)-2-[(*R*)-(Diphenylmethyl)sulfinyl]acetamide. *UNII-V63XWA605I*. *CAS-112111-43-0*. INN. *Wakefulness promoting agent*. ◇*CEP-10953*

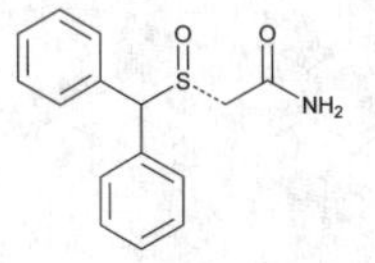

Arnolol. $C_{14}H_{23}NO_3$. 253.34. (±)-3-Amino-1-[*p*-(2-methoxyethyl)phenoxy]-3-methyl-2-butanol. *UNII-98HS077RUP*. *CAS-87129-71-3*. INN.

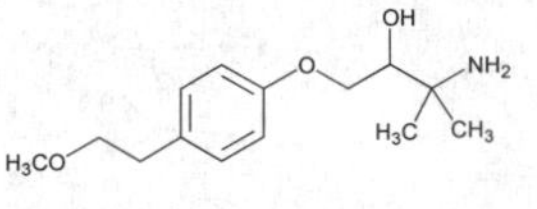

Arofylline [*1997*] (ar of′ i lin). $C_{14}H_{13}ClN_4O_2$. 304.73. 3-(*p*-Chlorophenyl)-1-propylxanthine. *UNII-87L38AY71R*. *CAS-136145-07-8*. INN; BAN. *Anti-asthmatic (type IV phosphodiesterase inhibitor); asthma prophylactic; bronchodilator*. ◇*LAS 31025*

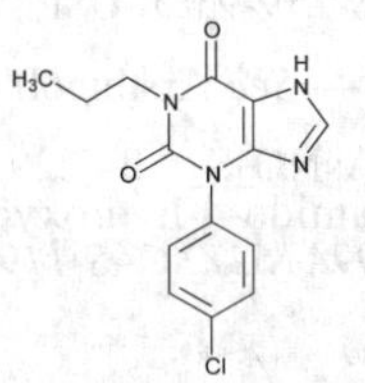

Aronixil. $C_{14}H_{15}ClN_4O_2$. 306.75. *N*-[4-Chloro-6-(2,3-xylidino)-2-pyrimidinyl]glycine. *UNII-15UTM533IP*. *CAS-86627-15-8*. INN.

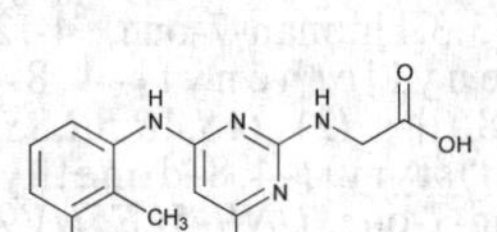

Arotinolol. $C_{15}H_{21}N_3O_2S_3$. 371.54. [Arotinolol Hydrochloride is JAN.] (±)-5-[2-[[3-(*tert*-Butylamino)-2-hydroxypropyl]thio]-4-thiazolyl]-2-thiophenecarboxamide. *UNII-394E3P3B99*. *CAS-68377-92-4*. INN; MI.

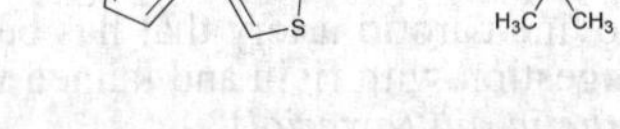

---

† Brand name formerly used, and/or firm no longer concerned with this product.

Arprinocid [*1977*] (ar prin′ oh sid). $C_{12}H_9ClFN_5$. 277.68. (1) 9*H*-Purin-6-amine, 9-[(2-chloro-6-fluorophenyl)methyl]-; (2) 9-(2-Chloro-6-fluorobenzyl)adenine. *CAS-55779-18-5.* INN; BAN. *Coccidiostat.* Arpocox (Merck)

Arpromidine. $C_{21}H_{25}FN_6$. 380.46. (±)-1-[3-(*p*-Fluorophenyl)-3-(2-pyridyl)propyl]-3-(3-imidazol-4-ylpropyl)guanidine. *UNII-85713MT0EH. CAS-106669-71-0.* INN.

Arsambide — *See* Carbarsone.

Arsanilic Acid (ar″ sa nil′ ik as′ id). **USP.** $C_6H_8AsNO_3$. 217.05. *p*-Aminobenzenearsonic acid. *UNII-UD-X9AKS7GM. CAS-98-50-0.* INN; BAN; MI. *Antibacterial (veterinary).* ◊*AS 101*

Arsenic Trioxide [*2001*] (ar′ se nik trye ox′ ide). As_2O_3. 197.84. (1) Arsenic oxide; (2) Diarsenic trioxide. *UNII-S7V92P67HO. CAS-1327-53-3.* JAN. *Treatment of acute promyelocytic leukemia.* Trisenox (Cephalon)

Arsphenamine. *CAS-139-93-5.* USP XIII; MI.

Arsthinenol (DCF) — *See* Arsthinol.

Arsthinol. $C_{11}H_{14}AsNO_3S_2$. 347.29. 3-Hydroxypropylene ester of 3-acetamido-4-hydroxydithiobenzenearsonous acid. *UNII-QNT09A162Y. CAS-119-96-0.* INN; MI.

Arteflene [*1995*] (ar′ te fleen). $C_{19}H_{18}F_6O_3$. 408.33. (1) 2,3-Dioxabicyclo[3.3.1]nonan-7-one, 4-[2-[2,4-bis(trifluoromethyl)phenyl]ethenyl]-4,8-dimethyl-[1*S*-[1α,4β(*Z*),5α,8β]]-; (2) (1*S*,4*R*,5*R*,8*S*)-4-[(*Z*)-2,4-Bis(trifluoromethyl)styryl]-4,8-dimethyl-2,3-dioxabicyclo[3.3.1]nonan-7-one. *UNII-5PE5HV9NF0. CAS-123407-36-3.* INN. *Antimalarial.* ◊*Ro 42-1611*

Artegraft [*1970*] (ar′ te graft). Arterial graft composed of a section of bovine carotid artery that has been subjected to enzymatic digestion with ficin and tanned with dialdehyde starch. *Prosthetic aid (arterial).*

Artemether [*2008*] (ar tem′ e ther). $C_{16}H_{26}O_5$. 298.37. (1) 3,12-Epoxy-12*H*-pyrano[4,3-*j*]-1,2-benzodioxepin, decahydro-10-methoxy-3,6,9-trimethyl-, (3*R*,5a*S*,6*R*,8a*S*,9*R*,10*S*,12*R*,12a*R*)-; (2) (3*R*,5a*S*,6*R*,8a*S*,9*R*,10*S*,12*R*,12a*R*)-10-Methoxy-3,6,9-trimethyldecahydro-3,12-epoxypyrano[4,3-*j*]-1,2-benzodioxepine. *UNII-C7D6T3H22J. CAS-71963-77-4.* INN; BAN; MI. *Antimalarial.*

Artemisinin. $C_{15}H_{22}O_5$. 282.33. (3*R*,5a*S*,6*R*,8a*S*,9*R*,12-*S*,12a*R*)-Octahydro-3,6,9-trimethyl-3,12-epoxy-12*H*-pyrano[4,3-*j*]-1,2-benzodioxepin-10(3*H*)-one. *UNII-9RMU91N5K2. CAS-63968-64-9.* INN; MI.

Artemisone. $C_{19}H_{31}NO_6S$. 401.52. 4-[(3*R*,5a*S*,6-*R*,8a*S*,9*R*,10*R*,12*R*,12a*R*)-3,6,9-Trimethyldecahydro-12*H*-3,12-epoxypyrano[4,3-*j*][1,2]benzodioxepin-10-yl]thiomorpholine-1,1-dione. *CAS-255730-18-8.* INN. *[Name previously used: Artemifone.]*

Artemotil. $C_{17}H_{28}O_5$. 312.40. (3*R*,5a*S*,6*R*,8a*S*,9*R*,10*S*,12-*R*,12a*R*)-10-Ethoxydecahydro-3,6,9-trimethyl-3,12-epoxy-12*H*-pyrano[4,3-*j*]-1,2-benzodioxepin. *UNII-XGL7GFB9YI. CAS-75887-54-6.* INN.

Artenimol. $C_{15}H_{24}O_5$. 284.35. (3*R*,5a*S*,6*R*,8a*S*,9*R*,10*S*,12-*R*,12a*R*)-Decahydro-3,6,9-trimethyl-3,12-epoxy-12*H*-pyrano[4,3-*j*]-1,2-benzodioxepin-10-ol. *CAS-81496-81-3.* INN.

Arterolane. $C_{22}H_{36}N_2O_4$. 392.53. *N*-(2-Amino-2-methylpropyl)-2-{*cis*-dispiro[adamantane-2,3′-[1,2,4]trioxolane-5′,1″-cyclohexan]-4″-yl}acetamide. *CAS-664338-39-0.* INN.

Artesunate [*2002*] (ar tes′ oo nate). $C_{19}H_{28}O_8$. 384.42. (1) Butanedioic acid, mono[(3*R*,5a*S*,6*R*,8a*S*,9*R*,10*S*,12-*R*,12a*R*)-decahydro-3,6,9-trimethyl-3,12-epoxy-12*H*-pyrano[4,3-*j*]-1,2-benzodioxepin-10-yl] ester; (2) 4-Oxo-4-[[(3*R*,5a*S*,6*R*,8a*S*,9*R*,10*S*,12*R*,12a*R*)-3,6,9-trimethyldecahydro-3,12-epoxypyrano[4,3-*j*]-1,2-benzodioxepin-10-yl hydrogen butanedioate. *UNII-60W3249T9M. CAS-182824-33-5; CAS-88495-63-0* [replaced]. INN; BAN; MI. *Antimalarial therapy.* Arsumax (Knoll, Switzerland)

Articaine. $C_{13}H_{20}N_2O_3S$. 284.37. 4-Methyl-3-[2-(propylamino)propionamido]-2-thiophenecarboxylic acid, methyl ester. *UNII-D3SQ406G9X. CAS-23964-58-1.* INN; BAN. *[Name previously used: Carticaine.]* ◇40 045; Hoe 045

Articaine Hydrochloride [*1998*] (ar′ ti kane hye″ droe klor′ ide). $C_{13}H_{20}N_2O_3S.HCl$. 320.84. (1) 2-Thiophenecarboxylic acid, 4-methyl-3-[[1-oxo-2-(propylamino)propyl]amino]-, methyl ester, monohydrochloride; (2) Methyl 4-methyl-3-[2-(propylamino)propionamido]-2-thiophenecarboxylate, monohydrochloride. *UNII-QS9014Q792. CAS-23964-57-0. Local-anesthetic.* Septanest (Cilag-Chemie, Switzerland); Septocaine (Cilag-Chemie, Switzerland); Ultracaine (Hoechst AG, Germany) ◇HOE 045; 40 045

Artilide Fumarate [*1992*] (ar′ ti lide fue′ ma rate). $[C_{19}H_{34}N_2O_3S]_2.C_4H_4O_4$. 857.17. [Artilide is INN.] (1) Methanesulfonamide, *N*-[4-[4-(dibutylamino)-1-hydroxybutyl]phenyl]-, (*R*)-, (*E*)-2-butenedioate (2:1) (salt); (2) (+)-4′-[(*R*)-4-(Dibutylamino)-1-hydroxybutyl]methanesulfonanilide fumarate (2:1) (salt). *UNII-H5L34MU3TQ* [artilide]. *CAS-133267-20-6; CAS-133267-19-3* [artilide]. *Cardiac depressant (anti-arrhythmic).* ◇U-88943E

Arundic Acid. $C_{11}H_{22}O_2$. 186.29. (2*R*)-2-Propyloctanoic acid. *UNII-F2628ZD0FO. CAS-185517-21-9.* INN.

Arzoxifene. $C_{28}H_{29}NO_4S$. 475.60. 2-(*p*-Methoxyphenyl)-3-[*p*-(2-piperidinoethoxy)phenoxy]benzo[*b*]thiophene-6-ol. *UNII-E569WG6E60. CAS-182133-25-1.* INN.

Arzoxifene Hydrochloride [*1998*] (ar zox′ i feen hye″ droe klor′ ide). $C_{28}H_{29}NO_4S.HCl$. 512.06. (1) 2-(4-Methoxyphenyl)-3-[4-[2-(1-piperidinyl)ethoxy]phenoxy]benzo[*b*]thiophene-6-ol hydrochloride; (2) 2-(*p*-Methoxyphenyl)-3-[*p*-(2-piperidinoethoxy)phenoxy]benzo[*b*]thiophene-6-ol hydrochloride. *CAS-182133-27-3. Treatment of symptoms associated with uterine fibroids, endometriosis, and dysfunctional uterine bleeding; in the treatment of estrogen receptor positive recurrent/metastatic breast cancer; as an adjuvant to breast cancer therapy (selective estrogen receptor modulator).* ◇SERM 3; LY353381.HCl

[74]As — *See* Sodium Arsenate As 74.

Ascorbic Acid (as kore′ bik as′ id). **USP.** $C_6H_8O_6$. 176.12. (1) L-Ascorbic acid; (2) L-Ascorbic acid. *UNII-PQ6CK8PD0R. CAS-50-81-7.* INN; BAN; JAN. *Vitamin (antiscorbutic); acidifier (urinary).* Ascorbicap (ICN†); Cebione (Abbott†); Cecon (Abbott); Cenolate (Abbott); Cetane (Forest†); Cetane-Caps TC (Forest†); Cevalin (Lilly); Cevex (Marion Merrell Dow†)

Ascorbyl Gamolenate. $C_{24}H_{36}O_7$. 436.54. 1) L-Ascorbic acid, 6-[(6Z,9Z,12Z)-6,9,12-octadecatrienoate]; 2) 6-*O*-[(6Z,9Z,12Z)-Octadeca-6,9,12-trienoyl]-L-*threo*-hex-2-enono-1,4-lactone. *UNII-0ZIP7YM8DI. CAS-109791-32-4.* BAN; INN. ◇SC103

Ascorbyl Palmitate (as kore′ bil pal′ mi tate). **NF.** $C_{22}H_{38}O_7$. 414.53. (1) L-Ascorbic acid, 6-hexadecanoate; (2) L-Ascorbic acid 6-palmitate. *CAS-137-66-6. Pharmaceutic aid (antioxidant).*

Aselizumab. Immunoglobulin G4, anti-(L-selectin) (human-mouse monoclonal HuDreg-55 heavy chain), disulfide with human-mouse monoclonal HuDreg-55 light chain, dimer. *CAS-395639-53-9.* INN.

Asenapine Maleate [*2002*] (a sen′ a peen mal′ ee ate). $C_{17}H_{16}ClNO.C_4H_4O_4$. 401.84. [Asenapine is INN and BAN.] (1) 1*H*-Dibenz[2,3:6,7]oxepino[4,5-*c*]pyrrole, 5-chloro-2,3,3a,12b-tetrahydro-2-methyl-, (3a*R*,12b*R*)-*rel*-, (2*Z*)-2-butenedioate (1:1); (2) (3a*RS*,12b*RS*)-5-Chloro-2-methyl-2,3,3a,12b-tetrahydro-1*H*-dibenzo[2,3:6,7]oxepino[4,5-*c*]pyrrole (2*Z*)-2-butenedioate (1:1). *UNII-CU9463U2E2; UNII-JKZ19V908O* [asenapine]. *CAS-85650-56-2; CAS-65576-45-6* [asenapine]. *Treatment of psychosis (dopamine/serotonin antagonist with antagonism to D_1, D_2, D_3, and D_4 and 5-HT_{1A}, 5-HT_{2A}, 5-HT_{2C}, 5-HT_6, and 5-HT_7 receptors as well as histamine H_1 and α_1 and α_2 adrenergic receptors).* ◇*Org 5222*

Aseripide. $C_{26}H_{30}FN_3O_6S$. 531.60. (2*R*,4*R*)-3-[*N*-[[3-[(*S*)-1-carboxyethyl]phenyl]carbamoyl]glycyl]-2-(*o*-fluorophenyl)-4-thiazolidinecarboxylic acid, 4-*tert*-butylester. *UNII-G2M24F1I2A. CAS-153242-02-5.* INN.

Asimadoline. $C_{27}H_{30}N_2O_2$. 414.54. *N*-[(α*S*)-α-[[(3*S*)-3-Hydroxy-1-pyrrolidinyl]methyl]benzyl]-*N*-methyl-2,2-diphenylacetamide. *UNII-D0VK52NV5M. CAS-153205-46-0.* INN.

Asobamast. $C_{13}H_{15}N_3O_5S$. 325.34. 2-Ethoxyethyl [4-(3-methyl-5-isoxazolyl)-2-thiazolyl]oxamate. *UNII-F0R68O7C4V. CAS-104777-03-9.* INN; BAN.

Asocainol. $C_{27}H_{31}NO_3$. 417.54. (±)-6,7,8,9-Tetrahydro-2,12-dimethoxy-7-methyl-6-phenethyl-5*H*-dibenz[*d,f*]azonin-1-ol. *UNII-J40338OKKT. CAS-77400-65-8.* INN.

Asoprisnil [*2002*] (as oh pris′ nil). $C_{28}H_{35}NO_4$. 449.58. (1) Benzaldehyde, 4-[(11β,17β)-17-methoxy-17-(methoxymethyl)-3-oxoestra-4,9-dien-11-yl]-, 1-oxime, [*C*(*E*)]-; (2) 11β-[4-[(*E*)-(Hydroxyimino)methyl]phenyl]-17β-methoxy-17-(methoxymethyl)estra-4,9-dien-3-one. *CAS-199396-76-4.* INN; BAN. *Treatment of endometriosis and uterine fibroids; possible adjunct to hormone replacement therapy.* ◇*J867*

Asoprisnil Ecamate. $C_{31}H_{40}N_2O_5$. 520.66. 11β-{4-[(*E*)-(Ethylcarbamoyloxyimino)methyl]phenyl}-17β-methoxy-17α-(methoxymethyl)estra-4,9-dien-3-one. *CAS-222732-94-7.* INN.

Aspalon. An extract of glycyrrhiza. JAN.

Asparaginase [*1970*] (as par′ a jin ase). [Colaspase is BAN; L-Asparaginase is JAN.] Enzyme isolated from *Escherichia coli*, or obtained from other sources. (1) Asparaginase; (2) L-Asparagine amidohydrolase; (3) L-Asparaginase. *UNII-G4FQ3CKY5R. CAS-9015-68-3. Antineoplastic.* Crasnitin (Bayer†); Elspar (Merck) ◇*NSC-109229*

L-Asparaginase (JAN) — *See* Asparaginase.

Asparagine. **NF.** $C_4H_8N_2O_3.H_2O$. 150.13. (1) L-Asparagine; (2) L-ga-Aminosuccinamic acid, monohydrate. *CAS-5794-13-8; CAS-70-47-3* [anhydrous].

Aspartame [*1971*] (as′ par tame). **NF.** $C_{14}H_{18}N_2O_5$. 294.30. (1) L-Phenylalanine, *N*-L-α-aspartyl-, 1-methyl ester; (2) 3-Amino-*N*-(α-carboxyphenethyl)succinamic acid *N*-methyl ester. *UNII-Z0H242BBR1. CAS-22839-47-0; CAS-53906-69-7* [replaced]. INN; BAN. *Sweetener.* ◇*SC-18862; APM*

Aspartame Acesulfame (as′ par tame a″ se sul′ fame). **NF.** $C_{18}H_{23}O_9N_3S$. 457.45. (1) Aspartame acesulfame salt; (2) [2-Carboxy-β-(*N*-b-methoxycarbonyl-2-phenyl)ethylcarbamoyl)]ethanaminium 6-methyl-4-oxo-1,2,3-oxathiazin-3-ide-2,2-dioxide; (3) L-Phenylalanine, L-α-aspartyl-2-methyl ester compound with 6-methyl-1,2,3-oxathiazin-4(3*H*)-one 2,2-dioxide (1:1). *CAS-106372-55-8.*

L-Aspartate Potassium (JAN) — *See* Potassium Aspartate.

Aspartic Acid [*1979*] (as par′ tik as′ id). **USP.** C₄H₇NO₄. 133.10. [L-Aspartic Acid is JAN.] (1) L-Aspartic acid; (2) L-Aspartic acid. *UNII-30KYC7MIAI. CAS-6899-03-2; CAS-56-84-8* [L]. INN; MI. *Amino acid.*

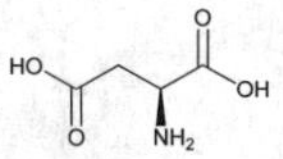

L-Aspartic Acid (JAN) — *See* Aspartic Acid.

Aspartocin [*1963*] (as″ par toe′ sin). C₄₂H₆₄N₁₂O₁₂S₂. 993.16. Antibiotic produced by *Streptomyces griseus.* (1) Oxytocin, 4-L-asparagine-; (2) Aspartocin. *CAS-4117-65-1; CAS-1402-89-7* [replaced]. INN. *Antibacterial.* ◇*A 8999*

Asperkinase. *Aspergillus oryzae* proteinase. *CAS-9000-99-1.* CA, Vol. 62. Megazyme (SmithKline Beecham†)

Asperlin [*1966*] (as′ per lin). C₁₀H₁₂O₅. 212.20. Antibiotic produced by *Aspergillus nidulans.* (1) 2*H*-Pyran-2-one, 5-(acetyloxy)-5,6-dihydro-6-(3-methyloxiranyl)-; (2) 6-(1,2-Epoxypropyl)-5,6-dihydro-5-hydroxy-2*H*-pyran-2-one acetate; (3) 6,7-Epoxy-4,5-dihydroxy-2-octenoic acid δ-lactone acetate. *CAS-30387-51-0. Antibacterial; antineoplastic.* ◇*U-13,933; NSC-93158*

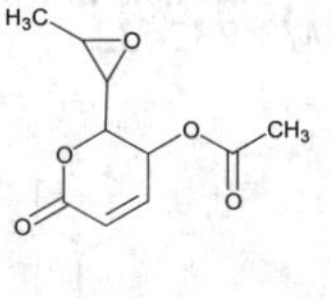

Aspidosperma. *CAS-1398-11-4.* USP IX; MI.

Aspirin (as′ pir in). **USP.** C₉H₈O₄. 180.16. (1) Benzoic acid, 2-(acetyloxy)-; (2) Salicylic acid acetate. *UNII-R16CO5Y76E. CAS-50-78-2.* BAN; JAN. *Analgesic; antipyretic; antirheumatic.* [*Name previously used: Acetylsalicylic Acid.*]

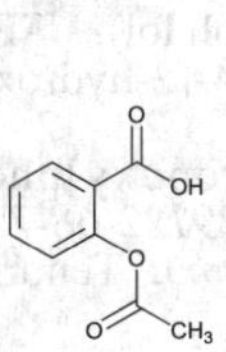

Aspirin Aluminum. *UNII-E33TS05V6B. CAS-23413-80-1.* NF XIII; JAN.

Aspirin DL-Lysine. C₉H₈O₄·C₆H₁₄N₂O₂. 326.34. DL-Lysine-acetylsalicylate. *CAS-62952-06-1.* JAN.

Aspoxicillin. C₂₁H₂₇N₅O₇S. 493.53. (2*S*,5*R*,6*R*)-6-[(2*R*)-2-[(2*R*)-2-Amino-3-(methylcarbamoyl)propionamido]-2-(*p*-hydroxyphenyl)acetamido]-3,3-dimethyl-7-oxo-4-thia-1-azabicyclo[3.2.0]heptane-2-carboxylic acid. *UNII-0745KNO26J. CAS-63358-49-6.* INN; JAN; MI.

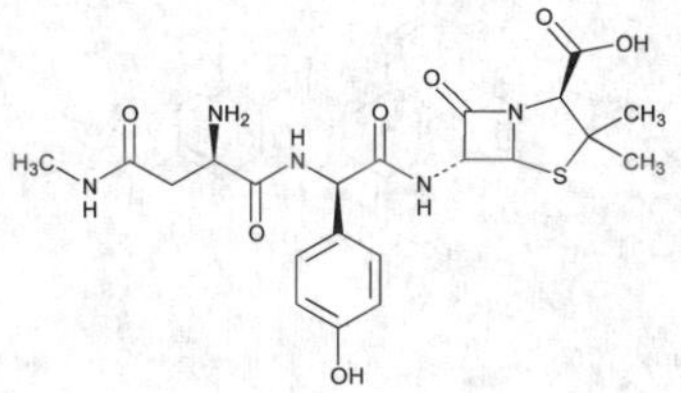

Astemizole [*1979*] (a stem′ i zole). **USP.** C₂₈H₃₁FN₄O. 458.57. (1) 1*H*-Benzimidazol-2-amine, 1-[(4-fluorophenyl)methyl]-*N*-[1-[2-(4-methoxyphenyl)ethyl]-4-piperidinyl]-; (2) 1-(*p*-Fluorobenzyl)-2-[[1-(*p*-methoxyphenethyl)-4-piperidyl]amino]benzimidazole. *CAS-68844-77-9.* INN; BAN; JAN. *Anti-allergic; antihistaminic.* Hismanal (Janssen) ◇*R 43,512*

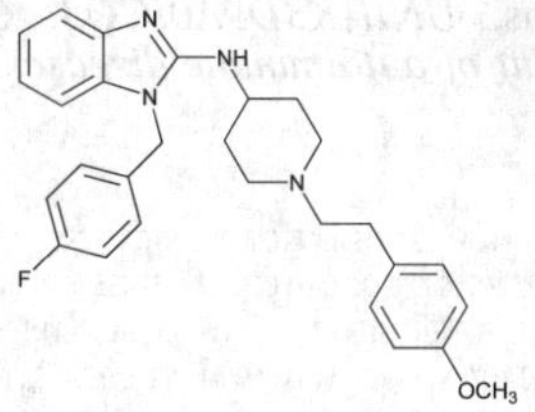

Asthremedin. JAN.

Astifilcon A [*1985*] (as″ ti fil′ kon). (C₅H₈O₂)ₓ(C₆H₉NO)ᵧ. (1) 2-Propenoic acid, 2-methyl-, methyl ester, polymer with 1-ethenyl-2-pyrrolidinone; (2) Methyl methacrylate polymer with 1-vinyl-2-pyrrolidinone. *CAS-25655-01-0. Contact lens material (hydrophilic).* Breath-O (Toray, Japan)

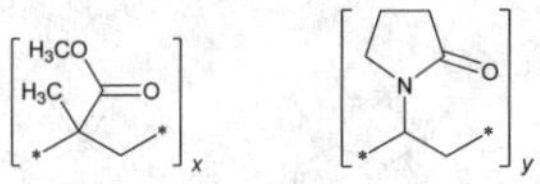

Astromicin Sulfate [*1980*] (as″ troe mye′ sin sul′ fate). C₁₇H₃₅N₅O₆·2H₂SO₄. 601.65. [Astromicin is INN.] Antibiotic produced by *Micromonospora.* (1) L-*chiro*-Inositol, 4-amino-1-[(aminoacetyl)methylamino]-1,4-dideoxy-3-*O*-(2,6-diamino-2,3,4,6,7-pentadeoxy-β-L-*lyxo*-heptopyranosyl)-6-*O*-methylsulfate (1:2) (salt); (2) 4-Amino-1-(2-amino-*N*-methylacetamido)-1,4-dideoxy-3-*O*-(2,6-diamino-2,3,4,6,7-pentadeoxy-β-L-*lyxo*-heptopyranosyl)-6-*O*-methyl-L-*chiro*-inositol sulfate (1:2) (salt). *UNII-POY3S0T3BD; UNII-7JHD84H15J* [astromicin]. *CAS-72275-67-3; CAS-66768-12-5* [*x*H₂SO₄]; *CAS-55779-06-1* [astromicin]. JAN. *Antibacterial.* [*Note—The base compound has been known as Fortimicin A.*] ◇*Abbott-44747*

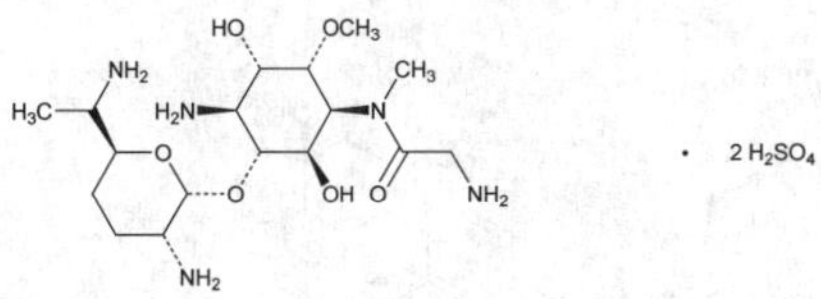

---

† Brand name formerly used, and/or firm no longer concerned with this product.

Asulacrine. $C_{24}H_{24}N_4O_4S$. 464.54. 9-[2-Methoxy-4-(methyl-sulfonylamino)anilino]-*N*,5-dimethylacridine-4-carboxa-mide. *UNII-S8P50T62B6. CAS-80841-47-0.* BAN. ◇*CI-921; NSC 343499*

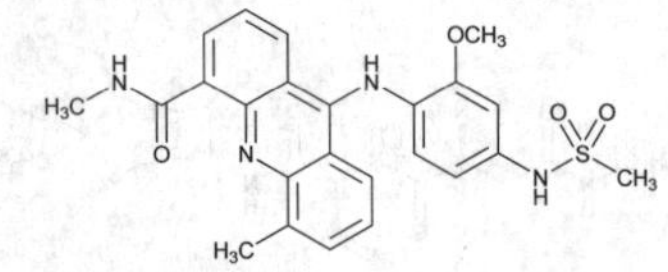

Asunaron. An extract obtained from *Japanese arborvitae.* JAN.

AT III — *See* Antithrombin III Human.

Atacicept [*2007*] (a ta′ si sept). $C_{3104}H_{4788}N_{856}O_{950}S_{44}$ (homodimer). Human Transmembrane Activator and CAML Interactor (TACI) - Immunoglobulin G_1 Fc Domain Fusion Protein (Fc5). Molecular weight is approximately 73,400 daltons. *UNII-K3D9A0ICQ3. CAS-845264-92-8.* INN. *Treatment of autoimmune diseases.* ◇*TACI-Fc5*

```
AMRSCPEEQY WDPLLGTCMS CKTICNHQSQ RTCAAFCRSL SCRKEQGKFY
DHLLRDCISC ASICGQHPKQ CAYFCENKLR SEPKSSDKTH TCPPCPAPEA
EGAPSVFLFP PKPKDTLMIS RTPEVTCVVV DVSHEDPEVK FNWYVDGVEV
HNAKTKPREE QYNSTYRVVS VLTVLHQDWL NGKEYKCKVS NKALPSSIEK
TISKAKGQPR EPQVYTLPPS RDELTKNQVS LTCLVKGFYP SDIAVEWESN
GQPENNYKTT PPVLDSDGSF FLYSKLTVDK SRWQQGNVFS CSVMHEALHN
HYTQKSLSLS PGK                                        2
```
* glycosylation site

Ataciguat. $C_{21}H_{19}Cl_2N_3O_6S_3$. 576.49. 5-Chloro-2-[(5-chloro-2-thienyl)sulfonylamino]-*N*-[4-(morpholin-4-ylsulfonyl)-phenyl]benzamide. *UNII-QP166M390Q. CAS-254877-67-3.* INN.

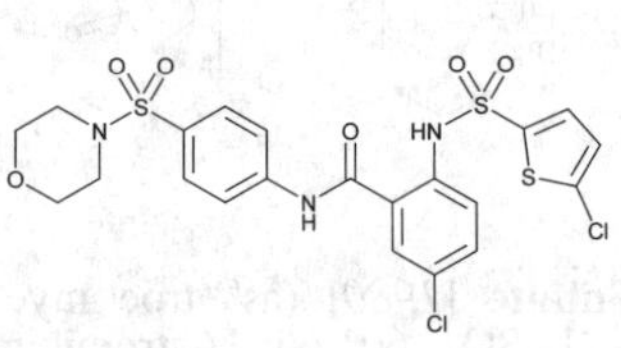

Ataluren [*2008*] (a″ ta lur′ en). $C_{15}H_9FN_2O_3$. 284.24. (1) Benzoic acid, 3-[5-(2-fluorophenyl)-1,2,4-oxadiazol-3-yl]- ; (2) 3-[5-(2-Fluorophenyl)-1,2,4-oxadiazol-3-yl]benzoic acid. *UNII-K16AME9I3V. CAS-775304-57-9. Treatment of disorders caused by nonsense (premature stop codon) mutations.* ◇*PTC124*

Atamestane. $C_{20}H_{26}O_2$. 298.42. 1-Methylandrosta-1,4-diene-3,17-dione. *CAS-96301-34-7.* INN.

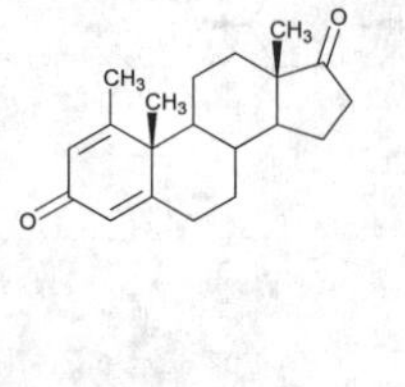

Ataprost. $C_{21}H_{32}O_4$. 348.48. (+)-(2*E*,3a*S*,4*R*,5*R*,6a*S*)-4-[(1*E*,3*S*)-3-Cyclopentyl-3-hydroxypropenyl]-3,3a,4,5,6,6a-hexahydro-5-hydroxy-$\Delta^{2(1H)}$,Δ-pentalenevaleric acid. *UNII-M41LMG25QB. CAS-83997-19-7.* INN.

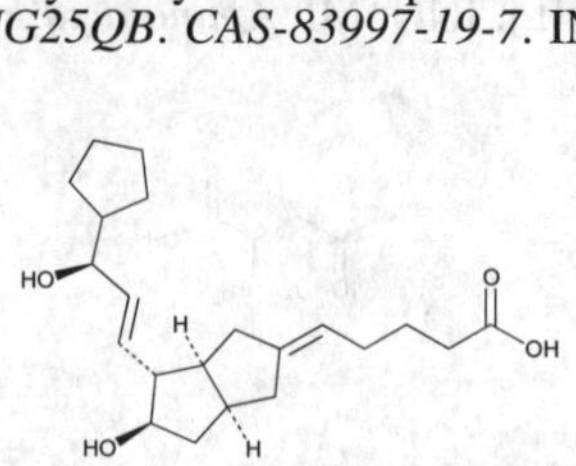

Ataquimast. $C_{11}H_{13}N_3O$. 203.24. 1-Ethyl-3-(methylamino)-2(1*H*)-quinoxalinone. *UNII-II3F5A2G0F. CAS-182316-31-0.* INN.

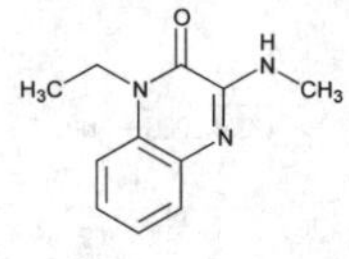

Atazanavir Sulfate [*2002*] (a″ ta zan′ a vir sul′ fate). $C_{38}H_{52}N_6O_7.H_2O_4S$. 802.93. [Atazanavir is INN and BAN.] (1) 2,5,6,10,13-Pentaazatetradecanedioic acid, 3-12-bis(1,1-dimethylethyl)-8-hydroxy-4,11-dioxo-9-(phenyl-methyl)-6-[[-4-(2-pyridinyl)phenyl]methyl]-, dimethyl es-ter, (3*S*,8*S*,9*S*,12*S*)-, sulfate (1:1) (salt); (2) Dimethyl (3*S*,8*S*,9*S*,12*S*)-9-benzyl-3,12,di-*tert*-butyl-8-hydroxy-4,11-dioxo-6-(*p*-2-pyridylbenzyl)-2,5,6,10,13-pentaazate-tradecanedioate, sulfate (1:1) (salt). *UNII-4MT4VIE29P; UNII-QZU4H47A3S* [atazanavir]. *CAS-229975-97-7; CAS-198904-31-3* [atazanavir]. *Treatment of acute and chronic HIV infection (HIV protease inhibitor).* Reyataz (Bristol-Myers Squibb) ◇*BMS-232632-05*

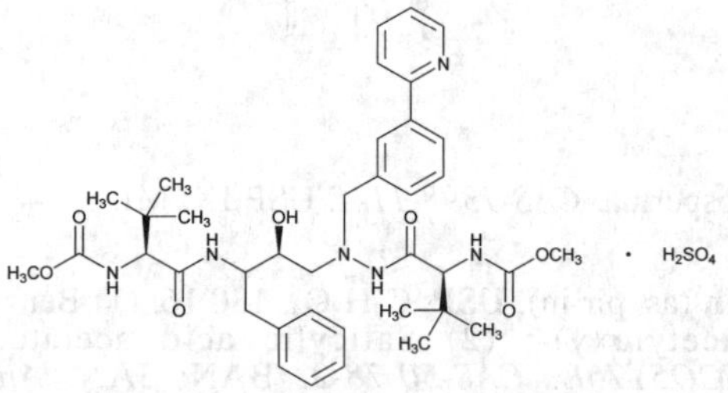

Atenolol [*1976*] (a ten′ oh lol). **USP.** $C_{14}H_{22}N_2O_3$. 266.34. (1) Benzeneacetamide, 4-[2-hydroxy-3-[(1-methylethyl)ami-no]propoxy]-; (2) 2-[*p*-[2-Hydroxy-3-(isopropylamino)propoxy]phenyl]acetamide. *UNII-50VV3VW0TI. CAS-29122-68-7.* INN; BAN; JAN. *Anti-adrenergic (β-receptor).* Tenormin (AstraZeneca) ◇*ICI 66,082*

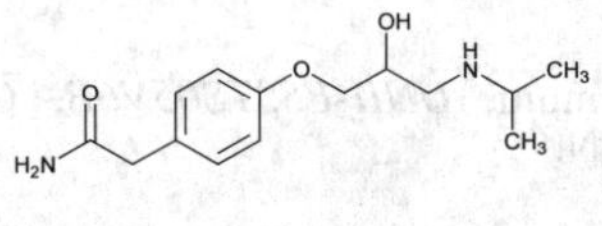

Atevirdine Mesylate [*1993*] (a″ te vir′ deen mes′ i late). $C_{21}H_{25}N_5O_2.CH_4O_3S$. 475.56. [Atevirdine is INN.] (1) Piperazine, 1-[3-(ethylamino)-2-pyridinyl]-4-[(5-methoxy-1*H*-indol-2-yl)carbonyl]-, monomethanesulfonate; (2) 1-[3-(Ethylamino)-2-pyridyl]-4-[(5-methoxyindol-2-yl)car-bonyl]piperazine monomethanesulfonate. *UNII-*

A948D8673W; UNII-N24015WC6D [atevirdine]. *CAS-138540-32-6; CAS-136816-75-6* [atevirdine]. *Antiviral.* ◇*U-87201E*

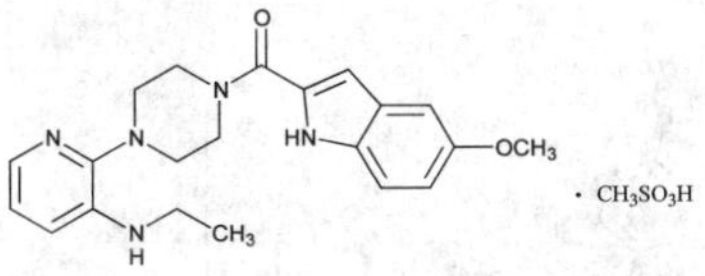

Atexakin Alfa. $C_{917}H_{1483}N_{255}O_{288}S_9$. 20,976.73. 1-(1-L-Alanyl-L-proline)interleukin 6 (human clone HGF15 protein moiety reduced), cyclic (44→50), (73→83)-bis(disulfide). *CAS-143631-61-2.* INN.

Athyromazole — *See* Carbimazole.

Atibeprone. $C_{17}H_{18}N_2O_3S$. 330.40. 7-[(5-Isopropyl-1,3,4-thiadiazol-2-yl)methoxy]-3,4-dimethylcoumarin. *UNII-PZV3P03F1U. CAS-153420-96-3.* INN.

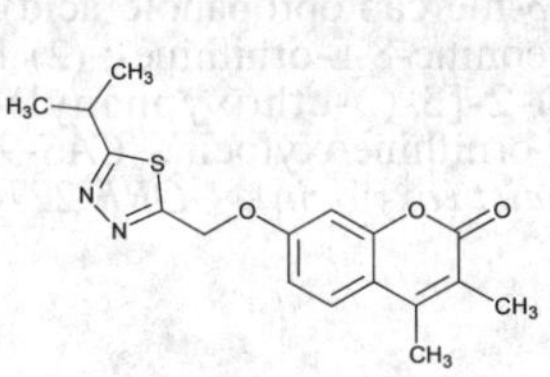

Atilmotin [*2004*] (a″ til moe′ tin). $C_{86}H_{135}N_{20}O_{19}^+$. 1753.00. (1) L-Lysinamide, *N*-[(2*S*)-1-oxo-3-phenyl-2-(trimethylammonio)propyl]-L-valyl-L-prolyl-L-isoleucyl-L-phenylalanyl-L-threonyl-L-tyrosylglycyl-L-α-glutamyl-L-leucyl-L-glutaminyl-D-arginyl-L-leucyl-; (2) *N*-[(2*S*)-3-Phenyl-2-(trimethylammonio)propanoyl]-L-valyl-L-prolyl-L-isoleucyl-L-phenylalanyl-L-threonyl-L-tyrosylglycyl-L-glutamyl-L-leucyl-L-glutaminyl-D-arginyl-L-leucyl-L-lysinamide. *UNII-4WQQ18VL49. CAS-533927-56-9.* INN. *Intended for use in the stimulation of gastrointestinal motility (GI prokinetic agent) (motilin receptor agonist).* ◇*MOT-288; OHM-11638; BAX-ACC-1638*

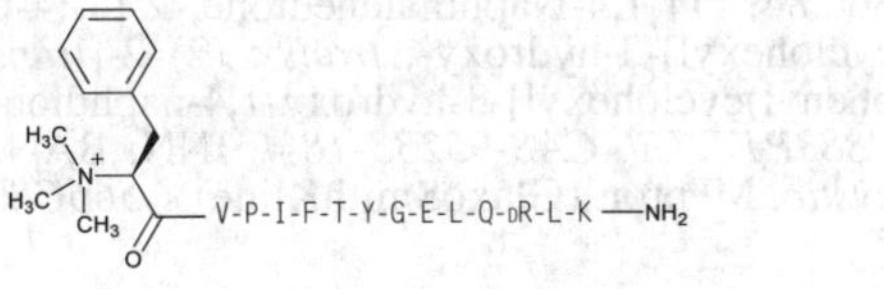

Atipamezole [*1989*] (a″ ti pam′ e zole). $C_{14}H_{16}N_2$. 212.29. (1) 1*H*-Imidazole, 4-(2-ethyl-2,3-dihydro-1*H*-inden-2-yl)-; (2) 4-(2-Ethyl-2-indanyl)imidazole. *UNII-03N9U5JAF6. CAS-104054-27-5.* INN; BAN. *Antagonist (α₂-receptor).* Antisedan (Farmos Group Ltd., Finland) ◇*MPV-1248*

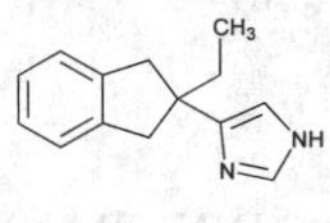

Atiprimod Dihydrochloride [*1996*] (a tip′ ri mod dye hye″ droe klor′ ide). $C_{22}H_{44}N_2 \cdot 2HCl$. 409.52. [Atiprimod is INN.] (1) 2-Azaspiro[4.5]decane-2-propanamine *N,N*-diethyl-8,8-dipropyl-, dihydrochloride; (2) 2-[3-(Diethylamino)propyl]-8,8-dipropyl-2-azaspiro[4.5]decane dihy-

drochloride. *UNII-O12I24570R. CAS-130065-61-1; CAS-123018-47-3* [atiprimod]. *Anti-arthritic; anti-inflammatory.* ◇*SK&F 106615-A2; SKF-106615-A2*

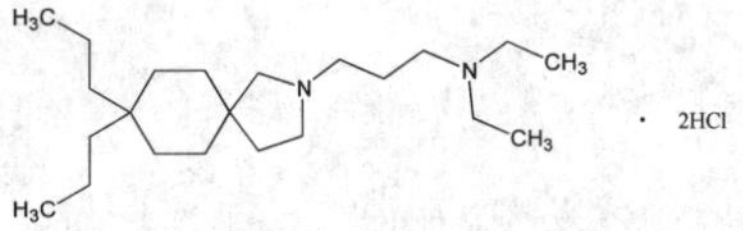

Atiprimod Dimaleate [*1997*] (a tip′ ri mod dye mal′ ee ate). $C_{22}H_{44}N_2 \cdot 2C_4H_4O_4$. 568.74. (1) 2-Azaspiro[4.5]decane-2-propanamine, *N,N*-diethyl,- 8,8-dipropyl-, (*Z*)-2-butenedioate (1:2); (2) 2-[3-(Diethylamino)propyl]-8,8-dipropyl-2-azaspiro[4.5]decane maleate (1:2). *UNII-YNU265SSR3. CAS-183063-72-1. Anti-arthritic; anti-inflammatory; immunomodulator.* ◇*SK&F 106615-I2*

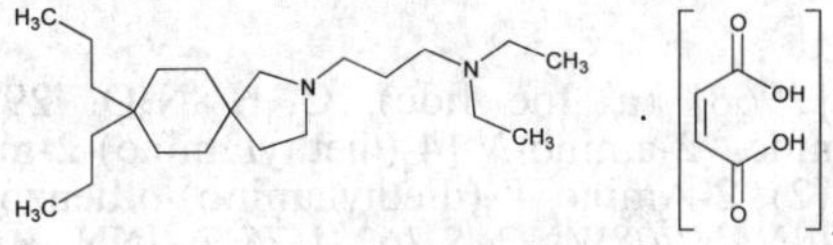

Atiprosin Maleate [*1986*] (a″ ti proe′ sin mal′ ee ate). $C_{20}H_{29}N_3 \cdot C_4H_4O_4$. 427.54. [Atiprosin is INN.] (1) Pyrazino[2′,3′:3,4]pyrido[1,2-*a*]indole, 1-ethyl-1,2,3,4,4a,5,6,12b-octahydro-12-methyl-4-(1-methylethyl)-, *trans*, (*Z*)-2-butenedioate (1:1); (2) *trans*-1-Ethyl-1,2,3,4,4a,5,6,12b-octahydro-4-isopropyl-12-methylpyrazino[2′,3′:3,4]pyrido[1,2-*a*]indole maleate (1:1). *UNII-50SZ4782J0. CAS-89303-64-0; CAS-89303-63-9* [atiprosin]. *Antihypertensive.* ◇*AY-28,228*

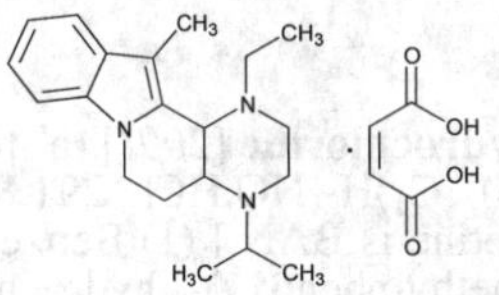

Atizoram [*1995*] (a ti zor′ am). $C_{18}H_{24}N_2O_3$. 316.39. Tetrahydro-5-[4-methoxy-3-[(1*S*,2*S*,4*R*)-2-norbomyloxy]-phenyl]-2(1*H*)-pyrimidinone. *CAS-135637-46-6.* INN.

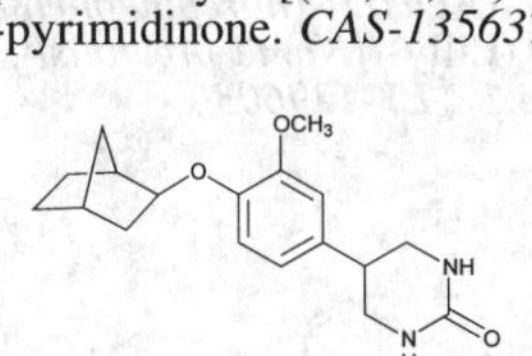

Atlafilcon A [*1989*] (at″ la fil′ kon). $(C_2H_4O)_y(C_5H_8O_2)_z$. (1) Ethenol, polymer with methyl 2-methyl-2-propenoate; (2) Vinyl alcohol, polymer with methyl methacrylate. *CAS-25214-48-6. Contact lens material (hydrophilic).*

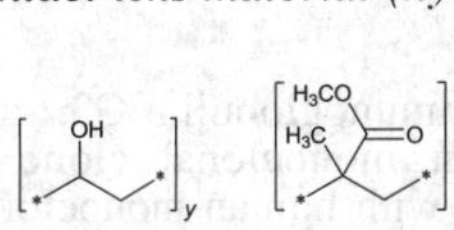

Atliprofen. $C_{13}H_{12}O_2S$. 232.30. (±)-*p*-3-Thienylhydratropic acid. *UNII-11YB79G1Y6. CAS-108912-17-0.* INN.

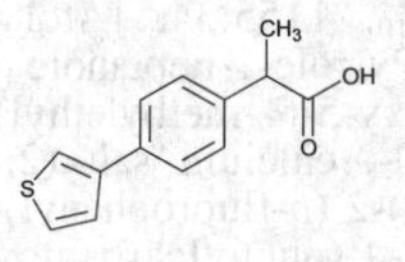

---

† Brand name formerly used, and/or firm no longer concerned with this product.

Atocalcitol. C$_{32}$H$_{46}$O$_4$. 494.71. (1*S*,3*R*,5*Z*,7*E*,20*R*)-20-[3-(2-Hydroxypropan-2-yl)benzyloxymethyl]-9,10-secopregna-5,7,10(19)-triene-1α,3gb-diol. *UNII-PR3292R3H7. CAS-302904-82-1.* INN.

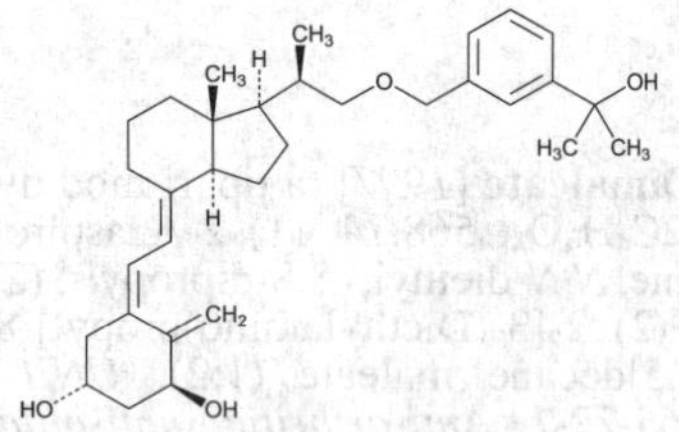

Atolide [*1968*] (a′ toe lide). C$_{18}$H$_{23}$N$_3$O. 297.39. (1) Benzamide, 2-amino-*N*-[4-(diethylamino)-2-methylphenyl]-; (2) 2-Amino-4′-(diethylamino)-*o*-benzotoluidide. *UNII-OBN5I4B08W. CAS-16231-75-7.* INN. *Anticonvulsant.* ◇*W 5733; Go 1213*

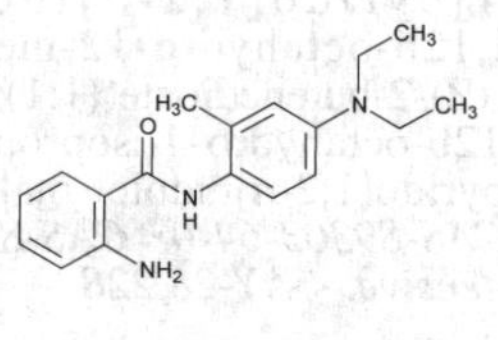

Atomoxetine Hydrochloride [*2001*] (a″ toe mox′ e teen hye″ droe klor′ ide). C$_{17}$H$_{21}$NO.HCl. 291.82. [Tomoxetine is INN; Atomoxetine is BAN.] (1) Benzenepropanamine, *N*-methyl-γ-(2-methylphenoxy)-, hydrochloride, (-); (2) (-)-*N*-Methyl-3-phenyl-3-(*o*-tolyloxy)propylamine hydrochloride. *UNII-57WVB6I2W0. CAS-82248-59-7; CAS-83015-26-3* [tomoxetine]. *Treatment of attention deficit hyperactivity disorder (ADHD) (norepinephrine reuptake inhibitor).* Strattera (Lilly) *[Name previously used: Tomoxetine Hydrochloride.]* ◇*LY-139603*

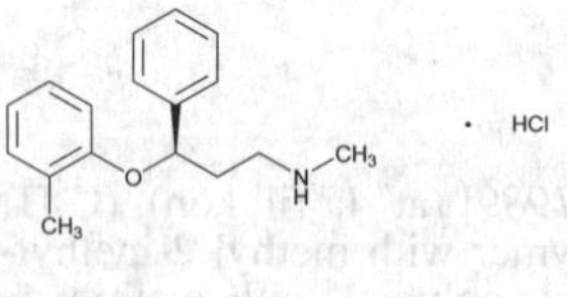

Atorolimumab. Immunoglobulin G3, anti-(human Rh(D) antigen) (human monoclonal clone P3x22914G4 γ3-chain), disulfide with human monoclonal P3x22914G4 κ-chain, dimer. *CAS-202833-08-7.* INN.

Atorvastatin Calcium [*1994*] (a tor″ va stat′ in kal′ see um). C$_{66}$H$_{68}$CaF$_2$N$_4$O$_{10}$. 1155.34. [Atorvastatin is INN and BAN.] (1) 1*H*-Pyrrole-1-heptanoic acid, 2-(4-fluorophenyl)-β,δ-dihydroxy-5-(1-methylethyl)-3-phenyl-4-[(phenylamino)carbonyl]-, calcium salt (2:1), [*R*-(*R**,*R**)]-; (2) Calcium (βR,δR)-2-(*p*-fluorophenyl)-β,δ-dihydroxy-5-isopropyl-3-phenyl-4-(phenylcarbamoyl)pyrrole-1-heptanoate (1:2). *UNII-48A5M73Z4Q; UNII-A0JWA85V8F*

[atorvastatin]. *CAS-134523-03-8; CAS-134523-00-5* [atorvastatin]. *Inhibitor (HMG-CoA reductase).* Lipitor (Pfizer) ◇*CI-981*

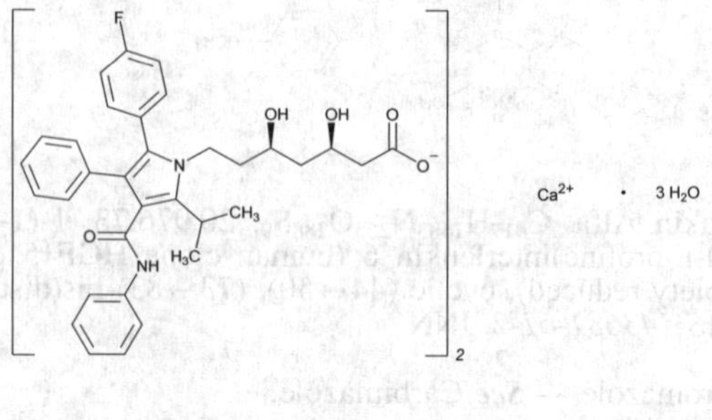

Atosiban [*1989*] (a toe′ si ban). C$_{43}$H$_{67}$N$_{11}$O$_{12}$S$_2$. 994.19. (1) Oxytocin, 1-(3-mercaptopropanoic acid)-2-(*O*-ethyl-D-tyrosine)-4-L-threonine-8-L-ornithine-; (2) 1-(3-Mercaptopropionic acid)-2-[3-(*p*-ethoxyphenyl)-D-alanine]-4-L-threonine-8-L-ornithineoxytocin. *CAS-90779-69-4.* INN; BAN. *Antagonist (oxytocin).* ◇*ORF 22164; RWJ 22164*

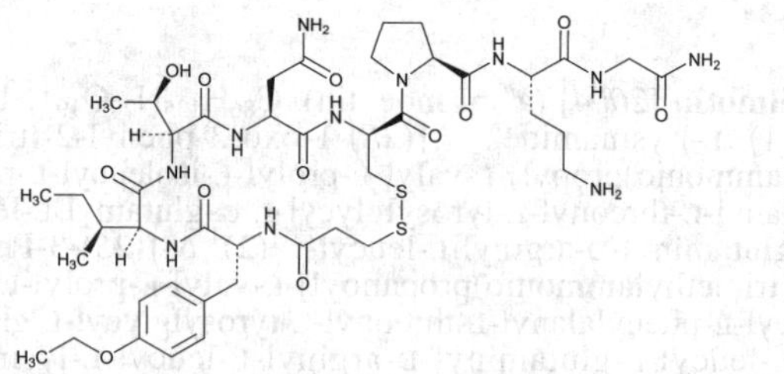

Atovaquone [*1993*] (a toe′ va kwone). **USP.** C$_{22}$H$_{19}$ClO$_3$. 366.84. (1) 1,4-Naphthalenedione, 2-[4-(4-chlorophenyl)-cyclohexyl]-3-hydroxy-, *trans*-; (2) 2-[*trans*-4-(*p*-Chlorophenyl)cyclohexyl]-3-hydroxy-1,4-naphthoquinone. *UNII-Y883P1Z2LT. CAS-95233-18-4.* INN; BAN. *Antipneumocystic.* Mepron (GlaxoSmithKline) ◇*566C80; 566C*

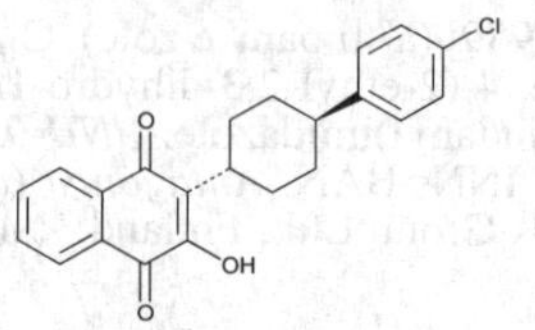

Atracurium Besilate (INN, BAN) — *See* Atracurium Besylate.

Atracurium Besylate [*1983*] (a tra kure′ ee um bes′ i late). **USP.** C$_{65}$H$_{82}$N$_2$O$_{18}$S$_2$. 1243.48. [Atracurium Besilate is INN and BAN.] (1) Isoquinolinium, 2,2′-[1,5-pentanediyl-bis[oxy(3-oxo-3,1-propanediyl)]]bis[1-[(3,4-dimethoxyphenyl)methyl]-1,2,3,4-tetrahydro-6,7-dimethoxy-2-methyl-, dibenzenesulfonate; (2) 2-(2-Carboxyethyl)-1,2,3,4-tetrahydro-6,7-dimethoxy-2-methyl-1-veratrylisoquinolinium benzenesulfonate, pentamethylene ester. *UNII-40AX66P76P. CAS-64228-81-5. Neuromuscular blocking agent.* Tracrium (Hospira) ◇*BW 33A*

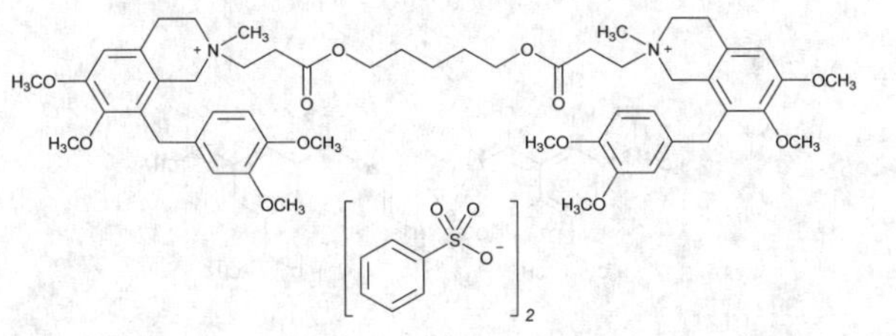

Atrasentan Hydrochloride [*2000*] (a″ tra sen′ tan hye″ droe klor′ ide). $C_{29}H_{38}N_2O_6 \cdot HCl$. 547.08. [Atrasentan is INN.] (1) 3-Pyrrolidinecarboxylic acid, 4-(1,3-benzodioxol-5-yl)-1-[2-(dibutylamino)-2-oxoethyl]-2-(4-methoxyphenyl)-, monohydrochloride, [2*R*-(2α,3β,4α)]; (2) (2*R*,3*R*,4*S*)-1-[(Dibutylcarbamoyl)methyl]-2-(*p*-methoxyphenyl)-4-[3,4-(methylenedioxy)phenyl]-3-pyrrolidinecarboxylic acid, monohydrochloride. *UNII-E4G31X93ZA; UNII-V6D7VK2215* [atrasentan]. *CAS-195733-43-8; CAS-173937-91-2* [atrasentan]. *Palliative treatment of bone pain due to metastatic prostate cancer and disease progression (endothelin (ET_A) receptor antagonist).* ◇*A-147627.1; ABT-627; Abbot-147627*

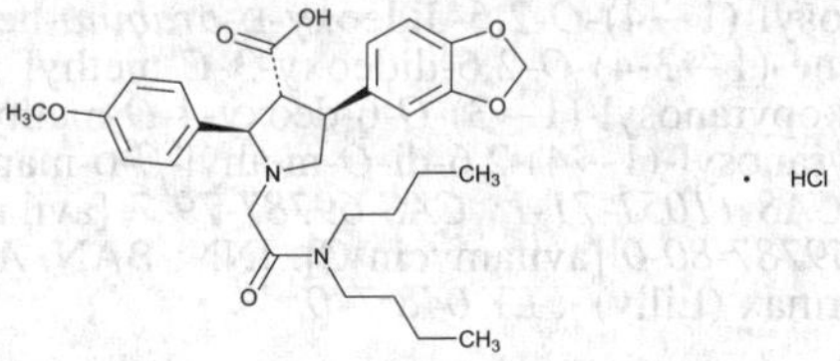

Atreleuton [*1997*] (a tre loo′ ton). $C_{16}H_{15}FN_2O_2S$. 318.37. 1-[(*R*)-3-[5-(*p*-Fluorobenzyl)-2-thienyl]-1-methyl-2-propynyl]-1-hydroxyurea. *UNII-U3O1T88E1M. CAS-154355-76-7.* INN. *Anti-asthmatic; inhibitor (5-lipoxygenase).* ◇*Abbott-85761; ABT-761; A-85761.0*

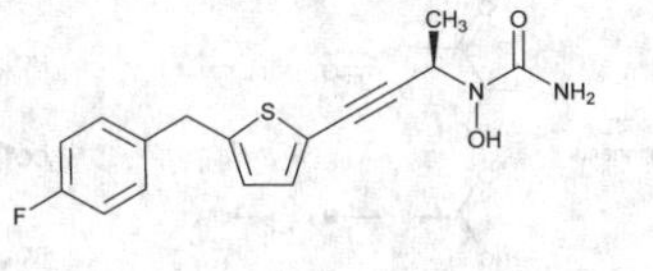

Atrimustine. $C_{41}H_{47}Cl_2NO_6$. 720.72. Estradiol 3-benzoate 17-glycolate, 4-[*p*-[bis(2-chloroethyl)amino]phenyl]butyrate. *UNII-XC0K09B7K4. CAS-75219-46-4.* INN.

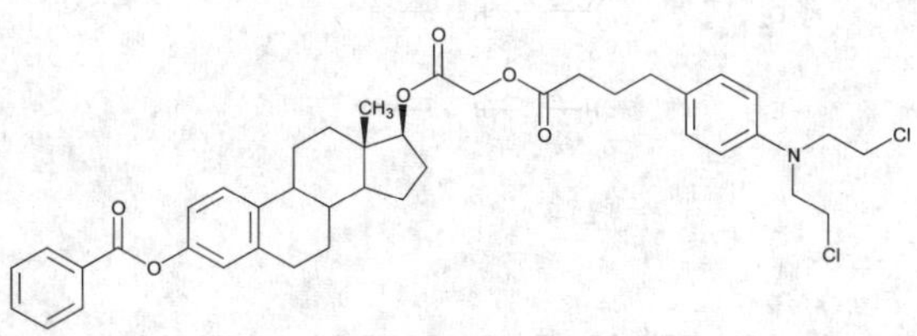

---

† Brand name formerly used, and/or firm no longer concerned with this product.

Atrinositol. $C_6H_{15}O_{15}P_3$. 420.10. D-*myo*-Inositol 1,2,6-tris(dihydrogen phosphate). *UNII-VYF3049W3N. CAS-28841-62-5.* INN.

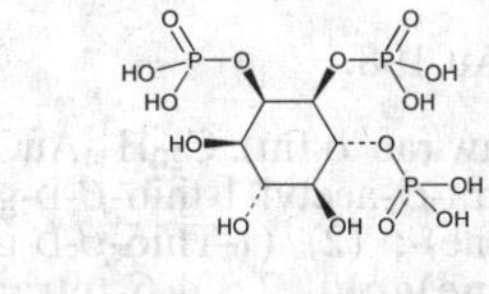

Atromepine. $C_{18}H_{25}NO_3$. 303.40. (-)-3α-Tropanyl 2-methyl-2-phenylhydracrylate. *UNII-9042592173. CAS-428-07-9.* INN; DCF.

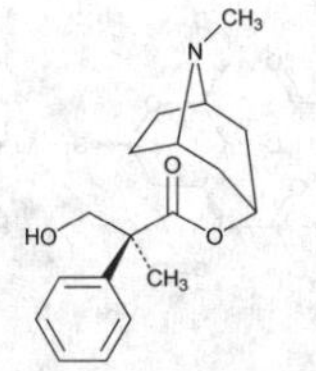

Atropine (at′ roe peen). **USP.** $C_{17}H_{23}NO_3$. 289.37. (1) Benzeneacetic acid, α-(hydroxymethyl)-8-methyl-8-azabicyclo[3.2.1]oct-3-yl ester, *endo*-(±)-; (2) 1α*H*,5α*H*-Tropan-3α-ol (±)-tropate (ester). *UNII-7C0697DR9I. CAS-51-55-8.* BAN. *Anticholinergic.* Atropen (Meridian)

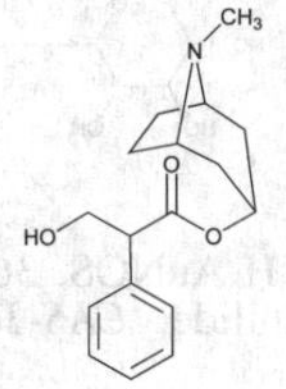

Atropine Methonitrate (INN, BAN, JAN) — *See* Methylatropine Nitrate.

Atropine Methylbromide. $C_{18}H_{26}BrNO_3$. 384.31. 3α-Hydroxy-8-methyl-1α*H*,5α*H*-tropanium bromide. *CAS-2870-71-5.* JAN.

Atropine Oxide Hydrochloride [*1962*] (at′ roe peen ox′ ide hye″ droe klor′ ide). $C_{17}H_{23}NO_4 \cdot HCl$. 341.83. [Atropine Oxide is INN.] (1) Benzeneacetic acid, α-(hydroxymethyl)-8-methyl-8-azabicyclo[3.2.1]oct-3-yl ester, 8-oxide, hydrochloride, *endo*-(±)-; (2) 1α*H*,5α*H*-Tropan-3α-ol (±)-tropate(ester) 8-oxide hydrochloride. *CAS-4574-60-1; CAS-4438-22-6* [atropine oxide]. *Anticholinergic.*

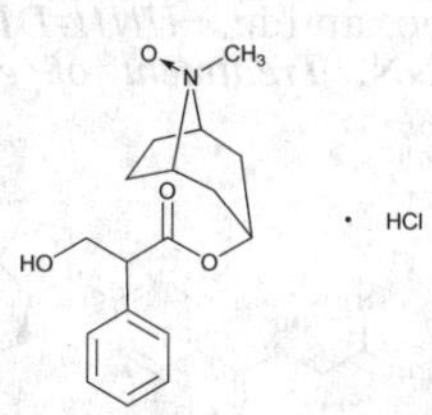

Atropine Sulfate (at′ roe peen sul′ fate). **USP.** $(C_{17}H_{23}NO_3)_2 \cdot H_2SO_4 \cdot H_2O$. 694.83. [Atropine Sulphate is BAN.] (1) Benzeneacetic acid, α-(hydroxymethyl)-, 8-methyl-8-azabicyclo[3.2.1]oct-3-yl ester, *endo*-(±)-, sulfate (2:1) (salt), monohydrate; (2) 1α*H*,5α*H*-Tropan-3α-ol (±)-tropate (ester), sulfate (2:1) (salt) monohydrate. *UNII-03J5ZE7KA5; UNII-7C0697DR9I* [atropine]. *CAS-5908-99-6; CAS-55-48-1* [anhydrous]; *CAS-51-55-8* [atropine]. JAN. *Anticholinergic (ophthalmic).*

Attapulgite, Activated (at″ a pul′ gite ak′ ti vay″ ted). **USP.** A highly heat-treated, processed, native magnesium aluminum silicate. *Pharmaceutic aid (suspending agent).* Parepectolin (Rhone-Poulenc Rorer†)

^{198}Au — *See* Gold Au 198.

Auranofin [*1976*] (aw ran′ o fin). $C_{20}H_{34}AuO_9PS$. 678.48. (1) Gold, (2,3,4,6-tetra-*O*-acetyl-1-thio-*β*-D-glucopyranosato-*S*)(triethylphosphine)-; (2) (1-Thio-*β*-D-glucopyranosato)(triethylphosphine)gold 2,3,4,6-tetraacetate. *UNII-3H04W2810V. CAS-34031-32-8.* INN; BAN; JAN. *Antirheumatic.* Ridaura (Promethus) ◇*SK&F 39162*

Aurothioglucose (aur″ oh thye″ oh gloo′ kose). **USP.** $C_6H_{11}AuO_5S$. 392.18. (1) Gold, (1-thio-D-glucopyranosato)-; (2) (1-Thio-D-glucopyranosato)gold. *CAS-12192-57-3. Antirheumatic.* Solganal (Schering)

Aurothioglycanide. C_8H_8AuNOS. 363.19. *S*-Gold derivative of 2-mercaptoacetanilide. *CAS-16925-51-2.* INN; DCF; MI.

Aurothiomalate Disodium — *See* Gold Sodium Thiomalate.

Avanafil [*2004*] (av an′ a fil). $C_{23}H_{26}ClN_7O_3$. 483.95. (1) 5-Pyrimidinecarboxamide, 4-[[(3-chloro-4-methoxyphenyl)methyl]amino]-2-[(2*S*)-2-(hydroxymethyl)-1-pyrrolidinyl]-*N*-(2-pyrimidinylmethyl)-; (2) 4-[[3-Chloro-4-methoxybenzyl)amino]-2-[(2*S*)-2-(hydroxymethyl)pyrrolidin-1-yl]-*N*-(pyrimidin-2-ylmethyl)pyrimidine-5-carboxamide; (3) (*S*)-4-(3-Chloro-4-methoxybenzylamino)-2-(2-hydroxymethylpyrrolidin-1-yl)-*N*-pyrimidin-2-ylmethyl-5-pyrimidinecarboxamide. *UNII-DR5S136IVO. CAS-330784-47-9.* INN. *Treatment of erectile dysfunction.* ◇*TA-1790*

Avasimibe [*1998*] (a va′ si mibe). $C_{29}H_{43}NO_4S$. 501.72. (1) *N*-[[2,6-Bis(1-methylethyl)phenoxy]sulfonyl]-2,4,6-tris(1-methylethyl)-benzeneacetamide; (2) 2,6-Diisopropylphenyl [(2,4,6-triisopropylphenyl)acetyl]sulfamate. *UNII-*

28LQ20T5RC. CAS-166518-60-1. INN. *Antiatherosclerotic; hypolipidemic (acyl-CoA: cholesterol acyltransferase [ACAT] inhibitor).* ◇*CI-1011*

Avicatonin. $C_{147}H_{243}N_{41}O_{46}$. 3320.75. 1-Butyric acid-2-L-alanine-3-L-serine-7-(L-2-aminobutyric acid)-26-L-aspartic acid-27-L-valine-29-L-alaninecalcitonin (salmon). *CAS-103451-84-9.* INN.

Avilamycin [*1986*] (a vil″ a mye′ sin). $C_{61}H_{88}Cl_2O_{32}$ (Avilamycin A). 1404.24. [Avilamycin A; Avilamycin C] *O*-(1*R*)-4-*C*-acetyl-6-deoxy-2,3-*O*-methylene-D-galactopyranosylidene-(1→3-4)-2-*O*-(2-methyl-1-oxopropyl)-*α*-L-lyxopyranosyl *O*-2,6-dideoxy-4-*O*-(3,5-dichloro-4-hydroxy-2-methoxy-6-methylbenzoyl)-*β*-D-*arabino*-hexopyranosyl-(1→4)-*O*-2,6-dideoxy-D-*arabino*-hexopyranosylidene-(1→3-4)-*O*-2,6-dideoxy-3-*C*-methyl-*β*-D-*arabino*-hexopyranosyl-(1→3)-*O*-6-deoxy-4-*O*-methyl-*β*-D-galactopyranosyl-(1→4)-2,6-di-*O*-methyl-*β*-D-mannopyranoside. *CAS-11051-71-1; CAS-69787-79-7 [avilamycin A]; CAS-69787-80-0 [avilamycin C].* INN; BAN. *Antibacterial.* Surmax (Lilly) ◇*LY 048 740*

Aviptadil. $C_{147}H_{238}N_{44}O_{42}S$. 3325.80. L-Histidyl-L-seryl-L-aspartyl-L-alanyl-L-valyl-L-phenylalanyl-L-threonyl-L-aspartyl-L-asparaginyl-L-tyrosyl-L-threonyl-L-arginyl-L-leucyl-L-arginyl-L-lysyl-L-glutaminyl-L-methionyl-L-alanyl-L-valyl-L-lysyl-L-lysyl-L-tyrosyl-L-leucyl-L-asparaginyl-L-seryl-L-isoleucyl-L-leucyl-L-asparagine. *CAS-40077-57-4.* INN; BAN.

Aviscumine. $C_{1251}H_{1956}N_{346}O_{374}S_5$ (A); $C_{1255}H_{1983}N_{363}O_{394}S_{15}$ (B). Toxin ML-I (mistletoe lectin I) (*Viscum album*). CAS-223577-45-5. INN.

```
MYERIRLRVT HQTTGEEYFR FITLLRDYVS SGSFSNEIPL LRQSTIPVSD
AQRFVLVELT VQGGDSITAA IDVTNLYVVA YQAGDQSYFL RDAPRGAETH
LFTGTTRSSL PFNGSYPDLE RYAGHRDQIP LGIDQLIQSV TALRFPGGST
RTQARSILIL IQMISEAARF NPILWRARQY INSGASFLPD VYMLELETSW
GQQSTQVQHS TDGVFNNPIR LAIPPGNFVT LTNVRDVIAS LAIMLFVCGE

MDDVTCSASE PRVRIVGRNG MCVDVRDDDF RDGNQIQLWP SKSNNDPNQL
WTIKRDGTIR SNGSCLTTYG YTAGVYVMIF CDNTAVREAT LWQIWGNGTI
INPRSNLVLA ASSGIKGTTL TVQTLDYTLG QGWLAGNDTA PREVTIYGFR
DLCMESNGGS VWVETCVSSQ KNQRWALYGD GSIRPKQNQD QCLTCGRDSV
STVINIVSCS AGSSGQRWVF TNEGAILNLK NGLAMDVAQA NPKLRRIIIY
PATGKPNQMW LPVP
```

Avitriptan Fumarate [*1997*] (a″ vi trip′ tan fue′ ma rate). $C_{22}H_{30}N_6O_3S.C_4H_4O_4$. 574.65. [Avitriptan is INN.] (1) 1*H*-Indole-5-methanesulfonamide, 3-[3-[4-(5-methoxy-4-pyrimidinyl)-1-piperazinyl]propyl]-*N*-methyl-, (*E*)-2-butenedioate (1:1); (2) 3-[3-[4-(5-Methoxy-4-pyrimidinyl)-1-piperazinyl]propyl]-*N*-methylindole-5-methanesulfonamide fumarate (1:1). *UNII-2G25KE3954. CAS-171171-42-9; CAS-151140-96-4* [avitriptan]. *Antimigraine.* ◇BMS-180048; BMS-180048-02

Avizafone. $C_{22}H_{27}ClN_4O_3$. 430.93. 2′-Benzoyl-4′-chloro-2-[(*S*)-2,6-diaminohexanamido]-*N*-methylacetanilide. *UNII-65NK71K78P. CAS-65617-86-9.* INN; BAN. ◇Ro 03-7355/000

Avobenzone [*1989*] (a″ voe ben′ zone). **USP.** $C_{20}H_{22}O_3$. 310.39. (1) 1,3-Propanedione, 1-[4-(1,1-dimethylethyl)-phenyl]-3-(4-methoxyphenyl)-; (2) 1-(*p-tert*-Butylphenyl)-3-(*p*-methoxyphenyl)-1,3-propanedione. *UNII-G63QQF2NOX. CAS-70356-09-1.* INN. *Sunscreen.* Parsol 1789 (Givaudan S.A., Switzerland)

Avoparcin [*1972*] (a″ voe par′ sin). Glycopeptide antibiotic obtained from *Streptomyces candidus.* (1) Avoparcin; (2) Avoparcin. *CAS-37332-99-3.* INN; BAN. *Antibacterial.* ◇CL 81,587

---

† Brand name formerly used, and/or firm no longer concerned with this product.

Avorelin. $C_{65}H_{85}N_{17}O_{12}$. 1296.48. 5-Oxo-L-prolyl-L-histidyl-L-tryptophyl-L-seryl-L-tyrosyl-2-methyl-D-tryptophyl-L-leucyl-L-arginyl-*N*-ethyl-L-prolinamide. *CAS-140703-49-7.* INN.

Avosentan. $C_{23}H_{21}N_5O_5S$. 479.51. *N*-[6-Methoxy-5-(2-methoxyphenoxy)-2-(pyridin-4-yl)pyrimidin-4-yl]-5-methylpyridine-2-sulfonamide. *UNII-L94KSX715K. CAS-290815-26-8.* INN.

Avotermin. $C_{1128}H_{1702}N_{296}O_{336}S_{20}$. 25,426.70. Transforming growth factor $\beta 3$ (human), dimer. *CAS-182212-66-4.* INN.

Avridine [*1983*] (a′ vri deen). $C_{43}H_{90}N_2O_2$. 667.19. (1) Ethanol, 2,2′-[[3-(dioctadecylamino)propyl]imino]bis-; (2) 2,2′-[[3-(Dioctadecylamino)propyl]imino]diethanol. *UNII-P9J7O7YNSW. CAS-35607-20-6.* INN. *Antiviral.* ◇CP-20,961

Axamozide. $C_{21}H_{22}ClN_3O_3$. 399.87. (±)-1-[1-(1,4-Benzodioxan-2-ylmethyl)-4-piperidyl]-5-chloro-2-benzimidazolinone. *UNII-MCG9O55T6K. CAS-85076-06-8.* INN.

Axitinib [*2005*] (ax i′ ti nib). $C_{22}H_{18}N_4OS$. 386.47. (1) Benzamide, *N*-methyl-2-[[3-[(1*E*)-2-(2-pyridinyl)ethenyl]-1*H*-indazol-6-yl]thio]-; (2) *N*-Methyl-2-[[3-[(1*E*)-2-(pyridin-2-yl)ethenyl]-1*H*-indazol-6-yl]sulfanyl]benzamide. *UNII-C9LVQ0YUXG. CAS-319460-85-0.* INN. *Antineoplastic, inhibitor of VEGF/PDGF tyrosine kinases.* ◇AG-013736

Axitirome [*1999*] (ax″ i tye′ rome). $C_{25}H_{24}FNO_6$. 453.46. (1) Ethyl (±)-[[4-[3-[(4-fluorophenyl)hydroxymethyl]-4-hydroxyphenoxy]-3,5-dimethylphenyl]amino]oxoacetate; (2)

Ethyl (±)-4′-[[α-(*p*-fluorophenyl)-α,4-dihydroxy-*m*-tolyl]oxy]-3′,5′-dimethyloxanilate. *UNII-V477CK910J. CAS-156740-57-7.* INN. *Hypolipidemic.* ◇CGS 26214

Axomadol [*2005*] (ax oh′ ma dol). $C_{16}H_{25}NO_3$. 279.37. (1) 1,3-Cyclohexanediol, 6-[(dimethylamino)methyl]-1-(3-methoxyphenyl)-, (1*R*,3*R*,6*R*)-*rel*-; (2) (1*RS*,3*RS*,6*RS*)-6-[(Dimethylamino)methyl]-1-(3-methoxyphenyl)cyclohexane-1,3-diol. *UNII-9J92U4CVS0. CAS-187219-99-4.* INN. *Treatment of pain, central analgesic.* ◇GRT151 base; BN110 base

Azabon [*1966*] (ay′ za bon). $C_{14}H_{20}N_2O_2S$. 280.39. (1) Benzenamine, 4-(3-azabicyclo[3.2.2]non-3-ylsulfonyl)-; (2) 3-Sulfanilyl-3-azabicyclo[3.2.2]nonane. *CAS-1150-20-5.* INN. *Stimulant (central).*

Azabuperone. $C_{17}H_{23}FN_2O$. 290.38. 4′-Fluoro-4-(hexahydropyrrolo[1,2-*a*]pyrazin-2(1*H*)-yl)butyrophenone. *UNII-9P043590EX. CAS-2856-81-7.* INN.

Azacitidine [*1978*] (ay za sye′ ti deen). $C_8H_{12}N_4O_5$. 244.20. (1) 1,3,5-Triazin-2(1*H*)-one, 4-amino-1-β-D-ribofuranosyl-; (2) 4-Amino-1-β-D-ribofuranosyl-*s*-triazin-2(1*H*)-one. *UNII-M801H13NRU. CAS-320-67-2.* INN. *Antineoplastic.* Vidaza (Pharmion) *[Name previously used: Ladakamycin.]* ◇U-18,496; NSC-102816

Azaclorzine Hydrochloride [*1977*] (ay″ za klor′ zeen hye″ droe klor′ ide). $C_{22}H_{24}ClN_3OS.2HCl$. 486.89. [Azaclorzine is INN.] (1) 10*H*-Phenothiazine, 2-chloro-10-[3-(hexahydropyrrolo[1,2-*a*]pyrazin-2(1*H*)-yl)-1-oxopropyl]-, dihydrochloride; (2) 2-Chloro-10-[3-(hexahydropyrrolo[1,2-*a*]pyrazin-2(1*H*)-yl)-propionyl]phenothiazine dihydrochloride. *UNII-7531I37BK3; UNII-7N4BHX8N3L* [az-

aclorzine]. *CAS-49780-10-1; CAS-49864-70-2* [azaclorzine]. *Vasodilator (coronary). [Name previously used: Nonachlazine.]* ◇AY-25,329

Azaconazole [*1981*] (ay″ za kon′ a zole). $C_{12}H_{11}Cl_2N_3O_2$. 300.14. (1) 1*H*-1,2,4-Triazole, 1-[[2-(2,4-dichlorophenyl)-1,3-dioxolan-2-yl]methyl]-; (2) 1-[[2-(2,4-Dichlorophenyl)-1,3-dioxolan-2-yl]methyl]-1*H*-1,2,4-triazole. *UNII-45683D94EU. CAS-60207-31-0.* INN. *Antifungal. [Name previously used: Azoconazole.]* ◇R-28,644

Azacosterol Hydrochloride [*1965*] (ay″ za kos′ ter ol hye″ droe klor′ ide). $C_{25}H_{44}N_2O.2HCl$. 461.55. [Azacosterol is INN.] (1) Androst-5-en-3-ol, 17-[[3-(dimethylamino)propyl]methylamino]-, dihydrochloride, (3β,17β)-; (2) 17β-[[3-(Dimethylamino)-propyl]methylamino]androst-5-en-3β-ol dihydrochloride; (3) 20,25-Diazacholesterol dihydrochloride. *UNII-B32804UAUQ. CAS-1249-84-9; CAS-313-05-3* [azacosterol]. *Chemosterilant, avian.* ◇SC-12937

Azacyclonol Hydrochloride. $C_{18}H_{21}NO.HCl$. 303.83. [Azacyclonol is INN and BAN.] α,α-Diphenyl-4-piperidinemethanol hydrochloride. *UNII-4BXX0XNP9R. CAS-1798-50-1; CAS-115-46-8* [azacyclonol]. NF XII; MI. Frenquel (Marion Merrell Dow†)

Azaepothilone B (trivial name) — *See* Ixabepilone.

Azaftozine. $C_{23}H_{24}F_3N_3OS$. 447.52. 10-[3-(Hexahydropyrrolo[1,2-*a*]pyrazin-2(1*H*)-yl)propionyl]-2-(trifluoromethyl)-phenothiazine. *UNII-8Y5377MMOO. CAS-54063-26-2.* INN.

Azalanstat Dihydrochloride [*1995*] (ay″ za lan′ stat dye hye″ droe klor′ ide). $C_{22}H_{24}ClN_3O_2S.2HCl$. 502.88. [Azalanstat is INN.] (1) Benzenamine, 4-[[[2-[2-(4-chlorophenyl)ethyl]-2-(1*H*-imidazol-1-ylmethyl)-1,3-dioxolan-4-yl]-

methyl]thio]-, dihydrochloride, (2*S*-*cis*)-; (2) 1-[[(2*S*,4*S*)-4-[[(*p*-Aminophenyl)thio]methyl]-2-(*p*-chlorophenethyl)-1,3-dioxolan-2-yl]methyl]imidazole dihydrochloride. *UNII-X30J960B4D; UNII-2NL79NI1WS* [azalanstat]. *CAS-143484-82-6; CAS-143393-27-5* [azalanstat]. *Hypolipidemic*. ✧*RS-21607-197*

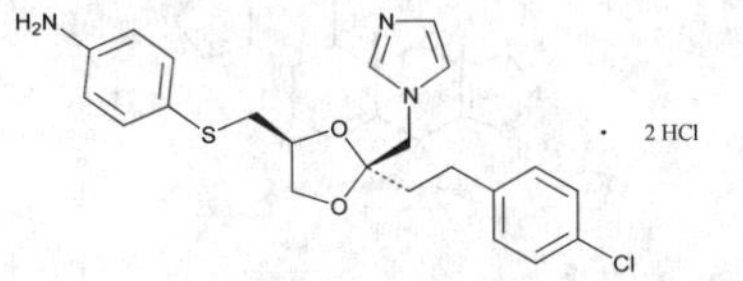

Azaline B (name previously used) — *See* Prazarelix Acetate.

Azalomycin. A mixture of related antibiotics produced by *Streptomyces hygroscopicus* var. *azalomyceticus* or the same substance obtained by any other means. *CAS-54182-65-9*. INN; BAN.

Azaloxan Fumarate [*1985*] (ay za lox′ an fue′ ma rate). $C_{18}H_{25}N_3O_3.C_4H_4O_4$. 447.48. [Azaloxan is INN.] (1) 2-Imidazolidinone, 1-[1-[2-(2,3-dihydro-1,4-benzodioxin-2-yl)ethyl]-4-piperidinyl]-, (*S*)-, (*E*)-2-butenedioate (1:1); (2) (*S*)-1-[1-[2-(1,4-Benzodioxan-2-yl)-ethyl]-4-piperidyl]-2-imidazolidinone fumarate (1:1). *UNII-8605L38D80; UNII-0O653FA999* [azaloxan]. *CAS-86116-60-1; CAS-72822-56-1* [azaloxan]. *Antidepressant*. ✧*CGS 7135A*

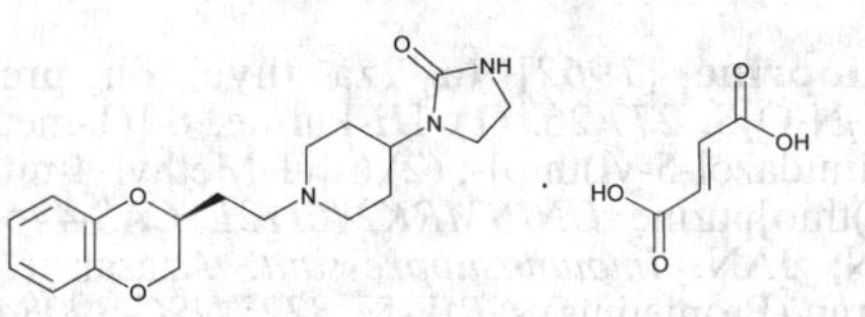

Azamethiphos. $C_9H_{10}ClN_2O_5PS$. 324.68. *S*-[(6-Chloro-2,3-dihydro-2-oxo-1,3-oxazolo-[4,5-*b*]pyridin-3-yl)methyl] *O,O*-dimethyl phosphorothioate. *UNII-9440R8149U*. *CAS-35575-96-3*. BAN. ✧*CGA 18809; OMS No 1825*

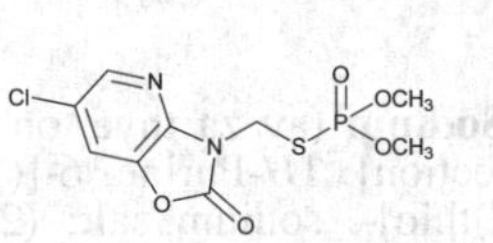

Azamethonium Bromide. $C_{13}H_{33}Br_2N_3$. 391.23. [(Methylimino)diethylene]bis(ethyldimethylammonium bromide). *UNII-4K6NEI0MSR; UNII-43XK6AW58D* [azamethonium]. *CAS-306-53-6; CAS-60-30-0* [azamethonium]. INN; BAN; MI.

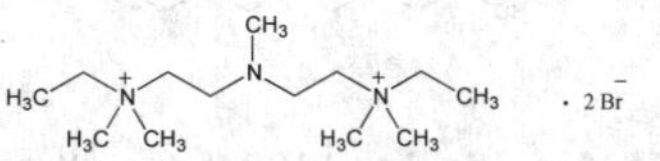

† Brand name formerly used, and/or firm no longer concerned with this product.

Azamulin. $C_{24}H_{38}N_4O_4S$. 478.65. [(5-Amino-*s*-triazol-3-yl)thio]acetic acid, 8-ester with (3a*S*,4*R*,5*S*,6*R*,8*R*,9-*R*,9a*R*,10*R*)-6-ethyloctahydro-5,8-dihydroxy-4,6,9,10-tetramethyl-3a,9-propano-3a*H*-cyclopentacycloocten-1(4*H*)-one. *CAS-76530-44-4*. INN.

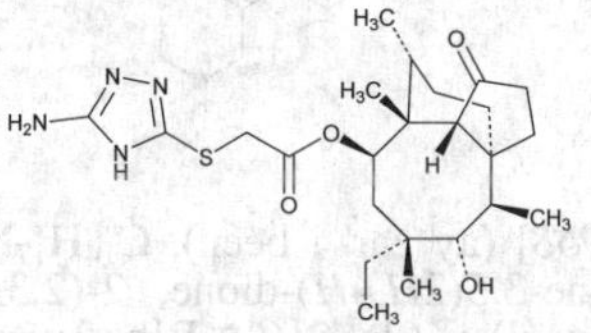

Azanator Maleate [*1974*] (ay zan′ a tor mal′ ee ate). $C_{18}H_{18}N_2O.C_4H_4O_4$. 394.42. [Azanator is INN.] (1) 5*H*-[1]Benzopyrano[2,3-*b*]pyridine, 5-(1-methyl-4-piperidinylidene)-, (*Z*)-2-butenedioate (1:1); (2) 5-(1-Methyl-4-piperidylidene)-5*H*-[1]benzopyrano[2,3-*b*]pyridine maleate (1:1). *UNII-63ISF1PDWX; UNII-699725286I* [azanator]. *CAS-39624-65-2; CAS-37855-92-8* [azanator]. *Bronchodilator*. ✧*Sch 15280*

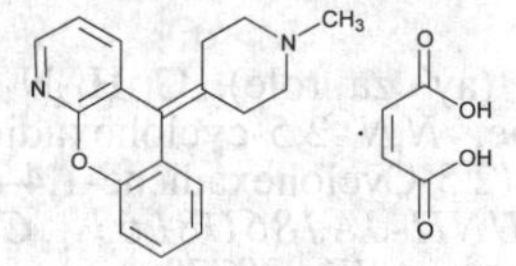

Azanidazole [*1977*] (ay″ za nye′ da zole). $C_{10}H_{10}N_6O_2$. 246.23. (1) 2-Pyrimidinamine, 4-[2-(1-methyl-5-nitro-1*H*-imidazol-2-yl)ethenyl]-, (*E*)-; (2) (*E*)-2-Amino-4-[2-(1-methyl-5-nitroimidazol-2-yl)vinyl]pyrimidine. *UNII-YP2Y0DRX4S*. *CAS-62973-76-6*. INN; BAN. *Antiprotozoal*.

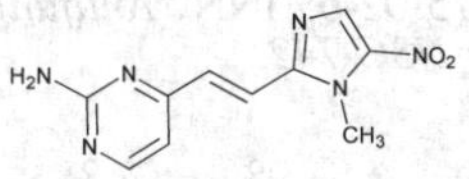

Azaperone [*1967*] (ay′ za per one). **USP**. $C_{19}H_{22}FN_3O$. 327.40. (1) 1-Butanone, 1-(4-fluorophenyl)-4-[4-(2-pyridinyl)-1-piperazinyl]-; (2) 4′-Fluoro-4-[4-(2-pyridyl)-1-piperazinyl]butyrophenone. *UNII-19BV78AK7W*. *CAS-1649-18-9*. INN; BAN. *Antipsychotic*. Stresnil (Janssen Pharmaceutica, Belgium); Suicalm (Janssen Pharmaceutica, Belgium) ✧*R 1929*

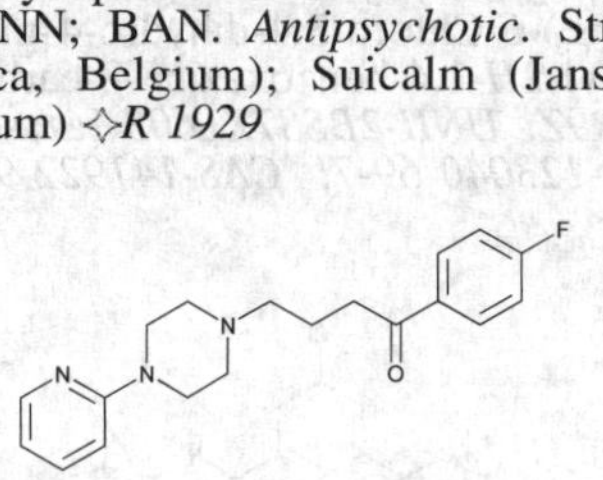

Azapetine Phosphate. [Azapetine is BAN.] *UNII-0N2U15U85W*. *CAS-130-83-6*. AMA-DE 1973. Ilidar (Hoffmann-LaRoche†)

Azaprocin. $C_{18}H_{24}N_2O$. 284.40. 3-Cinnamyl-8-propionyl-3,8-diazabicyclo[3.2.1]octan. *CAS-448-34-0*. INN.

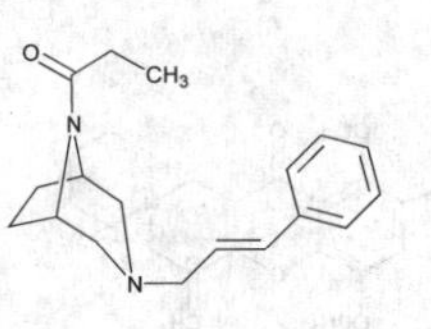

Azapropazone (INN, BAN, DCF) — *See* Apazone.

Azaquinzole. $C_{12}H_{16}N_2$. 188.27. 1,3,4,6,7,11b-Hexahydro-2*H*-pyrazino[2,1-*a*]isoquinoline. *UNII-T3H6486135. CAS-5234-86-6.* INN.

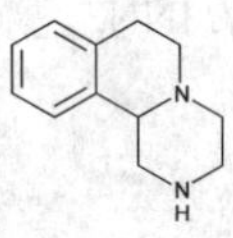

Azaribine [*1968*] (ay zar′ i been). $C_{14}H_{17}N_3O_9$. 371.30. (1) 1,2,4-Triazine-3,5(2*H,4H*)-dione, 2-(2,3,5-tri-*O*-acetyl-*β*-D-ribofuranosyl)-; (2) 2-*β*-D-Ribofuranosyl-*as*-triazine-3,5(2*H,4H*)-dione 2′,3′,5′-triacetate. *UNII-K1U80DO9EB. CAS-2169-64-4.* INN; BAN. *Antipsoriatic.* Triazure (Parke-Davis†) ◇*CB 304; NSC-67239*

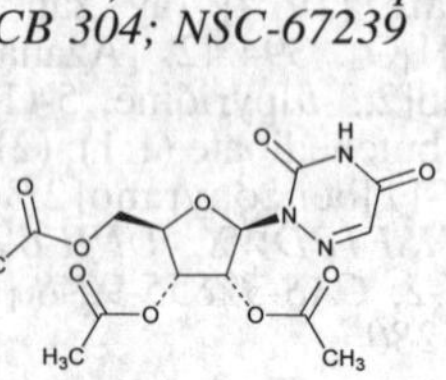

Azarole [*1979*] (ay′ za role). $C_{14}H_{12}N_4$. 236.27. (1) 1*H*-Pyrrol-1-amine, *N,N′*-2,5-cyclohexadiene-1,4-diylidene-bis-; (2) 1,1′-(2,5-Cyclohexadiene-1,4-diylidenedinitrilo)-dipyrrole. *UNII-JAJ86U8L6J. CAS-55872-82-7. Immunoregulator.* ◇*Win 38770*

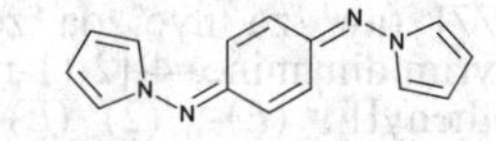

Azaserine [*1968*] (ay″ za ser′ een). $C_5H_7N_3O_4$. 173.13. (1) L-Serine, diazoacetate (ester); (2) L-Serine, diazoacetate (ester). *CAS-115-02-6.* INN. *Antifungal.* ◇*Cl 337; CN-15,757; P-165; NSC-742*

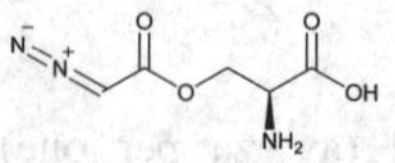

Azasetron. $C_{17}H_{20}ClN_3O_3$. 349.81. [Azasetron Hydrochloride is JAN.] (±)-6-Chloro-3,4-dihydro-4-methyl-3-oxo-*N*-3-quinuclidinyl-2*H*-1,4-benzoxazine-8-carboxamide. *UNII-77HC7URR9Z; UNII-2BSS7XL60S* [azasetron hydrochloride]. *CAS-123040-69-7; CAS-141922-90-9* [hydrochloride]. INN.

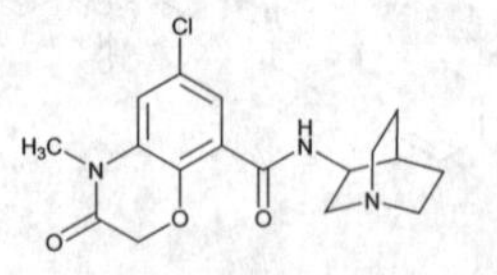

Azaspirium Chloride. $C_{22}H_{24}ClNO_5$. 417.88. 8,9-Dihydro-4,11-dimethoxy-9-methylene-5-oxospiro[5*H*-furo[3′,2′:6,7][1]benzopyrano[3,2-*c*]pyridine-7-(6*H*),1′-piperidinium]chloride. *UNII-8Y7H79TF0I. CAS-34959-30-3.* INN.

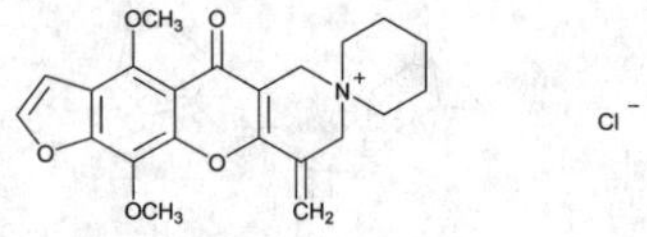

Azastene. $C_{23}H_{33}NO_2$. 355.51. (1) Androsta-2,5-dieno[2,3-*d*]isoxazol-17-ol, 4,4,17-trimethyl-, (17*β*)-; (2) 4,4,17-Trimethylandrosta-2,5-dieno[2,3-*d*]isoxazol-17*β*-ol. *UNII-1XA84ITL1H. CAS-13074-00-5.* [*Note—Azastene formerly was a USAN, from 1977 to 1981.*] ◇*Win 17625*

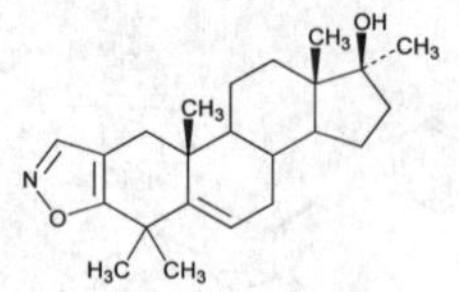

Azatadine Maleate [*1967*] (a za′ ta deen mal′ ee ate). **USP.** $C_{20}H_{22}N_2 \cdot 2C_4H_4O_4$. 522.55. [Azatadine is INN and BAN.] (1) 5*H*-Benzo[5,6]cyclohepta[1,2-*b*]pyridine, 6,11-dihydro-11-(1-methyl-4-piperidinylidene)-, (*Z*)-2-butenedioate (1:2); (2) 6,11-Dihydro-11-(1-methyl-4-piperidylidene)-5*H*-benzo[5,6]cyclohepta[1,2-*b*]pyridine maleate (1:2). *UNII-F3Q391WTX7; UNII-94Z39NID6C* [azatadine]. *CAS-3978-86-7; CAS-3964-81-6* [azatadine]. *Antihistaminic.* Optimine (Schering) ◇*Sch 10649*

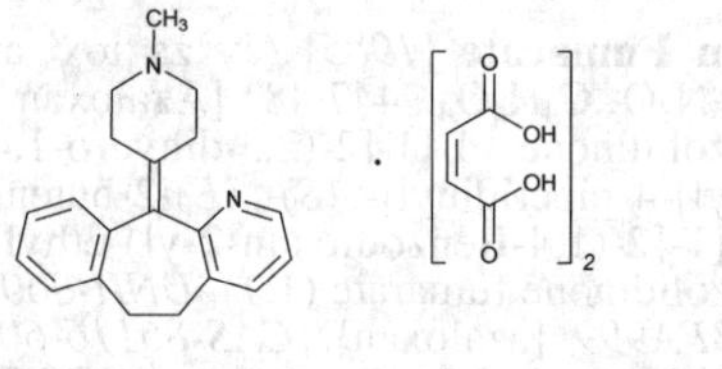

Azatepa (INN, BAN) — *See* Azetepa.

Azathioprine [*1962*] (ay za thye′ oh preen). **USP.** $C_9H_7N_7O_2S$. 277.26. (1) 1*H*-Purine, 6-[(1-methyl-4-nitro-1*H*-imidazol-5-yl)thio]-; (2) 6-[(1-Methyl-4-nitroimidazol-5-yl)thio]purine. *UNII-MRK240IY2L. CAS-446-86-6.* INN; BAN; JAN. *Immunosuppressant.* Azasan (Aaipharma); Imuran (Promethus) ◇*BW-57-322; NSC-39084*

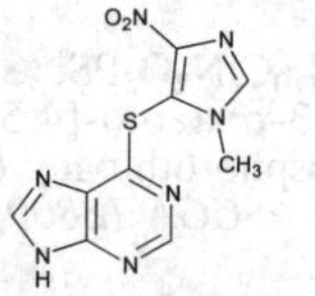

Azathioprine Sodium (ay za thye′ oh preen soe′ dee um). **USP** [for Injection]. 1*H*-Purine, 6-[(1-methyl-4-nitro-1*H*-imidazol-5-yl)thio]-, sodium salt; (2) 6-[(1-Methyl-4-nitroimidazol-5-yl)thio]purine sodium salt. *UNII-AM94R510MS. Immunosuppressant.*

Azelaic Acid [*1996*] (ay ze lay′ ik as′ id). $C_9H_{16}O_4$. 188.22. (1) Nonanedioic acid; (2) Azelaic acid. *UNII-F2VW3D43YT. CAS-123-99-9.* INN; MI. *Anti-acne.* Azelex (Allergan); Finacea (Intendis) ◇*ZK 62498*

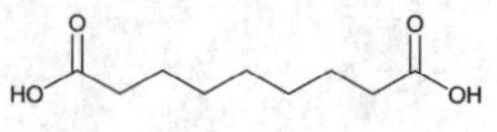

Azelastine Hydrochloride [*1984*] (a zel′ as teen hye″ droe klor′ ide). $C_{22}H_{24}ClN_3O \cdot HCl$. 418.36. [Azelastine is INN and BAN.] (1) 1(2*H*)-Phthalazinone, 4-[(4-chlorophenyl)-methyl]-2-(hexahydro-1-methyl-1*H*-azepin-4-yl)-, mono-hydrochloride; (2) 4-(*p*-Chlorobenzyl)-2-(hexahydro-1-methyl-1*H*-azepin-4-yl)-1(2*H*)-phthalazinone monohydrochloride. *UNII-0L591QR10I; UNII-ZQI909440X* [azelastine]. *CAS-79307-93-0; CAS-58581-89-8* [azelastine]. JAN. *Anti-allergic; anti-asthmatic*. Astelin (Medpointe); Optivar (Medpointe) ◇*A-5610; W-2979M; E-0659*

Azelnidipine. $C_{33}H_{34}N_4O_6$. 582.65. 3-[1-(Diphenylmethyl)-3-azetidinyl] 5-isopropyl (±)-2-amino-1,4-dihydro-6-methyl-4-(*m*-nitrophenyl)-3,5-pyridinedicarboxylate. *UNII-PV23P19YUG. CAS-123524-52-7.* INN.

Azepexole. $C_9H_{15}N_3O$. 181.23. 2-Amino-6-ethyl-5,6,7,8-tetrahydro-4*H*-oxazolo[4,5-*d*]azepine. *UNII-DGB112538O. CAS-36067-73-9.* INN; BAN.

Azepinamide — *See* Glypinamide.

Azepindole [*1978*] (ay ze pin′ dole). $C_{12}H_{14}N_2$. 186.25. (1) 1*H*-[1,4]Diazepino[1,2-*a*]indole, 2,3,4,5-tetrahydro-; (2) 2,3,4,5-Tetrahydro-1*H*-[1,4]diazepino[1,2-*a*]indole. *CAS-26304-61-0.* INN. *Antidepressant.* ◇*McN-2453*

Azetepa [*1962*] (ay ze tep′ a). $C_8H_{14}N_5OPS$. 259.27. [Azatepa is INN and BAN.] (1) Phosphinic amide, *P,P*-bis(1-aziridinyl)-*N*-ethyl-*N*-1,3,4-thiadiazol-2-yl-; (2) *P,P*-Bis(1-aziridinyl)-*N*-ethyl-*N*-1,3,4-thiadiazol-2-ylphosphinic amide. *UNII-D57I4Z650L. CAS-125-45-1.* *Antineoplastic.* ◇*CL 25477; NSC-64826*

Azetirelin. $C_{15}H_{20}N_6O_4$. 348.36. (-)-*N*-[[(2*S*)-4-Oxo-2-azetidinyl]carbonyl]-L-histidyl-L-prolinamide. *UNII-70J5AWG54Q. CAS-95729-65-0.* INN.

Azidamfenicol. $C_{11}H_{13}N_5O_5$. 295.25. D(-)-*threo*-2-Azido-*N*-[β-hydroxy-α-(hydroxymethyl)-*p*-nitrophenethyl]acetamide. *UNII-40257685LM. CAS-13838-08-9.* INN; BAN; DCF; MI.

Azidoamphenicol — *See* Azidamfenicol.

Azidocillin. $C_{16}H_{17}N_5O_4S$. 375.40. 6-(2-Azido-2-phenylacetamido)-3,3-dimethyl-7-oxo-4-thia-1-azabicyclo[3.2.0]-heptane-2-carboxylic acid. *UNII-R8XDP7L3SL. CAS-17243-38-8.* INN; BAN; MI. ◇*BRL 2534; SPC 297 D*

Azidothymidine (previously used name) — *See* Zidovudine.

Azilsartan [*2007*] (ay″ zil sar′ tan). $C_{25}H_{20}N_4O_5$. 456.45. (1) 1*H*-Benzimidazole-7-carboxylic acid, 1-[[2′-(2,5-dihydro-5-oxo-1,2,4-oxadiazol-3-yl)[1,1′-biphenyl]-4-yl]methyl]-2-ethoxy-; (2) 2-Ethoxy-1-{[2′-(5-oxo-4,5-dihydro-1,2,4-oxadiazol-3-yl)biphenyl-4-yl]methyl}-1*H*-benzimidazole-7-carboxylic acid. *UNII-F9NUX55P23. CAS-147403-03-0.* INN. *Treatment of hypertension.* ◇*TAK-536*

Azilsartan Kamedoxomil [*2007*] (ay″ zil sar′ tan kay″ me dox′ oh mil). $C_{30}H_{23}KN_4O_8$. 606.62. [Azilsartan Medoxomil is INN.] (1) 1*H*-Benzimidazole-7-carboxylic acid, 1-[[2′-(2,5-dihydro-5-oxo-1,2,4-oxadiazol-3-yl)[1,1′-biphenyl]-4-yl]methyl]-2-ethoxy-, (5-methyl-2-oxo-1,3-dioxol-4-yl)methyl ester, potassium salt; (2) Potassium 3-{4′-[(2-ethoxy-7-{[(5-methyl-2-oxo-1,3-dioxol-4-yl)methoxy]car-

---

† Brand name formerly used, and/or firm no longer concerned with this product.

bonyl}-1*H*-benzimidazol-1-yl)methyl]biphenyl-4-yl}-5-oxo-1,2,4-oxadiazol-4(5*H*)-ide. *UNII-WEC6I2K1FC. CAS-863031-24-7. Treatment of hypertension.* ◇*TAK-491*

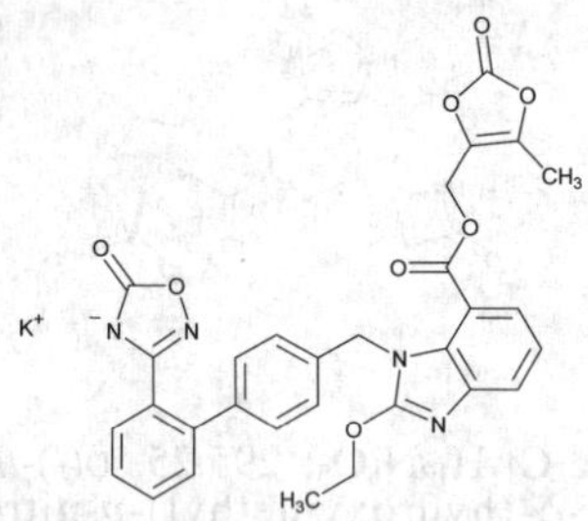

Azilsartan Medoxomil [*2007*] (ay″ zil sar′ tan me dox′ oh mil). $C_{30}H_{24}N_4O_8$. 568.53. (1) 1*H*-Benzimidazole-7-carboxylic acid, 1-[[2′-(2,5-dihydro-5-oxo-1,2,4-oxadiazol-3-yl)[1,1′-biphenyl]-4-yl]methyl]-2-ethoxy-, (5-methyl-2-oxo-1,3-dioxol-4-yl)methyl ester; (2) (5-Methyl-2-oxo-1,3-dioxol-4-yl)methyl 2-ethoxy-1-((2′-(5-oxo-4,5-dihydro-1,2,4-oxadiazol-3-yl)biphenyl-2-yl)methyl)-1*H*-benzo[d]imidazole-7-carboxylate. *UNII-LL0G25K7I2. CAS-863031-21-4.* INN. *Treatment of hypertension.* ◇*TAK-491*

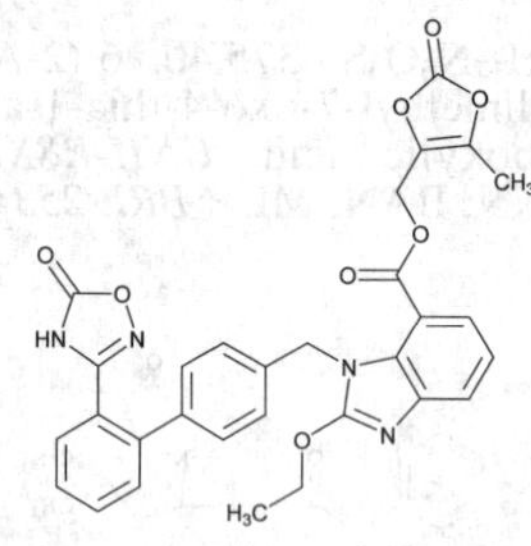

Azimexon. $C_9H_{14}N_4O$. 194.23. 1-[(1-(2-Cyano-1-aziridinyl)-1-methylethyl]-2-aziridinecarboxamide. *UNII-4NJ842U6BZ. CAS-64118-86-1.* INN.

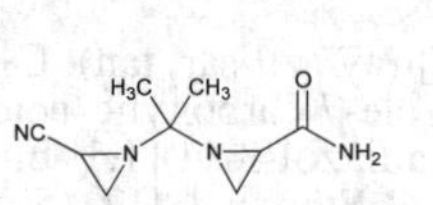

Azimilide Dihydrochloride [*1994*] (ay zim′ i lide dye hye″ droe klor′ ide). $C_{23}H_{28}ClN_5O_3$.2HCl. 530.88. [Azimilide is INN and BAN.] (1) 2,4-Imidazolidinedione, 1-[[5-(4-chlorophenyl)-2-furanyl]methylene]amino]-3-[4-(4-methyl-1-piperazinyl)butyl]-, dihydrochloride; (2) 1-[[5-(*p*-Chlorophenyl)furfurylidene]amino]-3-[4-(4-methyl-1-piperazinyl)butyl]hydantoin dihydrochloride. *UNII-6E6VJP68KR. CAS-149888-94-8; CAS-149908-53-2* [azimilide]. *Cardiac depressant (anti-arrhythmic).* ◇*NE-10064*

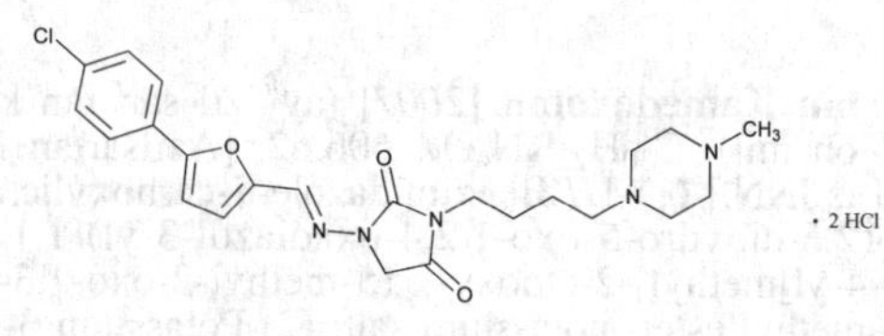

Azintamide. $C_{10}H_{14}ClN_3OS$. 259.76. 2-[(6-Chloro-3-pyridazinyl)thio]-*N,N*-diethylacetamide. *UNII-ACZ6L64B41. CAS-1830-32-6.* INN; MI. ◇*ST 9067*

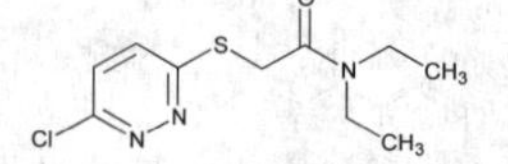

Azinthiamide — *See* Azintamide.

Azipramine Hydrochloride [*1976*] (ay zip′ ra meen hye″ droe klor′ ide). $C_{26}H_{26}N_2$.HCl. 402.96. [Azipramine is INN.] (1) Indolo[1,7-*ab*][1]benzazepine-1-ethanamine, 6,7-dihydro-*N*-methyl-*N*-(phenylmethyl)-, monohydrochloride; (2) 1-[2-(Benzylmethylamino)ethyl]-6,7-dihydroindolo[1,7-*ab*][1]benzazepine monohydrochloride. *UNII-U2508LW03T; UNII-1P9L1B4UIC* [azipramine]. *CAS-57529-83-6; CAS-58503-82-5* [azipramine]. *Antidepressant.* ◇*Pierrel-TQ 86*

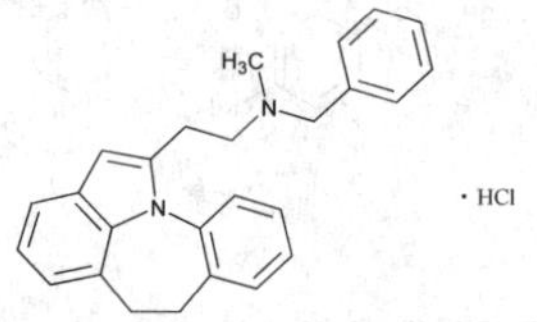

Azithromycin [*1987*] (ay zith″ roe mye′ sin). **USP**. $C_{38}H_{72}N_2O_{12}$.xH₂O. 748.98 (anhydrous). (1) 1-Oxa-6-azacyclopentadecan-15-one, 13-[(2,6-dideoxy-3-*C*-methyl-3-*O*-methyl-α-L-*ribo*-hexopyranosyl)oxy]-2-ethyl-3,4,10-trihydroxy-3,5,6,8,10,12,14-heptamethyl-11-[[3,4,6-trideoxy-3-(dimethylamino)-β-D-*xylo*-hexopyranosyl]oxy]-, [2*R*-(2*R**,3*S**,4*R**,5*R**,8*R**,10*R**,11*R**,12*S**,13*S**,14*R**)]-; (2) (2*R*,3*S*,4*R*,5*R*,8*R*,10*R*,11*R*,12*S*,13*S*,14*R*)-13-[(2,6-Dideoxy-3-*C*-methyl-3-*O*-methyl-α-L-*ribo*-hexopyranosyl)oxy]-2-ethyl-3,4,10-trihydroxy-3,5,6,8,10,12,14-heptamethyl-11-[[3,4,6-trideoxy-3-(dimethylamino)-β-D-*xylo*-hexopyranosyl]oxy]-1-oxa-6-azacyclopentadecan-15-one; (3) 9-Deoxo-9a-aza-9a-methyl-9a-homoerythromycin A. *UNII-F94OW58Y8V; UNII-5FD113117S* [azithromycin dihydrate]; *UNII-JTE4MNN1MD* [azithromycin monohydrate]. *CAS-83905-01-5* [anhydrous]; *CAS-121479-24-4* [monohydrate]; *CAS-117772-70-0* [dihydrate]. INN; BAN. *Antibacterial.* Zithromax (Pfizer); Zmax (Pfizer); Azasite (Inspire) ◇*CP-62,993; XZ-450*

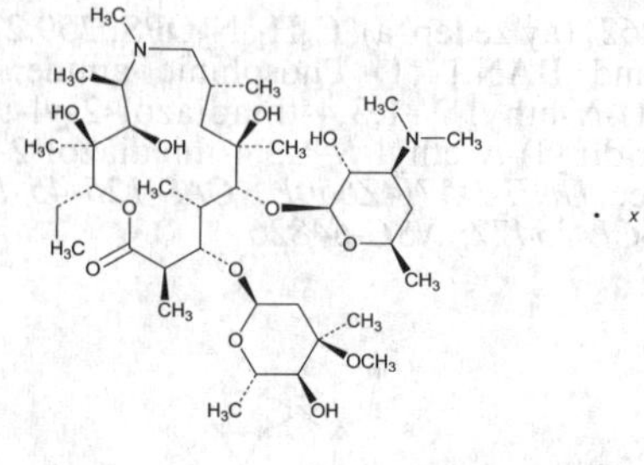

Azlocillin [*1976*] (az″ loe sil′ in). $C_{20}H_{23}N_5O_6S$. 461.49. (1) 4-Thia-1-azabicyclo[3.2.0]heptane-2-carboxylic acid, 3,3-dimethyl-7-oxo-6-[[[[(2-oxo-1-imidazolidinyl)carbonyl]amino]phenylacetyl]amino]-, [2*S*-[2α,5α,6β(*S**)]]-; (2) (2*S*,5*R*,6*R*)-3,3-Dimethyl-7-oxo-6-[(*R*)-2-(2-oxo-1-imidazolidinecarboxamido)-2-phenylacetamido]-4-thia-1-azabicyclo[3.2.0]heptane-2-carboxylic acid. *UNII-HUM6H389W0. CAS-37091-66-0.* INN; BAN. *Antibacterial.* Azlin (Bayer†)

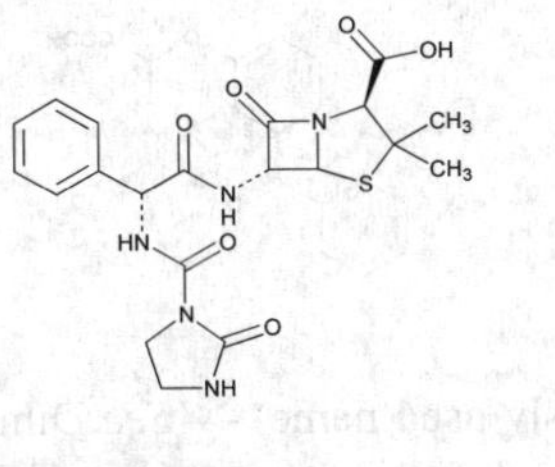

Azlocillin Sodium. $C_{20}H_{22}N_5NaO_6S$. 483.47. (1) 4-Thia-1-azabicyclo[3.2.0]heptane-2-carboxylic acid, 3,3-dimethyl-7-oxo-6-[[[[(2-oxo-1-imidazolidinyl)carbonyl]amino]phenylacetyl]amino]-, monosodium salt, [2*S*-[2α,5α,6β(*S**)]]-; (2) Sodium (2*S*,5*R*,6*R*)-3,3-dimethyl-7-oxo-6-[(*R*)-2-(2-oxo-1-imidazolidinecarboxamido)-2-phenylacetamido]-4-thia-1-azabicyclo[3.2.0]heptane-2-carboxylate. *UNII-DWV1EFW947. CAS-37091-65-9.* USP XXIII. *Antibacterial.* Azlin (Bayer)

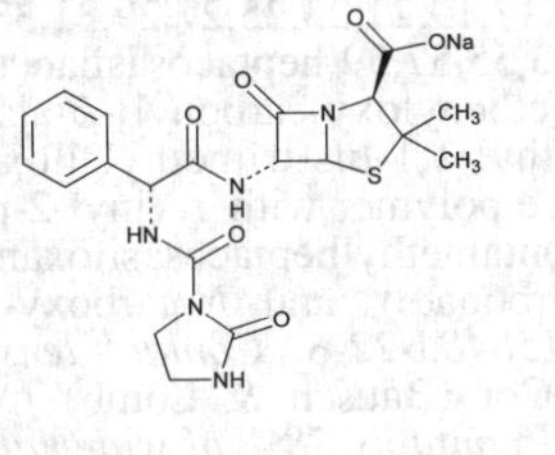

Azoconazole (previously used name) — *See* Azaconazole.

Azodisal Sodium (previously used name) — *See* Olsalazine Sodium.

Azolimine [*1974*] (ay zoe′ li meen). $C_{10}H_{11}N_3O$. 189.21. (1) 4-Imidazolidinone, 2-imino-3-methyl-1-phenyl-; (2) 2-Imino-3-methyl-1-phenyl-4-imidazolidinone. *UNII-DES29595KX. CAS-40828-45-3.* INN. *Diuretic.* ◇*CL 90,748*

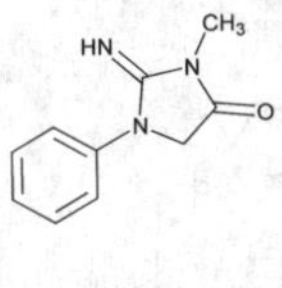

Azosemide [*1980*] (ay zoe′ se mide). $C_{12}H_{11}ClN_6O_2S_2$. 370.84. (1) Benzenesulfonamide, 2-chloro-5-(1*H*-tetrazol-5-yl)-4-[(2-thienylmethyl)amino]-; (2) 2-Chloro-5-(1*H*-tetrazol-5-yl)-*N*⁴-2-thenylsulfanilamide. *UNII-MR40VT1L8Z. CAS-27589-33-9.* INN; JAN. *Diuretic.*

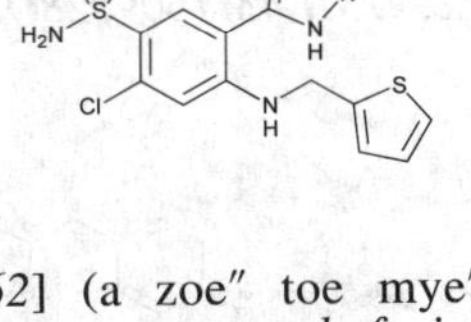

Azotomycin [*1962*] (a zoe″ toe mye′ sin). Antibiotic produced by *Streptomyces ambofaciens.CAS-7644-67-9.* INN. *Antineoplastic.* ◇*NSC-56654*

Azovan Blue (BAN) — *See* Evans Blue.

Azovan Sodium — *See* Evans Blue.

---

† Brand name formerly used, and/or firm no longer concerned with this product.

Azoximer Bromide. $[[C_8H_{15}BrN_2O_2]_x[C_6H_{12}N_2O]_y]_n$. Poly{[1-(carboxymethyl)piperazin-1-ium-1,4-diyl bromide]ethylene-co-[(piperazin-1,4-diyl 1-oxide)ethylene]}. *CAS-892497-01-7.* INN.

Aztreonam [*1983*] (az tree′ oh nam). USP. $C_{13}H_{17}N_5O_8S_2$. 435.43. (1) Propanoic acid, 2-[[[1-(2-amino-4-thiazolyl)-2-[(2-methyl-4-oxo-1-sulfo-3-azetidinyl)amino]-2-oxoethylidene]amino]oxy]-2-methyl-, [2*S*-[2α,3β(*Z*)]]-; (2) (*Z*)-2-[[[(2-Amino-4-thiazolyl)[[(2*S*,3*S*)-2-methyl-4-oxo-1-sulfo-3-azetidinyl]carbamoyl]methylene]amino]oxy]-2-methylpropionic acid. *UNII-G2B4VE5GH8. CAS-78110-38-0.* INN; BAN; JAN. *Antimicrobial.* Azactam (Bristol-Myers Squibb) ◇*SQ 26776*

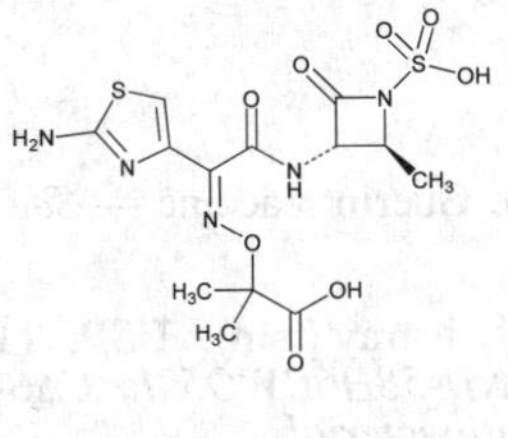

Aztreonam Lysine [*2005*] (az tree′ oh nam lye′ seen). $C_{13}H_{17}N_5O_8S_2 \cdot C_6H_{14}N_2O_2$. 581.62. (1) L-Lysine, mono[2-[[(*Z*)-[1-(2-amino-4-thiazolyl)-2-[[(2*S*,3*S*)-2-methyl-4-oxo-1-sulfo-3-azetidinyl]amino]-2-oxoethylidene]amino]oxy]-2-methylpropanoate]; (2) L-Lysine, mono[2-[[(*Z*)-[1-(2-aminothiazol-4-yl)-2-[[2*S*,3*S*)-2-methyl-4-oxo-1-sulfoazetidin-3-yl]amino]-2-oxoethylidene]amino]oxy]-2-methylpropanoate. *UNII-XNM7LT65NP. CAS-827611-49-4. Antimicrobial.* Cayston (Corus) ◇*Corus1020*

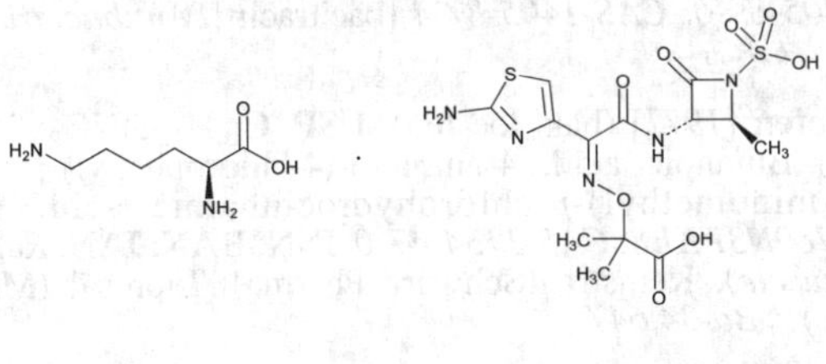

Azulene Sulfonate Sodium (JAN) — *See* Sodium Gualenate.

Azumolene Sodium [*1987*] (ay zoo′ moe leen soe′ dee um). $C_{13}H_8BrN_4NaO_3 \cdot 2H_2O$. 407.15. [Azumolene is INN.] (1) 2,4-Imidazolidinedione, 1-[[[5-(4-bromophenyl)-2-oxazolyl]methylene]amino]-, sodium salt, dihydrate; (2) 1-[[[5-(*p*-Bromophenyl)-2-oxazolyl]methylene]amino]hydantoin, sodium salt, dihydrate. *UNII-ISB31HSB8H; UNII-5U7IO9CV80* [azumolene]. *CAS-91524-18-4; CAS-64748-79-4* [azumolene]. *Relaxant (skeletal muscle).* ◇*EU-4093*

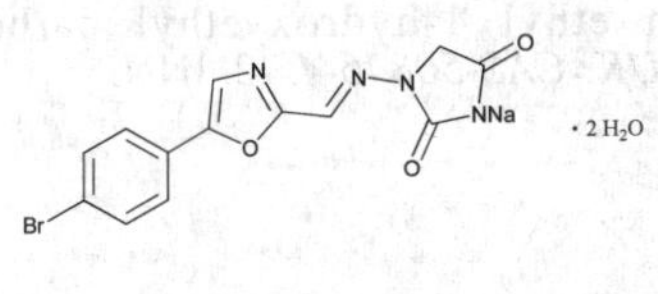

Azure A Carbacrylic Resin — *See* Azuresin.

Azuresin. $C_{14}H_{14}ClN_3S$. 291.80. 7-Aminophenothiazin-3-ylidene(dimethyl)ammonium chloride. *CAS-8050-34-8.* NF XIV; BAN. Diagnex Blue (Bristol-Myers Squibb†)

¹⁰B — *See* Borocaptate Sodium B 10.

Bacampicillin Hydrochloride [*1977*] (bak am′ pi sil′ in hye″ droe klor′ ide). USP. $C_{21}H_{27}N_3O_7S \cdot HCl$. 501.98. [Bacampicillin is INN and BAN.] (1) 4-Thia-1-azabicyclo[3.2.0]heptane-2-carboxylic acid, 6-[(aminophenylacetyl)amino]-3,3-dimethyl-7-oxo-, 1-[(ethoxycarbonyl)oxy]ethyl ester, monohydrochloride, [2*S*-[2α,5α,6β(*S**)]]-; (2) (2*S*,5*R*,6*R*)-6-[(*R*)-(2-Amino-2-phenylacetamido)]-3,3-dimethyl-7-oxo-4-thia-1-azabicyclo[3.2.0]heptane-2-carboxylic acid ester with ethyl 1-hydroxyethyl carbonate, monohydrochloride. *UNII-PM034U953T; UNII-8GM2J22278* [bacampicillin]. *CAS-37661-08-8; CAS-50972-17-3* [bacampicillin]. JAN. *Antibacterial.* Spectrobid (Pfizer)

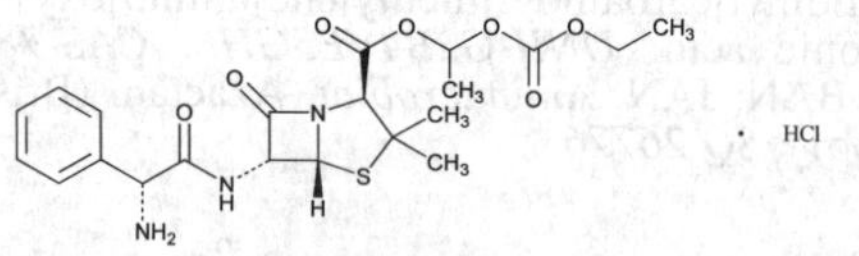

Bacillus Calmette-Guerin Vaccine — *See* BCG Vaccine.

Bacitracin (bas″ i tray′ sin). **USP.** (1) Bacitracin; (2) Bacitracin. *UNII-58H6RWO52I. CAS-1405-87-4.* INN; BAN; JAN. *Antibacterial.*

Bacitracin Methylene Disalicylate (bas″ i tray′ sin meth′ i leen dye″ sa lis′ i late). **USP** [Soluble]. A mixture of bacitracin methylene disalicylate and sodium bicarbonate. *Antibacterial; food additive (veterinary).*

Bacitracin Zinc (bas″ i tray′ sin zink). **USP.** (1) Bacitracins, zinc complex; (2) Bacitracins zinc complex. *UNII-89Y4M234ES; UNII-58H6RWO52I* [bacitracin]. *CAS-1405-89-6; CAS-1405-87-4* [bacitracin]. *Antibacterial.*

Baclofen [*1971*] (bak′ loe fen). **USP.** $C_{10}H_{12}ClNO_2$. 213.66. (1) Butanoic acid, 4-amino-3-(4-chlorophenyl)-; (2) β-(Aminomethyl)-*p*-chlorohydrocinnamic acid. *UNII-H789N3FKE8. CAS-1134-47-0.* INN; BAN; JAN. *Relaxant (muscle).* Kemstro (Schwarz Pharma); Lioresal (Medtronic) ◇*Ba-34,647*

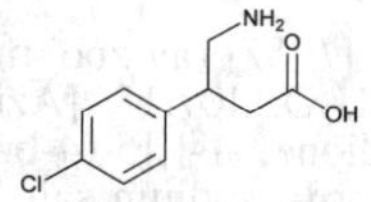

Bacmecillinam. $C_{20}H_{31}N_3O_6S$. 441.54. (2*S*,5*R*,6*R*)-6-[[(Hexahydro-1*H*-azepin-1-yl)methylene]amino]-3,3-dimethyl-7-oxo-4-thia-1-azabicyclo[3.2.0]heptane-2-carboxylic acid ester with ethyl 1-hydroxyethyl carbonate. *UNII-942B99D5UK. CAS-50846-45-2.* INN.

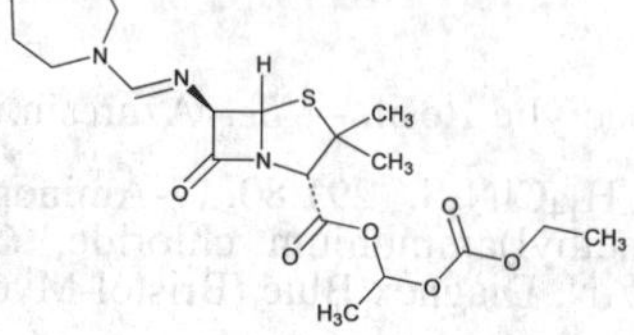

Bafetinib. $C_{30}H_{31}F_3N_8O$. 576.62. *N*-{3-[([5,5′-Bipyrimidin]-2-yl)amino]-4-methylphenyl}-4-{[(3*S*)-3-(dimethylamino)pyrrolidin-1-yl]methyl}-3-(trifluoromethyl)benzamide. *UNII-NVW4Z03I9B. CAS-887650-05-7.* INN.

Bakeprofen. $C_{16}H_{14}O_4$. 270.28. (±)-2-(*m*-Benzoylphenoxy)-propionic acid. *UNII-VMS3A207FA. CAS-117819-25-7.* INN.

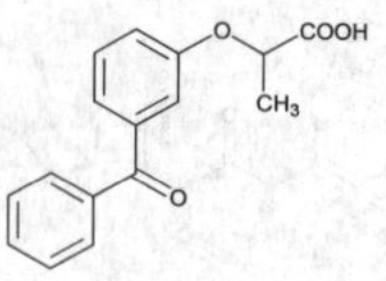

BAL (previously used name) — *See* Dimercaprol.

Balafilcon A [*1994*] (bal″ a fil′ kon). $(C_{15}H_{37}NO_5Si_4)_w(C_6H_9NO)_x(C_{68}H_{184}O_{32}Si_{27})_y(C_6H_9NO_4)_z$. (1) Carbamic acid, [3-[3,3,3-trimethyl-1,1-bis[[(trimethylsilyl)oxy]disiloxanyl]-propyl]-, ethenyl ester, polymer with 1-ethenyl-2-pyrrolidinone, ethenyl 7,7,9,9,11,11,13,13,15,15,17,17,-19,19,21,21,23,23,25,25,27,27,29,29,31,31,33,33,35,35,3-7,37,39,39,41,41,43,43,45,45,47,47,49,49,51,51,53,53,55,-55,57,57,59,59-tetrapentacontamethyl-65-oxo-2,8,10,12,14,16,18,20,22,24,26,28,30,32,34,36,38,40,42,4-4,46,48,50,52,54,56,58,64,66-nonacosaoxa-7,9,11,13,15,17,19,21,23,25,27,29,31,33,35,37,39,41,43,4-5,47,49,51,53,55,57,59-heptacosasilaoctahexacont-67-enoate, and *N*-[(ethenyloxy)carbonyl]-β-alanine; (2) Vinyl [3-[3,3,3-trimethyl-1,1-bis(trimethylsiloxy)disiloxanyl]propyl]carbamate polymer with 1-vinyl-2-pyrrolidinone, 4,4′-(tetrapentacontamethylheptacosasiloxanylene)di-1-butanol bis(vinyl carbonate), and *N*-carboxy-β-alanine *N*-vinyl ester. *CAS-158483-22-8. Contact lens material (hydrophilic).* OxyCor (Bausch & Lomb) [*Note—This contact lens material contains 38% of water at ambient temperature (23±2°C).*]

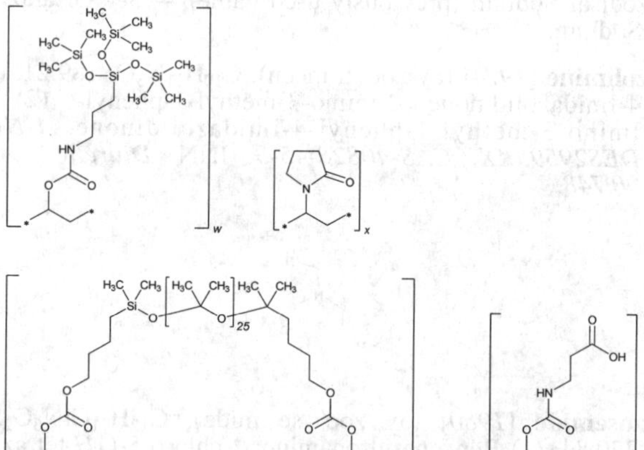

Balaglitazone. $C_{20}H_{17}N_3O_4S$. 395.43. (±)-5-[*p*-[(3,4-Dihydro-3-methyl-4-oxo-2-quinazolinyl)methoxy]benzyl]-2,4-thiazolidinedione. *UNII-4M1609828O. CAS-199113-98-9.* INN.

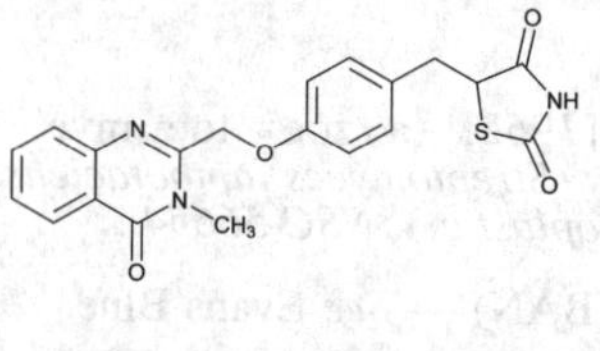

Balamapimod [*2006*] (bal″ a map′ i mod). $C_{30}H_{32}ClN_7OS$. 574.14. (1) 3-Quinolinecarbonitrile, 4-[[3-chloro-4-[(1-methyl-1*H*-imidazol-2-yl)thio]phenyl]amino]-6-methoxy-7-[4-(1-pyrrolidinyl)-1-piperidinyl]-; (2) 4-[[3-Chloro-4-[(1-methyl-1*H*-imidazol-2-yl)sulfanyl]phenyl]amino]-6-

methoxy-7-[4-(pyrrolidin-1-yl)piperidin-1-yl]quinoline-3-carbonitrile. *UNII-7Y0IV7N95Q. CAS-863029-99-6.* INN. *Oncology.* ◇*MKI-833*

Balazipone. $C_{13}H_{11}NO_2$. 213.23. *m*-(2-Acetyl-3-oxo-1-butenyl)benzonitrile. *UNII-GLI733V999. CAS-137109-71-8.* INN.

Balicatib. $C_{23}H_{33}N_5O_2$. 411.54. *N*-{1-[(Cyanomethyl)carbamoyl]cyclohexyl}-4-(4-propylpiperazin-1-yl)benzamide. *UNII-E00MVC7O57. CAS-354813-19-7.* INN.

Balipramine (previously used name) — *See* Depramine.

Balofloxacin. $C_{20}H_{24}FN_3O_4$. 389.42. (±)-1-Cyclopropyl-6-fluoro-1,4-dihydro-8-methoxy-7-[3-(methylamino)piperidino]-4-oxo-3-quinolinecarboxylic acid. *UNII-Q022B63JPM. CAS-127294-70-6.* INN.

Balsalazide Disodium [*1994*] (bal sal′ a zide dye soe′ dee um). $C_{17}H_{13}N_3Na_2O_6.2H_2O$. 437.31. [Balsalazide is INN and BAN.] (1) Benzoic acid, 5-[[4-[[(2-carboxyethyl)amino]carbonyl]phenyl]azo]-2-hydroxy-, disodium salt, dihydrate, (*E*)-; (2) (*E*)-5-[[*p*-[(2-Carboxyethyl)carbamoyl]phenyl]azo]salicylic acid, disodium salt, dihydrate. *UNII-1XL6BJI034; UNII-P80AL8J7ZP* [balsalazide]. *CAS-150399-21-6; CAS-80573-04-2* [balsalazide]. *Anti-inflammatory (gastrointestinal).* Colazal (Salix) ◇*BX661A*

Balsalazine — *See* Balsalazide Disodium.

---

† Brand name formerly used, and/or firm no longer concerned with this product.

Bamaluzole. $C_{14}H_{12}ClN_3O$. 273.72. 4-[(*o*-Chlorobenzyl)oxy]-1-methyl-1*H*-imidazo[4,5-*c*]pyridine. *UNII-GX1Q848LV4. CAS-87034-87-5.* INN.

Bamaquimast. $C_{16}H_{21}N_3O_3$. 303.36. 3-(3-Hydroxypropyl)-1-propyl-2(1*H*)-quinoxalinone methylcarbamate (ester). *UNII-5MZ70CT96H. CAS-135779-82-7.* INN.

Bambermycin (INN, BAN) — *See* Bambermycins.

Bambermycins [*1972*] (bam″ ber mye′ sins). [Bambermycin is INN and BAN.] Antibiotic complex, containing mainly moenomycin A and C, obtained from cultures of *Streptomyces bambergiensis*, or the same substance obtained by any other means. Bambermycin. *CAS-11015-37-5. Antibacterial.* Flavomycin (Hoechst-Roussel)

Bambuterol. $C_{18}H_{29}N_3O_5$. 367.44. (±)-5-[2-(*tert*-Butylamino)-1-hydroxyethyl]-*m*-phenylene bis(dimethylcarbamate). *CAS-81732-65-2.* INN; BAN; MI.

Bamethan Sulfate [*1965*] (bam′ e than sul′ fate). $(C_{12}H_{19}NO_2)_2.H_2SO_4$. 516.65. [Bamethan is INN and BAN.] (1) Benzenemethanol, α-[(butylamino)methyl]-4-hydroxy-, sulfate (2:1) (salt); (2) α-[(Butylamino)methyl]-*p*-hydroxybenzyl alcohol sulfate (2:1) (salt). *UNII-W2L3E1W827; UNII-Y08ZFJ9TFK* [bamethan]. *CAS-5716-20-1; CAS-3703-79-5* [bamethan]. JAN. *Vasodilator.*

Bamifylline Hydrochloride [*1966*] (bam if′ i lin hye″ droe klor′ ide). $C_{20}H_{27}N_5O_3.HCl$. 421.92. [Bamifylline is INN and BAN.] (1) 1*H*-Purine-2,6-dione, 7-[2-[ethyl(2-hydroxyethyl)amino]ethyl]-3,7-dihydro-1,3-dimethyl-8-(phenylmethyl)-, monohydrochloride; (2) 8-Benzyl-7-[2-[ethyl(2-hydroxyethyl)amino]ethyl]theophylline monohydrochloride. *UNII-66466QLM3S; UNII-ZTY15D026H* [bamifylline]. *CAS-20684-06-4; CAS-2016-63-9* [bamifylline]. *Bronchodilator.* ◇*AC 3810; 8102 CB; BAX 2739Z*

Baminercept Alfa [*2007*] (bam in′ er sept al′ fa). $C_{4074}H_{6282}N_{1134}O_{1274}S_{68}$. (1) β-Lymphotoxin receptor (human extracellular domain-containing fragment) fusion protein with immunoglobulin G1 (human γ1-chain Fc fragment); (2) Human tumor necrosis factor receptor superfamily member 3 (lymphotoxin-β receptor, TNF C receptor)-(2-195)-peptide (fragment of extracellular domain) fusion protein with human immunoglobulin heavy constant γ1 chain Fc fragment [227 residues, hinge (195-205) des-(1-4),C5>V, CH2 (206-315), CH3 (316-421) des-K[107]]dimer (201-201′:204-204′)-bisdisulfide, glycosolated. Molecular weight is approximately 93,710 daltons *UNII-HTV56CD308. CAS-909110-25-4.* INN. *Treatment of rheumatoid arthritis.* ◇*BG 9924*

```
AVPPYASENQ TCRDQEKEYY EPQHRICCSR CPPGTYVSAK CSRIRDTVCA
TCAENSYNEH WNYLTICQLC RPCDPVMGLE EIAPCTSKRK TQCRCQPGMF
CAAWALECTH CELLSDCPPG TEAELKDEVG KGNNHCVPCK AGHFQNTSSP
SARCQPHTRC ENQGLVEAAP GTAQSDTTCK NPLEPLPPEM SGTMVDKTHT
CPPCPAPELL GGPSVFLFPP KPKDTLMISR TPEVTCVVVD VSHEDPEVKF
NWYVDGVEVH NAKTKPREEQ YNSTYRVVSV LTVLHQDWLN GKEYKCKVSN
KALPAPIEKT ISKAKGQPRE PQVYTLPPSR DELTKNQVSL TCLVKGFYPS
DIAVEWESNG QPENNYKTTP PVLDSDGSFF LYSKLTVDKS RWQQGNVFSC
SVMHEALHNH YTQKSLSLSP G
```

Bamipine. $C_{19}H_{24}N_2$. 280.41. 4-(*N*-Benzylanilino)-1-methylpiperidine. *UNII-Y6BHZ28O92. CAS-4945-47-5.* INN; BAN; DCF; MI.

Bamirastine. $C_{31}H_{37}N_5O_3$. 527.66. 2-[6-({3-[4-(Diphenylmethoxy)piperidin-1-yl]propyl}amino)imidazo[1,2-b]pyridazin-2-yl]-2-methylpropanoic acid. *UNII-SIG10953FN. CAS-215529-47-8.* INN.

Bamnidazole [*1976*] (bam nye′ da zole). $C_7H_{10}N_4O_4$. 214.18. (1) 1*H*-Imidazole-1-ethanol, 2-methyl-5-nitro-, carbamate (ester); (2) 2-Methyl-5-nitroimidazole-1-ethanol carbamate (ester). *UNII-4X7Y0185J3. CAS-31478-45-2.* INN. *Antiprotozoal (Trichomonas).* ◇*R.P. 20 578*

Banoxantrone. $C_{22}H_{28}N_4O_6$. 444.48. 1,4-Bis[2-(dimethylazinoyl)ethylamino]-5,8-dihydroxy-9,10-anthraquinone. *UNII-W5H7E45YT3. CAS-136470-65-0.* INN; BAN.

Bapineuzumab [*2004*] (bap″ i nooz′ oo mab). $C_{6466}H_{10018}N_{1734}O_{2026}S_{44}$ (peptide). Immunoglobulin G1, anti-(human β-amyloid)(human-mouse monoclonal heavy chain), disulfide with human-mouse monoclonal light chain, dimer. Molecular weight of major glycoform is approximately 148,800 daltons. *UNII-NC11WKO35D. CAS-648895-38-9.* INN. *Treatment of prevention of Alzheimer's disease.* ◇*AAB-001, humanized 3D-6 monoclonal antibody*

Baquiloprim. $C_{17}H_{20}N_6$. 308.38. 5-[(2,4-Diamino-5-pyrimidinyl)methyl]-8-(dimethylamino)-7-methylquinoline. *UNII-3DE766VIG6. CAS-102280-35-3.* INN; BAN. ◇*1380U*

Barbexaclone. $C_{12}H_{12}N_2O_3 \cdot C_{10}H_{21}N$. 387.52. (-)-*N,$\alpha$*-Dimethylcyclohexaneethylamine compound with 5-ethyl-5-phenylbarbituric acid. *UNII-291GX1YB65. CAS-4388-82-3.* INN. Maliasin (Knoll†)

Barbital. $C_8H_{12}N_2O_3$. 184.19. 5,5-Diethylbarbituric acid. *UNII-5WZ53ENE2P. CAS-57-44-3.* NF XI; INN; BAN; JAN; MI. [*Name previously used: Barbitone.*]

Barbital Sodium. $C_8H_{11}N_2NaO_3$. 206.17. Sodium derivative of 5,5-diethylbarbituric acid. *UNII-275L5M93QS; UNII-5WZ53ENE2P* [barbital]. *CAS-144-02-5; CAS-57-44-3* [barbital]. NF XI; INN; MI. [*Name previously used: Barbital, Soluble.*]

Barbital, Soluble (previously used name) — *See* Barbital Sodium.

Barbitone (previously used name) — *See* Barbital.

Barbitone Sodium (BAN) — *See* Barbital Sodium.

Barium Hydroxide Lime (bar′ ee um hye drox′ ide lyme). **USP**. A mixture of barium hydroxide octahydrate and calcium hydroxide. *CAS-17194-00-2. Carbon dioxide absorbant.*

Barium Sulfate (bar′ ee um sul′ fate). **USP**. $BaSO_4$. 233.39. (1) Sulfuric acid, barium salt (1:1); (2) Barium sulfate (1:1). *UNII-25BB7EKE2E. CAS-7727-43-7*. JAN. *Diagnostic aid (radiopaque medium).* Baricon (Mallinckrodt†); Bar-test (Glenwood); Barocat (Mallinckrodt†); Barosperse (Mallinckrodt†); Barosperse II (Mallinckrodt†); Barotrast (Rhone-Poulenc Rorer†); Epi-C (Mallinckrodt†); Epi-Stat 57 (Mallinckrodt†); Epi-Stat 61 (Mallinckrodt†); Esophotrast (Rhone-Poulenc Rorer†); Oratrast (Rhone-Poulenc Rorer†)

Barixibat. $C_{42}H_{55}N_5O_8$. 757.91. 11-(D-Gluconamido)-*N*-{2-[(1*S*,2*R*,3*S*)-3-hydroxy-3-phenyl-2-(2-pyridyl)-1-(2-pyridylamino)propyl]phenyl}undecanamide. *CAS-263562-28-3.* INN.

Barmastine [*1991*] (bar mas′ teen). $C_{27}H_{29}N_7O_2$. 483.56. (1) 4*H*-Pyrido[1,2-*a*]pyrimidin-4-one, 3-[2-[4-[[3-(2-furanylmethyl)-3*H*-imidazo[4,5-*b*]pyridin-2-yl]amino]-1-piperidinyl]ethyl]-2-methyl-; (2) 3-[2-[4-[(3-Furfuryl-3*H*-imidazo[4,5-*b*]pyridin-2-yl)amino]piperidino]ethyl]-2-methyl-4*H*-pyrido[1,2-*a*]pyrimidin-4-one. *UNII-UIF43N1HSV. CAS-99156-66-8.* INN. *Antihistaminic.* ◇R 57959

Barnidipine. $C_{27}H_{29}N_3O_6$. 491.54. [Barnidipine Hydrochloride is JAN.] (+)-(3′*S*,4*S*)-1-Benzyl-3-pyrrolidinyl methyl 1,4-dihydro-2,6-dimethyl-4-(*m*-nitrophenyl)-3,5-pyridinedicarboxylate. *UNII-2VBY96ASWJ. CAS-104713-75-9.* INN.

Barucainide. $C_{22}H_{30}N_2O_2$. 354.49. 4-Benzyl-1,3-dihydro-7-[4-(isopropylamino)butoxy]-6-methylfuro[3,4-*c*]pyridine. *UNII-14NFL30YOH. CAS-79784-22-8.* INN.

Barusiban. $C_{40}H_{63}N_9O_8S$. 830.05. $C^{4,6},S^1$-Cyclo[*N*-(3-sulfanylpropanoyl)-D-tryptophyl-L-isoleucyl-L-alloisoleucyl-L-asparaginyl-L-2-aminobutanoyl-*N*-methyl-L-ornithinol]. *CAS-285571-64-4.* INN.

BAS — *See* Benanserin Hydrochloride.

Basifungin [*1995*] (ba″ si fun′ jin). $C_{60}H_{92}N_8O_{11}$. 1101.42. (1) Aureobasidin A; (2) *N*-[(2*R*,3*R*)-2-Hydroxy-3-methylvaleryl]-*N*-methyl-L-valyl-L-phenylalanyl-*N*-methyl-L-phenylalanyl-L-prolyl-L-alloisoleucyl-*N*-methyl-L-valyl-L-leucyl-3-hydroxy-*N*-methyl-L-valine α_1-lactone. *CAS-127785-64-2.* INN. *Antifungal.* ◇LY295337; NK 204; R106-1

Basiliximab [*1998*] (ba″ si lix′ i mab). (1) Immunoglobulin G1, anti-(human interleukin 2 receptor) (human-mouse monoclonal CHI621 γ1-chain), disulfide with human-mouse monoclonal CHI621 light chain, dimer; (2) Immunoglobulin G1 (human-mouse monoclonal CHI621 heavy chain antihuman interleukin 2 receptor), disulfide with human-mouse monoclonal CHI621 light chain, dimer. *UNII-9927MT646M. CAS-179045-86-4.* INN; BAN. *Immunosuppressant (monoclonal antibody).* Simulect (Novartis) ◇SDZ-CHI-621

Batabulin [*2006*] (ba″ ta bue′ lin). $C_{13}H_7F_6NO_3S$. 371.25. (1) Benzenesulfonamide, 2,3,4,5,6-pentafluoro-*N*-(3-fluoro-4-methoxyphenyl)-; (2) 2,3,4,5,6-Pentafluoro-*N*-(3-fluoro-4-methoxyphenyl)benzenesulfonamide. *UNII-T4NP8G3K6Q. CAS-195533-53-0. Treatment of various advanced refractory cancers (binds to β-tubulin).* ◇T138067; T67; TL 057

---

† Brand name formerly used, and/or firm no longer concerned with this product.

Batabulin Sodium [*2003*] (ba″ ta bue′ lin soe′ dee um). $C_{13}H_6F_6NNaO_3S$. 393.24. [Batabulin is INN.] (1) Benzenesulfonamide, 2,3,4,5,6-pentafluoro-*N*-(3-fluoro-4-methoxyphenyl)-, sodium salt; (2) Sodium 2,3,4,5,6-pentafluoro-*N*-(3-fluoro-4-methoxyphenyl)benzenesulfonamidate; (3) 2-Fluoro-1-methoxy-4-pentafluorophenylsulfonamidobenzene, sodium salt. *UNII-G04B77F772; UNII-T4NP8G3K6Q* [batabulin]. *CAS-195533-98-3; CAS-195533-53-0* [batabulin]. *Treatment of various refractory cancers, including hepatocellular carcinoma, breast, colon and non-small cell lung cancer.* ◇*T138067-sodium*

Batanopride Hydrochloride [*1990*] (ba tan′ oh pride hye″ droe klor′ ide). $C_{17}H_{26}ClN_3O_3 \cdot HCl$. 392.32. [Batanopride is INN.] (1) Benzamide, 4-amino-5-chloro-*N*-[2-(diethylamino)ethyl]-2-(1-methyl-2-oxopropoxy)-, monohydrochloride; (2) 4-Amino-5-chloro-*N*-[2-(diethylamino)ethyl]-2-[(1-methylacetonyl)oxy]benzamide monohydrochloride. *UNII-00L331RFEC. CAS-102670-59-7; CAS-102670-46-2* [batanopride]. *Anti-emetic.* ◇*BMY-25801-01*

Batebulast. $C_{19}H_{29}N_3O_2$. 331.45. *p-tert*-Butylphenyl *trans*-4-(guanidinomethyl)cyclohexanecarboxylate. *UNII-311WUU3BVY. CAS-81907-78-0.* INN.

Batelapine Maleate [*1990*] (ba tel′ a peen mal′ ee ate). $C_{16}H_{20}N_6 \cdot C_4H_4O_4$. 412.44. [Batelapine is INN.] (1) 11*H*-[1,2,4]Triazolo[1,5-*c*][1,3]benzodiazepine, 2-methyl-5-(4-methyl-1-piperazinyl)-, (*Z*)-2-butenedioate (1:1); (2) 2-Methyl-5-(4-methyl-1-piperazinyl)-11*H*-*s*-triazolo[1,5-*c*][1,3]benzodiazepine maleate (1:1). *UNII-66K342SF4G; UNII-P71TE299SG* [batelapine]. *CAS-120360-10-3; CAS-95634-82-5* [batelapine]. *Antipsychotic.* ◇*CGS 13429A*

Batilol. $C_{21}H_{44}O_3$. 344.57. 3-(Octadecyloxy)-1,2-propanediol. *CAS-544-62-7.* INN.

Batimastat [*1994*] (ba tim′ a stat). $C_{23}H_{31}N_3O_4S_2$. 477.64. (1) Butanediamide, N^4-hydroxy-N^1-[2-(methylamino)-2-oxo-1-(phenylmethyl)ethyl]-2-(2-methylpropyl)-3-[(2-thienylthio)methyl]-, [2*R*-[1(*S**),2*R**,3*S**]]-; (2) (2*S*,3*R*)-5-Methyl-3-[[(α*S*)-α-(methylcarbamoyl)phenethyl]carbamoyl]-2-[(2-thienylthio)methyl]hexanohydroxamic acid. *UNII-BK349F52C9. CAS-130370-60-4.* INN; BAN. *Antineoplastic.* ◇*BB-94*

Batoprazine. $C_{13}H_{14}N_2O_2$. 230.26. 8-(1-Piperazinyl)coumarin. *UNII-EZY3PL8Q0M. CAS-105685-11-8.* INN.

Batroxobin. Thrombin-like enzyme obtained from the venom of *Bothrops atrox.CAS-9039-61-6.* INN; JAN; MI.

Batyl Alcohol — *See* Batilol.

Batylol — *See* Batilol.

Bavituximab [*2006*] (bav″ i tux′ i mab). $C_{6446}H_{9946}N_{1702}O_{2042}S_{32}$. Immunoglobulin G1, anti-(phosphatidylserine)(human-mouse monoclonal ch3G4 heavy chain), disulfide with human-mouse monoclonal ch3G4 κ-chain, dimer. Molecular weight is approximately 145,300 daltons. *UNII-Q16CT95N25. CAS-648904-28-3.* INN. *Anti-cancer and anti-viral.*

Baxitozine. $C_{13}H_{14}O_6$. 266.25. (*E*)-3-(3,4,5-Trimethoxybenzoyl)acrylic acid. *UNII-A89J34472U. CAS-84386-11-8.* INN.

Bazedoxifene Acetate [*2002*] (ba″ ze dox′ i feen as′ e tate). $C_{30}H_{34}N_2O_3 \cdot C_2H_4O_2$. 530.65. [Bazedoxifene is INN.] (1) 1*H*-Indol-5-ol, 1-[[4-[2-(hexahydro-1*H*-azepin-1-yl)ethoxy]phenyl]methyl]-2-(4-hydroxyphenyl)-3-methyl-, monoacetate (salt); (2) 1-[*p*-[2-(Hexahydro-1*H*-azepin-1-yl)ethoxy]benzyl]-2-(*p*-hydroxyphenyl)-3-methylindol-5-ol monoacetate (salt). *UNII-J70472UD3D; UNII-Q16TT9C5BK* [bazedoxifene]. *CAS-198481-33-3; CAS-198481-32-2* [bazedoxifene]. JAN. *Prevention and treatment of osteoporosis (estrogen receptor modulator).* ◇*WAY-140424*

Bazinaprine. $C_{17}H_{19}N_5O$. 309.37. 3-[(2-Morpholinoethyl)a-mino]-6-phenyl-4-pyridazinecarbonitrile. *UNII-NU8Y4C529J. CAS-94011-82-2.* INN.

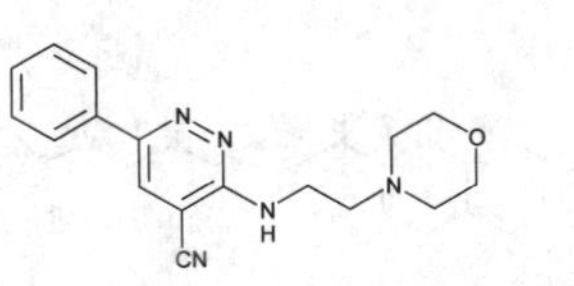

BCG Live. USP. A freeze-dried preparation of attenuated live bacteria derived from a culture of Bacillus Calmette-Guérin (*Mycobacterium bovis*, var. BCG).

BCG Vaccine. USP. A dried, living culture of the bacillus Calmette-Guérin strain of *Mycobacterium tuberculosis* var. *bovis*, grown in a suitable medium from a seed strain of known history that has been maintained to preserve its capacity for conferring immunity. *Immunizing agent (active).* Tice BCG (Organon)

Becampanel. $C_{10}H_{11}N_4O_7P$. 330.19. [(7-Nitro-2,3-dioxo-1,2,3,4-tetrahydroquinoxalin-5-yl)methylamino]methyl-phosphonic acid. *UNII-X3D0O800AJ. CAS-188696-80-2.* INN.

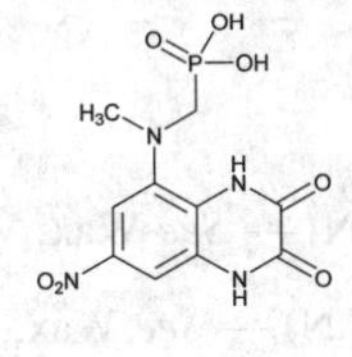

Becanthone Hydrochloride [*1965*] (be kan′ thone hye″ droe klor′ ide). $C_{22}H_{28}N_2O_2S.HCl$. 421.00. [Becantone is INN.] (1) 9*H*-Thioxanthen-9-one, 1-[[2-[ethyl(2-hydroxy-2-methoxypropyl)amino]ethyl]amino]-4-methyl-, monohy-drochloride; (2) 1-[[2-[Ethyl(2-hydroxy-2-methylpropyl)a-mino]ethyl]amino]-4-methylthioxanthen-9-one monohy-drochloride. *UNII-63T152J867. CAS-5591-22-0; CAS-15351-04-9* [becanthone]. *Antischistosomal.* Loranil (Ster-ling Winthrop†) ◇*Win 13820; NSC-15796*

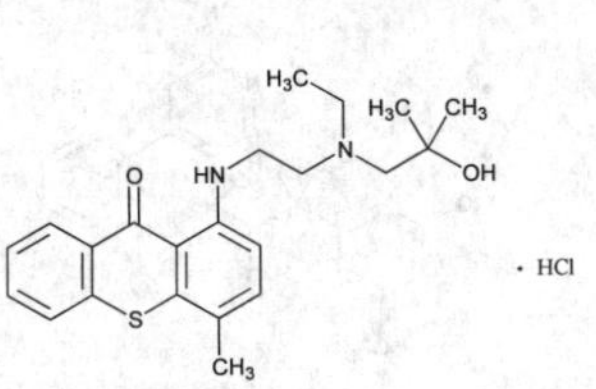

Becantone (INN) Hydrochloride — *See* Becanthone Hydro-chloride.

Becaplermin [*1995*] (be kap′ ler min). Recombinant human platelet-derived growth factor B. A recombinant protein produced by genetically engineered *Saccharomyces cere-visiae* cells, that is similar in amino acid composition and biological activity to the endogenous human PDGF-BB homodimer. Apparent molecular weight of approximately 30,000 daltons (SDS-PAGE determined). *CAS-165101-51-*

9. INN; BAN. *Chronic dermal ulcers treatment (promotes the proliferation of mesenchymally-derived cells).* Regran-ex (Johnson & Johnson) ◇*RWJ 60235*

```
SLGSLTIAEP   AMIAECKTRT   EVFEISRRLI   DRTNANFLVW   PPCVEVQRCS
GCCNNRNVQC   RPTQVQLRPV   QVRKIEIVRK   KPIFKKATVT   LEDHLACKCE
TVAAARPVT
```

Becatecarin [*2004*] (be″ ka tek′ ar in). $C_{33}H_{34}Cl_2N_4O_7$. 669.55. (1) 5*H*-Indolo[2,3-*a*]pyrrolo[3,4-*c*]carbazole-5,7(6*H*)-dione, 1,11-dichloro-6-[2-(diethylamino)ethyl]-12,13-dihydro-12-(4-*O*-methyl-β-D-glucopyranosyl)-; (2) 1,11-Dichloro-6-[2-(diethylamino)ethyl]-12-(4-*O*-methyl-β-D-glucopyranosyl)-12,13-dihydro-5*H*-indolo[2,3-*a*]pyr-rolo[3,4-*c*]carbazole-5,7(6*H*)-dione. *UNII-A60X6MBU6G. CAS-119673-08-4.* INN. *Antineoplastic (rebeccamycin analogue).* ◇*XL119; BMS-181176; BMY-27557; NSC-655649*

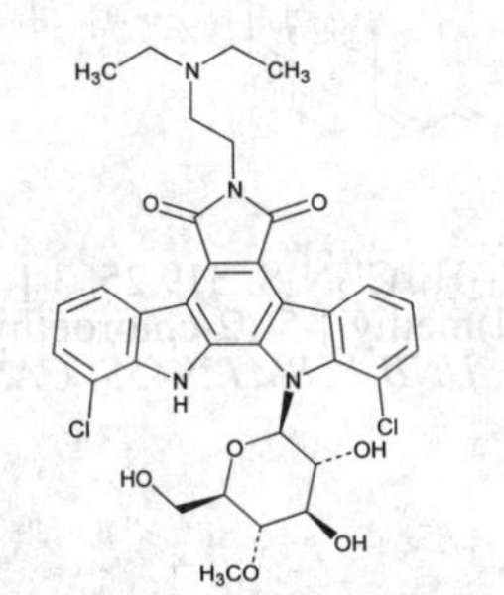

Beciparcil. $C_{12}H_{13}NO_3S_2$. 283.37. *p*-[(5-Thio-β-D-xylopyra-nosyl)thio]benzonitrile. *UNII-K90ZOR23P1. CAS-130782-54-6.* INN.

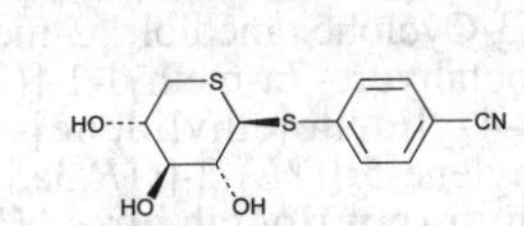

Beclamide. $C_{10}H_{12}ClNO$. 197.66. *N*-Benzyl-3-chloropropio-namide. *UNII-F5N0ALI65V. CAS-501-68-8.* INN; BAN; DCF; MI.

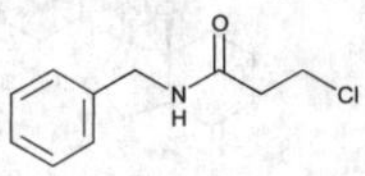

Becliconazole. $C_{18}H_{12}Cl_2N_2O$. 343.21. (±)-1-[*o*-Chloro-α-(5-chloro-2-benzofuranyl)benzyl]imidazole. *UNII-5361814USE. CAS-112893-26-2.* INN.

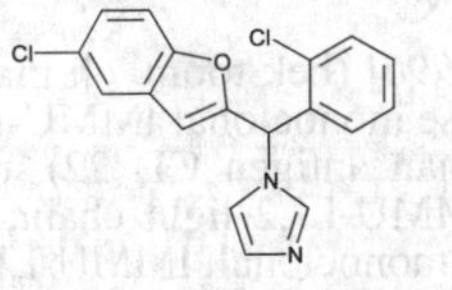

Beclobrate. $C_{20}H_{23}ClO_3$. 346.85. Ethyl (±)-2-[[α-(*p*-chloro-phenyl)-*p*-tolyl]oxy]-2-methylbutyrate. *UNII-USZ5-MY269R. CAS-55937-99-0.* INN; BAN; MI.

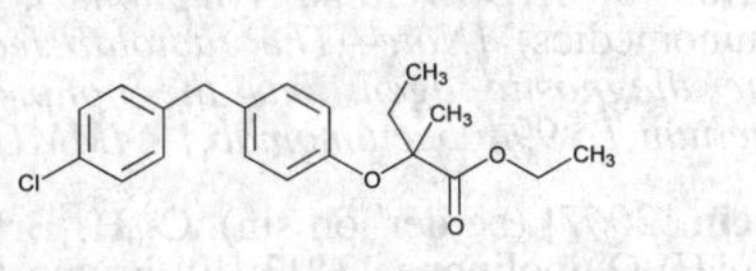

Beclometasone (INN) — *See* Beclomethasone Dipropionate.

---

† Brand name formerly used, and/or firm no longer concerned with this product.

Beclometasone Dipropionate (JAN) — *See* Beclomethasone Dipropionate.

Beclomethasone Dipropionate [*1973*] (be″ kloe meth′ a sone dye proe′ pee oh nate). **USP.** $C_{28}H_{37}ClO_7$. 521.04. [Beclometasone is INN and BAN; Beclomethasone Dipropionate is JAN.] (1) Pregna-1,4-diene-3,20-dione, 9-chloro-11-hydroxy-16-methyl-17,21-bis(1-oxopropoxy)-, $(11\beta,16\beta)$-; (2) 9-Chloro-11β,17,21-trihydroxy-16β-methylpregna-1,4-diene-3,20-dione 17,21-dipropionate. *UNII-5B307S63B2; UNII-KGZ1SLC28Z* [beclomethasone]. *CAS-5534-09-8; CAS-4419-39-0* [beclomethasone]. *Glucocorticoid.* Beclovent (GlaxoSmithKline); Beconase (GlaxoSmithKline); Vancenase (Schering); Vanceril (Schering) ◇*Sch 18020W*

Beclotiamine. $C_{12}H_{16}Cl_2N_4S$. 319.25. 3-[(4-Amino-2-methyl-5-pyrimidinyl)methyl]-5-(2-chloroethyl)-4-methylthiazolium chloride. *UNII-858M12945S. CAS-13471-78-8*. INN; MI.

Becocalcidiol [*2004*] (be″ koe kal″ si dye′ ol). $C_{23}H_{36}O_2$. 344.53. (1) 1,3-Cyclohexanediol, 2-methylene-5-[(2*E*)-[(1*R*,3a*S*,7a*R*)-octahydro-7a-methyl-1-[(1*S*)-1-methylpropyl]-4*H*-inden-4-ylidene]ethylidene]-, (1*R*,3*R*)-; (2) (1*R*,3*R*)-2-Methylene-5-[(2*E*)-2-[(1*R*,3a*S*,7a*R*)-7a-methyl-1-[(1*S*)-1-methylpropyl]octahydro-4*H*-inden-4-ylidene]ethylidene]cyclohexane-1,3-diol. *UNII-N75R59YD0F. CAS-524067-21-8*. INN. *Treatment of psoriasis (vitamin D analog).* ◇*QRX 101*

Bectumomab [*1996*] (bek toom′ oh mab). (1) Immunoglobulin G2a (mouse monoclonal IMMU-LL2 Fab′ fragment γ-chain anti-human antigen CD 22), disulfide with mouse monoclonal IMMU-LL2 light chain; (2) Immunoglobulin G 2a (mouse monoclonal IMMU-LL2 Fab′ fragment γ-chain anti-human antigen CD 22), disulfide with mouse monoclonal IMMU-LL2 light chain. Molecular weight is 48,000–50,000 daltons. *CAS-158318-63-9*. INN. *Monoclonal antibody (diagnosis of non-Hodgkin's lymphoma and detection of AIDS-related lymphoma).* Lympho Scan (Immunomedics) [*Note—The radiolabeled product used as the diagnostic agent has the nonproprietary name technetium Tc 99m bectumomab.*] ◇*IMMU-LL2*

Bederocin [*2007*] (be der′ oh sin). $C_{20}H_{21}BrFN_3OS$. 450.37. (1) 4(1*H*)-Quinolinone, 2-[[3-[[[4-bromo-5-(1-fluoroethenyl)-3-methyl-2-thienyl]methyl]amino]propyl]amino]-; (2) 2-[[3-[[[4-Bromo-5-(1-fluoroethenyl)-3-methylthiophen-2-yl]methyl]amino]propyl]amino]quinolin-4(1*H*)-one. *UNII-YV7QD1SJ9O. CAS-757942-43-1*. INN. *Antibacterial agent.* ◇*REP 8839*

Bedoradrine Sulfate [*2006*] (bed or′ a dreen sul′ fate). $2C_{24}H_{32}N_2O_5.H_2O_4S$. 955.12. [Bedoradrine is INN.] (1) Acetamide, *N,N*-dimethyl-2-[[(7*S*)-5,6,7,8-tetrahydro-7-[[(2*R*)-2-hydroxy-2-[4-hydroxy-3-(2-hydroxyethyl)phenyl]ethyl]amino]-2-naphthalenyl]oxy]-, sulfate; (2) Bis[2-[[(7*S*)-7-[[(2*R*)-2-hydroxy-2-[4-hydroxy-3-(2-hydroxyethyl)phenyl]ethyl]amino]-5,6,7,8-tetrahydronaphthalen-2-yl]oxy]-*N,N*-dimethylacetamide] sulfate. *UNII-P875C0DV2V; UNII-4EAR229231* [bedoradrine]. *CAS-194785-31-4; CAS-194785-19-8* [bedoradrine]. *Tocolytic for the acute management of imminent pre-term birth.* ◇*KUR-1246; MN-221*

Beef Tallow. JAN.

Beeswax, White (JAN) — *See* Wax, White.

Beeswax, Yellow (JAN) — *See* Wax, Yellow.

Befetupitant [*2005*] (bef″ et ue′ pi tant). $C_{29}H_{29}F_6N_3O_2$. 565.55. (1) Benzeneacetamide, *N,α,α*-trimethyl-*N*-[4-(2-methylphenyl)-6-(4-morpholinyl)-3-pyridinyl]-3,5-bis(trifluoromethyl)-; (2) 2-(3,5-Bis(trifluoromethyl)phenyl)-*N*-[4-[2-methylphenyl]-6-(morpholin-4-yl)pyridin-3-yl]-*N*-methylisobutyramide. *UNII-RSH7NDI7MI. CAS-290296-68-3*. INN. *Treatment of depression.* ◇*Ro 67-5930*

Befiperide. $C_{25}H_{31}N_3O_2$. 405.53. *N*-[2-[4-(7-Benzofuranoyl)-1-piperazinyl]ethyl]-*p*-isopropyl-*N*-methylbenzamide. *UNII-Q6353VLJ8E. CAS-100927-14-8*. INN.

Befiradol. $C_{20}H_{22}ClF_2N_3O$. 393.86. (3-Chloro-4-fluorophenyl)[4-fluoro-4-({[(5-methylpyridin-2-yl)methyl]amino}-methyl)piperidin-1-yl]methanone. *CAS-208110-64-9*. INN.

Befloxatone. $C_{15}H_{18}F_3NO_5$. 349.30. (*R*)-5-(Methoxymethyl)-3-[*p*-[(*R*)-4,4,4-trifluoro-3-hydroxybutoxy]phenyl]-2-oxazolidinone. *UNII-4H75PAD8M3. CAS-134564-82-2.* INN.

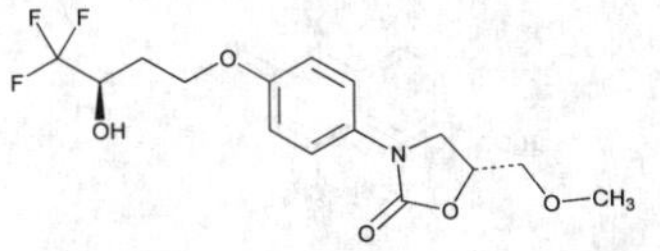

Befunolol. $C_{16}H_{21}NO_4$. 291.34. [Befunolol Hydrochloride is JAN.] 7-[2-Hydroxy-3-(isopropylamino)propoxy]-2-benzofuranyl methyl ketone. *UNII-418546MT3A. CAS-39552-01-7.* INN; MI.

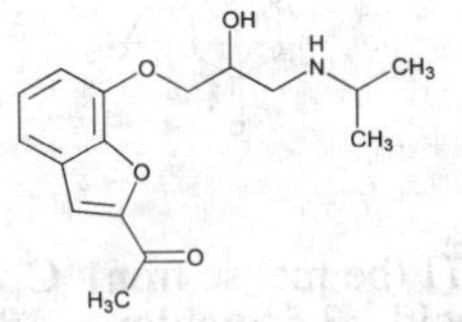

Befuraline. $C_{20}H_{20}N_2O_2$. 320.39. 1-(2-Benzofuranylcarbonyl)-4-benzylpiperazine. *UNII-787AQ35GHR. CAS-41717-30-0.* INN.

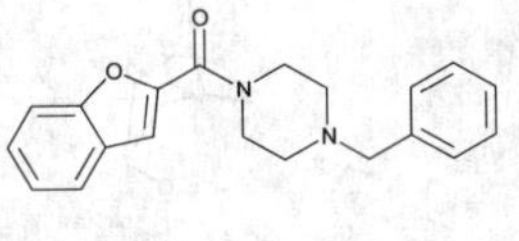

Begacestat [*2006*] (be gas′ e stat). $C_9H_8ClF_6NO_3S_2$. 391.74. (1) 2-Thiophenesulfonamide, 5-chloro-*N*-[(1*S*)-3,3,3-trifluoro-1-(hydroxymethyl)-2-(trifluoromethyl)propyl]-; (2) 5-Chloro-*N*-[(1*S*)-3,3,3-trifluoro-1-(hydroxymethyl)-2-(trifluoromethyl)propyl]thiophene-2-sulfonamide. *UNII-3666C56BBU. CAS-769169-27-9.* INN. *Treatment of Alzheimer's disease.* ◇*GSI-953*

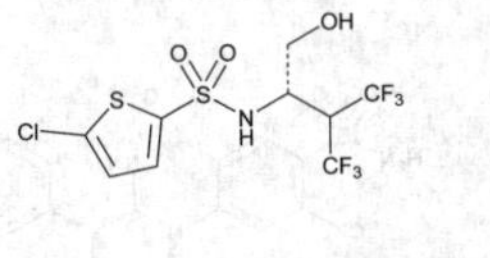

Behenyl Alcohol — *See* Docosanol.

Bekanamycin. $C_{18}H_{37}N_5O_{10}$. 483.51. [Bekanamycin Sulfate is JAN.] Antibiotic derived from *Streptomyces kanamyceticus.* Kanamycin B. *UNII-15JT14C3GI. CAS-4696-76-8.* INN; MI. ◇*NK 1006*

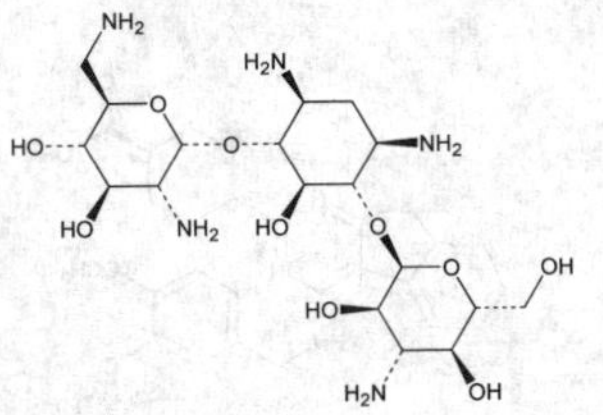

Belagenpumatucel-L [*2006*] (bel″ a jen″ pum a too′ sel - el). Allogeneic vaccine cocktail of TGF-β blocked, whole non-small cell lung cancer tumor cells. *Cell therapy treatment of non-small cell lung cancer.* Lucanix (NovaRx)

Belaperidone. $C_{22}H_{22}FN_3O_2$. 379.43. (+)-3-[2-[(1*S*,5*R*,6*S*)-6-(*p*-Fluorophenyl)-3-azabicyclo[3.2.0]hept-3-yl]ethyl]-2,4(1*H*,3*H*)-quinazolinedione. *UNII-4DN0TK4892. CAS-156862-51-0.* INN.

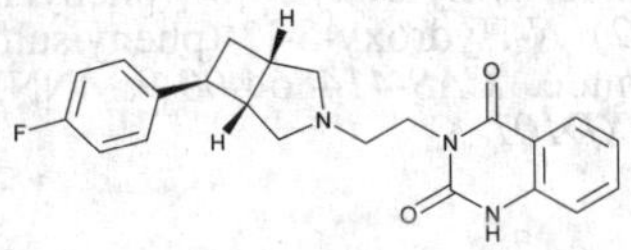

Belarizine. $C_{24}H_{26}N_2O$. 358.48. α-[4-(Diphenylmethyl)-1-piperazinyl]-*p*-cresol. *UNII-C4W7I532MX. CAS-52395-99-0.* INN.

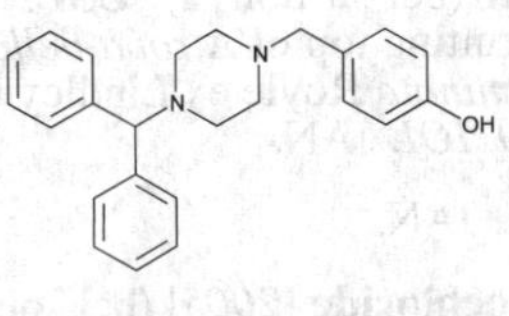

Belatacept [*2005*] (bel at′ a sept). $C_{3508}H_{5440}N_{922}O_{1096}S_{32}$. 91,500 daltons. (1) CTLA-4 (antigen) [29-tyrosine,104-glutamic acid] (human extracellular domain-containing fragment) fusion protein with immunoglobulin G1 (human monoclonal Fc domain-containing fragment), bimol. (120→120′)-disulfide; (2) [Tyr^{29},Glu^{104},Gln^{125},Ser^{130},-^{29},Glu^{104},Gln^{125},Ser^{130},Ser^{136},Ser^{139},Ser^{148}](CTLA-4 (antigen)-[3-126]-peptide (human extracellular domain-containing fragment) fusion protein with immunoglobulin G1-[233 *C*-terminal residues of the heavy chain]-peptide (human monoclonal Fc domain-containing fragment)) bimolecular (120→120′)-disulfide. *UNII-E3B2GI648A. CAS-706808-37-9.* INN. *Prevention of allograft rejection in recipients of solid organ transplants; prevention of graft-vs.-host disease following bone marrow transplantation; treatment of autoimmune diseases and conditions such as rheumatoid arthritis and Type 1 diabetes.* ◇*BMS-224818*

```
MHVAQPAVVL ASSRGIASFV CEYASPGKYT EVRVTVLRQA DSQVTEVCAA
TYMMGNELTF LDDSICTGTS SGNQVNLTIQ GLRAMDTGLY ICKVELMYPP
PYYEGIGNGT QIYVIDPEPC PDSDQEPKSS DKTHTSPPSP APELLGGSSV
FLFPPKPKDT LMISRTPEVT CVVVDVSHED PEVKFNWYVD GVEVHNAKTK
PREEQYNSTY RVVSVLTVLH QDWLNGKEYK CKVSNKALPA PIEKTISKAK
GQPREPQVYT LPPSRDELTK NQVSLTCLVK GFYPSDIAVE WESNGQPENN
YKTTPPVLDS DGSFFLYSKL TVDKSRWQQG NVFSCSVMHE ALHNHYTQKS
LSLSPGK
```
2

* - glycosylation site

Belfosdil [*1990*] (bel fos′ dil). $C_{27}H_{50}O_7P_2$. 548.63. (1) Phosphonic acid, [2-(2-phenoxyethyl)-1,3-propanediyl]-bis-, tetrabutyl ester; (2) Tetrabutyl [2-(2-phenoxyethyl)-trimethylene]diphosphonate. *UNII-W91CMS1V7Z. CAS-103486-79-9.* INN. *Antihypertensive (calcium channel blocker).* ◇*BMY-21891; SR-7037*

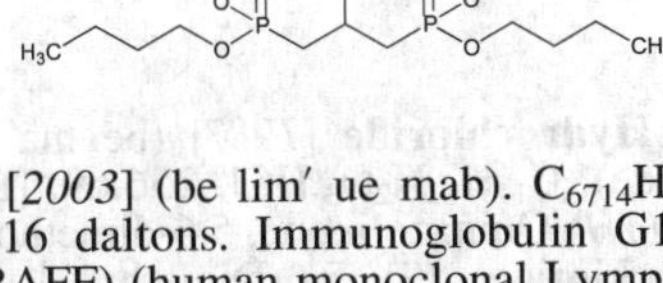

Belimumab [*2003*] (be lim′ ue mab). $C_{6714}H_{10428}N_{1816}O_{2102}S_{52}$. 151,716 daltons. Immunoglobulin G1, anti-(human cytokine BAFF) (human monoclonal LymphoStatB heavy chain), disulfure with human monoclonal LymphoStatB λ-chain, dimer. *CAS-356547-88-1.* INN. *Treatment of auto-immune disease.* LymphoStat-B (Human Genome Sciences)

Belinostat [*2006*] (be lin′ oh stat). $C_{15}H_{14}N_2O_4S$. 318.35. (1) 2-Propenamide, *N*-hydroxy-3-[3-[(phenylamino)sulfonyl]-phenyl]-; (2) *N*-Hydroxy-3-[3-(phenylsulfamoyl)phenyl]-prop-2-enamide. *CAS-414864-00-9.* INN. *Treatment of cancer.* ◇*PXD101*

Belladonna Leaf (bel″ a don′ a). **USP.** The dried leaf and flowering or fruiting top of *Atropa belladonna* Linné or of its variety *acuminata* Royle ex Lindley (Fam. Solanaceae). *UNII-6GZW20TIOI.* JAN.

Belladonna Root. JAN.

Belotecan Hydrochloride [*2005*] (bel″ oh tee′ kan hye″ droe klor′ ide). $C_{25}H_{27}N_3O_4$·HCl. 469.96. [Belotecan is INN.] (1) 1*H*-Pyrano[3′,4′:6,7]indolizino[1,2-*b*]quinoline-3,14(4*H*,12*H*)-dione, 4-ethyl-4-hydroxy-11-[2-[(1-methylethyl)amino]ethyl]-, monohydrochloride, (4*S*)-; (2) (4*S*)-4-Ethyl-4-hydroxy-11-[2-[(1-methylethyl)amino]ethyl]-1,12-dihydro-14*H*-pyrano[3′,4′:6,7]indolizino[1,2-*b*]quino-line-3,14(4*H*)-dione hydrochloride. *UNII-01DZ4127G7; UNII-27Z82M2G1N* [belotecan]. *CAS-213819-48-8; CAS-256411-32-2* [belotecan]. *Antineoplastic (DNA topoisomerase I inhibitor).* ◇*CKD-602*

Beloxamide [*1970*] (bel ox′ a mide). $C_{18}H_{21}NO_2$. 283.36. (1) Acetamide, *N*-(phenylmethoxy)-*N*-(3-phenylpropyl)-; (2) *N*-(Benzyloxy)-*N*-(3-phenylpropyl)acetamide. *UNII-S4YR4X39CA.* *CAS-15256-58-3.* INN. *Antihyperlipoproteinemic.* ◇*W-1372*

Beloxepin [*1997*] (bel ox′ e pin). $C_{19}H_{21}NO_2$. 295.38. (±)-*cis*-1,3,4,13b-Tetrahydro-2,10-dimethyldibenz[2,3:6,7]oxepi-no[4,5-*c*]pyridin-4a(2*H*)-ol. *UNII-G905IN29U4.* *CAS-135928-30-2.* INN. *Antidepressant.* ◇*Org 4428*

Bemarinone Hydrochloride [*1987*] (be ma′ ri none hye″ droe klor′ ide). $C_{11}H_{12}N_2O_3$·HCl. 256.69. [Bemarinone is INN.] (1) 2(1*H*)-Quinazolinone, 5,6-dimethoxy-4-methyl-, monohydrochloride; (2) 5,6-Dimethyl-4-methyl-2(1*H*)-quinazolinone monohydrochloride. *UNII-0GSS0O37A8.*

CAS-101626-69-1; CAS-92210-43-0 [bemarinone]. *Cardiotonic (positive inotropic); cardiotonic (vasodilator).* ◇*ORF 16600; RWJ 16600*

Bemegride. $C_8H_{13}NO_2$. 155.19. 3-Ethyl-3-methylglutarimide. *UNII-57DQA39DO2.* *CAS-64-65-3.* USP XVII; INN; BAN; JAN; MI. Megimide (Abbott†)

Bemesetron [*1991*] (be me′ se tron). $C_{15}H_{17}Cl_2NO_2$. 314.21. (1) Benzoic acid, 3,5-dichloro-, 8-methyl-8-azabicy-clo[3.2.1]oct-3-yl ester, *endo*-; (2) 1α*H*,5α*H*-Tropan-3α-yl 3,5-dichlorobenzoate. *CAS-40796-97-2.* INN. *Anti-emetic.* ◇*MDL 72,222*

Bemetizide. $C_{15}H_{16}ClN_3O_4S_2$. 401.89. 6-Chloro-3,4-dihydro-3-(α-methylbenzyl)-2*H*-1,2,4-benzothiadiazine-7-sulfona-mide 1,1-dioxide. *UNII-EZN4D2O31B.* *CAS-1824-52-8.* INN; BAN.

Beminafil. $C_{25}H_{24}ClN_3O_3S$. 481.99. *trans*-4-{4-[(3-Chloro-4-methoxybenzyl)amino][1]benzothieno[2,3-*d*]pyrimidin-2-yl}cyclohexanecarboxylic acid. *UNII-R3IOR5299G.* *CAS-566906-50-1.* INN.

Bemiparin Sodium. Sodium salt of depolymerized heparin obtained by alkaline degradation of quaternary ammonium salt of heparin from pork intestinal mucosa; the majority of the components have a 2-*O*-sulfo-4-enepyranosuronic acid structure at the non-reducing end and a 2-*N*,6-*O*-disulfo-D-glucosamine structure at the reducing end of their chain; the average relative molecular mass is about 3600 (3000 to 4200); the degree of sulfatation is about 2 per disaccharidic unit. *CAS-9041-08-1.* INN; BAN.

Bemitradine [*1986*] (be mi′ tra deen). $C_{15}H_{17}N_5O$. 283.33. (1) [1,2,4]Triazolo[1,5-*c*]pyrimidin-5-amine, 8-(2-ethoxyethyl)-7-phenyl-; (2) 5-Amino-8-(2-ethoxyethyl)-7-phenyl-*s*-triazolo[1,5-*c*]pyrimidine. *UNII-LT9004D9N0. CAS-88133-11-3.* INN. *Antihypertensive; diuretic.* ◇SC-33643

Bemoradan [*1989*] (be moe′ ra dan). $C_{13}H_{13}N_3O_3$. 259.26. (1) 2*H*-1,4-Benzoxazin-3(4*H*)-one, 7-(1,4,5,6-tetrahydro-4-methyl-6-oxo-3-pyridazinyl)-; (2) 7-(1,4,5,6-Tetrahydro-4-methyl-6-oxo-3-pyridazinyl)-2*H*-1,4-benzoxazin-3(4*H*)-one. *UNII-G2S2V1ETBQ. CAS-112018-01-6.* INN. *Cardiotonic.* ◇ORF 22867

Bemotrizinol [*2004*] (be″ moe triz′ i nol). $C_{38}H_{49}N_3O_5$. 627.81. (1) Phenol, 2,2′-[6-(4-methoxyphenyl)-1,3,5-triazine-2,4-diyl]bis[5-[(2-ethylhexyl)oxy]; (2) 2,2′-[6-(4-Methoxyphenyl)-1,3,5-triazine-2,4-diyl]bis[5-[(2-ethylhexyl)oxy]phenol]. *UNII-PWZ1720CBH. CAS-187393-00-6.* INN. *UVA absorber (intended for use as a topical sunscreen).* Tinosorb S (Ciba Specialty Chemicals) *[Note— The International Nomenclature Cosmetic Ingredient Name (INCI) for bemotrizinol is bis-ethylhexyloxyphenol methoxyphenol triazine.]* ◇BEMT; FAT 70'884

Benactyzine. $C_{20}H_{25}NO_3$. 327.42. 2-Diethylaminoethyl benzilate. *UNII-595EG71R3F; UNII-26R628272Q* [benactyzine hydrochloride]. *CAS-302-40-9; CAS-57-37-4* [hydrochloride]. INN; BAN; MI.

Benafentrine. $C_{23}H_{27}N_3O_3$. 393.48. *cis*-4′-(1,2,3,4,4a,10b-Hexahydro-8,9-dimethoxy-2-methylbenzo[*c*][1,6]-naphthyridin-6-yl)acetanilide. *UNII-3DXB7KMD1F. CAS-35135-01-4.* INN.

Benanserin Hydrochloride. *UNII-86Q50C824Z. CAS-525-02-0; CAS-441-91-8* [benanserin]. MI.

Benaprizine (INN, BAN) — *See* Benapryzine Hydrochloride.

Benapryzine Hydrochloride [*1971*] (ben ap′ ri zeen hye″ droe klor′ ide). $C_{21}H_{27}NO_3 \cdot HCl$. 377.90. [Benaprizine is INN and BAN.] (1) Benzeneacetic acid, α-hydroxy-α-phenyl-, 2-(ethylpropylamino)ethyl ester hydrochloride; (2) 2-(Ethylpropylamino)ethyl benzilate hydrochloride. *UNII-LNV63FWR8M. CAS-3202-55-9; CAS-22487-42-9* [benapryzine]. *Anticholinergic.* ◇BRL-1288

Benaxibine. $C_{12}H_{15}NO_6$. 269.25. *p*-(D-Xylosylamino)benzoic acid. *UNII-6EEL176LGY. CAS-27661-27-4.* INN.

Benazepril Hydrochloride [*1987*] (ben az′ e pril hye″ droe klor′ ide). **USP.** $C_{24}H_{28}N_2O_5 \cdot HCl$. 460.95. [Benazepril is INN and BAN.] (1) 1*H*-1-Benzazepine-1-acetic acid, 3-[[1-(ethoxycarbonyl)-3-phenylpropyl]amino]-2,3,4,5-tetrahydro-2-oxo-, monohydrochloride, [*S*-(*R**,*R**)]-; (2) (3*S*)-3-[[(1*S*)-1-Carboxy-3-phenylpropyl]amino]-2,3,4,5-tetrahydro-2-oxo-1*H*-1-benzazepine-1-acetic acid, 3-ethyl ester, monohydrochloride. *UNII-N1SN99T69T; UNII-UDM7Q7QWP8* [benazepril]. *CAS-86541-74-4; CAS-86541-75-5* [benazepril]. JAN. *Enzyme inhibitor (angiotensin-converting).* Lotensin (Novartis) ◇CGS 14824A HCl

Benazeprilat [*1987*] (ben az′ e pril at). $C_{22}H_{24}N_2O_5$. 396.44. (1) 1*H*-1-Benzazepine-1-acetic acid, 3-[(1-carboxy-3-phenylpropyl)amino]-2,3,4,5-tetrahydro-2-oxo-, [*S*-(*R**,*R**)]-; (2) (3*S*)-3-[[(1*S*)-1-Carboxy-3-phenylpropyl]amino]-

---

† Brand name formerly used, and/or firm no longer concerned with this product.

2,3,4,5-tetrahydro-2-oxo-1*H*-1-benzazepine-1-acetic acid. *UNII-JRM708L703. CAS-86541-78-8.* INN. *Enzyme inhibitor (angiotensin-converting).* ◇*CGS 14831*

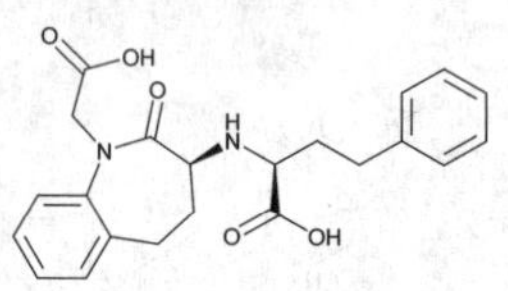

Bencianol. $C_{28}H_{22}O_6$. 454.47. (2*R*,3*S*)-3′,4′-[(Diphenylmethylene)dioxy]-3,5,7-flavantriol. *UNII-C4A4TVM56F. CAS-85443-48-7.* INN.

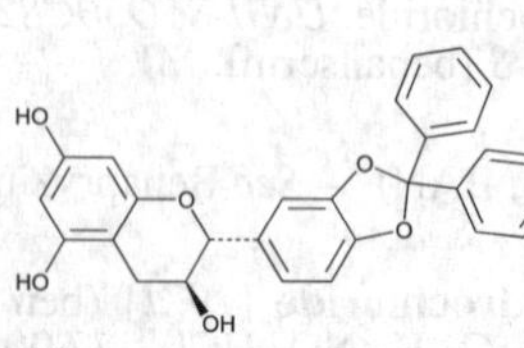

Bencisteine. $C_{15}H_{19}NO_4S$. 309.38. *N*-Acetyl-3-[(2-benzoylpropyl)thio]alanine. *UNII-9205LF98OL. CAS-42293-72-1.* INN; DCF.

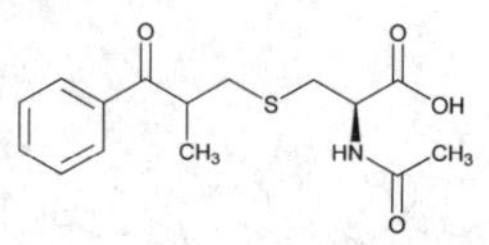

Benclonidine. $C_{16}H_{13}Cl_2N_3O$. 334.20. 1-Benzoyl-2-(2,6-dichloroanilino)-2-imidazoline. *UNII-1999398A3P. CAS-57647-79-7.* INN.

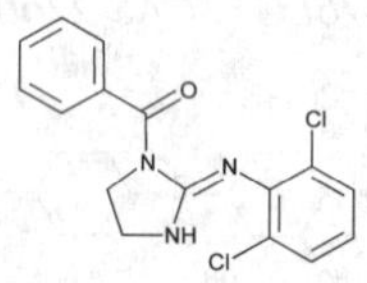

Bencyclane Fumarate. $C_{19}H_{31}NO.C_4H_4O_4$. 405.53. [Bencyclane is INN.] 3-[(1-Benzylcycloheptyl)oxy]-*N*,*N*-dimethylpropylamine fumarate. *UNII-OZN2MG334O; UNII-6I97Z6S135* [bencyclane]. *CAS-14286-84-1; CAS-2179-37-5* [bencyclane]. JAN; MI. ◇*EGYT 201*

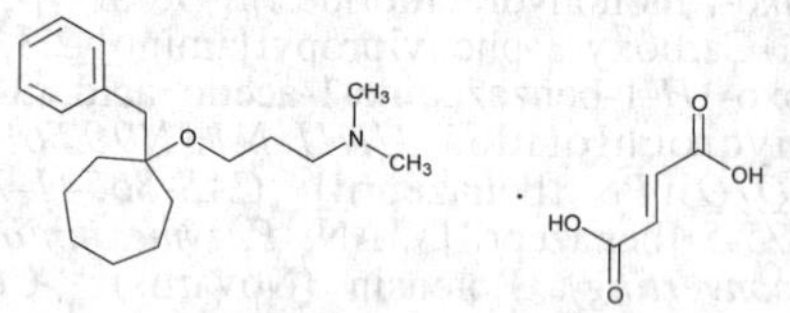

Bendacalol Mesylate [*1988*] (ben dak′ a lol mes′ i late). $C_{20}H_{23}NO_6.CH_4O_3S$. 469.51. (1) 1,4-Benzodioxin-2-methanol, α,α′-[iminobis(methylene)]bis[2,3-dihydro-, [2*R**[*S**[*R**(*S**)]]]-, methanesulfonate (salt); (2) (α*R*,α′*S*,2*S*,2′*R*)-α,α′-(Iminodimethylene)bis[1,4-benzodioxan-2-methanol]methanesulfonate (salt). *UNII-5KP3ZO1VLL; UNII-BQ0I558X42* [bendacalol]. *CAS-81737-62-4; CAS-81703-42-6* [bendacalol]. *Antihypertensive.* ◇*CGS 10078B*

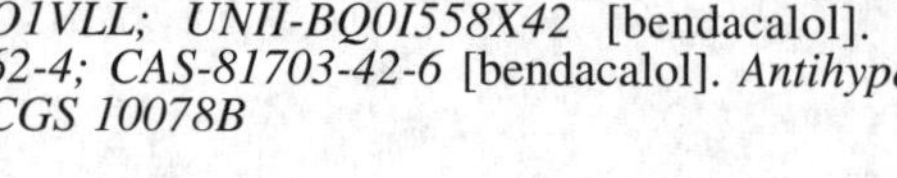

Bendamustine Hydrochloride [*2004*] (ben″ da mus′ teen hye″ droe klor′ ide). $C_{16}H_{21}Cl_2N_3O_2.HCl$. 394.72. [Bendamustine is INN.] (1) 1*H*-Benzimidazole-2-butanoic acid, 5-[bis(2-chloroethyl)amino]-1-methyl-, monohydrochloride; (2) 4-[5-[Bis(2-chloroethyl)amino]-1-methyl-1*H*-benzimidazole-2-yl]butanoic acid monohydrochloride. *UNII-981Y8SX18M; UNII-9266D9P3PQ* [bendamustine]. *CAS-3543-75-7; CAS-16506-27-7* [bendamustine]. JAN. *Treatment of hematologic cancer, especially non-Hodgkin's lymphoma.* Ribomustine (Amcis AG, Switzerland) ◇*SDX-105*

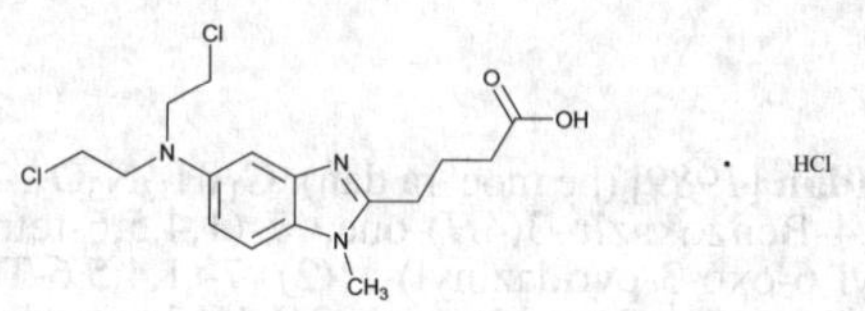

Bendazac [*1969*] (ben′ da zak). $C_{16}H_{14}N_2O_3$. 282.29. (1) Acetic acid, [[1-(phenylmethyl)-1*H*-indazol-3-yl]oxy]-; (2) [(1-Benzyl-1*H*-indazol-3-yl)oxy]acetic acid. *UNII-G4AG71204O. CAS-20187-55-7; CAS-81919-14-4* [lysine]. INN; BAN; JAN. *Anti-inflammatory.* ◇*AF 1934 [lysine]*

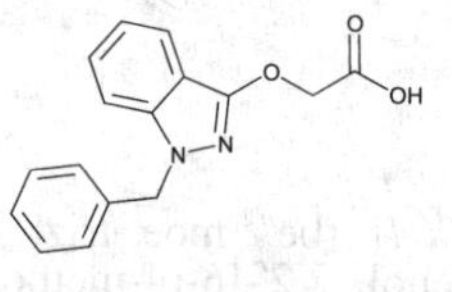

Bendazol. $C_{14}H_{12}N_2$. 208.26. 2-Benzylbenzimidazole. *UNII-26601THN1D. CAS-621-72-7.* INN; DCF; MI.

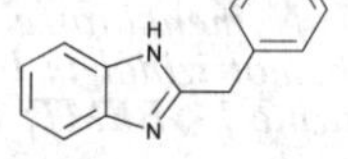

Benderizine. $C_{28}H_{34}N_2O_2$. 430.58. (*R*)-4-(Diphenylmethyl)-1,2-dimethyl-2-veratrylpiperazine. *UNII-KHV7ANE00E. CAS-59752-23-7.* INN.

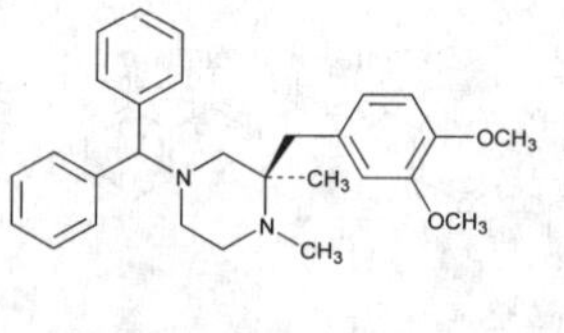

Bendrofluazide (former BAN) — *See* Bendroflumethiazide.

Bendroflumethiazide (ben″ droe floo″ me thye′ a zide). **USP**. $C_{15}H_{14}F_3N_3O_4S_2$. 421.41. (1) 2*H*-1,2,4-Benzothiadiazine-7-sulfonamide, 3,4-dihydro-3-(phenylmethyl)-6-(trifluoromethyl)-, 1,1-dioxide, (±)-; (2) (±)-3-Benzyl-3,4-dihydro-6-(trifluoromethyl)-2*H*-1,2,4-benzothiadiazine-7-sulfonamide 1,1-dioxide. *UNII-5Q52X6ICJI. CAS-73-48-3.* INN; BAN; JAN. *Diuretic; antihypertensive.* Naturetin (Apothecon)

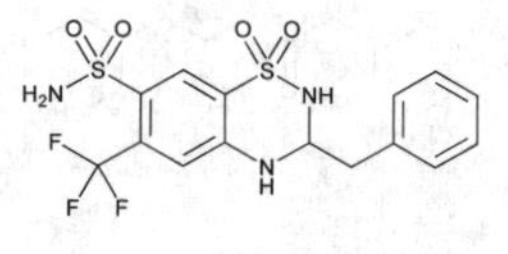

Benethamine Penicillin. $C_{16}H_{18}N_2O_4S.C_{15}H_{17}N$. 545.69. Benzylpenicillin salt of *N*-benzylphenethylamine. *UNII-O3S7RWT8R5. CAS-751-84-8.* INN; BAN.

Benexate. $C_{23}H_{27}N_3O_4$. 409.48. Benzyl salicylate, *trans*-4-(guanidinomethyl)cyclohexanecarboxylate. *UNII-O3PR2X907M. CAS-78718-52-2.* INN; MI.

Benexate Hydrochloride Betadex. $C_{23}H_{27}N_3O_4 \cdot HCl$. $C_{42}H_{70}O_{35}$. 1580.92. Benzyl 2-[*trans*-4-(guanidinomethyl)-cyclohexylcarbonyloxy]benzoate monohydrochloride β-cyclodextrin clathrate. JAN.

Benfluorex. $C_{19}H_{20}F_3NO_2$. 351.36. 2-[[α-Methyl-*m*-(trifluoromethyl)phenethyl]amino]ethanol benzoate (ester). *UNII-403FO0NQG3. CAS-23602-78-0.* INN; BAN; DCF; MI.

Benfosformin. $C_9H_{12}N_5Na_2O_3P \cdot H_2O$. 333.19. Disodium [(benzylamidino)amidino]phosphoramidate monohydrate. *UNII-49030P3C8S. CAS-52658-53-4; CAS-35282-33-8* [anhydrous]. INN; DCF. ◇*JAV 852*

Benfotiamine. $C_{19}H_{23}N_4O_6PS$. 466.45. *N*-[(4-Amino-2-methyl-5-pyrimidinyl)methyl]-*N*-(4-hydroxy-2-mercapto-1-methyl-1-butenyl)formamide *S*-benzoate *O*-phosphate. *CAS-22457-89-2.* INN; JAN; DCF; MI. ◇*8088 C.B.*

Benfurodil Hemisuccinate. $C_{19}H_{18}O_7$. 358.34. 2-(1-Hydroxyethyl)-β-(hydroxymethyl)-3-methyl-5-benzofuranacrylic acid γ-lactone hydrogen succinate. *UNII-Y4Z8D13662. CAS-3447-95-8.* INN; DCF; MI. ◇*4091 C.B.*

Benhepazone. $C_{15}H_{12}N_2O$. 236.27. 1-Benzyl-2(1*H*)-cyclo-heptimidazolone. *UNII-NBB4EM8UXC. CAS-363-13-3.* INN. ◇*RCH 314*

Benidipine. $C_{28}H_{31}N_3O_6$. 505.56. [Benidipine Hydrochloride is JAN.] ($\pm$)-(*R**)-3-[(*R**)-1-Benzyl-3-piperidyl] methyl 1,4-dihydro-2,6-dimethyl-4-(*m*-nitrophenyl)-3,5-pyridine-dicarboxylate. *CAS-105979-17-7.* INN.

Benmoxin. $C_{15}H_{16}N_2O$. 240.30. Benzoic acid 2-(α-methylbenzyl)hydrazide. *UNII-XC9FY2SGBG. CAS-7654-03-7.* INN; DCF; MI.

Benolizime. $C_{19}H_{26}N_2O_3$. 330.42. 1,2,3,4,4a,6,7,11b,12,13a-Decahydro-9,10-dimethoxy-13*H*-dibenzo[*a,f*]quinolizin-13-one oxime. *UNII-7RE4N644YF. CAS-61864-30-0.* INN.

Benorilate. $C_{17}H_{15}NO_5$. 313.30. 4-Acetamidophenyl salicylate acetate. *CAS-5003-48-5.* INN; BAN; DCF; MI. Benoral (Sterling Winthrop) *[Name previously used: Benorylate.]* ◇*Win 11450*

Benorterone [*1964*] (ben or′ ter one). $C_{19}H_{28}O_2$. 288.42. (1) *B*-Norandrost-4-en-3-one, 17-hydroxy-17-methyl-, (17β)-; (2) 17β-Hydroxy-17-methyl-*B*-norandrost-4-en-3-one. *UNII-J339Q7IM54. CAS-3570-10-3.* INN. *Anti-androgen.* ◇*SK&F 7690*

Benorylate (previously used name) — *See* Benorilate.

Benoxafos. $C_{12}H_{14}Cl_2NO_3PS_2$. 386.25. *S*-[(5,7-Dichlorobenzoxazol-2-yl)methyl] *O,O*-diethyl phosphorodithioate. *UNII-LF2DT5DL6H. CAS-16759-59-4.* INN.

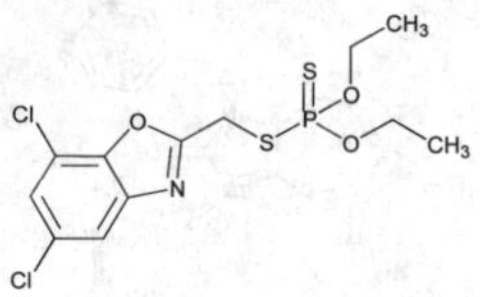

Benoxaprofen [*1976*] (ben ox″ a proe′ fen). $C_{16}H_{12}ClNO_3$. 301.72. (1) 5-Benzoxazoleacetic acid, 2-(4-chlorophenyl)-α-methyl, (±)-; (2) (±)-2-(*p*-Chlorophenyl)-α-methyl-5-benzoxazoleacetic acid. *UNII-17SZX404IM. CAS-51234-28-7.* INN; BAN. *Anti-inflammatory; analgesic.* Oraflex (Lilly†) ◇*Compound 90459*

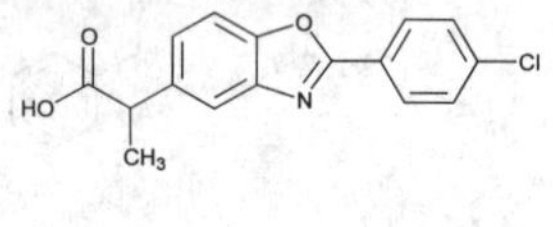

Benoxinate Hydrochloride (ben ox′ i nate hye″ droe klor′ ide). **USP.** $C_{17}H_{28}N_2O_3 \cdot HCl$. 344.88. [Oxybuprocaine is INN and BAN; Oxybuprocaine Hydrochloride is JAN.] (1) Benzoic acid, 4-amino-3-butoxy-, 2-(diethylamino)ethyl ester, monohydrochloride; (2) 2-(Diethylamino)ethyl 4-amino-3-butoxybenzoate monohydrochloride. *UNII-0VE4U49K15; UNII-AXQ0JYM303* [benoxinate]. *CAS-5987-82-6; CAS-99-43-4* [benoxinate]. *Anesthetic (topical).*

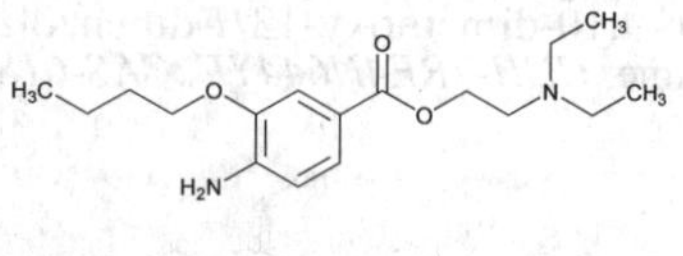

Benpenolisin. $C_{264}H_{350}K_{12}N_{48}O_{61}S_{12}$. 6025.85. N^6-[D-2-[(2*R*,4*S*)-4-Carboxy-5,5-dimethyl-2-thiazolidinyl]-*N*-(phenylacetyl)glycyl]-L-lysine monopotassium salt, dodecapeptide. *CAS-61990-92-9.* INN.

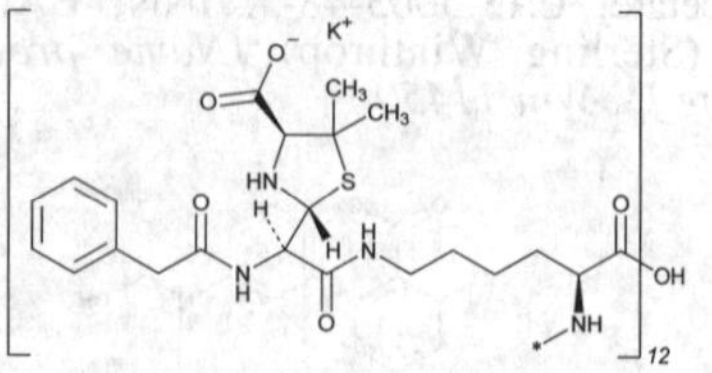

Benperidol [*1963*] (ben per′ i dol). $C_{22}H_{24}FN_3O_2$. 381.44. (1) 2*H*-Benzimidazol-2-one, 1-[1-[4-(4-fluorophenyl)-4-oxobutyl]-4-piperidinyl]-1,3-dihydro-; (2) 1-{1-[3-(*p*-Fluorobenzoyl)propyl]-4-piperidyl}-2-benzimidazolinone. *UNII-97O6X78C53. CAS-2062-84-2.* INN; BAN. *Antipsychotic.* ◇*McN-JR-4584; R-4584*

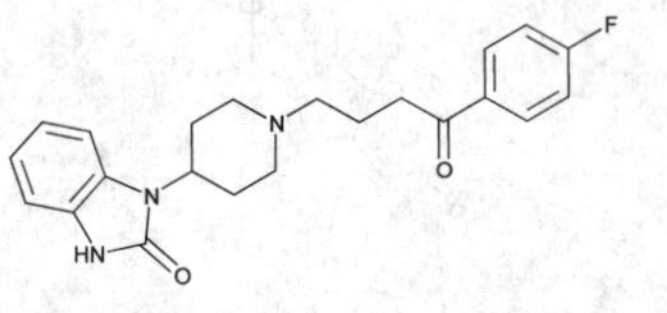

Benproperine. $C_{21}H_{27}NO$. 309.45. [Benproperine Phosphate is JAN.] 1-[2-(2-Benzylphenoxy)-1-methylethyl]piperidine. *UNII-3AA6IZ48YK. CAS-2156-27-6.* INN; MI. ◇*ASA ASA 158/5 [as phosphate]*

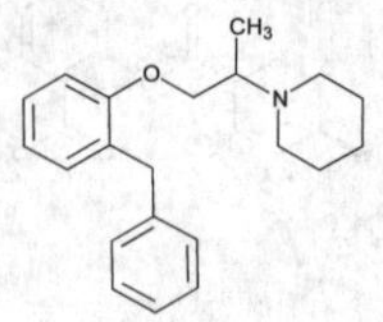

Benrixate. $C_{19}H_{30}N_2O_2$. 318.45. 4-Benzyl-1-piperidinecarboxylic acid, 2-(diethylamino)ethyl ester. *UNII-58NL35I27K. CAS-24671-26-9.* INN; DCF.

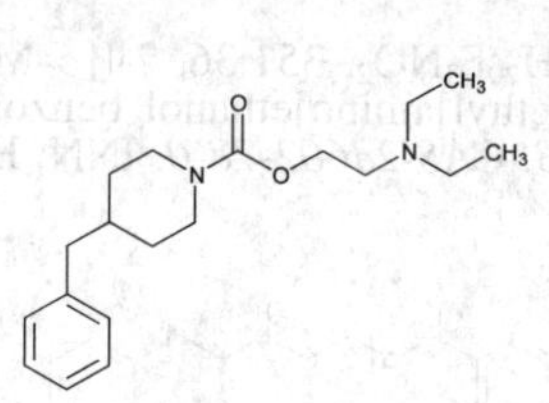

Bensalan [*1967*] (ben′ sa lan). $C_{14}H_{10}Br_3NO_2$. 463.95. (1) Benzamide, 3,5-dibromo-*N*-[(4-bromophenyl)methyl]-2-hydroxy-; (2) 3,5-Dibromo-*N*-(*p*-bromobenzyl)salicylamide. *CAS-15686-76-7.* INN. *Disinfectant.*

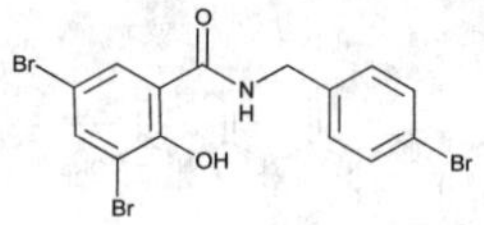

Benserazide [*1976*] (ben ser′ a zide). $C_{10}H_{15}N_3O_5$. 257.24. [Benserazide Hydrochloride is JAN.] (1) DL-Serine, 2-[(2,3,4-trihydroxyphenyl)methyl]hydrazide; (2) DL-Serine 2-(2,3,4-trihydroxybenzyl)hydrazide. *UNII-762OS3ZEJU. CAS-322-35-0.* INN; BAN. *Inhibitor (decarboxylase).* ◇*Ro 4-4602*

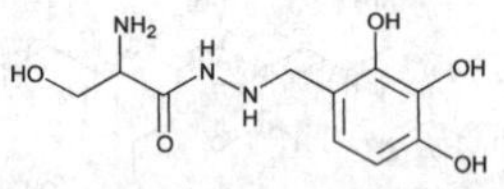

Bensuldazic Acid. $C_{12}H_{14}N_2O_2S_2$. 282.38. 5-Benzyldihydro-6-thioxo-2*H*-1,3,5-thiadiazine-3(4*H*)-acetic acid. *UNII-R8L0T98P0J; UNII-NC32G269EF* [sodium bensuldazate]. *CAS-1219-77-8; CAS-1950-15-8* [sodium bensuldazate]. INN; BAN.

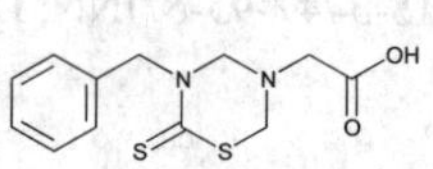

Bensylyte Hydrochloride — *See* Phenoxybenzamine Hydrochloride.

Bentamapimod. $C_{25}H_{23}N_5O_2S$. 457.55. 2-(1,3-Benzothiazol-2-yl)-2-[2-({4-[(morpholin-4-yl)methyl]phenyl}methoxy)-pyrimidin-4-yl]acetonitrile. *CAS-848344-36-5.* INN.

Bentazepam [*1977*] (ben taz′ e pam). $C_{17}H_{16}N_2OS$. 296.39. (1) 2*H*-[1]Benzothieno[2,3-*e*]-1,4-diazepin-2-one, 1,3,6,7,8,9-hexahydro-5-phenyl-; (2) 1,3,6,7,8,9-Hexahydro-5-phenyl-2*H*-[1]benzothieno[2,3-*e*]-1,4-diazepin-2-one. *UNII-66JKK43S1Z. CAS-29462-18-8*. INN. *Sedative-hypnotic.* ◇*CI-718*

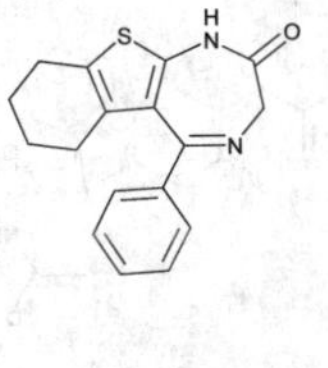

Bentemazole. $C_{11}H_{10}N_6$. 226.24. 5-(1-Benzylimidazol-2-yl)-1*H*-tetrazole. *UNII-P4QI4D1IUV. CAS-63927-95-7*. INN.

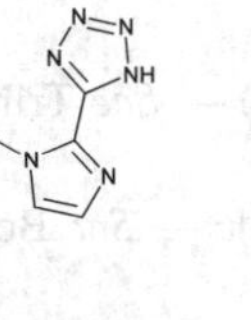

Bentiamine. $C_{26}H_{26}N_4O_4S$. 490.57. *N*-[(4-Amino-2-methyl-5-pyrimidinyl)methyl]-*N*-(4-hydroxy-2-mercapto-1-methyl-1-butenyl)formamide *O,S*-dibenzoate. *UNII-8PUY50JW-LU. CAS-299-88-7*. INN.

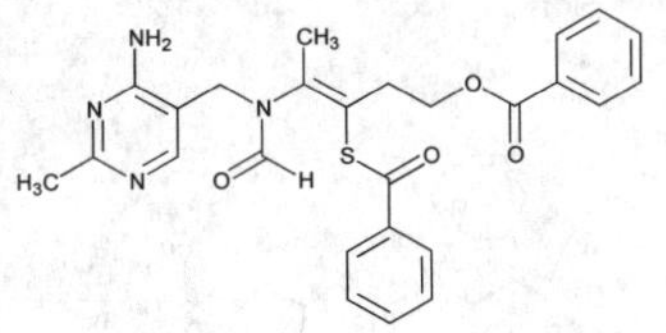

Bentipimine. $C_{27}H_{31}ClN_2S$. 451.07. 1-[2-[(*o*-Chloro-α-phenylbenzyl)thio]ethyl]-4-(*o*-methylbenzyl)piperazine. *UNII-768T9DK07R. CAS-17692-23-8*. INN.

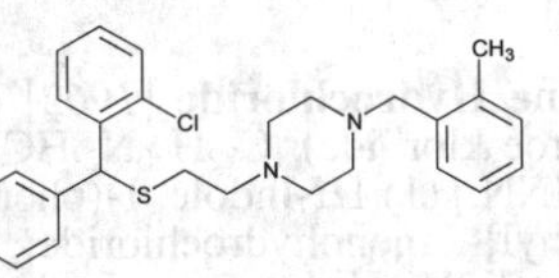

Bentiromide [*1979*] (ben tir′ oh mide). $C_{23}H_{20}N_2O_5$. 404.42. (1) Benzoic acid, 4-[[2-(benzoylamino)-3-(4-hydroxyphenyl)-1-oxopropyl]amino]-, (*S*)-; (2) (*S*)-*p*-(α-Benzamido-*p*-hydroxyhydrocinnamamido)benzoic acid. *UNII-239IF5W61J. CAS-37106-97-1*. INN; BAN; JAN. *Diagnostic aid (pancreas function determination).* Chymex (Savage) ◇*E-2663; BTPABA, PFT*

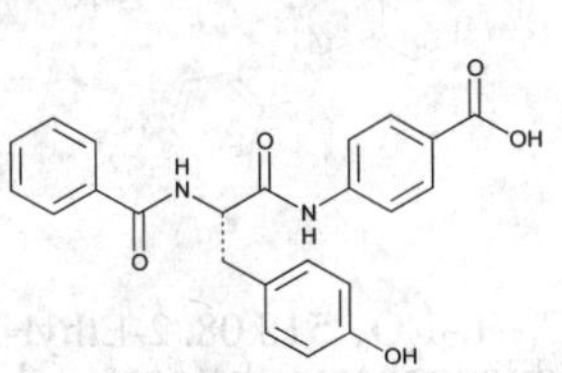

Bentonite (ben′ ton ite). **NF**. (1) Bentonite; (2) Bentonite. *UNII-A3N5ZCN45C. CAS-1302-78-9*. JAN. *Pharmaceutic aid (suspending agent).*

---

† Brand name formerly used, and/or firm no longer concerned with this product.

Bentoquatam [*1996*] (ben′ toe kwa″ tam). (1) Quaternium-18 bentonite; (2) Bis(hydrogenated tallow alkyl)dimethylammonium complex with sodium bentonite. *CAS-1340-69-8*. CID. *Barrier for the prevention of allergic contact dermatitis.* Ivy Block (Stand Homeopath)

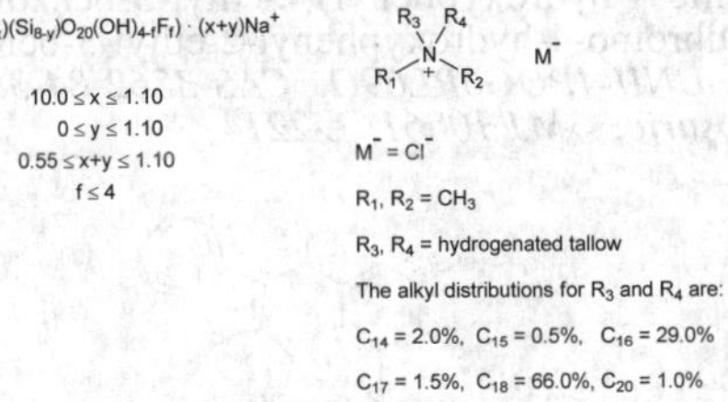

$$((Al_{4-x}Mg_x)(Si_{8-y})O_{20}(OH)_{4-f}F_f) \cdot (x+y)Na^+$$

$$10.0 \le x \le 1.10$$
$$0 \le y \le 1.10$$
$$0.55 \le x+y \le 1.10$$
$$f \le 4$$

$M^- = Cl^-$

$R_1, R_2 = CH_3$

R_3, R_4 = hydrogenated tallow

The alkyl distributions for R_3 and R_4 are:

C_{14} = 2.0%, C_{15} = 0.5%, C_{16} = 29.0%

C_{17} = 1.5%, C_{18} = 66.0%, C_{20} = 1.0%

Benurestat [*1974*] (ben ure′ e stat). $C_9H_9ClN_2O_3$. 228.63. (1) Benzamide, 4-chloro-*N*-[2-(hydroxyamino)-2-oxoethyl]-; (2) 2-(*p*-Chlorobenzamido)acetohydroxamic acid. *UNII-9RA9A22Z0W. CAS-38274-54-3*. INN. *Enzyme inhibitor (urease).* ◇*EU-2826*

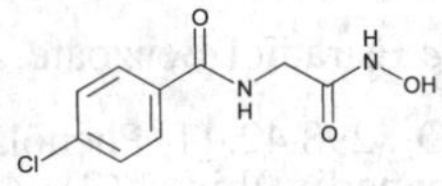

Benzaldehyde (ben zal′ de hyde). **NF**. C_7H_6O. 106.12. (1) Benzaldehyde; (2) Benzaldehyde. *UNII-TA269SD04T. CAS-100-52-7. Pharmaceutic aid (flavor).*

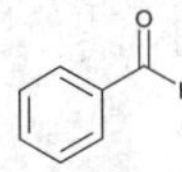

Benzalkonium Chloride (ben″ zal koe′ nee um klor′ ide). **NF**. (1) Ammonium, alkyldimethyl(phenylmethyl)-, chloride; (2) Alkylbenzyldimethylammonium chloride. *CAS-8001-54-5*. INN; BAN; JAN. *Pharmaceutic aid (preservative).* Roccal (Sterling Winthrop); Zephiran Chloride (Sterling Winthrop)

Benzaprinoxide. $C_{20}H_{20}ClNO$. 325.83. 1-Chloro-*N,N*-dimethyl-5*H*-dibenzo[*a,d*]cycloheptene-$\Delta^{5,\gamma}$-propylamine *N*-oxide. *UNII-8J11WBM781. CAS-52758-02-8*. INN.

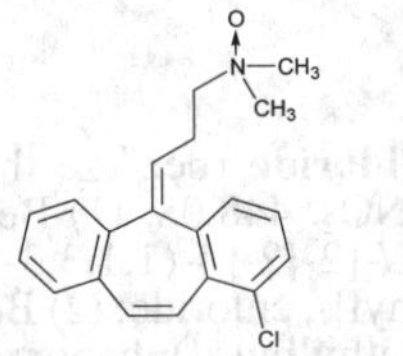

Benzarone. $C_{17}H_{14}O_3$. 266.29. 2-Ethyl-3-benzofuranyl *p*-hydroxyphenyl ketone. *UNII-23ZW4BG89C. CAS-1477-19-6*. INN; DCF; MI. ◇*L 2197*

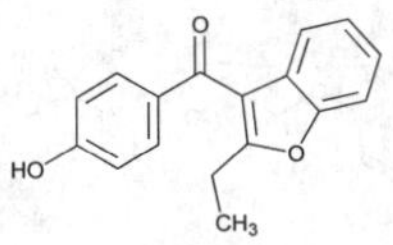

Benzathine Benzylpenicillin (INN, BAN) — *See* Penicillin G Benzathine.

Benzathine Penicillin (previously used name) — *See* Penicillin G Benzathine.

Benzatropine (INN, BAN) — *See* Benztropine Mesylate.

Benzazoline Hydrochloride — *See* Tolazoline Hydrochloride.

Benzbromaron (JAN) — *See* Benzbromarone.

Benzbromarone [*1976*] (benz broe' ma rone). $C_{17}H_{12}Br_2O_3$. 424.08. [Benzbromaron is JAN.] (1) Methanone, (3,5-dibromo-4-hydroxyphenyl)(2-ethyl-3-benzofuranyl)-; (2) 3,5-Dibromo-4-hydroxyphenyl-2-ethyl-3-benzofuranyl ketone. *UNII-4POG0RL69O. CAS-3562-84-3.* INN; BAN. *Uricosuric.* ◇*MJ 10061; L-2214*

Benzchinamide — *See* Benzquinamide.

Benzchlorpropamide — *See* Beclamide.

Benzene Hexachloride, Gamma (previously used name) — *See* Lindane.

Benzestrofol — *See* Estradiol Benzoate.

Benzestrol. $C_{20}H_{26}O_2$. 298.42. (1) Phenol, 4,4'-(1,2-diethyl-3-methyl-1,3-propanediyl)bis-; (2) 4,4'-(1,2-Diethyl-3-methyltrimethylene)diphenol. *UNII-A27512LR47. CAS-85-95-0.* USP XX; INN; BAN; MI.

Benzethacil — *See* Penicillin G Benzathine.

Benzethidine. $C_{23}H_{29}NO_3$. 367.48. 1-(2-Benzyloxyethyl)-4-phenylpiperidine-4-carboxylic acid ethyl ester. *UNII-X0I74BAR02. CAS-3691-78-9.* INN; BAN; DCF. ◇*NIH 7574*

Benzethonium Chloride (ben" ze thoe' nee um klor' ide). **USP.** $C_{27}H_{42}ClNO_2$. 448.08. (1) Benzenemethanaminium, *N,N*-dimethyl-*N*-[2-[2-[4-(1,1,3,3-tetramethylbutyl)phenoxy]ethoxy]ethyl]-, chloride; (2) Benzyldimethyl[2-[2-[*p*-(1,1,3,3-tetramethylbutyl)phenoxy]ethoxy]ethyl]ammonium chloride. *UNII-PH41D05744. CAS-121-54-0.* INN; BAN; JAN. *Anti-infective, topical; pharmaceutic aid (preservative).* Microklenz (Carrington); Phemerol Chloride (Parke-Davis)

Benzetimide Hydrochloride [*1969*] (ben zet' i mide hye" droe klor' ide). $C_{23}H_{26}N_2O_2$.HCl. 398.93. [Benzetimide is INN.] (1) [3,4'-Bipiperidine]-2,6-dione, 3-phenyl-1'-(phenylmethyl)-, monohydrochloride; (2) 2-(1-Benzyl-4-piperidyl)-2-phenylglutarimide monohydrochloride. *UNII-V6ERX20PHB; UNII-B987T0L5FX* [benzetimide]. *CAS-*

5633-14-7; CAS-119391-55-8 [benzetimide]. *Anticholinergic.* Dioxatrine (Janssen Pharmaceutica, Belgium) ◇*McN-JR-4929-11; Janssen R 4929*

Benzfetamine (INN, BAN) — *See* Benzphetamine Hydrochloride.

Benzhexol (BAN) — *See* Trihexyphenidyl Hydrochloride.

Benzilone Bromide — *See* Benzilonium Bromide.

Benzilonium Bromide [*1961*] (ben" zil oh' nee um broe' mide). $C_{22}H_{28}BrNO_3$. 434.37. (1) Pyrrolidinium, 1,1-diethyl-3-[(hydroxydiphenylacetyl)oxy]-, bromide; (2) 1,1-Diethyl-3-hydroxypyrrolidinium bromide benzilate. *UNII-EMB5M4GMHP. CAS-1050-48-2.* INN; BAN. *Anticholinergic.* Portyn (Parke-Davis†) ◇*CI-379; CN-20,172-3; PU-239*

Benzin, Petroleum. A mixture of low-boiling point hydrocarbons from petroleum. JAN.

Benzindopyrine Hydrochloride [*1962*] (ben zin" doe pye' reen hye" droe klor' ide). $C_{22}H_{20}N_2$.HCl. 348.87. [Benzindopyrine is INN.] (1) 1*H*-Indole, 1-(phenylmethyl)-3-[2-(4-pyridinyl)ethyl]-, monohydrochloride; (2) 1-Benzyl-3-[2-(4-pyridyl)ethyl]indole monohydrochloride. *UNII-G6G4YSZ601. CAS-5585-71-7. Antipsychotic.* ◇*IN 461; NSC-17789*

Benziodarone. $C_{17}H_{12}I_2O_3$. 518.08. 2-Ethyl-3-benzofuranyl 4-hydroxy-3,5-diiodophenyl ketone. *UNII-75CL65GTYR. CAS-68-90-6.* INN; BAN; JAN; DCF; MI. ◇*L 2329*

Benzmalecene. $C_{20}H_{19}Cl_2NO_3$. 392.28. N-[2,3-Bis(p-chlorophenyl)-1-methylpropyl]maleamic acid (α-form). *UNII-6ET4K804XA. CAS-148-07-2.* INN.

Benzmethoxazone — *See* Chlorthenoxazine.

Benznidazole. $C_{12}H_{12}N_4O_3$. 260.25. N-Benzyl-2-nitroimidazole-1-acetamide. *CAS-22994-85-0.* INN; MI.

Benzoaric Acid — *See* Ellagic Acid.

Benzobarbital. $C_{19}H_{16}N_2O_4$. 336.34. 1-Benzoyl-5-ethyl-5-phenylbarbituric acid. *UNII-YNJ78BD0AH. CAS-744-80-9.* INN.

Benzocaine (ben′ zoe kane). **USP**. $C_9H_{11}NO_2$. 165.19. [Ethyl Aminobenzoate is JAN.] (1) Benzoic acid, 4-amino-, ethyl ester; (2) Ethyl p-aminobenzoate. *UNII-U3RSY48JW5. CAS-94-09-7.* INN; BAN. *Anesthetic (topical).* Americaine (Fisons); Baby Anbesol (Whitehall-Robins) *[Name previously used: Ethyl Aminobenzoate.]*

Benzoclidine. $C_{14}H_{17}NO_2$. 231.29. 3-Quinuclidinol benzoate (ester). *UNII-G84189YY06. CAS-16852-81-6.* INN.

Benzoctamine Hydrochloride [*1968*] (ben zokt′ a meen hye″ droe klor′ ide). $C_{18}H_{19}N \cdot HCl$. 285.81. [Benzoctamine is INN and BAN.] (1) 9,10-Ethanoanthracene-9(10H)-methanamine, N-methyl-, hydrochloride; (2) N-Methyl-9,10-

ethanoanthracene-9(10H)-methylamine hydrochloride. *CAS-10085-81-1; CAS-17243-39-9* [benzoctamine]. *Relaxant (muscle); sedative-hypnotic.* ◇Ba-30803

Benzodepa [*1962*] (ben zoe dep′ a). $C_{12}H_{16}N_3O_3P$. 281.25. (1) Carbamic acid, [bis(1-aziridinyl)phosphinyl]-, phenylmethyl ester; (2) Benzyl[bis(1-aziridinyl)phosphinyl]carbamate. *CAS-1980-45-6.* INN. *Antineoplastic.* ◇AB-103; NSC-37096

Benzodiazepine Hydrochloride — *See* Medazepam Hydrochloride.

Benzododecinium Chloride. $C_{21}H_{38}ClN$. 339.99. Benzyldodecyldimethylammonium chloride. *UNII-Y5A751G47H. CAS-139-07-1; CAS-10328-35-5* [benzododecinium]. INN.

Benzogynestryl — *See* Estradiol Benzoate.

Benzoic Acid (ben zoe′ ik as′ id). **USP**. $C_7H_6O_2$. 122.12. (1) Benzoic acid; (2) Benzoic acid. *UNII-8SKN0B0MIM. CAS-65-85-0.* JAN. *Pharmaceutic aid (antifungal agent).*

Benzoin (ben′ zoin). **USP**. The balsamic resin obtained from *Styrax benzoin* Dryander or *Styrax paralleloneurus* Perkins, known in commerce as Sumatra Benzoin, or from *Styrax tonkinensis* (Pièrre) Craib ex Hartwich, or other species of the Section *Anthostyrax* of the genus *Styrax*, known in commerce as Siam Benzoin (Fam. Styraceae). *UNII-L7J6A1NE81. CAS-8050-35-9.* JAN. *Protectant (topical).*

Benzonatate (ben zoe′ na tate). **USP**. $C_{30}H_{53}NO_{11}$ (average). 603.74 (average). (1) Benzoic acid, 4-(butylamino)-, 2,5,8,11,14,17,20,23,26-nonaoxaoctacos-28-yl ester; (2) 2,5,8,11,14,17,20,23,26-Nonaoxaoctacosan-28-yl p-(butylamino)benzoate. *UNII-5P4DHS6ENR. CAS-104-31-4.* INN; BAN. *Antitussive.* Tessalon (Forest)

---

† Brand name formerly used, and/or firm no longer concerned with this product.

Benzopyrronium Bromide. $C_{20}H_{24}BrNO_3$. 406.31. 1,1-Dimethyl-3-hydroxypyrrolidinium bromide benzilate. *UNII-G4449OF7S3*. *CAS-13696-15-6*. INN.

Benzoquinonium Chloride. *UNII-O6HVT48T15*. *CAS-311-09-1; CAS-7554-16-7 [benzoquinonium]*. MI. Mytolon Chloride (Sterling Winthrop†)

Benzorphanol — *See* Levophenacylmorphan.

Benzosulfinide — *See* Saccharin.

Benzosulphinide Sodium — *See* Saccharin Sodium.

Benzotript. $C_{18}H_{15}ClN_2O_3$. 342.78. *N*-(*p*-Chlorobenzoyl)-L-tryptophan. *UNII-LS5O682BRO*. *CAS-39544-74-6*. INN.

Benzoxiquine [*1967*] (ben zox' i kwin). $C_{16}H_{11}NO_2$. 249.26. (1) 8-Quinolinol, benzoate (ester); (2) 8-Quinolinol benzoate (ester). *UNII-GRE0P19C3Z*. *CAS-86-75-9*. INN. *Disinfectant*. Dioxyline (Laboratoires Franca Inc., Canada) ◇*NSC-3951*

Benzoxonium Chloride. $C_{23}H_{42}ClNO_2$. 400.04. Benzyldodecylbis(2-hydroxyethyl)ammonium chloride. *UNII-12IM-O9R11X*. *CAS-19379-90-9*. INN; MI.

Benzoyl Peroxide [*1972*] (ben' zoe il per ox' ide). **USP**. $C_{14}H_{10}O_4$ (anhydrous). 242.23 (anhydrous). (1) Peroxide, dibenzoyl; (2) Benzoyl peroxide. *UNII-W9WZN9A0GM*. *CAS-94-36-0*. *Keratolytic*. Acne-Aid Cream (Stiefel†); Benoxyl (Stiefel); Benzac (Galderma); Benzac W (Galderma); Brevoxyl (Stiefel); Clear By Design (SmithKline Beecham†); Dry and Clear (Whitehall-Robins†); Epi-Clear (Bristol-Myers Squibb†); Fostex BPO Bar, Gel, and Wash (Bristol-Myers Products); Loroxide (Dermik); PanOxyl (Stiefel); Persa-Gel (Ortho Pharmaceutical); Vanoxide (Dermik) ◇*NSC-675*

Benzoylpas Calcium [*1961*] (ben zoe il' paz kal' see um). $C_{28}H_{20}CaN_2O_8 \cdot 5H_2O$. 642.62. [Calcium Benzamidosalicylate is INN and BAN.] (1) Benzoic acid, 4-(benzoylamino)-2-hydroxy-, calcium salt (2:1) pentahydrate; (2) Calcium 4-

benzamidosalicylate (1:2) pentahydrate. *UNII-DX586KL1YX; UNII-XEE879L727 [benzoylpas]*. *CAS-5631-00-5; CAS-528-96-1 [anhydrous]; CAS-13898-58-3 [benzoylpas]*. USP XX. *Antibacterial (tuberculostatic)*.

Benzoylthiamindisulfid — *See* Bisbentiamine.

Benzoylthiaminmonophosphat — *See* Benfotiamine.

Benzphetamine Chloride — *See* Benzphetamine Hydrochloride.

Benzphetamine Hydrochloride. $C_{17}H_{21}N \cdot HCl$. 275.82. [Benzfetamine is INN and BAN.] (+)-*N*-Benzyl-*N*,α-dimethylphenethylamine hydrochloride. *UNII-43DWT87QT7; UNII-0M3S43XK27 [benzphetamine]*. *CAS-5411-22-3; CAS-156-08-1 [benzphetamine]*. NF XIII; MI. Didrex (Pfizer)

Benzpiperylon. $C_{22}H_{25}N_3O$. 347.45. [Benzpiperylone is INN.] 4-Benzyl-1-(1-methyl-4-piperidinyl)-3-phenyl-3-pyrazolin-5-one. *CAS-53-89-4*. MI. Telon (Novartis†) ◇*KB 95*

Benzpiperylone (INN) — *See* Benzpiperylon.

Benzpyrinium Bromide. $C_{15}H_{17}BrN_2O_2$. 337.21. 1-Benzyl-3-hydroxypyridinium bromide dimethylcarbamate. *UNII-X0L78YB79M*. *CAS-587-46-2*. NF XII; INN; MI.

Benzquercin. $C_{50}H_{40}O_7$. 752.85. 3,3′,4′,5,7-Pentakis(benzyloxy)flavone. *UNII-499L7I0905*. *CAS-13157-90-9*. INN.

Benzquinamide [*1962*] (benz kwin' a mide). $C_{22}H_{32}N_2O_5$. 404.50. (1) 2*H*-Benzo[*a*]quinolizine-3-carboxamide, 2-(acetyloxy)-*N*,*N*-diethyl-1,3,4,6,7,11b-hexahydro-9,10-dimethoxy-; (2) *N*,*N*-Diethyl-1,3,4,6,7,11b-hexahydro-2-hydroxy-9,10-dimethoxy-2*H*-benzo[*a*]quinolizine-3-carboxamide acetate (ester). *UNII-0475EA27Q3*. *CAS-63-12-7*. INN; BAN. *Anti-emetic*. Emete-con (Roerig); Quantril (Roerig) ◇*P-2647; NSC-64375*

Benzthiazide. $C_{15}H_{14}ClN_3O_4S_3$. 431.94. (1) 2*H*-1,2,4-Benzothiadiazine-7-sulfonamide, 6-chloro-3-[[(phenylmethyl)thio]methyl]-, 1,1-dioxide; (2) 3-[(Benzylthio)methyl]-6-chloro-2*H*-1,2,4-benzothiadiazine-7-sulfonamide 1,1-dioxide. *UNII-1TD8J48L61*. *CAS-91-33-8*. USP XXIII; INN; BAN; JAN. *Diuretic; antihypertensive*. Aquatag (Solvay Pharmaceuticals); Exna (Robins)

Benztropine (former BAN) — *See* Benztropine Mesylate.

Benztropine Mesylate (benz′ troe peen mes′ i late). **USP**. $C_{21}H_{25}NO.CH_4O_3S$. 403.53. [Benzatropine is INN and BAN; Benztropine Mesilate is JAN.] (1) 8-Azabicyclo[3.2.1]octane, 3-(diphenylmethoxy)-, *endo*, methanesulfonate; (2) 3α-(Diphenylmethoxy)-1αH,5αH-tropane methanesulfonate. *UNII-WMJ8TL7510; UNII-1NHL2J4X8K* [benztropine]. *CAS-132-17-2; CAS-86-13-5* [benztropine]. *Antiparkinsonian*. Cogentin (Ovation)

Benzydamine Hydrochloride [*1965*] (ben zid′ a meen hye″ droe klor′ ide). $C_{19}H_{23}N_3O.HCl$. 345.87. [Benzydamine is INN and BAN.] (1) 1-Propanamine, *N,N*-dimethyl-3-[[1-(phenylmethyl)-1*H*-indazol-3-yl]oxy]-, monohydrochloride; (2) 1-Benzyl-3-[3-(dimethylamino)propoxy]-1*H*-indazole monohydrochloride. *CAS-132-69-4; CAS-642-72-8* [benzydamine]. JAN. *Analgesic; antipyretic; anti-inflammatory*. Tantum (Angelini Francesco, Italy) ◇*AF-864*

Benzydroflumethiazide — *See* Bendroflumethiazide.

---

† Brand name formerly used, and/or firm no longer concerned with this product.

Benzyl Alcohol (ben′ zil al′ ka hol). **NF**. C_7H_8O. 108.14. (1) Benzenemethanol; (2) Benzyl alcohol. *UNII-LKG8494WBH*. *CAS-100-51-6*. INN; JAN. *Pharmaceutic aid (antimicrobial agent)*.

Benzyl Antiserotonin — *See* Benanserin Hydrochloride.

Benzyl Benzoate (ben′ zil ben′ zoe ate). **USP**. $C_{14}H_{12}O_2$. 212.24. (1) Benzoic acid, phenylmethyl ester; (2) Benzyl benzoate. *UNII-N863NB338G*. *CAS-120-51-4*. JAN. *Pharmaceutic necessity for Dimercaprol [Injection]*.

Benzyl Nicotinate. $C_{13}H_{11}NO_2$. 213.23. *CAS-94-44-0*. JAN.

Benzylamide — *See* Beclamide.

Benzylhydrochlorothiazide. $C_{14}H_{14}ClN_3O_4S_2$. 387.86. 3-Benzyl-3,4-dihydro-6-chlor-2*H*, 1,2,4-benzothiadiazine-7-sulfonamide 1,1-dioxide. *UNII-176437APQH*. *CAS-1824-50-6*. JAN.

p-Benzyloxyphenol — *See* Monobenzone.

Benzylpenicillin. $C_{16}H_{18}N_2O_4S$. 334.39. (2*S*,5*R*,6*R*)-3,3-Dimethyl-7-oxo-6-(2-phenylacetamido)-4-thia-1-azabicyclo[3.2.0]heptane-2-carboxylic acid. *UNII-Q42T66VG0C*. *CAS-61-33-6*. INN; BAN; MI.

Benzylpenicillin Benzathine (JAN) — *See* Penicillin G Benzathine.

Benzylpenicillin Potassium (BAN, JAN) — *See* Penicillin G Potassium.

Benzylpenicillin Procaine — *See* Penicillin G Procaine.

Benzylpenicillin Sodium (BAN) — *See* Penicillin G Sodium.

Benzylpenicilloyl Polylysine (ben″ zil pen″ i sil′ oh il pol″ ee lye′ seen). **USP**. A molar concentration of benzylpenicilloyl moiety ($C_{16}H_{19}N_2O_5S$) of 0.01625 ± 0.00375 M. *Diagnostic aid (penicillin sensitivity)*. Pre-Pen (Schwarz Pharma)

Benzylsulfamide. $C_{13}H_{14}N_2O_2S$. 262.33. *N*⁴-Benzylsulfanilamide. *UNII-AI9WDT80FQ*. *CAS-104-22-3*. INN; DCF; MI. ◇*46 R.P.*

Benzylsulfanilamide — *See* Benzylsulfamide.

Bepafant. $C_{23}H_{22}ClN_5O_2S$. 467.97. 4-[[6-(*o*-Chlorophenyl)-8,9-dihydro-1-methyl-4*H*,7*H*-cyclopenta[4,5]thieno[3,2-*f*]-*s*-triazolo[4,3-*a*][1,4]diazepin-8-yl]carbonyl]morpholine. *UNII-CKS724B66O. CAS-114776-28-2.* INN.

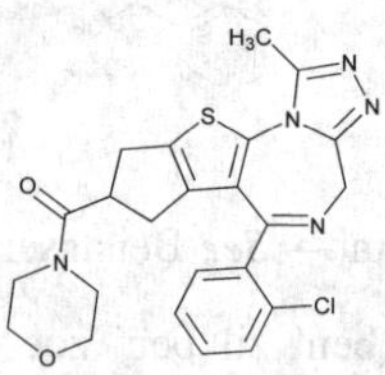

Beperidium Iodide. $C_{23}H_{34}IN_3O_3$. 527.44. *cis*-1-Ethyl-4-hydroxy-1-methylpiperidinium iodide (±)-α-(hexahydro-1*H*-azepin-1-yl)-, 1,2-benzisoxazole-3-acetate, mixture with *trans*-1-ethyl-4-hydroxy-1-methylpiperidinium iodide (±)-α-(hexahydro-1*H*-azepin-1-yl)-1,2-benzisoxazole-3-acetate (1:1). *UNII-25OIG0XCVX. CAS-86434-57-3.* INN.

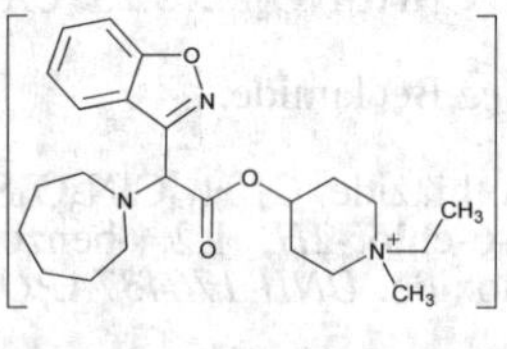

Beperminogene Perplasmid. Plasmid DNA containing human hepatocyte growth factor cDNA sequence driven by a cytomegalovirus promoter. *CAS-627861-07-8.* INN; JAN.

Bephene Oxinaphtoate — *See* Bephenium Hydroxynaphthoate.

Bephenium Embonate — *See* Bephenium Hydroxynaphthoate.

Bephenium Hydroxynaphthoate. $C_{28}H_{29}NO_4$. 443.53. (1) Benzenemethanaminium, *N,N*-dimethyl-*N*-(2-phenoxyethyl)-, salt with 3-hydroxy-2-naphthalenecarboxylic acid (1:1); (2) Benzyldimethyl(2-phenoxyethyl)ammonium 3-hydroxy-2-naphthoate (1:1). *UNII-47RU9546DX. CAS-3818-50-6; CAS-7181-73-9* [bephenium]. USP XXI; INN; BAN; MI.

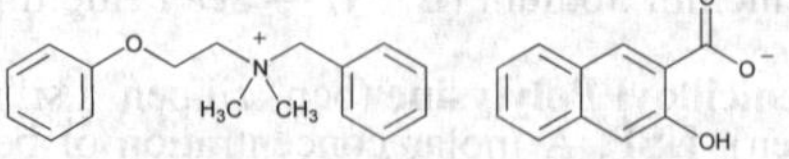

Bepiastine. $C_{16}H_{17}N_3OS$. 299.39. 6-[2-(Dimethylamino)ethyl]pyrido[2,3-*b*][1,5]benzothiazepin-5(6*H*)-one. *UNII-35QK773Y96. CAS-10189-94-3.* INN; DCF. ◇*UP 107*

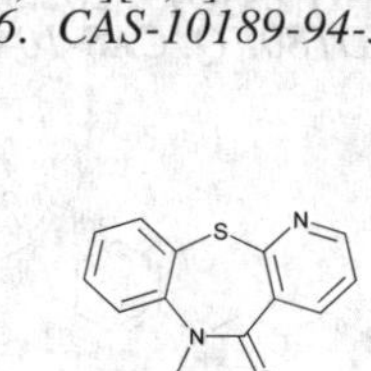

Bepotastine. $C_{21}H_{25}ClN_2O_3$. 388.89. (+)-4-[[(*S*)-*p*-Chloro-α-2-pyridylbenzyl]oxy]-1-piperidinebutyric acid. *UNII-HYD2U48IAS. CAS-125602-71-3.* INN.

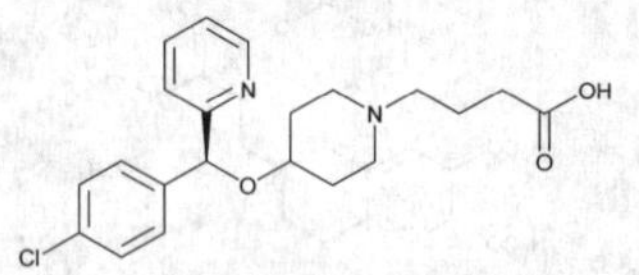

Bepridil Hydrochloride [*1981*] (bep′ ri dil hye″ droe klor′ ide). $C_{24}H_{34}N_2O \cdot HCl \cdot H_2O$. 421.02. [Bepridil is INN and BAN.] (1) 1-Pyrrolideneethanamine, β-[(2-methylpropoxy)methyl]-*N*-phenyl-*N*-(phenylmethyl)-, monohydrochloride, monohydrate; (2) 1-[2-(*N*-Benzylanilino)-1-(isobutoxymethyl)ethyl]-pyrrolidine monohydrochloride monohydrate. *UNII-4W2P15D93M. CAS-74764-40-2.* JAN. *Vasodilator.* Bepadin (Medpointe); Vascor (Johnson & Johnson) ◇*CERM 1978*

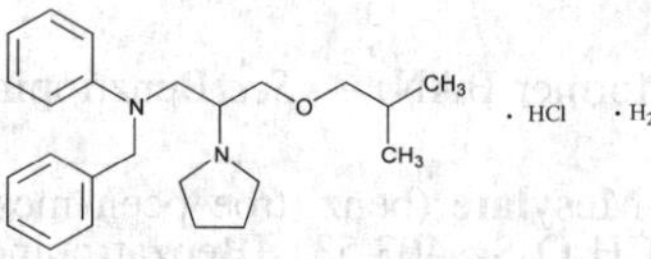

Beractant [*1989*] (ber ak′ tant). A modified bovine lung extract containing mostly phospholipids, modified by the addition of dipalmitoylphosphatidylcholine (DPPC), palmitic acid, and tripalmitin. (1) Beractant; (2) Beractant. *UNII-S866O45PIG. CAS-108778-82-1.* BAN. *Pulmonary surfactant.* Survanta (Ross) ◇*A-60386X*

Beraprost [*1991*] (ber′ a prost). $C_{24}H_{30}O_5$. 398.49. (1) 1*H*-Cyclopenta[*b*]benzofuran-5-butanoic acid, 2,3,3a,8b-tetrahydro-2-hydroxy-1-(3-hydroxy-4-methyl-1-octen-6-ynyl)-; (2) (±)-(1*R*,2*R*,3a*S*,8b*S*)-2,3,3a,8b-Tetrahydro-2-hydroxy-1-[(*E*)-(3*S*,4*RS*)-3-hydroxy-4-methyl-1-octen-6-ynyl]-1*H*-cyclopenta[*b*]benzofuran-5-butyric acid. *UNII-35E3NJJ4O6. CAS-88430-50-6.* INN. *Platelet aggregation inhibitor.* ◇*ML-1229; MDL-201229*

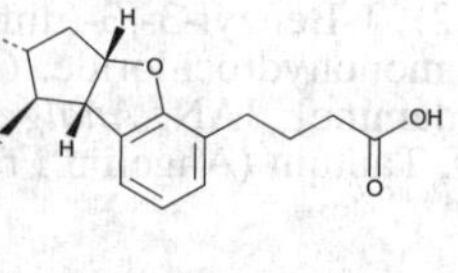

Beraprost Sodium [*1991*] (ber′ a prost soe′ dee um). $C_{24}H_{29}NaO_5$. 420.47. (1) 1*H*-Cyclopenta[*b*]benzofuran-5-butanoic acid, 2,3,3a,8b-tetrahydro-2-hydroxy-1-(3-hydroxy-4-methyl-1-octen-6-ynyl)-, monosodium salt; (2) Sodium (±)-(1*R*,2*R*,3a*S*,8b*S*)-2,3,3a,8b-tetrahydro-2-hydroxy-1-[(*E*)-(3*S*,4*RS*)-3-hydroxy-4-methyl-1-octen-6-ynyl]-1*H*-cyclopenta[*b*]benzofuran-5-butyrate. *UNII-15K99VDU5F; UNII-35E3NJJ4O6* [beraprost]. *CAS-88475-69-8; CAS-88430-50-6* [beraprost]. JAN. *Platelet aggregation inhibitor.* ◇*TRK-100; ML-1129; MDL-201129*

Berberine Chloride. $C_{20}H_{18}ClNO_4 \cdot xH_2O$. 371.81 (anhydrous). 5,6-Dihydro-9,10-dimethoxybenzo[*g*]-1,3-benzodioxolo[5,6-*a*]quinolizinium chloride hydrate. *CAS-633-65-8; CAS-2086-83-1* [berberine]. JAN.

Berberine Sulfate. $[C_{20}H_{18}NO_4]_2 \cdot SO_4 \cdot xH_2O$. 768.79 (anhydrous). 5,6-Dihydro-9,10-dimethoxybenzo[*g*]-1,3-benzodioxolo[5,6-*a*]quinolizinium sulfate. *CAS-633-66-9*. JAN.

Berberine Tannate. 5,6-Dihydro-9,10-dimethoxybenzo[*g*]-1,3-benzodioxolo[5,6-*a*]quinolizinium tannate. JAN.

Berefrine [*1993*] (ber ef' rin). $C_{14}H_{21}NO_2$. 235.32. (1) Phenol, 3-[2-(1,1-dimethylethyl)-3-methyl-5-oxazolidinyl]-; (2) *m*-[(2*R*,5*R*)-2-*tert*-butyl-3-methyl-5-oxazolidinyl]phenol mixture with *m*-[(2*S*,5*R*)-2-*tert*-butyl-3-methyl-5-oxazolidinyl]phenol. *CAS-105567-83-7*. INN. *Mydriatic. [Name previously used: Burefrine]*

Bergenin. $C_{14}H_{16}O_9$. 328.27. 3,4,4*a*,10*b*-Tetrahydro-3,4,8,10-tetrahydroxy-2-(hydroxymethyl)-9-methoxypyrano[3,2-*c*][2]benzopyran-6(*H*)-one. *UNII-L84RBE4IDC. CAS-477-90-7*. JAN.

Berlafenone. $C_{19}H_{25}NO_2$. 299.41. (±)-1-(2-Biphenylyloxy)-3-(*tert*-butylamino)-2-propanol. *UNII-4MYE3XA3GV. CAS-18965-97-4*. INN.

Bermastine — *See* Barmastine.

Bermoprofen. $C_{18}H_{16}O_4$. 296.32. (±)-10,11-Dihydro-α,8-dimethyl-11-oxodibenz[*b*,*f*]oxepin-2-acetic acid. *UNII-CWU66767HF. CAS-72619-34-2*. INN.

Beroctocog Alfa. $C_{3821}H_{5813}N_{1003}O_{1139}S_{35}$ + $C_{3547}H_{5400}N_{956}O_{1033}S_{35}$. Human blood-coagulation factor VIII-(1-740)-peptide complex with human blood-coagulation factor VIII-(1649-2332)-peptide. *CAS-9001-27-8*. INN.

Bertilimumab. Immunoglobulin G4, anti-(human eotaxin 1) (human monoclonal CAT-213 γ4-chain), disulfide with human monoclonal CAT 213 γ-chain, dimer. *CAS-375348-49-5*. INN; BAN.

Bertosamil. $C_{19}H_{36}N_2$. 292.50. 3'-Isobutyl-7'-isopropylspiro[cyclohexane-1,9'-[3,7]diazabicyclo[3.3.1]nonane]. *CAS-126825-36-3*. INN.

Berubicin Hydrochloride [*2007*] (be roo' bi sin hye" droe klor' ide). $C_{34}H_{35}NO_{11} \cdot HCl$. 670.10. [Berubicin is INN.] (1) 5,12-Naphthacenedione, 10-[[3-amino-2,3,6-trideoxy-4-*O*-(phenylmethyl)-α-L-*lyxo*-hexopyranosyl]oxy]-7,8,9,10-tetrahydro-6,8,11-trihydroxy-8-(hydroxyacetyl)-1-methoxy-, hydrochloride, (8*S*,10*S*)-; (2) (8*S*,10*S*)-10-[(3-Amino-4-*O*-benzyl-2,3,6-trideoxy-α-L-*lyxo*-hexopyranosyl)oxy]-6,8,11-trihydroxy-8-(hydroxyacetyl)-1-methoxy-7,8,9,10-tetrahydrotetracene-5,12-dione hydrochloride. *UNII-7BA3X03948. CAS-293736-67-1; CAS-677017-23-1* [berubicin]. *Treatment of cancer.* ◇*RTA 744; WP744*

Berupipam. $C_{19}H_{19}BrClNO_2$. 408.72. (+)-(5*S*)-5-(5-Bromo-2,3-dihydro-7-benzofuranyl)-8-chloro-2,3,4,5-tetrahydro-3-methyl-1*H*-3-benzazepin-7-ol. *CAS-150490-85-0*. INN.

Bervastatin. $C_{28}H_{31}FO_5$. 466.54. Ethyl $(\pm)$-$(3R^*,5S^*,6E)$-7-[4-(p-fluorophenyl)spiro[2H-1-benzopyran-2,1′-cyclopentan]-3-yl]-3,5-dihydroxy-6-heptenoate. *UNII-057SF9C1UZ. CAS-132017-01-7.* INN.

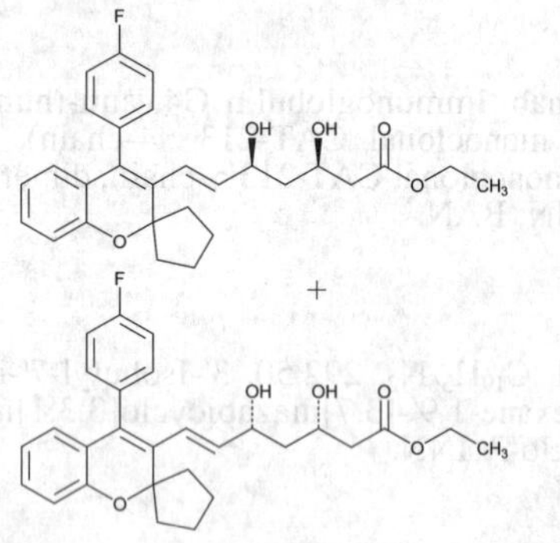

Berythromycin [*1971*] (be rith″ roe mye′ sin). $C_{37}H_{67}NO_{12}$. 717.93. (1) Erythromycin, 12-deoxy-; (2) 12-Deoxyerythromycin; (3) Erythromycin B. *CAS-527-75-3.* INN. *Antiamebic; antibacterial.* ◇Abbott-24091

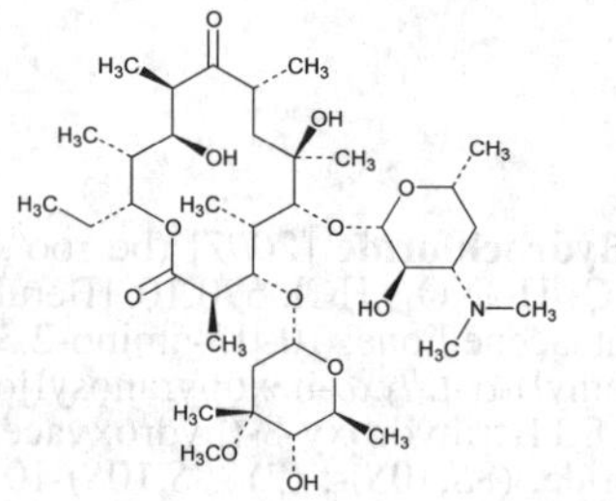

Besifloxacin Hydrochloride [*2007*] (be″ si flox′ a sin hye″ droe klor′ ide). $C_{19}H_{21}ClFN_3O_3 \cdot HCl$. 430.30. [Besifloxacin is INN.] (1) 3-Quinolinecarboxylic acid, 7-[(3R)-3-aminohexahydro-1H-azepin-1-yl]-8-chloro-1-cyclopropyl-6-fluoro-1,4-dihydro-4-oxo-, monohydrochloride; (2) (+)-7-[(3R)-3-Aminohexahydro-1H-azepin-1-yl]-8-chloro-1-cyclopropyl-6-fluoro-4-oxo-1,4-dihydroquinoline-3-carboxylic acid hydrochloride. *UNII-7506A6J57T. CAS-405165-61-9; CAS-141388-76-3* [besifloxacin]. *Anti-infective.* ◇SS734; BOL-303224-A

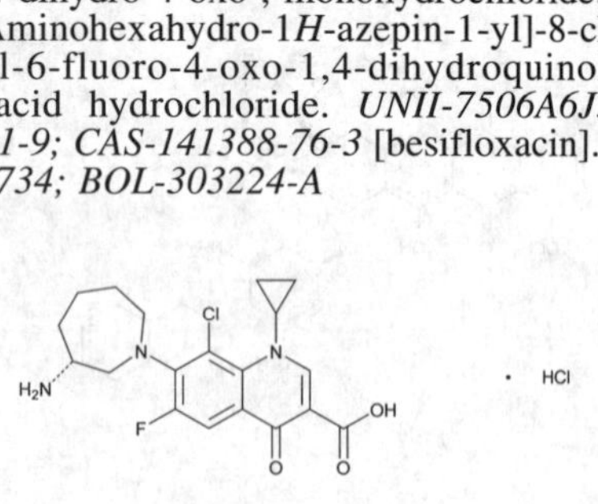

Besigomsin. $C_{23}H_{28}O_7$. 416.46. (+)-(6S,7S, biar-R)-5,6,7,8-Tetrahydro-1,2,3,13-tetramethoxy-6,7-dimethylbenzo[3,4]cycloocta[1,2-f][1,3]benzodioxol-6-ol. *UNII-L5U70J87J8. CAS-58546-54-6.* INN.

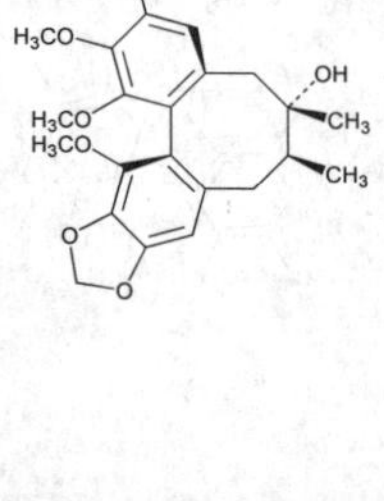

Besilesomab. Immunoglobulin G1, anti-(human CEA (carcinoembryonic antigen)-related antigen) (mouse monoclonal BW 250/183 heavy chain), disulfide with mouse monoclonal BW 250/183 κ-chain, dimer. *CAS-537694-98-7.* INN.

Besipirdine Hydrochloride [*1994*] (be si′ pir deen hye″ droe klor′ ide). $C_{16}H_{17}N_3 \cdot HCl$. 287.79. [Besipirdine is INN.] (1) 1H-Indol-1-amine, N-propyl-N-4-pyridinyl-, monohydrochloride; (2) 1-(Propyl-4-pyridylamino)indole monohydrochloride. *CAS-130953-69-4; CAS-119257-34-0* [besipirdine]. *Alzheimer's disease treatment (cognition enhancer).* ◇HP 749

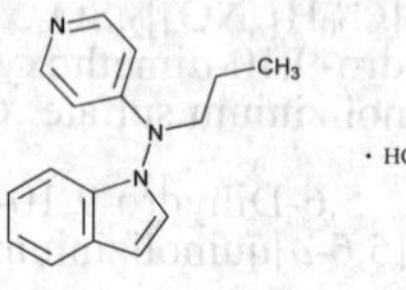

Besonprodil [*2002*] (be″ son proe′ dil). $C_{21}H_{23}FN_2O_3S$. 402.48. (1) 2(3H)-Benzoxazolone, 6-[[2-[4-[(4-fluorophenyl)methyl]-1-piperidinyl]ethyl]sulfinyl]; (2) 6-[2-[4-(4-Fluorobenzyl)-piperidin-1-yl]-ethanesulfinyl]-3H-benzoxazol-2-one. *CAS-253450-09-8. Treatment of Parkinson's Disease (NMDA receptor antagonist).* ◇CI-1041; PD 0196860; Co 200461

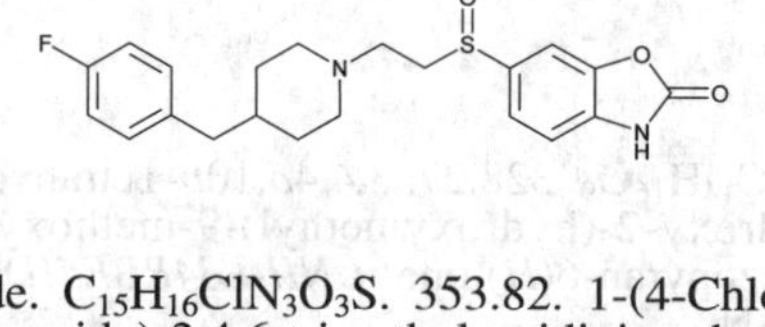

Besulpamide. $C_{15}H_{16}ClN_3O_3S$. 353.82. 1-(4-Chloro-3-sulfamoylbenzamido)-2,4,6-trimethylpyridinium hydroxide, inner salt. *UNII-048UJ2MM65. CAS-90992-25-9.* INN.

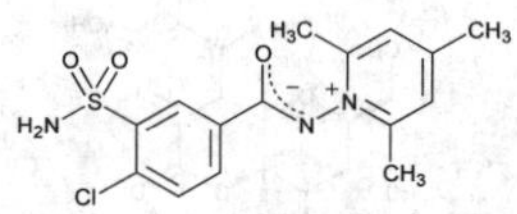

Besunide. $C_{18}H_{22}N_2O_4S$. 362.44. 3-(Butylamino)-α-phenyl-5-sulfamoyl-p-toluic acid. *UNII-P70VF8D9JJ. CAS-36148-38-6.* INN.

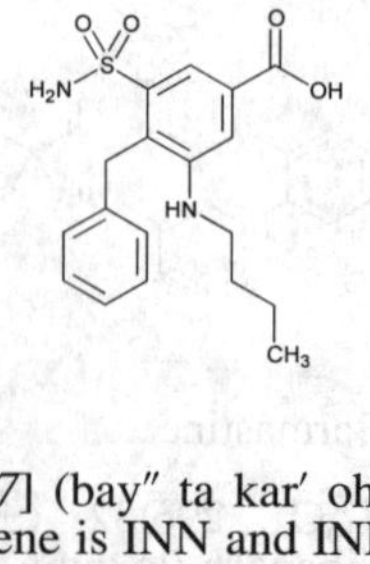

Beta Carotene [*1977*] (bay″ ta kar′ oh teen). **USP**. $C_{40}H_{56}$. 536.87. [Betacarotene is INN and INN.] (1) β,β-Carotene; (2) all-trans-β-Carotene; (3) (all-E)-1,1′-(3,7,12,16-Tetramethyl-1,3,5,7,9,11,13,15,17-octadecanonaene-1,18-diyl)-bis[2,6,6-trimethylcyclohexene]. *UNII-01YAE03M7J. CAS-7235-40-7. Ultraviolet screen.* BetaVit (BASF); Lucaratin (BASF); Solatene (Hoffmann-LaRoche)

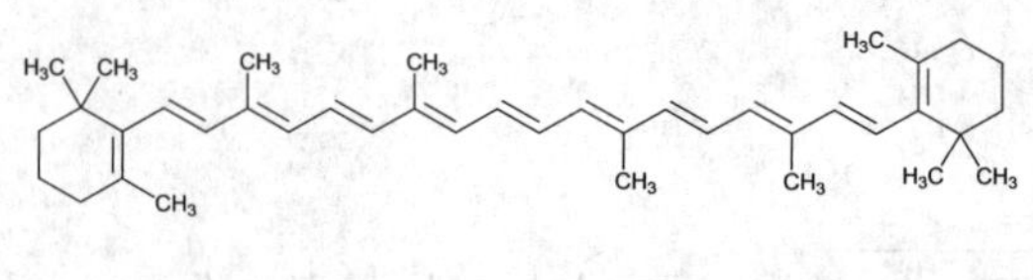

Betacarotene (INN) — *See* Beta Carotene.

Betacetylmethadol. $C_{23}H_{31}NO_2$. 353.50. (3*S*,6*R*)-3-Acetoxy-6-dimethylamino-4,4-diphenylheptane. *UNII-905GLN509G. CAS-17199-59-6.* INN; BAN.

Betadex [*1997*] (bay′ ta dex). **NF.** $C_{42}H_{70}O_{35}$. 1134.98. β-Cyclodextrin. *UNII-JV039JZZ3A. CAS-7585-39-9.* INN; BAN. *Pharmaceutic aid (sequestering agent). [Name previously used: Beta Cyclodextrin.]*

Beta-Estradiol Benzoate — *See* Estradiol Benzoate.

Betaeucaine Hydrochloride (previously used name) — *See* Eucaine Hydrochloride.

Betahistine Hydrochloride [*1962*] (bay″ ta his′ teen hye″ droe klor′ ide). **USP.** $C_8H_{12}N_2.2HCl$. 209.12. [Betahistine is INN and BAN; Betahistine Mesilate is JAN.] (1) 2-Pyridineethanamine, *N*-methyl-, dihydrochloride; (2) 2-[2-(Methylamino)ethyl]pyridine dihydrochloride. *UNII-49K58SMZ7U. CAS-5579-84-0; CAS-5638-76-6* [betahistine]. *Vasodilator.* Serc (Unimed) ◇*PT-9*

Betaine Hydrochloride (bee′ ta een hye″ droe klor′ ide). **USP.** $C_5H_{11}NO_2.HCl$. 153.61. (1) Methanaminium, 1-carboxy-*N,N,N*-trimethyl-, chloride; (2) Betaine hydrochloride; (3) (Carboxymethyl)trimethylammonium chloride. *CAS-590-46-5; CAS-141-58-2* [replaced]; *CAS-107-43-7* [betaine]. *Replenisher adjunct (electrolyte).* Cystadane (Rare)

Betameprodine. $C_{17}H_{25}NO_2$. 275.39. β-3-Ethyl-1-methyl-4-phenyl-4-propionyloxypiperidine. *UNII-4XS533X38C. CAS-468-50-8.* INN; BAN; DCF. ◇*Nu-1932*

Betamethadol. $C_{21}H_{29}NO$. 311.46. (3*S*,6*R*)-6-Dimethylamino-4,4-diphenyl-3-heptanol. *UNII-57ANR1Z628. CAS-17199-55-2.* INN; BAN; DCF.

---

† Brand name formerly used, and/or firm no longer concerned with this product.

Betamethasone [*1962*] (bay″ ta meth′ a sone). **USP.** $C_{22}H_{29}FO_5$. 392.46. (1) Pregna-1,4-diene-3,20-dione, 9-fluoro-11,17,21-trihydroxy-16-methyl-, (11β,16β)-; (2) 9-Fluoro-11β,17,21-trihydroxy-16β-methylpregna-1,4-diene-3,20-dione. *UNII-9842X06Q6M. CAS-378-44-9.* INN; BAN; JAN. *Glucocorticoid.* Celestone (Schering) ◇*Sch 4831; NSC-39470*

Betamethasone Acetate (bay″ ta meth′ a sone as′ e tate). **USP.** $C_{24}H_{31}FO_6$. 434.50. (1) Pregna-1,4-diene-3,20-dione, 9-fluoro-11,17-dihydroxy-16-methyl-21-(acetyloxy)-, (11β,16β)-; (2) 9-Fluoro-11β,17,21-trihydroxy-16β-methylpregna-1,4-diene-3,20-dione 21-acetate. *UNII-TI05AO53L7. CAS-987-24-6.* JAN. *Glucocorticoid.*

Betamethasone Acibutate. $C_{28}H_{37}FO_7$. 504.59. 9-Fluoro-11β,17,21-trihydroxy-16β-methylpregna-1,4-diene-3,20-dione 21-acetate 17-isobutyrate. *UNII-90I96070LY. CAS-5534-05-4.* INN; BAN.

Betamethasone Benzoate [*1969*] (bay″ ta meth′ a sone ben′ zoe ate). **USP.** $C_{29}H_{33}FO_6$. 496.57. (1) Pregna-1,4-diene-3,20-dione, 17-(benzoyloxy)-9-fluoro-11,21-dihydroxy-16-methyl-, (11β,16β)-; (2) 9-Fluoro-11β,17,21-trihydroxy-16β-methylpregna-1,4-diene-3,20-dione 17-benzoate. *UNII-877K0XW47A. CAS-22298-29-9. Glucocorticoid.* Uticort (Pfizer) ◇*W 5975*

Betamethasone Butyrate Propionate. $C_{29}H_{39}FO_7$. 518.61. (+)-9-Fluoro-11β,17,21-trihydroxy-16β-methylpregna-1,4-diene-3,20-dione 17-butyrate 21-propionate. *UNII-50FH5AG9RW. CAS-5534-02-1.* JAN.

Betamethasone Dipropionate [*1974*] (bay″ ta meth′ a sone dye proe′ pee oh nate). **USP.** $C_{28}H_{37}FO_7$. 504.59. (1) Pregna-1,4-diene-3,20-dione, 9-fluoro-11-hydroxy-16-methyl-17,21-bis(1-oxopropoxy)-, (11β,16β); (2) 9-Fluoro-11β,17,21-trihydroxy-16β-methylpregna-1,4-diene-3,20-dione 17,21-dipropionate. *UNII-826Y60901U. CAS-5593-20-4.* JAN. *Glucocorticoid.* Alphatrex (Savage); Diprolene (Schering); Diprosone (Schering) ◇*Sch 11460*

Betamethasone Sodium Phosphate (bay″ ta meth′ a sone soe′ dee um fos′ fate). **USP.** $C_{22}H_{28}FNa_2O_8P$. 516.40. (1) Pregna-1,4-diene-3,20-dione, 9-fluoro-11,17-dihydroxy-16-methyl-21-(phosphonooxy)-, disodium salt, (11β,16β)-; (2) 9-Fluoro-11β,17,21-trihydroxy-16β-methylpregna-1,4-diene-3,20-dione 21-(disodium phosphate). *UNII-7BK02SCL3W. CAS-151-73-5; CAS-360-63-4* [betamethasone dihydrogen phosphate]. JAN. *Glucocorticoid.* Celestone (Schering)

Betamethasone Valerate [*1969*] (bay″ ta meth′ a sone val′ er ate). **USP.** $C_{27}H_{37}FO_6$. 476.58. (1) Pregna-1,4-diene-3,20-dione, 9-fluoro-11,21-dihydroxy-16-methyl-17-[(1-oxopentyl)oxy]-, (11β,16β)-; (2) 9-Fluoro-11β,17,21-trihydroxy-16β-methylpregna-1,4-diene-3,20-dione 17-valerate. *UNII-9IFA5XM7R2. CAS-2152-44-5.* JAN. *Glucocorticoid.* Beta-val (Teva); Betaderm (Roaco); Betatrex (Savage); Dermabet (Taro); Luxiq (Connetics); Valisone (Schering); Valnac (Actavis)

Betamicin Sulfate [*1974*] (bay″ ta mye′ sin sul′ fate). $C_{19}H_{38}N_4O_{10}.xH_2SO_4$. 482.53 (base). [Betamicin is INN.] (1) D-Streptamine, *O*-6-amino-6-deoxy-α-D-glucopyranosyl-(1→4)-*O*-[3-deoxy-4-*C*-methyl-3-(methylamino)-β-L-arabinopyranosyl-(1→6)]-2-deoxy-, sulfate; (2) *O*-6-Amino-6-deoxy-α-D-glucopyranosyl-(1→4)-*O*-[3-deoxy-4-*C*-methyl-3-(methylamino)-β-L-arabinopyranosyl-(1→6)]-2-deoxy-D-streptamine sulfate. *UNII-FO90AO023F. CAS-43169-50-2; CAS-36889-15-3* [betamicin]. *Antibacterial.* ◇*Sch 14342*

Betamipron. $C_{10}H_{11}NO_3$. 193.20. *N*-Benzoyl-β-alanine. *UNII-3W0M245736. CAS-3440-28-6.* INN; JAN.

Betanaphthol. *UNII-P2Z71CIK5H. CAS-135-19-3.* NF XI.

Betanidine (INN, BAN) — *See* Bethanidine Sulfate.

Betanidine Sulfate (JAN) — *See* Bethanidine Sulfate.

Betaprodine. $C_{16}H_{23}NO_2$. 261.36. β-1,3-Dimethyl-4-phenyl-4-propionyloxypiperidine. *UNII-21J54X4Z4Z. CAS-468-59-7.* INN; BAN; DCF. ◇*Nu-1779*

Betasizofiran. $(C_{24}H_{40}O_{20})_n$. Scleroglucan or poly[→3(*O*-β-D-glucopyranosyl-(1→3)-*O*-[β-D-glucopyranosyl-(1→6)]-*O*-β-D-glucopyranosyl-(1→3)-*O*-β-D-glucopyranosyl-(1→] produced by *Sclerotium rolfsii*. Relative molecular mass is about 5.10^6. *CAS-39464-87-4.* INN.

Betaxolol Hydrochloride [*1983*] (be tax′ oh lol hye″ droe klor′ ide). **USP.** $C_{18}H_{29}NO_3.HCl$. 343.89. [Betaxolol is INN and BAN.] (1) 2-Propanol, 1-[4-[2-(cyclopropylmethoxy)ethyl]phenoxy]-3-[(1-methylethyl)amino]-, hydrochloride, (±)-; (2) (±)-1-[*p*-[2-(Cyclopropylmethoxy)ethyl]phenoxy]-3-(isopropylamino)-2-propanol hydrochloride. *UNII-6X97D2XT0O; UNII-O0ZR1R6RZ2* [betaxolol]. *CAS-63659-19-8; CAS-63659-18-7* [betaxolol]. JAN. *Anti-anginal; antihypertensive.* Betoptic (Alcon); Kerlone (Sanofi Aventis) ◇*SL 75.212-10; ALO 1401-02*

Betazole Hydrochloride. $C_5H_9N_3.2HCl$. 184.07. [Betazole is INN; Ametazole is BAN.] (1) 1*H*-Pyrazole-3-ethanamine, dihydrochloride; (2) 3-(2-Aminoethyl)pyrazole dihydrochloride. *UNII-66ABP6C83F; UNII-1C065P542O* [betazole]. *CAS-138-92-1; CAS-105-20-4* [betazole]. USP XX; JAN; MI. Histalog (Lilly)

Betazolium Chloride — *See* Betazole Hydrochloride.

Bethanechol Chloride (be than′ e kol klor′ ide). **USP.** $C_7H_{17}ClN_2O_2$. 196.68. (1) 1-Propanaminium, 2-[(aminocarbonyl)oxy]-*N,N,N*-trimethyl-, chloride, (±)-; (2) (±)-(2-Hydroxypropyl)trimethylammonium chloride carbamate. *UNII-H4QBZ2LO84. CAS-590-63-6; CAS-674-38-4* [bethanechol]. BAN; JAN. *Cholinergic.* Duvoid (WellSpring); Myotonachol (Glenwood); Urecholine (Odyssey)

Bethanidine Sulfate [*1962*] (be than′ i deen sul′ fate). $C_{10}H_{15}N_3.\frac{1}{2}H_2SO_4$. 226.29. [Betanidine is INN and BAN; Betanidine Sulfate is JAN.] (1) Guanidine, *N,N*′-dimethyl-*N*″-(phenylmethyl)-, sulfate (2:1); (2) 1-Benzyl-2,3-dimethylguanidine sulfate (1:½). *UNII-J4THI5N7O2. CAS-114-85-2; CAS-55-73-2* [bethanidine]. *Antihypertensive.* ◇*BW-467-C-60; NSC-106563*

Betiatide [*1990*] (be tye′ a tide). $C_{15}H_{17}N_3O_6S$. 367.38. (1) Glycine, *N*-[*N*-[*N*-[(benzoylthio)acetyl]glycyl]glycyl]-; (2) *N*-[*N*-[*N*-(Mercaptoacetyl)glycyl]glycyl]glycine benzoate (ester); (3) Thiobenzoic acid, *S*-ester with *N*-[*N*-[*N*-(mercaptoacetyl)glycyl]glycyl]glycine. *UNII-9NV2SR34P8. CAS-103725-47-9.* INN; BAN. *Pharmaceutic aid.* ◇*MP-600*

Betoxycaine Hydrochloride. $C_{19}H_{32}N_2O_4$·HCl. 388.93. [Betoxycaine is INN.] 2-[2-(Diethylamino)ethoxy]ethyl 3-amino-4-butoxybenzoate hydrochloride. *UNII-8II47759Z3; UNII-03DB58Y9DO* [betoxycaine]. *CAS-5003-47-4; CAS-3818-62-0* [betoxycaine]. MI.

Betrixaban [*2007*] (be trix′ a ban). $C_{23}H_{22}ClN_5O_3$. 451.91. (1) Benzamide, *N*-(5-chloro-2-pyridinyl)-2-[[4-[(dimethylamino)iminomethyl]benzoyl]amino]-5-methoxy-; (2) *N*-(5-Chloropyridin-2-yl)-2-[[4-(*N,N*-dimethylcarbamimidoyl)-benzoyl]amino]-5-methoxybenzamide. *UNII-74RWP7W0J9. CAS-330942-05-7.* INN. *Antithrombotic, prevention of deep vein thrombosis and pulmonary embolism after surgery.* ◇*PRT054021*

Betula Oil — *See* Methyl Salicylate.

Bevacizumab [*1999*] (bev″ a siz′ oo mab). $C_{6638}H_{10160}N_{1720}O_{2108}S_{44}$. Immunoglobulin G 1 (human-mouse monoclonal rhuMAb-VEGF γ-chain anti-human vascular endothelial growth factor), disulfide with human-mouse monoclonal rhuMAb-VEGF light chain, dimer. *UNII-2S9ZZM9Q9V. CAS-216974-75-3.*

Bevantolol Hydrochloride [*1980*] (be van′ toe lol hye″ droe klor′ ide). $C_{20}H_{27}NO_4$·HCl. 381.89. [Bevantolol is INN and BAN.] (1) 2-Propanol, 1-[[2-(3,4-dimethoxyphenyl)ethyl]amino]-3-(3-methylphenoxy)-, (±)-; (2) (±)-1-[(3,4-Dimethoxyphenethyl)amino]-3-(*m*-tolyloxy)-2-propanol hydrochloride. *UNII-34ZXW6ZV21. CAS-*

42864-78-8; CAS-59170-23-9 [bevantolol]. JAN. *Antianginal; antihypertensive; cardiac depressant (anti-arrhythmic).* Vantol (Parke-Davis†) ◇*Cl-775*

Bevasiranib Sodium [*2007*] (bev″ a sir′ a nib soe′ dee um). $C_{401}H_{463}N_{153}Na_{40}O_{290}P_{40}$. 14,224.00. [Bevasiranib is INN.] (1) RNA, (A-C-C-U-C-A-C-C-A-A-G-G-C-C-A-G-C-A-C-dT-dT), eicosasodium salt, complex with RNA (G-U-G-C-U-G-G-C-C-U-U-G-G-U-G-A-G-G-U-dT-dT) eicosasodium salt (1:1); (2) Duplex of thymidylyl-(3′→5′)-thymidylyl-(3′→5′)-uridylyl-(3′→5′)-guanylyl-(3′→5′)-guanylyl-(3′→5′)-adenylyl-(3′→5′)-guanylyl-(3′→5′)-uridylyl-(3′→5′)-guanylyl-(3′→5′)-guanylyl-(3′→5′)-uridylyl-(3′→5′)-uridylyl-(3′→5′)-cytidylyl-(3′→5′)-cytidylyl-(3′→5′)-guanylyl-(3′→5′)-guanylyl-(3′→5′)-uridylyl-(3′→5′)-cytidylyl-(3′→5′)-guanylyl-(3′→5′)-uridylyl-(3′→5′)-guanosine and thymidylyl-(3′→5′)-thymidylyl-(3′→5′)-cytidylyl-(3′→5′)-adenylyl-(3′→5′)-cytidylyl-(3′→5′)-guanylyl-(3′→5′)-adenylyl-(3′→5′)-cytidylyl-(3′→5′)-cytidylyl-(3′→5′)-guanylyl-(3′→5′)-guanylyl-(3′→5′)-adenylyl-(3′→5′)-adenylyl-(3′→5′)-cytidylyl-(3′→5′)-cytidylyl-(3′→5′)-adenylyl-(3′→5′)-cytidylyl-(3′→5′)-uridylyl-(3′→5′)-cytidylyl-(3′→5′)-cytidylyl-(3′→5′)-adennosine, tetracontasodium salt. *CAS-849758-52-7; CAS-959961-96-7* [bevasiranib]. *Treatment of wet age-related macular degeneration.* ◇*Cand5*

Bevirimat Dimeglumine [*2006*] (be vir′ i mat di me′ gloo meen). $C_{36}H_{56}O_6$·$2C_7H_{17}NO_5$. 975.25. [Bevirimat is INN.] (1) Lup-20(29)-en-28-oic acid, 3-(3-carboxy-3-methyl-1-oxobutoxy)-, (3β)-, compd. with 1-deoxy-1-(methylamino)-D-glucitol (1:2); (2) Bis[1-deoxy-1-(methylamino)-D-glucitol] 3β-(3-carboxylato-3-methylbutanoyloxy)lup-20(29)-en-28-oate. *UNII-O6DDV91W1M. CAS-823821-85-8; CAS-174022-42-5* [bevirimat]. *Treatment of HIV infection.* ◇*PA-457; PA-457N; PA103001; PA103001-01; PA103001-04; PA-457 di-NMG; DSB*2NMG*

Bevonium Metilsulfate. $C_{23}H_{31}NO_7S$. 465.56. [Bevonium Methylsulfate is JAN.] 2-(Hydroxymethyl)-1,1-dimethyl-piperidinium methyl sulfate benzilate. *UNII-UW-C15E373Z; UNII-34B0471E08* [bevonium]. *CAS-5205-82-3; CAS-33371-53-8* [bevonium]. INN; BAN; MI. *[Name previously used: Bevonium Methylsulphate.]* ◇*CG 201*

Bexarotene [*1998*] (bex ar′ oh teen). $C_{24}H_{28}O_2$. 348.48. (1) 4-[1-(5,6,7,8-Tetrahydro-3,5,5,8,8-pentamethyl-2-naphthalenyl)ethenyl]benzoic acid; (2) *p*-[1-(5,6,7,8-Tetrahydro-

―――――――――

† Brand name formerly used, and/or firm no longer concerned with this product.

3,5,5,8,8-pentamethyl-2-naphthyl)vinyl]benzoic acid. *UNII-A61RXM4375*. *CAS-153559-49-0*. INN; BAN. *Antineoplastic used in the treatment of cutaneous T-cell lymphoma; antidiabetic.* Targretin (Eisai Medical Research) ◇*LGD1069; LG100069*

Bexlosteride [*1998*] (bex loe′ ster ide). $C_{14}H_{16}ClNO$. 249.74. (1) Benzo[*f*]quinolin-3(2*H*)-one, 8-chloro-1,4,4a,5,6,10b-hexahydro-4-methyl-, (4a*R-trans*); (2) (4a*R*,10b*R*)-8-Chloro-1,4,4a,5,6,10b-hexahydro-4-methylbenzo[*f*]quinolin-3(2*H*)-one. *CAS-148905-78-6*. INN. *Treatment of prostate cancer (inhibits human type I isoform of 5α-reductase).* ◇*LY300502*

Bezafibrate [*1978*] (be″ za fye′ brate). $C_{19}H_{20}ClNO_4$. 361.82. (1) Propanoic acid, 2-[4-[2-[(4-chlorobenzoyl)amino]ethyl]phenoxy]-2-methyl-; (2) 2-[*p*-[2-(*p*-Chlorobenzamido)ethyl]phenoxy]-2-methylpropionic acid. *CAS-41859-67-0*. INN; BAN; JAN. *Antihyperlipoproteinemic.* ◇*BM 15.075*

Bezitramide. $C_{31}H_{32}N_4O_2$. 492.61. 1-(3-Cyano-3,3-diphenyl-propyl)-4-(2-oxo-3-propionyl-1-benzimidazolinyl)piperidine. *UNII-3KXW0Y310I*. *CAS-15301-48-1*. INN; BAN; DCF; MI. ◇*R 4845*

Bialamicol Hydrochloride [*1962*] (bye″ a lam′ i kol hye″ droe klor′ ide). $C_{28}H_{40}N_2O_2$·2HCl. 509.55. [Bialamicol is INN and BAN.] (1) [1,1′-Biphenyl]-4,4′-diol, 3,3′-bis[(-diethylamino)methyl]-5,5′-di-2-propenyl-, dihydrochloride; (2) 5,5′-Diallyl-α,α′-bis(diethylamino)-*m,m*′-bitolyl-4,4′-diol dihydrochloride. *UNII-VIQ3X36S8C*. *CAS-3624-*

96-2; *CAS-493-75-4* [bialamicol]. *Anti-amebic.* Camoform Hydrochloride (Parke-Davis†) ◇*CAM-807; CI-301; PAA-701; NSC-6386*

Biantrazole (previously used name for the free base) — *See* Losoxantrone Hydrochloride.

Biapenem [*1993*] (bye″ a pen′ em). $C_{15}H_{18}N_4O_4S$. 350.39. (1) 5*H*-Pyrazolo[1,2-a][1,2,4]triazol-4-ium, 6-[[2-carboxy-6-(1-hydroxyethyl)-4-methyl-7-oxo-1-azabicyclo[3.2.0]hept-2-en-3-yl]thio]-6,7-dihydro-, hydroxide, inner salt, [4*R*-[4α,5β,6β(*R**)]]-; (2) 6-[[(4*R*,5*S*,6*S*)-2-Carboxy-6-[(1*R*)-1-hydroxyethyl]-4-methyl-7-oxo-1-azabicyclo[3.2.0]hept-2-en-3-yl]thio]-6,7-dihydro-5*H*-pyrazolo[1,2-*a*]-*s*-triazol-4-ium hydroxide, inner salt. *UNII-YR5U3L9ZH1*. *CAS-120410-24-4*. INN. *Antibacterial.* ◇*LJ C10,627; L-627; CL 186,815*

Bibapcitide [*1997*] (bye bap′ si tide). $C_{112}H_{162}N_{36}O_{43}S_{10}$·3021.35. 13,13′-[Oxybis[methylene(2,5-dioxo-1,3-pyrrolidinediyl)]]bis[*N*-(mercaptoacetyl)-D-tyrosyl-*S*-(3-amino-propyl)-L-cysteinylglycyl-L-α-aspartyl-L-cysteinylglycyl glycyl-*S*-(acetamidomethyl)-L-cysteinylglycyl-*S*-(acetamidomethyl)-L-cysteinyl glycylglycyl-L-cysteinamide, cyclic (1→5), (1→5′)-bis(sulfide). *CAS-153507-46-1*. INN; BAN. *Radionuclide carrier. [Note—Bibapcitide is the starting material which combines with the radiodiagnostic sodium pertechnetate to yield technetium Tc 99m apcitide.]* ◇*P280*

Bibenzonium Bromide. $C_{19}H_{26}BrNO$. 364.32. [2-(1,2-Diphenylethoxy)ethyltrimethyl]ammonium bromide. *UNII-4455J9277Q; UNII-34YTZ517S2* [bibenzonium]. *CAS-15585-70-3; CAS-59866-76-1* [bibenzonium]. INN; BAN; MI.

Bibrocathin — *See* Bibrocathol.

Bibrocathol. $C_6HBiBr_4O_3$. 649.67. Bismuth derivative of tetrabromopyrocatechol. *UNII-0KJ20H1BLJ*. *CAS-6915-57-7*. INN; DCF; MI.

Bicalutamide [*1994*] (bye″ ka loo′ ta mide). $C_{18}H_{14}F_4N_2O_4S$. 430.37. (1) Propanamide, *N*-[4-cyano-3-(trifluoromethyl)-phenyl]-3-[(4-fluorophenyl)sulfonyl]-2-hydroxy-2-methyl-, (±)-; (2) (±)-4′-Cyano-α,α,α-trifluoro-3-[(*p*-fluorophenyl)sulfonyl]-2-methyl-*m*-lactotoluidide. *UNII-A0Z3NAU9DP. CAS-90357-06-5.* INN; BAN. *Antineoplastic.* Casodex (AstraZeneca) ◇*ICI 176,334*

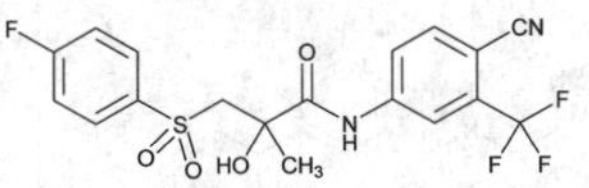

Bicifadine Hydrochloride [*1979*] (bye sif′ a deen hye″ droe klor′ ide). $C_{12}H_{15}N.HCl.$ 209.72. [Bicifadine is INN.] (1) 3-Azabicyclo[3.1.0]hexane, 1-(4-methylphenyl)-, hydrochloride, (±)-; (2) (±)-1-*p*-Tolyl-3-azabicyclo[3.1.0]hexane hydrochloride. *UNII-OE6G20P68T. CAS-66504-75-4; CAS-71195-57-8* [bicifadine]. *Analgesic.* ◇*CL 220,075*

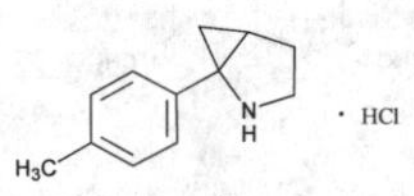

Bicillin V₂. Phenoxymethylpenicillin benzathine compound with phenoxymethylpenicillin potassium. JAN.

Biciromab [*1993*] (bye sir′ oh mab). (1) Immunoglobulin G (mouse monoclonal T2G1s Fab′ fragment anti-human fibrin II β-chain), disulfide with mouse monoclonal T2G1s light chain; (2) Immunoglobulin G (mouse monoclonal T2G1s Fab′ fragment anti-human fibrin II β-chain), disulfide with mouse monoclonal T2G1s light chain. Molecular weight is approximately 50,000 daltons. *CAS-138783-13-8; CAS-138783-14-9* [technetium Tc 99m biciromab]. INN; BAN. *Monoclonal antibody (antifibrin).* Fibriscint (Centocor†) *[Note—The radiolabeled product used in the diagnosis of deep vein thrombosis has the nonproprietary name technetium Tc 99m biciromab.]* ◇*T2G1s*

Biclodil Hydrochloride [*1984*] (bye′ kloe dil hye″ droe klor′ ide). $C_8H_8Cl_2N_4O.HCl.$ 283.54. [Biclodil is INN.] (1) Urea, [[[(2,6-dichlorophenyl)amino]iminomethyl]-, monohydrochloride; (2) [(2,6-Dichlorophenyl)amidino]urea monohydrochloride. *UNII-S9RZW428WX. CAS-75564-40-8; CAS-85125-49-1* [biclodil]. *Antihypertensive (vasodilator).* ◇*WHR-1051B*

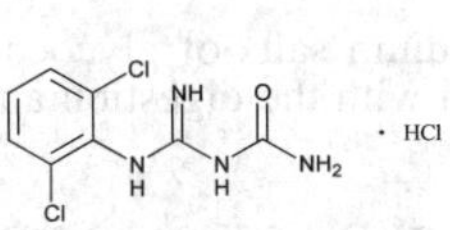

Biclofibrate. $C_{20}H_{21}Cl_2NO_4.$ 410.29. Bis(*p*-chlorophenoxy)-acetic acid, 1-methyl-2-pyrrolidinylmethyl ester. *UNII-73U81R979T. CAS-54063-27-3.* INN; DCF.

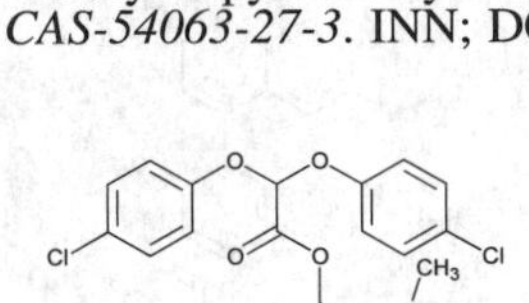

Biclotymol. $C_{21}H_{26}Cl_2O_2.$ 381.34. 2,2′-Methylenebis(6-chlorothymole). *UNII-W4K0AE8XW9. CAS-15686-33-6.* INN; DCF.

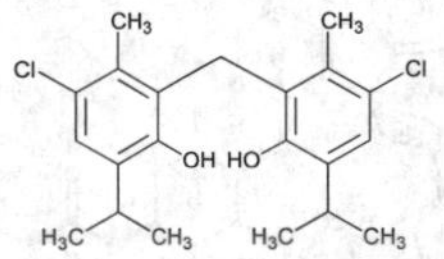

Bicozamicin. $C_{12}H_{18}N_2O_7.$ 302.28. Bicyclomycin. *CAS-38129-37-2.* INN; MI.

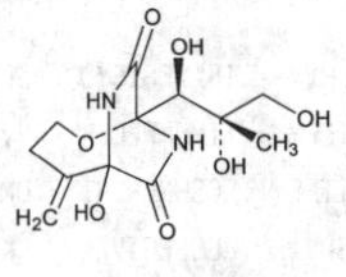

Bidimazium Iodide. $C_{26}H_{25}IN_2S.$ 524.46. 4-(4-Biphenylyl)-2-[*p*-(dimethylamino)styryl]-3-methylthiazolium iodide. *UNII-2D4432ZP6M. CAS-21817-73-2.* INN; BAN. ◇*65-318*

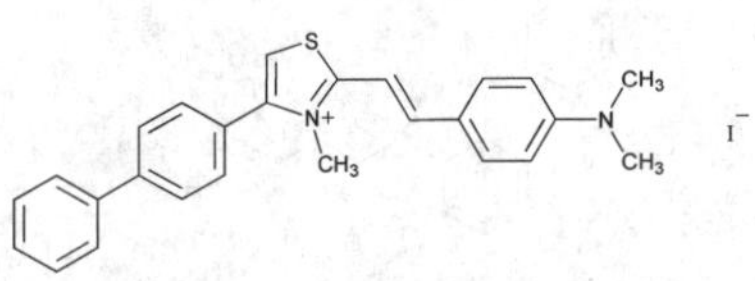

Bidisomide [*1990*] (bye dis′ oh mide). $C_{22}H_{34}ClN_3O_2.$ 407.98. (1) 1-Piperidinebutanamide, α-[2-[acetyl(1-methylethyl)amino]ethyl]-α-(2-chlorophenyl)-, (±)-; (2) (±)-α-(*o*-Chlorophenyl)-α-[2-(*N*-isopropylacetamido)ethyl]-1-piperidinebutyramide. *CAS-103810-45-3.* INN. *Cardiac depressant (anti-arrhythmic).* ◇*SC-40230*

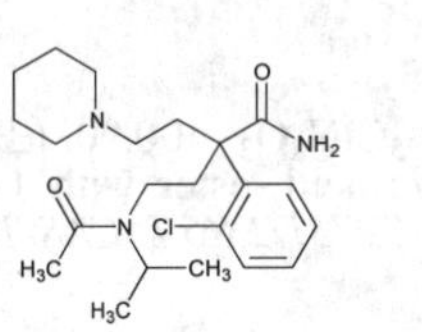

Biebrich Scarlet Red — *See* Scarlet Red.

Bietamiverine Hydrochloride. $C_{19}H_{30}N_2O_2.HCl.$ 354.91. [Bietamiverine is INN.] 2-Diethylaminoethyl α-phenyl-1-piperidineacetate hydrochloride. *UNII-646WTQ0G3E. CAS-479-81-2* [bietamiverine]. MI.

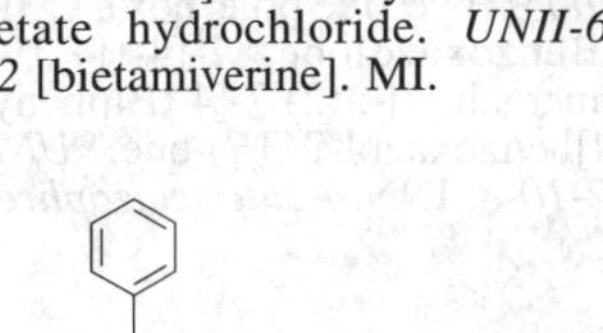

Bietaserpine. $C_{39}H_{53}N_3O_9.$ 707.85. (1) Methyl 13-[2-(diethylamino)ethyl]-1,2,3,4,4aα,5,7,8,13,13bβ,14,14aα-dodecahydro-2α,11-dimethoxy-3β-[(3,4,5-trimethoxybenzoyl)oxy]benz[*g*]indolo[2,3-*a*]quinolizine-1β-carboxylate; (2) Methyl 1-[2-(diethylamino)ethyl]-18β-hydroxy-11,17α-di-

---

methoxy-3β,20α-yohimban-16β-carboxylate, 3,4,5-trimethoxybenzoate (ester). *UNII-0P5B94FVD5. CAS-53-18-9.* INN; DCF; MI. ◇*DL 152; S-1210*

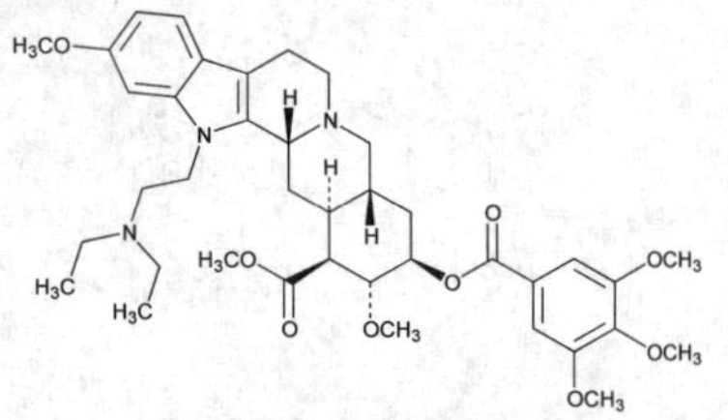

Bifarcept. $C_{1100}H_{1673}N_{271}O_{337}S_{10}$. Interferon α/β receptor (human isoform p40 precursor). *CAS-163796-60-9.* INN.

```
MLLSQNAFIV   RSLNLVLMVY   ISLVFGISYD   SPDYTDESCT   FKISLRNFRS
ILSWELKNHS   IVPTHYTLLY   TIMSKPEDLK   VVKNCANTTR   SFCDLTDEWR
STHEAYVTVL   EGFSGNTTLF   SCSHNFWLAI   DMSFEPPEFE   IVGFTNHINV
MVKFPSIVEE   ELQFDLSLVI   EEQSEGIVKK   HKPEIKGNMS   GNFTYIIDKL
IPNTNYCVSV   YLEHSDEQAV   IKSPLKCTLL   PPGQESEFS
```

Bifemelane. $C_{18}H_{23}NO$. 269.38. [Bifemelane Hydrochloride is JAN.] *N*-Methyl-4-[(α-phenyl-*o*-tolyl)oxy]butylamine. *CAS-90293-01-9.* INN; MI.

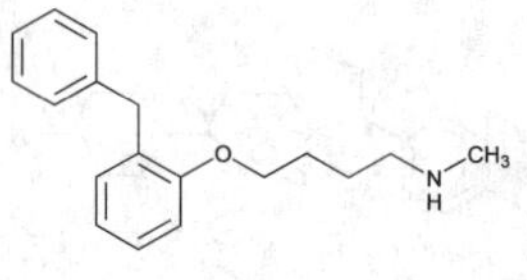

Bifepramide. $C_{21}H_{28}N_2O$. 324.46. (±)-*N*-[2-(Diethylamino)ethyl]-α-methyl-4-biphenylacetamide. *UNII-B1H2FS2WPP. CAS-70976-76-0.* INN.

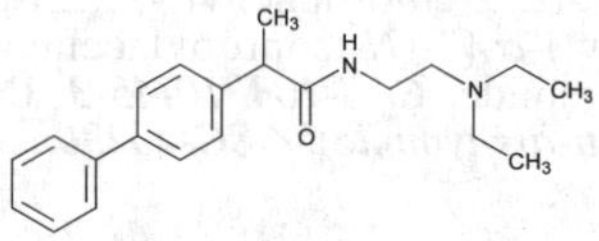

Bifeprofen. $C_{22}H_{25}ClN_2O_3$. 400.90. (±)-2′-Chloro-α-methyl-4-biphenylacetic acid, ester with 1-glycoloyl-4-methylpiperazine. *UNII-99731EX5X. CAS-108210-73-7.* INN.

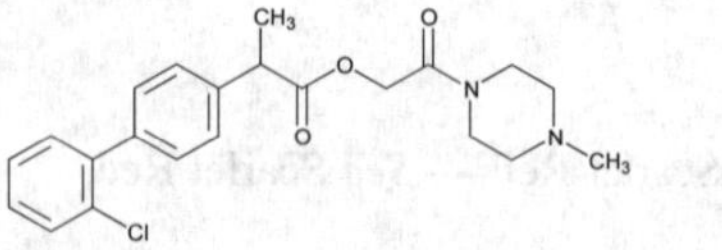

Bifeprunox [*2005*] (bye″ fee prue′ nox). $C_{24}H_{23}N_3O_2$. 385.46. (1) 2(3*H*)-Benzoxazolone, 7-[4-([1,1′-biphenyl]-3-yl-methyl)-1-piperazinyl]-; (2) 7-[4-(Biphenyl-3-ylmethyl)piperazin-1-yl]benzoxazol-2(3*H*)-one. *UNII-AP69E83Z79. CAS-350992-10-8.* INN. *Acute schizophrenia.*

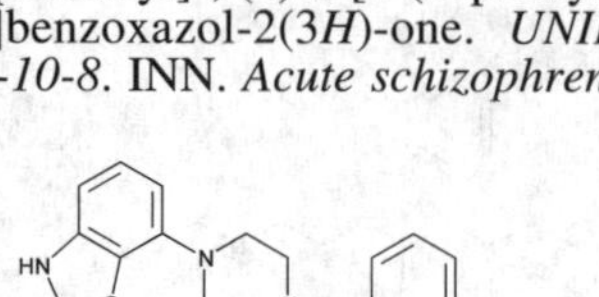

Bifeprunox Mesylate [*2005*] (bye″ fee prue′ nox mes′ i late). $C_{24}H_{23}N_3O_2 \cdot CH_4O_3S$. 481.56. (1) 2(3*H*)-Benzoxazolone, 7-[4-([1,1′-biphenyl]-3-ylmethyl)-1-piperazinyl]-, monomethanesulfonate; (2) 7-[4-(Biphenyl-3-ylmethyl)pipera-

zin-1-yl]benzoxazol-2(3*H*)-one methanesulfonate. *CAS-350992-13-1. Treatment of acute schizophrenia (partial D₂antagonist/5HT₁Aagonist).* ◇*DU127090*

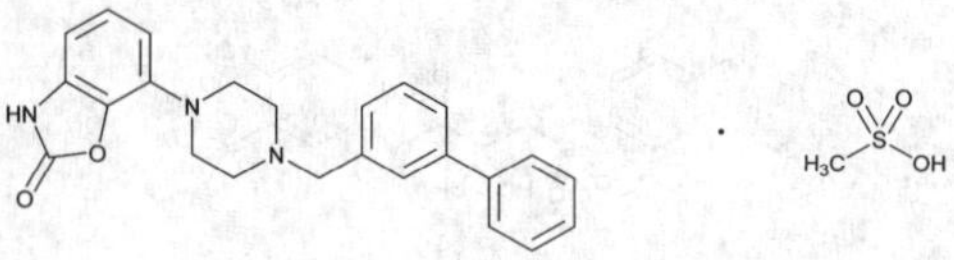

Bifluranol. $C_{17}H_{18}F_2O_2$. 292.32. *erythro*-4,4′-(1-Ethyl-2-methylethylene)-bis[2-fluorophenol]. *UNII-47602X79JF. CAS-34633-34-6.* INN; BAN; MI. ◇*BX 341*

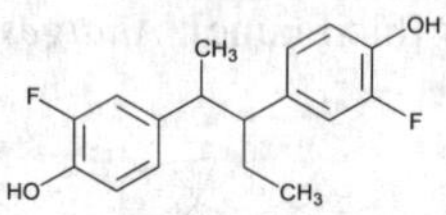

Bifonazole [*1981*] (bye fone′ a zole). $C_{22}H_{18}N_2$. 310.39. (1) 1*H*-Imidazole, 1-([1,1′-biphenyl]-4-ylphenylmethyl)-, (±)-; (2) (±)-1-(*p*,α-Diphenylbenzyl)imidazole. *CAS-60628-96-8.* INN; BAN; JAN. *Antifungal.* Mycospor (Bayer†) ◇*Bay h 4502*

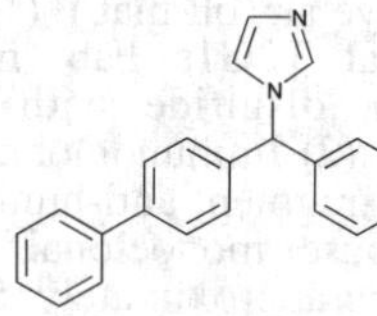

Bilastine. $C_{28}H_{37}N_3O_3$. 463.61. *p*-[2-[4-[1-(2-Ethoxyethyl)-2-benzimidazolyl]piperidino]ethyl]-α-methylhydratropic acid. *UNII-PA1123N395. CAS-202189-78-4.* INN.

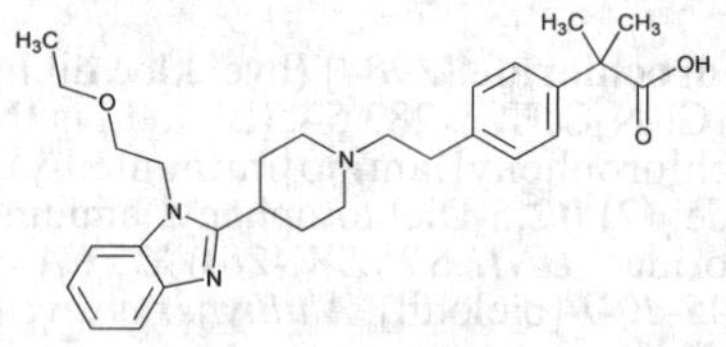

Bile Salts. The sodium salts of glycocholic and taurocholic acids, concerned with the digestion and absorption of fats. BAN.

Bimakalim. $C_{17}H_{14}N_2O_2$. 278.31. 2,2-Dimethyl-4-(2-oxo-1-(2*H*)-pyridyl)-2*H*-1-benzopyran-6-carbonitrile. *CAS-117545-11-6.* INN.

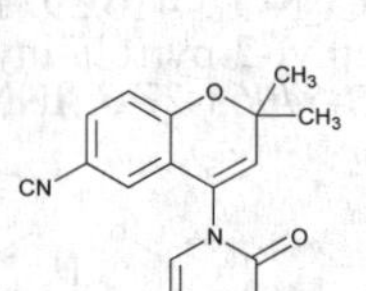

Bimatoprost [*2001*] (bye mat′ oh prost). $C_{25}H_{37}NO_4$. 415.57. (1) 5-Heptenamide, 7-[3,5-dihydroxy-2-(3-hydroxy-5-phenyl-1-pentenyl)cyclopentyl]-*N*-ethyl-, [1*R*-1[α(*Z*),2β(1*E*,3*S**)3α,5α]]-; (2) (*Z*)-7-[(1*R*,2*R*,3*R*,5*S*)-3,5-Dihydroxy-2-[(1*E*,3*S*)-3-hydroxy-5-phenyl-1-pentenyl]cyclopentyl]-*N*-ethyl-5-heptenamide. *UNII-QXS94885MZ. CAS-155206-00-1.* INN; BAN; JAN. *Lowers intraocular*

pressure (IOP) in patients with open angle glaucoma or ocular hypertension (synthetic prostamide analog). Lumigan (Allergan) ◇*AGN 192024*

Bimethadol — *See* Dimepheptanol.

Bimethoxycaine Lactate. *UNII-C4V95L5P6A. CAS-24407-55-4.* JAMA 149:1399 (1952).

Bimoclomol. $C_{14}H_{20}ClN_3O_2$. 297.78. ($\pm$)-*N*-(2-Hydroxy-3-piperidinopropoxy)nicotinimidoyl chloride. *CAS-130493-03-7.* INN.

Bimosiamose. $C_{46}H_{54}O_{16}$. 862.91. [Hexane-1,6-diylbis[6'-(α-D-mannopyranosyloxy)biphenyl-3',3-diyl]]diacetic acid. *UNII-97B5KCW80W. CAS-187269-40-5.* INN.

Bimosiamose Disodium [*2000*] (bye″ moe sye′ a mose dye soe′ dee um). $C_{46}H_{52}Na_2O_{16}$. 906.88. (1) [1,1'-Biphenyl]-3-acetic acid, 3',3'''-(1,6-hexanediyl)bis[6'-(α-D-mannopyranosyloxy)-, disodium salt; (2) Disodium 3',3'''-hexamethylenebis[6'-α-D-mannopyranosyloxy)-3-biphenylacetate). *UNII-7AK2FKB9AW. CAS-187269-60-9. Antiinflammatory (treatment of asthma; organ reperfusion injury in transplant or coronary revascularization; treatment of psoriasis).* ◇*TBC1269z*

Bindarit [*1992*] (bin′ da rit). $C_{19}H_{20}N_2O_3$. 324.37. (1) Propanoic acid, 2-methyl-2-[[1-(phenylmethyl)-1*H*-indazol-3-yl]methoxy]-; (2) 2-[(1-Benzyl-1*H*-indazol-3-yl)methoxy]-2-methylpropionic acid. *CAS-130641-38-2.* INN. *Antirheumatic.* ◇*AF 2838*

Bindazac — *See* Bendazac.

Binedaline. $C_{19}H_{23}N_3$. 293.41. 1-[[2-(Dimethylamino)ethyl]methylamino]-3-phenylindole. *UNII-3AVG9P140R. CAS-60662-16-0.* INN; MI.

Binetrakin [*1999*] (bin e′ tra kin). Interleukin 4 (human). Molecular weight is approximately 14,900 daltons. *CAS-207137-56-2.* INN. *Treatment of gastrointestinal carcinoma, rheumatoid arthritis and dendritic cell activation (immunomodulatory activities on B cells, macrophages, eosinophils and other hematopoietic cells).* ◇*SCH 39400*

```
HKCDITLQEI IKTLNSLTEQ KTLCTELTVT DIFAASKNTT EKETFCRAAT
VLRQFYSHHE KDTRCLGATA QQFHRHKQLI RFLKRLDRNL WGLAGLNSCP
VKEANQSTLE NFLERLKTIM REKYSKCSS
```

Binfloxacin [*1989*] (bin flox′ a sin). $C_{19}H_{22}FN_3O_3$. 359.39. (1) 3-Quinolinecarboxylic acid, 7-(1,4-diazabicyclo[3.2.2]-non-4-yl)-1-ethyl-6-fluoro-1,4-dihydro-4-oxo-; (2) 7-(1,4-Diazabicyclo[3.2.2]non-4-yl)-1-ethyl-6-fluoro-1,4-dihydro-4-oxo-3-quinolinecarboxylic acid. *UNII-78VM28ZA2H. CAS-108437-28-1.* INN. *Antibacterial (veterinary).* ◇*CP-73,049*

Binifibrate. $C_{25}H_{23}ClN_2O_7$. 498.91. 2-(*p*-Chlorophenoxy)-2-methylpropionic acid ester with 1,3-dinicotininoyloxy-2-propanol. *UNII-9NGZ4GPE20. CAS-69047-39-8.* INN; MI.

Biniramycin [*1969*] (bin ir″ a mye′ sin). Antibiotic produced by *Streptomyces bikiniensis* variant. (1) Biniramycin; (2) Biniramycin. *CAS-11056-11-4.* INN. *Antibacterial.* ◇*Antibiotic 241a*

Binizolast. $C_{18}H_{23}N_5O$. 325.41. 1-(Piperidinomethyl)-4-propyl-*s*-triazolo[4,3-*a*]quinazolin-5(4*H*)-one. *UNII-W2KGP0434Y. CAS-86662-54-6.* INN.

Binodaline — *See* Binedaline.

Binodenoson [*2002*] (bin″ oh den′ oh son). $C_{17}H_{25}N_7O_4$. 391.42. (1) Adenosine, 2-[(cyclohexylmethylene)hydrazino]-; (2) 2-[2-(Cyclohexylmethylene)diazanyl]-9-*β*-D-ribofuranosyl-9*H*-purin-6-amine. *CAS-144348-08-3.* INN; BAN. *Coronary vasodilator used in the diagnosis of coronary heart disease (adenosine A₂A agonist).* ◊*MRE0470*

Binospirone Mesylate [*1991*] (bin″ oh spye′ rone mes′ i late). $C_{20}H_{26}N_2O_4 \cdot CH_4O_3S$. 454.54. [Binospirone is INN.] (1) 8-Azaspiro[4.5]decane-7,9-dione, 8-[2-[[(2,3-dihydro-1,4-benzodioxin-2-yl)methyl]amino]ethyl]-, (±)-, monomethanesulfonate; (2) (±)-*N*-[2-[(1,4-Benzodioxan-2-ylmethyl)amino]ethyl]-1,1-cyclopentanediacetimide monomethanesulfonate. *UNII-155R3B9K8H. CAS-124756-23-6; CAS-102908-59-8* [binospirone]. *Anti-anxiety agent.* ◊*MDL 73,005EF*

Bioallethrin. $C_{19}H_{26}O_3$. 302.41. (*RS*)-3-Allyl-2-methyl-4-oxocyclopent-2-enyl (1*R*,3*R*)-2,2-dimethyl-3-(2-methylprop-1-enyl)cyclopropanecarboxylate. *CAS-584-79-2.* BAN.

Bioresmethrin. $C_{22}H_{26}O_3$. 338.44. (5-Benzyl-3-furyl)methyl (+)-*trans*-2,2-dimethyl-3-(2-methylpropenyl)cyclopropanecarboxylate. *UNII-YPP8YQZ13B. CAS-28434-01-7.* INN; MI.

Biosynthetic Human Parathyroid Hormone (1-34) [PTH(1-34)] — *See* Teriparatide.

Biosynthetic Human Parathyroid Hormone (1-34) [PTH(1-34)] — *See* Teriparatide Acetate.

Biotin (bye′ oh tin). **USP.** $C_{10}H_{16}N_2O_3S$. 244.31. (1) 1*H*-Thieno[3,4-*d*]imidazole-4-pentanoic acid, hexahydro-2-oxo-, [3a*S*-(3a*α*,4*β*,6a*α*)]-; (2) (3a*S*,4*S*,6a*R*)-Hexahydro-2-oxo-1*H*-thieno[3,4-*d*]imidazole-4-valeric acid. *UNII-6SO6U10H04. CAS-58-85-5.* INN; JAN. *Vitamin.* Bioepiderm (Sterling Winthrop†)

Bipenamol Hydrochloride [*1985*] (bye pen′ a mol hye″ droe klor′ ide). $C_{14}H_{15}NOS \cdot HCl$. 281.80. [Bipenamol is INN.] (1) Benzenemethanol, 2-[[2-(aminomethyl)phenyl]thio]-, hydrochloride; (2) *o*-[(*α*-Amino-*o*-tolyl)thio]benzyl alcohol hydrochloride. *UNII-49DCB7156W* [bipenamol]. *CAS-62220-58-0; CAS-79467-22-4* [bipenamol]. *Antidepressant.* ◊*BW 647U hydrochloride*

Biperiden (bye per′ i den). **USP.** $C_{21}H_{29}NO$. 311.46. (1) 1-Piperidinepropanol, *α*-bicyclo[2.2.1]hept-5-en-2-yl-*α*-phenyl-; (2) *α*-5-Norbornen-2-yl-*α*-phenyl-1-piperidinepropanol. *UNII-0FRP6G56LD. CAS-514-65-8.* INN; BAN; JAN. *Anticholinergic; antiparkinsonian.* Akineton (Knoll)

Biperiden Hydrochloride (bye per′ i den hye″ droe klor′ ide). **USP.** $C_{21}H_{29}NO \cdot HCl$. 347.92. (1) 1-Piperidinepropanol, *α*-bicyclo[2.2.1]hept-5-en-2-yl-*α*-phenyl-, hydrochloride; (2) *α*-5-Norbornen-2-yl-*α*-phenyl-1-piperidinepropanol hydrochloride. *UNII-K35N76CUHF; UNII-0FRP6G56LD* [biperiden]. *CAS-1235-82-1; CAS-514-65-8* [biperiden]. BAN; JAN. *Anticholinergic; antiparkinsonian.* Akineton (Abbott)

Biperiden Lactate (bye per′ i den lak′ tate). **USP** [Injection]. $C_{21}H_{29}NO \cdot C_3H_6O_3$. 401.54. (1) 1-Piperidinepropanol, *α*-bicyclo[2.2.1]hept-5-en-2-yl-*α*-phenyl-, compd. with 2-hydroxypropanoic acid (1:1); (2) *α*-5-Norbornen-2-yl-*α*-phenyl-1-piperidinepropanol lactate (salt). *UNII-09TD6C5147; UNII-0FRP6G56LD* [biperiden]. *CAS-7085-45-2; CAS-514-65-8* [biperiden]. BAN; JAN. *Anticholinergic; antiparkinsonian.* Akineton (Abbott)

Biphenamine Hydrochloride [*1962*] (bye fen′ a meen hye″ droe klor′ ide). $C_{19}H_{23}NO_3 \cdot HCl$. 349.85. [Xenysalate is INN and BAN.] (1) [1,1′-Biphenyl]-3-carboxylic acid, 2-hydroxy-2-(diethylamino)ethyl ester, hydrochloride; (2) 2-(Diethylamino)ethyl 2-hydroxy-3-biphenylcarboxylate hydrochloride. *UNII-0WN4KYJ0C0. CAS-5560-62-3; CAS-3572-52-9* [biphenamine]. *Anesthetic (topical); antibacterial; antifungal.*

Biprofenide — *See* Bifepramide.

Birch Oil, Sweet — *See* Methyl Salicylate.

Biricodar. $C_{34}H_{41}N_3O_7$. 603.71. 4-(3-Pyridyl)-1-[3-(3-pyridyl)propyl]butyl(S)-1-[(3,4,5-trimethoxyphenyl)glyoxyloyl]pipecolate. *UNII-3KG76X4KJK. CAS-159997-94-1.* INN.

Biricodar Dicitrate [*1997*] (bye″ ri koe′ dar dye sit′ rate). $C_{34}H_{41}N_3O_7.2C_6H_8O_7$. 987.95. (1) 4-(3-Pyridinyl)-1-[3-(3-pyridinyl)propyl]butyl (S)-1-[oxo(3,4,5-trimethoxyphenyl)acetyl]-2-piperidinecarboxylate 2-hydroxy-1,2,3-propanetricarboxylate (1:2); (2) 4-(3-Pyridyl)-1-[3-(3-pyridyl)propyl]butyl (S)-1-[(3,4,5-trimethoxyphenyl)glyoxyloyl]pipecolate, citrate (1:2). *UNII-9WQP0L619L. CAS-174254-13-8. Adjuvant chemotherapy (multidrug resistance inhibitor).* ◇VX-710-3

Biriperone. $C_{24}H_{26}FN_3O$. 391.48. (±)-4′-Fluoro-4-(3,4,6,7,12,12a-hexahydropyrazino[1′,2′:1,6]pyrido[3,4-*b*]indol-2(1*H*)-yl)butyrophenone. *UNII-5776HBV7UD. CAS-41510-23-0.* INN.

Bisacodyl (bis ak′ oh dil). **USP.** $C_{22}H_{19}NO_4$. 361.39. (1) Phenol, 4,4′-(2-pyridinylmethylene)bis-, diacetate (ester); (2) 4,4′-(2-Pyridylmethylene)diphenol diacetate (ester). *UNII-10X0709Y6I. CAS-603-50-9.* INN; BAN; JAN. *Laxative.* Correctol Tablets, Caplets (Schering-Plough Health-Care); Dulcolax (Boehringer Ingelheim); Evac-Q-Tabs (Savage); Feen-a-Mint Tablets (Schering-Plough Health-Care); Modane (Savage); SK-Bisacodyl (SmithKline Beecham†); Theralax (SmithKline Beecham†)

Bisacodyl Tannex [*1963*] (bis ak′ oh dil tan′ ex). Water-soluble complex of bisacodyl and tannic acid. (1) Phenol, 4,4′-(2-pyridinylmethylene)bis-, diacetate (ester), complex with tannic acid; (2) 4,4′-(2-Pyridylmethylene)diphenol diacetate (ester) complex with tannic acid. *UNII-10X0709Y6I* [bisacodyl]. *CAS-1336-29-4; CAS-603-50-9* [bisacodyl]. *Laxative.* Clysodrast (Rhone-Poulenc Rorer†)

Bisantrene Hydrochloride [*1981*] (bis′ an treen hye″ droe klor′ ide). $C_{22}H_{22}N_8.2HCl$. 471.39. [Bisantrene is INN.] (1) 9,10-Anthracenedicarboxaldehyde, bis[(4,5-dihydro-1*H*-imidazol-2-yl)hydrazone], dihydrochloride; (2) 9,10-Anthracenedicarboxaldehyde bis(2-imidazolin-2-ylhydrazone) dihydrochloride. *UNII-74GNV897RO. CAS-71439-68-4; CAS-78186-34-2* [bisantrene]. *Antineoplastic.* ◇CL 216,942

Bisaramil. $C_{17}H_{23}ClN_2O_2$. 322.83. *syn*-3-Ethyl-7-methyl-3,7-diazabicyclo[3.3.1]non-9-yl *p*-chlorobenzoate. *UNII-FVT2ESG270. CAS-89194-77-4.* INN.

Bisbendazole. $C_{28}H_{28}N_6S_4$. 576.82. Bis[1-(1-methyl-2-benzimidazolyl)ethyl] tetrathio-*p*-benzenedicarbamate. *UNII-WUI089UONU. CAS-32195-33-8.* INN.

Bisbentiamine. $C_{38}H_{42}N_8O_6S_2$. 770.92. *N,N*′-[Dithiobis[2-(2-benzoyloxyethyl)-1-methylvinylene]]bis[*N*-[(4-amino-2-methyl-5-pyrimidinyl)methyl]formamide]. *UNII-MEI78-CAM16. CAS-2667-89-2.* INN; JAN; MI.

Bisbutiamine — *See* Bisbutytiamine.

Bisbutytiamine. $C_{32}H_{46}N_8O_6S_2$. 702.89. *O*-Butyrylthiamine disulfide. *UNII-6A8BO41Z90. CAS-18481-23-7.* JAN.

Bisdequalinium Diacetate. $C_{44}H_{64}N_4O_4$. 713.00. 6,7,8,9,10,11,12,13,14,15,16,17,24,25,26,27,28,29,30,31,-32,33-Docosahydro-35,37-dimethyl-5,34:18,23-diethenodibenzo[*b,r*][1,5,16,20]tetraazacyclotriacontine-23,24-diium diacetate. *UNII-48RW3M5575. CAS-3785-44-2.* JAN.

Bisdisulizole Disodium [*2006*] (bis″ dye sul′ i zole dye soe′ dee um). $C_{20}H_{12}N_4Na_2O_{12}S_4$. 674.57. (1) 1*H*-Benzimidazole-4,6-disulfonic acid, 2,2′-(1,4-phenylene)bis-, disodium salt; (2) Disodium dihydrogen 2,2′-(1,4-phenylene)bis(1*H*-benzimidazole-4,6-disulfonate). *UNII-Z99XUY03BK. CAS-180898-37-7. Sunscreen.* Neo Heliopan AP (Symrise GmbH)

Bisfenazone. $C_{25}H_{29}N_5O_2$. 431.53. 3-[[(2,3-Dimethyl-5-oxo-1-phenyl-3-pyrazolin-4-yl)amino]methyl]-4-isopropyl-2-methyl-1-phenyl-3-pyrazolin-5-one. *UNII-3OA32ZIB31. CAS-55837-24-6.* INN; DCF.

Bisfentidine. $C_{14}H_{18}N_4$. 242.32. *N*-Isopropyl-*N*′-[*p*-(2-methylimidazol-4-yl)phenyl]formamidine. *CAS-96153-56-9.* INN.

Bishydroxycoumarin (previously used name) — *See* Dicumarol.

Bisibuthiamine (JAN) — *See* Sulbutiamine.

Bismucatebrol — *See* Bibrocathol.

Bismuth Aluminate [*1988*] (biz′ muth a loo′ mi nate). $Al_6Bi_2O_{12}$. 771.84. Aluminum bismuth oxide.

Bismuth Betanaphthol. *UNII-P2Z71CIK5H* [betanaphthol]. *CAS-8039-60-9; CAS-135-19-3* [betanaphthol]. USP IX.

Bismuth Carbonate [*1988*] (biz′ muth kar′ bo nate). *[Note— See also Bismuth Subcarbonate.]*

Bismuth Citrate (biz′ muth sit′ rate). **USP.** $BiC_6H_5O_7$. 398.08. 1,2,3-Propanetricarboxylic acid, 2-hydroxy-, bismuth(3+) salt (1:1). *UNII-N04867Y76N. CAS-813-93-4.* USP VIII.

Bismuth Glycollylarsanilate (previously used name) — *See* Glycobiarsol.

Bismuth Magnesium Aluminosilicate. JAN.

Bismuth Potassium Tartrate. *UNII-2XCW01A0N5. CAS-5798-41-4.* NF X; MI.

Bismuth Sodium Triglycollamate. *CAS-5798-43-6; CAS-139-13-9* [triglycollamic acid]. USP XVI; MI.

Bismuth Subcarbonate [*1988*] (biz′ muth sub kar′ bo nate). **USP.** Basic bismuth carbonate. *UNII-M41L2IN55T. CAS-5892-10-4.* JAN. *Protectant (topical).*

Bismuth Subcitrate Potassium [*2007*] (biz′ muth sub sit′ rate poe tas′ ee um). $C_{12}H_{14}BiK_5O_{17}$. 834.70. (1) 1,2,3-Propanetricarboxylic acid, 2-hydroxy-, bismuth(3+) potassium salt (2:1:5); (2) Bismuth pentapotassium dihydroxide bis(2-hydroxypropane-1,2,3-tricarboxylate hydrate. *CAS-880149-29-1. Treatment of H. pylori when used in combination with metronidazole and tetracycline hydrochloride.* ◇1001277

Bismuth Subgallate [*1988*] (biz′ muth sub gal′ ate). **USP.** $C_7H_5BiO_6$. 394.09. (1) Gallic acid bismuth basic salt; (2) Basic bismuth gallate. *UNII-YIW503MI7V. CAS-99-26-3; CAS-149-91-7* [gallic acid]. JAN.

Bismuth Subnitrate (biz′ muth sub nye′ trate). **USP.** $Bi_5O(OH)_9(NO_3)_4$. 1461.99. (1) Bismuth hydroxide nitrate oxide [$Bi_5O(OH)_9(NO_3)_4$]; (2) Bismuth hydroxide nitrate oxide [$Bi_5O(OH)_9(NO_3)_4$]. *UNII-H19J064BA5. CAS-1304-85-4.* JAN. *Pharmaceutic necessity.* Mammol (Abbott)

Bismuth Subsalicylate [*1988*] (biz′ muth sub″ sa lis′ i late). **USP.** $C_7H_5BiO_4$. 362.09. (1) (2-Hydroxybenzoato-*O*^{1})-oxobismuth; (2) 2-Hydroxybenzoic acid bismuth (3+) salt, basic. *UNII-62TEY51RR1. CAS-14882-18-9; CAS-87-27-4* [replaced]. JAN. *Antidiarrheal; antacid; anti-ulcerative.*

Bisnafide Dimesylate [*1995*] (bis′ na fide dye mes′ i late). $C_{32}H_{28}N_6O_8 \cdot 2CH_4O_3S$. 816.81. [Bisnafide is INN.] (1) 1*H*-Benz[*de*]isoquinoline-1,3(2*H*)-dione, 2,2′-[1,2-ethanediylbis[imino(1-methyl-2,1-ethanediyl)]]bis[5-nitro-, [*R*-(*R**,*R**)]-, dimethanesulfonate; (2) *N*,*N*′-[Ethylenebis[imino[(*R*)-1-methylethylene]]]bis[3-nitronaphthalimide]dimethanesulfonate. *UNII-J301BO0LMA; UNII-62H4W26906* [bisnafide]. *CAS-145124-30-7; CAS-144849-63-8* [bisnafide]. *Antineoplastic.* VersaLuma (DuPont Merck) ◇DMP 840

Bisobrin Lactate [*1969*] (bis′ oh brin lak′ tate). $C_{26}H_{36}N_2O_4 \cdot 2C_3H_6O_3$. 620.73. [Bisobrin is INN.] (1) Propanoic acid, 2-hydroxy-, compd. with (*R**,*S**)-1,1′-(1,4-butanediyl)bis[1,2,3,4-tetrahydro-6,7-dimethoxyisoquinoline] (2:1); (2) *meso*-1,1′-Tetramethylenebis[1,2,3,4-

tetrahydro-6,7-dimethoxyisoquinoline] dilactate. *CAS-24233-80-5; CAS-22407-74-5* [bisobrin]. *Fibrinolytic.* ◇*EN-1661L*

Bisoctrizole [*2004*] (bis′ tri zole). **USP.** $C_{41}H_{50}N_6O_2$. 658.87. (1) Phenol, 2,2′-methylenebis[6-(2*H*-benzotriazol-2-yl)-4-(1,1,3,3-tetramethylbutyl)]-; (2) 2,2′-Methylene-bis[6-(2*H*-benzotriazol-2-yl)-4-(1,1,3,3-tetramethylbutyl)-phenol]. *UNII-8NT850T0YS. CAS-103597-45-1.* INN. *UVA absorber (intended for use as a topical sunscreen).* Tinosorb M (Ciba Specialty Chemicals) *[Note—The International Nomenclature Cosmetic Ingredient Name (INCI) for bisoctrizole is methylene bis-benzotriazolyl tetramethylbutylphenol.]* ◇*MBBT; FAT 75′634*

Bisoprolol [*1987*] (bis″ oh proe′ lol). $C_{18}H_{31}NO_4$. 325.44. (1) 2-Propanol, 1-[4-[[2-(1-methylethoxy)ethoxy]methyl]phenoxy]-3-[(1-methylethyl)amino]-, (±)-; (2) (±)-1-[[α-(2-Isopropoxyethoxy)-*p*-tolyl]oxy]-3-(isopropylamino)-2-propanol. *UNII-Y41JS2NL6U. CAS-66722-44-9.* INN; BAN. *Antihypertensive (β-blocker).* ◇*CL 297,939; EMD 33 512*

Bisoprolol Fumarate [*1987*] (bis″ oh proe′ lol fue′ ma rate). **USP.** $(C_{18}H_{31}NO_4)_2 \cdot C_4H_4O_4$. 766.96. (1) 2-Propanol, 1-[4-[[2-(1-methylethoxy)ethoxy]methyl]phenoxy]-3-[(1-methylethyl)amino]-, (±)-, (*E*)-2-butenedioate (2:1) (salt); (2) (±)-1-[[α-(2-Isopropoxyethoxy)-*p*-tolyl]oxy]-3-(isopropylamino)-2-propanol fumarate (2:1) (salt). *UNII-UR59KN573L. CAS-104344-23-2.* JAN. *Antihypertensive (β-blocker).* Zebeta (Duramed) ◇*CL 297,939*

Bisorcic. $C_9H_{16}N_2O_4$. 216.23. N^2,N^5-Diacetyl-L-ornithine. *UNII-3V77J79MIF. CAS-39825-23-5.* INN.

Bisoxatin Acetate [*1967*] (bis ox′ a tin as′ e tate). $C_{24}H_{19}NO_6$. 417.41. [Bisoxatin is INN and BAN.] (1) 2*H*-1,4-Benzoxazin-3(4*H*)-one, 2,2-bis[4-(acetyloxy)phenyl]-; (2) 2,2-Bis(*p*-hydroxyphenyl)-2*H*-1,4-benzoxazin-3(4*H*)-one diacetate. *CAS-14008-48-1; CAS-17692-24-9* [bisoxatin]. JAN. *Laxative.* ◇*Wy-8138*

Bispyrithione Magsulfex [*1987*] (bis″ pir i thye′ one mag sul′ fex). $C_{10}H_8MgN_2O_6S_3 \cdot 3H_2O$. 426.73. (1) Magnesium, [2,2′-dithiobis[pyridine] 1,1′-dioxide-*O,O′,S*][sulfato(2-)-*O*]-, (*T*-4)-; (2) (2,2′-Dithiodipyridine 1,1′-dioxide)sulfato-magnesium trihydrate. *CAS-67182-81-4. Antibacterial; antidandruff; antifungal.* Omadine MDS (Olin)

Bithionol. $C_{12}H_6Cl_4O_2S$. 356.05. 2,2′-Thiobis(4,6-dichloro-phenol). *UNII-AMT77LS62O. CAS-97-18-7.* NF XII; INN; BAN; JAN; MI. Lorothidol (Sterling Winthrop†)

Bithionolate Sodium [*1962*] (bye thye′ oh noe late soe′ dee um). $C_{12}H_4Cl_4Na_2O_2S$. 400.02. [Sodium Bitionolate is INN.] (1) Phenol, 2,2′-thiobis[4,6-dichloro-, disodium salt; (2) 2,2′-Thiobis[4,6-dichlorophenol] disodium salt. *UNII-AMT77LS62O* [bithionol]. *CAS-6385-58-6; CAS-97-18-7* [bithionol]. *Anti-infective, topical.*

Bithionoloxide. $C_{12}H_6Cl_4O_3S$. 372.05. 2,2′-Sulfinylbis[4,6-dichlorophenol]. *UNII-6PL3DO2B30. CAS-844-26-8.* INN.

---

† Brand name formerly used, and/or firm no longer concerned with this product.

Bitipazone. $C_{20}H_{38}N_8S_2$. 454.70. 2,3-Butanedione bis[4-(2-piperidinoethyl)thiosemicarbazone]. *CAS-13456-08-1.* INN.

Bitolterol Mesylate [*1975*] (bye tol′ ter ol mes′ i late). $C_{28}H_{31}NO_5 \cdot CH_4O_3S$. 557.66. [Bitolterol is INN and BAN; Bitolterol Mesilate is JAN.] (1) Benzoic acid, 4-methyl-, 4-[2-[(1,1-dimethylethyl)amino]-1-hydroxyethyl]-1,2-phenylene ester methanesulfonate (salt); (2) 4-[2-(*tert*-Butylamino)-1-hydroxyethyl]-*o*-phenylene di-*p*-toluate methanesulfonate (salt); (3) α[[(*tert*-Butylamino)methyl]-3,4-dihydroxybenzyl alcohol 3,4-di-*p*-toluate methanesulfonate (salt). *UNII-4E53T3611U; UNII-9KY0QXD6LI* [bitolterol]. *CAS-30392-41-7; CAS-30392-40-6* [bitolterol]. *Bronchodilator.* Tornalate (Sanofi Aventis) ◇*Win 32,784*

Bitoscanate. $C_8H_4N_2S_2$. 192.26. *p*-Phenylene bis(isothiocyanate). *UNII-6D1R3P86GX. CAS-4044-65-9.* INN; MI. ◇*16842*

Bitter Tincture. Ethanol solution containing alcoholic extracts of a mixture of bitter orange peel, swertia herb and zanthoxylum fruit. JAN.

Bivalirudin [*1994*] (bye val′ i roo din). $C_{98}H_{138}N_{24}O_{33}$. 2180.29. (1) L-Leucine, D-phenylalanyl-L-prolyl-L-arginyl-L-prolylglycylglycylglycylglycyl-L-asparaginylglycyl-L-α-aspartyl-L-phenylalanyl-L-α-glutamyl-L-α-glutamyl-L-isoleucyl-L-prolyl-L-α-glutamyl-L-α-glutamyl-L-tyrosyl-; (2) D-Phenylalanyl-L-prolyl-L-arginyl-L-prolylglycylglycylglycylglycyl-L-asparaginylglycyl-L-α-aspartyl-L-phenylalanyl-L-α-glutamyl-L-α-glutamyl-L-isoleucyl-L-prolyl-L-α-glutamyl-L-α-glutamyl-L-tyrosyl-L-leucine. *UNII-TN9BEX005G. CAS-128270-60-0.* INN; BAN. *Anticoagulant; antithrombotic.* Angiomax (The Medicines Company) ◇*BG8967*

Bivatuzumab. Immunoglobulin G1 (human-mouse monoclonal BIWA4 γ1-chain anti-human antigen CD44v6), disulfide with human-mouse monoclonal BIWA4 κ-chain, dimer. *CAS-214559-60-1.* INN.

Bizelesin [*1992*] (bye zel′ e sin). $C_{43}H_{36}Cl_2N_8O_5$. 815.70. (1) Benzo[1,2-*b*:4,3-*b*′]dipyrrol-4-ol, 6,6′-[carbonylbis(imino-1*H*-indole-5,2-diylcarbonyl)]bis[8-(chloromethyl)-3,6,7,8-tetrahydro-1-methyl-, [*S*-(*R**,*R**)]-; (2) 1,3-Bis[2-[[(*S*)-1-(chloromethyl)-1,6-dihydro-5-hydroxy-8-methylbenzo[1,2-*b*:4,3-*b*′]dipyrrol-3(2*H*)-yl]carbonyl]indol-5-yl]-urea. *CAS-129655-21-6.* INN. *Antineoplastic.* ◇*U-77779*

Blastomycin. *CAS-1362-89-6.* NF XIV.

Bleomycin Sulfate [*1971*] (blee″ oh mye′ sin sul′ fate). **USP**. [Bleomycin is INN and BAN; Bleomycin Hydrochloride is JAN.] The sulfate salt of bleomycin, a mixture of basic cytotoxic glycopeptides produced by the growth of *Streptomyces verticillus*, or produced by other means. (1) Bleomycin sulfate (salt); (2) Bleomycin sulfate (salt). *UNII-7DP3NTV15T; UNII-40S1VHN69B* [bleomycin]. *CAS-9041-93-4; CAS-11056-06-7* [bleomycin]. JAN. *Antineoplastic.* Blenoxane (Bristol-Myers Squibb)

Major component: Bleomycin A₂

Blinatumomab [*2008*] (blin″ a toom′ oh mab). $C_{2367}H_{3577}N_{649}O_{772}S_{19}$. (1) Immunoglobulin, anti-(human CD19 (antigen)) (single-chain) fusion protein with immunoglobulin, anti-(human CD3 (antigen)) (clone 1 single-chain); (2) Immunoglobulin, anti-(human B-lymphocyte antigen CD19 (Leu-12)) mouse monoclonal scFv fragment {IGKV-IGKJ-tetraglycyl-L-seryltetraglycyl-L-seryltetraglycyl-L-seryl-IGHV-IGHJ} fusion protein with tetraglycyl-L-serine fusion protein with immunoglobulin, anti-(human T-cell surface glycoprotein CD3 ε chain (Leu-4)) mouse monoclonal scFv fragment {IGHV-IGHJ-L-valyl-L-glutamyltetrakis[diglycyl-L-seryl]diglycyl-L-valyl-L-aspartyl-IGKV-IGKJ} fusion protein with hexa-L-histamine. Molecular weight is approximately 54,100 daltons. *CAS-853426-35-4. Treatment of cancer.* ◇*MEDI-538; MT-103*

Blonanserin. $C_{23}H_{30}FN_3$. 367.50. 2-(4-Ethyl-1-piperazinyl)-4-(*p*-fluorophenyl)-5,6,7,8,9,10-hexahydrocycloocta[*b*]pyridine. *CAS-132810-10-7.* INN.

Blood Cells, Human Red (previously used name) — *See* Blood Cells, Red.

Blood Cells, Red (blud sels red). **USP**. The portion of blood that contains hemoglobin and is derived from human whole blood. *Blood replenisher. [Name previously used: Blood Cells, Human Red.]*

Blood Group Specific Substances A and B (previously used name) — *See* Blood Group Specific Substances A, B, and AB.

Blood Group Specific Substances A, B, and AB. USP XXVII. *Blood neutralizer. [Name previously used: Blood Group Specific Substances A and B.]*

Blood Grouping Serum, Anti-A (blud). **USP**. A sterile, liquid or dried preparation containing the particular blood group antibodies derived from high-titered blood plasma or serum of human subjects. It agglutinates human red cells containing A-antigens, i.e., blood groups A and AB (including subgroups A_1, A_2, A_1B, and A_2B but not necessarily weaker subgroups). *Diagnostic aid (blood, in vitro).*

Blood Grouping Serum, Anti-B (blud). **USP**. A sterile, liquid or dried preparation containing the particular blood group antibodies derived from high-titered blood plasma or serum of human subjects. It agglutinates human red cells containing B-antigens, i.e., blood groups B and AB (including subgroups A_1B, and A_2B). *Diagnostic aid (blood, in vitro).*

Blood Grouping Serums (blud). **USP**. A sterile, liquid or dried preparation containing one or more of the particular blood group antibodies derived from high-titered blood plasma or serum of human subjects. It causes either directly, or indirectly by the antiglobulin test, the visible agglutination of human red cells containing the particular antigen(s) for which it is specific.

Blood Grouping Serums Anti-D, Anti-C, Anti-E, Anti-c, Anti-e (blud). **USP**. Anti-Rh Blood Grouping Serums. *Diagnostic aid (blood, in vitro). [Name previously used: Anti-Rh Typing Serums]*

Blood, Whole (blud). **USP**. (1) ACD Whole Blood; (2) CPD Whole Blood; (3) CPDA-1 Whole Blood; (4) Heparin Whole Blood. *Blood replenisher. [Name previously used: Blood, Whole Human.]*

Blood, Whole Human (previously used name) — *See* Blood, Whole.

Bluensomycin. $C_{21}H_{39}N_5O_{14}$. 585.56. Antibiotic obtained from cultures of *Streptomyces verticillus*, or the same substance produced by any other means. *CAS-11011-72-6.* INN. ◇*U-12898*

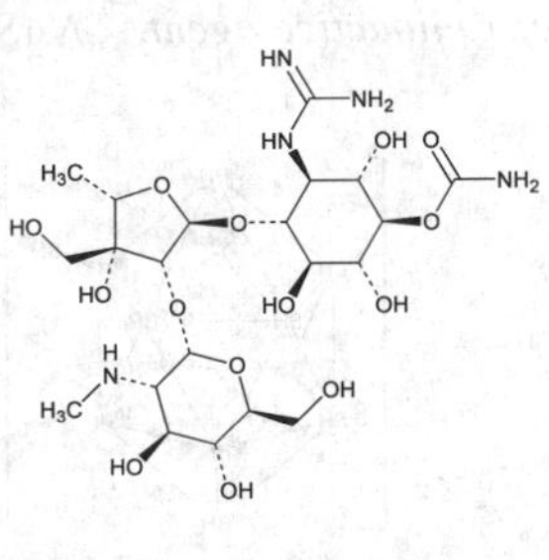

Boceprevir [*2007*] (boe se′ pre vir). $C_{27}H_{45}N_5O_5$. 519.68. (1) 3-Azabicyclo[3.1.0]hexane-2-carboxamide, *N*-[3-amino-1-(cyclobutylmethyl)-2,3-dioxopropyl]-3-[(2*S*)-2-[[[(1,1-dimethylethyl)amino]carbonyl]amino]-3,3-dimethyl-1-oxobutyl]-6,6-dimethyl-, (1*R*,2*S*,5*S*)-; (2) (1*R*,2*S*,5*S*)-*N*-[3-Amino-1-(cyclobutylmethyl)-2,3-dioxopropyl]-3-[(2*S*)-2-[[(1,1-dimethylethyl)carbamoyl]amino]-3,3-dimethylbuta-

noyl]-6,6-dimethyl-3-azabicyclo[3.1.0]hexane-2-carboxamide. *CAS-394730-60-0.* INN. *Treatment of hepatitis C infection.* ◇*SCH 503034*

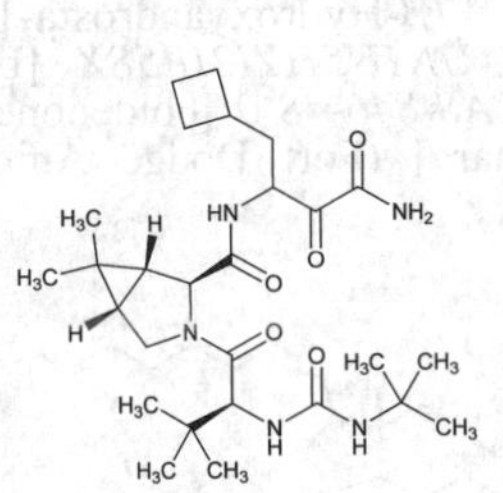

Boforsin — *See* Colforsin.

Bofumustine. $C_{18}H_{21}ClN_4O_9$. 472.83. 1-(2-Chloroethyl)-3-(2,3-*O*-isopropylidene-D-ribofuranosyl)-1-nitrosourea 5′-(*p*-nitrobenzoate). *UNII-6P52D0J76B.* *CAS-55102-44-8.* INN.

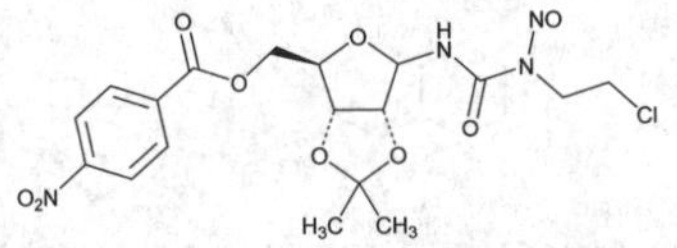

Bolandiol Dipropionate [*1965*] (bole″ an dye′ ol dye proe′ pee oh nate). $C_{24}H_{36}O_4$. 388.54. [Bolandiol is INN.] (1) Estr-4-ene-3,17-diol dipropanoate, (3*β*,17*β*)-; (2) Estr-4-ene-3*β*,17*β*-diol dipropionate. *UNII-595CNE7RHB.* *CAS-1986-53-4.* JAN. *Anabolic.* ◇*SC-7525*

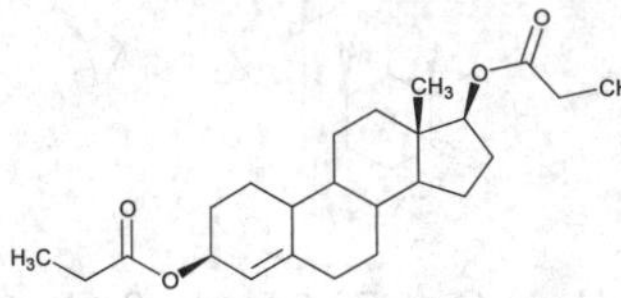

Bolasterone [*1964*] (bole as′ ter one). $C_{21}H_{32}O_2$. 316.48. (1) Androst-4-en-3-one, 17-hydroxy-7,17-dimethyl-, (7*α*,17*β*)-; (2) 17*β*-Hydroxy-7*α*,17-dimethylandrost-4-en-3-one; (3) 7*α*,17-Dimethyltestosterone. *UNII-T7ZM08F7FU.* *CAS-1605-89-6.* INN. *Anabolic.* ◇*U-19763; NSC-66233*

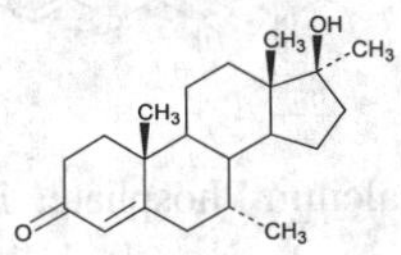

Bolazine. $C_{40}H_{64}N_2O_2$. 604.95. 17*β*-Hydroxy-2*α*-methyl-5*α*-androstan-3-one azine. *UNII-508ISH42Z9.* *CAS-4267-81-6.* INN.

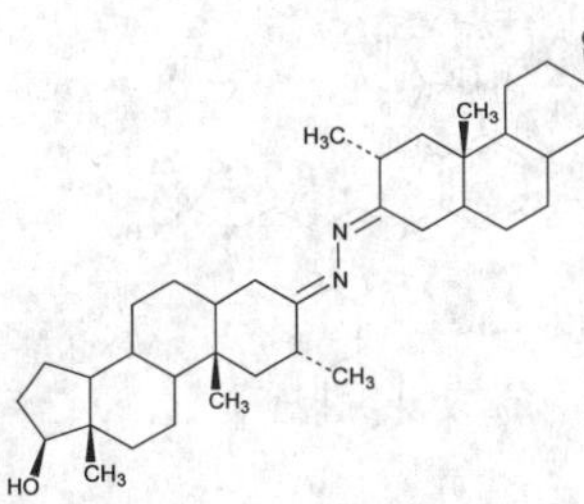

Boldenone Undecylenate [*1968*] (bole′ de none un de′ sil en ate). C₃₀H₄₄O₃. 452.67. [Boldenone is INN and BAN.] (1) Androsta-1,4-diene-3-one, 17-[(1-oxo-10-undecenyl)oxy]-, (17β)-; (2) 17β-Hydroxyandrosta-1,4-dien-3-one 10-undecenoate. *UNII-5H7121P58X* [boldenone]. *CAS-13103-34-9; CAS-846-48-0* [boldenone]. *Anabolic.* Equipoise [Veterinary] (Fort Dodge Animal Health) ◇*Ba-29038*

Bolenol [*1968*] (bole′ e nol). C₂₀H₃₂O. 288.47. (1) 19-Norpregn-5-en-17-ol, (17α)-; (2) 19-Nor-17α-pregn-5-en-17-ol. *CAS-16915-78-9.* INN. *Anabolic.*

Bolmantalate [*1965*] (bole man′ ta late). C₂₉H₄₀O₃. 436.63. (1) Estr-4-en-3-one, 17-[(tricyclo[3.3.1.1³,⁷]dec-1-ylcarbonyl)oxy]-, (17β)-; (2) 17β-Hydroxyestr-4-en-3-one 1-adamantanecarboxylate. *CAS-1491-81-2.* INN; BAN. *Anabolic.* ◇*38851*

Bometolol. C₂₅H₃₂N₂O₇. 472.53. (±)-8-(Acetonyloxy)-5-[3-[(3,4-dimethoxyphenethyl)amino]-2-hydroxypropoxy]-3,4-dihydrocarbostyril. *UNII-55QM6Y09ZY. CAS-65008-93-7.* INN.

Bone Ash — *See* Calcium Phosphate, Tribasic.

Bone Powder, Purified — *See* Calcium Phosphate, Tribasic.

Bopindolol. C₂₃H₂₈N₂O₃. 380.48. [Bopindolol Malonate is JAN.] (±)-1-(*tert*-Butylamino)-3-[(2-methylindol-4-yl)oxy]-2-propanol benzoate (ester). *CAS-62658-63-3; CAS-62658-64-4* [malonate]. INN; MI.

Boracic Acid — *See* Boric Acid.

Boric Acid (bor′ ik as′ id). **NF.** H₃BO₃. 61.83. (1) Boric acid (H₃BO₃); (2) Boric acid (H₃BO₃). *UNII-R57ZHV85D4. CAS-10043-35-3.* JAN. *Pharmaceutic necessity.*

Bornaprine. C₂₁H₃₁NO₂. 329.48. 3-(Diethylamino)propyl 2-phenyl-2-norbornanecarboxylate. *CAS-20448-86-6.* INN; BAN.

Bornaprolol. C₁₉H₂₉NO₂. 303.44. 1-(Isopropylamino)-3-(*o*-2-*exo*-norbornylphenoxy)-2-propanol. *CAS-66451-06-7.* INN.

Bornelone [*1979*] (bor′ ne lone). C₁₄H₂₀O. 204.31. (1) 3-Penten-2-one, 5-(3,3-dimethylbicyclo[2.2.1]hept-2-ylidene)-; (2) 5-(3,3-Dimethyl-2-norbornylidene)-3-penten-2-one. *UNII-LU86E5P72A. CAS-2226-11-1.* INN. *Ultraviolet screen.*

Bornyl Acetate [*1988*] (bor′ nil as′ e tate). C₁₂H₂₀O₂. 196.29. 1,7,7-Trimethylbicyclo[2.2.1]heptan-2-ol acetate; borneol acetate.

Borocaptate Sodium B 10 [*1989*] (bor″ oh kap′ tate soe′ dee um). ¹⁰B₁₂H₁₂Na₂S. [Sodium Borocaptate (¹⁰B) is INN.] (1) Dodecaborate(2-)-¹⁰B₁₂, 1,2,3,4,5,6,7,8,9,10,11-undecahydro-12-mercapto-, disodium; (2) Disodium undecahydromercaptododecaborate(2-)-¹⁰B₁₂. *CAS-103831-41-0. Antineoplastic; radioactive agent.* ◇*NASH; BSH*

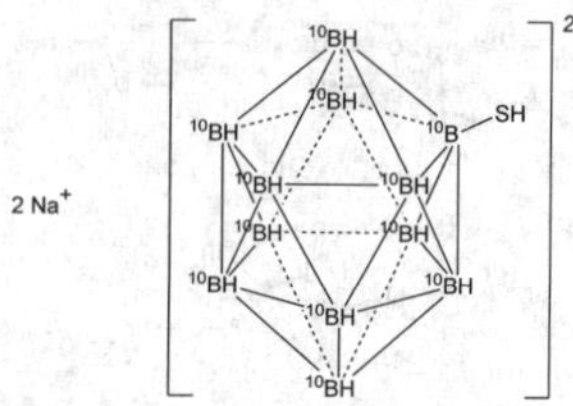

Boroglycerin. NF III.

Bortezomib [*2002*] (bor tez′ oh mib). C₁₉H₂₅BN₄O₄. 384.24. (1) Boronic acid, [(1*R*)-3-methyl-1-[[(2*S*)-1-oxo-3-phenyl-2-[(pyrazinylcarbonyl)amino]propyl]amino]butyl]-; (2) [(1*R*)-3-Methyl-1-[[(2*S*)-3-phenyl-2-[(pyrazinylcarbonyl)amino]propanoyl]amino]butyl]boronic acid; (3) *N*-[(1*S*)-1-Benzyl-2-[[(1*R*)-1-(dihydroxyboranyl)-3-methylbutyl]amino]-2-oxoethyl]pyrazinecarboxamide. *UNII-69G8BD63PP. CAS-179324-69-7.* INN; BAN. *Treatment of multiple cancers, including multiple myeloma, chronic* *lymphocytic leukemia, non-Hodgkins lymphoma, and pancreatic, colon, lung, and prostate cancers (proteasome inhibitor).* Velcade (Millennium) ◇*PS-341; LDP-341*

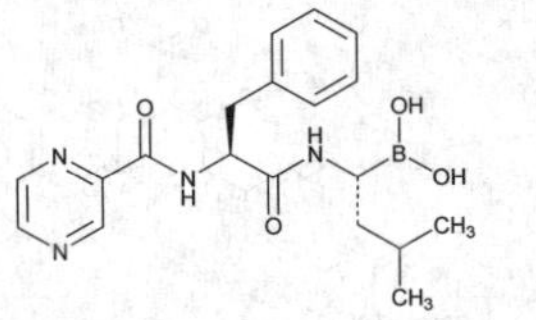

Bosentan [*1995*] (boe sen′ tan). $C_{27}H_{29}N_5O_6S.H_2O$. 569.63. (1) Benzenesulfonamide, 4-(1,1-dimethylethyl)-*N*-[6-(2-hydroxyethoxy)-5-(2-methoxyphenoxy)[2,2′-bipyrimidin]-4-yl]-, monohydrate; (2) *p-tert*-Butyl-*N*-[6-(2-hydroxyethoxy)-5-(*o*-methoxyphenoxy)-2-(2-pyrimidinyl)-4-pyrimidinyl]benzenesulfonamide monohydrate. *UNII-Q326023R30. CAS-157212-55-0; CAS-147536-97-0* [anhydrous]. INN; BAN. *Antagonist (endothelin receptor).* Tracleer (Actelion) ◇*Ro 47-0203/029*

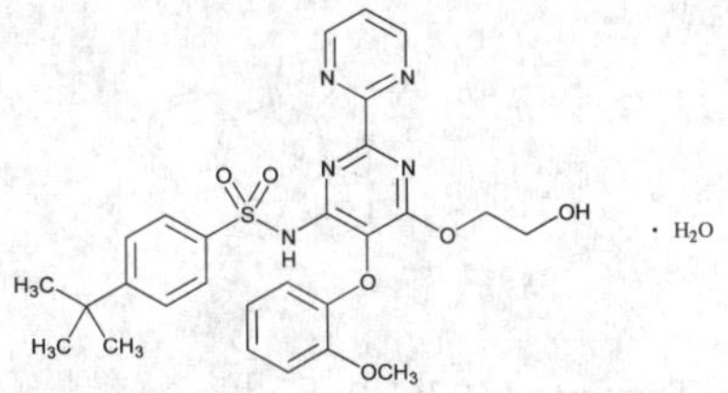

Bosutinib [*2005*] (boe sue′ ti nib). $C_{26}H_{29}Cl_2N_5O_3$. 530.45. (1) 3-Quinolinecarbonitrile, 4-[(2,4-dichloro-5-methoxyphenyl)amino]-6-methoxy-7-[3-(4-methyl-1-piperazinyl)propoxy]-; (2) 4-[(2,4-Dichloro-5-methoxyphenyl)amino]-6-methoxy-7-[3-(4-methylpiperazin-1-yl)propoxy]quinoline-3-carbonitrile. *UNII-5018V4AEZ0. CAS-380843-75-4.* INN. *Antineoplastic (Src kinase inhibitor).* ◇*SKI-606*

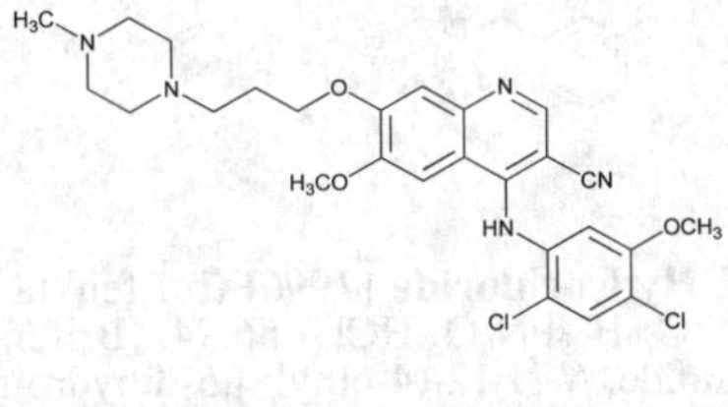

Botiacrine. $C_{20}H_{24}N_2OS$. 340.48. *S*-[2-(Dimethylamino)ethyl]-9,9-dimethyl-10-acridancarbothioate. *UNII-032WJR708Q. CAS-4774-53-2.* INN.

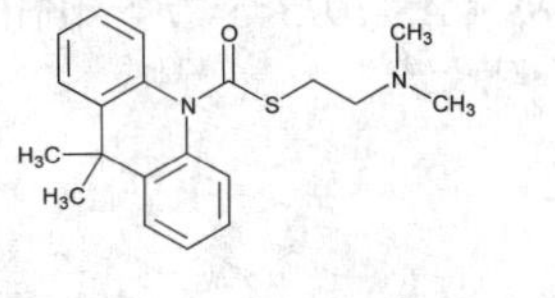

Botulism Antitoxin (bot′ ue lizm an″ tee tox′ in). **USP.** A sterile, nonpyrogenic solution of the refined and concentrated antitoxic antibodies, chiefly globulins, obtained from the blood of healthy horses that have been immunized against the toxins produced by the type A and type B and/or type E strains of *Clostridium botulinum. Immunizing agent (passive).*

Bovactant. An extract of bovine lung containing about 92% of phospholipids, 3.2% of cholesterol, 0.6% of surfactant-associated hydrophobic proteins and 0.4% of free fatty acid. Mean relative molecular mass of phospholipids, about 760 Daltons. BAN. ◇*SF-R11*

Bovine Fibrin. An insoluble plasma protein obtained by the action of bovine thrombin on bovine fibrinogen. BAN.

Boxidine [*1967*] (box′ i deen). $C_{19}H_{20}F_3NO$. 335.36. (1) Pyrrolidine, 1-[2-[[4′-(trifluoromethyl)[1,1′-biphenyl]-4-yl]oxy]ethyl]-; (2) 1-[2-[[4′-(Trifluoromethyl)-4-biphenylyl]oxy]ethyl]pyrrolidine. *CAS-10355-14-3.* INN. *Antihyperlipoproteinemic.* ◇*CL 65205*

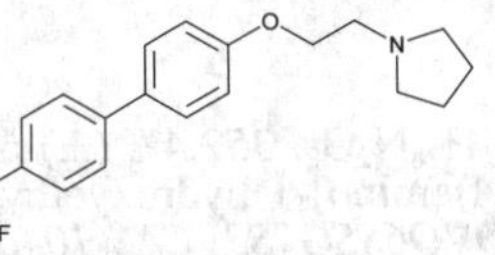

Brallobarbital. $C_{10}H_{11}BrN_2O_3$. 287.11. 5-Allyl-5-(2-bromoallyl)barbituric acid. *UNII-D0N7A2M3MU. CAS-561-86-4.* INN; MI.

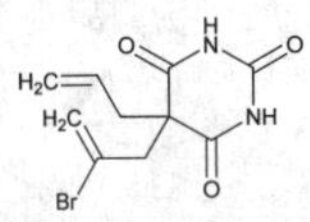

Brasofensine. $C_{16}H_{20}Cl_2N_2O$. 327.25. 3β-(3,4-Dichlorophenyl)-1αH,5αH-tropane-2α-carboxaldehyde (*E*)-(*O*-methyloxime). *UNII-1YP2S94RVH. CAS-171655-91-7.* INN.

Brasofensine Maleate [*1997*] (bra″ soe fen′ seen mal′ ee ate). $C_{16}H_{20}Cl_2N_2O.C_4H_4O_4$. 443.32. (1) [1*R*-(2-*endo*,3-*exo*)]-3-(3,4-Dichlorophenyl)-8-methyl-8-azabicyclo[3.2.1]octane-2-carboxaldehyde *O*-methyloxime, (*Z*)-2-butenedioate (1:1); (2) 3β-(3,4-Dichlorophenyl)-1αH,5αH-tropane-2α-carboxaldehyde (*E*)-(*O*-methyloxime), maleate (1:1). *UNII-S35880HLHZ. CAS-173830-14-3. Antiparkinsonian (dopamine reuptake inhibitor).* ◇*BMS-204756-07; NS 2214*

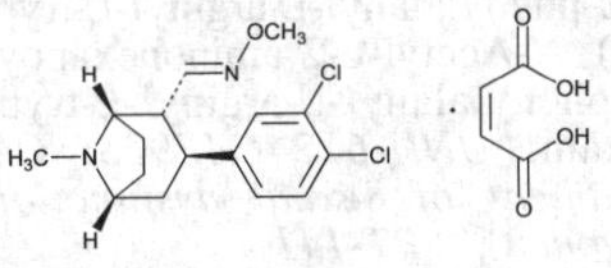

Brazergoline. $C_{23}H_{30}BrN_3O_2$. 460.41. 2-Bromo-6-methylergoline-8β-methanol hexahydro-1*H*-azepine-1-carboxylate (ester). *UNII-C9734VZR4O. CAS-60019-20-7.* INN.

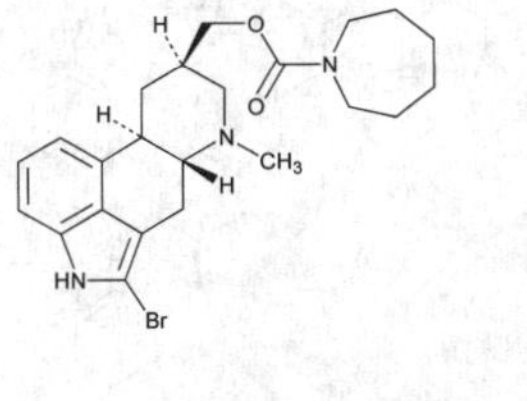

Brecanavir [*2005*] (bre kan′ a vir). $C_{33}H_{41}N_3O_{10}S_2$. 703.82. (1) Carbamic acid, [(1*S*,2*R*)-3-[(1,3-benzodioxol-5-ylsulfonyl)(2-methylpropyl)amino]-2-hydroxy-1-[[4-[(2-methyl-4-thiazolyl)methoxy]phenyl]methyl]propyl]-, (3*R*,3a*S*,6a*R*)-hexahydrofuro[2,3-*b*]furan-3-yl ester; (2) (3*R*,3a*S*,6a*R*)-Hexahydrofuro[2,3-*b*]furan-3-yl [(1*S*,2*R*)-3-[(1,3-benzodioxol-5-ylsulfonyl)(2-methylpropyl)amino]-2-hydroxy-1-[4-[(2-methylthiazol-4-yl)methoxy]benzyl]-

---

† Brand name formerly used, and/or firm no longer concerned with this product.

propyl]carbamate. *UNII-E367I8C7FI. CAS-313682-08-5.* INN. *Treatment of HIV infection in combination with other antiretroviral agents.* ◇*GW64085X*

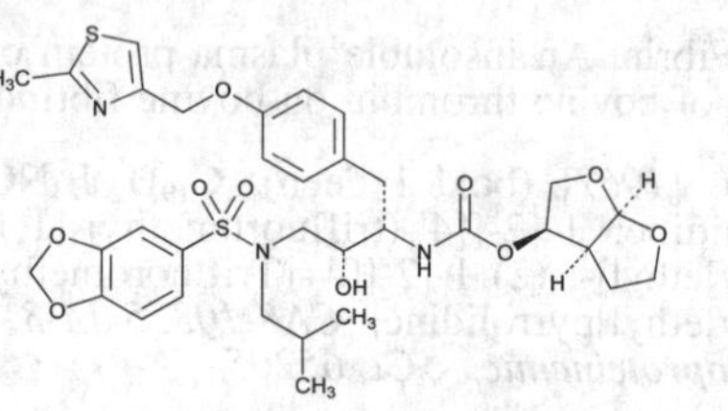

Brefonalol. $C_{22}H_{28}N_2O_2$. 352.47. (±)-6-[2-[(1,1-Dimethyl-3-phenylpropyl)amino]-1-hydroxyethyl]-3,4-dihydrocarbostyril. *UNII-DVO6SSG9S3. CAS-104051-20-9.* INN.

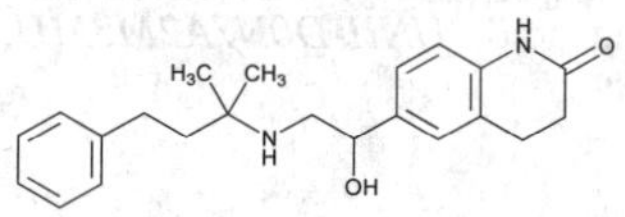

Bremazocine. $C_{20}H_{29}NO_2$. 315.45. 6-Ethyl-1,2,3,4,5,6-hexahydro-3-[(1-hydroxycyclopropyl)methyl]-11,11-dimethyl-2,6-methano-3-benzazocin-8-ol. *CAS-71990-00-6.* INN.

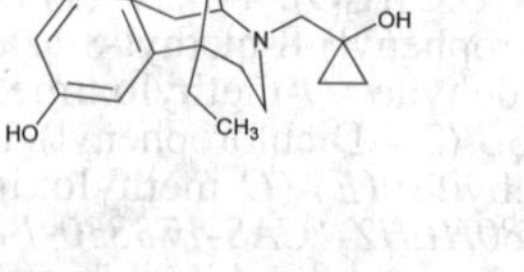

Bremelanotide [*2006*] (bre″ mel an′ oh tide). $C_{50}H_{68}N_{14}O_{10}$. 1025.16. (1) L-Lysine, N-acetyl-L-norleucyl-L-α-aspartyl-L-histidyl-D-phenylalanyl-L-arginyl-L-tryptophyl-, (2→7)-lactam; (2) N-Acetyl-L-2-aminohexanoyl-L-α-aspartyl-L-histidyl-D-phenylalanyl-L-arginyl-L-tryptophyl-L-lysine-(2→7)-lactam. *UNII-6Y24O4F92S. CAS-189691-06-3.* INN. *Treatment of sexual dysfunction (melanocortin receptor agonist).* ◇*PT-141*

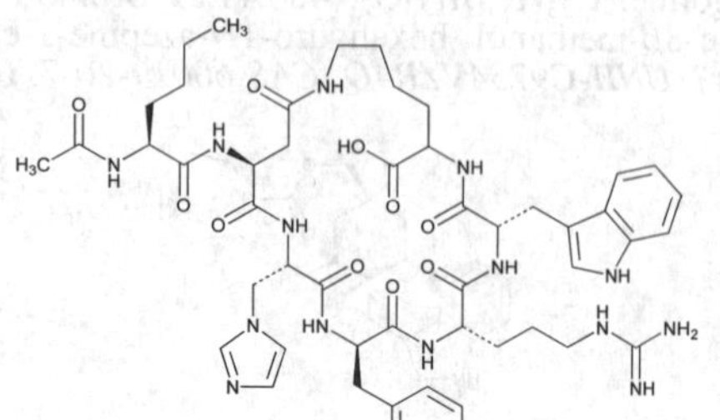

Brequinar Sodium [*1987*] (bre′ kwin ar soe′ dee um). $C_{23}H_{14}F_2NNaO_2$. 397.35. [Brequinar is INN.] (1) 4-Quinolinecarboxylic acid, 6-fluoro-2-(2′-fluoro[1,1′-biphenyl]-4-yl)-3-methyl-, sodium salt; (2) Sodium 6-fluoro-2-(2′-fluoro-4-biphenylyl)-3-methyl-4-quinolinecarboxylate.

UNII-49EEF6HRUS; UNII-5XL19F49H6 [brequinar]. *CAS-96201-88-6; CAS-96187-53-0* [brequinar]. *Antineoplastic.* ◇*Dup 785; NSC-368390*

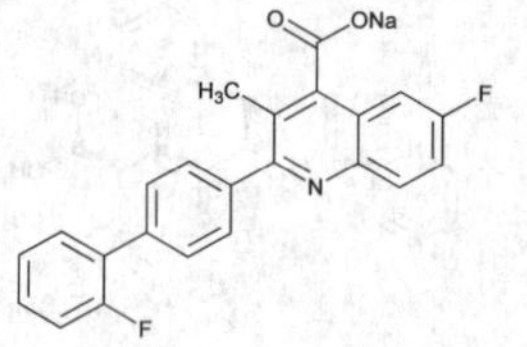

Bretazenil [*1990*] (bre taz′ e nil). $C_{19}H_{20}BrN_3O_3$. 418.28. (1) 9H-Imidazo[1,5-a]pyrrolo[2,1-c][1,4]benzodiazepine-1-carboxylic acid, 8-bromo-11,12,13,13a-tetrahydro-9-oxo-, 1,1-dimethylethyl ester, (S)-; (2) *tert*-Butyl (S)-8-bromo-11,12,13,13a-tetrahydro-9-oxo-9H-imidazo[1,5-a]pyrrolo[2,1-c][1,4]benzodiazepine-1-carboxylate. *UNII-OSZ0E9DGOJ. CAS-84379-13-5.* INN. *Anti-anxiety agent.* ◇*Ro 16-6028/000*

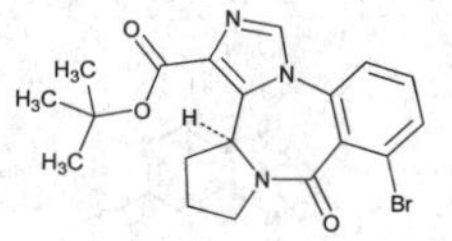

Bretylium Tosylate [*1976*] (bre til′ ee um tos′ i late). **USP.** $C_{18}H_{24}BrNO_3S$. 414.36. [Bretylium Tosilate is INN and BAN.] (1) Benzenemethanaminium, 2-bromo-N-ethyl-N,N-dimethyl-, salt with 4-methylbenzenesulfonic acid (1:1); (2) (o-Bromobenzyl)ethyldimethylammonium p-toluenesulfonate. *UNII-78ZP3YR353. CAS-61-75-6; CAS-59-41-6* [bretylium]. *Anti-adrenergic; cardiac depressant (anti-arrhythmic).* ◇*ASL-603*

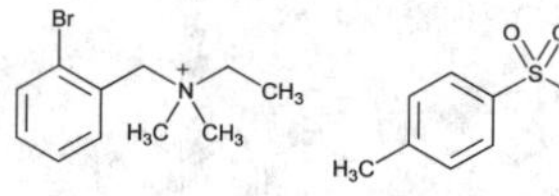

Brifentanil Hydrochloride [*1990*] (bri fen′ ta nil hye″ droe klor′ ide). $C_{20}H_{29}FN_6O_3 \cdot HCl$. 456.94. [Brifentanil is INN.] (1) Acetamide, N-[1-[2-(4-ethyl-4,5-dihydro-5-oxo-1H-tetrazol-1-yl)ethyl]-3-methyl-4-piperidinyl]-N-(2-fluorophenyl)-2-methoxy-, monohydrochloride, cis-(±)-; (2) (±)-cis-N-[1-[2-(4-Ethyl-5-oxo-2-tetrazolin-1-yl)ethyl]-3-methyl-4-piperidyl]-2′-fluoro-2-methoxyacetanilide monohydrochloride. *UNII-6GDT77PQBW* [brifentanil]. *CAS-117268-95-8; CAS-101345-71-5* [brifentanil]. *Analgesic (narcotic).* ◇*A-3331*

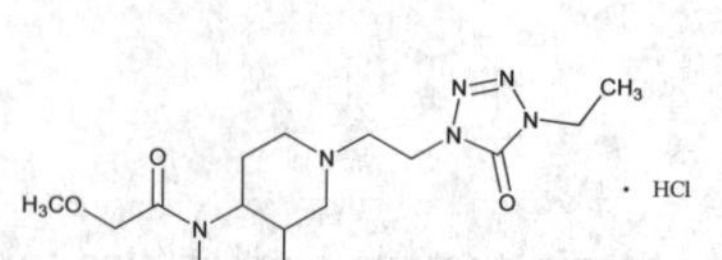

Brimonidine Tartrate [*1991*] (bri moe′ ni deen tar′ trate). $C_{11}H_{10}BrN_5 \cdot C_4H_6O_6$. 442.22. [Brimonidine is INN and BAN.] (1) 6-Quinoxalinamine, 5-bromo-N-(4,5-dihydro-1H-imidazol-2-yl)-, [S-(R*,R*)]-2,3-dihydroxybutanedioate (1:1); (2) 5-Bromo-6-(2-imidazolin-2-ylamino)quinoxaline D-tartrate (1:1). *UNII-4S9CL2DY2H; UNII-*

E6GNX3HHTE [brimonidine]. *CAS-79570-19-7; CAS-59803-98-4* [brimonidine]. *Adrenergic (ophthalmic).* Alphagan (Allergan) ◇*UK-14304-18; AGN 190342-LF*

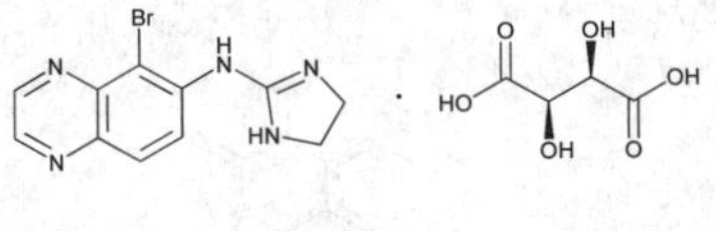

Brinase (INN) — *See* Brinolase.

Brinazarone. $C_{25}H_{32}N_2O_2$. 392.53. *p*-[3-(*tert*-Butylamino)propoxy]phenyl 2-isopropyl-3-indolizinyl ketone. *UNII-UC0DRK4OE0. CAS-89622-90-2.* INN.

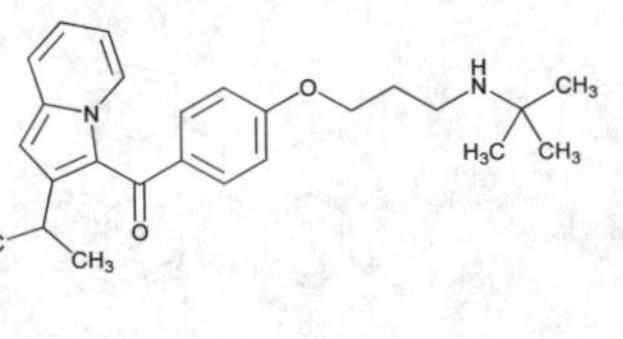

Brindoxime. $C_{18}H_{19}Br_2N_5O_2$. 497.18. 2-[[(6,8-Dibromo-9*H*-indeno[2,1-*d*]pyrimidin-9-ylidene)amino]oxy]-*N*-[2-(dimethylamino)ethyl]propionamide. *UNII-5CA81DKM2L. CAS-55837-17-7.* INN.

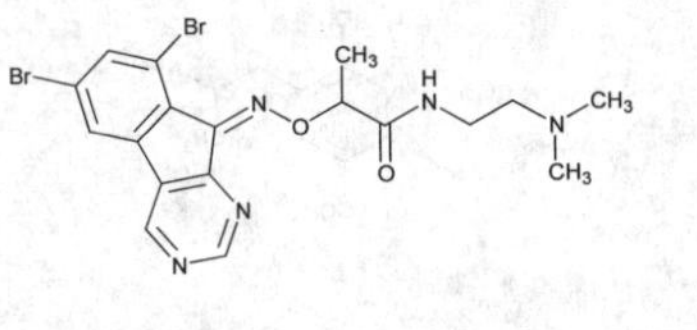

Brineurin (previously used name) — *See* Abrineurin.

Brinolase [*1971*] (brin′ oh lase). [Brinase is INN.] Fibrinolytic enzyme produced by *Aspergillus oryzae.* (1) Proteinase, Aspergillus oryzae, fibrinolytic; (2) Fibrinolytic enzyme of *Aspergillus oryzae. CAS-42615-60-1. Fibrinolytic.* ◇*CA-7; Protease 1*

Brinzolamide [*1997*] (brin zoe′ la mide). **USP.** $C_{12}H_{21}N_3O_5S_3$. 383.51. (1) 2*H*-Thieno[3,2-*e*]-1,2-thiazine-6-sulfonamide, 4-(ethylamino)-3,4-dihydro-2-(3-methoxypropyl)-, 1,1-dioxide, (*R*)-; (2) (*R*)-4-(Ethylamino)-3,4-dihydro-2-(3-methoxypropyl)-2*H*-thieno[3,2-*e*]-1,2-thiazine-6-sulfonamide 1,1-dioxide. *UNII-9451Z89515. CAS-138890-62-7.* INN; BAN. *Antiglaucoma agent.* Azopt (Alcon) ◇*AL-4862*

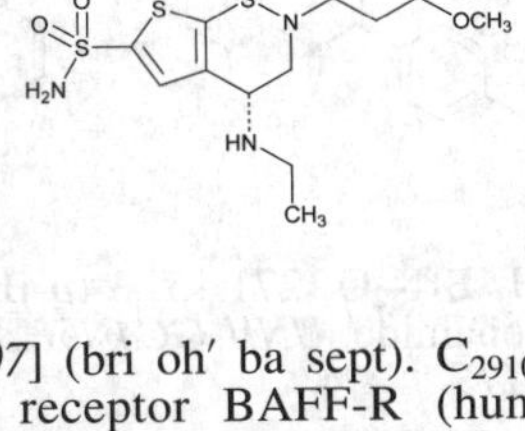

Briobacept [*2007*] (bri oh′ ba sept). $C_{2910}H_{4542}N_{814}O_{878}S_{24}$. (1) Cytokine receptor BAFF-R (human extracellular domain-containing fragment BR3) fusion protein with immunoglobulin G1 (human Fc domain-containing fragment), dimer; (2) Aspartyl[1-valine,20-asparagine,27-proline](human tumor necrosis factor receptor superfamily member 13C (BAFF receptor, BlyS receptor 3 or CD268 antigen)-(1-71)-peptidyl (part of the extracellular domain))valyl(human immunoglobulin G1 Fc fragment, *Homo sapiens* IGHG1-(104-329)-peptide), dimer (79-

79′:82-82′)-bisdisulfide. Molecular weight is approximately 65,750 daltons. *CAS-869881-54-9.* INN. *Treatment of autoimmune diseases.* ◇*BR-3-FC*

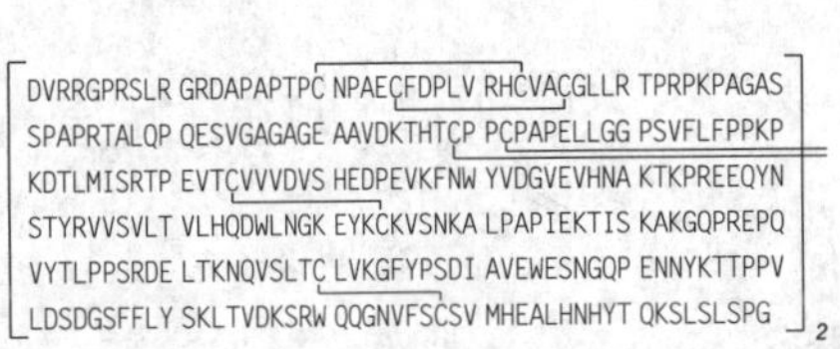

```
DVRRGPRSLR GRDAPAPTPC NPAECFDPLV RHCVACGLLR TPRPKPAGAS
SPAPRTALQP QESVGAGAGE AAVDKTHTCP PCPAPELLGG PSVFLFPPKP
KDTLMISRTP EVTCVVVDVS HEDPEVKFNW YVDGVEVHNA KTKPREEQYN
STYRVVSVLT VLHQDWLNGK EYKCKVSNKA LPAPIEKTIS KAKGQPREPQ
VYTLPPSRDE LTKNQVSLTC LVKGFYPSDI AVEWESNGQP ENNYKTTPPV
LDSDGSFFLY SKLTVDKSRW QQGNVFSCSV MHEALHNHYT QKSLSLSPG
```

Brivanib Alaninate [*2006*] (briv′ a nib al″ a nin′ ate). $C_{22}H_{24}FN_5O_4$. 441.46. (1) L-Alanine, (1*R*)-2-[[4-[(4-fluoro-2-methyl-1*H*-indol-5-yl)oxy]-5-methylpyrrolo[2,1-*f*][1,2,4]triazin-6-yl]oxy]-1-methylethyl ester; (2) (1*R*)-2-[[4-[(4-Fluoro-2-methyl-1*H*-indol-5-yl)oxy]-5-methylpyrrolo[2,1-*f*][1,2,4]triazin-6-yl]oxy]-1-methylethyl (2*S*)-2-aminopropanoate. *UNII-U2Y5OFN795. CAS-649735-63-7.* INN. *Antineoplastic; angiogenesis inhibitor.* ◇*BMS-582664*

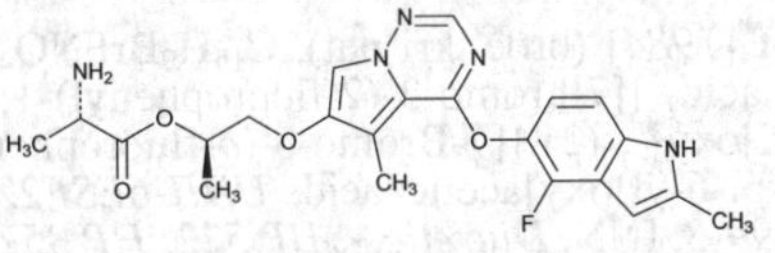

Brivaracetam [*2004*] (briv″ a ra′ se tam). $C_{11}H_{20}N_2O_2$. 212.29. (1) 1-Pyrrolidineacetamide, α-ethyl-2-oxo-4-propyl-, (α*S*,4*R*)-; (2) (2*S*)-2-[(4*R*)-2-Oxo-4-propylpyrrolidin-1-yl]butanamide. *UNII-U863JGG2IA. CAS-357336-20-0.* INN. *Treatment of epilepsy, neuropathic pain and essential tremor.* ◇*ucb 34714*

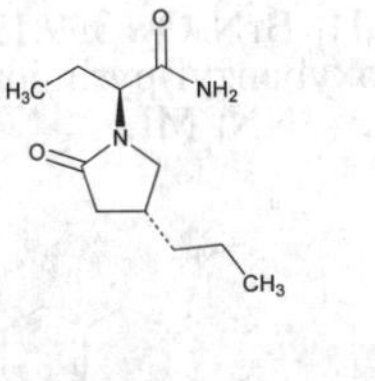

Brivudine. $C_{11}H_{13}BrN_2O_5$. 333.14. (*E*)-5-(2-Bromovinyl)-2′-deoxyuridine. *UNII-2M3055079H. CAS-69304-47-8.* INN.

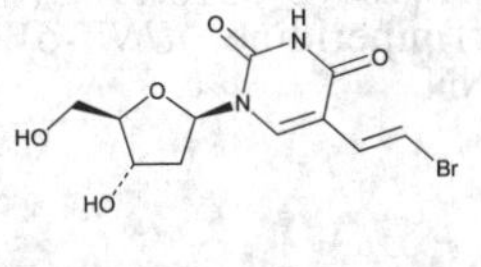

Brobactam. $C_8H_{10}BrNO_3S$. 280.14. (2*S*,5*R*,6*R*)-6-Bromo-3,3-dimethyl-7-oxo-4-thia-1-azabicyclo[3.2.0]heptane-2-carboxylic acid. *UNII-6I6JCF8EOE. CAS-26631-90-3.* INN.

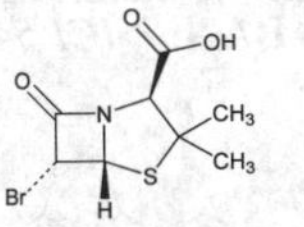

Brobenzoxaldine — *See* Broxaldine.

---

† Brand name formerly used, and/or firm no longer concerned with this product.

Broclepride. $C_{20}H_{23}BrClN_3O_2$. 452.77. 4-Amino-5-bromo-*N*-[1-(*p*-chlorobenzyl)-4-piperidyl]-*o*-anisamide. *UNII-CY5E0946P1. CAS-71195-56-7.* INN.

Brocresine [*1967*] (broe′ kre seen). $C_7H_8BrNO_2$. 218.05. (1) Phenol, 5-[(aminooxy)methyl]-2-bromo-; (2) α-(Aminooxy)-6-bromo-*m*-cresol. *UNII-11F6O06WN0. CAS-555-65-7.* INN; BAN. *Inhibitor (histidine decarboxylase).* ◇*NSD 1055; CL 54998; CL 108,756*

Brocrinat [*1984*] (broe′ kri nat). $C_{15}H_9BrFNO_4$. 366.14. (1) Acetic acid, [[7-bromo-3-(2-fluorophenyl)-1,2-benzisoxazol-6-yl]oxy]-; (2) [[7-Bromo-3-(*o*-fluorophenyl)-1,2-benzisoxazol-6-yl]oxy]acetic acid. *UNII-6ESF2Z39VZ. CAS-72481-99-3.* INN. *Diuretic.* ◇*HP 522; HP 3522; P 78 3522*

Brodimoprim. $C_{13}H_{15}BrN_4O_2$. 339.19. 2,4-Diamino-5-(4-bromo-3,5-dimethoxybenzyl)pyrimidine. *UNII-V1YC7T6LLI. CAS-56518-41-3.* INN; MI.

Brofaromine. $C_{14}H_{16}BrNO_2$. 310.19. 4-(7-Bromo-5-methoxy-2-benzofuranyl)piperidine. *UNII-6WV4B8Q07H. CAS-63638-91-5.* INN.

Brofezil. $C_{12}H_{10}BrNO_2S$. 312.18. 4-(*p*-Bromophenyl)-α-methyl-2-thiazoleacetic acid. *UNII-E375EMI4HW. CAS-17969-45-8.* INN; BAN. ◇*ICI 54,594 [as sodium salt]*

Brofoxine [*1976*] (broe fox′ een). $C_{10}H_{10}BrNO_2$. 256.10. (1) 2*H*-3,1-Benzoxazin-2-one, 6-bromo-1,4-dihydro-4,4-dimethyl-; (2) 6-Bromo-1,4-dihydro-4,4-dimethyl-2*H*-3,1-benzoxazin-2-one. *CAS-21440-97-1.* INN. *Antipsychotic.* ◇*F.I. 6820*

Brolaconazole. $C_{17}H_{15}BrN_2$. 327.22. ($\pm$)-1-(*p*-Bromo-β-phenylphenethyl)imidazole. *UNII-6CHG505391. CAS-108894-40-2.* INN.

Brolamfetamine. $C_{11}H_{16}BrNO_2$. 274.15. ($\pm$)-4-Bromo-2,5-dimethoxy-α-methylphenethylamine. *UNII-67WJC4Y2QY. CAS-64638-07-9.* INN.

Bromacrylide. $C_7H_{11}BrN_2O_2$. 235.08. *N*-[(3-Bromopropionamido)methyl]acrylamide. *UNII-173648DEO8. CAS-4213-51-8.* INN.

Bromadoline Maleate [*1983*] (brom ad′ oh leen mal′ ee ate). $C_{15}H_{21}BrN_2O.C_4H_4O_4$. 441.32. [Bromadoline is INN.] (1) Benzamide, 4-bromo-*N*-[2-(dimethylamino)cyclohexyl]-, *trans*-, (*Z*)-2-butenedioate (1:1); (2) *trans*-*p*-Bromo-*N*-[2-(dimethylamino)cyclohexyl]benzamide maleate (1:1). *UNII-R8DWN01P1M* [bromadoline]. *CAS-81447-81-6; CAS-67579-24-2* [bromadoline]. *Analgesic.* ◇*U-47,931E*

Bromamid. $C_{11}H_{15}BrN_2O$. 271.15. 3-(*p*-Bromoanilino)-*N,N*-dimethylpropionamide. *UNII-GC4N5H35P2. CAS-332-69-4.* INN. ◇*NA-119*

Bromanylpromide — *See* Bromamid.

Bromauric Acid. Hydrogen tetrabromoaurate(1-). NF V.

Bromazepam [*1969*] (broe maz′ e pam″). $C_{14}H_{10}BrN_3O$. 316.15. (1) 2*H*-1,4-Benzodiazepin-2-one, 7-bromo-1,3-dihydro-5-(2-pyridinyl)-; (2) 7-Bromo-1,3-dihydro-5-(2-

pyridyl)-2*H*-1,4-benzodiazepin-2-one. *CAS-1812-30-2.*
INN; BAN; JAN. *Tranquilizer (minor).* Lectopam (Roche,
Puerto Rico) ◇*Ro 5-3350*

Bromazine (INN, BAN, DCF) Hydrochloride — *See*
Bromodiphenhydramine Hydrochloride.

Brombenzonium — *See* Bromhexine Hydrochloride.

Bromchlorenone [*1961*] (brome klor′ e none).
$C_7H_3BrClNO_2$. 248.46. (1) 2(3*H*)-Benzoxazolone, 6-bro-
mo-5-chloro-; (2) 6-Bromo-5-chloro-2-benzoxazolinone.
UNII-A221572SK5. CAS-5579-85-1. INN. *Anti-infective,
topical.* ◇*NSC-24970*

Bromebric Acid. $C_{11}H_9BrO_4$. 285.09. (*E*)-3-*p*-Anisoyl-3-
bromoacrylic acid. *UNII-FGE8818GWA. CAS-5711-40-0.*
INN; BAN.

Bromelains [*1962*] (broe′ me laynz). [Bromelain is JAN.] A
concentrate of proteolytic enzymes derived from the
pineapple plant, *Ananas sativus.* (1) Bromelain; (2)
Bromelain. *CAS-9001-00-7.* INN; BAN. *Anti-inflammatory.*

Bromelin — *See* Bromelains.

Bromerguride. $C_{20}H_{25}BrN_4O$. 417.34. 3-(2-Bromo-9,10-dide-
hydro-6-methylergolin-8α-yl)-1,1-diethylurea. *UNII-
HX58M2377W. CAS-83455-48-5.* INN.

Brometenamine. $CHBr_3.C_6H_{12}N_4$. 392.92. Equimolecular
complex of bromoform and hexamethylenetetramine.
UNII-VW6613KQ0H. CAS-15585-71-4. INN; DCF.

Bromfenac Sodium [*1986*] (brome′ fen ak soe′ dee um).
$C_{15}H_{11}BrNNaO_3.1\frac{1}{2}H_2O$. 383.17. [Bromfenac is INN.] (1)
Benzeneacetic acid, 2-amino-3-(4-bromobenzoyl)-, monosodium salt, sesquihydrate; (2) Sodium [2-amino-3-(*p*-
bromobenzoyl)phenyl]acetate sesquihydrate. *UNII-*

8ECV571Y37; UNII-864P0921DW [bromfenac]. *CAS-
120638-55-3; CAS-91714-94-2* [bromfenac]. *Analgesic.*
Xibrom (Ista) ◇*AHR-10282B*

Bromhexine Hydrochloride [*1969*] (brom hex′ een hye″
droe klor′ ide). $C_{14}H_{20}Br_2N_2.HCl$. 412.59. [Bromhexine is
INN and BAN.] (1) Benzenemethanamine, 2-amino-3,5-
dibromo-*N*-cyclohexyl-*N*-methyl-, monohydrochloride; (2)
3,5-Dibromo-N^α-cyclohexyl-N^α-methyltoluene-α,2-di-
amine monohydrochloride. *CAS-611-75-6; CAS-3572-43-8*
[bromhexine]. JAN. *Expectorant; mucolytic.* ◇*NA 274*

Bromindione [*1961*] (broe″ min dye′ one). $C_{15}H_9BrO_2$.
301.13. (1) 1*H*-Indene-1,3(2*H*)-dione, 2-(4-bromophen-
yl)-; (2) 2-(*p*-Bromophenyl)-1,3-indandione. *CAS-1146-
98-1.* INN; BAN. *Anticoagulant.*

Bromisoval (INN) — *See* Bromisovalum.

Bromisovalum. $C_6H_{11}BrN_2O_2$. 223.07. [Bromisoval is INN;
Bromvalerylurea is JAN.] 2-Bromo-3-methylbutyrylurea.
UNII-469GW8R486. CAS-496-67-3. NF XI; MI. Bromural
(Knoll†)

Bromocamphor — *See* Camphor, Monobromated.

Bromociclen. $C_8H_5BrCl_6$. 393.75. 5-(Bromomethyl)-
1,2,3,4,7,7-hexachloro-2-norbornene. *UNII-J28T4D661G.
CAS-1715-40-8.* INN; BAN. *[Name previously used:
Bromocyclen.]*

Bromocriptine [*1976*] (broe″ moe krip′ teen). $C_{32}H_{40}BrN_5O_5$.
654.59. (1) Ergotaman-3′,6′,18-trione, 2-bromo-12′-hy-
droxy-2′-(1-methylethyl)-5′-(2-methylpropyl)-, (5′α)-; (2)

---

† Brand name formerly used, and/or firm no longer
concerned with this product.

2-Bromo-α-ergocryptine. *UNII-3A64E3G5ZO. CAS-25614-03-3.* INN; BAN. *Enzyme inhibitor (prolactin).* ◇*CB-154*

Bromocriptine Mesylate [*1977*] (broe″ moe krip′ teen mes′ i late). **USP.** $C_{32}H_{40}BrN_5O_5.CH_4SO_3$. 750.70. [Bromocriptine is BAN; Bromocriptine Mesilate is JAN.] (1) Ergotaman-3′,6′,18-trione, 2-bromo-12′-hydroxy-2′-(1-methylethyl)-5′-(2-methylpropyl)-, monomethanesulfonate (salt), (5′α)-; (2) 2-Bromoergocryptine monomethanesulfonate (salt). *UNII-FFP983J3OD; UNII-3A64E3G5ZO* [bromocriptine]. *CAS-22260-51-1; CAS-25614-03-3* [bromocriptine]. *Enzyme inhibitor (prolactin).* Parlodel (Novartis) ◇*CB-154 mesylate*

Bromodiethylacetylurea — *See* Carbromal.

Bromodiphenhydramine Hydrochloride (broe″ moe dye″ fen hye′ dra meen hye″ droe klor′ ide). **USP.** $C_{17}H_{20}BrNO.HCl$. 370.71. [Bromazine is INN and BAN.] (1) Ethanamine, 2-[(4-bromophenyl)phenylmethoxy]-*N,N*-dimethyl-, hydrochloride; (2) 2-[(*p*-Bromo-α-phenylbenzyl)oxy]-*N,N*-dimethylethylamine hydrochloride. *UNII-202J683U97; UNII-T032BI7727* [bromodiphenhydramine]. *CAS-1808-12-4; CAS-118-23-0* [bromodiphenhydramine]. *Antihistaminic.* Ambodryl (Pfizer)

Bromofenofos. $C_{12}H_7Br_4O_5P$. 581.77. 3,3′,5,5′-Tetrabromo-2,2′-biphenyldiol mono(dihydrogen phosphate). *UNII-XTH861Q3CR. CAS-21466-07-9.* INN; MI.

Bromoform. *UNII-TUT9J99IMU. CAS-75-25-2.* USP IX; MI.

Bromofos. $C_8H_8BrCl_2O_3PS$. 366.00. *O*-(4-Bromo-2,5-dichlorophenyl) *O,O*-dimethyl phosphorothioate. *UNII-74A4TNE8C3. CAS-2104-96-3.* INN.

Bromophenol Blue. *CAS-115-39-9.*

Bromophos — *See* Bromofos.

Bromopride. $C_{14}H_{22}BrN_3O_2$. 344.25. 4-Amino-5-bromo-*N*-[2-(diethylamino)ethyl]-*o*-anisamide. *UNII-75473V2YZK. CAS-4093-35-0.* INN; DCF; MI.

Bromovaluree (DCF) — *See* Bromisovalum.

Bromoxanide [*1974*] (broe mox′ a nide). $C_{19}H_{18}BrF_3N_2O_4$. 475.26. (1) Benzamide, *N*-[4-bromo-2-(trifluoromethyl)phenyl]-3-(1,1-dimethylethyl)-2-hydroxy-6-methyl-5-nitro-; (2) 4′-Bromo-3-*tert*-butyl-α′,α′,α′-trifluoro-5-nitro-2,6-cresoto-*o*-toluidide. *UNII-9MM438AA0G. CAS-41113-86-4.* INN. *Anthelmintic.* ◇*SK&F 61636*

Bromperidol [*1975*] (brom per′ i dol). $C_{21}H_{23}BrFNO_2$. 420.32. (1) 1-Butanone, 4-[4-(4-bromophenyl)-4-hydroxy-1-piperidinyl]-1-(4-fluorophenyl)-; (2) 4-[4-(*p*-Bromophenyl)-4-hydroxypiperidino]-4′-fluorobutyrophenone. *UNII-LYH6F7I22E. CAS-10457-90-6.* INN; BAN; JAN. *Antipsychotic.* ◇*R 11,333*

Bromperidol Decanoate [*1981*] (brom per′ i dol dek″ a noe′ ate). $C_{31}H_{41}BrFNO_3$. 574.56. (1) Decanoic acid, 4-(4-bromophenyl)-1-[4-(4-fluorophenyl)-4-oxobutyl]-4-piperidinyl ester; (2) 4-[4-(*p*-Bromophenyl)-4-hydroxypiperidinol]-4′-fluorobutyrophenone decanoate (ester). *UNII-LYH6F7I22E* [bromperidol]. *CAS-75067-66-2; CAS-10457-90-6* [bromperidol]. BAN. *Antipsychotic.* ◇*R-46,541*

Brompheniramine Maleate (brome″ fen ir′ a meen mal′ ee ate). **USP.** $C_{16}H_{19}BrN_2.C_4H_4O_4$. 435.31. [Brompheniramine is INN and BAN.] (1) 2-Pyridinepropanamine, γ-(4-bromophenyl)-*N,N*-dimethyl-, (±)-, (*Z*)-butenedioate (1:1); (2) (±)-2-*p*-Bromo-α-2-(dimethylamino)ethylbenzylpyridine maleate (1:1). *UNII-IXA7C9ZN03; UNII-*

H57G17P2FN [brompheniramine]. *CAS-980-71-2; CAS-86-22-6* [brompheniramine]. *Antihistaminic.* Dimetane (Wyeth)

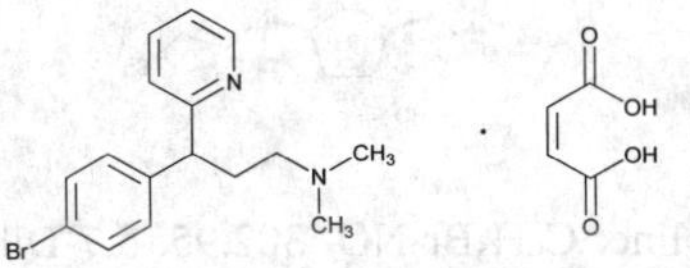

Bromvalerylurea (JAN) — *See* Bromisovalum.

Broncasma Berna. A sterile suspension of a killed strain of various bacteria. JAN.

Bronopol. $C_3H_6BrNO_4$. 199.99. 2-Bromo-2-nitro-1,3-propanediol. *UNII-6PU1E16C9W. CAS-52-51-7.* INN; BAN; JAN; MI.

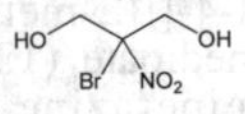

Broparestrol. $C_{22}H_{19}Br$. 363.29. 1-Bromo-2-*p*-(ethylphenyl)-1,2-diphenylethylene. *UNII-7U06D381UQ. CAS-479-68-5.* INN; DCF; MI. ◇*L.N. 107*

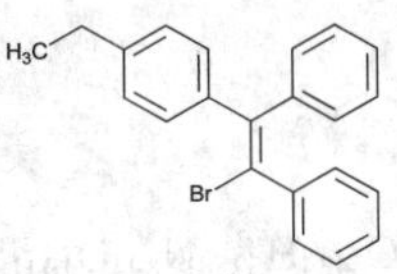

Broperamole [*1979*] (broe per′ a mole). $C_{15}H_{18}BrN_5O$. 364.24. (1) Piperidine, 1-[3-[5-(3-bromophenyl)-2*H*-tetrazol-2-yl]-1-oxopropyl]-; (2) 1-[3-[5-(*m*-Bromophenyl)-2*H*-tetrazol-2-yl]-propionyl]piperidine. *UNII-G5MIG3753N. CAS-33144-79-5.* INN. *Anti-inflammatory.* ◇*TR-2378*

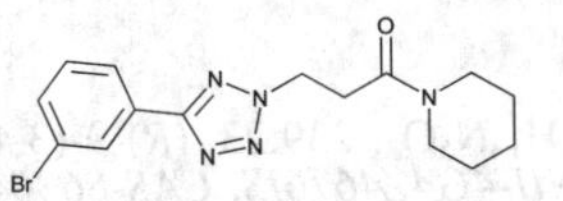

Bropirimine [*1986*] (broe pir′ i meen). $C_{10}H_8BrN_3O$. 266.09. (1) 4(3*H*)-Pyrimidinone, 2-amino-5-bromo-6-phenyl-; (2) 2-Amino-5-bromo-6-phenyl-4(3*H*)-pyrimidinone. *UNII-J57CTF25XJ. CAS-56741-95-8.* INN; BAN. *Antineoplastic; antiviral.* ◇*U-54,461*

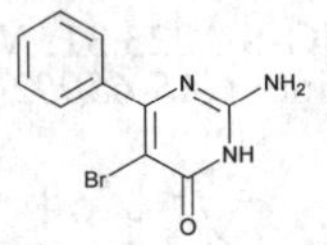

Broquinaldol. $C_{10}H_7Br_2NO$. 316.98. 5,7-Dibromo-2-methyl-8-quinolinol. *UNII-519JDS089K. CAS-15599-52-7.* INN.

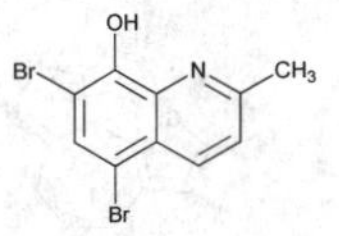

Brosotamide. $C_8H_8BrNO_2$. 230.06. 5-Bromo-2,3-cresotamide. *UNII-49NMI30XY2. CAS-40912-73-0.* INN; DCF.

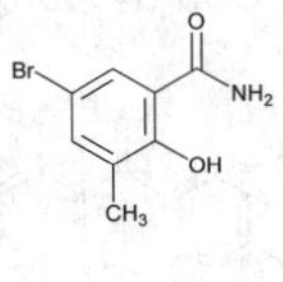

Brostallicin. $C_{30}H_{35}BrN_{12}O_5$. 723.58. 4-(2-Bromoacrylamido)-*N‴*-(2-guanidinoethyl)-1,1′,1″,1‴-tetramethyl-*N*,4′:*N*′,4″:*N*″,4‴-quater[pyrrole-2-carboxamide]. *CAS-203258-60-0.* INN.

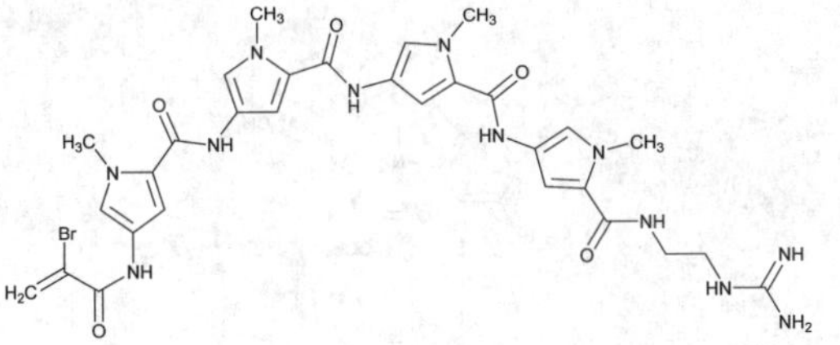

Brosuximide. $C_{10}H_8BrNO_2$. 254.08. 2-(*m*-Bromophenyl)succinimide. *UNII-MH88D3N73W. CAS-22855-57-8.* INN.

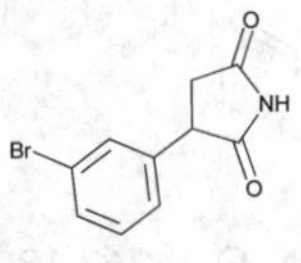

Brotianide. $C_{15}H_{10}Br_2ClNO_2S$. 463.57. 3,4′-Dibromo-5-chlorothiosalicylanilide acetate (ester). *UNII-30OGU6XH7S. CAS-23233-88-7.* INN; BAN. ◇*BAY 4059 Va; FBA 4059*

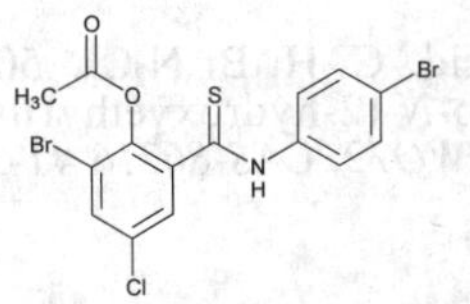

Brotizolam [*1983*] (broe tiz′ oh lam). $C_{15}H_{10}BrClN_4S$. 393.69. (1) 6*H*-Thieno[3,2-*f*][1,2,4]triazolo[4,3-*a*][1,4]diazepine, 2-bromo-4-(2-chlorophenyl)-9-methyl-; (2) 2-Bromo-4-(*o*-chlorophenyl)-9-methyl-6*H*-thieno[3,2-*f*]-*s*-

---

† Brand name formerly used, and/or firm no longer concerned with this product.

triazolo[4,3-*a*][1,4]diazepine. *CAS-57801-81-7.* INN; BAN; JAN. *Sedative-hypnotic.* Lendorm (Boehringer Ingelheim†) ◇*We 941*

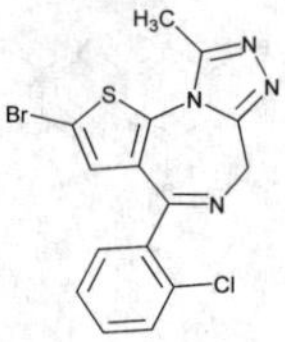

Brovanexine. $C_{24}H_{28}Br_2N_2O_4$. 568.30. 2′,4′-Dibromo-α-(cyclohexylmethylamino)-*o*-vanillotoluidide acetate (ester). *UNII-Y00SD533IW. CAS-54340-61-3.* INN.

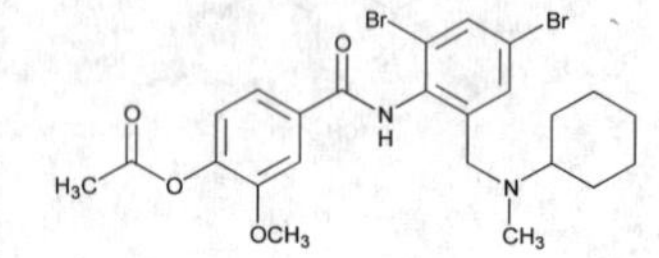

Brovavir — *See* Sorivudine.

Brovincamine. $C_{21}H_{25}BrN_2O_3$. 433.34. [Brovincamine Fumarate is JAN.] 11-Bromovincamine. *UNII-AYN5T18K5R. CAS-57475-17-9.* INN; MI.

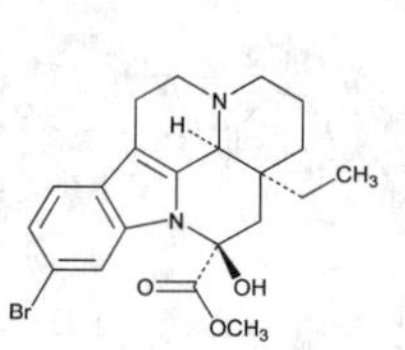

Broxaldine. $C_{17}H_{11}Br_2NO_2$. 421.08. 5,7-Dibromo-2-methyl-8-quinolinol benzoate ester. *UNII-6308U1DL5F. CAS-3684-46-6.* INN; DCF.

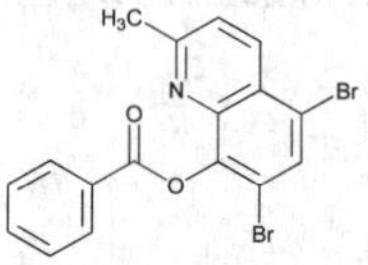

Broxaterol. $C_9H_{15}BrN_2O_2$. 263.13. (±)-3-Bromo-α-[(*tert*-butylamino)methyl]-5-isoxazolemethanol. *UNII-ZE4IRB4-DUC. CAS-76596-57-1.* INN.

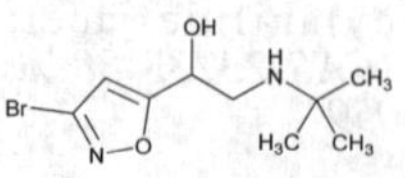

Broxitalamic Acid. $C_{12}H_{11}Br_3N_2O_5$. 502.94. 5-Acetamido-2,4,6-tribromo-*N*-(2-hydroxyethyl)isophthalamic acid. *UNII-CX05Q7WO72. CAS-86216-41-3.* INN.

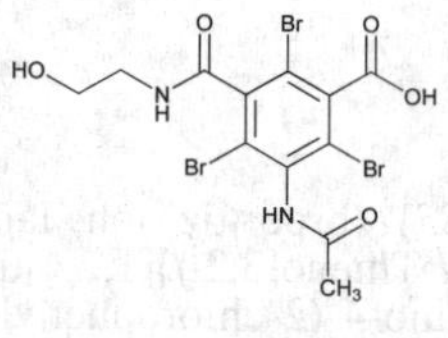

Broxuridine. $C_9H_{11}BrN_2O_5$. 307.10. 5-Bromo-2′-deoxy-uridine. *CAS-59-14-3.* INN; JAN.

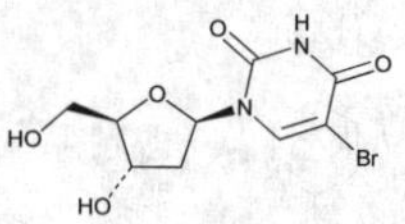

Broxyquinoline. $C_9H_5Br_2NO$. 302.95. 5,7-Dibromo-8-quinolinol. *UNII-UK4C618C8T. CAS-521-74-4.* INN; DCF; MI.

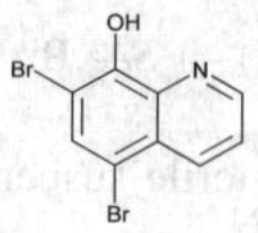

Brucine Sulfate. *CAS-4845-99-2; CAS-357-57-3* [brucine]. NF IX; MI.

Bucainide Maleate [*1976*] (bue′ ka nide mal′ ee ate). $C_{21}H_{35}N_3.2C_4H_4O_4$. 561.67. [Bucainide is INN.] (1) Piperazine, 1-hexyl-4-[[(2-methylpropyl)imino]phenyl-methyl]-, (*Z*)-2-butenedioate (1:2); (2) 1-Hexyl-4-(*N*-iso-butylbenzimidoyl)piperazine maleate (1:2). *UNII-F0D4M5RASG* [bucainide]. *CAS-51481-63-1; CAS-51481-62-0* [bucainide]. *Cardiac depressant (anti-arrhythmic).*

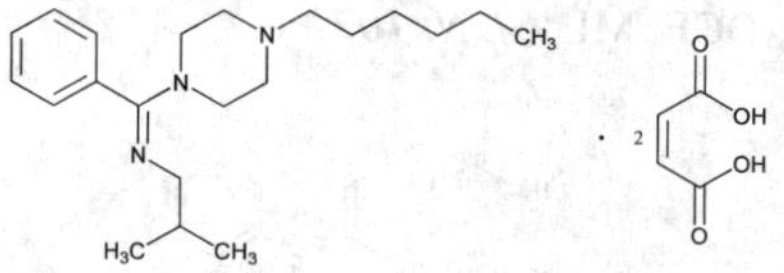

Bucelipase Alfa. $C_{3434}H_{5258}N_{894}O_{1041}S_{17}$. Human bile-salt-activated lipase (cholesterol esterase, EC 3.1.1.13), glyco-form alfa (recombinant hBSSL). *CAS-9026-00-0.* INN.

Bucetin. $C_{12}H_{17}NO_3$. 223.27. 3-Hydroxy-*p*-butyropheneti-dide. *UNII-6M7CVQ8PF8. CAS-1083-57-4.* INN; BAN; JAN; MI.

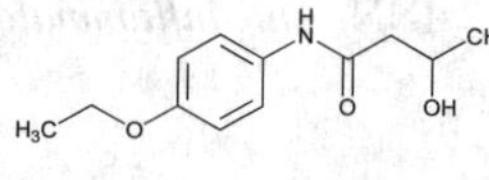

Buciclovir. $C_9H_{13}N_5O_3$. 239.23. (*R*)-9-(3,4-Dihydroxybutyl)-guanine. *UNII-4G4Z4676IS. CAS-86304-28-1.* INN.

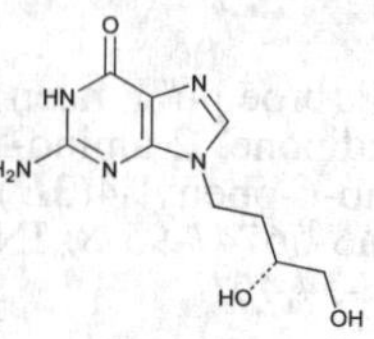

Bucillamine. $C_7H_{13}NO_3S_2$. 223.31. *N*-(2-Mercapto-2-methyl-propionyl)-L-cysteine. *CAS-65002-17-7.* INN; JAN; MI.

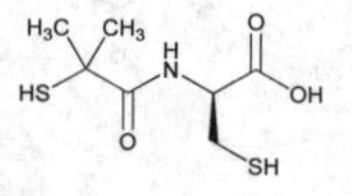

Bucindolol Hydrochloride [*1979*] (bue sin′ doe lol hye″ droe klor′ ide). $C_{22}H_{25}N_3O_2.HCl$. 399.91. [Bucindolol is INN and BAN.] (1) Benzonitrile, 2-[2-hydroxy-3-[[2-(1*H*-indol-

3-yl)-1,1-dimethylethyl]amino]propoxy]-, monohydrochloride; (2) *o*-[2-Hydroxy-3-[[2-indol-3-yl-1,1-dimethylethyl)amino]propoxy]benzonitrile monohydrochloride. *UNII-E9UO06K7CE* [bucindolol]. *CAS-70369-47-0; CAS-71119-11-4* [bucindolol]. *Antihypertensive.* ◇*MJ 13,105-1*

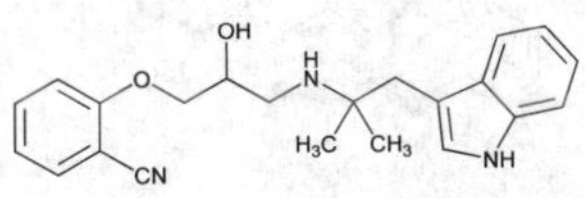

Bucladesine. $C_{18}H_{24}N_5O_8P$. 469.39. [Bucladesine Sodium is JAN.] *N*-(9-β-D-Ribofuranosyl)-9*H*-purin-6-yl)butyramide cyclic 3′,5′-(hydrogen phosphate) 2′-butyrate. *CAS-362-74-3*. INN; MI.

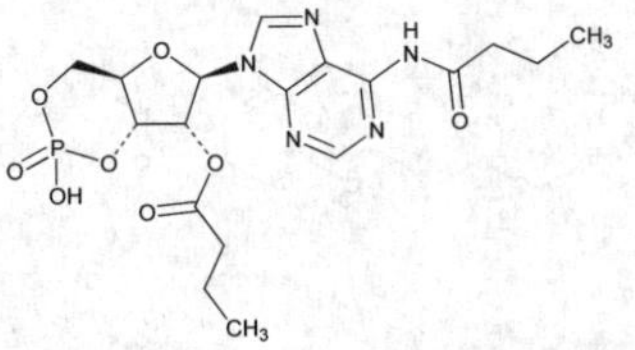

Buclizine Hydrochloride [*1962*] (bue′ kli zeen hye″ droe klor′ ide). $C_{28}H_{33}ClN_2 \cdot 2HCl$. 505.95. [Buclizine is INN and BAN.] (1) Piperazine, 1-[(4-chlorophenyl)phenylmethyl]-4-[[4-(1,1-dimethylethyl)phenyl]methyl]-, dihydrochloride; (2) 1-(*p-tert*-Butylbenzyl)-4-(*p*-chloro-α-phenylbenzyl)piperazine dihydrochloride. *UNII-58FQD093NU; UNII-0C94V6X681* [buclizine]. *CAS-129-74-8; CAS-82-95-1* [buclizine]. *Antinauseant.* Bucladin (Stuart) ◇*UCB 4445; NSC-25141*

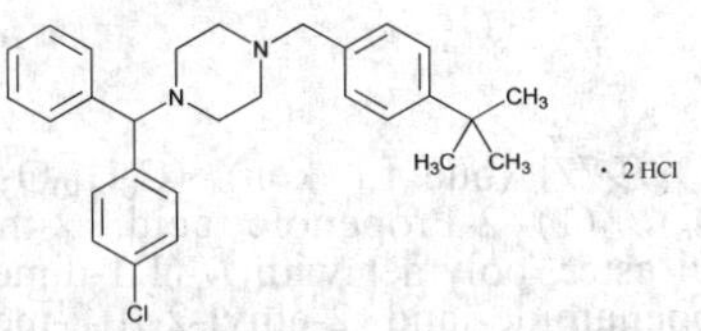

Buclosamide. $C_{11}H_{14}ClNO_2$. 227.69. *N*-Butyl-4-chlorosalicylamide. *UNII-O52NM0A9YL. CAS-575-74-6.* INN; BAN; DCF; MI.

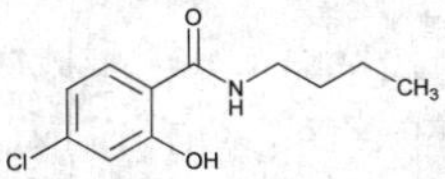

Bucloxic Acid. $C_{16}H_{19}ClO_3$. 294.77. 3-(3-Chloro-4-cyclohexylbenzoyl)propionic acid. *UNII-KV89R7ELF8. CAS-32808-51-8.* INN; DCF; MI. ◇*CB 804*

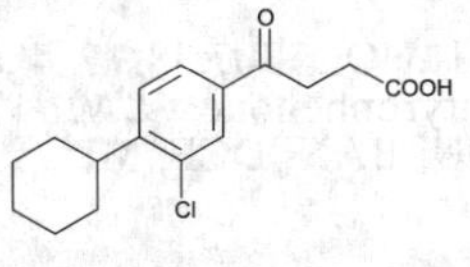

Bucolome. $C_{14}H_{22}N_2O_3$. 266.34. 5-Butyl-1-cyclohexylbarbituric acid. *UNII-9T08RAL174. CAS-841-73-6.* INN; JAN; MI.

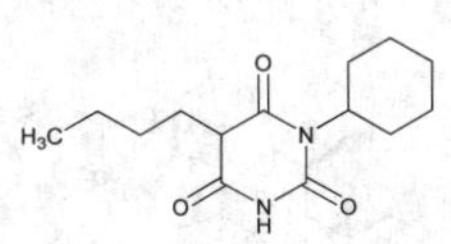

Bucricaine. $C_{17}H_{22}N_2$. 254.37. 9-(Butylamino)-1,2,3,4-tetrahydroacridine. *UNII-HUC352BGYM. CAS-316-15-4.* INN.

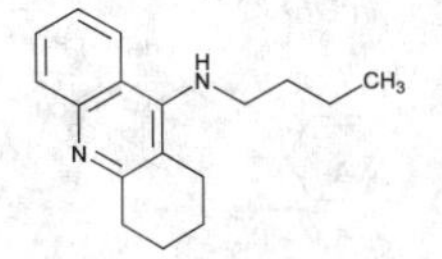

Bucrilate (INN) — *See* Bucrylate.

Bucromarone [*1986*] (bue kroe′ ma rone). $C_{29}H_{37}NO_4$. 463.61. (1) 4*H*-1-Benzopyran-4-one, 2-[4-[3-(dibutylamino)propoxy]-3,5-dimethylbenzoyl]-; (2) 2-[4-[3-(Dibutylamino)propoxyl]-3,5-dimethylbenzoyl]chromone. *UNII-JI688O846T. CAS-78371-66-1.* INN. *Cardiac depressant (anti-arrhythmic).*

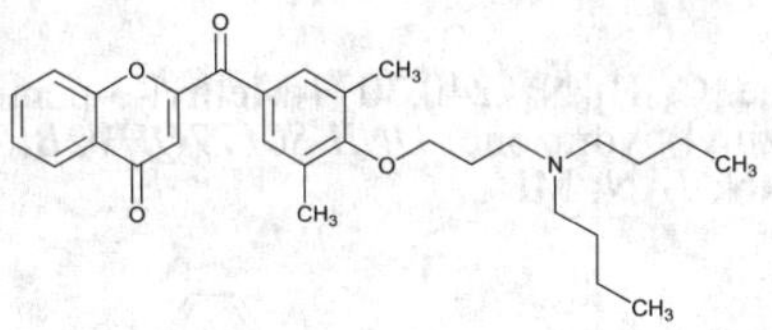

Bucrylate [*1969*] (bue′ kri late). $C_8H_{11}NO_2$. 153.18. [Bucrilate is INN.] (1) 2-Propenoic acid, 2-cyano-, 2-methylpropyl ester; (2) Isobutyl 2-cyanoacrylate. *CAS-1069-55-2. Surgical aid (tissue adhesive).* ◇*IBC*

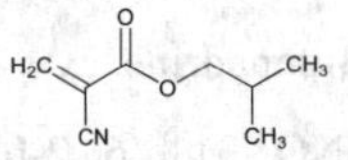

Bucumolol. $C_{17}H_{23}NO_4$. 305.37. [Bucumolol Hydrochloride is JAN.] 8-[3-(*tert*-Butylamino)-2-hydroxypropoxy]-5-methylcoumarin. *UNII-U8WVJ3501L. CAS-58409-59-9.* INN; MI.

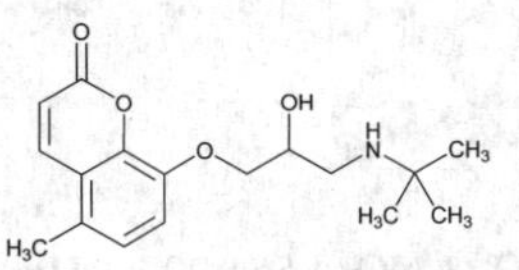

Budesonide [*1979*] (bue des′ oh nide). **USP.** $C_{25}H_{34}O_6$. 430.53. [Note—Budesonide is a mixture of two isomers; its content of [11β,16α(S)] may vary between 40% and 51%.] (1) Pregna-1,4-diene-3,20-dione, 16,17-butylidenebis(oxy)-11,21-dihydroxy-, [11β,16α(R)], and 16α,17-[(S)-Butylidenebis(oxy)]-11β,21-dihydroxypregna-1,4-diene-3,20-dione; (2) (*RS*)-11β,16α,17,21-Tetrahydroxypregna-1,4-diene-3,20-dione cyclic 16,17-acetal with butyraldehyde. *UNII-Q3OKS62Q6X. CAS-51333-22-3* [11β,16α]; *CAS-51372-29-3* [(11β,16α[*R*])]; *CAS-51372-28-2*

---

† Brand name formerly used, and/or firm no longer concerned with this product.

[(11β,16α[*S*])]. INN; BAN; JAN. *Anti-inflammatory.* Pulmicort (AstraZeneca); Rhinocort (AstraZeneca) ◇*S-1320*

Budipine. $C_{21}H_{27}N$. 293.45. 1-*tert*-Butyl-4,4-diphenylpiperidine. *UNII-L9026OPI2Z. CAS-57982-78-2.* INN; MI.

Budotitane. $C_{24}H_{28}O_6Ti$. 460.34. Diethoxybis(1-phenyl-1,3-butanedionato)titanium. *CAS-85969-07-9.* INN.

Budralazine. $C_{14}H_{16}N_4$. 240.30. 4-Methyl-3-penten-2-one (1-phthalazinyl)hydrazone. *UNII-S0177QHV2B. CAS-36798-79-5.* INN; JAN; MI.

Bufenadine — *See* Bufenadrine.

Bufenadrine. $C_{21}H_{29}NO$. 311.46. 2-[(*o-tert*-Butyl-α-phenylbenzyl)oxy]-*N,N*-dimethylethylamine. *UNII-9Y0T619B3U. CAS-604-74-0.* INN. ◇*B.S. 6534*

Bufeniode. $C_{19}H_{23}I_2NO_2$. 551.20. 4-Hydroxy-3,5-diiodo-α-[1[(1-methyl-3-phenylpropyl)amino]ethyl] benzyl alcohol. *UNII-JC82071PQS. CAS-22103-14-6.* INN; DCF; MI. ◇*HF 241*

Bufetolol. $C_{18}H_{29}NO_4$. 323.43. [Bufetolol Hydrochloride is JAN.] 1-(*tert*-Butylamino)-3-[*o*-[(tetrahydrofurfuryl)oxy]-phenoxy]-2-propanol. *UNII-WS1467RT9Z. CAS-53684-49-4.* INN; MI. ◇*Y 6124 [as hydrochloride]*

Bufexamac. $C_{12}H_{17}NO_3$. 223.27. 2-(*p*-Butoxyphenyl)-acetohydroxamic acid. *CAS-2438-72-4.* INN; BAN; JAN; DCF; MI. Anderm (Wyeth-Ayerst†); Paraderm (Wyeth-Ayerst); Parfenac (Wyeth-Ayerst) ◇*CP 1044 J3*

Bufezolac. $C_{21}H_{22}N_2O_2$. 334.41. 1-Isobutyl-3,4-diphenylpyrazole-5-acetic acid. *UNII-PUA774J9MP. CAS-50270-32-1.* INN.

Bufilcon A [*1977*] (bue fil′ kon). $(C_6H_{10}O_3)_x(C_9H_{15}NO_2)_y(C_{18}H_{26}O_6)_z$. (1) 2-Propenoic acid, 2-methyl-, 2-hydroxyethyl ester, polymer with *N*-(1,1-dimethyl-3-oxobutyl)-2-propenamide and 2-ethyl-2-[[(2-methyl-1-oxo-2-propenyl)oxy]methyl]-1,3-propanediyl bis(2-methyl-2-propenoate); (2) 2-Hydroxyethyl methacrylate polymer with *N*-(1,1-dimethyl-3-oxobutyl)acrylamide and 2-ethyl-2-(hydroxymethyl)-1,3-propanediol trimethacrylate. *CAS-56030-52-5. Contact lens material (hydrophilic).* ◇*80066*

Buflomedil. $C_{17}H_{25}NO_4$. 307.38. 2′,4′,6′-Trimethoxy-4-(1-pyrrolidinyl)butyrophenone. *UNII-V7I71DQ432. CAS-55837-25-7.* INN; BAN; DCF; MI.

Bufogenin. $C_{24}H_{32}O_4$. 384.51. 14,15β-Epoxy-3β-hydroxy-5β-bufa-20,22-dienolide. *UNII-3K654P2M4J. CAS-465-39-4.* INN; JAN; MI.

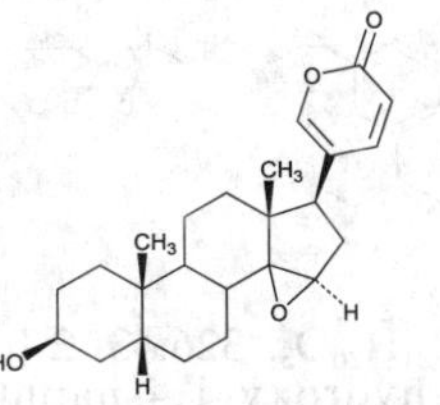

Buformin [*1965*] (bue for' min). $C_6H_{15}N_5$. 157.22. [Buformin Hydrochloride is JAN.] (1) Imidodicarbonimidic diamide, *N*-butyl-; (2) 1-Butylbiguanide. *CAS-692-13-7.* INN. *Antidiabetic.* ◇*DBV; W 37*

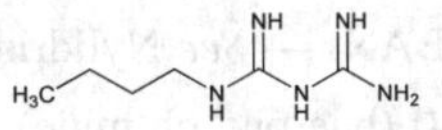

Bufrolin. $C_{18}H_{16}N_2O_6$. 356.33. 6-Butyl-1,4,7,10-tetrahydro-4,10-dioxo-1,7-phenanthroline-2,8-dicarboxylic acid. *UNII-46C1PX266N. CAS-54867-56-0.* INN; BAN.

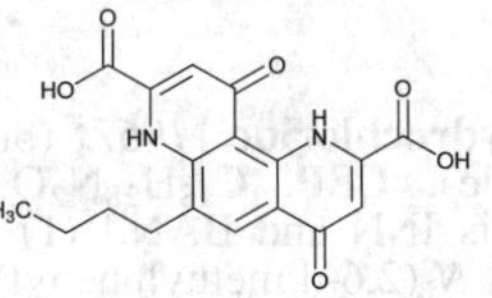

Bufuralol. $C_{16}H_{23}NO_2$. 261.36. α-[(*tert*-Butylamino)methyl]-7-ethyl-2-benzofuranmethanol. *UNII-891H89GFT4. CAS-54340-62-4.* INN; BAN; MI.

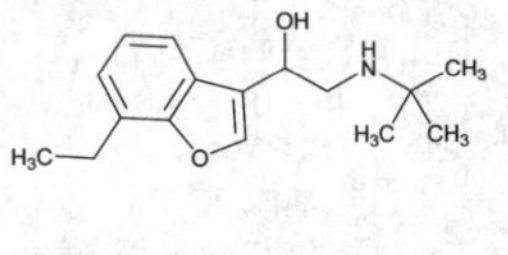

Bufylline (BAN and previously used name) — *See* Ambuphylline.

Bulaquine. $C_{21}H_{27}N_3O_3$. 369.46. Dihydro-3-[1-[[4-[(6-methoxy-8-quinolyl)amino]pentyl]amino]ethylidene]-2(3*H*)-furanone. *UNII-TSQ6U39Q3G. CAS-223661-25-4.* INN.

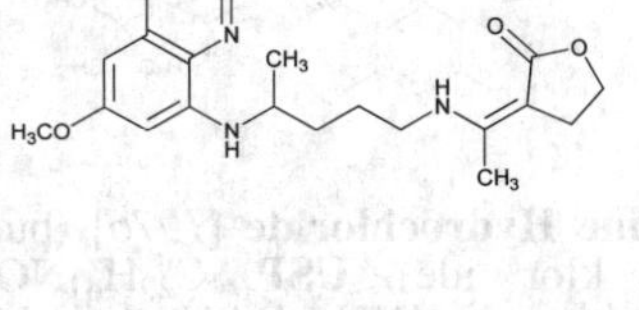

Bultal. A solution of chondroitin sulfate-iron colloid. JAN.

---

† Brand name formerly used, and/or firm no longer concerned with this product.

Bumadizone. $C_{19}H_{22}N_2O_3$. 326.39. Butylmalonic acid mono(1,2-diphenylhydrazide). *UNII-ATD81G944M. CAS-3583-64-0.* INN; DCF; MI.

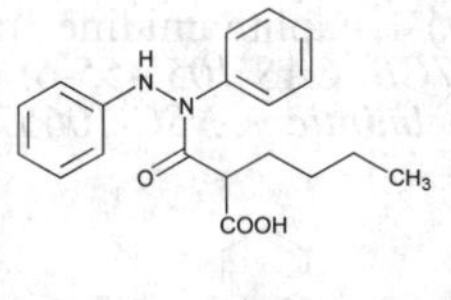

Bumecaine. $C_{18}H_{28}N_2O$. 288.43. 1-Butyl-2′,4′,6′-trimethyl-2-pyrrolidinecarboxanilide. *UNII-B77K612SPZ. CAS-30103-44-7.* INN.

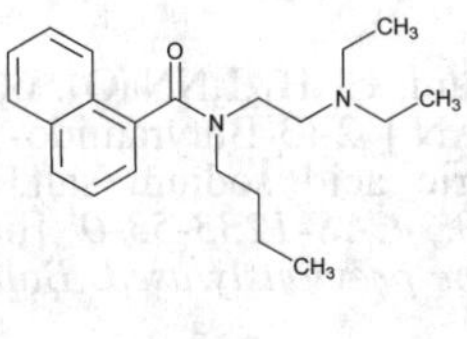

Bumepidil. $C_{12}H_{17}N_5$. 231.30. 8-*tert*-Butyl-7,8-dihydro-5-methyl-6*H*-pyrrolo[3,2-*e*]-*s*-triazolo[1,5-*a*]pyrimidine. *UNII-9FNZ7TFY4R. CAS-62052-97-5.* INN.

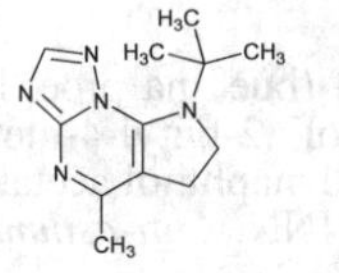

Bumetanide [*1976*] (bue met' a nide). **USP.** $C_{17}H_{20}N_2O_5S$. 364.42. (1) Benzoic acid, 3-(aminosulfonyl)-5-(butylamino)-4-phenoxy-; (2) 3-(Butylamino)-4-phenoxy-5-sulfamoylbenzoic acid. *UNII-0Y2S3XUQ5H. CAS-28395-03-1.* INN; BAN; JAN. *Diuretic.* Bumex (Roche) ◇*Ro 10-6338*

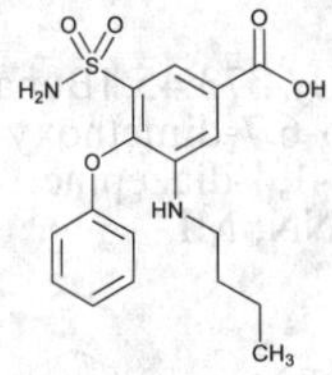

Bumetrizole [*1979*] (bue me' tri zole). $C_{17}H_{18}ClN_3O$. 315.80. (1) Phenol, 2-(5-chloro-2*H*-benzotriazol-2-yl)-6-(1,1-dimethylethyl)-4-methyl-; (2) 2-*tert*-Butyl-6-(5-chloro-2*H*-benzotriazol-2-yl)-*p*-cresol. *UNII-7ZF18Q354W. CAS-3896-11-5.* INN. *Ultraviolet screen.*

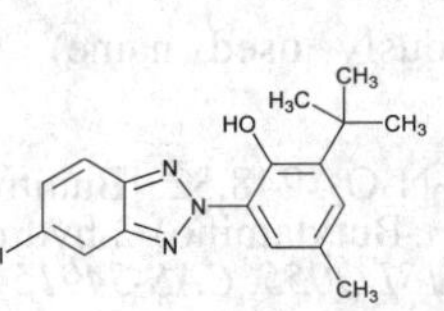

Bunaftine. $C_{21}H_{30}N_2O$. 326.48. *N*-Butyl-*N*-[2-(diethylamino)ethyl]-1-naphthamide. *UNII-GH09PRQ3FU. CAS-32421-46-8.* INN; MI.

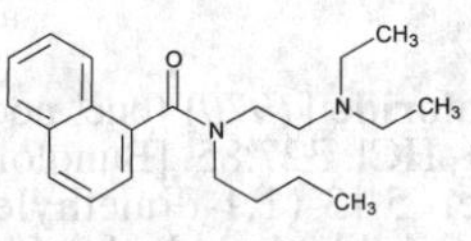

Bunamidine Hydrochloride [*1965*] (bue nam′ i deen hye″ droe klor′ ide). C$_{25}$H$_{38}$N$_2$O.HCl. 419.04. [Bunamidine is INN and BAN.] (1) 1-Naphthalenecarboximidamide, *N,N*-dibutyl-4-(hexyloxy)-, monohydrochloride; (2) *N,N*-Dibutyl-4-(hexyloxy)-1-naphthamidine monohydrochloride. *UNII-Y80LB0Q7CB. CAS-1055-55-6; CAS-3748-77-4* [bunamidine]. *Anthelmintic.* ◇*NSC-106571*

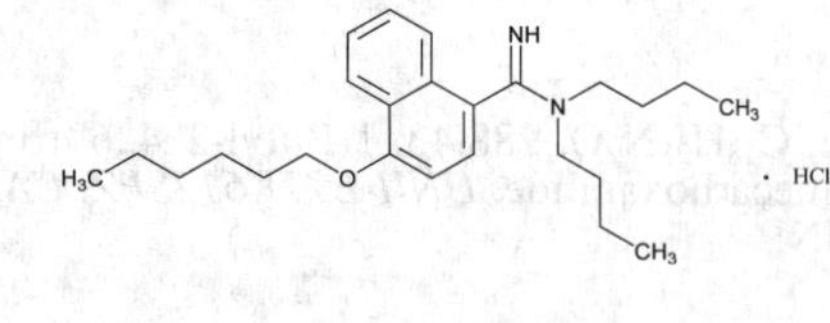

Bunamiodyl Sodium. C$_{15}$H$_{15}$I$_3$NNaO$_3$. 660.99. [Bunamiodyl is INN and BAN.] 2-(3-Butyramido-3,4,6-triiodophenyl-methylene)butyric acid sodium salt. *UNII-NTI7T2IEIE. CAS-1923-76-8; CAS-1233-53-0* [bunamiodyl]. NND 1964; MI. *[Name previously used: Buniodyl.]*

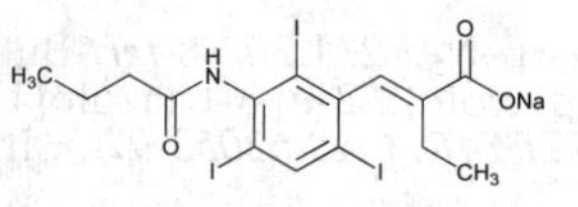

Bunaprolast [*1989*] (bue″ na proe′ last). C$_{17}$H$_{20}$O$_3$. 272.34. (1) 1-Naphthalenol, 2-butyl-4-methoxy-, acetate; (2) 2-Butyl-4-methoxy-1-naphthol acetate. *UNII-WKF2F316K6. CAS-99107-52-5.* INN. *Anti-asthmatic.* ◇*U-66858*

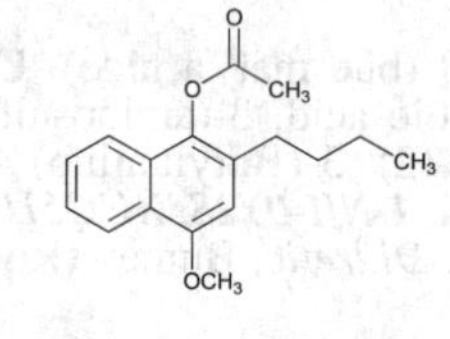

Bunazosin. C$_{19}$H$_{27}$N$_5$O$_3$. 373.45. [Bunazosin Hydrochloride is JAN.] 1-(4-Amino-6,7-dimethoxy-2-quinazolinyl)-4-butyrylhexahydro-1*H*-1,4-diazepine. *UNII-9UUW4V7G2H. CAS-80755-51-7.* INN; MI.

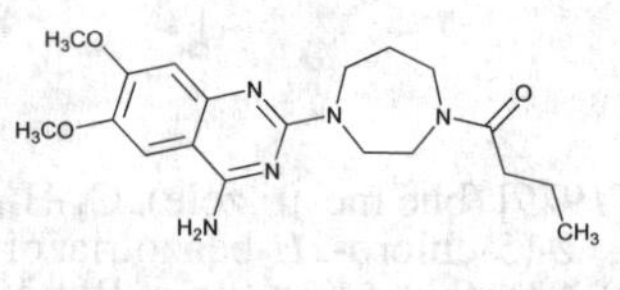

Bundlin (previously used name) — *See* Sedecamycin.

Buniodyl (previously used name) — *See* Bunamiodyl Sodium.

Bunitrolol. C$_{14}$H$_{20}$N$_2$O$_2$. 248.32. [Bunitrolol Hydrochloride is JAN.] *o*-[3-(*tert*-Butylamino)-2-hydroxypropoxy]benzonitrile. *UNII-F2613LO055. CAS-34915-68-9.* INN; MI. ◇*KO 1366*

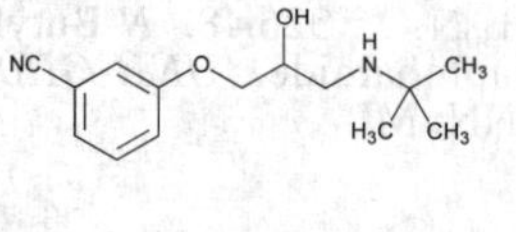

Bunolol Hydrochloride [*1970*] (bue′ noe lol hye″ droe klor′ ide). C$_{17}$H$_{25}$NO$_3$.HCl. 327.85. [Bunolol is INN.] (1) 1(2*H*)-Naphthalenone, 5-[3-(1,1-dimethylethyl)amino]-2-hydroxypropoxy]-3,4-dihydro-, hydrochloride (±); (2) (±)-5-[3-(*tert*-Butylamino)-2-hydroxypropoxy]-3,4-dihydro-

1(2*H*)-naphthalenone hydrochloride. *CAS-31969-05-8; CAS-27591-01-1* [bunolol]. *Anti-adrenergic (β-receptor).* ◇*W 6412A*

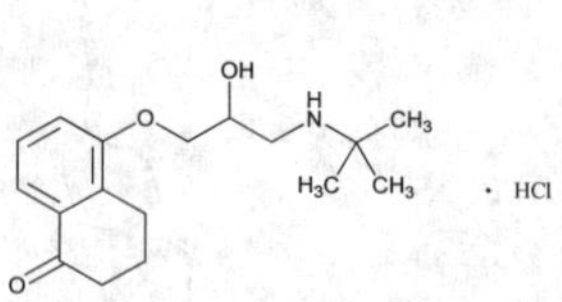

Buparvaquone. C$_{21}$H$_{26}$O$_3$. 326.43. 2-[(4-*tert*-Butylcyclohexyl)methyl]-3-hydroxy-1,4-naphthoquinone. *UNII-0354RT7LG4. CAS-88426-33-9.* INN; BAN; MI.

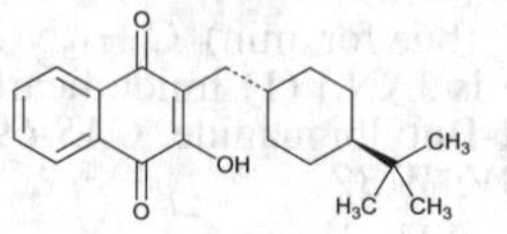

Buphenine (INN, BAN) — *See* Nylidrin Hydrochloride.

Bupicomide [*1974*] (bue pik′ oh mide). C$_{10}$H$_{14}$N$_2$O. 178.23. (1) 2-Pyridinecarboxamide, 5-butyl-; (2) 5-Butylpicolinamide. *CAS-22632-06-0.* INN. *Antihypertensive.* ◇*Sch 10595*

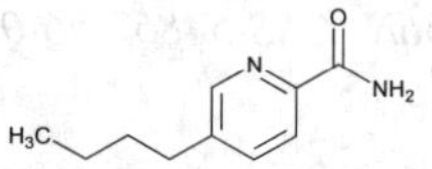

Bupivacaine Hydrochloride [*1967*] (bue piv′ a kane hye″ droe klor′ ide). USP. C$_{18}$H$_{28}$N$_2$O.HCl.H$_2$O. 342.90. [Bupivacaine is INN and BAN.] (1) 2-Piperidinecarboxamide, 1-butyl-*N*-(2,6-dimethylphenyl)-, monohydrochloride, monohydrate; (2) (±)-1-Butyl-2′,6′-pipecoloxylidide monohydrochloride, monohydrate. *UNII-7TQO7W3VT8; UNII-Y8335394RO* [bupivacaine]. *CAS-14252-80-3; CAS-2180-92-9* [bupivacaine]; *CAS-18010-40-7* [anhydrous]. JAN. *Anesthetic (local).* Marcaine (Hospira) ◇*Win 11,318; LAC-43*

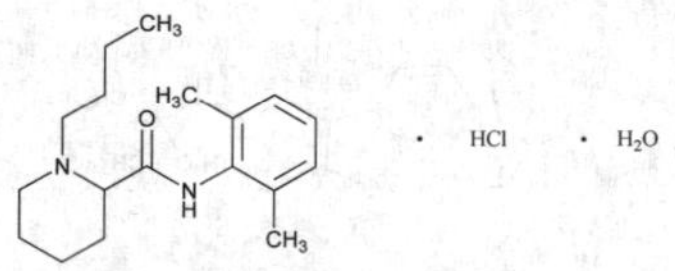

Bupranol — *See* Bupranolol.

Bupranolol. C$_{14}$H$_{22}$ClNO$_2$. 271.78. [Bupranolol Hydrochloride is JAN.] 1-(*tert*-Butylamino)-3-[(6-chloro-*m*-tolyl)oxy]-2-propanol. *UNII-858YGI5PIT. CAS-14556-46-8.* INN; DCF; MI. ◇*B 1312 [as hydrochloride]; KL-255 [as hydrochloride]*

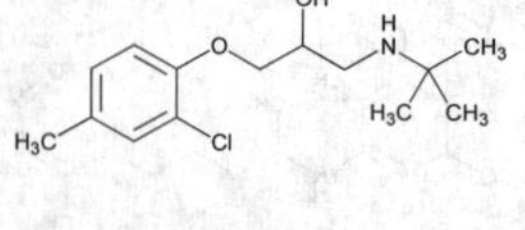

Buprenorphine Hydrochloride [*1976*] (bue″ pre nor′ feen hye″ droe klor′ ide). USP. C$_{29}$H$_{41}$NO$_4$.HCl. 504.10. [Buprenorphine is INN, BAN and JAN.] (1) 6,14-Ethenomorphinan-7-methanol, 17-(cyclopropylmethyl)-α-(1,1-dimethylethyl)-4,5-epoxy-18,19-dihydro-3-hydroxy-6-methoxy-α-methyl-, hydrochloride, [5α,7α(*S*)]-; (2) 21-Cyclopropyl-7α-[(*S*)-1-hydroxy-1,2,2-trimethylpropyl]-6,14-*endo*-ethano-6,7,8,14-tetrahydrooripavine hydrochloride. *UNII-56W8MW3EN1; UNII-40D3SCR4GZ* [buprenorphine]. *CAS-53152-21-9; CAS-52485-79-7* [buprenorphine]. JAN. *Analgesic.* Buprenex (Reckitt Benckiser); Subutex (Reckitt Benckiser) ◇*CL 112,302; RX 6029-M HCl; UM 952; NIH 8805*

Bupropion Hydrobromide [*2008*] (bue proe′ pee on hye″ droe broe′ mide). $C_{13}H_{18}ClNO.HBr$. 320.65. (1) 1-Propanone, 1-(3-chlorophenyl)-2-[(1,1-dimethylethyl)amino]-, hydrobromide (1:1); (2) (2*RS*)-1-(3-Chlorophenyl)-2-[(1,1-dimethylethyl)amino]propan-1-one hydrobromide. *UNII-E70G3G5863. CAS-905818-69-1. Treatment of major depressive disorder.*

Bupropion Hydrochloride [*1974*] (bue proe′ pee on hye″ droe klor′ ide). USP. $C_{13}H_{18}ClNO.HCl$. 276.20. [Bupropion is INN and BAN.] (1) 1-Propanone, 1-(3-chlorophenyl)-2-[(1,1-dimethylethyl)amino]-, hydrochloride, (±)-; (2) (±)-2-(*tert*-Butylamino)-3′-chloropropiophenone hydrochloride. *UNII-ZG7E5POY8O. CAS-31677-93-7; CAS-34911-55-2* [amfebutamone]. JAN. *Antidepressant.* Wellbutrin (GlaxoSmithKline); Zyban (GlaxoSmithKline) ◇*BW 323*

Buquineran. $C_{20}H_{29}N_5O_3$. 387.48. 1-Butyl-3-[1-(6,7-dimethoxy-4-quinazolinyl)-4-piperidyl]urea. *UNII-AWC1VMS3HC. CAS-59184-78-0.* INN; BAN.

Buquinolate [*1965*] (bue kwin′ oh late). $C_{20}H_{27}NO_5$. 361.43. (1) 3-Quinolinecarboxylic acid, 4-hydroxy-6,7-bis(2-methylpropoxy)-, ethyl ester; (2) Ethyl 4-hydroxy-6,7-diisobutoxy-3-quinolinecarboxylate. *UNII-MFL71K7PU4. CAS-5486-03-3.* INN. *Coccidiostat (for poultry).* ◇*EU-1093*

Buquiterine. $C_{18}H_{23}N_3O_3$. 329.39. 2-(*tert*-Butylamino)-6,7-dihydro-9,10-dimethoxy-4*H*-pyrimido[6,1-*a*]isoquinolin-4-one. *UNII-49YNN75I8N. CAS-76536-74-8.* INN.

Buramate [*1964*] (bue′ ra mate). $C_{10}H_{13}NO_3$. 195.22. (1) Carbamic acid, (phenylmethyl)-, 2-hydroxyethyl ester; (2) 2-Hydroxyethyl benzylcarbamate. *CAS-4663-83-6.* INN. *Anticonvulsant; antipsychotic.* ◇*AC-601; NSC-30223*

Burefrine (previously used name) — *See* Berefrine.

Burodiline. $C_{19}H_{29}NO_5$. 351.44. 1-Pyrrolidineethanol 4-butoxy-3,5-dimethoxybenzoate (ester). *UNII-4006BCR8NJ. CAS-36121-13-8.* INN.

Buserelin Acetate [*1979*] (bue″ se rel′ in as′ e tate). $C_{60}H_{86}N_{16}O_{13}.C_2H_4O_2$. 1299.48. [Buserelin is INN and BAN.] (1) Luteinizing hormone-releasing factor (pig), 6-[*O*-(1,1-dimethylethyl)-D-serine]-9-(*N*-ethyl-L-prolinamide)-10-deglycinamide-, monoacetate (salt); (2) 5-Oxo-L-prolyl-L-histidyl-L-tryptophyl-L-seryl-L-tyrosyl-*O-tert*-butyl-D-seryl-L-leucyl-L-arginyl-*N*-ethyl-L-prolinamide monoacetate (salt). *CAS-68630-75-1; CAS-57982-77-1* [buserelin]. JAN. *Gonad-stimulating principle.* Suprefact (Hoechst-Roussel†) ◇*HOE 766*

Buspirone Hydrochloride [*1973*] (bue spye′ rone hye″ droe klor′ ide). USP. $C_{21}H_{31}N_5O_2.HCl$. 421.96. [Buspirone is INN and BAN.] (1) 8-Azaspiro[4,5]decane-7,9-dione, 8-[4-[4-(2-pyrimidinyl)-1-piperazinyl]butyl]-, monohydrochloride; (2) *N*-[4-[4-(2-Pyrimidinyl)-1-piperazinyl]butyl]-1,1-cyclopentanediacetamide monohydrochloride. *UNII-207LT9J9OC; UNII-TK65WKS8HL* [buspirone]. *CAS-33386-08-2; CAS-36505-84-7* [buspirone]. *Tranquilizer (minor).* Buspar (Bristol-Myers Squibb) ◇*MJ 9022-1*

Busulfan (bue sul′ fan). USP. $C_6H_{14}O_6S_2$. 246.30. (1) 1,4-Butanediol, dimethanesulfonate; (2) 1,4-Butanediol dimethanesulfonate. *UNII-G1LN9045DK. CAS-55-98-1.*

---

† Brand name formerly used, and/or firm no longer concerned with this product.

INN; BAN; JAN. *Antineoplastic*. Busulfex (PDL Biopharma); Myleran (GlaxoSmithKline) *[Name previously used: Busulphan.]* ◇NSC-750

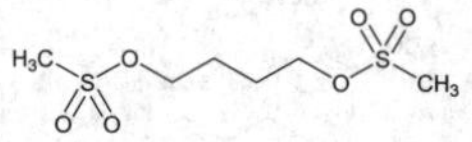

Butabarbital (bue″ ta bar′ bi tal). **USP**. $C_{10}H_{16}N_2O_3$. 212.25. [Secbutabarbital is BAN.] (1) 2,4,6(1*H*,3*H*,5*H*)-Pyrimidinetrione, 5-ethyl-5-(1-methylpropyl)-; (2) 5-*sec*-Butyl-5-ethylbarbituric acid. *UNII-P0078O25A9. CAS-125-40-6. Sedative-hypnotic.*

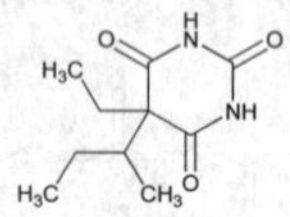

Butabarbital Sodium (bue″ ta bar′ bi tal soe′ dee um). **USP**. $C_{10}H_{15}N_2NaO_3$. 234.23. [Secbutabarbital Sodium is INN.] (1) 2,4,6(1*H*,3*H*,5*H*)-Pyrimidinetrione, 5-ethyl-5-(1-methylpropyl)-, monosodium salt; (2) Sodium 5-*sec*-butyl-5-ethylbarbiturate. *UNII-9WTD50I918; UNII-P0078O25A9* [butabarbital]. *CAS-143-81-7; CAS-125-40-6* [butabarbital]. *Sedative-hypnotic.* Butalan (Lannett); Butisol Sodium (Medpointe); Sarisol (Halsey)

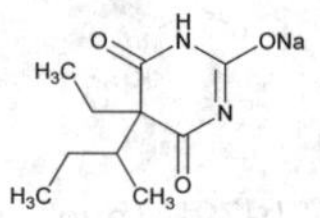

Butacaine Sulfate. $(C_{18}H_{30}N_2O_2)_2.H_2SO_4$. 710.96. [Butacaine is INN and BAN.] (1) 1-Propanol, 3-(dibutylamino)-, 4-aminobenzoate (ester), sulfate (salt) (2:1); (2) 3-(Dibutylamino)-1-propanol *p*-aminobenzoate (ester) sulfate (2:1). *UNII-PAU39W3CVB. CAS-149-15-5; CAS-149-16-6* [butacaine]. USP XX; MI. Butyn (Abbott†)

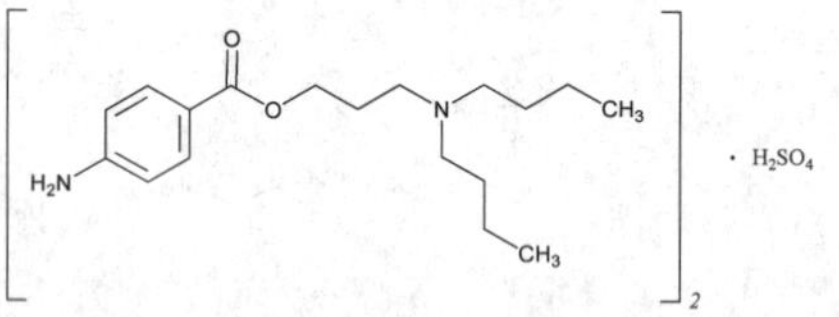

Butacetin [*1964*] (bue ta′ se tin). $C_{12}H_{17}NO_2$. 207.27. (1) Acetamide, *N*-[4-(1,1-dimethylethoxy)phenyl]-; (2) 4′-*tert*-Butoxyacetanilide. *CAS-2109-73-1. Analgesic; antidepressant.* ◇BW 63-90; NSC-106564

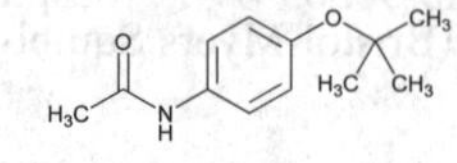

Butacetoluide — *See* Butanilicaine.

Butaclamol Hydrochloride [*1973*] (bue″ ta kla′ mol hye″ droe klor′ ide). $C_{25}H_{31}NO.HCl$. 397.98. [Butaclamol is INN.] (1) 1*H*-Benzo[6,7]cyclohepta[1,2,3-*de*]-pyrido[2,1-*a*]isoquinolin-3-ol, 3-(1,1-dimethylethyl)-2,3,4,4a,8,9,13b,14-octahydro-, hydrochloride, (3α,4aα,13bβ)-(±)-; (2) (±)-3α-*tert*-Butyl-2,3,4,4aβ,8,9,13bα,14-octahydro-1*H*-benzo[6,7]-cyclo-

hepta[1,2,3-*de*]pyrido[2,1-*a*]isoquinolin-3-ol hydrochloride. *UNII-8TUG8SF12T. CAS-36504-94-6; CAS-51152-91-1* [butaclamol]. *Antipsychotic.* ◇AY-23,028

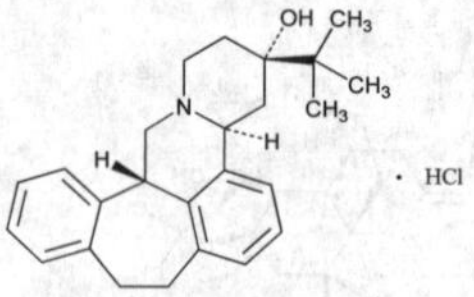

Butadiazamide. $C_{12}H_{14}ClN_3O_2S_2$. 331.84. *N*-(5-Butyl-1,3,4-thiadiazol-2-yl)-*p*-chlorobenzenesulfonamide. *CAS-7007-88-7.* INN.

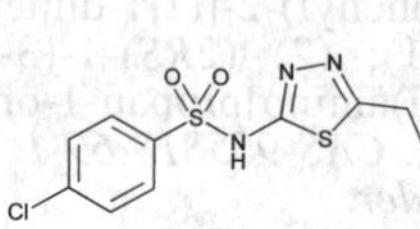

Butafosfan. $C_7H_{18}NO_2P$. 179.20. [1-(Butylamino)-1-methylethyl]phosphinic acid. *UNII-3Q2LQ1149L. CAS-17316-67-5.* INN; BAN.

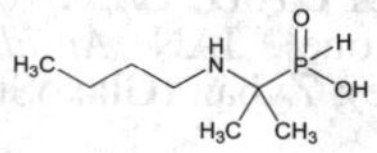

Butalamine. $C_{18}H_{28}N_4O$. 316.44. 5-{[2-(Dibutylamino)ethyl]amino}-3-phenyl-1,2,4-oxadiazole. *UNII-140T9JTG43. CAS-22131-35-7.* INN; BAN; MI. ◇*LA 1221 [as hydrochloride]*

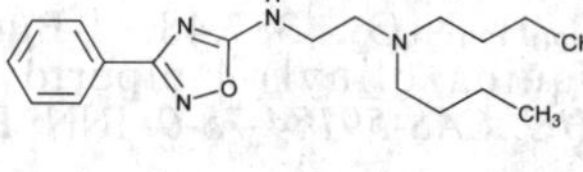

Butalbital [*1966*] (bue tal′ bi tal). **USP**. $C_{11}H_{16}N_2O_3$. 224.26. (1) 2,4,6(1*H*,3*H*,5*H*)-Pyrimidinetrione, 5-(2-methylpropyl)-5-(2-propenyl)-; (2) 5-Allyl-5-isobutylbarbituric acid. *UNII-KHS0AZ4JVK. CAS-77-26-9.* INN. *Sedative-hypnotic.* Sandoptal (Novartis†) *[Name previously used: Allylbarbituric Acid.]*

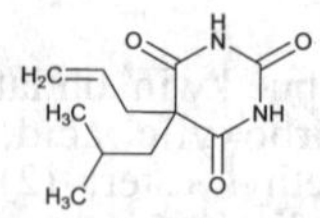

Butallylonal. *CAS-1142-70-7.* NF X; MI.

Butamben [*1975*] (bue tam′ ben). **USP**. $C_{11}H_{15}NO_2$. 193.24. (1) Benzoic acid, 4-amino-, butyl ester; (2) Butyl *p*-aminobenzoate. *UNII-EFW857872Q. CAS-94-25-7. Anesthetic (topical).* Butesin (Abbott) *[Name previously used: Butyl Aminobenzoate.]*

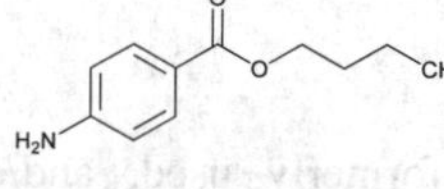

Butamben Picrate [*1981*] (bue tam′ ben pik′ rate). $(C_{11}H_{15}NO_2)_2 \cdot C_6H_3N_3O_7$. 615.59. (1) Benzoic acid, 4-amino-, butyl ester, compound with 2,4,6-trinitrophenol (2:1); (2) Butyl *p*-aminobenzoate, picrate (2:1). *CAS-577-48-0. Anesthetic (topical).* ◇*Abbott-34842*

Butamirate Citrate [*1972*] (bue ta mye′ rate sit′ rate). $C_{18}H_{29}NO_3 \cdot C_6H_8O_7$. 499.55. [Butamirate is INN and BAN.] (1) Benzeneacetic acid, α-ethyl-2-[2-(diethylamino)ethoxy]ethyl ester, 2-hydroxy-1,2,3-propanetricarboxylate (1:1); (2) 2-[2-(Diethylamino)ethoxy]ethyl 2-phenylbutyrate citrate (1:1). *CAS-18109-81-4; CAS-18109-80-3* [butamirate]. *Antitussive.* *[Name previously used: Butamyrate.]* ◇*Abbott-36581; HH 197*

Butamisole Hydrochloride [*1975*] (bue tam′ i sole hye″ droe klor′ ide). $C_{15}H_{19}N_3OS \cdot HCl$. 325.86. [Butamisole is INN.] (1) Propanamide, 2-methyl-*N*-[3-(2,3,5,6-tetrahydroimidazo[2,1-*b*]thiazol-6-yl)phenyl]-, monohydrochloride, (-)-; (2) (-)-2-Methyl-3′-(2,3,5,6-tetrahydroimidazo[2,1-*b*]thiazol-6-yl)propionanilide monohydrochloride. *UNII-QGM18599H5. CAS-54400-62-3; CAS-54400-59-8* [butamisole]. *Anthelmintic (veterinary).* ◇*CL 206,214*

Butamiverine — *See* Butaverine.

Butamoxane. $C_{13}H_{19}NO_2$. 221.30. 2-(Butylaminomethyl)-1,4-benzodioxane. *UNII-7725983GSD. CAS-4442-60-8.* INN.

Butamyrate (previously used name) — *See* Butamirate Citrate.

Butane (bue′ tane). **NF.** C_4H_{10}. 58.12. *n*-Butane. *UNII-6LV4FOR43R. CAS-106-97-8. Aerosol propellant.*

Butanilicaine. $C_{13}H_{19}ClN_2O$. 254.76. 2-(Butylamino)-6′-chloro-*o*-acetoluidide. *CAS-3785-21-5.* INN; BAN; MI.

Butanixin. $C_{16}H_{18}N_2O_2$. 270.33. 2-(*p*-Butanilino)nicotinic acid. *UNII-FZ99TBX0LI. CAS-55285-35-3.* INN.

Butanserin. $C_{24}H_{26}FN_3O_3$. 423.48. 3-[4-[4-(*p*-Fluorobenzoyl)piperidino]butyl]-2,4(1*H*,3*H*)quinazolinedione. *UNII-4I933V848G. CAS-87051-46-5.* INN.

Butantrone. $C_{18}H_{16}O_4$. 296.32. 10-Butyryl-1,8-dihydroxyanthrone. *UNII-9P148IBA8M. CAS-75464-11-8.* INN.

Butaperazine [*1962*] (bue″ ta per′ a zeen). $C_{24}H_{31}N_3OS$. 409.59. (1) 1-Butanone, 1-[10-[3-(4-methyl-1-piperazinyl)propyl]-10*H*-phenothiazin-2-yl]-; (2) 1-{10-[3-(4-Methyl-1-piperazinyl)propyl]phenothiazin-2-yl}-1-butanone. *UNII-TXP4T9106S. CAS-653-03-2.* INN. *Antipsychotic.* ◇*AHR-3000; Bayer 1362; Riker 595*

Butaperazine Maleate [*1969*] (bue″ ta per′ a zeen mal′ ee ate). $C_{24}H_{31}N_3OS \cdot 2C_4H_4O_4$. 641.73. (1) 1-Butanone, 1-[10-[3-(4-methyl-1-piperazinyl)propyl]-10*H*-phenothiazin-2-yl]-, (*Z*)-2-butenedioate (1:2); (2) 1-[10-[3-(4-Methyl-1-piperazinyl)propyl]phenothiazin-2-yl]-1-butanone maleate (1:2). *UNII-22VUW43J2H. CAS-1063-55-4. Antipsychotic.*

Butaprost [*1987*] (bue′ ta prost). $C_{24}H_{40}O_5$. 408.57. (1) Cyclopentaneheptanoic acid, 3-hydroxy-2-[4-hydroxy-4-(1-propylcyclobutyl)-1-butenyl]-5-oxo-, methyl ester, [1*R*-[1α,2β(1*E*,4*R***),3α]]-; (2) Methyl (1*R*,2*R*,3*R*)-3-hydroxy-2-[(1*E*,4*R*)-4-hydroxy-4-(1-propylcyclobutyl)-1-butenyl]-5-oxocyclopentaneheptanoate; (3) Methyl (13*E*,16*R*)-11α,16-dihydroxy-9-oxo-17,17-trimethylene-prost-13-en-1-oate. *UNII-HP16WVP23Y. CAS-69648-38-0.* INN; BAN. *Bronchodilator.* ◇*TR-4979; Bay q 4218*

---

† Brand name formerly used, and/or firm no longer concerned with this product.

Butaverine. $C_{18}H_{27}NO_2$. 289.41. Butyl 3-phenyl-3-(1-piperidyl)propionate. *UNII-1I5O5WIU8X. CAS-55837-14-4.* INN; DCF; MI.

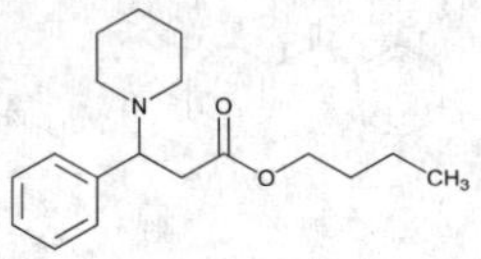

Butaxamine (INN, BAN) — *See* Butoxamine Hydrochloride.

Butedronate Tetrasodium [*1988*] (bue″ te droe′ nate tet″ ra soe′ dee um). $C_5H_6Na_4O_{10}P_2$. 380.00. (1) Butanedioic acid, (diphosphonomethyl)-, tetrasodium salt, (±)-; (2) (±)-(Diphosphonomethyl)succinic acid, tetrasodium salt. *CAS-97772-98-0. Diagnostic aid (bone imaging).* Teceos (Hoechst-Roussel†) ◇*Tc 924 (DPD)*

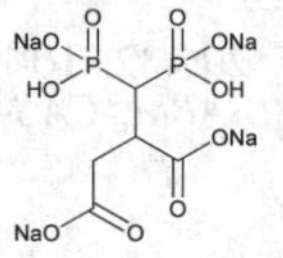

Butedronic Acid. $C_5H_{10}O_{10}P_2$. 292.07. (Diphosphonomethyl)succinic acid. *UNII-26PB1U68YF. CAS-51395-42-7.* INN; MI.

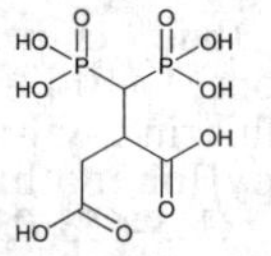

Butenafine Hydrochloride [*1997*] (bue ten′ a feen hye″ droe klor′ ide). $C_{23}H_{27}N·HCl$. 353.93. [Butenafine is INN and BAN.] (1) 1-Naphthalenemethanamine, *N*-[[4-(1,1-dimethylethyl)phenyl]methyl]-*N*-methyl-, hydrochloride; (2) *N*-(*p-tert*-Butylbenzyl)-*N*-methyl-1-naphthalenemethylamine hydrochloride. *UNII-R8XA2029ZI; UNII-91Y494NL0X* [butenafine]. *CAS-101827-46-7; CAS-101828-21-1* [butenafine]. JAN. *Antifungal.* Lotrimin (Schering); Mentax (Mylan Bertek) ◇*KP-363*

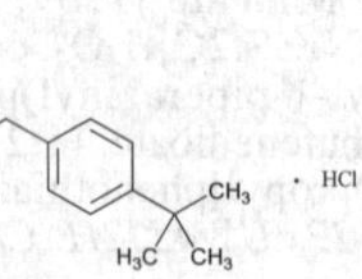

Butenemal — *See* Vinbarbital.

Buterizine [*1979*] (bue ter′ i zeen). $C_{31}H_{38}N_4$. 466.66. (1) 1*H*-Benzimidazole, 2-butyl-5-[[4-(diphenylmethyl)-1-piperazinyl]methyl]-1-ethyl-; (2) 2-Butyl-5-[[4-(diphenylmethyl)-1-piperazinyl]methyl]-1-ethylbenzimidazole. *UNII-N8516V0WOM. CAS-68741-18-4.* INN. *Vasodilator (peripheral).* ◇*R 38,198*

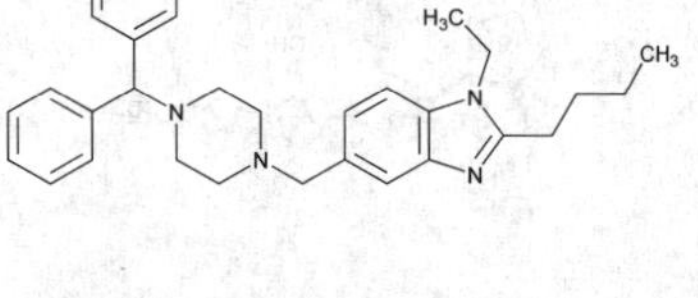

Butetamate. $C_{16}H_{25}NO_2$. 263.38. 2-(Diethylamino)ethyl 2-phenylbutyrate. *UNII-2VO6TC90PU. CAS-14007-64-8.* INN; BAN; MI. *[Name previously used: Butethamate.]* ◇*HH105*

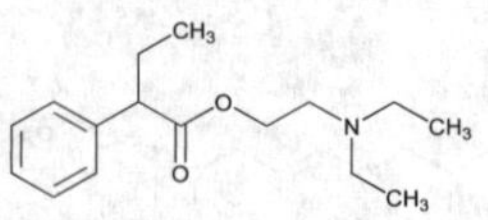

Butethal. $C_{10}H_{16}N_2O_3$. 212.25. [Butobarbital is BAN.] 5-Butyl-5-ethylbarbituric acid. *CAS-77-28-1.* NF X; MI. Neonal (Abbott†) *[Name previously used: Butobarbitone.]*

Butethamine Hydrochloride. *UNII-0M63DKI91K. CAS-553-68-4; CAS-2090-89-3* [butethamine]. NF XIII; MI.

Buthalital Sodium. A mixture of 100 parts by weight of the monosodium derivative of 5-allyl-5-isobutyl-2-thiobarbituric acid and 6 parts by weight of exsiccated sodium carbonate. *CAS-510-90-7.* INN; BAN; MI. *[Name previously used: Buthalitone Sodium.]*

Buthiazide [*1967*] (bue thye′ a zide). $C_{11}H_{16}ClN_3O_4S_2$. 353.85. [Butizide is INN.] (1) 2*H*-1,2,4-Benzothiadiazine-7-sulfonamide, 6-chloro-3,4-dihydro-3-(2-methylpropyl)-, 1,1-dioxide; (2) 6-Chloro-3,4-dihydro-3-isobutyl-2*H*-1,2,4-benzothiadiazine-7-sulfonamide 1,1-dioxide. *CAS-2043-38-1. Diuretic; antihypertensive.*

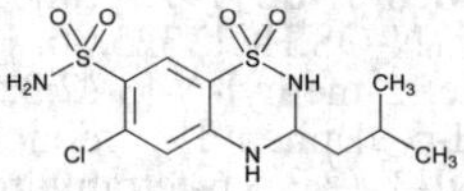

Butibufen. $C_{14}H_{20}O_2$. 220.31. 2-(*p*-Isobutylphenyl)butyric acid. *UNII-JSS1TEM917. CAS-55837-18-8.* INN; MI.

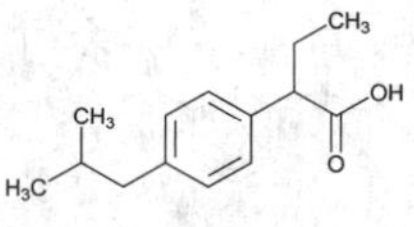

Butidrine. $C_{16}H_{25}NO$. 247.38. α-[(*sec*-Butylamino)methyl]-5,6,7,8-tetrahydro-2-naphthalene-methanol. *UNII-N2S0PKP5L5. CAS-7433-10-5.* INN; DCF; MI. ◇*CO 405*

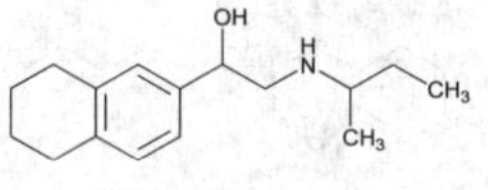

Butikacin [*1978*] (bue″ ti kay′ sin). $C_{22}H_{45}N_5O_{12}$. 571.62. (1) D-Streptamine, *O*-3-amino-3-deoxy-α-D-glucopyranosyl-(1→6)-*O*-[6-amino-6-deoxy-α-D-glucopyranosyl-(1→4)]-N^1-[(*S*)-4-amino-2-hydroxybutyl]-2-deoxy-; (2) *O*-3-Amino-3-deoxy-α-D-glucopyranosyl-(1→6)-*O*-[6-amino-6-deoxy-α-D-glucopyranosyl-(1→4)]-N^1-[(*S*)-4-amino-2-hydroxybutyl]-2-deoxy-D-streptamine. *CAS-59733-86-7.* INN; BAN. *Antibacterial.* ◇*UK-18,892*

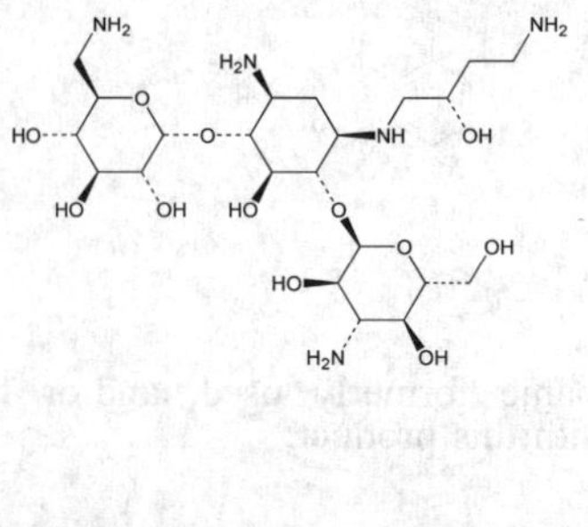

Butilfenin [*1979*] (bue″ til fen′ in). $C_{16}H_{22}N_2O_5$. 322.36. (1) Glycine, *N*-[2-[(4-butylphenyl)amino]-2-oxoethyl]-*N*-(carboxymethyl)-; (2) [[[(*p*-Butylphenyl)carbamoyl]methyl]imino]diacetic acid. *CAS-66292-52-2.* INN. *Diagnostic aid (hepatic function determination).* ◇*p*-BIDA

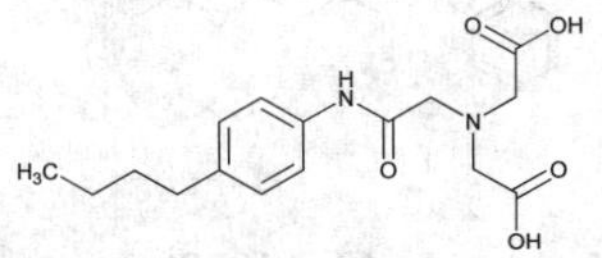

Butinazocine. $C_{18}H_{23}NO_2$. 285.38. (±)-3-(3-Butynyl)-1,2,3,4,5,6-hexahydro-11,11-dimethyl-2,6-methano-3-benzazocine-6,8-diol. *UNII-W11ET455ZI. CAS-93821-75-1.* INN.

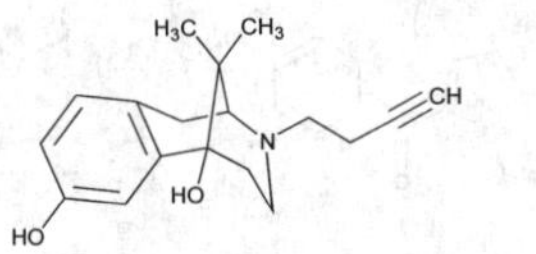

Butinoline. $C_{20}H_{21}NO$. 291.39. 1,1-Diphenyl-4-pyrrolidino-1′-yl but-2-yn-1-ol. *UNII-G216926E9T. CAS-968-63-8.* INN.

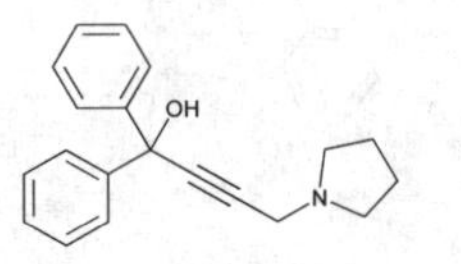

Butirosin Sulfate [*1976*] (bue tir′ oh sin sul′ fate). $C_{21}H_{41}N_5O_{12}.2H_2SO_4.2H_2O$. 787.76. [Butirosin is INN; Butirosin Sulphate is BAN.] Antibiotic produced by *Bacillus circulans.* (1) Butirosin sulfate; (2) D-Streptamine, *O*-2,6-diamino-2,6-dideoxy-α-D-glucopyranosyl-(1→4)-*O*-[β-D-xylofuranosyl-(1→5)]-*N*¹-(4-amino-2-hydroxy-1-oxobutyl)-2-deoxy-, (*S*)-; sulfate (1:2) (salt) dihydrate mixture with *O*-2,6-diamino-2,6-dideoxy-α-D-glucopyranosyl-(1→4)-*O*-[β-D-ribofuranosyl-(1→5)]-*N*¹-[(*S*)-4-amino-2-hydroxy-1-oxobutyl]-2-deoxy-D-streptamine sulfate (1:2) (salt) dihydrate; (3) *O*-2,6-Diamino-2,6-dideoxy-α-D-glucopyranosyl-(1→4)-*O*-[β-D-xylofuranosyl-(1→5)]-*N*¹-(4-amino-L-2-hydroxybutyryl)-2-deoxy-D-streptamine sulfate (1:2) (salt) dihydrate mixture with *O*-2,6-diamino-2,6-dideoxy-α-D-glucopyranosyl-(1→4)-*O*-[β-D-ribofuranosyl-(1→5)]-*N*¹-(4-amino-L-2-hydroxybutyryl)-2-deoxy-D-streptamine sulfate (1:2) (salt) dihydrate. *CAS-51022-98-*

1; *CAS-57549-48-1* [anhydrous]; *CAS-12772-35-9* [butirosin]. *Antibacterial.* [*Note—Butirosin Sulfate is a mixture of A and B forms.*] ◇CI-642

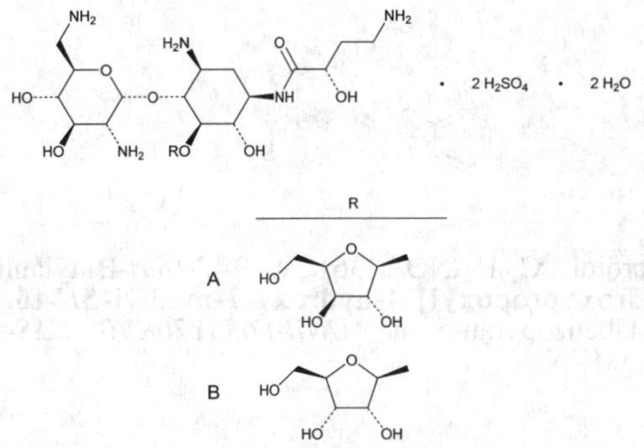

Butixirate [*1981*] (bue tix′ i rate). $C_{16}H_{16}O_2.C_{12}H_{17}N$. 415.57. (1) [1,1′-Biphenyl]-4-acetic acid, α-ethyl-, (±)-, compound with *trans*-4-phenylcyclohexanamine (1:1); (2) (±)-α-Ethyl-4-biphenylacetic acid, compound with *trans*-4-phenylcyclohexylamine (1:1). *UNII-82CYO8A460. CAS-19992-80-4.* INN. *Analgesic; antirheumatic.* Flectar (Maggioni Farmaceutici S.p.A., Italy) ◇*M.G. 5771*

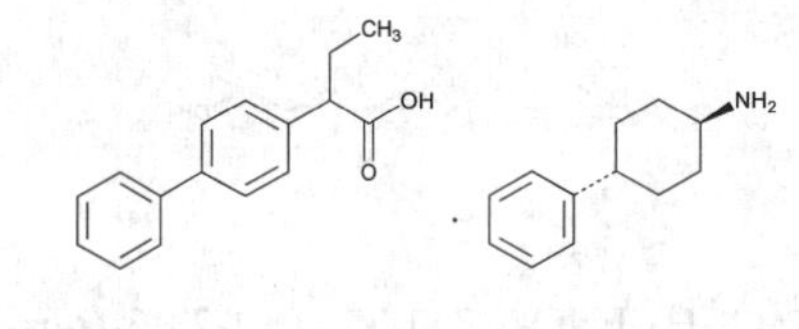

Butixocort. $C_{25}H_{36}O_5S$. 448.62. 11β,17-Dihydroxy-21-mercaptopregn-4-ene-3,20-dione 17-butyrate. *CAS-120815-74-9.* INN.

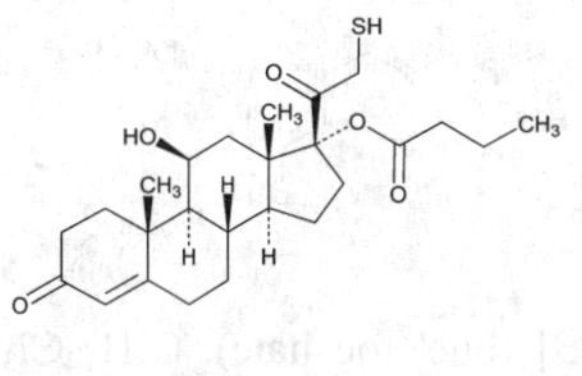

Butizide (INN) — *See* Buthiazide.

Butobarbital (BAN) — *See* Butethal.

Butobarbitone (previously used name) — *See* Butethal.

Butobendine. $C_{32}H_{48}N_2O_{10}$. 620.73. (+)-(*S*,*S*)-Ethylenebis[(-methylimino)(2-ethylethylene)]bis(3,4,5-trimethoxybenzoate). *UNII-RP2J52327K. CAS-55769-65-8.* INN; MI.

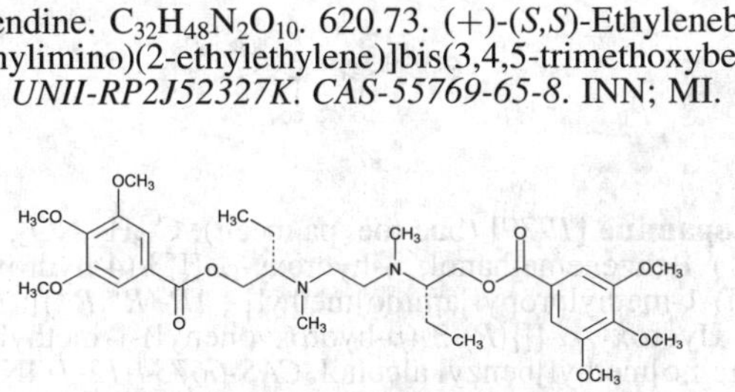

Butoconazole Nitrate [*1978*] (bue″ toe kon′ a zole nye′ trate). **USP.** $C_{19}H_{17}Cl_3N_2S.HNO_3$. 474.79. [Butoconazole is INN and BAN.] (1) 1*H*-Imidazole, 1-[4-(4-chlorophenyl)-2-[(2,6-dichlorophenyl)thio]butyl]-, mononitrate, (±)-; (2) (±)-1-[4-(*p*-Chlorophenyl)-2-[(2,6-dichlorophenyl)thio]butyl]imidazole mononitrate. *UNII-4805237NP5. CAS-*

---

† Brand name formerly used, and/or firm no longer concerned with this product.

64872-77-1; *CAS-64872-76-0* [butoconazole]. *Antifungal.* Femstat (Roche); Gynazole (KV Pharmaceutical) ◇*RS-35887; RS-35887-00-10-3*

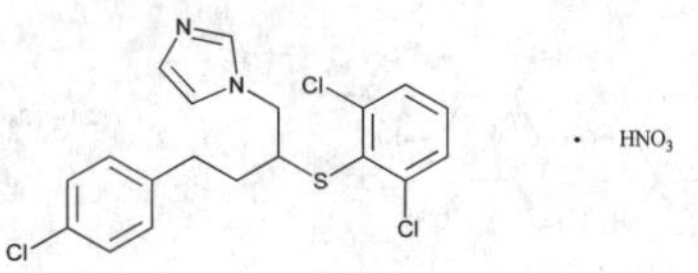

Butocrolol. $C_{19}H_{23}NO_6$. 361.39. 9-[3-(*tert*-Butylamino)-2-hydroxypropoxyl]-4-hydroxy-7-methyl-5*H*-furo[3,2-g][1]benzopyran-5-one. *UNII-F63SY70KV0. CAS-55165-22-5.* INN.

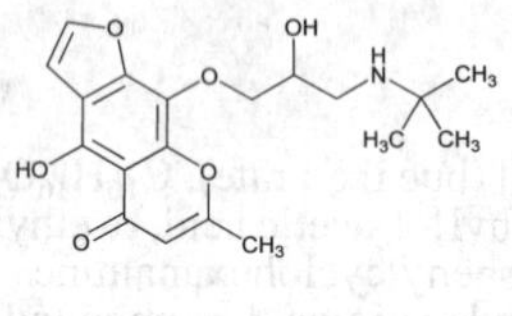

Butoctamide. $C_{12}H_{25}NO_2$. 215.33. [Butoctamide Semisuccinate is JAN.] *N*-(2-Ethylhexyl)-3-hydroxybutyramide. *UNII-6MDC25LQSR. CAS-32838-26-9.* INN; MI.

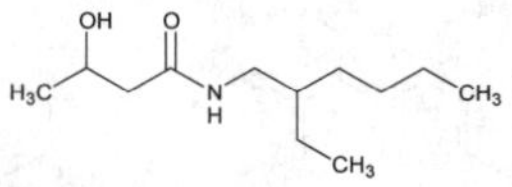

Butofilolol. $C_{17}H_{26}FNO_3$. 311.39. (±)-2′-[3-(*tert*-Butylamino)-2-hydroxypropoxyl-5′-fluorobutyrophenone. *UNII-4AZC6Y5A8G. CAS-64552-17-6.* INN; MI.

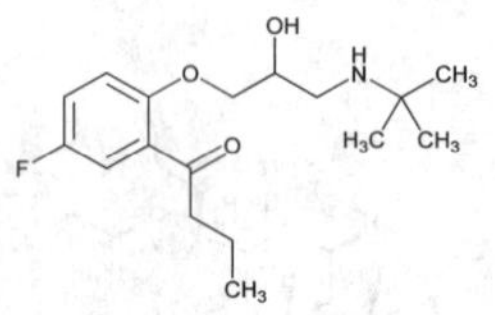

Butonate [*1973*] (bue′ toe nate). $C_8H_{14}Cl_3O_5P$. 327.53. (1) Butanoic acid, 2,2,2-trichloro-1-(dimethoxyphosphinyl)ethyl ester; (2) Butyric acid, ester with dimethyl (2,2,2-trichloro-1-hydroxyethyl)phosphonate; (3) *O,O*-Dimethyl (2,2,2-trichloro-1-*n*-butyryloxyethyl)phosphonate. *UNII-39M9R3Q494. CAS-126-22-7.* INN. *Anthelmintic.* ◇*ENT-20852*

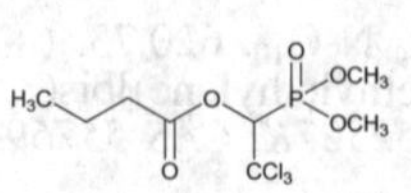

Butopamine [*1979*] (bue toe′ pa meen). $C_{18}H_{23}NO_3$. 301.38. (1) Benzenemethanol, 4-hydroxy-α-[[[3-(4-hydroxyphenyl)-1-methylpropyl]amino]methyl]-, [*R-(R*,R*)]; (2) (*R*)-*p*-Hydroxy-α-[[[(*R*)-3-(*p*-hydroxyphenyl)-1-methylpropyl]amino]methyl]benzyl alcohol. *CAS-66734-12-1.* INN. *Cardiotonic.* ◇*Compound LY 131126*

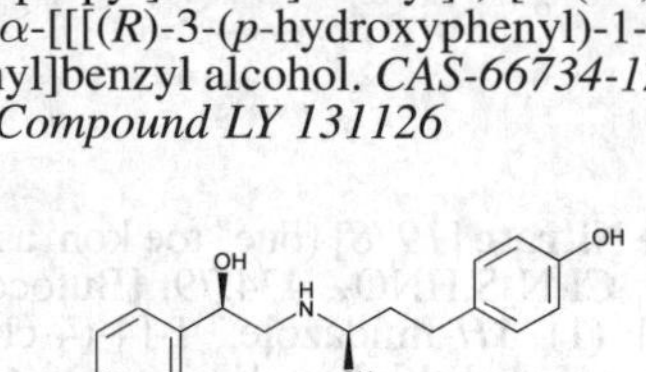

Butopiprine. $C_{19}H_{29}NO_3$. 319.44. 2-Butoxyethyl α-phenyl-1-piperidineacetate. *UNII-EHX04MU69R. CAS-55837-15-5.* INN; DCF. ◇*LD 2351 [as hydrobromide]*

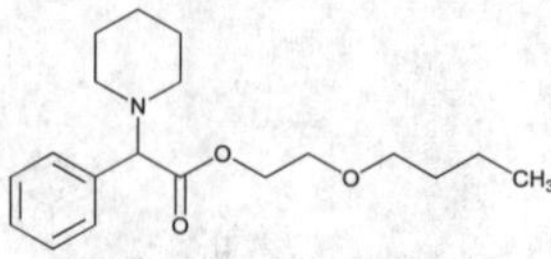

Butoprozine Hydrochloride [*1978*] (bue toe′ proe zeen hye″ droe klor′ ide). $C_{28}H_{38}N_2O_2$·HCl. 471.07. [Butoprozine is INN.] (1) Methanone, [4-[3-(dibutylamino)-propoxy]phenyl](2-ethyl-3-indolizinyl)-, monohydrochloride; (2) *p*-[3-(Dibutylamino)propoxy]phenyl 2-ethyl-3-indolizinyl ketone monohydrochloride. *UNII-H3H80F5CTY. CAS-62134-34-3; CAS-62228-20-0* [butoprozine]. *Cardiac depressant (anti-arrhythmic); anti-anginal.* ◇*L-9394*

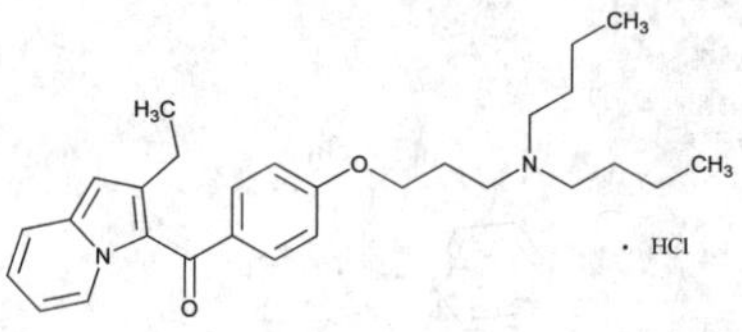

Butopyrammonium Iodide. $C_{17}H_{26}IN_3O$. 415.31. Butyldimethyl(2,3-dimethyl-5-oxo-1-phenyl-3-pyrazolin-4-yl)ammonium iodide. *UNII-M3PZW4O91B. CAS-7077-30-7.* INN.

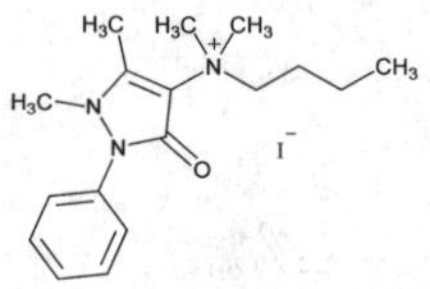

Butopyronoxyl. *UNII-4I5PG5VZ0V. CAS-532-34-3.* USP XV; MI.

Butorphanol [*1974*] (bue tor′ fa nol). $C_{21}H_{29}NO_2$. 327.46. (1) Morphinan-3,14-diol, 17-(cyclobutylmethyl)-; (2) (-)-17-(Cyclobutylmethyl)morphinan-3,14-diol. *UNII-QV897JC36D. CAS-42408-82-2.* INN; BAN. *Analgesic; antitussive.* ◇*levo-BC-2627*

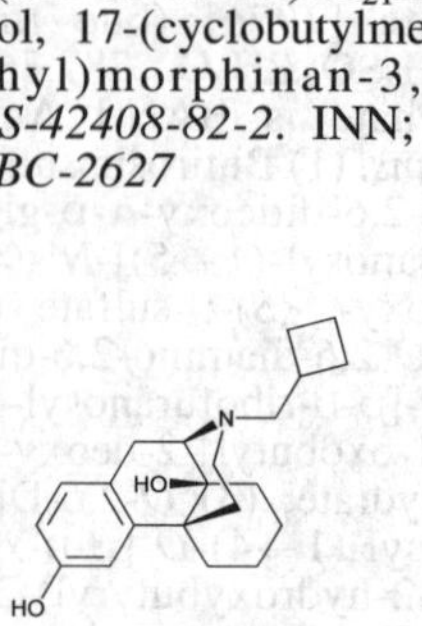

Butorphanol Tartrate [*1976*] (bue tor′ fa nol tar′ trate). **USP**. $C_{21}H_{29}NO_2$·$C_4H_6O_6$. 477.55. (1) Morphinan-3,14-diol, 17-(cyclobutylmethyl)-, (-)-, [*S-(R*,R*)*]-2,3-dihydroxybutanedioate (1:1) (salt); (2) (-)-17-(Cyclobutylmethyl)morphinan-3,14-diol D-(-)-tartrate (1:1) (salt). *UNII-2L7I72RUHN; UNII-QV897JC36D* [butorphanol]. *CAS-*

58786-99-5; CAS-42408-82-2 [butorphanol]. BAN; JAN. *Analgesic; antitussive.* Stadol (Apothecon) ◇*levo-BC-2627 tartrate*

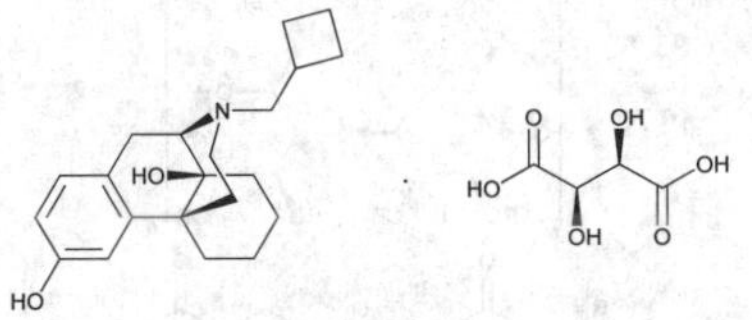

Butoxamine Hydrochloride [*1965*] (bue tox′ a meen hye″ droe klor′ ide). $C_{15}H_{25}NO_3 \cdot HCl$. 303.82. [Butaxamine is INN and BAN.] (1) Benzenemethanol, α-[1-[(1,1-dimethylethyl)amino]ethyl]-2,5-dimethoxy-, $(R*,S*)$-, hydrochloride, ($\pm$)-; (2) α-[1-(*tert*-Butylamino)ethyl]-2,5-dimethoxybenzyl alcohol hydrochloride. *CAS-5696-15-1; CAS-2922-20-5* [butaxamine]. *Antidiabetic; antihyperlipoproteinemic.* ◇*BW 64-9; NSC-106565*

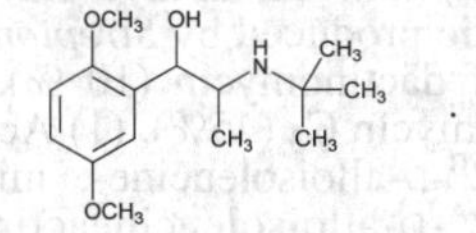

β-Butoxyethyl Nicotinate (JAN) — *See* Nicoboxil.

Butoxylate. $C_{32}H_{36}N_2O_2$. 480.64. Butyl 1-(3-cyano-3,3-diphenylpropyl)-4-phenylpiperidine-4-carboxylate. *UNII-13H7H1ET2J. CAS-15302-05-3.* INN.

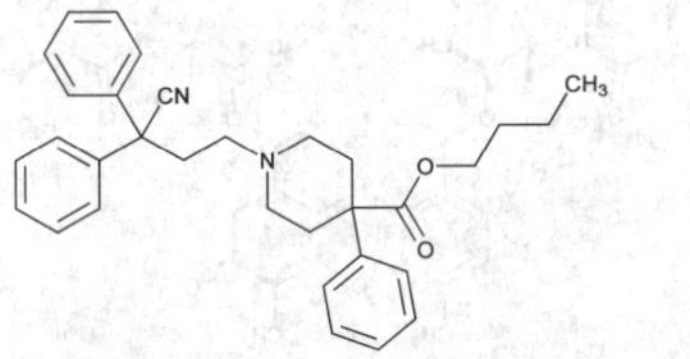

Butoxyphenylacethydroxamic Acid — *See* Bufexamac.

Butriptyline Hydrochloride [*1965*] (bue trip′ ti leen hye″ droe klor′ ide). $C_{21}H_{27}N \cdot HCl$. 329.91. [Butriptyline is INN and BAN.] (1) 5*H*-Dibenzo[*a,d*]cycloheptene-5-propanamine, 10,11-dihydro-*N,N,β*-trimethyl-, hydrochloride, ($\pm$)-; (2) ($\pm$)-10,11-Dihydro-*N,N,β*-trimethyl-5*H*-dibenzo[*a,d*]cycloheptene-5-propylamine hydrochloride. *UNII-LIJ2H8658W. CAS-5585-73-9; CAS-35941-65-2* [butriptyline]. *Antidepressant.* ◇*AY-62014*

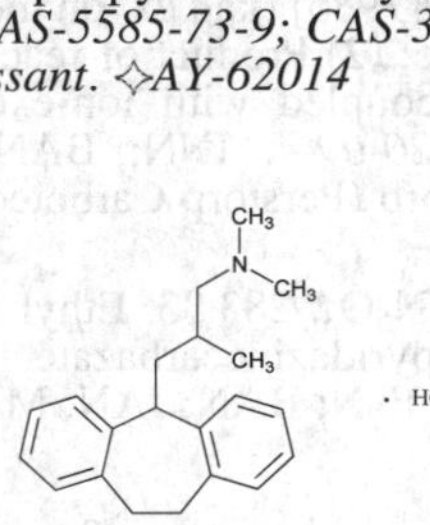

---

† Brand name formerly used, and/or firm no longer concerned with this product.

Butropium Bromide. $C_{28}H_{38}BrNO_4$. 532.51. 8-(*p*-Butoxybenzyl)-3α-hydroxy-1αH,5αH-tropanium bromide (-)-tropate. *CAS-29025-14-7.* INN; JAN; MI.

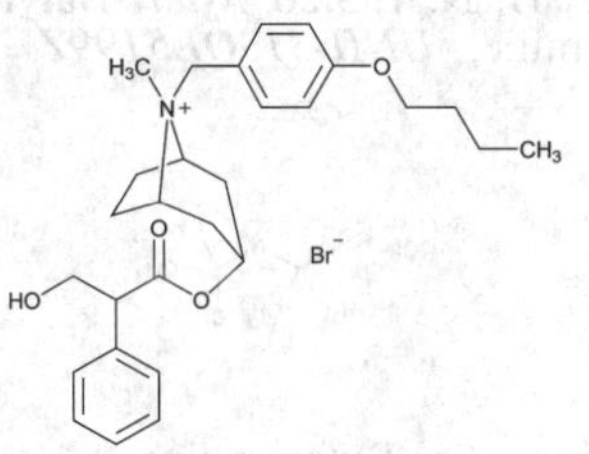

Butydrine — *See* Butidrine.

Butyl Alcohol (bue′ til al′ ka hol). **NF.** $C_4H_{10}O$. 74.12. (1) *n*-Butanol; (2) *n*-Butyl Alcohol. *CAS-71-36-3. Pharmaceutic aid (solvent).*

Butyl Aminobenzoate (previously used name) — *See* Butamben.

Butyl Chloride. *UNII-ZP7R667SGD. CAS-109-69-3.* NF XII; MI.

Butyl Methoxydibenzoylmethane — *See* Avobenzone.

Butyl Parahydroxybenzoate (JAN) — *See* Butylparaben.

p-Butylaminobenzoyldiethylaminoethyl Hydrochloride. $C_{17}H_{28}N_2O_2 \cdot HCl$. 328.88. 2-(Diethylamino)ethyl *p*-(butylamino)benzoate hydrochloride. *CAS-16488-48-5.* JAN.

Butylated Hydroxyanisole (bue′ ti lay″ ted hye drox″ ee an′ i sole). **NF.** $C_{11}H_{16}O_2$. 180.24. (1) Phenol, (1,1-dimethylethyl)-4-methoxy-; (2) *tert*-Butyl-4-methoxyphenol. *UNII-REK4960K2U. CAS-25013-16-5.* BAN. *Pharmaceutic aid (antioxidant).*

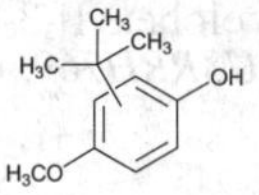

Butylated Hydroxytoluene (bue′ ti lay″ ted hye drox″ ee tol′ ue een). **NF.** $C_{15}H_{24}O$. 220.35. (1) Phenol, 2,6-bis(1,1-dimethylethyl)-4-methyl-; (2) 2,6-Di-*tert*-butyl-*p*-cresol. *UNII-1P9D0Z171K. CAS-128-37-0.* BAN. *Pharmaceutic aid (antioxidant).*

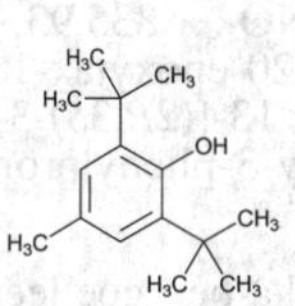

Butyl *p*-Hydroxybenzoate — *See* Butylparaben.

Butylparaben (bue″ til par′ a ben). **NF.** $C_{11}H_{14}O_3$. 194.23. [Butyl Parahydroxybenzoate is JAN.] (1) Benzoic acid, 4-hydroxy-, butyl ester; (2) Butyl *p*-hydroxybenzoate. *CAS-94-26-8. Pharmaceutic aid (antifungal agent).*

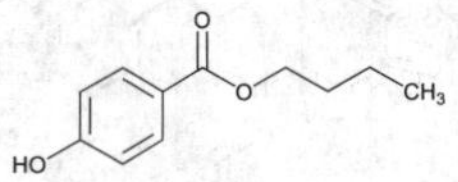

Butylphenamide. *UNII-4Q9N876YAJ. CAS-131-90-8.* J. Invest. Dermat. 27 (3), Sept. 1956.

Butylscopolamine Bromide. C$_{21}$H$_{30}$BrNO$_4$. 440.37. Scopolamine *N-n*-butylbromide. *UNII-0GH9JX37C8. CAS-149-64-4.* JAN.

Butynamine. C$_{10}$H$_{19}$N. 153.26. *N-tert*-Butyl-*N*,1,1-trimethyl-2-propynylamine. *UNII-313QE5199Z. CAS-3735-65-7.* INN.

Butyrylperazine — *See* Butaperazine.

Butyvinyl — *See* Vinylbital.

Buzepide Metiodide. C$_{23}$H$_{31}$IN$_2$O. 478.41. 1-(3-Carbamoyl-3,3-diphenylpropyl)perhydro-1-methylazepinium iodide. *UNII-5A9SS67K16. CAS-15351-05-0.* INN; DCF; MI. ◇*F.I. 6146; R 661*

BV-araU — *See* Sorivudine.

^{11}C — *See* Carbon Monoxide C 11.

^{11}C — *See* Methionine C 11.

^{11}C — *See* Sodium Acetate C 11.

^{45}Ca — *See* Calcium Chloride Ca 45.

^{47}Ca — *See* Calcium Chloride Ca 47.

Cabastine. C$_{26}$H$_{29}$FN$_2$O$_2$. 420.52. (±)-*trans*-1-[*cis*-4-Cyano-4-(*p*-fluorophenyl)cyclohexyl]-3-methyl-4-phenylisonipecotic acid. *UNII-COU3RRH769. CAS-79449-98-2.* INN.

Cabazitaxel. C$_{45}$H$_{57}$NO$_{14}$. 835.93. 1-Hydroxy-7β,10β-dimethoxy-9-oxo-5β,20-epoxytax-11-ene-2α,4,13α-triyl 4-acetate 2-benzoate 13-[(2*R*,3*S*)-3-{[(*tert*-butoxy)carbonyl]amino}-2-hydroxy-3-phenylpropanoate]. *CAS-183133-96-2.* INN.

Cabergoline [*1996*] (ka ber′ goe leen). C$_{26}$H$_{37}$N$_5$O$_2$. 451.60. (1) Ergoline-8β-carboxamide, *N*-[3-(dimethylamino)propyl]-*N*-[(ethylamino)carbonyl]-6-(2-propenyl)-; (2) 1-[(6-Allylergolin-8β-yl)carbonyl]-1-[3-(dimethylamino)propyl]-3-ethylurea. *UNII-LL60K9J05T. CAS-81409-90-7.* INN; BAN. *Antidyskinetic; antihyperprolactinemic; dopamine agonist.* Dostinex (Pfizer) ◇*FCE 21336*

Cabis Bromatum — *See* Bibrocathol.

Cabufocon A [*1976*] (kab″ ue foe′ kon). (1) Cellulose, acetate, butanoate; (2) Cellulose acetate butyrate. *CAS-9004-36-8. Contact lens material (hydrophobic).*

Cabufocon B [*1979*] (kab″ ue foe′ kon). (1) Cellulose, acetate, butanoate; (2) Cellulose acetate butyrate. *CAS-9004-36-8. Contact lens material (hydrophobic). [Note— Graphic formula same as for Cabufocon A.]* ◇*Tenite Butyrate Formula 264 H4*

Cacao Butter. JAN.

Cactinomycin [*1965*] (kak″ tin oh mye′ sin). [Actinomycin C is BAN.] Antibiotic produced by *Streptomyces chrysomallus.* A mixture of dactinomycin (10 %), actinomycin C$_2$ (45%), and actinomycin C$_3$ (45%). (1) Actinomycin D, 2^A-D-alloisoleucine-2^B-D-alloisoleucine-, mixt. with actinomycin D and 2^A-D-alloisoleucineactinomycin D; (2) Cactinomycin. *CAS-8052-16-2.* INN. *Antineoplastic.* [*Name previously used: Actinomycin C.*] ◇*H.B.F. 386; NSC-18268*

Cadexomer. Carboxymethylated microspheres produced by reaction of partially hydrolysed starch with epichlorhydrin; slowly degradable by amylase (with a half-life of more than 120 minutes). INN; MI.

Cadexomer Iodine [*1986*] (kad ex′ oh mer eye″ oh dine). (1) Cadexomer iodine; (2) Product of reaction of dextrin with epichlorohydrin coupled with ion-exchange groups and iodine. *CAS-94820-09-4.* INN; BAN. *Antiseptic; antiulcerative.* Iodosorb (Perstorp Carbotec, Sweden)

Cadralazine. C$_{12}$H$_{21}$N$_5$O$_3$. 283.33. Ethyl 6-[ethyl(2-hydroxypropyl)amino]-3-pyridazinecarbazate. *UNII-8T96I3U713. CAS-64241-34-5.* INN; BAN; JAN; MI.

Cadrofloxacin. $C_{19}H_{20}F_3N_3O_4$. 411.38. (-)-1-Cyclopropyl-8-(difluoromethoxy)-6-fluoro-1,4-dihydro-7-[(*S*)-3-methyl-1-piperazinyl]-4-oxo-3-quinolinecarboxylic acid. *UNII-1YOQ7J9ACY. CAS-153808-85-6.* INN.

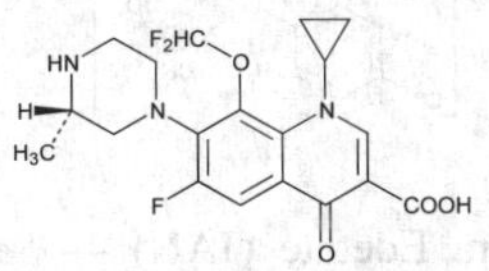

Cafaminol. $C_{11}H_{17}N_5O_3$. 267.28. 8-[(2-Hydroxyethyl)methylamino]caffeine. *UNII-0L1S25NC1L. CAS-30924-31-3.* INN; MI.

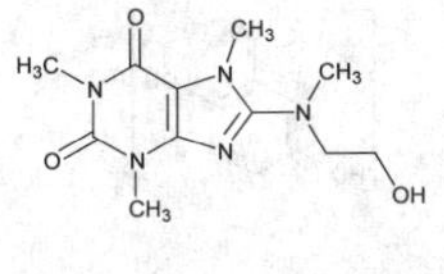

Cafedrine. $C_{18}H_{23}N_5O_3$. 357.41. 7-[2-(2-Hydroxy-1-methylphenethylamino)ethyl]theophylline. *UNII-0UYY5V4U2Q. CAS-58166-83-9.* INN; BAN.

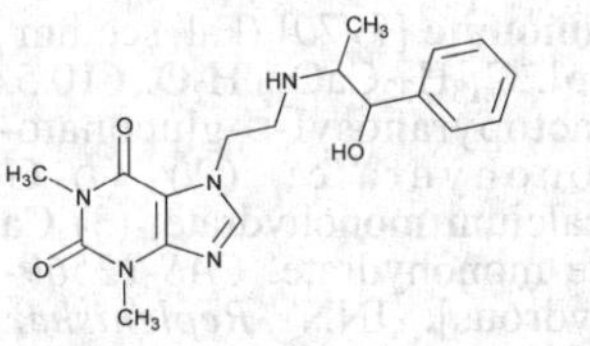

Caffeine (kaf' een). **USP**. $C_8H_{10}N_4O_2$. 194.19. (1) 1*H*-Purine-2,6-dione, 3,7-dihydro-1,3,7-trimethyl-; (2) 1,3,7-Trimethylxanthine. *UNII-3G6A5W338E. CAS-58-08-2; CAS-5743-12-4* [monohydrate]. BAN; JAN. *Stimulant (central).* NoDoz Caplets and Chewable Tablets (Bristol-Myers Products)

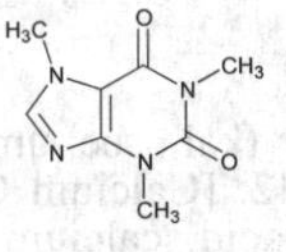

Caffeine Citrate (kaf' een sit' rate). **USP**. $C_{14}H_{18}N_4O_9$. 386.31. (1) 1*H*-Purine-2,6-dione, 3,7-dihydro-1,3,7-trimethyl-, 2-hydroxypropane-1,2,3-tricarboxylate; (2) 3,7-Dihydro-1,3,7-trimethyl-1*H*-purine-2,6-dione citrate. *UNII-U26EO4675Q. CAS-69-22-7.* Cafcit (Bristol-Myers Squibb)

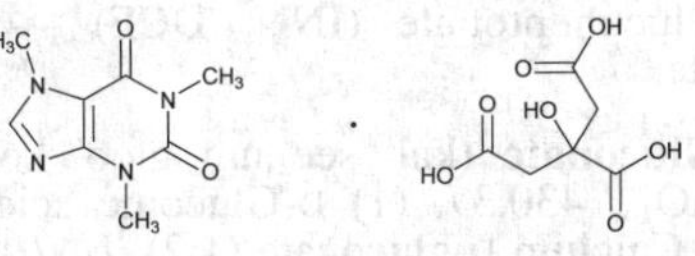

Caffeine, Citrated. *UNII-3G6A5W338E* [caffeine]. *CAS-69-22-7; CAS-58-08-2* [caffeine]; *CAS-5743-12-4* [caffeine monohydrate]. NF XIII; MI.

Calamine (kal' a mine). **USP**. (1) Iron oxide (Fe_2O_3), mixture with zinc oxide; (2) Calamine (pharmaceutical preparation). *CAS-8011-96-9.* JAN. *Protectant (topical).*

---

† Brand name formerly used, and/or firm no longer concerned with this product.

Calcidiol — *See* Calcifediol.

Calcifediol [*1975*] (kal" sif e dye' ol). **USP**. $C_{27}H_{44}O_2 \cdot H_2O$. 418.65. (1) 9,10-Secocholesta-5,7,10(19)-triene-3,25-diol monohydrate, (3β,5Z,7E)-; (2) 25-Hydroxycholecalciferol monohydrate. *UNII-P6YZ13C99Q. CAS-63283-36-3; CAS-19356-17-3* [anhydrous]. INN; BAN. *Regulator (calcium).* Calderol (Organon) ◇*U-32,070E*

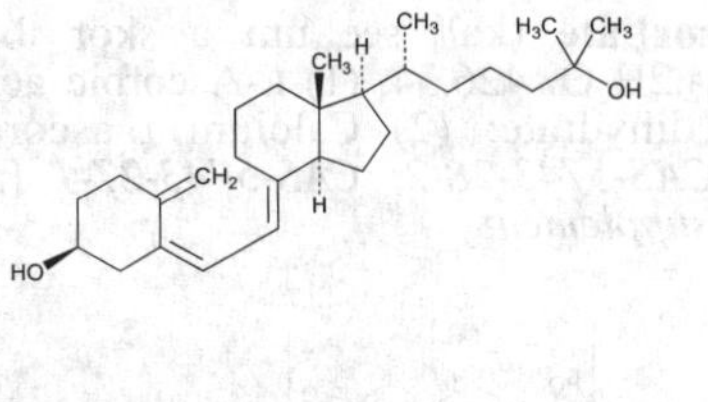

Calciferol (previously used name) — *See* Ergocalciferol.

Calcipotriene [*1992*] (kal" si poe trye' een). $C_{27}H_{40}O_3$. 412.60. [Calcipotriol is INN and BAN.] (1) 9,10-Secochola-5,7,10(19),22-tetraene-1,3,24-triol, 24-cyclopropyl-, (1α,3β,5Z,7E,22E,24S)-; (2) (5Z,7E,22E,24S)-24-Cyclopropyl-9,10-secochola-5,7,10(19),22-tetraene-1α,3β,24-triol. *UNII-143NQ3779B. CAS-112965-21-6. Antipsoriatic.* Dovonex (Warner Chilcott) ◇*MC 903*

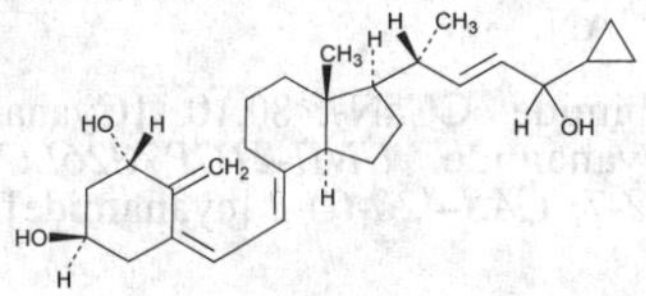

Calcipotriol (INN, BAN) — *See* Calcipotriene.

Calcitonin [*1967*] (kal" si toe' nin). **USP**. $C_{145}H_{240}N_{44}O_{48}S_2$ (salmon); $C_{151}H_{226}N_{40}O_{45}S_3$ (human). 3432 daltons. A polypeptide hormone that lowers the calcium concentration in the plasma of mammals; or the same substance obtained by synthesis. The source of the product (salmon, swine, etc.) must be indicated in the labeling. (1) Calcitonin (source); (2) Thyrocalcitonin (source). *UNII-7SFC6U2VI5* [salmon]; *UNII-I0IO929019* [human]. *CAS-47931-85-1* [salmon]; *CAS-21215-62-3* [human]; *CAS-9007-12-9.* INN; BAN; JAN. *Regulator (calcium).* Calcimar (Rhone-Poulenc Rorer); Cibacalcin (Ciba-Geigy†); Forcaltonin (Unigene); Fortical (Unigene)

CSNLSTCVLG KLSQELHKLQ TYPRTNTGSG TP——NH₂

Calcitriol [*1978*] (kal" si trye' ol). **USP**. $C_{27}H_{44}O_3$. 416.64. (1) 9,10-Secocholesta-5,7,10(19)-triene-1,3,25-triol, (1α,3β,5Z,7E)-; (2) (5Z,7E)-9,10-Secocholesta-5,7,10(19)-triene-1α,3β,25-triol. *UNII-FXC9231JVH. CAS-32222-06-3; CAS-77326-95-5* [monohydrate]. INN; BAN; JAN. *Regulator (calcium).* Calcijex (Abbott); Rocaltrol (Roche) *[Names previously used: 1α,25-dihydroxyvitamin D₃; 1α,25-dihydroxycholecalciferol.]* ◇*Ro 21-5535*

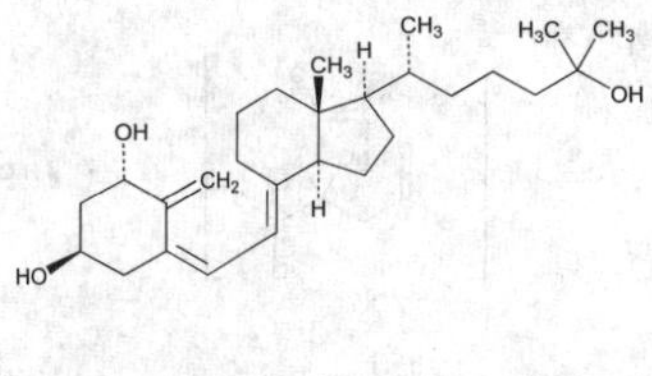

Calcium Acetate (kal′ see um as′ e tate). **USP**. $C_4H_6CaO_4$. 158.17. (1) Acetic acid, calcium salt; (2) Calcium acetate. *UNII-Y882YXF34X. CAS-62-54-4*. JAN. *Pharmaceutic aid (buffering agent)*. Phoslo (Fresenius)

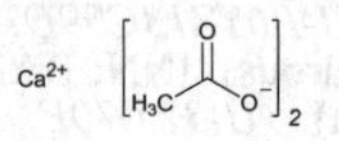

Calcium Ascorbate (kal′ see um a skor′ bate). **USP**. $C_{12}H_{14}CaO_{12}.2H_2O$. 426.34. (1) L-Ascorbic acid, calcium salt (2:1), dihydrate; (2) Calcium L-ascorbate (1:2), dihydrate. *CAS-5743-28-2; CAS-5743-27-1* [anhydrous]. *Nutritional supplement*.

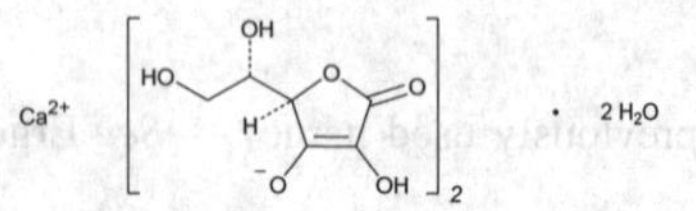

Calcium L-Aspartate. $C_8H_{12}CaN_2O_8.3H_2O$. 358.31. Calcium-L-aspartate. *CAS-21059-46-1*. JAN.

Calcium Benzamidosalicylate (INN, BAN) — *See* Benzoyl-pas Calcium.

Calcium Bromide. $CaBr_2$. 199.89. *UNII-87CNY2EEBH. CAS-7789-41-5*. JAN.

Calcium Carbimide. $CCaN_2$. 80.10. [Cyanamide is JAN.] Calcium cyanamide. *UNII-21CP7826LC* [cyanamide]. *CAS-156-62-7; CAS-420-04-2* [cyanamide]. INN.

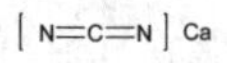

Calcium Carbonate (kal′ see um kar′ bo nate). **USP**. $CaCO_3$. 100.09. [Precipitated Calcium Carbonate is JAN.] (1) Carbonic acid, calcium salt (1:1); (2) Calcium carbonate (1:1). *UNII-H0G9379FGK. CAS-471-34-1. Antacid*. Cal-Sup (3M Pharmaceuticals); Children's Mylanta Upset Stomach Relief (Johnson & Johnson-Merck Consumer); Chooz (Schering-Plough HealthCare); Mylanta Soothing Lozenges (Johnson & Johnson-Merck Consumer) *[Name previously used: Calcium Carbonate, Precipitated.]*

Calcium Chloride (kal′ see um klor′ ide). **USP**. $CaCl_2.2H_2O$. 147.01. (1) Calcium chloride, dihydrate; (2) Calcium chloride dihydrate. *UNII-M4I0D6VV5M. CAS-10035-04-8; CAS-10043-52-4* [anhydrous]. JAN. *Replenisher (calcium)*.

Calcium Chloride Ca 45 [*1963*] (kal′ see um klor′ ide). $^{45}CaCl_2$. (1) Calcium chloride ($^{45}CaCl_2$); (2) Calcium chloride ($^{45}CaCl_2$). *CAS-14336-71-1. Radioactive agent*.

Calcium Chloride Ca 47 [*1963*] (kal′ see um klor′ ide). $^{47}CaCl_2$. (1) Calcium chloride ($^{47}CaCl_2$); (2) Calcium chloride ($^{47}CaCl_2$). *Radioactive agent*.

Calcium Citrate (kal′ see um sit′ rate). **USP**. $C_{12}H_{10}Ca_3O_{14}.4H_2O$. 570.49. (1) 1,2,3-Propanetricarboxylic acid, 2-hydroxy-, calcium salt (2:3), tetrahydrate; (2) Calcium citrate (3:2), tetrahydrate. *CAS-5785-44-4. Supplement (calcium)*. Citracal (Mission Pharmacal)

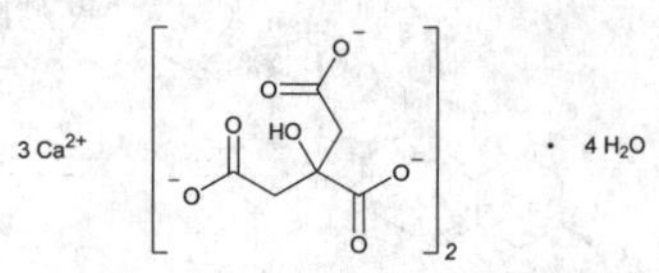

Calcium Clofibrate. $C_{20}H_{20}CaCl_2O_6$. 467.35. Calcium 2-(*p*-chlorophenoxy)-2-methylpropionate. *UNII-TT85QFR500. CAS-39087-48-4; CAS-882-09-7* [clofibric acid]. INN.

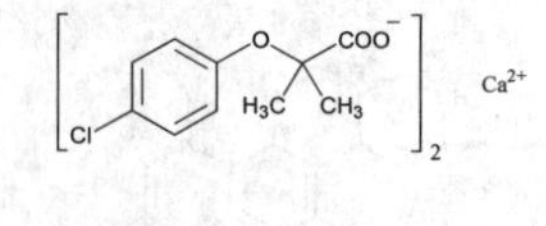

Calcium Disodium Edetate (JAN) — *See* Edetate Calcium Disodium.

Calcium Dobesilate. $C_{12}H_{10}CaO_{10}S_2$. 418.41. Calcium 2,5-dihydroxybenzenesulfonate. *CAS-20123-80-2; CAS-88-46-0* [dobesilic acid]. INN. ◇*205 E*

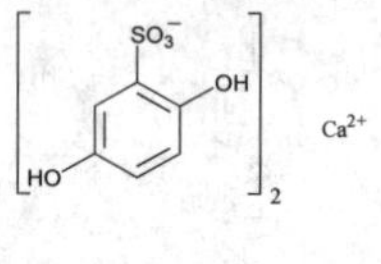

Calcium Doxybensylate — *See* Calcium Dobesilate.

Calcium Folinate (INN, BAN, JAN) — *See* Leucovorin Calcium.

Calcium Glubionate [*1970*] (kal′ see um gloo bye′ oh nate). **USP** [Syrup]. $C_{18}H_{32}CaO_{19}.H_2O$. 610.53. (1) Calcium, (4-*O*-β-D-galactopyranosyl-D-gluconato-O^1)(D-gluconato-O^1)-, monohydrate; (2) (D-Gluconato)(lactobionato)calcium monohydrate; (3) Calcium D-gluconate lactobionate monohydrate. *CAS-12569-38-9; CAS-31959-85-0* [anhydrous]. INN. *Replenisher (calcium)*. Neo-Calglucon (Novartis)

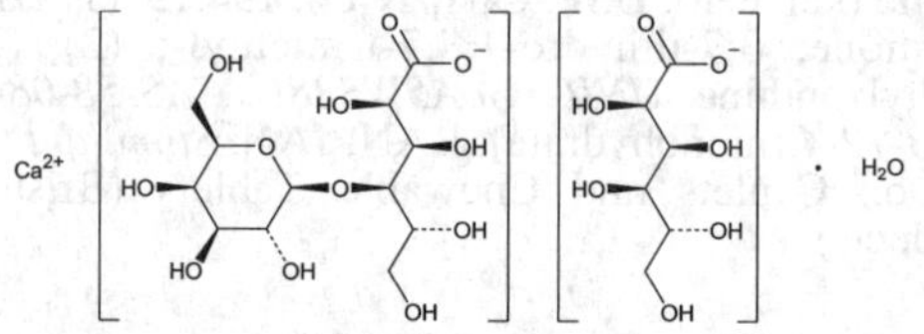

Calcium Gluceptate (kal′ see um gloo sep′ tate). **USP**. $C_{14}H_{26}CaO_{16}$. 490.42. [Calcium Glucoheptonate is INN.] (1) Glucoheptonic acid, calcium salt (2:1); (2) Calcium glucoheptonate (1:2). *UNII-L11651398J. CAS-29039-00-7. Replenisher (calcium)*.

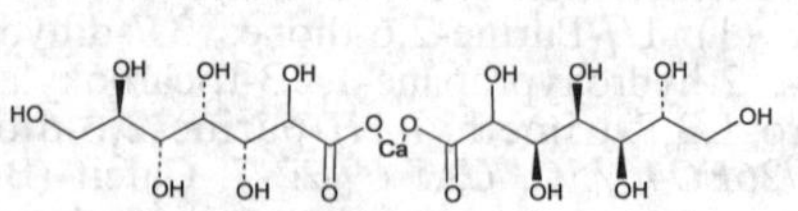

Calcium Glucoheptonate (INN, DCF) — *See* Calcium Gluceptate.

Calcium Gluconate (kal′ see um gloo′ koe nate). **USP**. $C_{12}H_{22}CaO_{14}$. 430.37. (1) D-Gluconic acid, calcium salt (2:1); (2) Calcium D-gluconate (1:2). *UNII-SQE6VB453K. CAS-299-28-5* [anhydrous]; *CAS-526-95-4* [D-gluconic acid]. JAN. *Replenisher (calcium)*. Calglucon (Novartis†)

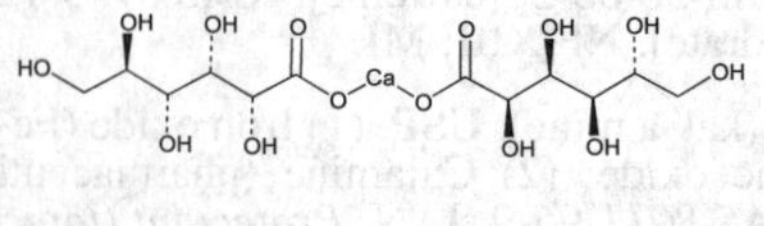

Calcium Glycerinophosphate — *See* Calcium Glycerophosphate.

Calcium Glycerophosphate. *CAS-27214-00-2; CAS-27082-31-1* [glycerophosphoric acid]. NF X; JAN; MI.

Calcium Hopantenate. $C_{20}H_{36}CaN_2O_{10} \cdot \frac{1}{2}H_2O$. 513.59. Calcium D-(+)-4-(2,4-dihydroxy-3,3-dimethylbutylamido)butyrate ½ hydrate. *CAS-17097-76-6* [anhydrous]. JAN.

Calcium Hydroxide (kal′ see um hye drox′ ide). **USP**. $Ca(OH)_2$. 74.09. (1) Calcium hydroxide; (2) Calcium hydroxide. *UNII-PF5DZW74VN. CAS-1305-62-0. Astringent.*

Calcium Hypophosphite. *UNII-CUI83R2732. CAS-7789-79-9.* NF X; MI.

Calcium Lactate (kal′ see um lak′ tate). **USP**. $C_6H_{10}CaO_6 \cdot x$-H_2O. 218.22 (anhydrous). (1) Propanoic acid, 2-hydroxy-, calcium salt (2:1), hydrate; (2) Calcium lactate (1:2) hydrate; (3) Calcium lactate (1:2) pentahydrate. *UNII-2URQ2N32W3. CAS-814-80-2* [anhydrous]; *CAS-41372-22-9* [hydrate]; *CAS-5743-47-5* [pentahydrate]. JAN. *Replenisher (calcium).* Prequist Powder (Parke-Davis)

Calcium Lactobionate (kal′ see um lak″ toe bye′ oh nate). **USP**. $C_{24}H_{42}CaO_{24} \cdot 2H_2O$. 790.68. (1) D-Gluconic acid, 4-O-β-D-galactopyranosyl-, calcium salt (2:1), dihydrate; (2) Lactobionic acid, calcium salt (2:1), dihydrate; (3) Calcium lactobionate (1:2), dihydrate. *CAS-110638-68-1. Supplement (calcium).*

Calcium Lactophosphate. *UNII-0LT9MW24NY. CAS-7546-28-3; CAS-18365-82-7* [lactophosphoric acid]. NF V.

Calcium Levofolinate (INN, BAN) — *See* Levoleucovorin Calcium.

Calcium Levulate — *See* Calcium Levulinate.

Calcium Levulinate (kal′ see um lev″ ue lin′ ate). **USP**. $C_{10}H_{14}CaO_6 \cdot 2H_2O$. 306.32. (1) Pentanoic acid, 4-oxo-, calcium salt (2:1), dihydrate; (2) Calcium levulinate (1:2) dihydrate. *UNII-T6133SO781. CAS-5743-49-7; CAS-591-64-0* [anhydrous]; *CAS-123-76-2* [levulinic acid]. BAN. *Replenisher (calcium).*

Calcium Mandelate. *UNII-29CS07FZII; UNII-NH496X0UJX* [mandelic acid]. *CAS-134-95-2; CAS-90-64-2* [mandelic acid]. USP XV.

Calcium Pantothenate (kal′ see um pan toe′ then ate). **USP**. $C_{18}H_{32}CaN_2O_{10}$. 476.53. [Pantothenic Acid is BAN.] (1) β-Alanine, *N*-(2,4-dihydroxy-3,3-dimethyl-1-oxobutyl)-, calcium salt (2:1), (*R*)-; (2) Calcium D-pantothenate (1:2). *UNII-568ET80C3D; UNII-19F5HK2737* [pantothenic acid]. *CAS-137-08-6; CAS-79-83-4* [pantothenic acid]. INN; JAN. *Vitamin (enzyme co-factor).* Calpan (BASF); Pantholin (Lilly†)

Calcium Pantothenate, Racemic (kal′ see um pan toe′ then ate ray see′ mik). **USP**. $C_{18}H_{32}CaN_2O_{10}$. 476.53. (1) β-Alanine, *N*-(2,4-dihydroxy-3,3-dimethyl-1-oxobutyl)-, calcium salt (2:1), (±)-; (2) Calcium DL-pantothenate (1:2). *CAS-6381-63-1; CAS-599-54-2* [DL-pantothenic acid]. *Vitamin (enzyme co-factor).*

Calcium Para-aminosalicylate (JAN) — *See* Aminosalicylate Calcium.

Calcium Phosphate Dihydrate, Dibasic (kal′ see um fos′ fate dye hye′ drate dye bay′ sik). **USP**. $CaHPO_4 \cdot 2H_2O$. 172.09. (1) Phosphoric acid, calcium salt (1:1); (2) Calcium phosphate, dihydrate (1:1). *UNII-O7TSZ97GEP; UNII-L11K75P92J* [calcium phosphate (1:1)]. *CAS-7789-77-7; CAS-7757-93-9* [calcium phosphate (1:1)]. JAN. *Replenisher (calcium); pharmaceutic aid (tablet base).* CalStar (FMC); D.C.P. (Parke-Davis†)

Calcium Phosphate, Tribasic (kal′ see um fos′ fate trye bay′ sik). **NF**. $Ca_5(OH)(PO_4)_3$. 502.31. (1) Calcium hydroxide phosphate ($Ca_5(OH)(PO_4)_3$); (2) Calcium hydroxide phosphate ($Ca_5(OH)(PO_4)_3$); (3) Hydroxyapatite or Hydroxylapatite. *CAS-12167-74-7. Replenisher (calcium).*

Calcium Polycarbophil [*1965*] (kal′ see um pol″ ee kar′ boe fil). **USP**. Calcium polycarbophil. *UNII-8F049NKY49. CAS-9003-97-8. Laxative.* Mitrolan (Robins); Noveon CA-1 (Goodrich); Noveon CA-2 (Goodrich); Sorboquel (Schering†) ◊*Wl 140*

Calcium Polystyrene Sulfonate. Calcium salt of sulfonated styrene polymer. *CAS-37286-92-3.* JAN.

Calcium Saccharate (kal′ see um sak′ a rate). **USP**. $C_6H_8CaO_8 \cdot 4H_2O$. 320.26. (1) D-Glucaric acid, calcium salt (1:1) tetrahydrate; (2) Calcium D-glucarate (1:1), tetrahydrate. *CAS-5793-89-5; CAS-87-73-0* [saccharic acid]. INN. *Pharmaceutic aid (stabilizer).*

Calcium Silicate (kal′ see um sil′ i kate). **NF**. A compound of not less than 4% calcium oxide and not more than 35% silicon dioxide. *Pharmaceutic aid (tablet excipient).*

Calcium Sodium Ferriclate (INN) — *See* Ferriclate Calcium Sodium.

Calcium Stearate (kal′ see um steer′ ate). **NF**. (1) Octadecanoic acid, calcium salt; (2) Calcium stearate. *UNII-776XM7047L. CAS-1592-23-0.* JAN. *Pharmaceutic aid (tablet and/or capsule lubricant).*

Calcium Sulfate (kal′ see um sul′ fate). **NF**. $CaSO_4$. 136.14. (1) Sulfuric acid, calcium salt (1:1); (2) Calcium sulfate (1:1). *UNII-WAT0DDB505; UNII-4846Q921YM* [calcium sulfate dihydrate]. *CAS-7778-18-9; CAS-10101-41-4* [dihydrate]. *Pharmaceutic aid (tablet and capsule diluent).*

---

† Brand name formerly used, and/or firm no longer concerned with this product.

Calcium Tetracemine Disodium — *See* Edetate Calcium Disodium.

Calcium Trisodium Pentetate (BAN) — *See* Pentetate Calcium Trisodium.

Calcium Undecylenate [*1988*] (kal′ see um un de′ sil en ate). **USP**. $C_{22}H_{38}O_4Ca$. 406.61. (1) 10-Undecenoic acid, calcium(2+) salt; (2) Calcium 10-undecenoate. *UNII-77YW1RTU8V. CAS-1322-14-1. Antifungal.*

Calciumedetate Sodium — *See* Edetate Calcium Disodium.

Calcobutrol. $C_{18}H_{32}CaN_4O_9$. 488.55. Calcium hydrogen 10-[(1*RS*,2*SR*)-2,3-dihydroxy-1-(hydroxymethyl)propyl]-1,4,7,10-tetraazacyclododecane-1,4,7-triacetate. *UNII-J1A8830GE7. CAS-151878-23-8.* INN.

Caldaret. $C_{11}H_{16}N_2O_3S$. 256.32. 5-Methyl-2-(piperazin-1-yl)benzenesulfonic acid. *UNII-9L3Y3IJ2HI. CAS-133804-44-1.* INN.

Caldiamide Sodium [*1990*] (kal dye′ a mide soe′ dee um). $C_{16}H_{26}CaN_5NaO_8 \cdot xH_2O$. 479.47 (anhydrous). [Caldiamide is INN.] (1) Calciate(1-), [5,8-bis(carboxymethyl)-11-[2-(methylamino)-2-oxoethyl]-3-oxo-2,5,8,11-tetraazatridecan-13-oato(3-)]-, sodium, hydrate; (2) Sodium [*N,N*-bis[2-[(carboxymethyl)[(methylcarbamoyl)methyl]amino]ethyl]-glycinato(3-)]calciate(1-), hydrate. *CAS-122760-91-2; CAS-128326-81-8* [caldiamide]. BAN. *Pharmaceutic aid.*

Calfactant [*1997*] (kal fak′ tant). Calfactant. An unmodified calf lung lavage extract containing mostly phospholipids and surfactant specific proteins (SP-B and SP-C). *UNII-Q4K217VGA9. CAS-183325-78-2.* BAN. *Prevention and treatment of neonatal respiratory distress syndrome (pulmonary surfactant).* Infasurf (Ony)

Calioben — *See* Iodobehenate Calcium.

Calomel. *UNII-J2D46N657D. CAS-10112-91-1.* NF XII; MI.

Caloxetic Acid. $C_{23}H_{31}CaN_3O_{11}$. 565.58. Trihydrogen [*N*-[(2*S*)-2-[bis(carboxymethyl)amino]-3-(*p*-ethoxyphenyl)-propyl]-*N*-[2-[bis(carboxymethyl)amino]ethyl]glycinato(5-)]calciate(3-). *UNII-PZ0O26OD9U. CAS-135306-78-4.* INN.

Calteridol Calcium [*1990*] (kal ter′ i dol kal′ see um). $C_{34}H_{58}Ca_3N_8O_{14}$. 923.10. [Calteridol is INN.] (1) Calciate(1-), [10-(2-hydroxypropyl)-1,4,7,10-tetraazacyclododecane-1,4,7-triacetato(3-)-$N^1,N^4,N^7,N^{10},O^1,O^4,O^7,O^{10}$]-, calcium (2:1); (2) (±)-Calcium bis[[10-(2-hydroxypropyl)-1,4,7,10-tetraazacyclododecane-1,4,7-triacetato(3-)]calciate(1-)]. *CAS-121915-83-1; CAS-132722-73-7* [calteridol]. BAN. *Pharmaceutic aid.* ◇SQ 33,248

Calusterone [*1970*] (kal us′ ter one). $C_{21}H_{32}O_2$. 316.48. (1) Androst-4-en-3-one, 17-hydroxy-7,17-dimethyl-, (7β,17β)-; (2) 17β-Hydroxy-7β,17-dimethylandrost-4-en-3-one; (3) 7β,17α-Dimethyltestosterone. *UNII-0678G6Q58A. CAS-17021-26-0.* INN. *Antineoplastic.* ◇U-22,550; NSC-88536

Camazepam. $C_{19}H_{18}ClN_3O_3$. 371.82. 7-Chloro-1,3-dihydro-3-hydroxy-1-methyl-5-phenyl-2*H*-1,4-benzodiazepin-2-one dimethylcarbamate (ester). *CAS-36104-80-0.* INN; MI.

Cambendazole [*1970*] (kam ben′ da zole). $C_{14}H_{14}N_4O_2S$. 302.35. (1) Carbamic acid, [2-(4-thiazolyl)-1*H*-benzimidazol-5-yl]-, 1-methylethyl ester; (2) Isopropyl 2-(4-triazolyl)-5-benzimidazolecarbamate. *UNII-079X63S3DU. CAS-26097-80-3.* INN; BAN. *Anthelmintic.* Camdan (Merck); Camvet [Veterinary] (Merial)

Camellia Oil. *UNII-T1PE06G0VE.* JAN.

Camiglibose [*1992*] (kam″ i glye′ bose). $C_{13}H_{25}NO_9.1\frac{1}{2}H_2O$. 366.36. (1) α-D-Glucopyranoside, methyl 6-deoxy-6-[3,4,5-trihydroxy-2-(hydroxymethyl)-1-piperidinyl]-, sesquihydrate, [2R-(2α,3β,4α,5β)]-; (2) Methyl 6-deoxy-6-[(2R,3R,4R,5S)-3,4,5-trihydroxy-2-(hydroxymethyl)piperidino]-α-D-glucopyranoside sesquihydrate. *UNII-XSD3N36UID. CAS-132438-21-2.* INN. *Antidiabetic.* ◇*MDL 73,945*

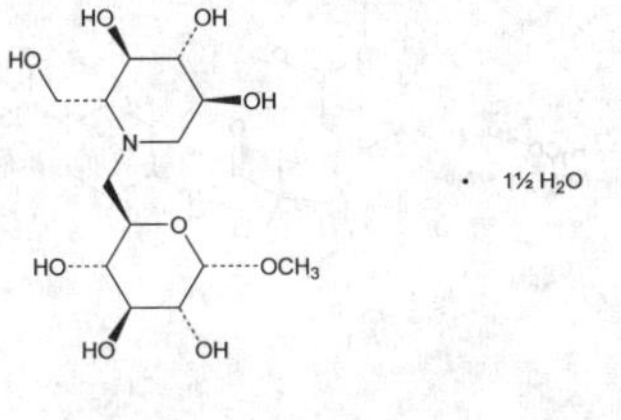

Camiverine. $C_{19}H_{30}N_2O_2$. 318.45. 2-Phenyl-*N*-[2-(1-pyrrolidinyl)ethyl]glycine isopentyl ester. *UNII-S5D373PRDG. CAS-54063-28-4.* INN.

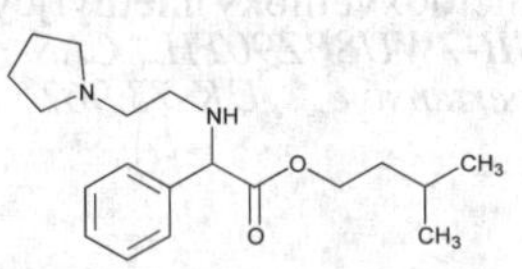

Camobucol [*2006*] (kam″ oh bue′ kol). $C_{33}H_{50}O_4S_2$. 574.88. (1) Acetic acid, [4-[[1-[[3,5-bis(1,1-dimethylethyl)-4-hydroxyphenyl]thio]-1-methylethyl]thio]-2,6-bis(1,1-dimethylethyl)phenoxy]-; (2) [4-[[1-[[3,5-Bis(1,1-dimethylethyl)-4-hydroxyphenyl]sulfanyl]-1-methylethyl]sulfanyl]-2,6-bis(1,1-dimethylethyl)phenoxy]acetic acid. *UNII-FZ7798X3IR. CAS-216167-92-9.* INN. *Treatment of inflammatory diseases.* ◇*AGIX-4207*

Camonagrel. $C_{15}H_{16}N_2O_3$. 272.30. (±)-5-(2-Imidazol-1-ylethoxy)-1-indancarboxylic acid. *UNII-XM930M133O. CAS-105920-77-2.* INN.

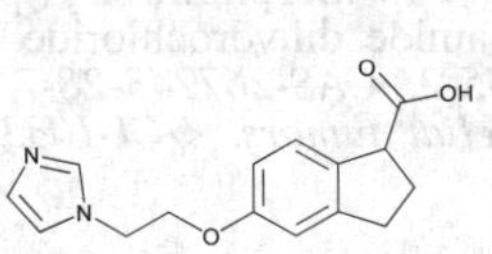

Camostat. $C_{20}H_{22}N_4O_5$. 398.41. [Camostat Mesilate is JAN.] *p*-Guanidinobenzoic acid, ester with (*p*-hydroxyphenyl)acetic acid, ester with *N,N*-dimethylglycolamide. *UNII-0FD207WKDU. CAS-59721-28-7.* INN; MI.

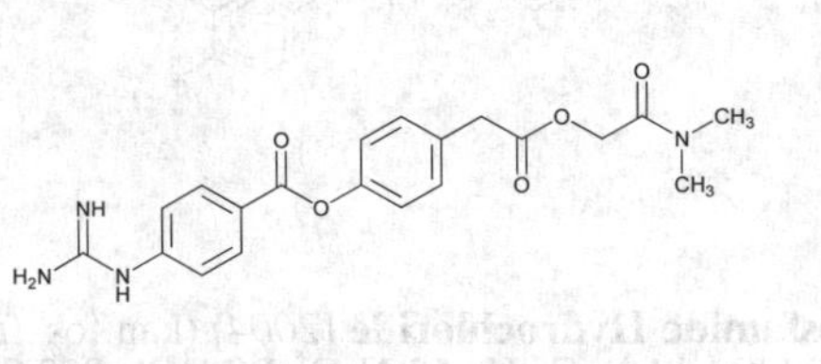

Camphetamide — *See* Camphotamide.

---

† Brand name formerly used, and/or firm no longer concerned with this product.

Camphor (kam′ for). **USP.** $C_{10}H_{16}O$. 152.23. [*d*-Camphor, *dl*-Camphor, and *trans*-π-Oxocamphor are JAN.] (1) Bicyclo[2.2.1]heptane-2-one, 1,7,7-trimethyl-; (2) Camphor; (3) 2-Bornanone. *CAS-76-22-2. Antipruritic.*

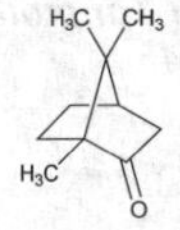

d-**Camphor** (JAN) — *See* Camphor.

dl-**Camphor** (JAN) — *See* Camphor.

Camphor, Monobromated. *CAS-76-29-9.* USP IX.

Camphorated Opium Tincture (previously used name) — *See* Paregoric.

Camphoric Acid. 1,2,2-Trimethyl-1,3-cyclopentanedicarboxylic acid. USP VIII; MI.

Camphotamide. $C_{21}H_{32}N_2O_5S$. 424.55. 3-Diethylcarbamoyl-1-methylpyridinium camphorsulfonate. *UNII-724377908B. CAS-4876-45-3.* INN; DCF; MI.

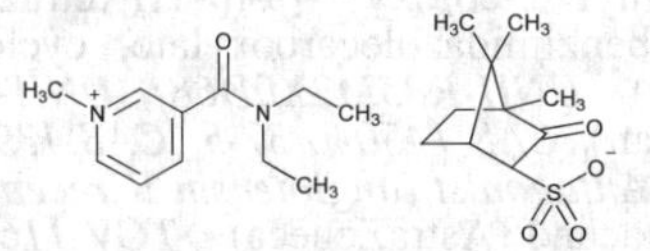

Camylofin. $C_{19}H_{32}N_2O_2$. 320.47. [Acamylophenine Hydrochloride is JAN.] *N*-[2-(Diethylamino)ethyl]-2-phenylglycine, isopentyl ester. *CAS-54-30-8.* INN; DCF; MI.

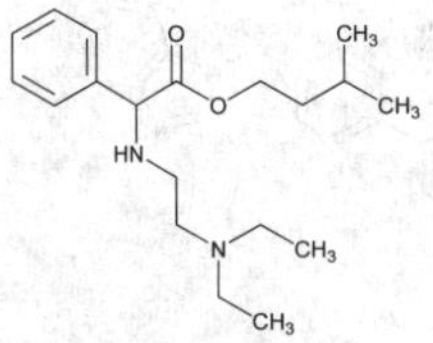

Canakinumab [*2008*] (kan″ a kin′ ue mab). $C_{6452}H_{9958}N_{1722}O_{2010}S_{42}$. (1) Immunoglobulin G1, anti-(human interleukin 1β) (human clone ACZ885 heavy chain V region); (2) Immunoglobulin G1, anti-(human interleukin-1 beta (IL-1β)) human monoclonal ACZ885; (1Glu>Glp)-γ1 heavy chain (221-214′)-disulfide with kappa light chain, dimer (227-227″:230-230″)-bisdisulfide. Molecular weight is approximately 145,200 daltons. *UNII-37CQ2C7X93. CAS-402710-27-4* [variable light κ chain]; *CAS-402710-25-2* [variable heavy γ1 chain]. INN. *Muckle-Wells syndrome, rheumatoid arthritis, other inflammatory conditions.* ◇*ACZ885*

Canbisol. $C_{24}H_{38}O_3$. 374.56. (±)-3-(1,1-Dimethylheptyl)-6aβ,7,8,9,10,10aα-hexahydro-6,6-dimethyl-6*H*-dibenzo[*b,d*]pyran-1,9-diol. *CAS-56689-43-1.* INN.

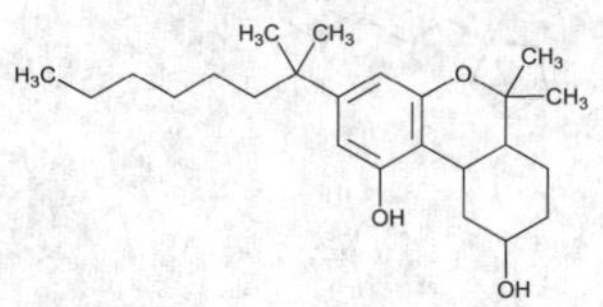

Candelilla Wax (kan″ de lil′ la). **NF.** The purified wax obtained from the leaves of the candelilla plant, *Euphorbia antisyphilitica. CAS-8006-44-8.*

Candesartan [*1997*] (kan″ de sar′ tan). $C_{24}H_{20}N_6O_3$. 440.45. (1) 1*H*-Benzimidazole-7-carboxylic acid, 2-ethoxy-1-[[2′-(1*H*-tetrazol-5-yl)[1,1′-biphenyl]-4-yl]methyl]-; (2) 2-Ethoxy-1-[*p*-(*o*-1*H*-tetrazol-5-ylphenyl)benzyl]-7-benzimidazolecarboxylic acid. *UNII-S8Q36MD2XX. CAS-139481-59-7. INN. Antagonist (angiotensin II receptor); antihypertensive.* ◇*CV-11974*

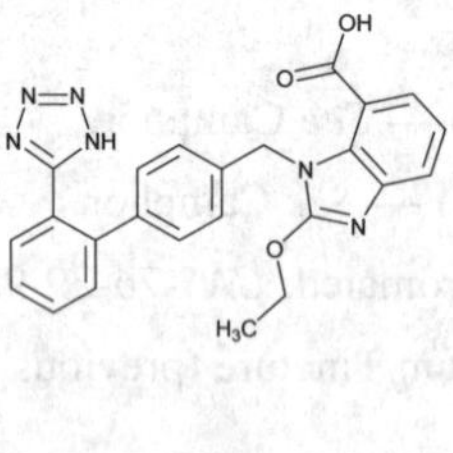

Candesartan Cilexetil [*1997*] (kan″ de sar′ tan sye lex′ e til). $C_{33}H_{34}N_6O_6$. 610.66. [Candesartan is BAN.] (1) 1*H*-Benzimidazole-7-carboxylic acid, 2-ethoxy-1-[[2′-(1*H*-tetrazol-5-yl)[1,1′-biphenyl]-4-yl]methyl]-, 1-[[(cyclohexyloxy)carbonyl]oxy]ethyl ester, (±)-; (2) (±)-1-Hydroxyethyl 2-ethoxy-1-[*p*-(*o*-1*H*-tetrazol-5-ylphenyl)-benzyl]-7-benzimidazolecarboxylate, cyclohexyl carbonate (ester). *UNII-R85M2X0D68; UNII-S8Q36MD2XX* [candesartan]. *CAS-145040-37-5; CAS-139481-59-7* [candesartan]. *Antagonist (angiotensin II receptor); antihypertensive.* Atacand (AstraZeneca) ◇*TCV-116*

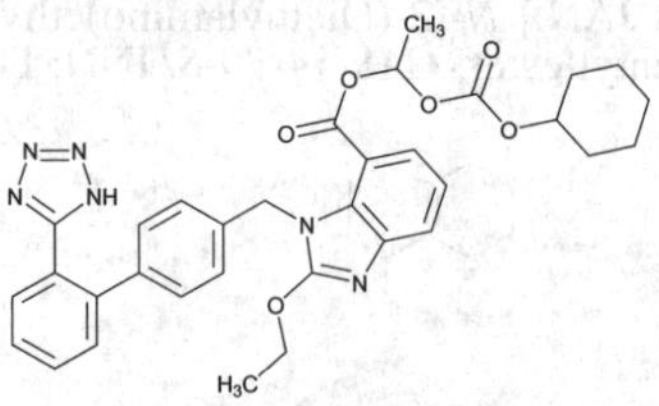

Candicidin [*1965*] (kan″ di sye′ din). (1) Candicidin; (2) Candicidin. *CAS-1403-17-4.* USP XXIII; INN; BAN. *Antifungal.* Vanobid (Sanofi Aventis) ◇*NSC-94219*

Candocuronium Iodide. $C_{26}H_{46}I_2N_2$. 640.47. 17a,17a-Dimethyl-3β-(1-methylpyrrolidinio)-17a-azonia-D-homo-androst-5-ene diiodide *UNII-SC80GNP08C. CAS-54278-85-2.* INN.

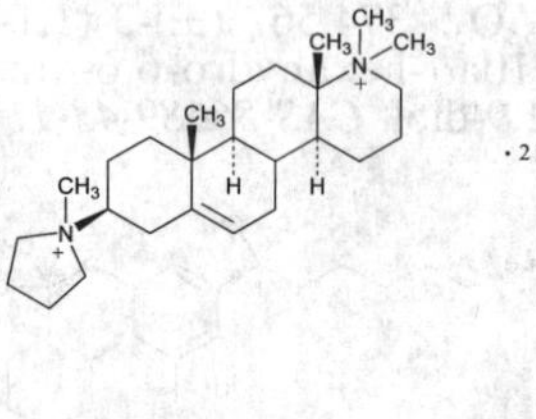

Candoxatril [*1993*] (kan dox′ a tril). $C_{29}H_{41}NO_7$. 515.64. (1) Cyclohexanecarboxylic acid, 4-[[[1-[3-[(2,3-dihydro-1*H*-inden-5-yl)oxy]-2-[(2-methoxyethoxy)methyl]-3-oxopropyl]cyclopentyl]carbonyl]amino]-, [4(*S*)-*cis*]-; (2) (αS)-1-[(*cis*-4-Carboxycyclohexyl)carbamoyl]-α-[(2-methoxy-

ethoxy)methyl]cyclopentanepropionic acid, α-5-indanyl ester. *CAS-123122-55-4.* INN; BAN. *Antihypertensive.* ◇*UK-79,300*

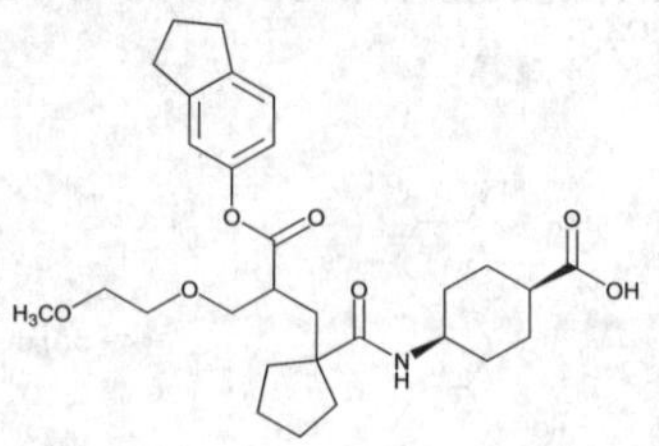

Candoxatrilat [*1993*] (kan dox′ a tril at). $C_{20}H_{33}NO_7$. 399.48. (1) Cyclohexanecarboxylic acid, 4-[[[1-[2-carboxy-3-(2-methoxyethoxy)propyl]cyclopentyl]carbonyl]amino]-, [4(*S*)-*cis*]-; (2) (αS)-1-[(*cis*-4-Carboxycyclohexyl)carbamoyl]-α-[(2-methoxyethoxy)methyl]cyclopentanepropionic acid. *UNII-7WU8BZ90TH. CAS-123122-54-3.* INN; BAN. *Antihypertensive.* ◇*UK-73,967*

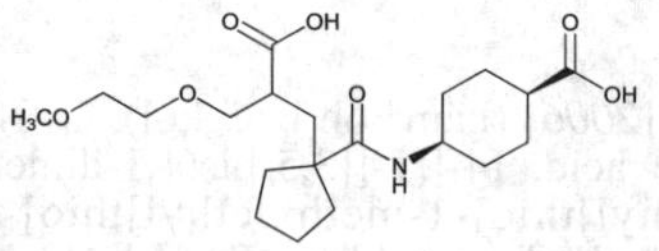

Canertinib Dihydrochloride [*2002*] (kan er′ ti nib dye hye″ droe klor′ ide). $C_{24}H_{25}ClFN_5O_3 \cdot 2HCl$. 558.86. [Canertinib is INN and BAN.] (1) 2-Propenamide, *N*-[4-[(3-chloro-4-fluorophenyl)amino]-7-[3-(4-morpholinyl)propoxy]-6-quinazolinyl]-, dihydrochloride; (2) *N*-[4-(3-Chloro-4-fluorophenyl)amino]-7-(3-morpholin-4-yl)propoxy]quinazolin-6-yl]prop-2-enamide dihydrochloride. *UNII-ICJ93X8X90. CAS-289499-45-2; CAS-267243-28-7* [canertinib]. *Treatment of epithelial tumors.* ◇*CI-1033; PD-183805; PD-0183805*

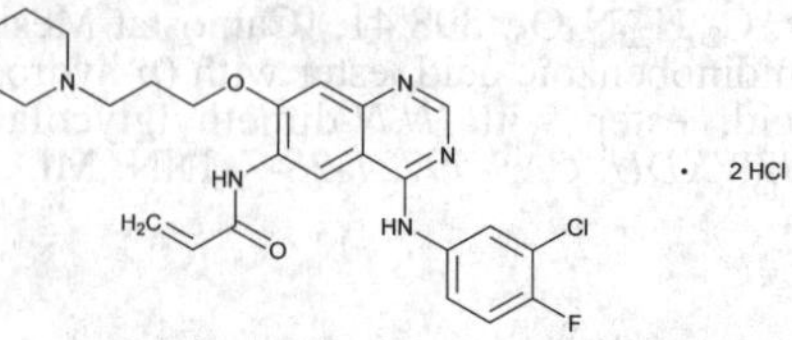

Canfosfamide Hydrochloride [*2004*] (kan fos′ fa mide hye″ droe klor′ ide). $C_{26}H_{40}Cl_4N_5O_{10}PS \cdot HCl$. 823.94. [Canfosfamide is INN.] (1) Glycine, L-γ-glutamyl-3-[[2-[[bis[bis(2-chloroethyl)amino]phosphinyl]oxy]ethyl]sulfonyl]-L-alanyl-2-phenyl-, monohydrochloride, (2*R*)-; (2) (2*S*)-2-Amino-5-[[(1*R*)-1-[[[2-[[bis[bis(2-chloroethyl)amino]phosphinyl]oxy]ethyl]sulfonyl]methyl]-2-[[(*R*)-carboxyphenylmethyl]amino]-2-oxoethyl]amino]-5-oxopentanoic acid monohydrochloride. *CAS-439943-59-6; CAS-158382-

37-7 [canfosfamide]. *Antineoplastic (activated by glutathione S-transferase (GST P1-1)).* Telcyta (Telik) ◇*TLK286; TER286*

Cangrelor [*2005*] (kan′ grel or). $C_{17}H_{25}Cl_2F_3N_5O_{12}P_3S_2$. 776.36. (1) 5′-Adenylic acid, *N*-[2-(methylthio)ethyl]-2-[(3,3,3-trifluoropropyl)thio]-, monoanhydride with (dichloromethylene)bis[phosphonic acid]; (2) (Dichloromethylene)diphosphonic *N*-[2-(methylsulfanyl)ethyl]-2-[(3,3,3-trifluoropropyl)sulfanyl-5′-adenylic monoanhydride. *UNII-6AQ1Y404U7. CAS-163706-06-7.* INN; BAN. *Anti-platelet agent.* ◇*AR-C69931XX*

Cangrelor Tetrasodium [*2005*] (kan′ grel or tet″ ra soe′ dee um). $C_{17}H_{21}Cl_2F_3N_5Na_4O_{12}P_3S_2$. 864.29. (1) 5′-Adenylic acid, *N*-[2-(methylthio)ethyl]-2-[(3,3,3-trifluoropropyl)thio]-, monoanhydride with (dichloromethylene)bis[phosphonic acid], tetrasodium salt; (2) *N*-[2-(Methylthio)ethyl]-2-[(3,3,3-trifluoropropyl)thio]-5′-adenylic acid, monoanhydride with (dichloromethylene)diphosphonic acid tetrasodium salt. *UNII-2144G00Y7W. CAS-163706-36-3. Antiplatelet agent.* ◇*AR-C69931MX*

Cannabinol. $C_{21}H_{26}O_2$. 310.43. 6,6,9-Trimethyl-3-pentyl-6*H*-dibenzo[*b,d*]pyran-1-ol. Product derived from *Cannabis sativa.CAS-521-35-7.* INN; BAN; MI.

Canola Oil. NF. (1) Low erucic acid rapeseed oil; (2) LEAR oil.

Canrenoate Potassium [*1967*] (kan ren′ oh ate poe tas′ ee um). $C_{22}H_{29}KO_4$. 396.56. [Potassium Canrenoate is JAN; Canrenoic Acid is INN and BAN.] (1) Pregna-4,6-diene-21-carboxylic acid, 17-hydroxy-3-oxo-, monopotassium salt (17α)-; (2) Potassium 17-hydroxy-3-oxo-17α-pregna-

4,6-diene-21-carboxylate. *UNII-M671F9NLEA. CAS-2181-04-6; CAS-4138-96-9* [canrenoic acid]. *Aldosterone antagonist.* ◇*SC-14266*

Canrenoic Acid (INN, BAN) — *See* Canrenoate Potassium.

Canrenone [*1967*] (kan′ re none). $C_{22}H_{28}O_3$. 340.46. (1) Pregna-4,6-diene-21-carboxylic acid, 17-hydroxy-3-oxo-, γ-lactone (17α)-; (2) 17-Hydroxy-3-oxo-17α-pregna-4,6-diene-21-carboxylic acid γ-lactone; (3) 17α-(2-Carboxyethyl)-17β-hydroxyandrosta-4,6-dien-3-one lactone. *CAS-976-71-6.* INN. *Aldosterone antagonist.* ◇*SC-9376*

Cantharides Tincture. Tincture prepared from the cantharides (the beetles of *Epicauta gorhami* Marseul *Meloidae*). JAN.

Cantuzumab Mertansine [*2002*] (kan tooz′ oo mab mer tan′ seen). $C_{35}H_{48}ClN_3O_{10}S$. 738.29. (1) Immunoglobulin G1, anti-(mucin CanAg) (human-mouse monoclonal C242 heavy chain), disulfide with human-mouse monoclonal C242 light chain, dimer, compound with $N^{2'}$-deacetyl-$N^{2'}$-(3-mercapto-1-oxopropyl)maytansine (1:4); (2) Immunoglobulin G1, anti-(mucin CanAg) human-mouse monoclonal C242 heavy chain), disulfide with human-mouse monoclonal C242 light chain, dimer, compound with $N^{2'}$-deacetyl-$N^{2'}$-(3-sulfanylpropanoyl)maytansine. *CAS-400010-39-1.* INN. *Treatment of colorectal cancer, pancreatic cancer and other solid tumor types that express the C242 antigen.* ◇*SB-408075; huC242-DM1*

Capadenoson. $C_{25}H_{18}ClN_5O_2S_2$. 520.03. 2-Amino-6-({[2-(4-chlorophenyl)-1,3-thiazol-4-yl]methyl}sulfanyl)-4-[4-(2-hydroxyethoxy)phenyl]pyridine-3,5-dicarbonitrile. *CAS-544417-40-5.* INN.

Capecitabine [*1995*] (kap″ e sye′ ta been). **USP.** $C_{15}H_{22}FN_3O_6$. 359.35. (1) Carbamic acid, [1-(5-deoxy-β-D-ribofuranosyl)-5-fluoro-1,2-dihydro-2-oxo-4-pyrimidinyl]-, pentyl ester; (2) Pentyl 1-(5-deoxy-β-D-ribofurano-

---

† Brand name formerly used, and/or firm no longer concerned with this product.

syl)-5-fluoro-1,2-dihydro-2-oxo-4-pyrimidinecarbamate. *UNII-6804DJ8Z9U. CAS-154361-50-9.* INN; BAN. *Antineoplastic.* Xeloda (Roche) ◇*Ro 09-1978/000*

Capeserod. $C_{23}H_{25}ClN_4O_4$. 456.92. 5-(8-Amino-7-chloro-2,3-dihydro-1,4-benzodioxin-5-yl)-3-[1-(2-phenylethyl)piperidin-4-yl]-1,3,4-oxadiazol-2(3*H*)-one. *UNII-8163770L8P. CAS-769901-96-4.* INN.

Capimorelin Tartrate (previously used name) — *See* Capromorelin Tartrate.

Capmul 8210 — *See* Monoctanoin.

Capobenate Sodium [*1971*] (kap″ oh ben′ ate soe′ dee um). $C_{16}H_{22}NNaO_6$. 347.34. (1) Hexanoic acid, 6-[(3,4,5-trimethoxybenzoyl)amino]-, monosodium salt; (2) Sodium 6-(3,4,5-trimethoxybenzamido)hexanoate. *UNII-505434F98H. CAS-27276-25-1; CAS-21434-91-3* [capobenic acid]. *Cardiac depressant (anti-arrhythmic).* ◇*C-3*

Capobenic Acid [*1971*] (kap″ oh ben′ ik as′ id). $C_{16}H_{23}NO_6$. 325.36. (1) Hexanoic acid, 6-[(3,4,5-trimethoxybenzoyl)amino]-; (2) 6-(3,4,5-Trimethoxybenzamido) hexanoic acid. *UNII-3R77T835TA. CAS-21434-91-3.* INN. *Cardiac depressant (anti-arrhythmic).* ◇*C-3*

Capravirine [*1999*] (kap″ ra vir′ een). $C_{20}H_{20}Cl_2N_4O_2S$. 451.37. (1) 1*H*-Imidazole-2-methanol, 5-[(3,5-dichlorophenyl)thio]-4-(1-methylethyl)-1-(4-pyridinylmethyl)-, carbamate (ester); (2) 5-[(3,5-Dichlorophenyl)thio]-4-isopropyl-1-(4-pyridylmethyl)imidazole-2-methanol carbamate (ester). *UNII-VHC779598X. CAS-178979-85-6.* INN. *Antiviral (reverse transcriptase inhibitor).* ◇*S-1153*

Capreomycin Sulfate [*1962*] (kap″ ree oh mye′ sin sul′ fate). **USP**. Antibiotic produced by *Streptomyces capreolus.* [Capreomycin is INN and BAN.] (1) Capreomycin sulfate; (2) Capreomycin sulfate. *UNII-9H8D3J7V21; UNII-*

232HYX66HC [capreomycin]. *CAS-1405-37-4; CAS-11003-38-6* [capreomycin]. JAN. *Antibacterial (tuberculostatic).* Capastat Sulfate (Lilly) ◇*34977*

Capromab Pendetide [*1994*] (kap′ roe mab pen′ de tide). [Capromab is INN and BAN.] (1) Immunoglobulin G 1 (mouse monoclonal 7E11-C5.3 anti-human prostatic carcinoma cell), disulfide with mouse monoclonal 7E11-C5.3 light chain, dimer, N^6-[*N*-[2-[[2-[bis(carboxymethyl)amino]ethyl](carboxymethyl)amino]ethyl]-*N*-(carboxymethyl)glycyl]-N^2-(*N*-glycyl-L-tyrosyl)-L-lysine conjugate; (2) Immunoglobulin G 1 (mouse monoclonal 7E11-C5.3 anti-human prostatic carcinoma cell), disulfide with mouse monoclonal 7E11-C5.3 light chain, dimer, N^6-[*N*-[2-[[2-[bis(carboxymethyl)amino]ethyl](carboxymethyl)amino]ethyl]-*N*-(carboxymethyl)glycyl]-N^2-(*N*-glycyl-L-tyrosyl)-L-lysine conjugate. Molecular weight is approximately 150,000 daltons. *CAS-145464-28-4; CAS-151763-64-3* [capromab]. *Monoclonal antibody.* ◇*CYT-356*

Capromorelin Tartrate [*1999*] (kap″ roe moe rel′ in tar′ trate). $C_{28}H_{35}N_5O_4 \cdot C_4H_6O_6$. 655.70. [Capromorelin is INN.] (1) Propanamide, 2-amino-*N*-[2-[2,3,3a,4,6,7-hexahydro-2-methyl-3-oxo-3a-(phenylmethyl)-5*H*-pyrazolo[4,3-*c*]pyridin-5-yl]-2-oxo-1-[(phenylmethoxy)methyl]ethyl]-2-methyl-, [*R*-(*R**,*R**)]-, [*R*-(*R**,*R**)]-2,3-dihydroxybutanedioate (1:1); (2) 2-Amino-*N*-[(1*R*)-1-[[(3a*R*)-3a-benzyl-2,3,3a,4,6,7-hexahydro-2-methyl-3-oxo-5*H*-pyrazolo[4,3-*c*]pyridin-5-yl]carbonyl]-2-(benzyloxy)ethyl]-2-methylpropionamide L-(+)-tartrate (1:1). *UNII-4150VMF5EP. CAS-193273-69-7; CAS-193273-66-4* [capromorelin]. *Treatment and prevention of frailty; treatment of congestive heart failure; treatment of catabolic illness (growth hormone secretagogue).[Name previously used: Capimorelin Tartrate.]* ◇*CP-424,391-18*

Caproxamine. $C_{15}H_{25}N_3O$. 263.38. 3′-Amino-4′-methylhexanophenone *O*-(2-aminoethyl)oxime. *UNII-7YQT311430. CAS-24047-16-3.* INN; BAN. ◇*DU 22550 [as sulfate]*

Caprylocaproyl Polyoxylglycerides. **NF**. Mixtures of monoesters, diesters, and triesters of glycerol and monoesters and diesters of polyethylene glycols with a mean relative molecular weight between 200 and 400.

Capsaicin (kap say′ sin). **USP**. $C_{18}H_{27}NO_3$. 305.41. (1) 6-Nonenamide, (*E*)-*N*-[(4-hydroxy-3-methoxy-phenyl)-methyl]-8-methyl; (2) (*E*)-8-Methyl-*N*-vanillyl-6-nonenamide. *UNII-S07O44R1ZM. CAS-404-86-4. Antineuralgic, specific pain syndromes, topical; analgesic (topical).*

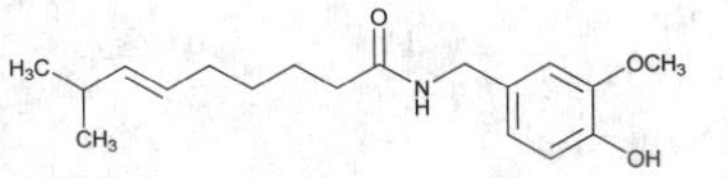

Capsicum (kap′ si kum). **USP**. The dried ripe fruit of *Capsicum frutescens* Linné, known in commerce as African Chillies, or of *Capsicum annuum* Linné var. *connoides* Irish, known in commerce as Tabasco Pepper, or *Capsicum annuum* var. *longum* Sendt, known in commerce as Louisiana Long Pepper, or of a hybrid between the Honka variety of Japanese Capsicum and the Old Louisiana Sport Capsicum known in commerce as Louisiana Sport Pepper (Fam. Solanaceae). JAN. *Carminative; counterirritant (external); stomachic.*

Capsicum Oleoresin (kap′ si kum oh″ lee oh rez′ in). **USP**. An alcoholic extract of the dried ripe fruits of *Capsicum annum* var. *minimum* and small fruited varieties of *C. fruiscons* (Solanaceae). *Carminative; counterirritant (external); stomachic.*

Captamine Hydrochloride [*1967*] (kap′ ta meen hye″ droe klor′ ide). $C_4H_{11}NS.HCl$. 141.66. [Captamine is INN.] (1) Ethanethiol, 2-(dimethylamino)-, hydrochloride; (2) 2-(Dimethylamino)ethanethiol hydrochloride; (3) *N*-(2-Mercaptoethyl)dimethylamine hydrochloride. *CAS-13242-44-9; CAS-108-02-1* [captamine]. *Depigmentor.* ◇*NSC-45463*

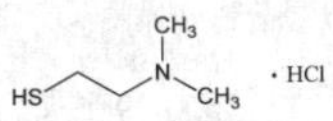

Captodiame Hydrochloride. $C_{21}H_{29}NS_2.HCl$. 396.05. [Captodiame is INN and BAN.] 2-[*p*-(Butylthio)-α-phenylbenzylthio]-*N*,*N*-dimethylethylamine hydrochloride. *UNII-9I7N9PR9J2. CAS-904-04-1; CAS-486-17-9* [captodiame]. MI.

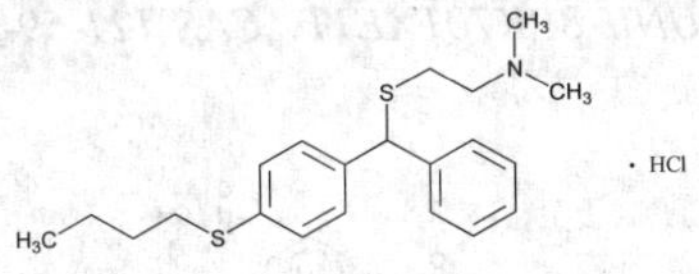

Captodiamine Hydrochloride — *See* Captodiame Hydrochloride.

Captopril [*1978*] (kap′ toe pril). **USP**. $C_9H_{15}NO_3S$. 217.29. (1) L-Proline, 1-[(2*S*)-3-mercapto-2-methyl-1-oxopropyl]-; (2) 1-[(2*S*)-3-Mercapto-2-methylpropionyl]-L-proline. *UNII-9G64RSX1XD. CAS-62571-86-2. INN; BAN; JAN. Antihypertensive; enzyme inhibitor (angiotensin-converting).* Capoten (Par) ◇*SQ 14,225*

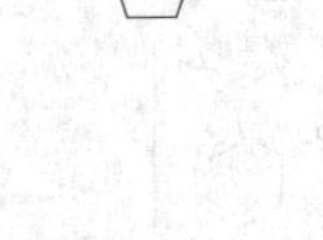

Capuride [*1963*] (kap′ ure ide). $C_9H_{18}N_2O_2$. 186.25. (1) Pentanamide, *N*-(aminocarbonyl)-2-ethyl-3-methyl-; (2) (2-Ethyl-3-methylvaleryl)urea. *CAS-5579-13-5.* INN. *Sedative-hypnotic.* Pacinox (Ortho-McNeil†) ◇*McN-X-94; NSC-27178*

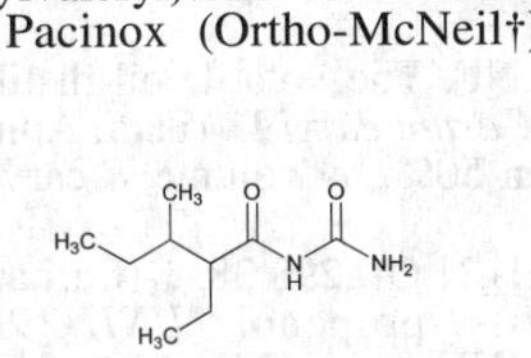

Carabersat. $C_{20}H_{20}FNO_4$. 357.38. (1) *N*-[(3*R*,4*S*)-6-Acetyl-3-hydroxy-2,2-dimethyl-4-chromanyl]-*p*-flurobenzamide; (1) *N*-[(3*R*,4*S*)-6-Acetyl-3-hydroxy-2,2-dimethylchroman-4-yl]-4-fluorobenzamide. *UNII-K9R83652CK. CAS-184653-84-7.* INN; BAN. ◇*SB-204269-EO*

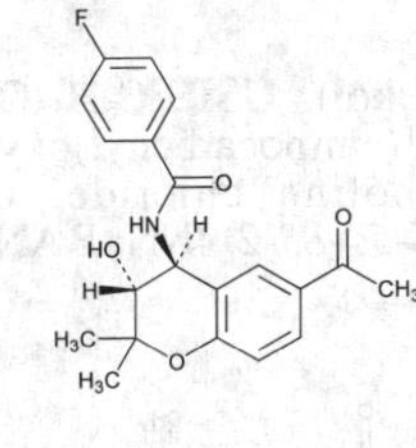

Caracemide [*1983*] (kar a′ se mide). $C_6H_{11}N_3O_4$. 189.17. (1) Acetamide, *N*-[(methylamino)carbonyl]-*N*-[(methylamino)carbonyl]oxy]-; (2) *N*-Acetyl-*N*,*O*-bis(methylcarbamoyl)hydroxylamine. *CAS-81424-67-1.* INN. *Antineoplastic.* ◇*NSC-253272*

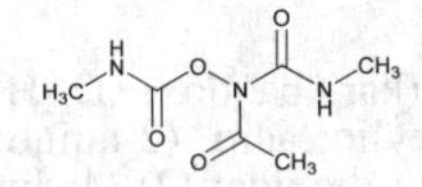

Carafiban. $C_{24}H_{27}N_5O_5$. 465.50. Ethyl (*S*)-β-[2-[(*S*)-4-(*p*-amidinophenyl)-4-methyl-2,5-dioxo-1-imidazolidinyl]acetamido]hydrocinnamate. *UNII-39IWK4M2UW. CAS-177563-40-5.* INN.

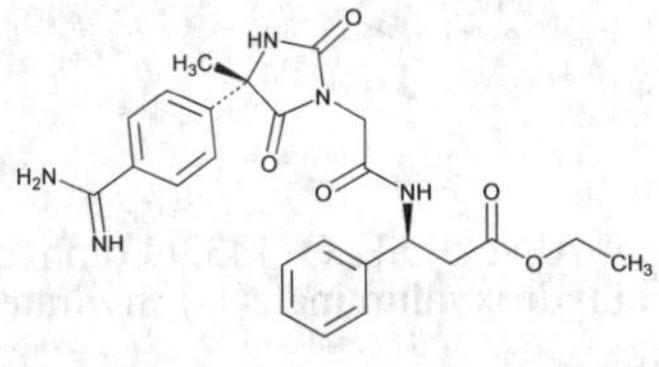

Caramel (kar′ a mel). **NF**. A concentrated solution of the product obtained by heating sugar or glucose until the sweet taste is destroyed and a uniform brown mass results, a small amount of alkali or of alkaline carbonate or a trace of mineral acid being added while heating. *CAS-8028-89-5. Pharmaceutic aid (color).*

Caramiphen Hydrochloride. $C_{18}H_{27}NO_2.HCl$. 325.87. [Caramiphen is INN and BAN.] 2-Diethylaminoethyl 1-phenylcyclopentane-1-carboxylate hydrochloride. *UNII-4858SN190E. CAS-125-85-9; CAS-77-22-5* [caramiphen]. MI.

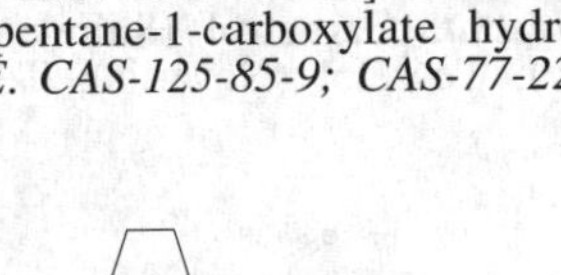

---

† Brand name formerly used, and/or firm no longer concerned with this product.

Caraway (kar′ a way). **NF**. The dried, ripe fruit of *Carum carvi* L. (Fam. Apiaceae). *UNII-W2FH8O2BBE*. *CAS-8000-42-8* [oil]. MI. *Pharmaceutic aid (flavor)*.

Caraway Oil. **NF**. The volatile oil distilled from the dried, ripe fruit of *Carum carvi* L. (Fam. Apiaceae) that contains not more than 50%, by volume, *d*-carvone ($C_{10}H_{14}O$).

Carazolol. $C_{18}H_{22}N_2O_2$. 298.38. 1-(Carbazol-4-yloxy)-3-(iso-propylamino)-2-propanol. *UNII-29PW75S82A*. *CAS-57775-29-8*. INN; BAN; MI. ◊*BM 51052*

Carbachol (kar′ ba kol). **USP**. $C_6H_{15}ClN_2O_2$. 182.65. (1) Ethanaminium, 2-[(aminocarbonyl)oxy]-*N,N,N*-trimethyl-, chloride; (2) Choline chloride, carbamate. *UNII-8Y164V895Y*. *CAS-51-83-2*. INN; BAN; JAN. *Cholinergic (ophthalmic)*.

Carbacholine Chloride (DCF) — *See* Carbachol.

Carbadipimidine Hydrochloride — *See* Carpipramine Dihydrochloride.

Carbadox [*1968*] (kar′ ba dox). $C_{11}H_{10}N_4O_4$. 262.22. (1) Hydrazinecarboxylic acid (2-quinoxalinylmethylene)-, methyl ester N^1,N^4-dioxide; (2) Methyl 3-(2-quinoxalinylmethylene)carbazate N^1,N^4-dioxide. *UNII-M2X04R2E2Y*. *CAS-6804-07-5*. INN; BAN. *Antibacterial*. Mecadox (Pfizer) ◊*GS-6244*

Carbaldrate. $CH_2AlNaO_5.nH_2O$. 143.99 (anhydrous). Sodium (carbonato)dihydroxyaluminate(1-) hydrate. *CAS-41342-54-5*. INN.

Carbamazepine [*1965*] (kar″ ba maz′ e peen). **USP**. $C_{15}H_{12}N_2O$. 236.27. (1) 5*H*-Dibenz[*b,f*]azepine-5-carboxamide; (2) 5*H*-Dibenz[*b,f*]azepine-5-carboxamide. *UNII-33CM23913M*. *CAS-298-46-4*. INN; BAN; JAN. *Analgesic; anticonvulsant*. Carbatrol (Shire); Epitol (Teva); Equetro (Shire); Tegretol (Novartis); Teril (Taro) ◊*G-32883*

Carbamide Peroxide (kar′ ba mide per ox′ ide). **USP**. $CH_6N_2O_3$. 94.07. (1) Urea, compd. with hydrogen peroxide (1:1); (2) Urea compound with hydrogen peroxide (1:1). *UNII-31PZ2VAU81*. *CAS-124-43-6*. *Anti-infective, topical (dental)*. Murine Ear Drops (Ross)

Carbamoylcholine Chloride — *See* Carbachol.

Carbamylmethylcholine Chloride — *See* Bethanechol Chloride.

Carbantel Lauryl Sulfate [*1976*] (kar ban′ tel lawr′ il sul′ fate). $C_{12}H_{16}ClN_3O.C_{12}H_{26}O_4S$. 520.13. [Carbantel is INN.] (1) Pentanimidamide, *N*-[[(4-chlorophenyl)amino]carbonyl]-, compd. with dodecyl hydrogen sulfate (1:1); (2) 1-(*p*-Chlorophenyl)-3-valerimidoylurea compound with dodecyl hydrogen sulfate (1:1). *UNII-0DMO75HN8B*. *CAS-54644-15-4; CAS-22790-84-7* [carbantel]. *Anthelmintic*. ◊*Win 29194-6*

Carbaril. $C_{12}H_{11}NO_2$. 201.22. [Carbaryl is BAN.] 1-Naphthyl methylcarbamate. *UNII-R890C8J3N1*. *CAS-63-25-2*. INN; MI. ◊*ENT-23969*

Carbarsone. $C_7H_9AsN_2O_4$. 260.08. (1) Arsonic acid, [4-[(aminocarbonyl)amino]phenyl]-; (2) *N*-Carbamoylarsanilic acid. *UNII-8PK70TXE1T*. *CAS-121-59-5*. USP XXI; INN; MI.

Carbaryl (BAN) — *See* Carbaril.

Carbasalate Calcium (INN, BAN) — *See* Carbaspirin Calcium.

Carbaspirin Calcium [*1963*] (karb as′ pir in kal′ see um). $C_{19}H_{18}CaN_2O_9$. 458.43. [Carbasalate Calcium is INN and BAN.] (1) Benzoic acid, 2-(acetyloxy)-, calcium salt, compd. with urea (1:1); (2) Salicylic acid acetate calcium salt, compound with urea (1:1) complex. *CAS-5749-67-7*. *Analgesic*.

Carbazeran [*1980*] (kar ba′ ze ran). $C_{18}H_{24}N_4O_4$. 360.41. (1) Carbamic acid, ethyl-, 1-(6,7-dimethoxy-1-phthalazinyl)-4-piperidinyl ester; (2) 1-(6,7-Dimethoxy-1-phthalazinyl)-4-piperidyl ethylcarbamate. *UNII-0N4I6K95P2. CAS-70724-25-3.* INN. *Cardiotonic.* ◇*UK-31,557*

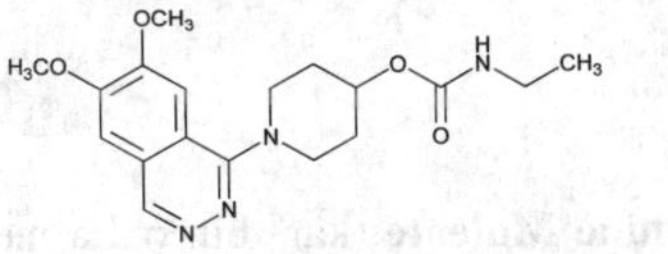

Carbazochrome. $C_{10}H_{12}N_4O_3$. 236.23. 3-Hydroxy-1-methyl-5,6-indolinedione semicarbazone. *UNII-81F061RQS4. CAS-69-81-8.* INN; JAN.

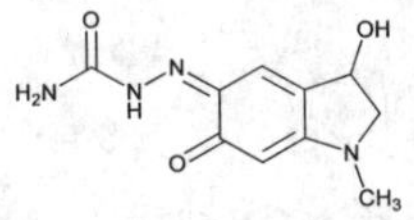

Carbazochrome Salicylate. $C_{10}H_{12}N_4O_3.C_7H_5NaO_3$. 396.33. Adenochrome semicarbazone, mixture with sodium salicylate. *UNII-3H4OD401LF. CAS-13051-01-9.* INN; MI.

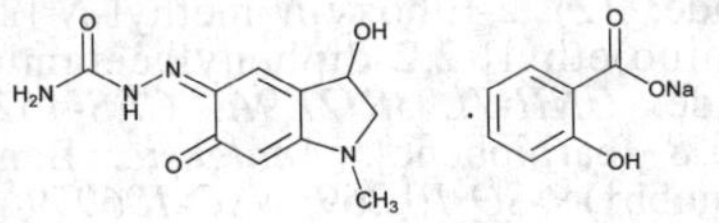

Carbazochrome Sodium Sulfonate. $C_{10}H_{11}N_4NaO_5S$. 322.27. Sodium salt of 5,6-dihydro-1-methyl-5,6-dioxo-3-indoline sulfonic acid 5-semicarbazone. *CAS-51460-26-5.* INN; JAN; MI.

Carbazocine. $C_{22}H_{28}N_2$. 320.47. 14-(Cyclopropylmethyl)-1,2,3,4,4a,5,6,11-octahydro-5,11b-iminoethano-11b*H*-benzo[a]carbazole. *CAS-15686-38-1.* INN.

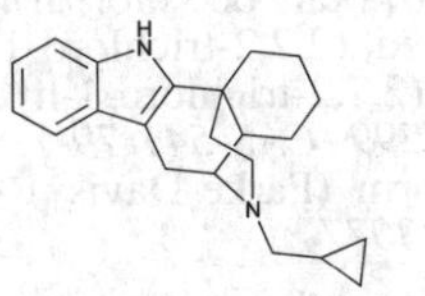

Carbenicillin Disodium [*1969*] (kar″ ben i sil′ in dye soe′ dee um). USP. $C_{17}H_{16}N_2Na_2O_6S$. 422.36. [Carbenicillin is INN and BAN; Carbenicillin Sodium is JAN.] (1) 4-Thia-1-azabicyclo[3.2.0]heptane-2-carboxylic acid, 6-[(carboxyphenylacetyl)amino]-3,3-dimethyl-7-oxo, disodium salt, [2*S*-(2α,5α,6β)]-; (2) *N*-(2-Carboxy-3,3-dimethyl-7-oxo-4-thia-1-azabicyclo[3.2.0]-hept-6-yl)-2-phe-

nylmalonamic acid disodium salt. *UNII-9TS4B3H261. CAS-4800-94-6; CAS-4697-36-3* [carbenicillin]. *Antibacterial.* ◇*CP-15-639-2; BRL-2064; NSC-111071*

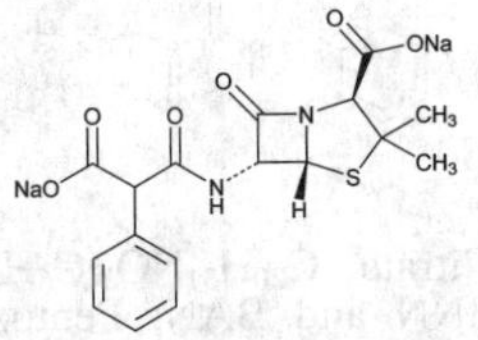

Carbenicillin Indanyl Sodium [*1972*] (kar″ ben i sil′ in in′ da nil soe′ dee um). USP. $C_{26}H_{25}N_2NaO_6S$. 516.54. [Carindacillin is INN and BAN; Carindacillin Sodium is JAN.] (1) 4-Thia-1-azabicyclo[3.2.0]heptane-2-carboxylic acid, 6-[[3-[(2,3-dihydro-1*H*-inden-5-yl)oxy]-1,3-dioxo-2-phenylpropyl]amino]-3,3-dimethyl-7-oxo-, monosodium salt, [2*S*-(2α,5α,6β)]-; (2) 1-(5-Indanyl)(2*S*,5*R*,6*R*)-*N*-(2-carboxy-3,3-dimethyl-7-oxo-4-thia-1-azabicyclo[3.2.0]hept-6-yl)-2-phenylmalonamate monosodium salt. *UNII-4OUL81K2RT. CAS-26605-69-6; CAS-35531-88-5* [carbenicillin indanyl]. *Antibacterial.* Geocillin (Pfizer) ◇*CP-15,464-2*

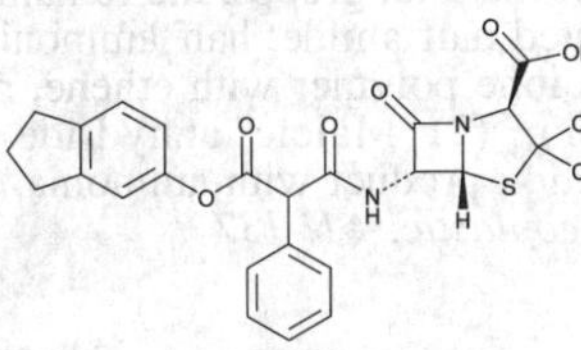

Carbenicillin Phenyl Sodium [*1973*] (kar″ ben i sil′ in fen′ il soe′ dee um). $C_{23}H_{21}N_2NaO_6S$. 476.48. [Carfecillin is INN and BAN; Carfecillin Sodium is JAN.] (1) 4-Thia-1-azabicyclo[3.2.0]heptane-2-carboxylic acid, 6-[(1,3-dioxo-3-phenoxy-2-phenylpropyl)amino]-3,3-dimethyl-7-oxo-, monosodium salt, [2*S*-(2α,5α,6β)]; (2) *N*-(2-Carboxy-3,3-dimethyl-7-oxo-4-thia-1-azabicyclo[3.2.0]hept-6-yl)-2-phenylmalonamic acid 1-phenyl ester sodium salt. *UNII-18N5JP36GY. CAS-21649-57-0; CAS-27025-49-6* [carbenicillin phenyl]. *Antibacterial.* ◇*BRL-3475*

Carbenicillin Potassium [*1968*] (kar″ ben i sil′ in poe tas′ ee um). $C_{17}H_{17}KN_2O_6S$. 416.49. (1) 4-Thia-1-azabicyclo[3.2.0]heptane-2-carboxylic acid, 6-[(carboxyphenylacetyl)amino]-3,3-dimethyl-7-oxo-, monopotassium salt, [6*S*-(2α,5α,6β)]-; (2) *N*-(2-Carboxy-3,3-dimethyl-7-oxo-4-thia-1-azabicyclo[3.2.0]hept-6-yl)-2-phenylmalonamic acid 2-(potassium salt). *UNII-3UX6B304L3; UNII-G42ZU72N5G* [carbenicillin]. *CAS-17230-86-3; CAS-4697-36-3* [carbenicillin]. *Antibacterial.* ◇*GS-3159*

Carbenoxolone Sodium [*1974*] (kar″ ben ox′ oh lone soe′ dee um). $C_{34}H_{48}Na_2O_7$. 614.72. [Carbenoxolone is INN and BAN.] (1) Olean-12-en-29-oic acid, 3-(3-carboxy-1-oxopropoxy)-11-oxo, disodium salt, (3β,20β)-; (2) 3β-Hydroxy-11-oxoolean-12-en-30-oic acid hydrogen succinate disodium salt. *CAS-7421-40-1; CAS-5697-56-3* [carbenoxolone]. JAN. *Glucocorticoid.*

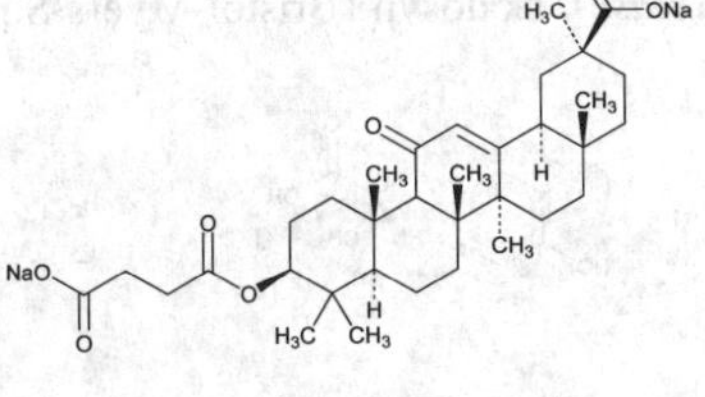

---

† Brand name formerly used, and/or firm no longer concerned with this product.

Carbenzide. $C_{11}H_{16}N_2O_2$. 208.26. Ethyl-3-(α-methylbenzyl)-carbazate. *CAS-3240-20-8.* INN.

Carbetapentane Citrate. $C_{20}H_{31}NO_3.C_6H_8O_7$. 525.59. [Pentoxyverine is INN and BAN; Pentoxyverine Citrate is JAN.] 2-[2-(Diethylamino)ethoxy]ethyl 1-phenylcyclopentanecarboxylate citrate (1:1). *UNII-4SH0MFJ5HJ. CAS-23142-01-0; CAS-77-23-6* [carbetapentane]. NF XIII; MI. Toclase (Pfizer)

Carbetimer [*1984*] (kar bet′ i mer). (In the graphic formula, *A* + *B* represents 100% of repeating groups, and *A* represents 14% to 25% of the total groups; the remaining substituents are unsubstituted half amide, half ammonium salt groups. (1) 2,5-Furandione polymer with ethene, reaction product with ammonia; (2) Maleic anhydride polymer with ethylene, reaction product with ammonia. *CAS-82230-03-3.* INN. *Antineoplastic.* ◇*N-137*

Carbetocin. $C_{45}H_{69}N_{11}O_{12}S$. 988.16. 1-Butyric acid-2-[3-(*p*-methoxyphenyl)-L-alanine]oxytocin. *CAS-37025-55-1.* INN; BAN; MI.

Carbidopa [*1972*] (kar″ bi doe′ pa). USP. $C_{10}H_{14}N_2O_4.H_2O$. 244.24. (1) Benzenepropanoic acid, α-hydrazino-3,4-dihydroxy-α-methyl-, monohydrate, (*S*)-; (2) (-)-L-α-Hydrazino-3,4-dihydroxy-α-methylhydrocinnamic acid monohydrate. *UNII-MNX7R8C5VO. CAS-38821-49-7; CAS-28860-95-9* [anhydrous]. INN; BAN; JAN. *Inhibitor (decarboxylase).* Lodosyn (Bristol-Myers Squibb)

Carbifene (INN, BAN) — *See* Carbiphene Hydrochloride.

Carbimazole. $C_7H_{10}N_2O_2S$. 186.23. Ethyl 3-methyl-2-thioimidazoline-1-carboxylate. *CAS-22232-54-8.* INN; BAN; DCF; MI.

Carbinoxamine Maleate (kar″ bin ox′ a meen mal′ ee ate). USP. $C_{16}H_{19}ClN_2O.C_4H_4O_4$. 406.86. [Carbinoxamine is INN and BAN.] (1) Ethanamine, 2-[(4-chlorophenyl)-2-pyridinylmethoxy]-*N,N*-dimethyl-, (*Z*)-2-butenedioate (1:1); (2) 2-[*p*-Chloro-α-[2-(dimethylamino)ethoxy]benzyl]pyridine maleate (1:1). *UNII-02O55696WH; UNII-982A7M02H5* [carbinoxamine]. *CAS-3505-38-2; CAS-486-16-8* [carbinoxamine]. JAN. *Antihistaminic.* Clistin (McNeil)

Carbiphene Hydrochloride [*1967*] (kar′ bi feen hye″ droe klor′ ide). $C_{28}H_{34}N_2O_2.HCl$. 467.04. [Carbifene is INN and BAN.] (1) Benzeneacetamide, α-ethoxy-*N*-methyl-*N*-[2-[methyl(2-phenylethyl)amino]ethyl]-α-phenyl-, monohydrochloride; (2) 2-Ethoxy-*N*-methyl-*N*-[2-(methylphenethylamino)ethyl]-2,2-diphenylacetamide monohydrochloride. *UNII-7L93SJ2K9A. CAS-467-22-1; CAS-15687-16-8* [carbiphene]. *Analgesic.* Bandol (Bristol-Myers Squibb†) ◇*SQ 10,269; NSC-106959*

Carbocistein (JAN) — *See* Carbocysteine.

Carbocisteine (INN, BAN) — *See* Carbocysteine.

Carbocloral [*1966*] (kar″ boe klor′ al). $C_5H_8Cl_3NO_3$. 236.48. (1) Carbamic acid, (2,2,2-trichloro-1-hydroxyethyl)-, ethyl ester; (2) Ethyl (2,2,2-trichloro-1-hydroxyethyl)carbamate. *UNII-K0KA807799. CAS-541-79-7.* INN; BAN. *Sedative-hypnotic.* Prodorm (Parke-Davis†) ◇*CI-336; CN-16146; HY-185; NSC-33077*

Carbocromen (INN, DCF) — *See* Chromonar Hydrochloride.

Carbocromen Hydrochloride (JAN) — *See* Chromonar Hydrochloride.

Carbocysteine [*1975*] (kar″ boe sis′ te een). $C_5H_9NO_4S$. 179.19. [Carbocisteine is INN and BAN; Carbocistein is JAN.] (1) Cysteine, *S*-(carboxymethyl)-; (2) 3-[(Carboxymethyl)thio]alanine. *CAS-2387-59-9. Mucolytic.* Loviscol (Wyeth-Ayerst); Mucofan (Wyeth-Ayerst) ◇*AHR-3053; LJ 206*

Carbodimid Calcium — *See* Calcium Carbimide.

Carbofenoton. $C_{11}H_{16}ClO_2PS_3$. 342.87. [Carbophenothion is BAN.] *S*-[[(*p*-Chlorophenyl)thio]methyl] *O,O*-diethyl phosphorodithioate. *CAS-786-19-6.* INN. ◇*R 1303*

Carbolic Acid — *See* Phenol.

Carbolonium Bromide (prevously used name) — *See* Hexcarbacholine Bromide.

Carbomer 910 [*1980*] (kar′ boe mer). [Carbomer is INN and BAN.] The viscosity of a neutralized 1.0% aqueous dispersion of Carbomer 910 is between 3000 and 7000 centipoises. (1) Polymer of 2-propenoic acid, cross-linked with allyl ethers of pentaerythritol; (2) Polymer of acrylic acid, cross-linked with allyl ethers of pentaerythritol. Molecular weight is approximately 750,000. *CAS-9003-01-4.* NF XXII. *Pharmaceutic aid (emulsifying agent); pharmaceutic aid (suspending agent).* Carbopol 910 (Noveon)

Carbomer 934 [*1980*] (kar′ boe mer). **NF.** The viscosity of a neutralized 0.5% aqueous dispersion of Carbomer 934 is between 30,500 and 39,400 centipoises. (1) Polymer of 2-propenoic acid, cross-linked with allyl ethers of sucrose; (2) Polymer of acrylic acid, cross-linked with allyl ethers of sucrose. Molecular weight is approximately 3,000,000. *CAS-9003-01-4. Pharmaceutic aid (emulsifying agent); pharmaceutic aid (suspending agent).* Carbopol 934 (Noveon)

Carbomer 934P [*1975*] (kar′ boe mer). **NF.** The viscosity of a neutralized 0.5% aqueous dispersion of Carbomer 934P is between 29,400 and 39,400 centipoises. (1) Polymer of 2-propenoic acid, cross-linked with allyl ethers of sucrose or pentaerythritol; (2) Polymer of acrylic acid, cross-linked with allyl ethers of sucrose or pentaerythritol. Molecular weight is approximately 3,000,000. *CAS-9003-01-4. Pharmaceutic aid (emulsifying agent); pharmaceutic aid (suspending and/or viscosity agent); pharmaceutic aid (thickening agent).* Carbopol 934P (Noveon); Carbopol 974P (Noveon) *[Name previously used: Carpolene.]*

Carbomer 940 [*1978*] (kar′ boe mer). **NF.** The viscosity of a neutralized 0.5% aqueous dispersion of Carbomer 940 is between 40,000 and 60,000 centipoises. (1) Polymer of 2-propenoic acid, cross-linked with allyl ethers of pentaerythritol; (2) Polymer of acrylic acid, cross-linked with allyl ethers of pentaerythritol. *CAS-9003-01-4. Pharmaceutic aid (emulsifying agent); pharmaceutic aid (suspending agent).* Carbopol 940 (Noveon); Carbopol 980 (Noveon)

Carbomer 941 [*1980*] (kar′ boe mer). **NF.** The viscosity of a neutralized 0.5% aqueous dispersion of Carbomer 941 is between 4,000 and 11,000 centipoises. (1) Polymer of 2-propenoic acid, cross-linked with allyl ethers of pentaerythritol; (2) Polymer of acrylic acid, cross-linked with allyl

ethers of pentaerythritol. Molecular weight is approximately 1,250,000. *CAS-9003-01-4. Pharmaceutic aid (emulsifying agent); pharmaceutic aid (suspending agent).* Carbopol 941 (Noveon); Carbopol 971P (Noveon); Carbopol 981 (Noveon)

Carbomer 1342 (kar′ boe mer). **NF.** The viscosity of a neutralized 1.0% aqueous dispersion of Carbomer 1342 is between 9,500 and 26,500 centipoises. *CAS-9003-01-4. Pharmaceutic aid (emulsifying agent); pharmaceutic aid (suspending agent).* Carbopol 1342 (Noveon); Pemulen TR-1 (Noveon); Pemulen TR-2 (Noveon)

Carbomer Copolymer (kar′ boe mer koe pol′ i mer). **NF.** A high molecular weight copolymer of acrylic acid and a long chain alkyl methacrylate cross-linked with allyl ethers of polyalcohols.

Carbomer Homopolymer (kar′ boe mer hoe″ moe pol′ i mer). **NF.** A high molecular weight polymer of acrylic acid cross-linked with allyl ethers of polyalcohols.

Carbomer Interpolymer (kar′ boe mer in″ ter pol′ i mer). **NF.** A carbomer homopolymer or copolymer that contains a block copolymer of polyethylene glycol and a long chain alkyl acid ester.

Carbomycin. An antibiotic obtained from cultures of *Streptomyces halstedii*, or the same substance produced by any other means. *CAS-4564-87-8.* INN; MI. Magnamycin (Pfizer) ◇*NSC-51001*

Carbon, Activated. Darco (ICI Americas†)

Carbon Dioxide. USP. CO_2. 44.01. (1) Carbon dioxide; (2) Carbon dioxide. *UNII-142M471B3J. CAS-124-38-9. Stimulant (respiratory).*

Carbon, Medicinal (JAN) — *See* Charcoal, Activated.

Carbon Monoxide [*2007*] (kar′ bon mon ox′ ide). CO. 28.01. Carbon Monoxide. *UNII-7U1EE4V452. CAS-630-08-0. Prophylaxis of graft dysfunction, in patients receiving allogenic kidney transplants.*

Carbon Monoxide C 11 [*1992*] (kar′ bon mon ox′ ide). **USP.** ^{11}CO. (1) Carbon-^{11}C monoxide; (2) [^{11}C]Carbon monoxide. *CAS-10456-04-9. Diagnostic aid (blood volume determination); radioactive agent.* [Notes—*The positron-emitting radiopharmaceutical is prepared in a cyclotron in individual medical centers only. Molecular weight is not applicable as only a portion of the molecules are labeled with carbon monoxide C 11.*]

Carbon Tetrachloride. CCl_4. 153.82. (1) Methane, tetrachloro-; (2) Carbon tetrachloride. *UNII-CL2T97X0V0. CAS-56-23-5.* NF XVII.

Carbophenothion (BAN) — *See* Carbofenotion.

Carboplatin [*1983*] (kar″ boe pla′ tin). **USP.** $C_6H_{12}N_2O_4Pt$. 371.25. (1) Platinum, diammine[1,1-cyclobutanedicarboxylato(2-)-*O,O*′]-, (*SP*-4-2); (2) *cis*-Diammine(1,1-cyclobutanedicarboxylato)platinum. *UNII-BG3F62OND5. CAS-41575-94-4.* INN; BAN; JAN. *Antineoplastic.* Paraplatin (Bristol-Myers Squibb) ◇*JM-8; NSC-241240*

---

† Brand name formerly used, and/or firm no longer concerned with this product.

Carboprost [*1976*] (kar′ boe prost). $C_{21}H_{36}O_5$. 368.51. (1) Prosta-5,13-dien-1-oic acid, 9,11,15-trihydroxy-15-methyl-, (5Z,9α,11α,13E,15S)-; (2) (E,Z)-(1R,2R,3R,5S)-7-[3,5-Dihydroxy-2-[(3S)-(3-hydroxy-3-methyl-1-octenyl)]cyclopentyl]-5-heptenoic acid; (3) (15S)-15-Methylprostaglandin $F_{2\alpha}$. *UNII-7B5032XT6O. CAS-35700-23-3.* INN; BAN. *Oxytocic.* ◇*U-32,921*

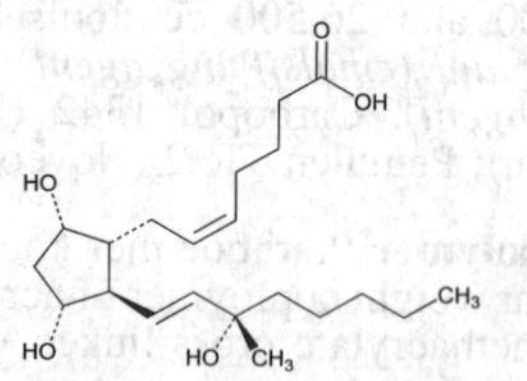

Carboprost Methyl [*1977*] (kar′ boe prost meth′ il). $C_{22}H_{38}O_5$. 382.53. (1) Prosta-5,13-dien-1-oic acid, 9,11,15-trihydroxy-15-methyl-, methyl ester, (5Z,9α,11α,13R,15S)-; (2) Methyl (Z)-7-[(1R,2R,3R,5S)-3,5-dihydroxy-2-[(E)-(3S)-3-hydroxy-3-methyl-1-octenyl]cyclopentyl]-5-heptenoate; (3) (15S)-15-Methylprostaglandin $F_{2\alpha}$ methyl ester. *CAS-35700-21-1. Oxytocic.* ◇*U-36,384*

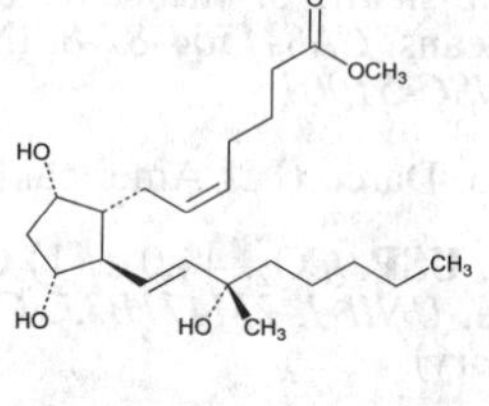

Carboprost Tromethamine [*1977*] (kar′ boe prost troe meth′ a meen). **USP.** $C_{21}H_{36}O_5 \cdot C_4H_{11}NO_3$. 489.64. [Carboprost Trometanol is BAN.] (1) Prosta-5,13-dien-1-oic acid, 9,11,15-trihydroxy-15-methyl-, (5Z,9α,11α,13E,15S)-, compound with 2-amino-2-(hydroxymethyl)-1,3-propanediol (1:1); (2) (Z)-7-[(1R,2R,3R,5S)-3,5-Dihydroxy-2-[(E)-(3S)-3-hydroxy-3-methyl-1-octenyl]cyclopentyl]-5-heptenoic acid compound with 2-amino-2-(hydroxymethyl)-1,3-propanediol (1:1); (3) (15S)-15-Methylprostaglandin $F_{2\alpha}$ tromethamine. *UNII-U4526F86FJ; UNII-7B5032XT6O* [carboprost]. *CAS-58551-69-2; CAS-35700-23-3* [carboprost]. *Oxytocic.* Hemabate (Pfizer) ◇*U-32,921E*

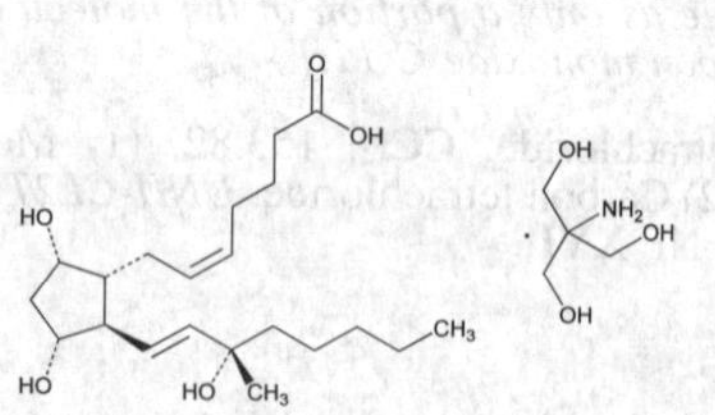

Carboquone. $C_{15}H_{19}N_3O_5$. 321.33. 2,5-Bis(1-aziridinyl)-3-(2-hydroxy-1-methoxyethyl)-6-methyl-*p*-benzoquinone carbamate (ester). *UNII-1CB0HBT12C. CAS-24279-91-2.* INN; JAN; MI.

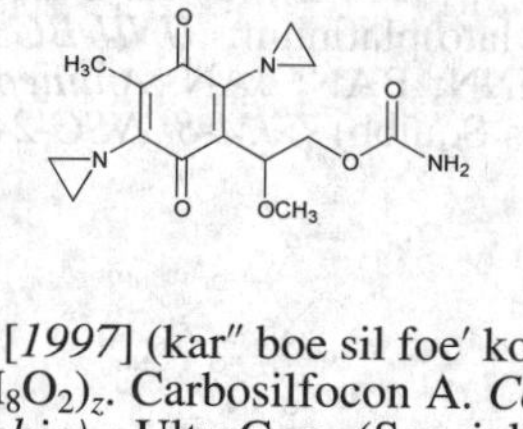

Carbosilfocon A [*1997*] (kar″ boe sil foe′ kon). $(C_{16}H_{14}O_3)_x(C_2H_6OSi)_y(C_5H_8O_2)_z$. Carbosilfocon A. *Contact lens material (hydrophobic).* UltraCon (Specialty UltraVision); Epicon (Specialty UltraVision) [*Note—The water content*

of the contact lens material is < 0.5% at ambient temperature (23±2°C), and the oxygen permeability is 50 × 10⁻¹¹(cm²/sec)(ml O₂/ml × mm Hg) at 35°C (Dk value).]

Carboxyimamidate — *See* Carbetimer.

Carboxymethylcellulose Calcium (kar box″ ee meth″ il sel′ ue lose kal′ see um). **NF.** [Carmellose is INN and JAN; Carmellose Calcium is BAN and JAN.] (1) Cellulose, carboxymethyl ether, calcium salt; (2) Cellulose carboxymethyl ether calcium salt. *CAS-9050-04-8. Pharmaceutic aid (tablet disintegrant).*

Carboxymethylcellulose Sodium (kar box″ ee meth″ il sel′ ue lose soe′ dee um). **USP.** [Carmellose Sodium is BAN and JAN.] (1) Cellulose, carboxymethyl ether, sodium salt; (2) Cellulose carboxymethyl ether sodium salt. *CAS-9004-32-4; CAS-9000-11-7* [cellulose carboxymethyl ether]. *Pharmaceutic aid (suspending agent); pharmaceutic aid (tablet excipient); pharmaceutic aid (viscosity-increasing agent).* Celluvisc (Allergan); Refresh Plus, Cellufresh Formula (Allergan)

Carboxymethylcellulose Sodium 12 (kar box″ ee meth″ il sel′ ue lose soe′ dee um). **NF.** The sodium salt of a polycarboxymethyl ether of cellulose; 12% sodium. *Pharmaceutic aid (suspending agent); pharmaceutic aid (viscosity-increasing agent).*

Carboxymethylcellulose Sodium, Low-Substituted (kar box″ ee meth″ il sel′ ue lose soe′ dee um). **NF.** (1) Cellulose, carboxymethyl ether, sodium salt, low-substituted; (2) Carmellose sodium, low-substituted. *CAS-9004-32-4.*

Carbromal. $C_7H_{13}BrN_2O_2$. 237.09. 2-Bromo-2-ethylbutyrylurea. *UNII-0Y299JY9V3. CAS-77-65-6.* INN; BAN; DCF; NF XI; MI. Adalin (Sterling Winthrop†)

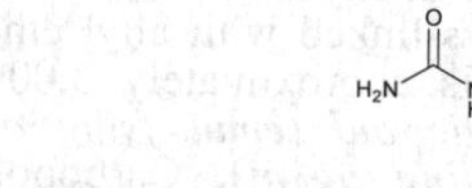

Carbubarb. $C_{11}H_{17}N_3O_5$. 271.27. 5-Butyl-5-(2-carbamoyloxyethyl)barbituric acid. *UNII-SIW4YR11ST. CAS-960-05-4.* INN; MI.

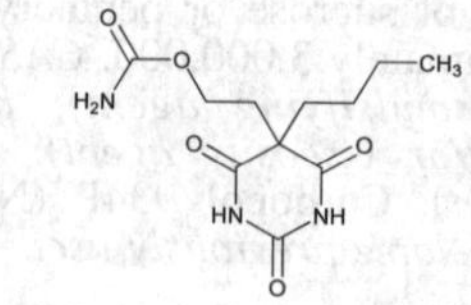

Carbubarbital (DCF) — *See* Carbubarb.

Carburazepam. $C_{17}H_{16}ClN_3O_2$. 329.78. 7-Chloro-1,2,3,5-tetrahydro-1-methyl-2-oxo-5-phenyl-4*H*-1,4-benzodiazepine-4-carboxamide. *UNII-41622NK45V. CAS-59009-93-7.* INN.

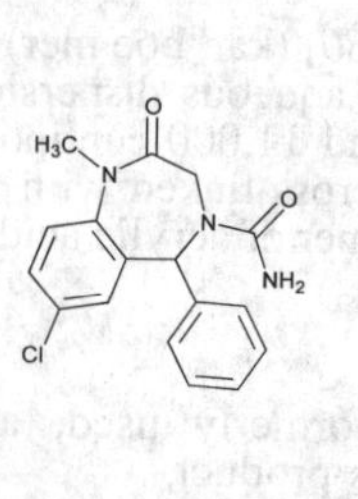

Carbutamide. $C_{11}H_{17}N_3O_3S$. 271.34. 1-Butyl-3-sulfanilylurea. *CAS-339-43-5*. INN; BAN; MI. *✧BZ 55; U-6987; Ca 1022*

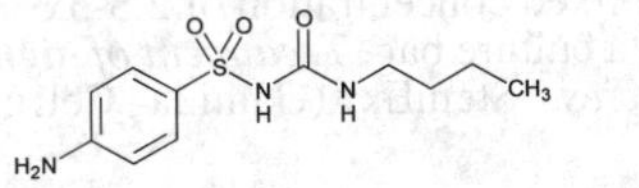

Carbuterol Hydrochloride [*1973*] (kar bue′ ter ol hye″ droe klor′ ide). $C_{13}H_{21}N_3O_3.HCl$. 303.79. [Carbuterol is INN and BAN.] (1) Urea, [5-[2-[(1,1-dimethylethyl)amino]-1-hydroxyethyl]-2-hydroxyphenyl]-, monohydrochloride; (2) [5-[2-(*tert*-Butylamino)-1-hydroxyethyl]-2-hydroxyphenyl]urea monohydrochloride. *UNII-G8F3U654FU*. *CAS-34866-46-1; CAS-34866-47-2* [carbuterol]. *Bronchodilator*. Bronsecur [as the base] (SmithKline Beecham†) *✧SK&F 40383*

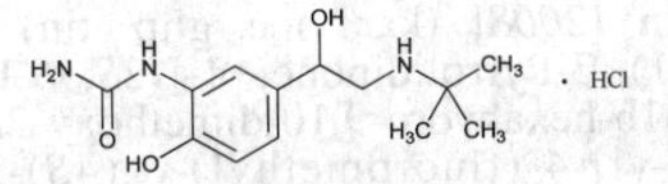

Carcainium Chloride. $C_{18}H_{22}ClN_3O_2$. 347.84. Dimethylbis[(phenylcarbamoyl)methyl]ammonium chloride. *UNII-SM0DJQ1HBT*. *CAS-1042-42-8*. INN.

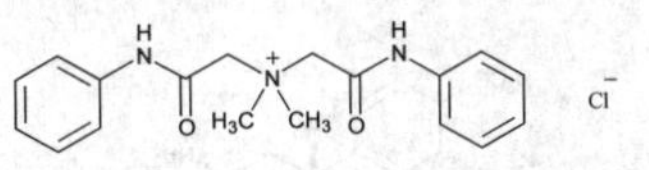

Cardamom Oil. NF. The volatile oil distilled from the seed of *Elettaria cardamomum* (L.) Maton (Fam. Zingiberaceae).

Cardamom Seed. NF. The dried ripe seed of *Elettaria cardamomum* (L.) Maton (Fam. Zingiberaceae).

Carebastine. $C_{32}H_{37}NO_4$. 499.64. *p*-[4-[4-(Diphenylmethoxy)piperidino]butyryl]-α-methylhydratropic acid. *UNII-75DLN707DO*. *CAS-90729-42-3*. INN.

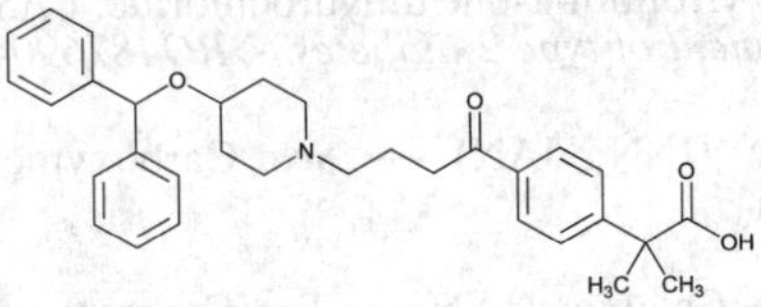

Carfecillin (INN, BAN) — *See* Carbenicillin Phenyl Sodium.

Carfecillin Sodium (JAN) — *See* Carbenicillin Phenyl Sodium.

Carfenazine (INN, BAN) — *See* Carphenazine Maleate.

Carfentanil Citrate [*1978*] (kar fen′ ta nil sit′ rate). $C_{24}H_{30}N_2O_3.C_6H_8O_7$. 586.63. [Carfentanil is INN.] (1) 4-Piperidinecarboxylic acid, 4-[(1-oxopropyl)phenylamino]-1-(2-phenylethyl)-, methyl ester, 2-hydroxy-1,2,3-propanetricarboxylate (1:1); (2) Methyl 1-phenethyl-4-(*N*-phenylpropionamido)isonipecotate citrate (1:1). *UNII-7LG286J8GV*. *CAS-61380-27-6; CAS-59708-52-0* [carfentanil]. *Analgesic (narcotic)*. *✧R 33,799*

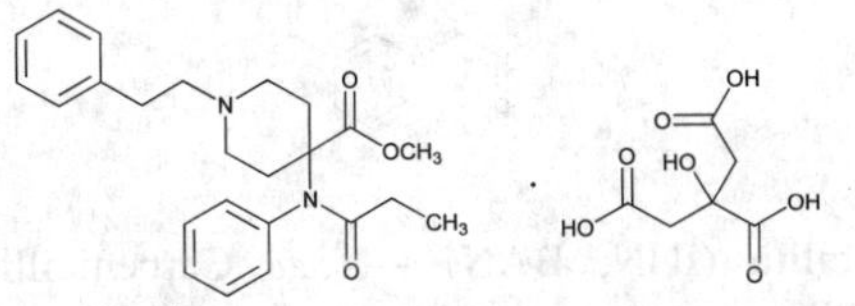

Carfilzomib [*2006*] (kar fil′ zoe mib). $C_{40}H_{57}N_5O_7$. 719.91. (1) L-Phenylalaninamide, (α*S*)-α-[(4-morpholinylacetyl)amino]benzenebutanoyl-L-leucyl-*N*-[(1*S*)-3-methyl-1-[[(2*R*)-2-methyloxiranyl]carbonyl]butyl]-; (2) (2*S*)-*N*-[(1*S*)-1-Benzyl-2-[[(1*S*)-3-methyl-1-[[(2*R*)-2-methyloxiran-2-yl]carbonyl]butyl]amino]-2-oxoethyl]-4-methyl-2-[[(2*S*)-2-[(morpholin-4-ylacetyl)amino]-4-phenylbutanoyl]amino]pentanamide. *CAS-868540-17-4*. INN. *Treatment of cancer*. *✧PR-171*

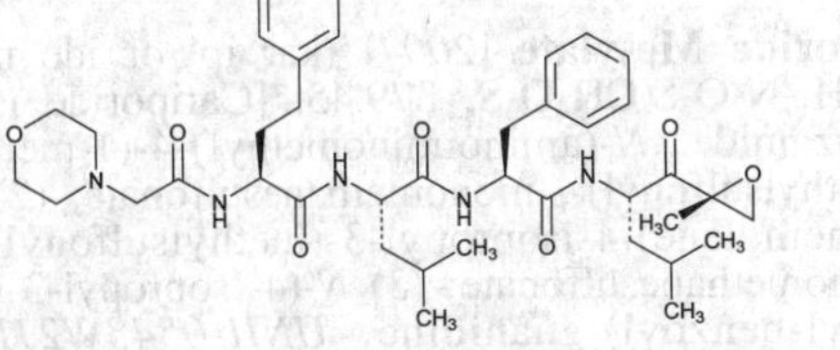

Carfimate. $C_{10}H_9NO_2$. 175.18. 1-Phenyl-2-propynyl carbamate. *UNII-X9N1XKR2OS*. *CAS-3567-38-2*. INN; MI.

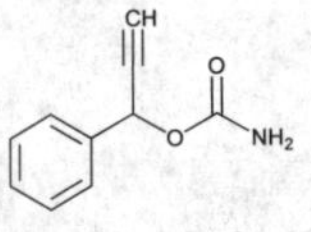

Carglumic Acid. $C_6H_{10}N_2O_5$. 190.15. *N*-Carbamoyl-L-glutamic acid. *UNII-5L0HB4V1EW*. *CAS-1188-38-1*. INN.

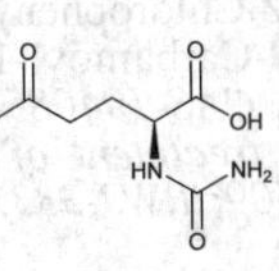

Cargutocin. $C_{42}H_{65}N_{11}O_{12}$. 916.03. 1-Butyric acid-6-(L-2-aminobutyric acid)-7-glycineoxytocin. *CAS-33605-67-3*. INN; JAN; MI.

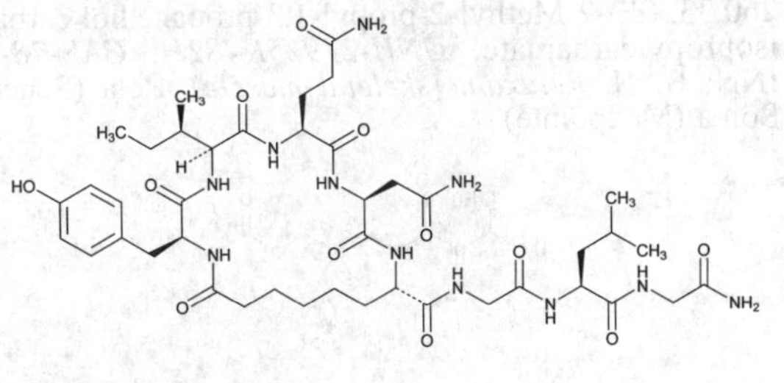

† Brand name formerly used, and/or firm no longer concerned with this product.

Caricotamide. $C_8H_{11}N_3O_2$. 181.19. 1-(2-Amino-2-oxoethyl)-1,4-dihydropyridine-3-carboxamide. *UNII-MC09H30MFS. CAS-64881-21-6.* INN.

Carindacillin (INN, BAN) — *See* Carbenicillin Indanyl Sodium.

Carindacillin Sodium (JAN) — *See* Carbenicillin Indanyl Sodium.

Cariporide. $C_{12}H_{17}N_3O_3S$. 283.35. *N*-(Diaminomethylene)-4-isopropyl-3-(methylsulfonyl)benzamide. *UNII-7E3392891K. CAS-159138-80-4.* INN.

Cariporide Mesylate [*2004*] (kar ip' or ide mes' i late). $C_{12}H_{17}N_3O_3S.CH_4O_3S$. 379.45. [Cariporide is INN.] (1) Benzamide, *N*-(aminoiminomethyl)-4-(1-methylethyl)-3-(methylsulfonyl)-, monomethanesulfonate; (2) *N*-(Diaminomethylene)-4-isopropyl-3-(methylsulfonyl)benzamide monomethanesulfonate; (3) *N*-(4-Isopropyl-3-methanesulfonyl-benzoyl)-guanidine. *UNII-0543W2JFRZ. CAS-159138-81-5; CAS-159138-80-4* [cariporide]. *Reduction of death and non-fatal myocardial infarction in patients undergoing CABG surgery.* ◇*HOE 642*

Cariprazine. $C_{21}H_{32}Cl_2N_4O$. 427.41. 3-(*trans*-4-{2-[4-(2,3-Dichlorophenyl)piperazin-1-yl]ethyl}cyclohexyl)-1,1-dimethylurea. *CAS-839712-12-8.* INN.

Carisbamate [*2006*] (kar" is bam' ate). $C_9H_{10}ClNO_3$. 215.63. (1) 1,2-Ethanediol, 1-(2-chlorophenyl)-, 2-carbamate, (1*S*)-; (2) (+)-(2*S*)-2-(2-Chlorophenyl)-2-hydroxyethyl carbamate; (3) (*S*)-2-*O*-Carbamoyl-1-o-chlorophenyl-ethanol. *UNII-P7725I9V3Z. CAS-194085-75-1.* INN. *Novel neuromodulator for the treatment of epilepsy and other CNS disorders.* ◇*YKP-509; RWJ-333369; JNJ-10234094*

Carisoprodol (kar eye" soe proe' dol). USP. $C_{12}H_{24}N_2O_4$. 260.33. (±)-2-Methyl-2-propyl-1,3-propanediol carbamate isopropylcarbamate. *UNII-21925K482H. CAS-78-44-4.* INN; BAN. *Relaxant (skeletal muscle).* Rela (Schering); Soma (Medpointe)

Carlecortemcel-L [*2007*] (kar" le kor tem' sel - el). StemEx is a suspension of human umbilical cord blood -derived, *ex vivo* expanded CD133+ cells in an infusion solution, composed of PBS buffer containing 1 mM EDTA and 0.5% HSA, to a fixed concentration of 2.3-3.3 × 10^6 cells/ml and packed in a culture bag. *Treatment of high risk hematologic malignancies.* StemEx (Gamida Cell); StemEx (Teva, Israel)

Carmantadine [*1973*] (kar man' ta deen). $C_{14}H_{21}NO_2$. 235.32. (1) 2-Azetidinecarboxylic acid, 1-tricyclo[3.3.1.1^{3,7}]dec-1-yl-; (2) 1-(1-Adamantyl)-2-azetidinecarboxylic acid. *CAS-38081-67-3.* INN. *Antiparkinsonian.* ◇*Sch 15427*

Carmegliptin [*2008*] (kar" me glip' tin). $C_{20}H_{28}FN_3O_3$. 377.45. (1) 2-Pyrrolidinone, 1-[(2*S*,3*S*,11b*S*)-2-amino-1,3,4,6,7,11b-hexahydro-9,10-dimethoxy-2*H*-benzo[*a*]quinolizin-3-yl]-4-(fluoromethyl)-, (4*S*)-; (2) (4*S*)-1-[(2*S*,3*S*,11b*S*)-2-Amino-9,10-dimethoxy-1,3,4,6,7,11b-hexahydro-2*H*-pyrido[2,1-*a*]isoquinolin-3-yl]-4-(fluoromethyl)pyrrolidin-2-one. *UNII-9Z723VGH7J. CAS-813452-18-5.* INN. *Treatment of type 2 diabetes.* ◇*RO4876904; R1579*

Carmegliptin Dihydrochloride [*2008*] (kar" me glip' tin dye hye" droe klor' ide). $C_{20}H_{28}FN_3O_3.2HCl$. 450.37. (1) 2-Pyrrolidinone, 1-[(2*S*,3*S*,11b*S*)-2-amino-1,3,4,6,7,11b-hexahydro-9,10-dimethoxy-2*H*-benzo[*a*]quinolizin-3-yl]-4-(fluoromethyl)-, dihydrochloride, (4*S*)-; (2) (4*S*)-1-[(2*S*,3*S*,11b*S*)-2-Amino-9,10-dimethoxy-1,3,4,6,7,11b-hexahydro-2*H*-pyrido[2,1-*a*]isoquinolin-3-yl]-4-(fluoromethyl)pyrrolidin-2-one dihydrochloride. *CAS-813452-14-1. Treatment of type 2 diabetes.* ◇*RO4876904-001*

Carmellose (INN, JAN) — *See* Carboxymethylcellulose Calcium.

Carmellose Calcium (JAN) — *See* Carboxymethylcellulose Calcium.

Carmellose Sodium (BAN, JAN) — *See* Carboxymethylcellulose Sodium.

Carmetizide. $C_{10}H_{12}ClN_3O_6S_2$. 369.80. Methyl 6-chloro-3,4-dihydro-2-methyl-7-sulfamoyl-2*H*-1,2,4-benzothiadiazine-3-carboxylate 1,1-dioxide. *CAS-42583-55-1.* INN.

Carminomycin Hydrochloride (previously used name) — *See* Carubicin Hydrochloride.

Carmofur. $C_{11}H_{16}FN_3O_3$. 257.26. 5-Fluoro-*N*-hexyl-3,4-dihydro-2,4-dioxo-1(2*H*)-pyrimidinecarboxamide. *UNII-HA82M3RAB2. CAS-61422-45-5.* INN; JAN; MI.

Carmoterol. $C_{21}H_{24}N_2O_4$. 368.43. 8-Hydroxy-5-[(1*R*)-1-hydroxy-2-{[(1*R*)-2-(4-methoxyphenyl)-1-methylethyl]amino}ethyl]quinolin-2(1*H*)-one. *CAS-147568-66-9.* INN.

Carmoxirole. $C_{24}H_{26}N_2O_2$. 374.48. 3-[4-(3,6-Dihydro-4-phenyl-1(2*H*)-pyridyl)butyl]indole-5-carboxylic acid. *CAS-98323-83-2.* INN.

Carmustine [*1970*] (kar mus′ teen). $C_5H_9Cl_2N_3O_2$. 214.05. (1) Urea, *N,N*′-bis(2-chloroethyl)-*N*-nitroso-; (2) 1,3-Bis(2-chloroethyl)-1-nitrosourea. *UNII-U68WG3173Y. CAS-154-93-8.* INN; BAN. *Antineoplastic.* Bicnu (Bristol-Myers Squibb); Gliadel (MGI Pharma) ◇*BCNU; NSC-409962*

Carnidazole [*1974*] (kar nye′ da zole). $C_8H_{12}N_4O_3S$. 244.27. (1) Carbamothioic acid, [2-(2-methyl-5-nitro-1*H*-imidazol-1-yl)ethyl]-, *O*-methyl ester; (2) *O*-Methyl [2-(2-methyl-5-nitroimidazol-1-yl)ethyl]thiocarbamate. *UNII-RH5KI819JG. CAS-42116-76-7.* INN; BAN. *Antiprotozoal.* ◇*R 28,096 [as hydrochloride]; R 25,831 [as the free base]*

Carnitine. $C_7H_{15}NO_3$. 161.20. [Carnitine Chloride is JAN.] (3-Carboxy-2-hydroxypropyl)trimethylammonium hydroxide inner salt. *CAS-461-06-3.* INN; MI.

Carocainide. $C_{18}H_{25}N_3O_5$. 363.41. 1-[4,7-Dimethoxy-6-[2-(1-pyrrolidinyl)ethoxy]-5-benzofuranyl]-3-methylurea. *UNII-T643E80J9K. CAS-66203-00-7.* INN.

Caroverine. $C_{22}H_{27}N_3O_2$. 365.47. 1-[2-(Diethylamino)ethyl]-3-(*p*-methoxybenzyl)-2(1*H*)-quinoxalinone. *UNII-XJ73B0K6KB. CAS-23465-76-1.* INN; MI.

Caroxazone [*1976*] (kar ox′ a zone). $C_{10}H_{10}N_2O_3$. 206.20. (1) 2*H*-1,3-Benzoxazine-3(4*H*)-acetamide, 2-oxo-; (2) 2-Oxo-2*H*-1,3-benzoxazine-3(4*H*)-acetamide. *UNII-807N226MNL. CAS-18464-39-6.* INN. *Antidepressant.* ◇*F.I. 6654*

Carperidine. $C_{17}H_{24}N_2O_3$. 304.38. Ethyl 1-(2-carbamoylethyl)-4-phenylpiperidine-4-carboxylate. *CAS-7528-13-4.* INN; BAN.

Carperitide [*2004*] (kar per′ i tide). $C_{127}H_{203}N_{45}O_{39}S_3$. 3080.44. (1) Atrial natriuretic peptide-28 (human); (2) L-Seryl-L-leucyl-L-arginyl-L-arginyl-L-seryl-L-seryl-L-cysteinyl-L-phenylalanylglycylglycyl-L-arginyl-L-methionyl-L-aspartyl-L-arginyl-L-isoleucylglycyl-L-alanyl-L-glutaminyl-L-serylglycyl-L-leucylglycyl-L-cysteinyl-L-asparaginyl-L-seryl-L-phenylalanyl-L-arginyl-L-tyrosine cyclic (7→23)-disulfide; (3) Atrial natriuretic peptide (human, 1-28); (4) α-Humanatrial natriuretic peptide. *CAS-89213-87-6.* INN. *Treatment of decompensated congestive heart failure.* (Daiichi Suntory, Japan) ◇*SUN 4936*

Carperone. $C_{19}H_{27}FN_2O_3$. 350.43. Isopropylcarbamic acid ester with 4′-fluoro-4-(4-hydroxypiperidino)butyrophenone. *UNII-Q3AP22Z9FJ. CAS-20977-50-8.* INN. ◇*AL-1021*

---

† Brand name formerly used, and/or firm no longer concerned with this product.

Carphenazine (previously used name) — *See* Carphenazine Maleate.

Carphenazine Maleate [*1962*] (kar fen′ a zeen mal′ ee ate). $C_{24}H_{31}N_3O_2S.2C_4H_4O_4$. 657.73. [Carfenazine is INN and BAN.] (1) 1-Propanone, 1-[10-[3-[4-(2-hydroxyethyl)-1-piperazinyl]propyl]-10*H*-phenothiazin-2-yl]-, (*Z*)-2-butenedioate (1:2); (2) 1-[10-[3-[4-(2-Hydroxyethyl)-1-piperazinyl]propyl]phenothiazin-2-yl]-1-propanone maleate (1:2). *UNII-0HX1Z0A2MC; UNII-CLY16Y8Z7E* [carphenazine]. *CAS-2975-34-0; CAS-2622-30-2* [carphenazine]. USP XXII. *Antipsychotic*. Proketazine (Wyeth) ◇*Wy-2445; NSC-71755*

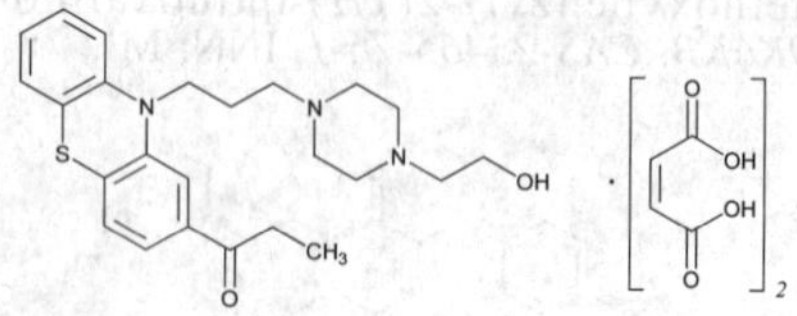

Carpindolol. $C_{19}H_{28}N_2O_4$. 348.44. Isopropyl (±)-4-[3-(*tert*-butylamino)-2-hydroxypropoxy]indole-2-carboxylate. *UNII-W8F97XP38W. CAS-39731-05-0.* INN.

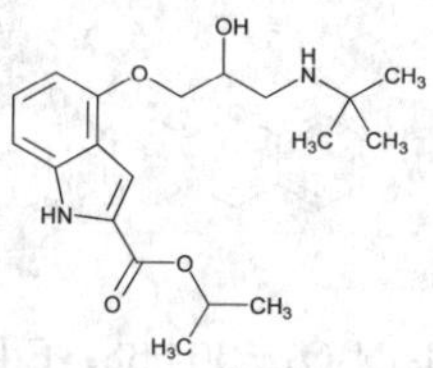

Carpipramine Dihydrochloride. $C_{28}H_{38}N_4O.2HCl.H_2O$. 537.56. [Carpipramine is INN; Carpipramine Hydrochloride and Carpipramine Maleate are JAN.] 1′-[3-(10,11-Dihydro-5*H*-dibenz[*b,f*]azepin-5-yl)propyl]-(1,4′-bipiperidine)-4′-carboxamide dihydrochloride monohydrate. *UNII-53X71X3I1W. CAS-7075-03-8; CAS-5942-95-0* [carpipramine]. MI. ◇*PZ 1511*

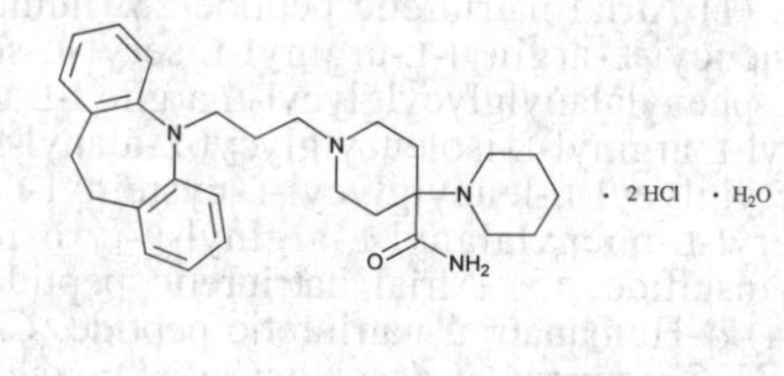

Carpolene (previously used name) — *See* Carbomer 934P.

Carprazidil. $C_{12}H_{13}N_5O_4$. 291.26. Methyl 5-(3,6-dihydro-1(2*H*)-pyridyl)-2-oxo-2*H*-[1,2,4]oxadiazolo[2,3-*a*]pyrimidine-7-carbamate. *UNII-O55EMK06L9. CAS-68020-77-9.* INN.

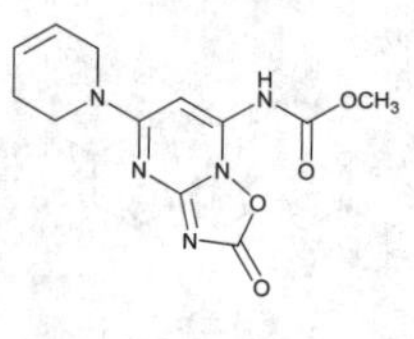

Carprofen [*1976*] (kar proe′ fen). **USP**. $C_{15}H_{12}ClNO_2$. 273.71. (1) 9*H*-Carbazole-2-acetic acid, 6-chloro-α-methyl-, (±)-; (2) (±)-6-Chloro-α-methylcarbazole-2-acetic acid. *UNII-FFL0D546HO. CAS-53716-49-7.* INN; BAN. *Anti-inflammatory*. Rimadyl (Roche) ◇*Ro 20-5720/000*

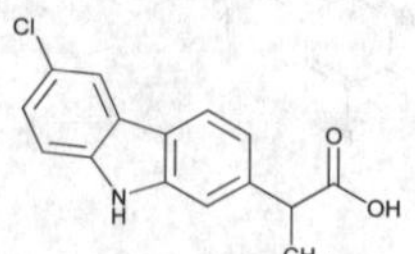

Carpronium Chloride. $C_8H_{18}ClNO_2$. 195.69. (3-Carboxypropyl)trimethylammonium chloride, methyl ester. *UNII-1R01BKB74A. CAS-13254-33-6.* INN; JAN; MI.

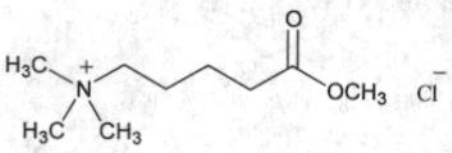

Carrageenan (kar″ a gee′ nan). **NF**. (1) Carrageenan; (2) Carrageenan. *CAS-9000-07-1. Pharmaceutic aid (suspending agent); pharmaceutic aid (viscosity-increasing agent)*. Marine Colloids (FMC)

Carsalam. $C_8H_5NO_3$. 163.13. 2*H*-1,3-Benzoxazine-2,4(3*H*)-dione. *UNII-685H843ULU. CAS-2037-95-8.* INN; BAN; DCF; MI.

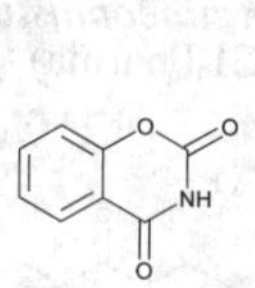

Carsatrin Succinate [*1992*] (kar sa′ trin sux′ i nate). $C_{25}H_{26}F_2N_6OS.C_4H_6O_4$. 614.66. [Carsatrin is INN.] (1) 1-Piperazineethanol, 4-[bis(4-fluorophenyl)methyl]-α-[(9*H*-purin-6-ylthio)methyl]-, (±)-, butanedioate (1:1) (salt); (2) (±)-4-[Bis(*p*-fluorophenyl)methyl]-α-[(9*H*-purin-6-ylthio)methyl]-1-piperazineethanol succinate (1:1) (salt). *UNII-YAZ544QOFD. CAS-132199-13-4; CAS-125363-87-3* [carsatrin]. *Cardiotonic*. ◇*RWJ 24517*

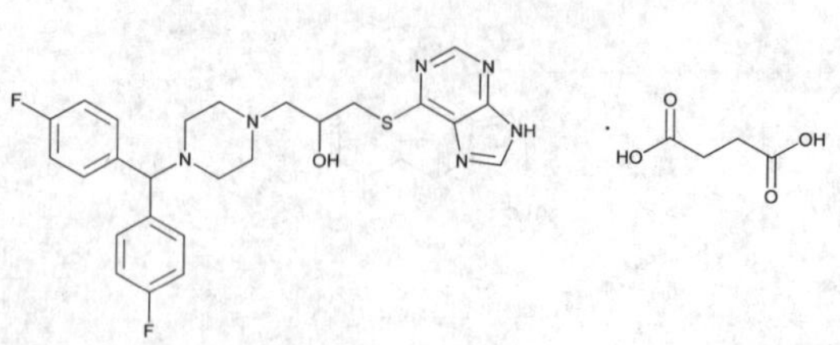

Cartasteine. $C_9H_{14}N_2O_4S_2$. 278.35. (*S*)-3-[*N*-[(*R*)-2-Mercaptopropionyl]glycyl]-4-thiazolidinecarboxylic acid. *UNII-E3N11DY0TA. CAS-149079-51-6.* INN.

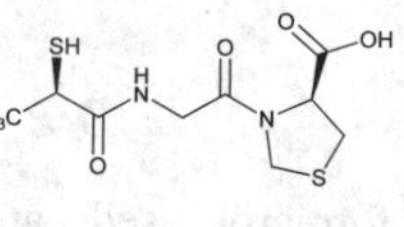

Cartazolate [*1975*] (kar taz′ oh late). C$_{15}$H$_{22}$N$_4$O$_2$. 290.36. (1) 1*H*-Pyrazolo[3,4-*b*]pyridine-5-carboxylic acid, 4-(butylamino)-1-ethyl-, ethyl ester; (2) Ethyl 4-(butylamino)-1-ethyl-1*H*-pyrazolo[3,4-*b*]-pyridine-5-carboxylate. *CAS-34966-41-1.* INN. *Antidepressant.* ⋄*SQ 65396*

Carteolol Hydrochloride [*1976*] (kar tee′ oh lol hye″ droe klor′ ide). **USP.** C$_{16}$H$_{24}$N$_2$O$_3$.HCl. 328.83. [Carteolol is INN and BAN.] (1) 2(1*H*)-Quinolinone, 5-[3-[(1,1-dimethylethyl)amino]-2-hydroxypropoxy]-3,4-dihydro-, monohydrochloride; (2) 5-[3-(*tert*-Butylamino)-2-hydroxypropoxy]-3,4-dihydrocarbostyril monohydrochloride. *UNII-4797W6I0T4; UNII-8NF31401XG* [carteolol]. *CAS-51781-21-6; CAS-51781-06-7* [carteolol]. JAN. *Anti-adrenergic (β-receptor).* Cartrol (Abbott); Ocupress (Novartis) ⋄*Abbott-43326; OPC-1085*

Carticaine (previously used name) — *See* Articaine.

Carubicin Hydrochloride [*1978*] (ka roo′ bi sin hye″ droe klor′ ide). C$_{26}$H$_{27}$NO$_{10}$.HCl. 549.95. [Carubicin is INN.] (1) 5,12-Naphthacenedione, 8-acetyl-10-[(3-amino-2,3,6-trideoxy-α-L-*lyxo*-hexopyranosyl)oxy]-7,8,9,10-tetrahydro-1,6,8,11-tetrahydroxy-, hydrochloride, (8*S-cis*)-; (2) (1*S*,3*S*)-3-Acetyl-1,2,3,4,6,11-hexahydro-3,5,10,12-tetrahydroxy-6,11-dioxo-1-naphthacenyl 3-amino-2,3,6-trideoxy-α-L-*lyxo*-hexopyranoside hydrochloride. *UNII-4V3R166MB3. CAS-52794-97-5; CAS-50935-04-1* [carubicin]. *Antineoplastic.* [*Name previously used: Carminomycin Hydrochloride.*]

Carumonam Sodium [*1985*] (kar oo′ moe nam soe′ dee um). C$_{12}$H$_{12}$N$_6$Na$_2$O$_{10}$S$_2$. 510.37. [Carumonam is INN and BAN.] (1) Acetic acid, [[[2-[[2-[[(aminocarbonyl)oxy]methyl]-4-oxo-1-sulfo-3-azetidinyl]amino]-1-(2-amino-4-thiazolyl)-2-oxoethylidene]amino]oxy]-, disodium salt, [2*S*-[2α,3α(*Z*)]]-; (2) (*Z*)-[[[(2-Amino-4-thiazolyl)[[(2*S*,3*S*)-2-(hydroxymethyl)-4-oxo-1-sulfo-3-azetidinyl]carbamoyl]methylene]amino]oxy]acetic acid,

carbamate (ester), disodium salt. *UNII-B4J4M4939D. CAS-86832-68-0; CAS-87638-04-8* [carumonam]. JAN. *Antibacterial.* ⋄*Ro 17-2301/006; AMA 1080(2Na)*

Carvedilol [*1988*] (kar ve′ dil ol). C$_{24}$H$_{26}$N$_2$O$_4$. 406.47. (1) 2-Propanol, 1-(9*H*-carbazol-4-yloxy)-3-[[2-(2-methoxyphenoxy)ethyl]amino]-, (±)-; (2) (±)-1-Carbazol-4-yloxy)-3-[[2-(*o*-methoxyphenoxy)ethyl]amino]-2-propanol. *UNII-0K47UL67F2. CAS-72956-09-3.* INN; BAN; JAN. *Antianginal; antihypertensive.* ⋄*BM 14.190*

Carvedilol Phosphate [*2004*] (kar ve′ dil ol fos′ fate). C$_{24}$H$_{26}$N$_2$O$_4$.H$_3$O$_4$P.½H$_2$O. 513.48. (1) 2-Propanol, 1-(9*H*-carbazol-4-yloxy)-3-[[2-(2-methoxyphenoxy)ethyl]amino]-, phosphate (salt), hydrate (2:2:1); (2) (2*RS*)-1-(9*H*-Carbazol-4-yloxy)-3-[[2-(2-methoxyphenoxy)ethyl]amino]propan-2-ol phosphate salt (1:1) hemihydrate. *UNII-EQT531S367. CAS-610309-89-2. Treatment of congestive heart failure, left ventricular dysfunction following myocardial infarction, and management of hypertension.* ⋄*SK&F-105517-D*

Carvotroline Hydrochloride [*1992*] (kar voe′ troe leen hye″ droe klor′ ide). C$_{18}$H$_{18}$FN$_3$.HCl. 331.81. [Carvotroline is INN.] (1) 1*H*-Pyrido[4,3-*b*]indole, 8-fluoro-2,3,4,5-tetrahydro-2-[2-(4-pyridinyl)ethyl]-, monohydrochloride; (2) 8-Fluoro-2,3,4,5-tetrahydro-2-[2-(4-pyridyl)ethyl]-1*H*-pyrido[4,3-*b*]indole monohydrochloride. *UNII-1Q63WWP8G5* [carvotroline]. *CAS-136777-43-0; CAS-107266-08-0* [carvotroline]. *Antipsychotic.* ⋄*WY-47791 HCl*

Carzelesin [*1992*] (kar zel′ e sin). C$_{41}$H$_{37}$ClN$_6$O$_5$. 729.22. (1) 2-Benzofurancarboxamide, *N*-[2-[[1-(chloromethyl)-1,6-dihydro-8-methyl-5-[[(phenylamino)carbonyl]oxy]benzo[1,2-*b*:4,3-*b*′]dipyrrol-3(2*H*)-yl]carbonyl]-1*H*-indol-5-yl]-6-(diethylamino)-, (*S*)-; (2) *N*-[2-[[(*S*)-1-(Chloromethyl)-1,6-dihydro-5-hydroxy-8-methylbenzo[1,2-*b*:4,3-*b*′]dipyrrol-3(2*H*)-yl]carbonyl]indol-5-yl]-6-(diethylami-

---

† Brand name formerly used, and/or firm no longer concerned with this product.

no)-2-benzofurancarboxamide carbanilate (ester). *UNII-668UF07O1P*. *CAS-119813-10-4*. INN. *Antineoplastic.* ◇*U-80244*

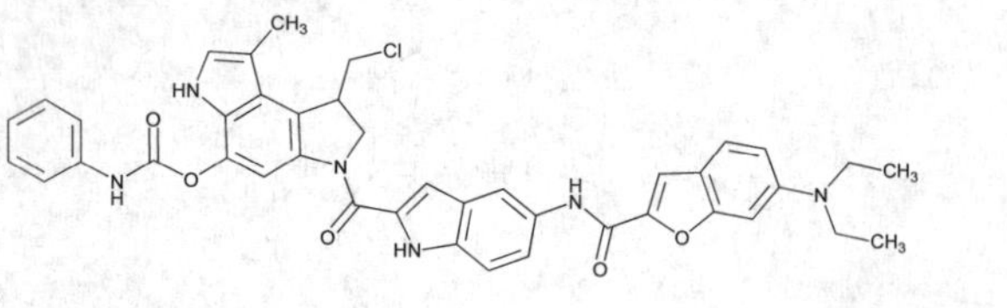

Carzenide. $C_7H_7NO_4S$. 201.20. *p*-Sulfamoylbenzoic acid. *CAS-138-41-0*. INN; MI.

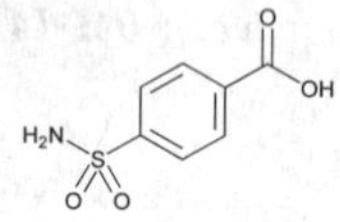

CAS [Chemical Abstracts Service] Registry Numbers — *See* Appendix III.

Casanthranol [*1962*] (ka san′ thra nol). **USP**. A purified mixture of the anthranol glycosides derived from *Cascara sagrada*. (1) Casanthranol; (2) Casanthranol. *CAS-8024-48-4*. *Laxative.*

Cascara Sagrada (kas kar′ a sa gra′ da). **USP**. [Cascara Sagrada Fluidextract is JAN.] The dried bark of *Rhamnus purshiana* De Candolle (Fam. Rhamnaceae).

Casokefamide. $C_{33}H_{40}N_6O_7$. 632.71. L-Tyrosyl-D-alanyl-L-phenylalanyl-D-alanyl-L-tyrosinamide. *UNII-B453T1E8MP. CAS-98815-38-4.* INN.

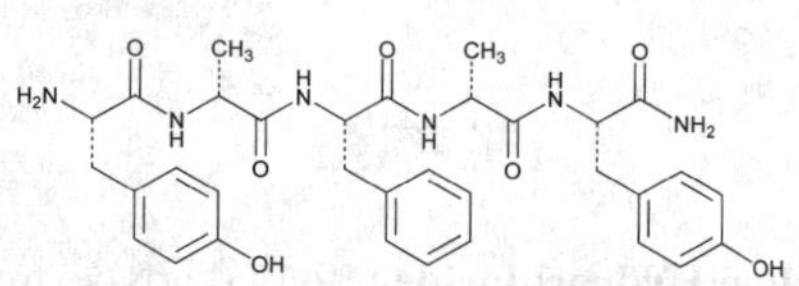

Casopitant Mesylate [*2005*] (kas oh′ pi tant mes′ i late). $C_{30}H_{35}F_7N_4O_2.CH_3SO_3H$. 712.72. [Casopitant is INN.] (1) 1-Piperidinecarboxamide, 4-(4-acetyl-1-piperazinyl)-*N*-{(1*R*)-1-[3,5-bis(trifluoromethyl)phenyl]ethyl}-2-(4-fluoro-2-methylphenyl)-*N*-methyl-, (2*R*,4*S*)-, monomethanesulfonate; (2) (2*R*,4*S*)-4-(4-Acetylpiperazin-1-yl)-*N*-[(1*R*)-1-[3,5-bis(trifluoromethyl)phenyl]ethyl]-2-(4-fluoro-2-methylphenyl)-*N*-methylpiperidine-1-carboxamide methanesulfonate. *UNII-7VSV9BL497; UNII-3B03KPM27L* [casopitant]. *CAS-414910-30-8; CAS-414910-27-3* [casopitant]. *Treatment of unipolar depression, anxiety, and insomnia disorders; prevention and treatment of nausea and vomiting; treatment of functional dyspepsia, irritable bowel syndrome, gastroesophageal reflux disease, and overactive bladder disease.* ◇*GW679769B*

Caspofungin. $C_{52}H_{88}N_{10}O_{15}$. 1093.31. (4*R*,5*S*)-5-[(2-Aminoethyl)amino]-*N*²-(10,12-dimethyltetradecanoyl)-4-hydroxy-L-ornithyl-L-threonyl-*trans*-4-hydroxy-L-prolyl-(*S*)-4-hydroxy-4-(*p*-hydroxyphenyl)-L-threonyl-*threo*-3-hy-

droxy-L-ornithyl-*trans*-3-hydroxy-L-proline cyclic (6→1)-peptide. *UNII-F0XDI6ZL63. CAS-162808-62-0.* INN; BAN.

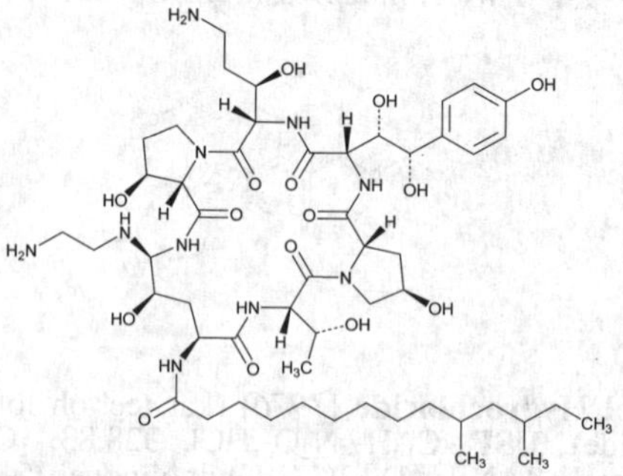

Caspofungin Acetate [*1998*] (kas″ poe fun′ jin as′ e tate). $C_{52}H_{88}N_{10}O_{15}.2C_2H_4O_2$. 1213.42. (1) 1-[(4*R*,5*S*)-5-[(2-Aminoethyl)amino]-*N*²-(10,12-dimethyl-1-oxotetradecyl)-4-hydroxy-L-ornithine]-5-[(3*R*)-3-hydroxy-L-ornithine]pneumocandin B₀, diacetate (salt); (2) (4*R*,5*S*)-5-[(2-Aminoethyl)amino]-*N*²-(10,12-dimethyltetradecanoyl)-4-hydroxy-L-ornithyl-L-threonyl-*trans*-4-hydroxy-L-prolyl-(*S*)-4-hydroxy-4-(*p*-hydroxyphenyl)-L-threonyl-*threo*-3-hydroxy-L-ornithyl-*trans*-3-hydroxy-L-proline cyclic (6→1)-peptide, diacetate (salt). *UNII-VUW370O5QE. CAS-179463-17-3.* BAN. *Antifungal (β-1,3-glucan synthesis inhibitor).* Cancidas (Merck) ◇*MK-0991*

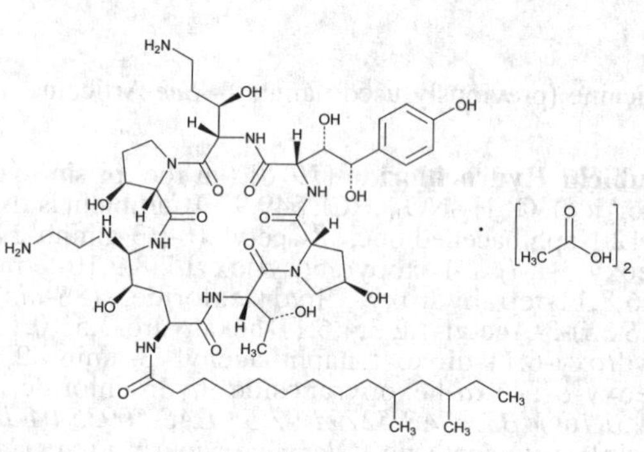

Cassia Oil — *See* Cinnamon Oil.

Castor Oil (kas′ tor). **USP**. The fixed oil obtained from the seed of *Ricinus communis* Linné (Fam. Euphorbiaceae). *UNII-D5340Y2I9G. CAS-8001-79-4.* JAN. *Laxative.*

Castor Oil, Hydrogenated (kas′ tor). **NF**. The refined, bleached, hydrogenated, and deodorized Castor Oil, consisting mainly of the triglyceride of hydroxystearic acid.

Cathine. $C_9H_{13}NO$. 151.21. (+)-Norpseudoephedrine. *UNII-E1L4ZW2F8O. CAS-492-39-7.* INN.

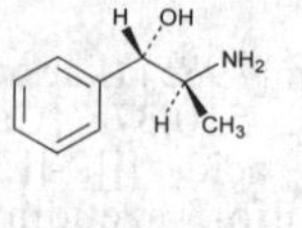

Cathinone. $C_9H_{11}NO$. 149.19. (*S*)-2-Aminopropiophenone. *CAS-71031-15-7.* INN; MI.

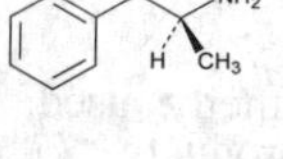

Catramilast [*2006*] (ka tra′ mi last). $C_{17}H_{22}N_2O_3$. 302.37. (1) 2*H*-Imidazol-2-one, 1-[2-[3-(cyclopropylmethoxy)-4-methoxyphenyl]propyl]-1,3-dihydro-, (*S*)-; (2) 1-[(2*S*)-2-[3-(Cyclopropylmethoxy)-4-methoxyphenyl]propyl]-1,3-dihydro-2*H*-imidazol-2-one. *UNII-QVZ4XA556B*. *CAS-183659-72-5*. INN. *Treatment of atopic dermatitis.* ◇*R115500*

Catridecacog. $C_{3708}H_{5735}N_{1013}O_{1111}S_{28}$. Human Factor XIII [$A_2$] homodimer (allele F13A*1B), recombinant DNA origin. *CAS-606138-08-3*. INN.

Catumaxomab. Immunoglobulin G2a, anti-(human antigen 17-1A) (mouse monoclonal Ho-3/TP-A-01/TPBs01 heavy chain), disulfide with mouse monoclonal Ho-3/TP-A-01/TPBs01 light chain, disulfide with immunoglobulin G2b anti-(human CD3 (antigen)) (rat monoclonal 26/II/6-1.2/TPBs01 heavy chain), disulfide with rat monoclonal 26/II/6-1.2/TPBs01 light chain. *CAS-509077-98-9*. INN.

CDP-Cholin — *See* Citicoline Sodium.

Cebaracetam. $C_{16}H_{18}ClN_3O_3$. 335.79. (±)-4-[[4-(*p*-Chlorophenyl)-2-oxo-1-pyrrolidinyl]acetyl]-2-piperazinone. *UNII-Q25MNP6OC1*. *CAS-113957-09-8*. INN.

Cedefingol [*1994*] (sed″ e fin′ gol). $C_{20}H_{41}NO_3$. 343.54. (1) Acetamide, *N*-[2-hydroxy-1-(hydroxymethyl)heptadecyl]-, [*S*-(*R**,*R**)]-; (2) *N*-[(1*S*,2*S*)-2-Hydroxy-1-(hydroxymethyl)heptadecyl]acetamide. *UNII-81HH79X39W*. *CAS-35301-24-7*. INN. *Antineoplastic (adjunct); antipsoriatic.* ◇*SPC-101210*

Cedelizumab [*1996*] (sed″ e liz′ oo mab). (1) Immunoglobulin G4 (human-mouse monoclonal OKTcdr4a complementary determining region-grafted γ-chain anti-human CD4 antigen), disulfide with human-mouse monoclonal OKTcdr4a complementary determining region-grafted κ-chain, dimer; (2) Immunoglobulin G4 (human-mouse monoclonal OKTcdr4a complementary determining region-grafted γ-chain anti-human CD4 antigen), disulfide with human-mouse monoclonal OKTcdr4a complementary determining region-grafted κ-chain, dimer. *CAS-156586-90-2*. INN. *Monoclonal antibody; immunosuppressant.* ◇*RWJ 49004*

Cediranib [*2007*] (se dir′ a nib). $C_{25}H_{27}FN_4O_3$. 450.51. (1) 4-[(4-Fluoro-2-methyl-1*H*-indol-5-yl)oxy]-6-methoxy-7-[3-(pyrrolidin-1-yl)propoxy]quinazoline; (2) Quinazoline, 4-[(4-fluoro-2-methyl-1*H*-indol-5-yl)oxy]-6-methoxy-7-[3-(1-pyrrolidinyl)propoxy]-. *UNII-NQU9IPY4K9*. *CAS-288383-20-0*. INN. *Treatment of cancer.* Recentin (AstraZeneca) ◇*AZD2171*

Cediranib Maleate [*2007*] (se dir′ a nib mal′ ee ate). $C_{25}H_{27}FN_4O_3 \cdot C_4H_4O_4$. 566.58. (1) Quinazoline, 4-[(4-fluoro-2-methyl-1*H*-indol-5-yl)oxy]-6-methoxy-7-[3-(1-pyrrolidinyl)propoxy]-, (2*Z*)-2-butenedioate (1:1); (2) 4-[(4-Fluoro-2-methyl-1*H*-indol-5-yl)oxy]-6-methoxy-7-[3-(pyrrolidin-1-yl)propoxy]quinazoline (2*Z*)-but-2-enedioate. *UNII-68AYS9A614*. *CAS-857036-77-2*. *Treatment of cancer.* Recentin (AstraZeneca) ◇*AZD2171 maleate*

Cefacetrile (INN, BAN) — *See* Cephacetrile Sodium.

Cefacetrile Sodium (JAN) — *See* Cephacetrile Sodium.

Cefaclor [*1976*] (sef′ a klor). **USP.** $C_{15}H_{14}ClN_3O_4S \cdot H_2O$. 385.82. (1) 5-Thia-1-azabicyclo[4.2.0]oct-2-ene-2-carboxylic acid, 7-[(aminophenylacetyl)amino]-3-chloro-8-oxo-, monohydrate, [6*R*-[6α,7β(*R**)]]-; (2) (6*R*,7*R*)-7-[(*R*)-2-Amino-2-phenylacetamido]-3-chloro-8-oxo-5-thia-1-azabicyclo[4.2.0]oct-2-ene-2-carboxylic acid monohydrate; (3) 3-Chloro-7-D-(2-phenylglycinamido)-3-cephem-4-carboxylic acid monohydrate. *UNII-69K7K19H4L*. *CAS-70356-03-5*; *CAS-53994-73-3* [anhydrous]. INN; BAN; JAN. *Antibacterial.* Ceclor (Lilly); Raniclor (Ranbaxy) ◇*Compound 99638*

Cefadroxil [*1974*] (sef″ a drox′ il). **USP.** $C_{16}H_{17}N_3O_5S \cdot H_2O$. 381.40. (1) 5-Thia-1-azabicyclo[4.2.0]oct-2-ene-2-carboxylic acid, 7-[[amino(4-hydroxyphenyl)acetyl]amino]-3-methyl-8-oxo-, monohydrate, [6*R*-[6α,7β(*R**)]]-; (2) (6*R*,7*R*)-7-[(*R*)-2-Amino-2-(*p*-hydroxyphenyl)acetamido]-3-methyl-8-oxo-5-thia-1-azabicyclo[4.2.0]oct-2-ene-2-carboxylic acid monohydrate. *UNII-280111G160*. *CAS-66592-87-8*; *CAS-50370-12-2* [anhydrous]; *CAS-119922-85-9* [hemihydrate]. INN; BAN; JAN. *Antibacterial.* Duricef (Warner Chilcott); Ultracef (Bristol Labs†) ◇*BL-S578; MJF 11567-3*

Cefalexin (INN, BAN, JAN) — *See* Cephalexin.

Cefaloglycin (INN, BAN, JAN) — *See* Cephaloglycin.

Cefalonium. $C_{20}H_{18}N_4O_5S_2$. 458.51. 3-(4-Carbamoylpyridylmethyl)-8-oxo-7-[*a*-(thien-2-yl)acetamido]-5-thia-1-azabicyclo[4.2.0]oct-2-ene-2-carboxylic acid. *CAS-5575-21-3*. INN; BAN. ◇*41071*

Cefaloram. $C_{18}H_{18}N_2O_6S$. 390.41. 3-(Acetoxymethyl)-8-oxo-7-(phenylacetamido)-5-thia-1-azabicyclo[4.2.0]oct-2-ene-2-carboxylic acid. *UNII-K3086GQJ9Z. CAS-859-07-4.* INN; BAN.

Cefaloridine (INN, BAN, JAN, DCF) — *See* Cephaloridine.

Cefalotin (INN, BAN) — *See* Cephalothin Sodium.

Cefalotin Sodium (JAN) — *See* Cephalothin Sodium.

Cefamandole [*1973*] (sef″ a man′ dole). $C_{18}H_{18}N_6O_5S_2$. 462.50. (1) 5-Thia-1-azabicyclo[4.2.0]oct-2-ene-2-carboxylic acid, 7-[[(hydroxyphenylacetyl)amino]-3-[[(1-methyl-1*H*-tetrazol-5-yl)thio]methyl]-8-oxo-, [6*R*-[6α,7β(*R**)]]-; (2) (6*R*,7*R*)-7-(*R*)-Mandelamido-3-[[(1-methyl-1*H*-tetrazol-5-yl)thio]methyl]-8-oxo-5-thia-1-azabicyclo[4.2.0]oct-2-ene-carboxylic acid; (3) 7-D-Mandelamido-3-[[(1-methyl-1*H*-tetrazol-5-yl)thio]methyl]-3-cephem-4-carboxylic acid. *UNII-5CKP8C2LLI. CAS-34444-01-4.* INN; BAN. *Antibacterial.* ◇*Compound 83405*

Cefamandole Nafate [*1975*] (sef″ a man′ dole naf′ ate). **USP.** $C_{19}H_{17}N_6NaO_6S_2$. 512.49. (1) 5-Thia-1-azabicyclo[4.2.0]oct-2-ene-2-carboxylic acid, 7-[[(formyloxy)phenylacetyl]amino]-3-[[(1-methyl-1*H*-tetrazol-5-yl)thio]methyl]-8-oxo-, monosodium salt, [6*R*-[6α,7β(*R**)]]-; (2) Sodium (6*R*,7*R*)-7-(*R*)-mandelamido-3-[[(1-methyl-1*H*-tetrazol-5-yl)thio]methyl]-8-oxo-5-thia-1-azabicyclo[4.2.0]oct-2-ene-2-carboxylate formate (ester). *UNII-8HDO7941DO; UNII-5CKP8C2LLI* [cefamandole]. *CAS-42540-40-9; CAS-34444-01-4* [cefamandole]. BAN. *Antibacterial.* Mandol (Lilly) ◇*106223*

Cefamandole Sodium. $C_{18}H_{17}N_6NaO_5S_2$. 484.48. (1) 5-Thia-1-azabicyclo[4.2.0]oct-2-ene-2-carboxylic acid, 7-[(hydroxyphenylacetyl)amino]-3-[[(1-methyl-1*H*-tetrazol-5-yl)thio]methyl]-8-oxo-, [6*R*-[6α,7β(*R**)]]-, monosodium salt; (2) Monosodium (6*R*,7*R*)-7-(*R*)-mandelamido-3-[[(1-methyl-1-*H*-tetrazol-5-yl)thio]methyl]-8-oxo-5-thia-1-azabicyclo[4.2.0]oct-2-ene-2-carboxylate. *UNII-IY6234ODVR. CAS-30034-03-8.* USP XXIII; JAN. *Antibacterial.*

Cefaparole [*1975*] (sef′ a pa role). $C_{19}H_{19}N_5O_5S_3$. 493.58. (1) 5-Thia-1-azabicyclo[4.2.0]oct-2-ene-carboxylic acid, 7-[[amino(4-hydroxyphenyl)acetyl]amino]-3-[[(5-methyl-1,3,4-thiadiazol-2-yl)thio]methyl]-8-oxo-, [6*R*-[6α,7β(*R**)]]-; (2) (6*R*,7*R*)-7-[(*R*)-2-Amino-2-(*p*-hydroxyphenyl)acetamido]-3-[[(5-methyl-1,3,4-thiadiazol-2-yl)thio]methyl]-8-oxo-5-thia-1-azabicyclo[4.2.0]oct-2-ene-2-carboxylic acid; (3) 7-[2-Amino-2-(*p*-hydroxyphenyl)acetamido]-3-[[(5-methyl-1,3,4-thiadiazol-2-yl)thio]methyl]-3-cephem-4-carboxylic acid. *CAS-51627-20-4.* INN. *Antibacterial.* ◇*110264*

Cefapirin (INN, BAN) — *See* Cephapirin Sodium.

Cefatrizine [*1975*] (sef″ a trye′ zeen). $C_{18}H_{18}N_6O_5S_2$. 462.50. (1) 5-Thia-1-azabicyclo[4.2.0]oct-2-ene-2-carboxylic acid, 7-[[amino(4-hydroxyphenyl)acetyl]amino]-8-oxo-3-[(1*H*-1,2,3-triazol-4-ylthio)methyl]-, [6*R*-[6α,7β(*R**)]]-; (2) (6*R*,7*R*)-7-[(*R*)-2-Amino-2-(*p*-hydroxyphenyl)acetamido]-8-oxo-3-[(*v*-triazol-4-ylthio)methyl]-5-thia-1-azabicyclo[4.2.0]oct-2-ene-2-carboxylic acid. *UNII-8P4W949T8K. CAS-51627-14-6.* INN; BAN. *Antibacterial.* ◇*BL-S640*

Cefazaflur Sodium [*1976*] (sef a′ za flur soe′ dee um). $C_{13}H_{12}F_3N_6NaO_4S_3$. 492.45. [Cefazaflur is INN.] (1) 5-Thia-1-azabicyclo[4.2.0]oct-2-ene-2-carboxylic acid, 3-[[(1-methyl-1*H*-tetrazol-5-yl)thio]methyl]-8-oxo-7-[[[(trifluoromethyl)thio]acetyl]amino]-, monosodium salt (6*R*-*trans*)-; (2) Sodium (6*R*,7*R*)-3-[[(1-methyl-1*H*-tetrazol-5-yl)thio]methyl]-8-oxo-7-[2-[(trifluoromethyl)thio]acetamido]-5-thia-1-azabicyclo[4.2.0]oct-2-ene-2-carboxylate. *UNII-8NJ5RWV39D. CAS-52123-49-6; CAS-58665-96-6* [cefazaflur]. *Antibacterial.* ◇*SK&F 59962*

Cefazedone. $C_{18}H_{15}Cl_2N_5O_5S_3$. 548.44. (6*R*,7*R*)-7-[2-(3,5-Dichloro-4-oxo-1(4*H*)-pyridyl)acetamido]-3-[[(5-methyl-1,3,4-thiadiazol-2-yl)thio]methyl]-8-oxo-5-thia-1-azabicyclo[4.2.0]-oct-2-ene-2-carboxylic acid. *UNII-7Y86X0D799. CAS-56187-47-4.* INN; BAN; MI.

Cefazolin (sef a′ zoe lin). **USP.** $C_{14}H_{14}N_8O_4S_3$. 454.51. (1) 5-Thia-1-azabicyclo[4.2.0]oct-2-ene-2-carboxylic acid, 3-[[(5-methyl-1,3,4-thiadiazol-2-yl)thio]methyl]-8-oxo-7-[[(1*H*-tetrazol-1-yl)acetyl]amino]-(6*R*-*trans*); (2) (6*R*,7*R*)-3-[[(5-Methyl-1,3,4-thiadiazol-2-yl)thio]methyl]-8-oxo-7-

[2-(1*H*-tetrazol-1-yl)acetamido]5-thia-1-azabicyclo[4.2.0]oct-2-ene-2-carboxylic acid. *UNII-IHS69L0Y4T. CAS-25953-19-9.* INN, BAN. *Antibacterial (systemic).*

Cefazolin Sodium [*1972*] (sef a′ zoe lin soe′ dee um). **USP.** $C_{14}H_{13}N_8NaO_4S_3$. 476.49. [Cefazolin is BAN.] (1) 5-Thia-1-azabicyclo[4.2.0]oct-2-ene-2-carboxylic acid, 3-[[(5-methyl-1,3,4-thiadiazol-2-yl)thio]methyl]-8-oxo-7-[[(1*H*-tetrazol-1-yl)acetyl]amino]-, monosodium salt (6*R-trans*)-; (2) Monosodium (6*R*,7*R*)-3-[[(5-methyl-1,3,4-thiadiazol-2-yl)thio]methyl]-8-oxo-7-[2-(1*H*-tetrazol-1-yl)acetamido]-5-thia-1-azabicyclo[4.2.0]oct-2-ene-2-carboxylate; (3) 3-[[(5-Methyl-1,3,4-thiadiazol-2-yl)thio]methyl]-7-[2-(1*H*-tetrazol-1-yl)acetamido]-3-cephem-4-carboxylate. *UNII-P380M0454Z. CAS-27164-46-1.* JAN. *Antibacterial (systemic).* Ancef (GlaxoSmithKline); Kefzol (Lilly) ◇*SK&F 41558; 46083*

Cefbuperazone [*1984*] (sef″ bue per′ a zone). $C_{22}H_{29}N_9O_9S_2$. 627.65. [Cefbuperazone Sodium is JAN.] (1) 5-Thia-1-azabicyclo[4.2.0]oct-2-ene-2-carboxylic acid, 7-[[2-[[(4-ethyl-2,3-dioxo-1-piperazinyl)carbonyl]amino]-3-hydroxy-1-oxobutyl]amino]-7-methoxy-3-[[(1-methyl-1*H*-tetrazol-5-yl)thio]methyl]-8-oxo-, [6*R*-[6α,7α,7(2*R**,3*S**)]]-; (2) (6*R*,7*S*)-7-[(2*R*,3*S*)-2-(4-Ethyl-2,3-dioxo-1-piperazinecarboxamido)-3-hydroxybutyramido]-7-methoxy-3-[[(1-methyl-1*H*-tetrazol-5-yl)thio]methyl]-8-oxo-5-thia-1-azabicyclo[4.2.0]oct-2-ene-2-carboxylic acid. *UNII-T0785J3X40. CAS-76610-84-9.* INN. *Antibacterial.* ◇*BMY-25182; T-1982*

Cefcanel. $C_{19}H_{18}N_4O_5S_3$. 478.57. (6*R*,7*R*)-7-[(*R*)-Mandelamido]-3-[[(5-methyl-1,3,4-thiadiazol-2-yl)thio]methyl]-8-oxo-5-thia-1-azabicyclo[4.2.0]oct-2-ene-2-carboxylic acid. *UNII-2F5V2R6VX8. CAS-41952-52-7.* INN.

Cefcanel Daloxate. $C_{27}H_{27}N_5O_9S_3$. 661.73. 2,3-Dihydroxy-2-butenyl (6*R*,7*R*)-7-[(*R*)-mandelamido]-3-[[(5-methyl-1,3,4-thiadiazol-2-yl)thio]methyl]-8-oxo-5-thia-1-azabicy-

---

† Brand name formerly used, and/or firm no longer concerned with this product.

clo[4.2.0]oct-2-ene-2-carboxylate, cyclic 2,3-carbonate, ester with L-alanine. *UNII-D9693UHF82. CAS-97275-40-6.* INN.

Cefcapene. $C_{17}H_{19}N_5O_6S_2$. 453.49. (6*R*,7*R*)-7-[(*Z*)-2-(2-Amino-4-thiazolyl)-2-pentenamido]-3-(hydroxymethyl)-8-oxo-5-thia-1-azabicyclo[4.2.0]oct-2-ene-2-carboxylic acid, carbamate (ester). *UNII-4D5D3422MW. CAS-135889-00-8.* INN.

Cefclidin. $C_{21}H_{26}N_8O_6S_2$. 550.61. (+)-1-[[(6*R*,7*R*)-7-[2-(5-Amino-1,2,4-thiadiazol-3-yl)glyoxylamido]-2-carboxy-8-oxo-5-thia-1-azabicyclo[4.2.0]oct-2-en-3-yl]methyl]-4-carbamoylquinuclidinium hydroxide, inner salt, 7^2-(*Z*)-(*O*-methyloxime). *CAS-105239-91-6.* INN.

Cefdaloxime. $C_{14}H_{15}N_5O_6S_2$. 413.43. (+)-(6*R*,7*R*)-7-[2-(2-Amino-4-thiazolyl)glyoxylamido]-3-(methoxymethyl)-8-oxo-5-thia-1-azabicyclo[4.2.0]oct-2-ene-2-carboxylic acid, 7^2-(*Z*)-oxime. *UNII-6856HDT30F. CAS-80195-36-4.* INN.

Cefdinir [*1991*] (sef′ di nir). $C_{14}H_{13}N_5O_5S_2$. 395.41. (1) 5-Thia-1-azabicyclo[4.2.0]oct-2-ene-2-carboxylic acid, 7-[[(2-amino-4-thiazolyl) (hydroxyimino)acetyl]amino]-3-ethenyl-8-oxo-, [6*R*-[6α,7β(*Z*)]]-; (2) (-)-(6*R*,7*R*)-7-[2-(2-Amino-4-thiazolyl)glyoxylamido]-8-oxo-3-vinyl-5-thia-1-

azabicyclo[4.2.0]oct-2-ene-2-carboxylic acid, 7^2-(Z)-oxime. *UNII-CI0FAO63WC. CAS-91832-40-5.* INN; BAN. *Antibacterial.* Omnicef (Abbott) ◇*CI-983; FK 482*

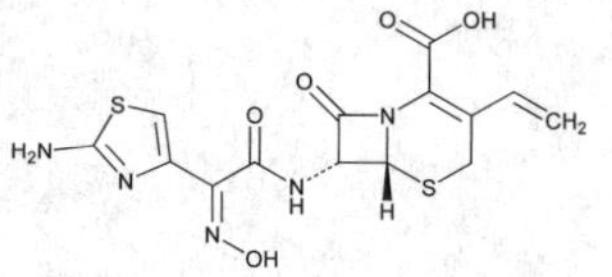

Cefditoren. $C_{19}H_{18}N_6O_5S_3$. 506.58. [Cefditoren Pivoxil is JAN.] (+)-(6R,7R)-7-[2-(2-Amino-4-thiazolyl)glyoxylamido]-3-[(Z)-2-(4-methyl-5-thiazolyl)vinyl]-8-oxo-5-thia-1-azabicyclo[4.2.0]oct-2-ene-2-carboxylic acid, 7^2-(Z)-(O-methyloxime). *UNII-81QS09V3YW. CAS-104145-95-1; CAS-117467-28-4* [pivoxil]. INN.

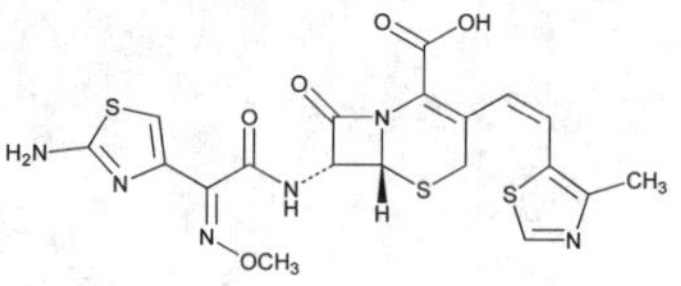

Cefedrolor. $C_{16}H_{16}ClN_3O_5S$. 397.83. (6R,7R)-7-[(R)-2-Amino-2-(3-chloro-4-hydroxyphenyl)acetamido]-3-methyl-8-oxo-5-thia-1-azabicyclo[4.2.0]oct-2-ene-2-carboxylic acid. *UNII-O3TY87KJII. CAS-57847-69-5.* INN.

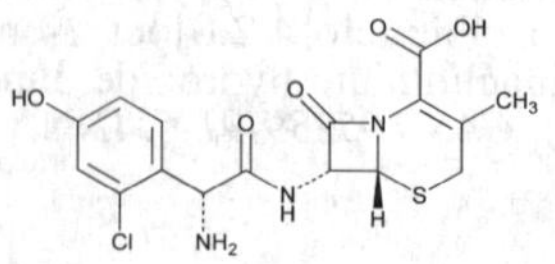

Cefempidone. $C_{22}H_{21}N_7O_6S_2$. 543.58. 1-[[(6R,7R)-7-[2-(2-Amino-5-thiazolyl)glyoxylamido]-2-carboxy-8-oxo-5-thia-1-azabicyclo[4.2.0]oct-2-en-3-yl]methyl]pyridinium hydroxide, inner salt, 7^2-(E)-[O-(2-oxo-3-pyrrolidinyl)oxime]. *UNII-3YUZ4494BQ. CAS-103238-57-9.* INN; BAN. ◇*GR 50692; TA 5901*

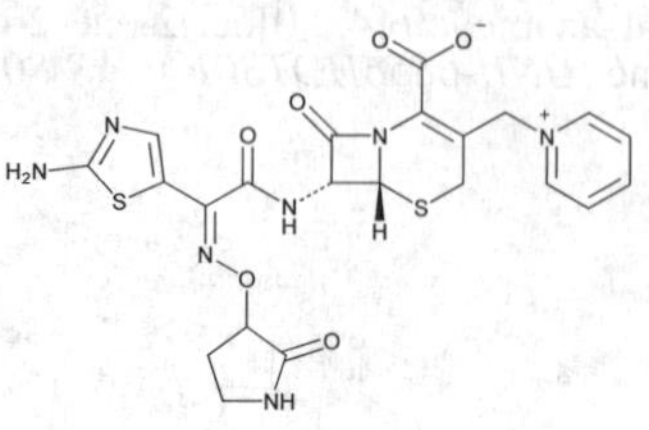

Cefepime [*1987*] (sef′ e peem). $C_{19}H_{24}N_6O_5S_2$. 480.56. (1) Pyrrolidinium, 1-[[7-[[(2-amino-4-thiazolyl)(methoxyimino)acetyl]amino]-2-carboxy-8-oxo-5-thia-1-azabicyclo[4.2.0]oct-2-en-3-yl]methyl]-1-methyl-, hydroxide, inner salt, [6R-[6α,7β(Z)]]-; (2) 1-[[(6R,7R)-7-[2-(2-Amino-4-thiazolyl)glyoxylamido]-2-carboxy-8-oxo-5-thia-1-azabicyclo[4.2.0]oct-2-en-3-yl]methyl]-1-methyl-

pyrrolidinium hydroxide, inner salt, 7^2-(Z)-(O-methyloxime). *UNII-807PW4VQE3. CAS-88040-23-7.* INN; BAN. *Antibacterial.* Maxipime (Squibb) ◇*BMY-28142*

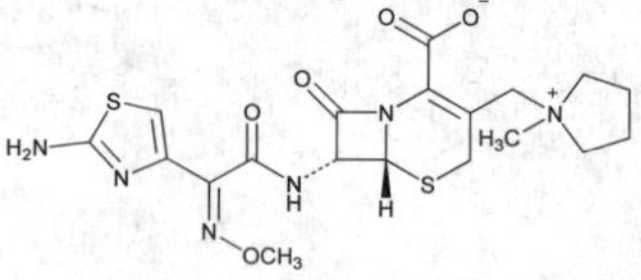

Cefepime Hydrochloride [*1993*] (sef′ e peem hye″ droe klor′ ide). USP. $C_{19}H_{25}ClN_6O_5S_2.HCl.H_2O$. 571.50. (1) Pyrrolidinium, 1-[[7-[[(2-amino-4-thiazolyl)(methoxyimino)acetyl]amino]-2-carboxy-8-oxo-5-thia-1-azabicyclo[4.2.0]oct-2-en-3-yl]methyl]-1-methyl-, chloride, monohydrochloride, monohydrate, [6R-[6α,7β(Z)]]-; (2) 1-[[(6R,7R)-7-[2-(2-Amino-4-thiazolyl)glyoxylamido]-2-carboxy-8-oxo-5-thia-1-azabicyclo[4.2.0]oct-2-en-3-yl]methyl]-1-methylpyrrolidinium chloride, 7^2-(Z)-(O-methyloxime), monohydrochloride, monohydrate. *UNII-I8X1O0607P. CAS-123171-59-5.* *Antibacterial.* ◇*BMY-28142 2HCl.H_2O*

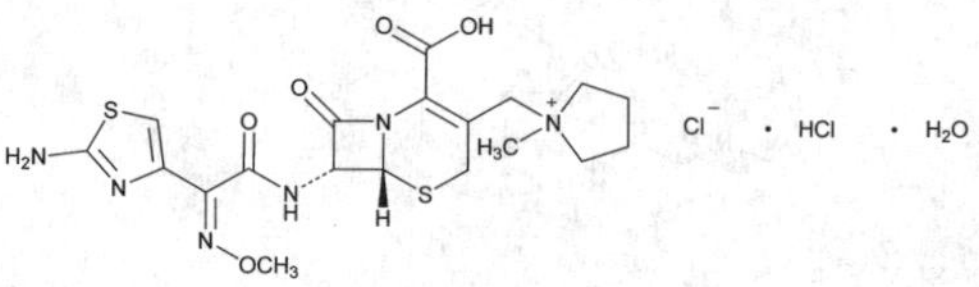

Cefetamet [*1983*] (sef et′ a met). $C_{14}H_{15}N_5O_5S_2$. 397.43. [Cefetamet Pivoxil Hydrochloride is JAN.] (1) 5-Thia-1-azabicyclo[4.2.0]oct-2-ene-2-carboxylic acid, 7-[[(2-amino-4-thiazolyl)(methoxyimino)acetyl]amino]-3-methyl-8-oxo-, [6R-[6α,7β(Z)]]-; (2) (6R,7R)-7-[2-(2-Amino-4-thiazolyl)glyoxylamido]-3-methyl-8-oxo-5-thia-1-azabicyclo[4.2.0]oct-2-ene-2-carboxylic acid, 7^2-(Z)-(O-methyloxime). *UNII-4R5TV783X3. CAS-65052-63-3.* INN. *Antibacterial (veterinary).* ◇*LY097964*

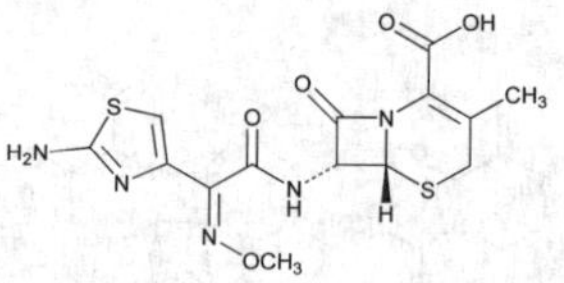

Cefetecol [*1990*] (sef et′ e kol). $C_{20}H_{17}N_5O_9S_2.4H_2O$. 607.57. (1) 5-Thia-1-azabicyclo[4.2.0]oct-2-ene-2-carboxylic acid, 7-[[(2-amino-4-thiazolyl)[[carboxy(3,4-dihydroxyphenyl)methoxy]imino]acetyl]amino]-8-oxo-, tetrahydrate, [6R-[6α,7β[Z(S*)]]]-; (2) (6R,7R)-7-[2-(2-Amino-4-thiazolyl)glyoxylamido]-8-oxo-5-thia-1-azabicyclo[4.2.0]oct-2-ene-2-carboxylic acid, 7^2-(Z)-[O-[(S)-α-carboxy-3,4-dihydroxybenzyl]oxime], tetrahydrate. *UNII-ST0WR0R5X1. CAS-127182-67-6.* INN; BAN. *Antibacterial.* ◇*GR 69153X*

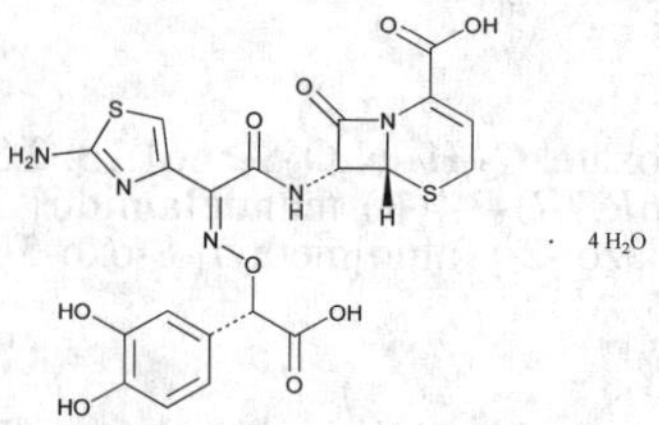

Cefetrizole. $C_{16}H_{15}N_5O_4S_3$. 437.52. (6R,7R)-8-Oxo-7-[2-(2-thienyl)acetamido]-3-[(*s*-triazol-3-ylthio)methyl]-5-thia-1-azabicyclo[4.2.0]oct-2-ene-2-carboxylic acid. *UNII-61K37E446T. CAS-65307-12-2.* INN.

Cefivitril. $C_{15}H_{15}N_7O_4S_3$. 453.52. (6R,7R)-7-[2-[[(Z)-2-Cyanovinyl]thio]acetamido]-3-[[(1-methyl-1*H*-tetrazol-5-yl)thio]methyl]-8-oxo-5-thia-1-azabicyclo[4.2.0]oct-2-ene-2-carboxylic acid. *UNII-776E09GMHQ. CAS-66474-36-0.* INN.

Cefixime [*1987*] (sef ix′ eem). **USP.** $C_{16}H_{15}N_5O_7S_2.3H_2O$. 507.50. (1) 5-Thia-1-azabicyclo[4.2.0]oct-2-ene-2-carboxylic acid, 7-[[(2-amino-4-thiazolyl)[(carboxymethoxy)imino]acetyl]amino]-3-ethenyl-8-oxo-, trihydrate, [6R-[6α,7β(Z)]]-; (2) (6R,7R)-7-[2-(2-Amino-4-thiazolyl)glyoxylamido]-8-oxo-3-vinyl-5-thia-1-azabicyclo[4.2.0]oct-2-ene-2-carboxylic acid, 7²-(Z)-[O-(carboxymethyl)oxime]trihydrate. *UNII-97I1C92E55. CAS-79350-37-1.* INN; BAN; JAN. *Antibacterial.* Suprax (Lupin) ◇*CL 284,635; FR 17027; FK 027*

Cefluprenam. $C_{20}H_{25}FN_8O_6S_2$. 556.59. (-)-[(E)-3-[(6R,7R)-7-[2-(5-Amino-1,2,4-thiadiazol-3-yl)glyoxylamido]-2-carboxy-8-oxo-5-thia-1-azabicyclo [4.2.0]oct-2-en-3-yl]allyl](carbamoylmethyl)ethylmethylammonium hydroxide, inner salt, 7²-(Z)-[O-(fluoromethyl)oxime]. *UNII-098633Q42P. CAS-116853-25-9.* INN.

Cefmatilen. $C_{15}H_{14}N_8O_5S_4$. 514.58. (-)-(6R,7R)-7-[2-(2-Amino-4-thiazolyl)glyoxylamido]-8-oxo-3-[[(*v*-trizol-4-ylthio)methyl]thio]-5-thia-1-azabicyclo[4.2.0]oct-2-ene-2-carboxylic acid, 7²-(Z)-oxime. *UNII-T750UM24H8. CAS-140128-74-1.* INN.

Cefmenoxime Hydrochloride [*1981*] (sef″ men ox′ eem hye″ droe klor′ ide). **USP.** $(C_{16}H_{17}N_9O_5S_3)_2.HCl$. 1059.58. [Cefmenoxime is INN.] (1) 5-Thia-1-azabicyclo[4.2.0]oct-2-ene-2-carboxylic acid, 7-[[(2-amino-4-thiazolyl)(methoxyimino)acetyl]amino]-3-[[(1-methyl-1*H*-tetrazol-5-yl)thio]methyl]-8-oxo-, hydrochloride (2:1), [6R-[6α,7β(Z)]]-; (2) (6R,7R)-7-[2-(2-Amino-4-thiazolyl)glyoxylamido]-3-[[(1-methyl-1*H*-tetrazol-5-yl)thio]methyl]-8-oxo-5-thia-1-azabicyclo[4.2.0]oct-2-ene-2-carboxylic acid 7²-(Z)-(O-methyloxime), hydrochloride (2:1). *UNII-NON736D32W; UNII-KBZ4844CXN* [cefmenoxime]. *CAS-75738-58-8; CAS-65085-01-0* [cefmenoxime]. JAN. *Antibacterial.* Cefmax (TAP) ◇*Abbott-50192 (HCl); SCE-1365 (Takeda) (base)*

Cefmepidium Chloride. $C_{23}H_{25}ClN_6O_8S_3$. 645.13. 4-[[[(6R,7R)-7-[2-(2-Amino-4-thiazolyl)glyoxylamido]-2-carboxy-8-oxo-5-thia-1-azabicyclo[4.2.0]oct-2-en-3-yl]methyl]thio]-1-methylpyridinium chloride 7²-(Z)-[O-(1-carboxy-1-methylethyl)oxime] S-oxide. *UNII-726233N8L3. CAS-107452-79-9.* INN.

Cefmetazole [*1992*] (sef met′ a zole). **USP.** $C_{15}H_{17}N_7O_5S_3$. 471.53. (1) 5-Thia-1-azabicyclo[4.2.0]oct-2-ene-2-carboxylic acid, 7-[[[(cyanomethyl)thio]acetyl]amino]-7-methoxy-3-[[(1-methyl-1*H*-tetrazol-5-yl)thio]methyl]-8-oxo-, (6R-*cis*)-; (2) (6R,7S)-7-[2-[(Cyanomethyl)thio]acetamido]-7-methoxy-3-[[(1-methyl-1*H*-tetrazol-5-yl)thio]methyl]-8-oxo-5-thia-1-azabicyclo[4.2.0]oct-2-ene-2-carboxylic acid. *UNII-3J962UJT8H. CAS-56796-20-4.* INN. *Antibacterial.* ◇*U-72791*

Cefmetazole Sodium [*1987*] (sef met′ a zole soe′ dee um). **USP.** $C_{15}H_{16}N_7NaO_5S_3$. 493.52. (1) 5-Thia-1-azabicyclo[4.2.0]oct-2-ene-2-carboxylic acid, 7-

[[[(cyanomethyl)thio]acetyl]amino]-7-methoxy-3-[[(1-methyl-1*H*-tetrazol-5-yl)thio]methyl]-8-oxo-, monosodium salt, (6*R-cis*)-; (2) Sodium (6*R*,7*S*)-7-[2-[(cyanomethyl)thio]acetamido]-7-methoxy-3-[[(1-methyl-1*H*-tetrazol-5-yl)thio]methyl]-8-oxo-5-thia-1-azabicyclo[4.2.0]oct-2-ene-2-carboxylate. *UNII-37Y9VR4W7A. CAS-56796-39-5*. JAN. *Antibacterial*. Zefazone (Pfizer) ◇*U-72791A*

Cefminox. $C_{16}H_{21}N_7O_7S_3$. 519.58. [Cefminox Sodium is JAN.] (6*R*,7*S*)-7-[2-[[(*S*)-2-Amino-2-carboxyethyl]thio]acetamido]-7-methoxy-3-[[(1-methyl-1*H*-tetrazol-5-yl)thio]methyl]-8-oxo-5-thia-1-azabicyclo[4.2.0]oct-2-ene-2-carboxylic acid. *UNII-PW08Y13465. CAS-75481-73-1*. INN; MI.

Cefodizime. $C_{20}H_{20}N_6O_7S_4$. 584.67. [Cefodizime Sodium is JAN.] (6*R*,7*R*)-7-[2-(2-Amino-4-thiazolyl)glyoxylamido]-3-[[[5-(carboxymethyl)-4-methyl-2-thiazolyl]thio]methyl]-8-oxo-5-thia-1-azabicyclo[4.2.0]oct-2-ene-2-carboxylic acid 7²-(*Z*)-(*O*-methyloxime). *CAS-69739-16-8; CAS-86329-79-5* [as sodium]. INN; BAN; MI. ◇*HR 221 [as sodium]; THR 221 [as sodium]; S 77 1221 B [as sodium]*

Cefonicid Monosodium [*1984*] (sef on' i sid mon" oh soe' dee um). $C_{18}H_{17}N_6NaO_8S_3$. 564.55. [Cefonicid is INN and BAN.] (1) 5-Thia-1-azabicyclo[4.2.0]oct-2-ene-2-carboxylic acid, 7-[(hydroxyphenylacetyl)amino]-8-oxo-3-[[[1-(sulfomethyl)-1*H*-tetrazol-5-yl]thio]methyl]-, monosodium salt, [6*R*-[6α,7β(*R**)]]-; (2) (6*R*,7*R*)-7-[(*R*)-Mandelamido]-8-oxo-3-[[[1-(sulfomethyl)-1*H*-tetrazol-5-yl]thio]methyl]-5-thia-1-azabicyclo[4.2.0]oct-2-ene-2-carboxylic acid, *S*-sodium salt. *UNII-QD9G66C5UF; UNII-6532B86WFG* [cefonicid]. *CAS-71420-79-6; CAS-61270-58-4* [cefonicid]. *Antibacterial*. ◇*SK&F D-75073-Z*

Cefonicid Sodium [*1979*] (sef on' i sid soe' dee um). USP. $C_{18}H_{16}N_6Na_2O_8S_3$. 586.53. (1) 5-Thia-1-azabicyclo[4.2.0]oct-2-ene-2-carboxylic acid, 7-[(hydroxyphenyl-acetyl)amino]-8-oxo-3-[[[1-(sulfomethyl)-1*H*-tetrazol-5-yl]thio]methyl]disodium salt, [6*R*-[6α,7β(*R**)]]-; (2) (6*R*,7*R*)-7-[(*R*)-Mandelamido]-8-oxo-3-[[[1-(sulfomethyl)-1-*H*-tetrazol-5-yl]thio]methyl]-5-thia-1-azabicy-

clo[4.2.0]oct-2-ene-2-carboxylic acid, disodium salt. *UNII-F74MFL78A1. CAS-61270-78-8*. *Antibacterial*. Monocid (GlaxoSmithKline) ◇*SK&F D-75073-Z₂*

Cefoperazone Sodium [*1979*] (sef" oh per' a zone soe' dee um). USP. $C_{25}H_{26}N_9NaO_8S_2$. 667.65. [Cefoperazone is INN and BAN.] (1) 5-Thia-1-azabicyclo[4.2.0]oct-2-ene-2-carboxylic acid, 7-[[[[(4-ethyl-2,3-dioxo-1-piperazinyl)-carbonyl]amino](4-hydroxyphenyl)acetyl]amino]-3-[[(1-methyl-1*H*-tetrazol-5-yl)thio]methyl]-8-oxo, monosodium salt, [6*R*-[6α,7β(*R**)]]-; (2) Sodium (6*R*,7*R*)-7-[(*R*)-2-(4-ethyl-2,3-dioxo-1-piperazinecarboxamido)-2-(*p*-hydroxyphenyl)acetamido-3-[[(1-methyl-1*H*-tetrazol-5-yl)thio]methyl]-8-oxo-5-thia-1-azabicyclo[4.2.0]oct-2-ene-2-carboxylate. *UNII-5FQG9774WD; UNII-7U75I1278D* [cefoperazone]. *CAS-62893-20-3; CAS-62893-19-0* [cefoperazone]. JAN. *Antibacterial*. Cefobid (Pfizer) ◇*T-1551; CP-52,640-2*

Ceforanide [*1978*] (sef or' a nide). USP. $C_{20}H_{21}N_7O_6S_2$. 519.55. (1) 5-Thia-1-azabicyclo[4.2.0]oct-2-ene-2-carboxylic acid, 7-[[[2-(aminomethyl)phenyl]acetyl]amino]-3-[[[1-(carboxymethyl)-1*H*-tetrazol-5-yl]thio]methyl]-8-oxo-, (6*R-trans*)-; (2) (6*R*,7*R*)-7-[2-(α-Amino-*o*-tolyl)acetamido]-3-[[[1-(carboxymethyl)-1*H*-tetrazol-5-yl]thio]methyl]-8-oxo-5-thia-1-azabicyclo[4.2.0]oct-2-ene-2-carboxylic acid; (3) 7-[*o*-(Aminomethyl)phenylacetamido]-3-[[[1-(carboxymethyl)-1*H*-tetrazol-5-yl]thio]methyl]-3-cephem-4-carboxylic acid. *UNII-8M1YF8951V. CAS-60925-61-3*. INN; BAN. *Antibacterial*. Precef (Apothecon) ◇*BL-S786*

Cefoselis. $C_{19}H_{22}N_8O_6S_2$. 522.56. (-)-5-Amino-2-[[(6*R*,7*R*)-7-[2-(2-amino-4-thiazolyl)glyoxylamido]-2-carboxy-8-oxo-5-thia-1-azabicyclo[4.2.0]oct-2-en-3-yl]methyl]-1-(2-hydroxyethyl)pyrazolium hydroxide, inner salt, 7²-(*Z*)-(*O*-methyloxime). *UNII-0B50MLU3H1. CAS-122841-10-5*. INN.

Cefotaxime Sodium [*1979*] (sef″ oh tax′ eem soe′ dee um). **USP.** $C_{16}H_{16}N_5NaO_7S_2$. 477.45. [Cefotaxime is INN and BAN.] (1) 5-Thia-1-azabicyclo[4.2.0]oct-2-ene-2-carboxylic acid, 3-[(acetyloxy)methyl]-7-[[(2-amino-4-thiazolyl)(methoxyimino)acetyl]amino]-8-oxo-, monosodium salt, [6*R*-[6α,7β(*Z*)]]-; (2) Sodium (6*R*,7*R*)-7-[2-(2-amino-4-thiazolyl)glyoxylamido]-3-(hydroxymethyl)-8-oxo-5-thia-1-azabicyclo[4.2.0]oct-2-ene-2-carboxylate 7^2-(*Z*)-(*O*-methyloxime), acetate (ester). *UNII-258J72S7TZ; UNII-N2GI8B1GK7* [cefotaxime]. *CAS-64485-93-4; CAS-63527-52-6* [cefotaxime]. JAN. *Antibacterial.* Cefotaxime (Abraxis); Claforan (Sanofi Aventis) ◇*HR 756; RU 24756*

Cefotetan [*1983*] (sef″ oh tee′ tan). **USP.** $C_{17}H_{17}N_7O_8S_4$. 575.62. (1) 5-Thia-1-azabicyclo[4.2.0]oct-2-ene-2-carboxylic acid, 7-[[[4-(2-amino-1-carboxy-2-oxoethylidene)-1,3-dithietan-2-yl]carbonyl]amino]-7-methoxy-3-[[(1-methyl-1*H*-tetrazol-5-yl)thio]methyl]-8-oxo-, [6*R*-(6α,7α)]-; (2) (6*R*,7*S*)-4-[[2-Carboxy-7-methoxy-3-[[(1-methyl-1*H*-tetrazol-5-yl)thio]methyl]-8-oxo-5-thia-1-azabicyclo[4.2.0]oct-2-en-7-yl]carbamoyl]-1,3-dithietane-$\Delta^{2,\alpha}$-malonamic acid; (3) (6*R*,7*S*)-7-[4-(Carbamoylcarboxymethylene)-1,3-dithiethane-2-carboxamido]-7-methoxy-3-[[(1-methyl-1*H*-tetrazol-5-yl)thio]methyl]-8-oxo-5-thia-1-azabicyclo[4.2.0]oct-2-ene-2-carboxylic acid. *UNII-48SPP0PA9Q. CAS-69712-56-7.* INN; BAN. *Antibacterial.* Cefotan (Zeneca) ◇*ICI 156,834*

Cefotetan Disodium [*1983*] (sef″ oh tee′ tan dye soe′ dee um). **USP.** $C_{17}H_{15}N_7Na_2O_8S_4$. 619.58. [Cefotetan Sodium is JAN.] (1) 5-Thia-1-azabicyclo[4.2.0]oct-2-ene-2-carboxylic acid, 7-[[[4-(2-amino-1-carboxy-2-oxoethylidene)-1,3-dithietan-2-yl]carbonyl]amino]-7-methoxy-3-[[(1-methyl-1*H*-tetrazol-5-yl)thio]methyl]-8-oxo-, disodium salt, [6*R*-(6α,7α)]-; (2) (6*R*,7*S*)-4-[[2-Carboxy-7-methoxy-3-[[(1-methyl-1*H*-tetrazol-5-yl)thio]methyl]-8-oxo-5-thia-1-azabicyclo[4.2.0]oct-2-en-7-yl]carbamoyl]-1,3-dithietane-$\Delta^{2,\alpha}$-malonamic acid, disodium salt; (3) (6*R*,7*S*)-7-[4-(Carbamoylcarboxymethylene)-1,3-dithietane-2-carboxamido]-7-methoxy-3-[[(1-methyl-1*H*-tetrazol-5-yl)thio]methyl]-8-oxo-5-thia-1-azabicyclo[4.2.0]oct-

---

† Brand name formerly used, and/or firm no longer concerned with this product.

2-ene-2-carboxylic acid, disodium salt. *UNII-0GXP746VXB. CAS-74356-00-6. Antibacterial.* Cefotan (AstraZeneca) ◇*YM-09330*

Cefotiam Hydrochloride [*1979*] (sef″ oh tye′ am hye″ droe klor′ ide). **USP.** $C_{18}H_{23}N_9O_4S_3$.2HCl. 598.55. [Cefotiam is INN and BAN; Cefotiam Hexetil Hydrochloride is JAN.] (1) 5-Thia-1-azabicyclo[4.2.0]oct-2-ene-2-carboxylic acid, 7-[[(2-amino-4-thiazolyl)acetyl]-amino]-3-[[[1-[2-(dimethylamino)ethyl]-1*H*-tetrazol-5-yl]-thio]methyl]-8-oxo-, hydrochloride, (6*R-trans*)-; (2) (6*R*,7*R*)-7-[2-(2-Amino-4-thiazolyl)acetamido]-3-[[[1-[2-(dimethylamino)ethyl]-1*H*-tetrazol-5-yl]thio]methyl]-8-oxo-5-thia-1-azabicyclo[4.2.0]oct-2-ene-2-carboxylic acid dihydrochloride; (3) 7(*R*)-[2-(2-Amino-4-thiazolyl)acetamido]-3-[[[1-[2-(dimethylamino)ethyl]-1*H*-tetrazol-5-yl]thio]methyl]-3-cephem-4-carboxylic acid dihydrochloride. *UNII-H7V12WDZ93; UNII-91W6Z2N718* [cefotiam]. *CAS-66309-69-1; CAS-61622-34-2* [cefotiam]. JAN. *Antibacterial.* Ceradon (Takeda) ◇*Abbott-48999; CGP-14221/E; SCE 963*

Cefovecin Sodium [*2002*] (sef″ oh vee′ sin soe′ dee um). $C_{17}H_{18}N_5NaO_6S_2$. 475.47. [Cefovecin is INN.] (1) 5-Thia-1-azabicyclo[4.2.0]oct-2-ene-2-carboxylic acid, 7-[[(2-amino-4-thiazolyl)(methoxyimino)acetyl]amino]-8-oxo-3-(tetrahydro-2-furanyl)-, monosodium salt, [6*R*-[3(*S**),6α,7β(*Z*)]]-; (2) Sodium (6*R*,7*R*)-7-[[(2*Z*)-(2-aminothiazol-4-yl)(methoxyimino)acetyl]amino]-8-oxo-3-[(2*S*)-tetrahydrofuran-2-yl]-5-thia-1-azabicyclo[4.2.0]oct-2-ene-2-carboxylate. *UNII-DL8Q24959P. CAS-141195-77-9; CAS-234096-34-5* [cefovecin]. *Antibacterial (intended for veterinary use).* ◇*UK-287,074-02*

Cefoxazole. $C_{21}H_{18}ClN_3O_7S$. 491.90. (6*R*,7*R*)-7-[3-(*o*-Chlorophenyl)-5-methyl-4-isoxazolecarboxamido]-3-(hydroxymethyl)-8-oxo-5-thia-1-azabicyclo[4.2.0]oct-2-ene-2-carboxylic acid acetate (ester). *UNII-BN10X2TL6I. CAS-36920-48-6.* INN; BAN.

Cefoxitin [*1973*] (sef ox′ i tin). $C_{16}H_{17}N_3O_7S_2$. 427.45. (1) 5-Thia-1-azabicyclo[4.2.0]oct-2-ene-2-carboxylic acid, 3-[[(aminocarbonyl)oxy]methyl]-7-methoxy-8-oxo-7-[(2-

thienylacetyl)amino]-, (6*R-cis*)-; (2) (6*R*,7*S*)-3-(Hydroxymethyl)-7-methoxy-8-oxo-7-[2-(2-thienyl)acetamido]-5-thia-1-azabicyclo[4.2.0]oct-2-ene-2-carboxylic acid carbamate (ester). *UNII-6OEV9DX57Y. CAS-35607-66-0.* INN; BAN. *Antibacterial.*

Cefoxitin Sodium [*1979*] (sef ox′ i tin soe′ dee um). **USP.** $C_{16}H_{16}N_3NaO_7S_2$. 449.43. (1) 5-Thia-1-azabicyclo[4.2.0]oct-2-ene-2-carboxylic acid, 3-[[(aminocarbonyl)oxy]methyl]-7-methoxy-8-oxo-7-[(2-thienylacetyl)amino]-, sodium salt, (6*R-cis*)-; (2) Sodium (6*R*,7*S*)-3-(hydroxymethyl)-7-methoxy-8-oxo-7-[2-(2-thienyl)acetamido]-5-thia-1-azabicyclo[4.2.0]oct-2-ene-2-carboxylate carbamate (ester). *UNII-Q68050H03T; UNII-6OEV9DX57Y* [cefoxitin]. *CAS-33564-30-6; CAS-35607-66-0* [cefoxitin]. BAN; JAN. *Antibacterial.* Mefoxin (Merck)

Cefozopran. $C_{19}H_{17}N_9O_5S_2$. 515.53. (-)-1-[[(6*R*,7*R*)-7-[2-(5-Amino-1,2,4-thiadiazol-3-yl)glyoxylamido]-2-carboxy-8-oxo-5-thia-1-azabicyclo[4.2.0]oct-2-en-3-yl]methyl]-1*H*-imidazo[1,2-*b*]pyridazin-4-ium hydroxide inner salt, 7²-(Z)-(O-methyloxime). *UNII-1LG87K28LW. CAS-113359-04-9.* INN.

Cefpimizole [*1984*] (sef pim′ i zole). $C_{28}H_{26}N_6O_{10}S_2$. 670.67. (1) Pyridinium, 1-[[2-carboxy-7-[[[[(5-carboxy-1*H*-imidazol-4-yl)carbonyl]amino]phenylacetyl]amino]-8-oxo-5-thia-1-azabicyclo[4.2.0]oct-2-en-3-yl]methyl]-4-(2-sulfoethyl)-, hydroxide, inner salt, [6*R*-[6α,7β(*R**)]]-; (2) 1-[[(6*R*,7*R*)-2-Carboxy-7-[(*R*)-2-(5-carboxyimidazole-4-carboxamido)-2-phenylacetamido]-8-oxo-5-thia-1-azabicyclo[4.2.0]oct-2-en-3-yl]methyl]-4-(2-sulfoethyl)pyridinium hydroxide, inner salt. *UNII-24S58UHU7N. CAS-84880-03-5.* INN. *Antibacterial.* ◇*U-63,196; AC 1370*

Cefpimizole Sodium [*1984*] (sef pim′ i zole soe′ dee um). $C_{28}H_{25}N_6NaO_{10}S_2$. 692.65. (1) Pyridinium, 1-[[2-carboxy-7-[[[[(5-carboxy-1*H*-imidazol-4-yl)carbonyl]amino]phenylacetyl]amino]-8-oxo-5-thia-1-azabicyclo[4.2.0]oct-2-en-3-yl]methyl]-4-(2-sulfoethyl)-, hydroxide, inner salt, monosodium salt, [6*R*-[6α,7β(*R**)]]-; (2) 1-[[(6*R*,7*R*)-2-Carboxy-7-[(*R*)-2-(5-carboxyimidazole-

4-carboxamido)-2-phenylacetamido]-8-oxo-5-thia-1-azabicyclo[4.2.0]oct-2-en-3-yl]methyl]-4-(2-sulfoethyl)pyridinium hydroxide, inner salt, monosodium salt. *UNII-X4628IMC52; UNII-24S58UHU7N* [cefpimizole]. *CAS-85287-61-2; CAS-84880-03-5* [cefpimizole]. JAN. *Antibacterial.* ◇*U-63,196E*

Cefpiramide [*1987*] (sef pir′ a mide). **USP.** $C_{25}H_{24}N_8O_7S_2$. 612.64. (1) 5-Thia-1-azabicyclo[4.2.0]oct-2-ene-2-carboxylic acid, 7-[[[[(4-hydroxy-6-methyl-3-pyridinyl)carbonyl]amino](4-hydroxyphenyl)acetyl]amino]-3-[[(1-methyl-1*H*-tetrazol-5-yl)thio]methyl]-8-oxo-, [6*R*-[6α,7β(*R**)]]-; (2) (6*R*,7*R*)-7-[(*R*)-2-(4-Hydroxy-6-methylnicotinamido)-2-(*p*-hydroxyphenyl)acetamido]-3-[[(1-methyl-1*H*-tetrazol-5-yl)thio]methyl]-8-oxo-5-thia-1-azabicyclo[4.2.0]oct-2-ene-2-carboxylic acid. *UNII-P936YA152N. CAS-70797-11-4.* INN. *Antibacterial.* ◇*WY-44,635*

Cefpiramide Sodium [*1987*] (sef pir′ a mide soe′ dee um). $C_{25}H_{23}N_8NaO_7S_2$. 634.62. (1) 5-Thia-1-azabicyclo[4.2.0]oct-2-ene-2-carboxylic acid, 7-[[[[(4-hydroxy-6-methyl-3-pyridinyl)carbonyl]amino](4-hydroxyphenyl)acetyl]amino]-3-[[(1-methyl-1*H*-tetrazol-5-yl)thio]methyl]-8-oxo-, monosodium salt, [6*R*-[6α,7β(*R**)]]-; (2) Sodium (6*R*,7*R*)-7-[(*R*)-2-(4-hydroxy-6-methylnicotinamido)-2-(*p*-hydroxyphenyl)acetamido]-3-[[(1-methyl-1*H*-tetrazol-5-yl)thio]methyl]-8-oxo-5-thia-1-azabicyclo[4.2.0]oct-2-ene-2-carboxylate. *UNII-137KB7GYKB. CAS-74849-93-7.* JAN. *Antibacterial.* ◇*WY-44,635 sodium*

Cefpirome Sulfate [*1989*] (sef′ pir ome sul′ fate). $C_{22}H_{22}N_6O_5S_2.H_2SO_4$. 612.66. [Cefpirome is INN and BAN.] (1) 5*H*-1-Pyrindinium, 1-[[7-[[(2-amino-4-thiazolyl)(methoxyimino)acetyl]amino]-2-carboxy-8-oxo-5-thia-1-azabicyclo[4.2.0]oct-2-en-3-yl]methyl]-6,7-dihydro-, hydroxide, inner salt, [6*R*-[6α,7β(*Z*)]]-, sulfate (1:1); (2) 1-[[(6*R*,7*R*)-7-[2-(2-Amino-4-thiazolyl)glyoxylamido]-2-carboxy-8-oxo-5-thia-1-azabicyclo[4.2.0]oct-2-en-3-yl]methyl]-6,7-dihydro-5*H*-1-pyrindinium hydroxide, inner salt, 7²-(*Z*)-(*O*-methyloxime), sulfate (1:1). *UNII-BA5ALU2ZT9. CAS-98753-19-6; CAS-84957-29-9* [cefpirome]. JAN. *Antibacterial.* Cefrom (Hoechst-Roussel†) ◇*HR 810 sulfate*

Cefpodoxime Proxetil [*1988*] (sef″ poe dox′ eem prox′ e til). **USP.** $C_{21}H_{27}N_5O_9S_2$. 557.60. [Cefpodoxime is INN and BAN.] (1) 5-Thia-1-azabicyclo[4.2.0]oct-2-ene-2-carboxylic acid, 7-[[(2-amino-4-thiazolyl)(methoxyimino)acetyl]amino]-3-(methoxymethyl)-8-oxo-, 1-[[(1-methylethoxy)carbonyl]oxy]ethyl ester, [6*R*-[6α,7β(*Z*)]]-; (2) (±)-1-Hydroxyethyl (+)-(6*R*,7*R*)-7-[2-(2-amino-4-thiazolyl)glyoxylamido]-3-(methoxymethyl)-8-oxo-5-thia-1-azabicyclo[4.2.0]oct-2-ene-2-carboxylate, 7²-(*Z*)-(*O*-methyloxime), isopropyl carbonate (ester); (3) (*RS*)-1-[(Isopropoxycarbonyl)oxy]ethyl (+)-(6*R*,7*R*)-7-[2-(2-amino-4-thiazolyl)-2-[(*Z*)-methoxyimino]acetamido]-3-(methoxymethyl)-8-oxo-5-thia-1-azabicyclo[4.2.0]oct-2-ene-2-carboxylate. *UNII-2TB00A1Z7N; UNII-7R4F94TVGY* [cefpodoxime]. *CAS-87239-81-4; CAS-80210-62-4* [cefpodoxime]. JAN. *Antibacterial.* Vantin (Pfizer) ◇*U-76252; CS-807*

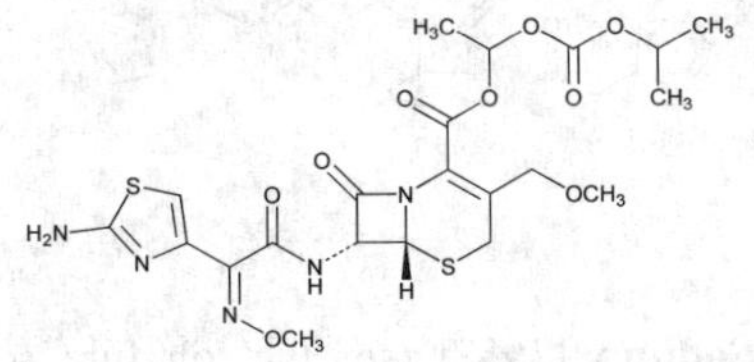

Cefprozil [*1990*] (sef proe′ zil). **USP.** C$_{18}$H$_{19}$N$_3$O$_5$S.H$_2$O. 407.44. (1) 5-Thia-1-azabicyclo[4.2.0]oct-2-ene-2-carboxylic acid, 7-[[amino(4-hydroxyphenyl)acetyl]amino]-8-oxo-3-(1-propenyl)-, monohydrate, [6*R*-[6α,7β(*R**)]]-; (2) (6*R*,7*R*)-7-[(*R*)-2-Amino-2-(*p*-hydroxyphenyl)acetamido]-8-oxo-3-propenyl-5-thia-1-azabicyclo[4.2.0]oct-2-ene-2-carboxylic acid. *UNII-4W0459ZA4V. CAS-121123-17-9; CAS-92665-29-7* [anhydrous]. INN; BAN. *Antibacterial.* Cefzil (Bristol-Myers Squibb) ◇*BMY-28100-03-800*

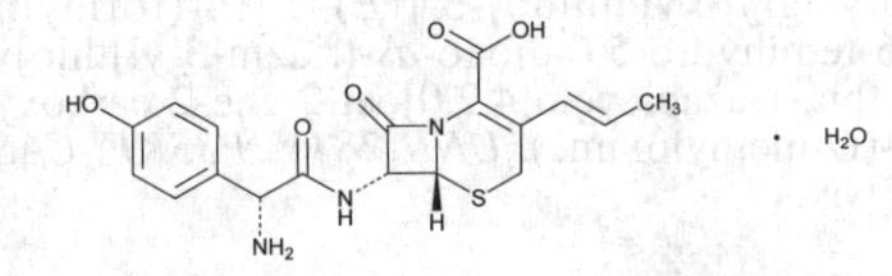

Cefquinome Sulfate [*1995*] (sef′ kwi nome sul′ fate). C$_{23}$H$_{24}$N$_6$O$_5$S$_2$.H$_2$SO$_4$. 626.68. [Cefquinome is INN and BAN.] (1) Quinolinium, 1-[[7-[[(2-amino-4-thiazolyl)(methoxyimino)acetyl]amino]-2-carboxy-8-oxo-5-thia-1-azabicyclo[4.2.0]oct-2-en-3-yl]methyl]-5,6,7,8-tetrahydro-, hydroxide, inner salt, [6*R*-[6α,7β(*Z*)]]-, sulfate (1:1); (2) 1-[[(6*R*,7*R*)-7-[2-(2-Amino-4-thiazolyl)glyoxylamido]-2-carboxy-8-oxo-5-thia-1-azabicyclo[4.2.0]oct-2-en-3-yl]methyl]-5,6,7,8-tetrahydroquinolinium hydroxide, inner salt, 7^2-(*Z*)-(*O*-methyloxime), sulfate (1:1). *UNII-3858K104DQ. CAS-118443-89-3; CAS-84957-30-2* [cefquinome]. *Antibacterial (veterinary).* ◇*HR111V-sulfate*

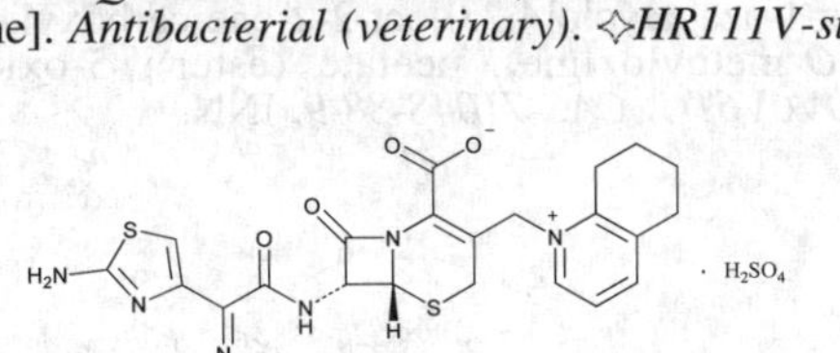

Cefradine (INN, BAN, JAN) — *See* Cephradine.

Cefrotil. C$_{20}$H$_{22}$N$_4$O$_4$S. 414.48. (6*R*,7*R*)-3-Methyl-8-oxo-7-[2-[*p*-(1,4,5,6-tetrahydro-2-pyrimidinyl)phenyl]acetamido]-5-thia-1-azabicyclo[4.2.0]oct-2-ene-2-carboxylic acid. *UNII-44P98H0A27. CAS-52231-20-6.* INN.

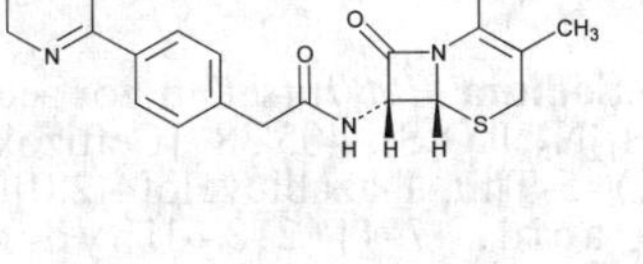

Cefroxadine [*1981*] (sef rox′ a deen). C$_{16}$H$_{19}$N$_3$O$_5$S. 365.40. (1) 5-Thia-1-azabicyclo[4.2.0]oct-2-ene-2-carboxylic acid, 7-[(amino-1,4-cyclohexadien-1-ylacetyl)amino]-3-methoxy-8-oxo-, [6*R*-[6α,7β(*R**)]]-; (2) (6*R*,7*R*)-7-[(*R*)-2-Amino-2-(1,4-cyclohexadien-1-yl)acetamido]-3-methoxy-8-oxo-5-thia-1-azabicyclo[4.2.0]oct-2-ene-2-carboxylic acid. *UNII-B908C4MV2R. CAS-51762-05-1.* INN; JAN. *Antibacterial.* ◇*CGP 9000*

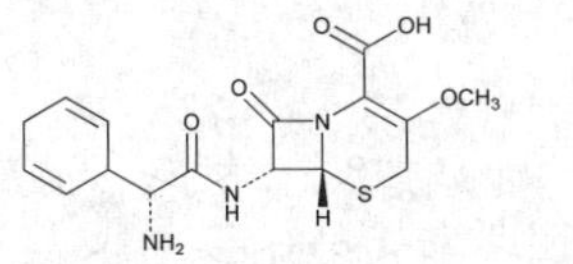

Cefsulodin Sodium [*1979*] (sef sul′ oh din soe′ dee um). C$_{22}$H$_{19}$N$_4$NaO$_8$S$_2$. 554.53. [Cefsulodin is INN and BAN.] (1) Pyridinium, 4-(aminocarbonyl)-1-[[2-carboxy-8-oxo-7-[(phenylsulfoacetyl)amino]-5-thia-1-azabicyclo[4.2.0]oct-2-en-3-yl]methyl]-, hydroxide, inner salt, monosodium salt, [6*R*-[6α,7β(*R**)]]; (2) 4-Carbamoyl-1-[[(6*R*,7*R*)-2-carboxy-8-oxo-7-[(2*R*)-2-phenyl-2-sulfoacetamido]-5-thia-1-azabicyclo[4.2.0]oct-2-en-3-yl]methylpyridinium hydroxide, inner salt, monosodium salt. *CAS-52152-93-9; CAS-62587-73-9* [cefsulodin]. JAN. *Antibacterial.* Cefomonil (TAP†) ◇*Abbott-46811; CGP-7174/E*

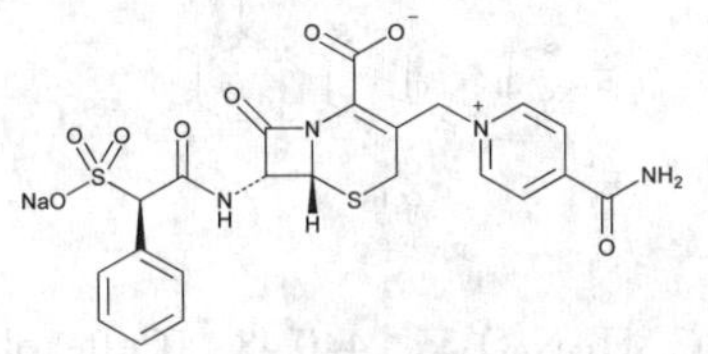

Cefsumide. C$_{17}$H$_{20}$N$_4$O$_6$S$_2$. 440.49. (6*R*,7*R*)-7-[(2*R*)-2-Amino-2-(*m*-methanesulfonamidophenyl)acetamido]-3-methyl-8-oxo-5-thia-1-azabicyclo[4.2.0]oct-2-ene-2-carboxylic acid. *UNII-3642W81J7A. CAS-54818-11-0.* INN.

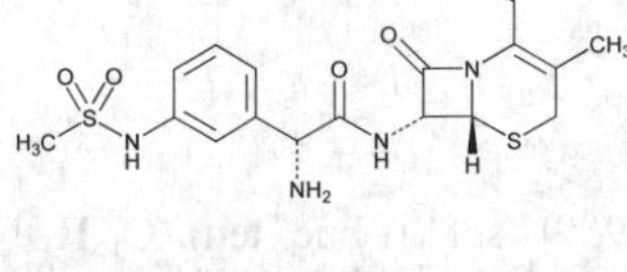

Ceftaroline Fosamil [*2006*] (sef tar′ oh leen fos′ a mil). C$_{22}$H$_{21}$N$_8$O$_8$PS$_4$.C$_2$H$_4$O$_2$.H$_2$O. 762.75. (1) Pyridinium, 4-[2-[[(6*R*,7*R*)-2-carboxy-7-[[(2*Z*)-(ethoxyimino)[5-(phosphonoamino)-1,2,4-thiadiazol-3-yl]acetyl]amino]-8-oxo-5-thia-1-azabicyclo[4.2.0]oct-2-en-3-yl]thio]-4-thiazolyl]-1-methyl-, inner salt, monoacetate, monohydrate; (2) (6*R*,7*R*)-7-[[(2*Z*)-(Ethoxyimino)[5-(phosphonoamino)-1,2,4-thiadiazol-3-yl]acetyl]amino]-3-[[4-(1-methylpyridinium-4-yl)thiazol-2-yl]sulfanyl]-8-oxo-5-thia-1-azabicyclo[4.2.0]oct-2-en-2-carboxylate monoacetate monohydrate. *UNII-P9VXV1408Y. CAS-866021-48-9.* INN. *Antibacterial agent.* ◇*TAK 599; PPI-0903*

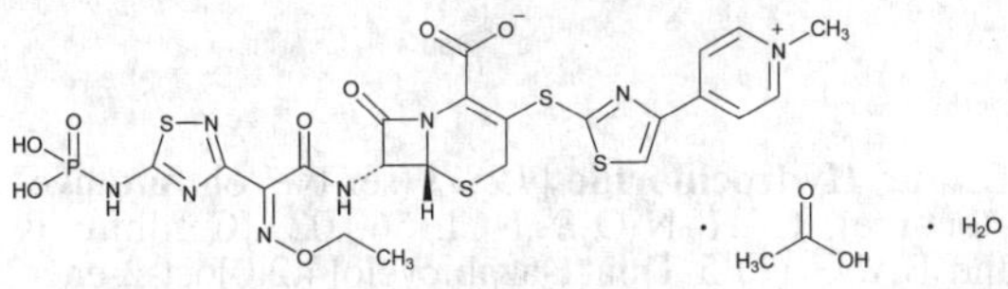

Ceftazidime [*1980*] (sef taz′ i deem). **USP.** C$_{22}$H$_{22}$N$_6$O$_7$S$_2$.5H$_2$O. 636.65. (1) Pyridinium, 1-[[7-[[(2-amino-4-thiazolyl)[(1-carboxy-1-methylethoxy)imino]acetyl]amino]-2-carboxy-8-oxo-5-thia-1-azabicy-

---

clo[4.2.0]oct-2-en-3-yl]methyl]-, hydroxide, inner salt, pentahydrate, [6*R*-[6α,7β(*Z*)]]-; (2) 1-[[(6*R*,7*R*)-7-[2-(2-Amino-4-thiazolyl)glyoxylamido]-2-carboxy-8-oxo-5-thia-1-azabicyclo[4.2.0]oct-2-en-3-yl]methyl]pyridinium hydroxide, inner salt, 7²-(*Z*)-[*O*-(1-carboxy-1-methylethyl)oxime], pentahydrate. *UNII-9M416Z9QNR. CAS-78439-06-2; CAS-72558-82-8* [anhydrous]. INN; BAN; JAN. *Antibacterial.* Fortaz (GlaxoSmithKline); Tazicef (Hospira); Tazidime (Lilly) ◇*GR 20263; LY 139381*

Cefteram. $C_{16}H_{17}N_9O_5S_2$. 479.49. [Cefteram Pivoxil is JAN.] (+)-(6*R*,7*R*)-7-[2-(2-Amino-4-thiazolyl)glyoxylamido]-3-[(5-methyl-2*H*-tetrazol-2-yl)methyl]-8-oxo-5-thia-1-azabicyclo[4.2.0]oct-2-ene-2-carboxylic acid, 7²-(*Z*)-(*O*-methyloxime). *UNII-74CQ4Q3N63. CAS-82547-58-8.* INN; MI.

Ceftezole. $C_{13}H_{12}N_8O_4S_3$. 440.48. [Ceftezole Sodium is JAN.] (6*R*,7*R*)-8-Oxo-7-[2-(1*H*-tetrazol-1-yl)acetamido]-3-[(1,3,4-thiadiazol-2-ylthio)methyl]-5-thia-1-azabicyclo[4.2.0]oct-2-ene-2-carboxylic acid. *UNII-2Z86SYP11W. CAS-26973-24-0.* INN; MI.

Ceftibuten [*1989*] (sef″ ti bue′ ten). $C_{15}H_{14}N_4O_6S_2$. 410.42. (1) 5-Thia-1-azabicyclo[4.2.0]oct-2-ene-2-carboxylic acid, 7-[[2-(2-amino-4-thiazolyl)-4-carboxy-1-oxo-2-butenyl]amino]-8-oxo-, [6*R*-[6α,7β(*Z*)]]-; (2) (+)-(6*R*,7*R*)-7-[(*Z*)-2-(2-Amino-4-thiazolyl)-4-carboxycrotonamido]-8-oxo-5-thia-1-azabicyclo[4.2.0]oct-2-ene-2-carboxylic acid. *UNII-IW71N46B4Y. CAS-97519-39-6.* INN; BAN. *Antibacterial.* Cedax (Schering) ◇*Sch 39720; 7432-S*

Ceftiofur Hydrochloride [*1987*] (sef tye′ oh fure hye″ droe klor′ ide). $C_{19}H_{17}N_5O_7S_3$.HCl. 560.02. [Ceftiofur is INN and BAN.] (1) 5-Thia-1-azabicyclo[4.2.0]oct-2-ene-2-carboxylic acid, 7-[[(2-amino-4-thiazolyl)(methoxyimino)acetyl]amino]-3-[[(2-furanylcarbonyl)thio]methyl]-8-oxo-, monohydrochloride, [6*R*-[6α,7β(*Z*)]]-; (2) (6*R*,7*R*)-7-[2-(2-Amino-4-thiazolyl)glyoxylamido]-3-(mercaptomethyl)-8-oxo-5-thia-1-azabicyclo[4.2.0]oct-2-ene-2-carboxylic acid, 7²-(*Z*)-(*O*-methyloxime), 2-furoate (ester), monohy-

drochloride. *UNII-6822A07436. CAS-80370-57-6* [ceftiofur]; *CAS-103980-44-5. Antibacterial (veterinary).* ◇*U-64279A*

Ceftiofur Sodium [*1987*] (sef tye′ oh fure soe′ dee um). $C_{19}H_{16}N_5NaO_7S_3$. 545.54. [Ceftiofur is BAN.] (1) 5-Thia-1-azabicyclo[4.2.0]oct-2-ene-2-carboxylic acid, 7-[[(2-amino-4-thiazolyl)(methoxyimino)acetyl]amino]-3-[[(2-furanylcarbonyl)thio]methyl]-8-oxo-, monosodium salt, [6*R*-[6α,7β(*Z*)]]-; (2) Sodium (6*R*,7*R*)-7-[2-(2-amino-4-thiazolyl)glyoxylamido]-3-(mercaptomethyl)-8-oxo-5-thia-1-azabicyclo[4.2.0]oct-2-ene-2-carboxylate, 7²-(*Z*)-(*O*-methyloxime), 2-furoate (ester). *UNII-NHI34IS56E. CAS-104010-37-9. Antibacterial (veterinary).* ◇*CM 31-916; U-64279E*

Ceftiolene. $C_{20}H_{18}N_8O_8S_3$. 594.60. (6*R*,7*R*)-7-[2-(2-Amino-4-thiazolyl)glyoxylamido]-3-[(*E*)-2-[[4-(formylmethyl)-1,4,5,6-tetrahydro-5,6-dioxo-*as*-triazin-3-yl]thio]vinyl]-8-oxo-5-thia-1-azabicyclo[4.2.0]oct-2-ene-2-carboxylic acid 7²-(*Z*)-(*O*-methyloxime). *UNII-28TV2P33KF. CAS-77360-52-2.* INN.

Ceftioxide. $C_{16}H_{17}N_5O_8S_2$. 471.46. (5*S*,6*R*,7*R*)-7-[2-(2-Amino-4-thiazolyl)glyoxylamido]-3-(hydroxymethyl)-8-oxo-5-thia-1-azabicyclo[4.2.0]oct-2-2-ene-carboxylic acid 7²-(*Z*)-(*O*-methyloxime), acetate (ester), 5-oxide. *UNII-6Z9DV0V6TG. CAS-71048-88-9.* INN.

Ceftizoxime Alapivoxil. $C_{22}H_{28}N_6O_8S_2$. 568.62. (+)-(Pivaloyloxy)methyl (6*R*,7*R*)-7-[2-[2-(L-alanylamino)thiazol-4-yl]glyoxylamido]-8-oxo-5-thia-1-azabicyclo[4.2.0]oct-2-ene-2-carboxylate 7²-(*Z*)-(*O*)-methyloxime). *CAS-135821-54-4.* INN.

Ceftizoxime Sodium [*1980*] (sef″ ti zox′ eem soe′ dee um). USP. $C_{13}H_{12}N_5NaO_5S_2$. 405.38. [Ceftizoxime is INN and BAN.] (1) 5-Thia-1-azabicyclo[4.2.0]oct-2-ene-2-carboxylic acid, 7-[[(2,3-dihydro-2-imino-4-thiazolyl)(methoxyimino)acetyl]amino]-8-oxomonosodium salt, [6*R*-[6α,7β(*Z*)]]-; (2) Sodium (6*R*,7*R*)-7-[2-(2-imino-4-thiazolin-4-yl)glyoxylamido]-8-oxo-5-thia-1-azabicyclo[4.2.0]oct-2-ene-2-carboxylate 7²-(*Z*)-(*O*-methyloxime). *UNII-26337D5X88; UNII-C43C467DPE* [ceftizoxime]. *CAS-68401-82-1; CAS-68401-81-0* [cefti-zoxime]. JAN. *Antibacterial.* Cefizox (Astellas) ◇*FK 749; FR 13749; SK&F 88373-Z*

Ceftobiprole [*2006*] (sef″ toe bye′ prole). $C_{20}H_{22}N_8O_6S_2$. 534.57. (1) 5-Thia-1-azabicyclo[4.2.0]oct-2-ene-2-car-boxylic acid, 7-[[(2Z)-(5-amino-1,2,4-thiadiazol-3-yl)(hydroxyimino)acetyl]amino]-8-oxo-3-[(E)-[(3′R)-2-oxo[1,3′-bipyrrolidin]-3-ylidene]methyl]-, (6R,7R)-; (2) (6R,7R)-7-[(2Z)-2-(5-Amino-1,2,4-thiadiazol-3-yl)-2-(hydroxyimino)acetamido]-8-oxo-3-[(E){(3′R)-2-oxo-[1,3′-bipyrrolidin]-3-ylidene}methyl]-5-thia-1-azabicy-clo[4.2.0]oct-2-ene-2-carboxylic acid. *UNII-5T97333YZK. CAS-209467-52-7.* INN. *Broad spectrum antibiotic.* ◇*BAL9141-000; Ro 63-9141*

Ceftobiprole Medocaril [*2006*] (sef″ toe bye′ prole me dok′ a ril). $C_{26}H_{25}N_8NaO_{11}S_2$. 712.64. (1) 5-Thia-1-azabicy-clo[4.2.0]oct-2-ene-2-carboxylic acid, 7-[[(2Z)-(5-amino-1,2,4-thiadiazol-3-yl) (hydroxyimino)acetyl]amino]-3-[(E)-[(3′R)-1′-[[(5-methyl-2-oxo-1,3-dioxol-4-yl)methox-y]carbonyl]-2-oxo[1,3′-bipyrrolidin]-3-ylidene]methyl]-8-oxo-, monosodium salt, (6R,7R)-; (2) (6R,7R)-7-[(2Z)-2-(5-Amino-1,2,4-thiadiazol-3-yl)-2-(hydroxyimino)ac-etamido]-3-[(E)[(3′R)-1′-[(5-methyl-2-oxo-1,3-dioxol-4-yl)methoxycarbonyl]-2-oxo-[1,3′-bipyrrolidin]-3-ylidene]-methyl]-8-oxo-5-thia-1-azabicyclo[4.2.0]oct-2-ene-2-car-boxylic acid monosodium salt. *UNII-N99027V28J. CAS-252188-71-9; CAS-376653-43-9.* INN. *Broad spectrum antibiotic.* ◇*BAL5788; BAL5788-001; Ro 65-5788*

Ceftriaxone Sodium [*1981*] (sef″ trye ax′ one soe′ dee um). **USP**. $C_{18}H_{16}N_8Na_2O_7S_3$·3½$H_2O$. 661.60. [Ceftriaxone is INN and BAN.] (1) 5-Thia-1-azabicyclo[4.2.0]oct-2-ene-2-carboxylic acid, 7-[[(2-amino-4-thiazolyl)(methoxyimino)-acetyl]amino]-8-oxo-3-[[(1,2,5,6-tetrahydro-2-methyl-5,6-dioxo-1,2,4-triazin-3-yl)thio]methyl]-, disodium salt, [6R-[6α,7β(Z)]]-, hydrate (2:7); (2) (6R,7R)-7-[2-(2-Amino-4-thiazolyl)glyoxylamido]-8-oxo-3-[[(1,2,5,6-tetrahydro-2-methyl-5,6-dioxo-*as*-triazin-3-yl)thio]methyl]-5-thia-1-azabicyclo[4.2.0]oct-2-ene-2-carboxylic acid, 7^2-(Z)-(O-methyloxime), disodium salt, sesquaterhydrate. *UNII-*

023Z5BR09K; UNII-75J73V1629 [ceftriaxone]. *CAS-104376-79-6; CAS-73384-59-5* [ceftriaxone]. JAN. *Anti-bacterial.* Rocephin (Roche) ◇*Ro 13-9904*

Cefuracetime. $C_{17}H_{17}N_3O_8S$. 423.40. (6R,7R)-7-[2-(2-Furyl)-glyoxylamido]-3-(hydroxymethyl)-8-oxo-5-thia-1-azabi-cyclo[4.2.0]oct-2-ene-2-carboxylic acid 7^2-(Z)-(O-methyloxime), acetate (ester). *UNII-F69EA18270. CAS-39685-31-9.* INN; BAN. ◇*640/1*

Cefuroxime [*1984*] (sef″ ue rox′ eem). $C_{16}H_{16}N_4O_8S$. 424.39. (1) 5-Thia-1-azabicyclo[4.2.0]oct-2-ene-2-carboxylic acid, 3-[[(aminocarbonyl)oxy]methyl]-7-[[2-furanyl(methoxyimino)acetyl]amino]-8-oxo-, [6R-[6α,7β(Z)]]-; (2) (6R,7R)-7-[2-(2-Furyl)glyoxylamido]-3-(hydroxymethyl)-8-oxo-5-thia-1-azabicyclo[4.2.0]oct-2-ene-2-carboxylic acid 7^2-(Z)-(O-methyloxime) carbamate (ester). *UNII-O1R9FJ93ED. CAS-55268-75-2.* INN; BAN. *Antibacterial.* ◇*640/359*

Cefuroxime Axetil [*1983*] (sef″ ue rox′ eem ax′ e til). **USP**. $C_{20}H_{22}N_4O_{10}S$. 510.47. (1) 5-Thia-1-azabicyclo[4.2.0]oct-2-ene-2-carboxylic acid, 3-[[(aminocarbonyl)oxy]methyl]-7-[[2-furanyl(methoxyimino)acetyl]amino]-8-oxo-, 1-(acetyloxy)ethyl ester, [6R-[6α,7β(Z)]]-; (2) (RS)-1-Hydro-xyethyl (6R,7R)-7-[2-(2-furyl)glyoxylamido]-3-(hydroxy-methyl)-8-oxo-5-thia-1-azabicyclo[4.2.0]oct-2-ene-2-car-boxylate, 7^2-(Z)-(O-methyloxime), 1-acetate 3-carbamate. *UNII-Z49QDT0J8Z; UNII-O1R9FJ93ED* [cefuroxime]. *CAS-64544-07-6; CAS-55268-75-2* [cefuroxime]. BAN; JAN. *Antibacterial.* Ceftin (GlaxoSmithKline) ◇*CCI 15641*

Cefuroxime Pivoxetil [*1989*] (sef″ ue rox′ eem piv ox′ e til). $C_{23}H_{28}N_4O_{11}S$. 568.55. (1) 5-Thia-1-azabicyclo[4.2.0]oct-2-ene-2-carboxylic acid, 3-[[(aminocarbonyl)oxy]methyl]-7-[[2-furanyl(methoxyimino)acetyl]amino]-8-oxo-, 1-(2-methoxy-2-methyl-1-oxopropoxy)ethyl ester, [6R-[6α,7β(Z)]]-; (2) 1-Hydroxyethyl (6R,7R)-7-[2-(2-furyl)-glyoxylamido]-3-(hydroxymethyl)-8-oxo-5-thia-1-azabi-cyclo[4.2.0]oct-2-ene-2-carboxylate, 7^2-(Z)-(O-

---

† Brand name formerly used, and/or firm no longer concerned with this product.

methyloxime), 3-carbamate 1-(2-methoxy-2-methylpropionate). *UNII-LR90117565. CAS-100680-33-9*. BAN. *Antibacterial.* ◇CCI 23628

Cefuroxime Sodium (sef″ ue rox′ eem soe′ dee um). **USP**. $C_{16}H_{15}N_4NaO_8S$. 446.37. (1) 5-Thia-1-azabicyclo[4.2.0]oct-2-ene-2-carboxylic acid, 3-[[(aminocarbonyl)oxy]methyl]-7-[[2-furanyl(methoxyimino)acetyl]amino]-8-oxo-, monosodium salt [$6R$-[$6\alpha,7\beta(Z)$]]-; (2) Sodium ($6R,7R$)-7-[2-(2-furyl)glyoxylamido]-3-(hydroxymethyl)-8-oxo-5-thia-1-azabicyclo[4.2.0]oct-2-ene-2-carboxylate, 7^2-(Z)-(O-methyloxime), carbamate (ester). *UNII-R8A7M9MY61. CAS-56238-63-2.* BAN; JAN. *Antibacterial.* Kefurox (Lilly); Zinacef (GlaxoSmithKline)

Cefuzonam. $C_{16}H_{15}N_7O_5S_4$. 513.59. [Cefuzonam Sodium is JAN.] (-)-($6R,7R$)-7-[2-(2-Amino-4-thiazolyl)glyoxylamido]-8-oxo-3-[(1,2,3-thiadiazol-5-ylthio)methyl]-5-thia-1-azabicyclo[4.2.0]oct-2-ene-2-carboxylic acid, 7^2-(Z)-(O-methyloxime). *UNII-860MT00T7T. CAS-82219-78-1.* INN; MI.

Celecoxib [*1998*] (sel″ e kox′ ib). $C_{17}H_{14}F_3N_3O_2S$. 381.37. (1) 4-[5-(4-Methylphenyl)-3-(trifluoromethyl)-1H-pyrazol-1-yl]benzenesulfonamide; (2) p-[5-p-tolyl-3-(trifluoromethyl)pyrazol-1-yl]benzenesulfonamide. *UNII-JCX84Q7J1L. CAS-169590-42-5.* INN; BAN. *Anti-inflammatory and analgesic (cyclooxygenase-2 inhibitor).* Celebrex (Pfizer) ◇SC-58635

Celgosivir Hydrochloride [*1997*] (sel goe′ si vir hye″ droe klor′ ide). $C_{12}H_{21}NO_5$.HCl. 295.76. [Celgosivir is INN.] (1) Butanoic acid, octahydro-1,7,8-trihydroxy-6-indolizinyl ester, hydrochloride, [1S-(1$\alpha,6\beta,7\alpha,8\beta,8a\beta$)]-; (2) (1$S,6S,7S,8R$,8a$R$)-Octahydro-1,7,8-trihydroxy-6-indolizi-

nyl butyrate, hydrochloride. *UNII-70U2NQU0FP. CAS-141117-12-6; CAS-121104-96-9* [celgosivir]. *Antiviral; inhibitor (α-glucosidase).* ◇MDL 28,574A

Celiprolol Hydrochloride [*1981*] (sel″ i proe′ lol hye″ droe klor′ ide). $C_{20}H_{33}N_3O_4$.HCl. 415.95. [Celiprolol is INN and BAN.] (1) Urea, N'-[3-acetyl-4-[3-[(1,1-dimethylethyl)amino]-2-hydroxypropoxy]phenyl]-N,N-diethyl-, monohydrochloride; (2) 3-[3-Acetyl-4-[3-(*tert*-butylamino)-2-hydroxypropoxy]phenyl]-1,1-diethylurea monohydrochloride. *UNII-G1M3398594. CAS-57470-78-7; CAS-56980-93-9* [celiprolol]. *Anti-adrenergic (β-receptor).* Selecor (Rhone-Poulenc Rorer)

Celivarone. $C_{34}H_{47}NO_4$. 533.74. Isopropyl 2-butyl-3-{4-[3-(dibutylamino)propyl]benzoyl}-1-benzofuran-5-carboxylate. *UNII-K45001587E. CAS-401925-43-7.* INN.

Cellaburate (sel ab′ ure ate). **NF**. (1) Cellulose acetate butanoate; (2) Cellulose acetate butyrate; (3) Acetylbutyrylcellulose; (4) Cellulose butyrate acetate; (5) Cellulose acetate butyrate. *CAS-9004-36-8.*

Cellacefate (sel as′ e fate). **NF**. (1) Cellulose, acetate, 1,2-benzenedicarboxylate; (2) Cellulose acetate phthalate. *CAS-9004-38-0.* INN; BAN; JAN. *Pharmaceutic aid (tablet coating agent).* "EASTMAN" C-A-P (Eastman) *[Names previously used: Cellulose Acetate Phthalate; Cellacephate.]*

Cellacephate (previously used name) — *See* Cellacefate.

Cellulase [*1962*] (sel′ ue lase). A concentrate of cellulose-splitting enzymes derived from *Aspergillus niger* and other sources. (1) Cellulase; (2) Cellulase. *CAS-9012-54-8. Enzyme (digestant adjunct).*

Cellulose, Absorbable — *See* Cellulose, Oxidized.

Cellulose Acetate (sel′ ue lose as′ e tate). **NF**. (1) Cellulose acetate; (2) Cellulose, acetate; (3) Cellulose, diacetate; (4) Cellulose, triacetate. *CAS-9004-35-7; CAS-9035-69-2* [diacetate]; *CAS-9012-09-3* [triacetate]. *Pharmaceutic aid (coating agent); polymer membrane, insoluble.* "EASTMAN" Cellulose Acetate CA 398-10NF (Eastman)

Cellulose Acetate Phthalate (previously used name) — *See* Cellacefate.

Cellulose, Crystalline (JAN) — *See* Cellulose, Microcrystalline.

Cellulose, Dispersible (BAN) — *See* Cellulose, Microcrystalline.

Cellulose, Microcrystalline (sel′ ue lose mye″ kroe kris′ ta lin). **NF.** [Dispersible Cellulose is BAN; Crystalline Cellulose is JAN.] (1) Cellulose; (2) Cellulose. *CAS-9004-34-6. Pharmaceutic aid (tablet and capsule diluent).* Avicel PH (FMC)

Cellulose, Oxidized (sel′ ue lose ox′ i dized). **USP.** Contains $20.0 \pm 4.0\%$ of carboxyl groups (COOH), calculated on the dried basis. JAN. *Hemostatic (local).*

Cellulose, Oxidized Regenerated (sel′ ue lose ox′ i dized). **USP.** Contains $21.0 \pm 3.0\%$ of carboxyl groups (COOH), calculated on the dried basis. *Hemostatic (local).* Surgicel Absorbable Hemostat (Ethicon); Surgicel Fibrillar Absorbable Hemostat (Ethicon); Surgicel Nu-Knit Absorbable Hemostat (Ethicon)

Cellulose Sodium Phosphate [*1985*] (sel′ ue lose soe′ dee um fos′ fate). **USP.** An insoluble, nonabsorbable ion-exchange resin made by phosphorylation of cellulose. It contains approximately 34% of inorganic phosphate and approximately 11% of sodium. (1) Cellulose, dihydrogen phosphate, disodium salt; (2) Cellulose disodium phosphate. *CAS-68444-58-6. Anti-urolithic.* Calcibind (Mission)

Celmoleukin. $C_{693}H_{1118}N_{178}O_{203}S_7$. 15,415.83. Interleukin 2 (human clone pTIL2-21a, protein moiety). *CAS-94218-72-1.* INN.

Celucloral. Cellulose 2-hydroxyethyl ether reaction product with chloral. INN; BAN. ◇*ML 1034*

Cemadotin. $C_{35}H_{56}N_6O_5$. 640.86. *N,N*-Dimethyl-L-valyl-L-valyl-*N*-methyl-L-valyl-L-prolyl-*N*-benzyl-L-prolinamide. *UNII-6SQ8M7ZSFV. CAS-159776-69-9.* INN.

Cenersen Sodium [*2006*] (sen′ er sen soe′ dee um). $C_{187}H_{226}N_{62}Na_{19}O_{103}P_{19}S_{19}$. 6624.69. [Cenersen is INN.] (1) DNA, d(*P*-thio)(C-C-C-T-G-C-T-C-C-C-C-C-T-G-G-C-T-C-C), nonadecasodium salt; (2) 2′-Deoxy-*P*-thiocytidylyl-(3′→5′)-2′-deoxy-*P*-thiocytidylyl-(3′→5′)-2′-deoxy-*P*-thiocytidylyl-(3′→5′)-*P*-thiothymidylyl-(3′→5′)-2′-deoxy-*P*-thioguanylyl-(3′→5′)-2′-deoxy-*P*-thiocytidylyl-(3′→5′)-*P*-thiothymidylyl-(3′→5′)-2′-deoxy-*P*-thiocytidylyl-(3′→5′)-2′-deoxy-*P*-thiocytidylyl-(3′→5′)-2′-deoxy-*P*-thiocytidylyl-(3′→5′)-2′-deoxy-*P*-thiocytidylyl-(3′→5′)-2′-deoxy-*P*-thiocytidylyl-(3′→5′)-*P*-thiothymidylyl-(3′→5′)-2′-deoxy-*P*-thioguanylyl-(3′→5′)-2′-deoxy-*P*-thioguanylyl-(3′→5′)-2′-deoxy-*P*-thiocytidylyl-(3′→5′)-*P*-thiothymidylyl-(3′→5′)-2′-deoxy-*P*-thiocytidylyl-(3′→5′)-2′-deoxycytidine nonadecasodium salt. *CAS-872847-66-0. Treatment of cancer.* ◇*OL(1)p53; EL625*

PS-d(CCCTGCTCCCCCCTGGCTCC)

Centrazene — *See* Simtrazene.

Centrophenoxine — *See* Meclofenoxate.

---

† Brand name formerly used, and/or firm no longer concerned with this product.

Cephacetrile Sodium [*1970*] (sef a′ se trile soe′ dee um). $C_{13}H_{12}N_3NaO_6S$. 361.31. [Cefacetrile is INN and BAN; Cefacetrile Sodium is JAN.] (1) 5-Thia-1-azabicyclo[4.2.0]oct-2-ene-2-carboxylic acid, 3-[(acetyloxy)methyl]-7-[(cyanoacetyl)amino]-8-oxo-, monosodium salt (6*R-trans*)-; (2) Monosodium (6*R*,7*R*)-7-(2-cyanoacetamido)-3-(hydroxymethyl)-8-oxo-5-thia-1-azabicyclo[4.2.0]oct-2-ene-2-carboxylate acetate (ester). *UNII-87TH1FJY1N. CAS-23239-41-0; CAS-10206-21-0* [cephacetrile]. USP XX. *Antibacterial.* ◇*BA 36278A*

Cephalexin [*1967*] (sef″ a lex′ in). **USP.** $C_{16}H_{17}N_3O_4S.H_2O$. 365.40. [Cefalexin is INN, BAN and JAN.] (1) 5-Thia-1-azabicyclo[4.2.0]oct-2-ene-2-carboxylic acid, 7-[(aminophenylacetyl)amino]-3-methyl-8-oxo-, monohydrate [6*R*-[6α,7β(*R**)]]-; (2) (6*R*,7*R*)-7-[(*R*)-2-Amino-2-phenylacetamido]-3-methyl-8-oxo-5-thia-1-azabicyclo[4.2.0]oct-2-ene-2-carboxylic acid monohydrate; (3) 7-(D-α-Amino-α-phenylacetamido)-3-methyl-8-oxo-3-cephem-4-carboxylic acid monohydrate. *UNII-OBN7UDS42Y. CAS-23325-78-2; CAS-15686-71-2* [anhydrous]. *Antibacterial.* Keflet (Lilly); Keflex (Middlebrook) ◇*66873*

Cephalexin Hydrochloride [*1987*] (sef″ a lex′ in hye″ droe klor′ ide). **USP.** $C_{16}H_{17}N_3O_4S.HCl.H_2O$. 401.87. (1) 5-Thia-1-azabicyclo[4.2.0]oct-2-ene-2-carboxylic acid, 7-[(aminophenylacetyl)amino]-3-methyl-8-oxo-, monohydrochloride, monohydrate, [6*R*-[6α,7β(*R**)]]-; (2) (6*R*,7*R*)-7-[(2*R*)-2-Amino-2-phenylacetamido]-3-methyl-8-oxo-5-thia-1-azabicyclo[4.2.0]oct-2-ene-2-carboxylic acid, monohydrochloride, monohydrate; (3) 7-(D-2-Amino-2-phenylacetamido)-3-methyl-3-cephem-4-carboxylic acid hydrochloride monohydrate. *UNII-6VJE5G3D98. CAS-105879-42-3. Antibacterial.* Keftab (Lilly) ◇*LY061188*

Cephaloglycin [*1965*] (sef″ a loe glye′ sin). $C_{18}H_{19}N_3O_6S.2H_2O$. 441.46. [Cefaloglycin is INN, BAN and JAN.] (1) 5-Thia-1-azabicyclo[4.2.0]oct-2-ene-carboxylic acid, 3-[(acetyloxy)methyl]-7-[(aminophenylacetyl)amino]-8-oxo-, [6*R*-[6α,7β(*R**)]], dihydrate; (2) (6*R*,7*R*)-7-[(*R*)-2-Amino-2-phenylacetamido]-3-(hydroxymethyl)-8-oxo-5-thia-1-azabicyclo[4.2.0]oct-2-ene-2-carboxylic acid acetate (ester) dihydrate; (3) 7-(D-α-Aminophenylacetamido)-cephalosporanic acid dihydrate. *UNII-NE7R11LA95; UNII-HD2D469W6U* [cephaloglycin anhydrous]. *CAS-22202-75-1; CAS-3577-01-3* [anhydrous]. USP XX. *Antibacterial.* Kafocin (Lilly) ◇*39435*

Cephalonium (previously used name) — *See* Cefalonium.

Cephaloram (previously used name) — *See* Cefaloram.

Cephaloridine [*1964*] (sef″ a lore′ i deen). $C_{19}H_{17}N_3O_4S_2$. 415.49. [Cefaloridine is INN, BAN and JAN.] (1) Pyridinium, 1-[[2-carboxy-8-oxo-7-[(2-thienylacetyl)amino]-5-thia-1-azabicyclo[4.2.0]-oct-2-en-3-yl]-methyl]-, hydroxide, inner salt, (6*R-trans*)-; (2) (6*R*,7*R*)-1-[[2-Carboxy-8-oxo-7-[2-(2-thienyl)acetamido]-5-thia-1-azabicyclo[4.2.0]oct-2-en-3-yl]methyl]pyridinium hydroxide, inner salt; (3) 7-[α-(2-Thienyl)acetamido]-3-(1-pyridylmethyl)-3-cephem-4-carboxylic acid betaine. *UNII-LVZ1VC61HB.* *CAS-50-59-9.* USP XX. *Antibacterial.* Kefloridin (Lilly†); Loridine (Lilly†) ◇*40602*

Cephalosporin C. 7-(5-Amino-5-carboxyvaleramido)cephalosporanic acid. *CAS-61-24-5.* BAN.

Cephalosporin N — *See* Adicillin.

Cephalothin Sodium [*1965*] (sef a′ loe thin soe′ dee um). **USP.** $C_{16}H_{15}N_2NaO_6S_2$. 418.42. [Cefalotin is INN and BAN; Cefalotin Sodium is JAN.] (1) 5-Thia-1-azabicyclo[4.2.0]oct-2-ene-2-carboxylic acid, 3-[(acetyloxy)-methyl]-8-oxo-7-[(2-thienylacetyl)amino]-, monosodium salt, (6*R-trans*)-; (2) Monosodium (6*R*,7*R*)-3-(hydroxymethyl)-8-oxo-7-[2-(2-thienyl)acetamido]-5-thia-1-azabicyclo[4.2.0]oct-2-ene-2-carboxylate acetate (ester). *UNII-C22G6EYP8B; UNII-R72LW146E6* [cephalothin]. *CAS-58-71-9; CAS-153-61-7* [cephalothin]. *Antibacterial.* Keflin (Lilly); Seffin (GlaxoSmithKline) ◇*38253*

Cephamandole (previously used name) — *See* Cefamandole.

Cephamandole Nafate (previously used name) — *See* Cefamandole Nafate.

Cephapirin Benzathine (sef a pye′ rin ben′ za theen). **USP.** $(C_{17}H_{17}N_3O_6S_2)_2 \cdot C_{16}H_{20}N_2$. 1087.27. (1) 5-Thia-1-azabicyclo[4.2.0]oct-2-ene-2-carboxylic acid, 3-[(acetyloxy)-methyl]-8-oxo-7-[[(4-pyridinylthio)acetyl]amino]-, (6*R-trans*)-, compd. with *N,N′*-bis(phenylmethyl)-1,2-ethanediamine (2:1); (2) (6*R*,7*R*)-3-(Hydroxymethyl)-8-oxo-7-[2-(4-pyridylthio)acetamido]-5-thia-1-azabicyclo[4.2.0]oct-2-ene-2-carboxylic acid compound with *N,N′*-dibenzylethylenediamine (2:1). *UNII-90G868409O.* *CAS-97468-37-6.*

Cephapirin Sodium [*1970*] (sef a pye′ rin soe′ dee um). **USP.** $C_{17}H_{16}N_3NaO_6S_2$. 445.45. [Cefapirin is INN and BAN; Sodium Cefapirin is JAN.] (1) 5-Thia-1-azabicyclo[4.2.0]oct-2-ene-2-carboxylic acid, 3-[(acetyloxy)-methyl]-8-oxo-7-[[(4-pyridylthio)acetyl]amino]-, monosodium salt, (6*R-trans*)-; (2) Monosodium (6*R*,7*R*)-3-(hydroxymethyl)-8-oxo-7-[2-(4-pyridylthio)acetamido]-5-thia-1-azabicyclo[4.2.0]oct-2-ene-2-carboxylate acetate (ester); (3) 7-[α-(4-Pyridylthio)acetamido]cephalosporanic

acid sodium salt. *UNII-431LFF7I7J. CAS-24356-60-3; CAS-21593-23-7* [cephapirin]. *Antibacterial.* Cefadyl (Apothecon) ◇*BL-P 1322*

Cepharanthine. $C_{37}H_{38}N_2O_6$. 606.71. 6′,12′-Dimethoxy-2,2′-dimethyl-6,7-[methylenebis(oxy)]oxyacanthan. *CAS-481-49-2.* JAN.

Cephazolin (previously used name) — *See* Cefazolin.

Cephoxazole (previously used name) — *See* Cefoxazole.

Cephradine [*1971*] (sef′ ra deen). **USP.** $C_{16}H_{19}N_3O_4S$. 349.40. [Note—The first two code designations listed herein apply to a non-stoichiometric hydrate containing up to 6% of water. The USAN for this compound, regardless of the state of hydration, is Cephradine. For labeling purposes, where not otherwise qualified, Cephradine is understood to be the non-stoichiometric hydrate form. Products containing the dihydrate form so indicate by appropriate labeling on each package, e.g., ''Each capsule contains *x* mg of cephradine as the dihydrate'' on a dosage-form package or ''cephradine as the dihydrate'' on each label of a bulk shipment of the compound.] [Cefradine is INN, BAN and JAN.] (1) 5-Thia-1-azabicyclo[4.2.0]oct-2-ene-2-carboxylic acid, 7-[(amino-1,4-cyclohexadien-1-yl-acetyl)amino]-3-methyl-8-oxo-, [6*R*-[6α,7β(*R**)]]-; (2) (6*R*,7*R*)-7-[(*R*)-2-Amino-2-(1,4-cyclohexadien-1-yl)acetamido]-3-methyl-8-oxo-5-thia-1-azabicyclo[4.2.0]oct-2-ene-2-carboxylic acid. *UNII-F1BC02I72W; UNII-56PPJ9MMPE* [cephradine dihydrate]. *CAS-38821-53-3* [anhydrous]; *CAS-58456-86-3* [dihydrate]; *CAS-31828-50-9* [non-stoichiometric hydrate]. *Antibacterial.* Anspor (GlaxoSmithKline); Velosef (Apothecon) ◇*SK&F D-39304; SQ 11436; SQ 22022* [*dihydrate*]

Cericlamine. $C_{12}H_{17}Cl_2NO$. 262.18. (±)-3-(3,4-Dichlorophenyl)-2-(dimethylamino)-2-methyl-1-propanol. *UNII-VES82D23IB. CAS-112922-55-1.* INN.

Cerium Oxalate. *CAS-139-42-4.* USP IX; MI.

Cerivastatin Sodium [*1996*] (se ri″ va stat′ in soe′ dee um). $C_{26}H_{33}FNNaO_5$. 481.53. [Cerivastatin is INN and BAN.] (1) 6-Heptanoic acid, 7-[4-(4-fluorophenyl)-5-(methoxymethyl)-2,6-bis(1-methylethyl)-3-pyridinyl]-3,5-dihydroxy-[*S*-[*R**,*S**-(*E*)]]-, sodium salt; (2) (+)-Sodium (3*R*,5*S*,6*E*)-7-[4-(*p*-fluorophenyl)-2,6-diisopropyl-5-(methoxymethyl)-3-pyridyl]-3,5-dihydroxy-6-heptenoate. *UNII-6Q18G1060S; UNII-AM91H2KS67* [cerivastatin].

CAS-143201-11-0; CAS-145599-86-6 [cerivastatin]. *Antihyperlipidemic; inhibitor (HMG-CoA reductase).* Baycol (Bayer) ◇*BAY w 6228*

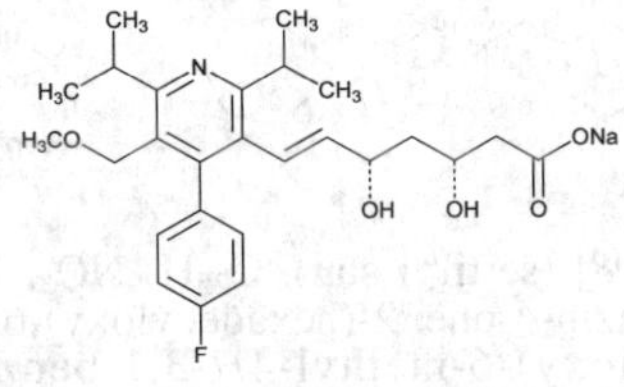

Cernitin Pollen Extract. JAN.

Ceronapril [*1990*] (se roe′ na pril). $C_{21}H_{33}N_2O_6P$. 440.47. (1) L-Proline, 1-[6-amino-2-[[hydroxy(4-phenylbutyl)phosphinyl]oxy]-1-oxohexyl]-, (S)-; (2) 1-[(2S)-6-Amino-2-hydroxyhexanoyl]-L-proline, hydrogen (4-phenylbutyl) phosphonate (ester). *CAS-111223-26-8.* INN. *Antihypertensive.* ◇*SQ 29,852*

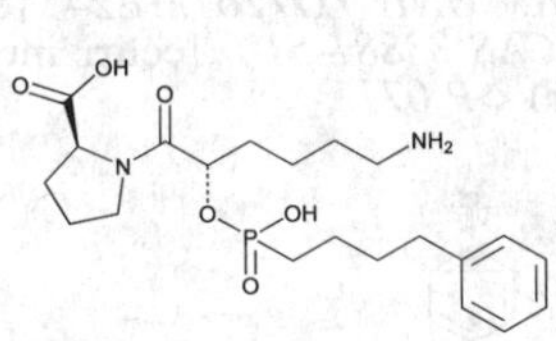

Certolizumab Pegol [*2003*] (ser″ toe liz′ oo mab peg′ ol). $C_{2115}H_{3252}N_{556}O_{673}S_{16}$ (peptide). Immunoglobulin, anti-(human tumor necrosis factor α) Fab′ fragment (human-mouse monoclonal CDP870 heavy chain), disulfide with human-mouse monoclonal CDP870 light chain, pegylated. Molecular weight is 47,696 daltons (unpegylated moiety). *UNII-UMD07X179E. CAS-428863-50-7.* INN; BAN; JAN. *Treatment of rheumatoid arthritis and inflammatory bowel disease, specifically Crohn's disease.* ◇*CDP870; PHA-738144*

Certoparin Sodium. Sodium salt of depolymerized heparin obtained by isoamyl nitrite degradation of heparin from pork intestinal mucosa; the majority of the components have a 2-*O*-sulfo-α-L-idopyranosuronic acid structure at the nonreducing end and a 6-*O*-sulfo-2,5-anhydro-D-mannose structure at the reducing end of their chain. The average relative molecular mass is 5,000 to 7,000; at least 70% less than 10,000. The degree of sulfation is 2 to 2.5 per disaccharide unit. INN; BAN.

Ceruletide [*1980*] (se roo′ le tide). $C_{58}H_{73}N_{13}O_{21}S_2$. 1352.40. (1) Caerulein; (2) 5-Oxo-L-prolyl-L-glutaminyl-L-α-aspartyl-*O*-sulfo-L-tyrosyl-L-threonylglycyl-L-tryptophyl-L-methionyl-L-α-aspartyl-L-phenylalaninamide; (3) 5-Oxo-L-prolyl-L-glutaminyl-L-aspartyl-L-tyrosyl-L-threonylglycyl-L-tryptophyl-L-methionyl-L-aspartylphenyl-L-alanina-

---

† Brand name formerly used, and/or firm no longer concerned with this product.

mide 4-(hydrogen sulfate) (ester). *UNII-888Y08971B. CAS-17650-98-5.* INN; BAN. *Stimulant (gastric secretory).*

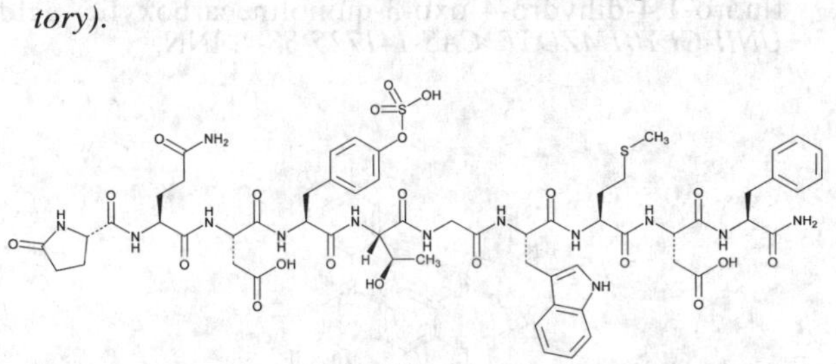

Ceruletide Diethylamine [*1980*] (se roo′ le tide dye eth′ il a meen). $C_{58}H_{73}N_{13}O_{21}S_2 \cdot xC_4H_{11}N$. (1) Caerulein compound with *N*-ethylethanamine; (2) Caerulein compound with diethylamine; (3) 5-Oxo-L-prolyl-L-glutaminyl-L-α-aspartyl-*O*-sulfo-L-tyrosyl-L-threonylglycyl-L-tryptophyl-L-methionyl-L-α-aspartyl-L-phenylalaninamide compound with *N*-ethylethanamine; (4) 5-Oxo-L-prolyl-L-glutaminyl-L-aspartyl-L-tyrosyl-L-threonylglycyl-L-tryptophyl-L-methionyl-L-aspartyl-phenyl-L-alaninamide 4-(hydrogen sulfate) (ester) compound with diethylamine. *UNII-4E1MIA8QQL. CAS-71247-25-1* [x salt]. JAN. *Stimulant (gastric secretory).* Tymtran (Pfizer) [*Note—The formation of the diethylamine salt is not a true stoichiometric reaction and the salt may exist with 1–3 moles of diethylamine.*]

Cesium Chloride Cs 131 [*1966*] (see′ zee um klor′ ide). $^{131}CsCl$. [Cesium (^{131}Cs) Chloride is INN.] *CAS-15690-63-8. Radioactive agent.* Cescan-131 (Abbott†)

Cetaben Sodium [*1978*] (see′ ta ben soe′ dee um). $C_{23}H_{38}NNaO_2$. 383.54. [Cetaben is INN.] (1) Benzoic acid, 4-(hexadecylamino)-, sodium salt; (2) Sodium *p*-(hexadecylamino)benzoate. *UNII-433YPU24B8; UNII-DTL5W0113X* [cetaben]. *CAS-64059-66-1; CAS-55986-43-1* [cetaben]. *Antihyperlipoproteinemic.* ◇*CL 203,821*

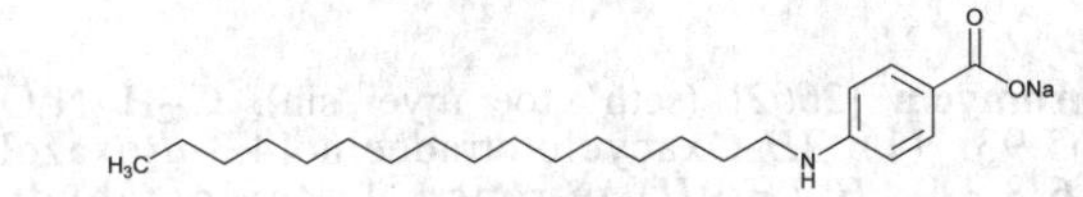

Cetalkonium Chloride [*1964*] (see″ tal koe′ nee um klor′ ide). $C_{25}H_{46}ClN$. 396.09. (1) Benzenemethanaminium, *N*-hexadecyl, *N,N*-dimethyl-, chloride; (2) Benzylhexadecyldimethylammonium chloride. *UNII-85474O1N9D. CAS-122-18-9.* INN; BAN. *Anti-infective, topical.* Zettyn (Sterling Winthrop†) ◇*NSC-32942*

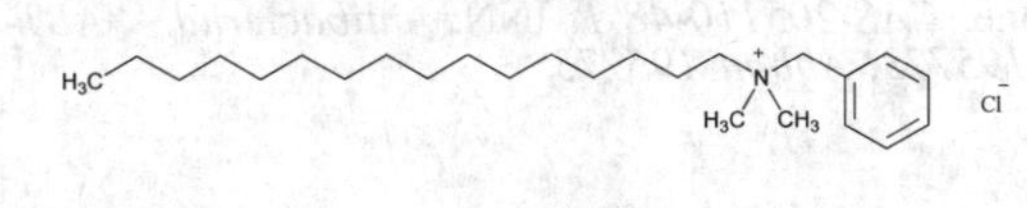

Cetamolol Hydrochloride [*1981*] (se tam′ oh lol hye″ droe klor′ ide). $C_{16}H_{26}N_2O_4 \cdot HCl$. 346.85. [Cetamolol is INN.] (1) Acetamide, 2-[2-[3-[(1,1-dimethylethyl)amino]-2-hydroxypropoxy]phenoxy]-*N*-methyl-, monohydrochloride, (±)-; (2) (±)-2-[*o*-[3-(*tert*-Butylamino)-2-hydroxypropoxy]phenoxy]-*N*-methylacetamide monohydrochloride. *UNII-5UNK5C6QM5. CAS-77590-95-5; CAS-34919-98-7* [cetamolol]. *Anti-adrenergic (β-receptor).* ◇*AI-27,303*

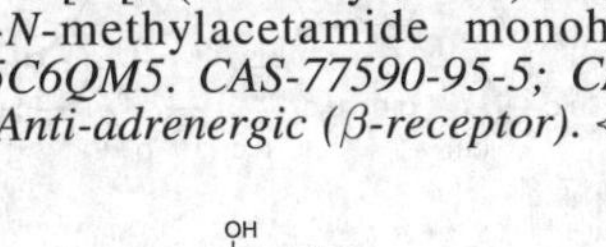

Cetanol (JAN) — *See* Cetyl Alcohol.

Cetefloxacin. $C_{20}H_{16}F_3N_3O_3$. 403.35. (-)-7-[(2*S*,3*R*)-3-Amino-2-methyl-1-azetidinyl]-1-(2,4-difluorophenyl)-6-fluoro-1,4-dihydro-4-oxo-3-quinolinecarboxylic acid. *UNII-CFY01MZD5T. CAS-141725-88-4*. INN.

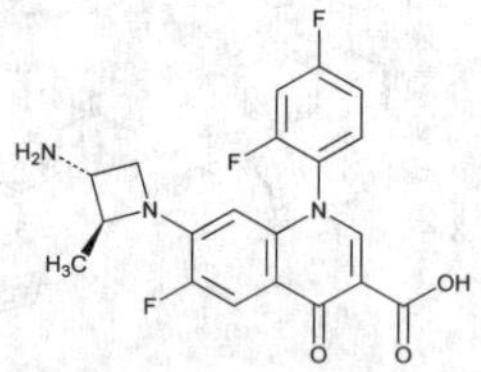

Cetermin. $C_{1132}H_{1716}N_{298}O_{330}S_{20}$. 25,420.87. Transforming growth factor β2 (human). *CAS-157238-32-9*. INN.

```
ALDAAYCFRN VQDNCCLRPL YIDFKRDLGW KWIHEPKGYN ANFCAGACPY
LWSSDTQHSR VLSLYNTINP EASASPCCVS QDLEPLTILY YIGKTPKIEQ
LSNMIVKSCK CS                                          ⎤
                                                       ⎦₂
```

Cethexonium Chloride. $C_{24}H_{50}ClNO$. 404.11. Hexadecyl(2-hydroxycyclohexyl)dimethylammonium chloride. *UNII-4F44UQX9EV. CAS-58703-78-9*. INN.

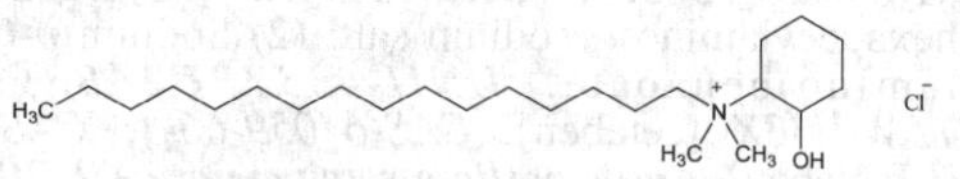

Cethromycin [*2002*] (seth″ roe mye′ sin). $C_{42}H_{59}N_3O_{10}$. 765.93. (1) 2*H*-Oxacyclotetradecino[4,3-*d*]oxazole-2,6,8,14(1*H*,7*H*,9*H*)-tetrone, 4-ethyloctahydro-3a,7,9,11,13,15-hexamethyl-11-[[3-(3-quinolinyl)-2-propenyl]oxy]-10-[[3,4,6-trideoxy-3-(dimethylamino)-β-D-xylo-hexopyranosyl]oxy]-, (3a*S*,4*R*,7*R*,9*R*,10*R*,11*R*,13*R*,15*R*,15a*R*)-; (2) (3a*S*,4*R*,7*R*,9*R*,10*R*,11*R*,13*R*,15*R*,15a*R*)-4-Ethyl-3a,7,9,11,13,15-hexamethyl-11-[[3-(quinolin-3-yl)prop-2-enyl]oxy]-10-[[3,4,6-trideoxy-3-(dimethylamino)-β-D-*xylo*-hexopyranosyl]oxy]octahydro-2*H*-oxacyclotetradecino[4,3-*d*]oxazole-2,6,8,14(1*H*,7*H*,9*H*)-tetrone. *CAS-205110-48-1*. INN. *Antibacterial*. ◇*ABT-773; A-195773; Abbott-195773*

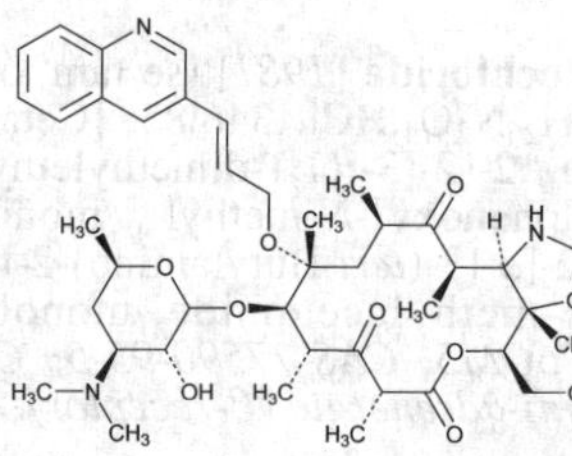

Cetiedil Citrate [*1978*] (se tye′ a dil sit′ rate). $C_{20}H_{31}NO_2S.C_6H_8O_7$. 541.65. [Cetiedil is INN.] (1) 3-Thiopheneacetic acid, α-cyclohexyl-, 2-(hexahydro-1*H*-azepin-1-yl)ethyl ester, 2-hydroxy-1,2,3-propanetricarboxylate (1:1); (2) 2-(Hexahydro-1*H*-azepin-1-yl)ethyl α-cyclohexyl-3-thiopheneacetate citrate (1:1). *UNII-IE65P4OE02. CAS-16286-69-4; CAS-14176-10-4* [cetiedil]. *Vasodilator (peripheral)*. Celsis (Ortho-McNeil†)

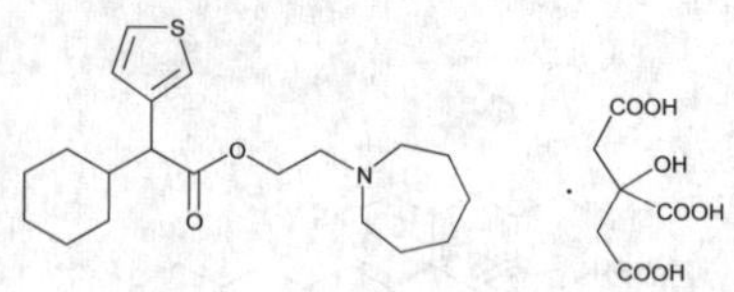

Cetilistat [*2008*] (se til′ i stat). $C_{25}H_{39}NO_3$. 401.58. (1) 4*H*-3,1-Benzoxazin-4-one, 2-(hexadecyloxy)-6-methyl-; (2) 2-(Hexadecyloxy)-6-methyl-4*H*-3,1-benzoxazin-4-one. *UNII-LC5G1JUA39. CAS-282526-98-1*. INN; BAN. *Treatment of obesity*. ◇*ATL-962*

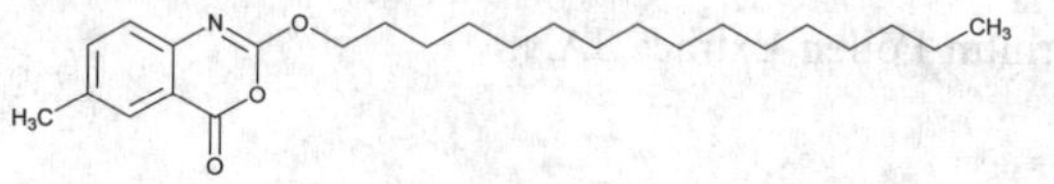

Cetirizine Hydrochloride [*1985*] (se tir′ i zeen hye″ droe klor′ ide). $C_{21}H_{25}ClN_2O_3.2HCl$. 461.81. [Cetirizine is INN and BAN.] (1) Acetic acid, [2-[4-[(4-chlorophenyl)phenylmethyl]-1-piperazinyl]ethoxy]-, dihydrochloride, ($\pm$)-; (2) ($\pm$)-[2-[4-(*p*-Chloro-α-phenylbenzyl)-1-piperazinyl]ethoxy]acetic acid, dihydrochloride. *UNII-64O047KTOA; UNII-YO7261ME24* [cetirizine]. *CAS-83881-52-1; CAS-83881-51-0* [cetirizine]. *Antihistaminic*. Zyrtec (Pfizer) ◇*P 071*

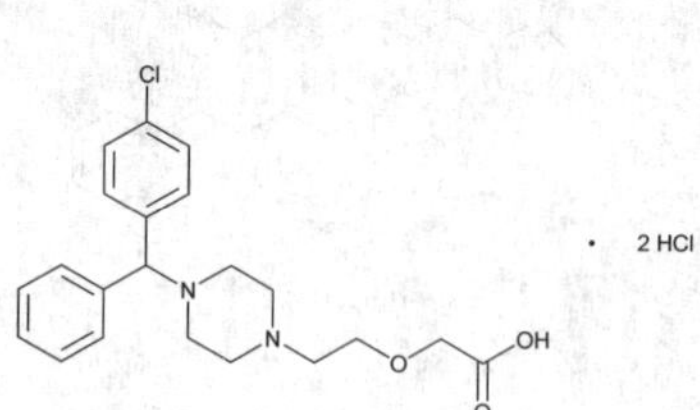

Cetobemidone (DCF) — *See* Ketobemidone.

Cetocycline Hydrochloride [*1977*] (see″ toe sye′ kleen hye″ droe klor′ ide). $C_{22}H_{21}NO_7.HCl$. 447.87. [Cetocycline is INN.] (1) 1,12(4*H*,5*H*)-Naphthacenedione, 2-acetyl-4-amino-4a,12a-dihydro-3,10,11,12a-tetrahydroxy-6,9-dimethyl-, hydrochloride, [4*R*-(4α,4aβ,12aβ)]-; (2) (4*R*,4a*S*,12a*S*)-2-Acetyl-4-amino-4a,12a-dihydro-3,10,11,12a-tetrahydroxy-6,9-dimethyl-1,12-(4*H*,5*H*)-naphthacenedione hydrochloride. *CAS-56433-46-6; CAS-53274-41-2* [4α,4aβ,12aβ]; *CAS-29144-42-1* [cetocycline]. *Antibacterial*. [*Name previously used: Cetotetrine Hydrochloride.*] ◇*Abbott-40728*

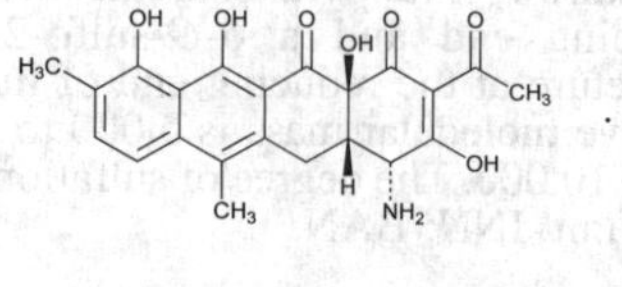

Cetofenicol (INN) — *See* Cetophenicol.

Cetohexazine. $C_6H_8N_2O$. 124.14. 4,6-Dimethyl-3(2*H*)-pyridazinone. *UNII-NS7PP85V4C. CAS-7007-92-3*. INN.

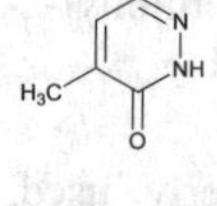

Cetomacrogol 1000. Polyethylene glycol 1000 monocetyl ether. *CAS-9004-95-9.* INN; BAN.

Cetophenicol [*1967*] (see″ toe fen′ i kol). $C_{13}H_{15}Cl_2NO_4$. 320.17. [Cetofenicol is INN.] (1) Acetamide, *N*-[2-(4-acetylphenyl)-2-hydroxy-1-(hydroxymethyl)ethyl]-2,2-dichloro-, [*R*-(*R**,*R**)]-; (2) D-*threo*-*N*-[*p*-Acetyl-β-hydroxy-α-(hydroxymethyl)phenethyl]-2,2-dichloroacetamide. *CAS-735-52-4. Antibacterial.* ◇W 3746

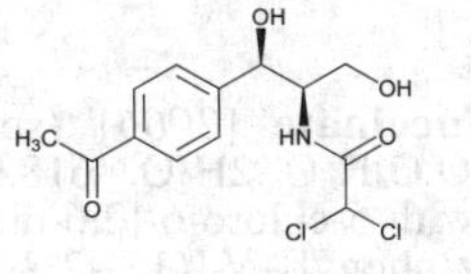

Cetophenylbutazone — *See* Kebuzone.

Cetostearyl Alcohol (see″ toe steer′ il al′ ka hol). **NF**. Contains not less than 40.0% of stearyl alcohol ($C_{18}H_{38}O$), and the sum of the stearyl alcohol content and the cetyl alcohol ($C_{16}H_{34}O$) content is not less than 90.0%. *Pharmaceutic aid (emulsifying agent).*

Cetotetrine Hydrochloride (previously used name) — *See* Cetocycline Hydrochloride.

Cetotiamine. $C_{18}H_{26}N_4O_6S$. 426.49. [Cetotiamine Hydrochloride is JAN.] *S*-Ester of *O*-ethyl thiocarbonate with *N*-[(4-amino-2-methyl-5-pyrimidinyl)methyl]-*N*-(4-hydroxy-2-mercapto-1-methyl-1-butenyl)formamide ethyl carbonate. *CAS-137-76-8.* INN; MI.

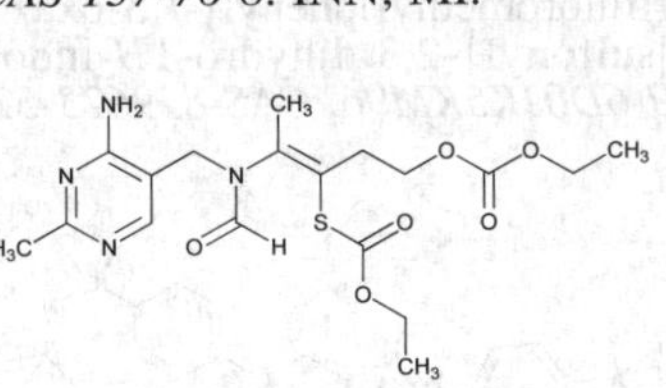

Cetoxime Hydrochloride. $C_{15}H_{17}N_3O \cdot HCl$. 291.78. [Cetoxime is INN and BAN.] 2-*N*-Benzylanilinoacetamidoxime hydrochloride. *CAS-22204-29-1; CAS-25394-78-9* [cetoxime]. MI.

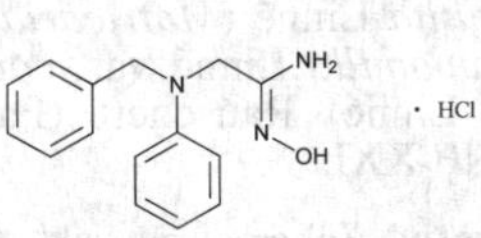

Cetraxate Hydrochloride [*1982*] (se trax′ ate hye″ droe klor′ ide). $C_{17}H_{23}NO_4 \cdot HCl$. 341.83. [Cetraxate is INN.] (1) Benzenepropanoic acid, 4-[[[4-(aminomethyl)cyclohexyl]carbonyl]oxy]-, hydrochloride, *trans*-; (2) *p*-Hydroxyhydrocinnamic acid *trans*-4-(aminomethyl)cyclohexanecarboxylate, hydrochloride. *UNII-08IT6P8VHY. CAS-27724-96-5; CAS-34675-84-8* [cetraxate]. JAN. *Anti-ulcerative (gastrointestinal).* ◇DV-1006

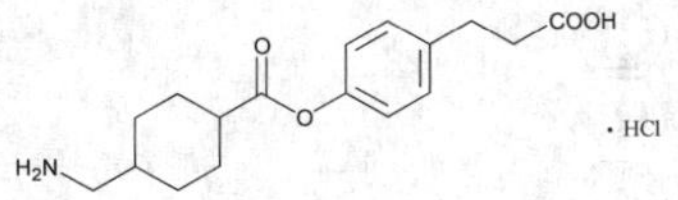

Cetrimide. A mixture consisting chiefly of tetradecyltrimethylammonium bromide together with smaller amounts of dodecyltrimethylammonium bromide and hexadecyltrimethylammonium bromide. *CAS-8044-71-1.* INN; BAN; JAN.

Cetrimonium Bromide (se″ tri moe′ nee um broe′ mide). **NF**. $C_{19}H_{42}BrN$. 364.45. Hexadecyltrimethylammonium bromide. *UNII-L64N7M9BWR. CAS-57-09-0; CAS-6899-10-1* [cetrimonium]. INN; BAN; MI.

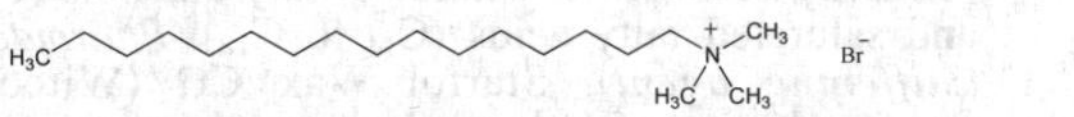

Cetrorelix. $C_{70}H_{92}ClN_{17}O_{14}$. 1431.04. *N*-Acetyl-3-(2-naphthyl)-D-alanyl-*p*-chloro-D-phenylalanyl-3-(3-pyridyl)-D-alanyl-L-seryl-L-tyrosyl-N^5-carbamoyl-D-ornithyl-L-leucyl-L-arginyl-L-prolyl-D-alaninamide. *UNII-OON1HFZ4-BA. CAS-120287-85-6.* INN; BAN. Cetrotide (Serono)

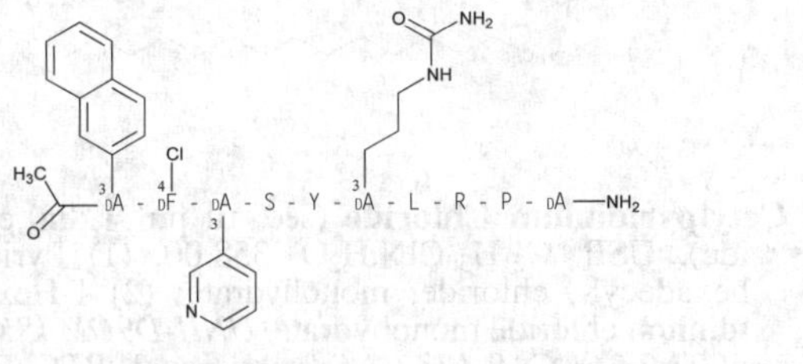

Cetrorelix Acetate [*2000*] (se″ troe rel′ ix as′ e tate). $C_{70}H_{92}ClN_{17}O_{14} \cdot xC_2H_4O_2$. 1431.06 (base). (1) D-Alaninamide, *N*-acetyl-3-(2-naphthalenyl)-D-alanyl-4-chloro-D-phenylalanyl-3-(3-pyridinyl)-D-alanyl-L-seryl-L-tyrosyl-N^5-(aminocarbonyl)-D-ornithyl-L-leucyl-L-arginyl-L-prolyl-, acetate (salt); (2) *N*-Acetyl-3-(2-naphthyl)-D-alanyl-*p*-chloro-D-phenylalanyl-3-(3-pyridyl)-D-alanyl-L-seryl-L-tyrosyl-N^5-carbamoyl-D-ornithyl-L-leucyl-L-arginyl-L-prolyl-D-alaninamide acetate (salt). *UNII-W9Y8L7GP4C. CAS-145672-81-7. Prevention of premature LH surges in patients undergoing controlled ovarian stimulation; antineoplastic (LHRH antagonist).* Cetrotide (Degussa A. G., Germany) ◇D-20761; SB-075 acetate; NS-75A

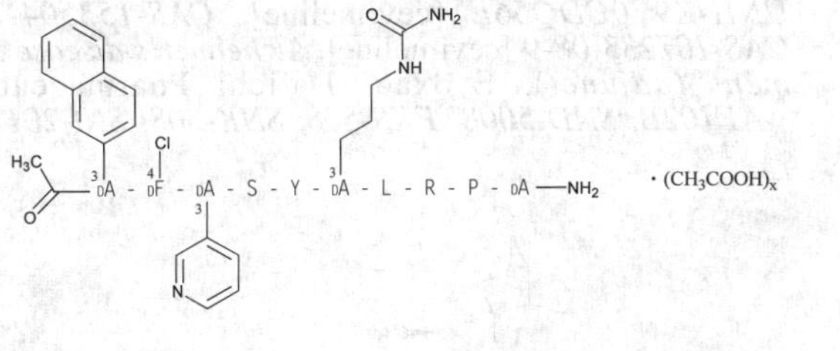

Cetuximab [*1999*] (se tux′ i mab). (1) Immunoglobulin G1, anti-(human epidermal growth factor receptor) (human-mouse monoclonal C225 γ1-chain), disulfide with human-mouse monoclonal C225 κ-chain, dimer; (2) Immunoglobulin G1 (human-mouse monoclonal C225 γ1-chain anti-human epidermal growth factor receptor), disulfide with human-mouse monoclonal C225 κ-chain, dimer. Molecular weight is approximately 170,000 daltons. *UNII-PQX0D8J21J. CAS-205923-56-4.* INN. *Treatment of EGF receptor-expressing cancers (monoclonal antibody).* ◇C225

---

† Brand name formerly used, and/or firm no longer concerned with this product.

Cetyl Alcohol (see′ til al′ ka hol). **NF**. $C_{16}H_{34}O$. 242.44. [Cetanol is JAN.] (1) 1-Hexadecanol; (2) 1-Hexadecanol. *UNII-936JST6JCN. CAS-124-29-8; CAS-36653-82-4. Pharmaceutic aid (emulsifying and stiffening agent).*

Cetyl Esters Wax (see′ til es′ ters). **NF**. A mixture consisting primarily of esters of saturated fatty alcohols (C_{14} to C_{18}) and saturated fatty acids (C_{14} to C_{18}). *Pharmaceutic aid (stiffening agent).* Starfol Wax CG (Witco) *[Name previously used: Synthetic Spermaceti.]*

Cetyl Palmitate (see′ til pal′ mi tate). **NF**. $C_{32}H_{64}O_2$. 480.85. (1) Hexadecanoic acid hexadecyl ester; (2) Cetyl palmitate. *UNII-5ZA2S6B08X. CAS-540-10-3.*

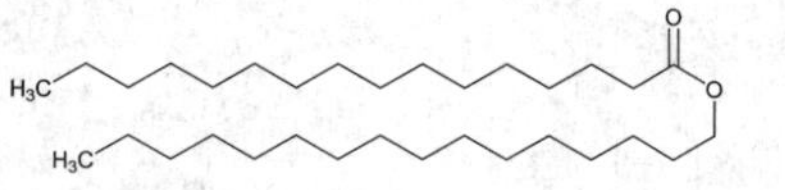

Cetylpyridinium Chloride (see″ til pir″ i din′ ee um klor′ ide). **USP**. $C_{21}H_{38}ClN.H_2O$. 358.00. (1) Pyridinium, 1-hexadecyl-, chloride, monohydrate; (2) 1-Hexadecylpyridinium chloride monohydrate. *UNII-D9OM4SK49P. CAS-6004-24-6; CAS-123-03-5 [anhydrous].* INN; BAN; JAN. *Anti-infective, topical; pharmaceutic aid (preservative).* Ceepryn (Marion Merrell Dow†); Cepacol (Marion Merrell Dow†)

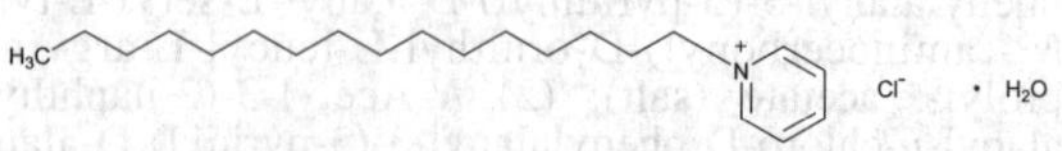

Cevimeline Hydrochloride [*1997*] (se vi′ me leen hye″ droe klor′ ide). $C_{10}H_{17}NOS.HCl.½H_2O$. 244.78. [Cevimeline is INN.] (1) Spiro[1-azabicyclo[2.2.2]octane-3,5′-[1,3]oxathiolane], 2′-methyl-, hydrochloride, hydrate (2:1), *cis*-; (2) (±)-*cis*-2-Methylspiro[1,3-oxathiolane-5,3′-quinuclidine] hydrochloride, hemihydrate. *UNII-P81Q6V85NP; UNII-K9V0CDQ56E [cevimeline]. CAS-153504-70-2; CAS-107233-08-9 [cevimeline]. Alzheimer's disease treatment (adjunct).* Evoxac (Daiichi Pharmaceutical) ◇*AF102B; SND-5008; FKS-508; SNK-508; SNI-2011*

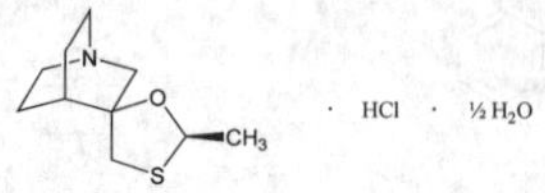

Cevipabulin Fumarate [*2006*] (se vip″ a bue′ lin fue′ ma rate). $C_{18}H_{18}ClF_5N_6O.C_4H_4O_4.2H_2O$. 616.92. [Cevipabulin is INN.] (1) [1,2,4]Triazolo[1,5-*a*]pyrimidin-7-amine, 5-chloro-6-[2,6-difluoro-4-[3-(methylamino)propoxy]phenyl]-*N*-[(1*S*)-2,2,2-trifluoro-1-methylethyl]-, (2*E*)-2-butenedioate (1:1), dihydrate; (2) 5-Chloro-6-[2,6-difluoro-4-[3-(methylamino)propoxy]phenyl]-*N*-[(1*S*)-2,2,2-trifluoro-1-methylethyl]-[1,2,4]triazolo[1,5-*a*]pyrimidin-7-amine (2E)-but-2-enedioate (1:1) dihydrate. *UNII-Q380BYV049;*

UNII-P14M0DWS2J [cevipabulin]. *CAS-849550-69-2; CAS-849550-05-6* [cevipabulin]. *Treatment of cancer.* ◇*TTI-237*

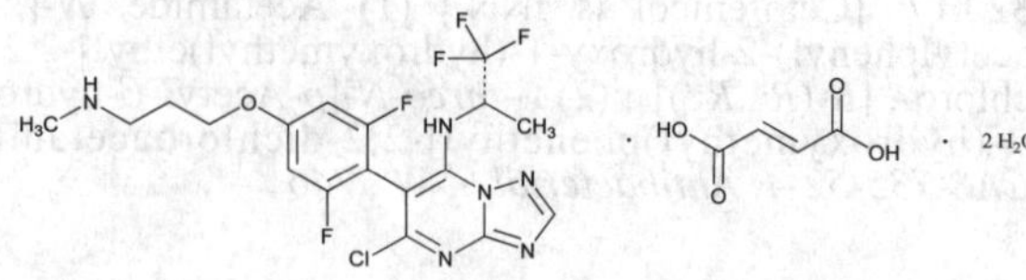

Cevipabulin Succinate [*2006*] (se vip″ a bue′ lin). $C_{18}H_{18}ClF_5N_6O.C_4H_6O_4.2H_2O$. 618.94. (1) Butanedioic acid, compd. with 5-chloro-6-[2,6-difluoro-4-[3-(methylamino)propoxy]phenyl]-*N*-[(1*S*)-2,2,2-trifluoro-1-methylethyl][1,2,4]triazolo[1,5-*a*]pyrimidin-7-amine (1:1), dihydrate; (2) 5-Chloro-6-[2,6-difluoro-4-[3-(methylamino)propoxy]phenyl]-*N*-[(1*S*)-2,2,2-trifluoro-1-methylethyl]-[1,2,4]triazolo[1,5-*a*]pyrimidin-7-amine butanedioate dihydrate. *CAS-852954-81-5. Anticancer.* ◇*TTI-237*

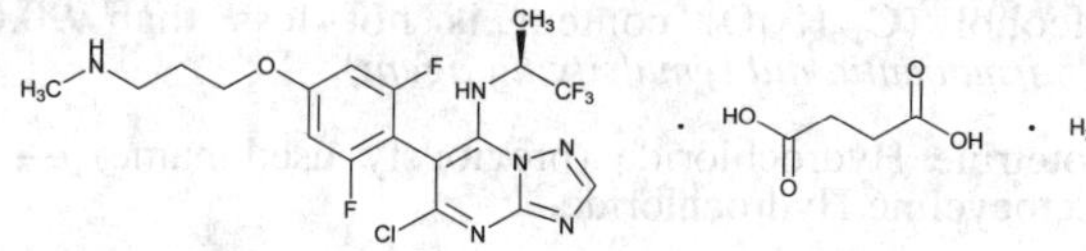

Cevitamic Acid — *See* Ascorbic Acid.

Cevoglitazar. $C_{27}H_{21}F_3N_2O_6S$. 558.53. (2*R*)-1-{[4-({5-Methyl-2-[4-(trifluoromethyl)phenyl]-1,3-oxazol-4-yl}methoxy)phenyl]sulfonyl}-2,3-dihydro-1*H*-indole-2-carboxylic acid. *UNII-6D0JK5KM96. CAS-839673-52-8.* INN.

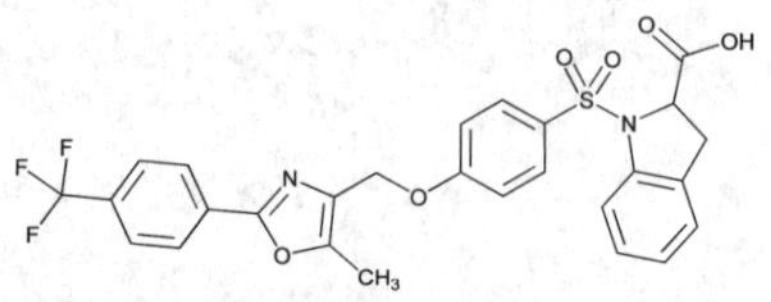

Chalk, Precipitated — *See* Calcium Carbonate.

Chamomile. Chamomile consists of the dried flower heads of *Matricaria recutita* Linné (*Matricaria chamomilla* Linné, *Matricaria chamomilla* Linné var. *courrantiana*, *Chamomilla recutita* Linné) Rauschert (Fam. Asteraceae alt. Compositae). NF XXI.

Charcoal, Activated (char′ kole ak′ ti vay″ ted). **USP**. [Medicinal Carbon is JAN.] The residue from the destructive distillation of various organic materials, treated to increase its absorptive power. *CAS-16291-96-6. Antidote (general purpose); pharmaceutic aid (adsorbant).*

Chaulmosulfone. $C_{48}H_{76}N_2O_4S$. 777.19. 4′,4″-Sulfonylbis(cyclopentanetridecananilide). *UNII-1S50W1WU8T. CAS-473-32-5.* INN; DCF.

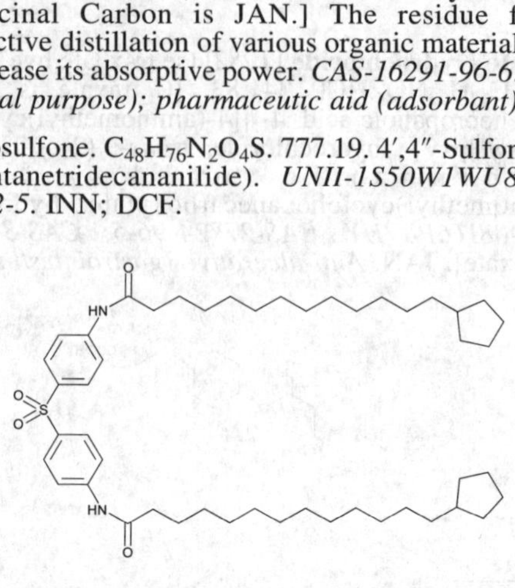

Chenic Acid (previously used name) — *See* Chenodiol.

Chenodeoxycholic Acid (INN, BAN, JAN) — *See* Chenodiol.

Chenodiol [*1978*] (kee″ noe dye′ ol). $C_{24}H_{40}O_4$. 392.57. [Chenodeoxycholic Acid is INN, BAN, and JAN.] (1) Cholan-24-oic acid, 3,7-dihydroxy-, $(3\alpha,5\beta,7\alpha)$-; (2) $3\alpha,7\alpha$-Dihydroxy-5β-cholan-24-oic acid. *UNII-0GEI24LG0J*. *CAS-474-25-9*. *Anticholelithogenic*. Chenix (Axcan Scandipharm) [*Name previously used: Chenic Acid.*]

Cherry Juice. **NF**. The liquid expressed from the fresh ripe fruit of *Prunus cerasus* L. (Fam. Rosaceae). *Pharmaceutic aid (flavor)*.

Chillifolinum — *See* Quillifoline.

Chinethazone — *See* Quinethazone.

Chiniofon. A mixture of four parts by weight of 8-hydroxy-7-iodo-5-quinolinesulfonic acid and one part by weight of sodium bicarbonate. *UNII-98F8Y85B6W*. *CAS-8002-90-2*. INN; DCF; NF XI.

Chlophedianol Hydrochloride [*1961*] (kloe″ fe dye′ a nol hye″ droe klor′ ide). $C_{17}H_{20}ClNO.HCl$. 326.26. [Clofedanol is INN and BAN; Clofedanol Hydrochloride is JAN.] (1) Benzenemethanol, 2-chloro-α-[2-(dimethylamino)ethyl]-α-phenyl-, hydrochloride; (2) 2-Chloro-α-[2-(dimethylamino)ethyl]benzhydrol hydrochloride. *UNII-69QQ58998Y; UNII-42C50P12AP* [chlophedianol]. *CAS-511-13-7; CAS-791-35-5* [chlophedianol]. *Antitussive*. Ulo (3M Pharmaceuticals) ◇*SL 501*

Chlophenadione — *See* Clorindione.

Chloquinate — *See* Cloquinate.

Chloracyzine. $C_{19}H_{21}ClN_2OS$. 360.90. 2-Chloro-10-(3-diethylaminopropionyl)phenothiazine. *UNII-TZ913SWN6M*. *CAS-800-22-6*. INN; DCF; MI.

Chloral Betaine [*1963*] (klor″ al bee′ ta een). $C_7H_{14}Cl_3NO_4$. 282.55. [Cloral Betaine is INN and BAN.] (1) Methanaminium, 1-carboxy-N,N,N-trimethyl-, hydroxide, inner salt, compd. with 2,2,2-trichloro-1,1-ethanediol (1:1); (2) Chloral hydrate betaine (1:1) compound. *CAS-2218-68-0*. NF XIV. *Sedative-hypnotic*. ◇*5107*

Chloral Hydrate (klor′ al hye′ drate). **USP**. $C_2H_3Cl_3O_2$. 165.40. (1) 1,1-Ethanediol, 2,2,2-trichloro-; (2) Chloral hydrate. *UNII-418M5916WG*. *CAS-302-17-0*. BAN; JAN. *Sedative-hypnotic*. Noctec (Bristol-Myers Squibb†); SK-Chloral Hydrate (SmithKline Beecham†)

Chloralformamide. *UNII-9YX16459LE*. *CAS-515-82-2*. USP VIII; MI.

Chloralodol (INN; BAN) — *See* Chlorhexadol.

Chloralose. $C_8H_{11}Cl_3O_6$. 309.53. α-Chloralose. *CAS-15879-93-3*. INN; DCF; MI.

Chlorambucil (klor am′ bue sil). **USP**. $C_{14}H_{19}Cl_2NO_2$. 304.21. (1) Benzenebutanoic acid, 4-[bis(2-chloroethyl)amino]-; (2) 4-[p-[Bis(2-chloroethyl)amino]phenyl]butyric acid. *UNII-18D0SL7309*. *CAS-305-03-3*. INN; BAN. *Antineoplastic*. Leukeran (GlaxoSmithKline) ◇*NSC-3088*

Chloramidobenzol — *See* Clofenamide.

Chloramine (previously used name) — *See* Chloramine-T.

Chloramine-T. $C_7H_7ClNNaO_2S$. 227.64. [Tosylchloramide Sodium is INN and BAN.] Sodium derivative of N-chloro-p-toluenesulfonamide trihydrate. *UNII-4IU6VSV0EI*. *CAS-127-65-1*. NF X; MI. [*Name previously used: Chloramine.*]

Chloramiphene — *See* Clomiphene Citrate.

Chloramphenicol (klor″ am fen′ i kol). **USP**. $C_{11}H_{12}Cl_2N_2O_5$. 323.13. (1) Acetamide, 2,2-dichloro-N-[2-hydroxy-1-(hydroxymethyl)-2-(4-nitrophenyl)ethyl]-, [R-(R^*,R^*)]-; (2) D-*threo*-(-)-2,2-Dichloro-N-[β-hydroxy-α-(hydroxy-

---

methyl)-*p*-nitrophenethyl]acetamide. *UNII-66974FR9Q1. CAS-56-75-7*. INN; BAN; JAN. *Antibacterial; antirickettsial*. Chloromycetin (Pfizer)

Chloramphenicol Palmitate (klor″ am fen′ i kol pal′ mi tate). **USP**. $C_{27}H_{42}Cl_2N_2O_6$. 561.54. (1) Hexadecanoic acid, 2-[(2,2-dichloroacetyl)amino]-3-hydroxy-3-(4-nitrophenyl)-propyl ester, [*R*-(*R**,*R**)]-; (2) D-*threo*-(-)-2,2-Dichloro-*N*-[β-hydroxy-α-(hydroxymethyl)-*p*-nitrophenethyl]acetamide α-palmitate. *UNII-43VU4207NW. CAS-530-43-8*. BAN; JAN. *Antibacterial; antirickettsial*. Chloromycetin Palmitate (Pfizer)

Chloramphenicol Pantothenate Complex [*1962*] (klor″ am fen′ i kol pan toe′ then ate). $(C_{11}H_{12}Cl_2N_2O_5)_4(C_{18}H_{32}Ca-N_2O_{10})$. 1769.05. [Cloramfenicol Pantotenate Complex is INN.] (1) β-Alanine, *N*-(2,4-dihydroxy-3,3-dimethyl-1-oxobutyl)-, calcium salt, (2:1), (*R*)-, compd. with [*R*-(*R**,*R**)]-2,2-dichloro-*N*-[2-hydroxy-1-(hydroxymethyl)-2-(4-nitrophenyl)ethyl]acetamide (1:4); (2) Pantothenic acid calcium salt (2:1) compound with D-threo-(-)-2,2-dichloro-*N*-[β-hydroxy-α-(hydroxymethyl)-*p*-nitrophenethyl]acetamide (1:4). *CAS-31342-36-6*. *Antibacterial; antirickettsial*. Pantofenicol (Pluriquimica, Portugal)

Chloramphenicol Sodium Succinate (klor″ am fen′ i kol soe′ dee um sux′ i nate). **USP**. $C_{15}H_{15}Cl_2N_2NaO_8$. 445.18. (1) Butanedioic acid, mono[2-[(2,2-dichloroacetyl)amino]-3-hydroxy-3-(4-nitrophenyl)propyl] ester, monosodium salt, [*R*-(*R**,*R**)]-; (2) D-*threo*-(-)-2,2-Dichloro-*N*-[β-hydroxy-α-(hydroxymethyl)-*p*-nitrophenethyl]acetamide α-(sodium succinate). *UNII-872109HX6B. CAS-982-57-0; CAS-56-75-7* [chloramphenicol]. BAN; JAN. *Antibacterial; antirickettsial*. Chloromycetin (Pfizer)

Chloranautine — *See* Dimenhydrinate.

Chlorazanil Hydrochloride. $C_9H_8ClN_5$.HCl. 258.11. [Chlorazanil is INN.] 2-Amino-4-*p*-chloroanilino-*s*-triazine hydrochloride. *UNII-9961SL881J. CAS-2019-25-2; CAS-500-42-5* [chlorazanil]. MI. Daquin (3M Pharmaceuticals†)

Chlorazodin (INN, DCF) — *See* Chloroazodin.

Chlorbenzoxamine Hydrochloride. $C_{27}H_{31}ClN_2O$.2HCl. 507.92. [Chlorbenzoxamine is INN.] 1-[2-(*o*-Chloro-α-phenylbenzyloxy)ethyl]-4-*o*-methylbenzylpiperazine dihydrochloride. *UNII-I898I67K6S. CAS-5576-62-5; CAS-522-18-9* [chlorbenzoxamine]. MI. ◇*UCB 1474*

Chlorbetamide. $C_{11}H_{11}Cl_4NO_2$. 331.02. 2,2-Dichloro-*N*-2,4-dichlorobenzyl-*N*-2-hydroxyethyl-acetamide. *UNII-3S489RFX0J. CAS-97-27-8*. INN; BAN; DCF; MI. Mantomide (Sterling Winthrop†)

Chlorbutin — *See* Chlorambucil.

Chlorbutol (BAN) — *See* Chlorobutanol.

Chlorcinnazine — *See* Clocinizine.

Chlorcyclizine Hydrochloride. $C_{18}H_{21}ClN_2$.HCl. 337.29. [Chlorcyclizine is INN and BAN.] (1) Piperazine, 1-[(4-chlorophenyl)phenylmethyl]-4-methyl-, monohydrochloride; (2) 1-(*p*-Chloro-α-phenylbenzyl)-4-methylpiperazine monohydrochloride. *UNII-NPB7A7874U. CAS-1620-21-9; CAS-82-93-9* [chlorcyclizine]. USP XXI; MI. Di-Paralene (Abbott†)

Chlordantoin [*1961*] (klor dan′ toin; klor dan′ toe in). $C_{11}H_{17}Cl_3N_2O_2S$. 347.69. [Clodantoin is INN and BAN.] (1) 2,4-Imidazolidinedione, 5-(1-ethylpentyl)-3-[(trichloromethyl)thio]-; (2) 5-(1-Ethylpentyl)-3-[(trichloromethyl)thio]hydantoin. *UNII-W14Z7581PA. CAS-5588-20-5. Antifungal*.

Chlordiazepoxide (klor″ dye az″ e pox′ ide). **USP**. $C_{16}H_{14}ClN_3O$. 299.75. (1) 3*H*-1,4-Benzodiazepin-2-amine, 7-chloro-*N*-methyl-5-phenyl-, 4-oxide; (2) 7-Chloro-2-(methylamino)-5-phenyl-3*H*-1,4-benzodiazepine 4-oxide. *UNII-6RZ6XEZ3CR. CAS-58-25-3*. INN; BAN; JAN. *Tranquilizer (minor)*.

Chlordiazepoxide Hydrochloride [*1963*] (klor″ dye az″ e pox′ ide hye″ droe klor′ ide). **USP**. $C_{16}H_{14}ClN_3O$.HCl. 336.22. (1) 3*H*-1,4-Benzodiazepin-2-amine, 7-chloro-*N*-methyl-5-phenyl-, 4-oxide, monohydrochloride; (2) 7-Chloro-2-(methylamino)-5-phenyl-3*H*-1,4-benzodiazepine 4-oxide monohydrochloride. *UNII-MFM6K1XWDK;*

UNII-6RZ6XEZ3CR [chlordiazepoxide]. *CAS-438-41-5; CAS-58-25-3* [chlordiazepoxide]. BAN; JAN. *Sedative-hypnotic.* Librium (Valeant) ◇*Ro 5-0690; NSC-115748*

Chlordimorine. $C_{19}H_{22}ClNO_2$. 331.84. 4-[3-(3-Chloro-4-biphenylyloxy)propyl]morpholine. *UNII-3SHS7PS4PL. CAS-494-14-4.* INN.

Chlorethate — *See* Clorethate.

Chlorfenisate — *See* Clofibrate.

Chlorhexadol. $C_8H_{15}Cl_3O_3$. 265.56. [Chloralodol is INN and BAN.] 2-Methyl-4-(2,2,2-trichloro-1-hydroxyethoxy)pentan-2-ol. *CAS-3563-58-4.* MI. Lora (Wallace†)

Chlorhexidine Gluconate [*1977*] (klor hex′ i deen gloo′ koe nate). **USP.** $C_{22}H_{30}Cl_2N_{10}\cdot2C_6H_{12}O_7$. 897.76. [Chlorhexidine is INN and BAN.] (1) 2,4,11,13-Tetraazatetradecanediimidamide, *N,N″*-bis(4-chlorophenyl)-3,12-diimino-, di-D-gluconate; (2) 1,1′-Hexamethylenebis[5-(*p*-chlorophenyl)biguanide] di-D-gluconate. *UNII-MOR84MUD8E; UNII-R4KO0DY52L* [chlorhexidine]. *CAS-18472-51-0; CAS-55-56-1* [chlorhexidine]. JAN. *Antimicrobial.* Cidastat (Ecolab); Dyna-hex (Xttrium); Hibiclens (Regent); Hibistat (Regent); Microderm (Johnson & Johnson); Peridex (3M Pharmaceuticals); Periochip (Dexcel); Periogard (Colgate); Pharmaseal Scrub Care (Pharmaseal); Prevacare (Johnson & Johnson)

Chlorhexidine Hydrochloride [*1963*] (klor hex′ i deen hye″ droe klor′ ide). $C_{22}H_{30}Cl_2N_{10}\cdot2HCl$. 578.37. (1) 2,4,11,13-Tetraazatetradecanediimidamide, *N,N″*-bis(4-chlorophenyl)-3,12-diimino-, dihydrochloride; (2) 1,1′-Hexamethylenebis[5-(*p*-chlorophenyl)biguanide] dihydrochloride. *UNII-E64XL9U38K. CAS-3697-42-5; CAS-55-56-1* [chlorhexidine]. BAN; JAN. *Anti-infective, topical.* ◇*AY-5312*

Chlorhexidine Phosphanilate [*1988*] (klor hex′ i deen fos fan′ i late). $C_{22}H_{30}Cl_2N_{10}\cdot2C_6H_8NO_3P$. 851.66. (1) 2,4,11,13-Tetraazatetradecanediimidamide, *N,N″*-bis(4-chlorophenyl)-3,12-diimino-, (4-aminophenyl)phospho-

nate (1:2); (2) 1,1′-Hexamethylenebis[5-(*p*-chlorophenyl)-biguanide] (*p*-aminophenyl)phosphonate (1:2). *CAS-77146-42-0. Antibacterial.* ◇*BMY-30120; CHP; WP-973*

Chlorimiphenin — *See* Imiclopazine.

Chlorimpiphenine — *See* Imiclopazine.

Chlorindanol [*1963*] (klor in′ da nol). C_9H_9ClO. 168.62. [Clorindanol is INN.] (1) 1*H*-Inden-4-ol, 7-chloro-2,3-dihydro-; (2) 7-Chloro-4-indanol. *UNII-7902N03BH0. CAS-145-94-8. Spermaticide.* ◇*NSC-158565*

Chloriodized Oil. Chlorinated and iodinated peanut oil. *CAS-8006-45-9.* USP XVI.

Chlorisondamine Chloride. $C_{14}H_{20}Cl_6N_2$. 429.04. 4,5,6,7-Tetrachloro-2-(2-dimethylaminoethyl)-2-methylisoindolinum chloride methochloride. *UNII-7B58W7756G. CAS-69-27-2.* INN; BAN; MI.

Chlorisondamone Chloride — *See* Chlorisondamine Chloride.

Chlormadinone Acetate [*1964*] (klor ma′ di none as′ e tate). $C_{23}H_{29}ClO_4$. 404.93. [Chlormadinone is INN and BAN.] (1) Pregna-4,6-diene-3,20-dione, 17-(acetyloxy)-6-chloro-; (2) 6-Chloro-17-hydroxypregna-4,6-diene-3,20-dione acetate. *UNII-0SY050L61N. CAS-302-22-7; CAS-1961-77-9* [chlormadinone]. NF XIII; JAN. *Progestin.* ◇*NSC-92338*

Chlormerodrin. $C_5H_{11}ClHgN_2O_2$. 367.20. [3-(Chloromercuri)-2-methoxypropyl)]urea. *UNII-99T5TWO621. CAS-62-37-3.* NF XIII; INN; BAN; MI. Mercloran (Parke-Davis†); Neohydrin (Marion Merrell Dow†)

Chlormerodrin Hg 197 [*1963*] (klor mer′ oh drin). $C_5H_{11}Cl^{197}HgN_2O_2$. [Chlormerodrin (^{197}Hg) is INN.] (1) Mercury-^{197}Hg,[3-[(aminocarbonyl)amino]-2-methoxypropyl]chloro-; (2) Chloro(2-methoxy-3-ureidopropyl)mer-

---

† Brand name formerly used, and/or firm no longer concerned with this product.

cury-^{197}Hg. *CAS-10375-56-1. USP XX. Diagnostic aid (renal function determination); radioactive agent.* Neohydrin-197 (Abbott†)

Chlormerodrin Hg 203 [*1963*] (klor mer′ oh drin). $C_5H_{11}Cl^{203}HgN_2O_2$. (1) Mercury-$^{203}Hg$,[3-[(aminocarbonyl)amino]-2-methoxypropyl]chloro-; (2) Chloro(2-methoxy-3-ureidopropyl)mercury-^{203}Hg. *CAS-2042-50-4. USP XX. Diagnostic aid (renal function determination); radioactive agent.* Neohydrin-203 (Abbott†)

Chlormeroprin — *See* Chlormerodrin.

Chlormethazanone — *See* Chlormezanone.

Chlormethine (INN, BAN) Hydrochloride — *See* Mechlorethamine Hydrochloride.

Chlormethylencycline — *See* Clomocycline.

Chlormezanone. $C_{11}H_{12}ClNO_3S$. 273.74. 2-(*p*-Chlorophenyl)-tetrahydro-3-methyl-4*H*-1,3-thiazin-4-one 1,1-dioxide. *UNII-GP568V9G19. CAS-80-77-3.* INN; BAN; JAN; MI. Trancopal (Sanofi Aventis)

Chlormidazole. $C_{15}H_{13}ClN_2$. 256.73. 1-*p*-Chlorobenzyl-2-methylbenzimidazole. *UNII-8IKK64FJVX. CAS-3689-76-7.* INN; BAN; MI.

Chlornaphazine. $C_{14}H_{15}Cl_2N$. 268.18. *N,N*-Bis(2-chloroethyl)-2-naphthylamine. *UNII-U46E473275. CAS-494-03-1.* INN; DCF; MI. ◇*CB 1048; R 48*

Chloroazodin. $C_2H_4Cl_2N_6$. 183.00. [Chlorazodin is INN.] (1) Diazenedicarboximidamide, *N,N″*-dichloro; (2) 1,1′-Azobis[*N*-chloroformamidine]. *UNII-SEF8X7MXO4. CAS-502-98-7.* USP XX; MI.

Chlorobutanol (klor″ oh bue′ ta nol). **NF.** $C_4H_7Cl_3O$. 177.46. [Chlorbutol is BAN.] (1) 2-Propanol, 1,1,1-trichloro-2-methyl-; (2) 1,1,1-Trichloro-2-methyl-2-propanol. *UNII-*

HM4YQM8WRC. CAS-57-15-8; CAS-6001-64-5 [hemihydrate]. INN; JAN. *Pharmaceutic aid (antimicrobial agent).* Chloretone (Parke-Davis)

Chlorochine — *See* Chloroquine.

Chlorocresol [*1980*] (klor″ oh kree′ sol). **NF.** C_7H_7ClO. 142.58. (1) Phenol, 4-chloro-3-methyl-; (2) 4-Chloro-*m*-cresol. *UNII-36W53O7109. CAS-59-50-7.* INN. *Antiseptic; disinfectant.*

Chlorodeoxylincomycin — *See* Clindamycin.

Chloroethane — *See* Ethyl Chloride.

Chloroform. $CHCl_3$. 119.38. (1) Methane, trichloro-; (2) Trichloromethane. *UNII-7V31YC746X. CAS-67-66-3.* NF XVII.

Chloroguanide Hydrochloride. $C_{11}H_{16}ClN_5$·HCl. 290.19. [Proguanil is INN and BAN.] 1-(*p*-Chlorophenyl)-5-isopropylbiguanide hydrochloride. *UNII-R71Y86M0WT. CAS-637-32-1; CAS-500-92-5* [chloroguanide]. USP XIV. Paludrine (Zeneca)

Chloroguanide Triazine Pamoate — *See* Cycloguanil Pamoate.

Chlorolincomycin — *See* Clindamycin.

Chloromethapyrilene Citrate — *See* Chlorothen Citrate.

Chlorophenothane. $C_{14}H_9Cl_5$. 354.49. [Clofenotane is INN.] 1,1,1-Trichloro-2,2-bis(*p*-chlorophenyl)ethane. *UNII-CIW5S16655. CAS-50-29-3.* NF XIV.

Chlorophenoxamide — *See* Clefamide.

Chlorophyllin Copper Complex [*1980*] (klor″ oh fil′ in kop′ er). Obtained from chlorophyll by replacing the methyl and phytyl ester groups with alkali (usually sodium but sometimes sodium and potassium) and replacing the magnesium with copper. *Deodorant.*

Chlorophyllin Copper Complex Sodium (klor″ oh fil′ in kop′ er). **USP.** [Chlorophyllin Copper Complex Sodium Salt is JAN.] Contains sodium salts of copper-chelated chlorophyll derivatives. Chloresium (Rystan); Derifil (Rystan)

Chloroprednisone Acetate. $C_{23}H_{27}ClO_6$. 434.91. [Chloroprednisone is INN.] 6α-Chloro-17,21-dihydroxypregna-1,4-diene-3,11,20-trione 21-acetate. *UNII-Z243A6BHCS*. *CAS-14066-79-6; CAS-52080-57-6* [chloroprednisone]. MI.

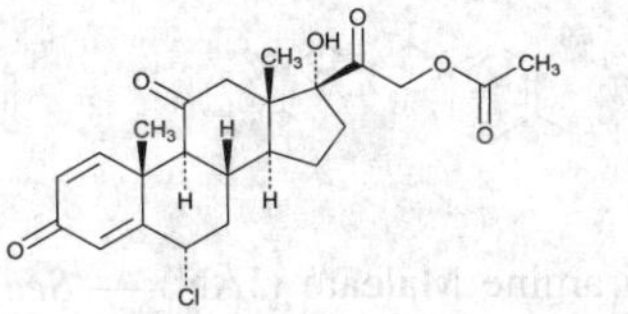

Chloroprocaine Hydrochloride (klor″ oh proe′ kane hye″ droe klor′ ide). **USP**. $C_{13}H_{19}ClN_2O_2$·HCl. 307.22. [Chloroprocaine is INN.] (1) Benzoic acid, 4-amino-2-chloro-, 2-(diethylamino)ethyl ester, monohydrochloride; (2) 2-(Diethylamino)ethyl 4-amino-2-chlorobenzoate monohydrochloride. *UNII-LT7Z1YW11H; UNII-5YVB0POT2H* [chloroprocaine]. *CAS-3858-89-7; CAS-133-16-4* [chloroprocaine]. *Anesthetic (local)*. Nesacaine (Abraxis)

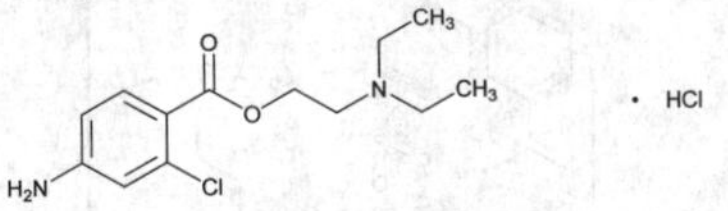

Chloropyramine. $C_{16}H_{20}ClN_3$. 289.80. 2-[(*p*-Chlorobenzyl)(2-dimethylaminoethyl)amino]pyridine. *UNII-2K3L8O9SOV. CAS-59-32-5*. INN; BAN; DCF; MI. *[Name previously used: Halopyramine.]*

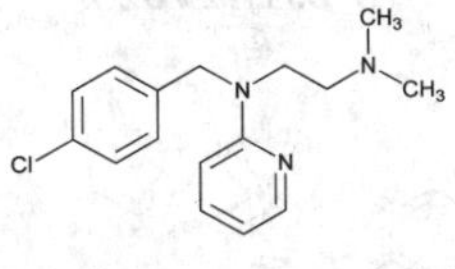

Chloropyrilene (INN, BAN) — *See* Chlorothen Citrate.

Chloroquine (klor′ oh kwin). **USP**. $C_{18}H_{26}ClN_3$. 319.87. (1) 1,4-Pentanediamine, N^4-(7-chloro-4-quinolinyl)-N^1,N^1-diethyl-; (2) 7-Chloro-4-[[4-(diethylamino)-1-methylbutyl]amino]quinoline. *UNII-886U3H6UFF. CAS-54-05-7*. INN; BAN. *Anti-amebic; antimalarial.*

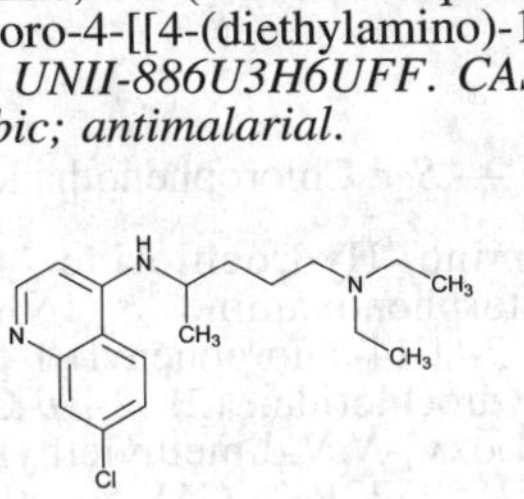

Chloroquine Diphosphate — *See* Chloroquine Phosphate.

Chloroquine Hydrochloride (klor′ oh kwin hye″ droe klor′ ide). **USP** [Injection]. $C_{18}H_{26}ClN_3$·2HCl. 392.79. [Chloroquine is BAN.] (1) 1,4-Pentanediamine, N^4-(7-chloro-4-quinolinyl)-N^1,N^1-diethyl-, dihydrochloride; (2) 7-(Chloro-4-[[4-diethylamino)-1-methylbutyl]amino]quinoline dihydrochloride. *UNII-NT0J0815S5. CAS-3545-67-3; CAS-54-05-7* [chloroquine]. *Anti-amebic; antimalarial.* Aralen Hydrochloride (Sanofi Aventis)

† Brand name formerly used, and/or firm no longer concerned with this product.

Chloroquine Phosphate (klor′ oh kwin fos′ fate). **USP**. $C_{18}H_{26}ClN_3$·$2H_3PO_4$. 515.86. (1) 1,4-Pentanediamine, N^4-(7-chloro-4-quinolinyl)-N^1,N^1-diethyl-, phosphate (1:2); (2) 7-Chloro-4-[[4-(diethylamino)-1-methylbutyl]amino]-quinoline phosphate (1:2). *UNII-6E17K3343P. CAS-50-63-5; CAS-54-05-7* [chloroquine]. BAN. *Antimalarial; anti-amebic; suppressant (lupus erythematosus).* Aralen (Sanofi Aventis)

Chloroserpidine. $C_{32}H_{37}ClN_2O_8$. 613.10. 10-Chlorodeserpidine. *UNII-98138WON55. CAS-7008-24-4*. INN; DCF.

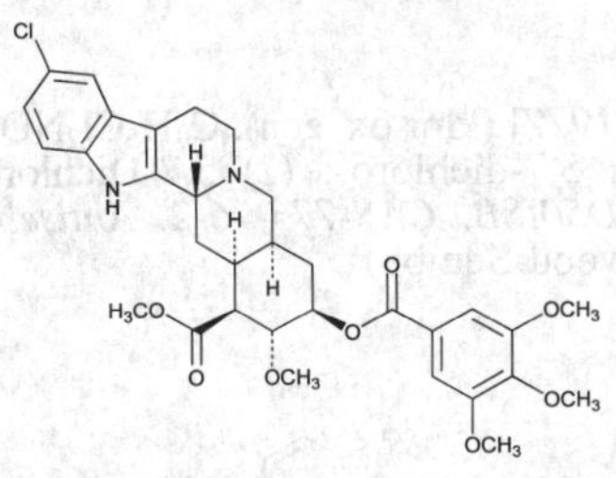

Chlorothen Citrate. $C_{14}H_{18}ClN_3S$·$C_6H_8O_7$. 487.95. [Chloropyrilene is INN and BAN.] 2-[(5-Chloro-2-thenyl)[2-(dimethylamino)ethyl]amino]pyridine citrate (1:1). *UNII-0X60R85C0J. CAS-148-64-1; CAS-148-65-2* [chlorothen]. NF XIII; MI.

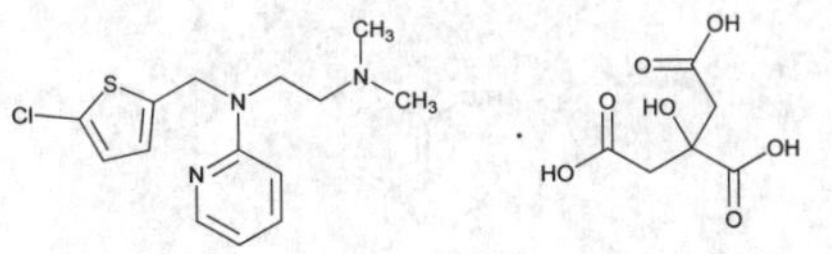

Chlorothenium Citrate — *See* Chlorothen Citrate.

Chlorothiazide (klor″ oh thye′ a zide). **USP**. $C_7H_6ClN_3O_4S_2$. 295.72. (1) 2*H*-1,2,4-Benzothiadiazine-7-sulfonamide, 6-chloro-, 1,1-dioxide; (2) 6-Chloro-2*H*-1,2,4-benzothiadiazine-7-sulfonamide 1,1-dioxide. *UNII-77W477J15H. CAS-58-94-6*. INN; BAN. *Diuretic.* Diuril (Merck)

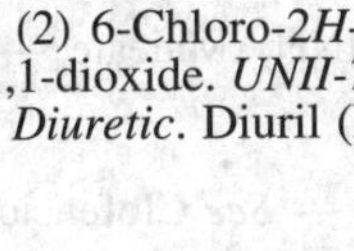

Chlorothiazide Sodium [*1964*] (klor″ oh thye′ a zide soe′ dee um). **USP** [for Injection]. $C_7H_5ClN_3NaO_4S_2$. 317.71. (1) 2*H*-1,2,4-Benzothiadiazine-7-sulfonamide, 6-chloro-, 1,1-dioxide, monosodium salt; (2) 6-Chloro-2*H*-1,2,4-benzothiadiazine-7-sulfonamide, 1,1-dioxide, monosodium salt. *UNII-SN86FG7N2K; UNII-77W477J15H* [chlorothiazide]. *CAS-7085-44-1; CAS-58-94-6* [chlorothiazide]. *Diuretic; antihypertensive.* Diuril (Ovation)

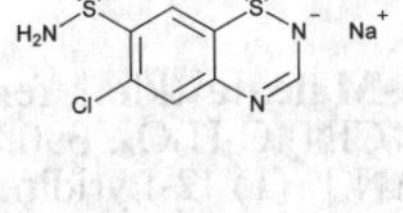

Chlorothymol. *UNII-LJ25TI0CVT. CAS-89-68-9*. NF XII; MI.

Chlorotrianisene. C$_{23}$H$_{21}$ClO$_3$. 380.86. (1) Benzene, 1,1',1''-(1-chloro-1-ethenyl-2-ylidene)tris[4-methoxy]-; (2) Chlorotris(*p*-methoxyphenyl)ethylene. *UNII-6V5034L121. CAS-569-57-3.* USP XXIII Supplement 1; INN; BAN. *Estrogen.* Tace (Sanofi Aventis) ◇*NSC-10108*

Chloroxine [*1977*] (klor ox' een). C$_9$H$_5$Cl$_2$NO. 214.05. (1) 8-Quinolinol, 5,7-dichloro-; (2) 5,7-Dichloro-8-quinolinol. *UNII-2I8BD50I8B. CAS-773-76-2. Antiseborrheic.* Capitrol (Westwood-Squibb)

Chloroxylenol [*1973*] (klor'' oh zye' le nol). **USP.** C$_8$H$_9$ClO. 156.61. (1) Phenol, 4-chloro-3,5-dimethyl-; (2) 4-Chloro-3,5-xylenol. *UNII-0F32U78V2Q. CAS-88-04-0.* INN; BAN. *Antibacterial.*

Chlorozone — *See* Chloramine-T.

Chlorpenthixol — *See* Clopenthixol.

Chlorphenamine (INN) Maleate — *See* Chlorpheniramine Maleate.

Chlorphenecyclane — *See* Clofenciclan.

Chlorphenesin Carbamate [*1963*] (klor fen' e sin). C$_{10}$H$_{12}$ClNO$_4$. 245.66. [Chlorphenesin is INN and BAN.] (1) 1,2-Propanediol, 3-(4-chlorophenoxy)-, 1-carbamate; (2) 3-(*p*-Chlorophenoxy)-1,2-propanediol 1-carbamate. *UNII-57U5YI11WP. CAS-886-74-8; CAS-104-29-0* [chlorphenesin]. JAN. *Relaxant (skeletal muscle).* Maolate (Pfizer) ◇*U-19,646*

Chlorphenindione — *See* Clorindione.

Chlorpheniramine Maleate (klor'' fen ir' a meen mal' ee ate). **USP.** C$_{16}$H$_{19}$ClN$_2$·C$_4$H$_4$O$_4$. 390.86. [Chlorphenamine is INN and BAN.] (1) 2-Pyridinepropanamine, γ-(4-chlorophenyl)-*N,N*-dimethyl-, (*Z*)-2-butenedioate (1:1); (2) 2-[*p*-Chloro-α-[2-(dimethylamino)ethyl]benzyl]pyridine maleate (1:1). *UNII-V1Q0O9OJ9Z; UNII-*

3U6IO1965U [chlorpheniramine]. *CAS-113-92-8; CAS-132-22-9* [chlorpheniramine]. JAN. *Antihistaminic.* Chlor-Trimeton (Schering-Plough); Teldrin (GlaxoSmithKline)

d-Chlorpheniramine Maleate (JAN) — *See* Dexchlorpheniramine Maleate.

Chlorpheniramine Polistirex [*1987*] (klor'' fen ir' a meen pol'' ee stye' rex). (1) Benzene, diethenyl-, polymer with ethenylbenzene, sulfonated, complex with γ-(4-chlorophenyl)-*N,N*-dimethyl-2-pyridinepropanamine; (2) Sulfonated styrene-divinylbenzene copolymer complex with 2-[*p*-chloro-α-[2-(dimethylamino)ethyl]benzyl]pyridine. *UNII-783AHI015X. Antihistaminic.*

Chlorphenoctium Amsonate. C$_{31}$H$_{41}$Cl$_2$N$_3$O$_5$S$_2$. 670.71. [(2,4-Dichlorophenoxy)methyl]dimethyl-*n*-octylammonium amsonate. *UNII-BJ1N2V028P. CAS-7168-18-5.* INN; BAN.

Chlorphenotane — *See* Chlorophenothane.

Chlorphenoxamine Hydrochloride. C$_{18}$H$_{22}$ClNO·HCl. 340.29. [Chlorphenoxamine is INN and BAN.] (1) Ethenamine, 2-[1-(4-chlorophenyl)-1-phenylethoxy]-*N,N*-dimethyl-, hydrochloride; (2) 2-[(*p*-Chloro-α-methyl-α-phenylbenzyl)oxy]-*N,N*-dimethylethylamine hydrochloride. *UNII-5I159322PY. CAS-562-09-4; CAS-77-38-3* [chlorphenoxamine]. USP XXI; MI. Phenoxene (Marion Merrell Dow†)

Chlorphentermine Hydrochloride [*1963*] (klor fen' ter meen hye'' droe klor' ide). C$_{10}$H$_{14}$ClN·HCl. 220.14. [Chlorphentermine is INN and BAN.] (1) Benzeneethanamine, 4-chloro-α,α-dimethyl-, hydrochloride; (2) *p*-Chloro-α,α-dimethylphenethylamine hydrochloride. *UNII-RL11HOJ7DM; UNII-NHW07912O7* [chlorphentermine]. *CAS-151-06-4; CAS-461-78-9* [chlorphentermine]. *Anorexic.* Pre-Sate (Parke-Davis) ◇*S-62; W 2426; NSC-76098*

Chlorphenylindandione — *See* Clorindione.

Chlorprocaine Chloride — *See* Chloroprocaine Hydrochloride.

Chlorproethazine Hydrochloride. $C_{19}H_{23}ClN_2S.HCl$. 383.38. [Chlorproethazine is INN.] 2-Chloro-10-(3-diethylaminopropyl)phenothiazine hydrochloride. *UNII-520P4U8V2Z. CAS-4611-02-3; CAS-84-01-5* [chlorproethazine]. MI. ◇*4909 RP*

Chlorproguanil Hydrochloride. $C_{11}H_{15}Cl_2N_5.HCl$. 324.64. [Chlorproguanil is INN and BAN.] 1-(3,4-Dichlorophenyl)-5-isopropylbiguanide hydrochloride. *UNII-6T04V14CU9. CAS-15537-76-5; CAS-537-21-3* [chlorproguanil]. MI.

Chlorpromazine (klor proe′ ma zeen). **USP**. $C_{17}H_{19}ClN_2S$. 318.86. [Chlorpromazine Hibenzate, Chlorpromazine Phenolphthalinate, and Chlorpromazine Tannate are JAN.] (1) 10*H*-Phenothiazine-10-propanamine, 2-chloro-*N,N*-dimethyl-; (2) 2-Chloro-10-[3-(dimethylamino)propyl]phenothiazine. *UNII-U42B7VYA4P. CAS-50-53-3.* INN; BAN. *Anti-emetic; antipsychotic.* Thorazine (GlaxoSmithKline)

Chlorpromazine Hydrochloride (klor proe′ ma zeen hye″ droe klor′ ide). **USP**. $C_{17}H_{19}ClN_2S.HCl$. 355.33. (1) 10*H*-Phenothiazine-10-propanamine, 2-chloro-*N,N*-dimethyl-, monohydrochloride; (2) 2-Chloro-10-[3-(dimethylamino)propyl]phenothiazine monohydrochloride. *UNII-9WP59609J6; UNII-U42B7VYA4P* [chlorpromazine]. *CAS-69-09-0; CAS-50-53-3* [chlorpromazine]. BAN; JAN. *Anti-emetic; antipsychotic.* Sonazine (Sandoz); Thorazine (GlaxoSmithKline)

---

† Brand name formerly used, and/or firm no longer concerned with this product.

Chlorpropamide (klor proe′ pa mide). **USP**. $C_{10}H_{13}ClN_2O_3S$. 276.74. (1) Benzenesulfonamide, 4-chloro-*N*-[(propylamino)carbonyl]-; (2) 1-[(*p*-Chlorophenyl)sulfonyl]-3-propylurea. *UNII-WTM2C3IL2X. CAS-94-20-2.* INN; BAN; JAN. *Antidiabetic.* Diabinese (Pfizer); Glucamide (Teva)

Chlorprophenpyridamine Maleate — *See* Chlorpheniramine Maleate.

Chlorprothixene [*1962*] (klor″ proe thix′ een). $C_{18}H_{18}ClNS$. 315.86. (1) 1-Propanamine, 3-(2-chloro-9*H*-thioxanthen-9-ylidene)-*N,N*-dimethyl-, (*Z*)-; (2) (*Z*)-2-Chloro-*N,N*-dimethylthioxanthene-$\Delta^{9,\gamma}$-propylamine. *UNII-9S7OD60EWP. CAS-113-59-7.* USP XXIII; INN; BAN; JAN. *Antipsychotic.* Taractan (Roche) ◇*N-714; Ro 4-0403*

Chlorpyrifos. *O,O*-Diethyl *O*-3,5,6-trichloro-2-pyridyl phosphorothioate. *CAS-2921-88-2.* BAN; MI.

Chlorquinaldol. $C_{10}H_7Cl_2NO$. 228.07. 5,7-Dichloro-2-methyl-8-quinolinol. *UNII-D6VHC87LLS. CAS-72-80-0.* INN; BAN; DCF; MI.

Chlortalidone (INN, BAN, JAN) — *See* Chlorthalidone.

Chlortetracycline Bisulfate (klor″ tet ra sye′ kleen bye sul′ fate). **USP**. [Chlortetracycline is INN and BAN.] 2-Naphthacenecarboxamide, 7-chloro-4-(dimethylamino)-1,4,4a,5,5a,6,11,12a-octahydro-3,6,10,12,12a-pentahydroxy-6-methyl-1,11-dioxo-, (4*S*,4a*S*,5a*S*,6*S*,12a*S*)-, sulfate (1:1); (2) 7-Chloro-4-(dimethylamino)-1,4,4a,5,5a,6,11,12a-octahydro-3,6,10,12,12a-pentahydroxy-6-methyl-1,11-dioxo-2-naphthacenecarboxamide bisulfate. *UNII-1D06KZ672I. CAS-27823-62-7; CAS-57-62-5* [chlortetracycline]. MI. *Antibacterial; antiprotozoal.*

Chlortetracycline Calcium. 7-Chloro-4-(dimethylamino)-1,4,4a,5,5a,6,11,12a-octahydro-3,6,10,12,12a-pentahydroxy-6-methyl-1,11-dioxo-2-naphthacenecarboxamide calcium salt. *UNII-NR4B2SX17S.* NND 1963.

Chlortetracycline Hydrochloride (klor″ tet ra sye′ kleen hye″ droe klor′ ide). **USP**. $C_{22}H_{23}ClN_2O_8.HCl$. 515.34. (1) 2-Naphthacenecarboxamide, 7-chloro-4-(dimethylamino)-1,4,4a,5,5a,6,11,12a-octahydro-3,6,10,12,12a-pentahydroxy-6-methyl-1,11-dioxo-, monohydrochloride [4*S*-(4α,4aα,5aα,6β,12aα)]-; (2) 7-Chloro-4-(dimethylamino)-1,4,4a,5,5a,6,11,12a-octahydro-3,6,10,12,12a-pentahydroxy-6-methyl-1,11-dioxo-2-naphthacenecarboxamide monohydrochloride. *UNII-O1GX33ON8R. CAS-64-72-2.* BAN. *Antibacterial; antiprotozoal.* Aureomycin (Lederle)

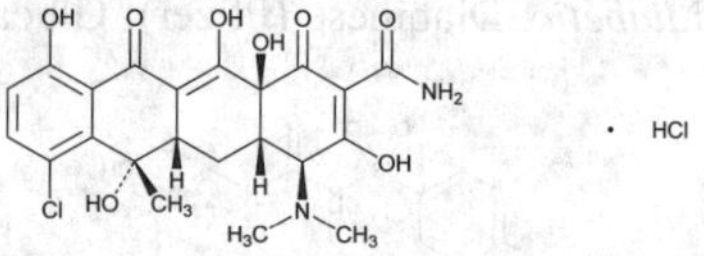

Chlorthalidone [*1961*] (klor thal′ i done). **USP.** $C_{14}H_{11}ClN_2O_4S$. 338.77. [Chlortalidone is INN, BAN and JAN.] (1) Benzenesulfonamide, 2-chloro-5-(2,3-dihydro-1-hydroxy-3-oxo-1*H*-isoindol-1-yl)-; (2) 2-Chloro-5-(1-hydroxy-3-oxo-1-isoindolinyl)benzenesulfonamide. *UNII-Q0MQD1073Q. CAS-77-36-1. Diuretic.* Hygroton (Sanofi Aventis); Thalitone (Monarch) ◇*G-33182; NSC-69200*

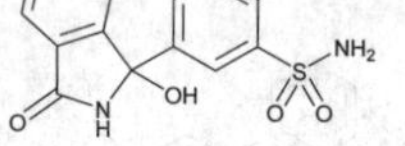

Chlorthenoxazine. $C_{10}H_{10}ClNO_2$. 211.64. 2-(2-Chloroethyl)-2,3-dihydro-4*H*-1,3-benzoxazin-4-one. *UNII-KA0B657LV3. CAS-132-89-8.* INN; BAN; MI. *[Name previously used: Chlorthenoxazin.]* ◇*AP 67*

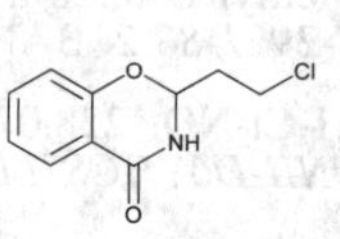

Chlorthiazide — *See* Chlorothiazide.

Chlortrianisestrol — *See* Chlorotrianisene.

Chlorzoxazone (klor zox′ a zone). **USP.** $C_7H_4ClNO_2$. 169.57. (1) 2(3*H*)-Benzoxazolone, 5-chloro-; (2) 5-Chloro-2-benzoxazolinone. *UNII-H0DE420U8G. CAS-95-25-0.* INN; BAN; JAN. *Relaxant (skeletal muscle).* Paraflex (Ortho-McNeil); Parafon (Ortho-McNeil); Strifon (Ferndale)

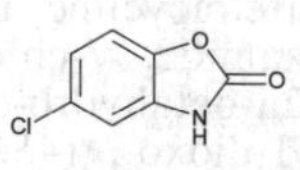

Chlosudimeprimylum — *See* Clopamide.

Chocolate (chok′ oh lat). **NF.** A powder prepared from the roasted, cured kernels of the ripe seed of *Theobroma cacao* L. (Fam. Sterculiaceae).

Cholecalciferol (koe″ le kal sif′ er ol). **USP.** $C_{27}H_{44}O$. 384.64. [Colecalciferol is INN and BAN.] (1) 9,10-Secocholesta-5,7,10(19)-trien-3-ol, (3β,5Z,7E)-; (2) Cholecalciferol. *UNII-1C6V77QF41. CAS-67-97-0.* BAN; JAN. *Vitamin (antirachitic).* [*Name previously used: 7-Dehydrocholesterol, Activated.*]

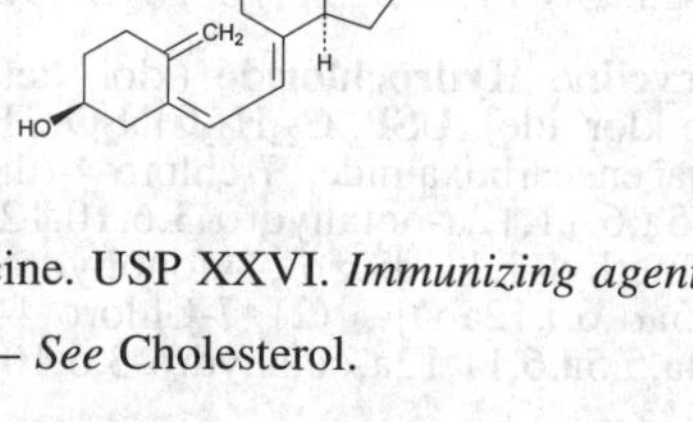

Cholera Vaccine. USP XXVI. *Immunizing agent (active).*

Cholesterin — *See* Cholesterol.

Cholesterol (koe les′ ter ol). **NF.** $C_{27}H_{46}O$. 386.65. (1) Cholest-5-en-3-ol, (3β)-; (2) Cholest-5-en-3β-ol. *UNII-97C5T2UQ7J. CAS-57-88-5.* BAN; JAN. *Pharmaceutic aid (emulsifying agent).*

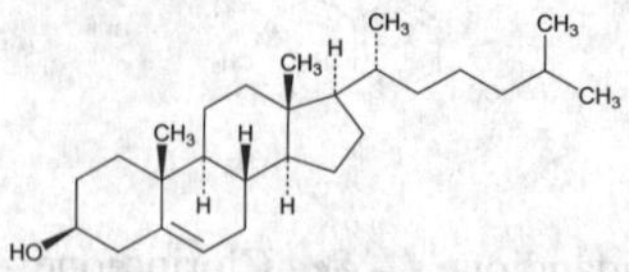

Cholestrin — *See* Cholesterol.

Cholestyramine Resin (koe″ le stye′ ra meen rez′ in). **USP.** [Colestyramine is INN, BAN and JAN.] (1) Cholestyramine; (2) Cholestyramine. *CAS-11041-12-6. Antihyperlipidemic; ion-exchange resin (bile salts).* Cholybar (Parke-Davis†); Duolite AP143 Resin (Rohm and Haas); Questran (Bristol Labs); Questran Light (Bristol Labs)

Choline Alfoscerate. $C_8H_{20}NO_6P$. 257.22. Choline hydroxide, (*R*)-2,3-dihydroxypropyl hydrogen phosphate, inner salt. *CAS-28319-77-9.* INN.

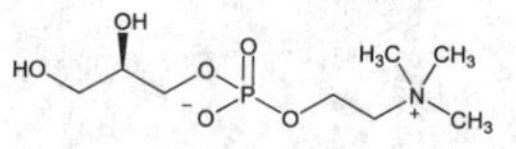

Choline Bitartrate. $C_9H_{19}NO_7$. 253.25. (1) 2-Hydroxyethanaminium,-*N,N,N*-trimethyl-, [*R*-(*R**,*R**)]-2,3-dihydroxybutanedioate (1:1); (2) (2-Hydroxyethyl)trimethylammonium-L-(+)-tartrate salt (1:1). *UNII-6K2W7T9V6Y. CAS-87-67-2; CAS-62-49-7* [choline].

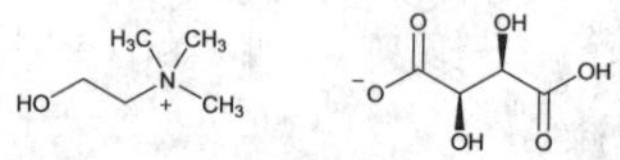

Choline Chloride. $C_5H_{14}ClNO$. 139.62. (1) (2-Hydroxyethyl)-trimethylammonium chloride; (2) 2-Hydroxy-*N,N,N*,-trimethylethanaminium chloride. *UNII-45I14D8O27. CAS-67-48-1; CAS-62-49-7* [choline]. INN; MI.

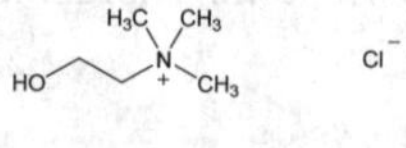

Choline Dihydrogen Citrate. *UNII-N91BDP6H0X* [choline]. *CAS-77-91-8; CAS-62-49-7* [choline]. NF XI; MI.

Choline Fenofibrate [*2006*] (koe′ leen fen″ oh fye′ brate). $C_5H_{14}NO^+.C_{17}H_{14}ClO_4^-$. 421.91. (1) Ethanaminium, 2-hydroxy-*N,N,N*-trimethyl-, salt with 2-[4-(4-chlorobenzoyl)phenoxy]-2-methylpropanoic acid (1:1); (2) 2-Hydroxy-*N,N,N*-trimethylethanaminium 2-[4-(4-chlorobenzoyl)phenoxy]-2-methylpropanoate. *UNII-4BMH7IZT98. CAS-856676-23-8.* INN. *Lipid-lowering agent.* ◇*ABT-335*

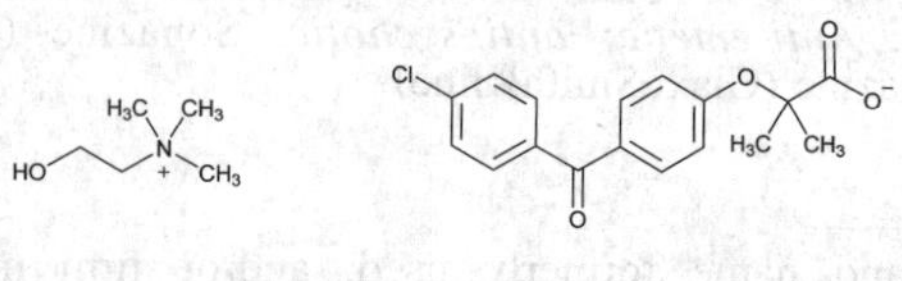

Choline Gluconate. $C_{11}H_{25}NO_8$. 299.32. (2-Hydroxyethyl)-trimethylammonium D-gluconate. *CAS-507-30-2*. INN.

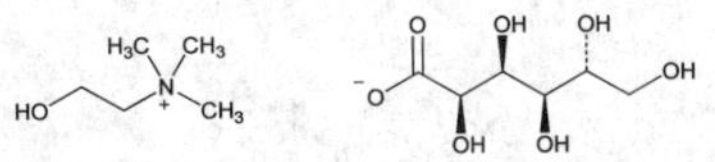

Choline Glycerophosphate — *See* Choline Alfoscerate.

Choline Salicylate [*1988*] (koe′ leen sa lis′ i late). $C_{12}H_{19}NO_4$. 241.28. (2-Hydroxyethyl)trimethylammonium salicylate. *UNII-KD510K1IQW*. *CAS-2016-36-6*. INN; BAN; JAN. Arthropan (Purdue Frederick)

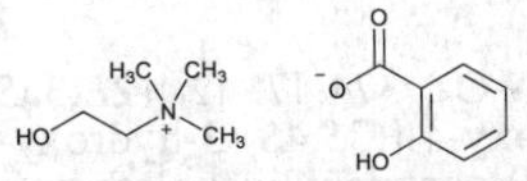

Choline Theophyllinate (INN, BAN) — *See* Oxtriphylline.

Choline Theophylline (JAN) — *See* Oxtriphylline.

Chondroitin 4-Sulfate — *See* Danaparoid Sodium.

Chondroitin 6-Sulfate — *See* Danaparoid Sodium.

Chondroitin Sulfate Sodium. $(C_{14}H_{19}NO_{14}SNa_2)_n$. Sodium chondroitin sulfate. *CAS-24967-93-9*. NF XXI; JAN.

Choriogonadotropin Alfa [*2000*] (kore″ ee oh goe nad″ oh troe′ pin al′ fa). $C_{437}H_{682}N_{122}O_{134}S_{13}$ (α-subunit); $C_{668}H_{1090}N_{196}O_{203}S_{13}$ (β-subunit). (1) Gonadotropin, chorionic (human α-subunit protein moiety reduced), complex with chorionic gonadotropin (human β-subunit protein moiety reduced); (2) Human chorionic gonadotropin (α-subunit protein moiety reduced), complex with human chorionic gonadotropin (β-subunit protein moiety reduced). Molecular weight is 38,000 daltons. *UNII-6413W06WR3*. *CAS-177073-44-8*; *CAS-56832-30-5* [α-subunit]; *CAS-56832-34-9* [β-subunit]. INN; BAN. *Treatment of infertility; cryptorchidism therapy adjuvant (recombinant human chorionic gonadotropin (rhCG))*. Ovidrel (Serono) ◇*ATC Code G03 GA Gonadotropins*

α - subunit

APDVQDCPEC TLQENPFFSQ PGAPILQCMG CCFSRAYPTP LRSKKTMLVQ
KNVTSESTCC VAKSYNRVTV MGGFKVENHT ACHCSTCYYH KS

β - subunit

SKEPLRPRCR PINATLAVEK EGCPVCITVN TTICAGYCPT MTRVLQGVLP
ALPQVVCNYR DVRFESIRLP GCPRGVNPVV SYAVALSCQC ALCRRSTTDC
GGPKDHPLTC DDPRFQDSSS SKAPPPSLPS PSRLPGPSDT PILPQ

* glycosylation sites

Chromic Chloride (krome′ ik klor′ ide). **USP**. $CrCl_3.6H_2O$. 266.45. (1) Chromium chloride ($CrCl_3$) hexahydrate; (2) Chromium(3+) chloride hexahydrate. *UNII-KB1PCR9DMW*. *CAS-10060-12-5*; *CAS-10025-73-7* [anhydrous]. *Supplement (trace mineral)*.

Chromic Chloride Cr 51 [*1963*] (krome′ ik klor′ ide). $^{51}CrCl_3$. (1) Chromium chloride ($^{51}CrCl_3$); (2) Chromium chloride ($^{51}CrCl_3$). *UNII-U4M5Y13FGM*. *CAS-16284-59-6*. *Radioactive agent*.

Chromic Phosphate Cr 51 [*1964*] (krome′ ik fos′ fate). $^{51}CrPO_4$. (1) Phosphoric acid, chromium(3+)-^{51}Cr salt; (2) Chromium(3+)-^{51}Cr phosphate. *Radioactive agent*.

Chromic Phosphate P 32 [*1963*] (krome′ ik fos′ fate). **USP** [Suspension]. $Cr^{32}PO_4$. (1) Phosphoric-^{32}P acid, chromium(3+) salt (1:1); (2) Chromium(3+) phosphate-^{32}P (1:1). *UNII-QHO02LZ4H2*. *CAS-24381-60-0*. *Radioactive agent*. Chromphosphotope (Bristol-Myers Squibb†); Phosphocol P32 (Mallinckrodt)

Chromium Cr 51 Edetate. **USP** [Injection]. (1) Glycine, *N,N*′-1,2-ethanediylbis[*N*-(carboxymethyl)-, chromium-51 complex; (2) (Ethylenedinitrilo)tetraacetic acid, chromium-51 complex. *CAS-27849-89-4*.

Chromium Picolinate. $C_{18}H_{12}N_3O_6Cr$. 418.30. Chromium Tripicolinate. *CAS-14639-25-9*. NF XXI.

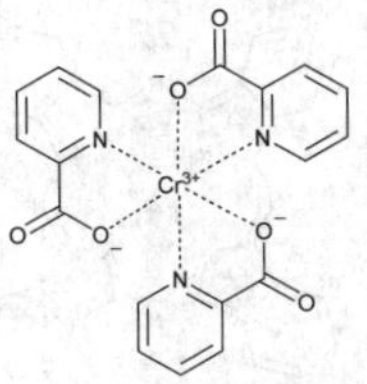

Chromocarb. $C_{10}H_6O_4$. 190.15. 4-Oxo-4*H*-1-benzopyran-2-carboxylic acid. *UNII-FY38S0790W*. *CAS-4940-39-0*. INN; DCF; MI.

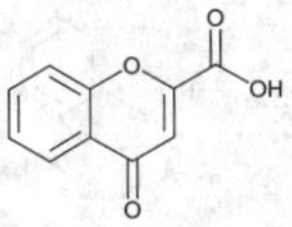

Chromomycin A$_3$. $C_{57}H_{82}O_{26}$. 1183.25. *CAS-7059-24-7*. JAN.

Chromonar Hydrochloride [*1965*] (kroe′ moe nar hye″ droe klor′ ide). $C_{20}H_{27}NO_5$.HCl. 397.89. [Carbocromen is INN; Carbocromen Hydrochloride is JAN.] (1) Acetic acid, [[3-[2-(diethylamino)ethyl]-4-methyl-2-oxo-2*H*-1-benzopyran-7-yl]oxy]-, ethyl ester, hydrochloride; (2) [[3-[2-(Diethylamino)ethyl]-4-methyl-2-oxo-2*H*-1-benzopyran-7-yl]oxy]acetic acid ethyl ester hydrochloride. *UNII-R0C9NIE5JJ* [chromonar]. *CAS-655-35-6*; *CAS-804-10-4* [chromonar]. *Vasodilator (coronary)*. Intensain (Abbott†) ◇*AG-3; A-27053; NSC-110430*

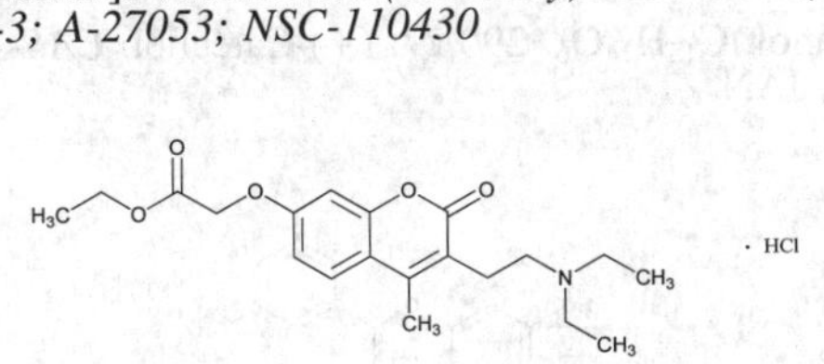

Chrysazin — *See* Danthron.

Chymopapain [*1971*] (kye″ moe pa pay′ in). Proteolytic enzyme isolated from papaya latex, differing from papain in electrophoretic mobility, solubility, and substrate specificity. Molecular weight is approximately 27,000. (1) Chymopapain; (2) Chymopapain. *UNII-1UK146T40N*. *CAS-9001-09-6*. INN; BAN. *Enzyme (proteolytic)*. Chymodiactin (Abbott); Discase (Abbott) ◇*BAX 1526; NSC-107079*

Chymotrypsin (kye″ moe trip′ sin). **USP**. (1) Chymotrypsin; (2) Chymotrypsin. *UNII-BVS505O332*. *CAS-9004-07-3*. INN; BAN; JAN. *Enzyme (proteolytic)*. Catarase (Novartis); Zolyse (Alcon)

---

† Brand name formerly used, and/or firm no longer concerned with this product.

Ciadox. $C_{12}H_9N_5O_3$. 271.23. Cyanoacetic acid (2-quinoxalinylmethylene)hydrazide, N^1,N^4-dioxide. *CAS-65884-46-0*. INN.

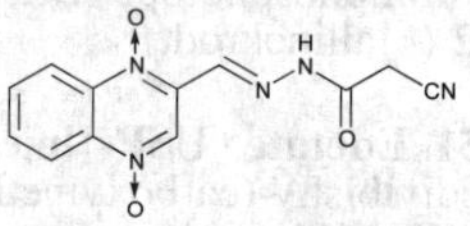

Ciaftalan Zinc. $C_{32}H_{16}N_8Zn$. 577.90. (*SP*-4-1)-[Phthalocyaninato(2-)-$N^{29},N^{30},N^{31},N^{32}$]zinc. *UNII-243KJ527MC. CAS-14320-04-8*. INN.

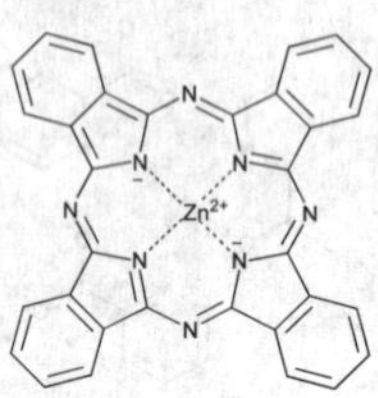

Ciamexon. $C_{11}H_{13}N_3O$. 203.24. (±)-1-[(2-Methoxy-6-methyl-3-pyridyl)methyl]-2-aziridinecarbonitrile. *UNII-325PG708LF. CAS-75985-31-8*. INN; BAN. ◇*BM 41.332*

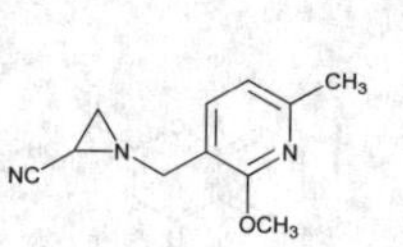

Cianergoline. $C_{19}H_{22}N_4O$. 322.40. (α-*RS*)-α-Cyano-6-methylergoline-8β-propionamide. *UNII-6337Z9RO7D. CAS-74627-35-3*. INN.

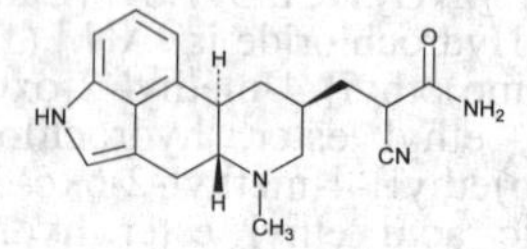

Cianidanol. $C_{15}H_{14}O_6$. 290.27. (+)-Catechol. *CAS-154-23-4*. INN; JAN.

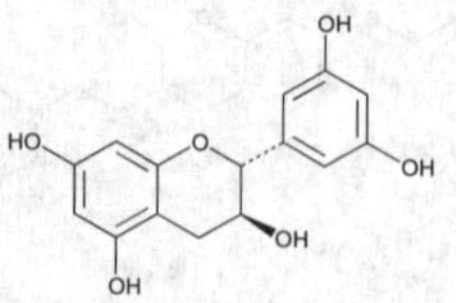

Cianidol — *See* Cianidanol.

Cianopramine. $C_{20}H_{23}N_3$. 305.42. 5-[3-(Dimethylamino)propyl]-10,11-dihydro-5*H*-dibenz[*b,f*]azepine-3-carbonitrile. *UNII-02MNR4P2PM. CAS-66834-24-0*. INN.

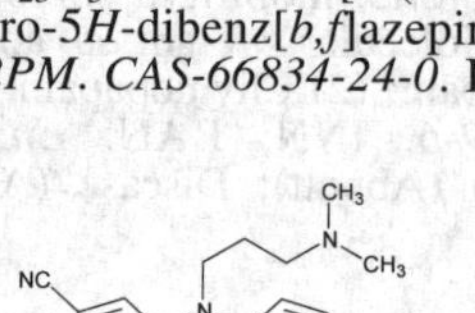

Ciapilome. $C_7H_6N_4O_2$. 178.15. *N*-(5-Cyano-4-oxo-1(4*H*)-pyrimidinyl)acetamide. *UNII-BX2MKR427K. CAS-53131-74-1*. INN.

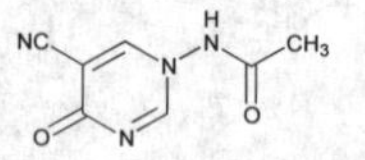

Cibenzoline (INN, BAN, and previously used name) — *See* Cifenline.

Cibenzoline Succinate (JAN) — *See* Cifenline.

Cicaprost. $C_{22}H_{30}O_5$. 374.47. [2-[(2*E*,3a*S*,4*S*,5*R*,6a*S*)-Hexahydro-5-hydroxy-4-[(3*S*,4*S*)-3-hydroxy-4-methyl-1,6-nonadiynyl]-2(1*H*)-pentalenylidene]ethoxy]acetic acid. *UNII-NE94J8CAMD. CAS-95722-07-9*. INN.

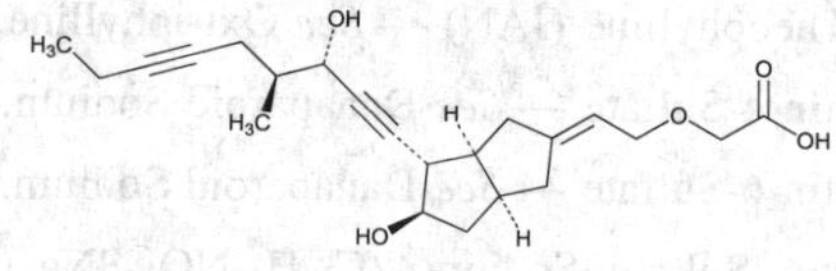

Cicarperone. $C_{20}H_{27}FN_2O_3$. 362.44. 4'-Fluoro-4-(octahydro-4-hydroxy-1(2*H*-quinolyl)butyrophenone carbamate (ester). *UNII-C65T2BG75L. CAS-54063-29-5*. INN.

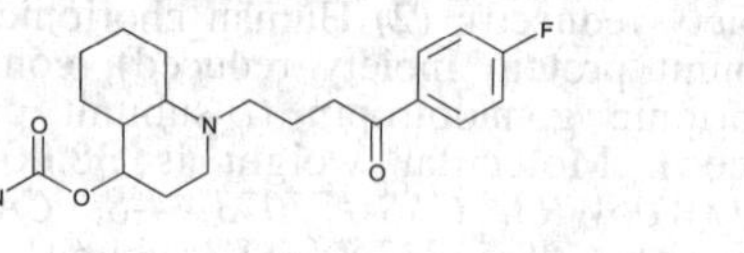

Ciclacillin (INN, BAN, JAN) — *See* Cyclacillin.

Ciclactate. $C_{12}H_{22}O_3$. 214.30. 3,3,5-Trimethylcyclohexyl lactate. *UNII-MYS6082G8G. CAS-15145-14-9*. INN.

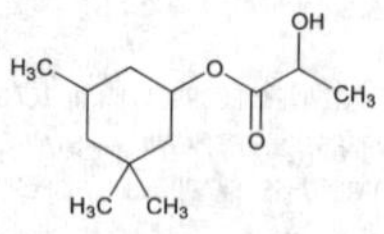

Ciclafrine Hydrochloride [*1975*] (sye klaf′ rin hye″ droe klor′ ide). $C_{15}H_{21}NO_2 \cdot HCl$. 283.79. [Ciclafrine is INN.] (1) Phenol, 3-(1-oxa-4-azaspiro[4.6]undec-2-yl)-, hydrochloride; (2) *m*-1-Oxa-4-azaspiro[4.6]undec-2-ylphenol hydrochloride. *UNII-E8MZK2U45W. CAS-51222-36-7; CAS-55694-98-9* [ciclafrine]. *Antihypotensive.* ◇*W 43026A; Go 3026A*

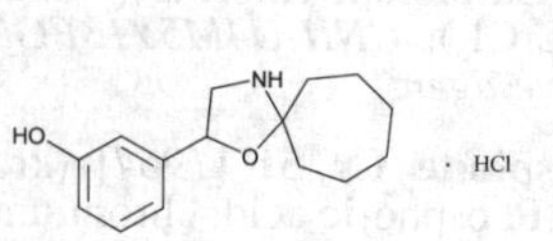

Ciclazindol [*1986*] (sye klaz′ in dol). $C_{17}H_{15}ClN_2O$. 298.77. (1) Pyrimido[1,2-*a*]indol-10-ol, 10-(3-chlorophenyl)-2,3,4,10-tetrahydro-; (2) 10-(*m*-Chlorophenyl)-2,3,4,10-

tetrahydropyrimido[1,2-*a*]indol-10-ol. *UNII-Y3I9520J7P. CAS-37751-39-6.* INN; BAN. *Antidepressant.* ◇WY-23,409

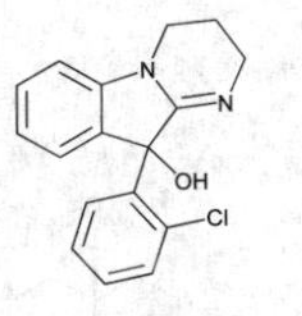

Ciclesonide [*2004*] (sye kles′ oh nide). $C_{32}H_{44}O_7$. 540.69. (1) Pregna-1,4-diene-3,20-dione, 16,17-[[(*R*)-cyclohexyl-methylene] bis(oxy)]-11-hydroxy-21-(2-methyl-1-oxopropoxy)-, (11β,16α); (2) 2*H*-Naphth [2′,1′:4,5] indeno [1,2-d][1,3] dioxole, pregna-1,4-diene-3,20-dione deriv. *UNII-S59502J185. CAS-126544-47-6; CAS-141845-82-1.* INN. *Treatment of asthma as prophylactic therapy in adults and adolescents.* Omnaris (Altana) ◇RPR251526

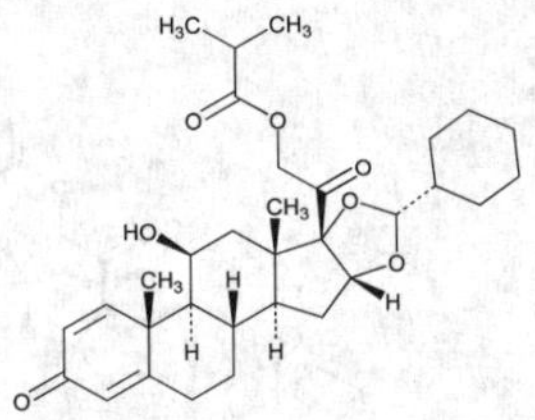

Cicletanine [*1990*] (sye klet′ a neen). $C_{14}H_{12}ClNO_2$. 261.70. (1) Furo[3,4-*c*]pyridin-7-ol, 3-(4-chlorophenyl)-1,3-dihydro-6-methyl-, (±)-; (2) (±)-3-(*p*-Chlorophenyl)-1,3-dihydro-6-methylfuro[3,4-*c*]pyridin-7-ol. *UNII-CHG7QC509W. CAS-89943-82-8; CAS-82747-56-6* [cicletanine hydrochloride]. INN; BAN. *Antihypertensive.* ◇(±)-BN-1270; Win 90,000

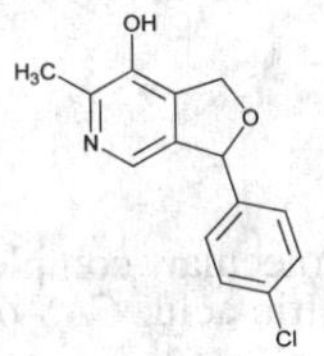

Ciclindole (INN) — *See* Cyclindole.

Cicliomenol. $C_{14}H_{19}IO$. 330.20. 2-Cyclohexyl-4-iodo-3,5-xylenol. *UNII-GYU56H6EBV. CAS-10572-34-6.* INN; DCF.

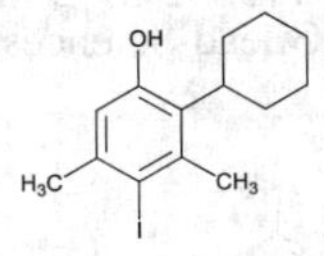

Ciclobendazole (INN and BAN) — *See* Cyclobendazole.

Ciclofenazine (INN) Hydrochloride — *See* Cyclophenazine Hydrochloride.

Cicloheximide (INN) — *See* Cycloheximide.

---

† Brand name formerly used, and/or firm no longer concerned with this product.

Ciclonicate. $C_{15}H_{21}NO_2$. 247.33. *trans*-3,3,5-Trimethylcyclohexyl nicotinate. *UNII-7H634NXI03. CAS-53449-58-4.* INN; MI.

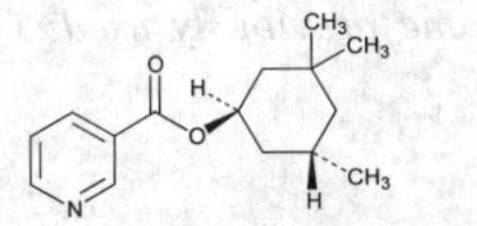

Ciclonium Bromide. $C_{22}H_{34}BrNO$. 408.42. Diethylmethyl{2-[(α-methyl-α-5-norbornen-2-ylbenzyl)oxy]ethyl} ammonium bromide. *CAS-29546-59-6.* INN. ◇Asta 3746

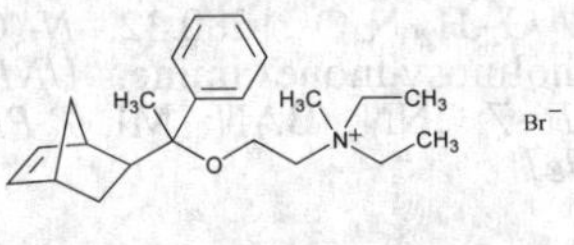

Ciclopirox [*1992*] (sye″ kloe pir′ ox). **USP.** $C_{12}H_{17}NO_2$. 207.27. (1) 2(1*H*)-Pyridinone, 6-cyclohexyl-1-hydroxy-4-methyl-; (2) 6-Cyclohexyl-1-hydroxy-4-methyl-2(1*H*)-pyridone. *UNII-19W019ZDRJ. CAS-29342-05-0.* INN; BAN. *Antifungal.* Loprox (Medicis) ◇HOE 296b

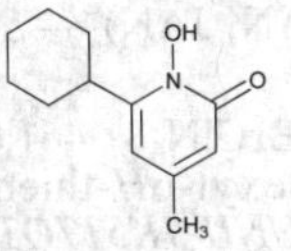

Ciclopirox Olamine [*1975*] (sye″ kloe pir′ ox ole′ a meen). **USP.** $C_{12}H_{17}NO_2 \cdot C_2H_7NO$. 268.35. (1) 2(1*H*)-Pyridinone, 6-cyclohexyl-1-hydroxy-4-methyl-, compound with 2-aminoethanol (1:1); (2) 6-Cyclohexyl-1-hydroxy-4-methyl-2(1*H*)-pyridone compound with 2-aminoethanol (1:1). *UNII-50MD4SB4AP. CAS-41621-49-2.* JAN. *Antifungal.* Loprox (Hoechst-Roussel) ◇HOE 296

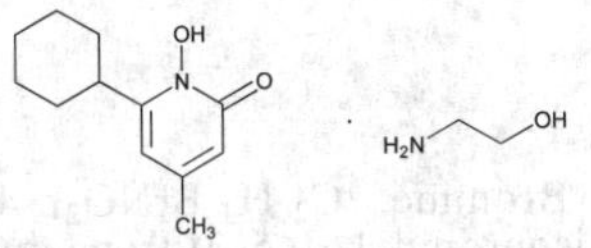

Ciclopramine. $C_{18}H_{20}N_2$. 264.36. 2,3,7,8-Tetrahydro-3-(methylamino)-1*H*-quino[1,8-*ab*][1]benzazepine. *UNII-BXS8X8APGS. CAS-33545-56-1.* INN.

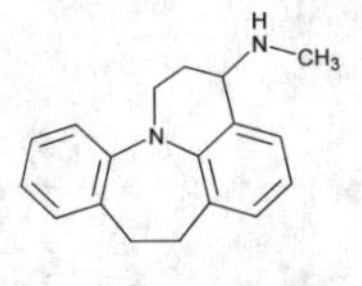

Cicloprofen [*1974*] (sye″ kloe proe′ fen). $C_{16}H_{14}O_2$. 238.28. (1) 9*H*-Fluorene-2-acetic acid, α-methyl-; (2) α-Methylfluorene-2-acetic acid. *CAS-36950-96-6.* INN; BAN. *Anti-inflammatory.* ◇SQ 20824

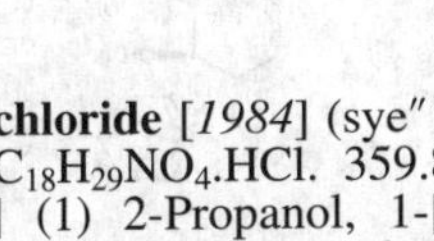

Cicloprolol Hydrochloride [*1984*] (sye″ kloe proe′ lol hye″ droe klor′ ide). $C_{18}H_{29}NO_4 \cdot HCl$. 359.89. [Cicloprolol is INN and BAN.] (1) 2-Propanol, 1-[4-[2-(cyclopropylmethoxy)ethoxy]phenoxy]-3-[(1-methylethyl)amino]-, hydrochloride, (±)-; (2) (±)-1-[*p*-[2-(Cyclopropylmethoxy)ethoxy]phenoxy]-3-(isopropylamino)-2-propanol hydrochloride. *UNII-1K2ACH4U3R* [cicloprolol]. *CAS-63686-79-3; CAS-63659-12-1* [cicloprolol]. *Anti-adrenergic (β-receptor). [Name previously used: Cycloprolol.]* ◇*SL 75 177-10*

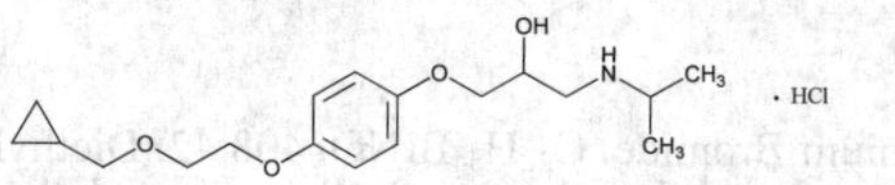

Ciclosidomine. $C_{13}H_{20}N_4O_3$. 280.32. *N*-(Cyclohexylcarbonyl)-3-morpholinosydnone imine. *UNII-S7P608OW2O. CAS-66564-16-7.* INN; BAN; MI. ◇*PR-G 138-CL [as hydrochloride]*

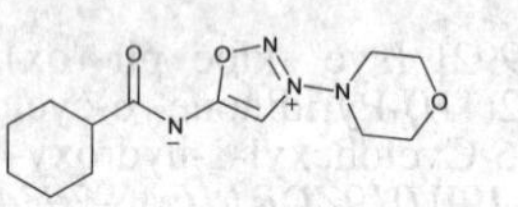

Ciclosporin (INN, BAN, JAN) — *See* Cyclosporine.

Ciclotizolam. $C_{20}H_{18}BrClN_4S$. 461.81. 2-Bromo-4-(*o*-chlorophenyl)-9-cyclohexyl-6*H*-thieno[3,2-*f*]-*s*-triazolo[4,3-*a*][1,4]diazepine. *UNII-JK517QTN4Q. CAS-58765-21-2.* INN; BAN. ◇*We 973-BS*

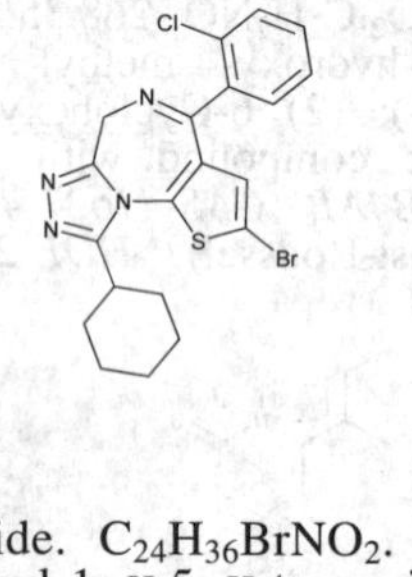

Ciclotropium Bromide. $C_{24}H_{36}BrNO_2$. 450.45. (8*r*)-3α-Hydroxy-8-isopropyl-1α*H*,5α*H*-tropanium bromide, α-phenylcyclopentaneacetate. *CAS-85166-20-7.* INN.

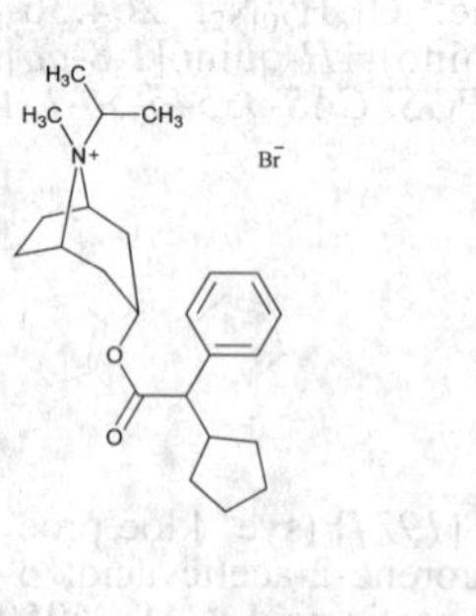

Cicloxilic Acid. $C_{13}H_{16}O_3$. 220.26. *cis*-2-Hydroxy-2-phenylcyclohexanecarboxylic acid. *UNII-18WJ167MZN. CAS-57808-63-6.* INN.

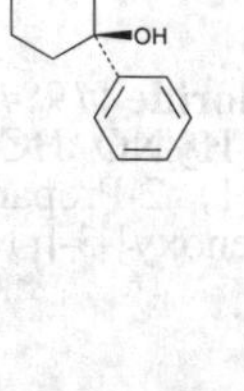

Cicloxolone. $C_{38}H_{56}O_7$. 624.85. 3β-Hydroxy-11-oxoolean-12-en-30-oic acid hydrogen *cis*-1,2-cyclohexanedicarboxylate. *UNII-3F85I03NLO. CAS-52247-86-6.* INN; BAN. ◇*BX 363A [as disodium salt]*

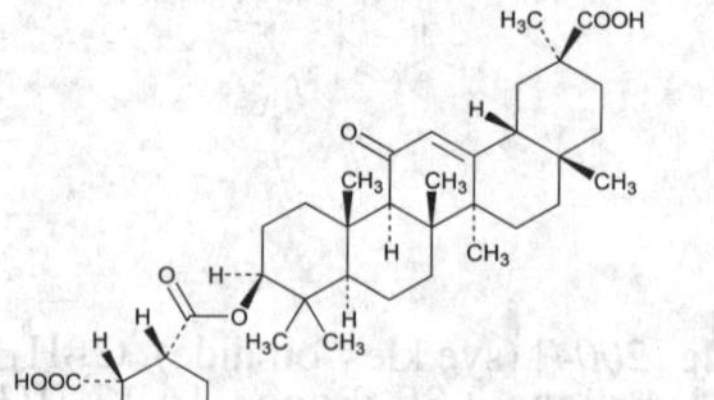

Cicortonide. $C_{29}H_{37}ClFNO_7$. 566.06. 3-(2-Chloroethoxy)-9-fluoro-11β,16α,17,21-tetrahydroxy-20-oxopregna-3,5-diene-6-carbonitrile, cyclic 16,17-acetal with acetone, 21-acetate. *UNII-UL947A614K. CAS-19705-61-4.* INN.

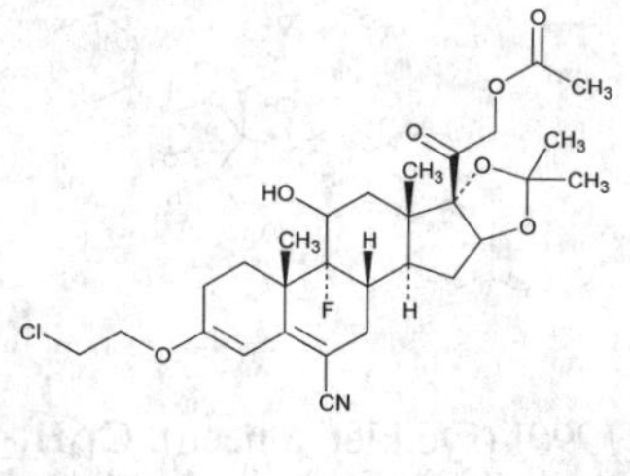

Cicrotoic Acid. $C_{10}H_{16}O_2$. 168.23. β-Methylcyclohexaneacrylic acid. *CAS-25229-42-9.* INN; DCF; MI. ◇*AD 106*

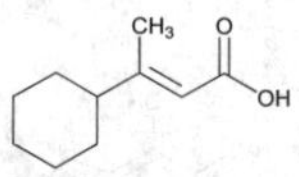

Cideferron. Macromolecular complex of ferric hydroxide with dextrin and citric acid. *CAS-64440-87-5.* INN; JAN.

Cidofovir [*1994*] (sye dof' oh vir). $C_8H_{14}N_3O_6P.2H_2O$. 315.22. (1) Phosphonic acid, [[2-(4-amino-2-oxo-1(2*H*)-pyrimidinyl)-1-(hydroxymethyl)ethoxy]methyl]-, dihydrate, (*S*)-; (2) [[(*S*)-2-(4-Amino-2-oxo-1(2*H*)-pyrimidinyl)-1-(hydroxymethyl)ethoxy]methyl]phosphonic acid, dihydrate; (3) 1-[(*S*)-3-Hydroxy-2-(phosphonomethoxy)propyl]cytosine dihydrate. *UNII-JIL713Q00N. CAS-149394-66-1; CAS-113852-37-2* [anhydrous]. INN; BAN. *Antiviral.* Vistide (Gilead Sciences) ◇*GS-0504*

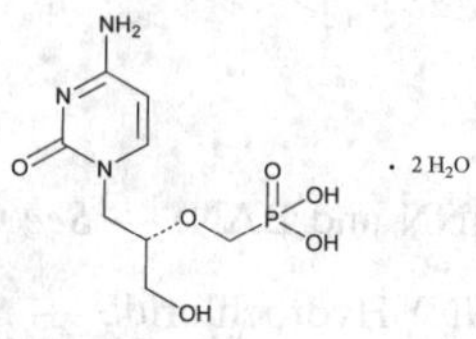

Cidoxepin Hydrochloride [*1967*] (sye dox' e pin hye″ droe klor' ide). $C_{19}H_{21}NO.HCl$. 315.84. [Cidoxepin is INN.] (1) 1-Propanamine, 3-dibenz[*b,e*]oxepin-11(6*H*)-ylidene-*N,N*-dimethyl-, hydrochloride, (*Z*)-; (2) (*Z*)-*N,N*-Dimethyldibenz[*b,e*]oxepin-Δ$^{11(6H),\gamma}$-propylamine hydrochloride.

UNII-XI27WMG8QK; UNII-F96TTB8728 [cidoxepin]. *CAS-25127-31-5; CAS-3607-18-9* [cidoxepin]. *Antidepressant.* ◇*P-4599*

Cifenline [*1981*] (sye fen′ leen). $C_{18}H_{18}N_2$. 262.35. [Cibenzoline is INN and BAN; Cibenzoline Succinate is JAN.] (1) 1*H*-Imidazole, 2-(2,2-diphenylcyclopropyl)-4,5-dihydro-, (±)-; (2) (±)-2-(2,2-Diphenylcyclopropyl)-2-imidazoline. *CAS-53267-01-9. Cardiac depressant (anti-arrhythmic). [Name previously used: Cibenzoline.]* ◇*Ro 22-7796*

Cifenline Succinate [*1987*] (sye fen′ leen sux′ i nate). $C_{18}H_{18}N_2.C_4H_6O_4$. 380.44. [Cibenzoline is BAN.] (1) 1*H*-Imidazole, 2-(2,2-diphenylcyclopropyl)-4,5-dihydro-, (±)-, butanedioate (1:1); (2) (±)-2-(2,2-Diphenylcyclopropyl)-2-imidazoline succinate (1:1). *CAS-100678-32-8. Cardiac depressant (anti-arrhythmic).* ◇*Ro 22-7796/001*

Cifostodine. $C_9H_{12}N_3O_7P$. 305.18. Cytidine cyclic 2′,3′-(hydrogen phosphate). *UNII-74B4VJV0WV. CAS-633-90-9.* INN.

Ciglitazone [*1983*] (sye gli′ ta zone). $C_{18}H_{23}NO_3S$. 333.45. (1) 2,4-Thiazolidinedione, 5-[[4-[(1-methylcyclohexyl)methoxy]phenyl]methyl]-, (±)-; (2) (±)-5-[p-[(1-Methylcyclohexyl)methoxy]benzyl]-2,4-thiazolidinedione. *UNII-U8QXS1WU8G. CAS-74772-77-3.* INN. *Antidiabetic.* ◇*ADD-3878; U-63287*

Ciheptolane. $C_{20}H_{23}NO_2$. 309.40. 10,11-Dihydro-*N,N*-dimethylspiro[5*H*-dibenzo[*a,d*]cycloheptene-5,2′-[1,3]dioxolane]-4′-methylamine. *UNII-NLD2X0VD2U. CAS-34753-46-3.* INN.

Ciladopa Hydrochloride [*1984*] (sye″ la doe′ pa hye″ droe klor′ ide). $C_{21}H_{26}N_2O_4.HCl$. 406.90. [Ciladopa is INN and BAN.] (1) 2,4,6-Cycloheptatrien-1-one, 2-[4-[2-(3,4-dimethoxyphenyl)-2-hydroxyethyl]-1-piperazinyl]-, monohydrochloride, (*S*)-; (2) (-)-(*S*)-2-[4-(β-Hydroxy-3,4-dimethoxyphenethyl)-1-piperazinyl]-2,4,6-cycloheptatrien-1-one monohydrochloride. *UNII-D09L486R3J* [ciladopa]. *CAS-83529-09-3; CAS-80109-27-9* [ciladopa]. *Antiparkinsonian; dopaminergic agent.* Tremerase (Wyeth-Ayerst) ◇*AY-27,110*

Cilansetron [*2005*] (sye lan′ se tron). $C_{20}H_{21}N_3O$. 319.40. (1) 4*H*-Pyrido[3,2,1-jk] carbazol-11 (8*H*)-one, 5,6,9,10-tetrahydro-10-[(2-methyl-1*H*-imidazol-1-yl) methyl]-, (10*R*)-; (2) (10*R*)-5,6,9,10-Tetrahydro-10[(2-methylimidazol-1-yl)methyl]-4*H*-pyrido[3,2,1-jk]carbazol-11(8*H*)-one. *UNII-2J6DQ1U5B5. CAS-120635-74-7.* INN. *Treatment of irritable bowel syndrome.* ◇*KC-9946*

Cilansetron Hydrochloride [*2005*] (sye lan′ se tron hye″ droe klor′ ide). $C_{20}H_{21}N_3O.HCl.H_2O$. 373.88. (1) 4*H*-Pyrido[3,2,1-jk] carbazol-11-(8*H*)-one, 5,6,9,10-tetrahydro-10-[(2-methyl-1*H*-imidazol-1-yl) methyl]-, monohydrochloride monohydrate (10*R*)-; (2) (10*R*)-5,6,9,10-Tetrahydro-10[(2-methylimidazol-1-yl)methyl)-4*H*-pyrido[3,2,1-jk]carbazol-11(8*H*)-one monohydrochloride, monohydrate. *UNII-40JL785VD0. CAS-209859-87-0; CAS-120635-74-7* [cilansetron]. *Treatment of Irritable Bowel Syndrome (IBS) with diarrhea predominance.* ◇*DU123265; KC-9946*

Cilastatin Sodium [*1984*] (sye″ la stat′ in soe′ dee um). **USP**. $C_{16}H_{25}N_2NaO_5S$. 380.43. [Cilastatin is INN and BAN.] (1) 2-Heptenoic acid, 7-[(2-amino-2-carboxyethyl)thio]-2-[[(2,2-dimethylcyclopropyl)carbonyl]amino]-, monosodium salt, [*R*-[*R*,S*-(Z)*]]-; (2) Sodium (*Z*)-7-[[(*R*)-2-amino-2-carboxyethyl]thio]-2-[(*S*)-2,2-dimethylcyclopropanecarboxamido]-2-heptenoate. *UNII-5428WXZ74M; UNII-141A6AMN38* [cilastatin]. *CAS-81129-83-1; CAS-82009-34-5* [cilastatin]. JAN. *Enzyme inhibitor.* ◇*MK-791*

Cilazapril [*1986*] (sye laz′ a pril). $C_{22}H_{31}N_3O_5 \cdot H_2O$. 435.51. (1) 6*H*-Pyridazino[1,2-*a*][1,2]diazepine-1-carboxylic acid, 9-[[1-(ethoxycarbonyl)-3-phenylpropyl]amino]octahydro-10-oxo-, monohydrate, [1*S*-[1α,9α(*R**)]]-; (2) (1*S*,9*S*)-9-[[(*S*)-1-Carboxy-3-phenylpropyl]amino]octahydro-10-oxo-6*H*-pyridazino[1,2-*a*][1,2]diazepine-1-carboxylic acid 9-ethyl ester monohydrate. *UNII-19KW7PI29F. CAS-92077-78-6; CAS-88768-40-5* [anhydrous]. INN; BAN; JAN. *Antihypertensive.* Inhibace (Hoffmann-LaRoche) ◇*Ro 31-2848/006*

Cilazaprilat. $C_{20}H_{27}N_3O_5$. 389.45. *N*-[(1*S*,9*S*)-1-Carboxy-10-oxoperhydropyridazino-[1,2-α][1,2]diazepin-9-yl]-4-phenyl-L-homoalanine. *UNII-WBL76FH528. CAS-90139-06-3.* INN; BAN. ◇*Ro 31-3113*

Cilengitide [*2001*] (sye len′ ji tide). $C_{27}H_{40}N_8O_7$. 588.66. Cyclo(L-arginylglycyl-L-α-aspartyl-D-phenylalanyl-*N*-methyl-L-valyl). *CAS-188968-51-6.* INN. *Angiogenesis inhibitor.*

Cilexetil [*1995*] (sye lex′ e til). $C_9H_{15}O_3$. 171.21. 1-[[(Cyclohexyloxy)carbonyl]oxy]ethyl. INN. *[Note—The radical designation, cilexetil, has been used in conjunction with sanfetrinem.]*

Cilmostim [*1996*] (sil′ moe stim). $C_{2198}H_{3424}N_{588}O_{704}S_{28}$ (protein moiety). 74kD–97kD (ca., determined by SDS-PAGE). (1) 1-223-Colony-stimulating factor 1 (human clone p3ACSF-69 protein moiety), cyclic (7→90), (48→139), (102→146)-tris(disulfide) dimer, cyclic (31→31′), (157→157′), (159→159′)-tris(disulfide); (2) 1-223-Colony-stimulating factor 1 (human clone p3ACSF-69 protein moiety), dimer, cyclic (7→90), (7′→90′), (31→31′), (48→139), (48′→139′), (102→146), (102′→146′), (157→157′), (159→159′)-nonakis(disulfide). *CAS-148637-05-2.* INN. *Hematopoietic (macrophage colony-stimulating factor).* Macstim (Genetics Institute) *[Names previously used: rhM-CSF, M-CSF, and CSF-1.]*

EEVSEYCSHM	IGSGHLQSLQ	RLIDSQMETS	CQITFEFVDQ	EQLKDPVCYL
KKAFLLVQDI	MEDTMRFRDN	TPNAIAIVQL	QELSLRLKSC	FTKDYEEHDK
ACVRTFYETP	LQLLEKVKNV	FNETKNLLDK	DWNIFSKNCN	NSFAECSSQD
VVTKPDCNCL	YPKAIPSSDP	ASVSPHQPLA	PSMAPVAGLT	WEDSEGTEGS
SLLPGEQPLH	TVDPGSAKQR	PPR		

(subscript 2)

Cilnidipine. $C_{27}H_{28}N_2O_7$. 492.52. (±)-(*E*)-Cinnamyl 2-methoxyethyl 1,4-dihydro-2,6-dimethyl-4-(*m*-nitrophenyl)-3,5-pyridinedicarboxylate. *UNII-97T5AZ1JIP. CAS-132203-70-4.* INN.

Cilobamine Mesylate [*1981*] (sye loe′ ba meen mes′ i late). $C_{17}H_{23}Cl_2NO \cdot CH_4O_3S$. 424.38. [Cilobamine is INN.] (1) Bicyclo[2.2.2]octan-2-ol, 2-(3,4-dichlorophenyl)-3-[(1-methylethyl)amino]-, *cis*-, methanesulfonate (salt); (2) *cis*-2-(3,4-Dichlorophenyl)-3-(isopropylamino)bicyclo[2.2.2]octan-2-ol methanesulfonate (salt). *UNII-SZ83PVQ06I. CAS-69429-85-2; CAS-69429-84-1* [cilobamine]. *Antidepressant. [Name previously used: Clobamine Mesylate.]* ◇*RMI 81,182EF*

Cilobradine. $C_{28}H_{38}N_2O_5$. 482.61. (+)-(*S*)-3-[[1-(3,4-Dimethoxyphenethyl)-3-piperidyl]methyl]-1,3,4,5-tetrahydro-7,8-dimethoxy-2*H*-3-benzazepin-2-one. INN.

Cilofungin [*1989*] (sye″ loe fun′ jin). $C_{49}H_{71}N_7O_{17}$. 1030.12. (1) Echinocandin B, 1-[(4*R*,5*R*)-4,5-dihydroxy-*N*²-[4-(octyloxy)benzoyl]-L-ornithine]-; (2) 1-[(4*R*,5*R*)-4,5-Dihydroxy-*N*²-[*p*-(octyloxy)benzoyl]-L-ornithine]echinocandin B; (3) (4*R*,5*R*)-4,5-Dihydroxy-*N*²-[*p*-(octyloxy)benzoyl]-L-ornithyl-L-threonyl-*trans*-4-hydroxy-L-prolyl-(*S*)-4-hydroxy-4-(*p*-hydroxyphenyl)-L-threonyl-L-threonyl-(3*S*,4*S*)-3-hydroxy-4-methyl-L-proline cyclic (6→1)-peptide. *CAS-79404-91-4*. INN. *Antifungal*. *✧LY121019*

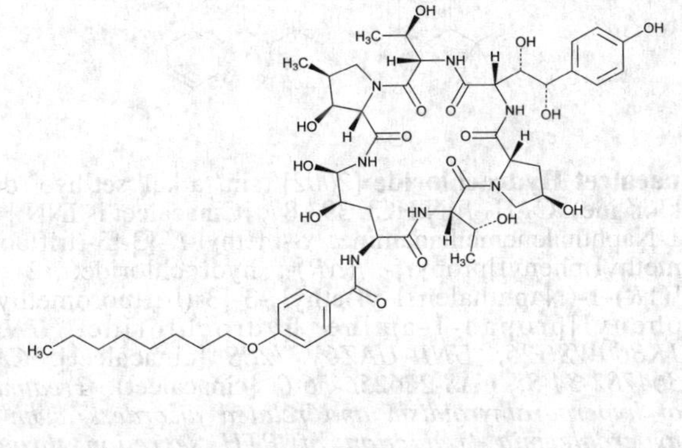

Cilomilast [*1999*] (sye loe′ mi last). $C_{20}H_{25}NO_4$. 343.42. *cis*-4-Cyano-4-[3-(cyclopentyloxy)-4-methoxyphenyl]cyclohexanecarboxylic acid. *CAS-153259-65-5*. INN. *Treatment of asthma, COPD, arthritis, atopic dermatitis, and multiple sclerosis (phosphodiesterase IV inhibitor)*. *✧SB 207499*

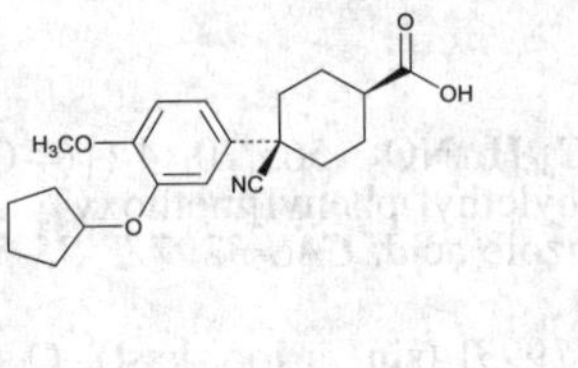

Ciloprost — *See* Iloprost.

Cilostamide. $C_{20}H_{26}N_2O_3$. 342.43. *N*-Cyclohexyl-4-[(1,2-dihydro-2-oxo-6-quinolyl)oxy]-*N*-methylbutyramide. *UNII-45S5605Q18*. *CAS-68550-75-4*. INN.

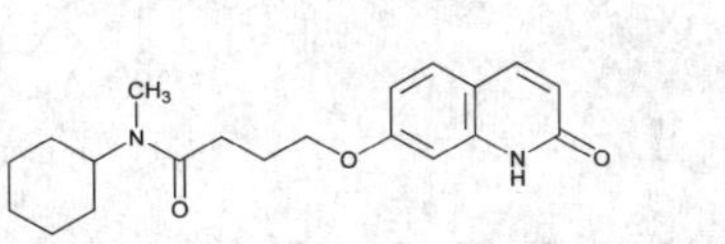

Cilostazol [*1997*] (sye loe′ sta zol). **USP**. $C_{20}H_{27}N_5O_2$. 369.46. (1) 2(1*H*)-Quinolinone, 6-[4-(1-cyclohexyl-1*H*-tetrazol-5-yl)butoxy]-3,4-dihydro-; (2) 6-[4-(1-Cyclohexyl-1*H*-tetrazol-5-yl)butoxy]-3,4-dihydrocarbostyril. *UNII-N7Z035406B*. *CAS-73963-72-1*. INN; BAN; JAN. *Vasodilator; inhibitor (platelet); antithrombotic*. Pletal (Otsuka) *✧OPC-13013; OPC-21*

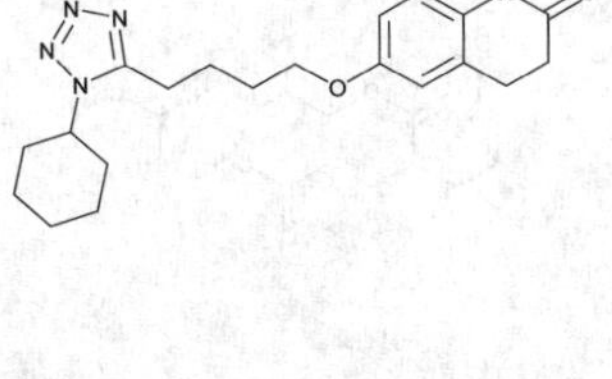

† Brand name formerly used, and/or firm no longer concerned with this product.

Ciltoprazine. $C_{23}H_{29}ClN_4O_3$. 444.95. 1-(5-Chloro-2-methoxybenzoyl)-3-[3-(4-*m*-tolyl-1-piperazinyl)propyl]urea. *UNII-91G29CI904*. *CAS-54063-30-8*. INN.

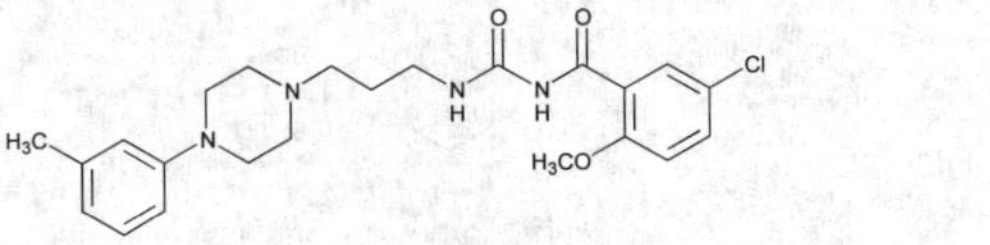

Ciluprevir [*2004*] (sye loo′ pre vir). $C_{40}H_{50}N_6O_8S$. 774.93. (1) Cyclopropa[*e*]pyrrolo[1,2-*a*][1,4]diazacyclopentadecine-14a(5*H*)-carboxylic acid, 6-[[(cyclopentyloxy)carbonyl]amino]-1,2,3,6,7,8,9,10,11,13a,14,15,16,16a-tetradecahydro-2-[[7-methoxy-2-[2-[(1-methylethyl)amino]-4-thiazolyl]-4-quinolinyl]oxy]-5,16-dioxo-, (2*R*,6*S*,12*Z*,13a*S*,14a*R*,16a*S*)-; (2) (2*R*,6*S*,12*Z*,13a*S*,14a*R*,16a*S*)-6-[[(Cyclopentyloxy)carbonyl]amino]-2-[[7-methoxy-2-[2-[(1-methylethyl)amino]thiazol-4-yl]quinolin-4-yl]oxy]-5,16-dioxo-1,2,3,6,7,8,9,10,11,13a,14,15,16,16a-tetradecahydrocyclopropa[*e*]pyrrolo[1,2-*a*][1,4]diazacyclopentadecine-14a(5*H*)-carboxylic acid. *UNII-75C8DU40T0*. *CAS-300832-84-2*. INN. *Treatment of Hepatitis C infection*. *✧BILN 2061 ZW*

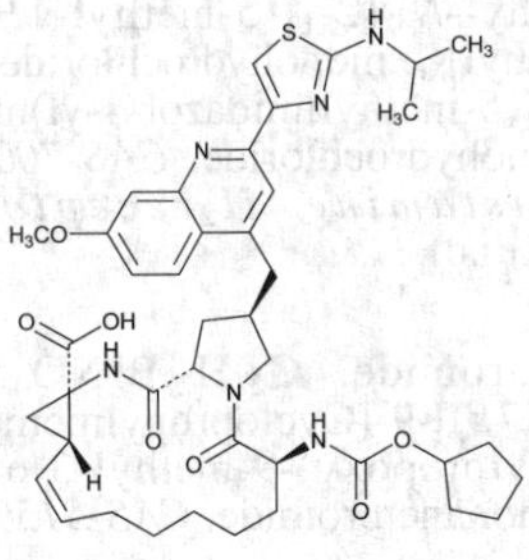

Cilutazoline. $C_{14}H_{18}N_2O$. 230.31. 2-[[(6-Cyclopropyl-*m*-tolyl)oxy]methyl]-2-imidazoline. *UNII-ZL910H358R*. *CAS-104902-08-1*. INN.

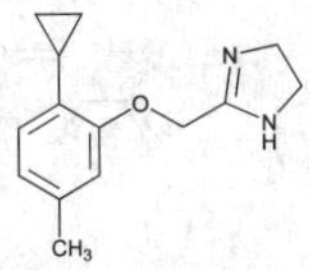

Cimaterol [*1986*] (sye ma′ ter ol). $C_{12}H_{17}N_3O$. 219.28. (1) Benzonitrile, 2-amino-5-[1-hydroxy-2-[(1-methylethyl)amino]ethyl]-, (±)-; (2) (±)-5-[1-Hydroxy-2-(isopropylamino)ethyl]anthranilonitrile. *UNII-ZPY8VRF0GB*. *CAS-54239-37-1*. INN. *Repartitioning agent*. *✧AC 263,780; AB-A 663*

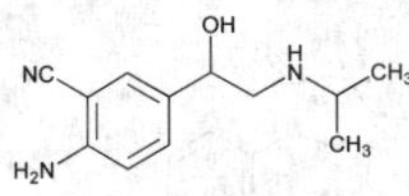

Cimemoxin. $C_7H_{16}N_2$. 128.22. (Cyclohexylmethyl)hydrazine. *UNII-584QS921R2*. *CAS-3788-16-7*. INN; DCF. *✧SD 286-03*

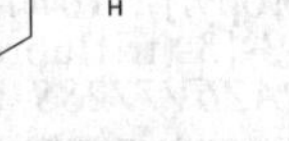

Cimepanol. $C_{10}H_{20}O$. 156.27. α-Isopropylcyclohexanemethanol. *UNII-1R7T67JP3G. CAS-29474-12-2.* INN.

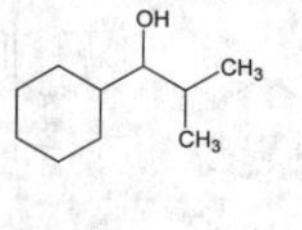

Cimetidine [*1975*] (sye me′ ti deen). **USP.** $C_{10}H_{16}N_6S$. 252.34. (1) Guanidine, N''-cyano-N-methyl-N'-[2-[[(5-methyl-1H-imidazol-4-yl)methyl]thio]ethyl]-; (2) 2-Cyano-1-methyl-3-[2-[[(5-methylimidazol-4-yl)-methyl]thio]ethyl]guanidine. *CAS-51481-61-9.* INN; BAN; JAN. *Antagonist (to histamine H_2receptors).* Tagamet (GlaxoSmithKline)

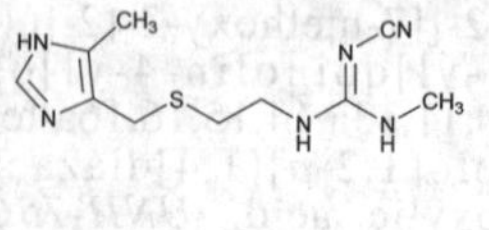

Cimetidine Hydrochloride [*1987*] (sye me′ ti deen hye″ droe klor′ ide). **USP.** $C_{10}H_{16}N_6S.HCl$. 288.80. (1) Guanidine, N''-cyano-N-methyl-N'-[2-[[(5-methyl-1H-imidazol-4-yl)-methyl]thio]ethyl]-, monohydrochloride; (2) 2-Cyano-1-methyl-3-[2-[[(5-methylimidazol-4-yl)methyl]thio]ethyl]-guanidine monohydrochloride. *CAS-70059-30-2. Antagonist (to histamine H_2receptors).* Tagamet (GlaxoSmithKline)

Cimetropium Bromide. $C_{21}H_{28}BrNO_4$. 438.36. [7(S)-(1α,2β,4β,5α,7β)]-9-(Cyclopropylmethyl)-7-(3-hydroxy-1-oxo-2-phenylpropoxy)-9-methyl-3-oxa-9-azoniatricyclo[3.3.1.0^{2,4}]nonane bromide. *CAS-51598-60-8.* INN; MI.

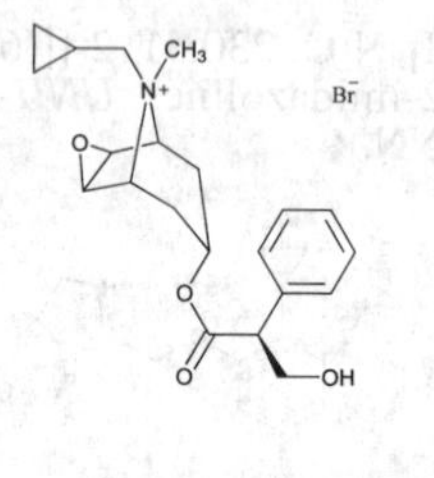

Cimicoxib. $C_{16}H_{13}ClFN_3O_3S$. 381.81. 4-[4-Chloro-5-(3-fluoro-4-methoxyphenyl)-1H-imidazol-1-yl]benzenesulfonamide. *UNII-W7FHJ107MC. CAS-265114-23-6.* INN.

Cimoxatone. $C_{19}H_{18}N_2O_4$. 338.36. α-[p-[5-(Methoxymethyl)-2-oxo-3-oxazolidinyl]phenoxy]-m-tolunitrile. *CAS-73815-11-9.* INN.

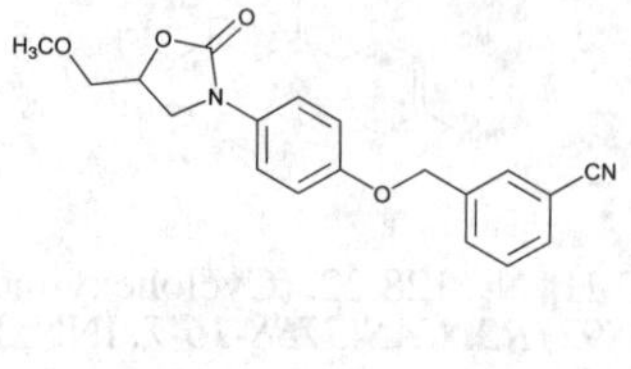

Cinacalcet [*2004*] (sin″ a kal′ set). $C_{22}H_{22}F_3N$. 357.41. (1) 1-Naphthalenemethanamine, α-methyl-N-[3-[3-(trifluoromethyl)phenyl]propyl]-, (αR)-; (2) N-[(1R)-1-(Naphthalen-1-yl)ethyl]-3-[3-(trifluoromethyl)phenyl]propan-1-amine. *UNII-UAZ6V7728S. CAS-226256-56-0.* BAN. *Treatment of hyperparathyroidism and related disorders,*

such as hypercalcemia (reduction of PTH secretion through modulation of calcium ion receptors on parathyroid cells). Sensipar (Amgen) ◇*AMG073*

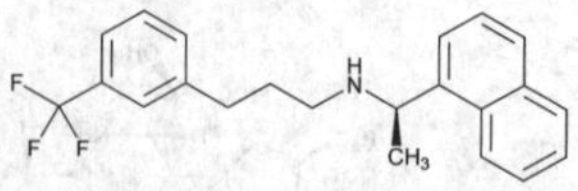

Cinacalcet Hydrochloride [*2002*] (sin″ a kal′ set hye″ droe klor′ ide). $C_{22}H_{22}F_3N.HCl$. 393.87. [Cinacalcet is INN.] (1) 1-Naphthalenemethanamine, α-methyl-N-[3-[3-(trifluoromethyl)phenyl]propyl]-, (αR)-, hydrochloride; (2) N-[(1R)-1-(Naphthalen-1-yl)ethyl]-3-[3-(trifluoromethyl)-phenyl]propan-1-amine hydrochloride. *UNII-1K860WSG25; UNII-UAZ6V7728S* [cinacalcet]. *CAS-364782-34-3; CAS-226256-56-0* [cinacalcet]. *Treatment of hyperparathyroidism and related disorders, such as hypercalcemia (reduction of PTH secretion through modulation of calcium ion receptors on parathyroid cells).* Sensipar (Amgen) ◇*AMG073 HCl*

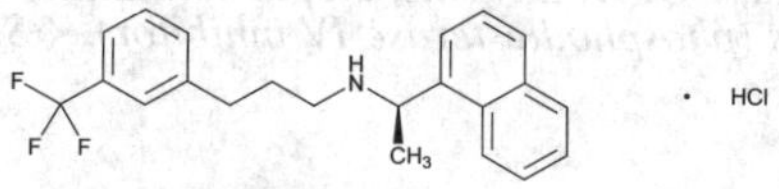

Cinaciguat. $C_{36}H_{39}NO_5$. 565.70. 4-({{(4-Carboxybutyl)[2-(2-{[4-(2-phenylethyl)phenyl]methoxy}phenyl)ethyl]amino}-methyl)benzoic acid. *CAS-329773-35-5.* INN.

Cinalukast [*1993*] (sin″ a loo′ kast). $C_{23}H_{28}N_2O_3S$. 412.55. (1) Butanoic acid, 4-[[3-[2-(4-cyclobutyl-2-thiazolyl)ethenyl]phenyl]amino]-2,2-diethyl-4-oxo-, (E)-; (2) 3′-[(E)-2-(4-Cyclobutyl-2-thiazolyl)vinyl]-2,2-diethylsuccinanilic acid. *CAS-128312-51-6.* INN. *Anti-asthmatic (leukotriene antagonist).* ◇*Ro 24-5913*

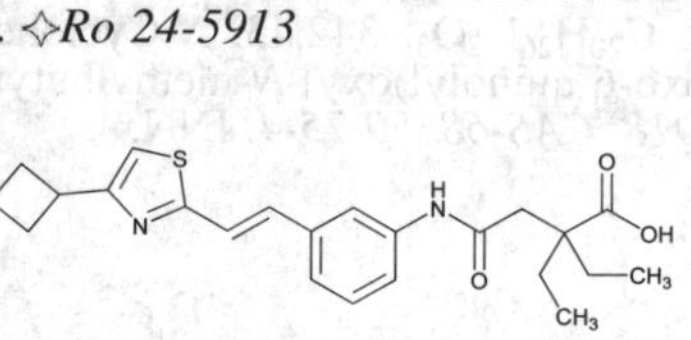

Cinametic Acid. $C_{12}H_{14}O_5$. 238.24. 4-(2-Hydroxyethoxy)-3-methoxycinnamic acid. *UNII-3E3106052Y. CAS-35703-32-3.* INN; DCF; MI.

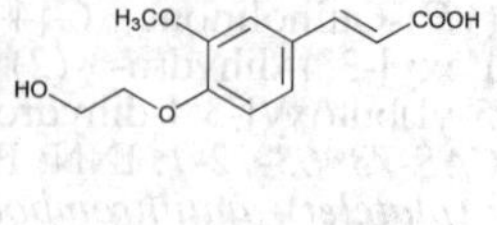

Cinamolol. $C_{16}H_{23}NO_4$. 293.36. Methyl (E)-o-[2-hydroxy-3-(isopropylamino)propoxy]cinnamate. *UNII-7531Q8398Y. CAS-39099-98-4.* INN.

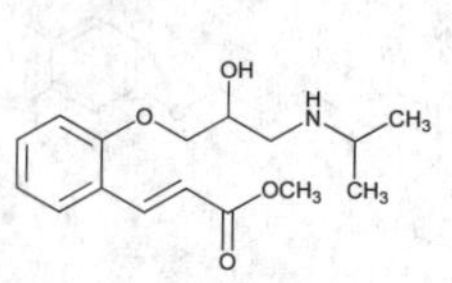

Cinanserin Hydrochloride [*1966*] (sin an′ ser in hye″ droe klor′ ide). $C_{20}H_{24}N_2OS.HCl$. 376.94. [Cinanserin is INN.] (1) 2-Propenamide, N-[2-[[3-(dimethylamino)propyl]thio]-phenyl]-3-phenyl-, monohydrochloride; (2) 2′-[[3-(Dimethylamino)propyl]thio]cinnamanilide monohydrochloride. *CAS-54-84-2; CAS-1166-34-3* [cinanserin]. *Serotonin inhibitor. ✧SQ 10,643; NSC-125717*

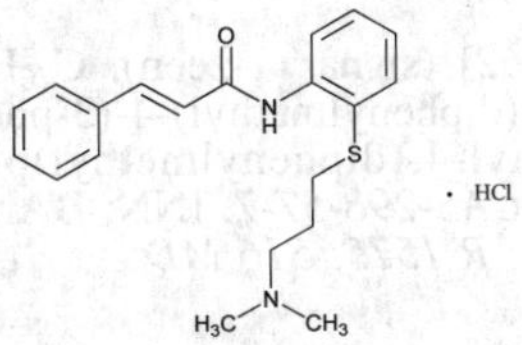

Cinaproxen. $C_{19}H_{21}NO_5S$. 375.44. *N*-Acetyl-L-cysteine (+)-(*S*)-6-methoxy-α-methyl-2-naphthaleneacetate (ester). *UNII-1J0E0I69E9. CAS-89163-44-0.* INN.

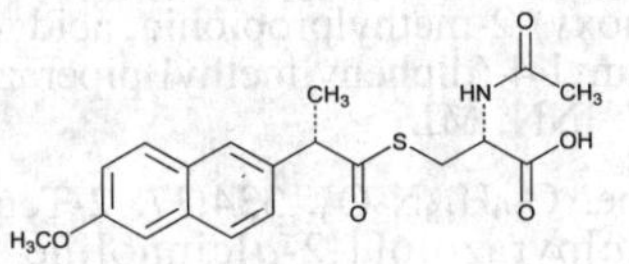

Cincaine Chloride — *See* Dibucaine Hydrochloride.

Cinchocaine (INN, BAN) — *See* Dibucaine.

Cinchonidine Sulfate. Cinchonidine sulfate (2:1). NF IX; MI.

Cinchonine Sulfate. *UNII-342JR840KF. CAS-5949-16-6; CAS-118-10-5* [cinchonine]. NF IX; MI.

Cinchophen. $C_{16}H_{11}NO_2$. 249.26. 2-Phenylcinchoninic acid. *CAS-132-60-5.* NF X; INN; BAN; MI. *[Name previously used: Phenylcinchoninic Acid.]*

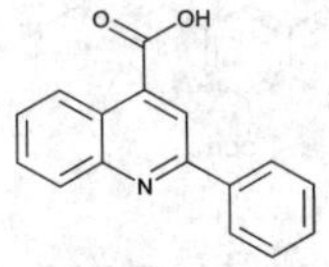

Cinecromen. $C_{34}H_{41}N_3O_{10}$. 651.70. 3,4,5-Trimethoxycinnamic acid ester with 3-(2-hydroxy-3-morpholinopropyl)-4-methyl-7-(4-morpholinecarboxamido)coumarin. *CAS-62380-23-8.* INN.

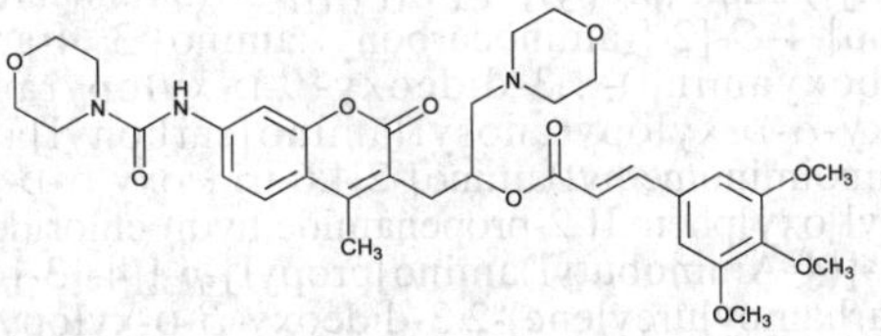

† Brand name formerly used, and/or firm no longer concerned with this product.

Cinepaxadil. $C_{29}H_{36}N_2O_9$. 556.60. α-[[(8-Acetyl-1,4-benzodioxan-5-yl)oxy]methyl]-4-(3,4,5-trimethoxycinnamoyl)-1-piperazineethanol. *CAS-69118-25-8.* INN.

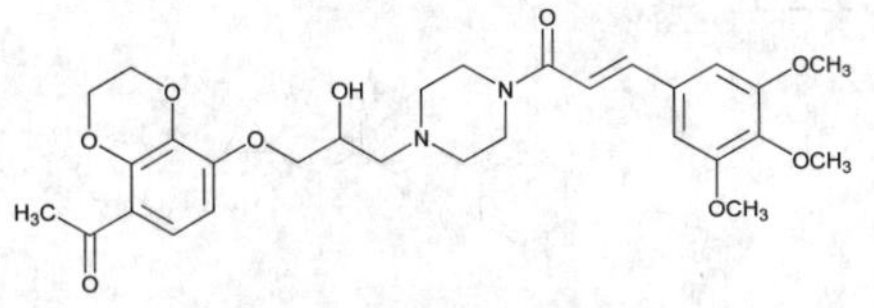

Cinepazet Maleate [*1975*] (sin″ e paz′ et mal′ ee ate). $C_{20}H_{28}N_2O_6.C_4H_4O_4$. 508.52. [Cinepazet is INN and BAN.] (1) 1-Piperazineacetic acid, 4-[1-oxo-3-(3,4,5-trimethoxyphenyl)-2-propenyl]-, ethyl ester, (*Z*)-2-butenedioate (1:1); (2) Ethyl 4-(3,4,5-trimethoxycinnamoyl)-1-piperazineacetate maleate (1:1). *CAS-50679-07-7; CAS-23887-41-4* [cinepazet]. *Anti-anginal.*

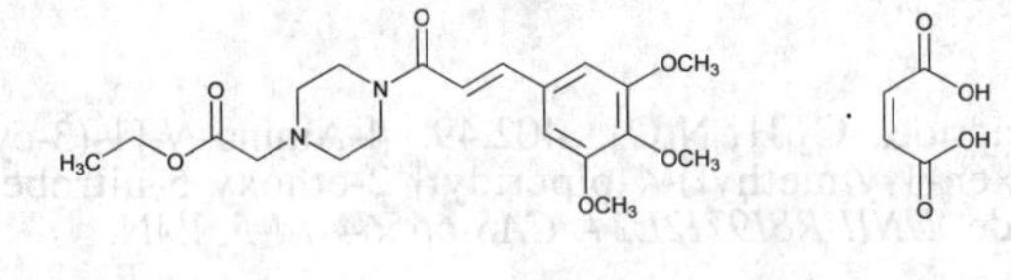

Cinepazic Acid. $C_{18}H_{24}N_2O_6$. 364.39. 4-(3,4,5-Trimethoxycinnamoyl)-1-piperazineacetic acid. *CAS-54063-23-9.* INN.

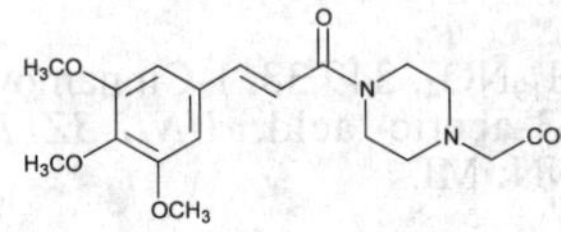

Cinepazide. $C_{22}H_{31}N_3O_5$. 417.50. [Cinepazide Maleate is JAN.] 1-[(1-Pyrrolidinylcarbonyl)methyl]-4-(3,4,5-trimethoxycinnamoyl)piperazine. *CAS-23887-46-9.* INN; BAN; DCF; MI. *✧MD 67350 [as maleate]*

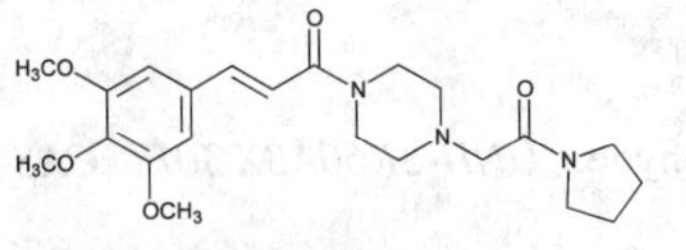

Cinfenine. $C_{25}H_{27}NO$. 357.49. (*E*)-*N*-[2-(Diphenylmethoxy)ethyl]-*N*-methylcinnamylamine. *UNII-P26FL0O04P. CAS-54141-87-6.* INN.

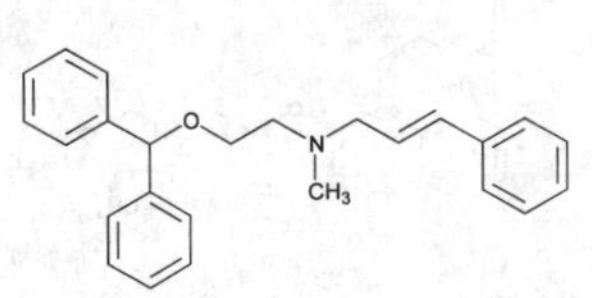

Cinfenoac. $C_{18}H_{14}O_6$. 326.30. *p*-[2-(α-Carboxy-*p*-anisoyl)vinyl]benzoic acid. *CAS-66984-59-6.* INN; BAN.

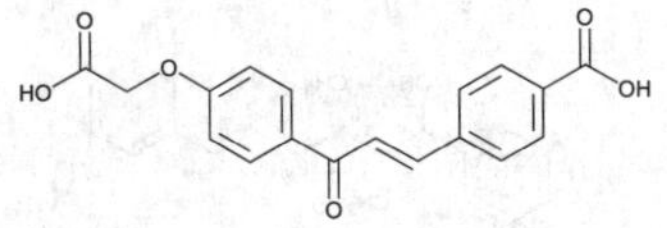

Cinflumide [*1985*] (sin′ floo mide). $C_{12}H_{12}FNO$. 205.23. (1) 2-Propenamide, *N*-cyclopropyl-3-(3-fluorophenyl)-, (*E*)-; (2) (*E*)-*N*-Cyclopropyl-*m*-fluorocinnamamide. *UNII-F0XVL451MO. CAS-64379-93-7.* INN. *Relaxant (muscle).* ◇*BW 532U*

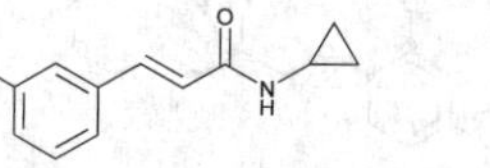

Cingestol [*1968*] (sin jes′ tol). $C_{20}H_{28}O$. 284.44. (1) 19-Norpregn-5-en-20-yn-17-ol, (17α)-; (2) 19-Nor-17α-pregn-5-en-20-yn-17-ol. *CAS-16915-71-2.* INN. *Progestin.*

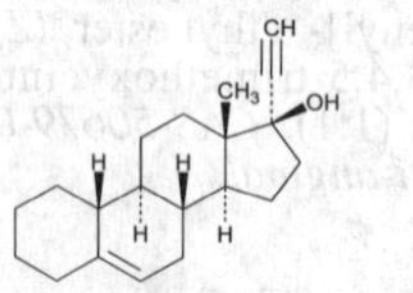

Cinitapride. $C_{21}H_{30}N_4O_4$. 402.49. 4-Amino-*N*-[1-(3-cyclohexen-1-ylmethyl)-4-piperidyl]-2-ethoxy-5-nitrobenzamide. *UNII-R8I97I2L24. CAS-66564-14-5.* INN.

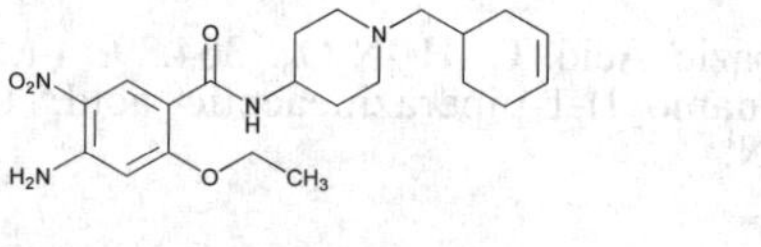

Cinmetacin. $C_{21}H_{19}NO_4$. 349.38. 1-Cinnamoyl-5-methoxy-2-methylindole-3-acetic acid. *UNII-3ZLI4719J9. CAS-20168-99-4.* INN; MI.

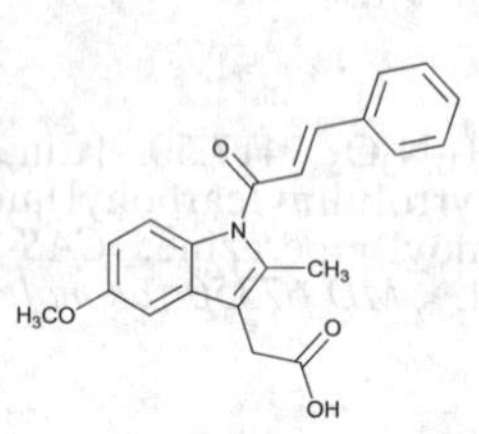

Cinnamaldehyde. *UNII-SR60A3XG0F. CAS-104-55-2.* NF IX; MI.

Cinnamaverine. $C_{21}H_{25}NO_2$. 323.43. 2-Diethylaminoethyl 2,3-diphenylacrylate. *UNII-M7R15X2683. CAS-1679-75-0.* INN; DCF.

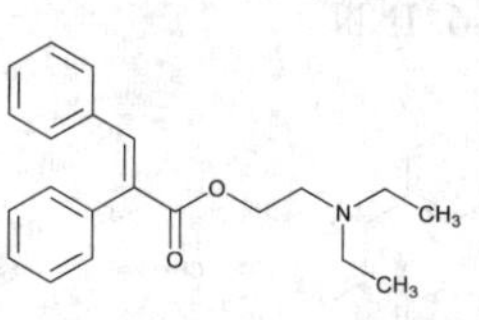

Cinnamedrine [*1967*] (sin″ a med′ rin). $C_{19}H_{23}NO$. 281.39. (1) Benzenemethanol, α-[1-[methyl(3-phenyl-2-propenyl)amino]ethyl]-; (2) α-[1-(Cinnamylmethylamino)ethyl]-benzyl alcohol. *CAS-90-86-8.* INN. *Relaxant (smooth muscle).*

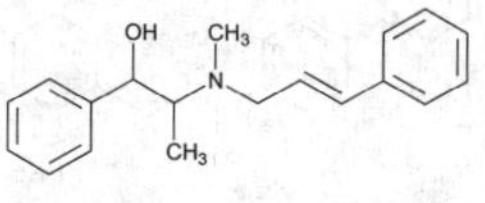

Cinnamic Aldehyde — *See* Cinnamaldehyde.

Cinnamon. *UNII-5S29HWU6QB.* NF XVI; MI.

Cinnamon Oil. *UNII-E5GY4I6YCZ. CAS-8007-80-5.* NF XVI; JAN.

Cinnarizine [*1962*] (si nar′ i zeen). $C_{26}H_{28}N_2$. 368.51. (1) Piperazine, 1-(diphenylmethyl)-4-(3-phenyl-2-propenyl)-; (2) 1-Cinnamyl-4-(diphenylmethyl)piperazine. *UNII-3DI2E1X18L. CAS-298-57-7.* INN; BAN; JAN. *Antihistaminic.* ◇*R 516; R 1575; 516 MD*

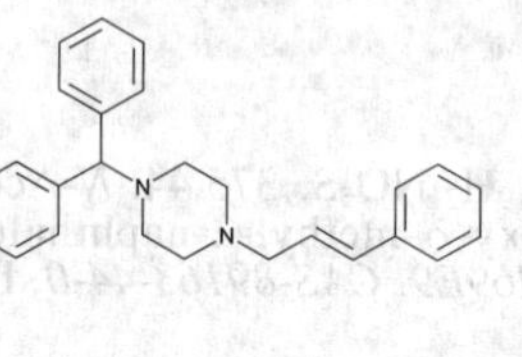

Cinnarizine Clofibrate. $C_{26}H_{28}N_2 \cdot C_{10}H_{11}ClO_3$. 583.16. 2-(*p*-Chlorophenoxy)-2-methylpropionic acid compound with (*E*)-1-cinnamyl-4-(diphenylmethyl)piperazine (1:1). *CAS-60763-49-7.* INN; MI.

Cinnofuradione. $C_{20}H_{18}N_2O_3$. 334.37. 2-Tetrahydrofurfuryl-1*H*-benzo[*c*]pyrazolo[1,2-*a*]cinnoline-1,3(2*H*)-dione. *UNII-1MO25S4CZP. CAS-477-80-5.* INN.

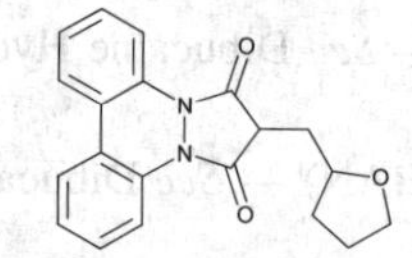

Cinnofuron — *See* Cinnofuradione.

Cinnopentazone (INN) — *See* Cintazone.

Cinnopropazone — *See* Apazone.

Cinoctramide. $C_{19}H_{27}NO_4$. 333.42. Octahydro-1-(3,4,5-trimethoxycinnamoyl)azocine. *UNII-69J8AO72Q3. CAS-28598-08-5.* INN.

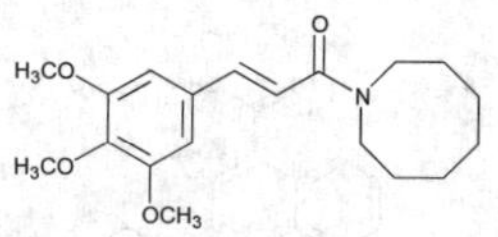

Cinodine Hydrochloride [*1979*] (sin′ oh deen hye″ droe klor′ ide). $C_{37}H_{59}N_{13}O_{13} \cdot x$HCl (each component). 893.94 (each component). (1) 2-Propenamide, *N*-[3-[(4-aminobutyl)amino]-propyl]-3-[4-[[4-[[[[2-[(aminocarbonyl)amino]-4-*O*-[2-[(aminocarbonyl)amino]-2¹,3²-anhydro-3-(carboxyamino)-2,3-dideoxy-β-D-xylopyranosyl]-2-deoxy-α-D-xylopyranosyl]amino]carbonyl]amino]-2-[(aminoiminomethyl)amino]-2,4,6-trideoxy-α-D-glucopyranosyl]oxy]phenyl]-, hydrochloride, (*E*)-, mixture with (*E*)-*N*-[3-[(4-aminobutyl)amino]propyl]-3-[4-[[4-[[[[2-[(aminocarbonyl)amino]-4-*O*-[2-[(aminocarbonyl)amino]-3²,4-anhydro-3-(carboxyamino)-2,3-dideoxy-β-D-xylopyranosyl]-2-deoxy-α-D-xylopyranosyl]amino]carbonyl]amino]-2-[(aminoiminomethyl)amino]-2,4,6-trideoxy-α-D-glucopyranosyl]oxy]phenyl]-2-propenamide hydrochloride; (2) (*E*)-*N*-[3-[(4-Aminobutyl)amino]propyl]-*p*-[[4-[3-[4-*O*-[2,3-(1-carbamoylureylene)-2,3-dideoxy-β-D-xylopyranosyl]-2-deoxy-2-ureido-α-D-xylopyranosyl]ureido]-2,4,6-trideoxy-2-guanidino-α-D-glucopyranosyl]oxy]cinnamamide hydrochloride mixture with (*E*)-*N*-[3-(4-aminobutyl)amino]propyl]-*p*-[[4-[3-[4-*O*-[3-(carboxyamino)-2,3-dideoxy-2-ureido-β-D-xylopyranosyl]-2-deoxy-2-ureido-α-D-xylopyranosyl]ureido]-2,4,6-trideoxy-2-guanidino-α-D-glucopyranosyl]oxy]cinnamamide intramolecular 3‴,4‴-ester hydrochloride; (3) Antibiotic BM 123γ hydrochloride. *CAS-68782-58-1; CAS-52932-64-6* [antibiotic BM 123γ]. *Antibacterial (veterinary).* ◇*CL 98984*

Cinolazepam. C₁₈H₁₃ClFN₃O₂. 357.77. 7-Chloro-5-(*o*-fluorophenyl)-2,3-dihydro-3-hydroxy-2-oxo-1*H*-1,4-benzodiazepine-1-propionitrile. *UNII-68P0556B0U. CAS-75696-02-5.* INN.

Cinoquidox. C₁₃H₁₂N₄O₃. 272.26. *N*-(2-Cyanoethyl)-3-methyl-2-quinoxalinecarboxamide 1,4-dioxide. *UNII-5743F6U086. CAS-64557-97-7.* INN.

Cinoxacin [*1974*] (sin ox′ a sin). **USP.** C₁₂H₁₀N₂O₅. 262.22. (1) [1,3]Dioxolo[4,5-*g*]cinnoline-3-carboxylic acid, 1-ethyl-1,4-dihydro-4-oxo-; (2) 1-Ethyl-1,4-dihydro-4-oxo[1,3]dioxolo[4,5-*g*]cinnoline-3-carboxylic acid. *UNII-LMK22VUH23. CAS-28657-80-9.* INN; BAN; JAN. *Antibacterial.* Cinobac (Lilly) ◇*64716*

Cinoxate [*1969*] (sin ox′ ate). C₁₄H₁₈O₄. 250.29. (1) Propenoic acid, 3-(4-methoxyphenyl)-, 2-ethoxyethyl ester; (2) 2-Ethoxyethyl *p*-methoxycinnamate. *UNII-5437O7N5BH. CAS-104-28-9.* USP XXV; INN. *Ultraviolet screen.*

Cinoxolone. C₄₁H₅₆O₅. 628.88. Cinnamyl 3β-hydroxy-11-oxoolean-12-en-30-oate acetate. *UNII-3LNU79AO9S. CAS-31581-02-9.* INN; BAN. ◇*Bx 311*

Cinoxopazide. C₂₀H₂₅N₃O₄. 371.43. 1-[(*E*)-3,4-Methylenedioxy)cinnamoyl]-4-[(1-pyrrolidinylcarbonyl)methyl]piperazine. *UNII-3T56HEP4NI. CAS-88053-05-8.* INN.

Cinperene [*1967*] (sin′ pe reen). C₂₅H₂₈N₂O₂. 388.50. (1) [3,4′-Bipiperidine]-2,6-dione, 3-phenyl-1′-(3-phenyl-2-propenyl)-; (2) 2-(1-Cinnamyl-4-piperidyl)-2-phenylglutarimide. *CAS-14796-24-8.* INN. *Antipsychotic.* ◇*R 5046*

Cinprazole. C₃₀H₃₂N₄O. 464.60. 3-[2-[[(4-Cinnamyl-1-piperazinyl)methyl]benzimidazol-1-yl]propiophenone. *UNII-601OJW5ILI. CAS-51493-19-7.* INN.

Cinpropazide. C₂₁H₃₁N₃O₅. 405.49. *N*-Isopropyl-4-(3,4,5-trimethoxycinnamoyl)-1-piperazineacetamide. *UNII-CX9T97T0XH. CAS-23887-47-0.* INN.

Cinromide [*1977*] (sin′ roe mide). C₁₁H₁₂BrNO. 254.12. (1) 2-Propenamide, 3-(3-bromophenyl)-, (*E*)-; (2) (*E*)-*m*-Bromo-*N*-ethylcinnamamide. *CAS-58473-74-8.* INN. *Anticonvulsant.*

Cintazone [*1969*] (sin′ ta zone). C₂₂H₂₂N₂O₂. 346.42. [Cinnopentazone is INN.] (1) 1*H*-Pyrazolo[1,2-*a*]cinnoline-1,3(2*H*)-dione,2-pentyl-6-phenyl-; (2) 2-Pentyl-6-phenyl-1*H*-pyrazolo[1,2-*a*]cinnoline-1,3(2*H*)-dione. *UNII-0BI682BR2D. CAS-2056-56-6. Anti-inflammatory.* ◇*AHR-3015; Scha-306; NSC-102825*

Cintramide (INN) — *See* Cintriamide.

Cintredekin Besudotox [*2004*] (sin″ tre dek′ in be soo′ doe tox). $C_{2234}H_{3512}N_{650}O_{682}S_{10}$. (1) Toxin hIL13-PE8QQR (plasmid phuIL13-Tx); (2) [Met[17],His[18]]human interleukin-13 precursor-(17-132)-peptide (132→246′)-protein with des-Ala[365],Asp[366],Val[367],Val[368],Ser[369],Leu[370],Thr[371], Cys[372],Pro[373],Val[374],Ala[375],Ala[376],Gly[377],Glu[378],Cys[379], Ala[380]-[Lys[246],Ala[247],Ser[248],Gly[249],Gly[250],Asn[364],Val[407], Ser[515],Gln[590],Gln[606],Arg[613]]exotoxin A (*Pseudomonas aeruginosa*)-(246-613)-peptide. Molecular weight is approximately 50,700 daltons. *CAS-372075-36-0.* INN. *Treatment of malignant glioma, including glioblastoma multiforme and anaplastic astrocytoma.* (Neopharm) ◇*IL13-PE38*

```
MHSPGPVPPS TALRELIEEL VNITQNQKAP LCNGSMVWSI NLTAGMYCAA
LESLINVSGC SAIEKTQRML SGFCPHKVSA GQFSSLHVRD TKIEVAQFVK
DLLLHLKKLF REGRFNKASG GPEGGSLAAL TAHQACHLPL ETFTRHRQPR
GWEQLEQCGY PVQRLVALYL AARLSWNQVD QVIRNALASP GSSGDLGEAI
REQPEQARLA LTLAAAESER FVRQGTGNDE AGAANGPADS GDALLERNYP
TGAEFLGDGG DVSFSTRGTQ NWTVERLLQA HRQLEERGYV FVGYHGTFLE
AAQSIVFGGV RARSQDLDAI WRGFYIAGDP ALAYGYAQDQ EPDARGRIRN
GALLRVYVPR SSLPGFYRTS LTLAAPEAAG EVERLIGHPL PLRLDAITGP
EEEGGRLETI LGWPLAERTV VIPSAIPTDP RNVGGDLDPS SIPDQEQAIS
ALPDYASQPG QPPREDLR
```

Cintriamide [*1963*] (sin trye′ a mide). $C_{12}H_{15}NO_4$. 237.25. [Cintramide is INN.] (1) 2-Propenamide, 3-(3,4,5-trimethoxyphenyl)-; (2) 3,4,5-Trimethoxycinnamamide. *CAS-5588-21-6. Antipsychotic.*

Cinuperone. $C_{23}H_{24}FN_3O$. 377.45. 4′-Fluoro-4-[4-(3-isoquinolyl)-1-piperazinyl]butyrophenone. *CAS-82117-51-9.* INN.

Cioteronel [*1992*] (sye″ oh ter′ oh nel). $C_{16}H_{28}O_2$. 252.39. (1) 2(1*H*)-Pentalenone, hexahydro-4-(5-methoxyheptyl)-; (2) (±)-Hexahydro-4-(5-methoxyheptyl)-2(1*H*)-pentalenone. *UNII-1RTH95874Z. CAS-89672-11-7.* INN. *Anti-androgen.*

Cipamfylline [*1994*] (sye pam′ fi lin). $C_{13}H_{17}N_5O_2$. 275.31. (1) 1*H*-Purine-2,6-dione, 8-amino-1,3-bis(cyclopropylmethyl)-3,7-dihydro-; (2) 8-Amino-1,3-bis(cyclopropylmethyl)xanthine. *CAS-132210-43-6.* INN. *Antiviral.* ◇*BRL 61063*

Cipemastat [*2000*] (sye pem′ a stat). $C_{22}H_{36}N_4O_5$. 436.55. (1) 1-Piperidinebutanamide, β-(cyclopentylmethyl)-*N*-hydroxy-γ-oxo-α-[(3,4,4-trimethyl-2,5-dioxo-1-imidazolidinyl)methyl]-, [*R*-(*R**,*R**)]-; (2) (α*R*,β*R*)-β-(Cyclopentylmethyl)-γ-oxo-α-[(3,4,4-piperidinebutyrohydroxamic acid. *CAS-190648-49-8.* INN. *Cartilage protective agent in rheumatoid arthritis (matrix metalloproteinase inhibitor).* Trocade (Hoffmann-LaRoche) ◇*Ro 32-3555/000*

Ciprafamide. $C_{21}H_{24}N_2O$. 320.43. *N*-(*cis*-2,*trans*-3-Diphenylcyclopropyl)-1-pyrrolidineacetamide. *UNII-PU98C417NB. CAS-35452-73-4.* INN.

Cipralisant. $C_{14}H_{20}N_2$. 216.32. 4-[(1*R*,2*R*)-2-(5,5-Dimethylhex-1-ynyl)cyclopropyl]-1*H*-imidazole. *UNII-309713XSKW. CAS-213027-19-1.* INN.

Cipralisant Maleate [*2001*] (sye pral′ i sant mal′ ee ate). $C_{14}H_{20}N_2 \cdot C_4H_4O_4$. 332.39. (1) 1*H*-Imidazole, 4-[(1*R*,2*R*)-2-(5,5-dimethyl-1-hexynyl)cyclopropyl]-, (2*Z*)-2-butenedioate (1:1); (2) 4-[(1*R*,2*R*)-2-(5,5-Dimethyl-1-hexynyl)cyclopropyl]imidazole maleate (1:1). *UNII-7ENI812SZS. CAS-223420-20-0. Treatment of attention deficit hyperactive disorders (ADHD), age related memory dysfunction, and other cognitive disorders (histamine H₃antagonist).* Perceptin (Gliatech) ◇*GT-2331*

Ciprazafone. $C_{19}H_{18}Cl_2N_2O_2$. 377.26. 4'-Chloro-2'-(*o*-chlorobenzoyl)-2-(cyclopropylamino)-*N*-methylacetanilide. *UNII-8RSD11181G. CAS-75616-03-4.* INN.

Ciprefadol Succinate [*1978*] (sye pref' a dol sux' i nate). $C_{19}H_{27}NO.C_4H_6O_4$. 403.51. [Ciprefadol is INN.] (1) Phenol, 3-[2-(cyclopropylmethyl)octahydro-4a(2*H*)-isoquinolinyl-, *trans*, (-)-, butanedioate (1:1) (salt); (2) (-)-*m*-[2-(Cyclopropylmethyl)-1,3,4,5,6,7,8,8aα-octahydro-4aβ(2*H*)-isoquinolyl]phenol succinate (1:1) (salt). *UNII-68ENP3YGUF. CAS-60719-85-9; CAS-59889-36-0* [ciprefadol]. *Analgesic.* ◇*Compound 113878*

Ciprocinonide [*1977*] (sip" roe sin' oh nide). $C_{28}H_{34}F_2O_7$. 520.56. (1) Pregna-1,4-diene-3,20-dione, 21-[(cyclopropylcarbonyl)oxy]-6,9-difluoro-11-hydroxy-16,17-[(1-methylethylidene)bis(oxy)]-, (6α,11β,16α)-; (2) 6α,9-Difluoro-11β,16α,17,21-tetrahydroxypregna-1,4-diene-3,20-dione cyclic 16,17-acetal with acetone, 21-cyclopropanecarboxylate. *CAS-58524-83-7.* INN. *Adrenocortical steroid.* ◇*RS-2386*

Ciprofibrate [*1976*] (sip" roe fye' brate). $C_{13}H_{14}Cl_2O_3$. 289.15. (1) Propanoic acid, 2-[4-(2,2-dichlorocyclopropyl)phenoxy]-2-methyl-; (2) 2-[*p*-(2,2-Dichlorocyclopropyl)phenoxy]-2-methylpropionic acid. *CAS-52214-84-3.* INN; BAN. *Antihyperlipoproteinemic.* ◇*Win 35833*

Ciprofloxacin [*1987*] (sip" roe flox' a sin). **USP**. $C_{17}H_{18}FN_3O_3$. 331.34. (1) 3-Quinolinecarboxylic acid, 1-cyclopropyl-6-fluoro-1,4-dihydro-4-oxo-7-(1-piperazinyl)-; (2) 1-Cyclopropyl-6-fluoro-1,4-dihydro-4-oxo-7-(1-pi-

perazinyl)-3-quinolinecarboxylic acid. *UNII-5E8K9I0O4U. CAS-85721-33-1.* INN; BAN. *Antibacterial.* Cipro (Bayer) ◇*Bay q 3939*

Ciprofloxacin Hydrochloride [*1987*] (sip" roe flox' a sin hye" droe klor' ide). **USP**. $C_{17}H_{18}FN_3O_3.HCl.H_2O$. 385.82. (1) 3-Quinolinecarboxylic acid, 1-cyclopropyl-6-fluoro-1,4-dihydro-4-oxo-7-(1-piperazinyl)-, monohydrochloride, monohydrate; (2) 1-Cyclopropyl-6-fluoro-1,4-dihydro-4-oxo-7-(1-piperazinyl)-3-quinolinecarboxylic acid, monohydrochloride, monohydrate. *UNII-4BA73M5E37. CAS-86393-32-0.* JAN. *Antibacterial.* Ciloxan (Alcon); Cipro (Bayer); Proquin (Esprit) ◇*Bay o 9867 monohydrate*

Ciprokiren. $C_{37}H_{55}N_5O_8S$. 729.93. (αS)-*N*-[(1*S*,2*R*,3*S*)-1-(Cyclohexylmethyl)-3-cyclopropyl-2,3-dihydroxypropyl]-α-[(αS)-α-[[[1-methyl-1-(morpholinocarbonyl)ethyl]sulfonyl]methyl]hydrocinnamamido]imidazole-4-propionamide. *UNII-K259Z4O1B3. CAS-143631-62-3.* INN.

Cipropride. $C_{17}H_{25}N_3O_4S$. 367.46. *N*-[[1-(Cyclopropylmethyl)-2-pyrrolidinyl]methyl]-5-sulfamoyl-*o*-anisamide. *UNII-0D2VUO6DCN. CAS-68475-40-1.* INN.

Ciproquazone. $C_{19}H_{18}N_2O_2$. 306.36. 1-(Cyclopropylmethyl)-6-methoxy-4-phenyl-2(1*H*)-quinazolinone. *UNII-P8S0GE5Q4I. CAS-33453-23-5.* INN.

Ciproquinate (INN) — *See* Cyproquinate.

Ciprostene Calcium [*1985*] (sye pros' teen kal' see um). $C_{44}H_{70}CaO_8$. 767.10. [Ciprostene is INN.] (1) Pentanoic acid, 5-[hexahydro-5-hydroxy-6-(3-hydroxy-1-octenyl)-3a-methyl-2(1*H*)-pentalenylidene, calcium salt (2:1),[3a*S*-[2*Z*,3aα,5β,6α(1*E*,3*R**),6aα]]-; (2) Calcium (*Z*)-

---

† Brand name formerly used, and/or firm no longer concerned with this product.

(3a*S*,5*R*,6*R*,6a*R*)-hexahydro-5-hydroxy-6-[(*E*)-(3*S*)-3-hydroxy-1-octenyl]-3a-methyl-Δ²(1*H*),δ-pentalenevalerate (1:2). *UNII-KZ075BHY4P* [ciprostene]. *CAS-81703-55-1; CAS-81845-44-5* [ciprostene]. *Platelet aggregation inhibitor.* ◇*U-61,431F*

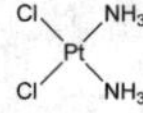

Ciproximide (INN) — *See* **Cyproximide.**

Ciramadol [*1978*] (sir a′ ma dol). C$_{15}$H$_{23}$NO$_2$. 249.35. (1) Phenol, 3-[(dimethylamino)(2-hydroxycyclohexyl)methyl]-, [1*R*-[1α(*R**),2α]]-(-)-; (2) (-)-(1*R*,2*R*)-2-[(*R*)-α-(Dimethylamino)-*m*-hydroxybenzyl]cyclohexanol. *UNII-9NQ109OW0G. CAS-63269-31-8.* INN. *Analgesic.* ◇*WY-15,705*

Ciramadol Hydrochloride [*1984*] (sir a′ ma dol hye″ droe klor′ ide). C$_{15}$H$_{23}$NO$_2$.HCl. 285.81. (1) Phenol, 3-[(dimethylamino)(2-hydroxycyclohexyl)methyl]-, hydrochloride, [1*R*-[1α(*R**),2α]]- (-)-; (2) (-)-(1*R*,2*R*)-2-[(*R*)-α-(Dimethylamino)-*m*-hydroxybenzyl]cyclohexanol hydrochloride. *UNII-090XO8449J. CAS-63323-46-6; CAS-63269-31-8* [ciramadol]. *Analgesic.* ◇*WY-15,705 HCl*

Cirazoline. C$_{13}$H$_{16}$N$_2$O. 216.28. 2-[(*o*-Cyclopropylphenoxy)methyl]-2-imidazoline. *UNII-QK318GVY3Y. CAS-59939-16-1.* INN.

Cirolemycin [*1968*] (sir oh″ le mye′ sin). A substance produced by *Streptomyces bellus* var. *cirolerosus* var. *nova.* (1) Cirolemycin; (2) Cirolemycin. *CAS-11056-12-5.* INN. *Antineoplastic; antibacterial.* ◇*U-12,241*

Cisapride [*1983*] (sis′ a pride). C$_{23}$H$_{29}$ClFN$_3$O$_4$. 465.95. (1) Benzamide, 4-amino-5-chloro-*N*-[1-[3-(4-fluorophenoxy)propyl]-3-methoxy-4-piperidinyl]-2-methoxy-, *cis*-; (2) *cis*-4-Amino-5-chloro-*N*-[1-[3-(*p*-fluorophenoxy)propyl]-3-methoxy-4-piperidyl]-*o*-anisamide. *UNII-UVL329170W. CAS-81098-60-4.* INN; BAN; JAN. *Stimulant (peristaltic).* Propulsid (Janssen) ◇*R-51,619*

Cisatracurium Besilate (INN, BAN) — *See* **Cisatracurium Besylate.**

Cisatracurium Besylate [*1995*] (sis at″ ra kure′ ee um bes′ i late). C$_{65}$H$_{82}$N$_2$O$_{18}$S$_2$. 1243.48. [Cisatracurium Besilate is INN and BAN.] (1) Isoquinolinium, 2,2′-[1,5-pentanediylbis[oxy(3-oxo-3,1-propanediyl)]]bis[1-[(3,4-dimethoxyphenyl)methyl]-1,2,3,4-tetrahydro-6,7-dimethoxy-2-methyl-, dibenzenesulfonate, [1*R*-[1α,2α(1′*R**,2′*R**)]]-; (2)

(1*R*,2*R*)-2-(2-Carboxyethyl)-1,2,3,4-tetrahydro-6,7-dimethoxy-2-methyl-1-veratrylisoquinolinium benzenesulfonate, pentamethylene ester. *UNII-80YS8O1MBS. CAS-96946-42-8. Neuromuscular blocking agent.* Nimbex (Abbott) ◇*51W89*

Cisclomiphene (previously used name) — *See* **Enclomiphene.**

Cisconazole [*1988*] (sis kon′ a zole). C$_{19}$H$_{15}$F$_3$N$_2$OS. 376.40. (1) 1*H*-Imidazole, 1-[[3-[(2,6-difluorophenyl)methoxy]-5-fluoro-2,3-dihydrobenzo[*b*]thien-2-yl]methyl]-, *cis*-(±)-; (2) (±)-*cis*-1-[[3-[(2,6-Difluorobenzyl)oxy]-5-fluoro-2,3-dihydrobenzo[*b*]thien-2-yl]methyl]imidazole. *CAS-104456-79-3.* INN. *Antifungal.* ◇*Sch 35852*

Cismadinone. C$_{21}$H$_{27}$ClO$_3$. 362.89. 6α-Chloro-17-hydroxypregna-1,4-diene-3,20-dione. *UNII-O00XM1O6TV. CAS-54063-31-9.* INN.

Cisplatin [*1977*] (sis pla′ tin). **USP.** Cl$_2$H$_6$N$_2$Pt. 300.05. (1) Platinum, diamminedichloro-, (*SP*-4-2)-; (2) *cis*-Diamminedichloroplatinum. *UNII-Q20Q21Q62J. CAS-15663-27-1.* INN; BAN; JAN. *Antineoplastic.* Platinol (Bristol-Myers Squibb) *[Name previously used: cis-Platinum II.]* ◇*Cis-DDP; NSC-119875*

Cistinexine. $C_{50}H_{60}Br_4N_6O_6S_2$. 1224.79. Dibenzyl [dithiobis[(R)-1-[[4,6-dibromo-α-(cyclohexylmethylamino)-o-tolyl]carbamoyl]ethylene]]dicarbamate. *UNII-62VR67FK8E*. *CAS-86042-50-4*. INN.

Citalopram (sye tal' oh pram). **USP.** $C_{20}H_{21}FN_2O$. 324.39. 1-[3-(Dimethylamino)propyl]-1-(p-fluorophenyl)-5-phthalancarbonitrile. *UNII-0DHU5B8D6V*. *CAS-59729-33-8*. INN; BAN; MI.

Citalopram Hydrobromide [*1998*] (sye tal' oh pram hye″ droe broe' mide). **USP.** $C_{20}H_{21}FN_2O \cdot HBr$. 405.30. (1) 5-Isobenzofurancarbonitrile, 1-[3-(dimethylamino)propyl]-1-(4-fluorophenyl)-1,3-dihydro-, monohydrobromide; (2) 1-[3-(Dimethylamino)propyl]-1-(p-fluorophenyl)-5-phthalancarbonitrile monohydrobromide. *UNII-I1E9D14F36*. *CAS-59729-32-7*. *Antidepressant (selective serotonin reuptake inhibitor).* Celexa (Forest) ◇*Lu 10-171-B*

Citatepine. $C_{20}H_{18}N_2S$. 318.44. 2,3,4,5-Tetrahydro-3-methyl-1H-dibenzo[2,3:6,7]thiepino[4,5-d]azepine-7-carbonitrile. *UNII-92S48G7U0W*. *CAS-65509-66-2*. INN.

Citatuzumab Bogatox. $C_{3455}H_{5371}N_{921}O_{1060}S_{18}$. Immunoglobulin Fab fusion protein, anti-[*Homo sapiens* tumor-associated calcium signal transducer 1 (TACSTD1, gastrointestinal tumor-associated protein 2, GA733-2, epithelial glycoprotein 2, EGP-2, epithelial cell adhesion molecule Ep-CAM, KSA, KS1/4 antigen, M4S, tumor antigen 17-1A, CD326)], humanized Fab fused with *Bougainvillea spectabilis Willd* rRNA N-glycosidase [type I ribosome inactivating protein (RIP), bouganin], VB6-845; gamma1 heavy chain fragment (1-225) [hexahistidyl (1-6) -humanized VH from 4D5MOC-B (*Homo sapiens* FR/*Mus musculus* CDR, *Homo sapiens* IGHJ4*01, V124>L) [8.8.9] (7-122) -*Homo sapiens* IGHG1*01 CH1-hinge fragment EPKSC (123-225)], (225-219′)-disulfide with kappa fusion chain (1′-481′) [humanized V-KAPPA from clone 4D5MOC-B (*Homo sapiens* FR/*Mus musculus* CDR, *Homo sapiens* IGKJ1*01, I126>L) [11.3.9] (1′-112′) -*Homo sapiens* IGKC*01 (113′-219′) -12-mer furin linker (proteolytic cleavage spacer from Pseudomonas exotoxin A) (220′-231′) -*Bougainvillea spectabilis Willd* bouganin fragment (27-276 from precursor, V354′>A, D358′>A, Y364′>N, I383′>A) (232′-481′)]. *CAS-945228-49-9*. INN.

Citenamide [*1968*] (sye ten' a mide). $C_{16}H_{13}NO$. 235.28. (1) 5H-Dibenzo[a,d]cycloheptene-5-carboxamide; (2) 5H-Dibenzo[a,d]cycloheptene-5-carboxamide. *CAS-10423-37-7*. INN. *Anticonvulsant.* ◇*AY-15,613*

Citenazone. $C_7H_6N_4S_2$. 210.28. 5-Formyl-2-thiophenecarbonitrile thiosemicarbazone. *CAS-21512-15-2*. INN. ◇*Hoe 105*

Citicoline Sodium [*1994*] (sye tik' oh leen soe' dee um). $C_{14}H_{25}N_4NaO_{11}P_2$. 510.31. [Citicoline is INN and JAN.] (1) Cytidine 5′-(trihydrogen diphosphate), P'-[2-(trimethylammonio)ethyl] ester, inner salt, monosodium salt; (2) Choline hydroxide, 5′-ester with cytidine 5′-(sodium dihydrogen diphosphate), inner salt. *CAS-33818-15-4; CAS-987-78-0* [citicoline]; *CAS-1477-47-0* [citicoline, replaced]. *Post-stroke and post-head trauma treatment.* CerAxon (Interneuron) ◇*IP 302 sodium*

Citiolone. $C_6H_9NO_2S$. 159.21. N-(Tetrahydro-2-oxo-3-thienyl)acetamide. *UNII-70JKL15MUH*. *CAS-1195-16-0*. INN; DCF; MI.

Citric Acid, Anhydrous (sit' rik as' id an hye' drus). **USP.** $C_6H_8O_7$. 192.12. (1) 1,2,3-Propanetricarboxylic acid, 2-hydroxy-; (2) Citric acid. *UNII-XF417D3PSL; UNII-2968PHW8QP* [monohydrate]. *CAS-77-92-9; CAS-5949-29-1* [monohydrate]. JAN.

---

† Brand name formerly used, and/or firm no longer concerned with this product.

Citric Acid Monohydrate (sit′ rik as′ id mon″ oh hye′ drate). **USP.** $C_6H_8O_7 \cdot H_2O$. 210.14. 1,2,3-Propanetricarboxylic acid, 2 hydroxy-, monohydrate. *CAS-5949-29-1.*

Citrovorum Factor — *See* Leucovorin Calcium.

Cixutumumab [*2008*] (six″ ue toom′ ue mab). $C_{6500}H_{10052}N_{1724}O_{2036}S_{44}$. (1) Immunoglobulin G1, anti-(human insulin-like growth factor I receptor) (human monoclonal IMC-A12 γ-chain), disulfide with human monoclonal IMC-A12 λ-chain, dimer; (2) Immunoglobulin G1, anti-(human insulin-like growth factor 1 receptor (EC 2.7.10.1 or CD221 antigen)); human monoclonal IMC-A12 γ1 heavy chain (233-213′)-disulfide with human mono-clonal IMC-A12 λ light chain (211′T>A), (239-239″:242-242″)-bisdisulfide dimer. Molecular weight is approximately 146,300 daltons. *UNII-2285XW22DR. CAS-947687-12-9. Treatment of solid tumors.* ◇*IMC-A12*

Cizolirtine. $C_{15}H_{21}N_3O$. 259.35. (±)-5-[α-[2-(Dimethylamino)ethoxy]benzyl]-1-methylpyrazole. *UNII-SMP167WV5D. CAS-142155-43-9.* INN.

Cladaribine (previously used name) — *See* Cladribine.

Cladribine [*1992*] (klad′ ri been). **USP.** $C_{10}H_{12}ClN_5O_3$. 285.69. (1) Adenosine, 2-chloro-2′-deoxy-; (2) 2-Chloro-2′-deoxyadenosine. *UNII-47M74X9YT5. CAS-4291-63-8.* INN; BAN. *Antineoplastic.* Leustatin (Ortho Biotech) *[Name previously used: Cladaribine.]* ◇*RWJ 26251*

Clamidoxic Acid. $C_{15}H_{11}Cl_2NO_4$. 340.16. [2-(3,4-Dichlorobenzamido)phenoxy]acetic acid. *UNII-4H4JU6738Q. CAS-6170-69-0.* INN; BAN. ◇*SNR 1804*

Clamikalant. $C_{19}H_{22}ClN_3O_5S_2$. 471.98. 1-[[5-[2-(5-Chloro-*o*-anisamido)ethyl]-2-methoxyphenyl]sulfonyl]-3-methyl-2-thiourea. *UNII-94301K998R. CAS-158751-64-5.* INN.

Clamoxyquin Hydrochloride [*1965*] (klam ox′ i kwin hye″ droe klor′ ide). $C_{17}H_{24}ClN_3O \cdot 2HCl$. 394.77. [Clamoxy-quine is INN and BAN.] (1) 8-Quinolinol, 5-chloro-7-[[[3-(diethylamino)propyl]amino]methyl]-, dihydrochloride; (2) 5-Chloro-7-[[[3-(diethylamino)propyl]amino]methyl]-8-quinolinol dihydrochloride. *UNII-SQ922M93PI. CAS-4724-59-8; CAS-2545-39-3* [clamoxyquin]. *Anti-amebic.* Clamoxyl (Parke-Davis†) ◇*CI-433; CN-17,900-2B; PAA-3854; NSC-20246*

Clanfenur. $C_{16}H_{15}ClFN_3O_2$. 335.76. 1-(*p*-Chlorophenyl)-3-(6-fluoro-*N,N*-dimethylanthraniloyl)urea. *UNII-KAM54NKT1Q. CAS-51213-99-1.* INN.

Clanobutin. $C_{18}H_{18}ClNO_4$. 347.79. 4-[*p*-Chloro-*N*-(*p*-methoxyphenyl)benzamido]butyric acid. *UNII-W6Y945055S. CAS-30544-61-7.* INN; MI.

Clantifen. $C_{11}H_7Cl_2NO_2S$. 288.15. 4-(2,6-Dichloroanilino)-3-thiophenecarboxylic acid. *UNII-677Z1OCG11. CAS-16562-98-4.* INN.

Clarithromycin [*1988*] (kla rith″ roe mye′ sin). **USP.** $C_{38}H_{69}NO_{13}$. 747.95. (1) Erythromycin, 6-*O*-methyl-; (2) 6-*O*-Methylerythromycin. *UNII-H1250JIK0A. CAS-81103-11-9.* INN; BAN; JAN. *Antibacterial.* Biaxin (Abbott) ◇*Abbott-56268; TE-031*

Clavulanate Potassium [*1986*] (klav′ ue la nate poe tas′ ee um). **USP.** $C_8H_8KNO_5$. 237.25. (1) 4-Oxa-1-azabicyclo[3.2.0]heptane-2-carboxylic acid, 3-(2-hydroxyethylidene)-7-oxo-, monopotassium salt, [2R-(2α,3Z,5α)]-; (2) Potassium (*Z*)-(2*R*,5*R*)-3-(2-hydroxyethylidene)-7-oxo-4-

oxa-1-azabicyclo[3.2.0]heptane-2-carboxylate. *UNII-Q42OMW3AT8. CAS-61177-45-5.* JAN. *Inhibitor (β-lactamase).* ◇*BRL 14151K*

Clavulanic Acid. $C_8H_9NO_5$. 199.16. (*Z*)-(2*R*,5*R*)-3-(2-Hydroxyethylidene)-7-oxo-4-oxa-1-azabicyclo[3.2.0]heptane-2-carboxylic acid. *UNII-23521W1S24. CAS-58001-44-8.* INN; BAN; MI. ◇*BRL 14151*

Clazolam [*1972*] (klaz′ oh lam). $C_{18}H_{17}ClN_2O$. 312.79. (1) Isoquino[2,1-*d*][1,4]benzodiazepin-6(7*H*)-one, 2-chloro-5,9,10,14b-tetrahydro-5-methyl-; (2) 2-Chloro-5,9,10,14b-tetrahydro-5-methylisoquino[2,1-*d*][1,4]-benzodiazepin-6(7*H*)-one. *CAS-7492-29-7.* INN. *Tranquilizer (minor).* ◇*41-123*

Clazolimine [*1974*] (klaz oh′ li meen). $C_{10}H_{10}ClN_3O$. 223.66. (1) 4-Imidazolidinone, 1-(4-chlorophenyl)-2-imino-3-methyl-; (2) 1-(*p*-Chlorophenyl)-2-imino-3-methyl-4-imidazolidinone. *UNII-C3XSG3DLPA. CAS-40828-44-2.* INN. *Diuretic.* ◇*CL 88,893*

Clazosentan. $C_{25}H_{23}N_9O_6S$. 577.57. *N*-{6-(2-Hydroxyethoxy)-5-(2-methoxyphenoxy)-2-[2-(1*H*-tetrazol-5-yl)-pyridin-4-yl]pyrimidin-4-yl}-5-methylpyridine-2-sulfonamide. *UNII-3DRR0X4728. CAS-180384-56-9.* INN.

Clazuril [*1988*] (klaz′ ue ril). $C_{17}H_{10}Cl_2N_4O_2$. 373.19. (1) Benzeneacetonitrile, 2-chloro-α-(4-chlorophenyl)-4-(4,5-dihydro-3,5-dioxo-1,2,4-triazin-2(3*H*)-yl)-; (2) [2-Chloro-4-(4,5-dihydro-3,5-dioxo-*as*-triazin-2(3*H*)-yl)phenyl](*p*-

---

† Brand name formerly used, and/or firm no longer concerned with this product.

chlorophenyl)acetonitrile. *UNII-O8W0R05772. CAS-101831-36-1.* INN; BAN. *Coccidiostat (for pigeons).* ◇*R62,690*

Clebopride [*1987*] (kleb′ oh pride). $C_{20}H_{24}ClN_3O_2$. 373.88. [Clebopride Malate is JAN.] (1) Benzamide, 4-amino-5-chloro-2-methoxy-*N*-[1-(phenylmethyl)-4-piperidinyl]-; (2) 4-Amino-*N*-(1-benzyl-4-piperidyl)-5-chloro-*o*-anisamide. *CAS-55905-53-8.* INN; BAN. *Anti-emetic.* Cleboril (Grupo Farmacéutico Almirall S.A., Spain) ◇*LAS 9273*

Clefamide. $C_{17}H_{16}Cl_2N_2O_5$. 399.23. 2,2-Dichloro-*N*-(2-hydroxyethyl)-*N*-[*p*-(*p*-nitrophenoxy)benzyl]acetamide. *UNII-4AZ2V8K4EK. CAS-3576-64-5.* INN; BAN.

Clemastine [*1969*] (kle mas′ teen). $C_{21}H_{26}ClNO$. 343.89. (1) Pyrrolidine, 2-[2-[1-(4-chlorophenyl)-1-phenylethoxy]ethyl]-1-methyl-, [*R*-(*R**,*R**)]-; (2) (+)-(2*R*)-2-[2-[[(*R*)-*p*-Chloro-α-methyl-α-phenylbenzyl]oxy]ethyl]-1-methyl-pyrrolidine. *UNII-95QN29S1ID. CAS-15686-51-8.* BAN. *Antihistaminic.* ◇*HS-592*

Clemastine Fumarate [*1977*] (kle mas′ teen fue′ ma rate). USP. $C_{21}H_{26}ClNO \cdot C_4H_4O_4$. 459.96. (1) Pyrrolidine, 2-[2-[1-(4-chlorophenyl)-1-phenylethoxy]ethyl]-1-methyl-, [*R*-(*R**,*R**)]-, (*E*)-2-butenedioate (1:1); (2) (+)-(2*R*)-2-[2-[[(*R*)-*p*-Chloro-α-methyl-α-phenylbenzyl]oxy]ethyl]-1-methylpyrrolidine fumarate (1:1). *UNII-19259EGQ3D; UNII-95QN29S1ID* [clemastine]. *CAS-14976-57-9; CAS-15686-51-8* [clemastine]. BAN; JAN. *Antihistaminic.* Tavist (Novartis)

Clemeprol. $C_{17}H_{20}ClNO$. 289.80. *m*-Chloro-α-[(dimethylamino)methyl]-β-phenylphenetyl alcohol. *UNII-R3TC4SE-W5A*. *CAS-71827-56-0*. INN; BAN.

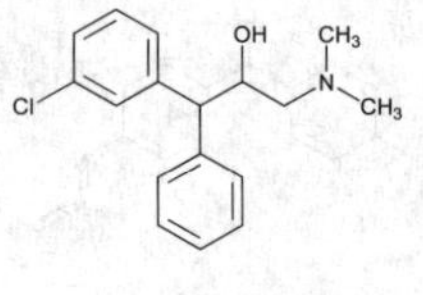

Clemizole. $C_{19}H_{20}ClN_3$. 325.84. [Clemizole Hydrochloride is JAN.] 1-*p*-Chlorobenzyl-2-(1-pyrrolidinylmethyl)benzimidazole. *UNII-T97CB3796L; UNII-85W6I13D8M* [hydrochloride]. *CAS-442-52-4; CAS-1163-36-6* [hydrochloride]. INN; BAN; MI. ◇*AL 20 [as hydrochloride]*

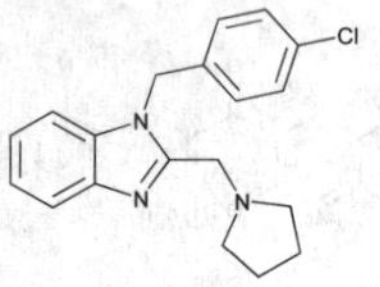

Clemizole Penicillin. Benzylpenicillin combined with 1-*p*-chlorobenzyl-2-(1-pyrrolidinylmethyl)benzimidazole. *UNII-5UL276H6TF*. *CAS-6011-39-8*. INN; BAN.

Clenbuterol. $C_{12}H_{18}Cl_2N_2O$. 277.19. [Clenbuterol Hydrochloride is JAN.] 4-Amino-α-[(*tert*-butylamino)methyl]-3,5-dichlorobenzyl alcohol. *UNII-XTZ6AXU7KN*. *CAS-37148-27-9*. INN; BAN; MI. ◇*NAB 365*

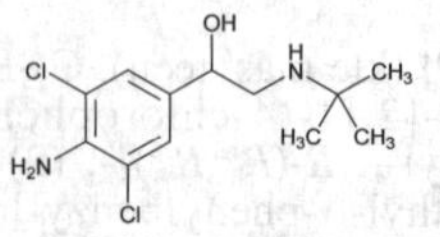

Clenoliximab. Immunoglobulin G 4 (human-Macaca monoclonal CE9γ4PE γ4-chain anti-human antigen CD 4), disulfide with human-Macaca monoclonal CE9γ4PE κ-chain, dimer. INN.

Clenpirin. $C_{14}H_{18}Cl_2N_2$. 285.21. [Clenpyrin is BAN.] 1-Butyl-2-[(3,4-dichlorophenyl)imino]pyrrolidine. *UNII-PFM79PGI92*. *CAS-27050-41-5*. INN. ◇*FBB 6896*

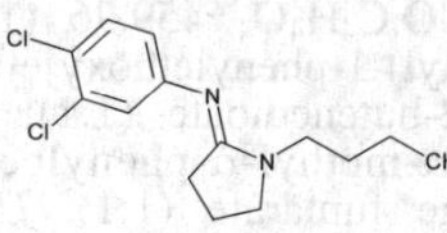

Clenpyrin (BAN) — *See* Clenpirin.

Clentiazem Maleate [*1989*] (klen tye′ a zem mal′ ee ate). $C_{22}H_{25}ClN_2O_4S.C_4H_4O_4$. 565.04. [Clentiazem is INN.] (1) 1,5-Benzothiazepin-4(5*H*)-one, 3-(acetyloxy)-8-chloro-5-[2-(dimethylamino)ethyl]-2,3-dihydro-2-(4-methoxyphenyl)-, (2*S-cis*)-, (Z)-2-butenedioate (1:1); (2) (+)-(2*S*,3*S*)-8-Chloro-5-[2-(dimethylamino)ethyl]-2,3-dihydro-3-hydroxy-2-(*p*-methoxyphenyl)-1,5-benzothiazepin-4(5*H*)-

one acetate (ester), maleate (1:1). *UNII-40DK034DRC* [clentiazem]. *CAS-96128-92-6; CAS-96125-53-0* [clentiazem]. *Antagonist (calcium channel).* ◇*TA-3090*

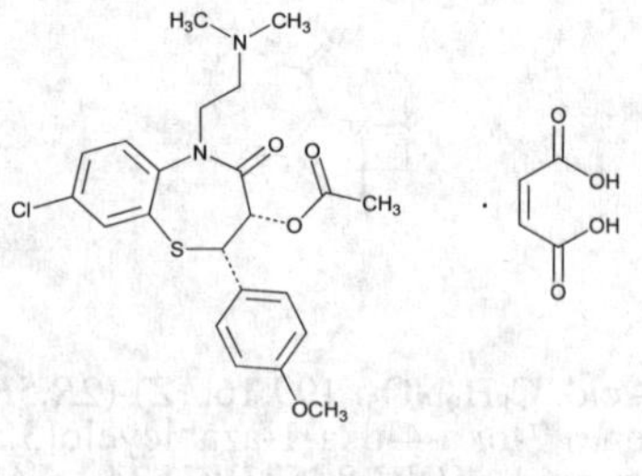

Cletoquine. $C_{16}H_{22}ClN_3O$. 307.82. 2-[[4-[(7-Chloro-4-quinolyl)amino]pentyl]amino]ethanol. *UNII-83CVD213TU*. *CAS-4298-15-1*. INN; BAN.

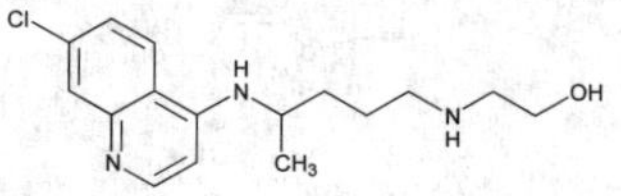

Clevidipine Butyrate [*2006*] (klev id′ i peen bue′ ti rate). $C_{21}H_{23}Cl_2NO_6$. 456.32. [Clevidipine is INN.] (1) 3,5-Pyridinedicarboxylic acid, 4-(2,3-dichlorophenyl)-1,4-dihydro-2,6-dimethyl-, methyl (1-oxobutoxy)methyl ester; (2) (Butanoyloxy)methyl methyl (4*RS*)-4-(2,3-dichlorophenyl)-2,6-dimethyl-1,4-dihydropyridine-3,5-dicarboxylate. *UNII-19O2GP3B7Q*. *CAS-167221-71-8; CAS-166432-28-6* [clevidipine]. *Antihypertensive.* Clevelox (The Medicines Company) ◇*H324/38*

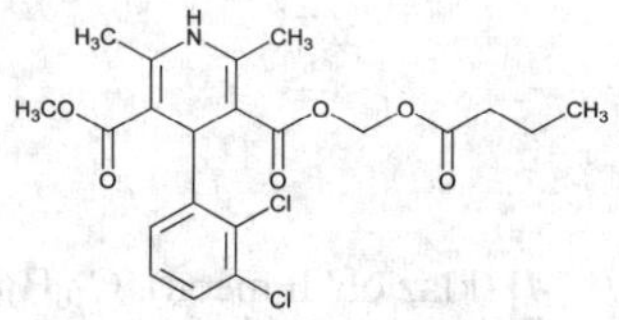

Clevudine [*1998*] (klev′ ue deen). $C_{10}H_{13}FN_2O_5$. 260.22. (1) 2,4(1*H*,3*H*)-Pyrimidinedione, 1-(2-deoxy-2-fluoro-β-L-arabinofuranosyl)-5-methyl-; (2) 1-(2-Deoxy-2-fluoro-β-L-arabinofuranosyl)thymine. *CAS-163252-36-6*. INN. *Antiviral used in the treatment of hepatitis B infection.* ◇*L-FMAU*

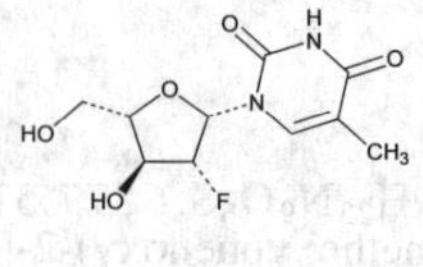

Clibucaine. $C_{15}H_{20}Cl_2N_2O$. 315.24. 2′,4′-Dichloro-β-piperidinobutyranilide. *UNII-NB2ZOX88RR*. *CAS-15302-10-0*. INN.

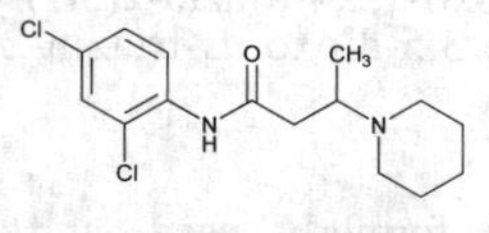

Clidafidine. $C_9H_8Cl_2N_2O$. 231.08. 2-[(2,6-Dichlorophenyl)-imino]oxazolidine. *CAS-33588-20-4.* INN.

Clidanac. $C_{16}H_{19}ClO_2$. 278.77. 6-Chloro-5-cyclohexyl-1-indancarboxylic acid. *UNII-UA6HM01WAK. CAS-34148-01-1.* INN; JAN; MI.

Clidinium Bromide [*1961*] (kli din' ee um broe' mide). **USP**. $C_{22}H_{26}BrNO_3$. 432.35. (1) 1-Azoniabicyclo[2.2.2]octane, 3-[(hydroxydiphenylacetyl)oxy]-1-methyl-, bromide, (±)-; (2) (±)-3-Hydroxy-1-methylquinuclidinium bromide benzilate. *UNII-91ZQW5JF1Z. CAS-3485-62-9.* INN; BAN. *Anticholinergic.* Quarzan (Roche) ◇*Ro 2-3773*

Climazolam. $C_{18}H_{13}Cl_2N_3$. 342.22. 8-Chloro-6-(*o*-chlorophenyl)-1-methyl-4*H*-imidazo[1,5-*a*][1,4]benzodiazepine. *UNII-O9KZB9HG1Y. CAS-59467-77-5.* INN.

Climbazole. $C_{15}H_{17}ClN_2O_2$. 292.76. 1-(*p*-Chlorophenoxy)-1-imidazol-1-yl-3,3-dimethyl-2-butanone. *UNII-9N42CW7I54. CAS-38083-17-9.* INN; BAN.

Climiqualine. $C_{18}H_{12}ClN_3$. 305.76. 3-Chloro-1-imidazol-1-yl-4-phenylisoquinoline. *UNII-M2I27EKQ47. CAS-55150-67-9.* INN.

---

† Brand name formerly used, and/or firm no longer concerned with this product.

Clinafloxacin Hydrochloride [*1992*] (klin″ a flox′ a sin hye″ droe klor′ ide). $C_{17}H_{17}ClFN_3O_3$.HCl. 402.25. [Clinafloxacin is INN.] (1) 3-Quinolinecarboxylic acid, 7-(3-amino-1-pyrrolidinyl)-8-chloro-1-cyclopropyl-6-fluoro-1,4-dihydro-4-oxo-, monohydrochloride, (±)-; (2) (±)-7-(3-Amino-1-pyrrolidinyl)-8-chloro-1-cyclopropyl-6-fluoro-1,4-dihydro-4-oxo-3-quinolinecarboxylic acid, monohydrochloride. *UNII-G17M59V0FY; UNII-8N86XTF9QD* [clinafloxacin]. *CAS-105956-99-8; CAS-105956-97-6* [clinafloxacin]. *Antibacterial.* ◇*CI-960 HCl*

Clindamycin [*1968*] (klin″ da mye′ sin). $C_{18}H_{33}ClN_2O_5S$. 424.98. (1) L-*threo*-α-D-*galacto*-Octopyranoside, methyl 7-chloro-6,7,8-trideoxy-6-[[(1-methyl-4-propyl-2-pyrrolidinyl)carbonyl]amino]-1-thio-, (2*S-trans*)-; (2) Methyl 7-chloro-6,7,8-trideoxy-6-(1-methyl-*trans*-4-propyl-L-2-pyrrolidinecarboxamido)-1-thio-L-*threo*-α-D-*galacto*-octopyranoside; (3) 7(*S*)-Chloro-7-deoxylincomycin. *UNII-3U02EL437C. CAS-18323-44-9.* INN; BAN. *Antibacterial.* Cleocin (Pharmacia & Upjohn) ◇*U-21,251*

Clindamycin Hydrochloride (klin″ da mye′ sin hye″ droe klor′ ide). **USP**. $C_{18}H_{33}ClN_2O_5S$.HCl. 461.44. (1) L-*threo*-α-D-*galacto*-Octopyranoside, methyl 7-chloro-6,7,8-trideoxy-6-[[(1-methyl-4-propyl-2-pyrrolidinyl)carbonyl]amino]-1-thio-, (2*S-trans*)-, monohydrochloride; (2) Methyl 7-chloro-6,7,8-trideoxy-6-(1-methyl-*trans*-4-propyl-L-2-pyrrolidinecarboxamido)-1-thio-L-*threo*-α-D-*galacto*-octopyranoside monohydrochloride. *UNII-T20OQ1YN1W; UNII-3U02EL437C* [clindamycin]. *CAS-21462-39-5; CAS-58207-19-5* [monohydrate]; *CAS-18323-44-9* [clindamycin]. BAN; JAN. *Antibacterial.* Cleocin (Pfizer)

Clindamycin Palmitate Hydrochloride [*1974*] (klin″ da mye′ sin pal′ mi tate hye″ droe klor′ ide). **USP**. $C_{34}H_{63}ClN_2O_6S$.HCl. 699.85. (1) L-*threo*-α-D-*galacto*-Octopyranoside, methyl 7-chloro-6,7,8-trideoxy-6-[[(1-methyl-4-propyl-2-pyrrolidinyl)carbonyl]amino]-1-thio-2-hexadecanoate, monohydrochloride, (2*S-trans*)-; (2) Methyl 7-chloro-6,7,8-trideoxy-6-(1-methyl-*trans*-4-propyl-L-2-pyrrolidinecarboxamido)-1-thio-L-*threo*-α-D-*galacto*-octopyranoside 2-palmitate monohydrochloride. *UNII-VN9A8JM7M7. CAS-25507-04-4; CAS-36688-78-5* [clindamycin palmitate]. JAN. *Antibacterial.* Cleocin (Pfizer) ◇*U-25,179 E*

Clindamycin Phosphate [*1972*] (klin″ da mye′ sin fos′ fate). **USP**. $C_{18}H_{34}ClN_2O_8PS$. 504.96. (1) L-*threo*-α-D-*galacto*-Octopyranoside, methyl 7-chloro-6,7,8-trideoxy-6-[[(1-methyl-4-propyl-2-pyrrolidinyl)carbonyl]amino]-1-thio-,

2-(dihydrogen phosphate), (2*S*-*trans*)-; (2) Methyl 7-chloro-6,7,8-trideoxy-6-(1-methyl-*trans*-4-propyl-L-2-pyrrolidinecarboxamido)-1-thio-L-*threo*-α-D-*galacto*-octopyranoside 2-(dihydrogen phosphate); (3) 7(*S*)-Chloro-7-deoxylincomycin 2-phosphate. *UNII-EH6D7113I8; UNII-3U02EL437C* [clindamycin]. *CAS-24729-96-2; CAS-18323-44-9* [clindamycin]. JAN. *Antibacterial.* Cleocin (Pfizer); Clindagel (Galderma); Clindesse (KV Pharmaceutical); Evoclin (Connetics) ◇*U-28,508*

Clinofibrate. $C_{28}H_{36}O_6$. 468.58. 2,2′-[Cyclohexylidenebis(*p*-phenyleneoxy)]bis[2-methylbutyric acid]. *UNII-0374EZJ8CU. CAS-30299-08-2.* INN; JAN; MI.

Clinolamide. $C_{24}H_{43}NO$. 361.60. *N*-Cyclohexyllinoleamide. *UNII-G90E14A6I6. CAS-3207-50-9.* INN.

Clinprost. $C_{22}H_{36}O_4$. 364.52. (+)-Methyl-(3a*S*,5*R*,6*R*,6a*S*)-1,3a,4,5,6,6a-hexahydro-5-hydroxy-6-[(*E*)-(3*S*)-3-hydroxy-1-octenyl]-2-pentalenevalerate. *UNII-6GRI2J11N5. CAS-88931-51-5.* INN.

Clioquinol (klye″ oh kwin′ ol). **USP.** C_9H_5ClINO. 305.50. (1) 8-Quinolinol, 5-chloro-7-iodo-; (2) 5-Chloro-7-iodo-8-quinolinol. *UNII-7BHQ856EJ5. CAS-130-26-7.* INN; BAN. *Anti-amebic; anti-infective, topical.* Domeform-HC (Bayer†); Quin-O-Creme (Marion Merrell Dow†); Rheaform Boluses [Veterinary] (Fort Dodge Animal Health†); Vioform (Ciba-Geigy†) *[Name previously used: Iodochlorhydroxyquin.]*

Clioxanide [*1968*] (klye ox′ a nide). $C_{15}H_{10}ClI_2NO_3$. 541.51. (1) Benzamide, 2-(acetyloxy)-*N*-(4-chlorophenyl)-3,5-diiodo-; (2) 4′-Chloro-3,5-diiodosalicylanilide acetate. *UNII-2Q9A409N0B. CAS-14437-41-3.* INN; BAN. *Anthelmintic.* ◇*CI-633; CN 59,567; SYD-230*

Clipoxamine — *See* Cliropamine.

Cliprofen [*1974*] (klye proe′ fen). $C_{14}H_{11}ClO_3S$. 294.75. (1) Benzeneacetic acid, 3-chloro-α-methyl-4-(2-thienylcarbonyl)-; (2) 3-Chloro-4-(2-thenoyl)hydratropic acid. *UNII-BB27ZR25WO. CAS-51022-75-4.* INN. *Anti-inflammatory.* ◇*R-25,160*

Cliropamine. $C_{19}H_{25}NO_2$. 299.41. (±)-(α*R**)-3-Hydroxy-4-methyl-α-[(1*S**)-1-[(3-phenylpropyl)amino]ethyl]benzyl alcohol. *UNII-87V8H2Q8IH. CAS-109525-44-2.* INN.

Clobamine Mesylate (previously used name) — *See* Cilobamine Mesylate.

Clobazam [*1975*] (kloe′ ba zam). $C_{16}H_{13}ClN_2O_2$. 300.74. (1) 1*H*-1,5-Benzodiazepine-2,4(3*H*,5*H*)-dione, 7-chloro-1-methyl-5-phenyl-; (2) 7-Chloro-1-methyl-5-phenyl-1*H*-1,5-benzodiazepine-2,4-(3*H*,5*H*)-dione. *UNII-2MRO291-B4U. CAS-22316-47-8.* INN; BAN. *Tranquilizer (minor).* Urbanyl (Hoechst-Roussel†) ◇*HR 376; H 4723; LM 2717*

Clobedolum — *See* Clonitazene.

Clobenoside. $C_{25}H_{32}Cl_2O_6$. 499.42. Ethyl 5,6-bis-*O*-(*p*-chlorobenzyl)-3-*O*-propyl-D-glucofuranoside. *UNII-8427MP5VHD. CAS-29899-95-4.* INN; MI. ◇*43853*

Clobenzepam. $C_{17}H_{18}ClN_3O$. 315.80. 7-Chloro-10-[2-(dimethylamino)ethyl]-5,10-dihydro-11*H*-dibenzo[*b,e*][1,4]diazepin-11-one. *UNII-0O6W0NP518. CAS-1159-93-9.* INN; MI.

Clobenzorex. $C_{16}H_{18}ClN$. 259.77. (+)-*N*-(*o*-Chlorobenzyl)-α-methylphenethylamine. *UNII-4A5352XI2A. CAS-13364-32-4.* INN; DCF; MI. ◇*SD 271-12*

Clobenztropine. $C_{21}H_{24}ClNO$. 341.87. 3-[(*p*-Chloro-α-phenylbenzyl)oxy]tropane. *CAS-5627-46-3.* INN; MI.

Clobetasol Propionate [*1983*] (kloe bay′ ta sol proe′ pee oh nate). **USP.** $C_{25}H_{32}ClFO_5$. 466.97. [Clobetasol is INN and BAN.] (1) Pregna-1,4-diene-3,20-dione, 21-chloro-9-fluoro-11-hydroxy-16-methyl-17-(1-oxopropoxy)-, (11β,16β)-; (2) 21-Chloro-9-fluoro-11β,17-dihydroxy-16β-methylpregna-1,4-diene-3,20-dione 17-propionate. *UNII-7796I9577M; UNII-ADN79D536H* [clobetasol]. *CAS-25122-46-7; CAS-25122-41-2* [clobetasol]. JAN. *Anti-inflammatory.* Clobex (Galderma); Cormax (Healthpoint); Embeline (Healthpoint); Olux (Connetics); Temovate (Altana) ◇*CCI 4725; GR 2/925*

Clobetasone Butyrate [*1983*] (kloe bay′ ta sone bue′ ti rate). $C_{26}H_{32}ClFO_5$. 478.98. [Clobetasone is INN and BAN.] (1) Pregna-1,4-diene-3,11,20-trione, 21-chloro-9-fluoro-16-methyl-17-(1-oxobutoxy)-, (16β)-; (2) 21-Chloro-9-fluoro-17-hydroxy-16β-methylpregna-1,4-diene-3,11,20-trione butyrate. *UNII-8U0H6XI6EO. CAS-25122-57-0; CAS-54063-32-0* [clobetasone]. JAN. *Anti-inflammatory.* ◇*CCI 5537; GR 2/1214*

---

† Brand name formerly used, and/or firm no longer concerned with this product.

Clobutinol. $C_{14}H_{22}ClNO$. 255.78. [Clobutinol Hydrochloride is JAN.] *p*-Chloro-α-[2-(dimethylamino)-1-methylethyl]-α-methylphenethyl alcohol. *UNII-1NY2IX043A. CAS-14860-49-2.* INN; MI. ◇*KAT 256 [as hydrochloride]*

Clobuzarit. $C_{17}H_{17}ClO_3$. 304.77. 2-[(4′-Chloro-4-biphenylyl)methoxy]-2-methylpropionic acid. *UNII-W3D7B06505. CAS-22494-47-9.* INN; BAN; MI. ◇*ICI 55,897*

Clocanfamide. $C_{18}H_{24}ClNO_2$. 321.84. *p*-Chloro-*N*-(2-hydroxyethyl)-*N*-[(3-methyl-2-norbornyl)methyl]benzamide. *UNII-21Q62BRI9U. CAS-18966-32-0.* INN.

Clocapramine. $C_{28}H_{37}ClN_4O$. 481.07. [Clocapramine Hydrochloride is JAN.] 1′-[3-(3-Chloro-10,11-dihydro-5*H*-dibenz[*b,f*]azepin-5-yl)propyl][1,4′-bipiperidine]-4′-carboxamide. *UNII-6EELlGB72K. CAS-47739-98-0.* INN; MI. ◇*Y 4153 [as hydrochloride]*

Clociguanil. $C_{12}H_{15}Cl_2N_5O$. 316.19. 4,6-Diamino-1-[(3,4-dichlorobenzyl)oxy]-1,2-dihydro-2,2-dimethyl-*s*-triazine. *UNII-32W4ZSE0X7. CAS-3378-93-6.* INN; BAN.

Clocinizine. $C_{26}H_{27}ClN_2$. 402.96. 1-(*p*-Chloro-α-phenylbenzyl)-4-cinnamylpiperazine. *UNII-8HQJ711KH8. CAS-298-55-5.* INN; DCF; MI.

Clocortolone Acetate [*1965*] (kloe kor′ toe lone as′ e tate). $C_{24}H_{30}ClFO_5$. 452.94. [Clocortolone is INN.] (1) Pregna-1,4-diene-3,20-dione, 21-(acetyloxy)-9-chloro-6-fluoro-11-hydroxy-16-methyl-, (6α,11β,16α)-; (2) 9-Chloro-6α-fluoro-11β,21-dihydroxy-16α-methylpregna-1,4-diene-

3,20-dione 21-acetate. *UNII-85061HTR8T; UNII-N8ZUB7XE0H* [clocortolone]. *CAS-4258-85-9; CAS-4828-27-7* [clocortolone]. *Glucocorticoid.* ◇*SH 818*

Clocortolone Pivalate [*1972*] (kloe kor′ toe lone piv′ a late). **USP.** $C_{27}H_{36}ClFO_5$. 495.02. (1) Pregna-1,4-diene-3,20-dione, 9-chloro-21-(2,2-dimethyl-1-oxopropoxy)-6-fluoro-11-hydroxy-16-methyl-, (6α,11β,16α)-; (2) 9-Chloro-6α-fluoro-11β,21-dihydroxy-16α-methylpregna-1,4-diene-3,20-dione 21-pivalate. *UNII-QBL8IZH14X. CAS-34097-16-0. Glucocorticoid.* Cloderm (Coria) ◇*SH 863*

Clocoumarol. $C_{21}H_{21}ClO_3$. 356.84. 3-[*p*-(2-Chloroethyl)-α-propylbenzyl]-4-hydroxycoumarin. *UNII-M9K14Z7S3L. CAS-35838-63-2.* INN.

Clodacaine. $C_{16}H_{26}ClN_3O$. 311.85. 2′-Chloro-2-[[2-(diethylamino)ethyl]ethylamino]acetanilide. *UNII-H743H7R6YE. CAS-5626-25-5.* INN.

Clodanolene [*1976*] (kloe dan′ oh leen). $C_{14}H_9Cl_2N_3O_3$. 338.15. (1) 2,4-Imidazolidinedione, 1-[[[5-(3,4-dichloro-phenyl)-2-furanyl]methylene]amino]-; (2) 1-[[5-(3,4-Di-chlorophenyl)furfurylidene]amino]hydantoin. *CAS-14796-28-2.* INN. *Relaxant (skeletal muscle).* ◇*F-413; F-605 (as the sodium)*

Clodantoin (INN, BAN) — *See* Chlordantoin.

Clodazon Hydrochloride [*1971*] (kloe′ da zone hye″ droe klor′ ide). $C_{18}H_{20}ClN_3O \cdot HCl \cdot H_2O$. 384.30. [Clodazon is INN.] (1) 2*H*-Benzimidazol-2-one,5-chloro-1-[3-(dimethyl-lamino)propyl]-1,3-dihydro-3-phenyl-, monohydrochlor-

ide, monohydrate; (2) 5-Chloro-1-[3-(dimethylamino)propyl]-3-phenyl-2-benzimidazolinone monohydrochloride monohydrate. *UNII-FSF9L5AH4G. CAS-31959-88-3; CAS-4913-61-5* [anhydrous]; *CAS-4755-59-3* [clodazon]. *Antidepressant.* ◇*HUF-2446; AW-14′2446*

Clodoxopone. $C_{21}H_{21}ClN_2O_3$. 384.86. 4-(*p*-Chlorophenyl)-5-[2-(4-phenyl-1-piperazinyl)ethyl]-1,3-dioxol-2-one. *UNII-F94O7Q5JLM. CAS-71923-34-7.* INN.

Clodronate Disodium [*2001*] (kloe droe′ nate dye soe′ dee um). $CH_2Cl_2Na_2O_6P_2 \cdot 4H_2O$. 360.92. (1) Phosphonic acid, (dichloromethylene)bis-, disodium salt tetrahydrate; (2) (Dichloromethylene)bisphosphonate disodium tetrahydrate. *UNII-N030400H8J. CAS-22560-50-5* [anhydrous]. *Bone calcium regulator.* Bonefos (Leiras Oy, Finland) ◇*177501; ZK 00091106*

Clodronic Acid [*1977*] (kloe dron′ ik as′ id). $CH_4Cl_2O_6P_2$. 244.89. (1) Phosphonic acid, (dichloromethylene)bis-; (2) (Dichloromethylene)diphosphonic acid; (3) Dichloro-methanediphosphonic acid. *UNII-0813BZ6866. CAS-10596-23-3.* INN; BAN. *Regulator (calcium).*

Clofarabine [*2003*] (kloe far′ a been). $C_{10}H_{11}ClFN_5O_3$. 303.68. (1) 9*H*-Purin-6-amine, 2-chloro-9-(2-deoxy-2-fluoro-β-D-arabinofuranosyl)-; (2) 2-Chloro-9-(2-deoxy-2-fluoro-β-D-arabinofuranosyl)-9*H*-purin-6-amine. *UNII-762RDY0Y2H. CAS-123318-82-1.* INN; BAN. *Treatment of primary refractory or relapsed acute myelogenous leukemia (AML) or acute lymphoblastic leukemia (ALL) in pediatric and adult patients.* Clolar (Genzyme)

Clofazimine [*1967*] (kloe faz′ i meen). **USP.** $C_{27}H_{22}Cl_2N_4$. 473.40. (1) 2-Phenazinamine, *N*,5-bis(4-chlorophenyl)-3,5-dihydro-3-[(1-methylethyl)imino]-; (2) 3-(*p*-Chloroanili-no)-10-(*p*-chlorophenyl)-2,10-dihydro-2-(isopropylimino)-

phenazine. *UNII-D959AE5USF. CAS-2030-63-9.* INN; BAN. *Antibacterial (tuberculostatic); antibacterial (leprostatic).* Lamprene (Novartis) ◇*G 30320; NSC-141046*

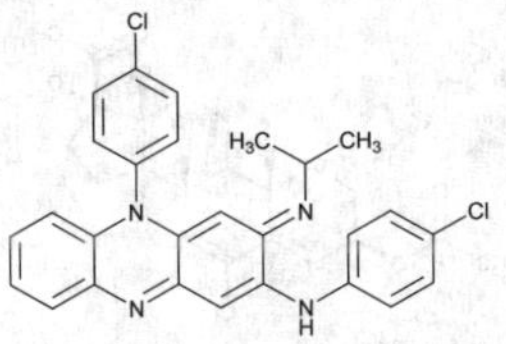

Clofedanol (INN; BAN) — *See* Chlophedianol Hydrochloride.

Clofedanol Hydrochloride (JAN) — *See* Chlophedianol Hydrochloride.

Clofenamic Acid. $C_{13}H_9ClNO_2$. 246.67. *N*-(2,3-Dichlorophenyl)anthranilic acid. *UNII-1X0MUE4C19. CAS-4295-55-0.* INN.

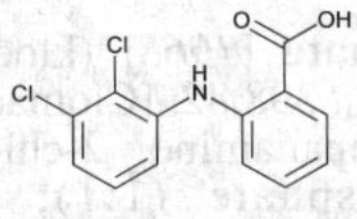

Clofenamide. $C_6H_7ClN_2O_4S_2$. 270.71. 4-Chloro-*m*-benzenedisulfonamide. *UNII-582ILN204B. CAS-671-95-4.* INN; JAN; MI.

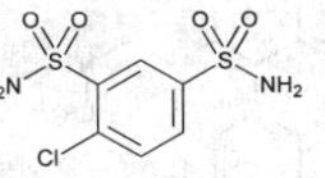

Clofenciclan. $C_{18}H_{28}ClNO$. 309.87. 2-[[1-(*p*-Chlorophenyl)cyclohexyl]oxy]triethylamine. *UNII-P4BVX0D2MX. CAS-5632-52-0.* INN; MI.

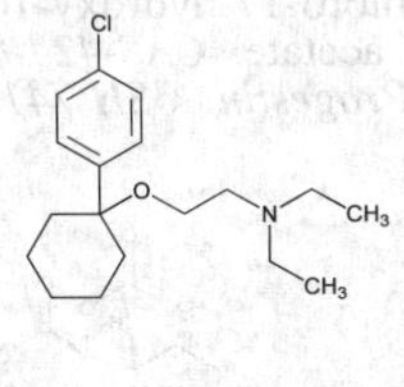

Clofenetamine Hydrochloride. $C_{20}H_{26}ClNO \cdot HCl$. 368.34. [Clofenetamine is INN.] 2-(*p*-Chloro-α-methyl-α-phenylbenzyloxy)triethylamine hydrochloride. *CAS-2019-16-1; CAS-511-46-6* [clofenetamine].

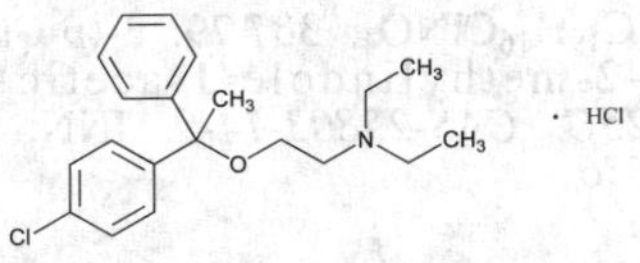

Clofenotane (INN) — *See* Chlorophenothane.

---

† Brand name formerly used, and/or firm no longer concerned with this product.

Clofenoxyde. $C_{16}H_{12}Cl_2O_3$. 323.17. 4,4′-Oxybis(2-chloroacetophenone). *UNII-1B2Zl1L2P8. CAS-3030-53-3.* INN; DCF.

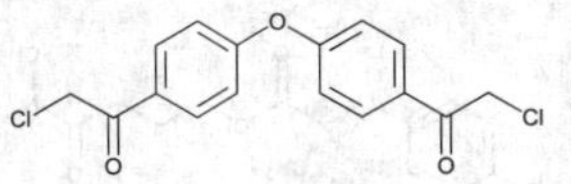

Clofenpyride — *See* Nicofibrate.

Clofeverine. $C_{16}H_{16}ClNO_3$. 305.76. 1-[(*p*-Chlorophenoxy)methyl]-1,2,3,4-tetrahydro-6,7-isoquinolinediol. *UNII-584A0O55XM. CAS-54340-63-5.* INN.

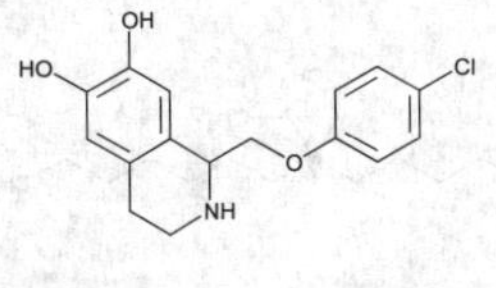

Clofexamide. $C_{14}H_{21}ClN_2O_2$. 284.78. 2-(*p*-Chlorophenoxy)-*N*-[2-(diethylamino)ethyl]acetamide. *UNII-071P4J77HF. CAS-1223-36-5.* INN; DCF. ◇*ANP 246*

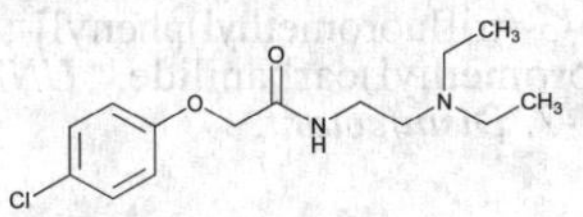

Clofezone. $C_{14}H_{21}ClN_2O_2 \cdot C_{19}H_{20}N_2O_2 \cdot 2H_2O$. 629.19. Equimolar combination of Clofexamide and Phenylbutazone. *UNII-TPT3MH65LD. CAS-60104-29-2.* INN; JAN; DCF. ◇*ANP 3260*

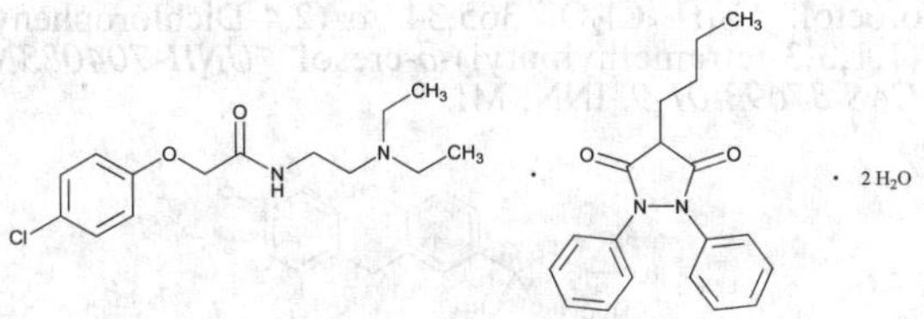

Clofibrate [*1963*] (kloe fye′ brate). **USP.** $C_{12}H_{15}ClO_3$. 242.70. (1) Propanoic acid, 2-(4-chlorophenoxy)-2-methyl-, ethyl ester; (2) Ethyl 2-(*p*-chlorophenoxy)-2-methylpropionate. *UNII-HPN91K7FU3. CAS-637-07-0.* INN; BAN; JAN. *Antihyperlipidemic.* Atromid (Wyeth) ◇*AY-61123; ICI 28257; NSC-79389*

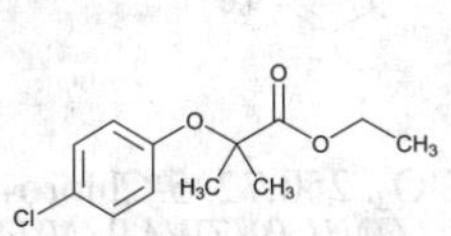

Clofibric Acid. $C_{10}H_{11}ClO_3$. 214.65. 2-(*p*-Chlorophenoxy)-2-methylpropionic acid. *CAS-882-09-7.* INN; DCF; MI.

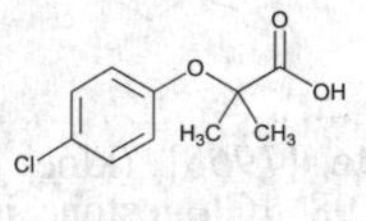

Clofibride. $C_{16}H_{22}ClNO_4$. 327.80. 2-(*p*-Chlorophenoxy)-2-methylpropionic acid, ester with 4-hydroxy-*N,N*-dimethylbutyramide. *UNII-0S9SLS3L93. CAS-26717-47-5.* INN; DCF.

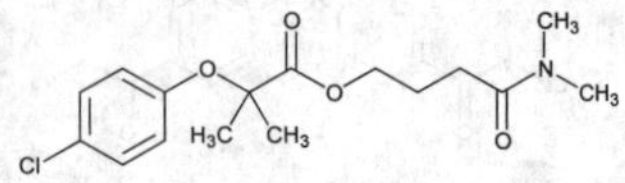

Clofilium Phosphate [*1979*] (kloe fil' ee um fos' fate). $C_{21}H_{39}ClNO_4P$. 435.97. (1) Benzenebutanaminium, 4-chloro-*N,N*-diethyl-*N*-heptyl-, phosphate (1:1); (2) [4-(*p*-Chlorophenyl)butyl]diethylheptylammonium phosphate (1:1). *CAS-68379-03-3.* INN. *Cardiac depressant (antiarrhythmic).* ◇*LY 150378*

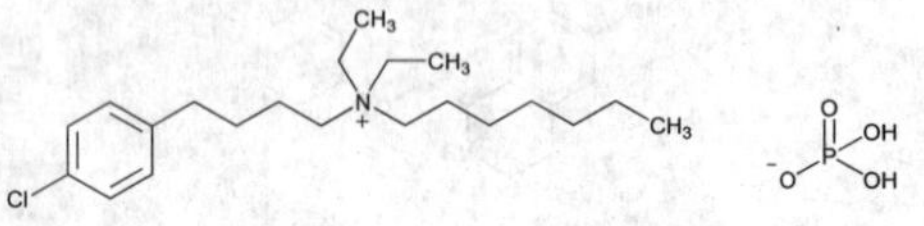

Clofinol — *See* Nicofibrate.

Cloflucarban [*1965*] (kloe" floo kar' ban). $C_{14}H_9Cl_2F_3N_2O$. 349.14. [Halocarban is INN.] (1) Urea, *N*-(4-chlorophenyl)-*N'*-[4-chloro-3-(trifluoromethyl)phenyl]-; (2) 4,4'-Dichloro-3-(trifluoromethyl)carbanilide. *UNII-I5ZZY3DC5G. CAS-369-77-7. Disinfectant.*

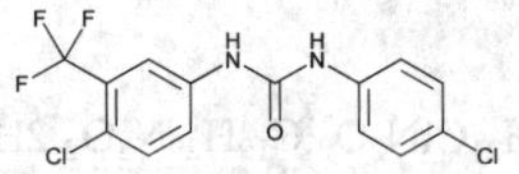

Clofluperol (INN, BAN) — *See* Seperidol Hydrochloride.

Clofoctol. $C_{21}H_{26}Cl_2O$. 365.34. α-(2,4-Dichlorophenyl)-4-(1,1,3,3-tetramethylbutyl)-*o*-cresol. *UNII-704083NI0R. CAS-37693-01-9.* INN; MI.

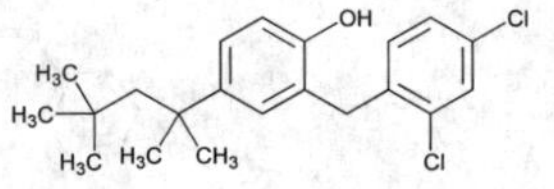

Cloforex. $C_{13}H_{18}ClNO_2$. 255.74. Ethyl (*p*-chloro-α,α-dimethylphenethyl)carbamate. *CAS-14261-75-7.* INN; MI. ◇*D 237*

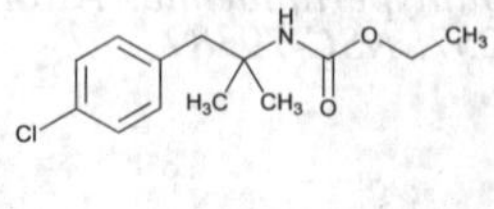

Clofurac. $C_{14}H_{15}ClO_2$. 250.72. 5-Chloro-6-cyclohexyl-2(3*H*)-benzofuranone. *UNII-0V7WAB3NV4. CAS-60986-89-2.* INN.

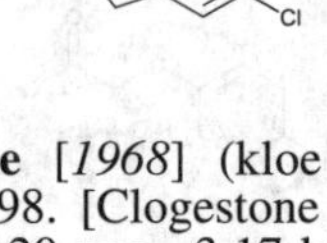

Clogestone Acetate [*1968*] (kloe jes' tone as' e tate). $C_{25}H_{33}ClO_5$. 448.98. [Clogestone is INN and BAN.] (1) Pregna-4,6-diene-20-one, 3,17-bis(acetyloxy)-6-chloro-,

(3β)-; (2) 6-Chloro-3β,17-dihydroxypregna-4,6-dien-20-one diacetate. *CAS-3044-32-4; CAS-20047-75-0* [clogestone]. *Progestin.* ◇*AY-11,440*

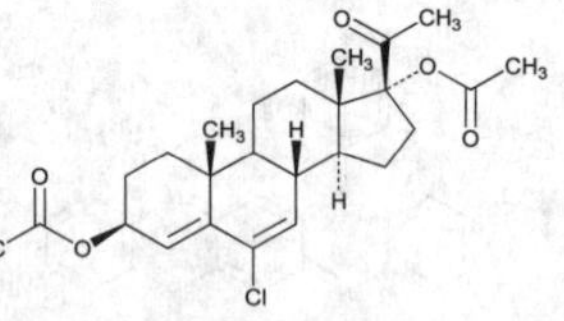

Cloguanamil. $C_9H_8ClN_5O$. 237.65. 1-Amidino-3-(3-chloro-4-cyanophenyl)urea. *CAS-21702-93-2.* INN; BAN. ◇*57C65*

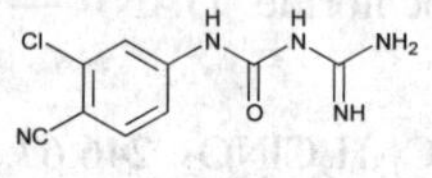

Cloguanamile (BAN) — *See* Cloguanamil.

Clomacran Phosphate [*1968*] (kloe' ma kran fos' fate). $C_{18}H_{21}ClN_2·H_3PO_4$. 398.82. [Clomacran is INN and BAN.] (1) 9-Acridinepropanamine, 2-chloro-9,10-dihydro-*N,N*-dimethyl-, phosphate (1:1); (2) 2-Chloro-9-[3-(dimethylamino)propyl]acridan phosphate (1:1). *CAS-22199-46-8; CAS-5310-55-4* [clomacran]. *Antipsychotic.* Devryl (SmithKline Beecham†); Olaxin (SmithKline Beecham†) ◇*SK&F 14336*

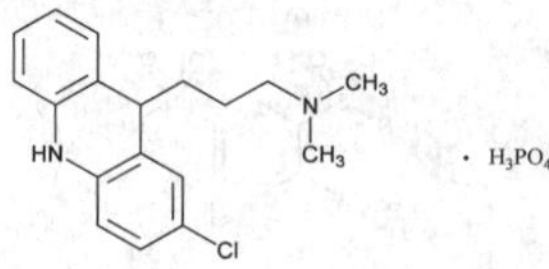

Clomegestone Acetate [*1968*] (kloe" me jes' tone as' e tate). $C_{24}H_{31}ClO_4$. 418.95. [Clomegestone is INN.] (1) Pregna-4,6-diene-3,20-dione, 17-(acetyloxy)-6-chloro-16-methyl-, (16α)-; (2) 6-Chloro-17-hydroxy-16α-methylpregna-4,6-diene-3,20-dione acetate. *CAS-424-89-5; CAS-5367-84-0* [clomegestone]. *Progestin.* ◇*SH 741*

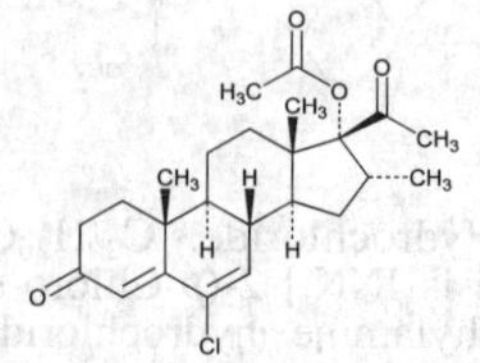

Clometacin. $C_{19}H_{16}ClNO_4$. 357.79. 3-(*p*-Chlorobenzoyl)-6-methoxy-2-methylindole-1-acetic acid. *UNII-L9M34YK25C. CAS-25803-14-9.* INN; DCF; MI. ◇*R 3959; C 1656*

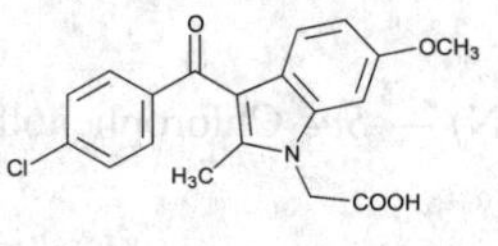

Clometerone (INN) — *See* Clometherone.

Clometherone [*1964*] (kloe meth′ er one). $C_{22}H_{31}ClO_2$. 362.93. [Clometerone is INN.] (1) Pregn-4-ene-3,20-dione, 6-chloro-16-methyl-, (6α,16α)-; (2) 6α-Chloro-16α-methylpregn-4-ene-3,20-dione. *UNII-01L3E93T4C. CAS-5591-27-5. Anti-estrogen.* ◇*38000*

Clomethiazole. C_6H_8ClNS. 161.65. 5-(2-Chloroethyl)-4-methylthiazole. *CAS-533-45-9.* INN; BAN; MI. ◇*SCTZ* [*as edisylate*]

Clometocillin. $C_{17}H_{18}Cl_2N_2O_5S$. 433.31. (3,4-Dichloro-α-methoxybenzyl)penicillin. *UNII-YI8LL014GF. CAS-1926-49-4.* INN; DCF; MI.

Clomide — *See* Aklomide.

Clomifene (INN) — *See* Clomiphene Citrate.

Clomifene Citrate (JAN) — *See* Clomiphene Citrate.

Clomifenoxide. $C_{26}H_{28}ClNO_2$. 421.96. 2-[*p*-(2-Chloro-1,2-diphenylvinyl)phenoxy]triethylamine *N*-oxide. *CAS-97642-74-5.* INN.

Clominorex [*1963*] (kloe min′ oh rex). $C_9H_9ClN_2O$. 196.63. (1) 2-Oxazolamine, 5-(4-chlorophenyl)-4,5-dihydro-; (2) 2-Amino-5-(*p*-chlorophenyl)-2-oxazoline. *UNII-O1R2462WA0. CAS-3876-10-6.* INN. *Anorexic.* ◇*McN-1107*

Clomiphene (BAN) — *See* Clomiphene Citrate.

Clomiphene Citrate [*1964*] (kloe′ mi feen sit′ rate). **USP.** $C_{26}H_{28}ClNO \cdot C_6H_8O_7$. 598.08. [Clomifene is INN and BAN; Clomifene Citrate is JAN.] (1) Ethanamine, 2-[4-(2-chloro-1,2-diphenylethenyl)phenoxy]-*N,N*-diethyl-, 2-hydroxy-1,2,3-propanetricarboxylate (1:1); (2) 2-[*p*-(2-Chloro-1,2-diphenylvinyl)phenoxy]triethylamine citrate (1:1). *UNII-1B8447E7YI; UNII-1HRS458QU2* [clomiphene]. *CAS-50-41-9; CAS-911-45-5* [clomiphene]. *Anti-estrogen.* Clomid (Sanofi Aventis); Milophene (Milex) ◇*MRL-41; MER-41; NSC-35770*

Clomipramine Hydrochloride [*1970*] (kloe mip′ ra meen hye″ droe klor′ ide). **USP.** $C_{19}H_{23}ClN_2 \cdot HCl$. 351.31. [Clomipramine is INN and BAN.] (1) 5*H*-Dibenz[*b,f*]azepine-5-propanamine, 3-chloro-10,11-dihydro-*N,N*-dimethyl-, monohydrochloride; (2) 3-Chloro-5-[3-(dimethylamino)propyl]-10,11-dihydro-5*H*-dibenz[*b,f*]azepine monohydrochloride. *UNII-2LXW0L6GWJ; UNII-NUV44L116D* [clomipramine]. *CAS-17321-77-6; CAS-303-49-1* [clomipramine]. JAN. *Antidepressant.* Anafranil (Tyco) ◇*G 34586*

Clomocycline. $C_{23}H_{25}ClN_2O_9$. 508.91. 7-Chloro-4-(dimethylamino)-1,4,4a,5,5a,6,11,12a-octahydro-3,6,10,12,12a-pentahydroxy-*N*-(hydroxymethyl)-6-methyl-1,11-dioxo-2-naphthacenecarboxamide. *UNII-YP0241BU76. CAS-1181-54-0.* INN; BAN; MI.

Clomoxir. $C_{14}H_{17}ClO_3$. 268.74. (±)-2-[5-(*p*-Chlorophenyl)-pentyl]glycidic acid. *UNII-PD884XOZ9F. CAS-88431-47-4.* INN.

Clonazepam [*1969*] (kloe naz′ e pam). **USP.** $C_{15}H_{10}ClN_3O_3$. 315.71. (1) 2*H*-1,4-Benzodiazepin-2-one, 5-(2-chlorophenyl)-1,3-dihydro-7-nitro-; (2) 5-(*o*-Chlorophenyl)-1,3-dihydro-7-nitro-2*H*-1,4-benzodiazepin-2-one. *UNII-5PE9FDE8GB. CAS-1622-61-3.* INN; BAN; JAN. *Anticonvulsant.* Klonopin (Roche) ◇*Ro 5-4023*

---

† Brand name formerly used, and/or firm no longer concerned with this product.

Clonazoline. $C_{14}H_{13}ClN_2$. 244.72. 2-(4-Chloro-1-naphthyl-methyl)-2-imidazoline. *UNII-YH9K692U9S. CAS-17692-28-3.* INN.

Clonidine [*1984*] (kloe′ ni deen). **USP.** $C_9H_9Cl_2N_3$. 230.09. (1) Benzenamine, 2,6-dichloro-*N*-2-imidazolidinylidene-; (2) 2-[(2,6-Dichlorophenyl)imino]imidazolidine. *UNII-MN3L5RMN02. CAS-4205-90-7.* INN; BAN. *Antihypertensive.* Catapres (Boehringer Ingelheim) ◇*ST-155-BS*

Clonidine Hydrochloride [*1969*] (kloe′ ni deen hye″ droe klor′ ide). **USP.** $C_9H_9Cl_2N_3 \cdot HCl$. 266.55. (1) Benzenamine, 2,6-dichloro-*N*-2-imidazolidinylidene-, monohydrochloride; (2) 2-[(2,6-Dichlorophenyl)imino]imidazolidine monohydrochloride. *UNII-W76I6XXF06; UNII-MN3L5RMN02* [clonidine]. *CAS-4205-91-8; CAS-4205-90-7* [clonidine]. BAN; JAN. *Antihypertensive.* Catapres (Boehringer Ingelheim); Duraclon (Xanodyne) ◇*ST-155*

Clonitazene. $C_{20}H_{23}ClN_4O_2$. 386.88. 2-(*p*-Chlorobenzyl)-1-(2-diethylaminoethyl)-5-nitrobenzimidazole. *UNII-S90R21A2V2. CAS-3861-76-5.* INN; BAN; DCF; MI.

Clonitrate [*1962*] (kloe nye′ trate). $C_3H_5ClN_2O_6$. 200.53. (1) 1,2-Propanediol, 3-chloro-, dinitrate; (2) 3-Chloro-1,2-propanediol dinitrate. *CAS-2612-33-1.* INN. *Vasodilator (coronary).*

Clonixeril [*1969*] (kloe nix′ er il). $C_{16}H_{17}ClN_2O_4$. 336.77. (1) 3-Pyridinecarboxylic acid, 2-[(3-chloro-2-methylphenyl)amino]-, 2,3-dihydroxypropyl ester; (2) 2,3-Dihydroxypropyl 2-(3-chloro-*o*-toluidino)nicotinate. *CAS-21829-22-1.* INN. *Analgesic.* ◇*Sch 12707*

Clonixin [*1969*] (kloe nix′ in). $C_{13}H_{11}ClN_2O_2$. 262.69. (1) 3-Pyridinecarboxylic acid, 2-[(3-chloro-2-methylphenyl)amino]-; (2) 2-(3-Chloro-*o*-toluidino)nicotinic acid. *UNII-V7DXN0M42R. CAS-17737-65-4.* INN. *Analgesic.* ◇*Sch 10304*

Clopamide [*1964*] (kloe′ pa mide). $C_{14}H_{20}ClN_3O_3S$. 345.84. (1) Benzamide, 3-(aminosulfonyl)-4-chloro-*N*-(2,6-dimethyl-1-piperidinyl)-, *cis*-; (2) 4-Chloro-*N*-(2,6-dimethylpiperidino)-3-sulfamoylbenzamide. *UNII-17S83WON0I. CAS-636-54-4.* INN; BAN. *Antihypertensive; diuretic.* Aquex (Novartis†) ◇*DT-327*

Clopenthixol [*1965*] (kloe″ pen thix′ ol). $C_{22}H_{25}ClN_2OS$. 400.96. (1) 1-Piperazineethanol, 4-[3-(2-chloro-9*H*-thioxanthen-9-ylidene)propyl]-; (2) 4-[3-(2-Chlorothioxanthen-9-ylidene)propyl]-1-piperazineethanol. *CAS-982-24-1.* INN; BAN. *Antipsychotic.* ◇*AY-62021; N-746; NSC-64087*

Cloperastine. $C_{20}H_{24}ClNO$. 329.86. [Cloperastine Fendizoate and Cloperastine Hydrochloride are JAN.] 1-{2-[(*p*-Chloro-α-phenylbenzyl)oxy]ethyl}piperidine. *UNII-69M5L7BXEK. CAS-3703-76-2.* INN; MI. ◇*HT-11*

Cloperidone Hydrochloride [*1966*] (kloe per′ i done hye″ droe klor′ ide). $C_{21}H_{23}ClN_4O_2 \cdot HCl$. 435.35. [Cloperidone is INN.] (1) 2,4(1*H*,3*H*)-Quinazolinedione, 3-[3-[4-(3-chlorophenyl)-1-piperazinyl]propyl]-, monohydrochloride; (2) 3-[3-[4-(*m*-Chlorophenyl)-1-piperazinyl]propyl]-2,4-

(1*H*,3*H*)-quinazolinedione monohydrochloride. *UNII-17682058OP. CAS-525-26-8; CAS-4052-13-5* [cloperidone]. *Sedative-hypnotic.* ◇*MA 1337*

Clophenoxate — *See* Meclofenoxate.

Clopidogrel Bisulfate [*1997*] (kloe pid′ oh grel bye sul′ fate). **USP.** $C_{16}H_{16}ClNO_2S.H_2SO_4$. 419.90. [Clopidogrel is INN and BAN.] (1) Thieno[3,2-*c*]pyridine-5(4*H*)-acetic acid, α-(2-chlorophenyl)-6,7-dihydro-, methyl ester, (*S*)-, sulfate (1:1); (2) Methyl (+)-(*S*)-α-(*o*-chlorophenyl)-6,7-dihydrothieno[3,2-*c*]pyridine-5(4*H*)-acetate, sulfate (1:1). *UNII-08I79HTP27; UNII-A74586SNO7* [clopidogrel]. *CAS-120202-66-6; CAS-113665-84-2* [clopidogrel]. *Inhibitor (platelet).* Plavix (Sanofi Aventis) ◇*SR 25990C*

Clopidol [*1968*] (kloe′ pi dol). $C_7H_7Cl_2NO$. 192.04. (1) 4-Pyridinol, 3,5-dichloro-2,6-dimethyl-; (2) 3,5-Dichloro-2,6-dimethyl-4-pyridinol. *UNII-8J763HFF5N. CAS-2971-90-6.* INN; BAN. *Coccidiostat (for poultry).*

Clopimozide [*1975*] (kloe pim′ oh zide). $C_{28}H_{28}ClF_2N_3O$. 495.99. (1) 2*H*-Benzimidazol-2-one, 1-[1-[4,4-bis(4-fluorophenyl)butyl]-4-piperidinyl]-5-chloro-1,3-dihydro-; (2) 1-[1-[4,4-Bis(*p*-fluorophenyl)butyl]-4-piperidyl]-5-chloro-2-benzimidazolinone. *UNII-7C6TA32SD2. CAS-53179-12-7.* INN. *Antipsychotic.* ◇*R 29,764*

Clopipazan Mesylate [*1978*] (kloe pi′ pa zan mes′ i late). $C_{19}H_{18}ClNO.CH_4O_3S$. 407.91. [Clopipazan is INN.] (1) Piperidine 4-(2-chloro-9*H*-xanthen-9-ylidene)-1-methyl-, methanesulfonate; (2) 4-(2-Chloroxanthen-9-ylidene)-1-methylpiperidine methanesulfonate. *UNII-4ZXX17M1C4. CAS-60086-22-8; CAS-60085-78-1* [clopipazan]. *Antipsychotic.* ◇*SK&F 69634*

Clopirac [*1975*] (kloe′ pir ak). $C_{14}H_{14}ClNO_2$. 263.72. (1) 1*H*-Pyrrole-3-acetic acid, 1-(4-chlorophenyl)-2,5-dimethyl-; (2) 1-(*p*-Chlorophenyl)-2,5-dimethylpyrrole-3-acetic acid. *UNII-J23127WJYB. CAS-42779-82-8.* INN; BAN. *Anti-inflammatory.* ◇*BRL 13856; CP 172 AP*

Cloponone. $C_{11}H_9Cl_4NO_2$. 329.01. (±)-2,2-Dichloro-*N*-[*p*-chloro-α-(chloromethyl)phenacyl]acetamide. *UNII-V51W472X6D. CAS-15301-50-5.* INN; BAN.

Clopoxide — *See* Chlordiazepoxide.

Clopoxide Chloride — *See* Chlordiazepoxide Hydrochloride.

Cloprednol [*1974*] (kloe pred′ nol). $C_{21}H_{25}ClO_5$. 392.87. (1) Pregna-1,4,6-triene-3,20-dione, 6-chloro-11,17,21-trihydroxy-, (11β)-; (2) 6-Chloro-11β,17,21-trihydroxypregna-1,4,6-triene-3,20-dione. *CAS-5251-34-3.* INN; BAN. *Glucocorticoid.* Cloradryn (Syntex) ◇*RS-4691*

Cloprostenol Sodium [*1976*] (kloe prost′ e nol soe′ dee um). $C_{22}H_{28}ClNaO_6$. 446.90. [Cloprostenol is INN and BAN.] (1) 5-Heptenoic acid, 7-[2-[4-(3-chlorophenoxy)-3-hydroxy-1-butenyl]-3,5-dihydroxycyclopentyl]-, [1α(*Z*),2β(1*E*,3*R**),3α,5α]-, sodium salt, (±)-; (2) (±)-Sodium (*Z*)-7-[(1*R**,2*R**,3*R**,5*S**)-2-[(*E*)-(3*R**)-4-(*m*-chlorophenoxy)-3-hydroxy-1-butenyl]-3,5-dihydroxycyclopentyl]-5-heptenoate. *UNII-886SAV9675. CAS-55028-72-3; CAS-40665-92-7* [cloprostenol]. *Prostaglandin.* Estrumate (Bayer Animal Health) ◇*ICI 80,996*

Cloprothiazole. $C_7H_{10}ClNS$. 175.68. 5-(3-Chloropropyl)-4-methylthiazole. *UNII-GKA5F0J75P. CAS-6469-36-9.* INN; DCF.

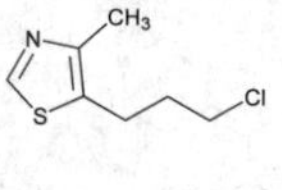

Cloquinate. $C_{18}H_{26}ClN_3.(C_9H_6INO_4S)_2$. 1022.11. 7-Chloro-4-[(4-diethylamino-1-methylbutyl)amino]quinoline di[8-hydroxy-7-iodo-5-quinolinesulfonate]. *UNII-KI24A9FF7S. CAS-7270-12-4.* INN; BAN.

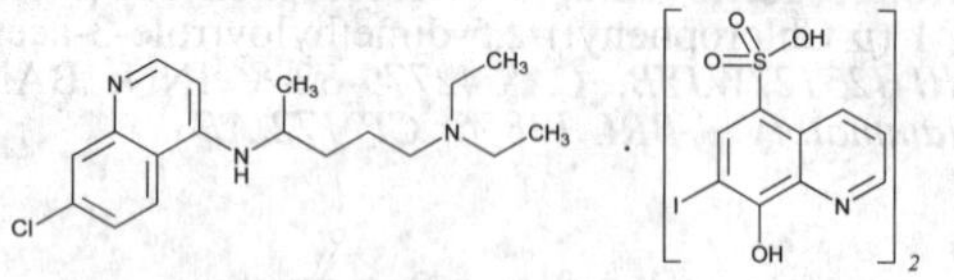

Cloquinozine. $C_{16}H_{22}ClN$. 263.81. 3-(*p*-Chlorobenzyl)octahydroquinolizine. *CAS-5220-68-8.* INN. ◇*QB-1*

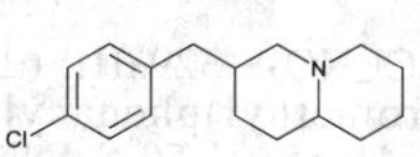

Cloracetadol. $C_{10}H_{10}Cl_3NO_3$. 298.55. β,β,β-Trichloro-α-hydroxy-*p*-acetophenetidide. *UNII-41Z22TQD48. CAS-15687-05-5.* INN; DCF.

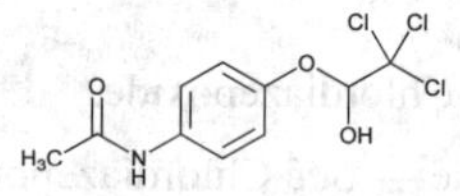

Cloral Betaine (INN; BAN) — *See* Chloral Betaine.

Cloramfenicol Pantotenate Complex (INN) — *See* Chloramphenicol Pantothenate Complex.

Cloranolol. $C_{13}H_{19}Cl_2NO_2$. 292.20. 1-(*tert*-Butylamino)-3-(2,5-dichlorophenoxy)-2-propanol. *UNII-Q3U058H86V. CAS-39563-28-5.* INN; MI.

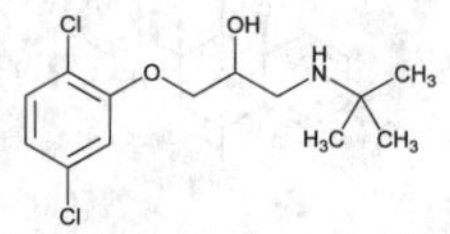

Clorazepate Dipotassium [*1969*] (klor az′ e pate dye″ poe tas′ ee um). **USP.** $C_{16}H_{11}ClK_2N_2O_4$. 408.92. [Dipotassium Clorazepate is INN.] (1) 1*H*-1,4-Benzodiazepine-3-carboxylic acid, 7-chloro-2,3-dihydro-2-oxo-5-phenyl-, potassium salt compound with potassium hydroxide (1:1); (2) Potassium 7-chloro-2,3-dihydro-2-oxo-5-phenyl-1*H*-1,4-benzodiazepine-3-carboxylate compound with potassium hydroxide (1:1). *UNII-63FN7G03XY; UNII-D51WO0G0L4* [clorazepic acid]. *CAS-57109-90-7; CAS-20432-69-3* [clorazepic acid]. JAN. *Tranquilizer (minor)*. Gen-xene (Alra); Tranxene (Ovation) ◇*4306 CB; Abbott-35616*

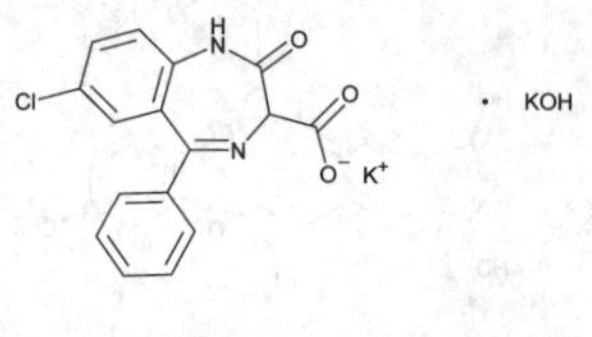

Clorazepate Monopotassium [*1976*] (klor az′ e pate mon″ oh poe tas′ ee um). $C_{16}H_{10}ClKN_2O_3$. 352.81. (1) 1*H*-1,4-Benzodiazepine-3-carboxylic acid, 7-chloro-2,3-dihydro-2-oxo-5-phenyl-, potassium salt; (2) Potassium 7-chloro-2,3-dihydro-2-oxo-5-phenyl-1*H*-1,4-benzodiazepine-3-carboxylate. *UNII-MS63G8NQUI; UNII-D51WO0G0L4* [clorazepic acid]. *CAS-5991-71-9; CAS-20432-69-3* [clorazepate]. *Tranquilizer (minor)*. ◇*4311 CB; Abbott-39083*

Clorazepic Acid. 7-Chloro-2,3-dihydro-2,2-dihydroxy-5-phenyl-1*H*-1,4-benzodiazepine-3-carboxylic acid. *UNII-D51WO0G0L4. CAS-20432-69-3.* BAN.

Cloretate (INN) — *See* Clorethate.

Clorethate [*1964*] (klor′ e thate). $C_5H_4Cl_6O_3$. 324.80. [Cloretate is INN.] (1) Ethanol, 2,2,2-trichloro-, carbonate (2:1); (2) Bis(2,2,2-trichloroethyl)carbonate. *CAS-5634-37-7. Sedative-hypnotic.* ◇*SK&F 12866*

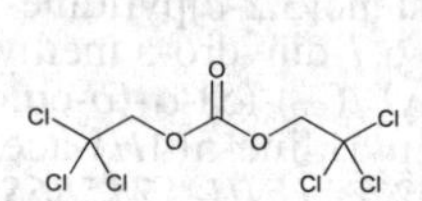

Clorexolone [*1967*] (klor ex′ oh lone). $C_{14}H_{17}ClN_2O_3S$. 328.81. (1) 1*H*-Isoindole-5-sulfonamide, 6-chloro-2-cyclohexyl-2,3-dihydro-3-oxo-; (2) 6-Chloro-2-cyclohexyl-3-oxo-5-isoindolinesulfonamide. *CAS-2127-01-7.* INN; BAN. *Diuretic.*

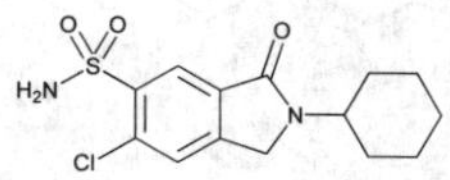

Clorfenvinfos. $C_{12}H_{14}Cl_3O_4P$. 359.57. [Clofenvinfos is BAN.] 2-Chloro-1-(2,4-dichlorophenyl)vinyl diethyl phosphate. *CAS-470-90-6.* INN. *[Name previously used: Chlorfenvinphos.]* ◇*SD 7859*

Clorgiline. $C_{13}H_{15}Cl_2NO$. 272.17. *N*-[3-(2,4-Dichlorophenoxy)propyl]-*N*-methyl-2-propynylamine. *UNII-LYJ16FZU9Q. CAS-17780-72-2.* INN; BAN. ◇*M&B 9302*

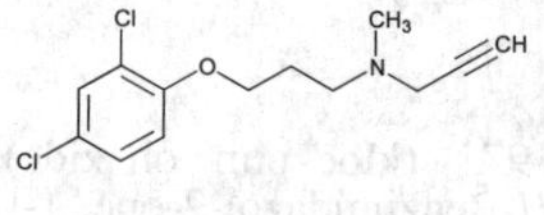

Clorgyline (BAN) — *See* Clorgiline.

Cloricromen. $C_{20}H_{26}ClNO_5$. 395.88. Ethyl [[8-chloro-3-[2-(diethylamino)ethyl]-4-methyl-2-oxo-2*H*-1-benzopyran-7-yl]oxy]acetate. *UNII-B9454PE93C. CAS-68206-94-0.* INN.

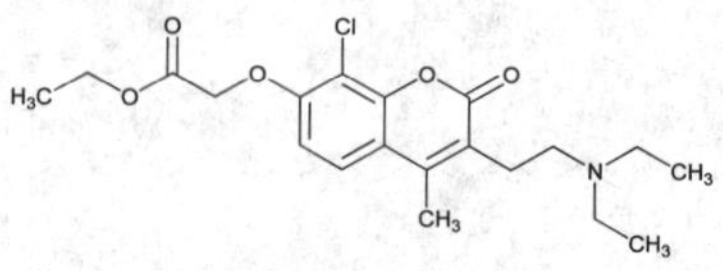

Cloridarol. $C_{15}H_{11}ClO_2$. 258.70. α-(*p*-Chlorophenyl)-2-benzofuranmethanol. *UNII-2L2063955H. CAS-3611-72-1.* INN.

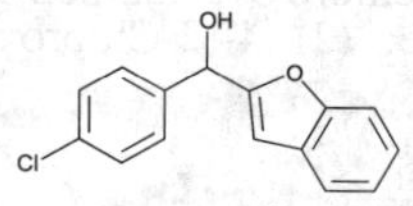

Clorindanic Acid. $C_{10}H_9ClO_3$. 212.63. 7-Chloro-4-hydroxy-5-indancarboxylic acid. *UNII-72531373MH. CAS-153-43-5.* INN; DCF. ◇*Win 19356*

Clorindanol (INN) — *See* Chlorindanol.

Clorindione. $C_{15}H_9ClO_2$. 256.68. 2-(*p*-Chlorophenyl)-1,3-indandione *UNII-541C7WS64R. CAS-1146-99-2.* INN; BAN; MI. ◇*G-25766*

Clormecaine. $C_{11}H_{15}ClN_2O_2$. 242.70. 2-(Dimethylamino)ethyl 3-amino-4-chlorobenzoate ester. *UNII-RR5R8BAX26. CAS-13930-34-2.* INN.

Clorofene (INN) — *See* Clorophene.

Cloroperone Hydrochloride [*1977*] (klor oh′ per one hye″ droe klor′ ide). $C_{22}H_{23}ClFNO_2.HCl$. 424.34. [Cloroperone is INN.] (1) 1-Butanone, 4-[4-(4-chlorobenzoyl)-1-piperidinyl]-1-(4-fluorophenyl)-, hydrochloride; (2) 4-[4-(*p*-Chlorobenzoyl)piperidino]-4′-fluorobutyrophenone hydrochloride. *UNII-95U4NV3X82. CAS-55695-56-2; CAS-61764-61-2* [cloroperone]. *Antipsychotic.* ◇*AHR-6134*

Clorophene [*1965*] (klor′ oh feen). $C_{13}H_{11}ClO$. 218.68. [Clorofene is INN.] (1) Phenol, 4-chloro-2-(phenylmethyl)-; (2) 4-Chloro-α-phenyl-*o*-cresol. *UNII-7560BB0BO3. CAS-120-32-1. Disinfectant.* ◇*NSC-59989*

Cloroqualone. $C_{16}H_{12}Cl_2N_2O$. 319.19. 3-(2,6-Dichlorophenyl)-2-ethyl-4(3*H*)-quinazolinone. *UNII-172D4Q6LOW. CAS-25509-07-3.* INN; DCF.

Clorotepine. $C_{19}H_{21}ClN_2S$. 344.90. 1-(8-Chloro-10,11-dihydrodibenzo[*b,f*]thiepin-10-yl)-4-methylpiperazine. *UNII-E65W20MU7A. CAS-13448-22-1.* INN.

Clorprenaline Hydrochloride [*1963*] (klor pren′ a leen hye″ droe klor′ ide). $C_{11}H_{16}ClNO.HCl.H_2O$. 268.18. [Clorprenaline is INN and BAN.] (1) Benzenemethanol, 2-chloro-α-[[(1-methylethyl)amino]methyl]-, hydrochloride, monohydrate; (2) *o*-Chloro-α[(isopropylamino)methyl]benzyl alcohol hydrochloride monohydrate. *UNII-T6CRE6WE0W. CAS-5588-22-7; CAS-6933-90-0* [anhydrous]; *CAS-3811-25-4* [clorprenaline]. JAN. *Bronchodilator.* ◇*20025*

Clorquinaldol — *See* Chlorquinaldol.

Clorsulon [*1983*] (klor′ sul on). **USP.** $C_8H_8Cl_3N_3O_4S_2$. 380.66. (1) 1,3-Benzenedisulfonamide, 4-amino-6-(trichloroethenyl)-; (2) 4-Amino-6-(trichlorovinyl)-*m*-benzenedisulfonamide. *UNII-EG1ZDO6LRD. CAS-60200-06-8.* INN; BAN. *Antiparasitic; fasciolicide.* Curatrem [Veterinary] (Merial) ◇*MK-401*

Clortermine Hydrochloride [*1969*] (klor′ ter meen hye″ droe klor′ ide). $C_{10}H_{14}ClN.HCl$. 220.14. [Clortermine is INN.] (1) Benzeneethanamine, 2-chloro-α,α-dimethyl-, hydrochloride; (2) *o*-Chloro-α,α-dimethylphenethylamine hydrochloride. *UNII-4FA88HM3IX* [clortermine]. *CAS-10389-72-7; CAS-10389-73-8* [clortermine]. *Anorexic.* ◇*Su-10568*

Closantel [*1976*] (kloe san′ tel). $C_{22}H_{14}Cl_2I_2N_2O_2$. 663.07. (1) Benzamide, *N*-[5-chloro-4-[(4-chlorophenyl)cyanomethyl]-2-methylphenyl]-2-hydroxy-3,5-diiodo-; (2) 5′-

---

Chloro-α^4-(*p*-chlorophenyl)-α^4-cyano-3,5-diiodo-2′,4′-salicyloxylidide. *UNII-EUL532EI54. CAS-57808-65-8.* INN; BAN. *Anthelmintic.* ◇*R 31,520*

Closiramine Aceturate [*1969*] (kloe sir′ a meen a set′ ue rate). $C_{18}H_{21}ClN_2 \cdot C_4H_7NO_3$. 417.93. [Closiramine is INN.] (1) Glycine, *N*-acetyl-, compd. with 8-chloro-6,11-dihydro-*N,N*-dimethyl-5*H*-benzo[5,6]cyclohepta[1,2-*b*]pyridine-11-ethanamine (1:1); (2) 8-Chloro-11-[2-(dimethylamino)ethyl]-6,11-dihydro-5*H*-benzo[5,6]cyclohepta[1,2-*b*]pyridine compound with *N*-acetylglycine (1:1). *UNII-00T9G32ZVH* [closiramine]. *CAS-23256-09-9; CAS-47135-88-6* [closiramine]. *Antihistaminic.* ◇*Sch 12169*

Clostebol. $C_{19}H_{27}ClO_2$. 322.87. [Clostebol Acetate is BAN.] 4-Chloro-17β-hydroxyandrost-4-en-3-one. *UNII-Z7D4G976SH. CAS-1093-58-9.* INN; MI.

Clothiapine [*1966*] (kloe thye′ a peen). $C_{18}H_{18}ClN_3S$. 343.87. [Clotiapine is INN and JAN.] (1) Dibenzo[*b,f*][1,4]thiazepine, 2-chloro-11-(4-methyl-1-piperazinyl)-; (2) 2-Chloro-11-(4-methyl-1-piperazinyl)dibenzo[*b,f*][1,4]thiazepine. *CAS-2058-52-8.* BAN. *Antipsychotic.* ◇*HF-2159*

Clothixamide Maleate [*1964*] (kloe thix′ a mide mal′ ee ate). $C_{24}H_{28}ClN_3OS \cdot 2C_4H_4O_4$. 674.16. [Clotixamide is INN.] (1) 1-Piperazinepropanamide, 4-[3-(2-chloro-9*H*-thioxanthen-9-ylidene)propyl]-*N*-methyl-, (*Z*)-2-butenedioate (1:2); (2) 4-[3-(2-Chlorothioxanthen-9-ylidene)propyl]-*N*-methyl-1-piperazinepropionamide maleate (1:2). *CAS-4434-20-2; CAS-4177-58-6* [clothixamide]. *Antipsychotic.* ◇*P-4385B; NSC-78714*

Clotiapine (INN, JAN, DCF) — *See* Clothiapine.

Clotiazepam. $C_{16}H_{15}ClN_2OS$. 318.82. 5-(*o*-Chlorophenyl)-7-ethyl-1,3-dihydro-1-methyl-2*H*-thieno[2,3-*e*]-1,4-diazepin-2-one. *CAS-33671-46-4.* INN; JAN; MI.

Cloticasone Propionate [*1984*] (kloe tik′ a sone proe′ pee oh nate). $C_{25}H_{31}ClF_2O_5S$. 517.03. [Cloticasone is INN and BAN.] (1) Androsta-1,4-diene-17-carbothioic acid, 6,9-difluoro-11-hydroxy-16-methyl-3-oxo-17-(1-oxopropoxy)-, *S*-(chloromethyl) ester, (6α,11β,16α,17α)-; (2) *S*-(Chloromethyl) 6α,9-difluoro-11β,17-dihydroxy-16α-methyl-3-oxoandrosta-1,4-diene-17β-carbothioate, 17-propionate. *CAS-80486-69-7; CAS-87556-66-9* [cloticasone]. *Anti-inflammatory.* ◇*CCI 18773*

Clotioxone. $C_9H_5Cl_3N_2O_2S$. 311.57. 2-Phenyl-4-[(trichloromethyl)thio]-Δ^2-1,3,4-oxadiazolin-5-one. *UNII-D7ID553901. CAS-1856-34-4.* INN; DCF. ◇*RP 13607*

Clotixamide (INN) Maleate — *See* Clothixamide Maleate.

Clotrimazole [*1970*] (kloe trim′ a zole). **USP.** $C_{22}H_{17}ClN_2$. 344.84. (1) 1*H*-Imidazole, 1-[(2-chlorophenyl)diphenylmethyl]-; (2) 1-(*o*-Chloro-α,α-diphenylbenzyl)imidazole. *UNII-G07GZ97H65. CAS-23593-75-1.* INN; BAN; JAN. *Antifungal.* Gyne-lotrimin (Schering-Plough); Lotrimin (Schering-Plough); Mycelex (Bayer) ◇*BAY 5097*

Clove Oil (klove). **NF.** The volatile oil distilled with steam from the dried flower buds of *Syzygium aromaticum* (L.) Merr. and L. M. Perry (Fam. Myrtaceae). *UNII-578389D6D0. CAS-8000-34-8.* MI. *Pharmaceutic aid (flavor).*

Clover, Red. The dried inflorescence of *Trifolium pratense* L. (Fam. Fabacear). NF XXI (Supplement 1).

Clovoxamine. $C_{14}H_{21}ClN_2O_2$. 284.78. 4′-Chloro-5-methoxy-valerophenone (E)-O-(2-aminoethyl)oxime. *UNII-7I22J7RY2A. CAS-54739-19-4.* INN.

Cloxacepride. $C_{22}H_{27}Cl_2N_3O_4$. 468.37. 5-Chloro-4-[2-(p-chlorophenoxy)acetamido]-N-[2-(diethylamino)ethyl]-o-anisamide. *UNII-Z4J6TAJ4FX. CAS-65569-29-1.* INN.

Cloxacillin Benzathine (klox″ a sil′ in ben′ za theen). **USP**. $(C_{19}H_{18}ClN_3O_5S)_2.C_{16}H_{20}N_2$. 1112.11. [Cloxacillin is INN and BAN.] (1) 4-Thia-1-azabicyclo[3.2.0]heptane-2-carboxylic acid, 6-[[[3-(2-chlorophenyl)-5-methyl-4-isoxazolyl]carbonyl]amino]-3,3-dimethyl-7-oxo-, [2S-$(2\alpha,5\alpha,6\beta)$]-, compd. with N,N'-bis(phenylmethyl)-1,2-ethanediamine (2:1); (2) (2S,5R,6R)-6-[3-(o-Chlorophenyl)-5-methyl-4-isoxazolecarboxamido]-3,3-dimethyl-7-oxo-4-thia-1-azabicyclo[3.2.0]heptane-2-carboxylic acid compound with N,N'-dibenzylethylenediamine (2:1). *UNII-AC79L7PV2G; UNII-O6X5QGC2VB* [cloxacillin]. *CAS-23736-58-5; CAS-61-72-3* [cloxacillin]. *Antibacterial.*

Cloxacillin Sodium [*1963*] (klox″ a sil′ in soe′ dee um). **USP**. $C_{19}H_{17}ClN_3NaO_5S.H_2O$. 475.88. (1) 4-Thia-1-azabicyclo[3.2.0]heptane-2-carboxylic acid, 6-[[[3-(2-chlorophenyl)-5-methyl-4-isoxazolyl]carbonyl]amino]-3,3-dimethyl-7-oxo-, monosodium salt, monohydrate, [2S-$(2\alpha,5\alpha,6\beta)$]-; (2) Monosodium (2S,5R,6R)-6-[3-(o-chlorophenyl)-5-methyl-4-isoxazolecarboxamido]-3,3-dimethyl-7-oxo-4-thia-1-azabicyclo[3.2.0]heptane-2-carboxylate monohydrate. *UNII-65LCB00B4Y. CAS-7081-44-9; CAS-642-78-4* [anhydrous]. JAN. *Antibacterial.* Cloxapen (GlaxoSmithKline); Tegopen (Apothecon) ◇*BRL-1621; P-25*

Cloxazolam. $C_{17}H_{14}Cl_2N_2O_2$. 349.21. 10-Chloro-11b-(o-chlorophenyl)-2,3,7,11b-tetrahydro-oxazolo[3,2-d][1,4]benzodiazepin-6(5H)-one. *UNII-GYL649Z0HY. CAS-24166-13-0.* INN; JAN; MI.

Cloxestradiol. $C_{20}H_{25}Cl_3O_3$. 419.77. 17β-(2,2,2-Trichloro-1-hydroxyethoxy)estra-1,3,5(10)-trien-3-ol. *UNII-42R9MZG1DL. CAS-54063-33-1.* INN.

Cloxifenol — *See* Triclosan.

Cloximate. $C_{14}H_{19}ClN_2O_3$. 298.77. 2-(Dimethylamino)ethyl (E)-[[(p-chloro-α-methylbenzylidene)amino]oxy]acetate. *UNII-544MD72T3H. CAS-58832-68-1.* INN.

Cloxiquine (INN) — *See* Cloxyquin.

Cloxotestosterone. $C_{21}H_{29}Cl_3O_3$. 435.81. 17β-(2,2,2-Trichloro-1-hydroxyethoxy)androst-4-en-3-one. *UNII-8422DH508N. CAS-53608-96-1.* INN.

Cloxphendyl — *See* Cloxypendyl.

Cloxypendyl. $C_{20}H_{25}ClN_4OS$. 404.96. 4-[3-(3-Chloro-10H-pyrido[3,2-b][1,4]benzothiazin-10-yl)propyl]-1-piperazine ethanol. *UNII-8BK5DLR67A. CAS-15311-77-0.* INN. ◇*D-1262*

---

† Brand name formerly used, and/or firm no longer concerned with this product.

Cloxyquin [*1973*] (klox′ i kwin). C₉H₆ClNO. 179.60. [Cloxiquine is INN.] (1) 8-Quinolinol, 5-chloro-; (2) 5-Chloro-8-quinolinol. *UNII-BPF36H1G6S. CAS-130-16-5. Antibacterial.*

Clozapine [*1969*] (kloe′ za peen). **USP.** C₁₈H₁₉ClN₄. 326.82. (1) 5*H*-Dibenzo[*b,e*][1,4]diazepine, 8-chloro-11-(4-methyl-1-piperazinyl)-; (2) 8-Chloro-11-(4-methyl-1-piperazinyl)-5*H*-dibenzo[*b,e*][1,4]diazepine. *UNII-J60AR2IKIC. CAS-5786-21-0.* INN; BAN. *Antipsychotic.* Clozaril (Novartis); Fazaclo (Azur) ◇*HF 1854*

⁵⁷Co — *See* Cobaltous Chloride Co 57.

⁵⁷Co — *See* Cyanocobalamin Co 57.

⁵⁸Co — *See* Cyanocobalamin Co 58.

⁶⁰Co — *See* Cobaltous Chloride Co 60.

⁶⁰Co — *See* Cyanocobalamin Co 60.

Coal Tar (kole tar). **USP.** The tar obtained as a by-product during the destructive distillation of bituminous coal at temperatures in the range of 900° to 1100°. *Anti-eczematic (topical).* AquaTar (Allergan Herbert); Fototar (ICN); Ionil-T (Galderma†); Ionil-T-Plus (Galderma†); Vanseb-T (Allergan Herbert); Zetar (Dermik)

Co-amilofruse. Amiloride Hydrochloride and Frusemide (Furosemide) in the proportions, by weight, 1 part to 8 parts, respectively. BAN.

Co-amilozide (koe″ a mil′ oh zide). PEN for Amiloride Hydrochloride and Hydrochlorothiazide. Amiloride Hydrochloride and Hydrochlorothiazide in the proportions, by weight, 1 part to 10 parts, respectively. BAN.

Co-amoxiclav (koe″ a mox′ i klav). PEN for Amoxicillin and Clavulanate Potassium. Amoxycillin (as the trihydrate or as the sodium salt) and Clavulanic Acid (as Potassium Clavulanate); the proportions are expressed in the form *x/y*, where *x* and *y* are the strengths in milligrams of Amoxycillin and Clavulanic Acid, respectively. BAN.

Cobalamin Concentrate. USP XXI.

Cobaltous Chloride Co 57 [*1963*] (koe bawl′ tus klor′ ide). ⁵⁷CoCl₂. (1) Cobalt chloride (⁵⁷CoCl₂); (2) Cobalt chloride (⁵⁷CoCl₂). *UNII-ZL40NE83QQ. CAS-16413-89-1. Radioactive agent.* Cobatope-57 (Bristol-Myers Squibb†)

Cobaltous Chloride Co 60 [*1963*] (koe bawl′ tus klor′ ide). ⁶⁰CoCl₂. (1) Cobalt chloride (⁶⁰CoCl₂); (2) Cobalt chloride (⁶⁰CoCl₂). *UNII-7812FUQ8VK. CAS-14543-09-0. Radioactive agent.* Cobatope-60 (Bristol-Myers Squibb†)

Cobamamide. C₇₂H₁₀₀CoN₁₈O₁₇P. 1579.58. Inner salt of the *Co*-(5′-deoxyadenosine-5′) derivative of the 3′-ester of cobinamide phosphate with 5,6-dimethyl-1-α-D-ribofuranosylbenzimidazole. *CAS-13870-90-1.* INN; JAN; MI. ◇*LM 176*

Co-beneldopa. Benserazide [as the hydrochloride] and Levodopa in the proportions, by weight, 1 part to 4 parts, respectively. BAN.

Cobiprostone [*2007*] (koe″ bi prost′ one). C₂₁H₃₄F₂O₅. 404.49. (1) Cyclopenta[*b*]pyran-5-heptanoic acid, 2-[(3*S*)-1,1-difluoro-3-methylpentyl]octahydro-2-hydroxy-6-oxo-, (2*R*,4a*R*,5*R*,7a*R*)-; (2) 7-[(2*R*,4a*R*,5*R*,7a*R*)-2-[(3*S*)-1,1-Difluoro-3-methylpentyl]-2-hydroxy-6-oxooctahydrocyclopenta[*b*]pyran-5-yl]heptanoic acid. *UNII-IL870Q3Z8I. CAS-333963-42-1.* INN. *Treatment of gastrointestinal disorders.* ◇*SPI-8811*

Co-bucafAPAP (koe″ bue kaf′ a pap). PEN for Butalbital, Acetaminophen, and Caffeine.

Cocaine (koe kane′). **USP.** C₁₇H₂₁NO₄. 303.35. (1) 8-Azabicyclo[3.2.1]octane-2-carboxylic acid, 3-(benzoyloxy)-8-methyl-, methyl ester, [1*R*-(*exo,exo*)]-; (2) Methyl 3β-hydroxy-1α*H*,5α*H*-tropane-2β-carboxylate benzoate (ester). *CAS-50-36-2.* BAN. *Anesthetic (topical).*

Cocaine Hydrochloride (koe kane′ hye″ droe klor′ ide). **USP.** C₁₇H₂₁NO₄·HCl. 339.81. (1) 8-Azabicyclo[3.2.1]octane-2-carboxylic acid, 3-(benzoyloxy)-8-methyl-, methyl ester, hydrochloride, [1*R*-(*exo,exo*)]-; (2) Methyl 3β-hydroxy-1α*H*,5α*H*-tropan-2β-carboxylate, benzoate (ester) hydrochloride. *CAS-53-21-4; CAS-50-36-2* [cocaine]. JAN. *Anesthetic (topical).*

Cocarboxylase. $C_{12}H_{20}N_4O_8P_2S$. 442.32. Pyrophosphoric ester of thiamine. *CAS-154-87-0.* INN; BAN; JAN; DCF; MI.

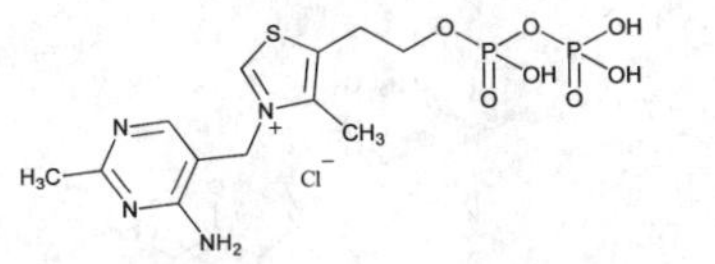

Co-careldopa (koe″ kar el doe′ pa). PEN for Carbidopa and Levodopa. Carbidopa and Levodopa; the proportions are expressed in the form *x/y*, where *x* and *y* are the strengths in milligrams of Carbidopa and Levodopa, respectively. BAN.

Coccidioidin (kok sid″ ee oi′ din). **USP.** A sterile solution containing the antigens obtained from the by-products of mycelial growth or from the spherules of the fungus *Coccidioides immitis. Diagnostic aid (dermal reactivity indicator).*

Cocculin — *See* Picrotoxin.

Co-climasone (koe klim′ a sone). PEN for Clotrimazole and Betamethasone Dipropionate.

Cocoa. NF XVI; MI.

Cocoa Butter (koe′ koe). **NF.** The fat obtained from the seed of *Theobroma cacao* Linné (Fam. Sterculiaceae). *CAS-8002-31-1. Pharmaceutic aid (suppository base).*

Co-codamol. Codeine Phosphate and Paracetamol (Acetaminophen); the proportions are expressed in the form *x/y*, where *x* and *y* are the strengths in milligrams of Codeine Phosphate and Paracetamol (Acetaminophen), respectively. BAN.

Co-codAPAP (koe koe′ da pap). PEN for Acetaminophen and Codeine Phosphate.

Co-codaprin (koe koe′ da prin). PEN for Aspirin and Codeine Phosphate. Codeine Phosphate and Aspirin in the proportions, by weight, 1 part to 50 parts, respectively. BAN.

Coconut Oil. NF. (1) Coconut oil; (2) Coconut oil. *UNII-Q9L0O73W7L. CAS-8001-31-8.*

Co-cyprindiol. Cyproterone Acetate and Ethinyloestradiol (Ethinyl Estradiol) in the proportions by weight, 2000 parts to 35 parts, respectively. BAN.

Cod Liver Oil (kod liv′ er). **USP.** The partially destearinated fixed oil obtained from fresh livers of *Gadus morrhua* Linné and other species of Fam. Gadidae. *UNII-BBL281NWFG.* BAN; JAN. *Vitamins A and D, source of.*

Cod Liver Oil, Nondestearinated. NF XIII.

Codactide. $C_{101}H_{158}N_{30}O_{23}S$. 2192.59. 1-D-Serine-17-L-lysine-18-L-lysinamide-α^{1-18}-corticotropin. *CAS-22572-04-9.* INN; BAN. ◇*Ba-41795*

Co-danthramer. Danthron and Poloxamer 188; the proportions are expressed in the form *x/y*, where *x* and *y* are the strengths in milligrams of Danthron and Poloxamer, respectively. The definition of *Co-danthramer* has been modified to include combinations of Danthron and Poloxamer 188 in the proportions 3 parts to 40 parts, respectively. This particular combination was previously known as *Strong Co-danthramer.* BAN.

Co-danthrusate. Danthron and Docusate Sodium in the proportions by weight, 5 parts to 6 parts, respectively. BAN.

Codeine (koe′ deen). **USP.** $C_{18}H_{21}NO_3.H_2O$. 317.38. (1) Morphinan-6-ol, 7,8-didehydro-4,5-epoxy-3-methoxy-17-methyl-, monohydrate, (5α,6α)-; (2) 7,8-Didehydro-4,5α-epoxy-3-methoxy-17-methylmorphinan-6α-ol monohydrate. *UNII-Q830PW7520. CAS-6059-47-8; CAS-76-57-3* [anhydrous]. BAN. *Antitussive; analgesic (narcotic).*

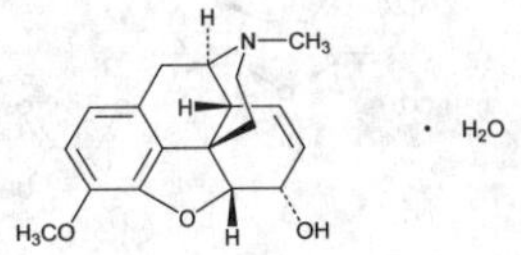

Codeine Phosphate (koe′ deen fos′ fate). **USP.** $C_{18}H_{21}NO_3.H_3PO_4.\frac{1}{2}H_2O$. 406.37. (1) Morphinan-6-ol, 7,8-didehydro-4,5-epoxy-3-methoxy-17-methyl-, (5α,6α)-, phosphate (1:1) (salt), hemihydrate; (2) 7,8-Didehydro-4,5α-epoxy-3-methoxy-17-methylmorphinan-6α-ol phosphate (1:1) (salt) hemihydrate. *UNII-GSL05Y1MN6. CAS-41444-62-6; CAS-52-28-8* [anhydrous]; *CAS-6059-47-8* [codeine]. BAN; JAN. *Antitussive; analgesic (narcotic).* Ambenyl Cough Syrup (Parke-Davis†); Colrex Compound (Solvay Pharmaceuticals†)

Codeine Polistirex [*1987*] (koe′ deen pol″ ee stye′ rex). (1) Benzene, diethenyl-, polymer with ethenylbenzene, sulfonated, complex with (5α,6α)-7,8-didehydro-4,5-epoxy-3-methoxy-17-methylmorphinan-6-ol; (2) Sulfonated styrene-divinylbenzene copolymer complex with 7,8-didehydro-4,5α-epoxy-3-methoxy-17-methylmorphinan-6α-ol. *UNII-SS85U8K5ZN. Antitussive.*

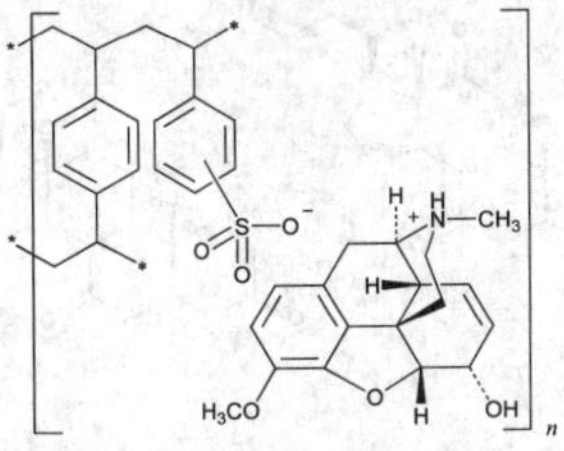

Codeine Sulfate (koe′ deen sul′ fate). **USP.** $(C_{18}H_{21}NO_3)_2.H_2SO_4.3H_2O$. 750.85. (1) Morphinan-6-ol, 7,8-didehydro-4,5-epoxy-3-methoxy-17-methyl-, (5α,6α)-, sulfate (2:1) (salt), trihydrate; (2) 7,8-Didehydro-4,5α-epoxy-3-methoxy-17-methylmorphinan-6α-ol sulfate (2:1) (salt) trihydrate. *CAS-6854-40-6; CAS-1420-53-7* [anhydrous]; *CAS-6059-47-8* [codeine]. *Analgesic (narcotic); antitussive.*

Co-dergocrine Mesylate (BAN) — *See* Ergoloid Mesylates.

Codorphone (previously used name) — *See* Conorphone Hydrochloride.

---

† Brand name formerly used, and/or firm no longer concerned with this product.

Codoxime [*1966*] (koe dox′ eem). $C_{20}H_{24}N_2O_5$. 372.41. (1) Acetic acid, [[(4,5-epoxy-3-methoxy-17-methylmorphinan-6-ylidene)amino]oxy]-, (5α)-; (2) [[(4,5α-Epoxy-3-methoxy-17-methylmorphinan-6-ylidene)amino]oxy] acetic acid; (3) Dihydrocodeinone *O*-(carboxymethyl)oxime. *CAS-7125-76-0.* INN. *Antitussive.*

Co-dydramol. Dihydrocodeine Tartrate and Paracetamol (Acetaminophen) in the proportions, by weight, 1 part to 50 parts, respectively. BAN.

Co-erynsulfisox (koe″ er in sul′ fi sox). PEN for Erythromycin Ethylsuccinate and Sulfisoxazole Acetyl.

Coffeine — *See* Caffeine.

Cofisatin. $C_{68}H_{79}NO_{11}$. 1086.35. 3,3-Bis(*p*-hydroxyphenyl)-2-indolinone 3,7,12-trioxo-5β-cholan-24-oic acid diester. *CAS-54063-34-2.* INN; DCF.

Cofisatine (DCF) — *See* Cofisatin.

Co-fluampicil. Flucloxacillin (Floxacillin) and Ampicillin in equal proportions by weight. BAN.

Co-flumactone. Hydroflumethiazide and Spironolactone in equal proportions by weight. BAN.

Cogazocine. $C_{21}H_{31}NO$. 313.48. 3-(Cyclobutylmethyl)-6-ethyl-1,2,3,4,5,6-hexahydro-11,11-dimethyl-2,6-methano-3-benzazocin-8-ol. *UNII-6GKB76713M. CAS-57653-29-9.* INN.

Co-hycodAPAP (koe″ hye koe′ da pap). PEN for Hydrocodone Bitartrate and Acetaminophen.

Colaspase (BAN) — *See* Asparaginase.

Colchamine — *See* Demecolcine.

Colchicine (kol′ chi seen). **USP**. $C_{22}H_{25}NO_6$. 399.44. (1) Acetamide, *N*-(5,6,7,9-tetrahydro-1,2,3,10-tetramethoxy-9-oxobenzo[*a*]heptalen-7-yl)-, (*S*)-; (2) Colchicine. *UNII-SML2Y3J35T. CAS-64-86-8.* JAN. *Suppressant (gout).*

Cold Cream. USP XXI.

Colecalciferol (INN, BAN) — *See* Cholecalciferol.

Coleneuramide [*2008*] (kol″ e nure′ a mide). $C_{39}H_{68}N_2O_8$. 692.97. (1) α-Neuraminamide, N^5-acetyl-N^1-[(3α,5α)-cholestan-3-yl]-2-*O*-methyl-; (2) 5-Acetamido-*N*-(5α-cholestan-3α-yl)-3,5-dideoxy-2-*O*-methyl-D-*glycero*-α-D-*galacto*-non-2-ulopyranosonamide. *CAS-204200-47-5. Treatment of diabetic neuropathy.* ◇MCC-257

Colesevelam Hydrochloride [*1997*] (koe″ le sev′ e lam hye″ droe klor′ ide). $(C_3H_7N)_m(C_3H_5ClO)_n(C_{12}H_{27}ClN_2)_o(C_{13}H_{27}N)_p.x$HCl. [Colesevelam is INN.] (1) 2-Propen-1-amine polymer with (chloromethyl)oxirane, *N,N,N*-trimethyl-6-(2-propenylamino)-1-hexanaminium chloride, and *N*-2-propenyl-1-decanamine, hydrochloride; (2) Allylamine polymer with 1-chloro-2,3-epoxypropane, [6-(allylamino)hexyl]trimethylammonium chloride and *N*-allyldecylamine, hydrochloride. *UNII-P4SG24WI5Q. CAS-182815-44-7; CAS-182815-43-6* [colesevelam]. *Antihyperlipidemic.* Welchol (Sankyo) ◇GT31-104HB

Colestilan. $(C_4H_6N_2.C_3H_5ClO)n$. 174.63. 2-Methylimidazole polymer with 1-chloro-2,3-epoxypropane. *CAS-95522-45-5.* INN. *[Name previously used: Colestimide.]*

Colestilan Chloride [*2007*] (koe les′ ti lan). $(C_7H_{11}N_2O.Cl)n$. [Colestilan is INN.] (1) 1*H*-Imidazole, 2-methyl-, polymer with (chloromethyl)oxirane; (2) Oxirane, (chloromethyl)-, polymer with 2-methyl-1*H*-imidazole. *CAS-95522-45-5. Treatment of hyperphosphatemia and hypercholesterole-*

mia in patients with chronic kidney disease on dialysis. Cholebine (Japan) (Mitsubishi Pharma) *[Name previously used: Colestimide.]* ◇MCI-196

Colestimide (previously used name) — *See* Colestilan.

Colestimide (previously used name) — *See* Colestilan Chloride.

Colestipol Hydrochloride [*1969*] (koe les′ ti pol hye″ droe klor′ ide). **USP.** [Colestipol is INN and BAN.] Because of the highly cross-linked and insoluble nature of this basic anion-exchange resin, no graphic formula has been assigned, and no molecular weight information is available. (1) Colestipol hydrochloride; (2) Copolymer of diethylene-triamine and 1-chloro-2,3-epoxypropane, hydrochloride (with approximately 1 out of 5 amine nitrogens proto-nated). *UNII-X7D10K905G. CAS-37296-80-3; CAS-26658-42-4* [colestipol]. *Antihyperlipidemic.* Colestid (Pfizer)

Colestolone [*1989*] (koe les′ toe lone). $C_{27}H_{44}O_2$. 400.64. (1) Cholest-8(14)-en-15-one, 3-hydroxy-, $(3\beta,5\alpha)$-; (2) 3β-Hydroxy-5α-cholest-8(14)-en-15-one. *CAS-50673-97-7.* INN. *Hypolipidemic.* ◇CL 274,471

Colestyramine (INN, BAN, JAN) — *See* Cholestyramine Resin.

Colextran. Dextran 2-(diethylamino)ethyl ether. *CAS-9015-73-0.* INN.

Colfenamate. $C_{16}H_{13}F_3N_2O_3$. 338.28. N-$(\alpha,\alpha,\alpha$-Trifluoro-m-tolyl)anthranilic acid, ester with glycolamide. *UNII-N0V0Q7845W. CAS-30531-86-3.* INN.

Colforsin [*1986*] (kol for′ sin). $C_{22}H_{34}O_7$. 410.50. (1) $1H$-Naphtho[2,1-b]pyran-1-one, 5-(acetyloxy)-3-ethenyldo-decahydro-6,10,10b-trihydroxy-3,4a,7,7,10a-pentameth-yl-, [$3R$-($3\alpha,4a\beta,5\beta,6\beta,6a\alpha,10\alpha,10a\beta,10b\alpha$)]-; (2) ($3R,4aR,5S,6S,6aS,10S,10aR,10bS$)-Dodecahydro-

5,6,10,10b-tetrahydroxy-3,4a,7,7,10a-pentamethyl-3-vi-nyl-$1H$-naphtho[2,1-b]pyran-1-one 5-acetate. *CAS-66575-29-9.* INN. *Antiglaucoma agent.* ◇HL 362; L 75 1362B

Colfosceril Palmitate [*1991*] (kol fos′ e ril pal′ mi tate). $C_{40}H_{80}NO_8P$. 734.04. (1) 3,5,9-Trioxa-4-phosphapentac-osan-1-aminium, 4-hydroxy-N,N,N-trimethyl-10-oxo-7-[(1-oxohexadecyl)oxy]-, hydroxide, inner salt, 4-oxide, (R)-; (2) Choline hydroxide, dihydrogen phosphate, inner salt, ester with L-1,2-dipalmitin; (3) 1,2-Dipalmitoyl-sn-glycero-3-phosphocholine. *UNII-319X2NFW0A. CAS-63-89-8.* INN; BAN. *Pulmonary surfactant.* ◇129Y83

Colimecycline. $C_{122}H_{172}N_{22}O_{40}$ (Nominal). 2586.79. Reaction product of one molecule of colistin with three molecules of oxytetracycline in presence of formaldehyde. $N,N′,N″$-Tris[[4-(dimethylamino)-1,4,4a,5,5a,6,11,12a-octahydro-3,5,6,10,12,12a-hexahydroxy-6-methyl-1,11-dioxo-2-naphthacenecarboxamido]methyl]polymyxin E (nominal). *CAS-58298-92-3.* INN; DCF.

Colistimethate Sodium [*1963*] (koe lis″ ti meth′ ate soe′ dee um). **USP.** $C_{58}H_{105}N_{16}Na_5O_{28}S_5$ (colistin A component). 1749.82; $C_{57}H_{103}N_{16}Na_5O_{28}S_5$ (colistin B component). 1735.79. [Colistin Sodium Methanesulfonate is JAN.] (1) Colistimethate sodium; (2) Pentasodium colistinmethane-sulfonate. *UNII-XW0E5YS77G. CAS-8068-28-8; CAS-*

---

† Brand name formerly used, and/or firm no longer concerned with this product.

21362-08-3 [replaced]. INN; BAN. *Antibacterial.* Colymycin (King) *[Name previously used: Colistin Sulphomethate.]* ◇*W 1929*

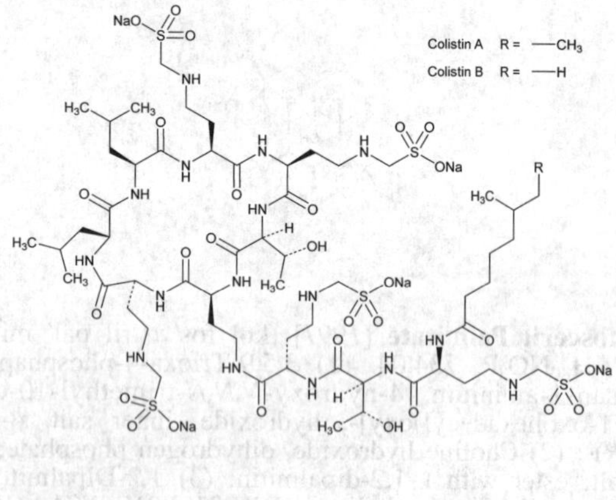

Colistin Sodium Methanesulfonate (JAN) — *See* Colistimethate Sodium.

Colistin Sulfate (koe lis′ tin sul′ fate). **USP**. [Colistin is INN and BAN.] (1) Colistin, sulfate; (2) Colistins sulfate. *UNII-WP15DXU577; UNII-Z67X93HJG1* [colistin]. *CAS-1264-72-8; CAS-1066-17-7* [colistin]. JAN. *Antibacterial.* Colymycin (King)

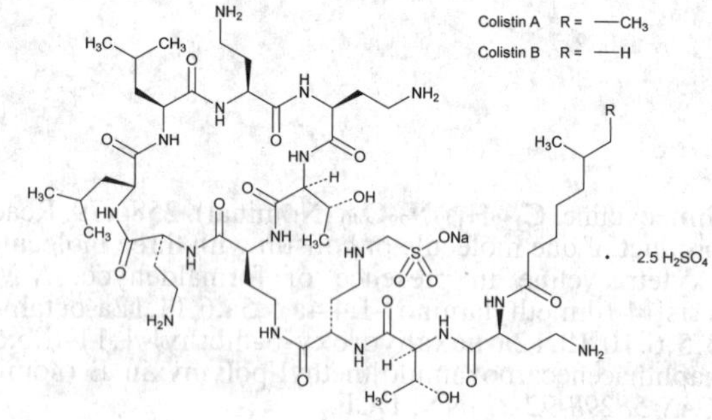

Colistin Sulphomethate (previously used name) — *See* Colistimethate Sodium.

Collodion (koe loe′ dee on). **USP**. A mixture of Pyroxylin, Ether and Alcohol. *Protectant (topical).*

Colloidal Gold (^{198}Au) **Injection** (JAN) — *See* Gold Au 198.

Colloidal Oatmeal. **USP**. The powder resulting from the grinding and further processing of whole oat grain meeting U.S. Standards for Number 1 or Number 2 oats (7 CFR 810.1001). *Antipruritic (topical).*

Colterol Mesylate [*1976*] (kol′ ter ol mes′ i late). $C_{12}H_{19}NO_3 \cdot CH_4O_3S$. 321.39. [Colterol is INN.] (1) 1,2-Benzenediol, 4-[2-[(1,1-dimethylethyl)amino]-1-hydroxyethyl]-, methanesulfonate (salt), (±)-; (2) (±)-α-[(*tert*-Butylamino)methyl]-3,4-dihydroxybenzyl alcohol methanesulfonate (salt). *UNII-25CJR2TJPW. CAS-17605-73-1; CAS-18866-78-9* [colterol]. *Bronchodilator.* ◇*Win 5563-3*

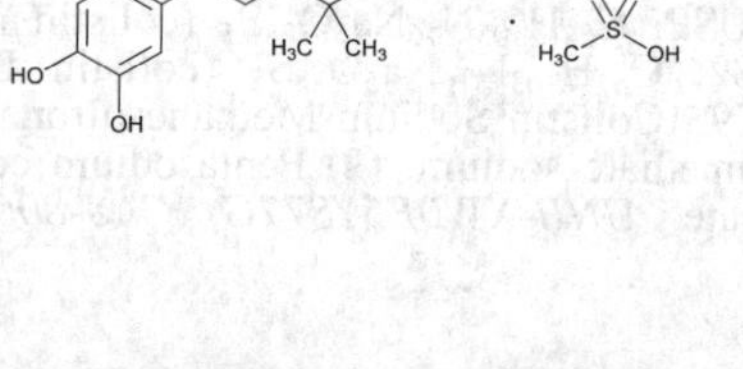

Coluracetam. $C_{19}H_{23}N_3O_3$. 341.40. *N*-(2,3-Dimethyl-5,6,7,8-tetrahydrofuro[2,3-*b*]quinolin-4-yl)-2-(2-oxopyrrolidin-1-yl)acetamide. *UNII-V6FL6O5GR7. CAS-135463-81-9*. INN.

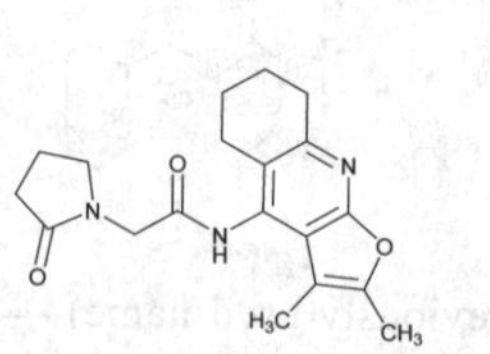

Co-magaldrox. Magnesium Hydroxide and Aluminium (Aluminum) Hydroxide; the proportions are expressed in the form *x*/*y* where *x* and *y* are the strengths in milligrams per unit dose of Magnesium Hydroxide and Aluminium (Aluminum) Hydroxide, respectively. BAN.

Co-methiamol. DL-Methionine and Paracetamol (Acetaminophen); the proportions are expressed in the form *x*/*y* where *x* and *y* are the strength in milligrams of DL-Methionine and Paracetamol (Acetaminophen) respectively. BAN.

Complex A/16686 — *See* Ramoplanin.

Complex A-16686 — *See* Ramoplanin.

Conatumumab [*2007*] (kon″ a toom′ ue mab). $C_{6466}H_{10006}N_{1730}O_{2024}S_{40}$. (1) Immunoglobulin G1, anti-(human cytokine receptor DR5 (death receptor 5)) (human monoclonal XG1-048 v w heavy chain), disulfide with human monoclonal XG1-048 v w light chain, dimer; (2) Immunoglobulin G1, anti-(human tumor necrosis factor receptor superfamily member 10B (death receptor 5, TRAIL-R2, CD262 antigen)); human monoclonal XG1-048 [Arg^{219},Glu^{361},Met^{365}]γ1 heavy chain (225-215′)-disulfide with κ light chain (231-231″:234-234″)-bisdisulfide dimer. Molecular weight is approximately 145,650 daltons. *CAS-896731-82-1*. INN. *Treatment of cancer.* ◇*AMG 655; TRAIL-R2 mAb*

Heavy chain

```
QVQLQESGPG LVKPSQTLSL TCTVSGGSIS SGDYFWSWIR QLPGKGLEWI
GHIHNSGTTY YNPSLKSRVT ISVDTSKKQF SLRLSSVTAA DTAVYYCARD
RGGDYYYGMD VWGQGTTVTV SSASTKGPSV FPLAPSSKST SGGTAALGCL
VKDYFPEPVT VSWNSGALTS GVHTFPAVLQ SSGLYSLSSV VTVPSSSLGT
QTYICNVNHK PSNTKVDKRV EPKSCDKTHT CPPCPAPELL GGPSVFLFPP
KPKDTLMISR TPEVTCVVVD VSHEDPEVKF NWYVDGVEVH NAKTKPREEQ
YNSTYRVVSV LTVLHQDWLN GKEYKCKVSN KALPAPIEKT ISKAKGQPRE
PQVYTLPPSR EEMTKNQVSL TCLVKGFYPS DIAVEWESNG QPENNYKTTP
PVLDSDGSFF LYSKLTVDKS RWQQGNVFSC SVMHEALHNH YTQKSLSLSP
GK
```

Light chain

```
EIVLTQSPGT LSLSPGERAT LSCRASQGIS RSYLAWYQQK PGQAPSLLIY
GASSRATGIP DRFSGSGSGT DFTLTISRLE PEDFAVYYCQ QFGSSPWTFG
QGTKVEIKRT VAAPSVFIFP PSDEQLKSGT ASVVCLLNNF YPREAKVQWK
VDNALQSGNS QESVTEQDSK DSTYSLSSTL TLSKADYEKH KVYACEVTHQ
GLSSPVTKSF NRGEC
```

* glycosylation site

Condurango Fluidextract. JAN.

Conessine Hydrobromide. $C_{24}H_{40}N_2.2HBr$. 518.41. [Conessine is INN.] Alkaloid obtained from the seeds of *Holarrhena antidysenterica* Linné. *UNII-N9EQE108I5. CAS-5913-82-6; CAS-546-06-5* [conessine]. MI.

Conestat Alfa. $C_{2355}H_{3745}N_{613}O_{728}S_{17}$. Human plasma protease C1 inhibitor (C1 esterase inhibitor) (*N,O*-glycosylated recombinant protein expressed in the mammary gland of transgenic rabbits), glycoform α. *CAS-80295-38-1*. INN.

Congazone Sodium — *See* Congo Red.

Congo Red. *CAS-573-58-0*. USP XV; MI.

Conivaptan. $C_{32}H_{26}N_4O_2$. 498.57. 4″-[(4,5-Dihydro-2-methylimidazo[4,5-*d*][1]benzazepin-6(1*H*)-yl)carbonyl]-2-biphenylcarboxanilide. *UNII-0NJ98Y462X. CAS-210101-16-9*. INN.

Conivaptan Hydrochloride [*1999*] (koe″ ni vap′ tan hye″ droe klor′ ide). $C_{32}H_{26}N_4O_2.HCl$. 535.04. (1) [1,1′-Biphenyl]-2-carboxamide, *N*-[4-[(4,5-dihydro-2-methylimidazo[4,5-*d*][1]benzazepin-6(1*H*)-yl)carbonyl]phenyl]-, monohydrochloride; (2) 4″-[(4,5-Dihydro-2-methylimidazo[4,5-*d*][1]benzazepin-6(1*H*)-yl)carbonyl]-2-biphenylcarboxanilide monohydrochloride. *UNII-75L57R6X36. CAS-168626-94-6. Hyponatremia and congestive heart failure (vasopressin antagonist)*. Vaprisol (Astellas) ◇*CI-1025; YM087*

Conorfone (INN) Hydrochloride — *See* Conorphone Hydrochloride.

Conorphone Hydrochloride [*1980*] (koe nor′ fone hye″ droe klor′ ide). $C_{23}H_{29}NO_3.HCl$. 403.94. [Conorfone is INN.] (1) Morphinan-6-one, 17-(cyclopropylmethyl)-4,5-epoxy-8-ethyl-3-methoxy-, hydrochloride, $(5\alpha,8\beta)$-; (2) 17-(Cyclopropylmethyl)-4,5α-epoxy-8β-ethyl-3-methoxymorphinan-6-one hydrochloride. *UNII-NN00W8BQ8N. CAS-70865-14-4; CAS-72060-05-0* [conorphone]. *Analgesic.* [*Name previously used: Codorphone.*] ◇*TR-5109*

Contusugene Ladenovec [*2006*] (kon too′ soo jeen la den′ oh vek). A modified human adenovirus 5 vector containing a cytomegalovirus promoter and a human p53 gene spliced into the DNA genome in place of the adenovirus E1A and E1B genes. *CAS-600735-73-7*. INN. *Treatment of solid tumors or neoplasms.* Advexin (Introgen Therapeutics) ◇*Ad5CMV-p53; INGN 201*

Co-oxycodAPAP (koe″ ox i koe′ da pap). PEN for Oxycodone and Acetaminophen.

COP — *See* Creatinolfosfate.

Co-phenotrope. Diphenoxylate Hydrochloride and Atropine Sulphate (Sulfate) in the proportions, by weight, 100 parts to 1 part, respectively. BAN.

Copovidone. NF. $(C_6H_9NO)_n + (C_4H_6O_2)_m$. (1) Acetic acid ethenyl ester polymer with 1-ethenyl-2-pyrrolidone; (2) 1-Vinyl-2-pyrrolidone polymer with vinyl acetate. *UNII-D9C330MD8B. CAS-25086-89-9*. BAN.

Copovithane. Copolymer of 2-methylenetrimethylene bis-(methylcarbamate) and 1-vinyl-2-pyrrolidone in the approximate ratio of 1 part to 4 parts, respectively. *CAS-68045-74-9*. BAN. ◇*BAY i 7433*

Copper Gluconate (kop′ er gloo′ koe nate). **USP**. $C_{12}H_{22}CuO_{14}$. 453.84. (1) Copper, bis (D-gluconato-O^1,O^2)-; (2) Copper D-gluconate (1:2). *CAS-527-09-3*. *Supplement (trace mineral).*

Copper Tetramibi Tetrafluoroborate. $C_{24}H_{44}BCuF_4N_4O_4$. 602.98. Tetrakis(2-methoxy-2-methylpropyl isocyanide-κN)copper(I) tetrafluoroborate. BAN.

---

† Brand name formerly used, and/or firm no longer concerned with this product.

Copper Undecylenate [*1988*] (kop′ er un de′ sil en ate). $C_{22}H_{38}O_4Cu$. 430.08. 10-Undecenoic acid, copper(2+) salt; Copper 10-undecenoate. *UNII-1LM0WKL73J*.

Co-prenozide. Oxprenolol Hydrochloride and Cyclopenthiazide in the proportions, by weight, 640 parts to 1 part, respectively. BAN.

Co-proxamol. Dextroproxyphene (Propoxyphene) Hydrochloride and Paracetamol (Acetaminophen) in the proportions, by weight, 1 part to 10 parts, respectively. BAN.

Co-proxAPAP (koe prox′ a pap). PEN for Propoxyphene Napsylate and Acetaminophen.

Corbadrine (INN and DCF) — *See* Levonordefrin.

Coriander Oil (kor″ ee an′ der). **NF**. The volatile oil obtained by steam distillation from the dried ripe fruit of *Coriandrum sativum* L. (Fam. Apiaceae). *UNII-7626GC95E5*. MI.

Corifollitropin Alfa [*1998*] (kor″ i fol″ i troe′ pin al′ fa). The substance is a heterodimer glycoprotein consisting of non-covalently associated α- and β-subunits. Site-directed mutagenesis and gene transfer techniques were used to add the C-terminal peptide of the β-subunit of human chorionic gonadotropin to the β-chain of human FSH. Hence, the α-subunit (92 amino acids) is identical to that of hFSH whereas the β-subunit is composed of the hFSH β-subunit (111 amino acids) and the last 28 amino acids of the C-terminal of the hCG β-subunit. The glycoprotein contains 4 N-linked carbohydrate chains at positions α52, α78, β7, and β24; O-glycosylation occurs at residues β115, β121, β126, and β132 on the C-terminal peptide. Molecular weight is approximately 38,000 to 62,000 daltons on SDS-PAGE. *CAS-195962-23-3*. INN. *Gonadotropin.* ◇Org 36286

```
APDVQDCPEC   TLQENPFFSQ   PGAPILQCMG   CCFSRAYPTP
LRSKKTMLVQ   KNVTSESTCC   VAKSYNRVTV   MGGFKVENHT
ACHCSTCYYH   KS

NSCELTNITI   AIEKEECRFC   ISINTTWCAG   YCYTRDLVYK
DPARPKIQKT   CTFKELVYET   VRVPGCAHHA   DSLYTYPVAT
QCHCGKCDSD   STDCTVRGLG   PSYCSFGEMK   ESSSSKAPPP
SLPSPSRLPG   PSDTPILPQ
```

       * glycosylation sites
       * sites de glycosylation
       * posiciónes de glicosilación

Cormetasone (INN) **Acetate** — *See* Cormethasone Acetate.

Cormethasone Acetate [*1973*] (kor meth′ a sone as′ e tate). $C_{24}H_{29}F_3O_6$. 470.48. [Cormetasone is INN.] (1) Pregna-1,4-diene-3,20-dione, 21-(acetyloxy)-6,6,9-trifluoro-11,17-dihydroxy-16-methyl-, (11β,16α)-; (2) 6,6,9-Trifluoro-11β,17,21-trihydroxy-16α-methylpregna-1,4-diene-3,20-dione 21-acetate. *CAS-35135-67-2; CAS-35135-68-3* [cormethasone]. *Anti-inflammatory (topical).* ◇RS-3694R

Corn Oil (korn). **NF**. The refined fixed oil obtained from the embryo of *Zea mays* Linné (Fam. Gramineae). *Pharmaceutic aid (solvent).*

Corn Starch (JAN) — *See* Starch.

Corn Syrup, High Fructose. NF. A sweet, nutritive saccharide mixture prepared as a clear, aqueous solution from high dextrose equivalent corn starch hydrolysate by the partial enzymatic conversion of dextrose to fructose, using an insoluble glucose isomerase enzyme preparation that complies with 21 CFR 184.1372.

Corn Syrup Solids (korn sir′ up). **NF**. A dried mixture of saccharides obtained by partial hydrolysis of edible corn starch by food grade acids and/or enzymes; 20% sugars expressed as D-glucose.

Corticorelin. $C_{208}H_{344}N_{60}O_{63}S_2$ (human). 4757.45 (human); $C_{205}H_{339}N_{59}O_{63}S$ (ovine). 4670.31 (ovine). Corticotropin-releasing factor. The source of the material should be indicated. INN.

Corticorelin Acetate [*2004*] (kor″ ti koe rel′ in as′ e tate). $C_{208}H_{344}N_{60}O_{63}S_2$. 4757.45. (1) Corticotropin-releasing factor (human); (2) Human corticotropin-releasing factor. *UNII-2YF82QN5RY. CAS-86784-80-7. Treatment of symptoms associated with peritumoral edema in brain tumor patients.* Xerecept (Hollister-Stier) *[Note—The source of the product (human, porcine, etc.) must be indicated in the labeling.]* ◇NEU 3002

```
SEEPPISLDL TFHLLREVLE MARAEQLAQQ AHSNRKLMEI I——NH2
```

Corticorelin Ovine Triflutate [*1990*] (kor″ ti koe rel′ in oh′ vine trye floo′ tate). $C_{205}H_{339}N_{59}O_{63}S.xC_2HF_3O_2$. (1) Corticotropin-releasing factor (sheep), trifluoroacetate (salt); (2) Corticotropin-releasing factor (sheep), trifluoroacetate (salt). *UNII-56X54T817Q. CAS-121249-14-7.* INN. *Diagnostic aid (adrenocortical insufficiency); diagnostic aid (Cushing's syndrome); hormone (corticotropin-releasing).* Acthrel (Ferring Pharmaceuticals)

```
SEQGEPPISLDL TFHLLREVLE MTKADQLAQQ AHSNRKLLDI A——NH2  · [ trifluoroacetate ]x

x = 4.1 - 8.2
```

Corticotrophin Zinc Hydroxide — *See* Corticotropin Zinc Hydroxide.

Corticotropin (kor″ ti koe troe′ pin). **USP** [Injection]. (1) Corticotropin; (2) Corticotropin. *UNII-K0U68Q2TXA. CAS-9002-60-2.* INN; BAN. *Hormone (adrenocorticotropic); glucocorticoid; diagnostic aid (adrenocortical insufficiency).* Acthar (Sanofi Aventis); Cortrophin (Organon) *[Name previously used: Corticotrophin.]*

Corticotropin, Repository (kor″ ti koe troe′ pin). **USP** [Injection]. (1) Corticotropin; (2) Corticotropin. *CAS-9002-60-2. Hormone (adrenocorticotropic); glucocorticoid; diagnostic aid (adrenocortical insufficiency).* Cortigel (Savage†); H.P. Acthar Gel (Rhone-Poulenc Rorer)

Corticotropin Tetracosapeptide — *See* Cosyntropin.

Corticotropin Zinc Hydroxide (kor″ ti koe troe′ pin zink hye drox′ ide). **USP** [Suspension, Injectable]. (1) Corticotropin zinc hydroxide; (2) Corticotropin zinc hydroxide. *CAS-9050-75-3.* INN. *Hormone (adrenocorticotropic); glucocorticoid; diagnostic aid (adrenocortical insufficiency).* Cortrophin Zinc ACTH (Organon†)

Cortisol — *See* Hydrocortisone.

Cortisone Acetate (kor′ ti sone as′ e tate). **USP**. $C_{23}H_{30}O_6$. 402.48. [Cortisone is INN and BAN.] (1) Pregn-4-ene-3,11,20-trione, 21-(acetyloxy)-17-hydroxy-; (2) 17,21-Dihydroxypregn-4-ene-3,11,20-trione 21-acetate. *UNII-883WKN7W8X; UNII-V27W9254FZ* [cortisone]. *CAS-50-04-4; CAS-53-06-5* [cortisone]. JAN. *Glucocorticoid.* Cortone (Merck)

Cortisuzol. $C_{37}H_{40}N_2O_8S$. 672.79. 11β,17,21-Trihydroxy-6,16α-dimethyl-2′-phenyl-2′*H*-pregna-2,4,6-trieno[3,2-*c*]pyrazol-20-one 21-(*m*-sulfobenzoate). *UNII-1PA76K-J99Y. CAS-50801-44-0.* INN; DCF.

Cortivazol [*1970*] (kor ti′ va zol). $C_{32}H_{38}N_2O_5$. 530.65. (1) 2′*H*-Pregna-2,4,6-trieno[3,2-*c*]pyrazol-20-one, 21-(acetyloxy)-11,17-dihydroxy-6,16-dimethyl-2′-phenyl-, (11β,16α)-; (2) 11β,17,21-Trihydroxy-6,16α-dimethyl-2′-phenyl-2′*H*-pregna-2,4,6-trieno[3,2-*c*]pyrazol-20-one 21-acetate. *CAS-1110-40-3.* INN. *Glucocorticoid.* ◇*NSC-80998*

Cortodoxone [*1966*] (kor″ toe dox′ one). $C_{21}H_{30}O_4$. 346.46. (1) Pregn-4-ene-3,20-dione, 17,21-dihydroxy-; (2) 17,21-Dihydroxypregn-4-ene-3,20-dione. *CAS-152-58-9.* INN; BAN. *Anti-inflammatory.* ◇*SK&F 3050; NSC-18317*

Co-simalcite. Activated Dimethicone and Hydrotalcite; the proportions are expressed in the form *x/y*, where *x* and *y* are the strengths in milligrams of activated Dimethicone and Hydrotalcite, respectively. BAN.

Cositecan [*2008*] (koe″ si tee′ kan). $C_{25}H_{28}N_2O_4Si$. 448.59. (1) 1*H*-Pyrano[3′,4′:6,7]indolizino[1,2-*b*]quinoline-3,14(4*H*,12*H*)-dione, 4-ethyl-4-hydroxy-11-[2-(trimethylsilyl)ethyl]-, (4*S*)-; (2) (4*S*)-4-Ethyl-4-hydroxy-11-[2-(trimethylsilyl)ethyl]-1,12-dihydro-14*H*-pyrano[3′,4′:6,7]in-

dolizino[1,2-*b*]quinoline-3,14(4*H*)-dione. *CAS-203923-89-1. Antineoplastic agent.* Karenitecin (BioNumerik) ◇*BNP1350*

Co-spironozide (koe″ spye ro noe′ zide). PEN for Spironolactone and Hydrochlorothiazide.

Cosyntropin [*1968*] (koe″ sin troe′ pin). $C_{136}H_{210}N_{40}O_{31}S$. 2933.44. [Tetracosactide is INN and BAN; Tetracosactide Acetate is JAN.] (1) α^{1-24}-Corticotropin; (2) L-Seryl-L-tyrosyl-L-seryl-L-methionyl-L-glutamyl-L-histidyl-L-phenylalanyl-L-arginyl-L-tryptophylglycyl-L-lysyl-L-prolyl-L-valylglycyl-L-lysyl-L-lysyl-L-arginyl-L-arginyl-L-prolyl-L-valyl-L-lysyl-L-valyl-L-tyrosyl-L-proline. *UNII-72YY86EA29. CAS-16960-16-0. Hormone (adrenocorticotropic).* Cortrosyn (Amphastar) *[Name previously used: Tetracosactrin.]*

SYSMEHFRWG KPVGKKRRPV KVYP

Cotarnine Chloride. *UNII-03F6B8N3QN. CAS-10018-19-6; CAS-82-54-2* [cotarnine]. NF VIII; MI.

Cotarnine Hydrochloride — *See* Cotarnine Chloride.

Co-tenidone. PEN for Atenolol and Chlorthalidone. Atenolol and Chlorthalidone in the proportions, by weight, 4 parts to 1 part, respectively. BAN.

Co-tetroxazine. Tetroxoprim and Sulphadiazine (Sulfadiazine) in the proportions, by weight, 2 parts to 5 parts, respectively. BAN.

Cotinine Fumarate [*1963*] (koe′ ti neen fue′ ma rate). $(C_{10}H_{12}N_2O)_2 \cdot C_4H_4O_4$. 468.50. [Cotinine is INN.] (1) 2-Pyrrolidinone, 1-methyl-5-(3-pyridinyl)-, (*S*)-, (*E*)-2-butenedioate (2:1); (2) (-)-1-Methyl-5-(3-pyridyl)-2-pyrrolidinone fumarate (2:1). *CAS-5695-98-7; CAS-486-56-6* [cotinine]. *Antidepressant.*

Co-triamterzide (koe″ trye am′ ter zide). PEN for Triamterene and Hydrochlorothiazide. Triamterene and Hydrochlorothiazide in the proportions, by weight, 2 parts to 1 part, respectively. BAN.

Co-trifamole. Trimethoprim and Sulphamoxole (Sulfamoxole) in the proportions, by weight, 1 part to 5 parts, respectively. BAN.

Co-trimazine. Trimethoprim and Sulphadiazine (Sulfadiazine) in the proportions, by weight, of 1 part to 5 parts, respectively. BAN.

Co-trimoxazole (koe″ trye mox′ a zole). PEN for Sulfamethoxazole and Trimethoprim. Trimethoprim and Sulphamethoxazole (Sulfamethoxazole) in the proportions, by weight, of 1 part to 5 parts, respectively. BAN.

Cotriptyline. $C_{20}H_{21}NO$. 291.39. 1-(Dimethylamino)-3-(10,11-dihydro-5*H*-dibenzo[*a,d*]cyclohepten-5-ylidene)-2-propanone. *UNII-KQJ4QI511C. CAS-34662-67-4.* INN; DCF.

---

† Brand name formerly used, and/or firm no longer concerned with this product.

Cotton, Purified (kot' un). **USP**. [Absorbent Cotton, Purified, is JAN.] The hair of the seed of cultivated varieties of *Gossypium hirsutum* Linné, or of other species of *Gossypium* Fam. Malvaceae), freed from adhering impurities, deprived of fatty matter, bleached, and sterilized. *Surgical aid.*

Cottonseed Oil (kot' un seed). **NF**. The refined fixed oil obtained from the seed of cultivated plants of various varieties of *Gossypium hirsutum* Linné or of other species of *Gossypium* (Fam. Malvaceae). *CAS-8001-29-4. Pharmaceutic aid (solvent).*

Coumafos (INN, BAN) — *See* Coumaphos.

Coumamycin (INN) — *See* Coumermycin.

Coumaphos. $C_{14}H_{16}ClO_5PS$. 362.77. [Coumafos is INN and BAN.] *O*-3-Chloro-4-methyl-7-coumarinyl *O,O*-diethyl phosphorothioate. *UNII-L08SZ5Z5JC. CAS-56-72-4.* MI. Baymix (Bayer Animal Health†); Meldane (Bayer Animal Health†) ◇*Bayer 21199*

Coumarin. *UNII-A4VZ22K1WT. CAS-91-64-5.* NF X; MI.

Coumazoline. $C_{14}H_{16}N_2O$. 228.29. 2-[(2-Ethylbenzofuran-3-yl)methyl]-2-imidazoline. *UNII-TR7Y641235. CAS-37681-00-8.* INN. ◇*L 5818 [as hydrochloride]*

Coumermycin [1965] (koo″ mer mye′ sin). $C_{55}H_{59}N_5O_{20}$. 1110.08. [Coumamycin is INN.] (1) 1*H*-Pyrrole-2-carboxylic acid, 5-methyl-, diester with *N,N′*-bis[7-[(6-deoxy-5-*C*-methyl-4-*O*-methyl-α-L-*lyxo*-hexopyranosyl)oxy]-4-hydroxy-8-methyl-2-oxo-2*H*-1-benzopyran-3-yl]-3-methyl-1*H*-pyrrole-2,4-dicarboxamide; (2) 5-Methylpyrrole-2-carboxylic acid, diester with 3,3′-[(3-methylpyrrole-2,4-diyl)bis(carbonylimino)]bis[4-hydroxy-8-methyl-7-[(tetrahydro-3,4-dihydroxy-5-methoxy-6,6-dimethylpyran-2-yl)oxy]coumarin]. *CAS-4434-05-3. Antibacterial.* ◇*NSC-107412*

Coumermycin Sodium [1984] (koo″ mer mye′ sin soe′ dee um). $C_{55}H_{57.6}N_5Na_{1.4}O_{20}$. 1140.85. (1) 1*H*-Pyrrole-2-carboxylic acid, 5-methyl-3,3′-diester with *N,N′*-bis[7-[(6-deoxy-5-*C*-methyl-4-*O*-methyl-α-L-*lyxo*-hexopyranosyl) oxy]-4-hydroxy-8-methyl-2-oxo-2*H*-1-benzopyran-3-yl]-3-methyl-1*H*-pyrrole-2,4-dicarboxamide, sodium salt (5:7); (2) 5-Methylpyrrole-2-carboxylic acid, 3″,3‴-diester with 3,3′-[(3-methylpyrrole-2,4-diyl)bis(carbonylimino)]-bis[7-(5,5-di-*C*-methyl-4-*O*-methyl-α-L-lyxopyranosyl) oxy]-4-hydroxy-8-methylcoumarin], sodium salt (5:7). *CAS-87901-11-9. Antibacterial.* ◇*Ro 5-4645/010*

Coumetarol. $C_{21}H_{16}O_7$. 380.35. 3,3′-(2-Methoxyethylidene)-bis(4-hydroxycoumarin). *UNII-UO1VQB3SPZ. CAS-4366-18-1.* INN; BAN; DCF; MI. *[Name previously used: Cumetharol.]*

Co-zidocapt. BAN for hydrochlorothiazide and captopril in the proportions, by weight, 1 part to 2 parts respectively.

[51]Cr — *See* Albumin, Chromated Cr 51 Serum.

[51]Cr — *See* Chromic Chloride Cr 51.

[51]Cr — *See* Chromic Phosphate Cr 51.

[51]Cr — *See* Sodium Chromate Cr 51.

Cranberry Liquid Preparation. A bright red juice derived from the fruits of *Vaccinium macrocarpon* Ait. or *Vaccinium oxycoccos* Linné (Fam. Ericaceae). NF XXI.

Creatinine (kree at′ i neen). **NF**. $C_4H_7N_3O$. 113.12. (1) Imidazolidin-4-one, 2-imino-1-methyl; (2) 2-Imino-1-methylimidazolidin-4-one. *UNII-AYI8EX34EU. CAS-60-27-5. Bulking agent for freeze drying.*

Creatinolfosfate. $C_4H_{12}N_3O_4P$. 197.13. 1-(2-Hydroxyethyl)-1-methylguanidine dihydrogen phosphate (ester). *UNII-5O564RN1QD. CAS-6903-79-3.* INN.

Creosote Carbonate. [Creosote is JAN.] *CAS-8001-59-0.* USP IX; MI.

Cresol (kree′ sol). **NF**. C_7H_8O. 108.14. (1) Phenol, methyl-; (2) Cresol. *CAS-1319-77-3.* JAN. *Disinfectant.*

Cresotamide. $C_8H_9NO_2$. 151.16. 2,3-Cresotamide. *UNII-5748P7L6IT. CAS-14008-60-7.* INN; DCF.

Cresoxydiol — *See* Mephenesin.

Crestomycin Sulfate — *See* Paromomycin Sulfate.

Cridanimod. $C_{15}H_{11}NO_3$. 253.25. 9-Oxo-10-acridanacetic acid. *UNII-X91E9EME19. CAS-38609-97-1.* INN.

Crilanomer. Starch polymer with acrylonitrile. INN.

Crilvastatin [*1992*] (kril″ va stat′ in). $C_{14}H_{23}NO_3$. 253.34. (1) L-Proline, 5-oxo-, 3,3,5-trimethylcyclohexyl ester; (2) 5-Oxo-L-proline, (±)-*cis*-3,3,5-trimethylcyclohexyl ester. *CAS-120551-59-9*. INN. *Antihyperlipidemic.* ◇*PMD-387*

Crisantaspase. L-Asparagine amidohydrolase obtained from cultures of *Erwinia chrysanthemi* (syn. *E. carotovora*). *CAS-9015-68-3*. BAN. *[See also Asparaginase.]*

Crisnatol Mesylate [*1988*] (kris′ na tol mes′ i late). $C_{23}H_{23}NO_2 \cdot CH_4O_3S$. 441.54. [Crisnatol is INN.] (1) 1,3-Propanediol, 2-[(6-chrysenylmethyl)amino]-2-methyl-, methanesulfonate (salt); (2) 2-[(6-Chrysenylmethyl)amino]-2-methyl-1,3-propanediol methanesulfonate (salt). *UNII-R6D31YA2WK*. *CAS-96389-69-4; CAS-96389-68-3* [crisnatol]. *Antineoplastic.* ◇*BW A770U mesylate*

Crobenetine. $C_{25}H_{33}NO_2$. 379.54. (2*R*,6*S*)-3-[(2*S*)-2-(Benzyloxy)propyl]-1,2,3,4,5,6-hexahydro-6,11,11-trimethyl-2,6-methano-3-benzazocin-10-ol. *CAS-221019-25-6*. INN.

Croconazole. $C_{18}H_{15}ClN_2O$. 310.78. [Croconazole Hydrochloride is JAN.] 1-[1-[*o*-[(*m*-Chlorobenzyl)oxy]phenyl]vinyl]imidazole. *UNII-446254H55G*. *CAS-77175-51-0*. INN.

Crofelemer [*1998*] (kroe fel′ e mer). Oligomeric proanthocyanidin from the latex of *Croton lechleri*. Crofelemer. Average molecular weight of approximately 2300 daltons. *CAS-148465-45-6*. *Antidiarrheal; antiviral.* Provir (Shaman); Virend (Shaman) ◇*SP-303*

Crofilcon A [*1974*] (kroe fil′ kon). $(C_7H_{12}O_4)_x(C_5H_8O_2)_y$. (1) 2-Propenoic acid, 2-methyl-, 2,3-dihydroxypropyl ester, polymer with methyl 2-methyl-2-propenoate; (2) 2,3-Dihydroxypropyl methacrylate polymer with methyl methacrylate. *CAS-50450-03-8*. *Contact lens material (hydrophilic).* ◇*CS-151*

Cromakalim. $C_{16}H_{18}N_2O_3$. 286.33. (±)-*trans*-3-Hydroxy-2,2-dimethyl-4-(2-oxo-1-pyrrolidinyl)-6-chromancarbonitrile. *UNII-0G4X367WA3*. *CAS-94470-67-4*. INN; BAN. ◇*BRL 34915*

Cromitrile Sodium [*1981*] (kroe′ mi trile soe′ dee um). $C_{20}H_{14}N_5NaO_5$. 427.35. [Cromitrile is INN.] (1) Benzonitrile, 4-[2-hydroxy-3-[[4-oxo-2-(1*H*-tetrazol-5-yl)-4*H*-1-benzopyran-5-yl]oxy]propoxy]-, monosodium salt, (±)-; (2) (±)-*p*-[2-Hydroxy-3-[[4-oxo-2-(1*H*-tetrazol-5-yl)-4*H*-1-benzopyran-5-yl]oxy]propoxy]benzonitrile monosodium salt. *CAS-53736-52-0; CAS-53736-51-9* [cromitrile]. *Antiasthmatic.* ◇*TR-2855*

Cromoglicate Lisetil. $C_{33}H_{36}N_2O_{12}$. 652.65. Diethyl 5,5′-[(2-hydroxytrimethylene)dioxy]bis[4-oxo-4*H*-1-benzopyran-2-carboxylate], ester with L-lysine. *UNII-VOZ07VZP8G*. *CAS-110816-79-0*. INN.

Cromoglicic Acid (INN) — *See* Cromolyn Sodium.

Cromoglycic Acid (BAN) — *See* Cromolyn Sodium.

Cromolyn Sodium [*1968*] (kroe′ mo lin soe′ dee um). **USP**. $C_{23}H_{14}Na_2O_{11}$. 512.33. [Cromoglicic Acid is INN and BAN; Sodium Cromoglicate is JAN.] (1) 4*H*-1-Benzopyran-2-carboxylic acid, 5,5′-[(2-hydroxy-1,3-propanediyl)bis(oxy)]bis[4-oxo-, disodium salt]; (2) Disodium 5,5′-[(2-

<hr>

† Brand name formerly used, and/or firm no longer concerned with this product.

hydroxytrimethylene)dioxy]bis[4-oxo-4*H*-1-benzopyran-2-carboxylate]. *UNII-Q2WXR1I0PK; UNII-Y0TK0FS77W* [cromolyn]. *CAS-15826-37-6; CAS-16110-51-3* [cromolyn]. *Anti-asthmatic (prophylactic)*. Crolom (Bausch & Lomb); Gastrocrom (Azur); Intal (King); Opticrom (Allergan) ◇*FPL.670*

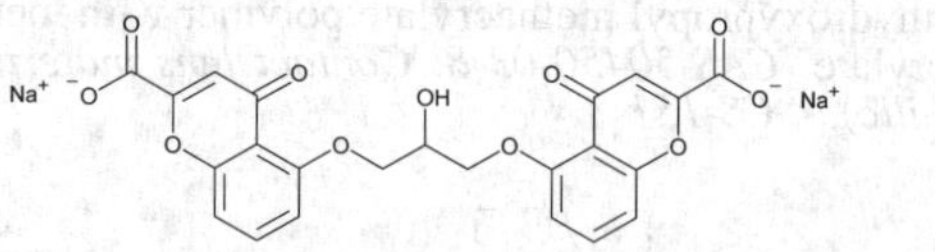

Cronidipine. $C_{30}H_{32}ClN_3O_8$. 598.04. [8-(*p*-Chlorophenyl)-1,4-dioxa-8-azaspiro[4,5]dec-2-yl]methyl methyl 1,4-dihydro-2,6-dimethyl-4-(*m*-nitrophenyl)-3,5-pyridinedicarboxylate. *UNII-7TXJ9MY5V9. CAS-113759-50-5*. INN.

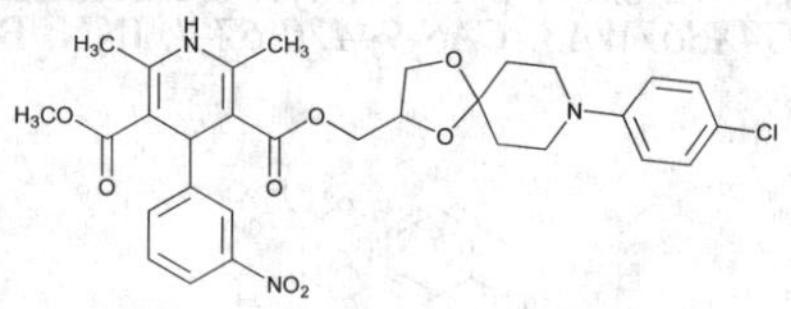

Cropropamide. $C_{13}H_{24}N_2O_2$. 240.34. *N*-[1-(Dimethylcarbamoyl)propyl]-*N*-propylcrotonamide. *CAS-3544-46-5* [*E*]; *CAS-633-47-6*. INN; BAN; MI.

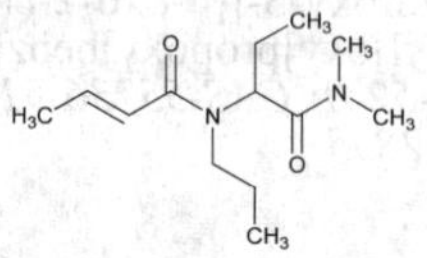

Croscarmellose Sodium [*1981*] (kros kar′ mel ose soe′ dee um). **NF**. [Croscarmellose is INN and BAN.] Carmellose (carboxymethylcellulose) sodium that has been internally cross-linked either by control of the reaction conditions or by the use of a cross-linking reagent. *Pharmaceutic aid (tablet disintegrant)*. Ac-Di-Sol (FMC); CLD 2 (Buckeye†) [*Names previously used: Cross-linked Carboxymethylcellulose Sodium and Modified Cellulose Gum.*]

Crospovidone (kros poe′ vi done). **NF**. $(C_6H_9NO)_n$. (1) 1-Ethenyl-2-pyrrolidinone, homopolymer; (2) 1-Vinyl-2-pyrrolidinone homopolymer. *CAS-9003-39-8*. INN; BAN. *Pharmaceutic aid (tablet excipient)*. Kollidon CL (BASF); Kollidon CLM (BASF); Polyplasdone (International Specialty Products)

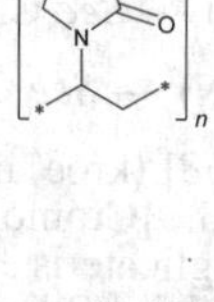

Cross-linked Carboxymethylcellulose Sodium (previously used name) — *See* Croscarmellose Sodium.

Crotamiton (kroe tam′ i ton). **USP**. $C_{13}H_{17}NO$. 203.28. (1) 2-Butenamide, *N*-ethyl-*N*-(2-methylphenyl)-; (2) *N*-Ethyl-*o*-crotonotoluidide. *UNII-D6S4O4XD0H. CAS-483-63-6*. INN; BAN; JAN. *Scabicide*. Crotan (Summers); Eurax (Westwood-Squibb)

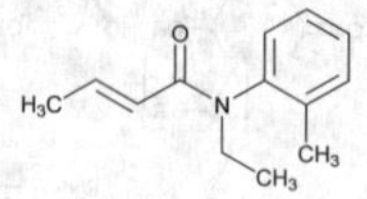

Crotetamide. $C_{12}H_{22}N_2O_2$. 226.32. *N*-[1-(Dimethylcarbamoyl)propyl]-*N*-ethylcrotonamide. *UNII-642I97LB5B. CAS-6168-76-9*. INN; BAN; MI. [*Name previously used: Crotethamide.*]

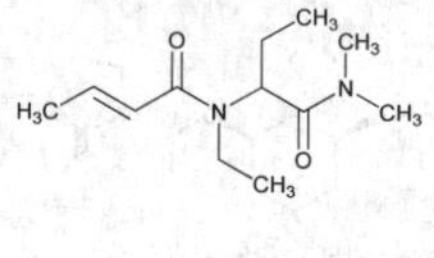

Crotethamide (previously used name) — *See* Crotetamide.

Crotoniazide. $C_{10}H_{11}N_3O$. 189.21. Isonicotinic acid 2-butenylidenehydrazide. *UNII-C4DT7VL6FU. CAS-7007-96-7*. INN; DCF.

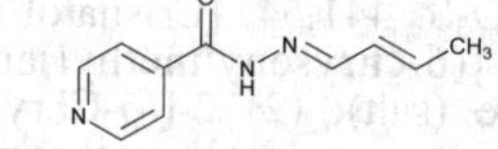

Crotonylidenisoniazid — *See* Crotoniazide.

Crotoxyfos. α-Methylbenzyl 3-(dimethoxyphosphinyloxy)-isocrotonate. *CAS-7700-17-6*. BAN; MI.

Crufomate [*1968*] (kroo′ foe mate). $C_{12}H_{19}ClNO_3P$. 291.71. (1) Phosphoramidic acid methyl-, 2-chloro-4-(1,1-dimethylethyl)phenyl methyl ester; (2) 4-*tert*-Butyl-2-chlorophenyl methyl methylphosphoramidate. *UNII-V82Q65924L. CAS-299-86-5*. INN; BAN. *Anthelmintic (veterinary)*.

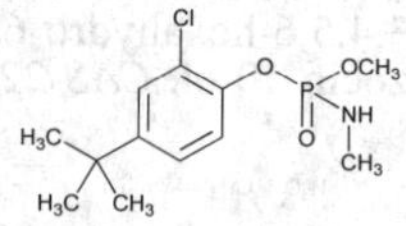

Cryopreserved Human Fibroblast-Derived Dermal Substitute. **USP**. A living monolayer skin substitute derived from neonatal foreskins.

Cryptenamine Acetates. NND 1964. Unitensen (Medpointe)

Crystal Violet — *See* Gentian Violet.

^{131}Cs — *See* Cesium Chloride Cs 131.

CSF-1 (previously used name) — *See* Cilmostim.

^{64}Cu — *See* Cupric Acetate Cu 64.

Cumetharol (previously used name) — *See* Coumetarol.

Cupric Acetate Cu 64 [*1963*] (kue′ prik as′ e tate). $C_4H_6{}^{64}CuO_4$. (1) Acetic acid, copper(2+)-^{64}Cu salt; (2) Copper(2+)-^{64}Cu acetate. *Radioactive agent*.

Cupric Chloride (kue′ prik klor′ ide). **USP**. $CuCl_2.2H_2O$. 170.48. (1) Copper chloride ($CuCl_2$) dihydrate; (2) Copper(2+) chloride dihydrate. *UNII-S2QG84156O. CAS-10125-13-0; CAS-7447-39-4* [anhydrous]. *Supplement (trace mineral)*.

Cupric Sulfate (kue′ prik sul′ fate). **USP**. $CuSO_4 \cdot 5H_2O$. 249.69. (1) Sulfuric acid, copper(2+) salt (1:1), pentahydrate; (2) Copper(2+) sulfate (1:1) pentahydrate. *UNII-LRX7AJ16DT. CAS-7758-99-8; CAS-7758-98-7* [anhydrous]. *Antidote (to phosphorus).*

Cuprimyxin [*1973*] (kue″ pri mix′ in). $C_{26}H_{18}CuN_4O_8$. 577.99. (1) Copper, bis(6-methoxy-1-phenazinol 5,10-dioxidato-O^1,O^{10})-; (2) Bis(6-methoxy-1-phenazinol 5,10-dioxidato) copper. *UNII-Q728680892. CAS-28069-65-0.* INN. *Antibacterial (veterinary); antifungal.* Unitop [Veterinary] (Hoffmann-LaRoche†) ◇*Ro 7-4488/1*

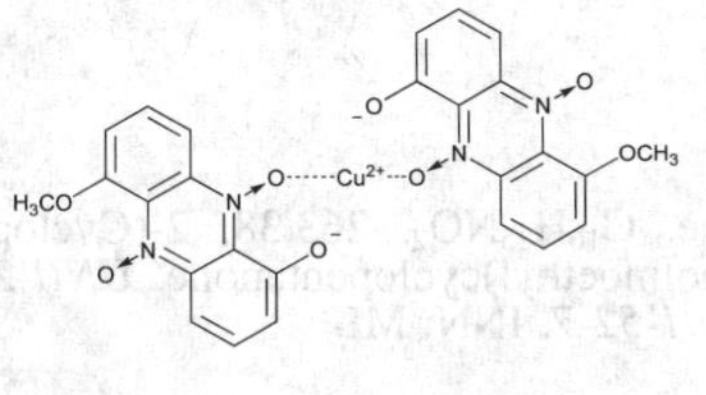

Cuproxoline. $C_{18}H_{12}CuN_2O_{14}S_4 \cdot 4C_4H_{11}N$. 964.65. Bis(dihydrogen 8-hydroxy-5,7-quinolinedisulfonato)copper, compound with diethylamine (1:4). *CAS-13007-93-7.* INN; BAN; MI.

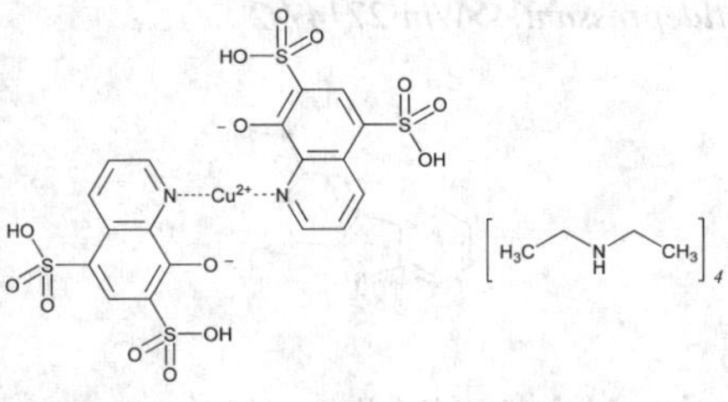

Custirsen Sodium [*2007*] (kus′ tir sen soe′ dee um). $C_{231}H_{292}N_{78}Na_{20}O_{119}P_{20}S_{20}$. 7785.81. [Custirsen is INN.] (1) DNA, d(*P*-thio)([2′-*O*-(2-methoxyethyl)]m5rC-[2′-*O*-(2-methoxyethyl)]rA-[2′-*O*-(2-methoxyethyl)]rG-[2′-*O*-(2-methoxyethyl)]m5rC-A-G-C-A-G-A-G-T-C-T-T-C-A-[2′-*O*-(2-methoxyethyl)]m5rU-[2′-*O*-(2-methoxyethyl)]m5rC-[2′-*O*-(2-methoxyethyl)]rA-[2′-*O*-(2-methoxyethyl)]m5-rU), eicosasodium salt; (2) 2′-*O*-(2-Methoxyethyl)-5-methyl-*P*-thiocytidylyl-(3′→5′)-2′-*O*-(2-methoxyethyl)-*P*-thioadenylyl-(3′→5′)-2′-*O*-(2-methoxyethyl)-*P*-thioguanylyl-(3′→5′)-2′-*O*-(2-methoxyethyl)-5-methyl-*P*-thiocytidylyl-(3′→5′)-2′-deoxy-*P*-thioadenylyl-(3′→5′)-2′-deoxy-*P*-thioguanylyl-(3′→5′)-2′-deoxy-*P*-thiocytidylyl-(3′→5′)-2′-deoxy-*P*-thioadenylyl-(3′→5′)-2′-deoxy-*P*-thioguanylyl-(3′→5′)-2′-deoxy-*P*-thioadenylyl-(3′→5′)-2′-deoxy-*P*-thioguanylyl-(3′→5′)-*P*-thiothymidylyl-(3′→5′)-2′-deoxy-*P*-thiocytidylyl-(3′→5′)-*P*-thiothymidylyl-(3′→5′)-*P*-thiothymidylyl-(3′→5′)-2′-deoxy-*P*-thiocytidylyl-(3′→5′)-2′-deoxy-*P*-thioadenylyl-(3′→5′)-2′-*O*-(2-methoxyethyl)-5-methyl-*P*-thiouridylyl-(3′→5′)-2′-*O*-(2-methoxyethyl)-5-methyl-*P*-thiocytidylyl-(3′→5′)-2′-*O*-(2-methoxyethyl)-*P*-thioadenylyl-(3′→5′)-2′-*O*-(2-methoxyethyl)-5-methyl-

P-thiouridine eicosasodium salt. *CAS-685922-56-9; CAS-903916-27-8* [custirsen]. *Treatment of cancer.* ◇*OGX-011; ISIS 112989*

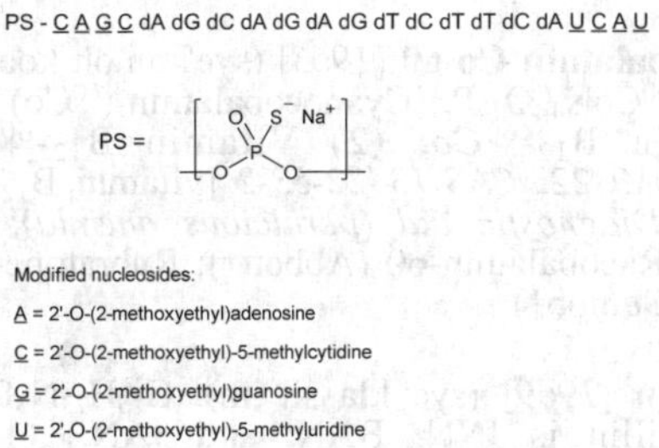

PS - C A G C dA dG dC dA dG dA dG dT dC dT dT dC dA U C A U

Modified nucleosides:

A = 2′-O-(2-methoxyethyl)adenosine

C = 2′-O-(2-methoxyethyl)-5-methylcytidine

G = 2′-O-(2-methoxyethyl)guanosine

U = 2′-O-(2-methoxyethyl)-5-methyluridine

Cyacetacide. $C_3H_5N_3O$. 99.09. Cyanoacetic acid hydrazide. *CAS-140-87-4.* INN; BAN; MI. *[Name previously used: Cyacetazide.]*

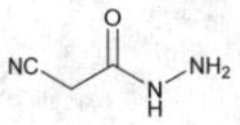

Cyamemazine. $C_{19}H_{21}N_3S$. 323.46. 10-[3-(Dimethylamino)-2-methylpropyl]phenothiazine-2-carbonitrile. *UNII-A2JGV5CNU4. CAS-3546-03-0.* INN; MI. ◇*RP 7204*

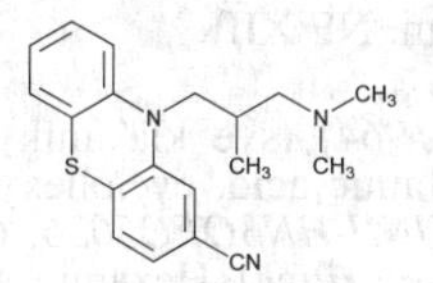

Cyamepromazine (DCF) — *See* Cyamemazine.

Cyanamide (JAN) — *See* Calcium Carbimide.

Cyanoacrylate (JAN) — *See* Mecrylate.

Cyanocobalamin (sye″ an oh koe bal′ a min). **USP**. $C_{63}H_{88}CoN_{14}O_{14}P$. 1355.37. (1) Vitamin B_{12}; (2) Vitamin B_{12}. *UNII-P6YC3EG204. CAS-68-19-9.* INN; BAN; JAN. *Vitamin (hematopoietic).* Berubigen (Pfizer); Betalin 12 (Lilly); Cobavite (Watson); Nascobal (QOL); Redisol (Merck); Rubramin (Bristol-Myers Squibb) *[Name previously used: Vitamin B_{12}.]*

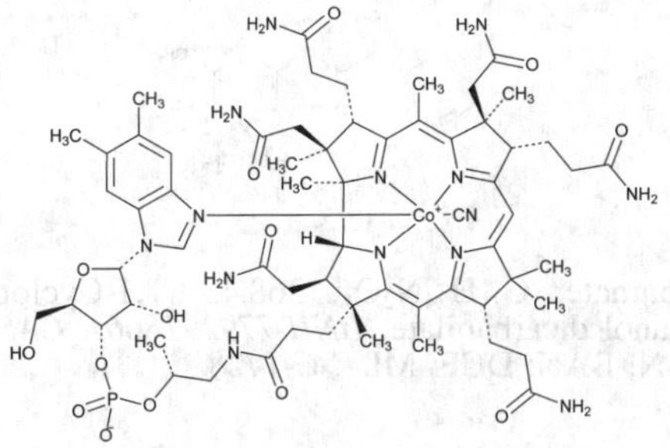

Cyanocobalamin Co 57 [*1963*] (sye″ an oh koe bal′ a min). **USP**. $C_{63}H_{88}{}^{57}CoN_{14}O_{14}P$. [Cyanocobalamin ($^{57}Co$) is INN.] (1) Vitamin B_{12}-^{57}Co; (2) Vitamin B_{12}-^{57}Co. *UNII-025P9I542Y. CAS-13115-03-2; CAS-41559-38-0. Diagnostic aid (pernicious anemia); radioactive agent.* Racobalamin-57 (Abbott†); Rubratope-57 (Bristol-Myers Squibb†)

---

† Brand name formerly used, and/or firm no longer concerned with this product.

Cyanocobalamin Co 58 (sye″ an oh koe bal′ a min). **USP** [Capsules]. $C_{63}H_{88}CoN_{14}O_{14}P$. 1355.37. (1) Vitamin B_{12}-^{58}Co; (2) Vitamin B_{12}-^{58}Co. *UNII-U0E93N6V2A. CAS-18195-32-9.* INN.

Cyanocobalamin Co 60 [*1963*] (sye″ an oh koe bal′ a min). $C_{63}H_{88}{}^{60}CoN_{14}O_{14}P$. [Cyanocobalamin ($^{60}Co$) is INN.] (1) Vitamin B_{12}-^{60}Co; (2) Vitamin B_{12}-^{60}Co. *UNII-562RS6MC22. CAS-13422-53-2* [vitamin B_{12}-^{60}Co]. USP XXII. *Diagnostic aid (pernicious anemia); radioactive agent.* Racobalamin-60 (Abbott†); Rubratope-60 (Bristol-Myers Squibb†)

Cyclacillin [*1969*] (sye kla sil′ in). $C_{15}H_{23}N_3O_4S$. 341.43. [Ciclacillin is INN, BAN, and JAN.] (1) 4-Thia-1-azabicyclo[3.2.0]heptane-2-carboxylic acid, 6-[[(1-amino-cyclohexyl)carbonyl]amino]-3,3-dimethyl-7-oxo-, [2S-(2α,5α,6β)]-; (2) 6-(1-Aminocyclohexanecarboxamido)-3,3-dimethyl-7-oxo-4-thia-1-azabicyclo[3.2.0]heptane-2-carboxylic acid. *UNII-72ZJ154X86. CAS-3485-14-1.* USP XXIII. *Antibacterial.* Cyclapen (Wyeth) ◇*Wy-4508*

Cyclamate Calcium. NF XIII.

Cyclamic Acid [*1964*] (sye kla′ mik as′ id). $C_6H_{13}NO_3S$. 179.24. (1) Sulfamic acid, cyclohexyl-; (2) Cyclohexane-sulfamic acid. *UNII-HN3OFO5036. CAS-100-88-9.* BAN. *Sweetener (non-nutritive).* Hexamic Acid (Abbott)

Cyclamide — *See* Glycyclamide.

Cyclandelate. USP. $C_{17}H_{24}O_3$. 276.37. (1) 3,3,5-Trimethyl-cyclohexanol α-phenyl-α-hydroxyacetate; (2) 1,5-*cis*-3,3,5-Trimethylcyclohexyl 2-hydroxy-2-phenyl acetate. *UNII-4139O1OAY2. CAS-456-59-7.* INN; BAN; JAN; MI. Cyclospasmol (Wyeth-Ayerst)

Cyclarbamate. $C_{21}H_{24}N_2O_4$. 368.43. 1,1-Cyclopentanedi-methanol dicarbanilate. *UNII-779291866J. CAS-5779-54-4.* INN; BAN; DCF; MI. ◇*C-1428*

Cyclazocine [*1965*] (sye klaz′ oh seen). $C_{18}H_{25}NO$. 271.40. (1) 2,6-Methano-3-benzazocin-8-ol, 3-(cyclopropyl-methyl)-1,2,3,4,5,6-hexahydro-6,11-dimethyl-; (2) 3-(Cy-clopropylmethyl)-1,2,3,4,5,6-hexahydro-6,11-dimethyl-2,6-methano-3-benzazocin-8-ol. *CAS-3572-80-3.* INN. *Analgesic.* ◇*Win 20,740; NSC-107429*

Cyclazodone. $C_{12}H_{12}N_2O_2$. 216.24. 2-(Cyclopropylamino)-5-phenyl-2-oxazolin-4-one. *CAS-14461-91-7.* INN; DCF.

Cyclexanone. $C_{16}H_{25}NO_2$. 263.38. 2-(Cyclopent-1-enyl)-2-(2-morpholinoethyl)cyclopentanone. *UNII-2OU4KS37EO. CAS-15301-52-7.* INN; MI.

Cyclindole [*1976*] (sye klin′ dole). $C_{14}H_{18}N_2$. 214.31. [Ciclindole is INN.] (1) 1*H*-Carbazol-3-amine, 2,3,4,9-tetrahydro-*N,N*-dimethyl-; (2) 3-(Dimethylamino)-1,2,3,4-tetrahydrocarbazole. *UNII-CXJ7G6BYD7. CAS-32211-97-5. Antidepressant.* ◇*Win 27147-2*

Cycliramine Maleate [*1963*] (sye klir′ a meen mal′ ee ate). $C_{18}H_{19}ClN_2 \cdot C_4H_4O_4$. 414.88. [Cycliramine is INN.] (1) Pyridine, 2-[(4-chlorophenyl)(1-methyl-4-piperidinylide-ne)methyl]-, (Z)-2-butenedioate (1:1); (2) 4-(p-Chloro-α-2-pyridylbenzylidene)-1-methylpiperidine maleate (1:1). *UNII-J542BCR0IQ. CAS-5781-37-3; CAS-47128-12-1* [cy-cliramine]. *Antihistaminic.* Prolergic (Schering†) ◇*Sch 2544; NSC-70933*

Cyclizine. $C_{18}H_{22}N_2$. 266.38. (1) Piperazine, 1-(diphenyl-methyl)-4-methyl-; (2) 1-(Diphenylmethyl)-4-methylpiper-azine. *UNII-QRW9FCR9P2. CAS-82-92-8.* USP XXIII; INN; BAN; DCF. *Antihistaminic.*

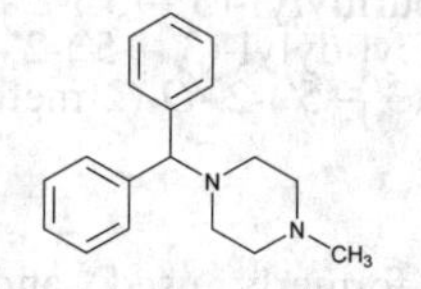

Cyclizine Hydrochloride (sye′ kli zeen hye″ droe klor′ ide). **USP**. $C_{18}H_{22}N_2.HCl$. 302.84. (1) Piperazine, 1-(diphenylmethyl)-4-methyl-, monohydrochloride; (2) 1-(Diphenylmethyl)-4-methylpiperazine monohydrochloride. *UNII-WOO1NHP4WE; UNII-QRW9FCR9P2* [cyclizine]. *CAS-303-25-3; CAS-82-92-8* [cyclizine]. BAN. *Anti-emetic.*

Cyclizine Lactate. $C_{18}H_{22}N_2.C_3H_6O_3$. 356.46. (1) Piperazine, 1-(diphenylmethyl)-4-methyl-, mono(2-hydroxypropanoate); (2) 1-(Diphenylmethyl)-4-methylpiperazine monolactate. *UNII-861R00J986; UNII-QRW9FCR9P2* [cyclizine]. *CAS-5897-19-8; CAS-82-92-8* [cyclizine]. USP XXIII; BAN. *Antinauseant.* Marezine (GlaxoSmithKline)

Cyclobarbital. $C_{12}H_{16}N_2O_3$. 236.27. 5-(1-Cyclohexen-1-yl)-5-ethylbarbituric acid. *UNII-0M8A98AD9H. CAS-52-31-3.* NF X; INN; BAN; MI. Phanodorn (Sterling Winthrop) *[Name previously used: Cyclobarbitone.]*

Cyclobarbital Calcium. *UNII-0HZN7FV25R. CAS-143-76-0.* NF XII; BAN. Phanodorn Calcium (Sterling Winthrop†)

Cyclobendazole [*1974*] (sye″ kloe ben′ da zole). $C_{13}H_{13}N_3O_3$. 259.26. [Ciclobendazole is INN and BAN.] (1) Carbamic acid, [5-(cyclopropylcarbonyl)-1*H*-benzimidazol-2-yl]-, methyl ester; (2) Methyl 5-(cyclopropylcarbonyl)-2-benzimidazolecarbamate. *UNII-JF3KQ40J31. CAS-31431-43-3. Anthelmintic.* ◊*R 17,147*

Cyclobenzaprine Hydrochloride [*1977*] (sye″ kloe ben′ za preen hye″ droe klor′ ide). **USP**. $C_{20}H_{21}N.HCl$. 311.85. [Cyclobenzaprine is INN.] (1) 1-Propanamine, 3-(5*H*-dibenzo[*a,d*]cyclohepten-5-ylidene)-*N,N*-dimethyl-, hydrochloride; (2) *N,N*-Dimethyl-5*H*-dibenzo[*a,d*]cycloheptene-$\Delta^{5,\gamma}$-propylamine hydrochloride. *UNII-0VE05JYS2P; UNII-69O5WQQ5TI* [cyclobenzaprine]. *CAS-6202-23-9; CAS-303-53-7* [cyclobenzaprine]. *Relaxant (muscle).* Flexeril (McNeil); Amrix (Cephalon) ◊*MK-130 [as the base]*

Cyclobutoic Acid. $C_{10}H_{18}O_3$. 186.25. β-Hydroxy-β-methylcyclohexanepropionic acid. *UNII-86KE25F200. CAS-17692-20-5.* INN; DCF.

Cyclobutyrol. $C_{10}H_{18}O_3$. 186.25. α-Ethyl-1-hydroxycyclohexaneacetic acid. *UNII-8T4L120N6M. CAS-512-16-3.* INN; DCF; MI.

Cyclocarbothiamine — *See* Cycotiamine.

Cyclocoumarol (BAN) — *See* Cyclocumarol.

Cyclocumarol. [Cyclocoumarol is BAN.] *UNII-725P8AW50M. CAS-518-20-7.* MI. Cumopyran (Abbott†)

Cyclofenil. $C_{23}H_{24}O_4$. 364.43. 4,4′-(Cyclohexylidenemethylene)diphenol diacetate ester. *UNII-J468V64WZ1. CAS-2624-43-3.* INN; BAN; JAN; DCF; MI. ◊*F 6066; ICI 48213*

Cyclofilcon A [*1979*] (sye″ kloe fil′ kon). $(C_6H_{10}O_3)_v$ $(C_4H_6O_2)_w(C_{18}H_{26}O_6)_x(C_8H_{14}O_2)_y(C_{10}H_{16}O_2)_z$. (1) 2-Propenoic acid, 2-methyl-, 2-hydroxyethyl ester, polymer with 2-methyl-2-propenoic acid, 2-ethyl-2-[[(2-methyl-1-oxo-2-propenyl)oxy]methyl]-1,3-propanediyl bis(2-methyl-2-propenoate), 2-methylpropyl 2-methyl-2-propenoate and cyclohexyl 2-methyl-2-propenoate; (2) 2-Hydroxyethyl methacrylate polymer with methacrylic acid, 2-ethyl-2-(hydroxymethyl)-1,3-propanediol trimethacrylate, isobutyl methacrylate and cyclohexyl methacrylate. *CAS-70145-52-7. Contact lens material (hydrophilic).*

Cycloguanil Embonate (INN, BAN) — *See* Cycloguanil Pamoate.

Cycloguanil Pamoate [*1964*] (sye″ kloe gwahn′ il pam′ oh ate). $(C_{11}H_{14}ClN_5)_2.C_{23}H_{16}O_6$. 891.80. [Cycloguanil Embonate is INN and BAN.] (1) 2-Naphthalenecarboxylic acid, 4,4′-methylenebis[3-hydroxy-, compd. with 1-(4-chlorophenyl)-1,6-dihydro-6,6-dimethyl-1,3,5-triazine-2,4-diamine (1:2); (2) 4,6-Diamino-1-(*p*-chlorophenyl)-1,2-dihydro-2,2-dimethyl-*s*-triazine compound (2:1) with 4,4′-methylenebis[3-hydroxy-2-naphthoic acid]. *UNII-*

---

† Brand name formerly used, and/or firm no longer concerned with this product.

26RM326WVN [cycloguanil]. *CAS-609-78-9; CAS-516-21-2* [cycloguanil]. *Antimalarial.* ◇*CI-501; CN-14,329-23A; PAM-MR-807-23a; NSC-77830*

Cyclohexanehexol — *See* Inositol.

Cycloheximide [*1978*] (sye″ kloe hex′ i mide). $C_{15}H_{23}NO_4$. 281.35. [Cicloheximide is INN.] (1) 2,6-Piperidinedione, 4-[2-(3,5-dimethyl-2-oxocyclohexyl)-2-hydroxyethyl]-, [1*S*-[1α(*S**),3α,5β]]-; (2) 3-[(*R*)-2-[(1*S*,3*S*,5*S*)-3,5-Dimethyl-2-oxocyclohexyl]-2-hydroxyethyl]glutarimide. *CAS-66-81-9. Antipsoriatic.* ◇*U-4527*

Cyclomenol. $C_{14}H_{20}O$. 204.31. 2-Cyclohexyl-3,5-xylenol. *UNII-TB885DRP1J. CAS-5591-47-9.* INN; DCF.

Cyclomethicone (sye″ kloe meth′ i kone). **NF.** $(C_2H_6OSi)_n$. (1) Cyclopolydimethylsiloxane; (2) Cyclomethicone. *CAS-69430-24-6. Pharmaceutic aid (wetting agent).* VS-7158 (Witco); VS-7207 (Witco); VS-7349 (Witco)

Cyclomethycaine Sulfate. $C_{22}H_{33}NO_3.H_2SO_4$. 457.58. [Cyclomethycaine is INN and BAN.] (1) Benzoic acid, 4-(cyclohexyloxy)-, 3-(2-methyl-1-piperidinyl)propyl ester sulfate (1:1); (2) 3-(2-Methylpiperidino)propyl *p*-(cyclohexyloxy)benzoate sulfate (1:1). *UNII-7323N7T136; UNII-15E9I74NZ8* [cyclomethycaine]. *CAS-50978-10-4; CAS-139-62-8* [cyclomethycaine]; *CAS-537-61-1* [hydrochloride]. USP XXI; MI. Surfacaine (Lilly†)

Cyclonium Iodide — *See* Oxapium Iodide.

Cyclopentamine Hydrochloride. $C_9H_{19}N.HCl$. 177.71. [Cyclopentamine is INN and BAN.] (1) Cyclopentaneethanamine, *N*-α-dimethyl-, hydrochloride; (2) *N*,α-Dimethylcyclopentaneethylamine hydrochloride. *UNII-*

F551446KF3. CAS-3459-06-1; CAS-102-45-4 [cyclopentamine, *N*,α-dimethylcyclopentaneethanamine]. USP XXI; MI. Clopane Hydrochloride (Lilly†)

Cyclopentaphene — *See* Cyclarbamate.

Cyclopenthiazide [*1962*] (sye″ kloe pen thye′ a zide). $C_{13}H_{18}ClN_3O_4S_2$. 379.88. (1) 2*H*-1,2,4-Benzothiadiazine-7-sulfonamide, 6-chloro-3-(cyclopentylmethyl)-3,4-dihydro-, 1,1-dioxide; (2) 6-Chloro-3-(cyclopentylmethyl)-3,4-dihydro-2*H*-1,2,4-benzothiadiazine-7-sulfonamide 1,1-dioxide. *CAS-742-20-1.* INN; BAN; JAN. *Antihypertensive.* ◇*Su-8341; NSC-107679*

Cyclopentolate Hydrochloride (sye″ kloe pen′ toe late hye″ droe klor′ ide). **USP.** $C_{17}H_{25}NO_3.HCl$. 327.85. [Cyclopentolate is INN and BAN.] (1) Benzeneacetic acid, α-(1-hydroxycyclopentyl)-, 2-(dimethylamino)ethyl ester, hydrochloride, (±)-; (2) 2-(Dimethylamino)ethyl (±)-1-hydroxy-α-phenylcyclopentaneacetate hydrochloride. *UNII-73I6I971TE; UNII-I76F4SHP7J* [cyclopentolate]. *CAS-5870-29-1; CAS-512-15-2* [cyclopentolate]. JAN. *Anticholinergic (ophthalmic).* Akpentolate (Akorn); Cyclogyl (Alcon); Pentolair (Bausch & Lomb)

Cyclophenazine Hydrochloride [*1967*] (sye″ kloe fen′ a zeen hye″ droe klor′ ide). $C_{23}H_{26}F_3N_3S.2HCl$. 506.45. [Ciclofenazine is INN.] (1) 10*H*-Phenothiazine, 10-[3-(4-cyclopropyl-1-piperazinyl)propyl]-2-(trifluoromethyl)-, dihydrochloride; (2) 10-[3-(4-Cyclopropyl-1-piperazinyl)propyl]-2-(trifluoromethyl)phenothiazine dihydrochloride. *UNII-H68VTK0LL9. CAS-15686-74-5; CAS-17692-26-1* [cyclophenazine]. *Antipsychotic.* ◇*60284*

Cyclophosphamide (sye″ kloe fos′ fa mide). **USP.** $C_7H_{15}Cl_2N_2O_2P.H_2O$. 279.10. (1) 2*H*-1,3,2-Oxazaphosphorin-2-amine, *N*,*N*-bis(2-chloroethyl)tetrahydro-, 2-oxide, monohydrate, (±); (2) (±)-2-[Bis(2-chloroethyl)amino]tetrahydro-2*H*-1,3,2-oxazaphosphorine 2-oxide monohydrate. *UNII-8N3DW7272P. CAS-6055-19-2; CAS-*

50-18-0 [anhydrous]. INN; BAN; JAN. *Antineoplastic; immunosuppressant.* Cytoxan (Bristol-Myers Squibb) ◇*NSC-26271*

Cyclopregnol. $C_{21}H_{32}O_2$. 316.48. 6β-Hydroxy-3,5-cyclopregnan-20-one. *UNII-Z06494074X. CAS-465-53-2.* INN; MI.

Cycloprolol (previously used name) — *See* Cicloprolol Hydrochloride.

Cyclopropane (sye″ kloe proe′ pane). **USP.** C_3H_6. 42.08. (1) Cyclopropane; (2) Cyclopropane. *CAS-75-19-4.* INN. *Anesthetic (inhalation).*

Cyclopyrronium Bromide. $C_{20}H_{30}BrNO_2$. 396.36. 1-Ethyl-3-hydroxy-1-methylpyrrolidinium bromide α-cyclopentylphenylacetate. *UNII-8C19ZXR2J2. CAS-15599-22-1.* INN.

Cycloserine (sye″ kloe ser′ een). **USP.** $C_3H_6N_2O_2$. 102.09. (1) 3-Isoxazolidinone, 4-amino-, (*R*)-; (2) (+)-4-Amino-3-isoxazolidinone. *UNII-95IK5KI84Z. CAS-68-41-7.* INN; BAN; JAN. *Antibacterial (tuberculostatic).* Seromycin (Lilly)

Cyclosporin A (previously used name) — *See* Cyclosporine.

Cyclosporine [*1981*] (sye″ kloe spor′ een). **USP.** $C_{62}H_{111}N_{11}O_{12}$. 1202.61. [Ciclosporin is INN, BAN and JAN.] (1) Cyclosporin A; (2) Cyclo[[(*E*)-(2*S*,3*R*,4*R*)-3-hydroxy-4-methyl-2-(methylamino)-6-octenoyl]-L-2-aminobutyryl-*N*-methylglycyl-*N*-methyl-L-leucyl-L-valyl-*N*-methyl-L-leucyl-L-alanyl-D-alanyl-*N*-methyl-L-leucyl-*N*-methyl-L-leucyl-*N*-methyl-L-valyl]; (3) [*R*-[*R**,*R**-(*E*)]]-Cyclic(L-alanyl-D-alanyl-*N*-methyl-L-leucyl-*N*-methyl-L-leucyl-*N*-methyl-L-valyl-3-hydroxy-*N*,4-dimethyl-L-2-amino-6-octenoyl-*N*-methylglycyl-*N*-methyl-L-leucyl-L-valyl-*N*-methyl-L-leucyl). *UNII-83HN0GTJ6D. CAS-59865-13-3. Immunosuppressant.*

---

† Brand name formerly used, and/or firm no longer concerned with this product.

Gengraf (Abbott); Neoral (Novartis); Restasis (Allergan); Sandimmune (Novartis) [*Names previously used: Cyclosporin A; Cyclosporin.*] ◇*27-400*

Cyclothiazide [*1963*] (sye″ kloe thye′ a zide). $C_{14}H_{16}ClN_3O_4S_2$. 389.88. (1) 2*H*-1,2,4-Benzothiadiazine-7-sulfonamide, 3-bicyclo[2.2.1]hept-5-en-2-yl-6-chloro-3,4-dihydro-, 1,1-dioxide; (2) 6-Chloro-3,4-dihydro-3-(5-norbornen-2-yl)-2*H*-1,2,4-benzothiadiazine-7-sulfonamide 1,1-dioxide. *UNII-P71U09G5BW. CAS-2259-96-3.* USP XXII; INN; BAN. *Diuretic; antihypertensive.* Anhydron (Lilly) ◇*35483*

Cyclovalone. $C_{22}H_{22}O_5$. 366.41. 2,6-Divanillylidenecyclohexanone. *CAS-579-23-7.* INN; MI.

Cycobemin — *See* Cyanocobalamin.

Cycotiamine. $C_{13}H_{16}N_4O_3S$. 308.36. [Cycotiamine Hydrochloride is JAN.] *N*-[1-(2-Oxo-1,3-oxathian-4-ylidene)ethyl]-*N*-[(4-amino-2-methyl-5-pyrimidinyl)methyl]-formamide. *UNII-FT8753F8R9. CAS-6092-18-8.* INN; JAN; MI.

Cycrimine Hydrochloride. $C_{19}H_{29}NO.HCl$. 323.90. [Cycrimine is INN and BAN.] (1) 1-Piperidinepropanol, α-cyclopentyl-α-phenyl-, hydrochloride; (2) α-Cyclopentyl-α-phenyl-1-piperidinepropanol hydrochloride. *UNII-9RB4L4K895; UNII-543567RFQQ* [cycrimine]. *CAS-126-02-3; CAS-77-39-4* [cycrimine]. USP XX; MI. Pagitane (Lilly)

Cyfluthrin. $C_{22}H_{18}Cl_2FNO_3$. 434.29. (*RS*)-α-Cyano-4-fluoro-3-phenoxybenzyl (1*RS*,3*RS*; 1*RS*,3*SR*)-3-(2,2-dichlorovinyl)-2,2-dimethylcyclopropanecarboxylate. *CAS-68359-37-5.* BAN; MI. ◇*Bay Vl 1704*

Cyhalothrin. $C_{23}H_{19}ClF_3NO_3$. 449.85. (*RS*)-α-Cyano-3-phenoxybenzyl (*Z*)-(1*RS*,3*RS*)-3-(2-chloro-3,3,3-trifluoropropenyl)-2,2-dimethylcyclopropanecarboxylate. *UNII-V0V73PEB8M. CAS-68085-85-8.* BAN; MI. ◇*PP 563*

Cyheptamide [*1966*] (sye hep′ ta mide). $C_{16}H_{15}NO$. 237.30. (1) 5*H*-Dibenzo[*a,d*]cycloheptene-5-carboxamide, 10,11-dihydro-; (2) 10,11-Dihydro-5*H*-dibenzo[*a,d*]cycloheptene-5-carboxamide. *CAS-7199-29-3.* INN. *Anticonvulsant.* ◇*AY-8682*

Cyheptropine. $C_{24}H_{27}NO_2$. 361.48. 10,11-Dihydro-5*H*-dibenzo[*a,d*]cycloheptene-5-carboxylic acid tropine ester. *CAS-602-40-4.* INN.

Cymemoxine (DCF) — *See* Cimemoxin.

Cynarine. $C_{25}H_{24}O_{12}$. 516.45. 3,4-Dihydroxycinnamic acid, 1-carboxy-4,5-dihydroxy-1,3-cyclohexylene ester. *CAS-1884-24-8.* INN; MI.

Cyoctol — *See* Cioteronel.

Cypenamine Hydrochloride [*1964*] (sye pen′ a meen hye″ droe klor′ ide). $C_{11}H_{15}N \cdot HCl$. 197.70. [Cypenamine is INN and BAN.] (1) Cyclopentanamine, 2-phenyl-, hydrochloride; (2) 2-Phenylcyclopentylamine hydrochloride. *CAS-5588-23-8; CAS-15301-54-9* [cypenamine]. *Antidepressant.*

Cypermethrin. (*RS*)-α-Cyano-3-phenoxybenzyl (1*RS*,3*RS*)-(1*RS*,3*RS*)-3-(2,2-dichlorovinyl)-2,2-dimethylcyclopropanecarboxylate. *UNII-1TR49121NP. CAS-52315-07-8.* BAN.

Cypothrin [*1978*] (sye′ poe thrin). $C_{28}H_{23}NO_3$. 421.49. (1) Spiro[cyclopropane-1,1′-[1*H*]indene]-2-carboxylic acid, 3,3-dimethyl-, cyano(3-phenoxyphenyl)methyl ester; (2) 3,3-Dimethylspiro[cyclopropane-1,1′-indene]-2-carboxylic acid, ester with *m*-phenoxymandelonitrile. *UNII-04X6A188YW. CAS-60148-52-9. Insecticide (veterinary).* ◇*CL 206,797*

Cyprazepam [*1971*] (sye praz′ e pam). $C_{19}H_{18}ClN_3O$. 339.82. (1) 3*H*-1,4-Benzodiazepin-2-amine, 7-chloro-*N*-(cyclopropylmethyl)-5-phenyl-, 4-oxide; (2) 7-Chloro-2-[(cyclopropylmethyl)amino]-5-phenyl-3*H*-1,4-benzodiazepine 4-oxide. *UNII-933N61G4SL. CAS-15687-07-7.* INN. *Sedative-hypnotic.* ◇*W 3623*

Cyprenorphine Hydrochloride. $C_{26}H_{33}NO_4 \cdot HCl$. 460.01. [Cyprenorphine is INN and BAN.] 6,7,8,14-*N*-(Cyclopropylmethyl)tetrahydro-7α-(1-hydroxy-1-methylethyl)-6,14-*endo*-ethenonororipavine hydrochloride. *CAS-16550-22-4; CAS-4406-22-8* [cyprenorphine]. MI. ◇*M 285*

Cyprodemanol (DCF) — *See* Cyprodenate.

Cyprodenate. $C_{13}H_{25}NO_2$. 227.34. 2-(Dimethylamino)ethyl cyclohexanepropionate. *UNII-I44VIC13P8. CAS-15585-86-1.* INN; DCF. ◇*LB 125; RD 406*

Cyproheptadine Hydrochloride (sye″ proe hep′ ta deen hye″ droe klor′ ide). **USP.** $C_{21}H_{21}N \cdot HCl \cdot 1\frac{1}{2}H_2O$. 350.88. [Cyproheptadine is INN and BAN.] (1) Piperidine, 4-(5*H*-dibenzo[*a,d*]cyclohepten-5-ylidene)-1-methyl-, hydrochloride, sesquihydrate; (2) 4-(5*H*-Dibenzo[*a,d*]cyclohepten-5-ylidene)-1-methylpiperidine hydrochloride sesquihydrate. *UNII-NJ82J0F8QC; UNII-2YHB6175DO* [cyproheptadine]. *CAS-41354-29-4; CAS-969-33-5* [anhydrous]; *CAS-129-03-3* [cyproheptadine]. JAN. *Antihistaminic; antipruritic.* Periactin (Merck)

Cyprolidol Hydrochloride [*1965*] (sye proe′ li dol hye″ droe klor′ ide). $C_{21}H_{19}NO.HCl.$ 337.84. [Cyprolidol is INN.] (1) Benzenemethanol, α-phenyl-α-[2-(4-pyridinyl)cyclopropyl]-, hydrochloride; (2) Diphenyl [2-(4-pyridyl)cyclopropyl]methanol hydrochloride. *CAS-2364-72-9; CAS-4904-00-1* [cyprolidol]. *Antidepressant.* ◇*IN 1060; NSC-84973*

Cyproquinate [*1968*] (sye″ proe kwin′ ate). $C_{20}H_{23}NO_5.$ 357.40. [Ciproquinate is INN.] (1) 3-Quinolinecarboxylic acid, 6,7-bis(cyclopropylmethoxy)-4-hydroxy-, ethyl ester; (2) Ethyl 6,7-bis(cyclopropylmethoxy)-4-hydroxy-3-quinolinecarboxylate. *CAS-19485-08-6. Coccidiostat (for poultry).* ◇*Su-18137*

Cyproterone Acetate [*1965*] (sye proe′ ter one as′ e tate). $C_{24}H_{29}ClO_4.$ 416.94. [Cyproterone is INN and BAN.] (1) 3′*H*-Cyclopropa[1,2]pregna-1,4,6-triene-3,20-dione, 17-(acetyloxy)-6-chloro-1,2-dihydro-, (1β,2β)-; (2) 6-Chloro-1β,2β-dihydro-17-hydroxy-3′*H*-cyclopropa[1,2]-pregna-1,4,6-triene-3,20-dione acetate. *UNII-E61Q31EK2F* [cyproterone]. *CAS-427-51-0; CAS-2098-66-0* [cyproterone]. JAN. *Anti-androgen. [Note—The free alcohol bears the code designation SH 881.]* ◇*SH 714; NSC-81430*

Cyproximide [*1967*] (sye prox′ i mide). $C_{11}H_8ClNO_2.$ 221.64. [Ciproximide is INN.] (1) 3-Azabicyclo[3.1.0]hexane-2,4-dione, 1-(4-chlorophenyl)-; (2) 1-(*p*-Chlorophenyl)-1,2-cyclopropanedicarboximide. *CAS-15518-76-0. Antipsychotic; antidepressant.* ◇*CL 53415*

Cyren A — *See* Diethylstilbestrol.

Cyromazine. $C_6H_{10}N_6.$ 166.18. *N*-Cyclopropyl-1,3,5-triazine-2,4,6-triamine. *UNII-CA49Y29RA9. CAS-66215-27-8.* INN; BAN; MI. ◇*CGA 72662*

Cysteamine [*1990*] (sis tee′ a meen). $C_2H_7NS.$ 77.15. [Mercaptamine is INN and BAN.] (1) Ethanethiol, 2-amino-; (2) 2-Aminoethanethiol. *UNII-5UX2SD1KE2. CAS-60-23-1. Anti-urolithic (cystine calculi).* ◇*MEA; L-1573*

Cysteamine Hydrochloride [*1991*] (sis tee′ a meen hye″ droe klor′ ide). $C_2H_7NS.HCl.$ 113.61. (1) Ethanethiol, 2-amino-, hydrochloride; (2) 2-Aminoethanethiol hydrochloride. *CAS-156-57-0. Anti-urolithic (cystine calculi).* ◇*CI-9148*

L-Cysteine (JAN) — *See* Cysteine Hydrochloride.

L-Cysteine Ethylester Hydrochloride (JAN) — *See* Cysteine Hydrochloride.

Cysteine Hydrochloride (sis′ te een hye″ droe klor′ ide). USP. $C_3H_7NO_2S.HCl.H_2O.$ 175.63. [Cysteine is INN; L-Cysteine, L-Cysteine Ethylester Hydrochloride, and L-Cysteinemethyl Hydrochloride are JAN.] (1) L-Cysteine hydrochloride monohydrate; (2) L-Cysteine hydrochloride monohydrate. *UNII-ZT934N0X4W; UNII-K848JZ4886* [cysteine]. *CAS-7048-04-6; CAS-52-89-1* [anhydrous]; *CAS-52-90-4* [cysteine]. *Amino acid.*

L-Cysteinemethyl Hydrochloride (JAN) — *See* Cysteine Hydrochloride.

Cystine [*1979*] (sis′ teen). $C_6H_{12}N_2O_4S_2.$ 240.30. L-Cystine. *UNII-48TCX9A1VT. CAS-56-89-3* [L]. INN. *Amino acid.*

Cytarabine [*1969*] (sye tayr′ a been). **USP.** C₉H₁₃N₃O₅. 243.22. (1) 2(1*H*)-Pyrimidinone, 4-amino-1-β-D-arabino-furanosyl-; (2) 1-β-D-Arabinofuranosylcytosine. *UNII-04079A1RDZ. CAS-147-94-4.* INN; BAN; JAN. *Antineo-plastic; antiviral.* Depocyt (Skyepharma) ✧*U-19,920*

Cytarabine Hydrochloride [*1964*] (sye tayr′ a been hye″ droe klor′ ide). C₉H₁₃N₃O₅.HCl. 279.68. (1) 2(1*H*)-Pyrimidinone, 4-amino-1-β-D-arabinofuranosyl-, monohy-drochloride; (2) 1-β-D-Arabinofuranosylcytosine monohy-drochloride. *UNII-33K3DB6591; UNII-04079A1RDZ* [cytarabine]. *CAS-69-74-9; CAS-147-94-4* [cytarabine]. *Antiviral. [Name previously used: Cytosine Arabinoside Hydrochloride.]* ✧*U-19920A; NSC-63878*

Cythioate. C₈H₁₂NO₅PS₂. 297.29. *O,O*-Dimethyl *O*-(4-sulfa-moylphenyl) phosphorothioate. *UNII-3OOH7Q4333. CAS-115-93-5.* BAN.

Cytochrome C. Cytochrome C. *CAS-9007-43-6.* JAN.

Cytosine Arabinoside Hydrochloride (previously used name) — *See* Cytarabine Hydrochloride.

D & C Brown No. 1 — *See* Resorcin Brown.

Dabelotine. C₁₅H₂₂N₂O₂. 262.35. (±)-1,2,3,4-Tetrahydro-1-methyl-8-(2-morpholinylmethoxy)quinoline. *UNII-6RY56RB98P. CAS-118976-38-8.* INN.

Dabigatran [*2008*] (da″ bi gat′ ran). C₂₅H₂₅N₇O₃. 471.51. (1) β-Alanine, *N*-[[2-[[[4-(aminoiminomethyl)phenyl]amino]-methyl]-1-methyl-1*H*-benzimidazol-5-yl]carbonyl]-*N*-2-pyridinyl-; (2) 3-{[(2-{[(4-Carbamimidoylphenyl)amino]-methyl}-1-methyl-1*H*-benzimidazol-5-yl)carbonyl](pyri-din-2-yl)amino}propanoic acid. *UNII-I0VM4M70GC. CAS-211914-51-1.* INN. *Deep vein thrombosis after surgery, venous thromboembolic events, stroke prevention in atrial fibrillation.* Pradaxa (Boehringer Ingelheim Pharma GmbH & Co. KG and Bidachem S.p.A.) ✧*BIBR 953 ZW*

Dabigatran Etexilate [*2008*] (da″ bi gat′ ran e tex′ i late). C₃₄H₄₁N₇O₅. 627.73. (1) β-Alanine, *N*-[[2-[[[4-[[[(hexy-loxy)carbonyl]amino]iminomethyl]phenyl]amino]methyl]-1-methyl-1*H*-benzimidazol-5-yl]carbonyl]-*N*-2-pyridinyl-, ethyl ester; (2) Ethyl 3-{[(2-{[(4-{[(hexyloxy)carbonyl]-carbamimidoyl}phenyl)amino]methyl}-1-methyl-1*H*-ben-zimidazol-5-yl)carbonyl](pyridin-2-yl)amino}propanoate. *UNII-2E18WX195X. CAS-211915-06-9.* INN. *Deep vein thrombosis after surgery, venous thromboembolic events,*

stroke prevention in atrial fibrillation. Pradaxa (Boehringer Ingelheim Pharma GmbH & Co. KG and Bidachem S.p.A.) ✧*BIBR 1048 BS RS1*

Dabigatran Etexilate Mesylate [*2008*] (da bye gat′ ran e tex′ i late mes′ i late). C₃₄H₄₁N₇O₅.*x*CH₄O₃S. (1) β-Alanine, *N*-[[2-[[[4-[[[(hexyloxy)carbonyl]amino]iminomethyl]pheny-l]amino]methyl]-1-methyl-1*H*-benzimidazol-5-yl]carbo-nyl]-*N*-2-pyridinyl-, ethyl ester, methanesulfonate; (2) Ethyl 3-{[(2-{[(4-{[(hexyloxy)carbonyl]carbamimidoyl}-phenyl)amino]methyl}-1-methyl-1*H*-benzimidazol-5-yl)-carbonyl](pyridin-2-yl)amino}propanoate, methanesulfo-nate. *CAS-593282-20-3. Deep vein thrombosis after surgery, venous thromboembolic events, stroke prevention in atrial fibrillation.* Pradaxa (Boehringer Ingelheim Pharma GmbH & Co. KG and Bidachem S.p.A.) ✧*BIBR 1048 MS*

Dabuzalgron Hydrochloride [*2004*] (da bue′ zal gron hye″ droe klor′ ide). C₁₂H₁₆ClN₃O₃S.HCl. 354.25. [Dabuzalgron is INN.] (1) Methanesulfonamide, *N*-[6-chloro-3-[(4,5-dihydro-1*H*-imidazol-2-yl)methoxy]-2-methylphenyl]-, monohydrochloride; (2) *N*-[6-Chloro-3-[(4,5-dihydro-1*H*-imidazol-2-yl)methoxy]-2-methylphenyl]methanesulfona-mide hydrochloride. *UNII-A7Q00A39MF; UNII-LGX4GZ74WO* [dabuzalgron]. *CAS-219311-43-0; CAS-219311-44-1* [dabuzalgron]. *Treatment of stress urinary incontinence.* ✧*RO115-1240/190*

Dacarbazine [*1972*] (da kar′ ba zeen). **USP.** C₆H₁₀N₆O. 182.18. (1) 1*H*-Imidazole-4-carboxamide, 5-(3,3-dimethyl-1-triazenyl)-; (2) 5-(3,3-Dimethyl-1-triazeno)imidazole-4-carboxamide. *UNII-7GR28W0FJI. CAS-4342-03-4.* INN; BAN; JAN. *Antineoplastic.* Dtic-Dome (Bayer) ✧*DIC; DTIC; NSC-45388*

Dacemazine. $C_{16}H_{16}N_2OS$. 284.38. 10-(*N,N*-Dimethylglycyl)phenothiazine. *UNII-88D34UY0QI. CAS-518-61-6.* INN.

Dacetuzumab [*2007*] (da″ se tooz′ oo mab). $C_{6452}H_{9964}N_{1732}O_{1998}S_{42}$. (1) Immunoglobulin G1, anti-(human CD40 (antigen)) (human-mouse monoclonal SGN-40 γ1-chain), disulfide with human-mouse monoclonal SGN-40 κ-chain, dimer; (2) Immunoglobulin G1, anti-[human Tumor Necrosis Factor receptor superfamily member 5 (B-cell surface antigen CD40)] humanized mouse monoclonal SGN-40 [Glu[353],Met[355]]γ1 heavy chain (217-219′)-disulfide with κ light chain (223-223″:226-226″)-bisdisulfide dimer. Molecular weight is approximately 145,100 daltons, for the peptide. *CAS-880486-59-9.* INN. *Treatment of CD40-positive cancers.* ◇*SGN-40; huS2C6*

Dacinostat. $C_{22}H_{25}N_3O_3$. 379.45. (2*E*)-*N*-Hydroxy-3-[4-({(2-hydroxyethyl)[2-(1*H*-indol-3-yl)ethyl]amino}methyl)phenyl]propenamide. *CAS-404951-53-7.* INN.

Dacisteine. $C_7H_{11}NO_4S$. 205.23. *N*-Acetyl-L-cysteine, acetate (ester). *UNII-WF970ATW3T. CAS-18725-37-6.* INN.

Dacliximab (previously used name) — *See* Daclizumab.

Daclizumab [*1997*] (dak liz′ oo mab). $C_{6394}H_{9888}N_{1696}O_{2012}S_{44}$ (protein moiety). Humanized anti-TAC monoclonal antibody comprised of four subunits, two heavy chains and two light chains. All four chains are linked via disulfide bridges. The molecule contains approximately 2% carbohydrate by weight. The antibody belongs to the IgG₁ subclass. The DNA sequence is 90% human origin and 10% mouse origin. The humanized anti-TAC is directed to the TAC receptor or high-affinity interleukin 2 receptor. Immunoglobulin G 1 (human-mouse monoclonal clone 1H4 γ-chain anti-human interleukin 2 receptor), disulfide with human-mouse monoclonal clone 1H4 light chain, dimer. Molecular weight is approximately 150,000 daltons. *CAS-152923-56-3.* BAN; INN. *Mono-*

clonal antibody (immunosuppressant). Zenapax (Hoffmann-LaRoche) *[Name previously used: Dacliximab]* ◇*Ro 24-7375*

Mature Humanized Heavy chain

```
QVQLVQSGAE VKKPGSSVKV SCKASGYTFT SYRMHWVRQA PGQGLEWIGY
INPSTGYTEY NQKFKDKATI TADESTNTAY MELSSLRSED TAVYYCARGG
GVFDYWGQGT LVTVSSASTK GPSVFPLAPS SKSTSGGTAA LGCLVKDYFP
EPVTVSWNSG ALTSGVHTFP AVLQSSGLYS LSSVVTVPSS SLGTQTYICN
VNHKPSNTKV DKKVEPKSCD KTHTCPPCPA PELLGGPSVF LFPPKPKDTL
MISRTPEVTC VVVDVSHEDP EVKFNWYVDG VEVHNAKTKP REEQYNSTYR
VVSVLTVLHQ DWLNGKEYKC KVSNKALPAP IEKTISKAKG QPREPQVYTL
PPSRDELTKN QVSLTCLVKG FYPSDIAVEW ESNGQPENNY KTTPPVLDSD
GSFFLYSKLT VDKSRWQQGN VFSCSVMHEA LHNHYTQKSL SLSPGK
```

Mature Humanized Light chain

```
DIQMTQSPST LSASVGDRVT ITCSASSSIS YMHWYQQKPG KAPKLLIYTT
SNLASGVPAR FSGSGSGTEF TLTISSLQPD DFATYYCHQR STYPLTFGQG
TKVEVKRTVA APSVFIFPPS DEQLKSGTAS VVCLLNNFYP REAKVQWKVD
NALQSGNSQE SVTEQDSKDS TYSLSSTLTL SKADYEKHKV YACEVTHQGL
SSPVTKSFNR GEC
```

Dacopafant. $C_{12}H_{11}N_3OS$. 245.30. (3*R*)-3-(3-Pyridyl)-1*H*,3*H*-pyrrolo[1,2-*c*]thiazole-7-carboxamide. *UNII-H1T03Z1G60. CAS-125372-33-0.* INN.

Dactinomycin [*1964*] (dak″ tin oh mye′ sin). **USP**. $C_{62}H_{86}N_{12}O_{16}$. 1255.42. [Actinomycin D is JAN.] (1) Actinomycin D; (2) Actinomycin D; (3) Specific stereoisomer of *N,N*′-[(2-amino-4,6-dimethyl-3-oxo-3*H*-phenoxazine-1,9-diyl)-bis[carbonylimino(2-hydroxypropylidene)-carbonyliminoisobutylidenecarbonyl-1,2-pyrrolidinediylcarbonyl(methylimino)methylenecarbonyl]]bis[*N*-methyl-L-valine] dilactone. *UNII-1CC1JFE158. CAS-50-76-0.* BAN. *Antineoplastic.* Cosmegen (Ovation) ◇*NSC-3053*

Dacuronium Bromide. $C_{33}H_{58}Br_2N_2O_3$. 690.63. 3α,17β-Dihydroxy-5α-androstan-2β,16β-ylene)bis-(1-methylpiperidinium)dibromide 3-acetate. *UNII-33482245B6. CAS-27115-86-2.* INN; BAN. ◇*NB 68*

---

† Brand name formerly used, and/or firm no longer concerned with this product.

Dagapamil. $C_{36}H_{56}N_2O_4$. 580.84. 2-[3-[(*m*-Methoxyphenethyl)methylamino]propyl]-2-(3,4,5-trimethoxyphenyl)-tetradecanenitrile. *UNII-64O87U613H. CAS-85247-76-3.* INN.

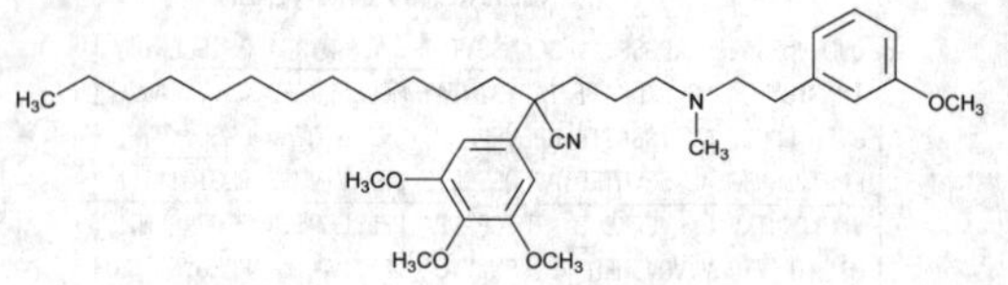

Daglutril. $C_{31}H_{38}N_2O_6$. 534.64. [(3*S*)-3-{1-[(2*R*)-2-Ethoxycarbonyl-4-phenylbutyl]cyclopentanecarboxamido}-2-oxo-2,3,4,5-tetrahydro-1*H*-1-benzazepin-1-yl]acetic acid. *UNII-KKV299446X. CAS-182821-27-8.* INN.

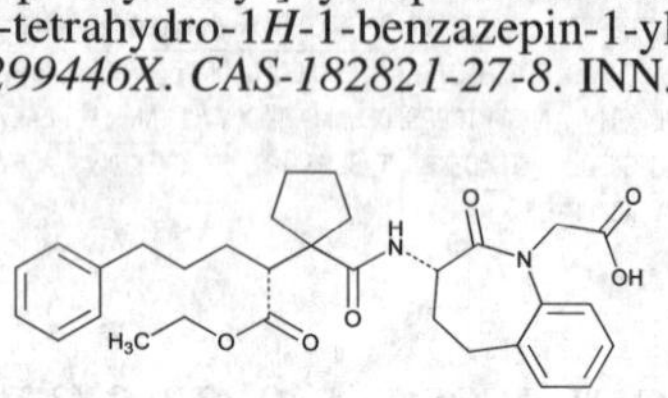

Dalanated Insulin — *See* Insulin, Dalanated.

Dalbavancin [*2004*] (dal″ ba van′ sin). $C_{88}H_{100}Cl_2N_{10}O_{28}$. 1816.69. (1) Ristomycin A aglycone, 5,31-dichloro-38-de(methoxycarbonyl)-7-demethyl-19-deoxy-56-*O*-[2-deoxy-2-[(10-methyl-1-oxoundecyl)amino]-β-D-glucopyranuronosyl]-38-[[[3-(dimethylamino)propyl]amino]carbonyl]-42-*O*-α-D-mannopyranosyl-N^{15}-methyl-; (2) 2-Deoxy-1-*O*-[(3*S*,15*R*,18*R*,34*R*,35*S*,38*S*,48*R*,50a*R*)-5,31-dichloro-38-[[3-(dimethylamino)propyl]carbamoyl]-6,11,34,40,44-pentahydroxy-42-(α-D-mannopyranosyloxy)-15-(methylamino)-2,16,36,50,51,59-hexaoxo-2,3,16,17,18,19,35,36,37,38,48,49,50,50a-tetradecahydro-20,23:30,33-dietheno-3,18:35,48-bis(iminomethano)-1*H*,15*H*-4,8:10,14:25,28:43,47-tetrameethno-34*H*-[1,14,6,22]dioxadiazacyclooctacosino[4,5-*m*][10,2,16]benzoxadiazacyclotetracosin-56-yl]-2-[(10-methylundecanoyl)amino]-β-D-glucopyranuronic acid (main component). *CAS-171500-79-1.* INN; BAN. *Antibiotic.* ◇BI397; MDL 64,397; A-A-1; VER001

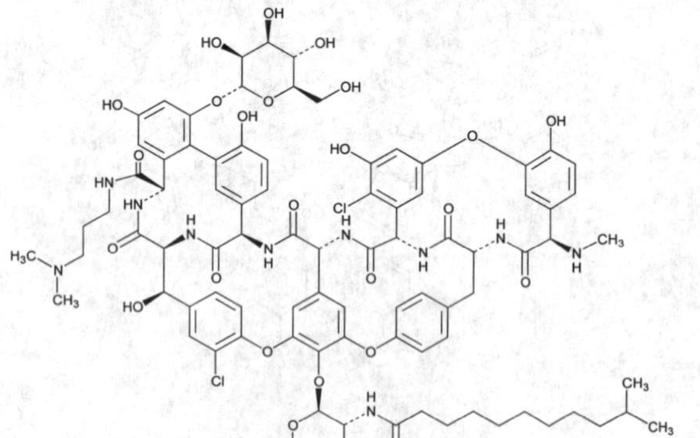

Dalbraminol. $C_{17}H_{26}N_4O_2$. 318.41. (±)-1-Phenoxy-3-[[2-[(1,3,5-trimethylpyrazol-4-yl)amino]ethyl]amino]-2-propanol. *UNII-7GDN12Q42M. CAS-81528-80-5.* INN.

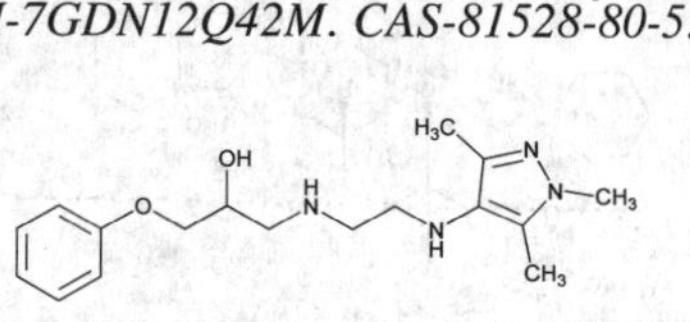

Dalcetrapib [*2007*] (dal set′ ra pib). $C_{23}H_{35}NO_2S$. 389.59. (1) Propanethioic acid, 2-methyl-, *S*-[2-[[[1-(2-ethylbutyl)cyclohexyl]carbonyl]amino]phenyl] ester; (2) *S*-[2-({[1-(2-Ethylbutyl)cyclohexyl]carbonyl}amino)phenyl] 2-methyl-propanethioate. *UNII-3D050LIQ3H. CAS-211513-37-0.* INN. *Preventing cardiovascular events in CHD patients and slowing progression of atherosclerosis.* ◇RO4607381

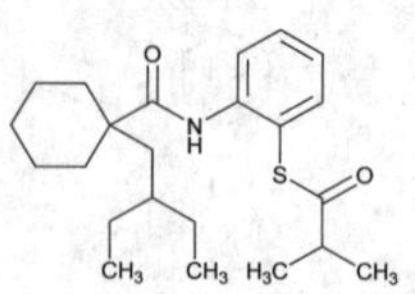

Dalcotidine. $C_{18}H_{29}N_3O_2$. 319.44. 1-Ethyl-3-[3-[(α-piperidino-*m*-tolyl)oxy]propyl]urea. *UNII-9968S2UKFJ. CAS-120958-90-9.* INN.

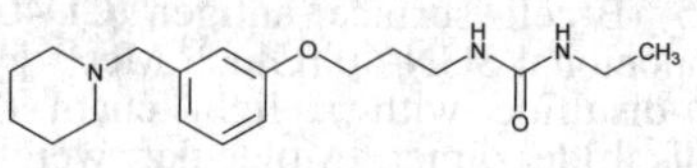

Daledalin Tosylate [*1970*] (dal ed′ a lin tos′ i late). $C_{19}H_{24}N_2 \cdot C_7H_8O_3S$. 452.61. [Daledalin is INN.] (1) 1*H*-Indole-3-propanamine, 2,3-dihydro-*N*,3-dimethyl-1-phenyl, mono(4-methylbenzenesulfonate); (2) 3-Methyl-3-[3-(methylamino)propyl]-1-phenylindoline mono-*p*-toluenesulfonate. *CAS-23226-37-1; CAS-30508-58-8* [replaced]; *CAS-22136-27-2* [daledalin]. *Antidepressant.* ◇UK-3557-15

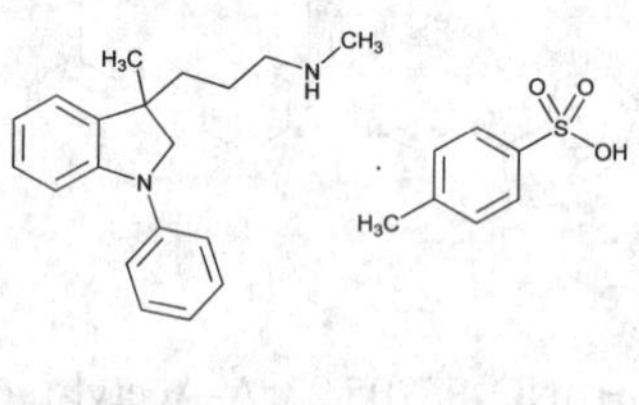

Dalfopristin [*1993*] (dal″ foe pris′ tin). $C_{34}H_{50}N_4O_9S$. 690.85. (1) Virginiamycin M_1, 26-[[2-(diethylamino)ethyl]sulfonyl]-26,27-dihydro-, (26*R*,27*S*)-; (2) (3*R*,4*R*,5*E*,10-*E*,12*E*,14*S*,26*R*,26a*S*)-26-[[2-(Diethylamino)ethyl]sulfonyl]-8,9,14,15,24,25,26,26a-octahydro-14-hydroxy-3-isopropyl-4,12-dimethyl-3*H*-21,18-nitrilo-1*H*,22*H*-pyrrolo[2,1-*c*][1,8,4,19]dioxadiazacyclotetracosine-1,7,16,22(4*H*,17*H*)-tetrone. *UNII-R9M4FJE48E. CAS-112362-50-2.* INN; BAN. *Antibacterial.* ◇RP 54476

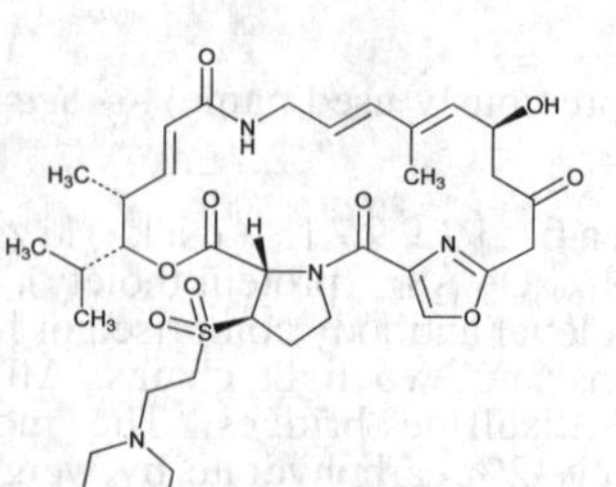

Dalteparin Sodium [*1993*] (dal″ te par′ in soe′ dee um; dal tep′ a rin soe′ dee um). Sodium salt of depolymerized heparin obtained by nitrous acid degradation of heparin from pork intestinal mucosa. The majority of the components have a 2-*O*-sulfo-α-L-idopyranosuronic acid structure at the non-reducing end and a 6-*O*-sulfo-2,5-anhydro-D-mannitol structure at the reducing end of their chain. The average relative molecular mass is about 5000, 90% of which ranges between 2000 and 9000. The degree of sulfation is 2 to 2.5 per disaccharide unit. *UNII-*

12M44VTJ7B. CAS-9041-08-1. INN; BAN. *Anticoagulant; antithrombotic.* Fragmin (Eisai Medical Research) ◇*Heparin Fragment Kabi 2165*

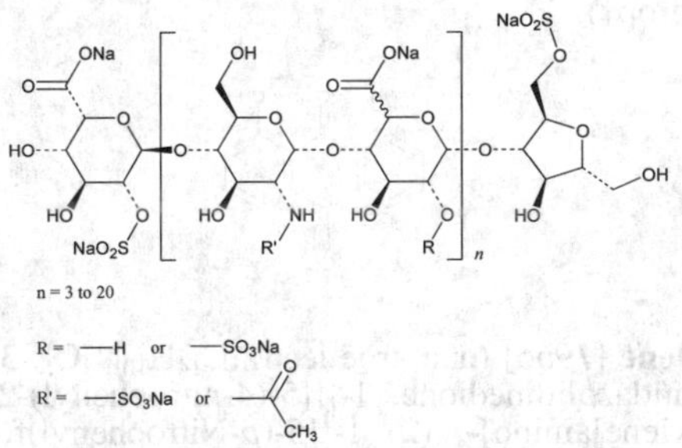

Daltroban [*1989*] (dal′ troe ban). $C_{16}H_{16}ClNO_4S$. 353.82. (1) Benzeneacetic acid, 4-[2-[[(4-chlorophenyl)sulfonyl]amino]ethyl]-; (2) [*p*-[2-(*p*-Chlorobenzenesulfonamido)ethyl]phenyl]acetic acid. *CAS-79094-20-5.* INN. *Immunosuppressant.* ◇*SK&F 96148; BM 13.505*

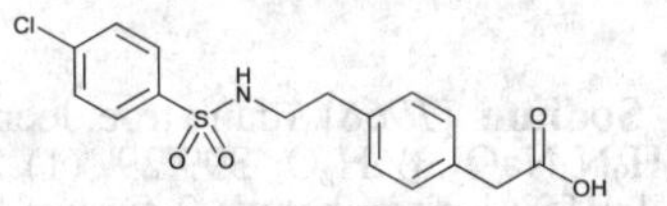

Dalvastatin [*1991*] (dal″ va stat′ in). $C_{24}H_{31}FO_3$. 386.50. (1) 2*H*-Pyran-2-one, 6-[2-[2-(4-fluoro-3-methylphenyl)-4,4,6,6-tetramethyl-1-cyclohexen-1-yl]ethenyl]tetrahydro-4-hydroxy-, [4α,6β(*E*)]-(±)-; (2) (±)-(4*R**,6*S**)-6-[(*E*)-2-[2-(4-Fluoro-*m*-tolyl)-4,4,6,6-tetramethyl-1-cyclohexen-1-yl]vinyl]tetrahydro-4-hydroxy-2*H*-pyran-2-one. *UNII-ZWE0X0IG9D. CAS-132100-55-1.* INN. *Antihyperlipidemic.* ◇*RG 12561*

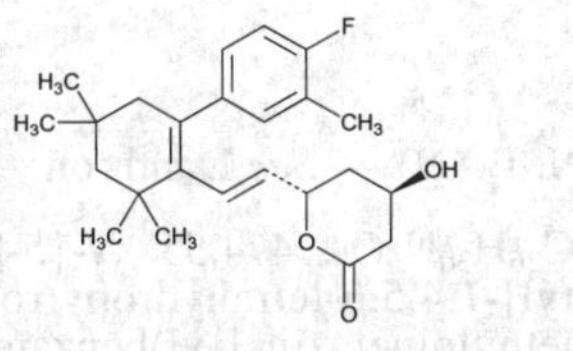

Dametralast. $C_6H_8N_6$. 164.17. 2,4-Diamino-7-methylpyrazolo[1,5-*a*]-*s*-triazine. *UNII-16992A3UUS. CAS-71680-63-2.* INN.

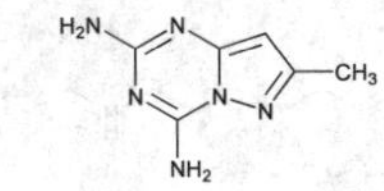

Damotepine. $C_{17}H_{17}NS$. 267.39. *N,N*-Dimethyldibenzo[*b,f*]thiepin-10-methylamine. *UNII-0V9VL751XU. CAS-1469-07-4.* INN; DCF.

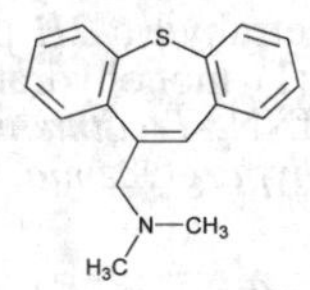

---

† Brand name formerly used, and/or firm no longer concerned with this product.

Danaparoid Sodium [*1992*] (dan ap′ a roid soe′ dee um). Danaparoid is a low molecular weight heparinoid, a mixture of the sodium salts of heparan sulfate (approximately 84%), dermatan sulfate (approximately 12%), and chondroitin sulfate (approximately 4%). It is derived from hog intestinal mucosa. Heparan Sulfate: (1) Heparitin, sulfate, sodium salt; (2) Heparitin, sulfate, sodium salt. Dermatan Sulfate: (1) Dermatan, 4-(hydrogen sulfate), sodium salt; (2) Dermatan 4-(sodium sulfate). Chondroitin 4-sulfate: (1) Chondroitin, 4-(hydrogen sulfate), sodium salt; (2) Chondroitin 4-(sodium sulfate). Chondroitin 6-sulfate: (1) Chondroitin, 6-(hydrogen sulfate), sodium salt; (2) Chondroitin 6-(sodium sulfate). *CAS-57459-72-0* [heparan, sulfate, sodium salt]; *CAS-54328-33-5* [dermatan, 4-(hydrogen sulfate), sodium salt]; *CAS-39455-18-0* [chondroitin, 4-(hydrogen sulfate), sodium salt]; *CAS-12678-07-8* [chondroitin, 6-(hydrogen sulfate), sodium salt]. INN; BAN. *Antithrombotic.* Orgaran (Organon) ◇*ORG 10172*

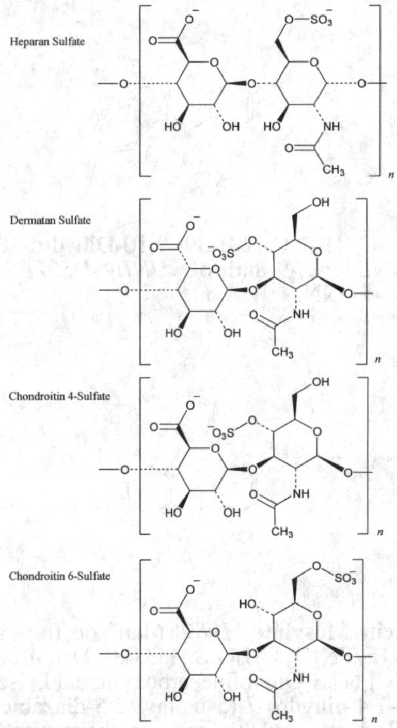

Danazol [*1968*] (dan′ a zol). USP. $C_{22}H_{27}NO_2$. 337.46. (1) Pregna-2,4-dien-20-yno[2,3-*d*]isoxazol-17-ol,(17α)-; (2) 17α-Pregna-2,4-dien-20-yno[2,3-*d*]isoxazol-17-ol. *UNII-N29QWW3BUO. CAS-17230-88-5.* INN; BAN; JAN. *Anterior pituitary suppressant.* Danocrine (Sanofi Aventis) ◇*Win 17,757*

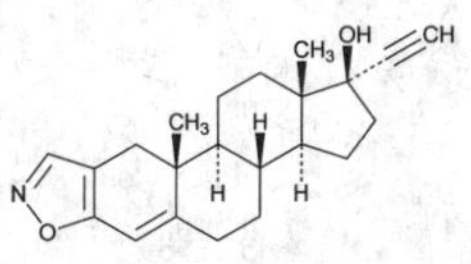

Daniplestim [*1997*] (dan ip′ le stim). $C_{564}H_{909}N_{161}O_{166}S_5$. 12,761.57. (1) 14-125-Interleukin 3 (human clone D11), 14-L-alanine-18-L-isoleucine-25-L-histidine-29-L-arginine-32-L-asparagine-37-L-proline-42-L-serine-45-L-methionine-51-L-arginine-55-L-threonine-59-L-leucine-62-L-valine-67-L-histidine-69-L-glutamic acid-73-glycine-76-L-alanine-79-L-arginine-82-L-glutamine-87-L-serine-93-L-serine-98-L-isoleucine-101-L-alanine-105-L-glutamine-109-L-glutamic acid-116-L-valine-120-L-glutamine-123-L-glutamic acid-; (2) 14-L-Alanine-18-L-isoleucine-25-L-histidine-29-L-arginine-32-L-asparagine-37-L-proline-42-L-serine-45-L-methionine-51-L-arginine-55-L-threonine-59-L-leucine-62-L-valine-67-L-histidine-69-L-glutamic acid-73-L-glycine-76-L-alanine-79-L-arginine-82-L-glutamine-87-L-serine-93-L-serine-98-L-isoleucine-101-L-alanine-105-L-glutamine-109-L-glutamic acid-116-L-valine-120-L-glutamine-123-L-glutamic acid-14-125-interleukin 3 (synthetic human variant). *CAS-161753-30-6*. INN. *Hematopoietic stimulant; antineutropenic.* ◇*SC-55494*

```
ANCSIMIDEI IHHLKRPPNP LLDPNNLNSE DMDILMERNL RTPNLLAFVR
AVKHLENASG IEAILRNLQP CLPSATAAPS RHPIIIKAGD WQEFREKLTF
YLVTLEQAQE QQ
```

Daniquidone. $C_{15}H_{11}N_3O$. 249.27. 8-Aminoisoindolo[1,2-*b*]quinazolin-12(10*H*)-one. *UNII-E780TX33D2. CAS-67199-66-0*. INN; BAN. ◇*BAY h 2049*

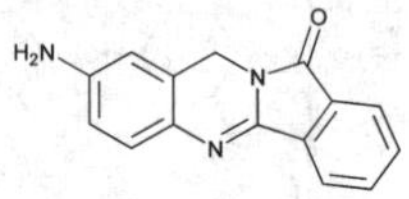

Danitracen. $C_{20}H_{21}NO$. 291.39. 9,10-Dihydro-10-(1-methyl-4-piperidylidene)-9-anthrol. *UNII-SD507F5T2W. CAS-31232-26-5*. INN. ◇*W-A 335*

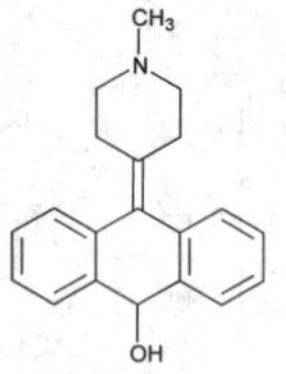

Danofloxacin Mesylate [*1989*] (dan″ oh flox′ a sin mes′ i late). $C_{19}H_{20}FN_3O_3.CH_4O_3S$. 453.48. [Danofloxacin is INN and BAN.] (1) 3-Quinolinecarboxylic acid, 1-cyclopropyl-6-fluoro-1,4-dihydro-7-(5-methyl-2,5-diazabicyclo[2.2.1]-hept-2-yl)-4-oxo-, (1*S*)-, monomethanesulfonate; (2) 1-Cyclopropyl-6-fluoro-1,4-dihydro-7-[(1*S*,4*S*)-5-methyl-2,5-diazabicyclo[2.2.1]hept-2-yl]-4-oxo-3-quinolinecarboxylic acid, monomethanesulfonate. *UNII-94F3SX3LEM; UNII-24CU1YS91D* [danofloxacin]. *CAS-119478-55-6; CAS-112398-08-0* [danofloxacin]. *Antibacterial (veterinary).* ◇*CP-76,136-27*

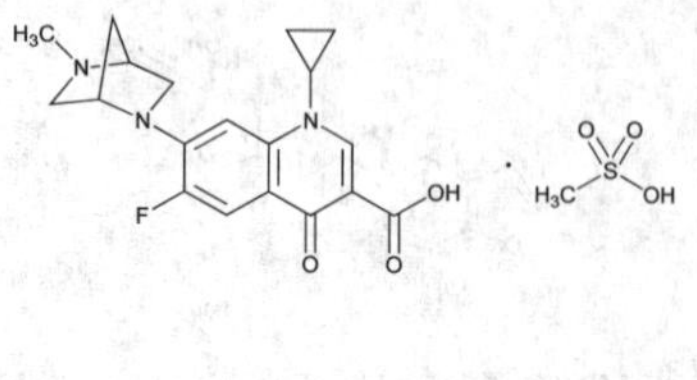

Danosteine. $C_5H_8O_4S$. 164.18. 3-[(Carboxymethyl)thio]propionic acid. *UNII-481GSD6F7Q. CAS-4938-00-5*. INN.

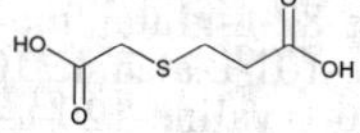

Danthron. $C_{14}H_8O_4$. 240.21. [Dantron is INN and BAN.] (1) 9,10-Anthracenedione, 1,8-dihydroxy-; (2) 1,8-Dihydroxyanthraquinone. *UNII-Z4XE6IBF3V. CAS-117-10-2*. USP XXI; MI. Dorbane (3M Pharmaceuticals†); Istizin (Sterling Winthrop†)

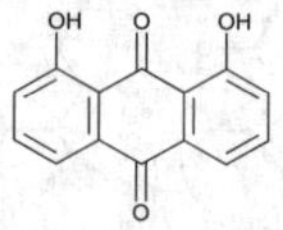

Dantrolene [*1966*] (dan′ troe leen). $C_{14}H_{10}N_4O_5$. 314.25. (1) 2,4-Imidazolidinedione, 1-[[[5-(4-nitrophenyl)-2-furanyl]-methylene]amino]-; (2) 1-[[5-(*p*-Nitrophenyl)furfurylidene]amino]hydantoin. *UNII-F64QU97QCR. CAS-7261-97-4*. INN; BAN. *Relaxant (skeletal muscle).* ◇*F-368*

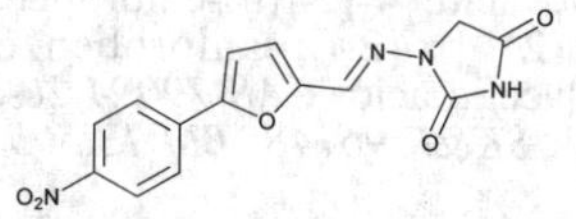

Dantrolene Sodium [*1968*] (dan′ troe leen soe′ dee um). **USP**. $C_{14}H_9N_4NaO_5.3½H_2O$. 399.29. (1) 2,4-Imidazolidinedione, 1-[[[5-(4-nitrophenyl)-2-furanyl]methylene]amino]-, sodium salt, hydrate (2:7); (2) 1-[[5-(*p*-Nitrophenyl)furfurylidene]amino]hydantoin sodium salt hydrate. *UNII-287M0347EV; UNII-F64QU97QCR* [dantrolene]. *CAS-24868-20-0; CAS-14663-23-1* [anhydrous]; *CAS-7261-97-4* [dantrolene]. BAN; JAN. *Relaxant (skeletal muscle).* Dantrium (Procter & Gamble) ◇*F-440*

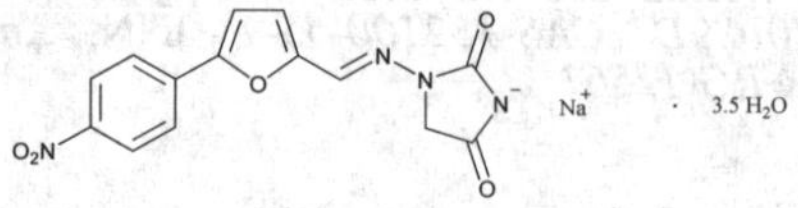

Dantron (INN, BAN) — *See* Danthron.

Danusertib. $C_{26}H_{30}N_6O_3$. 474.55. *N*-{5-[(2*R*)-2-Methoxy-2-phenylacetyl]-1,4,5,6-tetrahydropyrrolo[3,4-*c*]pyrazol-3-yl}-4-(4-methylpiperazin-1-yl)benzamide. *CAS-827318-97-8*. INN.

Dapabutan. $C_{19}H_{40}N_2O_2$. 328.53. (±)-3-[[3-(Dodecylamino)-propyl]amino]butyric acid. *UNII-1R0Y7O07NF. CAS-6582-31-6*. INN.

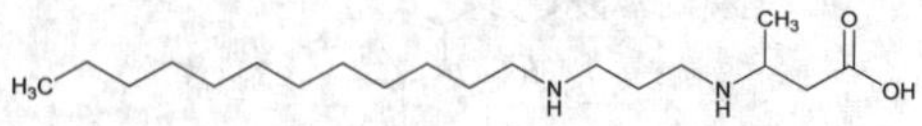

Dapagliflozin [*2008*] (dap″ a gli floe′ zin). $C_{21}H_{25}ClO_6.-C_3H_8O_2.H_2O$. 502.98. (1) D-Glucitol, 1,5-anhydro-1-*C*-[4-chloro-3-[(4-ethoxyphenyl)methyl]phenyl]-, (1*S*)-, compd. with (2*S*)-1,2-propanediol, hydrate (1:1:1); (2) (2*S*,3*R*,4*R*,5*S*,6*R*)-2-[4-Chloro-3-(4-ethoxybenzyl)phenyl]-6-(hydroxymethyl)tetrahydro-2*H*-pyran-3,4,5-triol, (2*S*)-propane-1,2-diol (1:1) monohydrate. *UNII-887K2391VH. CAS-960404-48-2*. INN. *Treatment of type 2 diabetes, or conditions causing hyperglycemia.* ◇*BMS-512148-05*

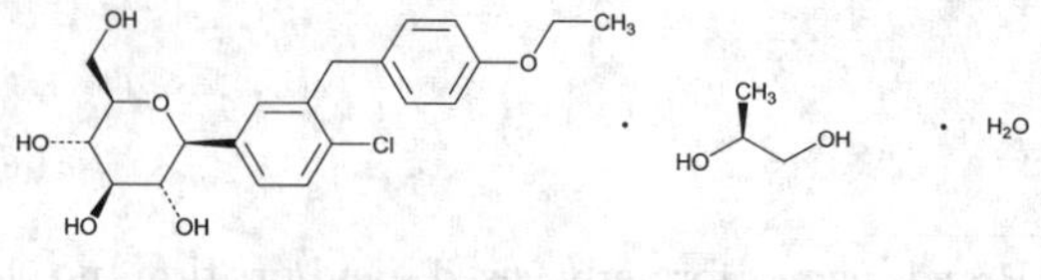

Dapiclermin [*2005*] (dap″ i kler′ min). $C_{945}H_{1482}N_{266}O_{278}S_3$. 21,114. (1) 2-185-Ciliary neurotrophic factor [17-alanine,63-arginine] (human isoform AXOKINE); (2) 2-185-[17-Alanine,63-arginine]ciliary neurotrophic factor-(2,185)-peptide (human isoform AXOKINE). *UNII-A3VLQ7024W. CAS-444069-80-1.* INN. *Treatment of overweight and obesity.* Axokine (Regeneron)

```
AFTEHSPLT PHRRDLASRS IWLARKIRSD LTALTESYVK HQGLNKNINL
DSADGMPVAS TDRWSELTEA ERLQENLQAY RTFHVLLARL LEDQQVHFTP
TEGDFHQAIH TLLLQVAAFA YQIEELMILL EYKIPRNEAD GMPINVGDGG
LFEKKLWGLK VLQELSQWTV RSIHDLRFIS SHQTG
```

Dapiprazole Hydrochloride [*1989*] (da pip′ ra zole hye″ droe klor′ ide). $C_{19}H_{27}N_5 \cdot HCl$. 361.91. [Dapiprazole is INN.] (1) 1,2,4-Triazolo[4,3-*a*]pyridine, 5,6,7,8-tetrahydro-3-[2-[4-(2-methylphenyl)-1-piperazinyl]ethyl]-, monohydrochloride; (2) 5,6,7,8-Tetrahydro-3-[2-(4-*o*-tolyl-1-piperazinyl)ethyl]-*s*-triazolo[4,3-*a*]pyridine monohydrochloride. *UNII-DS9UJN1I0X. CAS-72822-13-0; CAS-72822-12-9* [dapiprazole]. *Adrenergic (α-blocking); antiglaucoma agent; neuroleptic; psychotropic.* Rev-Eyes (Angelini) ◇*AF 2139*

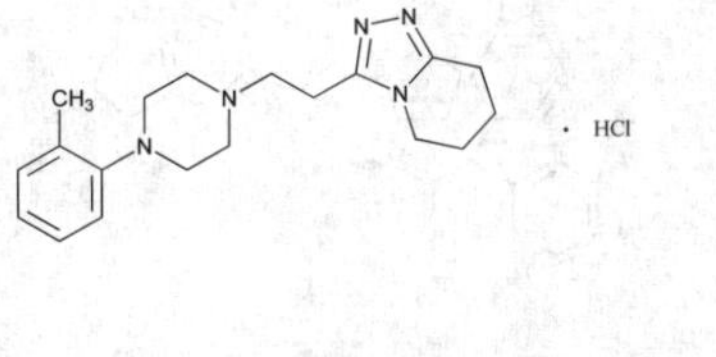

Dapitant. $C_{37}H_{39}NO_4$. 561.71. (3a*S*,4*S*,7a*S*)-Hexahydro-2-[(α*S*)-*o*-methoxyhydratropoyl]-4-(*o*-methoxyphenyl)-7,7-diphenyl-4-isoindolinol. *CAS-153438-49-4.* INN.

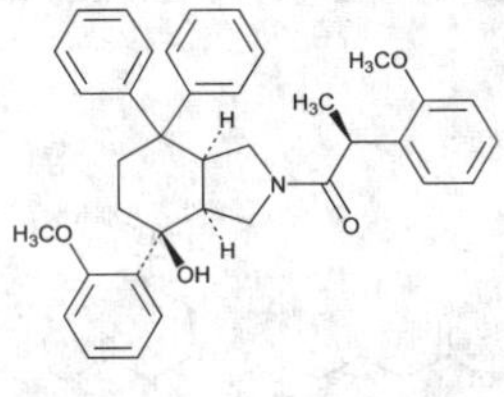

Dapivirine. $C_{20}H_{19}N_5$. 329.40. 4-[[4-[(2,4,6-Trimethylphenyl)amino]pyrimidin-2-yl]amino]benzonitrile. *UNII-TCN4MG2VXS. CAS-244767-67-7.* INN.

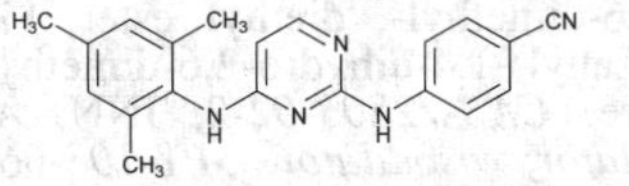

Daporinad. $C_{24}H_{29}N_3O_2$. 391.51. (2*E*)-*N*-[4-(1-Benzoylpiperidin-4-yl)butyl]-3-(pyridin-3-yl)prop-2-enamide. *CAS-201034-75-5.* INN.

Dapoxetine Hydrochloride [*1991*] (da pox′ e teen hye″ droe klor′ ide). $C_{21}H_{23}NO \cdot HCl$. 341.87. [Dapoxetine is INN.] (1) Benzenemethanamine, *N,N*-dimethyl-α-[2-(1-naphthalenyloxy)ethyl]-, hydrochloride, (*S*)-; (2) (+)-(*S*)-*N,N*-Dimethyl-α-[2-(1-naphthyloxy)ethyl]benzylamine hydro-

chloride. *UNII-U4OHT63MRI; UNII-GB2433A4M3* [dapoxetine]. *CAS-129938-20-1; CAS-119356-77-3* [dapoxetine]. *Antidepressant.* ◇*LY210448 HCl*

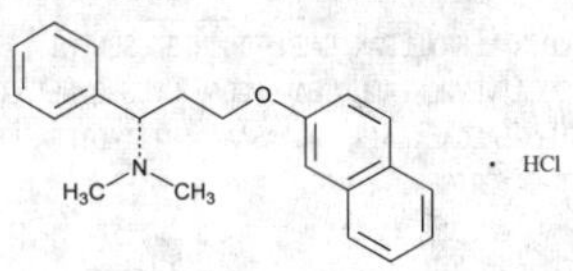

Daproterin — *See* Sapropterin Dihydrochloride.

Dapsone [*1963*] (dap′ sone). **USP.** $C_{12}H_{12}N_2O_2S$. 248.30. (1) Benzenamine, 4,4′-sulfonylbis-; (2) 4,4′-Sulfonyldianiline. *UNII-8W5C518302. CAS-80-08-0.* BAN. *Antibacterial (leprostatic); suppressant (dermatitis herpetiformis). [Name previously used: Diaminodiphenylsulfone.]* ◇*NSC-6091*

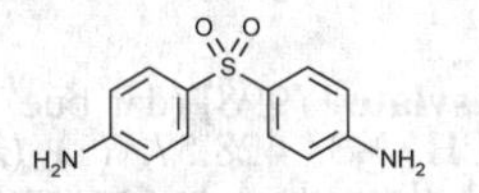

Daptomycin [*1989*] (dap″ toe mye′ sin). $C_{72}H_{101}N_{17}O_{26}$. 1620.67. (1) Daptomycin; (2) *N*-Decanoyl-L-tryptophyl-L-asparaginyl-L-aspartyl-L-threonylglycyl-L-ornithyl-L-aspartyl-D-alanyl-L-aspartylglycyl-D-seryl-*threo*-3-methyl-L-glutamyl-3-anthraniloyl-L-alanine ϵ_1-lactone. *UNII-NWQ5N31VKK. CAS-103060-53-3.* INN; BAN. *Antibacterial.* Cubicin (Cubist) ◇*LY 146032*

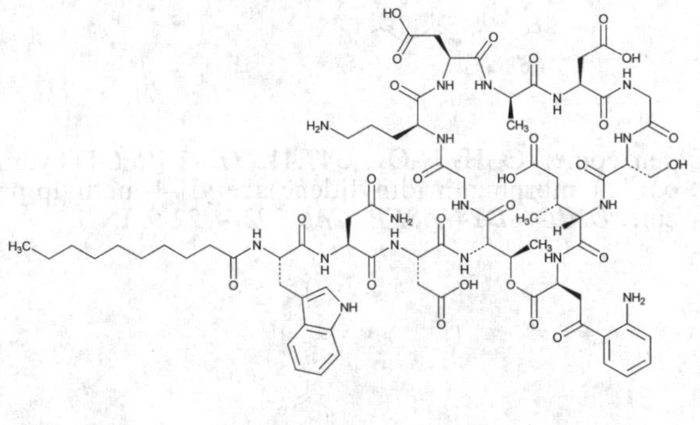

Darapladib [*2005*] (dar ap′ la dib). $C_{36}H_{38}F_4N_4O_2S$. 666.77. (1) 1*H*-Cyclopentapyrimidine-1-acetamide, *N*-[2-(diethylamino)ethyl]-2-[[(4-fluorophenyl)methyl]thio]-4,5,6,7-tetrahydro-4-oxo-*N*-[[4′-(trifluoromethyl)[1,1′-biphenyl]-4-yl]methyl]-; (2) *N*-[2-(Diethylamino)ethyl]-2-[2-[(4-fluorobenzyl)sulfanyl]-4-oxo-4,5,6,7-tetrahydro-1*H*-cyclopentapyrimidin-1-yl]-*N*-[[4′-(trifluoromethyl)biphenyl-4-yl]methyl]acetamide. *UNII-UI1U1MYH09. CAS-356057-34-6.* INN. *Treatment of atherosclerosis.* ◇*SB-480848*

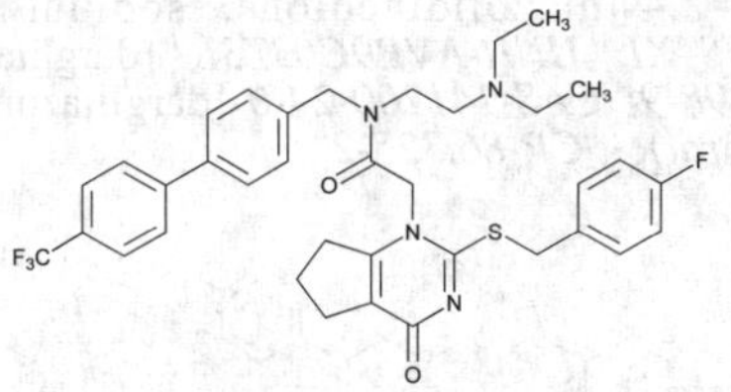

Darbepoetin Alfa [*2000*] (dar″ be poe′ e tin al′ fa). $C_{800}H_{1300}N_{228}O_{24}S_5$. 18,174 daltons. (1) Erythropoietin [30-asparagine, 32-threonine, 87-valine, 88-asparagine, 90-threonine] (human); (2) [30-L-Asparagine-32-L-threo-

---

nine-87-L-valine-88-L-asparagine-90-L-threonine]erythropoietin (human). *UNII-15UQ94PT4P. CAS-209810-58-2.* INN; BAN. *Treatment of anemia.* ◇*NESP*

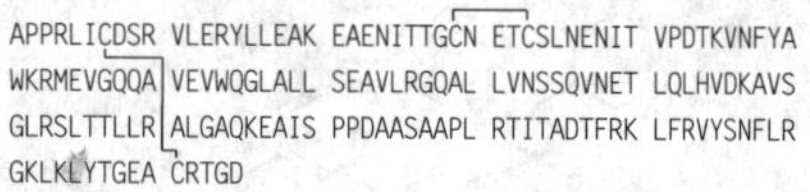

```
APPRLICDSR VLERYLLEAK EAENITTGCN ETCSLNENIT VPDTKVNFYA
WKRMEVGQQA VEVWQGLALL SEAVLRGQAL LVNSSQVNET LQLHVDKAVS
GLRSLTTLLR ALGAQKEAIS PPDAASAAPL RTITADTFRK LFRVYSNFLR
GKLKLYTGEA CRTGD
```

Darbufelone. $C_{18}H_{24}N_2O_2S$. 332.46. 5-[(Z)-3,5-Di-*tert*-butyl-4-hydroxybenzylidene]-2-imino-4-thiazolidinone. *UNII-72H8H6K34C. CAS-139226-28-1.* INN.

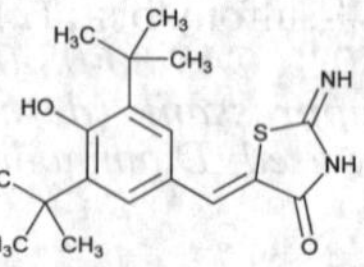

Darbufelone Mesylate [*1998*] (dar bue′ fel one mes′ i late). $C_{18}H_{24}N_2O_2S.CH_4O_3S$. 428.57. (1) (*Z*)-2-Amino-5-[[3,5-bis(1,1-dimethylethyl)-4-hydroxyphenyl]methylene]-4(5*H*)-thiazolone monomethanesulfonate (salt); (2) 5-[(Z)-3,5-Di-*tert*-butyl-4-hydroxybenzylidene]-2-imino-4-thiazolidinone monomethanesulfonate (salt). *UNII-5I2Y40C5PX. CAS-139340-56-0.* Anti-inflammatory; antiarthritic (dual cyclooxygenase and 5-lipoxygenase inhibitor). ◇*CI-1004*

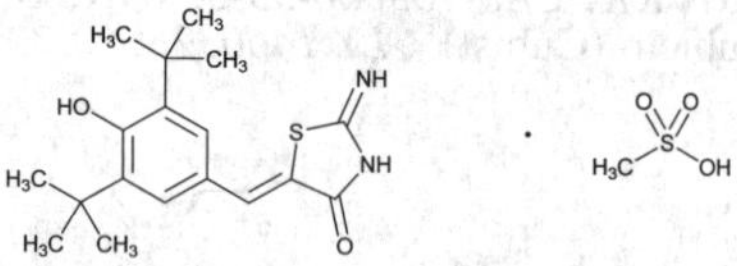

Darenzepine. $C_{21}H_{21}N_3O_2$. 347.41. (*E*)-1-[(5,6-Dihydro-6-oxo-11-morphanthridinylidene)acetyl]-4-methylpiperazine. *UNII-4SDY4L68FP. CAS-90274-22-9.* INN.

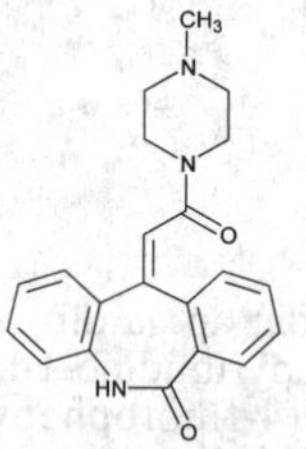

Darglitazone Sodium [*1993*] (dar gli′ ta zone soe′ dee um). $C_{23}H_{19}N_2NaO_4S$. 442.46. [Darglitazone is INN.] (1) 2,4-Thiazolidinedione, 5-[[4-[3-(5-methyl-2-phenyl-4-oxazolyl)-1-oxopropyl]phenyl]methyl]-, sodium salt, (±)-; (2) (±)-5-[*p*-[3-(5-Methyl-2-phenyl-4-oxazolyl)propionyl]benzyl]-2,4-thiazolidinedione, sodium salt. *UNII-A1P35HS4XI; UNII-AVP9C03Z3K* [darglitazone]. *CAS-141683-98-9; CAS-141200-24-0* [darglitazone]. *Hypoglycemic (oral).* ◇*CP-86,325-2*

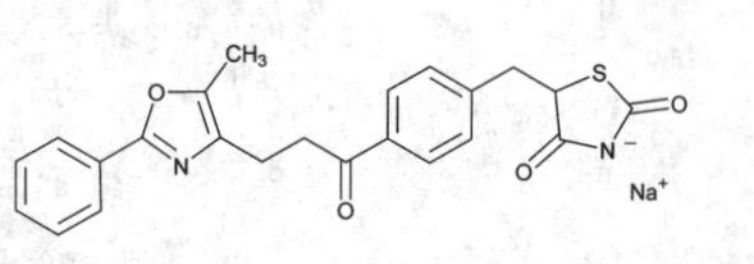

Darifenacin [*2005*] (dar″ i fen′ a sin). $C_{28}H_{30}N_2O_2$. 426.55. (1) 3-Pyrrolidineacetamide, 1-[2-(2,3-dihydro-5-benzofuranyl)ethyl]-α,α-diphenyl-, (3*S*)-; (2) 2-[(3*S*)-1-[2-(2,3-Di-

hydrobenzofuran-5-yl)ethyl]pyrrolidin-3-yl]-2,2-diphenylacetamide. *UNII-APG9819VLM. CAS-133099-04-4.* BAN. *Treatment for an overactive bladder.* ◇*UK-88525*

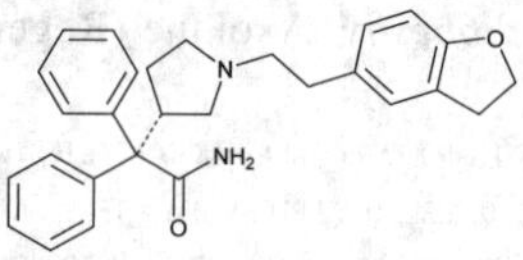

Darifenacin Hydrobromide [*2004*] (dar″ i fen′ a sin hye″ droe broe′ mide). $C_{28}H_{30}N_2O_2.HBr$. 507.46. [Darifenacin is INN and BAN.] (1) 3-Pyrrolidineacetamide, 1-[2-(2,3-dihydro-5-benzofuranyl)ethyl]-α,α-diphenyl-, monohydrobromide, (3*S*)-; (2) (*S*)-2-{1-[2-(2,3-Dihydrobenzofuran-5-yl)ethyl]-3-pyrrolidnyl}-2,2-diphenylacetamide hydrobromide. *UNII-CR02EYQ8GV; UNII-APG9819VLM* [darifenacin]. *CAS-133099-07-7; CAS-133099-04-4* [darifenacin]. *Treatment for an overactive bladder.* Enablex (Novartis) ◇*UK-88525-04 (hydrobromide)*

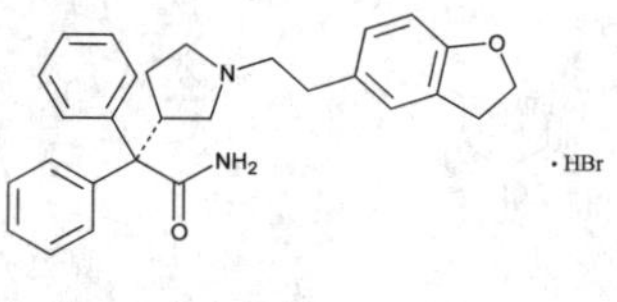

Darinaparsin [*2007*] (dar in″ a pars′ in). $C_{12}H_{22}AsN_3O_6S$. 411.31. (1) Glycine, L-γ-glutamyl-*S*-(dimethylarsino)-L-cysteinyl; (2) L-γ-Glutamyl-*S*-(dimethylarsanyl)-L-cysteinylglycine. *CAS-69819-86-9.* INN. *Antineoplastic.* ◇*ZIO-101*

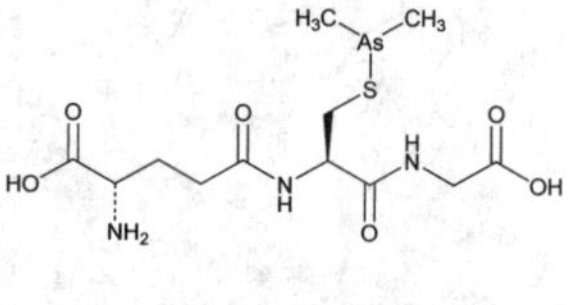

Darodipine [*1986*] (dar oh′ di peen). $C_{19}H_{21}N_3O_5$. 371.39. (1) 3,5-Pyridinedicarboxylic acid, 4-(4-benzofurazanyl)-1,4-dihydro-2,6-dimethyl-, diethyl ester; (2) Diethyl 4-(4-benzofurazanyl)-1,4-dihydro-2,6-dimethyl-3,5-pyridinedicarboxylate. *CAS-72803-02-2.* INN. *Antihypertensive; bronchodilator; vasodilator.* ◇*PY 108-068*

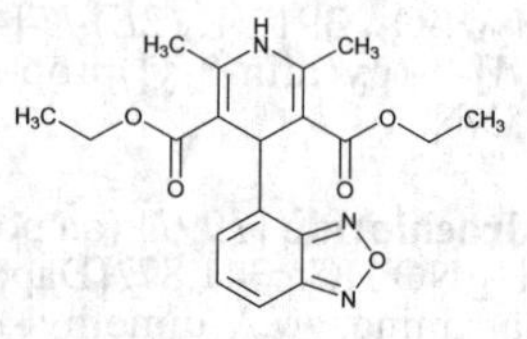

Darotropium Bromide [*2007*] (dar″ oh troe′ pee um). $C_{24}H_{29}BrN_2$. 425.40. (1) 8-Azoniabicyclo[3.2.1]octane, 3-(2-cyano-2,2-diphenylethyl)-8,8-dimethyl-, bromide, (3-*endo*)-; (2) (1*R*,3*r*,5*S*)-3-(2-Cyano-2,2-diphenylethyl)-8,8-

dimethyl-8-azoniabicyclo[3.2.1]octane bromide. *UNII-2W2V1U785A. CAS-850607-58-8.* INN. *Treatment of COPD.* ◇GSK233705B

Darsidomine. $C_9H_{16}N_4O$. 196.25. 3-(*cis*-2,6-Dimethylpiperidino)sydnone imine. *UNII-00I7BI3BB7. CAS-137500-42-6.* INN. *[Name previously used: Marsidomine.]*

Darunavir [*2005*] (dar ue′ na vir). $C_{27}H_{37}N_3O_7S$. 547.66. (1) [(1*S*,2*R*)-3-[[(4-Aminophenyl)sulfonyl](2-methylpropyl)amino]-2-hydroxy-1-(phenylmethyl)propyl]-carbamic acid (3*R*,3a*S*,6a*R*)-hexahydrofuro[2,3-*b*]furan-3-yl ester; (2) Carbamic acid, [(1*S*,2*R*)-3-[[(4-aminophenyl)sulfonyl](2-methylpropyl)amino]-2-hydroxy-1-(phenylmethyl)propyl]-, (3*R*,3a*S*,6a*R*)-hexahydrofuro[2,3-*b*]furan-3-yl ester. *UNII-YO603Y8113. CAS-206361-99-1.* INN. *Treatment of HIV infection.* ◇TMC 114

Darusentan. $C_{22}H_{22}N_2O_6$. 410.42. (+)-(*S*)-2-[(4,6-Dimethoxy-2-pyrimidinyl)oxy]-3-methoxy-3,3-diphenylpropionic acid. *CAS-171714-84-4.*

Dasantafil [*2004*] (da san′ ta fil). $C_{22}H_{28}BrN_5O_5$. 522.39. (1) 1*H*-Purine-2,6-dione, 7-[(3-bromo-4-methoxyphenyl)methyl]-1-ethyl-3,7-dihydro-8-[[(1*R*,2*R*)-2-hydroxycyclopentyl]amino]-3-(2-hydroxyethyl); (2) 7-(3-Bromo-4-methoxybenzyl)-1-ethyl-8-[[(1*R*,2*R*)-2-hydroxycyclopentyl]amino]-3-(2-hydroxyethyl)-3,7-dihydro-1*H*-purine-2,6-

---

† Brand name formerly used, and/or firm no longer concerned with this product.

dione. *UNII-48P711MI2G. CAS-569351-91-3.* INN. *Treatment of erectile dysfunction (phosphodiesterase (PDE) 5 isoenzyme inhibitor).* ◇SCH 446132

Dasatinib [*2005*] (da sa′ ti nib). $C_{22}H_{26}ClN_7O_2S.H_2O$. 506.02. (1) 5-Thiazolecarboxamide-*N*-(2-chloro-6-methylphenyl)-2-[[6-[4-(2-hydroxyethyl)-1-piperazinyl]-2-methyl-4-pyrimidinyl]amino]-, monohydrate; (2) *N*-(2-Chloro-6-methylphenyl)-2-[[6-[4-(2-hydroxyethyl)piperazin-1-yl]-2-methylpyrimidin-4-yl]amino]thiazole-5-carboxamide hydrate. *UNII-RBZ1571X5H. CAS-863127-77-9.* INN; JAN. *Anti-cancer.* Sprycel (Bristol-Myers Squibb) ◇BMS-354825-03

Datelliptium Chloride. $C_{23}H_{28}ClN_3O$. 397.94. 2-[2-(Diethylamino)ethyl]-9-hydroxy-5,11-dimethyl-6*H*-pyrido[4,3-*b*]carbazolium chloride. *UNII-V5QKF7Q20O. CAS-105118-14-7.* INN.

Daturine Hydrobromide — *See* Hyoscyamine Hydrobromide.

Daunorubicin Hydrochloride [*1976*] (daw″ noe roo′ bi sin hye″ droe klor′ ide). USP. $C_{27}H_{29}NO_{10}.HCl$. 563.98. [Daunorubicin is INN and BAN.] (1) 5,12-Naphthacenedione, 8-acetyl-10-[(3-amino-2,3,6-trideoxy-α-L-*lyxo*-hexopyranosyl)]oxy]-7,8,9,10-tetrahydro-6,8,11-trihydroxy-1-methoxy-, (8*S*-*cis*)-, hydrochloride; (2) (1*S*,3*S*)-3-Acetyl-1,2,3,4,6,11-hexahydro-3,5,12-trihydroxy-10-methoxy-6,11-dioxo-1-naphthacenyl 3-amino-2,3,6-trideoxy-α-L-*lyxo*-hexopyranoside hydrochloride. *UNII-UD984I04LZ; UNII-ZS7284E0ZP* [daunorubicin]. *CAS-23541-50-6; CAS-20830-81-3* [daunorubicin]. JAN. *Antineoplastic.* Cerubidine (Bedford); Daunoxome (Gilead Sciences) ◇FI 6339 *[as the base]; NDC 0082-4155; RP 13057 [as the base]; NSC-82151*

Davasaicin. $C_{22}H_{30}N_2O_3$. 370.49. 2-[4-(2-Aminoethoxy)-3-methoxyphenyl]-*N*-[3-(3,4-dimethylphenyl)propyl]acetamide. *CAS-147497-64-1.* INN.

Davunetide [*2008*] (dav ue′ ne tide). $C_{36}H_{60}N_{10}O_{12}$. 824.92. (1) L-Glutamine, L-asparaginyl-L-alanyl-L-prolyl-L-valyl-L-seryl-L-isoleucyl-L-prolyl-; (2) Human activity-dependent neuroprotective protein (ADNP)-(354-361)-peptide. *UNII-GF00K3IIWE. CAS-211439-12-2. Neuroprotection, treatment of cognitive impairment, treatment of neurodegeneration.* ◇*AL-108; AL-208*

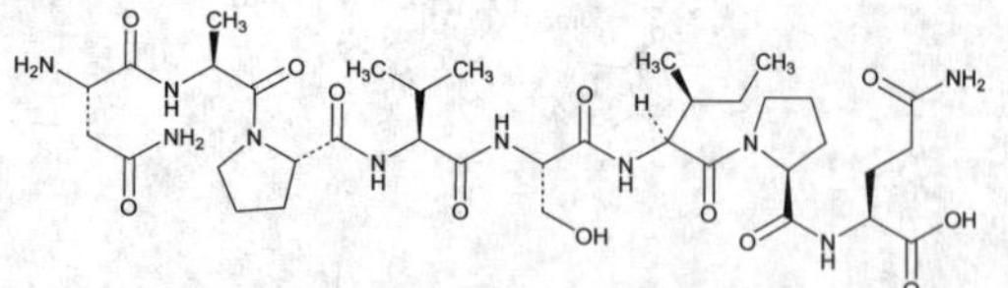

Daxalipram. $C_{14}H_{19}NO_4$. 265.30. (5*R*)-5-(4-Methoxy-3-propoxyphenyl)-5-methyl-1,3-oxazolidin-2-one. *CAS-189940-24-7.* INN.

Dazadrol Maleate [*1972*] (day′ za drol mal′ ee ate). $C_{15}H_{14}ClN_3O.C_4H_4O_4$. 403.82. [Dazadrol is INN.] (1) 2-Pyridinemethanol, α-(4-chlorophenyl)-α-(4,5-dihydro-1*H*-imidazol-2-yl)-, (*Z*)-2-butenedioate (1:1) (salt); (2) α-(*p*-Chlorophenyl)-α-2-imidazolin-2-yl-2-pyridinemethanol maleate (1:1) (salt). *CAS-25387-70-6; CAS-47029-84-5* [dazadrol]. *Antidepressant.* ◇*Sch 12650*

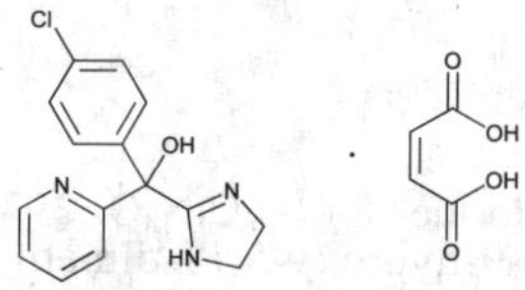

Dazepinil Hydrochloride [*1986*] (day zep′ i nil hye″ droe klor′ ide). $C_{17}H_{18}N_2.HCl$. 286.80. [Dazepinil is INN.] (1) 3*H*-1,3-Benzodiazepine, 4,5-dihydro-2,3-dimethyl-4-phenyl-, monohydrochloride, (±)-; (2) (±)-4,5-Dihydro-2,3-dimethyl-4-phenyl-3*H*-1,3-benzodiazepine monohydrochloride. *CAS-75991-49-0; CAS-75991-50-3* [dazepinil]. *Antidepressant.* ◇*HRP 543; P 76 2543*

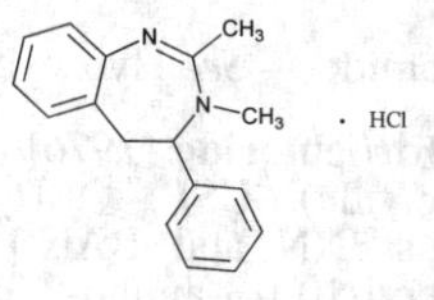

Dazidamine. $C_{19}H_{23}N_3S$. 325.47. 2-Benzyl-3-[[3-(dimethylamino)propyl]thio]-2*H*-indazole. *UNII-J191YXB819. CAS-75522-73-5.* INN.

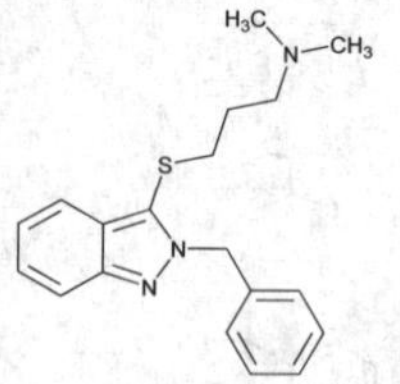

Dazmegrel [*1984*] (dayz′ me grel). $C_{16}H_{17}N_3O_2$. 283.33. (1) 1*H*-Indole-1-propanoic acid, 3-(1*H*-imidazol-1-ylmethyl)-2-methyl-; (2) 3-(Imidazol-1-ylmethyl)-2-methylindole-1-propionic acid. *CAS-76894-77-4.* INN; BAN. *Inhibitor (thromboxane synthetase).* ◇*UK-38,485*

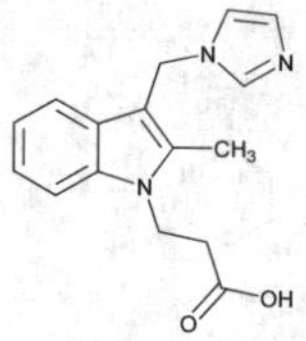

Dazolicine. $C_{17}H_{24}ClN_3S$. 337.91. 8-Chloro-3,4,5,6-tetrahydro-6-[(1-isopropyl-2-imidazolin-2-yl)methyl]-2*H*-1,6-benzothiazocine. *UNII-92KE01WH2P. CAS-61477-97-2.* INN.

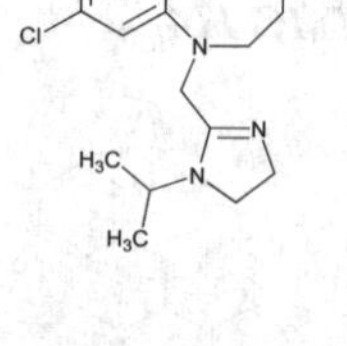

Dazopride Fumarate [*1984*] (day′ zoe pride fue′ ma rate). $C_{15}H_{23}ClN_4O_2.C_4H_4O_4$. 442.89. [Dazopride is INN.] (1) Benzamide, 4-amino-5-chloro-*N*-(1,2-diethyl-4-pyrazolidinyl)-2-methoxy-, (*E*)-2-butenedioate (1:1); (2) 4-Amino-5-chloro-*N*-(1,2-diethyl-4-pyrazolidinyl)-*o*-anisamide fumarate (1:1). *UNII-J8ZC30U6CH; UNII-CV07VSP2G8* [dazopride]. *CAS-81957-25-7; CAS-70181-03-2* [dazopride]. *Stimulant (peristaltic).* ◇*AHR-5531C*

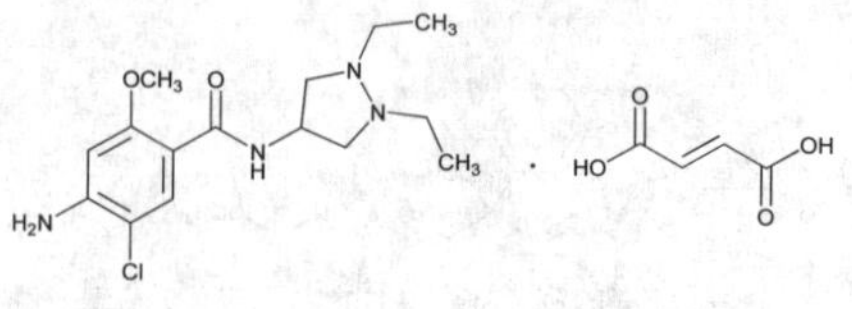

Dazoquinast. $C_{11}H_7N_3O_2$. 213.19. Imidazo[1,2-*a*]quinoxaline-2-carboxylic acid. *UNII-A16F9MIN3Z. CAS-76002-75-0.* INN.

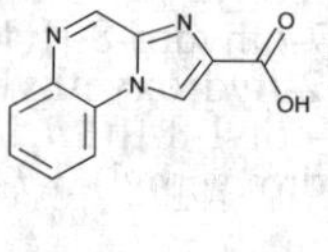

Dazoxiben Hydrochloride [*1981*] (day zox′ i ben hye″ droe klor′ ide). $C_{12}H_{12}N_2O_3.HCl$. 268.70. [Dazoxiben is INN and BAN.] (1) Benzoic acid, 4-[2-(1*H*-imidazol-1-yl)ethoxy]-, monohydrochloride; (2) *p*-(2-Imidazol-1-ylethoxy)benzoic acid monohydrochloride. *CAS-74226-22-5; CAS-78218-09-4* [dazoxiben]. *Antithrombotic.* ⬦*UK-37,248-01*

ddC (DDC) — *See* Zalcitabine.

o,p'-DDD (previously used name) — *See* Mitotane.

DDI — *See* Didanosine.

DDT — *See* Chlorophenothane.

17-Deacylnorgestimate — *See* Norelgestromin.

Deanol Aceglumate. $C_{11}H_{22}N_2O_6$. 278.30. [Deanol is BAN.] 2-(Dimethylamino)ethanol hydrogen *N*-acetylglutamate. *UNII-2PP737Z523. CAS-3342-61-8.* INN; MI.

Deanol Acetamidobenzoate. *UNII-JSQ17GL1CN.* MI. Deaner (3M Pharmaceuticals†)

Deboxamet. $C_{12}H_{14}N_2O_3$. 234.25. 5-Methoxy-2-methylindole-3-acetohydroxamic acid. *UNII-QJH0XA6AW9. CAS-34024-41-4.* INN.

Debrisoquin Sulfate [*1965*] (dee bris' oh kwin sul' fate). $(C_{10}H_{13}N_3)_2 \cdot H_2SO_4$. 448.54. [Debrisoquine is INN and BAN.] (1) 2(1*H*)-Isoquinolinecarboximidamide, 3,4-dihydro-, sulfate (2:1); (2) 3,4-Dihydro-2(1*H*)-isoquinolinecarboxamidine sulfate (2:1). *UNII-Q94064N9NW; UNII-X31CDK040E* [debrisoquin]. *CAS-581-88-4; CAS-1131-64-2* [debrisoquin]. *Antihypertensive.* Declinax (Hoffmann-LaRoche†) ⬦*RO 5-3307/1*

Debropol. $C_3H_6BrNO_3$. 183.99. (±)-2-Bromo-2-nitro-1-propanol. *UNII-28OQS360UJ. CAS-24403-04-1.* INN; BAN. ⬦*BTS 7706*

Decamethonium Bromide. $C_{16}H_{38}Br_2N_2$. 418.29. [Decamethonium Iodide is BAN.] (1) 1,10-Decanediaminium, *N,N,N,N',N',N'*-hexamethyl-, dibromide; (2) Decamethy-

lene bis[trimethylammonium] dibromide. *UNII-55C6RK944K. CAS-541-22-0; CAS-156-74-1* [decamethonium]. USP XX; INN; MI. Syncurine (GlaxoSmithKline)

Decamethonium Iodide (BAN) — *See* Decamethonium Bromide.

Decapinol — *See* Delmopinol.

Decavitamin. *CAS-8048-92-8.* USP XXI.

Decimemide. $C_{19}H_{31}NO_4$. 337.45. 4-(Decyloxy)-3,5-dimethoxybenzamide. *UNII-GAF9GJ18J5. CAS-14817-09-5.* INN; MI.

Decitabine [*1989*] (dee sye' ta been). $C_8H_{12}N_4O_4$. 228.21. (1) 1,3,5-Triazin-2(1*H*)-one, 4-amino-1-(2-deoxy-*β*-D-*erythro*-pentofuranosyl)-; (2) 4-Amino-1-(2-deoxy-*β*-D-*erythro*-pentofuranosyl)-*s*-triazin-2(1*H*)-one; (3) 5-Aza-2'-deoxycytidine. *UNII-776B62CQ27. CAS-2353-33-5.* INN; BAN. *Antineoplastic.* Dacogen (MGI Pharma) ⬦*DAC; NSC-127716*

Decitropine. $C_{23}H_{25}NO$. 331.45. 3*α*-(5*H*-Dibenzo[*a,d*]cyclohepten-5-yloxy)tropane. *CAS-1242-69-9.* INN.

Declaben (previously used name) — *See* Lodelaben.

Declenperone [*1979*] (dee klen' per one). $C_{22}H_{24}FN_3O_2$. 381.44. (1) 2*H*-Benzimidazol-2-one, 1-[3-[4-(4-fluorobenzoyl)-1-piperidinyl]propyl]-1,3-dihydro-; (2) 1-[3-[4-(*p*-Fluorobenzoyl)piperidino]propyl]-2-benzimidazolinone. *UNII-280VGV0X4H. CAS-63388-37-4.* INN. *Sedative (veterinary).* ⬦*R 33,204*

---

† Brand name formerly used, and/or firm no longer concerned with this product.

Declopramide. $C_{13}H_{20}ClN_3O$. 269.77. 4-Amino-3-chloro-N-[2-(diethylamino)ethyl]benzamide. *UNII-916GJF577D. CAS-891-60-1.* INN.

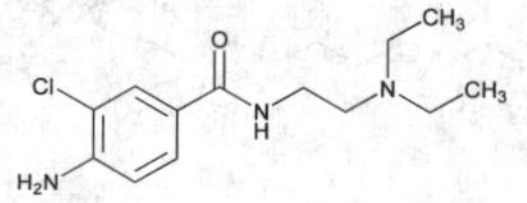

Decloxizine. $C_{21}H_{28}N_2O_2$. 340.46. 2-{2-[4-(Diphenylmethyl)-1-piperazinyl]ethoxy}ethanol. *UNII-919C49XAYD. CAS-3733-63-9.* INN. ◇*UCB 1402*

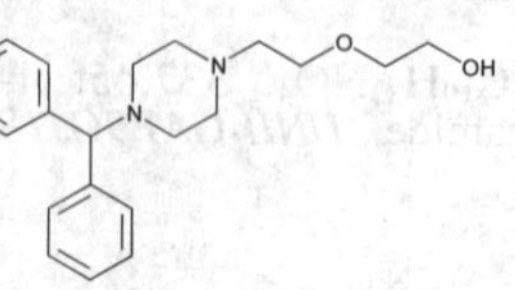

Decominol. $C_{13}H_{29}NO_2$. 231.37. 1-Amino-3-(decyloxy)-2-propanol. *UNII-4A3T9Z2TKX. CAS-60812-35-3.* INN.

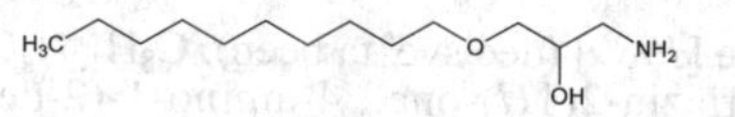

Decoquinate [*1968*] (dee″ koe kwin′ ate). **USP.** $C_{24}H_{35}NO_5$. 417.54. (1) 3-Quinolinecarboxylic acid, 6-(decyloxy)-7-ethoxy-4-hydroxy-, ethyl ester; (2) Ethyl 6-(decyloxy)-7-ethoxy-4-hydroxy-3-quinolinecarboxylate. *UNII-534I52PVWH. CAS-18507-89-6.* INN; BAN. *Coccidiostat (for poultry).* ◇*M&B 15497; HC 1528*

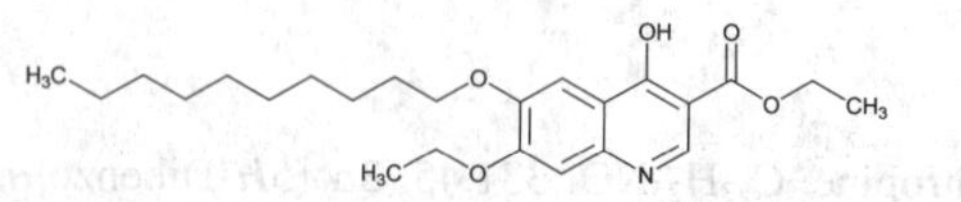

Dectaflur [*1973*] (dek′ ta flur). $C_{18}H_{37}N.HF$. 287.50. (1) 9-Octadecenylamine hydrofluoride; (2) 9-Octadecenylamine hydrofluoride. *CAS-36505-83-6* [nonstereospecific]; *CAS-1838-19-3* [9-octadecenylamine]. INN. *Dental caries prophylactic.* ◇*SK&F 38094*

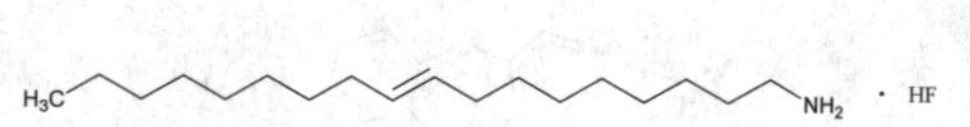

Deditonium Bromide. $C_{38}H_{66}Br_2N_2O_2$. 742.75. Decamethylenebis[dimethyl[2-(thymyloxy)ethyl]ammonium bromide]. *UNII-6BCE7KY501; UNII-B9JAY11T6C* [deditonium]. *CAS-2401-56-1; CAS-20462-53-7* [deditonium]. INN. ◇*249-16*

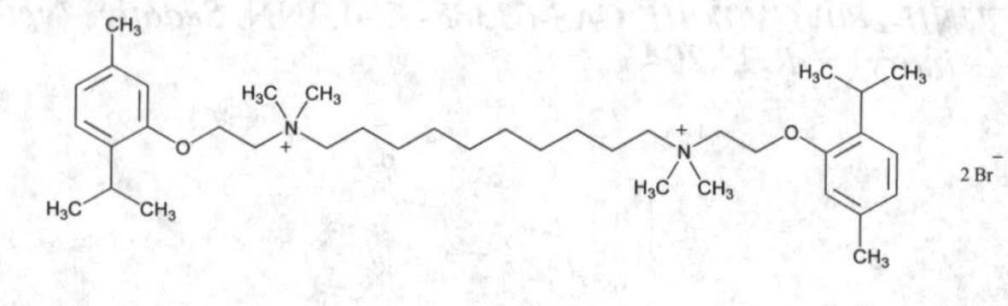

Deferasirox [*2004*] (dee fer′ a sir ox). $C_{21}H_{15}N_3O_4$. 373.36. (1) Benzoic acid, 4-[3,5-bis(2-hydroxyphenyl)-1H-1,2,4-triazol-1-yl]-; (2) 4-[3,5-Bis(2-hydroxyphenyl)-1H-1,2,4-triazol-1-yl]benzoic acid. *UNII-V8G4MOF2V9. CAS-201530-41-8.* INN; JAN. *Treatment of iron overload (iron chelator).* Exjade (Novartis) ◇*ICL670A*

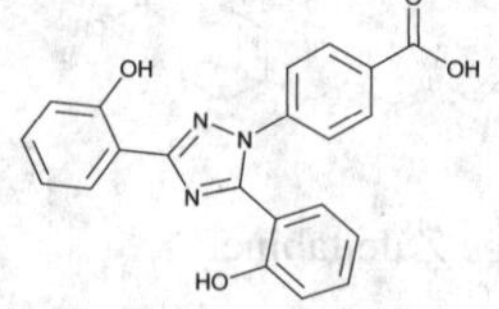

Deferiprone. $C_7H_9NO_2$. 139.15. 3-Hydroxy-1,2-dimethyl-4(1H)-pyridone. *UNII-2BTY8KH53L. CAS-30652-11-0.* INN; BAN. ◇*L1*

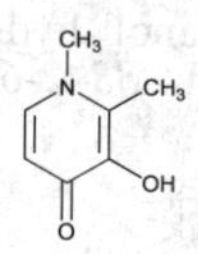

Deferitrin [*2004*] (dee fer′ i trin). $C_{11}H_{11}NO_4S$. 253.27. (1) 4-Thiazolecarboxylic acid, 2-(2,4-dihydroxyphenyl)-4,5-dihydro-4-methyl-, (4S)-; (2) (+)-(4S)-2-(2,4-Dihydroxyphenyl)-4-methyl-4,5-dihydrothiazole-4-carboxylic acid. *UNII-T69Y9LDN44. CAS-239101-33-8.* INN. *Tridentate oral chelator intended for use in the primary treatment of iron overload resulting from transfusion therapy.* ◇*GT56-252*

Deferoxamine [*1964*] (de fer ox′ a meen). $C_{25}H_{48}N_6O_8$. 560.68. [Desferrioxamine is BAN.] (1) Butanediamide, N'-[5-[[4-[[5-(acetylhydroxyamino)pentyl]amino]-1,4-dioxobutyl]hydroxyamino]pentyl]-N-(5-aminopentyl)-N-hydroxy-; (2) N-[5-{3-[(5-Aminopentyl)hydroxycarbamoyl] propionamido}pentyl]-3-{[5-(N-hydroxyacetamido)pentyl]carbamoyl}propionohydroxamic acid. *UNII-J06Y7MXW4D. CAS-70-51-9.* INN. *Chelating agent (iron).* ◇*NSC-527604*

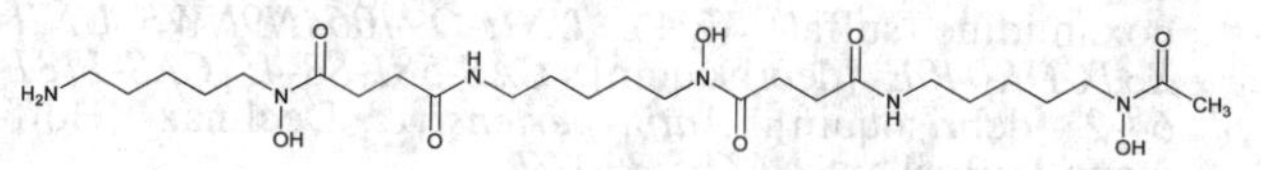

Deferoxamine Hydrochloride [*1966*] (de fer ox′ a meen hye″ droe klor′ ide). $C_{25}H_{48}N_6O_8.HCl$. 597.14. (1) Butanediamide, N'-[5-[[4-[[5-(acetylhydroxyamino)pentyl]amino]-1,4-dioxobutyl]hydroxyamino]pentyl]-N-(5-aminopentyl)-N-hydroxy- monohydrochloride; (2) N-[5-{3-[(5-Aminopentyl)hydroxycarbamoyl]propionamido}pentyl]-3-{[5-(N-hydroxyacetamido)pentyl]carbamoyl}propionohydroxamic acid monohydrochloride. *UNII-J06Y7MXW4D* [deferoxamine]. *CAS-1950-39-6; CAS-70-51-9* [deferoxamine]. ◇*Ba-29837*

Deferoxamine Mesylate [*1966*] (de fer ox′ a meen mes′ i late). **USP.** $C_{25}H_{48}N_6O_8.CH_4O_3S$. 656.79. [Deferoxamine Mesilate is JAN; Desferrioxamine Mesilate is BAN.] (1) Butanediamide, N'-[5-[[4-[[5-(acetylhydroxyamino)pentyl]amino]-1,4-dioxobutyl]hydroxyamino]pentyl]-N-(5-aminopentyl)-N-hydroxy-, monomethanesulfonate; (2) N-[5-[3-[(5-Aminopentyl)hydroxycarbamoyl]propionamido]pentyl]-3-[[5-(N-hydroxyacetamido)pentyl]carbamoyl]propionohydroxamic acid monomethanesulfonate (salt). *UNII-V9TKO7EO6K;*

UNII-J06Y7MXW4D [deferoxamine]. *CAS-138-14-7; CAS-70-51-9* [deferoxamine]. *Antidote (to iron poisoning); chelating agent.* Desferal (Novartis) ◇*Ba-33112*

Defibrotide. Polydeoxyribonucleotides from bovine lung or other mammalian organs with molecular weight between 15,000 and 30,000. INN; BAN; MI.

Deflazacort [*1986*] (dee flayz′ a kort). $C_{25}H_{31}NO_6$. 441.52. (1) 5′*H*-Pregna-1,4-dieno[17,16-*d*]oxazole-3,20-dione, 21-(acetyloxy)-11-hydroxy-2′-methyl-, (11β,16β)-; (2) 11β,21-Dihydroxy-2′-methyl-5′βH-pregna-1,4-dieno[17,16-*d*]oxazole-3,20-dione 21-acetate. *CAS-14484-47-0.* INN; BAN. *Anti-inflammatory.* ◇*MDL 458*

Deforolimus [*2007*] (dee″ for oh′ li mus). $C_{53}H_{84}NO_{14}P$. 990.21. (1) Rapamycin, 42-(dimethylphosphinate); (2) (1R,9S,12S,15R,16E,18R,19R,21R,23-S,24E,26E,28E,30S,32S,35R)-12-[(1R)-2-[(1S,3R,4R)-4-[(Dimethylphosphinoyl)oxy]-3-methoxycyclohexyl]-1-methylethyl]-1,18-dihydroxy-19,30-dimethoxy-15,17,21,23,29,35-hexamethyl-11,36-dioxa-4-azatricyclo[30.3.1.0^{4,9}]hexatriaconta-16,24,26,28-tetraene-2,3,10,14,20-pentone. *CAS-572924-54-0.* INN. *Antineoplastic.* ◇*AP23573*

Defosfamide. $C_9H_{20}Cl_3N_2O_3P$. 341.60. *N,N*-Bis(2-chloroethyl)-*N*′-(3-hydroxypropyl)phosphorodiamidic acid 2-chloroethyl ester. *UNII-0W33021S30. CAS-3733-81-1.* INN; MI.

Defoslimod. $C_{52}H_{100}N_2O_{20}P_2$. 1135.30. 2-Deoxy-6-*O*-[2-deoxy-2-[(*R*)-3-hydroxytetradecanamido]-β-D-glucopyranosyl]-2-[(*R*)-3-hydroxytetradecanamido]-α-D-glucopyranose 1,6′-bis(dihydrogen phosphate) 2′(3)-laurate. *CAS-171092-39-0.* INN.

Degarelix [*2007*] (deg″ a rel′ ix). $C_{82}H_{103}ClN_{18}O_{16}$. 1632.26. (1) D-Alaninamide, *N*-acetyl-3-(2-naphthalenyl)-D-alanyl-4-chloro-D-phenylalanyl-3-(3-pyridinyl)-D-alanyl-L-seryl-4-[[[(4S)-hexahydro-2,6-dioxo-4-pyrimidinyl]carbonyl]amino]-L-phenylalanyl-4-[(aminocarbonyl)amino]-D-phenylalanyl-L-leucyl-N^6-(1-methylethyl)-L-lysyl-L-prolyl-; (2) *N*-Acetyl-3-(naphthalen-2-yl)-D-alanyl-4-chloro-D-phenylalanyl-3-(pyridin-3-yl)-D-alanyl-L-seryl-4-({[(4S)-2,6-dioxo-hexahydropyrimidin-4-yl]carbonyl}amino)-L-phenylalanyl-4-(carbamoylamino)-D-phenylalanyl-L-leucyl-N^6-(1-methylethyl)-L-lysyl-L-prolyl-D-alaninamide. *CAS-214766-78-6.* INN. *Treatment of prostate cancer.* ◇*FE200486 (as acetate salt)*

Degarelix Acetate [*2008*] (deg″ a rel′ ix as′ e tate). $C_{82}H_{103}ClN_{18}O_{16} \cdot xC_2H_4O_2 \cdot nH_2O$. (1) D-Alaninamide, *N*-acetyl-3-(2-naphthalenyl)-D-alanyl-4-chloro-D-phenylalanyl-3-(3-pyridinyl)-D-alanyl-L-seryl-4-[[[(4S)-hexahydro-2,6-dioxo-4-pyrimidinyl]carbonyl]amino]-L-phenylalanyl-4-[(aminocarbonyl)amino]-D-phenylalanyl-L-leucyl-N^6-(1-methylethyl)-L-lysyl-L-prolyl, acetate, hydrate; (2) *N*-Acetyl-3-(naphthalen-2-yl)-D-alanyl-4-chloro-D-phenylalanyl-3-(pyridin-3-yl)-D-alanyl-L-seryl-4-({[(4S)-2,6-dioxohexahydropyrimidin-4-yl]carbonyl}amino)-L-phenylalanyl-4-(carbamoylamino)-D-phenylalanyl-L-leucyl-N^6-(1-methylethyl)-L-lysyl-L-prolyl-D-alaninamide acetate hydrate. *UNII-I18S89P20R. CAS-934246-14-7. Treatment of prostate cancer.* Firmagon (PolyPeptide) ◇*FE200486 (free base)*

Dehydroacetic Acid. $C_8H_8O_4$. 168.15. Keto form: (1) 2*H*-Pyran-2,4(3*H*)-dione, 3-acetyl-6-methyl-; (2) 3-Acetyl-6-methyl-2*H*-pyran-2,4(3*H*)-dione. Enol form: (1) 2*H*-Pyran-

2-one, 3-acetyl-4-hydroxy-6-methyl-; (2) 3-Acetyl-4-hy-droxy-6-methyl-2*H*-pyran-2-one. *CAS-520-45-6* [keto form]; *CAS-771-03-9* [enol form]. NF XVII.

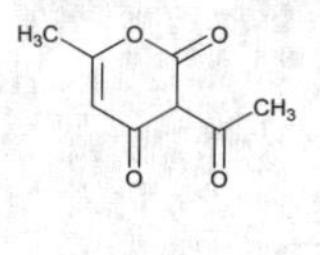

Dehydroandrosterone — *See* Prasterone.

Dehydrocholate Sodium. C$_{24}$H$_{33}$NaO$_5$. 424.51. [Sodium Dehydrocholate is INN.] (1) Cholan-24-oic acid, 3,7,12-trioxo-, sodium salt, (5β)-; (2) Sodium 3,7,12-trioxo-5β-cholan-24-oate. *UNII-W4193719XR. CAS-145-41-5; CAS-81-23-2* [dehydrocholic acid]. USP XXI. Decholin Sodium (Bayer†)

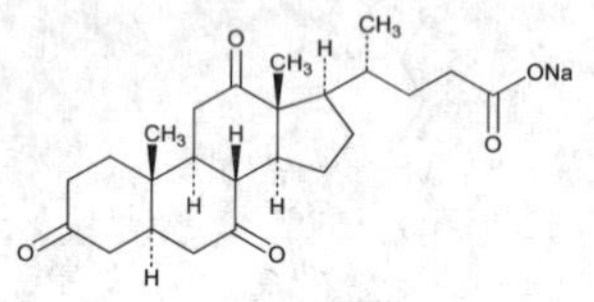

7-Dehydrocholesterol, Activated (previously used name) — *See* Cholecalciferol.

Dehydrocholic Acid (dee hye″ droe koe′ lik as′ id). **USP.** C$_{24}$H$_{34}$O$_5$. 402.52. (1) Cholan-24-oic acid, 3,7,12-trioxo-, (5β)-; (2) 3,7,12-Trioxo-5β-cholan-24-oic acid. *UNII-NH5000009I. CAS-81-23-2.* INN; BAN; JAN. *Choleretic.* Decholin (Bayer†); Dilabil (Sterling Winthrop†); Procholon (Bristol-Myers Squibb†)

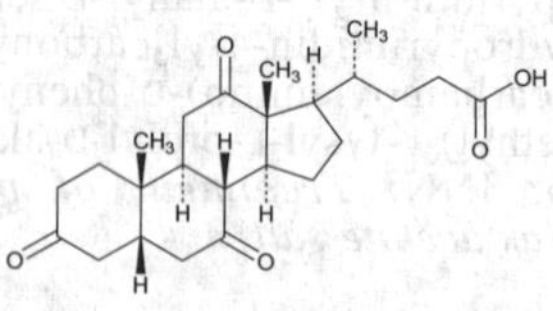

Dehydroemetine. C$_{29}$H$_{38}$N$_2$O$_4$. 478.62. 3-Ethyl-9,10-di-methoxy-1,6,7,11b-tetrahydro-2-[(1,2,3,4-tetrahydro-6,7-dimethoxy-1-isoquinolyl)methyl]-4*H*-benzo[*a*]quinolizine. *UNII-7S79QT1T91. CAS-4914-30-1.* INN; BAN; DCF; MI. ◇*Ro 1-9334/19*

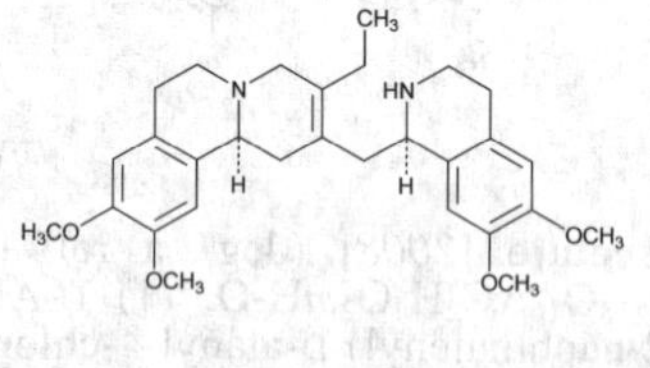

Delafloxacin [*2008*] (del″ a flox′ a sin). C$_{18}$H$_{12}$ClF$_3$N$_4$O$_4$. 440.76. (1) 3-Quinolinecarboxylic acid, 1-(6-amino-3,5-difluoro-2-pyridinyl)-8-chloro-6-fluoro-1,4-dihydro-7-(3-hydroxy-1-azetidinyl)-4-oxo-; (2) 1-(6-Amino-3,5-difluor-opyridin-2-yl)-8-chloro-6-fluoro-7-(3-hydroxyazetidin-1-yl)-4-oxo-1,4-dihydroquinoline-3-carboxylic acid. *UNII-6315412YVF. CAS-189279-58-1. Antibacterial.* ◇*RX-3341; WQ-3034; ABT-492*

Delafloxacin Meglumine [*2008*] (del″ a flox′ a sin me′ gloo meen). C$_{18}$H$_{12}$ClF$_3$N$_4$O$_4$.C$_7$H$_{17}$NO$_5$. 635.97. (1) D-Glucitol, 1-deoxy-1-(methylamino)-, 1-(6-amino-3,5-difluoro-2-pyridinyl)-8-chloro-6-fluoro-1,4-dihydro-7-(3-hydroxy-1-azetidinyl)-4-oxo-3-quinolinecarboxylate (salt); (2) 1-Deoxy-1-(methylamino)-D-glucitol 1-(6-amino-3,5-di-fluoropyridin-2-yl)-8-chloro-6-fluoro-7-(3-hydroxyazeti-din-1-yl)-4-oxo-1,4-dihydroquinoline-3-carboxylate (salt). *UNII-N7V53U4U4T. CAS-352458-37-8. Antibacterial.* ◇*RX-3341; WQ-3034; ABT-492*

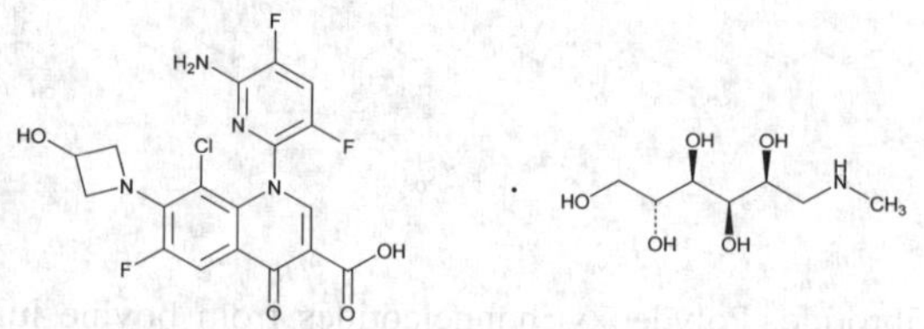

Delanterone. C$_{20}$H$_{28}$O. 284.44. 1α-Methylandrosta-4,16-dien-3-one. *UNII-AM2KZ47R0J. CAS-63014-96-0.* INN.

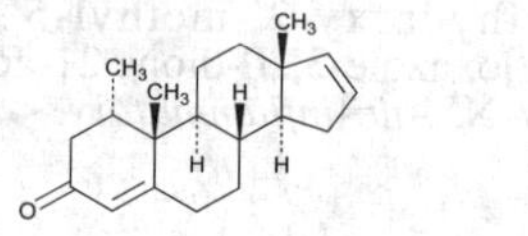

Delapril Hydrochloride [*1986*] (del′ a pril hye″ droe klor′ ide). C$_{26}$H$_{32}$N$_2$O$_5$.HCl. 489.00. [Delapril is INN.] (1) Glycine, *N*-(2,3-dihydro-1*H*-inden-2-yl)-*N*-[*N*-[1-(ethoxy-carbonyl)-3-phenylpropyl]-L-alanyl]-, monohydrochloride, (*S*)-; (2) Ethyl (*S*)-2-[[(*S*)-1-[(carboxymethyl)-2-indanyl-carbamoyl]ethyl]amino]-4-phenylbutyrate, monohy-drochloride. *UNII-2SMM3M5ZMH; UNII-W77UAL9THI* [delapril]. *CAS-83435-67-0; CAS-83435-66-9* [delapril]. JAN. *Antihypertensive; enzyme inhibitor (angiotensin-converting).* ◇*REV 6000A*

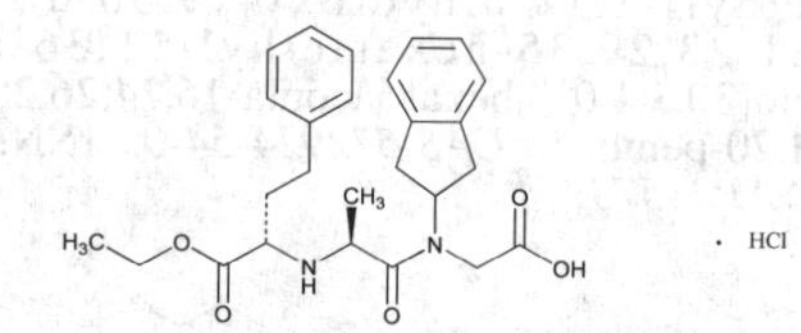

Delavirdine Mesylate [*1994*] (del″ a vir′ deen mes′ i late). C$_{22}$H$_{28}$N$_6$O$_3$S.CH$_4$O$_3$S. 552.67. [Delavirdine is INN.] (1) Piperazine, 1-[3-[(1-methylethyl)amino]-2-pyridinyl]-4-[[5-[(methylsulfonyl)amino]-1*H*-indol-2-yl]carbonyl]-, monomethanesulfonate; (2) 1-[3-(Isopropylamino)-2-pyri-dyl]-4-[(5-methanesulfonamidoindol-2-yl)carbonyl]piper-azine monomethanesulfonate. *UNII-421105KRQE; UNII-DOL5F9JD3E* [delavirdine]. *CAS-147221-93-0; CAS-136817-59-9* [delavirdine]. *Antiviral.* Rescriptor (Agouron) ◇*U-90152S*

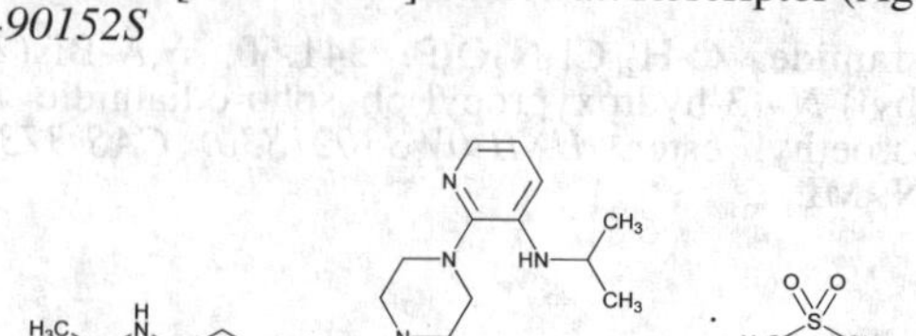

Delequamine Hydrochloride [*1994*] (del e′ kwa meen hye″ droe klor′ ide). C$_{18}$H$_{26}$N$_2$O$_3$S.HCl. 386.94. [Delequamine is INN.] (1) 6*H*-Isoquino[2,1-*g*][1,6]naphthyridine, 5,8,8a,9,10,11,12,12a,13,13a-decahydro-3-methoxy-12-(methylsulfonyl)-, monohydrochloride, [8a*R*-(8aα,12aα,13aα)]-; (2) (8a*R*,12a*S*,13a*S*)-5,8,8a,9,10,11,12,12a,13,13a-Decahydro-3-methoxy-12-(methylsulfonyl)-6*H*-isoquino[2,1-*g*][1,6]naphthyridine monohydrochloride. *CAS-119942-75-5; CAS-119905-05-4* [delequamine]. *Impotence therapy adjunct.* ◇*RS-15385-197*

Delergotrile. $C_{17}H_{19}N_3$. 265.35. 6-Methylergoline-8α-acetonitrile. *UNII-3U2FEE7NXX. CAS-59091-65-5.* INN.

Delfantrine. $C_{14}H_{22}N_4O_3S$. 326.41. *N′,N′-Dimethyl-3-[(4-methyl-1-piperazinyl)carbonyl]sulfanilamide. UNII-72C4702BMV. CAS-3436-11-1.* INN. ◇*Ba-32968*

Delfaprazine. $C_{18}H_{22}N_2$. 266.38. 1-(α²-Phenyl-2,5-xylyl)piperazine. *UNII-06YTS68E0H. CAS-117827-81-3.* INN.

Deligoparin Sodium [*2002*] (del″ i gope′ a rin soe′ dee um; del″ i goe par′ in soe′ dee um). Heparin, sodium salt. Molecular weight is approximately 3200 daltons ± 650 daltons. *CAS-9041-08-1.* INN. *Treatment of inflammatory bowel disease.* ◇*OP2000*

Delimotecan. [$C_{39}H_{46}N_6O_{14}[C_6H_{10}O_5]_x[C_8H_{12}O_7]_y]_n$. Poly{[2-*O*-(carboxymethyl)-α-D-glucopyranosyl-(1→6)]-*co*-[2-*O*-(15-{[(4*S*)-4,11-diethyl-4-hydroxy-3,14-dioxo-3,4,12,14-tetrahydro-1*H*-pyrano[3′,4′:6,7]indolizino[1,2-*b*]quinolin-9-yl]oxy}-2,5,8,11-tetraoxo-3,6,9,12-tetraazapentadecyl)-α-D-glucopyranosyl-(1→6)]-*co*-[α-D-glucopyranosyl-(1→6)]}. *CAS-187852-63-7* [for Na salt]. INN.

Delmadinone Acetate [*1970*] (del mad′ i none as′ e tate). $C_{23}H_{27}ClO_4$. 402.91. [Delmadinone is INN and BAN.] (1) Pregna-1,4,6-triene-3,20-dione, 17-(acetyloxy)-6-chloro-;

(2) 6-Chloro-17-hydroxypregna-1,4,6-triene-3,20-dione acetate. *CAS-13698-49-2; CAS-15262-77-8* [delmadinone]. *Progestin; anti-androgen; anti-estrogen.* ◇*RS-1301*

Delmetacin. $C_{18}H_{15}NO_3$. 293.32. 1-Benzoyl-2-methylindole-3-acetic acid. *UNII-I9Q51XHI1K. CAS-16401-80-2.* INN.

Delmitide Acetate [*2004*] (del′ mi tide as′ e tate). $C_{59}H_{105}N_{17}O_{11} \cdot C_2H_4O_2$. 1288.62. [Delmitide is INN.] (1) D-Tyrosinamide, D-arginyl-D-norleucyl-D-norleucyl-D-norleucyl-D-arginyl-D-norleucyl-D-norleucyl-D-norleucylglycyl-, monoacetate; (2) D-Arginyl-(2*R*)-2-aminohexanoyl-(2*R*)-2-aminohexanoyl-(2*R*)-2-aminohexanoyl-D-arginyl-(2*R*)-2-aminohexanoyl-(2*R*)-2-aminohexanoyl-(2*R*)-2-aminohexanoylglycyl-D-tyrosinamide monoacetate. *UNII-5Y1CNW44Y5. CAS-501019-16-5; CAS-287096-87-1* [delmitide]. *Treatment of chemotherapy-induced diarrhea (CID).* ◇*RSP58*

Delmopinol. $C_{16}H_{33}NO_2$. 271.44. (±)-3-(4-Propylheptyl)-4-morpholineethanol. *UNII-DT67WL708F. CAS-79874-76-3.* INN.

Delorazepam. $C_{15}H_{10}Cl_2N_2O$. 305.16. 7-Chloro-5-(*o*-chlorophenyl)-1,3-dihydro-2*H*-1,4-benzodiazepin-2-one. *CAS-2894-67-9.* INN.

---

† Brand name formerly used, and/or firm no longer concerned with this product.

Deloxolone. $C_{34}H_{52}O_6$. 556.77. 3β-Hydroxyolean-9(11)-en-30-oic acid, hydrogen succinate. *CAS-68635-50-7*. INN.

Delprostenate. $C_{23}H_{29}ClO_6$. 436.93. Methyl(2*E*,5*Z*)-7-[(1*R*,2*R*,3*R*,5*S*)-2-[(*E*)-(3*R*)-4-(*m*-chloro-phenoxy)-3-hydroxy-1-butenyl]-3,5-dihydroxycyclopentyl]-2,5-heptadienoate. *UNII-M99W4Q30OL. CAS-62524-99-6.* INN; BAN.

delta-9-Tetrahydrocannabinol — *See* Dronabinol.

delta-9-THC — *See* Dronabinol.

Deltafilcon A [*1978*] (del″ ta fil′ kon). $(C_6H_{10}O_3)_w$ $(C_4H_6O_2)_x(C_{18}H_{26}O_6)_y(C_8H_{14}O_2)_z$. (1) 2-Propenoic acid, 2-methyl-, 2-hydroxyethyl ester, polymer with 2-methyl-2-propenoic acid, 2-ethyl-2-[[(2-methyl-1-oxo-2-propenyl)oxy]methyl]-1,3-propanediyl bis(2-methyl-2-propenoate) and 2-methylpropyl 2-methyl-2-propenoate; (2) 2-Hydroxyethyl methacrylate polymer with methacrylic acid, 2-ethyl-2-(hydroxymethyl)-1,3-propanediol trimethacrylate and isobutyl methacrylate. *CAS-62906-34-7. Contact lens material (hydrophilic).*

Deltafilcon B [*1985*] (del″ ta fil′ kon). $(C_6H_{10}O_3)_w(C_4H_6O_2)_x$ $(C_{18}H_{26}O_6)_y(C_8H_{14}O_2)_z$. (1) 2-Propenoic acid, 2-methyl-, 2-hydroxyethyl ester, polymer with 2-methyl-2-propenoic acid, 2-ethyl-2-[[(2-methyl-1-oxo-2-propenyl)oxy]-methyl]-1,3-propanediyl bis(2-methyl-2-propenoate) and 2-methylpropyl 2-methyl-2-propenoate; (2) 2-Hydroxyethyl methacrylate polymer with methacrylic acid, 2-ethyl-2-(hydroxymethyl)-1,3-propanediol trimethacrylate and isobutyl methacrylate. *CAS-62906-34-7. Contact lens material (hydrophilic).* Amsof (Lombart); Amsof-Thin (Lombart); Aquasight (Lombart†); Aquasight-Thin (Lombart†) *[Note—Graphic formula same as for Deltafilcon A.]*

Deltamethrin. $C_{22}H_{19}Br_2NO_3$. 505.20. (*S*)-α-Cyano-3-phenoxybenzyl (1*R*,3*S*)-3-(2,2-dibromovinyl)-2,2-dimethylcyclopropanecarboxylate. *CAS-52918-63-5.* BAN.

Deltibant [*1996*] (del′ ti bant). $C_{128}H_{194}N_{40}O_{28}S_2$. 2805.29. (1) L-Arginine, D-arginyl-L-arginyl-L-prolyl-*trans*-4-hydroxy-L-prolylglycyl-L-phenylalanyl-*S*-[1-[6-(3-mercapto-2,5-dioxo-1-pyrrolidinyl)hexyl]-2,5-dioxo-3-pyrrolidinyl]-L-cysteinyl-D-phenylalanyl-L-leucyl-L-arginine, (7→7′)-sulfide with D-arginyl-L-arginyl-L-prolyl-*trans*-4-hydroxy-L-prolylglycyl-L-phenylalanyl-L-cysteinyl-D-phenylalanyl-L-leucyl-[*R*-(*R**,*S**)]-; (2) D-Arginyl-L-arginyl-L-prolyl-*trans*-4-hydroxy-L-prolylgylcyl-L-phenylalanyl-L-cysteinyl-D-phenylalanyl-L-leucyl-L-arginine, 7,7′-bis(sulfide) with (2*R*,2′*S*)-*N*,*N*′-hexamethylenebis[2-mercaptosuccinimide]. *CAS-140661-97-8.* INN. *Antagonist (bradykinin).* ◇*CP-0127*

Delucemine Hydrochloride [*2002*] (del ue′ se meen hye″ droe klor′ ide). $C_{16}H_{17}F_2N\cdot HCl$. 297.77. [Delucemine is INN.] (1) Benzenepropanamine, 3-fluoro-γ-(3-fluorophenyl)-*N*-methyl-, hydrochloride; (2) 3,3-Bis-(*m*-fluorophenyl)-*N*-methylpropylamine hydrochloride. *UNII-P110CQY44Z; UNII-124LSR3H2X* [delucemine]. *CAS-186495-99-8; CAS-186495-49-8* [delucemine]. *Neuroprotection (NMDA receptor antagonist).* ◇*NPS 1506·HCl*

Dembrexine. $C_{13}H_{17}Br_2NO_2$. 379.09. *trans*-4-[(3,5-Dibromosalicyl)amino]cyclohexanol. *UNII-4F61F502T5. CAS-83200-09-3.* INN; BAN.

Dembroxol — *See* Dembrexine.

Demecarium Bromide (dem″ e kar′ ee um broe′ mide). **USP**. $C_{32}H_{52}Br_2N_4O_4$. 716.59. (1) Benzenaminium, 3,3′-[1,10-decanediylbis[(methylimino)carbonyloxy]]bis[*N*,*N*,*N*-trimethyl-, dibromide; (2) (*m*-Hydroxyphenyl)trimethylammonium bromide decamethylenebis[methylcarbamate] (2:1). *UNII-61D5V4OKTP. CAS-56-94-0.* INN; BAN. *Cholinergic (ophthalmic).* Humorsol (Merck)

Demeclocycline (dem″ e kloe sye′ kleen). **USP**. $C_{21}H_{21}ClN_2O_8$. 464.85. [Demethylchlortetracycline is JAN.] (1) 2-Naphthacenecarboxamide, 7-chloro-4-(dimethylamino)-1,4,4a,5,5a,6,11,12a-octahydro-3,6,10,12,12a-pentahydroxy-1,11-dioxo-, [4*S*-(4α,4aα,5aα,6β,12aα)]-; (2) 7-Chloro-4-(dimethylamino)-1,4,4a,5,5a,6,11,12a-octahydro-3,6,10,12,12a-pentahydroxy-1,11-dioxo-2-naphthacenecarboxamide. *UNII-5R5W9ICI6O. CAS-127-33-3; CAS-13215-10-6* [sesquihydrate]. BAN. *Antibacterial. [Name previously used: Demethylchlortetracycline.]*

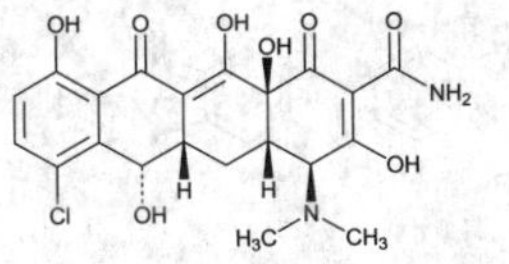

Demeclocycline Hydrochloride (dem″ e kloe sye′ kleen hye″ droe klor′ ide). **USP.** $C_{21}H_{21}ClN_2O_8 \cdot HCl$. 501.31. [Demethylchlortetracycline Hydrochloride is JAN.] (1) 2-Naphthacenecarboxamide, 7-chloro-4-(dimethylamino)-1,4,4a,5,5a,6,11,12a-octahydro-3,6,10,12,12a-pentahydroxy-1,11-dioxo-, monohydrochloride, [4*S*-(4α,4aα,5aα,6β,12aα)]-; (2) 7-Chloro-4-(dimethylamino)-1,4,4a,5,5a,6,11,12a-octahydro-3,6,10,12,12a-pentahydroxy-1,11-dioxo-2-naphthacenecarboxamide monohydrochloride. *UNII-29O079NTYT; UNII-5R5W9ICI6O* [demeclocycline]. *CAS-64-73-3; CAS-127-33-3* [demeclocycline]. BAN. *Antibacterial.* Declomycin (Stiefel)

Demecolcine. $C_{21}H_{25}NO_5$. 371.43. Deacetyl-*N*-methylcolchicine. *CAS-477-30-5.* INN; BAN; DCF; MI. ◇*C-12669; NSC-3096*

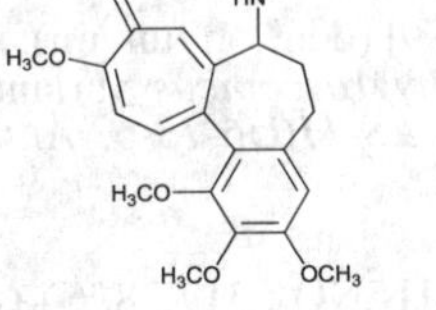

Demecycline [*1963*] (dem″ e sye′ kleen). $C_{21}H_{22}N_2O_8$. 430.41. (1) 2-Naphthacenecarboxamide, 4-(dimethylamino)-1,4,4a,5,5a,6,11,12a-octahydro-3,6,10,12,12a-pentahydroxy-1,11-dioxo-, [4*S*-(4α,4aα,5aα,6β,12aα)]-; (2) 4-(Dimethylamino)-1,4,4*a*,5,5a,6,11,12*a*-octahydro-3,6,10,12,12*a*-pentahydroxy-1,11-dioxo-2-naphthacenecarboxamide. *UNII-TV240CH11P. CAS-987-02-0.* INN. *Antibacterial.* ◇*A IX; CL 22415*

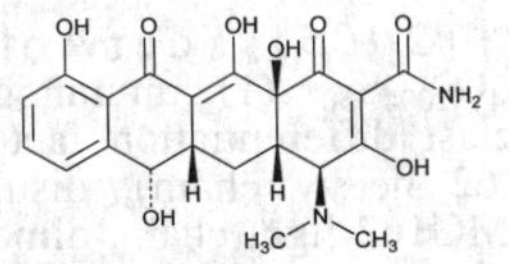

Demegestone. $C_{21}H_{28}O_2$. 312.45. 17-Methyl-19-norpregna-4,9-diene-3,20-dione. *UNII-6E89AM91SZ. CAS-10116-22-0.* INN; DCF; MI. ◇*R 2453*

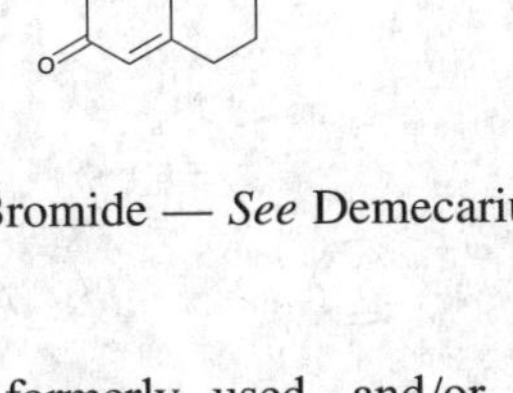

Demekastigmine Bromide — *See* Demecarium Bromide.

Demelverine. $C_{17}H_{21}N$. 239.36. *N*-Methyldiphenethylamine. *UNII-MX0B07OP8M. CAS-13977-33-8.* INN.

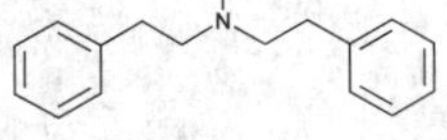

Demetacin — *See* Delmetacin.

Demethylchlortetracycline (JAN, DCF and previously used name) — *See* Demeclocycline.

Demethylchlortetracycline Hydrochloride (JAN) — *See* Demeclocycline Hydrochloride.

Demexiptiline. $C_{18}H_{18}N_2O$. 278.35. 5*H*-Dibenzo[*a,d*]cyclohepten-5-one *O*-[2-(methylamino)ethyl]oxime. *UNII-EYX738UZ5P. CAS-24701-51-7.* INN; MI.

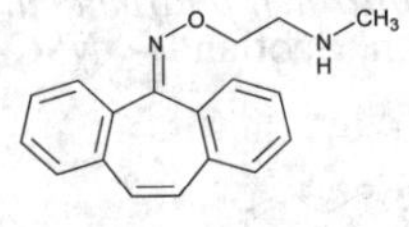

Demiditraz. $C_{13}H_{16}N_2$. 200.28. 2-[(1*S*)-1-(2,3-Dimethylphenyl)ethyl]-1*H*-imidazole. *CAS-944263-65-4.* INN.

Democonazole. $C_{19}H_{15}Cl_3N_2O_2$. 409.69. (*E*)-1-[2,4-Dichloro-β-[2-(*p*-chlorophenoxy)ethoxy]styryl]imidazole. *UNII-2Z4E7E087J. CAS-70161-09-0.* INN.

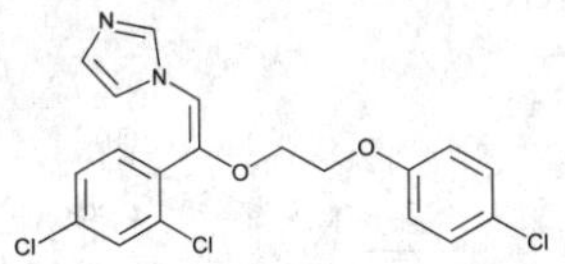

Demoxepam [*1970*] (dem ox′ e pam). $C_{15}H_{11}ClN_2O_2$. 286.71. (1) 2*H*-1,4-Benzodiazepin-2-one, 7-chloro-1,3-dihydro-5-phenyl-, 4-oxide; (2) 7-Chloro-1,3-dihydro-5-phenyl-2*H*-1,4-benzodiazepin-2-one 4-oxide. *CAS-963-39-3.* INN. *Tranquilizer (minor).* ◇*Ro 5-2092; NSC-46077*

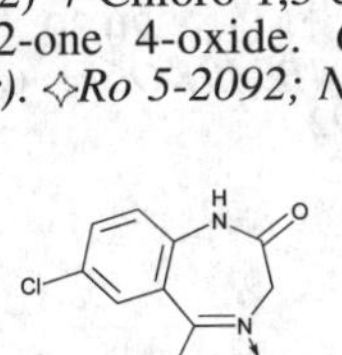

Demoxytocin. $C_{43}H_{65}N_{11}O_{12}S_2$. 992.17. 1-(3-Mercaptopropionic acid)-oxytocin. *CAS-113-78-0.* INN. Sandopart (Novartis†) ◇*ODA 914*

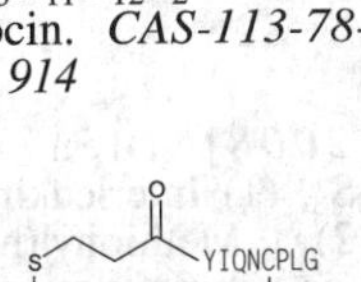

Denagliptin Tosylate [*2006*] (den″ a glip′ tin tos′ i late). $C_{20}H_{18}F_3N_3O \cdot C_7H_8O_3S$. 545.57. [Denagliptin is INN.] (1) 2-Pyrrolidinecarbonitrile, 1-[(2*S*)-2-amino-3,3-bis(4-fluorophenyl)-1-oxopropyl]-4-fluoro-, (2*S*,4*S*)-, mono(4-methylbenzenesulfonate); (2) (2*S*,4*S*)-1-[(2*S*)-2-Amino-3,3-bis(4-fluorophenyl)propanoyl]-4-fluoropyrrolidine-2-carbonitrile 4-methylbenzenesulfonate. *UNII-*

---

† Brand name formerly used, and/or firm no longer concerned with this product.

T47477CUF7; UNII-DOS9ZOT21L [denagliptin]. *CAS-811432-66-3; CAS-483369-58-0* [denagliptin]. *Treatment of Type 2 diabetes.* ◇*GW823093C*

Denatonium Benzoate [*1965*] (den″ a toe′ nee um ben′ zoe ate). **NF.** $C_{28}H_{34}N_2O_3 \cdot H_2O$. 464.60. (1) Benzenemethana-minium, *N*-[2-[(2,6-dimethylphenyl)amino]-2-oxoethyl]-*N,N*-diethyl-, benzoate, monohydrate; (2) Benzyl-diethyl[(2,6-xylylcarbamoyl)methyl]ammonium benzoate monohydrate. *UNII-4YK5Z54AT2. CAS-86398-53-0; CAS-3734-33-6* [anhydrous]. INN; BAN. *Pharmaceutic aid (alcohol denaturant); pharmaceutic aid (flavor).* Bitrex (Mac Farlan Smith, Scotland) ◇*NSC-157658*

Denaverine. $C_{24}H_{33}NO_3$. 383.52. 2-(Dimethylamino)ethyl (2-ethylbutoxy)diphenylacetate. *UNII-O14NF38MTL. CAS-3579-62-2.* INN.

Denbufylline. $C_{16}H_{24}N_4O_3$. 320.39. 7-Acetonyl-1,3-dibutyl-xanthine. *UNII-04B949KO6F. CAS-57076-71-8.* INN; BAN. ◇*BRL 30892*

Denenicokin [*2008*] (den″ en i koe′ kin). $C_{676}H_{1087}N_{205}O_{203}S_8$. (1) Interleukin 21 [methionyl] (syn-thetic human); (2) L-Methionyl(human interleukin-21). Molecular weight is approximately 15,590 daltons. *CAS-716840-32-3.* INN. *Treatment of cancer.* ◇*IL-21; rIL-21; recombinant human interleukin 21*

Denibulin Hydrochloride [*2006*] (den″ i bue′ lin hye″ droe klor′ ide). $C_{18}H_{19}N_5O_3S \cdot HCl$. 421.90. [Denibulin is INN.] (1) Carbamic acid, [5-[[4-[[(2*S*)-2-amino-1-oxopropyl]a-mino]phenyl]thio]-1*H*-benzimidazol-2-yl]-, methyl ester, monohydrochloride; (2) Methyl [5-[[4-[[(2*S*)-2-aminopro-panoyl]amino]phenyl]sulfanyl]-1*H*-benzimidazol-2-yl]car-

bamate monohydrochloride. *UNII-0U575HR16Q. CAS-779356-64-8; CAS-284019-34-7* [denibulin]. *Treatment of solid tumors.* ◇*MN-029*

Denileukin Diftitox [*1997*] (den″ i loo′ kin dif′ ti tox). $C_{2560}H_{4036}N_{678}O_{799}S_{17}$. *N*-L-Methionyl-387-L-histidine-388-L-alanine-1-388-toxin (*Corynebacterium diphtheriae* strain C7) (388→2′) protein with 2-133-interleukin 2 (human clone pTIL2-21a). *UNII-25E79B5CTM. CAS-173146-27-5.* INN; BAN. *Biological response modifier; antineoplastic.* ◇*LY335348; DAB$_{389}$IL2*

Denipride. $C_{18}H_{26}N_4O_5$. 378.42. (±)-4-Amino-5-nitro-*N*-[1-(tetrahydrofurfuryl)-4-piperidyl]-*o*-anisamide. *UNII-T5IBT2ZQS3. CAS-106972-33-2.* INN.

Denofungin [*1970*] (den″ oh fun′ jin). Antibiotic produced by *Streptomyces hygroscopicus* variant. (1) Denofungin; (2) Denofungin. *CAS-11056-13-6. Antifungal; antibacterial.* ◇*U-28,009*

Denopamine. $C_{18}H_{23}NO_4$. 317.38. (-)-(*R*)-α-[[(3,4-Dimethox-yphenethyl)amino]methyl]-*p*-hydroxybenzyl alcohol. *UNII-V5F60UPD8P. CAS-71771-90-9.* INN; JAN; MI.

Denosumab [*2005*] (den oh′ sue mab). $C_{6404}H_{9912}N_{1724}O_{2004}S_{50}$. (1) Immunoglobulin G2, anti-(human osteoclast differentiation factor) (human mono-clonal AMG162 heavy chain), disulfide with human monoclonal AMG162 light chain, dimer; (2) Immunoglo-bulin G2, anti-(human RANK ligand) (human monoclonal AMG162 heavy chain), disulfide with human monoclonal AMG162 light chain, dimer. Molecular weight is approxi-mately 144,700 daltons. *CAS-615258-40-7.* INN. *Preven-tion and treatment of all forms of osteoporosis or bone loss.* ◇*AMG 162*

Denotivir. $C_{18}H_{14}ClN_3O_2S$. 371.84. 5-Benzamido-4′-chloro-3-methyl-4-isothiazolecarboxanilide. *UNII-W656S9I00W. CAS-51287-57-1.* INN.

Denpidazone. $C_{20}H_{20}N_2O_3$. 336.38. 4-Butyl-1,2-dihydro-5-hydroxy-1,2-diphenyl-3,6-pyridazinedione. *UNII-E7N3FX2T1J. CAS-42438-73-3.* INN.

Denufosol Tetrasodium [*2004*] (den″ ue fos′ ol tet″ ra soe′ dee um). $C_{18}H_{23}N_5Na_4O_{21}P_4$. 861.25. [Denufosol is INN.] (1) Uridine 5′-(pentahydrogen tetraphosphate), P‴→5′-ester with ″-deoxycytidine, tetrasodium salt; (2) 2′-Deoxycytidine(5′)tetraphospho(5′)uridine tetrasodium salt. *UNII-5PC250KSSH* [denufosol]. *CAS-318250-11-2; CAS-211448-85-0* [denufosol]. *Treatment of rhinitis, URI and lung disease, cystic fibrosis, retinal detachment and edema.* ◇INS37217

Denzimol. $C_{19}H_{20}N_2O$. 292.37. (±)-α-(*p*-Phenethylphenyl)imidazole-1-ethanol. *UNII-9C78O7JATH. CAS-73931-96-1.* INN.

Deoxycorticosterone Acetate — *See* Desoxycorticosterone Acetate.

Deoxycortone (previously used name) — *See* Desoxycorticosterone Acetate.

15-Deoxyspergualin trihydrochloride — *See* Gusperimus Trihydrochloride.

Depelestat [*2004*] (de pel′ e stat). $C_{282}H_{412}N_{74}O_{75}S_6$. 6231.13. (1) Proteinase inhibitor M/NEI (synthetic human); (2) Human recombinant neutrophil elastase inhibitor, homologue of the second Kunitz domain of Inter-alpha-trypsin inhibitor light chain: [Glu285,Ile297,Phe300,Pro301,Arg302]AMBP protein precursor-(285-340)-peptide (human). *UNII-2M3V3B8OEA. CAS-506433-25-6.* INN. *Treatment of bronchopulmonary inflammatory damage, specifically Cystic Fibrosis.* ◇DX-890

```
EACNLPIVRG PCIAFFPRWA FDAVKGKCVL FPYGGCQGNG NKFYSEKECR
EYCGVP
```

Depramine. $C_{19}H_{22}N_2$. 278.39. 5-[3-(Dimethylamino)propyl]-5*H*-dibenz[*b,f*]azepine. *UNII-77C3T28736. CAS-303-54-8.* INN; BAN. [*Name previously used: Balipramine.*] ◇GP 31406

L-Deprenyl — *See* Selegiline Hydrochloride.

Depreotide [*1998*] (de pree′ oh tide). $C_{65}H_{96}N_{16}O_{12}S_2$. 1357.69. (1) Cyclo(L-homocysteinyl-*N*-methyl-L-phenylalanyl-L-tyrosyl-D-tryptophyl-L-lysyl-L-valyl) (1→1′)-sulfide with 3-[(mercaptoacetyl)amino]-L-alanyl-L-lysyl-L-cysteinyl-L-lysinamide; (2) Cyclo(L-homocysteinyl-*N*-methyl-L-phenylalanyl-L-tyrosyl-D-tryptophyl-L-lysyl-L-valyl), (1→1′)-sulfide with 3-(2-mercaptoacetamido)-L-alanyl-L-lysyl-L-cysteinyl-L-lysinamide. *CAS-161982-62-3.* INN. *Diagnostic aid (nuclear medicine imaging agent used in the detection and localization of somatostatin receptor expressing tumors).* ◇P829

Deprodone. $C_{21}H_{28}O_4$. 344.44. 11β,17-Dihydroxypregna-1,4-diene-3,20-dione. *UNII-Z380L7N00P. CAS-20423-99-8.* INN; BAN.

Deprostil [*1974*] (de prost′ il). $C_{21}H_{38}O_4$. 354.52. (1) Prostan-1-oic acid, 15-hydroxy-15-methyl-9-oxo-; (2) (1*R*,2*S*)-2-(3-Hydroxy-3-methyloctyl)-5-oxocyclopentaneheptanoic acid. *UNII-J651EHI78N. CAS-33813-84-2.* INN. *Antisecretory (gastric).* ◇AY 22,469

---

† Brand name formerly used, and/or firm no longer concerned with this product.

Deptropine Citrate. $C_{23}H_{27}NO.C_6H_8O_7$. 525.59. [Deptropine is INN and BAN.] 3-[10,11-Dihydro-5*H*-dibenzo[*a,d*]cyclohepten-5-yloxy]tropane citrate. *CAS-2169-75-7; CAS-604-51-3* [deptropine]. MI. ◇*BS 6987*

Dequalinium Chloride. $C_{30}H_{40}Cl_2N_4$. 527.57. 1,1'-Decamethylenebis(4-aminoquinaldinium chloride). *UNII-XYS8INN1I6. CAS-522-51-0; CAS-6707-58-0* [dequalinium]. INN; BAN; JAN; MI. ◇*BAQD 10*

Deracoxib [*1998*] (der″ a kox′ ib). $C_{17}H_{14}F_3N_3O_3S$. 397.37. 4-[3-(Difluoromethyl)-5-(3-fluoro-4-methoxyphenyl)-1*H*-pyrazol-1-yl]benzenesulfonamide. *UNII-VX29JB5XWV. CAS-169590-41-4.* INN. *Anti-inflammatory; analgesic (cyclooxygenase [COX-2] inhibitor).* ◇*SC-59046*

Deramciclane. $C_{20}H_{31}NO$. 301.47. *N,N*-Dimethyl-2-[[(1*R*,2*S*,4*R*)-2-phenyl-2-bornyl]oxy]ethylamine. *CAS-120444-71-5.* INN.

Deriglidole. $C_{16}H_{21}N_3$. 255.36. (+)-1,2,4,5-Tetrahydro-2-(2-imidazolin-2-yl)-2-propylpyrrolo[3,2,1-*hi*]indole. *UNII-68EP8R4PMV. CAS-122830-14-2.* INN.

Dermatan Sulfate — *See* Danaparoid Sodium.

Derpanicate. $C_{46}H_{54}N_8O_{12}S_2$. 975.10. Nicotinic acid, tetraester with *N,N*′-[dithiobis(ethyleneiminocarbonylethylene)]bis[(*R*)-2,4-dihydroxy-3,3-dimethylbutyramide]. *CAS-99518-29-3.* INN.

Derquantel [*2007*] (der kwon′ tel). $C_{28}H_{37}N_3O_4$. 479.61. (1) Spiro[4*H*,8*H*-[1,4]dioxepino[2,3-*g*]indole-8,7′(8′*H*)-[5*H*,6*H*-5a,9a](iminomethano)[1*H*]cyclopent[*f*]indolizin]-10′-one, 2′,3′,8′a,9,9′,10-hexahydro-1′-hydroxy-1′,4,4,8′,8′,11′-hexamethyl-, (1′*R*,5′a*S*,7′*R*,8′a*S*,9′a*R*)-; (2) (1′*R*,5′a*S*,7′*R*,8′a*S*,9′a*R*)-1′-Hydroxy-1′,4,4,8′,8′,11′-hexamethyl-2′,3′,8′a,9,9′,10-hexahydrospiro[4*H*,8*H*-[1,4]dioxepino[2,3-*g*]indole-8,7′(8′*H*)-[5*H*,6*H*-5a,9a](iminomethano)[1*H*]cyclopenta[*f*]indolizin]-10′-one; (3) (1*S*,6*R*,7*R*,9*S*,11*R*)-6-Hydroxy-4′,4′,6,10,10,13-hexamethyl-9′,10′-dihydro-4′*H*-spiro[3,13-diazatetracyclo[5.5.2.0^{1,9}.0^{3,7}]tetradecane-11,8′-[1,4]dioxepino[2,3-*g*]indol]-14-one. *UNII-0L0UGK6OOX. CAS-187865-22-1.* INN. *Anthelmintic.* ◇*PF-00520904*

Dersalazine. $C_{35}H_{32}N_6O_4$. 600.67. 2-Hydroxy-5-[[4-[(1*Z*)-3-[4-[(2-methyl-1*H*-imidazo[4,5-*c*]pyridin-1-yl)methyl]piperidin-1-yl]-3-oxo-1-phenylprop-1-enyl]phenyl]diazenyl]benzoic acid. *UNII-WS1IH75AJT. CAS-188913-58-8.* INN.

Desacetyl-Lanatoside C — *See* Deslanoside.

Desaglybuzole (DCF) — *See* Glybuzole.

Desamino-Oxytocin — *See* Demoxytocin.

Desaspidin. $C_{24}H_{30}O_8$. 446.49. 3′-[(5-Butyryl-2,4-dihydroxy-3,3-dimethyl-6-oxo-1,4-cyclohexadien-1-yl)methyl]-2′,6′-dihydroxy-4′-methoxybutyrophenone. *UNII-KV3495SGKS. CAS-114-43-2.* INN; MI.

Desciclovir [*1987*] (des sye′ kloe vir). $C_8H_{11}N_5O_2$. 209.21. (1) Ethanol, 2-[(2-amino-9*H*-purin-9-yl)methoxy]-; (2) 2-[(2-Amino-9*H*-purin-9-yl)methoxy]ethanol. *UNII-BHM1XXA2EZ. CAS-84408-37-7.* INN. *Antiviral.* ◇*BW A515U*

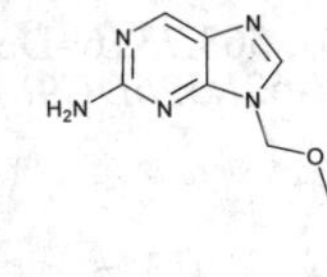

Descinolone Acetonide [*1966*] (des in′ oh lone a seet′ oh nide). $C_{24}H_{31}FO_5$. 418.50. [Descinolone is INN.] (1) Pregna-1,4-diene-3,20-dione, 9-fluoro-11-hydroxy-16,17-[(1-methylethylidene)bis(oxy)]-, (11*β*,16*α*)-; (2) 9-Fluoro-11*β*,16*α*,17-trihydroxypregna-1,4-diene-3,20-dione cyclic 16,17-acetal with acetone. *CAS-2135-14-0. Glucocorticoid.* ◇*CL 27,071; NSC-44827*

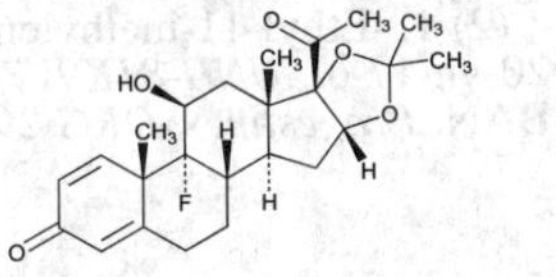

Deserpidine. $C_{32}H_{38}N_2O_8$. 578.65. (1) Methyl 17*α*-methoxy-18*β*-[(3,4,5-trimethoxybenzoyl)oxy]-3*β*,20*α*-yohimban-16*β*-carboxylate; (2) Methyl 18*β*-hydroxy-17*α*-methoxy-3*β*,20*α*-yohimban-16*β*-carboxylate, 3,4,5-trimethoxybenzoate (ester). *UNII-9016E3VB47. CAS-131-01-1.* INN; BAN; MI. Harmonyl (Abbott)

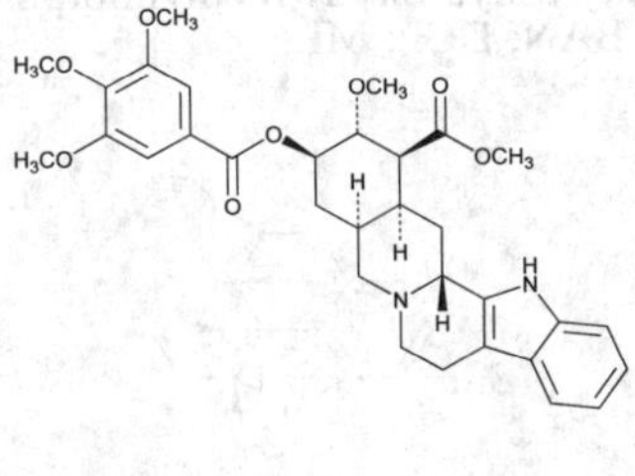

Desferrioxamine (BAN) — *See* Deferoxamine.

Desferrioxamine Mesilate (BAN) — *See* Deferoxamine Mesylate.

Desflurane [*1990*] (des floo′ rane). **USP**. $C_3H_2F_6O$. 168.04. (1) Ethane, 2-(difluoromethoxy)-1,1,1,2-tetrafluoro-, (±)-; (2) (±)-2-Difluoromethyl 1,2,2,2-tetrafluoroethyl ether. *UNII-CRS35BZ94Q. CAS-57041-67-5.* INN. *Anesthetic.* Suprane (Baxter Healthcare) ◇*I-653*

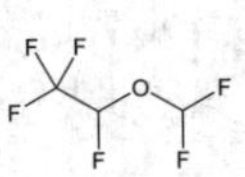

Desglugastrin. $C_{49}H_{61}N_9O_{13}$. 984.06. *N*-(4-Carboxybutyryl)-L-alanyl-L-tyrosylglycyl-L-tryptophyl-L-leucyl-L-*α*-aspartylphenyl-L-alaninamide. *CAS-51987-65-6.* INN.

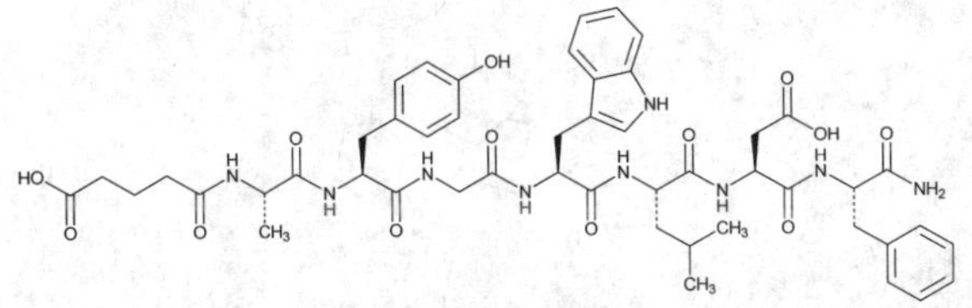

Desipramine Hydrochloride [*1962*] (des ip′ ra meen hye″ droe klor′ ide). **USP**. $C_{18}H_{22}N_2$.HCl. 302.84. [Desipramine is INN and BAN.] (1) 5*H*-Dibenz[*b,f*]azepine-5-propanamine, 10,11-dihydro-*N*-methyl-, monohydrochloride; (2) 10,11-Dihydro-5-[3-(methylamino)propyl]-5*H*-dibenz[*b,f*]azepine monohydrochloride. *UNII-1Y58DO4MY1; UNII-TG537D343B* [desipramine]. *CAS-58-28-6; CAS-50-47-5* [desipramine]. JAN. *Antidepressant.* Norpramin (Sanofi Aventis) ◇*G-35020; DMI; JB-8181; EX 4355; RMI 9,384A; NSC-114901*

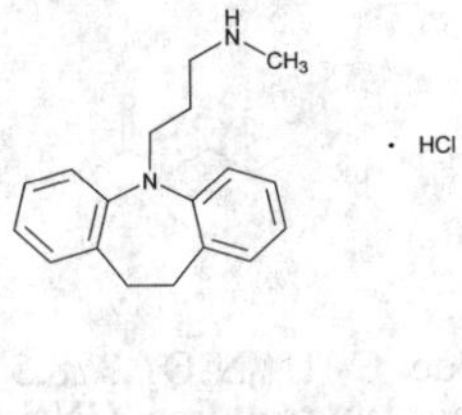

Desirudin [*1994*] (des″ i roo′ din). $C_{287}H_{440}N_{80}O_{110}S_6$. 6963.42. (1) Hirudin (*Hirudo medicinalis* isoform HV1), 63-desulfo-; (2) 63-Desulfohirudin (*Hirudo medicinalis* isoform HV1). *UNII-U0JZ726775. CAS-120993-53-5.* INN; BAN. *Anticoagulant.* ◇*CGP 39393*

```
VVYTDCTESG QNLCLCEGSN VCGQGNKCIL GSDGEKNQCV TGEGTPKPQS
HNDGDFEEIP EEYLQ
```

Deslanoside (des lan′ oh side). **USP**. $C_{47}H_{74}O_{19}$. 943.08. (1) Card-20(22)-enolide, 3-[(*O*-*β*-D-glucopyranosyl-(1→4)-*O*-2,6-dideoxy-*β*-D-*ribo*-hexopyranosyl-(1→4)-*O*-2,6-dideoxy-*β*-D-*ribo*-hexopyranosyl-(1→4)-2,6-dideoxy-*β*-D-*ribo*-hexopyranosyl)oxy]-12,14-dihydroxy-, (3*β*,5*β*,12*β*)-; (2) Deacetyllanatoside C. *UNII-YGY317RK75. CAS-17598-65-1.* INN; BAN; JAN. *Cardiotonic.* Cedilanid-D (Novartis)

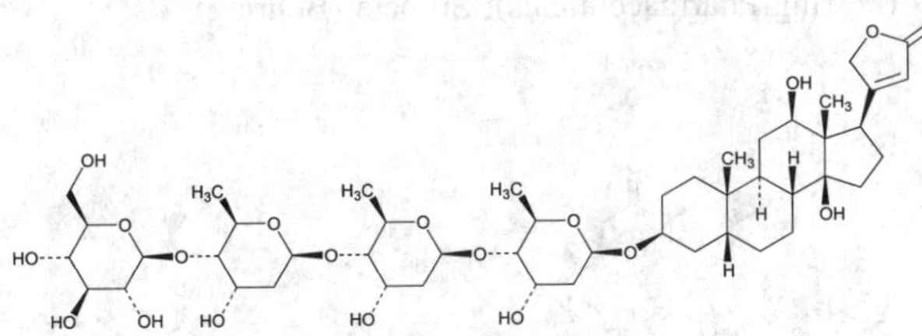

Desloratadine [*1998*] (des″ lor a′ ta deen). $C_{19}H_{19}ClN_2$. 310.82. (1) 8-Chloro-6,11-dihydro-11-(4-piperidinylidene)-5*H*-benzo[5,6]cyclohepta[1,2-*b*]pyridine; (2) 8-Chloro-6,11-dihydro-11-(4-piperidinylidene)-5*H*-benzo[5,6]cyclohepta[1,2-*b*]pyridine. *UNII-FVF865388R.*

---

† Brand name formerly used, and/or firm no longer concerned with this product.

CAS-100643-71-8. INN; BAN. *Treatment of seasonal allergic rhinitis (H₁receptor antagonist).* Clarinex (Schering-Plough) ◇*SCH 34117*

Deslorelin [*1989*] (des″ loe rel′ in). $C_{64}H_{83}N_{17}O_{12}$. 1282.45. (1) Luteinizing hormone-releasing factor (pig), 6-D-tryptophan-9-(*N*-ethyl-L-prolinamide)-10-deglycinamide-; (2) 5-Oxo-L-prolyl-L-histidyl-L-tryptophyl-L-seryl-L-tyrosyl-D-tryptophyl-L-leucyl-L-arginyl-*N*-ethyl-L-prolinamide. *CAS-57773-65-6.* INN; BAN. *LHRH agonist.* Somagard [as acetate] (Roberts Pharmaceutical) ◇*D-Trp LHRH-PEA*

Desmeninol. $C_5H_{10}O_3S$. 150.20. (±)-2-Hydroxy-4-(methylthio)butyric acid. *UNII-Z94465H1Y7. CAS-120-91-2.* INN.

Desmethylmoramide. $C_{24}H_{30}N_2O_2$. 378.51. 1-(4-Morpholino-2,2-diphenylbutyryl)pyrrolidine. *UNII-9B1Z1V29C3. CAS-1767-88-0.* INN.

Desmophosphamide — *See* Defosfamide.

Desmopressin Acetate [*1977*] (des″ moe pres′ in as′ e tate). **USP.** $C_{48}H_{68}N_{14}O_{14}S_2 \cdot 3H_2O$. 1183.31. [Desmopressin is INN and BAN.] (1) Vasopressin, 1-(3-mercaptopropanoic acid)-8-D-arginine-, monoacetate (salt), trihydrate; (2) 1-(3-Mercaptopropionic acid)-8-D-arginine-vasopressin monoacetate (salt) trihydrate. *UNII-XB13HYU18U; UNII-ENR1LLB0FP* [desmopressin]. *CAS-62357-86-2; CAS-62288-83-9* [anhydrous]; *CAS-16679-58-6* [desmopressin]. JAN. *Antidiuretic.* Ddavp (Sanofi Aventis); Minirin (Ferring Pharmaceuticals); Stimate (Behring)

Desmoteplase [*2003*] (des moe′ te plase). Plasminogen activator (Desmodus rotundus isoform α1 protein moiety reduced). Molecular weight is 55,000–58,000 daltons. *CAS-145137-38-8.* INN. *Treatment of acute myocardial infarction, acute ischemic stroke, pulmonary embolism and hemodialysis.* ◇*rDSPA alpha 1*

Desocriptine. $C_{32}H_{45}N_5O_4$. 563.73. 6′-Deoxo-9,10α-dihydro-β-ergocriptine. *UNII-62P526DC98. CAS-66759-48-6.* INN.

Desogestrel [*1990*] (des″ oh jes′ trel). $C_{22}H_{30}O$. 310.47. (1) 18,19-Dinorpregn-4-en-20-yn-17-ol, 13-ethyl-11-methylene-, (17α)-; (2) 13-Ethyl-11-methylene-18,19-dinor-17α-pregn-4-en-20-yn-17-ol. *UNII-81K9V7M3A3. CAS-54024-22-5.* INN; BAN. *Progestin.* ◇*ORG 2969*

Desolone — *See* Deprodone.

Desomorphine. $C_{17}H_{21}NO_2$. 271.35. Dihydrodeoxymorphine *or* 4,5-Epoxy-3-hydroxy-*N*-methylmorphinan. *CAS-427-00-9.* INN; BAN; DCF; MI.

Desonide [*1970*] (des′ oh nide). $C_{24}H_{32}O_6$. 416.51. (1) Pregna-1,4-diene-3,20-dione, 11,21-dihydroxy-16,17-[(1-methylethylidene)bis(oxy)]-, (11β,16α)-; (2) 11β,16α,17,21-Tetrahydroxypregna-1,4-diene-3,20-dione cyclic 16,17-acetal with acetone. *UNII-J280872D1O. CAS-638-94-8.* INN; BAN. *Anti-inflammatory.* Desowen (Galderma) ◇*D2083*

Desoximetasone [*1975*] (des ox″ i met′ a sone). **USP.** $C_{22}H_{29}FO_4$. 376.46. (1) Pregna-1,4-diene-3,20-dione, 9-fluoro-11,21-dihydroxy-16-methyl-, (11β,16α)-; (2) 9-Fluoro-11β,21-dihydroxy-16α-methylpregna-1,4-diene-3,20-dione. *UNII-4E07GXB7AU. CAS-382-67-2.* INN;

BAN. *Anti-inflammatory.* Topicort (Taro) *[Name previously used: Desoxymethasone.]* ◇*HOE 304; R 2113; A-41-304*

Desoxycorticosterone Acetate (des ox″ i kor″ ti koe ster′ one as′ e tate). **USP.** $C_{23}H_{32}O_4$. 372.50. [Desoxycortone is INN and BAN.] (1) Pregn-4-ene-3,20-dione, 21-(acetyloxy)-; (2) 11-Deoxycorticosterone acetate. *UNII-6E0A168OB8. CAS-56-47-3. Adrenocortical steroid (salt-regulating).* Doca (Organon); Percorten (Novartis) *[Name previously used: Deoxycortone.]*

Desoxycorticosterone Pivalate (des ox″ i kor″ ti koe ster′ one piv′ a late). **USP.** $C_{26}H_{38}O_4$. 414.58. (1) Pregn-4-ene-3,20-dione, 21-(2,2-dimethyl-1-oxopropoxy)-; (2) 11-Deoxycorticosterone pivalate. *UNII-16665T4A2X. CAS-808-48-0. Adrenocortical steroid (salt-regulating).* Percorten (Novartis)

Desoxycorticosterone Trimethylacetate. USP XVI.

Desoxycortone (INN; BAN) — *See* Desoxycorticosterone Acetate.

L-Desoxyephedrine (previously used name) — *See* Levmetamfetamine.

Desoxyephedrine Hydrochloride — *See* Methamphetamine Hydrochloride.

Destradiol — *See* Estradiol.

Desvenlafaxine Succinate [*2003*] (des ven″ la fax′ een sux′ i nate). $C_{16}H_{25}NO_2 \cdot C_4H_6O_4 \cdot H_2O$. 399.48. [Desvenlafaxine is INN and BAN.] (1) Butanedioic acid, compound with 4-[2-(dimethylamino)-1-(1-hydroxycyclohexyl)ethyl]phenol (1:1), monohydrate; (2) 1-[(1*RS*)-2-(Dimethylamino)-1-(4-hydroxyphenyl)ethyl]cyclohexanol hydrogen butanedioate monohydrate. *UNII-ZB22ENF0XR; UNII-NG99554ANW* [desvenlafaxine]. *CAS-386750-22-7; CAS-93413-62-8* [desvenlafaxine]. *Treatment of major depressive disorder.* ◇*Wy-45233*

Detajmium Bitartrate. $C_{31}H_{47}N_3O_9 \cdot H_2O$. 623.73. 4-[3-(Diethylamino)-2-hydroxypropyl]ajmalinium hydrogen tartrate monohydrate. *CAS-53862-81-0; CAS-33774-52-6* [anhydrous]. INN.

Detanosal. $C_{13}H_{19}NO_3$. 237.29. 2-(Diethylamino)ethyl salicylate. *UNII-Y09NU9DS9B. CAS-23573-66-2.* INN; DCF.

Deterenol Hydrochloride [*1970*] (de ter′ e nol hye″ droe klor′ ide). $C_{11}H_{17}NO_2 \cdot HCl$. 231.72. [Deterenol is INN.] (1) Benzenemethanol, 4-hydroxy-α-[[(1-methylethyl)amino]methyl]-, hydrochloride (±)-; (2) (±)-*p*-Hydroxy-α-[(isopropylamino)methyl]benzyl alcohol hydrochloride. *CAS-23239-36-3; CAS-3506-31-8* [deterenol]. *Adrenergic (ophthalmic).* ◇*AL 842*

Detirelix Acetate [*1987*] (de″ ti rel′ ix as′ e tate). $C_{78}H_{105}ClN_{18}O_{13} \cdot 2C_2H_4O_2$. 1658.34. [Detirelix is INN.] (1) D-Alaninamide, *N*-acetyl-3-(2-naphthalenyl)-D-alanyl-4-chloro-D-phenylalanyl-D-tryptophyl-L-seryl-L-tyrosyl-*N*⁶-[(ethylamino)(ethylimino)methyl]-D-lysyl-L-leucyl-L-arginyl-L-prolyl-, diacetate (salt); (2) *N*-Acetyl-3-(2-naphthyl)-D-alanyl-*p*-chloro-D-phenylalanyl-D-tryptophyl-L-seryl-L-tyrosyl-*N*⁶-(*N,N*′-diethylamidino)-D-lysyl-L-leucyl-L-arginyl-L-prolyl-D-alaninamide diacetate (salt). *CAS-89662-30-6* [detirelix]; *CAS-102583-46-0. Antagonist (LHRH).* ◇*RS-68439*

Detiviciclovir. $C_9H_{13}N_5O_2$. 223.23. 2-[(2-Amino-9*H*-purin-9-yl)methyl]propane-1,3-diol. *UNII-088W05943X. CAS-220984-26-9.* INN.

Detomidine Hydrochloride [*1988*] (de toe′ mi deen hye″ droe klor′ ide). $C_{12}H_{14}N_2 \cdot HCl$. 222.71. [Detomidine is INN and BAN.] (1) 1*H*-Imidazole, 4-[(2,3-dimethylphenyl)methyl]-, monohydrochloride; (2) 4-(2,3-Dimethylbenzy-

---

l)imidazole monohydrochloride. *UNII-95K4LKB6QE. CAS-90038-01-0; CAS-76631-46-4* [detomidine]. *Analgesic (veterinary); sedative-hypnotic.* ◇*MPV-253 AII*

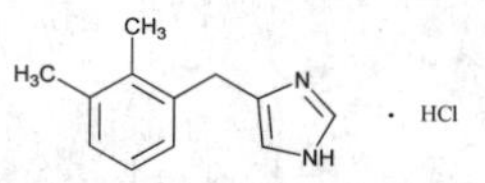

Detorubicin. $C_{33}H_{39}NO_{14}$. 673.66. Glyoxylic acid 3^2-ester with doxorubicin, 2-(diethyl acetal). *UNII-822EC3XEJZ. CAS-66211-92-5.* INN.

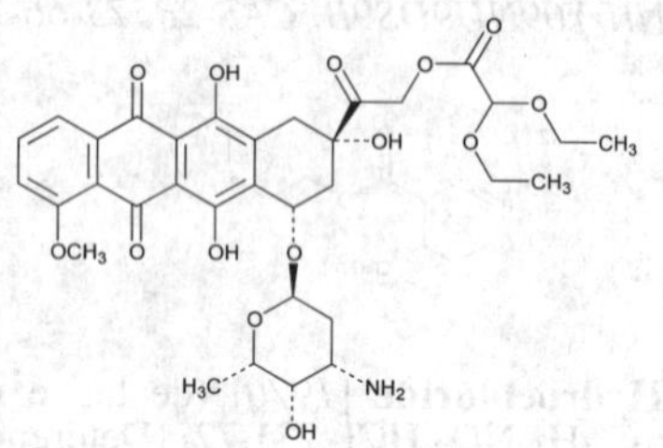

Detralfate. Dextran sulfate, sodium salt, aluminum complex. *CAS-37209-31-7.* INN.

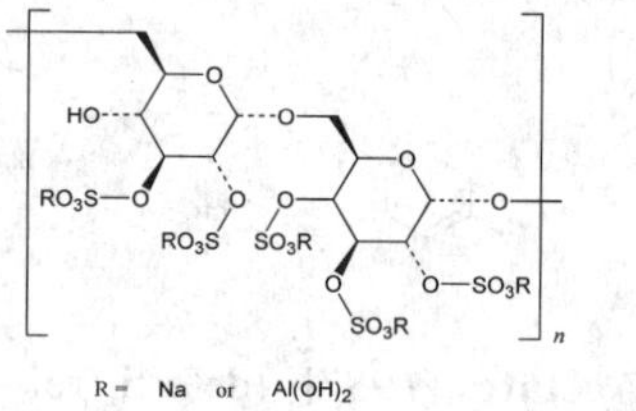

Detrothyronine. $C_{15}H_{12}I_3NO_4$. 650.97. D-3-[4-(4-Hydroxy-3-iodophenoxy)-3,5-diiodophenyl]-alanine. *CAS-5714-08-9.* INN. ◇*DT-3*

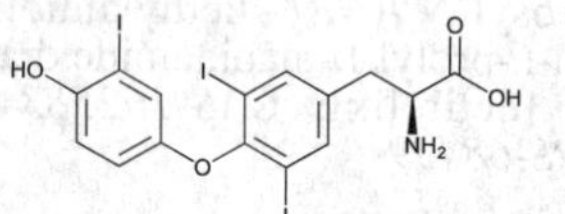

Detumomab. Immunoglobulin G1, anti-(human B lymphoma cell) (mouse monoclonal SPECIFID heavy chain), disulfide with mouse monoclonal SPECIFID light chain, dimer. *CAS-145832-33-3.* INN.

Deuterium Oxide [*1963*] (due teer′ ee um ox′ ide). Stable nuclide. (1) Water-d_2; (2) Heavy water (D$_2$O). *CAS-7789-20-0. Radioactive agent.* ◇^2H

Deutolperisone. $C_{16}H_{16}{}^2H_7NO$. 2-Methyl-1-{4-([$^2H_3$]methyl)[2,3,5,6-$^2H_4$]phenyl}-3-(piperidin-1-yl)propan-1-one. *CAS-474641-19-5.* INN.

Devapamil. $C_{26}H_{36}N_2O_3$. 424.58. 2-(3,4-Dimethoxyphenyl)-2-isopropyl-5-[(*m*-methoxyphenethyl)methylamino]valeronitrile. *UNII-M6142PTV7J. CAS-92302-55-1.* INN.

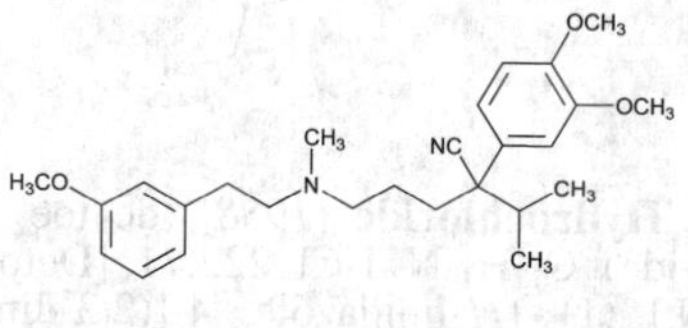

Devazepide [*1989*] (dev az′ e pide). $C_{25}H_{20}N_4O_2$. 408.45. (1) 1*H*-Indole-2-carboxamide, *N*-(2,3-dihydro-1-methyl-2-oxo-5-phenyl-1*H*-1,4-benzodiazepin-3-yl)-, (*S*)-; (2) (*S*)-*N*-(2,3-Dihydro-1-methyl-2-oxo-5-phenyl-1*H*-1,4-benzodiazepin-3-yl)indole-2-carboxamide. *CAS-103420-77-5.* INN. *Antagonist (cholecystokinin).* ◇*MK-329; L-364,718*

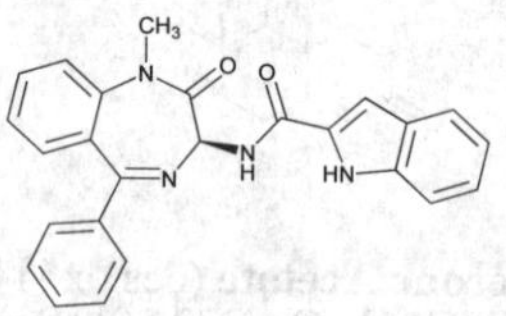

Dexamethasone (dex″ a meth′ a sone). **USP**. $C_{22}H_{29}FO_5$. 392.46. [Dexamethasone Metasulfobenzoate Sodium, Dexamethasone Palmitate, and Dexamethasone Valerate are JAN.] (1) Pregna-1,4-diene-3,20-dione, 9-fluoro-11,17,21-trihydroxy-16-methyl-, (11β,16α)-; (2) 9-Fluoro-11β,17,21-trihydroxy-16α-methylpregna-1,4-diene-3,20-dione. *UNII-7S5I7G3JQL. CAS-50-02-2.* INN; BAN; JAN. *Glucocorticoid.* Decadron (Merck); Dexone (Solvay Pharmaceuticals); Hexadrol (Organon); Maxidex (Alcon)

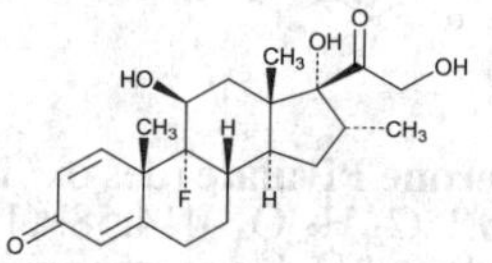

Dexamethasone Acefurate [*1987*] (dex″ a meth′ a sone a″ se fue′ rate). $C_{29}H_{33}FO_8$. 528.57. (1) Pregna-1,4-diene-3,20-dione, 21-(acetyloxy)-9-fluoro-17-[(2-furanylcarbonyl)oxy]-11-hydroxy-16-methyl-, (11β,16α)-; (2) 9-Fluoro-11β,17,21-trihydroxy-16α-methylpregna-1,4-diene-3,20-dione 21-acetate 17-(2-furoate). *UNII-W4N6E1T46B. CAS-83880-70-0.* INN. *Steroid (topical).* ◇*Sch 31353*

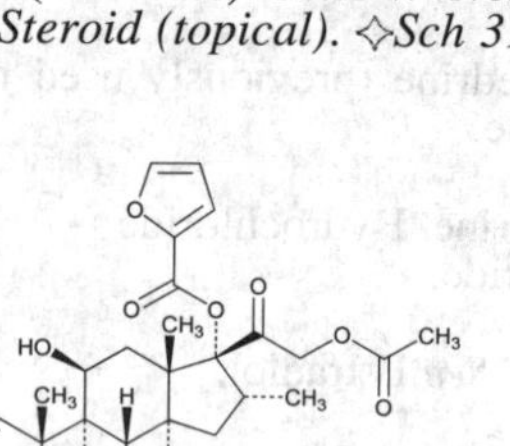

Dexamethasone Acetate [*1979*] (dex″ a meth′ a sone as′ e tate). **USP**. $C_{24}H_{31}FO_6$.H_2O. 452.51. (1) Pregna-1,4-diene-3,20-dione, 21-(acetyloxy)-9-fluoro-11,17-dihydroxy-16-methyl, monohydrate, (11β,16α)-; (2) 9-Fluoro-11β,17,21-trihydroxy-16α-methylpregna-1,4-diene-3,20-dione 21-acetate, monohydrate. *UNII-E2287TKU04; UNII-K7V8P532WP* [dexamethasone acetate anhydrous]. *CAS-55812-90-3; CAS-1177-87-3* [anhydrous]. BAN; JAN. *Adrenocortical steroid.* Decadron (Merck)

Dexamethasone Beloxil [*2003*] (dex″ a meth′ a sone bel ox′ il). $C_{29}H_{35}F_5$. 478.58. (1) (11β,16α)-9-Fluoro-3,17-dihydroxy-16-methyl-21-(phenylmethoxy)-pregna-1,4-diene-3,20-dione; (2) 21-(Benzyloxy)-9-fluoro-11β,17-dihydroxy-16α-methylpregna-1,4-diene-3,20-dione; (3) 21-*O*-Benzyldexamethasone. *UNII-V9T15U399I. CAS-150587-07-8. Anti-inflammatory used in the treatment of uveitis, iritis, keratitis, post-surgical inflammation, vernal keratoconjunctivitis, and giant papillary conjunctivitis.*

Dexamethasone Cipecilate. $C_{33}H_{43}FO_7$. 570.69. 9-Fluoro-11β-hydroxy-16α-methyl-3,20-dioxopregna-1,4-diene-17,21-diyl 21-cyclohexanecarboxylate 17-cyclopropanecarboxylate. *UNII-T51D685OXG. CAS-132245-57-9.* INN; JAN.

Dexamethasone Dipropionate [*1987*] (dex″ a meth′ a sone dye proe′ pee oh nate). $C_{28}H_{37}FO_7$. 504.59. [Dexamethasone Propionate is JAN.] (1) Pregna-1,4-diene-3,20-dione, 9-fluoro-11-hydroxy-16-methyl-17,21-bis(1-oxopropoxy)-, (11β,16α)-; (2) 9-Fluoro-11β,17,21-trihydroxy-16α-methylpregna-1,4-diene-3,20-dione 17,21-dipropionate. *UNII-K3UKR54YXW. CAS-55541-30-5. Anti-inflammatory (steroid).* ◇ST12

Dexamethasone Metasulfobenzoate Sodium (JAN) — *See* Dexamethasone.

Dexamethasone Palmitate (JAN) — *See* Dexamethasone.

Dexamethasone Sodium Phosphate (dex″ a meth′ a sone soe′ dee um fos′ fate). **USP**. $C_{22}H_{28}FNa_2O_8P$. 516.40. (1) Pregna-1,4-diene-3,20-dione, 9-fluoro-11,17-dihydroxy-16-methyl-21-(phosphonooxy)-, disodium salt, (11β, 16α)-; (2) 9-Fluoro-11β,17,21-trihydroxy-16α-methylpregna-1,4-diene-3,20-dione 21-(dihydrogen phosphate) disodium salt. *UNII-AI9376Y64P. CAS-2392-39-4; CAS-312-93-6* [dexamethasone 21-(dihydrogen phosphate)]. BAN; JAN. *Glucocorticoid.* Decadron (Merck); Hexadrol (Organon); Maxidex (Alcon)

Dexamethasone Valerate (JAN) — *See* Dexamethasone.

Dexamfetamine (INN, BAN) — *See* Dextroamphetamine.

Dexamisole [*1974*] (dex a′ mi sole). $C_{11}H_{12}N_2S$. 204.29. (1) Imidazo[2,1-*b*]thiazole, 2,3,5,6-tetrahydro-6-phenyl-, (*R*)-; (2) (+)-2,3,5,6-Tetrahydro-6-phenylimidazo[2,1-*b*]thiazole. *UNII-UMH46V5U01. CAS-14769-74-5.* INN. *Antidepressant.* ◇R 12,563 [as hydrochloride]

Dexamphetamine (DCF) — *See* Dextroamphetamine.

Dexbrompheniramine Maleate (dex″ brome fen ir′ a meen mal′ ee ate). **USP**. $C_{16}H_{19}BrN_2 \cdot C_4H_4O_4$. 435.31. [Dexbrompheniramine is INN and BAN.] (1) 2-Pyridinepropanamine, γ-(4-bromophenyl)-*N*,*N*-dimethyl-, (*S*)-, (*Z*)-2-butenedioate (1:1); (2) (+)-2-[*p*-Bromo-α-[2-(dimethylamino)ethyl]benzyl]pyridine maleate (1:1). *UNII-BPA9UT29BS; UNII-75T64B71RP* [dexbrompheniramine]. *CAS-2391-03-9; CAS-132-21-8* [dexbrompheniramine]. *Antihistaminic.* Disomer (Schering)

Dexbudesonide. $C_{25}H_{34}O_6$. 430.53. (*R*)-11β,16α,17,21-Tetrahydroxypregna-1,4-diene-3,20-dione 16,17-acetal with butyraldehyde. *UNII-Q3OKS62Q6X. CAS-51372-29-3.* INN.

Dexchlorpheniramine Maleate (dex″ klor fen ir′ a meen mal′ ee ate). **USP**. $C_{16}H_{19}ClN_2 \cdot C_4H_4O_4$. 390.86. [Dexchlorpheniramine is INN and BAN; *d*-Chlorpheniramine Maleate is JAN.] (1) 2-Pyridinepropanamine, γ-(4-chlorophenyl)-*N*,*N*-dimethyl-, (*S*)-, (*Z*)-2-butenedioate (1:1); (2) (+)-2-[*p*-Chloro-α-[2-(dimethylamino)ethyl]benzyl]pyridine maleate (1:1). *UNII-B10YD955QW; UNII-3Q9Q0B929N* [dexchlorpheniramine]. *CAS-2438-32-6; CAS-25523-97-1* [dexchlorpheniramine]. *Antihistaminic.* Mylaramine (Morton Grove); Polaramine (Schering)

Dexclamol Hydrochloride [*1975*] (dex′ kla mol hye″ droe klor′ ide). $C_{24}H_{29}NO \cdot HCl$. 383.95. [Dexclamol is INN.] (1) 1*H*-Benzo[6,7]cyclohepta[1,2,3-*de*]pyrido[2,1-*a*]isoquinolin-3-ol, 2,3,4,4a,8,9,13b,14-octahydro-3-(1-methylethyl)-, hydrochloride, (3α,4aα,13bβ)-(+)-; (2) (+)-2,3,4,4aβ,8,9,13bα,14-Octahydro-3α-isopropyl-1*H*-benzo[6,7]cyclohepta[1,2,3-*de*]pyrido[2,1-*a*]isoquinolin-3-ol hydrochloride. *CAS-52389-27-2; CAS-52340-25-7* [dexclamol]. *Sedative-hypnotic.* ◇AY-24,169

Dexecadotril. $C_{21}H_{23}NO_4S$. 385.48. (+)-N-[(R)-α-(Mercapto-methyl)hydrocinnamoyl]glycine, benzyl ester, acetate (ester). *UNII-5OFI9D9892. CAS-112573-72-5.* INN.

Dexefaroxan. $C_{13}H_{16}N_2O$. 216.28. (+)-(R)-2-(2-Ethyl-2,3-dihydro-2-benzofuranyl)-2-imidazoline. *UNII-F751MO69EV. CAS-143249-88-1.* INN.

Dexelvucitabine [*2006*] (dex″ el vue sye′ ta been). $C_9H_{10}FN_3O_3$. 227.19. (1) Cytidine, 2′,3′-didehydro-2′,3′-dideoxy-5-fluoro-; (2) (+)-4-Amino-5-fluoro-1-[(2R,5S)-5-(hydroxymethyl)-2,5-dihydrofuran-2-yl]pyrimidin-2(1H)-one. *UNII-KU8SPJ271W. CAS-134379-77-4.* INN. *Treatment of HIV-1 and HIV-2 infection.* Reverset (Incyte) ◇*INCB-8721; DPC-817; YZ-817*

Dexetimide [*1971*] (dex et′ i mide). $C_{23}H_{26}N_2O_2$. 362.46. (1) [3,4′-Bipiperidine]-2,6-dione, 3-phenyl-1′-(phenylmethyl)-, (S)-; (2) (+)-2-(1-Benzyl-4-piperidyl)-2-phenylglutarimide. *UNII-43477QYX3D. CAS-21888-98-2.* INN; BAN. *Anticholinergic.* ◇*R 16,470 [as hydrochloride]*

Dexetozoline. $C_{13}H_{20}N_2O_3S$. 284.37. (+)-Ethyl (Z)-(S)-3-methyl-4-oxo-5-piperidino-$\Delta^{2,\alpha}$-thiazolidineacetate. *UNII-KK9WYJ6556. CAS-77519-25-6.* INN.

Dexfenfluramine Hydrochloride [*1991*] (dex″ fen flur′ a meen hye″ droe klor′ ide). $C_{12}H_{16}F_3N.HCl$. 267.72. [Dexfenfluramine is INN and BAN.] (1) Benzeneethanamine, N-ethyl-α-methyl-3-(trifluoromethyl)-, hydrochloride, (S)-; (2) (+)-(S)-N-Ethyl-α-methyl-m-(trifluoromethyl)phenethylamine hydrochloride. *UNII-PM28L0FHNP. CAS-3239-45-0; CAS-3239-44-9 [dexfenfluramine].* *Appetite suppressant (systemic).* Redux (Interneuron) ◇*S 5614 HCl*

Dexfosfoserine. $C_3H_8NO_6P$. 185.07. (+)-L-Serine dihydrogen phosphate (ester). *CAS-407-41-0.* INN.

Dexibuprofen [*1997*] (dex″ eye bue proe′ fen). $C_{13}H_{18}O_2$. 206.28. (1) Benzeneacetic acid, α-methyl-4-(2-methylpropyl)-, (S)-; (2) (+)-(S)-p-Isobutylhydratropic acid. *CAS-51146-56-6.* INN; BAN. *Analgesic; anti-inflammatory.*

Dexibuprofen Lysine [*1989*] (dex″ eye bue proe′ fen lye′ seen). $C_{13}H_{18}O_2.C_6H_{14}N_2O_2.H_2O$. 370.48. (1) Benzeneacetic acid, α-methyl-4-(2-methylpropyl)-, (S)-, compd. with L-lysine (1:1) monohydrate; (2) (+)-(S)-p-Isobutylhydratropic acid, compound with L-lysine (1:1), monohydrate. *CAS-141505-32-0; CAS-113403-10-4 [anhydrous].* *Analgesic (cyclooxygenase inhibitor); anti-inflammatory.* Doctrin (Merck) ◇*L-669,455; MK-233*

Deximafen [*1974*] (dex im′ a fen). $C_{11}H_{13}N_3$. 187.24. (1) 1H-Imidazo[1,2-a]imidazole, 2,3,5,6-tetrahydro-5-(or-3)-phenyl-, (+)-; (2) (+)-2,3,5,6-Tetrahydro-5-(or-3-)phenyl-1H-imidazo[1,2-a]imidazole. *UNII-1V5135S169. CAS-42116-77-8; CAS-60719-87-1 [replaced].* INN. *Antidepressant.*

Dexindoprofen. $C_{17}H_{15}NO_3$. 281.31. (+)-(S)-p-(1-Oxo-2-isoindolinyl)hydratropic acid. *UNII-004T8726AU. CAS-53086-13-8.* INN.

Dexivacaine [*1968*] (dex iv′ a kane). $C_{15}H_{22}N_2O$. 246.35. (1) 2-Piperidinecarboxamide, N-(2,6-dimethylphenyl)-1-methyl-, (S)-; (2) (+)-1-Methyl-2′,6′-pipecoloxylidide. *UNII-QI846AL4NC. CAS-24358-84-7.* INN. *Anesthetic.*

Dexketoprofen. $C_{16}H_{14}O_3$. 254.28. (+)-(*S*)-*m*-Benzoylhydratropic acid. *CAS-22161-81-5.* INN; BAN.

Dexlansoprazole [*2006*] (dex″ lan soe′ pra zole). $C_{16}H_{14}F_3N_3O_2S$. 369.36. (1) 1*H*-Benzimidazole, 2-[(*R*)-[[3-methyl-4-(2,2,2-trifluoroethoxy)-2-pyridinyl]methyl]-sulfinyl]-; (2) (+)-2-[(*R*)-{[3-Methyl-4-(2,2,2-trifluoroethoxy)pyridin-2-yl]methyl}sulfinyl]-1*H*-benzimidazole; (3) 2-[(*R*)-[[3-Methyl-4-(2,2,2-trifluoroethoxy)-2-pyridinyl]methyl]sulfinyl]-1*H*-benzimidazole. *UNII-UYE4-T5I70X.* *CAS-138530-94-6.* INN. *Non-erosive GERD, healing of erosive esophagitis, and maintenance of healing of erosive esophagitis.* ◊*T-168390; TAK-390*

Dexlofexidine. $C_{11}H_{12}Cl_2N_2O$. 259.13. (+)-(*S*)-2-[1-(2,6-Dichlorophenoxy)ethyl]-2-imidazoline. *UNII-VXJ7Z24RN1.* *CAS-81447-79-2.* INN.

Dexloxiglumide. $C_{21}H_{30}Cl_2N_2O_5$. 461.38. (*R*)-4-(3,4-Dichlorobenzamido)-*N*-(3-methoxypropyl)-*N*-pentylglutaramic acid. *CAS-119817-90-2.* INN.

Dexmedetomidine [*1989*] (dex me″ de toe′ mi deen). $C_{13}H_{16}N_2$. 200.28. (1) 1*H*-Imidazole, 4-[1-(2,3-dimethylphenyl)ethyl]-, (*R*)-; (2) (+)-4-[(*S*)-α,2,3-Trimethylbenzyl]imidazole. *UNII-67VB76HONO.* *CAS-113775-47-6.* INN; BAN. *Tranquilizer.* Precedex (Hospira) ◊*MPV-1440*

Dexmedetomidine Hydrochloride [*1999*] (dex me″ de toe′ mi deen hye″ droe klor′ ide). $C_{13}H_{16}N_2$.HCl. 236.74. (1) 1*H*-Imidazole, 4-[1-(2,3-dimethylphenyl)ethyl]-, monohydrochloride, (*S*)-; (2) 4-[(*S*)-α,2,3-Trimethylbenzyl]imidazole monohydrochloride. *UNII-1018WH7F9I.* *CAS-145108-58-3. Sedative.*

Dexmethylphenidate Hydrochloride [*2002*] (dex meth″ il fen′ i date hye″ droe klor′ ide). $C_{14}H_{19}NO_2$.HCl. 269.77. [Dexmethylphenidate is INN.] (1) 2-Piperidineacetic acid, α-phenyl-, methyl ester, hydrochloride, (α*R*,2*R*)-; (2) Methyl (2*R*)-phenyl[(2*R*)-piperidin-2-yl]acetate hydrochloride. *UNII-1678OK0E08; UNII-M32RH9MFGP* [dexmethylphenidate]. *CAS-19262-68-1; CAS-40431-64-9* [dexmethylphenidate]. *Treatment of attention deficit/hyperactivity disorder (ADHD).* Focalin (Novartis)

Dexnafenodone. $C_{20}H_{23}NO$. 293.40. (+)-(*S*)-2-[2-(Dimethylamino)ethyl]-3,4-dihydro-2-phenyl-1(2*H*)-naphthalenone. *UNII-601X8G3PCW.* *CAS-92629-87-3.* INN.

Dexnebivolol. $C_{22}H_{25}F_2NO_4$. 405.44. (1*R*)-2-({(2*R*)-2-[(2*S*)-6-Fluoro-3,4-dihydro-2*H*-chromen-2-yl]-2-hydroxyethyl}amino)-1-[(2*R*)-6-fluoro-3,4-dihydro-2*H*-chromen-2-yl]ethanol. *CAS-118457-15-1.* INN.

Dexniguldipine. $C_{36}H_{39}N_3O_6$. 609.71. (+)-(*R*)-3-(4,4-Diphenylpiperidino)propyl methyl 1,4-dihydro-2,6-dimethyl-4-(*m*-nitrophenyl)-3,5-pyridinedicarboxylate. *CAS-120054-86-6.* INN.

Dexnorgestrel Acetime (previously used name) — *See* Norgestimate.

Dexormaplatin [*1990*] (dex or″ ma pla′ tin). $C_6H_{14}Cl_4N_2Pt$. 451.08. (1) Platinum, tetrachloro(1,2-cyclohexanediamine-*N*,*N*′)-, [*OC*-6-22-(1*R*-*trans*)]-; (2) (+)-*trans*-Tetrachloro(1,2-cyclohexanediamine)platinum. *CAS-96392-96-0.* INN. *Antineoplastic.* ◊*U-78,938*

Dexoxadrol Hydrochloride [*1962*] (dex ox′ a drol hye″ droe klor′ ide). $C_{20}H_{23}NO_2$.HCl. 345.86. [Dexoxadrol is INN.] (1) Piperidine, 2-(2,2-diphenyl-1,3-dioxolan-4-yl)-, hydro-

---

chloride; (2) (+)-2-(2,2-Diphenyl-1,3-dioxolan-4-yl)piper-idine hydrochloride. *UNII-T0C1IR71L8; UNII-JY5N9-F45AG* [dexoxadrol]. *CAS-631-06-1; CAS-4741-41-7* [dexoxadrol]. *Stimulant (central); analgesic.* ◇*CL-911C; U-22,559A; NSC-526062*

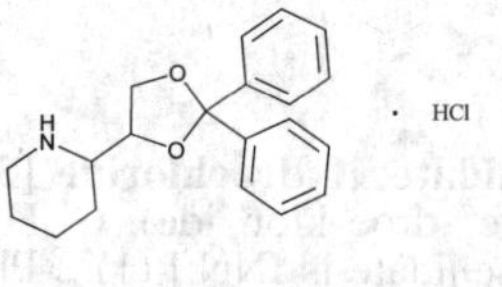

Dexpanthenol [*1970*] (dex pan' the nol). **USP.** $C_9H_{19}NO_4$. 205.25. (1) Butanamide, 2,4-dihydroxy-*N*-(3-hydroxypro-pyl)-3,3-dimethyl-, (*R*)-; (2) D-(+)-2,4-Dihydroxy-*N*-(3-hydroxypropyl)-3,3-dimethylbutyramide. *UNII-1O6C93RI7Z. CAS-81-13-0.* INN; BAN. *Cholinergic.* D-Panthenol 50 (BASF); Ilopan (Savage); Motilyn (Abbott†)

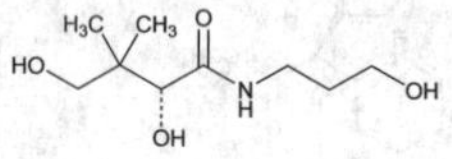

Dexpemedolac [*1994*] (dex″ pem ed' oh lak). $C_{22}H_{23}NO_3$. 349.42. (1) Pyrano[3,4-*b*]indole-1-acetic acid, 1-ethyl-1,3,4,9-tetrahydro-4-(phenylmethyl)-, (1*S-cis*)-; (2) (1*S*,4*R*)-4-Benzyl-1-ethyl-1,3,4,9-tetrahydropyrano[3,4-*b*]indole-1-acetic acid. *CAS-114030-44-3.* INN. *Analgesic.* ◇*WAY-PEM-420*

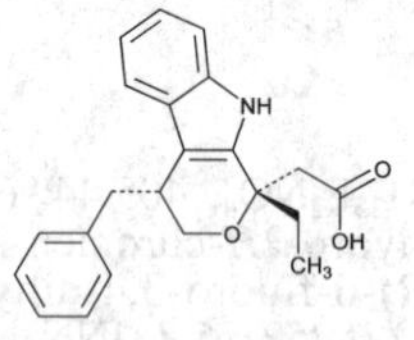

Dexpropranolol Hydrochloride [*1969*] (dex″ proe pran' oh lol hye″ droe klor' ide). $C_{16}H_{21}NO_2 \cdot HCl$. 295.80. [Dexpro-pranolol is INN and BAN.] (1) 2-Propanol, 1-[(1-methylethyl)-amino]-3-(1-naphthalenyloxy)-, hydrochlor-ide, (*R*)-; (2) (+)-1-(Isopropylamino)-3-(1-naphthyloxy)-2-propanol hydrochloride. *UNII-AB9DB0NX46. CAS-13071-11-9; CAS-5051-22-9* [dexpropranolol]. *Cardiac depressant (anti-arrhythmic); anti-adrenergic (β-recep-tor).* ◇*AY-20,694; I.C.I. 47,319*

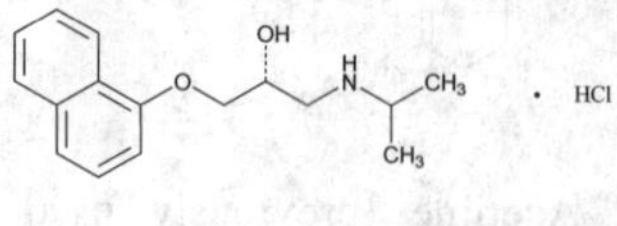

Dexproxibutene. $C_{22}H_{27}NO_2$. 337.46. (+)-3-[(Dimethylami-no)methyl]-1,2-diphenyl-3-buten-2-ol, propionate (ester). *UNII-ESH23ZBF8P. CAS-47419-52-3.* INN. ◇*44328*

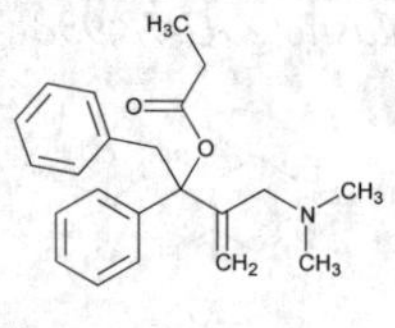

Dexrazoxane [*1990*] (dex ray zox' ane). $C_{11}H_{16}N_4O_4$. 268.27. (1) 2,6-Piperazinedione, 4,4'-(1-methyl-1,2-ethanediyl) bis-, (*S*)-; (2) (+)-(*S*)-4,4'-Propylenedi-2,6-piperazine-dione. *UNII-048L81261F. CAS-24584-09-6.* INN; BAN. *Cardioprotectant.* Zinecard (Pharmacia & Upjohn) ◇*ADR-529; ICRF-187; NSC-169780*

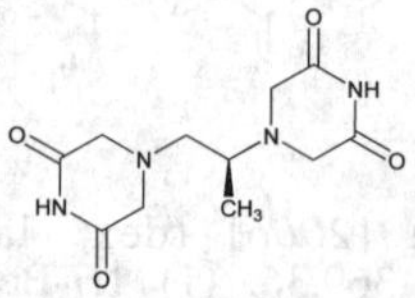

Dexsecoverine. $C_{22}H_{35}NO_2$. 345.52. (+)-(*S*)-1-Cyclohexyl-4-[ethyl(*p*-methoxy-α-methylphenethyl)amino]-1-butanone. *UNII-3O6AUX3I0J. CAS-90237-04-0.* INN.

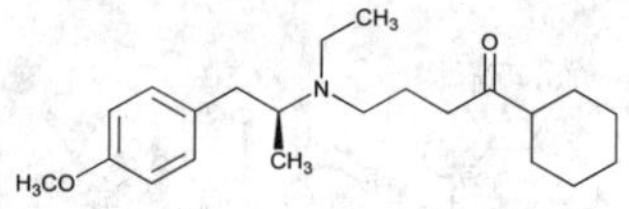

Dexsotalol Hydrochloride [*1995*] (dex soe' ta lol hye″ droe klor' ide). $C_{12}H_{20}N_2O_3S \cdot HCl$. 308.82. [Dexsotalol is INN.] (1) Methanesulfonamide, *N*-[4-[1-hydroxy-2-[(1-methyl-ethyl)amino]ethyl]phenyl]methanesulfonamide monohy-drochloride, (*S*)-; (2) (+)-(*S*)-4'-[1-Hydroxy-2-(isopropyl-amino)ethyl]methanesulfonanilide monohydrochloride. *CAS-4549-94-4; CAS-30236-32-9* [dexsotalol]. *Cardiac depressant (anti-arrhythmic).* ◇*BMY-05763-1-D*

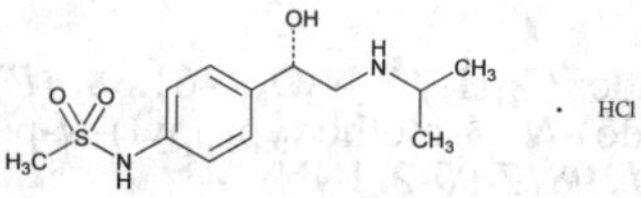

Dextilidine. $C_{17}H_{23}NO_2$. 273.37. (+)-Ethyl *trans*-2-(dimethy-lamino)-1-phenyl-3-cyclohexene-1-carboxylate. *UNII-2728MV084C. CAS-32447-90-8.* INN.

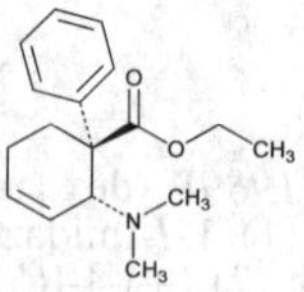

Dextiopronin. $C_5H_9NO_3S$. 163.19. *N*-[(*R*)-2-Mercaptopropio-nyl]glycine. *UNII-X294K8K2PF. CAS-29335-92-0.* INN.

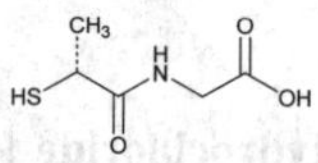

Dextofisopam [*2004*] (dex toe fis' oh pam). $C_{22}H_{26}N_2O_4$. 382.45. (1) 5*H*-2,3-Benzodiazepine, 1-(3,4-dimethoxyphe-nyl)-5-ethyl-7,8-dimethoxy-4-methyl-, (5*R*)-; (2) (+)-(5*R*)-1-(3,4-Dimethoxyphenyl)-5-ethyl-7,8-dimethoxy-4-methyl-5*H*-2,3-benzodiazepine. *UNII-EZ1515D6C1. CAS-82059-50-5*. INN. *Treatment of irritable bowel syndrome, Crohn's disease; anti-anxiety, anti-stress.* ◇*R-tofisopam*

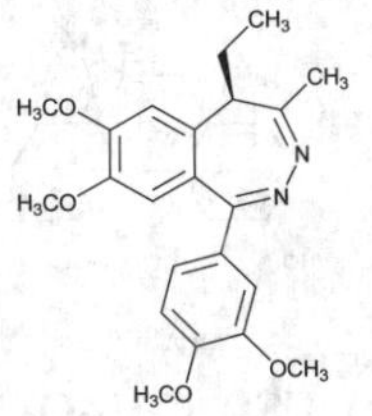

Dextran 1 (dex′ tran). **USP**. [Dextran is BAN.] A low molecular weight fraction of dextran, consisting of a mixture of isomaltooligosaccharides.

Dextran 40 [*1965*] (dex′ tran). **USP**. Dextran 40 is derived by controlled hydrolysis and fractionation of polysaccharides elaborated by the fermentative action of certain strains of *Leuconostoc mesenteroides* (NRRL, B.512 F; NCTC, 10817) on a sucrose substrate. It is a glucose polymer in which the linkages between glucose units are almost entirely of α-1:6 type. Its weight average molecular weight is in the 35,000 to 40,000 range. [Dextran is INN, BAN, and JAN.] (1) Dextrans; (2) Dextrans. *CAS-9004-54-0. Blood flow adjuvant; plasma volume extender.* Gentran 40 (Baxter Healthcare) ◇*LMWD; LMD; LVD*

Dextran 70 [*1966*] (dex′ tran). **USP**. Dextran 70 is derived by controlled hydrolysis and fractionation of polysaccharides elaborated by the fermentative action of certain appropriate strains of *Leuconostoc mesenteroides* (NRRL, B.512F; NCTC, 10817) on a sucrose substrate. It is a glucose polymer in which the linkages between glucose units are almost entirely of α-1:6 type. Its weight average molecular weight is in the 63,000 to 77,000 range. (1) Dextrans; (2) Dextrans. *Plasma volume extender.* Aquasite (Ciba Vision, US Ophthalmics)

Dextran 75 [*1965*] (dex′ tran). A polysaccharide produced by the action of *Leuconostoc mesenteroides* on sucrose. Average molecular weight: 75,000. (1) Dextrans; (2) Dextrans. *Plasma volume extender.* Gentran 75 (Baxter Healthcare)

Dextran Sulfate Sodium. Dextran sulfuric acid ester sodium salt. *CAS-9042-14-2*. JAN.

Dextranomer. Dextran 2,3-dihydroxypropyl 2-hydroxy-1,3-propanediyl ether. *CAS-56087-11-7*. INN; BAN; MI.

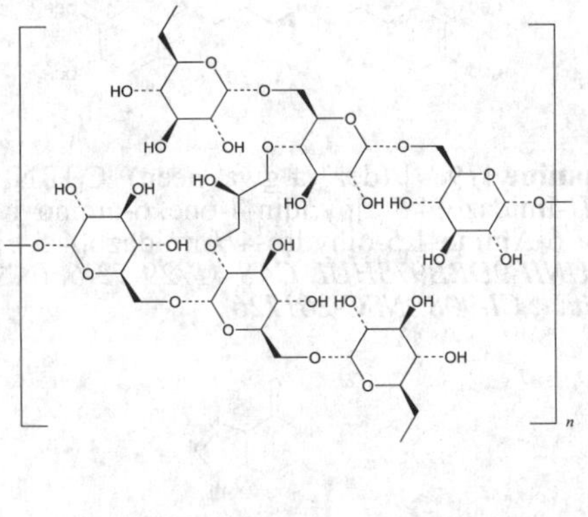

Dextrates [*1970*] (dex′ trates). **NF**. A mixture of sugars (approximately 92% dextrose monohydrate and 8% higher saccharides; dextrose equivalent is 95 to 97%) resulting from the controlled enzymatic hydrolysis of starch. *Pharmaceutic aid (tablet binder and diluent).*

Dextriferron. A colloidal solution of ferric hydroxide in complex with partially hydrolysed dextrin. *CAS-9004-51-7*. NF XIII; INN; BAN.

Dextrin (dex′ trin). **NF**. A starch, or partially hydrolyzed starch, modified by heating in a dry state, with or without acids, alkalies, or pH control agents. *CAS-9004-53-9*. BAN; JAN. *Pharmaceutic aid (suspending agent); pharmaceutic aid (viscosity-increasing agent); pharmaceutic aid (tablet binder); pharmaceutic aid (tablet and capsule diluent).*

Dextro Propoxyphene Hydrochloride — *See* Propoxyphene Hydrochloride.

Dextroamphetamine [*1964*] (dex″ troe am fet′ a meen). $C_9H_{13}N$. 135.21. [Dexamfetamine is INN and BAN.] (1) Benzeneethanamine, α-methyl-, (*S*)-; (2) (+)-α-Methyl-phenethylamine. *UNII-TZ47U051FI. CAS-51-64-9. Stimulant (central).* ◇*NSC-73713*

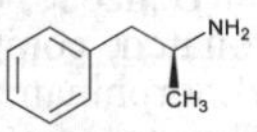

Dextroamphetamine Phosphate. $C_9H_{13}N.H_3PO_4$. 233.20. (1) Benzeneethanamine, α-methyl-, (*S*)-, phosphate (1:1); (2) (+)-α-Methylphenethylamine phosphate (1:1). *UNII-S76B51L5AM; UNII-TZ47U051FI* [dextroamphetamine]. *CAS-7528-00-9; CAS-6700-54-5* [replaced]; *CAS-51-64-9* [dextroamphetamine]. USP XX.

Dextroamphetamine Sulfate (dex″ troe am fet′ a meen sul′ fate). **USP**. $(C_9H_{13}N)_2.H_2SO_4$. 368.49. (1) Benzeneethanamine, α-methyl-, (*S*)-, sulfate (2:1); (2) (+)-α-Methylphenethylamine sulfate (2:1). *UNII-JJ768O327N. CAS-51-63-8; CAS-51-64-9* [dextroamphetamine]. *Stimulant (central).* Dexampex (Teva); Dexedrine (GlaxoSmithKline); Ferndex (Ferndale)

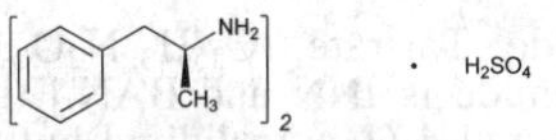

Dextrofemine. $C_{18}H_{23}NO$. 269.38. (+)-α-Methyl-*N*-(1-methyl-2-phenoxyethyl)phenethylamine. *UNII-WVB6I50566. CAS-15687-08-8*. INN; DCF.

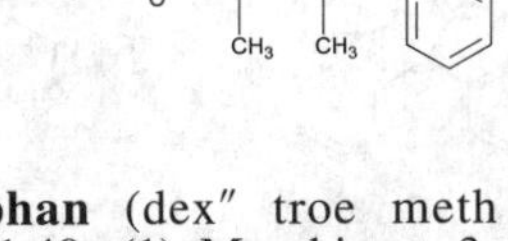

Dextromethorphan (dex″ troe meth or′ fan). **USP**. $C_{18}H_{25}NO$. 271.40. (1) Morphinan, 3-methoxy-17-methyl-, (9α,13α,14α)-; (2) 3-Methoxy-17-methyl-9α,13α,14α-morphinan. *UNII-7355X3ROTS. CAS-125-71-3*. INN; BAN. *Antitussive.*

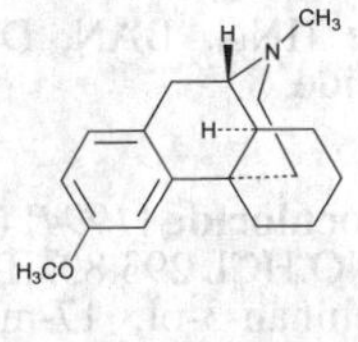

---

† Brand name formerly used, and/or firm no longer concerned with this product.

Dextromethorphan Hydrobromide (dex″ troe meth or′ fan hye″ droe broe′ mide). **USP.** $C_{18}H_{25}NO.HBr.H_2O$. 370.32. (1) Morphinan, 3-methoxy-17-methyl-, $(9\alpha,13\alpha,14\alpha)$-, hydrobromide, monohydrate; (2) 3-Methoxy-17-methyl-$9\alpha,13\alpha,14\alpha$-morphinan hydrobromide monohydrate. *UNII-9D2RTI9KYH; UNII-7355X3ROTS* [dextromethorphan]. *CAS-6700-34-1; CAS-125-69-9* [anhydrous]; *CAS-125-71-3* [dextromethorphan]. BAN; JAN. *Antitussive.* Benylin DM (Parke-Davis); Dextromethorphan Hydrobromide OROS Tablets (Ciba-Geigy); Drixoral Cough (Schering-Plough HealthCare†); PediaCare 1 (McNeil Consumer); Romilar (Hoffmann-LaRoche-International); St. Joseph Cough Syrup (Schering-Plough HealthCare†)

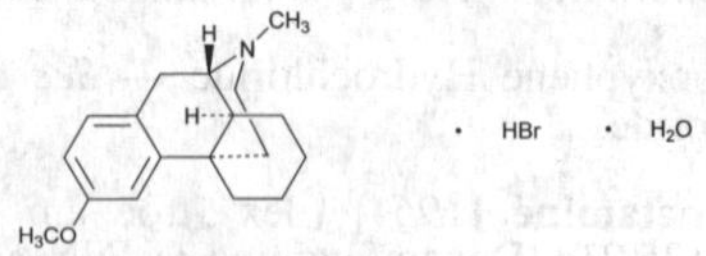

Dextromethorphan Polistirex [*1987*] (dex″ troe meth or′ fan pol″ ee stye′ rex). (1) Benzene, diethenyl-, polymer with ethenylbenzene, sulfonated, complex with $(9\alpha,13\alpha,14\alpha)$-3-methoxy-17-methylmorphinan; (2) Sulfonated styrene-divinylbenzene copolymer complex with 3-methoxy-17-methyl-$9\alpha,13\alpha,14\alpha$-morphinan. *Antitussive.* Delsym (Adams)

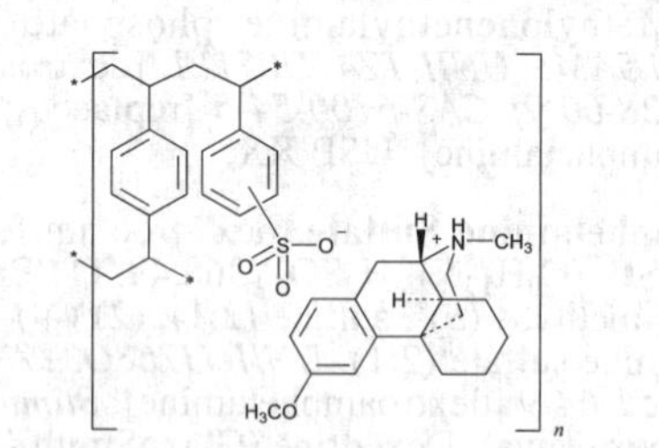

Dextromoramide Tartrate. $C_{25}H_{32}N_2O_2.C_4H_6O_6$. 542.62. [Dextromoramide is INN and BAN.] (+)-4-[2-Methyl-4-oxo-3,3-diphenyl-4-(1-pyrrolidinyl)butyl]morpholine bitartrate. *UNII-J778U505W5. CAS-2922-44-3; CAS-357-56-2* [dextromoramide]. MI. Dimorlin Tartrate (SmithKline Beecham†)

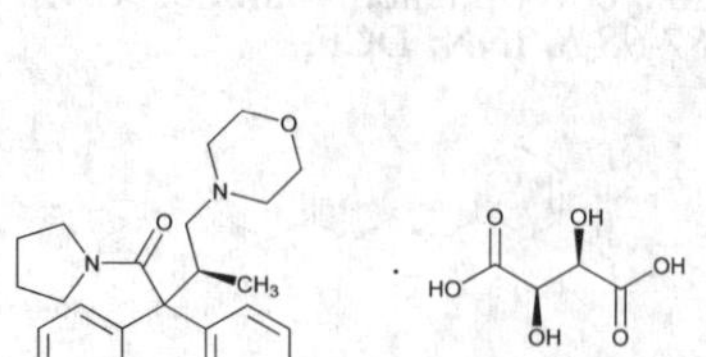

Dextropropoxiphene Chloride — *See* Propoxyphene Hydrochloride.

Dextropropoxyphene (INN, BAN, DCF) — *See* Propoxyphene Hydrochloride.

Dextrorphan Hydrochloride [*1994*] (dex tror′ fan hye″ droe klor′ ide). $C_{17}H_{23}NO.HCl$. 293.83. [Dextrorphan is INN and BAN.] (1) Morphinan-3-ol, 17-methyl-, hydrochloride, $(9\alpha,13\alpha,14\alpha)$-; (2) 17-Methyl-$9\alpha,13\alpha,14\alpha$-morphinan-3-

ol hydrochloride. *CAS-69376-27-8; CAS-125-73-5* [dextrorphan]. *Vasospastic therapy adjunct.* ◇*Ro 01-6794/706; Ro 1-6794 (dextrorphan)*

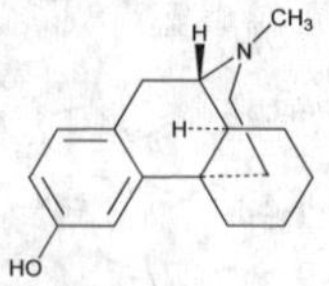

Dextrose (dex′ trose). **USP.** $C_6H_{12}O_6.H_2O$. 198.17. [Glucose is JAN.] (1) D-Glucose, monohydrate; (2) D-Glucose monohydrate. *UNII-IY9XDZ35W2. CAS-5996-10-1* [acyclic form]; *CAS-77029-61-9* [D-glucopyranose monohydrate]; *CAS-50-99-7* [D-glucose, anhydrous]; *CAS-2280-44-6* [D-glucopyranose, anhydrous]; *CAS-492-62-5* [α-D-glucopyranose, anhydrous]; *CAS-492-61-5* [β-D-glucopyranose, anhydrous]. *Replenisher (fluid and nutrient).*

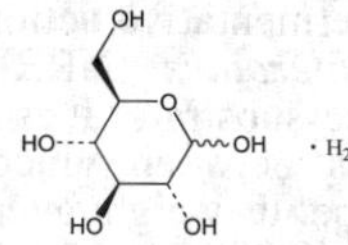

Dextrothyronine — *See* Detrothyronine.

Dextrothyroxine Sodium [*1962*] (dex″ troe thye rox′ een soe′ dee um). $C_{15}H_{10}I_4NNaO_4.xH_2O$. 798.85 (anhydrous). [Dextrothyroxine is BAN.] (1) D-Tyrosine, O-(4-hydroxy-3,5-diiodophenyl)-3,5-diiodo-, monosodium salt hydrate; (2) Monosodium D-thyroxine hydrate. *UNII-0H00N2AHSP; UNII-4W9K63FION* [dextrothyroxine]. *CAS-7054-08-2; CAS-137-53-1* [anhydrous]; *CAS-51-49-0* [dextrothyroxine]. USP XXI; INN. *Antihyperlipidemic.* Choloxin (Abbott)

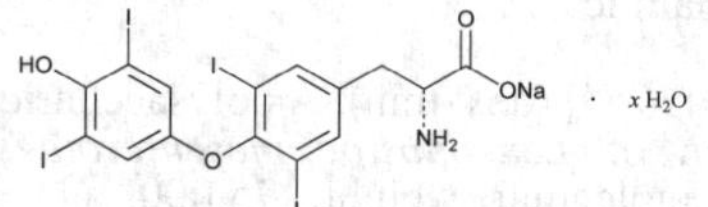

Dexverapamil. $C_{27}H_{38}N_2O_4$. 454.60. (+)-(R)-5-[(3,4-Dimethoxyphenethyl)methylamino]-2-(3,4-dimethoxyphenyl)-2-isopropylvaleronitrile. *UNII-QR5PYD126V. CAS-38321-02-7.* INN.

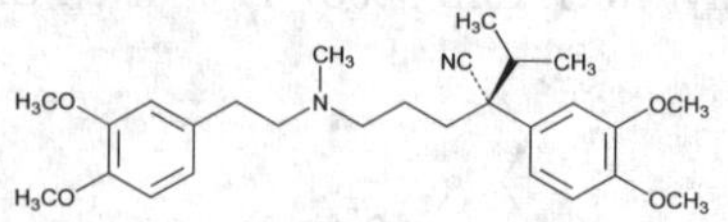

Dezaguanine [*1984*] (dez″ a gwa′ neen). $C_6H_6N_4O$. 150.14. (1) 4H-Imidazo[4,5-c]pyridin-4-one, 6-amino-1,5-dihydro-; (2) 6-Amino-1,5-dihydro-4H-imidazo[4,5-c]pyridin-4-one. *UNII-9DRB973HUI. CAS-41729-52-6.* INN. *Antineoplastic.* ◇*CI-908; NSC-261726*

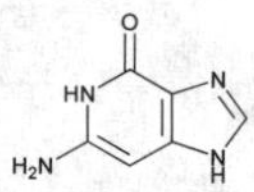

Dezaguanine Mesylate [*1984*] (dez″ a gwa′ neen mes′ i late). $C_7H_{10}N_4O_4S$. 246.24. (1) 4H-Imidazo[4,5-c]pyridin-4-one, 6-amino-1,5-dihydro-, monomethanesulfonate; (2) 6-Amino-1,5-dihydro-4*H*-imidazo[4,5-*c*]pyridin-4-one mono-methanesulfonate. *UNII-H56TJ4554M. CAS-87434-82-0. Antineoplastic.* ✧*CI-908 mesylate; PD 90,695-73*

Dezinamide [*1992*] (dez in′ a mide). C$_{11}$H$_{11}$F$_3$N$_2$O$_2$. 260.21. (1) 1-Azetidinecarboxamide, 3-[3-(trifluoromethyl)phenoxy]-; (2) 3-[(α,α,α-Trifluoro-*m*-tolyl)oxy]-1-azetidinecarboxamide. *CAS-91077-32-6.* INN. *Anticonvulsant.* ✧*AHR-11748; AN-051*

Dezocine [*1976*] (dez′ oh seen). C$_{16}$H$_{23}$NO. 245.36. (1) 5,11-Methanobenzocyclodecen-3-ol, 13-amino-5,6,7,8,9,10,11,12-octahydro-5-methyl-, (5α,11α,13*S**)-, (-)-; (2) (-)-13β-Amino-5,6,7,8,9,10,11α,12-octahydro-5α-methyl-5,11-methanobenzocyclodecen-3-ol. *UNII-VHX8K5SV4X. CAS-53648-55-8.* INN. *Analgesic.* Dalgan (AstraZeneca) ✧*WY-16,225*

DFMO HCl — *See* Eflornithine Hydrochloride.

Diacerein. C$_{19}$H$_{12}$O$_8$. 368.29. 9,10-Dihydro-4,5-dihydroxy-9,10-dioxo-2-anthroic acid, diacetate. *CAS-13739-02-1.* INN; MI.

Diacetamate. C$_{10}$H$_{11}$NO$_3$. 193.20. 4-Acetamidophenyl acetate. *UNII-BFG1TY61BG. CAS-2623-33-8.* INN; BAN.

Diacetolol Hydrochloride [*1979*] (dye a seet′ oh lol hye″ droe klor′ ide). C$_{16}$H$_{24}$N$_2$O$_4$·HCl. 344.83. [Diacetolol is INN and BAN.] (1) Acetamide, *N*-[3-acetyl-4-[2-hydroxy-3-[(1-methylethyl)amino]propoxy]phenyl]-, monohydrochloride, (±)-; (2) (±)-3′-Acetyl-4′-[2-hydroxy-3-(isopropylamino)propoxy]acetanilide monohydrochloride. *CAS-69796-04-9; CAS-22568-64-5* [diacetolol]. *Anti-adrenergic (β-receptor).* ✧*EU-4891; M&B 16942A*

Diacetylated Monoglycerides (dye″ a seet′ il ay″ ted mon″ oh glis′ er idze). **NF.** Glycerin esterified with edible fat-forming fatty acids and acetic acid. *Pharmaceutic aid (plasticizer).*

Diacetylmorphine Hydrochloride. [Diamorphine is BAN.] *CAS-1502-95-0; CAS-561-27-3* [diacetylmorphine]. USP IX; MI.

Diacetylnalorphine. C$_{23}$H$_{27}$NO$_5$. 397.46. (-)-(5*R*,6*S*)-9a-Allyl-4,5-epoxymorphin-7-en-3,6-diyldiacetate. *CAS-2748-74-5.* BAN.

Diacetylsalicylic Acid — *See* Dipyrocetyl.

Diacetyltannic Acid — *See* Acetyltannic Acid.

Diacetylthiamine — *See* Acetiamine.

Diallylbarbituric Acid (previously used name) — *See* Allobarbital.

Diallylnortoxiferene Dichloride — *See* Alcuronium Chloride.

Diallymal — *See* Allobarbital.

Diamfenetide. C$_{20}$H$_{24}$N$_2$O$_5$. 372.41. β,β′-Oxybis[*p*-acetophenetidide]. *UNII-U4TFJ7GB6T. CAS-36141-82-9.* INN; BAN; MI. [*Name previously used: Diamphenethide.*] ✧*Compound 68-198*

Diaminodiphenylsulfone (previously used name) — *See* Dapsone.

Diamocaine Cyclamate [*1969*] (dye a′ moe kane sye′ kla mate). C$_{37}$H$_{63}$N$_5$O$_7$S$_2$. 754.06. [Diamocaine is INN and BAN.] (1) Sulfamic acid, cyclohexyl-, compd. with 4-[2-(diethylamino)ethoxy]-*N*,4-diphenyl-1-piperidineethanamine (2:1); (2) 1-(2-Anilinoethyl)-4-[2-(diethylamino)ethoxy]-4-phenylpiperidine bis(cyclohexanesulfamate). *CAS-23469-05-8; CAS-27112-37-4* [diamocaine]. *Anesthetic (local).* ✧*R 10,948*

Diamorphine (BAN) — *See* Diacetylmorphine Hydrochloride.

Diamphenethide (previously used name) — *See* Diamfenetide.

Diampromide. C$_{21}$H$_{28}$N$_2$O. 324.46. *N*-[2-(Methylphenethylamino)propyl]propionanilide. *UNII-26G7YC77BU. CAS-552-25-0.* INN; BAN; DCF; MI.

Diamthazole. $C_{15}H_{23}N_3OS$. 293.43. [Dimazole is INN.] 6-(2-Diethylaminoethoxy)-2-dimethylaminobenzothiazol. *UNII-2KL01R8ZV1. CAS-95-27-2; CAS-136-96-9* [dihydrochloride]. BAN; MI. Asterol [as dihydrochloride] [Veterinary] (Hoffmann-LaRoche†)

Dianicline. $C_{13}H_{16}N_2O$. 216.28. (5a*S*,10a*R*)-6,7,9,10-Tetrahydro-5a*H*,11*H*-8,10a-methanopyrido[2′,3′:5,6]pyrano[2,3-*d*]azepine. *UNII-Y0SNM34C6O. CAS-292634-27-6.* INN.

Diapamide [*1967*] (dye ap′ a mide). $C_9H_{11}ClN_2O_3S$. 262.71. [Tiamizide is INN.] (1) Benzamide, 4-chloro-*N*-methyl-3-[(methylamino)sulfonyl]-; (2) 4-Chloro-*N*-methyl-3-(methylsulfamoyl)benzamide. *CAS-3688-85-5. Diuretic; antihypertensive.* ◇*CI-456; CN-36,337; D-1593*

Diaphenylsulfone (DCF) — *See* Dapsone.

Diaplasinin [*2005*] (dye″ a plas′ in in). $C_{32}H_{31}N_5O$. 501.62. (1) 1*H*-Indole, 3-pentyl-1-(phenylmethyl)-2-[6-(1*H*-tetrazol-5-ylmethoxy)-2-naphthalenyl]-; (2) 1-Benzyl-3-pentyl-2-[6-(1*H*-tetrazol-5-ylmethoxy)naphthalen-2-yl]-1*H*-indole. *UNII-NRL66AVH63. CAS-481631-45-2.* INN. *Treatment of fibrinolytic impairment diseases.* ◇*PAI-749*

Diarbarone. $C_{16}H_{20}N_2O_4$. 304.34. *N*-[2-(Diethylamino)ethyl]-4-hydroxy-2-oxo-2*H*-1-benzopyran-3-carboxamide. *UNII-IL298686U0. CAS-1233-70-1.* INN; DCF.

Diastase. An amylolytic enzyme mainly prepared from malt. *CAS-9000-92-4.* JAN.

Diathymosulfone. $C_{32}H_{34}N_4O_4S$. 570.70. Di[4-(4-hydroxy-2-methyl-5-isopropylphenylazo)phenyl]sulfone. *UNII-UK27RQ38IX. CAS-5964-62-5.* INN; DCF; MI.

Diatrizoate Meglumine (dye″ a trye zoe′ ate me′ gloo meen). **USP**. $C_{11}H_9I_3N_2O_4 \cdot C_7H_{17}NO_5$. 809.13. [Meglumine Amidotrizoate is BAN; Meglumine Amidotrizoate Injection is JAN.] (1) Benzoic acid, 3,5-bis(acetylamino)-2,4,6-triiodo-, compd. with 1-deoxy-1-(methylamino)-D-glucitol (1:1); (2) 1-Deoxy-1-(methylamino)-D-glucitol 3,5-diacetamido-2,4,6-triiodobenzoate (salt). *UNII-6HG8UB2MUY* [meglumine]. *CAS-131-49-7; CAS-117-96-4* [diatrizoic acid]; *CAS-6284-40-8* [meglumine]. *Diagnostic aid (radiopaque medium).* Cardiografin (Bracco); Cystografin (Bracco); Hypaque (GE Healthcare); Reno (Bracco) *[Note— Reno-M-30, Reno-M-60, Reno-M-DIP are also brand names for this drug.][Name previously used: Meglumine Diatrizoate.]*

Diatrizoate Methylglucamine — *See* Diatrizoate Meglumine.

Diatrizoate Sodium (dye″ a trye zoe′ ate soe′ dee um). **USP**. $C_{11}H_8I_3N_2NaO_4$. 635.90. [Meglumine Sodium Amidotrizoate Injection is JAN; Sodium Amidotrizoate is INN and BAN.] (1) Benzoic acid, 3,5-bis(acetylamino)-2,4,6-triiodo-, monosodium salt; (2) Monosodium 3,5-diacetamido-2,4,6-triiodobenzoate. *UNII-5UVC90J1LK* [diatrizoic acid]. *CAS-737-31-5; CAS-117-96-4* [diatrizoic acid]. *Diagnostic aid (radiopaque medium).* Hypaque (GE Healthcare); Md (Mallinckrodt); Urovist Sodium (Berlex) *[Name previously used: Sodium Diatrizoate.]* ◇*NSC-61815*

Diatrizoate Sodium I 125 [*1966*] (dye″ a trye zoe′ ate soe′ dee um). $C_{11}H_8{}^{125}I_3N_2NaO_4$. (1) Benzoic acid, 3,5-bis(acetylamino)-2,4,6-triiodo-, monosodium salt, labeled with iodine-125; (2) Monosodium 3,5-diacetamido-2,4,6-triiodobenzoate, labeled with iodine-125. *Radioactive agent.*

Diatrizoate Sodium I 131 [*1963*] (dye″ a trye zoe′ ate soe′ dee um). $C_{11}H_8{}^{131}I_3N_2NaO_4$. (1) Benzoic acid, 3,5-bis(acetylamino)-2,4,6-triiodo-, monosodium salt, labeled with iodine-131; (2) Monosodium 3,5-diacetamido-2,4,6-triiodobenzoate, labeled with iodine-131. *CAS-14855-77-7. Radioactive agent.*

Diatrizoic Acid [*1967*] (dye″ a trye zoe′ ik as′ id). **USP**. $C_{11}H_9I_3N_2O_4$. 613.91. [Amidotrizoic Acid is JAN and BAN.] (1) Benzoic acid, 3,5-bis(acetylamino)-2,4,6-triiodo-; (2) 3,5-Diacetamido-2,4,6-triiodobenzoic acid. *UNII-

5UVC90J1LK. CAS-117-96-4; CAS-50978-11-5 [dihydrate]. *Diagnostic aid (radiopaque medium).* ◇*NSC-262168*

Diaveridine [*1962*] (dye″ a ver′ i deen). $C_{13}H_{16}N_4O_2$. 260.29. (1) 2,4-Pyrimidinediamine, 5-[(3,4-dimethoxyphenyl)-methyl]-; (2) 2,4-Diamino-5-veratrylpyrimidine. *CAS-5355-16-8.* INN; BAN. *Antibacterial.* ◇*BW 49-210; NSC-408735*

Diazacholesterol Dihydrochloride — *See* Azacosterol Hydrochloride.

Diazepam [*1963*] (dye az′ e pam). **USP.** $C_{16}H_{13}ClN_2O$. 284.74. (1) 2*H*-1,4-Benzodiazepin-2-one, 7-chloro-1,3-dihydro-1-methyl-5-phenyl-; (2) 7-Chloro-1,3-dihydro-1-methyl-5-phenyl-2*H*-1,4-benzodiazepin-2-one. *UNII-Q3JTX2Q7TU. CAS-439-14-5.* INN; BAN; JAN. *Sedative-hypnotic.* Diastat (Valeant); Valium (Roche) ◇*LA III; Ro 5-2807; Wy-3467; NSC-77518*

Diazinon (previously used name) — *See* Dimpylate.

Diaziquone [*1981*] (dye az′ i kwone). $C_{16}H_{20}N_4O_6$. 364.35. (1) Carbamic acid, [2,5-bis(1-aziridinyl)-3,6-dioxo-1,4-cyclohexadiene-1,4-diyl]bis-, diethyl ester; (2) Diethyl 2,5-bis-(1-aziridinyl)-3,6-dioxo-1,4-cyclohexadiene-1,4-dicarbamate; (3) Aziridinyl benzoquinone. *CAS-57998-68-2.* INN. *Antineoplastic.* ◇*CI-904; AZQ; NSC-182986*

Diazoxide [*1962*] (dye″ az ox′ ide). **USP.** $C_8H_7ClN_2O_2S$. 230.67. (1) 2*H*-1,2,4-Benzothiadiazine, 7-chloro-3-methyl-, 1,1-dioxide; (2) 7-Chloro-3-methyl-2*H*-1,2,4-ben-

zothiadiazine 1,1-dioxide. *UNII-O5CB12L4FN. CAS-364-98-7.* INN; BAN; JAN. *Antihypertensive.* Proglycem (Baker Norton) ◇*SRG 95213; Sch 6783; NSC-64198*

Dibasol — *See* Bendazol.

Dibazol — *See* Bendazol.

Dibekacin. $C_{18}H_{37}N_5O_8$. 451.52. [Dibekacin Sulfate is JAN.] *O*-3-Amino-3-deoxy-α-D-glucopyranosyl-(1→4)-*O*-[2,6-diamino-2,3,4,6-tetradeoxy-α-D-*erythro*-hexopyranosyl-(1→6)]-2-deoxy-L-streptamine. *UNII-45ZFO9E525. CAS-34493-98-6.* INN; BAN; MI.

Dibemethine. $C_{15}H_{17}N$. 211.30. *N,N*-Dibenzylmethylamine. *UNII-67VKG5DY8W. CAS-102-05-6.* INN; DCF. ◇*L 566*

Dibencozide (DCF) — *See* Cobamamide.

Dibenthiamine (DCF) — *See* Bentiamine.

Dibenzathione — *See* Sulbentine.

Dibenzepin Hydrochloride [*1964*] (dye benz′ e pin hye″ droe klor′ ide). $C_{18}H_{21}N_3O\cdot HCl$. 331.84. [Dibenzepin is INN and BAN.] (1) 11*H*-Dibenzo[*b,e*][1,4]-diazepin-11-one, 10-[2-(dimethylamino)ethyl]-5,10-dihydro-5-methyl-, monohydrochloride; (2) 10-[2-(Dimethylamino)ethyl]-5,10-dihydro-5-methyl-11-*H*-dibenzo[*b,e*][1,4]diazepin-11-one monohydrochloride. *CAS-315-80-0; CAS-4498-32-2* [dibenzepin]. *Antidepressant.* ◇*HF 1927*

Dibenzothiophene [*1980*] (dye ben″ zoe thye′ oh feen). $C_{12}H_8S$. 184.26. (1) Dibenzothiophene; (2) Dibenzothiophene. *UNII-Z3D4AJ1R48. CAS-132-65-0. Keratolytic.*

Dibenzoylthiamin — *See* Bentiamine.

Dibenzthion — *See* Sulbentine.

Dibotermin Alfa [*2001*] (dye boe′ ter min al′ fa). Bone morphogenetic protein 2 (human recombinant rhBMP-2). Dibotermin alfa is a glycosylated (oligomannosidic), disulfide-linked dimeric protein consisting of all combinations of the two N-terminal processed subunits. The N-terminal glutamine may also exist as pyroglutamic acid, as a result of spontaneous cyclization of N-terminal glutamine to pyroglutamate. Molecular weights are approximately 28,000 to 33,000 daltons (dimer) or 14,000 to 17,000 daltons (monomer). *CAS-246539-15-1.* INN; BAN. *Osteoinductive agent for use in orthopaedic surgery, dental/craniofacial surgery, or spine surgery, as an adjunct to standard care or as a replacement for autogenous bone graft.*

```
 TFGHDGK   GHPLHKREKR   QAKHKQRKRL   KSSCKRHPLY   VDFSDVGWND
WIVAPPGYHA  FYCHGECPFP   LADHLNSTNH   AIVQTLVNSV   NSKIPKACCV
PTELSAISML  YLDENEKVVL   KNYQDMVVEG   CGCR
```

* glycosylation site

↓ NH₂-terminal processing sites

Dibromodulcitol — *See* Mitolactol.

Dibromohydroxyquinoline — *See* Broxyquinoline.

Dibrompropamidine. C₁₇H₁₈Br₂N₄O₂. 470.16. 4,4′-(Trimethylenedioxy)bis(3-bromobenzamidine). *UNII-269M3QL74S. CAS-496-00-4.* INN; BAN; MI. *[Name previously used: Dibromopropamidine.]*

Dibromsalan [*1963*] (dye brom′ sa lan). C₁₃H₉Br₂NO₂. 371.02. (1) Benzamide, 5-bromo-*N*-(4-bromophenyl)-2-hydroxy-; (2) 4′,5-Dibromosalicylanilide. *CAS-87-12-7.* INN. *Disinfectant.* ◇NSC-20527

Dibrospidium Chloride. C₁₈H₃₂Br₂Cl₂N₄O₂. 567.19. 3,12-Bis(3-bromopropionyl)-3,12-diaza-6,9-diazoniadispiro[5.2.5.2]hexadecane dichloride. *UNII-GRX5L9Y3Z3. CAS-86641-76-1.* INN.

Dibucaine (dye′ bue kane). **USP.** C₂₀H₂₉N₃O₂. 343.46. [Cinchocaine is INN and BAN.] (1) 4-Quinolinecarboxamide, 2-butoxy-*N*-[2-(diethylamino)ethyl]-; (2) 2-Butoxy-*N*-[2-(diethylamino)ethyl]cinchoninamide. *UNII-L6JW2TJG99. CAS-85-79-0.* Anesthetic (local). Nupercainal (Ciba-Geigy)

Dibucaine Hydrochloride (dye′ bue kane hye″ droe klor′ ide). **USP.** C₂₀H₂₉N₃O₂.HCl. 379.92. [Cinchocaine Hydrochloride is BAN.] (1) 4-Quinolinecarboxamide, 2-butoxy-*N*-[2-(diethylamino)ethyl]-, monohydrochloride; (2) 2-Butoxy-*N*-[2-(diethylamino)ethyl]cinchoninamide monohydrochloride. *UNII-Z97702A5DG; UNII-L6JW2TJG99* [dibucaine]. *CAS-61-12-1; CAS-85-79-0* [dibucaine]. JAN. *Anesthetic (local).* Nupercaine (Novartis)

Dibuprol. C₁₁H₂₄O₃. 204.31. 1,3-Dibutoxy-2-propanol. *UNII-1627CY4S8U. CAS-2216-77-5.* INN.

Dibupyrone. C₁₆H₂₂N₃NaO₄S. 375.42. Sodium (antipyrinylisobutylamino)methanesulfonate. *UNII-T99M8X4T54. CAS-1046-17-9.* INN; BAN.

Dibusadol. C₁₇H₂₆N₂O₃. 306.40. *N*-[4-(Diethylamino)butyl]salicylamide acetate (ester). *UNII-O55N96CWOW. CAS-24353-45-5.* INN.

Dibutoline Sulfate. *UNII-1W7R63X54A. CAS-532-49-0.* MI.

Dibutyl Phthalate (dye bue′ til thal′ ate). **NF.** C₁₆H₂₂O₄. 278.34. 1,2-Benzenedicarboxylic acid, dibutyl ester. *CAS-84-74-2.*

Dibutyl Sebacate (dye bue′ til seb′ a kate). **NF.** C₁₈H₃₄O₄. 314.46. (1) Sebacic acid; (2) Dibutyl decanedioate. *UNII-4W5IH7FLNY. CAS-109-43-3. Pharmaceutic aid (plasticizer).*

Dicarbine. C₁₃H₁₈N₂. 202.30. 2,3,4,4a,5,9b-Hexahydro-2,8-dimethyl-1*H*-pyrido[4,3-*b*]indole. *UNII-Y0EA50IJ3V. CAS-17411-19-7.* INN.

Dicarfen. C₁₉H₂₄N₂O₂. 312.41. 2-(Diethylamino)ethyl diphenylcarbamate ester. *UNII-P7MDS492AC. CAS-15585-88-3.* INN. ◇SD 25

Dichlofenthion. *o*-2,4-Dichlorophenyl *O,O*-diethyl phosphorothioate. *CAS-97-17-6.* BAN; MI. ◇V-C 13

Dichloralphenazone (dye″ klor al fen′ a zone). **USP**. $C_{15}H_{18}Cl_6N_2O_5$. 519.03. (1) 1,2-Dihydro-1,5-dimethyl-2-phenyl-3*H*-pyrazol-3-one, compd. with 2,2,2-trichloro-1,1-ethanediol (1:2); (2) Antipyrine, compound with chloral hydrate (1:2). *CAS-480-30-8*. BAN. *Sedative-hypnotic*.

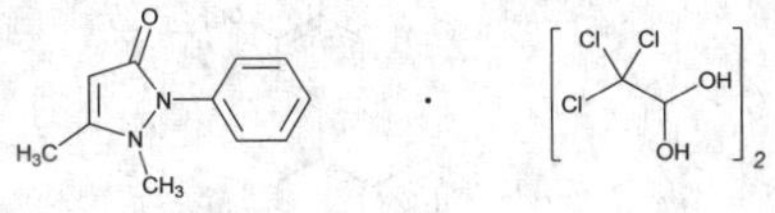

Dichloramine-T. *N,N*-Dichloro-*p*-toluenesulfonamide. NF VIII; MI.

Dichloranilino Imidazolin — *See* Clonidine Hydrochloride.

Dichlorisone Acetate. $C_{23}H_{28}Cl_2O_5$. 455.37. [Dichlorisone is INN.] 9α,11β-Dichloro-17α,21-dihydroxypregna-1,4-diene-3,20-dione 21-acetate. *UNII-AMW2MRV3OT* [dichlorisone]. *CAS-79-61-8; CAS-7008-26-6* [dichlorisone]. MI. Diloderm (Schering†)

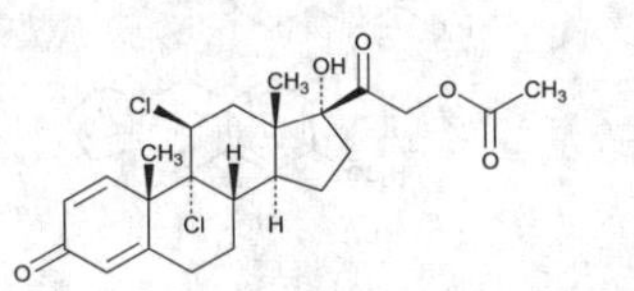

Dichlormethazanone — *See* Dichlormezanone.

Dichlormezanone. $C_{11}H_{11}Cl_2NO_3S$. 308.18. 2-(3,4-Dichlorophenyl)tetrahydro-3-methyl-4*H*-1,3-thiazin-4-one 1,1-dioxide. *UNII-TO4OC41XVI*. *CAS-5571-97-1*. INN.

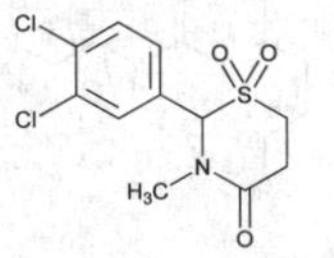

Dichlorodifluoromethane (dye klor″ oh dye floor″ oh meth′ ane). **NF**. CCl_2F_2. 120.91. (1) Methane, dichlorodifluoro-; (2) Dichlorodifluoromethane. *UNII-OFM06SG1KO*. *CAS-75-71-8*. *Pharmaceutic aid (aerosol propellant)*.

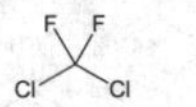

Dichlorometaxylenol — *See* Dichloroxylenol.

Dichlorophen. $C_{13}H_{10}Cl_2O_2$. 269.12. 2,2′-Methylenebis(4-chlorophenol). *UNII-T1J0JOU64O*. *CAS-97-23-4*. INN; BAN; DCF; MI. ◇*G-4*

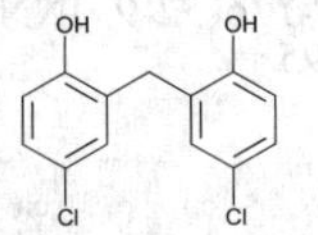

Dichlorophenarsine Hydrochloride. $C_6H_6AsCl_2NO.HCl$. 290.41. [Dichlorophenarsine is INN and BAN.] Dichlorophenarsinammonium chloride, 3-amino-4-hydroxyphenyldichloroarsine. *UNII-571850CM3R; UNII-*

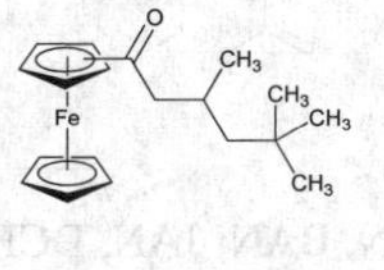

† Brand name formerly used, and/or firm no longer concerned with this product.

3WD5400T9N [dichlorophenarsine]. *CAS-536-29-8; CAS-455-83-4* [dichlorophenarsine]. USP XIV; MI. Dichlor-Mapharsen (Parke-Davis†)

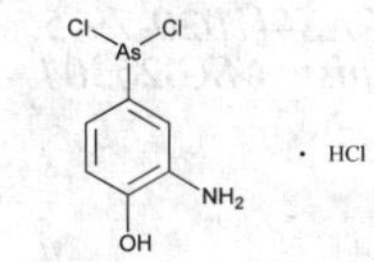

Dichlorotetrafluoroethane (dye klor″ oh te tra floor″ oh eth′ ane). **NF**. $C_2Cl_2F_4$. 170.92. [Cryofluorane is INN.] (1) Ethane, 1,2-dichloro-1,1,2,2-tetrafluoro-; (2) 1,2-Dichlorotetrafluoroethane. *UNII-6B5VVT93AR*. *CAS-76-14-2*. *Pharmaceutic aid (aerosol propellant)*.

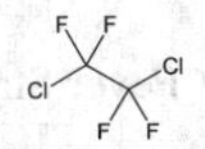

Dichloroxylenol. $C_8H_8Cl_2O$. 191.05. 2,4-Dichloro-3,5-xylenol. *UNII-51AC49OLT7*. *CAS-133-53-9*. INN; BAN; DCF; MI.

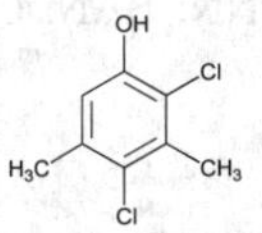

Dichlorphenamide (dye″ klor fen′ a mide). **USP**. $C_6H_6Cl_2N_2O_4S_2$. 305.16. [Diclofenamide is INN, BAN and JAN.] (1) 1,3-Benzenedisulfonamide, 4,5-dichloro-; (2) 4,5-Dichloro-*m*-benzenedisulfonamide. *UNII-VVJ6673MHY*. *CAS-120-97-8*. *Carbonic anhydrase inhibitor*. Daranide (Merck)

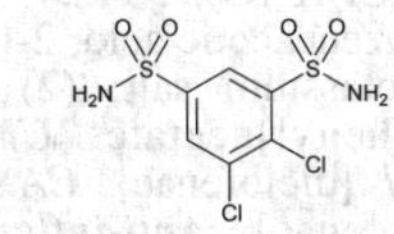

Dichlorvos [*1972*] (dye klor′ vos). $C_4H_7Cl_2O_4P$. 220.98. (1) Phosphoric acid, 2,2-dichloroethenyl dimethyl ester; (2) 2,2-Dichlorovinyl dimethyl phosphate. *UNII-7U370BPS14*. *CAS-62-73-7*. INN; BAN. *Anthelmintic*. Atgard (Boehringer Ingelheim Animal Health); Equigard (Boehringer Ingelheim Animal Health); Equigel (Boehringer Ingelheim Animal Health†); TASK Tabs (Boehringer Ingelheim Animal Health) ◇*SD 1750; DDVP; NSC-6738*

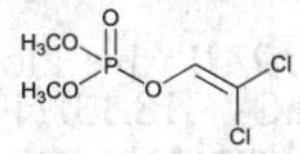

Dichromium Trioxide. Cr_2O_3. 151.99. Chromium(III) sesquioxide. *CAS-1308-38-9*. BAN.

Dichysterol — *See* Dihydrotachysterol.

Diciferron. $C_{19}H_{26}FeO$. 326.25. (3,5,5-Trimethylhexanoyl)-ferrocene. *CAS-65606-61-3*. INN.

Dicirenone [*1984*] (dye sye′ re none). $C_{26}H_{36}O_5$. 428.56. (1) Pregn-4-ene-7,21-dicarboxylic acid, 17-hydroxy-3-oxo-, γ-lactone, 1-methylethyl ester, $(7\alpha,17\alpha)$-; (2) 17-Hydroxy-3-oxo-17α-pregn-4-ene-7α,21-dicarboxylic acid, γ-lactone, isopropyl ester. *CAS-41020-79-5*. INN. *Hypotensive; aldosterone antagonist.* ◇*SC-26304*

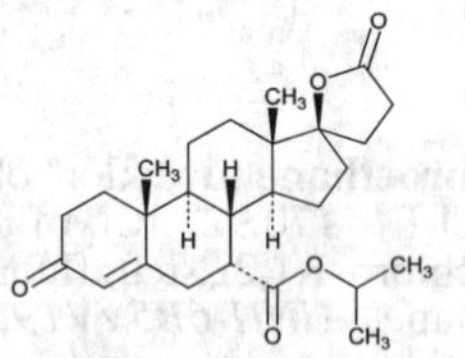

Dick Test — *See* Scarlet Fever Streptococcus Toxin.

Diclazuril [*1988*] (dye klaz′ ue ril). $C_{17}H_9Cl_3N_4O_2$. 407.64. (1) Benzeneacetonitrile, 2,6-dichloro-α-(4-chlorophenyl)-4-(4,5-dihydro-3,5-dioxo-1,2,4-triazin-2(3*H*)-yl)-; (2) (*p*-Chlorophenyl)[2,6-dichloro-4-(4,5-dihydro-3,5-dioxo-*as*-triazin-2(3*H*)-yl)phenyl]acetonitrile. *UNII-K110K1B1VE*. *CAS-101831-37-2*. INN; BAN. *Coccidiostat (for poultry).* ◇*R64,433*

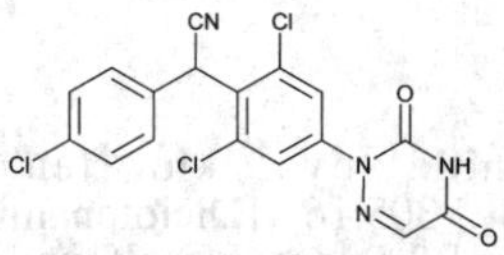

Diclofenac Potassium [*1992*] (dye kloe′ fen ak poe tas′ ee um). USP. $C_{14}H_{10}Cl_2KNO_2$. 334.24. [Diclofenac is INN and BAN.] (1) Benzeneacetic acid, 2-[(2,6-dichlorophenyl)amino]-, monopotassium salt; (2) Potassium [*o*-(2,6-dichloroanilino)phenyl]acetate. *UNII-L4D5UA6CB4; UNII-144O8QL0L1* [diclofenac]. *CAS-15307-81-0; CAS-15307-86-5* [diclofenac]. *Anti-inflammatory.* Cataflam (Novartis) ◇*CGP 45840B*

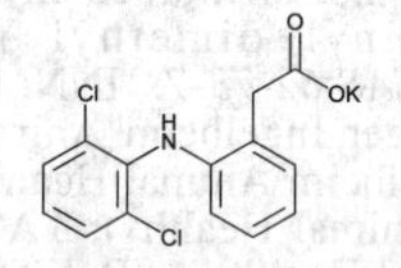

Diclofenac Sodium [*1973*] (dye kloe′ fen ak soe′ dee um). USP. $C_{14}H_{10}Cl_2NNaO_2$. 318.13. (1) Benzeneacetic acid, 2-[(2,6-dichlorophenyl)amino]-, monosodium salt; (2) Sodium [*o*-(2,6-dichloroanilino)phenyl]acetate. *UNII-QTG126297Q*. *CAS-15307-79-6*. JAN. *Anti-inflammatory.* Solaraze (Bioglan); Voltaren (Novartis) ◇*GP 45840*

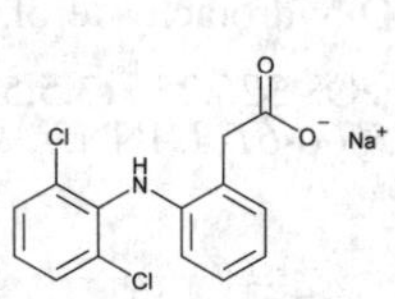

Diclofenamide (INN, BAN, JAN, DCF) — *See* Dichlorphenamide.

Diclofensine. $C_{17}H_{17}Cl_2NO$. 322.23. ($\pm$)-4-(3,4-Dichlorophenyl)-1,2,3,4-tetrahydro-7-methoxy-2-methylisoquinoline. *UNII-09HKW863J6*. *CAS-67165-56-4*. INN.

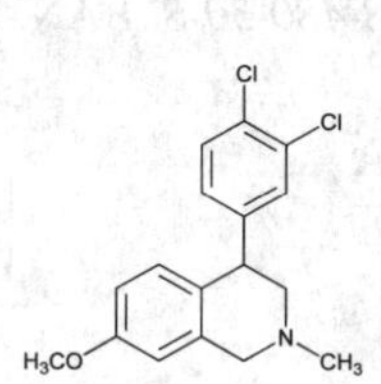

Diclofibrate — *See* Simfibrate.

Diclofurime. $C_{18}H_{22}Cl_2N_2O_3$. 385.28. 2,3-Dichloro-4-methoxyphenyl 2-furyl ketone (*E*)-*O*-[2-(diethylamino)ethyl]oxime. *UNII-D1FP3K444H*. *CAS-64743-08-4*. INN.

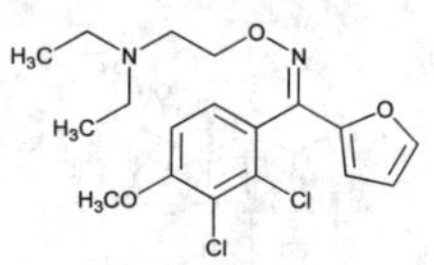

Diclometide. $C_{14}H_{20}Cl_2N_2O_2$. 319.23. 3,5-Dichloro-*N*-[2-(diethylamino)-ethyl]-*o*-anisamide. *UNII-05186J17EP*. *CAS-17243-49-1*. INN; DCF.

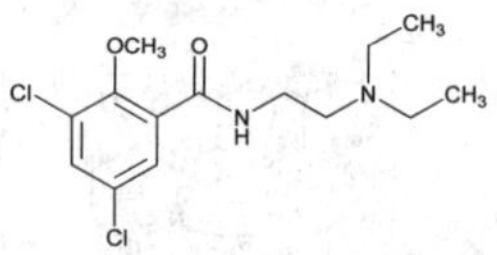

Diclonixin. $C_{12}H_8Cl_2N_2O_2$. 283.11. 2-(2,3-Dichloroanilino)-nicotinic acid. *UNII-357591W853*. *CAS-17737-68-7*. INN.

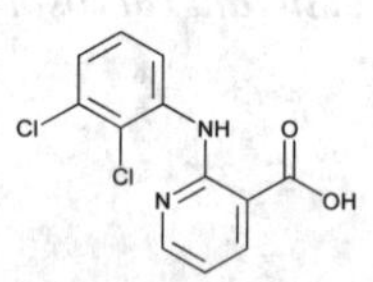

Dicloralurea [*1974*] (dye klor″ al ure ee′ a). $C_5H_6Cl_6N_2O_3$. 354.83. (1) Urea, *N,N*′-bis(2,2,2-trichloro-1-hydroxyethyl)-; (2) 1,3-Bis(2,2,2-trichloro-1-hydroxyethyl)urea. *UNII-9J3ZB93FIE*. *CAS-116-52-9*. INN. *Food additive (veterinary).* ◇*SK&F 1995*

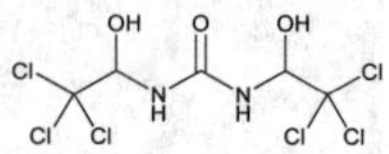

Dicloxacillin [*1965*] (dye klox″ a sil′ in). $C_{19}H_{17}Cl_2N_3O_5S$. 470.33. (1) 4-Thia-1-azabicyclo[3.2.0]heptane-2-carboxylic acid, 6-[[[3-(2,6-dichlorophenyl)-5-methyl-4-isoxazolyl]carbonyl]amino]-3,3-dimethyl-7-oxo-, [2*S*-(2α,5α,6β)]-; (2) 6-[3-(2,6-Dichlorophenyl)-5-methyl-4-isoxazolecarboxamido]-3,3-dimethyl-7-oxo-4-thia-1-azabicyclo[3.2.0]heptane-2-carboxylic acid. *UNII-COF19H7WBK. CAS-3116-76-5.* INN; BAN. *Antibacterial.* ◇*BRL-1702; R-13423*

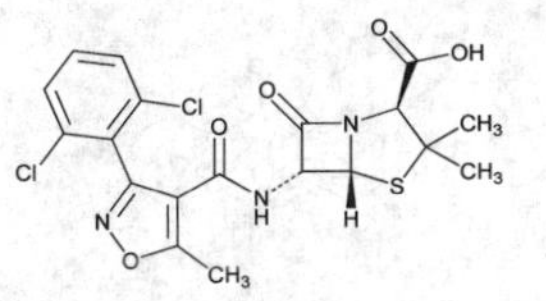

Dicloxacillin Sodium [*1968*] (dye klox″ a sil′ in soe′ dee um). **USP.** $C_{19}H_{16}Cl_2N_3NaO_5S.H_2O$. 510.32. (1) 4-Thia-1-azabicyclo[3.2.0]heptane-2-carboxylic acid, 6-[[[3-(2,6-dichlorophenyl)-5-methyl-4-isoxazolyl]carbonyl]amino]-3,3-dimethyl-7-oxo-, monosodium salt, monohydrate, [2*S*-(2α,5α,6β)]-; (2) Monosodium (2*S*,5*R*,6*R*)-6-[3-(2,6-dichlorophenyl)-5-methyl-4-isoxazolecarboxamido]-3,3-dimethyl-7-oxo-4-thia-1-azabicyclo[3.2.0]heptane-2-carboxylate monohydrate. *UNII-4HZT2V9KX0; UNII-COF19H7WBK* [dicloxacillin]. *CAS-13412-64-1; CAS-343-55-5* [anhydrous]; *CAS-3116-76-5* [dicloxacillin]. BAN; JAN. *Antibacterial.* Dynapen (Apothecon) ◇*P-1011*

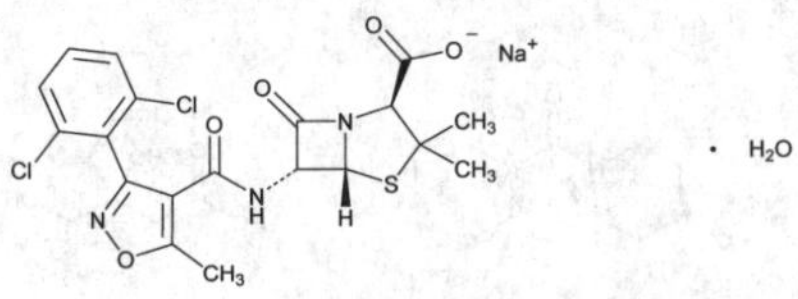

Dicobalt Edetate. $C_{10}H_{12}Co_2N_2O_8$. 406.08. Cobalt(2+)[(ethylenedinitrilo)tetraacetato]cobaltate(2-). *UNII-UKC6GH80QR. CAS-36499-65-7.* INN; BAN.

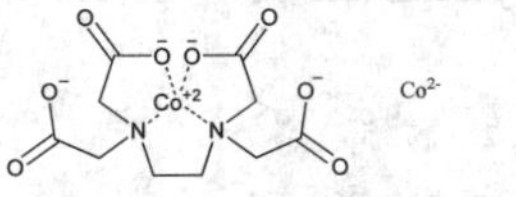

Dicolinium Iodide. $C_{16}H_{34}I_2N_2O_2$. 540.26. 2-Carboxy-1,1,6-trimethylpiperidinium iodide, ester with diethyl-(2-hydroxyethyl)methylammonium iodide. *UNII-4L6L92S51P. CAS-382-82-1.* INN; MI.

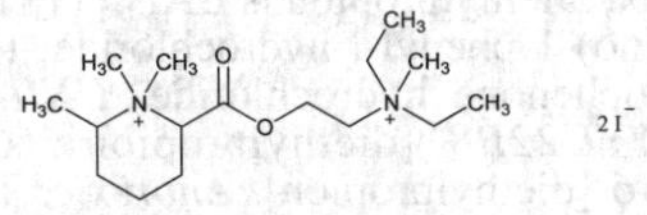

Dicophane (BAN) — *See* Chlorophenothane.

Dicoumarol (INN and DCF) — *See* Dicumarol.

Dicresulene. $C_{15}H_{16}O_8S_2$. 388.41. 3,3′-Methylenebis[6-hydroxy-*p*-toluenesulfonic acid]. *UNII-1I375617NG. CAS-78480-14-5.* INN.

Dicumarol [*1971*] (dye koo′ ma rol). $C_{19}H_{12}O_6$. 336.29. [Dicoumarol is INN.] (1) 2*H*-1-Benzopyran-2-one], 3,3′-Methylenebis[4-hydroxy-; (2) 3,3′-Methylenebis[4-hydroxycoumarin]. *UNII-7QID3E7BG7. CAS-66-76-2.* USP XXII. *Anticoagulant.* [Name previously used: Bishydroxycoumarin.]

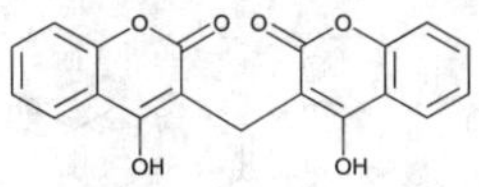

Dicyclomine Hydrochloride (dye sye′ kloe meen hye″ droe klor′ ide). **USP.** $C_{19}H_{35}NO_2.HCl$. 345.95. [Dicycloverine is INN and BAN; Dicycloverine Hydrochloride is JAN.] (1) [Bicyclohexyl]-1-carboxylic acid, 2-(diethylamino)ethyl ester, hydrochloride; (2) 2-(Diethylamino)ethyl [bicyclohexyl]-1-carboxylate hydrochloride. *UNII-CQ903KQA31; UNII-4KV4X8IF6V* [dicyclomine]. *CAS-67-92-5; CAS-77-19-0* [dicyclomine]. *Anticholinergic.* Bentyl (Axcan Scandipharm)

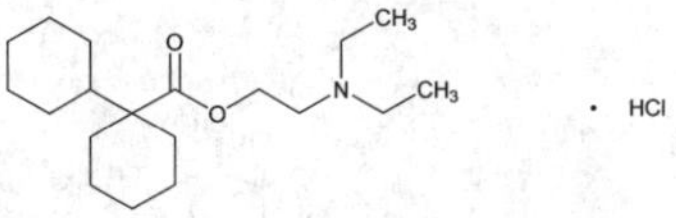

Dicycloverine (INN) — *See* Dicyclomine Hydrochloride.

Dicycloverine Hydrochloride (JAN) — *See* Dicyclomine Hydrochloride.

Didanosine [*1990*] (dye dan′ oh seen). **USP.** $C_{10}H_{12}N_4O_3$. 236.23. (1) Inosine, 2′,3′-dideoxy-; (2) 2′,3′-Dideoxyinosine. *UNII-K3GDH6OH08. CAS-69655-05-6.* INN; BAN. *Antiviral.* Videx (Bristol-Myers Squibb) ◇*BMY-40900*

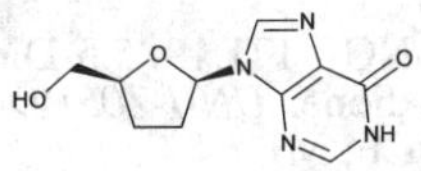

Dideoxycytidine — *See* Zalcitabine.

Dideoxyinosine (DDI) — *See* Didanosine.

Didrovaltrate. $C_{22}H_{32}O_8$. 424.48. 1,4a,5,7a-Tetrahydro-1,6-dihydroxyspiro[cyclopenta[*c*]pyran-7(6*H*),2′-oxirane]-4-methanol 6-acetate 1,4-diisovalerate. *UNII-KEN63D125F. CAS-18296-45-2.* INN.

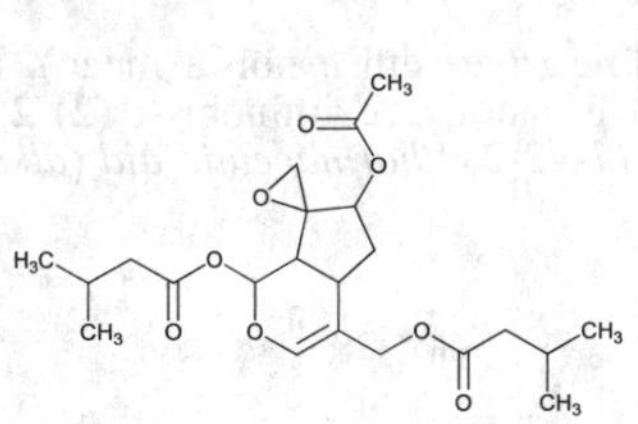

Dieldrin. $C_{12}H_8Cl_6O$. 380.91. A mixture containing 85% of 1,2,3,4,10,10-hexachloro-6,7-epoxy-1,4,4a,5,6,7,8,8a-octahydro-1,4-*exo*-5,8-*endo*-dimethanonaphthalene. *CAS-60-57-1.* INN; BAN; MI. ◇*Compound 497; HEOD*

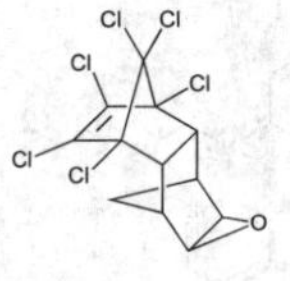

Diemal — *See* Barbital.

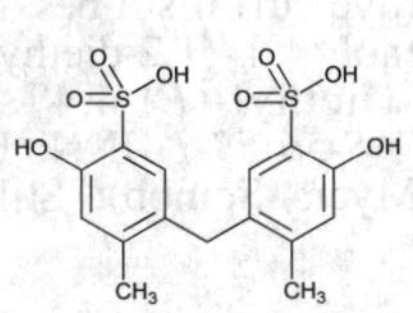

† Brand name formerly used, and/or firm no longer concerned with this product.

Dienestrol (dye″ en es′ trol). **USP.** $C_{18}H_{18}O_2$. 266.33. (1) Phenol, 4,4′-(1,2-diethylidene-1,2-ethanediyl)bis-, (*E,E*)-; (2) (*E,E*)-4,4′-(Diethylideneethylene)diphenol. *UNII-RRW32X4U1F. CAS-84-17-3; CAS-13029-44-2 [E,E].* INN; BAN. *Estrogen.* Dv (Sanofi Aventis); Estraguard (Solvay Pharmaceuticals) *[Name previously used: Dienoestrol.]*

Dienogest [*1999*] (dye en′ oh jest). $C_{20}H_{25}NO_2$. 311.42. (1) 19-Norpregna-4,9-diene-21-nitrile, 17-hydroxy-3-oxo-, (17α)-; (2) 17-Hydroxy-3-oxo-19-nor-17α-pregna-4,9-diene-21-nitrile. *CAS-65928-58-7.* INN; BAN. *Oral contraceptive; hormone replacement therapy.* Endometrion (Schering A.G., Germany) ◇*ZK 37659; STS 557; M 18575; MJR-35*

Dietamiphylline (DCF) — *See* Etamiphyllin.

Dietamiverine Hydrochloride — *See* Bietamiverine Hydrochloride.

Diethadione. $C_8H_{13}NO_3$. 171.19. 5,5-Diethyldihydro-2*H*-1,3-oxazine-2,4(3*H*)-dione. *UNII-Z0SPD4Z01X. CAS-702-54-5.* INN; BAN; DCF; MI.

Diethanolamine (dye″ eth a nol′ a meen). **NF.** $C_4H_{11}NO_2$. 105.14. (1) Ethanol, 2,2′-iminobis-; (2) 2,2′-Iminodiethanol. *CAS-111-42-2. Pharmaceutic aid (alkalizing agent).*

Diethazine Hydrochloride. $C_{18}H_{22}N_2S.HCl$. 334.91. [Diethazine is INN and BAN.] 10-(2-Diethylaminoethyl)phenothiazine hydrochloride. *UNII-S88072126Q. CAS-341-70-8; CAS-60-91-3 [diethazine].* MI. ◇*RP 2987*

Diethyl Phthalate (dye eth′ il thal′ ate). **NF.** $C_{12}H_{14}O_4$. 222.24. (1) 1,2-Benzenedicarboxylic acid, diethyl ester; (2) Diethyl phthalate. *UNII-UF064M00AF. CAS-84-66-2. Pharmaceutic aid (plasticizer).*

Diethylaminoethyl Diphenylhydroxypropionate Hydrochloride. $C_{21}H_{27}NO_3.HCl$. 377.90. 2-Diethylaminoethyl 3,3-diphenyl-3-hydroxypropionate. *CAS-53421-38-3.* JAN.

Diethylbarbituric Acid — *See* Barbital.

Diethylcarbamazine Citrate (dye eth″ il kar bam′ a zeen sit′ rate). **USP.** $C_{10}H_{21}N_3O.C_6H_8O_7$. 391.42. [Diethylcarbamazine is INN and BAN.] (1) 1-Piperazinecarboxamide, *N,N*-diethyl-4-methyl-, 2-hydroxy-1,2,3-propanetricarboxylate; (2) *N,N*-Diethyl-4-methyl-1-piperazinecarboxamide citrate (1:1). *UNII-OS1Z389K8S; UNII-V867Q8X3ZD [diethylcarbamazine]. CAS-1642-54-2; CAS-90-89-1 [diethylcarbamazine].* JAN. *Anthelmintic.* Hetrazan (Lederle)

Diethyldixanthogen — *See* Dixanthogen.

Diethylene Glycol Monoethyl Ether (dye eth′ il een glye′ kol mon″ oh eth″ il ee′ ther). **NF.** $C_6H_{14}O_3$. 134.17. 2-(2-Ethoxyethoxy)ethanol. *UNII-A1A1I8X02B. CAS-111-90-0.*

Diethylene Glycol Stearates (dye eth′ il een glye′ kol steer′ ates). **NF.** A mixture of diethylene glycol monoesters and diesters of stearic and palmitic acids.

Diethylpropion Hydrochloride (dye eth″ il proe′ pee on hye″ droe klor′ ide). **USP.** $C_{13}H_{19}NO.HCl$. 241.76. [Amfepramone is INN; Diethylpropion is BAN.] (1) 1-Propanone, 2-(diethylamino)-1-phenyl-, hydrochloride; (2) 2-(Diethylamino)propiophenone hydrochloride. *UNII-19V2PL39NG; UNII-Q94YYU22B8 [diethylpropion]. CAS-134-80-5; CAS-90-84-6 [diethylpropion]. Anorexic.* Tenuate (Sanofi Aventis); Tepanil (3M Pharmaceuticals)

Diethylstilbestrol (dye eth″ il stil bes′ trol). **USP.** $C_{18}H_{20}O_2$. 268.35. (1) Phenol 4,4′-(1,2-diethyl-1,2-ethenediyl)bis-, (*E*)-; (2) α,α′-Diethyl-(*E*)-4,4′-stilbenediol. *UNII-731DCA35BT. CAS-56-53-1.* INN; BAN. *Estrogen.* Stilbestrol (Bristol-Myers Squibb); Stilbetin (Bristol-Myers Squibb)

Diethylstilbestrol Diphosphate (dye eth″ il stil bes′ trol dye fos′ fate). **USP**. $C_{18}H_{22}O_8P_2$. 428.31. [Fosfestrol is INN, BAN, and JAN.] (1) Phenol, 4,4′-(1,2-diethyl-1,2-ethenediyl)bis-, bis(dihydrogen phosphate), (*E*)-; (2) α,α′-Diethyl-(*E*)-4,4′-stilbenediol bis(dihydrogen phosphate). *UNII-A0E0NMA80F*. *CAS-522-40-7*. *Estrogen*. Stilphostrol (Bayer)

Diethylstilbestrol Dipropionate. *UNII-Y98CK3J0OL*. *CAS-130-80-3*. NF XIV; MI. Dibestil (Sterling Winthrop†)

Diethylthiambutene. $C_{16}H_{21}NS_2$. 291.47. 3-Diethylamino-1,1-di-(2′-thienyl)-1-butene. *UNII-2Z91X9052O*. *CAS-86-14-6*. INN; BAN; DCF.

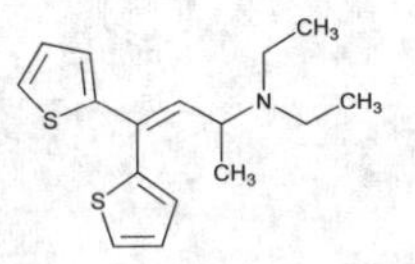

Diethyltoluamide (dye eth″ il tol ue′ a mide). **USP**. $C_{12}H_{17}NO$. 191.27. (1) Benzamide, *N,N*-diethyl-3-methyl-; (2) *N,N*-Diethyl-*m*-toluamide. *UNII-FB0C1XZV4Y*. *CAS-134-62-3*. INN; BAN. *Repellant, arthropod*.

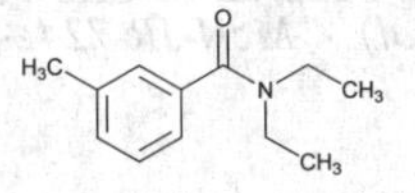

Dietifen. $C_{21}H_{27}NO_2$. 325.44. 4-[2-(Diethylamino)ethoxy]-phenyl phenethyl ketone. *UNII-UO003HH66V*. *CAS-3686-78-0*. INN.

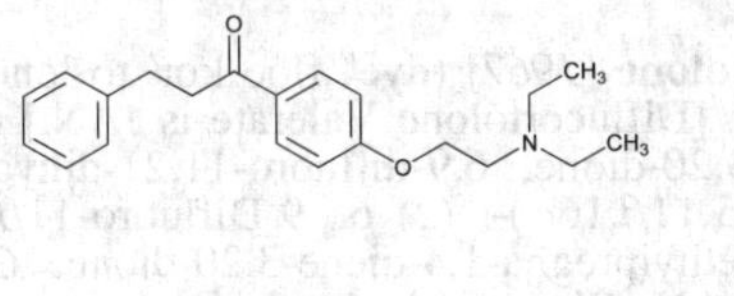

Dietroxine — *See* Diethadione.

Diexanthogen — *See* Dixanthogen.

Difebarbamate. $C_{28}H_{42}N_4O_9$. 578.65. 1,3-Bis(3-butoxy-2-hydroxypropyl)-5-ethyl-5-phenylbarbituric acid dicarbamate ester. *UNII-7EE4K616KK*. *CAS-15687-09-9*. INN; DCF.

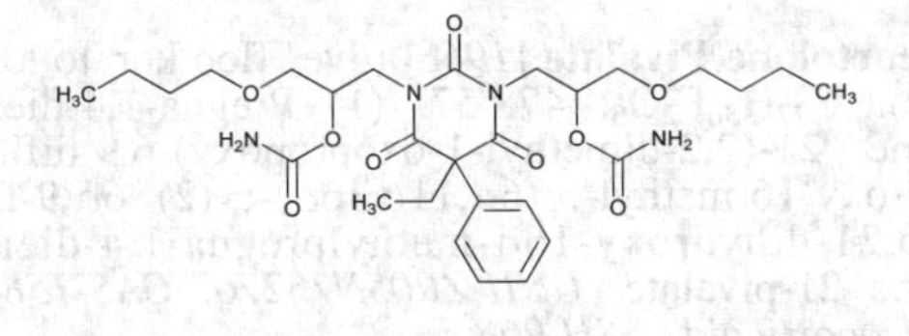

† Brand name formerly used, and/or firm no longer concerned with this product.

Difemerine Hydrochloride. $C_{20}H_{25}NO_3.HCl$. 363.88. [Difemerine is INN.] 2-(Dimethylamino)-1,1-dimethylethyl benzilate, hydrochloride. *UNII-00JM91Q28F*. *CAS-80387-96-8* [difemerine]. MI.

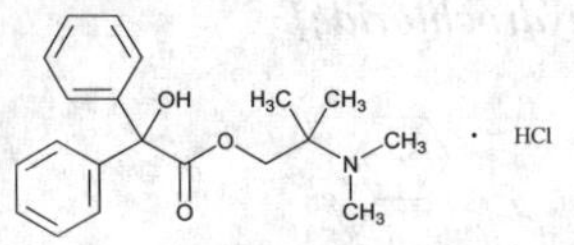

Difemetorex. $C_{20}H_{25}NO$. 295.42. 2-(Diphenylmethyl)-1-piperidineethanol. *UNII-O0417MPF6W*. *CAS-13862-07-2*. INN.

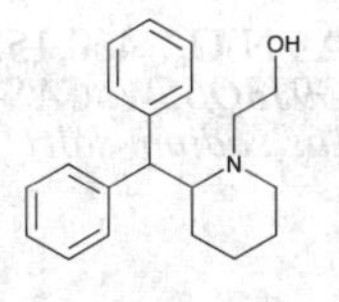

Difenamizole. $C_{20}H_{22}N_4O$. 334.41. 2-(Dimethylamino)-*N*-(1,3-diphenylpyrazol-5-yl)propionamide. *UNII-24MR6YLL3W*. *CAS-20170-20-1*. INN; MI.

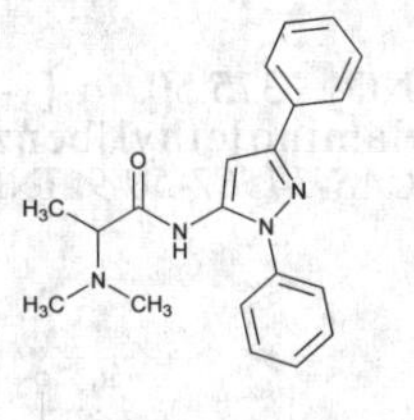

Difencloxazine Hydrochloride. $C_{19}H_{22}ClNO_2.HCl$. 368.30. [Difencloxazine is INN.] 4-[2-(*p*-Chloro-α-phenylbenzyloxy)ethyl]morpholine hydrochloride. *UNII-GH500BOX75; UNII-M277CV2CL8* [difencloxazine]. *CAS-1798-49-8; CAS-5617-26-5* [difencloxazine]. ✧*LD 2630*

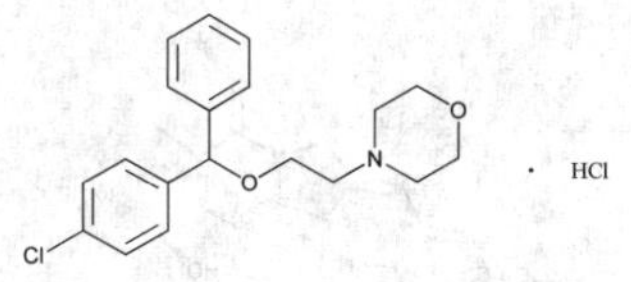

Difenidol (INN, BAN) — *See* Diphenidol.

Difenidol Hydrochloride (JAN) — *See* Diphenidol.

Difenoximide Hydrochloride [*1974*] (dye″ fen ox′ i mide hye″ droe klor′ ide). $C_{32}H_{31}N_3O_4.HCl$. 558.07. [Difenoximide is INN.] (1) 1-Piperidinebutanenitrile, 4-[[(2,5-dioxo-1-pyrrolidinyl)oxy]carbonyl]-α,α,4-triphenyl-, monohydrochloride; (2) *N*-[[1-(3-Cyano-3,3-diphenylpropyl)-4-phenylisonipecotoyl]oxy]succinimide monohydrochloride. *UNII-6GEY4W769K; UNII-8UG1323C03* [difenoximide]. *CAS-37800-79-6; CAS-47806-92-8* [difenoximide]. *Antiperistaltic*. ✧*SC-26100*

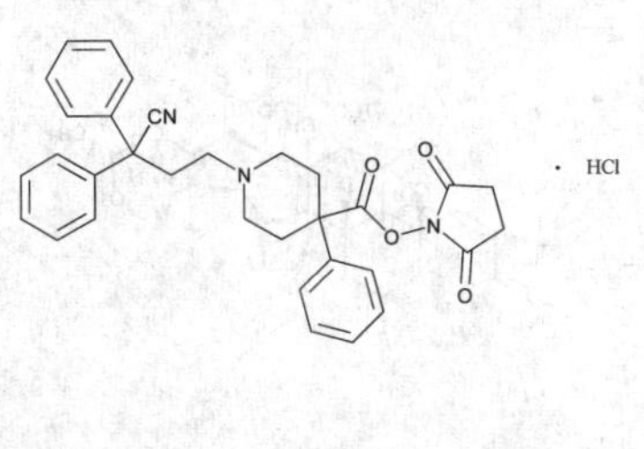

Difenoxin [*1971*] (dye″ fen ox′ in). $C_{28}H_{28}N_2O_2$. 424.53. (1) 4-Piperidinecarboxylic acid, 1-(3-cyano-3,3-diphenylpropyl)-4-phenyl-; (2) 1-(3-Cyano-3,3-diphenylpropyl)-4-phenylisonipecotic acid. *UNII-3ZZ5BJ9F2Q. CAS-28782-42-5.* INN; BAN. *Antiperistaltic.* ◇*McN-JR-15,403-11; R 15,403 [as hydrochloride]*

Difetarsone. $C_{14}H_{18}As_2N_2O_6$. 460.15. *N,N*-Ethylenediarsanilic acid. *UNII-G4G9J3Q65W. CAS-3639-19-8.* INN; BAN; DCF. ◇*RP 4763 [as sodium salt]*

Difeterol. $C_{25}H_{29}NO_2$. 375.50. α-[1-[[2-(Diphenylmethoxy)ethyl]methylamino]ethyl]benzyl alcohol. *UNII-A2P950OCL0. CAS-14587-50-9.* INN.

Diflomotecan. $C_{21}H_{16}F_2N_2O_4$. 398.36. (5*R*)-5-Ethyl-9,10-difluoro-1,4,5,13-tetrahydro-5-hydroxy-3*H*,15*H*-oxepino[3′,4′:6,7]indolizino[1,2-*b*]quinoline-3,15-dione. *CAS-220997-97-7.* INN.

Diflorasone Diacetate [*1973*] (dye flor′ a sone dye as′ e tate). USP. $C_{26}H_{32}F_2O_7$. 494.52. [Diflorasone is INN and BAN.] (1) Pregna-1,4-diene-3,20-dione, 17,21-bis(acetyloxy)-6,9-difluoro-11-hydroxy-16-methyl-, (6α,11β,16β)-; (2) 6α,9-Difluoro-11β,17,21-trihydroxy-16β-methylpregna-1,4-diene-3,20-dione 17,21-diacetate. *UNII-7W2J09SCWX; UNII-T2DHJ9645W [diflorasone]. CAS-33564-31-7; CAS-2557-49-5 [diflorasone].* JAN. *Anti-inflammatory (topical).* Florone (Pfizer); Psorcon (Sanofi Aventis) ◇*U-34,865*

Difloxacin Hydrochloride [*1986*] (dye flox′ a sin hye″ droe klor′ ide). $C_{21}H_{19}F_2N_3O_3.HCl$. 435.85. [Difloxacin is INN.] (1) 3-Quinolinecarboxylic acid, 6-fluoro-1-(4-fluorophenyl) 1,4-dihydro-7-(4-methyl-1-piperazinyl)-4-oxo-, monohydrochloride; (2) 6-Fluoro-1-(*p*-fluorophenyl)-1,4-dihydro-7-(4-methyl-1-piperazinyl)-4-oxo-3-quinolinecarboxylic acid monohydrochloride. *UNII-XJ0260HJ0O; UNII-5Z7OO9FNFD [difloxacin]. CAS-91296-86-5; CAS-98106-17-3 [difloxacin]. Anti-infective (DNA gyrase inhibitor).* ◇*Abbott-56619*

Difluanazine (INN) Hydrochloride — *See* Difluanine Hydrochloride.

Difluanine Hydrochloride [*1967*] (dye floo′ a neen hye″ droe klor′ ide). $C_{28}H_{33}F_2N_3.3HCl$. 558.96. [Difluanazine is INN.] (1) 1-Piperazineethanamine, 4-[4,4-bis(4-fluorophenyl)butyl]-*N*-phenyl-, trihydrochloride; (2) 1-(2-Anilinoethyl)-4-[4,4-bis(*p*-fluorophenyl)butyl]piperazine trihydrochloride. *CAS-5522-33-8; CAS-5522-39-4 [difluanine]. Stimulant (central).* ◇*McN-JR-7242-11; R 7242*

Diflucortolone [*1967*] (dye″ floo kor′ to lone). $C_{22}H_{28}F_2O_4$. 394.45. [Diflucortolone Valerate is JAN.] (1) Pregna-1,4-diene-3,20-dione, 6,9-difluoro-11,21-dihydroxy-16-methyl-, (6α,11β,16α)-; (2) 6α,9-Difluoro-11β,21-dihydroxy-16α-methylpregna-1,4-diene-3,20-dione. *CAS-2607-06-9.* INN; BAN. *Glucocorticoid.*

Diflucortolone Pivalate [*1968*] (dye″ floo kor′ to lone piv′ a late). $C_{27}H_{36}F_2O_5$. 478.57. (1) Pregna-1,4-diene-3,20-dione, 21-(2,2-dimethyl-1-oxopropoxy)-6,9-difluoro-11-hydroxy-16-methyl-, (6α,11β,16α)-; (2) 6α,9-Difluoro-11β,21-dihydroxy-16α-methylpregna-1,4-diene-3,20-dione 21-pivalate. *UNII-ZR05N78276. CAS-15845-96-2. Glucocorticoid.* ◇*SH 968*

Diflumidone Sodium [*1969*] (dye floo′ mi done soe′ dee um). $C_{14}H_{10}F_2NNaO_3S$. 333.29. [Diflumidone is INN and BAN.] (1) Methanesulfonamide, *N*-(3-benzoylphenyl)-1,1-difluoro-, sodium salt; (2) 3′-Benzoyl-1,1-difluoromethanesulfonanilide sodium salt. *UNII-E96467495S* [diflumidone]. *CAS-22737-01-5; CAS-22736-85-2* [diflumidone]. *Anti-inflammatory.* ◇*BA 4164-8; MBR-4164-8*

Diflunisal [*1975*] (dye floo′ ni sal). **USP.** $C_{13}H_8F_2O_3$. 250.20. (1) [1,1′-Biphenyl]-3-carboxylic acid, 2′,4′-difluoro-4-hydroxy-; (2) 2′,4′-Difluoro-4-hydroxy-3-biphenylcarboxylic acid. *UNII-7C546U4DEN. CAS-22494-42-4.* INN; BAN; JAN. *Anti-inflammatory; analgesic.* Dolobid (Merck)

Difluprednate [*1970*] (dye″ floo pred′ nate). $C_{27}H_{34}F_2O_7$. 508.55. (1) Pregna-1,4-diene-3,20-dione, 21-(acetyloxy)-6,9-difluoro-11-hydroxy-17-(1-oxobutoxy)-, (6α,11β)-; (2) 6α,9-Difluoro-11β,17,21-trihydroxypregna-1,4-diene-3,20-dione 21-acetate 17-butyrate. *CAS-23674-86-4.* INN; JAN. *Anti-inflammatory.* ◇*W 6309*

Difluromethylornithine — *See* Eflornithine Hydrochloride.

Difolliculin — *See* Estradiol Benzoate.

Diftalone [*1975*] (dif′ ta lone). $C_{16}H_{12}N_2O_2$. 264.28. (1) Phthalazino[2,3-*b*]phthalazine-5,12(7*H*,14*H*)-dione; (2) Phthalazino[2,3-*b*]phthalazine-5,12(7*H*,14*H*)-dione. *CAS-21626-89-1.* INN. *Anti-inflammatory.* ◇*L-5418*

Digalloyl Trioleate [*1988*] (dye gal′ loe il trye oh′ lee ate). $C_{68}H_{106}O_{12}$. 1115.56. (1) Gallic acid, 3-gallate, trioleate; (2) Oleic acid, triester with gallic acid, 3-ester with gallic acid. *UNII-PGQ9BY2MDE. CAS-17048-39-4.*

Digitalis (dij″ i tal′ is). **USP.** The dried leaf of *Digitalis purpurea* Linné (Fam. Scrophulariaceae). *UNII-F1T8QT9U8B. Cardiotonic.* Digifortis (Parke-Davis†); Digiglusin (Lilly†)

Digitoxin (dij″ i tox′ in). **USP.** $C_{41}H_{64}O_{13}$. 764.94. (1) Card-20(22)-enolide, 3-[(*O*-2,6-dideoxy-β-D-*ribo*-hexopyranosyl-(1→4)-*O*-2,6-dideoxy-β-D-*ribo*-hexopyranosyl-

---

(1→4)-2,6-dideoxy-β-D-*ribo*-hexopyranosyl)oxy]-14-hydroxy, (3β,5β)-; (2) Digitoxin. *UNII-E90NZP2L9U. CAS-71-63-6.* INN; BAN; JAN. *Cardiotonic.* Crystodigin (Lilly)

Digitoxoside — *See* Digitoxin.

Digoxin (di jox′ in). **USP.** $C_{41}H_{64}O_{14}$. 780.94. (1) Card-20(22)-enolide, 3-[(*O*-2,6-dideoxy-β-D-*ribo*-hexopyranosyl-(1→4)-*O*-2,6-dideoxy-β-D-*ribo*-hexopyranosyl-(1→4)-2,6-dideoxy-β-D-*ribo*-hexopyranosyl)oxy]-12,14-dihydroxy-, (3β,5β,12β)-; (2) Digoxin; (3) 3β-[(*O*-2,6-Dideoxy-β-D-*ribo*-hexopyranosyl-(1→4)-*O*-2,6-dideoxy-β-D-*ribo*-hexopyranosyl-(1→4)-2,6-dideoxy-β-D-*ribo*-hexopyranosyl)oxy]-12β,14-dihydroxy-5β-card-20(22)-enolide. *UNII-73K4184T59. CAS-20830-75-5.* INN; BAN; JAN. *Cardiotonic.* Lanoxin (GlaxoSmithKline)

Dihexyverine Hydrochloride [*1961*] (dye hex″ i ver′ een hye″ droe klor′ ide). $C_{20}H_{35}NO_2$.HCl. 357.96. [Dihexyverine is INN.] (1) [1,1′-Bicyclohexyl]-1-carboxylic acid, 2-(1-piperidinyl)ethyl ester hydrochloride; (2) 2-Piperidinoethyl ester of bicyclohexyl-1-carboxylic acid hydrochloride. *UNII-336704VYVB. CAS-5588-25-0; CAS-561-77-3* [dihexyverine]. *Anticholinergic.* ◇*JL-1078*

Dihydralazine Sulfate. $C_8H_{10}N_6$.H_2SO_4. 288.28. [Dihydralazine is INN and BAN.] 1,4-Dihydrazinophthalazine hydrogen sulfate. *UNII-1C2B1W91NK. CAS-7327-87-9; CAS-484-23-1* [dihydralazine]. MI.

Dihydrobenzthiazide — *See* Hydrobentizide.

Dihydrocodeine Bitartrate (dye hye″ droe koe′ deen bye tar′ trate). **USP.** $C_{18}H_{23}NO_3$.$C_4H_6O_6$. 451.47. [Dihydrocodeine is INN and BAN; Dihydrocodeine Phosphate is JAN.] (1) Morphinan-6-ol, 4,5-epoxy-3-methoxy-17-methyl-, (5α,6α)-2,3-dihydroxybutanedioate (1:1) (salt); (2) 4,5α-

Epoxy-3-methoxy-17-methylmorphinan-6α-ol (+)-tartrate (salt). *UNII-8LXS95BSA9. CAS-5965-13-9; CAS-125-28-0* [dihydrocodeine]. *Analgesic.* ◇*DF 118*

Dihydrocodeinone Bitartrate — *See* Hydrocodone Bitartrate.

Dihydroergotamine Mesylate [*1965*] (dye hye″ droe er got′ a meen mes′ i late). **USP.** $C_{33}H_{37}N_5O_5.CH_4O_3S$. 679.78. [Dihydroergotamine is INN and BAN; Dihydroergotamine Mesilate is JAN.] (1) Ergotoman-3′,6′,18-trione,9,10-dihydro-12′-hydroxy-2′-methyl-5′-(phenylmethyl)-, (5′α)-, monomethanesulfonate (salt); (2) Dihydroergotamine monomethanesulfonate. *UNII-81AXN7R2QT; UNII-436O5HM03C* [dihydroergotamine]. *CAS-6190-39-2; CAS-511-12-6* [dihydroergotamine]. *Anti-adrenergic.* D.H.E. 45 (Valeant); Migranal (Valeant)

Dihydroergotoxine Mesilate (JAN) — *See* Ergoloid Mesylates.

Dihydroergotoxine Mesylate (previously used name) — *See* Ergoloid Mesylates.

Dihydroergotoxine Methanesulfonate (previously used name) — *See* Ergoloid Mesylates.

Dihydroethaverine — *See* Drotaverine.

Dihydrogenated Ergot Alkaloids (previously used name) — *See* Ergoloid Mesylates.

Dihydroisoperparine — *See* Drotaverine.

Dihydromorphinone Hydrochloride (previously used name) — *See* Hydromorphone Hydrochloride.

Dihydroneopine — *See* Dihydrocodeine Bitartrate.

Dihydrostreptomycin Sulfate (dye hye″ droe strep″ toe mye′ sin sul′ fate). **USP.** $(C_{21}H_{41}N_7O_{12})_2.3H_2SO_4$. 1461.42. [Dihydrostreptomycin is INN and BAN.] Dihydrostreptomycin sulfate (2:3)(salt). *UNII-T7D4876IUE; UNII-P2I6R8W6UA* [dihydrostreptomycin]. *CAS-5490-27-7; CAS-128-46-1* [dihydrostreptomycin]. *Antibacterial.*

Dihydrostreptomycin-Streptomycin — *See* Streptoduocin.

Dihydrotachysterol (dye hye″ droe tak is′ ter ol). **USP.** $C_{28}H_{46}O$. 398.66. (1) 9,10-Secoergosta-5,7,22-trien-3-ol, (3β,5E,7E,10α,22E)-; (2) Dihydrotachysterol; (3) 9,10-Secoergosta-5,7,22-trien-3β-ol. *CAS-67-96-9.* INN; BAN; JAN. *Regulator (calcium).* Hytakerol (Sterling Winthrop)

Dihydrotheelin — *See* Estradiol.

1α,25-Dihydroxy-22-oxavitamin D_3 (previously used name) — *See* Maxacalcitol.

Dihydroxyacetone (dye″ hye drox″ ee as′ e tone). **USP.** $C_3H_6O_3$. 90.08. 1,3-Dihydroxy-2-propanone. *UNII-O10DDW6JOO. CAS-96-26-4.*

Dihydroxyaluminum Aminoacetate (dye″ hye drox″ ee a loo′ mi num a mee″ noe as′ e tate). **USP.** $C_2H_6AlNO_4.xH_2O$. 135.05 (anhydrous). (1) Aluminum, (glycinato-*N,O*)dihydroxy-, hydrate; (2) (Glycinato)dihydroxyaluminum hydrate. *CAS-41354-48-7; CAS-13682-92-3* [anhydrous]; *CAS-56-40-6* [aminoacetic acid]. *Antacid.* Alminate (Bristol-Myers Squibb)

Dihydroxyaluminum Sodium Carbonate (dye″ hye drox″ ee a loo′ mi num soe′ dee um kar′ bo nate). **USP.** $NaAl(OH)_2CO_3$. 143.99. (1) Aluminum, [carbonato(1-)-*O*]dihydroxy-, monosodium salt; (2) Sodium (*T*-4)-[carbonato(2-)-*O,O′*]dihydroxyaluminate(1-); (3) Sodium (carbonato)dihydroxyaluminate(1-). *CAS-12011-77-7; CAS-16482-55-6* [coordination complex]; *CAS-539-68-4* [replaced]. *Antacid.* Rolaids (Parke-Davis)

1α,25-dihydroxycholecalciferol (previously used name) — *See* Calcitriol.

24, 25-Dihydroxycholecalciferol — *See* Secalciferol.

Dihydroxyestrin — *See* Estradiol.

Dihydroxyprogesterone Acetophenide — *See* Algestone Acetophenide.

1α,25-dihydroxyvitamin D_3 (previously used name) — *See* Calcitriol.

Diiodobuphenine — *See* Bufeniode.

Diiodohydroxyquin (previously used name) — *See* Iodoquinol.

Diiodohydroxyquinoline (INN, BAN) — *See* Iodoquinol.

Diiodostearate Calcium. $C_{36}H_{66}CaI_4O_4$. 1110.60. Calcium 9,12-diiodostearate. JAN.

Diisobutylaminobenzoyloxypropyl Theophylline. $C_{25}H_{35}N_5O_4$. 469.58. 7-(3′-Diisobutylamino-2′-benzoyloxypropyl)theophylline. JAN.

Diisopromine Hydrochloride. $C_{21}H_{29}N$.HCl. 331.92. [Diisopromine is INN.] *N,N*-Diisopropyl-3,3-diphenylpropylamine hydrochloride. *UNII-9E8EN393AL. CAS-24358-65-4; CAS-5966-41-6* [diisopromine]. MI.

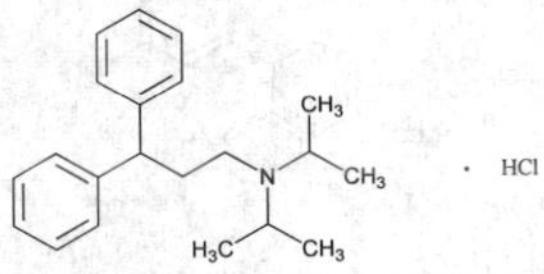

Diisopropanolamine. NF. $C_6H_{15}NO_2$. 133.19. (1) 2-Propanol, 1,1′-iminobis-; (2) 1,1′-Iminodi-2-propanol. *CAS-110-97-4.*

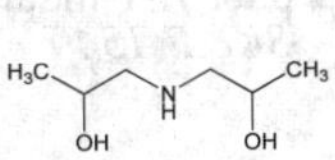

Diisopropylamine Dichloroacetate. $C_8H_{17}Cl_2NO_2$. 230.13. Dicloroacetic acid diisopropylammonium salt. *CAS-660-27-5.* JAN.

Dilazep. $C_{31}H_{44}N_2O_{10}$. 604.69. [Dilazep Dihydrochloride is JAN.] Tetrahydro-1*H*-1,4-diazepine-1,4(5*H*)-dipropanol 3,4,5-trimethoxybenzoate (diester). *UNII-F8KLC2BD5Z. CAS-35898-87-4.* INN; MI.

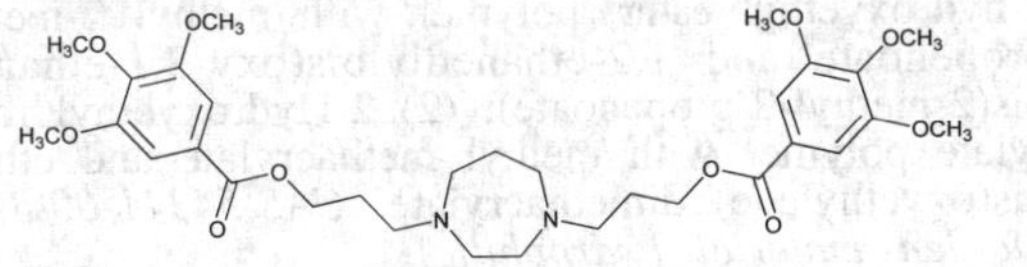

Dilevalol Hydrochloride [*1984*] (dye lev′ a lol hye″ droe klor′ ide). $C_{19}H_{24}N_2O_3$.HCl. 364.87. [Dilevalol is INN and BAN.] (1) Benzamide, 2-hydroxy-5-[1-hydroxy-2-[(1-methyl-3-phenylpropyl)amino]ethyl]-, monohydrochloride, [*R-(R*,R*)*]-; (2) (-)-5-[(1*R*)-1-Hydroxy-2-[[(1*R*)-1-methyl-3-phenylpropyl]amino]ethyl]salicylamide monohydrochloride. *UNII-P6629XE33T* [dilevalol]. *CAS-75659-08-4; CAS-75659-07-3* [dilevalol]. JAN. *Antihypertensive; anti-adrenergic (β-receptor).* ◇*Sch 19927*

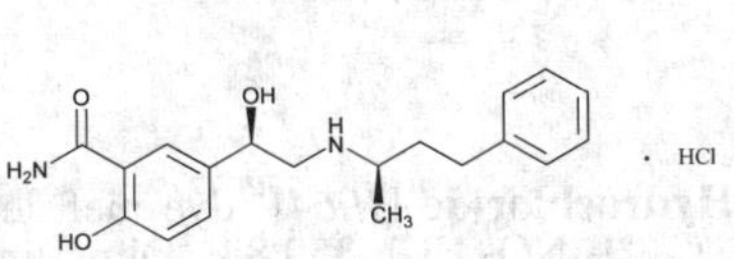

Dilmefone. $C_{16}H_{15}NO_3$. 269.30. 2′,4′-Dimethoxy-3-(4-pyridyl)acrylophenone. *UNII-QIO667518T. CAS-37398-31-5.* INN; DCF.

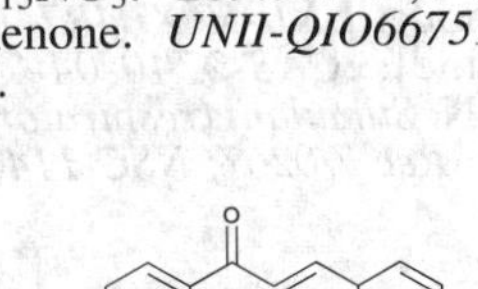

Dilopetine. $C_{13}H_{19}N_3OS$. 265.37. 2-[(2-Methyl-1*H*-pyrazol-3-yl)(thiophen-2-yl)methoxy]-*N,N*-dimethylethanamine. *CAS-247046-52-2.* INN.

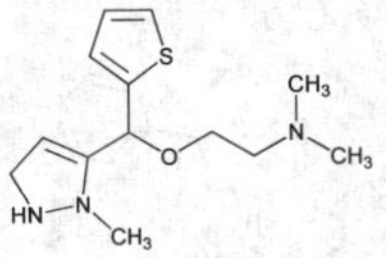

Diloxanide. $C_9H_9Cl_2NO_2$. 234.08. 2,2-Dichloro-4′-hydroxy-*N*-methylacetanilide. *UNII-89134SCM7M. CAS-579-38-4.* INN; BAN; DCF; MI.

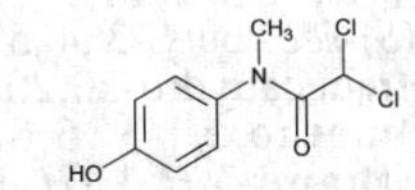

Diloxanide Furoate (dye lox′ a nide fure′ oh ate). **USP**. $C_{14}H_{11}Cl_2NO_4$. 328.15. (1) 4-(*N*-Methyl-2,2-dichloroacetamido)phenyl 2-furoate; (2) 2,2-Dichloroacetamido-4-*N*-methylphenyl 2-furoate. *CAS-3736-81-0.*

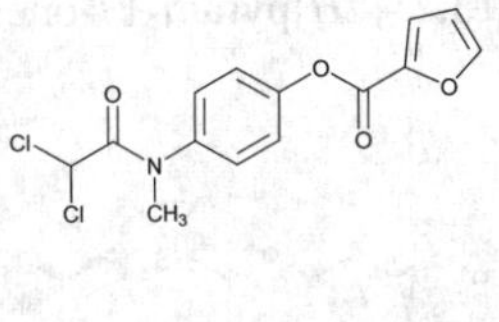

Diltiazem Hydrochloride [*1977*] (dil tye′ a zem hye″ droe klor′ ide). **USP**. $C_{22}H_{26}N_2O_4S$.HCl. 450.98. [Diltiazem is INN and BAN.] (1) 1,5-Benzothiazepin-4(5*H*)-one, 3-(acetyloxy)-5-[2-(dimethylamino)ethyl]-2,3-dihydro-2-(4-methoxyphenyl)-, monohydrochloride, (+)-*cis*-; (2) (+)-5-[2-(Dimethylamino)ethyl]-*cis*-2,3-dihydro-3-hydroxy-2-(*p*-methoxyphenyl)-1,5-benzothiazepin-4(5*H*)-one acetate (ester) monohydrochloride. *UNII-OLH94387TE; UNII-EE92BBP03H* [diltiazem]. *CAS-33286-22-5; CAS-42399-41-7* [diltiazem]. JAN. *Vasodilator (coronary).* Cardizem (Biovail); Dilacor (Watson); Tiazac (Biovail) ◇*RG 83606*

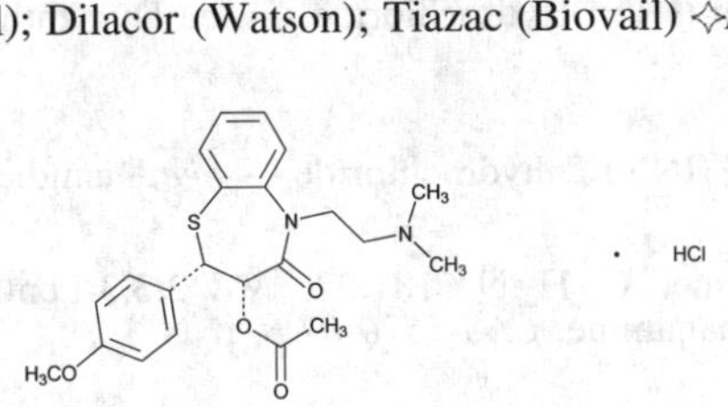

Diltiazem Malate [*1993*] (dil tye′ a zem mal′ ate). $C_{22}H_{26}N_2O_4S$.$C_4H_6O_5$. 548.61. (1) 1,5-Benzothiazepin-4(5*H*)-one, 3-(acetyloxy)-5-[2-(dimethylamino)ethyl]-2,3-dihydro-2-(4-methoxyphenyl)-, (2*S-cis*)-, (*S*)-hydroxybutanedioate (1:1); (2) (+)-(2*S*,3*S*)-5-[2-(Dimethylamino)ethyl]-2,3-dihydro-3-hydroxy-2-(*p*-methoxyphenyl)-1,5-benzothiazepin-4(5*H*)-one acetate (ester),(*S*)-malate (1:1). *UNII-14Y6444DRP. CAS-144604-00-2. Antihypertensive.* Tiamate (Merck) ◇*MK-793*

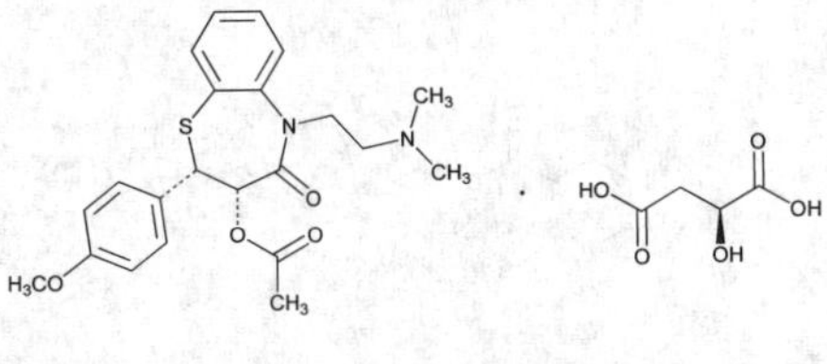

---

† Brand name formerly used, and/or firm no longer concerned with this product.

Dimabefylline. $C_{16}H_{19}N_5O_2$. 313.35. 7-[p-(Dimethylamino)-benzyl]theophylline. *UNII-L6V4Z7SX7S. CAS-1703-48-6.* INN; DCF.

Dimadectin. $C_{38}H_{58}O_{10}$ + $C_{37}H_{56}O_{10}$. 674.86. A mixture of (2a*E*,4*E*,5′*S*,6*S*,6′*R*,7*S*,8*E*,11*R*,13*R*,15*S*,17a*R*,20-*R*,20a*R*,20b*S*)-6′-(*S*)-*sec*-butyl-3′,4′,5′,6,6′,7,10,11,14,15,17a,20,20a,20b-tetradecahydro-20,20b-dihydroxy-7-[(2-methoxyethoxy)methoxy]-5′,6,8,19-tetramethyl-spiro[11,15-methano-2*H*,13*H*,17*H*-furo[4,3,2-*pq*][2,6]benzodioxacyclooctadecin-13,2′-[2*H*]pyran]-17-one (major component) and (2a*E*,4*E*,5′*S*,6*S*,6′*R*,7-*S*,8*E*,11*R*,13*R*,15*S*,17a*R*,20*R*,20a*R*,20b*S*)-3′,4′,5′,6,6′,7,10,11,14,15,17a,20,20a,20b-tetradecahydro-20,20b-dihydroxy-6′-isopropyl-7-[(2-methoxyethoxy)-methoxy]-5′,6,8,19-tetramethylspiro[11,15-methano-2*H*,13*H*,17*H*-furo[4,3,2-*pq*][2,6]benzodioxac-yclooctadecin-13,2′-[2*H*]pyran]-17-one. *CAS-156131-91-8.* INN.

Dimantine (INN) Hydrochloride — *See* Dymanthine Hydro-chloride.

Dimazole (INN) Dihydrochloride — *See* Diamthazole.

Dimecamine. $C_{12}H_{23}N$. 181.32. *N,N*-2,3,3-Pentamethyl-2-norbornanamine. *CAS-3570-07-8.* INN.

Dimecolonium Iodide. $C_{14}H_{30}I_2N_2O_2$. 512.21. Ester of 2-carboxy-1,1,6-trimethylpiperidinium iodide with (2-hydroxyethyl) trimethylammonium iodide. *UNII-4D4NC8MXLW. CAS-3425-97-6.* INN.

Dimecrotic Acid. $C_{12}H_{14}O_4$. 222.24. 2,4-Dimethoxy-β-methylcinnamic acid. *UNII-R46Y1C0ZR2. CAS-7706-67-4.* INN; DCF; MI.

Dimedrol — *See* Diphenhydramine Hydrochloride.

Dimefadane [*1963*] (dye mef′ a dane). $C_{17}H_{19}N$. 237.34. (1) 1*H*-Inden-1-amine, 2,3-dihydro-*N,N*-dimethyl-3-phenyl-; (2) *N,N*-Dimethyl-3-phenyl-1-indanamine. *CAS-5581-40-8.* INN. *Analgesic.* ◇*SK&F 1340*

Dimefilcon A [*1975*] (dye″ me fil′ kon). $(C_6H_{10}O_3)_x$.$(C_5H_8O_2)_y$.$(C_{14}H_{22}O_6)_z$. (1) 2-Propenoic acid, 2-methyl-, 2-hydroxyethyl ester, polymer with methyl 2-methyl-2-propenoate and 1,2-ethanediylbis(oxy-2,1-ethanediyl) bis(2-methyl-2-propenoate); (2) 2-Hydroxyethyl methacrylate polymer with methyl methacrylate and ethylene-bis(oxyethylene) dimethacrylate. *CAS-54341-00-3.* *Contact lens material (hydrophilic).*

Dimefline Hydrochloride [*1964*] (dye mef′ leen hye″ droe klor′ ide). $C_{20}H_{21}NO_3$.HCl. 359.85. [Dimefline is INN and BAN.] (1) 4*H*-1-Benzopyran-4-one, 8-[(dimethylamino)-methyl]-7-methoxy-3-methyl-2-phenyl-, hydrochloride; (2) 8-[(Dimethylamino)methyl]-7-methoxy-3-methylfla-vone hydrochloride. *UNII-H0XB4R74ID; UNII-9WII5M0-DU3* [dimefline]. *CAS-2740-04-7; CAS-1165-48-6* [dimefline]. JAN. *Stimulant (respiratory).* Remeflin (Wall-ace†) ◇*DW-62; Rec 7/0267; NSC-114650*

Dimefocon A [*1979*] (dye″ me foe′ kon). [(C₁₂H₁₀)OSi]*a*[C₂H₆OSi]*b*[C₃H₆OSi]*c*[C₄H₉OSi]*d*. (1) Dimefocon A; (2) Poly(diphenyl dimethyl methylvinyl dimethylvinyl siloxane). *Contact lens material (hydrophobic).*

Dimekolin — *See* Dimecolonium Iodide.

Dimelazine. C₁₉H₂₂N₂S. 310.46. 10-[(1,3-Dimethyl-3-pyrrolidinyl)methyl]phenothiazine. *UNII-7VI3P2OT72. CAS-15302-12-2.* INN.

Dimelin — *See* Dimecolonium Iodide.

Dimemorfan. C₁₈H₂₅N. 255.40. [Dimemorfan Phosphate is JAN.] (+)-3,17-Dimethylmorphinan. *UNII-623OAC38YU. CAS-36309-01-0.* INN; MI.

Dimenhydrinate (dye″ men hye′ dri nate). **USP.** C₁₇H₂₁NO.C₇H₇ClN₄O₂. 469.96. (1) 1*H*-Purine-2,6-dione, 8-chloro-3,7-dihydro-1,3-dimethyl-, compd. with 2-(diphenylmethoxy)-*N,N*-dimethylethanamine (1:1); (2) 8-Chlorotheophylline, compound with 2-(diphenylmethoxy)-*N,N*-dimethylethylamine (1:1). *UNII-JB937PER5C. CAS-523-87-5.* INN; BAN; JAN. *Anti-emetic.* Dramamine (Pfizer)

Dimenoxadol. C₂₀H₂₅NO₃. 327.42. 2-Dimethylaminoethyl 1-ethoxy-1,1-diphenylacetate. *UNII-4D65PBX0VK. CAS-509-78-4.* INN; BAN; DCF; MI. [*Name previously used: Dimenoxadole.*]

Dimepheptanol. C₂₁H₂₉NO. 311.46. 6-Dimethylamino-4,4-diphenyl-3-heptanol. *UNII-NNB4I01PA7. CAS-545-90-4.* INN; BAN; DCF; MI. ⬦*NIH 2933*

Dimepranol Acedoben [*1990*] (dye me′ pran ol a″ se doe′ ben). C₅H₁₃NO.C₉H₉NO₃. 282.34. [Dimepranol is INN.] (1) 2-Propanol, 1-(dimethylamino)-, (±)-, 4-(acetylamino)benzoate (salt); (2) (±)-1-(Dimethylamino)-2-propanol, *p*-acetamidobenzoate (salt). *UNII-1V339IMQ38. CAS-61990-51-0; CAS-53657-16-2* [dimepranol]. *Immunomodulator.*

Dimepregnen. C₂₃H₃₆O₂. 344.53. 3β-Hydroxy-6α,16α-dimethylpregn-4-en-20-one. *UNII-X08N6BOT8Y. CAS-21208-26-4.* INN; BAN. ⬦*St 1411*

Dimepropion (former BAN) — *See* Metamfepramone.

Dimeprozan. C₁₉H₂₁NO₂. 295.38. 2-Methoxy-*N,N*-dimethyl-Δ⁹,⁷-xanthenepropylamine. *UNII-C01407869B. CAS-6538-22-3.* INN.

Dimeprozinum — *See* Dimeprozan.

Dimercaprol (dye mer kap′ rol). **USP.** C₃H₈OS₂. 124.23. (1) 1-Propanol, 2,3-dimercapto; (2) 2,3-Dimercapto-1-propanol. *UNII-0CPP32S55X. CAS-59-52-9.* INN; BAN; JAN. *Antidote (to arsenic and gold and mercury poisoning).* Bal (Akorn) [*Name previously used: BAL.*]

Dimesna. C₄H₈Na₂O₆S₄. 326.34. Disodium 2,2′-dithiodiethanesulfonate. *CAS-16208-51-8.* INN.

Dimesone. $C_{23}H_{31}FO_4$. 390.49. 9α-Fluoro-11β,21-dihydroxy-16α,17-dimethylpregna-1,4-diene-3,20-dione. *CAS-25092-07-3*. INN; BAN.

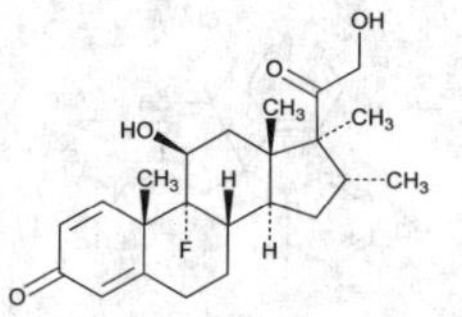

Dimetacrine. $C_{20}H_{26}N_2$. 294.43. 9,9-Dimethyl-10-[3-(dimethylamino)propyl]acridan. *CAS-4757-55-5*. INN; MI.

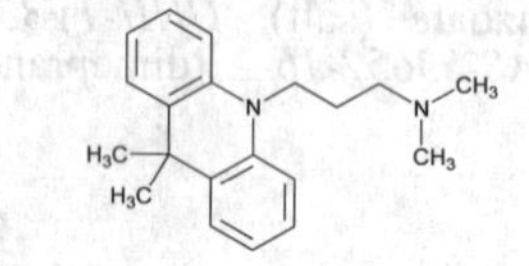

Dimetamfetamine. $C_{11}H_{17}N$. 163.26. (*S*)-*N*,*N*,α-Trimethyl-phenethylamine. *UNII-92M4C245D1*. *CAS-17279-39-9*. INN.

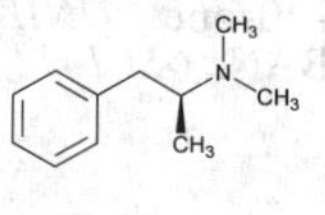

Dimethadione [*1965*] (dye meth a dye' one). $C_5H_7NO_3$. 129.11. (1) 2,4-Oxazolidinedione, 5,5-dimethyl-; (2) 5,5-Dimethyl-2,4-oxazolidinedione. *CAS-695-53-4*. INN. *Anticonvulsant.* ◇*BAX 1400Z; AC 1198; DMO; NSC-30152*

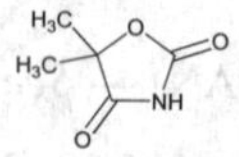

Dimethazan. $C_{11}H_{17}N_5O_2$. 251.28. 7-(2-Dimethylami-noethyl)theophylline. *CAS-519-30-2*. MI.

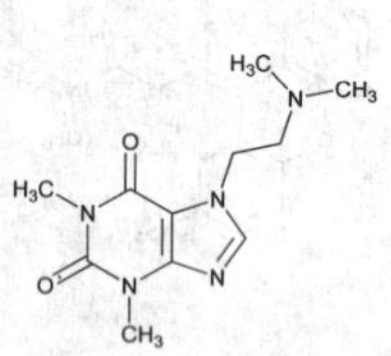

Dimethazine — *See* Mebolazine.

Dimethicone [*1982*] (dye meth' i kone). **NF.** [Dimeticone is INN, BAN and JAN.] (1) Dimethicone; (2) α-(Trimethyl-silyl)-ω-methylpoly[oxy(dimethylsilylene)]. *CAS-9006-65-9*. *Lubricant and hydrophobing agent; prosthetic aid (soft tissue)*. Sentry Dimethicone (Witco); Sentry Dimethicone Dispension (Witco)

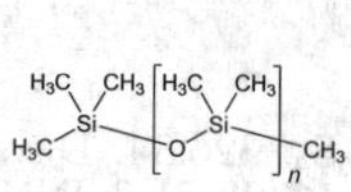

Dimethicone 350 [*1972*] (dye meth' i kone). A poly(di-methylsiloxane) fluid with a viscosity of 350 centistokes at 25° C. (1) Dimethicone 350; (2) α-(Trimethylsilyl)-ω-methylpoly[oxy(dimethylsilylene)]. *CAS-9006-65-9* [di-methicone]. *Prosthetic aid (soft tissue)*.

Dimethindene Maleate [*1962*] (dye meth' in deen mal' ee ate). $C_{20}H_{24}N_2$.$C_4H_4O_4$. 408.49. [Dimetindene is INN and BAN; Dimetindene Maleate is JAN.] (1) 1*H*-Indene-2-ethanamine, *N*,*N*-dimethyl-3-[1-(2-pyridinyl)ethyl]-, (*Z*)-2-butenedioate (1:1); (2) 2-[1-[2-[2-(Dimethylamino)ethy-l]inden-3-yl]ethyl]pyridine maleate (1:1). *UNII-6LL60J9E0O*. *CAS-3614-69-5; CAS-5636-83-9* [dimethin-dene]. USP XX. *Antihistaminic*. Forhistal Maleate (Ciba-Geigy†) ◇*Su-6518; NSC-107677*

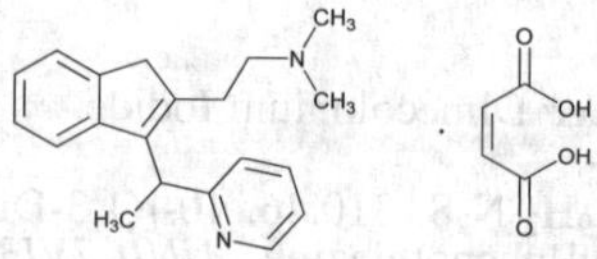

Dimethiodal Sodium. CHI_2NaO_3S. 369.88. Sodium diiodo-methanesulfonate. *UNII-F6Z53YN55N*. *CAS-124-88-9*. INN; DCF; MI.

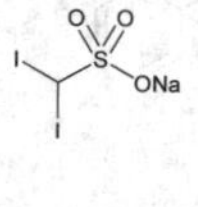

Dimethisoquin Hydrochloride [*1988*] (dye meth eye' soe kwin hye" droe klor' ide). $C_{17}H_{24}N_2O$.HCl. 308.85. [Quinisocaine is INN and BAN.] (1) Ethanamine, 2-[(3-butyl-1-isoquinolinyl)oxy]-*N*,*N*-dimethyl-, monohy-drochloride; (2) 3-Butyl-1-[2-(dimethylamino)ethoxy]iso-quinoline monohydrochloride. *UNII-SMP2689462; UNII-772EN3BH6I* [dimethisoquin]. *CAS-2773-92-4; CAS-86-80-6* [dimethisoquin].

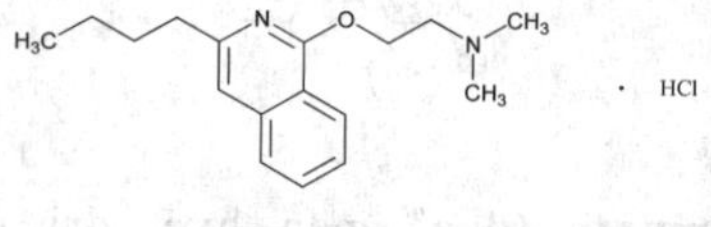

Dimethisteron (JAN) — *See* Dimethisterone.

Dimethisterone [*1965*] (dye meth is' ter one). $C_{23}H_{32}O_2$.H_2O. 358.51. [Dimethisteron is JAN.] (1) Androst-4-en-3-one, 17-hydroxy-6-methyl-17-(1-propynyl)-, monohydrate, (6α,17β)-; (2) 17β-Hydroxy-6-α-methyl-17-(1-propynyl)-androst-4-en-3-one monohydrate. *UNII-K4MZ02M175*. *CAS-41354-30-7; CAS-79-64-1* [anhydrous]. NF XIV; INN; BAN. *Progestin*. ◇*5048*

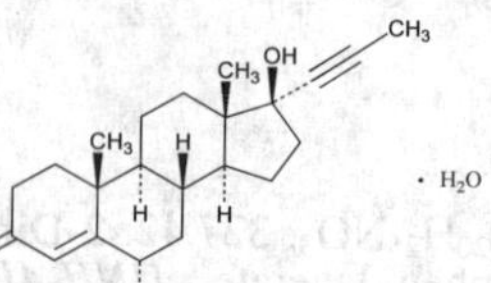

Dimetholizine. $C_{15}H_{24}N_2O_2$. 264.36. 1-(*o*-Methoxyphenyl)-4-(3-methoxypropyl)piperazine. *UNII-O6U9W3DMYT*. *CAS-7008-00-6*. INN.

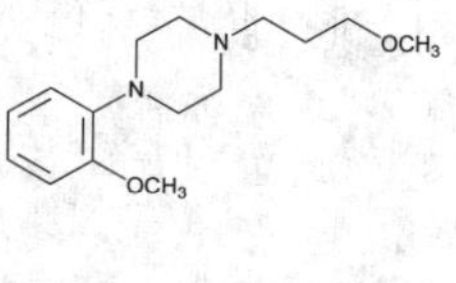

Dimethothiazine (previously used name) — *See* Fonazine Mesylate.

Dimethoxanate Hydrochloride. $C_{19}H_{22}N_2O_3S \cdot HCl$. 394.92. [Dimethoxanate is INN and BAN.] 2-(2-Dimethylaminoethoxy)ethyl phenothiazine-10-carboxylate hydrochloride. *UNII-N5I6SR31GJ. CAS-518-63-8; CAS-477-93-0* [dimethoxanate]. ND 1966; MI.

Dimethyl Fumarate [*2005*] (dye meth′ il fue′ ma rate). $C_6H_8O_4$. 144.13. (1) 2-Butenedioic acid, (2*E*)-, dimethyl ester; (2) Dimethyl (2*E*)-but-2-enedioate. *UNII-FO2303M-NI2. CAS-624-49-7. Immunomodulator.* ◇*AZL O 211089*

Dimethyl Ketone — *See* Acetone.

Dimethyl Phthalate. *UNII-08X7F5UDJM. CAS-131-11-3.* USP XV; MI.

Dimethyl Sulfoxide [*1965*] (dye meth′ il sul fox′ ide). **USP**. C_2H_6OS. 78.13. (1) Methane, sulfinylbis-; (2) Methyl sulfoxide. *UNII-YOW8V9698H. CAS-67-68-5.* INN; BAN. *Anti-inflammatory (topical).* Rimso-50 (Bioniche) ◇*DMSO; SQ 9453; NSC-763*

Dimethyl Tubocurarine Iodide (previously used name) — *See* Metocurine Iodide.

Dimethylaminoethyl Reserpilinate Dihydrochloride. $C_{26}H_{35}N_3O_5 \cdot 2HCl$. 542.50. Dimethylaminoethyl 16,17-didehydro-10,11-dimethoxy-19α-methyl-3β,20α-oxayohimban-16-carboxylate dihydrochloride. *CAS-3735-84-0.* JAN.

Dimethylcysteine — *See* Penicillamine.

Dimethylthiambutene. $C_{14}H_{17}NS_2$. 263.42. 3-Dimethylamino-1,1-di-(2′-thienyl)-1-butene. *UNII-915D88LM9O. CAS-524-84-5.* INN; BAN; DCF; MI.

Dimethyltubocurarine (BAN) — *See* Dimethyltubocurarinium Chloride.

Dimethyltubocurarinium Chloride. $C_{40}H_{48}Cl_2N_2O_6$. 723.72. [Dimethyltubocurarine is BAN.] *O,O*-Dimethyl-(+)-tubocurarine chloride. *CAS-33335-58-9.* INN.

Dimethylxanthine — *See* Theophylline.

Dimeticone (INN, BAN, JAN) — *See* Dimethicone.

Dimetindene (INN, BAN) — *See* Dimethindene Maleate.

Dimetindene Maleate (JAN) — *See* Dimethindene Maleate.

Dimetipirium Bromide. $C_{23}H_{30}BrNO_3$. 448.39. 1-(2-Hydroxyethyl)-1,2,5-trimethylpyrrolidinium bromide benzilate. *UNII-0WVM2U8MFI. CAS-51047-24-6.* INN.

Dimetofrine. $C_{11}H_{17}NO_4$. 227.26. 4-Hydroxy-3,5-dimethoxy-α-[(methylamino)methyl]benzyl alcohol. *UNII-BOM1J10QQM. CAS-22950-29-4.* INN; MI.

Dimetotiazine (INN, BAN) — *See* Fonazine Mesylate.

Dimetotiazine Mesilate (JAN) — *See* Fonazine Mesylate.

Dimetridazole. $C_5H_7N_3O_2$. 141.13. 1,2-Dimethyl-5-nitroimidazole. *UNII-K59P7XNB8X. CAS-551-92-8.* INN; BAN; MI. ◇*RP 8595*

Dimevamide (INN) Sulfate — *See* Aminopentamide Sulfate.

Diminazene. $C_{14}H_{15}N_7$. 281.32. 4,4′-(Diazoamino)benzamidine. *UNII-Y5G36EEA5Z. CAS-536-71-0.* INN; BAN; MI.

---

† Brand name formerly used, and/or firm no longer concerned with this product.

Dimiracetam. $C_6H_8N_2O_2$. 140.14. (±)-Dihydro-1*H*-pyrrolo[1,2-*a*]imidazole-2,5(3*H*,6*H*)-dione. *UNII-4AW7F70M-ZO. CAS-126100-97-8.* INN.

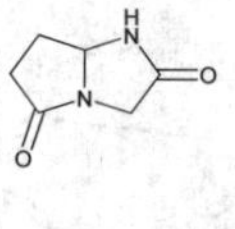

Dimorpholamine. $C_{20}H_{38}N_4O_4$. 398.54. *N,N'*-1,2-Ethanediyl-bis[*n*-butyl-4-morpholinecarboxamide]. *UNII-8YL4JT0L91. CAS-119-48-2.* JAN.

Dimoxamine Hydrochloride [*1977*] (dye mox′ a meen hye″ droe klor′ ide). $C_{13}H_{21}NO_2$·HCl. 259.77. (1) Benzeneethanamine, α-ethyl-2,5-dimethoxy-4-methyl-, hydrochloride, (*R*)-; (2) (*R*)-α-Ethyl-2,5-dimethoxy-4-methylphenethylamine hydrochloride. *CAS-52663-86-2; CAS-52842-59-8* [dimoxamine]. *Memory adjuvant.* ◇*BL-3912A*

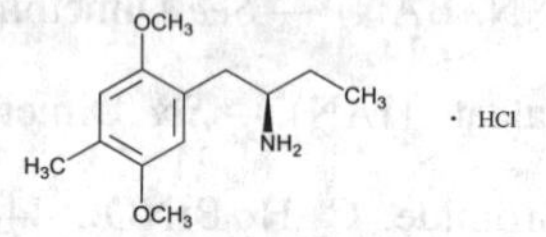

Dimoxaprost. $C_{21}H_{34}O_6$. 382.49. (*Z*)-7-[(1*RS*,2*RS*,3*RS*)-2-[(*E*)-(3*R*)-5-Ethoxy-3-hydroxy-4,4-dimethyl-1-pentenyl]-3-hydroxy-5-oxocyclopentyl]-5-heptenoic acid. *UNII-D3R9B47JTE. CAS-90243-98-4.* INN.

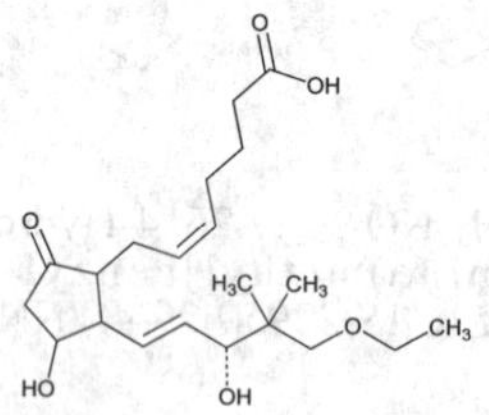

Dimoxyline. $C_{22}H_{25}NO_4$. 367.44. 1-(4-Ethoxy-3-methoxybenzyl)-6,7-dimethoxy-3-methylisoquinoline. *UNII-46X4C9TILS. CAS-147-27-3.* INN; MI.

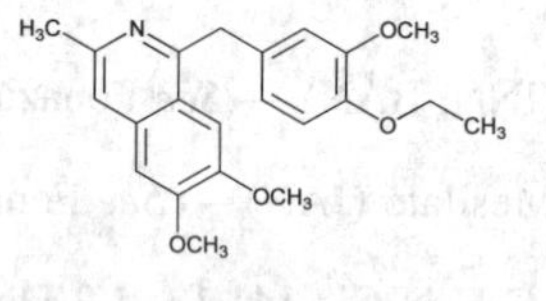

Dimpylate. $C_{12}H_{21}N_2O_3PS$. 304.35. *O,O*-Diethyl 2-isopropyl-6-methyl-4-pyrimidinylphosphorothioate. *CAS-333-41-5.* INN; BAN. *[Name previously used: Diazinon.]* ◇*G-24480*

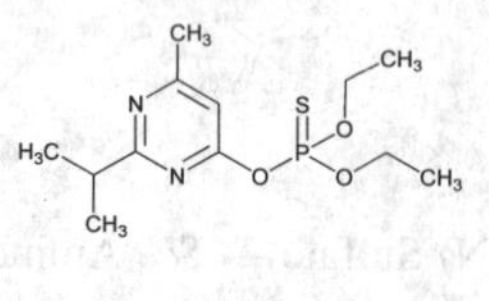

Dinaline. $C_{13}H_{13}N_3O$. 227.26. 2′,4-Diaminobenzanilide. *UNII-RG9G4Z82PY. CAS-58338-59-3.* INN.

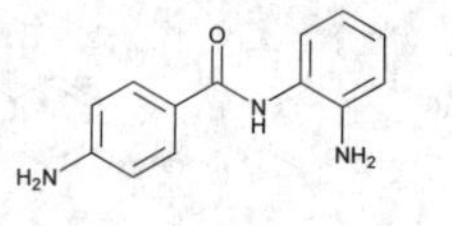

Dinazafone. $C_{20}H_{21}ClN_2O_2$. 356.85. 2′-Benzoyl-4′-chloro-*N*-methyl-2-[(2-methylallyl)amino]acetanilide. *UNII-411OG24QOU. CAS-71119-12-5.* INN.

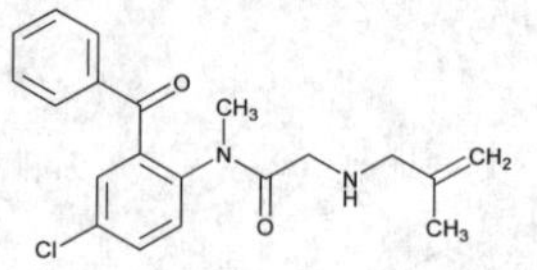

Diniprofylline. $C_{22}H_{20}N_6O_6$. 464.43. 7-(2,3-Dihydroxypropyl)theophylline bis(nicotinate ester). *UNII-2F70GCU00A. CAS-17692-30-7.* INN; DCF.

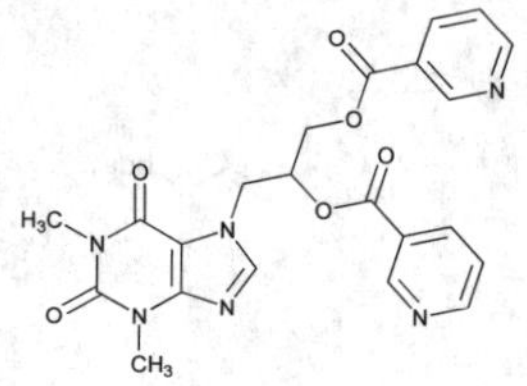

Dinitolmide. $C_8H_7N_3O_5$. 225.16. 3,5-Dinitro-*o*-toluamide. *UNII-AOX68RY4TV. CAS-148-01-6.* INN; BAN; MI.

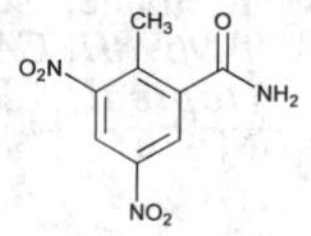

Dinitrotoluamide — *See* Dinitolmide.

Dinoprost [*1971*] (dye′ noe prost). $C_{20}H_{34}O_5$. 354.48. (1) Prosta-5,13-dien-1-oic acid, 9,11,15-trihydroxy-, (5*Z*,9α,11α,13*E*,15*S*)-; (2) (*E*,*Z*)-(1*R*,2*R*,3*R*,5*S*)-7-[3,5-Dihydroxy-2-[(3*S*)-(3-hydroxy-1-octenyl)]cyclopentyl]-5-heptenoic acid; (3) Prostaglandin F$_{2a}$. *UNII-B7IN85G1HY. CAS-551-11-1.* INN; BAN; JAN. *Oxytocic; prostaglandin.* ◇*U-14,583*

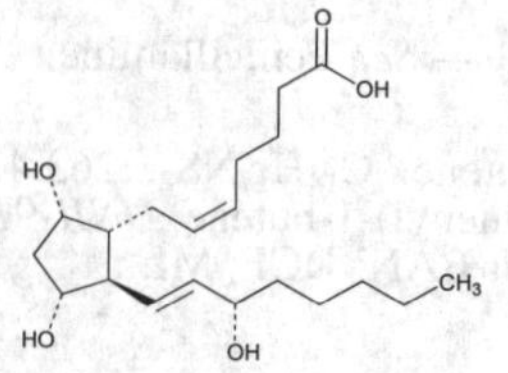

Dinoprost Trometamol (BAN) — *See* Dinoprost Tromethamine.

Dinoprost Tromethamine [*1973*] (dye′ noe prost troe meth′ a meen). **USP.** $C_{20}H_{34}O_5$·$C_4H_{11}NO_3$. 475.62. [Dinoprost Trometamol is BAN.] (1) Prosta-5,13-dien-1-oic acid, 9,11,15-trihydroxy-, (5*Z*,9α,11α,13*E*,15*S*)-, compd. with 2-amino-2-(hydroxymethyl)-1,3-propanediol (1:1); (2) (*E*,*Z*)-(1*R*,2*R*,3*R*,5*S*)-7-[3,5-Dihydroxy-2-[(3*S*)-(3-hydroxy-1-octenyl)]cyclopentyl]-5-heptenoic acid compound with 2-amino-2-(hydroxymethyl)-1,3-propanediol (1:1);

(3) Prostaglandin F_{2a} tromethamine. *UNII-CT6BBQ5A68. CAS-38562-01-5.* JAN. *Oxytocic; prostaglandin.* Prostin F2 Alpha (Pfizer) ◇*PGF₂α THAM; U-14,583E*

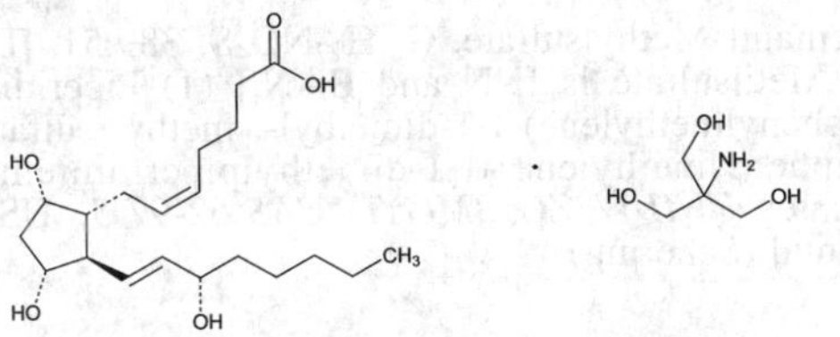

Dinoprostone [*1971*] (dye″ noe prost′ one). **USP.** $C_{20}H_{32}O_5$. 352.47. [Dinoprostone β-Cyclodextrin Clathrate is JAN.] (1) Prosta-5,13-dien-1-oic acid, 11,15-dihydroxy-9-oxo-, (5Z,11α,13E,15S)-; (2) (E,Z)-(1R,2R,3R)-7-[3-Hydroxy-2-[(3S)-(3-hydroxy-1-octenyl)]-5-oxocyclopentyl]-5-heptenoic acid; (3) Prostaglandin E_2. *UNII-K7Q1JQR04M. CAS-363-24-6.* INN; BAN; JAN. *Oxytocic; prostaglandin.* Prostin E2 (Pfizer) ◇*U-12,062*

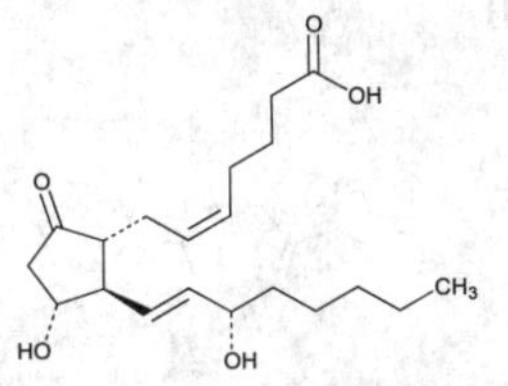

Dinoprostone β-Cyclodextrin Clathrate (JAN) — *See* Dinoprostone.

Dinsed [*1966*] (din′ sed). $C_{14}H_{14}N_4O_8S_2$. 430.41. (1) Benzenesulfonamide, *N,N′*-1,2-ethanediylbis[3-nitro-; (2) *N,N′*-Ethylenebis[3-nitrobenzenesulfonamide]. *CAS-96-62-8.* INN. *Coccidiostat (for poultry).* ◇*NSC-5109*

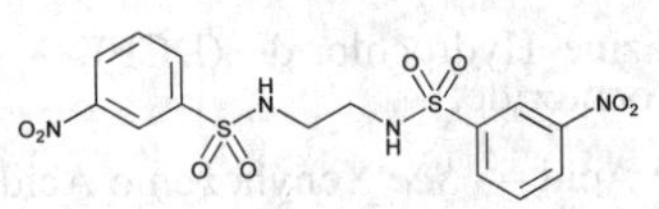

Dioctyl Calcium Sulfosuccinate (previously used name) — *See* Docusate Calcium.

Dioctyl Disodium Sulfosuccinate (JAN) — *See* Docusate Sodium.

Dioctyl Sodium Sulfosuccinate (previously used name) — *See* Docusate Sodium.

Diodone (INN) Injection — *See* Iodopyracet.

Diohippuric Acid I 125 [*1964*] (dye″ oh hip ure′ ik as′ id). $C_9H_7{}^{125}I_2NO_3$. (1) Glycine, *N*-[di(iodo-¹²⁵I)benzoyl]-; (2) Diiodo-¹²⁵I-hippuric acid. *Radioactive agent.*

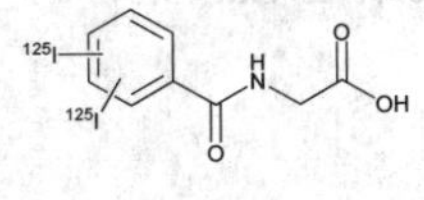

Diohippuric Acid I 131 [*1964*] (dye″ oh hip ure′ ik as′ id). $C_9H_7{}^{131}I_2NO_3$. (1) Glycine, *N*-[di(iodo-¹³¹I)benzoyl]-; (2) Diiodo-¹³¹I-hippuric acid. *Radioactive agent.*

---

† Brand name formerly used, and/or firm no longer concerned with this product.

Diosmin. $C_{28}H_{32}O_{15}$. 608.54. (1) 7-[[6-O-(6-Deoxy-ga-L-mannopyranosyl)-β-D-glucopyranosyl]oxy]-5-hydroxy-2-(3-hydroxy-4-methoxyphenyl)-4*H*-1-benzopyran-4-one; (2) Diosmin. *CAS-520-27-4.* INN; BAN; MI.

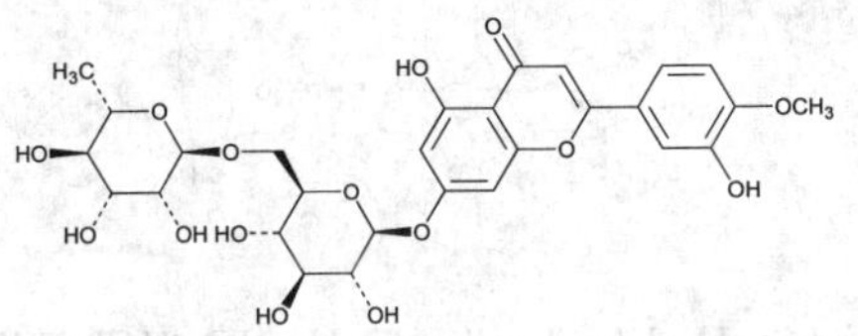

Diotyrosine I 125 [*1964*] (dye″ oh tye′ roe seen). $C_9H_9{}^{125}I_2NO_3$. (1) L-Tyrosine, 3,5-di(iodo-¹²⁵I)-; (2) 3,5-Diiodo-¹²⁵I-L-tyrosine. *Radioactive agent.*

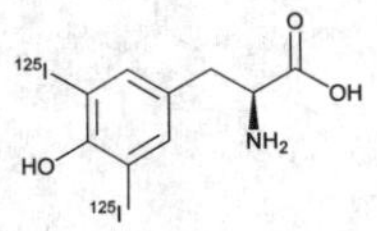

Diotyrosine I 131 [*1963*] (dye″ oh tye′ roe seen). $C_9H_9{}^{131}I_2NO_3$. (1) L-Tyrosine, 3,5-di(iodo-¹³¹I)-; (2) 3,5-Diiodo-¹³¹I-L-tyrosine. *CAS-14679-68-6. Radioactive agent.*

Dioxadilol. $C_{16}H_{25}NO_4$. 295.37. (±)-1-(1,4-Benzodioxan-2-ylmethoxy)-3-(*tert*-butylamino)-2-propanol. *UNII-G25Z4785LV. CAS-80743-08-4.* INN.

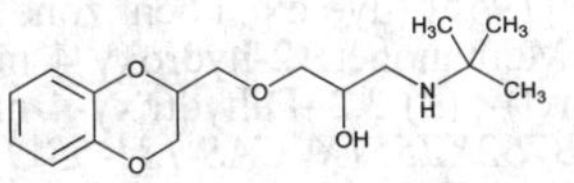

Dioxadrol Hydrochloride [*1962*] (dye ox′ a drol hye″ droe klor′ ide). $C_{20}H_{23}NO_2 \cdot HCl$. 345.86. [Dioxadrol is INN.] (1) Piperidine, 2-(2,2-diphenyl-1,3-dioxolan-4-yl)-, hydrochloride; (2) 2-(2,2-Diphenyl-1,3-dioxolan-4-yl)piperidine hydrochloride. *UNII-J14M291SAO. CAS-3666-69-1; CAS-6495-46-1* [dioxadrol]. *Antidepressant.* ◇*CL-639C*

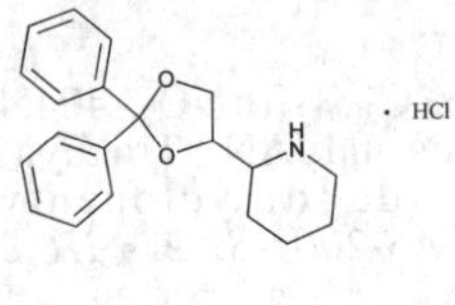

Dioxamate. $C_{15}H_{29}NO_4$. 287.40. (2-Methyl-2-nonyl-1,3-dioxolan-4-yl)methyl carbamate. *UNII-M084T66126. CAS-3567-40-6.* INN; BAN. ◇*A-2655*

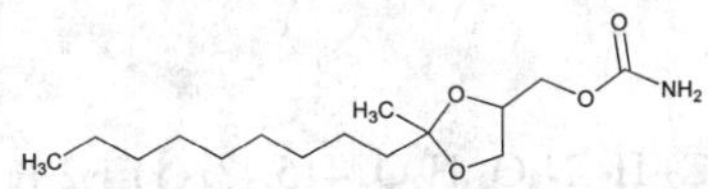

Dioxaphetyl Butyrate. $C_{22}H_{27}NO_3$. 353.45. Ethyl 4-morpholino-2,2-diphenylbutyrate. *UNII-G751H98FY4. CAS-467-86-7.* INN; BAN; MI.

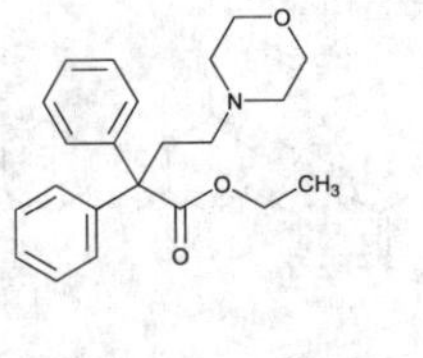

Dioxation. $C_{12}H_{26}O_6P_2S_4$. 456.54. A mixture consisting essentially of *cis-* and *trans-S,S′-5,5′-p*-dioxane-2,3-diyl bis(*O,O*-diethyl phosphorodithioate). *CAS-78-34-2.* INN; BAN; MI. *[Name previously used: Dioxathion.]* ◇AC-528

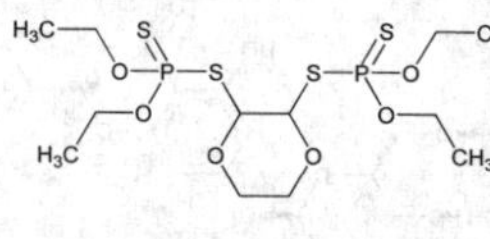

Dioxethedrin Hydrochloride. $C_{11}H_{17}NO_3$.HCl. 247.72. [Dioxethedrin is INN.] α-(1-Ethylaminoethyl)protocatechuyl alcohol hydrochloride. *UNII-82J92E653W* [dioxethedrin]. *CAS-497-75-6* [dioxethedrin]. MI.

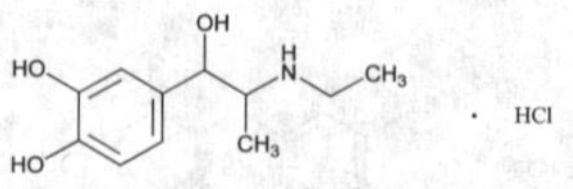

Dioxifedrine. $C_{10}H_{15}NO_3$. 197.23. 3,4-Dihydroxy-α-[1-(methylamino)ethyl]benzyl alcohol. *UNII-CF48QOH154.* *CAS-10329-60-9.* INN.

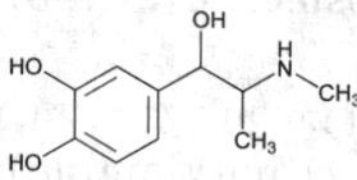

Dioxybenzone [*1965*] (dye ox″ i ben′ zone). **USP.** $C_{14}H_{12}O_4$. 244.24. (1) Methanone, (2-hydroxy-4-methoxyphenyl)(2-hydroxyphenyl)-; (2) 2,2′-Dihydroxy-4-methoxybenzophenone. *UNII-B762XZ551X.* *CAS-131-53-3.* INN. *Ultraviolet screen.* ◇NSC-56769

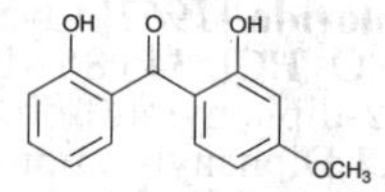

Dioxyline Phosphate. *CAS-5667-46-9.* Paveril Phosphate (Lilly†)

Dipenine Bromide. $C_{20}H_{38}BrNO_2$. 404.43. [Diponium Bromide is INN, BAN and JAN.] Triethyl(2-hydroxyethyl)ammonium bromide dicyclopentylacetate. *UNII-977A8K11XO.* *CAS-2001-81-2.* ◇HL 267; SA-267

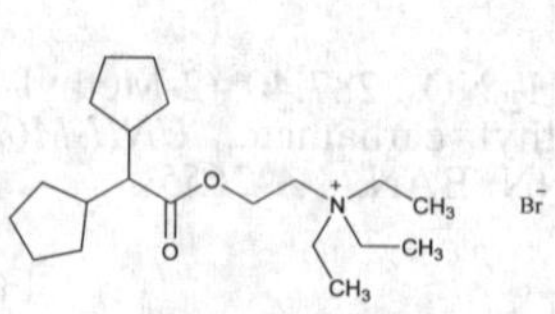

Diperodon. $C_{22}H_{27}N_3O_4$.H_2O. 415.48. (1) 1,2-Propanediol, 3-(1-piperidinyl)-, bis(phenylcarbamate) (ester), monohydrate; (2) 3-Piperidino-1,2-propanediol dicarbanilate (ester) monohydrate. *UNII-2456GO94TR.* *CAS-51552-99-9; CAS-101-08-6* [anhydrous]. USP XXII; INN; BAN.

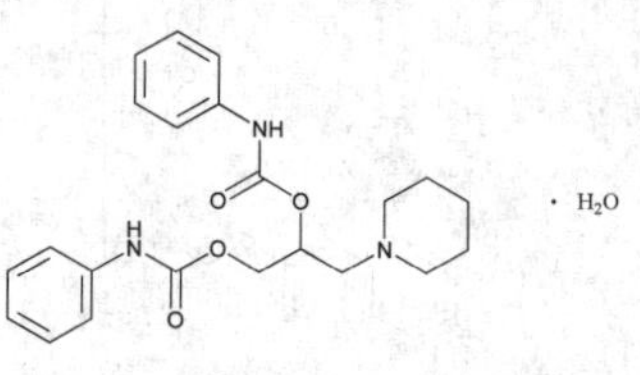

Diperodon Hydrochloride. *UNII-5YZ5R8I73Y; UNII-2456GO94TR* [diperodon]. *CAS-537-12-2; CAS-101-08-6* [diperodon]. MI. Diothane Hydrochloride (Marion Merrell Dow†)

Diphemanil Methylsulfate. $C_{21}H_{27}NO_4S$. 389.51. [Diphemanil Metilsulfate is INN and BAN.] (1) Piperidinium, 4-(diphenylmethylene)-1,1-dimethyl-, methyl sulfate; (2) 4-(Diphenylmethylene)-1,1-dimethylpiperidinium methyl sulfate. *UNII-W2ZG23MGYI.* *CAS-62-97-5.* USP XXII. Prantal (Schering)

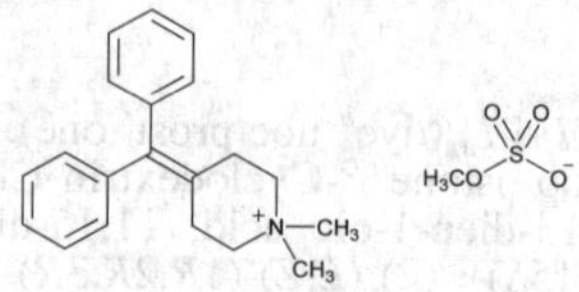

Diphenadione. $C_{23}H_{16}O_3$. 340.37. (1) 1*H*-Indene-1,3-(2*H*)-dione, 2-(diphenylacetyl)-; (2) 2-(Diphenylacetyl)-1,3-indandione. *UNII-54CA01C6JX.* *CAS-82-66-6.* USP XX; INN; BAN; MI.

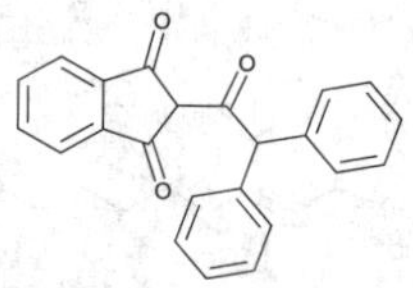

Diphenan. $C_{14}H_{13}NO_2$. 227.26. α-Phenyl-*p*-cresol carbamate. *UNII-U129BBY8DB.* *CAS-101-71-3.* INN; DCF; MI.

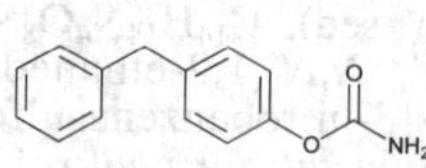

Diphenchloxazine Hydrochloride (DCF) — *See* Difencloxazine Hydrochloride.

Diphenesenic Acid — *See* Xenyhexenic Acid.

Diphenhydramine Citrate (dye″ fen hye′ dra meen sit′ rate). **USP.** $C_{17}H_{21}NO.C_6H_8O_7$. 447.48. [Diphenhydramine is INN, BAN, and JAN; Diphenhydramine Laurylsulfate and Diphenhydramine Tannate are JAN.] (1) Ethanamine, 2-(diphenylmethoxy)-*N,N*-dimethyl-, 2-hydroxy-1,2,3-propanetricarboxylate (1:1); (2) 2-(Diphenylmethoxy)-*N,N*-dimethylethylamine citrate (1:1). *UNII-8GTS82S83M* [diphenhydramine]. *CAS-88637-37-0; CAS-58-73-1* [diphenhydramine]. *Antihistaminic.*

Diphenhydramine Hydrochloride (dye″ fen hye′ dra meen hye″ droe klor′ ide). **USP.** $C_{17}H_{21}NO$.HCl. 291.82. (1) Ethanamine, 2-(diphenylmethoxy)-*N,N*-dimethyl-, hydrochloride; (2) 2-(Diphenylmethoxy)-*N,N*-dimethylethylamine hydrochloride. *UNII-TC2D6JAD40.* *CAS-147-24-0.* BAN; JAN. *Antihistaminic.* Benadryl (McNeil); Vicks Formula 44 (Procter & Gamble)

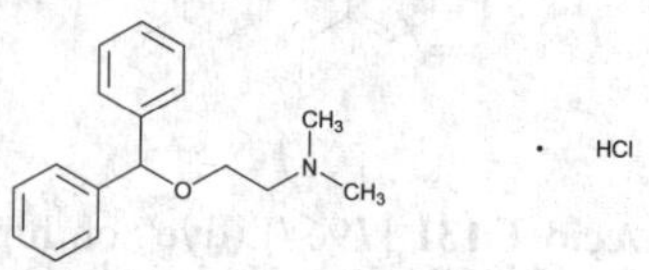

Diphenhydramine Laurylsulfate (JAN) — *See* Diphenhydramine Citrate.

Diphenhydramine Tannate (JAN) — *See* Diphenhydramine Citrate.

Diphenidol [*1963*] (dye fen′ i dol). $C_{21}H_{27}NO$. 309.45. [Difenidol is INN and BAN; Difenidol Hydrochloride is JAN.] (1) 1-Piperidinebutanol, α,α-diphenyl-; (2) α,α-Diphenyl-1-piperidinebutanol. *UNII-NQO8R319LY. CAS-972-02-1. Anti-emetic. ◇SK&F 478*

Diphenidol Hydrochloride [*1969*] (dye fen′ i dol hye″ droe klor′ ide). $C_{21}H_{27}NO.HCl$. 345.91. (1) 1-Piperidinebutanol, α,α-diphenyl, hydrochloride; (2) α,α-Diphenyl-1-piperidinebutanol hydrochloride. *UNII-DG355XWQ4T; UNII-NQO8R319LY* [diphenidol]. *CAS-3254-89-5; CAS-972-02-1* [diphenidol]. *Anti-emetic.* Vontrol (GlaxoSmithKline) ◇*SK&F 478-A*

Diphenidol Pamoate [*1969*] (dye fen′ i dol pam′ oh ate). $(C_{21}H_{27}NO)_2.C_{23}H_{16}O_6$. 1007.26. (1) 2-Naphthalenecarboxylic acid, 4,4′-methylenebis[3-hydroxy-, compd. with α,α-diphenyl-1-piperidinebutanol (1:2); (2) α,α-Diphenyl-1-piperidinebutanol compound with 4,4′-methylenebis[3-hydroxy-2-naphthoic acid] (2:1). *UNII-32021T3D6N; UNII-NQO8R319LY* [diphenidol]. *CAS-26363-46-2; CAS-972-02-1* [diphenidol]. *Anti-emetic.* ◇*SK&F 478-J*

Diphenoxylate Hydrochloride (dye″ fen ox′ i late hye″ droe klor′ ide). **USP.** $C_{30}H_{32}N_2O_2.HCl$. 489.05. [Diphenoxylate is INN and BAN.] (1) 4-Piperidinecarboxylic acid, 1-(3-cyano-3,3-diphenylpropyl)-4-phenyl-, ethyl ester, monohydrochloride; (2) Ethyl 1-(3-cyano-3,3-diphenylpropyl)-4-phenylisonipecotate monohydrochloride. *UNII-W24OD7YW48; UNII-73312P173G* [diphenoxylate]. *CAS-3810-80-8; CAS-915-30-0* [diphenoxylate]. *Antiperistaltic.*

Diphenylacetylindandione — *See* Diphenadione.

Diphenylbutazone — *See* Phenylbutazone.

Diphenylhydantoin (previously used name) — *See* Phenytoin.

Diphenylhydantoin Sodium (previously used name) — *See* Phenytoin Sodium.

Diphenylpiperidinomethyldioxolan Iodide. $C_{22}H_{28}INO_2$. 465.37. *N*-(2,2-Diphenyl-1,3-dioxolanyl-4-methyl)piperidium methyl iodide. *CAS-21216-78-4. JAN.*

Diphenylpyraline Hydrochloride. $C_{19}H_{23}NO.HCl$. 317.85. [Diphenylpyraline is INN and BAN; Diphenylpyraline Teoclate is JAN.] (1) Piperidine, 4-(diphenylmethoxy)-1-methyl-, hydrochloride; (2) 4-(Diphenylmethoxy)-1-methylpiperidine hydrochloride. *UNII-G9FU7F1E87;*

UNII-33361OE3AV [diphenylpyraline]. *CAS-132-18-3; CAS-147-20-6* [diphenylpyraline]. *USP XXI; JAN; MI.* Hispril (GlaxoSmithKline)

Diphenylpyraline Teoclate (JAN) — *See* Diphenylpyraline Hydrochloride.

Diphetarsone (DCF) — *See* Difetarsone.

Diphexamide Iodomethylate — *See* Buzepide Metiodide.

Diphosphopyridine Nucleotide (previously used name) — *See* Nadide.

Diphoxazide. $C_{17}H_{18}N_2O_3$. 298.34. 1-Acetyl-2-(3,3-diphenyl-3-hydroxypropionyl)hydrazine. *UNII-170ZT3R958. CAS-511-41-1.* INN.

Diphtheria Antitoxin. USP XXVI. *Immunizing agent (passive).*

Diphtheria Toxin, Diagnostic (previously used name) — *See* Diphtheria Toxin for Schick Test.

Diphtheria Toxin for Schick Test (dif theer′ ee a). USP XXX. *Diagnostic aid (dermal reactivity indicator). [Name previously used: Diphtheria Toxin, Diagnostic.]*

Diphtheria Toxin, Inactivated Diagnostic (previously used name) — *See* Schick Test Control.

Diphtheria Toxoid. USP XXVI. *Immunizing agent (active).*

Diphtheria Toxoid Adsorbed. USP XXVI. *Immunizing agent (active).*

Dipipanone Hydrochloride. $C_{24}H_{31}NO.HCl$. 385.97. [Dipipanone is INN and BAN.] 4,4-Diphenyl-6-piperidino-3-heptanone hydrochloride. *UNII-8VY00AJ0RL; UNII-X188638Y2V* [dipipanone]. *CAS-856-87-1; CAS-467-83-4* [dipipanone]. MI.

Dipiproverine Hydrochloride. $C_{20}H_{30}N_2O_2.2HCl$. 403.39. [Dipiproverine is INN.] 1-Piperidine-ethanol α-phenyl-1-piperidineacetate ester, as dihydrochloride. *UNII-8UYY5B89ZU; UNII-4XV7PTW3FZ* [dipiproverine]. *CAS-2404-18-4; CAS-117-30-6* [dipiproverine]. MI. ◇*LD 935*

Dipivalyl Epinephrine (previously used name) — *See* Dipivefrin.

Dipivefrin [*1978*] (dye″ piv ef′ rin). $C_{19}H_{29}NO_5$. 351.44. [Dipivefrine is INN and BAN.] (1) Propanoic acid, 2,2-dimethyl-, 4-[1-hydroxy-2-(methylamino)ethyl]-1,2-phenylene ester, (±)-; (2) (±)-3,4-Dihydroxy-α-[(methylamino)methyl]benzyl alcohol 3,4-dipivalate. *UNII-8Q1PVL543G. CAS-52365-63-6. Adrenergic (ophthalmic).* [*Name previously used: Dipivalyl Epinephrine.*] ◇DPE

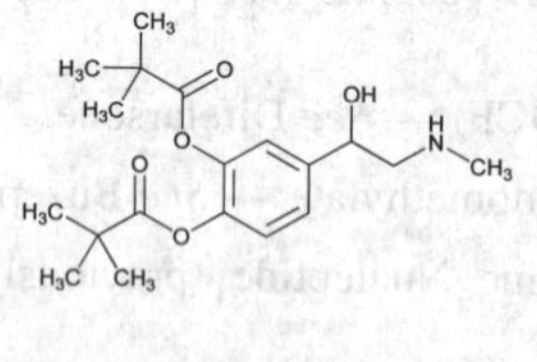

Dipivefrin Hydrochloride (dye″ piv ef′ rin hye″ droe klor′ ide). USP. $C_{19}H_{29}NO_5 \cdot HCl$. 387.90. (1) Propanoic acid, 2,2-dimethyl-, 4-[1-hydroxy-2-(methylamino)ethyl]-1,2-phenylene ester, hydrochloride, (±)-; (2) (±)-3,4-Dihydroxy-α-[(methylamino)methyl]benzyl alcohol 3,4-dipivalate hydrochloride. *UNII-5QTH9UHV0K. CAS-64019-93-8. JAN. Antiglaucoma agent.* Akpro (Akorn); Propine (Allergan)

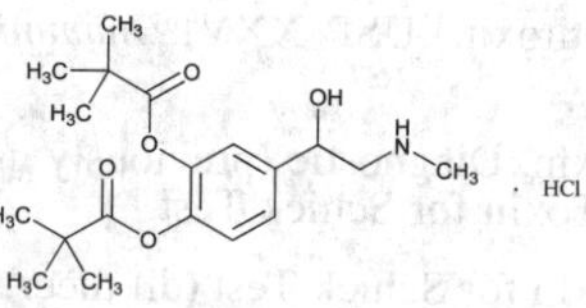

Dipivefrine (INN, BAN) — *See* Dipivefrin.

Diponium Bromide (INN, BAN, JAN) — *See* Dipenine Bromide.

Diprafenone. $C_{23}H_{31}NO_3$. 369.50. (±)-2′-[2-Hydroxy-3-(*tert*-pentylamino)propoxy]-3-phenylpropiophenone. *UNII-1P35MD5C1F. CAS-81447-80-5. INN.*

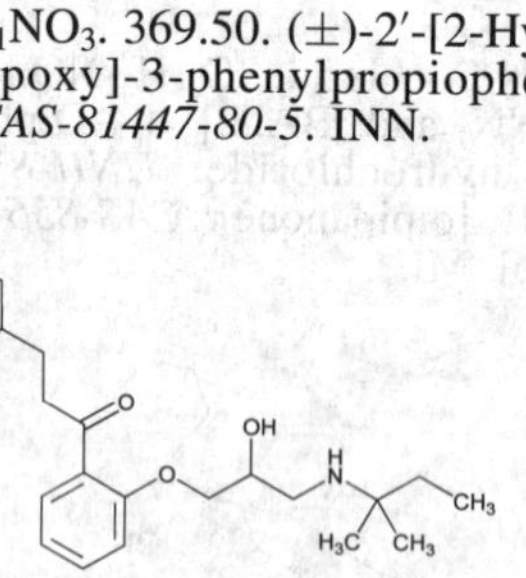

Diprenorphine. $C_{26}H_{35}NO_4$. 425.56. 21-Cyclopropyl-6,7,8,14-tetrahydro-7α-(1-hydroxy-1-methylethyl)-6,14-*endo*-ethanooripavine. *CAS-14357-78-9. INN; BAN; MI.* M50-50 Injection (Lemmon†) ◇M. 5050

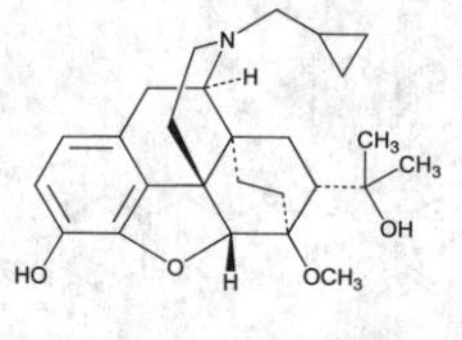

Diprobutine. $C_{10}H_{23}N$. 157.30. 1,1-Dipropylbutylamine. *UNII-5XE7IWD0JX. CAS-61822-36-4. INN; BAN.*

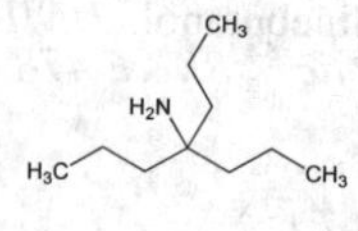

Diprofene. $C_{22}H_{29}NOS$. 355.54. 2-Dipropylaminoethyl diphenylthioacetate. *UNII-O99X77ZQ8E. CAS-5835-72-3. INN.*

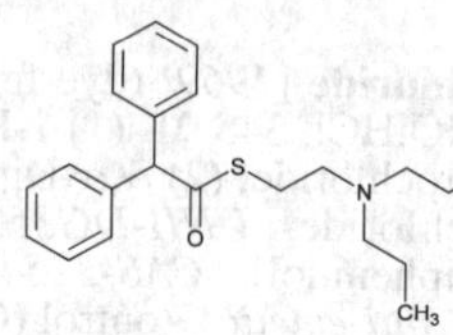

Diprogulic Acid. $C_{12}H_{18}O_7$. 274.27. 2,3:4,6-Di-*O*-isopropylidene-α-L-*xylo*-hexulofuranosonic acid. *UNII-3981541LXD. CAS-18467-77-1. INN.*

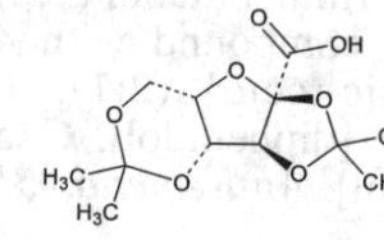

Diproleandomycin. $C_{41}H_{69}NO_{14}$. 799.98. Oleandomycin 4′,11-dipropionate. *CAS-14289-25-9. INN; DCF.*

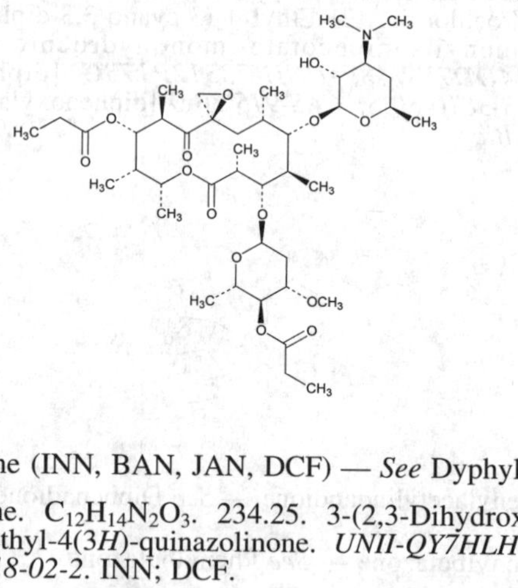

Diprophylline (INN, BAN, JAN, DCF) — *See* Dyphylline.

Diproqualone. $C_{12}H_{14}N_2O_3$. 234.25. 3-(2,3-Dihydroxypropyl)-2-methyl-4(3*H*)-quinazolinone. *UNII-QY7HLH8V4L. CAS-36518-02-2. INN; DCF.*

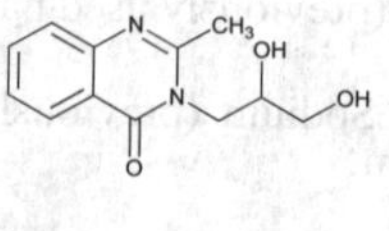

Diproteverine. $C_{26}H_{35}NO_4$. 425.56. 1-(3,4-Diethoxybenzyl)-3,4-dihydro-6,7-diisopropoxyisoquinoline. *UNII-8A5OIA91GT. CAS-69373-95-1. INN; BAN.* ◇BRL 40015

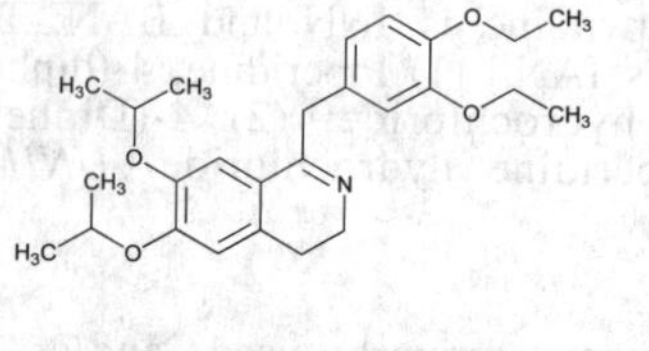

Diprothazine — *See* Dimelazine.

Diprotrizoate Sodium. $C_{13}H_{12}I_3N_2NaO_4$. 663.95. [Sodium Diprotrizoate is INN and BAN.] Sodium 3,5-dipropionamido-2,4,6-triiodobenzoate. *UNII-3XJY028PJZ; UNII-3CD7R3856C* [diprotrizoic acid]. *CAS-129-57-7; CAS-85-16-5* [diprotrizoic acid]. USP XVI; MI.

Diproxadol. $C_{12}H_{14}ClNO_4$. 271.70. 6-Chloro-4-(2,3-dihydroxypropyl)-2-methyl-2*H*-1,4-benzoxazin-3(4*H*)-one. *UNII-GC87H8686G. CAS-52042-24-7.* INN.

Dipyridamole [*1963*] (dye″ pir id′ a mole). **USP.** $C_{24}H_{40}N_8O_4$. 504.63. (1) Ethanol, 2,2′,2″,2‴-[(4,8-di-1-piperidinylpyrimido[5,4-*d*]pyrimidine-2,6-diyl)dinitrilo]tetrakis-; (2) 2,2′,2″,2‴-[(4,8-Dipiperidinopyrimido[5,4-*d*]pyrimidine-2,6-diyl)dinitrilo]tetraethanol. *UNII-64ALC7F90C. CAS-58-32-2.* INN; BAN; JAN. *Vasodilator (coronary).* Persantine (Boehringer Ingelheim) ◇*RA-8; NSC-515776*

Dipyrithione [*1972*] (dye pir″ i thye′ one). $C_{10}H_8N_2O_2S_2$. 252.31. (1) Pyridine, 2,2′-dithiobis- 1,1′-dioxide; (2) 2,2′-Dithiodipyridine 1,1′-dioxide. *UNII-9L87N86R9A. CAS-3696-28-4.* INN. *Antibacterial; antifungal.* ◇*OMDS*

Dipyrocetyl. $C_{11}H_{10}O_6$. 238.19. 2,3-Dihydroxybenzoic acid diacetate. *CAS-486-79-3.* INN; DCF; MI.

Dipyrone [*1962*] (dye pye′ rone). $C_{13}H_{16}N_3NaO_4S.H_2O$. 351.35. [Metamizole Sodium is INN; Sulpyrine is JAN.] (1) Methanesulfonic acid, [(2,3-dihydro-1,5-dimethyl-3-oxo-2-phenyl-1*H*-pyrazol-4-yl)methylamino]-, sodium salt, monohydrate; (2) Sodium (antipyrinylmethylamino)methanesulfonate monohydrate. *UNII-6429L0L52Y. CAS-5907-38-0; CAS-68-89-3* [anhydrous]. BAN. *Analgesic; antipyretic.* Diprofarn (Farmitalia, Societa Farmaceutici Italia, Italy); Novaldin (Sterling Winthrop) *[Name previously used: Methampyrone.]* ◇*NSC-73205*

Diquafosol Tetrasodium [*2003*] (dye kwa fos′ ol tet″ ra soe′ dee um). $C_{18}H_{22}N_4Na_4O_{23}P_4$. 878.23. [Diquafosol is INN and BAN.] (1) Uridine, 5′-(pentahydrogen tetraphosphate), P‴→5′-ester with uridine, tetrasodium salt; (2) Uridine(5′)-tetraphospho(5′)uridine tetrasodium salt. *UNII-X8T9SBH9LL; UNII-7828VC80FJ* [diquafosol]. *CAS-211427-08-6; CAS-59985-21-6* [diquafosol]. *Enhancement of mucosal hydration in the treatment of chronic dry eye (P2Y2 receptor antagonist).* ◇*INS365*

Dirithromycin [*1989*] (dye rith″ roe mye′ sin). **USP.** $C_{42}H_{78}N_2O_{14}$. 835.07. (1) Erythromycin, 9-deoxo-11-deoxy-9,11-[imino[2-(2-methoxyethoxy)ethylidene]oxy]-, [9*S*(*R*)]-; (2) (9*S*)-9-Deoxo-11-deoxy-9,11-[imino[(1*R*)-2-(2-methoxyethoxy)ethylidene]oxy]erythromycin. *UNII-1801D76STL. CAS-62013-04-1.* INN; BAN. *Antibacterial.* Dynabac (Lilly) ◇*LY 237216*

Dirlotapide [*2004*] (dir loe′ ta pide). $C_{40}H_{33}F_3N_4O_3$. 674.71. (1) 1*H*-Indole-2-carboxamide, 1-methyl-*N*-[(1*S*)-2-[methyl(phenylmethyl)amino]-2-oxo-1-phenylethyl]-5-[[[4′-(trifluoromethyl)[1,1′-biphenyl]-2-yl]carbonyl]amino]-; (2) *N*-[(1*S*)-2-(Benzylmethylamino)-2-oxo-1-phenylethyl]-1-methyl-5-[[[4′-(trifluoromethyl)biphenyl-2-yl]carbonyl]amino]-1*H*-indole-2-carboxamide. *UNII-578H0RMP25. CAS-481658-94-0.* INN. *Treatment of obesity in companion animals (dogs) (gut microsomal triglyceride transport protein (gMTP) inhibitor) .* ◇*CP-742,033*

____

† Brand name formerly used, and/or firm no longer concerned with this product.

Dirucotide [*2008*] (dye ruk′ oh tide). C$_{92}$H$_{141}$N$_{25}$O$_{26}$·2013.26. (1) L-Threonine, L-α-aspartyl-L-α-glutamyl-L-asparaginyl-L-prolyl-L-valyl-L-valyl-L-histidyl-L-phenylalanyl-L-phenylalanyl-L-lysyl-L-asparaginyl-L-isoleucyl-L-valyl-L-threonyl-L-prolyl-L-arginyl-; (2) Human myelin basic protein-(216-232)-peptide (major 18.5 kDa isoform-(82-98)-peptide). CAS-152074-97-0. *Treatment of multiple sclerosis.* ◇SF328; MBP8298

Dirucotide Acetate [*2008*] (dye ruk′ oh tide as′ e tate). C$_{92}$H$_{141}$N$_{25}$O$_{26}$·4C$_2$H$_4$O$_2$. 2253.46. (1) L-Threonine, L-α-aspartyl-L-α-glutamyl-L-asparaginyl-L-prolyl-L-valyl-L-valyl-L-histidyl-L-phenylalanyl-L-phenylalanyl-L-lysyl-L-asparaginyl-L-isoleucyl-L-valyl-L-threonyl-L-prolyl-L-arginyl-, tetraacetate (salt); (2) Human myelin basic protein-(216-232)-peptide (major 18.5 kDa isoform-(82-98)-peptide) tetraacetate (salt). UNII-48G1L28581. CAS-781666-30-6. *Treatment of multiple sclerosis.* ◇SF328

Disermolide. C$_{33}$H$_{55}$NO$_8$. 593.79. (3Z,5S,6S,7S,8R,9S,11Z,13S,14S,15S,16Z,18S)-8,14,18-Trihydroxy-19-[(2S,3R,4S,5R)-4-hydroxy-3,5-dimethyl-6-oxotetrahydro-2H-pyran-2-yl]-5,7,9,11,13,15-hexamethylnonadeca-1,3,11,16-tetraen-6-yl carbamate. CAS-127943-53-7. INN.

Disiquonium Chloride [*1987*] (dye″ see kwoe′ nee um klor′ ide). C$_{27}$H$_{60}$ClNO$_3$Si. 510.31. (1) 1-Decanaminium, N-decyl-N-methyl-N-[3-(trimethoxysilyl)propyl]-, chloride; (2) Didecylmethyl[3-(trimethoxysilyl)propyl]ammonium chloride. UNII-6G4NNS4CW4. CAS-68959-20-6. INN. *Antiseptic.*

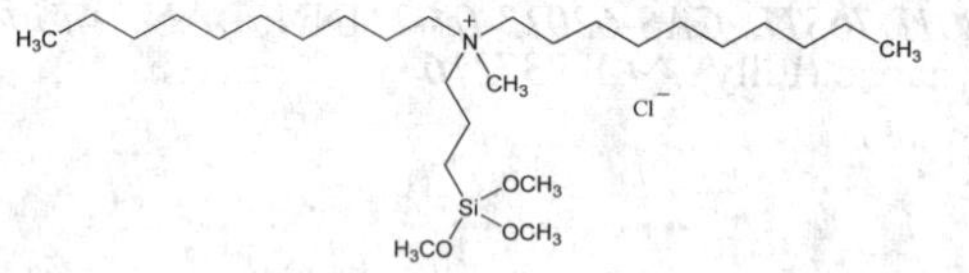

Disitertide. C$_{68}$H$_{109}$N$_{17}$O$_{22}$S$_2$. 1580.82. Human transforming growth factor-beta receptor type III-(710-723)-peptide. CAS-272105-42-7. INN.

Disobutamide [*1980*] (dye″ soe bue′ ta mide). C$_{23}$H$_{38}$ClN$_3$O. 408.02. (1) 1-Piperidinebutanamide, α-[2-[bis(1-methylethyl)amino]ethyl]-α-(2-chlorophenyl)-; (2) α-(o-Chlorophenyl)-α-[2-(diisopropylamino)ethyl]-1-piperidinebutyramide. CAS-68284-69-5. INN. *Cardiac depressant (anti-arrhythmic).* ◇SC-31828

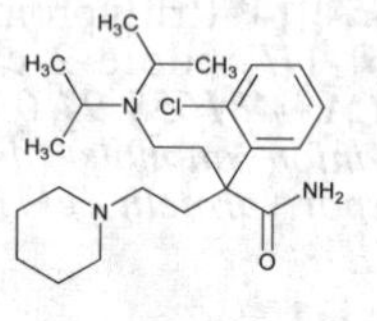

Disodium Edetate (BAN, JAN) — *See* Edetate Disodium.

Disodium Methylene Diphosphonate (previously used name) — *See* Medronate Disodium.

Disofenin [*1979*] (dye″ soe fen′ in). C$_{18}$H$_{26}$N$_2$O$_5$. 350.41. (1) Glycine, N-[2-[[2,6-bis(1-methylethyl)phenyl]amino]-2-oxoethyl]-N-(carboxymethyl)-; (2) [[[(2,6-Diisopropylphenyl)carbamoyl]methyl]imino]diacetic acid. CAS-65717-97-7. INN; BAN. *Diagnostic aid (carrier agent).*

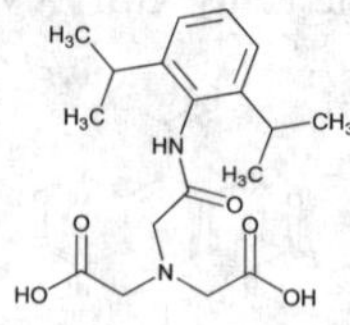

Disogluside. C$_{33}$H$_{52}$O$_8$. 576.76. (25R)-3β-(β-D-Glucopyranosyloxy)spirost-5-ene. UNII-8KI671F2NS. CAS-14144-06-0. INN.

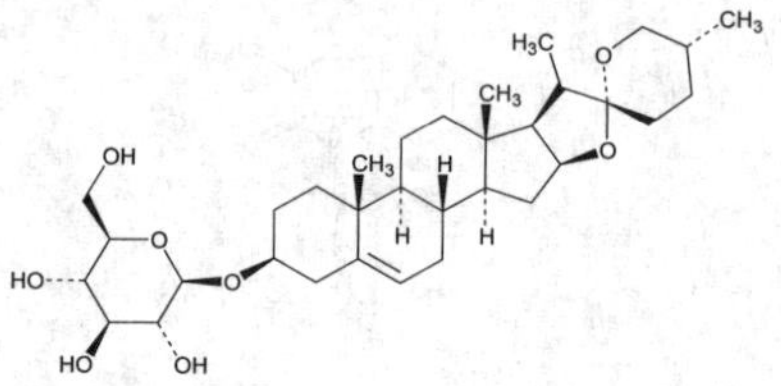

Disomotide [*2005*] (dye soe′ moe tide). C$_{47}$H$_{74}$N$_{10}$O$_{14}$S. 1035.21. (1) L-valine, L-isoleucyl-L-methionyl-L-α-aspartyl-L-glutaminyl-L-valyl-L-prolyl-L-phenylalanyl-L-seryl-; (2) [186-L-Methionine]melanocyte protein Pmel 17 (human melanoma-associated ME20 antigen)-(185-193)-peptide. UNII-8028PPX4PM. CAS-181477-43-0. INN. *Melanoma peptide vaccine.* ◇MPS-22

IMDQVPFSV

Disoprofol — *See* Propofol.

Disopromine Hydrochloride — *See* Diisopromine Hydrochloride.

Disopyramide [*1970*] (dye″ soe pir′ a mide). C$_{21}$H$_{29}$N$_3$O. 339.47. (1) 2-Pyridineacetamide, α-[2-[bis(1-methylethyl) amino]ethyl]-α-phenyl-; (2) α-[2-(Diisopropylamino)ethyl]-α-phenyl-2-pyridineacetamide. UNII-GFO928U8MQ. CAS-3737-09-5. INN; BAN; JAN. *Cardiac depressant (anti-arrhythmic).* ◇SC-7031

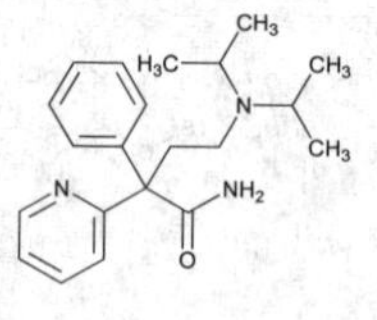

Disopyramide Phosphate [*1978*] (dye″ soe pir′ a mide fos′ fate). USP. C$_{21}$H$_{29}$N$_3$O·H$_3$PO$_4$. 437.47. (1) 2-Pyridineacetamide, α-[2-[bis(1-methylethyl)amino]ethyl]-α-phenyl-, (±)-, phosphate (1:1); (2) (±)-α-[2-(Diisopropylamino)ethyl]-α-phenyl-2-pyridineacetamide phosphate (1:1). UNII-N6BOM1935W; UNII-GFO928U8MQ [disopyramide]. CAS-22059-60-5; CAS-3737-09-5 [disopyramide]. BAN; JAN. *Cardiac depressant (anti-arrhythmic).* Norpace (Pfizer) ◇SC-13957

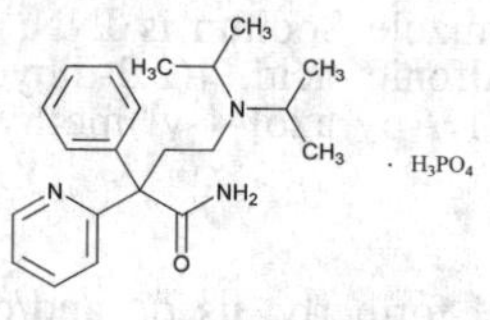

Disoxaril [*1987*] (dye sox′ a ril). $C_{20}H_{26}N_2O_3$. 342.43. (1) Isoxazole, 5-[7-[4-(4,5-dihydro-2-oxazolyl)phenoxy]heptyl]-3-methyl-; (2) 3-Methyl-5-[7-(*p*-2-oxazolin-2-ylphenoxy)heptyl]isoxazole. *UNII-FX8Q9PI4VP. CAS-87495-31-6.* INN. *Antiviral.* ◇*Win 51,711*

Distigmine Bromide. $C_{22}H_{32}Br_2N_4O_4$. 576.32. 3-Hydroxy-1-methylpyridinium bromide hexamethylenebis-(*N*-methylcarbamate). *CAS-15876-67-2.* INN; BAN; JAN; MI.

Disufenton Sodium [*2004*] (dye″ soo fen′ ton soe′ dee um). $C_{11}H_{13}NNa_2O_7S_2$. 381.33. (1) 1,3-Benzenedisulfonic acid, 4-[[(1,1-dimethylethyl)oxidoimino]methyl]-, disodium salt; (2) Disodium 4-*tert*-butyliminomethyl)benzene-,3-disulfonate *N*-oxide; (3) Disodium 4-[[(1,1-dimethylethyl)imino]methyl]benzene-1,3-disulfonate *N*-oxide. *UNII-7M1J3HN9VO. CAS-168021-79-2.* INN. *Neuroprotective agent used to treat ischemic stroke.* ◇*NXY-059*

Disulergine. $C_{17}H_{24}N_4O_2S$. 348.46. *N,N*-Dimethyl-*N′*-(6-methylergolin-8α-yl)sulfamide. *UNII-1Q3CYC1YR6. CAS-59032-40-5.* INN.

Disulfamide. $C_7H_9ClN_2O_4S_2$. 284.74. 5-Chlorotoluene-2,4-disulfonamide. *UNII-26POQ4GICP. CAS-671-88-5.* INN; BAN; MI. *[Name previously used: Disulphamide.]*

Disulfiram (dye sul′ fi ram). **USP.** $C_{10}H_{20}N_2S_4$. 296.54. (1) Thioperoxydicarbonic diamide [$(H_2N)C(S)]_2S_2$, tetraethyl-; (2) Bis(diethylthiocarbamoyl) disulfide. *UNII-TR3MLJ1UAI. CAS-97-77-8.* INN; BAN; JAN. *Alcohol deterrent.* Antabuse (Odyssey)

Disulphamide (previously used name) — *See* Disulfamide.

---

† Brand name formerly used, and/or firm no longer concerned with this product.

Disuprazole. $C_{16}H_{17}N_3OS_2$. 331.46. 2-[[[4-(Ethylthio)-3-methyl-2-pyridyl]methyl]sulfinyl]benzimidazole. *UNII-V81J4OO2OT. CAS-99499-40-8.* INN.

Ditazole. $C_{19}H_{20}N_2O_3$. 324.37. 2,2′-[(4,5-Diphenyl-2-oxazolyl)imino]diethanol. *UNII-H2BQI5Z8FT. CAS-18471-20-0.* INN; MI. ◇*S-222*

Ditekiren [*1989*] (dye te kye′ ren). $C_{50}H_{75}N_9O_8$. 930.19. (1) L-Histidinamide, 1-[(1,1-dimethylethoxy)carbonyl]-L-prolyl-L-phenylalanyl-*N*-[2-hydroxy-5-methyl-1-(2-methylpropyl)-4-[[[2-methyl-1-[[(2-pyridinylmethyl)amino]carbonyl]butyl]amino]carbonyl]hexyl]-*N*α-methyl-, [1*S*-[1*R**,2*R**,4*R**(1*R**,2*R**)]]-; (2) *tert*-Butyl (2*S*)-2-[[(α*S*)-α-[[(1*S*)-1-[[(1*S*,2*S*,4*S*)-4-hydroxy-1-isobutyl-5-methyl-4-[[(1*S*,2*S*)-2-methyl-1-[(2-pyridylmethyl)carbamoyl]butyl]carbamoyl]hexyl]carbamoyl]-2-imidazol-4-ylethyl]methylcarbamoyl]phenethyl]carbamoyl]-1-pyrrolidinecarboxylate. *CAS-103336-05-6.* INN. *Antihypertensive.* ◇*U-71038*

Ditercalinium Chloride. $C_{46}H_{50}Cl_2N_6O_2$. 789.83. 2,2′-([4,4′-Bipiperidine]-1,1′-diyldiethylene)bis[10-methoxy-7*H*-pyrido[4,3-*c*]carbazolium] dichloride. *UNII-40Z22S8DO8. CAS-74517-42-3.* INN.

Dithiazanine Iodide. $C_{23}H_{23}IN_2S_2$. 518.48. [Dithiazanine is BAN.] 3-Ethyl-2-[5-(3-ethyl-2-benzothiazolinylidene)-1,3-pentadienyl]benzothiazolium iodide. *UNII-8OEC3RA07X; UNII-5L7E7IY5EH* [dithiazanine]. *CAS-514-73-8; CAS-7187-55-5* [dithiazanine]. USP XVII; INN; MI. Abminthic (Pfizer†)

Dithranol (INN, BAN) — *See* Anthralin.

Ditiocade Sodium [*2003*] (dye tye′ oh kade soe′ dee um). $C_5H_{10}NNaOS_2 \cdot H_2O$. 205.27. (1) Carbamodithioic acid, ethoxyethyl-, sodium salt, monohydrate; (2) Sodium ethoxyethylcarbamodithioate monohydrate. *UNII-VIC0E207S4. CAS-444190-52-7. A final intermediate in the preparation of ^{99m}TcN-NOET, for in-vivo diagnosis of coronary artery disease.* Cisnoet (Berlex) ⋄*NOET*

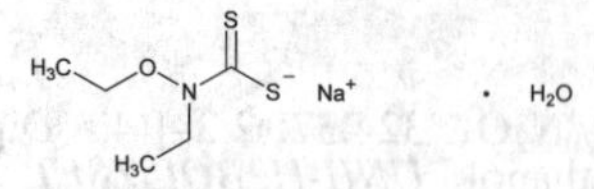

Ditiocarb Sodium. $C_5H_{10}NNaS_2$. 171.26. Sodium diethyl-dithiocarbamate. *CAS-148-18-5.* INN; MI.

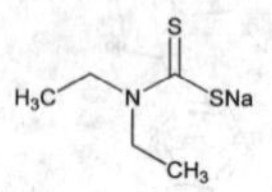

Ditiomustine. $C_{10}H_{18}Cl_2N_6O_4S_2$. 421.32. 1,1′-(Dithiodiethy-lene)bis[3-(2-chloroethyl)-1(or 3)-nitrosourea. *UNII-810O95170J. CAS-82599-22-2.* INN.

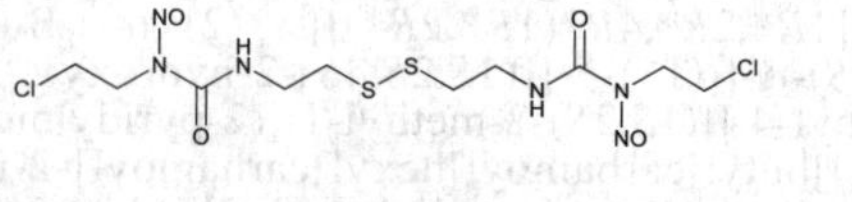

Ditolamide. $C_{13}H_{21}NO_2S$. 255.38. *N,N*-Dipropyl-*p*-toluene-sulfonamide. *UNII-AL8499KM94. CAS-723-42-2.* INN; DCF. ⋄*A-17624*

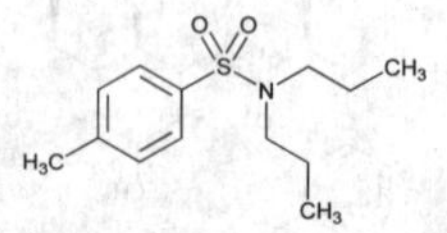

Ditophal. $C_{12}H_{14}O_2S_2$. 254.37. *S,S*-Diethyl ester of 1,3-dithioisophthalic acid. *UNII-40SR2754GL. CAS-584-69-0.* INN; BAN.

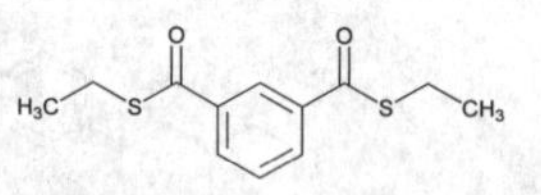

Divabuterol. $C_{22}H_{35}NO_5$. 393.52. (±)-5-[2-(*tert*-Butylamino)-1-hydroxyethyl]-*m*-phenylene dipivalate. *UNII-BVG9H4U2ZB. CAS-54592-27-7.* INN.

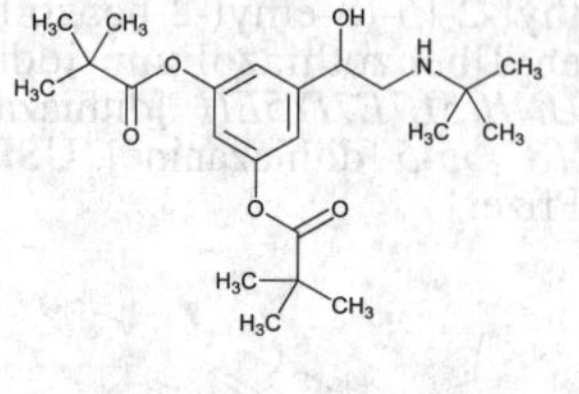

Divalproex Sodium [*1983*] (dye val′ proe ex soe′ dee um). USP. $(C_{16}H_{31}NaO_4)_n$. 310.41 (repeating unit molecular weight). [Valproate Semisodium is INN; Semisodium Valproate is BAN.] (1) Pentanoic acid, 2-propyl-, sodium salt (2:1); (2) Sodium hydrogen bis(2-propylvalerate), oligomer. *UNII-644VL95AO6. CAS-76584-70-8. Anticonvulsant.* Depakote (Abbott) ⋄*Abbott-50711*

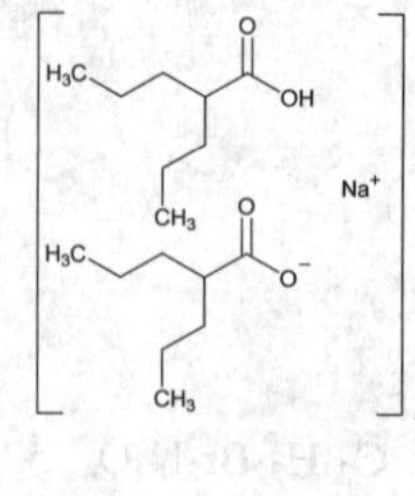

Divanilliden Cyclohexanone — *See* Cyclovalone.

Divaplon. $C_{17}H_{17}N_3O_2$. 295.34. 6-Ethyl-7-methoxy-5-methy-limidazo[1,2-*a*]pyrimidin-2-yl phenyl ketone. *UNII-4AOV43246G. CAS-90808-12-1.* INN.

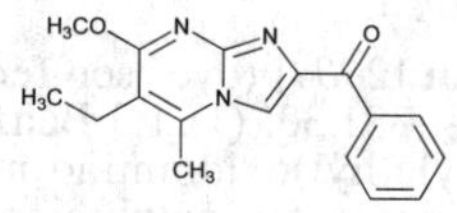

Diviminol — *See* Viminol.

Dixamone Bromide — *See* Methantheline Bromide.

Dixanthogen. $C_6H_{10}O_2S_4$. 242.40. *O,O*-Diethyl ester of dithiobis(thioformic acid). *CAS-502-55-6.* INN; DCF; MI.

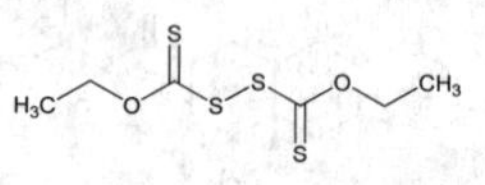

Dizatrifone. $C_{21}H_{21}N_3O_3$. 363.41. 2-(Cyclopropylmethyl)-5,6-bis(*p*-methoxyphenyl)-*as*-triazin-3(2*H*)-one. *UNII-913423W85V. CAS-92257-40-4.* INN.

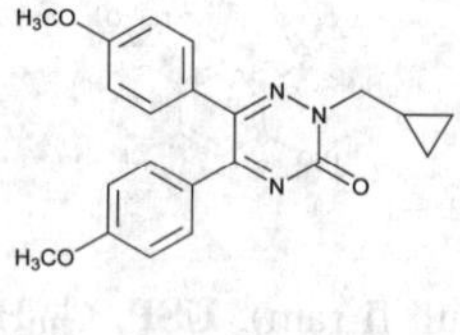

Dizocilpine Maleate [*1989*] (dye zoe′ sil peen mal′ ee ate). $C_{16}H_{15}N \cdot C_4H_4O_4$. 337.37. [Dizocilpine is INN.] (1) 5*H*-Dibenzo[*a,d*]cyclohepten-5,10-imine, 10,11-dihydro-5-methyl-, (+)-, (*Z*)-2-butenedioate (1:1); (2) (+)-10,11-Dihydro-5-methyl-5*H*-dibenzo[*a,d*]cyclohepten-5,10-imine maleate (1:1). *UNII-7PY8KH6811* [dizocilpine]. *CAS-77086-22-7; CAS-77086-21-6* [dizocilpine]. *Neuroprotective.* ⋄*MK-801*

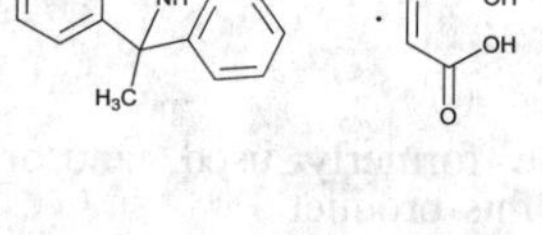

Dobupride. $C_{20}H_{30}ClN_3O_4$. 411.92. 4-Amino-2-butoxy-5-chloro-*N*-[1-(1,3-dioxolan-2-ylmethyl)-4-piperidyl]benzamide. *UNII-FW0Z2U7O23. CAS-106707-51-1.* INN.

Dobutamine [*1972*] (doe bue′ ta meen). **USP.** $C_{18}H_{23}NO_3$. 301.38. (1) 1,2-Benzenediol, 4-[2-[[3-(4-hydroxyphenyl)-1-methylpropyl]amino]ethyl]-, (±)-; (2) (±)-4-[2-[[3-(*p*-Hydroxyphenyl)-1-methylpropyl]amino]ethyl]pyrocatechol. *UNII-3S12J47372. CAS-34368-04-2.* INN; BAN. *Cardiotonic.* ◇*Compound 81929*

Dobutamine Hydrochloride [*1974*] (doe bue′ ta meen hye″ droe klor′ ide). **USP.** $C_{18}H_{23}NO_3 \cdot HCl$. 337.84. (1) 1,2-Benzenediol, 4-[2-[[3-(4-hydroxyphenyl)-1-methylpropyl]amino]ethyl]-, hydrochloride, (±)-; (2) (±)-4-[2-[[3-(*p*-Hydroxyphenyl)-1-methylpropyl]amino]ethyl]pyrocatechol hydrochloride. *UNII-0WR771DJXV; UNII-3S12J47372 [dobutamine]. CAS-49745-95-1; CAS-34368-04-2 [dobutamine].* BAN; JAN. *Cardiotonic.* Dobutrex (Lilly) ◇*46236*

Dobutamine Lactobionate [*1990*] (doe bue′ ta meen lak″ toe bye′ oh nate). $C_{18}H_{23}NO_3 \cdot C_{12}H_{22}O_{12}$. 659.68. (1) 1,2-Benzenediol, 4-[2-[[3-(4-hydroxyphenyl)-1-methylpropyl]amino]ethyl]-, (±)-, 4-*O*-β-D-galactopyranosyl-D-gluconate (salt); (2) (±)-4-[2-[[3-(*p*-Hydroxyphenyl)-1-methylpropyl]amino]ethyl]pyrocatechol lactobionate (salt). *CAS-104564-71-8. Cardiotonic.* ◇*LY207506*

Dobutamine Tartrate [*1987*] (doe bue′ ta meen tar′ trate). $C_{18}H_{23}NO_3 \cdot C_4H_6O_6$. 451.47. (1) 1,2-Benzenediol, 4-[2-[[3-(4-hydroxyphenyl)-1-methylpropyl]amino]ethyl]-, (±)-, [*S*-(*R**,*R**)]-2,3-dihydroxybutanedioate (1:1) (salt); (2)

(±)-4-[2-[[3-(*p*-Hydroxyphenyl)-1-methylpropyl]amino]ethyl]pyrocatechol D-tartrate (1:1) (salt). *UNII-5D1IB9AI6J. CAS-101626-66-8. Cardiotonic.* ◇*LY 174008*

Docarpamine. $C_{21}H_{30}N_2O_8S$. 470.54. (-)-(*S*)-2-Acetamido-*N*-(3,4-dihydroxyphenethyl)-4-(methylthio)butyramide bis(ethyl carbonate) (ester). *UNII-RPQ57D8S72. CAS-74639-40-0.* INN.

Docebenone [*1989*] (doe se′ be none). $C_{21}H_{26}O_3$. 326.43. (1) 2,5-Cyclohexadiene-1,4-dione, 2-(12-hydroxy-5,10-dodecadiynyl)-3,5,6-trimethyl-; (2) 2-(12-Hydroxy-5,10-dodecadiynyl)-3,5,6-trimethyl-*p*-benzoquinone. *UNII-2XRX3BD53M. CAS-80809-81-0.* INN. *Inhibitor (5-lipoxygenase).* ◇*AA-861; A-61589*

Docetaxel [*1994*] (doe″ se tax′ el). $C_{43}H_{53}NO_{14} \cdot 3H_2O$. 861.93. (1) Benzenepropanoic acid, β-[[(1,1-dimethylethoxy)carbonyl]amino]-α-hydroxy-, 12b-(acetyloxy)-12-(benzoyloxy)-2a,3,4,4a,5,6,9,10,11,12,12a,12b-dodecahydro-4,6,11-trihydroxy-4a,8,13,13-tetramethyl-5-oxo-7,11-methano-1*H*-cyclodeca[3,4]benz[1,2-*b*]oxet-9-yl ester trihydrate, [2a*R*-[2aα,4β,4aβ,6β,9α(α*R**,β*S**),11α,12α,12aα,12bα]]-; (2) (2*R*,3*S*)-*N*-Carboxy-3-phenylisoserine, *N-tert*-butyl ester, 13-ester with 5β,20-epoxy-1,2α,4,7β,10β,13α-hexahydroxytax-11-en-9-one 4-acetate 2-benzoate, trihydrate. *UNII-15H5577CQD. CAS-148408-66-6; CAS-114977-28-5 [anhydrous].* INN; BAN. *Antineoplastic.* Taxotere (Sanofi Aventis) ◇*RP 56976*

Doconazole [*1977*] (doe kon′ a zole). $C_{26}H_{22}Cl_2N_2O_3$. 481.37. (1) 1*H*-Imidazole, 1-[[4-[([1,1′-biphenyl]-4-yloxy)methyl]-2-(2,4-dichlorophenyl)-1,3-dioxolan-2-yl]methyl]-, *cis*-; (2) *cis*-1-[[4-[(4-Biphenyloxy)methyl]-2-(2,4-dichlorophe-

---

nyl)-1,3-dioxolan-2-yl]methyl]imidazole. *UNII-VR021VC9TY. CAS-59831-63-9.* INN. *Antifungal.* ◇*R 34,000*

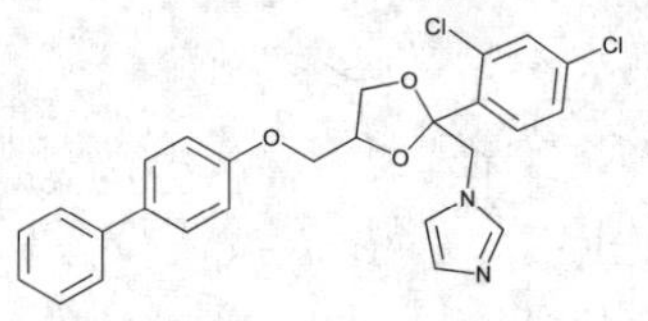

Doconexent. $C_{22}H_{32}O_2$. 328.49. [Omega-3 Marine Triglycerides is BAN.] (*all-Z*)-4,7,10,13,16,19-Docosahexaenoic acid. *UNII-ZAD9OKH9JC. CAS-6217-54-5.* INN.

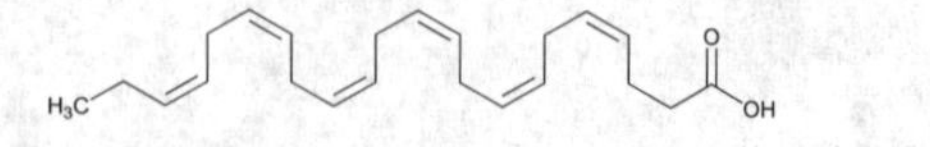

Docosanol [*1999*] (doe koe′ sa nol). $C_{22}H_{46}O$. 326.60. 1-Docosanol. *UNII-9G1OE216XY. CAS-661-19-8. Antiviral used in the treatment of herpes simplex labialis.* Abreva (GlaxoSmithKline) *[Note—The International Cosmetic Ingredient (ICNI) name for docosanol is behenyl alcohol.]*

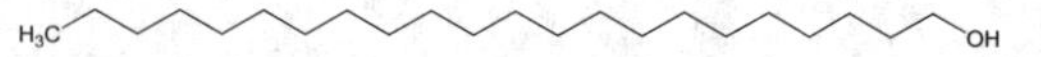

n-Docosanol — *See* Docosanol.

Docusate Calcium [*1980*] (dok′ ue sate kal′ see um). **USP.** $C_{40}H_{74}CaO_{14}S_2$. 883.22. (1) Butanedioic acid, sulfo-, 1,4-bis(2-ethylhexyl) ester, calcium salt; (2) 1,4-Bis(2-ethylhexyl) sulfosuccinate, calcium salt. *UNII-6K7YS503HC. CAS-128-49-4; CAS-10041-19-7* [1,4-bis(2-ethylhexyl)sulfosuccinate]. *Stool softener.* Surfak (Hoechst-Roussel†) *[Name previously used: Dioctyl Calcium Sulfosuccinate.]*

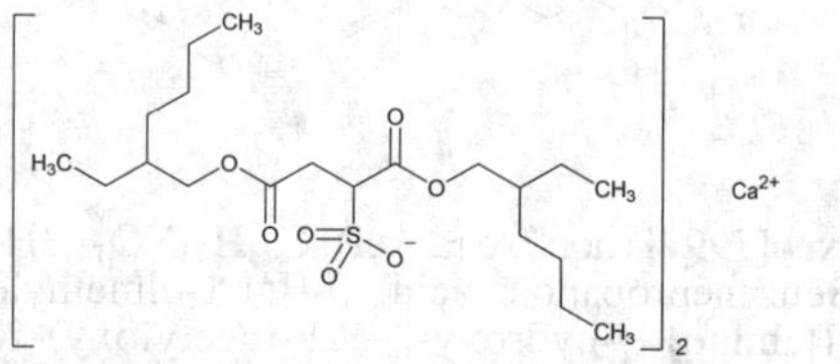

Docusate Potassium [*1980*] (dok′ ue sate poe tas′ ee um). **USP.** $C_{20}H_{37}KO_7S$. 460.67. (1) Butanedioic acid, sulfo-, 1,4-bis(2-ethylhexyl) ester, potassium salt; (2) Potassium 1,4-bis(2-ethylhexyl) sulfosuccinate. *UNII-CIK9F54ZHR. CAS-7491-09-0; CAS-10041-19-7* [docusate hydrogen]. *Stool softener.* Rectalad Enema (Wallace†)

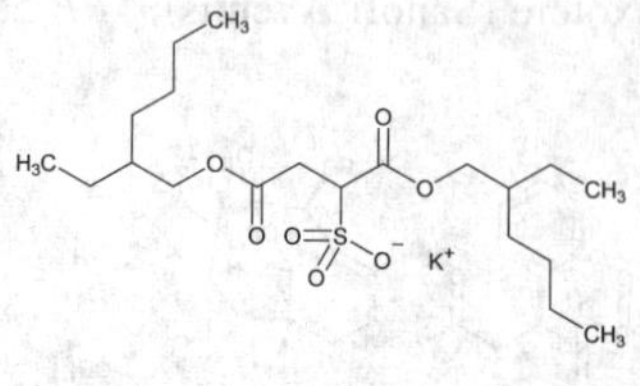

Docusate Sodium [*1980*] (dok′ ue sate soe′ dee um). **USP.** $C_{20}H_{37}NaO_7S$. 444.56. [Sodium Dioctyl Sulfosuccinate is INN; Dioctyl Disodium Sulfosuccinate is JAN.] (1) Butanedioic acid, sulfo-, 1,4-bis(2-ethylhexyl) ester, sodium salt; (2) Sodium 1,4-bis(2-ethylhexyl) sulfosuccinate. *UNII-F05Q2T2JA0. CAS-577-11-7; CAS-10041-19-7* [1,4-bis(2-ethylhexyl)sulfosuccinate]. BAN. *Stool softener; pharmaceutic aid (surfactant).* Colace (Roberts Pharmaceutical); Correctol Stool Softener Laxative (Schering-

Plough HealthCare); Dialose (Johnson & Johnson-Merck Consumer); Doxinate (Hoechst-Roussel†); D-S-S (Parke-Davis†); Modane Soft (Savage); Molofac (Bristol-Myers Squibb†) *[Name previously used: Dioctyl Sodium Sulfosuccinate.]*

Dodeclonium Bromide. $C_{22}H_{39}BrClNO$. 448.91. [2-(*p*-Chlorophenoxy)ethyl]dodecyldimethylammonium bromide. *UNII-XD8BU85ZLK. CAS-15687-13-5.* INN. ◇*GR 412*

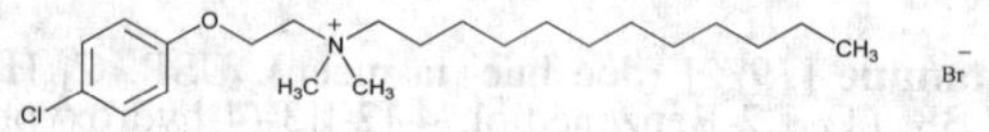

Dodicin. $C_{18}H_{39}N_3O_2$. 329.52. 3,6,9-Triazahenicosanoic acid. *UNII-72T37AL5JV. CAS-6843-97-6.* BAN.

Dofamium Chloride. $C_{25}H_{44}ClN_3O_2$. 454.09. Dimethyl[2-(*N*-methyldodecanamido)ethyl][(phenylcarbamoyl)methyl]ammonium chloride. *UNII-5504169OQ8. CAS-54063-35-3.* INN; BAN.

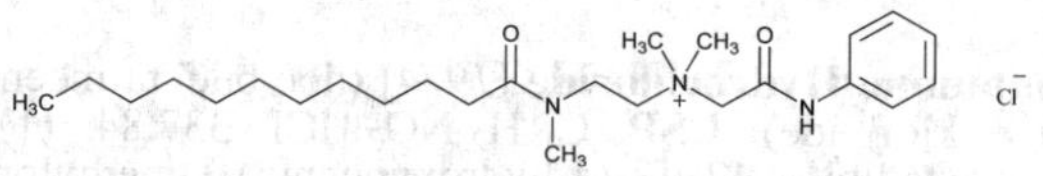

Dofequidar. $C_{30}H_{31}N_3O_3$. 481.59. 1-(Diphenylacetyl)-4-[(2*RS*)-2-hydroxy-3-(5-quinolyloxy)propyl]piperazine. *UNII-0BJK6B565B. CAS-129716-58-1.* INN.

Dofetilide [*1993*] (doe fet′ i lide). $C_{19}H_{27}N_3O_5S_2$. 441.56. (1) Methanesulfonamide, *N*-[4-[2-[methyl[2-[4-[(methylsulfonyl)amino]phenoxy]ethyl]amino]ethyl]phenyl]-; (2) *β*-[(*p*-Methanesulfonamidophenethyl)methylamino]methanesulfono-*p*-phenetidide. *UNII-R4Z9X1N2ND. CAS-115256-11-6.* INN; BAN. *Cardiac depressant (anti-arrhythmic).* Tikosyn (Pfizer) ◇*UK-68,798*

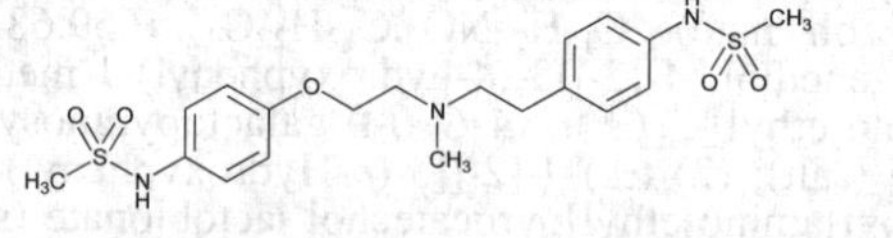

Dolasetron Mesylate [*1991*] (doe las′ e tron mes′ i late). **USP.** $C_{19}H_{20}N_2O_3.CH_4O_3S.H_2O$. 438.49. [Dolasetron is INN and BAN.] (1) 1*H*-Indole-3-carboxylic acid, octahydro-3-oxo-2,6-methano-2*H*-quinolizin-8-yl ester, (2α,6α,8α,9aβ)-, monomethanesulfonate; (2) Indole-3-carboxylic acid, ester with (8*r*)-hexahydro-8-hydroxy-2,6-methano-2*H*-quinolizin-3(4*H*)-one, monomethanesulfonate. *UNII-U3C8E5BWKR; UNII-82WI2L7Q6E* [dolasetron]. *CAS-115956-13-3; CAS-115956-12-2* [dolasetron]. *Anti-emetic; antimigraine.* Anzemet (Sanofi Aventis) ◇*MDL 73,147EF*

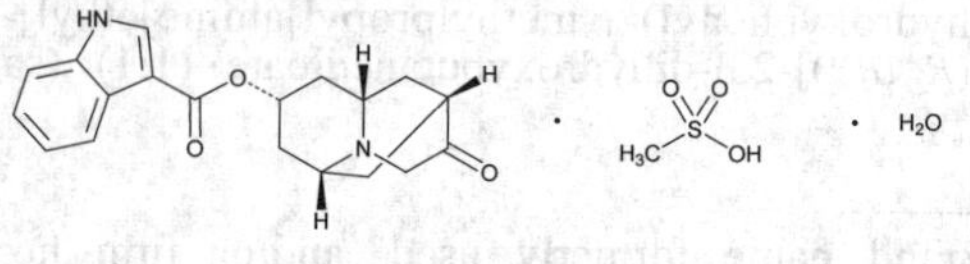

Doliracetam. $C_{16}H_{14}N_2O_2$. 266.29. (±)-2-Oxo-3-phenyl-1-indolineacetamide. *UNII-N70177JQTB. CAS-84901-45-1. INN.*

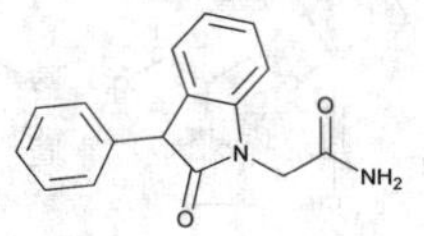

Domazoline Fumarate [*1973*] (doe maz′ oh leen fue′ ma rate). $C_{14}H_{20}N_2O_2.C_4H_4O_4$. 364.39. [Domazoline is INN.] (1) 1*H*-Imidazole,2-[(3,6-dimethoxy-2,4-dimethylphenyl)methyl]-4,5-dihydro-, (*E*)-2-butenedioate (1:1); (2) 2-(3,6-Dimethoxy-2,4-dimethylbenzyl)-2-imidazoline fumarate (1:1). *UNII-TQ4H2AG3JI; UNII-4FBV0WY9OG* [domazoline]. *CAS-35100-41-5; CAS-6043-01-2* [domazoline]. *Anticholinergic.* ◇*Sch 13166 D fumarate*

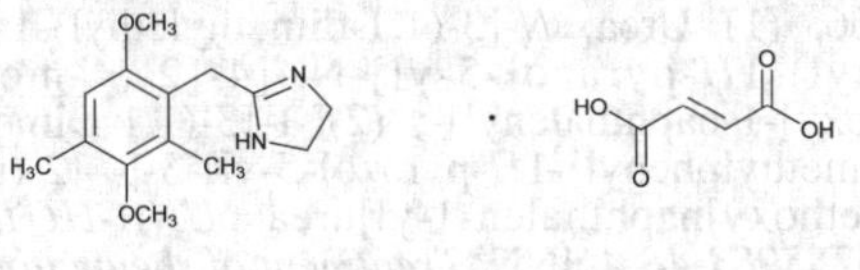

Domiodol [*1980*] (doe mye′ oh dol). $C_5H_9IO_3$. 244.03. (1) 1,3-Dioxolane-4-methanol, 2-(iodomethyl)-; (2) 2-(Iodomethyl)-1,3-dioxolane-4-methanol. *UNII-C1PXF8V06N. CAS-61869-07-6. INN. Mucolytic.* ◇*M.G. 13608*

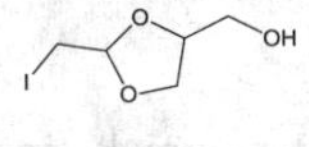

Domiphen Bromide [*1969*] (doe′ mi fen broe′ mide). $C_{22}H_{40}BrNO$. 414.46. (1) 1-Dodecanaminium, *N,N*-dimethyl-*N*-(2-phenoxyethyl)-, bromide; (2) Dodecyldimethyl(2-phenoxyethyl)ammonium bromide. *UNII-R4CY19YS7C. CAS-538-71-6; CAS-13900-14-6* [domiphen]. *BAN; JAN. Anti-infective, topical.* ◇*NSC-39415*

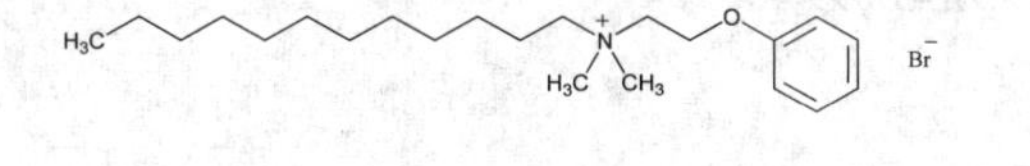

Domipizone. $C_{13}H_{16}N_2O_4$. 264.28. (±)-6-(3,4-Dimethoxyphenyl)-4,5-dihydro-5-(hydroxymethyl)-3(2*H*)-pyridazinone. *UNII-AV4229D6CH. CAS-95355-10-5. INN.*

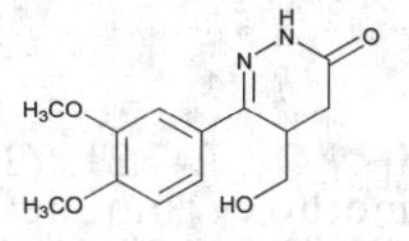

Domitroban. $C_{20}H_{27}NO_4S$. 377.50. (+)-(Z)-7-[(1*R*,2*S*,3*S*,4*S*)-3-Benzenesulfonamido-2-norbornyl]-5-heptenoic acid. *UNII-742F5K270Q. CAS-112966-96-8. INN.*

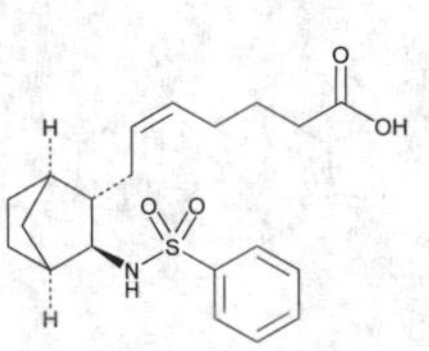

Domoprednate. $C_{26}H_{36}O_5$. 428.56. 11β,17a-Dihydroxy-*D*-homopregna-1,4-diene-3,20-dione 17a-butyrate. *UNII-910G0QIM2M. CAS-66877-67-6. INN.*

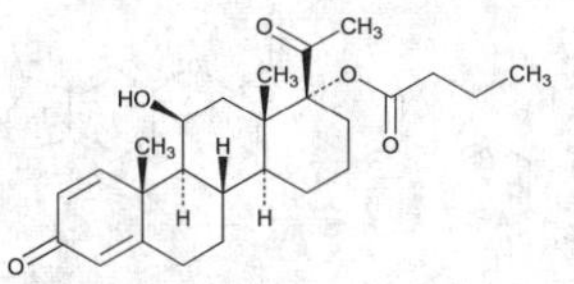

Domoxin. $C_{16}H_{18}N_2O_2$. 270.33. 1-(1,4-Benzodioxan-2-ylmethyl)-1-benzylhydrazine. *UNII-5C0K1GQB2L. CAS-61-74-5. INN.* ◇*IS 2596*

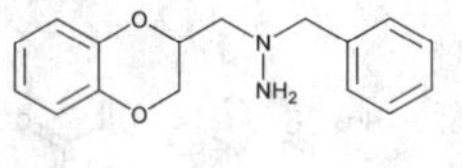

Domperidone [*1976*] (dome per′ i done). $C_{22}H_{24}ClN_5O_2$. 425.91. (1) 2*H*-Benzimidazol-2-one, 5-chloro-1-[1-[3-(2,3-dihydro-2-oxo-1*H*-benzimidazol-1-yl)propyl]-4-piperidinyl]-1,3-dihydro-; (2) 5-Chloro-1-[1-[3-(2-oxo-1-benzimidazolinyl)propyl]-4-piperidyl]-2-benzimidazolinone. *UNII-5587267Z69. CAS-57808-66-9. INN; BAN; JAN. Anti-emetic.* Motilium (Janssen) ◇*R 33,812*

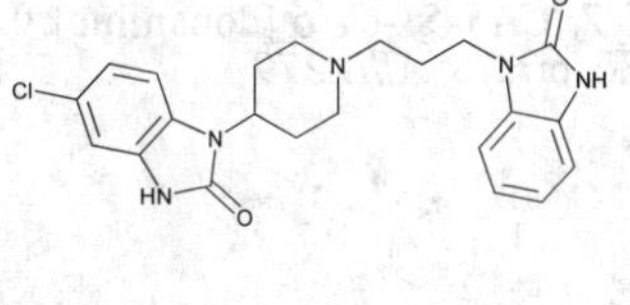

Donepezil Hydrochloride [*1997*] (doe nep′ e zil hye″ droe klor′ ide). $C_{24}H_{29}NO_3.HCl$. 415.95. [Donepezil is INN and BAN.] (±)-2-[(1-Benzyl-4-piperidyl)methyl]-5,6-dimethoxy-1-indanone hydrochloride. *UNII-3O2T2PJ89D; UNII-8SSC91326P* [donepezil]. *CAS-142057-77-0; CAS-120014-06-4* [donepezil]. *Alzheimer's disease treatment (adjunct); dementia symptoms treatment adjunct; cognition adjuvant; inhibitor (acetylcholinesterase).* Aricept (Eisai Medical Research) ◇*E2020; BNAG*

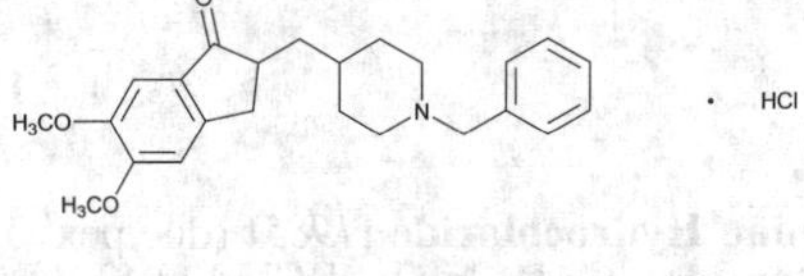

Donetidine [*1987*] (doe ne′ ti deen). $C_{20}H_{25}N_5O_3S$. 415.51. (1) 4(1*H*)-Pyrimidinone, 5-[(1,2-dihydro-2-oxo-4-pyridinyl)methyl]-2-[[2-[[[5-[(dimethylamino)methyl]-2-furanyl]methyl]thio]ethyl]amino]-; (2) 5-[(1,2-Dihydro-2-oxo-4-pyridyl)methyl]-2-[[2-[[5-[(dimethylamino)methyl]fur-

---

† Brand name formerly used, and/or firm no longer concerned with this product.

furyl]thio]ethyl]amino]-4(1*H*)-pyrimidinone. *UNII-E9730RXS4H. CAS-99248-32-5. INN; BAN. Antagonist (to histamine H₂receptors).* ✧*SK&F 93574*

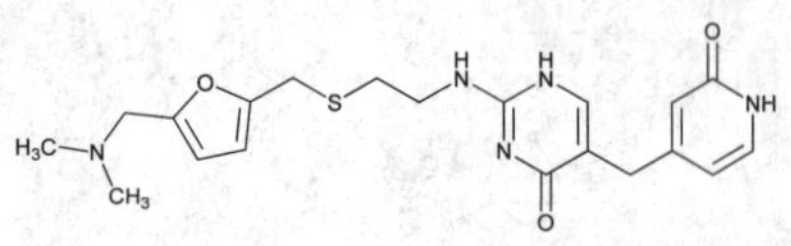

Donitriptan. C₂₃H₂₅N₅O₂. 403.48. 1-[[[3-(2-Aminoethyl)indol-5-yl]oxy]acetyl]-4-(*p*-cyanophenyl)piperazine. *UNII-70968BVH2J. CAS-170912-52-4. INN.*

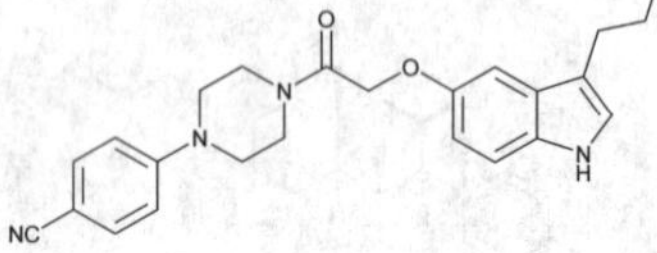

Dopamantine [*1974*] (doe″ pa man′ teen). C₁₉H₂₅NO₃. 315.41. (1) Tricyclo[3,3,1,1³,⁷]decane-1-carboxamide, *N*-[2-(3,4-dihydroxyphenyl)ethyl]-; (2) *N*-(3,4-Dihydroxyphenethyl)-1-adamantanecarboxamide. *CAS-39907-68-1.* INN. *Antiparkinsonian.* ✧*Sch 15507*

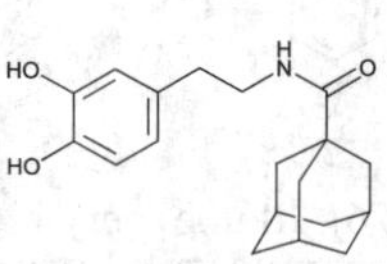

Dopamine Hydrochloride [*1969*] (doe′ pa meen hye″ droe klor′ ide). **USP.** C₈H₁₁NO₂.HCl. 189.64. [Dopamine is INN and BAN.] (1) 1,2-Benzenediol, 4-(2-aminoethyl)-, hydrochloride; (2) 4-(2-Aminoethyl)pyrocatechol hydrochloride. *UNII-7L3E358N9L; UNII-VTD58H1Z2X* [dopamine]. *CAS-62-31-7; CAS-51-61-6* [dopamine]. JAN. *Adrenergic.* Intropin (Hospira) ✧*ASL-279*

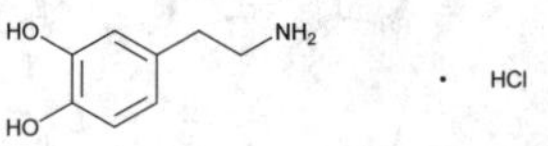

Dopexamine [*1985*] (doe pex′ a meen). C₂₂H₃₂N₂O₂. 356.50. (1) 1,2-Benzenediol, 4-[2-[[6-[(2-phenylethyl)amino]hexyl]amino]ethyl]-; (2) 4-[2-[[6-(Phenethylamino)hexyl]amino]ethyl]pyrocatechol. *UNII-398E7Z7JB5. CAS-86197-47-9.* INN; BAN. *Cardiovascular agent.* ✧*FPL 60278*

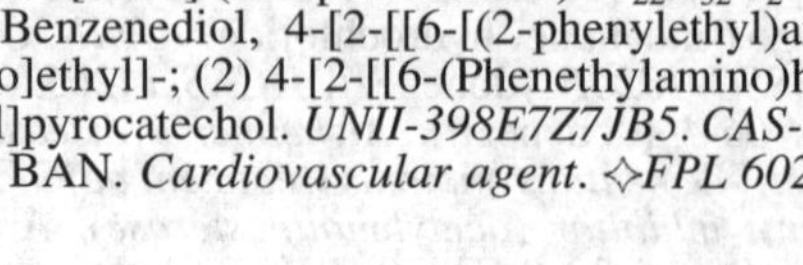

Dopexamine Hydrochloride [*1985*] (doe pex′ a meen hye″ droe klor′ ide). C₂₂H₃₂N₂O₂.2HCl. 429.42. (1) 1,2-Benzenediol, 4-[2-[[6-[(2-phenylethyl)amino]hexyl]amino]ethyl]-, dihydrochloride; (2) 4-[2-[[6-(Phenethylamino)hexyl]amino]ethyl]pyrocatechol dihydrochloride. *UNII-0VN909S60Y. CAS-86484-91-5.* BAN. *Cardiovascular agent.* Dopacard (Fisons†) ✧*FPL 60278AR*

Dopropidil. C₂₀H₃₅NO₂. 321.50. 1-[1-(Isobutoxymethyl)-2-[[1-(1-propynyl)cyclohexyl]oxy]ethyl]pyrrolidine. *UNII-Q9XQ7N7ZRD. CAS-79700-61-1. INN.*

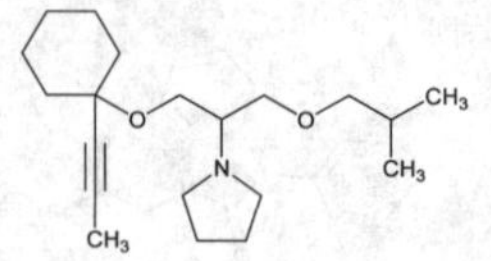

Doqualast. C₁₃H₈N₂O₃. 240.21. 11-Oxo-11*H*-pyrido[2,1-*b*]quinazoline-2-carboxylic acid. *UNII-N8F510M76F. CAS-64019-03-0. INN.*

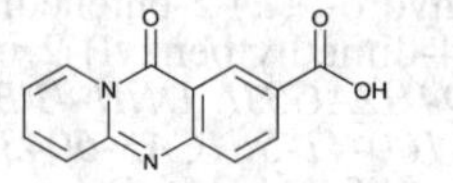

Doramapimod [*2002*] (dor″ a map′ i mod). C₃₁H₃₇N₅O₃. 527.66. (1) Urea, *N*-[3-(1,1-dimethylethyl)-1-(4-methylphenyl)-1*H*-pyrazol-5-yl]-*N*′-[4-[2-(4-morpholinyl)ethoxy]-1-naphthalenyl]-; (2) 1-[3-(1,1-Dimethylethyl)-1-(4-methylphenyl)-1*H*-pyrazol-5-yl]-3-[4-[2-(morpholin-4-yl)ethoxy]naphthalen-1-yl]urea. *UNII-HO1A8B3YVV. CAS-285983-48-4.* INN. *Treatment of rheumatoid arthritis, Crohn's disease and psoriasis.*

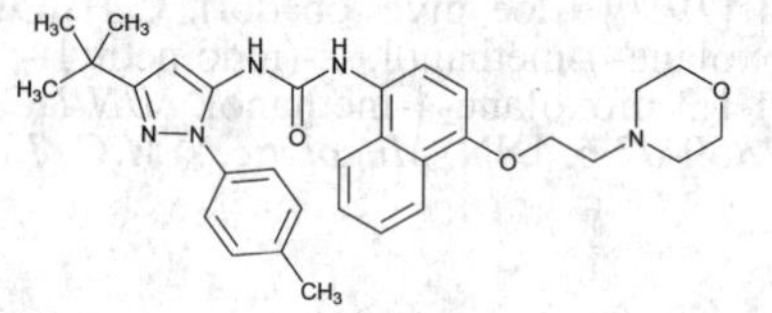

Doramectin [*1990*] (dor″ a mek′ tin). C₅₀H₇₄O₁₄. 899.11. (1) Avermectin A₁ₐ, 25-cyclohexyl-5-*O*-demethyl-25-de(1-methylpropyl)-; (2) (2*aE*,4*E*,8*E*)-(5′*S*,6*S*,6′*R*,7*S*,11*R*,13*S*,15*S*,17a*R*,20*R*,20a*R*,20b*S*)-6′-Cyclohexyl-5′,6,6′,7,10,11,14,15,17a,20,20a,20b-dodecahydro-20,20b-dihydroxy-5′,6,8,19-tetramethyl-17-oxospiro[11,15-methano-2*H*,13*H*,17*H*-furo[4,3,2-*pq*][2,6]benzodioxacyclooctadecin-13,2′-[2*H*]pyran]-7-yl 2,6-dideoxy-4-*O*-(2,6-dideoxy-3-*O*-methyl-α-ʟ-*arabino*-hexopyranosyl)-3-*O*-methyl-α-ʟ-*arabino*-hexopyranoside. *CAS-117704-25-3.* INN; BAN. *Antiparasitic (veterinary).* ✧*UK-67,994*

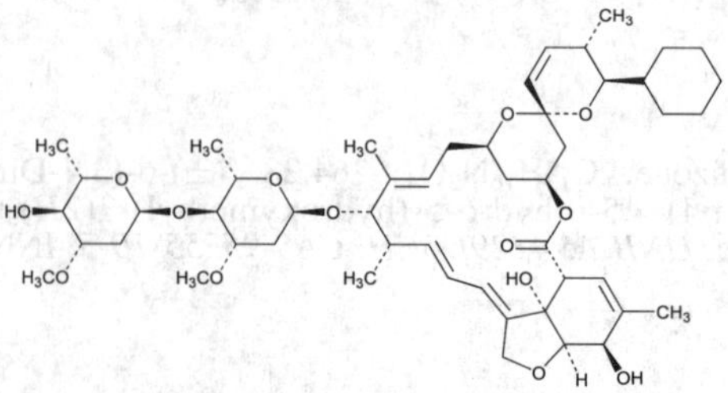

Doranidazole. C₈H₁₃N₃O₆. 247.21. (2*RS*,3*SR*)-3-{[2-Nitroimidazol-1-yl]methoxy}butane-1,2,4-triol. *UNII-911XR034RX. CAS-149838-23-3. INN.*

Dorastine Hydrochloride [*1970*] (dor as′ teen hye″ droe klor′ ide). C₂₀H₂₂ClN₃.2HCl. 412.78. [Dorastine is INN.] (1) 1*H*-Pyrido[4,3-*b*]indole, 8-chloro-2,3,4,5-tetrahydro-2-methyl-5-[2-(6-methyl-3-pyridinyl)ethyl]-, dihydrochloride; (2) 8-Chloro-2,3,4,5-tetrahydro-2-methyl-5-[2-(6-methyl-3-pyridiyl)ethyl]-1*H*-pyrido[4,3-*b*]indole dihydrochloride. *UNII-0M52541M8X. CAS-21228-28-4; CAS-21228-13-7* [dorastine]. *Antihistaminic.* ◇*Ro 5-9110/1*

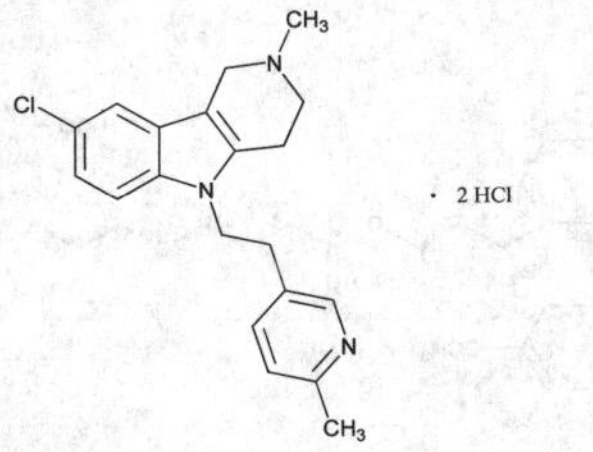

Doreptide. $C_{17}H_{24}N_4O_3$. 332.40. (2*S*)-*N*-[(α*R*)-α-[(Carbamoylmethyl)carbamoyl]-α-ethylbenzyl]-2-pyrrolidinecarboxamide. *UNII-51K3U6Q5ZN. CAS-90104-48-6.* INN.

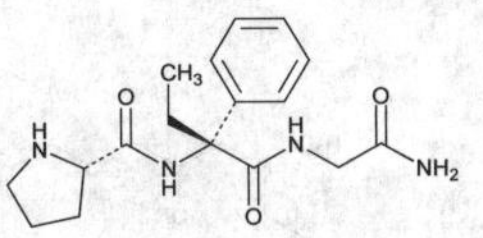

Doretinel [*1989*] (doe re′ ti nel). $C_{24}H_{30}O_2$. 350.49. (1) 2-Naphthalenol, 1,2,3,4-tetrahydro-7-[2-[4-(hydroxymethyl)phenyl]-1-methylethenyl]-1,1,4,4-tetramethyl-, (*E*)-; (2) *p*-[(*E*)-2-(5,6,7,8-Tetrahydro-7-hydroxy-5,5,8,8-tetramethyl-2-naphthyl)propenyl]benzyl alcohol. *UNII-G71TK93T5B. CAS-104561-36-6.* INN. *Antikeratinizing agent.* ◇*BASF 47011; ORF 20257; RWJ 20257*

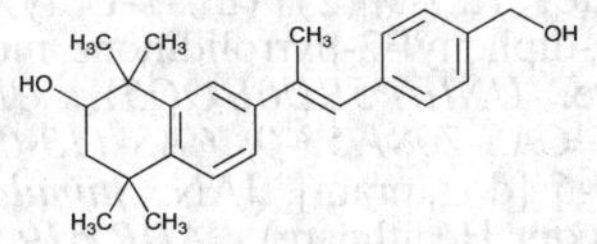

Doripenem [*2005*] (dor″ i pen′ em). $C_{15}H_{24}N_4O_6S_2$. 420.50. (1) 1-Azabicyclo[3.2.0]hept-2-ene-2-carboxylic acid, 3-[[(3*S*,5*S*)-5-[[(aminosulfonyl)amino]methyl]-3-pyrrolidinyl]thio]-6-[(1*R*)-1-hydroxyethyl]-4-methyl-7-oxo-, (4*R*,5*S*,6*S*)-; (2) (+)-(4*R*,5*S*,6*S*)-6-[(1*R*)-1-Hydroxyethyl]-4-methyl-7-oxo-3-[[(3*S*,5*S*)-5-[(sulfamoylamino)methyl]-3-pyrrolidinyl]thio]-1-azabicyclo[3.2.0]hept-2-ene-2-carboxylic acid. *UNII-BHV525JOBH. CAS-148016-81-3.* INN. *Antibiotic.* ◇*S-4661*

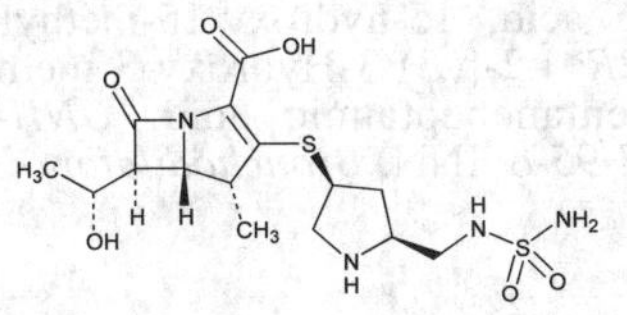

Dorlimomab Aritox. Ricin A chain-antibody ST 1 F(ab′)2 fragment immunotoxin. INN.

Dornase Alfa [*1997*] (dor′ nase al′ fa). $C_{1321}H_{1995}N_{339}O_{396}S_9$ (protein moiety). 29,249.62. Deoxyribonuclease (human clone 18-1 protein moiety). *UNII-953A26OA1Y. CAS-143831-71-4.* INN; BAN. *Cystic fibrosis therapy adjunct.* Pulmozyme (Genentech)

Dorzolamide Hydrochloride [*1992*] (dor zoe′ la mide hye″ droe klor′ ide). **USP.** $C_{10}H_{16}N_2O_4S_3$.HCl. 360.90. [Dorzolamide is INN and BAN.] (1) 4*H*-Thieno[2,3-*b*]thiopyran-2-sulfonamide, 4-(ethylamino)-5,6-dihydro-6-methyl-, 7,7-dioxide, monohydrochloride, (4*S-trans*)-; (2) (4*S*,6*S*)-4-(Ethylamino)-5,6-dihydro-6-methyl-4*H*-thieno[2,3-*b*]thiopyran-2-sulfonamide 7,7-dioxide, monohydrochloride. *UNII-QZO5366EW7; UNII-9JDX055TW1* [dorzolamide]. *CAS-130693-82-2; CAS-120279-96-1* [dorzolamide]. *Carbonic anhydrase inhibitor.* Trusopt (Merck) ◇*MK-507*

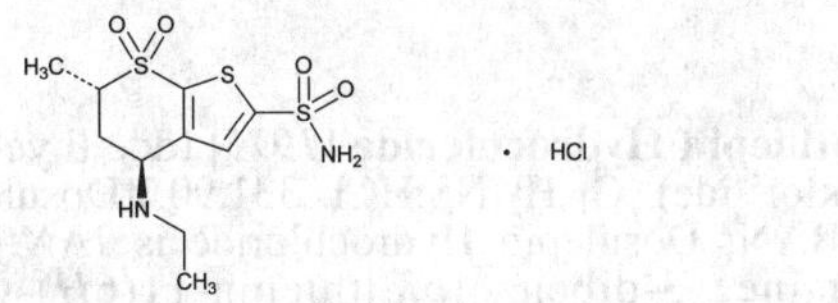

Dosergoside. $C_{34}H_{53}N_3O_3$. 551.80. *N*-[(1*S*,2*R*,3*E*)-2-Hydroxy-1-(hydroxymethyl)-3-heptadecenyl]-6-methylergoline-8β-carboxamide. *CAS-87178-42-5.* INN.

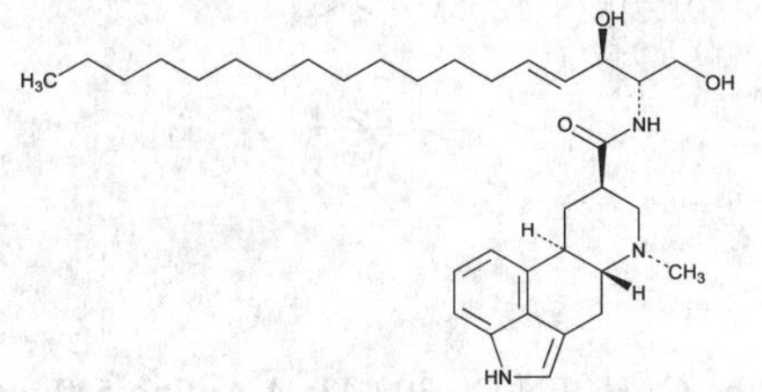

Dosmalfate. $C_{28}H_{60}Al_{14}O_{71}S_7$. 2134.93. [μ7-[[Diosmin heptasulfato](7-)]]tetracontahydroxytetradecaaluminum. *CAS-122312-55-4.* INN.

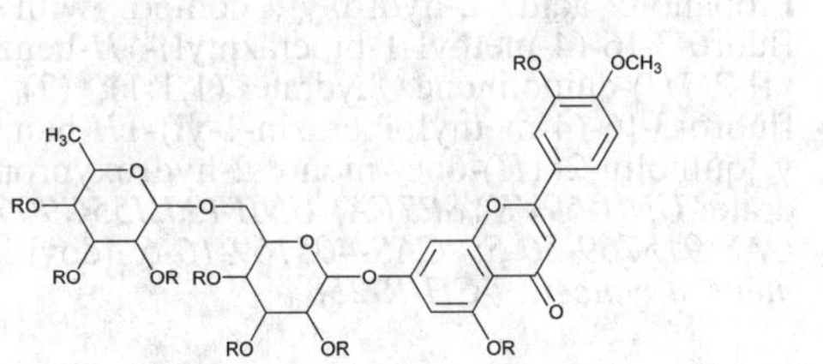

Dosulepin (INN) — *See* Dothiepin Hydrochloride.

Dosulepin Hydrochloride (JAN) — *See* Dothiepin Hydrochloride.

Dotarizine. $C_{29}H_{34}N_2O_2$. 442.59. 1-(Diphenylmethyl)-4-[3-(2-phenyl-1,3-dioxolan-2-yl)propyl]piperazine. *UNII-IO7663S6D3. CAS-84625-59-2.* INN.

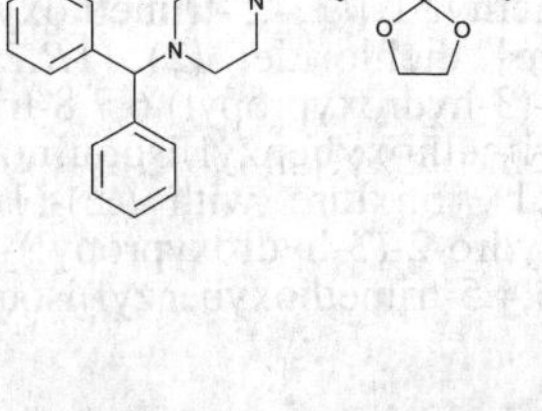

---

† Brand name formerly used, and/or firm no longer concerned with this product.

Dotefonium Bromide. $C_{20}H_{27}BrN_2O_2S$. 439.41. 1-Methyl-1-[2-(*N*-methyl-α-2-thienylmandelamido)ethyl]pyrrolidinium bromide. *UNII-D762286A5N. CAS-26058-50-4.* INN. ◇*H 4132*

Dothiepin Hydrochloride [*1975*] (doe thye′ e pin hye″ droe klor′ ide). $C_{19}H_{21}NS.HCl$. 331.90. [Dosulepin is INN and BAN; Dosulepin Hydrochloride is JAN.] (1) 1-Propanamine, 3-dibenzo[*b,e*]thiepin-11(6*H*)-ylidene-*N,N*-dimethyl-, hydrochloride; (2) *N,N*-Dimethyldibenzo[*b,e*]thiepin-Δ$^{11(6H),\gamma}$-propylamine hydrochloride. *UNII-3H0042311V; UNII-W13O82Z7HL* [dothiepin]. *CAS-897-15-4; CAS-113-53-1* [dothiepin]. *Antidepressant.*

Dovitinib. $C_{21}H_{21}FN_6O$. 392.43. 4-Amino-5-fluoro-3-[6-(4-methylpiperazin-1-yl)-1*H*-benzimidazole-2-yl]quinolin-2(1*H*)-one. *UNII-I35H55G906. CAS-405169-16-6.* INN.

Dovitinib Lactate [*2006*] (doe vi′ ti nib lak′ tate). $C_{21}H_{21}FN_6O.C_3H_6O_3.H_2O$. 500.52. [Dovitinib is INN.] (1) Propanoic acid, 2-hydroxy-, compd. with 4-amino-5-fluoro-3-[6-(4-methyl-1-piperazinyl)-1*H*-benzimidazol-2-yl]-2(1*H*)-quinolinone, hydrate (1:1:1); (2) 4-Amino-5-fluoro-3-[6-(4-methylpiperazin-1-yl)-1*H*-benzimidazol-2-yl]quinolin-2(1*H*)-one mono 2-hydroxypropanoate hydrate. *UNII-69VKY8P7EA; UNII-I35H55G906* [dovitinib]. *CAS-915769-50-5; CAS-405169-16-6* [dovitinib]. *Treatment of cancer.* ◇*CHIR-258*

Doxacurium Chloride [*1990*] (dox a kure′ ee um klor′ ide). $C_{56}H_{78}Cl_2N_2O_{16}$. 1106.13. (1) Isoquinolinium, 2,2′-[(1,4-dioxo-1,4-butanediyl)bis(oxy-3,1-propanediyl)]-bis[1,2,3,4-tetrahydro-6,7,8-trimethoxy-2-methyl-1-[(3,4,5-trimethoxyphenyl)methyl]-, dichloride, [1α,2β(1′*S**,2′*R**)]-, mixture with (±)-[1α,2β(1′*R**,2′*S**)]-2,2′-[(1,4-dioxo-1,4-butanediyl)bis(oxy-3,1-propanediyl)]bis[1,2,3,4-tetrahydro-6,7,8-trimethoxy-2-methyl-1-[(3,4,5-trimethoxyphenyl)methyl]isoquinolinium] dichloride; (2) (1*R*,2*S*;1*S*,2*R*)-1,2,3,4-Tetrahydro-2-(3-hydroxypropyl)-6,7,8-trimethoxy-2-methyl-1-(3,4,5-trimethoxybenzyl)isoquinolinium chloride, succinate (2:1), mixture with (±)-(1*R**,2*S**;1*R**,2*S**)-1,2,3,4-tetrahydro-2-(3-hydroxypropyl)-6,7,8-trimethoxy-2-methyl-1-(3,4,5-trimethoxybenzyl)isoquinolinium chlo-

ride, succinate (2:1). *UNII-M78TVM3G5Z. CAS-106819-53-8.* INN; BAN. *Neuromuscular blocking agent.* Nuromax (Abbott) ◇*BW A938U dichloride*

Doxaminol. $C_{26}H_{29}NO_3$. 403.51. 6,11-Dihydro-*N*-(2-hydroxy-3-phenoxypropyl)-*N*-methyldibenz[*b,e*]oxepin-11-ethylamine. *UNII-1RZ4ML637I. CAS-55286-56-1.* INN.

Doxapram Hydrochloride [*1962*] (dox′ a pram hye″ droe klor′ ide). **USP.** $C_{24}H_{30}N_2O_2.HCl.H_2O$. 432.98. [Doxapram is INN and BAN.] (1) 2-Pyrrolidinone, 1-ethyl-4-[2-(4-morpholinyl)ethyl]-3,3-diphenyl-, monohydrochloride, monohydrate, (±)-; (2) (±)-1-Ethyl-4-(2-morpholinoethyl)-3,3-diphenyl-2-pyrrolidinone monohydrochloride monohydrate. *UNII-P5RU6UOQ5Y; UNII-94F3830Q73* [doxapram]. *CAS-7081-53-0; CAS-113-07-5* [anhydrous]; *CAS-309-29-5* [doxapram]. JAN. *Stimulant (respiratory).* Dopram (Baxter Healthcare) ◇*AHR-619*

Doxaprost [*1975*] (dox′ a prost). $C_{21}H_{36}O_4$. 352.51. (1) Prost-13-en-1-oic acid, 15-hydroxy-15-methyl-9-oxo-, (13*E*)-; (2) (1*R**,2*R**)-2-[(*E*)-3-Hydroxy-3-methyl-1-octenyl]-5-oxocyclopentaneheptanoic acid. *UNII-W3G873MK03. CAS-51953-95-8.* INN. *Bronchodilator.* ◇*AY-24,559*

Doxazosin Mesylate [*1981*] (dox az′ oh sin mes′ i late). **USP.** $C_{23}H_{25}N_5O_5.CH_4O_3S$. 547.58. [Doxazosin is INN and BAN; Doxazosin Mesilate is JAN.] (1) Piperazine, 1-(4-amino-6,7-dimethoxy-2-quinazolinyl)-4-[(2,3-dihydro-1,4-benzodioxin-2-yl)carbonyl]-, monomethanesulfonate; (2) 1-(4-Amino-6,7-dimethoxy-2-quinazolinyl)-4-(1,4-benzodioxan-2-ylcarbonyl)piperazine monomethanesulfonate. *UNII-86P6PQK0MU; UNII-NW1291F1W8* [doxazosin]. *CAS-77883-43-3; CAS-74191-85-8* [doxazosin]. *Antihypertensive.* Cardura (Pfizer) ◇*UK-33,274-27*

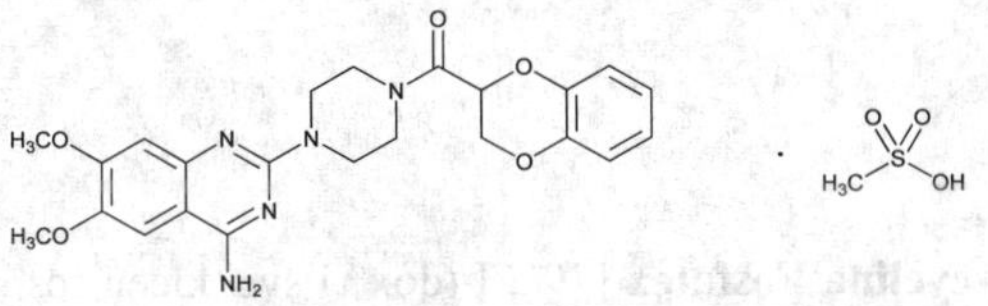

Doxefazepam. $C_{17}H_{14}ClFN_2O_3$. 348.76. 7-Chloro-5-(*o*-fluorophenyl)-1,3-dihydro-3-hydroxy-1-(2-hydroxyethyl)-2*H*-1,4-benzodiazepin-2-one. *UNII-231RV72C8L. CAS-40762-15-0.* INN; MI.

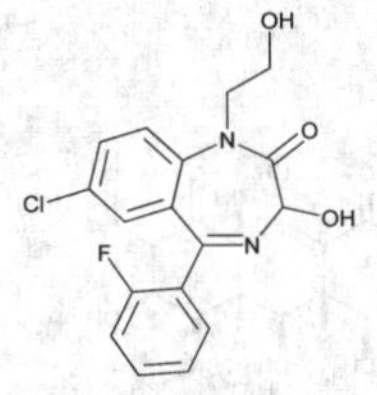

Doxenitoin. $C_{15}H_{14}N_2O$. 238.28. 5,5-Diphenyl-4-imidazolidinone. *CAS-3254-93-1.* INN; DCF; MI. ◇*SKF 2599*

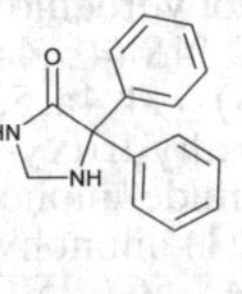

Doxepin Hydrochloride [*1964*] (dox′ e pin hye″ droe klor′ ide). **USP.** $C_{19}H_{21}NO.HCl$. 315.84. [Doxepin is INN and BAN.] (1) 1-Propanamine, 3-dibenz[*b,e*]oxepin-11(6*H*)ylidene-*N,N*-dimethyl-, hydrochloride; (2) *N,N*-Dimethyldibenz[*b,e*]oxepin-$\Delta^{11(6H),\gamma}$-propylamine hydrochloride. *UNII-3U9A0FE9N5; UNII-5ASJ6HUZ7D* [doxepin]. *CAS-1229-29-4; CAS-1668-19-5* [doxepin]; *CAS-4698-39-9* [(*E*)-isomer]; *CAS-25127-31-5* [(*Z*)-isomer]. *Antidepressant.* Sinequan (Pfizer); Zonalon (Bradley) [*Note—Doxepin Hydrochloride is a cis-trans (approximately 1:5) mixture.*] ◇*P-3693A; NSC-108160*

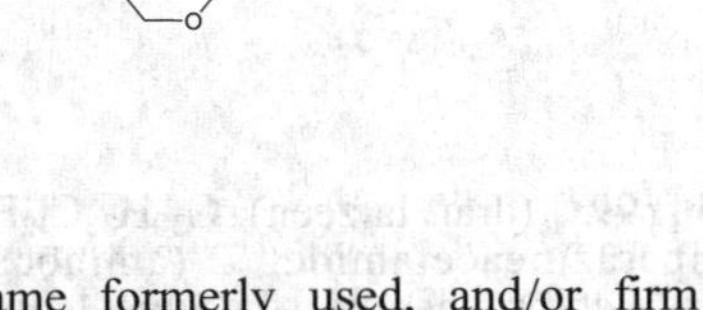

Doxercalciferol. $C_{28}H_{44}O_2$. 412.65. (5Z,7E,22E)-9,10-Secoergosta-5,7,10(19),22-tetraene-1α,3β-diol. *UNII-3DIZ9L-F5Y9. CAS-54573-75-0.* INN. Hectorol (Genzyme)

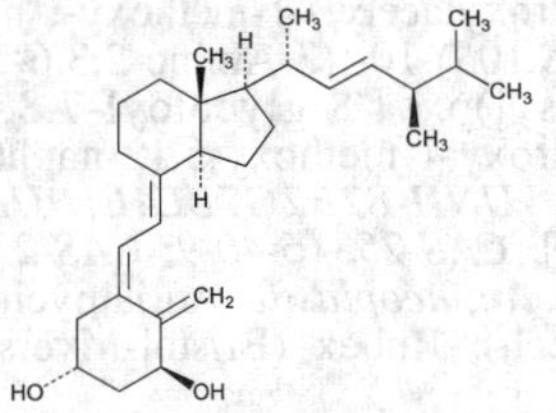

Doxibetasol. $C_{22}H_{29}FO_4$. 376.46. 9-Fluoro-11β,17-dihydroxy-16β-methylpregna-1,4-diene-3,20-dione. *UNII-0JS043FG0D. CAS-1879-77-2.* INN; BAN. [*Name previously used: Doxybetasol.*] ◇*GR 2/443 [as propionate]*

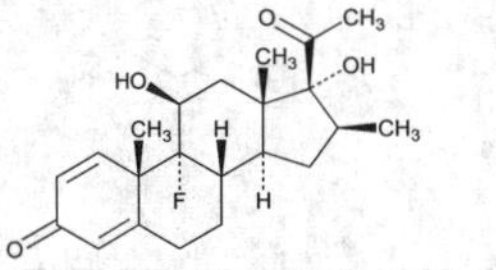

Doxifluridine. $C_9H_{11}FN_2O_5$. 246.19. 5′-Deoxy-5-fluorouridine. *UNII-V1JK16Y2JP. CAS-3094-09-5.* INN; JAN; MI.

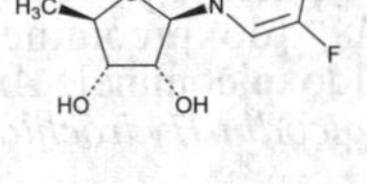

Doxofylline [*1990*] (dox of′ i lin). $C_{11}H_{14}N_4O_4$. 266.25. (1) 1*H*-Purine-2,6-dione, 7-(1,3-dioxolan-2-ylmethyl)-3,7-dihydro-1,3-dimethyl-; (2) 7-(1,3-Dioxolan-2-ylmethyl)theophylline. *UNII-MPM23GMO7Z. CAS-69975-86-6.* INN. *Bronchodilator.* Maxivent (Roberts Pharmaceutical) ◇*ABC 12/3*

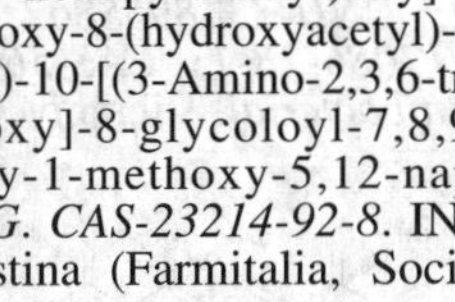

Doxorubicin [*1973*] (dox″ oh roo′ bi sin). $C_{27}H_{29}NO_{11}$. 543.52. (1) 5,12-Naphthacenedione, 10-[(3-amino-2,3,6-trideoxy-α-L-*lyxo*-hexopyranosyl)oxy]-7,8,9,10-tetrahydro-6,8,11-trihydroxy-8-(hydroxyacetyl)-1-methoxy-, (8*S-cis*)-; (2) (8*S*,10*S*)-10-[(3-Amino-2,3,6-trideoxy-α-L-*lyxo*-hexopyranosyl)oxy]-8-glycoloyl-7,8,9,10-tetrahydro-6,8,11-trihydroxy-1-methoxy-5,12-naphthacenedione. *UNII-80168379AG. CAS-23214-92-8.* INN; BAN. *Antineoplastic.* Adriblastina (Farmitalia, Societa Farmaceutici Italia, Italy)

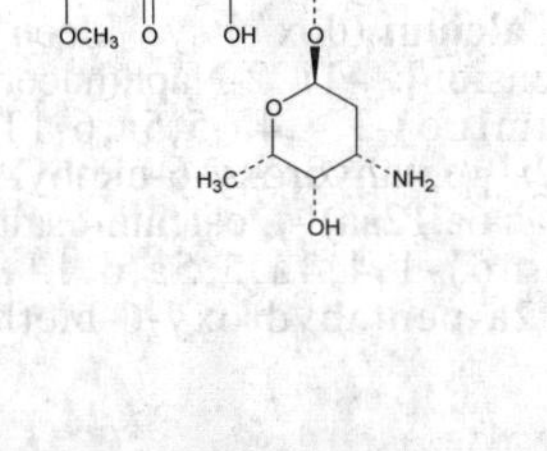

---

† Brand name formerly used, and/or firm no longer concerned with this product.

Doxorubicin Hydrochloride (dox″ oh roo′ bi sin hye″ droe klor′ ide). **USP.** $C_{27}H_{29}NO_{11}.HCl$. 579.98. (1) 5,12-Naphthacenedione, 10-[(3-amino-2,3,6-trideoxy-α-L-*lyxo*-hexopyranosyl)oxy]-7,8,9,10-tetrahydro-6,8,11-trihydroxy-8-(hydroxylacetyl)-1-methoxy-, hydrochloride (8S-*cis*)-; (2) (8S,10S)-10-[(3-Amino-2,3,6-trideoxy-α-L-*lyxo*-hexopyranosyl)oxy]-8-glycoloyl-7,8,9,10-tetrahydro-6,8,11-trihydroxy-1-methoxy-5,12-naphthacenedione hydrochloride. *UNII-82F2G7BL4E; UNII-80168379AG* [doxorubicin]. *CAS-25316-40-9; CAS-23214-92-8* [doxorubicin]. JAN. *Antineoplastic.* Adriamycin (Bedford); Doxil (Ortho Biotech); Rubex (Bristol-Myers Squibb) ◇*NSC-123127*

Doxpicodin Hydrochloride (previously used name) — *See* Doxpicomine Hydrochloride.

Doxpicomine Hydrochloride [*1980*] (dox pik′ oh meen hye″ droe klor′ ide). $C_{12}H_{18}N_2O_2.HCl$. 258.74. [Doxpicomine is INN.] (1) 3-Pyridinemethanamine, α-1,3-dioxan-5-yl-*N,N*-dimethyl-, monohydrochloride, (-)-; (2) (-)-3-[(Dimethylamino)-*m*-dioxan-5-ylmethyl]pyridine monohydrochloride. *UNII-9821373UA1* [doxpicomine]. *CAS-69494-04-8; CAS-62904-71-6* [doxpicomine]. *Analgesic. [Name previously used: Doxpicodin Hydrochloride.]* ◇*LY 108380*

Doxybetasol (previously used name) — *See* Doxibetasol.

Doxycycline [*1966*] (dox″ i sye′ kleen). **USP.** $C_{22}H_{24}N_2O_8.H_2O$. 462.45. [Doxycycline Hydrochloride is JAN.] (1) 2-Naphthacenecarboxamide, 4-(dimethylamino)-1,4,4a,5,5a,6,11,12a-octahydro-3,5,10,12,12a-pentahydroxy-6-methyl-1,11-dioxo-, [4S-(4α,4aα,5α,5aα,6α,12aα)]-, monohydrate; (2) 4-(Dimethylamino)-1,4,4a,5,5a,6,11,12a-octahydro-3,5,10,12,12a-pentahydroxy-6-methyl-1,11-dioxo-2-naphthacenecarboxamide monohydrate. *UNII-N12000U13O; UNII-334895S862* [doxycycline anhydrous]. *CAS-17086-28-1; CAS-564-25-0* [anhydrous]. INN; BAN. *Antibacterial.* Vibramycin (Pfizer) ◇*GS-3065*

Doxycycline Calcium (dox″ i sye′ kleen kal′ see um). **USP** [Oral Suspension]. (1) 2-Naphthacenecarboxamide, 4-(dimethylamino)-1,4,4a,5,5a,6,11,12a-octahydro-3,5,10,12,12a-pentahydroxy-6-methyl-1,11-dioxo-, [4S-(4a,4aa,5a,5aa,6a,12aa)]-, calcium salt (2:1); (2) 4-(Dimethylamino)-1,4,4a,5,5a,6,11,12a-octahydro-3,5,10,12,12a-pentahydroxy-6-methyl-1,11-dioxo-2-naphthacenecarboxamide calcium salt (2:1). *UNII-8ZL07I20SB. CAS-94088-85-4. Antibacterial; antiprotozoal.* Vibramycin (Pfizer)

Doxycycline Fosfatex [*1987*] (dox″ i sye′ kleen fos′ fa tex). $(C_{22}H_{24}N_2O_8)_3.NaPO_3.(HPO_3)_3$. 1675.21. (1) 2-Naphthacenecarboxamide, 4-(dimethylamino)-1,4,4a,5,5a,6,11,12a-octahydro-3,5,10,12,12a-pentahydroxy-6-methyl-1,11-dioxo-, [4S-(4α,4aα,5α,5aα,6α,12aα)]-, compound with metaphos-phoric acid ($H_4P_4O_{12}$) monosodium salt (3:1); (2) (4S,4aR,5S,5aR,6R,12aS)-4-(Dimethylamino)-1,4,4a,5,5a,6,11,12a-octahydro-3,5,10,12,12a-pentahydroxy-6-methyl-1,11-dioxo-2-naphthacenecarboxamide, compound with sodium trihydrogen metaphosphate ($H_3NaP_4O_{12}$) (3:1). *CAS-83038-87-3.* BAN. *Antibacterial.* ◇*AB08; DMSC*

Doxycycline Hyclate (dox″ i sye′ kleen hye′ klate). **USP.** $(C_{22}H_{24}N_2O_8.HCl)_2.C_2H_6O.H_2O$. 1025.87. (1) 2-Naphthacenecarboxamide, 4-(dimethylamino)-1,4,4a,5,5a,6,11,12a-octahydro-3,5,10,12,12a-pentahydroxy-6-methyl-1,11-dioxo-, monohydrochloride, compd. with ethanol (2:1), monohydrate, [4S-(4α,4aα,5α,5aα,6α,12aα)]-; (2) 4-(Dimethylamino)-1,4,4a,5,5a,6,11,12a-octahydro-3,5,10,12,12a-pentahydroxy-6-methyl-1,11-dioxo-2-naphthacenecarboxamide monohydrochloride, compound with ethyl alcohol (2:1), monohydrate. *UNII-19XTS3T51U. CAS-24390-14-5; CAS-564-25-0* [doxycycline]. *Antibacterial.* Atridox (Tolmar); Doryx (Warner Chilcott); Doxy (Abraxis); Periostat (CollaGenex); Vibramycin (Pfizer)

Doxylamine Succinate (dox il′ a meen sux′ i nate). **USP.** $C_{17}H_{22}N_2O.C_4H_6O_4$. 388.46. [Doxylamine is INN and BAN.] (1) Ethanamine, *N,N*-dimethyl-2-[1-phenyl-1-(2-pyridinyl)ethoxy]-, butanedioate (1:1); (2) 2-[α[2-(Dimethylamino)ethoxy]-α-methylbenzyl]pyridine succinate (1:1). *UNII-V9BI9B5YI2; UNII-95QB77JKPL* [doxylamine]. *CAS-562-10-7; CAS-469-21-6* [doxylamine]. *Antihistaminic.* Decapryn (Sanofi Aventis); Unisom (Pfizer)

Draflazine [*1993*] (draf′ la zeen). $C_{30}H_{33}Cl_2F_2N_5O_2$. 604.52. (1) 1-Piperazineacetamide, 2-(aminocarbonyl)-*N*-(4-amino-2,6-dichlorophenyl)-4-[5,5-bis(4-fluorophenyl)pentyl]-,(±)-; (2) (±)-4′-Amino-4-[5,5-bis(*p*-fluorophenyl) pentyl]-2-carbamoyl-2′,6′-dichloro-1-piperazineac-etanilide. *UNII-0Y25DT968Y*. *CAS-120770-34-5*. INN; BAN. *Cardioprotectant.* ◇*R 75231*

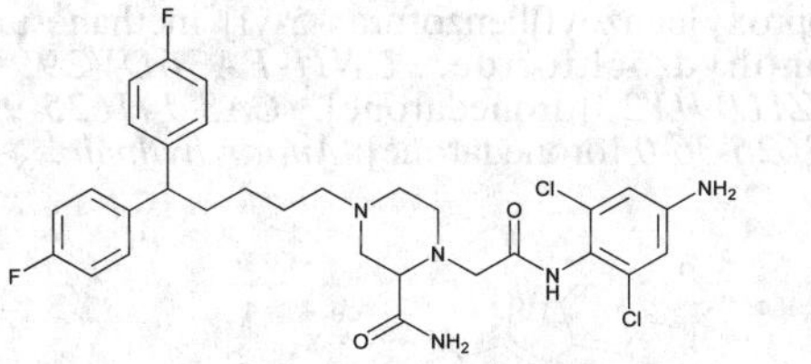

Dramedilol. $C_{20}H_{29}N_5O_4$. 403.48. Acetone (±)-[6-[3-[(3,4-dimethoxyphenethyl)amino]-2-hydroxypropoxy]-3-pyrida-zinyl]hydrazone. *UNII-8PW276HX8U*. *CAS-76953-65-6*. INN.

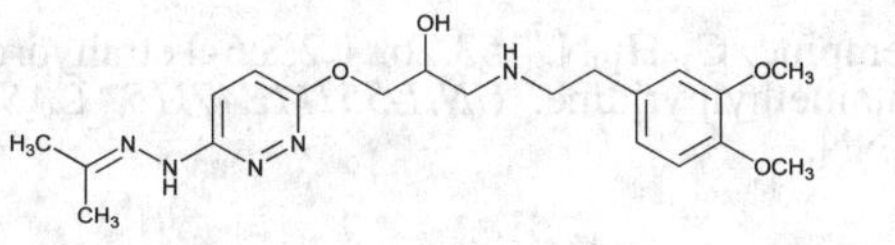

Draquinolol. $C_{24}H_{30}N_2O_4$. 410.51. 3-[*p*-[3-(*tert*-Butylamino)-2-hydroxypropoxy]phenyl]-7-methoxy-2-methylisocarbos-tyril. *UNII-K3B3L3Q0GV*. *CAS-67793-71-9*. INN.

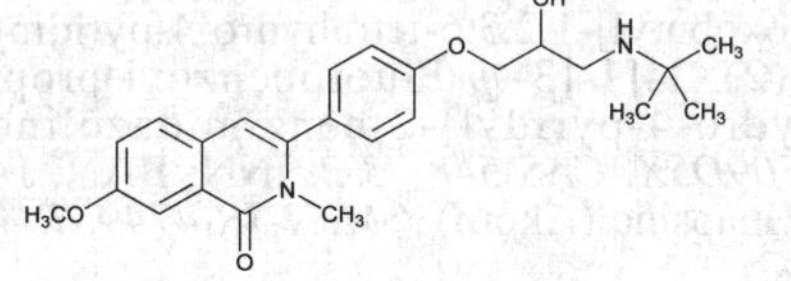

Drazidox. $C_{10}H_{10}N_4O_3$. 234.21. 3-Methyl-2-quinoxalinecar-boxylic acid hydrazide 1,4-dioxide. *UNII-W193003XW5*. *CAS-27314-77-8*. INN.

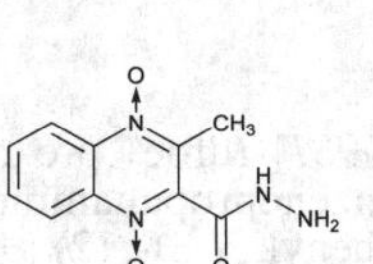

Dribendazole [*1983*] (drye ben′ da zole). $C_{15}H_{19}N_3O_2S$. 305.40. (1) Carbamic acid, [5-(cyclohexylthio)-1*H*-benzi-midazol-2-yl]-, methyl ester; (2) Methyl 5-(cyclohex-ylthio)-2-benzimidazolecarbamate. *UNII-5491IVP21O*. *CAS-63667-16-3*. INN. *Anthelmintic.* ◇*SK&F 63797*

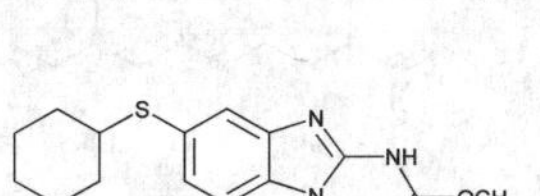

Drinabant. $C_{23}H_{20}Cl_2F_2N_2O_2S$. 497.38. *N*-{1-[Bis(4-chloro-phenyl)methyl]azetidin-3-yl}-*N*-(3,5-difluorophenyl)-methanesulfonamide. *CAS-358970-97-5*. INN.

---

† Brand name formerly used, and/or firm no longer concerned with this product.

Drinidene [*1976*] (drin′ i deen). $C_{10}H_9NO$. 159.18. (1) 1*H*-Inden-1-one, 2-(aminomethylene)-2,3-dihydro-; (2) 2-(Aminomethylene)-1-indanone. *CAS-53394-92-6*. INN. *Analgesic.* ◇*CP-24,877*

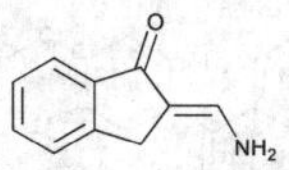

Drobuline [*1977*] (droe′ bue leen). $C_{19}H_{25}NO$. 283.41. (1) Benzenepropanol, α-[[(1-methylethyl)amino]methyl]-γ-phenyl-, (±)-; (2) (±)-1-(Isopropylamino)-4,4-diphenyl-2-butanol. *UNII-6LLN8EQ6TA*. *CAS-58473-73-7*. INN. *Car-diac depressant (anti-arrhythmic).* ◇*Compound 122587*

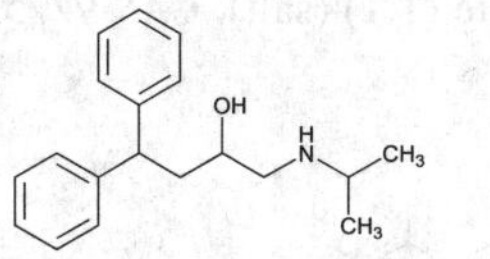

Drocarbil. *CAS-900-77-6*. NF XII; MI.

Drocinonide [*1973*] (droe sin′ oh nide). $C_{24}H_{35}FO_6$. 438.53. (1) Pregnane-3,20-dione, 9-fluoro-11,21-dihydroxy-16,17-[(1-methylethylidene)bis(oxy)]-, (5α,11β,16α)-; (2) 9-Fluoro-11β,16α,17,21-tetrahydroxy-5α-pregnane-3,20-dione cyclic 16,17-acetal with acetone. *CAS-36637-22-6*. INN. *Anti-inflammatory.*

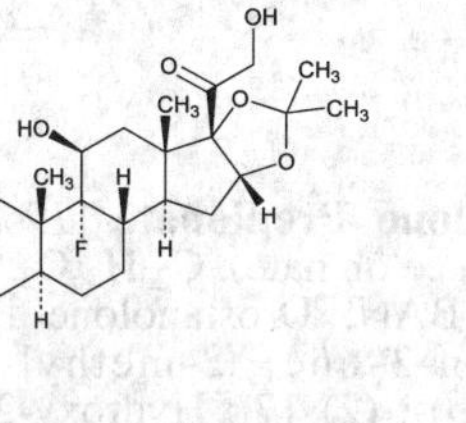

Droclidinium Bromide. $C_{22}H_{32}BrNO_3$. 438.40. 3-Hydroxy-1-methylquinuclidinium bromine α-phenylcyclohexanegly-colate. *UNII-Z4OYQ8EJO8*. *CAS-29125-56-2*. INN.

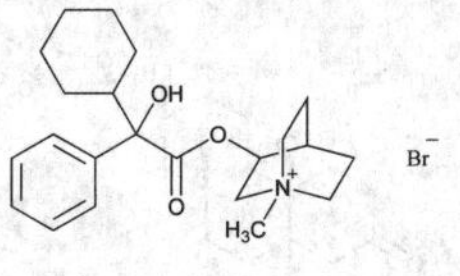

Drocode — *See* Dihydrocodeine Bitartrate.

Drofenine. $C_{20}H_{31}NO_2$. 317.47. 2-(Diethylamino)ethyl α-phenylcyclohexaneacetate. *UNII-4QWV355536*. *CAS-1679-76-1*. INN; MI.

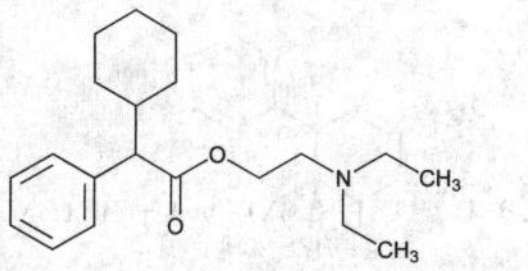

Droloxifene [*1994*] (droe lox′ i feen). $C_{26}H_{29}NO_2$. 387.51. (1) Phenol, 3-[1-[4-[2-(dimethylamino)ethoxy]phenyl]-2-phenyl-1-butenyl]-, (*E*)-; (2) (*E*)-α-[*p*-[2-(Dimethylamino)ethoxy]phenyl]-α′-ethyl-3-stilbenol. *UNII-0M67U6Z98F*. *CAS-82413-20-5*. INN. *Antineoplastic*.

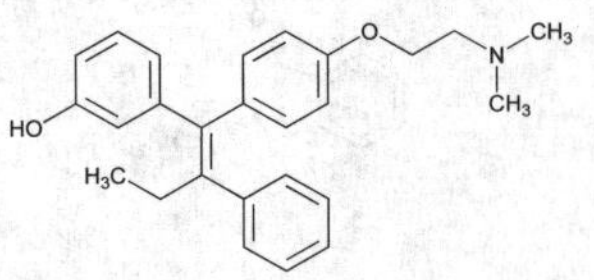

Droloxifene Citrate [*1994*] (droe lox′ i feen sit′ rate). $C_{26}H_{29}NO_2.C_6H_8O_7$. 579.64. (1) Phenol, 3-[1-[4-[2-(dimethylamino)ethoxy]phenyl]-2-phenyl-1-butenyl]-, (*E*)-, 2-hydroxy-1,2,3-propanetricarboxylate (1:1) (salt); (2) (*E*)-α-[*p*-[2-(Dimethylamino)ethoxy]phenyl]-α′-ethyl-3-stilbenol citrate (1:1) (salt). *CAS-97752-20-0*. *Antineoplastic*.

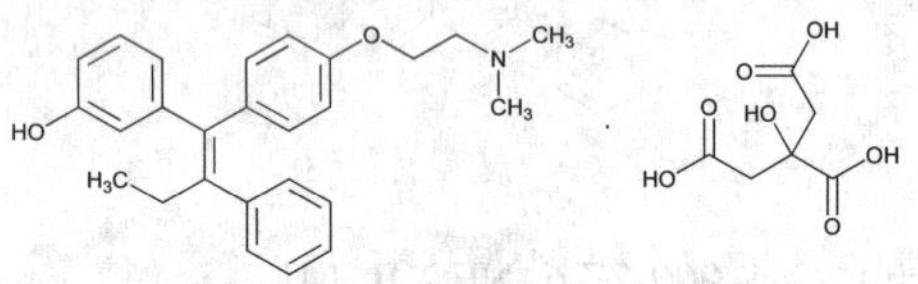

Drometrizole [*1979*] (droe me′ tri zole). $C_{13}H_{11}N_3O$. 225.25. (1) Phenol, 2-(2*H*-benzotriazol-2-yl)-4-methyl-; (2) 2-(2*H*-Benzotriazol-2-yl)-*p*-cresol. *UNII-5X93W9OFZL*. *CAS-2440-22-4*. INN. *Ultraviolet screen*.

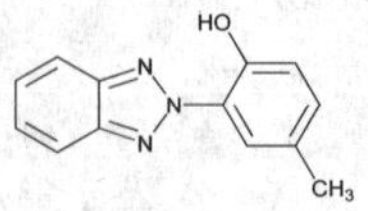

Dromostanolone Propionate [*1963*] (droe″ moe stan′ oh lone proe′ pee oh nate). $C_{23}H_{36}O_3$. 360.53. [Drostanolone is INN and BAN; Drostanolone Propionate is JAN.] (1) Androstan-3-one, 2-methyl-17-(1-oxopropoxy)-, (2α,5α,17β)-; (2) 17β-Hydroxy-2α-methyl-5α-androstan-3-one propionate. *UNII-X20UZ57G4O; UNII-7DR7H00HDT* [dromostanolone]. *CAS-521-12-0; CAS-58-19-5* [dromostanolone]. USP XX. *Antineoplastic*. Drolban (Lilly) ◇*32379; NSC-12198*

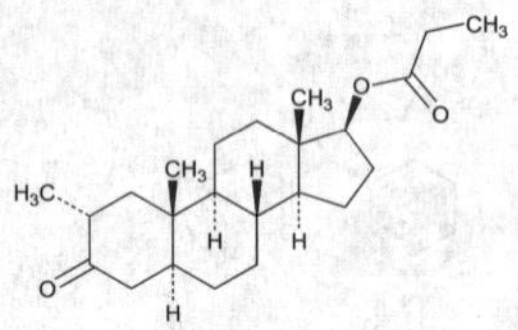

Dronabinol [*1984*] (droe nab′ i nol). USP. $C_{21}H_{30}O_2$. 314.46. (1) 6*H*-Dibenzo[*b,d*]pyran-1-ol, 6a,7,8,10a-tetrahydro-6,6,9-trimethyl-3-pentyl-, (6a*R-trans*)-; (2) (6a*R*,10a*R*)-6a,7,8,10a-Tetrahydro-6,6,9-trimethyl-3-pentyl-6*H*-dibenzo[*b,d*]pyran-1-ol. *UNII-7J8897W37S*. *CAS-1972-08-3*. INN. *Anti-emetic*. Marinol (Unimed) ◇*NSC-134454*

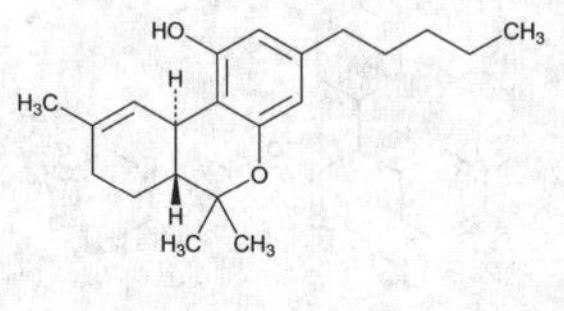

Dronedarone Hydrochloride [*2004*] (droe″ ne′ da rone hye″ droe klor′ ide). $C_{31}H_{44}N_2O_5S.HCl$. 593.22. [Dronedarone is INN.] (1) Methanesulfonamide, *N*-[2-butyl-3-[4-[3-(dibutylamino)propoxy]benzoyl]-5-benzofuranyl]-, monohydrochloride; (2) *N*-[2-Butyl-3-[4-[3-(dibutylamino)proproxy]benzoyl]benzofuran-5-yl] methanesulfonamide-, monohydrochloride. *UNII-FA36DV299Q; UNII-JQZ1L091Y2* [dronedarone]. *CAS-141625-93-6; CAS-141626-36-0* [dronedarone]. *Antiarrhythmic*. ◇*SR33598B*

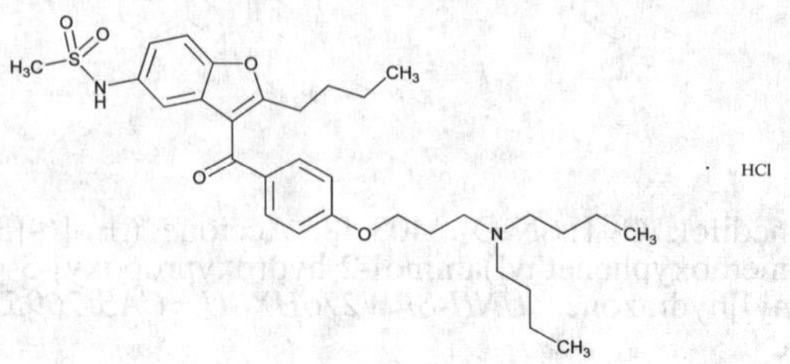

Dropempine. $C_{10}H_{19}N$. 153.26. 1,2,3,6-Tetrahydro-1,2,2,6,6-pentamethylpyridine. *UNII-551ME47I15*. *CAS-34703-49-6*. INN.

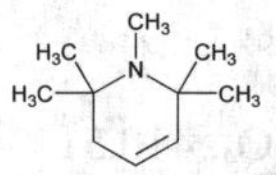

Droperidol [*1963*] (droe per′ i dol). USP. $C_{22}H_{22}FN_3O_2$. 379.43. (1) 2*H*-Benzimidazol-2-one, 1-[1-[4-(4-fluorophenyl)-4-oxobutyl]-1,2,3,6-tetrahydro-4-pyridinyl]-1,3-dihydro-; (2) 1-[1-[3-(*p*-Fluorobenzoyl)propyl]-1,2,3,6-tetrahydro-4-pyridyl]-2-benzimidazolinone. *UNII-O9U0F09D5X*. *CAS-548-73-2*. INN; BAN; JAN. *Antipsychotic*. Inapsine (Akorn) ◇*McN-JR-4749; R-4749*

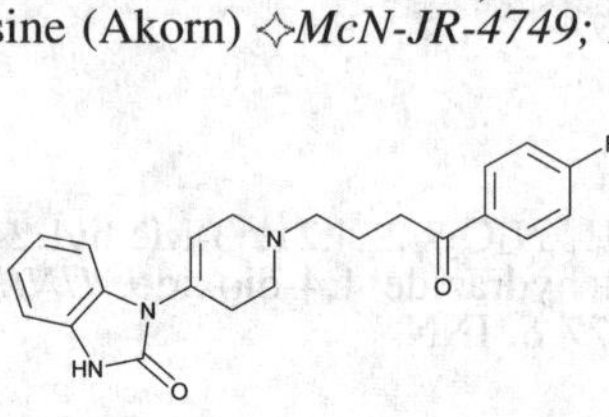

Droprenilamine [*1981*] (droe″ pre nil′ a meen). $C_{24}H_{33}N$. 335.53. (1) Benzenepropanamine, *N*-(2-cyclohexyl-1-methylethyl)-γ-phenyl-, (±)-; (2) (±)-*N*-(3,3-Diphenylpropyl)-α-methylcyclohexaneethylamine. *UNII-31IPX0ZD7R*. *CAS-57653-27-7*. INN. *Vasodilator (coronary)*. Valcor (Maggioni Farmaceutici S.p.A., Italy) ◇*M.G. 8926 [as hydrochloride]*

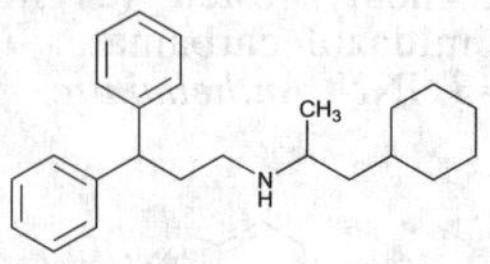

Dropropizine. $C_{13}H_{20}N_2O_2$. 236.31. 3-(4-Phenyl-1-piperazinyl)-1,2-propanediol. *UNII-U0K8WHL37U*. *CAS-17692-31-8*. INN; BAN; DCF; MI. ◇*UCB 1967*

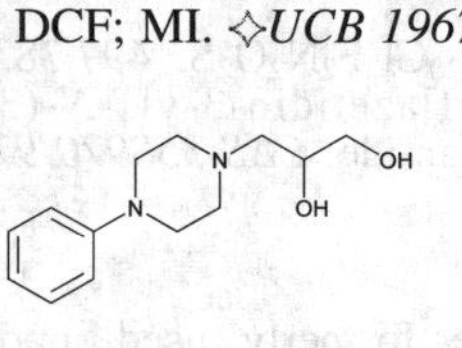

Drospirenone [*1997*] (droe spye′ re none). **USP.** $C_{24}H_{30}O_3$. 366.49. (1) (6*R*,7*R*,8*R*,9*S*,10*R*,13*S*,14*S*,15*S*,16*S*,17*S*)-1,3′,4′,6,6a,7,8,9,10,11,12,13,14,15,15a,16-Hexadecahydro-10,13-dimethylspiro-[17*H*-dicyclopropa[6,7:15,16]cyclopenta[*a*]phenanthrene-17,2′(5′*H*)-furan]-3,5′(2*H*)-dione; (2) 17-Hydroxy-6*β*,7*β*:15*β*,16*β*-dimethylene-3-oxo-17*α*-pregn-4-ene-21-carboxylic acid, *γ*-lactone. *UNII-N295J34A25. CAS-67392-87-4.* INN; BAN. *Aldosterone antagonist.* ◇*ZK 30595*

Drostanolone (INN, BAN) — *See* Dromostanolone Propionate.

Drostanolone Propionate (JAN) — *See* Dromostanolone Propionate.

Drotaverine. $C_{24}H_{31}NO_4$. 397.51. 1-(3,4-Diethoxybenzylidene)-6,7-diethoxy-1,2,3,4-tetrahydroisoquinoline. *UNII-98QS4N58TW. CAS-14009-24-6.* INN.

Drotebanol. $C_{19}H_{27}NO_4$. 333.42. [Oxymetebanol is JAN.] 3,4-Dimethoxy-17-methylmorphinan-6*β*,14-diol. *UNII-7RS2Q8MCK8. CAS-3176-03-2.* INN; BAN; DCF; MI.

Drotrecogin Alfa (activated) [*2000*] (droe tre koe′ gin al′ fa ak′ ti vay″ ted). $C_{2000}H_{3059}N_{559}O_{610}S_{31}$ (plus approximately 20% by weight Asn-linked carbohydrate). (1) Recombinant human activated protein C (rh-APC); (2) Blood coagulation factor XIV (human). Molecular weight is approximately 56,000 daltons. *UNII-JGH8MYC891. CAS-98530-76-8.* INN; BAN. *Antithrombotic; profibrinalytic; anti-inflam-*

matory used in the treatment of sepsis, stroke, and acute thrombotic diseases with high mortality and/or morbidity. ◇*LY203638*

```
ANSFLJJLRH   SSLJRLCIJJ   ICDFJJAKJI   FQNVDDTLAF   WSKHVDGDQC

LVLPLEHPCA   SLCCGHGTCI   BGIGSFSCDC   RSGWEGRFCQ   REVSFLNCSL*

DNGGCTHYCL   EEVGWRRCSC   APGYKLGDDL   LQCHPAVKFP   CGRPWKRMEK

KRSHL
                                                          DTE

DQEDQVDPRL   IDGKMTRRGD   SPWQVVLLDS   KKKLACGAVL   IHPSWVLTAA

HCMDESKKLL   VRLGEYDLRR   WEKWELDLDI   KEVFVHPNYS*  KSTTDNDIAL

LHLAQPATLS   QTIVPICLPD   SGLAERELNQ   AGQETLVTGW   GYHSSREKEA

KRNRTFVLNF*  IKIPVVPHNE*  CSEVMSNMVS   ENMLCAGILG   DRQDACEGDS

GGPMVASFHG   TWFLVGLVSW   GEGCGLLHNY   GVYTKVSRYL   DWIHGHIRDK

EAPQKSWAP
```

* glycosylation sites

Droxacin Sodium [*1976*] (drox′ a sin soe′ dee um). $C_{14}H_{12}NNaO_4$. 281.24. [Droxacin is INN.] (1) Furo[2,3-*g*]quinoline-7-carboxylic acid, 5-ethyl-2,3,5,8-tetrahydro-8-oxo-, sodium salt; (2) Sodium 5-ethyl-2,3,5,8-tetrahydro-8-oxofuro[2,3-*g*]quinoline-7-carboxylate. *UNII-3VOW3G2JQC; UNII-6XMB0871VB* [droxacin]. *CAS-57363-13-0; CAS-35067-47-1* [droxacin]. *Antibacterial.* ◇*SH 263*

Droxicainide. $C_{16}H_{24}N_2O_2$. 276.37. (±)-1-(2-Hydroxyethyl)-2′,6′-pipecoloxylidide. *UNII-J6W196LMV3. CAS-78421-12-2.* INN.

Droxicam. $C_{16}H_{11}N_3O_5S$. 357.34. 5-Methyl-3-(2-pyridyl)-2*H*,5*H*-1,3-oxazino[5,6-*c*][1,2]benzothiazine-2,4(3*H*)-dione 6,6-dioxide. *UNII-F24ADO1E2D. CAS-90101-16-9.* INN; MI.

Droxidopa [*2008*] (drox″ i doe′ pa). $C_9H_{11}NO_5$. 213.19. (1) L-Tyrosine, β,3-dihydroxy-, (βR)-; (2) (-)-(2S,3R)-2-Amino-3-(3,4-dihydroxyphenyl)-3-hydroxypropanoic acid. *UNII-J7A92W69L7. CAS-23651-95-8.* INN; JAN; MI. *Neurogenic hypotension.* ◇*DOPS; L-DOPS*

Droxifilcon A [*1977*] (drox″ i fil′ kon). $(C_6H_{10}O_3)_x$ $(C_{14}H_{22}O_6)_y(C_6H_9NO)_z$. (1) 2-Propenoic acid, 2-methyl-, 2-hydroxyethyl ester, polymer with 1,2-ethanediylbis(oxy-2,1-ethanediyl) bis(2-methyl-2-propenoate) and 1-ethenyl-2-pyrrolidinone; (2) 2-Hydroxyethyl methacrylate polymer with ethylenebis(oxyethylene) dimethacrylate and 1-vinyl-2-pyrrolidinone. *CAS-58503-81-4. Contact lens material (hydrophilic).*

Droxinavir Hydrochloride [*1995*] (drox in′ a vir hye″ droe klor′ ide). $C_{29}H_{51}N_5O_4{\cdot}HCl$. 570.21. [Droxinavir is INN.] (1) L-Valinamide, *N*-methylglycyl-*N*-[3-[[[(1,1-dimethylethyl)amino]carbonyl](3-methylbutyl)amino]-2-hydroxy-1-(phenylmethyl)propyl]-3-methyl-, monohydrochloride, [*R*-(*R**,*S**)]-; (2) 3-*tert*-Butyl-1-[(2R,3S)-3-[(2S)-3,3-dimethyl-2-[2-(methylamino)acetamido]butyramido]-2-hydroxy-4-phenylbutyl]-1-isopentylurea monohydrochloride. *UNII-7QZA627US7; UNII-3CF21QCB9J* [droxinavir]. *CAS-155662-50-3; CAS-159910-86-8* [droxinavir]. *Antiviral.* ◇*SC-55389A*

Droxypropine. $C_{18}H_{27}NO_3$. 305.41. 1-[1-[2-(2-Hydroxyethoxy)ethyl]-4-phenyl-4-piperidyl]-1-propanone. *UNII-94J1SMK20X. CAS-15599-26-5.* INN; BAN.

Dry Distillation Tar of Defatting Soybean. JAN.

Duazomycin [*1962*] (doo az″ oh mye′ sin). Antibiotic produced by *Streptomyces ambofaciens.* (1) Duazomycin; (2) Duazomycin. *CAS-1403-47-0.* INN. *Antineoplastic.* ◇*NSC-51097*

Dulanermin [*2007*] (doo″ la ner′ min). $C_{871}H_{1329}N_{243}O_{260}S_4$. (1) 114-281-Protein TRAIL (tumor necrosis factor-related apoptosis-inducing ligand) (synthetic human); (2) Human tumor necrosis factor ligand superfamily member 10 (TNF-related apoptosis-inducing ligand or Apo-2 ligand or CD253 antigen)-(114-281)-peptide (C-terminal part of the extracellular domain), noncovalent homotrimer. Molecular weight is approximately 19,500 daltons. *CAS-867153-61-5.* INN. *Treatment of metastatic non-small cell lung cancer.* ◇*Apo2L/TRAIL*

```
VRERGPQRVA AHITGTRGRS NTLSSPNSKN EKALGRKINS WESSRSGHSF
LSNLHLRNGE LVIHEKGFYY IYSQTYFRFQ EEIKENTKND KQMVQYIYKY
TSYPDPILLM KSARNSCWSK DAEYGLYSIY QGGIFELKEN DRIFVSVTNE
HLIDMDHEAS FFGAFLVG
```

Dulofibrate. $C_{16}H_{14}Cl_2O_3$. 325.19. *p*-Chlorophenyl 2-(*p*-chlorophenoxy)-2-methylpropionate. *UNII-5K0215OMQX. CAS-61887-16-9.* INN.

Duloxetine Hydrochloride [*1992*] (doo lox′ e teen hye″ droe klor′ ide). $C_{18}H_{19}NOS{\cdot}HCl$. 333.88. [Duloxetine is INN and BAN.] (1) 2-Thiophenepropanamine, *N*-methyl-γ-(1-naphthalenyloxy)-, hydrochloride, (*S*)-; (2) (+)-(*S*)-*N*-Methyl-γ-(1-naphthyloxy)-2-thiophenepropylamine hydrochloride. *UNII-9044SC542W; UNII-O5TNM5N07U* [duloxetine]. *CAS-136434-34-9; CAS-116539-59-4* [duloxetine]. *Antidepressant.* Cymbalta (Lilly) ◇*LY248686 HCl*

Dulozafone. $C_{20}H_{22}Cl_2N_2O_4$. 425.31. 2-[Bis(2-hydroxyethyl)amino]-4′-chloro-2′-(*o*-chlorobenzoyl)-*N*-methylacetanilide. *UNII-BK2633656Q. CAS-75616-02-3.* INN.

Dumorelin. $C_{218}H_{362}N_{72}O_{68}$. 5079.65. 27-L-Leucine-44a-glycine growth hormone-releasing factor (human). *CAS-105953-59-1.* INN.

```
YADAIFTNSY RKVLGQLSAR KLLQDIMSRQ QGESNQERGA RARLG
```

Duometacin. $C_{20}H_{19}NO_5$. 353.37. 3-(p-Anisoyl)-6-methoxy-2-methylindole-1-acetic acid. *UNII-L5WVJ201KN. CAS-25771-23-7.* INN; DCF. ◇*R 4444*

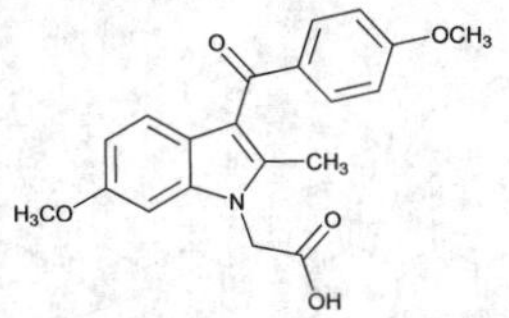

Duoperone Fumarate [*1986*] (doo oh′ per one fue′ ma rate). $C_{28}H_{26}F_4N_2OS.C_4H_4O_4$. 630.65. [Duoperone is INN.] (1) Methanone, (4-fluorophenyl)[1-[3-[2-(trifluoromethyl)-10H-phenothiazin-10-yl]propyl]-4-piperidinyl]-, (E)-2-butenedioate (1:1); (2) p-Fluorophenyl 1-[3-[2-(trifluoromethyl)phenothiazin-10-yl]propyl]-4-piperidyl ketone fumarate (1:1). *UNII-G7MM186D7U; UNII-E84FJ4KW3B* [duoperone]. *CAS-62030-89-1; CAS-62030-88-0* [duoperone]. *Neuroleptic.* ◇*AHR 6646*

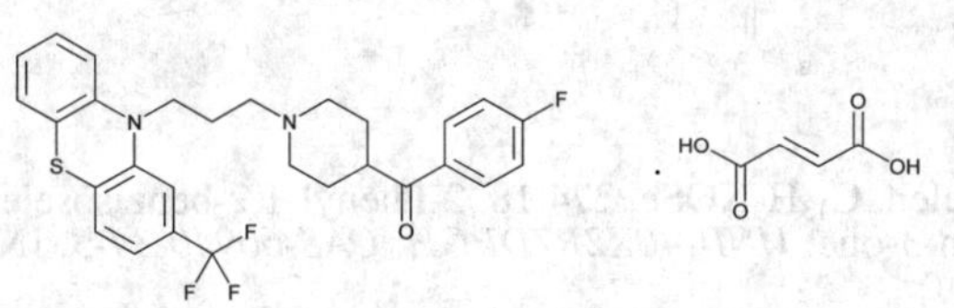

Dupracetam. $C_{12}H_{18}N_4O_4$. 282.30. 1,2-Bis[(2-oxo-1-pyrrolidinyl)acetyl]hydrazine. *UNII-BVM2UGN450. CAS-59776-90-8.* INN.

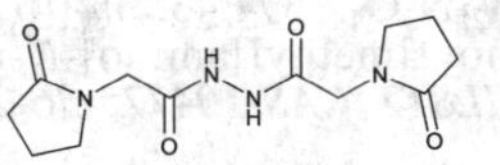

Durapatite [*1976*] (dur ap′ a tite). $Ca_5HO_{13}P_3$. 502.31. [Hydroxyapatite is BAN.] (1) Hydroxylapatite; (2) Hydroxylapatite. *CAS-1306-06-5. Prosthetic aid.* Alveograf (Sterling Winthrop); Periograf (Sterling Winthrop) ◇*Win 40350*

Dusting Powder, Absorbable. **USP**. An absorbable powder prepared by processing cornstarch and intended for use as a lubricant for surgical gloves. *Surgical glove lubricant.*

Dutacatib. $C_{23}H_{31}N_7O$. 421.54. N-({2-Cyano-4-[(2,2-dimethylpropyl)amino]pyrimidin-5-yl}methyl)-4-(4-methylpiperazin-1-yl)benzamide. *UNII-L3M76J6S37. CAS-501000-36-8.* INN.

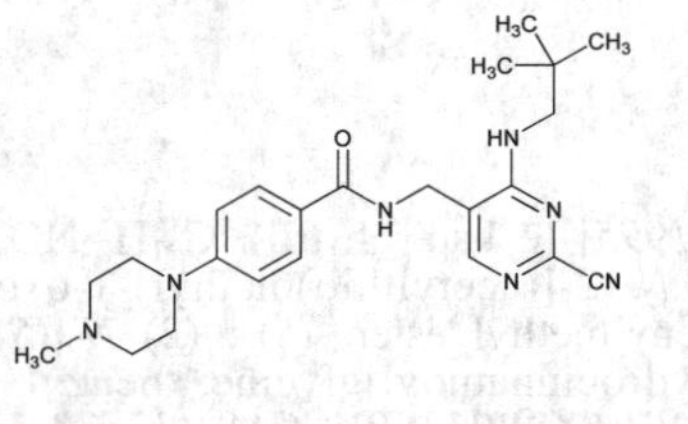

Dutasteride [*1997*] (doo tas′ ter ide). $C_{27}H_{30}F_6N_2O_2$. 528.53. (1) (5α,17β)-N-[2,5-Bis(trifluoromethyl)phenyl]-3-oxo-4-azaandrost-1-ene-17-carboxamide; (2) α,α,α,α′,α′,α′-Hexafluoro-3-oxo-4-aza-5α-androst-1-ene-17β-carboxy-2′,5′-xylidide. *UNII-O0J6XJN02I. CAS-164656-23-9.* INN;

BAN. *Treatment of benign prostatic hyperplasia (5α-reductase type 1 and 2 inhibitor).* Avodart (GlaxoSmithKline) ◇*GI 198745; GG-745*

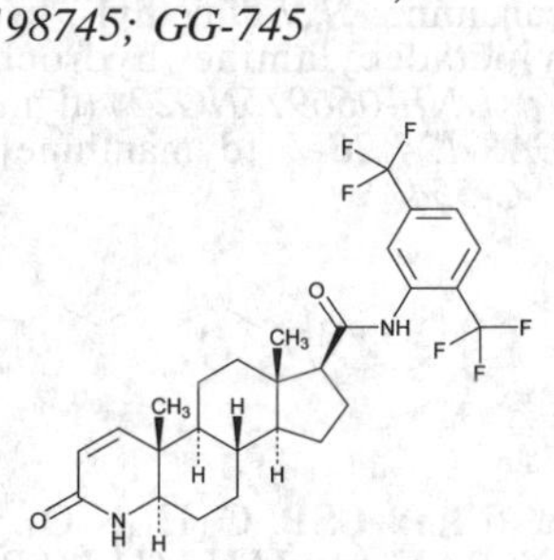

Duteplase. $C_{2736}H_{4174}N_{914}O_{824}S_{46}$. 64,529.12. 245-L-Methionineplasminogen activator (human tissue-type 2-chain form protein moiety). *CAS-120608-46-0.* INN; JAN.

Dutogliptin [*2008*] (doo″ toe glip′ tin). $C_{10}H_{20}BN_3O_3$. 241.10. (1) Boronic acid, [(2R)-1-[[(3R)-3-pyrrolidinylamino]acetyl]-2-pyrrolidinyl]-; (2) [(2R)-1-{[(3R)-Pyrrolidin-3-ylamino]acetyl}pyrrolidin-2-yl]boronic acid. *UNII-38EAO245ZX. CAS-852329-66-9. Treatment of type 2 diabetes.* ◇*PHX1149*

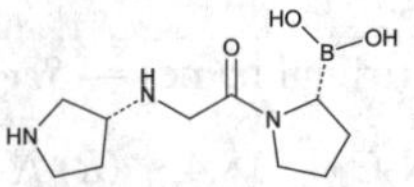

Dutogliptin Tartrate [*2008*] (doo″ toe glip′ tin). $C_{10}H_{20}BN_3O_3.C_4H_6O_6$. 391.18. (1) Boronic acid, [(2R)-1-[[(3R)-3-pyrrolidinylamino]acetyl]-2-pyrrolidinyl]-, (2R,3R)-2,3-dihydroxybutanedioate (1:1); (2) [(2R)-1-{N-[(3R)-Pyrrolidin-3-yl]glycyl}pyrrolidin-2-yl]boronic acid (2R,3R)-2,3-dihydroxybutanedioate (1:1). *UNII-79QH89EV9M. CAS-890402-81-0. Treatment of type 2 diabetes.* ◇*PHX-1149*

Dyclocaine (BAN) — *See* Dyclonine Hydrochloride.

Dyclonine Hydrochloride (dye′ kloe neen hye″ droe klor′ ide). **USP**. $C_{18}H_{27}NO_2.HCl$. 325.87. [Dyclonine is INN and BAN.] (1) 1-Propanone, 1-(4-butoxyphenyl)-3-(1-piperidinyl)-, hydrochloride; (2) 4′-Butoxy-3-piperidinopropiophenone hydrochloride. *UNII-ZEC193879Q; UNII-078A24Q30O* [dyclonine]. *CAS-536-43-6; CAS-586-60-7* [dyclonine]. *Anesthetic (topical).* Dyclone (AstraZeneca) *[Name previously used: Dyclocaine.]*

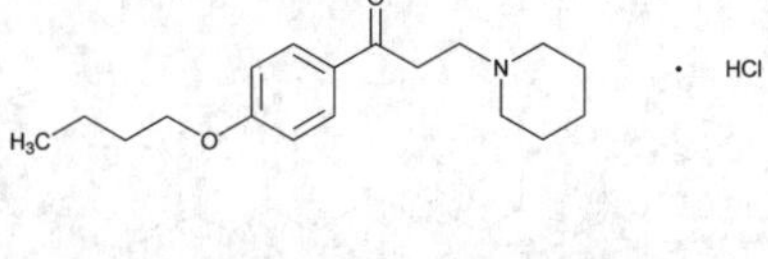

Dydrogesterone [*1962*] (dye″ droe jes′ ter one). **USP**. $C_{21}H_{28}O_2$. 312.45. (1) Pregna-4,6-diene-3,20-dione, (9β,10α)-; (2) 9β,10α-Pregna-4,6-diene-3,20-dione. *UNII-90I02KLE8K. CAS-152-62-5.* INN; BAN; JAN. *Progestin.* Gynorest (Solvay Pharmaceuticals) ◇*NSC-92336*

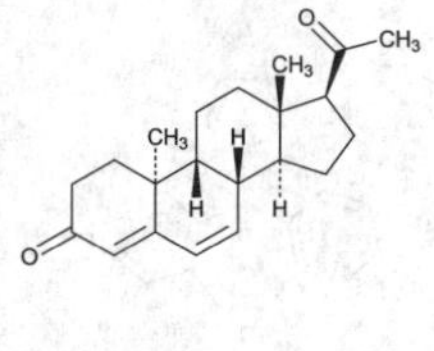

Dyflos (BAN) — *See* Isoflurophate.

---

† Brand name formerly used, and/or firm no longer concerned with this product.

Dymanthine Hydrochloride [*1963*] (dye man' theen hye" droe klor' ide). $C_{20}H_{43}N \cdot HCl$. 334.02. [Dimantine is INN.] (1) 1-Octadecanamine, *N,N*-dimethyl-, hydrochloride; (2) *N,N*-Dimethyloctadecylamine hydrochloride. *UNII-JAD662Q3U7; UNII-066975NG22* [dymanthine]. *CAS-1613-17-8; CAS-124-28-7* [dymanthine]. *Anthelmintic.* ◇*GS-1339; NSC-5547*

Dyphylline (dye' fi lin). **USP.** $C_{10}H_{14}N_4O_4$. 254.24. [Diprophylline is INN, BAN, and JAN.] (1) 1*H*-Purine-2,6-dione, 7-(2,3-dihydroxypropyl)-3,7-dihydro-1,3-dimethyl-, (±)-; (2) (±)-7-(2,3-Dihydroxypropyl)theophylline. *UNII-263T0E9RR9. CAS-479-18-5. Bronchodilator.* Lufyllin (Medpointe)

E2F Duplex Decoy (trivial name) — *See* Edifoligide Sodium.

Ebalzotan. $C_{19}H_{30}N_2O_2$. 318.45. (*R*)-*N*-Isopropyl-3-(isopropylpropylamino)-5-chromancarboxamide. *UNII-WV4B56N49H. CAS-149494-37-1.* INN.

Ebanicline Tosylate (previously used name) — *See* Tebanicline Tosylate.

Ebastine [*1987*] (e bas' teen). $C_{32}H_{39}NO_2$. 469.66. (1) 1-Butanone, 1-[4-(1,1-dimethylethyl)phenyl]-4-[4-(diphenylmethoxy)-1-piperidinyl]-; (2) 4'-*tert*-Butyl-4-[4-(diphenylmethoxy)piperidino]butyrophenone. *UNII-TQD7Q784P1. CAS-90729-43-4.* INN; BAN. *Antihistaminic.* Kestine (Rhone-Poulenc Rorer) ◇*LAS W-090; RP 64305*

Eberconazole. $C_{18}H_{14}Cl_2N_2$. 329.22. (±)-1-(2,4-Dichloro-10,11-dihydro-5*H*-dibenzo[*a,d*]cyclohepten-5-yl)imidazole. *UNII-V7O1U41C9B. CAS-128326-82-9.* INN.

Ebiratide. $C_{48}H_{73}N_{11}O_{10}S$. 996.23. L-Methionyl-L-glutamyl-L-histidyl-L-phenylalanyl-D-lysyl-*N*-(8-aminooctyl)-L-phenylalaninamide *S,S*-dioxide. *UNII-CM5J1V7AUT. CAS-105250-86-0.* INN.

Ebrotidine. $C_{14}H_{17}BrN_6O_2S_3$. 477.42. *p*-Bromo-*N*-[(*E*)-[[2-[[[2-[(diaminomethylene)amino]-4-thiazolyl]-methyl]thio]ethyl]amino]methylene]benzenesulfonamide. *UNII-TMZ3IBW2OW. CAS-100981-43-9.* INN.

Ebselen. $C_{13}H_9NOSe$. 274.18. 2-Phenyl-1,2-benzisoselenazolin-3-one. *UNII-40X2P7DPGH. CAS-60940-34-3.* INN.

Ecabapide. $C_{20}H_{25}N_3O_4$. 371.43. *m*-[[[(3,4-Dimethoxyphenethyl)carbamoyl]methyl]amino]-*N*-methylbenzamide. *UNII-4KA5WHL8T2. CAS-104775-36-2.* INN.

Ecabet. $C_{20}H_{28}O_5S$. 380.50. [Ecabet Sodium is JAN.] 13-Isopropyl-12-sulfopodocarpa-8,11,13-trien-15-oic acid. *UNII-2K02669KWP. CAS-33159-27-2.* INN.

Ecadotril [*1995*] (e kad' oh tril). $C_{21}H_{23}NO_4S$. 385.48. (1) Glycine, *N*-[2-[(acetylthio)methyl]-1-oxo-3-phenylpropyl]-, phenylmethyl ester, (*S*)-; (2) *N*-[(*S*)-α-(Mercaptomethyl)hydrocinnamoyl]glycine, benzyl ester, acetate (ester). *UNII-6XSR933SRK. CAS-112573-73-6.* INN. *Antihypertensive.* ◇*BAY y 7432; BP 1.02; S.049*

Ecalcidene [*2001*] (e kal′ si deen). $C_{29}H_{45}NO_3$. 455.67. Piperidine, 1-[(1α,3β,5Z,7E,20S)-1,3-dihydroxy-24-oxo-9,10-secochola-5,7,10(19)-trien-24-yl]-. *UNII-7RNN0MXE38. CAS-150337-94-3.* INN. *Treatment of psoriasis.[Note—Sponsor is Johnson & Johnson Consumer Products Worldwide.]*

Ecallantide [*2005*] (e kal′ lan tide). $C_{305}H_{442}N_{88}O_{91}S_8$. 7053.83. (1) Protein (synthetic human plasma kallikrein-inhibiting); (2) [Glu20,Ala21,Arg36,Ala38,His39,Pro40,Trp42]-tissue factor pathway inhibitor (human)-(20 79)-peptide (modified on reactive bond region Kunitz inhibitor 1 domain containing fragment); (3) Human plasma kallik-rein-inhibitor (synthetic protein). *UNII-5Q6TZN2HNM. CAS-460738-38-9.* INN. *Treatment of hereditary angioe-dema; reduction of blood loss during cardiothoracic surgery (plasma kallikrein inhibitor).* ◇*DX-88*

```
EAMHSFCAFK ADDGPCRAAH PRWFFNIFTR QCEEFIYGGC EGNQNRFESL
EECKKMCTRD
```

Ecamsule [*1997*] (e kam′ sool). $C_{28}H_{34}O_8S_2$. 562.69. (1) Bicyclo[2.2.1]heptane-1-methanesulfonic acid, 3,3′-(1,4-phenylenedimethylidyne)bis[7,7-dimethyl-2-oxo-; (2) (±)-(3E,3′E)-3,3′-(p-Phenylenedimethylidyne)bis[2-oxo-10-bornanesulfonic acid]. *CAS-92761-26-7.* INN. *Sunscreen.*

Ecarazine Hydrochloride — *See* Todralazine.

Ecastolol. $C_{26}H_{33}N_3O_6$. 483.56. (±)-4′-[3-[(3,4-Dimethoxy-phenethyl)amino]-2-hydroxypropoxy]-3′-(5-isoxazolyl)bu-tyranilide. *UNII-EEB95DS30P. CAS-77695-52-4.* INN.

Ecenofloxacin. $C_{19}H_{21}FN_4O_3$. 372.39. (+)-7-[(1R,5S,6S)-6-Amino-1-methyl-3-azabicyclo[3.2.0]hept-3-yl]-1-cyclo-propyl-6-fluoro-1,4-dihydro-4-oxo-1,8-naphthyridine-3-carboxylic acid. *UNII-3613ZY362L. CAS-162301-05-5.* INN.

Echinacea Angustifolia. *UNII-D982V7VT3P.* NF XXI.

Echinacea angustifolia, Powdered. NF XXI.

Echinacea pallida. *UNII-MGY2W95GWO.* NF XXI.

Echinacea pallida, Powdered. NF XXI.

Echinacea purpurea, Powdered. NF XXI.

Echinacea purpurea Root. NF XXI.

Echothiophate Iodide (ek″ oh thye′ oh fate eye′ oh dide). **USP**. $C_9H_{23}INO_3PS$. 383.23. [Ecothiopate Iodide is INN, BAN, and JAN.] (1) Ethanaminium, 2-[(diethoxypho-sphinyl)thio]-*N,N,N*-trimethyl-, iodide; (2) (2-Mercap-toethyl)trimethylammonium iodide *S*-ester with *O,O*-diethyl phosphorothioate. *UNII-BA9QH3P00T. CAS-513-10-0; CAS-6736-03-4* [echothiophate]. *Cholinergic (ophthalmic).* Phospholine Iodide (Wyeth)

Ecipramidil. $C_{29}H_{33}NO_5$. 475.58. 3-[[(2,2-Diphenylcyclopro-pyl)methyl]amino]propyl 3,4,5-trimethoxybenzoate. *UNII-6EJ6I44649. CAS-64552-16-5.* INN.

Eclanamine Maleate [*1986*] (e klan′ a meen mal′ ee ate). $C_{16}H_{22}Cl_2N_2O.C_4H_4O_4$. 445.34. [Eclanamine is INN.] (1) Propanamide, *N*-(3,4-dichlorophenyl)-*N*-[2-(dimethylami-no)cyclopentyl]-, *trans*-(±)-, (*Z*)-2-butenedioate (1:1); (2) (±)-*trans*-3′,4′-Dichloro-*N*-[2-(dimethylamino)cyclopen-tyl]propionanilide maleate (1:1). *UNII-J2C169J769. CAS-71027-14-0; CAS-71027-13-9* [eclanamine]. *Antidepres-sant.* ◇*U-48,753E*

---

† Brand name formerly used, and/or firm no longer concerned with this product.

Eclazolast [*1986*] (e klaz′ oh last). $C_{12}H_{12}ClNO_4$. 269.68. (1) 2-Benzoxazolecarboxylic acid, 5-chloro-, 2-ethoxyethyl ester; (2) 2-Ethoxyethyl 5-chloro-2-benzoxazolecarboxylate. *UNII-R5ELL4R7VD*. *CAS-80263-73-6*. INN. *Antiallergic; inhibitor (mediator release)*. ◇*RHC 2871*

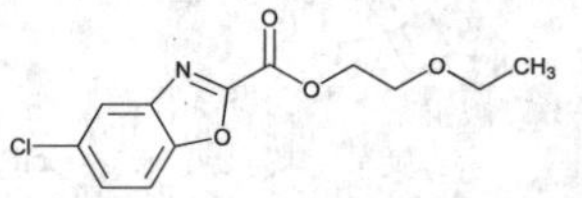

Ecogramostim. *N*-L-Methionylcolony-stimulating factor 2 (human U937 cell protein moiety reduced). *CAS-123120-99-0*. INN; BAN.

Ecomustine. $C_{10}H_{18}ClN_3O_6$. 311.72. Methyl 3-[3-(2-chloroethyl)-3-nitrosoureido]-2,3-dideoxy-α-D-*arabino*-hexapyranoside. *UNII-7369R4J7S2*. *CAS-98383-18-7*. INN.

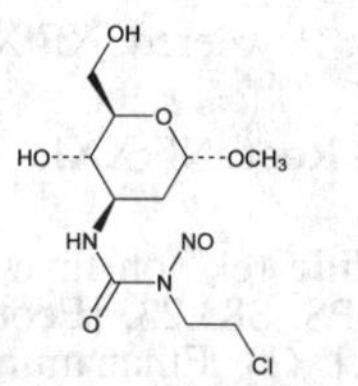

Econazole [*1972*] (e kon′ a zole). $C_{18}H_{15}Cl_3N_2O$. 381.68. (1) 1*H*-Imidazole, 1-[2-[(4-chlorophenyl)methoxy]-2-(2,4-dichlorophenyl)ethyl]-; (2) 1-[2,4-Dichloro-β-[(*p*-chlorobenzyl)oxy]phenethyl]imidazole. *UNII-6Z1Y2V4A7M*. *CAS-27220-47-9*. INN; BAN. *Antifungal.*

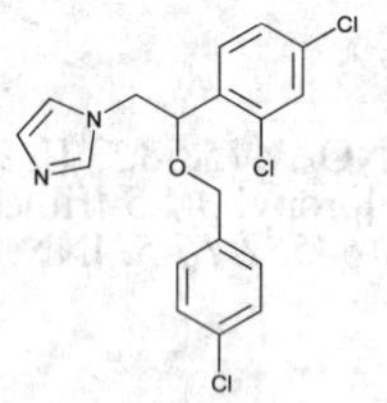

Econazole Nitrate [*1979*] (e kon′ a zole nye′ trate). **USP.** $C_{18}H_{15}Cl_3N_2O \cdot HNO_3$. 444.70. (1) 1*H*-Imidazole, 1-[2-[(4-chlorophenyl)methoxy]-2-(2,4-dichlorophenyl)ethyl]-, mononitrate, ($\pm$)-; (2) ($\pm$)-1-[2,4-Dichloro-β-[(*p*-chlorobenzyl)oxy]phenethyl]-imidazole mononitrate. *UNII-H438WYN10E; UNII-6Z1Y2V4A7M* [econazole]. *CAS-68797-31-9; CAS-27220-47-9* [econazole]. BAN; JAN. *Antifungal.* Spectazole (Johnson & Johnson) ◇*SQ 13050; R 14,827*

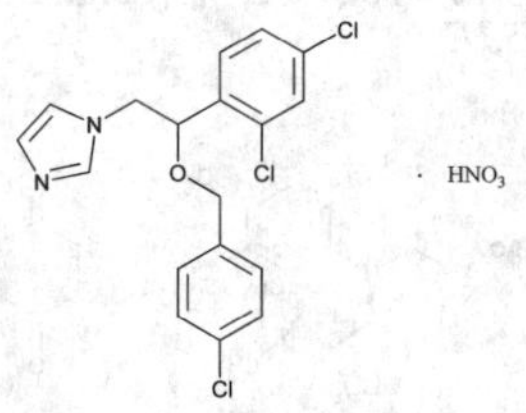

Ecopipam. $C_{19}H_{20}ClNO$. 313.82. (-)-(6a*S*,13b*R*)-11-Chloro-6,6a,7,8,9,13b-hexahydro-7-methyl-5*H*-benzo[*d*]-naphth[2,1-*b*]azepin-12-ol. *UNII-0X748O646K*. *CAS-112108-01-7*. INN.

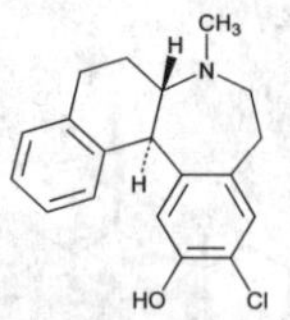

Ecopipam Hydrochloride [*1998*] (e″ koe pi′ pam hye″ droe klor′ ide). $C_{19}H_{20}ClNO \cdot HCl$. 350.28. (1) (6a*S-trans*)-11-Chloro-6,6a,7,8,9,13b-hexahydro-7-methyl-5*H*-benzo[*d*]-naphth[2,1-*b*]azepin-12-ol hydrochloride; (2) (-)-(6a*S*-13b*R*)-11-Chloro-6,6a,7,8,9,13b-hexahydro-7-methyl-5*H*-benzo[*d*]naphth[2,1-*b*]azepin-12-ol hydrochloride. *CAS-190133-94-9*. *Treatment of addiction disorders (selective dopamine receptor D₁/D₅antagonist)*. ◇*SCH 39166*

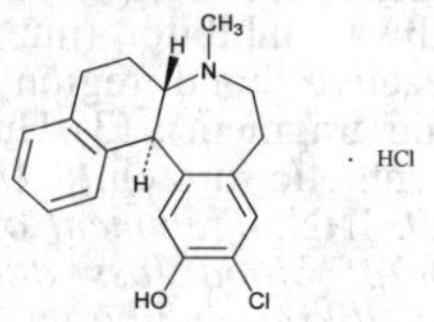

Ecopladib [*2004*] (e kop′ la dib). $C_{39}H_{33}Cl_3N_2O_5S$. 748.11. (1) Benzoic acid, 4-[2-[5-chloro-2-[2-[[[(3,4-dichlorophenyl)methyl]sulfonyl]amino]ethyl]-1-(diphenylmethyl)-1*H*-indol-3-yl]ethoxy]-; (2) 4-[2-[5-Chloro-2-[2-[[(3,4-dichlorobenzyl)sulfonyl]amino]ethyl]-1-(diphenylmethyl)-1*H*-indol-3-yl]ethoxy]benzoic acid. *UNII-48TI67E57Q*. *CAS-381683-92-7*. INN. *Treatment of pain and symptomatic management of arthritis*. ◇*PLA-725*

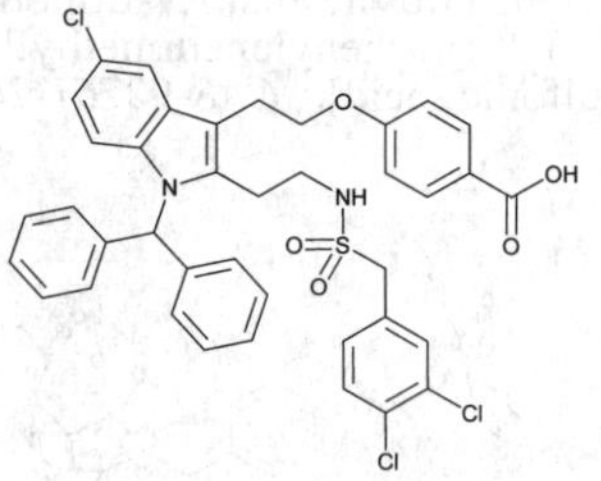

Ecostigmine Iodide — *See* Echothiophate Iodide.

Ecothiopate Iodide (INN, BAN, JAN) — *See* Echothiophate Iodide.

Ecraprost [*1999*] (e′ kra prost). $C_{28}H_{48}O_6$. 480.68. (1) Prosta-8,13-dien-1-oic acid, 11,15-dihydroxy-9-(1-oxobutoxy)-, butyl ester, (11α,13*E*,15*S*)-; (2) Butyl (4*R*,5*R*)-2,4-dihydroxy-5-[(1*E*,3*S*)-3-hydroxy-1-octenyl]-1-cyclopentene-1-heptanoate, 2-butyrate. *UNII-Q2XM6VR8DO*. *CAS-136892-64-3*. INN. *Treatment of peripheral arterial occlusive disease*. ◇*AS-013*

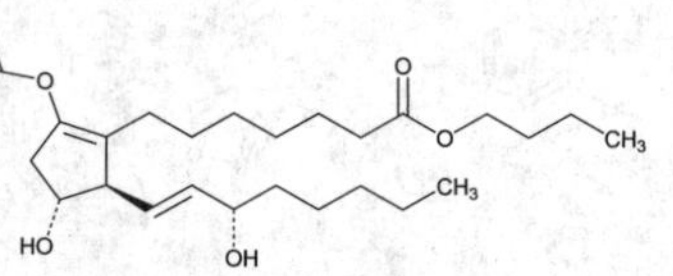

Ecromeximab [*2002*] (e″ kroe mex′ i mab). Immunoglobulin G1, anti-(GD3 ganglioside) (human-mouse monoclonal KM871 γ1-chain), disulfide with human-mouse monoclonal KM871 κ-chain, dimer. Molecular weight is approximately 145,255 daltons, according to the predicted amino acid sequence. *CAS-292819-64-8.* INN. *Treatment of malignant melanoma (monoclonal antibody).* ◇*KW-2871; KM871*

Ectylurea. $C_7H_{12}N_2O_2$. 156.18. *cis*-(2-Ethylcrotonyl)urea. *UNII-1U73ZZU4JK. CAS-95-04-5.* BAN; MI.

Eculizumab [*2002*] (e″ kue liz′ oo mab). Immunoglobulin, anti-(human complement C5 α-chain) (human-mouse monoclonal 5G1.1 heavy chain), disulfide with human-mouse monoclonal 5G1.1 light chain, dimer. Molecular weight is approximately 150,000 daltons. *UNII-A3ULP0F556. CAS-219685-50-4.* INN. *Treatment of autoimmune disease such as rheumatoid arthritis, membranous nephritis, lupus nephritis, dermatomyositis, and autoimmune hemolytic anemias.* ◇*h5G1.1; h5G1.1VHC+h5G1.1VLC*

Edaglitazone Sodium [*2005*] (e″ da gli′ ta zone soe′ dee um). $C_{24}H_{19}N_2NaO_4S_2$. 486.54. [Edaglitazone is INN.] (1) 2,4-Thiazolidinedione, 5-[[4-[2-(5-methyl-2-phenyl-4-oxazolyl)ethoxy]benzo[b]thien-7-yl]methyl]-, sodium salt; (2) Sodium(5*RS*)-5-[[4-[2-(5-methyl-2-phenyloxazol-4-yl)ethoxy]-1-benzothiophen-7-yl]methyl]-2,4-dioxothiazolidin-3-ide. *UNII-862MFS0O74; UNII-8GKF7V499B* [edaglitazone]. *CAS-369631-81-2; CAS-213411-83-7* [edaglitazone]. *Treatment of Type 2 diabetes.* ◇*RO2052349-602*

Edamine — *See* Ethylenediamine.

Edaravone. $C_{10}H_{10}N_2O$. 174.20. 3-Methyl-1-phenyl-2-pyrazolin-5-one. *UNII-S798V6YJRP. CAS-89-25-8.* INN.

Edathamil (previously used name for active moiety) — *See* Edetate Calcium Disodium.

Edatrexate [*1990*] (e″ da trex′ ate). $C_{22}H_{25}N_7O_5$. 467.48. (1) L-Glutamic acid, *N*-[4-[1-[(2,4-diamino-6-pteridinyl)-methyl]propyl]benzoyl]-; (2) *N*-[*p*-[1-[(2,4-Diamino-6-pteridinyl)methyl]propyl]benzoyl]-L-glutamic acid. *UNII-JT4X6Z1HRR. CAS-80576-83-6.* INN. *Antineoplastic.* ◇*CGP 30694*

Edelfosine. $C_{27}H_{58}NO_6P$. 523.73. Choline hydroxide, (±)-2-methoxy-3-(octadecyloxy)propyl hydrogen phosphate, inner salt. *UNII-1Y6SNA8L5S. CAS-70641-51-9.* INN.

Edetate Calcium Disodium [*1962*] (e′ de tate kal′ see um dye soe′ dee um). **USP.** $C_{10}H_{12}CaN_2Na_2O_8·xH_2O$. 374.27 (anhydrous). [Sodium Calcium Edetate is INN, BAN and JAN; Calcium Disodium Edetate is JAN.] (1) Calciate (2-), [[*N*,*N*′-1,2-ethanediylbis[*N*-(carboxymethyl)glycinato]](4-)-*N*,*N*′,*O*,*O*′,*O^N*,*O^N*′]-, disodium, hydrate, (*OC*-6-21)-; (2) Disodium[(ethylenedinitrilo)tetraacetato]calciate(2-) hydrate. *UNII-25IH6R4SGF; UNII-9G34HU7RV0* [edetic acid]. *CAS-23411-34-9; CAS-62-33-9* [anhydrous]; *CAS-60-00-4* [edetic acid]. *Chelating agent (metal).* Calcium Disodium Versenate (Graceway) *[Names previously used: Diazinon; Edathamil for active moiety.]*

Edetate Dipotassium [*1982*] (e′ de tate dye″ poe tas′ ee um). $C_{10}H_{14}K_2N_2O_8·2H_2O$. 404.45. (1) Glycine, *N*,*N*′-1,2-ethanediylbis[*N*-(carboxymethyl)-, dipotassium salt, dihydrate; (2) Dipotassium dihydrogen (ethylenedinitrilo)tetraacetate, dihydrate. *UNII-421KAV3DHT. CAS-25102-12-9; CAS-2001-94-7* [anhydrous]; *CAS-58167-76-3* [monohydrate]. *Pharmaceutic aid (chelating agent).* ◇*32-046*

Edetate Disodium (e′ de tate dye soe′ dee um). **USP.** $C_{10}H_{14}N_2Na_2O_8·2H_2O$. 372.24. [Disodium Edetate is BAN and JAN.] (1) Glycine, *N*,*N*′-1,2-ethanediylbis[*N*-(carboxymethyl)-, disodium salt, dihydrate; (2) Disodium (ethylenedinitrilo)tetraacetate dihydrate. *UNII-9G34HU7RV0* [edetic acid]. *CAS-6381-92-6; CAS-139-33-3* [anhydrous]; *CAS-60-00-4* [edetic acid]. *Chelating agent (metal); pharmaceutic aid (chelating agent).* Endrate (Hospira)

Edetate Sodium [*1966*] (e′ de tate soe′ dee um). $C_{10}H_{12}N_2Na_4O_8$. 380.17. (1) Glycine, *N*,*N*′-1,2-ethanediylbis[*N*-carboxymethyl-, tetrasodium salt; (2) Tetrasodium(ethylenedinitrilo)tetraacetate; (3) Tetrasodium ethylenediaminetetraacetate. *UNII-MP1J8420LU; UNII-9G34HU7RV0* [edetic acid]. *CAS-64-02-8; CAS-60-00-4* [edetic acid]. *Chelating agent.*

---

† Brand name formerly used, and/or firm no longer concerned with this product.

Edetate Trisodium [*1966*] (e' de tate trye soe' dee um). $C_{10}H_{13}N_2Na_3O_8$. 358.19. (1) Glycine, *N,N'*-1,2-ethanediyl-bis[*N*-carboxymethyl-, trisodium salt; (2) Trisodium hydrogen(ethylenedinitrilo)tetraacetate; (3) Trisodium hydrogen ethylenediaminetetraacetate. *UNII-420IP921MB; UNII-9G34HU7RV0* [edetic acid]. *CAS-150-38-9; CAS-60-00-4* [edetic acid]. *Chelating agent.*

Edetic Acid (e det' ik as' id). **NF**. $C_{10}H_{16}N_2O_8$. 292.24. (1) Glycine, *N,N'*-1,2-ethanediylbis[*N*-(carboxymethyl)-; (2) (Ethylenedinitrilo)tetraacetic acid. *UNII-9G34HU7RV0. CAS-60-00-4*. INN; BAN. *Pharmaceutic aid (chelating agent)*. Versene Acid (Dow Chemical)

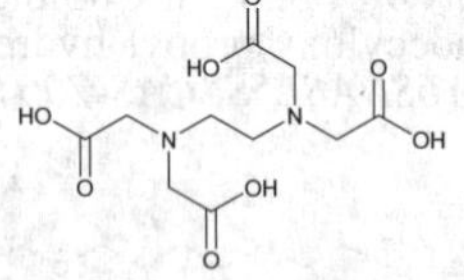

Edetol [*1983*] (e de tol'). $C_{14}H_{32}N_2O_4$. 292.41. (1) 2-Propanol, 1,1',1'',1'''-(1,2-ethanediyldinitrilo)tetrakis-; (2) 1,1',1'',1'''-(Ethylenedinitrilo)tetra-2-propanol. *UNII-Q4R969U9FR. CAS-102-60-3*. INN. *Pharmaceutic aid (alkalizing agent)*. Neutrol TE (BASF); Quadrol (BASF)

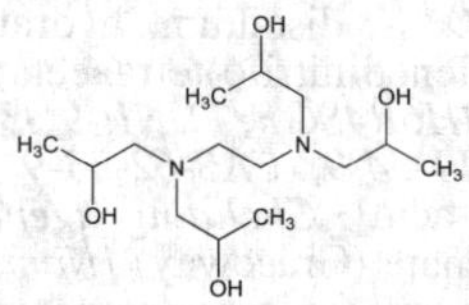

Edifoligide Sodium [*2003*] (e dif'' oh lig' ide soe' dee um). $C_{272}H_{318}N_{106}Na_{26}O_{138}P_{26}S_{26}$. 9516.80. [Edifoligide is INN.] (1) DNA, d(*P*-thio)(C-T-A-G-A-T-T-T-C-C-C-G-C-G), complex with DNA d(*P*-thio)(G-A-T-C-C-G-C-G-G-G-A-A-A-T) (1:1) hexacosodium salt; (2) 2'-Deoxy-*P*-thiocytidylyl-(3'→5')-*P*-thiothymidylyl-(3'→5')-2'-deoxy-*P*-thioadenylyl-(3'→5')-2'-deoxy-*P*-thioguanylyl-(3'→5')-2'-deoxy-*P*-thioadenylyl-(3'→5')-*P*-thiothymidylyl-(3'→5')-*P*-thiothymidylyl-(3'→5')-*P*-thiothymidylyl-(3'→5')-2'-deoxy-*P*-thiocytidylyl-(3'→5')-2'-deoxy-*P*-thiocytidylyl-(3'→5')-2'-deoxy-*P*-thiocytidylyl-(3'→5')-2'-deoxy-*P*-thioguanylyl-(3'→5')-2'-deoxy-*P*-thiocytidylyl-(3'→5')-2'-deoxy-*P*-thioguanine, complex with 2'-deoxy-*P*-thioguanylyl-(3'→5')-2'-deoxy-*P*-thioadenylyl-(3'→5')-*P*-thiothymidylyl-(3'→5')-2'-deoxy-*P*-thiocytidylyl-(3'→5')-2'-deoxy-*P*-thiocytidylyl-(3'→5')-2'-deoxy-*P*-thioguanylyl-(3'→5')-2'-deoxy-*P*-thiocytidylyl-(3'→5')-2'-deoxy-*P*-thioguanylyl-(3'→5')-2'-deoxy-*P*-thioguanylyl-(3'→5')-2'-deoxy-*P*-thioguanylyl-(3'→5')-2'-deoxy-*P*-thioadenylyl-(3'→5')-2'-deoxy-*P*-thioadenylyl-(3'→5')-*P*-thiothymidine, hexacosasodium salt. *CAS-328538-04-1* [for the base substance]. *Treatment autogenous vein grafts to prevent graft failure (oligonucleotide used with a pressure mediated device for ex vivo delivery to vein grafts).[Note—The trivial name, E2F Duplex Decoy, has appeared in literature.]* ◇*CGT003*

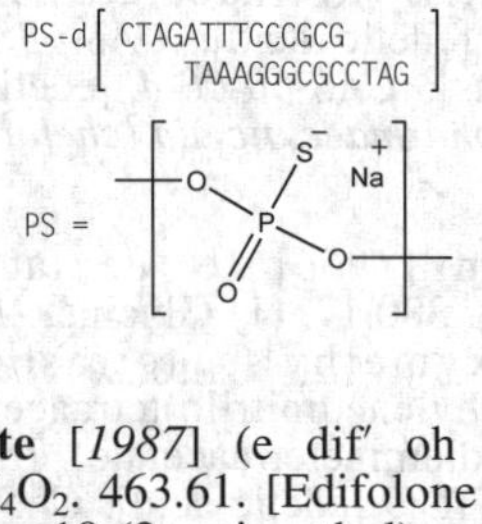

Edifolone Acetate [*1987*] (e dif' oh lone as' e tate). $C_{24}H_{37}NO_4.C_2H_4O_2$. 463.61. [Edifolone is INN.] (1) Estr-5-ene-3,17-dione, 10-(2-aminoethyl)-, cyclic bis(1,2-etha-

nediyl acetal), acetate; (2) 10-(2-Aminoethyl)estr-5-ene-3,17-dione, cyclic bis(ethylene acetal), acetate. *UNII-043L86G83X; UNII-4XE0U1P5FJ* [edifolone]. *CAS-90733-42-9; CAS-90733-40-7* [edifolone]. *Cardiac depressant (anti-arrhythmic).* ◇*SC-35135*

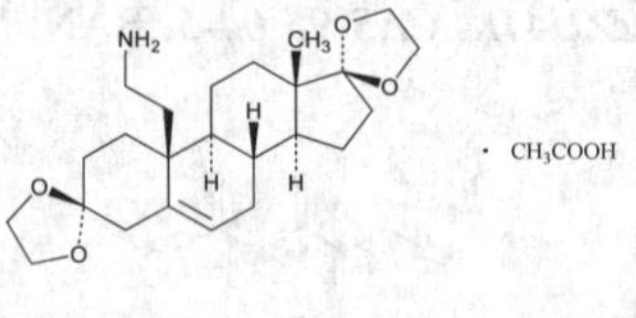

Edobacomab [*1993*] (e'' doe bak' oh mab). (1) Immunoglobulin M (mouse monoclonal XMMEN-OE5 anti-endotoxin), disulfide with mouse monoclonal XMMEN-OE5 light chain, pentameric dimer; (2) Immunoglobulin M (mouse monoclonal XMMEN-OE5 anti-endotoxin), disulfide with mouse monoclonal XMMEN-OE5 light chain, pentameric dimer. Molecular weight is approximately 1,000,000 daltons. *CAS-141410-98-2*. INN. *Monoclonal antibody (anti-endotoxin)*. E5 (Xoma)

Edodekin Alfa [*1998*] (e'' doe dek' in al' fa). Interleukin 12 (human). Molecular weight for glycosylated protein is 70,000-75,000 daltons. *CAS-187348-17-0*. INN. *Antiasthmatic.* ◇*Ro 24-7472/000*

40 kDa subunit of rHuIL-12

```
IWELKKDVYV VELDWYPDAP GEMVVLTCDT PEEDGITWTL DQSSEVLGSG
KTLTIQVKEF GDAGQYTCHK GGEVLSHSLL LLHKKEDGIW STDILKDQKE
PKNKTFLRCE AKNYSGRFTC WWLTTISTDL TFSVKSSRGS SDPQGVTCGA
ATLSAERVRG DNKEYEYSVE CQEDSACPAA EESLPIEVMV DAVHKLKYEN
YTSSFFIRDI IKPDPPKNLQ LKPLKNSRQV EVSWEYPDTW YTSSFFIRDI
IKPDPPKNLQ LKPLKNSRQV EVSWEYPDTW STPHSYFSLT FCVQVQGKSK
REKKDRVFTD KTSATVICRK NASISVRAQD RYYSSSWSEW ASVPCS
```

35 kDa subunit of rHuIL-12

```
RNLPVATPDP GMFPCLHHSQ NLLRAVSNML QKARQTLEFY PCTSEEIDHE
DITKDKTSTV EACLPLELTK NESCLNSRET SFITNGSCLA SRKTSFMMAL
CLSSIYEDLK MYQVEFKTMN AKLLMDPKRQ IFLDQNMLAV IDELMQALNF
NSETVPQKSS LEEPDFYKTK IKLCILLHAF RIRAVTIDRV TSYLNAS
```

Edogestrone. $C_{26}H_{38}O_5$. 430.58. 17-Hydroxy-6-methylpregn-5-ene-3,20-dione cyclic 3-(ethylene acetal) acetate. *UNII-9014UFK50C. CAS-809-01-8*. INN; BAN. ◇*PH 218*

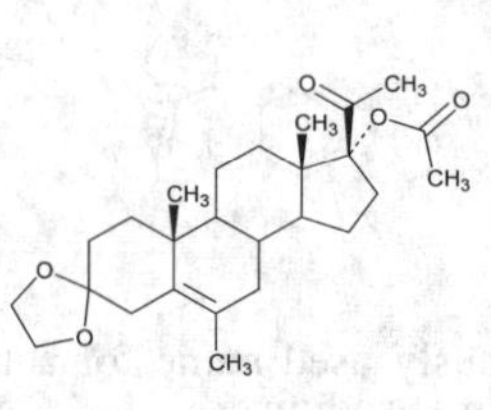

Edonentan [*2002*] (e don' en tan). $C_{28}H_{32}N_4O_5S.H_2O$. 554.66. (1) Butanamide, *N*-[[2'-[[(4,5-dimethyl-3-isoxazolyl) amino]sulfonyl]-4-(2-oxazolyl) [1,1'-biphenyl]-2-yl]methyl]-*N*,3,3-trimethyl-, monohydrate; (2) *N*-[2-[2-[(4,5-Dimethylisoxazol-3-yl)sulfamoyl]phenyl]-5-(oxazol-2-yl)benzyl]-*N*,3,3-trimethylbutanamide, monohydrate. *UNII-2CCC8CH216; UNII-S5016F5ZH4* [edonentan anhydrous]. *CAS-264609-13-4; CAS-210891-04-6* [anhydrous]. INN. *Treatment of heart failure (endothelin A(ET$_A$) inhibitor).* ◇*BMS-207940-02*

Edotecarin [*2005*] (e″ doe tek′ ar in). $C_{29}H_{28}N_4O_{11}$. 608.55. (1) 5*H*-Indolo[2,3-*a*]pyrrolo[3,4-*c*]carbazole-5,7(6*H*)-dione,12-β-D-glucopyranosyl-12,13-dihydro-2,10-dihydroxy-6-[[2-hydroxy-1-(hydroxymethyl)ethyl]amino]-; (2) 12-β-D-Glucopyranosyl-2,10-dihydroxy-6-[[2-hydroxy-1-(hydroxymethyl)ethyl]amino]-12,13-dihydro-6*H*-indolo[2,3-*a*]pyrrolo[3,4-*c*]carbazole-5,7-dione. *UNII-1V8X590XDP. CAS-174402-32-5.* INN. *Treatment of cancer.* ◇*PF-804950*

Edotreotide [*2002*] (e″ doe tree′ oh tide). $C_{65}H_{92}N_{14}O_{18}S_2$. 1421.64. (1) L-Cysteinamide, *N*-[[4,7,10-tris(carboxymethyl)-1,4,7,10-tetraazacyclodec-1-yl]acetyl]-D-phenylalanyl-L-cysteinyl-L-tyrosyl-D-tryptophyl-L-lysyl-L-threonyl-*N*-[(1*R*,2*R*)-2-hydroxy-1-(hydroxymethyl)propyl]-, cyclic(2→7)-disulfide; (2) *N*-[[4,7,10-Tris(carboxymethyl)-1,4,7,10-tetraazacycoldodec-1-yl]acetyl-D-phenylalanyl-L-cysteinyl-L-tyrosyl-D-tryprophyl-L-lysyl-L-threonyl-*N*-[(1*R*,2*R*)-2-hydroxy-1-(hydroxymethyl)propyl]-L-cysteinamide cyclic (2→7)-disulfide. *CAS-204318-14-9.* INN. *Diagnosis and staging of tumors expressing somatostatin receptors.* ◇*SMT 487*

Edoxaban. $C_{24}H_{30}ClN_7O_4S$. 548.06. *N*-(5-Chloropyridin-2-yl)-*N'*-[(1*S*,2*R*,4*S*)-4-(*N*,*N*-dimethylcarbamoyl)-2-(5-methyl-4,5,6,7-tetrahydro[1,3]thiazolo[5,4-*c*]pyridine-2-carboxamido)cyclohexyl]oxamide. *CAS-480449-70-5.* INN.

---

† Brand name formerly used, and/or firm no longer concerned with this product.

Edoxudine [*1984*] (e dox′ ue deen). $C_{11}H_{16}N_2O_5$. 256.26. (1) Uridine, 2′-deoxy-5-ethyl-; (2) 2′-Deoxy-5-ethyluridine. *CAS-15176-29-1.* INN. *Antiviral.* ◇*EDU; EUDR; ORF 15817; RWJ 15817*

Edratide [*2004*] (e′ dra tide). $C_{111}H_{149}N_{27}O_{28}$. 2309.53. L-Glycyl-L-tyrosyl- L-tyrosyl- L-tryptophyl-L-seryl-L-tryptophyl-L-isoleucyl-L-arginyl-L-glutaminyl-L-prolyl-L-prolyl-L-glycyl-L-lysyl-L-glycyl-L-glutamyl-L-glutamyl-L-tryptophyl-L-isoleucyl-L-glycine. *UNII-38PLP07BKC. CAS-433922-67-9.* INN; BAN. *Treatment of systemic lupus erythematosus.* ◇*TV-4710*

GYYWSWIRQP PGKGEEWIG

Edrecolomab [*1996*] (e″ dre kol′ oh mab). (1) Immunoglobulin G 2a (mouse monoclonal 17-1A γ-chain anti-human colon cancer tumor-associated antigen), disulfide with mouse monoclonal 17-1A light chain, dimer; (2) Immunoglobulin G 2a (mouse monoclonal 17-1A γ-chain anti-human colon cancer tumor-associated antigen), disulfide with mouse monoclonal 17-1A light chain, dimer. Molecular weight is approximately 148,000 daltons. *CAS-156586-89-9.* INN. *Monoclonal antibody (antineoplastic adjuvant).* Panorex (Centocor) ◇*C-1*

Edronocaine. $C_{15}H_{25}NO_2$. 251.36. *N*,1-Dimethyl-2′-(*m*-propoxyphenoxy)diethylamine. *UNII-6HWO3IJ4U9. CAS-190258-12-9.* INN.

Edrophone Chloride — *See* Edrophonium Chloride.

Edrophonium Chloride (e″ droe foe′ nee um klor′ ide). **USP**. $C_{10}H_{16}ClNO$. 201.69. (1) Benzenaminium, *N*-ethyl-3-hydroxy-*N*,*N*-dimethyl-, chloride; (2) Ethyl(*m*-hydroxyphenyl)dimethylammonium chloride. *UNII-QO611KSM5P. CAS-116-38-1; CAS-312-48-1* [edrophonium]. INN; BAN; JAN. *Antidote (to curare principles); diagnostic aid (myasthenia gravis).* Enlon (Baxter Healthcare); Tensilon (Valeant)

EDTA — *See* Edetic Acid.

EDTA Calcium — *See* Edetate Calcium Disodium.

Efalizumab [*2001*] (ef″ a liz′ oo mab). (1) Immunoglobulin G1, anti-(human CD11a (antigen) (human-mouse monoclonal hu1124 γ1-chain), disulfide with human-mouse monoclonal hu1124 light chain, dimer; (2) Immunoglobulin G 1 (human-mouse monoclonal hu1124 γ1-chain anti-human antigen CD 11a), disulfide with human-mouse monoclonal hu1124 light chain, dimer. Molecular weight is approximately 146,170 daltons. *UNII-XX2MN88N5D. CAS-214745-43-4.* INN. *Treatment of transplant rejections; antipsoriatic (immunomodulator monoclonal antibody which decreases the activation, migration, and adhesion of T-cells).* ◇*hu1124; anti-CD11a*

Efaproxiral [*2002*] (ef″ a prox′ ir al). $C_{20}H_{23}HO_4$. 328.40. (1) Propanoic acid, 2-[4-[2-[(3,5-dimethylphenyl)amino]-2-oxoethyl]phenoxy]-2-methyl-; (2) 2-[4-[(3,5-Dimethylphenyl)amino]-2-oxoethyl]phenoxy]-2-methylpropanic acid. *UNII-J81E81G364. CAS-131179-95-8.* INN. *Enhancement of radiation therapy (synthetic allosteric modifier of hemoglobin).* ◇*RSR13*

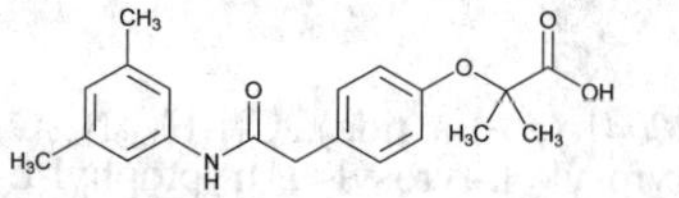

Efaproxiral Sodium [*2002*] (ef″ a prox′ ir al soe′ dee um). $C_{20}H_{22}NNaO_4$. 363.38. (1) Propanoic acid, 2-[4-[2-[(3,5-dimethylphenyl)amino]-2-oxoethyl]phenoxy]-2-methyl-, monosodium salt; (2) 2-[4-[2-[(3,5-Dimethylphenyl) amino]-2-oxoethyl]phenoxy]-2-methylpropanoic acid monosodium salt; (3) 2-[4((((3,5-Dimethylphenyl)amino) carbonyl)methyl)-phenoxy]-2-methyl propionic acid. *UNII-3L83QP52XI. CAS-170787-99-2. Treatment of clinical conditions characterized by tissue hypoxia including cardiovascular, surgical, and critical care conditions; adjunctive treatment in standard radiation therapy and chemotherapy (synthetic allosteric modifier of hemoglobin).* ◇*RSR13 sodium*

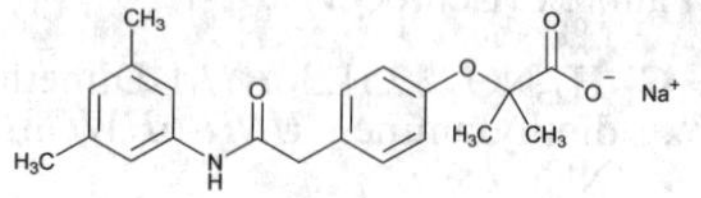

Efaroxan. $C_{13}H_{16}N_2O$. 216.28. (±)-2-(2-Ethyl-2,3-dihydro-2-benzofuranyl)-2-imidazoline. *UNII-G00490L21H. CAS-89197-32-0.* INN; BAN.

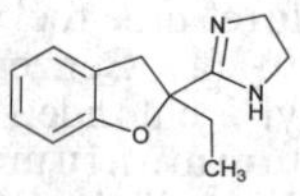

Efavirenz. $C_{14}H_9ClF_3NO_2$. 315.67. (*S*)-6-Chloro-4-(cyclopropylethynyl)-1,4-dihydro-4-(trifluoromethyl)-2*H*-3,1-benzoxazin-2-one. *UNII-JE6H2O27P8. CAS-154598-52-4.* INN; BAN. Sustiva (Bristol-Myers Squibb)

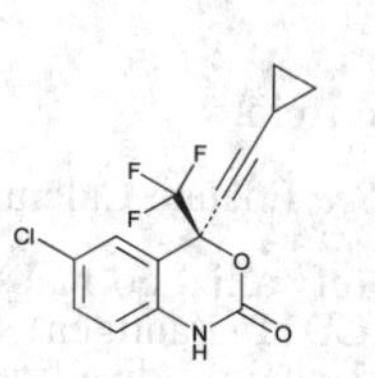

Efegatran Sulfate [*1994*] (ef″ e gat′ ran sul′ fate). $C_{21}H_{32}N_6O_3 \cdot H_2SO_4$. 514.60. [Efegatran is INN.] (1) L-Prolinamide, *N*-methyl-D-phenylalanyl-*N*-[4-[(aminoiminomethyl)amino]-1-formylbutyl]-, (*S*)-, sulfate (1:1); (2) *N*-Methyl-D-phenylalanyl-*N*-[(1*S*)-1-formyl-4-guanidinobutyl]-L-prolinamide sulfate (1:1). *UNII-VB4VCH77JV;*

UNII-VT0VK2474K [efegatran]. *CAS-126721-07-1; CAS-105806-65-3* [efegatran]. *Antithrombotic.* ◇*LY294468 sulfate*

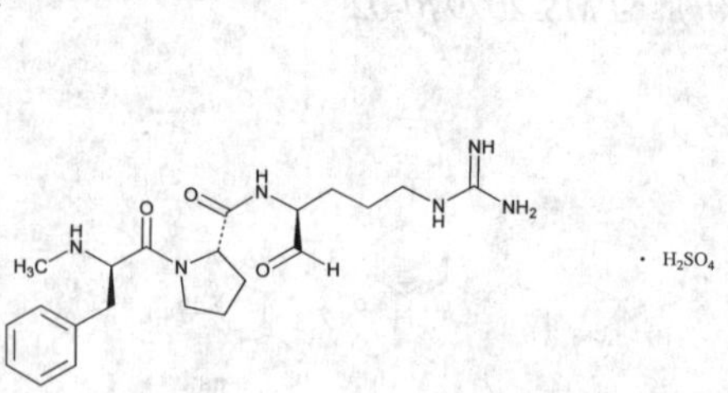

Efepristin. $C_{44}H_{52}N_8O_{10}$. 852.93. *N*-[(6*R*,9*S*,10*R*,13*S*,15a*S*, 22*S*,24a*S*)-6-Ethyldocosahydro-10,23-dimethyl-22-[*p*-(methylamino)benzyl]-5,8,12,15,17,21,24-heptaoxo-13-phenyl-12*H*-pyrido[2,1-*f*]pyrrolo[2,1-*l*][1,4,7,10,13,16]-oxapentaazacyclononadecin-9-yl]-3-hydroxypicolinamide. *CAS-57206-54-9.* INN.

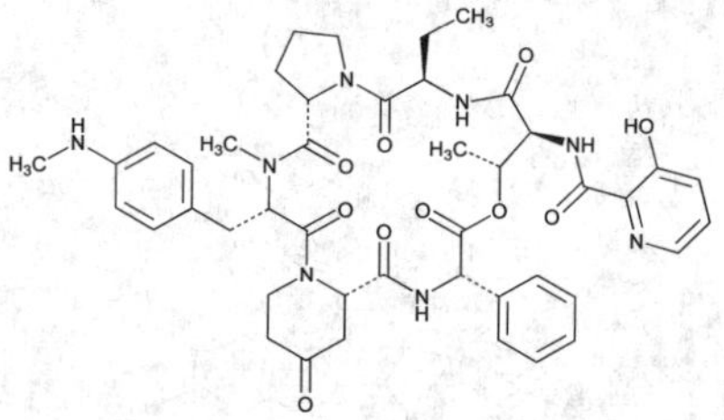

Efetozole. $C_{12}H_{14}N_2$. 186.25. (±)-2-Methyl-1-(α-methylbenzyl)imidazole. *UNII-MPI4B0COZ7. CAS-99500-54-6.* INN.

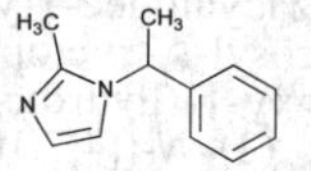

Efipladib [*2004*] (ef ip′ la dib). $C_{40}H_{35}Cl_3N_2O_4S$. 746.14. (1) Benzoic acid, 4-[3-[5-chloro-2-[2-[[[(3,4-dichlorophenyl)-methyl]sulfonyl]amino]ethyl]-1-(diphenylmethyl)-1*H*-indol-3-yl]propyl]-; (2) 4-[3-[5-Chloro-2-[2-[[(3,4-dichlorobenzyl)sulfonyl]amino]ethyl]-1-(diphenylmethyl)-1*H*-indol-3-yl]propyl]benzoic acid. *UNII-S97YUG2A91. CAS-381683-94-9.* INN. *Treatment of pain and symptomatic management of arthritis.* (Wyeth) ◇*PLA-902*

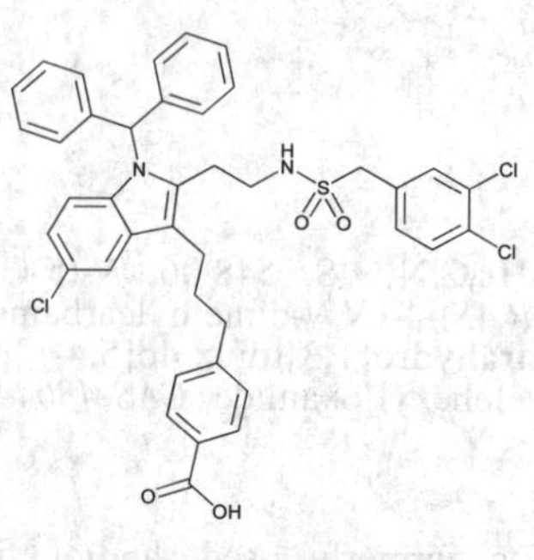

Efletirizine. $C_{21}H_{24}F_2N_2O_3$. 390.42. [2-[4-[Bis(*p*-fluorophenyl)methyl]-1-piperazinyl]ethoxy]acetic acid. *UNII-B6C301298G. CAS-150756-35-7.* INN.

Efletirizine Dihydrochloride [*2002*] (ef″ le tir′ i zeen dye hye″ droe klor′ ide). $C_{21}H_{24}F_2N_2O_3\cdot2HCl$. 463.35. (1) Acetic acid, [2-[4-[bis(4-fluorophenyl)methyl]-1-piperazinyl]ethoxy]-, dihydrochloride; (2) [2-[4-Bis(*p*-fluorophenyl)methyl)-1-piperazinyl]ethoxy]acetic acid, dihydrochloride. *UNII-JQ7ZT5MRA0. CAS-225367-66-8. Antihistaminic.* ◇*ucb 28754*

Eflornithine Hydrochloride [*1986*] (ef lor′ ni theen hye″ droe klor′ ide). $C_6H_{12}F_2N_2O_2\cdot HCl\cdot H_2O$. 236.64. [Eflornithine is INN and BAN.] (1) DL-Ornithine, 2-(difluoromethyl)-, monohydrochloride, monohydrate; (2) 2-(Difluoromethyl)-DL-ornithine monohydrochloride, monohydrate. *UNII-4NH22NDW9H; UNII-ZQN1G5V6SR* [eflornithine]. *CAS-96020-91-6; CAS-67037-37-0* [eflornithine]. *Antineoplastic; antiprotozoal.* Ornidyl (Sanofi Aventis); Vaniqa (Skinmedica) ◇*MDL 71,782 A*

Efloxate. $C_{19}H_{16}O_5$. 324.33. Ethyl-[(4-oxo-2-phenyl-4*H*-1-benzopyran-7-yl)oxy] acetate. *UNII-CZU6V3902K. CAS-119-41-5.* INN; JAN; MI.

Eflucimibe. $C_{29}H_{43}NO_2S$. 469.72. (*S*)-2-(Dodecylthio)-4′-hydroxy-2′,3′,5′-trimethyl-2-phenylacetanilide. *UNII-3DK1X2C37M. CAS-202340-45-2.* INN.

Eflumast. $C_{10}H_8FN_5O_3$. 265.20. 3′-Acetyl-5′-fluoro-2′-hydroxy-1*H*-tetrazole-5-carboxanilide. *UNII-3CIG2V70UB. CAS-70977-46-7.* INN.

Efonidipine. $C_{34}H_{38}N_3O_7P$. 631.66. [Efonidipine Hydrochloride is JAN.] 2-(*N*-Benzylanilino)ethyl (±)-1,4-dihydro-2,6-dimethyl-4-(*m*-nitrophenyl)-5-phosphononicotinate, cyclic 2,2-dimethyltrimethylene ester. *UNII-40ZTP2T37Q; UNII-3BR983K69O* [efonidipine hydrochloride]. *CAS-111011-63-3; CAS-111011-76-8* [hydrochloride]. INN.

Eformoterol (previously used name) — *See* Formoterol Fumarate.

Efrotomycin [*1985*] (ef″ roe toe mye′ sin). $C_{59}H_{88}N_2O_{20}$. 1145.33. (1) Mocimycin, 31-*O*-[6-deoxy-4-*O*-(6-deoxy-2,4-di-*O*-methyl-α-L-mannopyranosyl)-3-*O*-methyl-β-D-allopyranosyl]-1-methyl-; (2) (α*S*,2*R*,3*R*,4*R*,6*S*)-4-[[6-Deoxy-4-*O*-(6-deoxy-2,4-di-*O*-methyl-α-L-mannopyranosyl)-3-*O*-methyl-β-D-allopyranosyl]oxy]-*N*-[(2*E*,4*E*,6*S*,7*R*)-7-[(2*S*,3*S*,4*R*,5*R*)-5-[(1*E*,3*E*,5*E*)-6-(1,2-dihydro-4-hydroxy-1-methyl-2-oxonicotinoyl)-1,3,5-heptatrienyl]tetrahydro-3,4-dihydroxy-2-furyl]-6-methoxy-5-methyl-2,4-octadienyl]-α-ethyltetrahydro-2,3-dihydroxy-5,5-dimethyl-6-[(1*E*,3*Z*)-1,3-pentadienyl]-2*H*-pyran-2-acetamide. *CAS-56592-32-6.* INN; BAN. *Growth stimulant (veterinary).* Producil [Veterinary] (Merial) ◇*MK-621*

Efungumab [*2008*] (ef un′ gue mab). (1) Immunoglobulin, anti-(Candida heat-shock protein HSP 90) (human monoclonal HSP90mab fragment); (2) Immunoglobulin scFv fragment, anti-(heat shock protein 90 homolog from *Candida albicans* (yeast)), methionylalanyl-[human monoclonal HSP90mab VH domain (120 residues)]-tris[(tetra-

---

† Brand name formerly used, and/or firm no longer concerned with this product.

glycyl)seryl]-[human monoclonal HSP90mab V-KAPPA domain (107 residues)]-[arginyl-trialanyl-leucyl-glutamyl]-hexahistidine *immunomodulator*. Molecular weight is approximately 27,200 daltons. *CAS-762260-74-2*. INN. *Treatment of C. albicans infection.* Mycograb (Novartis) ◇*MYC123; MYC123A; MYC123B; MYC124; HSP90MAB*

Eganoprost. $C_{21}H_{34}O_6$. 382.49. Methyl (Z)-7-[(1R,2R,3R)-2-[(1E,3S,7R)-3,7-dihydroxy-1-octenyl]-3-hydroxy-5-oxocyclopentyl]-5-heptenoate. *UNII-KXG0PR9DIH. CAS-63266-93-3*. INN.

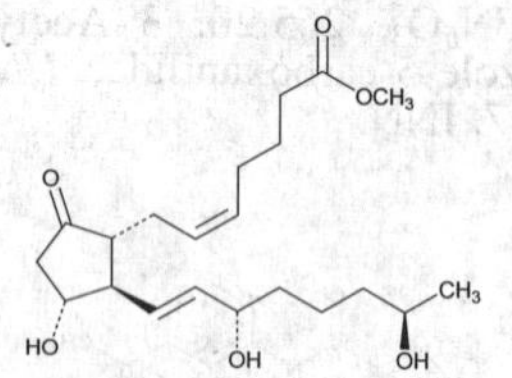

Eglumetad [*2004*] (e gloo′ me tad). $C_8H_{11}NO_4$. 185.18. (1) Bicyclo[3.1.0]hexane-2,6-dicarboxylic acid, 2-amino-, (1S,2S,5R,6S)-; (2) (+)-(1S,2S,5R,6S)-2-Aminobicyclo[3.1.0]hexane-2,6-dicarboxylic acid. *UNII-ONU5A67T2S. CAS-209216-09-1; CAS-176199-48-7* [anhydrous]. INN. *Treatment of general anxiety disorders and smoking cessation (metabotropic glutamate agonist).[- Name previously used: Eglumegad.]* ◇*LY354740*

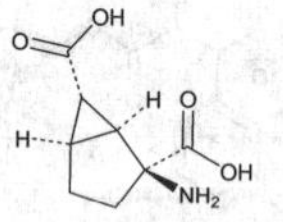

Egtazic Acid [*1983*] (eg tayz′ ik as′ id). $C_{14}H_{24}N_2O_{10}$. 380.35. (1) 6,9-Dioxa-3,12-diazatetradecanedioic acid, 3,12-bis (carboxymethyl)-; (2) [Ethylenebis(oxyethylenenitrilo)] tetraacetic acid. *UNII-526U7A2651. CAS-67-42-5*. INN. *Pharmaceutic aid.* ◇*EGTA*

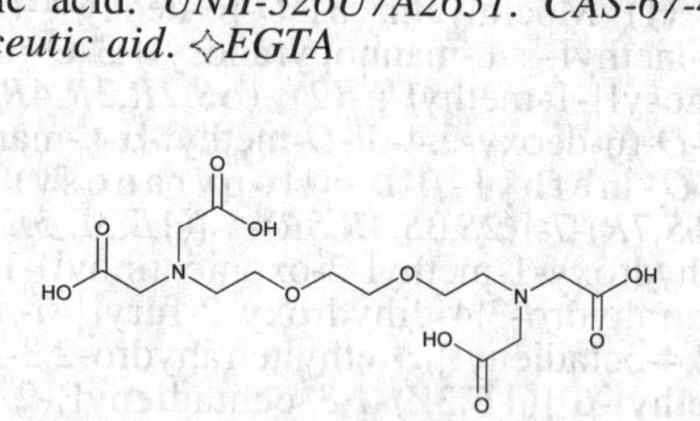

Egualen. $C_{15}H_{18}O_3S$. 278.37. 3-Ethyl-7-isopropyl-1-azulenesulfonic acid. *UNII-17VM9WN49U. CAS-99287-30-6*. INN.

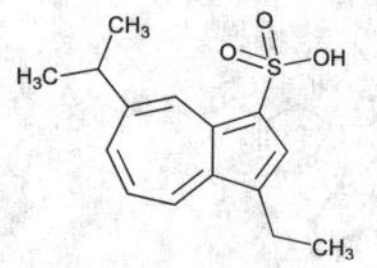

Elacridar Hydrochloride [*1997*] (el ak′ ri dar hye″ droe klor′ ide). $C_{34}H_{33}N_3O_5$.HCl. 600.10. [Elacridar is INN.] (1) 4-Acridinecarboxamide, N-[4-(2-(3,4-dihydro-6,7-dimethoxy-2(1H)-isoquinolinyl)ethyl]phenyl]-9,10-dihydro-5-methoxy-9-oxo-, monohydrochloride; (2) 4′-[2-(3,4-dihydro-6,7-dimethoxy-2(1H)-isoquinolyl)ethyl]-5-methoxy-9-oxo-4-acridancarboxanilide monohydrochloride.

UNII-NX2BHH1A5B; UNII-N488540F94 [elacridar]. *CAS-143851-98-3; CAS-143664-11-3* [elacridar]. *Antineoplastic (adjunct).* ◇*GF 120918A*

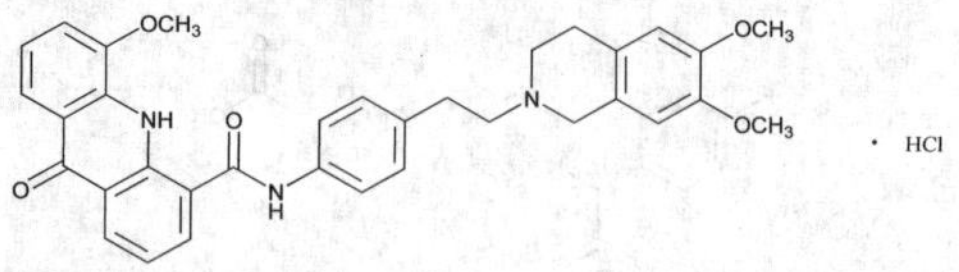

Elacytarabine. $C_{27}H_{45}N_3O_6$. 507.66. 4-Amino-1-{5-O-[(9E)-octadec-9-enoyl]-β-D-arabinofuranosyl}pyrimidin-2(1H)-one. *CAS-188181-42-2*. INN.

Elagolix [*2008*] (el″ a goe′ lix). $C_{32}H_{30}F_5N_3O_5$. 631.59. (1) Butanoic acid, 4-[[(1R)-2-[5-(2-fluoro-3-methoxyphenyl)-3-[[2-fluoro-6-(trifluoromethyl)phenyl]methyl]-3,6-dihydro-4-methyl-2,6-dioxo-1(2H)-pyrimidinyl]-1-phenylethyl]amino]-; (2) 4-{[[(1R)-2-(5-(2-Fluoro-3-methoxyphenyl)-3-{[2-fluoro-6-(trifluoromethyl)phenyl]methyl}-4-methyl-2,6-dioxo-3,6-dihydropyrimidin-1(2H)-yl]-1-phenylethyl]amino}butanoic acid. *UNII-5B2546MB5Z. CAS-834153-87-6*. INN. *Treatment of hormone-dependent diseases such as endometriosis, uterine fibroids, prostate cancer, and benign prostatic hyperplasia.* ◇*NBI-56418*

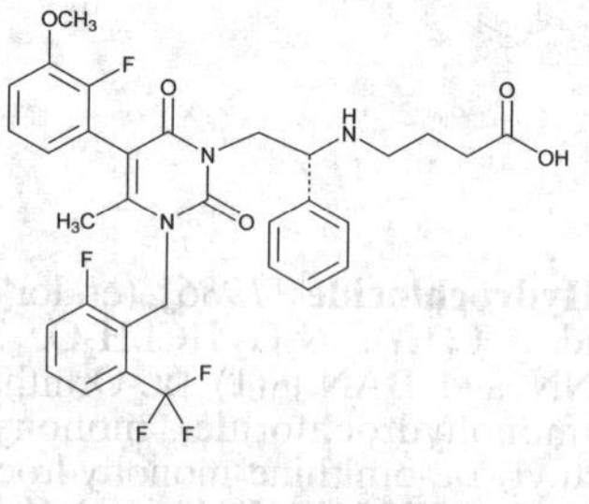

Elagolix Sodium [*2008*] (el″ a goe′ lix soe′ dee um). $C_{32}H_{29}F_5N_3NaO_5$. 653.57. (1) Butanoic acid, 4-[[(1R)-2-[5-(2-fluoro-3-methoxyphenyl)-3-[[2-fluoro-6-(trifluoromethyl)phenyl]methyl]-3,6-dihydro-4-methyl-2,6-dioxo-1(2H)-pyrimidinyl]-1-phenylethyl]amino]-, monosodium salt; (2) Sodium 4-}[(1R)-2-(5-(2-fluoro-3-methoxyphenyl)-3-{[2-fluoro-6-(trifluoromethyl)phenyl]methyl}-4-methyl-2,6-dioxo-3,6-dihydropyrimidin-1(2H)-yl)-1-phenylethyl]amino}butanoate. *UNII-5948VUI423. CAS-832720-36-2. Management of hormone-dependent diseases such as endometriosis, uterine fibroids, prostate cancer, and benign prostatic hyperplasia.* ◇*NBI-56418 Na*

Elantrine [*1972*] (el′ an treen). $C_{20}H_{24}N_2$. 292.42. (1) 1-Propanamine, 3-(5,6-dihydro-5-methyl-11H-dibenz[b,e]azepin-11-ylidene-N,N-dimethyl-; (2) 11-[3-(Dimethylamino)propylidene]-5,6-dihydro-5-methylmorphanthridine. *UNII-MV4FO7V23V. CAS-1232-85-5*. INN. *Anticholinergic.* ◇*EX 10-029-C; RMI 80,029*

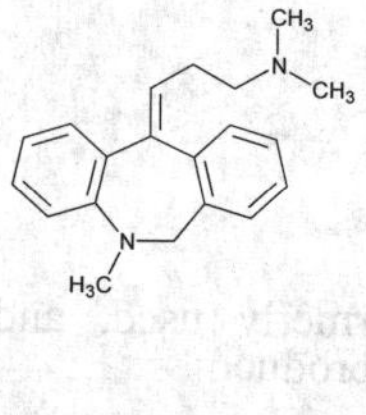

Elanzepine. $C_{19}H_{21}ClN_2$. 312.84. 3-Chloro-11-[3-(dimethylamino)propylidene]-5,6-dihydromorphanthridine. *UNII-95J02IOS74. CAS-6196-08-3.* INN.

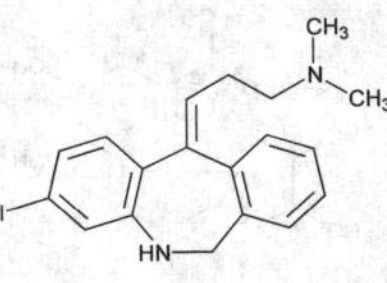

Elarofiban [*1999*] (el ar″ oh fye′ ban). $C_{22}H_{32}N_4O_4.H_2O$. 434.53. (1) 3-Pyridinepropanoic acid, *β*-[[[1-[1-oxo-3-(4-piperidinyl)propyl]-3-piperidinyl]carbonyl]amino]-, [*S*-(*R**,*S**)]-, monohydrate; (2) (*S*)-*β*-[(*R*)-1-[3-(4-Piperidyl)propionyl]nipecotamido]-3-pyridinepropionic acid, monohydrate. *UNII-6Y891C0JEV. CAS-221005-96-5; CAS-198958-88-2* [anhydrous]. INN. *Treatment of thrombotic disorders (platelet fibrinogen receptor [GPIIb/IIIa] antagonist). ✧RWJ-53308*

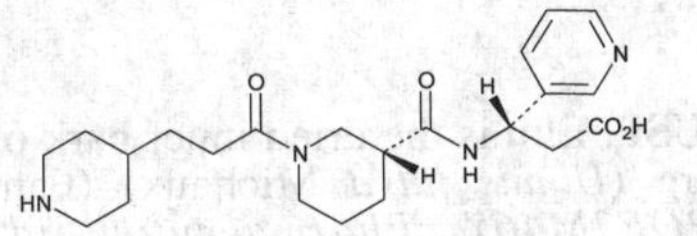

Elastase. Protease obtained from dried porcine pancreas. *CAS-9004-06-2.* JAN.

Elastofilcon A [*1980*] (e las″ toe fil′ kon). C_4H_9Si-$(C_2H_6OSi)_a(C_{12}H_{10}OSi)_b(C_3H_6OSi)_c$-$OSiC_4H_9$. (1) Elastofilcon A; (2) *α*-(Dimethylvinylsilyl)-*ω*-[(dimethylvinylsilyl)oxy]poly(dimethyldiphenyl methylvinyl siloxane). *Contact lens material (hydrophilic).* Silsoft Aphakic (Bausch & Lomb); Silsoft Super Plus (Bausch & Lomb); Sil-Tech (Bausch & Lomb†)

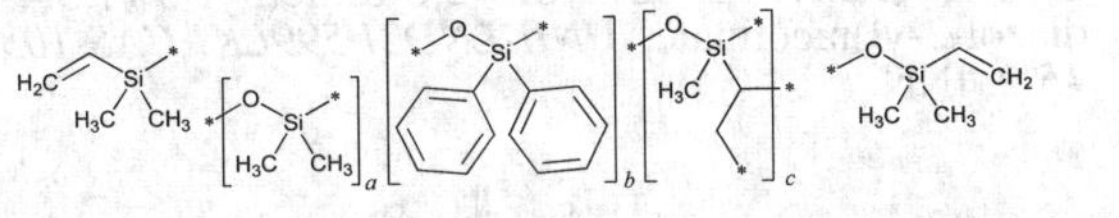

Elbanizine. $C_{26}H_{31}N_5O_2$. 445.56. 1-[2-[(2,6-Dimethyl-3-nitro-4-pyridyl)amino]ethyl]-4-(diphenylmethyl)piperazine. *UNII-S39YD087F9. CAS-110629-41-9.* INN.

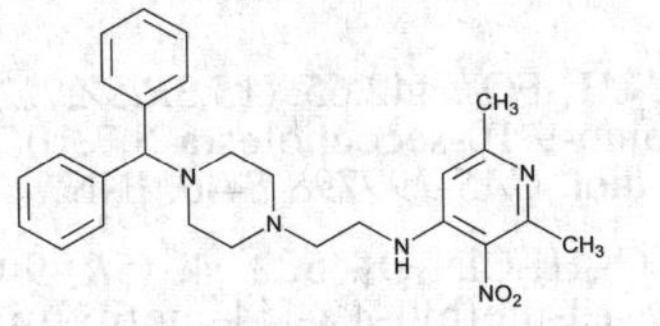

Elcatonin. $C_{148}H_{244}N_{42}O_{47}$. 3363.77. 1-Butyric acid-7-(L-2-aminobutyric acid)-26-L-aspartic acid-27-L-valine-29-L-alaninecalcitonin (salmon). *CAS-60731-46-6.* INN; JAN; MI.

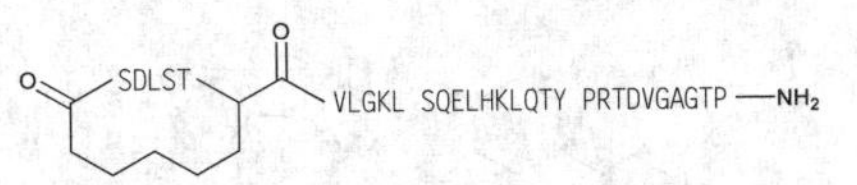

† Brand name formerly used, and/or firm no longer concerned with this product.

Eldacimibe [*1996*] (el da′ si mibe). $C_{39}H_{58}N_2O_5$. 634.89. (1) 1,3-Dioxane-4,6-dione, 5-[[[3,5-bis(1,1-dimethylethyl)-4-hydroxyphenyl]amino][[[4-(2,2-dimethylpropyl)phenyl]methyl]hexylamino]methylene]-2,2-dimethyl-; (2) Cyclic isopropylidene [(3,5-di-*tert*-butyl-4-hydroxyanilino)[hexyl(*p*-neopentylbenzyl)amino]methylene]malonate. *CAS-141993-70-6.* INN. *Antihyperlipidemic. ✧WAY-ACA-147*

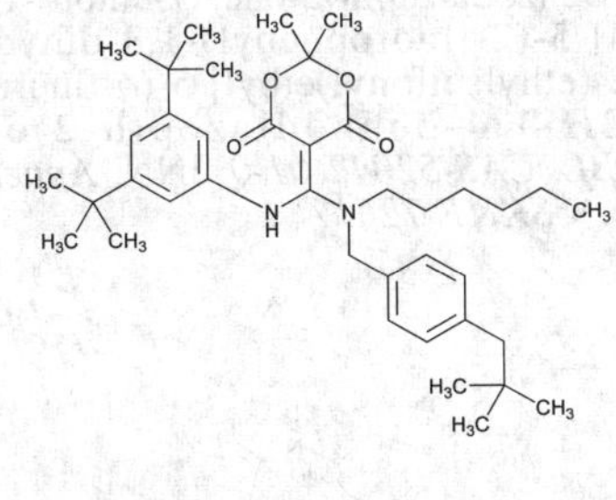

Eldecalcitol. $C_{30}H_{50}O_5$. 490.72. (5*Z*,7*E*)-2*β*-(3-Hydroxypropoxy)-9,10-secocholesta-5,7,10(19)-triene-1*α*,3*β*,25-triol. *CAS-104121-92-8.* INN.

Eldexomer. Microspheres produced by reaction of partially hydrolysed starch with epichlorhydrin, slowly degradable by amylase (with a half-life of more than 120 minutes). INN.

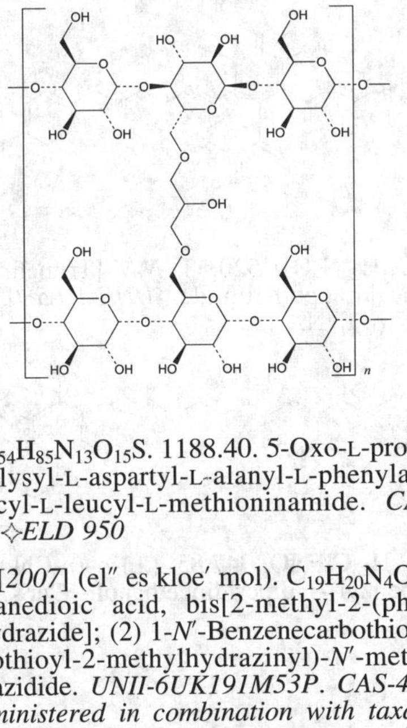

Eledoisin. $C_{54}H_{85}N_{13}O_{15}S$. 1188.40. 5-Oxo-L-prolyl-L-prolyl-L-seryl-L-lysyl-L-aspartyl-L-alanyl-L-phenylalanyl-L-isoleucylglycyl-L-leucyl-L-methioninamide. *CAS-69-25-0.* INN; MI. *✧ELD 950*

Elesclomol [*2007*] (el″ es kloe′ mol). $C_{19}H_{20}N_4O_2S_2$. 400.52. (1) Propanedioic acid, bis[2-methyl-2-(phenylthioxomethyl)hydrazide]; (2) 1-*N*′-Benzenecarbothioyl-3-(2-benzenecarbothioyl-2-methylhydrazinyl)-*N*′-methyl-oxopropanehydrazidide. *UNII-6UK191M53P. CAS-488832-69-5.* INN. *Administered in combination with taxanes for the treatment of solid-tumor cancer, non-small cell lung cancer, melanoma, sarcoma. ✧STA-4783*

Eletriptan. $C_{22}H_{26}N_2O_2S$. 382.52. 3-[[(*R*)-1-Methyl-2-pyrrolidinyl]methyl]-5-[2-(phenylsulfonyl)ethyl]indole. *UNII-22QOO9B8KI. CAS-143322-58-1.* INN; BAN. *✧UK-116,044; UK-116,044-04 [as hydrobromide]*

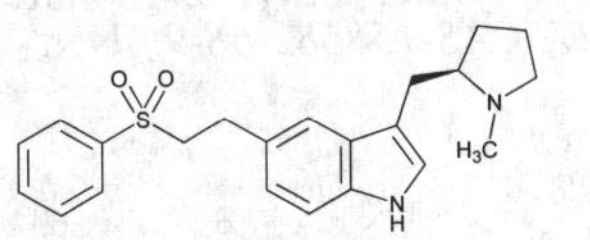

Eletriptan Hydrobromide [*1997*] (el″ e trip′ tan hye″ droe broe′ mide). $C_{22}H_{26}N_2O_2S.HBr$. 463.43. (1) (*R*)-3-[(1-Methyl-2-pyrrolidinyl)methyl]-5-[2-(phenylsulfonyl)ethyl]-1*H*-indole monohydrobromide; (2) 3-[[(*R*)-1-Methyl-2-pyrrolidinyl]methyl]-5-[2-(phenylsulfonyl)ethyl]indole, monohydrobromide. *UNII-M41W832TA3. CAS-177834-92-3. Antimigraine (5HT$_{1D}$-serotonin receptor agonist).* Relpax (Pfizer) ✧*UK-116,044-04*

Eleuthero. NF XXI.

Eleuthero, Powdered. NF XXI.

Elfazepam [*1976*] (el faz′ e pam). C$_{19}$H$_{18}$ClFN$_2$O$_3$S. 408.87. (1) *2H*-1,4-Benzodiazepin-2-one, 7-chloro-1-[2-(ethylsulfonyl)ethyl]-5-(2-fluorophenyl)-1,3-dihydro-; (2) 7-Chloro-1-[2-(ethylsulfonyl)ethyl]-5-(*o*-fluorophenyl)-1,3-dihydro-*2H*-1,4-benzodiazepin-2-one. *UNII-RM53R5R2BL. CAS-52042-01-0.* INN. *Appetite stimulant (veterinary).* ✧*SK&F 72517*

Elgodipine. C$_{29}$H$_{33}$FN$_2$O$_6$. 524.58. 2-[(*p*-Fluorobenzyl)methylamino]ethyl isopropyl (±)-1,4-dihydro-2,6-dimethyl-4-[2,3-(methylenedioxy)phenyl]-3,5-pyridinedicarboxylate. *UNII-3JI11Z5REF. CAS-119413-55-7.* INN.

Elinafide. C$_{31}$H$_{28}$N$_4$O$_4$. 520.58. *N,N′*-[Trimethylenebis(iminoethylene)]dinaphthalimide. *UNII-HL580335SI. CAS-162706-37-8.* INN.

Eliprodil. C$_{20}$H$_{23}$ClFNO. 347.85. (±)-α-(*p*-Chlorophenyl)-4-(*p*-fluorobenzyl)-1-piperidineethanol. *CAS-119431-25-3.* INN.

Elisartan. C$_{27}$H$_{29}$ClN$_6$O$_5$. 553.01. (±)-1-Hydroxyethyl 2-butyl-4-chloro-1-[*p*-(*o*-1*H*-tetrazol-5-ylphenyl)benzyl]imidazole-5-carboxylate, ethyl carbonate (ester). *UNII-WCC8Z95027. CAS-158682-68-9.* INN.

Ellagic Acid. C$_{14}$H$_6$O$_8$. 302.19. 2,3,7,8-Tetrahydroxy[1]benzopyrano[5,4,3-*cde*]-[1]benzopyran-5,10-dione. *UNII-19YRN3ZS9P. CAS-476-66-4.* INN; DCF; MI.

Elliptinium Acetate. C$_{20}$H$_{20}$N$_2$O$_3$. 336.38. 9-Hydroxy-2,5,11-trimethyl-6*H*-pyrido[4,3-*b*]carbazolium acetate. *CAS-58337-35-2.* INN; BAN; MI.

Elm (elm). **USP**. Elm is the dried inner bark of *Ulmus rubra* Muhlenberg (*Ulmus fulva* Michaux) (Fam. Ulmaceae). *UNII-63POE2M46Y. Pharmaceutic aid (suspending agent); demulcent.*

Elmustine. C$_5$H$_{10}$ClN$_3$O$_3$. 195.60. 1-(2-Chloroethyl)-3-(2-hydroxyethyl)-1-nitrosourea. *UNII-NAT2FD82D7. CAS-60784-46-5.* INN.

Elnadipine. C$_{19}$H$_{19}$Cl$_2$N$_3$O$_3$. 408.28. Isopropyl (-)-(*S*)-4-(2,3-dichlorophenyl)-1,4-dihydro-2,6-dimethyl-5-(1,3,4-oxadiazol-2-yl)nicotinate. *UNII-LND2P599LK. CAS-103946-15-2.* INN.

Elocalcitol. C$_{29}$H$_{43}$FO$_2$. 442.65. (1*S*,3*R*,5*Z*,7*E*,23*E*)-1-Fluoro-26,27-dihomo-9,10-secocholesta-5,7,10(19),16,23-pentaene-3,25-diol. *CAS-199798-84-0.* INN.

Elomotecan. C$_{29}$H$_{32}$ClN$_3$O$_4$. 522.04. (5*R*)-9-Chloro-5-ethyl-5-hydroxy-10-methyl-12-[(4-methylpiperidin-1-yl)methyl]-1,4,5,13-tetrahydro-3*H*,15*H*-oxepino[3′,4′:6,7]indolizino[1,2-b]quinoline-3,15-dione. *CAS-220998-10-7.* INN.

Elopiprazole. C$_{23}$H$_{22}$FN$_3$O. 375.44. 1-(7-Benzofuranyl)-4-[[5-(*p*-fluorophenyl)pyrrol-2-yl]methyl]piperazine. *UNII-419A0R564U. CAS-115464-77-2.* INN.

Elotuzumab [*2008*] (el″ oh tooz′ oo mab). C$_{6476}$H$_{9982}$N$_{1714}$O$_{2016}$S$_{42}$. (1) Immunoglobulin G1, anti-(human protein CS1) (human-mouse HuLuc63 heavy chain), disulfide with human-mouse HuLuc63 κ-chain, dimer; (2) Immunoglobulin G1, anti-(human SLAM family member 7 (CD2-like receptor activating cytotoxic cells, CD319 antigen)), humanized mouse monoclonal HuLuc63 gamma-1 heavy chain (222-214′)-disulfide with humanized mouse monoclonal HuLuc63 kappa light chain (228-228″;231-231″)-bisdisulfide dimer. Molecular weight is approximately 145,500 daltons. *UNII-1351PE5UGS. CAS-915296-00-3. Treatment of cancer.* ◇*HuLuc63; PDL063; PDL-063*

Elsamitrucin [*1990*] (el sam″ i troo′ sin). $C_{33}H_{35}NO_{13}$. 653.63. (1) Benzo[*h*][1]benzopyrano[5,4,3-*cde*][1]benzopyran-5,12-dione, 10-[[2-*O*-(2-amino-2,6-dideoxy-3-*O*-methyl-α-D-galactopyranosyl)-6-deoxy-3-*C*-methyl-β-D-galactopyranosyl]oxy]-6-hydroxy-1-methyl-; (2) Benzo[*h*][1]benzopyrano[5,4,3-*cde*][1]benzopyran-5,12-dione, 10-[[2-*O*-(2-amino-2,6-dideoxy-3-*O*-methyl-α-D-galactopyranosyl)-6-deoxy-3-*C*-methyl-β-D-galactopyranosyl]oxy]-6-hydroxy-1-methyl-; (3) 10-*O*-Elsaminosylelsarosylchartarin. *CAS-97068-30-9. INN. Antineoplastic.* ◇*BBM-2478A; BMY-28090*

Elsibucol [*2006*] (el″ si bue′ kol). $C_{35}H_{54}O_4S_2$. 602.93. (1) Butanoic acid, 4-[4-[[1-[[3,5-bis(1,1-dimethylethyl)-4-hydroxyphenyl]thio]-1-methylethyl]thio]-2,6-bis(1,1-dimethylethyl)phenoxy]-; (2) 4-[4-[[1-[[3,5-Bis(1,1-dimethylethyl)-4-hydroxyphenyl]sulfanyl]-1-methylethyl]sulfanyl]-2,6-bis(1,1-dimethylethyl)phenoxy]butanoic acid. *UNII-O7T92N1Y8T. CAS-216167-95-2. INN. Prevention of solid organ transplant rejection.* ◇*AGI-1096*

Elsilimomab. Immunoglobulin G1, anti-(human interleukin 6) (mouse monoclonal B-E8 heavy chain), disulfide with mouse monoclonal B-E8 κ-chain, dimer. *CAS-468715-71-1. INN.*

Eltanolone. $C_{21}H_{34}O_2$. 318.49. 3α-Hydroxy-5β-pregnan-20-one. *UNII-BXO86P3XXW. CAS-128-20-1. INN.*

Eltenac. $C_{12}H_9Cl_2NO_2S$. 302.18. 4-(2,6-Dichloroanilino)-3-thiopheneacetic acid. *UNII-A153L3JA99. CAS-72895-88-6. INN.*

Eltoprazine. $C_{12}H_{16}N_2O_2$. 220.27. 1-(1,4-Benzodioxan-5-yl)-piperazine. *UNII-510M006KO6. CAS-98224-03-4. INN.*

Eltrombopag Olamine [*2005*] (el trom′ boe pag ole′ a meen). $C_{25}H_{22}N_4O_4.2(C_2H_7NO)$. 564.63. [Eltrombopag is INN.] (1) [1,1′-Biphenyl]-3-carboxylic acid, 3′-[(2*Z*)-[1-(3,4-dimethylphenyl)-1,5-dihydro-3-methyl-5-oxo-4*H*-pyrazol-4-ylidene]hydrazino]-2′-hydroxy-, compound with 2-aminoethanol (1:2); (2) 3′-[(2*Z*)-2-[1-(3,4-Dimethylphenyl)-3-methyl-5-oxo-1,5-dihydro-4*H*-pyrazol-4-ylidene]diazanyl]-2′-hydroxybiphenyl-3-carboxylic acid compound with 2-aminoethanol (1:2). *UNII-4U07F515LG; UNII-S56D65XJ9G* [eltrombopag]. *CAS-496775-62-3; CAS-496775-61-2* [eltrombopag]. *JAN. Treatment of chemotherapy-induced thrombocytopenia and treatment of immune thrombocytopenic purpura.* ◇*SB-497115-GR*

Elucaine [*1973*] (el′ ue kane). $C_{19}H_{23}NO_2$. 297.39. (1) Benzenemethanol, α-[(diethylamino)methyl]-, benzoate (ester); (2) α-[(Diethylamino)methyl]benzyl alcohol benzoate (ester). *UNII-85EW9V00UL. CAS-25314-87-8. INN. Anticholinergic (gastric).*

Elvitegravir [*2007*] (el″ vi teg′ ra vir). $C_{23}H_{23}ClFNO_5$. 447.88. (1) 3-Quinolinecarboxylic acid, 6-[(3-chloro-2-fluorophenyl)methyl]-1,4-dihydro-1-[(1*S*)-1-(hydroxymethyl)-2-methylpropyl]-7-methoxy-4-oxo-; (2) 6-(3-Chloro-2-fluorobenzyl)-1-[(2*S*)-1-hydroxy-3-methylbutan-2-yl]-7-methoxy-4-oxo-1,4-dihydroquinoline-3-carboxylic acid. *UNII-4GDQ854U53. CAS-697761-98-1. INN. Treatment of HIV-1 infections.* ◇*GS-9137; JTK-303*

---

† Brand name formerly used, and/or firm no longer concerned with this product.

Elvucitabine [*2003*] (el″ vue sye′ ta been). C$_9$H$_{10}$FN$_3$O$_3$. 227.19. (1) 2(1*H*)-Pyrimidinone, 4-amino-1-[(2*S*,5*R*)-2,5-dihydro-5-(hydroxymethyl)-2-furanyl]-5-fluoro-; (2) 4-Amino-5-fluoro-1-[(2*S*,5*R*)-5-(hydroxymethyl)-2,5-dihydrofuran-2-yl]pyrimidin-2(1*H*)-one. *UNII-M09BUF90C0. CAS-181785-84-2.* INN. *Treatment of Hepatitis B virus (HBV) and Human Immunodeficiency virus (HIV) infection.* ◇*ACH-126,443*

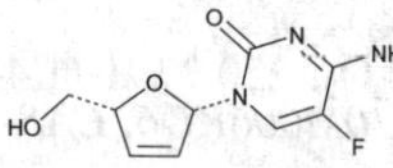

Elzasonan Citrate [*2002*] (el″ za sone′ an sit′ rate). C$_{22}$H$_{23}$Cl$_2$N$_3$OS.C$_6$H$_8$O$_7$. 640.53. [Elzasonan is INN.] (1) 3-Thiomorpholinone, 4-(3,4-dichlorphenyl)-2-[[2-(4-methyl-1-piperazinyl) phenyl]methylene]-, (2*Z*)-, 2-hydroxy-1,2,3-propanetricarboxylate (1:1); (2) (2*Z*)-4-(3,4-Dichlorphenyl)-2-[2-(4-methylpiperazin-1-yl)benzylidene]thiomorpholin-3-one citrate (1:1). *UNII-67JE11VN82; UNII-933PJL964R* [elzasonan]. *CAS-361343-20-6; CAS-361343-19-3* [elzasonan]. *Antidepressant (5-HT$_{1B/1D}$receptor antagonist).* ◇*CP-448,187-10*

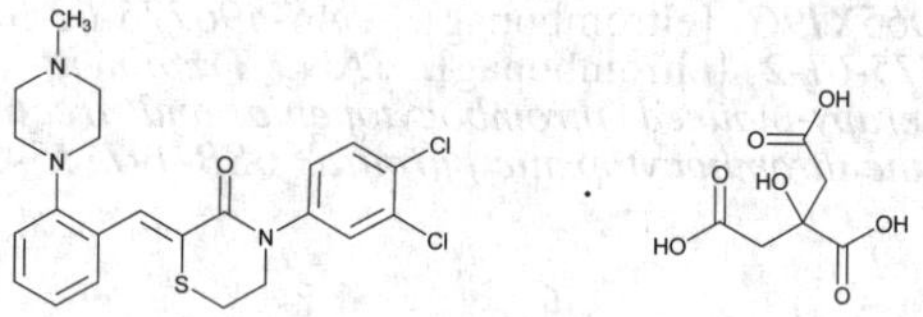

Elzasonan Hydrochloride [*2002*] (el″ za sone′ an hye″ droe klor′ ide). C$_{22}$H$_{23}$Cl$_2$N$_3$OS.HCl. 484.87. (1) 3-Thiomorpholinone, 4-(3,4-dichlorphenyl)-2-[[(2-(4-methyl-1-piperazinyl)phenyl]methylene]- monohydrochloride, (2*Z*)-; (2) (2*Z*)-4-(3,4-Dichlorphenyl)-2-[2-(4-methylpiperazin-1-yl)benzylidene]thiomorpholin-3-one monohydrochloride. *UNII-X38F62RR8L. CAS-220322-05-4. Antidepressant (5-HT$_{1B/1D}$receptor antagonist).* ◇*CP-448,187-01*

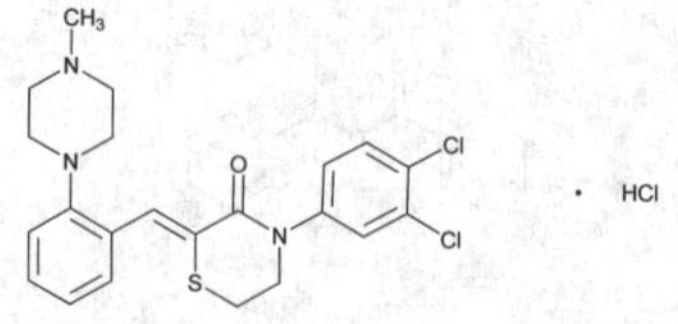

Elziverine. C$_{32}$H$_{37}$N$_3$O$_5$. 543.65. 6,7-Dimethoxy-4-[[4-(*o*-methoxyphenyl)-1-piperazinyl]methyl]-1-veratrylisoquinoline. *UNII-1I2BO46745. CAS-95520-81-3.* INN.

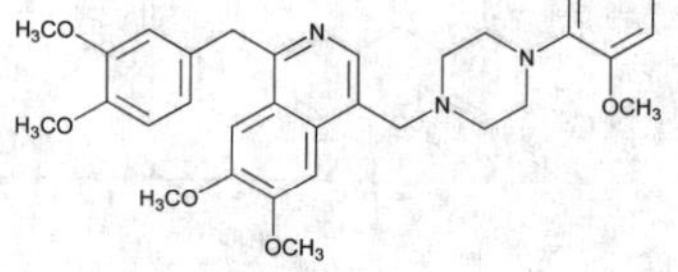

Emakalim. C$_{17}$H$_{16}$N$_2$O$_3$. 296.32. (-)-(3*S*,4*R*)-3-Hydroxy-2,2-dimethyl-4-(2-oxo-1(2*H*)-pyridyl)-6-chromancarbonitrile. *UNII-F1ZL87F3PM. CAS-129729-66-4.* INN.

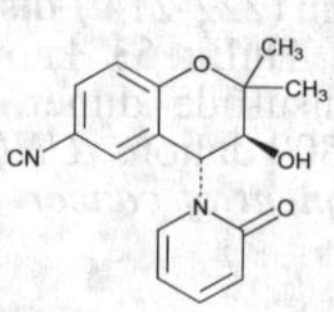

Emapunil. C$_{23}$H$_{23}$N$_5$O$_2$. 401.46. *N*-Benzyl-*N*-ethyl-2-(7-methyl-8-oxo-2-phenyl-7,8-dihydro-9*H*-purin-9-yl)acetamide. *CAS-226954-04-7.* [*Previously used INN.*]

Embeconazole. C$_{27}$H$_{25}$F$_3$N$_4$O$_3$S. 542.57. 4-{(1*E*,3*E*)-4-(*trans*-5-{[(2*R*,3*R*)-3-(2,4-Difluorophenyl)-3-hydroxy-4-(1*H*-1,2,4-triazol-1-yl)butan-2-yl]sulfanyl}-1,3-dioxan-2-yl)buta-1,3-dien-1-yl}-3-fluorobenzonitrile. *CAS-329744-44-7.* INN.

Embramine Hydrochloride. C$_{18}$H$_{22}$BrNO.HCl. 384.74. [Embramine is INN and BAN.] 2-[(*p*-Bromo-α-methyl-α-phenylbenzyl)oxy]-*N,N*-dimethylethylamine hydrochloride. *CAS-13977-28-1; CAS-3565-72-8* [embramine]. MI. Mebryl (SmithKline Beecham†)

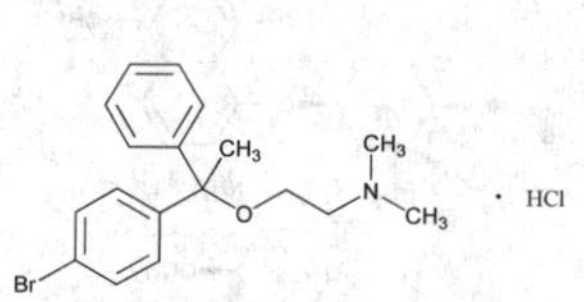

Embusartan. C$_{25}$H$_{24}$FN$_5$O$_3$. 461.49. Methyl 6-butyl-1-[2-fluoro-4-(*o*-1*H*-tetrazol-5-ylphenyl)benzyl]-1,2-dihydro-2-oxoisonicotinate. *CAS-156001-18-2.* INN.

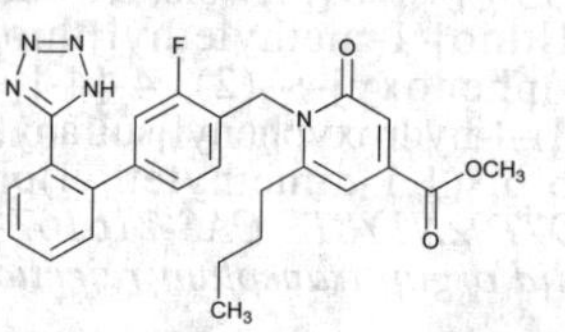

Embutramide [*1995*] (em bue′ tra mide). C$_{17}$H$_{27}$NO$_3$. 293.40. (1) Butanamide, *N*-[2-ethyl-2-(3-methoxyphenyl)-butyl]-4-hydroxy-; (2) *N*-(β,β-Diethyl-*m*-methoxyphenethyl)-4-hydroxybutyramide. *UNII-3P4TQG94T1. CAS-15687-14-6.* INN; BAN. *Anesthesia (general, veterinary).* Embutane (Hoechst-Roussel); T-61 (Hoechst-Roussel) ◇*HOE 18 680*

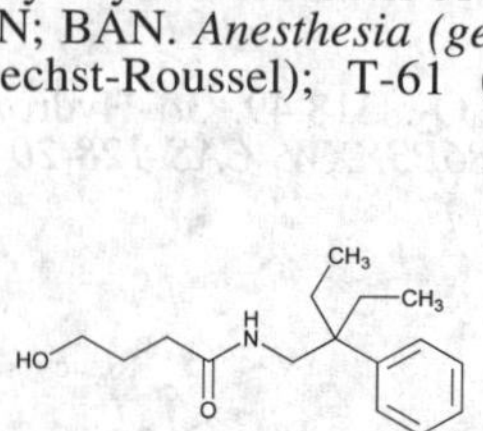

Emedastine Difumarate [*1996*] (em″ e das′ teen dye fue′ ma rate). **USP.** C$_{17}$H$_{26}$N$_4$O.2C$_4$H$_4$O$_4$. 534.56. [Emedastine is INN and BAN.] (1) 1*H*-Benzimidazole, 1-(2-ethoxyethyl)-2-(hexahydro-4-methyl-1*H*-1,4-diazepin-1-yl)-, (*E*)-2-butenedioate (1:2); (2) 1-(2-Ethoxyethyl)-2-(hexahydro-4-methyl-1*H*-1,4-diazepin-1-yl)benzimidazole fumarate (1:2). *UNII-42MB94QOSM; UNII-9J1H7Y9OJV* [emedastine]. *CAS-87233-62-3; CAS-87233-61-2* [emedastine]. JAN. *Antihistaminic, H$_1$-receptor; asthma prophylactic; anti-allergic.* Emadine (Alcon) ◇*AL-3432A*

Emepronium Bromide. C$_{20}$H$_{28}$BrN. 362.35. Ethyldimethyl(1-methyl-3,3-diphenylpropyl)ammonium bromide. *CAS-3614-30-0; CAS-27892-33-7* [emepronium]. INN; BAN; MI.

Emepronium Carrageenate. The ethyldimethyl(1-methyl-3,3-diphenylpropyl)ammonium salt of carrageenan, a linear polysaccharide of sulphated galactose and 3,6-anhydrogalactose residues existing in two principal fractions (κ- and λ-carrageenan). BAN.

Emetine Hydrochloride (em′ e teen hye″ droe klor′ ide). **USP.** C$_{29}$H$_{40}$N$_2$O$_4$.2HCl. 553.56. [Emetine is BAN.] (1) Emetan, 6′,7′,10,11-tetramethoxy-, dihydrochloride; (2) Emetine dihydrochloride. *CAS-316-42-7; CAS-483-18-1* [emetine]. *Anti-amebic.*

Emfilermin. Leukemia-inhibiting factor (human). *CAS-159075-60-2.* INN.

```
SPLPITPVNA TCAIRHPCHN NLMNQIRSQL AQLNGSANAL FILYYTAQGE
PFPNNLDKLC GPNVTDFPPF HANGTEKAKL VELYRIVVYL GTSLGNITRD
QKILNPSALS LHSKLNATAD ILRGLLSNVL CRLCSKYHVG HVDVTYGPDT
SGKDVFQKKK LGCQLLGKYK QIIAVLAQAF
```

Emideltide. C$_{35}$H$_{48}$N$_{10}$O$_{15}$. 848.81. L-Tryptophyl-L-alanylglycylglycyl-L-α-aspartyl-L-alanyl-L-serylglycyl-L-glutamic acid. *UNII-YN28Z5YZ73. CAS-62568-57-4.* INN.

```
WAGGDASGE
```

Emiglitate. C$_{17}$H$_{25}$NO$_7$. 355.38. Ethyl *p*-[2-[(2*R*,3*R*,4*R*,5*S*)-3,4,5-trihydroxy-2-(hydroxymethyl)piperidino]ethoxy]-benzoate. *CAS-80879-63-6.* INN; BAN. ◇*BAY o 1248*

Emilium Tosilate (INN) — *See* Emilium Tosylate.

Emilium Tosylate [*1977*] (em il′ i um tos′ i late). C$_{19}$H$_{27}$NO$_4$S. 365.49. [Emilium Tosylate is INN.] (1) Benzenemethanaminium, *N*-ethyl-3-methoxy-*N,N*-dimethyl-, salt with 4-methylbenzenesulfonic acid (1:1); (2) Ethyl(*m*-methoxybenzyl)dimethylammonium *p*-toluenesulfonate. *CAS-30716-01-9. Cardiac depressant (anti-arrhythmic).*

Emitefur [*1998*] (em it′ e fur). C$_{28}$H$_{19}$FN$_4$O$_8$. 558.47. (1) 3-[[3-(Ethoxymethyl)-5-fluoro-3,6-dihydro-2,6-dioxo-1(2*H*)-pyrimidinyl]carbonyl]benzoic acid, 6-(benzoyloxy)-3-cyano-2-pyridinyl ester; (2) *m*-[[3-(Ethoxymethyl)-5-fluoro-3,6-dihydro-2,6-dioxo-1(2*H*)-pyrimidinyl]carbonyl]benzoic acid, 2-ester with 2,6-dihydroxynicotinonitrile benzoate (ester). *CAS-110690-43-2.* INN. *Antineoplastic used in the treatment of stomach, colorectal, breast, non-small cell lung, and pancreatic cancers (inhibits DNA synthesis and RNA function).[Note—The Japanese tradename is Last-F.]* ◇*BOF-A2*

Emivirine [*1999*] (em″ i vir′ een). C$_{17}$H$_{22}$N$_2$O$_3$. 302.37. (1) 2,4(1*H*,3*H*)-Pyrimidinedione, 1-(ethoxymethyl)-5-(1-methylethyl)-6-(phenylmethyl)-; (2) 6-Benzyl-1-(ethoxymethyl)-5-isopropyluracil. *UNII-X87G8IX72O. CAS-149950-60-7.* INN. *Treatment of HIV-1 infections (nonnucleoside reverse transcriptase inhibitor).* Coactinon (Mitsubishi Chemical Corporation, Japan) ◇*MKC-442*

Emoctakin. C$_{372}$H$_{600}$N$_{106}$O$_{106}$S$_4$. 8381.65. Interleukin 8 (human). *CAS-142298-00-8.* INN.

```
SAKELRCQCI KTYSKPFHPK FIKELRVIES GPHCANTEII VKLSDGRELC
LDPKENWVQR VVEKFLKRAE NS
```

Emodepside. C$_{60}$H$_{90}$N$_6$O$_{14}$. 1119.39. Cyclo[(*R*)-lactoyl-*N*-methyl-L-leucyl-(*R*)-3-(*p*-morpholinophenyl)lactoyl-*N*-methyl-L-leucyl-(*R*)-lactoyl-*N*-methyl-L-leucyl-(*R*)-3-(*p*-morpholinophenyl)lactoyl-*N*-methyl-L-leucyl]. *CAS-155030-63-0*. INN.

Emonapride — *See* Nemonapride.

Emopamil. C$_{23}$H$_{30}$N$_2$. 334.50. 2-Isopropyl-5-(methylphenethylamino)-2-phenylvaleronitrile. *UNII-M514041RF7. CAS-78370-13-5*. INN.

Emorfazone. C$_{11}$H$_{17}$N$_3$O$_3$. 239.27. 4-Ethoxy-2-methyl-5-morpholino-3(2*H*)-pyridazinone. *UNII-V93U9DH62C. CAS-38957-41-4*. INN; JAN; MI.

Emricasan [*2007*] (em ri′ ka san). C$_{26}$H$_{27}$F$_4$N$_3$O$_7$. 569.50. (1) L-Alaninamide, *N*-[2-(1,1-dimethylethyl)phenyl]-2-oxoglycyl-*N*-[(1*S*)-1-(carboxymethyl)-2-oxo-3-(2,3,5,6-tetrafluorophenoxy)propyl]-; (2) (3*S*)-3-{*N*^{2}-[(2-*tert*-Butylphenyl)oxamoyl]-L-alaninamido}-4-oxo-5-(2,3,5,6-tetrafluorophenoxy)pentanoic acid. *UNII-P0GMS9N47Q. CAS-254750-02-2*. INN. *Prevention of fibrosis and inflammation in chronic liver disease.* ◇*PF 03491390; IDN 6556*

Emtricitabine [*1998*] (em″ trye sye′ ta been). C$_8$H$_{10}$FN$_3$O$_3$S. 247.25. (1) (2*R*-*cis*)-4-Amino-5-fluoro-1-[2-(hydroxymethyl)-1,3-oxathiolan-5-yl]-2(1*H*)-pyrimidinone; (2) 5-Fluoro-1-[(2*R*,5*S*)-2-(hydroxymethyl)-1,3-oxathiolan-5-yl]cytosine. *UNII-G70B4ETF4S. CAS-143491-57-0*. INN. *Antiviral (treatment of HIV-1 and hepatitis B infections).* Emtriva (Gilead Sciences) *[Note—Emtricitabine has appeared in the literature with the trivial names, (-)-FTC and FTC-(-).]* ◇*(-)-FTC; 524W91; BW-524W91; FTC-(-)*

Emylcamate. C$_7$H$_{15}$NO$_2$. 145.20. 3-Methyl-3-pentanol carbamate. *UNII-KCJ747D3R4. CAS-78-28-4*. INN; BAN; MI. ◇*KABI 925; MK-250*

Enadoline Hydrochloride [*1993*] (en ad′ oh leen hye″ droe klor′ ide). C$_{24}$H$_{32}$N$_2$O$_3$.HCl. 432.98. [Enadoline is INN.] (1) 4-Benzofuranacetamide, *N*-methyl-*N*-[7-(1-pyrrolidinyl)-1-oxaspiro[4.5]dec-8-yl]-, monohydrochloride, [5*R*-(5α,7α,8β)]-; (2) *N*-Methyl-*N*-[(5*R*,7*S*,8*S*)-7-(1-pyrrolidinyl)-1-oxaspiro[4.5]dec-8-yl]-4-benzofuranacetamide monohydrochloride. *CAS-124439-07-2; CAS-124378-77-4* [enadoline]. *Analgesic.* ◇*CI-977*

Enalapril Maleate [*1981*] (en al′ a pril mal′ ee ate). **USP**. C$_{20}$H$_{28}$N$_2$O$_5$.C$_4$H$_4$O$_4$. 492.52. [Enalapril is INN and BAN.] (1) L-Proline, 1-[*N*-[1-(ethoxycarbonyl)-3-phenylpropyl]-L-alanyl]-, (*S*)-, (*Z*)-2-butenedioate (1:1); (2) 1-[*N*-[(*S*)-1-Carboxy-3-phenylpropyl]-L-alanyl]-L-proline 1′-ethyl ester, maleate (1:1). *UNII-9O25354EPJ; UNII-69PN84IO1A* [enalapril]. *CAS-76095-16-4; CAS-75847-73-3* [enalapril]. JAN. *Antihypertensive.* Vasotec (Biovail)

Enalaprilat [*1984*] (en al′ a pril at″). **USP**. C$_{18}$H$_{24}$N$_2$O$_5$.2-H$_2$O. 384.42. (1) L-Proline, 1-[*N*-(1-carboxy-3-phenylpropyl)-L-alanyl]-, dihydrate, (*S*)-; (2) 1-[*N*-[(*S*)-1-Carboxy-3-phenylpropyl]-L-alanyl]-L-proline dihydrate. *UNII-GV0O7ES0R3. CAS-84680-54-6; CAS-76420-72-9* [anhydrous]. INN; BAN. *Antihypertensive.* Vasotec (Biovail) ◇*MK-422*

Enalkiren [*1989*] (en al kye′ ren). C$_{35}$H$_{56}$N$_6$O$_6$. 656.86. (1) L-Histidinamide, *N*-(3-amino-3-methyl-1-oxobutyl)-*O*-methyl-L-tyrosyl-*N*-[1-(cyclohexylmethyl)-2,3-dihydroxy-5-methylhexyl]-, [1*S*-(1*R**,2*S**,3*R**)]-; (2) (α*S*)-α-[(α*S*)-α-(3-Amino-3-methylbutyramido)-*p*-methoxyhydrocinnamamido]-*N*-[(1*S*,2*R*,3*S*)-1-(cyclohexylmethyl)-2,3-dihydroxy-5-methylhexyl]imidazole-4-propionamide. *CAS-113082-98-7*. INN. *Antihypertensive.* ◇*Abbott-64662*

Enallynymal Sodium — *See* Methohexital Sodium.

Enazadrem Phosphate [*1992*] (en az′ a drem fos′ fate). $C_{18}H_{25}N_3O.H_3O_4P$. 397.41. [Enazadrem is INN.] (1) 5-Pyrimidinol, 4,6-dimethyl-2-[(6-phenylhexyl)amino]-, phosphate (1:1) (salt); (2) 4,6-Dimethyl-2-[(6-phenylhexyl)amino]-5-pyrimidinol phosphate (1:1) (salt). *UNII-93VML10KA9; UNII-GDV807GKAD [enazadrem]. CAS-132956-22-0; CAS-107361-33-1 [enazadrem]. Antipsoriatic; inhibitor (5-lipoxygenase).* ◇*CP-70,490-09*

Enbucrilate. $C_8H_{11}NO_2$. 153.18. Butyl 2-cyanoacrylate. *CAS-6606-65-1. INN; BAN.*

Encainide Hydrochloride [*1978*] (en′ ka nide hye″ droe klor′ ide). $C_{22}H_{28}N_2O_2.HCl$. 388.93. [Encainide is INN and BAN.] (1) Benzamide, 4-methoxy-*N*-[2-[2-(1-methyl-2-piperidinyl)ethyl]phenyl]-, monohydrochloride, (±)-; (2) (±)-2′-[2-(1-Methyl-2-piperidyl)ethyl]-*p*-anisanilide monohydrochloride. *UNII-SY3J0147NB [encainide]. CAS-66794-74-9; CAS-37612-13-8 [encainide]. Cardiac depressant (anti-arrhythmic).* Enkaid (Bristol Labs†) ◇*MJ 9067-1*

Enciprazine Hydrochloride [*1989*] (en si′ pra zeen hye″ droe klor′ ide). $C_{23}H_{32}N_2O_6.2HCl$. 505.43. [Enciprazine is INN and BAN.] (1) 1-Piperazineethanol, 4-(2-methoxyphenyl)-α-[(3,4,5-trimethoxyphenoxy)methyl]-, dihydrochloride, (±)-; (2) (±)-4-(*o*-Methoxyphenyl)-α-[(3,4,5-trimethoxyphenoxy)methyl]-1-piperazineethanol dihydrochloride. *UNII-L6X660925G [enciprazine]. CAS-68576-88-5; CAS-68576-86-3 [enciprazine]. Tranquilizer (minor).* ◇*WY-48624*

Enclomifene (INN) — *See* Enclomiphene.

Enclomiphene [*1974*] (en kloe′ mi feen). $C_{26}H_{28}ClNO$. 405.96. [Enclomifene is INN.] (1) Ethanamine, 2-[4-(2-chloro-1,2-diphenylethenyl)phenoxy]-*N,N*-diethyl-, (*E*)-;

(2) (*E*)-2-[*p*-(2-Chloro-1,2-diphenylvinyl)phenoxy]triethylamine. *UNII-R6D2UI4FLS. CAS-15690-57-0. [Name previously used: Cisclomiphene.]* ◇*Isomer B; RMI 16,289*

Encyprate [*1965*] (en sye′ prate). $C_{13}H_{17}NO_2$. 219.28. (1) Carbamic acid, cyclopropyl(phenylmethyl)-, ethyl ester; (2) Ethyl *N*-benzylcyclopropanecarbamate. *CAS-2521-01-9. INN. Antidepressant.* ◇*MO-1255; A-19757*

Endiemal — *See* Metharbital.

Endixaprine. $C_{15}H_{15}Cl_2N_3O$. 324.21. 1-[6-(2,4-Dichlorophenyl)-3-pyridazinyl]-4-piperidinol. *UNII-V8674RM5KM. CAS-93181-85-2. INN.*

Endobenzyline Bromide. *CAS-8058-76-2.* MI. Ulcyn (Marion Merrell Dow†)

Endomide. $C_{17}H_{28}N_2O_2$. 292.42. (1*R*,2*S*,3*S*,4*S*)-*N,N,N′,N′*-Tetraethyl-5-norbornene-2,3-dicarboxamide. *UNII-BP0YBT71AK. CAS-4582-18-7. INN.*

Endomycin. Antibiotic obtained from cultures of *Streptomyces endus*, or the same substance produced by any other means. *CAS-1391-41-9.*

Endralazine Mesylate [*1981*] (en dral′ a zeen mes′ i late). $C_{14}H_{15}N_5O.CH_4O_3S$. 365.41. [Endralazine is INN and BAN.] (1) Pyrido[4,3-*c*]pyridazin-3(2*H*)-one, 6-benzoyl-5,6,7,8-tetrahydro-, hydrazone, monomethanesulfonate; (2) 6-Benzoyl-5,6,7,8-tetrahydropyrido[4,3-*c*]pyridazin-3(2*H*)-one hydrazone monomethanesulfonate. *UNII-333M5986I5. CAS-65322-72-7 [monomethanesulfonate]; CAS-39715-02-1 [endralazine]. Antihypertensive.* Migranal (Novartis) ◇*22-708*

Endrisone (INN) — *See* Endrysone.

Endrysone [*1973*] (en′ dri sone). $C_{22}H_{30}O_3$. 342.47. [Endrisone is INN.] (1) Pregna-1,4-diene-3,20-dione, 11-hydroxy-6-methyl-, (6α,11β)-; (2) 11β-Hydroxy-6α-methylpregna-1,4-diene-3,20-dione. *UNII-1QZ096EIEF. CAS-35100-44-8. Anti-inflammatory (topical, ophthalmic).*

Enecadin. $C_{21}H_{28}FN_3O$. 357.46. 4-(4-Fluorophenyl)-2-methyl-6-[[5-(piperidin-1-yl)pentyl]oxy]pyrimidine. *CAS-259525-01-4.* INN.

Enefexine. $C_{13}H_{19}N$. 189.30. 4-(*p*-Ethylphenyl)piperidine. *UNII-2JMM46GA2V. CAS-67765-04-2.* INN.

Enestebol. $C_{20}H_{28}O_3$. 316.43. 4,17β-Dihydroxy-17-methylandrosta-1,4-dien-3-one. *CAS-2320-86-7.* INN.

Enfenamic Acid. $C_{15}H_{15}NO_2$. 241.29. *N*-Phenethylanthranilic acid. *UNII-05KO5G76R2. CAS-23049-93-6.* INN; MI.

Enflufocon A [*1994*] (en″ floo foe′ kon). $(C_9H_{16}O_2)_r$ $(C_5H_8O_2)_s(C_{11}H_6F_{12}O_4)_t(C_{16}H_{38}O_5Si_4)_u(C_{13}H_{20}O_4)_v(C_{26}H_{58}O_9Si_6)_w(C_4H_6O_2)_x(C_6H_9NO)_y(C_{70}H_{188}O_{30}Si_{27})_z$. (1) 2,2-Dimethylpropyl 2-methyl-2-propenoate polymer with methyl 2-methyl-2-propenoate, bis[2,2,2-trifluoro-1-(trifluoromethyl)ethyl] methylenebutanedioate, 3-[3,3,3-trimethyl-1,1-bis[(trimethylsily)oxy]disiloxanyl]propyl 2-methyl-2-propenoate, 2,2-dimethyl-1,3-propanediyl bis(2-methyl-2-propenoate), [1,1,3,3-tetrakis[(trimethylsilyl)oxy]-1,3-disiloxanediyl]di-3,1-propanediyl bis(2-methyl-2-propenoate), 2-methyl-2-propenoic acid, 1-ethenyl-2-pyrrolidinone, and α-[dimethyl[4-[(2-methyl-1-oxopropenyl)oxy]butyl]silyl]-ω-[4-[(2-methyl-1-oxo-2-propenyl)oxy]butyl]poly[oxy(dimethylsilylene)]; (2) Neopentyl methacrylate polymer with methyl methacrylate, bis[2,2,2-trifluoro-1-(trifluoromethyl)ethyl] methylenesuccinate, 3-[3,3,3-trimethyl-1,1-bis(trimethylsiloxy)disiloxanyl]propyl methacrylate, 2,2-dimethyltrimethylene dimethacrylate, [1,1,3,3-tetrakis(trimethylsiloxy)disiloxanylene]bis(trimethylene) dimethacrylate, methacrylic acid, 1-vinyl-2-pyrrolidinone and (tetrapentacontamethylheptacosasiloxanylene)bis(tetramethylene) dimethacrylate. *Contact lens material (hydrophobic).* Boston 7/30 (Polymer Technology) [*Note—The oxygen permeability of the contact lens material is $36 \times 10^{-11}(cm^2/sec)(ml\ O_2/ml \times mm\ Hg)$ at $35°C$ (Dk value).*]

Enflufocon B [*1997*] (en″ floo foe′ kon). $(C_9H_{16}O_2)_r$ $(C_5H_8O_2)_s(C_{11}H_6F_{12}O_4)_t(C_{16}H_{38}O_5Si_4)_u(C_{13}H_{20}O_4)_v(C_{26}H_{58}O_9Si_6)_w(C_4H_6O_2)_x(C_6H_9NO)_y(C_{70}H_{188}O_{30}Si_{27})_z$. (1) 2,2-Dimethylpropyl 2-methyl-2-propenoate polymer with methyl 2-methyl-2-propenoate, bis[2,2,2-trifluoro-1-(trifluoromethyl)ethyl] methylenebutanedioate, 3-[3,3,3-trimethyl-1,1-bis[(trimethylsily)oxy]disiloxanyl]propyl 2-methyl-2-propenoate, 2,2-dimethyl-1,3-propanediyl bis(2-methyl-2-propenoate), [1,1,3,3-tetrakis[(trimethylsilyl)oxy]-1,3-disiloxanediyl]di-3,1-propanediyl bis(2-methyl-2-propenoate), 2-methyl-2-propenoic acid, 1-ethenyl-2-pyrrolidinone, and α-[dimethyl[4-[(2-methyl-1-oxopropenyl)oxy]butyl]silyl]-ω-[4-[(2-methyl-1-oxo-2-propenyl)oxy]butyl]poly[oxy(dimethylsilylene)]; (2) Neopentyl methacrylate polymer with methyl methacrylate, bis[2,2,2-trifluoro-1-(trifluoromethyl)ethyl] methylenesuccinate, 3-[3,3,3-trimethyl-1,1-bis(trimethylsiloxy)disiloxanyl]propyl methacrylate, 2,2-dimethyltrimethylene dimethacrylate, [1,1,3,3-tetrakis(trimethylsiloxy)disiloxanylene]bis(trimethylene) dimethacrylate, methacrylic acid, 1-vinyl-2-pyrrolidinone and (tetrapentacontamethylheptacosasiloxanylene)bis(tetramethylene) dimethacrylate. *CAS-156165-55-8. Contact lens material (hydrophobic).[Note—The water content of the contact lens material is < 1.0% at ambient temperature ($23±2°C$), and the oxygen permeability is $57±10 \times 10^{-11}(cm^2/sec)(ml\ O_2/ml \times mm\ Hg)$ at $35°C$ (Dk value).]*

Enflurane [*1970*] (en flur′ ane). **USP.** $C_3H_2ClF_5O$. 184.49. (1) Ethane, 2-chloro-1-(difluoromethoxy)-1,1,2-trifluoro-, (±)-; (2) (±)-2-Chloro-1,1,2-trifluoroethyl difluoromethyl ether. *UNII-91I69L5AY5. CAS-13838-16-9.* INN; BAN; JAN. *Anesthetic (inhalation).* Ethrane (Baxter Healthcare) ◇*Anesthetic Compound No. 347; NSC-115944*

Enfuvirtide [*2001*] (en fue′ vir tide). $C_{204}H_{301}N_{51}O_{64}$. 4491.88. (1) L-Phenylalaninamide, *N*-acetyl-L-tyrosyl-L-threonyl-L-seryl-L-leucyl-L-isoleucyl-L-histadyl-L-seryl-L-leucyl-L-isoleucyl-L-α-glutamyl-L-α-glutamyl-L-seryl-L-glutaminyl-L-asparaginyl-L-glutaminyl-L-glutaminyl-L-α-glutamyl-L-lysyl-L-asparaginyl-L-α-glutamyl-L-glutaminyl-L-α-glutamyl-L-leucyl-L-leucyl-L-α-glutamyl-L-leucyl-L-α-aspartyl-L-lysyl-L-tryptophyl-L-alanyl-L-seryl-L-leucyl-L-tryptophyl-L-asparaginyl-L-tryptophyl-; (2) *N*-Acetyl-L-tyrosyl-L-threonyl-L-seryl-L-leucyl-L-isoleucyl-L-histadyl-L-seryl-L-leucyl-L-isoleucyl-L-α-glutamyl-L-α-glutamyl-L-seryl-L-glutaminyl-L-asparaginyl-L-glutaminyl-L-glutaminyl-L-α-glutamyl-L-lysyl-L-asparaginyl-L-α-glutamyl-L-glutaminyl-L-α-glutamyl-L-leucyl-L-leucyl-L-α-glutamyl-L-leucyl-L-α-aspartyl-L-lysyl-L-tryptophyl-L-alanyl-L-seryl-L-leucyl-L-tryptophyl-L-asparaginyl-L-tryptophyl-L-phenylalaninamide. *UNII-19OWO1T3ZE. CAS-159519-65-0.* INN; BAN. *Antiviral (blockade of gp-41 mediated membrane fusion).* Fuzeon (Roche) [*Note—The trivial name, pentafuside, has appeared in literature.*] ◇*T20; DP178*

Englitazone Sodium [*1993*] (en gli′ ta zone soe′ dee um). $C_{20}H_{18}NNaO_3S$. 375.42. [Englitazone is INN.] (1) 2,4-Thiazolidinedione, 5-[[3,4-dihydro-2-(phenylmethyl)-2*H*-1-benzopyran-6-yl]methyl]-, sodium salt; (2) (-)-5-[[(2R)-

2-Benzyl-6-chromanyl]methyl]-2,4-thiazolidinedione, sodium salt. *UNII-VA5755GIJ8. CAS-109229-57-4; CAS-109229-58-5* [englitazone]. *Antidiabetic.* ◇*CP-72,467-2*

Enhexymal — *See* Hexobarbital.

Eniclobrate. $C_{24}H_{24}ClNO_3$. 409.91. 3-Pyridylmethyl (±)-2-[[α-(*p*-chlorophenyl)-*p*-tolyl]oxy]-2-methylbutyrate. *UNII-M469UFX48N. CAS-60662-18-2.* INN.

Enilconazole [*1980*] (en″ il kon′ a zole). $C_{14}H_{14}Cl_2N_2O$. 297.18. (1) 1*H*-Imidazole, 1-[2-(2,4-dichlorophenyl)-2-(2-propenyloxy)ethyl]-, (±)-; (2) (±)-1-[β-(Allyloxy)-2,4-dichlorophenethyl]-imidazole. *CAS-35554-44-0.* INN; BAN. *Antifungal.* ◇*R 23,979*

Enilospirone. $C_{15}H_{18}ClNO_3$. 295.76. (2*R*,5*RS*,6*R*)-6-(*m*-Chlorophenoxy)-2-methyl-1-oxa-4-azaspiro[4.5]decan-3-one. *UNII-WO31V62797. CAS-59798-73-1.* INN.

Eniluracil [*1997*] (en″ il ue′ ra sil; en″ il ure′ a sil). $C_6H_4N_2O_2$. 136.11. (1) 2,4(1*H*,3*H*)-Pyrimidinedione, 5-ethynyl-; (2) 5-Ethynyluracil. *UNII-2E2W0W5XIU. CAS-59989-18-3.* INN; BAN. *Antineoplastic (adjunct).* ◇*776C85*

Eniporide. $C_{14}H_{16}N_4O_3S$. 320.37. *N*-(Diaminomethylene)-5-(methylsulfonyl)-4-pyrrol-1-yl-*o*-toluamide. *CAS-176644-21-6.* INN.

Enisoprost [*1983*] (en eye′ soe prost). $C_{22}H_{36}O_5$. 380.52. (1) Prosta-4,13-dien-1-oic acid, 11,16-dihydroxy-16-methyl-9-oxo-, methyl ester, (4Z,11α,13E)-(±)-; (2) (±)-Methyl

(*Z*)-7-[(1*R*,2*R*,3*R*)-3-hydroxy-2-[(*E*)-(4*RS*)-4-hydroxy-4-methyl-1-octenyl]-5-oxocyclopentyl]-4-heptenoate. *CAS-81026-63-3.* INN. *Anti-ulcerative.* ◇*SC-34301*

Enlimomab [*1993*] (en lim′ oh mab). (1) Immunoglobulin G 2a (mouse monoclonal BI-RR-1 anti-human antigen CD 54), disulfide with mouse monoclonal BI-RR-1 light chain, dimer; (2) Immunoglobulin G 2a (mouse monoclonal BI-RR-1 anti-human antigen CD 54), disulfide with mouse monoclonal BI-RR-1 light chain, dimer. Molecular weight is approximately 150,000 daltons. *CAS-142864-19-5.* INN. *Anti-inflammatory; monoclonal antibody.* ◇*BI-RR-0001*

Enlimomab Pegol. Immunoglobulin G 2a (mouse monoclonal Bl-RR-1 anti-human antigen CD 54), disulfide with mouse monoclonal Bl-RR-1 light chain, dimer, reaction product with α-(2-carboxyethyl)-ω-methoxypoly(oxy-1,2-ethanediyl). *CAS-169802-84-0.* INN.

Enloplatin [*1991*] (en″ loe pla′ tin). $C_{13}H_{22}N_2O_5Pt$. 481.41. (1) Platinum, [1,1-cyclobutanedicarboxylato(2-)](tetrahydro-4*H*-pyran-4,4-dimethanamine-*N*,*N′*)-, (*SP*-4-2)-; (2) *cis*-(1,1-Cyclobutanedicarboxylato)[tetrahydro-4*H*-pyran-4,4-bis(methylamine)]platinum. *CAS-111523-41-2.* INN. *Antineoplastic.* ◇*CL 287,110*

Enocitabine. $C_{31}H_{55}N_3O_6$. 565.78. *N*-(1-β-D-Arabinofuranosyl-1,2-dihydro-2-oxo-4-pyrimidinyl)docosanamide. *UNII-9YVR68W306. CAS-55726-47-1.* INN; JAN; MI.

Enofelast [*1992*] (en oh′ fe last). $C_{16}H_{15}FO$. 242.29. (1) Phenol, 4-[2-(4-fluorophenyl)ethenyl]-2,6-dimethyl-, (*E*)-; (2) (*E*)-4′-Fluoro-3,5-dimethyl-4-stilbenol. *UNII-3T93TS0430. CAS-127035-60-3.* INN. *Anti-asthmatic.* ◇*BI-L-239*

Enolicam Sodium [*1981*] (e nol′ i kam soe′ dee um). $C_{17}H_{11}Cl_3NNaO_4S.H_2O$. 472.70. [Enolicam is INN.] (1) 1-Benzothiepin-4-carboxamide, 7-chloro-*N*-(3,4-dichlorophenyl)-2,3-dihydro-5-hydroxy-, 1,1-dioxide, monosodium salt, monohydrate; (2) 3′,4′,7-Trichloro-2,3-dihydro-5-hydroxy-1-benzothiepin-4-carboxanilide 1,1-dioxide, monosodium salt, monohydrate. *UNII-C3QYZ005LS; UNII-TEA6PI0H6H* [enolicam]. *CAS-73574-69-3* [monohy-

---

drate]; *CAS-59756-39-7* [anhydrous]; *CAS-59755-82-7* [enolicam]. *Anti-inflammatory; antirheumatic.* ◇*CGS 5391B (anhydrous)*

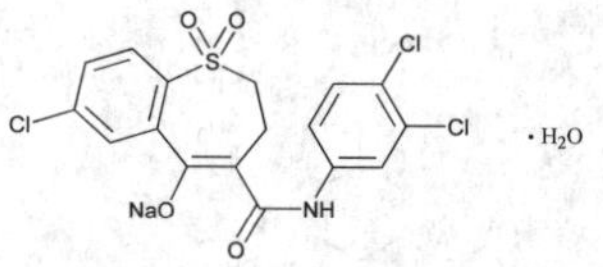

Enoxacin [*1984*] (en ox′ a sin). $C_{15}H_{17}FN_4O_3$. 320.32. (1) 1,8-Naphthyridine-3-carboxylic acid, 1-ethyl-6-fluoro-1,4-dihydro-4-oxo-7-(1-piperazinyl)-; (2) 1-Ethyl-6-fluoro-1,4-dihydro-4-oxo-7-(1-piperazinyl)-1,8-naphthyridine-3-carboxylic acid. *UNII-325OGW249P. CAS-74011-58-8.* INN; BAN; JAN. *Antibacterial.* Penetrex (Sanofi Aventis) ◇*AT-2266; CI-919; PD 107779*

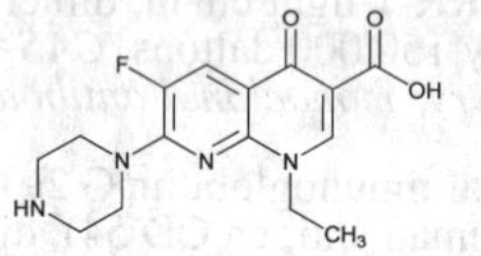

Enoxamast. $C_{13}H_{10}N_2O_5S$. 306.29. [4-(1,4-Benzodioxan-6-yl)-2-thiazolyl]oxamic acid. *UNII-08703R750L. CAS-74604-76-5.* INN.

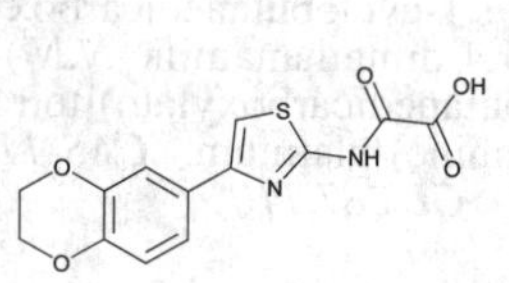

Enoxaparin Sodium [*1995*] (ee nox ap′ a rin soe′ dee um; ee nox″ a par′ in soe′ dee um). (1) Enoxaparin sodium; (2) Sodium salt of a low-molecular weight heparin obtained by alkaline depolymerization of the benzyl ester of heparin from porcine mucosa. *UNII-8NZ41MIK1O. CAS-679809-58-6.* INN; BAN; MI. *Antithrombotic intended for use in the treatment of deep vein thrombosis; prophylaxis of ischemic complications of unstable angina and non-Q-wave myocardial infarction, and treatment of acute deep vein thrombosis.* Lovenox (Sanofi Aventis) ◇*RP 54563; PK 10169*

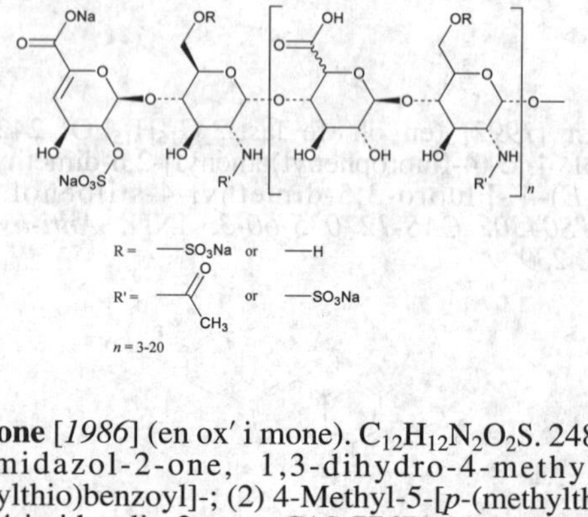

Enoximone [*1986*] (en ox′ i mone). $C_{12}H_{12}N_2O_2S$. 248.30. (1) 2*H*-Imidazol-2-one, 1,3-dihydro-4-methyl-5-[4-(methylthio)benzoyl]-; (2) 4-Methyl-5-[*p*-(methylthio)ben-zoyl]-4-imidazolin-2-one. *CAS-77671-31-9.* INN; BAN. *Cardiotonic.* Perfan (Marion Merrell Dow) ◇*MDL 17,043*

Enoxolone. $C_{30}H_{46}O_4$. 470.68. [Glycyrrhetic Acid is JAN.] 3β-Hydroxy-11-oxoolean-12-en-30-oic acid. *CAS-471-53-4.* INN; BAN; DCF; MI.

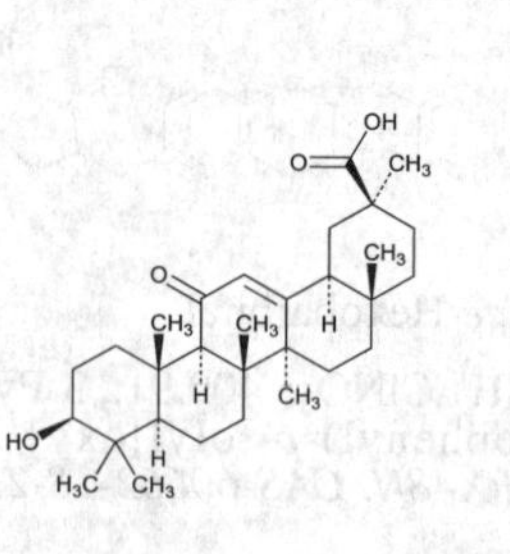

Enphenemal — *See* Mephobarbital.

Enpiprazole. $C_{16}H_{21}ClN_4$. 304.82. 1-(*o*-Chlorophenyl)-4-[2-(1-methylpyrazol-4-yl)ethyl]piperazine. *UNII-78G92X9EH7. CAS-31729-24-5.* INN; BAN.

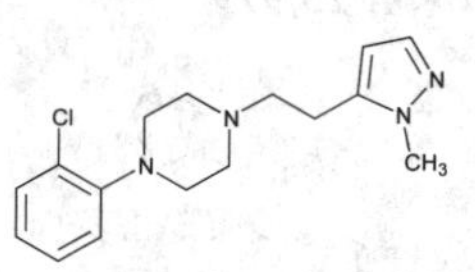

Enpiroline Phosphate [*1985*] (en pir′ oh leen fos′ fate). $C_{19}H_{18}F_6N_2O.H_3PO_4$. 502.34. [Enpiroline is INN.] (1) 4-Pyridinemethanol, α-(2-piperidinyl)-2-(trifluoromethyl)-6-[4-(trifluoromethyl)phenyl]-, (*R**,*R**)-(±)-, phosphate (1:1) (salt); (2) (±)-(*R**,*R**)-α-[2-(Trifluoromethyl)-6-(α,α,α-trifluoro-*p*-tolyl)-4-pyridyl]-2-piperidinemethanol phosphate (1:1) (salt). *UNII-QX39IR9V1D; UNII-8M7Y72EP9K* [enpiroline]. *CAS-66364-74-7; CAS-66364-73-6* [enpiroline]. *Antimalarial.* ◇*WR 180,409*

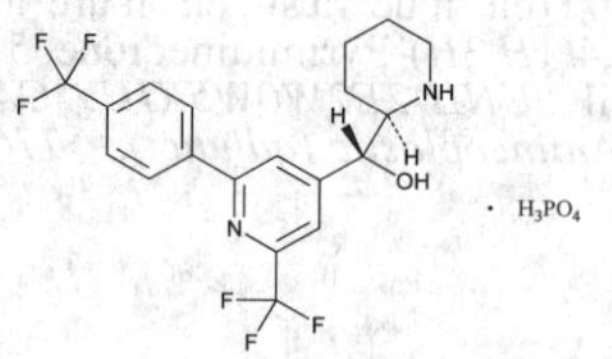

Enprazepine. $C_{20}H_{24}N_2$. 292.42. 5-[3-(Dimethylamino)pro-pyl]-5,6-dihydro-11-methylene-11*H*-dibenz[*b,e*]azepine. *UNII-L2H26JSV0I. CAS-47206-15-5.* INN.

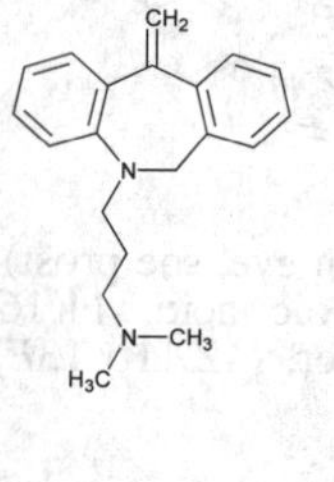

Enprofen (previously used name) — *See* Furaprofen.

Enprofylline [*1985*] (en prof′ i lin). $C_8H_{10}N_4O_2$. 194.19. (1) 1*H*-Purine-2,6-dione, 3,7-dihydro-3-propyl-; (2) 3-Propylxanthine. *UNII-DT7DT5E518. CAS-41078-02-8.* INN. *Bronchodilator.* ⬦*D 4028*

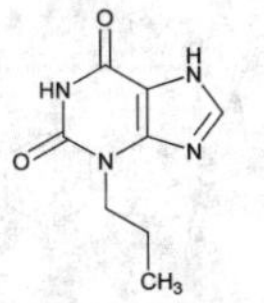

Enpromate [*1970*] (en′ proe mate). $C_{22}H_{23}NO_2$. 333.42. (1) Carbamic acid, cyclohexyl-, 1,1-diphenyl-2-propynyl ester; (2) 1,1-Diphenyl-2-propynyl cyclohexanecarbamate. *CAS-10087-89-5.* INN. *Antineoplastic.* ⬦*59156; NSC-112682*

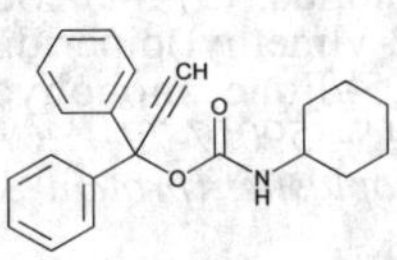

Enprostil [*1983*] (en prost′ il). $C_{23}H_{28}O_6$. 400.46. (1) 4,5-Heptadienoic acid, 7-[3-hydroxy-2-(3-hydroxy-4-phenoxy-1-butenyl)-5-oxocyclopentyl]-, methyl ester; (2) Methyl 7-[(1*R**,2*R**,3*R**)-3-hydroxy-2-[(*E*)-(3*R**)-3-hydroxy-4-phenoxy-1-butenyl]-5-oxocyclopentyl]-4,5-heptadienoate. *CAS-73121-56-9.* INN; BAN; JAN. *Antisecretory; antiulcerative.* Gardrin (Syntex) ⬦*RS-84135*

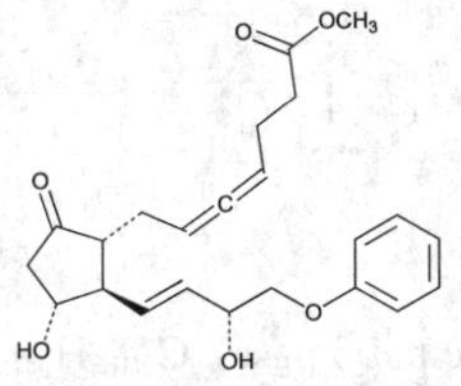

Enramycin. Antibiotic obtained from cultures of *Streptomyces fungicidicus* B 5477, or the same substance produced by any other means. *CAS-11115-82-5.* INN.

Enrasentan. $C_{29}H_{30}O_8$. 506.54. (1*S*,2*R*,3*S*)-3-[2-(2-Hydroxyethoxy)-4-methoxyphenyl]-1-[3,4-(methylenedioxy)phenyl]-5-propoxy-2-indancarboxylic acid. *CAS-167256-08-8.* INN.

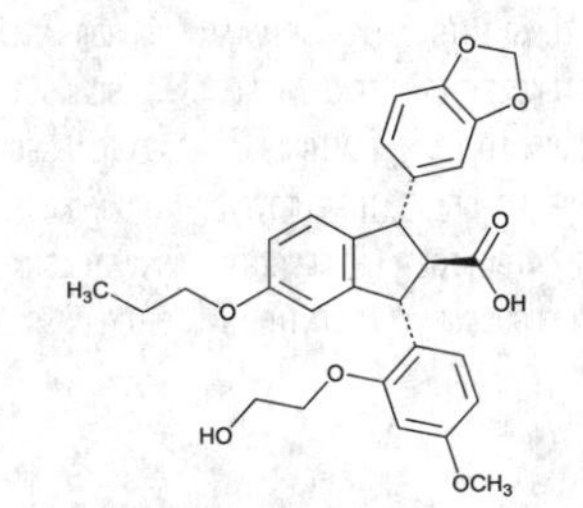

Enrofloxacin [*1988*] (en″ roe flox′ a sin). $C_{19}H_{22}FN_3O_3$. 359.39. (1) 3-Quinolinecarboxylic acid, 1-cyclopropyl-7-(4-ethyl-1-piperazinyl)-6-fluoro-1,4-dihydro-4-oxo-; (2) 1-Cyclopropyl-7-(4-ethyl-1-piperazinyl)-6-fluoro-1,4-dihydro-4-oxo-3-quinolinecarboxylic acid. *UNII-3DX3XEK1BN. CAS-93106-60-6.* INN; BAN. *Antibacterial (veterinary).* Baytril (Bayer Animal Health) ⬦*Bay Vp 2674*

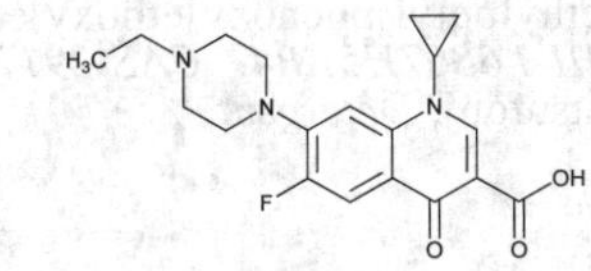

Ensaculin. $C_{26}H_{32}N_2O_5$. 452.54. 7-Methoxy-6-[3-[4-(*o*-methoxyphenyl)-1-piperazinyl]propoxy]-3,4-dimethylcoumarin. *UNII-869PGR00AT. CAS-155773-59-4.* INN.

Ensulizole [*1999*] (en sul′ i zole). **USP.** $C_{13}H_{10}N_2O_3S$. 274.30. (1) 1*H*-Benzimidazole-5-sulfonic acid-2-phenyl-; (2) 2-Phenylbenzimidazole-5-sulfonic acid. *CAS-27503-81-7.* INN. *[Name previously used: Phenylbenzimidazole Sulfonic Acid.] [Note—The International Cosmetic Ingredient (INCI) name ensulizole is phenylbenzimidazole sulfonic acid.]*

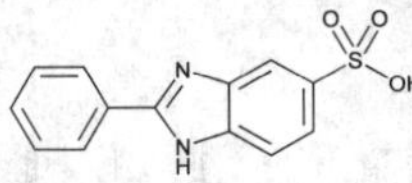

Entacapone [*1997*] (en tak′ a pone). $C_{14}H_{15}N_3O_5$. 305.29. (*E*)-α-Cyano-*N*,*N*-diethyl-3,4-dihydroxy-5-nitrocinnamamide. *UNII-4975G9NM6T. CAS-130929-57-6.* INN; BAN. *Antidyskinetic.* Comtan (Orion) ⬦*OR-611*

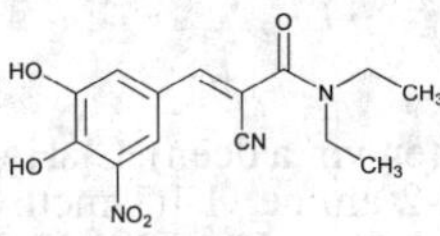

Entecavir [*1999*] (en tek′ a vir). $C_{12}H_{15}N_5O_3 \cdot H_2O$. 295.29. (1) 6*H*-Purin-6-one, 2-amino-1,9-dihydro-9-[(1*S*,3*R*,4*S*)-4-hydroxy-3-(hydroxymethyl)-2-methylenecyclopentyl]-monohydrate; (2) 9-[(1*S*,3*R*,4*S*)-4-Hydroxy-3-(hydroxymethyl)-2-methylenecyclopentyl]guanine monohydrate. *UNII-5968Y6H45M; UNII-NNU2O4609D* [entecavir anhydrous]. *CAS-209216-23-9; CAS-142217-69-4* [anhydrous]. INN. *Antiviral used in the treatment of hepatitis B infection.* Baraclude (Bristol-Myers Squibb) ⬦*BMS-200475-01; SQ34676*

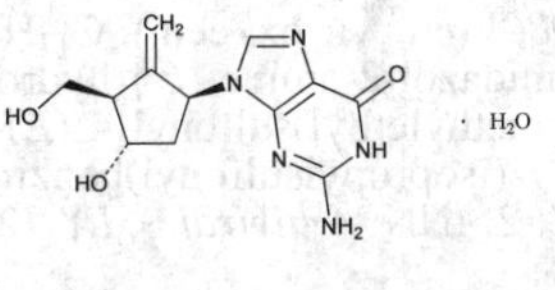

Entinostat [*2008*] (en tin′ oh stat). $C_{21}H_{20}N_4O_3$. 376.41. (1) Carbamic acid, *N*-[[4-[[(2-aminophenyl)amino]carbonyl]phenyl]methyl]-, 3-pyridinylmethyl ester; (2) Pyridin-3-ylmethyl ({4-[(2-aminophenyl)carbamoyl]phenyl}-methyl)carbamate. *CAS-209783-80-2.* INN. *Antineoplastic.* ⬦*SNDX-275*

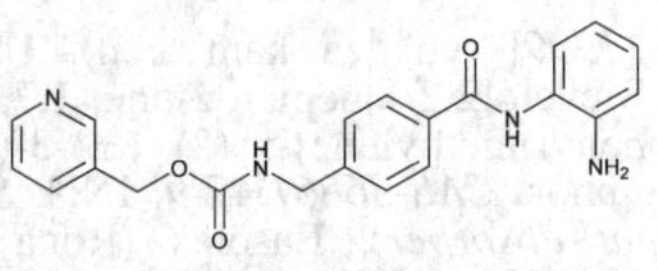

---

† Brand name formerly used, and/or firm no longer concerned with this product.

Entsufon Sodium [*1974*] (ent′ soo fon soe′ dee um). $C_{20}H_{33}NaO_6S$. 424.53. [Entsufon is INN.] (1) Ethanesulfonic acid, 2-[2-[2-[4-(1,1,3,3-tetramethylbutyl)phenoxy]ethoxy]ethoxy]-, sodium salt; (2) Sodium 2-[2-[2-[*p*-1,1,3,3-tetramethylbutyl)phenoxy]ethoxy]ethoxy]ethanesulfonate. *UNII-L6867H5FR4. CAS-2917-94-4; CAS-55837-16-6* [entsufon]. *Detergent.*

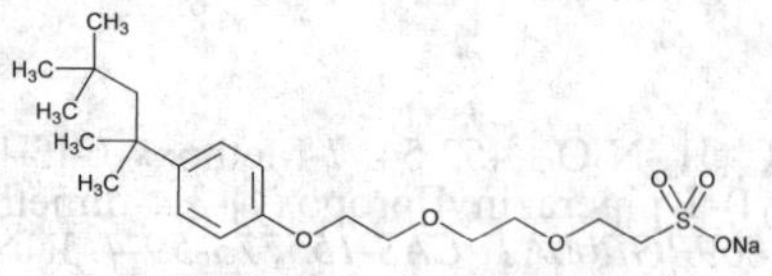

Enviomycin. $C_{25}H_{43}N_{13}O_{10}$. 685.69. [Enviomycin Sulfate is JAN.] Tuberactinomycin N; stereoisomer of [[15-(3,6-diamino-4-hydroxyhexanamido)-3-(hexahydro-2-imino-4-pyrimidinyl)-9,12-bis(hydroxymethyl-2,5,8,11,14-pentaoxo-1,4,7,10,13-pentaazacyclohexadec-6-ylidene]methyl]urea. *CAS-33103-22-9.* INN; MI.

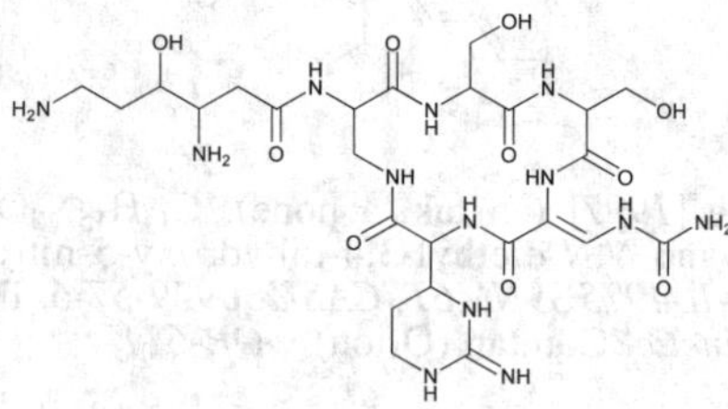

Enviradene [*1983*] (en vir′ a deen). $C_{19}H_{21}N_3O_2S$. 355.45. (1) 1*H*-Benzimidazol-2-amine, 1-[(1-methylethyl)sulfonyl]-6-(1-phenyl-1-propenyl)-, (*E*)-; (2) (*E*)-2-Amino-1-(isopropylsulfonyl)-6-(1-phenylpropenyl)benzimidazole. *UNII-9Q79A81839. CAS-80883-55-2.* INN. *Antiviral.* ◇*LY 127123*

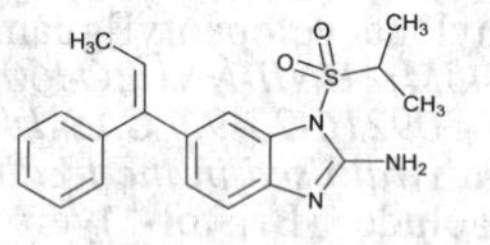

Enviroxime [*1980*] (en″ vir ox′ eem). $C_{17}H_{18}N_4O_3S$. 358.41. (1) 1*H*-Benzimidazol-2-amine, 6-[(hydroxyimino)phenylmethyl]-1-[(1-methylethyl)sulfonyl]-, (*E*)-; (2) (*E*)-2-Amino-6-benzoyl-1-(isopropylsulfonyl)benzimidazole oxime. *CAS-72301-79-2.* INN. *Antiviral.* ◇*LY 122772*

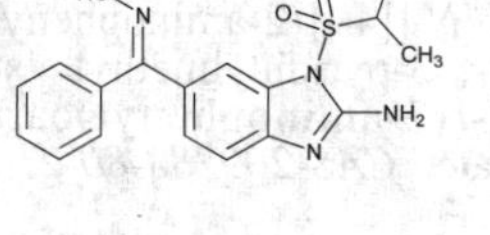

Enzacamene [*1999*] (en″ za kam′ een). USP. $C_{18}H_{22}O$. 254.37. (1) Bicyclo[2.2.1]heptan-2-one, 1,7,7-trimethyl-3-[(4-methylphenyl)methylene]-; (2) (±)-3-(*p*-Methylbenzylidene)camphor. *CAS-36861-47-9.* INN. *Sunscreen (ultraviolet light absorber).* Eusolex (Rona Laboratories, Great Britain); Neo Heliopan (Haarmann & Reimer, Germany) [*Note—The International Cosmetic Ingredient*

(ICNI) name for enzacamene is 4-methylbenzylidene camphor.] [Name previously used: Methyl Benzylidene Camphor.]

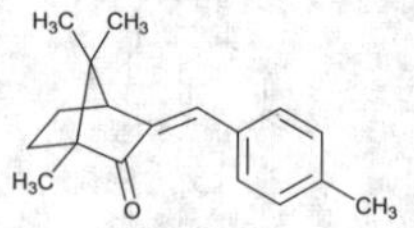

Enzastaurin Hydrochloride [*2003*] (en″ za staw′ rin hye″ droe klor′ ide). $C_{32}H_{29}N_5O_2 \cdot HCl$. 552.07. [Enzastaurin is INN.] (1) 1*H*-Pyrrole-2,5-dione, 3-(1-methyl-1*H*-indol-3-yl)-4-[1-[1-(2-pyridinylmethyl)-4-piperidinyl]-1*H*-indol-3-yl]-, monohydrochloride; (2) 3-(1-Methyl-1*H*-indol-3-yl)-4-[1-[1-(pyridin-2-ylmethyl)piperidin-4-yl]-1*H*-indol-3-yl]-1*H*-pyrrole-2,5-dione monohydrochloride. *UNII-KX7K68Z2UH. CAS-359017-79-1; CAS-170364-57-5* [enzastaurin]. *Antineoplastic (protein kinase C inhibitor).* ◇*LY317615*

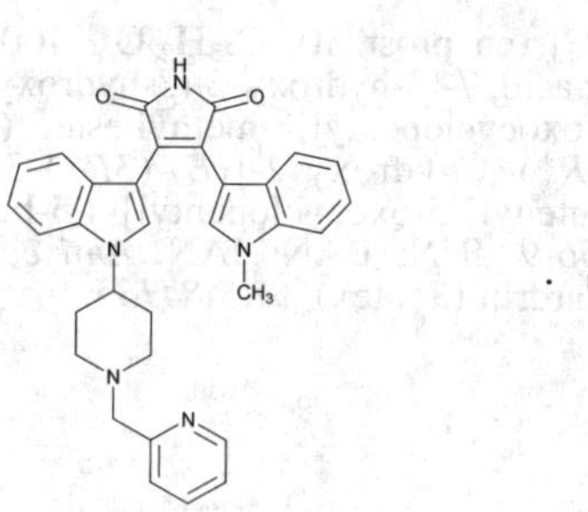

Epafipase [*1999*] (e paf′ i pase). $C_{2016}H_{3107}N_{545}O_{586}S_{14}$. (1) 6-400-Deacetylase, 1-alkyl-2-acetyllecithin (human); (2) 6-400-Deacetylase, 1-*O*-alkyl-2-acetyl-*sn*-glycero-3-phosphocholine (human). Molecular weight is approximately 44,799 daltons. *CAS-208576-22-1.* INN. *Antiallergenic; antiasthmatic (PAF antagonist [PAF acetylhydrolase]).* ◇*rPAF-AH*

AAASFGQTKI	PRGNGPYSVG	CTDLMFDHTN	KGTFLRLYYP	SQDNDRLDTL
WIPNKEYFWG	LSKFLGTHWL	MGNILRLLFG	SMTTPANWNS	PLRPGEKYPL
VVFSHGLGAF	RTLYSAIGID	LASHGFIVAA	VEHRDRSASA	TYYFKDQSAA
EIGDKSWLYL	RTLKQEEETH	IRNEQVRQRA	KECSQALSLI	LDIDHGKPVK
NALDLKFDME	QLKDSIDREK	IAVIGHSFGG	ATVIQTLSED	QRFRCGIALD
AWMFPLGDEV	YSRIPQPLFF	INSEYFQYPA	NIIKMKKCYS	PDKERKMITI
RGSVHQNFAD	FTFATGKIIG	HMLKLKGDID	SNVAIDLSNK	ASLAFLQKHL
GLHKDFDQWD	CLIEGDDENL	IPGTNINTTN	QHIMLQNSSG	IEKYN

Epalrestat. $C_{15}H_{13}NO_3S_2$. 319.40. 5-[(Z,E)-β-Methylcinnamylidene]-4-oxo-2-thioxo-3-thiazolidineacetic acid. *UNII-424DV0807X. CAS-82159-09-9.* INN; MI.

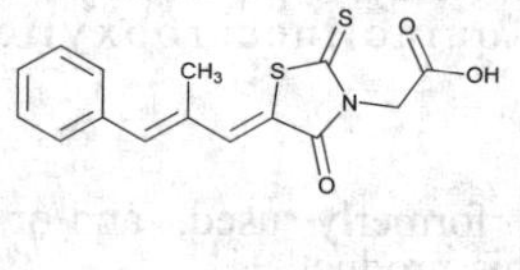

Epanolol [*1985*] (e pan′ oh lol). $C_{20}H_{23}N_3O_4$. 369.41. (±)-*N*-[2-[[3-(*o*-Cyanophenoxy)-2-hydroxypropyl]amino]ethyl]-2-(*p*-hydroxyphenyl)acetamide. *UNII-9KGC55KP6A*. *CAS-86880-51-5*. INN; BAN; MI. ◇*ICI 141,292*

Eperezolid [*1997*] (e″ per ez′ oh lid). $C_{18}H_{23}FN_4O_5$. 394.40. (1) Acetamide, *N*-[[3-[3-fluoro-4-[4-(hydroxyacetyl)-1-piperazinyl]phenyl]-2-oxo-5-oxazolidinyl]methyl]-, (*S*)-; (2) *N*-[[(*S*)-3-[3-fluoro-4-(4-glycoloyl-1-piperazinyl)phenyl]-2-oxo-5-oxazolidinyl]methyl]acetamide. *UNII-C460ZSU1OW*. *CAS-165800-04-4*. INN. *Antibacterial.* ◇*U-100,592*

Eperisone. $C_{17}H_{25}NO$. 259.39. [Eperisone Hydrochloride is JAN.] 4′-Ethyl-2-methyl-3-piperidinopropiophenone. *CAS-64840-90-0*. INN; MI.

Epervudine. $C_{12}H_{18}N_2O_5$. 270.28. 2′-Deoxy-5-isopropyluridine. *UNII-3G05PH9FAS*. *CAS-60136-25-6*. INN.

Epetirimod [*2007*] (e″ pe tir′ i mod). $C_{13}H_{15}N_5$. 241.29. (1) 1*H*-Imidazo[4,5-*c*][1,5]naphthyridin-4-amine, 1-(2-methylpropyl)-; (2) 1-(2-Methylpropyl)-1*H*-imidazo[4,5-*c*][1,5]naphthyridin-4-amine. *UNII-9P5MH9F521*. *CAS-227318-71-0*. INN. *Antiviral, antineoplastic.* ◇*851A; S-30563*

Epetirimod Esylate [*2008*] (e″ pe tir′ i mod es′ i late). $C_{13}H_{15}N_5 \cdot C_2H_6O_3S \cdot H_2O$. 369.44. (1) Ethanesulfonic acid, compd. with 1-(2-methylpropyl)-1*H*-imidazo[4,5-*c*][1,5]naphthyridin-4-amine, hydrate (1:1:1); (2) 1-(2-Methylpropyl)-1*H*-imidazo[4,5-*c*][1,5]naphthyridin-4-

amine monoethanesulfonate, monohydrate. *UNII-H92K6N217F*. *CAS-896444-34-1*. *Antiviral, antineoplastic.* ◇*851B; S-30563-35-65*

Ephedrine (e fed′ rin). **USP.** $C_{10}H_{15}NO$. 165.23. (1) Benzenemethanol, α-[1-(methylamino)ethyl]-, [*R*-(*R**,*S**)]-; (2) (-)-Ephedrine. *UNII-GN83C131XS*. *CAS-299-42-3* [(-)-ephedrine]; *CAS-50906-05-3* [hemihydrate]. BAN. *Bronchodilator.*

Ephedrine Hydrochloride (e fed′ rin hye″ droe klor′ ide). **USP.** $C_{10}H_{15}NO \cdot HCl$. 201.69. (1) Benzenemethanol, α-[1-(methylamino)ethyl]-, hydrochloride, [*R*-(*R**,*S**)]-; (2) (-)-Ephedrine hydrochloride. *UNII-NLJ6390P1Z*. *CAS-50-98-6* [(-)-ephedrine hydrochloride]; *CAS-299-42-3* [(-)-ephedrine]. BAN; JAN. *Bronchodilator.*

Ephedrine Sulfate (e fed′ rin sul′ fate). **USP.** $(C_{10}H_{15}NO)_2 \cdot H_2SO_4$. 428.54. [Ephedrine Sulphate is BAN.] (1) Benzenemethanol, α-[1-(methylamino)ethyl]-, [*R*-(*R**,*S**)]-, sulfate (2:1) (salt); (2) (-)-Ephedrine sulfate (2:1) (salt). *UNII-U6X61U5ZEG*. *CAS-134-72-5; CAS-299-42-3* [ephedrine]. *Adrenergic.* Isofedrol (Boehringer Mannheim GmbH, Germany)

Epicainide. $C_{21}H_{26}N_2O_2$. 338.44. *N*-[(1-Ethyl-2-pyrrolidinyl)methyl]benzilamide. *UNII-DZY7AR1B0U*. *CAS-66304-03-8*. INN.

Epicillin [*1970*] (ep i sil′ in). $C_{16}H_{21}N_3O_4S$. 351.42. (1) 4-Thia-1-azabicyclo[3.2.0]heptane-2-carboxylic acid, 6-[(amino-1,4-cyclohexadien-1-ylacetyl)amino]-3,3-dimethyl-7-oxo-, [2*S*-[2α,5α,6β(*S**)]]-; (2) 6-[D-2-Amino-2-(1,4-cyclohexadien-1-yl)acetamido]-3,3-dimethyl-7-oxo-4-thia-1-azabicyclo[3.2.0]heptane-2-carboxylic acid. *CAS-26774-90-3*. INN; BAN. *Antibacterial.* Dexacillin (Bristol-Myers Squibb†) ◇*SQ 11,302*

---

† Brand name formerly used, and/or firm no longer concerned with this product.

Epicriptine. $C_{32}H_{43}N_5O_5$. 577.71. 9,10α-Dihydro-13′-epi-β-ergocryptine. *UNII-5M64643B5U. CAS-88660-47-3.* INN.

Epidihydrocholesterin. $C_{27}H_{48}O$. 388.67. (3α,5α)-Cholestan-3-ol. *CAS-516-95-0.* JAN.

Epiestriol. $C_{18}H_{24}O_3$. 288.38. Estra-1,3,5(10)-triene-3,16β,17β-triol. *CAS-547-81-9.* INN; BAN; MI. *[Name previously used: Epioestriol.]*

Epilin — *See* Dietifen.

Epimestrol [*1969*] (ep″ i mes′ trol). $C_{19}H_{26}O_3$. 302.41. (1) Estra-1,3,5(10)-triene-16,17-diol, 3-methoxy-, (16α,17α)-; (2) 3-Methoxyestra-1,3,5(10)-triene-16α,17α-diol. *CAS-7004-98-0.* INN; BAN. *Anterior pituitary activator.* ◇*Org Org 817; NSC-55975*

Epinastine. $C_{16}H_{15}N_3$. 249.31. [Epinastine Hydrochloride is JAN.] 3-Amino-9,13b-dihydro-1*H*-dibenz[*c,f*]imidazo[1,5-*a*]azepine. *UNII-Q13WX941EF; UNII-GFM415S5XL* [epinastine hydrochloride]. *CAS-80012-43-7; CAS-80012-44-8* [hydrochloride]. INN.

Epinephrine (ep″ i nef′ rin). USP. $C_9H_{13}NO_3$. 183.20. [Adrenaline is BAN; Epinephrine Hydrochloride is JAN.] (1) 1,2-Benzenediol, 4-[1-hydroxy-2-(methylamino)ethyl]-, (*R*)-; (2) (-)-3,4-Dihydroxy-α-[(methylamino)methyl]benzyl alcohol. *UNII-YKH834O4BH. CAS-51-43-4.* INN; BAN; JAN. *Adrenergic (vasoconstrictor).* Epipen (Meridian); Adrenalin (King)

Epinephrine Bitartrate (ep″ i nef′ rin bye tar′ trate). USP. $C_9H_{13}NO_3 \cdot C_4H_6O_6$. 333.29. (1) 1,2-Benzenediol, 4-[1-hydroxy-2-(methylamino)ethyl]-, (*R*)-, [*R-(R**,*R**)]-2,3-dihydroxybutanedioate (1:1) (salt); (2) (-)-3,4-Dihydroxy-α-[(methylamino)methyl]benzyl alcohol (+)-tartrate (1:1) salt. *UNII-30Q7KI53AK; UNII-YKH834O4BH* [epinephr-

ine]. *CAS-51-42-3; CAS-51-43-4* [epinephrine]. JAN. *Adrenergic (ophthalmic).* Bronitin (Wyeth); Medihaler-epi (3M Pharmaceuticals)

Epinephryl Borate [*1964*] (ep″ i nef′ ril bore′ ate). USP [Ophthalmic Solution]. $C_9H_{12}BNO_4$. 209.01. (1) 1,3,2-Benzodioxaborole-5-methanol, 2-hydroxy-α-[(methylamino)methyl]-, (*R*)-; (2) (-)-3,4-Dihydroxy-α-[(methylamino)methyl]benzyl alcohol, cyclic 3,4-ester with boric acid. *CAS-5579-16-8. Adrenergic.* Epinal (Alcon); Eppy/N (Pilkington Barnes Hind)

Epioestriol (previously used name) — *See* Epiestriol.

Epipropidine [*1962*] (ep″ i proe′ pi deen). $C_{16}H_{28}N_2O_2$. 280.41. (1) 4,4′-Bipiperidine, 1,1′-bis(oxiranylmethyl)-; (2) 1,1′-Bis(2,3-epoxypropyl)-4,4′-bipiperidine. *UNII-T3RCY5OD7A. CAS-5696-17-3.* INN. *Antineoplastic.* ◇*28002; NSC-56308*

Epirizole [*1977*] (e pir′ i zole). $C_{11}H_{14}N_4O_2$. 234.25. (1) Pyrimidine, 4-methoxy-2-(5-methoxy-3-methyl-1*H*-pyrazol-1-yl)-6-methyl-; (2) 4-Methoxy-2-(5-methoxy-3-methylpyrazol-1-yl)-6-methylpyrimidine. *UNII-3B46O2FH8I. CAS-18694-40-1.* INN; JAN. *Analgesic; anti-inflammatory.* ◇*DA-398*

Epiroprim. $C_{19}H_{23}N_5O_2$. 353.42. 2,4-Diamino-5-(3,5-diethoxy-4-pyrrol-1-ylbenzyl)pyrimidine. *UNII-9G69D95443. CAS-73090-70-7.* INN.

Epirubicin Hydrochloride [*1984*] (ep″ i roo′ bi sin hye″ droe klor′ ide). $C_{27}H_{29}NO_{11} \cdot HCl$. 579.98. [Epirubicin is INN and BAN.] (1) 5,12-Naphthacenedione, 10-[(3-amino-2,3,6-trideoxy-α-L-*arabino*-hexopyranosyl)oxy]-7,8,9,10-tetrahydro-6,8,11-trihydroxy-8-(hydroxyacetyl)-1-methoxy-, hydrochloride, (8*S-cis*)-; (2) (1*S*,3*S*)-3-Glycoloyl-1,2,3,4,6,11-hexahydro-3,5,12-trihydroxy-10-methoxy-6,11-dioxo-1-naphthacenyl 3-amino-2,3,6-trideoxy-α-L-*arabino*-hexopyranoside hydrochloride. *UNII-

22966TX7J5; UNII-3Z8479ZZ5X [epirubicin]. *CAS-56390-09-1; CAS-56420-45-2* [epirubicin]. JAN. *Antineoplastic.* Ellence (Pfizer) ◇*IMI-28*

Epitetracycline Hydrochloride (ep″ i tet″ ra sye′ kleen hye″ droe klor′ ide). **USP.** $C_{22}H_{24}N_2O_8.HCl$. 480.90. (1) 2-Naphthacenecarboxamide, 4-(dimethylamino)-1,4,4a,5,5a,6,11,12a-octahydro-3,6,10,12,12a-pentahydroxy-6-methyl-1,11-dioxo-, monohydrochloride, [4*R*-(4α,4aβ,5aβ,6α,12aβ)]-; (2) (4*R*,4a*S*,5a*S*,6*S*,12a*S*)-4-(Dimethylamino)-1,4,4a,5,5a,6,11,12a-octahydro-3,6,10,12,12a-pentahydroxy-6-methyl-1,11-dioxo-2-naphthacenecarboxamide monohydrochloride. *CAS-23313-80-6. Antibacterial.*

Epithioandrostanol — *See* Epitiostanol.

Epitiostanol. $C_{19}H_{30}OS$. 306.51. 2α,3α-Epithio-5α-andro-stan-17β-ol. *CAS-2363-58-8.* INN; JAN; MI. ◇*10275-S*

Epitizide (INN, BAN) — *See* Epithiazide.

Epitumomab Cituxetan. Conjugate of 4-{(2*RS*)-2-[bis(carboxymethyl)amino]-3-({2-[bis(carboxymethyl)amino]ethyl}(carboxymethyl)amino)propyl}phe-nyl isothiocyanate forming a thiourea with the 6-amino of a lysine of immunoglobulin G1, anti-(human episialin) (mouse monoclonal HMFG-1 γ1-chain), disulfide with mouse monoclonal HMFG-1 light chain, dimer. *CAS-263547-71-3.* INN; BAN.

Epithiazide [*1962*] (ep″ i thye′ a zide). $C_{10}H_{11}ClF_3N_3O_4S_3$. 425.86. [Epitizide is INN and BAN.] (1) 2*H*-1,2,4-Benzothiadiazine-7-sulfonamide, 6-chloro-3,4-dihydro-3-[[(2,2,2-trifluoroethyl)thio]methyl]-, 1,1-dioxide; (2) 6-Chloro-3,4-dihydro-3{[(2,2,2-trifluoroethyl)thio]methyl}-2*H*-1,2,4-benzothiadiazine-7-sulfonamide 1,1-dioxide. *UNII-5B266B85J1. CAS-1764-85-8. Antihypertensive; diuretic.* ◇*P-2105; NSC-108164*

---

† Brand name formerly used, and/or firm no longer concerned with this product.

Eplerenone [*1997*] (e pler′ en one). $C_{24}H_{30}O_6$. 414.49. (1) Pregn-4-ene-7,21-dicarboxylic acid, 9,11-epoxy-17-hydroxy-3-oxo-, γ-lactone, methyl ester, (7α,11α,17α)-; (2) 9,11α-Epoxy-17-hydroxy-3-oxo-17α-pregn-4-ene-7α,21-dicarboxylic acid, γ-lactone, methyl ester. *UNII-6995V82D0B. CAS-107724-20-9.* INN. *Antihypertensive; aldosterone antagonist.* Inspra (Pfizer) ◇*SC-66110*

Eplivanserin. $C_{19}H_{21}FN_2O_2$. 328.38. (*E*)-2′-Fluoro-4-hydroxychalcone (*Z*)-*O*-[2-(dimethylamino)ethyl]oxime. *UNII-3CO94WO6DJ. CAS-130579-75-8.* INN; BAN.

Epoetin Alfa [*1990*] (e poe′ e tin al′ fa). $C_{809}H_{1301}N_{229}O_{240}S_5$ (amino acid sequence). 18,236.06. A 165 amino acid glycoprotein (approximately 62% protein and 38% carbohydrate by weight; total molecular weight of about 30,000 daltons) that regulates red blood cell production. Epoetin Alfa is produced by Chinese hamster ovary cells into which the human erythropoietin gene has been inserted. (1) 1-165-Erythropoietin (human clone λHEPOFL13 protein moiety), glycoform α; (2) 1-165-Erythropoietin (human clone λHEPOFL13 protein moiety), glycoform α. *UNII-64FS3BFH5W. CAS-113427-24-0.* INN; BAN; JAN. *Anti-anemic; hematinic.* Epogen (Amgen); Procrit (Ortho Biotech) ◇*EPO*

```
APPRLICDSR VLERYLLEAK EAENITTGCA EHCSLNENIT VPDTKVNFYA
WKRMEVGQQA VEVWQGLALL SEAVLRGQAL LVNSSQPWEP LQLHVDKAVS
GLRSLTTLLR ALGAQKEAIS PPDAASAAPL RTITADTFRK LFRVYSNFLR
GKLKLYTGEA CRTGD
```

Epoetin Beta [*1990*] (e poe′ e tin bay″ ta). $C_{809}H_{1301}N_{229}O_{240}S_5$ (amino acid sequence). 18,236.06. A 165 amino acid glycoprotein (approximately 62% protein and 38% carbohydrate by weight; total molecular weight of about 30,000 daltons) that regulates red blood cell production. Epoetin Beta is produced by the Chinese hamster ovary DN2-323 recombinant cell line. (1) 1-165-Erythropoietin (human clone λHEPOFL13 protein moiety) glycoform β; (2) 1-165-Erythropoietin (human clone λHEPOFL13 protein moiety), glycoform β. *UNII-64FS3BFH5W. CAS-122312-54-3.* INN; BAN; JAN. *Anti-anemic; hematinic.* Marogen (Chugai Pharmaceutical Co., Ltd., Japan) ◇*EPOCH; BM 06.019*

Epoetin Delta [*2001*] (e poe′ e tin del′ ta). $C_{809}H_{1301}N_{229}O_{240}S_5$. 1-165-Erythropoietin (human HMR4396), glycoform δ. Molecular weight is approximately 26,000 to 32,000 daltons (by MALDI-TOF analysis). *UNII-64FS3BFH5W. CAS-261356-80-3.* INN. *Treatment of anemia associated with chronic renal failure.* Dynepo (pending) (Aventis) ◇*HMR4396; GA-EPO*

```
APPRLICDSR VLERYLLEAK EAENITTGCA EHCSLNENIT VPDTKVNFYA
WKRMEVGQQA VEVWQGLALL SEAVLRGQAL LVNSSQPWEP LQLHVDKAVS
GLRSLTTLLR ALGAQKEAIS PPDAASAAPL RTITADTFRK LFRVYSNFLR
GKLKLYTGEA CRTGD
```

Epoetin Epsilon. $C_{809}H_{1301}N_{229}O_{240}S_5$. 18,235.72. 1-165-Erythropoietin (human clone λHEPOFL 13 protein moiety), glycoform ε. *UNII-64FS3BFH5W. CAS-154725-65-2.* INN.

Epoetin Gamma. $C_{809}H_{1301}N_{229}O_{240}S_5$ (for non-glycosylated protein). 18,235.72. 1-165-Erythropoietin (human clone λHEPOFL13 protein moiety), glycoform γ. *UNII-64FS3BFH5W. CAS-130455-76-4.* INN; BAN.

Epoetin Kappa. $C_{809}H_{1301}N_{229}O_{240}S_5$. 1-165-Erythropoietin (human JR-013), glycoform κ. *CAS-879555-13-2.* INN.

Epoetin Omega. $C_{809}H_{1301}N_{229}O_{240}S_5$. 18,235.72. 1-165-Erythropoietin (human clone λHEPOFL13 protein moiety), glycoform ω. *UNII-64FS3BFH5W. CAS-148363-16-0.* INN.

Epoetin Theta. $C_{809}H_{1301}N_{229}O_{240}S_5$. Human erythropoietin-(1-165)-peptide, glycoform ϑ. *CAS-762263-14-9.* INN.

Epoetin Zeta. $C_{809}H_{1301}N_{229}O_{240}S_5$. 1-165-Erythropoietin (human clone B03XA01), glycoform ζ. *CAS-604802-70-2.* INN.

Epoprostenol [*1979*] (e″ poe prost′ e nol). $C_{20}H_{32}O_5$. 352.47. (1) Prosta-5,13-dien-1-oic acid, 6,9-epoxy-11,15-dihydroxy-, (5Z,9α,11α,13E,15S)-; (2) (Z)-(3aR,4R,5R,6aS)-Hexahydro-5-hydroxy-4-[(E)-(3S)-3-hydroxy-1-octenyl]-2H-cyclopenta[b]furan-$\Delta^{2,\Delta}$-valeric acid. *UNII-DCR9Z582X0. CAS-35121-78-9.* INN. *Inhibitor (platelet).* [*Names previously used: Prostacyclin, PGI₂, Prostaglandin I₂, Prostaglandin X, PGX*] ◇*U-53,217*

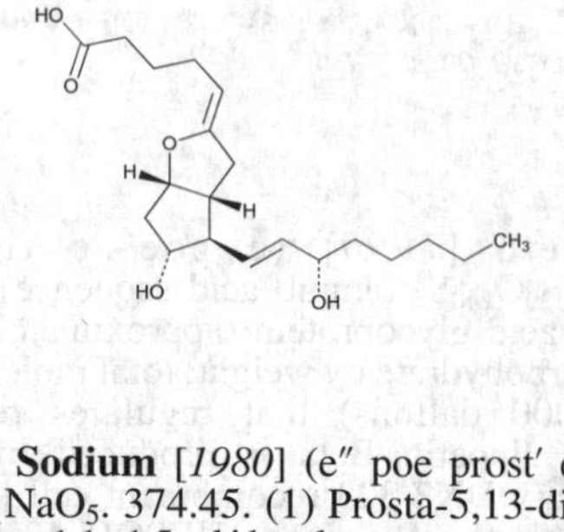

Epoprostenol Sodium [*1980*] (e″ poe prost′ e nol soe′ dee um). $C_{20}H_{31}NaO_5$. 374.45. (1) Prosta-5,13-dien-1-oic acid, 6,9-epoxy-11,15-dihydroxy-, sodium salt, (5Z,9α,11α,13E,15S)-; (2) Sodium (Z)-(3aR,4R,5R,6aS)-hexahydro-5-hydroxy-4-[(E)-(3S)-3-hydroxy-1-octenyl]-2H-cyclopenta[b]furan-$\Delta^{2,\Delta}$-valerate. *UNII-4K04IQ1OF4; UNII-DCR9Z582X0* [epoprostenol]. *CAS-61849-14-7; CAS-35121-78-9* [epoprostenol]. BAN. *Inhibitor (platelet).* Flolan (GlaxoSmithKline) ◇*U-53,217A*

Epostane [*1984*] (e′ poe stane). $C_{22}H_{31}NO_3$. 357.49. (1) Androst-2-ene-2-carbonitrile, 4,5-epoxy-3,17-dihydroxy-4,17-dimethyl-, (4α,5α,17β)-; (2) 4α,5-Epoxy-3,17β-dihy-droxy-4,17-dimethyl-5α-androst-2-ene-2-carbonitrile. *UNII-6375T36951. CAS-80471-63-2.* INN; BAN. *Interceptive.* ◇*Win 32,729*

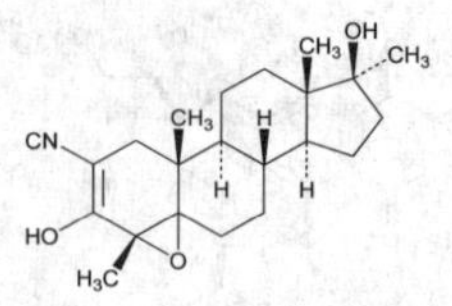

Epoxytropine Tropate Methylbromide — *See* Methscopolamine Bromide.

Epratuzumab [*1999*] (e″ pra tooz′ oo mab). (1) Immunoglobulin G, anti-(human CD22 (antigen)) (human-mouse monoclonal IMMU-hLL2 γ-chain), disulfide with human-mouse monoclonal IMMU-hLL2 κ-chain, dimer; (2) Immunoglobulin G (human-mouse monoclonal IMMU-hLL2 γ-chain anti-human antigen CD22), disulfide with human-mouse monoclonal IMMU-hLL2 κ-chain, dimer. Molecular weight is approximately 150,000 daltons. *CAS-205923-57-5.* INN. *Treatment of non-Hodgkin's B-cell lymphomas (monoclonal antibody).* Lymphocide (Immunomedics) ◇*IMMU-hLL2*

Eprazinone. $C_{24}H_{32}N_2O_2$. 380.52. [Eprazinone Hydrochloride is JAN.] 3-[4-(β-Ethoxyphenethyl)-1-piperazinyl]-2-methylpropiophenone. *UNII-883YNL63WU. CAS-10402-90-1.* INN; DCF; MI.

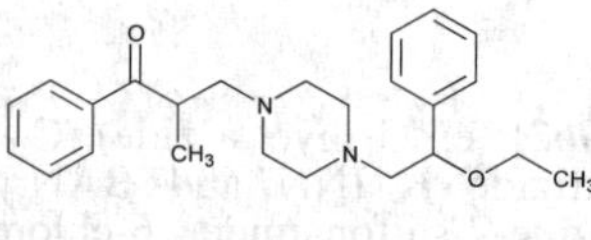

Eprinomectin [*1995*] (e prin″ oh mek′ tin). A mixture of two components having a ratio of 90% or more of Eprinomectin Component B_{1a} and 10% or less of Eprinomectin Component B_{1b}. *CAS-123997-26-2; CAS-133305-88-1* [component B_{1a}]; *CAS-133305-89-2* [component B_{1b}]. INN. *Antiparasitic (veterinary).* Eprinex [Veterinary] (Merial) ◇*MK-397*

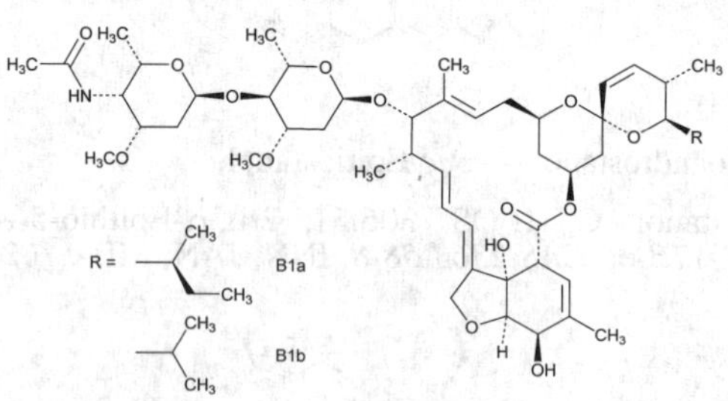

Eprinomectin Component B_{1a}. $C_{50}H_{75}NO_{14}$. 914.13. Component of Eprinomectin. (1) Avermectin A_{1a}, 4″-(acetylamino)-5-O-demethyl-4″-deoxy-, (4″R)-; (2) (2aE,4E,5′S,6S,6′R,7S,8E,11R,13S,15S,17aR,20R,20aR,20bS)-6′-(S)-sec-Butyl-5′,6,6′,7,10,11,14,15,17a,20,20a,20b-dodecahydro-20,20b-dihydroxy-5′,6,8,19-tetramethyl-17-oxo-spiro[11,15-methano-2H,13H,17H-furo[4,3,2-pq][2,6]benzodioxa-cyclooctadecin-13,2′-[2H]pyran]-7-yl-4-O-(4-acetamido-2,4,6-trideoxy-3-O-methyl-α-L-lyxo-hexopyranosyl)-2,6-dideoxy-3-O-methyl-α-L-arabino-hexopyranoside. *CAS-133305-88-1.*

Eprinomectin Component B_{1b}. $C_{49}H_{73}NO_{14}$. 900.10. Component of Eprinomectin. (1) Avermectin A_{1a}, 4″-(acetylamino)-5-O-demethyl-25-de(1-methylpropyl)-4″-deoxy-25-(1-methylethyl)-, (4″R)-; (2) (2aE,4E,5′S,6S,6′R,7S,8E,11R,13S,15S,17aR,20R,20aR,20bS)-5′,6,6′,7,10,11,14,15,17a,20,20a,20b-Dodecahydro-20,20b-dihydroxy-6′-isopropyl-

5′,6,8,19-tetramethyl-17-oxospiro[11,15-methano-2*H*,13*H*,17*H*-furo[4,3,2-*pq*][2,6]benzodioxacyclooctadecin-13,2′-[2*H*]pyran]-7-yl 4-*O*-(4-acetamido-2,4,6-trideoxy-3-*O*-methyl-α-L-*lyxo*-hexopyranosyl)-2,6-dideoxy-3-*O*-methyl-α-L-*arabino*-hexopyranoside. *CAS-133305-89-2.*

Epristeride [*1992*] (e pris′ ter ide). $C_{25}H_{37}NO_3$. 399.57. (1) Androsta-3,5-diene-3-carboxylic acid, 17-[[(1,1-dimethylethyl)amino]carbonyl]-, (17β)-; (2) 17β-(*tert*-Butylcarbamoyl)androsta-3,5-diene-3-carboxylic acid. *UNII-39517A04PS. CAS-119169-78-7.* INN; BAN. *Inhibitor (alpha reductase).* ◇*SK&F 105657*

Eprobemide. $C_{14}H_{19}ClN_2O_2$. 282.77. *p*-Chloro-*N*-(3-morpholinopropyl)benzamide. *UNII-URX5F7RDER. CAS-87940-60-1.* INN.

Eprodisate Disodium [*2005*] (e proe′ di sate dye soe′ dee um). $C_3H_6Na_2O_6S_2$. 248.19. [Eprodisate is INN.] (1) 1,3-Propanedisulfonic acid, disodium salt; (2) Disodium propane-1,3-disulfonate. *UNII-5X0D9H16IU. CAS-36589-58-9; CAS-21668-77-9* [eprodisate]. *Treatment of secondary (AA) amyloidosis.* ◇*NC-503*

Eprosartan [*1994*] (ep″ roe sar′ tan). $C_{23}H_{24}N_2O_4S$. 424.51. (1) 2-Thiophenepropanoic acid, α-[[2-butyl-1-[(4-carboxyphenyl)methyl]-1*H*-imidazol-5-yl]methylene]-, (*E*)-; (2) (*E*)-2-Butyl-1-(*p*-carboxybenzyl)-α-2-thenylimidazole-5-acrylic acid. *UNII-2KH13Z0S0Y. CAS-133040-01-4.* INN; BAN. *Antihypertensive.* ◇*SK&F 108566*

Eprosartan Mesylate [*1994*] (ep″ roe sar′ tan mes′ i late). $C_{23}H_{24}N_2O_4S\cdot CH_4O_3S$. 520.62. (1) 2-Thiophenepropanoic acid, α-[[2-butyl-1-[(4-carboxyphenyl)methyl]-1*H*-imidazol-5-yl]methylene]-, (*E*)-, monomethanesulfonate; (2) (*E*)-2-Butyl-1-(*p*-carboxybenzyl)-α-2-thenylimidazole-5-

---

† Brand name formerly used, and/or firm no longer concerned with this product.

acrylic acid, monomethanesulfonate. *UNII-8N2L1NX8S3. CAS-144143-96-4.* BAN. *Antihypertensive.* Teveten (Abbott) ◇*SK&F 108566-J*

Eprotirome. $C_{18}H_{17}Br_2NO_5$. 487.14. 3-({3,5-Dibromo-4-[4-hydroxy-3-(propan-2-yl)phenoxy]phenyl}amino)-3-oxopropanoic acid. *CAS-355129-15-6.* INN.

Eprovafen. $C_{18}H_{22}O_2S$. 302.43. 5-(3-Phenylpropyl)-2-thiophenevaleric acid. *UNII-4C9310B127. CAS-101335-99-3.* INN.

Eproxindine. $C_{23}H_{29}N_3O_3$. 395.49. (±)-*N*-[3-(Diethylamino)-2-hydroxypropyl]-3-methoxy-1-phenylindole-2-carboxamide. *CAS-83200-08-2.* INN.

Eprozinol. $C_{22}H_{30}N_2O_2$. 354.49. 4-(β-Methoxyphenethyl)-α-phenyl-1-piperazinepropanol. *UNII-IJ21AK8IVJ. CAS-32665-36-4.* INN; DCF; MI.

Epsiprantel. $C_{20}H_{26}N_2O_2$. 326.43. (±)-2-(Cyclohexylcarbonyl)-2,3,6,7,8,12b-hexahydropyrazino[2,1-*a*][2]benzazepin-4(1*H*)-one. *UNII-0C1SPQ0FSR. CAS-98123-83-2.* INN; BAN. Cestex (SmithKline Beecham Animal Health) ◇*BRL 38705*

Epsom Salt — *See* Magnesium Sulfate.

Eptacog Alfa. $C_{1982}H_{3054}N_{560}O_{618}S_{28}$. 45,512.71. [Eptacog Alfa (Activated) is BAN.] Blood-coagulation factor VII (human clone λHVII2463 protein moiety). *CAS-102786-61-8.* INN.

Eptaloprost. $C_{24}H_{34}O_5$. 402.52. 4-[2-[(2E,3aS,4S,5R,6aS)-Hexahydro-5-hydroxy-4-[(3S,4S)-3-hydroxy-4-methyl-1,6-nonadiynyl]-2(1H)-pentalenylidene]ethoxy]butyric acid. *UNII-93X6A56W84. CAS-90693-76-8.* INN.

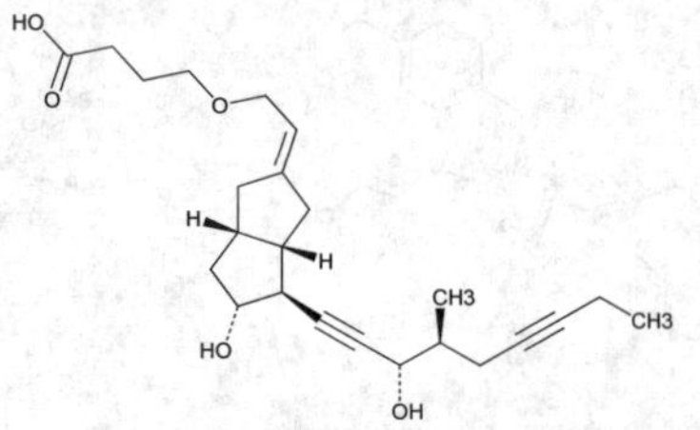

Eptamestrol — *See* Etamestrol.

Eptapirone. $C_{16}H_{23}N_7O_2$. 345.40. 4-Methyl-2-[4-[4-(2-pyrimidinyl)-1-piperazinyl]butyl]-*as*-triazine-3,5(2H,4H)-dione. *UNII-3M824XRO8N. CAS-179756-85-5.* INN.

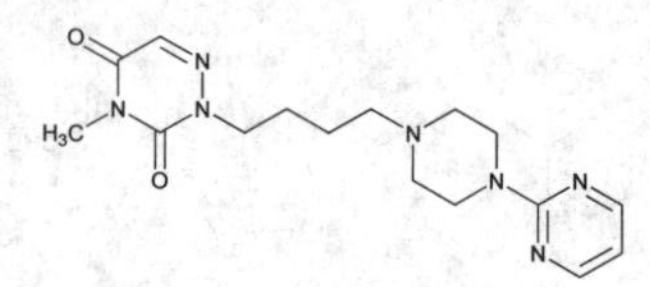

Eptaplatin. $C_{11}H_{20}N_2O_6Pt$. 471.37. *cis*-[(4R,5R)-2-Isopropyl-1,3-dioxolane-4,5-bis(methylamine)-N,N'][malonato(2-)-O,O']platinum. *CAS-146665-77-2.* INN.

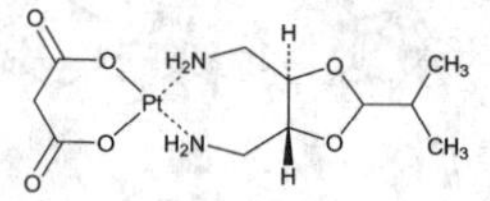

Eptaprost — *See* Eptaloprost.

Eptastatin Sodium — *See* Pravastatin Sodium.

Eptastigmine. $C_{21}H_{33}N_3O_2$. 359.51. *N*-Demethyl-*N*-heptylphysostigmine. *UNII-6PZZ52D76Q. CAS-101246-68-8.* INN.

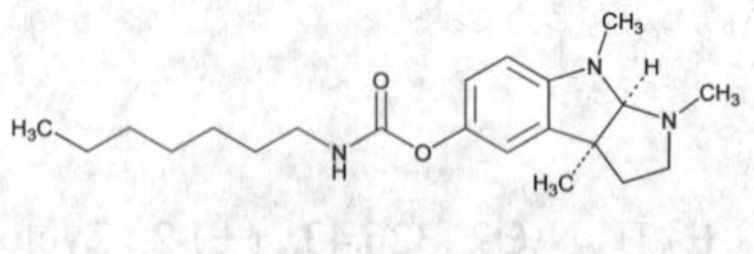

Eptazocine. $C_{15}H_{21}NO$. 231.33. [Eptazocine Hydrobromide is JAN.] (-)-(1S,6S)-2,3,4,5,6,7-Hexahydro-1,4-dimethyl-1,6-methano-1H-4-benzazonin-10-ol. *UNII-2208ZLI77S. CAS-72522-13-5.* INN; MI.

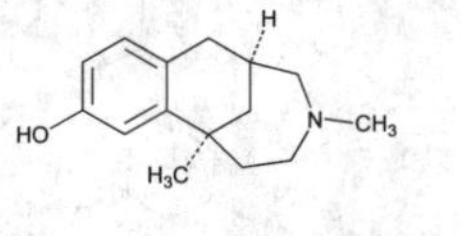

Eptifibatide. $C_{35}H_{49}N_{11}O_9S_2$. 831.96. N^6-Amidino-N^2-(3-mercaptopropionyl)-L-lysylglycyl-L-α-aspartyl-L-tryptophyl-L-prolyl-L-cysteinamide, cyclic(1-6)-disulfide. *UNII-NA8320J834. CAS-148031-34-9.* INN; BAN. *Integrilin* (Schering)

Eptotermin Alfa. $[C_{683}H_{1061}N_{197}O_{208}S_{10}]_2$. Human recombinant bone morphogenetic protein 7 (hrBMP-7) or osteogenic protein-1 (OP-1). *CAS-129805-33-0.* INN.

Equilin (ek' wi lin). **USP.** $C_{18}H_{20}O_2$. 268.35. (1) Estra-1,3,5(10),7-tetraen-17-one, 3-hydroxy-; (2) 3-Hydroxyestra-1,3,5(10),7-tetraen-17-one. *CAS-474-86-2. Estrogen.*

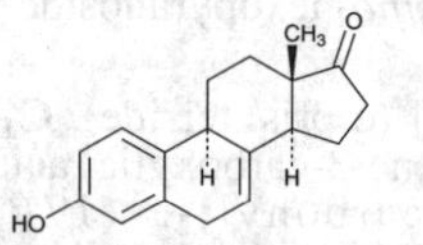

Erbulozole [*1991*] (er bue' loe zole). $C_{24}H_{27}N_3O_5S$. 469.55. (1) Carbamic acid, [4-[[[2-(1H-imidazol-1-ylmethyl)-2-(4-methoxyphenyl)-1,3-dioxolan-4-yl]methyl]thio]phenyl]-, ethyl ester, *cis*-(±)-; (2) Ethyl (±)-*cis*-*p*-[[[2-(imidazol-1-ylmethyl)-2-(*p*-methoxyphenyl)-1,3-dioxolan-4-yl]methyl]thio]carbanilate. *UNII-78XGN2K5RX. CAS-124784-31-2.* INN; BAN. *Antineoplastic (adjunct).* ◇R 55104

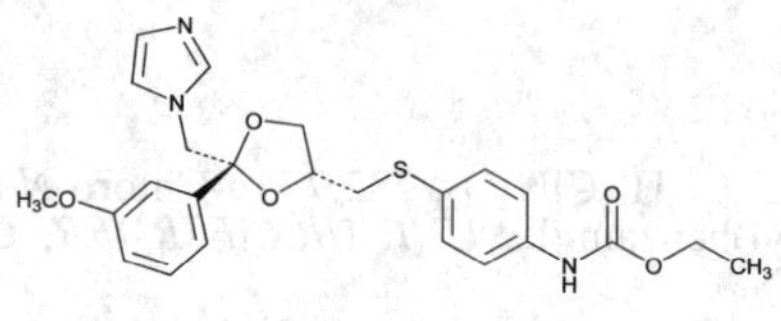

Erdosteine. $C_8H_{11}NO_4S_2$. 249.31. (±)-[[[(Tetrahydro-2-oxo-3-thienyl)carbamoyl]methyl]thio]acetic acid. *UNII-76J0853EKA. CAS-84611-23-4.* INN.

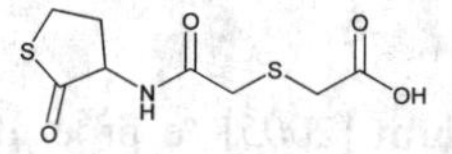

Ergocalciferol (er″ goe kal sif' er ol). **USP.** $C_{28}H_{44}O$. 396.65. (1) 9,10-Secoergosta-5,7,10(19),22-tetraen-3-ol, (3β,5Z,7E,22E)-; (2) Ergocalciferol. *UNII-VS041H42XC. CAS-50-14-6.* INN; BAN; JAN. *Vitamin (antirachitic).* Deltalin (Lilly); Drisdol (Sanofi Aventis) *[Names previously used: Oleovitamin D, Synthetic; Calciferol.]*

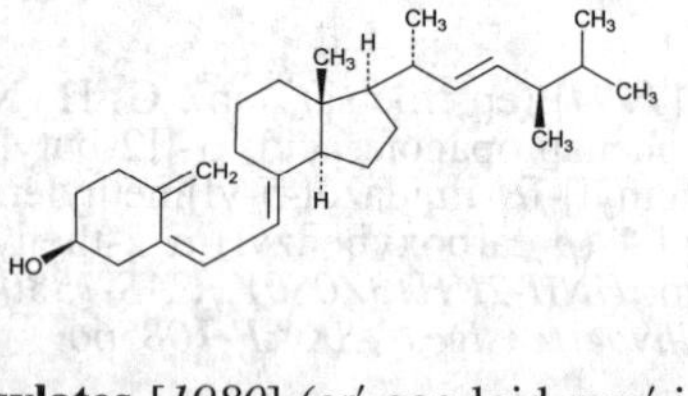

Ergoloid Mesylates [*1980*] (er' goe loid mes' i lates). **USP.** $C_{31}H_{41}N_5O_5 \cdot CH_4O_3S$ (dihydroergocornine mesylate). 659.79; $C_{35}H_{41}N_5O_5 \cdot CH_4O_3S$ (dihydroergocristine mesylate). 707.84; $C_{32}H_{43}N_5O_5 \cdot CH_4O_3S$ (dihydro-α-ergocryptine mesylate). 673.82; $C_{32}H_{43}N_5O_5 \cdot CH_4O_3S$ (dihydro-β-ergocryptine mesylate). 673.82. [Codergocrine Mesilate is BAN; Dihydroergotoxine Mesilate is JAN.] (1) Ergotaman-3′,6′,18-trione, 9,10-dihydro-12′-hydroxy-2′,5′-bis(1-methylethyl)-, (5′α,10α)-, monomethanesulfonate (salt) mixture with 9,10α-dihydro-12′-hydroxy-2′-(1-methylethyl)-5′α-(phenylmethyl)ergotaman-3′,6′,18-trione monomethanesulfonate (salt), 9,10α-dihydro-12′-hydroxy-2′-(1-methylethyl)-5′α-(2-methylpropyl)ergotaman-3′,6′,18-trione monomethanesulfonate (salt), and 9,10α-dihydro-12′-hydroxy-2′-(1-methylethyl)-5′α-(1-methylpropyl)ergotaman-3′,6′,18-trione monomethanesulfonate (salt); (2) Dihydroergotoxine monomethanesulfonate (salt); (3) An equiproportional mixture of dihydroergocornine mesylate, dihydroergocristine mesylate, and ratio of dihydro-α-ergocryptine mesylate to dihydro-β-ergocryptine mesylate is 1.5-2.5:1. *UNII-X3S33EX3KW. CAS-8067-24-1; CAS-11032-41-0* [dihydroergotoxine]. *Cognition adjuvant.* Alkergot (Sandoz); Circanol (3M Pharmaceuticals); Deapril (Bristol-Myers Squibb); Gerimal (Watson); Hydergine (Novartis) *[Names previously used: Dihydroergotoxine Mesylate; Dihydroergotoxine Methanesulfonate; Dihydrogenated Ergot Alkaloids; Hydrogenated Ergot Alkaloids.]*

Dihydroergocomine

Dihydroergocristine

Dihydro-alpha-ergocryptine

Dihydro-beta-ergocryptine

Ergometrine (INN, BAN) — *See* Ergonovine Maleate.

Ergometrine Maleate (JAN) — *See* Ergonovine Maleate.

Ergonovine Maleate (er″ goe noe′ veen mal′ ee ate). **USP.** $C_{19}H_{23}N_3O_2.C_4H_4O_4$. 441.48. [Ergometrine is INN and BAN; Ergometrine Maleate is JAN.] (1) Ergoline-8-carboxamide, 9,10-didehydro-*N*-(2-hydroxy-1-methylethyl)-6-methyl-, [8β(*S*)]-, (*Z*)-2-butenedioate (1:1) (salt); (2) 9,10-Didehydro-*N*-[(*S*)-2-hydroxy-1-methylethyl]-6-methylergoline-8β-carboxamide maleate (1:1) (salt). *UNII-YMH3D0ZJWV; UNII-WH41D8433D* [ergonovine]. *CAS-129-51-1; CAS-60-79-7* [ergonovine]. *Oxytocic.* Ergotrate Maleate (Lilly)

Ergotamine Tartrate (er got′ a meen tar′ trate). **USP.** $(C_{33}H_{35}N_5O_5)_2.C_4H_6O_6$. 1313.41. [Ergotamine is INN and BAN.] (1) Ergotaman-3′,6′,18-trione, 12′-hydroxy-2′-methyl-5′-(phenylmethyl)-, (5′α)-, [*R*-(*R**,*R**)]-2,3-dihydroxybutanedioate (2:1) (salt); (2) Ergotamine tartrate (2:1) (salt). *UNII-MRU5XH3B48; UNII-PR834Q503T* [ergotamine]. *CAS-379-79-3; CAS-113-15-5* [ergotamine]. JAN. *Analgesic (specific in migraine).* Ergostat (Pfizer); Wigrettes (Organon)

---

† Brand name formerly used, and/or firm no longer concerned with this product.

Eribaxaban [*2007*] (er″ i bax′ a ban). $C_{24}H_{22}ClFN_4O_4$. 484.91. (1) 1,2-Pyrrolidinedicarboxamide, N^1-(4-chlorophenyl)-N^2-[2-fluoro-4-(2-oxo-1(2*H*)-pyridinyl)phenyl]-4-methoxy-, (2*R*,4*R*)-; (2) (2*R*,4*R*)-N^1-(4-Chlorophenyl)-N^2-[2-fluoro-4-(2-oxopyridin-1(2*H*)-yl)phenyl]-4-methoxypyrrolidine-1,2-dicarboxamide. *UNII-5FCH6YDY7Z. CAS-536748-46-6.* INN. *Treatment and prevention of thromboembolic disorders.* ◇*PD 348,292*

Eribulin Mesylate [*2006*] (er″ i bue′ lin mes′ i late). $C_{40}H_{59}NO_{11}.CH_4O_3S$. 826.00. [Eribulin is INN.] (1) 11,15:18,21:24,28-Triepoxy-7,9-ethano-12,15-methano-9*H*,15*H*-furo[3,2-*i*]furo[2′,3′:5,6]pyrano[4,3-*b*][1,4]dioxacyclopentacosin-5(4*H*)-one, 2-[(2*S*)-3-amino-2-hydroxypropyl]hexacosahydro-3-methoxy-26-methyl-20,27-bis(methylene)-, (2*R*,3*R*,3a*S*,7*R*,8a*S*,9-*S*,10a*R*,11*S*,12*R*,13a*R*,13b*S*,15*S*,18*S*,21*S*,24*S*,26*R*,28-*R*,29a*S*)-, methanesulfonate (salt); (2) (2*R*,3*R*,3a*S*,7*R*,8a*S*,9*S*,10a*R*,11*S*,12-*R*,13a*R*,13b*S*,15*S*,18*S*,21*S*,24*S*,26*R*,28*R*,29a*S*)-2-[(2*S*)-3-Amino-2-hydroxypropyl]-3-methoxy-26-methyl-20,27-dimethylidenehexacosahydro-11,15:18,21:24,28-triepoxy-7,9-ethano-12,15-methano-9*H*,15*H*-furo[3,2-*i*]furo[2′,3′:5,6]pyrano[4,3-*b*][1,4]dioxacyclopentacosin-5(4*H*)-one methanesulfonate (salt). *UNII-AV9U0660CW. CAS-441045-17-6; CAS-253128-41-5* [eribulin]. *Antineoplastic.* ◇*E7389*

Ericolol. $C_{18}H_{24}ClNO_3$. 337.84. (±)-3-[2-[3-(*tert*-Butylamino)-2-hydroxypropoxy]-4-chlorophenyl]-2-cyclopenten-1-one. *UNII-38R2P4PIEI. CAS-85320-67-8.* INN.

Eriodictyon. *UNII-2Y7TIQ135H. CAS-8013-08-9.* NF XVI; MI.

Eritoran Tetrasodium [*2004*] (er″ i tor′ an tet″ ra soe′ dee um). $C_{66}H_{122}N_2Na_4O_{19}P_2$. 1401.58. [Eritoran is INN.] (1) α-D-Glucopyranose, 3-*O*-decyl-2-deoxy-6-*O*-[2-deoxy-3-*O*-[(3*R*)-3-methoxydecyl]-6-*O*-methyl-2-[[(11*Z*)-1-oxo-11-octadecenyl]amino]-4-*O*-phosphono-β-D-glucopyranosyl]-2-[(1,3-dioxotetradecyl)amino]-, 1-(dihydrogen phosphate), tetrasodium salt; (2) 3-*O*-Decyl-2-deoxy-6-*O*-[2-deoxy-3-*O*-[(3*R*)-3-methoxydecyl]-6-*O*-methyl-2-[(11*Z*)-octadec-11-enoylamino]-4-*O*-phosphonato-β-D-glucopyranosyl]-2-[(3-oxotetradecanoyl)amino]-α-D-glucopyranosyl tetrasodium phosphate. *CAS-185954-98-7; CAS-185955-*

34-4 [eritoran]. *Treatment of sepsis and other diseases due to reaction to bacterial endotoxin (endotoxin antagonist).* ◇*E5564; B1287*

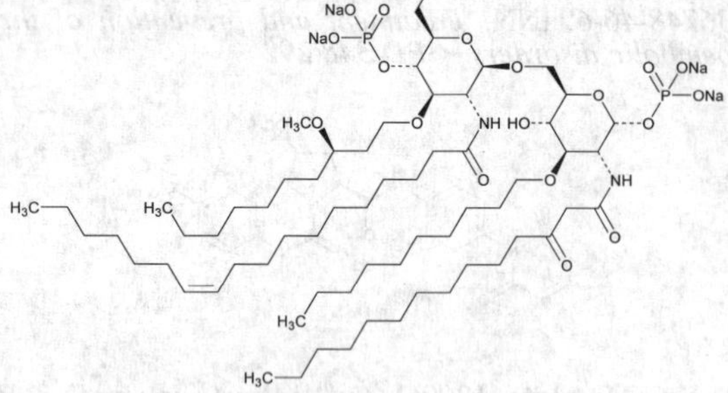

Eritrityl Tetranitrate (INN) — *See* Erythrityl Tetranitrate.

Erizepine. $C_{20}H_{22}N_2$. 290.40. 1,2,3,4,5,10-Hexahydro-3,10-dimethylazepino[4,5-*d*]dibenz[*b,f*]azepine. *UNII-7N7IQB45VO. CAS-96645-87-3.* INN.

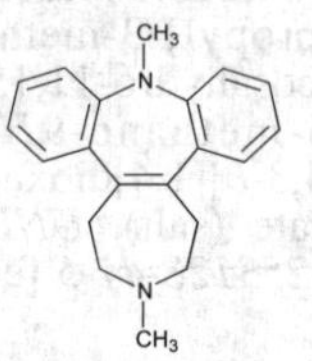

Erlizumab [*2000*] (er liz′ oo mab). (1) Immunoglobulin G1, anti-(human integrin *β*2) F(ab′)2 fragment (human-mouse monoclonal *γ*1-chain), disulfide with human-mouse monoclonal light chain, dimer; (2) Immunoglobulin G1 (human-mouse monoclonal F(ab′)₂ fragment *γ*1-chain anti-human antigen CD18), disulfide with human-mouse monoclonal light chain, dimer. Molecular weight is 98,598 daltons. *CAS-211323-03-4.* INN. *Adjunctive treatment to reperfusion therapy in acute myocardial infarction or other types of reperfusion therapy (monoclonal antibody).* ◇*rhuMAb CD18*

Erlosamide (previously used name) — *See* Lacosamide.

Erlotinib Hydrochloride [*2001*] (er loe′ ti nib hye″ droe klor′ ide). $C_{22}H_{23}N_3O_4$.HCl. 429.90. [Erlotinib is INN.] (1) 4-Quinazolinamine, *N*-(3-ethynylphenyl)-6,7-bis(2-methoxyethoxy)-, monohydrochloride; (2) 4-(*m*-Ethynylanilino)-6,7-bis(2-methoxyethoxy)quinazoline monohydrochloride. *UNII-DA87705X9K; UNII-J4T82NDH7E* [erlotinib]. *CAS-183319-69-9; CAS-183321-74-6* [erlotinib]. INN. *Treatment of proliferative neoplastic and malignant diseases, including multiple forms of solid tumors and psoriasis (inhibitor of epidermal growth factor receptor (EGFR; erb1) tyrosine kinase activity).* Tarceva (Genentech) ◇*CP-358,774-01; OSI-774*

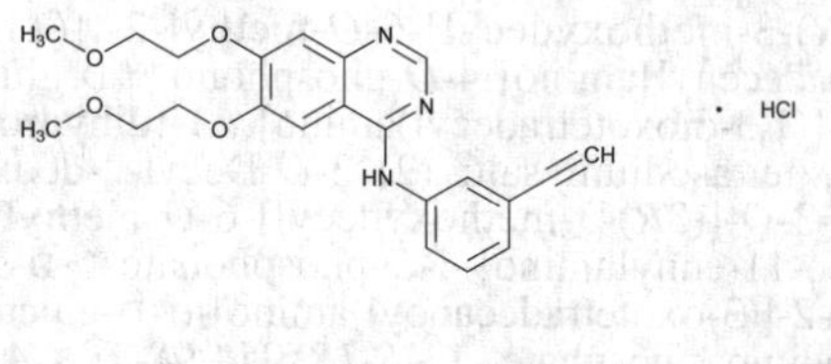

Erocainide. $C_{22}H_{33}ClN_2O$. 376.96. (*E*)-2-(*p*-Chlorobenzylidene)cyclohexanone (*E*)-*O*-[3-(diisopropylamino)propyl]oxime. *UNII-EJ9QI3Q1LT. CAS-85750-38-5.* INN.

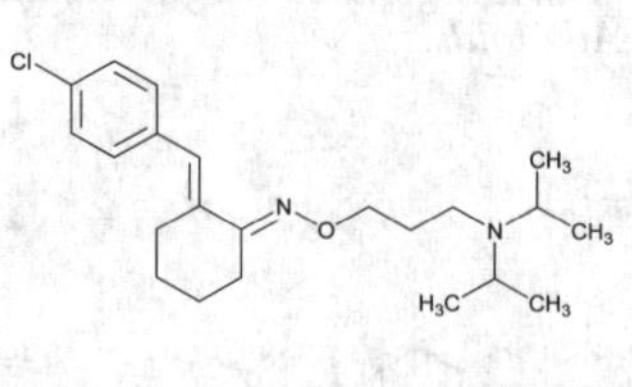

Ersentilide. $C_{21}H_{26}N_4O_5S$. 446.52. 4′-[(2*S*)-2-Hydroxy-3-[[2-(*p*-imidazol-1-ylphenoxy)ethyl]amino]propoxy]methanesulfonanilide. *UNII-L2JY6Z298S. CAS-125279-79-0.* INN.

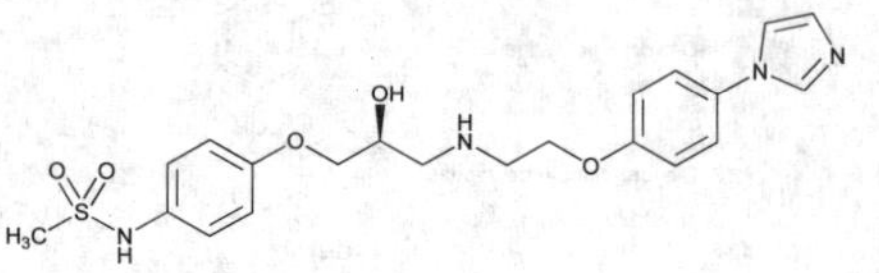

Ersofermin [*1992*] (er″ soe fer′ min). $C_{775}H_{1220}N_{220}O_{223}S_7$. 17,411.79 kD. Recombinant human basic fibroblast growth factor (bFGF) is an 157 amino acid, non-glycosylated protein isolated from human placenta and cloned and expressed in *E. coli.* (1) Fibroblast growth factor, basic (human clone *λ*KB7/*λ*HFL1 precursor reduced) *N*-(*N*-glycyl-L-threonyl)-; (2) *N*-(*N*-Glycyl-L-threonyl)basic fibroblast growth factor (human clone *λ*KB7/*λ*HFL1 precursor reduced). *CAS-111212-85-2.* INN. *Wound healing agent.* Trofak (Synergen) [*Note—Peptide maps have confirmed that there are four cysteines in the molecular backbone: two are disulfide bonded to exogenous cysteines (80 and 98).*]

```
GTMAAGSITT LPALPEDGGS GAFPPGHFKD PKRLYCKNGG FFLRIHPDGR
VDGVREKSDP HIKLQLQAEE RGVVSIKGVC ANRYLAMKED GRLLASKCVT
DECFFFERLE SNNYNTYRSR KYTSWYVALK RTGQYKLGSK TGPGQKAILF
LPMSAKS
```

Ertapenem Sodium [*2000*] (er″ ta pen′ em soe′ dee um). $C_{22}H_{24}N_3NaO_7S$. 497.50. [Ertapenem is INN and BAN.] (1) 1-Azabicyclo[3.2.0]hept-2-ene-2-carboxylic acid, 3-[[5-[[(3-carboxyphenyl)amino]carbonyl]-3-pyrrolidinyl]thio]-6-(1-hydroxyethyl)-4-methyl-7-oxo-, monosodium salt, [4*R*-[3(3*S**,5*S**), 4*α*,5*β*,6*β*(*R**)]]-; (2) (4*R*,5*S*,6*S*)-3-[[(3*S*,5*S*)-5-[(*m*-Carboxyphenyl)carbamoyl]-3-pyrrolidinyl]thio]-6-[(1*R*)-1-hydroxyethyl]-4-methyl-7-oxo-1-azabicyclo[3.2.0]hept-2-ene-2-carboxylic acid, monosodium salt. *UNII-2T90KE67L0; UNII-G32F6EID2H* [ertapenem]. *CAS-153832-38-3; CAS-153832-46-3* [ertapenem]. INN. *Antibacterial.* Invanz (Merck) ◇*MK-0826*

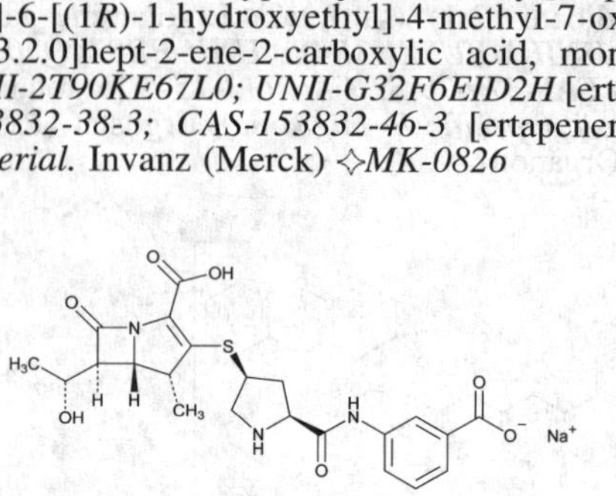

Ertiprotafib [*2002*] (er″ ti proe′ ta fib). $C_{31}H_{27}BrO_3S$. 559.51. (1) Benzenepropanoic acid, *α*-[4-(9-bromo-2,3-dimethylnaphtho[2,3-*b*]thien-4-yl)-2,6-dimethylphenoxy]-, (*αR*)-; (2) (2*R*)-2-[4-(9-Bromo-2,3-dimethylnaphtho[2,3-*b*]thiophen-4-yl)-2,6-dimethylphenoxy]-3-phenylpropionic acid.

UNII-5TPM2EB426. CAS-251303-04-5. INN. *Treatment of non-insulin dependent diabetes (protein tyrosine phosphatase 1B inhibitor).* ✧*PTP-112*

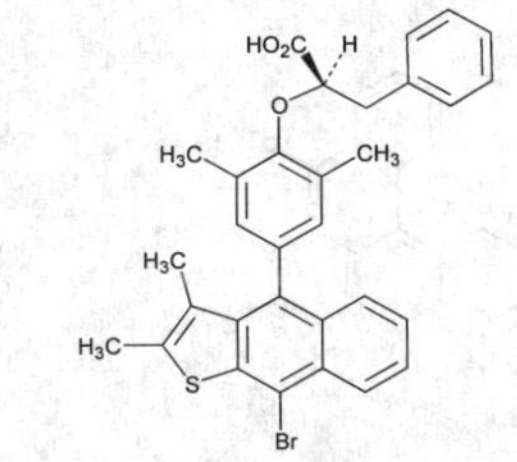

Ertumaxomab. Immunoglobulin G2a, anti-(human neu (receptor)) (mouse monoclonal 2502A/TP-A-02/TPBs03 heavy chain), disulfide with mouse monoclonal 2502A/TP-A-02/TPBs03 light chain, disulfide with immunoglobulin G2b anti-(human CD3 (antigen)) (rat monoclonal 26/II/6-1.2/TPBs03 heavy chain), bidisulfide with rat monoclonal 26/II/6-1.2/TPBs03 light chain. *CAS-509077-99-0.* INN.

Erythritol. **NF**. $C_4H_{10}O_4$. 122.12. (1) 1,2,3,4-Butanetetrol; (2) Butane 1,2,3,4-tetrol (*meso*-erythritol). *CAS-149-32-6.*

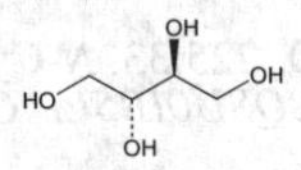

Erythrityl Tetranitrate [*1963*] (e rith′ ri til tet″ ra nye′ trate). $C_4H_6N_4O_{12}$. 302.11. [Eritrityl Tetranitrate is INN.] (1) 1,2,3,4-Butanetetrol, tetranitrate, (R^*,S^*)-; (2) Erythritol tetranitrate. *CAS-7297-25-8.* USP XXIII. *Vasodilator (coronary).* Cardilate (Glaxo Wellcome†) *[Name previously used: Erythrol Tetranitrate.]* ✧*NSC-106566*

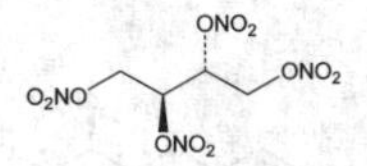

Erythrol Tetranitrate (previously used name) — *See* Erythrityl Tetranitrate.

Erythromycin (e rith″ roe mye′ sin). **USP**. $C_{37}H_{67}NO_{13}$. 733.93. (1) Erythromycin; (2) Erythromycin; (3) ($3R^*,4S^*,5S^*,6R^*,7R^*,9R^*,11R^*,12R^*,13S^*,14R^*$)-4-[(2,6-Dideoxy-3-*C*-methyl-3-*O*-methyl-α-L-*ribo*-hexopyranosyl)oxy]-14-ethyl-7,12,13-trihydroxy-3,5,7,9,11,13-hexamethyl-6-[[3,4,6-trideoxy-3-(dimethylamino)-β-D-*xylo*-hexopyranosyl]oxy]oxacyclotetradecane-2,10-dione. *UNII-63937KV33D. CAS-114-07-8.* INN; BAN; JAN. *Antibacterial.* E-mycin (Abbott); Emgel (Altana); Eryc (Warner Chilcott); Eryderm (Abbott); Erygel (Merz); Erymax (Merz); Ilotycin (Dista)

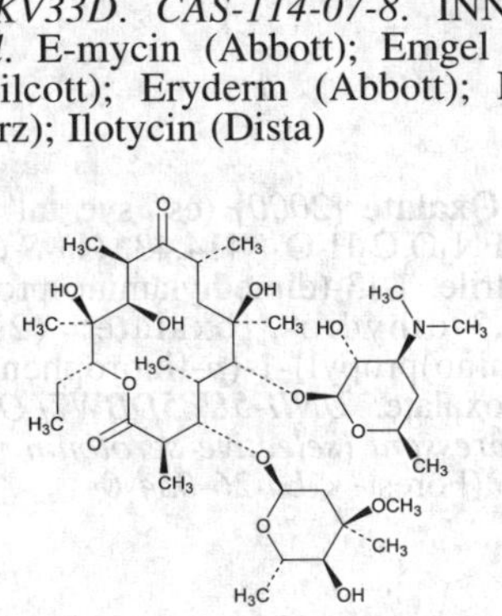

† Brand name formerly used, and/or firm no longer concerned with this product.

Erythromycin Acistrate [*1989*] (e rith″ roe mye′ sin a sis′ trate). $C_{39}H_{69}NO_{14}.C_{18}H_{35}O_2$. 1059.43. (1) Erythromycin, 2′-acetate, octadecanoate (salt); (2) Erythromycin 2′-acetate, stearate (salt). *CAS-96128-89-1.* INN. *Antibacterial.* Erasis (Orion Pharmaceutica, Finland)

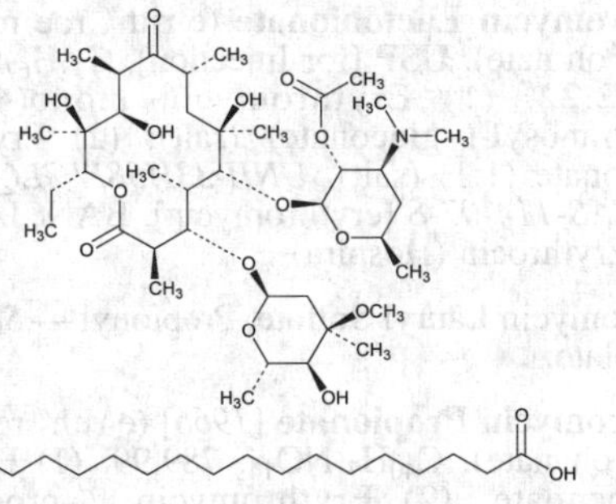

Erythromycin Estolate [*1962*] (e rith″ roe mye′ sin es′ toe late). **USP**. $C_{40}H_{71}NO_{14}.C_{12}H_{26}O_4S$. 1056.39. (1) Erythromycin, 2′-propanoate, dodecyl sulfate (salt); (2) Erythromycin 2′-propionate dodecyl sulfate (salt). *UNII-XRJ2P631HP; UNII-63937KV33D* [erythromycin]. *CAS-3521-62-8; CAS-114-07-8* [erythromycin]. BAN; JAN. *Antibacterial.* Ilosone (Dista) *[Name previously used: Erythromycin Propionate Lauryl Sulfate.]*

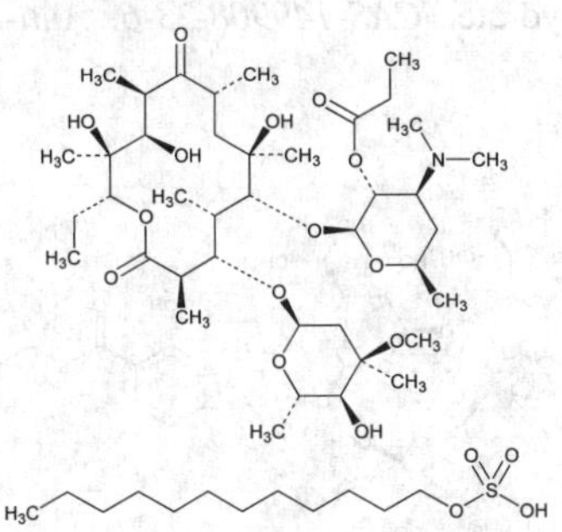

Erythromycin Ethylcarbonate. *UNII-D2JUE6GD5A.* USP XVIII.

Erythromycin Ethylsuccinate (e rith″ roe mye′ sin eth″ il sux′ i nate). **USP**. $C_{43}H_{75}NO_{16}$. 862.05. [Erythromycin Ethyl Succinate is BAN.] (1) Erythromycin 2′-(ethyl butanedioate); (2) Erythromycin 2′-(ethyl succinate). *UNII-1014KSJ86F. CAS-1264-62-6; CAS-114-07-8* [erythromycin]. JAN. *Antibacterial.* E-mycin (Pfizer); E.e.s. (Abbott); Eryped (Abbott); Pediamycin (Ross); Wyamycin (Wyeth)

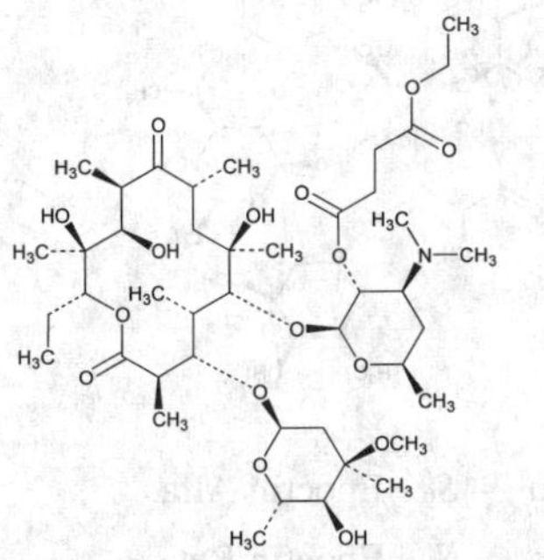

Erythromycin Gluceptate (e rith″ roe mye′ sin gloo sep′ tate). **USP** [Sterile]. $C_{37}H_{67}NO_{13}.C_7H_{14}O_8$. 960.11. (1) Erythromycin monoglucoheptonate (salt); (2) Erythromycin glucoheptonate (1:1) (salt). *UNII-2AY21R0U64. CAS-23067-13-2; CAS-114-07-8* [erythromycin]. *Antibacterial.* Ilotycin (Dista)

Erythromycin Glucoheptonate — *See* Erythromycin Gluceptate.

Erythromycin Lactobionate (e rith″ roe mye′ sin lak″ toe bye′ oh nate). **USP** [for Injection]. $C_{37}H_{67}NO_{13}.C_{12}H_{22}O_{12}$. 1092.22. (1) Erythromycin mono(4-*O*-β-D-galactopyranosyl-D-gluconate) (salt); (2) Erythromycin lactobionate (1:1) (salt). *UNII-33H58I7GLQ. CAS-3847-29-8; CAS-114-07-8* [erythromycin]. BAN; JAN. *Antibacterial.* Erythrocin (Hospira)

Erythromycin Lauryl Sulfate, Propionyl — *See* Erythromycin Estolate.

Erythromycin Propionate [*1966*] (e rith″ roe mye′ sin proe′ pee oh nate). $C_{40}H_{71}NO_{14}$. 789.99. (1) Erythromycin 2′-propanoate; (2) Erythromycin 2′-propionate. *UNII-63937KV33D* [erythromycin]. *CAS-134-36-1; CAS-114-07-8* [erythromycin]. *Antibacterial.*

Erythromycin Propionate Lauryl Sulfate (previously used name) — *See* Erythromycin Estolate.

Erythromycin Salnacedin [*1995*] (e rith″ roe mye′ sin sal na′ se din). $C_{37}H_{67}NO_{13}.C_{12}H_{13}NO_5S.2H_2O$. 1053.26. (1) Erythromycin, compound with *N*-acetyl-L-cysteine 2-hydroxybenzoate (ester) (1:1), dihydrate; (2) Erythromycin, compound with *N*-acetyl-L-cysteine salicylate (ester) (1:1), dihydrate. *CAS-149908-23-6. Anti-acne.* ◇*G-101, SCY-Er*

Erythromycin Stearate (e rith″ roe mye′ sin steer′ ate). **USP.** $C_{37}H_{67}NO_{13}.C_{18}H_{36}O_2$. 1018.40. (1) Erythromycin octadecanoate (salt); (2) Erythromycin stearate (salt). *UNII-LXW024X05M. CAS-643-22-1; CAS-114-07-8* [erythromycin]. BAN; JAN. *Antibacterial.* Bristamycin (Bristol-Myers Squibb); Erythrocin (Abbott)

Erythromycin Stinoprate. $C_{40}H_{71}NO_{14}.C_5H_9NO_3S$. 953.18. Erythromycin 2′-propionate, compound with *N*-acetyl-L-cysteine (1:1). *CAS-84252-03-9.* INN.

Erythropoietin — *See* Epoetin Alfa.

Erythropoietin — *See* Epoetin Beta.

Erythrosine Sodium. $C_{20}H_6I_4Na_2O_5.H_2O$. 897.87. (1) Spiro[isobenzofuran-1(3*H*),9′-[9*H*]xanthen]-3-one, 3′,6′-dihydroxy-2′,4′,5′,7′-tetraiodo-, disodium salt, monohydrate; (2) 2′,4′,5′,7′-Tetraiodofluorescein disodium salt monohy-

drate. *UNII-PN2ZH5LOQY. CAS-49746-10-3; CAS-568-63-8* [anhydrous, open form]; *CAS-16423-68-0* [anhydrous, closed form]; *CAS-15905-32-5* [erythrosine, phenolic]. USP XXII.

Esafloxacin. $C_{15}H_{17}FN_4O_3$. 320.32. (±)-7-(3-Amino-1-pyrrolidinyl)-1-ethyl-6-fluoro-1,4-dihydro-4-oxo-1,8-naphthyridine-3-carboxylic acid. *UNII-A6NT0I9X0K. CAS-79286-77-4.* INN.

Esaprazole. $C_{12}H_{23}N_3O$. 225.33. *N*-Cyclohexyl-1-piperazineacetamide. *UNII-38QSU0IB5L. CAS-64204-55-3.* INN; MI.

Esatenolol. $C_{14}H_{22}N_2O_3$. 266.34. 2-[*p*-[(2*S*)-2-Hydroxy-3-(isopropylamino)propoxy]phenyl]acetamide. *CAS-93379-54-5.* INN.

Escitalopram. $C_{20}H_{21}FN_2O$. 324.39. (+)-(*S*)-1-[3-(Dimethylamino)propyl]-1-(*p*-fluorophenyl)-5-phthalancarbonitrile. *UNII-4O4S742ANY. CAS-128196-01-0.* INN; BAN.

Escitalopram Oxalate [*2000*] (es″ sye tal′ oh pram ox′ a late). $C_{20}H_{21}FN_2O.C_2H_2O_4$. 414.43. (1) *S*-(+)-5-Isobenzofurancarbonitrile, 1-[3-(dimethylamino)propyl]-1-(4-fluorophenyl)-1,3-dihydro-, oxalate; (2) *S*-(+)-1-[3-(Dimethylamino)propyl]-1-(*p*-fluorophenyl)-5-phthalancarbonitrile oxalate. *UNII-5U85DBW7LO. CAS-219861-08-2. Antidepressant (selective serotonin reuptake inhibitor).* Lexapro (Forest) ◇*Lu 26-054-0*

Esculamine. $C_{15}H_{19}NO_6$. 309.31. 8-[[Bis(2-hydroxyethyl)a-mino]methyl]-6,7-dihydroxy-4-methylcoumarin. *UNII-4V7NMO33X6. CAS-2908-75-0.* INN.

Eseridine. $C_{15}H_{21}N_3O_3$. 291.35. (4a*S*,9a*S*)-2,3,4,4a,9,9a-Hex-ahydro-2,4a,9-trimethyl-1,2-oxazino[6,5-*b*]indol-6-yl-methylcarbamate. *UNII-LW9S78L4M8. CAS-25573-43-7.* INN; MI.

Eserine — *See* Physostigmine.

Eserine Salicylate — *See* Physostigmine Salicylate.

Esflurbiprofen. $C_{15}H_{13}FO_2$. 244.26. (*S*)-2-Fluoro-α-methyl-4-biphenylacetic acid. *CAS-51543-39-6.* INN; BAN. ◇*BTS 24332*

Esketamine. $C_{13}H_{16}ClNO$. 237.73. (*S*)-2-(*o*-Chlorophenyl)-2-(methylamino)cyclohexanone. *CAS-33643-46-8.* INN; BAN.

Eslicarbazepine. $C_{15}H_{14}N_2O_2$. 254.28. (10*S*)-10-Hydroxy-10,11-dihydro-5*H*-dibenzo[*b,f*]azepin-5-carboxamide. *CAS-104746-04-5.* INN.

Esmirtazapine. $C_{17}H_{19}N_3$. 265.35. (14b*S*)-2-Methyl-1,2,3,4,10,14b-hexahydropyrazino[2,1-*a*]pyrido[2,3-*c*][2]benzazepine. *UNII-4685R51V7M. CAS-61337-87-9.* INN.

Esmirtazapine Maleate [*2005*] (es″ mir taz′ a peen mal′ ee ate). $C_{17}H_{19}N_3 \cdot C_4H_4O_4$. 381.43. (1) Pyrazino[2,1-*a*]pyri-do[2,3-*c*][2]benzazepine, 1,2,3,4,10,14b-hexahydro-2-methyl-, (14b*S*)-, (2*Z*)-butenedioate (1:1); (2) (+)-(14b*S*)-2-Methyl-1,2,3,4,10,14b-hexahydropyrazino[2,1-*a*]pyri-do[2,3-*c*][2]benzazepine (2*Z*)-butenedioate. *UNII-I2U18E6JKA. CAS-680993-85-5. Treatment of moderate to severe vasomotor symptoms associated with menopause; treatment of primary insomnia.* ◇*Org 50081*

Esmolol Hydrochloride [*1983*] (es′ moe lol hye″ droe klor′ ide). $C_{16}H_{25}NO_4 \cdot HCl$. 331.83. [Esmolol is INN and BAN.] (1) Benzenepropanoic acid, 4-[2-hydroxy-3-[(1-methyl-ethyl)amino]propoxy]-, methyl ester, hydrochloride, (±)-; (2) (±)-Methyl *p*-[2-hydroxy-3-(isopropylamino)propox-y]hydrocinnamate hydrochloride. *UNII-V05260LC8D; UNII-MDY902UXSR* [esmolol]. *CAS-81161-17-3; CAS-103598-03-4* [esmolol]. *Anti-adrenergic (β-receptor).* Bre-vibloc (Baxter Healthcare) ◇*ASL-8052*

Esomeprazole. $C_{17}H_{19}N_3O_3S$. 345.42. 5-Methoxy-2-[(*S*)-[(4-methoxy-3,5-dimethyl-2-pyridyl)methyl]sulfinyl]benzimi-dazole. *UNII-N3PA6559FT. CAS-119141-88-7.* INN; BAN.

Esomeprazole Magnesium [*1999*] (es″ oh mep′ ra zole mag nee′ zee um). $C_{34}H_{36}MgN_6O_6S_2 \cdot 3H_2O$. 767.17. (1) 1*H*-Benzimidazole, 5-methoxy-2-[(*S*)-[(4-methoxy-3,5-di-methyl-2-pyridinyl)methyl]sulfinyl]-, magnesium salt, tri-hydrate; (2) 5-Methoxy-2-[(*S*)-[(4-methoxy-3,5-dimethyl-2-pyridyl)methyl]sulfinyl]benzimidazole, magnesium salt (2:1), trihydrate. *UNII-R6DXU4WAY9. CAS-217087-09-7. Gastric acid secretion inhibitor.* Nexium (AstraZeneca) ◇*H199/18 magnesium trihydrate*

Esomeprazole Potassium [*2007*] (es″ oh mep′ ra zole poe tas′ ee um). $C_{17}H_{18}KN_3O_3S$. 383.51. (1) 1*H*-Benzimidazole, 6-methoxy-2-[(*S*)-[(4-methoxy-3,5-dimethyl-2-pyridinyl)-methyl]sulfinyl]-, potassium salt (1:1); (2) (-)-5-Methoxy-2-{(*S*)-[(4-methoxy-3,5-dimethylpyridin-2-yl)methyl]sul-

____

finyl}-1*H*-benzimidazole potassium salt. *UNII-F37S7G37O2. CAS-161796-84-5. Treatment of GERD patients with a history of erosive esophagitis.*

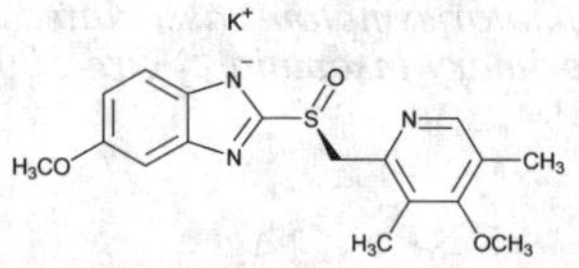

Esomeprazole Sodium [*2003*] (es″ oh mep′ ra zole soe′ dee um). $C_{17}H_{19}N_3NaO_3S$. 368.41. (1) 1*H*-Benzimidazole, 5-methoxy-2-[(*S*)-[(4-methoxy-3,5-dimethyl-2-pyridinyl)methyl]sulfinyl]-, sodium salt; (2) 5-Methoxy-2-[(*S*)-[(4-methoxy-3,5-dimethyl-2-pyridyl)methyl]sulfinyl]-1*H*-benzimidazole, sodium salt. *UNII-L2C9GWQ43H. CAS-161796-78-7. Gastric acid secretion inhibitor.* Nexium (AstraZeneca) ◇*H199/18 sodium*

Esonarimod. $C_{14}H_{16}O_4S$. 280.34. (±)-3-Mercapto-2-(*p*-methylphenacyl)propionic acid acetate. *UNII-PF4079THQO. CAS-101973-77-7.* INN.

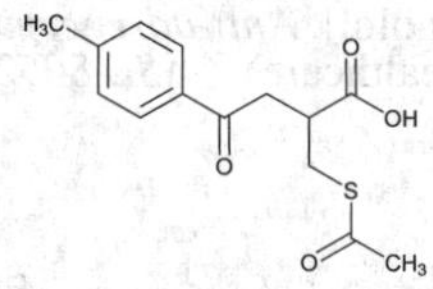

Esorubicin Hydrochloride [*1987*] (es″ oh roo′ bi sin hye″ droe klor′ ide). $C_{27}H_{29}NO_{10}.HCl$. 563.98. [Esorubicin is INN.] (1) 5,12-Naphthacenedione, 10-[(4-aminotetrahydro-6-methyl-2*H*-pyran-2-yl)oxy]-7,8,9,10-tetrahydro-6,8,11-trihydroxy-8-(hydroxyacetyl)-1-methoxy-, hydrochloride, [2*S*-[2α(8*R**,10*R**),4β,6β]]-; (2) (8*S*,10*S*)-10-[[(2*S*,4*R*,6*S*)-4-Aminotetrahydro-6-methyl-2*H*-pyran-2-yl]oxy]-8-glycoloyl-7,8,9,10-tetrahydro-6,8,11-trihydroxy-1-methoxy-5,12-naphthacenedione hydrochloride. *UNII-2UB1JJT82D. CAS-63950-06-1; CAS-63521-85-7* [esorubicin]. *Antineoplastic.* ◇*IMI 58*

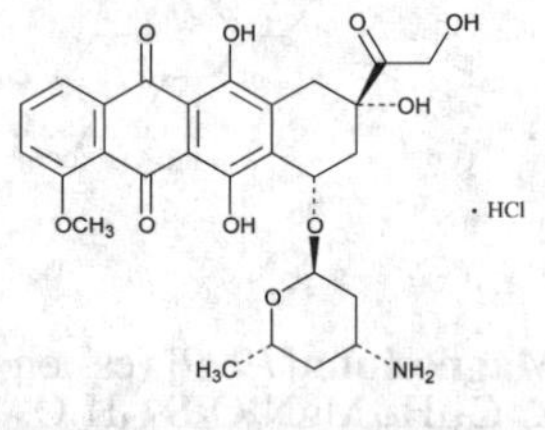

Esoxybutynin Chloride [*2003*] (es″ ox i bue′ ti nin klor′ ide). $C_{22}H_{31}NO_3.HCl$. 393.95. [Esoxybutynin is INN.] (1) Benzeneacetic acid, α-cyclohexyl-α-hydroxy-, 4-(diethylamino)-2-butynyl ester, hydrochloride, (α*S*)-; (2) 4-(Diethylamino)but-2-ynyl (2*S*)-cyclohexylhydroxyphenylacetate hydrochloride. *UNII-S547MDN7WX. CAS-230949-16-3; CAS-119618-22-3* [esoxybutynin]. *Treats overactive bladder symptoms of urgency, frequency and urinary incontinence (anti-spasmodic/anti-cholinergic).*

Espatropate. $C_{19}H_{23}N_3O_3$. 341.40. (*R*)-3-Quinuclidinyl (*R*)-α-(hydroxymethyl)-α-phenylimidazole-1-acetate. *UNII-13MIU3750H. CAS-132829-83-5.* INN; BAN. ◇*UK-88060*

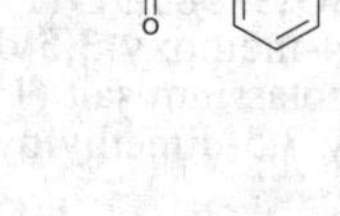

Esproquin Hydrochloride [*1974*] (es′ proe kwin hye″ droe klor′ ide). $C_{14}H_{21}NOS.HCl$. 287.85. [Esproquine is INN.] (1) Isoquinoline, 2-[3-(ethylsulfinyl)propyl]-1,2,3,4-tetrahydro-, hydrochloride; (2) 2-[3-(Ethylsulfinyl)propyl]-1,2,3,4-tetrahydroisoquinoline hydrochloride. *UNII-1P9E5C9137; UNII-3JYK9XFM9K* [esproquin]. *CAS-23486-22-8; CAS-37517-33-2* [esproquin]. *Adrenergic.* ◇*NC-7197*

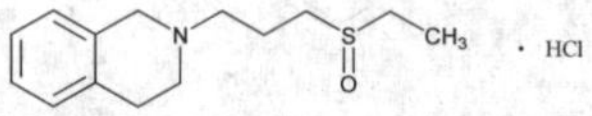

Esproquine (INN) — *See* Esproquin Hydrochloride.

Esreboxetine [*2007*] (es″ re box′ e tine). $C_{19}H_{23}NO_3$. 313.39. (1) Morpholine, 2-[(*S*)-(2-ethoxyphenoxy)phenylmethyl]-, (2*S*)-; (2) (+)-(2*S*)-2-[(*S*)-(2-Ethoxyphenoxy)phenylmethyl]morpholine. *UNII-L8S50ZY490. CAS-98819-76-2.* INN. *Treatment of depression.* ◇*reboxetine*

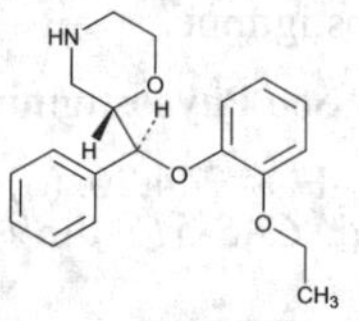

Esreboxetine Succinate [*2007*] (es″ re box′ e teen sux′ i nate). $C_{19}H_{23}NO_3.C_4H_6O_4$. 431.48. (1) Butanedioic acid, compd. with (2*S*)-2-[(*S*)-(2-ethoxyphenoxy)phenylmethyl]morpholine (1:1); (2) (+)-(2*S*)-2-[(*S*)-(2-Ethoxyphenoxy)phenylmethyl]morpholine hydrogen butanedioate. *UNII-XQO13W6OCH. CAS-635724-55-9. Treatment of chronic neuropathic pain.* ◇*PNU-165442G*

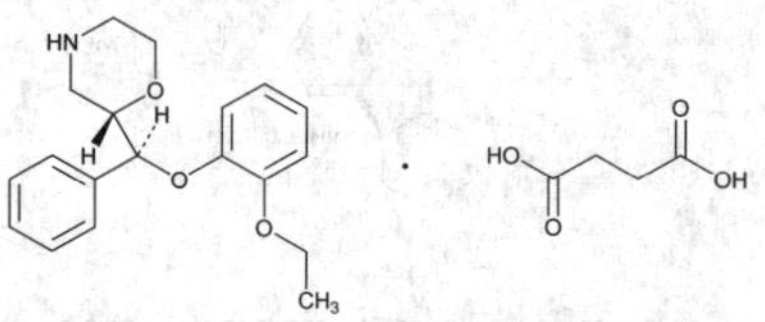

Estazolam [*1990*] (es taz′ oh lam). $C_{16}H_{11}ClN_4$. 294.74. (1) 4*H*-[1,2,4]Triazolo[4,3-*a*][1,4]benzodiazepine, 8-chloro-6-phenyl-; (2) 8-Chloro-6-phenyl-4*H*-*s*-triazolo[4,3-*a*][1,4]benzodiazepine. *UNII-36S3EQV54C. CAS-29975-16-4.* INN; JAN. *Sedative-hypnotic.* Prosom (Abbott) ◇*Abbott-47631*

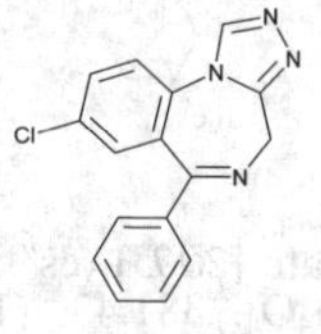

Esterifilcon A [*1982*] (es ter″ i fil′ kon). $(C_8H_{14}O_2)_x$ $(C_7H_{12}O_2)_y(C_{10}H_{14}O_4)_z$. (1) 2-Propenoic acid, 2-methyl-, butyl ester, polymer with butyl 2-propenoate and 1,2-

ethanediyl bis(2-methyl-2-propenoate); (2) Butyl methacrylate polymer with butyl acrylate and ethylene dimethacrylate. *Contact lens material (hydrophilic).*

Estomycin Sulfate — *See* Paromomycin Sulfate.

Estradiol (es″ tra dye′ ol). **USP.** $C_{18}H_{24}O_2$. 272.38. (1) Estra-1,3,5(10)-triene-3,17-diol, (17β)-; (2) Estra-1,3,5(10)-triene-3,17β-diol. *UNII-4TI98Z838E. CAS-50-28-2.* INN; BAN. *Estrogen.* Alora (Watson); Climara (Bayer); Estrace (Warner Chilcott); Estraderm (Novartis); Estring (Pfizer); Estrogel (Ascend Therapeutics); Fempatch (Pfizer); Gynodiol (Duramed); Innofem (Novo Nordisk); Menostar (Bayer); Vagifem (Novo Nordisk); Vivelle (Novartis); Elestrim (Bradley) *[Name previously used: Oestradiol.]* ◇*NSC-9895; NSC-20293 [as the alpha form]*

Estradiol Acetate [*2002*] (es″ tra dye′ ol as′ e tate). $C_{29}H_{26}O_3$. 422.51. (1) Estra-1,3,5(10)-triene-3,17-diol, (17β)-, 3-acetate; (2) 17β-Hydroxyestra-1,3,5(10)-trien-3-yl acetate. *UNII-5R97F5H93P. CAS-4245-41-4. Estrogen replacement therapy.* Femring (Warner Chilcott); Femtrace (Warner Chilcott) ◇*estradiol-3-acetate; E3A*

Estradiol Benzoate. $C_{25}H_{28}O_3$. 376.49. (1) Estra-1,3,5(10)-triene-3,17-diol, (17β)-, 3-benzoate; (2) Estradiol 3-benzoate. *UNII-1S4CJB5ZGN. CAS-50-50-0.* USP XX; INN; BAN; JAN; MI. *[Name previously used: Oestradiol Benzoate.]* ◇*NSC-9566*

Estradiol Cypionate (es″ tra dye′ ol sip′ ee oh nate). **USP.** $C_{26}H_{36}O_3$. 396.56. (1) Estra-1,3,5(10)-triene-3,17-diol, (17β)-, 17-cyclopentanepropanoate; (2) Estradiol 17-cyclopentanepropionate. *UNII-7E1DV054LO. CAS-313-06-4. Estrogen.* Depo (Pfizer)

Estradiol Dipropionate. *UNII-NIG5418BXB. CAS-113-38-2.* NF XIV; JAN.

---

† Brand name formerly used, and/or firm no longer concerned with this product.

Estradiol Enanthate [*1966*] (es″ tra dye′ ol e nan′ thate). $C_{25}H_{36}O_3$. 384.55. (1) Estra-1,3,5(10)-triene-3,17-diol (17β)-, 17-heptanoate; (2) Estradiol 17-heptanoate. *UNII-PAP315WZIA. CAS-4956-37-0. Estrogen.* ◇*SQ 16,150*

Estradiol Monobenzoate — *See* Estradiol Benzoate.

Estradiol Undecylate [*1965*] (es″ tra dye′ ol un de′ sil ate). $C_{29}H_{44}O_3$. 440.66. (1) Estra-1,3,5(10)-triene-3,17-diol (17β)-, 17-undecanoate; (2) Estradiol 17-undecanoate. *CAS-3571-53-7.* INN. *Estrogen.* Delestrec (Bristol-Myers Squibb†) ◇*SQ 9993*

Estradiol Valerate (es″ tra dye′ ol val′ er ate). **USP.** $C_{23}H_{32}O_3$. 356.50. (1) Estra-1,3,5(10)-triene-3,17-diol(17β)-, 17-pentanoate; (2) Estradiol 17-valerate. *UNII-OKG364O896. CAS-979-32-8.* INN; BAN; JAN. *Estrogen.* Delestrogen (King) *[Name previously used: Oestradiol Valerate.]* ◇*NSC-17590*

Estramustine [*1978*] (es″ tra mus′ teen). $C_{23}H_{31}Cl_2NO_3$. 440.40. (1) Estra-1,3,5(10)-triene-3,17-diol, 3-[bis(2-chloroethyl)carbamate], (17β)-; (2) Estradiol 3-[bis(2-chloroethyl)carbamate]. *UNII-35LT29625A. CAS-2998-57-4.* INN; BAN. *Antineoplastic.* ◇*Ro 22-2296/000*

Estramustine Phosphate Sodium [*1978*] (es″ tra mus′ teen fos′ fate soe′ dee um). $C_{23}H_{30}Cl_2NNa_2O_6P$. 564.35. (1) Estra-1,3,5(10)-triene-3,17-diol (17β)-, 3-[bis(2-chloroethyl)carbamate] 17-(dihydrogen phosphate), disodium salt; (2) Estradiol 3-[bis(2-chloroethyl)carbamate] 17-(dihydrogen phosphate), disodium salt. *UNII-75F375MT2N. CAS-52205-73-9.* BAN; JAN. *Antineoplastic.* Emcyt (Pfizer) ◇*Ro 21-8837/001*

Estrapronicate. $C_{27}H_{31}NO_4$. 433.54. Estradiol 17-nicotinate 3-propionate. *UNII-BC621AC03L. CAS-4140-20-9.* INN.

Estrazinol Hydrobromide [*1967*] (es traz′ i nol hye″ droe broe′ mide). $C_{20}H_{25}NO_2$·HBr. 392.33. [Estrazinol is INN.] (1) 8-Aza-19-norpregna-1,3,5(10)-trien-20-yn-17-ol, 3-methoxy-, hydrobromide, (17α)-(±)-; (2) (±)-3-Methoxy-8-aza-19-nor-17α-pregna-1,3,5(10)-trien-20-yn-17-ol hydrobromide. *UNII-P1NC244SOF; UNII-9KLU2E3573* [estrazinol]. *CAS-15179-97-2; CAS-5941-36-6* [estrazinol]. *Estrogen.* ◇*W 4454A*

Estriol (es′ tree ol). **USP.** $C_{18}H_{24}O_3$. 288.38. [Estriol Acetate Benzoate and Estriol Propionate are JAN; Estriol Succinate is INN.] (1) Estra-1,3,5(10)-triene-3,16,17-triol, (16α,17β)-; (2) Estriol. *CAS-50-27-1; CAS-514-68-1* [as succinate]. BAN; JAN. *Estrogen.* Theelol (Parke-Davis†) *[Name previously used: Oestriol.]*

Estriol Sodium Succinate. $C_{26}H_{30}Na_2O_9$. 532.49. Disodium 3-hydroxy-estra-1,3,5(10)-triene-16α,17β-diyl disuccinate. *CAS-113-22-4.* BAN.

Estrobene — *See* Diethylstilbestrol.

Estrofurate [*1971*] (es″ troe fure′ ate). $C_{24}H_{26}O_4$. 378.46. (1) 19,24-Dinorchola-1,3,5(10),7,20,22-hexaene-3,17-diol, 21,23-epoxy-, 3-acetate, (17α)-; (2) 21,23-Epoxy-19,24-dinor-17α-chola-1,3,5(10),7,20,22-hexaene-3,17-diol 3-acetate. *UNII-0CDE7T54KW. CAS-10322-73-3.* INN. *Estrogen.* ◇*AY-11,483*

Estrogenic Substances, Conjugated — *See* Estrogens, Conjugated.

Estrogenine — *See* Diethylstilbestrol.

Estrogens, Conjugated (es′ troe jenz kon′ joo gay″ ted). **USP.** A mixture of sodium estrone sulfate and sodium equilin sulfate. *UNII-IU5QR144QX.* JAN. *Estrogen.* Premarin (Wyeth)

Estrogens, Esterified (es′ troe jenz es ter′ i fide). **USP.** A mixture of the sodium salts of the sulfate esters of the estrogenic substances, principally estrone. *Estrogen.* Amnestrogen (Bristol-Myers Squibb); Estratab (Solvay Pharmaceuticals); Menest (King)

Estromenin — *See* Diethylstilbestrol.

Estrone (es′ trone). **USP.** $C_{18}H_{22}O_2$. 270.37. (1) Estra-1,3,5(10)-trien-17-one, 3-hydroxy-; (2) 3-Hydroxyestra-1,3,5(10)-triene-17-one. *UNII-2DI9HA706A. CAS-53-16-7.* INN; BAN. *Estrogen.* Theelin (Parkdale) *[Name previously used: Oestrone.]*

Estrone Sodium Sulfate. *UNII-6K6FDA543A. CAS-438-67-5; CAS-481-97-0* [estrone hydrogen sulfate]. AMA-DE 1973.

Estropipate (es″ troe pip′ ate). **USP.** $C_{18}H_{22}O_5S.C_4H_{10}N_2$. 436.56. (1) Estra-1,3,5(10)-trien-17-one, 3-(sulfooxy)-, compd. with piperazine (1:1); (2) Estrone hydrogen sulfate compound with piperazine (1:1). *UNII-SVI38UY019. CAS-7280-37-7; CAS-481-97-0* [estrone hydrogen sulfate]. BAN. *Estrogen.* Ogen (Pfizer); Ortho-est (Sun) *[Name previously used: Piperazine Estrone Sulfate.]*

Esuprone. $C_{13}H_{14}O_5S$. 282.31. 7-Hydroxy-3,4-dimethylcoumarin ethanesulfonate. *UNII-K7EB9E48ZE. CAS-91406-11-0.* INN.

Eszopiclone [*2002*] (es″ zoe pik′ lone). $C_{17}H_{17}ClN_6O_3$. 388.81. (1) 1-Piperazinecarboxylic acid, 4-methyl-, (5S)-6-(5-chloro-2-pyridinyl)-6,7-dihydro-7-oxo-5H-pyrrolo[3,4-b]pyrazin-5-yl ester; (2) (+)-(5S)-6-(5-Chloropyridin-2-yl)-7-oxo-6,7-dihydro-5H-pyrrolo[3,4-b]pyrazin-5-yl 4-methylpiperazine-1-carboxylate. *UNII-UZX80K71OE. CAS-138729-47-2.* INN. *Treatment of insomnia.* Lunesta (Sepracor) ◇*(S)-Zopiclone*

Etabenzarone. $C_{23}H_{27}NO_3$. 365.47. *p*-[2-(Diethylamino)ethoxy]phenyl-2-ethyl-3-benzofuranyl ketone. *UNII-DA25635W9D. CAS-15686-63-2.* INN. ◇*L 2642*

Etacepride. $C_{17}H_{24}N_2O_3$. 304.38. 5-Acetyl-*N*-[(1-ethyl-2-pyrrolidinyl)methyl]-*o*-anisamide. *UNII-199HW12728. CAS-68788-56-7.* INN.

Etacrynic Acid (INN, JAN, DCF) — *See* Ethacrynic Acid.

Etafedrine Hydrochloride [*1963*] (e ta fed′ rin hye″ droe klor′ ide). $C_{12}H_{19}NO$·HCl. 229.75. [Etafedrine is INN and BAN.] (1) Benzenemethanol, α-[1-(ethylmethylamino)ethyl]-, hydrochloride; (2) α-[1-(Ethylmethylamino)ethyl]benzyl alcohol hydrochloride. *UNII-Y134VQ304Y. CAS-5591-29-7; CAS-7681-79-0* [etafedrine]. *Adrenergic.* Nethamine (Marion Merrell Dow†)

Etafenone. $C_{21}H_{27}NO_2$. 325.44. [Etafenone Hydrochloride is JAN.] 2′-[2-(Diethylamino)ethoxy]-3-phenylpropiophenone. *UNII-0I14K589E7. CAS-90-54-0.* INN; MI.

Etafilcon A [*1977*] (e″ ta fil′ kon). $(C_6H_{10}O_3)_x(C_4H_5NaO_2)_y(C_{18}H_{26}O_6)_z$. (1) 2-Propenoic acid, 2-methyl-, 2-hydroxyethyl ester, polymer with sodium 2-methyl-2-propenoate and 2-ethyl-2-[[(2-methyl-1-oxo-2-propenyl)oxy]methyl]-1,3-propanediyl bis(2-methyl-2-propenoate); (2) 2-Hydroxyethyl methacrylate polymer with sodium methacrylate and 2-ethyl-2-(hydroxymethyl)-1,3-propanediol trimethacrylate. *CAS-61463-79-4. Contact lens material (hydrophilic).* ACUVUE (Vistakon); 1-Day ACUVUE (Vistakon); SUREVUE (Vistakon)

Etalocib [*2004*] (e tal′ oh kib). $C_{33}H_{33}FO_6$. 544.61. (1) Benzoic acid, 2-[3-[3-[(5-ethyl-4′-fluoro-2-hydroxy[1,1′-biphenyl]-4-yl)oxy]propoxy]-2-propylphenoxy]-; (2) 2-[3-[3-[(5-Ethyl-4′-fluoro-2-hydroxybiphenyl-4-yl)oxy]propoxy]-2-propylphenoxy]benzoic acid. *UNII-THY6R-IW44R. CAS-161172-51-6.* INN. *Antineoplastic (inhibits formation of 5-LO, LTB₄, LTC₄, and thromboxane $B_2(TxB_2)$; activates PPARγ nuclear receptors).* ◇*LY293111*

Etamestrol. $C_{35}H_{34}O_5$. 534.64. 7α-Methyl-19-nor-17α-pregna-1,3,5(10)-trien-20-yne-1,3,17-triol 1,3-dibenzoate. *UNII-VM88TV4OS5. CAS-73764-72-4.* INN.

Etaminile. $C_{15}H_{22}N_2$. 230.35. 4-Dimethylamino-2-ethyl-2-phenylvaleronitrile. *UNII-R3TGX0K69Z. CAS-15599-27-6.* INN. ◇*OM-977*

Etamiphyllin. $C_{13}H_{21}N_5O_2$. 279.34. [Etamiphylline is BAN.] 7-(2-Diethylaminoethyl)theophylline. *UNII-221A91BQ2S. CAS-314-35-2.* INN; MI.

Etamiphyllin Methesculetol — *See* Metescufylline.

Etamivan (INN, BAN, DCF) — *See* Ethamivan.

Etamocycline. $C_{50}H_{60}N_6O_{16}$. 1001.04. *N,N,*-{Ethylenebis[(-methylimino)methylene]}bis-[4′-(dimethylamino)-1,4,4a,5,5a,6,11,12a-octahydro-3,6,10,12,12a-pentahy-droxy-6-methyl-1,11-dioxo-2-naphthacenecarboxamide]. *UNII-96D1L38S9Q. CAS-15590-00-8.* INN; DCF.

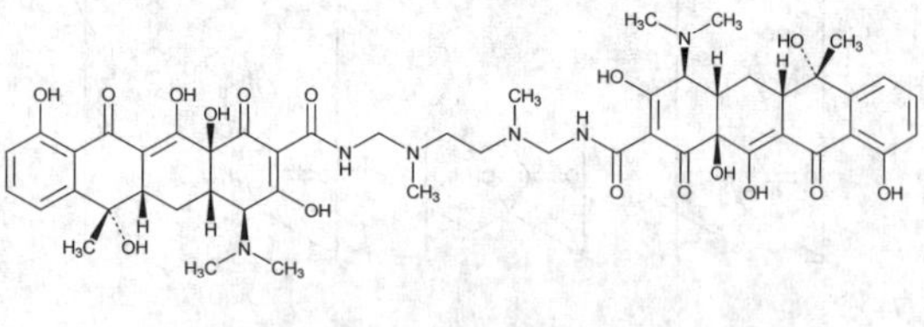

Etamsylate (INN, BAN, JAN) — *See* Ethamsylate.

Etanercept [*1998*] (ee tan′ er sept). $C_{2224}H_{3472}N_{618}O_{701}S_{36}$ (monomer). 51,238 daltons (non-glycosylated protein, monomer). 1-235-Tumor necrosis factor receptor (human) fusion protein with 236-467-immunoglobulin G1 (human γ1-chain Fc fragment), dimer. *UNII-OP401G7OJC. CAS-185243-69-0.* INN; BAN. *To decrease signs and symptoms of rheumatoid arthritis.* Enbrel (Immunex) ◇*rhu TNFR:Fc*

```
LPQVAFTPY APEPGSTCRL REYYDQTAQM CCSKCSPGQH AKVFCTKTSD
TVCDSCEDST YTQLWNWVPE CLSCGSRCSS DQVETQACTR EQNRICTCRP
GWYCALSKQE GCRLCAPLRK CRPGFGVARP GTETSDVVCK PCAPGTFSNT
TSSTDICRPH QICNVVAIPG NASMDAVCTS TSPTRSMAPG AVHLPQPVST
RSQHTQPTPE PSTAPSTSFL LPMGPSPPAE GSTGDEPKSC DKTHTCPPCP
APELLGGPSV FLFPPKPKDT LMISRTPEVT CVVVDVSHED PEVKFNWYVD
GVEVHNAKTK PREEQYNSTY RVVSVLTVLH QDWLNGKEYK CKVSNKALPA
PIEKTISKAK GQPREPQVYT LPPSREEMTK NQVSLTCLVK GFYPSDIAVE
WESNGQPENN YKTTPPVLDS DGSFFLYSKL TVDKSRWQQG NVFSCSVMHE
ALHNHYTQKS LSLSPGK
```

Etanidazole [*1987*] (e″ ta nye′ da zole). $C_7H_{10}N_4O_4$. 214.18. (1) 1*H*-Imidazole-1-acetamide, *N*-(2-hydroxyethyl)-2-nitro-; (2) *N*-(2-Hydroxyethyl)-2-nitroimidazole-1-acetamide. *CAS-22668-01-5.* INN. *Antineoplastic (hypoxic cell radiosensitizer).* Radinyl (Roberts Pharmaceutical) ◇*SR 2508; NSC-301467*

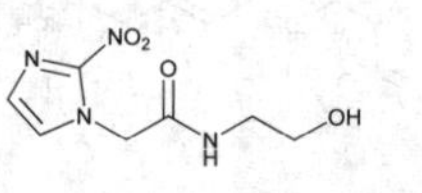

Etanterol. $C_{18}H_{24}N_2O_3$. 316.39. 5-Amino-α-[[(*p*-hydroxy-α-methylphenethyl)amino]methyl]-*m*-xylene-α,α′-diol. *UNII-1597304395. CAS-93047-39-3.* INN.

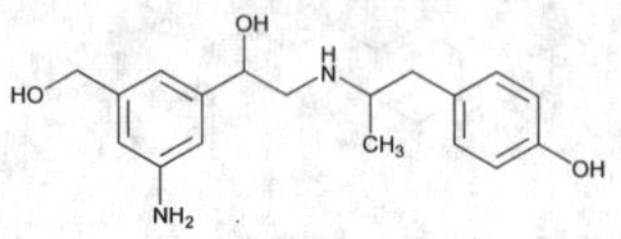

Etaperazine — *See* Perphenazine.

Etaqualone. $C_{17}H_{16}N_2O$. 264.32. 3-(*o*-Ethylphenyl)-2-methyl-4(3*H*)-quinazolinone. *UNII-HFS3HB32J7. CAS-7432-25-9.* INN; MI.

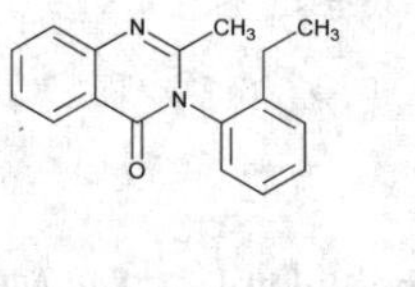

Etaracizumab [*2007*] (e tar″ a siz′ oo mab). $C_{6392}H_{9908}N_{1732}O_{1996}S_{42}$. (1) Immunoglobulin G1 (synthetic mouse NSO cell heavy chain variable region fragment), complex with immunoglobulin G1 (synthetic mouse NSO cell light chain variable region fragment); (2) Immunoglo-bulin G1, anti-[human alphaVbeta3 (CD51/CD61, CD51/GPIIIa, CD51/platelet membrane glycoprotein IIIa, vitro-nectin receptor)] humanized monoclonal antibody MEDI-522 (hLM609); gamma1 heavy chain [humanized VH (*Homo sapiens* FR/*Mus musculus* CDR from clone LM609)-*Homo sapiens* IGHG1*03] (220-214′)-disulfide with kappa light chain [humanized V-KAPPA (*Homo sapiens* FR/*Mus musculus* CDR from clone LM609)-*Homo sapiens* IGKC*01]; (226-226″:229-229″)-bisdisulfide di-mer; (3) A fully humanized, recombinant IgG kappa monoclonal antibody. Molecular weight is approximately 144,300 daltons. *CAS-892553-42-3.* INN. *Treatment of metastatic melanoma, prostate cancer.* Abegrin (MedIm-mune) ◇*MEDI-522*

Etarotene [*1990*] (e tar′ oh teen). $C_{25}H_{32}O_2S$. 396.59. (1) Naphthalene, 6-[2-[4-(ethylsulfonyl)phenyl]-1-methyl-ethenyl]-1,2,3,4-tetrahydro-1,1,4,4-tetramethyl-, (*E*)-; (2) 6-[(*E*)-*p*-(Ethylsulfonyl)-α-methylstyryl]-1,2,3,4-tetrahy-dronaphthalene. *CAS-87719-32-2.* INN. *Keratolytic.* ◇*Ro 15-1570/000*

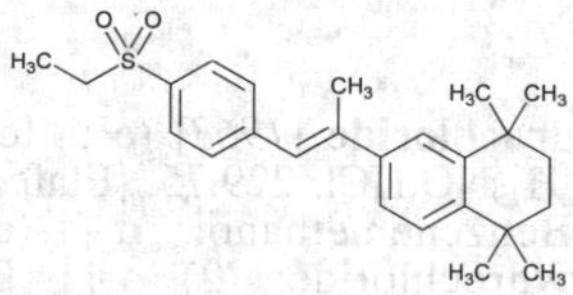

Etasuline. $C_{16}H_{15}ClN_2S$. 302.82. 6-Chloro-2-(ethylamino)-4-phenyl-4*H*-3,1-benzothiazine. *UNII-J4LUG3IAAN. CAS-16781-39-8.* INN.

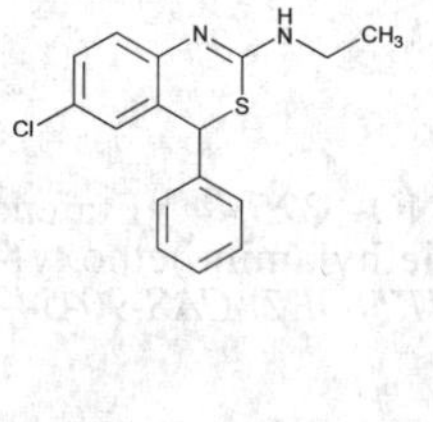

Etazepine. $C_{17}H_{17}NO_2$. 267.32. (±)-11-Ethoxy-5,11-dihydro-5-methyl-6*H*-dibenz[*b,e*]azepin-6-one. *UNII-SBC76K7XWC. CAS-88124-27-0.* INN.

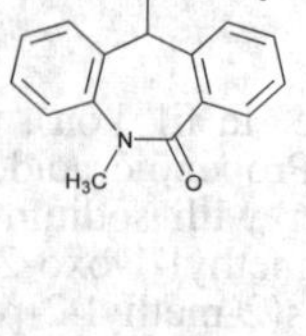

Etazolate Hydrochloride [*1975*] (e taz′ oh late hye″ droe klor′ ide). $C_{14}H_{19}N_5O_2$·HCl. 325.79. [Etazolate is INN.] (1) 1*H*-Pyrazolo[3,4-*b*]pyridine-5-carboxylic acid, 1-ethyl-4-[(1-methylethylidene)hydrazino]-, ethyl ester, monohy-drochloride; (2) Ethyl 1-ethyl-4-(isopropylidenehydrazi-no)-1*H*-pyrazolo[3,4-*b*]pyridine-5-carboxylate monohydrochloride. *UNII-7YO3254Y6B; UNII-I89Y79062L* [etazolate]. *CAS-35838-58-5; CAS-51022-77-6* [etazolate]. *Antipsychotic.* ◇*SQ 20009*

Etebenecid. C₁₁H₁₅NO₄S. 257.31. *p*-Diethylsulfamoylbenzoic acid. *UNII-443I5098G. CAS-1213-06-5.* INN; BAN. *[Name previously used: Ethebenecid.]*

Etenzamide (previously used name) — *See* Ethenzamide.

Eterobarb [*1974*] (e ter′ oh barb). C₁₆H₂₀N₂O₅. 320.34. (1) 2,4,6(1*H*,3*H*,5*H*)-Pyrimidinetrione, 5-ethyl-1,3-bis(-methoxymethyl)-5-phenyl-; (2) 5-Ethyl-1,3-bis(methoxymethyl)-5-phenylbarbituric acid. *UNII-432SI047GA. CAS-27511-99-5.* INN; BAN. *Anticonvulsant.* Antilon (Marion Merrell Dow†) ◇*EX 12-095; RMI 16,238*

Etersalate. C₁₉H₁₉NO₆. 357.36. Salicylic acid acetate, ester with β-hydroxy-*p*-acetophenetidide. *UNII-653GN04T2G. CAS-62992-61-4.* INN; MI.

Ethacridine Lactate. C₁₅H₁₅N₃O.C₃H₆O₃.H₂O. 361.39. [Ethacridine is INN and BAN; Acrinol is JAN.] 6,9-Diamino-2-ethoxyacridine lactate monohydrate. *CAS-1837-57-6; CAS-442-16-0* [ethacridine]. MI. Antidiar 200 (Hoechst-Roussel†); Rivanol (Hoechst-Roussel†)

Ethacrynate Sodium [*1966*] (eth″ a krin′ ate soe′ dee um). **USP** [for Injection]. C₁₃H₁₁Cl₂NaO₄. 325.12. (1) Acetic acid, [2,3-dichloro-4-(2-methylene-1-oxobutyl)phenoxy]-, sodium salt; (2) Sodium [2,3-dichloro-4-(2-

methylenebutyryl)phenoxy]acetate. *UNII-K41MYV7MPM; UNII-M5DP350VZV* [ethacrynic acid]. *CAS-6500-81-8; CAS-58-54-8* [ethacrynic acid]. *Diuretic.* Edecrin (Aton)

Ethacrynic Acid [*1963*] (eth a krin′ ik as′ id). **USP**. C₁₃H₁₂Cl₂O₄. 303.14. [Etacrynic Acid is INN, BAN and JAN.] (1) Acetic acid, [2,3-dichloro-4-(2-methylene-1-oxobutyl)phenoxy]-; (2) [2,3-Dichloro-4-(2-methylenebutyryl)phenoxy]acetic acid. *UNII-M5DP350VZV. CAS-58-54-8. Diuretic.* Edecrin (Aton) ◇*MK-595; NSC-85791*

Ethambutol Hydrochloride [*1963*] (eth am′ bue tol hye″ droe klor′ ide). **USP**. C₁₀H₂₄N₂O₂.2HCl. 277.23. [Ethambutol is INN and BAN.] (1) 1-Butanol, 2,2′-(1,2-ethanediyldiimino)bis-, dihydrochloride, [*S*-(*R**,*R**)]-; (2) (+)-2,2′-(Ethylenediimino)-di-1-butanol dihydrochloride. *UNII-QE4VW5FO07; UNII-8G167061QZ* [ethambutol]. *CAS-1070-11-7; CAS-74-55-5* [ethambutol]. JAN. *Antibacterial (tuberculostatic).* Myambutol (Stat Trade) ◇*CL 40881*

Ethamivan [*1961*] (eth am′ i van). C₁₂H₁₇NO₃. 223.27. [Etamivan is INN and BAN.] (1) Benzamide, *N,N*-diethyl-4-hydroxy-3-methoxy-; (2) *N,N*-Diethylvanillamide. *UNII-M44O63YPV9. CAS-304-84-7.* USP XX. *Stimulant (central and respiratory).* Vandid (3M Pharmaceuticals†) ◇*NSC-406087*

Ethamsylate [*1964*] (eth am′ si late). C₆H₆O₅S.C₄H₁₁N. 263.31. [Etamsylate is INN, BAN and JAN.] (1) Benzenesulfonic acid, 2,5-dihydroxy-, compd. with *N*-ethylethanamine (1:1); (2) 2,5-Dihydroxybenzenesulfonic acid compound with diethylamine (1:1). *CAS-2624-44-4. Hemostatic.* ◇*MD 141; E 141*

Ethanol (JAN) — *See* Alcohol.

Ethanolamine Oleate [*1987*] (eth″ a nol′ a meen oh′ lee ate). C₁₈H₃₄O₂.C₂H₇NO. 343.54. (1) 9-Octadecenoic acid (*Z*)-, compound with 2-aminoethanol (1:1); (2) Oleic acid

---

† Brand name formerly used, and/or firm no longer concerned with this product.

compound with 2-aminoethanol (1:1). *UNII-U4RY8MRX7C. CAS-2272-11-9. Sclerosing agent.* Ethamolin (QOL)

Ethaverine Hydrochloride. C$_{24}$H$_{29}$NO$_4$.HCl. 431.95. [Ethaverine is INN.] 1-(3,4-Diethoxybenzyl)-6,7-diethoxyisoquinoline hydrochloride. *UNII-6Z6T599E49; UNII-2H2HC19DYZ [ethaverine]. CAS-985-13-7; CAS-486-47-5 [ethaverine]. MI.* Ethaquin (Ascher†)

Ethchlorvynol (eth klor′ vi nol). **USP.** C$_7$H$_9$ClO. 144.60. (1) 1-Penten-4-yn-3-ol, 1-chloro-3-ethyl-; (2) 1-Chloro-3-ethyl-1-penten-4-yn-3-ol. *UNII-6EIM3851UZ. CAS-113-18-8. INN; BAN. Sedative-hypnotic.* Placidyl (Abbott)

Ethebenecid (previously used name) — *See* Etebenecid.

Ethenzamide. C$_9$H$_{11}$NO$_2$. 165.19. *o*-Ethoxybenzamide. *CAS-938-73-8. INN; BAN; JAN; MI. [Name previously used: Etenzamide.]*

Ether (ee′ ther). **USP.** C$_4$H$_{10}$O. 74.12. (1) Ethane, 1,1′-oxybis-; (2) Ethyl ether. *UNII-0F5N573A2Y. CAS-60-29-7. JAN. Anesthetic (inhalation).*

Ethiazide. C$_9$H$_{12}$ClN$_3$O$_4$S$_2$. 325.79. 6-Chloro-3-ethyl-3,4-dihydro-2*H*-1,2,4-benzothiadiazine-7-sulfonamide 1,1-dioxide. *UNII-EK9LSW731R. CAS-1824-58-4. INN; BAN; JAN; MI.*

Ethidium Bromide — *See* Homidium Bromide.

Ethinamate. C$_9$H$_{13}$NO$_2$. 167.21. (1) Cyclohexanol, 1-ethynyl-, carbamate; (2) 1-Ethynylcyclohexanol carbamate. *UNII-IAN371PP48. CAS-126-52-3.* USP XXII; INN; BAN; JAN. Valmid (Dista)

Ethinyl Estradiol (eth′ i nil es″ tra dye′ ol). **USP.** C$_{20}$H$_{24}$O$_2$. 296.40. [Ethinylestradiol is INN, BAN and JAN.] (1) 19-Norpregna-1,3,5(10)-trien-20-yne-3,17-diol, (17α)-; (2) 19-Nor-17α-pregna-1,3,5(10)-trien-20-yne-3,17-diol. *UNII-423D2T571U. CAS-57-63-6. Estrogen.* Estinyl (Schering); Feminone (Pfizer); Lynoral (Organon) *[Name previously used: Ethinyloestradiol.]* ◇NSC-10973

Ethinylestradiol (INN, BAN, JAN) — *See* Ethinyl Estradiol.

Ethinyloestradiol (previously used name) — *See* Ethinyl Estradiol.

Ethiodized Oil (eth eye′ oh dyzd). **USP** [Injection]. An iodine addition product of the ethyl ester of the fatty acids of poppyseed oil, containing 37.05 ± 1.85% of organically combined iodine. *CAS-8008-53-5. Diagnostic aid (radiopaque medium).* Ethiodol (Savage)

Ethiodized Oil I 131 [*1965*] (eth eye′ oh dyzd). [Ethiodized Oil (^{131}I) is INN.] An iodine addition product of the ethyl ester of the fatty acid of poppyseed oil, containing 475 mg per ml (37% by weight) of iodine. (A part of the iodine is the radioactive isotope, ^{131}I.) *Antineoplastic; radioactive agent.* Ethiodol-131 (Abbott†)

Ethiofos (previously used USAN) — *See* Amifostine.

Ethionamide [*1961*] (e thye on′ a mide). **USP.** C$_8$H$_{10}$N$_2$S. 166.24. (1) 4-Pyridinecarbothioamide, 2-ethyl-; (2) 2-Ethylthioisonicotinamide. *UNII-OAY8ORS3CQ. CAS-536-33-4. INN; BAN; JAN. Antibacterial (tuberculostatic).* Trecator (Wyeth) ◇1314 TH

Ethisterone. C$_{21}$H$_{28}$O$_2$. 312.45. 17-Ethynyl-17β-hydroxyandrost-4-en-3-one. *UNII-P201BVY1MJ. CAS-434-03-7.* NF XIII; INN; BAN; MI. Ora-Lutin (Parke-Davis†); Pranone (Schering†); Syngestrotabs (Pfizer); Trosinone (Abbott†) *[Name previously used: Anhydrohydroxyprogesterone.]* ◇NSC-9565

Ethmozine — *See* Moricizine.

Ethoglucid (previously used name) — *See* Etoglucid.

Ethoheptazine Citrate. $C_{16}H_{23}NO_2 \cdot C_6H_8O_7$. 453.48. [Ethoheptazine is BAN.] Ethyl hexahydro-1-methyl-4-phenyl-1H-azepine-4-carboxylate citrate (1:1). *UNII-LXK8EE245D. CAS-2085-42-9; CAS-77-15-6* [ethoheptazine]. NF XIII; INN; MI.

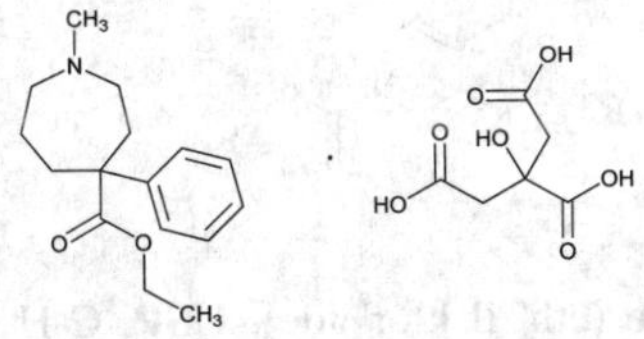

Ethohexadiol. *UNII-M9JGK7U88V. CAS-94-96-2.* USP XVIII; MI.

Ethomoxane Hydrochloride. $C_{15}H_{23}NO_3 \cdot HCl$. 301.81. [Ethomoxane is INN and BAN.] ($\pm$)-2-(Butylaminomethyl)-8-ethoxy-1,4-benzodioxan hydrochloride. *CAS-6038-78-4; CAS-3570-46-5* [ethomoxane].

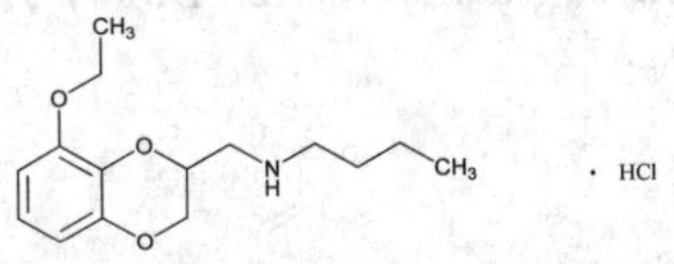

Ethonam Nitrate [*1967*] (eth′ oh nam nye′ trate). $C_{16}H_{18}N_2O_2 \cdot HNO_3$. 333.34. [Etonam is INN.] (1) 1H-Imidazole-5-carboxylic acid, 1-(1,2,3,4-tetrahydro-1-naphthalenyl)-, ethyl ester, mononitrate; (2) Ethyl 1-(1,2,3,4-tetrahydro-1-naphthyl)imidazole-5-carboxylate mononitrate. *UNII-OT5Z8RA5RQ; UNII-G84P716Z93* [ethonam]. *CAS-15037-55-5; CAS-15037-44-2* [ethonam]. *Antifungal.* ◇*R 10.100*

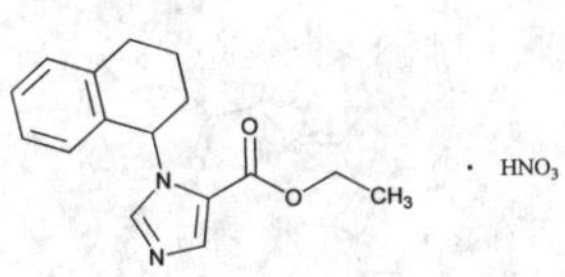

Ethopabate (eth″ oh pab′ ate). **USP.** $C_{12}H_{15}NO_4$. 237.25. (1) Benzoic acid, 4-(acetylamino)-2-ethoxy-, methyl ester; (2) Methyl 4-acetamido-2-ethoxybenzoate. *UNII-F4X3L6068O. CAS-59-06-3.* BAN; MI.

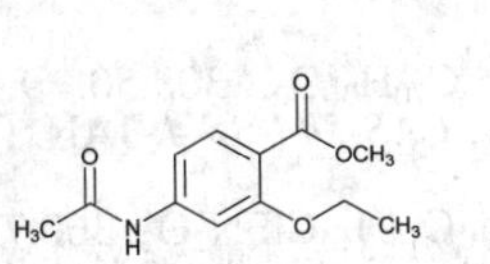

Ethopropazine Hydrochloride. $C_{19}H_{24}N_2S \cdot HCl$. 348.93. [Profenamine is INN and BAN; Profenamine Hibenzate and Profenamine Hydrochloride are JAN.] (1) 10H-Phenothiazine-10-ethanamine, N,N-diethyl-α-methyl-, monohydrochloride; (2) 10-[2-(Diethylamino)propyl]phenothiazine monohydrochloride. *UNII-O00T111VRN;*

UNII-7WI4P02YN1 [ethopropazine]. *CAS-1094-08-2; CAS-522-00-9* [ethopropazine]. USP XXIII. *Antiparkinsonian.* Parsidol (Pfizer)

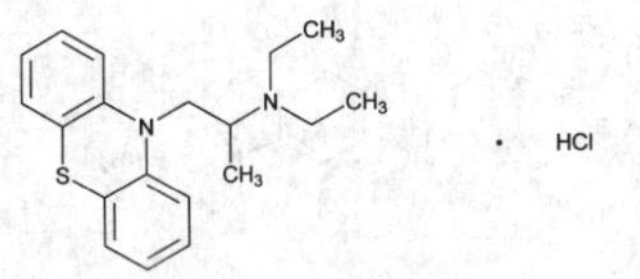

Ethosalamide (previously used name) — *See* Etosalamide.

Ethosuximide [*1962*] (eth″ oh sux′ i mide). **USP.** $C_7H_{11}NO_2$. 141.17. (1) 2,5-Pyrrolidinedione, 3-ethyl-3-methyl-, ($\pm$)-; (2) ($\pm$)-2-Ethyl-2-methylsuccinimide. *UNII-5SEH9X1D1D. CAS-77-67-8.* INN; BAN; JAN. *Anticonvulsant.* Zarontin (Pfizer) ◇*CI-366; CN-10,395; PM-671; NSC-64013*

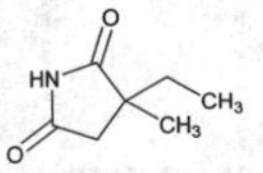

Ethotoin (eth′ oh toin; eth′ oh toe in). **USP.** $C_{11}H_{12}N_2O_2$. 204.23. (1) 2,4-Imidazolidinedione, 3-ethyl-5-phenyl-, ($\pm$)-; (2) ($\pm$)-3-Ethyl-5-phenylhydantoin. *UNII-46QG38NC4U. CAS-86-35-1.* INN; BAN; JAN. *Anticonvulsant.* Peganone (Ovation)

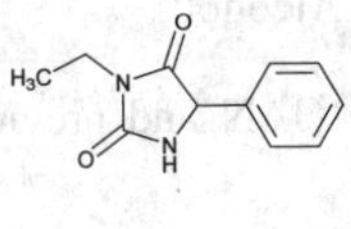

Ethoxarutine — *See* Ethoxazorutoside.

Ethoxazene Hydrochloride [*1963*] (eth ox′ a zeen hye″ droe klor′ ide). $C_{14}H_{16}N_4O \cdot HCl$. 292.76. [Etoxazene is INN.] (1) 1,3-Benzenediamine, 4-[(4-ethoxyphenyl)azo]-, monohydrochloride; (2) 4-[(p-Ethoxyphenyl)azo]-m-phenylenediamine monohydrochloride. *UNII-5C90PJN6E5. CAS-2313-87-3; CAS-94-10-0* [ethoxazene]. *Analgesic.* Serenium (Bristol-Myers Squibb†) ◇*SQ 2128; NSC-7214*

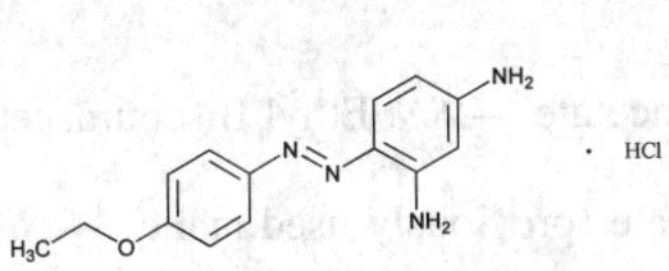

Ethoxazorutoside. $C_{33}H_{41}NO_{17}$. 723.68. 2-Morpholinoethylrutin. *CAS-30851-76-4.* INN; DCF.

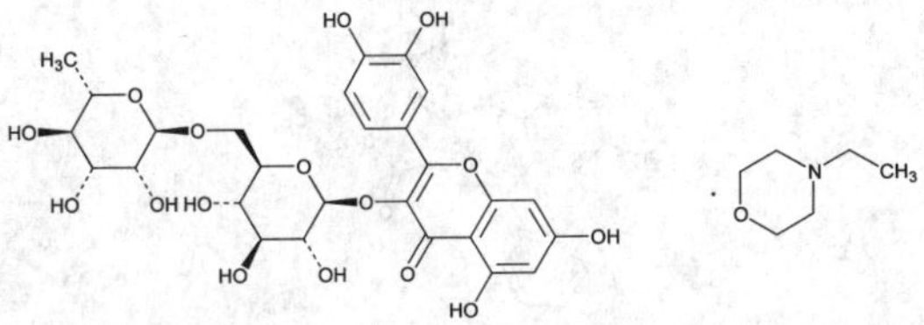

---

† Brand name formerly used, and/or firm no longer concerned with this product.

Ethoxzolamide. $C_9H_{10}N_2O_3S_2$. 258.32. (1) 2-Benzothiazolesulfonamide, 6-ethoxy-; (2) 6-Ethoxy-2-benzothiazolesulfonamide. *UNII-Z52H4811WX. CAS-452-35-7.* USP XX; MI. Cardrase (Pfizer); Ethamide (Allergan)

Ethybenztropine [*1962*] (eth″ i benz′ troe peen). $C_{22}H_{27}NO$. 321.46. [Etybenzatropine is INN and BAN.] (1) 8-Azabicyclo[3.2.1]octane, 3-(diphenylmethoxy)-8-ethyl-, *endo*-; (2) 3α-(Diphenylmethoxy)-8-ethyl-1αH,5αH-nortropane. *UNII-G1X2X9N95N. CAS-524-83-4. Anticholinergic.* Panolid (Novartis†) ◇*UK-738*

Ethyl Acetate (eth′ il as′ e tate). **NF**. $C_4H_8O_2$. 88.11. (1) Acetic acid, ethyl ester; (2) Ethyl acetate. *UNII-76845O8NMZ. CAS-141-78-6. Pharmaceutic aid (solvent).*

Ethyl Alcohol — *See* Alcohol.

Ethyl Aminobenzoate (JAN and previously used name) — *See* Benzocaine.

Ethyl Biscoumacetate. $C_{22}H_{16}O_8$. 408.36. Ethyl bis(4-hydroxy-2-oxo-2H-1-benzopyran-3-yl)acetate. *UNII-08KL644731. CAS-548-00-5.* NF XIII; INN; BAN; MI.

Ethyl Biscumacetate — *See* Ethyl Biscoumacetate.

Ethyl Carbamate (previously used name) — *See* Urethane.

Ethyl Carfluzepate. $C_{20}H_{17}ClFN_3O_4$. 417.82. Ethyl 7-chloro-5-(o-fluorophenyl)-2,3-dihydro-1-(methylcarbamoyl)-2-oxo-1H-1,4-benzodiazepine-3-carboxylate. *UNII-36M73UIK01. CAS-65400-85-3.* INN.

Ethyl Cartrizoate. $C_{15}H_{15}I_3N_2O_6$. 700.00. (3,5-Diacetamido-2,4,6-triiodobenzoyloxy)acetic acid ethylester. *UNII-8FVI4DU91L. CAS-5714-09-0.* INN.

Ethyl Chloride (eth′ il klor′ ide). **USP**. C_2H_5Cl. 64.51. (1) Ethane, chloro-; (2) Chloroethane. *CAS-75-00-3. Anesthetic (topical).*

Ethyl Dibunate [*1962*] (eth′ il dye′ bue nate). $C_{20}H_{28}O_3S$. 348.50. (1) 1-Naphthalenesulfonic acid, 3,6-bis(1,1-dimethylethyl)-, ethyl ester; (2) Ethyl 3,6-di-*tert*-butyl-1-naphthalenesulfonate. *CAS-5560-69-0.* INN; BAN. *Antitussive.* Neodyne (Marion Merrell Dow†) ◇*NDR 304*

Ethyl Dihydroxypropyl PABA — *See* Roxadimate.

Ethyl Dirazepate. $C_{18}H_{14}Cl_2N_2O_3$. 377.22. Ethyl 7-chloro-5-(o-chlorophenyl)-2,3-dihydro-2-oxo-1H-1,4-benzodiazepine-3-carboxylate. *UNII-74FAA305EW. CAS-23980-14-5.* INN.

Ethyl Ether — *See* Ether.

Ethyl Icosapentate. $C_{22}H_{34}O_2$. 330.50. Ethyl all-*cis*-5,8,11,14,17-icosapentaenoic acid. *UNII-6GC8A4PAYH. CAS-73310-10-8.* JAN.

Ethyl Linoleate. $C_{20}H_{36}O_2$. 308.50. 9,12-Octadecadienoic acid ethyl ester. *CAS-544-35-4.* JAN.

Ethyl Loflazepate. $C_{18}H_{14}ClFN_2O_3$. 360.77. Ethyl 7-chloro-5-(o-fluorophenyl)-2,3-dihydro-2-oxo-1H-1,4-benzodiazepine-3-carboxylate. *UNII-VJB5FW9W9J. CAS-29177-84-2.* INN; JAN; MI.

Ethyl Nitrite [Spirit]. *CAS-109-95-5.* NF XI; MI.

Ethyl Oleate (eth′ il oh′ lee ate). **NF**. $C_{20}H_{38}O_2$. 310.51. (1) 9-Octadecenoic acid, (Z)-, ethyl ester; (2) Ethyl oleate. *UNII-Z2Z439864Y. CAS-111-62-6. Pharmaceutic aid (vehicle).*

Ethyl Oxide — *See* Ether.

Ethyl Parahydroxybenzoate (JAN) — *See* Ethylparaben.

Ethyl Piperidinoacetylaminobenzoate. $C_{16}H_{22}N_2O_3$. 290.36. *p*-(Piperidinoacetamide)benzoic acid ethyl ester. *UNII-6M452G7O1F. CAS-41653-21-8.* JAN.

Ethyl Pyrophosphate. $C_8H_{20}O_7P_2$. 290.19. Tetraethyl pyrophosphate. BAN.

Ethyl Vanillin (eth′ il va nil′ in). **NF**. $C_9H_{10}O_3$. 166.17. (1) Benzaldehyde, 3-ethoxy-4-hydroxy-; (2) 3-Ethoxy-4-hydroxybenzaldehyde. *UNII-YC9ST449YJ. CAS-121-32-4. Pharmaceutic aid (flavor).*

Ethylcellulose (eth″ il sel′ ue lose). **NF**. (1) Cellulose, ethyl ester; (2) Cellulose ethyl ether. *CAS-9004-57-3.* INN. *Pharmaceutic aid (tablet binder).* Aquacoat ECD (FMC); Ethocel (Dow Chemical)

Ethylchlordiphene — *See* Etofamide.

Ethyldicoumarol — *See* Ethyl Biscoumacetate.

Ethylene. *UNII-91GW059KN7. CAS-74-85-1.* NF XIII; MI.

Ethylene Glycol Stearates (eth′ i leen glye′ kol steer′ ates). **NF**. A mixture of ethylene glycol monoesters and diesters of stearic and palmitic acids.

Ethylenediamine (eth″ i leen dye′ a meen). **USP**. $C_2H_8N_2$. 60.10. (1) 1,2-Ethanediamine; (2) Ethylenediamine. *UNII-60V9STC53F. CAS-107-15-3.* JAN. Component of Aminophylline Injection. *[Note—Edamine is the recommended contraction for the ethylenediamine radical.]*

Ethylenediaminetetraacetate — *See* Edetate Disodium.

Ethylenedinitrilotetraacetate Disodium — *See* Edetate Disodium.

Ethylestrenol [*1962*] (eth″ il es′ tre nol). $C_{20}H_{32}O$. 288.47. [Ethylnandrol is JAN.] (1) 19-Norpregn-4-en-17-ol, (17α)-; (2) 19-Nor-17α-pregn-4-en-17β-ol. *UNII-ADC79EK5Q8. CAS-965-90-2.* INN; BAN. *Anabolic.* Maxibolin (Organon) *[Name previously used: Ethyloestrenol.]*

Ethylhexanediol — *See* Ethohexadiol.

Ethylhydrocupreine Hydrochloride. *CAS-3413-58-9; CAS-522-60-1* [ethylhydrocupreine]. NF VIII; MI.

Ethylmethylthiambutene. $C_{15}H_{19}NS_2$. 277.45. 3-Ethylmethylamino-1,1-di-(2′-thienyl)-1-butene. *UNII-722BFZ899Q. CAS-441-61-2.* INN; BAN; DCF; MI.

Ethylmorphine Hydrochloride. [Ethylmorphine is BAN.] *UNII-MFM5450P3T. CAS-125-30-4; CAS-76-58-4* [ethylmorphine]. NF XIII; JAN; MI.

Ethylnandrol (JAN) — *See* Ethylestrenol.

Ethylnorepinephrine Hydrochloride. $C_{10}H_{15}NO_3$·HCl. 233.69. (1) 1,2-Benzenediol, 4-(2-amino-1-hydroxybutyl)-, hydrochloride; (2) α-(1-Aminopropyl)-3,4-dihydroxybenzyl alcohol hydrochloride. *UNII-X94OZJ468Y. CAS-3198-07-0; CAS-536-24-3* [ethylnorepinephrine]. USP XXII. Bronkephrine (Sterling Winthrop)

Ethyloestrenol (previously used name) — *See* Ethylestrenol.

Ethylpapaverine Hydrochloride — *See* Ethaverine Hydrochloride.

Ethylparaben (eth″ il par′ a ben). **NF**. $C_9H_{10}O_3$. 166.17. [Ethyl Parahydroxybenzoate is JAN.] (1) Benzoic acid, 4-hydroxy-, ethyl ester; (2) Ethyl *p*-hydroxybenzoate. *UNII-14255EXE39. CAS-120-47-8. Pharmaceutic aid (antifungal agent).*

Ethylphenacemide — *See* Pheneturide.

Ethylstibamine. $C_{10}H_{19}N_2O_3Sb$. 337.03. [Stibosamine is INN.] (1) Diethylamine *p*-aminobenzenestibonate; (2) Dihydroxyphenylstibine oxide compound with diethylamine. MI.

Ethynerone [*1965*] (e thye′ ner one). $C_{20}H_{23}ClO_2$. 330.85. (1) 19-Norpregna-4,9-dien-20-yn-3-one, 21-chloro-17-hydroxy-, (17α)-; (2) 21-Chloro-17-hydroxy-19-nor-17α-pregna-4,9-dien-20-yn-3-one. *UNII-CKM4S0R7LX. CAS-3124-93-4.* INN. *Progestin.*

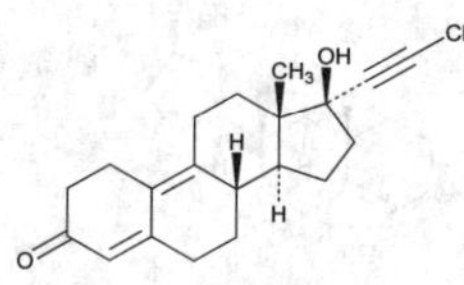

Ethynodiol Diacetate [*1962*] (e thye″ noe dye′ ol dye as′ e tate). **USP.** $C_{24}H_{32}O_4$. 384.51. [Etynodiol is INN and BAN; Etynodiol Acetate is JAN.] (1) 19-Norpregn-4-en-20-yne-3,17-diol, diacetate, (3β,17α)-; (2) 19-Nor-17α-pregn-4-en-20-yne-3β,17-diol diacetate. *UNII-62H10A1236; UNII-9E01C36A9S* [ethynodiol]. *CAS-297-76-7; CAS-1231-93-2* [ethynodiol]. *Progestin.* ◇*SC 11800*

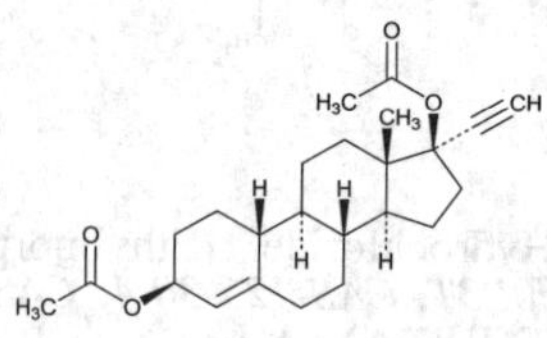

Ethypicone. $C_{10}H_{15}NO_2$. 181.23. 3,3-Diethyl-5-methyl-2,4(1*H*,3*H*)-pyridinedione. *UNII-2PO3M8FE7C. CAS-467-90-3.* INN.

Ethypropymal Sodium — *See* Probarbital Sodium.

Etibendazole [*1983*] (e″ ti ben′ da zole). $C_{18}H_{16}FN_3O_4$. 357.34. (1) Carbamic acid, [5-[2-(4-fluorophenyl)-1,3-dioxolan-2-yl]-1*H*-benzimidazol-2-yl]-, methyl ester; (2) Methyl 5-[2-(*p*-fluorophenyl)-1,3-dioxolan-2-yl]-2-benzimidazolecarbamate. *UNII-1XU086MM3H. CAS-64420-40-2.* INN. *Anthelmintic.* ◇*R-34,803*

Eticlopride. $C_{17}H_{25}ClN_2O_3$. 340.85. (-)-(*S*)-5-Chloro-3-ethyl-*N*-[(1-ethyl-2-pyrrolidinyl)methyl]-6-methoxysalicylamide. *UNII-J8M468HBH4. CAS-84226-12-0.* INN.

Eticyclidine. $C_{14}H_{21}N$. 203.32. *N*-Ethyl-1-phenylcyclohexylamine. *UNII-O8I1LL6A89. CAS-2201-15-2.* INN.

Etidocaine [*1973*] (e tye′ doe kane). $C_{17}H_{28}N_2O$. 276.42. (1) Butanamide, *N*-(2,6-dimethylphenyl)-2-(ethylpropylamino)-, (±)-; (2) (±)-2-(Ethylpropylamino)-2′,6′-butyroxylidide. *UNII-I6CQM0F31V. CAS-36637-18-0.* INN; BAN. *Anesthetic (local).* Duranest [as hydrochloride] (Astra) ◇*W-19053 [as hydrochloride]*

Etidronate Disodium [*1977*] (e ti droe′ nate dye soe′ dee um). **USP.** $C_2H_6Na_2O_7P_2$. 249.99. (1) Phosphonic acid, (1-hydroxyethylidene)bis-, disodium salt; (2) Disodium dihydrogen (1-hydroxyethylidene)diphosphonate. *UNII-M16PXG993G; UNII-M2F465ROXU* [etidronic acid]. *CAS-7414-83-7; CAS-2809-21-4* [etidronic acid]. JAN. *Bone resorption inhibitor.* Didronel (Procter & Gamble) [*Note—Other etidronic acid sodium salts are designated as etidronate monosodium, etidronate trisodium, and etidronate tetrasodium. The term etidronate sodium is to be used only where the salt cannot be identified more precisely.*]

Etidronic Acid [*1970*] (e ti dron′ ik as′ id). $C_2H_8O_7P_2$. 206.03. (1) Phosphonic acid, (1-hydroxyethylidene)bis-; (2) (1-Hydroxyethylidene)diphosphonic acid. *UNII-M2F465ROXU. CAS-2809-21-4.* INN; BAN. *Regulator (calcium).*

Etifelmine. $C_{17}H_{19}N$. 237.34. 2-(Diphenylmethylene)butylamine. *UNII-1ZFB1FR98E. CAS-341-00-4.* INN; MI.

Etifenin [*1980*] (e″ ti fen′ in). $C_{16}H_{22}N_2O_5$. 322.36. (1) Glycine, *N*-(carboxymethyl)-*N*-[2-[(2,6-diethylphenyl)amino]-2-oxoethyl]-; (2) [[[(2,6-Diethylphenyl)carbamoyl]methyl]imino]diacetic acid. *CAS-63245-28-3*. INN; BAN. *Diagnostic aid.*

Etifoxine. $C_{17}H_{17}ClN_2O$. 300.78. 6-Chloro-2-(ethylamino)-4-methyl-4-phenyl-4*H*-3,1-benzoxazine. *CAS-21715-46-8*. INN; BAN; DCF; MI. ◇*36-801; HOE 36801*

Etilamfetamine. $C_{11}H_{17}N$. 163.26. *N*-Ethyl-α-methylphenethylamine. *CAS-457-87-4*. INN.

Etilefrine. $C_{10}H_{15}NO_2$. 181.23. [Etilefrine Hydrochloride is JAN.] α-[(Ethylamino)methyl]-*m*-hydroxybenzyl alcohol. *UNII-ZB6F8MY53V. CAS-709-55-7*. INN; BAN; MI.

Etilefrine Pivalate. $C_{15}H_{23}NO_3$. 265.35. (±)-*m*-[(Ethylamino)-1-hydroxyethyl]phenyl pivalate. *UNII-3RLD929C4S. CAS-85750-39-6*. INN.

Etilevodopa [*2001*] (e″ ti lee″ voe doe′ pa). $C_{11}H_{15}NO_4$. 225.24. (1) L-Tyrosine, 3-hydroxy-, ethyl ester; (2) (-)-3,4-Dihydroxy-L-phenylalanine, ethyl ester. *UNII-895X917GYE. CAS-37178-37-3*. INN. *Antiparkisonian.* ◇*TV-1203*

Etintidine Hydrochloride [*1980*] (e tin′ ti deen hye″ droe klor′ ide). $C_{12}H_{16}N_6S·HCl$. 312.82. [Etintidine is INN.] (1) Guanidine, *N″*-cyano-*N*-[2-[[(5-methyl-1*H*-imidazol-4-yl)methyl]thio]ethyl]-*N′*-2-propynyl-, monohydrochloride; (2) 2-Cyano-1-[2-[[(5-methylimidazol-4-yl)methyl]thio]ethyl]-3-(2-propynyl)guanidine monohydrochloride. *CAS-71807-56-2; CAS-69539-53-3* [etintidine]. *Antagonist (to histamine H_2 receptors).* ◇*BL-5641A*

Etipirium Iodide. $C_{21}H_{26}INO_3$. 467.34. 1-(2-Hydroxyethyl)-1-methylpyrrolidinium iodide benzilate (ester). *UNII-D6FH7ALQ18. CAS-3478-15-7*. INN.

Etiprednol Dicloacetate [*2002*] (e ti pred′ nol dye″ kloe as′ e tate). $C_{24}H_{30}Cl_2O_6$. 485.40. (1) Androsta-1,4-diene-17-carboxylic acid, 17-[(dichloroacetyl)oxy]-11-hydroxy-3-oxo-, ethyl ester, (11β,17α)-; (2) Ethyl 17-[(dichloroacetyl)oxy]-11β-hydroxy-3-oxoandrosta-1,4-diene-17β-carboxylate. *CAS-199331-40-3*. INN; BAN. *Anti-inflammatory corticosteroid.* ◇*BNP-166*

Etiproston. $C_{24}H_{32}O_7$. 432.51. (*Z*)-7-[(1*R*,2*R*,3*R*,5*S*)-3,5-Dihydroxy-2-[(*E*)-2-[2-(phenoxymethyl)-1,3-dioxolan-2-yl]vinyl]cyclopentyl]-5-heptenoic acid. *UNII-TCU22W0APY. CAS-59619-81-7*. INN; MI.

Etiracetam. $C_8H_{14}N_2O_2$. 170.21. (±)-α-Ethyl-2-oxo-1-pyrrolidineacetamide. *UNII-230447L0GL. CAS-33996-58-6*. INN.

Etiroxate. $C_{18}H_{17}I_4NO_4$. 818.95. α-Methyl-DL-thyroxine ethyl ester. *UNII-0S3LDN5P7H. CAS-17365-01-4*. INN; MI.

Etisazole. $C_9H_{10}N_2S$. 178.25. 3-(Ethylamino)-1,2-benzisothiazole. *UNII-G0WB531332. CAS-7716-60-1*. INN; BAN; MI. ◇*Bay VA 9387*

Etisomicin. $C_{20}H_{39}N_5O_7$. 461.55. *O*-3-Deoxy-3-(ethylamino)-4-*C*-methyl-*β*-L-arabinopyranosyl-(1→4)-*O*-[2,6-diamino-2,3,4,6-tetradeoxy-*α*-D-*glycero*-hex-4-enopyranosyl-(1→6)]-2-deoxy-L-streptamine. *UNII-0BZK9FE5DE. CAS-70639-48-4*. INN; BAN. ◇*BAY V1 4718*

Etisulergine. $C_{19}H_{28}N_4O_2S$. 376.52. *N,N*-Diethyl-*N′*-(6-methylergolin-8*α*-yl)sulfamide. *UNII-28N73Q6O7Y. CAS-64795-23-9*. INN.

Etizolam. $C_{17}H_{15}ClN_4S$. 342.85. 4-(*o*-Chlorophenyl)-2-ethyl-9-methyl-6*H*-thieno[3,2-*f*]-*s*-triazolo[4,3-*a*][1,4]diazepine. *UNII-A76XI0HL37. CAS-40054-69-1*. INN; JAN; MI.

Etobedolum — *See* Etonitazene.

Etocarlide. $C_{17}H_{20}N_2O_2S$. 316.42. 4,4′-Diethoxythiocarbanilide. *UNII-46V3V5EQAM. CAS-1234-30-6*. INN.

Etocrilene (INN) — *See* Etocrylene.

Etocrylene [*1979*] (e″ toe krye′ leen). $C_{18}H_{15}NO_2$. 277.32. [Etocrilene is INN.] (1) 2-Propenoic acid, 2-cyano-3,3-diphenyl-, ethyl ester; (2) Ethyl 2-cyano-3,3-diphenylacrylate. *CAS-5232-99-5*. *Ultraviolet screen.*

Etodolac [*1975*] (e toe′ doe lak). **USP.** $C_{17}H_{21}NO_3$. 287.35. [Etodolic Acid is INN.] (1) Pyrano[3,4-*b*]indole-1-acetic acid, 1,8-diethyl-1,3,4,9-tetrahydro-(±)-; (2) (±)-1,8-Diethyl-1,3,4,9-tetrahydropyrano[3,4-*b*]indole-1-acetic acid. *UNII-2M36281008. CAS-41340-25-4*. INN; BAN. *Anti-inflammatory.* Lodine (Wyeth) ◇*AY-24,236*

Etodolic Acid (INN) — *See* Etodolac.

Etodroxizine. $C_{23}H_{31}ClN_2O_3$. 418.96. 2-{2-[2-[4-(*p*-Chloro-*α*-phenylbenzyl)-1-piperazinyl]ethoxy]ethoxy} ethanol. *UNII-CI1S3XAK7O. CAS-17692-34-1*. INN; MI.

Etofamide. $C_{19}H_{20}Cl_2N_2O_5$. 427.28. 2,2-Dichloro-*N*-(2-ethoxyethyl)-*N*-[(*p*-nitrophenoxy)benzyl]-acetamide. *UNII-03F36JH21U. CAS-25287-60-9*. INN.

Etofenamate [*1987*] (e″ toe fen′ a mate). $C_{18}H_{18}F_3NO_4$. 369.34. (1) Benzoic acid, 2-[[3-(trifluoromethyl)phenyl]amino]-, 2-(2-hydroxyethoxy)ethyl ester; (2) 2-(2-Hydroxyethoxy)ethyl *N*-(*α,α,α*-trifluoro-*m*-tolyl)anthranilate. *CAS-30544-47-9*. INN; BAN. *Analgesic; anti-inflammatory.* ◇*WHR-5020; TVX485; Bay d 1107*

Etofenprox. $C_{25}H_{28}O_3$. 376.49. *α*-[(*p*-Ethoxy-*β,β*-dimethylphenethyl)oxy]-*m*-phenoxytoluene. *UNII-0LD7P9153C. CAS-80844-07-1*. INN.

Etofibrate. $C_{18}H_{18}ClNO_5$. 363.79. 2-Hydroxyethyl nicotinate 2-(*p*-chlorophenoxy)-2-methylpropionate (ester). *UNII-23TF67G79M. CAS-31637-97-5*. INN; MI.

Etoformin Hydrochloride [*1975*] (e″ toe for′ min hye″ droe klor′ ide). $C_8H_{19}N_5$·HCl. 221.73. [Etoformin is INN.] (1) Imidodicarbonimidic diamide, *N*-butyl-*N″*-ethyl-, monohydrochloride; (2) 1-Butyl-2-ethylbiguanide monohydrochloride. *UNII-19HR3G3ESA; UNII-630F8M4Q1D* [etoformin]. *CAS-53597-26-5; CAS-45086-03-1* [etoformin]. *Antidiabetic.* ◇*SH E 199*

Etofuradine. $C_{18}H_{21}N_3O$. 295.38. *N*-(Benzofuran-2-yl-methyl)-*N*-2-pyridyl-*N′,N′*-dimethylethylenediamine. *UNII-DQ61UZ670G. CAS-17692-35-2.* INN.

Etofylline. $C_9H_{12}N_4O_3$. 224.22. 7-(2-Hydroxyethyl)theophylline. *CAS-519-37-9.* INN; BAN; MI.

Etofylline Clofibrate (INN) — *See* Theofibrate.

Etoglucid. $C_{12}H_{22}O_6$. 262.30. 1,2:15,16-Diepoxy-4,7,10,13-tetraoxahexadecane. *CAS-1954-28-5.* INN; BAN; MI. *[Name previously used: Ethoglucid.]* ◇*ICI 32865*

Etolorex. $C_{12}H_{18}ClNO$. 227.73. 2-[(*p*-Chloro-α,α-dimethyl-phenethyl)amino]ethanol. *UNII-449NCX1P03. CAS-54063-36-4.* INN.

Etolotifen. $C_{24}H_{29}NO_4S$. 427.56. 4,9-Dihydro-4-[1-[2-[2-(2-hydroxyethoxy)ethoxy]ethyl]-4-piperidylidene]-10*H*-benzo[4,5]cyclohepta[1,2-*b*]thiophen-10-one. *UNII-U64HJ4AK57. CAS-82140-22-5.* INN.

Etoloxamine. $C_{19}H_{25}NO$. 283.41. 2-[(α-Phenyl-*o*-tolyl)oxy]-triethylamine. *UNII-NEZ417265P. CAS-1157-87-5.* INN.

Etomidate [*1975*] (e tom′ i date). $C_{14}H_{16}N_2O_2$. 244.29. (1) 1*H*-Imidazole-5-carboxylic acid, 1-(1-phenylethyl)-, ethyl ester, (+)-; (2) (+)-Ethyl 1-(α-methylbenzyl)imidazole-5-carboxylate. *UNII-Z22628B598. CAS-33125-97-2.* INN; BAN. *Sedative-hypnotic.* Amidate (Hospira)

Etomidoline. $C_{23}H_{29}N_3O_2$. 379.50. 2-Ethyl-3-(β-piperidino-*p*-phenetidino)phthalimidine. *UNII-WFS7G78GYJ. CAS-21590-92-1.* INN; JAN; MI.

Etomoxir. $C_{17}H_{23}ClO_4$. 326.82. Ethyl (+)-(*R*)-2-[6-(*p*-chloro-phenoxy)hexyl]glycidate. *CAS-124083-20-1.* INN.

Etonam (INN) Nitrate — *See* Ethonam Nitrate.

Etonitazene. $C_{22}H_{28}N_4O_3$. 396.48. 1-(2-Diethylaminoethyl)-2-(*p*-ethoxybenzyl)-5-nitrobenzimidazole. *UNII-9U3GT3353T. CAS-911-65-9.* INN; BAN; DCF; MI. ◇*Ba-20684; NIH 7607*

Etonogestrel [*1993*] (e toe noe jes′ trel). $C_{22}H_{28}O_2$. 324.46. (1) 18,19-Dinor-17α-pregn-4-en-20-yn-3-one, 13-ethyl-17-hydroxy-11-methylene-; (2) 13-Ethyl-17-hydroxy-11-

---

methylene-18,19-dinor-17α-pregn-4-en-20-yn-3-one. *UNII-304GTH6RNH. CAS-54048-10-1.* INN; BAN. *Progestin.* Implanon (Organon) ◇ORG 3236

Etoperidone Hydrochloride [*1988*] (e″ toe per′ i done hye″ droe klor′ ide). C$_{19}$H$_{28}$ClN$_5$O.HCl. 414.37. [Etoperidone is INN.] (1) 3*H*-1,2,4-Triazol-3-one, 2-[3-[4-(3-chlorophenyl)-1-piperazinyl]propyl]-4,5-diethyl-2,4-dihydro-, monohydrochloride; (2) 1-[3-[4-(*m*-Chlorophenyl)-1-piperazinyl]propyl]-3,4-diethyl-Δ^2-1,2,4-triazolin-5-one monohydrochloride. *UNII-2FSU2FR80J; UNII-KAI6M-VO39Z* [etoperidone]. *CAS-57775-22-1; CAS-52942-31-1* [etoperidone]. *Antidepressant.* Etonin (Ortho-McNeil†) ◇McN-A-2673-11

Etoposide [*1978*] (e toe′ poe side). **USP.** C$_{29}$H$_{32}$O$_{13}$. 588.56. (1) Furo[3′,4′:6,7]naphtho[2,3-*d*]-1,3-dioxol-6(5a*H*)-one-, 9-[(4,6-*O*-ethylidene-β-D-glucopyranosyl)oxy]5,8,8a,9-tetrahydro-5-(4-hydroxy-3,5-dimethoxyphenyl), [5*R*-[5α,5aβ,8aα,9β(*R**)]]-; (2) 4′-Demethylepipodophyllotoxin 9-[4,6-*O*-(*R*)-ethylidene-β-D-glucopyranoside]. *UNII-6PLQ3CP4P3. CAS-33419-42-0.* INN; BAN; JAN. *Antineoplastic.* Vepesid (Bristol-Myers Squibb) ◇VP-16-213

Etoposide Phosphate [*1992*] (e toe′ poe side fos′ fate). C$_{29}$H$_{33}$O$_{16}$P. 668.54. (1) Furo[3′,4′:6,7]naphtho[2,3-*d*]-1,3-dioxol-6(5a*H*)-one, 5-[3,5-dimethoxy-4-(phosphonooxy)phenyl]-9-[(4,6-*O*-ethylidene-β-D-glucopyranosyl)oxy]-5,8,8a,9-tetrahydro-, [5*R*-[5α,5aβ,8aα,9β(*R**)]]-; (2) 4′-Demethylepipodophyllotoxin 9-[4,6-*O*-(*R*)-ethylidene-β-D-glucopyranoside], 4′-(dihydrogen phosphate). *UNII-528XYJ8L1N. CAS-117091-64-2. Antineoplastic.* Etopophos (Bristol-Myers Squibb) ◇BMY 40481

Etoprindole. C$_{15}$H$_{21}$N$_3$O. 259.35. 1-[2-(Dimethylamino)ethyl]indol-3-yl ethyl ketone oxime. *UNII-LBU97HVE51. CAS-54063-37-5.* INN; DCF.

Etoprine [*1977*] (e′ toe preen). C$_{12}$H$_{12}$Cl$_2$N$_4$. 283.16. (1) 2,4-Pyrimidinediamine, 5-(3,4-dichlorophenyl)-6-ethyl-; (2) 2,4-Diamino-5-(3,4-dichlorophenyl)-6-ethylpyrimidine. *UNII-406PGU9KGI. CAS-18588-57-3. Antineoplastic.*

Etoricoxib [*2000*] (e toe″ ri kox′ ib). C$_{18}$H$_{15}$ClN$_2$O$_2$S. 358.84. (1) 2,3′-Bipyridine, 5-chloro-6′-methyl-3-[4-(methylsulfonyl)phenyl]-; (2) 5-Chloro-6′-methyl-3-[*p*-(methylsulfonyl)phenyl]-2,3′-bipyridine. *CAS-202409-33-4.* INN; BAN. *Anti-inflammatory; analgesic used in the treatment of osteoarthritis and rheumatoid arthritis (COX-2 inhibitor).* ◇MK-0663

Etorphine. C$_{25}$H$_{33}$NO$_4$. 411.53. 6,7,8,14-Tetrahydro-7α-(1-hydroxy-1-methylbutyl)-6,14-*endo*-ethenooripavine. *CAS-14521-96-1.* INN; BAN; MI. M99 Injection (Lemmont†) ◇M. 99 [as hydrochloride]

Etosalamide. C$_{11}$H$_{15}$NO$_3$. 209.24. *o*-(2-Ethoxyethoxy)benzamide. *UNII-1PU994YJUH. CAS-15302-15-5.* INN; BAN. [*Name previously used: Ethosalamide.*]

Etoxadrol Hydrochloride [*1970*] (e tox′ a drol hye″ droe klor′ ide). C$_{16}$H$_{23}$NO$_2$.HCl. 297.82. [Etoxadrol is INN.] (1) Piperidine, 2-(2-ethyl-2-phenyl-1,3-dioxolan-4-yl), hydrochloride; (2) (+)-2-(2-Ethyl-2-phenyl-1,3-dioxolan-4-yl)-piperidine hydrochloride. *CAS-23239-37-4; CAS-28189-85-7* [etoxadrol]. *Anesthetic.* ⋄*CL-1848C*

Etoxazene (INN) Hydrochloride — *See* Ethoxazene Hydrochloride.

Etoxeridine. $C_{18}H_{27}NO_4$. 321.41. 1-[2-(2-Hydroxyethoxy)ethyl]-4-phenylpiperidine-4-carboxylic acid ethyl ester. *UNII-RHW35E1G7E. CAS-469-82-9.* INN; BAN. ⋄*UCB 2073; Wy-2039*

Etozolin [*1965*] (e″ toe zoe′ lin). $C_{13}H_{20}N_2O_3S$. 284.37. (1) Acetic acid, [3-methyl-4-oxo-5-(1-piperidinyl)-2-thiazolidinylidene]-, ethyl ester; (2) 3-Methyl-4-oxo-5-piperidino-$\Delta^{2,a}$-thiazolidineacetic acid ethyl ester. *UNII-UEO8UW9V1Z. CAS-73-09-6.* INN. *Diuretic.* ⋄*W 2900A*

Etrabamine. $C_8H_{12}N_2S$. 168.26. 4,5,6,7-Tetrahydro-6-(methylamino)benzothiazole. *UNII-V55R69267Q. CAS-70590-58-8.* INN.

Etravirine [*2005*] (e″ tra vir′ een). $C_{20}H_{15}BrN_6O$. 435.28. (1) Benzonitrile, 4-[[6-amino-5-bromo-2-[(4-cyanophenyl)amino]-4-pyrimidinyl]oxy]-3,5-dimethyl-; (2) 4-[[6-Amino-5-bromo-2-[(4-cyanophenyl)amino]-4-pyrimidinyl]oxy]-3,5-dimethyl-benzonitrile. *UNII-0C50HW4FO1. CAS-269055-15-4.* INN; JAN. *Treatment of HIV infection.* ⋄*TMC 125*

Etretin — *See* Acitretin.

Etretinate [*1979*] (e tret′ i nate). $C_{23}H_{30}O_3$. 354.48. (1) 2,4,6,8-Nonatetraenoic acid, 9-(4-methoxy-2,3,6-trimethylphenyl)-, ethyl ester, (*all-E-*); (2) Ethyl (*all-E*)-9-(4-methoxy-2,3,6-trimethylphenyl)-3,7-dimethyl-2,4,6,8-nonatetraenoate. *UNII-65M2UDR9AG. CAS-54350-48-0.* INN; BAN; JAN. *Antipsoriatic.* Tegison (Roche) ⋄*Ro 10-9359*

Etriciguat. $C_{22}H_{16}FN_7$. 397.41. 2-[1-(2-Fluorobenzyl)-1*H*-pyrazolo[3,4-*b*]pyridin-3-yl]-5-(4-pyridyl)pyrimidin-4-amine. *UNII-E3ZEH4F4CA. CAS-402595-29-3.* INN.

Etryptamine Acetate [*1961*] (e trip′ ta meen as′ e tate). $C_{12}H_{16}N_2 \cdot C_2H_4O_2$. 248.32. [Etryptamine is INN and BAN.] (1) 1*H*-Indole-3-ethanamine, α-ethyl-, monoacetate; (2) 3-(2-Aminobutyl)indole monoacetate. *UNII-3RY07R55EE; UNII-GR181O3R32* [etryptamine]. *CAS-118-68-3; CAS-2235-90-7* [etryptamine]. *Stimulant (central).* ⋄*U-17312E; NSC-63963*

Etybenzatropine (INN, BAN, DCF) — *See* Ethybenztropine.

Etymemazine Hydrochloride. $C_{20}H_{26}N_2S \cdot HCl$. 362.96. [Etymemazine is INN.] 10-[3-(Dimethylamino)-2-methylpropyl]-2-ethylphenothiazine hydrochloride. *UNII-A7002E7T2Z; UNII-861J4K81C7* [etymemazine]. *CAS-3737-33-5; CAS-523-54-6* [etymemazine]. MI. ⋄*RP 6484*

Etynodiol (INN, BAN) — *See* Ethynodiol Diacetate.

Etynodiol Acetate (JAN) — *See* Ethynodiol Diacetate.

Etyprenaline — *See* Isoetharine.

Eucaine Hydrochloride. *UNII-73NDV3S9Y7. CAS-555-28-2; CAS-500-34-5* [β-eucaine]. NF VIII; MI. *[Name previously used: Betaeucaine Hydrochloride.]*

Eucalyptol [*1988*] (ue″ ka lip′ tol). **USP.** $C_{10}H_{18}O$. 154.25. (1) 1,3,3-Trimethyl-2-oxabicyclo[2.2.2]octane; (2) 1,8-Epoxy-*p*-menthane. *UNII-RV6J6604TK. CAS-470-82-6.*

Eucalyptus Oil. *UNII-2R04ONI662. CAS-8000-48-4.* NF XVI; JAN; MI.

Eucatropine Hydrochloride (ue kat′ roe peen hye″ droe klor′ ide). **USP.** $C_{17}H_{25}NO_3 \cdot HCl$. 327.85. [Eucatropine is INN and BAN.] (1) Benzeneacetic acid, α-hydroxy-, 1,2,2,6-tetramethyl-4-piperidinyl ester hydrochloride; (2) 1,2,2,6-

---

† Brand name formerly used, and/or firm no longer concerned with this product.

Tetramethyl-4-piperidyl mandelate hydrochloride. *CAS-536-93-6; CAS-100-91-4* [eucatropine]. *Anticholinergic (ophthalmic).*

Eufauserase. $C_{1170}H_{1764}N_{300}O_{387}S_{14}$. A broad-spectrum, monocomponent serine-protease enzyme, extracted and purified from *Euphausia superba* (Antarctic krill). INN; BAN. ◇*PHM-101*

```
AVENCGPVAP   RNK

IVGGMEVTPH   AYPWQVGLFI   DDMYFCGGSI   ISDEWVLTAH
CMDGAGFVEV   VMGAHSIHDE   TEATQVRATS   TDFFTHENWN
SFTLSNDLAL   IKMPAPIEFN   DVIQPVCLPT   YTDASDDFVG
ESVTLTGWGK   PSDSAFGIAE   QLREVDVTTI   TTADCQAYYG
IVTDKILCID   SEGGHGSCNG   DSGGPMNYVT   GGVTQTRGIT
SFGSSTGCET   GYPDGYTRVT   SYLDWIESNT   GIAIDP
```

Eugenol (ue' je nol). **USP.** $C_{10}H_{12}O_2$. 164.20. (1) Phenol, 2-methoxy-4-(2-propenyl)-; (2) 4-Allyl-2-methoxyphenol. *CAS-97-53-0. Analgesic (dental).*

Euphausia Extract. A purified extract from *Euphausia superba* (Antarctic krill) containing water-extractable macromolecules, mainly proteins in the molecular weight range 10-60 kDa; the main action is due to the serine-proteases present with a molecular weight range of 20-40 kDa. BAN.

Euprocin Hydrochloride [*1969*] (ue' proe sin hye" droe klor' ide). $C_{24}H_{34}N_2O_2$.2HCl. 455.46. [Euprocin is INN.] (1) Cinchonan-9-ol, 10,11-dihydro-6'-(3-methylbutoxy)-, dihydrochloride, (8α,9R)-; (2) $O^{6'}$-Isopentylhydrocupreine-dihydrochloride. *UNII-EVA0339N2N. CAS-18984-80-0; CAS-1301-42-4* [euprocin]. *Anesthetic (topical).* ◇*WI 287*

Euquinine — *See* Quinine Ethylcarbonate.

Evandamine. $C_{11}H_{16}N_4S$. 236.34. (±)-2-(3-Amino-5-methyl-2-pyrazolin-1-yl)-4,5,6,7-tetrahydrobenzothiazole. *UNII-ZG2L2878MD. CAS-100035-75-4.* INN.

Evans Blue. $C_{34}H_{24}N_6Na_4O_{14}S_4$. 960.81. [Azovan Blue is BAN.] (1) 1,3-Naphthalenedisulfonic acid, 6,6'-[(3,3'-dimethyl[1,1'-biphenyl]-4,4'-diyl)bis(azo)]bis[4-amino-5-hydroxy]-, tetrasodium salt; (2) C.I. direct blue 53 tetrasodium salt. *UNII-45PG892GO1. CAS-314-13-6; CAS-179472-53-8* [replaced]. USP XXII.

Evernimicin [*1999*] (e″ ver ni mye' sin). $C_{70}H_{97}Cl_2NO_{38}$. 1631.41. (1) *O*-(1*R*)-4-*O*-(2,4-Dihydroxy-6-methylbenzoyl)-2,3-*O*-methylene-D-xylopyranosylidene-(1→3-4)-α-L-lyxopyranosyl *O*-2,3,6-trideoxy-3-*C*-methyl 4-*O*-methyl-3-nitro-α-L-*arabino*-hexopyranosyl-(1→3)-*O*-2,6-dideoxy-4-*O*-(3,5-dichloro-4-hydroxy-2-methoxy-6-methylbenzoyl)-β-D-*arabino*-hexopyranosyl-(1→4)-*O*-(1*R*)-2,6-dideoxy-D-*arabino*-hexopyranosylidene-(1→3-4)-*O*-6-deoxy-3-*C*-methyl-β-D-mannopyranosyl-(1→3)-*O*-6-deoxy-4-*O*-methyl-β-D-galactopyranosyl-(1→4)-2,6-di-*O*-methyl-β-D-mannopyranoside; (2) *O*-(1*R*)-2,3-*O*-Methylene-4-*O*-(6-methyl-β-resorcyloyl)-D-xylopyranosylidene-(1→3-4)-α-L-lyxopyranosyl *O*-2,3,6-trideoxy-3-*C*-methyl 4-*O*-methyl-3-nitro-α-L-*arabino*-hexopyranosyl-(1→3)-*O*-2,6-dideoxy-4-*O*-(3,5-dichloro-6-methoxy-4,2-cresotoyl)-β-D-*arabino*-hexopyranosyl-(1→4)-*O*-(1*R*)-2,6-dideoxy-D-*arabino*-hexopyranosylidene-(1→3-4)-*O*-6-deoxy-3-*C*-methyl-β-D-mannopyranosyl-(1→3)-*O*-6-deoxy-4-*O*-methyl-β-D-galactopyranosyl-(1→4)-2,6-di-*O*-methyl-β-D-mannopyranoside. *CAS-109545-84-8.* INN. *Antibacterial.* Ziracin (Schering-Plough HealthCare) ◇*SCH 27899*

Everolimus [*2003*] (e″ ver oh' li mus). $C_{53}H_{83}NO_{14}$. 958.22. (1) (1*R*,9*S*,12*S*,15*R*,16*E*,18*R*,19*R*,21*R*,23-*S*,24*E*,26*E*,28*E*,30*S*,32*S*,35*R*)-1,18-Dihydroxy-12-[(1*R*)-2-[(1*S*,3*R*,4*R*)-4-(2-hydroxyethoxy)-3-methoxycyclohexyl]-1-methylethyl]-19,30-dimethoxy-15,17,21,23,29,35-hexamethyl-11,36-dioxa-4-azatricyclo[30.3.1.0⁴,⁹]hexatriaconta-16,24,26,28-tetraene-2,3,10,14,20-pentaone; (2) (3*S*,6*R*,7*E*,9*R*,10*R*,12*R*,14*S*,15*E*,17*E*,19*E*,21*S*,23*S*,26*R*,27-*R*,34a*S*)-9,10,12,13,14,21,22,23,24,25,26,27,32,33,34,34a-Hexadecahydro-9,27-dihydroxy-3-[(1*R*)-2-[(1*S*,3*R*,4*R*)-4-(2-hydroxyethoxy)-3-methoxycyclohexyl]-1-methylethyl]-10,21-dimethoxy-6,8,12,14,20,26-hexamethyl-23,27-epoxy-3*H*-pyrido[2,1-*c*][1,4]oxaazacyclohentriacontine-1,5,11,28,29(4*H*,6*H*,31*H*)-pentone; (3) 42-*O*-(2-Hydroxyethyl)rapamycin. *CAS-159351-69-6.* INN. *Immunosuppressant.* ◇*RAD001*

Evicromil. $C_{14}H_{12}O_5$. 260.24. 8-Ethyl-5-hydroxy-4-oxo-6-vinyl-4*H*-chromene-2-carboxylic acid. *UNII-MKO1PH93P2. CAS-62571-88-4.* BAN.

Exalamide. $C_{13}H_{19}NO_2$. 221.30. *o*-(Hexyloxy)benzamide. *UNII-7JEC65JCG2. CAS-53370-90-4.* INN; JAN; MI.

Exametazime [*1990*] (ex″ a met′ a zeem). $C_{13}H_{28}N_4O_2$. 272.39. (1) 2-Butanone, 3,3′-[(2,2-dimethyl-1,3-propane-diyl)diimino]bis-, dioxime, [*R**,*R**-(*E*,*E*)]-(±)-; (2) (±)-(3*RS*,3′*RS*)-3,3′-[(2,2-Dimethyltrimethylene)diimino]di-2-butanone (*E*,*E*)-dioxime. *UNII-G29272NCKL. CAS-105613-48-7; CAS-100551-63-1* [replaced]. INN; BAN; JAN. *Diagnostic aid (regional cerebral perfusion imaging). [Name previously used: Hexametazine.]* ◇*dl HM-PAO*

Examorelin. $C_{47}H_{58}N_{12}O_6$. 887.04. L-Histidyl-2-methyl-D-tryptophyl-L-alanyl-L-tryptophyl-D-phenylalanyl-L-lysinamide. *UNII-09QF37C617. CAS-140703-51-1.* INN.

Exaprolol Hydrochloride [*1981*] (ex″ a proe′ lol hye″ droe klor′ ide). $C_{18}H_{29}NO_2 \cdot HCl$. 327.89. [Exaprolol is INN.] (1) 2-Propanol, 1-(2-cyclohexylphenoxy)-3-[(1-methylethyl)amino]-, hydrochloride, (±)-; (2) (±)-1-(*o*-Cyclohexylphenoxy)-3-(isopropylamino)-2-propanol hydrochloride. *UNII-FGT82HNC7L; UNII-Q4XX54I93R* [exaprolol]. *CAS-59333-90-3* [monohydrochloride]; *CAS-55837-19-9* [exaprolol]. *Anti-adrenergic (β-receptor).* ◇*M.G. 8823*

Exatecan. $C_{24}H_{22}FN_3O_4$. 435.45. (1*S*,9*S*)-1-Amino-9-ethyl-5-fluoro-1,2,3,9,12,15-hexahydro-9-hydroxy-4-methyl-10*H*,13*H*-benzo[*de*]pyrano[3′,4′:6,7]indolizino[1,2-*b*]quinoline-10,13-dione. *UNII-OC71PP0F89. CAS-171335-80-1.* INN.

Exatecan Alideximer. Exatecan linked via the tetrapeptide (glycylglycyl-L-phenylalanylglycyl) to poly[oxy(2-hydroxymethylethylene)oxy(hydroxymethylmethylene)] partly *O*-substituted with carboxymethyl groups with some carboxy groups amide linked to the tetrapeptide. INN.

Exatecan Mesylate [*1998*] (ex″ a tee′ kan mes′ i late). $C_{24}H_{22}FN_3O_4 \cdot CH_4O_3S \cdot 2H_2O$. 567.58. (1) (1*S-trans*)-1-Amino-9-ethyl-5-fluoro-1,2,3,9,12,15-hexahydro-9-hydroxy-4-methyl-10*H*, 13*H*-benzo[*de*]pyrano[3′,4′:6,7]indolizino[1,2-*b*]quinoline-10,13-dione monomethanesulfonate (salt), dihydrate; (2) (1*S*,9*S*)-1-Amino-9-ethyl-5-fluoro-1,2,3,9,12,15-hexahydro-9-hydroxy-4-methyl-10*H*, 13*H*-benzo[*de*]pyrano[3′,4′:6,7]indolizino[1,2-*b*]quinoline-10,13-dione monomethanesulfonate (salt), dihydrate. *CAS-197720-53-9. Antineoplastic.* ◇*DX-8951f*

Exbivirumab. $C_{6416}H_{9924}N_{1732}O_{1982}S_{44}$. Immunoglobulin G, anti-(hepatitis B surface antigen) (human monoclonal 19.79.5 heavy chain), disulfide with human monoclonal 19.79.5 λ chain, dimer. *CAS-569658-80-6.* INN.

Exemestane [*1999*] (ex″ e mes′ tane). $C_{20}H_{24}O_2$. 296.40. (1) Androsta-1,4-diene-3,17-dione, 6-methylene-; (2) 6-Methyleneandrosta-1,4-diene-3,17-dione. *UNII-NY22HMQ4BX. CAS-107868-30-4.* INN; BAN. *Antineoplastic used to treat advanced breast cancer (aromatase inhibitor).* Aromasin (Pfizer) ◇*PNU-155971; FCE24304*

Exenatide [*2003*] (ex en′ a tide). $C_{184}H_{282}N_{50}O_{60}S$. 4186.57 (peptide). (1) Exendin 4; (2) L-Histidylglycyl-L-glutamyl-glycyl-L-threonyl-L-phenylalanyl-L-threonyl-L-seryl-L-aspartyl-L-leucyl-L-seryl-L-lysyl-L-glutaminyl-L-methionyl-L-glutamyl-L-glutamyl-L-glutamyl-L-alanyl-L-valyl-L-arginyl-L-leucyl-L-phenylalanyl-L-isoleucyl-L-glutamyl-L-tryptophyl-L-leucyl-L-lysyl-L-asparaginylglycylglycyl-L-prolyl-L-seryl-L-serylglycyl-L-alanyl-L-prolyl-L-prolyl-L-prolyl-L-serinamide. *UNII-9P1872D4OL. CAS-141732-76-5; CAS-141758-74-9.* INN; BAN; JAN. *Antidiabetic.* ◇*AC002993; AC2993A; AC2993; AC 2993; AC-2993; LY2148568*

HGEGTFTSDL SKQMEEEAVR LFIEWLKNGG PSSGAPPPS

Exepanol. $C_{11}H_{15}NO_2$. 193.24. (±)-*cis*-2,3,4,5-Tetrahydro-3-(methylamino)-1-benzoxepin-5-ol. *CAS-77416-65-0.* INN.

Exifone. $C_{13}H_{10}O_7$. 278.21. 2,3,3′,4,4′,5′-Hexahydroxybenzophenone. *CAS-52479-85-3.* INN; MI.

Exiproben. $C_{16}H_{24}O_5$. 296.36. *o*-[3-(Hexyloxy)-2-hydroxy-propoxy]benzoic acid. *UNII-SID40G6U6D. CAS-26281-69-6.* INN; MI. ◇*DCH 21 [as sodium salt]*

Exisulind. $C_{20}H_{17}FO_4S$. 372.41. 5-Fluoro-2-methyl-1-[(*Z*)-*p*-(methylsulfonyl)benzylidene]indene-3-acetic acid. *CAS-59973-80-7.* INN.

Ezatiostat Hydrochloride [*2007*] (ez″ a tye′ oh stat hye″ droe klor′ ide). $C_{27}H_{35}N_3O_6$·HCl. 534.04. [Ezatiostat is INN.] (1) Glycine, L-γ-glutamyl-*S*-(phenylmethyl)-L-cysteinyl-2-phenyl-, diethyl ester, monohydrochloride, (2*R*)-; (2) Ethyl (2*R*)-[(4*S*)-4-amino-5-ethoxy-5-oxopentanoyl]-*S*-benzyl-L-cysteinyl-2-phenylglycinate hydrochloride. *UNII-D59N834676. CAS-286942-97-0; CAS-168682-53-9* [ezatiostat]. *Treatment of disorders of bone marrow cellular growth and differentiation.* Telintra (Telik) ◇*TLK199; TER199*

Ezetimibe [*1999*] (e zet′ i mide). $C_{24}H_{21}F_2NO_3$. 409.43. (1) 2-Azetidinone, 1-(4-fluorophenyl)-3-[3-(4-fluorophenyl)-3-hydroxypropyl]-4-(4-hydroxyphenyl)-, [3*R*-[3α(*S**),4β]]-; (2) (3*R*,4*S*)-1-(*p*-Fluorophenyl)-3-[(3*S*)-3-(*p*-fluorophenyl)-3-hydroxypropyl]-4-(*p*-hydroxyphenyl)-2-azetidinone. *UNII-EOR26LQQ24. CAS-163222-33-1.* INN; BAN. *Antihyperlipidemic (intestinal cholesterol absorption inhibitor).* Zetia (Merck/Schering-Plough) ◇*SCH58235*

Ezlopitant [*1999*] (ez loe′ pi tant). $C_{31}H_{38}N_2O$. 454.65. (1) 1-Azabicyclo[2.2.2]octan-3-amine, 2-(diphenylmethyl)-*N*-[[2-methoxy-5-(1-methylethyl)phenyl]methyl]-, (2*S*-*cis*)-; (2) (2*S*,3*S*)-2-(Diphenylmethyl)-3-[(5-isopropyl-2-meth-

oxybenzyl)amino]quinuclidine. *CAS-147116-64-1.* INN. *Treatment of emesis, pain, and inflammation (substance P [NK-1] receptor antagonist).* ◇*CJ-11, 974*

^{18}F — *See* Fludeoxyglucose F 18.

^{18}F — *See* Fluorodopa F 18.

^{18}F — *See* Sodium Fluoride F 18.

Fabesetron. $C_{18}H_{19}N_3O$. 293.36. (+)-(*R*)-8,9-Dihydro-10-methyl-7-[(5-methylimidazol-4-yl)methyl]pyrido[1,2-*a*]indol-6(7*H*)-one. *UNII-QU72HVX338. CAS-129300-27-2.* INN.

Factor IX Complex (fak′ tor). **USP.** [Factor IX Fraction is BAN.] A sterile, freeze-dried powder consisting of partially purified Factor IX fraction, as well as concentrated Factors II, VII and X fractions, of venous plasma. *Hemostatic.* AlphaNine (Alpha Therapeutic†); AlphaNine SD (Alpha Therapeutic); Konyne 80 (Bayer); Mononine (Centeon); Profilnine (Alpha Therapeutic†); Profilnine SD (Alpha Therapeutic); Proplex T (Hyland)

Factor IX Fraction (BAN) — *See* Factor IX Complex.

Factor VIII (rDNA). [Octocog Alfa is BAN.] Recombinant human antihemophilic factor VIII (without von Willebrand factor) derived from a cloned human factor VIII gene produced from genetically engineered baby hamster kidney (bhk) cells. ◇*BAY w 6240*

Fadolmidine. $C_{13}H_{14}N_2O$. 214.26. 3-(Imidazol-4-ylmethyl)-5-indanol. *UNII-WLN5FGH1CY. CAS-189353-31-9.* INN. *[Name previously used: Radolmidine.]*

Fadolmidine Hydrochloride [*2002*] (fa dol′ mi deen hye″ droe klor′ ide). $C_{13}H_{14}N_2O$·HCl. 250.72. (1) 1*H*-Inden-5-ol, 2,3-dihydro-3-(1*H*-imidazol-4-ylmethyl)-, monohydrochloride; (2) 3-(Imidazol-4-ylmethyl)-5-indanol monohydrochloride. *UNII-S3709T25V6. CAS-189353-32-0. Spinal analgesic ($α_2$-adrenoreceptor agonist).[Name previously used: Radolmidine Hydrochloride.]* ◇*MPV-2426*

Fadrozole Hydrochloride [*1990*] (fad′ roe zole hye″ droe klor′ ide). $C_{14}H_{13}N_3$·HCl. 259.73. [Fadrozole is INN.] (1) Benzonitrile, 4-(5,6,7,8-tetrahydroimidazo[1,5-*a*]pyridin-

5-yl)-, monohydrochloride, (±)-; (2) (±)-*p*-(5,6,7,8-Tetra-hydroimidazo[1,5-*a*]pyridin-5-yl)benzonitrile monohy-drochloride. *CAS-102676-96-0; CAS-102676-47-1* [fadrozole]. *Antineoplastic.* ◇*CGS 16949A*

Falecalcitriol. $C_{27}H_{38}F_6O_3$. 524.58. (+)-(5*Z*,7*E*)-26,26,26,27,27,27-Hexafluoro-9,10-secocholesta-5,7,10(19)-triene-1α,3β,25-triol. *CAS-83805-11-2.* INN. *[Name previously used: Flocalcitriol.]*

Falimarev (CEA, MUC-1, fowlpox virus) [*2005*] (fa lim′ a rev). Panvac-f. Molecular weight is approximately 290,000 ± 50,000 daltons. *CAS-685563-14-8. Treatment of pancreatic cancer, CEA-bearing tumors.* Panvac (Therion Biologics)

Falintolol. $C_{12}H_{24}N_2O_2$. 228.33. Cyclopropyl methyl ketone, (±)-(*EZ*)-*O*-[3-(*tert*-butylamino)-2-hydroxypropyl]oxime. *UNII-733BXR9780. CAS-90581-63-8.* INN.

Falipamil. $C_{24}H_{32}N_2O_5$. 428.52. 2-[3-[(3,4-Dimethoxyphene-tyl)methylamino]propyl]-5,6-dimethoxyphthalimidine. *UNII-N6A93ZMN7U. CAS-77862-92-1.* INN.

Falnidamol. $C_{18}H_{19}ClFN_7$. 387.84. 8-(3-Chloro-4-fluoroani-lino)-2-[(1-methyl-4-piperidyl)amino]pyrimido[5,4-*d*]py-rimidine. *CAS-196612-93-8.* INN.

Famciclovir [*1992*] (fam sye′ kloe vir). $C_{14}H_{19}N_5O_4$. 321.33. (1) 1,3-Propanediol, 2-[2-(2-amino-9*H*-purin-9-yl)ethyl]-, diacetate (ester); (2) 2-[2-(2-Amino-9*H*-purin-9-yl)ethyl]-1,3-propanediol diacetate (ester). *UNII-QIC03ANI02. CAS-104227-87-4.* INN; BAN. *Antiviral.* Famvir (Novartis) ◇*BRL-42810*

Famiraprinium Chloride. $C_{15}H_{18}ClN_3O_2$. 307.78. 6-Amino-1-(3-carboxypropyl)-5-methyl-3-phenylpyridazinium chloride. *UNII-TKL72421ZD. CAS-108894-41-3.* INN.

Famotidine [*1984*] (fam oh′ ti deen). **USP**. $C_8H_{15}N_7O_2S_3$. 337.45. (1) Propanimidamide, *N*′-(aminosulfonyl)-3-[[[2-[(diaminomethylene)amino]-4-thiazolyl]methyl]thio]-; (2) [1-Amino-3-[[[2-[(diaminomethylene)amino]-4-thiazolyl]methyl]thio]propylidene]sulfamide. *UNII-5QZO15J2Z8. CAS-76824-35-6.* INN; BAN; JAN. *Antagonist (to histamine H_2receptors).* Fluxid (Schwarz Pharma); Pepcid (Merck) ◇*MK-208*

Famotine Hydrochloride [*1969*] (fam′ oh teen hye″ droe klor′ ide). $C_{16}H_{14}ClNO·HCl$. 308.20. [Famotine is INN.] (1) Isoquinoline, 1-[(4-chlorophenoxy)methyl]-3,4-dihydro-, hydrochloride; (2) 1-[(*p*-Chlorophenoxy)methyl]-3,4-dihydroisoquinoline hydrochloride. *UNII-7L9H348XUO. CAS-10500-82-0; CAS-18429-78-2* [famotine]. *Antiviral.* ◇*UK-2054*

Fampridine [*1994*] (fam′ pri deen). $C_5H_6N_2$. 94.11. (1) 4-Pyridinamine; (2) 4-Aminopyridine. *UNII-BH3B64OKL9. CAS-504-24-5.* INN. *Multiple sclerosis symptomatic treatment.* Neurelan (Élan) ◇*EL-970*

---

† Brand name formerly used, and/or firm no longer concerned with this product.

Famprofazone. $C_{24}H_{31}N_3O$. 377.52. 4-Isopropyl-2-methyl-3-{[methyl(α-methylphenethyl)amino]methyl}-1-phenyl-3-pyrazolin-5-one. *UNII-HN0NCX453C. CAS-22881-35-2.* INN; BAN.

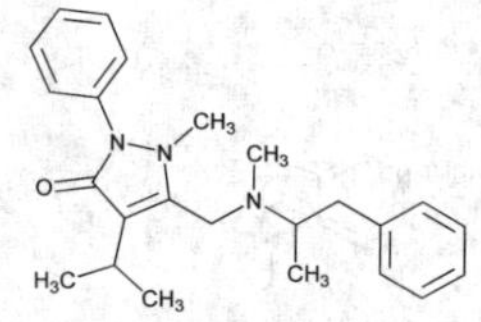

Fampronil. $C_{16}H_6Cl_3F_3N_6$. 445.61. 2-{5-Chloro-1-[2,6-dichloro-4-(trifluoromethyl)phenyl]-3-methyl-1*H*-pyrazol-4-yl}-1*H*-imidazole-4,5-dicarbonitrile. *CAS-134183-95-2.* INN.

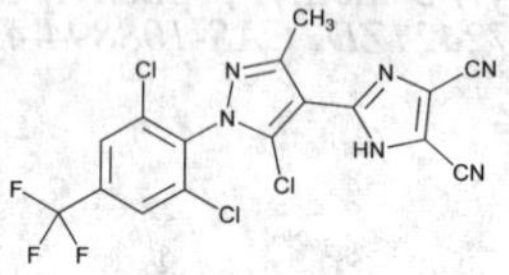

Fananserin [*1996*] (fan an' ser in). $C_{23}H_{24}FN_3O_2S$. 425.52. (1) 2*H*-Naphth[1,8-*cd*]isothiazole, 2-[3-[4-(4-fluorophenyl)-1-piperazinyl]propyl]-, 1,1-dioxide; (2) 2-[3-[4-(*p*-Fluorophenyl)-1-piperazinyl]propyl]-2*H*-naphth[1,8-*cd*]isothiazole 1,1-dioxide. *CAS-127625-29-0.* INN. *Antipsychotic.* ◇RP 62203

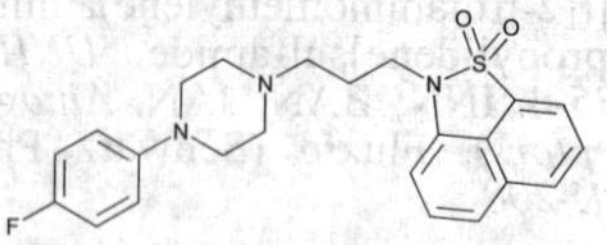

Fanapanel. $C_{14}H_{15}F_3N_3O_6P$. 409.25. [[3,4-Dihydro-7-morpholino-2,3-dioxo-6-(trifluoromethyl)-1(2*H*)-quinoxalinyl]methyl]phosphonic acid. *UNII-E3AP71EM0O. CAS-161605-73-8.* INN.

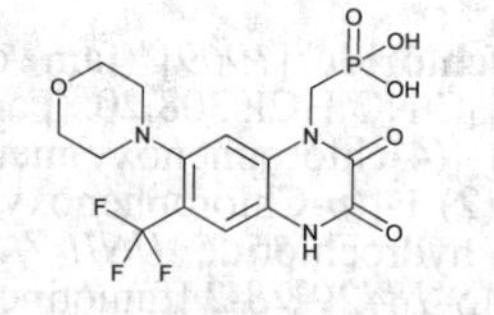

Fandofloxacin. $C_{20}H_{18}F_2N_4O_3$. 400.38. 6-Fluoro-1-(5-fluoro-2-pyridyl)-1,4-dihydro-7-(4-methyl-1-piperazinyl)-4-oxo-3-quinolinecarboxylic acid. *UNII-16406OC637. CAS-164150-99-6.* INN.

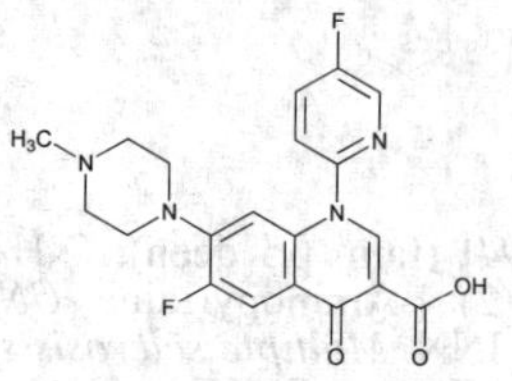

Fandosentan Potassium [*2002*] (fan" doe sen' tan poe tas' ee um). $C_{25}H_{17}F_3KNO_5S$. 539.56. [Fandosentan is INN.] (1) 2*H*-1,2-Benzothiazine-3-carboxylic acid, 4-(7-ethyl-1,3-benzodioxol-5-yl)-2-[2-(trifluoromethyl)phenyl]-, 1,1-dioxide, potassium salt; (2) Potassium 4-(7-ethyl-1,3-benzodioxol-5-yl)-2-[2-(trifluoromethyl)phenyl]-2*H*-1,2-benzothiazine-3-carboxylate 1,1-dioxide. *UNII-14U0D2SA4K; UNII-771E5ELJ7N* [fandosentan]. *CAS-221246-12-4; CAS-221241-63-0* [fandosentan]. *Treats pulmonary hypertension.* ◇CI-1034; PD 180988; PD 180988-0016

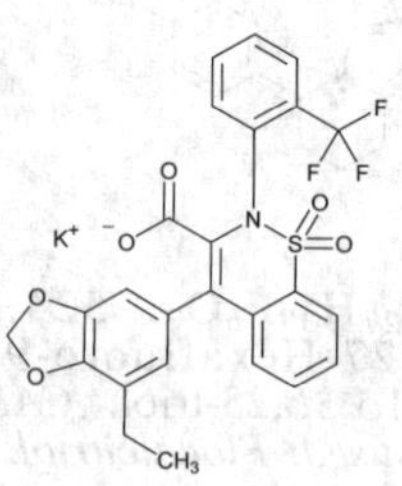

Fanetizole Mesylate [*1983*] (fan et' i zole mes' i late). $C_{17}H_{16}N_2S.CH_4O_3S$. 376.49. [Fanetizole is INN and BAN.] (1) 2-Thiazolamine, 4-phenyl-*N*-(2-phenylethyl)-, monomethanesulfonate; (2) 2-(Phenethylamino)-4-phenylthiazole monomethanesulfonate. *UNII-D3OG7B0G4M; UNII-BH48F620JA* [fanetizole]. *CAS-79069-95-7; CAS-79069-94-6* [fanetizole]. *Immunoregulator.* ◇CP-48,810-27

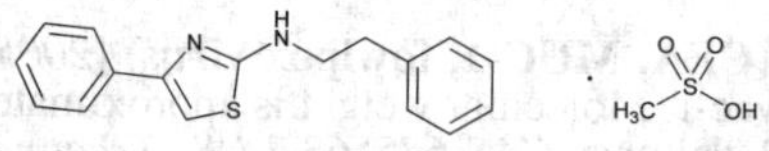

Fanthridone (previously used name) — *See* Fantridone Hydrochloride.

Fantofarone. $C_{13}H_{38}N_2O_5S$. 334.52. 1-[[*p*-[3-[(3,4-Dimethoxyphenethyl)methylamino]propoxy]phenyl]sulfonyl]-2-isopropylindolizine. *UNII-KU213XYO69. CAS-114432-13-2.* INN; BAN. ◇SR 33557

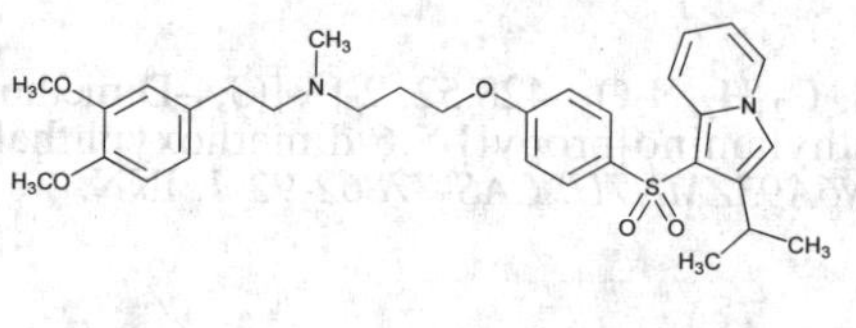

Fantridone Hydrochloride [*1969*] (fan' tri done hye" droe klor' ide). $C_{18}H_{20}N_2O.HCl.H_2O$. 334.84. [Fantridone is INN and BAN.] (1) 6(5*H*)-Phenanthridinone, 5-[3-(dimethylamino)propyl]-, monohydrochloride, monohydrate; (2) 5-[3-(Dimethylamino)propyl]-6(5*H*)-phenanthridinone monohydrochloride monohydrate. *UNII-DU65LYP662. CAS-24390-12-3; CAS-22461-13-8* [anhydrous]; *CAS-17692-37-4* [fantridone]. *Antidepressant. [Name previously used: Fanthridone.]* ◇AGN 616

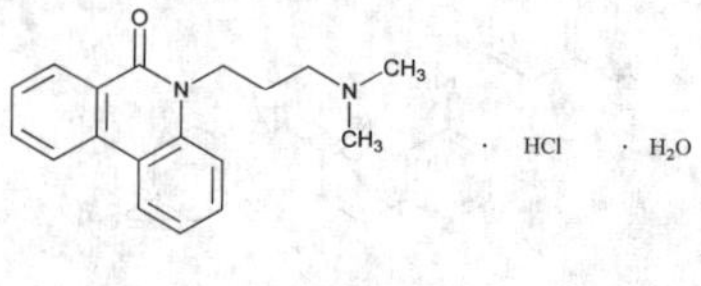

Faralimomab. Immunoglobulin G1, anti-(human interferon type I receptor) (mouse monoclonal 64G12 γ1-chain), disulfide with mouse monoclonal 64G12 light chain, dimer. *CAS-167816-91-3.* INN.

Farampator [*2005*] (far am' pa tor). $C_{12}H_{13}N_3O_2$. 231.25. (1) Piperidine, 1-(2,1,3-benzoxadiazol-5-ylcarbonyl)-; (2) 1-(2,1,3-Benzoxadiazol-5-ylcarbonyl)piperidine. *UNII-7X6P5N8K2L. CAS-211735-76-1*. INN. *Treatment of schizophrenia.* ◇*Org 24448; CX691*

Farglitazar [*2000*] (far gli' ta zar). $C_{34}H_{30}N_2O_5$. 546.61. (1) L-Tyrosine, *N*-(2-benzoylphenyl)-*o*-[2-(5-methyl-2-phenyl-4-oxazolyl)ethyl]-; (2) *N*-(*o*-Benzoylphenyl)-*O*-[2-(5-methyl-2-phenyl-4-oxazolyl)ethyl]-L-tyrosine. *CAS-196808-45-4*. INN. *Treatment of Type II diabetes (insulin action enhancer).* ◇*GI262570X*

Farletuzumab [*2008*] (far″ le tooz' oo mab). $C_{6466}H_{9928}N_{1716}O_{2020}S_{42}$. (1) Immunoglobulin G1, anti-(human receptor FR-α (folate receptor α)) (human-mouse monoclonal MORAb-003 heavy chain), disulfide with human-mouse monoclonal MORAb-003 κ-chain, dimer; (2) Immunoglobulin G1, anti-(human folate receptor alpha (ovarian tumor-associated antigen Mov18)); humanized mouse monoclonal MORAb-003 γ1 heavy chain (222-217′)-disulfide with humanized mouse monoclonal MORAb-003 κ light chain (228-228″:231-231″)-bisdisulfide dimer. Molecular weight is approximately 145,400 daltons. *UNII-2O09BG0OWA. CAS-896723-44-7. Treatment of cancer.* ◇*MORAb-003*

Faropenem Medoxomil [*2006*] (far″ oh pen' em me dox' oh mil). $C_{17}H_{19}NO_8S$. 397.40. [Faropenem is INN.] (1) 4-Thia-1-azabicyclo[3.2.0]hept-2-ene-2-carboxylic acid, 6-[(1*R*)-1-hydroxyethyl]-7-oxo-3-[(2*R*)-tetrahydro-2-furanyl]-, (5-methyl-2-oxo-1,3-dioxol-4-yl)methyl ester, (5*R*,6*S*); (2) (5-Methyl-2-oxo-1,3-dioxol-4-yl)methyl (5*R*,6*S*)-6-[(1*R*)-1-hydroxyethyl]-7-oxo-3-[(2*R*)-tetrahydrofuran-2-yl]-4-thia-1-azabicyclo[3.2.0]hept-2-ene-2-carboxylate. *UNII-5OK523O4FU; UNII-F52Y83BGH3* [faropenem]. *CAS-141702-36-5; CAS-106560-14-9* [faropenem]. *Treatment of bacterial infections.[Name previously used: Fropenem.]* ◇*A0026*

Fasidotril. $C_{23}H_{25}NO_6S$. 443.51. *N*-[(*S*)-α-(Mercaptomethyl)-3,4-(methylenedioxy)hydrocinnamoyl]-L-alanine, benzyl ester acetate (ester). *UNII-BIB7HG2V9E. CAS-135038-57-2*. INN.

Fasiplon. $C_{13}H_{15}N_5O_2$. 273.29. 6-Ethyl-7-methoxy-5-methyl-2-(5-methyl-1,2,4-oxadiazol-3-yl)imidazo[1,2-*a*]pyrimidine. *UNII-XCA050IPGB. CAS-106100-65-6*. INN.

Fasobegron. $C_{24}H_{24}ClNO_4$. 4'-(2-{[(2*R*)-2-(3-Chlorophenyl)-2-hydroxyethyl]amino}ethyl)-3-methoxy-[1,1'-biphenyl]-4-carboxylic acid. *CAS-643094-49-9*. INN.

Fasoracetam. $C_{10}H_{16}N_2O_2$. 196.25. (+)-1-[[(*R*)-5-Oxo-2-pyrrolidinyl]carbonyl]piperidine. *UNII-42O8UF5CJB. CAS-110958-19-5*. INN.

Fasudil. $C_{14}H_{17}N_3O_2S$. 291.37. Hexahydro-1-(5-isoquinolylsulfonyl)-1*H*-1,4-diazepine. *UNII-Q0CH43PGXS. CAS-103745-39-7*. INN.

Fat, Hard (fat). **NF**. A mixture of glycerides of saturated fatty acids. *Pharmaceutic aid (suppository base).*

Favipiravir. $C_5H_4FN_3O_2$. 157.10. 6-Fluoro-3-hydroxypyrazine-2-carboxamide. *CAS-259793-96-9*. INN.

Faxeladol [*2008*] (fax el' a dol). $C_{15}H_{23}NO$. 233.35. (1) Phenol, 3-[(1*R*,2*R*)-2-[(dimethylamino)methyl]cyclohexyl]-; (2) 3-{(1*R*,2*R*)-2-[(Dimethylamino)methyl]cyclohexyl}phenol. *UNII-C04V6SGK8H. CAS-433265-65-7*. INN. *Analgesic agent.* ◇*GRTA9906; GRTA0009906; EM906; GRT-TA300; GCR9905*

Fazadinium Bromide. $C_{28}H_{24}Br_2N_6$. 604.34. 1,1'-Azobis[3-methyl-2-phenyl-1*H*-imidazo[1,2-*a*]pyridin-4-ium] dibromide. *CAS-49564-56-9*. INN; BAN; MI. ◇*AH 8165D*

---

† Brand name formerly used, and/or firm no longer concerned with this product.

Fazarabine [*1987*] (faz ar′ a been). $C_8H_{12}N_4O_5$. 244.20. (1) 1,3,5-Triazin-2(1*H*)-one, 4-amino-1-β-D-arabinofuranosyl-; (2) 4-Amino-1-β-D-arabinofuranosyl-*s*-triazin-2(1*H*)-one. *UNII-5V71D8JOKK. CAS-65886-71-7.* INN. *Antineoplastic.* ◇*ara-AC; 5-azacytosine arabinoside; NSC-281272*

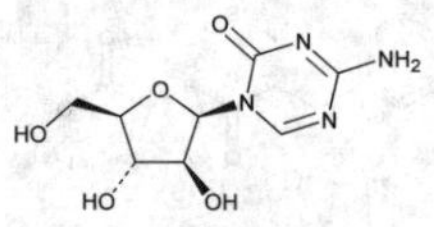

FD&C Red No. 2 — *See* Amaranth.

FD&C Red No. 3 — *See* Erythrosine Sodium.

[59]Fe — *See* Ferric Chloride Fe 59.

[59]Fe — *See* Ferric Citrate (^{59}Fe) [Injection].

[59]Fe — *See* Ferrous Citrate Fe 59.

[59]Fe — *See* Ferrous Sulfate Fe 59.

Febantel [*1977*] (fe ban′ tel). $C_{20}H_{22}N_4O_6S$. 446.48. (1) Carbamic acid, [[2-[(methoxyacetyl)amino]-4-(phenylthio)phenyl]carbonimidoyl]bis-, dimethyl ester; (2) Dimethyl [[2-(2-methoxyacetamido)-4-(phenylthio)phenyl]imidocarbonyl]dicarbamate. *UNII-S75C401OS1. CAS-58306-30-2.* INN; BAN. *Anthelmintic (veterinary).* Combotel (Bayer Animal Health†); Negabot Plus Paste (Bayer Animal Health†); Oratel (Bayer Animal Health†); Rintal (Bayer Animal Health) ◇*BAY Vh 5757; Bay h 5757*

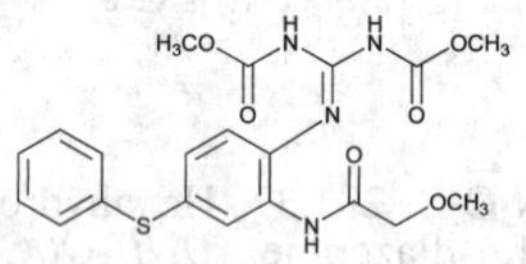

Febarbamate. $C_{20}H_{27}N_3O_6$. 405.44. 1-(3-Butoxy-2-hydroxypropyl)-5-ethyl-5-phenylbarbituric acid carbamate ester. *UNII-5Z48ONN38P. CAS-13246-02-1.* INN; DCF; MI. ◇*Go-560*

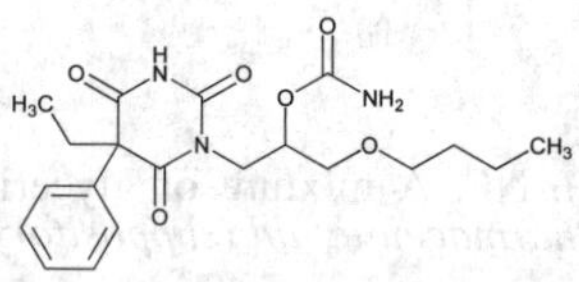

Febuprol. $C_{13}H_{20}O_3$. 224.30. 1-Butoxy-3-phenoxy-2-propanol. *UNII-B5RKR9Y63Y. CAS-3102-00-9.* INN; MI.

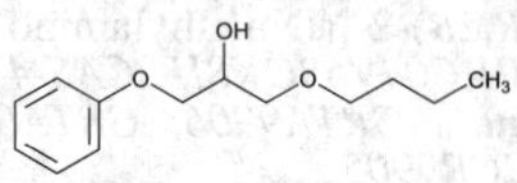

Febuverine. $C_{28}H_{38}N_2O_4$. 466.61. 1,4-Piperazinediethanol di(2-phenylbutyrate ester). *UNII-AX03A96739. CAS-7077-33-0.* INN. ◇*PG 430*

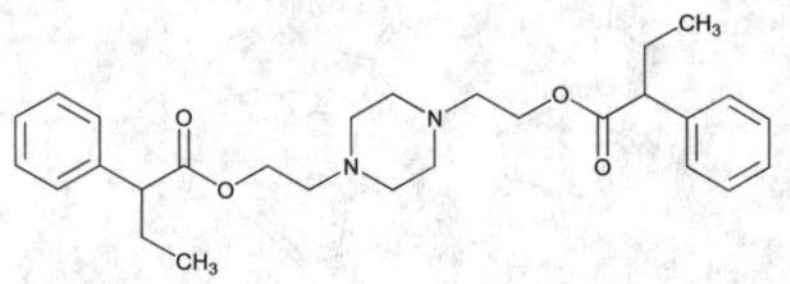

Febuxostat [*2002*] (feb ux′ oh stat). $C_{16}H_{16}N_2O_3S$. 316.37. (1) 5-Thiazolecarboxylic acid, 2-[3-cyano-4-(2-methylpropoxy)phenyl]-4-methyl-; (2) 2-(3-Cyano-4-(2-methylpropoxy)phenyl]-4-methylthiazole-5-carboxylic acid. *UNII-101V0R1N2E. CAS-144060-53-7.* INN. *Management of hyperuricemia in patients with gout (xanthine oxidase/xanthine dehydrogenase inhibitor).* ◇*TMX-67*

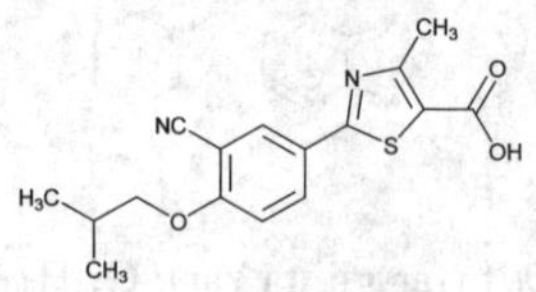

Feclemine. $C_{24}H_{42}N_2$. 358.60. 2-(α-Cyclohexylbenzyl)-*N,N,N′,N′*-tetraethyl-1,3-propanediamine. *UNII-5P7U986QGO. CAS-3590-16-7.* INN; MI.

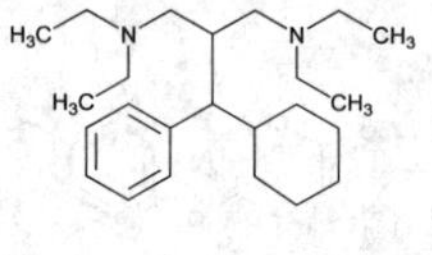

Feclobuzone. $C_{27}H_{25}ClN_2O_4$. 476.95. *p*-Chlorobenzoic acid, ester with 4-butyl-4-(hydroxymethyl)-1,2-diphenyl-3,5-pyrazolidinedione. *UNII-R6889JIL5D. CAS-23111-34-4.* INN. ◇*AE-9*

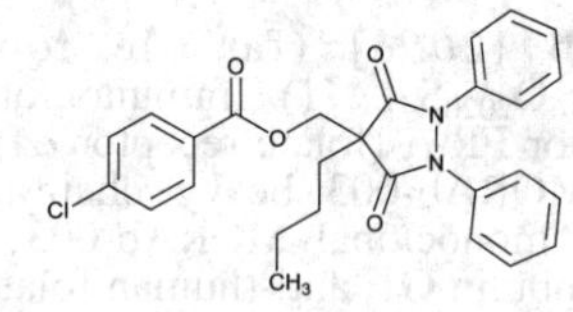

Fedotozine. $C_{22}H_{31}NO_4$. 373.49. (+)-(*R*)-α-Ethyl-*N,N*-dimethyl-α-[[(3,4,5-trimethoxybenzyl)oxy]methyl]benzylamine. *CAS-123618-00-8.* INN.

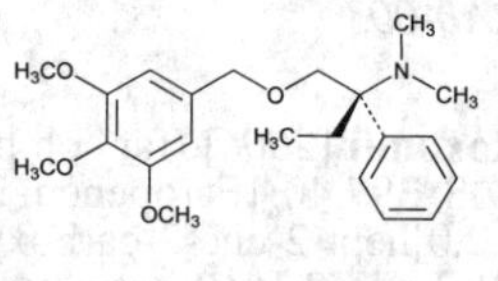

Fedrilate. $C_{20}H_{29}NO_4$. 347.45. 1-Methyl-3-morpholinopropyl tetrahydro-4-phenyl-2*H*-pyran-4-carboxylate. *CAS-23271-74-1.* INN; DCF. ◇*UCB 3928*

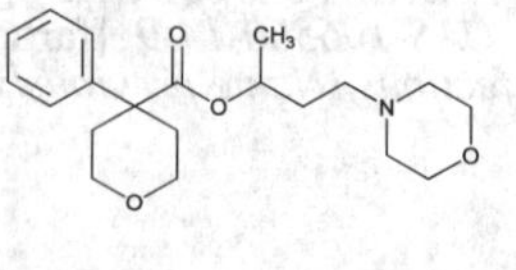

Felbamate [*1992*] (fel bam′ ate). $C_{11}H_{14}N_2O_4$. 238.24. (1) 1,3-Propanediol, 2-phenyl-, dicarbamate; (2) 2-Phenyl-1,3-propanediol dicarbamate. *UNII-X72RBB02N8. CAS-25451-15-4.* INN. *Anti-epileptic.* Felbatol (Medpointe) ◇*W-554*

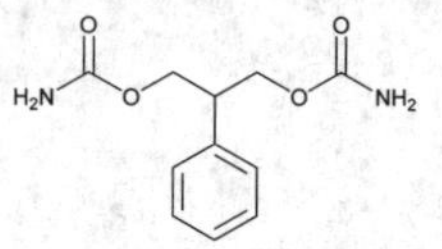

Felbinac [*1987*] (fel′ bi nak). $C_{14}H_{12}O_2$. 212.24. [Felbinac Ethyl is JAN.] (1) [1,1′-Biphenyl]-4-acetic acid; (2) 4-Biphenylacetic acid. *CAS-5728-52-9*. INN; BAN; JAN. *Anti-inflammatory*. Dolinac (Wyeth-Ayerst); Flexfree (Wyeth-Ayerst); Napageln (Wyeth-Ayerst†); Target (Wyeth-Ayerst); Traxam (Wyeth-Ayerst) ◇*CL 83,544; LJC 10,141*

Felipyrine. $C_{15}H_{20}N_2O$. 244.33. 1-Phenyl-3-piperidino-2-pyrrolidinone. *UNII-D9FU86687U*. *CAS-1980-49-0*. INN.

Felodipine [*1985*] (fe loe′ di peen). **USP.** $C_{18}H_{19}Cl_2NO_4$. 384.25. (1) 3,5-Pyridinedicarboxylic acid 4-(2,3-dichlorophenyl)-1,4-dihydro-2,6-dimethyl-, ethyl methyl ester, (±)-; (2) (±)-Ethyl methyl 4-(2,3-dichlorophenyl)-1,4-dihydro-2,6-dimethyl-3,5-pyridinedicarboxylate. *UNII-OL961R6O2C*. *CAS-72509-76-3; CAS-86189-69-7*. INN; BAN. *Vasodilator*. Plendil (AstraZeneca) ◇*H 154/82*

Feloprentan. $C_{31}H_{32}N_2O_6$. 528.60. (2S)-3-[2-(3,4-Dimethoxyphenyl)ethoxy]-2-[(4,6-dimethylpyrimidin-2-yl)oxy]-3,3-diphenylpropanoic acid. *CAS-204267-33-4*. INN.

Felvizumab [*1997*] (fel viz′ oo mab). (1) Immunoglobulin G 1 (human-mouse monoclonal, γ-chain anti-respiratory syncytial virus), disulfide with human-mouse monoclonal κ-chain, dimer; (2) Immunoglobulin G 1 (human-mouse monoclonal, γ-chain anti-respiratory syncytial virus), disulfide with human-mouse monoclonal κ-chain, dimer. Molecular weight is theoretically 146 kDa. *CAS-167747-20-8*. INN. *Antiviral; monoclonal antibody (antiviral)*. ◇*SB 209763*

Felypressin [*1965*] (fel″ i pres′ in). $C_{46}H_{65}N_{13}O_{11}S_2$. 1040.22. (1) Vasopressin, 2-L-phenylalanine-8-L-lysine-; (2) 2-(L-Phenylalanine)-8-L-lysinevasopressin; (3) L-Cysteinyl-L-phenylalanyl-L-phenylalanyl-L-glutaminyl-L-asparaginyl-

L-cysteinyl-L-prolyl-L-lysylglycinamide cyclic (1→6)disulfide. *UNII-17N2918V6G*. *CAS-56-59-7*. INN; BAN. *Vasoconstrictor*. PLV-2 (Novartis†)

CFFQNCPKG

Femoxetine. $C_{20}H_{25}NO_2$. 311.42. (+)-*trans*-3-[(*p*-Methoxyphenoxy)methyl]-1-methyl-4-phenylpiperidine. *CAS-59859-58-4*. INN; MI.

Fenabutene. $C_{12}H_{14}O_2$. 190.24. *p*-(1-Methylpropenyl)phenyl acetate. *UNII-Q0VL46026O*. *CAS-5984-83-8*. INN; DCF. ◇*CB 309*

Fenacetinol. $C_{10}H_{13}NO_3$. 195.22. *p*-Glycolophenetidide. *UNII-SP28AL52TM*. *CAS-22521-79-5*. INN; DCF. ◇*PM-1952*

Fenaclon. $C_{11}H_{14}ClNO$. 211.69. 3-Chloro-*N*-phenethylpropionamide. *UNII-6M4IR9QY13*. *CAS-306-20-7*. INN.

Fenadiazole. $C_8H_6N_2O_2$. 162.15. *o*-1,3,4-Oxadiazol-2-ylphenol. *UNII-8YX6HIZ0IP*. *CAS-1008-65-7*. INN; DCF; MI. ◇*JL 512*

Fenaftic Acid. $C_{24}H_{31}NO_4$. 397.51. 1-(Diethylcarbamoyl)-1,2,3,4,5,6,7,8-octahydro-6,6-dimethyl-8-oxo-3-phenyl-2-naphthoic acid. *UNII-V628N5FTX8*. *CAS-27736-80-7*. INN; DCF.

---

† Brand name formerly used, and/or firm no longer concerned with this product.

Fenalamide [*1967*] (fen al′ a mide). $C_{19}H_{30}N_2O_3$. 334.45. (1) Benzeneacetic acid, α-[[[2-(diethylamino)ethyl]amino]carbonyl]-α-ethyl-, ethyl ester; (2) Ethyl *N*-[2-(diethylamino)ethyl]-2-ethyl-2-phenylmalonamate. *CAS-4551-59-1.* INN. *Relaxant (smooth muscle).*

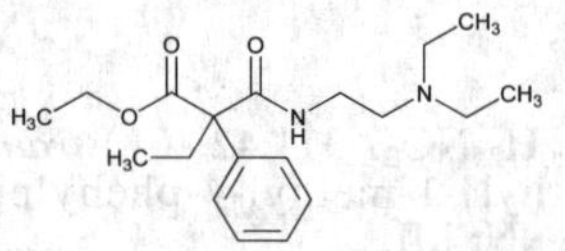

Fenalcomine. $C_{20}H_{27}NO_2$. 313.43. α-Ethyl-*p*-[2-[(α-methylphenethyl)amino]ethoxy]benzyl alcohol. *UNII-1TBQ3A47P8. CAS-34616-39-2.* INN; DCF; MI.

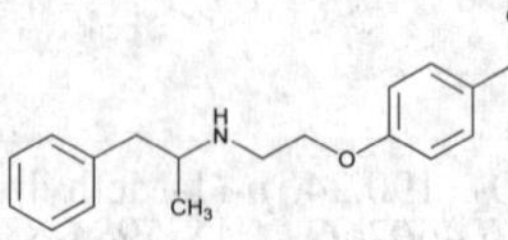

Fenamifuril. $C_{14}H_{17}NO_5$. 279.29. Tetrahydrofurfuryl (2-carbamoylphenoxy)acetate. *UNII-55408BLV3G. CAS-735-64-8.* INN.

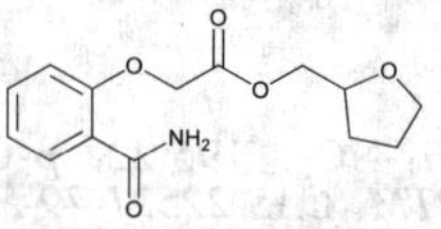

Fenamisal (INN, BAN) — *See* Phenyl Aminosalicylate.

Fenamole [*1965*] (fen′ a mole). $C_7H_7N_5$. 161.16. (1) 1*H*-Tetrazol-5-amine, 1-phenyl-; (2) 5-Amino-1-phenyl-1*H*-tetrazole. *CAS-5467-78-7.* INN. *Anti-inflammatory.* ◇AL 0559; P-463; PAT; NSC-25413

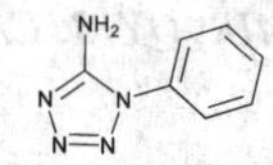

Fenaperone. $C_{21}H_{29}FN_2O_3$. 376.46. 4-[3-(*p*-Fluorobenzoyl)propyl]-1-piperazinecarboxylic acid, cyclohexyl ester. *UNII-V6W7F1R86P. CAS-54063-38-6.* INN.

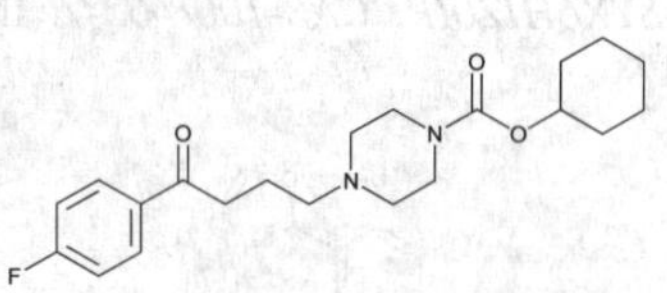

Fenarsone — *See* Carbarsone.

Fenasprate — *See* Benorilate.

Fenbendazole [*1975*] (fen ben′ da zole). **USP.** $C_{15}H_{13}N_3O_2S$. 299.35. (1) Carbamic acid, [5-(phenylthio)-1*H*-benzimidazol-2-yl]-, methyl ester; (2) Methyl 5-(phenylthio)-2-benzimidazolecarbamate. *UNII-621BVT9M36. CAS-43210-67-9.* INN; BAN. *Anthelmintic.* Panacur (Hoechst-Roussel) ◇*Hoe 881V*

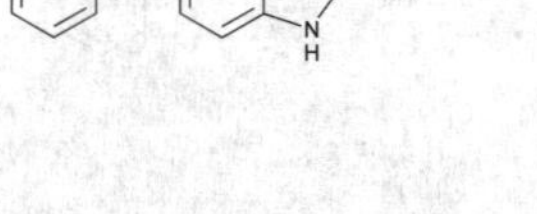

Fenbenicillin. $C_{22}H_{22}N_2O_5S$. 426.49. (α-Phenoxybenzyl)penicillin. *UNII-641EDA6X6L. CAS-1926-48-3.* INN; BAN; MI. *[Name previously used: Phenbenicillin.]*

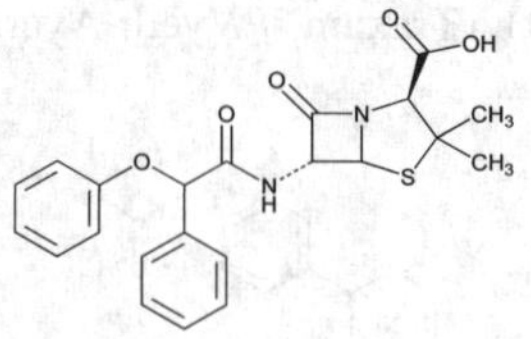

Fenbufen [*1973*] (fen bue′ fen). $C_{16}H_{14}O_3$. 254.28. (1) [1,1′-Biphenyl]-4-butanoic acid, γ-oxo-; (2) 3-(4-Biphenylylcarbonyl)propionic acid. *CAS-36330-85-5.* INN; BAN; JAN. *Anti-inflammatory.* ◇CL 82,204

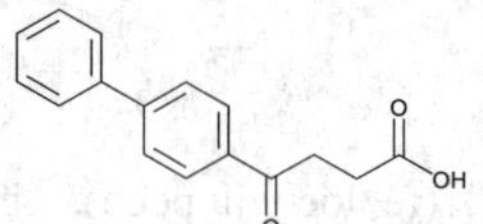

Fenbutrazate. $C_{23}H_{29}NO_3$. 367.48. 2-(3-Methyl-2-phenylmorpholino)ethyl 2-phenylbutyrate. *UNII-BKY8H56395. CAS-4378-36-3.* INN; BAN; MI. *[Name previously used: Phenbutrazate.]*

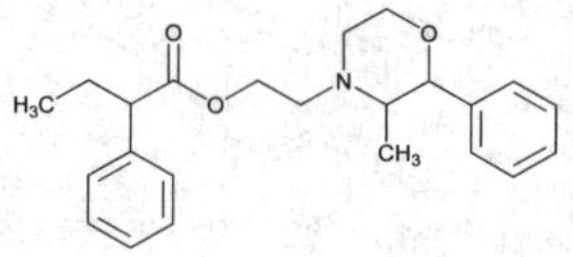

Fencamfamin Hydrochloride. $C_{15}H_{21}N \cdot HCl$. 251.79. [Fencamfamin is INN and BAN.] 3-Phenyl-*N*-ethyl-2-norbornanamine hydrochloride. *UNII-0M1J60BWEX. CAS-2240-14-4; CAS-1209-98-9 [fencamfamin].* MI.

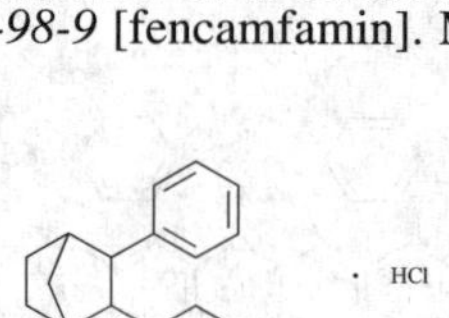

Fencarbamide (INN, DCF) — *See* Phencarbamide.

Fenchlorphos (previously used name) — *See* Ronnel.

Fencibutirol [*1983*] (fen″ si bue′ ti rol). $C_{16}H_{22}O_3$. 262.34. (1) Cyclohexaneacetic acid, α-ethyl-1-hydroxy-4-phenyl-, (±)-; (2) (±)-α-Ethyl-1-hydroxy-4-phenylcyclohexaneacetic acid. *UNII-H2V165956A. CAS-5977-10-6.* INN. *Choleretic.* Verecolene (Maggioni Farmaceutici S.p.A., Italy) ◇*Mg 4833*

Fenclexonium Metilsulfate. $C_{22}H_{35}NO_4S$. 409.58. 1-[3-(1-Cyclohexenyl)-3-phenylpropyl]-1-methylpiperidinium methylsulfate. *UNII-88M0X6627K; UNII-BV3N6F82WN* [fenclexonium]. *CAS-30817-43-7; CAS-27112-40-9* [fenclexonium]. INN.

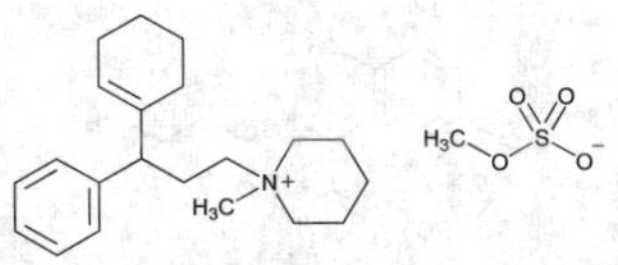

Fenclofenac [*1978*] (fen kloe′ fen ak). $C_{14}H_{10}Cl_2O_3$. 297.13. (1) Benzeneacetic acid, 2-(2,4-dichlorophenoxy)-; (2) [*o*-(2,4-Dichlorophenoxy)phenyl]acetic acid. *UNII-Y01JW64D01. CAS-34645-84-6.* INN; BAN. *Anti-inflammatory.* ✧*Rx 67408; R 67408*

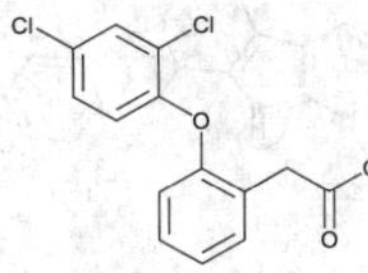

Fenclofos (INN) — *See* Ronnel.

Fenclonine [*1967*] (fen′ kloe neen). $C_9H_{10}ClNO_2$. 199.63. (1) Alanine, 3-(4-chlorophenyl)-, DL-; (2) DL-3-(*p*-Chlorophenyl)alanine. *CAS-7424-00-2.* INN. *Serotonin inhibitor.* ✧*CP-10,188; NSC-77370*

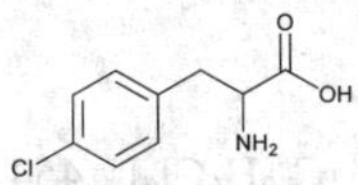

Fenclorac [*1975*] (fen′ klor ak). $C_{14}H_{16}Cl_2O_2$. 287.18. (1) Benzeneacetic acid, α,3-dichloro-4-cyclohexyl-; (2) Chloro(3-chloro-4-cyclohexylphenyl)acetic acid. *UNII-5458S22S8I. CAS-36616-52-1.* INN. *Anti-inflammatory.* ✧*WHR-539*

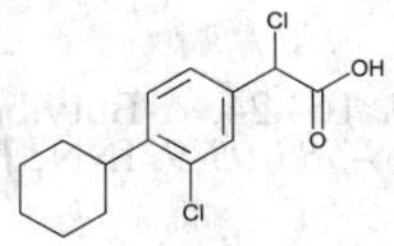

Fenclorfos (BAN) — *See* Ronnel.

Fenclozic Acid. $C_{11}H_8ClNO_2S$. 253.70. 2-(*p*-Chlorophenyl)-4-thiazoleacetic acid. *UNII-58SRQ4DV53. CAS-17969-20-9.* INN; BAN; MI. ✧*I.C.I. 54,450*

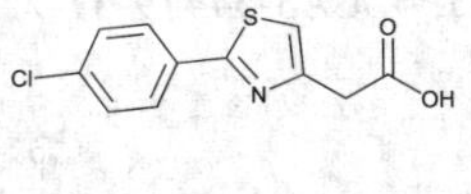

† Brand name formerly used, and/or firm no longer concerned with this product.

Fendiline. $C_{23}H_{25}N$. 315.45. *N*-(3,3-Diphenylpropyl)-α-methylbenzylamine. INN; MI.

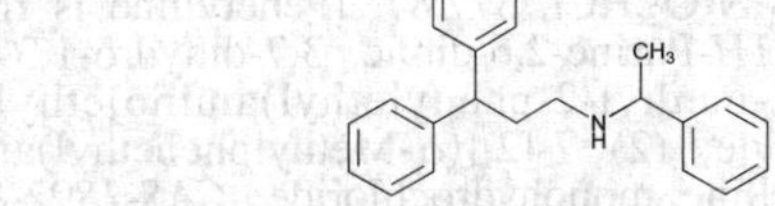

Fendizoate. 2-[(6-Hydroxybiphenyl-3-yl)carbonyl]benzoate. INN.

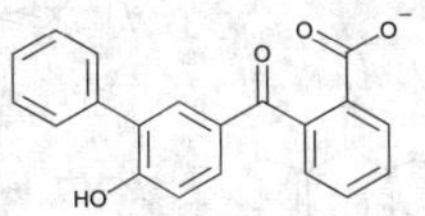

Fendosal [*1976*] (fen′ doe sal). $C_{25}H_{19}NO_3$. 381.42. (1) Benzoic acid, 5-(4,5-dihydro-2-phenyl-3*H*-benz[*e*]indol-3-yl)-2-hydroxy-; (2) 5-(4,5-Dihydro-2-phenyl-3*H*-benz[*e*]indol-3-yl)salicylic acid. *CAS-53597-27-6.* INN; BAN. *Anti-inflammatory.* Alnovin (Hoechst-Roussel†) ✧*P 71-0129*

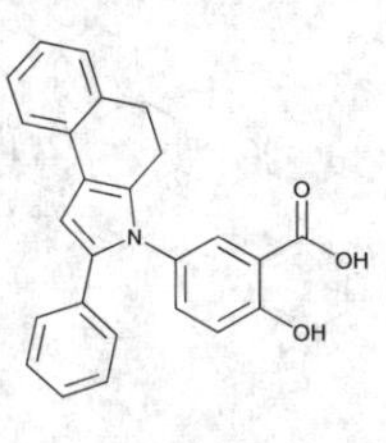

Feneritrol. $C_{45}H_{52}O_8$. 720.89. Pentaerythritol tetrakis(2-phenylbutyrate). *CAS-15301-67-4.* INN; DCF. ✧*SD 149-01*

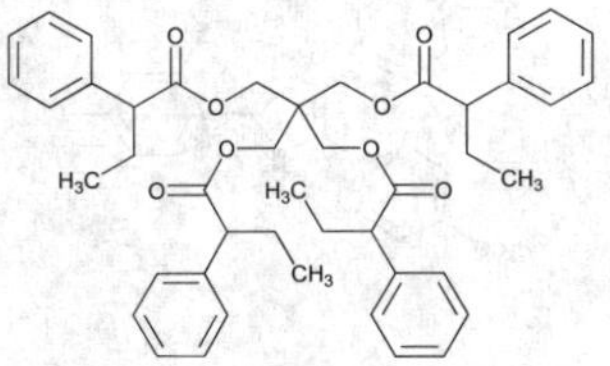

Fenestrel [*1967*] (fen es′ trel). $C_{16}H_{20}O_2$. 244.33. (1) 3-Cyclohexene-1-carboxylic acid, 5-ethyl-6-methyl-4-phenyl-; (2) 5-Ethyl-6-methyl-4-phenyl-3-cyclohexene-1-carboxylic acid. *CAS-7698-97-7.* INN. *Estrogen.*

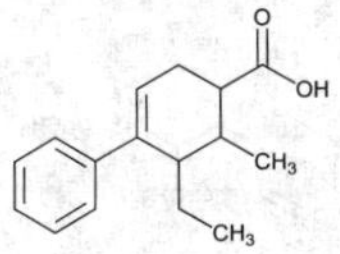

Fenethazine. $C_{16}H_{18}N_2S$. 270.39. 10-(2-Dimethylaminoethyl)phenothiazine. *UNII-8J97CUZ4HX. CAS-522-24-7.* INN; DCF; MI.

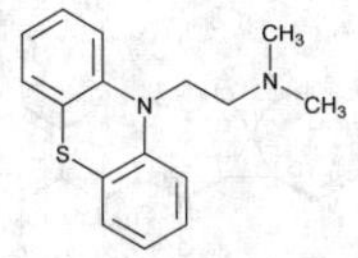

Fenethylline (previously used name) — *See* Fenethylline Hydrochloride.

Fenethylline Hydrochloride [*1966*] (fen eth' i lin hye" droe klor' ide). $C_{18}H_{23}N_5O_2 \cdot HCl$. 377.87. [Fenetylline is INN and BAN.] (1) 1*H*-Purine-2,6-dione, 3,7-dihydro-1,3-dimethyl-7-[2-[(1-methyl-2-phenylethyl)amino]ethyl]-, monohydrochloride; (2) 7-[2-[(α-Methylphenethyl)amino]ethyl]theophylline monohydrochloride. *CAS-1892-80-4; CAS-3736-08-1* [fenethylline]. *Stimulant (central).* [*Name previously used: Fenethylline.*]

Fenetradil. $C_{22}H_{36}N_2O_3$. 376.53. 1-(Isobutoxymethyl)-2-(4-methyl-1-piperazinyl)ethyl 2-phenylbutyrate. *UNII-9GXY5Z0873. CAS-54063-39-7*. INN; DCF.

Fenflumizole. $C_{23}H_{18}F_2N_2O_2$. 392.40. 2-(2,4-Difluorophenyl)-4,5-bis(*p*-methoxyphenyl)imidazole. *UNII-PD0931191Q. CAS-73445-46-2*. INN.

Fenfluramine Hydrochloride [*1965*] (fen flur' a meen hye" droe klor' ide). $C_{12}H_{16}F_3N \cdot HCl$. 267.72. [Fenfluramine is INN and BAN.] (1) Benzeneethanamine, *N*-ethyl-α-methyl-3-(trifluoromethyl)-, hydrochloride; (2) *N*-Ethyl-α-methyl-*m*-(trifluoromethyl)phenethylamine hydrochloride. *UNII-3KC089243P. CAS-404-82-0; CAS-458-24-2* [fenfluramine]. *Anorexic.* Pondimin (Robins) ◇*AHR-3002*

Fenfluthrin. $C_{15}H_{11}Cl_2F_5O_2$. 389.14. 2,3,4,5,6-Pentafluorobenzyl (1*R*,3*S*)-3-(2,2-dichlorovinyl)-2,2-dimethylcyclopropanecarboxylate. *UNII-416P10SE9G. CAS-75867-00-4*. INN; BAN. ◇*Bay Vn 6528; BAYNAC*

Fengabine [*1987*] (fen' ga been). $C_{17}H_{17}Cl_2NO$. 322.23. (1) Phenol, 2-[(butylimino)(2-chlorophenyl)methyl]-4-chloro-, (*Z*)-; (2) (*Z*)-2-(*N*-Butyl-*o*-chlorobenzimidoyl)-4-chlorophenol. *UNII-YQG0NJI5A7. CAS-80018-06-0*. INN; BAN. *Mood regulator.* ◇*SL 79.229-00*

Fenharmane. $C_{18}H_{18}N_2$. 262.35. 1-Benzyl-2,3,4,9-tetrahydro-1*H*-pyrido[3,4-*b*]indole. *UNII-9E96TNX6EZ. CAS-3851-30-7*. INN.

Fenimide [*1966*] (fen' i mide). $C_{13}H_{15}NO_2$. 217.26. (1) 2,5-Pyrrolidinedione, 4-ethyl-3-methyl-3-phenyl-; (2) 3-Ethyl-2-methyl-2-phenylsuccinimide. *CAS-60-45-7*. INN; BAN. *Antipsychotic.* ◇*CI-419; PM 1807*

Feniodium Chloride. $C_{12}H_6Cl_5I$. 454.35. Bis(2,4-dichlorophenyl)iodonium chloride. *UNII-L32B98BGJS. CAS-34563-73-0*. INN.

Fenipentol. $C_{11}H_{16}O$. 164.24. α-Butylbenzyl alcohol. *UNII-X3FZE77O60. CAS-583-03-9*. INN; JAN; MI.

Fenirofibrate. $C_{17}H_{17}ClO_4$. 320.77. ($\pm$)-2-[[α-(*p*-Chlorophenyl)-α-hydroxy-*p*-tolyl]oxy]-2-methylpropionic acid. *UNII-2VG7825GP4. CAS-54419-31-7*. INN.

Fenisorex [*1972*] (fen eye' soe rex). $C_{16}H_{16}FNO$. 257.30. (1) 1*H*-2-Benzopyran-3-methanamine, 7-fluoro-3,4-dihydro-1-phenyl-, *cis*-; (2) *cis*-7-Fluoro-1-phenyl-3-isochroman-methylamine. *UNII-C0P8MP2SR5. CAS-34887-52-0.* INN; BAN. *Anorexic*.

Fenitrothion. $C_9H_{12}NO_5PS$. 277.23. *O,O*-Dimethyl *O*-4-nitro-*m*-tolyl phosphorothioate. *UNII-W8M4X3Y7ZY. CAS-122-14-5.* BAN.

Fenleuton [*1994*] (fen loo' ton). $C_{17}H_{15}FN_2O_3$. 314.31. (1) Urea, *N*-[3-[3-(4-fluorophenoxy)phenyl]-1-methyl-2-propynyl]-*N*-hydroxy-, (±)-; (2) (±)-1-[3-[*m*-(*p*-Fluorophenoxy)phenyl]-1-methyl-2-propynyl]-1-hydroxyurea. *UNII-LG64454O6I. CAS-141579-54-6.* INN. *Inhibitor (5-lipoxygenase, veterinary)*. LoFrin (Abbott) ◇*Abbott-76745*

Fenmetozole Hydrochloride [*1974*] (fen met' oh zole hye" droe klor' ide). $C_{10}H_{10}Cl_2N_2O \cdot HCl$. 281.57. [Fenmetozole is INN.] (1) 1*H*-Imidazole, 2-[(3,4-dichlorophenoxy)methyl]-4,5-dihydro-, monohydrochloride; (2) 2-[(3,4-Dichlorophenoxy)methyl]-2-imidazoline monohydrochloride. *CAS-23712-05-2; CAS-41473-09-0* [fenmetozole]. *Antidepressant; antagonist (to narcotics)*. ◇*DH-524*

Fenmetramide [*1963*] (fen met' ra mide). $C_{11}H_{13}NO_2$. 191.23. (1) 3-Morpholinone, 5-methyl-6-phenyl-; (2) 5-Methyl-6-phenyl-3-morpholinone. *CAS-5588-29-4.* INN; BAN. *Antidepressant*. ◇*McN-1075*

Fennel Oil (fen' el). **NF.** The volatile oil distilled with steam from the dried, ripe fruit of *Foeniculum vulgare* Mill. (Fam. Apiaceae). *UNII-59AAO5F6HT.* JAN; MI. *Pharmaceutic aid (flavor)*.

Fenobam [*1978*] (fen' oh bam). $C_{11}H_{11}ClN_4O_2$. 266.68. (1) Urea monohydrate, *N*-(3-chlorophenyl)-*N'*-(4,5-dihydro-1-methyl-4-oxo-1*H*-imidazol-2-yl)-; (2) 1-(*m*-Chlorophen-yl)-3-(1-methyl-4-oxo-2-imidazolin-2-yl)urea monohydrate. *CAS-63540-28-3.* INN. *Sedative-hypnotic*. ◇*McN-3377-98*

Fenocinol. $C_{16}H_{18}O_3$. 258.31. 2,4-Dimethoxy-α-methylbenzhydrol *UNII-UPY9RD84AG. CAS-3671-05-4.* INN; DCF.

Fenoctimine Sulfate [*1982*] (fen ok' ti meen sul' fate). $C_{27}H_{38}N_2 \cdot H_2SO_4 \cdot ½H_2O$. 497.69. [Fenoctimine is INN.] (1) Piperidine, 4-(diphenylmethyl)-1-[(octylimino)methyl]-, sulfate (1:1), hemihydrate; (2) 4-(Diphenylmethyl)-1-(*N*-octylformimidoyl)piperidine sulfate (1:1), hemihydrate. *UNII-448AZ2116G; UNII-B45CF873F8* [fenoctimine]. *CAS-69365-66-8; CAS-69365-67-9* [anhydrous]; *CAS-69365-65-7* [fenoctimine]. *Antisecretory (gastric)*. ◇*McN-4097-12-98*

Fenofibrate [*1976*] (fen" oh fye' brate). **USP.** $C_{20}H_{21}ClO_4$. 360.83. Isopropyl 2-[*p*-(*p*-chlorobenzoyl)phenoxy]-2-methylpropionate. *UNII-U202363UOS. CAS-49562-28-9.* INN; BAN; MI. *Antihyperlipidemic*. Antara (Reliant); Lipofen (Proethic); Tricor (Abbott); Triglide (Skyepharma)

Fenoldopam Mesylate [*1984*] (fee nol' doe pam mes' i late). **USP.** $C_{16}H_{16}ClNO_3 \cdot CH_4SO_3$. 401.86. [Fenoldopam is INN and BAN.] (1) 1*H*-3-Benzazepine-7,8-diol, 6-chloro-2,3,4,5-tetrahydro-1-(4-hydroxyphenyl)-, methanesulfonate (salt); (2) 6-Chloro-2,3,4,5-tetrahydro-1-(*p*-hydroxyphenyl)-1*H*-3-benzazepine-7,8-diol methanesulfonate (salt). *UNII-HA3R0MY016; UNII-INU8H2KAWG* [fenoldopam]. *CAS-67227-57-0; CAS-67227-56-9* [fenoldopam]. *Antihypertensive; dopamine agonist*. Corlopam (Hospira) ◇*SK&F 82526-J*

---

† Brand name formerly used, and/or firm no longer concerned with this product.

Fenoprofen [*1971*] (fen″ oh proe′ fen). $C_{15}H_{14}O_3$. 242.27. (1) Benzeneacetic acid, α-methyl-3-phenoxy-, ($\pm$)-; (2) ($\pm$)-*m*-Phenoxyhydratropic acid. *UNII-RA33EAC7KY. CAS-31879-05-7*. INN; BAN. *Anti-inflammatory; analgesic.* ◇*53858*

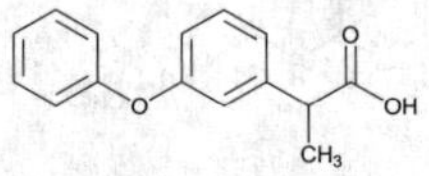

Fenoprofen Calcium [*1974*] (fen″ oh proe′ fen kal′ see um). **USP.** $C_{30}H_{26}CaO_6 \cdot 2H_2O$. 558.63. (1) Benzeneacetic acid, α-methyl-3-phenoxy-, calcium salt dihydrate, ($\pm$)-; (2) Calcium ($\pm$)-*m*-phenoxyhydratropate dihydrate. *UNII-0X2CW1QABJ; UNII-RA33EAC7KY* [fenoprofen]. *CAS-53746-45-5; CAS-34597-40-5* [anhydrous]; *CAS-31879-05-7* [fenoprofen]. BAN; JAN. *Anti-inflammatory; analgesic.* Nalfon (Pedinol) ◇*69323*

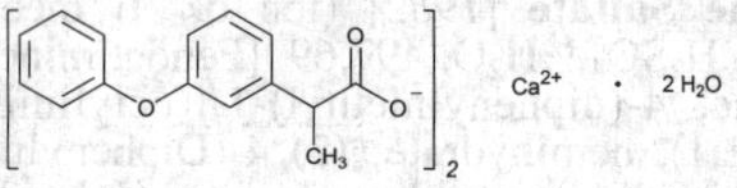

Fenoterol [*1971*] (fen oh′ ter ol). $C_{17}H_{21}NO_4$. 303.35. [Fenoterol Hydrobromide is JAN.] (1) 1,3-Benzenediol, 5-[1-hydroxy-2-[[2-(4-hydroxyphenyl)-1-methylethyl]amino]ethyl]-; (2) 3,5-Dihydroxy-α-[[(*p*-hydroxy-α-methylphenethyl)amino]methyl]benzyl alcohol. *UNII-22M9P70OQ9. CAS-13392-18-2*. INN; BAN. *Bronchodilator.* Berotec [as hydrobromide] (Boehringer Ingelheim) ◇*TH 1165a [as hydrobromide salt]*

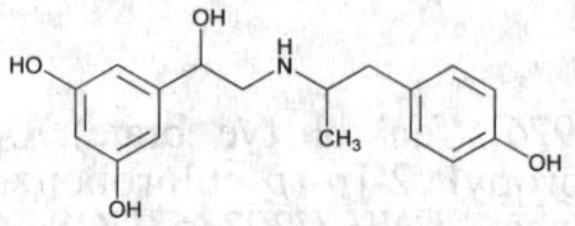

Fenoverine. $C_{26}H_{25}N_3O_3S$. 459.56. 10-[(4-Piperonyl-1-piperazinyl)acetyl]phenothiazine. *UNII-N274ZQ6PZJ. CAS-37561-27-6*. INN; DCF; MI.

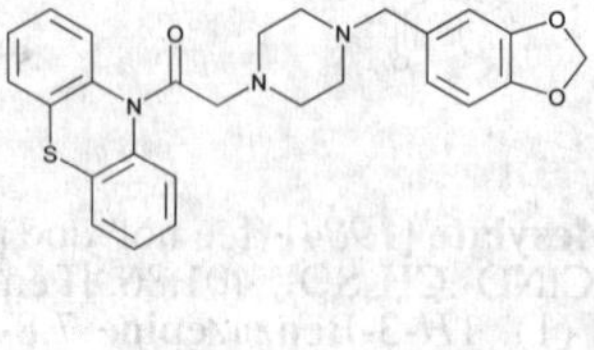

Fenoxazol — *See* Pemoline.

Fenoxazoline Hydrochloride. $C_{13}H_{18}N_2O \cdot HCl$. 254.76. [Fenoxazoline is INN.] 2-(2-Isopropylphenoxymethyl)-2-imidazoline hydrochloride. *UNII-6K28Y098S7; UNII-97JJW1W1R3* [fenoxazoline]. *CAS-21370-21-8; CAS-4846-91-7* [fenoxazoline]. MI.

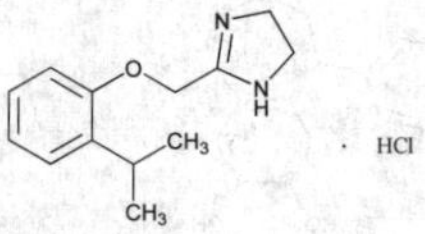

Fenoxedil. $C_{28}H_{42}N_2O_5$. 486.64. 2-(*p*-Butoxyphenoxy)-*N*-(2,5-diethoxyphenyl)-*N*-[2-(diethylamino)ethyl]acetamide. *UNII-ABX8234H6M. CAS-54063-40-0*. INN; DCF; MI.

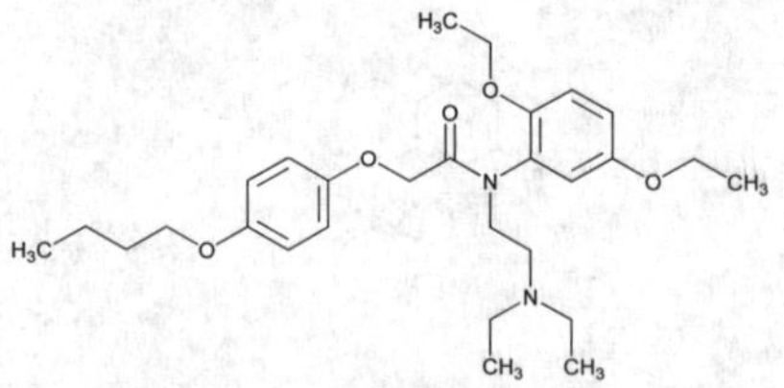

Fenoxypropazine (INN, BAN) — *See* Phenoxypropazine.

Fenozolone. $C_{11}H_{12}N_2O_2$. 204.23. 2-Ethylamino-4-oxo-5-phenyl-2-oxazolin. *UNII-1NZI4LMU6G. CAS-15302-16-6*. INN; DCF; MI. ◇*LD 3394*

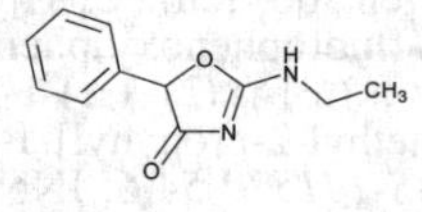

Fenpentadiol. $C_{12}H_{17}ClO_2$. 228.72. 2-(*p*-Chlorophenyl)-4-methyl-2,4-pentanediol. *UNII-BLO7300903. CAS-15687-18-0*. INN; DCF; MI. ◇*Rd 292*

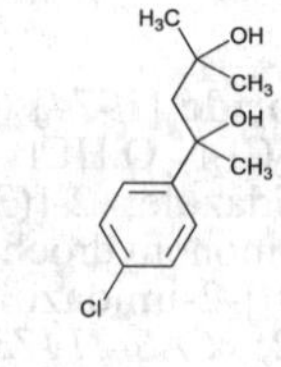

Fenperate. $C_{25}H_{31}NO_4$. 409.52. 2-Piperidinoethyl α-benzyl-α-hydroxyhydrocinnamate acetate (ester). *UNII-1NJ4DG390G. CAS-55837-26-8*. INN.

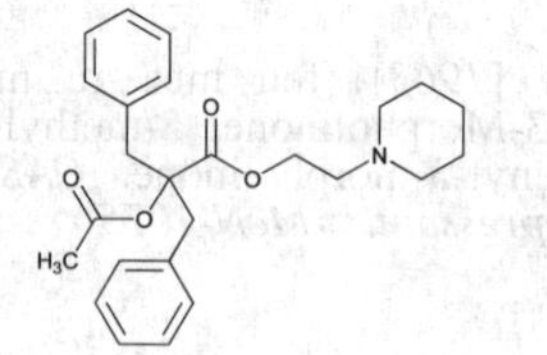

Fenpipalone [*1974*] (fen pip′ a lone). $C_{17}H_{22}N_2O_2$. 286.37. (1) 2-Oxazolidinone, 5-[2-(3,6-dihydro-4-phenyl-1(2*H*)-pyridinyl)ethyl]-3-methyl-; (2) 5-[2-(3,6-Dihydro-4-phenyl-1(2*H*)-pyridyl)ethyl]-3-methyl-2-oxazolidinone. *CAS-21820-82-6*. INN. *Anti-inflammatory.* ◇*AHR-1680*

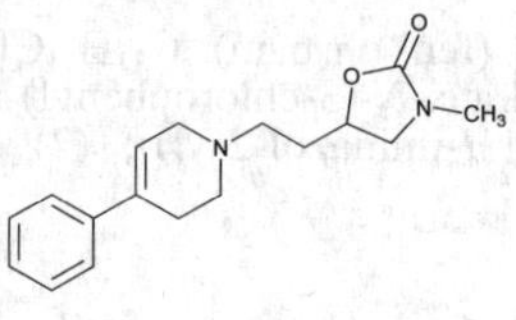

Fenpipramide. $C_{21}H_{26}N_2O$. 322.44. α,α-Diphenyl-1-piperidi-nebutyramide. *UNII-88445508X3; UNII-KJ2V75P034* [fenpipramide hydrochloride]. *CAS-77-01-0; CAS-14007-53-5* [hydrochloride]. INN; BAN.

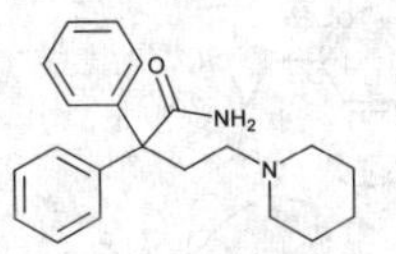

Fenpiprane Hydrochloride. $C_{20}H_{25}N$.HCl. 315.88. [Fenpi-prane is INN and BAN.] 1-(3,3-Diphenylpropyl)piperidine hydrochloride. *UNII-684N1BF96B; UNII-S2FVB1RL5X* [fenpiprane]. *CAS-3329-14-4; CAS-3540-95-2* [fenpi-prane].

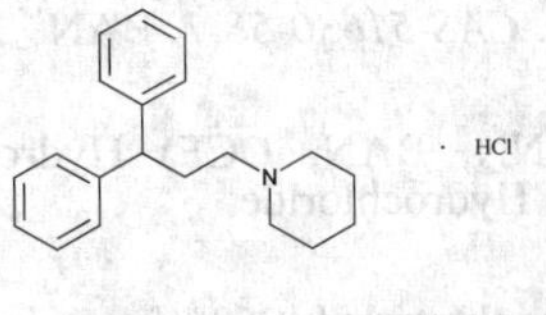

Fenpiverinium Bromide. $C_{22}H_{29}BrN_2O$. 417.38. 1-(3-Carba-moyl-3,3-diphenylpropyl)-1-methylpiperidinium bromide. *UNII-36479UA8GL. CAS-125-60-0*. INN; MI.

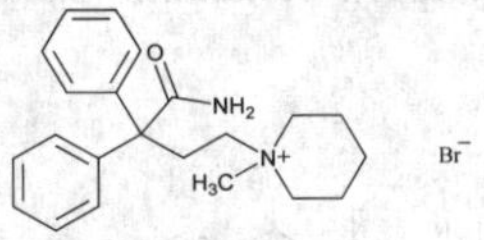

Fenprinast Hydrochloride [*1982*] (fen′ pri nast hye″ droe klor′ ide). $C_{16}H_{16}ClN_5O$.HCl.H_2O. 384.26. [Fenprinast is INN.] (1) 9*H*-Imidazo[1,2-*a*]purin-9-one, 4-[(4-chlorophe-nyl)methyl]-1,4,6,7-tetrahydro-6,6-dimethyl-, monohy-drochloride, monohydrate; (2) 4-(*p*-Chlorobenzyl)-1,4,6,7-tetrahydro-6,6-dimethyl-9*H*-imidazo[1,2-*a*]purin-9-one monohydrochloride monohydrate. *CAS-77482-47-4; CAS-75184-94-0* [fenprinast]. *Bronchodilator (anti-aller-gic).* ◇*MJ 13401-1-3*

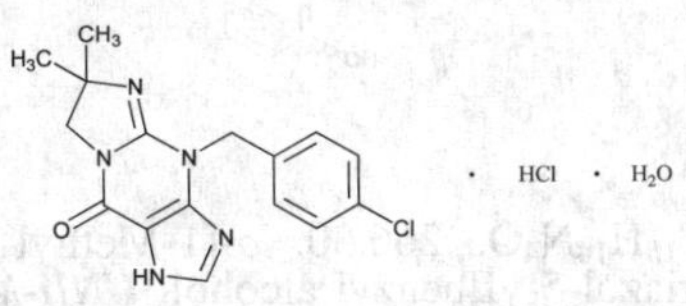

Fenproporex. $C_{12}H_{16}N_2$. 188.27. ($\pm$)-3-[(α-Methylphenethy-l)amino]propionitrile. *UNII-W0194S5FOA. CAS-15686-61-0*. INN; DCF; MI.

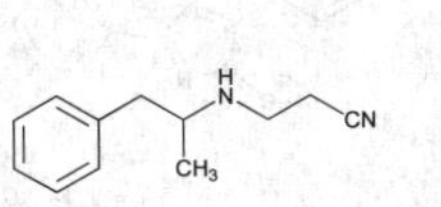

Fenprostalene [*1979*] (fen prost′ a leen). $C_{23}H_{30}O_6$. 402.48. (1) 4,5-Heptadienoic acid, 7-[3,5-dihydroxy-2-(3-hydroxy-4-phenoxy-1-butenyl)cyclopentyl]-, methyl ester; (2) Methyl ($\pm$)-7-[(1*R**,2*R**,3*R**,5*S**)-3,5-dihydroxy-2-[(*E*)-(3*R**)-3-hydroxy-4-phenoxy-1-butenyl]cyclopentyl]-4,5-

heptadienoate. *UNII-X8I39OJF4P. CAS-69381-94-8.* INN; BAN. *Luteolysin.* Synchrocept B [Veterinary] (Syntex) ◇*RS-84043*

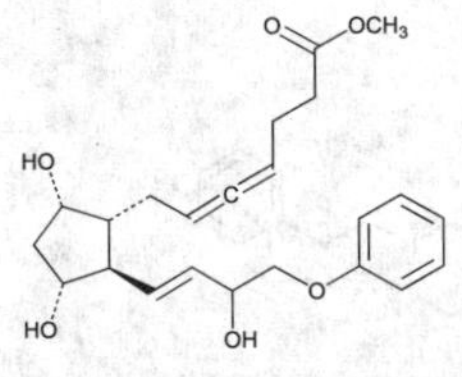

Fenquizone [*1981*] (fen′ kwi zone). $C_{14}H_{12}ClN_3O_3S$. 337.78. (1) 6-Quinazolinesulfonamide, 7-chloro-1,2,3,4-tetrahy-dro-4-oxo-2-phenyl-, ($\pm$)-; (2) ($\pm$)-7-Chloro-1,2,3,4-tetra-hydro-4-oxo-2-phenyl-6-quinazolinesulfonamide. *UNII-LJ1U13R8IK*. *CAS-20287-37-0*. INN. *Diuretic*. Idrolone (Maggioni Farmaceutici S.p.A., Italy) ◇*M.G. 13054*

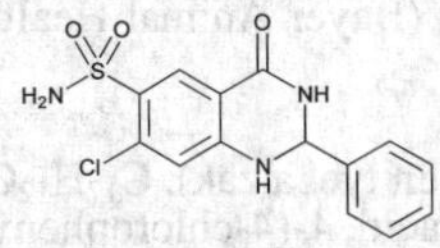

Fenretinide [*1984*] (fen ret′ i nide). $C_{26}H_{33}NO_2$. 391.55. (1) Retinamide, *N*-(4-hydroxyphenyl)-; (2) *all-trans*-4′-Hydro-xyretinanilide. *CAS-65646-68-6*. INN. *Antineoplastic.* ◇*McN-R-1967*

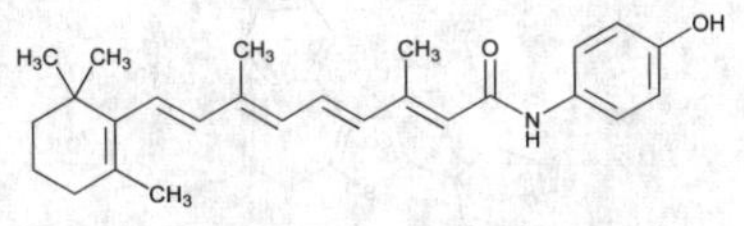

Fenspiride Hydrochloride [*1969*] (fen′ spir ide hye″ droe klor′ ide). $C_{15}H_{20}N_2O_2$.HCl. 296.79. [Fenspiride is INN.] (1) 1-Oxa-3,8-diazaspiro[4,5]decan-2-one, 8-(2-pheny-lethyl)-, monohydrochloride; (2) 8-Phenethyl-1-oxa-3,8-diazaspiro[4.5]decan-2-one monohydrochloride. *CAS-5053-08-7; CAS-5053-06-5* [fenspiride]. *Bronchodilator; anti-adrenergic (α-receptor).* ◇*NAT-333; NDR-5998A*

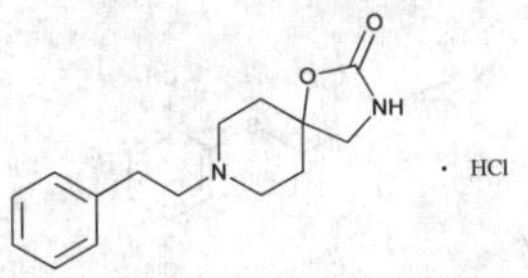

Fentanyl [*2006*] (fen′ ta nil). $C_{22}H_{28}N_2O$. 336.47. (1) Propanamide, *N*-phenyl-*N*-[1-(2-phenylethyl)-4-piperidi-nyl]; (2) *N*-(1-Phenethylpiperidin-4-yl)-*N*-phenylpropiona-mide. *UNII-UF599785JZ. CAS-437-38-7.* BAN. *Analgesic.* Duragesic (ALZA)

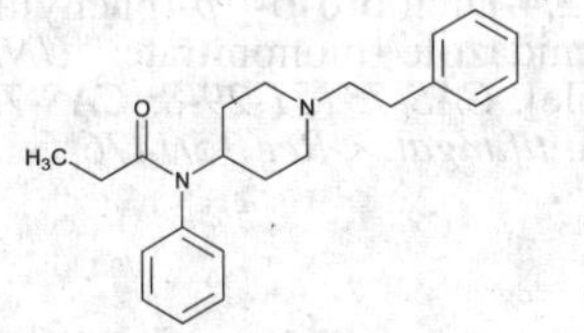

Fentanyl Citrate [*1963*] (fen′ ta nil sit′ rate). **USP.** $C_{22}H_{28}N_2O.C_6H_8O_7$. 528.59. [Fentanyl is INN.] (1) Propa-namide, *N*-phenyl-*N*-[1-(2-phenylethyl)-4-piperidinyl]-, 2-hydroxy-1,2,3-propanetricarboxylate (1:1); (2) *N*-(1-Phe-nethyl-4-piperidyl)propionanilide citrate (1:1). *UNII-*

---

† Brand name formerly used, and/or firm no longer concerned with this product.

MUN5LYG46H; UNII-UF599785JZ [fentanyl]. *CAS-990-73-8; CAS-437-38-7* [fentanyl]. BAN; JAN. *Analgesic (narcotic).* Actiq (Cephalon); Fentora (Cephalon); Sublimaze (Akorn) ◇*McN-JR-4263-49; R-4263*

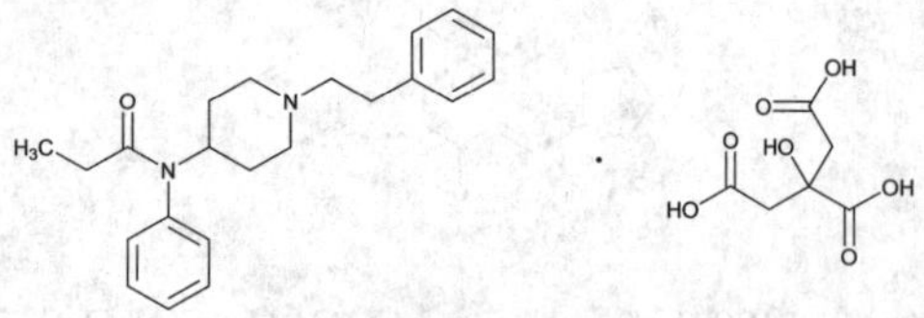

Fenthion. *O,O*-Dimethyl *O*-4-methylthio-*m*-tolyl phosphorothioate. *UNII-BL0L45OVKT. CAS-55-38-9.* BAN; MI. Pro-Spot (Bayer Animal Health); Spotton (Bayer Animal Health); Tiguvon (Bayer Animal Health)

Fentiazac [*1984*] (fen tye′ a zak). $C_{17}H_{12}ClNO_2S$. 329.80. (1) 5-Thiazoleacetic acid, 4-(4-chlorophenyl)-2-phenyl-; (2) 4-(*p*-Chlorophenyl)-2-phenyl-5-thiazoleacetic acid. *CAS-18046-21-4.* INN; BAN; JAN. *Anti-inflammatory.* ◇*WY-21,894*

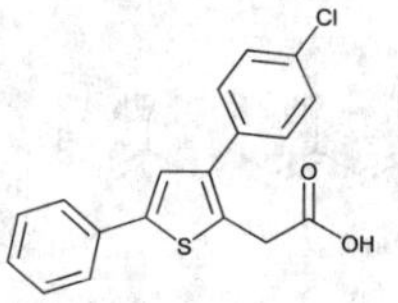

Fenticlor [*1970*] (fen′ ti klor). $C_{12}H_8Cl_2O_2S$. 287.16. (1) Phenol, 2,2′-thiobis[4-chloro-; (2) 2,2′-Thiobis[4-chlorophenol]. *UNII-D61659OVD0. CAS-97-24-5.* INN; BAN. *Anti-infective, topical.* ◇*S 7; NSC-4112*

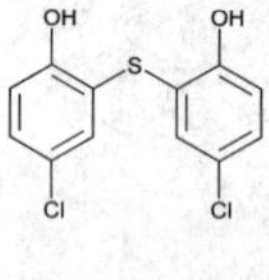

Fenticonazole Nitrate [*1982*] (fen″ ti kon′ a zole nye′ trate). $C_{24}H_{20}Cl_2N_2OS.HNO_3$. 518.41. [Fenticonazole is INN and BAN.] (1) 1*H*-Imidazole, 1-[2-(2,4-dichlorophenyl)-2-[[4-(phenylthio)phenyl]methoxy]ethyl]-, (±)-, mononitrate; (2) (±)-1-[2,4-Dichloro-β-[[*p*-(phenylthio)benzyl]oxy]-phenethyl]imidazole mononitrate. *UNII-QG05NRB077* [fenticonazole]. *CAS-73151-29-8; CAS-72479-26-6* [fenticonazole]. *Antifungal.* ◇*Rec 15/1476*

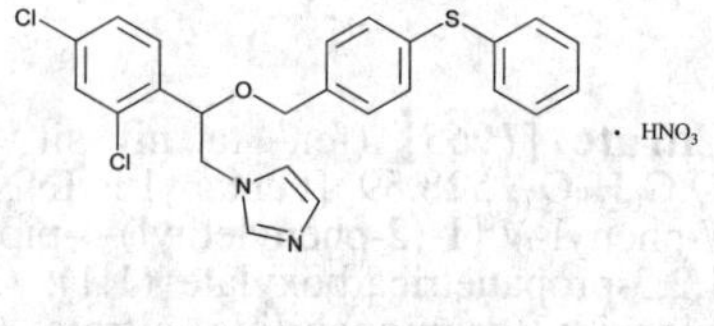

Fentonium Bromide. $C_{31}H_{34}BrNO_4$. 564.51. 3α-Hydroxy-8-(*p*-phenylphenacyl)-1αH,5αH-tropanium bromide (-)-tropate. *CAS-5868-06-4.* INN; MI. ◇*Z 326; Fa 402*

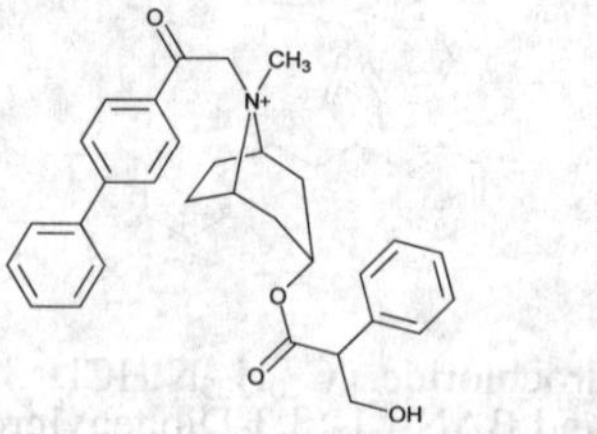

Fenvalerate. $C_{25}H_{22}ClNO_3$. 419.90. (*RS*)-α-Cyano-3-phenoxybenzyl (*RS*)-2-(4-chloro-phenyl)-3-methylbutyrate. *UNII-Z6MXZ39302. CAS-51630-58-1.* BAN.

Fenyramidol (INN, BAN, DCF) Hydrochloride — *See* Phenyramidol Hydrochloride.

Fenyripol Hydrochloride [*1963*] (fen ir′ i pol hye″ droe klor′ ide). $C_{12}H_{13}N_3O.HCl$. 251.71. [Fenyripol is INN.] (1) Benzenemethanol, α-[(2-pyrimidinylamino)methyl]-, monohydrochloride; (2) α-[(2-Pyrimidinylamino)methyl]-benzyl alcohol monohydrochloride. *CAS-2441-88-5; CAS-3607-24-7* [fenyripol]. *Relaxant (skeletal muscle).* ◇*IN 836; NSC-43183*

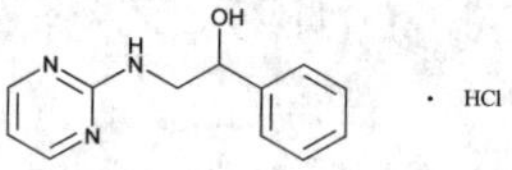

Fepentolic Acid. $C_{12}H_{16}O_4$. 224.25. α-Butyl-α-hydroxy-4,3-cresotic acid. *UNII-2Y3Q6049LX. CAS-17243-33-3.* INN; DCF. ◇*RCM 258*

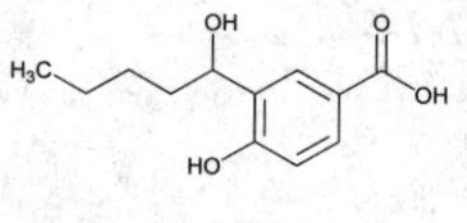

Fepitrizol. $C_{15}H_{14}N_4O$. 266.30. *o*-[1-Methyl-3-(3-pyridyl)-1*H*-1,2,4-triazol-5-yl]benzyl alcohol. *UNII-M9C5T4Q638. CAS-53415-46-6.* INN.

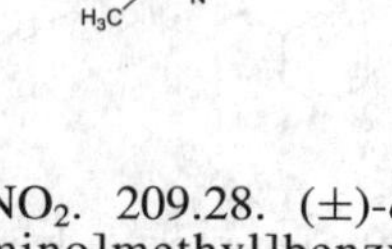

Fepradinol. $C_{12}H_{19}NO_2$. 209.28. (±)-α-[[(2-Hydroxy-1,1-dimethylethyl)amino]methyl]benzyl alcohol. *UNII-860MHI4WBA. CAS-63075-47-8.* INN.

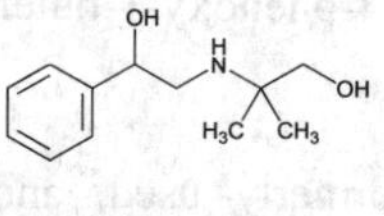

Feprazone. $C_{20}H_{20}N_2O_2$. 320.39. 4-(3-Methyl-2-butenyl)-1,2-diphenyl-3,5-pyrazolidinedione. *UNII-7BVX6J0CGR. CAS-30748-29-9.* INN; BAN; JAN; MI. ◇*DA 2370*

Fepromide. $C_{23}H_{30}N_2O_5$. 414.49. 3,4,5-Trimethoxy-*N*-[1-(phenoxymethyl)-2-(1-pyrrolidinyl)ethyl] benzamide. *UNII-6XXK617AU2. CAS-54063-41-1.* INN; DCF. ◇*1875 CERM*

Feprosidnine. $C_{11}H_{13}N_3O$. 203.24. 3-(α-Methylphenethyl)-sydnone imine. *UNII-1G4W8NR1PT. CAS-22293-47-6.* INN.

Fermagate. $CH_{12}Fe_2Mg_4O_{15}$·$4H_2O$. 545.07. Diiron(III) tetra-magnesium carbonate dodecahydroxide—water (1/4). *CAS-119175-48-3.* INN.

Ferpifosate Sodium. $C_{21}H_{21}FeNa_6N_3O_{18}P_3$. 890.11. Hexasodium tris[(4,5-dihydroxy-6-methyl-3-pyridinemethanol 3-phosphato)(3-)-O^3,O^3,O^5]ferrate(6-). *UNII-4S9081543Q. CAS-138708-32-4.* INN.

Ferric Ammonium Citrate (fer′ ik a moe′ nee um sit′ rate). **USP**. Ammonium iron(3+) citrate. Ferriseltz (Otsuka)

Ferric Ammonium Sulfate. *CAS-7783-83-7.*

Ferric Cacodylate. *CAS-5968-84-3; CAS-75-60-5* [cacodylic acid]. NF X.

Ferric Carboxymaltose [*2006*] (fer′ ik kar box″ ee mawl′ tose). $Fe^{III}{}_w([C_6H_{10}O_5]_aC_6H_{11}O_7)_x(OH)_yO_z$·$nH_2O$. (1) Iron Dextri-Maltose; (2) Iron(3+) hydroxide oxide poly-(1→4)-α-D-glucopyranosyl-(1→4)-D-gluconate hydrate; (3) Polynuclear iron (III)-hydroxide 4(*R*)-(poly-(1→4)-*O*-α-D-glucopyranosyl)-oxy-2(*R*),3(*S*),5(*R*), 6-tetrahydroxy-hexanoate. *CAS-9007-72-1.* INN. *Hematinic; Iron carbohydrate complex for the treatment of patients with iron deficiency anemia.* ◇*VIT-45*

Ferric Chloride. *UNII-U38V3ZVV3V. CAS-10025-77-1.* MI.

Ferric Chloride Fe 59 [*1963*] (fer′ ik klor′ ide). $^{59}FeCl_3$. (1) Iron chloride ($^{59}FeCl_3$); (2) Iron chloride ($^{59}FeCl_3$). *CAS-18497-67-1. Radioactive agent.*

Ferric Citrate (^{59}Fe) [Injection]. A sterile solution containing radioactive iron (^{59}Fe) in the ferric state, 1% w/v of sodium citrate, and sufficient sodium chloride to make the solution isotonic with blood. *CAS-54063-42-2.* INN; JAN.

Ferric Citrochloride Tincture. Iron(3+) chloride citrate. NF XI.

Ferric Fructose [*1968*] (fer′ ik fruk′ tose). $(C_6H_{10}FeO_7)_nK_{n/2}$ (n = 2 to 100). (1) D-Fructose, iron(3+)-contg. complex, potassium salt (2:1); (2) Fructose iron complex, compound with potassium (2:1). *CAS-12286-76-9.* INN. *Hematinic.* ◇*CB 302*

Ferric Gluconate. $[C_6H_{11}O_7]_3Fe$·$3H_2O$. 695.33. JAN.

Ferric Glycerophosphate. *CAS-1301-70-8; CAS-27082-31-1* [glycerophosphoric acid]. NF X.

Ferric Hydroxide Sucrose Complex (previously used name) — *See* Iron Sucrose.

Ferric Hypophosphite. *UNII-A75SB6QHEG. CAS-7783-84-8.* NF X; MI.

Ferric Oxide (fer′ ik ox′ ide). **NF**. [Ferric Oxide, Saccharated is JAN.] Contains 98.75 ± 1.75% of Fe_2O_3, calculated on the ignited basis. *Pharmaceutic aid (color).*

Ferric Oxide, Red. *UNII-1K09F3G675.* NF XVI.

Ferric Oxide, Yellow. *UNII-EX438O2MRT.* NF XVI.

Ferric Pyrophosphate, Soluble. *CAS-1332-96-3.* NF VII; MI.

Ferric Subsulfate (fer′ ik sub sul′ fate). **USP** [Solution]. $Fe_4(OH)_2(SO_4)_5$. 737.71. (1) Basic ferric sulfate solution; (2) Monsel′s Solution. *CAS-8053-12-1; CAS-1310-45-8.* NF XI; MI.

Ferric Sulfate (fer′ ik sul′ fate). **USP**. $Fe_2(SO_4)_3$·xH_2O. 399.88 (anhydrous). (1) Ferric persulfate; (2) Ferric sesquisulfate; (3) Ferric tersulfate. *CAS-10028-22-5* [ferric tersulfate]; *CAS-142906-29-4* [hydrate].

Ferricholinate — *See* Ferrocholinate.

Ferriclate Calcium Sodium [*1973*] (fer′ i klate kal′ see um soe′ dee um). $C_{12}H_{44}CaFe_6Na_4O_{36}$. 1231.56. [Calcium Sodium Ferriclate is INN.] (1) Ferrate(3-), pentaaqua[D-gluconato(4-)-O^2,O^4,O^5]tetra-μ-hydroxydihydroxytri-, calcium sodium (2:1:4); (2) Monocalcium tetrasodium bis-[pentaaqua[D-gluconato(4-)]-tetra-μ-hydroxydioxotriferrate-(3-)]. *CAS-34150-62-4. Hematinic.* Kelfer (Laboratorio Mauricio Villela S. A., Brazil)

Ferristene [*1994*] (fer ris′ teen). $C_8H_{11}NO_3S$·$(Fe_2O_3)_{0.725}$. (1) Ferristene; (2) Iron ferrite with carrier particles of monosized spheres of crosslinked poly(ammonium styrenesulfonate). *CAS-155773-56-1.* BAN. *Diagnostic aid (paramagnetic).* Dynospheres M-035 (Dyno Particles AS, Norway)

Ferrocholate — *See* Ferrocholinate.

Ferrocholinate. $C_{11}H_{20}FeNO_9$. 366.12. Chelate prepared by reacting equimolar quantities of freshly precipitated ferric hydroxide with choline dihydrogen citrate. *UNII-LWI5ZJ8WVL. CAS-1336-80-7.* INN; MI.

Ferropolimaler. $(C_7H_8FeO_5)_n$. [Iron Polymalether is JAN.] Maleic acid polymer with methyl vinyl ether, iron(2+) salt. *CAS-54063-44-4.* INN.

Ferroquine. $C_{23}H_{24}ClFeN_3$. 433.75. *N'*-(7-Chloroquinolin-4-yl)-*N*,*N*-dimethyl-*C*,*C'*-(ferrocene-1,2-diyl)dimethanamine. *CAS-185055-67-8.* INN.

Ferrotrenine. $C_{12}H_{24}FeN_2O_8$. 380.17. Hydrogen bis(*N*-ethylidenethreoninato) diaquoferrate (II). *CAS-15339-50-1.* INN; JAN.

Ferrous Citrate Fe 59 [*1963*] (fer′ us sit′ rate). $C_{12}H_{10}{}^{59}Fe_3O_{14}$. (1) 1,2,3-Propanetricarboxylic acid, 2-hydroxy-, iron(2+)-^{59}Fe salt; (2) Iron(2+)-^{59}Fe citrate. *CAS-64521-35-3.* USP XXII. *Radioactive agent.* Ferrutope (Bristol-Myers Squibb†)

Ferrous Fumarate (fer′ us fue′ ma rate). **USP.** $C_4H_2FeO_4$. 169.90. (1) 2-Butenedioic acid, (*E*)-, iron(2+) salt; (2) Iron(2+) fumarate. *UNII-R5L488RY0Q; UNII-88XHZ13131* [fumaric acid]. *CAS-141-01-5; CAS-110-17-8* [fumaric acid]. JAN. *Hematinic.* Feostat (Forest); Toleron (Mallinckrodt)

Ferrous Gluconate (fer′ us gloo′ koe nate). **USP.** $C_{12}H_{22}FeO_{14}.2H_2O$. 482.17. (1) D-Gluconic acid, iron(2+) salt (2:1), dihydrate; (2) Iron(2+) gluconate (1:2) dihy-

drate. *CAS-12389-15-0; CAS-299-29-6* [anhydrous]; *CAS-526-95-4* [D-gluconic acid]. *Hematinic.* Fergon (Sterling Health U.S.A.)

Ferrous Lactate. Iron(2+) lactate. *UNII-5JU4C2L5A0.* NF V; MI. Ferro Drops (Parke-Davis†)

Ferrous Orotate. $Fe(C_5H_3O_4N_2)_2.7\frac{1}{2}H_2O$. 501.14. Ferrous orotate heptahemihydrate. JAN.

Ferrous Sulfate (fer′ us sul′ fate). **USP.** $FeSO_4.7H_2O$. 278.01. (1) Sulfuric acid, iron(2+) salt (1:1), heptahydrate; (2) Iron(2+) sulfate (1:1) heptahydrate. *UNII-39R4TAN1VT. CAS-7782-63-0; CAS-7720-78-7* [anhydrous]. JAN. *Hematinic.* Feosol (SmithKline Beecham); Fero-Gradumet (Abbott†); Mol-Iron (Schering-Plough HealthCare†); Natabec (Parke-Davis†); Slow-Fe (Ciba-Geigy†)

Ferrous Sulfate, Dried (fer′ us sul′ fate). **USP.** $FeSO_4.xH_2O$. 151.91 (anhydrous). (1) Sulfuric acid, iron(2+) salt (1:1), hydrate; (2) Iron(2+)sulfate (1:1) hydrate. *CAS-13463-43-9; CAS-7720-78-7* [anhydrous]. *Anti-anemic.*

Ferrous Sulfate Fe 59 [*1963*] (fer′ us sul′ fate). $^{59}FeSO_4$. (1) Sulfuric acid, iron(2+)-^{59}Fe salt; (2) Iron(2+)-^{59}Fe sulfate. *Radioactive agent.*

Fertirelin Acetate [*1988*] (fer″ ti rel′ in as′ e tate). $C_{55}H_{76}N_{16}O_{12}.C_2H_4O_2$. 1213.34. [Fertirelin is INN and BAN.] (1) Luteinizing hormone-releasing factor (pig), 9-(*N*-ethyl-L-prolinamide)-10-deglycinamide-, monoacetate (salt); (2) 5-Oxo-L-prolyl-L-histidyl-L-tryptophyl-L-seryl-L-tyrosylglycyl-L-leucyl-L-arginyl-*N*-ethyl-L-prolinamide monoacetate (salt). *CAS-106756-71-2; CAS-38234-21-8* [fertirelin]. *Hormone (gonadotropin-releasing, veterinary).* ◇*U-69689E; TAP 031 (as the base)*

Ferucarbotran [*1997*] (fer″ ue kar′ boe tran). A nonstoichiometric polycrystalline mixture of iron (II) and iron (III) oxides (magnetite Fe_3O_4 and maghemite-γ Fe_2O_3) in which iron (II) oxide is specified to be less than 5%. A colloidal aqueous suspension of superparamagnetic iron oxide particles coated with carboxydextran. According to TEM electron microscopy measurements, the iron oxide core has a diameter of 3 to 5 nm. The hydrodynamic diameter of the coated particles measured by PCS (photon correlation spectroscopy) is 45 to 65 nm. In the colloidal aqueous suspension, the carboxydextran coat has a thickness of about 25 nm (calculated from PCS measurements). Molecular weight is approximately 20,000 daltons. BAN. *Diagnostic aid (paramagnetic).* ◇*ZK 132281*

Ferumoxides [*1992*] (fer″ ue mox′ ides). **USP** [Injection]. $(Fe_2O_3)_m(FeO)_n$. (1) Iron oxide crystal is inverse spinel (X-ray data); (2) Fe(II) and Fe(III) are present (Mössbauer Spectroscopy; (3) Physical form is a colloidal particle of nonstoichiometric magnetite. *UNII-G6N3J05W84. CAS-119683-68-0.* BAN. *Diagnostic aid (paramagnetic).* Feridex (Advanced Magnetics) ◇*AMI-25*

Ferumoxsil [*1992*] (fer″ ue mox′ sil). **USP** [Oral Suspension]. Silicone polymer bonded to colloidal particles of superparamagnetic, nonstoichiometric magnetite. (1) Iron oxide crystal is inverse spinel (X-ray data); (2) Fe (II) and Fe(III) are present (Mössbauer Spectroscopy); (3) Physical form is a colloidal particle of nonstoichiometric magnetite with a silicone polymer bonded to the iron oxide. *UNII-6HJV9H13XS.* BAN. *Diagnostic aid (paramagnetic).* Gastromark (Advanced Magnetics) ◇*AMI-121*

Ferumoxtran-10 [*1997*] (fer″ ue mox′ tran). (FeO).₁ (Fe₂O₃).₄₅(C₆H₁₀O₅).₄₁ (average formula). A superparamagnetic iron oxide [a mixed iron Fe(II) and Fe(III) oxide] covered with low molecular weight dextran (dextran T-10). The iron oxide is a superparamagnetic form of a non-stoichiometric magnetite which is 43-60 A in diameter. In solution, a colloidal particle has a Stokes diameter of 170 to 210 A by size exclusion chromatography. The colloidal particle consists of crystals of iron oxide with a covering of dextran (60-75 A thick). Ferumoxtran-10. *CAS-189047-99-2. Diagnostic aid (paramagnetic).* Combidex (Advanced Magnetics) ◇*Code 7227; BMS 180549*

Ferumoxytol [*2003*] (fer″ ue mox′ i tol). FeO₁.₄₉ (approximately); C₃₉₈H₆₄₆O₃₃₇ (coating). Polyglucose sorbitol carboxymethyl ether-coated non-stoichiometric magnetite. Ferumoxytol is a superparamagnetic iron oxide that is coated with a low molecular weight semi-synthetic carbohydrate, polyglucose sorbitol carboxymethyl ether. The iron oxide is a superparamagnetic form of non-stoichiometric magnetite with crystal size of 6.2 to 7.3 nm. In solution, the colloidal particle of ferumoxytol has a Stokes diameter of 18-20 nm. Molecular weight is approximately 308,000. *CAS-1309-38-2. Diagnostic aid, magnetic resonance imaging (MRI); treatment of iron deficiency.* ◇*Code 7228*

Fesoterodine Fumarate [*2004*] (fes″ oh ter′ oh deen fue′ ma rate). C₂₆H₃₇NO₃.C₄H₄O₄. 527.65. [Fesoterodine is INN.] (1) Propanoic acid, 2-methyl-, 2-[(1*R*)-3-[bis(1-methylethyl)amino]-1-phenylpropyl]-4-(hydroxymethyl)phenyl ester, (2*E*)-2-butenedioate (1:1) (salt); (2) 2-[(1*R*)-3-[Bis(1-methylethyl)amino]-1-phenylpropyl]-4-(hydroxymethyl)-phenyl 2-methylpropanoate hydrogen (2*E*)-butenedioate (salt). *UNII-EOS72165S7. CAS-286930-03-8.* JAN. *Treatment of overactive bladder (muscarinic antagonist).* (Schwarz Pharma Limited, Ireland) ◇*SPM 907; SPM 8272*

Fetoxilate (INN, BAN) — *See* Fetoxylate Hydrochloride.

Fetoxylate (previously used name) — *See* Fetoxylate Hydrochloride.

Fetoxylate Hydrochloride [*1969*] (fe tox′ i late hye″ droe klor′ ide). C₃₆H₃₆N₂O₃.HCl. 581.14. [Fetoxilate is INN and BAN.] (1) 4-Piperidinecarboxylic acid, 1-(3-cyano-3,3-diphenylpropyl)-4-phenyl-, 2-phenoxyethyl ester, monohydrochloride; (2) 2-Phenoxyethyl 1-(3-cyano-3,3-diphenylpropyl)-4-phenylisonipecotate monohydrochloride. *CAS-*

23607-71-8; *CAS-54063-45-5* [fetoxylate]. *Relaxant (smooth muscle). [Name previously used: Fetoxylate.]* ◇*McN-JR-13,558-11; R 13,558*

Feverfew. The dried leaves of *Tanacetum parthenium* (Linné) Schultz-Bip. (Fam. Asteraceae), collected when the plant is in flower. NF XXI.

Fexicaine. C₂₅H₃₄N₂O₄. 426.55. 2-(*p*-Butoxyphenoxy)-*N*-(*o*-methoxyphenyl)-*N*-[2-(1-pyrrolidinyl)ethyl]acetamide. *UNII-5N2K83R1L2. CAS-54063-46-6.* INN; DCF.

Fexinidazole. C₁₂H₁₃N₃O₃S. 279.31. 1-Methyl-2-[[*p*-(methylthio)phenoxy]methyl]-5-nitroimidazole. *UNII-306ERL82IR. CAS-59729-37-2.* INN.

Fexofenadine Hydrochloride [*1995*] (fex″ oh fen′ a deen hye″ droe klor′ ide). USP. C₃₂H₃₉NO₄.HCl. 538.12. [Fexofenadine is INN and BAN.] (1) Benzeneacetic acid, 4-[1-hydroxy-4-[4-(hydroxydiphenylmethyl)-1-piperidinyl]butyl]-α,α-dimethyl-, hydrochloride, (±)-; (2) (±)-*p*-[1-Hydroxy-4-[4-(hydroxydiphenylmethyl)piperidino]butyl]-α-methylhydratropic acid, hydrochloride. *UNII-2S068B75ZU; UNII-E6582LOH6V* [fexofenadine]. *CAS-153439-40-8; CAS-138452-21-8* [replaced]; *CAS-83799-24-0* [fexofenadine]. *Antihistaminic.* Allegra (Sanofi Aventis) ◇*MDL 16,455A*

Fezatione. C₁₇H₁₄N₂S₂. 310.44. 3-[(*p*-Methylbenzylidene)-amino]-4-phenyl-4-thiazoline-2-thione. *CAS-15387-18-5.* INN.

Fezolamine Fumarate [*1984*] (fe zol′ a meen fue′ ma rate). $C_{20}H_{23}N_3 \cdot C_4H_4O_4$. 421.49. [Fezolamine is INN.] (1) 1*H*-Pyrazole-1-propanamine, *N,N*-dimethyl-3,4-diphenyl-, (*E*)-2-butenedioate (1:1); (2) 1-[3-(Dimethylamino)propyl]-3,4-diphenylpyrazole fumarate (1:1). *UNII-11GX0BGV7P; UNII-1133E05F6C* [fezolamine]. *CAS-80410-37-3; CAS-80410-36-2* [fezolamine]. *Antidepressant.* ◇*Win 41528-2*

FIAC — *See* Fiacitabine.

Fiacitabine [*1991*] (fye a sye′ ta been). $C_9H_{11}FIN_3O_4$. 371.10. (1) 2(1*H*)-Pyrimidinone, 4-amino-1-(2-deoxy-2-fluoro-*β*-D-arabinofuranosyl)-5-iodo-; (2) 1-(2-Deoxy-2-fluoro-*β*-D-arabinofuranosyl)-5-iodocytosine. *UNII-4058H365ZB.* *CAS-69123-90-6.* INN. *Antiviral.*

Fialuridine [*1992*] (fye″ al ure′ i deen). $C_9H_{10}FIN_2O_5$. 372.09. (1) 2,4(1*H*,3*H*)-Pyrimidinedione, 1-(2-deoxy-2-fluoro-*β*-D-arabinofuranosyl)-5-iodo-; (2) 1-(2-Deoxy-2-fluoro-*β*-D-arabinofuranosyl)-5-iodouracil. *UNII-53T7IN77LC.* *CAS-69123-98-4.* INN. *Antiviral.*

FIAU — *See* Fialuridine.

Fibracillin. $C_{26}H_{28}ClN_3O_6S$. 546.04. D-6-[2-[2-(*p*-Chlorophenoxy)-2-methylpropionamido]-2-phenylacetamido]-3,3-dimethyl-7-oxo-4-thia-1-azabicyclo[3.2.0]heptane-2-carboxylic acid. *UNII-VSM36G5OTK.* *CAS-51154-48-4.* INN.

Fibrin. An insoluble plasma protein obtained by the action of thrombin on fibrinogen. INN; MI.

Fibrinogen (^{125}I) (INN) — *See* Fibrinogen I 125.

Fibrinogen, Human. USP XIX; MI. Fibrogen (Marion Merrell Dow†)

Fibrinogen I 125 [*1978*] (fye brin′ oh jen). [Fibrinogen (^{125}I) is INN.] A preparation of fibrinogen (human) labeled with ^{125}I. Less than 5% of the radioiodine is not bound to protein; there is less than 0.38 mcg of protein-bound iodine per mg of fibrinogen. (1) Fibrinogen labeled with iodine-125; (2) Fibrinogen labeled with iodine-125. *Diagnostic aid (vascular patency); radioactive agent.* Ibrin (Nycomed Amersham†); Sensor (Abbott†)

Fibrinolysin, Human. Enzyme obtained from human plasma by conversion of profibrinolysin with streptokinase to fibrinolysin. *CAS-9004-09-5.* INN; BAN. Actase (Ortho Pharmaceutical†) *[Name previously used: Plasmin.]*

Fibroblast Interferon (previously used name) — *See* Interferon Beta.

Fidarestat. $C_{12}H_{10}FN_3O_4$. 279.22. (+)-(2*S*,4*S*)-6-Fluoro-2′,5′-dioxospiro[chroman-4,4′-imidazolidine]-2-carboxamide. *CAS-136087-85-9.* INN.

Fidaxomicin [*2008*] (fye dax″ oh mye′ sin). $C_{52}H_{74}Cl_2O_{18}$. 1058.04. (1) Oxacyclooctadeca-3,5,9,13,15-pentaen-2-one, 3-[[[6-deoxy-4-*O*-(3,5-dichloro-2-ethyl-4,6-dihydroxybenzoyl)-2-*O*-methyl-*β*-D-mannopyranosyl]oxy]methyl]-12-[[6-deoxy-5-*C*-methyl-4-*O*-(2-methyl-1-oxopropyl)-*β*-D-*lyxo*-hexopyranosyl]oxy]-11-ethyl-8-hydroxy-18-[(1*R*)-1-hydroxyethyl]-9,13,15-trimethyl-, (3*E*,5*E*,8*S*,9*E*,11*S*,12-*R*,13*E*,15*E*,18*S*)-; (2) (3*E*,5*E*,8*S*,9*E*,11*S*,12-*R*,13*E*,15*E*,18*S*)-3-({[6-Deoxy-4-*O*-(3,5-dichloro-2-ethyl-4,6-dihydroxybenzoyl)-2-*O*-methyl-*β*-D-mannopyranosyl]oxy}methyl)-12-{[6-deoxy-5-*C*-methyl-4-*O*-(2-methylpropanoyl)-*β*-D-*lyxo*-hexopyranosyl]oxy}-11-ethyl-8-hydroxy-18-[(1*R*)-1-hydroxyethyl]-9,13,15-trimethyloxacyclooctadeca-3,5,9,13,15-pentaen-2-one. *CAS-873857-62-6.* *Treatment and prevention of Clostridium difficile Infections (CDI) or Clostridium difficile-Associated Diarrhea (CDAD).* ◇*PAR-101; OPT-80*

Fidexaban [*2004*] (fye dex′ a ban). $C_{25}H_{24}F_2N_6O_5$. 526.49. (1) Glycine, *N*-[2-[5-(aminoiminomethyl)-2-hydroxyphenoxy]-6-[3-(4,5-dihydro-1-methyl-1*H*-imidazol-2-yl)phenoxy]-3,5-difluoro-4-pyridinyl]-*N*-methyl-; (2) [[2-(5-Carbamimidoyl-2-hydroxyphenoxy)-3,5-difluoro-6-[3-(1-methyl-4,5-dihydro-1*H*-imidazol-2-yl)phenoxy]pyridin-4-yl]methylamino]acetic acid. *UNII-10NHF3008V.* *CAS-183305-24-0.* INN. *Anticoagulant (Factor Xa inhibitor).* ◇*ZK 807834*

Fiduxosin. $C_{30}H_{29}N_5O_4S$. 555.65. 8-Phenyl-3-[4-[(3a*R*,9b*R*)-1,3a,4,9b-tetrahydro-9-methoxy[1]benzopyrano[3,4-*c*]pyrrol-2(3*H*)-yl]butyl]pyrazino[2′,3′:4,5]thieno[3,2-*d*]pyrimidine-2,4(1*H*,3*H*)-dione. *UNII-W9O92HYT6I.* *CAS-208993-54-8.* INN.

Fiduxosin Hydrochloride [*1999*] (fye dux′ oh sin hye″ droe klor′ ide). $C_{30}H_{29}N_5O_4S \cdot HCl$. 592.11. (1) Pyrazino[2′,3′:4,5]thieno[3,2-*d*]pyrimidine-2,4(1*H*,3*H*)-dione, 8-phenyl-3-[4-[(3a*R*,9b*R*)-1,3a,4,9b-tetrahydro-9-methoxy[1]benzopyrano[3,4-*c*]pyrrol-2(3*H*)-yl]butyl]-, monohydrochloride; (2) 8-Phenyl-3-[4-[(3a*R*,9b*R*)-1,3a,4,9b-tetrahydro-9-methoxy[1]benzopyrano[3,4-*c*]pyrrol-2(3*H*)-yl]butyl]pyrazino[2′,3′:4,5]thieno[3,2-*d*]pyrimidine-

2,4(1*H*,3*H*)-dione monohydrochloride. *CAS-208992-74-9. Treatment of benign prostatic hyperplasia (α_{1a}-adreno-ceptor antagonist).* ◇*A-185980.1; ABT-980*

Figitumumab [*2008*] (fig″ i toom′ ue mab). $C_{6462}H_{9948}N_{1736}O_{2020}S_{54}$. (1) Immunoglobulin G2, anti-(human insulin-like growth factor I receptor) (human monoclonal CP-751,871 clone 2.13.2 heavy chain) disulfide with human monoclonal CP-751,871 clone 2.13.2 light chain, dimer; (2) Immunoglobulin G2, anti-(human insulin-like growth factor 1 receptor (EC.2.7.10.1 or CD221 antigen)); human monoclonal CP-751,871 clone 2.13.2 γ2 heavy chain (139-214′)-disulfide with human monoclonal CP-751,871 clone 2.13.2 κ light chain, dimer (227-227″:228-228″:231-231″:234-234″)-tetrakisdisulfide. Molecular weight is approximately 146,000 daltons. *CAS-943453-46-1. Treatment of cancer.* ◇*CP-751,871*

Figopitant. $C_{27}H_{31}F_6N_3O$. 527.54. (*S*)-*N*-[Bis(3,5-trifluoro-methyl)phenethyl]-4-(cyclopropylmethyl)-*N*-methyl-α-phenyl-1-piperazineacetamide. *CAS-502422-74-4.* INN.

Filaminast [*1996*] (fil am′ i nast). $C_{15}H_{20}N_2O_4$. 292.33. (1) Ethanone, 1-[3-(cyclopentyloxy)-4-methoxyphenyl]-, *O*-(aminocarbonyl)oxime, (*E*)-; (2) 3′-(Cyclopentyloxy)-4′-methoxyacetophenone (*E*)-*O*-carbamoyloxime. *CAS-141184-34-1.* INN. *Anti-asthmatic (selective phosphodies-terase IV inhibitor).* ◇*WAY-PDA-641*

Filenadol. $C_{14}H_{19}NO_4$. 265.30. (±)-*erythro*-α-Methyl-β-[3,4-(methylenedioxy)phenyl]-4-morpholineethanol. *UNII-YFT8T83CF9. CAS-78168-92-0.* INN.

Filgrastim [*1990*] (fil gra′ stim). $C_{845}H_{1339}N_{223}O_{243}S_9$. 18,800 daltons. A single chain, 175 amino acid polypeptide, nonglycosylated, expressed by *E. coli*. (1) Colony-stimu-lating factor (human clone 1034), *N*-L-methionyl-; (2) *N*-L-

Methionylcolony-stimulating factor (human clone 1034). *UNII-PVI5M0M1GW. CAS-121181-53-1.* INN; BAN. *Anti-neutropenic; hematopoietic stimulant.* Neupogen (Amgen) ◇*r-metHuG-CSF*

```
MTPLGPASSL PQSFLLKSLE QVRKIQGSGA ALQEKLCATY KLCHPEELVL
LGHSLGIPWA PLSSCPSQAL QLAGCLSQLH SGLFLYQGLL QALEGISPEL
GPTLDTLQLD VADFATTIWQ QMEELGMAPA LQPTQGAMPA FASAFQRRAG
GVLVASHLQS FLEVSYRVLR HLAQP
```

Filipin [*1968*] (fil′ i pin). $C_{35}H_{58}O_{11}$. 654.83. (1) Filipin III; (2) Oxacyclooctacosa-17,19,21,23,25-pentaen-2-one, 4,6,8,10,12,14,16,27-octahydroxy-3-(1-hydroxyhexyl)-17,28-dimethyl-. *CAS-480-49-9.* INN. *Antifungal.* ◇*U-5956; NSC-3364*

Fimasartan. $C_{27}H_{31}N_7OS$. 501.65. 2-({2-Butyl-4-methyl-6-oxo-1-{[2′-(1*H*-tetrazol-5-yl)biphenyl-4-yl]methyl}-1,6-dihydropyrimidin-5-yl})-*N*,*N*-dimethylthioacetamide. *CAS-247257-48-3.* INN.

Finafloxacin. $C_{20}H_{19}FN_4O_4$. 398.39. (-)-8-Cyano-1-cyclopro-pyl-6-fluoro-7-[(4a*S*,7a*S*)-hexahydropyrrolo[3,4-*b*]-1,4-oxazin-6(2*H*)-yl]-4-oxo-1,4-dihydroquinoline-3-car-boxylic acid. *CAS-209342-40-5.* INN.

Finasteride [*1989*] (fin as′ ter ide). **USP**. $C_{23}H_{36}N_2O_2$. 372.54. (1) 4-Azaandrost-1-ene-17-carboxamide, *N*-(1,1-dimethylethyl)-3-oxo-, (5α,17β)-; (2) *N-tert*-Butyl-3-oxo-4-aza-5α-androst-1-ene-17β-carboxamide. *UNII-57GNO57U7G. CAS-98319-26-7.* INN; BAN. *Inhibitor (alpha reductase).* Propecia (Merck); Proscar (Merck) ◇*MK-906*

---

† Brand name formerly used, and/or firm no longer concerned with this product.

Fingolimod Hydrochloride [*2005*] (fin gol′ i mod hye″ droe klor′ ide). $C_{19}H_{33}NO_2.HCl$. 343.93. [Fingolimod is INN.] (1) 1,3-Propanediol, 2-amino-2-[2-(4-octylphenyl)ethyl]-, hydrochloride; (2) 2-Amino-2-[2-(4-octylphenyl)ethyl]propane-1,3-diol hydrochloride. *UNII-G926EC510T; UNII-3QN8BYN5QF* [fingolimod]. *CAS-162359-56-0; CAS-162359-55-9* [fingolimod]. *Prophylaxis of organ rejection in patients receiving allogenic renal transplants (sphingosine-1-phosphate receptor).* ◇*FTY720*

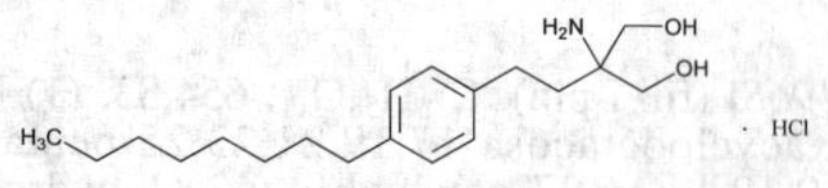

Finrozole. $C_{18}H_{15}FN_4O$. 322.34. *p*-[(1*RS*,2*SR*)-3-(*p*-Fluorophenyl)-2-hydroxy-1-(1*H*-1,2,4-triazol-1-yl)propyl]benzonitrile. *CAS-160146-17-8.* INN.

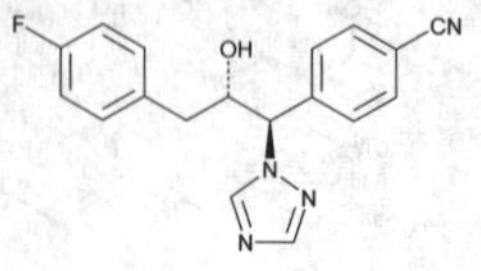

Fipamezole. $C_{14}H_{15}FN_2$. 230.28. 4-[(2*RS*)-2-Ethyl-5-fluoroindan-2-yl]-1*H*-imidazole. *UNII-T5RCK09KHV. CAS-150586-58-6.* INN.

Fipexide. $C_{20}H_{21}ClN_2O_4$. 388.84. 1-[(*p*-Chlorophenoxy)acetyl]-4-piperonylpiperazine. *UNII-TG44VME01D. CAS-34161-24-5.* INN; DCF; MI.

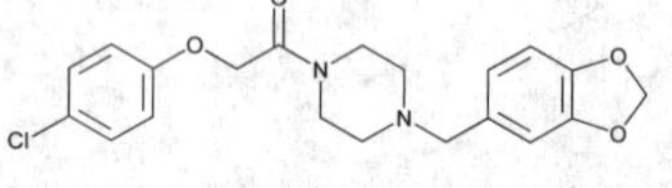

Fipronil. $C_{12}H_4Cl_2F_6N_4OS$. 437.15. (*RS*)-5-Amino-1-(2,6-dichloro-4-trifluoromethylphenyl)-4-(trifluoromethylsulfinyl)pyrazole-3-carbonitrile. *UNII-QGH063955F. CAS-120068-37-3.* BAN. ◇*RM 1601; MB 46030*

Firategrast [*2006*] (fir a′ te grast). $C_{27}H_{27}F_2NO_6$. 499.50. (1) [1,1′-Biphenyl]-4-propanoic acid, α-[(2,6-difluorobenzoyl)amino]-4′-(ethoxymethyl)-2′,6′-dimethoxy-, (α*S*)-; (2) (2*S*)-2-[(2,6-Difluorobenzoyl)amino]-3-[4′-(ethoxymethyl)-2′,6′-dimethoxybiphenyl-4-yl]propanoic acid. *UNII-OJY3SK9H5F. CAS-402567-16-2.* INN. *Treatment of multiple sclerosis and inflammatory bowel disease.* ◇*SB-683699*

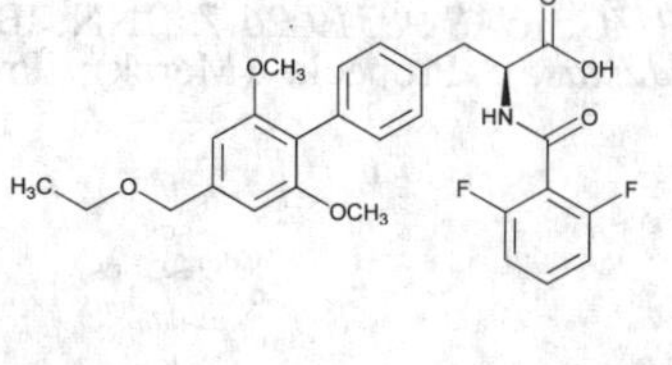

Firocoxib [*2003*] (fir″ oh kox′ ib). $C_{17}H_{20}O_5S$. 336.40. (1) 2(5*H*)-Furanone, 3-(cyclopropylmethoxy)-5,5-dimethyl-4-[4-(methylsulfonyl)phenyl]-; (2) 3-(Cyclopropylmethoxy)-5,5-dimethyl-4-[4-(methylsulfonyl)phenyl]furan-2(5*H*)-one; (3) 3-(Cyclopropylmethoxy)-4-(4-methylsulfonyl)-

phenyl)-5,5-dimethylfuranone. *UNII-Y6V2W4S4WT. CAS-189954-96-9.* INN. *Treatment of pain, inflammation and fever.* Equioxx (Merial) ◇*ML-1,785,713*

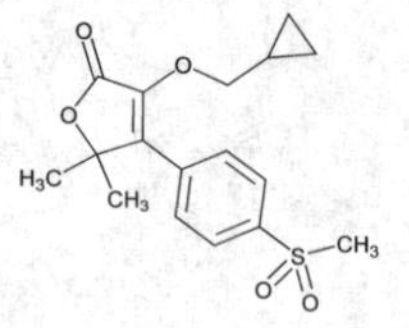

Fisalamine — *See* Mesalamine.

Fispemifene [*2006*] (fis pem′ i feen). $C_{26}H_{27}ClO_3$. 422.94. (1) Ethanol, 2-[2-[4-[(1*Z*)-4-chloro-1,2-diphenyl-1-butenyl]phenoxy]ethoxy]-; (2) 2-[2-[4-[(1*Z*)-4-Chloro-1,2-diphenylbut-1-enyl]phenoxy]ethoxy]ethanol. *UNII-3VZ2833V08. CAS-341524-89-8.* INN. *Male hypogonadism, male urinary tract symptoms.* ◇*HM-101; HM-101a*

Flamenol. $C_7H_8O_3$. 140.14. 5-Methoxyresorcinol. *UNII-6201E0JIF3. CAS-2174-64-3.* INN; DCF.

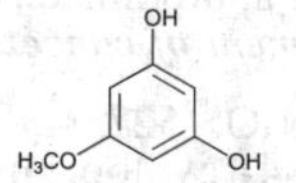

Flavamine. $C_{21}H_{23}NO_2$. 321.41. 6-[(Diethylamino)methyl]-3-methylflavone. *UNII-QL5Z51GXKI. CAS-15686-60-9.* INN.

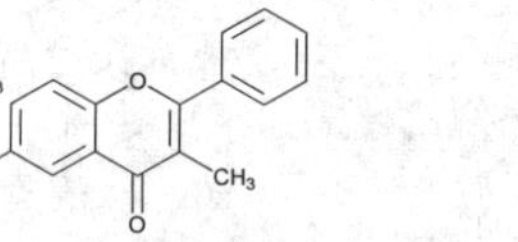

Flavin Adenin Dinucleotide. $C_{27}H_{33}N_9O_{15}P_2$. 785.55. *CAS-146-14-5.* JAN.

Flavodic Acid. $C_{19}H_{14}O_8$. 370.31. [(4-Oxo-2-phenyl-4*H*-1-benzopyran-5,7-diyl)dioxy]diacetic acid. *UNII-2Z9V171UEM. CAS-37470-13-6.* INN; DCF.

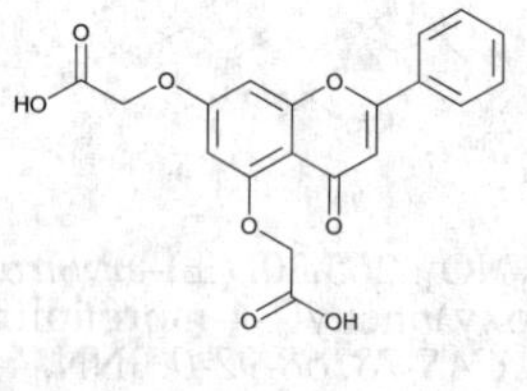

Flavodilol Maleate [*1983*] (flay″ voe dil′ ol mal′ ee ate). $C_{21}H_{23}NO_4.C_4H_4O_4$. 469.48. [Flavodilol is INN.] (1) 4*H*-1-Benzopyran-4-one, 7-[2-hydroxy-3-(propylamino)propoxy]-2-phenyl-, (±)-, (*Z*)-2-butenedioate (1:1) (salt); (2) (±)-7-[2-Hydroxy-3-(propylamino)propoxy]flavone maleate (1:1) (salt). *UNII-M8FR1KL85J* [flavodilol]. *CAS-79619-32-2; CAS-79619-31-1* [flavodilol]. *Antihypertensive.* ◇*PR-877-530L*

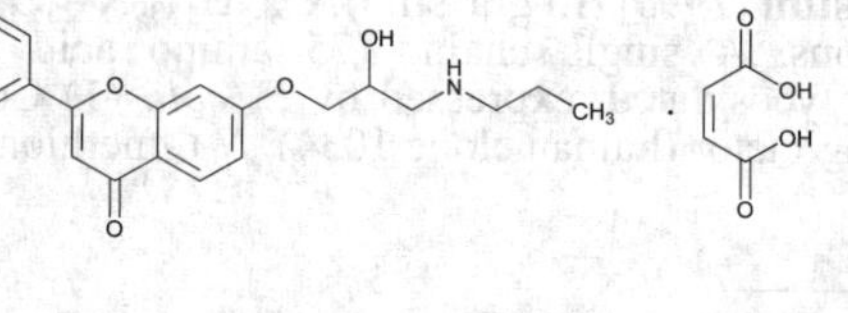

Flavonoid — *See* Troxerutin.

Flavopiridol (trivial name) — *See* Alvocidib.

Flavoxate Hydrochloride [*1968*] (flay vox′ ate hye″ droe klor′ ide). $C_{24}H_{25}NO_4 \cdot HCl$. 427.92. [Flavoxate is INN and BAN.] (1) 4*H*-1-Benzopyran-8-carboxylic acid, 3-methyl-4-oxo-2-phenyl-, 2-(1-piperidinyl)ethyl ester, hydrochloride; (2) 2-Piperidinoethyl 3-methyl-4-oxo-2-phenyl-4*H*-1-benzopyran-8-carboxylate hydrochloride. *UNII-9C05J6089W; UNII-3E74Y80MEY* [flavoxate]. *CAS-3717-88-2; CAS-15301-69-6* [flavoxate]. JAN. *Relaxant (smooth muscle).* Urispas (Ortho-McNeil) ◇*DW-61; NSC-114649*

Flazalone [*1971*] (flay′ za lone). $C_{19}H_{19}F_2NO_2$. 331.36. (1) (4-Fluorophenyl)[4-(4-fluorophenyl)-4-hydroxy-1-methyl-3-piperidinyl]methanone; (2) *p*-Fluorophenyl 4-(*p*-fluorophenyl)-4-hydroxy-1-methyl-3-piperidyl ketone. *CAS-21221-18-1.* INN; BAN. *Anti-inflammatory.* ◇*NSC-102629*

Flecainide Acetate [*1977*] (flek′ a nide as′ e tate). **USP**. $C_{17}H_{20}F_6N_2O_3 \cdot C_2H_4O_2$. 474.39. [Flecainide is INN and BAN.] (1) Benzamide, *N*-(2-piperidinylmethyl)-2,5-bis(2,2,2-trifluoroethoxy)-, monoacetate; (2) *N*-(2-Piperidylmethyl)-2,5-bis(2,2,2-trifluoroethoxy)benzamide monoacetate. *UNII-M8U465Q1WQ; UNII-K94FTS1806* [flecainide]. *CAS-54143-56-5; CAS-54143-55-4* [flecainide]. JAN. *Cardiac depressant (anti-arrhythmic).* Tambocor (3M Pharmaceuticals)

Flerobuterol. $C_{12}H_{18}FNO$. 211.28. α-[(*tert*-Butylamino)-methyl]-*o*-fluorobenzyl alcohol. *UNII-F05RR5M463. CAS-82101-10-8.* INN.

Fleroxacin [*1987*] (fler ox′ a sin). $C_{17}H_{18}F_3N_3O_3$. 369.34. (1) 3-Quinolinecarboxylic acid, 6,8-difluoro-1-(2-fluoroethyl)-1,4-dihydro-7-(4-methyl-1-piperazinyl)-4-oxo-; (2) 6,8-Difluoro-1-(2-fluoroethyl)-1,4-dihydro-7-(4-methyl-1-piperazinyl)-4-oxo-3-quinolinecarboxylic acid. *UNII-*

---

† Brand name formerly used, and/or firm no longer concerned with this product.

N804LDH51K. CAS-79660-72-3. INN; BAN; JAN. *Antibacterial.* Megalone (Hoffmann-LaRoche) ◇*Ro 23-6240/000*

Flesinoxan. $C_{22}H_{26}FN_3O_4$. 415.46. (+)-(*S*)-*p*-Fluoro-*N*-[2-[4-[2-(hydroxymethyl)-1,4-benzodioxan-5-yl]-1-piperazinyl]-ethyl]benzamide. *CAS-98206-10-1.* INN.

Flestolol Sulfate [*1985*] (fles′ toe lol sul′ fate). $C_{15}H_{22}FN_3O_4 \cdot H_2SO_4$. 425.43. [Flestolol is INN.] (1) Benzoic acid, 2-fluoro-, 3-[[2-[(aminocarbonyl)amino]-1,1-dimethylethyl]amino]-2-hydroxypropyl ester, (±)-, sulfate (1:1) (salt); (2) *o*-Fluorobenzoic acid, 3-ester with (±)-[2-[(2,3-dihydroxypropyl)amino]-2-methylpropyl]urea, sulfate (1:1) (salt). *UNII-T5MWT8445U; UNII-LI02075E1W* [flestolol]. *CAS-88844-73-9; CAS-87721-62-8* [flestolol]. *Anti-adrenergic (β-receptor).* ◇*ACC-9089*

Fletazepam [*1974*] (fle taz′ e pam). $C_{17}H_{13}ClF_4N_2$. 356.75. (1) 1*H*-1,4-Benzodiazepine, 7-chloro-5-(2-fluorophenyl)-2,3-dihydro-1-(2,2,2-trifluoroethyl)-; (2) 7-Chloro-5-(*o*-fluorophenyl)-2,3-dihydro-1-(2,2,2-trifluoroethyl)-1*H*-1,4-benzodiazepine. *CAS-34482-99-0.* INN; BAN. *Relaxant (skeletal muscle).* ◇*Sch 15698*

Flezelastine. $C_{29}H_{30}FN_3O$. 455.57. (±)-4-(*p*-Fluorobenzyl)-2-(hexahydro-1-phenethyl-1*H*-azepin-4-yl)-1(2*H*)-phthalazinone. *UNII-77K18757UK. CAS-135381-77-0.* INN.

Flibanserin [*1997*] (flib an′ ser in). $C_{20}H_{21}F_3N_4O$. 390.40. (1) 1,3-Dihydro-1-[2-[4-[3-(trifluoromethyl)phenyl]-1-piperazinyl]ethyl]-2*H*-benzimidazol-2-one; (2) 1-[2-[4-(α,α,α-

Trifluoro-*m*-tolyl)-1-piperazinyl]ethyl]-2-benzimidazoli-
none. *CAS-167933-07-5*. INN. *Antidepressant (5-HT$_{1a}$a-
gonist and 5-HT$_2$antagonist).* ◇*BIMT 17 BS; BIMT 17*

Flindokalner [*2002*] (flin″ doe kal′ ner). $C_{16}H_{10}ClF_4NO_2$.
359.70. (1) 2*H*-Indol-2-one, 3-(5-chloro-2-methoxyphe-
nyl)-3-fluoro-1,3-dihydro-6-(trifluoromethyl)-, (3*S*)-; (2)
(3*S*)-3-(5-Chloro-2-methoxyphenyl)-3-fluoro-6-(trifluoromethyl)-1,3-dihydro-2*H*-indol-2-one. *UNII-J57O328W4W*.
CAS-187523-35-9. INN. *Neuroprotectant (opener of large
conductance, calcium-activated (maxi-K) K$^+$channels.*
MaxiPost (Bristol-Myers Squibb) ◇*BMS-204352*

Flocalcitriol (previously used name) — *See* Falecalcitriol.

Floctafenine [*1977*] (flok″ ta fen′ een). $C_{20}H_{17}F_3N_2O_4$.
406.36. (1) Benzoic acid, 2-[[8-(trifluoromethyl)-4-quino-
linyl]amino]-, 2,3-dihydroxypropyl ester; (2) 2,3-
Dihydroxypropyl *N*-[8-(trifluoromethyl)-4-quinolyl]an-
thranilate. *CAS-23779-99-9*. INN; BAN; JAN. *Analgesic.*
Idarac (Hoechst-Roussel†) ◇*R 4318; Ru 15750*

Flomoxef. $C_{15}H_{18}F_2N_6O_7S_2$. 496.47. [Flomoxef Sodium is
JAN.] (-)-(6*R*,7*R*)-7-[2-[(Difluoromethyl)thio]acetamido]-
3-[[[1-(2-hydroxyethyl)-1*H*-tetrazol-5-yl]thio]methyl]-7-
methoxy-8-oxo-5-oxa-1-azabicyclo[4.2.0]oct-2-ene-2-car-
boxylic acid. *UNII-V9E5U5XF42*. *CAS-99665-00-6*. INN;
MI.

Flopristin. $C_{28}H_{38}FN_3O_6$. 531.62. (3*R*,4*R*,5*E*,10*E*,12*E*,14*S*,16-
R,26a*R*)-16-Fluoro-14-hydroxy-4,12-dimethyl-3-(propan-
2-yl)-3,4,8,9,14,15,16,17,24,25,26,26a-dodecahydro-
1*H*,7*H*,22*H*-21,18-azenopyrrolo[2,1-*c*][1,8,4,19]dioxadiaz-
acyclotetracosine-1,7,22-trione. *CAS-318498-76-9*. INN.

Flopropione. $C_9H_{10}O_4$. 182.17. 2′,4′,6′-Trihydroxypropiophe-
none. *UNII-05V5NVB5Y1*. *CAS-2295-58-1*. INN; DCF;
JAN; MI.

Florantyrone. $C_{20}H_{14}O_3$. 302.32. γ-Oxo-8-fluoranthenebuty-
ric acid. *UNII-UZ5LMI200P*. *CAS-519-95-9*. INN; BAN;
MI.

Flordipine [*1983*] (flor′ di peen). $C_{26}H_{33}F_3N_2O_5$. 510.55. (1)
3,5-Pyridinedicarboxylic acid, 1,4-dihydro-2,6-dimethyl-1-
[2-(4-morpholinyl)ethyl]-4-[2-(trifluoromethyl)phenyl]-,
diethyl ester; (2) Diethyl 1,4-dihydro-2,6-dimethyl-1-(2-
morpholinoethyl)-4-(α,α,α-trifluoro-*o*-tolyl)3,5-pyridine-
dicarboxylate. *CAS-77590-96-6*. INN. *Antihypertensive.*
◇*RHC 2906*

Floredil. $C_{16}H_{25}NO_4$. 295.37. 4-[2-(3,5-Diethoxyphenoxy)
ethyl]morpholine. *UNII-LHX2B2R19F*. *CAS-53731-36-5*.
INN; DCF; MI.

Floretione — *See* Fluoresone.

Florfenicol [*1986*] (flor fen′ i kol). $C_{12}H_{14}Cl_2FNO_4S$. 358.21.
(1) Acetamide, 2,2-dichloro-*N*-[1-(fluoromethyl)-2-hy-
droxy-2-[4-(methylsulfonyl)phenyl]ethyl]-, [*R*-(*R**,*S**)]-;
(2) 2,2-Dichloro-*N*-[(α*S*,β*R*)-α-(fluoromethyl)-β-hy-
droxy-*p*-(methylsulfonyl)phenethyl]acetamide; (3) D-
threo-2,2-Dichloro-*N*-[α-(fluoromethyl)-β-hydroxy-*p*-
(methylsulfonyl)phenethyl]acetamide. *UNII-9J97307Y1H*.
CAS-76639-94-6. INN; BAN. *Antibacterial (veterinary).*
Nuflor [Veterinary] (Schering-Plough Animal Health)
◇*Sch 25298*

Florifenine. $C_{23}H_{22}F_3N_3O_2$. 429.43. 2-(1-Pyrrolidinyl)ethyl
N-[7-(trifluoromethyl)-4-quinolyl]anthranilate. *UNII-
S7UT8VQG94*. *CAS-83863-79-0*. INN.

Floropipamide (previously used name) — *See* Pipamperone.

Floropipeton — *See* Propyperone.

Flosatidil. $C_{26}H_{34}F_3N_3O_3S$. 525.63. Isobutyl [2-(dimethyla-mino)ethyl][[[*o*-(methylthio)phenyl][*m*-(trifluoromethyl)-benzyl]carbamoyl]methyl]carbamate. *UNII-19S89CMO38. CAS-113593-34-3.* INN.

Flosequinan [*1989*] (floe se′ kwin an). $C_{11}H_{10}FNO_2S$. 239.27. (1) 4(1*H*)-Quinolinone, 7-fluoro-1-methyl-3-(methylsulfi-nyl)-; (2) 7-Fluoro-1-methyl-3-(methylsulfinyl)-4(1*H*)-qui-nolone. *UNII-6NB119DLU7. CAS-76568-02-0.* INN; BAN. *Antihypertensive (vasodilator).* ◇BTS 49 465

Flosulide. $C_{16}H_{13}F_2NO_4S$. 353.34. *N*-[6-(2,4-Difluorophe-noxy)-1-oxo-5-indanyl]methanesulfonamide. *UNII-GVR41S4ZHJ. CAS-80937-31-1.* INN.

Flotrenizine. $C_{31}H_{38}F_2N_2O$. 492.64. (±)-4-[Bis(*p*-fluorophe-nyl)methyl]-α-(*p-tert*-butylphenyl)-1-piperazinebutanol. *UNII-A4JO90697G. CAS-82190-92-9.* INN.

Flovagatran. $C_{27}H_{36}BN_3O_7$. 525.40. (1*R*)-1-{*N*-[(Benzylox-y)carbonyl]-D-phenylalanyl-L-prolinamido}butylboronic acid. *CAS-871576-03-3.* INN.

Floverine. $C_{10}H_{14}O_4$. 198.22. 2-(3,5-Dimethoxyphenox-y)ethanol. *UNII-S77YM77P92. CAS-27318-86-1.* INN; DCF.

Floxacillin [*1972*] (flox″ a sil′ in). $C_{19}H_{17}ClFN_3O_5S$. 453.87. [Flucloxacillin is INN and BAN; Flucloxacillin Sodium is JAN.] (1) 4-Thia-1-azabicyclo[3.2.0]heptane-2-carboxylic acid, 6-[[[3-(2-chloro-6-fluorophenyl)-5-methyl-4-isoxa-zolyl]carbonyl]amino]-3,3-dimethyl-7-oxo-, [2*S*(2α,5α,6β)]; (2) 6-[3-(2-Chloro-6-fluorophenyl)-5-methyl-4-isoxazolecarboxamido]-3,3-dimethyl-7-oxo-4-thia-1-azabicyclo[3.2.0]heptane-2-carboxylic acid; (3) 3-(2-Chloro-6-fluorophenyl)-5-methyl-4-isoxazolylpenicil-lin. *CAS-5250-39-5. Antibacterial.* Floxapen (Beecham Research Laboratories, England) ◇BRL 2039

Floxacrine. $C_{20}H_{13}ClF_3NO_3$. 407.77. 7-Chloro-3,4-dihydro-10-hydroxy-3-(α,α,α-trifluoro-*p*-tolyl)-1,9(2*H*)acridan-dione. *UNII-V09GC6329G. CAS-53966-34-0.* INN.

Floxuridine [*1965*] (flox ure′ i deen). **USP**. $C_9H_{11}FN_2O_5$. 246.19. (1) Uridine, 2′-deoxy-5-fluoro-; (2) 2′-Deoxy-5-fluorouridine. *UNII-039LU4415M. CAS-50-91-9.* INN. *Antiviral; antineoplastic.* ◇FUDR; NSC-27640

Fluacizine. $C_{20}H_{21}F_3N_2OS$. 394.45. 10-[3-(Diethylamino)pro-pionyl]-2-(trifluoromethyl)phenothiazine. *UNII-E2M3325B1R. CAS-30223-48-4.* INN; MI.

---

† Brand name formerly used, and/or firm no longer concerned with this product.

Flualamide. C$_7$H$_{23}$F$_3$N$_2$O$_2$. 224.26. 2-(Allyloxy)-*N*-[2-(diethylamino)ethyl]-α,α,α-trifluoro-*p*-toluamide. *UNII-57F7CWY79K. CAS-5107-49-3.* INN; DCF.

Fluanisone. C$_{21}$H$_{25}$FN$_2$O$_2$. 356.43. 4′-Fluoro-4-[4-(*o*-methoxyphenyl)-1-piperazinyl]butyrophenone. *UNII-1D0W98U1I4. CAS-1480-19-9.* INN; BAN; DCF; MI. ◇*MD 2028; R 2028; R 2167*

Fluazacort [*1974*] (floo az′ a kort). C$_{25}$H$_{30}$FNO$_6$. 459.51. (1) 5′*H*-Pregna-1,4-dieno[17,16-*d*]oxazole-3,20-dione, 21-(acetyloxy)-9-fluoro-11-hydroxy-2′-methyl-, (5′β,11β)-; (2) 9-Fluoro-11β,21-dihydroxy-2′-methyl-5′βH-pregna-1,4-dieno[17,16-*d*]oxazole-3,20-dione 21-acetate. *CAS-19888-56-3.* INN. *Anti-inflammatory.* ◇*L-6400*

Fluazuron. C$_{20}$H$_{10}$Cl$_2$F$_5$N$_3$O$_3$. 506.21. 1-[4-Chloro-3-[[3-chloro-5-(trifluoromethyl)-2-pyridyl]oxy]phenyl]-3-(2,6-difluorobenzoyl)urea. *UNII-VB0PV6I7L6. CAS-86811-58-7.* INN.

Flubanilate Hydrochloride [*1965*] (floo ban′ i late hye″ droe klor′ ide). C$_{14}$H$_{19}$F$_3$N$_2$O$_2$·HCl. 340.77. [Flubanilate is INN.] (1) Carbamic acid, [2-(dimethylamino)ethyl][3-(trifluoromethyl)phenyl]-, ethyl ester, monohydrochloride; (2) Ethyl *N*-[2-(dimethylamino)ethyl]-*m*-(trifluoromethyl)carbanilate monohydrochloride. *UNII-GG0009389P; UNII-G510OWF4F4* [flubanilate]. *CAS-967-48-6; CAS-847-20-1* [flubanilate]. *Stimulant (central).*

Flubendazole [*1976*] (floo ben′ da zole). C$_{16}$H$_{12}$FN$_3$O$_3$. 313.28. (1) Carbamic acid, [5-(4-fluorobenzoyl)-1*H*-benzimidazol-2-yl]-, methyl ester; (2) Methyl 5-(*p*-fluorobenzoyl)-2-benzimidazolecarbamate. *UNII-R8M46911LR. CAS-31430-15-6.* INN; BAN. *Antiprotozoal.* ◇*R 17,889*

Flubenisolone — *See* Betamethasone.

Flubepride. C$_{20}$H$_{24}$FN$_3$O$_4$S. 421.49. *N*-[[1-(*p*-Fluorobenzyl)-2-pyrrolidinyl]methyl]-5-sulfamoyl-*o*-anisamide. *UNII-UU4X6T9FT5. CAS-56488-61-0.* INN.

Flubuperone — *See* Melperone.

Flucarbril. C$_{11}$H$_8$F$_3$NO. 227.18. 1-Methyl-2-oxo-6-(trifluoromethyl)quinoline. *CAS-2261-94-1.* INN.

Flucetorex. C$_{20}$H$_{21}$F$_3$N$_2$O$_3$. 394.39. α-[[α-Methyl-*m*-(trifluoromethyl)phenethyl]carbamoyl]-*p*-acetanisidide. *UNII-0JJT8MQ49S. CAS-40256-99-3.* INN; DCF. ◇*PM-3944*

Flucindole [*1977*] (floo sin′ dole). C$_{14}$H$_{16}$F$_2$N$_2$. 250.29. (1) 1*H*-Carbazol-3-amine, 6,8-difluoro-2,3,4,9-tetrahydro-*N,N*-dimethyl-; (2) 3-(Dimethylamino)-6,8-difluoro-1,2,3,4-tetrahydrocarbazole. *UNII-5CYU0D0S8M. CAS-40594-09-0.* INN. *Antipsychotic.* ◇*Win 35150*

Fluciprazine. C$_{21}$H$_{29}$FN$_2$O$_2$. 360.47. α-[[(1-Ethynylcyclohexyl)oxy]methyl]-4-(*p*-fluorophenyl)-1-piperazineethanol. *UNII-ZBD6Y9UT6T. CAS-54340-64-6.* INN; DCF.

Fluclorolone Acetonide (INN, BAN) — *See* Flucloronide.

Flucloronide [*1970*] (floo klor′ oh nide). $C_{24}H_{29}Cl_2FO_5$. 487.39. [Fluclorolone Acetonide is INN and BAN.] (1) Pregna-1,4-diene-3,20-dione, 9,11-dichloro-6-fluoro-21-hydroxy-16,17-[(1-methylethylidene)bis(oxy)]-, (6α,11β,16α)-; (2) 9,11β-Dichloro-6α-fluoro-16α,17,21-trihydroxypregna-1,4-diene-3,20-dione cyclic 16,17-acetal with acetone. *CAS-3693-39-8. Glucocorticoid.* ◇*RS-2252*

Flucloxacillin (INN, BAN) — *See* Floxacillin.

Flucloxacillin Sodium (JAN) — *See* Floxacillin.

Fluconazole [*1988*] (floo kon′ a zole). **USP**. $C_{13}H_{12}F_2N_6O$. 306.27. (1) 1*H*-1,2,4-Triazole-1-ethanol, 1-(2,4-difluorophenyl)-1-(1*H*-1,2,4-triazol-1-ylmethyl)-; (2) 2,4-Difluoro-1′,1′-bis(1*H*-1,2,4-triazol-1-ylmethyl)benzyl alcohol. *UNII-8VZV102JFY. CAS-86386-73-4.* INN; BAN; JAN. *Antifungal.* Diflucan (Pfizer) ◇*UK-49,858*

Flucrilate (INN) — *See* Flucrylate.

Flucrylate [*1969*] (floo′ kri late). $C_7H_6F_3NO_2$. 193.12. [Flucrilate is INN.] (1) 2-Propenoic acid, 2-cyano-, 2,2,2-trifluoro-1-methylethyl ester; (2) 2,2,2-Trifluoro-1-methylethyl 2-cyanoacrylate. *CAS-23023-91-8. Surgical aid (tissue adhesive).* ◇*BA 4197; MBR-4197*

Flucytosine [*1969*] (floo sye′ toe seen). **USP**. $C_4H_4FN_3O$. 129.09. (1) Cytosine, 5-fluoro-; (2) 5-Fluorocytosine. *UNII-D83282DT06. CAS-2022-85-7.* INN; BAN; JAN. *Antifungal.* Ancobon (Valeant) ◇*Ro 2-9915*

Fludalanine [*1977*] (floo dal′ a neen). $C_3H_5DFNO_2$. 125.07. (1) D-Alanine-2-*d*, 3-fluoro-; (2) 3-Fluoro-D-alanine-2-*d*. *CAS-35523-45-6.* INN. *Antibacterial.*

Fludarabine Phosphate [*1982*] (floo dayr′ a been fos′ fate). **USP**. $C_{10}H_{13}FN_5O_7P$. 365.21. [Fludarabine is INN.] (1) 9*H*-Purin-6-amine, 2-fluoro-9-(5-*O*-phosphono-β-D-arabinofuranosyl)-; (2) 9-β-D-Arabinofuranosyl-2-fluoroadenine 5′-(dihydrogen phosphate). *UNII-1X9VK9O1SC; UNII-P2K93U8740* [fludarabine]. *CAS-75607-67-9; CAS-21679-14-1* [fludarabine]. BAN. *Antineoplastic.* Fludara (Bayer) ◇*NSC-312887*

Fludazonium Chloride [*1976*] (floo″ da zoe′ nee um klor′ ide). $C_{26}H_{20}Cl_5FN_2O_2$. 588.71. (1) 1*H*-Imidazolium, 1-[2-(2,4-dichlorophenyl)-2-[(2,4-dichlorophenyl)methoxy]ethyl]-3-[2-(4-fluorophenyl)-2-oxoethyl]-, chloride; (2) 1-[2,4-Dichloro-β-[(2,4-dichlorobenzyl)oxy]phenethyl]-3-(*p*-fluorophenacyl)imidazolium chloride. *UNII-039G8U30HE. CAS-53597-28-7.* INN. *Anti-infective, topical.* ◇*R 23,633*

Fludeoxyglucose F 18 [*1989*] (floo″ de ox″ i gloo′ kose). **USP** [Injection]. $C_6H_{11}{}^{18}FO_5$. [Fludeoxyglucose (^{18}F) is INN.] (1) α-D-Glucopyranose, 2-deoxy-2-(fluoro-^{18}F)-; (2) 2-Deoxy-2-fluoro-^{18}F-α-D-glucopyranose. *CAS-105851-17-0. Diagnostic aid; radioactive agent.* ◇^{18}FDG

Fludiazepam. $C_{16}H_{12}ClFN_2O$. 302.73. 7-Chloro-5-(*o*-Fluorophenyl)-1,3-dihydro-1-methyl-2*H*-1,4-benzodiazepin-2-one. *UNII-7F64A2K16Z. CAS-3900-31-0.* INN; JAN; MI.

Fludorex [*1967*] (floo′ doe rex). $C_{11}H_{14}F_3NO$. 233.23. (1) Benzeneethanamine, β-methoxy-*N*-methyl-3-(trifluoromethyl)-; (2) β-Methoxy-*N*-methyl-*m*-(trifluoromethyl)phenethylamine. *CAS-15221-81-5.* INN. *Anorexic; antiemetic.* ◇*Win 11,464*

---

† Brand name formerly used, and/or firm no longer concerned with this product.

Fludoxopone. $C_{21}H_{21}FN_2O_3$. 368.40. 4-(*p*-Fluorophenyl)-5-[2-(4-phenyl-1-piperazinyl)ethyl]-1,3-dioxol-2-one. *UNII-2KN23X015H. CAS-71923-29-0.* INN.

Fludrocortisone Acetate (floo″ droe kor′ ti sone as′ e tate). **USP.** $C_{23}H_{31}FO_6$. 422.49. [Fludrocortisone is INN and BAN.] (1) Pregn-4-ene-3,20-dione, 21-(acetyloxy)-9-fluoro-11,17-dihydroxy-, (11β)-; (2) 9-Fluoro-11β,17,21-trihydroxypregn-4-ene-3,20-dione 21-acetate. *UNII-V47IF0PVH4; UNII-U0476M545B* [fludrocortisone]. *CAS-514-36-3; CAS-127-31-1* [fludrocortisone]. JAN. *Adrenocortical steroid (salt-regulating).*

Fludroxicortide — *See* Flurandrenolide.

Fludroxycortide (INN, BAN, JAN, DCF) — *See* Flurandrenolide.

Flufenamic Acid [*1962*] (floo″ fen am′ ik as′ id). $C_{14}H_{10}F_3NO_2$. 281.23. (1) Benzoic acid, 2-[[3-(trifluoromethyl)phenyl]amino]-; (2) *N*-(α,α,α-Trifluoro-*m*-tolyl)anthranilic acid. *CAS-530-78-9.* INN; BAN; JAN. *Anti-inflammatory.* Arlef (Parke-Davis†) ◇*CI 440; CN-27,554; INF-1837; NSC-82699*

Flufenisal [*1969*] (floo fen′ i sal). $C_{15}H_{11}FO_4$. 274.24. (1) [1,1′-Biphenyl]-3-carboxylic acid, 4-(acetyloxy)-4′-fluoro-; (2) 4′-Fluoro-4-hydroxy-3-biphenylcarboxylic acid acetate. *CAS-22494-27-5.* INN. *Analgesic.*

Flufosal. $C_8H_6F_3O_6P$. 286.10. α,α,α-Trifluoro-2,4-cresotic acid dihydrogen phosphate. *UNII-GK3KFF4TIW. CAS-65708-37-4.* INN.

Flufylline. $C_{21}H_{24}FN_5O_3$. 413.45. 7-[2-[4-(*p*-Fluorobenzoyl)piperidino]ethyl]theophylline. *UNII-O8G173034U. CAS-82190-91-8.* INN.

Flugestone (INN and BAN) Acetate — *See* Flurogestone Acetate.

Fluindarol. $C_{16}H_9F_3O_2$. 290.24. 2-(α,α,α-Trifluoro-*p*-tolyl)indan-1,3-dione. *UNII-22Z9Q44OIG. CAS-6723-40-6.* INN.

Fluindione. $C_{15}H_9FO_2$. 240.23. 2-(*p*-Fluorophenyl)-1,3-indandione. *UNII-EQ35YMS20Q. CAS-957-56-2.* INN; MI.

Flumazenil [*1987*] (floo maz′ e nil). **USP.** $C_{15}H_{14}FN_3O_3$. 303.29. (1) 4*H*-Imidazo[1,5-*a*][1,4]benzodiazepine-3-carboxylic acid, 8-fluoro-5,6-dihydro-5-methyl-6-oxo-, ethyl ester; (2) Ethyl 8-fluoro-5,6-dihydro-5-methyl-6-oxo-4*H*-imidazo[1,5-*a*][1,4]benzodiazepine-3-carboxylate. *UNII-40P7XK9392. CAS-78755-81-4.* INN; BAN. *Antagonist (to benzodiazepine).* Romazicon (Roche) ◇*Ro 15-1788/000*

Flumazenil C 11 (floo maz′ e nil). **USP** [injection]. (1) 4*H*-Imidazo[1,5-*a*][1,4]benzodiazepine-3-carboxylic acid, 8-fluoro-5,6-dihydro-5-[^{11}C]methyl-6-oxo-, ethyl ester; (2) Ethyl 8-fluoro-5,6-dihydro-5-[^{11}C]methyl-6-oxo-4*H*-imidazo[1,5-*a*][1,4]benzodiazepine-3-carboxylate.

Flumazepil — *See* Flumazenil.

Flumecinol. $C_{16}H_{15}F_3O$. 280.28. α-Ethyl-3-(trifluoromethyl)-benzhydrol. *CAS-56430-99-0*. INN; MI.

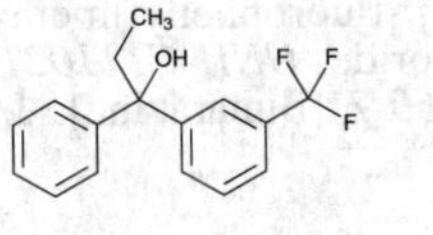

Flumedroxone. $C_{22}H_{29}F_3O_3$. 398.46. 17-Hydroxy-6α-(trifluoromethyl)pregn-4-ene-3,20-dione. *UNII-K80185F39X*. *CAS-15687-21-5*. INN; BAN; MI. ✧*WG 537 [as acetate]*

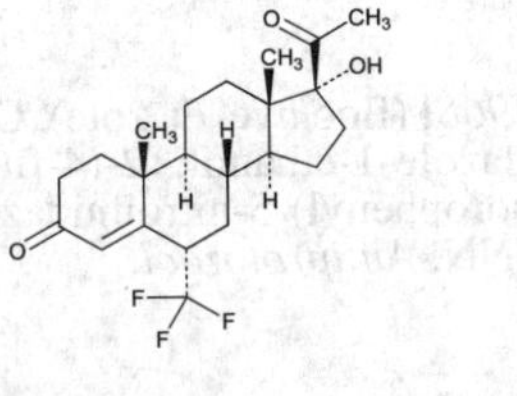

Flumequine [*1975*] (floo' me kwin). $C_{14}H_{12}FNO_3$. 261.25. (1) 1*H*,5*H*-Benzo[*ij*]quinolizine-2-carboxylic acid, 9-fluoro-6,7-dihydro-5-methyl-1-oxo-; (2) 9-Fluoro-6,7-dihydro-5-methyl-1-oxo-1*H*,5*H*-benzo[*ij*]quinolizine-2-carboxylic acid. *UNII-UVG8VSP2SJ*. *CAS-42835-25-6*. INN; BAN. *Antibacterial*.

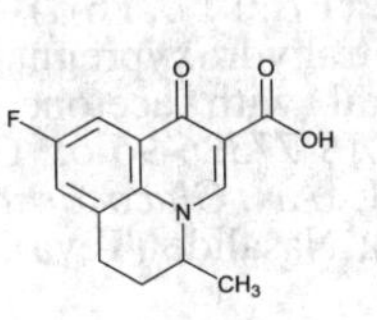

Flumeridone [*1981*] (floo mer' i done). $C_{22}H_{23}ClFN_5O_2$. 443.90. (1) 2*H*-Benzimidazol-2-one, 1-[3-[4-(5-chloro-2,3-dihydro-2-oxo-1*H*-benzimidazol-1-yl)-1-piperidinyl]propyl]-5-fluoro-1,3-dihydro-; (2) 5-Chloro-1-[1-[3-(5-fluoro-2-oxo-1-benzimidazolinyl)propyl]-4-piperidyl]-2-benzimidazolinone. *UNII-7ZZN46QU1N*. *CAS-75444-64-3*. INN; BAN. *Anti-emetic*. ✧*R-45,486*

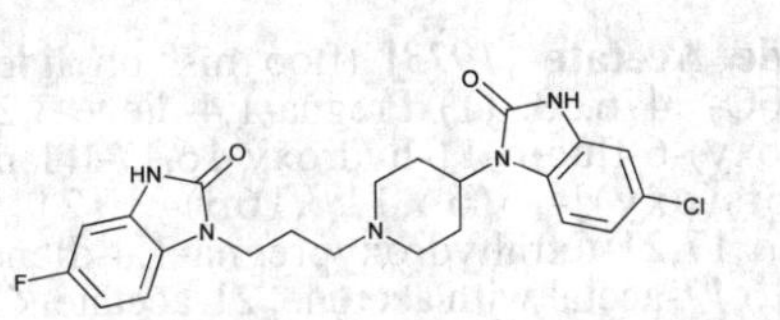

Flumetasone (INN, BAN, DCF) — *See* Flumethasone.

Flumetasone Pivalate (BAN, JAN) — *See* Flumethasone Pivalate.

Flumethasone [*1963*] (floo meth' a sone). $C_{22}H_{28}F_2O_5$. 410.45. [Flumetasone is INN and BAN.] (1) Pregna-1,4-diene-3,20-dione, 6,9-difluoro-11,17,21-trihydroxy-16-methyl-, (6α,11β,16α)-; (2) 6α,9-Difluoro-11β,17,21-trihydroxy-16α-methylpregna-1,4-diene-3,20-dione. *UNII-LR3CD8SX89*. *CAS-2135-17-3*. *Glucocorticoid*. Flucort [Veterinary] (Syntex) ✧*U-10,974; NSC-54702*

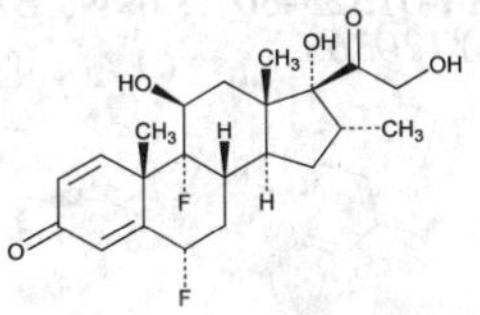

Flumethasone Pivalate [*1963*] (floo meth' a sone piv' a late). **USP**. $C_{27}H_{36}F_2O_6$. 494.57. [Flumetasone Pivalate is BAN and JAN.] (1) Pregna-1,4-diene-3,20-dione, 21-(2,2-dimethyl-1-oxopropoxy)-6,9-difluoro-11,17-dihydroxy-16-methyl-, (6α,11β,16α)-; (2) 6α,9-Difluoro-11β,17,21-trihydroxy-16α-methylpregna-1,4-diene-3,20-dione 21-pivalate. *UNII-0DV09X6F21; UNII-LR3CD8SX89* [flumethasone]. *CAS-2002-29-1; CAS-2135-17-3* [flumethasone]. *Glucocorticoid*. Locorten (Novartis) ✧*NSC-107680*

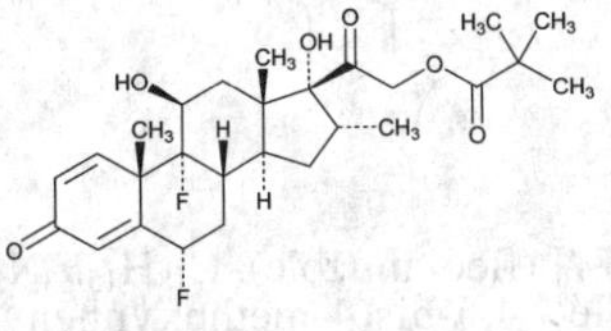

Flumethiazide. $C_8H_6F_3N_3O_4S_2$. 329.28. 6-(Trifluoromethyl)-2*H*-1,2,4-benzothiadiazine-7-sulfonamide 1,1-dioxide. *UNII-3PA0CDS0M5*. *CAS-148-56-1*. INN; BAN; MI. Ademol (Bristol-Myers Squibb†)

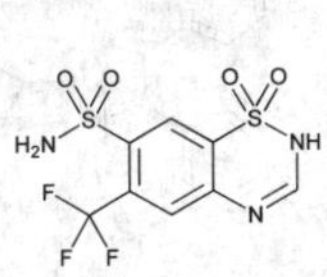

Flumethrin. $C_{28}H_{22}Cl_2FNO_3$. 510.38. α-Cyano-4-fluoro-3-phenoxybenzyl-3-(β,4-dichlorosytryl)-2,2-dimethylcyclopropanecarboxylate. BAN; MI. ✧*BAY V1 6045*

Flumetramide [*1966*] (floo met' ra mide). $C_{11}H_{10}F_3NO_2$. 245.20. (1) 3-Morpholinone, 6-[4-(trifluoromethyl)phenyl]-; (2) 6-(α,α,α-Trifluoro-*p*-tolyl)-3-morpholinone. *CAS-7125-73-7*. INN. *Relaxant (skeletal muscle)*. Duraflex (Ortho-McNeil†) ✧*McN-1546*

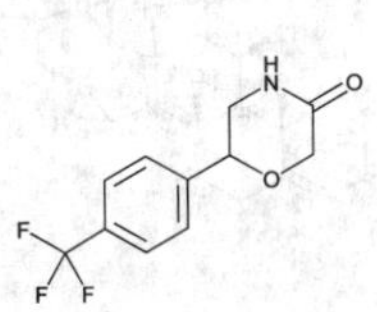

Flumexadol. $C_{11}H_{12}F_3NO$. 231.21. 2-(α,α,α-Trifluoro-*m*-tolyl)morpholine. *UNII-V9783UEL0F*. *CAS-30914-89-7*. INN.

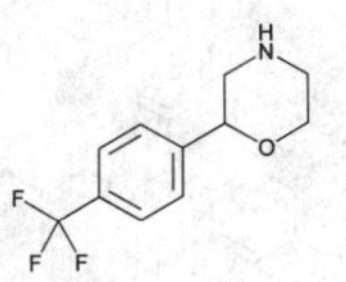

† Brand name formerly used, and/or firm no longer concerned with this product.

Flumezapine [*1981*] (floo mez′ a peen). $C_{17}H_{19}FN_4S$. 330.42. (1) 10*H*-Thieno[2,3-*b*][1,5]benzodiazepine, 7-fluoro-2-methyl-4-(4-methyl-1-piperazinyl)-; (2) 7-Fluoro-2-methyl-4-(4-methyl-1-piperazinyl)-10*H*-thieno[2,3-*b*][1,5]benzodiazepine. *CAS-61325-80-2*. INN; BAN. *Antipsychotic; neuroleptic.* ◇*LY120363*

Fluminorex [*1963*] (floo min′ oh rex). $C_{10}H_9F_3N_2O$. 230.19. (1) 2-Oxazolamine, 4,5-dihydro-5-[4-(trifluoromethyl)phenyl]-; (2) 2-Amino-5-(α,α,α-trifluoro-*p*-tolyl)-2-oxazoline. *UNII-LUO2Z7954T*. *CAS-720-76-3*. INN. *Anorexic.* ◇*McN-1231*

Flumizole [*1974*] (floo′ mi zole). $C_{18}H_{15}F_3N_2O_2$. 348.32. (1) 1*H*-Imidazole, 4,5-bis(4-methoxyphenyl)-2-(trifluoromethyl)-; (2) 4,5-Bis(*p*-methoxyphenyl)-2-(trifluoromethyl)imidazole. *CAS-36740-73-5*. INN. *Anti-inflammatory.* ◇*CP-22,665*

Flumoxonide [*1977*] (floo mox′ oh nide). $C_{26}H_{34}F_2O_7$. 496.54. (1) Pregna-1,4-diene-3,20-dione, 6,9-difluoro-11-hydroxy-21,21-dimethoxy-16,17-[(1-methylethylidene)bis(oxy)]-, (6α,11β,16α)-; (2) 6α,9-Difluoro-11β,16α,17-trihydroxy-3,20-dioxopregna-1,4-dien-21-al 21-(dimethyl acetal) cyclic 16,17-acetal with acetone. *CAS-60135-22-0*. INN. *Adrenocortical steroid.* ◇*RS-40584*

Flunamine. $C_{15}H_{15}F_2NO$. 263.28. 2-[Bis(*p*-fluorophenyl)methoxy]ethylamine. *UNII-IZ1GXE233H*. *CAS-50366-32-0*. INN.

Flunarizine Hydrochloride [*1970*] (floo nar′ i zeen hye″ droe klor′ ide). $C_{26}H_{26}F_2N_2$.2HCl. 477.42. [Flunarizine is INN and BAN.] (1) Piperazine, 1-[bis(4-fluorophenyl)methyl]-4-(3-phenyl-2-propenyl)-, dihydrochloride, (*E*)-; (2) (*E*)-1-[Bis-(*p*-fluorophenyl)methyl]-4-cinnamylpiperazine dihydrochloride. *UNII-C11102TO53*. *CAS-30484-77-6*; *CAS-52468-60-7* [flunarazine]. JAN. *Vasodilator.* ◇*R 14,950*

Flunidazole [*1968*] (floo nye′ da zole). $C_{11}H_{10}FN_3O_3$. 251.21. (1) 1*H*-Imidazole-1-ethanol, 2-(4-fluorophenyl)-5-nitro-; (2) 2-(*p*-Fluorophenyl)-5-nitroimidazole-1-ethanol. *CAS-4548-15-6*. INN. *Antiprotozoal.*

Flunisolide [*1974*] (floo nis′ oh lide). USP. $C_{24}H_{31}FO_6$.½-H_2O. 443.51. (1) Pregna-1,4-diene-3,20-dione, 6-fluoro-11,21-dihydroxy-16,17-[(1-methylethylidene)bis(oxy)]-, hemihydrate, (6α,11β,16α)-; (2) 6α-Fluoro-11β,16α,17,21-tetrahydroxypregna-1,4-diene-3,20-dione cyclic 16,17-acetal with acetone, hemihydrate. *UNII-QK4DYS664X*. *CAS-77326-96-6*; *CAS-3385-03-3* [anhydrous]. INN; BAN; JAN. *Glucocorticoid.* Aerobid (Roche); Aerospan (Forest); Nasalide (Teva); Nasarel (Teva) ◇*RS-3999*

Flunisolide Acetate [*1973*] (floo nis′ oh lide as′ e tate). $C_{26}H_{33}FO_7$. 476.53. (1) Pregna-1,4-diene-3,20-dione, 21-(acetyloxy)-6-fluoro-11-hydroxy-16,17-[(1-methylethylidene)bis(oxy)]-, (6α,11β,16α)-; (2) 6α-Fluoro-11β,16α,17,21-tetrahydroxypregna-1,4-diene-3,20-dione cyclic 16,17-acetal with acetone, 21-acetate. *CAS-4533-89-5*. *Anti-inflammatory.* ◇*RS-1320*

Flunitrazepam [*1976*] (floo″ nye traz′ e pam). $C_{16}H_{12}FN_3O_3$. 313.28. (1) 2*H*-1,4-Benzodiazepin-2-one, 5-(2-fluorophenyl)-1,3-dihydro-1-methyl-7-nitro-; (2) 5-(*o*-Fluorophenyl)-1,3-dihydro-1-methyl-7-nitro-2*H*-1,4-benzodiazepin-2-one. *CAS-1622-62-4*. INN; BAN; JAN. *Sedative-hypnotic.* Rohypnol (Roche, Puerto Rico†) ◇*Ro 5-4200*

Flunixin [*1973*] (floo nix′ in). $C_{14}H_{11}F_3N_2O_2$. 296.24. (1) 3-Pyridinecarboxylic acid, 2-[[2-methyl-3-(trifluoromethyl)phenyl]amino]-; (2) 2-($\alpha^3,\alpha^3,\alpha^3$-Trifluoro-2,3-xylidino)nicotinic acid. *UNII-356IB1O400*. *CAS-38677-85-9*. INN; BAN. *Anti-inflammatory; analgesic.* ◇*Sch 14714*

Flunixin Meglumine [*1974*] (floo nix′ in me′ gloo meen). **USP**. $C_{14}H_{11}F_3N_2O_2 \cdot C_7H_{17}NO_5$. 491.46. (1) 3-Pyridinecarboxylic acid, 2-[[2-methyl-3-(trifluoromethyl)phenyl]amino]-, compd. with 1-deoxy-1-(methylamino)-D-glucitol (1:1); (2) 2-($\alpha^3,\alpha^3,\alpha^3$-Trifluoro-2,3-xylidino)nicotinic acid compound with 1-deoxy-1-(methylamino)-D-glucitol (1:1). *UNII-8Y3JK0JW3U; UNII-356IB1O400* [flunixin]; *UNII-6HG8UB2MUY* [meglumine]. *CAS-42461-84-7; CAS-38677-85-9* [flunixin]; *CAS-6284-40-8* [meglumine]. *Anti-inflammatory; analgesic.* Banamine [Veterinary] (Schering-Plough Animal Health) ◇*Sch 14714 meglumine*

Flunoprost. $C_{22}H_{29}FO_5$. 392.46. (*Z*)-7-[(1*R*,2*R*,3*R*,5*R*)-5-Fluoro-3-hydroxy-2-[(*E*)-(3*R*)-3-hydroxy-4-phenoxy-1-butenyl]cyclopentyl]-5-heptenoic acid. *UNII-8MF6L4447J*. *CAS-86348-98-3*. INN.

Flunoxaprofen. $C_{16}H_{12}FNO_3$. 285.27. (+)-2-(*p*-Fluorophenyl)-α-methyl-5-benzoxazoleacetic acid. *UNII-UKU5U19W9M*. *CAS-66934-18-7*. INN; MI.

Fluocinolide (previously used name) — *See* Fluocinonide.

Fluocinolone Acetonide [*1962*] (floo″ oh sin′ oh lone a seet′ oh nide). **USP**. $C_{24}H_{30}F_2O_6$. 452.49. [Fluocinolone is BAN.] (1) Pregna-1,4-diene-3,20-dione, 6,9-difluoro-11,21-dihydroxy-16,17-[(1-methylethylidene)bis(oxy)]-, (6α,11β,16α)-; (2) 6α,9-Difluoro-11β,16α,17,21-tetrahydroxypregna-1,4-diene-3,20-dione, cyclic 16,17-acetal with acetone. *UNII-0CD5FD6S2M*. *CAS-67-73-2*. INN;

JAN. *Glucocorticoid.* Derma-Smoothe/FS (Hill Dermac); Fluocet (Alpharma); Fluonid (Allergan); Fluotrex (Savage); FS Shampoo (Galderma); Retisert (Bausch & Lomb); Synalar (Medicis) ◇*NSC-92339*

Fluocinonide [*1970*] (floo″ oh sin′ oh nide). **USP**. $C_{26}H_{32}F_2O_7$. 494.52. (1) Pregna-1,4-diene-3,20-dione, 21-(acetyloxy)-6,9-difluoro-11-hydroxy-16,17-[(1-methylethylidene)bis(oxy)]-, (6α,11β,16α)-; (2) 6α,9-Difluoro-11β,16α,17,21-tetrahydroxypregna-1,4-diene-3,20-dione, cyclic 16,17-acetal with acetone, 21-acetate. *UNII-2W4A77YPAN*. *CAS-356-12-7*. INN; BAN; JAN. *Glucocorticoid.* Lidex (Medicis); Vanos (Medicis) *[Name previously used: Fluocinolide.]* ◇*NSC-101791*

Fluocortin Butyl [*1974*] (floo″ oh kor′ tin bue′ til). $C_{26}H_{35}FO_5$. 446.55. [Fluocortin is INN.] (1) Pregna-1,4-dien-21-oic acid, 6-fluoro-11-hydroxy-16-methyl-3,20-dioxo-, butyl ester (6α,11β,16α)-; (2) Butyl 6α-fluoro-11β-hydroxy-16α-methyl-3,20-dioxopregna-1,4-dien-21-oate. *CAS-41767-29-7; CAS-33124-50-4* [fluocortin]. BAN. *Anti-inflammatory.* ◇*SH K 203*

Fluocortolone [*1965*] (floo″ oh kor′ toe lone). $C_{22}H_{29}FO_4$. 376.46. (1) Pregna-1,4-diene-3,20-dione, 6-fluoro-11,21-dihydroxy-16-methyl-, (6α,11β,16α)-; (2) 6α-Fluoro-11β,21-dihydroxy-16α-methylpregna-1,4-diene-3,20-dione. *UNII-65VXC1MH0J*. *CAS-152-97-6*. INN; BAN. *Glucocorticoid.* ◇*SH 742*

Fluocortolone Caproate [*1966*] (floo″ oh kor′ toe lone kap′ roe ate). $C_{28}H_{39}FO_5$. 474.60. (1) Pregna-1,4-diene-3,20-dione, 6-fluoro-11,21-dihydroxy-16-methyl-21-[(1-oxohexyl)oxy]-, (6α,11β,16α)-; (2) 6α-Fluoro-11β,21-dihydroxy-16α-methylpregna-1,4-diene-3,20-dione 21-hexanoate. *CAS-303-40-2*. *Glucocorticoid.* ◇*SH 770*

Fluopromazine (previously used name) — *See* Triflupromazine.

Fluoracizine — *See* Fluacizine.

Fluorescein (floor′ a seen). **USP.** $C_{20}H_{12}O_5$. 332.31. (1) Spiro[isobenzofuran-1(3*H*),9′-[9*H*]xanthen]-3-one,3′6′-dihydroxy-; (2) Fluorescein. *UNII-TPY09G7XIR. CAS-2321-07-5.* BAN; JAN. *Diagnostic aid (corneal trauma indicator).* Fluorescite (Alcon)

Fluorescein Lisicol. $C_{51}H_{63}N_3O_{11}S$. 926.12. N^6-({3′,6′-Dihydroxy-3-oxospiro[isobenzofuran-1(3*H*),9′-xanthen]-5-yl}thiocarbamoyl)-N^2-(3α,7α,12α-trihydroxy-5β-cholan-24-oyl)-L-lysine. *CAS-140616-46-2.* INN.

Fluorescein Sodium (flure′ a seen soe′ dee um). **USP.** $C_{20}H_{10}Na_2O_5$. 376.27. (1) Spiro[isobenzofuran-1(3*H*),9′-[9*H*]xanthene]-3-one, 3′6′-dihydroxy, disodium salt; (2) Fluorescein disodium salt. *UNII-93X55PE38X; UNII-TPY09G7XIR* [fluorescein]. *CAS-518-47-8; CAS-2321-07-5* [fluorescein]. BAN; JAN. *Diagnostic aid (corneal trauma indicator).* Fluorescite (Alcon); Funduscein (Novartis) *[Name previously used: Fluorescein, Soluble.]*

Fluorescein, Soluble (previously used name) — *See* Fluorescein Sodium.

Fluoresone. $C_8H_9FO_2S$. 188.22. Ethyl *p*-fluorophenyl sulfone. *UNII-343BH0S0XR. CAS-2924-67-6.* INN; DCF; MI.

Fluorhydrocortisone Acetate — *See* Fludrocortisone Acetate.

Fluorine F 18 Fluorodeoxyglucose — *See* Fludeoxyglucose F 18.

Fluormethylprednisolone — *See* Dexamethasone.

Fluorodeoxyglucose F 18 — *See* Fludeoxyglucose F 18.

Fluorodopa F 18 [*1990*] (floor″ oh doe′ pa). **USP** [Injection]. $C_9H_{10}^{18}FNO_4$. (1) L-Tyrosine, 2-(fluoro-^{18}F)-5-hydroxy-; (2) 3-(2-Fluoro-^{18}F-4,5-dihydroxyphenyl)-L-alanine. *CAS-92812-82-3.* INN. *Diagnostic aid (brain imaging); radioactive agent. [Note—This radiopharmaceutical, labeled with a cyclotron-generated radionuclide, is prepared in individual nuclear medical centers.]*

Fluorometholone (floor″ oh meth′ oh lone). **USP.** $C_{22}H_{29}FO_4$. 376.46. (1) Pregna-1,4-diene-3,20-dione, 9-fluoro-11,17-dihydroxy-6-methyl-, (6α,11β)-; (2) 9-Fluoro-11β,17-dihydroxy-6α-methylpregna-1,4-diene-

3,20-dione. *UNII-SV0CSG527L. CAS-426-13-1.* INN; BAN; JAN. *Glucocorticoid.* Fml (Allergan); Oxylone (Pfizer)

Fluorometholone Acetate [*1984*] (floor″ oh meth′ oh lone as′ e tate). **USP.** $C_{24}H_{31}FO_5$. 418.50. (1) Pregna-1,4-diene-3,20-dione, 17-(acetyloxy)-9-fluoro-11-hydroxy-6-methyl-, (6α,11β)-; (2) 9-Fluoro-11β,17-dihydroxy-6α-methylpregna-1,4-diene-3,20-dione 17-acetate. *UNII-9I50C3I3OK; UNII-SV0CSG527L* [fluorometholone]. *CAS-3801-06-7; CAS-426-13-1* [fluorometholone]. *Antiinflammatory.* Flarex (Alcon) ◇*U-17,323*

Fluorosalan [*1966*] (floor oh′ sa lan). $C_{14}H_8Br_2F_3NO_2$. 439.02. [Flusalan is INN.] (1) Benzamide, 3,5-dibromo-2-hydroxy-*N*-[3-(trifluoromethyl)phenyl]-; (2) 3,5-Dibromo-α,α,α-trifluoro-*m*-salicylotoluidide; (3) 3,5-Dibromo-3′-(trifluoromethyl)salicylanilide. *CAS-4776-06-1. Disinfectant.*

Fluorouracil [*1962*] (floor″ oh ure′ a sil). **USP.** $C_4H_3FN_2O_2$. 130.08. (1) 2,4(1*H*,3*H*)-Pyrimidinedione, 5-fluoro-; (2) 5-Fluorouracil. *UNII-U3P01618RT. CAS-51-21-8.* INN; BAN; JAN. *Antineoplastic.* Adrucil (Pfizer); Carac (Sanofi Aventis); Efudex (Valeant); Fluoroplex (Allergan) ◇*Ro 2-9757; 5-FU; NSC-19893*

Fluoruridine Deoxyribose — *See* Floxuridine.

Fluostigmine — *See* Isoflurophate.

Fluotracen Hydrochloride [*1977*] (floo oh tray′ sen hye″ droe klor′ ide). $C_{21}H_{24}F_3N$.HCl. 383.88. [Fluotracen is INN.] (1) 9-Anthracenepropanamine, 9,10-dihydro-*N*,*N*,10-trimethyl-2-(trifluoromethyl)-, *cis*-(±)-, hydrochloride; (2) (±)-*cis*-9,10-Dihydro-*N*,*N*,10-trimethyl-2-(trifluoromethyl)-9-anthracenepropylamine hydrochloride. *CAS-57363-14-1; CAS-35764-73-9* [fluotracen]. *Antipsychotic; antidepressant.* ◇*SK&F 28175*

Fluoxetine [*1975*] (floo ox′ e teen). $C_{17}H_{18}F_3NO$. 309.33. (1) Benzenepropanamine, *N*-methyl-γ-[4-(trifluoromethyl)-phenoxy]-, (±)-; (2) (±)-*N*-Methyl-3-phenyl-3-[(α,α,α-trifluoro-*p*-tolyl)oxy]propylamine. *UNII-01K63SUP8D*. *CAS-54910-89-3*. INN; BAN. *Antidepressant.*

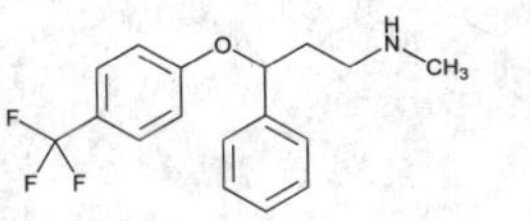

Fluoxetine Hydrochloride [*1988*] (floo ox′ e teen hye″ droe klor′ ide). USP. $C_{17}H_{18}F_3NO.HCl$. 345.79. (1) Benzene-propanamine, *N*-methyl-γ-[4-(trifluoromethyl)phenoxy]-, hydrochloride, (±)-; (2) (±)-*N*-Methyl-3-phenyl-3-[(α,α,α-trifluoro-*p*-tolyl)oxy]propylamine, hydrochloride. *UNII-I9W7N6B1KJ*. *CAS-59333-67-4*. *Antidepressant.* Prozac (Lilly); Sarafem (Warner Chilcott) ◇*LY110140*

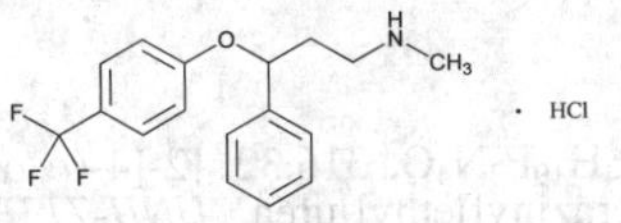

Fluoximesterone — *See* Fluoxymesterone.

Fluoxiprednisolone — *See* Triamcinolone.

Fluoxymesterone (floo ox″ i mes′ ter one). USP. $C_{20}H_{29}FO_3$. 336.44. (1) Androst-4-en-3-one, 9-fluoro-11,17-dihydroxy-17-methyl-, (11β,17β)-; (2) 9-Fluoro-11β,17β-dihydroxy-17-methylandrost-4-en-3-one. *UNII-9JU12S4YFY*. *CAS-76-43-7*. INN; BAN; JAN. *Androgen.* Android (Valeant); Halotestin (Pfizer); Ora-testryl (Bristol-Myers Squibb) ◇*NSC-12165*

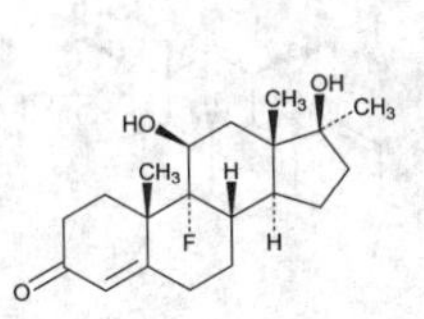

Fluparoxan Hydrochloride [*1989*] (floo″ pa rox′ an hye″ droe klor′ ide). $C_{10}H_{10}FNO_2.HCl.\frac{1}{2}H_2O$. 240.66. [Fluparoxan is INN and BAN.] (1) 1*H*-[1,4]Benzodioxino[2,3-*c*]pyrrole, 5-fluoro-2,3,3a,9a-tetrahydro-, hydrochloride, hemihydrate, (3a*S-trans*)-; (2) (3a*S*,9a*S*)-5-Fluoro-2,3,3a,9a-tetrahydro-1*H*-[1,4]benzodioxino[2,3-*c*]pyrrole hydrochloride, hemihydrate. *CAS-111793-41-0; CAS-105182-45-4* [fluparoxan]. *Antidepressant.* ◇*GR50360A*

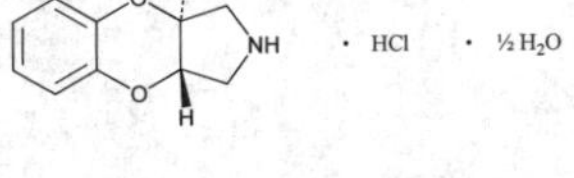

---

† Brand name formerly used, and/or firm no longer concerned with this product.

Flupentixol. $C_{23}H_{25}F_3N_2OS$. 434.52. 2-Trifluoromethyl-9-[3-[4-(2-hydroxyethyl)piperazin-1-yl]propylidene]thiox-anthene. *UNII-FA0UYH6QUO*. *CAS-2709-56-0*. INN; BAN; DCF; MI. [*Name previously used: Flupenthixol.*] ◇*N-7009; LC 44*

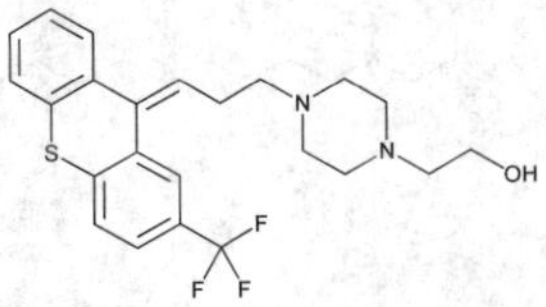

Fluperamide [*1975*] (floo per′ a mide). $C_{30}H_{32}ClF_3N_2O_2$. 545.04. (1) 1-Piperidinebutanamide, 4-[4-chloro-3-(trifluoromethyl)phenyl]-4-hydroxy-*N,N*-dimethyl-α,α-diphenyl-; (2) 4-(4-Chloro-α,α,α-trifluoro-*m*-tolyl)-4-hydroxy-*N,N*-dimethyl-α,α-diphenyl-1-piperidinebutyramide. *UNII-6H13T09362*. *CAS-53179-10-5*. INN. *Antiperistaltic.* ◇*R 18,910*

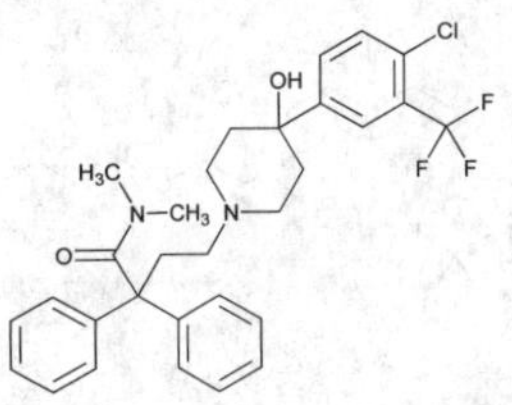

Fluperlapine. $C_{19}H_{20}FN_3$. 309.38. 3-Fluoro-6-(4-methyl-1-piperazinyl)morphanthridine. *UNII-EWG253M961*. *CAS-67121-76-0*. INN.

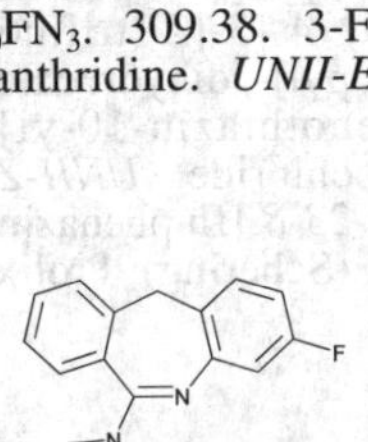

Fluperolone Acetate [*1962*] (floo per′ oh lone as′ e tate). $C_{24}H_{31}FO_6$. 434.50. [Fluperolone is INN and BAN.] (1) Androsta-1,4-dien-3-one, 17-[2-(acetyloxy)-1-oxopropyl]-9-fluoro-11,17-dihydroxy-, [11β,17α,17(*S*)]-; (2) 9-Fluoro-11β,17α-dihydroxy-17-(*S*)-lactoylandrosta-1,4-dien-3-one 17β-acetate. *CAS-2119-75-7; CAS-3841-11-0* [fluperolone]. *Glucocorticoid.* Methral (Pfizer) ◇*P-1742*

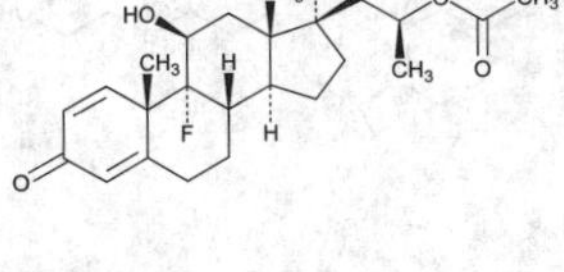

Fluphenazine Decanoate (floo fen′ a zeen dek″ a noe′ ate). USP. (1) Decanoic acid, 2-[4-[3-[2-(trifluoromethyl)-10*H*-Decanoate phenothiazin-10-yl]propyl]-1-piperazinyl]ethyl ester; (2) 2-[4-[3-[2-(Trifluoromethyl)phenothiazin-10-yl]-

propyl]-1-piperazinyl]ethyl decanoate. *UNII-FMU62K1L3C. CAS-5002-47-1.* BAN; JAN. *Antipsychotic.*

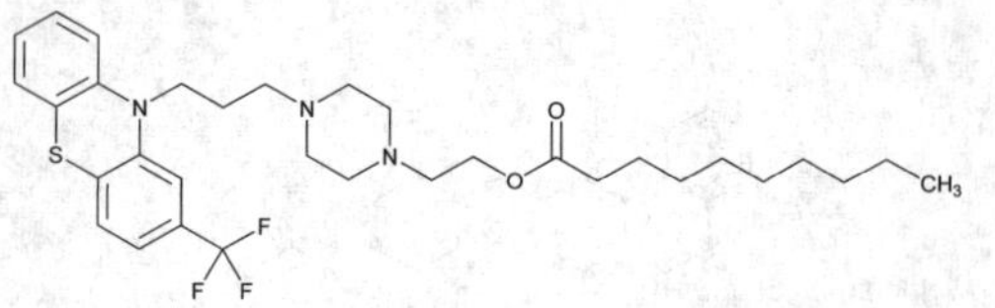

Fluphenazine Enanthate (floo fen′ a zeen e nan′ thate). **USP.** $C_{29}H_{38}F_3N_3O_2S$. 549.69. [Fluphenazine is INN; Fluphenazine Enantate is BAN; Fluphenazine Maleate is JAN.] (1) Heptanoic acid, 2-[4-[3-[2-(trifluoromethyl)-10*H*-phenothiazin-10-yl]propyl]-1-piperazinyl]ethyl ester; (2) 2-[4-[3-[2-(Trifluoromethyl)phenothiazin-10-yl]propyl]-1-piperazinyl]ethyl heptanoate. *UNII-QSB34YF0W9. CAS-2746-81-8; CAS-69-23-8* [fluphenazine]. JAN. *Antipsychotic.* Prolixin (Apothecon)

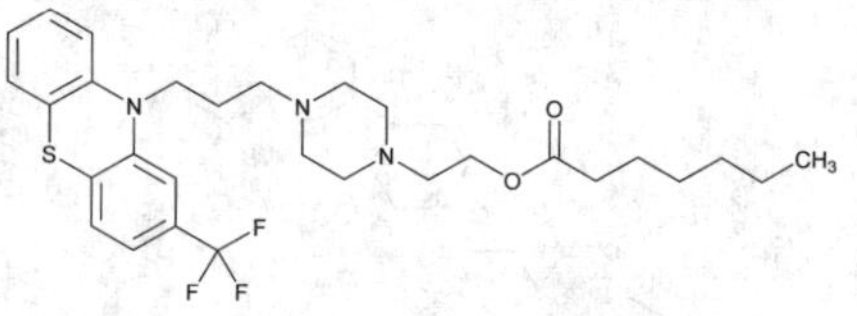

Fluphenazine Hydrochloride (floo fen′ a zeen hye″ droe klor′ ide). **USP.** $C_{22}H_{26}F_3N_3OS{\cdot}2HCl$. 510.44. (1) 1-Piperazineethanol, 4-[3-[2-(trifluoromethyl)-10*H*-phenothiazin-10-yl]propyl]-, dihydrochloride; (2) 4-[3-[2-(Trifluoromethyl)phenothiazin-10-yl]propyl]-1-piperazineethanol dihydrochloride. *UNII-ZOU145W1XL. CAS-146-56-5; CAS-69-23-8* [fluphenazine]. BAN; JAN. *Antipsychotic.* Permitil (Schering); Prolixin (Apothecon)

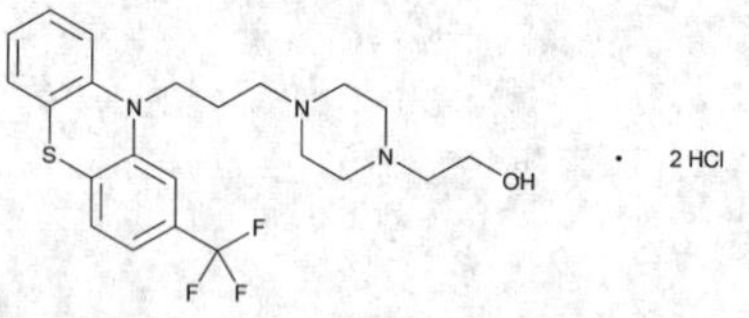

Flupimazine. $C_{23}H_{27}F_3N_2O_2S$. 452.53. 2-[[1-[3-[2-(Trifluoromethyl)phenothiazin-10-yl]propyl]-4-piperidyl]oxy]ethanol. *UNII-AZJ60Y1VSK. CAS-47682-41-7.* INN.

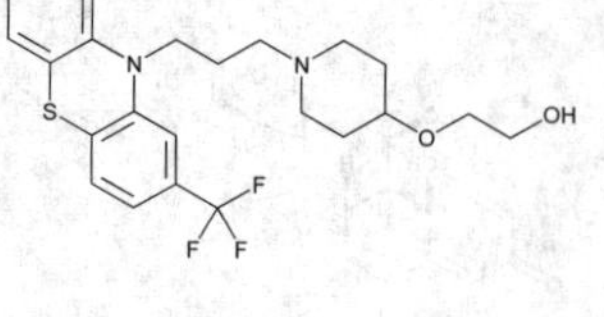

Flupirtine Maleate [*1984*] (floo pir′ teen mal′ ee ate). $C_{15}H_{17}FN_4O_2{\cdot}C_4H_4O_4$. 420.39. [Flupirtine is INN and BAN.] (1) Carbamic acid, [2-amino-6-[[(4-fluorophenyl)methyl]amino]-3-pyridinyl]-, ethyl ester, (Z)-2-butenedioate (1:1); (2) Ethyl 2-amino-6-[(*p*-fluorobenzyl)amino]-3-pyridinecarbamate maleate (1:1). *UNII-0VCI53PK4A; UNII-MOH3ET196H* [flupirtine]. *CAS-75507-68-5; CAS-56995-20-1* [flupirtine]. *Analgesic.* ◇*W-2964M; D-9998*

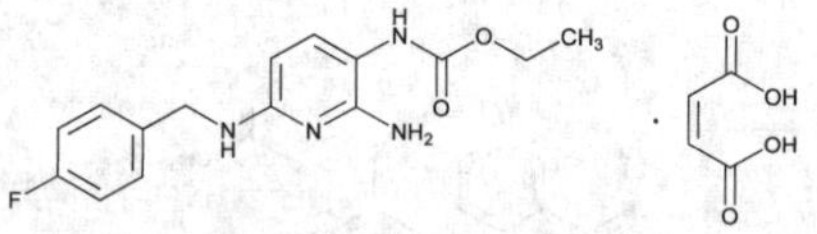

Flupranone. $C_{20}H_{24}FN_3O_2$. 357.42. 3-[4-(*p*-Fluorophenyl)-3,6-dihydro-1(2*H*)-pyridyl]-1-[1-(2-hydroxyethyl)-5-methylpyrazol-4-yl]-1-propanone. *UNII-N0U9G33XKT. CAS-21686-10-2.* INN.

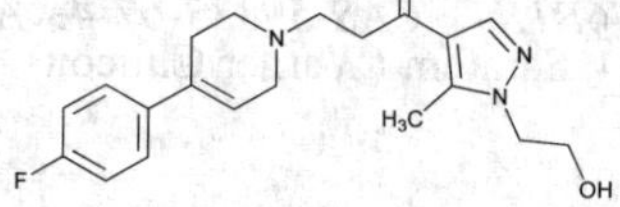

Fluprazine. $C_{14}H_{19}F_3N_4O$. 316.32. [2-[4-(α,α,α-Trifluoro-*m*-tolyl)-1-piperazinyl]ethyl]urea. *UNII-713BBL6840. CAS-76716-60-4.* INN.

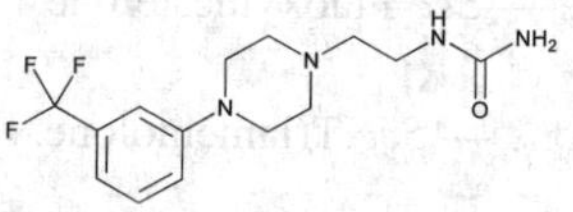

Fluprednidene. $C_{22}H_{27}FO_5$. 390.45. 9-Fluoro-11β,17,21-trihydroxy-16-methylenepregna-1,4-diene-3,20-dione. *UNII-FA517NS3N7. CAS-2193-87-5.* INN; BAN; MI.

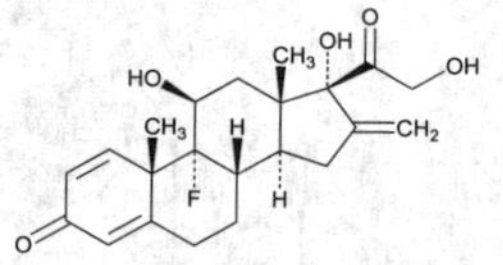

Fluprednisolone [*1962*] (floo″ pred nis′ oh lone). $C_{21}H_{27}FO_5$. 378.43. (1) Pregna-1,4-diene-3,20-dione, 6-fluoro-11,17,21-trihydroxy-, (6α,11β)-; (2) 6α-Fluoro-11β,17,21-trihydroxypregna-1,4-diene-3,20-dione. *UNII-9H05937G3X. CAS-53-34-9.* INN; NF XIII; BAN. *Glucocorticoid.* Alphadrol (Pfizer) ◇*U-7800; NSC-47439*

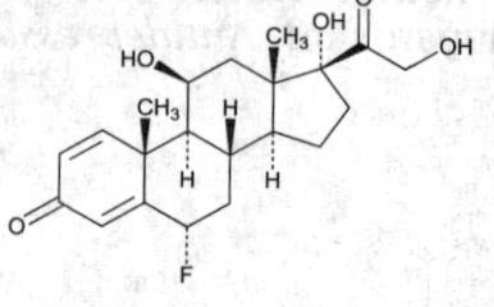

Fluprednisolone Valerate [*1968*] (floo″ pred nis′ oh lone val′ er ate). $C_{26}H_{35}FO_6$. 462.55. (1) Pregna-1,4-diene-3,20-dione, 6-fluoro-11,21-dihydroxy-17[[(1-oxopentyl)oxy]-, (6α,11β)-; (2) 6α-Fluoro-11β,17,21-trihydroxypregna-1,4-diene-3,20-dione 17-valerate. *UNII-PH7R4L7SNF. CAS-23257-44-5. Glucocorticoid.*

Fluprofen. $C_{15}H_{13}FO_2$. 244.26. 2-(3′-Fluoro-4-biphenylyl)-propionic acid. *UNII-P69N9N4Y9Y*. *CAS-17692-38-5*. INN; BAN. ◇*RD 17345; BTS 17345*

Fluprofylline. $C_{22}H_{26}FN_5O_3$. 427.47. 7-[3-[4-(*p*-Fluorobenzoyl)piperidino]propyl]theophylline. *UNII-6Y42K4JRBJ*. *CAS-85118-43-0*. INN.

Fluproquazone [*1981*] (floo proe′ kwa zone). $C_{18}H_{17}FN_2O$. 296.34. (1) 2(1*H*)-Quinazolinone, 4-(4-fluorophenyl)-7-methyl-1-(1-methylethyl)-; (2) 4-(*p*-Fluorophenyl)-1-isopropyl-7-methyl-2(1*H*)-quinazolinone. *CAS-40507-23-1*. INN; BAN. *Analgesic*. Tormosyl (Novartis†) ◇*46-790*

Fluprostenol Sodium [*1976*] (floo prost′ e nol soe′ dee um). $C_{23}H_{28}F_3NaO_6$. 480.45. [Fluprostenol is INN and BAN.] (1) 5-Heptenoic acid, 7-[3,5-dihydroxy-2-[3-hydroxy-4-[3-(trifluoromethyl)phenoxy]-1-butenyl]cyclopentyl]-; [1α(Z),2β(1*E*,3*R**),3α,5α]-, sodium salt, (±)-; (2) (±) Sodium (*Z*)-7-[(1*R**,2*R**,3*R**,5*S**)-3,5-dihydroxy-2-[(*E*)-(3*R**)-3-hydroxy-4-[(α,α,α-trifluoro-*m*-tolyl)oxy]-1-butenyl]cyclopentyl]-5-heptenoate. *UNII-6H4ZY4O7NA; UNII-358S7VUE5N* [fluprostenol]. *CAS-55028-71-2; CAS-40666-16-8* [fluprostenol]. *Prostaglandin*. Equimate (Bayer Animal Health†) ◇*ICI 81,008; ICI 80,008 [as sodium salt]*

Fluquazone [*1977*] (floo′ kwa zone). $C_{16}H_{10}ClF_3N_2O$. 338.71. (1) 2(1*H*)-Quinazolinone, 6-chloro-4-phenyl-1-(2,2,2-trifluoroethyl)-; (2) 6-Chloro-4-phenyl-1-(2,2,2-trifluoroethyl)-2(1*H*)-quinazolinone. *UNII-31YX4A42L4*. *CAS-37554-40-8*. INN. *Anti-inflammatory*. ◇*EN-970*

Fluracil — *See* Fluorouracil.

Fluradoline Hydrochloride [*1982*] (flur ad′ oh leen hye″ droe klor′ ide). $C_{17}H_{16}FNOS·HCl$. 337.84. [Fluradoline is INN.] (1) Ethanamine, 2-[(8-fluorodibenz[*b,f*]oxepin-10-yl)thio]-*N*-methyl-, hydrochloride; (2) 2-[(8-Fluorodibenz[*b,f*]oxepin-10-yl)thio]-*N*-methylethylamine hydrochloride. *CAS-77590-97-7; CAS-71316-84-2* [fluradoline]. *Analgesic*. ◇*HP 494; P 76 2494A*

Flurandrenolide [*1969*] (flur″ an dren′ oh lide). **USP**. $C_{24}H_{33}FO_6$. 436.51. [Fludroxycortide is INN, BAN and JAN.] (1) Pregn-4-ene-3,20-dione, 6-fluoro-11,21-dihydroxy-16,17-[(1-methylethylidene)bis(oxy)]-, (6α,11β,16α)-; (2) 6α-Fluoro-11β,16α,17,21-tetrahydroxypregn-4-ene-3,20-dione, cyclic 16,17-acetal with acetone. *UNII-8EUL29XUQT*. *CAS-1524-88-5*. *Glucocorticoid*. Cordran (Oclassen) *[Name previously used: Flurandrenolone.]* ◇*33379*

Flurandrenolone (previously used name) — *See* Flurandrenolide.

Flurantel. $C_{19}H_{12}F_6N_2O_7$. 494.30. 2,6-Dihydroxy-3-nitro-3′,5′-bis(trifluoromethyl)benzanilide diacetate (ester). *UNII-3Q14SL1C0O*. *CAS-30533-89-2*. INN.

Flurazepam Hydrochloride [*1968*] (flur az′ e pam hye″ droe klor′ ide). **USP**. $C_{21}H_{23}ClFN_3O·2HCl$. 460.80. [Flurazepam is INN, BAN, and JAN.] (1) 2*H*-1,4-Benzodiazepin-2-one, 7-chloro-1-[2-(diethylamino)ethyl]-5-(2-fluorophenyl)-1,3-dihydro-, dihydrochloride; (2) 7-Chloro-1-[2-(diethylamino)ethyl]-5-(*o*-fluorophenyl)-1,3-dihydro-2*H*-1,4-benzodiazepin-2-one dihydrochloride. *UNII-756RDM536M;*

---

† Brand name formerly used, and/or firm no longer concerned with this product.

UNII-IHP475989U [flurazepam]. *CAS-1172-18-5; CAS-17617-23-1* [flurazepam]. JAN. *Anticonvulsant; relaxant (muscle); sedative-hypnotic.* Dalmane (Valeant) ◇*Ro 5-6901; NSC-78559*

Flurbiprofen [*1976*] (flur″ bi proe′ fen). **USP.** $C_{15}H_{13}FO_2$. 244.26. (1) [1,1′-Biphenyl]-4-acetic acid, 2-fluoro-α-methyl-, (±)-; (2) (±)-2-Fluoro-α-methyl-4-biphenylacetic acid; (3) (±)-2-(2-Fluoro-4-biphenylyl)propionic acid. *UNII-5GRO578KLP. CAS-5104-49-4.* INN; BAN; JAN. *Analgesic; anti-inflammatory.* Ansaid (Pfizer) ◇*U-27,182; BTS 18,322*

Flurbiprofen Sodium (flur″ bi proe′ fen soe′ dee um). **USP.** $C_{15}H_{12}FNaO_2 \cdot 2H_2O$. 302.27. (1) [1,1′-Biphenyl]-4-acetic acid, 2-fluoro-α-methyl, sodium salt dihydrate, (±)-; (2) Sodium (±)-2-(2-fluoro-4-biphenylyl)propionate dihydrate. *UNII-Z5B97MU9K4. CAS-56767-76-1. Inhibitor (prostaglandin synthesis).* Ocufen (Allergan)

Fluretofen [*1978*] (flur″ e toe′ fen). $C_{14}H_9F$. 196.22. (1) 1,1′-Biphenyl, 4′-ethynyl-2-fluoro-; (2) 4′-Ethynyl-2-fluorobiphenyl. *CAS-56917-29-4.* INN. *Anti-inflammatory; antithrombotic.* ◇*Compound 93819*

Flurfamide (previously used name) — *See* Flurofamide.

Flurithromycin. $C_{37}H_{66}FNO_{13}$. 751.92. (8S)-8-Fluoroerythromycin. *UNII-56C9DTE69V. CAS-82664-20-8.* INN.

Flurocitabine [*1977*] (flur″ oh sye′ ta been). $C_9H_{10}FN_3O_4$. 243.19. (1) 6H-Furo[2′,3′;4,5]oxazolo[3,2-a]pyrimidine-2-methanol, 7-fluoro-2,3,3a,9a-tetrahydro-3-hydroxy-6-imino-, [2R-(2α,3β,3aβ,9aβ)]-; (2) (2R,3R,3aS,9aR)-7-Fluoro-2,3,3a,9a-tetrahydro-3-hydroxy-6-imino-6H-furo[2′,3′:4,5]oxazolo[3,2-a]pyrimidine-2-methanol; (3) 2,2′-Anhydro-5-fluoro-1-β-D-arabinofuranosylcytosine. *UNII-89TPE33M27. CAS-37717-21-8.* INN. *Antineoplastic.* ◇*Ro 21-0702; AAFC*

Flurofamide [*1980*] (flur oh′ fa mide). $C_7H_9FN_3O_2P$. 217.14. (1) Benzamide, *N*-(diaminophosphinyl)-4-fluoro-; (2) *N*-(Diaminophosphinyl)-*p*-fluorobenzamide. *CAS-70788-28-2.* INN. *Enzyme inhibitor (urease). [Name previously used: Flurfamide.]* ◇*EU-4534*

Flurogestone Acetate [*1965*] (flur″ oh jes′ tone as′ e tate). $C_{23}H_{31}FO_5$. 406.49. [Flugestone is INN and BAN.] (1) Pregn-4-ene-3,20-dione, 17-(acetyloxy)-9-fluoro-11-hydroxy-, (11β)-; (2) 9-Fluoro-11β,17-dihydroxypregn-4-ene-3,20-dione 17-acetate. *UNII-X60881643X. CAS-2529-45-5. Progestin.* ◇*SC-9880; NSC-65411*

Flurothyl [*1962*] (flur′ oh thil). $C_4H_4F_6O$. 182.06. [Flurotyl is INN and BAN.] (1) Ethane, 1,1′-oxybis[2,2,2-trifluoro-; (2) Bis(2,2,2-trifluoroethyl) ether. *UNII-9Z467FG2YK. CAS-333-36-8.* USP XXI. *Stimulant (central).* Indoklon (Ohmeda) ◇*SK&F 6539*

Flurotyl (INN, BAN) — *See* Flurothyl.

Fluroxene [*1961*] (flur ox′ een). $C_4H_5F_3O$. 126.08. (1) Ethene, (2,2,2-trifluoroethoxy)-; (2) 2,2,2-Trifluoroethyl vinyl ether. *UNII-FO7JHA3G03. CAS-406-90-6.* NF XIV; INN. *Anesthetic (inhalation).* Fluoromar (Ohmeda)

Fluroxyspiramine — *See* Spiramide.

Flusalan (INN) — *See* Fluorosalan.

Flusilfocon A [*1989*] (floo″ sil foe′ kon). $(C_{16}H_{38}O_6Si_4)_t(C_{26}H_{58}O_9Si_6)_u(C_5H_8O_2)_v(C_6H_7F_3O_2)_w(C_4H_6O_2)_x(C_9H_{15}NO_2)_y(C_{14}H_{22}O_6)_z$. (1) 3-[[3,3,3-Trimethyl-1,1-bis[(trimethylsilyl)oxy]disiloxanyl]oxy]propyl 2-methyl-2-propenoate polymer with [1,1,3,3-tetrakis[(trimethylsilyl)oxy]-1,3-disiloxanediyl]di-3,1-propanediyl bis(2-methyl-2-propenoate), methyl 2-methyl-2-propenoate, 2,2,2-trifluoroethyl 2-methyl-2-propenoate, 2-methyl-2-propenoic acid, *N*-(1,1-dimethyl-3-oxobutyl)-2-propenamide and 1,2-

ethanediylbis(oxy-2,1-ethanediyl) bis(2-methyl-2-propenoate); (2) 3-[3,3,3-Trimethyl-1,1-bis(trimethylsiloxy)disiloxanoxy]propyl methacrylate polymer with [tetrakis(trimethylsiloxy)disiloxanylene]bis(trimethylene) dimethacrylate, methyl methacrylate, 2,2,2-trifluoroethyl methacrylate, methacrylic acid, *N*-(1,1-dimethyl-3-oxobutyl)acrylamide and triethylene glycol dimethacrylate. *Contact lens material (hydrophobic).* Fluorex 700 (G.T. Laboratories) *[Note—The water content of the contact lens material is < 1.0% at ambient temperature (23±2°C), and the oxygen permeability is 70 × 10^{-11}(cm²/sec)(ml O₂/ml × mm Hg) at 35°C (Dk value).]*

Flusilfocon B *[1989]* (floo″ sil foe′ kon). ($C_{16}H_{38}O_6$ $Si_4)_t(C_{26}H_{58}O_9Si_6)_u(C_5H_8O_2)_v(C_6H_7F_3O_2)_w(C_4H_6O_2)_x(C_9H_{15}$ $NO_2)_y(C_{14}H_{22}O_6)_z$. (1) 3-[[3,3,3-Trimethyl-1,1-bis[(trimethylsilyl)oxy]disiloxanyl]oxy]propyl 2-methyl-2-propenoate polymer with [1,1,3,3-tetrakis[(trimethylsilyl)oxy]-1,3-disiloxanediyl]di-3,1-propanediyl bis(2-methyl-2-propenoate), methyl 2-methyl-2-propenoate, 2,2,2-trifluoroethyl 2-methyl-2-propenoate, 2-methyl-2-propenoic acid, *N*-(1,1-dimethyl-3-oxobutyl)-2-propenamide and 1,2-ethanediylbis(oxy-2,1-ethanediyl) bis(2-methyl-2-propenoate); (2) 3-[3,3,3-Trimethyl-1,1-bis(trimethylsiloxy)disiloxanoxy]propyl methacrylate polymer with [tetrakis(trimethylsiloxy)disiloxanylene]bis(trimethylene) dimethacrylate, methyl methacrylate, 2,2,2-trifluoroethyl methacrylate, methacrylic acid, *N*-(1,1-dimethyl-3-oxobutyl)acrylamide and triethylene glycol dimethacrylate. *Contact lens material (hydrophobic).* Fluorex 500 (G.T. Laboratories) *[Note—The water content of the contact lens material is < 1.0% at ambient temperature (23±2°C), and the oxygen permeability is 50 × 10^{-11}(cm²/sec)(ml O₂/ml × mm Hg) at 35°C (Dk value).]*

Flusilfocon C *[1989]* (floo″ sil foe′ kon). ($C_{16}H_{38}O_6$ $Si_4)_t(C_{26}H_{58}O_9Si_6)_u(C_5H_8O_2)_v(C_6H_7F_3O_2)_w(C_4H_6O_2)_x(C_9H_{15}$ $NO_2)_y(C_{14}H_{22}O_6)_z$. (1) 3-[[3,3,3-Trimethyl-1,1-bis[(trimethylsilyl)oxy]disiloxanyl]oxy]propyl 2-methyl-2-propenoate polymer with [1,1,3,3-tetrakis[(trimethylsilyl)oxy]-1,3-disiloxanediyl]di-3,1-propanediyl bis(2-methyl-2-propenoate), methyl 2-methyl-2-propenoate, 2,2,2-trifluoroethyl 2-methyl-2-propenoate, 2-methyl-2-propenoic acid, *N*-(1,1-dimethyl-3-oxobutyl)-2-propenamide and 1,2-ethanediylbis(oxy-2,1-ethanediyl) bis(2-methyl-2-propenoate); (2) 3-[3,3,3-Trimethyl-1,1-bis(trimethylsiloxy)disiloxanoxy]propyl methacrylate polymer with [tetrakis(trimethylsiloxy)disiloxanylene]bis(trimethylene) dimethacrylate, methyl methacrylate, 2,2,2-trifluoroethyl methacrylate, methacrylic acid, *N*-(1,1-dimethyl-3-oxobutyl)acrylamide and triethylene glycol dimethacrylate. *Contact lens material (hydrophobic).* Fluorex 300 (G.T. Laboratories) *[Note—The water content of the contact lens material is < 1.0% at ambient temperature (23±2°C), and the oxygen permeability is 30 × 10^{-11}(cm²/sec)(ml O₂/ml × mm Hg) at 35°C (Dk value).]*

Flusilfocon D *[1989]* (floo″ sil foe′ kon). ($C_{16}H_{38}O_6$ $Si_4)_t(C_{26}H_{58}O_9Si_6)_u(C_5H_8O_2)_v(C_6H_7F_3O_2)_w(C_4H_6O_2)_x(C_9H_{15}$ $NO_2)_y(C_{14}H_{22}O_6)_z$. (1) 3-[[3,3,3-Trimethyl-1,1-bis[(trimethylsilyl)oxy]disiloxanyl]oxy]propyl 2-methyl-2-propenoate polymer with [1,1,3,3-tetrakis[(trimethylsilyl)oxy]-1,3-disiloxanediyl]di-3,1-propanediyl bis(2-methyl-2-propenoate), methyl 2-methyl-2-propenoate, 2,2,2-trifluoroethyl 2-methyl-2-propenoate, 2-methyl-2-propenoic acid, *N*-(1,1-dimethyl-3-oxobutyl)-2-propenamide and 1,2-ethanediylbis(oxy-2,1-ethanediyl) bis(2-methyl-2-propenoate); (2) 3-[3,3,3-Trimethyl-1,1-bis(trimethylsiloxy)disiloxanoxy]propyl methacrylate polymer with [tetrakis(trimethylsiloxy)disiloxanylene]bis(trimethylene) dimethacrylate, methyl methacrylate, 2,2,2-trifluoroethyl methacrylate, methacrylic acid, *N*-(1,1-dimethyl-3-

oxobutyl)acrylamide and triethylene glycol dimethacrylate. *Contact lens material (hydrophobic).* Fluorex 900 (G.T. Laboratories) *[Note—The water content of the contact lens material is < 1.0% at ambient temperature (23±2°C), and the oxygen permeability is 86 × 10^{-11}(cm²/sec)(ml O₂/ml × mm Hg) at 35°C (Dk value).]*

Flusilfocon E *[1995]* (floo″ sil foe′ kon). ($C_{16}H_{38}O_6$ $Si_4)_t(C_{26}H_{58}O_9Si_6)_u(C_5H_8O_2)_v(C_6H_7F_3O_2)_w(C_4H_6O_2)_x(C_9H_{15}$ $NO_2)_y(C_{14}H_{22}O_6)_z$. (1) 3-[[3,3,3-Trimethyl-1,1-bis[(trimethylsilyl)oxy]disiloxanyl]oxy]propyl 2-methyl-2-propenoate polymer with [1,1,3,3-tetrakis[(trimethylsilyl)oxy]-1,3-disiloxanediyl]di-3,1-propanediyl bis(2-methyl-2-propenoate), methyl 2-methyl-2-propenoate, 2,2,2-trifluoroethyl 2-methyl-2-propenoate, 2-methyl-2-propenoic acid, *N*-(1,1-dimethyl-3-oxobutyl)-2-propenamide and 1,2-ethanediylbis(oxy-2,1-ethanediyl) bis(2-methyl-2-propenoate); (2) 3-[3,3,3-Trimethyl-1,1-bis(trimethylsiloxy)disiloxanoxy]propyl methacrylate polymer with [tetrakis(trimethylsiloxy)disiloxanylene]bis(trimethylene) dimethacrylate, methyl methacrylate, 2,2,2-trifluoroethyl methacrylate, methacrylic acid, *N*-(1,1-dimethyl-3-oxobutyl)acrylamide and triethylene glycol dimethacrylate. *CAS-169590-40-3. Contact lens material (hydrophobic).* Fluorex 600 (G.T. Laboratories) *[Note—The water content of the contact lens material is < 1.0% at ambient temperature (23±2°C), and the oxygen permeability is 60 × 10^{-11}(cm²/sec)(ml O₂/ml × mm Hg) at 35°C (Dk value).]*

Flusoxolol. $C_{22}H_{30}FNO_4$. 391.48. (*S*)-1-[*p*-[2-[(*p*-Fluorophenethyl)oxy]ethoxy]phenoxy]-3-(isopropylamino)-2-propanol. *UNII-1GPL60IRCI. CAS-84057-96-5.* INN; BAN.

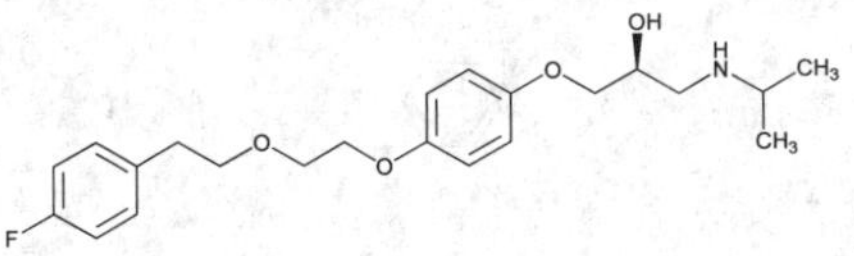

Fluspiperone *[1976]* (floo spi′ per one). $C_{23}H_{25}F_2N_3O_2$. 413.46. (1) 1,3,8-Triazaspiro[4.5]decan-4-one, 1-(4-fluorophenyl)-8-[4-(4-fluorophenyl)-4-oxobutyl]-; (2) 8-[3-(*p*-Fluorobenzoyl)propyl]-1-(*p*-fluorophenyl)-1,3,8-triazaspiro[4.5]decan-4-one. *UNII-V0Q53N427T. CAS-54965-22-9.* INN. *Antipsychotic.* ◇*R 28,930*

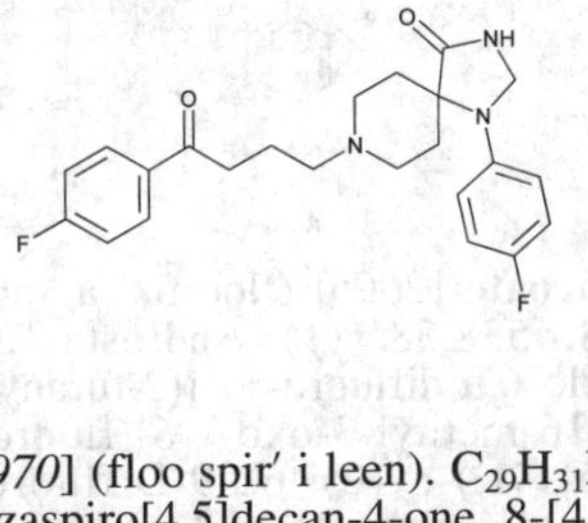

Fluspirilene *[1970]* (floo spir′ i leen). $C_{29}H_{31}F_2N_3O$. 475.57. (1) 1,3,8-Triazaspiro[4.5]decan-4-one, 8-[4,4-bis(4-fluorophenyl)butyl]-1-phenyl-; (2) 8-[4,4-Bis(*p*-fluorophenyl)butyl]-1-phenyl-1,3,8-triazaspiro-[4.5]decan-4-one. *CAS-1841-19-6.* INN; BAN. *Antipsychotic.* Imap (Ortho-McNeil†) ◇*McN-JR-6218; R 6218*

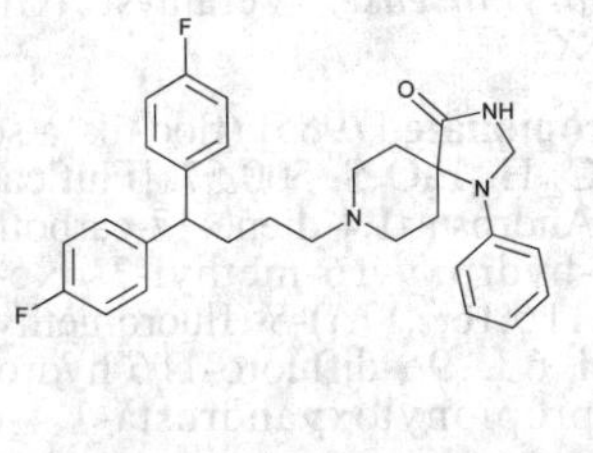

Flutamide [*1975*] (floo′ ta mide). **USP.** $C_{11}H_{11}F_3N_2O_3$. 276.21. (1) Propanamide, 2-methyl-*N*-[4-nitro-3-(trifluoromethyl)phenyl]-; (2) α,α,α-Trifluoro-2-methyl-4′-nitro-*m*-propionotoluidide. *UNII-76W6J0943E. CAS-13311-84-7.* INN; BAN. Eulexin (Schering) ◇*Sch 13521*

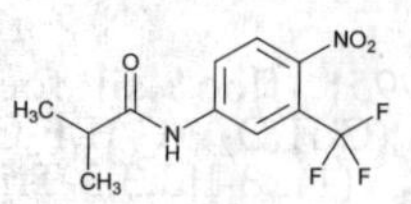

Flutazolam. $C_{19}H_{18}ClFN_2O_3$. 376.81. 10-Chloro-11b-(*o*-fluorophenyl)-2,3,7,11b-tetrahydro-7-(2-hydroxyethyl)oxazolo[3,2-*d*][1,4]benzodiazepin-6(5*H*)-one. *UNII-5G2K7O5D8S. CAS-27060-91-9.* INN; JAN; MI.

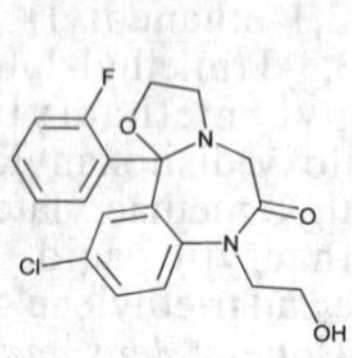

Flutemazepam. $C_{16}H_{12}ClFN_2O_2$. 318.73. 7-Chloro-5-(*o*-fluorophenyl)-1,3-dihydro-3-hydroxy-1-methyl-2*H*-1,4-benzodiazepin-2-one. *UNII-J8U5694BCW. CAS-52391-89-6.* INN.

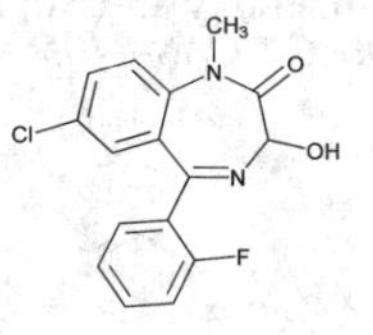

Flutiazin [*1969*] (floo tye′ a zin). $C_{14}H_8F_3NO_2S$. 311.28. (1) 10*H*-Phenothiazine-1-carboxylic acid, 8-(trifluoromethyl)-; (2) 8-(Trifluoromethyl)phenothiazine-1-carboxylic acid. *CAS-7220-56-6.* INN. *Anti-inflammatory (veterinary).*

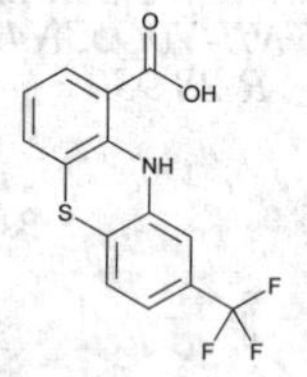

Fluticasone Furoate [*2006*] (floo tik′ a sone fure′ oh ate). $C_{27}H_{29}F_3O_6S$. 538.58. (1) Androsta-1,4-diene-17-carbothioic acid, 6,9-difluoro-17-[(2-furanylcarbonyl)oxy]-11-hydroxy-16-methyl-3-oxo-, *S*-(fluoromethyl) ester, (6α,11β,16α,17α)-; (2) 6α,9-Difluoro-17-[[(fluoromethyl)sulfanyl]carbonyl]-11β-hydroxy-16α-methyl-3-oxoandrosta-1,4-dien-17α-yl furan-2-carboxylate; (3) (6α,11β,16α,17α)-6,9-Difluoro-17-(((fluoromethyl)thio)carbonyl)-11-hydroxy-16-methyl-3-oxoandrosta-1,4-dien-17-yl-2-furancarboxylate. *UNII-JS86977WNV. CAS-397864-44-7.* INN. *Asthma, allergy, and chronic obstructive pulmonary disease.* Veramyst (GlaxoSmithKline) ◇*GW685698X*

Fluticasone Propionate [*1985*] (floo tik′ a sone proe′ pee oh nate). **USP.** $C_{25}H_{31}F_3O_5S$. 500.57. [Fluticasone is INN and BAN.] (1) Androsta-1,4-diene-17-carbothioic acid, 6,9-difluoro-11-hydroxy-16-methyl-3-oxo-17-(1-oxopropoxy)-, (6α,11β,16α,17α)-*S*-(fluoromethyl) ester; (2) *S*-Fluoromethyl 6α, 9α-difluoro-11β-hydroxy-16α-methyl-3-oxo-17α-propionyloxyandrosta-1,4-diene-17β-car-

bothioate. *UNII-O2GMZ0LF5W. CAS-80474-14-2; CAS-90566-53-3* [fluticasone]. *Anti-inflammatory.* Cutivate (Altana); Flonase (GlaxoSmithKline); Flovent (GlaxoSmithKline) ◇*CCI 18781*

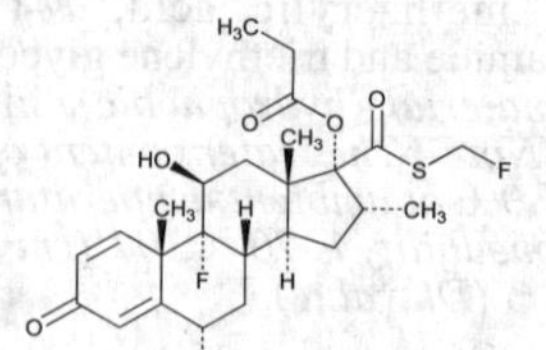

Flutizenol. $C_{20}H_{24}F_3N_3OS_2$. 443.55. 4-[3-[6-Trifluoromethyl-4*H*-thieno[2,3-*b*][1,4]benzothiazin-4-yl]propyl]-1-piperazineethanol. *UNII-0P1AN6K49Q. CAS-10202-40-1.* INN.

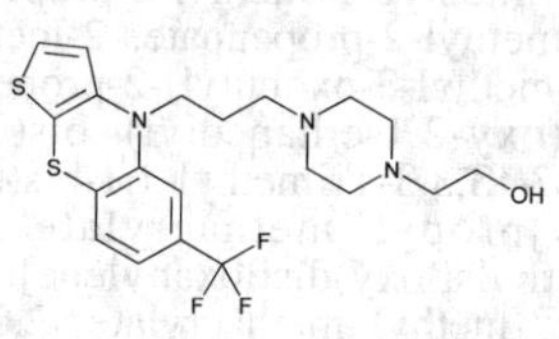

Flutomidate. $C_{14}H_{15}FN_2O_2$. 262.28. Ethyl (±)-1-(*p*-fluoro-α-methylbenzyl)imidazole-5-carboxylate. *UNII-CX3RPB4DVF. CAS-84962-75-4.* INN.

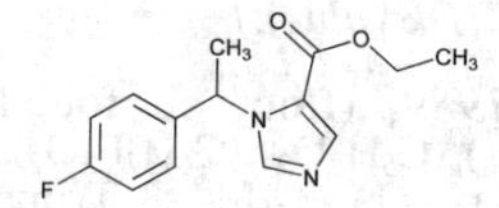

Flutonidine. $C_{10}H_{12}FN_3$. 193.22. 2-(5-Fluoro-*o*-toluidino)-2-imidazoline. *UNII-ZCC19F3X8K. CAS-28125-87-3.* INN. ◇*ST 600*

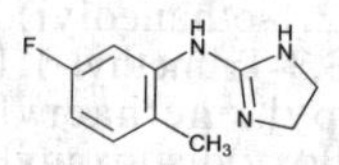

Flutoprazepam. $C_{19}H_{16}ClFN_2O$. 342.79. 7-Chloro-1-(cyclopropylmethyl)-5-(*o*-fluorophenyl)-1,3-dihydro-2*H*-1,4-benzodiazepin-2-one. *UNII-2GHY1101MM. CAS-25967-29-7.* INN; JAN; MI.

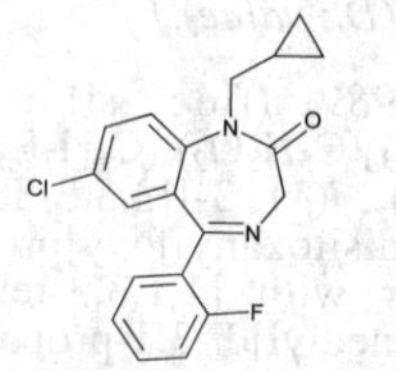

Flutrimazole. $C_{22}H_{16}F_2N_2$. 346.37. 1-[*o*-Fluoro-α-(*p*-fluorophenyl)-α-phenylbenzyl]imidazole. *CAS-119006-77-8.* INN; BAN. ◇*UR-4056*

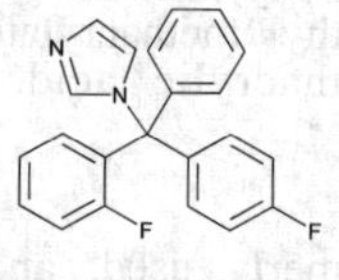

Flutroline [*1980*] (floo′ troe leen). $C_{27}H_{25}F_3N_2O$. 450.50. (1) 2*H*-Pyrido[4,3-*b*]indole-2-butanol, 8-fluoro-α,5-bis(4-fluorophenyl)-1,3,4,5-tetrahydro-, ($\pm$)-; (2) ($\pm$)-8-Fluoro-α,5-bis(*p*-fluorophenyl)-1,3,4,5-tetrahydro-2*H*-pyrido[4,3-*b*]indole-2-butanol. *CAS-70801-02-4*. INN. *Antipsychotic.* ◇*CP-36,584*

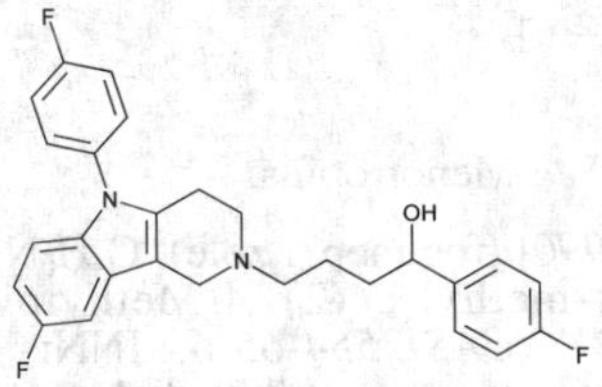

Flutropium Bromide. $C_{24}H_{29}BrFNO_3$. 478.39. (8*r*)-8-(2-Fluoroethyl)-3α-hydroxy-1αH,5αH-tropanium bromide, benzilate. *UNII-K3V6HB0M57. CAS-63516-07-4*. INN; JAN; MI.

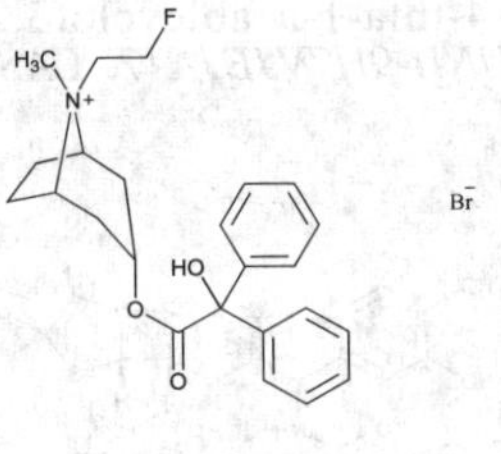

Fluvastatin Sodium [*1989*] (floo″ va stat′ in soe′ dee um). **USP**. $C_{24}H_{25}FNNaO_4$. 433.45. [Fluvastatin is INN and BAN.] (1) 6-Heptenoic acid, 7-[3-(4-fluorophenyl)-1-(1-methylethyl)-1*H*-indol-2-yl]-3,5-dihydroxy-, monosodium salt, [*R**,*S**-(*E*)]-($\pm$)-; (2) Sodium ($\pm$)-(3*R**,5*S**,6*E*)-7-[3-(*p*-fluorophenyl)-1-isopropylindol-2-yl]-3,5-dihydroxy-6-heptenoate. *UNII-PYF7O1FV7F; UNII-4L066368AS* [fluvastatin]. *CAS-93957-55-2; CAS-93957-54-1* [fluvastatin]. *Antihyperlipidemic; inhibitor (HMG-CoA reductase).* Lescol (Novartis) ◇*XU 62-320*

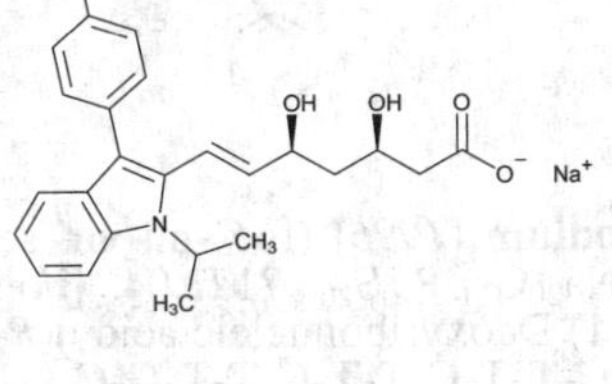

Fluvoxamine Maleate [*1995*] (floo vox′ a meen mal′ ee ate). **USP**. $C_{15}H_{21}F_3N_2O_2.C_4H_4O_4$. 434.41. [Fluvoxamine is INN and BAN.] (1) 1-Pentanone, 5-methoxy-1-[4-(trifluoromethyl)phenyl]-, *O*-(2-aminoethyl)oxime, (*E*)-, (*Z*)-2-butenedioate (1:1); (2) 5-Methoxy-4′-(trifluoromethyl)valerophenone (*E*)-*O*-(2-aminoethyl)oxime, maleate (1:1). *UNII-5LGN83G74V; UNII-O4L1XPO44W* [fluvoxamine].

---

† Brand name formerly used, and/or firm no longer concerned with this product.

CAS-61718-82-9; CAS-54739-18-3 [fluvoxamine]. *Antiobsessional agent.* Luvox (Solvay Pharmaceuticals) ◇*DU23000*

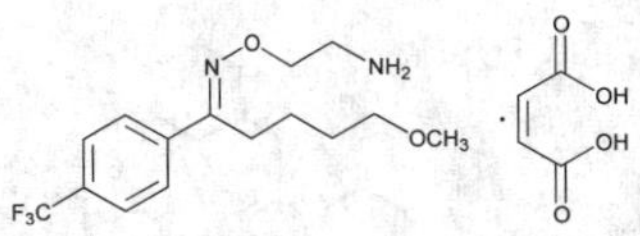

Fluzinamide [*1984*] (floo zin′ a mide). $C_{12}H_{13}F_3N_2O_2$. 274.24. (1) 1-Azetidinecarboxamide, *N*-methyl-3-[3-(trifluoromethyl)phenoxy]-; (2) *N*-Methyl-3-[(α,α,α-trifluoro-*m*-tolyl)oxy]-1-azetidinecarboxamide. *CAS-76263-13-3*. INN. *Anticonvulsant.* ◇*AHR-8559*

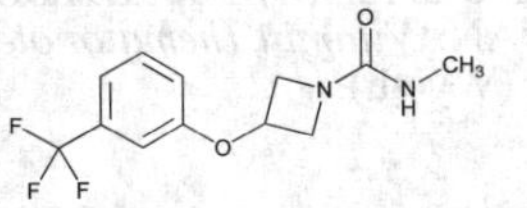

Fluzoperine. $C_{15}H_{19}FN_2O_2$. 278.32. 5-[2-(Diethylamino)-ethyl]-4-(*p*-fluorophenyl)-4-oxazolin-2-one. *UNII-5909OF92EF. CAS-52867-77-3*. INN.

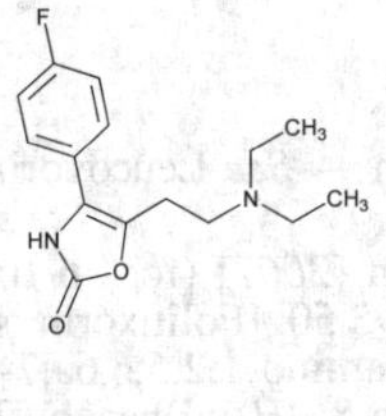

Focofilcon A [*1985*] (foe″ koe fil′ kon). $(C_6H_{10}O_3)_x$ $(C_4H_6O_2)_y$. (1) 2-Propenoic acid, 2-methyl-, 2-hydroxyethyl ester, polymer with 2-methyl-2-propenoic acid; (2) 2-Hydroxyethyl methacrylate polymer with methacrylic acid. *CAS-31693-08-0. Contact lens material (hydrophilic).* FRE-FLEX (Optech) *[Note—This contact lens material contains 55% of water.]*

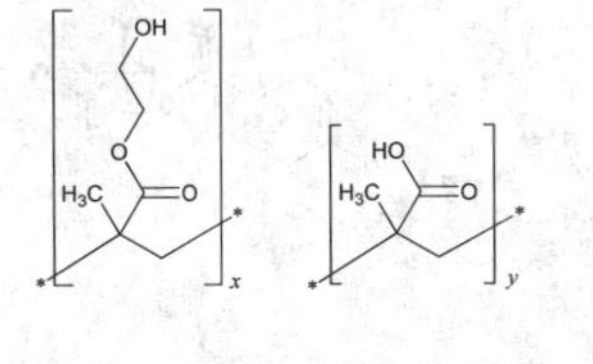

Fodipir [*1994*] (foe′ di pir). $C_{22}H_{32}N_4O_{14}P_2$. 638.46. (1) *N,N*′-1,2-Ethanediylbis[*N*-[[3-hydroxy-2-methyl-5-[(phosphonooxy)methyl]-4-pyridinyl]methyl]glycine]; *N,N*′-Ethylenebis[*N*-[[3-hydroxy-5-(hydroxymethyl)-2-methyl-4-pyridyl]methyl]glycine] 5,5′-bis(dihydrogen phosphate). *CAS-118248-91-2*. INN. *Excipient.* ◇*DPDP*

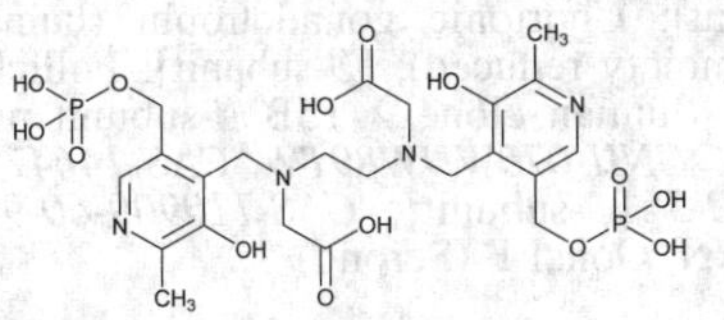

Folacin — *See* Folic Acid.

Folate Sodium. *UNII-935E97BOY8* [folic acid]. *CAS-6484-89-5; CAS-59-30-3* [folic acid].

410 FOLES–FOMIV

Folescutol. $C_{14}H_{15}NO_5$. 277.27. 6,7-Dihydroxy-4-(morpholinomethyl)coumarin. *UNII-D32TNF4T6G. CAS-15687-22-6.* INN; DCF; MI. ◇*LD 2988*

Folic Acid (foe′ lik as′ id). **USP.** $C_{19}H_{19}N_7O_6$. 441.40. (1) L-Glutamic acid, *N*-[4-[[(2-amino-1,4-dihydro-4-oxo-6-pteridinyl)methyl]amino]benzoyl]-; (2) Folic acid; (3) *N*-[*p*-[[(2-Amino-4-hydroxy-6-pteridinyl)methyl]amino]benzoyl]-L-glutamic acid. *UNII-935E97BOY8. CAS-59-30-3.* INN; BAN; JAN. *Vitamin (hematopoietic).* Folicet (Mission); Folvite (Wyeth)

Folinate-SF Calcium — *See* Leucovorin Calcium.

Folitixorin Calcium [*2007*] (foe″ li tix′ or in kal′ see um). $C_{20}H_{21}CaN_7O_6$. 495.50. [Folitixorin is INN.] (1) L-Glutamic acid, *N*-[4-(3-amino-1,2,5,6,6a,7-hexahydro-1-oxoimidazo[1,5-*f*]pteridin-8(9*H*)-yl)benzoyl]-, calcium salt (1:1); (2) Calcium (2*S*)-2-[[4-(3-amino-1-oxo-1,4,5,6,6a,7-hexahydroimidazo[1,5-*f*]pteridin-8(9*H*)-yl)benzoyl]amino]pentanedioate. *CAS-133978-75-3; CAS-3432-99-3* [folitixorin]. *Antineoplastic enhancing drug.* ◇*ANX-510; CoFactor*

Follicle Stimulating Hormone (BAN) — *See* Menotropins.

Follidrin — *See* Estradiol Benzoate.

Follitropin Alfa. $C_{437}H_{682}N_{122}O_{134}S_{13}$ (α-subunit). 10,205.69 (α-subunit); $C_{538}H_{833}N_{145}O_{171}S_{13}$ (β-subunit). 12,485.10 (β-subunit). Follicle-stimulating hormone, glycoform α. [α-subunit]: Chorionic gonadotropin (human α-subunit protein moiety reduced); [β-subunit]: Follicle-stimulating hormone (human clone λ 15B β-subunit protein moiety reduced). *UNII-076WHW89TW. CAS-146479-72-3; CAS-56832-30-5* [α-subunit]; *CAS-110909-60-9* [β-subunit]. INN; BAN. Gonal-F (Serono)

Follitropin Beta. $C_{437}H_{682}N_{122}O_{134}S_{13}$ (α-subunit). 10,205.69 (α-subunit); $C_{538}H_{833}N_{145}O_{171}S_{13}$ (β-subunit). 12,485.10 (β-subunit). Follicle-stimulating hormone, glycoform β. [α-subunit]: Chorionic gonadotropin (human α-subunit protein moiety reduced); [β-subunit]: Follicle-stimulating hormone (human β-subunit protein moiety reduced). *UNII-076WHW89TW. CAS-146479-72-3; CAS-150490-84-9* [replaced]; *CAS-56832-30-5* [α-subunit]; *CAS-110909-60-9* [β-subunit]. INN; BAN.

```
APDVQDCPEC TLQENPFFSQ PGAPILQCMG CCFSRAYPTP LRSKKTMLVQ
KNVTSESTCC VAKSYNRVTV MGGFKVENHT ACHCSTCYYH KS

NSCELTNITI AIEKEECRFC ISINTTWCAG YCYTRDLVYK DPARPKIQKT
CTFKELVYET VRVPGCAHHA DSLYTYPVAT QCHCGKCDSD STDCTVRGLG
PSYCSFGEMK E
```

Follotropin — *See* Menotropins.

Fomepizole [*1990*] (foe mep′ i zole). $C_4H_6N_2$. 82.10. (1) 1*H*-Pyrazole, 4-methyl-; (2) 4-Methylpyrazole. *UNII-83LCM6L2BY. CAS-7554-65-6.* INN; BAN. *Antidote (alcohol dehydrogenase inhibitor).* Antizol (Jazz) ◇*4-MP*

Fomidacillin. $C_{24}H_{28}N_6O_{10}S$. 592.58. (2*S*,5*R*,6*R*)-6-[(*R*)-2-(3,4-Dihydroxyphenyl)-2-(4-ethyl-2,3-dioxo-1-piperazinecarboxamido)acetamido]-6-formamido-3,3-dimethyl-7-oxo-4-thia-1-azabicyclo[3.2.0]heptane-2-carboxylic acid. *UNII-9H7VJE7A17. CAS-98048-07-8.* INN; BAN.

Fominoben. $C_{21}H_{24}ClN_3O_3$. 401.89. [Fominoben Hydrochloride is JAN.] 3′-Chloro-α-[methyl[(morpholinocarbonyl)methyl]amino]-*o*-benzotoluidide. *CAS-18053-31-1.* INN; MI. ◇*PB 89 [as hydrochloride]*

Fomivirsen Sodium [*1996*] (foe″ mi vir′ sen soe′ dee um). $C_{204}H_{243}N_{63}Na_{20}O_{114}P_{20}S_{20}$. 7122.04. [Fomivirsen is INN and BAN.] (1) Deoxyribonucleic acid d(*P*-thio)(G-C-G-T-T-T-G-C-T-C-T-T-C-T-T-C-T-T-G-C-G), eicosasodium salt; (2) 2′-Deoxy-*P*-thioguanylyl-(5′→3′)-2′-deoxy-*P*-thiocytidylyl-(5′→3′)-2′-deoxy-*P*-thioguanylyl-(5′→3′)-2′-deoxy-*P*-thiothymidylyl-(5′→3′)-2′-deoxy-*P*-thiothymidylyl-(5′→3′)-2′-deoxy-*P*-thiothymidylyl-(5′→3′)-2′-deoxy-*P*-thioguanylyl-(5′→3′)-2′-deoxy-*P*-thiocytidylyl-(5′→3′)-2′-deoxy-*P*-thiothymidylyl-(5′→3′)-2′-deoxy-*P*-thiocytidylyl-(5′→3′)-2′-deoxy-*P*-thiothymidylyl-(5′→3′)-2′-deoxy-*P*-thiothymidylyl-(5′→3′)-2′-deoxy-*P*-thiocytidylyl-(5′→3′)-2′-deoxy-*P*-thiothymidylyl-(5′→3′)-2′-deoxy-*P*-thiothymidylyl-(5′→3′)-2′-deoxy-*P*-thiocytidylyl-(5′→3′)-2′-deoxy-*P*-thiothymidylyl-(5′→3′)-2′-deoxy-*P*-thiothymidylyl-(5′→3′)-2′-deoxy-*P*-thioguanylyl-(5′→3′)-2′-deoxy-*P*-thiocytidylyl-(5′→3′)-2′-deoxyguanosine, eicosasodium salt. *UNII-3Z6W3S36X5. CAS-160369-77-7; CAS-144245-

52-3 [fomivirsen]. *Antisense antiviral used in the therapy of cytomegalovirus retinitis.* Vitravene (Novartis) *[Note—The following structure is positioned vertically due to space limitations.]* ◇ISIS 2922

PS-d(GCGTTTGCTCTTCTTCTTGCG)

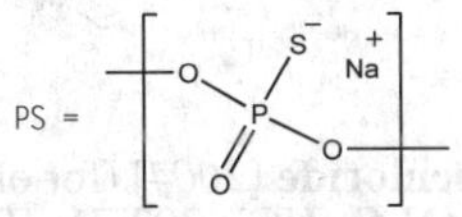

Fomocaine. $C_{20}H_{25}NO_2$. 311.42. 4-[3-(α-Phenoxy-*p*-tolyl)-propyl]morpholine. *UNII-4XO7A09HQM. CAS-17692-39-6.* INN; BAN; MI.

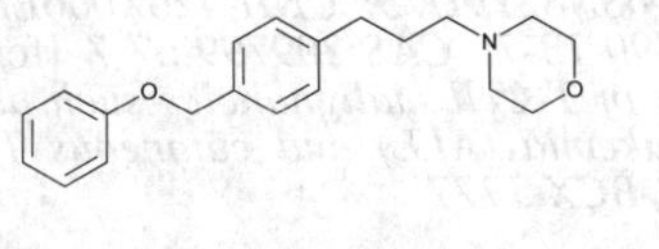

Fonatol — *See* Diethylstilbestrol.

Fonazine Mesylate [*1967*] (foe′ na zeen mes′ i late). $C_{20}H_{29}N_3O_5S_3$. 487.66. [Dimetotiazine is INN and BAN; Dimetotiazine Mesilate is JAN.] (1) 10*H*-Phenothiazine-2-sulfonamide, 10-[2-(dimethylamino)propyl]-*N,N*-dimethyl-, monomethanesulfonate; (2) 10-[2-(Dimethylamino)propyl]-*N,N*-dimethylphenothiazine-2-sulfonamide monomethanesulfonate. *UNII-B28V86NGNK. CAS-7455-39-2; CAS-7456-24-8* [fonazine]. *Serotonin inhibitor. [Name previously used: Dimethothiazine.]* ◇IL-6302 mesylate; 8599 R.P. mesylate

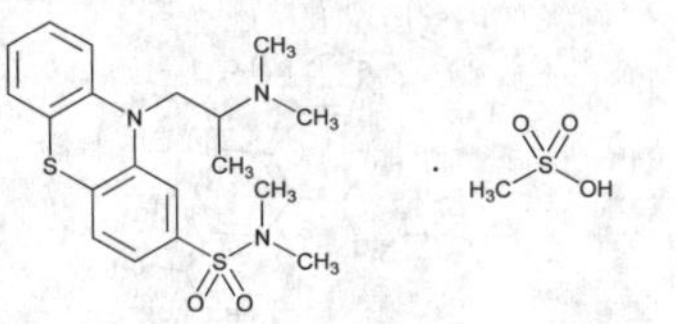

Fondaparinux Sodium [*2001*] (fon dap′ a rin ux soe′ dee um; fon″ da par′ in ux soe′ dee um). $C_{31}H_{43}N_3Na_{10}O_{49}S_8$. 1728.08. (1) α-D-Glucopyranoside, methyl *O*-2-deoxy-6-*O*-sulfo-2-(sulfoamino)-α-D-glucopyranosyl-(1→4)-*O*-β-D-glucopyranuronosyl-(1→4)-*O*-2-deoxy-3,6-di-*O*-sulfo-2-(sulfoamino)-α-D-glucopyranosyl-(1→4)-*O*-2-*O*-sulfo-α-L-idopyranuronosyl-(1→4)-2-deoxy-2-(sulfoamino)-, 6-(hydrogen sulfate), decasodium salt; (2) Methyl *O*-2-deoxy-6-*O*-sulfo-2-(sulfoamino)-α-D-glucopyranosyl-(1→4)-*O*-β-D-glucopyranuronosyl-(1→4)-*O*-2-deoxy-3,6-di-*O*-sulfo-2-(sulfoamino)-α-D-glucopyranosyl-(1→4)-*O*-2-*O*-sulfo-α-L-idopyranuronosyl-(1→4)-2-deoxy-6-*O*-sulfo-2-(sulfoamino)-α-D-glucopyranoside, decasodium salt. *UNII-X0Q6N9USOZ. CAS-114870-03-0.* INN; BAN. *Antithrombotic (indirect and selective synthetic factor Xa inhibitor).* Arixtra (GlaxoSmithKline) ◇SR 90107A; ORG 31540

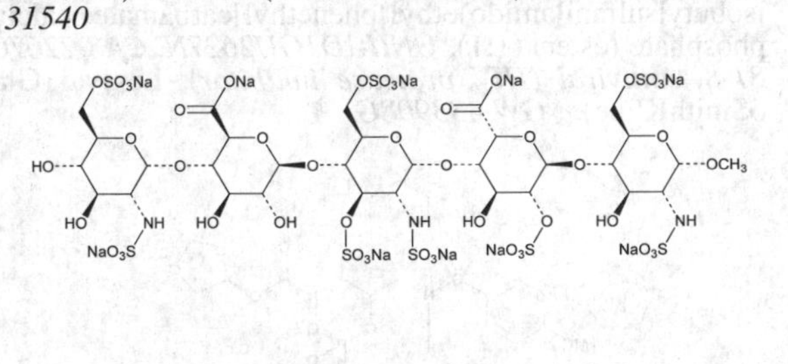

Fontolizumab [*2002*] (fon″ toe liz′ oo mab). Immunoglobulin G1, anti-(human interferon γ) (human-mouse monoclonal HuZAF γ1-chain), disulfide with human-mouse monoclonal HuZAF light chain, dimer. Molecular weight is approximately 150,000 daltons. *UNII-6J92H2439Z. CAS-326859-36-3.* INN; BAN. *Immunoregulatory agent to treat auto-immune diseases.* ◇HuZAF

Fopirtoline. $C_{11}H_{15}ClN_2OS$. 258.77. 4-[2-[(6-Chloro-2-pyridyl)thio]ethyl]morpholine. *UNII-C7B0AH4986. CAS-22514-23-4.* INN.

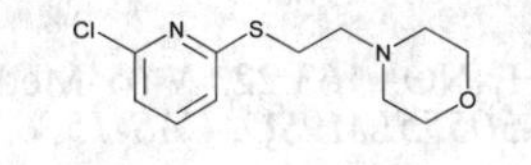

Forasartan [*1995*] (for″ a sar′ tan). $C_{23}H_{28}N_8$. 416.52. (1) Pyridine, 5-[(3,5-dibutyl-1*H*-1,2,4-triazol-1-yl)methyl]-2-[2-(1*H*-tetrazol-5-yl)phenyl]-; (2) 5-[(3,5-Dibutyl-1*H*-1,2,4-triazol-1-yl)methyl]-2-(*o*-1*H*-tetrazol-5-ylphenyl)-pyridine. *UNII-065F7WPT0B. CAS-145216-43-9.* INN. *Antihypertensive.* ◇SC-52458

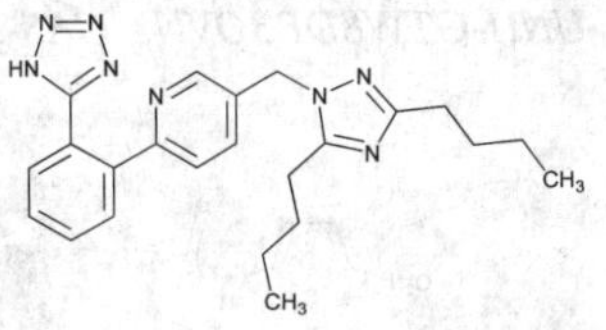

Foravirumab. $C_{6400}H_{9908}N_{1716}O_{1998}S_{44}$. Immunoglobulin G1, anti-[rabies virus glycoprotein], *Homo sapiens* monoclonal antibody, CR4098; gamma1 heavy chain (1-448) [*Homo sapiens* VH (IGHV3-33-(IGHD)-IGHJ4*01) [8.8.12] (1-119) - IGHG1*03, CH3 K130>del (120-448)], (222-214′)-disulfide with kappa light chain (1′-214′) [*Homo sapiens* V-KAPPA (IGKV1-17-IGKJ4*01) [6.3.9] (1′-107′) - IGKC*01 (108′-214′)]; (228-228″:231-231″)-bisdisulfide dimer. *CAS-944548-38-3.* INN.

Forfenimex. $C_9H_{11}NO_4$. 197.19. (+)-(*S*)-2-(α,3-Dihydroxy-*p*-tolyl)glycine. *UNII-EL461OY152. CAS-72973-11-6.* INN.

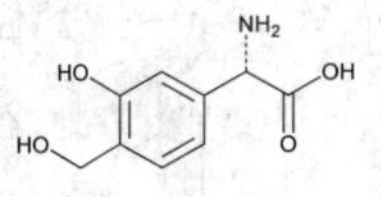

Formaldehyde (for mal′ de hyde). **USP** [Solution]. CH_2O. 30.03. [Formalin is JAN.] (1) Formaldehyde; (2) Formaldehyde. *UNII-1HG84L3525. CAS-50-00-0. Disinfectant.*

Formalin (JAN) — *See* Formaldehyde.

Formebolone. $C_{21}H_{28}O_4$. 344.44. 11α,17β-Dihydroxy-17-methyl-3-oxoandrosta-1,4-diene-2-carboxaldehyde. *UNII-Z2MMV08KUQ. CAS-2454-11-7.* INN; BAN.

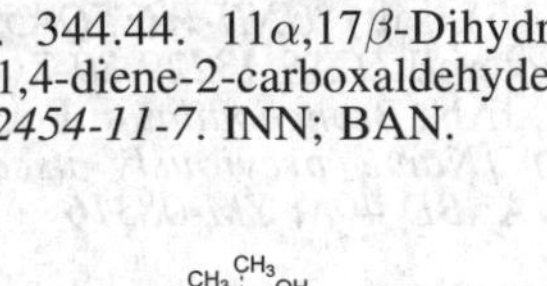

---

† Brand name formerly used, and/or firm no longer concerned with this product.

Formestane. $C_{19}H_{26}O_3$. 302.41. 4-Hydroxyandrost-4-ene-3,17-dione. *CAS-566-48-3.* INN; BAN. ◇*CGP 32349*

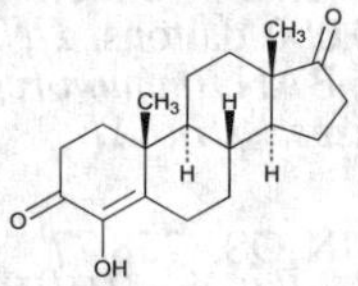

Formetamide — *See* Formetorex.

Formetorex. $C_{10}H_{13}NO$. 163.22. *N*-(α-Methylphenethyl)formamide. *UNII-30555LM9SQ. CAS-15302-18-8.* INN.

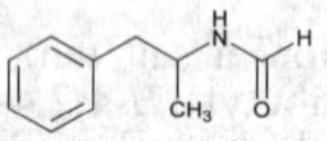

Formidacillin — *See* Fomidacillin.

Forminitrazole. $C_4H_3N_3O_3S$. 173.15. 2-Formamido-5-nitrothiazole. *UNII-GTW8DB3OVN. CAS-500-08-3.* INN; BAN; MI.

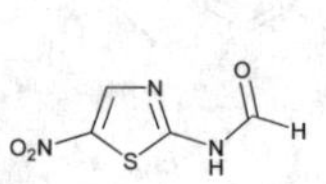

Formocortal [*1969*] (for″ moe kor′ tal). $C_{29}H_{38}ClFO_8$. 569.06. (1) Pregna-3,5-diene-6-carboxaldehyde, 21-(acetyloxy)-3-(2-chloroethoxy)-9-fluoro-11-hydroxy-16,17-[(1-methylethylidene)bis(oxy)]-20-oxo-, (11β,16α)-; (2) 3-(2-Chloroethoxy)-9-fluoro-11β,16α,17,21-tetrahydroxy-20-oxo-pregna-3,5-diene-6-carboxaldehyde, cyclic 16,17-acetal with acetone, 21-acetate. *CAS-2825-60-7.* INN; BAN. *Glucocorticoid.* Deflamene (Farmitalia, Societa Farmaceutici Italia, Italy); Fluderma (Farmitalia, Societa Farmaceutici Italia, Italy)

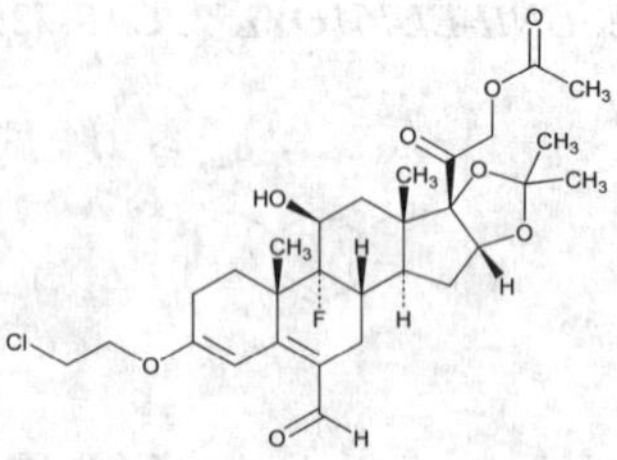

Formoterol Fumarate [*1997*] (for moe′ ter ol fue′ ma rate). $(C_{19}H_{24}N_2O_4)_2 \cdot C_4H_4O_4$. 804.88. [Formoterol is INN and BAN.] ($\pm$)-2′-Hydroxy-5′-[($R*$)-1-hydroxy-2-[[($R*$)-p-methoxy-α-methylphenethyl]amino]ethyl]formanilide fumarate (2:1) (salt). *UNII-P3T5QA5J9N; UNII-5ZZ84GCW8B* [formoterol]. *CAS-43229-80-7; CAS-73573-87-2* [formoterol]. JAN. *Bronchodilator.* Foradil (Novartis); Performist (Dey) *[Name previously used: Eformoterol.]* ◇*CGP 25827A; BD 40A; YM-08316*

Forodesine [*2004*] (for oh′ de seen). $C_{11}H_{14}N_4O_4$. 266.25. (1) 4*H*-Pyrrolo[3,2-*d*]pyrimidin-4-one, 7-[(2*S*,3*S*,4*R*,5*R*)-3,4-dihydroxy-5-(hydroxymethyl)-2-pyrrolidinyl]-1,5-dihydro-; (2) (-)-7-[(2*S*,3*S*,4*R*,5*R*)-3,4-Dihydroxy-5-(hydroxymethyl)pyrrolidin-2-yl]-1,5-dihydro-4*H*-pyrrolo[3,2-*d*]pyrimidin-4-one. *UNII-426X066ELK. CAS-209799-67-7.*

Treatment of T-Cell malignancies such as acute lymphoblastic leukemia (ALL) and cutaneous T-cell lymphoma (CTCL). Fodosine (BioCryst) ◇*BCX-1777*

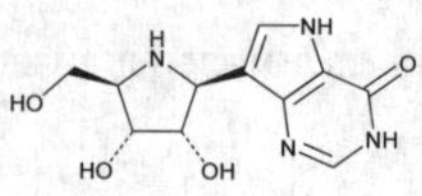

Forodesine Hydrochloride [*2004*] (for oh′ de seen hye″ droe klor′ ide). $C_{11}H_{14}N_4O_4 \cdot HCl$. 302.71. [Forodesine is INN.] (1) 4*H*-Pyrrolo[3,2-*d*]pyrimidin-4-one, 7-[(2*S*,3*S*,4*R*,5*R*)-3,4-dihydroxy-5-(hydroxymethyl)-2-pyrrolidinyl]-1,5-dihydro-, monohydrochloride; (2) (-)-7-[(2*S*,3*S*,4*R*,5*R*)-3,4-Dihydroxy-5-(hydroxymethyl)pyrrolidin-2-yl]-1,5-dihydro-4*H*-pyrrolo[3,2-*d*]pyrimidin-4-one monohydrochloride. *UNII-6SN82Y9U73; UNII-426X066ELK* [forodesine]. *CAS-284490-13-7; CAS-209799-67-7* [forodesine]. JAN. *Treatment of T-Cell malignancies such as acute lymphoblastic leukemia (ALL) and cutaneous T-cell lymphoma (CTCL).* ◇*BCX-1777*

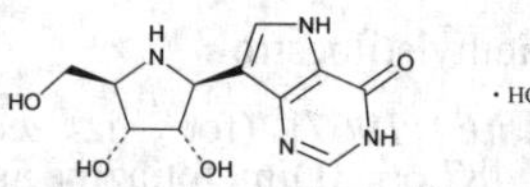

Foropafant. $C_{28}H_{40}N_4S$. 464.71. 3-[[[2-(Dimethylamino)ethyl][4-(2,4,6-triisopropylphenyl)-2-thiazolyl]amino]methyl]pyridine. *UNII-VWJ2QVH41J. CAS-136468-36-5.* INN.

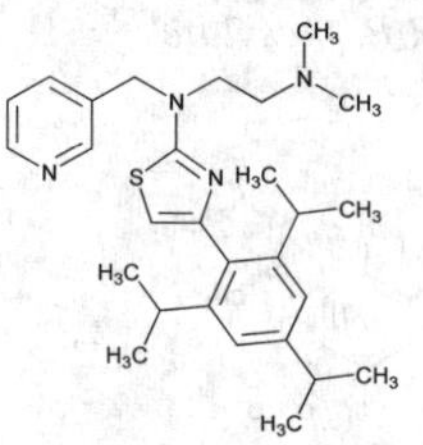

Forskolin — *See* Colforsin.

Fortimicin A — *See* Astromicin Sulfate.

Fosalvudine Tidoxil. $C_{35}H_{64}FN_2O_8PS$. 722.93. (2*RS*)-2-(Decyloxy)-3-[(dodecyl)sulfanyl]propyl [(2*R*,3*S*,5*R*)-3-fluoro-5-(5-methyl-2,4-dioxo-3,4-dihydropyrimidin-1(2*H*)-yl)tetrahydrofuran-2-yl]methyl hydrogen phosphate. *CAS-763903-67-9.* INN.

Fosamprenavir Calcium [*2000*] (fos″ am pren′ a vir kal′ see um). $C_{25}H_{36}CaN_3O_9PS$. 625.68. (1) Carbamic acid, [(1*S*,2*R*)-3-[[(4-aminophenyl)sulfonyl](2-methylpropyl)amino]-1-(phenylmethyl)-2-(phosphonooxy)propyl]-, *C*-[(3*S*)-tetrahydro-3-furanyl] ester, calcium salt (1:1); (2) (3*S*)-Tetrahydro-3-furyl [(α*S*)-α-[(1*R*)-1-hydroxy-2-(N^1-isobutylsulfanilamido)ethyl]phenethyl]carbamate, calcium phosphate (ester) (1:1). *UNII-ID1GU2627N. CAS-226700-81-8. Antiviral (HIV protease inhibitor).* Lexiva (GlaxoSmithKline) ◇*GW 433908G*

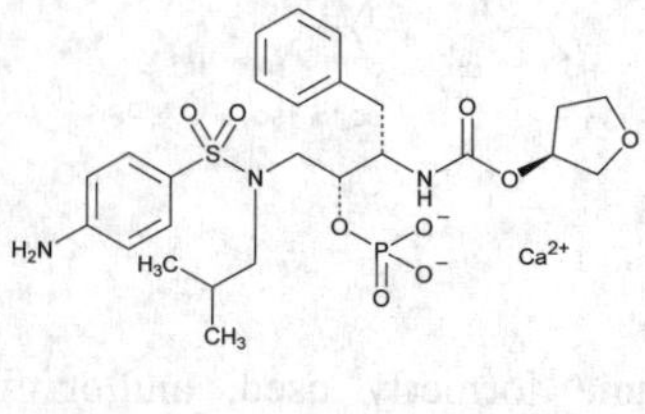

Fosamprenavir Sodium [*1999*] (fos″ am pren′ a vir soe′ dee um). $C_{25}H_{34}N_3Na_2O_9PS$. 629.57. [Fosamprenavir is INN.] (1) Carbamic acid, [(1*S*,2*R*)-3-[[(4-aminophenyl)sulfonyl](2-methylpropyl)amino]-1-(phenylmethyl)-2-(phosphonooxy)propyl]-, *C*-[(3*S*)-tetrahydro-3-furanyl] ester, disodium salt; (2) (3*S*)-Tetrahydro-3-furyl [(α*S*)-α-[(1*R*)-1-hydroxy-2-(*N*¹-isobutylsulfanilamido)ethyl]phenethyl]-carbamate, disodium phosphate (ester). *UNII-XSG28FSA0W*. *CAS-226700-80-7*; *CAS-226700-79-4* [fosamprenavir]. *Antiviral (HIV protease inhibitor).* ◇*GW 433908A*

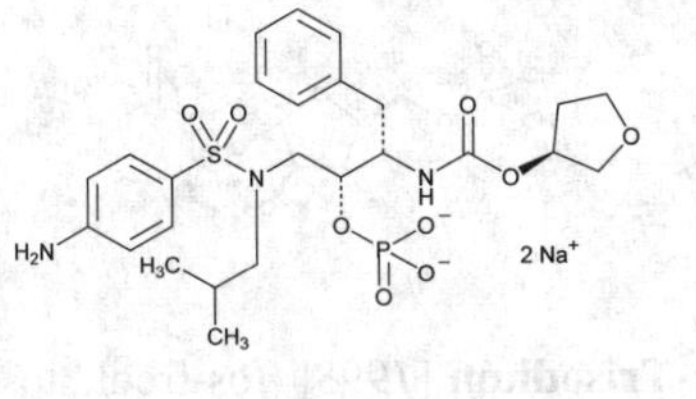

Fosaprepitant Dimeglumine [*2005*] (fos″ a pre′ pi tant di me′ gloo meen). $C_{23}H_{22}F_7N_4O_6P.2C_7H_{17}NO_5$. 1004.83. [Fosaprepitant is INN.] (1) D-Glucitol, 1-deoxy-1-(methylamino)-, [3-[[(2*R*,3*S*)-2-[(1*R*)-1-[3,5-bis(trifluoromethyl)phenyl]ethoxy]-3-(4-fluorophenyl)-4-morpholinyl]methyl]-2,5-dihydro-5-oxo-1*H*-1,2,4-triazol-1-yl]phosphonate (2:1) (salt); (2) Bis(1-deoxy-1-(methylamino)-D-Glucitol) [3-[[(2*R*,3*S*)-2-[(1*R*)-1-[3,5-bis(trifluoromethyl)phenyl]ethoxy]-3-(4-fluorophenyl)-4-morpholinyl]methyl]-2,5-dihydro-5-oxo-1*H*-1,2,4-triazol-1-yl]phosphonate. *UNII-D35FM8T64X*; *UNII-6L8OF9XRDC* [fosaprepitant]. *CAS-265121-04-8*; *CAS-172673-20-0* [fosaprepitant]. *Antiemetic.* ◇*MK-0517*

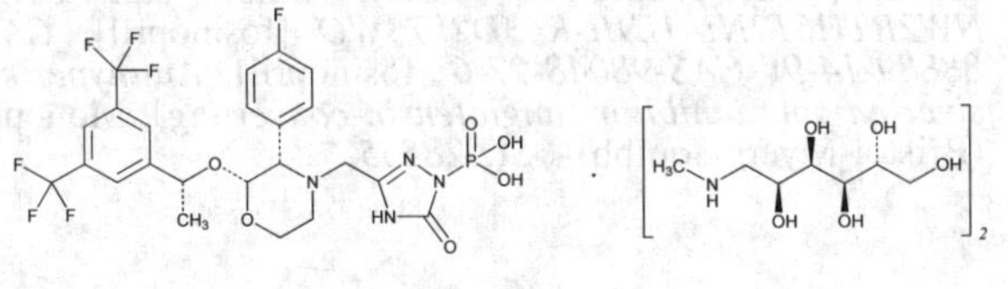

Fosarilate [*1985*] (fos ar′ i late). $C_{17}H_{28}ClO_5P$. 378.83. (1) Phosphonic acid, [6-(2-chloro-4-methoxyphenoxy)hexyl]-, diethyl ester; (2) Diethyl [6-(2-chloro-4-methoxyphenoxy)hexyl]phosphonate. *UNII-GM8PQW6Q2J*. *CAS-73514-87-1*. INN. *Antiviral.* ◇*Win 42,202*

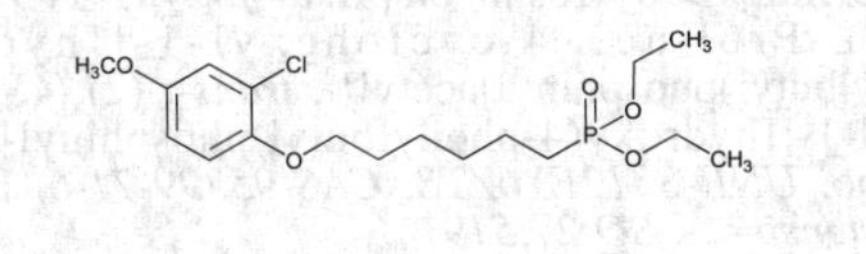

Fosazepam [*1975*] (fos az′ e pam). $C_{18}H_{18}ClN_2O_2P$. 360.77. (1) 2*H*-1,4-Benzodiazepin-2-one, 7-chloro-1-[(dimethylphosphinyl)methyl]-1,3-dihydro-5-phenyl-; (2) 7-Chloro-1-[(dimethylphosphinyl)methyl]-1,3-dihydro-5-phenyl-2*H*-1,4-benzodiazepin-2-one. *CAS-35322-07-7*. INN; BAN. *Sedative-hypnotic.* ◇*HR 930*

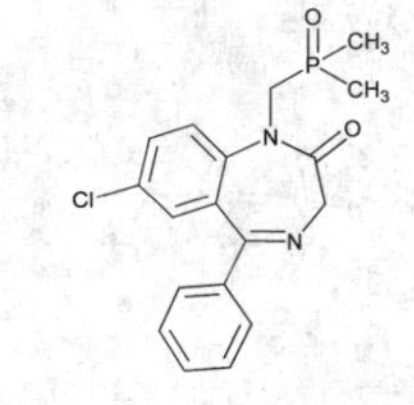

Fosbretabulin Disodium [*2008*] (fos″ bre ta bue′ lin dye soe′ dee um). $C_{18}H_{19}Na_2O_8P$. 440.29. (1) Phenol, 2-methoxy-5-[(1*Z*)-2-(3,4,5-trimethoxyphenyl)ethenyl]-, dihydrogen phosphate, disodium salt; (2) 2-Methoxy-5-[(1*Z*)-2-(3,4,5-trimethoxyphenyl)ethenyl]phenyl disodium phosphate. *UNII-702RHR475O*. *CAS-222030-63-9*. *Treatment of cancer and ocular vascular proliferative disorders.* ◇*CA4DP*

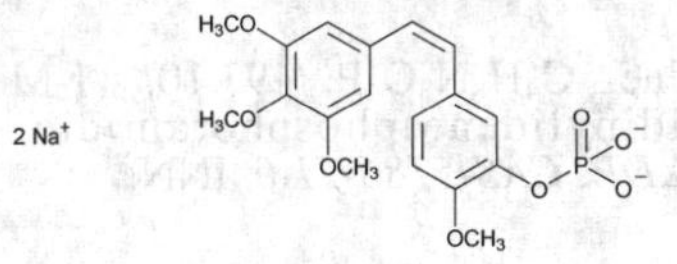

Foscarnet Sodium [*1985*] (fos kar′ net soe′ dee um). CNa_3O_5P. 191.95. (1) Phosphinecarboxylic acid, dihydroxy-, oxide, trisodium salt; (2) Phosphonoformic acid, trisodium salt. *UNII-964YS0OOG1*. *CAS-63585-09-1*. INN; BAN. *Antiviral.* Foscavir (AstraZeneca) ◇*EHB 776*

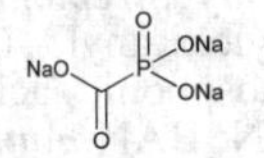

Foscolic Acid. $C_{16}H_{11}O_8P$. 362.23. 2,2′-Phosphinicodilactic acid. *CAS-2398-95-0*. INN. ◇*PDLA*

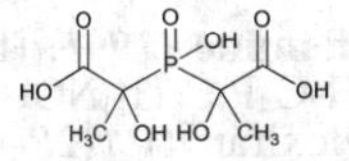

Fosenazide. $C_{14}H_{15}N_2O_2P$. 274.25. (Diphenylphosphinyl)acetic acid, hydrazide. *UNII-16C19Z7F4I*. *CAS-16543-10-5*. INN.

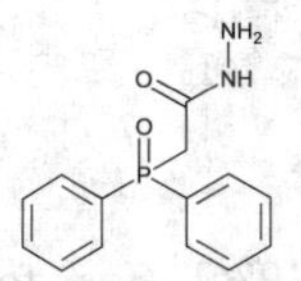

Fosenopril Sodium — *See* Fosinopril Sodium.

Fosfestrol (INN, BAN, JAN) — *See* Diethylstilbestrol Diphosphate.

Fosfluconazole. $C_{13}H_{13}F_2N_6O_4P$. 386.25. (1) 2,4-Difluoro-α,α-bis(1*H*-1,2,4-triazol-1-ylmethyl)benzyl alcohol, dihydrogen phosphate (ester); (2) 1-(2,4-Difluorophenyl)-2-

---

† Brand name formerly used, and/or firm no longer concerned with this product.

(1*H*-1,2,4-triazol-1-yl)-1-[(1*H*-1,2,4-triazol-1-yl)methyl]ethyl dihydrogen phosphate. *UNII-3JIJ299EWH. CAS-194798-83-9*. INN; BAN. ◇*UK-292,663*

Fosfluridine Tidoxil. $C_{34}H_{62}FN_2O_{10}PS$. 740.90. 5-Fluorouridine 5′-[(2*RS*)-2-(decyloxy)-3-(dodecylsulfanyl)propyl hydrogen phosphate]. *CAS-174638-15-4*. INN.

Fosfocreatinine. $C_4H_8N_3O_4P$. 193.10. (1-Methyl-4-oxo-2-imidazolidinylidene)phosphoramidic acid. *UNII-RG2371KXDE. CAS-5786-71-0*. INN.

Fosfomycin [*1970*] (fos″ foe mye′ sin). $C_3H_7O_4P$. 138.06. [Fosfomycin Calcium and Fosfomycin Sodium are JAN.] Antibiotic produced by *Streptomyces fradiae*. (1) Phosphonic acid, (3-methyloxiranyl)-, (2*R-cis*)-; (2) (-)-(1*R*,2*S*)-(1,2-Epoxypropyl)phosphonic acid. *UNII-2N81MY12TE. CAS-23155-02-4*. INN; BAN. *Antibacterial.*

Fosfomycin Tromethamine [*1991*] (fos″ foe mye′ sin troe meth′ a meen). $C_3H_7O_4P.C_4H_{11}NO_3$. 259.19. (1) Phosphonic acid, (3-methyloxiranyl)-, (2*R-cis*)-, compd. with 2-amino-2-(hydroxymethyl)-1,3-propanediol (1:1); (2) (1*R*,2*S*)-(1,2-Epoxypropyl)phosphonic acid, compound with 2-amino-2-(hydroxymethyl)-1,3-propanediol (1:1). *UNII-7FXW6U30GY. CAS-78964-85-9*. *Antibacterial*. Monurol (Zambon) ◇*Z 1282*

Fosfonet Sodium [*1976*] (fos′ foe net soe′ dee um). $C_2H_3Na_2O_5P.H_2O$. 202.01. (1) Phosphonoacetic acid, disodium salt, monohydrate; (2) Disodium phosphonoacetate monohydrate. *UNII-BY5RLE340B. CAS-54870-27-8; CAS-36983-81-0* [anhydrous]; *CAS-4408-78-0* [phosphonoacetic acid]. INN. *Antiviral*. ◇*Abbott-38642*

Fosfosal. $C_7H_7O_6P$. 218.10. Salicylic acid dihydrogen phosphate. *UNII-124X2V25W4. CAS-6064-83-1*. INN; MI.

Fosfructose. $C_6H_{14}O_{12}P_2$. 340.12. D-Fructose 1,6-bis(dihydrogen phosphate). *CAS-488-69-7*. INN.

Fosfructose Trisodium [*1998*] (fos frook′ tose trye soe′ dee um; fos fruk′ tose trye soe′ dee um). $C_6H_{11}Na_3O_{12}P_2.8H_2O$. 550.18. D-Fructose 1,6-bis(dihydrogen phosphate), trisodium salt, octahydrate. *CAS-81028-91-3. Cardioprotectant for ischemic disorders.* ◇*CPC-111*

Fosinopril Sodium [*1986*] (fos in′ oh pril soe′ dee um). **USP**. $C_{30}H_{45}NNaO_7P$. 585.64. [Fosinopril is INN and BAN.] (1) L-Proline, 4-cyclohexyl-1-[[[2-methyl-1-(1-oxopropoxy)propoxy](4-phenylbutyl)phosphinyl]acetyl]-, sodium salt, [1[*S**(*R**)],2α,4β]-; (2) (4*S*)-4-Cyclohexyl-1-[(*R*)-[(*S*)-1-hydroxy-2-methylpropoxy](4-phenylbutyl)phosphinyl]acetyl-L-proline propionate (ester), sodium salt. *UNII-NW2RTH6T2N; UNII-R43D2573WO* [fosinopril]. *CAS-88889-14-9; CAS-98048-97-6* [fosinopril]. *Antihypertensive; enzyme inhibitor (angiotensin-converting)*. Monopril (Bristol-Myers Squibb) ◇*SQ 28555*

Fosinoprilat [*1990*] (fos in′ oh pril at″). $C_{23}H_{34}NO_5P$. 435.49. (1) L-Proline, 4-cyclohexyl-1-[[hydroxy(4-phenylbutyl)phosphinyl]acetyl]-, *trans*-; (2) (4*S*)-4-Cyclohexyl-1-[[hydroxy(4-phenylbutyl)phosphinyl]acetyl]-L-proline. *UNII-S312EY6ZT8. CAS-95399-71-6*. INN. *Antihypertensive*. ◇*SQ 27,519*

Fosmenic Acid. $C_7H_{13}O_3P$. 176.15. (3-Cyclohexen-1-ylhydroxymethyl)phosphinic acid. *UNII-VD27I23138. CAS-13237-70-2.* INN.

Fosmidomycin. $C_4H_{10}NO_5P$. 183.10. [3-(*N*-Hydroxyformamido)propyl]phosphonic acid. *UNII-5829E3D9I9. CAS-66508-53-0.* INN.

Fosopamine. $C_9H_{14}NO_5P$. 247.18. 4-[2-(Methylamino)ethyl]-pyrocatechol 1-(dihydrogen phosphate). *UNII-50Q2Q042YR. CAS-103878-96-2.* INN.

Fosphenytoin Sodium [*1993*] (fos fen′ i toin soe′ dee um; fos fen′ i toe in soe′ dee um). **USP.** $C_{16}H_{13}N_2Na_2O_6P$. 406.24. [Fosphenytoin is INN and BAN.] (1) 2,4-Imidazolidinedione, 5,5-diphenyl-3-[(phosphonooxy)methyl]-, disodium salt; (2) 3-(Hydroxymethyl)-5,5-diphenylhydantoin, disodium phosphate (ester). *UNII-7VLR55452Z; UNII-B4SF212641* [fosphenytoin]. *CAS-92134-98-0; CAS-93390-81-9* [fosphenytoin]. *Anticonvulsant.* Cerebyx (Pfizer) ◇*ACC-9653-010 (sodium salt); CI-982*

Fospirate [*1968*] (fos′ pi rate). $C_7H_7Cl_3NO_4P$. 306.47. (1) Phosphoric acid, dimethyl 3,5,6-trichloro-2-pyridinyl ester; (2) Dimethyl 3,5,6-trichloro-2-pyridyl phosphate. *CAS-5598-52-7.* INN. *Anthelmintic (veterinary).*

Fospropofol Disodium [*2005*] (fos proe poe′ fol dye soe′ dee um). $C_{13}H_{19}Na_2O_5P$. 332.24. [Fospropofol is INN.] (1) Methanol, [2,6-bis(1-methylethyl)phenoxy]-, dihydrogen phosphate, disodium salt; (2) [2,6-Bis(1-methylethyl)phenoxy]methyl disodium phosphate; (3) 2,6-Diisopropylphenoxymethyl phosphate, disodium salt. *UNII-30868AY0IF;*

UNII-LZ257RZP7K [fospropofol]. *CAS-258516-87-9; CAS-258516-89-1* [fospropofol]. *Procedural sedation.* Aquavan (Guilford)

Fosquidone [*1990*] (fos′ kwi done). $C_{28}H_{22}NO_6P$. 499.45. (1) Phosphoric acid, mono(phenylmethyl) mono(5,8,13,14-tetrahydro-14-methyl-8,13-dioxobenz[5,6]isoindolo[2,1-*b*]isoquinolin-9-yl) ester, (±)-; (2) Benzyl (±)-5,8,13,14-tetrahydro-14-methyl-8,13-dioxobenz[5,6]isoindolo[2,1-*b*]isoquinolin-9-yl hydrogen phosphate. *UNII-FD6QP9BP8U. CAS-114517-02-1.* INN; BAN. *Antineoplastic.* ◇*GR 63178K*

Fostamatinib [*2008*] (fos″ ta ma′ ti nib). $C_{23}H_{26}FN_6O_9P$. 580.46. (1) 2*H*-Pyrido[3,2-*b*]-1,4-oxazin-3(4*H*)-one, 6-[[5-fluoro-2-[(3,4,5-trimethoxyphenyl)amino]-4-pyrimidinyl]amino]-2,2-dimethyl-4-[(phosphonooxy)methyl]-; (2) [6-({5-Fluoro-2-[(3,4,5-trimethoxyphenyl)amino]pyrimidin-4-yl}amino)-2,2-dimethyl-3-oxo-2,3-dihydro-4*H*-pyrido[3,2-*b*]-1,4-oxazin-4-yl]methyl dihydrogen phosphate. *CAS-901119-35-5. Treatment of rheumatoid arthritis, immune thrombocytopenic purpura, and B-cell lymphoma.* ◇*R935788 free acid; R788 free acid*

Fostamatinib Disodium [*2008*] (fos″ ta ma′ ti nib dye soe′ dee um). $C_{23}H_{24}FN_6Na_2O_9P \cdot 6H_2O$. 732.51. (1) 2*H*-Pyrido[3,2-*b*]-1,4-oxazin-3(4*H*)-one, 6-[[5-fluoro-2-[(3,4,5-trimethoxyphenyl)amino]-4-pyrimidinyl]amino]-2,2-dimethyl-4-[(phosphonooxy)methyl]-, disodium salt, hexahydrate; (2) [6-({5-Fluoro-2-[(3,4,5-trimethoxyphenyl)amino]pyrimidin-4-yl}amino)-2,2-dimethyl-3-oxo-2,3-dihydro-4*H*-pyrido[3,2-*b*]-1,4-oxazin-4-yl]methyl disodium phosphate hexahydrate. *UNII-86EEZ49YVB. CAS-914295-16-2. Treatment of rheumatoid arthritis, immune thrombocytopenic purpura, and B-cell lymphoma.* ◇*R935788 sodium; R788 sodium*

---

† Brand name formerly used, and/or firm no longer concerned with this product.

Fostedil [*1984*] (fos′ te dil). $C_{18}H_{20}NO_3PS$. 361.40. (1) Phosphonic acid, [[4-(2-benzothiazolyl)phenyl]methyl]-, diethyl ester; (2) Diethyl (*p*-2-benzothiazolylbenzyl)phosphonate. *CAS-75889-62-2.* INN. *Vasodilator (calcium channel blocker).* ◇*A-53986; KB-944*

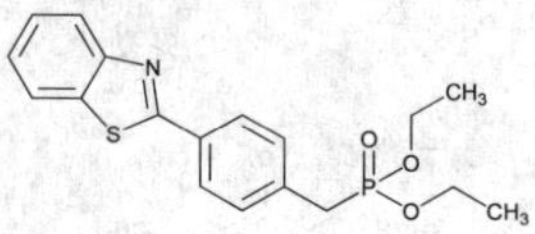

Fostriecin Sodium [*1986*] (fos′ trye e sin soe′ dee um). $C_{19}H_{26}NaO_9P$. 452.37. [Fostriecin is INN.] (1) 2*H*-Pyran-2-one, 5,6-dihydro-6-[3,6,13-trihydroxy-3-methyl-4-(phosphonooxy)-1,7,9,11-tridecatetraenyl]-, monosodium salt; (2) 5,6-Dihydro-6-[3,4,6,13-tetrahydroxy-3-methyl-1,7,9,11-tridecatetraenyl]-2*H*-pyran-2-one 4-(sodium hydrogen phosphate). *CAS-87860-39-7; CAS-87810-56-8* [fostriecin]. *Antineoplastic.* ◇*CI-920*

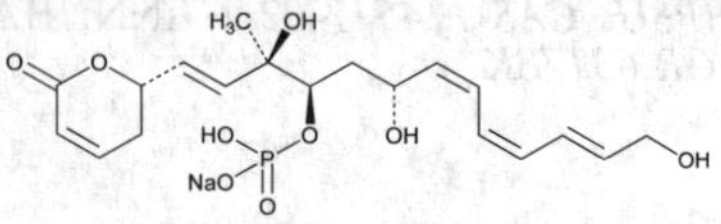

Fosveset [*1999*] (fos′ ve set). $C_{33}H_{44}N_3O_{14}P$. 737.69. (1) 2-Oxa-6,9-diaza-1-phosphaundecan-11-oic acid, 4-[bis(carboxymethyl)amino]-6,9-bis(carboxymethyl)-1-[(4,4-diphenylcyclohexyl)oxy]-1-hydroxy-, 1-oxide; (2) *N*-[2-[Bis(carboxymethyl)amino]ethyl]-*N*-[(*R*)-2-[bis(carboxymethyl)amino]-3-hydroxypropyl]glycine, 4,4-diphenylcyclohexyl hydrogen phosphate (ester). *CAS-193901-91-6.* INN. *Ligant excipient.* ◇*MS 325168A*

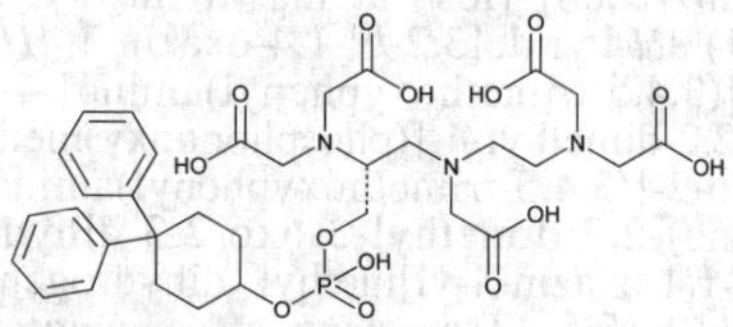

Fotemustine. $C_9H_{19}ClN_3O_5P$. 315.69. (±)-Diethyl [1-[3-(2-chloroethyl)-3-nitrosoureido]ethyl]phosphonate. *CAS-92118-27-9.* INN; BAN; MI. ◇*S 10036*

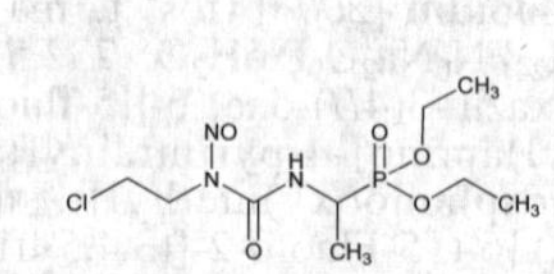

Fotretamine. $C_{14}H_{28}N_9OP_3$. 431.35. 2,2,4,4,6-Pentakis(1-aziridinyl)-2,2,4,4,6,6-hexahydro-6-morpholino-1,3,5,2,4,6-triazatriphosphorine. *UNII-7Z7670589C. CAS-37132-72-2.* INN.

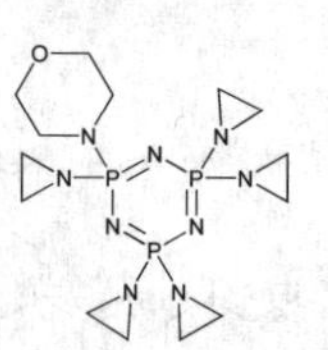

Fouchet's Reagent [Solution]. A solution of trichloroacetic acid, ferric chloride, and purified water.

Fozivudine Tidoxil. $C_{35}H_{64}N_5O_8PS$. 745.95. (2*RS*)-2-(Decyloxy)-3-(dodecylthio)propyl hydrogen 3′-azido-3′-deoxy-5′-thymidylate. *CAS-141790-23-0.* INN.

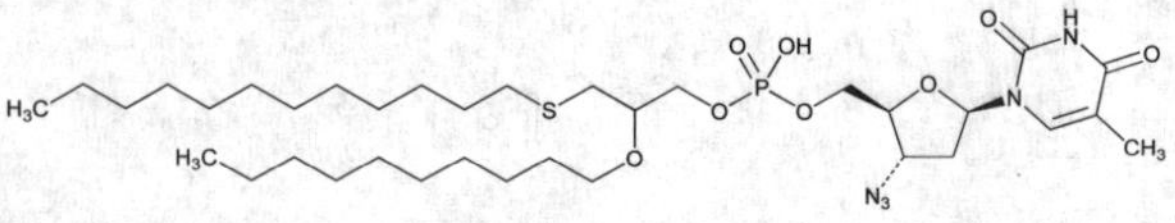

Frabuprofen. $C_{26}H_{33}F_3N_2O_2$. 462.55. 2-[4-(α,α,α-Trifluoro-*m*-tolyl)-1-piperazinyl]ethyl (±)-*p*-isobutylhydratropate. *UNII-K0T69WUD4Z. CAS-86696-88-0.* INN.

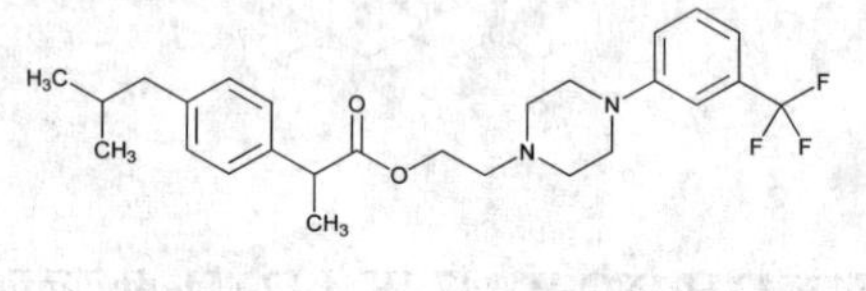

Fradafiban. $C_{20}H_{21}N_3O_4$. 367.40. (3*S*,5*S*)-5-[[(4′-Amidino-4-biphenylyl)oxy]methyl]-2-oxo-3-pyrrolidineacetic acid. *UNII-DQ0H2B8YKN. CAS-148396-36-5.* INN.

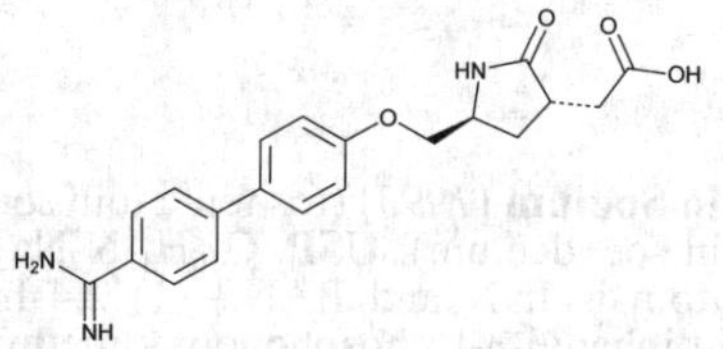

Fradiomycin Sulfate (JAN) — *See* Neomycin Sulfate.

Frakefamide. $C_{30}H_{34}FN_5O_5$. 563.62. L-Tyrosyl-D-alanyl-*p*-fluoro-L-phenylalanyl-L-phenylalaninamide. *UNII-DM32B4GU70. CAS-188196-22-7.* INN.

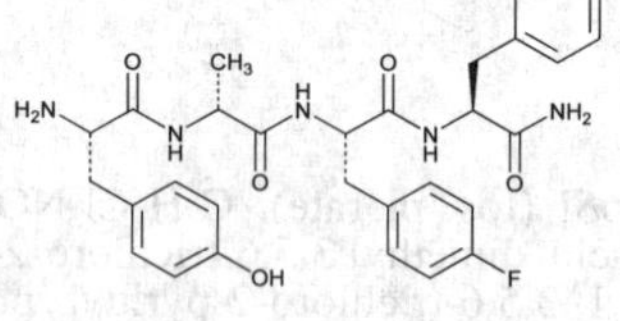

Framycetin. $C_{23}H_{46}N_6O_{13}$. 614.64. Antibiotic produced by *Streptomyces decaris.* Neomycin B. *UNII-4BOC774388. CAS-119-04-0.* INN; BAN; DCF.

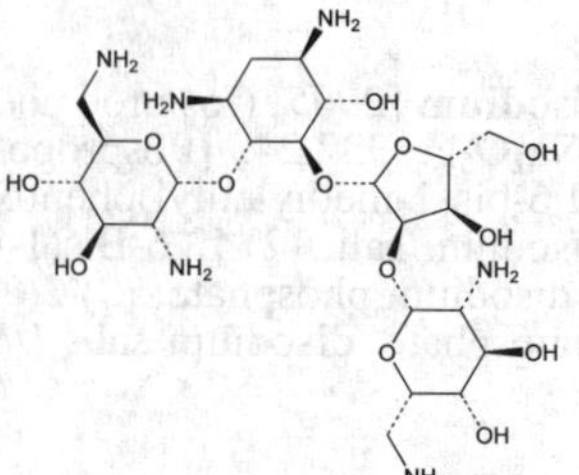

Frentizole [*1976*] (fren′ ti zole). $C_{15}H_{13}N_3O_2S$. 299.35. (1) Urea, *N*-(6-methoxy-2-benzothiazolyl)-*N*′-phenyl-; (2) 1-(6-Methoxy-2-benzothiazolyl)-3-phenylurea. *CAS-26130-02-9*. INN; BAN. *Immunoregulator.* ◇*Compound 53616*

Freselestat. $C_{23}H_{28}N_6O_4$. 452.51. 2-[5-Amino-6-oxo-2-phenylpyrimidin-1(6*H*)-yl]-*N*-[(1*RS*)-1-(5-*tert*-butyl-1,3,4-oxadiazol-2-yl)-3-methyl-1-oxobutan-2-yl]acetamide. *CAS-208848-19-5*. INN.

Fronepidil. $C_{21}H_{31}NO_2$. 329.48. 1-[1-(Isobutoxymethyl)-2-[(1-methyl-1-phenyl-2-propynyl)oxy]ethyl]pyrrolidine. *UNII-94JPL25DUK*. *CAS-79700-63-3*. INN.

Fropenem (previously used name) — *See* Faropenem Medoxomil.

Frovatriptan. $C_{14}H_{17}N_3O$. 243.30. (*R*)-5,6,7,8-Tetrahydro-6-(methylamino)carbazole-3-carboxamide. *UNII-H82Q2D5WA7*. *CAS-158747-02-5*. INN; BAN.

Frovatriptan Succinate [*1997*] (froe″ va trip′ tan sux′ i nate). $C_{14}H_{17}N_3O.C_4H_6O_4.H_2O$. 379.41. (1) (+)-(*R*)-2,3,4,9-Tetrahydro-3-(methylamino)-1*H*-carbazole-6-carboxamide butanedioate (1:1), monohydrate; (2) (+)-(*R*)-5,6,7,8-Tetrahydro-6-(methylamino)carbazole-3-carboxamide succinate (1:1), monohydrate. *UNII-D28J6W18HY*. *CAS-158930-17-7*. *Antimigraine (5-HT$_{1D}$agonist)*. Frova (Endo) ◇*SB 209509-AX; VML 251*

Froxiprost. $C_{24}H_{29}F_3O_6$. 470.48. Methyl (2*E*,5*Z*)-7-[(1*R*,2*R*,3*R*,5*S*)-3,5-dihydroxy-2-[(*E*)-(3*R*)-3-hydroxy-4-[(α,α,α-trifluoro-*m*-tolyl)oxy]-1-butenyl]cyclopentyl]-2,5-heptadienoate. *UNII-EOS1G6F668*. *CAS-62559-74-4*. INN.

Fructose (fruk′ tose; frook′ tose). **USP**. $C_6H_{12}O_6$. 180.16. (1) D-Fructose; (2) D-Fructose. *UNII-6YSS42VSEV*. *CAS-57-48-7*. JAN. *Nutrient.*

Frusemide (previously used name) — *See* Furosemide.

Ftalofyne (INN) — *See* Phthalofyne.

Ftaxilide. $C_{16}H_{15}NO_3$. 269.30. 2′,6′-Dimethylphthalanilic acid. *UNII-7Z71845H3F*. *CAS-19368-18-4*. INN; DCF; MI.

(-)-FTC (trivial name) — *See* Emtricitabine.

FTC-(-) (trivial name) — *See* Emtricitabine.

Ftivazide. $C_{14}H_{13}N_3O_3$. 271.27. Isonicotinic acid vanillylidenehydrazide. *UNII-40Q4C3O4V0*. *CAS-149-17-7*. INN.

Ftormetazine. $C_{21}H_{22}F_3N_3OS$. 421.48. 10-[3-(4-Methyl-1-piperazinyl)propionyl]-2-(trifluoromethyl)phenothiazine. *UNII-1P441EE1PH*. *CAS-33414-30-1*. INN.

---

† Brand name formerly used, and/or firm no longer concerned with this product.

Ftorpropazine. $C_{22}H_{24}F_3N_3O_2S$. 451.51. 10-[3-[4-(2-Hydroxyethyl)-1-piperazinyl]propionyl]-2-(trifluoromethyl)phenothiazine. *UNII-CU0X85F735*. *CAS-33414-36-7*. INN.

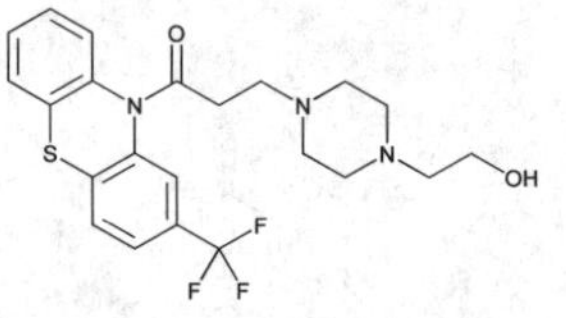

Fubrogonium Iodide. $C_{14}H_{23}BrINO_3$. 460.15. Diethyl (3-hydroxybutyl)methylammonium iodide 5-bromo-2-furoate. *UNII-4791MN0PVE*. *CAS-3690-58-2*. INN.

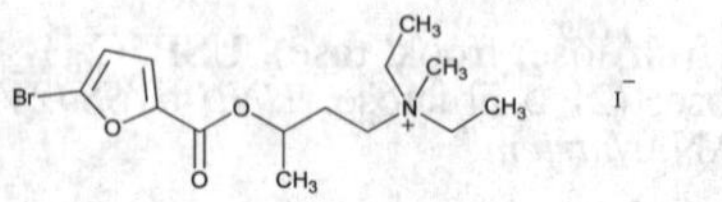

Fuchsin, Basic (fook′ sin). **USP**. $C_{20}H_{19}N_3$.HCl. 301.39 (rosaniline form); $C_{19}H_{17}N_3$.HCl. 287.36 (pararosaniline form). (1) Benzenamine, 4-[(4-aminophenyl)(4-imino-2,5-cyclohexadien-1-ylidene)methyl]-2-methyl-, monohydrochloride; (2) C.I. Basic Violet 14 monohydrochloride. *CAS-632-99-5*. *Anti-infective, topical.*

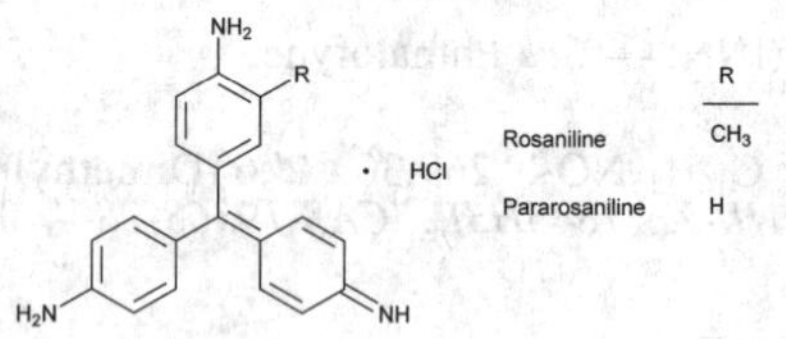

Fudosteine. $C_6H_{13}NO_3S$. 179.24. (-)-3-[(3-Hydroxypropyl)thio]-L-alanine. *UNII-UR9VPI71PT*. *CAS-13189-98-5*. INN.

Fuladectin. A mixture of Fuladectin Component A_4 and Fuladectin Component A_3 (80:20). INN.

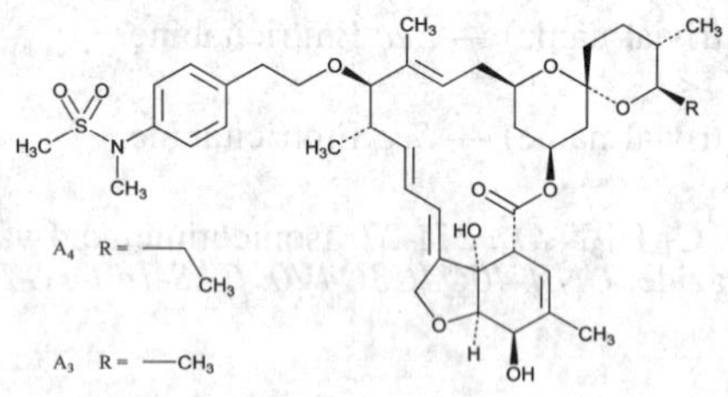

Fuladectin Component A_3. $C_{41}H_{57}NO_{10}S$. 755.96. 4′-[2-[[(2a*E*,4*E*,5′*S*,6*S*,6′*R*,7*R*,8*E*,11*R*,13*R*,15*S*,17a*R*,20-*R*,20a*R*,20b*S*)-3′,4′,5′,6,6′,7,10,11,14,15,17a,20,20a,20b-Tetradecahydro-20,20b-dihydroxy-5′,6,6′,8,19-pentamethyl-17-oxospiro[11,15-methano-2*H*,13*H*,17*H*-furo[4,3,2-*pq*][2,6]benzodioxacyclooctadecin-13,2′-[2*H*]pyran]-7-yl]oxy]ethyl]-*N*-methylmethanesulfonanilide. *CAS-150702-33-3*. INN.

Fuladectin Component A_4. $C_{42}H_{59}NO_{10}S$. 769.98. 4′-[2-[[(2a*E*,4*E*,5′*S*,6*S*,6′*R*,7*R*,8*E*,11*R*,13*R*,15*S*,17a*R*,20-*R*,20a*R*,20b*S*)-6′-Ethyl-3′,4′,5′,6,6′,7,10,11,14,15,17a,-20,20a,20b-tetradecahydro-20,20b-dihydroxy-5′,6,8,19-tetramethyl-17-oxospiro[11,15-methano-2*H*,13*H*,17*H*-furo[4,3,2-*pq*][2,6]benzodioxacyclooctadecin-13,2′-[2*H*]pyran]-7-yl]oxy]ethyl]-*N*-methylmethanesulfonanilide. *CAS-150702-32-2*. INN.

Fulmicoton — *See* Pyroxylin.

Fulvestrant [*1998*] (ful ves′ trant). $C_{32}H_{47}F_5O_3S$. 606.77. (1) Estra-1,3,5(10)-triene-3,17-diol, 7-[9-[(4,4,5,5,5-pentafluoropentyl)sulfinyl]nonyl]-, (7α,17β)-; (2) 7α-[9-[(4,4,5,5,-Pentafluoropentyl)sulfinyl]nonyl]estra-1,3,5(10)-triene-3,17β-diol. *UNII-22X328QOC4*. *CAS-129453-61-8*. INN; BAN. *Treatment of breast cancer (antiestrogen).* Faslodex (AstraZeneca) ◇*ICI 182,780; ZD9238*

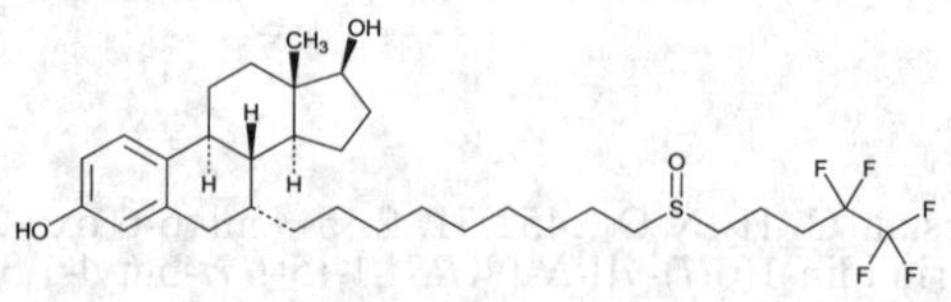

Fumagillin. $C_{26}H_{34}O_7$. 458.54. Antibiotic obtained from cultures of *Aspergillus fumigatus*, or the same substance produced by any other means. *UNII-7OW73204U1*. *CAS-23110-15-8*. INN; BAN; DCF; MI. Fumidil (Abbott†)

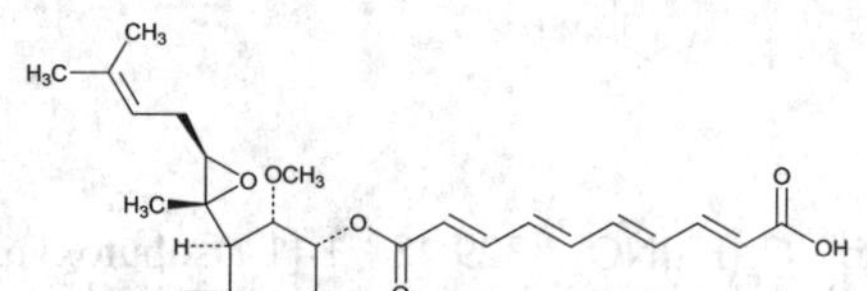

Fumaric Acid (fue mar′ ik as′ id). **NF**. $C_4H_4O_4$. 116.07. (1) 2-Butenedioic acid, [*E*]-; (2) Fumaric acid. *UNII-88XHZ13131*. *CAS-110-17-8*. *Acidifier.*

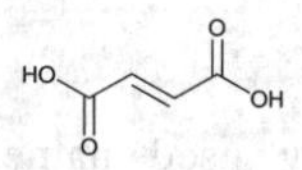

Fumoxicillin [*1984*] (fue mox″ i sil′ in). $C_{21}H_{21}N_3O_6S$. 443.47. (1) 4-Thia-1-azabicyclo[3.2.0]heptane-2-carboxylic acid, 6-[[[(2-furanylmethylene)amino](4-hydroxyphenyl)acetyl]amino]-3,3-dimethyl-7-oxo-, [2*S*-[2α,5α,6β(*S**)]]-; (2) (2*S*,5*R*,6*R*)-6-[(*R*)-2-(Furfurylideneamino)-2-(*p*-hydroxyphenyl)acetamido]-3,3-dimethyl-7-oxo-4-thia-1-azabicyclo[3.2.0]heptane-2-carboxylic acid. *UNII-C7H9M9492J*. *CAS-78186-33-1*. INN. *Antibacterial.* ◇*FU-02*

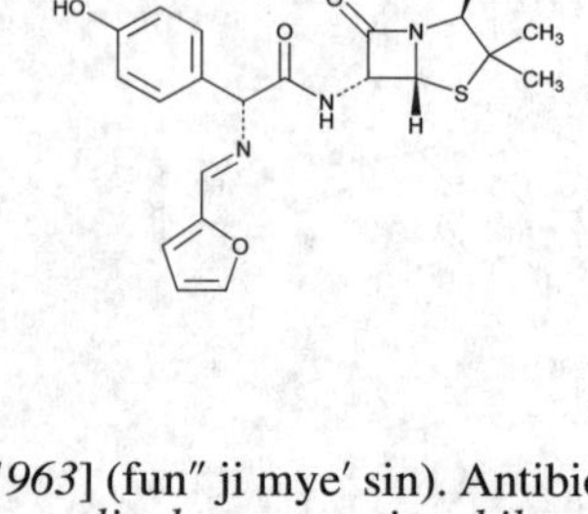

Fungimycin [*1963*] (fun″ ji mye′ sin). Antibiotic produced by *Streptomyces coelicolor* var. *aminophilus*. (1) Fungimycin; (2) Fungimycin. *CAS-1404-87-1*. *Antifungal.* ◇*NC-1968; WX 2412*

Fuprazole. $C_{28}H_{30}N_4O_2$. 454.56. 3-[2-[[(4-Cinnamyl-1-piper-azinyl)methyl]-1-benzimidazolyl]-1-(2-furyl)-1-propanone. *UNII-47JUM7D622. CAS-60248-23-9.* INN.

Furacilin — *See* Nitrofurazone.

Furacrinic Acid. $C_{15}H_{14}O_4$. 258.27. 6-Methyl-5-(2-methylenebutyryl)-2-benzofurancarboxylic acid. *CAS-23580-33-8.* INN; BAN. ◇48-674

Furafylline. $C_{12}H_{12}N_4O_3$. 260.25. 3-Furfuryl-1,8-dimethylxanthine. *UNII-C2087G0XX3. CAS-80288-49-9.* INN.

Furalazine. $C_9H_7N_5O_3$. 233.18. 3-Amino-6-[2-(5-nitro-2-furyl)vinyl]-*as*-triazine. *UNII-2133JVQ6VE. CAS-556-12-7.* INN.

Furaltadone. $C_{13}H_{16}N_4O_6$. 324.29. (±)-5-(Morpholinomethyl)-3-[(5-nitrofurfurylidene)amino]-2-oxazolidinone. *UNII-5X4V82ZN30. CAS-139-91-3.* INN; BAN; MI.

Furaprofen [*1979*] (fure″ a proe′ fen). $C_{17}H_{14}O_3$. 266.29. (1) 7-Benzofuranacetic acid, α-methyl-3-phenyl-, (±)-; (2) (±)-α-Methyl-3-phenyl-7-benzofuranacetic acid. *UNII-T9G78A1R21. CAS-67700-30-5.* INN. *Anti-inflammatory.* [*Name previously used: Enprofen*] ◇R-803

Furazabol. $C_{20}H_{30}N_2O_2$. 330.46. 17-Methyl-5α-androstano[2,3-*c*]furazan-17β-ol. *UNII-2W07HSP5PX. CAS-1239-29-8.* INN; JAN; MI.

Furazolidone (fure″ a zol′ i done). **USP.** $C_8H_7N_3O_5$. 225.16. (1) 2-Oxazolidinone, 3-[[(5-nitro-2-furanyl)methylene]amino]-; (2) 3-[(5-Nitrofurfurylidene)amino]-2-oxazolidinone. *UNII-5J9CPU3RE0. CAS-67-45-8.* INN; BAN. *Anti-infective, topical; antiprotozoal (Trichomonas, topical).* Furoxone (Shire)

Furazolium Chloride [*1964*] (fure″ a zoe′ lee um klor′ ide). $C_9H_8ClN_3O_3S$. 273.70. (1) 5*H*-Imidazo[2,1-*b*]thiazol-4-ium, 6,7-dihydro-3-(5-nitro-2-furanyl)-, chloride; (2) 6,7-Dihydro-3-(5-nitro-2-furyl)-5*H*-imidazo[2,1-*b*]thiazolium chloride. *CAS-5118-17-2.* INN. *Antibacterial.* ◇NF-963

Furazolium Tartrate [*1968*] (fure″ a zoe′ lee um tar′ trate). $C_{13}H_{13}N_3O_9S$. 387.32. (1) 5*H*-Imidazo[2,1-*b*]thiazol-4-ium, 6,7-dihydro-3-(5-nitro-2-furanyl)-, [*R*-(*R**,*R**)]-2,3-dihydroxybutanedioate (1:1); (2) 6,7-Dihydro-3-(5-nitro-2-furyl)-5*H*-imidazo[2,1-*b*]thiazolium hydrogen tartrate. *CAS-17692-15-8. Antibacterial.* ◇NF-1425

Furbucillin. $C_{19}H_{24}N_2O_7S$. 424.47. 6-[(*R*)-2-Hydroxy-4-methylvaleramido]-3,3-dimethyl-7-oxo-4-thia-1-azabicyclo[3.2.0]heptane-2-carboxylic acid 2-furoate (ester). *UNII-104NHK678E. CAS-54340-65-7.* INN.

Furcloprofen. $C_{15}H_{11}ClO_3$. 274.70. (+)-8-Chloro-α-methyl-3-dibenzofuranacetic acid. *UNII-V52IY042L9. CAS-58012-63-8.* INN.

Furegrelate Sodium [*1985*] (fure eg′ re late soe′ dee um). $C_{15}H_{10}NNaO_3 \cdot H_2O$. 293.25. [Furegrelate is INN.] (1) 2-Benzofurancarboxylic acid, 5-(3-pyridinylmethyl)-, sodium salt, monohydrate; (2) Sodium 5-(3-pyridylmethyl)-2-benzofurancarboxylate monohydrate. *UNII-*

---

† Brand name formerly used, and/or firm no longer concerned with this product.

KX4D9BZA6X [furegrelate]. *CAS-87463-91-0; CAS-85666-24-6* [furegrelate]. *Inhibitor (thromboxane synthetase).* ◇*U-63,557A*

Furethidine. $C_{21}H_{31}NO_4$. 361.48. 1-(2-Tetrahydrofurfuryloxyethyl)-4-phenylpiperidine-4-carboxylic acid ethyl ester. *UNII-6U9XA4JOD4. CAS-2385-81-1.* INN; BAN; DCF; MI.

Furfenorex. $C_{15}H_{19}NO$. 229.32. (+)-*N*-Methyl-*N*-(α-methylphenethyl)furfurylamine. *UNII-X83CZ0Y5TF. CAS-3776-93-0.* INN; DCF. ◇*SD 27115 [as cyclamate]; E-106-E [as cyclamate]*

Furidarone. $C_{13}H_{10}I_2O_3$. 468.03. 2,5-Dimethyl-3-furyl-4-hydroxy-3,5-diiodophenyl ketone. *UNII-F93C12LM0D. CAS-4662-17-3.* INN.

Furmethoxadone. $C_9H_9N_3O_5$. 239.18. 5-Methyl-3-(5-nitrofurfurylideneamino)-2-oxazolidinone. *UNII-G31553PPJU. CAS-6281-26-1.* INN.

Furnidipine. $C_{21}H_{24}N_2O_7$. 416.42. (±)-Methyl tetrahydrofurfuryl,1,4-dihydro-2,6-dimethyl-4-(*o*-nitrophenyl)-3,5-pyridinedicarboxylate. *UNII-AJ6J4424XT. CAS-138661-03-7.* INN.

Furobufen [*1973*] (fure″ oh bue′ fen). $C_{16}H_{12}O_4$. 268.26. (1) 2-Dibenzofuranbutanoic acid, γ-oxo-; (2) γ-Oxo-2-dibenzofuranbutyric acid. *CAS-38873-55-1.* INN. *Anti-inflammatory.* ◇*AY-21,367*

Furodazole [*1977*] (fure oh′ da zole). $C_{15}H_{11}N_3O_2 \cdot xH_2O$. 265.27 (anhydrous). (1) 1*H*-Imidazo[4,5-*f*]quinolin-9-ol, 2-(2-furanyl)-7-methyl-, hydrate; (2) 2-(2-Furyl)-7-methyl-1*H*-imidazo[4,5-*f*]quinolin-9-ol hydrate. *UNII-9745E7HEBG. CAS-56119-96-1* [anhydrous]. INN. *Anthelmintic.* ◇*F-691*

Furofenac. $C_{12}H_{14}O_3$. 206.24. 2-Ethyl-2,3-dihydro-5-benzofuranacetic acid. *UNII-86TB3JLD8A. CAS-56983-13-2.* INN.

Furomazine. $C_{24}H_{27}ClN_2O_3S$. 459.00. 3-[1-[3-(2-Chlorophenothiazin-10-yl)propyl]-4-hydroxy-4-piperidyl]dihydro-2(3*H*)-furanone. *UNII-4868V9LSKR. CAS-28532-90-3.* INN.

Furomine [*1995*] (fure′ oh meen). $C_{20}H_{32}N_2O_4$. 364.48. (1) 4,4′-[1,2-Ethanediylbis(iminomethylidyne)]bis[dihydro-2,2,5,5-tetramethyl-3(2*H*)-furanone; (2) 4,4′-[Ethylenebis(iminomethylidyne)]bis[dihydro-2,2,5,5-tetramethyl-3(2*H*)-furanone]. *UNII-T2GIP8IIG6. CAS-142996-66-5.* INN; BAN. *Ligand.* ◇*MP-1549*

Furosemide [*1964*] (fure oh′ se mide). **USP.** $C_{12}H_{11}ClN_2O_5S$. 330.74. (1) Benzoic acid, 5-(aminosulfonyl)-4-chloro-2-[(2-furanylmethyl)amino]-; (2) 4-Chloro-*N*-furfuryl-5-sulfamoylanthranilic acid. *UNII-7LXU5N7ZO5. CAS-54-31-9.* INN; BAN; JAN. *Diuretic.* Lasix (Sanofi Aventis) *[Name previously used: Frusemide.]* ◇*LB-502*

Furostilbestrol. $C_{28}H_{24}O_6$. 456.49. α,α'-Diethyl-4,4'-stilbene-diol di-2-furoate. *UNII-JN9M0YN4VL. CAS-549-40-6.* INN; DCF.

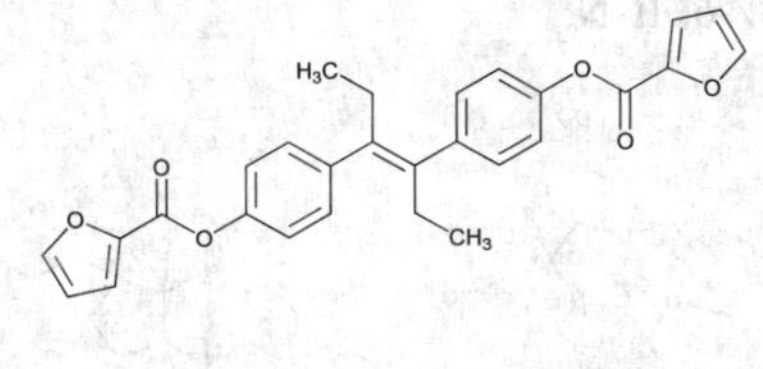

Furoxicillin — *See* Fumoxicillin.

Fursalan [*1967*] (fure′ sa lan). $C_{12}H_{13}Br_2NO_3$. 379.04. (1) Benzamide, 3,5-dibromo-2-hydroxy-*N*-[(tetrahydro-2-fur-anyl)methyl]-; (2) 3,5-Dibromo-*N*-(tetrahydrofurfuryl)sali-cylamide. *CAS-15686-77-8.* INN. *Disinfectant.*

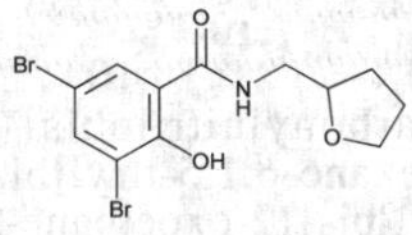

Fursultiamine. $C_{17}H_{26}N_4O_3S_2$. 398.54. [Fursultiamine Hydro-chloride is JAN.] *N*-[(4-Amino-2-methyl-5-pyrimidinyl)-methyl]-*N*-[4-hydroxy-1-methyl-2-[(tetrahydrofurfuryl)-dithio]-1-butenyl]formamide. *CAS-804-30-8.* INN; JAN; MI. ◇*TTFD*

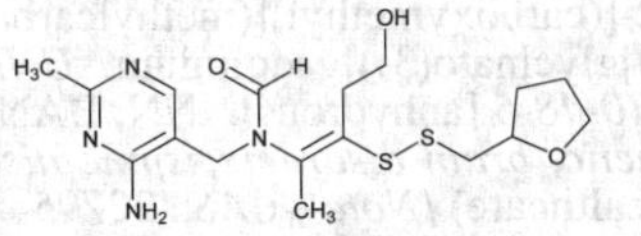

Furterene. $C_{10}H_9N_7O$. 243.22. 2,4,7-Triamino-6-(2-furyl)p-teridine. *UNII-TY1X1WG26A. CAS-7761-75-3.* INN; DCF; MI.

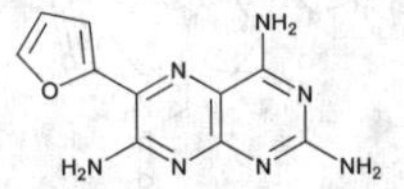

Furtrethonium Iodide. $C_8H_{14}INO$. 267.11. Furfuryltrimethy-lammonium iodide. *UNII-1D064NLD7G; UNII-AI-Q630U6XO* [furtrethonium]. *CAS-541-64-0; CAS-7618-86-2* [furtrethonium]. INN; MI. Furmethide Iodide (SmithKline Beecham†)

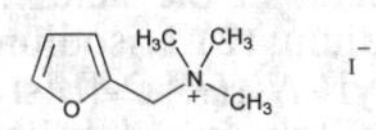

Furtrimethonium Iodide — *See* Furtrethonium Iodide.

Fusafungine. Antibiotic obtained from cultures of a *fusarium* belonging to *Lateritium Wr.* section, or the same substance produced by any other means. *CAS-1393-87-9.* INN; BAN; DCF; MI. ◇*S 314*

Fusidate Sodium [*1968*] (fue′ si date soe′ dee um). $C_{31}H_{47}NaO_4$. 506.69. [Sodium Fusidate is JAN.] (1) 29-Nordammara-17(20),24-dien-21-oic acid, 16-(acetyloxy)-3,11-dihydroxy-, monosodium salt, $(3\alpha,4\alpha,8\alpha,9\beta,11\alpha,13\alpha,14\beta,16\beta,17Z)$-; (2) Sodium $3\alpha,11\alpha,16\beta$-trihydroxy-29-nor-$8\alpha,9\beta,13\alpha,14\beta$-dammara-17(20),24-dien-21-oate 16-acetate; (3) Fusidic acid, so-dium salt. *UNII-J7P3696BCQ; UNII-59XE10C19C* [fusi-dic acid]. *CAS-751-94-0; CAS-6990-06-3* [fusidic acid]. *Antibacterial.* Fucidine (Bristol-Myers Squibb†) ◇*SQ 16360*

Fusidic Acid [*1967*] (fue sid′ ik as′ id). $C_{31}H_{48}O_6$. 516.71. (1) 29-Nordammara-17(20),24-dien-21-oic acid, 16-(acety-loxy)-3,11-dihydroxy-, $(3\alpha,4\alpha,8\alpha,9\beta,11\alpha,13\alpha,14\beta,16\beta,17Z)$-; (2) $3\alpha,11\alpha,16\beta$-Trihydroxy-29-nor-$8\alpha,9\beta,13\alpha,14\beta$-dammara-17(20),24-dien-21-oic acid 16-acetate; (3) Fusidic acid. *UNII-59XE10C19C. CAS-6990-06-3.* INN; BAN. *Antibacterial.* ◇*SQ 16,603*

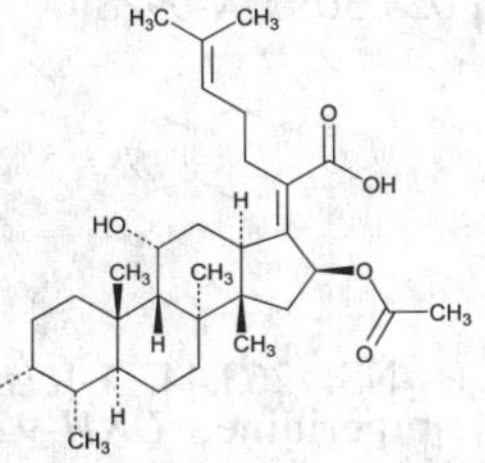

Fuzlocillin. $C_{25}H_{26}N_6O_8S$. 570.57. $(2S,5R,6R)$-6-[(2*R*)-2-[3-[(*E*)-Furfurylideneamino]-2-oxo-1-imidazolidinecarboxa-mido]-2-(*p*-hydroxyphenyl)acetamido]-3,3-dimethyl-7-oxo-4-thia-1-azabicyclo[3.2.0]heptane-2-carboxylic acid. *UNII-J6UQP7JHOT. CAS-66327-51-3.* INN; BAN. ◇*BAY BAY Vk 4999*

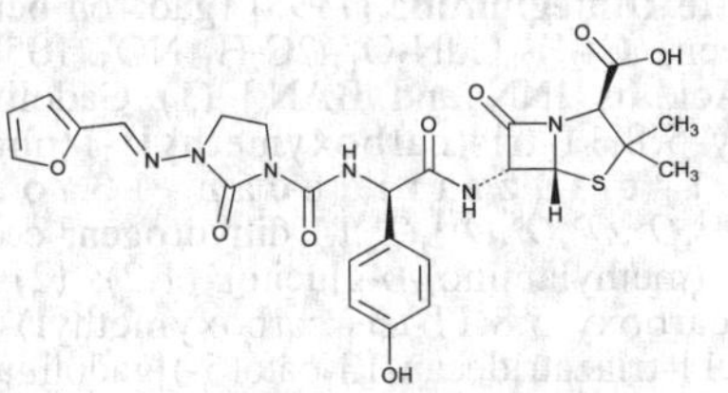

Fytic Acid (INN) — *See* Phytic Acid.

G6M — *See* Galamustine.

^{67}Ga — *See* Gallium Citrate Ga 67.

Gabapentin [*1989*] (gab″ a pen′ tin). **USP.** $C_9H_{17}NO_2$. 171.24. (1) Cyclohexaneacetic acid, 1-(aminomethyl)-; (2) 1-(Aminomethyl)cyclohexaneacetic acid. *UNII-6CW7F3G59X. CAS-60142-96-3.* INN; BAN. *Anticonvul-sant.* Neurontin (Pfizer) ◇*CI-945; GOE 3450*

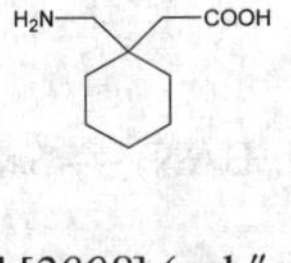

Gabapentin Enacarbil [*2008*] (gab″ a pen′ tin en″ a kar′ bil). $C_{16}H_{27}NO_6$. 329.39. (1) Cyclohexaneacetic acid, 1-[[[[1-(2-methyl-1-oxopropoxy)ethoxy]carbonyl]amino]methyl]-; (2) (1-{[({(1*RS*)-1-[(2-Methylpropanoyl)oxy]ethoxy}carbonyl)amino]methyl}cyclohexyl)acetic acid. *UNII-75OCL1SPBQ. CAS-478296-72-9.* INN. *Treatment of neuropathic pain and restless legs syndrome.* ◇*XP13512*

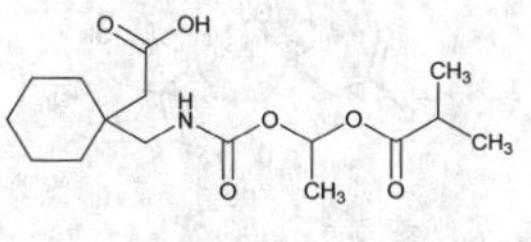

---

† Brand name formerly used, and/or firm no longer concerned with this product.

Gabexate. $C_{16}H_{23}N_3O_4$. 321.37. [Gabexate Mesilate is JAN.] Ethyl *p*-hydroxybenzoate 6-guanidinohexanoate. *UNII-4V7M9137X9. CAS-39492-01-8.* INN; MI.

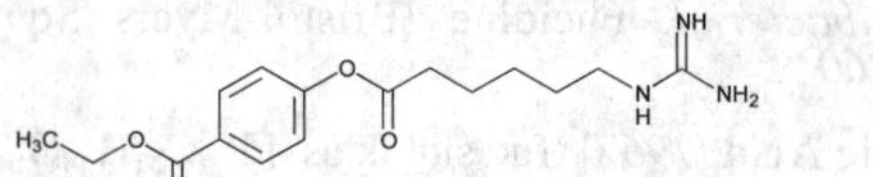

Gaboxadol [*2005*] (gab ox′ a dol). $C_6H_8N_2O_2$. 140.14. (1) Isoxazolo[5,4-*c*]pyridin-3(2*H*)-one, 4,5,6,7-tetrahydro-; (2) 4,5,6,7-Tetrahydroisoxazolo[5,4-*c*]pyridin-3(2*H*)-one. *UNII-K1M5RVL18S. CAS-64603-91-4.* INN. *Treatment of insomnia.* ◇*Lu 02-030; MK-0928*

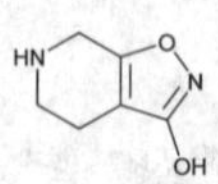

Gacyclidine. $C_{16}H_{25}NS$. 263.44. 1-[*cis*-2-Methyl-1-(2-thienyl)cyclohexyl]piperidine. *UNII-9290ND070R. CAS-68134-81-6.* INN.

Gadobenate Dimeglumine [*1993*] (gad″ oh ben′ ate di me′ gloo meen). $C_{22}H_{28}GdN_3O_{11} \cdot 2C_7H_{17}NO_5$. 1058.15. [Gadobenic Acid is INN and BAN.] (1) Gadolinate(2-), [4-carboxy-5,8,11-tris(carboxymethyl)-1-phenyl-2-oxa-5,8,11-triazatridecan-13-oato(5-)-$N^5,N^8,N^{11},O^4,O^5,O^8,O^{11},O^{13}$]-, dihydrogen, comp. with 1-deoxy-1-(methylamino)-D-glucitol (1:2); (2) Dihydrogen [(±)-4-carboxy-5,8,11-tris(carboxymethyl)-1-phenyl-2-oxa-5,8,11-triazatridecan-13-oato(5-)]gadolinate(2-), compound with 1-deoxy-1-(methylamino)-D-glucitol (1:2). *UNII-3Q6PPC19PO. CAS-127000-20-8; CAS-113662-23-0* [gadobenic acid]. *Diagnostic aid (paramagnetic).* Multihance (Bracco) ◇*B19036/7*

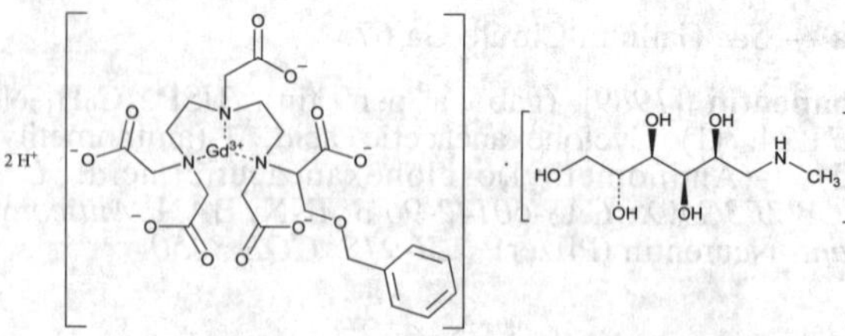

Gadobenic Acid (INN, BAN) — *See* Gadobenate Dimeglumine.

Gadobutrol. $C_{18}H_{31}GdN_4O_9$. 604.71. [10-[(1*RS*,2*SR*)-2,3-Dihydroxy-1-(hydroxymethyl)propyl]-1,4,7,10-tetraazacyclododecane-1,4,7-triacetato(3-)]gadolinium. *CAS-138071-82-6.* INN.

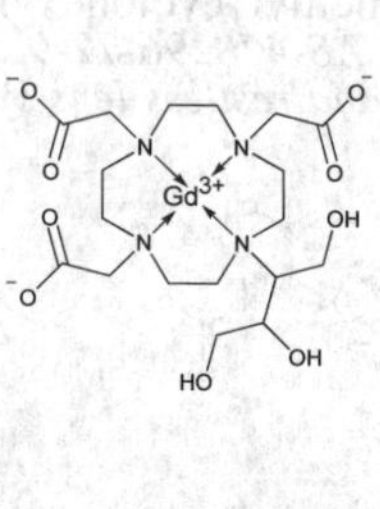

Gadocoletic Acid. $C_{41}H_{63}GdN_4O_{14}$. 993.21. Trihydrogen [3β-[[(4*S*)-4-[bis[2-[bis[(carboxy-κO)methyl]amino-κN]ethyl]amino-κN]-4-(carboxy-κO)butanoyl]amino]-12α-hydroxy-5β-cholan-24-oato(6-)]gadolinate(3-). *CAS-280776-87-6.* INN.

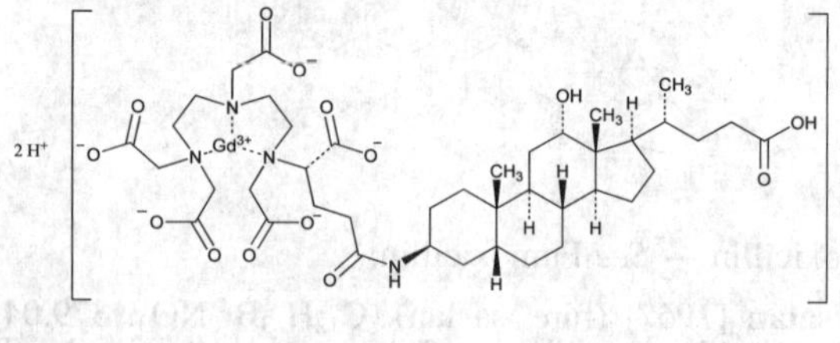

Gadodenterate. $C_{585}H_{927}Gd_{24}N_{165}O_{213}$. 10,10′,10″,10‴, 10⁗,10′″″,10″″″,10‴″″,10⁗″″,10′″″″″,10″″″″″, 10‴″″″″,10⁗″″″″,10′″″″″″,10″″″″″″,10‴″″″″″, 10⁗″″″″″,10′″″″″″″,10″″″″″″″,10‴″″″″″″, 10⁗″″″″″″,10′″″″″″″″,10″″″″″″″″,10‴″″″″″″″-{Benzene-1,3,5-triyltris(carbonylnitrilobis{(ethan-2,1-diylimino)[(5*S*)-6-oxohexane-6,1,5-triyl]bis(imino[(5*S*)-6-oxohexane-6,1,5-triyl]bis{(2-oxoethane-2,1-diyl)imino[(2*S*)-1-oxopropane-1,2-diyl]})]})}tetracosakis[1,4,7,10-tetraazacyclodecane-1,4,7-triacetato(3-)gadolinium(III)]. *CAS-544697-52-1.* INN.

Gadodiamide [*1990*] (gad″ oh dye′ a mide). **USP.** $C_{16}H_{26}GdN_5O_8$. 573.66 (anhydrous). (1) [5,8-Bis(carboxymethyl)-11-[2-(methylamino)-2-oxoethyl]-3-oxo-2,5,8,11-tetraazatridecan-13-oato(3-)]gadolinium; (2) [*N,N*-Bis[2-[(carboxymethyl)[(methylcarbamoyl)methyl]amino]ethyl]glycinato(3-)]gadolinium. *UNII-84F6U3J2R6. CAS-131410-48-5* [anhydrous]. INN; BAN. *Diagnostic aid (paramagnetic, brain disorders; spine disorders).* Omniscan (GE Healthcare) *[Note—CAS 122795-43-1 refers to the substance containing the water of coordination and multiple (x) waters of hydration.]* ◇*GdDTPA-BMA; S-041*

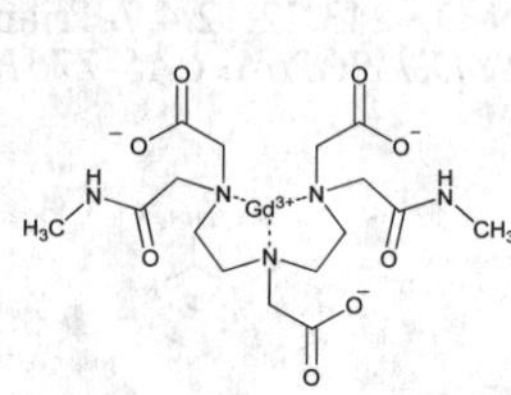

Gadofosveset Trisodium [*1999*] (gad″ oh fos′ ve set trye soe′ dee um). $C_{33}H_{40}GdN_3Na_3O_{15}P$. 975.87. [Gadofosveset is INN.] (1) Gadolinate(3-), aqua [[4-[bis[(carboxy-κO)methyl]amino-κN]-6,9-bis[(carboxy-κO)methyl]-1-[(4,4-diphenylcyclohexyl)oxy]-1-hydroxy-2-oxa-6,9-diaza-1-phosphaundecan-11-oic acid- $\kappa N6$, $\kappa N9$, $\kappa O11$] 1-oxidato(6-)]-, trisodium; (2) Trisodium [*N*-[2-[bis(carboxymethyl)amino]ethyl]-*N*-[(*R*)-2-[bis(carboxymethyl)amino]-3-hydroxypropyl]glycine 4,4-diphenylcyclohexyl hydrogen phosphato (6-)]gadolinate(3-). *CAS-211570-55-7; CAS-193901-90-5* [anhydrous]. *Diagnostic contrast agent for vascular enhancement of MRI scans.* ◇*MS 32520*

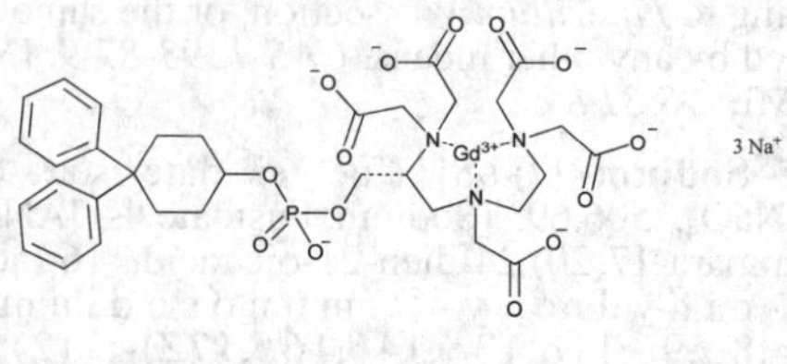

Gadomelitol. $C_{228}H_{313}Br_{12}GdN_{32}O_{116}$. 6474.17. Hydrogen [2,2′,2″,2‴-[1,4,7,10-tetraazacyclododecane-1,4,7,10-triyl]tetrakis[5-[[2-[[4-[[4-[[2-[[3,5-bis[bis[(2*S*,3*R*,4*R*,5*R*)-2,3,4,5,6-pentahydroxyhexyl-2,4,6-tribromo]carbamoyl]-

phenyl]amino]-2-oxoethyl]carbamoyl]phenyl]carbamoyl]-phenyl] amino]-2-oxoethyl]amino]-5-oxopentanoato] (4-)] gadolinate(1-). *CAS-227622-74-4.* INN.

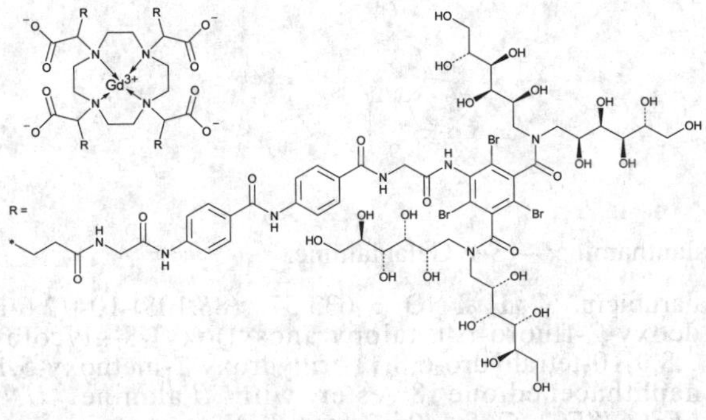

Gadopenamide. $C_{22}H_{34}GdN_5O_{10}$. 685.78. [*N,N*-Bis[2-[(carboxymethyl)[(morpholinocarbonyl)methyl]amino]ethyl]-glycinato(3-)]gadolinium. *UNII-VC7M3XD17L. CAS-117827-80-2.* INN.

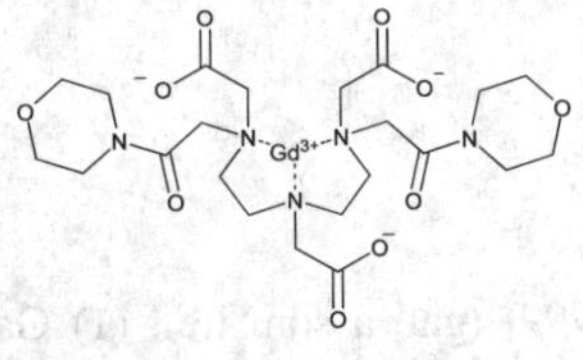

Gadopentetate Dimeglumine [*1988*] (gad″ oh pen′ te tate di me′ gloo meen). **USP** [Injection]. $C_{14}H_{20}GdN_3O_{10} \cdot 2C_7H_{17}NO_5$. 938.00. [Gadopentetic Acid is INN and BAN; Meglumine Gadopentetate is JAN.] (1) Gadolinate(2-), [*N,N*-bis[2-[bis(carboxymethyl)amino]ethyl]glycinato(5-)]-, dihydrogen, compd. with 1-deoxy-1-(methylamino)-D-glucitol (1:2); (2) Dihydrogen [*N,N*-bis[2-[bis(carboxymethyl)amino]ethyl]glycinato(5-)]gadolinate(2-), compound with 1-deoxy-1-(methylamino)-D-glucitol (1:2). *CAS-86050-77-3; CAS-80529-93-7* [gadopentetic acid]. *Diagnostic aid.* Magnevist (Bayer) ◇*SH L 451 A*

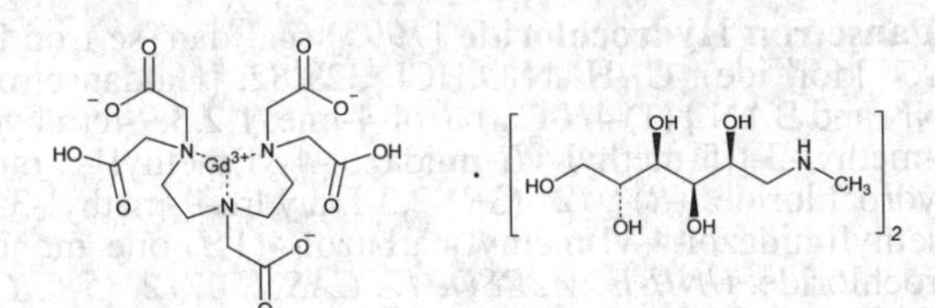

Gadoteric Acid. $C_{16}H_{25}GdN_4O_8$. 558.64. Hydrogen [1,4,7,10-tetraazacyclododecane-1,4,7,10-tetraacetato(4-)]gadolinate(1-). *UNII-QVF9Y6955W. CAS-72573-82-1.* INN; BAN.

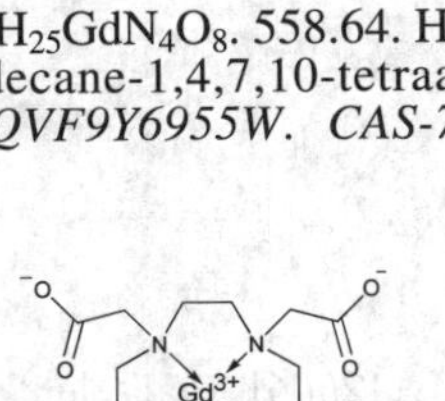

Gadoteridol [*1990*] (gad″ oh ter′ i dol). **USP.** $C_{17}H_{29}GdN_4O_7$. 558.68. (1) Gadolinium, [10-(2-hydroxypropyl)-1,4,7,10-tetraazacyclododecane-1,4,7-triacetato(3-)-

$N^1,N^4,N^7,N^{10},O^1,O^4,O^7,O^{10}$]-; (2) (±)-[10-(2-Hydroxypropyl)-1,4,7,10-tetraazacyclododecane-1,4,7-triacetato(3-)]gadolinium. *UNII-0199MV609F. CAS-120066-54-8.* INN; BAN; JAN. *Diagnostic aid (paramagnetic).* Prohance (Bracco) ◇*SQ 32,692*

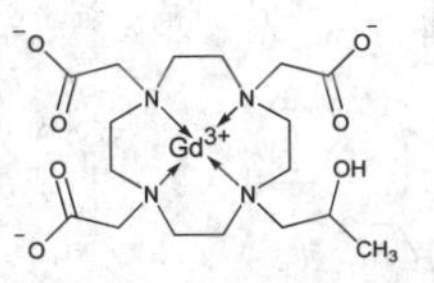

Gadoversetamide [*1994*] (gad″ oh ver set′ a mide). **USP.** $C_{20}H_{34}GdN_5O_{10}$. 661.76. (1) (Gadoversetamide) [8,11-bis(carboxymethyl)-14-[2-[(2-methoxyethyl)amino]-2-oxoethyl]-6-oxo-2-oxa-5,8,11,14-tetraazahexadecan-16-oato(3-)], gadolinium; (2) [*N,N*-Bis[2-[(carboxymethyl)[[(2-methoxyethyl)carbamoyl]methyl]amino]ethyl]glycinato(3-)]gadolinium. *UNII-RLM74T3Z9D. CAS-131069-91-5.* INN; BAN. *Diagnostic aid (paramagnetic, brain disorders; spine disorders).* Optimark (Mallinckrodt) ◇*MP-1177*

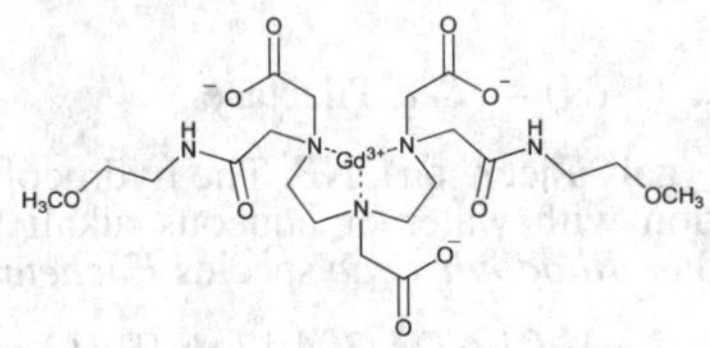

Gadoxanum [*1997*] (gad oh zan′ um). Gadolinium xanthan gum complex. (1) Gadoxanum; (2) Gadoxanum. *CAS-177072-49-0. Diagnostic aid.*

Gadoxetate Disodium [*2004*] (gad ox′ e tate dye soe′ dee um). $C_{23}H_{28}GdN_3Na_2O_{11}$. 725.71. (1) Gadolinate(2-), [*N*-[2-[bis[(carboxy-κ*O*)methyl]amino-κ*N*]-3-(4-ethoxyphenyl)propyl]-*N*-[2-[bis[(carboxy-κ*O*)methyl]amino-κ*N*]ethyl]glycinato(5-)-κ*N*,κ*O*]-, disodium, [SA-8-11252634-(*S*)]-; (2) Disodium [*N*-[(2*S*)-2-[bis(carboxymethyl)amino]-3-(*p*-ethoxyphenyl)propyl]-*N*-[2-[bis(carboxymethyl)amino]ethyl]glycinato(5-)]gadolinate(2-). *UNII-HOY74VZE0M. CAS-135326-22-6. Paramagnetic contrast agent for enhancement in magnetic resonance imaging (MRI).* ◇*ZK 139834*

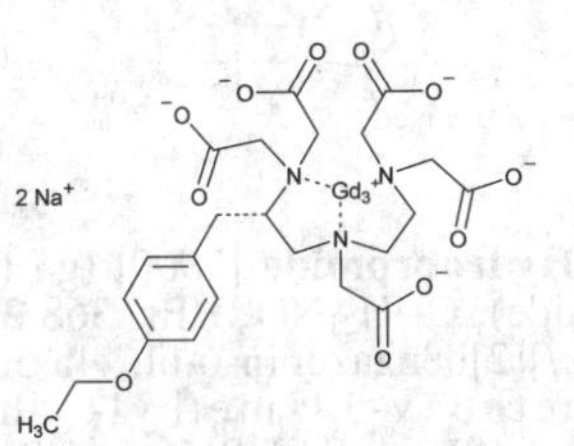

---

† Brand name formerly used, and/or firm no longer concerned with this product.

Gadoxetic Acid. $C_{23}H_{30}GdN_3O_{11}$. 681.75. Dihydrogen [*N*-[(2*S*)-2-[bis(carboxymethyl)amino]-3-(*p*-ethoxyphenyl)-propyl]-*N*-[2-[bis(carboxymethyl)amino]ethyl]glycinato(5-)]gadolinate(2-). *UNII-3QJA87N40S. CAS-135326-11-3.* INN.

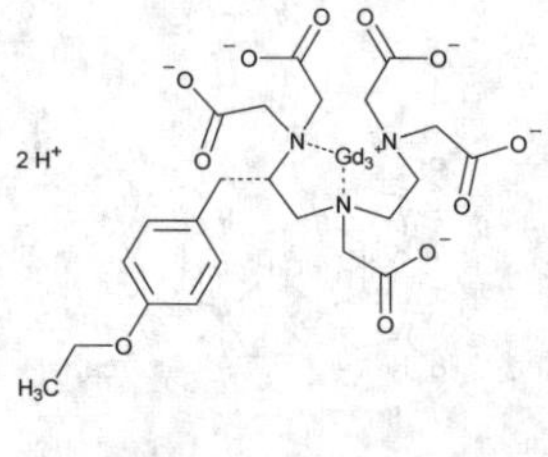

Gadozelite [*1997*] (gad oh zel′ ite). Gadolinium zeolite complex. (1) Gadozelite; (2) Gadozelite. *Diagnostic aid.*

Gaiactamine (DCF) — *See* Guaiactamine.

Gaietamine — *See* Guaiactamine.

Galactose [*2000*] (ga lak′ tose). **NF.** $C_6H_{12}O_6$. 180.16. α-D-Galactopyranose. *UNII-X2RN3Q8DNE. CAS-3646-73-9. Diagnostic aid (ultrasound contrast medium).*

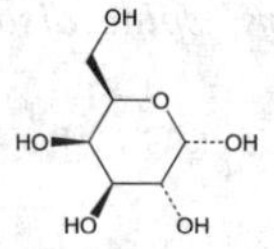

Galactosidase (JAN) — *See* Tilactase.

Galageenan (gal″ a jeen′ an). **NF.** The hydrocolloid obtained by extraction with water or aqueous alkali from the red seaweed class *Rhodophyceae* species *Eucheuma gelatinae.*

Galamustine. $C_{10}H_{19}Cl_2NO_5$. 304.17. 6-[Bis(2-chloroethyl)amino]-6-deoxy-D-galactopyranose. *UNII-P771FDQ1WJ. CAS-105618-02-8.* INN.

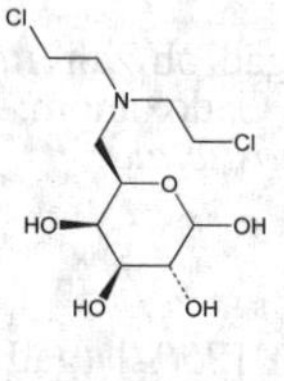

Galantamine [*2000*] (ga lan′ ta meen). $C_{17}H_{21}NO_3$. 287.35. (1) 6*H*-Benzofuro[3a,3,2-*ef*][2]benzazepin-6-ol, 4a,5,9,10,11,12-hexahydro-3-methoxy-11-methyl-, (4a*S*,6*R*,8a*S*)-; (2) (4a*S*,6*R*,8a*S*)-4a,5,9,10,11,12-Hexahydro-3-methoxy-11-methyl-6*H*-benzofuro[3a,3,2-*ef*][2]benzazepin-6-ol. *UNII-0D3Q044KCA. CAS-357-70-0.* INN; BAN; MI. *Treatment of Alzheimer's disease (cholinesterase inhibitor).* Reminyl (Janssen Pharmaceutica, Belgium)

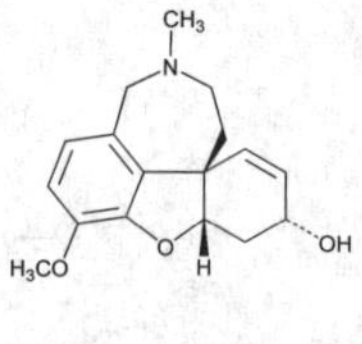

Galantamine Hydrobromide [*2000*] (ga lan′ ta meen hye″ droe broe′ mide). $C_{17}H_{21}NO_3 \cdot HBr$. 368.27. (1) 6*H*-Benzofuro[3a,3,2-*ef*][2]benzazepin-6-ol, 4a,5,9,10,11,12-hexahydro-3-methoxy-11-methyl-, hydrobromide, (4a*S*,6*R*,8a*S*)-; (2) (4a*S*,6*R*,8a*S*)-4a,5,9,10,11,12-hexahydro-3-methoxy-11-methyl-6*H*-benzofuro[3a,3,2-*ef*][2]ben-

zazepin-6-ol hydrobromide. *UNII-MJ4PTD2VVW. CAS-1953-04-4. Treatment of Alzheimer's disease (cholinesterase inhibitor).* Razadyne (Ortho-McNeil)

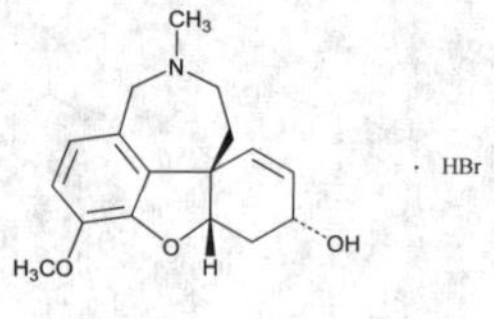

Galanthamine — *See* Galantamine.

Galarubicin. $C_{30}H_{32}FNO_{13}$. 633.57. (8*S*,10*S*)-10-[(2.6-Dideoxy-2-fluoro-α-L-talopyranosyl)oxy]-8-glycoloyl-7,8,9,10-tetrahydro-6,8,11-trihydroxy-1-methoxy-5,12-naphthacenedione 8^2-ester with β-alanine. *UNII-6F39648E92. CAS-140637-86-1.* INN.

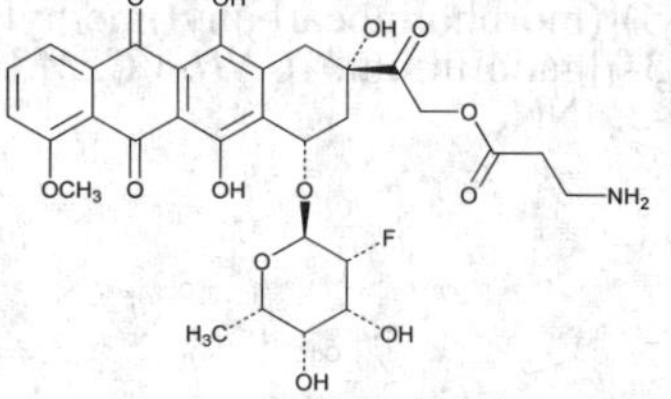

Galasomite [*1999*] (gal′ a som ite). (1) Galasomite; (2) 8-Carbamoyloctyl-4-*O*-(4-*O*-(α-D-galactopyranosyl)-β-D-galactopyranosyl)-β-D-glucopyranoside siloxylpropyl diatomite. *Treatment of verocytotoxogenic E. coli infections (adsorbent).* Synsorb Pk (Synsorb) ◇*SBI-0067*

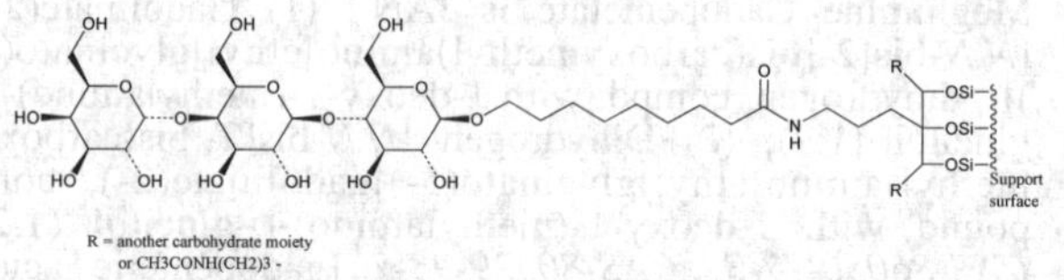

Galdansetron Hydrochloride [*1995*] (gal dan′ se tron hye″ droe klor′ ide). $C_{18}H_{19}N_3O \cdot HCl$. 329.82. [Galdansetron is INN and BAN.] (1) 4*H*-Carbazol-4-one, 1,2,3,9-tetrahydro-9-methyl-3-[(5-methyl-1*H*-imidazol-4-yl)methyl]-, monohydrochloride, (*R*)-; (2) (3*R*)-2,3-Dihydro-9-methyl-3-[(5-methylimidazol-4-yl)methyl]carbazol-4(1*H*)-one monohydrochloride. *UNII-E3M2R8Q947. CAS-156712-35-5; CAS-116684-92-5 [galdansetron]. Anti-emetic.* ◇*GR 81225C; GR 81225X [as the base]*

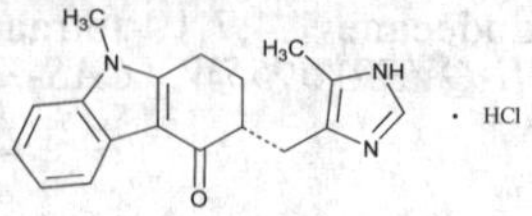

Galgenprostucel-L [*2006*] (gal″ jen pros too′ sel - el). *Galgenprostucel-L (CG1940) is one of two components of a prostate cancer cellular immunotherapy. CG1940 consists of a prostate adenocarcinoma cell line, PC-3, that has been modified to secrete human Granulocyte Macrophage Colony Stimulating Factor (GM-CSF) and irradiated to prevent cellular replication. Immunotherapy for the treatment of prostate cancer.* GVAX Prostate (Cell Genesys) ◇*CG1940*

Galiximab [*2003*] (ga lix′ i mab). Immunoglobulin G1, anti-(human CD80 (antigen)) (human-Macaca irus monoclonal IDEC-114 heavy chain), disulfide with human-Macaca irus monoclonal IDEC-114 λ-chain, dimer. *UNII-S9OX9692ZB. CAS-357613-77-5.* INN. *Treatment of psoriasis.* ◇*IDEC-114*

Gallamine Triethiodide (gal′ a meen trye″ eth eye′ oh dide). **USP.** $C_{30}H_{60}I_3N_3O_3$. 891.53. [Gallamine is BAN.] (1) Ethanaminium, 2,2′,2″-[1,2,3-benzenetriyltris(oxy)]-tris[*N,N,N*-triethyl]-, triiodide; (2) [*v*-Phenenyltris(oxyethylene)]tris[triethylammonium] triiodide. *UNII-Q3254X40X2. CAS-65-29-2; CAS-153-76-4* [gallamine]. INN. *Neuromuscular blocking agent.* Flaxedil (Davis & Geck)

Gallamone Triethiodide — *See* Gallamine Triethiodide.

Gallic Acid. *UNII-632XD903SP. CAS-149-91-7.* NF VII; MI.

Gallium Citrate Ga 67 [*1975*] (gal′ ee um sit′ rate). **USP** [Injection]. $C_6H_5{}^{67}GaO_7$. [Gallium (^{67}Ga) Citrate is INN.] (1) 1,2,3-Propanetricarboxylic acid, 2-hydroxy-, gallium-^{67}Ga (1:1) salt; (2) Gallium-^{67}Ga citrate (1:1). *UNII-4LJK511Z86. CAS-41183-64-6; CAS-52260-70-5* [replaced]. JAN. *Diagnostic aid (radiopaque medium); radioactive agent.* Neoscan (Medi-Physics)

Gallium Nitrate [*1992*] (gal′ ee um nye′ trate). $GaN_3O_9.9$-H_2O. 417.88. (1) Nitric acid, gallium salt, nonahydrate; (2) Gallium nitrate nonahydrate. *UNII-VRA0C6810N. CAS-135886-70-3; CAS-13494-90-1* [anhydrous]. *Regulator (calcium).* Ganite (Genta) ◇*NSC-15200*

Gallopamil. $C_{28}H_{40}N_2O_5$. 484.63. 5-[(3,4-Dimethoxyphenethyl)methylamino]-2-isopropyl-2-(3,4,5-trimethoxyphenyl)valeronitrile. *CAS-16662-47-8.* INN; BAN; MI.

Gallotannic Acid — *See* Tannic Acid.

---

† Brand name formerly used, and/or firm no longer concerned with this product.

Galocitabine. $C_{19}H_{22}FN_3O_8$. 439.39. *N*-[1-(5-Deoxy-β-D-ribofuranosyl)-5-fluoro-1,2-dihydro-2-oxo-4-pyrimidinyl]-3,4,5-trimethoxybenzamide. *UNII-X9788XI79O. CAS-124012-42-6.* INN.

Galosemide. $C_{15}H_{14}F_3N_3O_3S$. 373.35. *N*-[[4-(α,α,α-Trifluoro-*m*-toluidino)-3-pyridyl]sulfonyl]propionamide. *UNII-J8QB2W9908. CAS-52157-91-2.* INN.

Galsulfase [*2004*] (gal sul′ fase). $C_{2529}H_{3843}N_{689}O_{716}S_{16}$. [Galsulfase (genetical recombination) is JAN.] (1) Sulfatase, acetylgalactosamine 4- (human CSL4S-342 cell); (2) *N*-Acetylgalactosamine 4-sulfatase (human CSL4S-342 cell). Molecular weight is approximately 55,870 daltons. *UNII-59UA429E5G. CAS-552858-79-4.* INN; BAN. *Treatment of Marateaux-Lamy syndrome (Mucopolysaccharidosis MPS VI).* Aryplase (BioMarin)

```
AGASRPPHLV FLLADDLGWN DVGFHGSRIR TPHLDALAAG GVLLDNYYTQ
PLCTPSRSQL LTGRYQIRTG LQHQIIWPCQ PSCVPLDEKL LPQLLKEAGY
TTHMVGKWHL GMYRKECLPT RRGFDTYFGY LLGSEDYYSH ERCTLIDALN
VTRCALDFRD GEEVATGYKN MYSTNIFTKR AIALITNHPP EKPLFLYLAL
QSVHEPLQVP EEYLKPYDFI QDKNRHHYAG MVSLMDEAVG NVTAALKSSG
LWNNTVFIFS TDNGGQTLAG GNNWPLRGRK WSLWEGGVRG VGFVASPLLK
QKGVKNRELI HISDWLPTLV KLARGHTNGT KPLDGFDVWK TISEGSPSPR
IELLHNIDPN FVDSSPCPRN SMAPAKDDSS LPEYSAFNTS VHAAIRHGNW
KLLTGYPGCG YWFPPPSQYN VSEIPSSDPP TKTLWLFDID RDPEERHDLS
REYPHIVTKL LSRLQFYHKH SVPVYFPAQD PRCDPKATGV WGPWM
```

Galtifenin. $C_{16}H_{21}IN_2O_5$. 448.25. [[[(2,6-Diethyl-3-iodophenyl)carbamoyl]methyl]imino]diacetic acid. *UNII-XZ3FK6LC67. CAS-106719-74-8.* INN.

Galyfilcon A [*2002*] (gal″ ee fil′ kon). $(C_6H_{10}O_3)_a$ $(C_{17}H_{38}O_6Si_3)_b(C_5H_9NO)_c(C_6H_9NO)_d(C_{35}H_{92}O_{13}Si_{12})_e(C_{10}H_{14}O_4)_f$. (1) Siloxanes and Silicones, di-Me, Bu group- and 3-[(2-methyl-1-oxo-2-propenyl)oxy]propyl group-terminated (n=11), polymers with *N,N*-dimethyl-2-propenamide, ethylene dimethacrylate, 2-hydroxyethyl methacrylate, 2-hydroxy-3-[3-[1,3,3,3-tetramethyl-1-[(trimethylsilyl)oxy]-disiloxanyl]propoxy]propyl methacrylate and vinylpyrrolidone; (2) Copolymer of 3-(23-butyltetracosamethyldodecasiloxanyl)propyl 2-methylprop-2-enoate (n=11), *N,N*-dimethylprop-2-enamide, 1-ethenylpyrrolidin-2-one, ethylene bis(2-methylprop-2-enoate), 2-hydroxyethyl 2-methylprop-2-enoate and (2*RS*)-2-hydroxy-3-[3-[1,3,3,3-tetramethyl-1-[(trimethylsilyl)oxy]disiloxanyl]propoxy]-propyl 2-methylprop-2-enoate. *CAS-446264-97-7. Contact* *lens material (hydrophilic).[Note—The water content of the contact lens material is 47% at ambient temperature (23±2°C), the purity of 2-hydroxyethyl methacrylate (HEMA) is 99%, and the oxygen permeability is 60±2 × 10⁻¹¹(cm²/sec)(ml O₂/ml × mm Hg) at 35°C (Dk value).]*

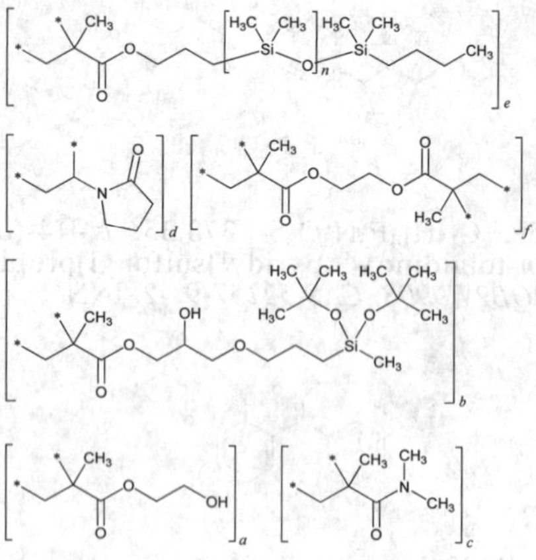

Gamfexine [*1966*] (gam fex′ een). $C_{17}H_{27}N$. 245.40. (1) Benzenepropanamine, γ-cyclohexyl-*N,N*-dimethyl-; (2) *N,N*-Dimethyl-γ-phenylcyclohexanepropylamine. *CAS-7273-99-6.* INN. *Antidepressant.* ◇*Win 1344*

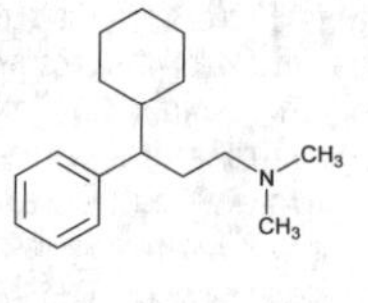

Gamithromycin [*2006*] (gam ith″ roe mye′ sin). $C_{40}H_{76}N_2O_{12}$. 777.04. (1) 1-Oxa-7-azacyclopentadecan-15-one, 13-[(2,6-dideoxy-3-*C*-methyl-3-*O*-methyl-α-L-*ribo*-hexopyranosyl)oxy]-2-ethyl-3,4,10-trihydroxy-3,5,8,10,12,14-hexamethyl-7-propyl-11-[[3,4,6-trideoxy-3-(dimethylamino)-β-D-xylo-hexopyranosyl]oxy]-, (2*R*,3*S*,4*R*,5*S*,8*R*,10*R*,11*R*,12*S*,13*S*,14*R*)-; (2) (2*R*,3*S*,4*R*,5*S*,8*R*,10*R*,11*R*,12*S*,13*S*,14*R*)-13-[(2,6-dideoxy-3-*C*-methyl-3-*O*-methyl-α-L-*ribo*-hexopyranosyl)oxy]-2-ethyl-3,4,10-trihydroxy-3,5,8,10,12,14-hexamethyl-7-propyl-11-[[3,4,6-trideoxy-3-(dimethylamino)-β-D-*xylo*-hexopyranosyl]oxy]-1-oxa-7-azacyclopentadecan-15-one. *CAS-145435-72-9.* INN. *Veterinary antibacterial.* ◇*ML-1,709,460*

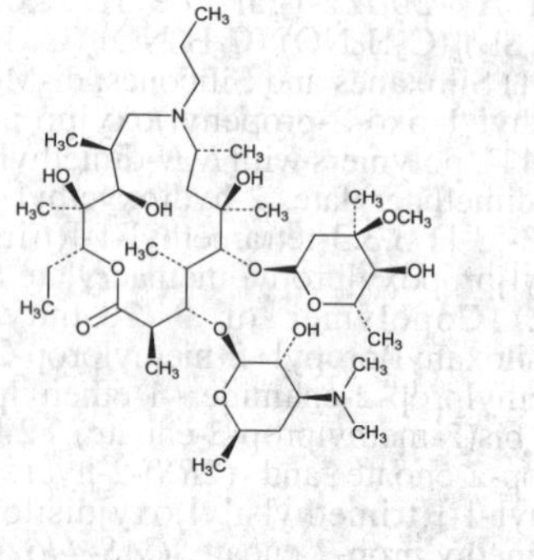

Gamma Oryzanol. $C_{40}H_{58}O_4$. 602.89. 9,19-Cyclo-9β-lanost-24-en-3β-ol 4-hydroxy-3-methoxycinamate. *UNII-SST9XCL51M. CAS-11042-64-1.* JAN.

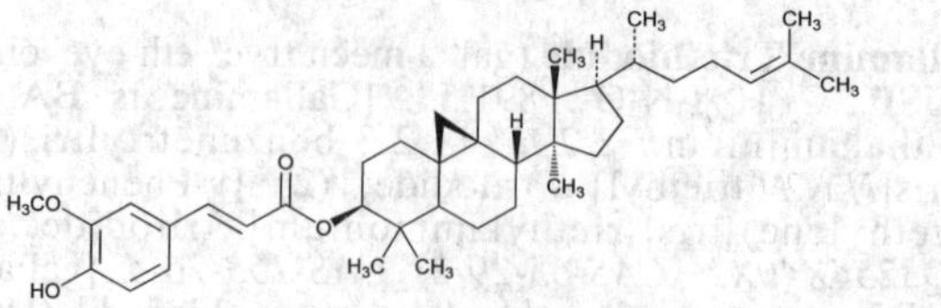

Gammaphos — *See* Amifostine.

Gamma-vinyl GABA — *See* Vigabatrin.

Gamolenic Acid. $C_{18}H_{30}O_2$. 278.43. (Z,Z,Z)-6,9,12-Octadecatrienoic acid. *CAS-506-26-3.* INN; BAN.

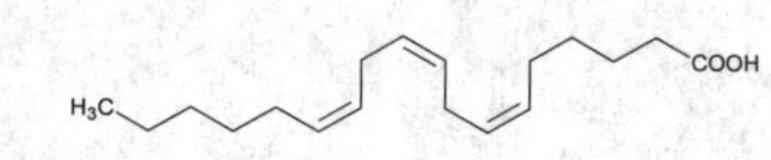

Ganaxolone [*1995*] (gan ax′ oh lone). $C_{22}H_{36}O_2$. 332.52. 3α-Hydroxy-3-methyl-5α-pregnan-20-one. *UNII-98WI44O-HIQ. CAS-38398-32-2.* INN. *Treatment of epilepsy and migraine.* ◇*CCD 1042*

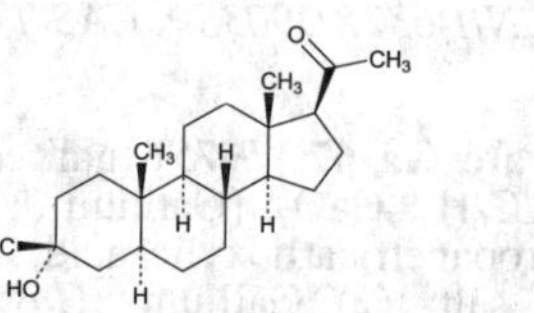

Ganciclovir [*1987*] (gan sye′ kloe vir). **USP.** $C_9H_{13}N_5O_4$. 255.23. (1) 6*H*-Purin-6-one, 2-amino-1,9-dihydro-9-[[2-hydroxy-1-(hydroxymethyl)ethoxy]methyl]-; (2) 9-[[2-Hydroxy-1-(hydroxymethyl)ethoxy]methyl]guanine. *UNII-P9G3CKZ4P5. CAS-82410-32-0.* INN; BAN; JAN. *Antiviral.* Cytovene (Roche); Vitrasert (Bausch & Lomb) ◇*BW 759U; RS-21592*

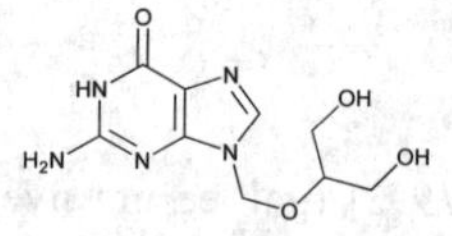

Ganciclovir Sodium [*1988*] (gan sye′ kloe vir soe′ dee um). $C_9H_{12}N_5NaO_4$. 277.21. [Ganciclovir is INN and BAN.] (1) 6*H*-Purin-6-one, 2-amino-1,9-dihydro-9-[[2-hydroxy-1-(hydroxymethyl)ethoxy]methyl]-, monosodium salt; (2) 9-[[2-Hydroxy-1-(hydroxymethyl)ethoxy]methyl]guanine, monosodium salt. *UNII-02L083W284; UNII-P9G3CKZ4P5* [ganciclovir]. *CAS-107910-75-8; CAS-82410-32-0* [ganciclovir]. *Antiviral.* ◇*RS-21592 sodium*

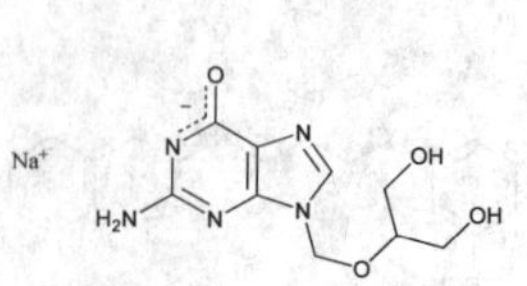

Ganefromycin. $C_{65}H_{95}NO_{21}$ [empirical molecular formula]. 1226.44. An antibiotic produced by *Streptomyces lydicus.* Ganefromycin is a complex antibiotic with two major components: α and β. [component α] (2*E*,4*E*,6*E*)-7-[(2*R**,3*R**,5*R**)-5-[7-[(3*E*,5*E*)-3-[[*O*-2,6-Dideoxy-3-*O*-methyl-α-*lyxo*-hexopyranosyl-(1→4)-*O*-2,6-dideoxy-3-*O*-methyl-β-*ribo*-hexopyranosyl-(1→4)-2,6-dideoxy-3-*O*-

methyl-α-*lyxo*-hexopyranosyl]oxy]-2-[(2*S**,3*S**,4*S**,6*R**)-tetrahydro-2,3,4-trihydroxy-5,5-dimethyl-6-[(1*E*,3*Z*)-1,3-pentadienyl]-2*H*-pyran-2-yl]propionamido]-2-methoxy-1,3 - dimethyl - 3,5 - heptadienyl]tetrahydro - 3 - hydroxy-2-furyl]-2,4,6-heptatrienoic acid, 2³-phenylacetate; [component β] (2*E*,4*E*,6*E*)-7-[(2*R**,3*R**,5*R**)-5-[7-[(3*E*,5*E*)-3-[[*O*-2,6-Dideoxy-3-*O*-methyl-α-*lyxo*-hexopyranosyl-(1→4)-*O*-2,6-dideoxy-3-*O*-methyl-β-*ribo*-hexopyranosyl-(1→4)-2,6-dideoxy-3-*O*-methyl-α-*lyxo*-hexopyranosyl]oxy]-2-[(2*S**,3*S**,4*S**,6*R**)-tetrahydro-2,3,4-trihydroxy-5,5-dimethyl-6-[(1*E*,3*Z*)-1,3-pentadienyl]-2*H*-pyran-2-yl]propionamido]-2-methoxy-1,3-dimethyl-3,5-heptadienyl]tetrahydro-3-hydroxy-2-furyl]-2,4,6-heptatrienoic acid, 2⁴-phenylacetate. *CAS-114451-31-9* [component α]; *CAS-114451-30-8* [component β]. INN.

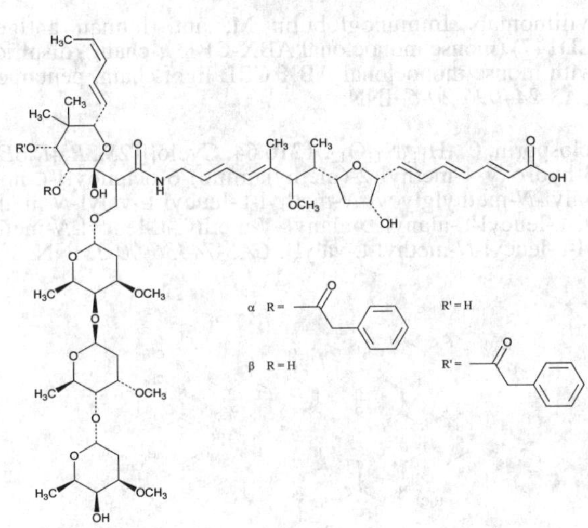

Ganglefene. $C_{20}H_{33}NO_3$. 335.48. 3-Diethylamino-1,2-dimethylpropyl *p*-isobutoxybenzoate. *CAS-299-61-6*. INN; MI.

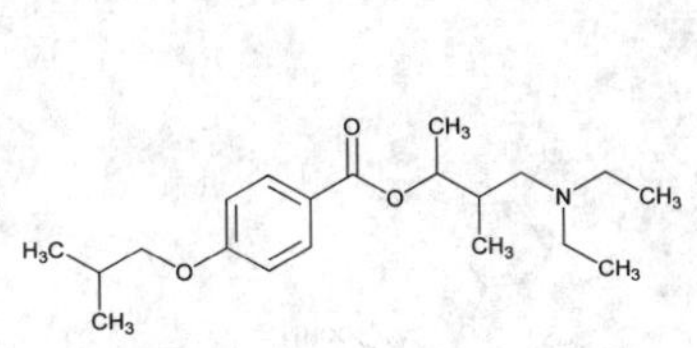

Ganirelix Acetate [*1991*] (ga″ ni rel′ ix as′ e tate). $C_{80}H_{113}ClN_{18}O_{13}\cdot2C_2H_4O_2$. 1690.42. [Ganirelix is INN and BAN.] (1) D-Alaninamide, *N*-acetyl-3-(2-naphthalenyl)-D-alanyl-4-chloro-D-phenylalanyl-3-(3-pyridinyl)-D-alanyl-L-seryl-L-tyrosyl-*N*⁶-[(ethylamino)(ethylimino)methyl]-D-lysyl-L-leucyl-*N*⁶-[(ethylamino)(ethylimino)methyl]-L-lysyl-L-prolyl-, diacetate (salt); (2) *N*-Acetyl-3-(2-naphthyl)-D-alanyl-*p*-chloro-D-phenylalanyl-3-(3-pyridyl)-D-alanyl-L-seryl-L-tyrosyl-*N*⁶-(*N*,*N*′-diethylamidino)-D-lysyl-L-leucyl-*N*⁶-(*N*,*N*′-diethylamidino)-L-lysyl-L-pro-

lyl-D-alaninamide diacetate (salt). *UNII-56U7906FQW*. *CAS-129311-55-3*; *CAS-124904-93-4* [ganirelix]. *Gonadstimulating principle.* ◇*RS-26306*

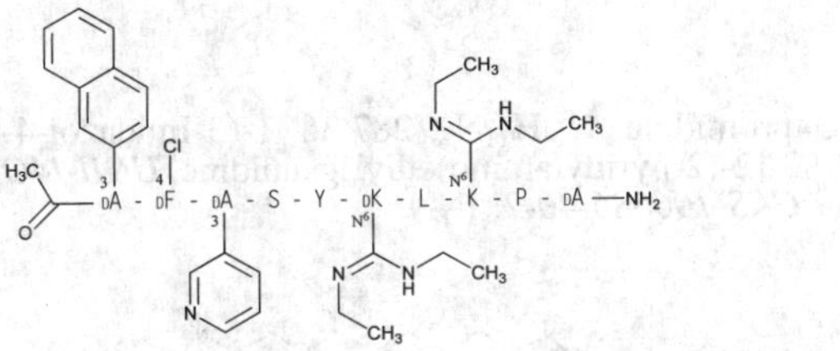

Ganstigmine. $C_{22}H_{27}N_3O_3$. 381.47. (4a*S*,9a*S*)-2,3,4,4a,9,9a-Hexahydro-2,4a,9-trimethyl-1,2-oxazino[6,5-*b*]indol-6-yl *o*-ethylcarbanilate. *CAS-457075-21-7*. INN.

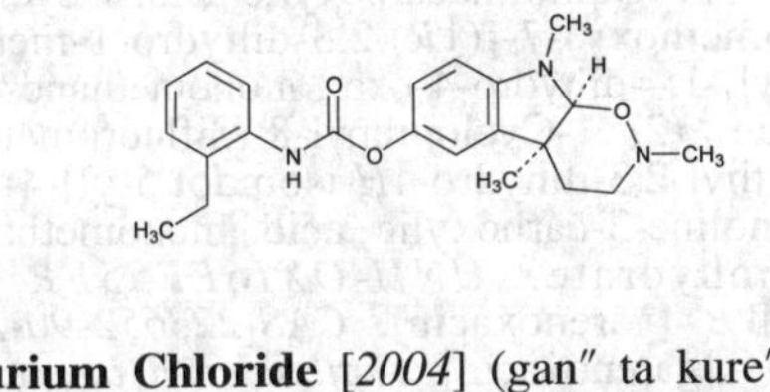

Gantacurium Chloride [*2004*] (gan″ ta kure′ ee um klor′ ide). $C_{53}H_{69}Cl_3N_2O_{14}$. 1064.48. (1) Isoquinolinium, 2-[3-[[(2*Z*)-2-chloro-1,4-dioxo-4-[3-[(1*S*,2*R*)-1,2,3,4-tetrahydro-6,7-dimethoxy-2-methyl-1-(3,4,5-trimethoxyphenyl)isoquinolinio]propoxy]-2-butenyl]oxy]propyl]-1,2,3,4-tetrahydro-6,7-dimethoxy-2-methyl-1-[(3,4,5-trimethoxyphenyl)methyl]-, dichloride, (1*R*,2*S*)-; (2) (1*R*,2*S*)-2-[3-[[(2*Z*)-2-Chloro-4-[3-[(1*S*,2*R*)-6,7-dimethoxy-2-methyl-1-(3,4,5-trimethoxyphenyl)-1,2,3,4-tetrahydroisoquinolinio]propoxy]-4-oxobut-2-enoyl]oxy]propyl]-6,7-dimethoxy-2-methyl-1-(3,4,5-trimethoxybenzyl)-1,2,3,4-tetrahydroisoquinolinium dichloride. *CAS-213998-46-0*. INN; BAN. *Induces muscle paralysis as a surgical adjunct (neuromuscular blocker).* ◇*GW-280430A*

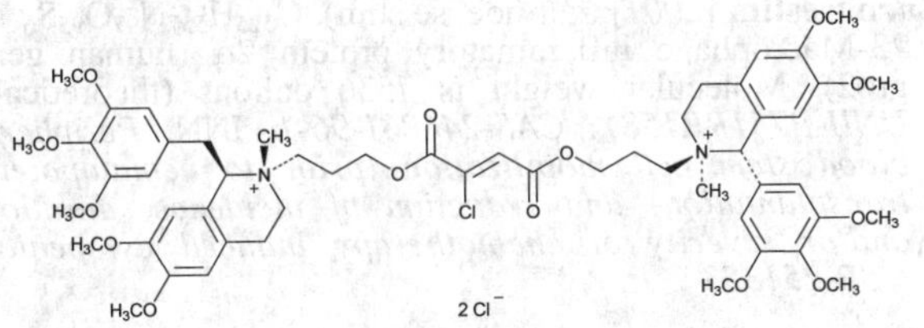

Gantenerumab [*2008*] (gan″ te ner′ ue mab). $C_{6496}H_{10072}N_{1740}O_{2024}S_{42}$. Immunoglobulin G1, anti-(human beta-amyloid proteins 42 and 40) human monoclonal antibody; γ1 heavy chain (*Homo sapiens* VH-IGHG1) (229-215′)-disulfide with κ light chain (*Homo sapiens* V-KAPPA-IGKC); (235-235″:238-238″)-bisdisulfide dimer. Molecular weight is approximately 146,300 daltons (peptide). *CAS-89957-37-9*. INN. *Treatment of Alzheimer's disease.* ◇*R1450; R04909832*

Gantofiban. $C_{21}H_{29}N_5O_6$. 447.48. 4-[[(5*R*)-3-[*p*-(Carboxyamidino)phenyl]-2-oxo-5-oxazolidinyl]methyl]-1-piperazineacetic acid, 1-ethyl methyl ester. *UNII-MRG9KH7HF6*. *CAS-183547-57-1*. INN.

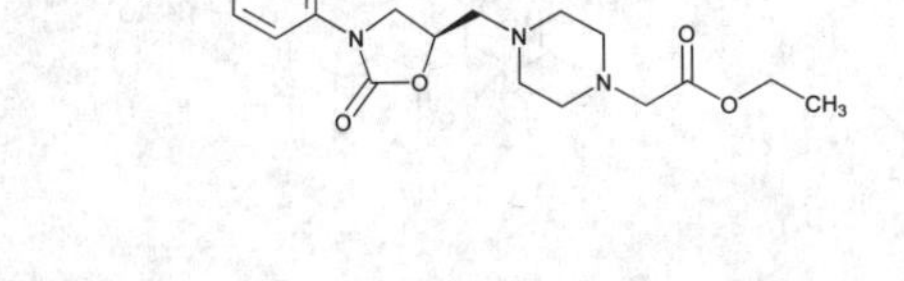

Gapicomine. $C_{12}H_{13}N_3$. 199.25. 4,4′-(Iminodimethylene)dipyridine. *UNII-WWW0P95393. CAS-1539-39-5.* INN.

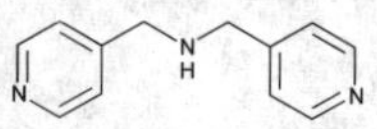

Gapromidine. $C_{14}H_{21}N_7$. 287.36. 1-(3-Imidazol-4-ylpropyl)-3-[2-(2-pyridylamino)ethyl]guanidine. *UNII-I4O62614HA. CAS-106686-40-2.* INN.

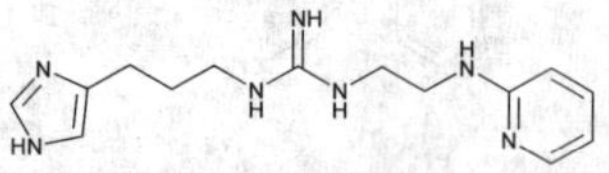

Garenoxacin Mesylate [*2002*] (gar″ en ox′ a sin mes′ i late). $C_{23}H_{20}F_2N_2O_4 \cdot CH_4O_3S \cdot H_2O$. 540.53. [Garenoxacin is INN and BAN.] (1) 3-Quinolinecarboxylic acid, 1-cyclopropyl-8-(difluoromethoxy)-7-[(1R)-2,3-dihydro-1-methyl-1H-isoindol-5-yl]-1,4-dihydro-4-oxo-, monomethanesulfonate, monohydrate; (2) 1-Cyclopropyl-8-(difluoromethoxy)-7-[(1R)-1-methyl-2,3-dihydro-1H-isoindol-5-yl]-4-oxo-1,4-dihydroquinoline-3-carboxylic acid monomethanesulfonate monohydrate. *UNII-OXI6EF55FR; UNII-V72H9867WB* [garenoxacin]. *CAS-223652-90-2; CAS-194804-75-6* [garenoxacin]. *Antibacterial agent.* ◇*BMS-284756-01; T-3811ME*

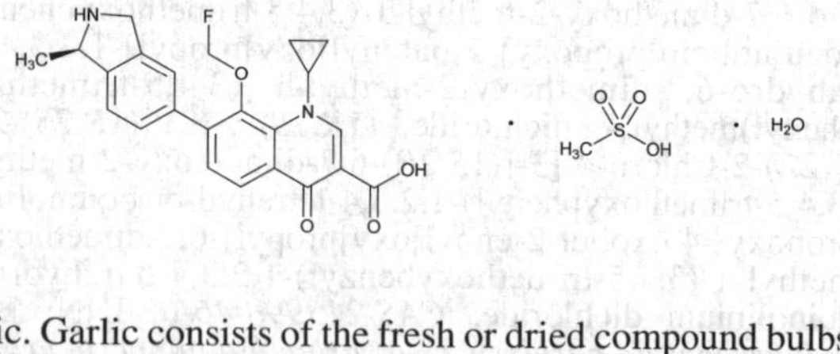

Garlic. Garlic consists of the fresh or dried compound bulbs of *Allium sativum* Linné (Fam. Liliaceae). *UNII-V1V998DC17.* NF XXI.

Garnocestim [*2001*] (gar noe′ se stim). $C_{325}H_{557}N_{97}O_{95}S_6$. 5-73-Macrophage inflammatory protein 2α (human gene gro2). Molecular weight is 7536 daltons (theoretical). *UNII-P751RR158Y. CAS-246861-96-1.* INN. *Peripheral blood stem cell mobilization (prior to hematopoietic transplantation) and reduction of incidence, duration, and/or severity of chemotherapy induced cytopenias.* ◇*SB-251353*

```
TELRCQ   CLQTLQGIHL   KNIQSVKVKS   PGPHCAQTEV
IATLKNGQKA   CLNPASPMVK   KIIEKMLKNG   KSN
```

Gas Gangrene Antitoxin, Pentavalent. [PHS: *Gas Gangrene Polyvalent Antitoxin*].

Gastric Mucin. High molecular weight glycoprotein precipitated by ethanol (60%) after pepsin/hydrochloric acid digestion of hogs' stomach linings. BAN.

Gatifloxacin [*1997*] (gat″ i flox′ a sin). $C_{19}H_{22}FN_3O_4 \cdot 1\frac{1}{2}H_2O$. 402.42. (±)-1-Cyclopropyl-6-fluoro-1,4-dihydro-8-methoxy-7-(3-methyl-1-piperazinyl)-4-oxo-3-quinolinecarboxylic acid, sesquihydrate. *UNII-L4618BD7KJ. CAS-180200-66-2.* INN. *Antibacterial.* Tequin (Bristol-Myers Squibb); Zymar (Allergan) ◇*BMS-206584-01; AM-1155*

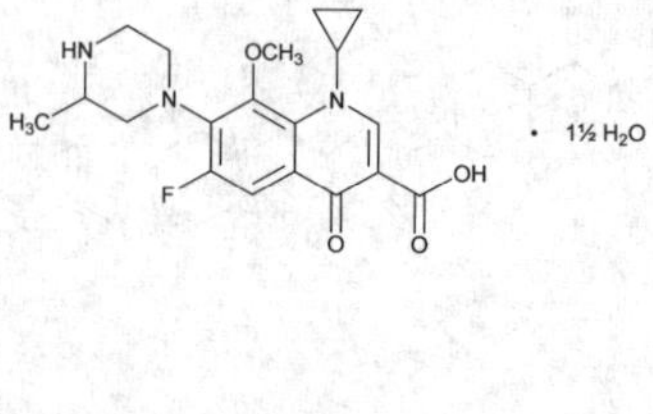

Gaultheria Oil — *See* Methyl Salicylate.

Gavestinel [*1998*] (gav es′ ti nel). $C_{18}H_{12}Cl_2N_2O_3$. 375.21. (1) (E)-4,6-Dichloro-3-[3-oxo-3-(phenylamino)-1-propenyl]-1H-indole-2-carboxylic acid; (2) 4,6-Dichloro-3-[(E)-2-(phenylcarbamoyl)vinyl]indole-2-carboxylic acid. *UNII-318X4QY113. CAS-153436-22-7.* INN; BAN. *Treatment of stroke (N-methyl-D-aspartate [NMDA] receptor antagonist).* ◇*GV 150526X*

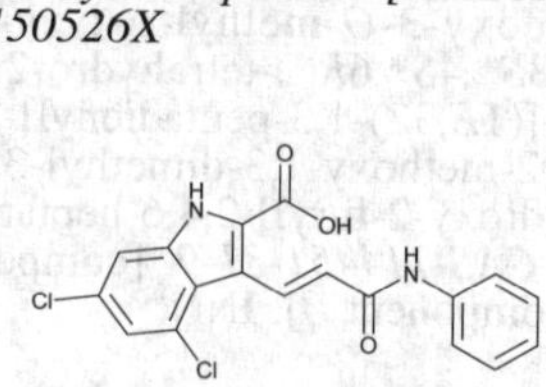

Gavilimomab. Immunoglobulin M, anti-(human antigen CD147) (mouse monoclonal ABX-CBL μ-chain), disulfide with mouse monoclonal ABX-CBL light chain, pentamer. *CAS-244096-20-6.* INN.

Geclosporin. $C_{63}H_{113}N_{11}O_{12}$. 1216.64. Cyclo[[(2S,3R,4R,6E)-3-hydroxy-4-methyl-2-(methylamino)-6-octenoyl]-L-norvalyl-N-methylglycyl-N-methyl-L-leucyl-L-valyl-N-methyl-L-leucyl-L-alanyl-D-alanyl-N-methyl-L-leucyl-N-methyl-L-leucyl-N-methyl-L-valyl]. *CAS-74436-00-3.* INN.

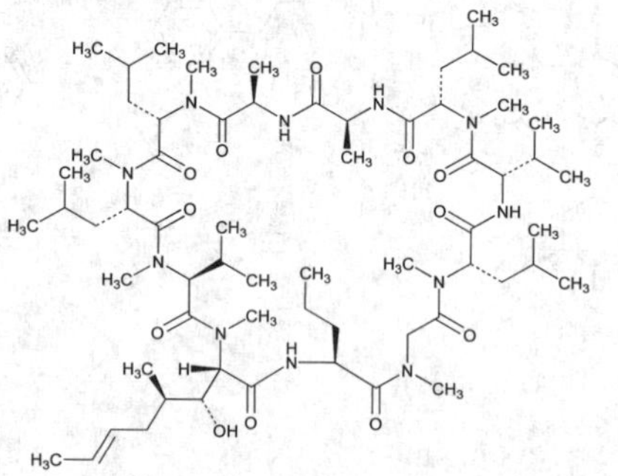

Gedocarnil. $C_{23}H_{21}ClN_2O_4$. 424.88. Isopropyl 5-(p-chlorophenoxy)-4-(methoxymethyl)-9H-pyrido[3,4-b]indole-3-carboxylate. *UNII-BWP53NPW3F. CAS-109623-97-4.* INN.

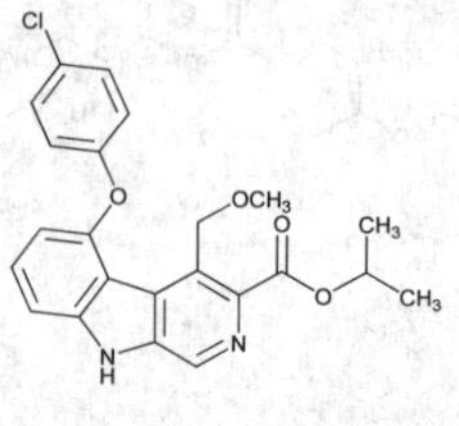

Gefarnate. $C_{27}H_{44}O_2$. 400.64. *trans*-3,7-Dimethyl-2,6-octadienyl 5,9,13-trimethyl-4,8,12-tetradecatrienoate. *UNII-1ISE2Y6ULA. CAS-51-77-4.* INN; BAN; JAN; MI. ◇*DA 688*

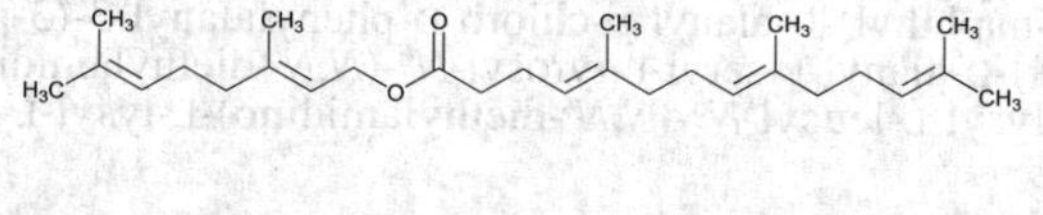

Gefitinib [*2002*] (ge fi′ ti nib). $C_{22}H_{24}ClFN_4O_3$. 446.90. 4-Quinazolinamine, N-(3-chloro-4-fluorophenyl)-7-methoxy-6-[3-4-morpholin)propoxy]-. *UNII-S65743JHBS. CAS-*

184475-35-2. INN; BAN. *Treatment of advanced non-small cell lung cancer, and a range of other major human solid tumor types.* Iressa (AstraZeneca) ◇*ZD1839*

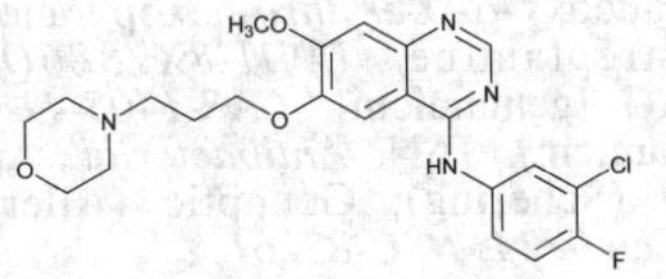

Gelatin (jel′ a tin). **NF**. A product obtained by the partial hydrolysis of collagen derived from the skin, white connective tissue, and bones of animals. *UNII-2G86QN327L. CAS-9000-70-8.* JAN. *Pharmaceutic aid (encapsulating agent); pharmaceutic aid (suspending agent); pharmaceutic aid (tablet binder); pharmaceutic aid (tablet coating agent).*

Gelatin Solution, Special Intravenous — *See* Polygeline.

Gellan Gum (jel′ an gum). **NF**. A high molecular weight polysaccharide gum produced by a pure-culture fermentation of a carbohydrate with *Pseudomonas elodea*, purified by recovery with isopropyl alcohol, and then dried and milled. *CAS-71010-52-1.*

Gemazocine. C₂₀H₂₉NO. 299.45. 3-(Cyclopropylmethyl)-6-ethyl-1,2,3,4,5,6-hexahydro-11,11-dimethyl-2,6-methano-3-benzazocin-8-ol. *CAS-54063-47-7.* INN.

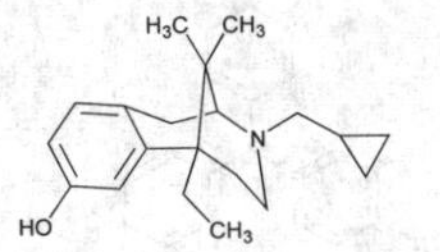

Gemcabene Calcium [*2002*] (jem′ ka been kal′ see um). C₁₆H₂₈CaO₅. 340.47. [Gemcabene is INN.] (1) Hexanoic acid, 6,6′-oxybis[2,2-dimethyl-, calcium salt (1:1); (2) Calcium 6,6′-oxybis(2,2-dimethylhexanoate). *UNII-Z9AM8GST2F; UNII-B96UX1DDKS* [gemcabene]. *CAS-209789-08-2; CAS-183293-82-5* [gemcabene]. *Atherosclerosis therapy; treatment of lipoprotein disorders.* ◇*CI-1027; PD-0072953*

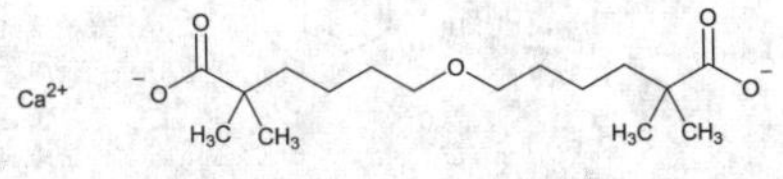

Gemcadiol [*1976*] (jem″ ka dye′ ol). C₁₄H₃₀O₂. 230.39. (1) 1,10-Decanediol, 2,2,9,9-tetramethyl-; (2) 2,2,9,9-Tetramethyl-1,10-decanediol. *CAS-35449-36-6.* INN. *Antihyperlipoproteinemic.* ◇*CI-720*

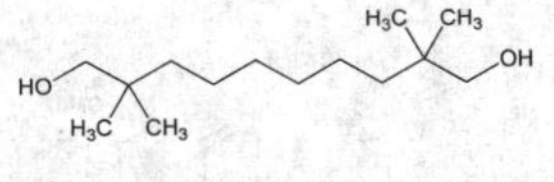

Gemcitabine [*1989*] (jem sye′ ta been). C₉H₁₁F₂N₃O₄. 263.20. (1) Cytidine, 2′-deoxy-2′,2′-difluoro-; (2) 2′-Deoxy-2′,2′-difluorocytidine. *UNII-B76N6SBZ8R. CAS-95058-81-4.* INN; BAN. *Antineoplastic.* ◇*LY188011*

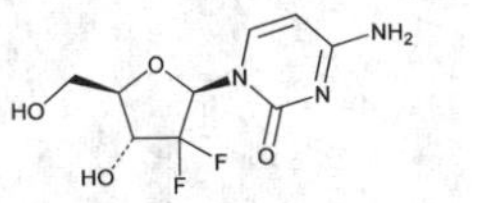

Gemcitabine Hydrochloride [*1990*] (jem sye′ ta been hye″ droe klor′ ide). **USP**. C₉H₁₁F₂N₃O₄.HCl. 299.66. (1) Cytidine, 2′-deoxy-2′,2′-difluoro-, monohydrochloride; (2) 2′-Deoxy-2′,2′-difluorocytidine monohydrochloride (β-isomer). *UNII-U347PV74IL. CAS-122111-03-9. Antineoplastic.* Gemzar (Lilly) ◇*LY188011 hydrochloride*

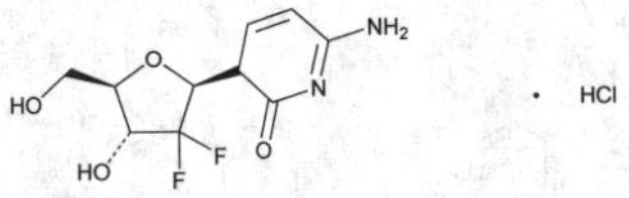

Gemeprost [*1983*] (jem′ e prost). C₂₃H₃₈O₅. 394.54. (1) Prosta-2,13-dien-1-oic acid, 11,15-dihydroxy-16,16-dimethyl-9-oxo-, methyl ester, (2*E*,11α,13*E*,15*R*)-; (2) Methyl (*E*)-7-[(1*R*,2*R*,3*R*)-3-hydroxy-2-[(*E*)-(3*R*)-3-hydroxy-4,4-dimethyl-1-octenyl]-5-oxocyclopentyl]-2-heptenoate. *CAS-64318-79-2.* INN; BAN; JAN. *Prostaglandin.* ◇*SC-37681*

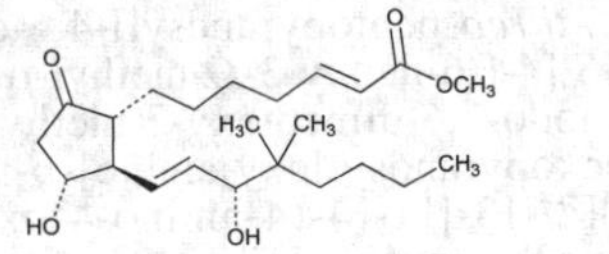

Gemfibrozil [*1980*] (jem fye′ broe zil). **USP**. C₁₅H₂₂O₃. 250.33. (1) Pentanoic acid, 5-(2,5-dimethylphenoxy)-2,2-dimethyl-; (2) 2,2-Dimethyl-5-(2,5-xylyloxy)valeric acid. *UNII-Q8X02027X3. CAS-25812-30-0.* INN; BAN. *Antihyperlipidemic.* Lopid (Pfizer) ◇*CI-719*

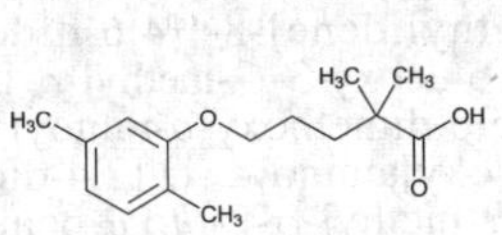

Gemifloxacin. C₁₈H₂₀FN₅O₄. 389.38. (±)-7-[3-(Aminomethyl)-4-oxo-1-pyrrolidinyl]-1-cyclopropyl-6-fluoro-1,4-dihydro-4-oxo-1,8-naphthyridine-3-carboxylic acid, 7⁴-(*Z*)-(*O*)-methyloxime). *UNII-OKR68Y0E4T. CAS-204519-64-2.* INN.

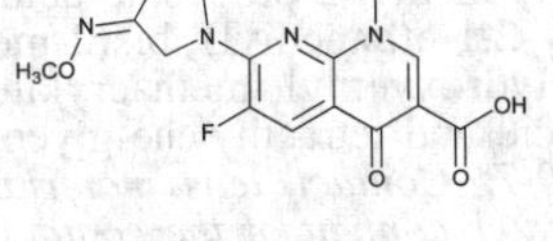

Gemifloxacin Mesylate [*1998*] (jem″ i flox′ a sin mes′ i late). C₁₈H₂₀FN₅O₄.CH₄O₃S. 485.49. (1) (*Z*)-7-[3-(Aminomethyl)-4-(methoxyimino)-1-pyrrolidinyl]-1-cyclopropyl-6-fluoro-1,4-dihydro-4-oxo-1,8-naphthyridine-3-carboxylic acid monomethanesulfonate; (2) (±)-7-[3-(Aminomethyl)-4-oxo-1-pyrrolidinyl]-1-cyclopropyl-6-fluoro-1,4-dihydro-4-oxo-1,8-naphthyridine-3-carboxylic acid,

---

† Brand name formerly used, and/or firm no longer concerned with this product.

7^4-(Z)-(*O*-methyloxime), monomethanesulfonate. *UNII-X4S9F8RL01. CAS-204519-65-3. Antibacterial.* Factive (Oscient) ◇*SB-265805-S; LB 20304a*

Gemopatrilat [*2000*] (jem″ oh pa′ tril at). $C_{19}H_{26}N_2O_4S$. 378.49. (1) 1*H*-Azepine-1-acetic acid, hexahydro-6-[[(2*S*)-2-mercapto-1-oxo-3-phenylpropyl]amino]-2,2-dimethyl-7-oxo-, (6*S*)-; (2) (6*S*)-Hexahydro-6-[(α*S*)-α-mercaptohydrocinnamamido]-2,2-dimethyl-7-oxo-1*H*-azepine-1-acetic acid. *CAS-160135-92-2. INN. Treatment of hypertension and congestive heart failure (vasopeptidase inhibitor).* ◇*BMS-189921*

Gemtuzumab Ozogamicin [*2000*] (jem tooz′ oo mab oh″ zoe ga mye′ sin). [Gemtuzumab is INN.] (1) Immunoglobulin G4, anti-(human CD33 (antigen)) (human-mouse monoclonal hP67.6 γ_4-chain), disulfide with human-mouse monoclonal hP67.6 κ-chain, dimer, methyl [(1*R*,4*Z*, 8*S*, 13*E*)-8-[[2-*O*-[4-(acetylethylamino)-2,4-dideoxy-3-*O*-methyl-α-L-*threo*-pentopyranosyl]-4,6-dideoxy-4-[[[2,6-dideoxy-4-*S*-[4-[(6-deoxy-3-*O*-methyl-α-L-mannopyranosyl)oxy]-3-iodo-5,6-dimethoxy-2-methylbenzoyl]-4-thio-β-D-*ribo*-hexopyranosyl]oxy]amino]-β-D-glucopyranosyl]oxy]-13-[2-[[3-[[1-[4-(4-amino-4-oxobutoxy)phenyl]ethylidene]hydrazino]-1,1-dimethyl-3-oxopropyl]-dithio]ethylidene]-1-hydroxy-11-oxobicyclo[7.3.1]trideca-4,9-diene-2,6-diyn-10-yl]carbamate conjugate; (2) Immunoglobulin G4 (human-mouse monoclonal hP67.6 γ_4-chain anti-human antigen CD33), disulfide with human-mouse monoclonal hP67.6 κ-chain, dimer, conjugate with methyl (1*R*, 4*Z*, 8*S*, 13*E*)-13-[2-[[2-[[[*p*-(3-carbamoylpropoxy)-α-methylbenzylidene]hydrazino]carbonyl]-1,1-dimethylethyl]dithio]ethylidene]-8-[[4,6-dideoxy-4-[[[2,6-dideoxy-4-*S*-[4-[(6-deoxy-3-*O*-methyl-α-L-mannopyranosyl)oxy]-3-iodo-5,6-dimethoxy-*o*-toluoyl]-4-thio-β-D-*ribo*-hexopyranosyl]oxy]amino]-2-*O*-[2,4-dideoxy-4-(*N*-ethylacetamido)-3-*O*-methyl-α-L-*threo*-pentopyranosyl]-β-D-glucopyranosyl]oxy]-1-hydroxy-11-oxobicyclo[7.3.1]trideca-4,9-diene-2,6-diyne-10-carbamate. Molecular weight is approximately 153,000 daltons. *UNII-8GZG754X6M. CAS-220578-59-6. Treatment of relapsed, acute myelogenous leukemia (cytotoxic calicheamicin derivative conjugated to a humanized monoclonal antibody).* Mylotarg (Wyeth) ◇*WAY-CMA-676; CMA-676; CDP-771*

Genfilcon A [*1996*] (jen fil′ kon). $(C_6H_{10}O_3)_x(C_4H_6O_2)_y$ $(C_{16}H_{26}O_7)_z$. (1) 2-Hydroxyethyl 2-methyl-2-propenoate polymer with 2-methyl-2-propenoic acid and oxybis(2,1-ethanediyloxy-2,1-ethanediyl) bis(2-methyl-2-propenoate); (2) 2-Hydroxyethyl methacrylate polymer with methacrylic acid and tetraethylene glycol dimethacrylate. *CAS-89558-90-7. Contact lens material (hydrophobic). [Note—The water content of the contact lens material is 48±0.2% at ambient temperature (23±2°C), the purity of 2-hydroxyethyl methacrylate (HEMA) is 99.5%, and the oxygen permeability is $13 \times 10^{-11}(cm^2/sec)(ml\ O_2/ml \times mm\ Hg)$ at 35°C (Dk value).]*

Gentamicin Sulfate [*1963*] (jen″ ta mye′ sin sul′ fate). **USP.** [Gentamicin is BAN.] Gentamicin Sulfate, produced by *Micromonospora purpurea* n. sp., is a complex antibiotic substance with three components, sulfates of gentamicin C_1, gentamicin C_2, and gentamicin C_{1A}. (1) Gentamicin sulfate (salt); (2) Gentamycin sulfate; (3) [Chemical name for gentamicin C_{1A}.] *O*-3-Deoxy-4-*C*-methyl-3-(methylamino)-β-L-arabinopyranosyl-(1→6)-*O*-[2,6-diamino-2,3,4,6-tetradeoxy-α-D-*erythro*-hexopyranosyl-(1→4)]-2-deoxy-D-streptamine. *UNII-8X7386QRLV; UNII-T6Z9V48IKG* [gentamicin]. *CAS-1405-41-0; CAS-1403-66-3* [gentamicin]. JAN. *Antibacterial.* Apogen (King); Garamycin (Schering); Genoptic (Allergan); Gentak (Akorn) ◇*Sch 9724; NSC-82261*

Gentian Violet (jen′ shun). **USP.** $C_{25}H_{30}ClN_3$. 407.98. [Methylrosanilinium Chloride is INN, BAN and JAN.] (1) Methanaminium, *N*-[4-[bis[4-(dimethylamino)phenyl]methylene]-2,5-cyclohexadien-1-ylidene]-*N*-methyl-, chloride; (2) C.I. Basic violet 3; (3) [4-[Bis[*p*-(dimethylamino)phenyl]methylene]-2,5-cyclohexadien-1-ylidene]-dimethylammonium chloride. *UNII-J4Z741D6O5. CAS-548-62-9. Anti-infective, topical.* Gvs (Savage) *[Name previously used: Methylrosaniline Chloride.]*

Gentisic Acid Ethanolamide. NF XVIII. *Pharmaceutic aid (complexing agent).*

Gepefrine. $C_9H_{13}NO$. 151.21. (+)-(*S*)-*m*-(2-Aminopropyl)-phenol. *UNII-V51RRX51VH. CAS-18840-47-6. INN; MI.*

Gepirone Hydrochloride [*1985*] (jep′ ir one hye″ droe klor′ ide). $C_{19}H_{29}N_5O_2$.HCl. 395.93. [Gepirone is INN.] (1) 2,6-Piperidinedione, 4,4-dimethyl-1-[4-[4-(2-pyrimidinyl)-1-piperazinyl]butyl]-, monohydrochloride; (2) 3,3-Dimethyl-1-[4-[4-(2-pyrimidinyl)-1-piperazinyl]butyl]glutarimide monohydrochloride. *UNII-80C9L8EP6V; UNII-JW5Y7B8Z18* [gepirone]. *CAS-83928-66-9; CAS-83928-76-1* [gepirone]. *Tranquilizer.* ◇*BMY 13805-1*

Geroquinol. $C_{16}H_{22}O_2$. 246.34. 2-Geranylhydroquinone. *UNII-4155989DN5. CAS-10457-66-6.* INN; DCF.

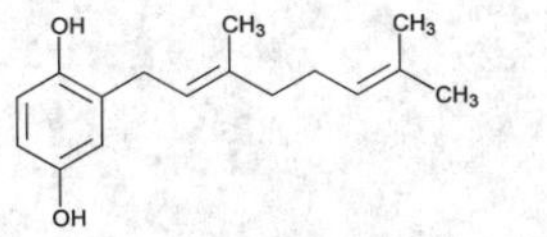

Gestaclone [*1969*] (jes′ ta klone). $C_{23}H_{27}ClO_2$. 370.91. (1) 3*H*-Dicyclopropa[1,2:16,17]cyclopenta[*a*]phenanthren-3-one, 17-acetyl-6-chloro-1,1a,2,8,9,10,11,12,13,14,15,16,16a,17-tetradecahydro-10,13-dimethyl-, (1α,2α,8α,9β,10α,13α,14β,16α,17α)-; (2) 17β-Acetyl-6-chloro-1β,1a,2β,8β,9α,10,11,12,13,14α,15,16β,16a,17-tetradecahydro-10β,13β-dimethyl-3*H*-dicycloprop-a[1,2:16,17]cyclopenta[*a*]-phenanthren-3-one; (3) 6-Chloro-1α,2α:16α,17-bismethylene-4,6-pregnadiene-3,20-dione. *CAS-19291-69-1.* INN. *Progestin. ♢SH 1040*

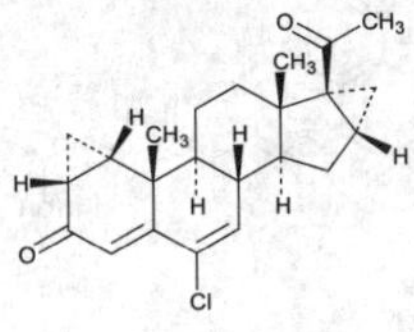

Gestadienol. $C_{20}H_{26}O_3$. 314.42. 17-Hydroxy-19-norpregna-4,6-diene-3,20-dione. *CAS-58769-17-8.* INN.

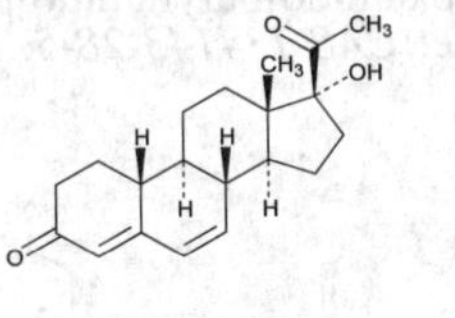

Gestodene [*1977*] (jes′ toe deen). $C_{21}H_{26}O_2$. 310.43. (1) Pregna-4,15-dien-20-yn-3-one, 13-ethyl-17-hydroxy-18,19-dinor-, (17α)-; (2) 13-Ethyl-17-hydroxy-18,19-dinor-17α-pregna-4,15-dien-20-yn-3-one. *CAS-60282-87-3.* INN; BAN. *Progestin. ♢SH B 331*

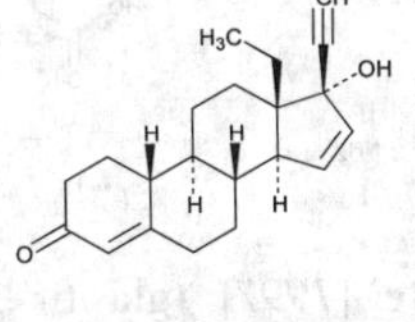

Gestonorone Caproate [*1965*] (jes toe′ nor one kap′ roe ate). $C_{26}H_{38}O_4$. 414.58. (1) 19-Norpregn-4-ene-3,20-dione, 17-[(1-oxohexyl)oxy]-; (2) 17-Hydroxy-19-norpregn-4-ene-3,20-dione hexanoate. *UNII-U38E620NS6. CAS-1253-28-7.* INN; BAN; JAN. *Progestin. [Name previously used: Gestronol; Gestonorone Hexanoate.] ♢SH 582; NSC-84054*

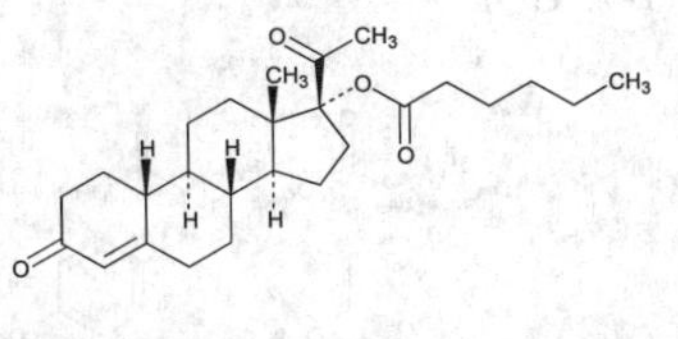

Gestonorone Hexanoate (previously used name) — *See* Gestonorone Caproate.

† Brand name formerly used, and/or firm no longer concerned with this product.

Gestrinone [*1978*] (jes′ tri none). $C_{21}H_{24}O_2$. 308.41. (1) Pregna-4,9,11-trien-20-yn-3-one, 13-ethyl-17-hydroxy-18,19-dinor-, (17α)-; (2) 13-Ethyl-17-hydroxy-18,19-dinor-17α-pregna-4,9,11-trien-20-yn-3-one. *CAS-16320-04-0; CAS-40542-65-2* [replaced]. INN; BAN. *Progestin. ♢R 2323; RU 2323; A 46 745*

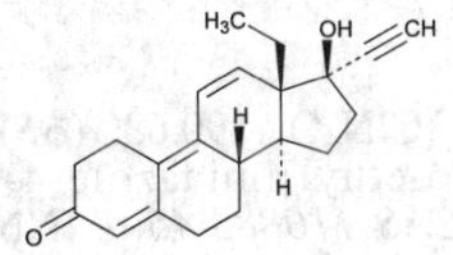

Gestronol (previously used name) — *See* Gestonorone Caproate.

Gevotroline Hydrochloride [*1990*] (jev oh′ troe leen hye″ droe klor′ ide). $C_{19}H_{20}FN_3.HCl$. 345.84. [Gevotroline is INN.] (1) 1*H*-Pyrido[4,3-*b*]indole, 8-fluoro-2,3,4,5-tetrahydro-2-[3-(3-pyridinyl)propyl]-, monohydrochloride; (2) 8-Fluoro-2,3,4,5-tetrahydro-2-[3-(3-pyridyl)propyl]-1*H*-pyrido[4,3-*b*]indole monohydrochloride. *CAS-112243-58-0; CAS-107266-06-8* [gevotroline]. *Antipsychotic. ♢WY-47384*

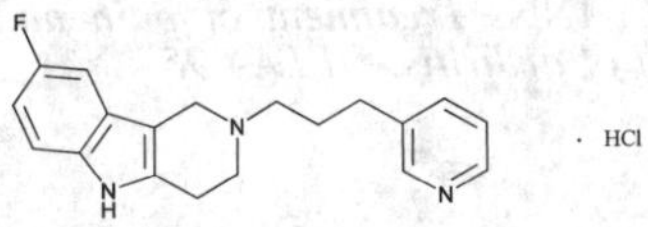

Gimatecan. $C_{25}H_{25}N_3O_5$. 447.48. (4*S*)-11-[(*E*)-[(1,1-Dimethylethoxy)imino]methyl]-4-ethyl-4-hydroxy-1,12-dihydro-14*H*-pyrano[3′,4′:6,7]indolizino[1,2-*b*]quinoline-3,14(4*H*)-dione. *UNII-7KKS9R192F. CAS-292618-32-7.* INN.

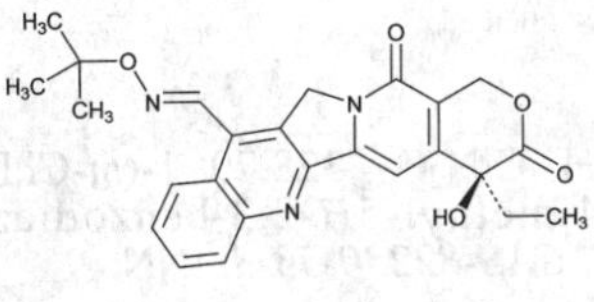

Gimeracil. $C_5H_4ClNO_2$. 145.54. 5-Chloro-2,4-pyridinediol. *UNII-UA8SE1325T. CAS-103766-25-2.* INN.

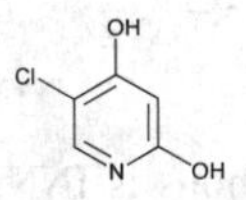

Ginger. The rhizome of *Zingiber officinale* Roscoe (Fam. Zingiberaceae), scraped or unscraped. *UNII-C5529G5JPQ.* NF XXI.

Ginger, Powdered. NF XXI.

Ginkgo. The dried leaf of *Ginkgo biloba* Linné (Fam. Ginkgoaceae). *UNII-19FUJ2C58T.* NF XXI.

Ginseng, American. NF XXI.

Ginseng, Asian. The dried roots of *Panax ginseng* C.A. Meyer (Fam. Araliaceae). NF XXI.

Giparmen. $C_{13}H_{10}O_3$. 214.22. 4-Methyl-7-(2-propynyloxy)-coumarin. *UNII-6272R7515Q. CAS-67268-43-3.* INN.

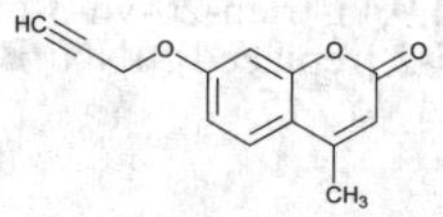

Giracodazole. $C_6H_{11}ClN_4O$. 190.63. (αS)-2-Amino-α-[(1S)-2-amino-1-chloroethyl]imidazole-4-methanol. *UNII-RU19QYB9WZ. CAS-110883-46-0.* INN.

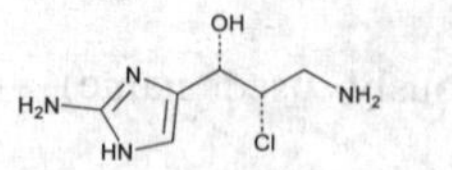

Giractide. $C_{100}H_{156}N_{34}O_{22}S$. 2218.59. 1-Glycine-18-L-argininamide-α^{1-18}-corticotropin. *CAS-24870-04-0.* INN; MI.

Giripladib [*2006*] (jir ip′ la dib). $C_{41}H_{36}ClF_3N_2O_4S$. 745.25. (1) Benzoic acid, 4-[3-[5-chloro-1-(diphenylmethyl)-2-[2-[[[[2-(trifluoromethyl)phenyl]methyl]sulfonyl]amino]ethyl]-1H-indol-3-yl]propyl]-; (2) 4-[3-[5-Chloro-1-(diphenylmethyl)-2-[2-[[[2-(trifluoromethyl)benzyl]sulfonyl]amino]ethyl]-1H-indol-3-yl]propyl]benzoic acid. *CAS-865200-20-0.* INN. *Treatment of pain and symptomatic management of arthritis.* ◇PLA-695

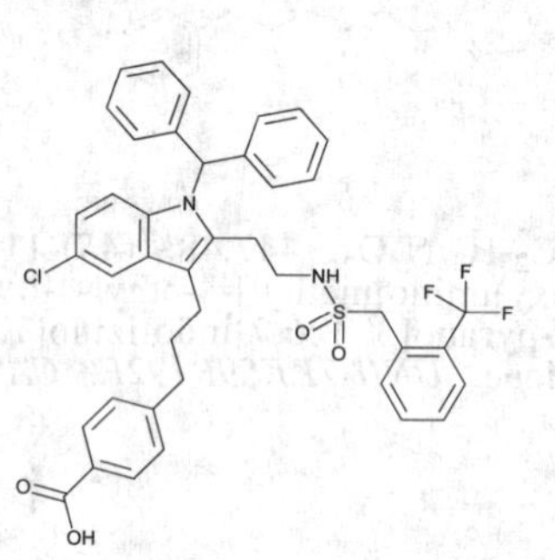

Girisopam. $C_{18}H_{17}ClN_2O_2$. 328.79. 1-(m-Chlorophenyl)-7,8-dimethoxy-4-methyl-5H-2,3-benzodiazepine. *UNII-2LP301A921. CAS-82230-53-3.* INN.

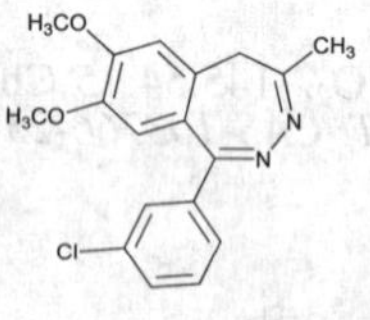

Gitalin. [Gitalin Amorphous is INN.] Glycosidal constituent obtained from *Digitalis purpurea* Linné (Fam. *Scrophulariaceae*). NF XIII; MI. Gitaligin (Schering†)

Gitaloxin. $C_{42}H_{64}O_{15}$. 808.95. Gitoxin 16-formate. *CAS-3261-53-8.* INN.

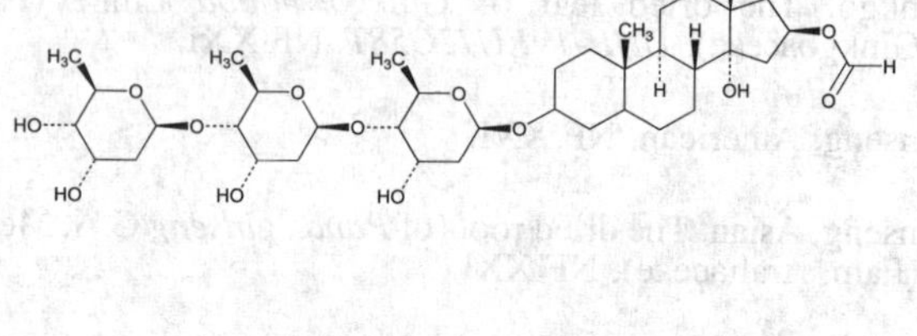

Gitoformate. $C_{46}H_{64}O_{19}$. 920.99. Gitoxin 3′,3″,3‴,4‴,16-pentaformate. *CAS-7685-23-6.* INN.

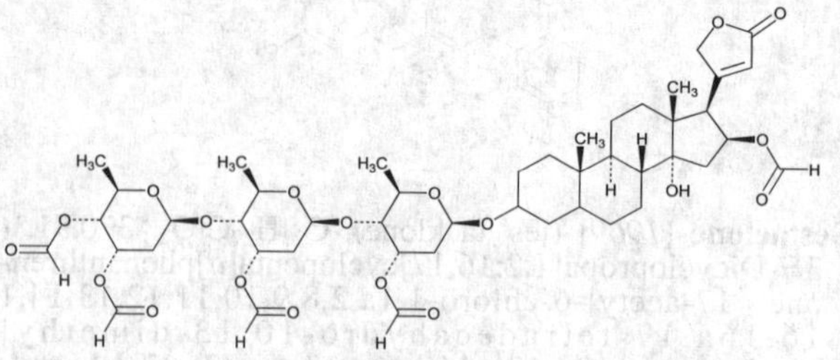

Glafenine. $C_{19}H_{17}ClN_2O_4$. 372.80. 2,3-Dihydroxypropyl N-(7-chloro-4-quinolyl) anthranilate. *UNII-46HL4I09AH. CAS-3820-67-5.* INN; DCF; JAN; MI. ◇R 1707

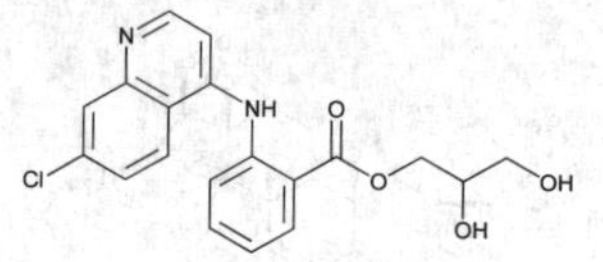

Glaphenine — *See* Glafenine.

Glaspimod. $C_{48}H_{74}N_{12}O_{22}$. 1171.17. $N^2,N^{2'}$-[(2S,7S)-2,7-Bis[(2S)-3-carboxy-2-[(2S)-4-carboxy-2-[(2S)-5-oxo-2-pyrrolidinecarboxamido]butyramido]propionamido]octanedioyl]di-L-lysine. *CAS-134143-28-5.* INN; BAN. ◇SK&F 107647

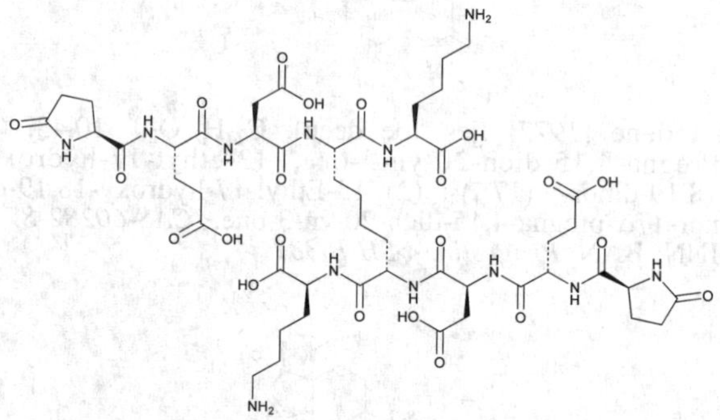

Glatiramer Acetate [*1997*] (gla tir′ a mer as′ e tate). $(C_5H_9NO_4 \cdot C_3H_7NO_2 \cdot C_6H_{14}N_2O_2 \cdot C_9H_{11}NO_3)_x \cdot xC_2H_4O_2$. The molar fraction of each amino acid residue ranges as follows: L-Glu 0.129-0.153, L-Ala 0.392-0.462, L-Tyr 0.086-0.100, and L-Lys 0.300-0.374. (1) L-Glutamic acid polymer with L-alanine, L-lysine and L-tyrosine, acetate (salt); (2) L-Glutamic acid peptide with L-alanine, L-lysine and L-tyrosine, acetate (salt). *UNII-5M691HL4BO. CAS-147245-92-9.* BAN. *Immunomodulator.* Copaxone (Teva) ◇Copolymer-1; COP-1

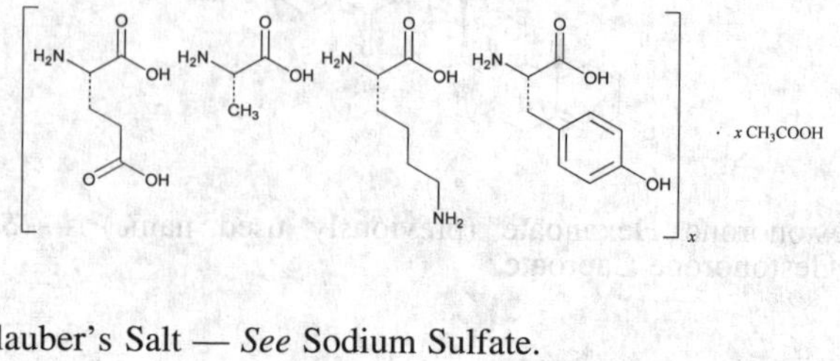

Glauber's Salt — *See* Sodium Sulfate.

Glaucarubin. *UNII-EH6H7VS52J.* MI. Glaumeba (Marion Merrell Dow†)

Glaze, Pharmaceutical. **NF**. A specially denatured alcoholic solution containing 38.5 ± 18.5% of anhydrous shellac and is made with either dehydrated alcohol or alcohol containing 5% of water by volume. *Pharmaceutic aid (tablet coating agent)*.

Glaziovine. $C_{18}H_{19}NO_3$. 297.35. (±)-Glaziovine. *UNII-KE7-J8A65P6. CAS-17127-48-9*. INN.

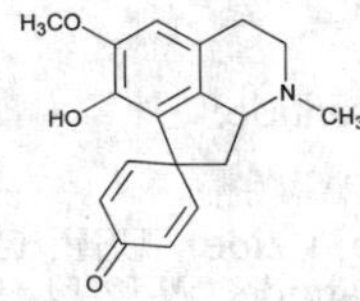

Glemanserin [*1992*] (gle man′ ser in). $C_{20}H_{25}NO$. 295.42. (1) 4-Piperidinemethanol, α-phenyl-1-(2-phenylethyl)-, (±)-; (2) (±)-1-Phenethyl-α-phenyl-4-piperidinemethanol. *CAS-132553-86-7* [(±)]; *CAS-107703-78-6.* INN. *Anti-anxiety agent.* ◇*MDL 11,939*

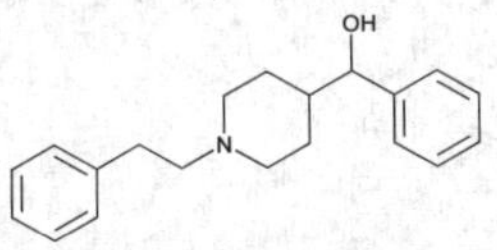

Glenvastatin. $C_{27}H_{26}FNO_3$. 431.50. (4*R*,6*S*)-6-[(*E*)-2-[4-(*p*-Fluorophenyl)-2-isopropyl-6-phenyl-3-pyridyl]vinyl]tetrahydro-4-hydroxy-2*H*-pyran-2-one. *UNII-X98U22RT62. CAS-122254-45-9*. INN.

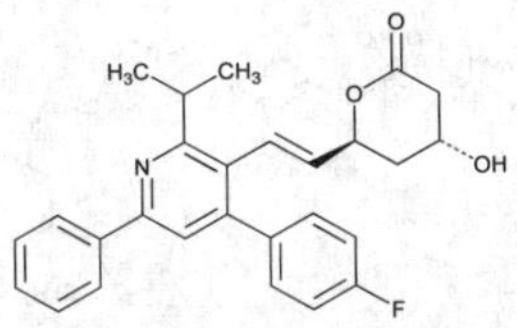

Gleptoferron [*1978*] (glep toe′ fer on). $(FeOOH)_m[HO-(C_6H_{10}O_5)_x\text{-}C_7H_{13}O_7]_n$. (1) Gleptoferron; (2) Gleptoferron. *UNII-898723IQHQ. CAS-57680-55-4.* INN; BAN. *Hematinic (veterinary).* Gleptosil (Fisons Pharmaceuticals Ltd., Great Britain); Heptomer (Fisons Pharmaceuticals Ltd., Great Britain) [*Note—Product has also been described as iron heptonate.*]

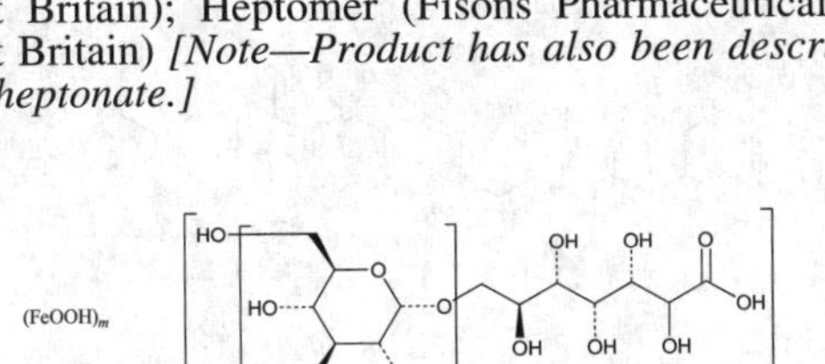

Gliamilide [*1975*] (glye am′ i lide). $C_{23}H_{33}N_5O_5S$. 491.60. (1) 3-Pyridinecarboxamide, *N*-[2-[1-[[[[(bicyclo[2.2.1]hept-5-en-2-ylmethyl)amino]carbonyl]amino]sulfonyl]-4-piperidinyl]ethyl]-2-methoxy-, *endo;* (2) *endo*-1-[[4-[2-(2-Meth-

oxynicotinamido)ethyl]piperidino]sulfonyl]-3-(5-norbornen-2-ylmethyl)urea. *CAS-51876-98-3*. INN. *Antidiabetic.* ◇*CP-27,634*

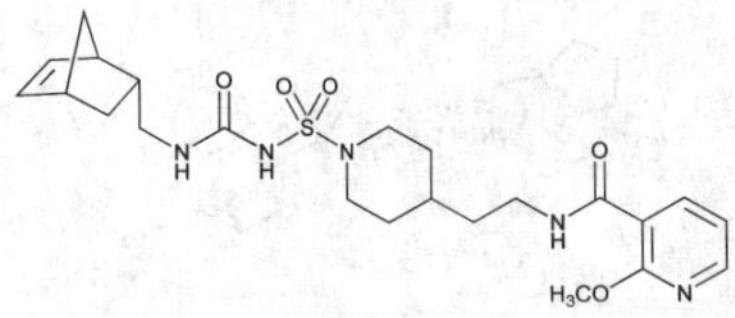

Glibenclamide (INN, BAN, JAN, DCF) — *See* Glyburide.

Glibornuride [*1971*] (glye born′ ure ide). $C_{18}H_{26}N_2O_4S$. 366.48. (1) Benzenesulfonamide, *N*-[[(3-hydroxy-4,7,7-trimethylbicyclo[2.2.1]hept-2-yl)amino]carbonyl]-4-methyl-, [1*S*-(*endo, endo*)]-; (2) *endo, endo*-1-[(1*R*)-(2-Hydroxy-3-bornyl)]-3-(*p*-tolylsulfonyl)urea. *CAS-26944-48-9.* INN; BAN. *Antidiabetic.* Glutril (Hoffmann-LaRoche†) ◇*Ro 6-4563*

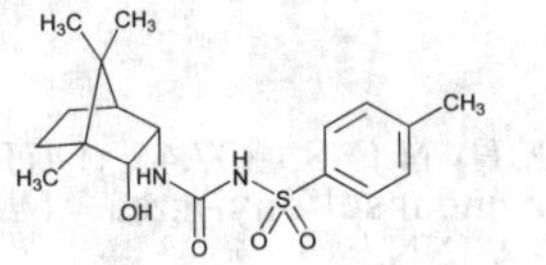

Glibutimine. $C_{21}H_{30}N_4O_3S$. 418.55. *N*-[*p*-[[3-(3-Cyclohexen-1-yl)-2-imino-1-imidazolidinyl]sulfonyl]phenethyl]butyramide. *CAS-25859-76-1.* INN. ◇*GP 51084*

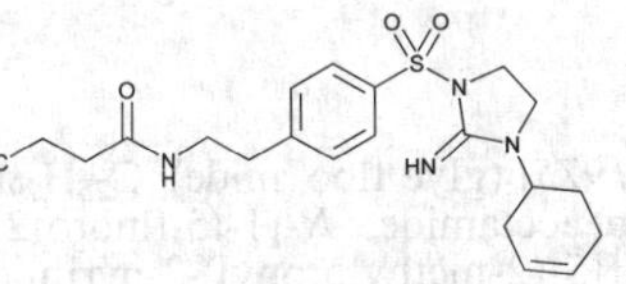

Glicaramide. $C_{30}H_{42}N_6O_5S$. 598.76. 1-Cyclohexyl-3-[[*p*-[2-[1-ethyl-4-(isopentyloxy)-3-methyl-1*H*-pyrazolo[3,4-*b*]pyridine-5-carboxamido]ethyl]phenyl]sulfonyl]urea. *UNII-UK5SR22C8Q. CAS-36980-34-4.* INN.

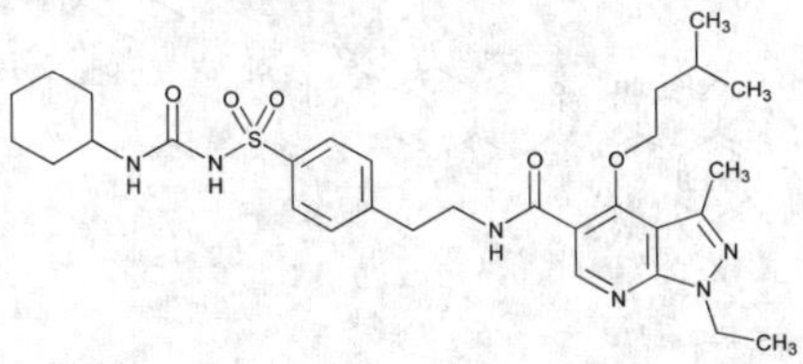

Glicetanile Sodium [*1977*] (glye set′ a nile soe′ dee um). $C_{23}H_{24}ClN_4NaO_4S$. 510.97. [Glicetanile is INN.] (1) Benzeneacetamide, *N*-(5-chloro-2-methoxyphenyl)-4-[[[5-(2-methylpropyl)-2-pyrimidinyl]amino]sulfonyl]-, monosodium salt; (2) 5′-Chloro-2-[*p*-[(5-isobutyl-2-pyrimidinyl)sulfamoyl]phenyl]-*o*-acetanisidide monosodium salt. *UNII-M3FU19R357; UNII-S39J3B52KS* [glicetanile]. *CAS-24428-71-5; CAS-24455-58-1* [glicetanile]. *Antidiabetic.* [*Name previously used: Glydanile Sodium.*] ◇*SH 1051*

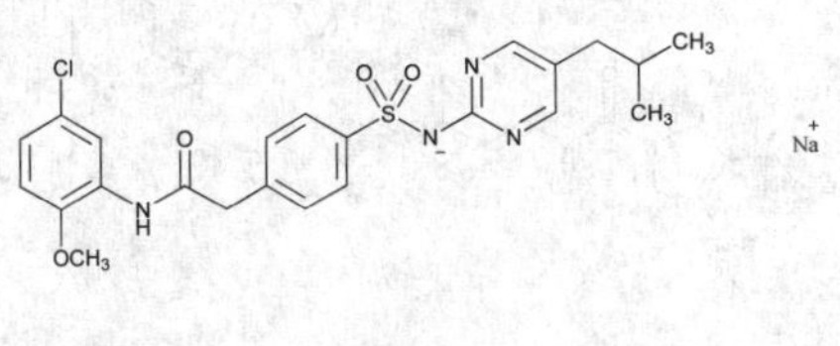

Gliclazide. C$_{15}$H$_{21}$N$_3$O$_3$S. 323.41. 1-(3-Azabicyclo[3.3.0]oct-3-yl)-3-(*p*-tolylsulfonyl)urea. *CAS-21187-98-4.* INN; BAN; JAN; DCF; MI. ◇*SE 1702*

Glicondamide. C$_{18}$H$_{20}$ClN$_3$O$_5$S. 425.89. 1-[[*p*-[2-(5-Chloro-*o*-anisamido)ethyl]phenyl]sulfonyl]-3-methylurea. *UNII-876SH4764F. CAS-52994-25-9.* INN.

Glidazamide. C$_{16}$H$_{23}$N$_3$O$_3$S. 337.44. 1-(Hexahydro-1*H*-azepin-1-yl)-3-(5-indansulfonyl)urea. *UNII-904C84L01N. CAS-3074-35-9.* INN.

Gliflumide [*1975*] (glye floo′ mide). C$_{25}$H$_{29}$FN$_4$O$_4$S. 500.59. (1) Benzeneacetamide, *N*-[1-(5-fluoro-2-methoxyphenyl)ethyl]-4-[[[5-(2-methylpropyl)-2-pyrimidinyl]amino]sulfonyl]-, (*S*)-(-)-; (2) (-)-(*S*)-*N*-(5-Fluoro-2-methoxy-α-methylbenzyl)-2-[*p*-[(5-isobutyl-2-pyrimidinyl)sulfamoyl]phenyl]acetamide. *UNII-USE67B01YN. CAS-35273-88-2.* INN. *Antidiabetic.* ◇*SH 3.1168*

Glimepiride [*1992*] (glye mep′ ir ide). **USP.** C$_{24}$H$_{34}$N$_4$O$_5$S. 490.62. (1) 1*H*-Pyrrole-1-carboxamide, 3-ethyl-2,5-dihydro-4-methyl-*N*-[2-[4-[[[[(4-methylcyclohexyl)amino]carbonyl]amino]sulfonyl]phenyl]ethyl]-2-oxo-, *trans*-; (2) 1-[[*p*-[2-(3-Ethyl-4-methyl-2-oxo-3-pyrroline-1-carboxamido)ethyl]phenyl]sulfonyl]-3-(*trans*-4-methylcyclohexyl)urea. *UNII-6KY687524K. CAS-93479-97-1.* INN; BAN. *Hypoglycemic.* Amaryl (Sanofi Aventis) ◇*HOE 490*

Glipalamide. C$_{12}$H$_{15}$N$_3$O$_3$S. 281.33. (±)-5-Methyl-*N*-(*p*-tolylsulfonyl)-2-pyrazoline-1-carboxamide. *UNII-W7J490CUHM. CAS-37598-94-0.* INN.

Glipentide — *See* Glisentide.

Glipizide [*1974*] (glip′ i zide). **USP.** C$_{21}$H$_{27}$N$_5$O$_4$S. 445.54. (1) Pyrazinecarboxamide, *N*-[2-[4-[[[(cyclohexylamino)carbonyl]amino]sulfonyl]phenyl]ethyl]-5-methyl-; (2) 1-Cyclohexyl-3-[[*p*-[2-(5-methylpyrazinecarboxamido)ethyl]phenyl]sulfonyl]urea. *UNII-X7WDT95N5C. CAS-29094-61-9.* INN; BAN. *Antidiabetic.* Glucotrol (Pfizer) ◇*CP-28,720; K 4024*

Gliquidone. C$_{27}$H$_{33}$N$_3$O$_6$S. 527.63. 1-Cyclohexyl-3-[[*p*-[2-(3,4-dihydro-7-methoxy-4,4-dimethyl-1,3-dioxo-2(1*H*)-isoquinolyl)ethyl]phenyl]sulfonyl]urea. *UNII-C7C2QDD75P. CAS-33342-05-1.* INN; BAN; MI. ◇*ARDF 26*

Glisamuride. C$_{23}$H$_{31}$N$_5$O$_4$S. 473.59. 1-Methyl-3-[*p*-[[3-(4-methylcyclohexyl)ureido]sulfonyl]phenethyl]-1-(2-pyridyl) urea. *UNII-T4C11E36L0. CAS-52430-65-6.* INN.

Glisentide. C$_{22}$H$_{27}$N$_3$O$_5$S. 445.53. 1-Cyclopentyl-3-[[*p*-[2-(*o*-anisamido)ethyl]phenyl]sulfonyl]urea. *UNII-392TQL1E2Z. CAS-32797-92-5.* INN.

Glisindamide. $C_{24}H_{28}N_4O_5S$. 484.57. 1-Cyclohexyl-3-[[*p*-[2-(1-oxo-2-isoindolinecarboxamido)ethyl]phenyl]sulfonyl]urea. *UNII-1928X5O3S5. CAS-71010-45-2.* INN.

Glisolamide. $C_{20}H_{26}N_4O_5S$. 434.51. 1-Cyclohexyl-3-[[*p*-[2-(5-methyl-3-isoxazolecarboxamido)ethyl]phenyl]sulfonyl]urea. *UNII-F83U6T74XR. CAS-24477-37-0.* INN.

Glisoxepide. $C_{20}H_{27}N_5O_5S$. 449.52. 1-(Hexahydro-1*H*-azepin-1-yl)-3-[[*p*-[2-(5-methyl-3-isoxazolecarboxamido)ethyl]phenyl]sulfonyl]urea. *UNII-H7SC0I332I. CAS-25046-79-1.* INN; BAN; DCF; MI. ⬦*BAY B 4231; FBB 4231; RP 22410*

Globulin, Immune (glob′ ue lin i mune′). **USP.** A sterile, nonpyrogenic solution of globulins that contains many antibodies normally present in adult human blood. *Immunizing agent (passive).* BayGam (Bayer); Gamimune N 5% (Bayer); Gamimune N 10% (Bayer); Gammagard (Hyland); Gammagee (Merck); Gammar (Centeon); Gammar-P I.V. (Centeon); Gamulin (Marion Merrell Dow†); Immu-G (Parke-Davis†); Immuglobin (Savage†); Sandoglobulin (Novartis); Venoglobulin-I (Alpha Therapeutic); Venoglobulin-S (Alpha Therapeutic) *[Name previously used: Globulin, Immune Human Serum.]*

Globulin, Immune Human Serum (previously used name) — *See* Globulin, Immune.

Globulin Serum, Anti-Human (glob′ ue lin). **USP.** A sterile, liquid preparation of serum produced by immunizing lower animals such as rabbits or goats with human serum or plasma, or with selected human plasma proteins. It is free from agglutinins and hemolysins to nonsensitized human red cells of all blood groups. It contains a suitable antimicrobial preservative.

Gloxazone [*1968*] (glox′ a zone). $C_8H_{16}N_6OS_2$. 276.38. (1) Hydrazinecarbothioamide, 2,2′-[1-(1-ethoxyethyl)-1,2-ethanediylidene]bis-; (2) 3-Ethoxy-2-oxobutyraldehyde bis(thiosemicarbazone); (3) (1-Ethoxyethyl)glyoxal bis(thiosemicarbazone). *UNII-OP8B49OL1J. CAS-2507-91-7.* INN; BAN. *Anaplasmodastat (veterinary).* Contrapar (Wellcome, Great Britain) ⬦*BW 356-C-61; NSC-82116*

Gloximonam [*1986*] (glox″ i moe′ nam). $C_{18}H_{25}N_5O_8S$. 471.48. (1) Acetic acid, [[3-[[(2-amino-4-thiazolyl)(methoxyimino)acetyl]amino]-2-methyl-4-oxo-1-azetidinyl]oxy]-, 2-(1,1-dimethylethoxy)-2-oxoethyl ester, [2*S*-[2α,3β(*Z*)]]-; (2) [[(2*S*,3*S*)-3-[(2-Amino-4-thiazolyl)glyoxylamido]-2-methyl-4-oxo-1-azetidinyl]oxy]acetic acid, ester with *tert*-butyl glycolate, 3^2-(*Z*)-(*O*-methyloxime). *UNII-9J68LNZ9ZL. CAS-90850-05-8.* INN. *Antibacterial.* ⬦*SQ 82531*

Glucagon (gloo′ ka gon). **USP.** $C_{153}H_{225}N_{43}O_{49}S$. 3482.75. (1) Glucagon (pig); (2) Glucagon. *UNII-76LA80IG2G. CAS-16941-32-5.* INN; BAN; JAN. *Antidiabetic.*

HSQGTFTSDY SKYLDSRRAQ DFVQWLMNT

Glucalox. Polymerized complex of glycerol and aluminum hydroxide. *CAS-12182-48-8.* INN; BAN. *[Name previously used: Glycalox.]*

Glucametacin. $C_{25}H_{27}ClN_2O_8$. 518.94. 2-[2-[1-(*p*-Chlorobenzoyl)-5-methoxy-2-methylindol-3-yl]acetamido]-2-deoxy-D-glucose. *UNII-N1EXE5EHAN. CAS-52443-21-7.* INN; MI.

Glucarpidase. $C_{1950}H_{3157}N_{543}O_{599}S_7$ (monomer). Recombinant glutamate carboxypeptidase (carboxypeptidase G2). *CAS-9074-87-7.* INN.

Gluceptate Sodium [*1978*] (gloo sep′ tate soe′ dee um). $C_7H_{13}NaO_8$. 248.16. (1) D-*glycero*-D-*gulo*-Heptonic acid, monosodium salt; (2) Monosodium D-*glycero*-D-*gulo*-

---

† Brand name formerly used, and/or firm no longer concerned with this product.

heptonate. *UNII-3D49LE7HM2. CAS-13007-85-7; CAS-87-74-1* [D-*glycero*-D-*gulo*-heptonic acid]. *Pharmaceutic aid.*

Gluconolactone (gloo kon″ oh lak′ tone). **USP.** $C_6H_{10}O_6$. 178.14. (1) D-Gluconic acid δ-lactone; (2) Glucono delta-lactone. *UNII-WQ29KQ9POT. CAS-90-80-2. Chelating agent.*

Glucosamine [*1971*] (gloo kose′ a meen). $C_6H_{13}NO_5$. 179.17. (1) D-Glucose, 2-amino-2-deoxy-; (2) 2-Amino-2-deoxy-β-D-glucopyranose. *CAS-3416-24-8.* NF XXI (tablets); INN. *Pharmaceutic aid.*

Glucosamine Hydrochloride. $C_6H_{13}NO_5$.HCl. 215.63. (1) D-Glucose, 2-amino-2-deoxy-, hydrochloride; (2) 2-Amino-2-deoxy-β-D-glucopyranose hydrochloride. *CAS-66-84-2.* NF XXI.

Glucosamine Sulfate Potassium Chloride. $(C_6H_{14}NO_5)_2$ $SO_4.2KCl$. 605.52. (1) Bis(D-Glucose, 2-amino-2-deoxy-), sulfate potassium chloride complex; (2) Bis(2-Amino-2-deoxy-β-D-glucopyranose) sulfate potassium chloride complex(-,-). *CAS-38899-05-7.* NF XXI.

Glucosamine Sulfate Sodium Chloride. $(C_6H_{14}NO_5)_2SO_4$. $2NaCl$. 573.31. (1) Bis(D-Glucose, 2-amino-2-deoxy-), sulfate sodium chloride complex; (2) Bis(2-Amino-2-deoxy-β-D-glucopyranose) sulfate sodium chloride complex (-,-). *CAS-38899-05-7.* NF XXI.

Glucose (JAN) — *See* Dextrose.

Glucose Enzymatic Test Strip (gloo′ kose en″ zi mat′ ik). **USP.** Consists of the enzymes glucose oxidase and horseradish peroxidase, a suitable substrate for the reaction of hydrogen peroxide catalyzed by peroxidase, and other inactive ingredients impregnated and dried on filter paper.

Glucose, Liquid (gloo′ kose). **NF.** A product obtained by the incomplete hydrolysis of starch. It consists chiefly of dextrose, dextrins, maltose, and water. *Pharmaceutic aid (tablet binder); pharmaceutic aid (tablet coating agent).* Glucose-40 (Ciba Vision, US Ophthalmics); Insta-Glucose (ICN)

Glucose Oxidase. Enzyme obtained from mycelia of fungi, such as *Aspergilli* and *Penicillia*. MI.

Glucosulfamide. $C_{13}H_{21}N_2NaO_{11}S_2$. 468.43. Glucose sodium bisulfite compound of N^1-hydroxymethylsulfanilamide. *CAS-7007-76-3.* INN.

Glucosulfone. $C_{24}H_{34}N_2Na_2O_{18}S_3$. 780.70. 4,4′-Diaminophe-nylsulfone-N,N-di(dextrose sodium sulfonate). *CAS-554-18-7.* INN; MI. ◊*SN-166* [*as the sodium salt*]

Glucurolactone. $C_6H_8O_6$. 176.12. [Glucuronolactone is JAN.] γ-Lactone of D-glucofuranuronic acid. *CAS-63-29-6.* INN; DCF; MI.

Glucuronamide. $C_6H_{11}NO_6$. 193.15. β-D-Glucopyranuron-amide. *CAS-61914-43-0.* INN; BAN; JAN.

Glucuronolactone (JAN) — *See* Glucurolactone.

Glufanide Disodium (previously used name) — *See* Oglufa-nide Disodium.

Glufosfamide. $C_{10}H_{21}Cl_2N_2O_7P$. 383.16. β-D-Glucopyranose 1-[N,N'-bis(2-chloroethyl)]phosphorodiamidate. *UNII-1W5N8SZD9A. CAS-132682-98-5.* INN.

Glunicate. $C_{36}H_{28}N_6O_{10}$. 704.64. 2-Deoxy-2-nicotinamido-β-D-glucopyranose 1,3,4,6-tetranicotinate. *CAS-80763-86-6.* INN.

Gluside — *See* Saccharin.

Gluside, Soluble — *See* Saccharin Sodium.

Glusoferron. D-Gluconic acid polymer with D-glucitol, iron(3+) salt. *CAS-56959-18-3.* INN.

Glutamate Sodium (JAN) — *See* Sodium Glutamate.

Glutamic Acid [*1988*] (gloo tam′ ik as′ id). $C_5H_9NO_4$. 147.13. *UNII-3KX376GY7L. CAS-6899-05-4; CAS-56-86-0* [L-glutamic acid]. INN.

Glutamine [*2002*] (gloo′ ta meen). **USP.** $C_5H_{10}N_2O_3$. 146.14. [L-Glutamine is JAN, Levoglutamide is DCF.] (1) L-Glutamine; (2) 2-Aminoglutaramic acid. *UNII-0RH81L854J. CAS-56-85-9.* INN. *Dietary supplement.* Nutrestore (Nutritional Restart) [*Name previously used: Levoglutamide.*]

Glutaral [*1973*] (gloo′ ta ral). **USP** [Concentrate]. $C_5H_8O_2$. 100.12. (1) Pentanedial; (2) Pentanedial; (3) Glutaraldehyde. *UNII-T3C89M417N. CAS-111-30-8.* INN; JAN. *Disinfectant.* Sonacide (Wyeth-Ayerst)

Glutathione. $C_{10}H_{17}N_3O_6S$. 307.32. *N*-(*N*-L-γ-Glutamyl-L-cysteinyl)glycine. *UNII-GAN16C9B8O. CAS-70-18-8.* BAN; JAN.

Glutaurine. $C_7H_{14}N_2O_6S$. 254.26. *N*-(2-Sulfoethyl)-L-glutamine. *UNII-B5T2Z06Y9N. CAS-56488-60-9.* INN.

Glutethimide. $C_{13}H_{15}NO_2$. 217.26. (1) 2,6-Piperidinedione, 3-ethyl-3-phenyl-; (2) 2-Ethyl-2-phenylglutarimide. *UNII-C8I4BVN78E. CAS-77-21-4.* USP XXIII; INN; BAN. *Sedative-hypnotic.* Doriden (Sanofi Aventis)

Glyburide [*1969*] (glye′ bure ide). **USP.** $C_{23}H_{28}ClN_3O_5S$. 494.00. [Glibenclamide is INN, BAN, and JAN.] (1) Benzamide, 5-chloro-*N*-[2-[4-[[[(cyclohexylamino)carbonyl]amino]sulfonyl]phenyl]ethyl]-2-methoxy-; (2) 1-[[*p*-[2-(5-Chloro-*o*-anisamido)ethyl]phenyl]sulfonyl]-3-cyclohexylurea. *UNII-SX6K58TVWC. CAS-10238-21-8. Antidiabetic.* Diabeta (Sanofi Aventis); Glynase (Pfizer); Micronase (Pfizer) ◇*HB 419; U-26,452*

Glybutamide (DCF) — *See* Carbutamide.

Glybuthiazol. $C_{12}H_{16}N_4O_2S_2$. 312.41. N^1-(5-*tert*-Butyl-1,3,4-thiadiazol-2-yl)sulfanilamide. *UNII-35421N8E8W. CAS-535-65-9.* INN; DCF; MI. ◇*RP 2259*

Glybuthizol — *See* Glybuthiazol.

Glybuzole. $C_{12}H_{15}N_3O_2S_2$. 297.40. *N*-(5-*tert*-butyl-1,3,4-thiadiazol-2-yl)benzenesulfonamide. *UNII-1DJ2B68M2C. CAS-1492-02-0.* INN; JAN; MI. ◇*RP 7891; AN 1324*

Glycalox (previously used name) — *See* Glucalox.

Glycerides Oleiques Polyoxyethylenes — *See* Peglicol 5 Oleate.

Glycerin (glis′ er in). **USP.** $C_3H_8O_3$. 92.09. [Glycerol is INN.] (1) 1,2,3-Propanetriol; (2) Glycerol. *UNII-PDC6A3C0OX. CAS-56-81-5.* JAN. *Pharmaceutic aid (humectant); pharmaceutic aid (solvent).* Ophthalgan (Wyeth-Ayerst); Optim (Dow Chemical); Osmoglyn (Alcon)

Glycerol (INN) — *See* Glycerin.

Glycerol, Iodinated [*1963*] (glis′ er ol eye′ oh di nay″ ted). $C_6H_{11}IO_3$. 258.05. Iodinated dimers of glycerol. (1) 1,3-Dioxolane-4-methanol, 2-(1-iodoethyl)-; (2) 2-(1-Iodoethyl)-1,3-dioxolane-4-methanol. *CAS-5634-39-9*. BAN. *Expectorant*. Organidin (Wallace)

Glyceryl Behenate (glis′ er il be hen′ ate). **NF**. A mixture of glycerides of fatty acids, mainly behenic acid. *Pharmaceutic aid (tablet and/or capsule lubricant).*

Glyceryl Borate — *See* Boroglycerin.

Glyceryl Distearate (glis′ er il dye steer′ ate). **NF**. A mixture of diglycerides, mainly glyceryl distearate, together with variable quantities of monoglycerides and triglycerides. *UNII-73071MW2KM. CAS-1323-83-7.*

Glyceryl Guaiacolate (previously used name) — *See* Guaifenesin.

Glyceryl Monolinoleate (glis′ er il mon″ oh lin oh′ lee ate). **NF**. A mixture of monoglycerides, mainly glyceryl monooleate and glyceryl monolinoleate, together with variable quantities of diglycerides and triglycerides. *CAS-26545-74-4.*

Glyceryl Monooleate (glis′ er il mon″ oh oh′ lee ate). **NF**. A mixture of monoglycerides, mainly glyceryl monooleate, together with variable quantities of diglycerides and triglycerides. *CAS-25496-72-4.*

Glyceryl Monostearate (glis′ er il mon″ oh steer′ ate). **NF**. (1) Octadecanoic acid, monoester with 1,2,3-propanetriol; (2) Monostearin. *CAS-31566-31-1*. JAN. *Pharmaceutic aid (emulsifying agent).* "EASTMAN" 600 (Eastman)

Glyceryl PABA — *See* Lisadimate.

Glyceryl Triacetate (previously used name) — *See* Triacetin.

Glyceryl Trinitrate (BAN and previously used name) — *See* Nitroglycerin.

Glycerylaminophenaquine — *See* Glafenine.

Glycine (glye′ seen). **USP**. $C_2H_5NO_2$. 75.07. [Aminoacetic Acid is JAN.] (1) Glycine; (2) Glycine. *UNII-TE7660X-O1C. CAS-56-40-6*. INN. Component of irrigating solution. Glycolixir (Bristol-Myers Squibb†) *[Name previously used: Aminoacetic Acid.]*

Glyclopyramide. $C_{11}H_{14}ClN_3O_3S$. 303.77. 1-[(p-Chlorophenyl)sulfonyl]-3-(1-pyrrolidinyl)urea. *UNII-KE474IKG1W. CAS-631-27-6*. INN; JAN.

Glycobiarsol. $C_8H_9AsBiNO_6$. 499.06. (1) Bismuth, [[4-[(hydroxyacetyl)amino]phenyl]arsonato(1-)]oxo-; (2) (Hydrogen *N*-glycoloylarsanilato)oxobismuth. *UNII-E3U8347QWJ. CAS-116-49-4*. USP XXI; INN; BAN; MI. *[Name previously used: Bismuth Glycollylarsanilate.]*

Glycocoll — *See* Glycine.

Glycol Distearate [*1981*] (glye′ kol dye steer′ ate). $C_{38}H_{74}O_4$ (Predominant). 594.99. It has an iodine value of less than 1, a saponification value of 190 to 200, and an acid value of less than 6. (1) Octadecanoic acid, 1,2-ethanediyl ester; (2) Ethylene distearate. *CAS-627-83-8*. CID. *Pharmaceutic aid (thickening agent).*

Glycophenylate — *See* Mepenzolate Bromide.

Glycopyrrolate [*1963*] (glye″ koe pir′ oh late). **USP**. $C_{19}H_{28}BrNO_3$. 398.33. [Glycopyrronium Bromide is INN, BAN, and JAN.] (1) Pyrrolidinium, 3-[(cyclopentylhydroxyphenylacetyl)oxy]-1,1-dimethyl-, bromide; (2) 3-Hydroxy-1,1-dimethylpyrrolidinium bromide α-cyclopentylmandelate. *UNII-V92SO9WP2I. CAS-596-51-0. Anticholinergic*. Robinul (Sciele) ◇AHR-504

Glycopyrrone Bromide — *See* Glycopyrrolate.

Glycopyrronium Bromide (INN, BAN, JAN) — *See* Glycopyrrolate.

Glycyclamide. $C_{14}H_{20}N_2O_3S$. 296.39. 1-Cyclohexyl-3-p-tolylsulfonylurea. *UNII-C40N4EJY68. CAS-664-95-9*. INN. ◇K-386; K-38

Glycyrrhetic Acid (JAN) — *See* Enoxolone.

Glycyrrhetinic Acid — *See* Glycyrrhizin.

Glycyrrhiza. NF XVI; JAN; MI.

Glycyrrhizin. $C_{42}H_{62}O_{16}$. 822.93. 20β-Carboxy-11-oxo-30-norolean-12-en-3β-yl-2-*O*-β-D-glucopyranuronosyl-α-D-glucopyranosiduronic acid. *CAS-1405-86-3*. JAN.

Glycyrrhizinate Dipotassium. $C_{42}H_{60}K_2O_{16}$. 899.11. Dipotassium (3β,20β)-20-carboxy-11-oxo-30-norolean-12-en-3-yl-2-*O*-β-D-glucopyranuronosyl-α-D-glucopyranosiduronate. JAN.

Glycyrrhizinic Acid — *See* Glycyrrhizin.

Glydanile Sodium (previously used name) — *See* Glicetanile Sodium.

Glyhexamide [*1965*] (glye hex′ a mide). $C_{16}H_{22}N_2O_3S$. 322.42. (1) 1*H*-Indene-5-sulfonamide, *N*-[(cyclohexylamino)carbonyl]-2,3-dihydro-; (2) 1-Cyclohexyl-3-(5-indanylsulfonyl)urea. *CAS-451-71-8*. INN. *Antidiabetic.* Subose (Bristol-Myers Squibb†) ◇*SQ 15,860; NSC-106960*

Glyhexylamide — *See* Metahexamide.

Glymidine Sodium [*1965*] (glye′ mi deen soe′ dee um). $C_{13}H_{14}N_3NaO_4S$. 331.32. (1) Benzenesulfonamide, *N*-[5-(2-methoxyethoxy)-2-pyrimidinyl]-, sodium salt; (2) [*N*-[5-(2-Methoxyethoxy)-2-pyrimidinyl]benzenesulfonamido] sodium salt. *UNII-4C5I4BQZ8F* [glymidine]. *CAS-3459-20-9; CAS-339-44-6* [glymidine]. INN; BAN; JAN. *Antidiabetic.* ◇*SH 717*

Glyoctamide [*1963*] (glye ok′ ta mide). $C_{16}H_{24}N_2O_3S$. 324.44. (1) Benzenesulfonamide, *N*-[(cyclooctylamino)carbonyl]-4-methyl-; (2) 1-Cyclooctyl-3-(*p*-tolylsulfonyl)urea. *CAS-1038-59-1*. INN. *Antidiabetic.*

Glyparamide [*1963*] (glye par′ a mide). $C_{15}H_{16}ClN_3O_3S$. 353.82. (1) Benzenesulfonamide, 4-chloro-*N*-[[[4-(dimethylamino)phenyl]amino]carbonyl]-; (2) 1-[(*p*-Chlorophenyl)sulfonyl]-3-[*p*-(dimethylamino)phenyl]urea. *UNII-9S339BH15E. CAS-5581-42-0. Antidiabetic.* ◇*P-1306*

Glyphylline — *See* Dyphylline.

Glypinamide. $C_{13}H_{18}ClN_3O_3S$. 331.82. 1-[(*p*-Chlorophenyl)sulfonyl]-3-(hexahydro-1*H*-azepin-1-yl)urea. *UNII-ORE084U8IP. CAS-1228-19-9*. INN; MI.

Glyprothiazol. $C_{11}H_{14}N_4O_2S_2$. 298.38. N^1-(5-Isopropyl-1,3,4-thiadiazol-2-yl)sulfanilamide. *UNII-1804FJN4MO. CAS-80-34-2*. INN; DCF. ◇*RP 2254; VK-57; IPTD; PASIT*

Glyprothizol — *See* Glyprothiazol.

Glysobuzole. $C_{13}H_{17}N_3O_3S_2$. 327.42. *N*-(5-Isobutyl-1,3,4-thiadiazol-2-yl)-*p*-methoxybenzenesulfonamide. *UNII-887VHL8899. CAS-3567-08-6*. INN; BAN; DCF. *[Name previously used: Isobuzole.]*

Gold Au 198 [*1963*] (golde). [Colloidal Gold (¹⁹⁸Au) Injection is JAN.] (1) Gold, isotope of mass 198; (2) Gold, isotope of mass 198. *CAS-10043-49-9*. USP XX. *Antineoplastic; diagnostic aid (liver imaging); radioactive agent.* Aurcoloid-198 (Abbott†); Aureotope (Bristol-Myers Squibb†); Auroscan-198 (Abbott†)

Gold Sodium Thiomalate (golde soe′ dee um thye″ oh mal′ ate). **USP.** $C_4H_3AuNa_2O_4S+C_4H_4AuNaO_4S$. 368.09. [Sodium Aurothiomalate is INN and JAN.] A mixture of the mono- and di-sodium salts of gold thiomalic acid. (1) Butanedioic acid, mercapto-, monogold(1+) sodium salt; (2) Mercaptosuccinic acid, monogold(1+) sodium salt. *CAS-12244-57-4; CAS-70-49-5* [thiomalic acid]. *Antirheumatic.* Myochrysine (Merck)

Gold Sodium Thiosulfate. $Na_3Au(S_2O_3)_2.2H_2O$. 526.22. [Sodium Aurotiosulfate is INN.] Sodium dithiosulfatoaurate (I). NF XII; MI.

Gold Thioglucose — *See* Aurothioglucose.

Goldenseal. NF XXI.

Goldenseal, Powdered. NF XXI.

Golimumab [*2004*] (goe lim′ ue mab). $C_{6530}H_{10068}N_{1752}O_{2026}S_{44}$. Immunoglobulin G1, anti-(human tumor necrosis factor α) (human monoclonal CNTO 148 γ1-chain), disulfide with human monoclonal CNTO 148 κ-chain, dimer. Molecular weight is approximately 147,000 daltons. *CAS-476181-74-5*. INN. *Treatment of inflammatory disorders; rheumatoid arthritis, uveitis, asthma and Crohn's disease.* ◇*CNTO 148*

---

† Brand name formerly used, and/or firm no longer concerned with this product.

Golotimod [*2007*] (goe lot' i mod). $C_{16}H_{19}N_4O_5$. 347.35. (1) D-γ-Glutamyl-L-Tryptophan; (2) (2*R*)-2-Amino-5-[[(1*S*)-1-carboxy-2-(1*H*-indol-3-yl)ethyl]amino]-5-oxopentanoic acid. *UNII-637C487Y09. CAS-229305-39-9.* INN. *Treatment of infectious disease.* ◇*SCV-07*

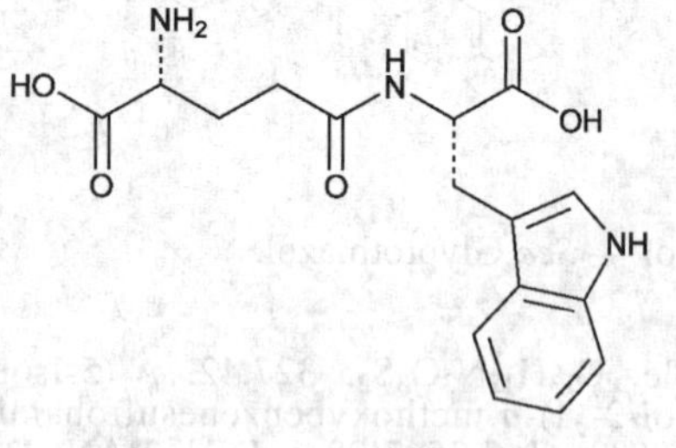

Gomiliximab [*2002*] (goe" mi lix' i mab). Immunoglobulin G1, anti-(human immunoglobulin E receptor type II) (human-Macaca irus monoclonal IDEC-152 γ1-chain), disulfide with human-Macaca irus monoclonal IDEC-152 κ-chain, dimer. *CAS-357613-86-6. Treatment of allergic asthma.* ◇*IDEC-152*

Gonadorelin Acetate [*1975*] (goe nad" oh rel' in as' e tate). **USP.** $C_{55}H_{75}N_{17}O_{13} \cdot xC_2H_4O_2 \cdot yH_2O$. [Gonadorelin is INN and BAN; Gonadorelin Diacetate is JAN.] Gonadorelin acetate is the diacetate salt (as the tetrahydrate) or a mixture of monoacetate and diacetate hydrates. (1) Luteinizing hormone-releasing factor acetate (salt) hydrate; (2) 5-Oxo-L-prolyl-L-histidyl-L-tryptophyl-L-seryl-L-tyrosylglycyl-L-leucyl-L-arginyl-L-prolylglycinamide acetate (salt) hydrate. *UNII-2RG1XQ1NYJ. CAS-52699-48-6; CAS-33515-09-2* [gonadorelin]. *Gonad-stimulating principle.* Lutrepulse (Ferring Pharmaceuticals) *[Name previously used: Luteinizing Hormone–releasing Factor Diacetate Tetrahydrate.]* ◇*Abbott-41070*

5-oxoP H W S Y G L R P G　　• *x* CH₃COOH　　• *y* H₂O

Gonadorelin Hydrochloride [*1975*] (goe nad" oh rel' in hye" droe klor' ide). **USP.** $C_{55}H_{75}N_{17}O_{13} \cdot 2HCl$. 1255.21. (1) Luteinizing hormone–releasing factor hydrochloride; (2) 5-Oxo-L-prolyl-L-histidyl-L-tryptophyl-L-seryl-L-tyrosylgly-cyl-L-leucyl-L-arginyl-L-prolylglycinamide hydrochloride. *Note—Gonadorelin Hydrochloride is the monohydrochloride or the dihydrochloride or as a mixture of these. UNII-3PFC574ITA. CAS-51952-41-1; CAS-33515-09-2* [gonadorelin]. *Gonad-stimulating principle.* Factrel (Baxter Healthcare) *[Name previously used: Luteinizing Hormone–releasing Factor Dihydrochloride.]* ◇*AY-24,031*

Gonadotrophin, Chorionic (INN, BAN, JAN) — *See* Gonadotropin, Chorionic.

Gonadotrophin, Serum (INN, BAN, JAN, DCF) — *See* Gonadotropin, Serum.

Gonadotropin, Chorionic (goe nad" oh troe' pin kor" ee on' ok). **USP.** [Gonadotrophin, Chorionic is INN, BAN, and JAN.] A gonad-stimulating polypeptide hormone obtained from the urine of pregnant women. *CAS-9002-61-3. Gonad-stimulating principle.* A.p.l. (Ferring Pharmaceuticals); Follutein (Bristol-Myers Squibb); Pregnyl (Organon)

Gonadotropin, Serum. [Gonadotrophin, Serum is INN, BAN, and JAN.] The follicle-stimulating substance obtained from the serum of pregnant mares. *CAS-9002-70-4.* Anteron (Schering†)

Goralatide. $C_{20}H_{33}N_5O_9$. 487.50. 1-[*N²*-[*N*-(*N*-Acetyl-L-seryl)-L-α-aspartyl]-L-lysyl]-L-proline. *CAS-120081-14-3.* INN.

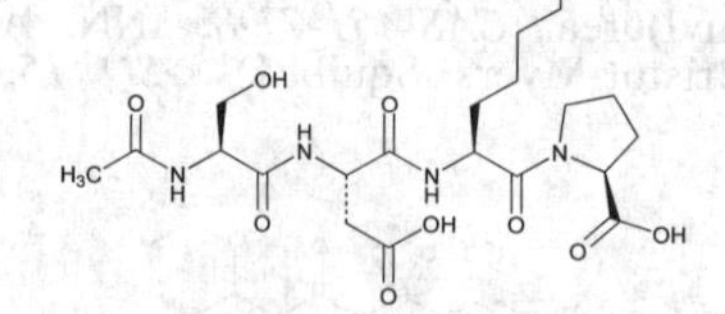

Goserelin [*1987*] (goe" se rel' in). $C_{59}H_{84}N_{18}O_{14}$. 1269.41. [Goserelin Acetate is JAN.] (1) Luteinizing hormone-releasing factor (pig), 6-[*O*-(1,1-dimethylethyl)-D-serine]-10-deglycinamide-, 2-(aminocarbonyl)hydrazide; (2) 1-(5-Oxo-L-prolyl-L-histidyl-L-tryptophyl-L-seryl-L-tyrosyl-*O*-*tert*-butyl-D-seryl-L-leucyl-L-arginyl-L-prolyl)semicarbazide. *UNII-0F65R8P09N. CAS-65807-02-5.* INN; BAN. *LHRH agonist.* Zoladex (Zeneca) ◇*ICI 118,630*

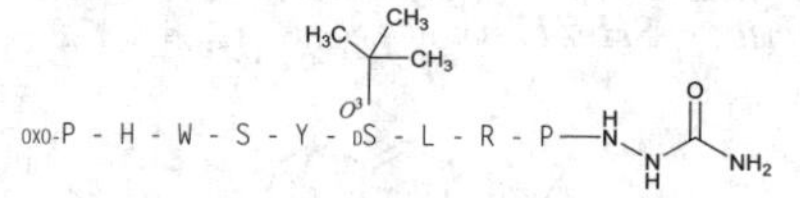

Govafilcon A [*1991*] (goe" va fil' kon). $(C_6H_{10}O_3)_v$ $(C_8H_{14}O_3)_w(C_4H_6O_2)_x(C_4H_6O_2)_y(C_{10}H_{14}O_4)_z$. (1) 2-Propenoic acid, 2-methyl-, 2-hydroxyethyl ester, polymer with (±)-2-hydroxybutyl 2-methyl-2-propenoate, ethenyl acetate, 2-methyl-2-propenoic acid and 1,2-ethanediyl bis(2-methyl-2-propenoate); (2) 2-Hydroxyethyl methacrylate polymer with (±)-2-hydroxybutyl methacrylate, vinyl acetate, methacrylic acid and ethylene dimethacrylate. *CAS-131517-13-0. Contact lens material (hydrophilic).*

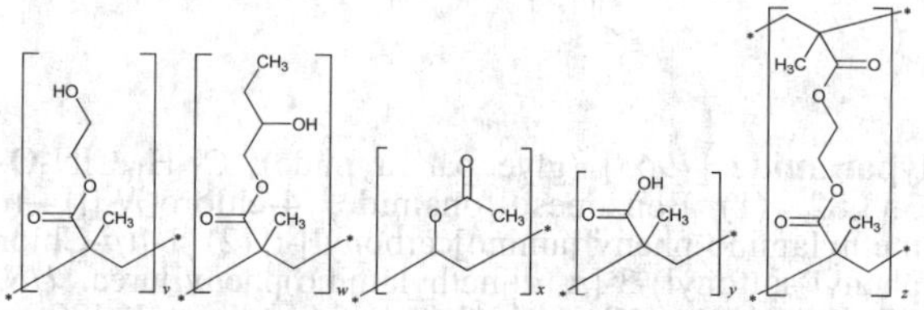

Goxalapladib [*2005*] (gox" a lap' la dib). $C_{40}H_{39}F_5N_4O_3$. 718.75. (1) 1,8-Naphthyridine-1(4*H*)-acetamide, 2-[2-(2,3-difluorophenyl)ethyl]-*N*-[1-(2-methoxyethyl)-4-piperidinyl]-4-oxo-*N*-[[4'-(trifluoromethyl)[1,1'-biphenyl]-4-yl]methyl]-; (2) 2-[2-[2-(2,3-Difluorophenyl)ethyl]-4-oxo-1,8-naphthyridin-1(4*H*)-yl]-*N*-[1-(2-methoxyethyl)piperidin-4-yl]-*N*-[[4'-(trifluoromethyl)biphenyl-4-yl]methyl]acetamide; (3) 2-{2-[2-(2,3-Difluorophenyl)ethyl]-4-oxo-1,8-naphthyridin-1(4*H*)-yl}-*N*-{1-(2-methoxyethyl)piperidin-4-yl}-*N*-[[4'-(trifluoromethyl)-1,1'-biphenyl-4-yl]methyl}acetamide. *UNII-GNG9ZD197L. CAS-412950-27-7.* INN. *Treatment of atherosclerosis.*

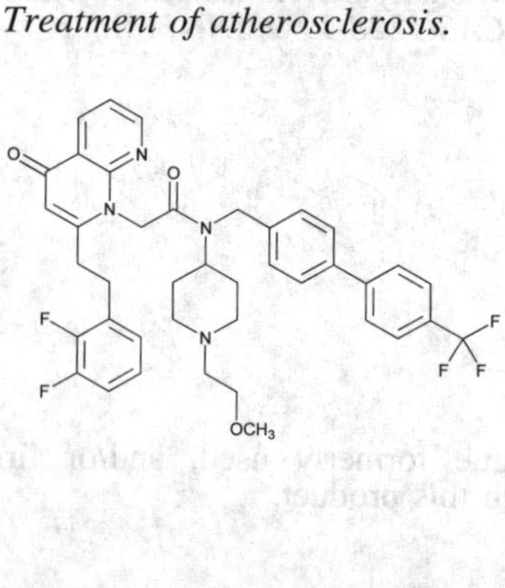

Graftskin. **USP**. A living, bilayered skin substitute derived from neonatal foreskins.

Gramicidin (gram i sye' din). **USP**. (1) Gramicidin; (2) Gramicidin. *UNII-5IE62321P4*. *CAS-1405-97-6*. INN; BAN. *Antibacterial*. Gramoderm (Schering†)

Gramicidin S. $C_{60}H_{92}N_{12}O_{10}$. 1141.45. Cyclo(L-valyl-L-ornithyl-L-leucyl-D-phenylalanyl-L-prolyl-L-valyl-L-ornithyl-L-leucyl-D-phenylalanyl-L-prolyl). *CAS-113-73-5*. INN; MI.

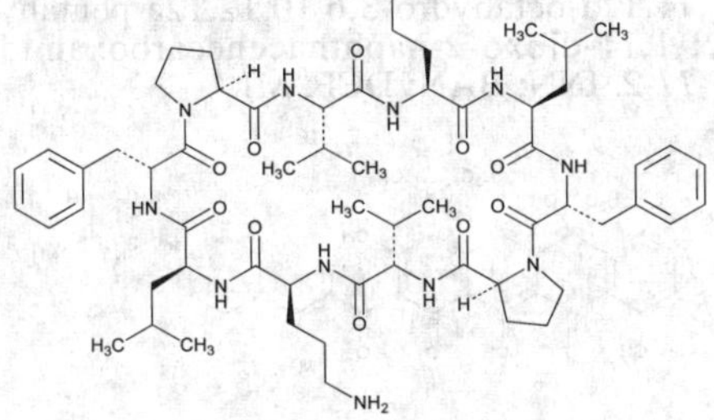

Granisetron [*1991*] (gra nis' e tron). $C_{18}H_{24}N_4O$. 312.41. (1) 1*H*-Indazole-3-carboxamide, 1-methyl-*N*-(9-methyl-9-azabicyclo[3.3.1]non-3-yl)-, *endo*-; (2) 1-Methyl-*N*-(9-methyl-*endo*-9-azabicyclo[3.3.1]non-3-yl)-1*H*-indazole-3-carboxamide. *UNII-WZG3J2MCOL*. *CAS-109889-09-0*. INN; BAN. *Anti-emetic*. ◇*BRL 43694*

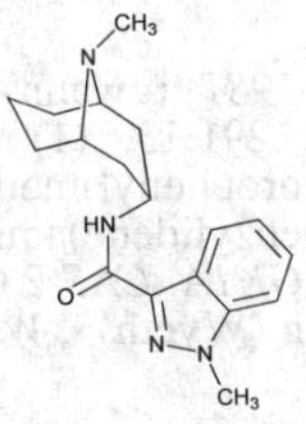

Granisetron Hydrochloride [*1992*] (gra nis' e tron hye" droe klor' ide). $C_{18}H_{24}N_4O{\cdot}HCl$. 348.87. (1) 1*H*-Indazole-3-carboxamide, 1-methyl-*N*-(9-methyl-9-azabicyclo[3.3.1]non-3-yl)-, monohydrochloride, *endo*-; (2) 1-Methyl-*N*-(9-methyl-*endo*-9-azabicyclo[3.3.1]non-3-yl)-1*H*-indazole-3-carboxamide monohydrochloride. *UNII-318F6L70J8*. *CAS-107007-99-8*. *Anti-emetic*. Kytril (Roche) ◇*BRL 43694A*

Grepafloxacin Hydrochloride [*1995*] (grep" a flox' a sin hye" droe klor' ide). $C_{19}H_{22}FN_3O_3{\cdot}HCl$. 395.86. [Grepafloxacin is INN and BAN.] (1) 3-Quinolinecarboxylic acid, 1-cyclopropyl-6-fluoro-1,4-dihydro-5-methyl-7-(3-methyl-1-piperazinyl)-4-oxo-, monohydrochloride, (±)-; (2) (±)-1-Cyclopropyl-6-fluoro-1,4-dihydro-5-methyl-7-(3-methyl-1-piperazinyl)-4-oxo-3-quinolinecarboxylic acid monohydrochloride. *UNII-A4ER1Z8N9N;*

UNII-L1M1U2HC31 [grepafloxacin]. *CAS-161967-81-3; CAS-119914-60-2* [grepafloxacin]. *Antibacterial*. Raxar (Otsuka) ◇*OPC-17116*

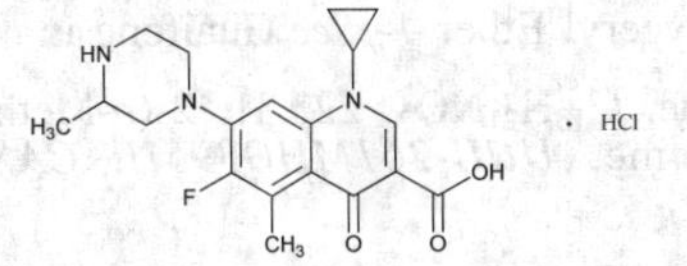

Griseofulvin (gris" ee oh ful' vin). **USP**. $C_{17}H_{17}ClO_6$. 352.77. (1) Spiro[benzofuran-2(3*H*),1'-[2]cyclohexene]-3,4'-dione, 7-chloro-2',4,6-trimethoxy-6'-methyl-, (1'*S-trans*)-; (2) 7-Chloro-2',4,6-trimethoxy-6'β-methylspiro[benzofuran-2(3*H*),1'-[2]cyclohexene]-3,4'-dione. *UNII-32HRV3E3D5*. *CAS-126-07-8*. INN; BAN; JAN. *Antifungal*. Fulvicin Bolus [Veterinary] (Schering-Plough Animal Health†); Fulvicin-P/G (Schering); Fulvicin-U/F (Schering); Fulvicin-U/F Powder and Tablets [Veterinary] (Schering-Plough Animal Health); Grifulvin V (Ortho Pharmaceutical); Grisactin (Wyeth-Ayerst); Gris-PEG (Allergan Herbert)

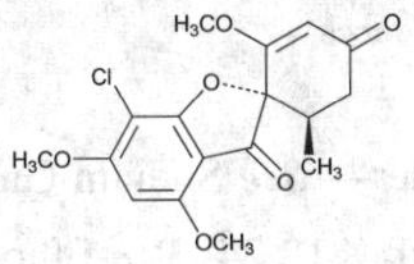

G-Strophanthin (JAN) — *See* Ouabain.

Guabenxan. $C_{10}H_{13}N_3O_2$. 207.23. (1,4-Benzodioxan-6-ylmethyl)guanidine. *UNII-SAW16W26X6*. *CAS-19889-45-3*. INN; DCF.

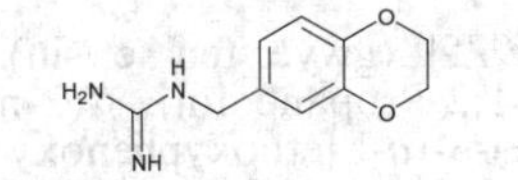

Guacetisal. $C_{16}H_{14}O_5$. 286.28. *o*-Methoxyphenyl salicylate acetate. *UNII-T6EKB9V2O2*. *CAS-55482-89-8*. INN.

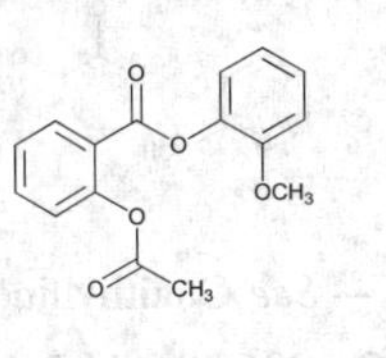

Guafecainol. $C_{16}H_{27}NO_4$. 297.39. 1-[2-(Diethylamino)-ethoxy]-3-(*o*-methoxyphenoxy)-2-propanol. *CAS-36199-78-7*. INN.

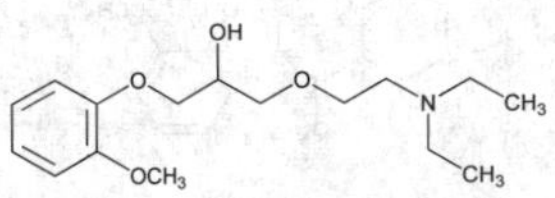

Guaiac. Gum or resin guaiac from wood of *Guajacum officinale* (Linné) or *G. sanctum* (Linné), Fam. *Zygophyllaceae*. MI.

Guaiacol. $C_7H_8O_2$. 124.14. 2-Methoxyphenol. *UNII-6JKA7-MAH9C*. *CAS-90-05-1*. NF X; JAN; MI.

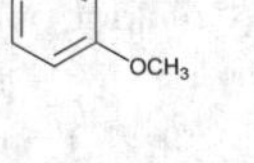

---

† Brand name formerly used, and/or firm no longer concerned with this product.

p-Guaiacol (previously used name) — *See* Mequinol.

Guaiacol Carbonate. *UNII-Q71XPQ6R29. CAS-553-17-3.* NF VII; MI.

Guaiacol Glyceryl Ether — *See* Guaifenesin.

Guaiactamine. $C_{13}H_{21}NO_2$. 223.31. 2-(*o*-Methoxyphenoxy)-triethylamine. *UNII-261MHO395H. CAS-15687-23-7.* INN; MI.

Guaiapate [*1981*] (gwye' a pate). $C_{18}H_{29}NO_4$. 323.43. (1) Piperidine, 1-[2-[2-[2-(2-methoxyphenoxy)ethoxy]ethoxy]ethyl]-; (2) 1-[2-[2-[2-(*o*-Methoxyphenoxy)ethoxy]ethoxy]ethyl]piperidine. *UNII-BDL7R8N38D. CAS-852-42-6.* INN. *Antitussive.* Klamar (Maggioni Farmaceutici S.p.A., Italy) ◇*M.G. 5454*

Guaiazulene Soluble — *See* Sodium Gualenate.

Guaietolin. $C_{11}H_{16}O_4$. 212.24. 3-(*o*-Ethoxyphenoxy)-1,2-propanediol. *CAS-63834-83-3.* INN.

Guaifenesin [*1975*] (gwye fen' e sin). **USP.** $C_{10}H_{14}O_4$. 198.22. (1) 1,2-Propanediol, 3-(2-methoxyphenoxy)-(±)-; (2) (±)-3-(*o*-Methoxyphenoxy)-1,2-propanediol. *UNII-495W7451VQ. CAS-93-14-1.* INN; BAN; JAN. *Expectorant.* Mucinex (Adams) [*Names previously used: Glyceryl Guaiacolate; Guaiphenesin.*]

Guaifylline (INN) — *See* Guaithylline.

Guaimesal. $C_{16}H_{14}O_5$. 286.28. (±)-2-(*o*-Methoxyphenoxy)-2-methyl-1,3-benzodioxan-4-one. *UNII-K43273G1CW. CAS-81674-79-5.* INN.

Guaiphenesin (previously used name) — *See* Guaifenesin.

Guaisteine. $C_{15}H_{19}NO_4S_2$. 341.45. Thioacetic acid, *S*-ester with (±)-3-(mercaptoacetyl)-2-[(*o*-methoxyphenoxy)-methyl]thiazolidine. *UNII-Y5PAQ48WOO. CAS-103181-72-2.* INN.

Guaithylline [*1965*] (gwye' thi lin). $C_7H_8N_4O_2 \cdot C_{10}H_{14}O_4$. 378.38. [Guaifylline is INN.] (1) 1*H*-Purine-2,6-dione, 3,7-dihydro-1,3-dimethyl-, compd. with 3-(2-methoxyphenoxy-1,2-propanediol (1:1); (2) Theophylline compound with 3-(*o*-methoxyphenoxy)-1,2-propanediol. *CAS-5634-38-8. Bronchodilator; expectorant.*

Guamecycline. $C_{29}H_{38}N_8O_8$. 626.66. *N*-[[4-(Amidinoamidino)-1-piperazinyl]methyl]-4-(dimethylamino)-1,4,4a,-5,5a,6,11,12a-octahydro-3,6,10,12,12a-pentahydroxy-6-methyl-1,11-dioxo-2-naphthacenecarboxamide. *CAS-16545-11-2.* INN; BAN; DCF; MI.

Guanabenz [*1971*] (gwahn' a benz). $C_8H_8Cl_2N_4$. 231.08. (1) Hydrazinecarboximidamide, 2-[(2,6-dichlorophenyl)-methylene]-; (2) [(2,6-Dichlorobenzylidene)amino]guanidine. *CAS-5051-62-7.* INN. *Antihypertensive.* ◇*Wy-8678; NSC-68982*

Guanabenz Acetate [*1981*] (gwahn' a benz as' e tate). **USP.** $C_8H_8Cl_2N_4 \cdot C_2H_4O_2$. 291.13. (1) Hydrazinecarboximidamide, 2-[(2,6-dichlorophenyl)methylene]-, monoacetate; (2) [(2,6-Dichlorobenzylidene)amino]guanidine monoacetate. *UNII-443O19GK1A. CAS-23256-50-0.* JAN. *Antihypertensive.* Wytensin (Wyeth) ◇*WY-8678 acetate*

Guanacline Sulfate [*1968*] (gwahn' a kleen sul' fate). $C_9H_{18}N_4 \cdot H_2SO_4 \cdot 2H_2O$. 316.38. [Guanacline is INN and BAN.] (1) Guanidine, [2-(3,6-dihydro-4-methyl-1(2*H*)-pyridinyl)ethyl]-, sulfate (1:1), dihydrate; (2) [2-(3,6-Dihydro-4-methyl-1(2*H*)-pyridyl)ethyl]guanidine sulfate (1:1) dihydrate. *CAS-23389-32-4; CAS-1562-71-6* [anhydrous]; *CAS-1463-28-1* [guanacline]. *Antihypertensive.* ◇*B 1464*

Guanadrel Sulfate [*1968*] (gwahn' a drel sul' fate). **USP.** $(C_{10}H_{19}N_3O_2)_2 \cdot H_2SO_4$. 524.63. [Guanadrel is INN.] (1) Guanidine (1,4-dioxaspiro[4.5]dec-2-ylmethyl)-, sulfate (2:1); (2) (1,4-Dioxaspiro[4.5]dec-2-ylmethyl)guanidine sulfate (2:1). *UNII-MT147RMO91; UNII-765C9332T4* [guanadrel]. *CAS-22195-34-2; CAS-40580-59-4* [guanadrel]. *Antihypertensive*. Hylorel (Pfizer) ◇*CL-1388R; U-28,288D*

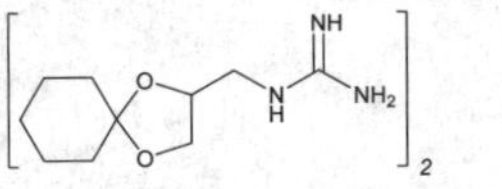

Guanazodine. $C_9H_{20}N_4$. 184.28. [(Octahydro-2-azocinyl)methyl]guanidine. *CAS-32059-15-7*. INN; MI.

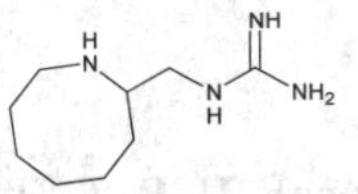

Guancidine (INN) — *See* Guancydine.

Guanclofine. $C_9H_{12}Cl_2N_4$. 247.12. [2-(2,6-Dichloroanilino)ethyl]guanidine. *UNII-9D89762N7C. CAS-55926-23-3*. INN.

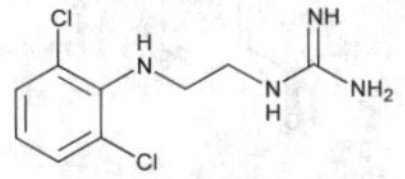

Guancydine [*1967*] (gwahn′ si deen). $C_7H_{14}N_4$. 154.21. [Guancidine is INN.] (1) Guanidine, *N″*-cyano-*N*-(1,1-dimethylpropyl)-; (2) 2-Cyano-1-*tert*-pentylguanidine. *CAS-1113-10-6*. *Antihypertensive*. ◇*CL 2422*

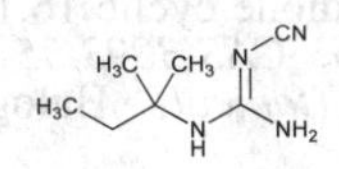

Guanethidine Monosulfate [*1966*] (gwahn eth′ i deen mon″ oh sul′ fate). **USP**. $C_{10}H_{22}N_4.H_2SO_4$. 296.39. [Guanethidine is INN and BAN.] (1) Guanidine, [2-(hexahydro-1(2*H*)-azocinyl)ethyl]-, sulfate (1:1); (2) [2-(Hexahydro-1(2*H*)-azocinyl)ethyl]guanidine sulfate (1:1). *UNII-5UBY8Y002G; UNII-ZTI6C33Q2Q* [guanethidine]. *CAS-645-43-2; CAS-55-65-2* [guanethidine]. *Antihypertensive*. Ismelin (Novartis)

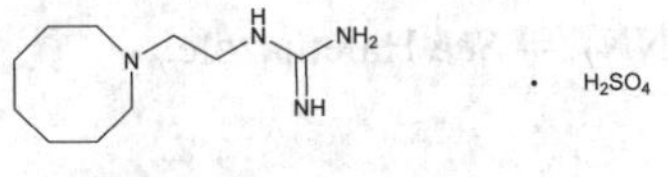

Guanethidine Sulfate [*1963*] (gwahn eth′ i deen sul′ fate). $(C_{10}H_{22}N_4)_2.H_2SO_4$. 494.70. (1) Guanidine, [2-(hexahydro-1(2*H*)-azocinyl)ethyl]-, sulfate (2:1); (2) [2-(Hexahydro-1(2*H*)-azocinyl)ethyl]guanidine sulfate (2:1). *UNII-8AQ60474G9; UNII-ZTI6C33Q2Q* [guanethidine]. *CAS-60-02-6; CAS-55-65-2* [guanethidine]. USP XXI; JAN. *Antihypertensive*. ◇*Su-5864; NSC-29863*

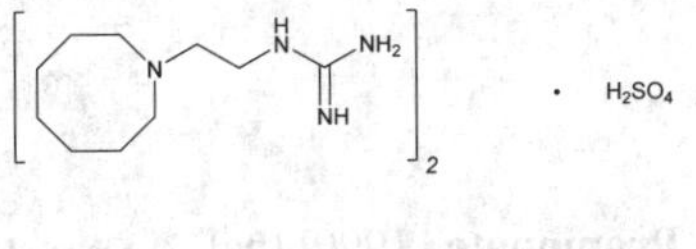

Guanfacine Hydrochloride [*1979*] (gwahn′ fa seen hye″ droe klor′ ide). **USP**. $C_9H_9Cl_2N_3O.HCl$. 282.55. [Guanfacine is INN and BAN.] (1) Benzeneacetamide, *N*-(aminoiminomethyl)-2,6-dichloro-, monohydrochloride; (2) *N*-Amidino-2-(2,6-dichlorophenyl)acetamide monohydrochloride. *UNII-PML56A160O; UNII-30OMY4G3MK* [guanfacine]. *CAS-29110-48-3; CAS-29110-47-2* [guanfacine]. JAN. *Antihypertensive*. Tenex (Dr. Reddy's) ◇*BS 100-141*

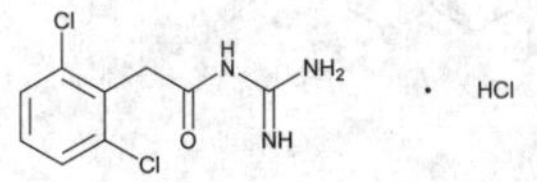

Guanisoquin Sulfate [*1964*] (gwahn eye′ soe kwin sul′ fate). $[C_{10}H_{12}BrN_3]_2.H_2SO_4$. 606.33. [Guanisoquine is INN.] (1) 2(1*H*)-Isoquinolinecarboximidamide, 7-bromo-3,4-dihydro-, sulfate (2:1); (2) 7-Bromo-3,4-dihydro-2(1*H*)-isoquinolinecarboxamide sulfate (2:1). *UNII-E4E8GE5LVJ; UNII-307YLU08D8* [guanisoquin]. *CAS-1212-83-5; CAS-154-73-4* [guanisoquin]. *Antihypertensive*. ◇*P-3896*

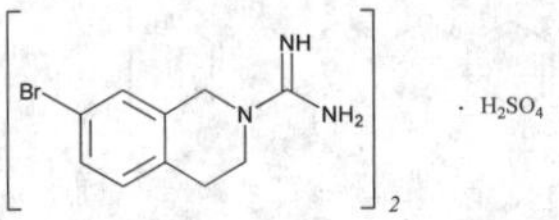

Guanoclor Sulfate [*1964*] (gwahn′ oh klor sul′ fate). $[C_9H_{12}Cl_2N_4O]_2.H_2SO_4$. 624.33. [Guanoclor is INN and BAN.] (1) Hydrazinecarboximidamide, 2-[2-(2,6-dichlorophenoxy)ethyl]-, sulfate (2:1); (2) {[2-(2,6-Dichlorophenoxy)ethyl]amino}guanidine sulfate (2:1). *UNII-Q1U97XK18R; UNII-M4HBT852YO* [guanoclor]. *CAS-551-48-4; CAS-5001-32-1* [guanoclor]. *Antihypertensive*. Vatensol (Pfizer) ◇*3-01029; NSC-108163*

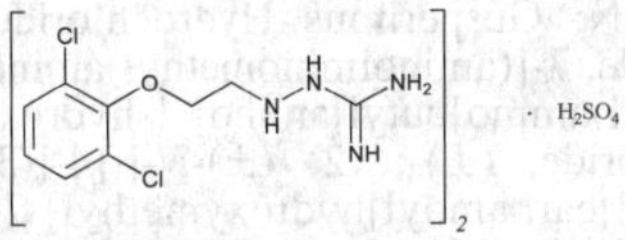

Guanoctine Hydrochloride [*1966*] (gwahn ok′ teen hye″ droe klor′ ide). $C_9H_{21}N_3.HCl$. 207.74. [Guanoctine is INN.] (1) Guanidine, (1,1,3,3-tetramethylbutyl)-, monohydrochloride; (2) (1,1,3,3-Tetramethylbutyl)guanidine monohydrochloride. *CAS-1070-95-7; CAS-3658-25-1* [guanoctine]. *Antihypertensive*. ◇*BP-1184; A-7283*

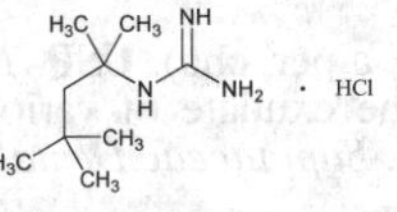

Guanoxabenz [*1974*] (gwahn ox′ a benz). $C_8H_8Cl_2N_4O$. 247.08. (1) Hydrazinecarboximidamide, 2-[(2,6-dichlorophenyl)methylene]-*N*-hydroxy-; (2) 1-[(2,6-Dichlorobenzylidene)amino]-3-hydroxyguanidine. *UNII-P9HIK5V7WK. CAS-24047-25-4*. INN. *Antihypertensive*. ◇*43-663*

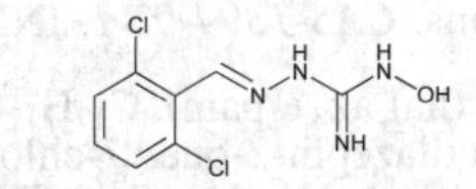

---

† Brand name formerly used, and/or firm no longer concerned with this product.

Guanoxan Sulfate [*1964*] (gwahn ox′ an sul′ fate). [$C_{10}H_{13}N_3O_2$]$_2$.H_2SO_4. 512.54. [Guanoxan is INN and BAN.] (1) Guanidine, (2,3-dihydro-1,4-benzodioxin-2-ylmethyl)-, sulfate (2:1); (2) 1,4-Benzodioxan-2-ylmethyl)-guanidine sulfate (2:1). *CAS-5714-04-5; CAS-2165-19-7* [guanoxan]. *Antihypertensive.* Envacar (Pfizer) ◇*3-01003*

Guanoxyfen Sulfate [*1965*] (gwahn ox′ i fen sul′ fate). ($C_{10}H_{15}N_3O$)$_2$.H_2SO_4. 484.57. [Guanoxyfen is INN.] (1) Guanidine, (3-phenoxypropyl)-, sulfate (2:1); (2) (3-Phenoxypropyl)quanidine sulfate (2:1). *UNII-47XBA61Y31; UNII-03HN50ZAF0* [guanoxyfen]. *CAS-1021-11-0; CAS-13050-83-4* [guanoxyfen]. *Antihypertensive; antidepressant.* ◇*CI-515; CN-34,799-5A; EA-166; HP 1598*

Guar Gum (gwahr gum). **NF**. A gum obtained from the ground endosperms of *Cyamopsis tetragonolobus* (Linné) Taub. (Fam. Leguminosae). *Pharmaceutic aid (tablet binder); pharmaceutic aid (tablet disintegrant).*

Gum Arabic — *See* Acacia.

Guncotton, Soluble — *See* Pyroxylin.

Gusperimus Trihydrochloride [*1993*] (gus per′ i mus trye hye″ droe klor′ ide). $C_{17}H_{37}N_7O_3$.3HCl. 496.90. [Gusperimus is INN; Gusperimus Hydrochloride is JAN.] (1) Heptanamide, 7-[(aminoiminomethyl)amino]-*N*-[2-[[4-[(3-aminopropyl)amino]butyl]amino]-1-hydroxy-2-oxoethyl]-, trihydrochloride, (±)-; (2) (±)-*N*-[[[4-[(3-Aminopropyl)amino]butyl]carbamoyl]hydroxymethyl]-7-guanidinoheptanamide trihydrochloride. *CAS-85468-01-5; CAS-104317-84-2* [gusperimus]; *CAS-84937-45-1* [hydrochloride]. *Immunosuppressant.* ◇*BMS-181173; BMY-42215-1; NKT-01; NSC-356894*

Gutta Percha (gut′ a per′ cha). **USP**. *Trans* isomer of rubber prepared from the exudate of various trees of the genus *Palaquium*, Fam. Sapotaceae.*Dental restoration agent.*

Gynergon — *See* Estradiol.

Gynoestryl — *See* Estradiol.

³H — *See* Water, Tritiated.

4HA (previously used name) — *See* Mequinol.

Hachimycin. [Trichomycin is JAN.] Antibiotic produced by *Streptomyces hachijoensis,* or the same substance produced by any other means. *CAS-1394-02-1.* INN; BAN; MI.

Halazepam [*1972*] (hal az′ e pam). $C_{17}H_{12}ClF_3N_2O$. 352.74. (1) 2*H*-1,4-Benzodiazepin-2-one, 7-chloro-1,3-dihydro-5-phenyl-1-(2,2,2-trifluoroethyl)-; (2) 7-Chloro-1,3-dihydro-5-phenyl-1-(2,2,2-trifluoroethyl)-2*H*-1,4-benzodiazepin-2-

one. *UNII-320YC168LF. CAS-23092-17-3.* USP XXII; INN; BAN. *Sedative-hypnotic.* Paxipam (Schering) ◇*Sch 12041*

Halazone (hal′ a zone). **USP**. $C_7H_5Cl_2NO_4S$. 270.09. (1) Benzoic acid, 4-[(dichloroamino)sulfonyl]-; (2) *p*-(Dichlorosulfamoyl)benzoic acid. *UNII-G359OL82VB. CAS-80-13-7.* INN. *Disinfectant.*

Halcinonide [*1973*] (hal sin′ oh nide). **USP**. $C_{24}H_{32}ClFO_5$. 454.96. (1) Pregn-4-ene-3,20-dione, 21-chloro-9-fluoro-11-hydroxy-16,17-[(1-methylethylidene)bis(oxy)]-, (11*β*,16*α*)-; (2) 21-Chloro-9-fluoro-11*β*,16*α*,17-trihydroxypregn-4-ene-3,20-dione cyclic 16,17-acetal with acetone. *UNII-SI86V6QNEG. CAS-3093-35-4.* INN; BAN; JAN. *Anti-inflammatory (topical).* Halog (Westwood-Squibb) ◇*SQ 18566*

Haletazole (INN) — *See* Halethazole.

Halethazole. $C_{19}H_{21}ClN_2OS$. 360.90. [Haletazole is INN.] 5-Chloro-2-[*p*-(2-diethylaminoethoxy)phenyl]benzothiazole. *UNII-U89MCO87LX. CAS-15599-36-7.* BAN; MI.

Halobetasol Propionate [*1990*] (hal″ oh bay′ ta sol proe′ pee oh nate). $C_{25}H_{31}ClF_2O_5$. 484.96. [Ulobetasol is INN.] (1) Pregna-1,4-diene-3,20-dione, 21-chloro-6,9-difluoro-11-hydroxy-16-methyl-17-(1-oxopropoxy)-, (6*α*,11*β*,16*β*)-; (2) 21-Chloro-6*α*,9-difluoro-11*β*,17-dihydroxy-16*β*-methylpregna-1,4-diene-3,20-dione 17-propionate. *UNII-

91A0K1TY3Z; UNII-9P6159HM7T [halobetasol]. *CAS-66852-54-8; CAS-98651-66-2* [halobetasol]. *Anti-inflammatory (topical).* ◇*BMY-30056; CGP-14,458*

Halocarban (INN) — *See* Cloflucarban.

Halocortolone. $C_{22}H_{27}ClF_2O_3$. 412.90. 9-Chloro-6α,11β-difluoro-21-hydroxy-16α-methylpregna-1,4-diene-3,20-dione. *CAS-24320-27-2.* INN.

Halocrinic Acid — *See* Brocrinat.

Halofantrine Hydrochloride [*1979*] (hal″ oh fan′ treen hye″ droe klor′ ide). $C_{26}H_{30}Cl_2F_3NO.HCl$. 536.88. [Halofantrine is INN and BAN.] (1) 9-Phenanthrenemethanol, 1,3-dichloro-α-[2-(dibutylamino)ethyl]-6-(trifluoromethyl)-, hydrochloride; (2) 1,3-Dichloro-α-[2-(dibutylamino)ethyl]-6-(trifluoromethyl)-9-phenanthrenemethanol hydrochloride. *UNII-H77DL0Y630; UNII-Q2OS4303HZ* [halofantrine]. *CAS-36167-63-2; CAS-69756-53-2* [halofantrine]; *CAS-66051-63-6* [[$\pm$]-halofantrine]. *Antimalarial.* Halfan (GlaxoSmithKline) ◇*WR-171669*

Halofenate [*1971*] (hal″ oh fen′ ate). $C_{19}H_{17}ClF_3NO_4$. 415.79. (1) Benzeneacetic acid, 4-chloro-α-[3-(trifluoromethyl)-phenoxy]-, 2-(acetylamino)ethyl ester; (2) (*p*-Chlorophenyl)[(α,α,α-trifluoro-*m*-tolyl)oxy]acetic acid ester with *N*-(2-hydroxyethyl)acetamide. *CAS-26718-25-2.* INN; BAN. *Antihyperlipoproteinemic; uricosuric.*

Halofuginone Hydrobromide [*1981*] (hal″ oh fue′ ji none hye″ droe broe′ mide). $C_{16}H_{17}BrClN_3O_3.HBr$. 495.59. [Halofuginone is INN and BAN.] (1) 4(3*H*)-Quinazolinone, 7-bromo-6-chloro-3-[3-(3-hydroxy-2-piperidyl)-2-oxo-propyl]-, hydrobromide, *trans*-($\pm$)-; (2) ($\pm$)-*trans*-7-Bro-

---

† Brand name formerly used, and/or firm no longer concerned with this product.

mo-6-chloro-3-[3-(3-hydroxy-2-piperidyl)-acetonyl]-4(3*H*)-quinazolinone monohydrobromide. *UNII-L31MM1385E* [halofuginone]. *CAS-64924-67-0; CAS-55837-20-2* [halofuginone]. *Antiprotozoal.* Stenorol (Roussel-UCLAF, France) ◇*RU-19110*

Halometasone. $C_{22}H_{27}ClF_2O_5$. 444.90. 2-Chloro-6α,9-difluoro-11β,17,21-trihydroxy-16α-methylpregna-1,4-diene-3,20-dione. *CAS-50629-82-8.* INN; MI.

Halonamine. $C_{15}H_{15}ClFNO$. 279.74. 2-[[*p*-Chloro-α-(*p*-fluorophenyl)benzyl]oxy]ethylamine. *CAS-50583-06-7.* INN.

Halopemide [*1977*] (hal oh′ pe mide). $C_{21}H_{22}ClFN_4O_2$. 416.88. (1) Benzamide, *N*-[2-[4-(5-chloro-2,3-dihydro-2-oxo-1*H*-benzimidazol-1-yl)-1-piperidinyl]ethyl]-4-fluoro-; (2) *N*-[2-[4-(5-Chloro-2-oxo-1-benzimidazolinyl)piperidino]ethyl]-*p*-fluorobenzamide. *UNII-65Q28TV0ZY.* *CAS-59831-65-1.* INN. *Antipsychotic.* ◇*R 34,301*

Halopenium Chloride. $C_{22}H_{30}BrCl_2NO$. 475.29. 4-Bromobenzyl[3-(4-chloro-5-methyl-2-isopropylphenoxy)propyl]-dimethylammonium chloride. *UNII-RT6K0322Q7.* *CAS-7008-13-1.* INN; BAN.

Haloperidol [*1965*] (hal″ oh per′ i dol). **USP.** $C_{21}H_{23}ClFNO_2$. 375.86. (1) 1-Butanone, 4-[4-(4-chlorophenyl)-4-hydroxy-1-piperidinyl]-1-(4-fluorophenyl)-; (2) 4-[4-(*p*-Chlorophenyl)-4-hydroxypiperidino]-4′-fluorobutyrophenone. *UNII-*

J6292F8L3D. CAS-52-86-8. INN; BAN; JAN. *Antidyskinetic (in Gilles de la Tourette's disease); antipsychotic.* Haldol (Ortho-McNeil) ◊*R-1625; McN-JR-1625*

Haloperidol Decanoate [*1980*] (hal″ oh per′ i dol dek″ a noe′ ate). $C_{31}H_{41}ClFNO_3$. 530.11. (1) Decanoic acid, 4-(4-chlorophenyl)-1-[4-(4-fluorophenyl)-4-oxobutyl]-4-piperidinyl ester; (2) Decanoic acid, ester with 4-[4-(*p*-chlorophenyl)-4-hydroxypiperidino]-4′-fluorobutyrophenone. *UNII-AC20PJ4101. CAS-74050-97-8.* BAN; JAN. *Antipsychotic.* Haldol (Ortho-McNeil) ◊*R-13,672*

Halopone Chloride — *See* Halopenium Chloride.

Halopredone Acetate [*1976*] (hal″ oh pred′ one as′ e tate). $C_{25}H_{29}BrF_2O_7$. 559.39. [Halopredone is INN.] (1) Pregna-1,4-diene-3,20-dione, 17,21-bis(acetyloxy)-2-bromo-6,9-difluoro-11-hydroxy-, (6β,11β)-; (2) 2-Bromo-6β,9-difluoro-11β,17,21-trihydroxypregna-1,4-diene-3,20-dione 17,21-diacetate. *CAS-57781-14-3; CAS-57781-15-4* [halopredone]. JAN. *Anti-inflammatory (topical).*

Haloprogesterone [*1962*] (hal″ oh proe jes′ ter one). $C_{21}H_{28}BrFO_2$. 411.35. (1) Pregn-4-ene-3,20-dione, 17-bromo-6-fluoro-, (6α)-; (2) 17-Bromo-6α-fluoropregn-4-ene-3,20-dione; (3) 17α-Bromo-6α-fluoroprogesterone. *UNII-803BIX5JG5. CAS-3538-57-6.* INN. *Progestin.*

Haloprogin [*1967*] (hal″ oh proe′ jin). $C_9H_4Cl_3IO$. 361.39. (1) Benzene, 1,2,4-trichloro-5-[(3-iodo-2-propynyl)oxy]-; (2) 3-Iodo-2-propynyl 2,4,5-trichlorophenyl ether. *UNII-AIU7053OWL. CAS-777-11-7.* USP XXIII; INN; JAN. *Antibacterial.* Halotex (Westwood-Squibb) ◊*M-1028 (Meiji); NSC-100071*

Halopyramine (previously used name) — *See* Chloropyramine.

Halothane (hal′ oh thane). **USP**. $C_2HBrClF_3$. 197.38. (1) Ethane, 2-bromo-2-chloro-1,1,1-trifluoro-, (±)-; (2) (±)-2-Bromo-2-chloro-1,1,1-trifluoroethane. *UNII-UQT9G45D1P. CAS-151-67-7.* INN; BAN; JAN. *Anesthetic (inhalation).* Fluothane (Wyeth)

Haloxazolam. $C_{17}H_{14}BrFN_2O_2$. 377.21. 10-Bromo-11b-(*o*-fluorophenyl)-2,3,7,11b-tetrahydrooxazolo[3,2-*d*][1,4]benzodiazepin-6(5*H*)-one. *CAS-59128-97-1.* INN; JAN; MI.

Haloxon. $C_{14}H_{14}Cl_3O_6P$. 415.59. 3-Chloro-7-hydroxy-4-methylcoumarin bis(2-chloroethyl)phosphate. *UNII-T8KXA37068. CAS-321-55-1.* INN; BAN; MI.

Halquinol (BAN) — *See* Halquinols.

Halquinols [*1964*] (hal′ kwin ols). [Halquinol is BAN.] (1) 8-Quinolinol, 5,7-dichloro-, mixt. with 5-chloro-8-quinolinol and 7-chloro-8-quinolinol; (2) 5,7-Dichloro-8-quinolinol mixt. with 5-chloro-8-quinolinol and 7-chloro-8-quinolinol; (3) 5,7-Dichloro-8-quinolinol, 5-chloro-8-quinolinol, and 7-chloro-8-quinolinol in proportions resulting naturally from chlorination of 8-quinolinol. *CAS-8067-69-4. Antiinfective, topical.* Quinolor (Bristol-Myers Squibb†) ◊*SQ 16,401*

Hamamelis — *See* Witch Hazel.

Hamycin [*1965*] (ha mye′ sin). Antibiotic derived from *Streptomyces pimprina.* (1) Hamycin; (2) Hamycin. *CAS-1403-71-0.* INN. *Antifungal.*

Hawthorn Leaf with Flower. NF XXI.

Hawthorn Leaf with Flower, Powdered. NF XXI.

HCTZ — *See* Hydrochlorothiazide.

Hedaquinium Chloride. $C_{34}H_{46}Cl_2N_2$. 553.65. 2,2′-Hexadecamethylenebis(isoquinolinium chloride). *CAS-4310-89-8.* INN; BAN; MI. ◊*B1Q 16*

Hefilcon A [*1997*] (he fil′ kon). $(C_6H_{10}O_3)_x(C_6H_9NO)_y$ $(C_{10}H_{14}O_4)_z$. (1) 2-Hydroxyethyl methacrylate polymer with 1-vinyl-2-pyrrolidinone and ethylene dimethacrylate;

(2) 2-Hydroxyethyl 2-methyl-2-propenoate polymer with 1-vinyl-2-pyrrolidinone and ethylene dimethacrylate; (3) 2-Propenoic acid, 2-methyl-, 2-hydroxyethyl ester, polymer with 1-ethenyl-2-pyrrolidinone and 1,2-ethanediyl bis(2-methyl-2-propenoate). *CAS-36425-29-3. Contact lens material (hydrophilic).* Crescent Bifocal (Bausch & Lomb†); Benz 42 (Benz Research and Development) *[Note—The water content of the contact lens material is 42%±2 at ambient temperature (23±2°C), the purity of 2-hydroxyethyl methacrylate (HEMA) is >99.5%, and the oxygen permeability is 11 × 10⁻¹¹(cm²/sec)(ml O₂/ml × mm Hg) at 35°C (Dk value).]*

Hefilcon B [*1979*] (he fil′ kon). $(C_6H_{10}O_3)_x(C_6H_9NO)_y(C_{10}H_{14}O_4)_z$. (1) 2-Hydroxyethyl methacrylate polymer with 1-vinyl-2-pyrrolidinone and ethylene dimethacrylate; (2) 2-Hydroxyethyl 2-methyl-2-propenoate polymer with 1-vinyl-2-pyrrolidinone and ethylene dimethacrylate; (3) 2-Propenoic acid, 2-methyl-, 2-hydroxyethyl ester, polymer with 1-ethenyl-2-pyrrolidinone and 1,2-ethanediyl bis(2-methyl-2-propenoate). *CAS-36425-29-3. Contact lens material (hydrophilic).* Criterion Ultra Toric (Bausch & Lomb†); Naturvus (Milton Roy); Optima Toric (Bausch & Lomb) *[Note—The chemical names, structural and molecular formula, and CAS Registry Number are identical for Hefilcon A, B and C.]*

Hefilcon C [*1998*] (he fil′ kon). $(C_6H_{10}O_3)_x(C_6H_9NO)_y(C_{10}H_{14}O_4)_z$. (1) 2-Hydroxyethyl methacrylate polymer with 1-vinyl-2-pyrrolidinone and ethylene dimethacrylate; (2) 2-Hydroxyethyl 2-methyl-2-propenoate polymer with 1-vinyl-2-pyrrolidinone and ethylene dimethacrylate; (3) 2-Propenoic acid, 2-methyl-, 2-hydroxyethyl ester, polymer with 1-ethenyl-2-pyrrolidinone and 1,2-ethanediyl bis(2-methyl-2-propenoate). *CAS-36425-29-3. Contact lens material (hydrophilic).* Gold Medalist Toric (Bausch & Lomb); Igel 56 (Igel Vision Care) *[Note—The water content of the contact lens material is 56.2% at ambient temperature (23±2°C), the purity of 2-hydroxyethyl methacrylate (HEMA) is 99.6%, and the oxygen permeability is 20 × 10⁻¹¹(cm²/sec)(ml O₂/ml × mm Hg) at 35°C (Dk value).][The chemical names, structural and molecular formula, and CAS Registry Number are identical for Hefilcon A, B and C.]*

Helenien (JAN) — *See* Xantofyl Palmitate.

Heliomycin. $C_{23}H_{18}O_6$. 390.39. Antibiotic obtained from cultures of *Actinomyces flavochromogenes* var. *heliomycini* or the same substance obtained by any other means. *UNII-7N3A092A5X. CAS-11029-70-2.* INN.

Helium (hee′ lee um). **USP.** He. 4.00. (1) Helium; (2) Helium. *CAS-7440-59-7. Gases, diluent for.*

Hemocoagulase. Enzyme obtained from the venom of the viper *Bothrops jararca.CAS-9001-13-2.* JAN.

Hemoglobin Crosfumaril [*1996*] (hee′ moe gloe″ bin kros fue′ ma ril). (1) Hemoglobin A₀ (human $\alpha_2\beta_2$ tetrameric subunit), α-chain 99,99′-diamide with (*E*)-2-butenoic acid; (2) Hemoglobin A₀ (human $\alpha_2\beta_2$ tetrameric subunit), α-chain 99,99′-diamide with fumaric acid. Molecular weight is approximately 64,500 daltons. *CAS-142261-03-8.* INN. *Perfusion deficit disorders treatment.* HemAssist (Baxter Healthcare) ◇*DCLHb*

Hemoglobin Glutamer-200 (Bovine) [*1997*] (hee′ moe gloe″ bin gloo′ ta mer boe′ vine). Hemoglobin-based oxygen carrier 301 is a solution of purified, glutaraldehyde-polymerized, bovine hemoglobin. The average polymer weight is 200,000 daltons. *CAS-192230-37-8. Oxygen carrier for veterinary use.* Oxyglobin Solution (Biopure) ◇*HBOC-301*

Hemoglobin Glutamer-250 (Bovine) [*1997*] (hee′ moe gloe″ bin gloo′ ta mer boe′ vine). [Hemoglobin glutamer is INN.] Hemoglobin-based oxygen carrier 201 is a solution of purified, glutaraldehyde-polymerized, bovine hemoglobin. The average polymer weight is 250,000 daltons. *CAS-192230-36-7. Oxygen carrier and blood substitute for human use.* Hemopure (Biopure) ◇*HBOC-201*

Hemoglobin Glutamer-256 (Human) [*2006*] (hee′ moe gloe″ bin gloo′ ta mer hue′ man). $C_{685}H_{1071}N_{187}O_{194}S_3$ (αHb) $C_{724}H_{1119}N_{195}O_{201}S_3$ (βHb). Hemoglobin Glutamer-256. *CAS-679404-95-6. Immediate replacement of lost oxygen-carrying capacity due to red blood cell loss.* PolyHeme (Northfield)

α Hb

```
VLSPADKTNV KAAWGKVGAH AGEYGAEALE RMFLSFPTTK TYFPHFDLSH
GSAQVKGHGK KVADALTNAV AHVDDMPNAL SALSDLHAHK LRVDPVNFKL
LSHCLLVTLA AHLPAEFTPA VHASLDKFLA SVSTVLTSKY R
```

β Hb

```
VHLTPEEKSA VTALWGKVNV DEVGGEALGR LLVVYPWTQR FFESFGDLST
PDAVMGNPKV KAHGKKVLGA FSDGLAHLDN LKGTFATLSE LHCDKLHVDP
ENFRLLGNVL VCVLAHHFGK EFTPPVQAAY QKVVAGVANA LAHKYH
```

Hemoglobin Raffimer [*2002*] (hee′ moe gloe″ bin raf′ fi mer). Hemoglobin raffimer is a solution of purified, *o*-raffinose cross-linked human hemoglobin A₀ in lactated Ringer's. For any given sample, the molecular weight is greater than 500,000 daltons for not more than 3% of the material, between 64,000 and 500,000 daltons for 54 to 62% of the material, approxiamtely 64,000 daltons for 34 to 43% of the material and approximately 32,000 daltons for 5% or less of the material. *CAS-197462-97-8.* INN; BAN. *Blood substitute, human derived hemoglobin based oxygen carrier (HBOC).* Hemolink (Hemosol, Canada)

Heparan Sulfate — *See* Danaparoid Sodium.

Heparin Calcium (hep′ a rin kal′ see um). **USP.** [Heparin is BAN.] The calcium salt of sulfated glycosaminoglycans present as a mixture of heterogeneous molecules of mixed mucopolysaccharide nature varying in molecular weights. JAN. *Anticoagulant.* Calciparine (Sanofi Aventis)

Heparin Sodium (hep′ a rin soe′ dee um). **USP.** The sodium salt of sulfated glycosaminoglycans present as a mixture of heterogeneous molecules varying in molecular weights. *UNII-ZZ45AB24CA; UNII-T2410KM04A* [heparin]. *CAS-9041-08-1; CAS-9005-49-6* [heparin]. INN; BAN; JAN. *Anticoagulant.* Lipo-hepin (3M Pharmaceuticals); Liquaemin Sodium (Organon); Panheprin (Hospira)

---

† Brand name formerly used, and/or firm no longer concerned with this product.

Hepatitis B Immune Globulin. **USP**. A sterile, nonpyrogenic solution free from turbidity, consisting of globulins derived from the blood plasma or human donors who have high titers of antibodies against hepatitis B surface antigen. *Immunizing agent (passive)*. BayHep B (Bayer); H-Big (Abbott†); Hep-B-Gammagee (Merck)

Hepatitis B Virus Vaccine Inactivated. USP XXX. *Immunizing agent (active)*. Engerix-B (SmithKline Beecham); H-B-Vax (Merck); Heptavax-B (Merck)

Hepronicate. $C_{28}H_{31}N_3O_6$. 505.56. 2-Hexyl-2-(hydroxymethyl)-1,3-propanediol trinicotinate. *UNII-E4RK86FAVR. CAS-7237-81-2*. INN; JAN; MI.

Heptabarb (INN, BAN) — *See* Heptabarbital.

Heptabarbital. $C_{13}H_{18}N_2O_3$. 250.29. [Heptabarb is INN and BAN.] 5-(1-Cyclohepten-1-yl)-5-ethylbarbituric acid. *UNII-V10R70ML23. CAS-509-86-4*. MI. *[Name previously used: Heptabarbitone.]*

Heptaminol Hydrochloride. $C_8H_{19}NO.HCl$. 181.70. [Heptaminol is INN and BAN.] 6-Amino-2-methyl-2-heptanol hydrochloride. *CAS-543-15-7; CAS-372-66-7* [heptaminol]. MI.

Heptaverine. $C_{18}H_{25}N$. 255.40. *N,N*-Dimethyl-γ-phenyl-$\Delta^{2,\gamma}$-norbornanepropylamine. *UNII-0035H8M4YL. CAS-54063-48-8*. INN.

Heptolamide. $C_{15}H_{22}N_2O_3S$. 310.41. 1-Cycloheptyl-3-*p*-tolylsulfonylurea. *CAS-1034-82-8*. INN.

Hepzidine. $C_{21}H_{25}NO$. 307.43. 4-(10,11-Dihydro-5*H*-dibenzo[*a,d*]cyclohepten-5-yloxy)-1-methylpiperidine. *UNII-72FH6333M6. CAS-1096-72-6*. INN.

Heroin Hydrochloride — *See* Diacetylmorphine Hydrochloride.

Hesperidin. $C_{28}H_{34}O_{15}$. 610.56. *UNII-E750O06Y6O. CAS-520-26-3*. MI.

Hetacillin [*1965*] (het″ a sil′ in). $C_{19}H_{23}N_3O_4S$. 389.47. (1) 4-Thia-1-azabicyclo[3.2.0]heptane-2-carboxylic acid, 6-(2,2-dimethyl-5-oxo-4-phenyl-1-imidazolidinyl)-3,3-dimethyl-7-oxo-, [2*S*-[2α,5α,6β(*S**)]]-; (2) 6-(2,2-Dimethyl-5-oxo-4-phenyl-1-imidazolidinyl)-3,3-dimethyl-7-oxo-4-thia-1-azabicyclo[3.2.0]heptane-2-carboxylic acid. *UNII-TN4JSC48CV. CAS-3511-16-8*. USP XXII; INN; BAN. *Antibacterial*. Versapen (Bristol-Myers Squibb) ◇*BRL-804; BL-P 804*

Hetacillin Potassium [*1968*] (het″ a sil′ in poe tas′ ee um). $C_{19}H_{22}KN_3O_4S$. 427.56. (1) 4-Thia-1-azabicyclo[3.2.0]heptane-2-carboxylic acid, 6-(2,2-dimethyl-5-oxo-4-phenyl-1-imidazolidinyl)-3,3-dimethyl-7-oxo-, monopotassium salt, [2*S*-[2α,5α,6β(*S**)]]-; (2) Potassium 6-(2,2-dimethyl-5-oxo-4-phenyl-1-imidazolidinyl)-3,3-dimethyl-7-oxo-4-thia-1-azabicyclo[3.2.0]heptane-2-carboxylate. *UNII-95PFX5932Y; UNII-TN4JSC48CV* [hetacillin]. *CAS-5321-32-4; CAS-3511-16-8* [hetacillin]. USP XXIII; JAN. *Antibacterial*. Versapen-K (Bristol-Myers Squibb)

Hetaflur [*1973*] (het′ a flur). $C_{16}H_{35}N.HF$. 261.46. (1) Hexadecylamine hydrofluoride; (2) Hexadecylamine hydrofluoride. *UNII-S58EH61Q1Y; UNII-O2H0Q02M4P* [hexadecylamine]. *CAS-3151-59-5; CAS-143-27-1* [hexadecylamine]. INN; BAN. *Dental caries prophylactic.* ◇*SK&F 2208*

Hetastarch [*1972*] (het′ a starch). [Hydroxyethylstarch is JAN.] A starch that is composed of more than 90% of amylopectin and that has been etherified to the extent that an average of 7 to 8 of the OH groups present in every 10 D-glucopyranose units of starch polymer have been converted into OCH_2CH_2OH groups. (1) Starch, 2-hydroxyethyl ether; (2) Starch 2-hydroxyethyl ether. *CAS-9005-27-0*. BAN. *Plasma volume extender*. Hespan (DuPont Merck)

15(*S*)-HETE — *See* Icomucret.

Heteronium Bromide [*1963*] (het″ er oh′ nee um broe′ mide). $C_{18}H_{22}BrNO_3S$. 412.34. (1) Pyrrolidinium, 3-[(hydroxyphenyl-2-thienylacetyl)oxy]-1,1-dimethyl-, bromide; (2) (±)-3-Hydroxy-1,1-dimethylpyrrolidinium bromide α-phenyl-2-thiopheneglycolate; (3) α+β-(±)-(1-Methyl-3-pyrrolidinyl) α-phenyl-α-(2-thienyl)glycolate methobromide. *CAS-7247-57-6.* INN; BAN. *Anticholinergic.* ◇*31814*

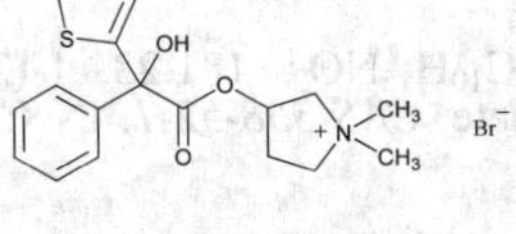

Hexachlorane — *See* Lindane.

Hexachlorophene (hex″ a klor′ oh feen). **USP.** $C_{13}H_6Cl_6O_2$. 406.90. (1) Phenol, 2,2′-methylenebis[3,4,6-trichloro-; (2) 2,2′-Methylenebis[3,4,6-trichlorophenol]. *UNII-IWW5FV6NK2. CAS-70-30-4.* INN; BAN. *Anti-infective, topical; detergent.* Dial (Dial); Gamophen (Arabrook); Germa-medica (Huntington); Phisohex (Sanofi Aventis); Pre-op (Davis & Geck); Septisol (Vestal); Turgex (Xttrium) *[Name previously used: Hexachlorophane.]*

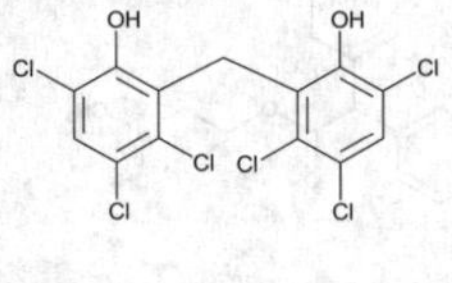

Hexacyclonate Sodium. $C_9H_{15}NaO_3$. 194.20. Sodium 1-(hydroxymethyl)cyclohexaneacetate. *CAS-7009-49-6; CAS-7491-42-1* [hexacyclonic acid]. INN; MI.

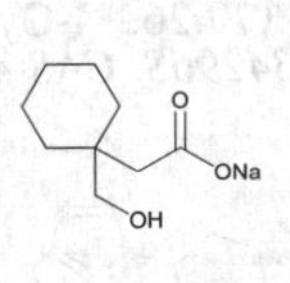

Hexacyprone. $C_{16}H_{20}O_3$. 260.33. 1-Benzyl-2-oxocyclo hexanepropionic acid. *CAS-892-01-3.* INN.

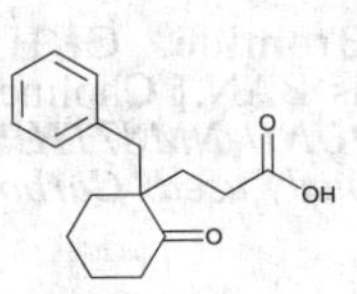

Hexadecanol — *See* Cetyl Alcohol.

Hexadiline. $C_{19}H_{33}N$. 275.47. 2-(2,2-Dicyclohexylvinyl)piperidine. *CAS-3626-67-3.* INN. ◇*MRL 38*

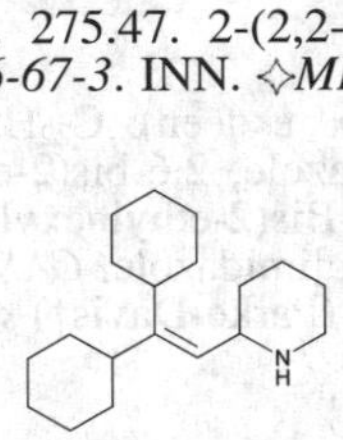

Hexadimethrine Bromide. $(C_{13}H_{30}Br_2N_2)n$. *N,N,N′,N′*-Tetramethyl-1,6-hexanediamine polymer with 1,3-dibromopropane. *CAS-9011-04-5.* INN; BAN; MI. Polybrene (Abbott†)

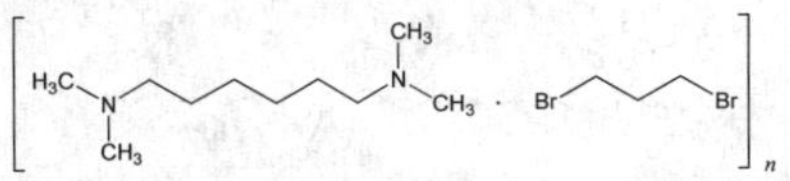

Hexadiphane — *See* Prozapine.

Hexadylamine — *See* Hexadiline.

Hexafluorenium Bromide [*1961*] (hex″ a floor en′ i um broe′ mide). $C_{36}H_{42}Br_2N_2$. 662.54. [Hexafluronium Bromide is INN.] (1) 1,6-Hexanediaminium, *N,N′*-di-9*H*-fluoren-9-yl-*N,N,N′,N′*-tetramethyl-, dibromide; (2) Hexamethylenebis [fluoren-9-yldimethylammonium] dibromide. *UNII-B64NJG83K2. CAS-317-52-2.* USP XXI. *Relaxant (skeletal muscle); synergist (succinylcholine).* Mylaxen (Medpointe) ◇*NSC-19477*

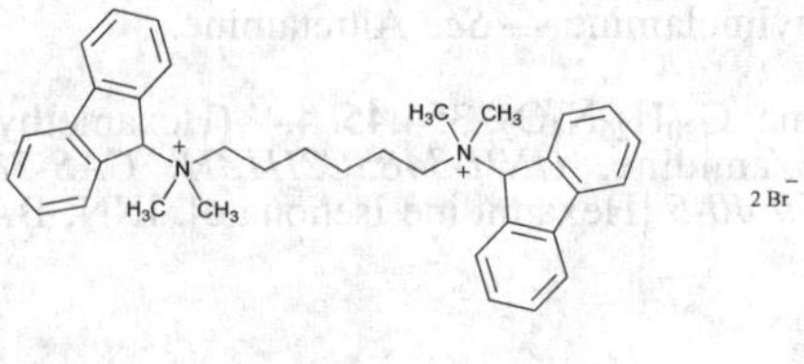

Hexafluorodiethyl Ether — *See* Flurothyl.

Hexaflurone Bromide — *See* Hexafluorenium Bromide.

Hexafluronium Bromide (INN) — *See* Hexafluorenium Bromide.

Hexafocon A [*1997*] (hex″ a foe′ kon). $(C_{16}H_{38}O_5Si_4)_v(C_7H_6F_6O_2)_w(C_4H_6O_2)_x(C_{13}H_{20}O_4)_y(C_{70}H_{188}O_{30}Si_{27})_x$. (1) 3-[3,3,3-Trimethyl-1,1-bis(trimethylsilyl)oxy]disiloxanyl] propyl 2-methyl-2-propenoate polymer with 2,2,2-trifluoro-1-(trifluoromethyl)ethyl 2-methyl-2-propenoate, 2-methyl-2-propenoic acid, 2,2-dimethyl-1,3-propanediyl bis(2-methyl-2-propenoate) and α-[dimethyl[4-[(2-methyl-1-oxo-2-propenyl)oxy]butyl]silyl]-gv-[[dimethyl[4-(2-methyl-1-oxo-2-propenyl)oxy]butyl]silyl]oxy]pentacosa[oxy(dimethylsilylene)]; (2) 3-[3,3,3-Trimethyl-1,1-bis(trimethylsiloxy)disiloxanyl]propyl methacrylate polymer with 2,2,2-trifluoro-1-(trifluoromethyl)ethyl methacrylate, methacrylic acid, 2,2-dimethyltrimethylene dimethacrylate and (tetrapentacontamethylheptacosasiloxanylene)bis(tetramethylene) dimethacrylate. *CAS-189385-65-7. Contact lens material (hydrophobic).* Quantum II (Polymer Technology) *[Note—The water content of the contact lens material is < 1.0% at ambient temperature (23±2°C), and the oxygen permeability is 135 ± 8 × 10^{-11}(cm²/sec)(ml O₂/ml × mm Hg) at 35°C (Dk value).]*

Hexamarium Bromide — *See* Distigmine Bromide.

Hexametazine (previously used name) — *See* Exametazime.

Hexamethone Bromide — *See* Hexamethonium Bromide.

---

† Brand name formerly used, and/or firm no longer concerned with this product.

Hexamethonium Bromide. $C_{12}H_{30}Br_2N_2$. 362.19. Hexamethylenebis(trimethylammonium bromide). *UNII-8J77X3S603; UNII-3C9PSP36Z2* [hexamethonium]. *CAS-55-97-0; CAS-60-26-4* [hexamethonium]. INN; BAN; JAN; MI. Bistrium Bromide (Bristol-Myers Squibb†)

Hexamethonium Iodide. $C_{12}H_{30}I_2N_2$. 456.19. *N,N*-Hexamethylenebis(trimethylammonium) di-iodide. *UNII-G2753KSN40. CAS-870-62-2.* BAN.

Hexamethonium Tartrate. $C_{20}H_{40}N_2O_{12}$. 500.54. *N,N*-Hexamethylenebis(trimethylammonium) di(hydrogen tartrate). *CAS-2079-78-9.* BAN.

Hexamethylenamine (previously used name) — *See* Methenamine.

Hexamethylenamine Mandelate — *See* Methenamine Mandelate.

Hexamethylenetetramine — *See* Methenamine.

Hexamethylmelamine — *See* Altretamine.

Hexamidine. $C_{20}H_{26}N_4O_2$. 354.45. 4,4′-(Hexamethylenedioxy)dibenzamidine. *UNII-3483C2H13H. CAS-3811-75-4; CAS-659-40-5* [Hexamidine Isetionate]. INN; BAN; DCF; MI.

Hexamine (JAN) — *See* Methenamine.

Hexamine Hippurate (previously used name) — *See* Methenamine Hippurate.

Hexamine Mandelate (JAN) — *See* Methenamine Mandelate.

Hexaminolevulinate Hydrochloride [*2003*] (hex a mee″ noe lev′ ue lin ate hye″ droe klor′ ide). $C_{11}H_{21}NO_3 \cdot HCl$. 251.75. (1) Pentanoic acid, 5-amino-4-oxo-, hexyl ester, hydrochloride; (2) Hexyl 5-amino-4-oxopentanoate hydrochloride. *UNII-D4F329SL1O. CAS-140898-91-5. Diagnostic agent for the diagnosis of bladder cancer.* ◇*P-1026*

Hexapradol. $C_{19}H_{25}NO$. 283.41. α-(1-Aminohexyl)benzhydrol. *CAS-15599-37-8.* INN.

Hexaprofen. $C_{15}H_{20}O_2$. 232.32. *p*-Cyclohexylhydratropic acid. *CAS-24645-20-3.* INN; BAN. ◇*BTS 13622*

Hexapropymate. $C_{10}H_{15}NO_2$. 181.23. 1-(2-Propynyl)cyclohexanol carbamate. *CAS-358-52-1.* INN; BAN; DCF; MI.

Hexasonium Iodide. $C_{18}H_{27}IO_2S$. 434.38. (2-Hydroxyethyl)dimethyl sulfonium iodide α-phenyl cyclohexaneacetate. *CAS-3569-59-3.* INN.

Hexavitamin. USP XXI. Hepicebrin [Tablets] (Lilly); Polytaxin (Sterling Winthrop†)

Hexazole. $C_{10}H_{17}N_3$. 179.26. 4-Cyclohexyl-3-ethyl-1,2,4-triazole. *UNII-9LVF34296S. CAS-4671-03-8.* BAN.

Hexcarbacholine Bromide. $C_{18}H_{40}Br_2N_4O_4$. 536.34. [Hexcarbacholine is BAN.] Choline bromide hexamethylenedicarbamate. *UNII-NM87THP11P. CAS-306-41-2.* INN. *[Name previously used: Carbolonium Bromide.]*

Hexedine [*1967*] (hex′ e deen). $C_{22}H_{45}N_3$. 351.61. (1) 1*H*-Imidazo[1,5-*c*]imidazole, 2,6-bis(2-ethylhexyl)hexahydro-7a-methyl-; (2) 2,6-Bis(2-ethylhexyl)-hexahydro-7a-methyl-1*H*-imidazo[1,5-*c*]imidazole. *CAS-5980-31-4.* INN. *Antibacterial.* Sterisol (Parke-Davis†) ◇*W 4701*

Hexemal — *See* Cyclobarbital.

Hexestrol. $C_{18}H_{22}O_2$. 270.37. [Hexestrol Diphosphate Sodium is JAN.] 4,4′-(1,2-Diethylethylene)diphenol. *UNII-10BI795R7D. CAS-5635-50-7.* NF XI; INN; MI. ◇*NSC-9894*

Hexetidine. $C_{21}H_{45}N_3$. 339.60. 5-Amino-1,3-bis(2-ethylhexyl)hexahydro-5-methylpyrimidine. *UNII-852A84Y8LS. CAS-141-94-6.* BAN; MI. Sterisil (Parke-Davis†)

Hexicide — *See* Lindane.

Hexinol — *See* Cyclomenol.

Hexobarbital. $C_{12}H_{16}N_2O_3$. 236.27. (1) 2,4,6(1*H*,3*H*,5*H*)-Pyrimidinetrione, 5-(1-cyclohexen-1-yl)-1,5-dimethyl; (2) 5-(1-Cyclohexen-1-yl)-1,5-dimethylbarbituric acid. *UNII-AL8Z8K3P6S. CAS-56-29-1.* USP XXI; INN; BAN; JAN; MI. Evipal (Sterling Winthrop†); Sombucaps (3M Pharmaceuticals†); Sombulex (3M Pharmaceuticals†) *[Name previously used: Hexobarbitone.]*

Hexobarbital Sodium. *UNII-I788X867K7; UNII-AL8Z8K3P6S* [hexobarbital]. *CAS-50-09-9; CAS-56-29-1* [hexobarbital]. NF XII. Evipal Sodium (Sterling Winthrop†)

Hexobendine [*1972*] (hex″ oh ben′ deen). $C_{30}H_{44}N_2O_{10}$. 592.68. (1) Benzoic acid, 3,4,5-trimethoxy-, 1,2-ethanediylbis[(methylimino)-3,1-propanediyl] ester; (2) 3,4,5-Trimethoxybenzoic acid, diester with 3,3′-[ethylenebis(methylimino)]di-1-propanol. *CAS-54-03-5.* INN; BAN. *Vasodilator.*

Hexocyclium Methylsulfate. $C_{21}H_{36}N_2O_5S$. 428.59. [Hexocyclium Metilsulfate is INN and BAN.] 4-(β-Cyclohexyl-β-hydroxyphenethyl)-1,1-dimethylpiperazinum methylsulfate. *UNII-84OPZ2Q0VB. CAS-115-63-9; CAS-6004-98-4* [hexocyclium]. AMA-DE 1973; ND 1966; MI. Tral (Abbott)

Hexoprenaline Sulfate [*1993*] (hex″ oh pren′ a leen sul′ fate). $C_{22}H_{32}N_2O_6 \cdot H_2SO_4$. 518.58. [Hexoprenaline is INN and BAN.] (1) 1,2-Benzenediol, 4,4′-[1,6-hexanediylbis[imino(1-hydroxy-2,1-ethanediyl)]]bis-, sulfate (1:1) (salt); (2) (±)-α,α′-[Hexamethylenebis(iminomethylene)]bis[3,4-dihydroxybenzyl alcohol] sulfate (1:1) (salt). *CAS-32266-10-7; CAS-3215-70-1* [hexoprenaline]. JAN; MI. *Bronchodilator; tocolytic.* Delaprem (Savage†) ◇*ST1512/SO4*

Hexopyrimidine — *See* Hexetidine.

Hexopyrrolate — *See* Hexopyrronium Bromide.

Hexopyrronium Bromide. $C_{20}H_{30}BrNO_3$. 412.36. 1,1-Dimethyl-3-hydroxy-pyrrolidinium bromide α-phenyl-cyclohexaneglycolate. *CAS-3734-12-1.* INN.

Hexydaline — *See* Methenamine Mandelate.

Hexylcaine Hydrochloride. $C_{16}H_{23}NO_2 \cdot HCl$. 297.82. [Hexylcaine is INN.] (1) 2-Propanol, 1-(cyclohexylamino)-, benzoate (ester), hydrochloride; (2) 1-(Cyclohexylamino)-2-propanol benzoate (ester) hydrochloride. *UNII-V00NQ7SDYI; UNII-5111U0826Z* [hexylcaine]. *CAS-532-76-3; CAS-532-77-4* [hexylcaine]. USP XXII. Cyclaine (Merck)

Hexylene Glycol (hex′ il een glye′ kol). **NF**. $C_6H_{14}O_2$. 118.17. (1) 2,4-Pentanediol, 2-methyl-; (2) 2-Methyl-2,4-pentanediol. *CAS-107-41-5. Pharmaceutic aid (humectant); pharmaceutic aid (solvent).*

---

† Brand name formerly used, and/or firm no longer concerned with this product.

Hexylresorcinol (hex″ il re sor′ si nol). **USP.** C$_{12}$H$_{18}$O$_2$. 194.27. (1) 1,3-Benzenediol, 4-hexyl-; (2) 4-Hexylresorcinol. *UNII-R9QTB5E82N. CAS-136-77-6.* BAN. *Anthelmintic.*

^{197}Hg — *See* Chlormerodrin Hg 197.

^{197}Hg — *See* Merisoprol Acetate Hg 197.

^{197}Hg — *See* Merisoprol Hg 197.

^{203}Hg — *See* Chlormerodrin Hg 203.

^{203}Hg — *See* Merisoprol Acetate Hg 203.

Hilafilcon A [*1997*] (hye″ la fil′ kon). (C$_6$H$_{10}$O$_3$)$_w$(C$_6$H$_9$NO)$_x$(C$_7$H$_{10}$O$_2$)$_y$(C$_{10}$H$_{14}$O$_4$)$_z$. 2-Hydroxyethyl methacrylate polymer with 1-vinyl-2-pyrrolidinone, allyl methacrylate and ethylene dimethacrylate. *CAS-188063-80-1. Contact lens material (hydrophilic).* Award (Bausch & Lomb) *[Note—The water content of the contact lens material is 70% at ambient temperature (23±2°C), the purity of 2-hydroxyethyl methacrylate (HEMA) is >97%, and the oxygen permeability is 35 × 10^{-11}(cm^2/sec)(ml O$_2$/ml × mm HG) at 35°C (Dk value).]*

Hilafilcon B [*2000*] (hye″ la fil′ kon). (C$_6$H$_{10}$O$_3$)$_w$(C$_6$H$_9$NO)$_x$(C$_7$H$_{10}$O$_2$)$_y$(C$_{10}$H$_{14}$O$_4$)$_z$. (1) 2-Propenoic acid, 2-methyl-, 1,2-ethanediyl ester, polymer with 1-ethenyl-2-pyrrolidinone, 2-hydroxyethyl 2-methyl-2-propenoate and 2-propenyl 2-methyl-2-propenoate); (2) 2-Hydroxyethyl methacrylate polymer with 1-vinyl-2-pyrrolidinone, allyl methacrylate and ethylene glycol dimethacrylate. *CAS-188063-80-1. Contact lens material (hydrophilic).* Award (Bausch & Lomb) *[Note—The water content of the contact lens material is 59% at ambient temperature (23±2°C), the purity of 2-hydroxyethyl methacrylate (HEMA) is >99%, and the oxygen permeability is 20 × 10^{-11}(cm^2/sec)(ml O$_2$/ml × mm Hg) at 35°C (Dk value).]*

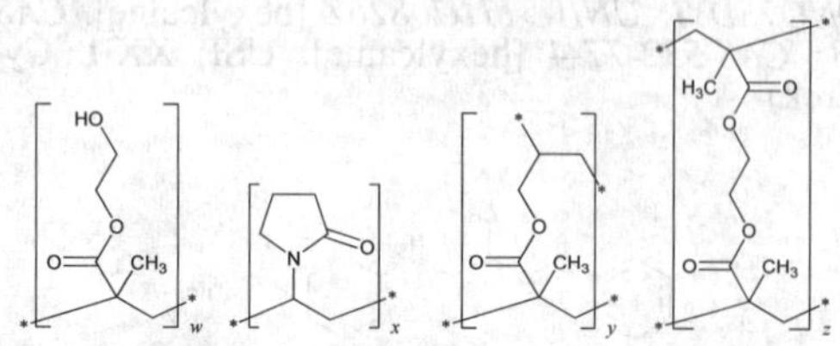

Hioxifilcon A [*1995*] (hye ox″ i fil′ kon). (C$_7$H$_{12}$O$_4$)$_x$(C$_6$H$_{10}$O$_3$)$_y$(C$_{10}$H$_{14}$O$_4$)$_z$. (1) 2-Propenoic acid, 2-methyl-, 2,3-dihydroxypropyl ester, polymer with 2-hydroxyethyl 2-methyl-2-propenoate, and 1,2-ethanediyl bis(2-methyl-2-propenoate); (2) 2,3-Dihydroxypropyl methacrylate polymer with 2-hydroxyethyl methacrylate and ethylene dimethacrylate. *CAS-82356-44-3. Contact lens material (hydrophilic).* Benz-G 5X (Benz Research and Development) *[Note—The water content of the contact lens material is 55-59% at ambient temperature (23±2°C),*

the purity of 2-hydroxyethyl methacrylate (HEMA) is >99%, and the oxygen permeability is 20 × 10^{-11}(cm^2/ sec)(ml O$_2$/ml × mm Hg) at 35°C (Dk value).]

Hioxifilcon D [*2005*] (hye ox″ i fil′ kon). (C$_7$H$_{12}$O$_4$)$_x$(C$_6$H$_{10}$O$_3$)$_y$ (C$_{10}$H$_{14}$O$_4$)$_z$. (1) 2-Propenoic acid, 2-methyl-, 2,3-dihydroxypropyl ester, polymer with 2-hydroxyethyl 2-methyl-2-propenoate, and 1,2-ethanediyl bis(2-methyl-2-propenoate); (2) 2,3-Dihydroxypropyl methacrylate polymer with 2-hydroxyethyl methacrylate and ethylene dimethacrylate. *CAS-82356-44-3. Contact lens material (hydrophilic).* Benz-G 4X (Benz Research and Development) *[Note—The water content of the contact lens material is 54 ± 2% at ambient temperature (23±2°C), and the oxygen permeability is 21 × 10^{-11}(cm^2/sec)(ml O$_2$/ ml × mm Hg) at 35°C (Dk value).]*

Histamine Dihydrochloride [*1988*] (his′ ta meen dye hye″ droe klor′ ide). C$_5$H$_9$N$_3$.2HCl. 184.07. *UNII-3POA0-Q644U; UNII-820484N8I3* [histamine]. *CAS-51-45-6* [histamine].

Histamine Phosphate (his′ ta meen fos′ fate). **USP.** C$_5$H$_9$N$_3$.2H$_3$PO$_4$. 307.14. (1) 1*H*-Imidazole-4-ethanamine, phosphate (1:2); (2) Histamine phosphate (1:2). *UNII-QWB37T4WZZ. CAS-51-74-1. Stimulant (gastric secretory).*

Histapyrrodine. C$_{19}$H$_{24}$N$_2$. 280.41. 1-(2-*N*-Benzylanilinoethyl)pyrrolidine. *UNII-0FYM61NG4D. CAS-493-80-1.* INN; DCF; MI.

Histidine [*1979*] (his′ ti deen). **USP.** C$_6$H$_9$N$_3$O$_2$. 155.15. (1) L-Histidine; (2) L-Histidine. *UNII-4QD397987E. CAS-71-00-1* [L]. INN. *Amino acid.*

Histidine Monohydrochloride. NF X; MI.

Histoplasmin (his″ toe plaz′ min). **USP.** A clear, colorless, sterile solution containing standardized culture filtrates of *Histoplasma capsulatum* grown on liquid synthetic medium. *CAS-9008-05-3. Diagnostic aid (dermal reactivity indicator).*

Histrelin [*1985*] (his trel′ in). C$_{66}$H$_{86}$N$_{18}$O$_{12}$. 1323.50. (1) Luteinizing hormone-releasing factor (pig), 6-[1-(phenylmethyl)-D-histidine]-9-(*N*-ethyl-L-prolinamide)-10-deglycinamide-; (2) 5-Oxo-L-prolyl-L-histidyl-L-tryptophyl-L-seryl-L-tyrosyl-*N*^{τ}-benzyl-D-histidyl-L-leucyl-L-arginyl-*N*-

ethyl-L-prolinamide. *UNII-H50H3S3W74. CAS-76712-82-8*. INN. *LHRH agonist*. Supprelin (Roberts Pharmaceutical) ◇*ORF 17070; RWJ 17070*

HN2 Hydrochloride — *See* Mechlorethamine Hydrochloride.

Hofocon A [2002] (hoe foe′ kon). $(C_6H_7F_3O_2)_u$ $(C_{16}H_{38}O_5Si_4)_v$ $(C_{26}H_{58}O_9Si_6)_w$ $(C_4H_6O_2)_x$ $(C_{10}H_{14}O_4)_y$ $(C_6H_9NO)_z$. (1) 2-Propenoic acid, 2-methyl-, polymer with 1,2,-ethanediyl bis(2-methyl-2-propenoate), 1-ethenyl-2-pyrrolidinone, [1,1,3,3-tetrakis[(trimethylsilyl)oxy]-1,3-disiloxanediyl]di-3,1-propanediyl bis(2-methyl-2-propenoate), 2,2,2-trifluoroethyl 2-methyl-2-propenoate and 3-[3,3,3-trimethyl-1,1-bis[(trimethylsilyl)oxy]disiloxanyl]propyl 2-methyl-2-propenoate; (2) 2,2,2-Trifluoroethyl methacrylate polymer with 3-[3,3,3-trimethyl-1,1-bis(trimethylsiloxy)disiloxanyl)propyl methacrylate, [1,1,3,3-tetrakis[(trimethylsilyl)oxy]-1,3-disiloxanediyl]di-3,1-propanediylbis(2-methyl-2-propenoate), methacrylic acid, ethylene dimethacrylate and 1-vinyl-2-pyrrolidinone. *CAS-242148-62-5. Contact lens material (hydrophobic).[Note—The water content of the contact lens material is <0.1% at ambient temperature (23±2°C), and the oxygen permeability is 73.7 × 10⁻¹¹ (cm²/sec)(ml O₂/ml × mm Hg) at 35°C (Dk value).]*

Homarylamine. $C_{10}H_{13}NO_2$. 179.22. *N*-Methyl-3,4-methylenedioxyphenethylamine. *UNII-6FJ4B5B368. CAS-451-77-4; CAS-533-10-8* [hydrochloride]. INN.

Homatropine Hydrobromide (hoe mat′ roe peen hye″ droe broe′ mide). **USP.** $C_{16}H_{21}NO_3 \cdot HBr$. 356.25. [Homatropine is BAN.] (1) Benzeneacetic acid, α-hydroxy-, 8-methyl-8-azabicyclo[3.2.1]oct-3-yl ester, hydrobromide, *endo*-(±)-; (2) 1αH,5αH-Tropan-3α-ol mandelate (ester) hydrobro-

mide. *UNII-BEW7469QZ0. CAS-51-56-9; CAS-87-00-3* [homatropine]. JAN. *Anticholinergic (ophthalmic)*. Isopto Homatropine (Alcon)

Homatropine Methylbromide (hoe mat′ roe peen meth″ il broe′ mide). **USP.** $C_{17}H_{24}BrNO_3$. 370.28. (1) 8-Azoniabicyclo[3.2.1]octane, 3-[(hydroxyphenylacetyl)oxy]-8,8-dimethyl-, bromide, *endo*-; (2) 3α-Hydroxy-8-methyl-1αH,5αH-tropanium bromide mandelate. *UNII-68JRS2HC1C. CAS-80-49-9; CAS-87-00-3* [homatropine]. INN; BAN. *Anticholinergic*. Equipin (Mission); Homapin (Mission)

Homidium Bromide. $C_{21}H_{20}BrN_3$. 394.31. 3,8-Diamino-5-ethyl-6-phenylphenanthridinium bromide. *UNII-059NUO2Z1L. CAS-1239-45-8*. INN; BAN; MI.

Homochlorcyclizine. $C_{19}H_{23}ClN_2$. 314.85. [Homochlorcyclizine Hydrochloride is JAN.] 1-(*p*-Chloro-α-phenylbenzyl)-hexahydro-4-methyl-1*H*-1,4-diazepine. *UNII-N5MVC31W2N. CAS-848-53-3*. INN; BAN; MI.

Homofenazine. $C_{23}H_{28}F_3N_3OS$. 451.55. Hexahydro-4-[3-[2-(trifluoromethyl)phenothiazin-10-yl]propyl]-1*H*-1,4-diazepine-1-ethanol. *UNII-PEL7G6VRZ2. CAS-3833-99-6*. INN; MI. ◇*D-775; HFZ*

Homomenthyl Salicylate (previously used name) — *See* Homosalate.

Homopipramol. $C_{24}H_{31}N_3O$. 377.52. 4-[3-(5*H*-Dibenz[*b,f*]azepin-5-yl)propyl]hexahydro-1*H*-1,4-diazepine-1-ethanol. *UNII-09YNW8E5CT. CAS-35142-68-8.* INN.

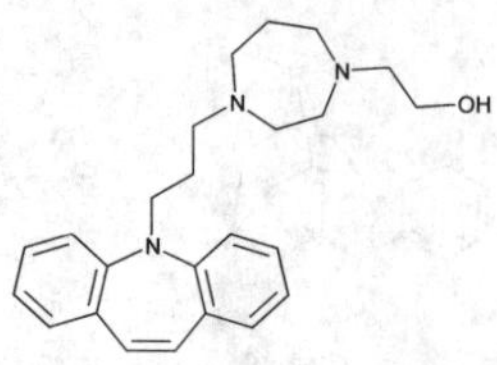

Homosalate [*1972*] (hoe″ moe sal′ ate). **USP.** $C_{16}H_{22}O_3$. 262.34. (1) Benzoic acid, 2-hydroxy-, 3,3,5-trimethylcyclohexyl ester; (2) 3,3,5-Trimethylcyclohexyl salicylate. *CAS-118-56-9.* INN. *Ultraviolet screen.* Eusolex (Rona Laboratories, Great Britain); Heliophan (Greeff) [*Name previously used: Homomenthyl Salicylate.*]

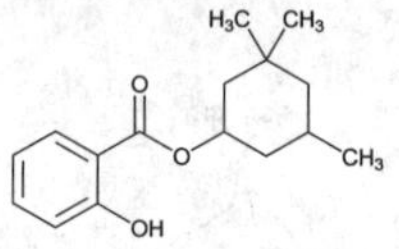

4-Homosulfanilamide — *See* Mafenide.

Homprenorphine. $C_{28}H_{37}NO_4$. 451.60. 22-Cyclopropyl-7α-((*R*)-1-hydroxy-1-methylpropyl)-6,14-*endo*-ethenotetrahydrothebaine. *CAS-16549-56-7.* INN; BAN. ◇*R&S 5205-M*

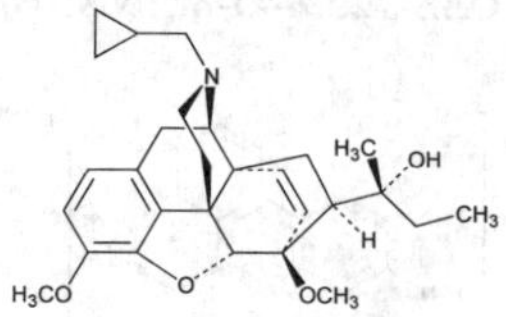

Honey. *UNII-Y9H1V576FH. CAS-8028-66-8.* JAN.

Honey, Purified. **NF**. Obtained by purification of honey from the comb of the bee, *Apis mellifera L.* and all subspecies of *Apis mellifera*.

Hopantenic Acid. $C_{10}H_{19}NO_5$. 233.26. D-(+)-4-(2,4-Dihydroxy-3,3-dimethylbutyramido)butyric acid. *CAS-18679-90-8.* INN; MI.

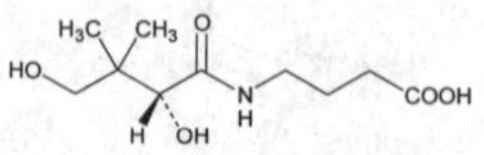

Hoquizil Hydrochloride [*1969*] (hoe′ kwi zil hye″ droe klor′ ide). $C_{19}H_{26}N_4O_5 \cdot HCl$. 426.89. [Hoquizil is INN.] (1) 1-Piperazinecarboxylic acid, 4-(6,7-dimethoxy-4-quinazolinyl)-, 2-hydroxy-2-methylpropyl ester, monohydrochloride; (2) 2-Hydroxy-2-methylpropyl 4-(6,7-dimethoxy-4-quinazolinyl)-1-piperazinecarboxylate monohydrochloride. *CAS-23256-28-2; CAS-21560-59-8* [hoquizil]. *Bronchodilator.* ◇*CP-14,185-1*

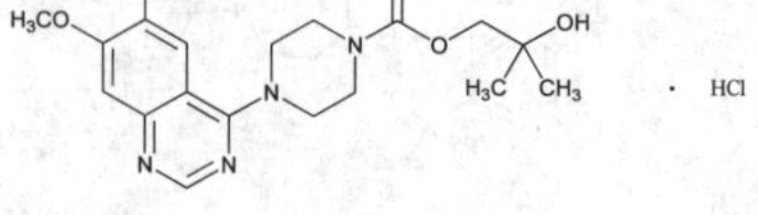

Horse Chestnut. The dried seeds of *Aesculus hippocastanum* L. (Fam. Hippocastanaceae). *UNII-2331W47PSX.* NF XXI.

Horse Chestnut Extract, Powdered. [Horse-chestnut Seed Extract is JAN.] NF XXI.

Horse Chestnut, Powdered. NF XXI.

Horse-chestnut Leaf Extract. JAN.

HQMME; Hydroxyquinone Methyl Ether (previously used name) — *See* Mequinol.

Human Follicle Stimulating Hormone (previously used name) — *See* Menotropins.

Human Growth Hormone (JAN) — *See* Somatropin.

Human Menopausal Gonadotrophins. Purified extract of human post-menopausal urine containing follicle-stimulating hormone (FSH) and luteinising hormone (LH); the relative *in-vivo* activity is designed as a ratio. BAN.

Human Serum Albumin Diethylenetriaminepentaacetic Acid Technetium (^{99m}Tc) Injection (JAN) — *See* Technetium Tc 99m Pentetate.

Human T-cell Inhibitor — *See* Muromonab-CD3.

Hyalosidase. Hyaluronoglucosaminidase. *CAS-37326-33-3.* INN; BAN.

Hyaluronate Sodium [*1986*] (hye″ al ure on′ ate soe′ dee um). $(C_{14}H_{20}NNaO_{11})_n$. [Hyaluronic Acid is BAN.] (1) Hyaluronic acid, sodium salt; (2) Sodium hyaluronate. *CAS-9067-32-7; CAS-9004-61-9* [hyaluronic acid]. JAN. *Synovitis agent (veterinary).* Equron [Veterinary] (Fort Dodge Animal Health); Legend (Bayer Animal Health); Synacid [Veterinary] (Schering-Plough Animal Health)

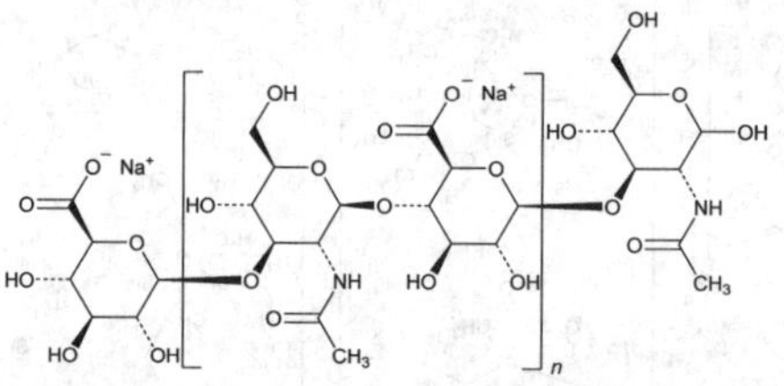

Hyaluronic Acid (BAN) — *See* Hyaluronate Sodium.

Hyaluronidase (Human Recombinant) [*2005*] (hye″ al ure on′ i dase hue′ man ree kom′ bi nant). $C_{2327}H_{3553}N_{589}O_{667}S_{20}$. (1) 36-482-Hyaluronoglucosaminidase PH20 (human); (2) Hyaluronidase 1 (human sperm surface protein PH-20)-(1-447)peptide. Molecular weight is approximately 51,106 daltons. *CAS-757971-58-7. Spreading agent.* Hylenex (Halozyme); Cumulase (Halozyme) ◇*rHuPH20*

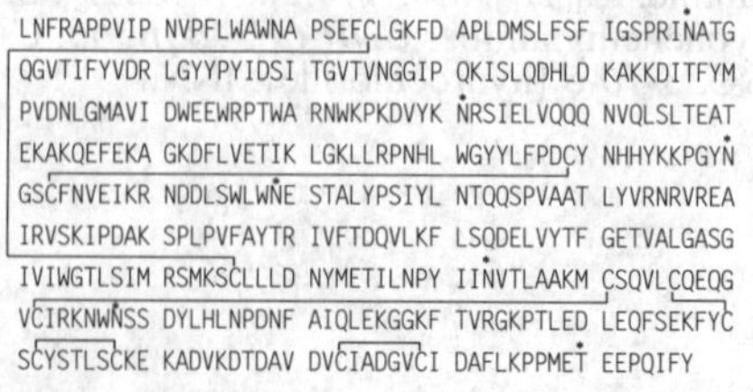

```
LNFRAPPVIP NVPFLWAWNA PSEFCLGKFD APLDMSLFSF IGSPRINATG
QGVTIFYVDR LGYYPYIDSI TGVTVNGGIP QKISLQDHLD KAKKDITFYM
PVDNLGMAVI DWEEWRPTWA RNWKPKDVYK NRSIELVQQQ NVQLSLTEAT
EKAKQEFEKA GKDFLVETIK LGKLLRPNHL WGYYLFPDCY NHHYKKPGYN
GSCFNVEIKR NDDLSLWLWN E STALYPSIYL NTQQSPVAAT LYVRNRVREA
IRVSKIPDAK SPLPVFAYTR IVFTDQVLKF LSQDELVYTF GETVALGASG
IVIWGTLSIM RSMKSCLLLD NYMETILNPY IINVTLAAKM CSQVLCQEQG
VCIRKNWNSS DYLHLNPDNF AIQLEKGGKF TVRGKPTLED LEQFSEKFYC
SCYSTLSCKE KADVKDTDAV DVCIADGVCI DAFLKPPMET EEPQIFY
```
* glycosylation sites

Hyaluronidase (Ovine) [*2004*] (hye″ al ure on′ i dase oh′ vine). **USP** [Injection]. $C_{2600}H_{4040}N_{696}O_{774}S_{23}$ (peptide). (1) Hyaluronidase (sheep testis isoenzyme); (2) Hyaluronidase (glycoprotein, sheep testis isoenzyme). Molecular weight is approximately 58,170 daltons. *UNII-64R4OHP8T0. CAS-488712-31-8; CAS-9001-54-1.* INN; BAN; JAN. *Spreading agent.* Diffusin (Ortho Pharmaceutical†); Enzodase (Bristol-Myers Squibb†); Hyazyme (Abbott†); Vitrase (Biozyme Laboratories Ltd., UK); Wydase (Wyeth-Ayerst) *[Note—The source of the product (ovine, porcine, etc.) must be indicated in the labeling.]* ◇*HYO6A*

```
LDFRAPPLIS NTSFLWAWNA PAERCVKIFK LPPDLRLFSV KGSPQKSATG
QFITLFYADR LGYYPHIDEK TGNTVYGGIP QLGNLKNHLE KAKKDIAYYI
PNDSVGLAVI DWENWRPTWA RNWKPKDVYR DESVELVLQK NPQLSFPEAS
KIAKVDFETA GKSFMQETLK LGKLLRPNHL WGYYLFPDCY NHNYNQPTYN
GNCSDLEKRR NDDLDWLWKE STALFPSVYL NIKLKSTPKA AFYVRNRVQE
AIRLSKIASV ESPLPVFVYH RPVFTDGSST YLSQGDLVNS VGEIVALGAS
GIIMWGSLNL SLTMQSCMNL GNYLNTTLNP YIINVTLAAK MCSQVLCHDE
GVCTRKQWNS SDYLHLNPMN FAIQTGKGGK YTVPGKVTLE DLQTFSDKFY
CSCYANINCK KRVDIKNVHS VNVCMAEDIC IEGPVKLQPS DHSSSQNEAS
TTTVSSISPS TTATTVSPCT PEKQSPECLK VRCLEAIANV TQTGCQGVKW
KNTSSQSSIQ NIKNQTTY
```

Hybufocon A [*2002*] (hye″ bue foe′ kon). $(C_{26}H_{58}O_9Si_6)_q$ $(C_{16}H_{38}O_5Si_4)_r(C_7H_{12}O_4)_s(C_7H_6F_6O_2)_t(C_6H_{10}O_3)_u(C_6H_7F_3$ $O_2)_v(C_{14}H_{22}O_6)_w(C_7H_{10}O_2)_x(C_5H_8O_2)_y(C_3H_4O_2)_z$. (1) 2-Propenoic acid, 2-methyl-, 1,2-ethanediylbis(oxy-2,1-ethanediyl) ester, polymer with 2,3-dihydroxypropyl 2-methyl-2-propenoate, 2-hydroxyethyl 2-methyl-2-propenoate, methyl 2-methyl-2-propenoate, 2-propenoic acid, 2-propenyl 2-methyl-2-propenoate, [1,1,3,3-tetrakis[(trimethylsilyl)oxy]- 1,3-disiloxanediyl]di-3,1-propanediyl bis(2-methyl-2-propenoate), 2,2,2-trifluoroethyl 2-methyl-2-propenoate, 2,2,2-trifluoro-1-(trifluoromethyl)ethyl 2-methyl-2-propenoate and 3-[3,3,3-trimethyl-1,1-bis[(trimethylsilyl)oxy]disiloxanyl]propyl 2-methyl-2-propenoate; (2) Ethylenebis(oxyethylene) bis(2-methylprop-2-enoate) polymer with 2,3-dihydroxypropyl 2-methylprop-2-enoate, 2-hydroxyethyl 2-methylprop-2-enoate, methyl 2-methylprop-2-enoate, prop-2-enoic acid, prop-2-enyl 2-methylprop-2-enoate, [1,1,3,3-tetrakis[(trimethylsilanyl)oxy]disiloxane-1,3-diyl]dipropane-3,1-diyl bis(2-methylprop-2-enoate), 2,2,2-trifluoroethyl 2-methylprop-2-enoate, 2,2,2-trifluoro-1-(trifluoromethyl)ethyl 2-methylprop-2-enoate and 3-[3,3,3-trimethyl-1,1-bis[(trimethylsilanyl)oxy]disiloxanyl]propyl 2-methylprop-2-enoate. *CAS-403483-39-6. Contact lens material (hydrophobic).* Hybrid FS (Contamac) *[Note—The water content of the contact lens material is < 1.0% at ambient temperature (23±2°C), and the oxygen permeability is 31 ± 2 × 10⁻¹¹(cm²/sec)(ml O₂/ml × mm Hg) at 35°C (Dk value).]*

Hycanthone [*1966*] (hye kan′ thone). $C_{20}H_{24}N_2O_2S$. 356.48. (1) 9*H*-Thioxanthen-9-one, 1-[[2-(diethylamino)ethyl]amino]-4-(hydroxymethyl)-; (2) 1-[[2-(Diethylamino)ethyl]amino]-4-(hydroxymethyl)thioxanthen-9-one. *CAS-3105-97-3.* INN. *Antischistosomal.* ◇*Win 24,933; NSC-134434*

Hycanthone Mesylate. *CAS-23255-93-8; CAS-3105-97-3* [hycanthone]. AMA-DE 1971; MI. Etrenol (Sterling Winthrop)

---

† Brand name formerly used, and/or firm no longer concerned with this product.

Hydracarbazine. $C_5H_7N_5O$. 153.14. 6-Hydrazino-3-pyridazinecarboxamide. *UNII-6CTK2FB9QM. CAS-3614-47-9.* INN; DCF; MI. ◇*TH-2151*

Hydralazine Hydrochloride (hye dral′ a zeen hye″ droe klor′ ide). USP. $C_8H_8N_4$.HCl. 196.64. [Hydralazine is INN and BAN.] (1) Phthalazine, 1-hydrazino-, monohydrochloride; (2) 1-Hydrazinophthalazine monohydrochloride. *UNII-FD171B778Y; UNII-26NAK24LS8* [hydralazine]. *CAS-304-20-1; CAS-86-54-4* [hydralazine]. JAN. *Antihypertensive.* Apresoline (Novartis); Dralzine (Teva)

Hydralazine Polistirex [*1987*] (hye dral′ a zeen pol″ ee stye′ rex). (1) Benzene, diethenyl-, polymer with ethenylbenzene, sulfonated, complex with 1-hydrazinophthalazine; (2) Sulfonated diethenylbenzene-ethenylbenzene copolymer complex with 1-hydrazinophthalazine. *Antihypertensive.*

Hydrargaphen. $C_{33}H_{24}Hg_2O_6S_2$. 981.85. Phenylmercuric 3,3′-methylenebis(2-naphthalenesulfonate). *CAS-14235-86-0.* INN; BAN; MI.

Hydrastine. $C_{21}H_{21}NO_6$. 383.39. (1) Phthalide (*S*)-6,7-dimethoxy-3-(*R*)-(5,6,7,8-tetrahydro-6-methyl-1,3-dioxolo(4,5-*g*)isoquinolin-5-yl)-; (2) (*S*)-6,7-Dimethoxy-3-(*R*)-(6-methyl-5,6,7,8-tetrahydro-[1,3]dioxolo[4,5-*g*]isoquinolin-5-yl)isobenzofuran-1(3*H*)-one. *UNII-8890V3217X. CAS-118-08-1.* USP IX; MI.

Hydrastine Hydrochloride. *UNII-562PDC2I9K. CAS-5936-28-7; CAS-118-08-1* [hydrastine]. USP IX.

Hydrastinine Hydrochloride. $C_{11}H_{13}NO_3 \cdot HCl$. 243.69. (1) 1,3-Dioxolo(4,5-*g*)isoquinolin-5-ol, hydrochloride; (2) 5,6,7,8-Tetrahydro-6-methyl-5,6,7,8-Tetrahydro-6-methyl-1,3-dioxolo(4,5-*g*)isoquinolin-5-ol, hydrochloride. *CAS-4884-68-8; CAS-6592-85-4* [hydrastinine]. NF VIII; MI.

Hydrazinoxane — *See* Domoxin.

Hydrobentizide. $C_{15}H_{16}ClN_3O_4S_3$. 433.95. 3-[(Benzylthio)methyl]-6-chloro-3,4-dihydro-2*H*-1,2,4-benzothiadiazine-7-sulfonamide 1,1-dioxide. *CAS-13957-38-5*. INN; DCF.

Hydrobutamine — *See* Butidrine.

Hydrochloric Acid (hye″ droe klor′ ik as′ id). **NF.** HCl. 36.46. (1) Hydrochloric acid; (2) Hydrochloric acid. *UNII-QTT17582CB. CAS-7647-01-0.* JAN. *Pharmaceutic aid (acidifying agent).*

Hydrochlorothiazide (hye″ droe klor″ oh thye′ a zide). **USP.** $C_7H_8ClN_3O_4S_2$. 297.74. (1) 2*H*-1,2,4-Benzothiadiazine-7-sulfonamide, 6-chloro-3,4-dihydro-, 1,1-dioxide; (2) 6-Chloro-3,4-dihydro-2*H*-1,2,4-benzothiadiazine-7-sulfonamide 1,1-dioxide. *UNII-0J48LPH2TH. CAS-58-93-5.* INN; BAN; JAN. *Diuretic.* Esidrix (Novartis); Hydrodiuril (Merck); Oretic (Abbott); Zide (Solvay Pharmaceuticals)

Hydrocodone Bitartrate [*1963*] (hye droe koe′ done bye tar′ trate). **USP.** $C_{18}H_{21}NO_3 \cdot C_4H_6O_6 \cdot 2\frac{1}{2}H_2O$. 494.49. [Hydrocodone is INN and BAN.] (1) Morphinan-6-one, 4,5-epoxy-3-methoxy-17-methyl-, (5α)-, [*R*-(*R**,*R**)]-2,3-dihydroxybutanedioate (1:1), hydrate (2:5); (2) 4,5α-Epoxy-3-methoxy-17-methylmorphinan-6-one tartrate (1:1) hydrate (2:5). *UNII-NO70W886KK; UNII-6YKS4Y3WQ7* [hydrocodone]. *CAS-34195-34-1; CAS-6190-38-1* [replaced]; *CAS-143-71-5* [anhydrous]; *CAS-125-29-1* [hydrocodone]. *Antitussive.* Dicodid (Knoll†); Mercodinone (Marion Merrell Dow†)

Hydrocodone Polistirex [*1987*] (hye droe koe′ done pol″ ee stye′ rex). (1) Benzene, diethenyl-, polymer with ethenylbenzene, sulfonated, complex with (5α)-4,5-epoxy-3-methoxy-17-methylmorphinan-6-one; (2) Sulfonated styr-

ene-divinylbenzene copolymer complex with 4,5α-epoxy-3-methoxy-17-methylmorphinan-6-one. *UNII-CO68M0Q897. Antitussive.*

Hydrocortamate Hydrochloride. $C_{27}H_{41}NO_6 \cdot HCl$. 512.08. [Hydrocortamate is INN.] 11β,17α,21-Trihydroxypregn-4-ene-3,20-dione 21-diethylaminoacetate hydrochloride. *UNII-9QM8U7R83W; UNII-Y3N00BK5WK* [hydrocortamate]. *CAS-125-03-1; CAS-76-47-1* [hydrocortamate]. AMA-DE 1973; ND 1965; MI. Magnacort (Pfizer)

Hydrocortisone (hye″ droe kor′ ti sone). **USP.** $C_{21}H_{30}O_5$. 362.46. (1) Pregn-4-ene-3,20-dione, 11,17,21-trihydroxy-, (11β)-; (2) Cortisol. *UNII-WI4X0X7BPJ. CAS-50-23-7.* INN; BAN; JAN. *Glucocorticoid.* Cortef (Pfizer); Cortril (Pfizer); Hydrocortone (Merck); Hytone (Dermik) ◇*NSC-10483*

Hydrocortisone Aceponate. $C_{26}H_{36}O_7$. 460.56. 11β,17,21-Trihydroxy pregn-4-ene-3,20-dione 21-acetate 17-propionate. *CAS-74050-20-7.* INN.

Hydrocortisone Acetate (hye″ droe kor′ ti sone as′ e tate). **USP.** $C_{23}H_{32}O_6$. 404.50. (1) Pregn-4-ene-3,20-dione, 21-(acetyloxy)-11,17-dihydroxy-, (11β)-; (2) Cortisol 21-acetate. *UNII-3X7931PO74. CAS-50-03-3.* BAN; JAN. *Glucocorticoid.* Cortef Acetate (Pfizer); Cortril (Pfizer); Hydrocortone (Merck)

Hydrocortisone Buteprate (previously used name) — *See* Hydrocortisone Probutate.

Hydrocortisone Butyrate [*1980*] (hye″ droe kor′ ti sone bue′ ti rate). **USP.** $C_{25}H_{36}O_6$. 432.55. (1) Pregn-4-ene-3,20-dione, 11,21-dihydroxy-17-(1-oxobutoxy)-, (11β)-; (2) Cortisol 17-butyrate; (3) 11β,17,21-Trihydroxypregn-4-

ene-3,20-dione 17-butyrate. *UNII-05RMF7YPWN. CAS-13609-67-1.* BAN; JAN. *Glucocorticoid.* Locoid (Yamanouchi)

Hydrocortisone Cyclopentylpropionate — *See* Hydrocortisone Cypionate.

Hydrocortisone Cypionate. $C_{29}H_{42}O_6$. 486.64. (1) Pregn-4-ene-3,20-dione, 21-(3-cyclopentyl-1-oxopropoxy)-11,17-dihydroxy-, (11β)-; (2) Cortisol 21-cyclopentanepropionate. *UNII-4XDY25L70B. CAS-508-99-6.* USP XXII. Cortef (Pfizer)

Hydrocortisone Hemisuccinate (hye″ droe kor′ ti sone hem″ ee sux′ i nate). **USP.** $C_{25}H_{34}O_8 \cdot H_2O$. 480.55. [Hydrocortisone Succinate is JAN.] (1) Pregn-4-ene-3,20-dione, 21-(3-carboxy-1-oxopropoxy)-11,17-dihydroxy-, (11β)-, monohydrate; (2) Cortisol 21-(hydrogen succinate) monohydrate. *UNII-LIU00Z1Z84. CAS-83784-20-7; CAS-2203-97-6* [anhydrous]. *Adrenocortical steroid.*

Hydrocortisone Probutate [*1997*] (hye″ droe kor′ ti sone proe bue′ tate). $C_{28}H_{40}O_7$. 488.61. [Hydrocortisone Butyrate Propionate is JAN.] (1) 11β-Hydroxy-17-(1-oxobutoxy)-21-(1-oxopropoxy)pregn-4-ene-3,20-dione; (2) $11\beta,17,21$-Trihydroxypregn-4-ene-3,20-dione 17-butyrate 21-propionate. *UNII-O6550D6K3A. CAS-72590-77-3. Glucocorticoid.* Pandel (Savage) *[Name previously used: Hydrocortisone Buteprate.]* ◇*TS 408*

Hydrocortisone Sodium Phosphate (hye″ droe kor′ ti sone soe′ dee um fos′ fate). **USP.** $C_{21}H_{29}Na_2O_8P$. 486.40. (1) Pregn-4-ene-3,20-dione, 11,17-dihydroxy-21-(phosphonooxy)-, disodium salt, (11β)-; (2) Cortisol 21-(disodium phosphate). *UNII-0388G963HY. CAS-6000-74-4; CAS-3863-59-0* [cortisol 21-(dihydrogen phosphate)]. BAN; JAN. *Glucocorticoid.* Hydrocortone (Merck)

Hydrocortisone Sodium Succinate (hye″ droe kor′ ti sone soe′ dee um sux′ i nate). **USP.** $C_{25}H_{33}NaO_8$. 484.51. (1) Pregn-4-ene-3,20-dione, 21-(3-carboxy-1-oxopropoxy)-11,17-dihydroxy-, monosodium salt, (11β)-; (2) Cortisol 21-(sodium succinate). *UNII-50LQB69S1Z. CAS-125-04-2; CAS-2203-97-6* [hydrocortisone succinate]. BAN; JAN. *Glucocorticoid.* A-hydrocort (Hospira); Solu-cortef (Pfizer)

Hydrocortisone Valerate [*1977*] (hye″ droe kor′ ti sone val′ er ate). **USP.** $C_{26}H_{38}O_6$. 446.58. (1) Pregn-4-ene-3,20-dione, 11,21-dihydroxy-17-[(1-oxopentyl)oxy]-, (11β)-; (2) Cortisol 17-valerate; (3) $11\beta,17,21$-Trihydroxypregn-4-ene-3,20-dione 17-valerate. *UNII-68717P8FUZ. CAS-57524-89-7. Glucocorticoid.*

Hydrocotarnine Hydrochloride. $C_{12}H_{15}NO_3 \cdot HCl \cdot H_2O$. 275.73. 5,6,7,8-Tetrahydro-4-methoxy-6-methyl-1,3-dioxolo[4,5-g]isoquinoline hydrochloride hydrate. *CAS-550-10-7.* JAN.

Hydrofilcon A [*1979*] (hye″ droe fil′ kon). $(C_6H_9NO)_x$ $(C_{12}H_{14}O_2)_y(C_9H_{14}O_3)_z$. (1) 2-Pyrrolidinone, 1-ethenyl-, polymer with 2-phenylethyl 2-methyl-2-propenoate and 2-(2-propenyloxy)ethyl 2-methyl-2-propenoate; (2) 1-Vinyl-2-pyrrolidinone polymer with phenethyl methacrylate and 2-(allyloxy)ethyl methacrylate. *CAS-58985-93-6. Contact lens material (hydrophilic).* ◇*WX 14822; AO-407*

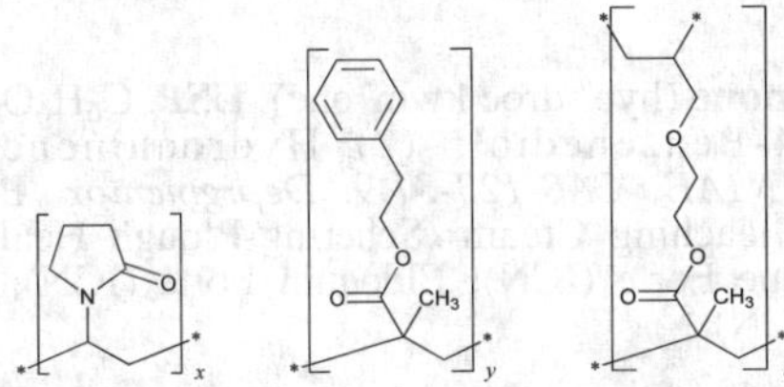

Hydroflumethiazide (hye″ droe floo″ me thye′ a zide). **USP.** $C_8H_8F_3N_3O_4S_2$. 331.29. (1) 2*H*-1,2,4-Benzothiadiazine-7-sulfonamide, 3,4-dihydro-6-(trifluoromethyl)-, 1,1-dioxide; (2) 3,4-Dihydro-6-(trifluoromethyl)-2*H*-1,2,4-benzothiadiazine-7-sulfonamide 1,1-dioxide. *UNII-501CFL162R. CAS-135-09-1.* INN; BAN; JAN. *Antihypertensive; diuretic.* Diucardin (Wyeth); Saluron (Shire)

Hydrogen Peroxide (hye′ droe jen per ox′ ide). **USP.** H_2O_2. 34.01. [Oxydol is JAN.] (1) Hydrogen peroxide; (2) Hydrogen peroxide. *UNII-BBX060AN9V. CAS-7722-84-1. Anti-infective, topical.*

Hydrogenated Ergot Alkaloids (previously used name) — *See* Ergoloid Mesylates.

Hydromadinone. $C_{21}H_{29}ClO_3$. 364.91. 6α-Chloro-17-hydroxyprogesterone. *CAS-16469-74-2.* INN.

Hydromorphinol. $C_{17}H_{21}NO_4$. 303.35. 14-Hydroxydihydromorphine. *CAS-2183-56-4.* INN; BAN; DCF.

Hydromorphone Hydrochloride (hye″ droe mor′ fone hye″ droe klor′ ide). **USP.** $C_{17}H_{19}NO_3 \cdot HCl$. 321.80. [Hydromorphone is INN and BAN.] (1) Morphinan-6-one, 4,5-epoxy-3-hydroxy-17-methyl-, hydrochloride, (5α)-; (2) $4,5\alpha$-Epoxy-3-hydroxy-17-methylmorphinan-6-one hydrochloride. *UNII-L960UP2KRW; UNII-Q812464R06* [hydromorphone]. *CAS-71-68-1; CAS-466-99-9* [hydromorphone]. *Analgesic (narcotic).* Dilaudid (Abbott) *[Name previously used: Dihydromorphinone Hydrochloride.]*

Hydromorphone Sulfate. AMA-DE 1973.

4-Hydroperoxycyclophosphamide — *See* Perfosfamide.

Hydroquinone (hye″ droe kwin′ one). **USP**. $C_6H_6O_2$. 110.11. (1) 1,4-Benzenediol; (2) Hydroquinone. *UNII-XV74C1N1AE. CAS-123-31-9. Depigmentor*. Black and White Bleaching Cream (Schering-Plough HealthCare†); Eldopaque Forte (ICN); Eldoquin Forte (ICN); Solaquin Forte (ICN)

Hydrotalcite. $Mg_6Al_2(OH)_{16}CO_3.4H_2O$. 603.98. Aluminum dimagnesium carbonate hexahydroxide tetrahydrate. *CAS-12304-65-3*. INN; BAN; JAN.

Hydroxamethocaine (previously used name) — *See* Hydroxytetracaine.

Hydroxidione Sodium Succinate — *See* Hydroxydione Sodium Succinate.

Hydroxindasate. $C_{21}H_{24}N_2O_3$. 352.43. 3-(2-Aminoethyl)-1-(*p*-methoxybenzyl)-2-methylindol-5-ol acetate ester. *UNII-U8687J667P. CAS-7008-14-2*. INN.

Hydroxindasol. $C_{19}H_{22}N_2O_2$. 310.39. 3-(2-Aminoethyl)-1-(*p*-methoxybenzyl)-2-methylindol-5-ol. *UNII-880XXO778K. CAS-7008-15-3*. INN.

Hydroxizine Chloride — *See* Hydroxyzine Hydrochloride.

Hydroxocobalamin [*1962*] (hye drox″ oh koe bal′ a min). **USP**. $C_{62}H_{89}CoN_{13}O_{15}P$. 1346.36. [Hydroxocobalamin Acetate is JAN.] (1) Cobinamide, dihydroxide, dihydrogen phosphate (ester), mono(inner salt), 3′-ester with 5,6-dimethyl-1-α-D-ribofuranosyl-1*H*-benzimidazole; (2) Cobinamide dihydroxide dihydrogen phosphate (ester), mono(inner salt), 3′-ester with 5,6-dimethyl-1-α-D-ribofur-

anosylbenzimidazole. *UNII-Q40X8H422O. CAS-13422-51-0*. INN; BAN; JAN. *Vitamin (hematopoietic)*. Alpharedisol (Merck)

Hydroxocobemine — *See* Hydroxocobalamin.

Hydroxyamfetamine (INN, BAN) — *See* Hydroxyamphetamine Hydrobromide.

Hydroxyamphetamine Hydrobromide (hye drox″ ee am fet′ a meen hye″ droe broe′ mide). **USP**. $C_9H_{13}NO.HBr$. 232.12. [Hydroxyamfetamine is INN and BAN.] (1) Phenol, 4-(2-aminopropyl)-, hydrobromide; (2) (±)-*p*-(2-Aminopropyl)-phenol hydrobromide. *UNII-59IG47SZ0E; UNII-FQR280JW2N* [hydroxyamphetamine]. *CAS-306-21-8; CAS-103-86-6* [hydroxyamphetamine]; *CAS-1518-86-1* [replaced]. *Adrenergic (ophthalmic)*. Paredrine (Akorn)

4-Hydroxyanisole (previously used name) — *See* Mequinol.

p-Hydroxyanisole (previously used name) — *See* Mequinol.

Hydroxyapatite — *See* Calcium Phosphate, Tribasic.

Hydroxyapatite (BAN) — *See* Durapatite.

Hydroxycarbamide (INN) — *See* Hydroxyurea.

Hydroxychloroquine Sulfate (hye drox″ ee klor′ oh kwin sul′ fate). **USP**. $C_{18}H_{26}ClN_3O.H_2SO_4$. 433.95. [Hydroxychloroquine is INN and BAN.] (1) Ethanol, 2-[[4-[(7-chloro-4-quinolinyl)amino]pentyl]ethyl]amino-, (±)-, sulfate (1:1) salt; (2) (±)-2-[[4-[(7-Chloro-4-quinolyl)amino]penty-l]ethylamino]ethanol sulfate (1:1) (salt). *UNII-8Q2869CNVH; UNII-4QWG6N8QKH* [hydroxychloroquine]. *CAS-747-36-4; CAS-118-42-3* [hydroxychloroquine]. *Antimalarial; suppressant (lupus erythematosus)*. Plaquenil (Sanofi Aventis)

Hydroxycincophene (DCF) — *See* Oxycinchophen.

Hydroxydione Sodium Succinate. $C_{25}H_{35}NaO_6$. 454.53. 21-Hydroxy-5β-pregnane-3,20-dione 21-(sodium succinate). *UNII-53J8I8O5EW. CAS-53-10-1; CAS-303-01-5* [hydroxydione]. INN; BAN; MI. Viadril (Pfizer)

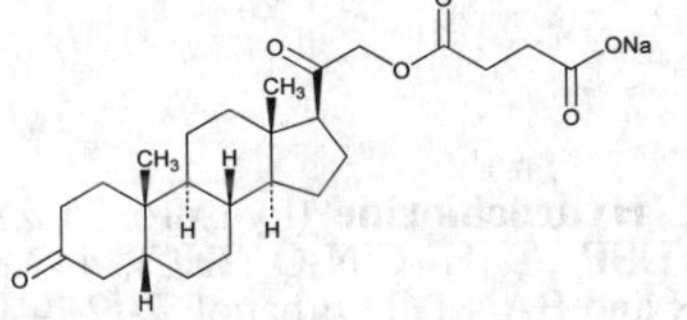

Hydroxyethyl Cellulose (hye drox″ ee eth′ il sel′ ue lose). **NF**. Cellulose, 2-hydroxyethyl ether. *CAS-9004-62-0. Pharmaceutic aid (suspending agent); pharmaceutic aid (viscosity-increasing agent).* Cellosize (Union Carbide)

Hydroxyethyl Starch 130/0.4 [*2008*] (hye drox″ ee eth′ il stahrch). (1) Starch 2-hydroxyethyl ether; (2) A starch composed of more than 90% amylopectin that has been etherified to the extend that an average of 3.8 to 4.5 of the OH groups present in every 10 D-glucopyranose units of the starch polymer have been converted into OCH_2CH_2OH groups. Molecular weight is approximately 130,000 daltons. *CAS-9005-27-0. Prophylaxis of hypervolemia.* Voluven (Fresenius Kabi Deutschland GmbH) ◇*HES 130/0.4*

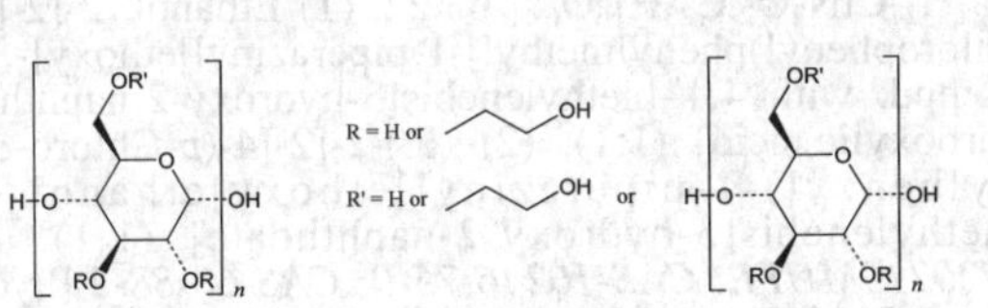

Hydroxyethylstarch (JAN) — *See* Hetastarch.

Hydroxyhexamide. *CAS-3168-01-2.*

Hydroxymesterone — *See* Medrysone.

Hydroxypethidine. $C_{15}H_{21}NO_3$. 263.33. 4-(*m*-Hydroxyphenyl)-1-methylpiperidine-4-carboxylic acid ethyl ester. *UNII-W1J43H2B3K. CAS-468-56-4.* INN; BAN; MI. ◇*Win 771*

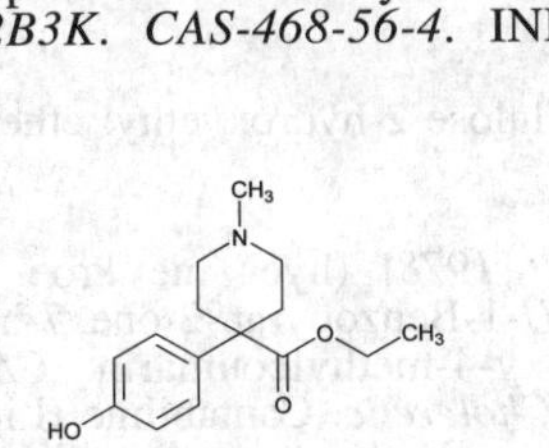

Hydroxyphenamate [*1962*] (hye drox″ ee fen′ a mate). $C_{11}H_{15}NO_3$. 209.24. [Oxyfenamate is INN.] (1) 1,2-Butanediol, 2-phenyl-, 1-carbamate; (2) 2-Phenyl-1,2-butanediol 1-carbamate. *UNII-MD0414799X. CAS-50-19-1. Tranquilizer (minor).* ◇*Al-0361; P-301; NSC-108034*

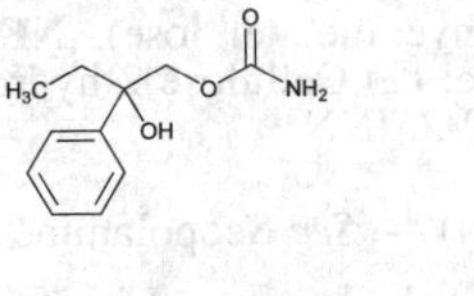

Hydroxyprocaine. $C_{13}H_{20}N_2O_3$. 252.31. 2-Diethylaminoethyl 4-aminosalicylate. *UNII-12LGO1XVPA. CAS-487-53-6.* INN; DCF; BAN; MI.

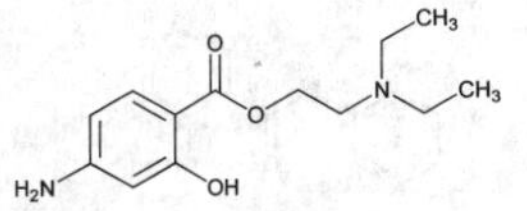

Hydroxyprogesterone Caproate (hye drox″ ee proe jes′ ter one kap′ roe ate). **USP**. $C_{27}H_{40}O_4$. 428.60. [Hydroxyprogesterone is INN and BAN.] (1) Pregn-4-ene-3,20-dione, 17-[(1-oxohexyl)oxy]-; (2) 17-Hydroxypregn-4-ene-3,20-dione hexanoate. *UNII-276F2O42F5. CAS-630-56-8; CAS-68-96-2* [hydroxyprogesterone]. INN; JAN. *Progestin.* Delalutin (Bristol-Myers Squibb) ◇*NSC-17592*

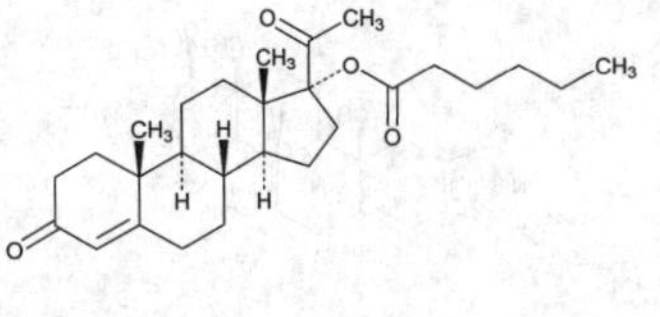

Hydroxypropyl Betadex (hye drox″ ee proe′ pil bay′ ta dex). **NF**. $C_{42}H_{70}O_{35}(C_3H_6O)_x$ where x ≈ 7 MS, MS being Molar Substitution. Beta cyclodextrin, 2-hydroxypropyl ether. *CAS-94035-02-6.*

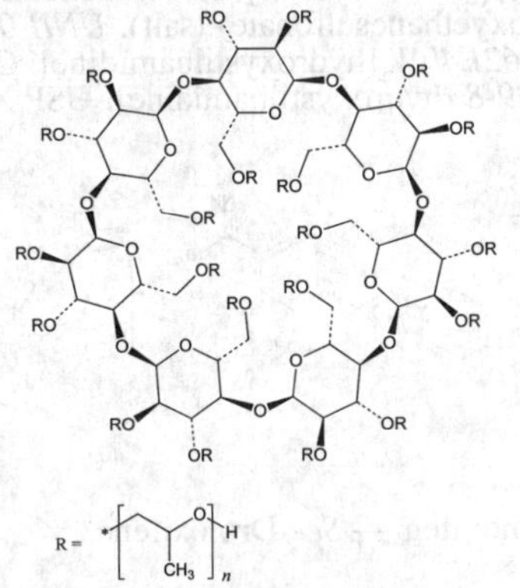

Hydroxypropyl Cellulose (hye drox″ ee proe′ pil sel′ ue lose). **NF**. [Hydroxypropylcellulose is JAN.] Cellulose, 2-hydroxypropyl ether. *UNII-RFW2ET671P. CAS-9004-64-2.* INN. *Protectant (topical); pharmaceutic aid (emulsifying agent); pharmaceutic aid (tablet coating agent).* Lacrisert (Aton)

Hydroxypropyl Methylcellulose (previously used name) — *See* Hypromellose.

Hydroxypropyl Methylcellulose 1828. (1) Cellulose, 2-hydroxypropyl methyl ether; (2) Cellulose hydroxypropyl methyl ether. *CAS-9004-65-3.* USP XX.

Hydroxypropyl Methylcellulose Phthalate (previously used name) — *See* Hypromellose Phthalate.

Hydroxypropyl Methylcellulose Phthalate 200731. NF 18.

Hydroxypropyl Methylcellulose Phthalate 220824. NF 18.

Hydroxypropylcellulose (JAN) — *See* Hydroxypropyl Cellulose.

Hydroxypropylmethylcellulose (JAN) — *See* Hypromellose.

Hydroxypropylmethylcellulose Phthalate (JAN) — *See* Hypromellose Phthalate.

---

† Brand name formerly used, and/or firm no longer concerned with this product.

Hydroxypyridine Tartrate. $C_9H_9NO_6$. 227.17. Tartaric ester of 3-hydroxypyridine. *CAS-7008-17-5; CAS-109-00-2* [3-pyridinol]. INN; DCF.

Hydroxystearin Sulfate. Sulfonated hydrogenated castor oil. *CAS-8031-45-6*. NF IX.

Hydroxystenozole. $C_{21}H_{30}N_2O$. 326.48. 17β-Hydroxy-17α-methylandrost-4-eno[3,2-c]pyrazole. *CAS-5697-57-4*. INN.

Hydroxystilbamidine Isethionate. $C_{16}H_{16}N_4O.2C_2H_6O_4S$. 532.59. [Hydroxystilbamidine is INN and BAN.] (1) Benzenecarboximidamide, 4-[2-[4-(aminoiminomethyl)-phenyl]ethenyl]-3-hydroxy-, bis(2-hydroxyethanesulfo-nate) (salt); (2) 2-Hydroxy-4,4′-stilbenedicarboxamidine bis(2-hydroxyethanesulfonate) (salt). *UNII-0163PVD2QZ; UNII-39J262E49W* [hydroxystilbamidine]. *CAS-533-22-2; CAS-495-99-8* [hydroxystilbamidine]. USP XXII.

3-Hydroxytamoxifen — *See* Droloxifene.

Hydroxytetracaine. $C_{15}H_{24}N_2O_3$. 280.36. 2-Dimethylami-noethyl 4-butylaminosalicylate. *UNII-8A96H4311N. CAS-490-98-2*. INN; BAN; DCF; MI. *[Name previously used: Hydroxamethocaine.]*

Hydroxytoluic Acid. $C_8H_8O_3$. 152.15. 2-Hydroxy-3-methyl-benzoic acid. *UNII-ZH3HEY032H. CAS-83-40-9*. INN; BAN. ◇*3 MS*

Hydroxyurea [*1965*] (hye drox″ ee ure ee′ a). **USP**. $CH_4N_2O_2$. 76.05. [Hydroxycarbamide is INN and BAN.] (1) Urea, hydroxy-; (2) Hydroxyurea. *UNII-*

X6Q56QN5QC. CAS-127-07-1. Antineoplastic. Droxia (Bristol-Myers Squibb); Hydrea (Bristol-Myers Squibb) ◇*SQ 1089; NSC-32065*

Hydroxyzine Hydrochloride (hye drox′ i zeen hye″ droe klor′ ide). **USP**. $C_{21}H_{27}ClN_2O_2.2HCl$. 447.83. [Hydroxy-zine is INN and BAN.] (1) Ethanol, 2-[2-[4-[(4-chlorophe-nyl)phenylmethyl]-1-piperazinyl]ethoxy]-, dihydrochlor-ide, ($\pm$)-; (2) ($\pm$)-2-[2-[4-(p-Chloro-α-phenylbenzyl)-1-piperazinyl]ethoxy]ethanol dihydrochloride. *UNII-76755771U3. CAS-2192-20-3; CAS-68-88-2* [hydroxy-zine]. JAN. *Tranquilizer (minor).* Atarax (Pfizer); Vistaril (Pfizer)

Hydroxyzine Pamoate (hye drox′ i zeen pam′ oh ate). **USP**. $C_{21}H_{27}ClN_2O_2.C_{23}H_{16}O_6$. 763.27. (1) Ethanol, 2-[2-[4-[(4-chlorophenyl)phenylmethyl]-1-piperazinyl]ethoxy]-, ($\pm$)-, compd. with 4,4′-methylenebis[3-hydroxy-2-naphthalene-carboxylic acid] (1:1); (2) ($\pm$)-2-[2-[4-(p-Chloro-α-phe-nylbenzyl)-1-piperazinyl]ethoxy]ethanol 4,4′-methylenebis[3-hydroxy-2-naphthoate] (1:1). *UNII-M20215MUFR. CAS-10246-75-0; CAS-68-88-2* [hydroxy-zine]. JAN. *Tranquilizer (minor).* Hy-Pam (Teva); Vistaril (Pfizer)

Hyetellose. Cellulose 2-hydroxyethyl ether. *CAS-9004-62-0*. INN.

Hymecromone [*1978*] (hye″ me kroe′ mone). $C_{10}H_8O_3$. 176.17. (1) 2H-1-Benzopyran-2-one, 7-hydroxy-4-methyl-; (2) 7-Hydroxy-4-methylcoumarin. *CAS-90-33-5*. INN; BAN; JAN. *Choleretic.* Cantabiline (Lipha, S.A., France) ◇*LM-94*

Hymetellose (hye me′ tel lose). **NF**. (1) Methylhydroxy-ethylcellulose; (2) Cellulose 2-hydroxyethyl methyl ether. *CAS-9032-42-2*. INN.

Hyoscine (BAN) — *See* Scopolamine Hydrobromide.

Hyoscine Hydrobromide (previously used name) — *See* Scopolamine Hydrobromide.

Hyoscine Methobromide (BAN) — *See* Methscopolamine Bromide.

Hyoscyamine (hye″ oh sye′ a meen). **USP.** $C_{17}H_{23}NO_3$. 289.37. (1) Benzeneacetic acid, α-(hydroxymethyl)-, 8-methyl-8-azabicyclo[3.2.1]oct-3-yl ester, [3(*S*)-*endo*]-; (2) 1αH,5αH-Tropan-3α-ol (-)-tropate (ester). *UNII-PX44XO846X. CAS-101-31-5. BAN. Anticholinergic.*

Hyoscyamine Hydrobromide (hye″ oh sye′ a meen hye″ droe broe′ mide). **USP.** $C_{17}H_{23}NO_3$.HBr. 370.28. (1) Benzeneacetic acid, α-(hydroxymethyl)-, 8-methyl-8-azabicyclo[3.2.1]oct-3-yl ester, hydrobromide [3(*S*)-*endo*]-; (2) 1αH,5αH-Tropan-3α-ol (-)-tropate (ester) hydrobromide. *UNII-IWT50P9S79. CAS-306-03-6; CAS-101-31-5* [hyoscyamine]. *Anticholinergic.*

Hyoscyamine Sulfate (hye″ oh sye′ a meen sul′ fate). **USP.** $(C_{17}H_{23}NO_3)_2$.H_2SO_4.$2H_2O$. 712.85. [Hyoscyamine Sulphate is BAN.] (1) Benzeneacetic acid, α-(hydroxymethyl)-, 8-methyl-8-azabicyclo[3.2.1]oct-3-yl ester, [3(*S*)-*endo*]-, sulfate (2:1), dihydrate; (2) 1αH,5αH-Tropan-3α-ol (-)-tropate (ester) sulfate (2:1) (salt) dihydrate. *UNII-F2R8V82B84. CAS-6835-16-1; CAS-620-61-1* [anhydrous]; *CAS-101-31-5* [hyoscyamine]. *Anticholinergic.* Anaspaz (Ascher); Levsin (Schwarz Pharma); Levsinex (Schwarz Pharma); Neoquess (Forest†)

Hypophosphorous Acid (hye″ poe fos′ for us as′ id). **NF.** H_3PO_2. 66.00. (1) Phosphinic acid; (2) Hypophosphorous acid. *CAS-6303-21-5. Pharmaceutic aid (antioxidant).*

Hyprolose — *See* Hydroxypropyl Cellulose.

Hyprolose. Cellulose 2-hydroxypropyl ether. *CAS-9004-64-2.* INN.

Hypromellose (hye proe′ me lose). **USP.** [Hydroxypropylmethylcellulose is JAN.] (1) Cellulose, 2-hydroxypropyl methyl ether; (2) Cellulose hydroxypropyl methyl ether. *UNII-3NXW29V3WO. CAS-9004-65-3.* INN; BAN. *Pharmaceutic aid (suspending agent); pharmaceutic aid (tablet excipient); pharmaceutic aid (viscosity-increasing agent).* GenTeal (Ciba Vision, US Ophthalmics); Goniosol (Ciba Vision, US Ophthalmics); Isopto Tears (Alcon); Methocel E, F, J, K (Dow Chemical); Tearisol (Ciba Vision, US Ophthalmics); Ultra Tears (Alcon) *[Name previously used: Hydroxypropyl Methylcellulose.]*

Hypromellose Acetate Succinate (hye proe′ me lose as′ e tate sux′ i nate). **NF.** (1) Hydroxypropyl methylcellulose acetate succinate; (2) Cellulose, 2-hydroxypropyl methyl ether, acetate hydrogen butanedioate; (3) Cellulose, 2-hydroxypropyl methyl ether, acetate succinate. *CAS-71138-97-1.*

Hypromellose Phthalate (hye proe′ me lose thal′ ate). **NF.** [Hydroxypropylmethylcellulose Phthalate is JAN.] A monophthalic acid ester of hydroxypropyl methylcellulose. *Pharmaceutic aid (coating agent).* "EASTMAN" HPMCP (Eastman) *[Name previously used: Hydroxypropyl Methylcellulose Phthalate.]*

¹²³I — *See* Iobenguane I 123.

¹²³I — *See* Iobenguane Sulfate I 123.

---

† Brand name formerly used, and/or firm no longer concerned with this product.

¹²³I — *See* Iocanlidic Acid I 123.

¹²³I — *See* Iodocetylic Acid I 123.

¹²³I — *See* Iodohippurate Sodium I 123.

¹²³I — *See* Iofetamine Hydrochloride I 123.

¹²³I — *See* Iolopride (¹²³I).

¹²³I — *See* Iomazenil (¹²³I).

¹²³I — *See* Sodium Iodide I 123.

¹²⁵I — *See* Iodinated I 125 Albumin.

¹²⁵I — *See* Albumin, Iodinated I 125 Serum.

¹²⁵I — *See* Diatrizoate Sodium I 125.

¹²⁵I — *See* Diohippuric Acid I 125.

¹²⁵I — *See* Diotyrosine I 125.

¹²⁵I — *See* Fibrinogen I 125.

¹²⁵I — *See* Insulin I 125.

¹²⁵I — *See* Iodohippurate Sodium I 125.

¹²⁵I — *See* Iodopyracet I 125.

¹²⁵I — *See* Iomethin I 125.

¹²⁵I — *See* Iothalamate Sodium I 125.

¹²⁵I — *See* Liothyronine I 125.

¹²⁵I — *See* Oleic Acid I 125.

¹²⁵I — *See* Povidone I 125.

¹²⁵I — *See* Rose Bengal Sodium I 125.

¹²⁵I — *See* Sodium Iodide I 125.

¹²⁵I — *See* Thyroxine I 125.

¹²⁵I — *See* Triolein I 125.

¹³¹I — *See* Iodinated I 131 Albumin Aggregated.

¹³¹I — *See* Albumin, Aggregated Iodinated I 131 Serum.

¹³¹I — *See* Iodinated I 131 Albumin.

¹³¹I — *See* Albumin, Iodinated I 131 Serum.

¹³¹I — *See* Diatrizoate Sodium I 131.

¹³¹I — *See* Diohippuric Acid I 131.

¹³¹I — *See* Diotyrosine I 131.

¹³¹I — *See* Ethiodized Oil I 131.

¹³¹I — *See* Insulin I 131.

¹³¹I — *See* Iobenguane I 131.

¹³¹I — *See* Iodipamide Sodium I 131.

¹³¹I — *See* Iodoantipyrine I 131.

¹³¹I — *See* Iodocholesterol I 131.

¹³¹I — *See* Iodohippurate Sodium I 131.

¹³¹I — *See* Iodopyracet I 131.

¹³¹I — *See* Iomethin I 131.

¹³¹I — *See* Iothalamate Sodium I 131.

¹³¹I — *See* Iotyrosine I 131.

¹³¹I — *See* Liothyronine I 131.

¹³¹I — *See* Macrosalb (¹³¹I).

¹³¹I — *See* Oleic Acid I 131.

[131]I — *See* Povidone I 131.

[131]I — *See* Rose Bengal Sodium I 131.

[131]I — *See* Sodium Iodide I 131.

[131]I — *See* Thyroxine I 131.

[131]I — *See* Tolpovidone I 131.

[131]I — *See* Triolein I 131.

Ibacitabine. $C_9H_{12}IN_3O_4$. 353.11. 2′-Deoxy-5-iodocytidine. *CAS-611-53-0.* INN.

Ibafloxacin [*1989*] (eye″ ba flox′ a sin). $C_{15}H_{14}FNO_3$. 275.27. (1) 1*H*,5*H*-Benzo[*ij*]quinolizine-2-carboxylic acid, 9-fluoro-6,7-dihydro-5,8-dimethyl-1-oxo-; (2) 9-Fluoro-6,7-dihydro-5,8-dimethyl-1-oxo-1*H*,5*H*-benzo[*ij*]quinolizine-2-carboxylic acid. *CAS-91618-36-9.* INN; BAN. *Antibacterial.* ◇S-25930; R-835

Ibalizumab [*2007*] (eye″ ba liz′ oo mab). Immunoglobulin G4, anti-(human CD4 (antigen)) (human-mouse monoclonal 5A8 γ4-chain), disulfide with human-mouse monoclonal 5A8 κ-chain, dimer. *CAS-680188-33-4.* INN. *Treatment of HIV/AIDS in HIV-1 infected patients.* ◇TNX-355

Heavy chain

```
QVQLQQSGPE VVKPGASVKM SCKASGYTFT SYVIHWVRQK PGQGLDWIGY
INPYNDGTDY DEKFKGKATL TSDTSTSTAY MELSSLRSED TAVYYCAREK
DNYATGAWFA YWGQGTLVTV SSASTKGPSV FPLAPCSRST SESTAALGCL
VKDYFPEPVT VSWNSGALTS GVHTFPAVLQ SSGLYSLSSV VTVPSSSLGT
KTYTCNVDHK PSNTKVDKRV ESKYGPPCPS CPAPEFLGGP SVFLFPPKPK
DTLMISRTPE VTCVVVDVSQ EDPEVQFNWY VDGVEVHNAK TKPREEQFNS
TYRVVSVLTV LHQDWLNGKE YKCKVSNKGL PSSIEKTISK AKGQPREPQV
YTLPPSQEEM TKNQVSLTCL VKGFYPSDIA VEWESNGQPE NNYKTTPPVL
DSDGSFFLYS RLTVDKSRWQ EGNVFSCSVM HEALHNHYTQ KSLSLSLGK
```
2

Light chain

```
DIVMTQSPDS LAVSLGERVT MNCKSSQSLL YSTNQKNYLA WYQQKPGQSP
KLLIYWASTR ESGVPDRFSG SGSGTDFTLT ISSVQAEDVA VYYCQQYYSY
RTFGGGTKLE IKTVAAPSVF IFPPSDEQLK SGTASVVCLL NNFYPREAKV
QWKVDNALQS GNSQESVTEQ DSKDSTYSLS STLTLSKADY EKHKVYACEV
THQGLSSPVT KSFNRGEC
```
2

Ibandronate Sodium [*1997*] (eye ban′ droe nate soe′ dee um). $C_9H_{22}NNaO_7P_2 \cdot H_2O$. 359.23. Sodium trihydrogen [1-hydroxy-3-(methylpentylamino)propylidene]diphosphonate, monohydrate. *UNII-J12U072QL0.* CAS-138926-19-9. JAN. *Bone resorption inhibitor; antihypercalcemic.* Boniva (Roche) ◇BM 21.0955 · Na · H2O

Ibandronic Acid. $C_9H_{23}NO_7P_2$. 319.23. [1-Hydroxy-3-(methylpentylamino)propylidene]diphosphonic acid. *UNII-UMD7G2653W. CAS-114084-78-5.* INN; BAN.

Ibazocine. $C_{20}H_{29}NO$. 299.45. 1,2,3,4,5,6-Hexahydro-6,11,11-trimethyl-3-(3-methyl-2-butenyl)-2,6-methano-3-benzazocin-8-ol. *CAS-57653-28-8.* INN.

Ibipinabant [*2007*] (eye″ bi pin′ a bant). $C_{23}H_{20}Cl_2N_4O_2S$. 487.40. (1) 1*H*-Pyrazole-1-carboximidamide, 3-(4-chlorophenyl)-*N*-[(4-chlorophenyl)sulfonyl]-4,5-dihydro-*N*′-methyl-4-phenyl-, (4*S*)-; (2) (*E*)-(4*S*)-3-(4-Chlorophenyl)-*N*′-[(4-chlorophenyl)sulfonyl]-*N*-methyl-4-phenyl-4,5-dihydro-1*H*-pyrazole-1-carboximidamide. *UNII-O5CSC6WH1T. CAS-464213-10-3.* INN. *Treatment of obesity.* ◇SLV-319; BMS-646256

Iboctadekin [*2004*] (eye bok″ ta de′ kin). $C_{801}H_{1264}N_{212}O_{252}S_{10}$. 18,217.00. (1) Human interleukin-18 (recombinant, expressed in *Escherichia coli*); (2) Purified iboctadekin is a recombinant human cytokine, interleukin-18 (IL-18) belonging to the IL-1 family, also known as interferon-γ-inducing factor (IGIF), expressed in a non-pathenogenic strain of *Escherichia coli*. Iboctadekin, consisting of 157 amino acids, is formed *in vivo* following the activation of proIL-18 by caspase-4 and consists of a single polypeptide chain that is not glycosylated. The protein contains four cysteine residues present as free sulfhydryl groups. *CAS-479198-61-3.* INN. *Treatment of disseminated solid tumors.* ◇SB-485232

```
YFGKLESKLS VIRNLNDQVL FIDQGNRPLF EDMTDSDCRD NAPRTIFIIS
MYKDSQPRGM AVTISVKCEK ISTLSCENKI ISFKEMNPPD NIKDTKSDII
FFQRSVPGHD NKMQFESSSY EGYFLACEKE RDLFKLILKK EDELGDRSIM
FTVQNED
```

Ibodutant. $C_{37}H_{48}N_4O_4S$. 644.87. 6-Methyl-*N*-{1-[({(1*R*)-1-[({1-[(Tetrahydro-2*H*-pyran-4-yl)methyl]piperidin-4-yl}-methyl)amino]-3-phenyl-1-oxopropan-2-yl}amino)carbonyl]cyclopentyl}-1-benzothiophene-2-carboxamide. *CAS-522664-63-7.* INN.

Ibopamine [*1981*] (eye boe′ pa meen). $C_{17}H_{25}NO_4$. 307.38.
(1) Propanoic acid, 2-methyl-, 4-[2-(methylamino)ethyl]-
1,2-phenylene ester; (2) 4-[2-(Methylamino)ethyl]-*o*-phenylene diisobutyrate. *UNII-8ZCA2I2L11. CAS-66195-31-1.*
INN; BAN. *Dopaminergic agent (peripheral).* ◇*SB 7505*

Ibritumomab Tiuxetan [*1998*] (eye″ bri toom′ oh mab tye
ux′ e tan). (1) Immunoglobulin G1, anti-(human CD20
(antigen)) (mouse monoclonal IDEC-Y2B8 γ1-chain),
disulfide with mouse monoclonal IDEC-Y2B8 κ-chain,
dimer, *N*-[2-[bis(carboxymethyl)amino]-3-(4-isothiocyanatophenyl)propyl]-*N*-[2-[bis(carboxymethyl)amino]propyl]glycine conjugate; (2) Immunoglobulin G1 (mouse
monoclonal IDEC-Y2B8 γ1-chain anti-human antigen
CD20), disulfide with mouse monoclonal IDEC-Y2B8 κ-
chain, dimer, *N*-[2-[bis(carboxymethyl)amino]-3-(*p*-isothiocyanatophenyl)propyl]-*N*-[2-[bis(carboxymethyl)amino]propyl]glycine conjugate. Molecular weight is
approximately 1500 daltons. *UNII-4Q52C550XK. CAS-
206181-63-7.* INN; BAN; JAN. *Antineoplastic (monoclonal antibody).[Note—Yttrium-labeled ibritumomab tiuxetan is used for the treatment of non-Hodgkin's B-cell
lymphoma, co-administered with rituximab.]* ◇*IDEC-
Y2B8; IDEC-129*

Ibrolipim [*2002*] (eye broe′ li pim). $C_{19}H_{20}BrN_2O_4P$. 451.25.
(1) Phosphonic acid, [[4-[[(4-bromo-2-cyanophenyl)amino]carbonyl]phenyl]methyl]-, diethyl ester; (2) Diethyl [4-
[(4-bromo-2-cyanophenyl)carbamoyl]benzyl]phosphonate.
UNII-07H1561618. CAS-133208-93-2. INN. *Antiatherogenic; antiobesity; antidyslipidemia; anticachexia; and
antidiabetes/syndrome X.* ◇*NO-1886; OPF 009*

Ibrotal — *See* Ibrotamide.

Ibrotamide. $C_7H_{14}BrNO$. 208.10. (1) Butanamide, 2-bromo-2-
ethyl-3-methyl-; (2) 2-Bromo-2-ethylisovaleramide. *CAS-
466-14-8.* INN; DCF; MI.

Ibudilast. $C_{14}H_{18}N_2O$. 230.31. 1-(2-Isopropylpyrazolo[1,5-
a]pyridin-3-yl)-2-methyl-1-propanone. *UNII-
M0TTH61XC5. CAS-50847-11-5.* INN; JAN; MI.

Ibufenac [*1966*] (eye bue′ fen ak). $C_{12}H_{16}O_2$. 192.25. (1)
Benzeneacetic acid, 4-(2-methylpropyl)-; (2) (*p*-
Isobutylphenyl)acetic acid. *CAS-1553-60-2.* INN; BAN.
Analgesic; anti-inflammatory. Dytransin (Boots, England)
◇*RD 11654*

Ibuprofen [*1968*] (eye″ bue proe′ fen). **USP.** $C_{13}H_{18}O_2$.
206.28. (1) Benzeneacetic acid, α-methyl-4-(2-methylpropyl), (±)-; (2) (±)-*p*-Isobutylhydratropic acid; (3) (±)-2-
(*p*-Isobutylphenyl)propionic acid. *UNII-WK2XYI10QM.
CAS-15687-27-1; CAS-58560-75-1* [± mixture]. INN;
BAN; JAN. *Anti-inflammatory.* Advil (Wyeth); Motrin
(McNeil) ◇*U-18,573*

Ibuprofen Aluminum [*1980*] (eye″ bue proe′ fen a loo′ mi
num). $C_{26}H_{35}AlO_5$. 454.53. (1) Aluminum, hydroxybis[α-
methyl-4-(2-methylpropyl)benzeneacetato-*O*]-, (±)-; (2)
(±)-Hydroxybis(*p*-isobutylhydratropato)aluminum. *UNII-
WK2XYI10QM* [ibuprofen]; *UNII-WK2XYI10QM* [ibuprofen]. *CAS-61054-06-6; CAS-15687-27-1* [ibuprofen]; *CAS-
58560-75-1* [(±)-ibuprofen]. *Anti-inflammatory.* ◇*U-
18,573G*

Ibuprofen Lysine [*2005*] (eye″ bue proe′ fen lye′ seen).
$C_6H_{14}N_2O_2$.$C_{13}H_{18}O_2$. 352.47. (1) L-Lysine, mono[α-methyl-4-(2-methylpropyl)benzeneacetate]; (2) L-Lysine
mono[(2*RS*)-2-[4-(2-methylpropyl)phenyl]propanoate.
*UNII-N01ORX9D6S. CAS-57469-77-9. Anti-inflammatory
(prostaglandin synthetase inhibitor).* Neoprofen (Ovation)

Ibuprofen Piconol [*1988*] (eye″ bue proe′ fen pik′ o nol).
$C_{19}H_{23}NO_2$. 297.39. (1) Benzeneacetic acid, α-methyl-4-
(2-methylpropyl)-, 2-pyridinylmethyl ester, (±)-; (2) 2-

Pyridylmethyl (±)-*p*-isobutylhydratropate. *UNII-B0F91K5U4N. CAS-112017-99-9.* JAN. *Anti-inflammatory (topical).* ◇*Be-100; U-75630*

Ibuproxam. $C_{13}H_{19}NO_2$. 221.30. *p*-Isobutylhydratropohydroxamic acid. *CAS-53648-05-8.* INN; MI.

Ibutamoren Mesylate [*1997*] (eye bue″ ta mor′ en mes′ i late). $C_{27}H_{36}N_4O_5S.CH_4O_3S$. 624.77. [Ibutamoren is INN.] 2-Amino-*N*-[(*R*)-2-(benzyloxy)-1-[[1-(methylsulfonyl)-spiro[indoline-3,4′-piperidin]-1′-yl]carbonyl]ethyl]-2-methylpropionamide monomethanesulfonate. *CAS-159752-10-0; CAS-159634-47-6* [ibutamoren]. *Growth hormone releasing factor.* ◇*MK-0677*

Ibuterol. $C_{20}H_{31}NO_5$. 365.46. 5-[2-(*tert*-Butylamino)-1-hydroxyethyl]-*m*-phenylene diisobutyrate. *CAS-53034-85-8.* INN.

Ibutilide Fumarate [*1990*] (eye bue′ ti lide fue′ ma rate). $(C_{20}H_{36}N_2O_3S)_2.C_4H_4O_4$. 885.23. [Ibutilide is INN and BAN.] (1) Methanesulfonamide, *N*-[4-[4-(ethylheptylamino)-1-hydroxybutyl]phenyl]-, (±)-, (*E*)-2-butenedioate (2:1) (salt); (2) (±)-4′-[4-(Ethylheptylamino)-1-hydroxybutyl]methanesulfonanilide fumarate (2:1) (salt). *UNII-9L5X4M5L6I; UNII-2436VX1U9B* [ibutilide]. *CAS-122647-32-9; CAS-122647-31-8* [ibutilide]. *Cardiac depressant (anti-arrhythmic).* Corvert (Pfizer) ◇*U-70226E*

Ibuverine. $C_{18}H_{26}O_3$. 290.40. Isobutyl α-phenylcyclohexane-glycolate. *CAS-31221-85-9.* INN.

Ibylcaine Chloride — *See* Butethamine Hydrochloride.

Icaridin. $C_{12}H_{23}NO_3$. 229.32. 1-Methylpropyl 2-(2-hydroxyethyl)piperidine-1-carboxylate. *CAS-119515-38-7.* INN.

Icatibant Acetate [*1993*] (eye kat′ i bant as′ e tate). $C_{59}H_{89}N_{19}O_{13}S.xC_2H_4O_2$. 1304.52 (as free base). [Icatibant is INN.] (1) L-Arginine, D-arginyl-L-arginyl-L-prolyl-*trans*-4-hydroxy-L-prolylglycyl-3-(2-thienyl)-L-alanyl-L-seryl-D-1,2,3,4-tetrahydro-3-isoquinolinecarbonyl-L-(2α,3aβ,7aβ)-octahydro-1*H*-indole-2-carbonyl-, acetate (salt); (2) (*R*)-Arginyl-(*S*)-arginyl-(*S*)-prolyl-(2*S*,4*R*)-(4-hydroxyprolyl)glycyl-(*S*)-[3-(2-thienyl)alanyl]-(*S*)-seryl-(*R*)-[(1,2,3,4-tetrahydro-3-isoquinolyl)carbonyl]-(2*S*,3a*S*,7a*S*)-[(hexahydro-2-indolinyl)carbonyl]-(*S*)-arginine acetate (salt). *CAS-138614-30-9; CAS-130308-48-4* [icatibant]. *Antagonist (bradykinin).* ◇*HOE 140*

Ichthammol (ik′ tha mol). **USP**. (1) Ichthammol; (2) Ichthammol. *CAS-8029-68-3.* BAN; JAN. *Anti-infective, topical.* Ichthymall (Mallinckrodt†)

Iclaprim [*2008*] (eye′ kla prim). $C_{19}H_{22}N_4O_3$. 354.40. (1) 2,4-Pyrimidinediamine, 5-[(2-cyclopropyl-7,8-dimethoxy-2*H*-1-benzopyran-5-yl)methyl]-; (2) 5-{[(2*RS*)-2-Cyclopropyl-7,8-dimethoxy-2*H*-1-benzopyran-5-yl]methyl}pyrimidine-2,4-diamine. *UNII-42445HUU0O. CAS-192314-93-5.* *Antibiotic.* ◇*AR-100*

Iclaprim Mesylate [*2008*] (eye′ kla prim mes′ i late). $C_{19}H_{22}N_4O_3.CH_4O_3S$. 450.51. [Iclaprim is INN.] (1) 2,4-Pyrimidinediamine, 5-[(2-cyclopropyl-7,8-dimethoxy-2*H*-1-benzopyran-5-yl)methyl]-, monomethanesulfonate; (2) 5-[[(2*RS*)-2-Cyclopropyl-7,8-dimethoxy-2*H*-1-benzopyr-an-5-yl]methyl]pyrimidine-2,4-diamine methanesulfonate. *UNII-7U972CJ5AT. CAS-474793-41-4; CAS-192314-93-5* [iclaprim]. *Anti-infective.* ◇*AR-100.001*

Iclazepam. $C_{21}H_{21}ClN_2O_2$. 368.86. 7-Chloro-1-[2-(cyclopropylmethoxy)ethyl]-1,3-dihydro-5-phenyl-2*H*-1,4-benzodiazepin-2-one. *UNII-FL061Q6NMC. CAS-57916-70-8.* INN.

Icodextrin [*2002*] (eye″ koe dex′ trin). $[C_6H_{10}O_5]_n$. (1) A complex polyglucopyranose produced by the enzymatic hydrolysis of corn. It is primarily composed of α-1,4-glucopyranose linkage with less that 10% α-1,6 linkage; (2) A complex α-D-glucopyranan produced by the enzymatic hydrolysis of corn. It is primarily composed of (1→4)-α-D-glucopyrano linkage with less than 10% $(1\rightarrow6)$-α linkage. Dextrin, having more than 85% of its molecules with molecular masses between 1640 and 45,000 with a claimed-average molecular mass of approximately 20,000. *UNII-2NX48Z0A9G. CAS-337376-15-5.* INN; BAN. *The osmotic agent in a peritoneal dialysis solution.* Extraneal (Baxter Healthcare)

Icodulinum. $C_{10}H_{10}N_2OS$. 206.26. 6-(2-Thiazolylamino)-*m*-cresol. *UNII-H91334173C. CAS-138511-81-6.* INN.

Icofungipen. $C_7H_{11}NO_2$. 141.17. (1*R*,2*S*)-2-Amino-4-methylenecyclopentane-1-carboxylic acid. *UNII-I20202Q8M8. CAS-198022-65-0.* INN.

Icometasone Enbutate. $C_{28}H_{37}ClO_7$. 521.04. 9-Chloro-11β,17,21-trihydroxy-16α-methylpregna-1,4-diene-3,20-dione 17-butyrate 21-acetate. *CAS-103466-73-5.* INN; BAN. *[Name previously used: Icomethasone Enbutate.]* ◇*CL09*

Icomucret [*2004*] (eye koe′ mue kret). $C_{20}H_{32}O_3$. 320.47. (1) 5,8,11,13-Eicosatetraenoic acid, 15-hydroxy-, (5*Z*,8*Z*,11*Z*,13*E*,15*S*)-; (2) (5*Z*,8*Z*,11*Z*,13*E*,15*S*)-15-Hydroxyicosa-5,8,11,13-tetraenoic acid. *UNII-44JHK6G39Q. CAS-54845-95-3.* INN. *Treatment of dry eye (stimulates glycoprotein secretion).* (Alcon Research) *[Note—The trivial name, 15(S)-HETE, has been used for icomucret in the literature.]* ◇*AL-12959*

Icopezil Maleate [*1996*] (eye koe′ pe zil mal′ ee ate). $C_{23}H_{25}N_3O_2 \cdot C_4H_4O_4$. 491.54. [Icopezil is INN.] (1) 6*H*-Pyrrolo[3,2-*f*]-1,2-benzisoxazol-6-one, 5,7-dihydro-3-[2-[1-(phenylmethyl)-4-piperidinyl]ethyl]-, (*Z*)-2-butenedioate (1:1); (2) 3-[2-(1-Benzyl-4-piperidyl)ethyl]-5,7-dihydro-6*H*-pyrrolo[3,2-*f*]-1,2-benzisoxazol-6-one maleate (1:1). *CAS-145815-98-1; CAS-145508-78-7* [icopezil]. *Alzheimer's disease treatment (cognition enhancer); cognition adjuvant; inhibitor (acetylcholinesterase).* ◇*CP-118,954-11*

Icosapent. $C_{20}H_{30}O_2$. 302.45. [Omega-3 Marine Triglycerides is BAN.] (*all-Z*)-5,8,11,14,17-Eicosapentaenoic acid. *CAS-10417-94-4.* INN.

Icospiramide. $C_{28}H_{31}F_2N_5O_2$. 507.57. 8-[*cis*-4-Cyano-4-(*p*-fluorophenyl)cyclohexyl]-1-(*p*-fluorophenyl)-4-oxo-1,3,8-triazaspiro[4.5]decane-3-acetamide. *UNII-H0N246YG4Y. CAS-79449-99-3.* INN.

Icotidine [*1985*] (eye koe′ ti deen). $C_{21}H_{25}N_5O_2$. 379.46. (1) 4(1*H*)-Pyrimidinone, 2-[[4-(3-methoxy-2-pyridinyl)butyl]amino]-5-[(6-methyl-3-pyridinyl)methyl]-; (2) 2-[[4-(3-Methoxy-2-pyridyl)butyl]amino]-5-[(6-methyl-3-pyridyl)methyl]-4(1*H*)-pyrimidinone. *UNII-25Y9G9575K. CAS-71351-79-6. Antagonist (to histamine H₂and H₁receptors).* ◇*SK&F 93319*

Icrocaptide. $C_{21}H_{40}N_8O_5$. 484.59. Glycyl-N^2-ethyl-L-lysyl-L-prolyl-L-arginine. *CAS-169543-49-1.* INN.

Ictasol [*1970*] (ik′ ta sol). $C_{28}H_{36}Na_2O_6S_3$ (Tentative). 610.76. Substance obtained by the destructive distillation of bituminous schists, sulfonation of the distillate, and neutralization with sodium hydroxide. The temperatures of distillation and sulfonation are controlled to prevent

---

† Brand name formerly used, and/or firm no longer concerned with this product.

excessive carbonization, and the product exhibits in aqueous solutions a light transmittance up to 50 times that of equivalent solutions of ichthammol. (1) Ictasol; (2) Ictasol. *CAS-12542-33-5. Disinfectant.*

Idarubicin Hydrochloride [*1987*] (eye″ da roo′ bi sin hye″ droe klor′ ide). **USP.** $C_{26}H_{27}NO_9 \cdot HCl$. 533.95. [Idarubicin is INN and BAN.] (1) 5,12-Naphthacenedione, 9-acetyl-7-[(3-amino-2,3,6-trideoxy-α-L-*lyxo*-hexopyranosyl)oxy]-7,8,9,10-tetrahydro-6,9,11-trihydroxyhydrochloride, (7*S*-*cis*)-; (2) (1*S*,3*S*)-3-Acetyl-1,2,3,4,6,11-hexahydro-3,5,12-trihydroxy-6,11-dioxo-1-naphthacenyl 3-amino-2,3,6-tri-deoxy-α-L-*lyxo*-hexopyranoside, hydrochloride. *UNII-5VV3MDU5IE; UNII-ZRP63D75JW* [idarubicin]. *CAS-57852-57-0; CAS-58957-92-9* [idarubicin]. INN. *Antineoplastic.* Idamycin (Bedford) ◇*IMI 30*

Idaverine. $C_{24}H_{39}N_3O_3$. 417.58. (+)-1-(4-{Ethyl[(*S*)-*p*-meth-oxy-α-methylphenethyl]amino}butyryl)-*N*,*N*-dimethyliso-nipecotamide. *CAS-100927-13-7.* INN.

Idazoxan. $C_{11}H_{12}N_2O_2$. 204.23. (±)-2-(1,4-Benzodioxan-2-yl)-2-imidazoline. *CAS-79944-58-4.* INN; BAN.

Idebenone. $C_{19}H_{30}O_5$. 338.44. 2-(10-Hydroxydecyl)-5,6-di-methoxy-3-methyl-*p*-benzoquinone. *UNII-HB6PN45W4J. CAS-58186-27-9.* INN; JAN; MI.

Idenast. $C_{28}H_{31}FN_4O_2$. 474.57. 2-[4-[4-(*p*-Fluorophenyl)-1-piperazinyl]butyl]-1-(*p*-methoxyphenyl)-3-indazolinone. *UNII-ABY1GJ356X. CAS-108674-88-0.* INN.

Idoxifene [*1996*] (eye dox′ i feen). $C_{28}H_{30}INO$. 523.45. (1) Pyrrolidine, 1-[2-[4-[1-(4-iodophenyl)-2-phenyl-1-buten-yl]phenoxy]ethyl-, (*E*)-; (2) 1-[2-[*p*-[(*E*)-β-Ethyl-α-(*p*-io-dophenyl)styryl]phenoxy]ethyl]pyrrolidine. *CAS-116057-*

75-1. INN; BAN. *Antineoplastic; hormone (replacement therapy, estrogen receptor antagonist); osteoporosis treat-ment and prevention.* ◇*CB 7432; SB-223030*

Idoxuridine [*1962*] (eye″ dox ure′ i deen). **USP.** $C_9H_{11}IN_2O_5$. 354.10. (1) Uridine, 2′-deoxy-5-iodo-; (2) 2′-Deoxy-5-iodouridine. *UNII-LGP81V5245. CAS-54-42-2.* INN; BAN; JAN. *Antiviral (ophthalmic).* Dendrid (Alcon); Herplex (Allergan); Stoxil (GlaxoSmithKline) ◇*Allergan 211; 5IUDR; IDU; SK&F 14287; NSC-39661*

Idrabiotaparinux Sodium. $C_{53}H_{79}N_4Na_9O_{51}S_8$. 2051.62. Non-asodium methyl (2-deoxy-3,4-di-*O*-methyl-2-{6-[5-(2-ox-ohexahydro-1*H*-thieno[3,4-*d*]imidazol-4-yl)pentanamido]-hexanamido}-6-*O*-sulfo-α-D-glucopyranosyl)-(1→4)-(2,3-di-*O*-methyl-β-D-glucopyranosyluronate)-(1→4)-(2,3,6-tri-*O*-sulfo-α-D-glucopyranoside)-(1→4)-(2,3-di-*O*-meth-yl-α-L-idopyranosyluronate)-(1→4)-2,3,6-tri-*O*-sulfo-α-D-glucopyranoside. *CAS-405159-59-3.* INN.

Idralfidine. $C_{11}H_{14}N_4O$. 218.26. 4,2-Cresotaldehyde 2-imida-zolin-2-ylhydrazone. *CAS-95668-38-5.* INN.

Idramantone. $C_{10}H_{14}O_2$. 166.22. 5-Hydroxy-2-adamantanone. *CAS-20098-14-0.* INN.

Idraparinux Sodium [*2004*] (eye drap′ a rin ux soe′ dee um; eye″ dra par′ in ux soe′ dee um). $C_{38}H_{55}Na_9O_{49}S_7$. 1727.18. (1) α-D-Glucopyranoside, methyl *O*-2,3,4-tri-*O*-methyl-6-*O*-sulfo-α-D-glucopyranosyl-(1→4)-*O*-2,3-di-*O*-methyl-β-D-glucopyranuronosyl-(1→4)-*O*-2,3,6-tri-*O*-sulfo-α-D-glucopyranosyl-(1→4)-*O*-2,3-di-*O*-methyl-α-L-idopyra-nuronosyl-(1→4)-,2,3,6-tris(hydrogen sulfate), nonaso-dium salt; (2) Methyl (sodium 2,3,4-tri-*O*-methyl-6-*O*-sulfonato-α-D-glucopyranosyl)-(1→4)-(sodium 2,3-di-*O*-methyl-β-D-glucopyranosylurate)-(1→4)-(trisodium 2,3,6-tri-*O*-sulfonato-α-D-glucopyranosyl)-(1→4)-(sodium -2,3-di-*O*-methyl-α-L-idopyranosyluronate)-(1→4)-(trisodium

2,3,6-tri-*O*-sulfonato-α-D-glucopyranoside). *CAS-149920-56-9.* INN. *Antithrombotic, indirect, selective, synthetic factor Xa inhibitor.* (Sanofi-Synthelabo) ◇*SANORG34006*

Idrapril. $C_{11}H_{18}N_2O_5$. 258.27. (1*S*,2*R*)-2-[[(Hydroxycarbamoyl)methyl]methylcarbamoyl]cyclohexanecarboxylic acid. *CAS-127420-24-0.* INN.

Idremcinal [*1998*] (eye drem′ si nal). $C_{39}H_{69}NO_{12}$. 743.96. (1) 8,9-Didehydro-*N*-demethyl-9-deoxo-6-deoxy-6,9-epoxy-*N*-(1-methylethyl)erthromycin; (2) 8,9-Didehydro-*N*-demethyl-9-deoxo-6-deoxy-6,9-epoxy-*N*-isopropylerythromycin. *CAS-110480-13-2.* INN. *Gastrointestinal prokinetic (motilin agonist).* ◇*EM574*

Idrobutamine — *See* Butidrine.

Idrocilamide. $C_{11}H_{13}NO_2$. 191.23. *N*-(2-Hydroxyethyl)cinnamamide. *UNII-6C816LUB1O. CAS-6961-46-2.* INN; DCF; MI.

Idronoxil [*2004*] (eye″ droe nox′ il). $C_{15}H_{12}O_3$. 240.25. (1) 2*H*-1-Benzopyran-7-ol, 3-(4-hydroxyphenyl)-; (2) 3-(4-Hydroxyphenyl)-2*H*-chromen-7-ol. *UNII-995FT1W541. CAS-81267-65-4.* INN. *Antineoplastic which acts as an*

---

† Brand name formerly used, and/or firm no longer concerned with this product.

antiproliferative, topoisomerase II inhibitor; 5α reductase inhibitor.[Note—The trivial name, phenoxodiol, has appeared in literature.] ◇*NV-06*

Idropranolol. $C_{16}H_{23}NO_2$. 261.36. 1-[(5,6-Dihydro-1-naphthyl)oxy]-3-(isopropylamino)-2-propanol. *CAS-27581-02-8.* INN; DCF.

Idursulfase [*2002*] (eye″ dur sul′ fase). $C_{2689}H_{4057}N_{699}O_{792}S_{14}$ (reduced peptide sequence). 61,880 daltons. (1) Sulfatase, L-idurono-; (2) α-L-Iduronate sulfate sulfatase. *UNII-5W8JGG2651. CAS-50936-59-9.* INN; BAN; JAN. *Treatment of Hunter Syndrome (enzyme that degrades the glycosaminoglycans heparan sulfate and dermatan sulfate).* ◇*EC 3.1.6.13*

SETQANSTTD	ALNVLLIIVD	DLRPSLGCYG	DKLVRSPNID	QLASHSLLFQ
NAFAQQAVCA	PSRVSFLTGR	RPDTTRLYDF	NSYWRVHAGN	FSTIPQYFKE
NGYVTMSVGK	VFHPGISSNH	TDDSPYSWSF	PPYHPSSEKY	ENTKTCRGPD
GELHANLLCP	VDVLDVPEGT	LPDKQSTEQA	IQLLEKMKTS	ASPFFLAVGY
HKPHIPFRYP	KEFQKLYPLE	NITLAPDPEV	PDGLPPVAYN	PWMDIRQRED
VQALNISVPY	GPIPVDFQRK	IRQSYFASVS	YLDTQVGRLL	SALDDLQLAN
STIIAFTSDH	GWALGEHGEW	AKYSNFDVAT	HVPLIFYVPG	RTASLPEAGE
KLFPYLDPFD	SASQLMEPGR	QSMDLVELVS	LFPTLAGLAG	LQVPPRCPVP
SFHVELCREG	KNLLKHFRFR	DLEEDPYLPG	NPRELIAYSQ	YPRPSDIPQW
NSDKPSLKDI	KIMGYSIRTI	DYRYTVWVGF	NPDEFLANFS	DIHAGELYFV
DSDPLQDHNM	YNDSQGGDLF	QLLMP		

Ifenprodil. $C_{21}H_{27}NO_2$. 325.44. [Ifenprodil Tartrate is JAN.] 4-Benzyl-α-(*p*-hydroxyphenyl)-β-methyl-1-piperidineethanol. *CAS-23210-56-2.* INN; DCF; MI. ◇*RC 61-91*

Iferanserin. $C_{23}H_{28}N_2O$. 348.48. (*E*)-2′-{2-[(2*S*)-1-Methyl-2-piperidyl]ethyl}cinnamanilide. *CAS-58754-46-4.* INN.

Ifetroban [*1994*] (eye fe′ troe ban). $C_{25}H_{32}N_2O_5$. 440.53. (1) Benzenepropanoic acid, 2-[[3-[4-[(pentylamino)carbonyl]-2-oxazolyl]-7-oxabicyclo[2.2.1]hept-2-yl]methyl]-, [1*S*-(*exo,exo*)]-; (2) *o*-[[1*S*,2*R*,3*S*,4*R*)-3-[4-(Pentylcarbamoyl)-

2-oxazolyl]-7-oxabicyclo[2.2.1]hept-2-yl]methyl]hydrocinnamic acid. *UNII-E833KT807K. CAS-143443-90-7.* INN. *Antithrombotic.* ◇BMS-180291

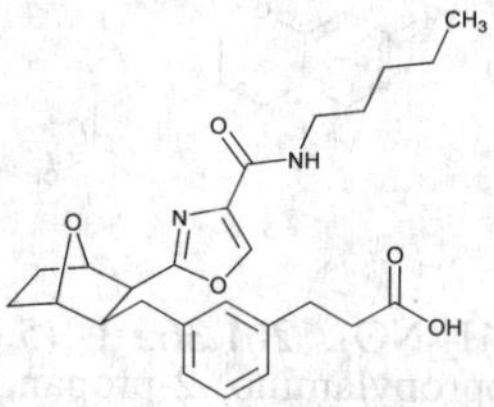

Ifetroban Sodium [*1994*] (eye fe′ troe ban soe′ dee um). $C_{25}H_{31}N_2NaO_5$. 462.51. (1) Benzenepropanoic acid, 2-[[3-[4-[(pentylamino)carbonyl]-2-oxazolyl]-7-oxabicyclo[2.2.1]hept-2-yl]methyl]-, monosodium salt, [1*S*-(*exo,exo*)]-; (2) Sodium *o*-[[(1*S*,2*R*,3*S*,4*R*)-3-[4-(pentylcarbamoyl)-2-oxazolyl]-7-oxabicyclo[2.2.1]hept-2-yl]methyl]hydrocinnamate. *UNII-48IJA0E92C. CAS-156715-37-6. Antithrombotic.* ◇BMS-180291-02

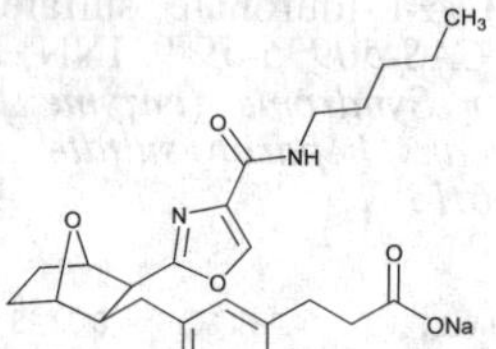

Ifosfamide [*1978*] (eye fos′ fa mide). **USP.** $C_7H_{15}Cl_2N_2O_2P$. 261.09. (1) 2*H*-1,3,2-Oxazaphosphorin-2-amine, *N*,3-bis(2-chloroethyl)tetrahydro-, 2-oxide; (2) 3-(2-Chloroethyl)-2-[(2-chloroethyl)amino]tetrahydro-2*H*-1,3,2-oxazaphosphorine 2-oxide. *UNII-UM20QQM95Y. CAS-3778-73-2.* INN; BAN; JAN. *Antineoplastic.* Ifex (Bristol-Myers Squibb) ◇MJF 9325; Z4942; NSC-109724

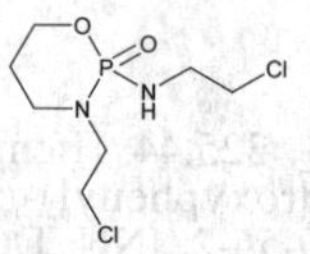

Ifoxetine. $C_{13}H_{19}NO_2$. 221.30. (±)-*cis*-4-(2,3-Xylyloxy)-3-piperidinol. *UNII-LHH887104B. CAS-66208-11-5.* INN.

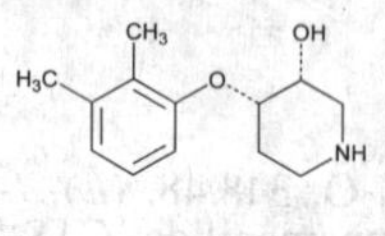

Iganidipine. $C_{28}H_{38}N_4O_6$. 526.62. (±)-3-(4-Allyl-1-piperazinyl)-2,2-dimethylpropyl methyl 1,4-dihydro-2,6-dimethyl-4-(*m*-nitrophenyl)-3,5-pyridinedicarboxylate. *UNII-9FPE98DLZ5. CAS-119687-33-1.* INN.

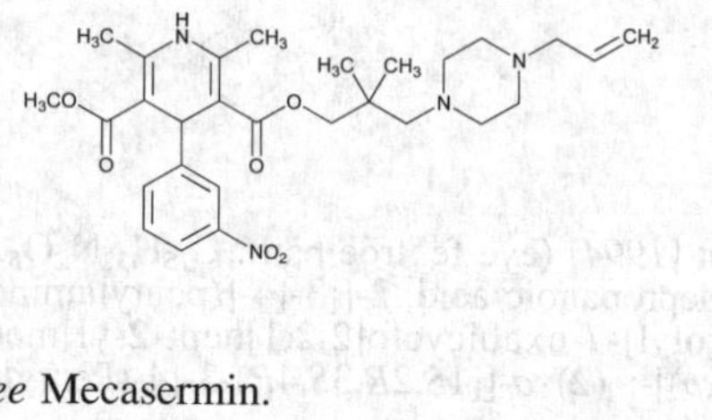

IGF-I — *See* Mecasermin.

Igmesine. $C_{23}H_{29}N$. 319.48. (+)-α-[(*E*)-Cinnamyl]-*N*-(cyclopropylmethyl)-α-ethyl-*N*-methylbenzylamine. *CAS-140850-73-3.* INN.

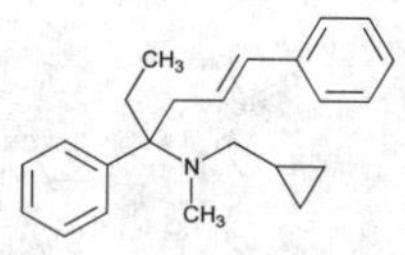

Igmesine Hydrochloride [*1997*] (ig′ mes een hye″ droe klor′ ide). $C_{23}H_{29}N \cdot HCl$. 355.94. (1) (+)-(*E*)-*N*-(Cyclopropylmethyl)-α-ethyl-*N*-methyl-α-(3-phenyl-2-propenyl)benzenemethanamine hydrochloride; (2) (+)-α-[(*E*)-Cinnamyl]-*N*-(cyclopropylmethyl)-α-ethyl-*N*-methylbenzylamine. *CAS-130152-35-1. Antidepressant (sigma receptor ligand).* ◇CI-1019; JO-1784

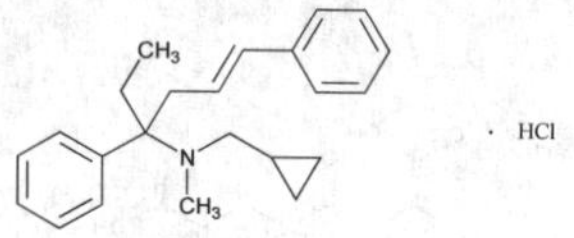

Igovomab. Immunoglobulin G1, anti-(human CA 125 (carbohydrate antigen)) F(ab′)₂ fragment (mouse monoclonal OC125F(AB′)₂ γ1-chain), disulfide with mouse monoclonal OC125F(AB′)₂ light chain, dimer. INN.

Iguratimod. $C_{17}H_{14}N_2O_6S$. 374.37. *N*-[7-[(Methylsulfonyl)amino]-4-oxo-6-phenoxy-4*H*-1-benzopyran-3-yl]formamide. *UNII-4IHY34Y2NV. CAS-123663-49-0.* INN.

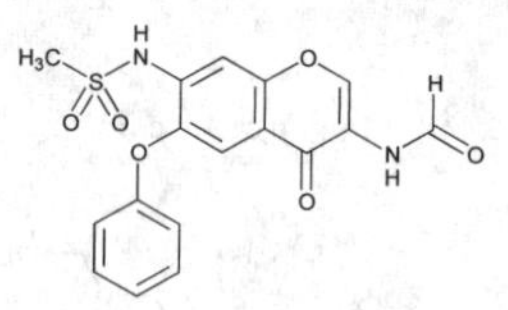

Ilaprazole. $C_{19}H_{18}N_4O_2S$. 366.44. 2-[(*RS*)-[(4-Methoxy-3-methylpyridin-2-yl)methyl]sulfinyl]-5-(1*H*-pyrrol-1-yl)-1*H*-benzimidazole. *UNII-776Q6XX45J. CAS-172152-36-2.* INN.

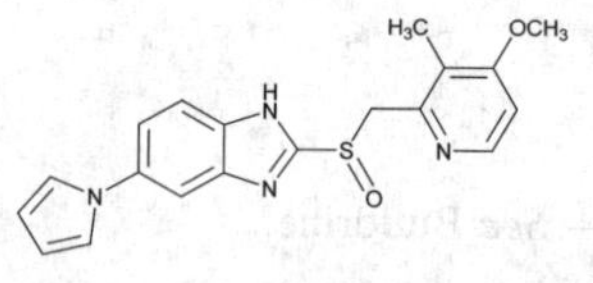

Ilatreotide. $C_{61}H_{86}N_{10}O_{20}S_2$. 1343.52. *N*-(1-Deoxy-4-*O*-α-D-glucopyranosyl-D-fructopyranos-1-yl)-D-phenylalanyl-L-cysteinyl-L-phenylalanyl-D-tryptophyl-L-lysyl-L-threonyl-*N*-[(1*R*,2*R*)-2-hydroxy-1-(hydroxymethyl)propyl]-L-cysteinamide cyclic (2→7)-disulfide. *CAS-119719-11-8.* INN.

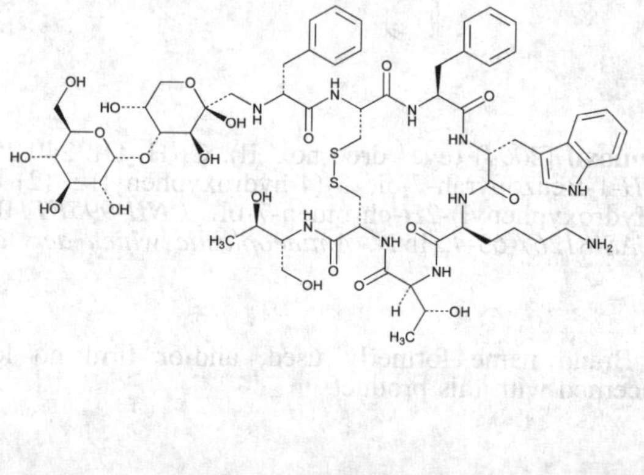

Ilepatril. $C_{22}H_{28}N_2O_5S$. 432.53. (4S,7S,12bR)-7-[(2S)-2-(Acetylsulfanyl)-3-methylbutanamido]-6-oxo-1,2,3,4,6,7,8,12b-octahydropyrido[2,1-a][2]benzazepine-4-carboxylic acid. *CAS-473289-62-2.* INN.

Ilepcimide [*1994*] (eye lep′ si mide). $C_{15}H_{17}NO_3$. 259.30. (1) Piperidine, 1-[3-(1,3-benzodioxol-5-yl)-1-oxo-2-propenyl]-, (E)-; (2) 1-[(E)-3,4-(Methylenedioxy)cinnamoyl]piperidine. *UNII-5ML58O200F. CAS-82857-82-7.* INN. *Anticonvulsant.* [*Name previously used: Antiepilepsirine.*]

Iliparcil. $C_{16}H_{18}O_6S$. 338.38. 4-Ethyl-7-[(5-thio-β-D-xylopyranosyl)oxy]coumarin. *CAS-137214-72-3.* INN.

Ilmofosine [*1990*] (il″ moe fos′ seen). $C_{26}H_{56}NO_5PS$. 525.77. (1) 3,5-Dioxa-9-thia-4-phosphapentacosan-1-aminium, 4-hydroxy-7-(methoxymethyl)-N,N,N-trimethyl-, hydroxide, inner salt, 4-oxide, (±)-; (2) Choline hydroxide, (±)-3-(hexadecylthio)-2-(methoxymethyl)propyl hydrogen phosphate, inner salt. *CAS-89315-55-9.* INN. *Antineoplastic.* ◇*BM 41.440*

Ilodecakin [*1998*] (eye″ loe dek′ a kin). Interleukin 10 (human clone pH15C). Molecular weight is approximately 18,647. *CAS-149824-15-7.* INN. *Treatment of Crohns' disease, ulcerative colitis, rheumatoid arthritis, psoriasis (immunomodulator).* Tenovil (Schering-Plough Research) ◇*SCH 52000*

```
SPGQGTQSEN   SCTHFPGNLP   NMLRDLRDAF   SRVKTFFQMK   DQLDNLLLKE
SLLEDFKGYL   GCQALSEMIQ   FYLEEVMPQA   ENQDPDIKAH   VNSLGENLKT
LRLRLRRCHR   FLPCENKSKA   VEQVKNAFNK   LQEKGIYKAM   SEFDIFINYI
EAYMTMKIRN
```

Ilomastat [*1994*] (eye loe′ ma stat). $C_{20}H_{28}N_4O_4$. 388.46. (1) [S-(R^*,S^*)]-N^4-Hydroxy-N^1-[1H-indol-3-ylmethyl)-2-(methylamino)-2-oxoethyl]-2-(2-methylpropyl)butanediamide; (2) (R)-N^1-Hydroxy-N-[(S)-2-indol-3-yl-1-(methylcarbamoyl)ethyl]-2-isobutylsuccinamide. *CAS-*

142880-36-2. INN. *Treatment of corneal ulcers, inflammatory conditions, and cancers (matrix metalloproteinase inhibitor).*

Ilonidap [*1994*] (eye lon′ i dap). $C_{14}H_8ClFN_2O_3S$. 338.74. (1) 1H-Indole-1-carboxamide, 6-chloro-5-fluoro-2,3-dihydro-3-(hydroxy-2-thienylmethylene)-2-oxo-, (Z)-; (2) 6-Chloro-5-fluoro-3-[(Z)-α-hydroxy-2-thienylidene]-2-oxo-1-indolinecarboxamide. *CAS-135202-79-8.* INN. *Anti-inflammatory.* ◇*CP-72,133*

Iloperidone [*1993*] (eye″ loe per′ i done). $C_{24}H_{27}FN_2O_4$. 426.48. (1) Ethanone, 1-[4-[3-[4-(6-fluoro-1,2-benzisoxazol-3-yl)-1-piperidinyl]propoxy]-3-methoxyphenyl]-; (2) 4′-[3-[4-(6-Fluoro-1,2-benzisoxazol-3-yl)piperidino]propoxy]-3′-methoxyacetophenone. *CAS-133454-47-4.* INN; BAN. *Antipsychotic.* ◇*HP 873*

Iloprost [*2004*] (eye′ loe prost). $C_{22}H_{32}O_4$. 360.49. (1) Pentanoic acid, 5-[(3aS,4R,5R,6aS)-hexahydro-5-hydroxy-4-[(1E,3S)-3-hydroxy-4-methyl-1-octen-6-ynyl]-2(1H)-pentalenylidene]-, (5E)-; (2) (5E)-[3aS,4R,5R,6aS)-5-Hydroxy-4-[(1E)-(3S,4RS)-3-hydroxy-4-methyloct-1-en-6-ynyl]-hexahydropentalen-2(1H)-ylidene]pentanoic acid. *UNII-JED5K35YGL. CAS-78919-13-8; CAS-73873-87-7[replaced].* INN; BAN. *Treatment of pulmonary hypertension (prostacyclin analogue).* Ventavis (Actelion) ◇*ZK 00036374*

Imafen Hydrochloride [*1976*] (im′ a fen hye″ droe klor′ ide). $C_{11}H_{13}N_3$·HCl. 223.70. [*Imafen is INN.*] (1) 1H-Imidazo[1,2-a]imidazole, 2,3,5,6-tetrahydro-5-(or-3-)-phenyl-, monohydrochloride; (2) 2,3,5,6-Tetrahydro-5-(or-3-)-phenyl-1H-imidazo[1,2-a]imidazole monohydrochloride.

---

† Brand name formerly used, and/or firm no longer concerned with this product.

UNII-W0X9P59ZQU; UNII-43S5D07K8G [imafen]. *CAS-53361-24-3; CAS-59198-18-4* [imafen]. *Antidepressant.* ◇*R 25,540*

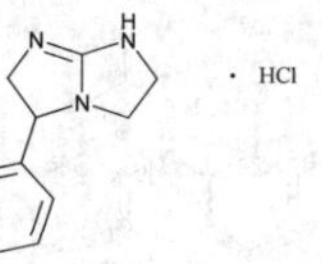

Imanixil. $C_{17}H_{17}F_3N_6O_2$. 394.35. 4-Amino-2-(4,4-dimethyl-2-oxo-1-imidazolidinyl)-α,α,α-trifluoro-5-pyrimidinecarboxy-*m*-toluidide. *UNII-8892KM4U61. CAS-75689-93-9.* INN.

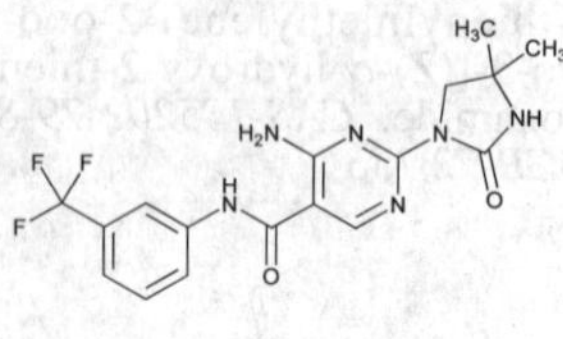

Imatinib. $C_{29}H_{31}N_7O$. 493.60. α-(4-Methyl-1-piperazinyl)-3′-[[4-(3-pyridyl)-2-pyrimidinyl]amino]-*p*-tolu-*p*-toluidide. *UNII-BKJ8M8G5HI. CAS-152459-95-5.* INN; BAN.

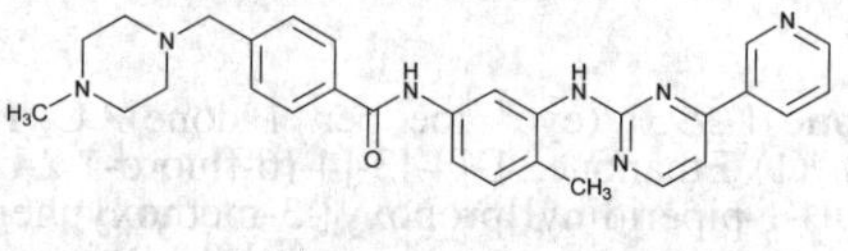

Imazodan Hydrochloride [*1986*] (im az′ oh dan hye″ droe klor′ ide). $C_{13}H_{12}N_4O \cdot HCl$. 276.72. [Imazodan is INN.] (1) 3(2*H*)-Pyridazinone, 4,5-dihydro-6-[4-(1*H*-imidazol-1-yl)-phenyl]-, monohydrochloride; (2) 4,5-Dihydro-6-(*p*-imidazol-1-ylphenyl)-3(2*H*)-pyridazinone monohydrochloride. *UNII-5EP74J9Q34. CAS-89198-09-4; CAS-84243-58-3* [imazodan]. *Cardiotonic.* ◇*CI-914*

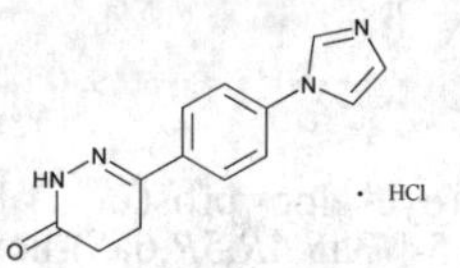

Imcarbofos [*1980*] (im karb′ oh fos). $C_{17}H_{30}N_4O_7P_2S_2$. 528.52. (1) Phosphoramidic acid, [(2-methoxy-1,4-phenylene)-bis(iminocarbonothioyl)]bis-, tetraethyl ester; (2) Tetraethyl [(2-methoxy-*p*-phenylene)bis[imino(thiocarbonyl)]]diphosphoramidate. *UNII-21H450VP7K. CAS-66608-32-0.* INN. *Anthelmintic (veterinary).* ◇*CL 217,658*

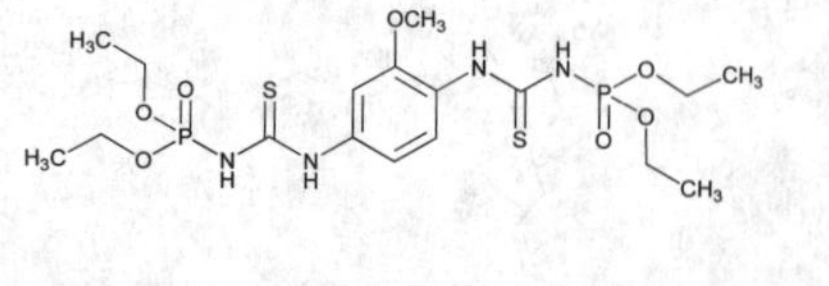

Imciromab Pentetate [*1993*] (im sir′ oh mab pen′ te tate). [Imciromab is INN.] (1) Immunoglobulin G 2a (mouse monoclonal R11D10 cell Fab fragment anti-human cardiac myosin heavy chain), disulfide with mouse monoclonal R11D10 cell κ-chain, *N*,*N*-bis[2-[bis(carboxymethyl)amino]ethyl]glycine conjugate; (2) Immunoglobulin G 2a (mouse monoclonal R11D10 cell Fab fragment anti-human cardiac myosin heavy chain), disulfide with mouse monoclonal R11D10 cell κ-chain, *N*,*N*-bis[2-[bis(carboxymethyl)amino]ethyl]glycine conjugate. Molecular weight is approximately 50,000 daltons. *CAS-138660-99-8; CAS-138661-00-4* [indium In 111 imciromab pentetate]. BAN. *Monoclonal antibody (antimyosin).* Myoscint (Centocor) [*Note—The radiolabeled product used as a cardiac imaging agent has the nonproprietary name indium In 111 imciromab pentetate.*] ◇*C-4*

Imeglimin. $C_6H_{13}N_5$. 155.20. (4*R*)-6-(Dimethylamino)-4-methyl-4,5-dihydro-1,3,5-triazin-2-amine. *CAS-775351-65-0.* INN.

Imepition. $C_{13}H_{14}ClN_3O_2$. 279.72. 1-(4-Chlorophenyl)-4-(morpholin-4-yl)-1,5-dihydro-2*H*-imidazol-2-one. *CAS-188116-07-6.* INN.

Imexon [*2005*] (eye mex′ on). $C_4H_5N_3O$. 111.10. (1) 1,3-Diazabicyclo[3.1.0]hex-3-en-2-one, 4-amino-; (2) (5*RS*)-4-Amino-1,3-diazabicyclo[3.1.0]hex-3-en-2-one. *UNII-8F63U28T2V. CAS-59643-91-3.* INN. *Cancer chemotherapy.* Amplimexon (Amplimed)

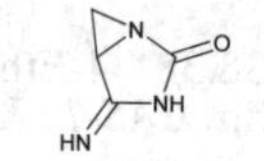

Imiclopazine. $C_{25}H_{32}ClN_5OS$. 486.07. 1-[2-[4-[3-(2-Chlorophenothiazin-10-yl)propyl]-1-piperazinyl]ethyl]-3-methyl-2-imidazolidinone. *UNII-WGL8B3MDAS. CAS-7224-08-0.* INN; MI.

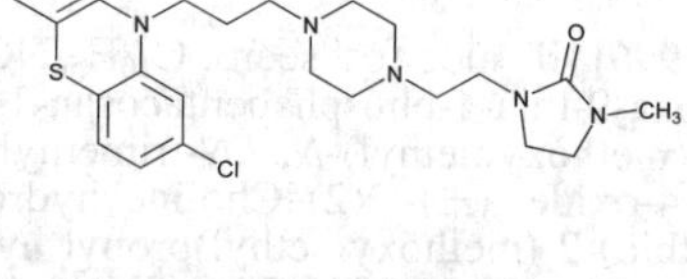

Imidafenacin. $C_{20}H_{21}N_3O$. 319.40. 4-(2-Methyl-1*H*-imidazol-1-yl)-2,2-diphenylbutanamide. *CAS-170105-16-5.* INN.

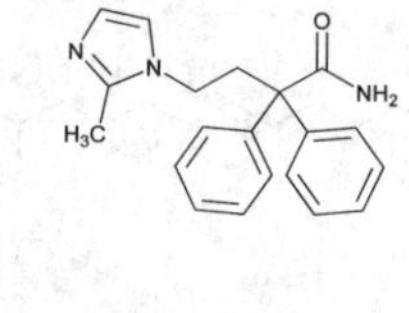

Imidapril. $C_{20}H_{27}N_3O_6$. 405.44. [Imidapril Hydrochloride is JAN.] (*S*)-3-(*N*-[(*S*)-1-Ethoxycarbonyl-3-phenylpropyl]-L-alanyl)-1-methyl-2-oxoimidazoline-4-carboxylic acid. *UNII-BW7H1TJS22. CAS-89371-37-9; CAS-89396-94-1* [hydrochloride]. INN; BAN.

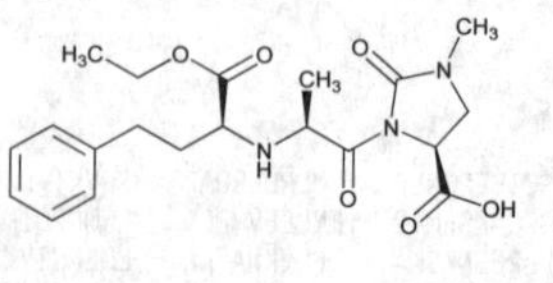

Imidaprilat. $C_{18}H_{23}N_3O_6$. 377.39. (4*S*)-3-[(2*S*)-*N*-[(1*S*)-1-Carboxy-3-phenylpropyl]alanyl]-1-methyl-2-oxo-4-imidazolidinecarboxylic acid. *UNII-WUU07Y30IA. CAS-89371-44-8.* INN; BAN. ◇*6366A*

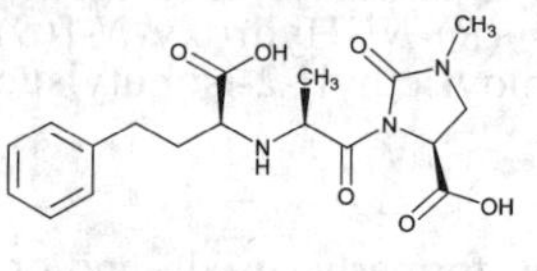

Imidazole Salicylate. $C_{10}H_{10}N_2O_3$. 206.20. Salicylic acid, compound with imidazole (1:1). *UNII-4JVD4X01MJ. CAS-36364-49-5.* INN; MI.

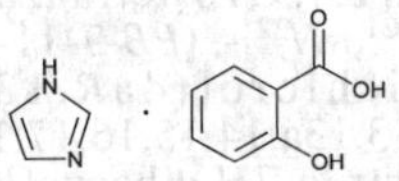

Imidecyl Iodine [*1964*] (im i′ de sil eye″ oh dine). Complex consisting of: 2-alkyl-(C_7H_{15} to $C_{17}H_{35}$)-1-(carboxymethyl)-1-(2-hydroxyethyl)-2-imidazolinium chloride; 3,6,9,12,15,18,21,24,27,30,33,36,39-tridecaoxadopentacontan-1-ol; and iodine. (1) Imidecyl iodine; (2) Imidecyl iodine. *CAS-1336-78-3. Anti-infective, topical.*

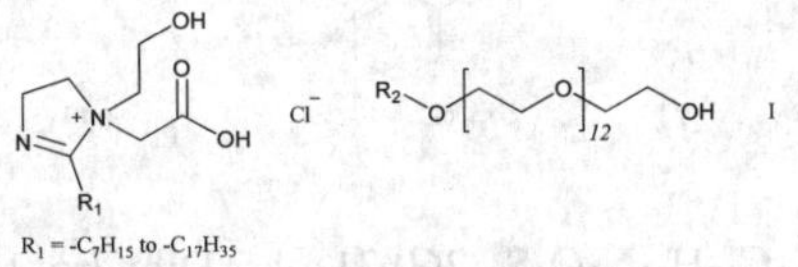

Imidocarb Hydrochloride [*1970*] (im i′ doe karb hye″ droe klor′ ide). $C_{19}H_{20}N_6O.2HCl$. 421.32. [Imidocarb is INN and BAN.] (1) Urea, *N,N′*-bis[3-(4,5-dihydro-1*H*-imidazol-2-yl)phenyl]-, dihydrochloride; (2) 3,3′-Di-2-imidazolin-2-ylcarbanilide dihydrochloride. *UNII-KCC1V76AH8. CAS-5318-76-3; CAS-27885-92-3* [imidocarb]. *Antiprotozoal (Babesia).* ◇*4A65*

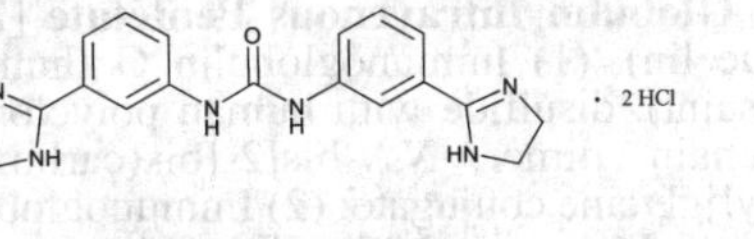

Imidoline Hydrochloride [*1965*] (im id′ oh leen hye″ droe klor′ ide). $C_{13}H_{18}ClN_3O.HCl$. 304.22. [Imidoline is INN.] (1) 2-Imidazolidinone, 1-(3-chlorophenyl)-3-[2-(dimethylamino)ethyl]-, monohydrochloride; (2) 1-(*m*-Chlorophenyl)-3-[2-(dimethylamino)ethyl]-2-imidazolidinone monohydrochloride. *CAS-5588-31-8; CAS-7303-78-8* [imidoline]. *Antipsychotic.* ◇*CL 48156*

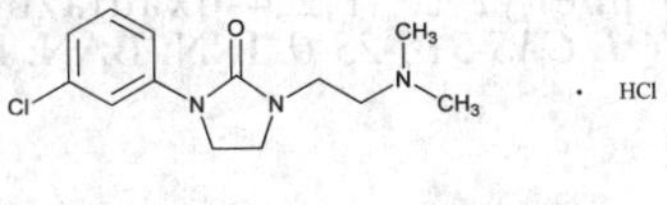

Imidurea (im id″ ue ree′ a; im id″ ure ee′ a). **NF.** $C_{11}H_{16}N_8O_8$. 388.29. (1) *N,N″*-Methylenebis[*N′*-[3-(hydroxymethyl)-2,5-dioxo-4-imidazolidinyl]urea]; (2) 1,1′-Methylenebis[3-[3-(hydroxymethyl)-2,5-dioxo-4-imidazolidinyl]urea]. *UNII-M629807ATL. CAS-39236-46-9. Antimicrobial.*

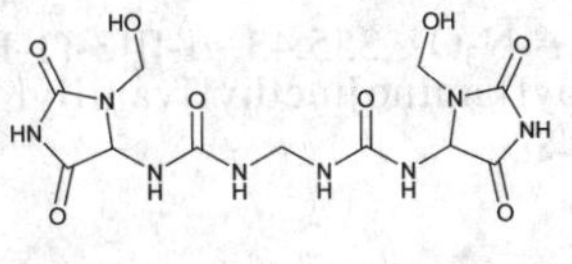

Imiglitazar. $C_{28}H_{26}N_2O_5$. 470.52. (*E*)-4-[({4-[(5-Methyl-2-phenyl-1,3-oxazol-4-yl)methoxy]phenyl}methoxy)imino]-4-phenylbutanoic acid. *CAS-250601-04-8.* INN.

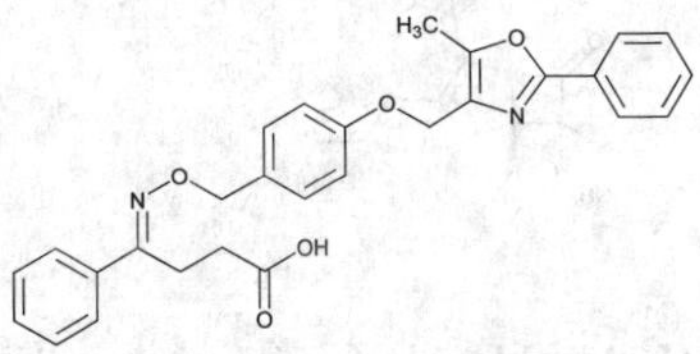

Imiglucerase [*1995*] (im″ i gloo′ ser ase). $C_{2532}H_{3843}N_{671}$ $O_{711}S_{16}$. 60,430 (determined by mass spectroscopy). 495-L-Histidineglucosylceramidase (human placenta isoenzyme protein moiety). *UNII-Q6U6J48BWY. CAS-154248-97-2.* INN; BAN. *Enzyme replenisher (glucocerebrosidase).* Cerezyme (Genzyme)

```
ARPCIPKSFG YSSVVCVCNA TYCDSFDPPT FPALGTFSRY ESTRSGRRME
LSMGPIQANH TGTGLLLTLQ PEQKFQKVKG FGGAMTDAAA LNILALSPPA
QNLLLKSYFS EEGIGYNIIR VPMASCDFSI RTYTYADTPD DFQLHNFSLP
EEDTKLKIPL IHRALQLAQR PVSLLASPWT SPTWLKTNGA VNGKGSLKGQ
PGDIYHQTWA RYFVKFLDAY AEHKLQFWAV TAENEPSAGL LSGYPFQCLG
FTPEHQRDFI ARDLGPTLAN STHHNVRLLM LDDQRLLLPH WAKVVLTDPE
AAKYVHGIAV HWYLDFLAPA KATLGETHRL FPNTMLFASE ACVGSKFWEQ
SVRLGSWDRG MQYSHSIITN LLYHVVGWTD WNLALNPEGG PNWVRNFVDS
PIIVDITKDT FYKQPMFYHL GHFSKFIPEG SQRVGLVASQ KNDLDAVALM
HPDGSAVVVV LNRSSKDVPL TIKDPAVGFL ETISPGYSIH TYLWHRQ
```

Imiloxan Hydrochloride [*1984*] (im″ i lox′ an hye″ droe klor′ ide). $C_{14}H_{16}N_2O_2.HCl$. 280.75. [Imiloxan is INN.] (1) 1*H*-Imidazole- 2-[(2,3-dihydro-1,4-benzodioxin-2-yl)methyl]-1-ethyl-, monohydrochloride, (±)-; (2) (±)-2-(1,4-Benzodioxan-2-ylmethyl)-1-ethylimidazole monohydrochloride; (3) (±)-2-[(1-Ethyl-2-imidazolyl)methyl]-1,4-benzodioxane hydrochloride. *CAS-86710-23-8; CAS-81167-16-0* [imiloxan]. *Antidepressant.* ◇*RS-21361*

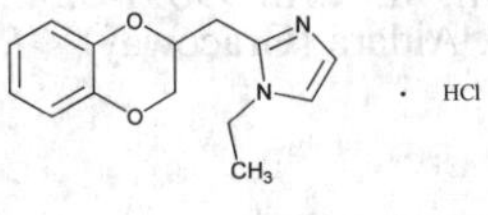

Iminophenimide. $C_{12}H_{14}N_2O_2$. 218.25. 3-Ethyl-3-phenylpiperazine-2,6-dione. *CAS-7008-18-6.* INN.

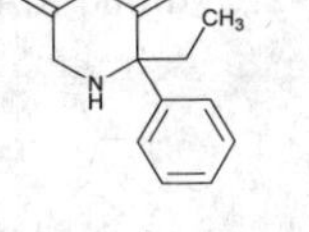

Imipemide (previously used name) — *See* Imipenem.

Imipenem [*1983*] (im″ i pen′ em). **USP.** $C_{12}H_{17}N_3O_4S.H_2O$. 317.36. (1) 1-Azabicyclo[3.2.0]hept-2-ene-2-carboxylic acid, 6-(1-hydroxyethyl)-3-[[2-[(iminomethyl)amino]ethyl]thio]-7-oxo-, monohydrate, [5*R*-[5α,6α(*R**)]]-; (2) (5*R*,6*S*)-3-[[2-(Formimidoylamino)ethyl]thio]-6-[(*R*)-1-hydroxyethyl]-7-oxo-1-azabicyclo[3.2.0]hept-2-ene-2-carboxylic acid monohydrate. *UNII-71OTZ9ZE0A. CAS-*

---

† Brand name formerly used, and/or firm no longer concerned with this product.

74431-23-5; CAS-64221-86-9 [anhydrous]. INN; BAN; JAN. *Antibacterial. [Name previously used: Imipemide.]* ◇*MK-0787*

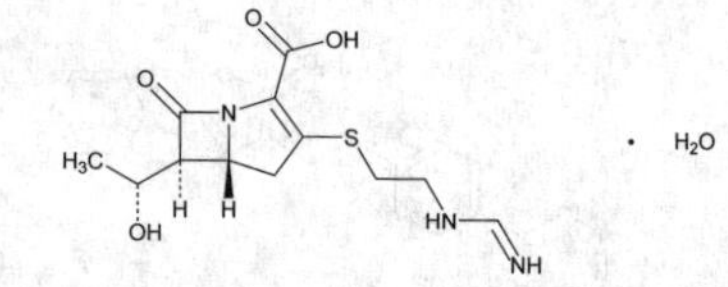

Imipramine Hydrochloride (im ip′ ra meen hye″ droe klor′ ide). **USP.** $C_{19}H_{24}N_2 \cdot HCl$. 316.87. [Imipramine is INN and BAN.] (1) 5*H*-Dibenz[*b,f*]azepine-5-propanamine, 10,11-dihydro-*N,N*-dimethyl-, monohydrochloride; (2) 5-[3-(Dimethylamino)propyl]-10,11-dihydro-5*H*-dibenz[*b,f*]azepine monohydrochloride. *UNII-BKE5Q1J60U; UNII-OGG85SX4E4* [imipramine]. *CAS-113-52-0; CAS-50-49-7* [imipramine]. JAN. *Antidepressant.* Tofranil (Tyco)

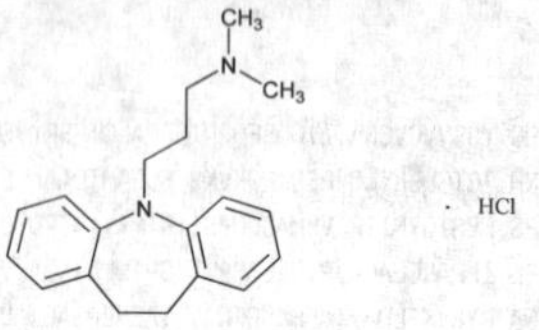

Imipraminoxide. $C_{19}H_{24}N_2O$. 296.41. 5-[3-(Dimethylamino)-propyl]-10,11-dihydro-5*H*-dibenz[*b,f*]azepine *N*-oxide. *UNII-8MKS280XJW. CAS-6829-98-7.* INN.

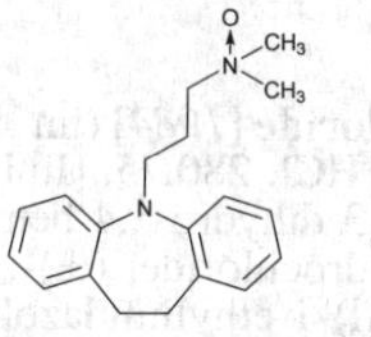

Imiquimod [*1991*] (im i′ kwi mod). $C_{14}H_{16}N_4$. 240.30. (1) 1*H*-Imidazo[4,5-*c*]quinolin-4-amine, 1-(2-methylpropyl)-; (2) 4-Amino-1-isobutyl-1*H*-imidazo[4,5-*c*]quinoline. *UNII-P1QW714R7M. CAS-99011-02-6.* INN; BAN. *Immunomodulator.* Aldara (Graceway) ◇*R-837; S26308*

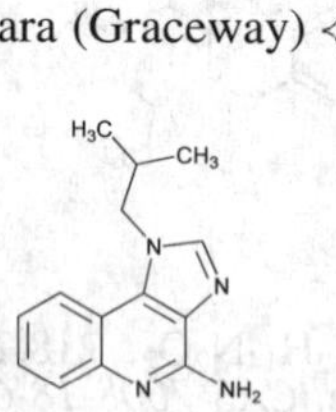

Imirestat. $C_{15}H_8F_2N_2O_2$. 286.23. 2,7-Difluorospiro[fluorene-9,4′-imidazolidine]-2′,5′-dione. *CAS-89391-50-4.* INN.

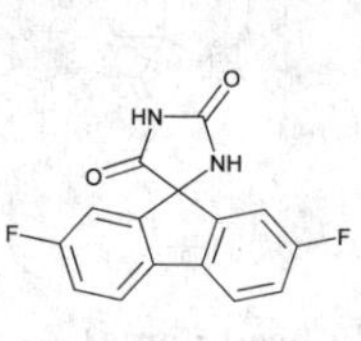

Imisopasem Manganese [*2005*] (im″ i soe′ pa sem man′ ga nees). $C_{21}H_{35}Cl_2MnN_5$. 483.38. (1) Manganese, dichloro[(4a*R*,13a*R*,17a*R*,21a*R*)-1,2,3,4,4a,5,6,12,13,13a,14,15,16,17,17a,18,19,20,21,21a-eicosahydro-11,7-nitrilo-7*H*-dibenzo[*b,h*][1,4,7,10]tetraazacycloheptadecine-$\kappa N^5,\kappa N^{13},\kappa N^{18},\kappa N^{21},\kappa N^{22}$]-, (*PB-7-11-2344′3′*)-; (2) (*PB-7-11-2344′3′*)-Dichloro[(4a*R*,13a*R*,17a*R*,21a*R*)-1,2,3,4,4a,5,6,12,13,13a,14,15,16,17,17a,18,19,20,21,21a-icosahydro-11,7-nitrilo-7*H*-dibenzo[*b,h*][1,4,7,10]tetraaz-acycloheptadecine-$\kappa N^5,\kappa N^{13},\kappa N^{18},\kappa N^{21},\kappa N^{22}$]-manganese. *CAS-218791-21-0.* INN. *Relief of pain and inflammation.* ◇*M40403; 403; SC-72325*

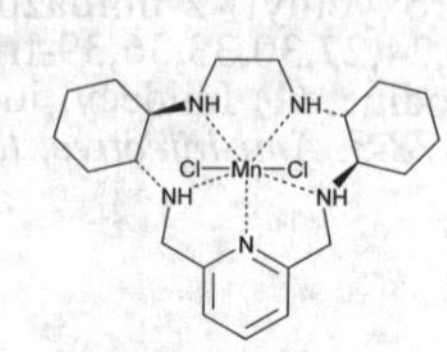

Imitrodast. $C_{13}H_{12}N_2O_2S$. 260.31. 4,5-Dihydro-2-(imidazol-1-ylmethyl)benzo[*b*]thiophene-6-carboxylic acid. *UNII-JCQ5G1KFHN. CAS-114686-12-3.* INN.

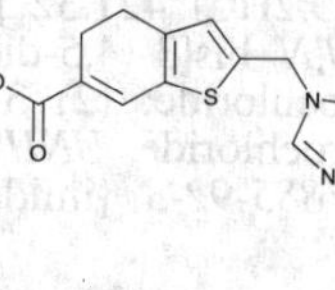

Immune Globulin Intravenous Pentetate [*1996*] (i mune′ glob′ ue lin). (1) Immunoglobulin G (human polyclonal Macroscint), disulfide with human polyclonal Macroscint light chain, dimer, *N,N*-bis[2-[bis(carboxymethyl)amino]ethyl]glycine conjugate; (2) Immunoglobulin G (human polyclonal Macroscint), disulfide with human polyclonal Macroscint light chain, dimer, *N,N*-bis[2-[bis(carboxy-methyl)amino]ethyl]glycine conjugate. *CAS-145464-27-3. Diagnostic aid.* Macroscint (Johnson & Johnson) *[Note—To be utilized as a radiodiagnostic imaging agent when labeled with Indium In 111 for the detection of focal sites of inflammation or infection.]* ◇*RWJ 28299*

Imolamine. $C_{14}H_{20}N_4O$. 260.33. 4-[2-(Diethylamino)ethyl]-5-imino-3-phenyl-Δ^2-1,2,4-oxadiazoline. *UNII-K5F4RU5VQJ. CAS-318-23-0.* INN; BAN; DCF; MI.

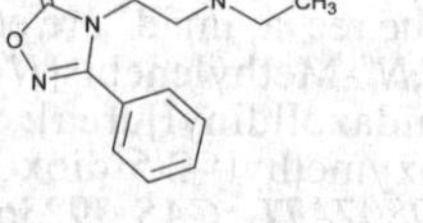

Imoxiterol. $C_{20}H_{25}N_3O_3$. 355.43. α-[[[3-(1-Benzimidazolyl)-1-methylpropyl]amino]methyl]vanillyl alcohol. *CAS-88578-07-8.* INN.

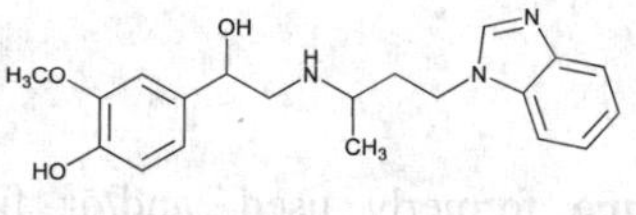

Impacarzine. $C_{28}H_{55}N_5O_2$. 493.77. *N,N*-Diethyl-4-[2-(2-oxo-3-tetradecyl-1-imidazolidinyl)ethyl]-1-piperazinecarboxamide. *UNII-25G65PH99M. CAS-41340-39-0.* INN.

IMPE — *See* Etipirium Iodide.

Implitapide. $C_{35}H_{37}N_3O_2$. 531.69. (αS)-α-[α-(2,4-Dimethyl-9*H*-pyrido[2,3-*b*]indol-9-yl)-*p*-tolyl]-*N*-[(αR)-α-(hydroxymethyl)benzyl]cyclopentaneacetamide. *UNII-Q70OH404HR. CAS-177469-96-4.* INN.

Impromidine Hydrochloride [*1979*] (im proe′ mi deen hye″ droe klor′ ide). $C_{14}H_{23}N_7S.3HCl$. 430.83. [Impromidine is INN and BAN.] (1) Guanidine, *N*-[3-(1*H*-imidazol-4-yl)propyl]-*N*′-[2-[[(5-methyl-1*H*-imidazol-4-yl)-methyl]thio]ethyl]-, trihydrochloride; (2) 1-(3-Imidazol-4-ylpropyl)-3-[2-[[(5-methylimidazol-4-yl)-methyl]thio]ethyl]guanidine trihydrochloride. *UNII-E57WP5Y41J; UNII-931L4X5WMM* [impromidine]. *CAS-65573-02-6; CAS-55273-05-7* [impromidine]. *Diagnostic aid (gastric secretion indicator).* ◇SK&F 92676-A₃

Improsulfan. $C_8H_{19}NO_6S_2$. 289.37. [Improsulfan Tosilate is JAN.] 3,3′-Iminodi-1-propanol dimethanesulfonate (ester). *CAS-13425-98-4.* INN; MI.

Imuracetam. $C_{11}H_{18}N_4O_3$. 254.29. 1,3-Bis[(2-oxo-1-pyrrolidinyl)methyl]urea. *UNII-972FNV35ZM. CAS-67542-41-0.* INN.

¹¹¹In — *See* Imciromab Pentetate.

¹¹¹In — *See* Immune Globulin Intravenous Pentetate.

¹¹¹In — *See* Indium In 111 Altumomab Pentetate.

¹¹¹In — *See* Indium In 111 Chloride.

¹¹¹In — *See* Indium In 111 Oxyquinoline.

¹¹¹In — *See* Indium In 111 Pentetreotide.

¹¹¹In — *See* Indium In 111 Satumomab Pendetide.

¹¹¹In — *See* Pentetate Indium Disodium In 111.

¹¹³ᵐIn — *See* Indium Chlorides In 113m.

Inakalant. $C_{23}H_{34}N_4O_5$. 446.54. *tert*-Butyl (2-{7-[(2*S*)-3-(4-cyanophenoxy)-2-hydroxypropyl]-9-oxa-3,7-diazabicyclo[3.3.1]nonan-3-yl}ethyl)carbamate. *CAS-335619-18-6.* INN.

Inalimarev (CEA, MUC-1, Vaccinia virus) [*2005*] (in″ a lim′ a rev vax in′ ee a). PANVAC-V. The genome size is approximately 290,000 ± 50,000. *CAS-685563-13-7.* *Treatment of pancreatic cancer, CEA-bearing tumors.* Panvac (Therion Biologics)

Inamrinone [*1999*] (eye nam′ ri none). **USP.** $C_{10}H_9N_3O$. 187.20. [Amrinone is INN, BAN, and JAN.] (1) [3,4′-Bipyridin]-6(1*H*)-one, 5-amino-; (2) 5-Amino[3,4′-bipyridin]-6(1*H*)-one. *UNII-JUT23379TN. CAS-60719-84-8.* *Cardiotonic.* Inocor (Sterling Winthrop) [*Name previously used: Amrinone.*] ◇Win 40680

Inaperisone. $C_{16}H_{23}NO$. 245.36. ($\pm$)-4′-Ethyl-2-methyl-3-(1-pyrrolidinyl)propiophenone. *UNII-0QAC3P785O. CAS-99323-21-4.* INN.

Incadronic Acid. $C_8H_{19}NO_6P_2$. 287.19. [(Cycloheptylamino)-methylene]diphosphonic acid *UNII-G5C4M8847E. CAS-124351-85-5.* INN.

Incyclinide [*2005*] (in sye′ kli nide). $C_{19}H_{17}NO_7$. 371.34. (1) 2-Naphthacenecarboxamide, 1,4,4a,5,5a,6,11,12a-octahydro-3,10,12,12a-tetrahydroxy-1,11-dioxo-, (4a*S*,5a*R*,12a*S*)-; (2) (4a*S*,5a*R*,12a*S*)-3,10,12,12a-Tetrahydroxy-1,11-dioxo-1,4,4a,5,5a,6,11,12a-octahydrotetracene-2-carboxamide. *UNII-21G64WZQ4I. CAS-15866-90-7.* INN. *Treatment of acne, rosacea, and acute respiratory distress syndrome.* Metastat (CollaGenex) ◇COL-3

Indacaterol [*2008*] (in″ da ka′ ter ol). $C_{24}H_{28}N_2O_3$. 392.49. (1) 2(1*H*)-Quinolinone, 5-[(1*R*)-2-[(5,6-diethyl-2,3-dihydro-1*H*-inden-2-yl)amino]-1-hydroxyethyl]-8-hydroxy-; (2) 5-{(1*R*)-2-[(5,6-Diethyl-2,3-dihydro-1*H*-inden-2-yl)a-

<hr>

mino]-1-hydroxyethyl}-8-hydroxyquinolin-2(1*H*)-one. *UNII-8OR09251MQ. CAS-312753-06-3.* INN. *Treatment of COPD.* ◇*QAB149*

Indacaterol Maleate [*2008*] (in″ da ka′ ter ol mal′ ee ate). C₂₄H₂₈N₂O₃.C₄H₄O₄. 508.56. (1) 2(1*H*)-Quinolinone, 5-[(1*R*)-2-[(5,6-diethyl-2,3-dihydro-1*H*-inden-2-yl)amino]-1-hydroxyethyl]-8-hydroxy-, (2*Z*)-2-butenedioate (1:1); (2) 5-{(1*R*)-2-[(5,6-Diethyl-2,3-dihydro-1*H*-inden-2-yl)ami-no]-1-hydroxyethyl}-8-hydroxyquinolin-2(1*H*)-one hydrogen (2*Z*)-2-butenedioate (salt). *UNII-2JEC1ITX7R. CAS-753498-25-8. Treatment of COPD.* ◇*QAB149-AFA*

Indacrinic Acid — *See* Indacrinone.

Indacrinone [*1979*] (in dak′ ri none). C₁₈H₁₄Cl₂O₄. 365.21. (1) Acetic acid, [(6,7-dichloro-2,3-dihydro-2-methyl-1-oxo-2-phenyl-1*H*-inden-5-yl)oxy]-, (±)-; (2) (±)-[(6,7-Dichloro-2-methyl-1-oxo-2-phenyl-5-indanyl)oxy]acetic acid. *UNII-B926Y9U4QN. CAS-57296-63-6.* INN. *Antihypertensive; diuretic.* ◇*MK-196*

Indalpine. C₁₅H₂₀N₂. 228.33. 3-[2-(4-Piperidyl)ethyl]indole. *CAS-63758-79-2.* INN; BAN; MI.

Indanazoline. C₁₂H₁₅N₃. 201.27. 2-(4-Indanylamino)-2-imidazoline. *UNII-L0U38EHD86. CAS-40507-78-6.* INN; MI.

Indanidine. C₁₁H₁₃N₅. 215.25. 4-(2-Imidazolin-2-ylamino)-2-methyl-2*H*-indazole. *UNII-MP564IFE34. CAS-85392-79-6.* INN.

Indanorex. C₁₂H₁₇NO. 191.27. 2-(1-Aminopropyl)-2-indanol. *CAS-16112-96-2.* INN.

Indantadol. C₁₁H₁₄N₂O. 190.24. 2-[(2,3-Dihydro-1*H*-inden-2-yl)amino]acetamide. *CAS-202844-10-8.* INN.

Indapamide [*1979*] (in dap′ a mide). **USP.** C₁₆H₁₆ClN₃O₃S. 365.83. (1) Benzamide, 3-(aminosulfonyl)-4-chloro-*N*-(2,3-dihydro-2-methyl-1*H*-indol-1-yl)-; (2) 4-Chloro-*N*-(2-methyl-1-indolinyl)-3-sulfamoylbenzamide. *UNII-F08910511L. CAS-26807-65-8.* INN; BAN; JAN. *Antihypertensive; diuretic.* Lozol (Sanofi Aventis)

Indatraline. C₁₆H₁₅Cl₂N. 292.20. (±)-*trans*-3-(3,4-Dichloro-phenyl)-*N*-methyl-1-indanamine. *CAS-86939-10-8.* INN.

Indecainide Hydrochloride [*1983*] (in dek′ a nide hye″ droe klor′ ide). C₂₀H₂₄N₂O.HCl. 344.88. [Indecainide is INN.] (1) 9*H*-Fluorene-9-carboxamide, 9-[3-[(1-methylethyl)amino]propyl]-, monohydrochloride; (2) 9-[3-(Isopropyl-amino)propyl]fluorene-9-carboxamide monohydrochloride. *UNII-M76V0B96L5; UNII-3AZF20DM1T* [indecainide]. *CAS-73681-12-6; CAS-74517-78-5* [indecainide]. *Cardiac depressant (anti-arrhythmic).* Decabid (Lilly) ◇*LY 135837*

Indeglitazar [*2008*] (in″ de gli′ ta zar). C₁₉H₁₉NO₆S. 389.42. (1) 1*H*-Indole-3-propanoic acid, 5-methoxy-1-[(4-methox-yphenyl)sulfonyl]-; (2) 3-{5-Methoxy-1-[(4-methoxyphe-nyl)sulfonyl]-1*H*-indol-3-yl}propanoic acid. *CAS-835619-41-5. Treatment of type II diabetes.* ◇*PPM-204*

Indeloxazine Hydrochloride [*1981*] (in″ del ox′ a zeen hye″ droe klor′ ide). C₁₄H₁₇NO₂.HCl. 267.75. [Indeloxazine is INN.] (1) Morpholine, 2-[(1*H*-inden-7-yloxy)methyl]-, hydrochloride, (±)-; (2) (±)-2-[(Inden-7-yloxy)methyl]-morpholine hydrochloride. *UNII-15QZ6NE84E. CAS-65043-22-3.* JAN. *Antidepressant.* ◇*CI-874*

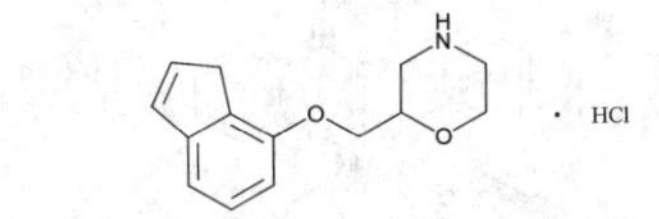

Indenolol. C$_{15}$H$_{21}$NO$_2$. 247.33. [Indenolol Hydrochloride is JAN.] 1-[Inden-4(*or* 7)-yloxy]-3-(isopropylamino)-2-propanol. *CAS-60607-68-3.* INN; BAN; MI. ◇*Sch 28316Z*

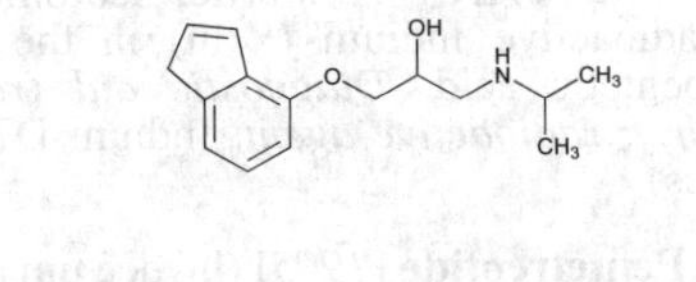

Indibulin [*2007*] (in″ di bue′ lin). C$_{22}$H$_{16}$ClN$_3$O$_2$. 389.83. (1) 1*H*-Indole-3-acetamide, 1-[(4-chlorophenyl)methyl]-α-oxo-*N*-4-pyridinyl-; (2) 2-{1-[(4-Chlorophenyl)methyl]-1*H*-indol-3-yl}-2-oxo-*N*-(pyridin-4-yl)acetamide. *UNII-80K4H2RB8P. CAS-204205-90-3.* INN. *Treatment of cancer.* ◇*ZIO-301; D-24851*

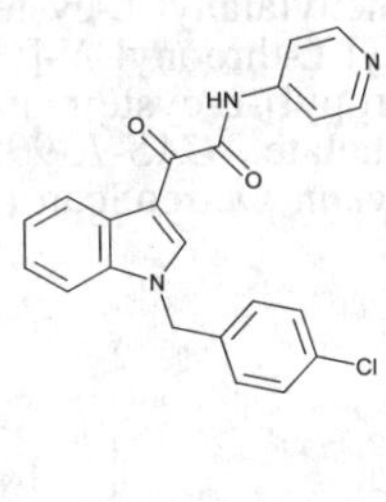

Indigocarmine (JAN) — *See* Indigotindisulfonate Sodium.

Indigotindisulfonate Sodium (in″ di goe″ tin dye sul′ foe nate soe′ dee um). **USP.** C$_{16}$H$_8$N$_2$Na$_2$O$_8$S$_2$. 466.35. [Indigocarmine is JAN.] (1) 1*H*-Indole-5-sulfonic acid, 2-(1,3-dihydro-3-oxo-5-sulfo-2*H*-indol-2-ylidene)-2,3-dihydro-3-oxo-, disodium salt; (2) Disodium 3,3′-dioxo-[Δ$^{2,2'}$-biindoline]-5,5′-disulfonate. *CAS-860-22-0; CAS-483-20-5* [5,5′-indigotindisulfonic acid]. *Diagnostic aid (cystoscopy).* Indigo Carmine (Becton Dickinson Microbiology†)

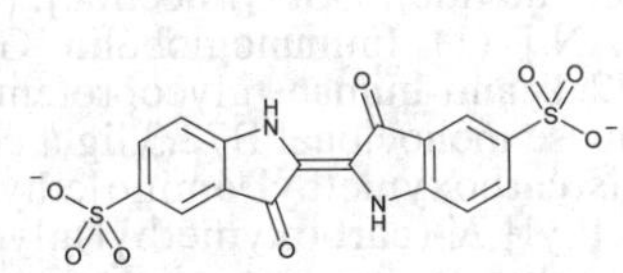

Indinavir [*1997*] (in din′ a vir). C$_{36}$H$_{47}$N$_5$O$_4$.H$_2$O. 631.80. (1) D-*erythro*-Pentonamide, 2,3,5-trideoxy-*N*-(2,3-dihydro-2-hydroxy-1*H*-inden-1-yl)-5-[2-[[(1,1-dimethylethyl)amino]carbonyl]-4-(3-pyridinylmethyl)-1-piperazinyl]-2-(phenylmethyl)-, monohydrate, [1(1*S*,2*R*),5(*S*)]-; (2) (α*R*,γ*S*,2*S*)-α-Benzyl-2-(*tert*-butylcarbamoyl)-γ-hydroxy-*N*-[(1*S*,2*R*)-2-hydroxy-1-indanyl]-4-(3-pyridylmethyl)-1-piperazinevaleramide monohydrate. *UNII-5W6YA9PKKH;*

UNII-9MG78X43ZT [indinavir anhydrous]. *CAS-180683-37-8; CAS-150378-17-9* [anhydrous]. INN; BAN. *Antiviral.*

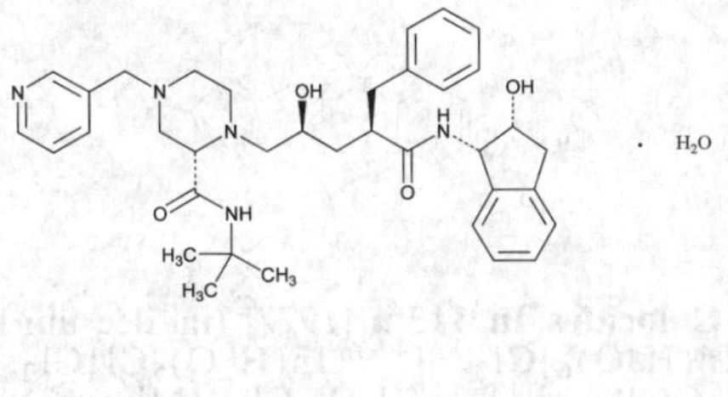

Indinavir Sulfate [*1995*] (in din′ a vir sul′ fate). **USP.** C$_{36}$H$_{47}$N$_5$O$_4$.H$_2$SO$_4$. 711.87. (1) D-*erythro*-Pentonamide, 2,3,5-trideoxy-*N*-(2,3-dihydro-2-hydroxy-1*H*-inden-1-yl)-5-[2-[[(1,1-dimethylethyl)amino]carbonyl]-4-(3-pyridinyl-methyl)-1-piperazinyl]-2-(phenylmethyl)-, [1(1*S*,2*R*,5(*S*)]-, sulfate (1:1) (salt); (2) (α*R*,γ*S*,2*S*)-α-Benzyl-2-(*tert*-butyl-carbamoyl)-γ-hydroxy-*N*-[(1*S*,2*R*)-2-hydroxy-1-indanyl]-4-(3-pyridylmethyl)-1-piperazinevaleramide sulfate (1:1) (salt). *UNII-771H53976Q. CAS-157810-81-6. Antiviral.* Crixivan (Merck) ◇*MK-639; L-735,524*

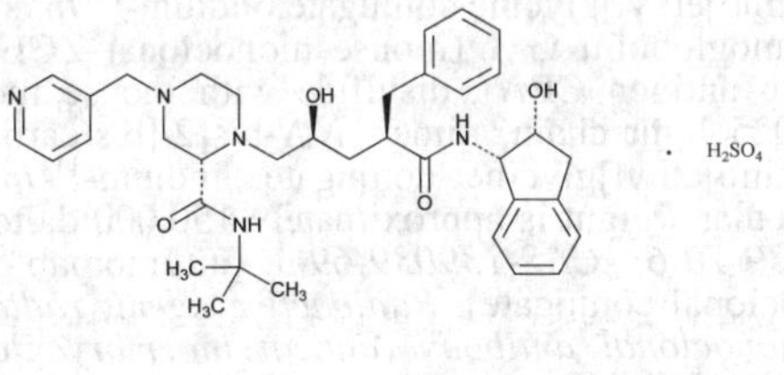

Indiplon [*2002*] (in′ di plon). C$_{20}$H$_{16}$N$_4$O$_2$S. 376.43. (1) *N*-Methyl-*N*-[3-[3-(2-thienylcarbonyl)-pyrazolo[1,5-*a*]pyrimidin-7-yl]phenyl]acetamide; (2) *N*-Methyl-*N*-[3-3-(thiophen-2-ylcarbonyl)pyrazolo[1,5-*a*]pyrimidin-7-yl]phenyl]-acetamide; (3) 3-(2-Thienylcarbonyl)-7-(3-*N*-methylacetamide)-pyrazolo[1,5-α]pyrimidine. *UNII-8BT63DA42E. CAS-325715-02-4.* INN. *Sedative/hypnotic (GABA$_A$ agonist).* ◇*NBI-34060*

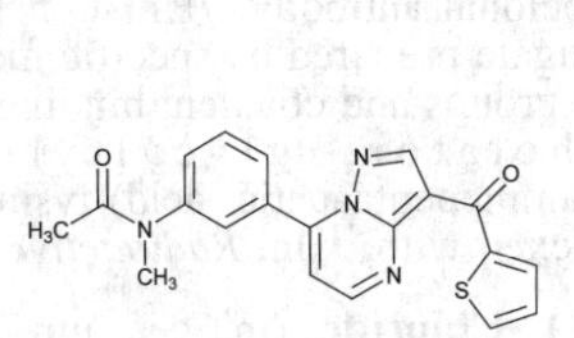

Indisetron. C$_{17}$H$_{23}$N$_5$O. 313.40. *N*-(3,9-Dimethyl-*endo*-3,9-diazabicyclo[3.3.1]non-7-yl)-1*H*-indazole-3-carboxamide. *UNII-89RBZ66NVC. CAS-141549-75-9.* INN.

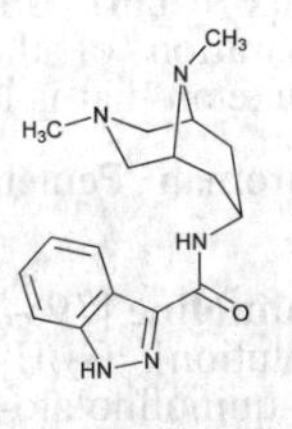

---

† Brand name formerly used, and/or firm no longer concerned with this product.

Indisulam [*2005*] (in″ di soo′ lam). $C_{14}H_{12}ClN_3O_4S_2$. 385.85. (1) *N*-(3-Chloro-1*H*-indol-7-yl)benzene-1,4-disulfonamide; (2) 1,4-Benzenedisulfonamide, *N*-(3-chloro-1*H*-indol-7-yl). *CAS-165668-41-7.* INN; BAN. *Antineoplastic.* ◇*E7070*

Indium Chlorides In 113m [*1977*] (in′ dee um klor′ ide). $[^{113m}In(H_2O)_6]Cl_3$, $[^{113m}In(H_2O)_5Cl]Cl_2$, $[^{113m}In(H_2O)_4Cl_2]Cl$, $^{113m}In(H_2O)_3Cl_3$ (Mixture). (1) Indium(3+)-^{113m}In, hexaaqua-, trichloride mixture with pentaaquachloroindium(2+)-^{113m}In dichloride, tetraaquadichloroindium(1+)-^{113m}In chloride, and triaquatrichloroindium-^{113m}In; (2) Hydrated indium(3+)-^{113m}In chlorides. USP XX. *Radioactive agent.*

Indium (^{111}In) Diethylenetriamine Pentaacetate Injection (JAN) — *See* Indium In 111 Pentetate.

Indium In 111 Altumomab Pentetate [*1993*] (in′ dee um al toom′ oh mab pen′ te tate). [Altumomab is INN.] (1) Immunoglobulin G 1 (mouse monoclonal ZCE025 anti-human antigen CEA), disulfide with mouse monoclonal ZCE025 light chain, dimer, *N,N*-bis[2-[bis(carboxymethyl)amino]ethyl]glycine conjugate, indium-^{111}In chelate; (2) Immunoglobulin G 1 (mouse monoclonal ZCE025 anti-human antigen CEA), disulfide with mouse monoclonal ZCE025 light chain, dimer, *N,N*-bis[2-[bis(carboxymethyl)amino]ethyl]glycine conjugate, indium-^{111}In chelate. Molecular weight is approximately 150,000 daltons. *CAS-139039-70-6; CAS-139039-69-3* [altumomab pentetate monoclonal conjugate]. *Radioactive agent; radiodiagnostic monoclonal antibody (anticarcinoembryonic antigen [CEA]).* Hybri-CEAker (Hybritech) *[Note—Altumomab is the USAN assigned to the monoclonal antibody; Altumomab Pentetate is the USAN assigned to the monoclonal conjugate, identified as Immunoglobulin G 1 (mouse monoclonal ZCE025 anti-human antigen CEA), disulfide with mouse monoclonal ZCE025 light chain, dimer, N,N-bis[2-[bis(carboxymethyl)amino]ethyl]glycine conjugate.]* ◇*MAB35; ZCE025*

Indium In 111 Capromab Pendetide (in′ dee um kap′ roe mab pen′ de tide). **USP** [Injection]. A sterile, nonpyrogenic, murine monoclonal antibody, 7E11-C 5.3, (CYT-351), an immunoconjugate prepared by specific modification of the carbohydrate groups and covalent binding to the tripeptide linker chelator, glycyltyrosyl-(*N*, *E*-diethylenetriaminepentaacetic acid)-lysine hydrochloride that is complexed with ^{111}In. *Radioactive agent.*

Indium In 111 Chloride (in′ dee um klor′ ide). **USP** [Solution]. [Indium (^{111}In) Chloride Injection is JAN.] (1) Indium Chloride ($^{111}InCl_3$); (2) Indium (^{111}In) trichloride. *CAS-10025-82-8. Radioactive agent.* INDICLOR (Nycomed Amersham)

Indium In 111 CYT-103 (previously used name) — *See* Indium In 111 Satumomab Pendetide.

Indium In 111 Ibritumomab Tiuxetan (in′ dee um eye″ bri toom′ oh mab tye ux′ e tan). **USP** [Injection]. A sterile, nonpyrogenic preparation of the immunoconjugate of ibritumomab and tiuxetan that is labeled with ^{111}In.

Indium In 111 Imciromab Pentetate — *See* Imciromab Pentetate.

Indium In 111 Oxyquinoline [*1984*] (in′ dee um ox″ i kwin′ oh leen). **USP** [Solution]. $C_{27}H_{18}^{111}InN_3O_3$. 543.45. (1) Indium-$^{111}In$, tris(8-quinolinolato-*N¹,O⁸*)-; (2) Tris(8-quinolinolato)indium-^{111}In. *UNII-LGX9OL562T. CAS-65389-*

08-4. Diagnostic aid; radioactive agent. Indium Oxine (Nycomed Amersham); Indium Oxine In 111 (Medi-Physics)

Indium In 111 Pentetate (in′ dee um pen′ te tate). **USP** [Injection]. [Indium (^{111}In) Diethylenetriamine Pentaacetate Injection is JAN.] A sterile, isotonic solution, containing radioactive indium (^{111}In) in the form of a chelate of pentetic acid. *Diagnostic aid (radionuclide cisternography); radioactive agent.* Indium DTPA In 111 (Medi-Physics)

Indium In 111 Pentetreotide [*1995*] (in′ dee um pen″ te tree′ oh tide). **USP** [Injection]. $C_{63}H_{84}^{111}InN_{13}O_{19}S_2$. (1) Indate (1-)-$^{111}In$,[*N*-[2-[[2-[bis(carboxymethyl)amino]ethyl](carboxymethyl)amino]ethyl]-*N*-(carboxymethyl)glycyl-D-phenylalanyl-L-cysteinyl-L-phenylalanyl-D-tryptophyl-L-lysyl-L-threonyl-*N*-[2-hydroxy-1-(hydroxymethyl)propyl]-L-cysteinamide cyclic (3→8)-disulfidato(4-)]-, hydrogen, [*R*-(*R**,*R**)]-; (2) *N*-[2-[[2-Bis(carboxymethyl)amino]ethyl](carboxymethyl)amino]ethyl]-*N*-(carboxymethyl)glycyl-D-phenylalanyl-L-cysteinyl-L-phenylalanyl-D-tryptophyl-L-lysyl-L-threonyl-*N*-[(1*R*,2*R*)-2-hydroxy-1-(hydroxymethyl)propyl]-L-cysteinamide, cyclic (3→8)-disulfide, [^{111}In]chelate. *CAS-139096-04-1. Diagnostic aid; radioactive agent.* OctreoScan (Mallinckrodt) ◇*MP-1727*

Indium In 111 Satumomab Pendetide [*1993*] (in′ dee um sa toom′ oh mab pen′ de tide). **USP** [Injection]. [Satumomab is INN and BAN.] (1) Immunoglobulin G 1 (mouse monoclonal B72.3 anti-human glycoprotein TAG-72), disulfide with mouse monoclonal B72.3 light chain, dimer, N^6-[*N*-[2-[[2-[bis(carboxymethyl)amino]ethyl](carboxymethyl)amino]ethyl]-*N*-(carboxymethyl)glycyl]-N^2-(*N*-glycyl-L-tyrosyl)-L-lysine conjugate, indium-^{111}In chelate; (2) Immunoglobulin G 1 (mouse monoclonal B72.3 anti-human glycoprotein TAG-72), disulfide with mouse monoclonal B72.3 light chain, dimer, N^6-[*N*-[2-[[2-[bis(carboxymethyl)amino]ethyl](carboxymethyl)amino]ethyl]-*N*-(carboxymethyl)glycyl]-N^2-(*N*-glycyl-L-tyrosyl)-L-lysine conjugate, indium-^{111}In chelate. *CAS-138955-27-8; CAS-138955-26-7* [satumomab pendetide monoclonal-linker/chelator]; *CAS-144058-40-2* [satumomab]. *Radioactive agent; radiodiagnostic monoclonal antibody (ovarian and colorectal carcinoma).* OncoScint CR/OV (Cytogen) *[Note—Satumomab is the USAN assigned to the monoclonal antibody and satumomab pendetide identifies the monoclonal-linker/chelator. Names previously used: Indium In 111 CYT-103 and Monab B72.3-GYK-DTPA-^{111}In.]* ◇*CYT-103^{111}In*

Indobufen. $C_{18}H_{17}NO_3$. 295.33. (±)-2-[*p*-(1-Oxo-2-isoindolinyl)phenyl]butyric acid. *CAS-63610-08-2.* INN; MI.

Indocate. $C_{22}H_{26}N_2O_2$. 350.45. 2-(Dimethylamino)ethyl 1-benzyl-2,3-dimethylindole-5-carboxylate. *UNII-78D9U89TBG. CAS-31386-25-1.* INN.

Indocyanine Green (in″ doe sye′ a neen). **USP.** $C_{43}H_{47}N_2NaO_6S_2$. 774.96. (1) 1*H*-Benz[*e*]indolium, 2-[7-[1,3-dihydro-1,1-dimethyl-3-(4-sulfobutyl)-2*H*-benz[*e*]indol-2-ylidene]-1,3,5-heptatrienyl]-1,1-dimethyl-3-(4-sulfobutyl)-, hydroxide, inner salt, sodium salt; (2) 2-[7-[1,1-Dimethyl-3-(4-sulfobutyl)benz[*e*]indolin-2-ylidene]-1,3,5-heptatrienyl]-1,1-dimethyl-3-(4-sulfobutyl)-1*H*-benz[*e*]indolium hydroxide, inner salt, sodium salt. *UNII-IX6J1063HV. CAS-3599-32-4.* JAN. *Diagnostic aid (cardiac output determination); diagnostic aid (hepatic function determination).* IC-Green (Akorn)

Indolapril Hydrochloride [*1984*] (in dol′ a pril hye″ droe klor′ ide). $C_{24}H_{34}N_2O_5$·HCl. 467.00. [Indolapril is INN.] (1) 1*H*-Indole-2-carboxylic acid, 1-[2-[[1-(ethoxycarbonyl)-3-phenylpropyl]amino]-1-oxopropyl]octahydro-, monohydrochloride, [2*S*-[1[*R**(*R**)],2α,3aβ,7aβ]]-; (2) (2*S*,3a*S*,7a*S*)-1-[(*S*)-*N*-[(*S*)-1-Carboxy-3-phenylpropyl]alanyl]hexahydro-2-indolinecarboxylic acid, 1-ethyl ester, monohydrochloride. *CAS-80828-32-6; CAS-80876-01-3* [indolapril]. *Antihypertensive.* ◇CI-907

Indolidan [*1987*] (in dol′ i dan). $C_{14}H_{15}N_3O_2$. 257.29. (1) 2*H*-Indol-2-one, 1,3-dihydro-3,3-dimethyl-5-(1,4,5,6-tetrahydro-6-oxo-3-pyridazinyl)-; (2) 3,3-Dimethyl-5-(1,4,5,6-tetrahydro-6-oxo-3-pyridazinyl)-2-indolinone. *CAS-100643-96-7.* INN; BAN. *Cardiotonic.* ◇LY 195115

Indometacin (INN, BAN, JAN, DCF) — *See* Indomethacin.

Indometacin Farnesil (JAN) — *See* Indomethacin.

Indomethacin [*1963*] (in″ doe meth′ a sin). **USP.** $C_{19}H_{16}ClNO_4$. 357.79. [Indometacin is INN, BAN and JAN; Indometacin Farnesil is JAN.] (1) 1*H*-Indole-3-acetic acid, 1-(4-chlorobenzoyl)-5-methoxy-2-methyl-; (2) 1-(*p*-Chlorobenzoyl)-5-methoxy-2-methylindole-3-acetic acid. *UNII-XXE1CET956. CAS-53-86-1. Anti-inflammatory.* Indocin (Merck)

Indomethacin Sodium [*1987*] (in″ doe meth′ a sin soe′ dee um). **USP.** $C_{19}H_{15}ClNNaO_4$·3H_2O. 433.82. (1) 1*H*-Indole-3-acetic acid, 1-(4-chlorobenzoyl)-5-methoxy-2-methyl-, sodium salt, trihydrate; (2) Sodium 1-(*p*-chlorobenzoyl)-5-methoxy-2-methylindole-3-acetate, trihydrate. *UNII-0IMX38M2GG. CAS-74252-25-8. Anti-inflammatory.* Indocin (Ovation)

Indopanolol. $C_{20}H_{23}ClN_2O_3$. 374.86. (±)-1-[(3-Chloro-2-methylindol-4-yl)oxy]-3-[(2-phenoxyethyl)amino]-2-propanol. *UNII-2JQ3661CAD. CAS-69907-17-1.* INN.

Indopine. $C_{23}H_{28}N_2$. 332.48. 3-[2-(1-Phenethyl-4-piperidyl)ethyl]indole. *UNII-J57707EKBI; UNII-CZ5QG07777* [indopine hydrochloride]. *CAS-3569-26-4; CAS-24361-13-5* [hydrochloride]. INN.

Indoprofen [*1976*] (in″ doe proe′ fen). $C_{17}H_{15}NO_3$. 281.31. (1) Benzeneacetic acid, 4-(1,3-dihydro-1-oxo-2*H*-isoindol-2-yl)-α-methyl-; (2) *p*-(1-Oxo-2-isoindolinyl)hydratropic acid. *CAS-31842-01-0*. INN; BAN. *Analgesic; anti-inflammatory.* ◇*K 4277*

Indoramin [*1971*] (in dor′ a min). $C_{22}H_{25}N_3O$. 347.45. (1) Benzamide, *N*-[1-[2-(1*H*-indol-3-yl)ethyl]-4-piperidinyl]-; (2) *N*-[1-(2-Indol-3-ylethyl)-4-piperidyl]benzamide. *UNII-0Z802HMY7H*. *CAS-26844-12-2*. INN; BAN. *Antihypertensive.* ◇*Wy 21901*

Indoramin Hydrochloride [*1984*] (in dor′ a min hye″ droe klor′ ide). $C_{22}H_{25}N_3O \cdot HCl$. 383.91. (1) Benzamide, *N*-[1-[2-(1*H*-indol-3-yl)ethyl]-4-piperidinyl]-, monohydrochloride; (2) *N*-[1-(2-Indol-3-ylethyl)-4-piperidyl]benzamide monohydrochloride. *CAS-38821-52-2*. BAN. *Antihypertensive.* ◇*WY-21,901 HCl*

Indorenate Hydrochloride [*1981*] (in dor′ en ate hye″ droe klor′ ide). $C_{13}H_{16}N_2O_3 \cdot HCl$. 284.74. [Indorenate is INN.] (1) 1*H*-Indole-3-acetic acid, α-(aminomethyl)-5-methoxy-, methyl ester, monohydrochloride, (±)-; (2) Methyl (±)-α-(aminomethyl)-5-methoxyindole-3-acetate monohydrochloride. *UNII-860O06CJWZ*. *CAS-72318-55-9*. *Antihypertensive.* ◇*TR-3369*

Indoxole [*1965*] (in dox′ ole). $C_{22}H_{19}NO_2$. 329.39. (1) 1*H*-Indole, 2,3-bis(4-methoxyphenyl)-; (2) 2,3-Bis(*p*-methoxyphenyl)indole. *CAS-5034-76-4*. INN. *Antipyretic; anti-inflammatory.* ◇*U-22020*

Indriline Hydrochloride [*1968*] (in′ dri leen hye″ droe klor′ ide). $C_{19}H_{21}N \cdot HCl$. 299.84. [Indriline is INN.] (1) 1*H*-Indene-1-ethanamine, *N,N*-dimethyl-1-phenyl-, hydrochloride; (2) *N,N*-Dimethyl-1-phenylindene-1-ethylamine hydrochloride. *CAS-2988-32-1; CAS-7395-90-6* [indriline]. *Stimulant (central).* ◇*MJ 1986*

Inecalcitol. $C_{26}H_{40}O_3$. 400.59. (7*E*)-19-Nor-9,10-seco-14β-cholesta-5,7-dien-23-yne-1α,3β,25-triol. *CAS-163217-09-2*. INN.

Infliximab [*1996*] (in flix′ i mab). Immunoglobulin G (human-mouse monoclonal cA2 heavy chain anti-human tumor necrosis factor), disulfide with human-mouse monoclonal cA2 light chain, dimer. *UNII-B72HH48FLU*. *CAS-170277-31-3*. INN; BAN.

Influenza Virus Vaccine (in″ floo en′ za). **USP.** A sterile, aqueous suspension of suitably inactivated influenza virus types A and B, either individually or combined, or virus sub-units prepared from the extra-embryonic fluid of influenza virus-infected chicken embryo. *Immunizing agent (active).* Fluogen (Parke-Davis†); FluShield (Lederle); Fluzone (Bristol-Myers Squibb†)

Ingenol Mebutate [*2008*] (in′ je nol meb′ ue tate). $C_{25}H_{34}O_6$. 430.53. (1) 2-Butenoic acid, 2-methyl-, (1a*R*,2*S*,5*R*,5a*S*,6-*S*,8a*S*,9*R*,10a*R*)-1a,2,5,5a,6,9,10,10a-octahydro-5,5a-dihydroxy-4-(hydroxymethyl)-1,1,7,9-tetramethyl-11-oxo-1*H*-2,8a-methanocyclopenta[*a*]cyclopropa[*e*]cyclodecen-6-yl ester, (2*Z*)-; (2) (1a*R*,2*S*,5*R*,5a*S*,6*S*,8a*S*,9*R*,10a*R*)-5,5a-Dihydroxy-4-(hydroxymethyl)-1,1,7,9-tetramethyl-11-oxo-1a,2,5,5a,6,9,10,10a-octahydro-1*H*-2,8a-methanocyclopenta[*a*]cyclopropa[*e*]cyclodecen-6-yl (2*Z*)-2-methylbut-2-enoate. *UNII-7686S50JAH*. *CAS-75567-37-2*. *Treatment of actinic keratosis and superficial basal cell carcinoma.* ◇*PEP-005*

Ingliforib [*2000*] (in″ gli foe′ rib). $C_{23}H_{24}ClN_3O_5$. 457.91. (1) 1*H*-Indole-2-carboxamide, 5-chloro-*N*-[(1*S*,2*R*)-3-[(3*R*,4*S*)-3,4-dihydroxy-1-pyrrolidinyl]-2-hydroxy-3-oxo-1-(phenylmethyl)propyl]-; (2) [*R*-[*R**,*S**-(*cis*)]]-5-Chloro-*N*-[3-(3,4-dihydroxy-1-pyrrolidinyl)-2-hydroxy-3-oxo-1-(phenylmethyl)propyl]-1*H*-indole-2-carboxamide. *UNII-UII7156WLU*. *CAS-186392-65-4*. INN. *Treatment of type 2 diabetes mellitus (glycogen phosphorylase inhibitor).* ◇*CP-368,296*

Inicarone. $C_{17}H_{15}NO_2$. 265.31. 2-Isopropyl-3-benzofuranyl 4-pyridyl ketone. *UNII-1EVW48QLUN*. *CAS-39178-37-5*. INN.

Inocoterone Acetate [*1989*] (in″ oh koe′ ter one as′ e tate). $C_{18}H_{26}O_3$. 290.40. [Inocoterone is INN.] (1) 7*H*-Benz[*e*]inden-7-one, 3-(acetyloxy)-6-ethyl-1,2,3,3a,4,5,8,9,9a,9b-decahydro-3a-methyl-, [3*S*-(3α,3aα,9aα,9bβ)]-; (2) 17β-

Hydroxy-2,5-*seco*-A-dinorestr-9-en-5-one acetate. *UNII-ONU02D116S. CAS-83646-86-0; CAS-83646-97-3* [inocoterone]. *Anti-acne.* ◇*RU 882; RU 38882*

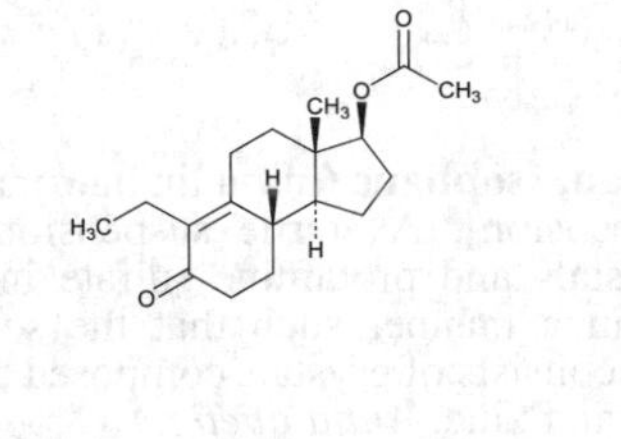

Inogatran. $C_{21}H_{38}N_6O_4$. 438.56. *N*-[(1*R*)-2-Cyclohexyl-1-[[(2*S*)-2-[(3-guanidinopropyl)carbamoyl]piperidino]carbonyl]ethyl]glycine. *CAS-155415-08-0.* INN.

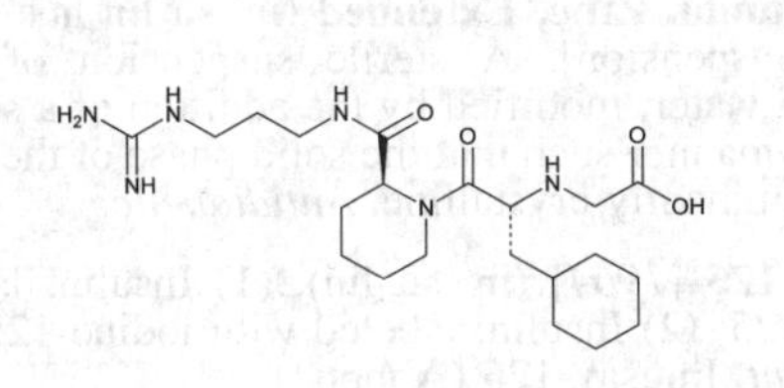

Inolimomab. Immunoglobulin G1, anti-(human interleukin 2 receptor α-chain) (mouse monoclonal B-B10 γl-chain), disulfide with mouse monoclonal B-B10 κ-chain, dimer. *CAS-152981-31-2.* INN.

Inolitazone. $C_{27}H_{26}N_4O_4S$. 502.58. *rac*-5-[(4-{[6-(4-Amino-3,5-dimethylphenoxy)-1-methyl-1*H*-benzimidazol-2-yl]methoxy}phenyl)methyl]-1,3-thiazolidine-2,4-dione. *CAS-223132-37-4.* INN.

Inosine. $C_{10}H_{12}N_4O_5$. 268.23. Inosine. *CAS-58-63-9.* INN; JAN; MI.

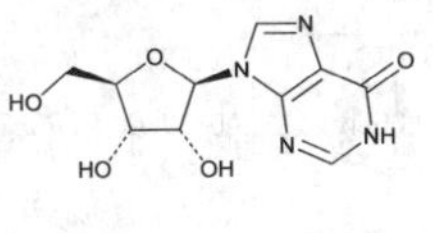

Inosine Pranobex. $C_{10}H_{12}N_4O_5 \cdot C_{14}H_{22}N_2O_4$. 550.56. Inosine-2-hydroxypropyldimethylammonium 4-acetamidobenzoate (1:3). *CAS-36703-88-5.* BAN; JAN; MI.

Inositol. *UNII-4L6452S749.* NF XII; MI.

Inositol Hexanicotinate (JAN) — *See* Inositol Niacinate.

Inositol Niacinate [*1962*] (in oh′ si tol nye′ a sin ate). $C_{42}H_{30}N_6O_{12}$. 810.72. [Inositol Nicotinate is INN and BAN; Inositol Hexanicotinate is JAN.] (1) *myo*-Inositol, hexa-3-pyridinecarboxylate; (2) *myo*-Inositol hexanicotinate; (3) 1,2,3,5/4,6 Cyclohexanehexol hexanicotinate. *UNII-A99MK953KZ. CAS-6556-11-2. Vasodilator (periph-*

eral). Hexopal (Sterling Winthrop); Linodil (Sterling Winthrop†); Palohex (Sterling Winthrop) ◇*Win 9154; NSC-49506*

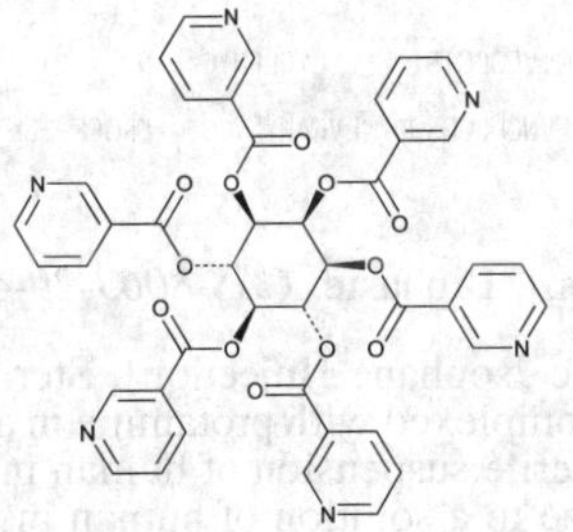

Inositol Nicotinate (INN, BAN) — *See* Inositol Niacinate.

Inotuzumab Ozogamicin [*2004*] (in″ oh tooz′ oo mab oh″ zoe ga mye′ sin). $C_{6518}H_{10002}N_{1738}O_{2036}S_{42}$. Immunoglobulin G4 (anti-(human CD22 (antigen)) (human-mouse monoclonal G544 heavy chain), disulfide with human-mouse monoclonal G544 κ-chain, dimer, methyl [(1*R*,4*Z*,8*S*,13*E*)-8-[[2-*O*-[4-(acetylethylamino)-2,4-dideoxy-3-*O*-methyl-α-L-*threo*-pentopyranosyl]-4,6-dideoxy-4-[[[2,6-dideoxy-4-*S*-[4-[(6-deoxy-3-*O*-methyl-α-L-mannopyranosyl)oxy]-3-iodo-5,6-dimethoxy-2-methylbenzoyl]-4-thio-β-D-*ribo*-hexopyranosyl]oxy]amino]-β-D-glucopyranosyl]oxy]-13-[2-[[3-[[1-[4-(4-amino-4-oxobutoxy)phenyl]ethylidene]hydrazino]-1,1-dimethyl-3-oxopropyl]dithio]ethylidene]-1-hydroxy-11-oxobicyclo[7.3.1]trideca-4,9-diene-2,6-diyn-10-yl]carbamate conjugate. Molecular weight is approximately 150,000 daltons. *CAS-635715-01-4.* INN. *Oncological treatment.* (Wyeth) ◇*CMC-544; WAY-207294*

Inprochone — *See* Inproquone.

Inproquone. $C_{16}H_{22}N_2O_4$. 306.36. 2,5-Bis(ethyleneimino)-3,6-dipropoxy-*p*-benzoquinone. *UNII-C6Y700V0M4. CAS-436-40-8.* INN; BAN. ◇*E 39; RP 6870; NSC-17261*

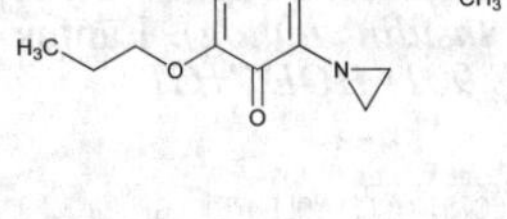

INSH — *See* Salinazid.

Insulin (in′ su lin). USP. $C_{256}H_{381}N_{65}O_{76}S_6$ (Insulin pig). 5777.54 (pig); $C_{254}H_{377}N_{65}O_{75}S_6$ (Insulin ox). 5733.49 (ox). [Pork] (1) Insulin (ox), 8^A-L-threonine-10^A-L-isoleucine-; (2) Insulin (dog); (3) Insulin (pig). [Beef] (1) Insulin (ox); (2) Insulin (ox). *CAS-12584-58-6* [pig]; *CAS-11070-73-8* [ox]. BAN; JAN. *Antidiabetic.*

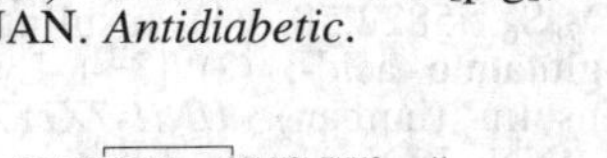

```
GIVEQCCTSI  CSLYQLENYC N
FVNQHLCGSH  LVEALYLVCG ERGFFYTPKA
```

Insulin Argine. $C_{269}H_{407}N_{73}O_{79}S_6$. 6119.94. 30^{B}a-L-Arginine-30^{B}b-L-arginineinsulin (human). *CAS-68859-20-1.* INN.

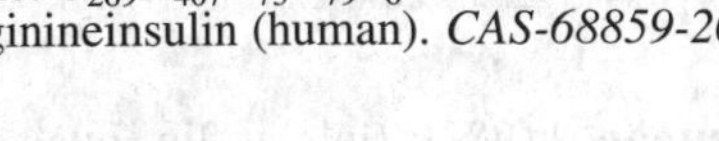

```
GIVEQCCTSI  CSLYQLENYC N
FVNQHLCGSH  LVEALYLVCG ERGFFYTPKT RR
```

---

† Brand name formerly used, and/or firm no longer concerned with this product.

Insulin Aspart [*1998*] (in′ su lin as′ part). $C_{256}H_{381}N_{65}O_{79}S_6$. 5825.54. 28^B-L-Aspartic acid-insulin (human). *UNII-D933668QVX. CAS-116094-23-6*. INN; BAN. *Antidiabetic.* ◇*Insulin X14; INA-X14; B28-Asp-Insulin*

```
GIVEQCCTSI  CSLYQLENYC  N
FVNQHLCGSH  LVEALYLVCG  ERGFFYTDKT
```

Insulin [Injection], Biphasic. *CAS-8063-29-4*. INN; BAN.

Insulin, Biphasic Isophane [Injection]. Sterile suspension of beef insulin complexed with protamine in a solution of pork insulin or a sterile suspension of human insulin complexed with protamine in a solution of human insulin. *CAS-8063-29-4*. BAN.

Insulin, Dalanated [*1963*] (in′ su lin dal′ a nay″ ted). Insulin derivative prepared by the removal of the C-terminal alanine from the B chain of insulin. (1) Insulin, dalanated; (2) Insulin, dalanated. *CAS-9004-12-0*. INN. *Antidiabetic.* ◇*S.N. 44*

Insulin Defalan. $C_{247}H_{372}N_{64}O_{75}S_6$ (porcine). 5630.37 (porcine); $C_{245}H_{368}N_{64}O_{74}S_6$ (bovine). 5586.32 (bovine). 1^B-de(L-Phenylalanine)insulin. *CAS-11091-62-6* [porcine]; *CAS-51798-72-2* [bovine]. INN.

Insulin Detemir [*1999*] (in′ su lin det′ e mir). $C_{267}H_{402}N_{64}O_{76}S_6$. 5916.82 daltons. (1) 29^B-[N^6-(1-Oxotetradecyl)-L-lysine]-(1^A-21^A),(1^B-29^B)-insulin (human); (2) 29^B-(N^6-Myristoyl-L-lysine)-30^B-de-L-threonineinsulin (human). *UNII-4FT78T86XV. CAS-169148-63-4*. INN; BAN. *Antidiabetic.* ◇*NN-304*

```
GIVEQCCTSI  CSLYQLENYC  N
FVNQHLCGSH  LVEALYLVCG  ERGFFYTPK
```

Insulin Glargine [*1999*] (in′ su lin glar′ jeen). $C_{267}H_{404}N_{72}O_{78}S_6$. 6062.89. (1) Insulin (human), 21^A-glycine-30^{B}a-L-arginine-30^{B}b-L-arginine-; (2) 21^A-Glycine-30^{B}a-L-arginine-30^{B}b-L-arginine insulin (human). *UNII-2ZM8CX04RZ. CAS-160337-95-1*. INN; BAN. *Antidiabetic (basal insulin analog).* Lantus (Hoechst Marion Roussel) ◇*HOE 901; HOE 71GT*

```
GIVEQCCTSI  CSLYQLENYC  G
FVKQHLCGSH  LVEALYLVCG  ERGFFYTPKT  RR
```

Insulin, Globin Zinc. [Globin Zinc Insulin Injection is INN.] (1) Insulin globin zinc; (2) Insulin globin zinc. USP XX.

Insulin Glulisine [*2003*] (in′ su lin gloo′ lis een). $C_{258}H_{384}N_{64}O_{78}S_6$. 5822.58. (1) Insulin (human),3^B-L-lysine,29^B-L-glutamic acid-; (2) [3^B-L-Lysine,29^B-L-glutamic acid]insulin (human). *UNII-7XIY785AZD. CAS-207748-29-6*. INN; JAN. *Treatment of type 1 and type 2 diabetes.* ◇*HMR 1964*

```
GIVEQCCTSI  CSLYQLENYC  N
FVKQHLCGSH  LVEALYLVCG  ERGFFYTPET
```

Insulin Human [*1983*] (in′ su lin hue′ man). **USP**. $C_{257}H_{383}N_{65}O_{77}S_6$. 5807.57. [Insulin Human (Biosynthesis) and Insulin Human (Synthesis) are JAN.] A protein that has the normal structure of the natural antidiabetic principle produced by the human pancreas. Insulin (human). *UNII-*

1Y17CTI5SR. CAS-11061-68-0. INN; BAN. *Antidiabetic.* Humulin (Lilly); Novolin (Novo Nordisk); Velosulin (Novo Nordisk)

```
GIVEQCCTSI  CSLYQLENYC  N
FVNQHLCGSH  LVEALYLVCG  ERGFFYTPKT
```

Insulin Human, Isophane (in′ su lin hue′ man eye′ soe fane). **USP** [Suspension]. A sterile suspension of zinc-insulin human crystals and protamine sulfate in buffered water, combined in a manner such that the solid phase of the suspension consists of crystals composed of insulin human, protamine, and zinc. *Antidiabetic.*

Insulin Human Zinc (in′ su lin hue′ man zink). **USP** [Suspension]. (1) Insulin zinc; (2) Insulin zinc. *CAS-8049-62-5*. *Antidiabetic.*

Insulin Human Zinc, Extended (in′ su lin hue′ man zink). **USP** [Suspension]. A sterile suspension of insulin in buffered water, modified by the addition of a suitable zinc salt in a manner such that the solid phase of the suspension is predominantly crystalline. *Antidiabetic.*

Insulin I 125 [*1964*] (in′ su lin). (1) Insulin, labeled with iodine-125; (2) Insulin, labeled with iodine-125. *Radioactive agent.* Imusay-125 (Abbott†)

Insulin I 131 [*1963*] (in′ su lin). (1) Insulin, labeled with iodine-131; (2) Insulin, labeled with iodine-131. *CAS-37294-43-2. Radioactive agent.* Imusay-131 (Abbott†)

Insulin, Isophane (in′ su lin eye′ soe fane). **USP** [Suspension]. [Insulin Injection, Isophane (Aqueous Suspension) is JAN.] A sterile suspension of zinc-insulin crystals and protamine sulfate in buffered water, combined in a manner such that the solid phase of the suspension consists of crystals composed of insulin, protamine, and zinc. *CAS-9004-17-5*. INN; BAN. *Antidiabetic.* NPH (Novo Nordisk); NPH Iletin (Lilly)

Insulin Lispro [*1994*] (in′ su lin lis′ pro). **USP**. $C_{257}H_{383}N_{65}O_{77}S_6$. 5807.57. (1) Insulin (human), 28^B-L-lysine-29^B-L-proline-; (2) 28^B-L-Lysine-29^B-L-prolineinsulin (human). *UNII-GFX7QIS1II. CAS-133107-64-9*. INN; BAN. *Antidiabetic.* ◇*LY275585*

```
GIVEQCCTSI  CSLYQLENYC  N
FVNQHLCGSH  LVEALYLVCG  ERGFFYTKPT
```

Insulin, Neutral [*1965*] (in′ su lin). [Neutral Insulin Injection is INN, BAN, and JAN.] A neutral, buffered solution of pork insulin. *CAS-9004-14-2. Antidiabetic.*

Insulin, Neutral [Injection] of Purified Porcine. $C_{256}H_{361}N_{65}O_{73}S_6$. 5709.39. A sterile solution of purified porcine insulin buffered at pH 7. JAN.

Insulin, Protamine Zinc. [Protamine Zinc Insulin Injection is INN; Insulin Zinc Protamine Injection (Aqueous Suspension) is JAN.] (1) Insulin protamine zinc; (2) Insulin protamine zinc. *CAS-9004-17-5*. USP XXII.

Insulin Zinc (in′ su lin zink). **USP** [Suspension]. [Insulin Zinc Suspension, Compound is INN; Insulin Zinc Injection (Aqueous Suspension) and Insulin Zinc Purified Porcine (Suspension) are JAN.] (1) Insulin zinc; (2) Insulin zinc. *CAS-8049-62-5*. BAN. *Antidiabetic.* Lente Iletin (Lilly); Lente (Novo Nordisk)

Insulin Zinc, Extended (in′ su lin zink). **USP** [Suspension]. [Insulin Zinc Suspension (Crystalline) is INN and BAN; Insulin Zinc Injection, Crystalline (Aqueous Suspension) is JAN.] A sterile suspension of insulin in buffered water, modified by the addition of a suitable zinc salt in a manner such that the solid phase of the suspension is predominantly crystalline. *Antidiabetic.* Ultralente (Novo Nordisk†); Ultralente Iletin (Lilly)

Insulin Zinc Injection (Aqueous Suspension) (JAN) — *See* Insulin Zinc.

Insulin Zinc Injection, Amorphous (Aqueous Suspension) (JAN) — *See* Insulin Zinc, Prompt.

Insulin Zinc Injection, Crystalline (Aqueous Suspension) (JAN) — *See* Insulin Zinc, Extended.

Insulin Zinc, Prompt (in′ su lin zink). **USP** [Suspension]. [Insulin Zinc Suspension (Amorphous) is INN and BAN; Insulin Zinc Injection, Amorphous (Aqueous Suspension) is JAN.] A sterile suspension of insulin in buffered water, modified by the addition of a suitable zinc salt in a manner such that the solid phase of the suspension is amorphous. *Antidiabetic.* Semilente Iletin (Lilly); Semilente (Novo Nordisk†)

Insulin Zinc Protamine Injection (Aqueous Suspension) (JAN) — *See* Insulin, Protamine Zinc.

Insulin Zinc, Purified Porcine (Suspension) (JAN) — *See* Insulin Zinc.

Insulin Zinc Suspension (Crystalline) (INN, BAN) — *See* Insulin Zinc, Extended.

Insulin Zinc Suspension (Amorphous) (INN, BAN) — *See* Insulin Zinc, Prompt.

Insulin Zinc Suspension, Compound (INN) — *See* Insulin Zinc.

Interferon. Proteins formed by the interaction of animal cells with viruses, capable of conferring on animal cells resistance to virus infection. *CAS-9008-11-1.* BAN.

Interferon Alfa. A glycoprotein of molecular weight 17,000–30,000 produced from human lymphoblastoid cells induced with *Sendai virus. CAS-74899-72-2.* BAN; JAN.

Interferon Alfa (BALL-1). A glycoprotein of molecular weight 13,000–21,000 produced from human lymphoblastoid cells (BALL-1) induced with *Sendai virus. CAS-74899-72-2.* JAN.

Interferon Alfa-2a [*1987*] (in″ ter feer′ on al′ fa). $C_{860}H_{1353}N_{227}O_{255}S_9$. 19,240.92. [Interferon Alfa-2a (Genetical Recombination) is JAN.] (1) Interferon αA (human leukocyte protein moiety reduced); (2) Interferon αA (human leukocyte protein moiety reduced). *UNII-47RRR83SK7. CAS-76543-88-9.* INN; BAN. *Antineoplastic; biological response modifier.* Roferon-A (Hoffmann-LaRoche) ◇*Ro 22-8181*

```
CDLPQTHSLG SRRTLMLLAQ MRKISLFSCL KDRHDFGFPQ EEFGNQFQKA
ETIPVLHEMI QQIFNLFSTK DSSAAWDETL LDKFYTELYQ QLNDLEACVI
QGVGVTETPL MKEDSILAVR KYFQRITLYL KEKKYSPCAW EVVRAEIMRS
FSLSTNLQES LRSKE
```

Interferon Alfa-2b [*1987*] (in″ ter feer′ on al′ fa). $C_{860}H_{1353}N_{229}O_{255}S_9$. 19,268.93. (1) Interferon α2b (human leukocyte clone Hif-SN206 protein moiety reduced); (2) Interferon α2b (human leukocyte clone Hif-SN206 protein moiety reduced). *UNII-43K1W2T1M6. CAS-99210-65-8.*

INN; BAN. *Antineoplastic; biological response modifier.* Intron A (Schering); Intron A HSA-free (Schering) ◇*Sch 30500*

```
CDLPQTHSLG SRRTLMLLAQ MRRISLFSCL KDRHDFGFPQ EEFGNQFQKA
ETIPVLHEMI QQIFNLFSTK DSSAAWDETL LDKFYTELYQ QLNDLEACVI
QGVGVTETPL MKEDSILAVR KYFQRITLYL KEKKYSPCAW EVVRAEIMRS
FSLSTNLQES LRSKE
```

Interferon Alfacon-1 [*1997*] (in″ ter feer′ on al′ fa kon). $C_{870}H_{1366}N_{236}O_{259}S_9$. 19,564.18. A non-naturally occurring type-1 interferon having 166 amino acids produced by recombinant technique using a synthetic DNA coding sequence. As expressed in *E. coli,* the product is nonglycosylated and has an *N*-terminal methionine. *N*-L-Methionyl-22-L-arginine-76-L-alanine-78-L-aspartic acid-79-L-glutamic acid-86-L-tyrosine-90-L-tyrosine-156-L-threonine-157-L-asparagine-158-L-leucineinterferon α1 (human lymphoblast reduced). *UNII-56588OP40D. CAS-118390-30-0.* INN; BAN. *Biological response modifier; antiviral.*

Interferon Alfa-n1 [*1987*] (in″ ter feer′ on al′ fa). Secreted proteins, known previously as leucocyte interferon or lymphoblastoid interferon, that are produced according to the information coded by interferon genes and that exert nonspecific antiviral activity at least in homologous cells through cellular metabolic processes involving synthesis of both ribonucleic acid and protein. (1) α-Interferons; (2) α-Interferons. INN; BAN. *Antineoplastic; biological response modifier.* Wellferon (Glaxo Wellcome)

Interferon Alfa-n3 [*1988*] (in″ ter feer′ on al′ fa). A mixture of natural interferon alfa proteins; secreted proteins that are produced according to the information coded by interferon genes and that exert nonspecific antiviral activity at least in homologous cells through cellular metabolic processes involving synthesis of both ribonucleic acid and proteins. (1) Interferons, α-; (2) α-Interferons. *Antineoplastic; biological response modifier.* Alferon LDO (Interferon Sciences); Alferon N Gel (Interferon Sciences); Alferon N Injection (Interferon Sciences) [*Name previously used: Leukocyte Interferon.*]

Interferon Beta. A secreted protein, known previously as fibroblast interferon, that is produced according to the information coded by a species of interferon gene. *CAS-74899-71-1.* BAN; JAN. [*Name previously used: Fibroblast Interferon.*]

Interferon Beta-1a [*1993*] (in″ ter feer′ on bay′ ta). $C_{908}H_{1406}N_{246}O_{252}S_7$ (protein moiety). 20,024.85 (protein moiety). Interferon beta-1a is a glycosylate polypeptide consisting of 166 amino acid residues produced from cultured Chinese Hamster ovary cells containing the engineered gene for human interferon beta. Glycosylation occurs at the asparagine (Asn) residue at position 80. The glycoprotein is approximately 89% protein and 11% carbohydrate by weight. (1) Interferon β1 (human fibroblast protein moiety); (2) Interferon β1 (human fibroblast protein moiety). *UNII-XRO4566Q4R. CAS-145258-61-3.* INN; BAN. *Antineoplastic; biological response modifier.* Neoferon (Biogen)

```
MSYNLLGFLQ RSSNFQCQKL LWQLNGRLEY CLKDRMNFDI PEEIKQLQQF
QKEDAALTIY EMLQNIFAIF RQDSSSTGWN ETIVENLLAN VYHQINHLKT
VLEEKLEKED FTRGKLMSSL HLKRYYGRIL HYLKAKEYSH CAWTIVRVEI
LRNFYFINRL TGYLRN
```

Interferon Beta-1b [*1994*] (in″ ter feer′ on bay′ ta). $C_{903}H_{1399}N_{245}O_{252}S_5$. 19,879.60. Interferon beta-1b is a non-glycosylated polypeptide produced in *E. coli* and consisting of 165 amino acid residues. (1) 2-166-Interferon β1 (human fibroblast reduced), 17-L-serine-; (2) 17-L-

---

† Brand name formerly used, and/or firm no longer concerned with this product.

Serine-2-166-interferon β1 (human fibroblast reduced). *UNII-TTD90R31WZ. CAS-145155-23-3.* INN; BAN. *Immunomodulator.* Betaseron (Berlex)

```
SYNLLGFLQ RSSNFQSQKL LWQLNGRLEY CLKDRMNFDI PEEIKQLQQF
QKEDAALTIY EMLQNIFAIF RQDSSSTGWN ETIVENLLAN VYHQINHLKT
VLEEKLEKED FTRGKLMSSL HLKRYYGRIL HYLKAKEYSH CAWTIVRVEI
LRNFYFINRL TGYLRN
```

Interferon Gamma-1a. $C_{761}H_{1206}N_{214}O_{225}S_6$. 17,145.42. Polypeptide consisting of 146 amino acid residues, produced in *E. coli* K-12 (C600) by expression interferon gamma-cDNA derived from human splenic lymphocyte-mRNA. *CAS-98059-18-8.* INN; BAN; JAN.

Interferon Gamma-1b [*1987*] (in″ ter feer′ on). $C_{734}H_{1166}N_{204}O_{216}S_5$. 16,464.69. (1) 1-139-Interferon γ (human lymphocyte protein moiety reduced), N^2-L-methionyl-; (2) N^2-L-Methionyl-1-139-interferon γ (human lymphocyte protein moiety reduced). *CAS-98059-61-1.* INN; BAN. *Antineoplastic; biological response modifier; immunoregulator.* Actimmune (Genentech)

```
                                                            M
QDPYVKEAEN LKKYFNAGHS DVADNGTLFL GILKNWKEES DRKIMQSQIV
SFYFKLFKNF KDDQSIQKSV ETIKEDMNVK FFNSNKKKRD DFEKLTNYSV
TDLNVQRKAI HELIQVMAEL SPAAKTGKRK RSQMLFRGR
```

Interferon Gamma-2a — *See* Interferon Gamma-1b.

Interleukin 2 — *See* Aldesleukin.

Intermedine. Active principle of the *pars intermedia* of the pituitary. *CAS-9002-79-3.* INN.

Intiquinatine. $C_{18}H_{14}BrNO_4$. 388.21. (2*R*)-2-{4-[(7-Bromoquinolin-2-yl)oxy]phenoxy}propanoic acid. *CAS-445041-75-8.* INN. *[Name previously used: Tiliquinatine.]*

Intoplicine. $C_{21}H_{24}N_4O$. 348.44. 11-[[3-(Dimethylamino)propyl]amino]-8-methyl-7*H*-benzo[*e*]pyrido[4,3-*b*]indol-3-ol. *UNII-FB2CIN6HMI. CAS-125974-72-3.* INN. ◇RP 60475

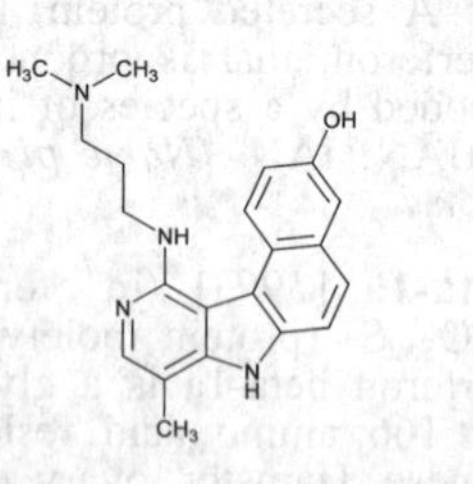

Intrazole [*1970*] (in′ tra zole). $C_{17}H_{12}ClN_5O$. 337.76. (1) 1*H*-Indole, 1-(4-chlorobenzoyl)-3-(1*H*-tetrazol-5-ylmethyl)-; (2) 1-(*p*-Chlorobenzoyl)-3-(1*H*-tetrazol-5-ylmethyl)indole. *CAS-15992-13-9.* INN. *Anti-inflammatory.* ◇BL-R 743

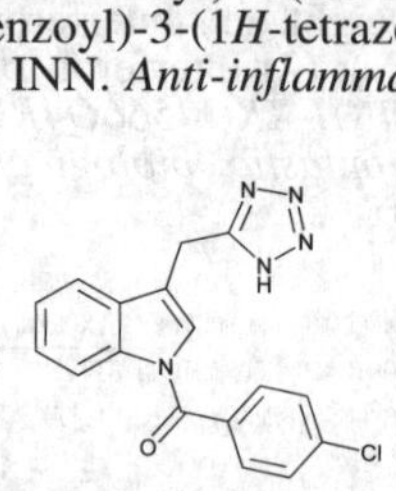

Intriptyline Hydrochloride [*1971*] (in trip′ ti leen hye″ droe klor′ ide). $C_{21}H_{19}N \cdot HCl$. 321.84. [Intriptyline is INN.] (1) 2-Butyn-1-amine, 4-(5-*H*-dibenzo[*a,d*]cyclohepten-5-ylidene)-*N,N*-dimethyl; (2) 4-(5*H*-Dibenzo[*a,d*]cyclohepten-5-ylidene)-*N,N*-dimethyl-2-butynylamine hydrochloride.

UNII-HK1HKT378E; UNII-GU9MLT8VE0 [intriptyline]. *CAS-27466-29-1; CAS-27466-27-9* [intriptyline]. *Antidepressant.* ◇AY-22,124

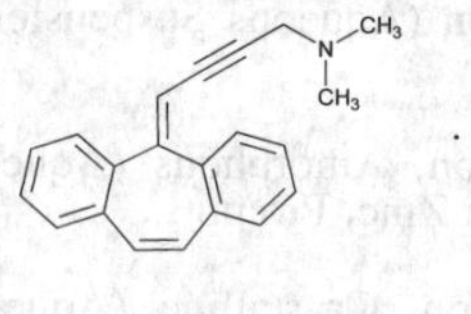

Inulin (in′ ue lin). **USP.** $C_6H_{11}O_5(C_6H_{10}O_5)_nOH$. (1) Inulin; (2) Inulin. *CAS-9005-80-5.* BAN. *Diagnostic aid (renal function determination).*

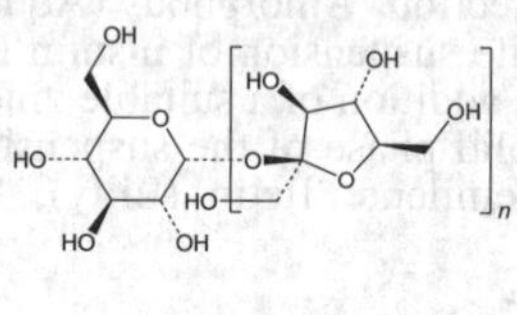

Iobenguane I 123 (eye″ oh ben′ gwane). **USP** [Injection]. $(C_8H_{10}{}^{123}IN_3)_2 \cdot H_2SO_4$. (1) [[3-(Iodo-^{123}I)-phenyl]methyl]-guanidine sulfate (2:1); (2) (*m*-Iodo-^{123}I)-benzyl)guanidine sulfate (2:1). *CAS-139755-80-9. Radioactive agent.*

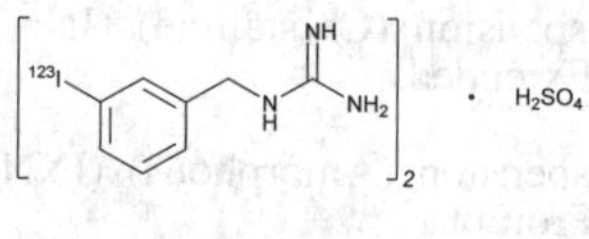

Iobenguane I 131 [*1997*] (eye″ oh ben′ gwane). **USP** [Injection]. $(C_8H_{10}{}^{131}IN_3)_2 \cdot H_2SO_4$. [Iobenguane (^{131}I) is INN.] (1) Guanidine, [[3-(iodo-^{131}I)phenyl]methyl]-; (2) (*m*-[^{131}I]Iodobenzyl)guanidine. *UNII-Q461L7AK4R. CAS-77679-27-7. Diagnostic aid; radioactive agent.*

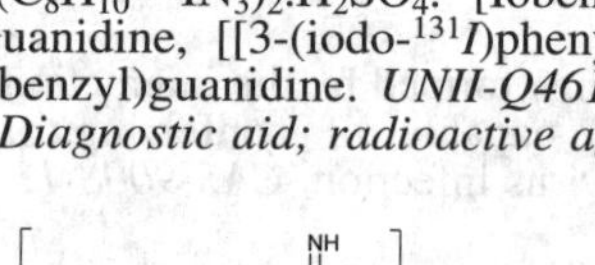

Iobenguane Sulfate I 123 [*1994*] (eye″ oh ben′ gwane sul′ fate). $(C_8H_{10}{}^{123}IN_3)_2 \cdot H_2SO_4$. (1) Guanidine, [[3-(iodo-^{123}*I*)phenyl]methyl]-, sulfate (2:1); (2) (*m*-Iodo-^{123}*I*-benzyl)guanidine sulfate (2:1). *UNII-23X1185WBO. CAS-139755-80-9; CAS-77679-27-7* [iobenguane (^{131}I)]. *Diagnostic aid (radioactive, adrenomedullary disorders and neuroendocrine tumors); radioactive agent. [Note—This radiopharmaceutical, labeled with a cyclotron-generated radionuclide, is prepared in individual nuclear medical centers.]*

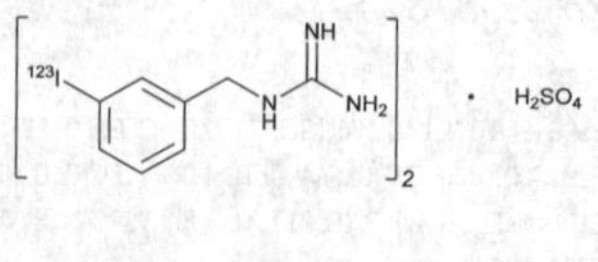

Iobenguane Sulfate I 131 [*1997*] (eye″ oh ben′ gwane sul′ fate). $(C_8H_{10}{}^{131}IN_3)_2 \cdot H_2SO_4$. (1) Guanidine, [[3-(iodo-^{131}*I*)phenyl]methyl]-, sulfate (2:1); (2) (*m*-[^{131}I]Iodobenzyl)guanidine sulfate (2:1). *UNII-M575VKV19N. CAS-149210-33-3. Diagnostic aid; radioactive agent.*

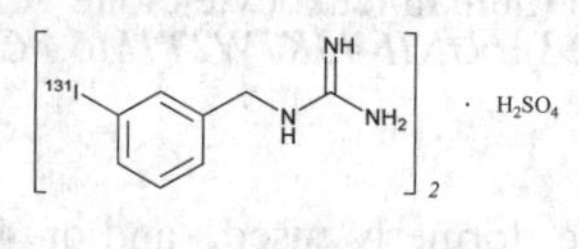

Iobenzamic Acid [*1968*] (eye″ oh ben zam′ ik as′ id). $C_{16}H_{13}I_3N_2O_3$. 662.00. (1) β-Alanine, *N*-(3-amino-2,4,6-triiodobenzoyl)-*N*-phenyl-; (2) *N*-(3-Amino-2,4,6-triiodobenzoyl)-*N*-phenyl-β-alanine. *CAS-3115-05-7*. INN; BAN; JAN. *Diagnostic aid (radiopaque medium, cholecystographic)*. Osbil (Mallinckrodt†)

Iobitridol. $C_{20}H_{28}I_3N_3O_9$. 835.16. *N,N′*-Bis(2,3-dihydroxypropyl)-5-[2-(hydroxymethyl)hydracrylamido]-2,4,6-triiodo-*N,N′*-dimethylisophthalamide. *CAS-136949-58-1*. INN; BAN.

Iobutoic Acid. $C_{15}H_{16}I_3NO_5$. 671.00. 4-[2,4,6-Triiodo-3-(morpholinocarbonyl)phenoxy]butyric acid. *UNII-ZJC1Z4E09L*. *CAS-13445-12-0*. INN; DCF.

Iocanlidic Acid (^{123}I) (INN) — *See* Iocanlidic Acid I 123.

Iocanlidic Acid I 123 [*1997*] (eye″ oh kan li′ dik as′ id). $C_{21}H_{33}{}^{123}IO_2$. [Iocanlidic Acid (^{123}I) is INN.] (1) Benzenepentadecanoic acid, 4-(iodo-^{123}I)-; (2) 15-(*p*-[^{123}I]Iodophenyl)pentadecanoic acid. *CAS-74855-17-7*. *Diagnostic aid (radioactive, cardiac disease)*.

Iocarmate Meglumine [*1977*] (eye″ oh kar′ mate me′ gloo meen). $C_{24}H_{20}I_6N_4O_8 \cdot 2C_7H_{17}NO_5$. 1644.29. [Meglumine Iocarmate is BAN.] (1) Benzoic acid, 3,3′-[(1,6-dioxo-1,6-hexanediyl)diimino]bis[2,4,6-triiodo-5-[(methylamino)carbonyl]-, compound with 1-deoxy-1-(methylamino)-D-glucitol (1:2); (2) 5,5′-(Adipoyldiimino)bis[2,4,6-triiodo-*N*-methylisophthalamic acid] compound with 1-deoxy-1-(methylamino)-D-glucitol (1:2). *UNII-2303MD51O1; UNII-82PB24K6TZ* [iocarmic acid]; *UNII-6HG8UB2MUY* [meglumine]. *CAS-54605-45-7; CAS-10397-75-8* [iocarmic acid]; *CAS-6284-40-8* [meglumine]. *Diagnostic aid (radiopaque medium)*. Dimeray (Mallinckrodt†) ◇*MP 2032-Meglumine*

Iocarmic Acid [*1973*] (eye″ oh kar′ mik as′ id). $C_{24}H_{20}I_6N_4O_8$. 1253.86. (1) Benzoic acid, 3,3′-[(1,6-dioxo-1,6-hexanediyl)diimino]bis[2,4,6-triiodo-5-[(methylamino)carbonyl]-; (2) 5,5′-(Adipoyldiimino)bis[2,4,6-triiodo-*N*-methylisophthalamic acid]. *UNII-82PB24K6TZ*. *CAS-10397-75-8*. INN; BAN. *Diagnostic aid (radiopaque medium)*. ◇*MP 2032*

Iocetamic Acid [*1969*] (eye′ oh see tam′ ik as′ id). $C_{12}H_{13}I_3N_2O_3$. 613.96. (1) Propanoic acid, 3-[acetyl(3-amino-2,4,6-triiodophenyl)amino]-2-methyl-; (2) *N*-Acetyl-*N*-(3-amino-2,4,6-triiodophenyl)-2-methyl-β-alanine. *UNII-FA675Q0E3E*. *CAS-16034-77-8*. USP XXIII; INN; BAN. *Diagnostic aid (radiopaque medium)*. Cholebrine (Mallinckrodt) ◇*MP-620*

Iodamide [*1968*] (eye oh′ da mide). $C_{12}H_{11}I_3N_2O_4$. 627.94. (1) Benzoic acid, 3-(acetylamino)-5-[(acetylamino)methyl]-2,4,6-triiodo-; (2) α,5-Diacetamido-2,4,6-triiodo-*m*-toluic acid. *UNII-4RII332OOR*. *CAS-440-58-4*. INN; BAN; JAN. *Diagnostic aid (radiopaque medium)*. Jodomiron (Bracco Industria Chimica S.p.A., Italy); Uromiro (Bracco Industria Chimica S.p.A., Italy); Uromiron (Bracco Industria Chimica S.p.A., Italy) ◇*B-4130; SH 926*

Iodamide Meglumine [*1977*] (eye oh′ da mide me′ gloo meen). $C_{12}H_{11}I_3N_2O_4 \cdot C_7H_{17}NO_5$. 823.15. [Meglumine Iodamide Injection and Meglumine Sodium Iodamide Injection are JAN.] (1) Benzoic acid, 3-(acetylamino)-5-[(acetylamino)methyl]-2,4,6-triiodo-, compound with 1-deoxy-1-(methylamino)-D-glucitol (1:1); (2) α,5-Diacetamido-2,4,6-triiodo-*m*-toluic acid compound with 1-deoxy-1-(methylamino)-D-glucitol (1:1). *UNII-6X283535A3; UNII-4RII332OOR* [iodamide]; *UNII-6HG8UB2MUY* [meglumine]. *CAS-18656-21-8; CAS-440-58-4* [iodamide]; *CAS-6284-40-8* [meglumine]. *Diagnostic aid (radiopaque medium)*. Renovue (Bracco)

---

† Brand name formerly used, and/or firm no longer concerned with this product.

Iodecimol. $C_{35}H_{44}I_6N_6O_{16}$. 1566.18. 5,5′-[Malonylbis[(2-hydroxyethyl)imino]]bis[*N,N*′-bis[2-hydroxy-1-(hydroxymethyl)ethyl]-2,4,6-triiodoisophthalamide]. *UNII-3SDG4RSP99. CAS-81045-33-2*. INN.

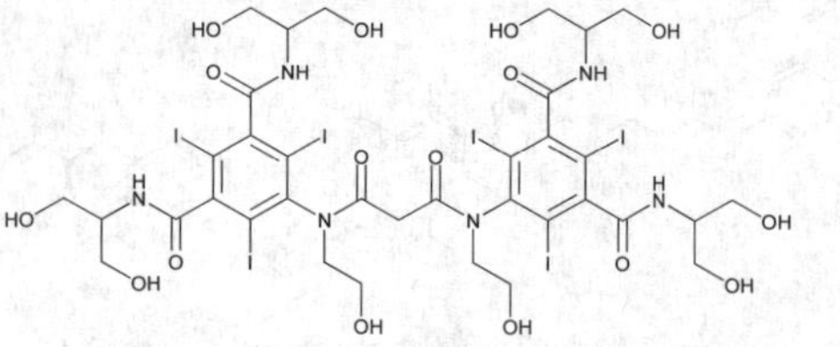

Iodecol — *See* Iodecimol.

Iodetryl. $C_{20}H_{38}I_2O_2$. 564.32. Ethyl 9,10-diiodo-octadecanoate. *CAS-7008-02-8*. INN; DCF.

Iodinated I 125 Albumin (eye′ oh di nay″ ted al bue′ min). **USP** [Injection]. Albumin labeled with iodine-125. *Diagnostic aid (blood volume determination); radioactive agent.*

Iodinated I 131 Albumin (eye′ oh di nay″ ted al bue′ min). **USP** [Injection]. Albumin labeled with iodine-131. *Diagnostic aid (blood volume determination); diagnostic aid (intrathecal imaging); radioactive agent.*

Iodinated I 131 Albumin Aggregated (eye′ oh di nay″ ted al bue′ min ag′ re gay″ ted). **USP** [Injection]. Albumin labeled with iodine-131. *Radioactive agent.*

Iodine (eye″ oh dine). **USP.** I_2. 253.81. (1) Iodine; (2) Iodine. *UNII-9679TC07X4. CAS-7553-56-2.* JAN. *Anti-infective, topical.*

Iodine Povacrylex [*2005*] (eye″ oh dine poe″ va krye′ lex). $[(C_5H_8O_2)_{n1}\cdot(C_6H_9NO)_{n2}\cdot(C_{11}H_{20}O_2)_{n3}]_x\cdot xNa.xI_2$. (1) 2-Propenoic acid, 2-methyl-, methyl ester, polymer with 1-ethenyl-2-pyrrolidinone and isooctyl 2-propenoate, compound with iodine and sodium iodide (NaI); (2) Methyl 2-methylprop-2-enoate polymer with 1-ethenylpyrrolidin-2-one and isooctyl prop-2-enoate compound with diiodine and sodium iodide. Molecular weight is approximately 520,000 daltons. *CAS-845736-10-9. Topical antiseptic.* Duraprep copolymer (3M Specialty Materials)

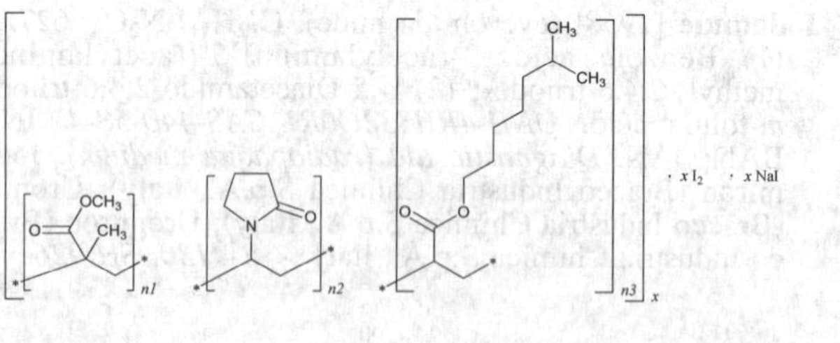

Iodipamide (eye″ oh dip′ a mide). **USP.** $C_{20}H_{14}I_6N_2O_6$. 1139.76. [Adipiodone is INN, BAN and JAN.] (1) Benzoic acid, 3,3′-[(1,6-dioxo-1,6-hexanediyl)diimino]bis[2,4,6-triiodo-; (2) 3,3′-(Adipoyldiimino)bis[2,4,6-triiodobenzoic acid]. *UNII-TKQ858A3VW. CAS-606-17-7.* Pharmaceutic necessity for Iodipamide Meglumine [Injection]. Cholografin (Bristol-Myers Squibb†)

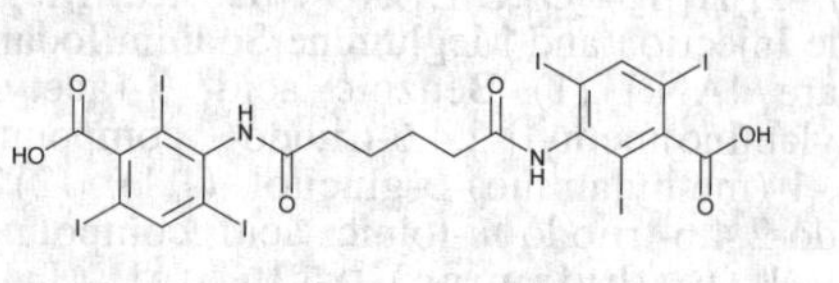

Iodipamide Meglumine (eye″ oh dip′ a mide me′ gloo meen). **USP** [Injection]. $C_{20}H_{14}I_6N_2O_6\cdot2C_7H_{17}NO_5$. 1530.19. [Adipiodone Meglumine Injection is JAN.] (1) Benzoic acid, 3,3′-[(1,6-dioxo-1,6-hexanediyl)diimino]bis[2,4,6-triiodo-, compd. with 1-deoxy-1-(methylamino)-D-glucitol (1:2); (2) 1-Deoxy-1-(methylamino)-D-glucitol 3,3′-(adipoyldiimino)bis[2,4,6-triiodobenzoate] (2:1) (salt). *UNII-6HG8UB2-MUY* [meglumine]. *CAS-3521-84-4; CAS-606-17-7* [iodipamide]; *CAS-6284-40-8* [meglumine]. *Diagnostic aid (radiopaque medium).* Cholografin Meglumine (Bracco)

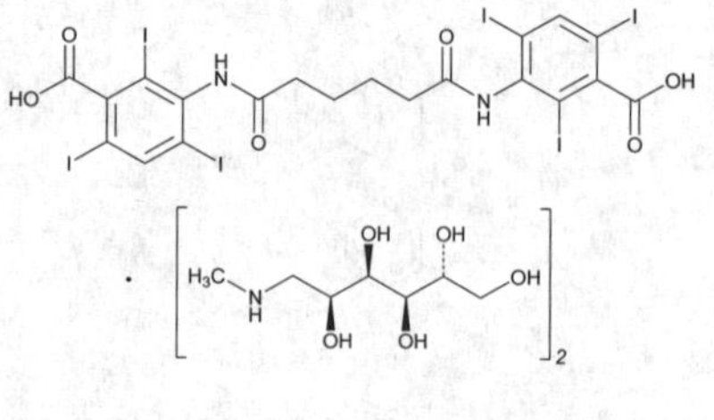

Iodipamide Methylglucamine Injection — *See* Iodipamide Meglumine.

Iodipamide Sodium. *UNII-3J6WZA9PXS. CAS-2618-26-0; CAS-606-17-7* [iodipamide]. USP XVIII. Cholografin Sodium (Bracco)

Iodipamide Sodium I 131 [*1963*] (eye″ oh dip′ a mide soe′ dee um). $C_{20}H_{12}{}^{131}I_6N_2Na_2O_6$. (1) Benzoic acid, 3,3′-[(1,6-dioxo-1,6-hexanediyl)diimino]bis[2,4,6-tri(iodo-^{131}I)-, disodium salt; (2) Disodium 3,3′-(adipoyldiimino)bis[2,4,6-triiodi-^{131}I-benzoate]. *CAS-24360-85-8. Radioactive agent.* Radio-Cholografin (Bristol-Myers Squibb†)

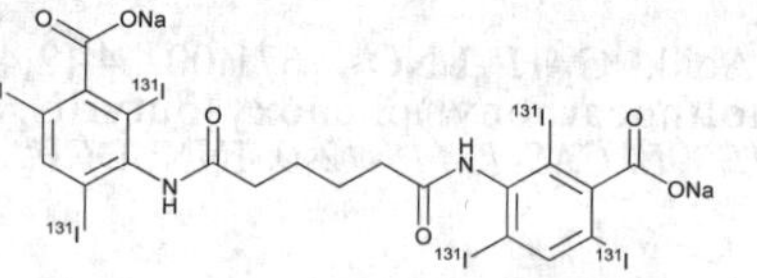

Iodisan — *See* Prolonium Iodide.

Iodixanol [*1990*] (eye″ oh dix′ a nol). **USP.** $C_{35}H_{44}I_6N_6O_{15}$. 1550.18. (1) 1,3-Benzenedicarboxamide, 5,5′-[(2-hydroxy-1,3-propanediyl)bis(acetylimino)]bis[*N,N*′-bis(2,3-dihydroxypropyl)-2,4,6-triiodo-; (2) 5,5′-[(2-Hydroxytrimethylene)bis(acetylimino)]bis[*N,N*′-bis(2,3-dihydroxypropyl)-2,4,6-triiodoisophthalamide]. *UNII-HW8W27HTXX. CAS-92339-11-2.* INN; BAN. *Diagnostic aid (radiopaque medium).* Visipaque (GE Healthcare) ◇2-5410-3A

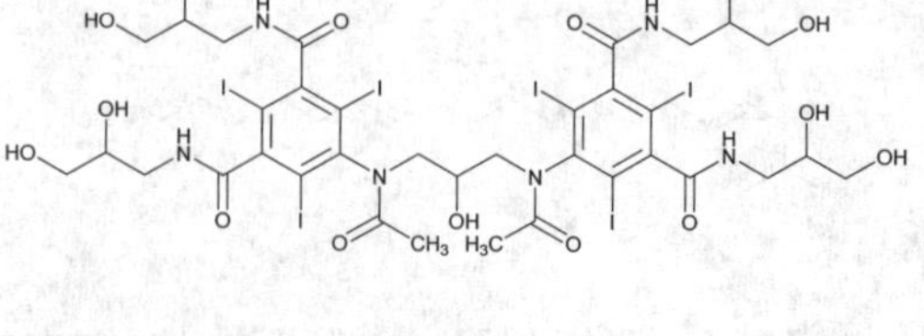

Iodized Oil. *CAS-8001-40-9.* NF XIII; MI.

Iodoalphionic Acid. $C_{15}H_{12}I_2O_3$. 494.06. [Pheniodol Sodium is INN.] 3-(4-Hydroxy-3,5-diiodophenyl)-2-phenylpropionic acid. *UNII-060B6580LL. CAS-577-91-3.* NF XII; MI. Priodax (Schering†)

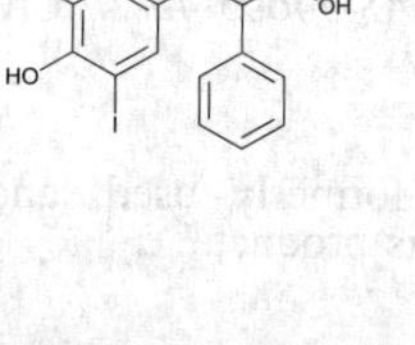

Iodoantipyrine I 131 [*1963*] (eye oh″ doe an″ tee pye′ reen). $C_{11}H_{11}{}^{131}IN_2O$. (1) 3*H*-Pyrazol-3-one, 1,2-dihydro-4-iodo-^{131}I-1,5-dimethyl-2-phenyl-; (2) 4-Iodo-^{131}I-antipyrine. *UNII-QR6HQ1U73Z. CAS-3791-63-7. Radioactive agent.*

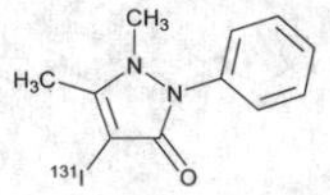

Iodobehenate Calcium. Calcium iododocosanoate. NF X.

Iodobenzylguanidine Sulfate I 123 — *See* Iobenguane Sulfate I 123.

Iodocetylic Acid I 123 [*1981*] (eye oh″ doe see′ til ik as′ id). $C_{16}H_{31}{}^{123}IO_2$. [Iodocetylic Acid (^{123}I) is INN.] (1) Hexadecanoic acid, 16-(iodo-^{123}I)-; (2) 16-Iodo-^{123}I-hexadecanoic acid. *CAS-54510-20-2. Diagnostic aid; radioactive agent.* ◇*RA-C-384*

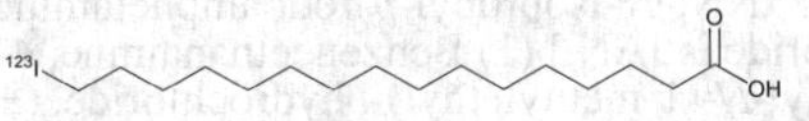

Iodochlorhydroxyquin (previously used name) — *See* Clioquinol.

Iodocholesterol (^{131}I) (INN) — *See* Iodocholesterol I 131.

Iodocholesterol I 131 [*1978*] (eye oh″ doe koe les′ ter ol). $C_{27}H_{45}{}^{131}IO$. [Iodocholesterol (^{131}I) is INN.] (1) Cholest-5-en-3-ol, 19(iodo-^{131}I)-, (3β)-; (2) 19-Iodo-^{131}Icholest-5-en-3β-ol. *CAS-42220-21-3. Radioactive agent.*

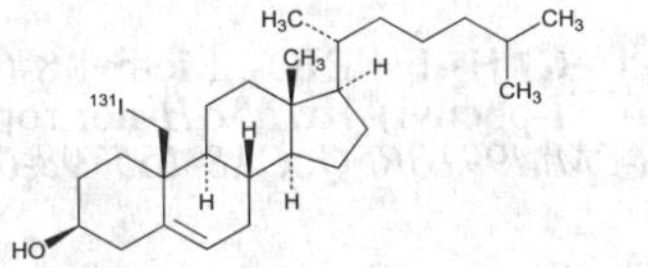

Iodofenphos. $C_8H_8Cl_2IO_3PS$. 413.00. *O*-(2,5-Dichloro-4-iodophenyl) *O,O*-dimethyl phosphorothioate. *UNII-SME6G1846X. CAS-18181-70-9.* BAN.

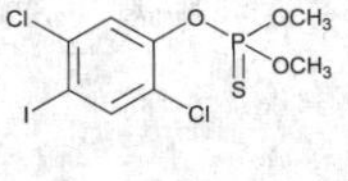

Iodofiltic Acid I 123 [*2006*] (eye″ oh doe fil′ tik as′ id). $C_{22}H_{35}[{}^{123}I]O_2$. 454.40. (1) Benzenepentadecanoic acid, 4-(iodo-^{123}I)-β-methyl-; (2) (3*RS*)-15-(4-[^{123}I]iodophenyl)-3-methylpentadecanoic acid. *UNII-0J7USQ749M. CAS-123748-56-1.* INN. *Metabolic imaging pharmaceutical for detection of ischemic myocardium.* Zemiva (Molecular Insight) ◇*BMIPP*

Iodoform (eye oh′ doe form). **USP.** CHI_3. 393.73. Triiodomethane. *UNII-KXI2J76489. CAS-75-47-8.* JAN; MI.

Iodohippurate Sodium I 123 [*1978*] (eye oh″ doe hip′ ure ate soe′ dee um). **USP** [Injection]. $C_9H_7{}^{123}INNaO_3$. [Sodium *o*-Iodo-^{123}I-Hippurate is JAN.] (1) Glycine, *N*-[2-(iodo-^{123}I)benzoyl]-, monosodium salt; (2) Sodium *o*-iodo-^{123}I-

hippurate. *UNII-4NW20GFQ7H. CAS-56254-07-0. Diagnostic aid (renal function determination); radioactive agent.* Nephroflow (Medi-Physics†)

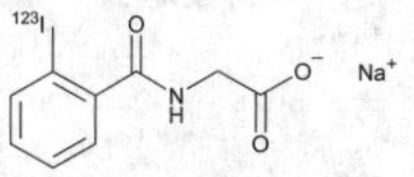

Iodohippurate Sodium I 125 [*1964*] (eye oh″ doe hip′ ure ate soe′ dee um). $C_9H_7{}^{125}INNaO_3$. (1) Glycine, *N*-[2-(iodo-^{125}I)benzoyl]-, monosodium salt; (2) Monosodium *o*-iodo-^{125}I-hippurate. *UNII-T5536Q4O60. CAS-7230-65-1. Radioactive agent.* Hippuran-125 (Abbott†); Hippuran I 125 (Mallinckrodt†); Hipputope I-125 (Bristol-Myers Squibb†)

Iodohippurate Sodium I 131 [*1963*] (eye oh″ doe hip′ ure ate soe′ dee um). **USP** [Injection]. $C_9H_7{}^{131}INNaO_3$. [Sodium Iodohippurate (^{131}I) is INN; Sodium Iodohippurate (^{131}I) Injection is JAN.] (1) Glycine, *N*-[2-(iodo-^{131}I)benzoyl]-, monosodium salt; (2) Monosodium *o*-iodo-^{131}I-hippurate. *UNII-9BRV734R3E. CAS-881-17-4. Diagnostic aid (renal function determination); radioactive agent.* Hippuran-131 (Abbott†); Hippuran I 131 (Mallinckrodt); Hipputope (Bristol-Myers Squibb†)

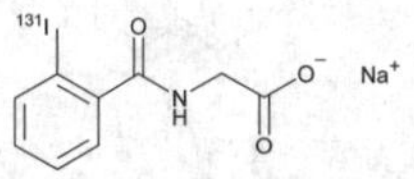

Iodol. C_4HI_4N. 570.68. 2,3,4,5-Tetraiodopyrrole. *UNII-35ZC5024YS. CAS-87-58-1.* USP VIII; MI.

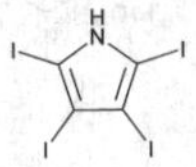

Iodolecithine. JAN.

Iodomethamate Sodium. $C_8H_3I_2NNa_2O_5$. 492.90. 1,4-Dihydro-3,5-diiodo-1-methyl-4-oxo-2,6-pyridinedicarboxylic acid, disodium salt. *UNII-EER9874LXT. CAS-519-26-6; CAS-1951-53-7* [iodomethamate]. NF XII. Neo-Iopax (Schering†)

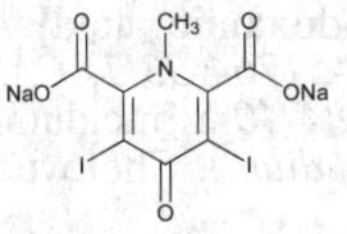

Iodopanoic Acid — *See* Iopanoic Acid.

Iodophthalein Sodium. $C_{20}H_8I_4Na_2O_4$. 865.87. Disodium salt of tetraiodophenolphthalein. *CAS-632-73-5; CAS-386-17-4* [iodophthalein]. NF XI; INN; MI. [*Name previously used: Iodophthalein, Soluble.*]

Iodophthalein, Soluble (previously used name) — *See* Iodophthalein Sodium.

Iodopyracet. $C_{11}H_{16}I_2N_2O_5$. 510.06. [Diodone is INN.] 3,5-Diiodo-4-oxo-1-(4*H*)-pyridineacetic acid 2,2′-iminodiethanol (1:1) compound. *UNII-ZTK4026YJ5.* NF XIII; MI. Diodrast (Sterling Winthrop†)

Iodopyracet I 125 [*1964*] (eye oh″ doe pye′ ra set). $C_{11}H_{16}{}^{125}I_2N_2O_5$. (1) 1(4*H*)-Pyridineacetic acid, 3,5-di(iodo-^{125}I)-4-oxo-, compd. with 2,2′-iminobis[ethanol] (1:1); (2) 3,5-Diiodo-^{125}I-4-oxo-1(4*H*)-pyridineacetic acid, compound with 2,2′-iminodiethanol (1:1). *Radioactive agent.*

Iodopyracet I 131 [*1963*] (eye oh″ doe pye′ ra set). $C_{11}H_{16}{}^{131}I_2N_2O_5$. (1) 1(4*H*)-Pyridineacetic acid, 3,5-di(iodo-^{131}I)-4-oxo-, compd. with 2,2′-iminobis[ethanol] (1:1); (2) 3,5-Diiodo-^{131}I-4-oxo-1(4*H*)-pyridineacetic acid, compound with 2,2′-iminodiethanol (1:1). *Radioactive agent.*

Iodoquinol [*1980*] (eye oh″ doe kwin′ ol). **USP.** $C_9H_5I_2NO$. 396.95. [Diiodohydroxyquinoline is INN and BAN.] (1) 8-Quinolinol, 5,7-diiodo-; (2) 5,7-Diiodo-8-quinolinol. *UNII-63W7IE88K8. CAS-83-73-8. Anti-amebic.* Ioquin (Abbott†); Quinadome (Bayer†); Yodoxin (Glenwood) *[Name previously used: Diiodohydroxyquin.]*

Iodothiouracil. $C_4H_3IN_2OS$. 254.05. 5-Iodo-2-thiouracil. *UNII-61O17612T5. CAS-5984-97-4. INN; BAN.*

Iodothymol — *See* Thymol Iodide.

Iodoxamate Meglumine [*1979*] (eye oh dox′ a mate me′ gloo meen). $C_{26}H_{26}I_6N_2O_{10}\cdot2C_7H_{17}NO_5$. 1678.35. (1) Benzoic acid, 3,3′-[(1,16-dioxo-4,7,10,13-tetraoxahexadecane-1,16-diyl)diimino]bis[2,4,6-triiodo-, compound with 1-deoxy-1-(methylamino)-D-glucitol (1:2); (2) 3,3′-[Ethylenebis(oxyethyleneoxyethylenecarbonylimino)]bis[2,4,6-triiodobenzoic acid] compound with 1-deoxy-1-(methylamino)-D-glucitol (1:2). *UNII-CIX5G6J9R1; UNII-NS1Y283HW4 [iodoxamic acid]; UNII-6HG8UB2MUY [meglumine]. CAS-51764-33-1; CAS-31127-82-9 [iodoxamic acid]; CAS-6284-40-8 [meglumine]. BAN. Diagnostic aid (radiopaque medium).* Cholovue (Bracco)

Iodoxamic Acid [*1974*] (eye″ oh dox am′ ik as′ id). $C_{26}H_{26}I_6N_2O_{10}$. 1287.92. (1) Benzoic acid, 3,3′-[(1,16-dioxo-4,7,10,13-tetraoxahexadecane-1,16-diyl)diimino]-bis[2,4,6-triiodo-; (2) 3,3′-[Ethylenebis(oxyethyleneoxyethylenecarbonylimino)]bis[2,4,6-triiodobenzoic acid]. *UNII-NS1Y283HW4. CAS-31127-82-9. INN; BAN; JAN. Diagnostic aid (radiopaque medium).* Endobil (Bracco

Industria Chimica S.p.A., Italy); Endomirabil (Bracco Industria Chimica S.p.A., Italy); Videocolangio (Bracco Industria Chimica S.p.A., Italy) ◇*SQ 21982; B 10610*

Iodoxyl — *See* Iodomethamate Sodium.

Iofendylate (INN, BAN) — *See* Iophendylate.

Iofetamine (^{123}I) (INN) — *See* Iofetamine Hydrochloride I 123.

Iofetamine Hydrochloride I 123 [*1984*] (eye″ oh fet′ a meen hye″ droe klor′ ide). $C_{12}H_{18}{}^{123}IN\cdot HCl$. 335.74. [Iofetamine ($^{123}I$) is INN; *N*-Isopropyl-*p*-Iodoamphetamine (^{123}I) Hydrochloride is JAN.] (1) Benzeneethanamine, 4-(iodo-^{123}I)-α-methyl-*N*-(1-methylethyl)-, hydrochloride, (±)-; (2) (±)-*p*-Iodo-^{123}I-*N*-isopropyl-α-methylphenethylamine hydrochloride; (3) [^{123}I](±)-*N*-Isopropyl-*p*-iodoamphetamine hydrochloride. *UNII-R5O1XB5L3M. CAS-85068-76-4. Diagnostic aid; radioactive agent.* ◇^{123}I-M123; ^{123}I labeled IMP

Ioflupane (^{123}I). $C_{18}H_{23}F^{123}INO_2$. Methyl 8-(3-fluoropropyl)-3β-(*p*-iodo-^{123}I-phenyl)-1α*H*,5α*H*-nortropane-2β-carboxylate. *UNII-3MM99T8R5Q. CAS-155798-07-5. INN; BAN.*

Iofratol. $C_{31}H_{36}I_6N_6O_{13}$. 1462.08. *N,N″*-(2-Hydroxytrimethylene)bis[*N′*-[2-hydroxy-1-(hydroxymethyl)ethyl]-2,4,6-triiodo-5-[(*S*)-lactamido]isophthalamide]. *CAS-141660-63-1. INN.*

Ioglicic Acid [*1975*] (eye″ oh gli′ sik as′ id). $C_{13}H_{12}I_3N_3O_5$. 670.96. (1) Benzoic acid, 3-(acetylamino)-2,4,6-triiodo-5-[[[2-(methylamino)-2-oxoethyl]amino]carbonyl]-; (2) 5-Acetamido-2,4,6-triiodo-*N*-[(methylcarbamoyl)methyl]isophthalamic acid. *UNII-3LGR5S8101. CAS-49755-67-1. INN; BAN. Diagnostic aid (radiopaque medium).* ✧*SH H 200 AB*

Ioglucol [*1979*] (eye″ oh gloo′ kol). $C_{18}H_{24}I_3N_3O_9$. 807.11. (1) D-Gluconamide, *N*-[3-[acetyl(2-hydroxyethyl)amino]-2,4,6-triiodo-5-[(methylamino)carbonyl]phenyl]-; (2) 3′-[*N*-(2-Hydroxyethyl)acetamido]-2′,4′,6′-triiodo-5′-(methyl-carbamoyl)-D-gluconanilide. *UNII-ZZU2X307FG. CAS-63941-73-1. INN. Diagnostic aid (radiopaque medium).* ✧*MP-6026*

Ioglucomide [*1979*] (eye″ oh gloo′ koe mide). $C_{20}H_{28}I_3N_3O_{13}$. 899.16. (1) D-Gluconamide, *N,N′*-[2,4,6-triiodo-5-[(methy-lamino)carbonyl]-1,3-phenylene]bis-; (2) *N,N′*-[2,4,6-Triiodo-5-(methylcarbamoyl)-*m*-phenylene]bis[D-glucona-mide]. *CAS-63941-74-2. INN. Diagnostic aid (radiopaque medium).* ✧*MP-8000*

Ioglunide. $C_{18}H_{24}I_3N_3O_9$. 807.11. 3′-[(2-Hydroxyethyl)car-bamoyl]-2′,4′,6′-triiodo-5′-(*N*-methylacetamido-D-gluco-anilide. *CAS-56562-79-9. INN.*

Ioglycamic Acid [*1964*] (eye″ oh glye kam′ ik as′ id). $C_{18}H_{10}I_6N_2O_7$. 1127.71. (1) Benzoic acid, 3,3′-[oxybis[(1-oxo-2,1-ethanediyl)imino]]bis[2,4,6-triiodo-; (2) 3,3′-(Di-glycoloyldiimino)bis[2,4,6-triiodobenzoic acid]. *UNII-ET36GPP4T7. CAS-2618-25-9. INN; BAN. Diagnostic aid (radiopaque medium, cholecystographic).* ✧*BE 419*

Iogulamide [*1981*] (eye″ oh gul′ a mide). $C_{20}H_{26}I_3N_3O_{12}$. 881.15. (1) 1,3-Benzenedicarboxamide, *N,N′*-bis(2,3-dihy-droxypropyl)-5-[(L-*xylo*-2-hexulosonoyl)amino]-2,4,6-triiodo-; (2) *N,N′*-Bis(2,3-dihydroxypropyl)-5-L-*xylo*-2-hexulosonamido-2,4,6-triiodoisophthalamide. *CAS-75751-89-2. Diagnostic aid (radiopaque medium).* ✧*MP-10013*

Iohexol [*1980*] (eye″ oh hex′ ol). **USP.** $C_{19}H_{26}I_3N_3O_9$. 821.14. (1) 1,3-Benzenedicarboxamide, 5-[acetyl(2,3-dihydroxy-propyl)amino]-*N,N′*-bis(2,3-dihydroxypropyl)-2,4,6-triio-do; (2) *N,N′*-Bis(2,3-dihydroxypropyl)-5-[*N*-(2,3-dihydroxypropyl)acetamido]-2,4,6-triiodoisophthalamide. *UNII-4419T9MX03. CAS-66108-95-0. INN; BAN; JAN. Diagnostic aid (radiopaque medium).* Omnipaque (GE Healthcare) ✧*Win 39424*

Iolidonic Acid. $C_{15}H_{16}I_3NO_3$. 639.01. α-Ethyl-2,4,6-triiodo-3-(2-oxo-1-pyrrolidinyl)hydrocinnamic acid. *UNII-B1H5V6OZSE. CAS-21766-53-0. INN.*

Iolixanic Acid. $C_{15}H_{18}I_3NO_5$. 673.02. 2-[2-[3-(*N*-Ethyl-acetamido)-2,4,6-triiodophenoxy]ethoxy]propionic acid. *CAS-22730-86-5. INN.*

Iolopride (^{123}I). $C_{15}H_{21}{}^{123}IN_2O_3$. *N*-[[(2*S*)-1-Ethyl-2-pyrroli-dinyl]methyl]-6-hydroxy-5-([^{123}I]iodo)-*o*-anisamide. *CAS-113716-48-6. INN.*

Iomazenil (^{123}I). $C_{15}H_{14}{}^{123}IN_3O_3$. Ethyl 5,6-dihydro-7-iodo-^{123}I-5-methyl-6-oxo-4H-imidazo[1,5-a][1,4]benzodiazepine-3-carboxylate. *CAS-127396-36-5*. INN.

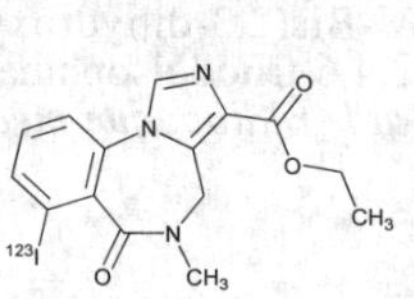

Iomeglamic Acid. $C_{12}H_{13}I_3N_2O_3$. 613.96. 3′-Amino-2′,4′,6′-triiodo-N-methylglutaranilic acid. *UNII-S4H62451TO*. *CAS-25827-76-3*. INN; MI. ◇$RG\ 270$

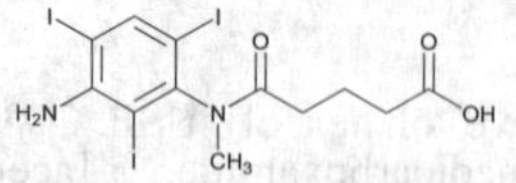

Iomeprol [*1989*] (eye″ oh me′ prole). $C_{17}H_{22}I_3N_3O_8$. 777.09. (1) 1,3-Benzenedicarboxamide, N,N'-bis(2,3-dihydroxypropyl)-5-[(hydroxyacetyl)methylamino]-2,4,6-triiodo-; (2) N,N'-Bis(2,3-dihydroxypropyl)-2,4,6-triiodo-5-(N-methylglycolamido)isophthalamide. *CAS-78649-41-9*. INN; BAN; JAN. *Diagnostic aid (radiopaque medium).*

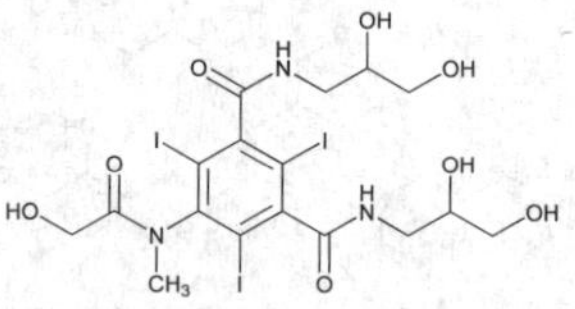

Iomethin I 125 [*1969*] (eye″ oh meth′ in). $C_{14}H_{18}{}^{125}IN_3$. Some of the iodine atoms are ^{125}I. [Iometin (^{125}I) is INN.] (1) 1,3-Propanediamine, N'-(7-iodo-^{125}I-4-quinolinyl)-N,N-dimethyl-; (2) 4-[[3-(Dimethylamino)propyl]amino]-7-iodo-^{125}I-quinoline. *CAS-17033-82-8*. *Diagnostic aid (neoplasm); radioactive agent.* ◇$125\ I\ NM$-113

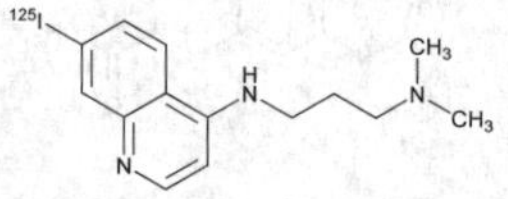

Iomethin I 131 [*1969*] (eye″ oh meth′ in). $C_{14}H_{18}{}^{131}IN_3$. Some of the iodine atoms are ^{131}I. [Iometin (^{131}I) is INN.] (1) 1,3-Propanediamine, N'-(7-iodo-^{131}I-4-quinolinyl)-N,N-dimethyl-; (2) 4-[[3-(Dimethylamino)propyl]amino]-7-iodo-^{131}I-quinoline. *CAS-17033-83-9*. *Diagnostic aid (neoplasm); radioactive agent.* ◇$131\ I\ NM$-113

Iometin (^{125}I) (INN) — *See* Iomethin I 125.

Iometin (^{131}I) (INN) — *See* Iomethin I 131.

Iometopane I 123 [*1997*] (eye″ oh me toe′ pane). $C_{16}H_{20}{}^{123}INO_2$. [Iometopane ^{123}I is INN.] (1) 8-Azabicyclo[3.2.1]octane-2-carboxylic acid, 3-[4-(iodo-^{123}I)phenyl]-8-methyl-, methyl ester, [1R-(exo,exo)]-; (2) Methyl 3β-(p-[^{123}I]iodophenyl-1αH,5αH-tropane-2β-carboxylate. *CAS-136794-86-0*. *Diagnostic aid.* Dopascan (Guilford) ◇GPI-200

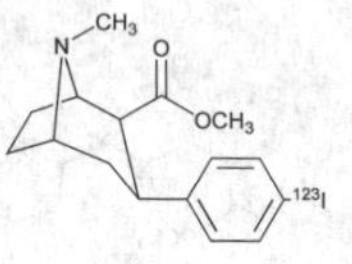

Iomorinic Acid. $C_{17}H_{20}I_3N_3O_4$. 711.07. 2-Methyl-N-[2,4,6-triiodo-3-[(1-morpholinoethylidene)amino]benzoyl]-β-alanine. *CAS-51934-76-0*. INN.

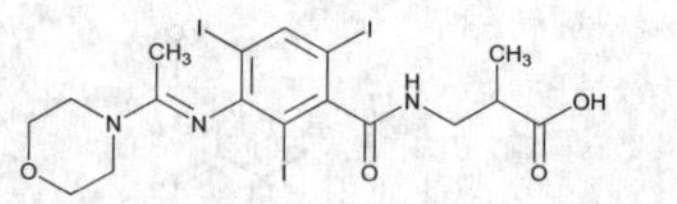

Iopamidol [*1979*] (eye″ oh pam′ i dol). **USP**. $C_{17}H_{22}I_3N_3O_8$. 777.09. (1) 1,3-Benzenedicarboxamide, N,N'-bis[2-hydroxy-1-(hydroxymethyl)ethyl]-5-[(2-hydroxy-1-oxopropyl)amino]-2,4,6-triiodo-, (S)-; (2) (S)-N,N'-bis[2-Hydroxy-1-(hydroxymethyl)ethyl]-2,4,6-triiodo-5-lactamidoisophthalamide. *UNII-JR13W81H44*. *CAS-60166-93-0*. INN; BAN; JAN. *Diagnostic aid (radiopaque medium).* Isovue (Bracco) ◇$SQ\ 13,396$

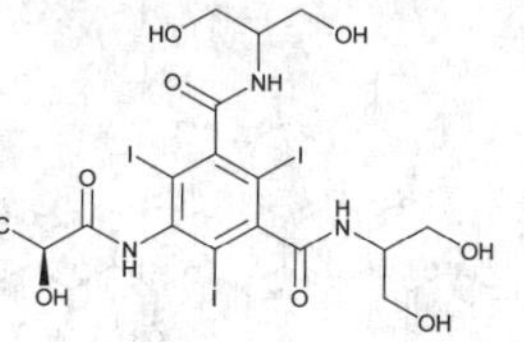

Iopanoic Acid (eye″ oh pa noe′ ik as′ id). **USP**. $C_{11}H_{12}I_3NO_2$. 570.93. (1) Benzenepropanoic acid, 3-amino-α-ethyl-2,4,6-triiodo-, ($\pm$)-; (2) (pm)-3-Amino-α-ethyl-2,4,6-triiodohydrocinnamic acid. *UNII-FE9794P71J*. *CAS-96-83-3*. INN; BAN; JAN. *Diagnostic aid (radiopaque medium).* Telepaque (GE Healthcare)

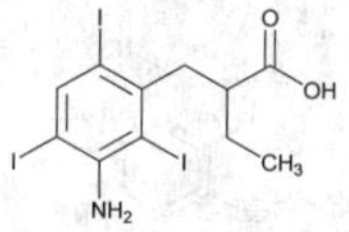

Iopentol [*1987*] (eye″ oh pen′ tol). $C_{20}H_{28}I_3N_3O_9$. 835.16. (1) 1,3-Benzenedicarboxamide, 5-[acetyl(2-hydroxy-3-methoxypropyl)amino]-N,N'-bis(2,3-dihydroxypropyl)-2,4,6-triiodo-; (2) N,N'-Bis(2,3-dihydroxypropyl)-5-[N-(2-hydroxy-3-methoxypropyl)acetamido]-2,4,6-triiodoisophthalamide. *CAS-89797-00-2*. INN; BAN. *Diagnostic aid (radiopaque medium).* ◇$Cpd.\ 5411$

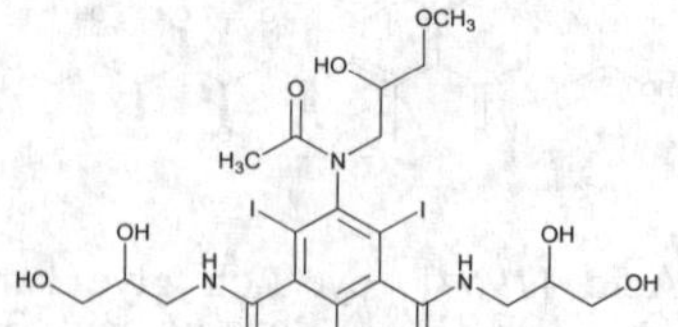

Iophendylate (eye″ oh fen′ di late). **USP**. $C_{19}H_{29}IO_2$. 416.34. [Iofendylate is INN and BAN.] (1) Benzenedecanoic acid, iodo-ι-methyl-, ethyl ester; (2) Ethyl 10-(iodophenyl)undecanoate. *CAS-1320-11-2*. *Diagnostic aid (radiopaque medium).* Pantopaque (Alcon)

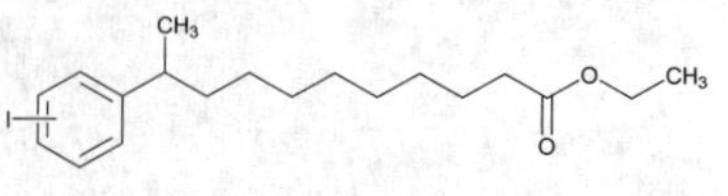

Iophenoic Acid (INN) — *See* Iophenoxic Acid.

Iophenoxic Acid. $C_{11}H_{11}I_3O_3$. 571.92. [Iophenoic Acid is INN.] α-Ethyl-3-hydroxy-2,4,6-triiodohydrocinnamic acid. *CAS-96-84-4*. USP XVI; MI. Teridax (Schering†)

Ioprocemic Acid [*1980*] (eye″ oh proe see′ mik as′ id). $C_{13}H_{14}I_3NO_3$. 612.97. (1) Benzenepropanoic acid, 3-(acetylethylamino)-2,4,6-triiodo-; (2) 3-(*N*-Ethylacetamido)-2,4,6-triiodohydrocinnamic acid. *UNII-BD20Y3892A. CAS-1456-52-6*. INN. *Diagnostic aid (radiopaque medium).* ◇*ZK 10 720*

Iopromide [*1995*] (eye oh′ proe mide). **USP.** $C_{18}H_{24}I_3N_3O_8$. 791.11. (1) 1,3-Benzenedicarboxamide, *N*,*N*′-bis(2,3-dihydroxypropyl)-2,4,6-triiodo-5-[(methoxyacetyl)amino]-*N*-methyl-; (2) *N*,*N*′-Bis(2,3-dihydroxypropyl)-2,4,6-triiodo-5-(2-methoxyacetamido)-*N*-methylisophthalamide. *UNII-712BAC33MZ. CAS-73334-07-3*. INN; BAN; MI. *Diagnostic aid (radiopaque medium).* Ultravist (Bayer) ◇*ZK 35760*

Iopronic Acid [*1974*] (eye″ oh proe′ nik as′ id). $C_{15}H_{18}I_3NO_5$. 673.02. (1) Butanoic acid, 2-[[2-[3-(acetylamino)-2,4,6-triiodophenoxy]ethoxy]methyl]-, (±)-; (2) (±)-2-[[2-(3-Acetamido-2,4,6-triiodophenoxy)ethoxy]methyl]butyric acid. *CAS-37723-78-7*. INN; BAN. *Diagnostic aid (radiopaque medium, cholecystographic).* Bilimiro (Bracco Industria Chimica S.p.A., Italy); Bilimiron (Bracco Industria Chimica S.p.A., Italy); Oravue (Bristol-Myers Squibb†); Videobil (Bracco Industria Chimica S.p.A., Italy) ◇*SQ 21983; B 11420*

Iopydol [*1963*] (eye″ oh pye′ dol). $C_8H_9I_2NO_3$. 420.97. (1) 4(1*H*)-Pyridinone, 1-(2,3-dihydroxypropyl)-3,5-diiodo-; (2) 1-(2,3-Dihydroxypropyl)-3,5-diiodo-4(1*H*)-pyridone. *UNII-T4661K682A. CAS-5579-92-0*. INN; BAN; JAN. *Diagnostic aid (radiopaque medium, bronchographic).*

Iopydone [*1963*] (eye″ oh pye′ done). $C_5H_3I_2NO$. 346.89. (1) 4(1*H*)-Pyridinone, 3,5-diiodo-; (2) 3,5-Diiodo-4(1*H*)-pyridone. *UNII-J6B56XB19T. CAS-5579-93-1*. INN; BAN; JAN. *Diagnostic aid (radiopaque medium, bronchographic).*

Iosarcol. $C_{21}H_{29}I_3N_4O_9$. 862.19. 3,5-Diacetamido-2,4,6-triiodo-*N*-methyl-*N*[[methyl(D-*gluco*-2,3,4,5,6-pentahydroxyhexyl)carbamoyl]methyl]benzamide. *CAS-97702-82-4*. INN.

Iosefamic Acid [*1964*] (eye″ oh sef am′ ik as′ id). $C_{28}H_{28}I_6N_4O_8$. 1309.97. (1) Benzoic acid, 3,3′-[(1,10-dioxo-1,10-decanediyl)diimino]bis[2,4,6-triiodo-5-[(methylamino)carbonyl]-; (2) 5,5′-(Sebacoyldiimino)bis[2,4,6-triiodo-*N*-methylisophthalamic acid]. *CAS-5591-33-3*. INN. *Diagnostic aid (radiopaque medium).* ◇*MP-271*

Ioseric Acid [*1975*] (eye″ oh ser′ ik as′ id). $C_{15}H_{16}I_3N_3O_7$. 731.02. (1) Benzoic acid, 3-[[[1-(hydroxymethyl)-2-(methylamino)-2-oxoethyl]amino]carbonyl]-2,4,6-triiodo-5-[(methoxyacetyl)amino]-; (2) *N*-[2-Hydroxy-1-(methylcarbamoyl)ethyl]-2,4,6-triiodo-5-(2-methoxyacetamido)isophthalamic acid. *UNII-6O7C9P18WG. CAS-51876-99-4*. INN. *Diagnostic aid (radiopaque medium).* ◇*SH H 239 AB*

Iosimenol [*2006*] (eye″ oh sim′ e nol). $C_{31}H_{36}I_6N_6O_{14}$. 1478.08. (1) 1,3-Benzenedicarboxamide, 5,5′-(1,3-dioxo-1,3-propanediyl)bis[(2,3-dihydroxypropyl)imino]]bis[*N*-(2,3-dihydroxypropyl)-2,4,6-triiodo-; (2) 5,5′-[Propanedioylbis[(2,3-dihydroxypropyl)imino]]bis[*N*-(2,3-dihydroxypropyl)-2,4,6-triiodoisophthalamide]. *CAS-181872-90-2.* INN. *Iodinated x-ray contrast agent.* ◇*MP-3047-04; BP-13; ICJ 3393*

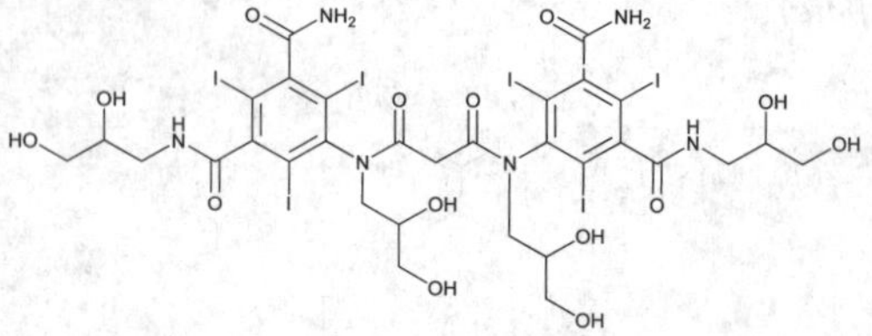

Iosimide. $C_{21}H_{30}I_3N_3O_9$. 849.19. *N,N,N′,N′,N″,N″-Hexakis(2-hydroxyethyl)-2,4,6-triiodo-1,3,5-benzenetricarboxamide. CAS-79211-10-2.* INN.

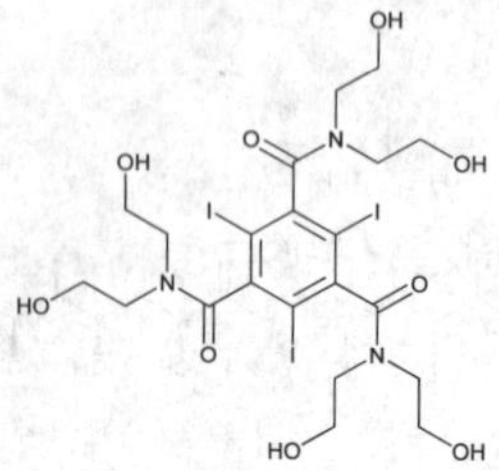

Iosulamide Meglumine [*1978*] (eye″ oh sul′ a mide me′ gloo meen). $C_{28}H_{28}I_6N_4O_{10}S.C_7H_{17}NO_5$. 1569.25. [Iosulamide is INN.] (1) Benzoic acid, 3,3′-[sulfonylbis[(1-oxo-3,1-propanediyl)imino]]bis[5-(acetylethylamino)-2,4,6-triiodo-, compd. with 1-deoxy-1-(methylamino)-D-glucitol (1:1); (2) 3,3′-[Sulfonylbis(ethylenecarbonylimino)]bis[5-(*N*-ethyl-acetamino)-2,4,6-triiodobenzoic acid] compound with 1-deoxy-1-(methylamino)-D-glucitol (1:1). *UNII-6HG8UB2-MUY* [meglumine]. *CAS-63534-64-5; CAS-23205-04-1* [iosulamide]; *CAS-6284-40-8* [meglumine]. *Diagnostic aid (radiopaque medium).*

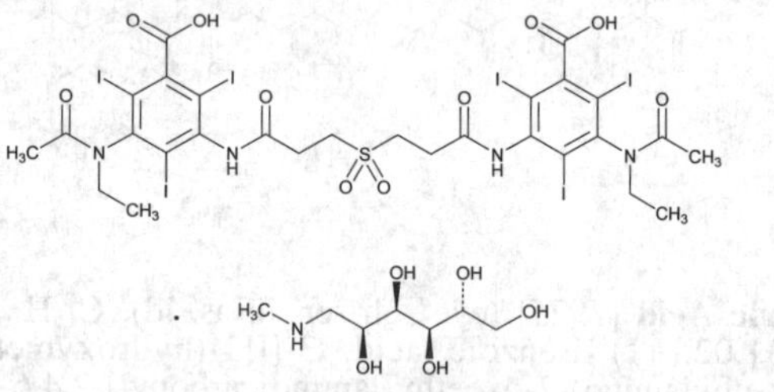

Iosumetic Acid [*1975*] (eye″ oh soo met′ ik as′ id). $C_{13}H_{15}I_3N_2O_3$. 627.98. (1) Butanoic acid, 4-[ethyl[2,4,6-triiodo-3-(methylamino)phenyl]amino]-4-oxo-; (2) *N*-Ethyl-2′,4′,6′-triiodo-3′-(methylamino)succinanilic acid. *UNII-8738M34B4Y. CAS-37863-70-0.* INN. *Diagnostic aid (radiopaque medium).*

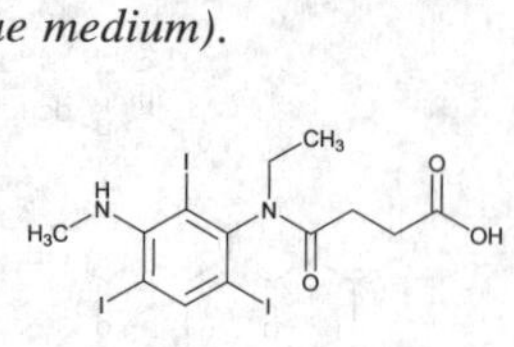

Iotalamic Acid (INN, BAN, JAN, DCF) — *See* Iothalamic Acid.

Iotasul [*1980*] (eye oh′ ta sul). $C_{38}H_{50}I_6N_6O_{14}S$. 1608.33. (1) 1,3-Benzenedicarboxamide, 5,5′-[thiobis[(1-oxo-3,1-propanediyl)imino]]bis[*N,N*-bis(2,3-dihydroxypropyl)-2,4,6-triiodo-*N,N*-dimethyl-; (2) 5,5′-[Thiobis(ethylenecarbony-

limino)]bis[*N,N*-bis(2,3-dihydroxypropyl)-2,4,6-triiodo-*N,N′*-dimethylisophthalamide]. *CAS-71767-13-0.* INN. *Diagnostic aid (radiopaque medium).* ◇*ZK 79 112*

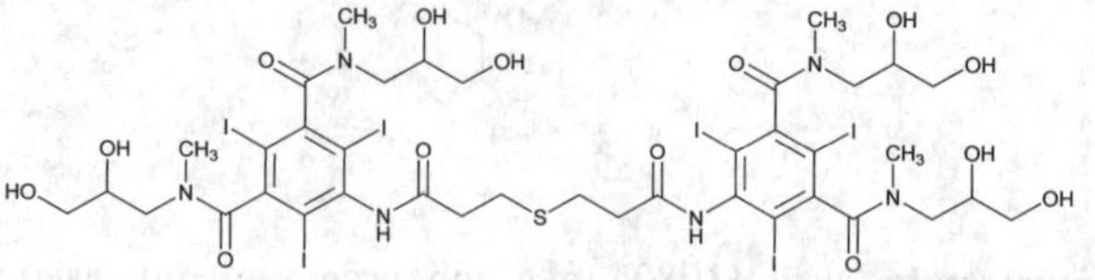

Iotetric Acid [*1977*] (eye″ oh te′ trik as′ id). $C_{24}H_{22}I_6N_2O_{10}$. 1259.87. (1) Benzoic acid, 3,3′-[(1,14-dioxo-3,6,9,12-tetraoxatetradecane-1,14-diyl)bis[2,4,6-triiodo-; (2) 3,3′-[Ethylenebis(oxyethyleneoxymethylenecarbonylimino)]bis[2,4,6-triiodobenzoic acid]. *UNII-JQ0A5VKV0Y. CAS-60019-19-4.* INN. *Diagnostic aid (radiopaque medium).* ◇*ZK 71 630*

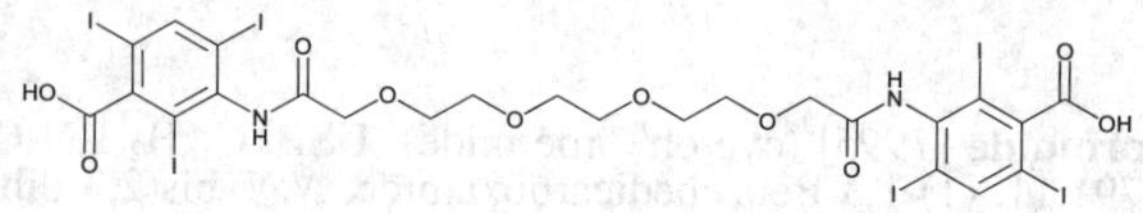

Iothalamate Meglumine (eye″ oh thal′ a mate me′ gloo meen). **USP** [Injection]. $C_{11}H_9I_3N_2O_4.C_7H_{17}NO_5$. 809.13. [Meglumine Iotalamate is BAN; Meglumine Iotalamate Injection is JAN.] (1) Benzoic acid, 3-(acetylamino)-2,4,6-triiodo-5-[(methylamino)carbonyl]-, compd. with 1-deoxy-1-(methylamino)-D-glucitol (1:1); (2) 1-Deoxy-1-(methylamino)-D-glucitol 5-acetamido-2,4,6-triiodo-*N*-methylisophthalamate (salt). *UNII-6HG8UB2MUY* [meglumine]. *CAS-13087-53-1; CAS-2276-90-6* [iothalamic acid]; *CAS-6284-40-8* [meglumine]. *Diagnostic aid (radiopaque medium).* Conray (Mallinckrodt)

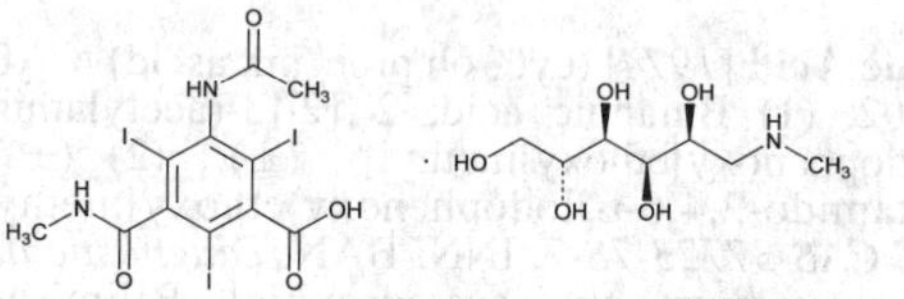

Iothalamate Sodium (eye″ oh thal′ a mate soe′ dee um). **USP** [Injection]. $C_{11}H_8I_3N_2NaO_4$. 635.90. [Sodium Iotalamate Injection is JAN.] (1) Benzoic acid, 3-(acetylamino)-2,4,6-triiodo-5-[(methylamino)carbonyl]-, monosodium salt; (2) Monosodium 5-acetamido-2,4,6-triiodo-*N*-methylisophthalamate. *UNII-16CHD79MIX* [iothalamic acid]. *CAS-1225-20-3; CAS-2276-90-6* [iothalamic acid]. *Diagnostic aid (radiopaque medium).* Conray (Mallinckrodt)

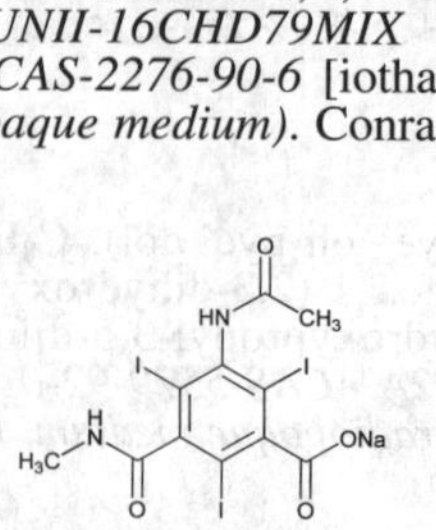

Iothalamate Sodium I 125 [*1967*] (eye″ oh thal′ a mate soe′ dee um). **USP** [Injection]. $C_{11}H_8{}^{125}I_3N_2NaO_4$. [Sodium Iotalamate (^{125}I) is INN; Sodium Iotalamate is BAN.] (1) Benzoic acid, 3-(acetylamino)diiodoiodo-^{125}I-5-[(methylamino)carbonyl]-, monosodium salt; (2) Monosodium 5-acetamido-triiodo-*N*-methylisophthalamate, labeled with iodine-125. *UNII-31J5U3Q9ZN. CAS-17692-74-9. Radioactive agent.* Glofil-125 (Abbott†)

Iothalamate Sodium I 131 [*1967*] (eye″ oh thal′ a mate soe′ dee um). $C_{11}H_8{}^{131}I_3N_2NaO_4$. [Sodium Iotalamate ($^{131}I$) is INN.] (1) Benzoic acid, 3-(acetylamino)diiodoiodo-^{131}*I*-5-[(methylamino)carbonyl]-, monosodium salt; (2) Monosodium 5-acetamido-triiodo-*N*-methylisophthalamate, labeled with iodine-131. *UNII-KDN276D83N. CAS-15845-98-4. Radioactive agent.* Conray I 131 (Mallinckrodt†); Glofil-131 (Abbott†)

Iothalamic Acid [*1962*] (eye″ oh thal am′ ik as′ id). **USP**. $C_{11}H_9I_3N_2O_4$. 613.91. [Iotalamic Acid is INN, BAN and JAN.] (1) Benzoic acid, 3-(acetylamino)-2,4,6-triiodo-5-[(methylamino)carbonyl]-; (2) 5-Acetamido-2,4,6-triiodo-*N*-methylisophthalamic acid. *UNII-16CHD79MIX. CAS-2276-90-6. Diagnostic aid (radiopaque medium). ◇MI-216*

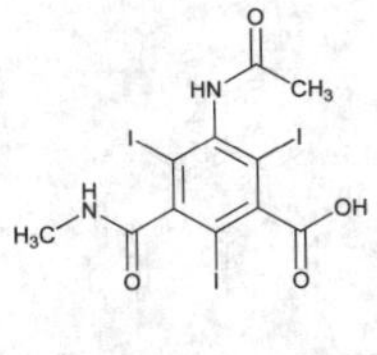

Iothiouracil Sodium. *UNII-Y3779XL39I.* NND 1964.

Iotranic Acid. $C_{24}H_{22}I_6N_2O_9$. 1243.87. 3,3′-[Oxybis(ethyleneoxyethylenecarbonylimino)]bis[2,4,6-triiodobenzoic acid]. *UNII-4F8YJZ690M. CAS-26887-04-7.* INN.

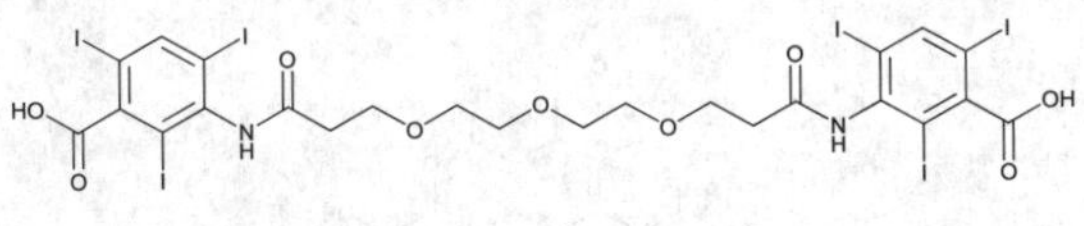

Iotriside. $C_{16}H_{20}I_3N_3O_7$. 747.06. (±)-*N,N′*-Bis(2,3-dihydroxypropyl)-2,4,6-triiodo-*N*-methyl-1,3,5-benzenetricarboxamide. *UNII-S0GPJ58I2D. CAS-79211-34-0.* INN.

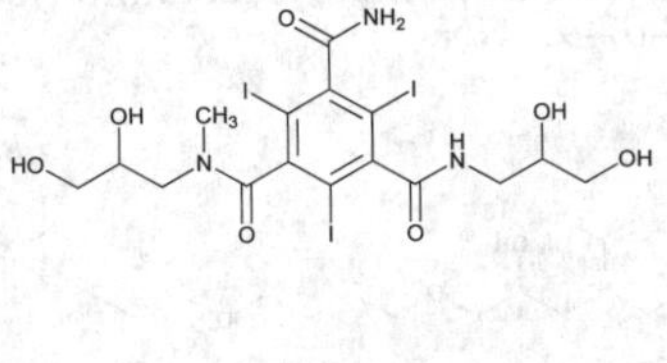

Iotrizoic Acid. $C_{18}H_{24}I_3NO_8$. 763.10. 2,4,6-Triiodo-3-[2-[2-[2-[2-(2-methoxy)ethoxy]ethoxy]ethoxy]acetamido]benzoic acid. *UNII-3184855T90. CAS-16024-67-2.* INN.

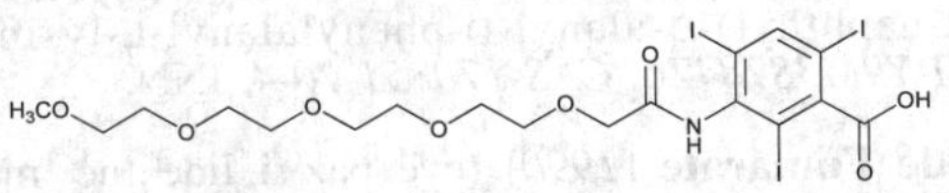

Iotrol (previously used name) — *See* Iotrolan.

Iotrolan [*1984*] (eye oh′ troe lan). $C_{37}H_{48}I_6N_6O_{18}$. 1626.23. (1) 1,3-Benzenedicarboxamide, 5,5′-[(1,3-dioxo-1,3-propanediyl)bis(methylimino)]bis[*N,N′*-bis[2,3-dihydroxy-1-(hydroxymethyl)propyl]-2,4,6-triiodo-; (2) 5,5′-[Malonylbis(methylimino)]bis[*N,N′*-bis[2,3-dihydroxy-1-(hydroxymethyl)propyl]-2,4,6-triiodoisophthalamide]. *UNII-16FL47B687. CAS-79770-24-4.* INN; BAN; JAN. *Diagnostic aid (radiopaque medium).* Osmovist (Bayer) *[Name previously used: Iotrol.] ◇ZK 39 482*

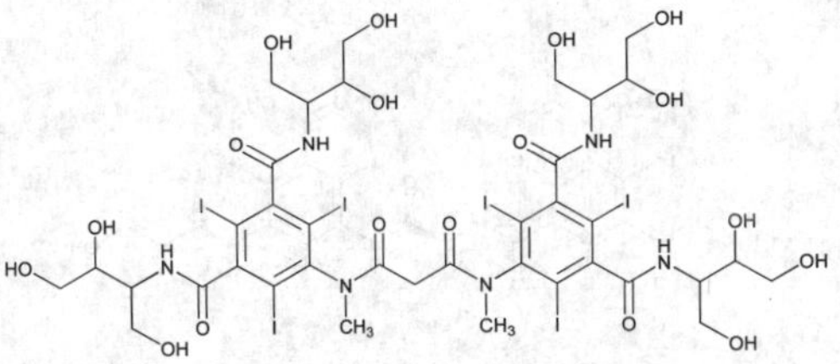

Iotroxate Meglumine. $C_{22}H_{18}I_6N_2O_9.2C_7H_{17}NO_5$. 1606.24. 3,3′-[Oxybis(ethyleneoxymethylenecarbonylimino)]-bis(2,4,6-triiodobenzoic acid) compound with meglumine. JAN.

Iotroxic Acid [*1974*] (eye″ oh trox′ ik as′ id). $C_{22}H_{18}I_6N_2O_9$. 1215.81. (1) Benzoic acid, 3,3′-[oxybis[2,1-ethanediyloxy(1-oxo-2,1-ethanediyl)imino]]bis[2,4,6, triiodo-; (2) 3,3′-[Oxybis(ethyleneoxymethylenecarbonylimino)]-bis[2,4,6-triiodobenzoic acid]; (3) 3,3′-(3,6,9-Trioxaundecanedioyldiamino)bis(2,4,6-triiodobenzoic acid). *UNII-84C5PTP9X6. CAS-51022-74-3.* INN; BAN; JAN. *Diagnostic aid (radiopaque medium). ◇SH 213 AB*

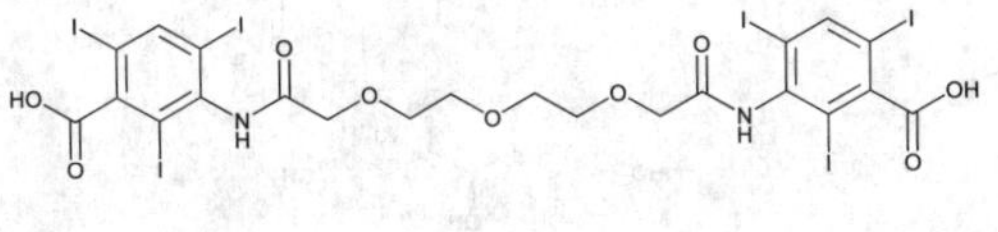

Iotyrosine I 131 [*1963*] (eye″ oh tye′ roe seen). $C_9H_{10}{}^{131}INO_3$. (1) L-Tyrosine, 3-(iodo-^{131}*I*)-; (2) 3-Iodo-^{131}*I*-L-tyrosine. *UNII-Q1M94GA18P. CAS-16624-40-1. Radioactive agent.*

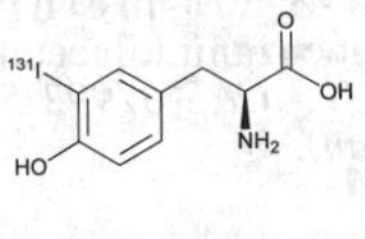

Ioversol [*1987*] (eye″ oh ver′ sol). **USP**. $C_{18}H_{24}I_3N_3O_9$. 807.11. (1) 1,3-Benzenedicarboxamide, *N,N′*-bis(2,3-dihydroxypropyl)-5-[(hydroxyacetyl)(2-hydroxyethyl)amino]-2,4,6-triiodo-; (2) *N,N′*-Bis(2,3-dihydroxypropyl)-5-[*N*-(2-hydroxyethyl)glycolamido]-2,4,6-triiodoisophthalamide. *UNII-N3RIB7X24K. CAS-87771-40-2.* INN; BAN. *Diagnostic aid (radiopaque medium).* Optiray (Mallinckrodt) *◇MP 328*

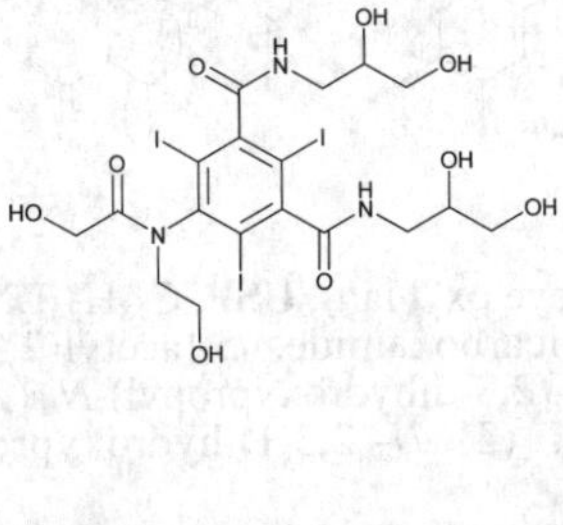

† Brand name formerly used, and/or firm no longer concerned with this product.

Ioxabrolic Acid. $C_{24}H_{21}Br_3I_3N_5O_8$. 1127.88. *N*-(2-Hydroxyethyl)-2,4,6-triiodo-5-[2-[2,4,6-tribromo-3-(*N*-methylacetamido)-5-(methylcarbamoyl)benzamido]acetamido]isophthalamic acid. *UNII-LP80S8XS18. CAS-96191-65-0*. INN.

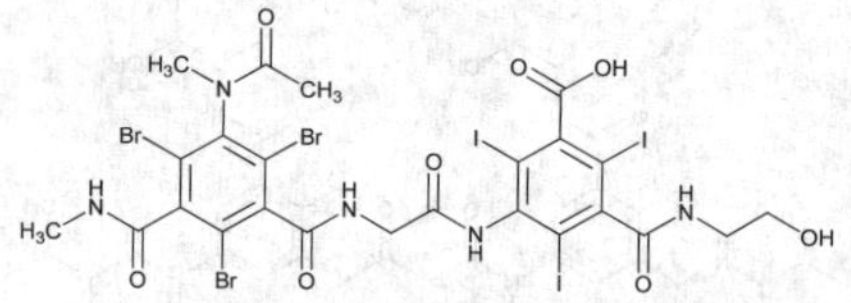

Ioxaglate Meglumine [*1982*] (eye″ ox ag′ late me′ gloo meen). $C_{24}H_{21}I_6N_5O_8 \cdot C_7H_{17}NO_5$. 1464.09. [Meglumine Ioxaglate is BAN.] (1) Benzoic acid, 3-[[[[3-(acetylmethylamino)-2,4,6-triiodo-5-[(methylamino)carbonyl]benzoyl]amino]acetyl]amino]-5-[[(2-hydroxyethyl)amino]carbonyl]-2,4,6-triiodo-, compound with 1-deoxy-1-(methylamino)-D-glucitol (1:1); (2) *N*-(2-Hydroxyethyl)-2,4,6-triiodo-5-[2-[2,4,6-triiodo-3-(*N*-methylacetamido)-5-(methylcarbamoyl)benzamido]acetamido]isophthalamic acid, compound with 1-deoxy-1-(methylamino)-D-glucitol (1:1). *UNII-75JR975T11. CAS-59018-13-2. Diagnostic aid (radiopaque medium)*. ◇*MP 302 (mixt. with Ioxaglate Sodium)*

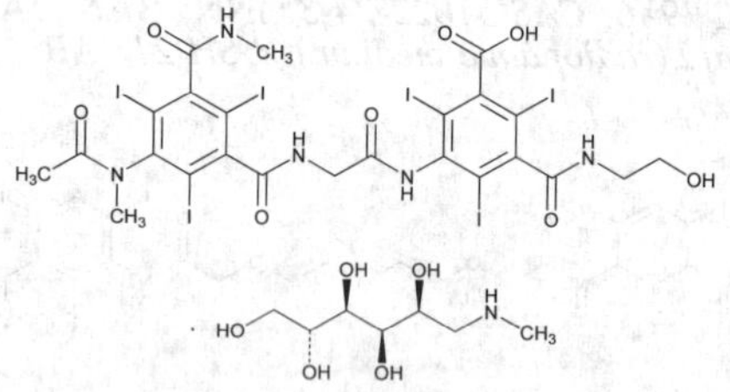

Ioxaglate Sodium [*1982*] (eye″ ox ag′ late soe′ dee um). $C_{24}H_{20}I_6N_5NaO_8$. 1290.86. [Sodium Ioxaglate is BAN.] (1) Benzoic acid, 3-[[[[3-(acetylmethylamino)-2,4,6-triiodo-5-[(methylamino)carbonyl]benzoyl]amino]acetyl]amino]-5-[[(2-hydroxyethyl)amino]carbonyl]-2,4,6-triiodo-, sodium salt; (2) Sodium *N*-(2-hydroxyethyl)-2,4,6-triiodo-5-[2-[2,4,6-triiodo-3-(*N*-methylacetamido)-5-(methylcarbamoyl)benzamido]acetamido]isophthalamate. *UNII-HQ43CN02U9. CAS-67992-58-9. Diagnostic aid (radiopaque medium)*.

Ioxaglic Acid [*1982*] (eye″ ox ag′ lik as′ id). **USP**. $C_{24}H_{21}I_6N_5O_8$. 1268.88. (1) Benzoic acid, 3-[[[[3-(acetylmethylamino)-2,4,6-triiodo-5-[(methylamino)carbonyl]benzoyl]amino]acetyl]amino]-5-[[(2-hydroxyethyl)amino]carbonyl]-2,4,6-triiodo-; (2) *N*-(2-Hydroxyethyl)-2,4,6-triiodo-5-[2-[2,4,6-triiodo-3-(*N*-methylacetamido)-5-(methylcarbamoyl)benzamido]acetamido]isophthalamic acid. *UNII-Z40X7EI2AF. CAS-59017-64-0*. INN; BAN; JAN. *Diagnostic aid (radiopaque medium)*. ◇*P-286*

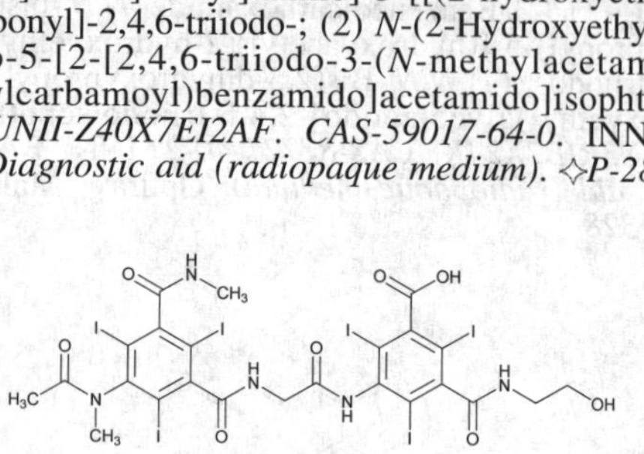

Ioxilan [*1989*] (eye ox′ i lan). **USP**. $C_{18}H_{24}I_3N_3O_8$. 791.11. (1) 1,3-Benzenedicarboxamide, 5-[acetyl(2,3-dihydroxypropyl)amino]-*N*-(2,3-dihydroxypropyl)-*N'*-(2-hydroxyethyl)-2,4,6-triiodo-; (2) *N*-(2,3-Dihydroxypropyl)-5-[*N*-(2,3-dihydroxypropyl)acetamido]-*N'*-(2-hydroxyethyl)-2,4,6-triiodoisophthalamide. *UNII-A4YJ7J11TG. CAS-107793-72-6*. INN. *Diagnostic aid*. Oxilan (Guerbet)

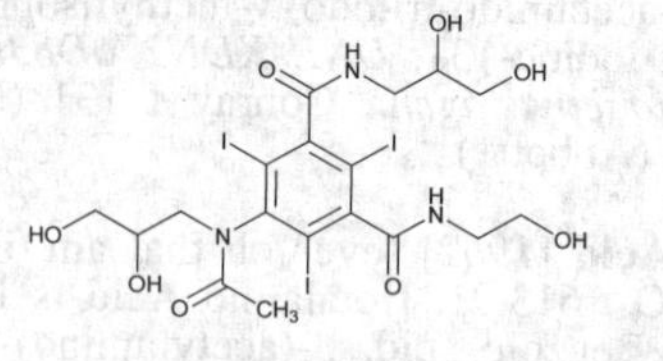

Ioxitalamic Acid. $C_{12}H_{11}I_3N_2O_5$. 643.94. 5-Acetamido-*N*-(2-hydroxyethyl)-2,4,6-triiodoisophthalamic acid. *UNII-967RDI7Z6K. CAS-28179-44-4*. INN; DCF. ◇*AG 58107*

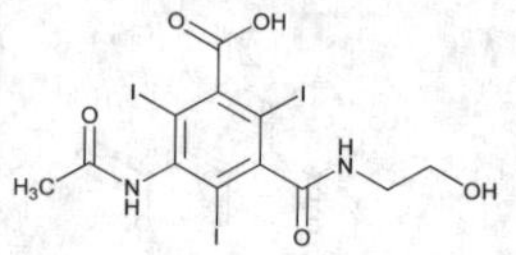

Ioxotrizoic Acid [*1975*] (eye ox″ oh trye zoe′ ik as′ id). $C_{11}H_9I_3N_2O_5$. 629.91. (1) Benzoic acid, 3-(acetylamino)-5-[(hydroxyacetyl)amino]-2,4,6-triiodo-; (2) 3-Acetamido-5-glycolamido-2,4,6-triiodobenzoic acid. *UNII-4H2LVB8X5O. CAS-19863-06-0*. INN. *Diagnostic aid (radiopaque medium)*. ◇*SH 2.1139/H 248 AB*

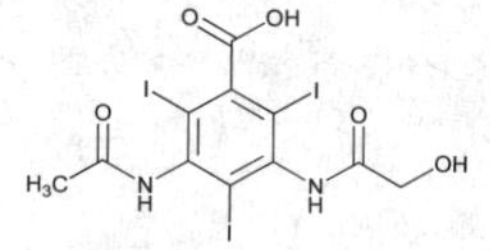

Iozomic Acid. $C_{34}H_{40}I_6N_4O_{12}$. 1458.13. 3,3′-[Tetramethylenebis[oxy(2-hydroxytrimethylene)acetylimino)]]-bis[2,4,6-triiodo-5-(*N*-methylacetamido)benzoic acid]. *CAS-31598-07-9*. INN.

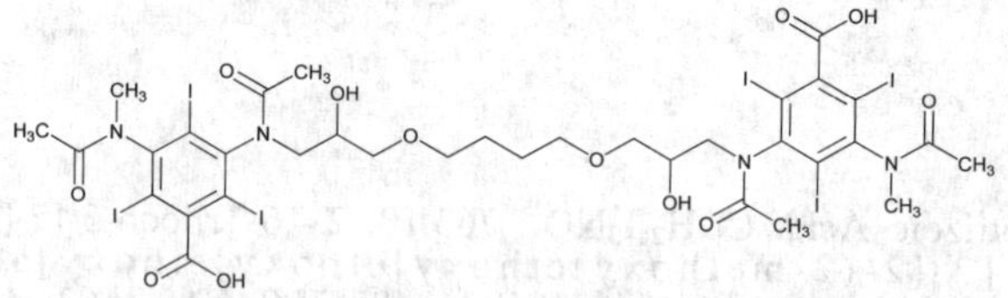

Ipamorelin. $C_{38}H_{49}N_9O_5$. 711.85. 2-Methylalanyl-L-histidyl-3-(2-naphthyl)-D-alanyl-D-phenylalanyl-L-lysinamide. *UNII-Y9M3S784Z6. CAS-170851-70-4*. INN.

Ipazilide Fumarate [*1990*] (eye paz′ i lide fue′ ma rate). $C_{24}H_{30}N_4O \cdot C_4H_4O_4$. 506.59. [Ipazilide is INN.] (1) 1*H*-Pyrazole-1-acetamide, *N*-[3-(diethylamino)propyl]-4,5-diphenyl-, (*E*)-2-butenedioate (1:1); (2) *N*-[3-(Diethylamino)propyl]-4,5-diphenylpyrazole-1-acetamide fumarate (1:1). *UNII-2MI60P494I. CAS-115436-74-3; CAS-115436-73-2 [ipazilide]. Cardiac depressant (anti-arrhythmic)*. ◇*Win 54,177-4*

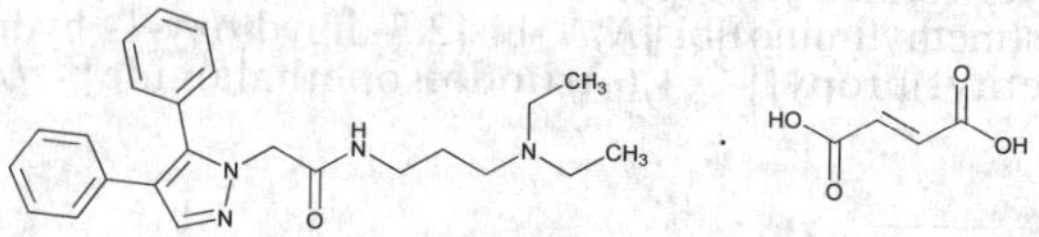

Ipecac (ip′ e kak). **USP.** Consists of the dried rhizome and roots of *Cephaëlis acuminata* Karsten, or of *Cephaëlis ipecacuanha* (Brotero) A. Richard (Fam. Rubiaceae). *UNII-62I3C8233L.* Emetic. Ipsatol (Key Pharmaceuticals†)

Ipenoxazone. $C_{22}H_{34}N_2O_2$. 358.52. (+)-(4*S*,5*R*)-3-[3-(Hexahydro-1*H*-azepin-1-yl)propyl]-4-isobutyl-5-phenyl-2-oxazolidinone. *UNII-839F26EVAQ. CAS-104454-71-9.* INN.

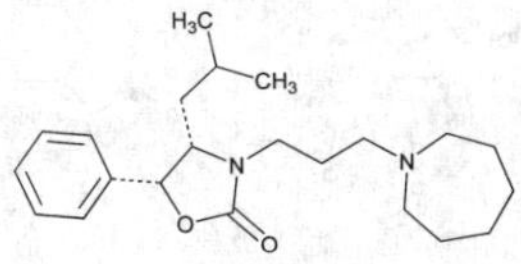

Ipexidine Mesylate [*1980*] (eye pex′ i deen mes′ i late). $C_{26}H_{54}N_{10}O_2 \cdot 2CH_4O_3S$. 730.98. [Ipexidine is INN.] (1) Urea, *N,N″*-[1,4-Piperazinediylbis(3,1-propanediyliminocarbonimidoyl)]bis[*N*′-hexyl-, dimethanesulfonate; (2) 1,1′-[1,4-Piperazinediylbis(trimethyleneiminoimidocarbonyl)]bis[3-hexylurea] dimethanesulfonate. *CAS-69017-90-9; CAS-69017-89-6* [ipexidine]. INN. *Dental caries prophylactic.* ◇*CK-0569 [as the base]*

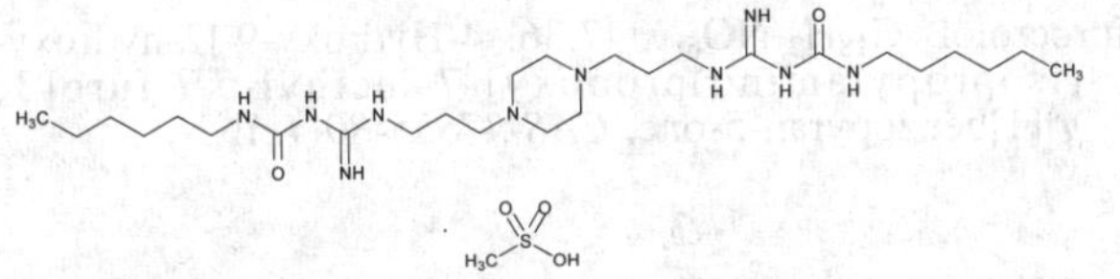

Ipidacrine. $C_{12}H_{16}N_2$. 188.27. 9-Amino-2,3,5,6,7,8-hexahydro-1*H*-cyclopenta[*b*]quinoline. *UNII-CV71VTP0VN. CAS-62732-44-9.* INN.

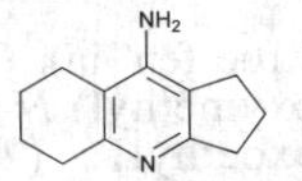

Ipilimumab [*2005*] (ip″ i lim′ ue mab). $C_{6472}H_{9972}N_{1732}O_{2004}S_{40}$. Immunoglobulin G1, anti-(human CTLA-4 (antigen)) (human γ1-chain), disulfide with human κ-chain, dimer. Molecular weight is approximately 145,400 daltons. *UNII-6T8C155666. CAS-477202-00-9.* INN. *Treatment of oncology disease and HIV infection.* ◇*MDX-010; MDX-CTLA-4*

Ipodate Calcium. $C_{24}H_{24}CaI_6N_4O_4$. 1233.98. (1) Benzenepropanoic acid, 3-[[(dimethylamino)methylene]amino]-2,4,6-triiodo-, calcium salt; (2) Calcium 3-[[(dimethylamino)methylene]amino]-2,4,6-triiodohydrocinnamate. *UNII-F604ZKI910* [ipodic acid]. *CAS-1151-11-7; CAS-5587-89-3* [ipodic acid]. USP XXIII. *Diagnostic aid (radiopaque medium).* Oragrafin Calcium (Bracco)

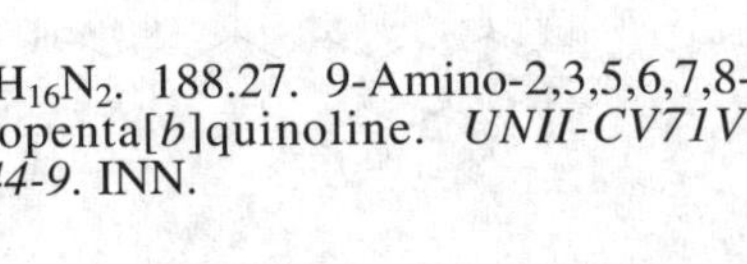

Ipodate Sodium [*1962*] (eye′ poe date soe′ dee um). **USP.** $C_{12}H_{12}I_3N_2NaO_2$. 619.94. [Sodium Iopodate is INN, BAN and JAN.] (1) Benzenepropanoic acid, 3-[[(dimethylamino)methylene]amino]-2,4,6-triiodo-, sodium salt; (2) Sodium 3-[[(dimethylamino)methylene]amino]-2,4,6-

triiodohydrocinnamate. *UNII-F604ZKI910* [ipodic acid]. *CAS-1221-56-3; CAS-5587-89-3* [ipodic acid]. *Diagnostic aid (radiopaque medium).* Oragrafin Sodium (Bracco) [*Name previously used: Sodium Ipodate.*] ◇*NSC-106962*

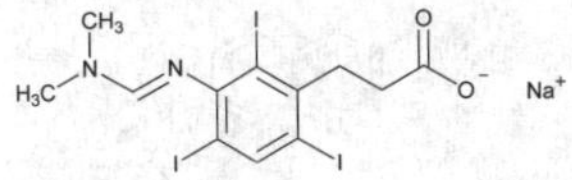

Ipragratine. $C_{20}H_{29}NO_3$. 331.45. 9-Isopropylgranatoline (±)-tropate (ester). *CAS-22150-28-3.* INN.

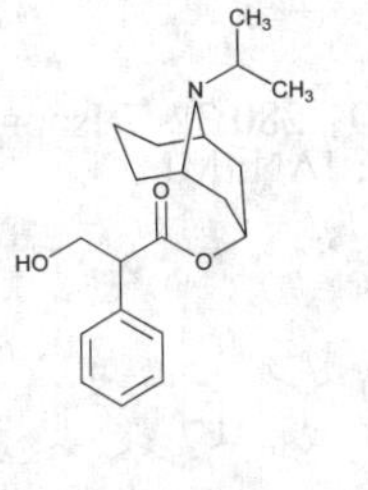

Ipramidil. $C_{10}H_{16}N_4O_4$. 256.26. *N,N*-Diisopropyl-3,4-furazandicarboxamide 2-oxide. *UNII-9ZPC9768EH. CAS-83656-38-6.* INN.

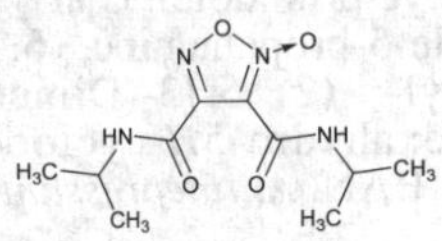

Ipratropium Bromide [*1977*] (ip″ ra troe′ pee um broe′ mide). $C_{20}H_{30}BrNO_3 \cdot H_2O$. 430.38. (1) 8-Azoniabicyclo[3.2.1]octane, 3-(3-hydroxy-1-oxo-2-phenylpropoxy)-8-methyl-8-(1-methylethyl)-, bromide, monohydrate(*endo,syn*)-, (±)-; (2) (8*r*)-3α-Hydroxy-8-isopropyl-1αH,5αH-tropanium bromide (±)-tropate monohydrate. *UNII-J697UZ2A9J. CAS-66985-17-9; CAS-22254-24-6* [anhydrous]. INN; BAN; JAN. *Bronchodilator.* Atrovent (Boehringer Ingelheim) ◇*Sch 1000-Br-monohydrate*

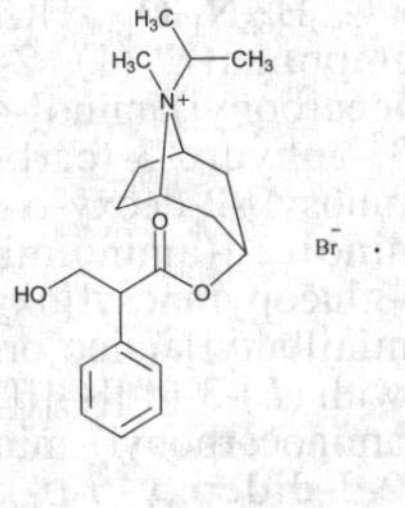

Ipravacaine. $C_{18}H_{26}N_2O$. 286.41. (2*RS*)-1-(Cyclopropylmethyl)-2′,6′-dimethyl-2-piperidinecarboxanilide. *CAS-166181-63-1.* INN.

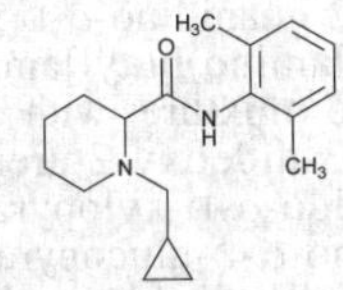

---

† Brand name formerly used, and/or firm no longer concerned with this product.

Iprazochrome. $C_{12}H_{16}N_4O_3$. 264.28. 3-Hydroxy-1-isopropyl-5,6-indolinedione 5-semicarbazone. *CAS-7248-21-7*. INN.

Iprazone — *See* Isoprazone.

Ipriflavone. $C_{18}H_{16}O_3$. 280.32. 7-Isopropoxyisoflavone. *CAS-35212-22-7*. INN; JAN; MI.

Iprindole [*1965*] (eye prin′ dole). $C_{19}H_{28}N_2$. 284.44. (1) 5*H*-Cyclooct[*b*]indole-5-propanamine, 6,7,8,9,10,11-hexahydro-*N,N*-dimethyl-; (2) 5-[3-(Dimethylamino)propyl]-6,7,8,9,10,11-hexahydro-5*H*-cyclooct[*b*]indole. *CAS-5560-72-5*. INN; BAN. *Antidepressant.* ◇Wy-3263

Iprocinodine Hydrochloride [*1979*] (ip″ roe sin′ oh deen hye″ droe klor′ ide). $C_{40}H_{65}N_{13}O_{13} \cdot x$HCl (each component). 936.02 (each component). (1) 2-Propenamide, 3-[4-[[4-[[[[2-[(aminocarbonyl)amino]-4-*O*-[2-](aminocarbonyl)amino]-$2^1,3^2$-anhydro-3-(carboxyamino)-2,3-dideoxy-β-D-xylopyranosyl]-2-deoxy-α-D-xylopyranosyl]amino]carbonyl]amino]-2-[(aminoiminomethyl)amino]-2,4,6-trideoxy-α-D-glucopyranosyl]oxy]phenyl]-*N*-[3-[[4-[(1-methylethyl)amino]butyl]amino]propyl]-, hydrochloride, (*E*)-, mixture with (*E*)-3-[4-[[4-[[[[2-[(aminocarbonyl)amino]-4-*O*-[2-[(aminocarbonyl)amino]-3^2,4-anhydro-3-(carboxyamino)-2,3-dideoxy-β-D-xylopyranosyl]-2-deoxy-α-D-xylopyranosyl]amino]carbonyl]amino]-2-[(aminoiminomethyl)amino]-2,4,6-trideoxy-α-D-glucopyranosyl]oxy]phenyl]-*N*-[3-[[4-[(1-methylethyl)amino]butyl]amino]propyl]-2-propenamide hydrochloride; (2) (*E*)-*p*-[[4-[3-[4-*O*-[2,3-(1-Carbamoylureylene)-2,3-dideoxy-β-D-xylopyranosyl]-2-deoxy-2-ureido-α-D-xylopyranosyl]ureido]-2,4,6-trideoxy-2-guanidino-α-D-glucopyranosyl]oxy]-*N*-[3-[[4-(isopropylamino)butyl]amino]propyl]cinnamamide hydrochloride mixture with (*E*)-*p*-[[4-[3-[4-*O*-[3-(carboxyamino)-2,3-dideoxy-2-ureido-β-D-xylopyranosyl]-2-deoxy-2-ureido-α-D-xylopyranosyl]ureido]-2,4,6-trideoxy-2-guanidino-α-D-glucopyranosyl]oxy]-*N*-[3-[[4-(isopropylamino)butyl]amino]propyl]cinnamamide intramolecular 3′′′,4′′′-ester hydrochloride; (3) *N*-(1-Methylethy-

l)antibiotic BM 123γ hydrochloride. *CAS-68782-59-2; CAS-67527-59-7* [*N*-(1-methylethyl)antibiotic BM 123γ]. *Antibacterial (veterinary).* ◇CL 205925

Iproclozide. $C_{11}H_{15}ClN_2O_2$. 242.70. (*p*-Chlorophenoxy)acetic acid 2-isopropylhydrazide. *UNII-1II9D6CB3J. CAS-3544-35-2*. INN; BAN; DCF; MI. ◇PC-603

Iprocrolol. $C_{18}H_{21}NO_6$. 347.36. 4-Hydroxy-9-[2-hydroxy-3-(isopropylamino)propoxy]-7-methyl-5*H*-furo[3,2-*g*][1]benzopyran-5-one. *CAS-37855-80-4*. INN.

Iprofenin [*1978*] (ip″ roe fen′ in). $C_{15}H_{20}N_2O_5$. 308.33. (1) Glycine, *N*-(carboxymethyl)-*N*-[2-[[4-(1-methylethyl)phenyl]amino]-2-oxoethyl]-; (2) [[(*p*-Cumenylcarbamoyl)methyl]imino]diacetic acid. *CAS-66292-53-3*. *Diagnostic aid (hepatic function determination).*

Iproheptine. $C_{11}H_{25}N$. 171.32. [Iproheptine Hydrochloride is JAN.] *N*-Isopropyl-1,5-dimethylhexylamine. *CAS-13946-02-6*. INN.

Iproniazid. $C_9H_{13}N_3O$. 179.22. Isonicotinic acid 2-isopropylhydrazide. *CAS-54-92-2; CAS-305-33-9* [as phosphate]. INN; BAN; DCF; MI.

Ipronidazole [*1969*] (ip″ roe nye′ da zole). $C_7H_{11}N_3O_2$. 169.18. (1) 1*H*-Imidazole, 1-methyl-2-(1-methylethyl)-5-nitro-; (2) 2-Isopropyl-1-methyl-5-nitroimidazole. *UNII-*

045BU63E23. CAS-14885-29-1. INN; BAN. *Antiprotozoal (Histomonas).* Ipropran [Veterinary] (Hoffmann-LaRoche†) ◇*Ro 7-1554; NSC-109212*

Ipropethidine — *See* Properidine.

Iproplatin [*1984*] (ip″ roe pla′ tin). $C_6H_{20}Cl_2N_2O_2Pt$. 418.23. (1) Platinum, dichlorodihydroxybis(2-propanamine)-, (*OC-6-33*); (2) *ab*-Dichloro-*ce*-dihydroxy-*df*-bis(isopropylamine)platinum. *CAS-62928-11-4.* INN; BAN. *Antineoplastic.* ◇*JM-9; NSC-256927*

Iprotiazem. $C_{37}H_{49}N_3O_5S$. 647.87. (+)-(*R*)-2-Isopropyl-4-methyl-2-[*o*-[4-[4-(3,4,5-trimethoxyphenethyl)-1-piperazinyl]butoxy]phenyl]-2*H*-1,4-benzothiazin-3(4*H*)-one. *UNII-3VPX99Q2D7. CAS-105118-13-6.* INN.

Iproveratril — *See* Verapamil.

Iproxamine Hydrochloride [*1975*] (eye prox′ a meen hye″ droe klor′ ide). $C_{18}H_{29}NO_4$·HCl. 359.89. [Iproxamine is INN.] (1) Carbonic acid, 4-[2-(dimethylamino)ethoxy]-2-methyl-5-(1-methylethyl)phenyl 1-methylethyl ester, hydrochloride; (2) 5-[2-(Dimethylamino)ethoxy]carvacryl isopropyl carbonate hydrochloride. *UNII-83L52U43TX; UNII-URR853YLZA* [iproxamine]. *CAS-51222-37-8; CAS-52403-19-7* [iproxamine]. *Vasodilator.* ◇*Go 2782; W 42782*

Iprozilamine. $C_{13}H_{22}ClN_5S$. 315.87. 4-Chloro-2-(isopropylamino)-6-(4-methyl-1-piperazinyl)-5-(methylthio)pyrimidine. *UNII-8WTG4RSP9Y. CAS-55477-19-5.* INN.

Ipsalazide. $C_{16}H_{13}N_3O_6$. 343.29. (*E*)-*p*-[(3-Carboxy-4-hydroxyphenyl)azo]hippuric acid. *UNII-499H4332KZ. CAS-80573-03-1.* INN; BAN. ◇*BX 650 A*

Ipsapirone Hydrochloride [*1988*] (ip″ sa pye′ rone hye″ droe klor′ ide). $C_{19}H_{23}N_5O_3S$·HCl. 437.94. [Ipsapirone is INN and BAN.] (1) 1,2-Benzisothiazol-3(2*H*)-one, 2-[4-[4-(2-pyrimidinyl)-1-piperazinyl]butyl]-, 1,1-dioxide, monohydrochloride; (2) 2-[4-[4-(2-Pyrimidinyl)-1-piperazinyl]butyl]-1,2-benzisothiazolin-3-one 1,1-dioxide, monohydrochloride. *UNII-08R5U8PYVO; UNII-6J9B11MN0K* [ipsapirone]. *CAS-92589-98-5; CAS-95847-70-4* [ipsapirone]. *Anti-anxiety agent.* ◇*BAY q 7821*

Iquindamine. $C_{15}H_{23}N_3$. 245.36. 1-[[2-(Diethylamino)ethyl]amino]-3,4-dihydroisoquinoline. *UNII-F2U67W4R4J. CAS-55299-11-1.* INN.

^{192}Ir — *See* Iridium Ir 192.

Iralukast. $C_{38}H_{37}F_3O_8S$. 710.76. 7-[[(1*S*,2*E*,4*Z*)-9-(4-Acetyl-3-hydroxy-2-propylphenoxy)-1-[(α*R*)-α-hydroxy-*m*-(trifluoromethyl)benzyl]-2,4-nonadienyl]thio-4-oxo-4*H*-1-benzopyran-2-carboxylic acid. *UNII-L1E28E0J8F. CAS-151581-24-7.* INN.

Irampanel. $C_{18}H_{19}N_3O_2$. 309.36. 5-[*o*-[2-(Dimethylamino)ethoxy]phenyl]-3-phenyl-1,2,4-oxadiazole. *UNII-R2GZD7LMYX. CAS-206260-33-5*. INN.

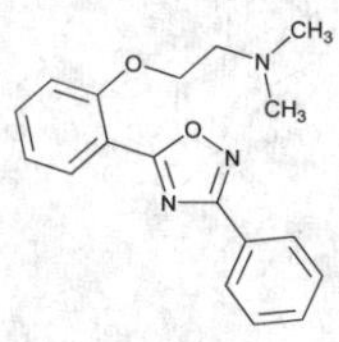

Iratumumab [*2005*] (ir″ a toom′ ue mab). $C_{6358}H_{9830}N_{1682}O_{1992}S_{38}$. Immunoglobulin G1, anti-(human CD30 (antigen)) (human monoclonal MDX-060 heavy chain), disulfide with human monoclonal MDX-060 light chain, dimer. Molecular weight is approximately 170,000 daltons. *CAS-640735-09-7*. INN. *Oncological diseases; treatment of relapsed or refractory CD30 positive lymphoma including Hodgkin's Disease.* ◇*MDX-060*

Irbesartan [*1996*] (ir″ be sar′ tan). **USP.** $C_{25}H_{28}N_6O$. 428.53. (1) 1,3-Diazaspiro[4.4]non-1-en-4-one, 2-butyl-3-[[2′-(1*H*-tetrazol-5-yl)[1,1′-biphenyl]-4-yl]methyl]-; (2) 2-Butyl-3-[*p*-(*o*-1*H*-tetrazol-5-ylphenyl)benzyl]-1,3-diazaspiro[4.4]-non-1-en-4-one. *UNII-J0E2756Z7N. CAS-138402-11-6.* INN; BAN. *Antihypertensive (angiotensin II receptor antagonist).* Avapro (Sanofi Aventis) ◇*BMS-186295; SR 47436*

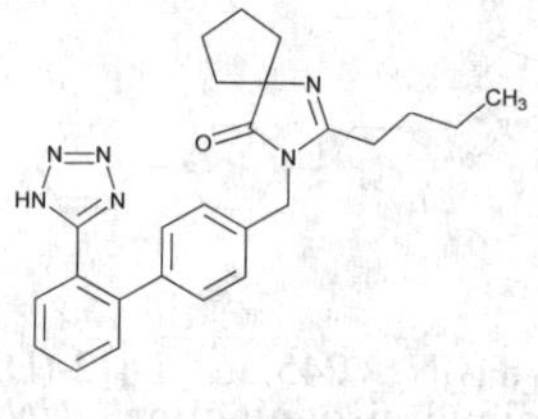

Iridium Ir 192 [*1963*] (ir id′ ee um). (1) Iridium, isotope of mass 192; (2) Iridium, isotope of mass 192. *CAS-14694-69-0. Radioactive agent.* Iriditope (Bristol-Myers Squibb†)

Irindalone. $C_{24}H_{29}FN_4O$. 408.51. (+)-(1*R*,3*S*)-1-[2-[4-[3-(*p*-Fluorophenyl)-1-indanyl]-1-piperazinyl]ethyl]-2-imidazolidinone. *UNII-4F39T8N10K. CAS-96478-43-2.* INN.

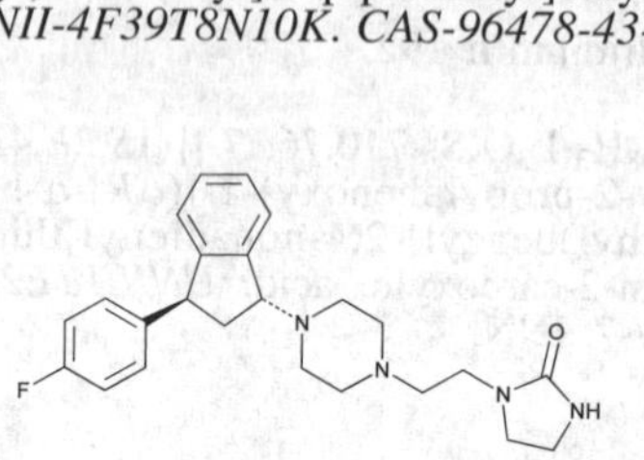

Irinotecan Hydrochloride [*1995*] (eye″ ri noe tee′ kan hye″ droe klor′ ide). $C_{33}H_{38}N_4O_6.HCl.3H_2O$. 677.18. [Irinotecan is INN and BAN.] (1) [1,4′-Bipiperidine]-1′-carboxylic acid, 4,11-diethyl-3,4,12,14-tetrahydro-4-hydroxy-3,14-dioxo-1*H*-pyrano[3′,4′:6,7]indolizino[1,2-*b*]quinolin-9-yl ester, monohydrochloride, trihydrate, (*S*)-; (2) (+)-7-Éthyl-10-hydroxycamptothecine 10-[1,4′-bipiperidine]-1′-carboxylate, monohydrochloride, trihydrate. *UNII-042LA-Q1IIS; UNII-7673326042* [irinotecan]. *CAS-136572-09-3;*

CAS-97682-44-5 [irinotecan]. JAN. *Antineoplastic (DNA topoisomerase 1 inhibitor).* Camptosar (Pfizer) ◇*U-101,440E*

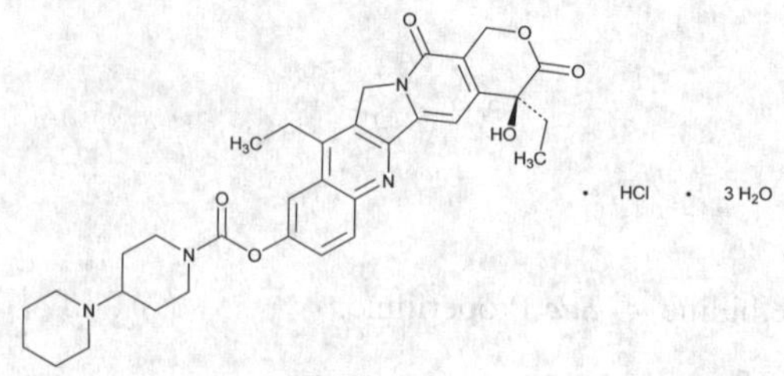

Irloxacin. $C_{16}H_{13}FN_2O_3$. 300.28. 1-Ethyl-6-fluoro-1,4-dihydro-4-oxo-7-pyrrol-1-yl-3-quinolinecarboxylic acid. *UNII-36SG77D21B. CAS-91524-15-1.* INN.

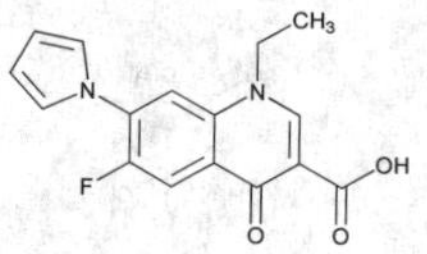

Irofulven [*1998*] (ir″ oh ful′ ven). $C_{15}H_{18}O_3$. 246.30. (*R*)-6′-Hydroxy-3′-(hydroxymethyl)-2′,4′,6′-trimethylspiro[cyclopropane-1,5′-[5*H*]inden]-7′(6′*H*)-one. *CAS-158440-71-2.* INN. *Antineoplastic (DNA synthesis inhibitor/apoptosis inducer).* ◇*MGI 114*

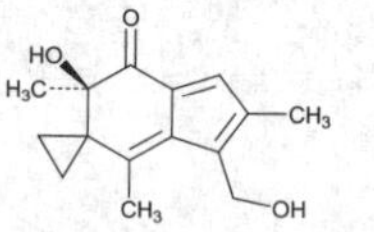

Irolapride. $C_{19}H_{28}N_2O_3$. 332.44. (±)-5-Butyryl-*N*-[(1-ethyl-2-pyrrolidinyl)methyl]-*o*-anisamide. *UNII-JS492IR8Z6. CAS-64779-98-2.* INN.

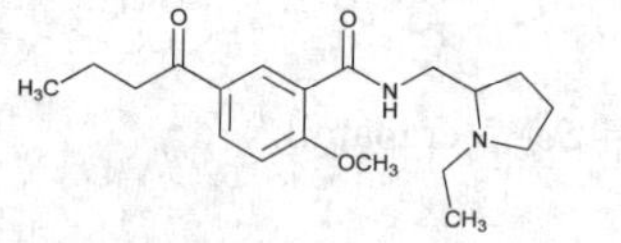

Iron Carbohydrate Complex — *See* Polyferose.

Iron Dextran (eye′ urn dex′ tran). **USP** [Injection]. A sterile, colloidal solution of ferric hydroxide in complex with partially hydrolyzed dextran of low molecular weight, in water. *UNII-95HR524N2M. CAS-9004-66-4. Hematinic.* Dexferrum (Luitpold); Infed (Watson); Proferdex (New River)

Iron Heptonate — *See* Gleptoferron.

Iron(III) hydroxide Sucrose Complex (previously used name) — *See* Iron Sucrose.

Iron Oxide Saccharated (previously used name) — *See* Iron Sucrose.

Iron Perchloride — *See* Ferric Chloride.

Iron Polymalether (JAN) — *See* Ferropolimaler.

Iron Saccharate (previously used name) — *See* Iron Sucrose.

Iron Sorbitex [*1965*] (eye′ urn sor′ bi tex). **USP** [Injection]. A sterile, colloidal solution of a complex of trivalent iron, sorbitol, and citric acid, stabilized with dextrin and sorbitol. (1) Iron sorbitex; (2) Iron sorbitex. *CAS-1338-16-5. Hematinic.* ◇*Astra 1572*

Iron Sucrose [*1998*] (eye′ urn soo′ krose). **USP** [Injection]. [Saccharated Ferric Oxide is JAN.] (1) Iron saccharate; (2) Sucrose, iron complex. *UNII-FZ7NYF5N8L. CAS-8047-67-4.* BAN. *Treatment of iron deficiency anemia and related indications (hematinic).* Venofer (American Regent) *[Names previously used: Iron Sugar, Iron Sucrose Complex, Iron Oxide Saccharated, Iron(III) hydroxide Sucrose Complex, Saccharated Iron, Saccharated Iron Oxide, Ferric Hydroxide Sucrose Complex, and Iron Saccharate.]* ◇*XI-921*

Iron Sucrose Complex (previously used name) — *See* Iron Sucrose.

Iron Sugar (previously used name) — *See* Iron Sucrose.

Iroplact. $C_{346}H_{585}N_{97}O_{102}S_5$. 7896.26. *N*-L-Methionyl blood platelet factor 4 (human subunit). *CAS-154248-96-1.* INN.

```
MEAEEDGDLQ CLCVKTTSQV RPRHITSLEV IKAGPHCPTA QLIATLKNGR
KICLDLQAPL YKKIIKKLLE S
```

Iroxanadine. $C_{14}H_{20}N_4O$. 260.33. (-)-5-(Piperidin-1-ylmethyl)-3-(pyridin-3-yl)-5,6-dihydro-2*H*-1,2,4-oxadiazine. *CAS-276690-58-5.* INN.

Irsogladine. $C_9H_7Cl_2N_5$. 256.09. [Irsogladine Maleate is JAN.] 2,4-Diamino-6-(2,5-dichlorophenyl)-*s*-triazine. *UNII-QBX79NZC1D. CAS-57381-26-7.* INN; MI.

Irtemazole [*1991*] (ir tem′ a zole). $C_{18}H_{16}N_4$. 288.35. (1) 1*H*-Benzimidazole, 5-(1*H*-imidazol-1-ylphenylmethyl)-2-methyl-, (±)-; (2) (±)-5-(α-Imidazol-1-ylbenzyl)-2-methylbenzimidazole. *UNII-AAK27WY74I. CAS-115574-30-6.* INN; BAN. *Uricosuric.* ◇*R 60844*

Isaglidole. $C_{11}H_{13}FN_4$. 220.25. 4-Fluoro-2-(2-imidazolin-2-ylamino)isoindoline. *UNII-B51UC955KQ. CAS-110605-64-6.* INN.

Isalmadol. $C_{22}H_{27}NO_4$. 369.45. 3-{(1*RS*,2*RS*)-2-[(Dimethylamino)methyl]-1-hydroxycyclohexyl}phenyl 2-hydroxybenzoate. *CAS-269079-62-1.* INN.

Isalsteine. $C_{14}H_{15}NO_6S$. 325.34. (±)-*N*-[2-[(2-Methyl-4-oxo-1,3-benzodioxan-2-yl)thio]propionyl]glycine. *UNII-K0YPY57FUQ. CAS-116818-99-6.* INN.

Isamfazone. $C_{22}H_{23}N_3O_2$. 361.44. (-)-*N*-Methyl-*N*-(α-methylphenethyl)-6-oxo-3-phenyl-1(6*H*)-pyridazineacetamide. *UNII-XUW8L8PW09. CAS-55902-02-8.* INN.

Isamoltan. $C_{16}H_{22}N_2O_2$. 274.36. (±)-1-(Isopropylamino)-3-(*o*-pyrrol-1-ylphenoxy)-2-propanol. *UNII-2TP37O5J17. CAS-116861-00-8.* INN.

Isamoxole [*1977*] (eye″ sa mox′ ole). $C_{12}H_{20}N_2O_2$. 224.30. (1) Propanamide, *N*-butyl-2-methyl-*N*-(4-methyl-2-oxazolyl)-; (2) *N*-Butyl-2-methyl-*N*-(4-methyl-2-oxazolyl)propionamide. *CAS-57067-46-6.* INN; BAN. *Anti-asthmatic.* ◇*Compound 90606*

Isatoribine [*1999*] (eye″ sa tore′ i been). $C_{10}H_{12}N_4O_6S.H_2O$. 334.31. 5-Amino-3-β-D-ribofuranosylthiazolo[4,5-*d*]pyrimidine-2,7(3*H*,6*H*)-dione monohydrate. *CAS-198832-38-1; CAS-122970-40-5* [anhydrous]. INN; BAN. *Immunomodulator (regulates cell growth by perturbing signal transduction).* Immusine (ICN) ◇*ICN-10146; N10146; NARI-10146*

---

† Brand name formerly used, and/or firm no longer concerned with this product.

Isavuconazole. $C_{22}H_{17}F_2N_5OS$. 437.47. 4-{2-[(2R,3R)-3-(2,5-Difluorophenyl)-3-hydroxy-4-(1H-1,2,4-triazol-1-yl)butan-2-yl]-1,3-thiazol-4-yl}benzonitrile. *CAS-241479-67-4.* INN.

Isavuconazonium Chloride. $C_{35}H_{35}ClF_2N_8O_5S$. 753.22. 1-{(2R,3R)-3-[4-(4-Cyanophenyl)-1,3-thiazol-2-yl]-2-(2,5-difluorophenyl)-2-hydroxybutyl}-4-{(1RS)-1-[methyl-(3-{[(methylamino)acetyloxy]methyl}pyridin-2-yl)carbamoyloxy]ethyl}-1,2,4-triazolium chloride. *CAS-338990-84-4.* INN.

Isaxonine. $C_7H_{11}N_3$. 137.18. 2-(Isopropylamino)pyrimidine. *UNII-883G6DMT63. CAS-4214-72-6.* INN; MI.

Isbogrel. $C_{18}H_{19}NO_2$. 281.35. (E)-7-Phenyl-7-(3-pyridyl)-6-heptenoic acid. *UNII-HGB7P08R36. CAS-89667-40-3.* INN.

Isbufylline. $C_{11}H_{16}N_4O_2$. 236.27. 7-Isobutyltheophylline. *UNII-9C8Z5F38D0. CAS-90162-60-0.* INN.

Iscotrizinol [*2007*] (is″ koe triz′ i nol). $C_{44}H_{59}N_7O_5$. 765.98. (1) Benzoic acid, 4,4′-[[6-[[4-[[(1,1-dimethylethyl)amino]carbonyl]phenyl]amino]-1,3,5-triazine-2,4-diyl]diimino]bis-, bis(2-ethylhexyl) ester; (2) Bis(2-ethylhexyl) 4,4′-[(6-{[4-(*tert*-butylcarbamoyl)phenyl]amino}-1,3,5-triazine-2,4-diyl)diimino]dibenzoate. *UNII-2UTZ0QC864. CAS-154702-15-5. Sunscreen.* Uvasorb HEB (3V) ◇*Diethylhexyl butamido triazone (INCI)*

Iseganan Hydrochloride [*2002*] (eye″ se gan′ an hye″ droe klor′ ide). $C_{78}H_{126}N_{30}O_{18}S_4 \cdot xHCl \cdot yH_2O$. 1900.29 (anhydrous base). [Iseganan is INN.] L-Argininamide, L-arginylglycylglycyl-L-leucyl-L-cysteinyl-L-tyrosyl-L-cysteinyl-L-arginylglycyl-L-arginyl-L-phenylalanyl-L-cysteinyl-L-valyl-L-cysteinyl-L-valylglycyl-, cyclic (5→14), (7→12)-bis(disulfide), hydrochloride, hydrate. *CAS-244015-05-2; CAS-257277-05-7* [iseganan]. INN. *Antimicrobial peptide intended for use in the reduction in the severity of oral mucositis; oral decontamination in*

ventilator-associated pneumonia; aerosol formulation for control of infections in patients with cystic fibrosis. ◇*IB-367-03*

RGGLCYCRGR FCVCVGR ·HCl ·H2O

Isepamicin [*1986*] (eye sep″ a mye′ sin). $C_{22}H_{43}N_5O_{12}$. 569.60. [Isepamicin Sulfate is JAN.] (1) D-Streptamine, O-6-amino-6-deoxy-α-D-glucopyranosyl-(1→4)-O-[3-deoxy-4-C-methyl-3-(methylamino)-β-L-arabinopyranosyl-(1→6)]-N^1-(3-amino-2-hydroxy-1-oxopropyl)-2-deoxy-, (S)-; (2) O-6-Amino-6-deoxy-α-D-glucopyranosyl-(1→4)-O-[3-deoxy-4-C-methyl-3-(methylamino)-β-L-arabinopyranosyl-(1→6)]-2-deoxy-N^1-[(S)-isoseryl]-D-streptamine. *CAS-58152-03-7.* INN; BAN. *Antibacterial (aminoglycoside).* ◇*Sch 21420*

Ismomultin Alfa [*2004*] (iz″ moe mul′ tin al′ fa). $C_{1827}H_{2785}N_{493}O_{530}S_{11}$. 40,489. (1) Glycoprotein gp 39 (human cartilage isoform Org 39141); (2) 47-261-Glycoprotein gp 39 (human clone CDM8-gp39 reduced). *CAS-457913-93-8.* INN. *Treatment of rheumatoid arthritis.* ◇*Org 39141*

```
YKLVCYYTSW SQYREGDGSC FPDALDRFLC THIIYSFANI SNDHIDTWEW
NDVTLYGMLN TLKNRNPNLK TLLSVGGWNF GSQRFSKIAS NTQSRRTFIK
SVPPFLRTHG FDGLDLAWLY PGRRDKQHFT TLIKEMKAEF IKEAQPGKKQ
LLLSAALSAG KVTIDSSYDI AKISQHLDFI SIMTYDFHGA WRGTTGHHSP
LFRGQEDASP DRFSNTDYAV GYMLRLGAPA SKLVMGIPTF GRSFTLASSE
TGVGAPISGP GIPGRFTKEA GTLAYYEICD FLRGATVHRI LGQQVPYATK
GNQWVGYDDQ ESVKSKVQYL KDRQLAGAMV WALDLDDFQG SFCGQDLRFP
LTNAIKDALA AT
```

Iso-alcoholic Elixir. *CAS-8030-62-4.* NF XV.

Isoaminile. $C_{16}H_{24}N_2$. 244.38. [Isoaminile Citrate is JAN.] 4-Dimethylamino-2-isopropyl-2-phenylvaleronitrile. *CAS-77-51-0.* INN; BAN; DCF; MI.

Isoamyl Methoxycinnamate (previously used name) — *See* Amiloxate.

Isobromindione. $C_{15}H_9BrO_2$. 301.13. (±)-5-Bromo-2-phenyl-1,3-indandione. *UNII-J1J87P409K. CAS-1470-35-5.* INN.

Isobucaine Hydrochloride. $C_{15}H_{23}NO_2 \cdot HCl$. 285.81. (1) 1-Propanol, 2-methyl-2-[(2-methylpropyl)amino]-, benzoate (ester), hydrochloride; (2) 2-(Isobutylamino)-2-methyl-1-

propanol benzoate (ester) hydrochloride. *UNII-0C78CV13XZ. CAS-3562-15-0; CAS-14055-89-1* [isobucaine]. USP XXI.

Isobutamben [*1977*] (eye″ soe bue tam′ ben). $C_{11}H_{15}NO_2$. 193.24. (1) Benzoic acid, 4-amino-, 2-methylpropyl ester; (2) Isobutyl *p*-aminobenzoate. *UNII-9566855ULN. CAS-94-14-4*. INN. *Anesthetic (topical)*.

Isobutane (eye″ soe bue′ tane). **NF**. C_4H_{10}. 58.12. Contains not less than 95.0% of isobutane (C_4H_{10}). *UNII-BXR49TP611. CAS-75-28-5. Aerosol propellant*.

Isobutylhydrochlorothiazide — *See* Buthiazide.

Isobuzole (previously used name) — *See* Glysobuzole.

Isocarboxazid. $C_{12}H_{13}N_3O_2$. 231.25. (1) 3-Isoxazolecarboxylic acid, 5-methyl-, 2-(phenylmethyl)hydrazide; (2) 5-Methyl-3-isoxazolecarboxylic acid 2-benzylhydrazide. *UNII-34237V843T. CAS-59-63-2*. USP XXIII; INN; BAN. *Antidepressant*.

Isoconazole [*1973*] (eye″ soe kon′ a zole). $C_{18}H_{14}Cl_4N_2O$. 416.13. [Isoconazole Nitrate is JAN.] (1) 1*H*-Imidazole, 1-[2-(2,4-dichlorophenyl)-2-[(2,6-dichlorophenyl)methoxy]ethyl]-; (2) 1-[2,4-Dichloro-β-[(2,6-dichlorobenzyl)oxy]phenethyl]imidazole. *CAS-27523-40-6*. INN; BAN. *Antibacterial; antifungal.* ◇*R-15,454 [as nitrate salt]*

Isocromil. $C_{19}H_{16}O_5$. 324.33. 2-(*o*-Isopropoxyphenyl)-4-oxo-4*H*-1-benzopyran-6-carboxylic acid. *UNII-0L7AR6G18O. CAS-57009-15-1*. INN.

Isodapamide — *See* Zidapamide.

Isoetarine (INN, BAN) — *See* Isoetharine.

Isoethadione — *See* Paramethadione.

Isoetharine [*1962*] (eye″ soe eth′ a reen). **USP** [Inhalation Solution]. $C_{13}H_{21}NO_3$. 239.31. [Isoetarine is INN and BAN.] (1) 1,2-Benzenediol, 4-(1-hydroxy-2-[(1-methylethyl)amino]butyl)-; (2) 3,4-Dihydroxy-α-[1-(isopropylamino)propyl]benzyl alcohol. *UNII-YV0SN3276Q. CAS-530-08-5; CAS-13725-16-1* [replaced]; *CAS-32095-14-0* [replaced]. *Bronchodilator.* ◇*Win 3406*

Isoetharine Hydrochloride (eye″ soe eth′ a reen hye″ droe klor′ ide). **USP**. $C_{13}H_{21}NO_3 \cdot HCl$. 275.77. (1) 1,2-Benzenediol, 4-[1-hydroxy-2-[(1-methylethyl)amino]butyl]-, hydrochloride; (2) 3,4-Dihydroxy-α-[1-(isopropylamino)propyl]benzyl alcohol hydrochloride. *UNII-51V8U784H3; UNII-YV0SN3276Q* [isoetharine]. *CAS-2576-92-3; CAS-530-08-5* [isoetharine]. *Bronchodilator.* Bronkosol (Sanofi Aventis)

Isoetharine Mesylate (eye″ soe eth′ a reen mes′ i late). **USP**. $C_{13}H_{21}NO_3 \cdot CH_4O_3S$. 335.42. (1) 1,2-Benzenediol, 4-[1-hydroxy-2-[(1-methylethyl)amino]-butyl]-, methanesulfonate (salt); (2) 3,4-Dihydroxy-α-[1-(isopropylamino)propyl]benzyl alcohol methanesulfonate (salt). *UNII-DV74WJ5PJB. CAS-7279-75-6; CAS-530-08-5* [isoetharine]. *Bronchodilator.* Bronkometer (Sanofi Aventis)

Isofezolac. $C_{23}H_{18}N_2O_2$. 354.40. 1,3,4-Triphenylpyrazole-5-acetic acid. *UNII-7K6U6T1360. CAS-50270-33-2*. INN; MI.

Isoflupredone Acetate [*1976*] (eye″ soe floo′ pred one as′ e tate). **USP**. $C_{23}H_{29}FO_6$. 420.47. [Isoflupredone is INN and BAN.] (1) Pregna-1,4-diene-3,20-dione, 21-(acetyloxy)-9-fluoro-11,17-dihydroxy-, (11β)-; (2) 9-Fluoro-11β,17,21-trihydroxypregna-1,4-diene-3,20-dione 21-acetate. *UNII-55P9TUL75S; UNII-HYS0B45Z2S* [isoflupredone]. *CAS-338-98-7; CAS-338-95-4* [isoflupredone]. *Anti-inflammatory.* ◇*U-6013*

Isoflurane [*1972*] (eye″ soe flur′ ane). **USP**. $C_3H_2ClF_5O$. 184.49. (1) Ethane, 2-chloro-2-(difluoromethoxy)-1,1,1-trifluoro-; (2) 1-Chloro-2,2,2-trifluoroethyl difluoromethyl ether. *UNII-CYS9AKD70P. CAS-26675-46-7.* INN; BAN; JAN. *Anesthetic (inhalation).* Forane (Baxter Healthcare) ◇*Compound 469*

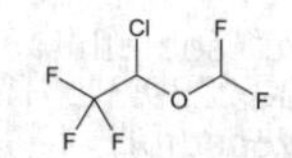

Isoflurophate (eye″ soe flur′ oh fate). **USP.** $C_6H_{14}FO_3P$. 184.15. [Dyflos is BAN.] (1) Phosphorofluoridic acid, bis(1-methylethyl) ester; (2) Diisopropyl phosphorofluoridate. *UNII-12UHW9R67N. CAS-55-91-4. Cholinergic (ophthalmic).* Floropryl (Merck)

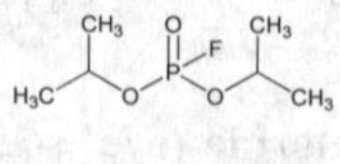

Isoleucine [*1980*] (eye″ soe loo′ seen). **USP.** $C_6H_{13}NO_2$. 131.17. [L-Isoleucine is JAN.] (1) L-Isoleucine; (2) L-Isoleucine. *UNII-04Y7590D77. CAS-73-32-5.* INN. *Amino acid.*

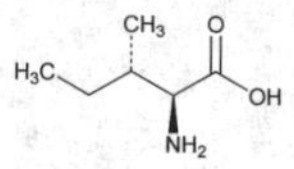

L-Isoleucine (JAN) — *See* Isoleucine.

Isomalt. NF. $CH_{24}O_{11}$. 212.19. (1) 6-*O*-α-Glucopyranosyl-D-sorbitol; (2) 6-*O*-α-D-Glucopyranosyl-D-glucitol. *CAS-64519-82-0* [dihydrate]. BAN. ◇*BAY i 3930*

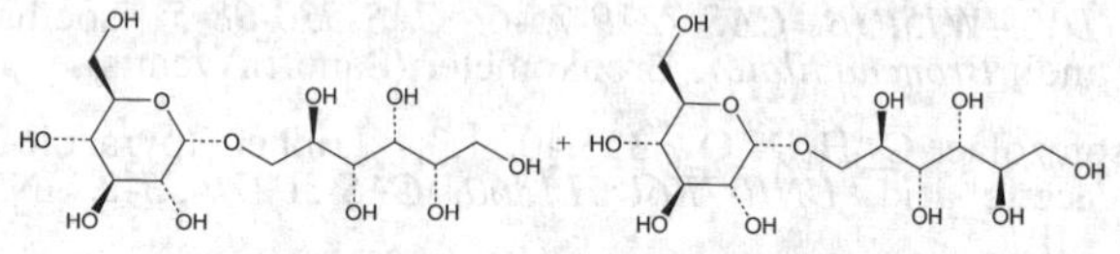

Isomazole Hydrochloride [*1986*] (eye soe′ ma zole hye″ droe klor′ ide). $C_{14}H_{13}N_3O_2S$·HCl. 323.80. [Isomazole is INN.] (1) 1*H*-Imidazo[4,5-*c*]pyridine, 2-[2-methoxy-4-(methylsulfinyl)phenyl]-, monohydrochloride; (2) 2-[2-Methoxy-4-(methylsulfinyl)phenyl]-1*H*-imidazo[4,5-*c*]pyridine monohydrochloride. *CAS-87359-33-9; CAS-86315-52-8* [isomazole]. *Cardiotonic.* ◇*LY 175326*

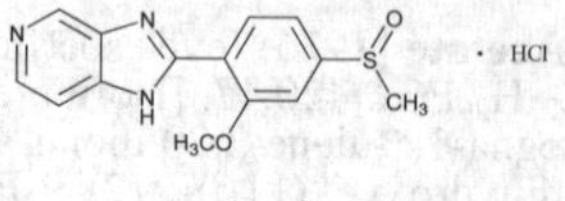

Isomerol [*1980*] (eye soe′ mer ol). C_7H_6HgO. 306.71. (1) (a) Mercury, [3-methylphenolato(2-)-*C²,O*]- and (b) [3-Methylphenolato(2-)-*C⁶,O*]mercury; (2) (a) 2-Methyl-7-oxa-8-mercurabicyclo[4.2.0]octa-1,3,5-triene and (b) 4-Methyl-7-oxa-8-mercurabicyclo[4.2.0]octa-1,3,5-triene. *CAS-72526-12-6* [a]; *CAS-72526-13-7* [b]. *Antiseptic.* [*Name previously used: Parahydrecin.*]

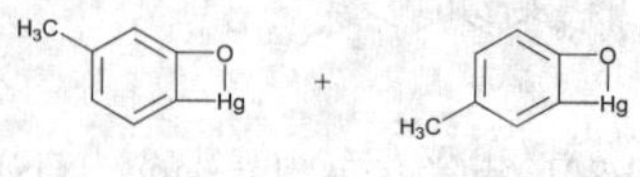

Isometamidium Chloride. $C_{28}H_{26}ClN_7$. 496.01. 8-[3-(*m*-Amidinophenyl)-2-triazeno]-3-amino-5-ethyl-6-phenyl-phenanthridinium chloride. *UNII-7NH28I651F. CAS-34301-55-8.* INN; BAN; MI. ◇*A-4180*

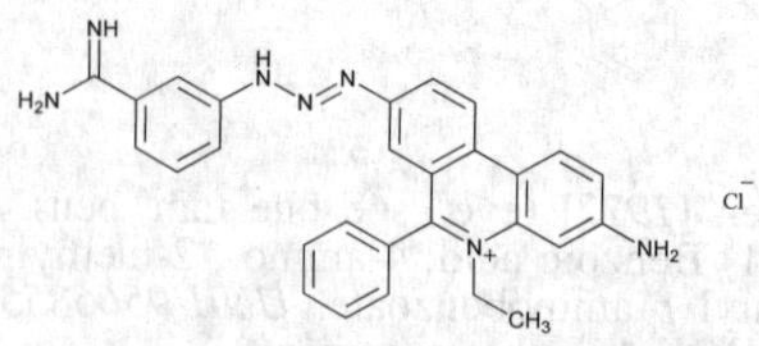

Isomethadone. $C_{21}H_{27}NO$. 309.45. 6-Dimethylamino-5-methyl-4,4-diphenyl-3-hexanone. *UNII-12L95QD6KV. CAS-466-40-0.* INN; BAN; DCF; MI. ◇*Win 1783*

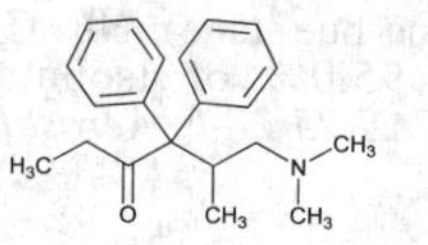

Isomethepdrine Chloride — *See* Isomethepgene Hydrochloride.

Isomethepdrine Chloride — *See* Isometheptene Hydrochloride.

Isometheptene Hydrochloride. $C_9H_{19}N$·HCl. 177.71. [Isometheptene is INN and BAN.] *N*,1,5-Trimethyl-4-hexenylamine hydrochloride. *UNII-9Z4CJC3O5F; UNII-Y7L24THH6T* [isometheptene]. *CAS-6168-86-1; CAS-503-01-5* [isometheptene]. NND 1964; MI. Octin (Knoll†)

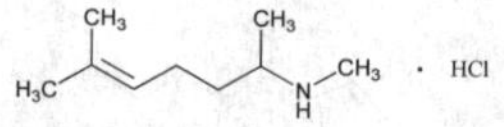

Isometheptene Mucate (eye″ soe meth ep′ teen mue′ kate). **USP.** $(C_9H_{19}N)_2$·$C_6H_{10}O_8$. 492.65. (1) Isometheptene, galactarate (2:1) (salt); (2) 6-Methylamino-2-methylheptene, tetrahydroxyadipic acid (2:1) (salt). *CAS-7492-31-1.*

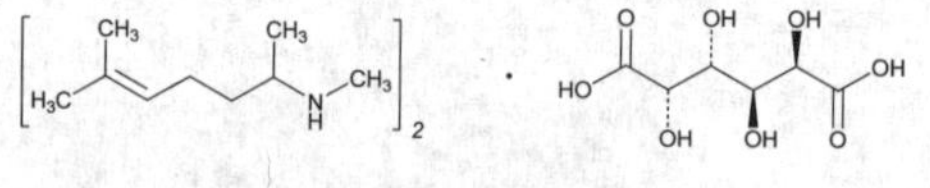

Isomolpan Hydrochloride [*1991*] (eye″ soe mol′ pan hye″ droe klor′ ide). $C_{15}H_{21}NO_2$·HCl. 283.79. [Isomolpan is INN.] (±)-*trans*-1,3,4,4a,5,10b-Hexahydro-4-propyl-2*H*-[1]benzopyrano[3,4-*b*]pyridin-9-ol hydrochloride. *CAS-121096-86-4; CAS-107320-86-5* [isomolpan]. *Antipsychotic (dopamine autoreceptor agonist).* ◇*CGS 15855A*

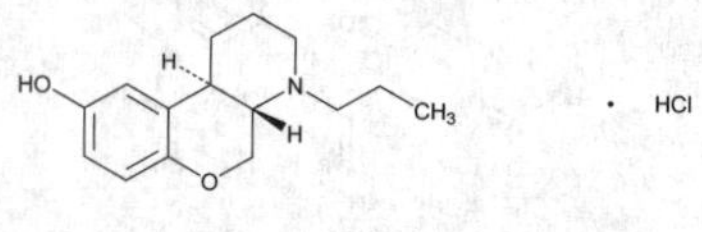

Isomylamine Hydrochloride [*1969*] (eye″ soe mil′ a meen hye″ droe klor′ ide). $C_{18}H_{35}NO_2$·HCl. 333.94. (1) Cyclohexanecarboxylic acid, 1-(3-methylbutyl)-, 2-(diethylamino)ethyl ester hydrochloride; (2) 2-(Diethylamino)ethyl 1-

isopentylcyclohexanecarboxylate hydrochloride. *UNII-8S4M0WS2UA. CAS-24357-98-0; CAS-28815-27-2* [isomylamine]. *Relaxant (smooth muscle).* ◇*NSC-78987*

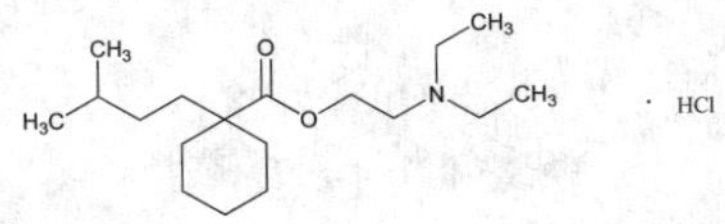

Isoniazid (eye″ soe nye′ a zid). **USP.** $C_6H_7N_3O$. 137.14. (1) 4-Pyridinecarboxylic acid, hydrazide; (2) Isonicotinic acid hydrazide. *UNII-V83O1VOZ8L. CAS-54-85-3.* INN; BAN; JAN. *Antibacterial (tuberculostatic).* Inh (Novartis); Nydrazid (Bristol-Myers Squibb)

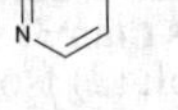

Isoniazid Glucuronate Sodium. $C_{12}H_{14}N_3NaO_7.2H_2O$. 371.28. Sodium glucuronate isonicotinyl hydrazone dihydrate. *CAS-25129-81-1* [anhydrous]. JAN.

Isoniazide Sodium Methanesulfonate (JAN) — *See* Methaniazide.

Isonicophen — *See* Aconiazide.

Isonicotinylhydrazine — *See* Isoniazid.

Isonixin. $C_{14}H_{14}N_2O_2$. 242.27. 2-Hydroxy-2′,6′-nicotinoxylidide. *UNII-BYX6E7M5QE. CAS-57021-61-1.* INN; MI.

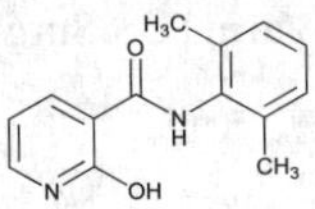

Isophenethanol — *See* Nifenalol.

Isoprazone. $C_{15}H_{18}N_2O$. 242.32. 1-(4-Amino-2-methyl-5-phenylpyrrol-3-yl)-2-methyl-1-propanone. *UNII-LB0T3NEB48. CAS-56463-68-4.* INN; BAN.

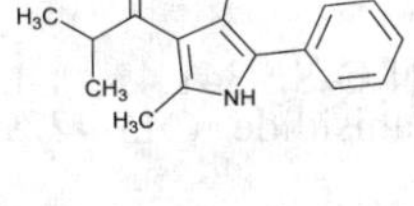

Isoprednidene. $C_{22}H_{28}O_5$. 372.45. 11β,17,21-Trihydroxy-16-methylenepregna-4,6-diene-3,20-dione. *CAS-17332-61-5.* INN; BAN.

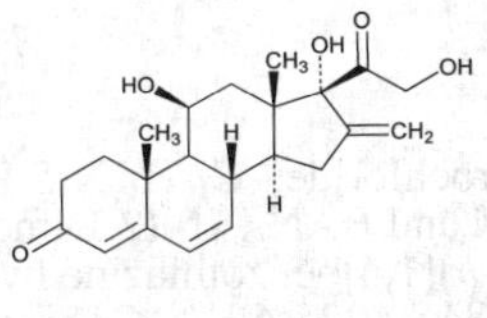

Isopregnenone — *See* Dydrogesterone.

Isoprenaline (INN, BAN) — *See* Isoproterenol Hydrochloride.

L-Isoprenaline — *See* Levisoprenaline.

---

† Brand name formerly used, and/or firm no longer concerned with this product.

l-Isoprenaline Hydrochloride (JAN) — *See* Isoproterenol Hydrochloride.

Isoprofen. $C_{15}H_{20}O_2$. 232.32. 2-Isopropyl-α-methyl-5-indanacetic acid. *CAS-57144-56-6.* INN.

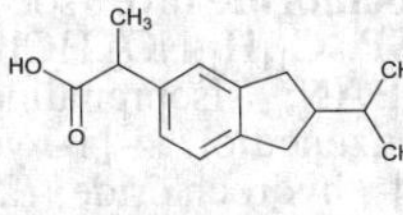

Isopropamide Iodide (eye″ soe proe′ pa mide eye′ oh dide). **USP.** $C_{23}H_{33}IN_2O$. 480.43. (1) Benzenepropanaminium, γ-(aminocarbonyl)-*N*-methyl-*N,N*-bis(1-methylethyl)-γ-phenyl-, iodide; (2) (3-Carbamoyl-3,3-diphenylpropyl)diisopropylmethylammonium iodide. *UNII-E0KNA372SZ; UNII-8B9I31H724* [isopropamide]. *CAS-71-81-8; CAS-7492-32-2* [isopropamide]. INN; BAN; JAN. *Anticholinergic.* Darbid (GlaxoSmithKline)

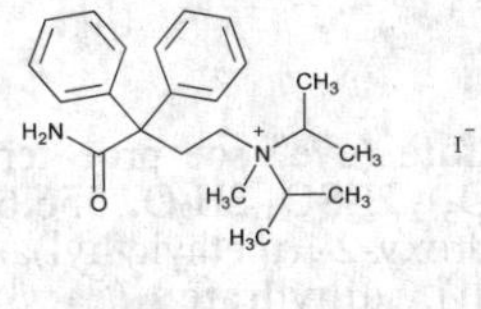

Isopropanol (JAN) — *See* Isopropyl Alcohol.

Isopropicillin. $C_{18}H_{22}N_2O_5S$. 378.44. (1-Methyl-1-phenoxyethyl)penicillin. *CAS-4780-24-9.* INN.

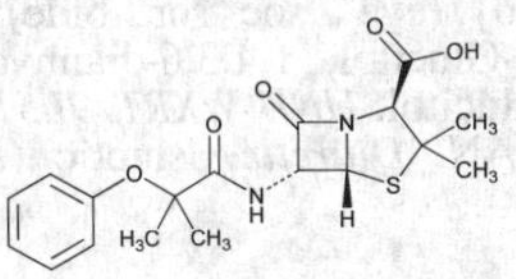

Isoproponum Iodide — *See* Isopropamide Iodide.

Isopropyl Alcohol (eye″ soe proe′ pil al′ ka hol). **USP.** C_3H_8O. 60.10. [Isopropanol is JAN.] (1) 2-Propanol; (2) Isopropyl alcohol. *UNII-ND2M416302. CAS-67-63-0. Anti-infective, topical; pharmaceutic aid (solvent).*

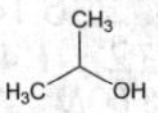

Isopropyl Myristate [*2005*] (eye″ soe proe′ pil mir′ is tate). **NF.** $C_{17}H_{34}O_2$. 270.45. (1) Tetradecanoic acid, 1-methylethyl ester; (2) Myristic acid, isopropyl alcohol ester. *UNII-0RE8K4LNJS. CAS-110-27-0. Pharmaceutic aid (emollient).* Estergel (Merck)

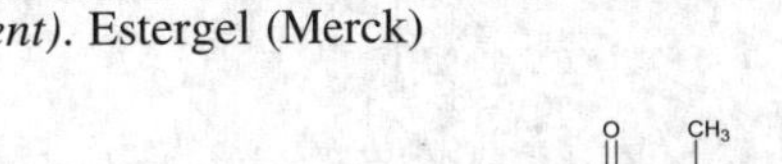

Isopropyl Palmitate (eye″ soe proe′ pil pal′ mi tate). **NF.** $C_{19}H_{38}O_2$. 298.50. (1) Hexadecanoic acid, 1-methylethyl ester; (2) Isopropyl palmitate. *UNII-8CRQ2TH63M. CAS-142-91-6. Pharmaceutic aid (vehicle, oleaginous).*

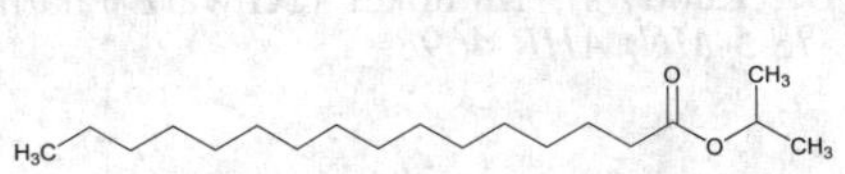

Isopropylantipyrine (JAN) — *See* Propyphenazone.

Isopropylarterenol Hydrochloride — *See* Isoproterenol Hydrochloride.

Isopropylarterenol Sulfate — *See* Isoproterenol Sulfate.

N-Isopropyl-*p*-Iodoamphetamine (^{123}I) Hydrochloride (JAN) — *See* Iofetamine Hydrochloride I 123.

Isoproterenol Hydrochloride (eye″ soe proe ter′ e nol hye″ droe klor′ ide). **USP.** $C_{11}H_{17}NO_3$.HCl. 247.72. [Isoprenaline is INN and BAN; *l*-Isoprenaline Hydrochloride is JAN.] (1) 1,2-Benzenediol, 4-[1-hydroxy-2-[(1-methylethyl)amino]ethyl]-, hydrochloride; (2) 3,4-Dihydroxy-α-[(isopropylamino)methyl]benzyl alcohol hydrochloride. *UNII-DIA2A74855; UNII-L628TT009W* [isoproterenol]. *CAS-51-30-9; CAS-7683-59-2* [isoproterenol]. *Bronchodilator*. Aerolone (Lilly); Isuprel (Sanofi Aventis); Norisodrine (Abbott)

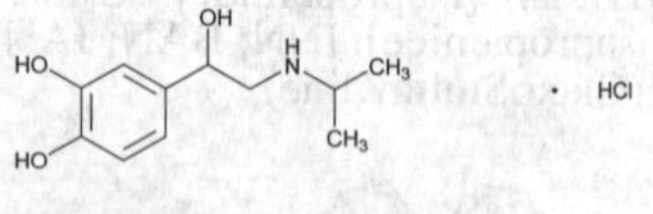

Isoproterenol Sulfate (eye″ soe proe ter′ e nol sul′ fate). **USP.** $(C_{11}H_{17}NO_3)_2$.H_2SO_4.$2H_2O$. 556.62. (1) 1,2-Benzenediol, 4-[1-hydroxy-2-[(methylethyl)amino]ethyl]-, sulfate (2:1) (salt), dihydrate; (2) 3,4-Dihydroxy-α-[(isopropylamino)methyl]benzyl alcohol sulfate (2:1) (salt) dihydrate. *UNII-925FX3X776. CAS-6700-39-6; CAS-299-95-6* [anhydrous]; *CAS-7683-59-2* [isoproterenol]. JAN. *Bronchodilator*. Norisodrine (Abbott)

Isosorbide [*1966*] (eye″ soe sor′ bide). **USP.** $C_6H_{10}O_4$. 146.14. (1) D-Glucitol, 1,4:3,6-dianhydro-; (2) 1,4:3,6-Dianhydro-D-glucitol. *UNII-WXR179L51S. CAS-652-67-5.* INN; BAN; JAN. *Diuretic*. Ismotic (Alcon) ◇*AT-101; NSC-40725*

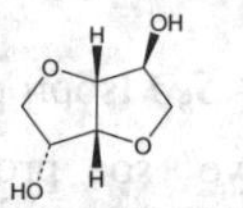

Isosorbide Dinitrate [*1966*] (eye″ soe sor′ bide dye nye′ trate). **USP.** $C_6H_8N_2O_8$. 236.14. (1) D-Glucitol, 1,4:3,6-dianhydro-, dinitrate; (2) 1,4:3,6-Dianhydro-D-glucitol dinitrate. *UNII-IA7306519N. CAS-87-33-2.* INN; BAN; JAN. *Vasodilator (coronary)*. Dilatrate (Schwarz Pharma); Isordil (Biovail); Sorbitrate (AstraZeneca)

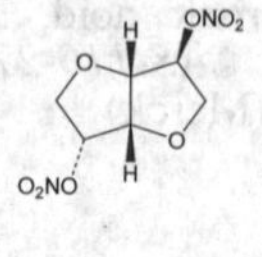

Isosorbide Mononitrate [*1988*] (eye″ soe sor′ bide mon″ oh nye′ trate). **USP.** $C_6H_9NO_6$. 191.14. (1) D-Glucitol, 1,4:3,6-dianhydro-, 5-nitrate; (2) 1,4:3,6-Dianhydro-D-glucitol 5-nitrate. *UNII-LX1OH63030. CAS-16051-77-7.* INN; BAN; JAN. *Vasodilator (coronary)*. Imdur (Schering-Plough); Ismo (Dr. Reddy's); Monoket (Schwarz Pharma) ◇*BM 22.145; IS 5-MN; AHR-4698*

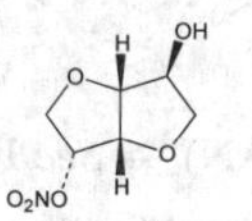

Isospaglumic Acid. $C_{11}H_{16}N_2O_8$. 304.25. *N*-(*N*-Acetyl-L-α-aspartyl)-L-glutamic acid. *CAS-3106-85-2.* INN.

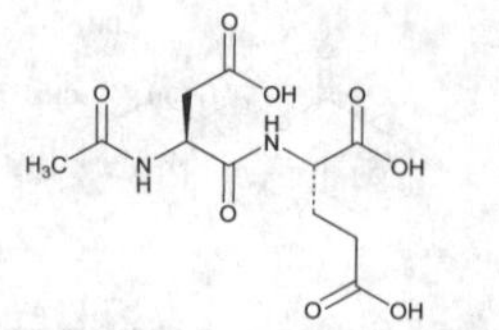

Isospirilene — *See* Spirilene.

Isostearyl Alcohol [*1980*] (eye″ soe steer′ il al′ ka hol). $C_{18}H_{38}O$. 270.49. A mixture of branched chain aliphatic 18 carbon alcohols, having an iodine value of 10 to 20, a saponification value of less than 3, and an acid value of less than 0.5. (1) Isooctadecanol; (2) Isooctadecyl alcohol. CID. *Pharmaceutic aid (emollient); pharmaceutic aid (solvent)*. Witcohol 66 (Witco)

Isosulfamerazine — *See* Sulfaperin.

Isosulfan Blue [*1979*] (eye″ soe sul′ fan). $C_{27}H_{31}N_2NaO_6S_2$. 566.66. [Sulphan Blue is BAN.] (1) Ethanaminium, *N*-[4-[[4-(diethylamino)phenyl](2,5-disulfophenyl)methylene]-2,5-cyclohexadien-1-ylidene]-*N*-ethyl-, hydroxide, inner salt, sodium salt; (2) [4-[α-[*p*-(Diethylamino)phenyl]-2,5-disulfobenzylidene]-2,5-cyclohexadien-1-ylidene]diethylammonium hydroxide, inner salt, sodium salt. *UNII-39N9K8S2A4. CAS-68238-36-8. Diagnostic aid (lymphangiography)*. Lymphazurin (US Surgical) ◇*P-4125; P-1888*

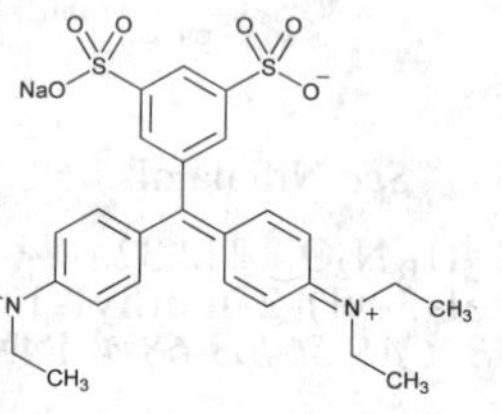

Isosulpride. $C_{15}H_{23}N_3O_4S$. 341.43. 1-Ethyl-5′-sulfamoyl-2-pyrrolidineacet-*o*-anisidide. *CAS-42792-26-7.* INN.

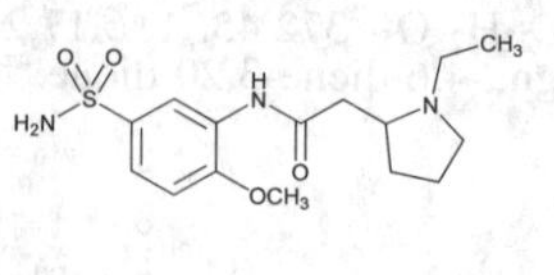

Isothipendyl Hydrochloride. $C_{16}H_{19}N_3S$.HCl. 321.87. [Isothipendyl is INN and BAN.] 10-(2-Dimethylaminopropyl)-10*H*-pyrido[3,2-*b*][1,4]benzothiazine hydrochloride. *UNII-953AP1LBV8. CAS-1225-60-1; CAS-482-15-5* [isothipendyl]. JAN; MI.

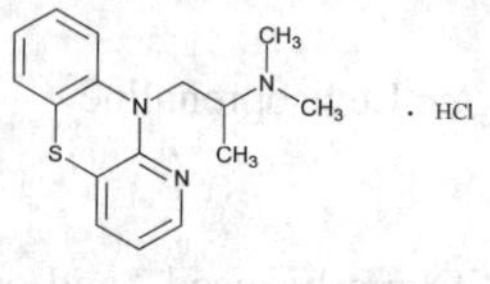

Isotiquimide [*1986*] (eye″ soe ti′ kwim ide). $C_{11}H_{14}N_2S$. 206.31. (1) 8-Quinolinecarbothioamide, 5,6,7,8-tetrahydro-4-methyl-, (±)-; (2) (±)-5,6,7,8-Tetrahydro-4-methylthio-8-quinolinecarboxamide. *UNII-EX1ND80X1I. CAS-56717-18-1*. INN; BAN. *Anti-ulcerative*. ◇*WY-24,377*

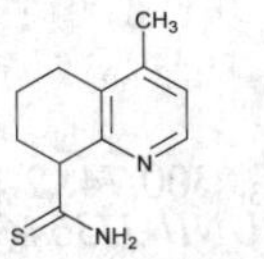

Isotretinoin [*1979*] (eye″ soe tret′ i noin). **USP**. $C_{20}H_{28}O_2$. 300.44. (1) Retinoic acid, 13-*cis*-; (2) 3,7-Dimethyl-9-(2,6,6-trimethyl-1-cyclohexen-1-yl)2-*cis*-4-*trans*-6-*trans*-8-*trans*-nonatetraenoic acid. *UNII-EH28UP18IF. CAS-4759-48-2*. INN; BAN. *Keratolytic*. Accutane (Roche); Amnesteem (Genpharm); Claravis (Barr); Sotret (Ranbaxy) ◇*Ro 4-3780*

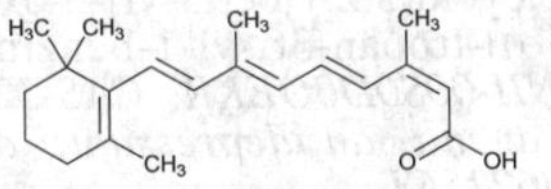

Isotretinoin Anisatil [*1997*] (eye″ soe tret′ i noin a ni′ sa til). $C_{29}H_{36}O_4$. 448.59. (1) Retinoic acid, 1-2-(4-methoxyphenyl)-2-oxoethyl ester, 13-*cis*-; (2) *p*-Methoxyphenacyl 13-*cis*-retinoate. *CAS-127471-94-7. Anti-acne*. ◇*GR 116526X*

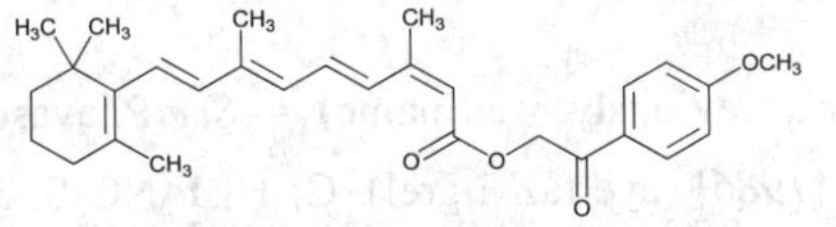

Isovaleramide [*2005*] (eye″ soe va ler′ a mide). $C_5H_{11}NO$. 101.15. (1) Butanamide, 3-methyl-; (2) 3-Methylbutanamide. *UNII-9CP4KB634M. CAS-541-46-8. Anxiolytic, anticonvulsant, antispastic, antimigraine, mood stabilizer and analgesic*. ◇*NFS1776*

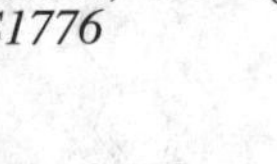

Isoxaprolol. $C_{19}H_{26}N_2O_3$. 330.42. (±)-(*E*)-1-(*tert*-Butylamino)-3-[*o*-[2-(3-methyl-5-isoxazolyl)vinyl]phenoxy]-2-propanol. *UNII-0Y84EU1HAA. CAS-75949-60-9*. INN.

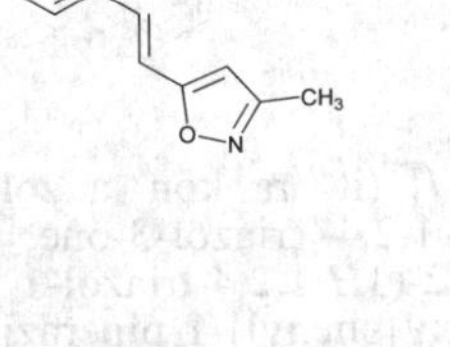

Isoxepac [*1977*] (eye sox′ e pak). $C_{16}H_{12}O_4$. 268.26. (1) Dibenz[*b,e*]oxepin-2-acetic acid, 6,11-dihydro-11-oxo-; (2) 6,11-Dihydro-11-oxodibenz[*b,e*]oxepin-2-acetic acid. *CAS-55453-87-7*. INN; BAN. *Anti-inflammatory*. Artil (Hoechst-Roussel†) ◇*HP 549; P 720549*

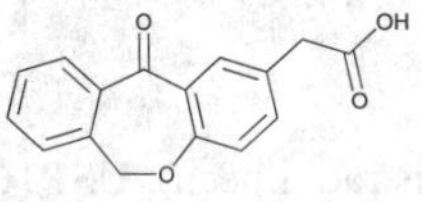

Isoxicam [*1974*] (eye sox′ i kam). $C_{14}H_{13}N_3O_5S$. 335.34. (1) 2*H*-1,2-Benzothiazine-3-carboxamide, 4-hydroxy-2-methyl-*N*-(5-methyl-3-isoxazolyl)-, 1,1-dioxide; (2) 4-Hydroxy-2-methyl-*N*-(5-methyl-3-isoxazolyl)-2*H*-1,2-benzothiazine-3-carboxamide 1,1-dioxide. *UNII-8XU734C4NG. CAS-34552-84-6*. INN; BAN. *Anti-inflammatory*. Maxicam (Parke-Davis†) ◇*W 8495*

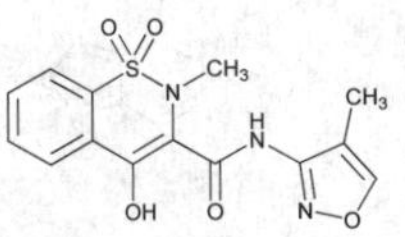

Isoxsuprine Hydrochloride (eye sox′ sue preen hye″ droe klor′ ide). **USP**. $C_{18}H_{23}NO_3 \cdot HCl$. 337.84. [Isoxsuprine is INN and BAN.] (1) Benzenemethanol, 4-hydroxy-α-[1-[(1-methyl-2-phenoxyethyl)amino]ethyl]-, hydrochloride, stereoisomer; (2) *p*-Hydroxy-α-[1-[(1-methyl-2-phenoxyethyl)amino]ethyl]benzyl alcohol hydrochloride; (3) (±)-(α*R**)-*p*-Hydroxy-α-[(1*S**)-1-[[(1*S**)-1-methyl-2-phenoxyethyl]amino]ethyl]benyl alcohol hydrochloride. *UNII-V74TEQ36CO; UNII-R15UI3245N* [isoxsuprine]. *CAS-579-56-6; CAS-34331-89-0; CAS-395-28-8* [isoxsuprine]. JAN. *Vasodilator*. Vasodilan (Apothecon)

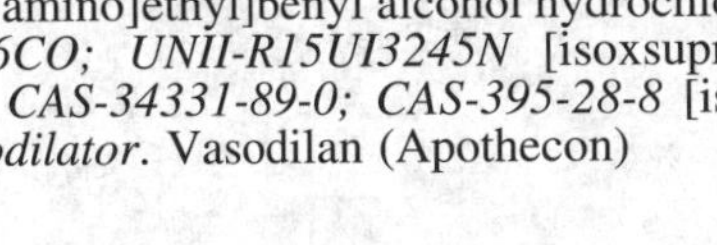

Ispinesib Mesylate [*2005*] (is pin′ e sib mes′ i late). $C_{30}H_{33}ClN_4O_2 \cdot CH_4O_3S$. 613.17. [Ispinesib is INN.] (1) Benzamide, *N*-(3-aminopropyl)-*N*-[(1*R*)-1-[7-chloro-3,4-dihydro-4-oxo-3-(phenylmethyl)-2-quinazolinyl]-2-methylpropyl]-4-methyl-, monomethanesulfonate; (2) *N*-(3-Aminopropyl)-*N*-[(1*R*)-1-(3-benzyl-7-chloro-4-oxo-3,4-dihydroquinazolin-2-yl)-2-methylpropyl]-4-methylbenzamide monomethanesulfonate. *UNII-R6ZMD4UH3D. CAS-514820-03-2; CAS-336113-53-2* [ispinesib]. *Antineoplastic (kinesin inhibitor)*. ◇*SB-715992-S; CK0238273*

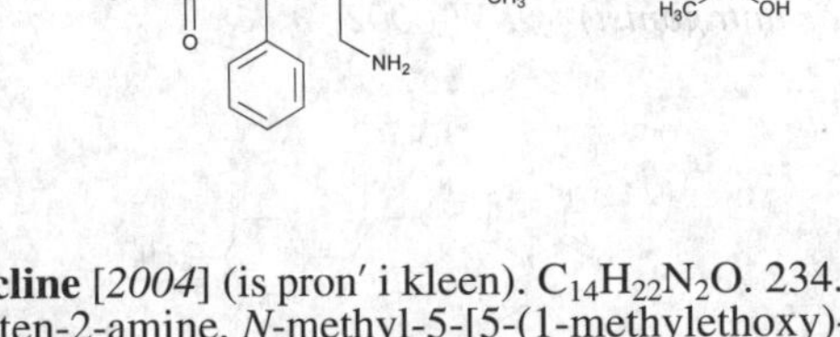

Ispronicline [*2004*] (is pron′ i kleen). $C_{14}H_{22}N_2O$. 234.34. (1) 4-Penten-2-amine, *N*-methyl-5-[5-(1-methylethoxy)-3-pyridinyl]-, (2*S*,4*E*)-; (2) (2*S*,4*E*)-*N*-Methyl-5-[5-(1-methylethoxy)pyridin-3-yl]pent-4-en-2-amine. *UNII-*

---

† Brand name formerly used, and/or firm no longer concerned with this product.

3E05NBH9V5. CAS-252870-53-4. INN. *Treatment of cognitive and memory disorders (neuronal nicotinic receptor partial agonist).* ◇*TC-01734*

Isradipine [*1987*] (is rad′ i peen). **USP.** $C_{19}H_{21}N_3O_5$. 371.39. (1) 3,5-Pyridinedicarboxylic acid, 4-(4-benzofurazanyl)-1,4-dihydro-2,6-dimethyl-, methyl 1-methylethyl ester, (±)-; (2) Isopropyl methyl (±)-4-(4-benzofurazanyl)-1,4-dihydro-2,6-dimethyl-3,5-pyridinedicarboxylate. *UNII-YO1UK1S598. CAS-75695-93-1.* INN; BAN. *Antagonist (calcium channel).* Dynacirc (Reliant) ◇*PN 200-110*

Israpafant. $C_{28}H_{29}ClN_4S$. 489.07. (±)-4-(*o*-Chlorophenyl)-2-(*p*-isobutylphenethyl)-6,9-dimethyl-6*H*-thieno[3,2-*f*]-*s*-triazolo[4,3-*a*][1,4]diazepine. *UNII-O3MCV749SW. CAS-117279-73-9.* INN.

Isrodipine — *See* Isradipine.

Istaroxime. $C_{21}H_{32}N_2O_3$. 360.49. 3-[(2-Aminoethoxy)imino]-5α-androstan-6,17-dione. *CAS-203737-93-3.* INN.

Istradefylline [*2003*] (is″ tra def′ i lin). $C_{20}H_{24}N_4O_4$. 384.43. (1) 1*H*-Purine-2,6-dione, 8-[(1*E*)-2-(3,4-dimethoxyphenyl)ethenyl]-1,3-diethyl-3,7-dihydro-7-methyl-; (2) 8-[(1*E*)-2-(3,4-Dimethoxyphenyl)ethenyl]-1,3-diethyl-7-methyl-3,7-dihydro-1*H*-purine-2,6-dione; (3) (*E*)-8-(3,4-Dimethoxystyryl)-1,3-diethyl-7-methyl-3,7-dihydro-1*H*-purine-2,6-dione. *UNII-2GZ0LIK7T4. CAS-155270-99-8.* INN. *Treatment of Parkinson's disease (adenosine A_{2A} receptor antagonist).* ◇*KW-6002*

Itameline. $C_{14}H_{15}ClN_2O_3$. 294.73. (*E*)-*p*-Chlorophenyl 3-formyl-5,6-dihydro-1(2*H*)-pyridinecarboxylate, *O*-methyloxime. *UNII-5VO597V509. CAS-121750-57-0.* INN.

Itanoxone. $C_{17}H_{13}ClO_3$. 300.74. 2-[*p*-(*o*-Chlorophenyl)phenacyl]acrylic acid. *UNII-11364Q5595. CAS-58182-63-1.* INN.

Itasetron [*1995*] (eye″ ta set′ ron). $C_{16}H_{20}N_4O_2$. 300.36. (1) 1*H*-Benzimidazole-1-carboxamide, 2,3-dihydro-*N*-(8-methyl-8-azabicyclo[3.2.1]oct-3-yl)-2-oxo, *endo*-; (2) 2-Oxo-*N*-1α*H*,5α*H*-tropan-3α-yl-1-benzimidazoline-1-carboxamide. *UNII-00S0D0OEKR. CAS-123258-84-4.* INN. *Anti-anxiety agent; antidepressant; anti-emetic.* ◇*U-98079A; DAU6215CL*

Itavastatin (previously used name) — *See* Pitavastatin.

Itazigrel [*1986*] (eye taz′ i grel). $C_{18}H_{14}F_3NO_2S$. 365.37. (1) Thiazole, 4,5-bis(4-methoxyphenyl)-2-(trifluoromethyl)-; (2) 4,5-bis(*p*-Methoxyphenyl)-2-(trifluoromethyl)thiazole. *CAS-70529-35-0.* INN. *Platelet aggregation inhibitor.* ◇*U-53,059*

Itazogrel — *See* Itazigrel.

Itobarbital — *See* Butalbital.

Itopride. $C_{20}H_{26}N_2O_4$. 358.43. *N*-[*p*-[2-(Dimethylamino)ethoxy]benzyl]veratramide. *UNII-81BMQ80QRL. CAS-122898-67-3.* INN.

Itraconazole [*1984*] (it″ ra kon′ a zole). $C_{35}H_{38}Cl_2N_8O_4$. 705.63. (1) 3*H*-1,2,4-Triazol-3-one, 4-[4-[4-[4-[[2-(2,4-dichlorophenyl)-2-(1*H*-1,2,4-triazol-1-ylmethyl)-1,3-dioxolan-4-yl]methoxy]phenyl]-1-piperazinyl]phenyl]-2,4-dihydro-2-(1-methylpropyl)-; (2) (±)-1-*sec*-Butyl-4-[*p*-[4-[*p*-[[(2*R**,4*S**)-2-(2,4-dichlorophenyl)-2-(1*H*-1,2,4-triazol-1-ylmethyl)-1,3-dioxolan-4-yl]methoxy]phenyl]-1-piperazinyl]phenyl]-Δ^2-1,2,4-triazolin-5-one. *UNII-304NUG5GF4. CAS-84625-61-6.* INN; BAN; JAN. *Antifungal.* Sporanox (Janssen) ✧*R 51,211*

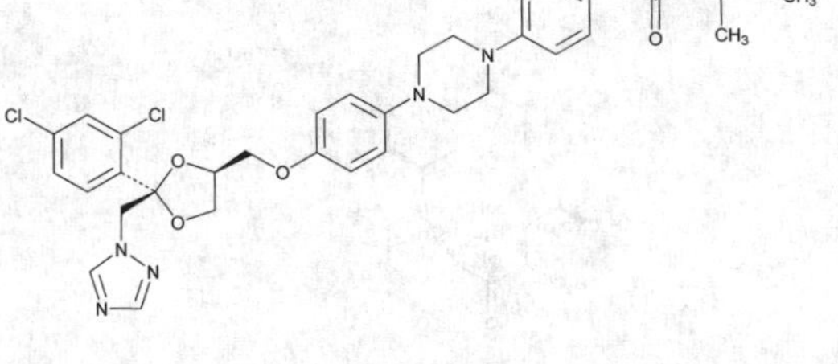

Itramin Tosilate (INN, BAN) — *See* Itramin Tosylate.

Itramin Tosylate. $C_2H_6N_2O_3.C_7H_8O_3S$. 278.28. [Itramin Tosilate is INN and BAN.] 2-Aminoethanol nitrate (ester) *p*-toluenesulfonate. *CAS-13445-63-1.* MI.

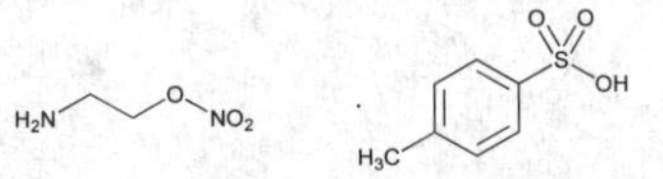

Itriglumide. $C_{33}H_{38}N_2O_4$. 526.67. (*R*)-2′-(8-Azaspiro[4,5]dec-8-ylcarbonyl)-4′,6′-dimethyl-3-(1-naphthyl)glutaranilic acid. *UNII-879A12466H. CAS-201605-51-8.* INN.

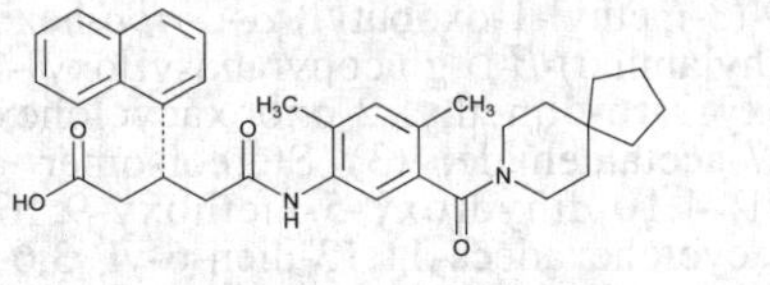

Itrocainide. $C_{23}H_{27}N_3O$. 361.48. *N*-[2-(Diethylamino)ethyl]-1-*o*-tolyl-4-isoquinolinecarboxamide. *UNII-79EDP2V-HY8. CAS-90828-99-2.* INN.

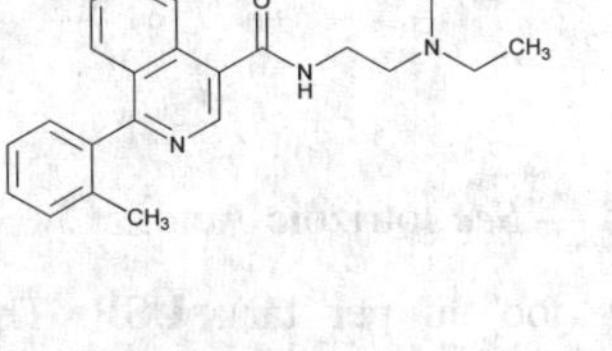

Itrocinonide. $C_{29}H_{38}F_2O_9$. 568.60. 6α,9-Difluoro-11β,16α,17-trihydroxy-3-oxoandrosta-1,4-diene-17β-carboxylic acid, ester with ethyl (*S*)-1-hydroxyethyl carbonate, cyclic (*R*)-16,17-acetal with butyraldehyde. *UNII-2ZW8NEP6PQ. CAS-106033-96-9.* INN.

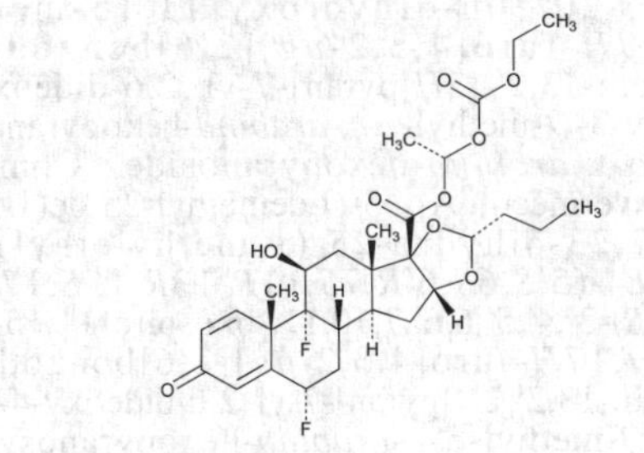

Iturelix [*2000*] (eye″ tue rel′ ix). $C_{82}H_{108}ClN_{17}O_{14}$. 1591.29. (1) D-Alaninamide, *N*-acetyl-3-(naphthalenyl)-D-alanyl-4-chloro-D-phenylalanyl-3-(3-pyridinyl)-D-alanyl-L-seryl-N^6-3-pyridinylcarbonyl)-L-lysyl-N^6-(3-pyridinylcarbonyl)-D-lysyl-L-leucyl-N^6-(1-methylethyl)-L-lysyl-L-prolyl-; (2) [*N*-Acetyl-3-(naphhalen-2-yl)-D-alanyl]-*p*-chloro-D-phenylalanyl-3-(3-pyridyl)-D-alanyl-L-seryl-N^6-nicotinyl-L-lysyl-N^6-nicotinyl-D-lysyl-L-leucyl-N^6-isopropyl-L-lysyl-L-prolyl-D-alaninamide. *CAS-112568-12-4.* INN. *Reversible inhibition of gonadotropin secretion and subsequent suppression of ovarian and testicular steroid secretion (gonadotropin releasing hormone antagonist).* ✧*Orf-32541*

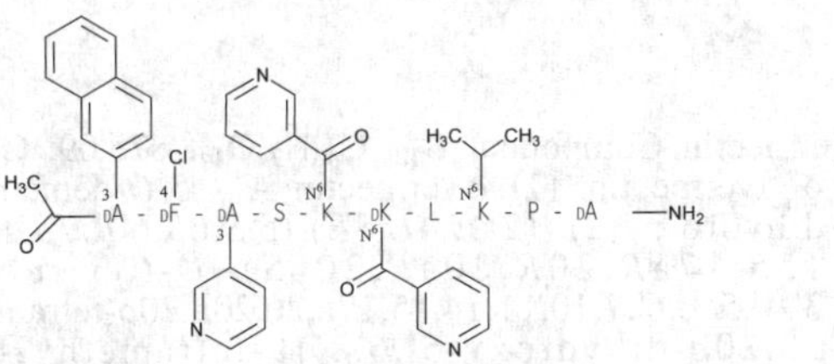

Ivabradine. $C_{27}H_{36}N_2O_5$. 468.59. 3-[3-[[[(7*S*)-3,4-Dimethoxybicyclo[4.2.0]octa-1,3,5-trien-7-yl]methyl]methylamino]propyl]-1,3,4,5-tetrahydro-7,8-dimethoxy-2*H*-3-benzazepin-2-one. *UNII-3H48L0LPZQ. CAS-155974-00-8.* INN.

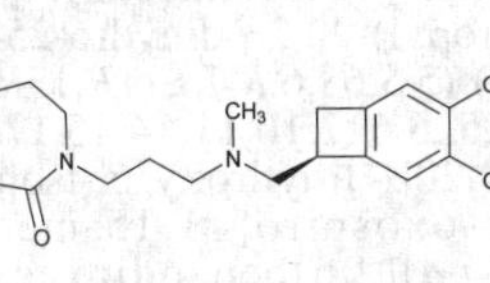

Ivarimod. $C_{30}H_{44}N_2O_5$. 512.68. 4-[[(3a*R*,3b*S*,5a*R*,6*R*,9a*R*,9b*R*,11*R*,11a*R*)-1,2,3,3a,4,5,5a,6,7,8,9,9a,9b,10,11,11a-Hexadecahydro-2-(2-hydroxyethyl)-12-isopropyl-6,9a-dimethyl-1,3-dioxo-3b,11-etheno-3b*H*-naphth[2,1-*e*]isoindol-6-yl]carbonyl]morpholine. *UNII-191NHP88M6. CAS-53003-81-9.* INN.

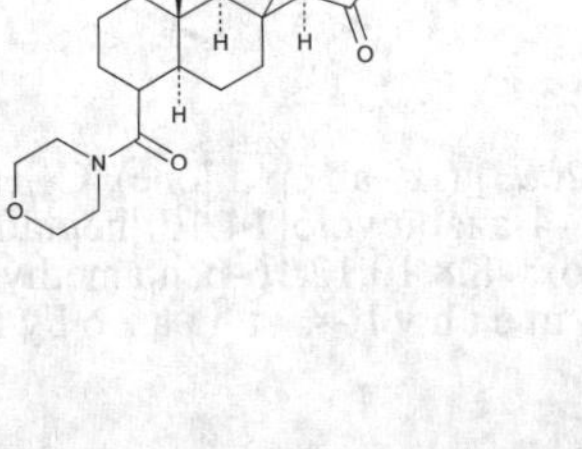

---

† Brand name formerly used, and/or firm no longer concerned with this product.

Ivermectin [*1979*] (eye″ ver mek′ tin). **USP.** C₄₈H₇₄O₁₄ (Component H₂B₁ₐ). 875.09; C₄₇H₇₂O₁₄ (Component H₂B₁ᵦ). 861.07. Component H₂B₁ₐ: (1) Avermectin A₁ₐ, 5-*O*-demethyl-22,23-dihydro-; (2) (2a*E*,4*E*,8*E*)-(5′*S*,6*S*,6′*R*,7*S*,11*R*,13*R*,15*S*,17a*R*,20*R*,20a*R*,20b*S*)-6′-(*S*)-*sec*-Butyl-3′,4′,5′,6,6′,7,10,11,14,15,17a,20,20a,20b-tetradecahydro-20,20b-dihydroxy[11,15-methano-2*H*,13*H*,17*H*-furo[4,3,2-*pg*][2,6]benzodioxacyclooctadecin-13,2′-[2*H*]pyran]-7-yl 2,6-dideoxy-4-*O*-(2,6-dideoxy-3-*O*-methyl-α-L-*arabino*-hexopyranosyl)-3-*O*-methyl-α-L-*arabino*-hexopyranoside. Component H₂B₁ᵦ: (1) Avermectin A₁ₐ, 5-*O*-demethyl-25-de(1-methylpropyl)-22,23-dihydro-25-(1-methylethyl)-; (2) (2a*E*,4*E*,8*E*)-(5′*S*,6*S*,6′*R*,7*S*,11*R*,13*R*,15*S*,17a*R*,20-*R*,20a*R*,20b*S*)-3′,4′,5′,6,6′,7,10,11,-oxospiro[11,15-methano-2*H*,13*H*,17*H*-furo[4,3,2-*pg*][2,6]benzodioxacyclooctadecin-13,2′[2*H*]pyran]-7-yl 2,6-dideoxy-4-*O*-(2,6-dideoxy-3-*O*-methyl-α-L-*arabino*-hexopyranosyl)-3-*O*-methyl-α-L-*arabino*-hexopyranoside. *UNII-8883YP2R6D. CAS-70288-86-7; CAS-70161-11-4* [component B₁ₐ]; *CAS-70209-81-3* [component B₁ᵦ]. INN; BAN. *Antiparasitic.* Stromectol (Merck)

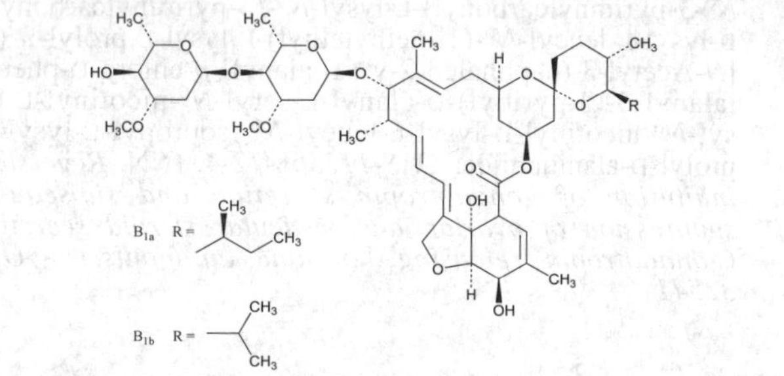

Ivermectin Component B₁ₐ. C₄₈H₇₄O₁₄. 875.09. Component of Ivermectin. (1) Avermectin A₁ₐ, 5-*O*-demethyl-22,23-dihydro-; (2) (2a*E*,4*E*,8*E*)-(5′*S*,6*S*,6′*R*,7*S*,11*R*,13*R*,-15*S*,17a*R*,20*R*,20a*R*,20b*S*)-6′-(*S*)-*sec*-Butyl-3′,4′,5′,6,6′,7,10,11,14,15,17a,20,20a,20b-tetradecahydro-20,20b-dihydroxy-5′,6,8,19-tetramethyl-17-oxo-spiro[11,15-methano-2*H*,13*H*,17*H*-furo[4,3,2-*pq*][2,6]benzodioxacyclooctadecin-13,2′-[2*H*]pyran]-7-yl 2,6-dideoxy-4-*O*-(2,6-dideoxy-3-*O*-methyl-α-L-*arabino*-hexopyranosyl)-3-*O*-methyl-α-L-*arabino*-hexopyranoside. *CAS-70161-11-4.* MI.

Ivermectin Component B₁ᵦ. C₄₇H₇₂O₁₄. 861.07. Component of Ivermectin. (1) Avermectin A₁ₐ, 5-*O*-demethyl-25-de(1-methylpropyl)-22,23-dihydro-25-(1-methylethyl)-; (2) (2a*E*,4*E*,8*E*)-(5′*S*,6*S*,6′*R*,7*S*,11*R*,13*R*,15*S*,17a*R*,20*R*,20a*R*,20b*S*)-3′,4′,5′,6,6′,7,10,11,14,15,17a,20,20a,20b-Tetradecahydro-20,20b-dihydroxy-6′-isopropyl-5′,6,8,19-tetramethyl-17-oxospiro[11,15-methano-2*H*,13*H*,17*H*-furo[4,3,2-*pq*][2,6]benzodioxacyclooctadecin-13,2′-[2*H*]pyran]-7-yl 2,6-dideoxy-4-*O*-(2,6-dideoxy-3-*O*-methyl-α-L-*arabino*-hexopyranosyl)-3-*O*-methyl-α-L-*arabino*-hexopyranoside. *CAS-70209-81-3.*

Ivoqualine. C₂₀H₂₆N₂O. 310.43. 6-Methoxy-4-[3-[(3*S*,4*R*)-3-vinyl-4-piperidyl]propyl]quinoline. *UNII-W0K2QLU43U. CAS-72714-75-1.* INN.

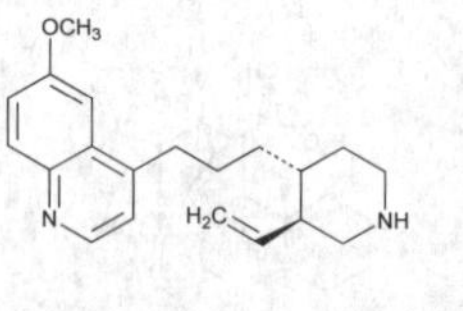

Ixabepilone [*2003*] (ix″ ab ep′ i lone). C₂₇H₄₂N₂O₅S. 506.70. (1) 17-Oxa-4-azabicyclo[14.1.0]heptadecane-5,9-dione, 7,11-dihydroxy-8,8,10,12,16-pentamethyl-3-[(1*E*)-1-methyl-2-(2-methyl-4-thiazolyl)ethenyl]-,

(1*S*,3*S*,7*S*,10*R*,11*S*,12*S*,16*R*)-; (2) (1*S*,3*S*,7*S*,10*R*,11*S*,12*S*,16*R*)-7,11-Dihydroxy-8,8,10,12,16-pentamethyl-3-[(1*E*)-1-methyl-2-(2-methylthiazol-4-yl)ethenyl]-17-oxa-4-azabicyclo[14.1.0]heptadecane-5,9-dione. *UNII-K27005NP0A. CAS-219989-84-1.* INN; JAN. *Antineoplastic; antimitotic.[Note—The trivial name, azaepothilone B, has appeared in literature.]* ◇BMS 247550-01

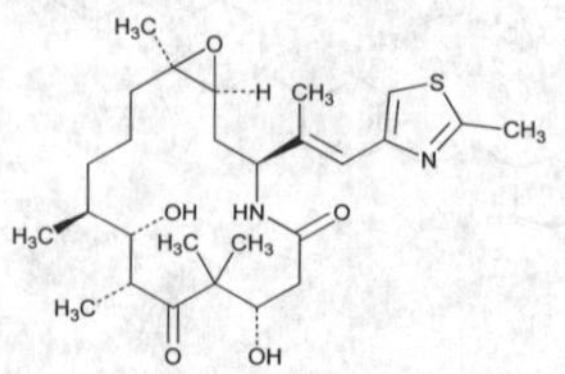

Izonsteride [*1998*] (eye zon′ ster ide). C₂₄H₂₆N₂OS₂. 422.61. (1) Benzo[*f*]quinolin-3(2*H*)-one, 8-[(4-ethyl-2-benzothiazolyl)thio]-1,4,4a,5,6,10b-hexahydro-4,10b-dimethyl-, (4a*R*-trans); (2) (4a*R*,10b*R*)-8-[(4-Ethyl-2-benzothiazolyl)thio]-1,4,4a,5,6,10b-hexahydro-4,10b-dimethylbenzo[*f*]quinolin-3-(2*H*)-one. *CAS-176975-26-1.* INN. *Treatment of prostate cancer (inhibits human type I and II isoforms of 5α-reductase).* ◇LY320236

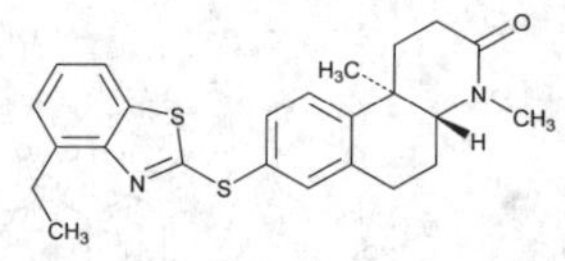

Jodphthalein Sodium — *See* Iodophthalein Sodium.

Jofendylate — *See* Iophendylate.

Jopanoic Acid — *See* Iopanoic Acid.

Josamycin [*1976*] (joe″ sa mye′ sin). C₄₂H₆₉NO₁₅. 827.99. [Josamycin Propionate is JAN.] (1) Leucomycin V, 3-acetate 4ᵝ-(3-methylbutanoate); (2) Stereoisomer of 4-(acetyloxy)-6-[[3,6-dideoxy-4-*O*-[2,6-dideoxy-3-*C*-methyl-4-*O*-(3-methyl-1-oxobutyl)-α-L-*ribo*-hexopyranosyl]-3-(dimethylamino)-β-D-glucopyranosyl]oxy]-10-hydroxy-5-methoxy-9,16-dimethyl-2-oxooxacyclohexadeca-11,13-diene-7-acetaldehyde; (3) Stereoisomer of 7-(formyl-methyl)-4,10-dihydroxy-5-methoxy-9,16-dimethyl-2-oxooxacyclohexadeca-11,13-dien-6-yl 3,6-dideoxy-4-*O*-(2,6-dideoxy-3-*C*-methyl-α-L-*ribo*-hexopyranosyl)-3-(dimethylamino)-β-D-glucopyranoside 4′-acetate 4″-isovalerate. *CAS-56689-45-3.* INN; BAN; JAN. *Antibacterial.* ◇EN-141

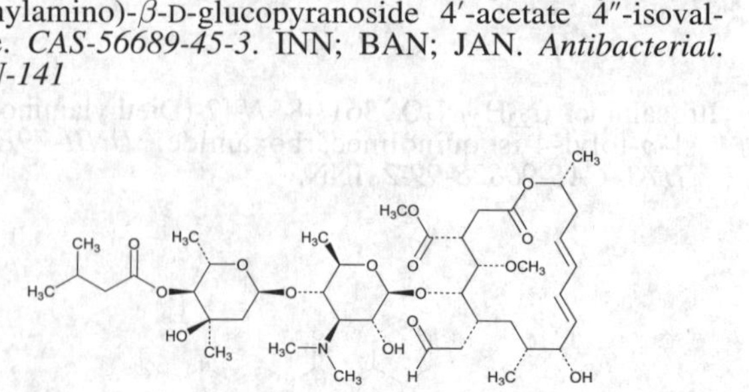

Jotrizoic Acid — *See* Iotrizoic Acid.

Juniper Tar (joo′ ni per tar). **USP.** The empyreumatic volatile oil obtained from the woody portions of *Juniperus oxycedrus* Linné (Fam. Pinaceae). *CAS-8013-10-3. Pharmaceutic necessity.*

⁴²K — *See* Potassium Chloride K 42.

Kainic Acid. $C_{10}H_{15}NO_4$. 213.23. 2-Carboxy-4-isopropenyl-3-pyrrolidineacetic acid. *UNII-SIV03811UC. CAS-487-79-6.* INN; JAN; MI.

Kalafungin [*1968*] (ka la fun' jin). $C_{16}H_{12}O_6$. 300.26. Antibiotic produced by *Streptomyces tanashiensis* strain *kala.* (1) 2*H*-Furo[3,2-*b*]naphtho[2,3-*d*]pyran-2,6,11-trione, 3,3a,5,11b-tetrahydro-7-hydroxy-5-methyl-; (2) Kalafungin. *CAS-11048-15-0.* INN. *Antifungal.* ◇*U-19,718; NSC-137443*

Kallidinogenase. Enzyme isolated from the pancreas or urine of mammals. *CAS-9001-01-8.* INN; BAN; JAN.

Kanamycin B — *See* Bekanamycin.

Kanamycin Sulfate (kan″ a mye′ sin sul′ fate). **USP**. $C_{18}H_{36}N_4O_{11} \cdot H_2SO_4$. 582.58. [Kanamycin is INN and BAN; Kanamycin Monosulfate is JAN.] (1) D-Streptamine, *O*-3-amino-3-deoxy-α-D-glucopyranosyl(1→6)-*O*-[6-amino-6-deoxy-α-D-glucopyranosyl(1→4)]-2-deoxy-, sulfate (1:1) (salt); (2) Kanamycin sulfate (1:1) (salt). *UNII-OW1N4G4R9W; UNII-RUC37XUP2P* [kanamycin]. *CAS-25389-94-0; CAS-133-92-6* [replaced]; *CAS-59-01-8* [kanamycin]. JAN. *Antibacterial.* Kantrex (Apothecon); Klebcil (King)

Kaolin (kay′ oh lin). **USP**. Native hydrated aluminum silicate, powdered and freed from gritty particles by elutriation. *CAS-1332-58-7.* JAN. *Adsorbant.* Vanclay (Vanderbilt)

Kasal [*1971*] (kay′ sal). Approximately $Na_8Al_2(OH)_2(PO_4)_4$ with about 30 % of dibasic sodium phosphate; Sodium aluminum phosphate, basic. *Food additive.*

---

† Brand name formerly used, and/or firm no longer concerned with this product.

Kebuzone. $C_{19}H_{18}N_2O_3$. 322.36. [Ketophenylbutazone is JAN.] 4-(3-Oxobutyl)-1,2-diphenyl-3,5-pyrazolidinedione. *UNII-4VD83UL6Y6. CAS-853-34-9.* INN; MI.

Keliximab. Immunoglobulin G1, anti-(human CD4 (antigen)) (human-macaca monoclonal CE9.1 γ1-chain), disulfide with human-macaca monoclonal CE9.1 λ-chain, dimer. *CAS-174722-30-6.* INN.

Kellofylline — *See* Visnafylline.

Keoxifene Hydrochloride (previously used name) — *See* Raloxifene Hydrochloride.

Keracyanin. $C_{27}H_{31}ClO_{15}$. 630.98. 3-[[6-*O*-(6-Deoxy-α-L-mannopyranosyl)-β-D-glucopyranosyl]oxy]-3′,4′,5,7-tetrahydroxyflavylium chloride. *UNII-V0N2VMB4FV. CAS-18719-76-1.* INN; DCF.

Ketamine Hydrochloride [*1966*] (kee′ ta meen hye″ droe klor′ ide). **USP**. $C_{13}H_{16}ClNO \cdot HCl$. 274.19. [Ketamine is INN and BAN.] (1) Cyclohexanone, 2-(2-chlorophenyl)-2-(methylamino)-, hydrochloride; (2) (±)-2-(*o*-Chlorophenyl)-2-(methylamino)cyclohexanone hydrochloride. *UNII-O18YUO0I83; UNII-690G0D6V8H* [ketamine]. *CAS-1867-66-9; CAS-6740-88-1* [ketamine]. JAN. *Anesthetic.* Ketalar (King) ◇*CI-581; CL 369; CN-52,372-2*

Ketanserin [*1981*] (kee tan′ ser in). $C_{22}H_{22}FN_3O_3$. 395.43. (1) 2,4(1*H*,3*H*)-Quinazolinedione, 3-[2-[4-(4-fluorobenzoyl)-1-piperidinyl]ethyl]-; (2) 3-[2-[4-(*p*-Fluorobenzoyl)piperidino]ethyl]-2,4-(1*H*,3*H*)-quinazolinedione. *CAS-74050-98-9.* INN; BAN. *Serotonin antagonist.* ◇*R-41,468*

Ketazocine [*1976*] (kee taz′ oh seen). $C_{18}H_{23}NO_2$. 285.38. (1) 2,6-Methano-3-benzazocin-1(2*H*)-one, 3-(cyclopropylmethyl)-3,4,5,6-tetrahydro-8-hydroxy-6,11-dimethyl-, (2α,6α,11S*)-; (2) (2R*,6S*,11S*)-3-(Cyclopropylmethyl)-3,4,5,6-tetrahydro-8-hydroxy-6,11-dimethyl-2,6-methano-3-benzazocin-1(2*H*)-one. *CAS-36292-69-0*. INN. *Analgesic.* ◇*Win 34,276*

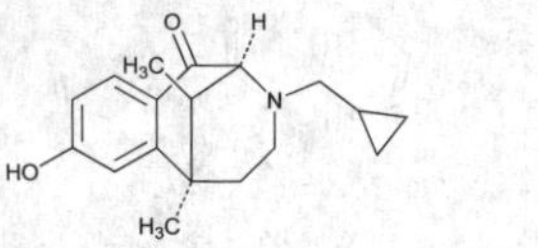

Ketazolam [*1971*] (kee taz′ oh lam). $C_{20}H_{17}ClN_2O_3$. 368.81. (1) 4*H*-[1,3]-Oxazino[3,2-*d*][1,4]benzodiazepine-4,7(6*H*)-dione, 11-chloro-8,12b-dihydro-2,8-dimethyl-; (2) 11-Chloro-8,12b-dihydro-2,8-dimethyl-12b-phenyl-4*H*-[1,3]-oxazino[3,2-*d*][1,4]benzodiazepine-4,7(6*H*)dione. *CAS-27223-35-4*. INN; BAN. *Tranquilizer (minor).* ◇*U-28,774*

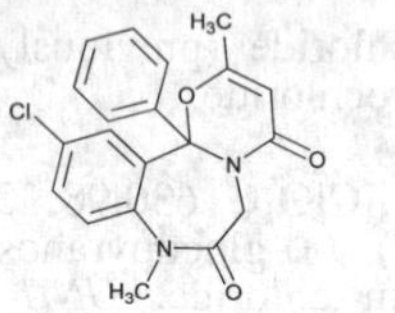

Kethoxal [*1969*] (kee thox′ al). $C_6H_{12}O_4$. 148.16. [Ketoxal is INN.] (1) 2-Butanone, 3-ethoxy-1,1-dihydroxy-; (2) 3-Ethoxy-1,1-dihydroxy-2-butanone. *CAS-27762-78-3*. *Antiviral.* ◇*U-2032*

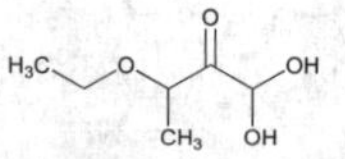

Ketimipramine (INN) Fumarate — *See* Ketipramine Fumarate.

Ketipramine Fumarate [*1968*] (kee tip′ ra meen fue′ ma rate). $C_{19}H_{22}N_2O.C_4H_4O_4$. 410.46. [Ketimipramine is INN.] (1) 10*H*-Dibenz[*b,f*]azepin-10-one, 5-[3-(dimethylamino)-propyl]-5,11-dihydro-, (*E*)-2-butenedioate (1:1); (2) 5-[3-(Dimethylamino)propyl]-5,11-dihydro-10*H*-dibenz[*b,f*]a-zepin-10-one fumarate (1:1). *CAS-17243-32-2; CAS-796-29-2* [ketipramine]. *Antidepressant.* ◇*G 35259*

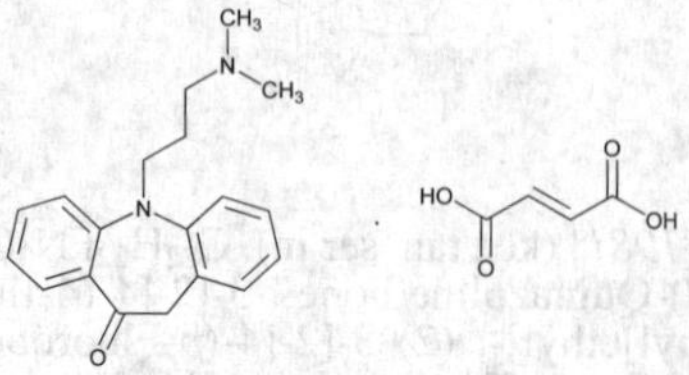

Ketobemidone. $C_{15}H_{21}NO_2$. 247.33. (1) 1-[4-(*m*-Hydroxy-phenyl)-1-methyl-4-piperidyl]-1-propanone; (2) 4-(*m*-Hy-droxyphenyl)-1-methyl-4-propionylpiperidine. *UNII-PQS1L514CF*. *CAS-469-79-4*. INN; BAN; MI.

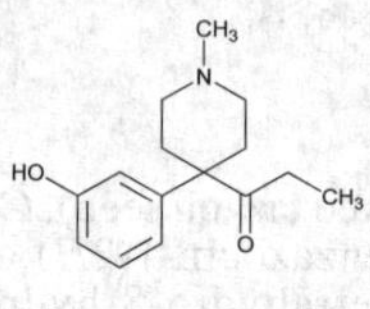

Ketocaine. $C_{18}H_{29}NO_2$. 291.43. 2′-[2-(Diisopropylami-no)ethoxy]butyrophenone. *UNII-WA1RT89G9X*. *CAS-1092-46-2*. INN.

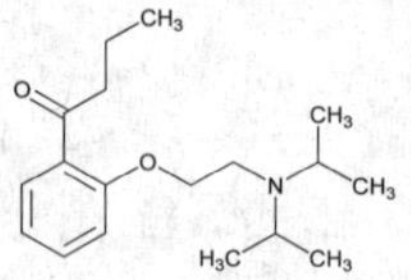

Ketocainol. $C_{18}H_{31}NO_2$. 293.44. *o*-[2-(Diisopropylami-no)ethoxy]-α-propylbenzyl alcohol. *UNII-UQG78PXR4W*. *CAS-7488-92-8*. INN.

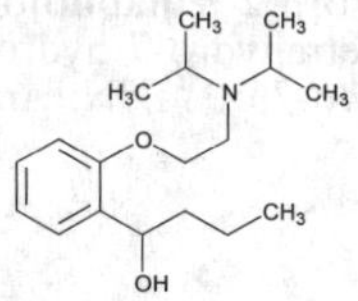

Ketoconazole [*1978*] (kee″ toe kon′ a zole). **USP**. $C_{26}H_{28}Cl_2N_4O_4$. 531.43. (1) Piperazine, 1-acetyl-4-[4-[[2-(2,4-dichlorophenyl)-2-(1*H*-imidazol-1-ylmethyl)-1,3-di-oxolan-4-yl]methoxy]phenyl]-, *cis*-; (2) (±)-*cis*-1-Acetyl-4-[*p*-[[2-(2,4-dichlorophenyl)-2-(imidazol-1-ylmethyl)-1,3-dioxolan-4-yl]methoxy]phenyl]piperazine. *UNII-R9400W927I*. *CAS-65277-42-1*. INN; BAN; JAN. *Antifun-gal.* Ketozole (Taro); Nizoral (Janssen); Nizoral (McNeil); Xolegel (Barrier) ◇*R 41,400*

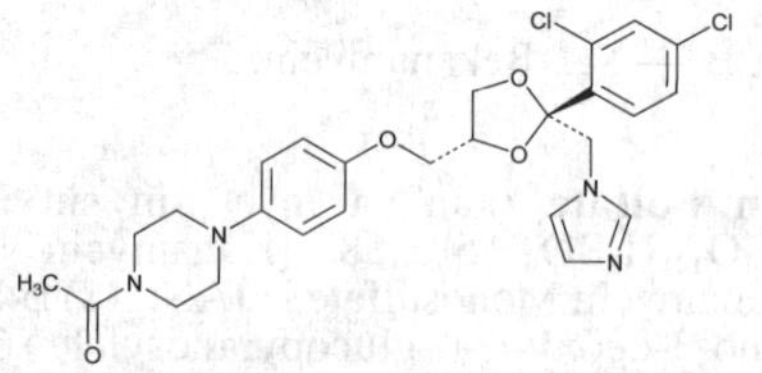

Ketohexazine — *See* Cetohexazine.

Ketophenylbutazone (JAN) — *See* Kebuzone.

Ketoprofen [*1972*] (kee″ toe proe′ fen). **USP**. $C_{16}H_{14}O_3$. 254.28. (1) Benzeneacetic acid, 3-benzoyl-α-methyl-, (±)-; (2) (±)-*m*-Benzoylhydratropic acid. *UNII-90Y4QC304K*. *CAS-22071-15-4*. INN; BAN; JAN. *Anti-inflammatory.* Actron (Bayer); Orudis (Wyeth); Oruvail (Wyeth) ◇*R.P. 19,583*

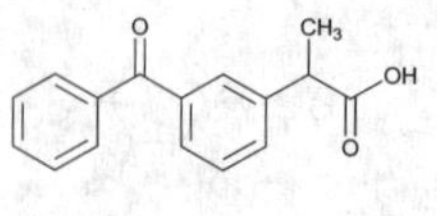

Ketorfanol [*1983*] (kee tor′ fa nol). $C_{20}H_{25}NO_2$. 311.42. (1) Morphinan-6-one, 17-(cyclopropylmethyl)-4-hydroxy-; (2) 17-(Cyclopropylmethyl)-4-hydroxymorphinan-6-one. *UNII-8Z0ZXE70XL*. *CAS-79798-39-3*. INN. *Analgesic.* ◇*SBW-22*

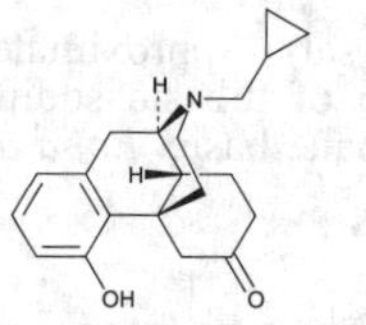

Ketorolac Tromethamine [*1984*] (kee″ toe role′ ak troe meth′ a meen). **USP.** $C_{15}H_{13}NO_3 \cdot C_4H_{11}NO_3$. 376.40. [Ketorolac is INN and BAN.] (1) 1*H*-Pyrrolizine-1-carboxylic acid, 5-benzoyl-2,3-dihydro, (±)-, compound with 2-amino-2-(hydroxymethyl)-1,3-propanediol (1:1); (2) (±)-5-Benzoyl-2,3-dihydro-1*H*-pyrrolizine-1-carboxylic acid, compound with 2-amino-2-(hydroxymethyl)-1,3-propanediol (1:1). *UNII-4EVE5946BQ; UNII-YZI5105V0L* [ketorolac]. *CAS-74103-07-4; CAS-74103-06-3* [ketorolac]. *Analgesic.* Acular (Allergan); Toradol (Roche)

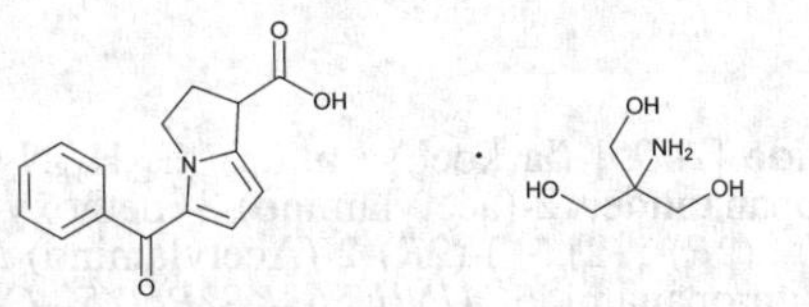

Ketotifen Fumarate [*1979*] (kee″ toe tye′ fen fue′ ma rate). $C_{19}H_{19}NOS \cdot C_4H_4O_4$. 425.50. [Ketotifen is INN and BAN.] (1) 10*H*-Benzo[4,5]cyclohepta[1,2-*b*]thiophen-10-one, 4,9-dihydro-4-(1-methyl-4-piperidinylidene)-, (*E*)-2-butenedioate (1:1); (2) 4,9-Dihydro-4-(1-methyl-4-piperidylidene)-10*H*-benzo[4,5]cyclohepta[1,2-*b*]thiophen-10-one fumarate (1:1). *UNII-HBD503WORO; UNII-X49220T18G* [ketotifen]. *CAS-34580-14-8; CAS-34580-13-7* [ketotifen]. JAN. *Anti-asthmatic.* Zaditor (Novartis) ◇*HC 20,511 fumarate*

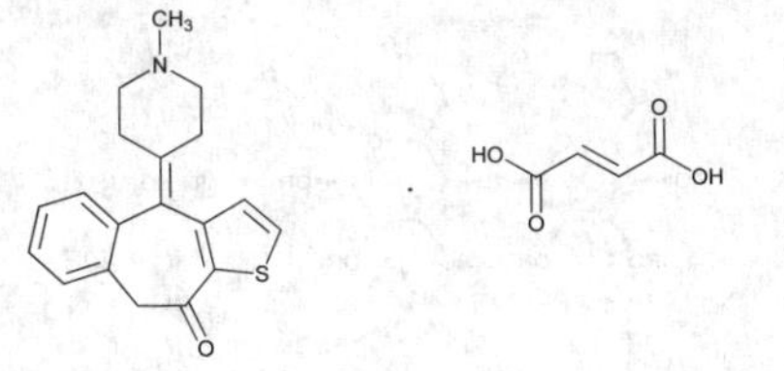

Ketotrexate. $C_{21}H_{27}N_7O_6$. 473.48. *N*-[*p*-[[2-(2-Amino-1,4,5,6,7,8-hexahydro-5-methyl-4-oxo-6-pteridinyl)ethyl]amino]benzoyl]-L-glutamic acid. *UNII-504RN634MM. CAS-52196-22-2.* INN.

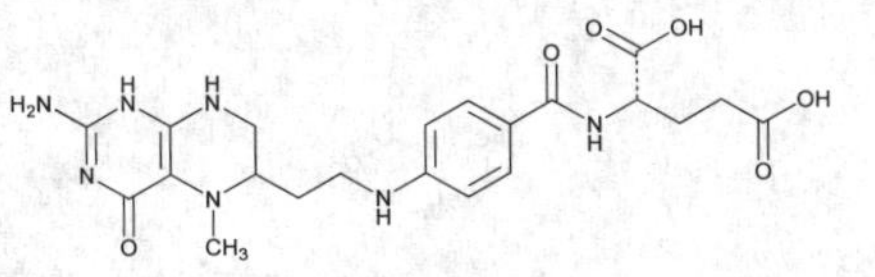

Ketoxal (INN) — *See* Kethoxal.

Khellin. $C_{14}H_{12}O_5$. 260.24. 4,9-Dimethoxy-7-methyl-5*H*-furo[3,2-*g*][1]benzopyran-5-one. *UNII-5G117T0TJZ. CAS-82-02-0.* INN; DCF; MI. Ammivin (Marion Merrell Dow†); Khelloyd (Hoechst-Roussel†)

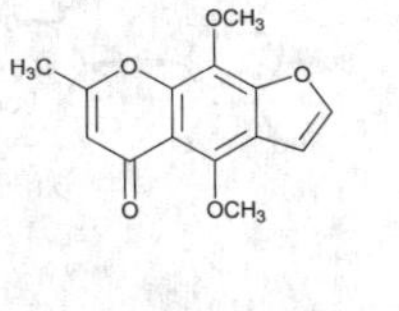

Khelloside. $C_{19}H_{20}O_{10}$. 408.36. 7-Hydroxymethyl-4-methoxy-5*H*-furo[3,2-*g*][1]benzopyran-5-one glucoside. *CAS-17226-75-4.* INN; DCF.

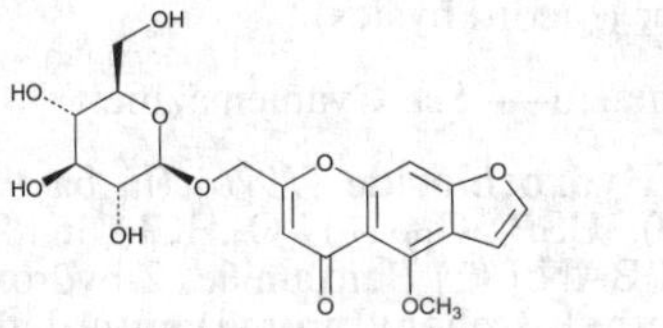

Kitasamycin [*1967*] (kit″ a sa mye′ sin). [Kitasamycin Tartrate is JAN; Acetylkitasamycin also is JAN.] Antibiotic produced by *Streptomyces kitasatoensis.* (1) Leucomycin; (2) Kitasamycin. *CAS-1392-21-8; CAS-37280-56-1* [tartrate]. INN; BAN; JAN. *Antibacterial.*

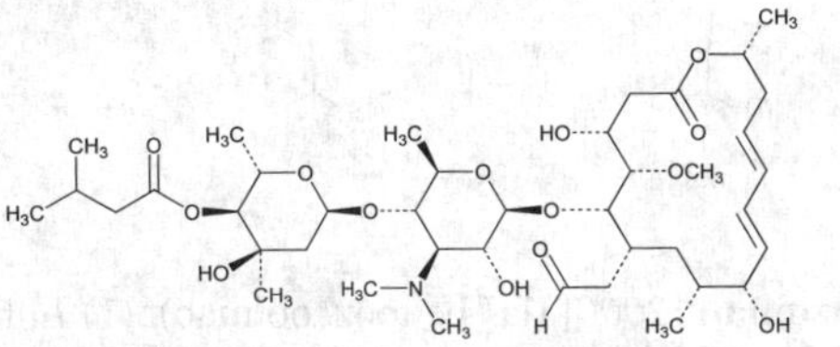

Kolfocon A [*1989*] (kol foe′ kon). $(C_{16}H_{38}O_5Si_4)_w(C_5H_8O_2)_x$ $(C_4H_6O_2)_y(C_{10}H_{14}O_4)_z$. [Gas permeability DK value: 18.0.] (1) 2-Propenoic acid, 2-methyl-, 3-[3,3,3-trimethyl-1,1-bis[(trimethylsilyl)oxy]disiloxanyl]propyl ester, polymer with methyl 2-methyl-2-propenoate, 2-methyl-2-propenoic acid and 1,2-ethanediyl bis(2-methyl-2-propenoate); (2) 3-[3,3,3-Trimethyl-1,1-bis(trimethylsiloxy)disiloxanyl]propyl methacrylate, polymer with methyl methacrylate, methacrylic acid and ethylene dimethacrylate. *CAS-113378-32-8. Contact lens material (hydrophobic).* Optacryl 60 (Paragon); Optikem 18 (Optacryl)

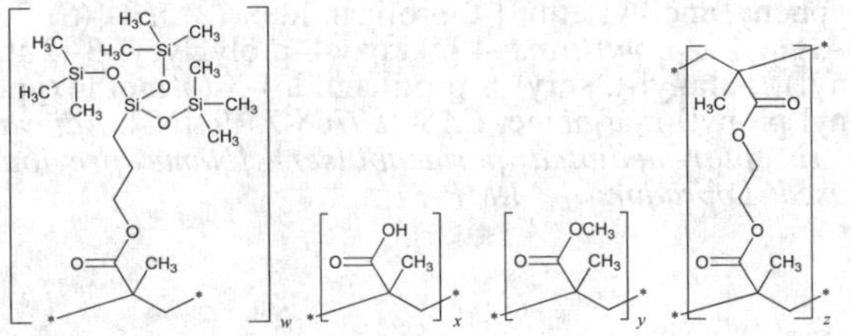

Kolfocon B [*1989*] (kol foe′ kon). [Gas permeability DK value: 32.0.] *Contact lens material (hydrophobic).* Optacryl K (Paragon); Optikem 32 (Optacryl) *[Note—The chemical names, structural and molecular formulas, and CAS Registry number are identical to Kolfocon A.]*

Kolfocon C [*1989*] (kol foe′ kon). [Gas permeability DK value: 59.0.] *Contact lens material (hydrophobic).* Optacryl Extra (Paragon) *[Note—The chemical names, structural and molecular formulas, and CAS Registry number are identical to Kolfocon A.]*

Kolfocon D [*1989*] (kol foe′ kon). [Gas permeability DK value: 84.0.] *Contact lens material (hydrophobic).* Optacryl Z (Paragon) *[Note—The chemical names, structural and molecular formulas, and CAS Registry number are identical to Kolfocon A.]*

[81m]Kr — *See* Krypton Kr 81m.

[85]Kr — *See* Krypton Clathrate Kr 85.

Krypton Clathrate Kr 85 [*1963*] (krip′ ton klath′ rate). *Radioactive agent.*

---

† Brand name formerly used, and/or firm no longer concerned with this product.

Krypton Kr 81m [*1978*] (krip′ ton). **USP**. Kr 81m. (1) Krypton, isotope of mass 81 (metastable); (2) Krypton, isotope of mass 81 (metastable). *UNII-68QN45K12N. CAS-15678-91-8. Radioactive agent.* Krypton Kr 81m Gas Generator (Medi-Physics)

Kyamepromazin — *See* Cyamemazine.

Labetalol Hydrochloride [*1976*] (la bayt′ a lol hye″ droe klor′ ide). **USP**. $C_{19}H_{24}N_2O_3 \cdot HCl$. 364.87. [Labetalol is INN and BAN.] (1) Benzamide, 2-hydroxy-5-[1-hydroxy-2-[(1-methyl-3-phenylpropyl)amino]ethyl]-, monohydrochloride; (2) 5-[1-Hydroxy-2-[(1-methyl-3-phenylpropyl)amino]ethyl]salicylamide monohydrochloride. *UNII-1GEV3BAW9J; UNII-R5H8897N95* [labetalol]. *CAS-32780-64-6; CAS-36894-69-6* [labetalol]. JAN. *Anti-adrenergic (α-receptor); anti-adrenergic (β-receptor).* Normodyne (Schering); Trandate (Promethus) ◊*Sch 15719W; AH 5158A*

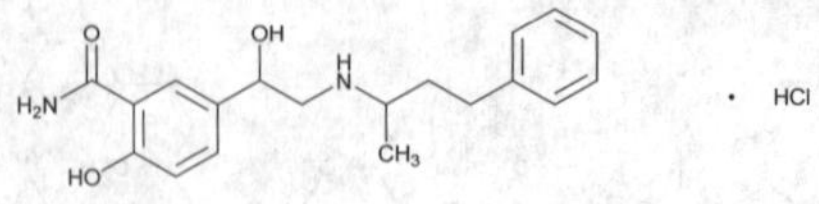

Labetuzumab [*2000*] (la″ be tooz′ oo mab). (1) Immunoglobulin G, anti-(human carcinoembryonic antigen) (human-mouse monoclonal hMN-14 γ-chain), disulfide with human-mouse monoclonal hMN-14 κ-chain, dimer; (2) Immunoglobulin G (human-mouse monoclonal hMN-14 γ-chain anti-human carcinoembryonic antigen), disulfide with human-mouse monoclonal hMN-14 κ-chain, dimer. Molecular weight is approximately 150,000 daltons *CAS-219649-07-7*. INN. *Treatment of colorectal cancer (humanized monoclonal antibody hMN-14 targeting CEA-positive cancers).* CEA-CIDE (Immunomedics) ◊*hMN-14*

Labradimil [*1999*] (la bray′ di mil). $C_{49}H_{75}N_{15}O_{12}S$. 1098.28. (1) [*S-(R*,R*)*]-L-Arginyl-L-prolyl-*trans*-4-hydroxy-L-prolylglycyl-3-(2-thienyl)-L-alanyl-L-seryl-*N*-[2-[[4-(aminoiminomethyl)amino]-1-carboxybutyl]amino]-1-[(4-methoxyphenyl)methyl]ethyl]-L-prolinamide; (2) N^2-[(S)-2-[L-Arginyl-L-prolyl-*trans*-4-hydroxy-L-prolylglycyl-3-(2-thienyl)-L-alanyl-L-seryl-L-prolinamido]-3-(*p*-methoxyphenyl)propyl]-L-arginine. *CAS-159768-75-9.* INN. *Adjuvant; "receptor-mediated permeabiliser".[Name previously used: Lobradimil.]* ◊*RMP-7*

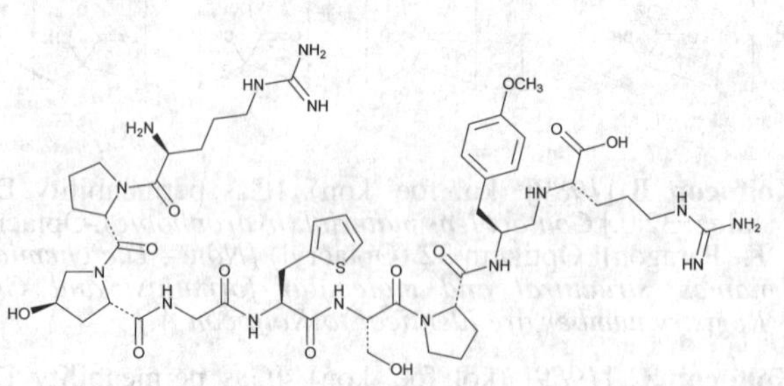

Lachesine Chloride. $C_{20}H_{26}ClNO_3$. 363.88. (2-Benziloyloxyethyl)ethyldimethylammonium chloride. *UNII-720J8565ZF. CAS-1164-38-1.* BAN.

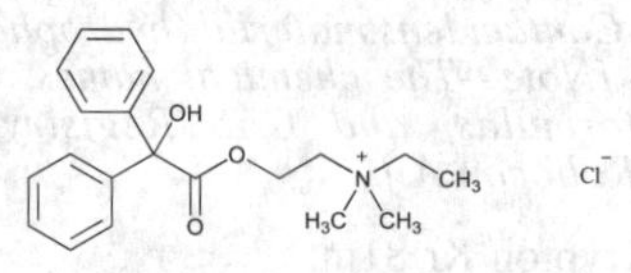

Lacidipine [*1989*] (la si′ di peen). $C_{26}H_{33}NO_6$. 455.54. (1) 3,5-Pyridinedicarboxylic acid, 4-[2-[3-(1,1-dimethylethoxy)-3-oxo-1-propenyl]phenyl]-1,4-dihydro-2,6-di-methyl-, diethyl ester, (*E*)-; (2) 4-[*o*-[(*E*)-2-Carboxyvinyl]phenyl]-1,4-dihydro-2,6-dimethyl-3,5-pyridinedicarboxylic acid, 4-*tert*-butyl diethyl ester. *UNII-260080034N. CAS-103890-78-4.* INN; BAN. *Antihypertensive.* ◊*GR 43659X*

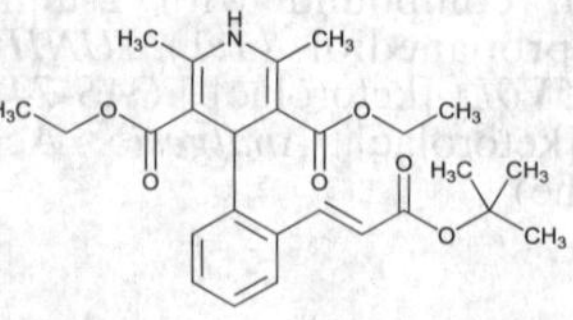

Lacosamide [*2005*] (la koe′ sa mide). $C_{13}H_{18}N_2O_3$. 250.29. (1) Propanamide, 2-(acetylamino)-3-methoxy-*N*-(phenylmethyl)-, (2*R*)-; (2) (+)-(2*R*)-2-(Acetylamino)-*N*-benzyl-3-methoxypropanamide. *UNII-563KS2PQY5. CAS-175481-36-4.* INN. *Treatment of epilepsy and neuropathic pain.[Name previously used: Erlosamide.]* ◊*SPM 927; ADD 243037*

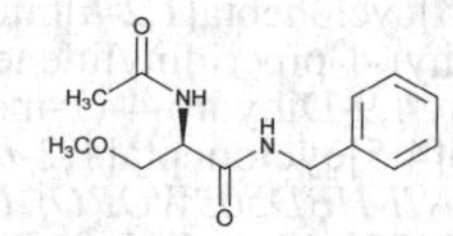

Lactalfate. $C_{12}H_{54}Al_{16}O_{75}S_8$. 2086.74. Lactose octakis(hydrogen sulfate), basic aluminum salt. *CAS-96427-12-2.* INN.

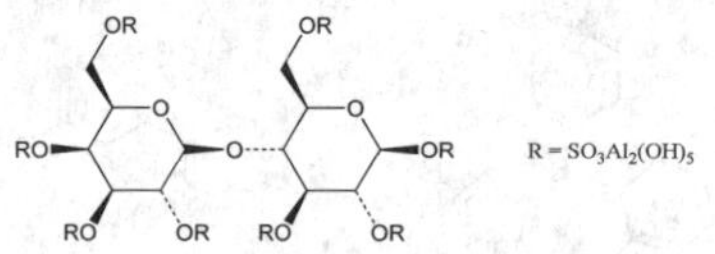

Lactase (lak′ tase). **USP**. Lactase (β-D-galactoside galactohydrolase) is a hydrolytic enzyme derived from the mold *Aspergillus oryzae*.

Lactic Acid (lak′ tik as′ id). **USP**. $C_3H_6O_3$. 90.08. (1) Propanoic acid, 2-hydroxy-; (2) Lactic acid. *UNII-33X04XA5AT. CAS-50-21-5.* JAN. *Pharmaceutic necessity for Sodium Lactate [Injection].*

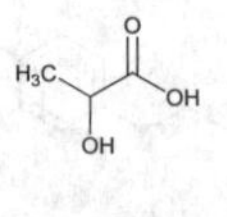

Lactitol (lak′ ti tol). **NF**. $C_{12}H_{24}O_{11}$. 344.31. 4-*O*-β-D-Galactopyranosyl-D-glucitol. *UNII-L2B0WJF7ZY; UNII-UH2K6W1Y64* [lactitol monohydrate]. *CAS-585-86-4; CAS-81025-03-8* [dihydrate]; *CAS-81025-04-9* [monohydrate]. INN; BAN.

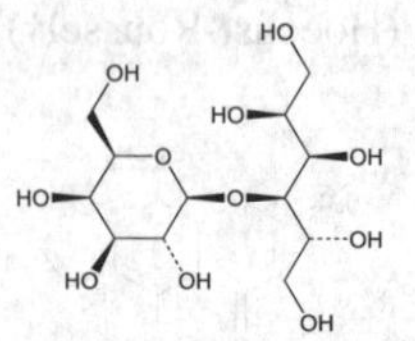

Lactobacillus Acidophilus. [Lactomin is JAN.] Preparation made from acid-producing bacterium.

Lactoflavin — *See* Riboflavin.

Lactomin (JAN) — *See* Lactobacillus Acidophilus.

Lactose, Anhydrous (lak′ tose an hye′ drus). **NF**. [Lactose is JAN.] Anhydrous Lactose is primarily beta lactose or a mixture of alpha and beta lactose. *Pharmaceutic aid (tablet and capsule diluent).*

Lactose Monohydrate (lak′ tose mon″ oh hye′ drate). **NF**. Lactose Monohydrate is a natural disaccharide, obtained from milk, which consists of one glucose and one galactose moiety. *UNII-EWQ57Q8I5X. Pharmaceutic aid (tablet and capsule diluent).*

Lactulose [*1965*] (lak′ tue lose). **USP**. $C_{12}H_{22}O_{11}$. 342.30. (1) D-Fructose, 4-*O*-β-D-galactopyranosyl-; (2) Lactulose; (3) 4-*O*-β-D-Galactopyranosyl-D-fructofuranose. *UNII-9U7D5QH5AE. CAS-4618-18-2.* INN; BAN; JAN. *Laxative.* Acilac (Technilab); Cholac (Alra); Constilac (Alra); Constulose (Actavis); Enulose (Actavis); Generlac (Morton Grove); Laxilose (Technilab)

Ladakamycin (previously used name) — *See* Azacitidine.

Ladirubicin. $C_{29}H_{31}NO_{11}S$. 601.62. (1*S*,3*S*-3-Acetyl-1,2,3,4,6,11,hexahydro-3,5,12-trihydroxy-6,11-dioxo-1-naphthacenyl 3-(1-aziridinyl)-2,3,6-trideoxy-4-*O*-(methylsulfonyl)-α-L-*lyxo*-hexopyranoside. *CAS-171047-47-5.* INN.

Ladostigil Tartrate [*2004*] (lad″ oh stij′ il tar′ trate). $_2(C_{16}H_{20}N_2O_2)\cdot C_4H_6O_6$. 694.77. [Ladostigil is INN.] (1) Carbamic acid, ethylmethyl-, (3*R*)-2,3-dihydro-3-(2-propynylamino)-1*H*-inden-5-yl ester, (2*R*,3*R*)-2,3-dihydroxybutanedioate (2:1); (2) (3*R*)-3-(Prop-2-ynylamino)-2,3-dihydro-1*H*-inden-5-yl ethylmethylcarbamate (2*R*,3*R*)-tartarate (2:1). *UNII-2J1346C51H. CAS-209394-46-7; CAS-209394-27-4* [ladostigil]. *Treatment of Alzheimer's disease*

(*an inhibitor of monoamine oxidase (MAO-A and B), an acetylcholinesterase inhibitor, and a neuroprotectant*). ◇*TV-3326*

Laflunimus. $C_{15}H_{13}F_3N_2O_2$. 310.27. (*Z*)α-Cyano-$\alpha^{4'}$,$\alpha^{4'}$,$\alpha^{4'}$-trifluoro-β-hydroxycyclopropaneacrylo-3′,4′-xylide. *UNII-44EH625IUS. CAS-147076-36-6.* INN.

Lafutidine. $C_{22}H_{29}N_3O_4S$. 431.55. ($\pm$)-2-(Furfurylsulfinyl)-*N*-[(*Z*)-4-[[4-(piperidinomethyl)-2-pyridyl]oxy]-2-butenyl]acetamide. *UNII-49S4O7ADLC. CAS-118288-08-7.* INN.

Lagatide. $C_{33}H_{58}N_{10}O_9$. 738.88. L-Prolyl-L-valyl-L-threonyl-L-lysyl-L-prolyl-L-glutaminyl-D-alaninamide. *CAS-157476-77-2.* INN.

P V T K P Q ᴅA

Laidlomycin Propionate Potassium [*1989*] (layd″ loe mye′ sin proe′ pee oh nate poe tas′ ee um). $C_{40}H_{65}KO_{13}$. 793.03. [Laidlomycin is INN and BAN.] (1) Monensin, 16-deethyl-3-*O*-demethyl-16-methyl-3-*O*-(1-oxopropyl)-, 26-propanoate, monopotassium salt; (2) Potassium (α*S*,β*R*,γ*S*,2*S*,5*R*,7*S*,8*R*,9*S*)-β,9-dihydroxy-α,γ,2,8-tetramethyl-2-[(2*R*,5*S*)-tetrahydro-5-methyl-5-[2*R*,3*S*,5*R*-tetrahydro-3-methyl-5-[(2*S*,3*S*,5*R*,6*R*)-tetrahydro-6-hydroxy-6-(hydroxymethyl)-3,5-dimethyl-2*H*-pyran-2-yl]-2-furyl]-2-furyl]-1,6-dioxaspiro[4.5]decane-7-butyrate, β,6‴¹-dipropionate. *UNII-05TAA9I0Z8. CAS-84799-02-0; CAS-56283-74-0* [laidlomycin]. *Growth stimulant (veterinary).* Cattlyst [Veterinary] (Syntex) ◇*RS-11988*

Lamifiban [*1995*] (la″ mi fye′ ban). $C_{24}H_{28}N_4O_6$. 468.50. (1) Acetic acid, [[1-[2-[[4-(aminoiminomethyl)benzoyl]amino]-3-(4-hydroxyphenyl)-1-oxopropyl]-4-piperidinyl]oxy]-, (*S*)-; (2) [[1-[*N*-(*p*-Amidinobenzoyl)-L-tyrosyl]-4-piperidyl]oxy]acetic acid. *CAS-144412-49-7.* INN. *Antithrombotic.* ◇*Ro 44-9883/000*

Lamifiban Hydrochloride [*2000*] (la″ mi fye′ ban hye″ droe klor′ ide). $C_{24}H_{28}N_4O_6 \cdot HCl.$ 504.96. (1) (*S*)-[[1-[2-[[4-(Aminoiminomethyl)benzoyl]amino]-3-(4-hydroxyphenyl)-1-oxopropyl]-4-piperidinyl]oxy]acetic acid monohydrochloride; (2) [[1-[*N*-(*p*-Amidinobenzoyl)-L-tyrosyl]-4-piperidyl]oxy]acetic acid monohydrochloride. *UNII-3UZ1CTQ989. CAS-243835-65-6. Fibrinogen receptor antagonist.* ◇*Ro 44-9883/023*

Lamivudine [*1992*] (la miv′ ue deen). **USP.** $C_8H_{11}N_3O_3S.$ 229.26. (1) 2(1*H*)-Pyrimidinone, 4-amino-1-[2-(hydroxymethyl)-1,3-oxathiolan-5-yl]-, (2*R-cis*)-; (2) (-)-1-[(2*R,5S*)-2-(Hydroxymethyl)-1,3-oxathiolan-5-yl]cytosine. *UNII-2T8Q726O95. CAS-134678-17-4.* INN; BAN. *Antiviral.* Epivir (GlaxoSmithKline) ◇*GR 109714X*

Lamotrigine [*1985*] (la moe′ tri jeen). $C_9H_7Cl_2N_5.$ 256.09. (1) 1,2,4-Triazine-3,5-diamine, 6-(2,3-dichlorophenyl)-; (2) 3,5-Diamino-6-(2,3-dichlorophenyl)-*as*-triazine. *UNII-U3H27498KS. CAS-84057-84-1.* INN; BAN. *Anticonvulsant.* Lamictal (GlaxoSmithKline) ◇*BW 430C*

Lamtidine. $C_{18}H_{28}N_6O.$ 344.45. 1-[*m*-[3-[(3-Amino-1-methyl-1*H*-1,2,4-triazol-5-yl)amino]propoxy]benzyl]piperidine. *UNII-BO55Z3JL5K. CAS-73278-54-3.* INN; BAN. ◇*AH 22216*

Lanatoside C. $C_{49}H_{76}O_{20}.$ 985.12. Glycoside obtained from the leaves of *Digitalis lanata* Ehrh. *CAS-17575-22-3.* NF XIII; INN; BAN; JAN; DCF; MI.

Lancovutide. $C_{89}H_{125}N_{23}O_{25}S_3.$ 2013.28. ($C^{3,15}R$)-$C^{3,15}$-Hydroxy[2-L-lysine,10-L-phenylalanine, 12-L-phenylalanine-,13-L-valine]lantibiotic ancovenin (*Streptomyces* sp). *CAS-1391-36-2.* INN.

Landiolol. $C_{25}H_{39}N_3O_8.$ 509.59. (-)-[(*S*)-2,2-Dimethyl-1,3-dioxolan-4-yl]methyl *p*-[(*S*)-2-hydroxy-3-[[2-(4-morpholinecarboxamido)ethyl]amino]propoxy]hydrocinnamate. *UNII-62NWQ924LH. CAS-133242-30-5.* INN.

Lanepitant. $C_{33}H_{45}N_5O_3.$ 559.74. *N*-[(*R*)-2-Indol-3-yl-1-[[*N*-(*o*-methoxybenzyl)acetamido]methyl]ethyl][1,4′-bipiperidine]-1′-acetamide. *UNII-17G8FN2E1F. CAS-170566-84-4.* INN.

Lanicemine. $C_{13}H_{14}N_2.$ 198.26. (+)-2-[(*S*)-β-Aminophenethyl]pyridine. *UNII-9TMU325RK3. CAS-153322-05-5.* INN.

Lanimostim [*2004*] (lan″ i moe′ stim). $C_{2146}H_{3346}N_{572}O_{686}S_{28} \cdot$ 49,033 daltons. (1) 4-221-Colony-stimulating factor 1 (human clone p3ACSF-69 reduced); (2) 4-221-Colony-stimulating factor 1 (human clone p3ACSF-69) (dimer). *CAS-117276-75-2.* INN. *Antineoplastic; anti-infective growth factor that acts on both progenitor and mature cells of the macrophage line.*

```
SEYÇSHM IGSGHLQSLQ RLIDSQMETS CQITFEFVDQ
EQLKDPVÇYL KKAFLLVQDI MEDTMRFRDN TPNAIAIVQL
QELSLRLKSC FTKDYEEHDK AÇVRTFYETP LQLLEKVKNV
FNETKNLLDK DWNIFSKNCN NSFAECSSQD VVTKPDCNCL
YPKAIPSSDP ASVSPHQPLA PSMAPVAGLT WEDSEGTEGS
SLLPGEQPLH TVDPGSAKQR P
```
$_2$

Laniquidar. $C_{37}H_{36}N_4O_3$. 584.71. Methyl 6,11-dihydro-11-[1-[2-[4-(-2-quinolylmethoxy)phenyl]ethyl]-4-piperidinylidene]-5*H*-imidazo[2,1-*b*][3]benzazepine-3-carboxylate. *UNII-K3FRN4DDOY. CAS-197509-46-9.* INN.

Lanoconazole. $C_{14}H_{10}ClN_3S_2$. 319.83. $(\pm)$-α-[(*E*)-4-(*o*-Chlorophenyl)-1,3-dithiolan-2-ylidene]imidazole-1-acetonitrile. *UNII-4E7858311F. CAS-101530-10-3.* INN.

Lanolin (lan′ oh lin). **USP.** [Purified Lanolin is JAN.] The purified, wax-like substance from the wool of sheep, *Ovis aries* Linné (Fam. Bovidae), that has been cleaned, decolorized, and deodorized. *Pharmaceutic aid (ointment base, absorbent). [Name previously used: Anhydrous Lanolin.]*

Lanolin Alcohols (lan′ oh lin al′ ka hols). **NF.** A mixture of aliphatic alcohols, triterpenoid alcohols, and sterols, obtained by the hydrolysis of lanolin. *Pharmaceutic aid (emulsifying agent).*

Lanolin, Anhydrous (previously used name) — *See* Lanolin.

Lanolin, Hydrous (JAN) — *See* Lanolin, Modified.

Lanolin, Modified (lan′ oh lin). **USP.** [Hydrous Lanolin is JAN.] The purified, wax-like substance from the wool of sheep, *Ovis aries* Linné (Fam. Bovidae), that has been processed to reduce the contents of free lanolin alcohols and detergent and pesticide residues. *Pharmaceutic aid (ointment base, absorbent).*

Lanolin, Purified (JAN) — *See* Lanolin.

Lanoteplase [*1997*] (lan oh′ te plase). $C_{2184}H_{3323}N_{633}O_{666}S_{29}$ (amino acid sequence). 50,032.53. A tissue plasminogen activator protein derived from human t-PA by deletion of the fibronectin-like and EGF-like domains and mutations of Asn-117 to Gln-117. The deletion removes native human t-PA residues Cys-6 through Ile-86. The protein is produced by expression in a mammalian host cell of a DNA sequence encoding the peptide sequence. The protein is the nonreduced form containing 12 disulfide bridges and two glycosylation sites. (1) (1-5)-(87-527)-Plasminogen activator (human tissue-type protein moiety), *N*-[*N²*-(*N*-glycyl-L-alanyl)-L-arginyl]-117-L-glutamine-245-L-methionine; (2) *N*-[*N²*-(*N*-Glycyl-L-alanyl)-L-arginyl]-117-L-glutamine-245-L-methionine-(1-5)-(87-527)-plasminogen ac-

tivator (human tissue-type protein moiety). *CAS-171870-23-8.* INN. *Plasminogen activator; thrombolytic.* ◇*BMS-200980; SUN 9216*

```
GARSYQVIDT RATCYEDQGI SYRGTWSTAE SGAECTNWQS SALAQKPYSG
RRPDAIRLGL GNHNYCRNPD RDSKPWCYVF KAGKYSSEFC STPACSEGNS
DCYFGNGSAY RGTHSLTESG ASCLPWNSMI LIGKVYTAQN PSAQALGLGK
HNYCRNPDGD AKPWCHMLKN RRLTWEYCDV PSCSTCGLRQ YSQPQFRIKG
GLFADIASHP WQAAIFAKHR RSPGERFLCG GILISSCWIL SAAHCFQERF
PPHHLTVILG RTYRVVPGEE EQKFEVEKYI VHKEFDDDTY DNDIALLQLK
SDSSRCAQES SVVRTVCLPP ADLQLPDWTE CELSGYGKHE ALSPFYSERL
KEAHVRLYPS SRCTSQHLLN RTVTDNMLCA GDTRSGGPQA NLHDACQGDS
GGPLVCLNDG RMTLVGIISW GLGCGQKDVP GVYTKVTNYL DWIRDNMRP
```

* glycosylation sites

Lanperisone. $C_{15}H_{18}F_3NO$. 285.30. (-)-(*R*)-2-Methyl-3-(1-pyrrolidinyl)-4′-(trifluoromethyl)propiophenone. *UNII-TO2JP2G53H. CAS-116287-14-0.* INN.

Lanproston. $C_{24}H_{31}ClO_7$. 466.95. (*Z*)-7-[(1*R*,2*R*,3*R*,5*S*)-2-[(*E*)-2-[2-[(*m*-Chlorophenoxy)methyl]-1,3-dioxolan-2-yl]vinyl]-3,5-dihydroxycyclopentyl]-5-heptenoic acid. *UNII-KC523G2996. CAS-105674-77-9.* INN; BAN.

Lanreotide Acetate [*1992*] (lan ree′ oh tide as′ e tate). $C_{54}H_{69}N_{11}O_{10}S_2 \cdot x(C_2H_4O_2)$. 1096.32 (base compound). [Lanreotide is INN and BAN.] (1) L-Threoninamide, 3-(2-naphthalenyl)-D-alanyl-L-cysteinyl-L-tyrosyl-D-tryptophyl-L-lysyl-L-valyl-L-cysteinyl-, cyclic (2→7)-disulfide, acetate (salt); (2) 3-(2-Naphthyl)-D-alanyl-L-cysteinyl-L-tyrosyl-D-tryptophyl-L-lysyl-L-valyl-L-cysteinyl-L-threoninamide, cyclic (2→7)-disulfide, acetate (salt). *UNII-IEU56G3J9C; UNII-0G3DE8943Y* [lanreotide]. *CAS-127984-74-1; CAS-108736-35-2* [lanreotide]. *Antineoplastic.* ◇*BIM-23014C*

Lansoprazole [*1989*] (lan soe′ pra zole). **USP.** $C_{16}H_{14}F_3N_3O_2S$. 369.36. (1) 1*H*-Benzimidazole, 2-[[[3-methyl-4-(2,2,2-trifluoroethoxy)-2-pyridinyl]methyl]sulfinyl]-; (2) 2-[[[3-Methyl-4-(2,2,2-trifluoroethoxy)-2-pyri-

---

† Brand name formerly used, and/or firm no longer concerned with this product.

dyl]methyl]sulfinyl]benzimidazole. *UNII-0K5C5T2QPG. CAS-103577-45-3.* INN; BAN. *Anti-ulcerative.* Prevacid (TAP) ◇*AG-1749; A-65006*

Lanthanum Carbonate [*2003*] (lan′ tha num kar′ bo nate). $La_2(CO_3)_3 \cdot_xH_2O$. 457.80 (anhydrous mass). [Lanthanum Carbonate Hydrate is JAN.] (1) Carbonic acid, lanthanum (3+) salt (3:2), hydrate; (2) Dilanthanum tricarbonate hydrate. *UNII-490D9F069T. CAS-54451-24-0. Treatment of hyperphosphataemia in patients with end stage renal disease.* Fosrenol (Shire)

Lapaquistat Acetate [*2006*] (la pa′ kwi stat as′ e tate). $C_{33}H_{41}ClN_2O_9$. 645.14. [Lapaquistat is INN.] (1) 4-Piperidineacetic acid, 1-[[(3*R*,5*S*)-1-[3-(acetyloxy)-2,2-dimethylpropyl]-7-chloro-5-(2,3-dimethoxyphenyl)-1,2,3,5-tetrahydro-2-oxo-4,1-benzoxazepin-3-yl]acetyl]-; (2) 2-(1-(2-((3*R*,5*S*)-1-(3-Acetoxy-2,2-dimethylpropyl)-7-chloro-5-(2,3-dimethoxyphenyl)-2-oxo-1,2,3,5-tetrahydrobenzo[e][1,4]oxazepin-3-yl)acetyl)piperidin-4-yl)acetic acid. *UNII-IUH3AY74O3. CAS-189060-13-7; CAS-189059-71-0* [lapaquistat]. JAN. *Cholesterol-lowering agent.* ◇*TAK 475*

Lapatinib Ditosylate [*2003*] (la pa′ ti nib dye tos′ i late). $C_{29}H_{26}ClFN_4O_4S \cdot 2C_7H_8O_3S \cdot H_2O$. 943.48. [Lapatinib is INN.] (1) 4-Quinazolinamine, *N*-[3-chloro-4-[(3-fluorophenyl)methoxy]phenyl]-6-[5-[[[2-(methylsulfonyl)ethyl]amino]methyl]-2-furanyl]-, bis(4-methylbenzenesulfonate), monohydrate; (2) *N*-[3-Chloro-4-[(3-fluorobenzyl)oxy]phenyl]-6-[5-[[[2-(methylsulfonyl)ethyl]amino]methyl]furan-2-yl]quinazolin-4-amine bis(4-methylbenzenesulfonate) monohydrate. *UNII-G873GX646R; UNII-0VUA21238F* [lapatinib]. *CAS-388082-78-8; CAS-231277-92-2* [lapatinib]. *Anti-neoplastic agent.* Tykerb (GlaxoSmithKline) ◇*GW572016F*

Lapirium Chloride (INN) — *See* Lapyrium Chloride.

Lapisteride. $C_{29}H_{40}N_2O_3$. 464.64. *N*-[1-(4-Methoxyphenyl)-1-methylethyl]-3-oxo-4-aza-5α-androst-1-ene-17β-carboxamide. *CAS-142139-60-4.* INN; BAN.

Laprafylline. $C_{29}H_{36}N_6O_2$. 500.64. 8-[2-[4-(Diphenylmethyl)-1-piperazinyl]ethyl]-3-isobutyl-1-methylxanthine. *CAS-90749-32-9.* INN.

Lapuleucel-T [*2005*] (la″ pu loo′ sel - tee). Product is a specific active immunotherapeutic composed of antigen-loaded autologous antigen presenting cells designed to stimulate a T cell immune response specific for the tumor-associated antigen Her2/neu. *Treatment of cancers overexpressing Her2/neu.* Neuvenge (Dendreon) ◇*APC8024*

Lapyrium Chloride [*1972*] (la pir′ ee um klor′ ide). $C_{21}H_{35}ClN_2O_3$. 398.97. [Lapirium Chloride is INN.] (1) Pyridinium, 1-[2-oxo-2-[[2-[(1-oxododecyl)oxy]ethyl]amino]ethyl]-, chloride; (2) 1-[[(2-Hydroxyethyl)carbamoyl]methyl]pyridinium chloride laurate (ester). *CAS-6272-74-8. Pharmaceutic aid (surfactant).* ◇*NSC-33659*

Laquinimod Sodium [*2007*] (la kwin′ i mod soe′ dee um). $C_{19}H_{17}ClN_2NaO_3$. 379.79. [Laquinimod is INN.] (1) 3-Quinolinecarboxamide, 5-chloro-*N*-ethyl-1,2-dihydro-4-hydroxy-1-methyl-2-oxo-*N*-phenyl-, sodium salt; (2) Sodium 5-chloro-3-(ethylphenylcarbamoyl)-1-methyl-2-oxo-1,2-dihydroquinolin-4-olate. *UNII-4H914M0CSP; UNII-908SY76S4G* [laquinimod]. *CAS-248282-07-7; CAS-248281-84-7* [laquinimod]. *Treatment of multiple sclerosis.* ◇*ABR-215062 sodium; TV-5600*

Laramycin — *See* Zorbamycin.

Larazotide [*2008*] (la raz′ oh tide). $C_{32}H_{55}N_9O_{10}$. 725.83. (1) Glycine, glycylglycyl-L-valyl-L-leucyl-L-valyl-L-glutaminyl-L-prolyl-; (2) Glycylglycyl-L-valyl-L-leucyl-L-valyl-L-glutaminyl-L-prolylglycine. *UNII-ZN3R5560ZV. CAS-258818-34-7.* INN. *Treatment of inflammatory and autoimmune diseases.* ◇*AT-2347*

Larazotide Acetate [2007] (la raz′ oh tide as′ e tate). $C_{32}H_{55}N_9O_{10} \cdot C_2H_4O_2$. 785.89. [Larazotide is INN.] (1) Glycine, glycylglycyl-L-valyl-L-leucyl-L-valyl-L-glutaminyl-L-prolyl-, monoacetate; (2) Glycylglycyl-L-valyl-L-leucyl-L-valyl-L-glutaminyl-L-prolylglycine acetate. *UNII-FO8S2IW40N. CAS-881851-50-9; CAS-258818-34-7* [larazotide]. *Treatment of Celiac disease and treatment of Inflammatory Bowel Disease.* ◇*AT-1001*

Lard. JAN.

Laromustine [2007] (lar″ oh mus′ teen). $C_6H_{14}ClN_3O_5S_2$. 307.78. (1) Methanesulfonic acid, 1-(2-chloroethyl)-2-[(methylamino)carbonyl]-2-(methylsulfonyl)hydrazide; (2) 2′-(2-Chloroethyl)-*N*-methyl-1′,2′-bis(methylsulfonyl)carbamohydrazide; (3) 1,2-Bis(methylsulfonyl)-1-(2-chloroethyl)-2-[(methylamino)carbonyl]hydrazine. *CAS-173424-77-6.* INN. *Antineoplastic; treatment of acute myeloid leukemia.* Cloretazine (Vion) ◇*VNP40101M; 101M*

Laronidase [2000] (lar on′ i dase). $C_{3567}H_{5645}N_{921}O_{1261}S_{12}P_4$. [Laronidase (genetical recombination) is JAN.] Iduronidase, α-L-[8-histidine] (human). Molecular weight is approximately 82,000 daltons. *CAS-210589-09-6.* INN. *Enzyme replacement in Mucopolysaccharidosis I (MPS I).*

AEAPHLVQVD	AARALWPLRR	FWRSTGFCPP	LPHSQADQYV	LSWDQQLNLA
YVGAVPHRGI	KQVRTHWLLE	LVTTRGSTGR	GLSYNFTHLD	GYLDLLRENQ
LLPGFELMGS	ASGHFTDFED	KQQVFEWKDL	VSSLARRYIG	RYGLAHVSKW
NFETWNEPDH	HDFDNVSMTM	QGFLNYYDAC	SEGLRAASPA	LRLGGPGDSF
HTPPRSPLSW	GLLRHCHDGT	NFFTGEAGVR	LDYISLHRKG	ARSSISILEQ
EKVVAQQIRQ	LFPKFADTPI	YNDEADPLVG	WSLPQPWRAD	VTYAAMVVKV
IAQHQNLLLA	NTTSAFPYAL	LSNDNAFLSY	HPHPFAQRTL	TARFQVNNTR
PPHVQLLRKP	VLTAMGLLAL	LDEEQLWAEV	SQAGTVLDSN	HTVGVLASAH
RPQGPADAWR	AAVLIYASDD	TRAHPNRSVA	VTLRLRGVPP	GPGLVYVTRY
LDNGLCSPDG	EWRRLGRPVF	PTAEQFRRMR	AAEDPVAAAP	RPLPAGGRLT
LRPALRLPSL	LLVHVCARPE	KPPGQVTRLR	ALPLTQGQLV	LVWSDEHVGS
KCLWTYEIQF	SQDGKAYTPV	SRKPSTFNLF	VFSPDTGAVS	GSYRVRALDY
WARPGPFSDP	VPYLEVPVPR	GPPSPGNP		

　　* glycosylation sites
　　↳ disulfide

Laropiprant [2006] (lar oh′ pi prant). $C_{21}H_{19}ClFNO_4S$. 435.90. (1) Cyclopent[*b*]indole-3-acetic acid, 4-[(4-chlorophenyl)methyl]-7-fluoro-1,2,3,4-tetrahydro-5-(methylsulfonyl)-, (3*R*)-; (2) (-)-[(3*R*)-4-(4-Chlorobenzyl)-7-fluoro-5-(methylsulfonyl)-1,2,3,4-tetrahydrocyclopenta[*b*]indol-3-yl]acetic acid. *UNII-G7N11T8O78. CAS-571170-77-9.* INN. *Treatment of atherosclerosis, dyslipidemia, and related conditions when administered with niacin.* ◇*MK-0524*

Larotaxel. $C_{45}H_{53}NO_{14}$. 831.90. 1-Hydroxy-9-oxo-5β,20-epoxy-7β,19-cyclotax-11-ene-2α,4,10β,13α-tetrayl 4,10-Diacetate 2-benzoate 13-{(2*R*,3*S*)-3-[(*tert*-butoxycarbonyl)amino]-2-hydroxy-3-phenylpropanoate}. *CAS-156294-36-9.* INN.

Lasalocid [1973] (la sal′ oh sid). $C_{34}H_{54}O_8$. 590.79. (1) Benzoic acid, 6-[7(*R*)-[5(*S*)-Ethyl-5-(5(*R*)-ethyltetrahydro-5-hydroxy-6(*S*)-methyl-2*H*-pyran-2(*R*)-yl)tetrahydro-3(*S*)-methyl-2(*S*)-furanyl]-4(*S*)-hydroxy-3(*R*),5(*S*)-dimethyl-6-oxononyl]-2-hydroxy-3-methyl-; (2) 6-[7(*R*)-[5(*S*)-Ethyl-5-(*R*)-ethyltetrahydro-5-hydroxy-6(*S*)-methyl-2*H*-pyran-2(*R*)-yl)tetrahydro-3(*S*)-methyl-2(*S*)-furyl]-4(*S*)-hydroxy-3(*R*),5(*S*)-dimethyl-6-oxononyl]-2,3-cresotic acid. *UNII-W7V2ZZ2FWB. CAS-25999-31-9.* INN; BAN. *Coccidiostat (for poultry).* Avatec [as sodium] [Veterinary] (Hoffmann-LaRoche); Bovatec [as sodium] [Veterinary] (Hoffmann-LaRoche) ◇*Ro 2-2985*

Lasinavir. $C_{35}H_{53}N_3O_9$. 659.81. *tert*-Butyl [(αS)-α-[(1*S*,3*R*)-1-hydroxy-3-[[(1*S*)-1-[(2-methoxyethyl)carbamoyl]-2-methylpropyl]carbamoyl]-4-(2,3,4-trimethoxyphenyl)butyl]phenethyl]carbamate. *UNII-0QGV823713. CAS-175385-62-3.* INN.

---

† Brand name formerly used, and/or firm no longer concerned with this product.

Lasofoxifene. $C_{28}H_{31}NO_2$. 413.55. (-)-*cis*-5,6,7,8-Tetrahydro-6-phenyl-5-[*p*-[2-(1-pyrrolidinyl)ethoxy]phenyl]-2-naphthol. *UNII-337G83N988. CAS-180916-16-9.* INN.

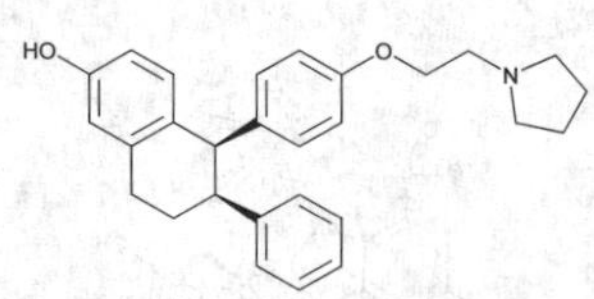

Lasofoxifene Tartrate [*1999*] (la″ soe fox′ i feen tar′ trate). $C_{28}H_{31}NO_2 \cdot C_4H_6O_6$. 563.64. (1) 2-Naphthalenol, 5,6,7,8-tetrahydro-6-phenyl-5-[4-[2-(1-pyrrolidinyl)ethoxy]phenyl]-, *cis*-(-)-, [*S*-(*R**,*R**)]-2,3-dihydroxybutanedioate (1:1) (salt); (2) (-)-*cis*-5,6,7,8-Tetrahydro-6-phenyl-5-[*p*-[2-(1-pyrrolidinyl)ethoxy]phenyl]-2-naphthol D-tartrate (1:1) (salt). *UNII-85X09V2GSO. CAS-190791-29-8. Treatment and prevention of osteoporosis and breast cancer; reduction of cardiovascular risk (tissue selective estrogen agonist/antagonist).* ◇*CP-336,156-CB*

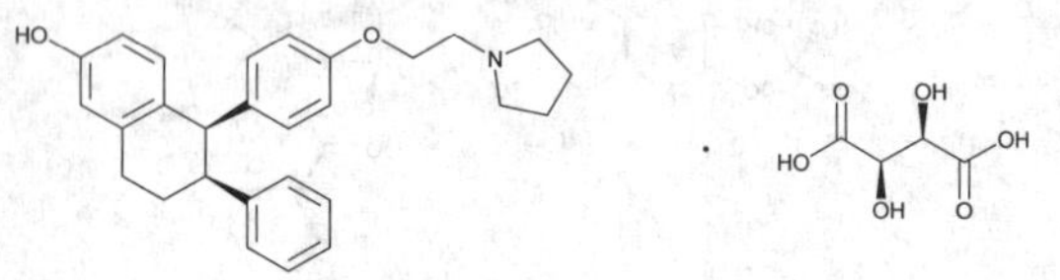

Latamoxef (INN, BAN) — *See* Moxalactam Disodium.

Latamoxef Sodium (JAN) — *See* Moxalactam Disodium.

Latanoprost [*1996*] (la tan′ oh prost). $C_{26}H_{40}O_5$. 432.59. (1) 5-Heptenoic acid, 7-[3,5-dihydroxy-2-(3-hydroxy-5-phenylpentyl)cyclopentyl]-1-methylethyl ester, [1*R*-[1α(*Z*),2β(*R**),3α,5α]]-; (2) Isopropyl (*Z*)-7-[(1*R*,2*R*,3*R*,5*S*)-3,5-dihydroxy-2-[(3*R*)-3-hydroxy-5-phenylpentyl]cyclopentyl]-5-heptenoate. *UNII-6Z5B6HVF6O. CAS-130209-82-4.* INN; BAN. *Antiglaucoma agent.* Xalatan (Pfizer) ◇*PHXA41; XA41*

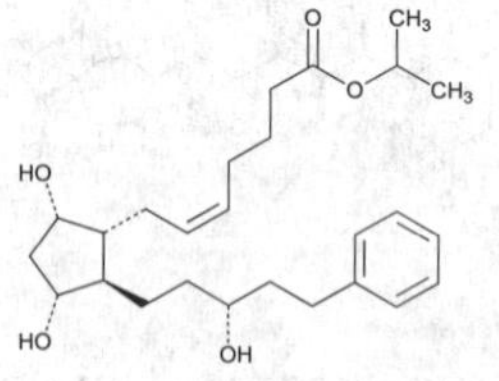

Latidectin. $C_{46}H_{61}NO_{11}$ (component A_3). 803.98; $C_{47}H_{63}NO_{11}$ (component A_4). 818.00. Mixture of components A_4 and A_3: component A_4, (2a¹*S*,2aE,4*E*,5′*S*,6*S*,6′*R*,7*R*,8*E*,11*R*,13*R*,15*S*,17a*R*,20*R*,20a*R*)-6′-ethyl-2a¹,20-dihydroxy-5′,6,8,19-tetramethyl-17-oxo-2a¹,3′,4′,5′,6,6′,7,10,11,14,15,17a,20,20a-tetradecahydro-2*H*,13*H*,17*H*-spiro[11,15-methanofuro[4,3,2-*pq*][2,6]benzodioxacyclooctadecine-13,2′-pyran]-7-yl 1-[4-(methoxyacetamido)phenyl]cyclopentanecarboxylate; component A_3, (2a¹*S*,2a*E*,4*E*,5′*S*,6*S*,6′*R*,7*R*,8*E*,11*R*,13*R*,15*S*,17a*R*,20*R*,20a*R*)-2a¹,20-dihydroxy-5′,6,6′,8,19-pentamethyl-17-oxo-2a¹,3′,4′,5′,6,6′,7,10,11,14,15,17a,20,20a-tetradecahydro-2*H*,13*H*,17*H*-spiro[11,15-methanofuro[4,3,2-*pq*][2,6]benzodioxacyclooctadecine-13,2′-[2*H*]pyran]-7-yl

1-[4-(methoxyacetamido)phenyl]cyclopentanecarboxylate. *CAS-371918-51-3* [component A_3]; *CAS-371918-44-4* [component A.i4]. INN.

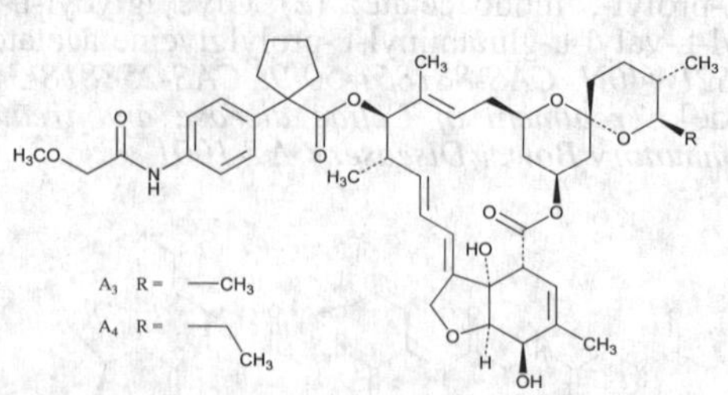

Laudexium Methylsulfate. $C_{54}H_{80}N_2O_{16}S_2$. 1077.35. [Laudexium Metilsulfate is INN and BAN.] 2,2′-Decamethylenebis(1,2,3,4-tetrahydro)-6,7-dimethoxy-2-methyl-1-veratrylisoquinolium methylsulfate. *CAS-3253-60-9.* MI. *[Name previously used: Laudexium Methylsulphate]*

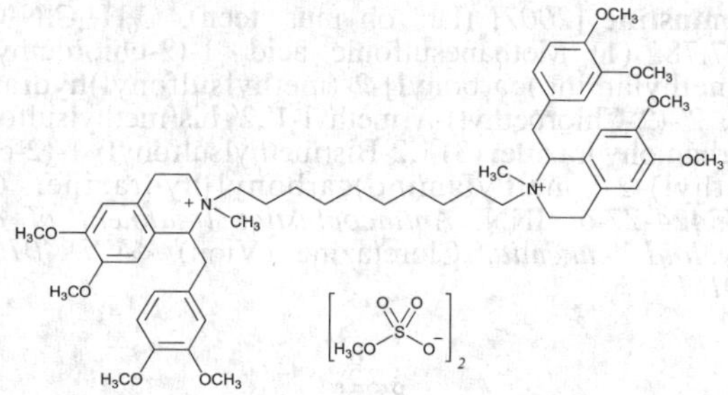

Laudexium Metilsulfate (INN, BAN) — *See* Laudexium Methylsulfate.

Lauralkonium Chloride. $C_{29}H_{44}ClNO_2$. 474.12. Benzyl[2-[*p*-(lauroyl)phenoxy]ethyl]dimethylammonium chloride. *CAS-19486-61-4.* INN; DCF.

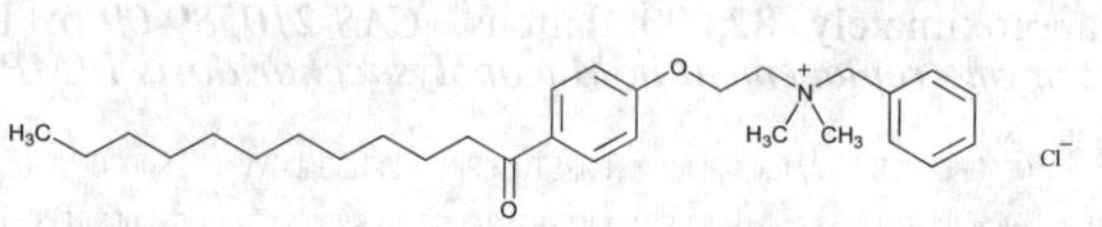

Laurcetium Bromide. $C_{18}H_{38}BrNO_2$. 380.40. (Carboxymethyl)dodecyldimethylammonium bromide, ethyl ester. *UNII-G1TGH6857X. CAS-1794-75-8.* INN.

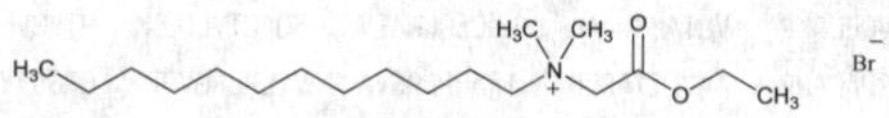

Laureth 4 [*1978*] (law′ reth). $C_{20}H_{42}O_5$. 362.54. (1) Poly(oxy-1,2-ethanediyl), α-dodecyl-ω-hydroxy-; (2) Polyethylene glycol monododecyl ether. *CAS-9002-92-0. Pharmaceutic aid (surfactant).* Brij 30 (ICI Americas)

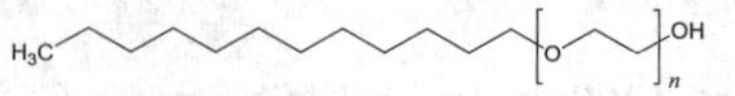

Laureth 9 [*1963*] (law′ reth). $C_{30}H_{62}O_{10}$ (average). 582.81 (average). A mixture of polyethylene glycol monododecyl ethers averaging about 9 ethylene oxide groups per molecule. (1) Poly(oxy-1,2-ethanediyl), α-dodecyl-ω-hydroxy-; (2) Polyethylene glycol monododecyl ether. *CAS-9002-92-0. Spermaticide; pharmaceutic aid (surfactant). [Note—Graphic formula same as for Laureth 4.]*

Laureth 10S [*1979*] (law′ reth). $C_{32}H_{66}O_{10}S$ (Approximate). 642.93. (In the graphic formula, *n*, which is indicative of the average chain length of the polymeric portion, is 10.) (1) Poly(oxy-1,2-ethanediyl),α-[2-(dodecylthio)ethyl]-ω-hydroxy-; (2) Polyethylene glycol mono[2-(dodecylthio)ethyl] ether; (3) α-[2-(Dodecylthio)ethyl]-ω-hydroxypoly(oxyethylene). *CAS-9014-89-5. Spermaticide.*

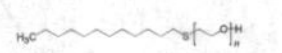

Laurixamine. $C_{15}H_{33}NO$. 243.43. 3-(Dodecyloxy)propylamine. *UNII-WY0R7196HP. CAS-7617-74-5.* INN.

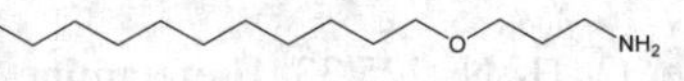

Laurocapram [*1984*] (law″ roe kay′ pram). $C_{18}H_{35}NO$. 281.48. (1) 2*H*-Azepin-2-one, 1-dodecylhexahydro-; (2) 1-Dodecylhexahydro-2*H*-azepin-2-one. *UNII-1F3X9DRV9X. CAS-59227-89-3.* INN. *Pharmaceutic aid (excipient).* ◇*N-0252*

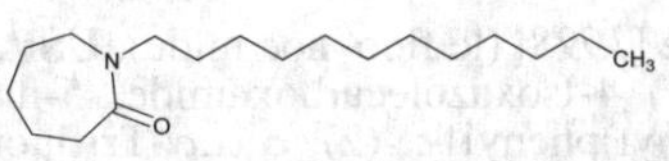

Lauroguadine. $C_{20}H_{36}N_6O$. 376.54. 1,1′-[4-(Dodecyloxy)-*m*-phenylene]diguanidine. *UNII-J587DZQ8YB. CAS-135-43-3.* INN; MI. ◇*P 7*

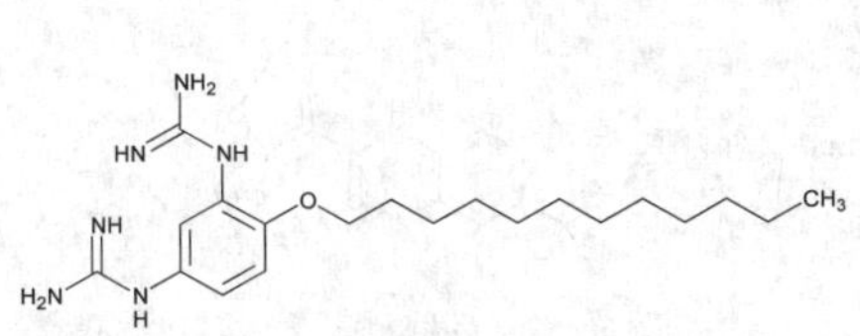

Laurolinium Acetate. $C_{24}H_{38}N_2O_2$. 386.57. 4-Amino-1-dodecylquinaldinium acetate. *UNII-R01EZP92PU. CAS-146-37-2.* INN; BAN; MI.

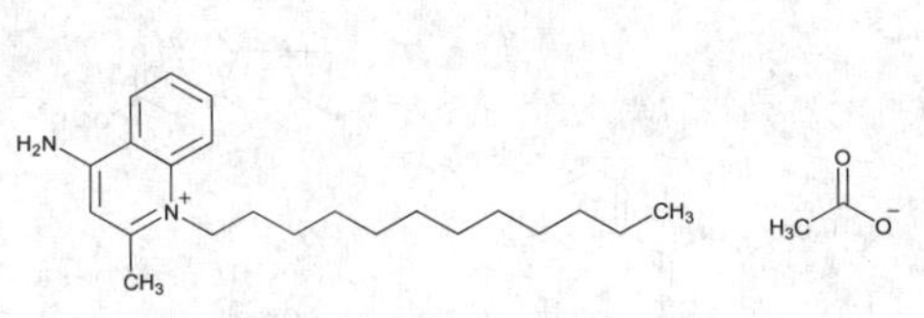

Lauromacrogol 400. [Lauromacrogol is BAN and JAN.] Polyethylene glycol monododecyl ether, the name is followed by a number (400) corresponding approximately to the average molecular mass of the polyethylene glycol portion. *CAS-9015-55-8.* INN.

Lauroyl Polyoxylglycerides. **NF.** Mixtures of monoesters, diesters, and triesters of glycerol and monoesters and diesters of polyethylene glycols with a mean relative molecular weight between 300 and 1500.

---

† Brand name formerly used, and/or firm no longer concerned with this product.

Lauryl Isoquinolinium Bromide [*1981*] (lawr′ il eye″ soe kwin″ oh lin′ i um broe′ mide). $C_{21}H_{32}BrN$. 378.39. (1) Isoquinolinium, 2-dodecyl-, bromide; (2) 2-Dodecylisoquinolinium bromide. *CAS-93-23-2. Anti-infective.*

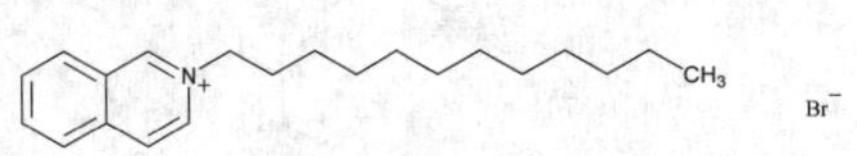

Lavender Oil. *CAS-8000-28-0.* NF XVI; JAN; MI.

Lavoltidine Succinate [*1989*] (lav ole′ ti deen sux′ i nate). $(C_{19}H_{29}N_5O_2)_2.C_4H_6O_4$. 837.02. [Lavoltidine is INN and BAN.] (1) 1*H*-1,2,4-Triazole-3-methanol, 1-methyl-5-[[3-[3-(1-piperidinylmethyl)phenoxy]propyl]amino]-, butanedioate (2:1) (salt); (2) 1-Methyl-5-[[3-[(α-piperidino-*m*-tolyl)oxy]propyl]amino]-1*H*-1,2,4-triazole-3-methanol succinate (2:1) (salt). *CAS-86160-82-9; CAS-76956-02-0* [lavoltidine]. *Anti-ulcerative (histamine H₂-receptor blocker).* [*Name previously used: Loxotidine.*] ◇*AH 23844A; AH 23844 [lavoltidine]*

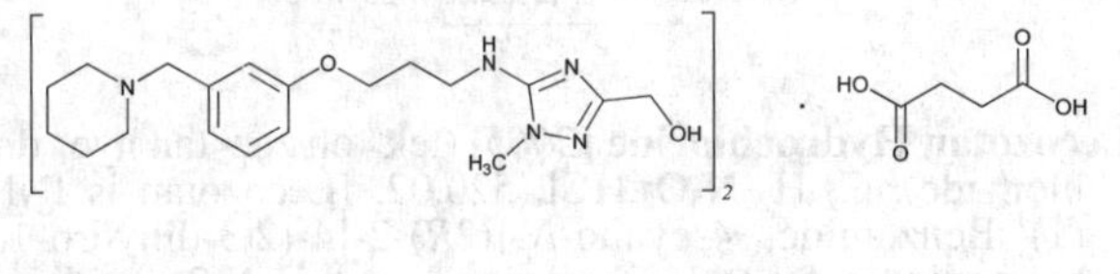

Lazabemide [*1992*] (laz a′ bem ide). $C_8H_{10}ClN_3O$. 199.64. (1) 2-Pyridinecarboxamide, *N*-(2-aminoethyl)-5-chloro-; (2) *N*-(2-Aminoethyl)-5-chloropicolinamide. *UNII-420HD787N9. CAS-103878-84-8.* INN; BAN. *Antiparkinsonian.* ◇*Ro 19-6327/000*

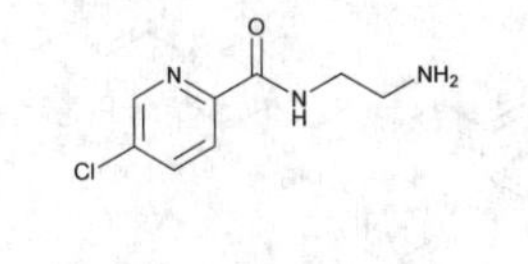

Lazabemide Hydrochloride [*1999*] (laz a′ bem ide hye″ droe klor′ ide). $C_8H_{10}ClN_3O.HCl$. 236.10. (1) 2-Pyridinecarboxamide, *N*-(2-aminoethyl)-5-chloro-, monohydrochloride; (2) *N*-(2-Aminoethyl)-5-chloropicolinamide monohydrochloride. *UNII-PI150J9ZX1. CAS-103878-83-7. Treatment of Alzheimer's disease.* Tempium (Hoffmann-LaRoche) ◇*Ro 19-6327/001*

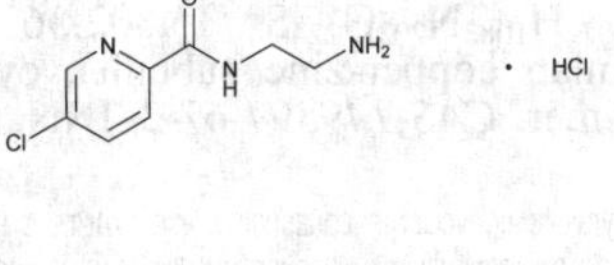

Lead Acetate. JAN.

Lecimibide [*1994*] (le sim′ i bide). $C_{34}H_{40}F_2N_4OS$. 590.77. (1) Urea, *N*′-(2,4-difluorophenyl)-*N*-[5-[(4,5-diphenyl-1*H*-imidazol-2-yl)thio]pentyl]-*N*-heptyl-; (2) 3-(2,4-Difluorophenyl)-1-[5-[(4,5-diphenylimidazol-2-yl)thio]pentyl]-1-heptylurea. *CAS-130804-35-2*. INN. *Antihyperlipidemic*. ◇*DuP 128*

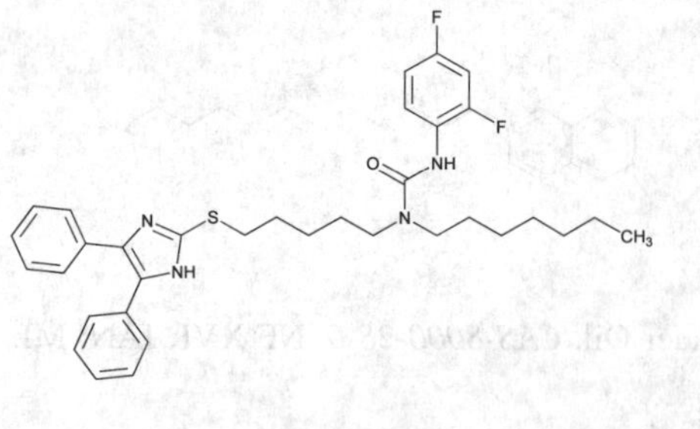

Lecithin (les′ i thin). **NF**. A complex mixture of acetone-insoluble phosphatides, which consist chiefly of phosphatidyl choline, phosphatidyl ethanolamine, phosphatidyl serine, and phosphatidyl inositol, combined with various amounts of other substances such as triglycerides, fatty acids, and carbohydrates, as separated from the crude vegetable oil source. *Pharmaceutic aid (emulsifying agent)*.

Leconotide. $C_{107}H_{179}N_{35}O_{36}S_7$. 2756.23. Omega-conopeptide MVIIA. *CAS-247207-64-3*. INN.

```
CKSKGAKCSK  LMYDCCSGSC  SGTVGRC
```

Lecozotan Hydrochloride [*2005*] (lek″ oh zoe′ tan hye″ droe klor′ ide). $C_{28}H_{29}N_5O_3$.HCl. 520.02. [Lecozotan is INN.] (1) Benzamide, 4-cyano-*N*-[(2*R*)-2-[4-(2,3-dihydro-1,4-benzodioxin-5-yl)-1-piperazinyl]propyl]-*N*-2-pyridinyl-, monohydrochloride; (2) 4-Cyano-*N*-[(2*R*)-2-[4-(2,3-dihydro-1,4-benzodioxin-5-yl)piperazin-1-yl]propyl]-*N*-(pyridin-2-yl)benzamide monohydrochloride. *UNII-23EDE20K1X; UNII-48854OTZ5E* [lecozotan]. *CAS-433282-68-9; CAS-434283-16-6* [lecozotan]. *Treatment of cognitive deficits associated with Alzheimer's disease (5-HT$_{1A}$receptor antagonist)*. ◇*SRA-333*

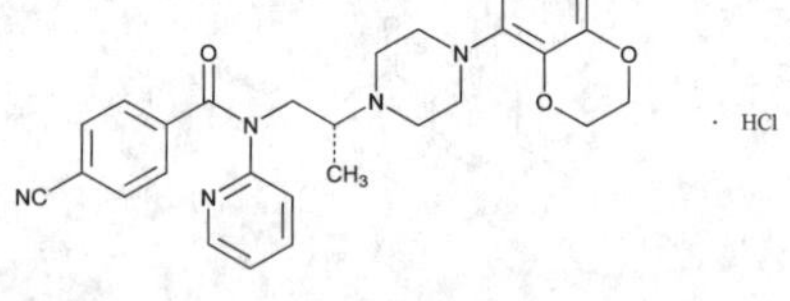

Ledazerol. $C_{11}H_{12}N_2O_2$. 204.23. 2-Hydroxy-3-(imidazol-4-ylmethyl)benzyl alcohol. *UNII-P13OO3FPZB. CAS-116795-97-2*. INN.

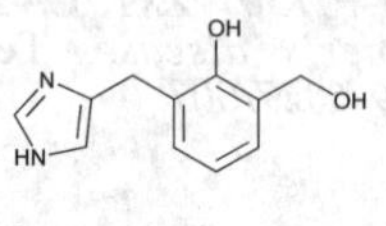

Ledismase. $C_{679}H_{1083}N_{203}O_{224}S_4$. 15,802.36. Superoxide dismutase (human copper-zinc subunit), cyclic (57→146)-disulfide, dimer. *CAS-149394-67-2*. INN.

```
ATKAVCVLKG DGPVQGIINF EQKESNGPVK VWGSIKGLTE GLHGFHVHEF
GDNTAGCTSA GPHFNPLSRK HGGPKDEERH VGDLGNVTAD KDGVADVSIE
DSVISLSGDH CIIGRTLVVH EKADDLGKGG NEESTKTGNA GSRLACGVIG
IAQ
```

Ledoxantrone Trihydrochloride [*1997*] (led ox′ an trone trye hye″ droe klor′ ide). $C_{21}H_{27}N_5OS$.3HCl. 506.92. [Ledoxantrone is INN.] 5-[(2-Aminoethyl)amino]-2-[2-(diethylamino)ethyl]-2*H*-[1]benzothiopyrano[4,3,2-*cd*]indazol-8-ol trihydrochloride. *CAS-119221-49-7; CAS-113457-05-9* [ledoxantrone]. *Antineoplastic (DNA topoisomerase II inhibitor)*. [*Note—Ledoxantrone Trihydrochloride supersedes Sedoxantrone Trihydrochloride.*] ◇*CI-958*

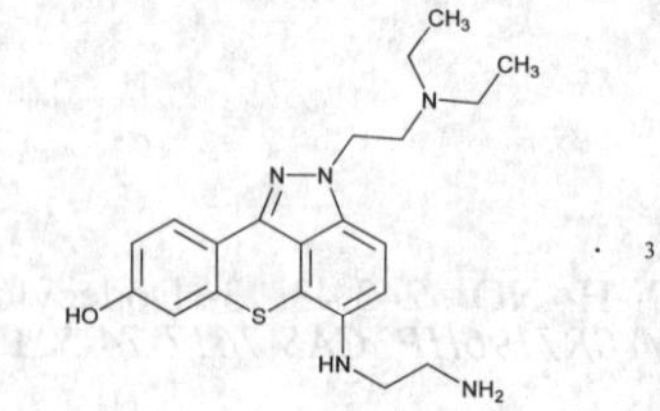

Lefetamine. $C_{16}H_{19}N$. 225.33. [Lefetamine Hydrochloride is JAN.] (-)-*N,N*-Dimethyl-1,2-diphenylethylamine. *UNII-4J9726V5Y9. CAS-7262-75-1*. INN; MI.

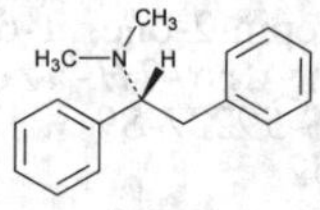

Leflunomide [*1998*] (le floo′ noe mide). **USP**. $C_{12}H_9F_3N_2O_2$. 270.21. (1) 4-Isoxazolecarboxamide, 5-methyl-*N*-[4-(trifluoromethyl)phenyl]-; (2) α,α,α-Trifluoro-5-methyl-4-isoxazolecarboxy-*p*-toluidide. *UNII-G162GK9U4W. CAS-75706-12-6*. INN; BAN. *Antineoplastic (blocks PDGF receptor function, inhibiting the growth and survival of human tumor cells when administered intravenously); used in the treatment of rheumatoid arthritis when administered orally*. Arava (Sanofi Aventis) ◇*SU101; HWA-486*

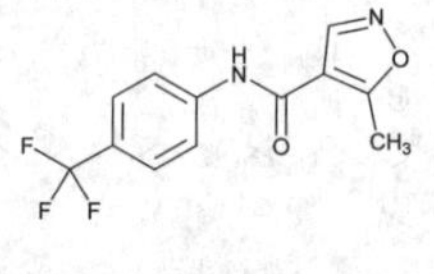

Lefradafiban. $C_{23}H_{25}N_3O_6$. 439.46. (3*S*,5*S*)-5-[[[4′-(Carboxyamidino)-4-biphenylyl]oxy]methyl]-2-oxo-3-pyrrolidineacetic acid, dimethyl ester. *UNII-0R4888YXR5. CAS-149503-79-7*. INN.

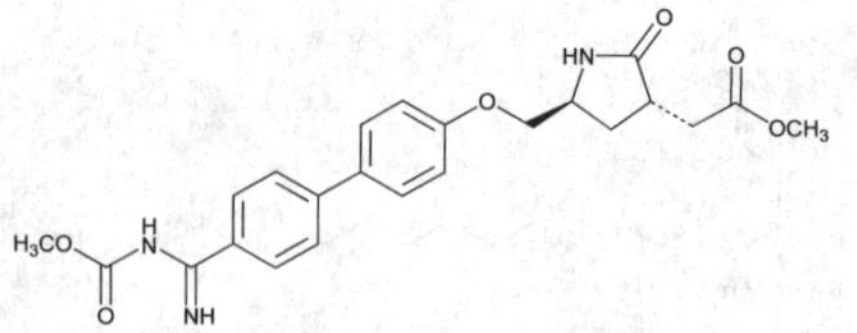

Leiopyrrole. $C_{23}H_{28}N_2O$. 348.48. 1-[*o*-[2-(Diethylamino)ethoxy]phenyl]-2-methyl-5-phenylpyrrole. *UNII-S1URO6678T. CAS-5633-16-9*. INN; DCF; MI.

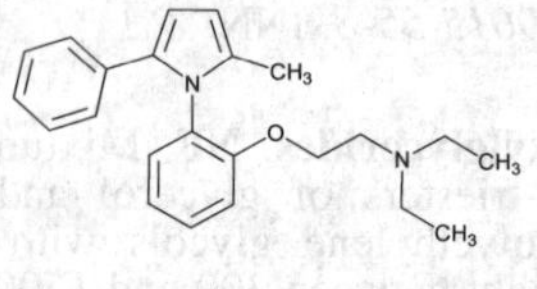

Lemalesomab. Immunoglobulin G1, anti-(human NCA-90 granulocyte cell antigen) (mouse monoclonal IMMU-MN3 γ1-chain), disulfide with mouse monoclonal IMMU-MN3 κ-chain, dimer. *CAS-250242-54-7*. INN.

Lemidosul. $C_{12}H_{19}NO_3S$. 257.35. α-Amino-4-*tert*-butyl-6-(methylsulfonyl)-*o*-cresol. *UNII-98C3QM4D0P. CAS-88041-40-1.* INN.

Lemildipine. $C_{20}H_{22}Cl_2N_2O_6$. 457.30. 3-Isopropyl 5-methyl ($\pm$)-4-(2,3-dichlorophenyl)-1,4-dihydro-2-(hydroxymethyl)-6-methyl-3,5-pyridinedicarboxylate, carbamate (ester). *CAS-125729-29-5.* INN.

Leminoprazole. $C_{19}H_{23}N_3OS$. 341.47. ($\pm$)-2-[[*o*-(Isobutylmethylamino)benzyl]sulfinyl]benzimidazole. *CAS-104340-86-5.* INN.

Lemon Oil (lem′ on). **NF**. The volatile oil obtained by expression, without the aid of heat, from the fresh peel of the fruit of *Citrus x limon* (L.) Osbeck (Fam. Rutaceae), with or without the previous separation of the pulp and the peel. *CAS-8008-56-8. Pharmaceutic aid (flavor).*

Lemon Tincture (lem′ on). **NF**. Prepared from lemon peel, which is the outer yellow rind of the fresh, ripe fruit of *Citrus x limon* (L.) Osbeck (Fam. Rutaceae).

Lemoxinol. $C_7H_6OCl_2(C_2H_4O)n$. α-(4,6-Dichloro-*m*-tolyl)-oxy-ω-hydroxypoly(oxyethylene). Each *lemoxinol* name is followed by a number indicating the approximate number of oxyethylene groups present (e.g. *lemoxinol 5*), and the individual chemical names may contain a specific numerical syllable for the same purpose. INN.

Lemuteporfin. $C_{44}H_{48}N_4O_{10}$. 792.87. Dimethyl ($2RS,2^1SR$)-8-ethenyl-13,17-bis[3-(2-hydroxyethoxycarbonyl)-3-oxopropyl]-2,7,12,18-tetramethyl-2,2^1-dihydrobenzo[b]porphyrin-2^1,2^2-dicarboxylate. *CAS-215808-49-4.* INN.

Lenalidomide [*2004*] (len″ a lid′ oh mide). $C_{13}H_{13}N_3O_3$. 259.26. (1) 2,6-Piperidinedione, 3-(4-amino-1,3-dihydro-1-oxo-2*H*-isoindol-2-yl)-; (2) 3-(4-Amino-1-oxo-1,3-dihydro-2*H*-isoindol-2-yl)piperidine-2,6-dione. *UNII-F0P408N6V4. CAS-191732-72-6.* INN; BAN. *Immunomulator intended for use in the treatment of multiple myeloma, myelodysplastic syndromes, solid tumors including glioma and metastatic melanoma, Crohn's disease, and heart failure.* Revlimid (Celgene) ◇*CC-5013; CDC-501*

Lenampicillin. $C_{21}H_{23}N_3O_7S$. 461.49. [Lenampicillin Hydrochloride is JAN.] 2,3-Dihydroxy-2-butenyl($2S,5R,6R$)-6-[(R)-2-amino-2-phenylacetamido]-3,3-dimethyl-7-oxo-4-thia-1-azabicyclo[3.2.0]heptane-2-carboxylate, cyclic carbonate. *CAS-86273-18-9.* INN; MI.

Lenapenem. $C_{18}H_{29}N_3O_5S$. 399.50. (+)-($4R,5S,6S$)-6-[(R)-1-Hydroxyethyl]-3-[[($3S,5S$)-5-[(R)-1-hydroxy-3-(methylamino)propyl]-3-pyrrolidinyl]thio]-4-methyl-7-oxo-1-azabicyclo[3.2.0]hept-2-ene-2-carboxylic acid. *UNII-D6NBQ3H12U. CAS-149951-16-6.* INN.

Lenefilcon A [*2001*] (len″ e fil′ kon). $(C_6H_{10}O_3)_x(C_7H_{12}O_4)_y(C_{16}H_{26}O_7)_z$. (1) 2-Hydroxyethyl 2-methyl-2-propenoate polymer with 2,3-dihydroxypropyl 2-methyl-2-propenoate and oxybis(2,1-ethanediyloxy-2,1-ethanediyl) bis(2-methyl-2-propenoate); (2) 2-Hydroxyethyl methacrylate polymer with 2,3-dihydroxypropyl methacrylate and oxybis(ethyleneoxyethylene) dimethacrylate. *CAS-131577-81-6. Contact lens material (hydrophilic).[Note—The water content of the contact lens material is $55\pm0.4\%$ at ambient temperature ($23\pm2°C$), the purity of 2-*

---

hydroxyethyl methacrylate (HEMA) is >99.5%, and the oxygen permeability is $16\pm0.6 \times 10^{-11}(cm^2/sec)(ml\ O_2/ml \times mm\ Hg)$ at 35°C (Dk value).]

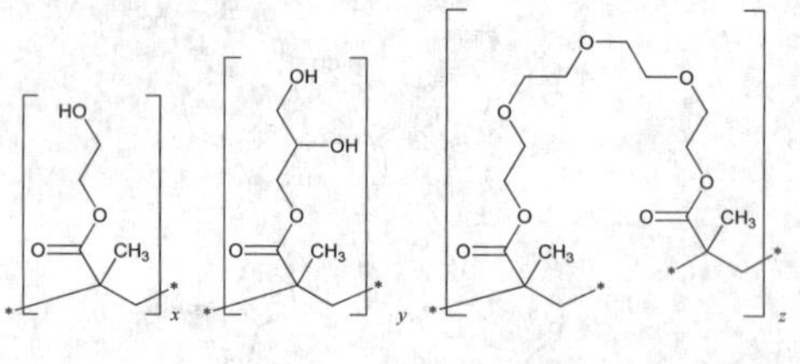

Lenercept [*1997*] (len′ er sept). $C_{1993}H_{3112}N_{562}O_{624}S_{34}$. 46,019.69. 1-182-Tumor necrosis factor receptor (human reduced), (182→104′)-protein with 104-330-immunoglobulin G 1 (human clone pTJ5 Cγ 1 reduced). *CAS-156679-34-4*. INN; BAN. *Immunomodulator.* ◇*Ro 45-2081*

Leniquinsin [*1967*] (len″ i kwin′ sin). $C_{20}H_{20}N_2O_4$. 352.38. (1) 4-Quinolinamine, *N*-[(3,4-dimethoxyphenyl)methylene]-6,7-dimethoxy-; (2) 6,7-Dimethoxy-4-(veratrylideneamino)quinoline. *CAS-10351-50-5*. INN. *Antihypertensive.* ◇*EU-1085*

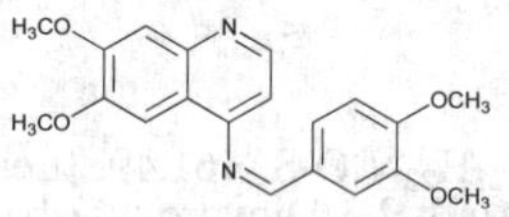

Lenograstim [*1992*] (len″ oh gra′ stim). A glycoprotein consisting of 174 amino acid residues, produced in Chinese hamster ovary cells by expression of a human granulocyte colony-stimulating factor-cDNA derived from a human oral cavity squamous cell line-mRNA. (1) [Component 1] Colony-stimulating factor (human clone 1034), 133-[*O*-[*O*-(*N*-acetyl-α-neuraminosyl)-(2→3)-*O*-β-D-galactopyranosyl-(1→3)-2-(acetylamino)-2-deoxy-β-D-galactopyranosyl]-L-threonine]-; [Component 2] Colony-stimulating factor (human clone 1034), 133-[*O*-[*O*-(*N*-acetyl-α-neuraminosyl)-(2→6)-*O*-[*O*-(*N*-acetyl-α-neuraminosyl)-(2→3)-β-D-galactopyranosyl-(1→3)]-2-(acetylamino)-2-deoxy-β-D-galactopyranosyl]-L-threonine]-; (2) 133-[*O*-[*O*-(*N*-Acetyl-α-neuraminosyl)-(2→3)-[*O*-β-D-galactopyranosyl-(1→3)]-2-acetamido-2-deoxy-β-D-galactopyranosyl]-L-threonine]colony-stimulating factor (human clone 1034) mixture with 133-[*O*-[*O*-(*N*-acetyl-α-neuraminosyl)-(2→6)-*O*-[*O*-(*N*-acetyl-α-neuraminosyl)-(2→3)-β-D-galactopyranosyl-(1→3)]-2-acetamido-2-deoxy-β-D-galactopyranosyl]-L-threonine]colony-stimulating factor (human clone 1034). *CAS-135968-09-1; CAS-130120-55-7* [component 1]; *CAS-130120-54-6* [component 2]. INN; BAN. *Antineutropenic; hematopoietic stimulant.* ◇*rG-CSF*

```
TPLGPASSLP QSFLLKCLEQ VRKIQGDGAA LQEKLQATYK LQHPEELVLL
GHSLGIPWAP LSSCPSQALQ LAGCLSQLHS GLFLYQGLLQ ALEGISPELG
PTLDTLQLDV ADFATTIWQQ MEELGMAPAL QPTQGAMPAF ASAFQRRAGG
VLVASHLQSF LEVSYRVLRH LAQP

* glycosylation site
```

Lenperone [*1972*] (len′ per one). $C_{22}H_{23}F_2NO_2$. 371.42. (1) 1-Butanone, 4-[4-(4-fluorobenzoyl)-1-piperidinyl]-1-(4-fluorophenyl)-; (2) 4′-Fluoro-4-[4-(*p*-fluorobenzoyl)piperidino]butyrophenone. *UNII-13P4GX22ES*. *CAS-24678-13-5*. INN. *Antipsychotic.* ◇*AHR-2277 [as hydrochloride]*

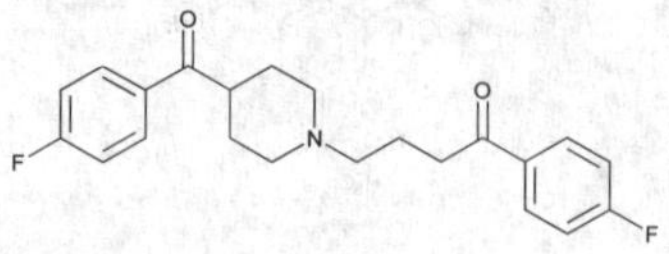

Lensiprazine. $C_{24}H_{27}FN_4O_2$. 422.50. (2*R*)-8-{4-[3-(5-Fluoro-1*H*-indol-3-yl)propyl]piperidin-1-yl}-2-methyl-2*H*-1,4-benzoxazin-3(4*H*)-one. *CAS-327026-93-7*. INN.

Lentinan. D-Glucan mainly composed of a β-(1→3)linkage obtained from the fruit body of *Lentinus edodes*. JAN.

Lepirudin. $C_{287}H_{440}N_{80}O_{111}S_6$. 6979.42. 1-L-Leucine-2-L-threonine-63-desulfohirudin (*Hirudo medicinalis* isoform HV1). *UNII-Y43GF64R34*. *CAS-138068-37-8*. INN; BAN.

```
LTYTDCTESG QNLCLCQGSN VCGQGNKCIL GSNGEKNQCV TGEGTPKPQS
HNDGDFEEIP EEYLQ
```

Leptacline. $C_{12}H_{23}N$. 181.32. 1-(Cyclohexylmethyl)piperidine. *UNII-5DXM29256P*. *CAS-5005-72-1*. INN; DCF.

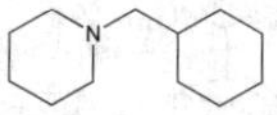

Lercanidipine Hydrochloride [*2002*] (ler″ ka nid′ i peen hye″ droe klor′ ide). $C_{36}H_{41}N_3O_6 \cdot HCl$. 648.19. [Lercanidipine is INN and BAN.] (1) 3,5-Pyridinedicarboxylic acid, 1,4-dihydro-2,6-dimethyl-4-(3-nitrophenyl)-, 2-[(3,3-diphenylpropyl)methylamino]-1,1-dimethylethyl methyl ester, monohydrochloride; (2) 2-[(3,3-Diphenylpropyl)methylamino]-1,1-dimethylethyl methyl (4*RS*)-2,6-dimethyl-4-(3-nitrophenyl)-1,4-dihydropyridine-3,5-dicarboxylate monohydrochloride. *UNII-OA8TFX68PE*. *CAS-132866-11-6; CAS-100427-26-7* [lercanidipine]. *Antihypertensive compound; calcium channel blocker.* Cardiovasc (Recordati, Italy); Carmen (Recordati, Italy); Corifeo (Recordati, Italy); Lercadip (Recordati, Italy); Lercan (Recordati, Italy); Lercapin (Recordati, Italy); Lercaton (Recordati, Italy); Lerkamen (Recordati, Italy); Lerzam (Recordati, Italy); Renovia (Recordati, Italy); Vasodip (Recordati, Italy); Zandip (Recordati, Italy); Zanicor (Recordati, Italy) ◇*Rec-15/2375*

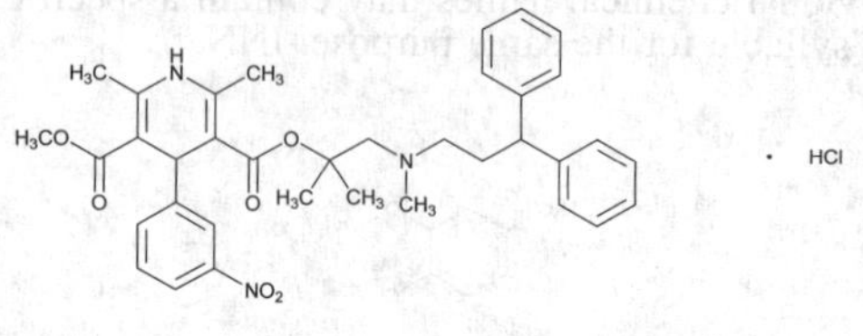

Lerdelimumab. Immunoglobulin G4, anti-(human transforming growth factor β2) (human monoclonal CAT-152 γ4-chain), disulfide with human monoclonal CAT-152 λ-chain, dimer. *CAS-285985-06-0*. INN.

Lergotrile [*1975*] (ler' goe trile). $C_{17}H_{18}ClN_3$. 299.80. (1) Ergoline-8-acetonitrile, 2-chloro-6-methyl-, (8β)-; (2) 2-Chloro-6-methylergoline-8β-acetonitrile. *UNII-O68JXU1W09. CAS-36945-03-6.* INN. *Enzyme inhibitor (prolactin).* ◇79907

Lergotrile Mesylate [*1975*] (ler' goe trile mes' i late). $C_{17}H_{18}ClN_3.CH_4O_3S$. 395.90. (1) Ergoline-8-acetonitrile, 2-chloro-6-methyl-, (8β)-, monomethanesulfonate; (2) 2-Chloro-6-methylergoline-8β-acetonitrile monomethanesulfonate. *UNII-1945N48N9E. CAS-51473-23-5; CAS-36945-03-6* [lergotrile]. *Enzyme inhibitor (prolactin).* ◇83636

Leridistim [*1998*] (ler id' i stim). $C_{1550}H_{2463}N_{425}O_{462}S_{12}$. (1) 14-125-Interleukin 3 [14-alanine, 50-aspartic acid] (human reduced) fusion protein with peptide (synthetic) fusion protein with granulocyte colony-stimulating factor [17-serine] (human reduced); (2) 14-L-Alanine-50-L-aspartic acid-14-125-interleukin 3 (human reduced) fusion protein with peptide (synthetic) linked fusion protein with 17-L-serinegranulocyte colony-stimulating factor (human reduced). Molecular weight is approximately 32,767 daltons. *CAS-193700-51-5.* INN. *Treatment of chemotherapy-induced neutropenia and thrombocytopenia (multifunctional agonist that activates both interleukin-3 and G-CSF receptors).* ◇SC-70935

```
ANCSNMIDEI ITHLKQPPLP LLDFNNLNGE DQDILMDNNL RRPNLEAFNR
AVKSLQNASA IESILKNLLP CLPLATAAPT RHPIHIKDGD WNEFRRKLTF
YLKTLENAQA QQYVEGGGGS PGEPSGPIST INPSPPSKES HKSPNMATPL
GPASSLPQSF LLKSLEQVRK IQGDGAALQE KLCATYKLCH PEELVLLGHS
LGIPWAPLSS CPSQALQLAG CLSQLHSGLF LYQGLLQALE GISPELGPTL
DTLQLDVADF ATTIWQQMEE LGMAPALQPT QGAMPAFASA FQRRAGGVLV
ASHLQSFLEV SYRVLRHLAQ P
```

Lerisetron. $C_{18}H_{20}N_4$. 292.38. 1-Benzyl-2-(1-piperazinyl)-benzimidazole. *UNII-Q36R82SXRG. CAS-143257-98-1.* INN.

Lesopitron. $C_{15}H_{21}ClN_6$. 320.82. 2-[4-[4-(4-Chloropyrazol-1-yl)butyl]-1-piperazinyl]pyrimidine. *UNII-H1CGM4755H. CAS-132449-46-8.* INN.

Lestaurtinib [*2004*] (le stawr' ti nib). $C_{26}H_{21}N_3O_4$. 439.46. (1) 9,12-Epoxy-1H-diindolo[1,2,3-fg:3',2',1'-kl]pyrrolo[3,4-i][1,6]benzodiazocin-1-one, 2,3,9,10,11,12-hexahydro-10-hydroxy-10-(hydroxymethyl)-9-methyl-, [9S-

(9α,10β,12α)]-; (2) (9S,10S,12R)-10-Hydroxy-10-(hydroxymethyl)-9-methyl-2,3,9,10,11,12-hexahydro-9,12-epoxy-1H-diindolo[1,2,3-fg:3',2',1'-kl]pyrrolo[3,4-i][1,6]benzodiazocin-1-one. *UNII-DO989GC5D1. CAS-111358-88-4.* INN. *Treatment of tumors such as prostate and pancreatic carcinomas (selective inhibitor of tyrosine kinase).* ◇CEP-701; A-154475.0; SP924; KT5555

Leteprinim. $C_{15}H_{13}N_5O_4$. 327.29. *p*-[3-(1,6-Dihydro-6-oxo-9H-purin-9-yl)propionamido]benzoic acid. *UNII-NBY3IU407M. CAS-138117-50-7.* INN.

Leteprinim Potassium [*1998*] (let" e prin im poe tas' ee um). $C_{15}H_{12}KN_5O_4$. 365.39. (1) Potassium 4-[[3-(1,6-dihydro-6-oxo-9H-purin-9-yl)-1-oxopropyl]amino]benzoate; (2) Potassium *p*-[3-(1,6-dihydro-6-oxo-9H-purin-9-yl)propionamido]benzoate. *UNII-Q06WU8JY4F. CAS-192564-13-9. Treatment of central neurodegenerative disease, i.e., Alzheimer's disease, spinal cord injury, and stroke.* Neotrofin (NeoTherapeutics) ◇AIT-082

Letimide Hydrochloride [*1970*] (let' i mide hye" droe klor' ide). $C_{14}H_{18}N_2O_3.HCl$. 298.77. [Letimide is INN.] (1) 2H-1,3-Benzoxazine-2,4(3H)-dione, 3-[2-(diethylamino)ethyl]-, monohydrochloride; (2) 3-[2-(Diethylamino)ethyl]-2H-1,3-benzoxazine-2,4(3H)-dione monohydrochloride. *UNII-S48955N1AL* [letimide]. *CAS-21791-39-9; CAS-26513-90-6* [letimide]. *Analgesic.* ◇MA-1443

Letogestin (previously used name) — *See* Tosagestin.

Letosteine. $C_{10}H_{17}NO_4S_2$. 279.38. 2-[2-[(Carboxymethyl)thio]ethyl]-4-thiazolidinecarboxylic acid 2-ethyl ester. *UNII-6MVF9U95DW. CAS-53943-88-7.* INN; MI.

Letrazuril. $C_{17}H_9Cl_2FN_4O_2$. 391.18. (±)-[2,6-Dichloro-4-(4,5-dihydro-3,5-dioxo-*as*-triazin-2(3*H*)-yl)phenyl](*p*-fluorophenyl)acetonitrile. *CAS-103337-74-2*. INN.

Letrozole [*1993*] (let′ roe zole). **USP.** $C_{17}H_{11}N_5$. 285.30. (1) Benzonitrile, 4,4′-(1*H*-1,2,4-triazol-1-ylmethylene)bis-; (2) 4,4′-(1*H*-1,2,4-Triazol-1-ylmethylene)dibenzonitrile. *UNII-7LKK855W8I. CAS-112809-51-5*. INN; BAN. *Antineoplastic*. Femara (Novartis) ◇*CGS 20267*

Leucarsone — *See* Carbarsone.

Leuciglumer. $(C_6H_{13}NO_2.C_6H_{11}NO_4)_n$. L-Leucine polymer with 5-methyl hydrogen L-glutamate. *CAS-41385-14-2*. INN.

Leucine [*1979*] (loo′ seen). **USP.** $C_6H_{13}NO_2$. 131.17. [L-Leucine is JAN.] (1) L-Leucine; (2) L-Leucine. *UNII-GMW67QNF9C. CAS-61-90-5* [L]. INN. *Amino acid*.

L-Leucine (JAN) — *See* Leucine.

Leucinocaine. $C_{17}H_{28}N_2O_2$. 292.42. 2-(Diethylamino)-4-methyl-1-pentanol *p*-aminobenzoate (ester). *UNII-64DXV166PH. CAS-92-23-9*. INN; MI.

Leucobasal (previously used name) — *See* Mequinol.

Leucocianidol. $C_{15}H_{14}O_7$. 306.27. 3,3′,4,4′,5,7-Flavanhexol. *UNII-RAP1D6110C. CAS-480-17-1*. INN; DCF.

Leucodine B (previously used name) — *See* Mequinol.

Leucovorin Calcium (loo″ koe voe′ rin kal′ see um). **USP.** $C_{20}H_{21}CaN_7O_7$. 511.50. [Calcium Folinate is INN and JAN; Folinic Acid is BAN.] (1) L-Glutamic acid, *N*-[4-[[(2-amino-5-formyl-1,4,5,6,7,8-hexahydro-4-oxo-6-pteridinyl)methyl]amino]benzoyl]-, calcium salt (1:1); (2) Calcium *N*-[*p*-[[[(6*RS*)-2-amino-5-formyl-5,6,7,8-tetrahydro-4-hydroxy-6-pteridinyl]methyl]amino]benzoyl]-L-glutamate (1:1). *UNII-RPR1R4COP4. CAS-1492-18-8; CAS-41927-89-3* [replaced]; *CAS-6035-45-6* [pentahydrate]; *CAS-58-05-9* [leucovorin]. *Anti-anemic (folate deficiency); antidote (to folic acid antagonists)*. Wellcovorin (GlaxoSmithKline) ◇*NSC-3590*

Leukocyte Interferon (previously used name) — *See* Interferon Alfa-n3.

Leukocyte Typing Serum. USP XXVII. *Diagnostic aid (blood, in vitro)*.

Leuprolide Acetate [*1981*] (loo′ proe lide as′ e tate). **USP.** $C_{59}H_{84}N_{16}O_{12}.(C_2H_4O_2)_n$ n 1 or 2. 1209.41 (as free base). [Leuprorelin is INN and BAN.] (1) Luteinizing hormone-releasing factor, 6-D-leucine-9-(*N*-ethyl-L-prolinamide)-10-deglycinamide acetate (salt); (2) 5-Oxo-L-prolyl-L-histidyl-L-tryptophyl-L-seryl-L-tyrosyl-D-leucyl-L-leucyl-L-arginyl-*N*-ethyl-L-prolinamide acetate (salt). *UNII-37JNS02E7V. CAS-74381-53-6. Antineoplastic; lHRH agonist*. Lupron (TAP); Viadur (ALZA) ◇*TAP-144; Abbott-43818*

Leuprorelin (INN, BAN) — *See* Leuprolide Acetate.

Leurubicin. $C_{33}H_{40}N_2O_{12}$. 656.68. (8*S*,10*S*)-10-[[3-[(*S*)-2-Amino-4-methylvaleramido]-2,3,6-trideoxy-α-L-*lyxo*-hexopyranosyl]oxy]-8-glycoloyl-7,8,9,10-tetrahydro-6,8,11-trihydroxy-1-methoxy-5,12-naphthacenedione. *UNII-1Z20MGK851. CAS-70774-25-3*. INN.

Levacetylmethadol (INN) — *See* Levomethadyl Acetate.

Levalbuterol Hydrochloride [*1997*] (lev″ al bue′ ter ol hye″ droe klor′ ide). C$_{13}$H$_{21}$NO$_3$.HCl. 275.77. (*R*)-α^1-[(*tert*-Butylamino)methyl]-4-hydroxy-*m*-xylene-α,α′-diol hydrochloride. *UNII-WDQ1526QJM. CAS-50293-90-8. Bronchodilator; asthma prophylactic.* Xopenex (Sepracor)

Levalbuterol Sulfate [*1997*] (lev″ al bue′ ter ol sul′ fate). C$_{13}$H$_{21}$NO$_3$.H$_2$SO$_4$. 337.39. (*R*)-α^1-[(*tert*-Butylamino)methyl]-4-hydroxy-*m*-xylene-α,α′-diol sulfate (2:1). *CAS-148563-16-0. Bronchodilator; asthma prophylactic.*

Levalbuterol Tartrate [*2004*] (lev″ al bue′ ter ol tar′ trate). 2(C$_{13}$H$_{21}$NO$_3$).C$_4$H$_6$O$_6$. 628.71. 1,3-Benzenedimethanol, α^1-[[(1,1-dimethylethyl)amino]methyl]-4-hydroxy-, (α^{1}R)-, (2R,3R)-2,3-dihydroxybutanedioate (2:1) (salt). *UNII-ADS4I3E22M. CAS-661464-94-4. Anti-asthmatic and bronchodilator (β$_2$-adrenergic receptor agonist).* Xopenex (Sepracor)

Levallorphan Tartrate. C$_{19}$H$_{25}$NO.C$_4$H$_6$O$_6$. 433.49. [Levallorphan is INN and BAN.] (1) Morphinan-3-ol, 17-(2-propenyl)-, [*R*-(*R**,*R**)]-2,3-dihydroxybutanedioate (1:1) (salt); (2) 17-Allylmorphinan-3-ol tartrate (1:1) (salt). *UNII-U0VSF7HTN0; UNII-353613BU4U* [levallorphan]. *CAS-71-82-9; CAS-152-02-3* [levallorphan]. USP XXI; JAN; MI. Lorfan (Roche)

Levamfetamine Succinate [*1962*] (lev″ am fet′ a meen sux′ i nate). C$_9$H$_{13}$N.C$_4$H$_6$O$_4$. 253.29. [Levamfetamine is INN and BAN.] (1) Butanedioic acid, compd. with (-)-(*R*)-α-methylbenzeneethanamine (1:1); (2) (-)-(*R*)-α-Methylphenethylamine succinate (1:1). *CAS-5634-40-2; CAS-156-34-3* [levamfetamine]. *Anorexic. [Name previously used: Levamphetamine.]*

Levamisole Hydrochloride [*1970*] (lee vam′ i sole hye″ droe klor′ ide). **USP.** C$_{11}$H$_{12}$N$_2$S.HCl. 240.75. [Levamisole is INN and BAN.] (1) Imidazo[2,1-*b*]thiazole, 2,3,5,6-tetrahydro-6-phenyl-, monohydrochloride, (*S*)-; (2) (-)-2,3,5,6-Tetrahydro-6-phenylimidazo[2,1-*b*]thiazole monohydrochloride. *UNII-DL9055K809; UNII-2880D3468G* [le-

vamisole]. *CAS-16595-80-5; CAS-14769-73-4* [levamisole]. *Biological response modifier.* Ergamisol (Janssen) ◇*R 12,564*

Levamlodipine Malate [*2006*] (lee″ vam loe′ di peen mal′ ate). C$_{20}$H$_{25}$ClN$_2$O$_5$.C$_4$H$_6$O$_5$. 542.96. [Levamlodipine is INN.] (1) 3,5-Pyridinedicarboxylic acid, 2-[(2-aminoethoxy)methyl]-4-(2-chlorophenyl)-1,4-dihydro-6-methyl-, 3-ethyl 5-methyl ester, (4*S*)-, (2*S*)-hydroxybutanedioate (1:1); (2) 3-Ethyl 5-methyl (4*S*)-2-[(2-aminoethoxy)methyl]-4-(2-chlorophenyl)-6-methyl-1,4-dihydropyridine-3,5-dicarboxylate (2*S*)-hydroxybutanedioate (1:1). *UNII-S0QL3IT20J. CAS-736178-83-9; CAS-103129-82-4* [levamlodipine]. *Hypertension, chronic stable angina, vasospastic angina.*

Levamphetamine (previously used name) — *See* Levamfetamine Succinate.

Levarterenol Bitartrate (previously used name) — *See* Norepinephrine Bitartrate.

Levcromakalim [*1993*] (leev kroe ma′ ka lim). C$_{16}$H$_{18}$N$_2$O$_3$. 286.33. (1) 2*H*-1-Benzopyran-6-carbonitrile, 3,4-dihydro-3-hydroxy-2,2-dimethyl-4-(2-oxo-1-pyrrolidinyl)-, (3*S*,*trans*)-; (2) (3*S*,4*R*)-3-Hydroxy-2,2-dimethyl-4-(2-oxo-1-pyrrolidinyl)-6-chromancarbonitrile. *CAS-94535-50-9.* INN; BAN. *Anti-asthmatic; antihypertensive.* ◇*BRL 38227*

Levcycloserine [*1990*] (leev sye″ kloe ser′ een). C$_3$H$_6$N$_2$O$_2$. 102.09. (1) 3-Isoxazolidinone, 4-amino-, (*S*)-; (2) (*S*)-4-Amino-3-isoxazolidinone. *UNII-AK7DRB7FMO. CAS-339-72-0.* INN. *Enzyme inhibitor (Gaucher's disease).*

Levdobutamine Lactobionate [*1991*] (lev″ doe bue′ ta meen lak″ toe bye′ oh nate). C$_{18}$H$_{23}$NO$_3$.C$_{12}$H$_{22}$O$_{12}$. 659.68. [Levdobutamine is INN.] (1) 1,2-Benzenediol, 4-[2-[[3-(4-hydroxyphenyl)-1-methylpropyl]amino]ethyl]-, (*S*)-, 4-*O*-β-D-galactopyranosyl-D- gluconate (salt); (2) 4-[2-[[(*S*)-3-(*p*-Hydroxyphenyl)-1-methylpropyl]amino]ethyl]pyrocate-

---

† Brand name formerly used, and/or firm no longer concerned with this product.

chol lactobionate (1:1) (salt). *CAS-129388-07-4; CAS-61661-06-1* [levdobutamine]. *Cardiotonic.* ◇*LY206243 lactobionate*

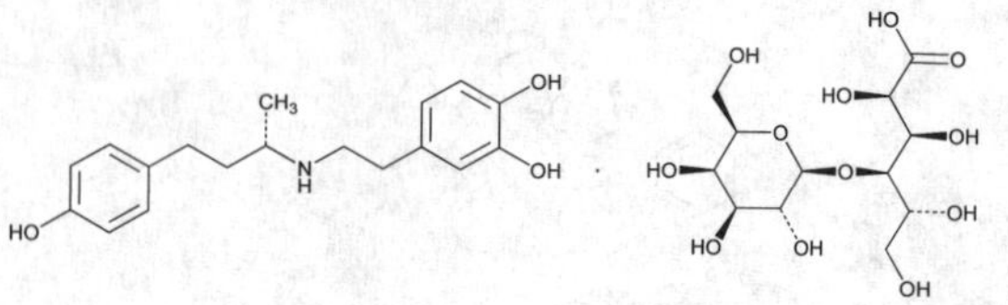

Levemopamil. $C_{23}H_{30}N_2$. 334.50. (-)-(*S*)-2-Isopropyl-5-(methylphenethylamino)-2-phenylvaleronitrile. *UNII-TDE8767O88. CAS-101238-51-1.* INN.

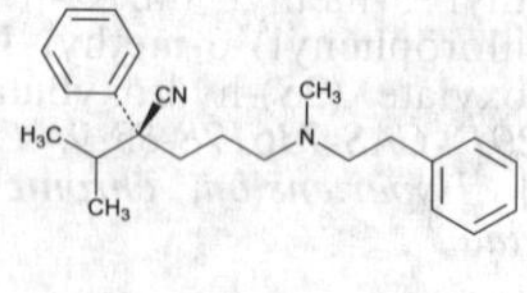

Levetiracetam [*1999*] (lee″ va tye ra′ se tam). $C_8H_{14}N_2O_2$. 170.21. (1) 1-Pyrrolidineacetamide, α-ethyl-2-oxo-, (α*S*)-; (2) (-)-(*S*)-α-Ethyl-2-oxo-1-pyrrolidineacetamide. *UNII-44YRR34555. CAS-102767-28-2.* INN; BAN. *Antiepileptic.* Keppra (UCB) ◇*ucb L059; ucb 22059*

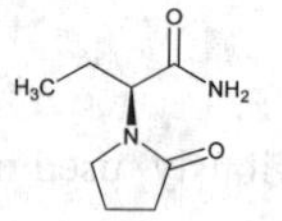

Levisoprenaline. $C_{11}H_{17}NO_3$. 211.26. (-)-(*R*)-α-(Isopropylaminomethyl)protocatechuyl alcohol. *UNII-588N0603CT. CAS-51-31-0.* INN; DCF.

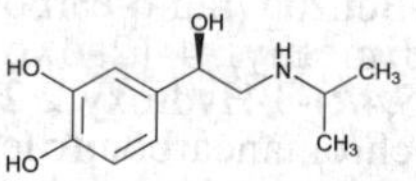

Levlofexidine. $C_{11}H_{12}Cl_2N_2O$. 259.13. (-)-(*R*)-2-[1-(2,6-Dichlorophenoxy)ethyl]-2-imidazoline. *UNII-5SPW497X0Z. CAS-81447-78-1.* INN.

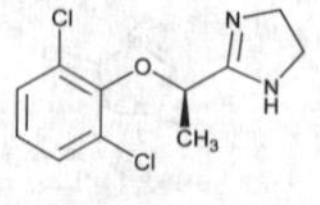

Levmetamfetamine [*1998*] (lev″ met am fet′ a meen). **USP**. $C_{10}H_{15}N$. 149.23. (1) Benzeneethanamine, *N*,α-dimethyl-, (*R*)-; (2) (-)-(*R*)-*N*,α-Dimethylphenethylamine. *UNII-Y24T9BT2Q2. CAS-33817-09-3.* INN. *Nasal decongestant.* [*Name previously used:* L-Desoxyephedrine.]

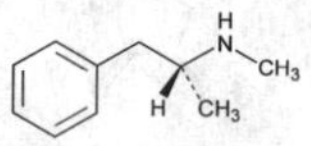

Levobetaxolol Hydrochloride [*1989*] (lee″ voe be tax′ oh lol hye″ droe klor′ ide). $C_{18}H_{29}NO_3 \cdot HCl$. 343.89. [Levobetaxolol is INN.] (1) 2-Propanol, 1-[4-[2-(cyclopropylmethoxy)ethyl]phenoxy]-3-[(1-methylethyl)amino]-, hydrochloride, (*S*)-; (2) (-)-(*S*)-1-[*p*-[2-(Cyclopropylmethoxy)ethyl]phenoxy]-3-(isopropylamino)-2-propanol hydrochloride.

UNII-8MR4W4O06J; UNII-75O9XHA4TU [levobetaxolol]. *CAS-116209-55-3; CAS-93221-48-8* [levobetaxolol]. *Anti-adrenergic (β-receptor).* Betaxon (Alcon) ◇*AL1577A*

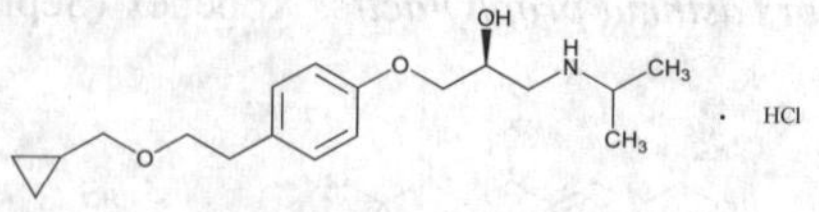

Levobunolol Hydrochloride [*1979*] (lee″ voe bue′ noe lol hye″ droe klor′ ide). **USP**. $C_{17}H_{25}NO_3 \cdot HCl$. 327.85. [Levobunolol is INN and BAN.] (1) 1(2*H*)-Naphthalenone, 5-[3-[(1,1-dimethylethyl)amino]-2-hydroxypropoxy]-3,4-dihydro-, hydrochloride, (-)-(*S*); (2) (-)-(*S*)-5-[3-(*tert*-Butylamino)-2-hydroxypropoxy]-3,4-dihydro-1(2*H*)-naphthalenone hydrochloride. *UNII-O90S49LDHH; UNII-G6317AOI7K* [levobunolol]. *CAS-27912-14-7; CAS-47141-42-4* [levobunolol]. *Anti-adrenergic (β-receptor).* Akbeta (Akorn); Betagan (Allergan) ◇*W 7000A*

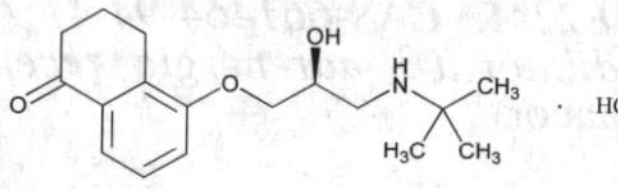

Levobupivacaine. $C_{18}H_{28}N_2O$. 288.43. (*S*)-1-Butyl-2′,6′-pipecoloxylidide. *UNII-J998RDZ5I1. CAS-27262-47-1.* INN; BAN.

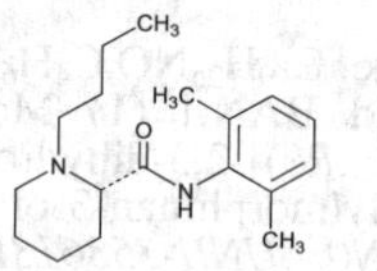

Levobupivacaine Hydrochloride [*1998*] (lee″ voe bue piv′ a kane hye″ droe klor′ ide). $C_{18}H_{28}N_2O \cdot HCl$. 324.89. (1) (*S*)-1-Butyl-*N*-(2,6-dimethylphenyl)-2-piperidinecarboxamide monohydrochloride; (2) (*S*)-1-Butyl-2′,6′-pipecoloxylidide monohydrochloride. *UNII-J998RDZ5I1. CAS-27262-48-2. Local anesthetic; analgesic.* Chirocaine (Purdue)

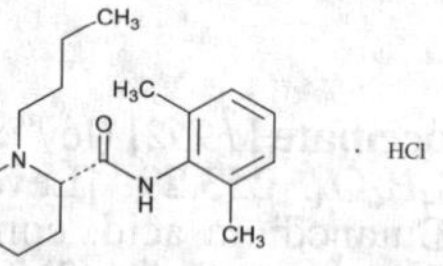

Levocabastine Hydrochloride [*1985*] (lee″ voe ka bas′ teen hye″ droe klor′ ide). **USP**. $C_{26}H_{29}FN_2O_2 \cdot HCl$. 456.98. [Levocabastine is INN and BAN.] (1) 4-Piperidinecarboxylic acid, 1-[4-cyano-4-(4-fluorophenyl)cyclohexyl]-3-methyl-4-phenyl-, monohydrochloride, (-)-[1(*cis*),3α,4β]-; (2) (-)-*trans*-1-[*cis*-4-Cyano-4-(*p*-fluorophenyl)cyclohexyl]-3-methyl-4-phenylisonipecotic acid monohydrochloride. *UNII-124XMA6YEI; UNII-H68BP06S81* [levocabastine]. *CAS-79547-78-7; CAS-79516-68-0* [levocabastine]. *Antihistaminic.* Livostin (Novartis) ◇*R 50,547*

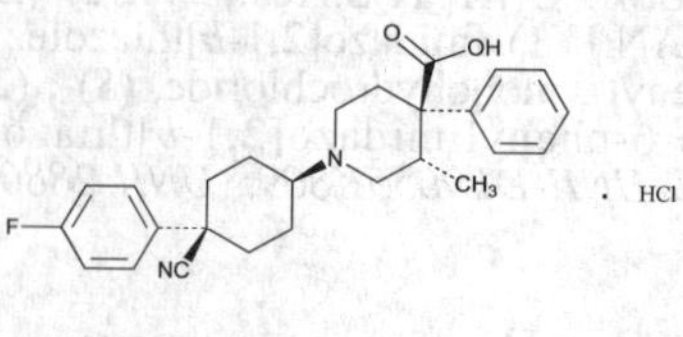

Levocarbinoxamine Tartrate — *See* Rotoxamine Tartrate.

Levocarnitine [*1987*] (lee″ voe kar′ ni teen). **USP.** $C_7H_{15}NO_3$. 161.20. [Levocarnitine Chloride is INN and JAN.] (1) 1-Propanaminium, 3-carboxy-2-hydroxy-*N,N,N*-trimethyl-, hydroxide, inner salt, (*R*)-; (2) (L-3-Carboxy-2-hydroxypropyl)trimethylammonium hydroxide, inner salt. *UNII-0G389FZZ9M. CAS-541-15-1.* INN; BAN. *Replenisher (carnitine).* Carnitor (Sigma-Tau)

Levocarnitine Propionate Hydrochloride [*2002*] (lee″ voe kar′ ni teen proe′ pee oh nate hye″ droe klor′ ide). $C_{10}H_{20}ClNO_4$. 253.72. (1) 1-Propanaminium, 3-carboxy-*N,N,N*-trimethyl-2-(1-oxopropoxy)-, chloride, (*R*)-; (2) (2*R*)-3-Carboxy-*N,N,N*-trimethyl-2-(propanoyloxy)propan-1-aminium chloride. *CAS-119793-66-7. Source of energy substrate in the Krebs cycle (anaplerotic action) and carnitine replenesher for use in the treatment of peripheral arterial disease.* Dromos (Biosint S.p.A.) ◇*ST 261*

Levocetirizine [*2007*] (lee″ voe se tir′ i zeen). $C_{21}H_{25}ClN_2O_3$. 388.89. (1) Acetic acid, [2-[4-[(*R*)-(4-chlorophenyl)phenylmethyl]-1-piperazinyl]ethoxy]-; (2) (2-{4-[(*R*)-(4-Chlorophenyl)phenylmethyl]piperazin-1-yl}ethoxy)acetic acid. *UNII-6U5EA9RT2O. CAS-130018-77-8.* INN; BAN. *Antihistamine.*

Levocetirizine Dihydrochloride [*2007*] (lee″ voe se tir′ a zeen). $C_{21}H_{25}ClN_2O_3$·2HCl. 461.81. (1) Acetic acid, [2-[4-[(*R*)-(4-chlorophenyl)phenylmethyl]-1-piperazinyl]ethoxy]-, dihydrochloride; (2) (2-{4-[(*R*)-(4-Chlorophenyl)phenylmethyl]piperazin-1-yl}ethoxy)acetic acid dihydrochloride. *UNII-SOD6A38AGA. CAS-130018-87-0. Antihistamine.* Xyzal (UCB) ◇*UCB 28556*

Levodopa [*1969*] (lee″ voe doe′ pa). **USP.** $C_9H_{11}NO_4$. 197.19. (1) L-Tyrosine, 3-hydroxy-; (2) (-)-3-(3,4-Dihydroxyphenyl)-L-alanine. *UNII-46627O600J. CAS-59-92-7.* INN; BAN; JAN. *Antiparkinsonian.* Bendopa (Valeant); Dopar (Shire); Larodopa (Roche)

Levodropropizine. $C_{13}H_{20}N_2O_2$. 236.31. (-)-(*S*)-3-(4-Phenyl-1-piperazinyl)-1,2-propanediol. *UNII-3O31P6T4G3. CAS-99291-25-5.* INN; BAN.

Levofacetoperane. $C_{14}H_{19}NO_2$. 233.31. (-)-α-Phenyl-2-piperidinemethanol acetate (ester). *UNII-3SZ9ZII529. CAS-634-08-2.* INN.

Levofenfluramine. $C_{12}H_{16}F_3N$. 231.26. (-)-(*R*)-*N*-Ethyl-α-methyl-*m*-(trifluoromethyl)phenethylamine. *CAS-37577-24-5.* INN.

Levofloxacin [*1996*] (lee″ voe flox′ a sin). $C_{18}H_{20}FN_3O_4$·½H₂O. 370.38. (1) 7*H*-Pyrido[1,2,3-*de*]-1,4-benzoxazine-6-carboxylic acid, 9-fluoro-2,3-dihydro-3-methyl-10-(4-methyl-1-piperazinyl)-7-oxo-hydrate (2:1), (*S*)-; (2) (-)-(*S*)-9-Fluoro-2,3-dihydro-3-methyl-10-(4-methyl-1-piperazinyl)-7-oxo-7*H*-pyrido[1,2,3-*de*]-1,4-benzoxazine-6-carboxylic acid, hemihydrate. *UNII-6GNT3Y5LMF. CAS-138199-71-0.* INN; BAN; JAN. *Antibacterial.* Levaquin (Ortho-McNeil); Quixin (Vistakon) ◇*DR-3355; RWJ-25213*

Levofuraltadone [*1965*] (lee″ voe fue ral′ ta done). $C_{13}H_{16}N_4O_6$. 324.29. (1) 2-Oxazolidinone, 5-(4-morpholinylmethyl)-3-[[(5-nitro-2-furanyl)methylene]amino]-, (-)-; (2) (-)-5-(Morpholinomethyl)-3-[(5-nitrofurfurylidene)amino]-2-oxazolidinone. *CAS-3795-88-8.* INN. *Antibacterial; antiprotozoal.* ◇*NF-602; NF-902 [as hydrochloride]; NSC-527986*

Levoglutamide (previously used name) — *See* Glutamine.

Levolansoprazole. $C_{16}H_{14}F_3N_3O_2S$. 369.36. (-)-2-[[(*S*)-{[3-Methyl-4-(2,2,2-trifluoroethoxy)pyridin-2-yl]methyl}sulfinyl]-1*H*-benzamidazole. *CAS-138530-95-7.* INN.

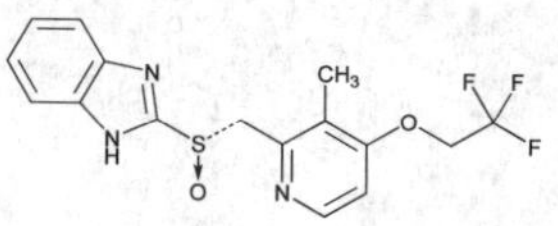

Levoleucovorin Calcium [*1991*] (lee″ voe loo″ koe voe′ rin kal′ see um). $C_{20}H_{21}CaN_7O_7$. 511.50. [Calcium Levofolinate is INN and BAN.] (1) L-Glutamic acid, *N*-[4-[[(2-amino-5-formyl-1,4,5,6,7,8-hexahydro-4-oxo-6-pteridinyl)methyl]amino]benzoyl]-, calcium salt (1:1), (*S*)-; (2) Calcium *N*-[*p*-[[[(6*S*)-amino-5-formyl-1,4,5,6,7,8-hexahydro-4-oxo-6-pteridinyl]methyl]amino]benzoyl]-L-glutamate (1:1). *UNII-778XL6VBS8. CAS-80433-71-2. Antidote (to folic acid antagonists).* ◇*CL 307,782*

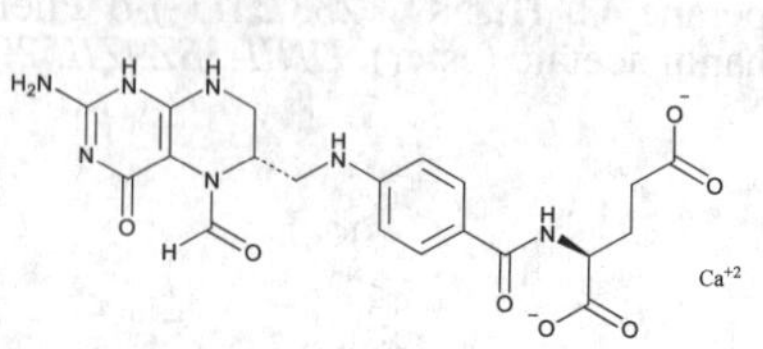

Levomefolate Calcium [*2008*] (lee″ voe me foe′ late). $C_{20}H_{23}CaN_7O_6$. 497.52. (1) L-Glutamic acid, *N*-[4-[[[(6*S*)-2-amino-1,4,5,6,7,8-hexahydro-5-methyl-4-oxo-6-pteridinyl]methyl]amino]benzoyl]-, calcium salt (1:1); (2) Calcium *N*-[4-({[(6*S*)-2-amino-5-methyl-4-oxo-1,4,5,6,7,8-hexahydropteridin-6-yl]methyl}amino)benzoyl]-L-glutamate. *CAS-151533-22-1. Treatment and prevention of folate deficiency.* Metafolin (Merck Eprova AG); Nutrifolin (Merck Eprova AG); Bodyfolin (Merck Eprova AG) *[Name previously used: Levomefolinate Calcium.]* ◇*LMCA*

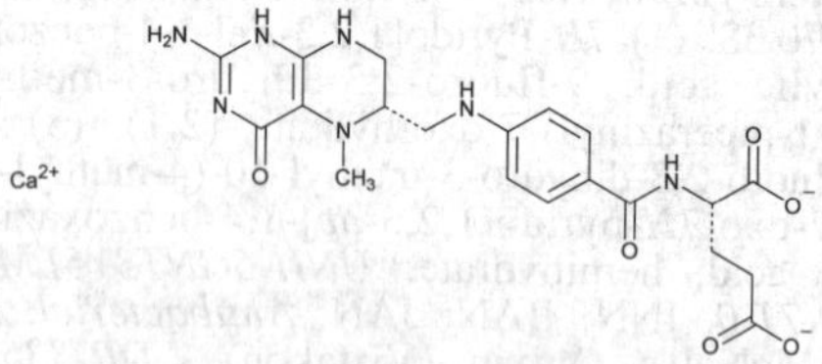

Levomefolic Acid [*2008*] (lee″ voe me foe′ lik). $C_{20}H_{25}N_7O_6$. 459.46. (1) L-Glutamic acid, *N*-[4-[[[(6*S*)-2-amino-3,4,5,6,7,8-hexahydro-5-methyl-4-oxo-6-pteridinyl]methyl]amino]benzoyl]-; (2) *N*-[4-({[(6*S*)-2-Amino-5-methyl-4-oxo-1,4,5,6,7,8-hexahydropteridin-6-yl]methyl}amino)benzoyl]-L-glutamic acid. *UNII-8S95DH25XC. CAS-31690-09-2.* INN. *Treatment and prevention of folate deficiency.* Metafolin (Merck Eprova AG); Nutrifolin (Merck Eprova AG); Bodyfolin (Merck Eprova AG) *[Name previously used: Levomefolinic Acid.]* ◇*LMSR*

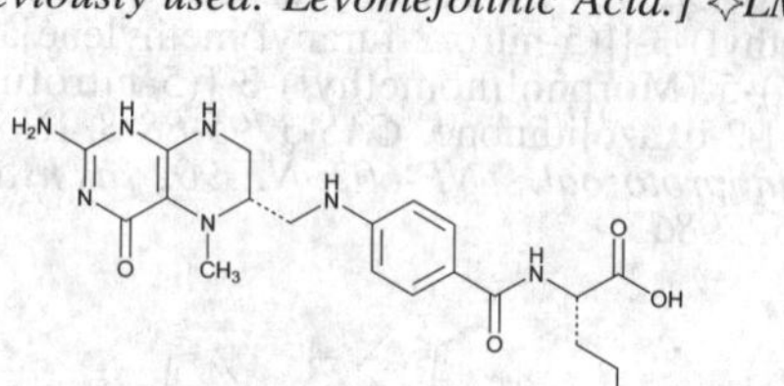

Levomenol. $C_{15}H_{26}O$. 222.37. (-)-6-Methyl-2-(4-methyl-3-cyclohexen-1-yl)-5-hepten-2-ol. *UNII-24WE03BX2T. CAS-23089-26-1.* INN.

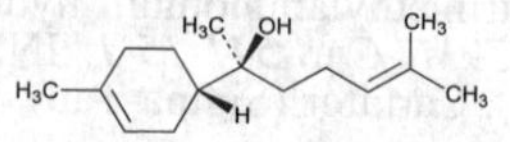

Levomenthol. $C_{10}H_{20}O$. 156.27. [*l*-Menthol is JAN.] (-)-(1*R*,3*R*,4*S*)-Menthol. *UNII-BZIR15MTK7. CAS-2216-51-5.* INN; BAN.

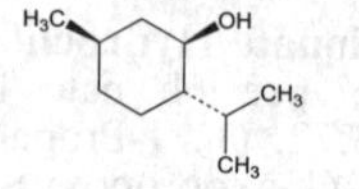

Levomepate — *See* Atromepine.

Levomepromazine [*2003*] (lee″ voe me proe′ ma zeen). $C_{19}H_{24}N_2OS$. 328.47. (1) 10*H*-Phenothiazine-10-propanamine, 2-methoxy-*N,N,β*-trimethyl-, (*βR*)-; (2) (-)-(2*R*)-3-(2-Methoxy-10*H*-phenothiazin-10-yl)-*N,N*,2-trimethylpropan-1-amine. *UNII-9G0LAW7ATQ. CAS-60-99-1.* INN; BAN; DCF. *Analgesic (central nervous system depressant).* Levoprome (Immunex) ◇*RP-7044; XP03*

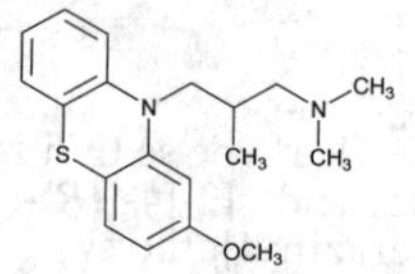

Levomepromazine Hydrochloride [*2003*] (lee″ voe me proe′ ma zeen hye″ droe klor′ ide). $C_{19}H_{24}N_2OS$.HCl. 364.93. (1) 10*H*-Phenothiazine-10-propanamine, 2-methoxy-*N,N,β*-trimethyl-, monohydrochloride, (*βR*)-; (2) (2*R*)-3-(2-Methoxy-10*H*-phenothiazin-10-yl)-*N,N*,2-trimethylpropan-1-amine hydrochloride. *UNII-42BB1Y2586. CAS-1236-99-3.* JAN. *Analgesic (central nervous system depressant).* Nozinan (Aventis)

Levomepromazine Maleate [*2003*] (lee″ voe me proe′ ma zeen mal′ ee ate). $C_{19}H_{24}N_2OS.C_4H_4O_4$. 444.54. (1) 10*H*-Phenothiazine-10-propanamine, 2-methoxy-*N,N,β*-trimethyl-, (*βR*)-, (2*Z*)-2-butenedioate (1:1); (2) (2*R*)-3-(2-Methoxy-10*H*-phenothiazin-10-yl)-*N,N*,2-trimethylpropan-1-amine hydrogen (2*Z*)-but-2-enedioate. *UNII-5KN5Y9V01K. CAS-7104-38-3.* JAN. *Analgesic (central nervous system depressant).* Nozinan (Aventis); Tisercin (Egis)

Levomethadone. $C_{21}H_{27}NO$. 309.45. (-)-(*R*)-6-(Dimethylamino)-4,4-diphenyl-3-heptanone. *CAS-125-58-6.* INN.

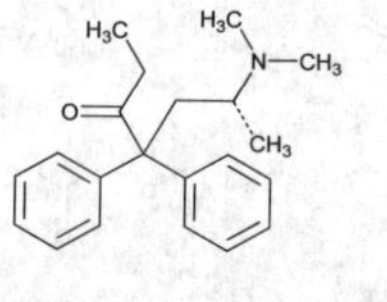

Levomethadyl Acetate [*1972*] (lee″ voe meth′ a dil as′ e tate). $C_{23}H_{31}NO_2$. 353.50. [Levacetylmethadol is INN.] (1) Benzeneethanol, *β*-[2-(dimethylamino)propyl]-*α*-ethyl-*β*-phenyl-, acetate (ester), (-)-; (2) (-)-6-(Dimethylamino)-

4,4-diphenyl-3-heptanol acetate (ester). *CAS-34433-66-4; CAS-1477-40-3* [levomethadyl]. *Analgesic (narcotic).* ◇*LAAM*

Levomethadyl Acetate Hydrochloride [*1994*] (lee″ voe meth′ a dil as′ e tate hye″ droe klor′ ide). $C_{23}H_{31}NO_2.HCl$. 389.96. (1) Benzeneethanol, β-[2-(dimethylamino)propyl]-α-ethyl-β-phenyl-, acetate (ester), hydrochloride, [S-(R^*,R^*)]-; (2) (-)-(3S,6S)-6-(Dimethylamino)-4,4-diphenyl-3-heptanol acetate (ester), hydrochloride. *UNII-B54CW5KG52. CAS-43033-72-3. Analgesic (narcotic).* Orlaam (Roxane) ◇*LAAM; MK790*

Levomethorphan. $C_{18}H_{25}NO$. 271.40. (-)-3-Methoxy-*N*-methylmorphinan. *CAS-125-70-2.* INN; BAN; DCF.

Levo-Methylaminoethanolcatechol — *See* Epinephrine.

Levometiomeprazine. $C_{19}H_{24}N_2S_2$. 344.54. (-)-10-[3-(Di-methylamino)-2-methylpropyl]-2-(methylthio)phenothia-zine. *CAS-1759-09-7.* INN; DCF.

Levomilnacipran. $C_{15}H_{22}N_2O$. 246.35. (1S,2R)-2-(Amino-methyl)-*N*,*N*-diethyl-1-phenylcyclopropanecarboxamide. *CAS-96847-55-1.* INN.

Levomoprolol. $C_{13}H_{21}NO_3$. 239.31. (-)-(S)-1-(Isopropylami-no)-3-(*o*-methoxyphenoxy)-2-propanol. *CAS-77164-20-6.* INN.

Levomoramide. $C_{25}H_{32}N_2O_2$. 392.53. (-)-4-[2-Methyl-4-oxo-3,3-diphenyl-4-(1-pyrrolidinyl)butyl]morpholine. *CAS-5666-11-5.* INN; BAN; DCF.

Levonadifloxacin. $C_{19}H_{21}FN_2O_4$. 360.38. (5S)-9-Fluoro-8-(4-hydroxypiperidin-1-yl)-5-methyl-1-oxo-6,7-dihydro-1H,5H-benzo[*ij*]quinolizine-2-carboxylic acid. *CAS-154357-42-3.* INN.

Levonantradol Hydrochloride [*1979*] (lee″ voe nan′ tra dol hye″ droe klor′ ide). $C_{27}H_{35}NO_4.HCl$. 474.03. [Levonan-tradol is INN and BAN.] (1) 1,9-Phenanthridinediol, 5,6,6a,7,8,9,10,10a-octahydro-6-methyl-3-(1-methyl-4-phenylbutoxy)-, 1-acetate, hydrochloride, [6S-[3(S^*),6α,6aα,9α,10aβ]]-; (2) (-)-(6S,6aR,9R,10aR)-5,6,6a,7,8,9,10,10a-Octahydro-6-methyl-3-[(R)-1-methyl-4-phenylbutoxy]-1,9-phenanthridinediol 1-acetate, hydro-chloride. *UNII-V92884KHRI. CAS-70222-86-5; CAS-71048-87-8* [levonantradol]. *Analgesic.* ◇*CP-50,556-1*

Levonebivolol. $C_{22}H_{25}F_2NO_4$. 405.44. (1S)-2-({(2S)-2-[(2R)-6-Fluoro-3,4-dihydro-2H-chromen-2-yl]-2-hydroxyethyl}amino)-1-[(2S)-6-fluoro-3,4-dihydro-2H-chromen-2-yl]ethanol. *CAS-118457-16-2.* INN.

Levonordefrin (lee″ voe nor def′ rin). **USP.** $C_9H_{13}NO_3$. 183.20. [Corbadrine is INN.] (1) 1,2-Benzenediol, 4-(2-amino-1-hydroxypropyl)-, [R-(R^*,S^*)]-; (2) (-)-α-(1-Ami-noethyl)-3,4-dihydroxybenzyl alcohol. *UNII-V008L6478D. CAS-829-74-3; CAS-18829-78-2* [replaced]. *Adrenergic (vasoconstrictor).* Neo-Cobefrin (Cook-Waite)

Levonorgestrel [*1980*] (lee″ voe nor jes′ trel). **USP.** $C_{21}H_{28}O_2$. 312.45. (1) 18,19-Dinorpregn-4-en-20-yn-3-one, 13-ethyl-17-hydroxy-, (17α)-(-)-; (2) (-)-13-Ethyl-17-hydroxy-18,19-dinor-17α-pregn-4-en-20-yn-3-one. *UNII-5W7SIA7YZW. CAS-797-63-7.* INN; BAN. *Proges-tin.* Mirena (Bayer); Norplant (Population Council); Plan B (Duramed) [*Former designation as the ''d-enantiomer of norgestrel'' or as ''d-norgestrel'' was incorrect and should have been* D-*norgestrel for configuration and levorotatory,* [α]$_D$= -33°, *for optical activity.*] ◇*WY-5104*

Levophenacylmorphan. $C_{24}H_{27}NO_2$. 361.48. (-)-3-Hydroxy-*N*-phenacylmorphinan. *CAS-10061-32-2.* INN; BAN; DCF.

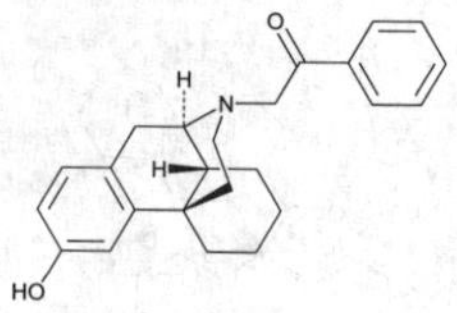

Levopropicillin (INN) Potassium — *See* Levopropylcillin Potassium.

Levopropoxyphene Napsylate [*1962*] (lee″ voe proe pox′ i feen nap′ si late). $C_{22}H_{29}NO_2.C_{10}H_8O_3S.H_2O$. 565.72. [Levopropoxyphene is INN and BAN.] (1) Benzeneethanol, α-[2-(dimethylamino)-1-methylethyl]-α-phenyl-, propanoate (ester), [*R*-(*R**,*S**)]-, compd. with 2-naphthalenesulfonic acid (1:1), monohydrate; (2) 2-Naphthalenesulfonic acid compound with (-)-α-[2-(dimethylamino)-1-methylethyl]-α-phenylphenethyl propionate (1:1) monohydrate. *CAS-55557-30-7; CAS-5714-90-9* [anhydrous]; *CAS-5667-69-6* [replaced]; *CAS-2338-37-6* [levopropoxyphene]. USP XXII. *Antitussive.* Novrad (Lilly†) ◇29866

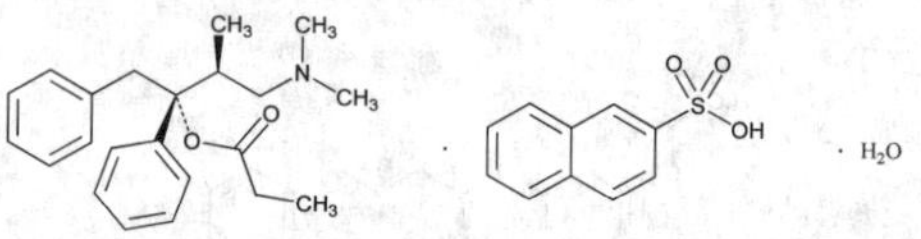

Levopropylcillin Potassium [*1962*] (lee″ voe proe″ pil sil′ in poe tas′ ee um). $C_{18}H_{21}KN_2O_5S$. 416.53. [Levopropicillin is INN.] (1) 4-Thia-1-azabicyclo[3.2.0]heptane-2-carboxylic acid, 3,3-dimethyl-7-oxo-6-[(1-oxo-2-phenoxybutyl)amino]-, monopotassium salt, [2*S*-[2α,5α,6β(*R**)]]-; (2) Potassium (2*S*,5*R*,6*R*)-3,3-dimethyl-7-oxo-6-[(2*S*)-phenoxybutyramido]-4-thia-1-azabicyclo[3.2.0]heptane-2-carboxylate. *CAS-4803-44-5; CAS-7245-75-2* [replaced]; *CAS-3736-12-7* [levopropylcillin]. *Antibacterial.* ◇BRL-284; P-248; 38389

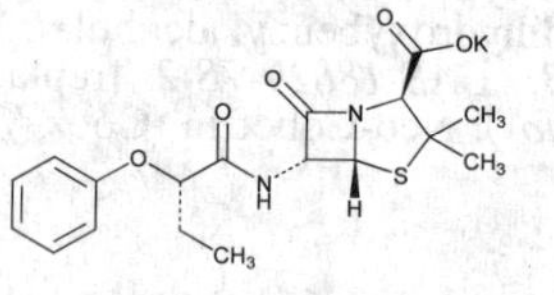

Levopropylhexedrine. $C_{10}H_{21}N$. 155.28. (-)-*N*,α-Dimethylcyclohexaneethylamine. *CAS-6192-97-8.* INN.

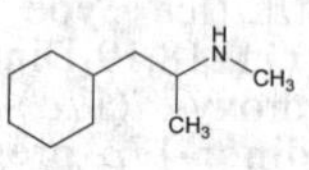

Levoprotiline. $C_{20}H_{23}NO$. 293.40. (-)-(*R*)-α-[(Methylamino)methyl]-9,10-ethanoanthracene-9(10*H*)-ethanol. *CAS-76496-68-9.* INN.

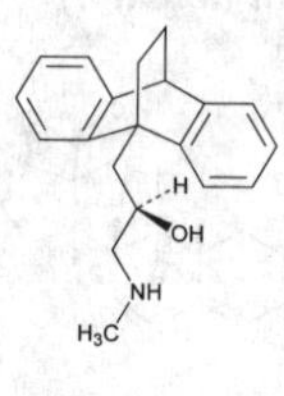

Levorin. Antibiotic of the polyene series, obtained from cultures of *Actinomyces levoris,* or the same substance produced by any other means. *CAS-11014-70-3.* INN.

Levormeloxifene. $C_{30}H_{35}NO_3$. 457.60. (-)-1-[2-[4-[(3*R*,4*R*)-7-Methoxy-2,2-dimethyl-3-phenyl-4-chromanyl)phenoxy]ethyl]pyrrolidine. *CAS-78994-23-7.* INN.

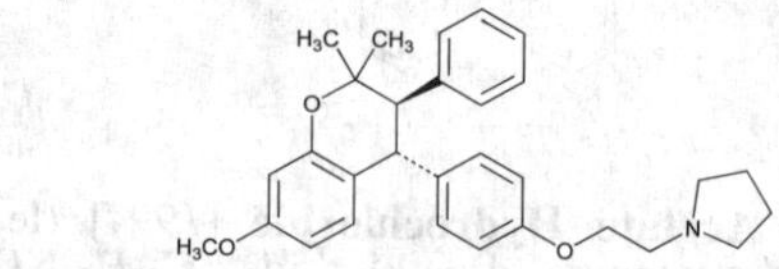

Levorphanol Tartrate (lee vor′ fa nol tar′ trate). **USP.** $C_{17}H_{23}NO.C_4H_6O_6.2H_2O$. 443.49. [Levorphanol is INN and BAN.] (1) Morphinan-3-ol, 17-methyl-, [*R*-(*R**,*R**)]-2,3-dihydroxybutanedioate (1:1) (salt), dihydrate; (2) 17-Methylmorphinan-3-ol, tartrate (1:1) (salt) dihydrate. *UNII-04WQU6T9QI; UNII-27618J1N2X* [levorphanol]. *CAS-5985-38-6; CAS-125-72-4* [anhydrous]; *CAS-6700-40-9* [replaced]; *CAS-77-07-6* [levorphanol]. *Analgesic (narcotic).* Levo-Dromoran (Valeant)

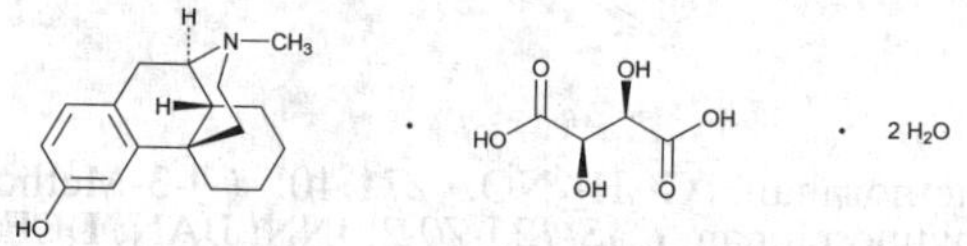

Levosalbutamol. $C_{13}H_{21}NO_3$. 239.31. (*R*)-α^1-[(*tert*-Butylamino)methyl]-4-hydroxy-*m*-xylene-α,α'-diol. *CAS-34391-04-3.* INN.

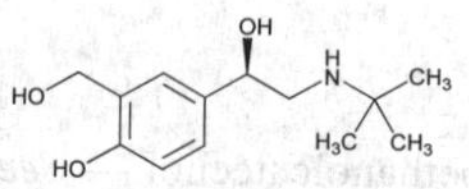

Levosemotiadil. $C_{29}H_{32}N_2O_6S$. 536.64. (-)-(*S*)-2-[5-Methoxy-2-[3-[methyl[2-[3,4-(methylenedioxy)phenoxy]ethyl]amino]propoxy]phenyl]-4-methyl-2*H*-1,4-benzothiazin-3(4*H*)-one. *CAS-116476-16-5.* INN.

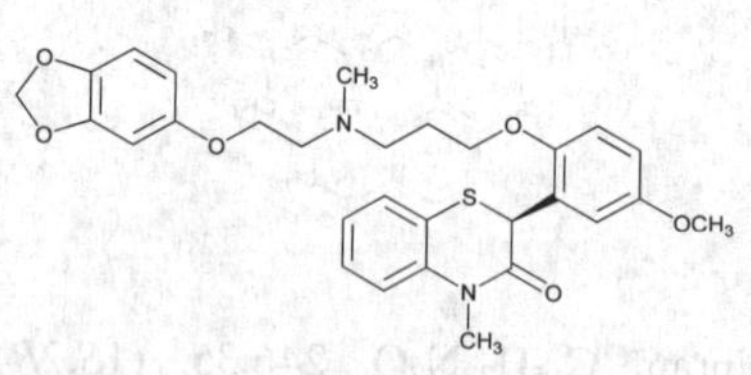

Levosimendan [*1998*] (lee″ voe si men′ dan). $C_{14}H_{12}N_6O$. 280.28. (1) (*R*)-[[4-(1,4,5,6-Tetrahydro-4-methyl-6-oxo-3-pyridazinyl]phenyl]hydrazono] propanedinitrile; (2) Mesoxalonitrile [*p*-[(*R*)-1,4,5,6-tetrahydro-4-methyl-6-oxo-pyridazinyl]phenyl]hydrazone. *CAS-141505-33-1.* INN. *Treatment of congestive heart failure (cardiotonic; positive inotrope; vasodilator).* Simdax (Orion Pharmaceutica, Finland) ◇(-)-OR-1259

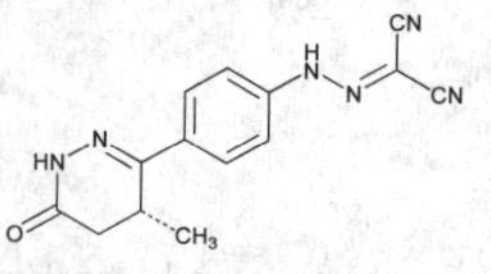

Levosulpiride. $C_{15}H_{23}N_3O_4S$. 341.43. (-)-*N*-[[(*S*)-1-Ethyl-2-pyrrolidinyl]methyl]-5-sulfamoyl-*o*-anisamide. *CAS-23672-07-3*. INN.

Levothyroxine Sodium (lee″ voe thye rox′ een soe′ dee um). **USP**. $C_{15}H_{10}I_4NNaO_4 \cdot xH_2O$. 798.85 (anhydrous). [Levothyroxine is BAN.] [*See also* Liotrix.] (1) L-Tyrosine, *O*-(4-hydroxy-3,5-diiodophenyl)-3,5-diiodo-, monosodium salt, hydrate; (2) Monosodium L-thyroxine hydrate. *UNII-9J765S329G. CAS-25416-65-3; CAS-55-03-8* [anhydrous]; *CAS-51-48-9* [L-thyroxine]. INN; JAN. *Thyroid hormone.* Levo-t (Alara); Levothroid (Lloyd); Levoxyl (King); Synthroid (Abbott); Unithroid (Stevens J)

Levotofisopam [*2004*] (lee″ voe toe fis′ oh pam). $C_{22}H_{26}N_2O_4$. 382.45. (1) 5*H*-2,3-Benzodiazepine, 1-(3,4-dimethoxyphenyl)-5-ethyl-7,8-dimethoxy-4-methyl-, (5*S*)-; (2) (-)-(5*S*)-1-(3,4-Dimethoxyphenyl)-5-ethyl-7,8-dimethoxy-4-methyl-5*H*-2,3-benzodiazepine. *UNII-11ZYL7QK34. CAS-82059-51-6*. INN. *Anxiolytic, autonomic instability.* ◇*(S)-tofisopam*

Levovir — *See* Clevudine.

Levoxadrol Hydrochloride [*1962*] (lee vox′ a drol hye″ droe klor′ ide). $C_{20}H_{23}NO_2 \cdot HCl$. 345.86. [Levoxadrol is INN.] (1) Piperidine, 2-(2,2-diphenyl-1,3-dioxolan-4-yl)-, hydrochloride; (2) (-)-2-(2,2-Diphenyl-1,3-dioxolan-4-yl)piperidine hydrochloride. *UNII-3ARD9VMM81; UNII-811X558HU0* [levoxadrol]. *CAS-23257-58-1; CAS-4792-18-1* [levoxadrol]. *Anesthetic (local); relaxant (smooth muscle).* ◇*CL-912C; NSC-526063*

Levulose (BAN) — *See* Fructose.

Lexacalcitol. $C_{29}H_{48}O_4$. 460.69. (5*Z*,7*E*,20*R*)-20-[(4-Ethyl-4-hydroxyhexyl)oxy]-9,10-secopregna-5,7,10(19)-triene-1α,3β-diol. *UNII-9G3DCA3958. CAS-131875-08-6*. INN.

Lexatumumab [*2006*] (lex″ a toom′ ue mab). $C_{6346}H_{9832}N_{1720}O_{2002}S_{42}$. (1) Immunoglobulin G1, anti-(human cytokine receptor TRAIL-R2) (human monoclonal HGS-ETR2 heavy chain), disulfide with human monoclonal HGS-ETR2 λ-chain, dimer; (2) Immunoglobulin G1, anti-(human tumor necrosis factor receptor superfamily member 10B (Death receptor 5 or TRAIL-R2)) (human monoclonal HGS-ETR2 heavy chain), disulfide with human monoclonal HGS-ETR2 λ-chain, dime. Molecular weight is approximately 143,600 daltons. *CAS-845816-02-6*. INN. *Treatment of cancer.* ◇*HGS-ETR2; HGS1018*

Lexgenleucel-T [*2007*] (lex″ jen loo′ sel - tee). Medicament comprises an autologous CD4+ T cell product transduced with a lentiviral vector carrying an HIV antisense sequence targeted to the HIV envelope gene. *Treatment of HIV/AIDS.* VRX496 (Virxsys) ◇*VRX496*

Lexipafant [*1994*] (lex i′ pa fant). $C_{23}H_{30}N_4O_4S$. 458.57. (1) L-Leucine, *N*-methyl-*N*-[[4-[(2-methyl-1*H*-imidazo[4,5-*c*]pyridin-1-yl)methyl]phenyl]sulfonyl]-, ethyl ester; (2) *N*-Methyl-*N*-[[α-(2-methyl-1*H*-imidazo[4,5-*c*]pyridin-1-yl)-*p*-tolyl]sulfonyl]-L-leucine, ethyl ester. *CAS-139133-26-9*. INN; BAN. *Platelet activating factor antagonist.* ◇*BB-882; DO6*

Lexithromycin [*1991*] (lex ith″ roe mye′ sin). $C_{38}H_{70}N_2O_{13}$. 762.97. (1) Erythromycin, 9-(*O*-methyloxime); (2) Erythromycin 9-(*O*-methyloxime). *CAS-53066-26-5*. INN. *Antibacterial.* ◇*Wy-48314*

---

† Brand name formerly used, and/or firm no longer concerned with this product.

Lexofenac. $C_{14}H_{14}O_3$. 230.26. [p-(3-Oxo-1-cyclohexen-1-yl)phenyl]acetic acid. *UNII-3578QN1B5H. CAS-41387-02-4.* INN.

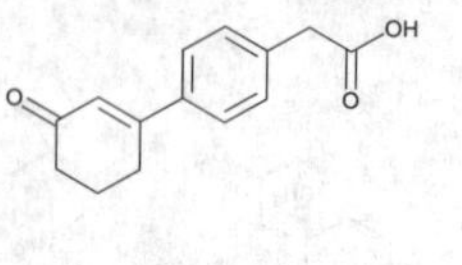

LHN-1 — *See* Tinzaparin Sodium.

Liarozole Fumarate [*1993*] (lye ar′ oh zole fue′ ma rate). $2C_{17}H_{13}ClN_4.3C_4H_4O_4$. 965.75. [Liarozole is INN and BAN.] (1) 1*H*-Benzimidazole, 5-[(3-chlorophenyl)-1*H*-imidazol-1-ylmethyl]-, (±)-, (*E*)-2-butenedioate (2:3); (2) (±)-5-(*m*-Chloro-α-imidazol-1-ylbenzyl)benzimidazole fumarate (2:3). *CAS-145858-52-2; CAS-115575-11-6* [liarozole]; *CAS-145858-51-1* [deleted]. *Antipsoriatic.* Liazal (Janssen) ◇*R 85246*

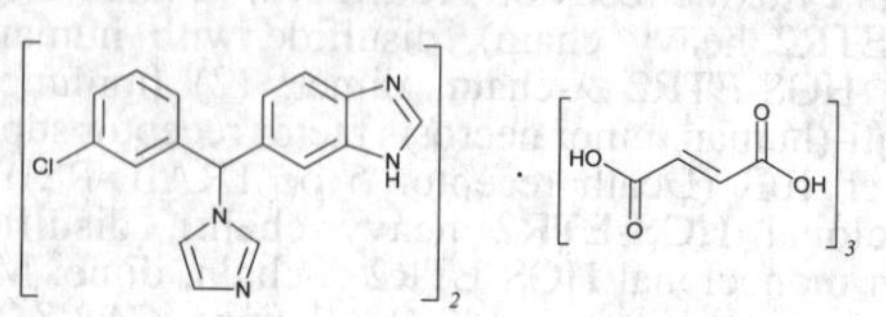

Liarozole Hydrochloride [*1993*] (lye ar′ oh zole hye″ droe klor′ ide). $C_{17}H_{13}ClN_4.HCl$. 345.23. (1) 1*H*-Benzimidazole, 5-[(3-chlorophenyl)-1*H*-imidazol-1-ylmethyl]-, monohydrochloride, (±)-; (2) (±)-5-(*m*-Chloro-α-imidazol-1-yl-benzyl)benzimidazole monohydrochloride. *CAS-145858-50-0. Antineoplastic.* ◇*R 75251*

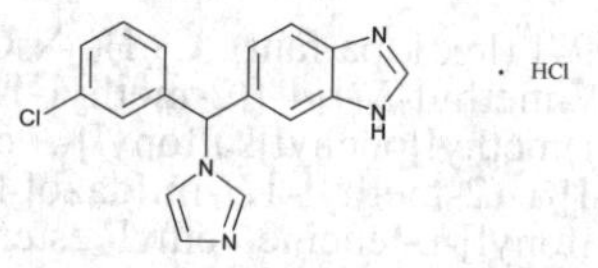

Liatermin [*1998*] (lye at′ er min). $C_{1290}H_{2210}N_{420}O_{394}S_{18}$. 30,000 daltons. (1) *N*-Methionylneurotrophic factor (human glial-derived), dimer; (2) *N*-Methionyl human glial cell line-derived neurotrophic factor. *CAS-188630-14-0.* INN. *Treatment of Parkinson's disease (promotion of dopaminergic neuronal process growth).*

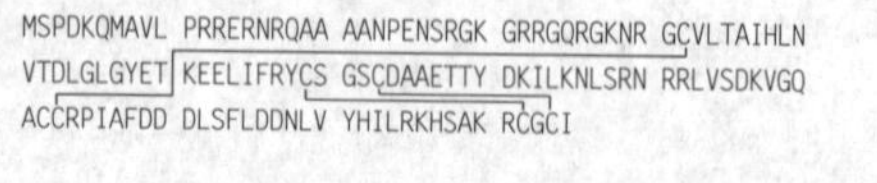

```
MSPDKQMAVL PRRERNRQAA AANPENSRGK GRRGQRGKNR GCVLTAIHLN
VTDLGLGYET KEELIFRYCS GSCDAAETTY DKILKNLSRN RRLVSDKVGQ
ACCRPIAFDD DLSFLDDNLV YHILRKHSAK RCGCI
```

Libecillide. $C_{23}H_{32}N_4O_7S$. 508.59. 2-[[(5-Carboxy-5-formamidopentyl)carbamoyl](2-phenylacetamido)methyl]-5,5-dimethyl-4-thiazolidinecarboxylic acid. *UNII-19ONH7KRJ3. CAS-27826-45-5.* INN.

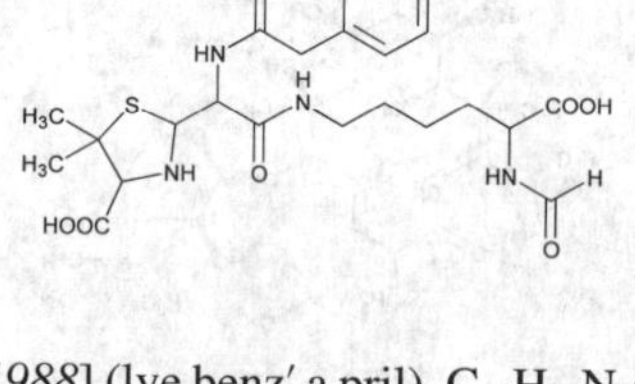

Libenzapril [*1988*] (lye benz′ a pril). $C_{18}H_{25}N_3O_5$. 363.41. (1) 1*H*-1-Benzazepine-1-acetic acid, 3-[(5-amino-1-carboxypentyl)amino]-2,3,4,5-tetrahydro-2-oxo-, [*S*-(*R**,*R**)]; (2) *N*-[(3*S*)-1-(Carboxymethyl)-2,3,4,5-tetrahydro-2-oxo-1*H*-

1-benzazepin-3-yl]-L-lysine. *UNII-QD8496WWYK. CAS-109214-55-3.* INN. *Enzyme inhibitor (angiotensin-converting).* ◇*CGS 16617*

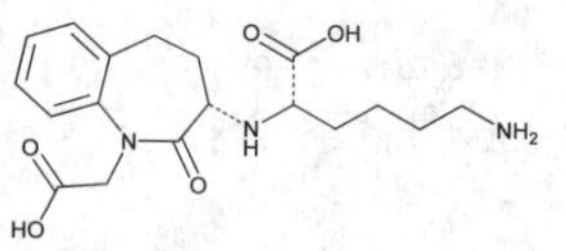

Libivirumab. $C_{6598}H_{10232}N_{1788}O_{2060}S_{46}$. Immunoglobulin G, anti- (hepatitis B surface antigen)(human monoclonal 17.1.41 heavy chain), disulfide with human monoclonal 17.1.41 κ-chain, dimer. *CAS-569658-79-3.* INN.

Licarbazepine. $C_{15}H_{14}N_2O_2$. 254.28. 10,11-Dihydro-10-hydroxy-5*H*-dibenz[*b,f*]azepine-5-carboxamide. *CAS-29331-92-8.* INN.

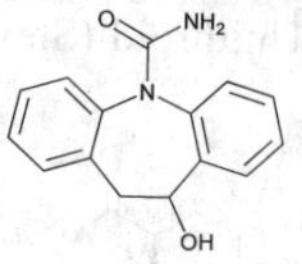

Licofelone. $C_{23}H_{22}ClNO_2$. 379.88. [6-(4-Chlorophenyl)-2,2-dimethyl-7-phenyl-2,3-dihydro-1*H*-pyrrolizin-5-yl]acetic acid. *UNII-P5T6BYS22Y. CAS-156897-06-2.* INN.

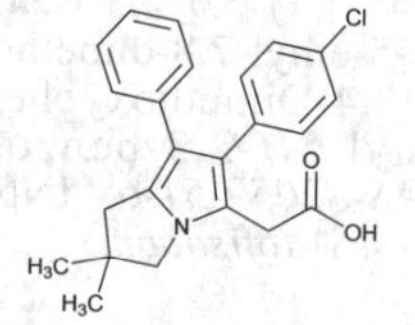

Licorice (lik′ o rish). **NF**. The roots, rhizomes, and stolons of *Glycyrrhiza glabra* Linné or *Glycyrrhiza uralensis* Fisher (Fam. Leguminosae).

Licostinel [*1997*] (lye kos′ ti nel). $C_8H_3Cl_2N_3O_4$. 276.03. 6,7-Dichloro-1,4-dihydro-5-nitro-2,3-quinoxalinedione. *UNII-3Z3037LJTC. CAS-153504-81-5.* INN. *NMDA antagonist.* ◇*ACEA 1021*

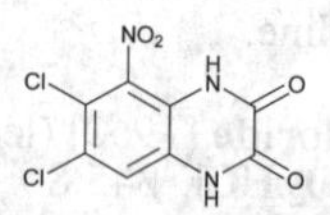

Licryfilcon A [*1981*] (lye″ kri fil′ kon). $(C_6H_{10}O_3)_x$ $(C_{10}H_{14}O_4)_y$. (1) 2-Propenoic acid, 2-methyl-, 2-hydroxyethyl ester, polymer with 1,2-ethanediyl bis(2-methyl-2-propenoate); (2) 2-Hydroxyethyl methacrylate polymer with ethylene dimethacrylate. *CAS-25053-81-0. Contact lens material (hydrophilic).* [Note—This contact lens material contains 55% water as 0.9% saline.]

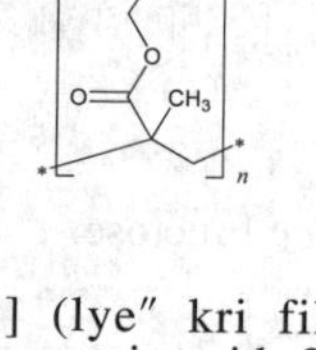

Licryfilcon B [*1981*] (lye″ kri fil′ kon). $(C_6H_{10}O_3)_x$ $(C_{10}H_{14}O_4)_y$. (1) 2-Propenoic acid, 2-methyl-, 2-hydroxyethyl ester, polymer with 1,2-ethanediyl bis(2-methyl-2-propenoate); (2) 2-Hydroxyethyl methacrylate polymer with ethylene dimethacrylate. *CAS-25053-81-0. Contact lens material (hydrophilic). [Note—This contact lens material contains 70% water as 0.9% saline. Graphic formula same as for Licryfilcon A.]*

Lidadronic Acid. $C_5H_{16}N_2O_6P_2$. 262.14. [1-Amino-3-(dimethylamino)propylidene]diphosphonic acid. *CAS-63132-38-7. INN.*

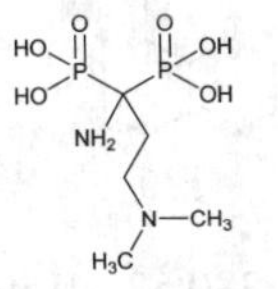

Lidakol — *See* Docosanol.

Lidamidine Hydrochloride [*1978*] (lye dam′ i deen hye″ droe klor′ ide). $C_{11}H_{16}N_4O.HCl$. 256.73. [Lidamidine is INN.] (1) Urea, *N*-(2,6-dimethylphenyl)-*N*′-[imino(methylamino)methyl]-, monohydrochloride; (2) 1-(Methylamidino)-3-(2,6-xylyl)urea monohydrochloride. *CAS-65009-35-0; CAS-66871-56-5 [lidamidine]. Antiperistaltic.* ◇*WHR-1142A*

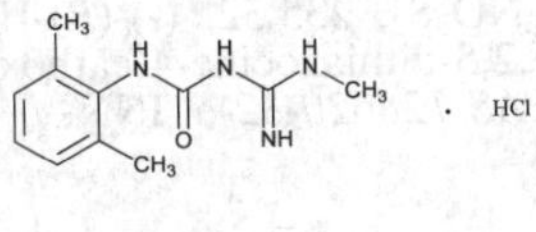

Lidanserin. $C_{26}H_{31}FN_2O_4$. 454.53. (±)-4-[3-[3-[4-(*p*-Fluorobenzoyl)piperidino]propoxy]-4-methoxyphenyl]-2-pyrrolidinone. *UNII-80O1E9JZLN. CAS-73725-85-6. INN.*

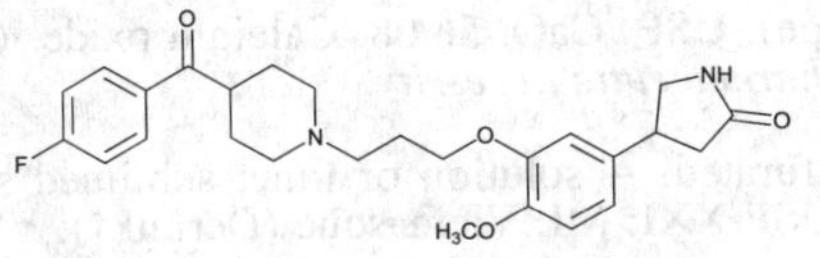

Lidimycin (INN) — *See* Lydimycin.

Lidocaine (lye′ doe kane). **USP.** $C_{14}H_{22}N_2O$. 234.34. (1) Acetamide, 2-(diethylamino)-*N*-(2,6-dimethylphenyl)-; (2) 2-(Diethylamino)-2′,6′-acetoxylidide. *UNII-98PI200987. CAS-137-58-6. INN; BAN; JAN. Anesthetic (topical).* Alphacaine (Carlisle); Lidoderm (Endo); Xylocaine (AstraZeneca)

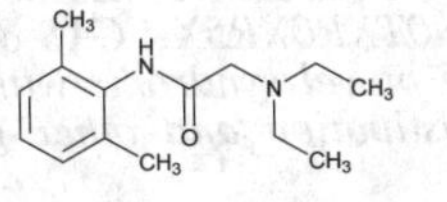

Lidocaine Benzyl Benzoate — *See* Denatonium Benzoate.

Lidocaine Hydrochloride (lye′ doe kane hye″ droe klor′ ide). **USP.** $C_{14}H_{22}N_2O.HCl.H_2O$. 288.81. (1) Acetamide, 2-(diethylamino)-*N*-(2,6-dimethylphenyl)-, monohydrochloride, monohydrate; (2) 2-(Diethylamino)-2′,6′-acetoxylidide monohydrochloride monohydrate. *UNII-V13007Z41A. CAS-6108-05-0; CAS-73-78-9 [anhydrous]; CAS-137-58-6 [lidocaine]. BAN; JAN. Anesthetic (local).* Lidopen (Meridian); Xylocaine (Abraxis); Zingo (Anesira)

---

† Brand name formerly used, and/or firm no longer concerned with this product.

Lidofenin [*1978*] (lye″ doe fen′ in). $C_{14}H_{18}N_2O_5$. 294.30. (1) Glycine, *N*-(carboxymethyl)-*N*-[2-[(2,6-dimethylphenyl)amino]-2-oxoethyl]-; (2) [[(2,6-Xylylcarbamoyl)methyl]imino]diacetic acid. *UNII-EK22QV7701. CAS-59160-29-1. INN. Diagnostic aid (hepatic function determination).* Hepato-Scan (Medi-Physics†) ◇*HIDA*

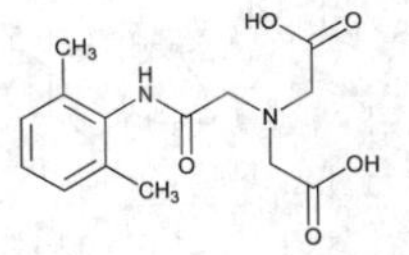

Lidofilcon A [*1977*] (lye″ doe fil′ kon). $(C_6H_9NO)_w(C_5H_8O_2)_x(C_7H_{10}O_2)_y(C_{10}H_{14}O_4)_z$. (1) 2-Pyrrolidinone, 1-ethenyl-, polymer with methyl 2-methyl-2-propenoate, 2-propenyl 2-methyl-2-propenoate and 1,2-ethanediyl bis(2-methyl-2-propenoate); (2) 1-Vinyl-2-pyrrolidinone polymer with methyl methacrylate, allyl methacrylate and ethylene dimethacrylate. *CAS-56551-60-1. Contact lens material (hydrophilic).* B & L 70 (Bausch & Lomb); FW Toric (Bausch & Lomb†); Medalist Toric (Bausch & Lomb†) *[Note—This contact lens material contains 70% of water. A contact lens material prepared from the same monomers but containing 79% of water is known as Lidofilcon B.]*

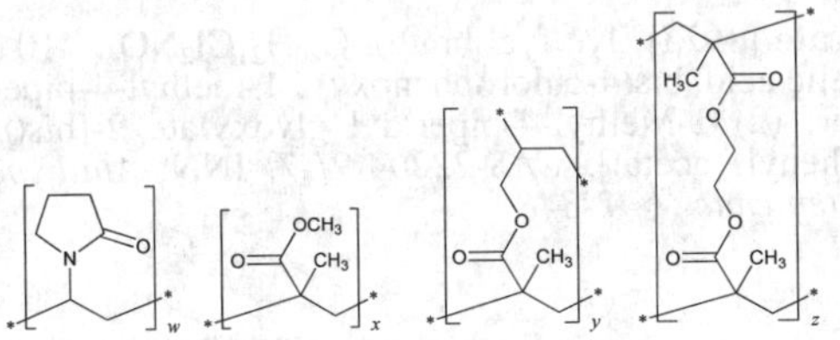

Lidofilcon B [*1977*] (lye″ doe fil′ kon). *CAS-56551-60-1. Contact lens material (hydrophilic). [Note—This contact lens material is prepared from the same monomers as Lidofilcon A; it contains 79% of water. Graphic formula same as for Lidofilcon A.]*

Lidoflazine [*1966*] (lye doe′ fla zeen). $C_{30}H_{35}F_2N_3O$. 491.62. (1) 1-Piperazineacetamide, 4-[4,4-bis(4-fluorophenyl)butyl]-*N*-(2,6-dimethylphenyl)-; (2) 4-[4,4-Bis(*p*-fluorophenyl)butyl]-1-piperazineaceto-2′,6′-xylidide. *UNII-J4ZHN3HBTE. CAS-3416-26-0. INN; BAN. Vasodilator (coronary).* Angex (Janssen†); Clinium (Ortho-McNeil†) ◇*McN-JR-7904; R 7904*

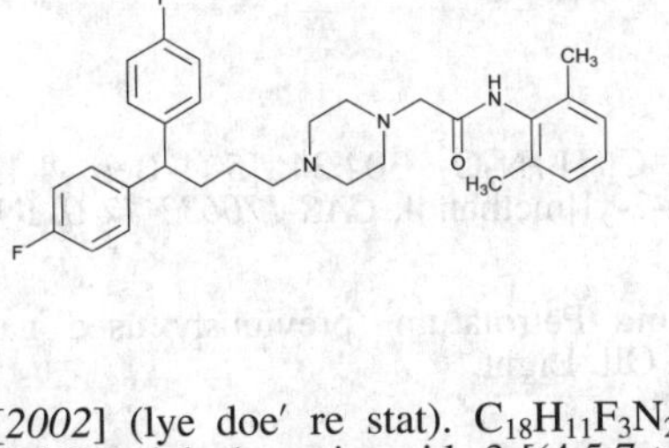

Lidorestat [*2002*] (lye doe′ re stat). $C_{18}H_{11}F_3N_2O_2S.H_2O$. 394.37. (1) 1*H*-Indole-1-acetic acid, 3-[(4,5,7-trifluoro-2-benzothiazolyl)methyl]-, monohydrate; (2) 3-[(4,5,7-Triflurobenzothiazol-2-yl)methyl]-1*H*-indol-1-yl]acetic acid, monohydrate. *UNII-9Z74BD3QPP. CAS-245116-90-9 [anhydrous]. INN. Treatment of diabetic complications,*

including neuropathy, retinopathy, cataracts, nephropathy (selective aldose reductase inhibitor). ◇*IDD-676; IDD-000676-01*

Lifarizine [*1991*] (lye far′ i zeen). $C_{29}H_{32}N_4$. 436.59. (1) Piperazine, 1-(diphenylmethyl)-4-[[5-methyl-2-(4-methylphenyl)-1*H*-imidazol-4-yl]methyl]-; (2) 1-(Diphenylmethyl)-4-[(5-methyl-2-*p*-tolylimidazol-4-yl)methyl]piperazine. *UNII-C37051245K. CAS-119514-66-8.* INN; BAN. *Platelet aggregation inhibitor.* ◇*RS-87476-000*

Lifibrate [*1973*] (lye fye′ brate). $C_{20}H_{21}Cl_2NO_4$. 410.29. (1) Acetic acid, bis(4-chlorophenoxy)-, 1-methyl-4-piperidinyl ester; (2) 1-Methyl-4-piperidyl glyoxylate 2-[bis(*p*-chlorophenyl) acetal]. *CAS-22204-91-7.* INN. *Antihyperlipoproteinemic.* ◇*42-348*

Lifibrol [*1994*] (lye fib′ rol). $C_{21}H_{26}O_4$. 342.43. (1) Benzoic acid, 4-[4-[4-(1,1-dimethylethyl)phenyl]-2-hydroxybutoxy]-, (±)-; (2) (±)-*p*-[4-(*p-tert*-Butylphenyl)-2-hydroxybutoxy]benzoic acid. *CAS-96609-16-4.* INN. *Hypocholesterolemic.* ◇*K 12148*

Lificiguat. $C_{19}H_{16}N_2O_2$. 304.34. [5-(1-Benzyl-1*H*-indazol-3-yl)furan-2-yl]methanol. *CAS-170632-47-0.* INN.

Light Liquid Petrolatum (previously used name) — *See* Mineral Oil, Light.

Lignocaine (former BAN) — *See* Lidocaine.

Lignocaine Hydrochloride (former BAN) — *See* Lidocaine Hydrochloride.

Lilopristone. $C_{29}H_{37}NO_3$. 447.61. 11β-[*p*-(Dimethylamino)phenyl]-17β-hydroxy-17-[(*Z*)-3-hydroxypropenyl]estra-4,9-dien-3-one. *UNII-3GL26H7N6T. CAS-97747-88-1.* INN.

Limaprost. $C_{22}H_{36}O_5$. 380.52. [Limaprost α-Cyclodextrin Clathrate is JAN.] (*E*)-7-[(1*R*,2*R*,3*R*)-3-Hydroxy-2-[(*E*)-(3*S*,5*S*)-3-hydroxy-5-methyl-1-nonenyl]-5-oxocyclopentyl]-2-heptenoic acid. *CAS-88852-12-4.* INN; MI.

Limazocic. $C_8H_{13}NO_3S_2$. 235.32. (-)-(*R*)-Hexahydro-7,7-dimethyl-6-oxo-1,2,5-dithiazocine-4-carboxylic acid. *UNII-FY2I4AJB16. CAS-128620-82-6.* INN.

Lime (lyme). USP. CaO. 56.08. Calcium oxide. *CAS-1305-78-8. Pharmaceutic necessity.*

Lime, Sulfurated. A solution of lime, sublimed sulfur, and water. USP XXI; MI. Vlemasque (Dermik†); Vlem-Dome (Bayer†)

d-**Limonene.** $C_{10}H_{16}$. 136.23. *d*(*R*)-4-Isopropenyl-1-methylcyclohexene. *UNII-GFD7C86Q1W. CAS-138-86-3* [Limonene]. JAN.

Linaclotide [*2007*] (lin ak′ loe tide). $C_{59}H_{79}N_{15}O_{21}S_6$. 1526.74. (1) L-Tyrosine, L-cysteinyl-L-cysteinyl-L-α-glutamyl-L-tyrosyl-L-cysteinyl-L-cysteinyl-L-asparaginyl-L-prolyl-L-alanyl-L-cysteinyl-L-threonylglycyl-L-cysteinyl-, cyclic (1→6),(2→10),(5→13)-tris(disulfide); (2) [9-L-Tyrosine]heat-stable enterotoxin (*Escherichia coli*)-(6-19)-peptide. *UNII-N0TXR0XR5X. CAS-851199-59-2. Treatment of irritable bowel syndrome with constipation (IBS-C), chronic constipation and other gastrointestinal disorders.*

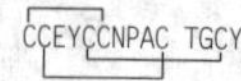

Linaclotide Acetate [*2006*] (lin ak′ loe tide as′ e tate). $C_{59}H_{79}N_{15}O_{21}S_6 \cdot C_2H_4O_2$. 1586.79. [Linaclotide is INN.] (1) L-Tyrosine, L-cysteinyl-L-cysteinyl-L-α-glutamyl-L-tyrosyl-L-cysteinyl-L-cysteinyl-L-asparaginyl-L-prolyl-L-alanyl-L-cysteinyl-L-threonylglycyl-L-cysteinyl-, cyclic (1→6),(2→10),(5→13)-tris(disulfide), monoacetate (salt); (2) L-Cysteinyl-L-cysteinyl-L-α-glutamyl-L-tyrosyl-L-cysteinyl-L-cysteinyl-L-asparaginyl-L-prolyl-L-alanyl-L-cysteinyl-L-threonylglycyl-L-cysteinyl-L-tyrosine cyclic (1→6),(2→10),(5→13)-tris(disulfide) monoacetate (salt). *UNII-NSF067KU1M. CAS-851199-60-5; CAS-851199-59-*

2 [linaclotide]. *Treatment of gastrointestinal disorders including irritable bowel syndrome with constipation (IBS-C) and chronic constipation (CC).* ◇*MM-416775*

Linagliptin. $C_{25}H_{28}N_8O_2$. 472.54. 8-[(3*R*)-3-Aminopiperidin-1-yl]-7-(but-2-yn-1-yl)-3-methyl-1-[(4-methylquinazolin-2-yl)methyl]-3,7-dihydro-1*H*-purine-2,6-dione. *CAS-668270-12-0.* INN.

Linaprazan. $C_{21}H_{26}N_4O_2$. 366.46. 8-{[(2,6-Dimethylphenyl)-methyl]amino}-*N*-(2-hydroxyethyl)-2,3-dimethylimidazo[1,2-*a*]pyridine-6-carboxamide. *CAS-248919-64-4.* INN.

Linarotene [*1991*] (lin ar′ oh teen). $C_{23}H_{30}N_2O_2S$. 398.56. (1) Ethanone, 1-(5,6,7,8-tetrahydro-5,5,8,8-tetramethyl-2-naphthalenyl)-, [4-(methylsulfonyl)phenyl]hydrazone, (*E*)-; (2) 5′,6′,7′,8′-Tetrahydro-5′,5′,8′,8′-tetramethyl-2′-acetonaphthone (*E*)-[*p*-(methylsulfonyl)phenyl]hydrazone. *UNII-S3WF2KTK27. CAS-127304-28-3.* INN. *Antikeratinizing agent.* ◇*RWJ 24834; BASF 52404*

Lincomycin [*1962*] (lin″ koe mye′ sin). $C_{18}H_{34}N_2O_6S$. 406.54. Antibiotic produced by *Streptomyces lincolnensis* variant. (1) D-*erythro*-α-D-*galacto*-Octopyranoside, methyl 6,8-dideoxy-6-[[(1-methyl-4-propyl-2-pyrrolidinyl)carbonyl]amino]-1-thio-, (2*S-trans*)-; (2) Methyl 6,8-dideoxy-6-*trans*-(1-methyl-4-propyl-L-2-pyrrolidinecarboxamido)-1-thio-D-*erythro*-α-D-*galacto*-octopyranoside. *UNII-BOD072YW0F. CAS-154-21-2.* INN; BAN. *Antibacterial.* ◇*U-10,149*

Lincomycin Hydrochloride (lin″ koe mye′ sin hye″ droe klor′ ide). USP. $C_{18}H_{34}N_2O_6S.HCl.H_2O$. 461.01. (1) D-*erythro*-α-D-*galacto*-Octopyranoside, methyl 6,8-dideoxy-6-[[(1-methyl-4-propyl-2-pyrrolidinyl)carbonyl]amino]-1-thio-, monohydrochloride, monohydrate, (2*S-trans*)-; (2) Methyl 6,8-dideoxy-6-(1-methyl-*trans*-4-propyl-L-2-pyrrolidinecarboxamido)-1-thio-D-*erythro*-α-D-*galacto*-octopyranoside monohydrochloride monohydrate. *UNII-M6T05Z2B68; UNII-BOD072YW0F* [lincomycin]. *CAS-*

7179-49-9; *CAS-859-18-7* [anhydrous]; *CAS-154-21-2* [lincomycin]. JAN. *Antibacterial.* Lincocin (Pfizer) ◇*NSC-70731*

Lindane [*1980*] (lin′ dane). USP. $C_6H_6Cl_6$. 290.83. (1) Cyclohexane, 1,2,3,4,5,6-hexachloro-, (1α,2α,3β,4α,5α,6β)-; (2) γ-1,2,3,4,5,6-Hexachlorocyclohexane. *UNII-59NEE7PCAB. CAS-58-89-9.* INN; BAN. *Pediculicide; scabicide.* Kwell (Reed & Carnrick); Scabene (Stiefel) *[Name previously used: Benzene Hexachloride, Gamma.]*

Linetastine. $C_{35}H_{40}N_2O_6$. 584.70. (2*E*,4*E*)-*N*-[2-[4-(Diphenylmethoxy)piperidino]ethyl]-5-(4-hydroxy-3-methoxyphenyl)-2,4-pentadienamide ethyl carbonate (ester). *UNII-7U248Z56LA. CAS-159776-68-8.* INN.

Linezolid [*1997*] (lin ayz′ oh lid). $C_{16}H_{20}FN_3O_4$. 337.35. (1) Acetamide, *N*-[[3-[3-fluoro-4-(4-morpholinyl)phenyl]-2-oxo-5-oxazolidinyl]methyl]-, (*S*)-; (2) *N*-[[(*S*)-3-(3-Fluoro-4-morpholinophenyl)-2-oxo-5-oxazolidinyl]methyl]acetamide. *UNII-ISQ9I6J12J. CAS-165800-03-3.* INN; BAN. *Antibacterial.* Zyvox (Pfizer) ◇*U-100,766*

Linogliride [*1986*] (lin oh′ glir ide). $C_{16}H_{22}N_4O$. 286.37. (1) 4-Morpholinecarboximidamide, *N*-(1-methyl-2-pyrrolidinylidene)-*N*′-phenyl-; (2) *N*-(1-Methyl-2-pyrrolidinylidene)-*N*′-phenyl-4-morpholinecarboxamidine. *UNII-7E521JYJ4X. CAS-75358-37-1.* INN. *Antidiabetic.* ◇*McN 3935*

Linogliride Fumarate [*1982*] (lin oh′ glir ide fue′ ma rate). $C_{16}H_{22}N_4O.C_4H_4O_4$. 402.44. (1) 4-Morpholinecarboximidamide, *N*-(1-methyl-2-pyrrolidinylidene)-*N*′-phenyl-, (*E*)-2-butenedioate (1:1); (2) *N*-(1-Methyl-2-pyrrolidinyli-

<hr>

† Brand name formerly used, and/or firm no longer concerned with this product.

dene)-*N'*-phenyl-4-morpholinecarboxamidine fumarate (1:1). *UNII-4326S15UIP. CAS-78782-47-5. Antidiabetic.* ◇*McN-3935*

Linoleoyl Polyoxylglycerides. NF. Mixtures of monoesters, diesters, and triesters of glycerol and monoesters and diesters of polyethylene glycols with a mean relative molecular weight between 300 and 400.

Linolexamide — *See* Clinolamide.

Linopirdine [*1992*] (lin oh′ per deen). $C_{26}H_{21}N_3O$. 391.46. (1) 2*H*-Indol-2-one, 1,3-dihydro-1-phenyl-3,3-bis(4-pyridinylmethyl)-; (2) 1-Phenyl-3,3-bis(4-pyridinylmethyl)-2-indolinone. *CAS-105431-72-9.* INN. *Alzheimer's disease treatment (cognition enhancer).* ◇*DuP 996*

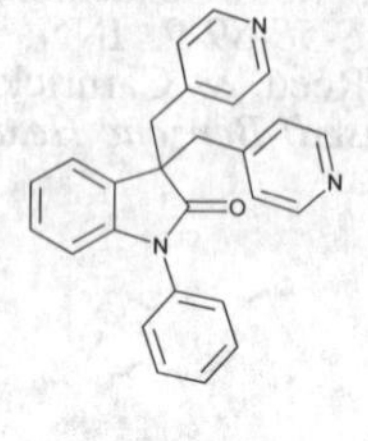

Linopristin. $C_{50}H_{63}N_9O_{10}$. 950.09. *N*-{(6*R*,9*S*,10*R*,13*S*,15a*S*,22*S*,24a*S*)-22-{[4-(dimethylamino)phenyl]methyl}-6-ethyl-10,23-dimethyl-18-[(morpholin-4-yl)methyl]-5,8,12,15,21,24-hexaoxo-13-phenyl-1,2,3,5,6,7,8,9,10,11,12,13,14,15,15a,16,19,21,22,23,24,24a-docosahydropyrido[2,1-*f*]pyrrolo[2,1-*l*][1,4,7,10,13,16]oxapentaazacyclononadecin-9-yl}-3-hydroxypyridine-2-carboxamide. *CAS-325965-23-9.* INN.

Linotroban. $C_{14}H_{15}NO_5S_2$. 341.40. [[5-(2-Benzenesulfonamidoethyl)-2-thienyl]oxy]acetic acid. *UNII-6O2O36OL57. CAS-120824-08-0.* INN.

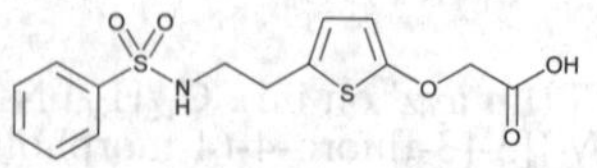

Linsidomine. $C_6H_{10}N_4O_2$. 170.17. 3-Morpholinosydnone imine. *UNII-5O5U71P6VQ. CAS-33876-97-0.* INN.

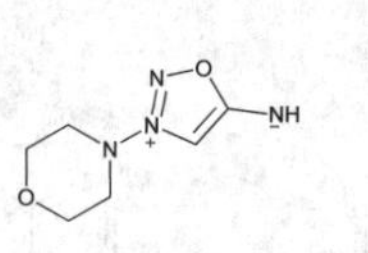

Lintitript. $C_{20}H_{14}ClN_3O_3S$. 411.86. 2-[[4-(*o*-Chlorophenyl)-2-thiazolyl]carbamoyl]indole-1-acetic acid. *UNII-3YFV00531K. CAS-136381-85-6.* INN.

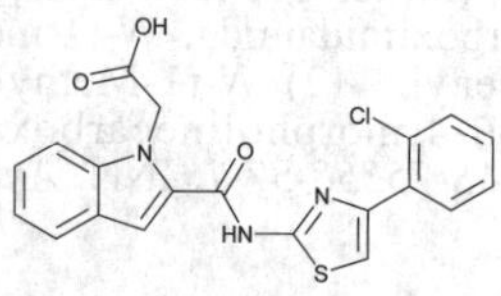

Lintopride. $C_{14}H_{19}ClN_4O_2$. 310.78. 4-Amino-5-chloro-*N*-[(1-ethyl-2-imidazolin-2-yl)methyl]-*o*-anisamide. *UNII-C2R0GEU722. CAS-107429-63-0.* INN.

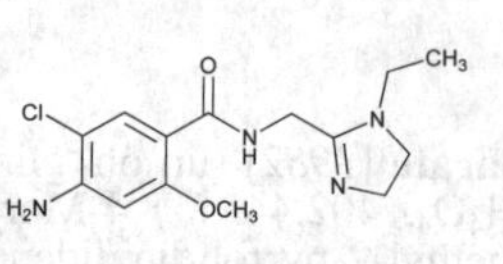

Lintuzumab. Immunoglobulin G1 anti-(human CD33 (antigen)) (human-mouse monoclonal HuM195 γ1-chain), disulfide with human monoclonal HuM195 κ-chain, dimer. *CAS-166089-32-3.* INN.

Liothyronine I 125 [*1964*] (lye″ oh thye′ roe neen). $C_{15}H_{12}{}^{125}I_3NO_4$. [Liothyronine is INN and BAN.] (1) L-Tyrosine, *O*-(4-Hydroxy-3-iodophenyl)-3,5-diiodo-, labeled with iodine-125; (2) L-Alanine, 3-[4-(4-hydroxy-3-iodophenoxy)-3,5-diiodophenyl]-, labeled with iodine-125. *UNII-S1UAI9MKMG; UNII-06LU7C9H1V* [liothyronine]. *CAS-24359-14-6; CAS-6893-02-3* [liothyronine]. *Radioactive agent.* Triomet-125 (Abbott†)

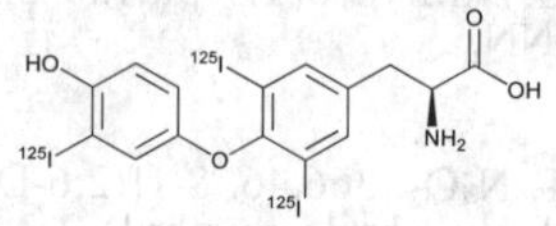

Liothyronine I 131 [*1963*] (lye″ oh thye′ roe neen). $C_{15}H_{12}{}^{131}I_3NO_4$. (1) L-Tyrosine, *O*-(4-hydroxy-3-iodophenyl)-3,5-diiodo-, labeled with iodine-131; (2) L-Alanine, 3-[4-(4-hydroxy-3-iodophenoxy)-3,5-diiodophenyl]-, labeled with iodine-131. *UNII-86AZ0G22V2; UNII-06LU7C9H1V* [liothyronine]. *CAS-20196-64-9; CAS-6893-02-3* [liothyronine]. *Radioactive agent.* Triomet-131 (Abbott†); Tri-Thyrotope (Bristol-Myers Squibb†)

Liothyronine Sodium (lye″ oh thye′ roe neen soe′ dee um). **USP.** $C_{15}H_{11}I_3NNaO_4$. 672.96. [*See also* Liotrix.] (1) L-Tyrosine, *O*-(4-hydroxy-3-iodophenyl)-3,5-diiodo-, monosodium salt; (2) Monosodium L-3-[4-(4-hydroxy-3-iodophenoxy)-3,5-diiodophenyl]alanine. *UNII-GCA9VV7D2N; UNII-06LU7C9H1V* [liothyronine]. *CAS-55-06-1; CAS-6893-02-3* [liothyronine]. BAN; JAN. *Thyroid hormone.* Cytomel (King)

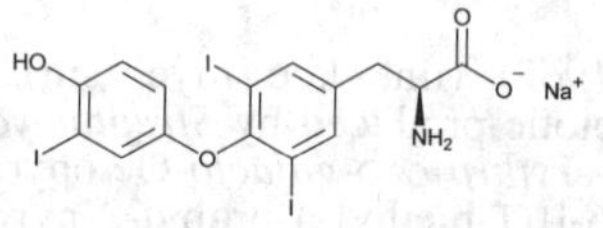

Liotrix [*1969*] (lye′ oh trix). **USP** [Tablets]. A mixture of liothyronine sodium ($C_{15}H_{11}I_3NNaO_4$) and levothyroxine sodium ($C_{15}H_{10}I_4NNaO_4 \cdot xH_2O$), in a ratio of 1:1 in terms of biological activity, or in a ratio of 1:4 in terms of weight. (1) L-Tyrosine, *O*-(4-hydroxy-3,5-diiodophenyl)-3,5-diiodo-, monosodium salt, hydrate, mixt. with *O*-(4-hydroxy-3-iodophenyl)-3,5-diiodo-L-tyrosine monosodium salt; (2) Monosodium L-thyroxine hydrate mixt. with monosodium L-3-[4-(4-hydroxy-3-iodophenoxy)-3,5-diiodophenyl]alanine. *CAS-8065-29-0. Thyroid hormone.* Euthroid (Parke-Davis†); Thyrolar (Forest)

Lipancreatin — *See* Pancrelipase.

Lipoic Acid, Alpha. $C_8H_{14}O_2S_2$. 206.33. (1) Thioctic Acid; (2) 1,2-Dithiolane-3-pentanoic acid; (3) 1,2-Dithiolane-3-valeric acid. *CAS-1077-28-7.* NF XXI.

Liprotamase [*2008*] (lye proe′ ta mase). $C_{2342}H_{3521}N_{597}O_{742}S_{18}$ (amylase). 52,480 (amylase); $C_{1465}H_{2300}N_{402}O_{468}S_3$ (lipase). 33,130 (lipase); $C_{1244}H_{1947}N_{347}O_{418}S$ (protease). 28,480 (protease). Amylase α-; Lipase, triacylglycerol; Proteinase, aspergillus alkaline. *CAS-884502-91-4. Treatment of malabsorption due to partial or complete pancreatic insufficiency (PI).* Theraclec (Altus); Trizytek (Altus) ◇*ALTU-135*

Lipstatin — *See* Orlistat.

Liquid Petrolatum (previously used name) — *See* Mineral Oil.

Liraglutide [*2007*] (lir″ a gloo′ tide). $C_{172}H_{265}N_{43}O_{51}$. 3751.20. (1) Glycine, L-histidyl-L-alanyl-L-α-glutamylglycyl-L-threonyl-L-phenylalanyl-L-threonyl-L-seryl-L-α-aspartyl-L-valyl-L-seryl-L-seryl-L-tyrosyl-L-leucyl-L-α-glutamylglycyl-L-glutaminyl-L-alanyl-L-alanyl-N^6-[N-(1-oxohexadecyl)-L-γ-glutamyl]-L-lysyl-L-α-glutamyl-L-phenylalanyl-L-isoleucyl-L-alanyl-L-tryptophyl-L-leucyl-L-valyl-L-arginylglycyl-L-arginyl-; (2) $N^{\epsilon 26}$-(N-Hexadecanoyl-L-γ-glutamyl)-[34-L-arginine]glucagon-like peptide 1-(7-37)-peptide; (3) Arg^{34}Lys^{26}-(N-ϵ-(γ-Glu(N-α-hexadecanoyl)))-GLP-1[7-37]. *CAS-204656-20-2.* INN; JAN. *Adjunctive therapy to improve glycemic control, with diet and exercise, in patients with type II diabetes.* ◇*NNC 90-1170; NN2211*

HAEG TFTSDVSSYL EGQAAKEFIA WLVRGRG

Liranaftate. $C_{18}H_{20}N_2O_2S$. 328.43. O-(5,6,7,8,-Tetrahydro-2-naphthyl) 6-methoxy-N-methylthio-2-pyridinecarbamate. *UNII-5253IGO5X3. CAS-88678-31-3.* INN.

Lirequinil. $C_{26}H_{25}ClN_2O_3$. 448.94. (3S)-1-[(10-Chloro-6,7-dihydro-4-oxo-3-phenyl-4H-benzo[a]quinolizin-1-yl)carbonyl]-3-ethoxypyrrolidine. *UNII-2VUW1087AD. CAS-143943-73-1.* INN.

Lirexapride. $C_{24}H_{36}ClN_3O_2$. 434.01. 4-Amino-5-chloro-α-cyclopropyl-N-[(1R,2R)-2-[(4-methylpiperidino)methyl]-cyclohexyl]-o-anisamide. *UNII-N33SZ2N85M. CAS-145414-12-6.* INN.

Lirimilast. $C_{17}H_{12}Cl_2N_2O_6S$. 443.26. 2-(2,4-Dichlorobenzoyl)-3-ureidobenzofuran-6-yl methanesulfonate. *CAS-329306-27-6.* INN.

Liroldine. $C_{20}H_{20}F_2N_4$. 354.40. 2,2′-[(3,3′-Difluoro-4,4′-biphenylylene)dinitrilo]dipyrrolidine. *UNII-H7H9M0ICD7. CAS-105102-20-3.* INN.

Lisadimate [*1990*] (lis ad′ i mate). $C_{10}H_{13}NO_4$. 211.21. (1) 1,2,3-Propanetriol, 1-(4-aminobenzoate), (±)-; (2) (±)-Glycerol 1-(p-aminobenzoate). *UNII-A886B5N5IM. CAS-136-44-7.* INN. *Sunscreen.*

Lisdexamfetamine Dimesylate [*2005*] (lis dex″ am fet′ a meen dye mes′ i late). $C_{15}H_{25}N_3O\cdot(CH_4O_3S)_2$. 455.59. [Lisdexamfetamine is INN.] (1) Hexanamide, 2,6-diamino-N-[(1S)-1-methyl-2-phenylethyl]-, (2S)-, dimethanesulfonate; (2) (2S)-2,6-Diamino-N-[(1S)-1-methyl-2-phenylethyl]hexanamide dimethanesulfonate. *UNII-SJT761GEGS; UNII-H645GUL8KJ* [lisdexamfetamine]. *CAS-608137-33-3; CAS-608137-32-2* [lisdexamfetamine]. *Treatment of attention deficit hyperactivity disorder (ADHD).* Vyvanse (Shire) ◇*NRP104*

Lisinopril [*1984*] (lye sin′ oh pril). **USP.** $C_{21}H_{31}N_3O_5\cdot2H_2O$. 441.52. (1) L-Proline, 1-[N^2-(1-carboxy-3-phenylpropyl)-L-lysyl]-, dihydrate, (S)-; (2) 1-[N^2-[(S)-1-Carboxy-3-phenylpropyl]-L-lysyl]-L-proline dihydrate. *UNII-E7199S1YWR. CAS-83915-83-7; CAS-76547-98-3* [anhydrous]. INN; BAN; JAN. *Antihypertensive.* Prinivil (Merck); Zestril (AstraZeneca) ◇*MK-521*

---

† Brand name formerly used, and/or firm no longer concerned with this product.

Lisofylline [*1994*] (lye sof′ i lin). $C_{13}H_{20}N_4O_3$. 280.32. (1) 1*H*-Purine-2,6-dione, 3,7-dihydro-1-(5-hydroxyhexyl)-3,7-dimethyl-, (*R*)-; (2) 1-[(*R*)-5-Hydroxyhexyl]theobromine. *UNII-L1F2Q2X956. CAS-100324-81-0.* INN. *Immunomodulator.* ProTec (Cell Therapeutics†) ◇*CT 1501R*

Lisuride. $C_{20}H_{26}N_4O$. 338.45. [Lisuride Maleate is JAN.] 3-(9,10-Didehydro-6-methylergolin-8α-yl)-1,1-diethylurea. *CAS-18016-80-3.* INN; BAN; MI. *[Name previously used: Lysuride.]*

Litenimod. $C_{256}H_{322}N_{95}O_{129}P_{25}S_{25}$. 8369.82. *P*-Thiothymidylyl-(3′→5′)-2′-deoxy-*P*-thioadenylyl-(3′→5′)-2′-deoxy-*P*-thioadenylyl-(3′→5′)-2′-deoxy-*P*-thioadenylyl-(3′→5′)-2′-deoxy-*P*-thiocytidylyl-(3′→5′)-2′-deoxy-*P*-thioguanylyl-(3′→5′)-*P*-thiothymidylyl-(3′→5′)-*P*-thiothymidylyl-(3′→5′)-2′-deoxy-*P*-thioadenylyl-(3′→5′)-*P*-thiothymidylyl-(3′→5′)-2′-deoxy-*P*-thioadenylyl-(3′→5′)-2′-deoxy-*P*-thioadenylyl-(3′→5′)-2′-deoxy-*P*-thiocytidylyl-(3′→5′)-2′-deoxy-*P*-thioguanylyl-(3′→5′)-*P*-thiothymidylyl-(3′→5′)-*P*-thiothymidylyl-(3′→5′)-2′-deoxy-*P*-thioadenylyl-(3′→5′)-*P*-thiothymidylyl-(3′→5′)-2′-deoxy-*P*-thioguanylyl-(3′→5′)-2′-deoxy-*P*-thioadenylyl-(3′→5′)-2′-deoxy-*P*-thiocytidylyl-(3′→5′)-2′-deoxy-*P*-thioguanylyl-(3′→5′)-*P*-thiothymidylyl-(3′→5′)-2′-deoxy-*P*-thiocytidylyl-(3′→5′)-2′-deoxy-*P*-thioadenylyl-(3′→5′)-thymidine. *CAS-852313-25-8.* INN.

Litgenprostucel-L [*2006*] (lit″ jen pros too′ sel - el). CG8711 is one of two components of a prostate cancer cellular immunotherapy consisting of a prostate adenocarcinoma cell line, LNCaP, that has been modified to secrete Granulocyte Macrophage Colony Stimulating Factor (GM-CSF) and irradiated to prevent tumor cell replication. *Cellular immunotherapy product for the treatment of prostate cancer.* GVAX Prostate (Cell Genesys) ◇*CG8711*

Lithium Benzoate. *UNII-R9Z042Z19E. CAS-553-54-8.* NF VIII; MI.

Lithium Carbonate [*1968*] (lith′ ee um kar′ bo nate). **USP.** Li_2CO_3. 73.89. (1) Carbonic acid, dilithium salt; (2) Dilithium carbonate. *UNII-2BMD2GNA4V. CAS-554-13-2.* JAN. *Antimanic.* Eskalith (JDS); Lithobid (JDS) ◇*CP-15,467-61; NSC-16895*

Lithium Citrate (lith′ ee um sit′ rate). **USP.** $C_6H_5Li_3O_7.4H_2O$. 281.98. (1) 1,2,3-Propanetricarboxylic acid, 2-hydroxy-trilithium salt tetrahydrate; (2) Trilithium citrate tetrahydrate. *UNII-5Z6E9K79YV. CAS-6080-58-6; CAS-919-16-4* [anhydrous]. *Antimanic.*

Lithium Hydroxide (lith′ ee um hye drox′ ide). **USP.** $LiOH.H_2O$. 41.96. (1) Lithium hydroxide monohydrate; (2) Lithium hydroxide monohydrate. *CAS-1310-66-3; CAS-1310-65-2* [anhydrous]. *Antimanic.*

Lithium Salicylate. *UNII-93F1SP6QIN.* NF VIII.

Litomeglovir. $C_{25}H_{30}N_4O_5S$. 498.59. 2-[[4-[[5-(Dimethylamino)-1-naphthyl]sulfonamido]phenyl]carbamoyl]-2-methylpropyl glycinate. *UNII-X2ZU9993TF. CAS-321915-31-5.* INN.

Litoxetine. $C_{16}H_{19}NO$. 241.33. 4-(2-Naphthylmethoxy)piperidine. *UNII-9980ST005G. CAS-86811-09-8.* INN.

Litracen. $C_{20}H_{23}N$. 277.40. 9-(3-Methylaminopropylidene)-10,10-dimethyl-9,10-dihydroanthracene. *UNII-2B3D399IVR. CAS-5118-30-9.* INN.

Livaraparin Calcium. Calcium salt of a low molecular mass heparin that is obtained by nitrous acid depolymerization of heparin from porcine intestinal mucosa; the majority of the components have a 2-*O*-sulfo-α-L-idopyranosuronic acid structure at the non-reducing end and a 6-*O*-sulfo-structure at the reducing end of their chain; the mass-average molecular mass ranges between 3000 and 5000 with 75% is less than 8000; the degree of sulfatation is approximately 2 per disaccharidic unit. INN.

Liver Extract. An extract of mammalian (usually pig) liver containing small amounts of cyanocobalamin, folic acid and, possibly, other hemopoietic factors; present in many preparations. BAN.

Lividomycin. $C_{29}H_{55}N_5O_{18}$. 761.77. *O*-2-Amino-2,3-dideoxy-α-D-*ribo*-hexopyranosyl-(1→4)-*O*-[*O*-α-D-mannopyranosyl-(1→4)-*O*-2,6-diamino-2,6-dideoxy-β-L-idopyranosyl-(1→3)-β-D-ribofuranosyl-(1→5)]-2-deoxy-D-streptamine. *CAS-36441-41-5.* INN; DCF.

Lixazinone Sulfate [*1988*] (lix az′ i none sul′ fate). $C_{21}H_{28}N_4O_3.H_2SO_4.H_2O$. 500.57. [Lixazinone is INN.] (1) Butanamide, *N*-cyclohexyl-*N*-methyl-4-[(1,2,3,5-tetrahydro-2-oxoimidazo[2,1-*b*]quinazolin-7-yl)oxy]-, sulfate (1:1), monohydrate; (2) *N*-Cyclohexyl-*N*-methyl-4-[(1,2,3,5-tetrahydro-2-oxoimidazo[2,1-*b*]quinazolin-7-

yl)oxy]butyramide sulfate (1:1), monohydrate. *CAS-101626-67-9; CAS-94192-59-3 [lixazinone]. Cardiotonic (phosphodiesterase inhibitor).* ◇*RS-82856*

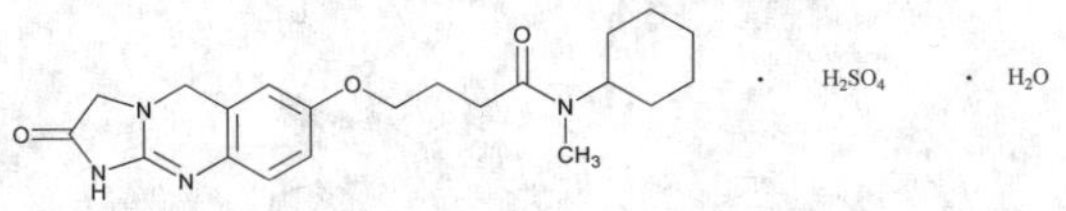

Lixisenatide. $C_{215}H_{347}N_{61}O_{65}S$. 4858.49. Des-38-proline-exendine-4 (*Heloderma suspectum*)-(1-39)-peptidylpenta-L-lysyl-L-lysinamide. *CAS-320367-13-3.* INN.

Lixivaptan [*1999*] (lix″ i vap′ tan). $C_{27}H_{21}ClFN_3O_2$. 473.93. (1) Benzamide, *N*-[3-chloro-4-(5*H*-pyrrolo[2,1-*c*][1,4]benzodiazepin-10(11*H*)-ylcarbonyl)phenyl]-5-fluoro-2-methyl-; (2) 3′-Chloro-5-fluoro-4′-(5*H*-pyrrolo[2,1-*c*][1,4]benzodiazepin-10(11*H*)-ylcarbonyl)-*o*-toluanilide. *UNII-8F5X4B082E. CAS-168079-32-1.* INN. *Treatment of nonhypovolemic hyponatremia (selective V2-receptor antagonist).* ◇*WAY-VPA-985*

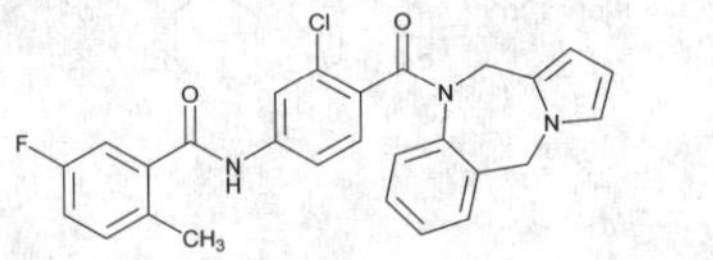

Lobaplatin. $C_9H_{18}N_2O_3Pt$. 397.33. *cis*-[*trans*-1,2-Cyclobutanebis(methylamine)][(*S*)-lactato-*O*¹,*O*¹]platinum. *CAS-135558-11-1.* INN.

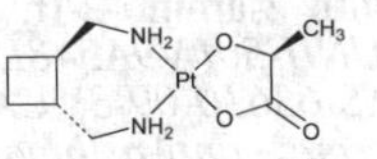

Lobeglitazone. $C_{24}H_{24}N_4O_5S$. 480.54. (5*RS*)-5{[4-(2-{[6-(4-Methoxyphenoxy)pyrimidin-4-yl]methylamino}ethoxy)-phenyl]methyl}-1,3-thiazolidine-2,4-dione. *CAS-607723-33-1.* INN.

Lobeline. $C_{22}H_{27}NO_2$. 337.46. [Lobeline Hydrochloride is JAN.] 2-[6-(*β*-Hydroxyphenethyl)-1-methyl-2-piperidyl]-acetophenone. *CAS-90-69-7.* INN; BAN; MI.

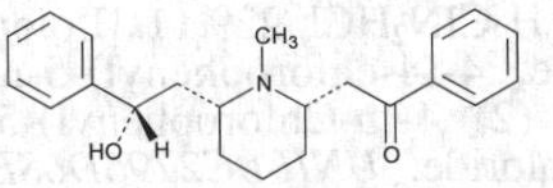

Lobendazole [*1972*] (loe ben′ da zole). $C_{10}H_{11}N_3O_2$. 205.21. (1) Carbamic acid, 1*H*-benzimidazol-2-yl-, ethyl ester; (2) Ethyl 2-benzimidazolecarbamate. *UNII-CMF6Z78SWL. CAS-6306-71-4.* INN. *Anthelmintic (veterinary).* ◇*SK&F 24529; NSC-42044*

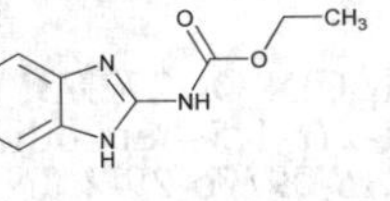

Lobenzarit Sodium [*1985*] (loe benz′ a rit soe′ dee um). $C_{14}H_8ClNNa_2O_4$. 335.65. [Lobenzarit is INN; Lobenzarit Disodium is JAN.] (1) Benzoic acid, 2-[(2-carboxypheny-

l)amino]-4-chloro-, disodium salt; (2) Disodium 4-chloro-2,2′-iminodibenzoate. *UNII-7Z9SP74BXF. CAS-64808-48-6; CAS-63329-53-3 [lobenzarit]. Antirheumatic.* ◇*CCA*

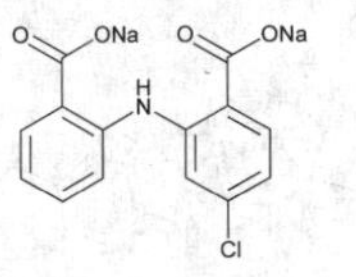

Lobradimil (previously used name) — *See* Labradimil.

Lobucavir [*1994*] (loe bue′ ka vir). $C_{11}H_{15}N_5O_3$. 265.27. (1) 6*H*-Purin-6-one, 2-amino-9-[2,3-bis(hydroxymethyl)cyclobutyl]-1,9-dihydro, [1*R*-(1*α*,2*β*,3*α*)]; (2) 9-[(1*R*,2*R*,3*S*)-2,3-Bis(hydroxymethyl)cyclobutyl]guanine. *CAS-127759-89-1.* INN. *Antiviral.* ◇*BMS-180194; SQ 34,514*

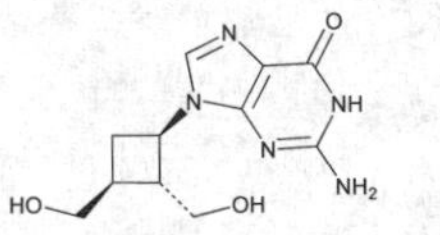

Lobuprofen. $C_{25}H_{33}ClN_2O_2$. 428.99. 2-[4-(*m*-Chlorophenyl)-1-piperazinyl]ethyl (±)-*p*-isobutylhydratropate. *UNII-X2T6O1TUNX. CAS-96128-90-4.* INN.

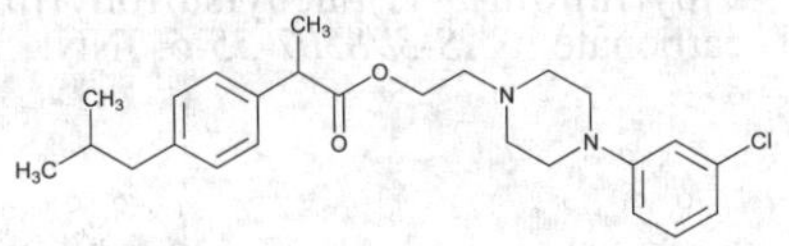

Locicortolone Dicibate. $C_{36}H_{50}Cl_2O_5$. 633.69. 9,11*β*-Dichloro-21-hydroxy-16*α*-methylpregna-1,4-diene-3,20-dione dicyclohexylmethyl carbonate. *UNII-G87210HO7A. CAS-78467-68-2.* INN.

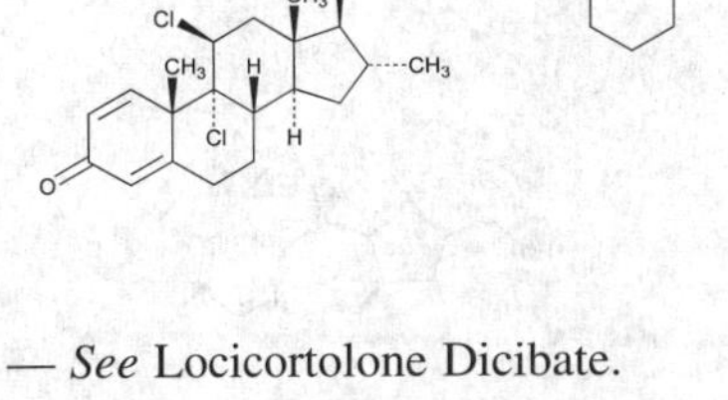

Locicortone — *See* Locicortolone Dicibate.

Lodaxaprine. $C_{15}H_{16}ClN_3O$. 289.76. 1-[6-(*o*-Chlorophenyl)-3-pyridazinyl]-4-piperidinol. *UNII-D59ZQ3VVMV. CAS-93181-81-8.* INN.

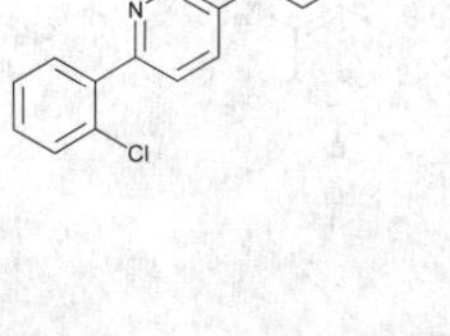

---

† Brand name formerly used, and/or firm no longer concerned with this product.

Lodazecar. $C_{22}H_{24}BrClN_4O_4$. 523.81. 1-[1,1-Bis(hydroxymethyl)ethyl]-3-[(S)-6-bromo-5-(o-chlorophenyl)-2,3-dihydro-1,3-dimethyl-2-oxo-1H-1,4-benzodiazepin-7-yl]urea. *UNII-T4D9016A00. CAS-87646-83-1.* INN.

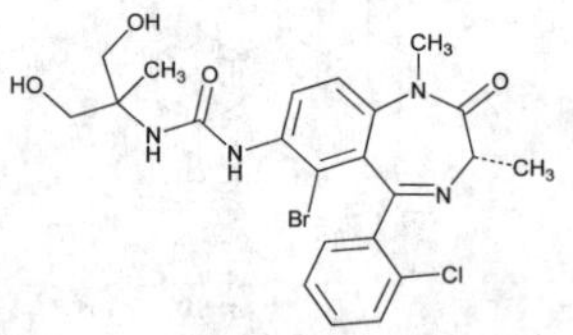

Lodelaben [*1989*] (loe del′ a ben). $C_{25}H_{41}ClO_3$. 425.04. (1) Benzoic acid, 2-chloro-4-(1-hydroxyoctadecyl)-, (±)-; (2) (±)-2-Chloro-4-(1-hydroxyoctadecyl)benzoic acid. *CAS-111149-90-7; CAS-93105-81-8* [replaced]. INN. *Antiarthritic; emphysema therapy adjunct. [Name previously used: Declaben.]* ◇SC-39026

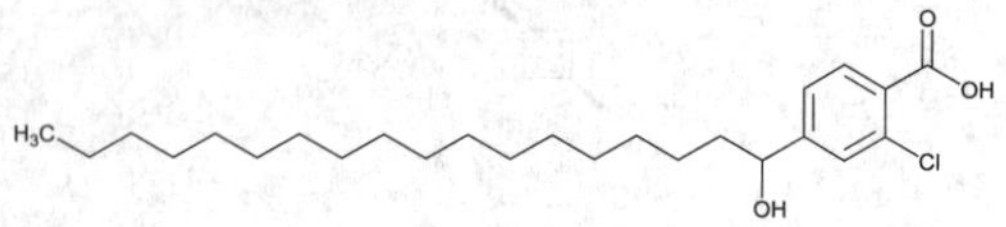

Lodenafil Carbonate. $C_{47}H_{62}N_{12}O_{11}S_2$. 1035.20. Bis(2-{4-[4-ethoxy-3-(1-methyl-7-oxo-3-propyl-4,7-dihydro-1H-pyrazolo[4,3-d]pyrimidin-5-yl)phenylsulfonyl]piperazin-1-yl}ethyl) carbonate. *CAS-398507-55-6.* INN.

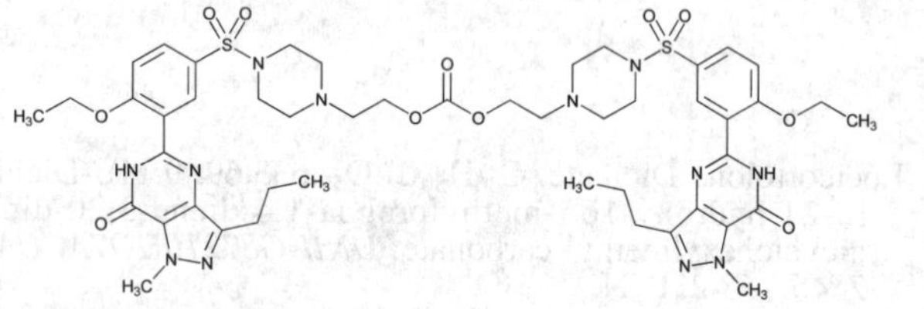

Lodenosine [*1997*] (loe den′ oh seen). $C_{10}H_{12}FN_5O_2$. 253.23. 9-(2,3-Dideoxy-2-fluoro-β-D-*threo*-pentofuranosyl) adenine. *CAS-110143-10-7.* INN. *Antiviral.* ◇F-ddA; NSC-613792

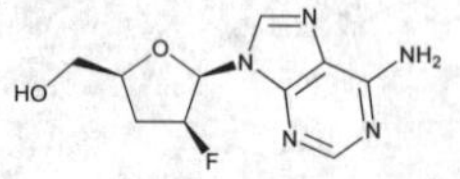

Lodinixil. $C_{14}H_{17}ClN_4$. 276.76. 4-Chloro-2-(dimethylamino)-6-(2,3-xylidino)pyrimidine. *UNII-P2I071P32B. CAS-86627-50-1.* INN.

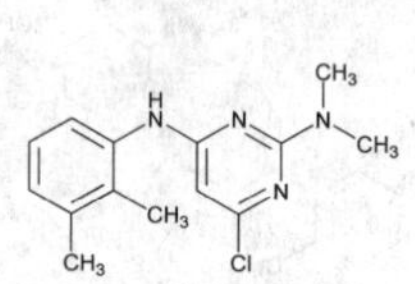

Lodiperone. $C_{21}H_{20}Cl_2FN_3O_2$. 436.31. 5-[2-[4-(3,5-Dichlorophenyl)-1-piperazinyl]ethyl]-4-(p-fluorophenyl)-4-oxazolin-2-one. *UNII-T8593BT7B4. CAS-72444-63-4.* INN.

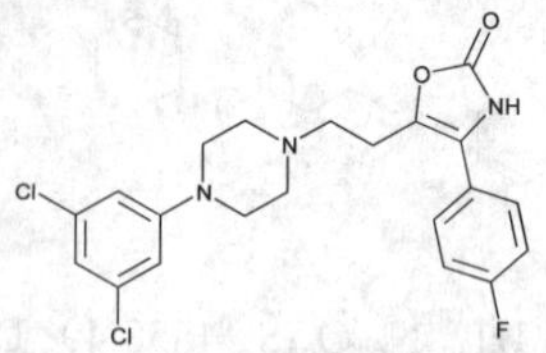

Lodoxamide Ethyl [*1978*] (loe dox′ a mide eth′ il). $C_{15}H_{14}ClN_3O_6$. 367.74. [Lodoxamide is INN and BAN.] (1) Acetic acid, 2,2′-[(2-chloro-5-cyano-1,3-phenylene)diimino]bis[2-oxo-, diethyl ester; (2) Diethyl N,N'-(2-chloro-5-cyano-m-phenylene)dioxamate. *UNII-SPU695OD73* [lodoxamide]. *CAS-53882-13-6; CAS-53882-12-5* [lodoxamide]. *Anti-allergic; anti-asthmatic.* ◇U-42,718

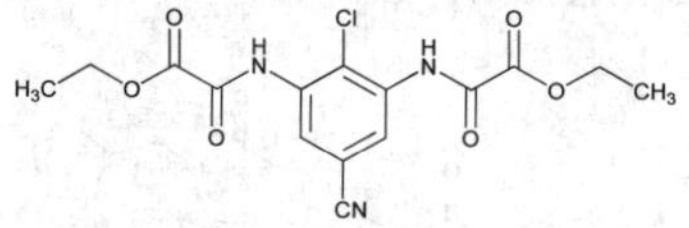

Lodoxamide Tromethamine [*1978*] (loe dox′ a mide troe meth′ a meen). $C_{11}H_6ClN_3O_6 \cdot 2C_4H_{11}NO_3$. 553.90. [Lodoxamide Trometamol is BAN.] (1) Acetic acid, 2,2′-[(2-chloro-5-cyano-1,3-phenylene)diimino]bis[2-oxo-, compound with 2-amino-2-(hydroxymethyl)-1,3-propanediol (1:2); (2) N,N'-(2-Chloro-5-cyano-m-phenylene)dioxamic acid compound with 2-amino-2-(hydroxymethyl)-1,3-propanediol (1:2). *UNII-50LV9A548L; UNII-SPU695OD73* [lodoxamide]. *CAS-63610-09-3; CAS-53882-12-5* [lodoxamide]. *Anti-allergic; anti-asthmatic.* Alomide (Alcon) ◇U-42,585E

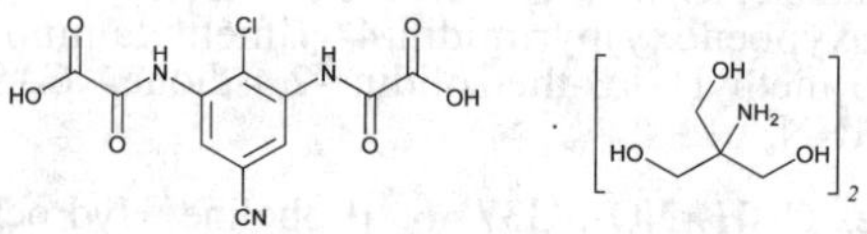

Lofemizole Hydrochloride [*1984*] (loe fem′ i zole hye″ droe klor′ ide). $C_{10}H_9ClN_2 \cdot HCl$. 229.11. [Lofemizole is INN.] (1) 1H-Imidazole, 4-(4-chlorophenyl)-5-methyl-, monohydrochloride; (2) 4-(p-Chlorophenyl)-5-methylimidazole monohydrochloride. *UNII-0C2796D6SB. CAS-70169-80-1; CAS-65571-68-8* [lofemizole]. *Anti-inflammatory; analgesic; antipyretic.*

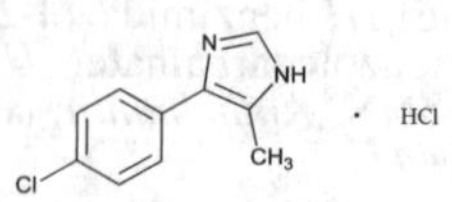

Lofendazam. $C_{15}H_{13}ClN_2O$. 272.73. 8-Chloro-1,3,4,5-tetrahydro-1-phenyl-2H-1,5-benzodiazepin-2-one. *UNII-V7O53S50SN. CAS-29176-29-2.* INN; BAN.

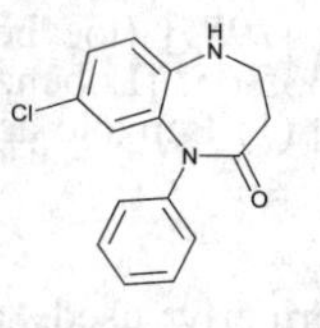

Lofentanil Oxalate [*1980*] (loe fen′ ta nil ox′ a late). $C_{25}H_{32}N_2O_3 \cdot C_2H_2O_4$. 498.57. [Lofentanil is INN and BAN.] (1) 4-Piperidinecarboxylic acid, 3-methyl-4-[(1-oxopropyl)phenylamino]-1-(2-phenylethyl)-, methyl ester, *cis*, (-)-, ethanedioate (1:1); (2) (-)-Methyl *cis*-3-methyl-1-phenethyl-4-(*N*-phenylpropionamido)isonipecotate oxalate (1:1). *UNII-6C1599T3OQ. CAS-61380-41-4; CAS-61380-40-3* [lofentanil]. *Analgesic (narcotic).* ◇*R 34,995*

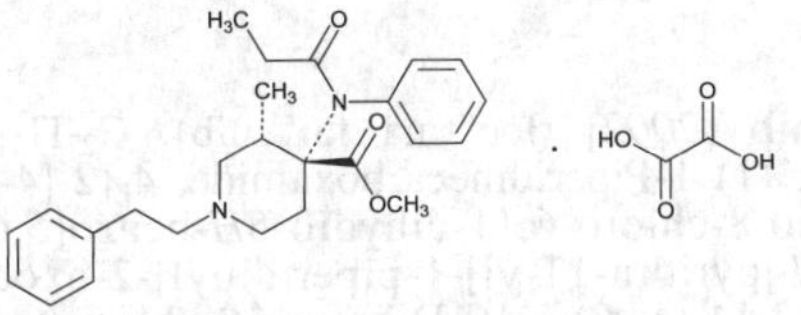

Lofepramine Hydrochloride [*1986*] (loe fep′ ra meen hye″ droe klor′ ide). $C_{26}H_{27}ClN_2O \cdot HCl$. 455.42. [Lofepramine is INN and BAN.] (1) Ethanone, 1-(4-chlorophenyl)-2-[[3-(10,11-dihydro-5*H*-dibenz[*b*,*f*]azepin-5-yl)propyl]methylamino]-, monohydrochloride; (2) 4′-Chloro-2-[[3-(10,11-dihydro-5*H*-dibenz[*b*,*f*]azepin-5-yl)propyl]methylamino]-acetophenone monohydrochloride. *CAS-26786-32-3; CAS-23047-25-8* [lofepramine]. JAN. *Antidepressant.* ◇*WHR-2908A*

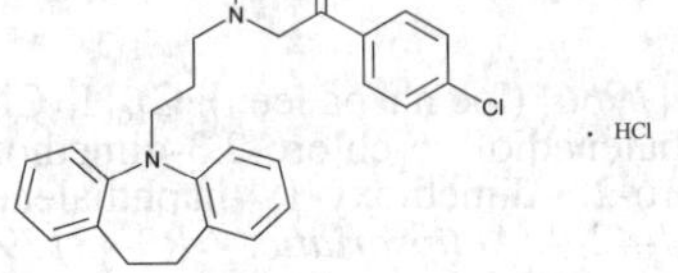

Lofexidine Hydrochloride [*1986*] (loe fex′ i deen hye″ droe klor′ ide). $C_{11}H_{12}Cl_2N_2O \cdot HCl$. 295.59. [Lofexidine is INN and BAN.] (1) 1*H*-Imidazole, 2-[1-(2,6-dichlorophenoxy)ethyl]-4,5-dihydro-, monohydrochloride; (2) 2-[1-(2,6-Dichlorophenoxy)ethyl]-2-imidazoline monohydrochloride. *CAS-21498-08-8; CAS-31036-80-3* [lofexidine]. *Antihypertensive.* Lofexidine (Rhone-Poulenc Rorer) ◇*MDL 14,042*

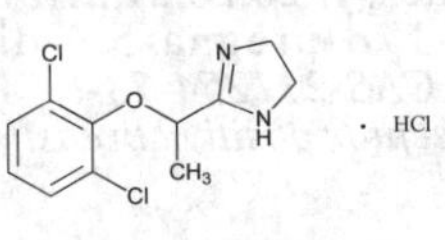

Loflucarban. $C_{13}H_9Cl_2FN_2S$. 315.19. 3,5-Dichloro-4′-fluorothiocarbanilide. *UNII-6QO0F8648P. CAS-790-69-2.* INN; MI.

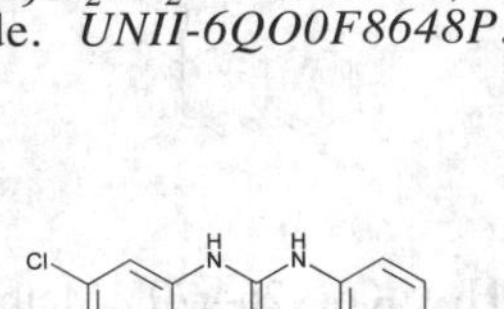

Lombazole. $C_{22}H_{17}ClN_2$. 344.84. (±)-1-(α-4-Biphenylyl-*o*-chlorobenzyl)imidazole. *UNII-ZHC772U9S3. CAS-60628-98-0.* INN; BAN.

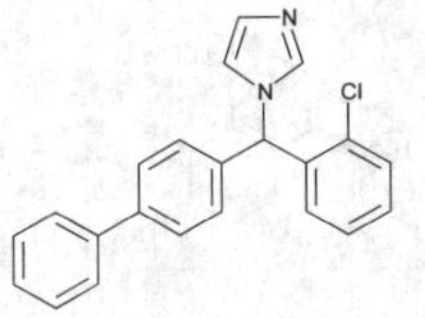

Lomefloxacin [*1988*] (loe″ me flox′ a sin). $C_{17}H_{19}F_2N_3O_3$. 351.35. (1) 3-Quinolinecarboxylic acid, 1-ethyl-6,8-difluoro-1,4-dihydro-7-(3-methyl-1-piperazinyl)-4-oxo-, (±)-; (2) (±)-1-Ethyl-6,8-difluoro-1,4-dihydro-7-(3-methyl-1-piperazinyl)-4-. *UNII-L6BR2WJD8V. CAS-98079-51-7.* INN; BAN. *Antibacterial.* ◇*SC-47111A*

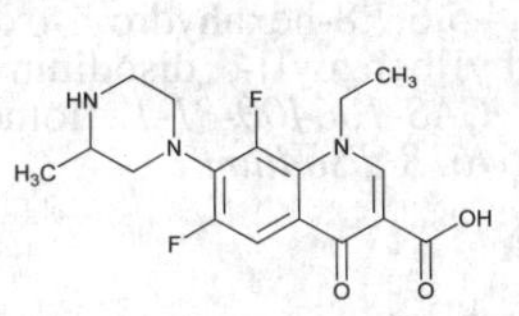

Lomefloxacin Hydrochloride [*1988*] (loe″ me flox′ a sin hye″ droe klor′ ide). $C_{17}H_{19}F_2N_3O_3 \cdot HCl$. 387.81. (1) 3-Quinolinecarboxylic acid, 1-ethyl-6,8-difluoro-1,4-dihydro-7-(3-methyl-1-piperazinyl)-4-oxo-, monohydrochloride, (±)-; (2) (±)-1-Ethyl-6,8-difluoro-1,4-dihydro-7-(3-methyl-1-piperazinyl)-4-oxo-3-quinolinecarboxylic acid, monohydrochloride. *UNII-9VC7S3ZXXB. CAS-98079-52-8.* JAN. *Antibacterial.* Maxaquin (Pfizer) ◇*NY-198; SC-47111*

Lomefloxacin Mesylate [*1989*] (loe″ me flox′ a sin mes′ i late). $C_{17}H_{19}F_2N_3O_3 \cdot CH_4O_3S$. 447.45. (1) 3-Quinolinecarboxylic acid, 1-ethyl-6,8-difluoro-1,4-dihydro-7-(3-methyl-1-piperazinyl)-4-oxo-, monomethanesulfonate, (±)-; (2) (±)-1-Ethyl-6,8-difluoro-1,4-dihydro-7-(3-methyl-1-piperazinyl)-4-oxo-3-quinolinecarboxylic acid, monomethanesulfonate. *UNII-6908F93PY1. CAS-114394-67-1.* *Antibacterial.* ◇*SC-47111B*

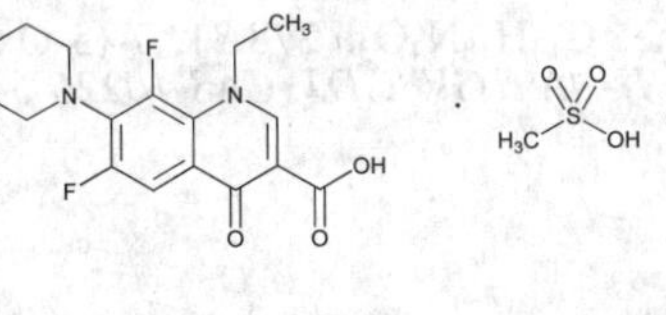

Lomeguatrib. $C_{10}H_8BrN_5OS$. 326.17. 6-[(4-Bromo-2-thienyl)methoxyl]purin-2-amine. *UNII-S79265T71M. CAS-192441-08-0.* INN; BAN.

Lomerizine. $C_{27}H_{30}F_2N_2O_3$. 468.54. 1-[Bis(*p*-fluorophenyl)methyl]-4-(2,3,4-trimethoxybenzyl)piperazine. *UNII-DEE37CY4VO. CAS-101477-55-8.* INN.

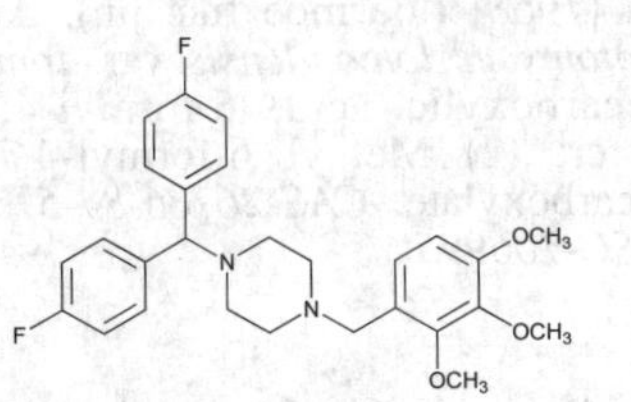

Lometraline Hydrochloride [*1972*] (loe me′ tra leen hye″ droe klor′ ide). $C_{13}H_{18}ClNO \cdot HCl$. 276.20. [Lometraline is INN.] (1) 1-Naphthalenamine, 8-chloro-1,2,3,4-tetrahydro-5-methoxy-*N,N*-dimethyl-, hydrochloride; (2) 8-Chloro-1,2,3,4-tetrahydro-5-methoxy-*N,N*-dimethyl-1-naphthyl-

---

† Brand name formerly used, and/or firm no longer concerned with this product.

amine hydrochloride. *UNII-T2OJ193WGR. CAS-34552-78-8; CAS-39951-65-0* [lometraline]. *Antipsychotic; antiparkinsonian.* ◇*CP-14,368-1*

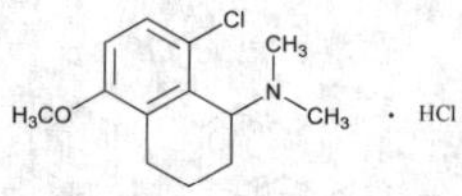

Lometrexol Sodium [*1990*] (loe″ me trex′ ol soe′ dee um). $C_{21}H_{23}N_5Na_2O_6$. 487.42. [Lometrexol is INN and BAN.] (1) L-Glutamic acid, *N*-[4-[2-(2-amino-3,4,5,6,7,8-hexahydro-4-oxopyrido[2,3-*d*]pyrimidin-6-yl)ethyl]benzoyl]-, disodium salt, (*R*)-; (2) Disodium *N*-[*p*-[2-[(*R*)-2-amino-3,4,5,6,7,8-hexahydro-4-oxopyrido[2,3-*d*]pyrimidin-6-yl]ethyl]benzoyl]-L-glutamate; (3) L-Glutamic acid, *N*-[4-[2-(2-amino-1,4,5,6,7,8-hexahydro-4-oxopyrido[2,3-*d*]pyrimidin-6-yl)ethyl]benzoyl]-, disodium salt, (*R*)-. *CAS-120408-07-3; CAS-106400-81-1* [lometrexol]. *Antineoplastic.* ◇*LY264618 disodium*

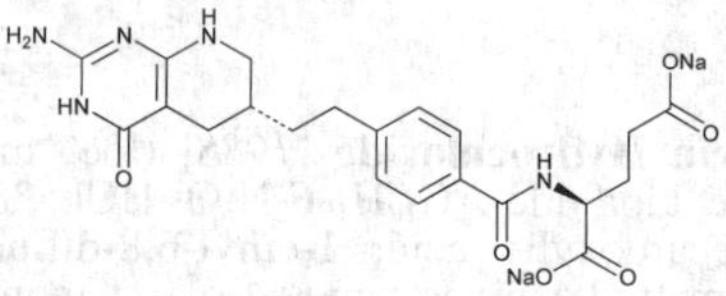

Lomevactone. $C_{18}H_{17}ClO_2$. 300.78. 4-(*p*-Chlorophenyl)tetrahydro-6-methyl-3-phenyl-2*H*-pyran-2-one. *UNII-TP71SPS85C. CAS-81478-25-3.* INN.

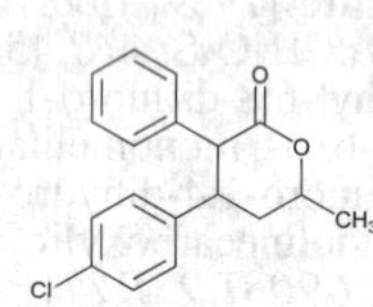

Lomifylline. $C_{13}H_{18}N_4O_3$. 278.31. 7-(5-Oxohexyl)theophylline. *UNII-NA91GV8GDJ. CAS-10226-54-7.* INN.

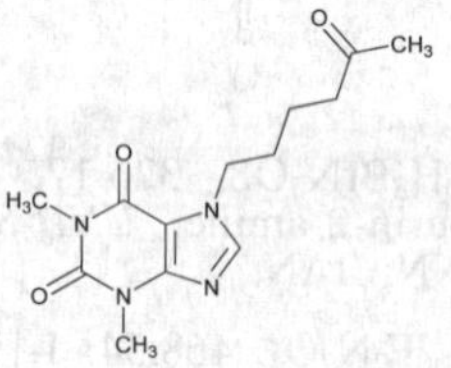

Lomofungin [*1968*] (loe moe fun′ jin). Antibiotic derived from *Streptomyces lomondensis* var. *lomondensis*. (1) 1-Phenazinecarboxylic acid, 6-formyl-4,7,9-trihydroxy-, methyl ester; (2) Methyl 6-formyl-4,7,9-trihydroxy-1-phenazinecarboxylate. *CAS-26786-84-5. Antifungal.* ◇*U-24,792; NSC-106995*

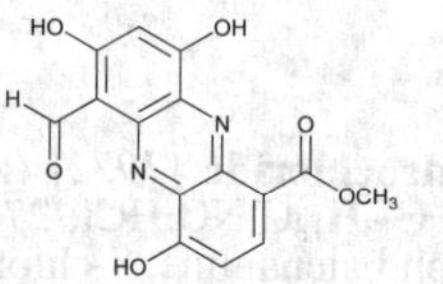

Lomustine [*1972*] (loe mus′ teen). $C_9H_{16}ClN_3O_2$. 233.70. (1) Urea, *N*-(2-chloroethyl)-*N*′-cyclohexyl-*N*-nitroso-; (2) 1-(2-Chloroethyl)-3-cyclohexyl-1-nitrosourea. *UNII-7BRF0Z81KG. CAS-13010-47-4.* INN; BAN. *Antineoplastic.* Ceenu (Bristol-Myers Squibb) ◇*CCNU; NSC-79037*

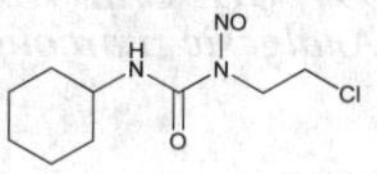

Lonafarnib [*2002*] (loe″ na far′ nib). $C_{27}H_{31}Br_2ClN_4O_2$. 638.82. (1) 1-Piperidinecarboxamide, 4-[2-[4-[(11*R*-3,10-dibromo-8-chloro-6,11-dihydro-5*H*-benzo[5,6]cyclohepta[1,2-*b*]pyridin-11-yl]-1-piperidinyl]-2-oxoethyl]-; (2) (+)-4-[2-[4-(11*R*)-3,10-Dibromo-8-chloro-6,11-dihydro-5*H*-benzo[5,6]cyclohepta[1,2-*b*]pyridin-11-yl)-piperidin-1-yl]]-2-oxoethyl]-piperidine-1-carboxamide. *UNII-IOW153004F. CAS-193275-84-2.* INN. *Chemotherapeutic (farnesyl transferase inhibitor).* ◇*SCH 66336*

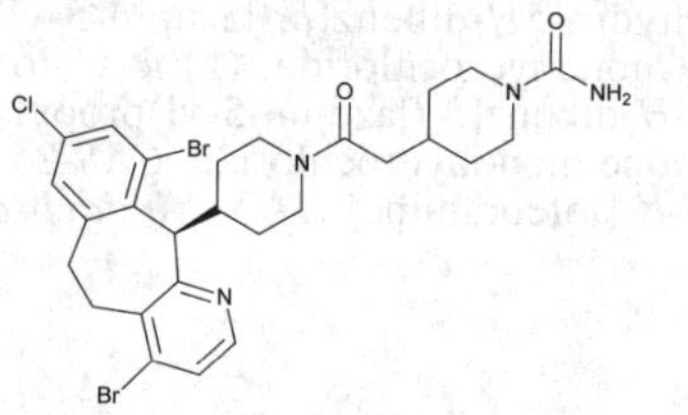

Lonapalene [*1986*] (loe na′ pa leen). $C_{16}H_{15}ClO_6$. 338.74. (1) 1,4-Naphthalenediol, 6-chloro-2,3-dimethoxy-, diacetate; (2) 6-Chloro-2,3-dimethoxy-1,4-naphthalenediol diacetate. *CAS-91431-42-4. Antipsoriatic.* ◇*RS-43179*

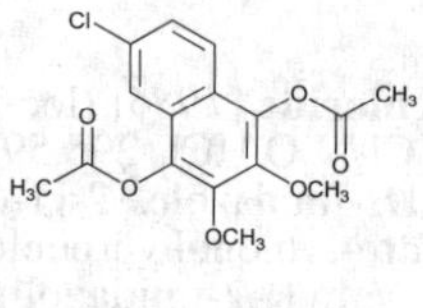

Lonaprisan [*2008*] (loe nap′ ri san). $C_{28}H_{29}F_5O_3$. 508.52. (1) 19-Norpregna-4,9-dien-3-one, 11-(4-acetylphenyl)-20,20,21,21,21-pentafluoro-17-hydroxy-, (11*β*,17*α*)-; (2) 11*β*-(4-Acetylphenyl)-20,20,21,21,21-pentafluoro-17-hydroxy-19-nor-17*α*-pregna-5,9-dien-3-one. *UNII-F5Z5EL4D26. CAS-211254-73-8.* INN. *Treatment of progesterone receptor positive breast cancer.* ◇*ZK 230211*

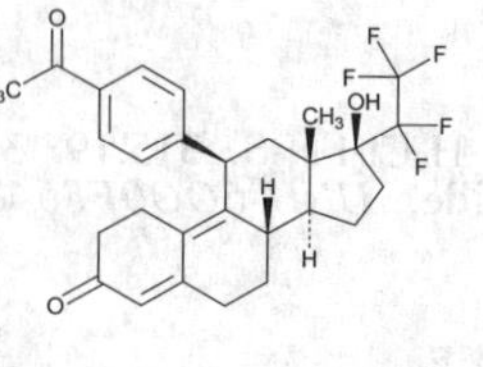

Lonaprofen. $C_{14}H_{13}ClO_3$. 264.70. Methyl 2-[(1-chloro-2-naphthyl)oxy]propionate. *UNII-4G86N0SVV3. CAS-41791-49-5.* INN.

Lonazolac. $C_{17}H_{13}ClN_2O_2$. 312.75. 3-(p-Chlorophenyl)-1-phenylpyrazole-4-acetic acid. *UNII-13097143QI. CAS-53808-88-1.* INN; MI.

Lonidamine. $C_{15}H_{10}Cl_2N_2O_2$. 321.16. 1-(2,4-Dichlorobenzyl)-1H-indazole-3-carboxylic acid. *CAS-50264-69-2.* INN; BAN; MI.

Lontucirev (Replicating Adenovirus) [*2004*] (lon too′ si rev). (1) DNA (human adenovirus ONYX-015); (2) E1B-55kDa gene-deleted adenovirus. *CAS-437981-77-6. Treatment of multiple cancers (E1-B deleted adenovirus; replication competent virus).* ◇*ONYX-015; CI-1042*

Loperamide Hydrochloride [*1975*] (loe per′ a mide hye″ droe klor′ ide). **USP.** $C_{29}H_{33}ClN_2O_2 \cdot HCl$. 513.50. [Loperamide is INN and BAN.] (1) 1-Piperidinebutanamide, 4-(4-chlorophenyl)-4-hydroxy-N,N-dimethyl-α,α-diphenyl-, monohydrochloride; (2) 4-(p-Chlorophenyl)-4-hydroxy-N,N-dimethyl-α,α-diphenyl-1-piperidinebutyramide monohydrochloride. *UNII-77TI35393C; UNII-6X9OC3H4II* [loperamide]. *CAS-34552-83-5; CAS-53179-11-6* [loperamide]. JAN. *Antiperistaltic.* Imodium (McNeil) ◇*R 18,553*

Loperamide Oxide. $C_{29}H_{33}ClN_2O_3$. 493.04. *trans*-4-(p-Chlorophenyl)-4-hydroxy-N,N-dimethyl-α,α-diphenyl-1-piperidinebutyramide 1-oxide. *CAS-106900-12-3.* INN; BAN. ◇*R58425*

Lopinavir [*1998*] (loe pin′ a vir). $C_{37}H_{48}N_4O_5$. 628.80. (1) [1S-[1R*(R*),3R*,4R*]]-N-[4-[[(2,6-Dimethylphenoxy)acetyl]amino]-3-hydroxy-5-phenyl-1-(phenylmethyl)pentyl]tetrahydro-α-(1-methylethyl)-2-oxo-1(2H)-pyrimidineacetamide; (2) (αS)-Tetrahydro-N-[(αS)-α-[(2S,3S)-2-hydroxy-4-phenyl-3-[2-(2,6-xylyloxy)acetamido]butyl]phenethyl]-α-isopropyl-2-oxo-1(2H)-pyrimidineacetamide. *UNII-2494G1JF75. CAS-192725-17-0.* INN; BAN. *Antiviral (HIV protease inhibitor).* ◇*ABT-378; A-157378.0*

Lopirazepam. $C_{14}H_9Cl_2N_3O_2$. 322.15. 7-Chloro-5-(o-chlorophenyl)-1,3-dihydro-3-hydroxy-2H-pyrido[3,2,-e]-1,4-diazepin-2-one. *UNII-8PDI6DY6GV. CAS-42863-81-0.* INN.

Lopobutan. $C_{19}H_{39}NO_3$. 329.52. ($\pm$)-3-[[3-(Dodecyloxy)propyl]amino]butyric acid. *UNII-L6IE0KAZ8O. CAS-6582-30-5.* INN.

Loprazolam. $C_{23}H_{21}ClN_6O_3$. 464.90. (Z)-6-(o-Chlorophenyl)-2,4-dihydro-2-[(4-methyl-1-piperazinyl)methylene]-8-nitro-1H-imidazo[1,2-a][1,4]benzodiazepin-1-one. *UNII-759N8462G8. CAS-61197-73-7.* INN; BAN; MI.

Lopremone (previously used name) — *See* Protirelin.

Loprodiol. $C_5H_{10}Cl_2O_2$. 173.04. 2,2-Bis(chloromethyl)-1,3-propanediol. *UNII-U1K5BS2ABA. CAS-2209-86-1.* INN.

Loracarbef [*1989*] (lor″ a kar′ bef). **USP.** $C_{16}H_{16}ClN_3O_4 \cdot H_2O$. 367.78. (1) 1-Azabicyclo[4.2.0]oct-2-ene-2-carboxylic acid, 7-[(aminophenylacetyl)amino]-3-chloro-8-oxo-, monohydrate, [6R-[6α,7β(R*)]]-; (2) (6R,7S)-7-[(R)-2-Amino-2-phenylacetamido]-3-chloro-8-oxo-1-azabicyclo[4.2.0]oct-2-ene-2-carboxylic acid, monohydrate. *UNII-3X11EVM5SU. CAS-121961-22-6; CAS-76470-66-1* [anhydrous]. INN; BAN. *Antibacterial.* Lorabid (King) ◇*LY163892 monohydrate*

---

† Brand name formerly used, and/or firm no longer concerned with this product.

Lorajmine Hydrochloride [*1976*] (lor aj′ meen hye″ droe klor′ ide). $C_{22}H_{27}ClN_2O_3 \cdot HCl$. 439.38. [Lorajmine is INN.] (1) Ajmalan-17,21-diol, 17-(chloroacetate), monohydrochloride, (17*R*,21α)-; (2) Ajmaline 17-(chloroacetate) monohydrochloride. *CAS-40819-93-0; CAS-47562-08-3* [lorajmine]. *Cardiac depressant (anti-arrhythmic).* ◇*Win 11831*

Lorapride. $C_{14}H_{22}ClN_3O_3S$. 347.86. 5-Chloro-*N*¹-[(1-ethyl-2-pyrrolidinyl)methyl]-2-methoxysulfanilamide. *UNII-549TIC7B4R. CAS-68677-06-5.* INN.

Loratadine [*1986*] (lor a′ ta deen). **USP.** $C_{22}H_{23}ClN_2O_2$. 382.88. (1) 1-Piperidinecarboxylic acid, 4-(8-chloro-5,6-dihydro-11*H*-benzo[5,6]cyclohepta[1,2-*b*]pyridin-11-ylidene)-, ethyl ester; (2) Ethyl 4-(8-chloro-5,6-dihydro-11*H*-benzo[5,6]cyclohepta[1,2-*b*]pyridin-11-ylidene)-1-piperidinecarboxylate. *UNII-7AJO3BO7QN. CAS-79794-75-5.* INN; BAN. *Antihistaminic.* Alavert (Wyeth); Claritin (Schering-Plough) ◇*Sch 29851*

Lorazepam [*1969*] (lor az′ e pam). **USP.** $C_{15}H_{10}Cl_2N_2O_2$. 321.16. (1) 2*H*-1,4-Benzodiazepin-2-one, 7-chloro-5-(2-chlorophenyl)-1,3-dihydro-3-hydroxy-, (±)-; (2) (±)-7-Chloro-5-(*o*-chlorophenyl)-1,3-dihydro-3-hydroxy-2*H*-1,4-benzodiazepin-2-one. *UNII-O26FZP769L. CAS-846-49-1.* INN; BAN; JAN. *Tranquilizer (minor).* Ativan (Biovail) ◇*Wy-4036*

Lorbamate [*1970*] (lor bam′ ate). $C_{12}H_{22}N_2O_4$. 258.31. (1) Carbamic acid, cyclopropyl-, 2-[[(aminocarbonyl)oxy]methyl]-2-methylpentyl ester; (2) 2-(Hydroxymethyl)-2-methylpentyl cyclopropanecarbamate carbamate (ester). *CAS-24353-88-6; CAS-30865-33-9* [replaced]. INN. *Relaxant (muscle).* ◇*Abbott-19957*

Lorcainide Hydrochloride [*1977*] (lor′ ka nide hye″ droe klor′ ide). $C_{22}H_{27}ClN_2O \cdot HCl$. 407.38. [Lorcainide is INN and BAN.] (1) Benzeneacetamide, *N*-(4-chlorophenyl)-*N*-[1-(1-methylethyl)-4-piperidinyl]-, monohydrochloride; (2) 4′-Chloro-*N*-(1-isopropyl-4-piperidyl)-2-phenylacetanilide monohydrochloride. *UNII-1T1S98ONM1. CAS-58934-46-6; CAS-59729-31-6* [lorcainide]. *Cardiac depressant (anti-arrhythmic).* ◇*R 15,889*

Lorcaserin Hydrochloride [*2006*] (lor ka′ ser in hye″ droe klor′ ide). $C_{11}H_{14}ClN \cdot HCl$. 232.15. [Lorcaserin is INN.] (1) 1*H*-3-Benzazepine, 8-chloro-2,3,4,5-tetrahydro-1-methyl-, hydrochloride, (1*R*)-; (2) (1*R*)-8-Chloro-1-methyl-2,3,4,5-tetrahydro-1*H*-3-benzazepine hydrochloride. *UNII-0QJF08GDPE. CAS-846589-98-8; CAS-616202-92-7* [lorcaserin]. *Anti-obesity (activate 5-HT₂c receptor).* ◇*APD356*

Lorcinadol [*1989*] (lor sin′ a dol). $C_{17}H_{19}ClN_4$. 314.81. (1) Pyridazine, 3-chloro-6-[4-(3-phenyl-2-propenyl)-1-piperazinyl]-, (*E*)-; (2) (*E*)-3-Chloro-6-(4-cinnamyl-1-piperazinyl)pyridazine. *UNII-S1IC65Y242. CAS-104719-71-3.* INN; BAN. *Analgesic.* ◇*R 62 818*

Loreclezole [*1991*] (lor ek′ le zole). $C_{10}H_6Cl_3N_3$. 274.53. (1) 1*H*-1,2,4-Triazole, 1-[2-chloro-2-(2,4-dichlorophenyl)ethenyl]-, (*Z*)-; (2) (*Z*)-1-(β,2,4-Trichlorostyryl)-1*H*-1,2,4-triazole. *UNII-6DJ32STZ5W. CAS-117857-45-1.* INN; BAN. *Anti-epileptic.* ◇*R 72063*

Lorglumide. $C_{22}H_{32}Cl_2N_2O_4$. 459.41. (±)-4-(3,4-Dichlorobenzamido)-*N*,*N*-dipentylglutaramic acid. *UNII-LAD1UQ73BE. CAS-97964-56-2.* INN.

Lormetazepam [*1980*] (lor me taz′ e pam). C₁₆H₁₂Cl₂N₂O₂. 335.18. (1) 2*H*-1,4-Benzodiazepin-2-one, 7-chloro-5-(2-chlorophenyl)-1,3-dihydro-3-hydroxy-1-methyl-; (2) 7-Chloro-5-(*o*-chlorophenyl)-1,3-dihydro-3-hydroxy-1-methyl-2*H*-1,4-benzodiazepin-2-one. *CAS-848-75-9.* INN; BAN; JAN. *Sedative-hypnotic.* ◇*WY-4082*

Lornoxicam [*1993*] (lor nox′ i kam). C₁₃H₁₀ClN₃O₄S₂. 371.82. (1) 2*H*-Thieno[2,3-*e*]-1,2-thiazine-3-carboxamide, 6-chloro-4-hydroxy-2-methyl-*N*-2-pyridinyl-, 1,1-dioxide; (2) 6-Chloro-4-hydroxy-2-methyl-*N*-2-pyridyl-2*H*-thieno[2,3-*e*]-1,2-thiazine-3-carboxamide 1,1-dioxide. *UNII-ER09126G7A.* CAS-70374-39-9. INN; BAN. *Analgesic; anti-inflammatory.* ◇*Ro 13-9297; CTX*

Lorpiprazole. C₂₁H₂₆F₃N₅. 405.46. (±)-*cis*-5,5a,6,7,8,8a-Hexahydro-3-[2-[4-(α,α,α-trifluoro-*m*-tolyl)-1-piperazinyl]ethyl]cyclopenta[3,4]pyrrolo[2,1-*c*]-*s*-triazole. *UNII-0M14O7T47Q.* CAS-108785-69-9. INN.

Lortalamine [*1986*] (lor tal′ a meen). C₁₅H₁₇ClN₂O₂. 292.76. (1) 4a,10-(Iminoethano)-4a*H*-[1]benzopyrano[3,2-*c*]pyridin-12-one, 8-chloro-1,2,3,4,10,10a-hexahydro-2-methyl-, (4aα,10α,10aα)-(±)-; (2) (±)-(4a*R**,10*R**,10a*S**)-8-Chloro-1,2,3,4,10,10a-hexahydro-2-methyl-4a,10-(iminoethano)-4a*H*-[1]benzopyrano[3,2-*c*]pyridin-12-one. *CAS-70384-91-7.* INN. *Antidepressant.* ◇*LM-1404*

Lorzafone [*1983*] (lor′ za fone). C₁₈H₁₇Cl₂N₃O₃.H₂O. 412.27. (1) Glycinamide, glycyl-*N*-[4-chloro-2-(2-chlorobenzoyl)-phenyl]-*N*-methyl-, monohydrate; (2) 2-(2-Aminoac-

etamido)-4′-chloro-2′-(*o*-chlorobenzoyl)-*N*-methylacetanilide monohydrate. *CAS-81603-65-8; CAS-59179-95-2* [anhydrous]. INN. *Tranquilizer (minor).* ◇*LY 123508*

Losartan Potassium [*1992*] (loe sar′ tan poe tas′ ee um). USP. C₂₂H₂₂ClKN₆O. 461.00. [Losartan is INN and BAN.] (1) 1*H*-Imidazole-5-methanol, 2-butyl-4-chloro-1-[[2′-(1*H*-tetrazol-5-yl)[1,1′-biphenyl]-4-yl]methyl]-, monopotassium salt; (2) 2-Butyl-4-chloro-1-[*p*-(*o*-1*H*-tetrazol-5-ylphenyl)benzyl]imidazole-5-methanol, monopotassium salt. *UNII-3ST302B24A; UNII-JMS50MPO89* [losartan]. *CAS-124750-99-8; CAS-114798-26-4* [losartan]. *Antihypertensive.* Cozaar (Merck) ◇*DuP 753*

Losigamone. C₁₂H₁₁ClO₄. 254.67. (5*R**)-5-[(α*S**)-*o*-Chloro-α-hydroxybenzyl]-4-methoxy-2(5*H*)-furanone. *CAS-112856-44-7.* INN.

Losindole. C₁₉H₂₀ClN. 297.82. (±)-(3aα,4α,9aα)-6-Chloro-3a,4,9,9a-tetrahydro-2-methyl-4-phenylbenz[*f*]isoindoline. *UNII-IX8TM6153H.* CAS-69175-77-5. INN.

Losmiprofen. C₁₇H₁₅ClO₄. 318.75. (±)-2-[[3-(*p*-Chlorobenzoyl)-*o*-tolyl]oxy]propionic acid. *UNII-GRY6X9550R.* CAS-74168-08-4. INN.

Losoxantrone Hydrochloride [*1992*] (loe sox′ an trone hye″ droe klor′ ide). C₂₂H₂₇N₅O₄.2HCl.½H₂O. 507.41. [Losoxantrone is INN and BAN.] (1) Anthra[1,9-*cd*]pyrazol-6(2*H*)-one, 7-hydroxy-2-[2-[(2-hydroxyethyl)amino]ethyl]-5-[[2-[(2-hydroxyethyl)amino]ethyl]amino]-, dihydrochloride, hydrate (2:1); (2) 7-Hydroxy-2-[2-[(2-hydroxyethyl)amino]ethyl]-5-[[2-[(2-hydroxyethyl)amino]ethyl]amino]anthra[1,9-*cd*]pyrazol-6(2*H*)-one, dihydrochloride, hemihydrate. *UNII-W6E2751URX.* CAS-

---

† Brand name formerly used, and/or firm no longer concerned with this product.

132937-89-4; CAS-88303-60-0 [losoxantrone]. Antineoplastic. [Name previously used for the free base: Biantrazole.] ◇*DUP 941; NSC-357885*

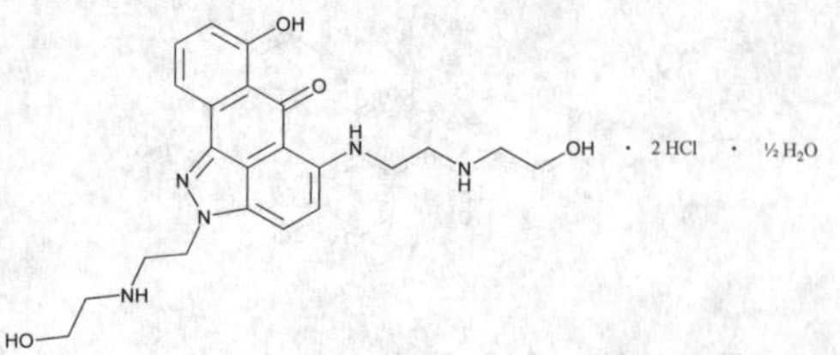

Losulazine Hydrochloride [*1984*] (loe sul′ a zeen hye″ droe klor′ ide). $C_{27}H_{22}F_4N_4O_3S.HCl$. 595.01. [Losulazine is INN.] (1) Piperazine, 1-[(4-fluorophenyl)sulfonyl]-4-[4-[[7-(trifluoromethyl)-4-quinolinyl]amino]benzoyl]-, monohydrochloride; (2) 1-[(*p*-Fluorophenyl)sulfonyl]-4-[*p*-[[7-(trifluoromethyl)-4-quinolyl]amino]benzoyl]piperazine monohydrochloride. *CAS-81435-67-8. Antihypertensive.* ◇*U-54,669F*

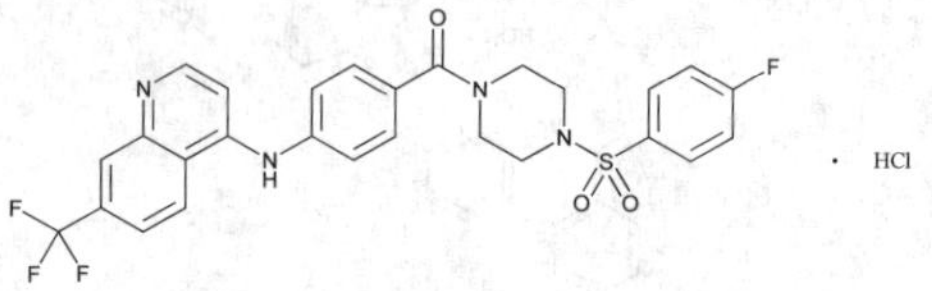

Loteprednol Etabonate [*1990*] (loe″ te pred′ nol et″ a boe′ nate). $C_{24}H_{31}ClO_7$. 466.95. [Loteprednol is INN and BAN.] (1) Androsta-1,4-diene-17-carboxylic acid, 17-[(ethoxycarbonyl)oxy]-11-hydroxy-3-oxo-, chloromethyl ester, (11β,17α)-; (2) Chloromethyl 11β,17-dihydroxy-3-oxo-androsta-1,4-diene-17β-carboxylate, 17-(ethyl carbonate). *UNII-YEH1EZ96K6; UNII-Z8CBU6KR16 [loteprednol]. CAS-82034-46-6; CAS-129260-79-3 [loteprednol]. Anti-inflammatory (topical).* Alrex (Bausch & Lomb); Lotemax (Bausch & Lomb) ◇*P-5604; HGP-1; CDDD 5604*

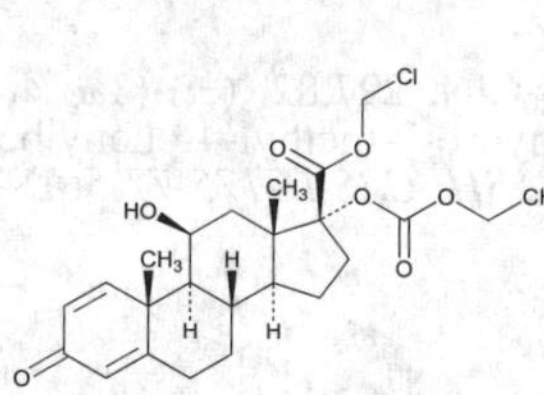

Lotifazole. $C_{12}H_9Cl_3N_2O_2S$. 351.64. 2,2,2-Trichloroethyl 4-phenyl-2-thiazolecarbamate. *UNII-1B3TF200TI. CAS-71119-10-3.* INN.

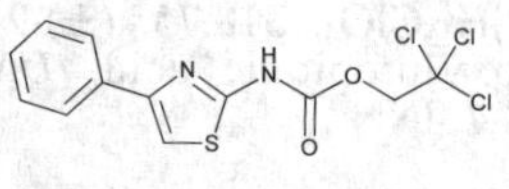

Lotifocon B [*1994*] (loe″ ti foe′ kon). $(C_{16}H_{38}O_5Si_4)_u(C_{26}H_{58}O_9Si_6)_v(C_5H_8O_2)_w(C_6H_7F_3O_2)_x(C_4H_6O_2)_y(C_{10}H_{14}O_4)_z$. (1) 3-[3,3,3-Trimethyl-1,1-bis[(trimethylsilyl)oxy]disiloxanyl]propyl 2-methyl-2-propenoate polymer with [1,1,3,3-tetrakis[(trimethylsilyl)oxy]-1,3-disiloxane-diyl]di-3,1-propanediyl bis(2-methyl-2-propenoate, methyl 2-methyl-2-propenoate, 2,2,2-trifluoroethyl 2-methyl-2-propenoate, 2-methyl-2-propenoic acid, and 1,2-ethanediyl bis(2-methyl-2-propenoate); (2) 3-[3,3,3-Trimethyl-1,1-bis(trimethylsiloxy)disiloxanyl]propyl methacrylate polymer with [1,1,3,3-tetrakis(trimethylsiloxy)disiloxanylene]-bis(trimethylene) dimethacrylate, methyl methacrylate, 2,2,2-trifluoroethyl methacrylate, methacrylic acid and ethylene dimethacrylate. *CAS-144031-34-5. Contact lens material (hydrophobic).* OP-2 (Sterling Winthrop) [*Note—The oxygen permeability of the contact lens material is 15 × $10^{-11}(cm^2/sec)(ml\ O_2/ml × mm\ Hg)$ at 35°C (Dk value).]*

Lotifocon C [*1994*] (loe″ ti foe′ kon). $(C_{16}H_{38}O_5Si_4)_u(C_{26}H_{58}O_9Si_6)_v(C_5H_8O_2)_w(C_6H_7F_3O_2)_x(C_4H_6O_2)_y(C_{10}H_{14}O_4)_z$. (1) 3-[3,3,3-Trimethyl-1,1-bis[(trimethylsilyl)oxy]disiloxanyl]propyl 2-methyl-2-propenoate polymer with [1,1,3,3-tetrakis[(trimethylsilyl)oxy]-1,3-disiloxane-diyl]di-3,1-propanediyl bis(2-methyl-2-propenoate, methyl 2-methyl-2-propenoate, 2,2,2-trifluoroethyl 2-methyl-2-propenoate, 2-methyl-2-propenoic acid, and 1,2-ethanediyl bis(2-methyl-2-propenoate); (2) 3-[3,3,3-Trimethyl-1,1-bis(trimethylsiloxy)disiloxanyl]propyl methacrylate polymer with [1,1,3,3-tetrakis(trimethylsiloxy)disiloxanylene]-bis(trimethylene) dimethacrylate, methyl methacrylate, 2,2,2-trifluoroethyl methacrylate, methacrylic acid and ethylene dimethacrylate. *CAS-144031-34-5. Contact lens material (hydrophobic).* OP-6 (Sterling Winthrop) [*Note—The oxygen permeability of the contact lens material is 58 × $10^{-11}(cm^2/sec)(ml\ O_2/ml × mm\ Hg)$ at 35°C (Dk value).]*

Lotrafiban Hydrochloride [*1997*] (loe″ tra fye′ ban hye″ droe klor′ ide). $C_{23}H_{32}N_4O_4.HCl$. 464.99. [Lotrafiban is INN.] (*S*)-2,3,4,5-Tetrahydro-4-methyl-3-oxo-7-[[4-(4-piperidyl)piperidino]carbonyl]-1*H*-1,4-benzodiazepine-2-acetic acid, monohydrochloride. *UNII-GSV7V79C63. CAS-179599-82-7; CAS-171049-14-2 [lotrafiban]. Antithrombotic; platelet aggregation inhibitor.* ◇*SB-214857-A*

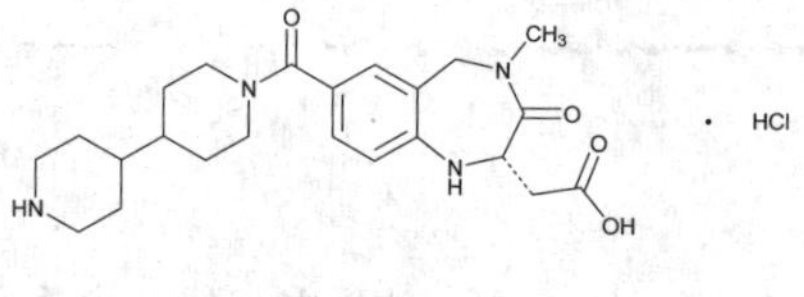

Lotrafilcon A [*1996*] (loe″ tra fil′ kon). $(C_{103}H_{217}N_3F_{36}O_{49}Si_{27})_x(C_5H_9NO)_y(C_{16}H_{38}O_5Si_4)_z$. (1) 2-Propenoic acid, 2-methyl-, 2-isocyanatoethyl ester, polymer with *N,N*-dimethyl-2-propenamide,Fomblin Z-DOL,α-[[3-(2-hydroxyethyl)propyl]dimethylsilyl]-ω-[[[3-(2-hydroxyethoxy)-propyl]dimethylsilyl]oxy]poly[oxy(dimethylsilylene)], 5-isocyanato-1-(isocyanatomethyl)-1,3,3-trimethylcyclohexane, and 3-[3,3,3-trimethyl-1,1-bis[trimethylsilyl)oxy]disiloxanyl]propyl 2-methyl-2-propenoate; (2) 2-Isocyanatoethyl methacrylate polymer with *N,N*-dimethylacrylamide, 2,2,4,4,6,6,8,8,10,10,12,12,14,14,16,16,17,17,19,19,20,20,22,22,23,23,25,25,26,26,28,28,29,29,31,31-hexatriacontafluoro-3,5,7,9,11,13,15,18,21,24,27,30-dodecaoxadotriacontane-1,32-diol, 2,2-[(tetrapentacontamethylheptacosasiloxanylene)bis(trimethyleneoxy)diethanol, 5-isocyanato-1-(isocyanatomethyl)-1,3,3-trimethylcyclohexane, and 3-[3,3,3-trimethyl-1,1-bis[trimethylsiloxy]disiloxanyl]propylmethacrylate. *CAS-203170-33-3. Contact lens material (hydrophilic).* See3 (Ciba Vision) [*Note—The water content of the contact lens material is 24% at ambient temperature (23±2°C), and the oxygen permeability is 140 × $10^{-11}(cm^2/sec)(ml\ O_2/ml × mm\ Hg)$ at 35°C (Dk intrinsic).]*

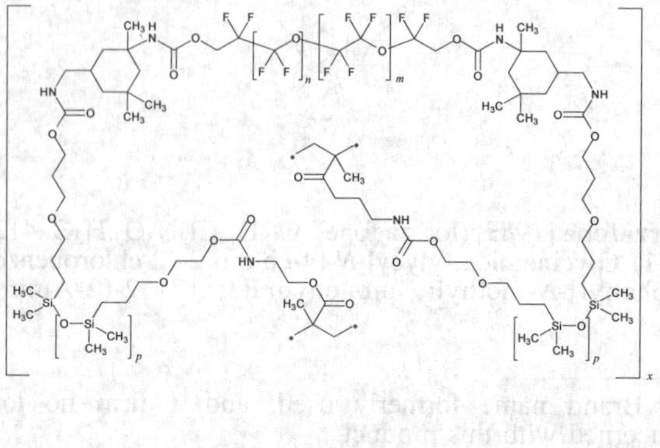

Lotrafilcon B [*2000*] (loe″ tra fil′ kon). ($C_{103}H_{217}N_3F_{36}O_{49}$-$Si_{27})_x(C_5H_9NO)_y(C_{16}H_{38}O_5Si_4)_z$. (1) 2-Propenoic acid, 2-methyl-, 2-isocyanatoethyl ester, polymer with *N,N*-dimethyl-2-propenamide,Fomblin Z-DOL,α-[[3-(2-hydroxyethyl)propyl]dimethylsilyl]-ω-[[[3-(2-hydroxyethoxy)propyl]dimethylsilyl]oxy]poly[oxy(dimethylsilylene)], 5-isocyanato-1-(isocyanatomethyl)-1,3,3-trimethylcyclohexane, and 3-[3,3,3-trimethyl-1,1-bis[trimethylsilyl]oxy]disiloxanyl]propyl 2-methyl-2-propenoate; (2) 2-Isocyanatoethyl methacrylate polymer with *N,N*-dimethylacrylamide, 2,2,4,4,6,6,8,8,10,10,12,12,14,14,16,16,17,17,19,19,20,20,22,22,23,23,25,25,26,26,28,28,29,29,31,31-hexatriacontafluoro-3,5,7,9,11,13,15,18,21,24,27,30-dodecaoxadotriacontane-1,32-diol, 2,2-[(tetrapentacontamethylheptacosasiloxanylene)bis(trimethyleneoxy)diethanol, 5-isocyanato-1-(isocyanatomethyl)-1,3,3-trimethylcyclohexane, and 3-[3,3,3-trimethyl-1,1-bis[trimethylsiloxy]disiloxanyl]propylmethacrylate. *CAS-203170-33-3. Contact lens material (hydrophilic).[Note— The water content of the contact lens material is 33% at ambient temperature (23±2°C), and the oxygen permeability is 110 ± 2 × 10⁻¹¹(cm²/sec)(ml O₂/ml × mm Hg) at 35°C (Dk intrinsic).]*

Lotrifen. $C_{16}H_{10}ClN_3$. 279.72. 2-(*p*-Chlorophenyl)-*s*-triazolo[5,1-*a*]isoquinoline. *UNII-K6J75G277H. CAS-66535-86-2.* INN; MI.

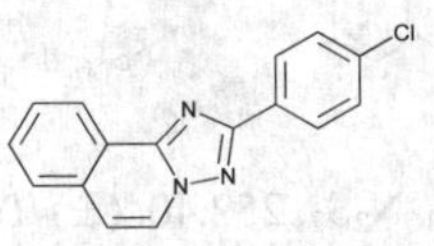

Lotucaine. $C_{18}H_{29}NO_2$. 291.43. 2,2,5,5-Tetramethyl-α-[(*o*-tolyloxy)methyl]-1-pyrrolidineethanol. *UNII-QCA39I2AP7. CAS-52304-85-5.* INN; DCF. ◇*MY-33-7 [as hydrochloride]*

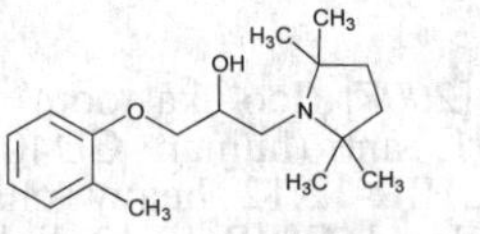

Lovastatin [*1987*] (loe″ va stat′ in). **USP.** $C_{24}H_{36}O_5$. 404.54. (1) Butanoic acid, 2-methyl-, 1,2,3,7,8,8a-hexahydro-3,7-dimethyl-8-[2-(tetrahydro-4-hydroxy-6-oxo-2*H*-pyran-2-yl)ethyl]-1-naphthalenyl ester, [1*S*-[1α(*R**),3α,7β,8β(2*S**,4*S**),8aβ]]-; (2) (*S*)-2-Methylbutyric acid, 8-ester with (4*R*,6*R*)-6-[2-[(1*S*,2*S*,6*R*,8*S*,8a*R*)-1,2,6,7,8,8a-hexahydro-8-hydroxy-2,6-dimethyl-1-naphthyl]ethyl]tetrahydro-4-hydroxy-2*H*-pyran-2-one. *UNII-9LHU78OQFD. CAS-75330-75-5.* INN; BAN. *Antihyperlipidemic; inhibitor (HMG-CoA reductase).* Altoprev (Teva); Mevacor (Merck) *[Name previously used: Mevinolin.]* ◇*MK-803*

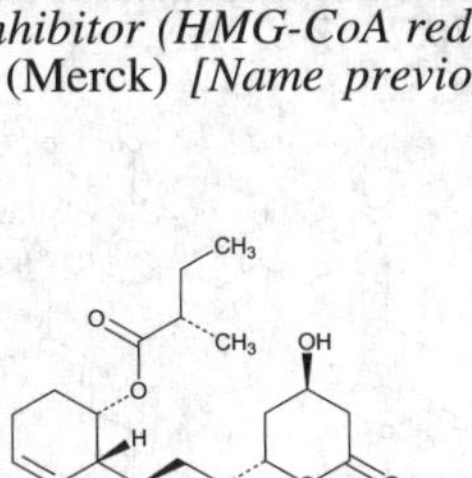

Loviride [*1997*] (loe′ vir ide). $C_{17}H_{16}Cl_2N_2O_2$. 351.23. (1) Benzeneacetamide, α-[(2-acetyl-5-methylphenyl)amino]-2,6-dichloro-, (±)-; (2) (±)-2-(6-Acetyl-*m*-toluidino)-2-(2,6-dichlorophenyl)acetamide. *CAS-147362-57-0.* INN; BAN. *Antiviral.* ◇*R-89439*

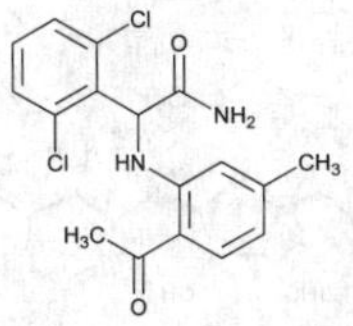

Loxanast. $C_{14}H_{26}O_2$. 226.36. *cis*-4-Isohexyl-1-methylcyclohexanecarboxylic acid. *UNII-746YWK1B07. CAS-69915-62-4.* INN.

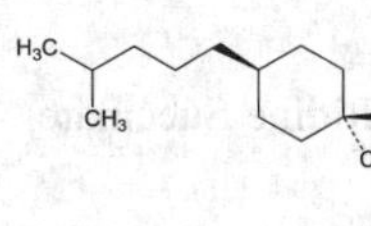

Loxapine [*1969*] (lox′ a peen). $C_{18}H_{18}ClN_3O$. 327.81. (1) Dibenz[*b,f*][1,4]oxazepine, 2-chloro-11-(4-methyl-1-piperazinyl)-; (2) 2-Chloro-11-(4-methyl-1-piperazinyl)dibenz[*b,f*][1,4]oxazepine. *UNII-LER583670J. CAS-1977-10-2.* INN; BAN. *Tranquilizer (minor).* Loxitane-C Oral Suspension [as hydrochloride] (Wyeth-Ayerst); Loxitane Intramuscular [as hydrochloride] (Wyeth-Ayerst) ◇*SUM 3170; CL 62,362*

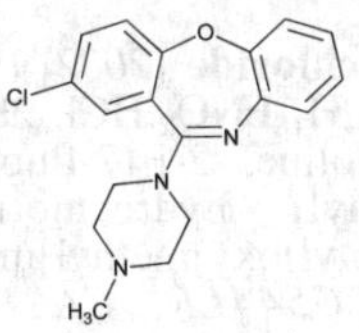

Loxapine Succinate [*1969*] (lox′ a peen sux′ i nate). **USP.** $C_{18}H_{18}ClN_3O.C_4H_6O_4$. 445.90. (1) Butanedioic acid, compd. with 2-chloro-11-(4-methyl-1-piperazinyl)dibenz[*b,f*][1,4]oxazepine (1:1); (2) 2-Chloro-11-(4-methyl-1-piperazinyl)dibenz[*b,f*][1,4]oxazepine succinate (1:1). *UNII-X59SG0MRYU; UNII-LER583670J. CAS-27833-64-3; CAS-1977-10-2 [loxapine]. Tranquilizer (minor).* Loxapine (Mylan); Loxitane (Watson) ◇*CL 71563*

Loxiglumide. $C_{21}H_{30}Cl_2N_2O_5$. 461.38. (±)-4-(3,4-Dichlorobenzamido)-*N*-(3-methoxypropyl)-*N*-pentylglutaramic acid. *CAS-107097-80-3.* INN.

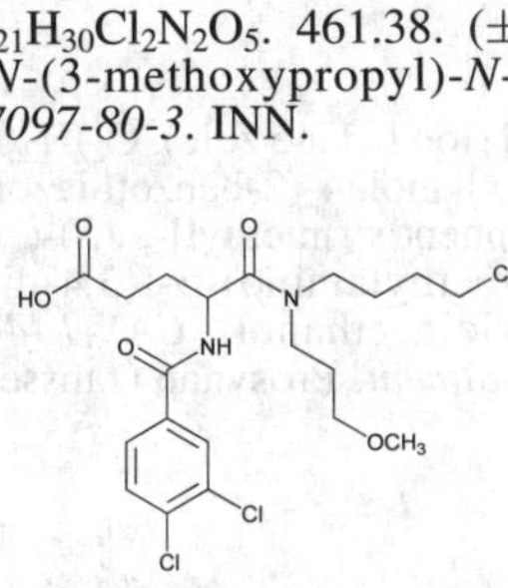

Loxoprofen. $C_{15}H_{18}O_3$. 246.30. [Loxoprofen Sodium is JAN.] (±)-*p*-[(2-Oxocyclopentyl)methyl]hydratropic acid. *UNII-3583H0GZAP. CAS-68767-14-6.* INN; MI.

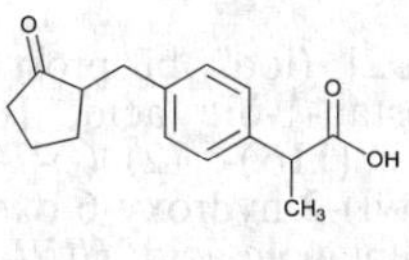

Loxoribine [*1990*] (lox or′ i been). $C_{13}H_{17}N_5O_6$. 339.30. (1) Guanosine, 7,8-dihydro-8-oxo-7-(2-propenyl)-; (2) 7-Allyl-2-amino-9-β-D-ribofuranosylpurine-6,8(1*H*,9*H*)-dione. *UNII-9CAS0V66OI. CAS-121288-39-9.* INN. *Immunostimulant; vaccine adjuvant.* ◇*RWJ 21757*

Loxotidine (previously used name) — *See* Lavoltidine Succinate.

Loxtidine — *See* Lavoltidine Succinate.

Lozilurea. $C_{10}H_{13}ClN_2O$. 212.68. 1-(*m*-Chlorobenzyl)-3-ethylurea. *UNII-677AYV0R9N. CAS-71475-35-9.* INN.

Lubazodone Hydrochloride [*2002*] (loo baz′ oh done hye″ droe klor′ ide). $C_{14}H_{18}FNO_2 \cdot HCl$. 287.76. [Lubazodone is INN.] (1) Morpholine, 2-[[(7-fluoro-2,3-dihydro-1*H*-inden-4-yl)oxy]methyl]-, hydrochloride (2*S*)-; (2) (*S*)-2-[[(7-Fluoro-4-indanyl)oxy]methyl]morpholine hydrochloride. *UNII-2KT2C544LR. CAS-161178-10-5; CAS-161178-07-0* [lubazodone]. *Antidepressant (selective serotonin (5-HT) reuptake inhibitor and 5-HT$_{2A}$antagonist).* ◇*YM992; YM-35992; SM-50C*

Lubeluzole [*1997*] (loo bel′ ue zole). $C_{22}H_{25}F_2N_3O_2S$. 433.51. (1) 1-Piperidineethanol, 4-(2-benzothiazolylmethylamino)-α-[(3,4-difluorophenoxy)methyl]-, (*S*)-; (2) (+)-(*S*)-4-(2-Benzothiazolylmethylamino)-α-[(3,4-difluorophenoxy)-methyl]-1-piperidineethanol. *CAS-144665-07-6.* INN; BAN. *Stroke treatment.* Prosynap (Janssen) ◇*R-87926*

Lubiprostone [*2002*] (loo″ bi prost′ one). $C_{20}H_{32}F_2O_5$. 390.46. (1) Prostan-1-oic acid, 16,16-difluoro-11-hydroxy-9,15-dioxo-, (11α)-; (2) (-)-7-[(2*R*,4a*R*,5*R*,7a*R*)-2-(1,1-Difluoropentyl)-2-hydroxy-6-oxooctahydrocyclopenta[*b*]pyran-5-yl]heptanoic acid. *UNII-7662KG2R6K. CAS-136790-76-6.* INN. *Treatment of constipation and bowel*

preparation. Amitiza (Takeda) *[Note—The CA Index name and CAS Registry number are given for the tautomeric monocyclic isomer.]* ◇*RU-0211*

Lucanthone Hydrochloride [*1962*] (loo kan′ thone hye″ droe klor′ ide). $C_{20}H_{24}N_2OS \cdot HCl$. 376.94. [Lucanthone is INN and BAN.] (1) 9*H*-Thioxanthen-9-one, 1-[[2-(diethylamino)ethyl]amino]-4-methyl-, monohydrochloride; (2) 1-[[2-(Diethylamino)ethyl]amino]-4-methylthioxanthen-9-one monohydrochloride. *UNII-918K9N56QZ. CAS-548-57-2; CAS-479-50-5* [lucanthone]. USP XVIII. *Antischistosomal.* ◇*79 T61; NSC-14574*

Lucartamide. $C_{12}H_{16}N_2S_2$. 252.40. ($\pm$)-Tetrahydro-*N*-methyl-2-(6-methyl-2-pyridyl)thio-2-thiophenecarboxamide. *UNII-610T1NWH34. CAS-76743-10-7.* INN.

Lucatumumab [*2007*] (loo″ ka toom′ ue mab). (1) Immunoglobulin G1, anti-(human CD40 (antigen)) (human monoclonal CHIR-12.12 heavy chain), disulfide with human monoclonal CHIR-12.12 light chain, dimer; (2) Fully human recombinant monoclonal antibody of the IgG1 isotype targeting the human CD40 protein. Polypeptide composed of 1336 amino acid residues and with a molecular weight of approximately 146,000 daltons. *CAS-903512-50-5.* INN. *Treatment of cancer.* ◇*CHIR-12.12; HCD-122*

Lucensomycin — *See* Lucimycin.

Lucimycin. Antibiotic obtained from cultures of *Streptomyces lucensis,* or the same substance produced by any other means. *CAS-13058-67-8.* INN.

Lucinactant [*2003*] (loo″ sin ak′ tant). Lucinactant. A surfactant formulation containing a mixture of synthetic phospholipids, fatty acid, and synthetic peptide. Lucinactant is comprised of sinapultide, colfosceril palmitate (dipalmitoylphosphatidylcholine [DPPC]), palmitoyloleaylphosphatidyl glycerol, sodium salt (POPG), and palmitic acid. *Treatment of respiratory distress syndrome (RDS) in adults; treatment and prevention of RDS in infants.* ◇*KL₄-surfactant; ATI 02*

Lufenuron. $C_{17}H_8Cl_2F_8N_2O_3$. 511.15. 1-[2,5-Dichloro-4-(1,1,2,3,3,3-hexafluoropropoxy)phenyl]-3-(2,6-difluoro-benzoyl)urea. *UNII-1R754M4918. CAS-103055-07-8.* INN; BAN.

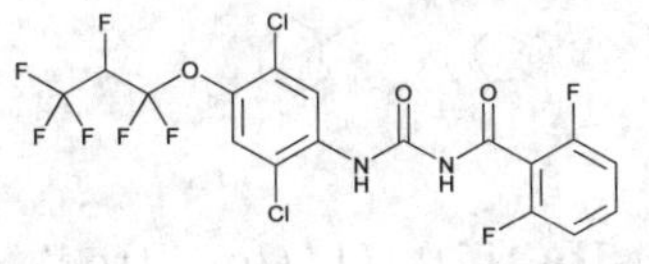

Lufironil [*1993*] (loo fir′ oh nil). $C_{13}H_{19}N_3O_4$. 281.31. (1) 2,4-Pyridinedicarboxamide,*N,N′*-bis(2-methoxyethyl)-; (2) *N,N′*-Bis(2-methoxyethyl)-2,4-pyridinedicarboxamide. *CAS-128075-79-6.* INN. *Inhibitor (collagen).* ◇*HOE 077*

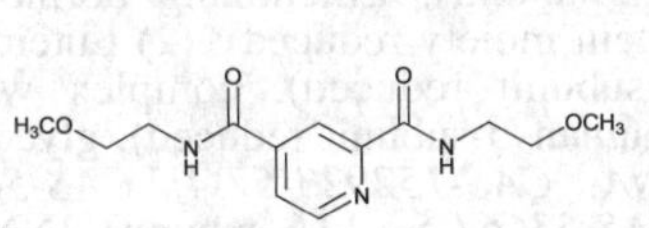

Lufuradom. $C_{22}H_{20}FN_3O_2$. 377.41. (±)-*N*-[(8-Fluoro-2,3-dihydro-1-methyl-5-phenyl-1*H*-1,4-benzodiazepin-2-yl)methyl]-3-furamide. *UNII-GS8D070P7W. CAS-85118-42-9.* INN.

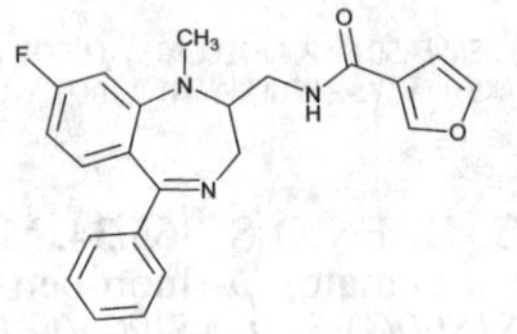

Luliconazole. $C_{14}H_9Cl_2N_3S_2$. 354.28. (-)-(*E*)-[(4*R*)-4-(2,4-Dichlorophenyl)-1,3-dithiolan-2-ylidene](1*H*-imidazol-1-yl)acetonitrile. *UNII-RE91AN4S8G. CAS-187164-19-8.* INN.

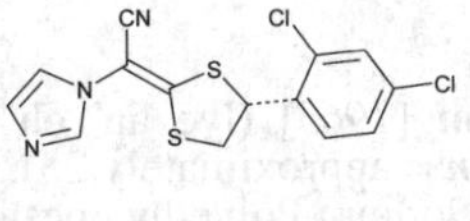

Lumefantrine [*2008*] (loo″ me fan′ treen). $C_{30}H_{32}Cl_3NO$. 528.94. (1) 9*H*-Fluorene-4-methanol, 2,7-dichloro-9-[(4-chlorophenyl)methylene]-α-[(dibutylamino)methyl]-, (9*Z*)-; (2) (1*RS*)-2-(Dibutylamino)-1-{(9*Z*)-2,7-dichloro-9-[(4-chlorophenyl)methylene]-9*H*-fluorene-4-yl}ethanol. *UNII-F38R0JR742. CAS-82186-77-4.* INN; BAN. *Antimalarial.*

Lumiliximab [*2003*] (loo″ mi lix′ i mab). $C_{6850}H_{10656}N_{1824}O_{2106}S_{50}$. Immunoglobulin G1, anti-(human immunoglobulin E receptor type II) (human-Macaca irus monoclonal IDEC-152 γ1-chain), disulfide with human-Macaca irus monoclonal IDEC-152 κ-chain, dimer. *CAS-357613-86-6.* INN. *Treatment of allergic asthma, allergic rhinitis, and chronic lymphocytic leukemia.* ◇*IDEC-152*

Lumiracoxib [*2002*] (loo mye″ ra kox′ ib). $C_{15}H_{13}ClFNO_2$. 293.72. (1) Benzeneacetic acid, 2-[(2-chloro-6-fluorophenyl)amino]-5-methyl-; (2) 2-[(2-Chloro-6-fluorophenyl)a-mino]-5-methylphenyl]acetic acid. *UNII-V91T9204HU. CAS-220991-20-8.* INN; BAN. *Treatment of rheumatoid arthritis, osteoarthritis, and pain prevention.* ◇*COX-189*

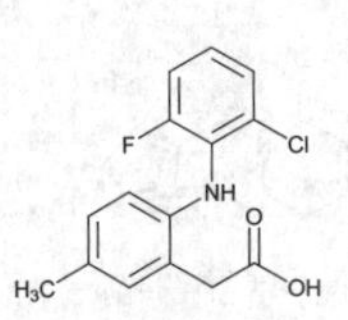

Lupitidine Hydrochloride [*1985*] (loo pi′ ti deen hye″ droe klor′ ide). $C_{21}H_{27}N_5O_2S.3HCl$. 522.92. [Lupitidine is INN.] (1) 4(1*H*)-Pyrimidinone, 2-[[2-[[[5-[(dimethylamino)-methyl]-2-furanyl]methyl]thio]ethyl]amino]-5-[(6-methyl-3-pyridinyl)methyl]-, trihydrochloride; (2) 2-[[2-[[5-[(Di-methylamino)methyl]furfuryl]thio]ethyl]amino]-5-[(6-methyl-3-pyridyl)methyl]-4-(1*H*)-pyrimidinone trihy-drochloride. *CAS-72716-75-7; CAS-83903-06-4* [lupiti-dine]. *Antagonist (to histamine H₂receptors, veterinary).* ◇*SK&F 93479*

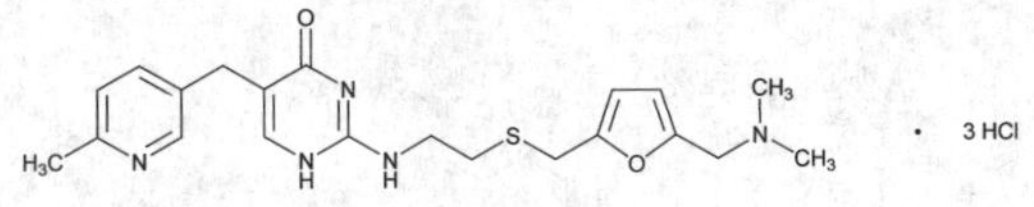

Luprostiol. $C_{21}H_{29}ClO_6S$. 444.97. (±)-(*Z*)-7-[(1*R**,2*S**,3*S**,5*R**)-2-[[(2*R**)-3-(*m*-Chlorophenoxy)-2-hy-droxypropyl]thio]-3,5-dihydroxycyclopentyl]-5-heptenoic acid. *UNII-HWR60H5GZB. CAS-67110-79-6.* INN; BAN; MI.

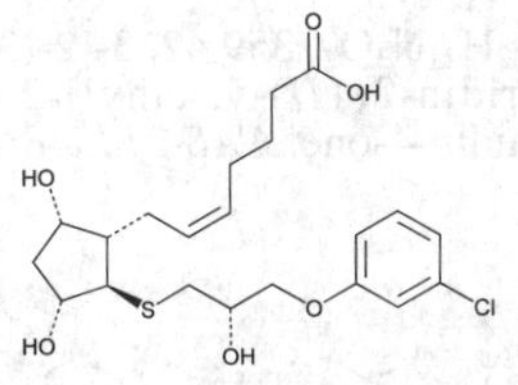

Lurasidone Hydrochloride [*2005*] (loo ras′ i done hye″ droe klor′ ide). $C_{28}H_{36}N_4O_2S.HCl$. 529.14. [Lurasidone is INN.] (1) 4,7-Methano-1*H*-isoindole-1,3(2*H*)-dione, 2-[[(1*R*,2*R*)-2-[[4-(1,2-benzisothiazol-3-yl)-1-piperazinyl]methyl]cy-clohexyl]methyl]hexahydro-, monohydrochloride (3a*R*,4*S*,7*R*,7a*S*)-; (2) (3a*R*,4*S*,7*R*,7a*S*)-2-{(1*R*,2*R*)-2-[1,2-Benzisothiazol-3-yl)piperazin-1-ylmethyl]cyclohexyl-methyl}hexahydro-4,7-methano-2*H*-isoindole-1,3-dione, hydrochloride. *UNII-O0P4I58511I. CAS-367514-88-3; CAS-367514-87-2* [lurasidone]. *Treatment of schizophre-nia (high-affinity agonist of serotonin 5-HT1A, 5-HT2, and 5-HT7 receptors as well as dopamine D2 receptors).* ◇*SM-13496*

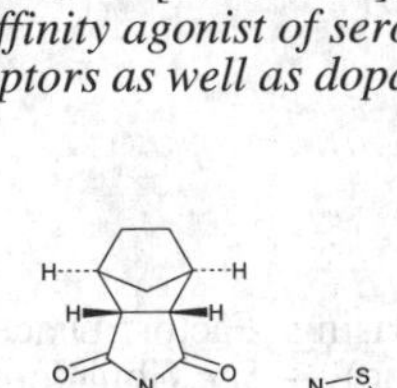

Lurosetron Mesylate [*1993*] (loo roe′ se tron mes′ i late). $C_{17}H_{17}FN_4O.CH_4O_3S$. 408.45. [Lurosetron is INN and BAN.] (1) 1*H*-Pyrido[4,3-*b*]indol-1-one, 6-fluoro-2,3,4,5-tetrahydro-5-methyl-2-[(5-methyl-1*H*-imidazol-4-yl)-methyl]-, monomethanesulfonate; (2) 6-Fluoro-2,3,4,5-tetrahydro-5-methyl-2-[(5-methylimidazol-4-yl)methyl]-

---

† Brand name formerly used, and/or firm no longer concerned with this product.

1*H*-pyrido[4,3-*b*]indol-1-one monomethanesulfonate. *CAS-143486-90-2; CAS-128486-54-4* [lurosetron]. *Antiemetic.* ◇*GR 87442 N*

Lurtotecan Dihydrochloride [*1996*] (loor″ toe tee′ kan dye hye″ droe klor′ ide). $C_{28}H_{30}N_4O_6 \cdot 2HCl$. 591.48. [Lurtotecan is INN.] (1) 11*H*-1,4-Dioxino[2,3-*g*]pyrano[3′,4′:6,7]indolizino[1,2-*b*]quinoline-9,12(8*H*,14*H*)-dione, 8-ethyl-2,3-dihydro-8-hydroxy-15-[(4-methyl-1-piperazinyl)methyl]-, dihydrochloride, (*S*); (2) (8*S*)-8-Ethyl-2,3-dihydro-8-hydroxy-15-[(4-methyl-1-piperazinyl)methyl]-11*H*-*p*-dioxino[2,3-*g*]pyrano[3′,4′:6,7]indolizino[1,2-*b*]quinoline-9,12(8*H*,14*H*)-dione dihydrochloride. *CAS-155773-58-3; CAS-149882-10-0* [lurtotecan]. *Antineoplastic (DNA topoisomerase I inhibitor).* ◇*GI147211C*

Lusaperidone. $C_{22}H_{21}N_3O_2$. 359.42. 3-[2-(3,4-Dihydrobenzofuro[3,2-*c*]pyridin-2(1*H*)-yl)ethyl]-2-methyl-4*H*-pyrido[1,2-*a*]pyrimidin-4-one. *CAS-214548-46-6.* INN.

Lusupultide [*2007*] (loo″ soo pul′ tide). $C_{182}H_{310}N_{40}O_{35} \cdot$ 3618.66. (1) 2-35-Lipoprotein SP-C (human pulmonary surfactant associated reduced), 5-L-phenylalanine-6-L-phenylalanine-33-L-isoleucine-; (2) [5-L-Phenylalanine,6-L-phenylalanine,33-L-isoleucine]human pulmonary surfactant-associated protein C-(2-35)-peptide. *UNII-6MCT347Y2B. CAS-200074-80-2.* INN. *Lung surfactant replacement.* ◇*B9420-001*

GIPFFPVHLK RLLIVVVVVV LIVVVIVGAL LIGL

Luteinizing Hormone-releasing Factor Diacetate Tetrahydrate (previously used name) — *See* Gonadorelin Acetate.

Luteinizing Hormone-releasing Factor Dihydrochloride (previously used name) — *See* Gonadorelin Hydrochloride.

Lutrelin Acetate [*1984*] (loo trel′ in as′ e tate). $C_{65}H_{85}N_{17}O_{12} \cdot C_2H_4O_2$. 1356.53. [Lutrelin is INN.] (1) Luteinizing hormone-releasing factor (pig), 6-D-tryptophan-7-(*N*-methyl-L-leucine)-9-(*N*-ethyl-L-prolinamide)-10-deglycinamide-, monoacetate (salt); (2) 5-Oxo-L-prolyl-L-histidyl-L-tryptophyl-L-seryl-L-tyrosyl-D-tryptophyl-*N*-methyl-L-leucyl-L-arginyl-*N*-ethyl-L-prolinamide monoacetate (salt). *CAS-83784-18-3; CAS-66866-63-5* [lutrelin]. *LHRH agonist.* ◇*WY-40,972*

Lutropin Alfa [*2001*] (loo troe′ pin al′ fa). $C_{437}H_{682}N_{122}O_{134}S_{13}$ (α-subunit). 10,205.67 (α-subunit); $C_{577}H_{929}N_{165}O_{161}S_{14}$ (β-subunit). 13,202.49 (β-subunit). (1) Luteinizing hormone (human α-subunit reduced complex human β-subunit reduced), glycoform α. [α-subunit]: Chorionic gonadotropin (human α-subunit protein moiety reduced); [β-subunit]: Luteinizing hormone (human β-subunit protein moiety reduced); (2) Luteinizing hormone (human α-subunit reduced), complex with luteinizing hormone (human β-subunit reduced), glycoform α. *UNII-3JGY52XJNA. CAS-152923-57-4; CAS-56832-30-5* [α-subunit]; *CAS-53664-53-2* [β-subunit]. INN; BAN. *Treatment of chronic anovulation due to hypogonadotropic hypogonadism.* Luveris (Serono) ◇*ATC G03 GA Gonadotropins*

```
SREPLRPWCH   PINAILAVEK   EGCPVCITVN   TTICAGYCPT   MMRVLQAVLP
PLPQVVCTYR   DVRFESIRLP   GCPRGVDPVV   SFPVALSCRC   GPCRRSTSDC
GGPKDHPLTC   DHPQLSGLLF   L

APDVQDCPEC   TLQENPFFSQ   PGAPILQCMG   CCFSRAYPTP   LRSKKTMLVQ
KNVTSESTCC   VAKSYNRVTV   MGGFKVENHT   ACHCSTCYYH   KS
```

Luxabendazole. $C_{15}H_{12}FN_3O_5S$. 365.34. Methyl 5-hydroxy-2-benzimidazolecarbamate, *p*-fluorobenzenesulfonate (ester). *UNII-34S1S00GV3. CAS-90509-02-7.* INN; BAN. ◇*HOE 216V*

Lyapolate Sodium [*1963*] (lye ap′ oh late soe′ dee um). $(C_2H_3NaO_3S)_n$ (*n* = approximately 25). [Sodium Apolate is INN and BAN; Sodium Polyethylenesulfonate is JAN.] (1) Ethenesulfonic acid, homopolymer, sodium salt; (2) Sodium ethenesulfonate polymer. *CAS-25053-27-4; CAS-26101-52-0* [ethenesulfonic acid homopolymer]. *Anticoagulant.* Peson (Hoechst-Roussel†)

Lycetamine [*1978*] (lye seet′ a meen). $C_{22}H_{47}N_3O$. 369.63. (1) Hexanamide, 2,6-diamino-*N*-hexadecyl-, (*S*)-; (2) L-2,6-Diamino-*N*-hexadecylhexanamide. *CAS-60209-20-3.* *Antimicrobial (topical).* ◇*P-71*

Lycine Hydrochloride — *See* Betaine Hydrochloride.

Lydimycin [*1968*] (lye″ di mye′ sin). $C_{10}H_{14}N_2O_3S$. 242.29. [Lidimycin is INN.] Antibiotic produced by *Streptomyces lydicus*. (1) 2-Pentenoic acid, 5-(hexahydro-2-oxo-1*H*-thieno[3,4-*d*]imidazol-4-yl)-, [3a*S*(3aα,4β,6aα)]-; (2) Lydimycin. *CAS-10118-85-1. Antifungal.* ◇*U-15,965*

Lymecycline. $C_{29}H_{38}N_4O_{10}$. 602.63. (+)-*N*-(5-Amino-5-carboxypentylaminomethyl)-4-dimethylamino-1,4,4a,5,5a,6,11,12a-octahydro-3,6,10,12,12a-pentahydroxy-6-methyl-1,11-dioxonaphthacene-2-carboxamide. *UNII-7D6EM3S13P. CAS-992-21-2.* INN; BAN; MI.

Lymphogranuloma Venereum Antigen. USP XXI. Lygranum (Bristol-Myers Squibb†)

Lynestrenol [*1962*] (lin es′ tre nol). $C_{20}H_{28}O$. 284.44. (1) 19 Norpregn-4-en-20-yn-17-ol, (17α)-; (2) 19-Nor-17α-pregn-4-en-20-yn-17-ol. *CAS-52-76-6.* INN; BAN; JAN. *Progestin.* ◇*NSC-37725*

Lynoestrenol (BAN) — *See* Lynestrenol.

Lypressin [*1965*] (lye pres′ in). **USP** [Nasal Solution]. $C_{46}H_{65}N_{13}O_{12}S_2$. 1056.22. (1) Vasopressin, 8-L-lysine-; (2) 8-L-Lysinevasopressin; (3) L-Cysteinyl-L-tyrosyl-L-phenylalanyl-L-glutaminyl-L-asparaginyl-L-cysteinyl-L-prolyl-L-lysylglycinamide cyclic (1→6)-disulfide. *UNII-7CZF3L922Y. CAS-50-57-7.* INN; BAN. *Antidiuretic; vasoconstrictor.* Diapid (Novartis) ◇*L-8*

Lysergic Acid Diethylamide — *See* Lysergide.

Lysergide. $C_{20}H_{25}N_3O$. 323.43. *N,N*-Diethyllysergamide. *UNII-8NA5SWF92O. CAS-50-37-3.* INN; BAN; DCF; MI. ◇*LSD*

Lysine [*1979*] (lye′ seen). $C_6H_{14}N_2O_2$. 146.19. (1) L-Lysine; (2) L-Lysine. *UNII-K3Z4F929H6. CAS-56-87-1* [L]. INN. *Amino acid.*

Lysine Acetate (lye′ seen as′ e tate). **USP**. $C_6H_{14}N_2O_2$.-$C_2H_4O_2$. 206.24. (1) L-Lysine monoacetate; (2) L-Lysine monoacetate. *UNII-TTL6G7LIWZ. CAS-57282-49-2. Amino acid.*

Lysine Hydrochloride [*1980*] (lye′ seen hye″ droe klor′ ide). **USP**. $C_6H_{14}N_2O_2$.HCl. 182.65. (1) L-Lysine monohydrochloride; (2) L-Lysine monohydrochloride. *UNII-JNJ23Q2COM. CAS-657-27-2; CAS-56-87-1* [L-lysine]. JAN. *Amino acid.*

Lysostaphin [*1966*] (lye″ soe staf′ in). Enzyme produced by *Staphylococcus staphylolyticus*. (1) Lysostaphin; (2) Lysostaphin. *CAS-9011-93-2. Antibacterial enzyme.*

Lysozyme Chloride. *CAS-9001-63-2* [lysozyme]. JAN.

Lysuride (previously used name) — *See* Lisuride.

Mabuprofen. $C_{15}H_{23}NO_2$. 249.35. (±)-*N*-(2-Hydroxyethyl)-*p*-isobutylhydratropamide. *UNII-02B8S6J90B. CAS-82821-47-4.* INN.

Mabuterol. $C_{13}H_{18}ClF_3N_2O$. 310.74. [Mabuterol Hydrochloride is JAN.] 4-Amino-α-[(*tert*-butylamino)methyl]-3-chloro-5-(trifluoromethyl)benzyl alcohol. *UNII-R4K19W6S7Q. CAS-56341-08-3.* INN; MI.

Macitentan. $C_{19}H_{20}Br_2N_6O_4S$. 588.27. *N*-[5-(4-Bromophenyl)-6-{2-[(5-bromopyrimidin-2-yl)oxi]ethoxy}pyrimidin-4-yl]-*N′*-propylsulfuric diamide. *CAS-441798-33-0.* INN.

Macrogol (BAN, JAN) — *See* Polyethylene Glycol.

Macrogol 8 Stearate (BAN) — *See* Polyoxyl 8 Stearate.

Macrogol 40 Stearate (BAN) — *See* Polyoxyl 40 Stearate.

Macrogol 4000 (INN) — *See* Polyethylene Glycol 4000.

Macrogol Ester 400 (INN) — *See* Polyoxyl 8 Stearate.

Macrogol Ester 2000 (INN) — *See* Polyoxyl 40 Stearate.

Macrophage-targeted β-glucocerebrosidase (previously used name) — *See* Alglucerase.

Macrosalb (^{131}I). Macroaggregated iodinated (^{131}I) human albumin. *CAS-54182-63-7.* INN; BAN.

---

† Brand name formerly used, and/or firm no longer concerned with this product.

Macrosalb (^{99m}Tc). [Technetium (^{99m}Tc) Labelled Macroaggregated Human Serum Albumin Injection is JAN.] Technetium (^{99m}Tc) labeled macroaggregated human serum albumin. *CAS-54277-47-3*. INN; BAN.

Maduramicin [*1985*] (ma dur″ a mye′ sin). $C_{47}H_{83}NO_{17}$. 934.16. (1) Lonomycin A, 23,27-didemethoxy-2,6,22-tridemethyl-11-*O*-demethyl-22-[(2,6-dideoxy-3,4-di-*O*-methyl-β-L-*arabino*-hexopyranosyl)oxy]-6-methoxy-, monoammonium salt, (3*R*,4*S*,5*S*,6*R*,7*S*,22*S*)-; (2) Ammonium (2*R*,3*S*,4*S*,5*R*,6*S*)-tetrahydro-2-hydroxy-6-[(*R*)-1-[(2*S*,5*R*,7*S*,8*R*,9*S*)-9-hydroxy-2,8-dimethyl-1-2-[(2*S*,2′*R*,3′*S*,5*R*,5′*R*)-octahydro-2-methyl-3′-[[(2*R*,4*S*,5*S*,6*S*)-tetrahydro-4,5-dimethoxy-6-methyl-2*H*-pyran-2-yl]oxy]-5′-[(2*S*,3*S*,5*R*,6*S*)-tetrahydro-6-hydroxy-3,5,6-trimethyl-2*H*-pyran-2-yl][2,2′-bifuran]-5-yl]-1,6-dioxaspiro[4.5]dec-7-yl]ethyl]-4,5-dimethoxy-3-methyl-2*H*-pyran-2-acetate. *CAS-84878-61-5*. INN; BAN. *Anticoccidal.* ◇CL 273,703

Mafenide [*1967*] (maf′ en ide). $C_7H_{10}N_2O_2S$. 186.23. (1) Benzenesulfonamide, 4-(aminomethyl)-; (2) α-Amino-*p*-toluenesulfonamide. *UNII-58447S8P4L*. *CAS-138-39-6*. INN; BAN. *Antibacterial.* Sulfamylon (Sterling Winthrop†) ◇NSC-34632

Mafenide Acetate (maf′ en ide as′ e tate). **USP**. $C_7H_{10}N_2O_2S.C_2H_4O_2$. 246.28. (1) Benzenesulfonamide, 4-(aminomethyl)-, monoacetate; (2) α-Amino-*p*-toluenesulfonamide monoacetate. *UNII-RQ6LP6Z0WY*. *CAS-13009-99-9*. JAN. *Anti-infective, topical.* Sulfamylon (UDL)

Mafenide Hydrochloride. *UNII-58447S8P4L* [mafenide]. *CAS-138-37-4; CAS-138-39-6* [mafenide]. MI; AMA-DE 1971.

Mafilcon A [*1977*] (ma fil′ kon). $(C_6H_{10}O_3)_v(C_9H_{16}O_2)_w$ $(C_4H_6O_2)_x(C_5H_8O_2)_y(C_{14}H_{12}O_3)_z$. (1) 2-Propenoic acid, 2-methyl-, 2-hydroxyethyl ester, polymer with pentyl 2-methyl-2-propenoate, ethenyl acetate, ethenyl propanoate, and 3-hydroxy-2-naphthalenyl 2-methyl-2-propenoate; (2) 2-Hydroxyethyl methacrylate polymer with pentyl meth-

acrylate, vinyl acetate, vinyl propionate, and 3-hydroxy-2-naphthyl methacrylate. *CAS-58167-74-1*. *Contact lens material (hydrophilic).*

Mafoprazine. $C_{22}H_{28}FN_3O_3$. 401.47. 4′-[3-[4-(*o*-Fluorophenyl)-1-piperazinyl]propoxy]-*m*-acetanisidide. *UNII-D7UUO54C6N*. *CAS-80428-29-1*. INN.

Mafosfamide. $C_9H_{19}Cl_2N_2O_5PS_2$. 401.27. ($\pm$)-2-[[2-[Bis(2-chloroethyl)amino]tetrahydro-2*H*-1,3,2-oxazaphosphorin-4-yl]thio]ethanesulfonic acid *P-cis*-oxide. *UNII-5970HH9923*. *CAS-88859-04-5*. INN.

Magaldrate [*1963*] (mag′ al drate). **USP**. $Al_5Mg_{10}(OH)_{31}(SP_4)_2.xH_2O$. 1097.38 (anhydrous). (1) Aluminum magnesium hydroxide sulfate ($Al_5Mg_{10}(OH)_{31}(SO_4)_2.xH_2O$); (2) Aluminum magnesium hydroxide sulfate, hydrate. [Formerly treated as $Al_2H_{14}.Mg_4O_{14}2H_2O$. *CAS-39366-43-3*.] *CAS-74978-16-8*. INN; BAN. *Antacid.* Riopan (Whitehall-Robins) ◇AY-5710

Magnesia, [Milk of] (mag nee′ zha). **USP**. $Mg(OH)_2$. 58.32. (1) Magnesium hydroxide; (2) Magnesium hydroxide. *CAS-1309-42-8*. *Antacid; laxative.* Mint-O-Mag (Bristol-Myers Squibb†) [*Name previously used: Magnesia Magma.*]

Magnesia Magma (previously used name) — *See* Magnesia, [Milk of].

Magnesium Aluminometasilicate (mag nee′ zee um a loo″ mi noe met″ a sil′ i kate). **NF**. A synthetic material that exists in two forms, Type I-A and Type I-B, having different pH requirements. The required contents for both forms are the same: $32.3 \pm 3.2\%$ aluminum oxide (Al_2O_3), $12.7 \pm 1.3\%$ magnesium oxide (MgO), and $32.4 \pm 3.2\%$ silicon dioxide (SiO_2), calculated on the dried basis.

Magnesium Aluminometasilicate (JAN) — *See* Silodrate.

Magnesium Aluminosilicate (mag nee′ zee um a loo″ mi noe sil′ i kate). **NF**. A synthesized material that contains $24.1 \pm 3.6\%$ of magnesium oxide (MgO), and $30.65 \pm 3.65\%$ of aluminum oxide (Al_2O_3), and $18.05 \pm 3.65\%$ of silicon dioxide (SiO_2), calculated on the dried basis. JAN.

Magnesium Aluminosilicate (JAN) — *See* Magnesium Aluminum Silicate.

Magnesium Aluminum Silicate (mag nee′ zee um a loo′ mi num sil′ i kate). **NF**. A blend of colloidal montmorillonite and saponite that has been processed to remove grit and nonswellable ore components. *Pharmaceutic aid (suspending agent)*. Veegum (Vanderbilt)

Magnesium Aspartate. $C_8H_{12}MgN_2O_8 \cdot 4H_2O$. 360.56. [See the entry for Potassium Aspartate and Magnesium Aspartate.]

Magnesium Carbonate (mag nee′ zee um kar′ bo nate). **USP**. (1) Carbonic acid, magnesium salt, basic; or, Carbonic acid, magnesium salt (1:1), hydrate. (2) Magnesium carbonate, basic; or, Magnesium carbonate (1:1) hydrate. *UNII-0E53J927NA*. *CAS-23389-33-5* [normal, dihydrate]; *CAS-39409-82-0* [basic]; *CAS-546-93-0* [anhydrous]. JAN. *Antacid*.

Magnesium Chloride (mag nee′ zee um klor′ ide). **USP**. $MgCl_2 \cdot 6H_2O$. 203.30. (1) Magnesium chloride, hexahydrate; (2) Magnesium chloride hexahydrate. *UNII-02F3473H9O*; *UNII-59XN63C8VM* [magnesium chloride anhydrous]. *CAS-7791-18-6*; *CAS-7786-30-3* [anhydrous]. *Replenisher (electrolyte)*.

Magnesium Citrate (mag nee′ zee um sit′ rate). **USP**. $C_{12}H_{10}Mg_3O_{14}$. 451.11. (1) 1,2,3-Propanetricarboxylic acid, hydroxy-, magnesium salt (2:3); (2) Magnesium citrate (3:2). *CAS-3344-18-1*. *Laxative*.

Magnesium Clofibrate. $C_{20}H_{20}Cl_2MgO_6$. 451.58. Bis[2-(*p*-chlorophenoxy)-2-methylpropionato]magnesium. *UNII-Y11SP157PJ*. *CAS-14613-30-0*. INN.

Magnesium Gluconate (mag nee′ zee um gloo′ koe nate). **USP**. $C_{12}H_{22}MgO_{14} \cdot xH_2O$. 414.60 (anhydrous). (1) D-Gluconic acid, magnesium salt (2:1), hydrate; (2) Magnesium D-gluconate (1:2) hydrate; (3) Magnesium D-gluconate (1:2) dihydrate. *CAS-59625-89-7* [dihydrate]; *CAS-3632-91-5* [anhydrous]. *Replenisher (magnesium)*. Almora (Forest†)

Magnesium Glycinate [*1988*] (mag nee′ zee um glye′ sin ate). $C_4H_8MgN_2O_4$. 172.42. *UNII-IFN18A4Y6B*. *CAS-14783-68-7*.

Magnesium Hydroxide (mag nee′ zee um hye drox′ ide). **USP**. $Mg(OH)_2$. 58.32. (1) Magnesium hydroxide; (2) Magnesium hydroxide. *UNII-NBZ3QY004S*. *CAS-1309-42-8*. JAN. *Antacid; laxative*. Oxaine M (Wyeth-Ayerst†); Phillips Magnesia Tablets (Sterling Health U.S.A.); Phillips Milk of Magnesia Liquid (Sterling Health U.S.A.)

Magnesium Oxide (mag nee′ zee um ox′ ide). **USP**. MgO. 40.30. (1) Magnesium oxide; (2) Magnesium oxide. *UNII-3A3U0GI71G*. *CAS-1309-48-4*. JAN. *Pharmaceutic aid (sorbent)*.

Magnesium Phosphate (mag nee′ zee um fos′ fate). **USP**. $Mg_3(PO_4)_2 \cdot 5H_2O$. 352.93. (1) Phosphoric acid, magnesium salt (2:3), pentahydrate; (2) Magnesium phosphate (3:2) pentahydrate. *CAS-10233-87-1*; *CAS-7757-87-1* [anhydrous]. *Antacid*.

Magnesium Salicylate (mag nee′ zee um sa lis′ i late). **USP**. $C_{14}H_{10}MgO_6 \cdot 4H_2O$. 370.59. (1) Magnesium, bis(2-hydroxybenzoato-O^1,O^2)-, tetrahydrate; (2) Magnesium salicylate (1:2), tetrahydrate. *UNII-41728CY7UX*. *CAS-18917-95-8*; *CAS-18917-89-0* [anhydrous]. *Analgesic; antipyretic; antirheumatic*. Backache Caplets (Bristol-Myers Products); Bayer Select Backache (Sterling Health U.S.A.); Magan (Savage); Mobidin (Ascher); Momentum (Whitehall-Robins)

Magnesium Silicate (mag nee′ zee um sil′ i kate). **NF**. A compound that contains not less than 15.0% of magnesium oxide (MgO) and not less than 67.0% of silicon dioxide (SiO_2), calculated on the ignited basis. JAN. *Pharmaceutic aid (tablet excipient)*.

Magnesium Stearate (mag nee′ zee um steer′ ate). **NF**. (1) Octadecanoic acid, magnesium salt; (2) Magnesium stearate. *UNII-70097M6I30*. *CAS-557-04-0*. JAN. *Pharmaceutic aid (tablet and/or capsule lubricant)*.

Magnesium Sulfate (mag nee′ zee um sul′ fate). **USP**. $MgSO_4 \cdot 7H_2O$. 246.47. (1) Sulfuric acid magnesium salt (1:1), heptahydrate; (2) Magnesium sulfate (1:1) heptahydrate. *UNII-DE08037SAB*. *CAS-10034-99-8*; *CAS-7487-88-9* [anhydrous]. JAN. *Anticonvulsant; laxative; replenisher (electrolyte)*.

Magnesium Trisilicate (mag nee′ zee um trye sil′ i kate). **USP**. $2MgO \cdot 3SiO_2 \cdot xH_2O$. 260.86 (anhydrous). (1) Silicic acid ($H_4Si_3O_8$), magnesium salt (1:2), hydrate; (2) Magnesium silicate hydrate ($Mg_2Si_3O_8 \cdot xH_2O$). *UNII-C2E1CI501T*. *CAS-39365-87-2*; *CAS-14987-04-3* [anhydrous]. *Antacid*. Trimax (Sterling Winthrop)

Maitansine (INN) — *See* Maytansine.

Malathion (mal″ a thye′ on). **USP**. $C_{10}H_{19}O_6PS_2$. 330.36. (1) Butanedioic acid, [(dimethoxyphosphinothioyl)-thio]-, diethyl ester, (±)-; (2) Diethyl (±)-mercaptosuccinate, *S*-ester with *O,O*-dimethyl phosphorodithioate. *UNII-U5N7SU872W*. *CAS-121-75-5*. BAN. *Pediculicide*. Ovide (Taro)

Maleic Acid. NF. $C_4H_4O_4$. 116.07. (1) (*Z*)-Butenedioic acid; (2) *Cis*-Butenedioic acid. *UNII-91XW058U2C. CAS-110-16-7.*

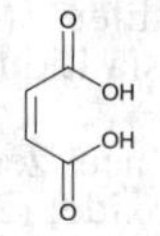

Maletamer (INN; BAN) — *See* Malethamer.

Malethamer [*1963*] (mal eth′ a mer). [Maletamer is INN and BAN.] High molecular weight copolymer of ethylene with maleic anhydride, cross-linked with 1 to 2 %, by weight, of vinyl crotonate. (1) 2-Butenoic acid, ethenyl ester, polymer with ethene and 2,5-furandione; (2) Maleic anhydride polymer with ethylene and vinyl crotonate. *CAS-67832-40-0; CAS-29535-27-1[replaced]; CAS-9011-01-2 [replaced].* *Antiperistaltic.* ◊*21679-CH*

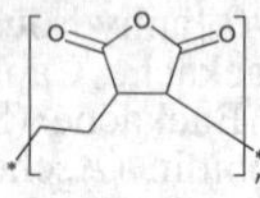

Maleylsulfathiazole. $C_{13}H_{11}N_3O_5S_2$. 353.37. 4′-(2-Thiazolyl-sulfamoyl)maleanilic acid. *UNII-N7T6304257. CAS-515-57-1.* INN; DCF.

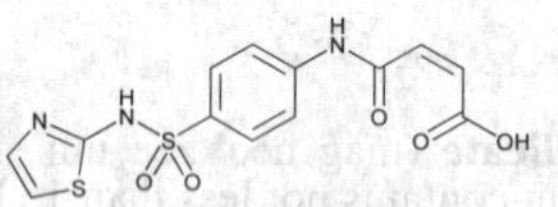

Malic Acid (mal′ ik as′ id). **NF.** $C_4H_6O_5$. 134.09. (1) Hydroxybutanedioic acid, (±)-; (2) (±)-Malic acid; (3) (±)-Hydroxysuccinic acid. *CAS-617-48-1. Pharmaceutic aid (acidifying agent).*

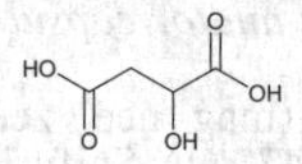

Mallotus Japonicus Extract. JAN.

Malotilate [*1988*] (mal oh′ ti late). $C_{12}H_{16}O_4S_2$. 288.38. (1) Propanedioic acid, 1,3-dithiol-2-ylidene-, bis(1-methyl-ethyl) ester; (2) Diisopropyl 1,3-dithiole-$\Delta^{2,\alpha}$-malonate. *CAS-59937-28-9.* INN; JAN. *Liver disorder treatment.* ◊*NKK-105*

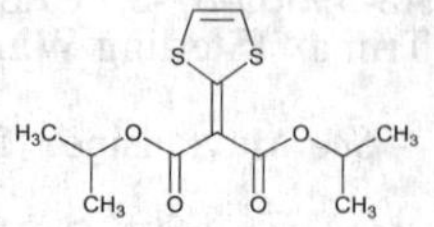

Malt Extract. JAN.

Maltitol (mawl′ ti tol). **NF.** $C_{12}H_{24}O_{11}$. 344.31. D-Glucopyr-anosyl-D-glucitol. *UNII-D65DG142WK. CAS-585-88-6.* BAN. *Sweetener.*

Maltodextrin (mawl″ toe dex′ trin). **NF.** A nonsweet, nutritive saccharide mixture of polymers that consists of D-glucose units, with a Dextrose Equivalent less than 20. *Pharmaceutic aid (coating agent); pharmaceutic aid (tablet binder); pharmaceutic aid (tablet and capsule diluent); pharmaceutic aid (viscosity-increasing agent).*

Maltol. NF. $C_6H_6O_3$. 126.11. 3-Hydroxy-2-methyl-4-pyrone. *UNII-3A9RD92BS4. CAS-118-71-8.*

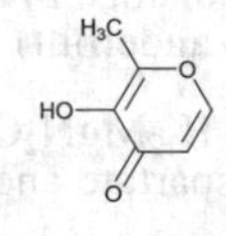

Maltose (mawl′ tose). **NF.** $C_{12}H_{22}O_{11}$. 342.30. 4-*O*-α-D-Glucopyranosyl-*β*-D-glucopyranose. *CAS-69-79-4.* JAN.

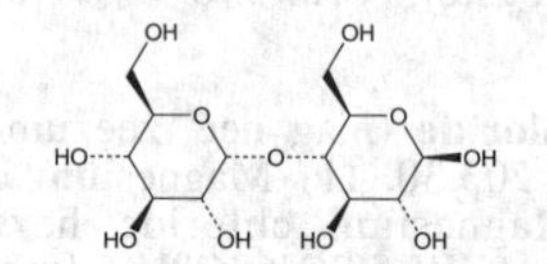

Managlinat Dialanetil. $C_{21}H_{33}N_4O_6PS$. 500.55. Diethyl *N,N′*-{5-[2-amino-5-(2-methylpropyl)-1,3-thiazol-4-yl]furan-2-ylphosphonoyl}di-L-alaninate. *CAS-280782-97-0.* INN.

Mandelic Acid. $C_8H_8O_3$. 152.15. (1) α-Hydroxyphenylacetic acid; (2) Phenylacetic acid, α-hydroxy-. *UNII-NH496X0UJX. CAS-90-64-2.* USP XXV.

Mangafodipir. $C_{22}H_{30}MnN_4O_{14}P_2$. 691.38. Hexahydrogen (*OC*-6-13)-[[*N,N′*-ethylenebis[*N*-[[3-hydroxy-5-(hydroxy-methyl)-2-methyl-4-pyridyl]methyl]glycine] 5,5′-bis(phos-phato)](8-)]manganate(6-). *CAS-155319-91-8.* INN; BAN.

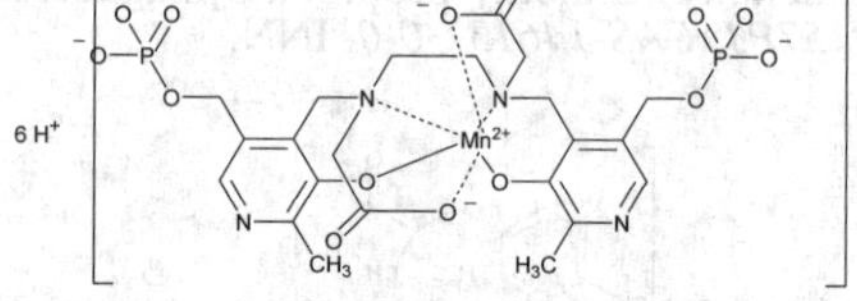

Mangafodipir Trisodium [*1994*] (man″ ga foe′ di pir trye soe′ dee um). **USP.** $C_{22}H_{27}MnN_4Na_3O_{14}P_2$. 757.32. (1) Trisodium trihydrogen (*OC*-6-13)-[[*N,N′*-1,2-ethanediyl-bis[*N*-[[3-hydroxy-2-methyl-5-[(phosphonooxy)methyl]-4-pyridinyl]methyl]glycinato]](8-)-manganate(6-); (2) Triso-dium trihydrogen (*OC*-6-13)-[[*N,N′*-ethylenebis[*N*-[[3-hy-droxy-5-(hydroxymethyl)-2-methyl-4-pyridyl]methyl]gly-cine] 5,5′-bis(phosphato)](8-)]manganate(6-). *UNII-129FW80TG4. CAS-140678-14-4. Diagnostic (paramag-netic contrast agent).* Teslascan (GE Healthcare) ◊*WIN 59010*

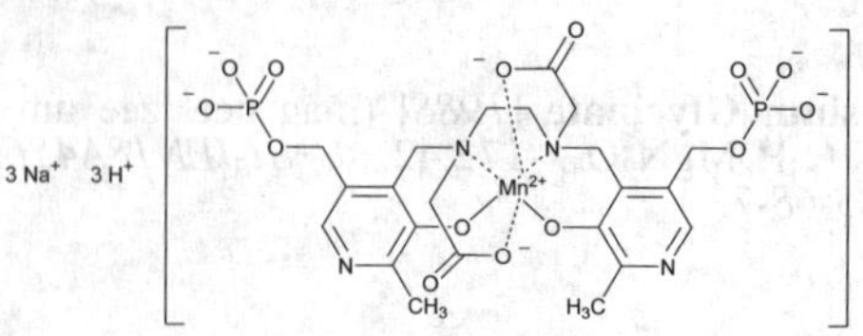

Manganese Chloride (man′ ga nees klor′ ide). **USP.** $MnCl_2 \cdot 4H_2O$. 197.91. (1) Manganese chloride ($MnCl_2$) tetrahydrate; (2) Manganese(2+) chloride tetrahydrate. *UNII-6YB4901Y90* [manganese chloride anhydrous]. *CAS-13446-34-9; CAS-7773-01-5* [anhydrous]. *Supple-ment (trace mineral).*

Manganese Gluconate (man′ ga nees gloo′ koe nate). **USP**. $C_{12}H_{22}MnO_{14}$. 445.23. (1) Bis(D-gluconato-O^1,O^2) manganese; (2) Manganese D-gluconate (1:2). *CAS-6485-39-8; CAS-84368-35-4* [replaced]. *Supplement (trace mineral).*

Manganese Glycerophosphate. Glycerol phosphate manganese salt. NF X.

Manganese Hypophosphite. Manganese(2+) phosphinate. NF X; MI.

Manganese Sulfate (man′ ga nees sul′ fate). **USP**. $MnSO_4.$-H_2O. 169.02. (1) Sulfuric acid, manganese(2+) salt (1:1) monohydrate; (2) Manganese(2+) sulfate (1:1) monohydrate. *UNII-W00LYS4T26; UNII-IGA15S9H40* [manganese sulfate anhydrous]. *CAS-10034-96-5; CAS-7785-87-7* [anhydrous]; *CAS-6485-39-8; CAS-84368-35-4* [replaced]. *Supplement (trace mineral).*

Manidipine 6300. $C_{35}H_{38}N_4O_6$. 610.70. [Manidipine Hydrochloride is JAN.] 2-[4-(Diphenylmethyl)-1-piperazinyl]ethyl methyl (±)-1,4-dihydro-2,6-dimethyl-4-(*m*-nitrophenyl)-3,5-pyridinecarboxylate. *UNII-6O4754US88. CAS-120092-68-4.* INN.

Manifaxine. $C_{12}H_{15}F_2NO_2$. 243.25. (2*S*,3*S*,5*R*)-2-(3,5-Difluorophenyl)-3,5-dimethylmorpholin-2-ol. *UNII-J8IE53-G2IV. CAS-135306-39-7.* INN; BAN.

Manitimus. $C_{15}H_{11}F_3N_2O_2$. 308.26. (2*Z*)-2-Cyano-3-hydroxy-*N*-[4-(trifluoromethyl)phenyl]hept-2-en-6-ynamide. *CAS-202057-76-9.* INN.

Manna Sugar — *See* Mannitol.

Mannite — *See* Mannitol.

Mannitol (man′ i tol). **USP**. $C_6H_{14}O_6$. 182.17. [D-Mannitol is JAN.] (1) D-Mannitol; (2) D-Mannitol. *UNII-3OWL53-L36A. CAS-69-65-8. Diagnostic aid (renal function determination); diuretic.* Osmitrol (Baxter Healthcare); Resectisol (B Braun)

D-**Mannitol (JAN)** — *See* Mannitol.

Mannitol Hexanitrate. $C_6H_8N_6O_{18}$. 452.16. Hexanitrate of D-mannitol. *CAS-15825-70-4.* INN; MI. Nitranitol (Marion Merrell Dow†)

Mannityl Nitrate — *See* Mannitol Hexanitrate.

Mannomustine. $C_{10}H_{22}Cl_2N_2O_4$. 305.20. 1,6-Bis[(2-chloroethyl)amino]-1,6-dideoxy-D-mannitol. *UNII-E60VWA40D2. CAS-576-68-1.* INN; BAN; DCF; MI. ◇BCM; *NSC-9698 [as hydrochloride]*

Mannosulfan. $C_{10}H_{22}O_{14}S_4$. 494.53. D-Mannitol 1,2,5,6-tetramethanesulfonate. *CAS-7518-35-6.* INN. ◇*R-52*

Manozodil. $C_{10}H_{16}N_2S$. 196.31. 4,5,6,7-Tetrahydro-2-methyl-5-[(methylamino)methyl]benzothiazole. *UNII-GZM2484VQ4. CAS-77528-67-7.* INN.

Mantabegron. $C_{19}H_{27}NO_2$. 301.42. (2*RS*)-1-(Adamantan-1-ylamino)-3-phenoxypropan-2-ol. *CAS-36144-08-8.* INN.

Mapatumumab [*2005*] (ma″ pa toom′ ue mab). $C_{6388}H_{9856}N_{1712}O_{1998}S_{46}$. (1) Immunoglobulin G1, anti-(human cytokine receptor DR4 (death receceptor 4)) (human monoclonal TRM-1 heavy chain), disulfide with human monoclonal TRM-1 λ-chain, dimer; (2) Immunoglobulin G1, anti-(human TRAIL-R1) (human monoclonal

TRM-1 heavy chain), disulfide with human monoclonal TRM-1 λ-chain, dimer. *CAS-658052-09-6.* INN. *Treatment of cancer.* ◇*TRAIL-R1 mAb; TRM-1; HGS-ETR1*

Mapinastine. $C_{23}H_{34}N_6O$. 410.56. 1-(2-Ethoxyethyl)-2-[[4-(4-pyrazol-1-ylbutyl)-1-piperazinyl]methyl]benzimidazole. *UNII-62LN840SFZ. CAS-140945-32-0.* INN.

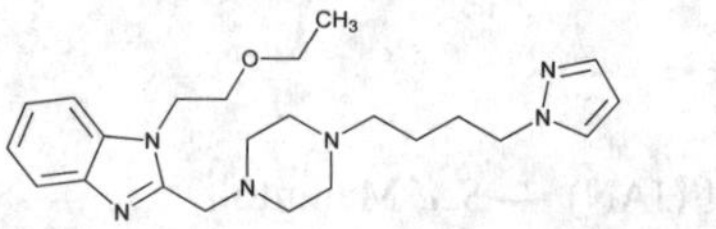

Maprotiline [*1971*] (ma proe′ ti leen). $C_{20}H_{23}N$. 277.40. (1) 9,10-Ethanoanthracene-9(10*H*)-propanamine, *N*-methyl-; (2) *N*-Methyl-9,10-ethanoanthracene-9(10*H*)-propylamine. *UNII-2U1W68TROF. CAS-10262-69-8.* INN; BAN. *Antidepressant.* ◇*Ba-34,276 [as hydrochloride]*

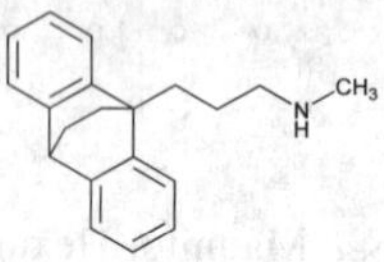

Maprotiline Hydrochloride (ma proe′ ti leen hye″ droe klor′ ide). **USP.** $C_{20}H_{23}N$·HCl. 313.86. (1) 9,10-Ethanoanthracene-9(10*H*)-propanamine, *N*-methyl-, hydrochloride; (2) *N*-Methyl-9,10-ethanoanthracene-9(10*H*)-propylamine hydrochloride. *UNII-7C8J54PVFI. CAS-10347-81-6.* JAN. *Antidepressant.* Ludiomil (Novartis)

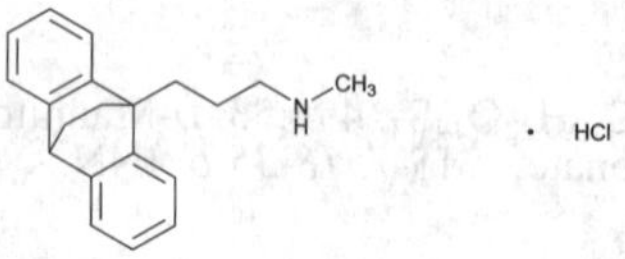

Maraviroc (mar″ a vir′ ok). $C_{29}H_{41}F_2N_5O$. 513.67. 4,4-Difluoro-*N*-[(1*S*)-3-{(1*R*,3*S*,5*S*)-3-[3-methyl-5-(propan-2-yl)-4*H*-1,2,4-triazol-4-yl]-8-azabicyclo[3.2.1]octan-8-yl}-1-phenylpropyl]cyclohexanecarboxamide. *UNII-MD6P741W8A. CAS-376348-65-1.* INN; JAN.

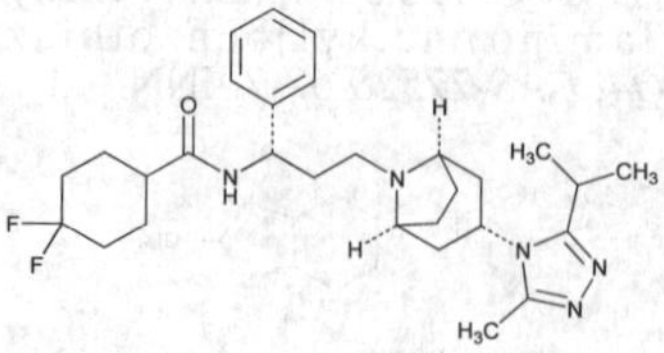

Marbofloxacin. $C_{17}H_{19}FN_4O_4$. 362.36. 9-Fluoro-2,3-dihydro-3-methyl-10-(4-methyl-1-piperazinyl)-7-oxo-7*H*-pyrido[3,2,1-*ij*][4,1,2]benzoxadiazine-6-carboxylic acid. *UNII-8X09WU898T. CAS-115550-35-1.* INN; BAN.

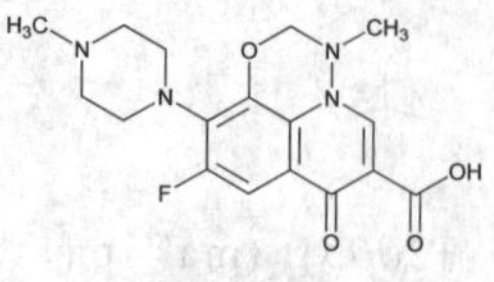

Maribavir [*1998*] (ma rye′ ba vir). $C_{15}H_{19}Cl_2N_3O_4$. 376.24. (1) 5,6-Dichloro-*N*-(1-methylethyl)-1-β-L-ribofuranosyl-1*H*-benzimidazol-2-amine; (2) 5,6-Dichloro-2-(isopropyl-amino)-1-β-L-ribofuranosylbenzimidazole. *CAS-176161-24-3.* INN; BAN. *Treatment of cytomegalovirus infections (antiviral).* ◇*1263W94*

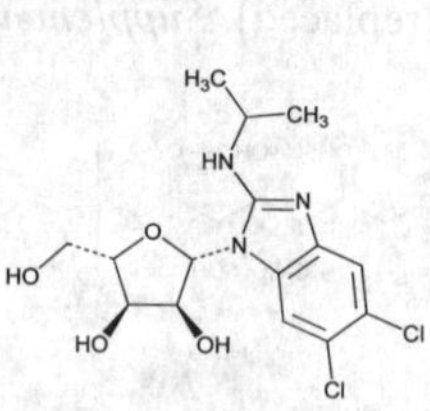

Maridomycin. $C_{41}H_{67}NO_{16}$. 829.97. 10-(Formylmethyl)-7,13-dihydroxy-8-methoxy-3,12-dimethyl-5-oxo-4,17-dioxabicyclo[14.1.0]heptadec-14-en-9-yl 3,6-dideoxy-4-*O*-(2,6-dideoxy-3-*C*-methyl-α-L-*ribo*-hexopyranosyl)-3-(dimethylamino)-β-D-glucopyranoside 4″,7′-dipropionate (ester). *CAS-35775-82-7.* INN.

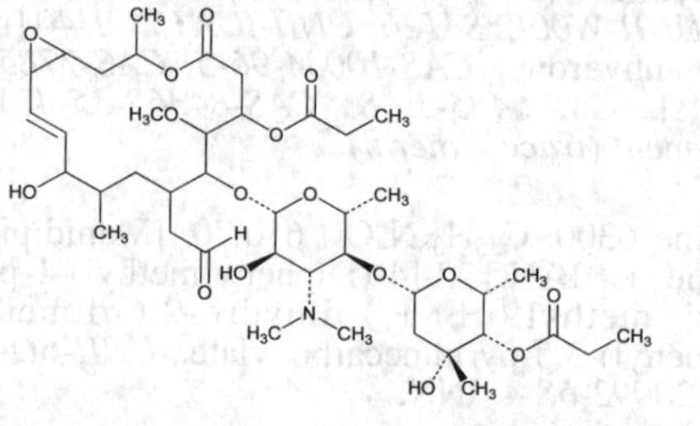

Marimastat [*1996*] (ma rim′ a stat). $C_{15}H_{29}N_3O_5$. 331.41. (1) Butanediamide, N^4-[2,2-dimethyl-1-[(methylamino)carbonyl]propyl]-N^1,2-dihydroxy-3-(2-methylpropyl)-, [2*S*-[N^4(*R**),2*R**,3*S**]]-; (2) (2*S*,3*R*)-3-[[(1*S*)-2,2-Dimethyl-1-(methylcarbamoyl)propyl]carbamoyl]-2-hydroxy-5-methylhexanohydroxamic acid. *CAS-154039-60-8.* INN; BAN. *Antineoplastic (matrix metalloproteinase inhibitor).* ◇*BB-2516*

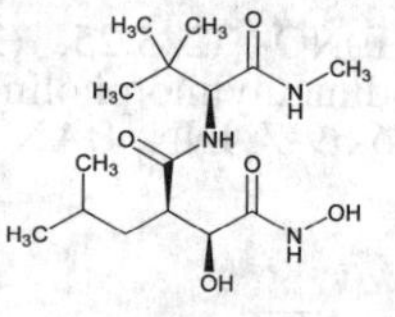

Mariptiline. $C_{18}H_{18}N_2O$. 278.35. 1a,10b-Dihydro-dibenzo[*a,e*]cyclopropa[*c*]cyclohepten-6(1*H*)-one *O*-(2-aminoethyl)oxime. *CAS-60070-14-6.* INN.

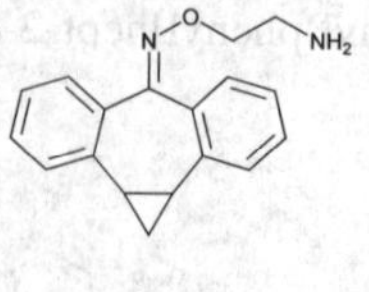

Maritime Pine. NF XXI.

Maritime Pine Extract. NF XXI.

Maropitant Citrate [*2004*] (mar oh′ pi tant sit′ rate). $C_{32}H_{40}N_2O·C_6H_8O_7·H_2O$. 678.81. [Maropitant is INN.] (1) 1-Azabicyclo[2.2.2]octan-3-amine, *N*-[[5-(1,1-dimethylethyl)-2-methoxyphenyl]methyl]-2-(diphenylmethyl)-, (2*S*,3*S*)-, 2-hydroxy-1,2,3-propanetricarboxylate (1:1), monohydrate; (2) (2*S*,3*S*)-*N*-[5-(1,1-Dimethylethyl)-2-methoxybenzyl]-2-(diphenylmethyl)-1-azabicyclo[2.2.2]octan-3-amine 2-hydroxy-1,2,3-propanetricarboxylate (1:1), monohydrate. *UNII-LXN6S3999X. CAS-359875-09-5; CAS-147116-67-4* [maropitant]. *Anti-emetic.* ◇*CJ-11,972*

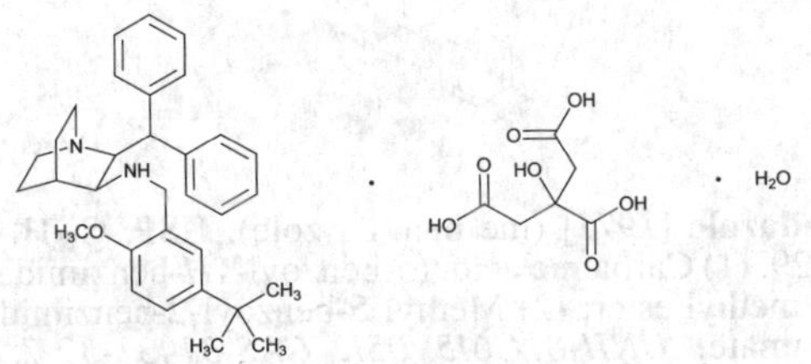

Maroxepin. $C_{19}H_{19}NO$. 277.36. 2,3,4,5-Tetrahydro-3-methyl-1*H*-dibenz[2,3:6,7]oxepino[4,5-*d*]azepine. *UNII-XG4094G0OY. CAS-65509-24-2.* INN.

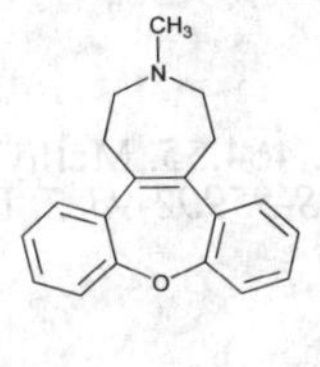

Marsidomine (previously used name) — *See* Darsidomine.

Masilukast. $C_{31}H_{32}F_3N_3O_5S$. 615.66. 3-[(2-Methoxy-4-{[(2-methylphenyl)sulfonyl]carbamoyl}phenyl)methyl]-1-methyl-*N*-[(2*R*)-4,4,4-trifluoro-2-methylbutyl]-1*H*-indole-5-carboxamide. *CAS-136564-68-6.* INN.

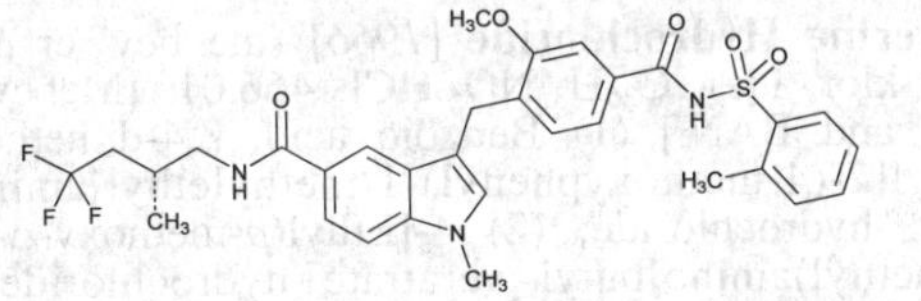

Masitinib. $C_{28}H_{30}N_6OS$. 498.64. 4-[(4-Methylpiperazin-1-yl)methyl]-*N*-(4-methyl-3-{[4-(pyridin-3-yl)-1,3-thiazol-2-yl]amino}phenyl)benzamide. *CAS-790299-79-5.* INN.

Maslimomab. Mouse monoclonal immunoglobulin G2b, anti-human T-cell receptor α/β chain. *CAS-127757-92-0.* INN.

Masoprocol [*1990*] (ma soe′ pro kol). $C_{18}H_{22}O_4$. 302.36. (1) 1,2-Benzenediol, 4,4′-(2,3-dimethyl-1,4-butanediyl)bis-, (*R**,*S**)-; (2) *meso*-4,4′-(2,3-Dimethyltetramethylene)dipyrocatechol. *UNII-7BO8G1BYQU. CAS-27686-84-6.* INN. *Antineoplastic.* Actinex (University Of Arizona Cancer Center) ◇*CHX-100; meso-NDGA*

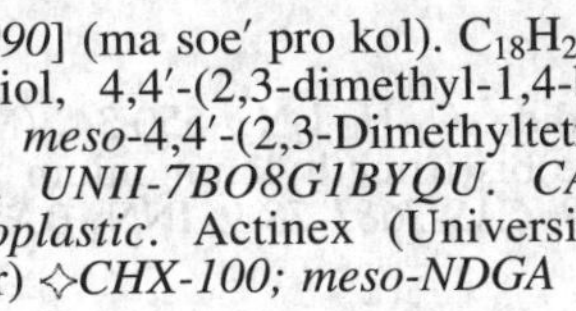

Matuzumab. Immunoglobulin G1, anti-(human epidermal growth factor receptor) (humanized MAb 425 γ1 chain), disulfide with humanized MAb 425 κ-chain, dimer. *CAS-339186-68-4.* INN.

Mavacoxib [*2005*] (ma″ va kox′ ib). $C_{16}H_{11}F_4N_3O_2S$. 385.34. (1) Benzenesulfonamide, 4-[5-(4-fluorophenyl)-3-(trifluoromethyl)-1*H*-pyrazol-1-yl]-; (2) 4-[5-(4-Fluorophenyl)-3-

(trifluoromethyl)-1*H*-pyrazol-1-yl]benzenesulfonamide. *UNII-YFT7X7SR77. CAS-170569-88-7.* INN. *Treatment of pain, inflammation, and fever.* ◇*PHA 739,521*

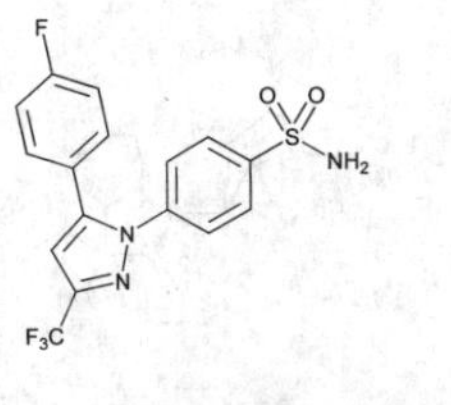

Maxacalcitol [*1998*] (max a kal′ si tol). $C_{26}H_{42}O_4$. 418.61. (1) [1*S*-[1α(*R**),3aβ,4*E*(1*S**,3*R**,5*Z*),7aα]]-4-Methylene-5-[2-[octahydro-1-[1-(3-hydroxy-3-methylbutoxy)ethyl]-7a-methyl-4*H*-inden-4-ylidene]ethylidene]-1,3-cyclohexanediol; (2) (+)-(5*Z*,7*E*,20*S*)-20-(3-Hydroxy-3-methylbutoxy)-9,10-secopregna-5,7,10(19)-triene-1α,3β-diol. *CAS-103909-75-7.* INN. *Antipsoriatic (vitamin D analogue which inhibits proliferation of cultured keratinocytes and induces terminal differentiation).* Prezios (Chugai Pharmaceutical Co., Ltd., Japan) *[Names previously used: 22-Oxacalcitriol and 1α,25-Dihydroxy-22-oxavitamin D3.]* ◇*OCT; SCH 209579*

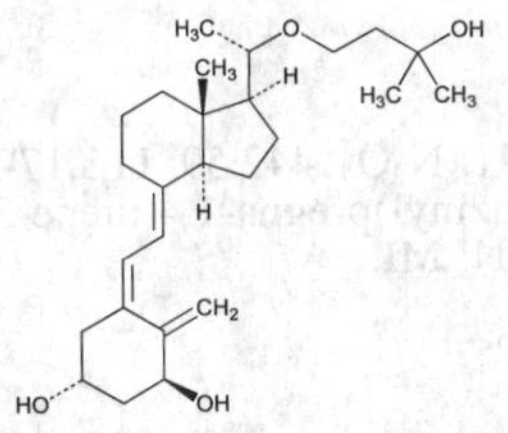

Maytansine [*1978*] (may tan′ seen). $C_{34}H_{46}ClN_3O_{10}$. 692.20. [Maitansine is INN.] Compound derived from *Maytenus* species. (1) Maytansine; (2) *N*-Acetyl-*N*-methyl-L-alanine[1*S*-(1*R**,2*S**,3*R**,5*R**,6*R**,16*E*,18*E*,20*S**,21*R**)]-11-chloro-21-hydroxy-12,20-dimethoxy-2,5,9,16-tetramethy-8,23-dioxo-4,24-dioxa-9,22-diazatetracyclo[19.3.1.1^{10,14}.0^{3,5}]hexacosa-10,12,14(26),16,18-pentaen-6-yl ester. *CAS-35846-53-8. Antineoplastic.* ◇*NSC-153858*

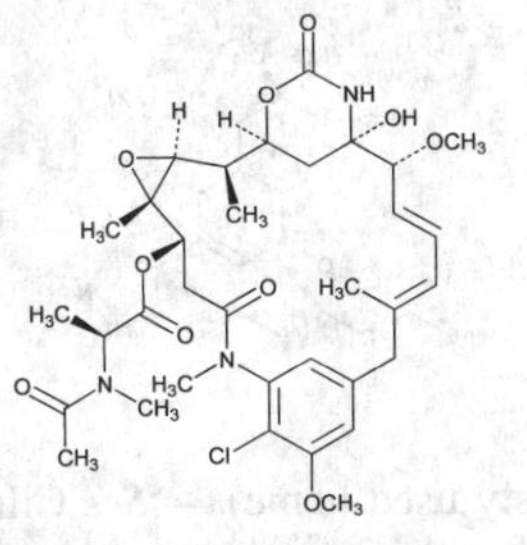

Mazapertine Succinate [*1994*] (ma″ za per′ teen sux′ i nate). $C_{26}H_{35}N_3O_2 \cdot C_4H_6O_4$. 539.66. [Mazapertine is INN.] (1) Piperidine, 1-[3-[[4-[2-(1-methylethoxy)phenyl]-1-piperazinyl]methyl]benzoyl]-, butanedioate (1:1); (2) 1-[α-[4-(*o*-Isopropoxyphenyl)-1-piperazinyl]-*m*-toluoyl]piperidine succinate (1:1). *CAS-134208-18-7; CAS-134208-17-6* [mazapertine]. *Antipsychotic.* ◇*RWJ 37796*

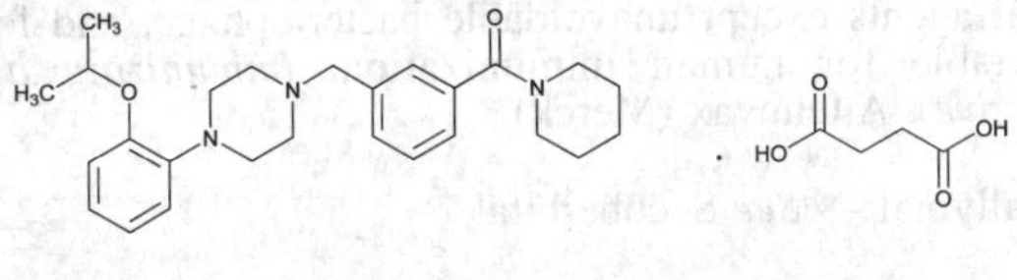

---

† Brand name formerly used, and/or firm no longer concerned with this product.

Mazaticol. $C_{21}H_{27}NO_3S_2$. 405.57. [Mazaticol Hydrochloride is JAN.] 6,6,9-Trimethyl-9-azabicyclo[3.3.1]non-3β-yl di-2-thienylglycolate. *CAS-42024-98-6.* INN. ◇*PG-501*

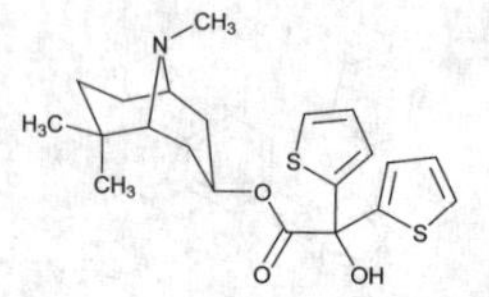

Mazindol [*1970*] (may′ zin dol). **USP**. $C_{16}H_{13}ClN_2O$. 284.74. (1) 3*H*-Imidazo[2,1-*a*]isoindol-5-ol, 5-(4-chlorophenyl)-2,5-dihydro-, (±)-; (2) (±)-5-(*p*-Chlorophenyl)-2,5-dihydro-3*H*-imidazo[2,1-*a*]isoindol-5-ol. *UNII-C56709M5NH. CAS-22232-71-9.* INN; BAN. *Anorexic.* Mazanor (Wyeth); Sanorex (Novartis) ◇*42-548*

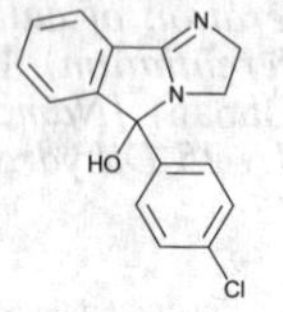

Mazipredone. $C_{26}H_{38}N_2O_4$. 442.59. 11β,17-Dihydroxy-21-(4-methyl-1-piperazinyl)pregna-1,4-diene-3,20-dione. *CAS-13085-08-0.* INN; MI.

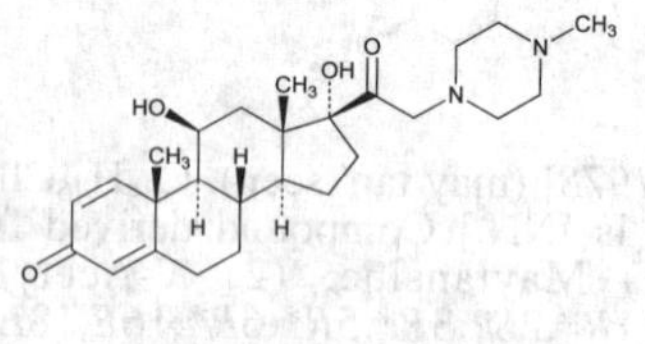

Mazokalim. $C_{23}H_{28}N_6O_6$. 484.51. Ethyl 5-[(3*S*,4*R*)-4-[(1,6-dihydro-6-oxo-3-pyridazinyl)oxy]-3-hydroxy-2,2,3-trimethyl-6-chromanyl]-1*H*-tetrazole-1-butyrate. *CAS-164178-54-5.* INN; BAN.

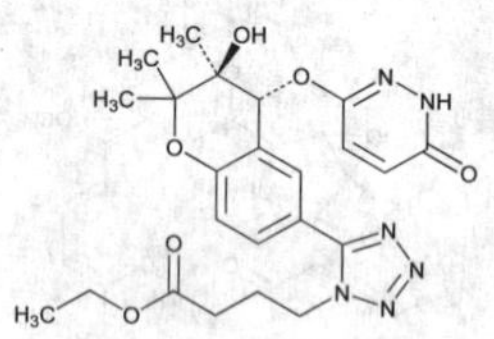

M-CSF (previously used name) — *See* Cilmostim.

MDP — *See* Medronate Disodium.

Measles Immune Globulin. [PHS: *Measles Immune Globulin (Human)*]. USP XVIII.

Measles Virus Vaccine Live (mee′ zulz). **USP**. A bacterially sterile preparation of live virus derived from a strain of measles virus tested for neurovirulence in monkeys, and for immunogenicity, free from all demonstrable viable microbial agents except unavoidable bacteriophage, and found suitable for human immunization. *Immunizing agent (active).* Attenuvax (Merck)

Meballymal — *See* Secobarbital.

Mebamoxine — *See* Benmoxin.

Mebanazine. $C_8H_{12}N_2$. 136.19. α-Methylbenzylhydrazine. *UNII-Z5R55CJ4CG. CAS-65-64-5.* INN; BAN.

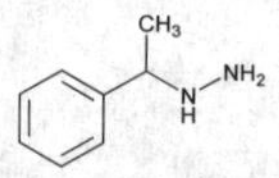

Mebendazole [*1971*] (me ben′ da zole). **USP**. $C_{16}H_{13}N_3O_3$. 295.29. (1) Carbamic acid, (5-benzoyl-1*H*-benzimidazol-2-yl)-, methyl ester; (2) Methyl 5-benzoyl-2-benzimidazole-carbamate. *UNII-81G6I5V05I. CAS-31431-39-7.* INN; BAN; JAN. *Anthelmintic.* ◇*R 17,635*

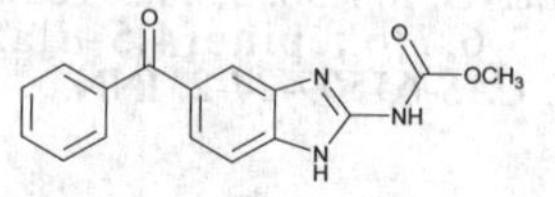

Mebenoside. $C_{28}H_{32}O_6$. 464.55. Methyl 3,5,6-tri-*O*-benzyl-D-glucofuranoside. *CAS-55902-93-7.* INN; DCF.

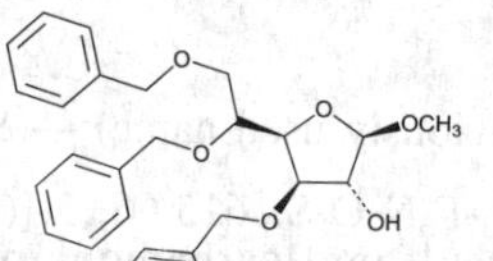

Mebeverine Hydrochloride [*1966*] (me bev′ er een hye″ droe klor′ ide). $C_{25}H_{35}NO_5 \cdot HCl$. 466.01. [Mebeverine is INN and BAN.] (1) Benzoic acid, 3,4-dimethoxy-, 4-[ethyl[2-(4-methoxyphenyl)-1-methylethyl]amino]butyl ester, hydrochloride; (2) 4-[Ethyl(*p*-methoxy-α-methyl-phenethyl)amino]butyl veratrate hydrochloride. *UNII-15VZ5AL4JN. CAS-2753-45-9; CAS-3625-06-7* [mebeverine]. *Relaxant (smooth muscle).* ◇*CSAG-144*

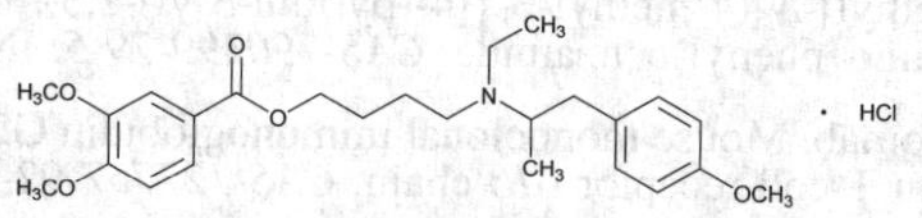

Mebezonium Iodide. $C_{19}H_{40}I_2N_2$. 550.34. (Methylenedi-1,4-cyclohexylene)bis(trimethylammonium iodide). *UNII-7GVF119EM8. CAS-7681-78-9.* INN; BAN.

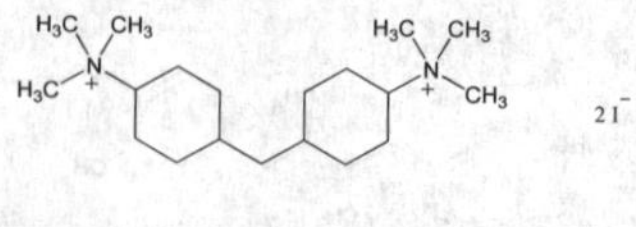

Mebhydrolin. $C_{19}H_{20}N_2$. 276.38. [Mebhydrolin Napadisylate is JAN.] 5-Benzyl-1,3,4,5-tetrahydro-2-methyl-2*H*-pyrido[4,3-*b*]indole. *UNII-9SUK9B7XVY. CAS-524-81-2.* INN; BAN; MI.

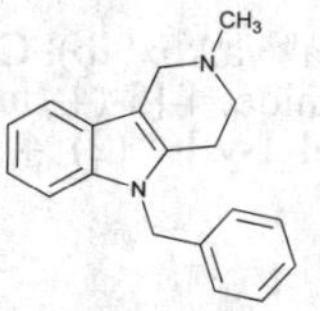

Mebiquine. $C_{10}H_{10}BiNO_3$. 401.17. Dihydroxy(6-methyl-8-quinolinolato)bismuth. *UNII-DBE10Q8QF6. CAS-23910-07-8.* INN; DCF; MI.

Mebolazine. $C_{42}H_{68}N_2O_2$. 633.00. 17β-Hydroxy-2α,17-dimethyl-5α-androstan-3-one azine. *CAS-3625-07-8.* INN.

Mebrofenin [*1981*] (me″ broe fen′ in). **USP.** $C_{15}H_{19}BrN_2O_5$. 387.23. (1) Glycine, *N*-[2-[(3-bromo-2,4,6-trimethylphenyl)amino]-2-oxoethyl]-*N*-(carboxymethyl)-; (2) [[[(3-Bromomesityl)carbamoyl]methyl]imino]diacetic acid. *UNII-7PV0B6ED98. CAS-78266-06-5.* INN; BAN. *Diagnostic aid (hepatobiliary function determination).* ⬦*SQ 26962*

Mebrophenhydramine Hydrochloride — *See* Embramine Hydrochloride.

Mebubarbital — *See* Pentobarbital.

Mebumal — *See* Pentobarbital.

Mebutamate [*1961*] (me bue′ ta mate). $C_{10}H_{20}N_2O_4$. 232.28. (1) 1,3-Propanediol, 2-methyl-2-(1-methylpropyl)-, dicarbamate; (2) 2-*sec*-Butyl-2-methyl-1,3-propanediol dicarbamate. *UNII-5H8F175RER. CAS-64-55-1.* INN; BAN; JAN. *Antihypertensive.* Dormate (Medpointe) ⬦*W-583*

Mebutizide. $C_{13}H_{20}ClN_3O_4S_2$. 381.90. 6-Chloro-3,4-dihydro-3-(1,2-dimethylbutyl)-2*H*-1,2,4-benzothiadiazine-7-sulfonamide 1,1-dioxide. *CAS-3568-00-1.* INN; DCF.

Mecamylamine Hydrochloride (me″ ka mil′ a meen hye″ droe klor′ ide). **USP.** $C_{11}H_{21}N.HCl$. 203.75. [Mecamylamine is INN and BAN.] (1) Bicyclo[2.2.1]heptan-2-amine, *N*,2,3,3-tetramethyl-, hydrochloride; (2) *N*,2,3,3-Tetramethyl-2-norbornanamine hydrochloride. *UNII-4956DJR58O; UNII-6EE945D3OK* [mecamylamine]. *CAS-826-39-1; CAS-60-40-2* [mecamylamine]. *Antihypertensive.* Inversine (Targacept)

Mecarbinate. $C_{13}H_{15}NO_3$. 233.26. Ethyl 5-hydroxy-1,2-dimethylindole-3-carboxylate. *UNII-Z927X3UJ2W. CAS-15574-49-9.* INN.

Mecarbine — *See* Mecarbinate.

Mecasermin [*1997*] (me ka′ ser min). $C_{331}H_{512}N_{94}O_{101}S_7$. 7648.63 daltons. Insulin-like growth factor I (human). *UNII-7GR9I2683O. CAS-68562-41-4.* INN; BAN. *Treatment of amyotrophic lateral sclerosis; treatment of diabetes mellitus (types I and II); treatment of growth hormone insensitivity (GHIS).* Myotrophin (Cephalon-Chiron) [*Note—Mecasermin has appeared in the literature as somatomedin-C, IGF-I, and rhIGF-1.*] ⬦*CEP-151*

```
GPETLCGAEL VDALQFVCGD RGFYFNKPTG YGSSSRRAPQ TGIVDECCFR
SCDLRRLEMY CAPLKPAKSA
```

Mecasermin Rinfabate [*2004*] (me ka′ ser min rin′ fa bate). $C_{1231}H_{1967}N_{371}O_{384}S_{20}$. 36,304. (1) Insulin-like growth factor I (human), complex with insulin-like growth factor-binding protein IGFBP-3 (human); (2) Complex of recombinant human insulin-like growth factor I (somatomedin C) with recombinant human insulin-like growth factor-binding protein 3. *CAS-478166-15-3.* INN. *Antidiabetic.* Somatokine (Avecia, UK) ⬦*rhIGF-I/rhIGFBP-3*

```
GPETLCGAEL VDALQFVCGD RGFYFNKPTG YGSSSRRAPQ TGIVDECCFR
SCDLRRLEMY CAPLKPAKSA

GASSAGLGPV VRCEPCDARA LAQCAPPPAV CAELVREPGC GCCLTCALSE
GQPCGIYTER CGSGLRCQPS PDEARPLQAL LDGRGLCVNA SAVSRLRAYL
LPAPPAPGNA SESEEDRSAG SVESPSVSST HRVSDPKFHP LHSKIIIIKK
GHAKDSQRYK VDYESQSTDT QNFSSESKRE TEYGPCRREM EDTLNHLKFL
NVLSPRGVHI PNCDKKGFYK KKQCRPSKGR KRGFCWCVDK YGQPLPGYTT
KGKEIHCYSM QSK
```

Mecetronium Ethylsulfate [*1984*] (me se troe′ nee um eth″ il sul′ fate). $C_{22}H_{49}NO_4S$. 423.69. [Mecetronium Etilsulfate is INN and BAN.] (1) 1-Hexadecanaminium, *N*-ethyl-*N*,*N*-dimethyl-, ethyl sulfate; (2) Ethylhexadecyldimethylammonium ethyl sulfate. *UNII-QM95LPV3CA. CAS-3006-10-8. Antiseptic.* [*Name previously used: Mecetronium Ethylsulphate.*]

---

† Brand name formerly used, and/or firm no longer concerned with this product.

Mechinolum (previously used name) — *See* Mequinol.

Mechlorethamine Hydrochloride (me″ klor eth′ a meen hye″ droe klor′ ide). **USP.** $C_5H_{11}Cl_2N.HCl$. 192.51. [Chlormethine is INN and BAN; Nitrogen Mustard *N*-Oxide Hydrochloride is JAN.] (1) Ethanamine, 2-chloro-*N*-(2-chloroethyl)-*N*-methyl-, hydrochloride; (2) 2,2′-Dichloro-*N*-methyldiethylamine hydrochloride. *UNII-L0MR697HHI; UNII-50D9XSG0VR* [mechlorethamine]. *CAS-55-86-7; CAS-51-75-2* [mechlorethamine]. *Antineoplastic.* Mustargen (Ovation) *[Name previously used: Mustine.]* ◇NSC-762

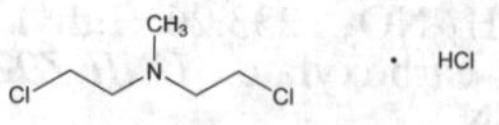

Meciadanol. $C_{16}H_{16}O_6$. 304.29. (2*R*,3*S*)-3-Methoxy-3′,4′,5,7-flavantetrol. *CAS-65350-86-9.* INN.

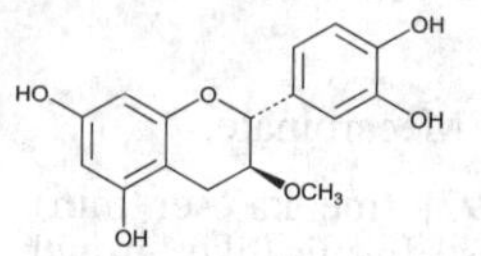

Mecillinam (INN, BAN) — *See* Amdinocillin.

Mecinarone. $C_{24}H_{27}NO_6$. 425.47. 1-[6-[2-(Dimethylamino)-ethoxy]-4,7-dimethoxy-5-benzofuranyl]-3-(*p*-methoxyphenyl)-2-propen-1-one. *CAS-26225-59-2.* INN.

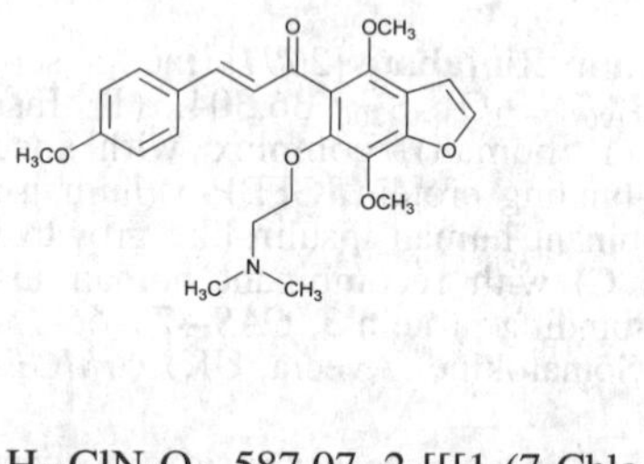

Meclinertant. $C_{32}H_{31}ClN_4O_5$. 587.07. 2-[[[1-(7-Chloroquinolin-4-yl)-5-(2,6-dimethoxyphenyl)-1*H*-pyrazol-3-yl]carbonyl]amino]tricyclo[3.3.1.1³,⁷]decane-2-carboxylic acid. *CAS-146362-70-1.* INN. *[Name previously used: Reminertant.]*

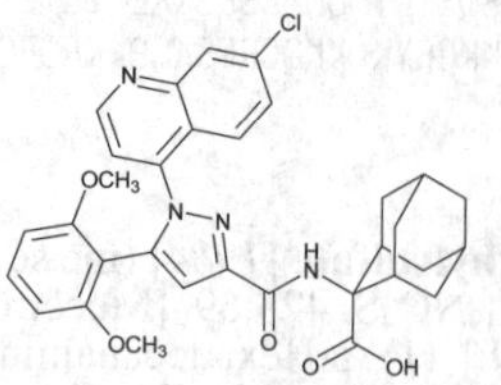

Meclizine Hydrochloride (mek′ li zeen hye″ droe klor′ ide). **USP.** $C_{25}H_{27}ClN_2.2HCl.H_2O$. 481.89. [Meclozine is INN and BAN.] (1) Piperazine, 1-[(4-chlorophenyl)phenylmethyl]-4-[(3-methylphenyl)methyl]-, dihydrochloride, monohydrate; (2) 1-(*p*-Chloro-α-phenylbenzyl)-4-(*m*-methylbenzyl)piperazine dihydrochloride monohydrate.

UNII-HDP7W44CIO; UNII-3L5TQ84570 [meclizine]. *CAS-31884-77-2; CAS-1104-22-9* [anhydrous]; *CAS-569-65-3* [meclizine]. JAN. *Anti-emetic.* Antivert (Pfizer)

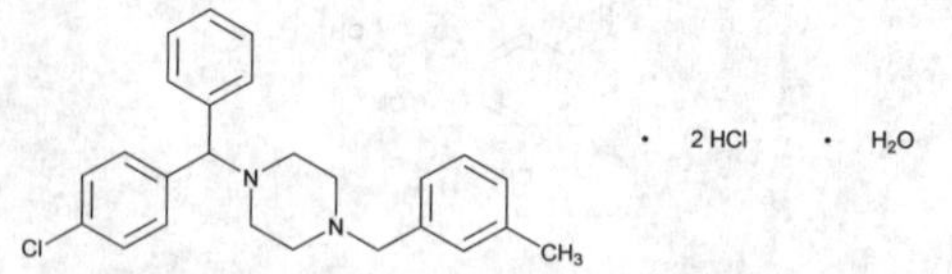

Meclocycline [*1963*] (me″ kloe sye′ kleen). $C_{22}H_{21}ClN_2O_8$. 476.86. (1) 2-Naphthacenecarboxamide, 7-chloro-4-(dimethylamino)-1,4,4a,5,5a,6,11,12a-octahydro-3,5,10,12,12a-pentahydroxy-6-methylene-1,11-dioxo-, [4*S*-(4α,4aα,5α,5aα,12aα)]-; (2) 7-Chloro-4-(dimethylamino)-1,4,4a,5,5a,6,11,12a-octahydro-3,5,10,12,12a-pentahydroxy-6-methylene-1,11-dioxo-2-naphthacenecarboxamide. *UNII-23Q8M2HE6S. CAS-2013-58-3.* INN; BAN. *Antibacterial.* ◇GS-2989; NSC-78502

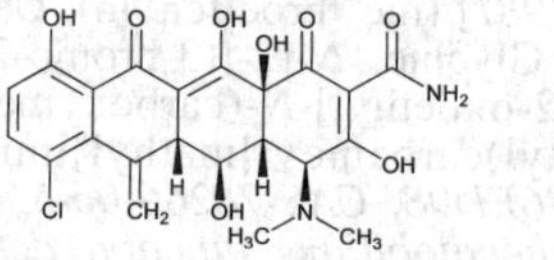

Meclocycline Sulfosalicylate [*1980*] (me″ kloe sye′ kleen sul″ foe sa lis′ i late). **USP.** $C_{22}H_{21}ClN_2O_8.C_7H_6O_6S$. 695.05. (1) 2-Naphthacenecarboxamide, 7-chloro-4-(dimethylamino)-1,4,4a,5,5a,6,11,12a-octahydro-3,5,10,12,12a-pentahydroxy-6-methylene-1,11-dioxo-, [4*S*-(4α,4aα,5α,5aα,12aα)]-, mono(2-hydroxy-5-sulfobenzoate) (salt); (2) (4*S*,4a*R*,5*S*,5a*R*,12a*S*)-7-Chloro-4-(dimethylamino)-1,4,4a,5,5a,6,11,12a-octahydro-3,5,10,12,12a-pentahydroxy-6-methylene-1,11-dioxo-2-naphthacenecarboxamide mono(5-sulfosalicylate) (salt). *UNII-46VZA7RX2B. CAS-73816-42-9; CAS-2013-58-3* [meclocycline]. *Antibacterial.* Meclan (Johnson & Johnson)

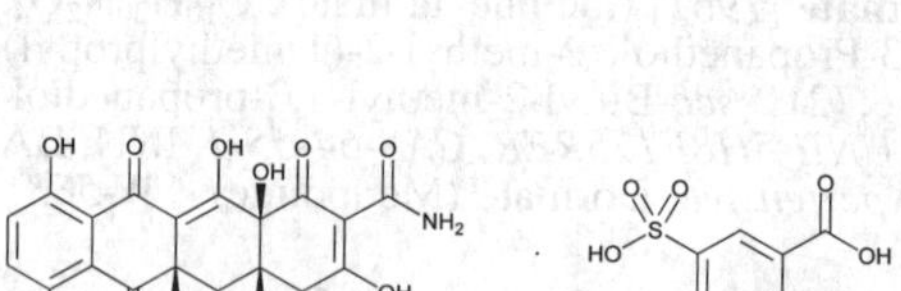

Meclofenamate Sodium [*1978*] (mek″ loe fen′ a mate soe′ dee um). **USP.** $C_{14}H_{10}Cl_2NNaO_2.H_2O$. 336.15. (1) Benzoic acid, 2-[(2,6-dichloro-3-methylphenyl)amino]-, monosodium salt, monohydrate; (2) Monosodium *N*-(2,6-dichloro-*m*-tolyl)anthranilate monohydrate. *UNII-94NJ818U2W; UNII-48I5LU4ZWD* [meclofenamic acid]. *CAS-6385-02-0; CAS-644-62-2* [meclofenamic acid]. *Anti-inflammatory.* Meclomen (Pfizer) ◇Cl-583.Na salt

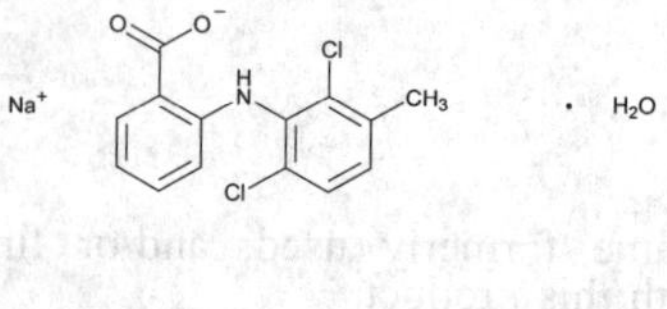

Meclofenamic Acid [*1976*] (mek″ loe fen am′ ik as′ id). $C_{14}H_{11}Cl_2NO_2$. 296.15. (1) Benzoic acid, 2-[(2,6-dichloro-3-methylphenyl)amino]-; (2) *N*-(2,6-Dichloro-*m*-tolyl)anthranilic acid. *UNII-48I5LU4ZWD. CAS-644-62-2.* INN; BAN. *Anti-inflammatory.* ◇*CI-583; INF 4668*

Meclofenoxate. $C_{12}H_{16}ClNO_3$. 257.71. [Meclofenoxate Hydrochloride is JAN.] 2-(Dimethylamino)ethyl(*p*-chlorphenoxy)acetate. *CAS-51-68-3.* INN; BAN; DCF; MI.

Meclonazepam. $C_{16}H_{12}ClN_3O_3$. 329.74. (+)-(*S*)-5-(*o*-Chlorophenyl)-1,3-dihydro-3-methyl-7-nitro-2*H*-1,4-benzodiazepin-2-one. *CAS-58662-84-3.* INN.

Mecloqualone [*1968*] (me″ kloe kwah′ lone). $C_{15}H_{11}ClN_2O$. 270.71. (1) 4(3*H*)-Quinazolinone, 3-(2-chlorophenyl)-2-methyl-; (2) 3-(*o*-Chlorophenyl)-2-methyl-4(3*H*)-quinazolinone. *CAS-340-57-8.* INN. *Sedative-hypnotic.* ◇*W 4744; NSC-142005*

Mecloralurea. $C_4H_7Cl_3N_2O_2$. 221.47. 1-Methyl-3-(2,2,2-trichloro-1-hydroxyethyl)urea. *CAS-1954-79-6.* INN; DCF; MI.

Meclorisone Dibutyrate [*1978*] (me klor′ i sone dye bue′ ti rate). $C_{30}H_{40}Cl_2O_6$. 567.54. [Meclorisone is INN and BAN.] (1) Pregna-1,4-diene-3,20-dione, 9,11-dichloro-16-methyl-17,21-bis(1-oxobutoxy)-, (11β,16α)-; (2) 9,11β-

Dichloro-17,21-dihydroxy-16α-methylpregna-1,4-diene-3,20-dione dibutyrate. *CAS-10549-91-4; CAS-4732-48-3* [meclorisone]. *Anti-inflammatory (topical).* ◇*Sch 11572*

Mecloxamine. $C_{19}H_{24}ClNO$. 317.85. 2-[(*p*-Chloro-α-methyl-α-phenylbenzyl)oxy]-*N,N*-dimethylpropylamine. *CAS-5668-06-4.* INN; MI.

Meclozine (INN, BAN) — *See* Meclizine Hydrochloride.

Mecobalamin [*1972*] (me″ koe bal′ a min). $C_{63}H_{91}Co\cdot N_{13}O_{14}P$. 1344.38. (1) Cobinamide, Co-methyl derivative, hydroxide, dihydrogen phosphate (ester), inner salt, 3′-ester with 5,6-dimethyl-1-α-D-ribofuranosylbenzimidazole; (2) Cobinamide, Co-methyl derivative, hydroxide, dihydrogen phosphate (ester), inner salt, 3′-ester with 5,6-dimethyl-1-α-D-ribofuranosylbenzimidazole. *CAS-13422-55-4.* INN; BAN; JAN. *Vitamin (hematopoietic).*

Mecrilate (INN) — *See* Mecrylate.

Mecrylate [*1969*] (me′ kri late). $C_5H_5NO_2$. 111.10. [Mecrilate is INN; Cyanoacrylate is JAN.] (1) 2-Propenoic acid, 2-cyano-, methyl ester; (2) Methyl 2-cyanoacrylate. *CAS-137-05-3. Surgical aid (tissue adhesive).*

Mecysteine. $C_4H_9NO_2S$. 135.18. Methyl ester of cysteine. *UNII-RQ6L463N3B. CAS-2485-62-3; CAS-18598-63-5* [hydrochloride]. INN; BAN; MI. *[Name previously used: Methyl Cysteine.]*

Medazepam Hydrochloride [*1968*] (me daz′ e pam hye″ droe klor′ ide). $C_{16}H_{15}ClN_2$·HCl. 307.22. [Medazepam is INN, BAN, and JAN.] (1) 1*H*-1,4-Benzodiazepine, 7-chloro-2,3-dihydro-1-methyl-5-phenyl, monohydrochloride; (2) 7-Chloro-2,3-dihydro-1-methyl-5-phenyl-1*H*-1,4-benzodiazepine monohydrochloride. *UNII-ETM878JC9K; UNII-P0J3387W3S* [medazepam]. *CAS-2898-11-5; CAS-2898-12-6* [medazepam]. *Tranquilizer (minor)*. Nobrium (Hoffmann-LaRoche†) ◇*Ro 5-4556*

Medazomide. $C_6H_9N_3O_2$. 155.15. 1,4,5,6-Tetrahydro-1-methyl-6-oxo-3-pyridazinecarboxamide. *UNII-4Q1Q4V31K8. CAS-300-22-1.* INN. ◇*L-1777*

Medazonamide — *See* Medazomide.

Medetomidine Hydrochloride [*1987*] (me″ de toe′ mi deen hye″ droe klor′ ide). $C_{13}H_{16}N_2$.HCl. 236.74. [Medetomidine is INN and BAN.] (1) 1*H*-Imidazole, 4-[1-(2,3-dimethylphenyl)ethyl]-, monohydrochloride, (±)-; (2) (±)-4-(α,2,3-Trimethylbenzyl)imidazole monohydrochloride. *UNII-BH210P244U.* CAS-86347-15-1; CAS-86347-14-0 [medetomidine]. *Analgesic (veterinary); sedative (veterinary).* ◇*MPV-785*

Medibazine. $C_{25}H_{26}N_2O_2$. 386.49. 1-(Diphenylmethyl)-4-piperonylpiperazine. *UNII-7NFK89B690. CAS-53-31-6.* INN; DCF; MI. ◇*S 4105*

Medifoxamine. $C_{16}H_{19}NO_2$. 257.33. (Dimethylamino)acetaldehyde diphenyl acetal. *CAS-32359-34-5.* INN; DCF; MI.

Medigoxin (former BAN) — *See* Metildigoxin.

Medorinone [*1988*] (me doe′ ri none). $C_9H_8N_2O$. 160.17. (1) 1,6-Naphthyridin-2(1*H*)-one, 5-methyl-; (2) 5-Methyl-1,6-naphthyridin-2(1*H*)-one. *UNII-80X61Y4X0B. CAS-88296-61-1.* INN. *Cardiotonic.* ◇*Win 49,016*

Medorubicin. $C_{26}H_{27}NO_{10}$. 513.49. (1*S*,3*S*)-3-Glycoloyl-1,2,3,4,6,11-hexahydro-3,5,12-trihydroxy-6,11-dioxo-1-naphthacenyl 3-amino-2,3,6-trideoxy-α-L-*lyxo*-hexopyranoside. *CAS-64314-52-9.* INN.

Medrogestone [*1964*] (me″ droe jes′ tone). $C_{23}H_{32}O_2$. 340.50. (1) Pregna-4,6-diene-3,20-dione, 6,17-dimethyl-; (2) 6,17-Dimethylpregna-4,6-diene-3,20-dione. *CAS-977-79-7.* INN; BAN. *Progestin.* ◇*AY-62022; NSC-123018*

Medronate Disodium [*1977*] (me′ droe nate dye soe′ dee um). $CH_4Na_2O_6P_2$. 219.97. (1) Phosphonic acid, methylenebis-, disodium dihydrogen salt; (2) Disodium dihydrogen methylenediphosphonate. *UNII-HAY5MT18L3. CAS-25681-89-4. Pharmaceutic aid. [Names previously used: Disodium Methylene Diphosphonate; MDP.]*

Medronic Acid [*1978*] (me dron′ ik as′ id). $CH_6O_6P_2$. 176.00. (1) Phosphonic acid, methylenebis-; (2) Methylenediphosphonic acid. *UNII-73OS0QIN3O. CAS-1984-15-2.* INN; BAN. *Pharmaceutic aid.*

Medroxalol [*1979*] (me drox′ a lol). $C_{20}H_{24}N_2O_5$. 372.41. (1) Benzamide, 5-[2-[[3-(1,3-benzodioxol-5-yl)-1-methylpropyl]amino]-1-hydroxyethyl]-2-hydroxy-; (2) 5-[1-Hydroxy-2-[[1-methyl-3-[3,4-(methylenedioxy)phenyl]propyl]amino]ethyl]salicylamide. *CAS-56290-94-9.* INN; BAN. *Antihypertensive.* ◇*RMI 81,968*

Medroxalol Hydrochloride [*1979*] (me drox′ a lol hye″ droe klor′ ide). $C_{20}H_{24}N_2O_5$·HCl. 408.88. (1) Benzamide, 5-[2-[[3-(1,3-benzodioxol-5-yl)-1-methylpropyl]amino]-1-hydroxyethyl]-2-hydroxy-, monohydrochloride; (2) 5-[1-Hydroxy-2-[[1-methyl-3-[3,4-(methylenedioxy)phenyl]propyl]amino]ethyl]salicylamide monohydrochloride. *CAS-70161-10-3; CAS-56290-94-9* [medroxalol]. *Antihypertensive.* ◇*RMI 81,968 A*

Medroxiprogesterone Acetate — *See* Medroxyprogesterone Acetate.

Medroxyprogesterone Acetate (me drox″ ee proe jes′ ter one as′ e tate). **USP.** $C_{24}H_{34}O_4$. 386.52. [Medroxyprogesterone is INN and BAN.] (1) Pregn-4-ene-3,20-dione, 17-(acetyloxy)-6-methyl-, (6α)-; (2) 17-Hydroxy-6α-methylpregn-4-ene-3,20-dione acetate. *UNII-C2QI4IOI2G; UNII-HSU1C9YRES* [medroxyprogesterone]. *CAS-71-58-9; CAS-520-85-4* [medroxyprogesterone]. JAN. *Progestin.* Provera (Pfizer) ◇*NSC-26386*

Medrylamine. $C_{18}H_{23}NO_2$. 285.38. 2-(*p*-Methoxy-α-phenylbenzyloxy)-*N,N*-dimethylethylamine. *UNII-5R003655CR. CAS-524-99-2.* INN; DCF; MI.

Medrysone [*1965*] (me′ dri sone). $C_{22}H_{32}O_3$. 344.49. (1) Pregn-4-ene-3,20-dione, 11-hydroxy-6-methyl-, (6α,11β)-; (2) 11β-Hydroxy-6α-methylpregn-4-ene-3,20-dione. *UNII-D2UFC189XF. CAS-2668-66-8.* USP XXII; INN. *Glucocorticoid.* Hms (Allergan) ◇*U-8471; NSC-63278*

Mefeclorazine. $C_{20}H_{25}ClN_2O_2$. 360.88. 1-*o*-Chlorophenyl-4-(3,4-dimethoxyphenethyl)piperazine. *UNII-IM840F32VV. CAS-1243-33-0.* INN; DCF.

Mefenamic Acid [*1962*] (mef″ e nam′ ik as′ id). **USP.** $C_{15}H_{15}NO_2$. 241.29. (1) Benzoic acid, 2-(2,3-dimethylphenyl)amino-; (2) *N*-2,3-Xylylanthranilic acid. *UNII-*367589PJ2C. CAS-61-68-7.* INN; BAN; JAN. *Anti-inflammatory; analgesic.* Ponstel (Sciele) ◇*CI-473; CN-35355; INF-3355*

Mefenidil [*1982*] (me fen′ i dil). $C_{12}H_{11}N_3$. 197.24. (1) 1*H*-Imidazole-4-acetonitrile, 5-methyl-2-phenyl-; (2) 5-Methyl-2-phenylimidazole-4-acetonitrile. *UNII-74WY8560J7. CAS-58261-91-9.* INN. *Vasodilator (cerebral).* ◇*McN-2378*

Mefenidil Fumarate [*1983*] (me fen′ i dil fue′ ma rate). $C_{12}H_{11}N_3$·$C_4H_4O_4$. 313.31. (1) 1*H*-Imidazole-4-acetonitrile, 5-methyl-2-phenyl-, (*E*)-2-butanedioate (1:1); (2) 5-Methyl-2-phenylimidazole-4-acetonitrile fumarate (1:1). *UNII-5QH19BF6YG. CAS-83153-38-2; CAS-58261-91-9* [mefenidil]. *Vasodilator (cerebral).* ◇*McN-2378-46*

Mefenidramium Metilsulfate. $C_{19}H_{27}NO_5S$. 381.49. [2-(Diphenylmethoxy)ethyl]trimethylammonium methyl sulfate. *UNII-TF9FPB4V3Y. CAS-4858-60-0.* INN.

Mefenorex Hydrochloride [*1968*] (me fen′ oh rex hye″ droe klor′ ide). $C_{12}H_{18}ClN$·HCl. 248.19. [Mefenorex is INN.] (1) Benzeneethanamine, *N*-(3-chloropropyl)-α-methyl-, hydrochloride; (2) *N*-(3-Chloropropyl)-α-methylphenethylamine hydrochloride. *UNII-6X1N18AU15. CAS-5586-87-8; CAS-17243-57-1* [mefenorex]. *Anorexic.* ◇*Ro 4-5282*

Mefeserpine. $C_{32}H_{38}N_2O_8$. 578.65. Methyl reserpate ester of (*p*-methoxyphenoxy)acetic acid. *CAS-3735-85-1.* INN.

---

† Brand name formerly used, and/or firm no longer concerned with this product.

Mefexamide [*1967*] (me fex′ a mide). $C_{15}H_{24}N_2O_3$. 280.36. (1) Acetamide, *N*-[2-(diethylamino)ethyl]-2-(4-methoxyphenoxy)-; (2) *N*-[2-(Diethylamino)ethyl]-2-(*p*-methoxyphenoxy)acetamide. *CAS-1227-61-8*. INN. *Stimulant (central)*.

Mefloquine [*1975*] (me′ floe kwin). $C_{17}H_{16}F_6N_2O$. 378.31. (1) 4-Quinolinemethanol, α-2-piperidinyl-2,8-bis(trifluoromethyl)-, (*R**,*S**)-(±)-; (2) (DL-*erythro*-α-2-Piperidyl-2,8-bis(trifluoromethyl)-4-quinolinemethanol. *UNII-TML814419R*. *CAS-53230-10-7*. INN; BAN. *Antimalarial*. ◇*WR 142,490; Ro 21-5998*

Mefloquine Hydrochloride [*1984*] (me′ floe kwin hye″ droe klor′ ide). USP. $C_{17}H_{16}F_6N_2O \cdot HCl$. 414.77. (1) 4-Quinolinemethanol, α-2-piperidinyl-2,8-bis(trifluoromethyl)-, monohydrochloride, (*R**,*S**)- (±)-; (2) DL-*erythro*-α-2-Piperidyl-2,8-bis(trifluoromethyl)-4-quinolinemethanol monohydrochloride. *UNII-5Y9L3636O3*. *CAS-51773-92-3*. *Antimalarial*. Lariam (Roche) ◇*Ro 21-5998/001*

Mefruside [*1967*] (me′ froo side). $C_{13}H_{19}ClN_2O_5S_2$. 382.88. (1) 1,3-Benzenedisulfonamide, 4-chloro-N^1-methyl-N^1-[(tetrahydro-2-methyl-2-furanyl)methyl]-; (2) 4-Chloro-N^1-methyl-N^1-(tetrahydro-2-methylfurfuryl)-*m*-benzenedisulfonamide. *CAS-7195-27-9*. INN; BAN; JAN. *Diuretic*. ◇*BAY 1500*

Megalomicin Potassium Phosphate [*1977*] (me ga loe mye′ sin poe tas′ ee um fos′ fate). $C_{44}H_{80}N_2O_{15} \cdot 2KH_2PO_4$. 1149.28. [Megalomicin is INN.] (1) Megalomicin A compound with potassium dihydrogen phosphate (1:2); (2) (3*R*,4*S*,5*S*,6*R*,7*R*,9*R*,11*R*,12*R*,13*R*,14*R*)-4-[(2,6-Dideoxy-3-*C*-methyl-α-L-*ribo*-hexopyranosyl)oxy]-14-ethyl-12,13-dihydroxy-3,5,7,9,11,13-hexamethyl-7-[[2,3,6-trideoxy-3-(dimethylamino)-α-L-*ribo*-hexopyranosyl]oxy]-6-[[3,4,6-trideoxy-3-(dimethylamino)-β-D-*xylo*-hexopyranosyl]oxy]oxacyclotetradecane-2,10-dione, com-

pound with potassium dihydrogen phosphate (1:2). *CAS-51481-68-6; CAS-28022-11-9* [megalomicin]. *Antibacterial*. ◇*Sch 13430.2KH₂PO₄*

Megestrol Acetate [*1963*] (me jes′ trol as′ e tate). USP. $C_{24}H_{32}O_4$. 384.51. [Megestrol is INN and BAN.] (1) Pregna-4,6-diene-3,20-dione, 17-(acetyloxy)-6-methyl-; (2) 17-Hydroxy-6-methylpregna-4,6-diene-3,20-dione acetate. *UNII-TJ2M0FR8ES; UNII-EA6LD1M70M* [megestrol]. *CAS-595-33-5; CAS-3562-63-8* [megestrol]. *Antineoplastic*. Megace (Bristol-Myers Squibb) ◇*BDH 1298; SC 10363; 5071; NSC-71423*

Meglitinide. $C_{17}H_{16}ClNO_4$. 333.77. *p*-[2-(5-Chloro-*o*-anisamido)ethyl]benzoic acid. *UNII-8V6OK1I088*. *CAS-54870-28-9*. INN.

Meglucycline. $C_{29}H_{37}N_3O_{13}$. 635.62. 2-Deoxy-2-[[[4-(dimethylamino)-1,4,4a,5,5a,6,11,12a-octahydro-3,6,-10,12,12a-pentahydroxy-6-methyl-1,11-dioxo-2-naphthacene-carboxamido]methyl]amino]-β-D-glucopyranose. *CAS-31770-79-3*. INN.

Meglumine (me′ gloo meen). USP. $C_7H_{17}NO_5$. 195.21. (1) D-Glucitol, 1-deoxy-1-(methylamino)-; (2) 1-Deoxy-1-(methylamino)-D-glucitol. *UNII-6HG8UB2MUY*. *CAS-6284-40-8*. INN; BAN; JAN. *Diagnostic aid (radiopaque medium)*.

Meglumine Amidotrizoate (BAN) — *See* Diatrizoate Meglumine.

Meglumine Amidotrizoate Injection (JAN) — *See* Diatrizoate Meglumine.

Meglumine Diatrizoate (previously used name) — *See* Diatrizoate Meglumine.

Meglumine Gadopentetate (JAN) — *See* Gadopentetate Dimeglumine.

Meglumine Iocarmate (BAN) — *See* Iocarmate Meglumine.

Meglumine Iodamide Injection (JAN) — *See* Iodamide Meglumine.

Meglumine Iotalamate Injection (JAN) — *See* Iothalamate Meglumine.

Meglumine Sodium Amidotrizoate Injection (JAN) — *See* Diatrizoate Sodium.

Meglumine Sodium Iodamide Injection (JAN) — *See* Iodamide Meglumine.

Meglutol [*1978*] (me′ gloo tol). $C_6H_{10}O_5$. 162.14. (1) Pentanedioic acid, 3-hydroxy-3-methyl-; (2) 3-Hydroxy-3-methylglutaric acid. *CAS-503-49-1*. INN. *Antihyperlipoproteinemic*. ◇*CB-337*

Mel B — *See* Melarsoprol.

Mel W — *See* Melarsonyl Potassium.

Meladrazine. $C_{11}H_{23}N_7$. 253.35. 2,4-Bis(diethylamino)-6-hydrazino-*s*-triazine. *UNII-2V6Z0JG2X0. CAS-13957-36-3*. INN; BAN. ◇*Ba 13155 [as tartrate]*

Melafocon A [*1988*] (mel″ a foe′ kon). $(C_{16}H_{38}O_5Si_4)_v$ $(C_7H_6F_6O_2)_w(C_6H_9NO)_x(C_4H_6O_2)_y(C_{10}H_{14}O_4)_z$. (1) 2-Propenoic acid, 2-methyl-, 3-[3,3,3-trimethyl-1,1-bis[[(trimethylsilyl)oxy]disiloxanyl]propyl ester, polymer with 2,2,2-trifluoro-1-(trifluoromethyl)ethyl 2-methyl-2-propenoate, 1-ethenyl-2-pyrrolidinone, 2-methyl-2-propenoic acid and 1,2-ethanediyl bis(2-methyl-2-propenoate); (2) 3-[3,3,3-Trimethyl-1,1-bis(trimethylsiloxy)disiloxanyl]propyl methacrylate polymer with 2,2,2-trifluoro-1-(trifluoromethyl)ethyl methacrylate, 1-vinyl-2-pyrrolidinone, methacrylic acid ethylene dimethacrylate. *CAS-107078-89-7. Contact lens material (hydrophobic).*

Melagatran. $C_{22}H_{31}N_5O_4$. 429.51. *N*-[(*R*)-[[(2*S*)-2-[(*p*-Amidinobenzyl)carbamoyl]-1-azetidinyl]carbonyl]cyclohexylmethyl]glycine. *UNII-2A9QP32MD4. CAS-159776-70-2.* INN.

Melarsomine. $C_{13}H_{21}AsN_8S_2$. 428.41. bis(2-Aminoethyl) *p*-[(4,6-diamino-*s*-triazin-2-yl)amino]dithiobenzenearsonite. *UNII-374GJ0S41A. CAS-128470-15-5.* INN.

Melarsonyl Potassium. $C_{13}H_{11}AsK_2N_6O_4S_2$. 532.51. Potassium 2-[*p*-[(4,6-diamino-*s*-triazin-2-yl)amino]phenyl]-1,3,2-dithiarsolane-4,5-dicarboxylate. *CAS-13355-00-5; CAS-37526-80-0* [melarsonyl]. INN; BAN; DCF. ◇*RP 9955*

Melarsoprol. $C_{12}H_{15}AsN_6OS_2$. 398.34. 2-[*p*-(4,6-Diamino-*s*-triazin-2-ylamino)phenyl]-1,3,2-dithiarsolane-4-methanol. *CAS-494-79-1*. INN; BAN; DCF; MI. ◇*RP 3854*

Meldonium. $C_6H_{14}N_2O_2$. 146.19. 3-(2,2,2-Trimethyldiazaniumyl)propanoate. *UNII-73H7UDN6EC. CAS-76144-81-5.* INN.

Melengestrol Acetate [*1963*] (mel″ en jes′ trol as′ e tate). **USP.** $C_{25}H_{32}O_4$. 396.52. [Melengestrol is INN and BAN.] (1) Pregna-4,6-diene-3,20-dione, 17-(acetyloxy)-6-methyl-16-methylene-; (2) 17-Hydroxy-6-methyl-16-methylene-pregna-4,6-diene-3,20-dione acetate. *UNII-4W5HDS3936. CAS-2919-66-6; CAS-5633-18-1* [melengestrol]. *Antineoplastic; progestin.* ◇*BDH 1921; 5373; NSC-70968*

---

† Brand name formerly used, and/or firm no longer concerned with this product.

Meletimide. $C_{24}H_{28}N_2O_2$. 376.49. (±)-2-[1-(*p*-Methylbenzyl)-4-piperidyl]-2-phenylglutarimide. *UNII-NZP1W4BK07. CAS-14745-50-7.* INN.

Melevodopa. $C_{10}H_{13}NO_4$. 211.21. (-)-3,4-Dihydroxy-L-phenylalanine, methyl ester. *CAS-7101-51-1.* INN.

Melfalan — *See* Melphalan.

Melilot Extract. JAN.

Melinamide. $C_{26}H_{41}NO$. 383.61. *N*-(α-Methylbenzyl)linoleamide. *CAS-14417-88-0.* INN; JAN; MI.

Melitracen Hydrochloride [*1968*] (mel i tray′ sen hye″ droe klor′ ide). $C_{21}H_{25}N \cdot HCl$. 327.89. [Melitracen is INN.] (1) 1-Propanamine, 3-(10,10-dimethyl-9(10*H*)-anthracenylidene)-*N*,*N*-dimethyl-, hydrochloride; (2) *N*,*N*,10,10-Tetramethyl-$\Delta^{9(10H),\gamma}$-anthracenepropylamine hydrochloride. *CAS-10563-70-9; CAS-5118-29-6* [melitracen]. JAN. *Antidepressant.* ◇*U-24,973A*

Melizame [*1974*] (mel′ i zame). $C_7H_6N_4O_2$. 178.15. (1) Phenol, 3-(1*H*-tetrazol-5-yloxy)-; (2) 5-(*m*-Hydroxyphenoxy)-1*H*-tetrazole. *UNII-292N180GYN. CAS-26921-72-2.* INN. *Sweetener.* ◇*Compound 56063*

Melogliptin. $C_{15}H_{21}FN_6O$. 320.37. (2*S*,4*S*)-4-Fluoro-1-[2-({(1*R*,3*S*)-3-[(1*H*-1,2,4-triazol-1-yl)methyl]cyclopentyl}amino)acetyl]pyrrolidine-2-carbonitrile. *CAS-868771-57-7.* INN.

Meloxicam [*1997*] (mel ox′ i kam). **USP.** $C_{14}H_{13}N_3O_4S_2$. 351.40. 4-Hydroxy-2-methyl-*N*-(5-methyl-2-thiazolyl)-2*H*-1,2-benzothiazine-3-carboxamide 1,1-dioxide. *UNII-*

VG2QF83CGL. CAS-71125-38-7. INN; BAN. *Anti-inflammatory (nonsteroidal).* Mobic (Boehringer Ingelheim) ◇*UH-AC 62XX*

Melperone. $C_{16}H_{22}FNO$. 263.35. 4′-Fluoro-4-(4-methylpiperidino)butyrophenone. *UNII-J8WA3K39B7. CAS-3575-80-2.* INN; BAN; DCF; MI. ◇*FG 5111*

Melphalan [*1963*] (mel′ fa lan). **USP.** $C_{13}H_{18}Cl_2N_2O_2$. 305.20. (1) L-Phenylalanine, 4-[bis(2-chloroethyl)amino]-; (2) L-3-[*p*-[Bis(2-chloroethyl)amino]phenyl]alanine. *UNII-Q41OR9510P. CAS-148-82-3.* INN; BAN; JAN. *Antineoplastic.* Alkeran (GlaxoSmithKline) ◇*CB 3025; NSC-8806 [as hydrochloride]*

Melquinast. $C_{15}H_{16}N_4O_3$. 300.31. Ethyl 6-ethyl-5,6-dihydro-9-methyl-5-oxo-*s*-triazolo[1,5-*c*]quinazoline-2-carboxylate. *UNII-0RO0SEU9AY. CAS-87611-28-7.* INN.

Meluadrine. $C_{12}H_{18}ClNO_2$. 243.73. (-)-(*R*)-α-[(*tert*-Butylamino)methyl]-2-chloro-4-hydroxybenzyl alcohol. *UNII-FYC8314117. CAS-134865-33-1.* INN.

Memantine. $C_{12}H_{21}N$. 179.30. 3,5-Dimethyl-1-adamantanamine. *UNII-W8O17SJF3T. CAS-19982-08-2.* INN; BAN; MI.

Memantine Hydrochloride [*2003*] (me man′ teen hye″ droe klor′ ide). $C_{12}H_{21}N \cdot HCl$. 215.76. (1) Tricyclo[3.3.1.1^{3,7}]decan-1-amine, 3,5-dimethyl-, hydrochloride; (2) 3,5-Dimethyltricyclo[3.3.1.1^{3,7}]decan-1-amine hydrochloride;

(3) 3,5-Dimethyl-1-adamantanamine hydrochloride; (4) 1-Amino-3,5-dimethyladamantane hydrochloride. *UNII-JY0WD0UA60. CAS-41100-52-1. Treatment of Alzheimer's disease.* Namenda (Forest)

Memotine Hydrochloride [*1969*] (mem' oh teen hye" droe klor' ide). $C_{17}H_{17}NO_2 \cdot HCl$. 303.78. [Memotine is INN.] (1) Isoquinoline, 3,4-dihydro-1-(4-methoxyphenoxy)methyl]-, hydrochloride; (2) 3,4-Dihydro-1-[(*p*-methoxyphenoxy)-methyl]isoquinoline hydrochloride. *CAS-10540-97-3; CAS-18429-69-1* [memotine]. *Antiviral.* ◇*UK-2371*

Menabitan Hydrochloride [*1983*] (men ab' i tan hye" droe klor' ide). $C_{37}H_{56}N_2O_3 \cdot 2HCl$. 649.77. [Menabitan is INN.] (1) 1-Piperidinebutanoic acid, α,2-dimethyl-, 8-(1,2-dimethylheptyl)-1,3,4,5-tetrahydro-5,5-dimethyl-2-(2-propynyl)-2*H*-[1]benzopyrano[4,3-*c*]pyridin-10-yl ester, dihydrochloride, (±)-; (2) (±)-8-(1,2-Dimethylheptyl)-1,3,4,5-tetrahydro-5,5-dimethyl-2-(2-propynyl)-2*H*-[1]benzopyrano[4,3-*c*]pyridin-10-yl α,2-dimethyl-1-piperidinebutyrate, dihydrochloride. *CAS-58019-50-4; CAS-83784-21-8* [menabitan]. *Analgesic.* ◇*SP-204*

Menadiol Sodium Diphosphate (men" a dye' ol soe' dee um dye fos' fate). **USP.** $C_{11}H_8Na_4O_8P_2 \cdot 6H_2O$. 530.17. [Menadiol is BAN.] (1) 1,4-Naphthalenediol, 2-methyl-, bis(dihydrogen phosphate), tetrasodium salt, hexahydrate; (2) 2-Methyl-1,4-naphthalenediol bis(dihydrogen phosphate) tetrasodium salt, hexahydrate. *UNII-2OVL75B30W; UNII-VQ093653DO* [menadiol]. *CAS-6700-42-1; CAS-131-13-5* [anhydrous]; *CAS-84-98-0* [menadiol bis(dihydrogen phosphate)]; *CAS-481-85-6* [menadiol]. *Vitamin (prothrombogenic).* Kappadione (Lilly); Synkayvite (Roche)

Menadiol Sodium Sulfate. $C_{11}H_8Na_2O_8S_2$. 378.29. [Menadiol Potassium Sulfate is BAN.] 2-Methyl-1,4-naphthalenediol bis(hydrogen sulfate) disodium salt. *UNII-LCF9984C2K. CAS-1612-30-2.* INN. *[Name previously used: Potassium Menaphthosulphate.]*

Menadione (men" a dye' one). **USP.** $C_{11}H_8O_2$. 172.18. (1) 1,4-Naphthalenedione, 2-methyl-; (2) 2-Methyl-1,4-naphthoquinone. *UNII-723JX6CXY5. CAS-58-27-5.* BAN. *Vitamin (prothrombogenic).* Kayquinone (Abbott)

Menadione Sodium Bisulfite. $C_{11}H_9NaO_5S \cdot 3H_2O$. 330.29. (1) 2-Naphthalenesulfonic acid, 1,2,3,4-tetrahydro-2-methyl-1,4-dioxo-, sodium salt, trihydrate; (2) Sodium 1,2,3,4-tetrahydro-2-methyl-1,4-dioxo-2-naphthalenesulfonate trihydrate. *UNII-723JX6CXY5* [menadione]. *CAS-6147-37-1; CAS-130-37-0* [anhydrous]; *CAS-58-27-5* [menadione]. USP XX; INN; MI. Hykinone (Abbott†); Klotogen (Abbott†)

Menadoxime. $C_{13}H_{14}N_2O_4$. 262.26. Ammonium salt of 2-methylnaphthoquinone 4-oxime *O*-carboxymethyl ether. *CAS-6146-99-2.* BAN.

Menaphthene — *See* Menadione.

Menaphthone — *See* Menadione.

Menaphthone Sodium Bisulfite — *See* Menadione Sodium Bisulfite.

Menatetrenone. $C_{31}H_{40}O_2$. 444.65. 2-Methyl-3-(3,7,11,15-tetramethyl-2,6,10,14-hexadecatetraenyl)-1,4-naphthoquinone. *UNII-27Y876D139. CAS-863-61-6.* INN; JAN.

Menbutone. $C_{15}H_{14}O_4$. 258.27. 3-(4-Methoxy-1-naphthoyl)-propionic acid. *UNII-341YM32546. CAS-3562-99-0.* INN; BAN; MI. ◇*SC 1749 [as sodium salt]*

Menfegol. $(C_2H_4O)_nC_{16}H_{24}O$. α-[*p*-(*p*-Menthyl)phenyl]-ω-hydroxypoly(oxyethylene). *CAS-57821-32-6.* INN.

Menglytate. $C_{14}H_{26}O_3$. 242.35. *p*-Menth-3-yl ethoxyacetate. *CAS-579-94-2.* INN.

Menichlopholan — *See* Niclofolan.

Meningococcal Polysaccharide Vaccine Group A. USP XXVI. *Immunizing agent (active).*

Meningococcal Polysaccharide Vaccine Group C. USP XXVI. *Immunizing agent (active).*

Menitrazepam. $C_{16}H_{17}N_3O_3$. 299.32. 5-(1-Cyclohexen-1-yl)-1,3-dihydro-1-methyl-7-nitro-2*H*-1,4-benzodiazepin-2-one. *UNII-1243654WZK. CAS-28781-64-8.* INN; DCF. $\diamond$*CB 4857*

Menoctone [*1967*] (men ok′ tone). $C_{24}H_{32}O_3$. 368.51. (1) 1,4-Naphthalenedione, 2-(8-cyclohexyloctyl)-3-hydroxy-; (2) 2-(8-Cyclohexyloctyl)-3-hydroxy-1,4-naphthoquinone. *UNII-QP1A5BD6K9. CAS-14561-42-3.* INN. *Antimalarial.* $\diamond$*Win 11,530; NSC-103336*

Menogaril [*1986*] (men′ oh ga ril). $C_{28}H_{31}NO_{10}$. 541.55. (1) 2,6-Epoxy-2*H*-naphthaceno[1,2-*b*]oxocin-9,16-dione, 4-(dimethylamino)-3,4,5,6,11,12,13,14-octahydro-3,5,8,10,13-pentahydroxy-11-methoxy-6,13-dimethyl-, [2 *R* - (2 α, 3 β, 4 α, 5 β, 6 α, 1 1 α, 1 3 α)] - ; (2) (2*R*,3*S*,4*R*,5*R*,6*R*,11*R*,13*R*)-4-(Dimethylamino)-3,4,5,6,11,12,13,14-octahydro-3,5,8,10,13-pentahydroxy-11-methoxy-6,13-dimethyl-2,6-epoxy-2*H*-naphthac-

eno[1,2-*b*]oxocin-9,16-dione. *UNII-8JSV4O30HQ. CAS-71628-96-1.* INN. *Antineoplastic.* $\diamond$*U-52,047; NSC-269148*

Menotrophin (BAN) — *See* Menotropins.

Menotropins [*1967*] (men″ oh troe′ pins). USP. [Menotrophin is BAN.] An extract of human post-menopausal urine containing both follicle-stimulating hormone and luteinizing hormone. (1) Follicle stimulating hormone; (2) Follicle stimulating hormone. *CAS-9002-68-0. Gonad-stimulating principle.* Humegon (Organon); Pergonal (Serono) *[Name previously used: Human Follicle Stimulating Hormone.]* $\diamond$*FSH; HMG*

Mentha Oil. JAN.

l-Menthol (JAN) — *See* Levomenthol.

Menthol (men′ thol). USP. $C_{10}H_{20}O$. 156.27. [*dl*-Menthol is JAN.] Cyclohexanol, 5-methyl-2-(1-methylethyl)-. *CAS-1490-04-6. Antipruritic (topical).* Fisherman's Friend Lozenges (Bristol-Myers Products); Therapeutic Mineral Ice (Bristol-Myers Products)

Menthyl Anthranilate — *See* Mequinol.

Menthyl Anthranilate (previously used name) — *See* Meradimate.

Meobentine Sulfate [*1977*] (mee″ oh ben′ teen sul′ fate). $(C_{11}H_{17}N_3O)_2 \cdot H_2SO_4$. 512.62. [Meobentine is INN.] (1) Guanidine, *N*-[(4-methoxyphenyl)methyl]-*N′,N″*-dimethyl-, sulfate (2:1); (2) 1-(*p*-Methoxybenzyl)-2,3-dimethyl-guanidine sulfate (2:1). *CAS-58503-79-0; CAS-46464-11-3* [meobentine]. *Cardiac depressant (anti-arrhythmic).*

Mepacrine (INN, BAN) — *See* Quinacrine Hydrochloride.

Meparfynol. $C_6H_{10}O$. 98.14. [Methylpentynol is INN and BAN.] 3-Methyl-1-pentyn-3-ol. *UNII-B017BC5B1N. CAS-77-75-8.* MI. Dormison (Schering†)

Mepartricin [*1975*] (me″ par trye′ sin). A methyl ester of partricin, which is a mixture in a constant ratio (about 1:1) of two polyene (heptaene) substances with very similar structure (not yet fully elucidated) and very similar biological properties. (1) Partricin, methyl-; (2) Methylpartricin. *CAS-11121-32-7.* INN; BAN. *Antifungal; antiprotozoal.* ◇*SPA-S-160; SN 654*

Mepazine Acetate. $C_{19}H_{22}N_2S.C_2H_4O_2$. 370.51. [Pecazine is INN and BAN.] 10-[(1-Methyl-3-piperidyl)methyl]phenothiazine. *UNII-U42703EIIO. CAS-24360-97-2; CAS-60-89-9* [mepazine]. NND 1964.

Mepenzolate Bromide. $C_{21}H_{26}BrNO_3$. 420.34. (1) Piperidinium, 3-[(hydroxydiphenylacetyl)oxy]-1,1-dimethyl-, bromide; (2) 3-Hydroxy-1,1-dimethylpiperidinium bromide benzilate. *UNII-APX8D32IX1. CAS-76-90-4; CAS-25990-43-6* [mepenzolate]. USP XXIII Supplement 1; INN; BAN; JAN. *Anticholinergic.* Cantil (Sanofi Aventis)

Mepenzolate Methylbromide — *See* Mepenzolate Bromide.

Mepenzolone Bromide — *See* Mepenzolate Bromide.

Meperidine Hydrochloride (me per′ i deen hye″ droe klor′ ide). **USP.** $C_{15}H_{21}NO_2.HCl$. 283.79. [Pethidine is INN and BAN; Pethidine Hydrochloride is JAN.] (1) 4-Piperidinecarboxylic acid, 1-methyl-4-phenyl-, ethyl ester, hydrochloride; (2) Ethyl 1-methyl-4-phenylisonipecotate hydrochloride. *UNII-N8E7F7Q170; UNII-9E338QE28F* [meperidine]. *CAS-50-13-5; CAS-57-42-1* [meperidine]. *Analgesic (narcotic).* Demerol (Hospira); Demerol (Sanofi Aventis)

Mephenesin. $C_{10}H_{14}O_3$. 182.22. 3-(*o*-Methylphenoxy)-1,2-propanediol. *UNII-7B8PIR2954. CAS-59-47-2.* NF XII; INN; BAN; MI. Tolserol (Bristol-Myers Squibb†)

Mephenhydramine — *See* Moxastine.

---

† Brand name formerly used, and/or firm no longer concerned with this product.

Mephenoxalone. $C_{11}H_{13}NO_4$. 223.23. 5-[(*o*-Methylphenoxy)methyl]-2-oxazolidinone. *CAS-70-07-5.* INN; DCF; AMADE 1971; MI. Lenetran (Marion Merrell Dow†)

Mephentermine Sulfate. $(C_{11}H_{17}N)_2.H_2SO_4$. 424.60. [Mephentermine is INN and BAN.] (1) Benzeneethanamine, *N,α,α*-trimethyl-, sulfate (2:1); (2) *N,α,α*-Trimethylphenethylamine sulfate (2:1). *UNII-580655Z8RR; UNII-TEZ91L71V4* [mephentermine]. *CAS-1212-72-2; CAS-6190-60-9* [dihydrate]; *CAS-100-92-5* [mephentermine]. USP XXIII. *Adrenergic (vasoconstrictor).* Wyamine Sulfate (Baxter Healthcare)

Mephenytoin [*1962*] (me fen′ i toin; me fen′ i toe in). **USP.** $C_{12}H_{14}N_2O_2$. 218.25. (1) 2,4-Imidazolidinedione, 5-ethyl-3-methyl-5-phenyl-, (±)-; (2) (±)-5-Ethyl-3-methyl-5-phenylhydantoin. *UNII-R420KW629U. CAS-50-12-4.* INN; BAN. *Anticonvulsant.* Mesantoin (Novartis) *[Name previously used: Methoin.]* ◇*NSC-34652*

Mephobarbital (mef″ oh bar′ bi tal). **USP.** $C_{13}H_{14}N_2O_3$. 246.26. [Methylphenobarbital is INN and BAN.] (1) 2,4,6(1*H*,3*H*,5*H*)-Pyrimidinetrione, 5-ethyl-1-methyl-5-phenyl-; (2) 5-Ethyl-1-methyl-5-phenylbarbituric acid. *UNII-5NC67NU76B. CAS-115-38-8.* JAN. *Anticonvulsant; sedative-hypnotic.* Mebaral (Sterling Winthrop); Menta-Bal (Marion Merrell Dow†) *[Name previously used: Methylphenobarbitone.]*

Mepicycline — *See* Pipacycline.

Mepindolol. $C_{15}H_{22}N_2O_2$. 262.35. 1-(Isopropylamino)-3-[(2-methylindol-4-yl)oxy]-2-propanol. *CAS-23694-81-7.* INN; BAN; MI.

Mepiperphenidol Bromide. *CAS-520-20-7.*

Mepiprazole. $C_{16}H_{21}ClN_4$. 304.82. 1-(*m*-Chlorophenyl)-4-[2-(5-methylpyrazol-3-yl)ethyl]piperazine. *UNII-977BAL0NR7. CAS-20326-12-9.* INN; BAN; MI.

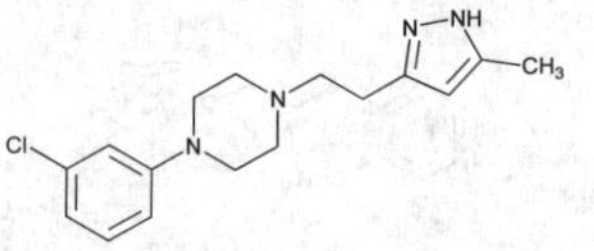

Mepirizole — *See* Epirizole.

Mepiroxol. $C_6H_7NO_2$. 125.13. 3-Pyridinemethanol 1-oxide. *UNII-BR2Z22465M. CAS-6968-72-5.* INN; DCF.

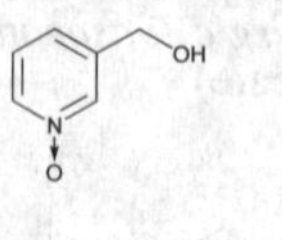

Mepitiostane. $C_{25}H_{40}O_2S$. 404.65. Cyclopentanone $2\alpha,3\alpha$-epithio-5α-androstan-17β-yl methyl acetal. *CAS-21362-69-6.* INN; JAN; MI.

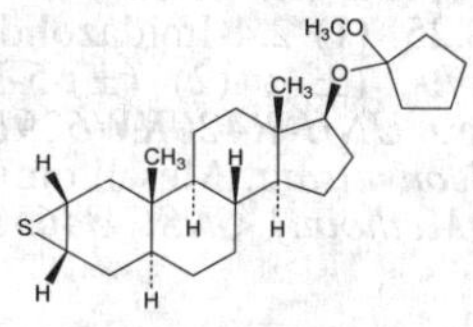

Mepivacaine Hydrochloride (me piv′ a kane hye″ droe klor′ ide). **USP.** $C_{15}H_{22}N_2O\cdot HCl$. 282.81. [Mepivacaine is INN and BAN.] (1) 2-Piperidinecarboxamide, *N*-(2,6-dimethylphenyl)-1-methyl-, monohydrochloride, (±)-; (2) (±)-1-Methyl-2′,6′-pipecoloxylidide monohydrochloride. *UNII-4VFX2L7EM5; UNII-B6E06QE59J* [mepivacaine]. *CAS-1722-62-9; CAS-96-88-8* [mepivacaine]. JAN. *Anesthetic (local).* Carbocaine (Hospira); Polocaine (Abraxis)

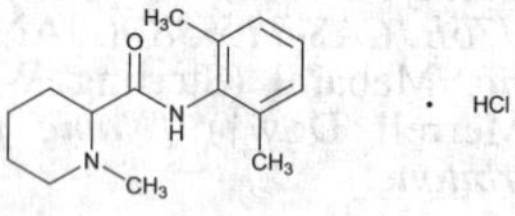

Mepixanox. $C_{20}H_{21}NO_3$. 323.39. 3-Methoxy-4-(piperidinomethyl)xanthen-9-one. *UNII-7419T4YQQW. CAS-17854-59-0.* INN; MI.

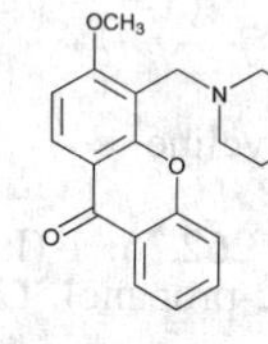

Mepolizumab [*1998*] (me″ poe liz′ oo mab). (1) Immunoglobulin G1, anti-(human interleukin 5) (human-mouse monoclonal SB-240563 γ1-chain), disulfide with human-mouse monoclonal SB-240563 κ-chain, dimer; (2) Immunoglobulin G1 (human-mouse monoclonal SB-240563 γ1-chain anti-human interleukin 5), disulfide with human-mouse monoclonal SB-240563 κ-chain, dimer. Molecular weight is approximately 146,000 daltons. *CAS-196078-29-2.* INN. *Immunomodulator (monoclonal antibody).* ◇SB-240563

Mepramidil. $C_{28}H_{33}NO_5$. 463.57. 3,4,5-Trimethoxybenzoic acid, 3-[(3,3-diphenylpropyl)amino]propyl ester. *UNII-5C8KR48J61. CAS-23891-60-3.* INN. ◇PF-26

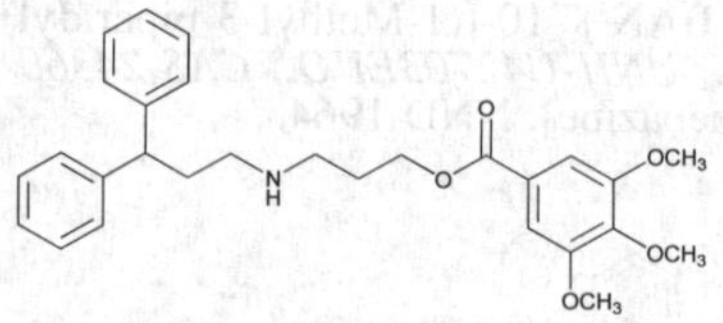

Meprednisone [*1965*] (me pred′ ni sone). **USP.** $C_{22}H_{28}O_5$. 372.45. (1) Pregna-1,4-diene-3,11,20-trione, 17,21-dihydroxy-16-methyl-, (16β)-; (2) 17,21-Dihydroxy-16β-methylpregna-1,4-diene-3,11,20-trione. *UNII-67U96J8P35. CAS-1247-42-3.* INN. Betapar (Schering) ◇Sch 4358; NSC-527579

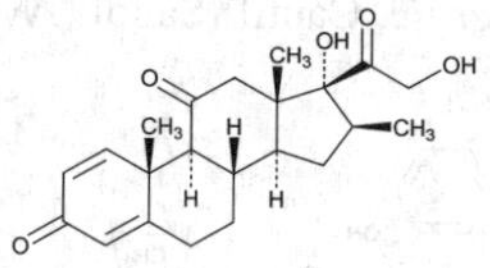

Meprobamate (me″ proe bam′ ate). **USP.** $C_9H_{18}N_2O_4$. 218.25. (1) 1,3-Propanediol, 2-methyl-2-propyl-, dicarbamate; (2) 2-Methyl-2-propyl-1,3-propanediol dicarbamate. *UNII-9I7LNY769Q. CAS-57-53-4.* INN; BAN; JAN. *Sedative-hypnotic.* Equanil (Wyeth); Miltown (Medpointe)

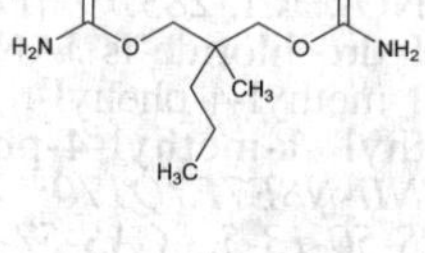

Meprochol. $C_7H_{16}BrNO$. 210.11. (2-Methoxyprop-2-enyl)trimethylammonium bromide. *UNII-7K2B1728PB. CAS-590-31-8.* BAN.

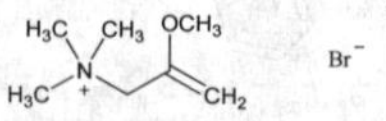

Meproscillarin. $C_{31}H_{44}O_8$. 544.68. 3β-[(6-Deoxy-4-*O*-methyl-α-L-mannopyranosyl)oxy]-14-hydroxybufa-4,20,22-trienolide. *CAS-33396-37-1.* INN; BAN.

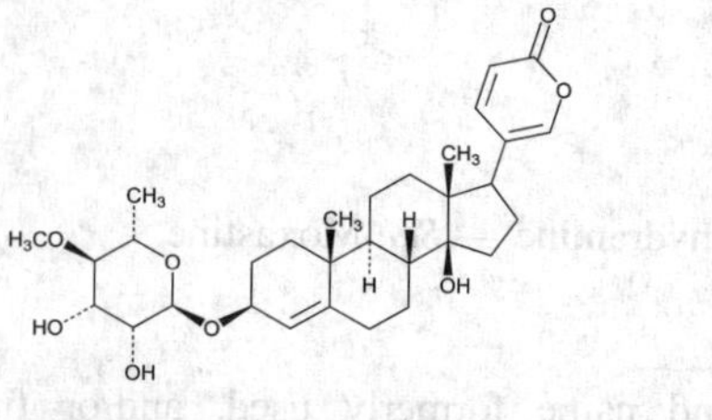

Meprotixol. $C_{19}H_{23}NO_2S$. 329.46. 9-[3-(Dimethylamino)pro-pyl]-2-methoxy-thioxanthene-9-ol. *CAS-4295-63-0.* INN; BAN. *[Name previously used: Meprothixol.]* ◇*N-7020*

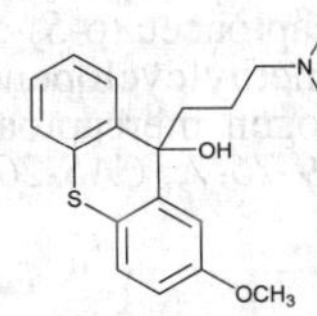

Meprylcaine Hydrochloride. $C_{14}H_{21}NO_2.HCl$. 271.78. [Me-prylcaine is INN.] (1) 1-Propanol-2-methyl-2-(propylami-no)-, benzoate (ester), hydrochloride; (2) 2-Methyl-2-(propylamino)-1-propanol benzoate (ester) hydrochloride. *UNII-VR843X5GXG. CAS-956-03-6; CAS-495-70-5* [me-prylcaine]. USP XXII.

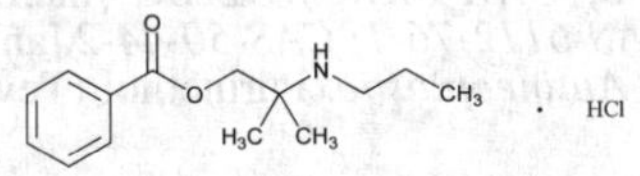

Meptazinol Hydrochloride [*1984*] (mep taz′ i nol hye″ droe klor′ ide). $C_{15}H_{23}NO.HCl$. 269.81. [Meptazinol is INN and BAN.] (1) Phenol, 3-(3-ethylhexahydro-1-methyl-1*H*-aze-pin-3-yl)-, hydrochloride; (2) *m*-(3-Ethylhexahydro-1-methyl-1*H*-azepin-3-yl)phenol hydrochloride. *CAS-59263-76-2; CAS-54340-58-8* [meptazinol]. *Analgesic.* ◇*WY 22811 HCl; IL 22811 HCl*

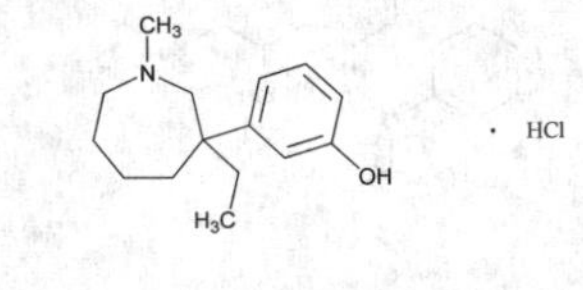

Mepyramine (INN, BAN) — *See* Pyrilamine Maleate.

Mepyrium — *See* Amprolium.

Mepyrrotazine — *See* Dimelazine.

Mequidox [*1968*] (me′ kwi dox). $C_{10}H_{10}N_2O_3$. 206.20. (1) 2-Quinoxalinemethanol, 3-methyl-, 1,4-dioxide; (2) 3-Meth-yl-2-quinoxalinemethanol 1,4-dioxide. *CAS-16915-79-0.* INN. *Antibacterial.* ◇*GS-7443*

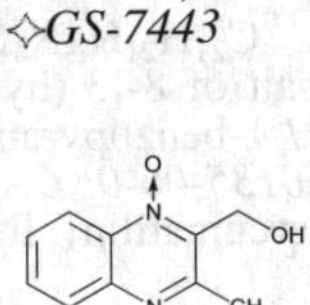

Mequinol [*1999*] (me′ kwin ol). $C_7H_8O_2$. 124.14. (1) Phenol, 4-methoxy-; (2) *p*-Methoxyphenol. *UNII-6HT8U7K3AM. CAS-150-76-5.* INN; DCF. *Treatment of hyperpigmenta-tion.[Names previously used: 4-Methoxyphenol, 4-Hydro-xyanisole, HQMME; Hydroxyquinone Methyl Ether, p-Guaiacol, Leucobasal, Leucodine B, Mechinolum, Novo-*

Dermoquinona, 4HA, and p-Hydroxyanisole. Note—The International Cosmetic Ingredient (INCI) name is p-hydroxyanisole.] ◇*BMS-181158*

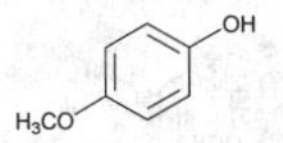

Mequitamium Iodide. $C_{21}H_{25}IN_2S$. 464.41. (±)-1-Methyl-3-(phenothiazin-10-ylmethyl)quinuclidinium iodide. *CAS-101396-42-3.* INN.

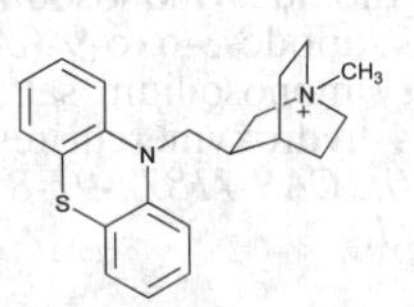

Mequitazine. $C_{20}H_{22}N_2S$. 322.47. 10-(3-Quinuclidinyl-methyl)phenothiazine. *CAS-29216-28-2.* INN; BAN; JAN; DCF; MI.

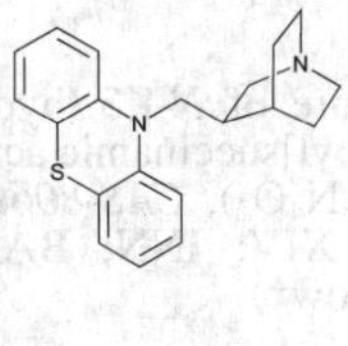

Mequitazium Iodide — *See* Mequitamium Iodide.

Meradimate [*1999*] (mer ad′ i mate). **USP.** $C_{17}H_{25}NO_2$. 275.39. (1) Cyclohexanol, 5-methyl-2-(1-methylethyl)-, 2-aminobenzoate; (2) Anthranilic acid, *p*-menth-3-yl ester. *CAS-134-09-8.* INN. *Sunscreen (ultraviolet A absorber).* Neo Heliopan (H & R Florasynth) *[Name previously used: Menthyl Anthranilate.] [Note—The International Cosmetic Ingredient (INCI) name for meradimate is menthyl anthranilate.]*

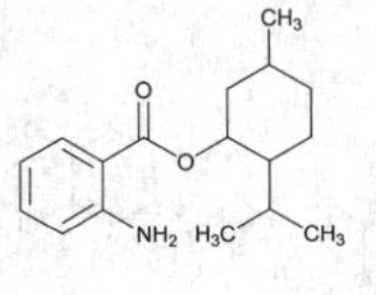

Merafloxacin. $C_{19}H_{23}F_2N_3O_3$. 379.40. (±)-1-Ethyl-7-[3-[(ethylamino)methyl]-1-pyrrolidinyl]-6,8-difluoro-1,4-di-hydro-4-oxo-3-quinolinecarboxylic acid. *CAS-110013-21-3.* INN.

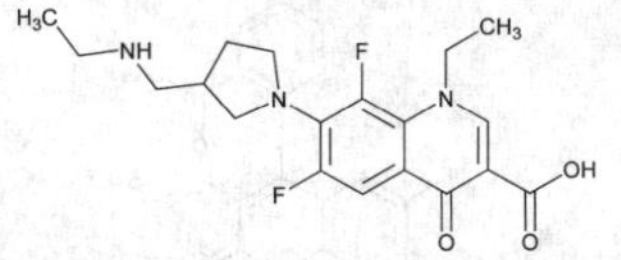

Meragidone Sodium. $C_{10}H_{12}HgNNaO_5.C_7H_8N_4O_2$. 629.95. (1) Mercurate(1-), (3-(5-carboxylato-1,2-dihydro-2-oxo-1-pyridinyl)-2-methoxypropyl)hydroxy-, sodium, compd. with 3,7-dihydro-1,3-dimethyl-1*H*-purine-2,6-dione; (2)

---

† Brand name formerly used, and/or firm no longer concerned with this product.

Sodium (3-(5-carboxylato-2-oxopyridin-1(2*H*)-yl)-2-methoxypropyl)(hydroxy) mercury compd. with theophylline. *CAS-7097-62-3.* Merdroxone Sodium (Sterling Winthrop†)

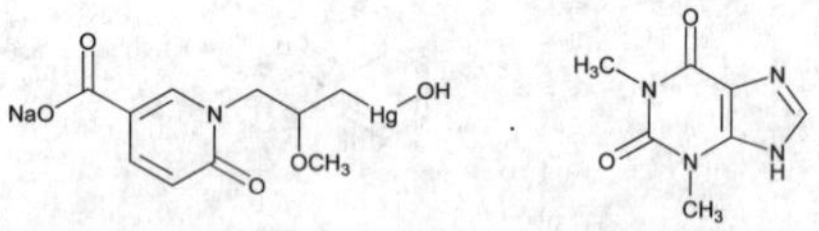

Meralein Sodium [*1962*] (mer′ a leen soe′ dee um). $C_{19}H_9HgI_2NaO_7S$. 858.72. (1) Mercury, (3′,6′-dihydroxy-2′,7′-diiodospiro[3*H*-2,1-benzoxathiole-3,9′-[9*H*]xanthen]-5′-yl)hydroxy-, *S,S*-dioxide, monosodium salt; (2) Hydroxy[6-hydroxy-2,7-diiodo-3-oxo-9-(*o*-sulfophenyl)-3*H*-xanthen-5-yl]mercury monosodium salt; (3) Monosodium salt of 2,7-diiodo-4-hydroxymercuriresorcinsulfonphthalein. *CAS-4386-35-0; CAS-71872-91-8* [meralein]. INN. *Anti-infective, topical.*

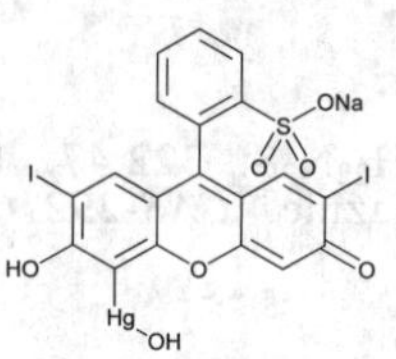

Meralluride. A mixture of *N*-[[3-(hydroxymercuri)-2-methoxypropyl]carbamoyl]succinamic acid ($C_9H_{16}HgN_2O_6$) and theophylline ($C_7H_8N_4O_2$). *CAS-8069-64-5; CAS-129-99-7* [as sodium]. NF XIV; INN; BAN; MI. Mercuhydrin (Marion Merrell Dow†)

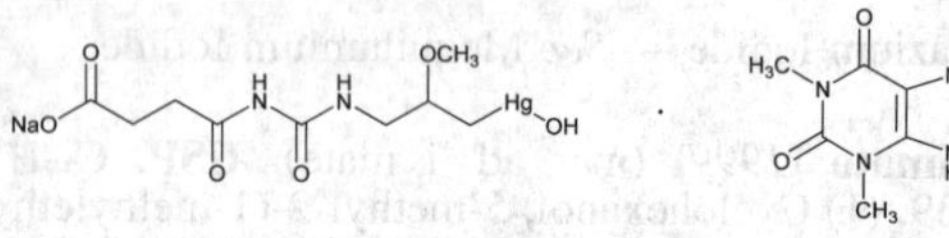

Merbaphen. $C_{16}H_{16}ClHgN_2NaO_6$. 591.34. (1) Mercury(1-), (4-(carboxymethoxy)-3-chlorophenyl)(5,5-diethyl-2,4,6(1*H*,3*H*,5*H*)-pyrimidinetrionato-*O*²)-, monosodium salt; (2) Sodium (4-(carboxylatomethoxy)-3-chlorophenyl)(5,5-diethyl-4,6-dioxo-1,4,5,6-tetrahydropyrimidin-2-yloxy)mercury. USP XI.

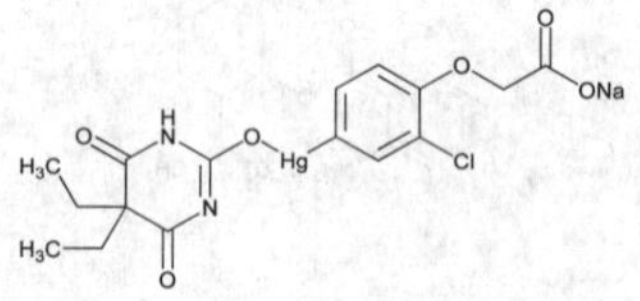

Merbromin. $C_{20}H_8Br_2HgNa_2O_6$. 750.65. [Mercurochrome is JAN.] Disodium salt of 2,7-dibromo-4-hydroxymercurifluoresceine. *CAS-129-16-8.* NF XII; INN; MI.

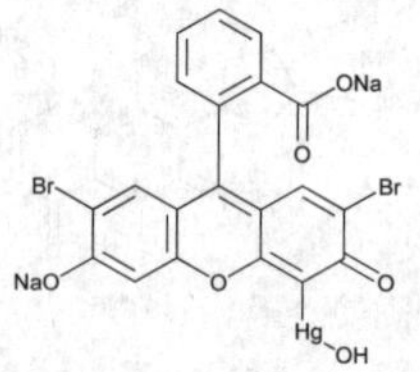

Mercaptamine (INN, BAN, DCF) — *See* Cysteamine.

Mercaptoarsenical — *See* Arsthinol.

Mercaptoarsenol — *See* Arsthinol.

Mercaptomerin Sodium. $C_{16}H_{25}HgNNa_2O_6S$. 606.01. [Mercaptomerin is INN and BAN.] (1) Mercury, [3-[[(3-carboxy-2,2,3-trimethylcyclopentyl)carbonyl]amino]-2-methoxypropyl](mercaptoacetato-*S*)-, disodium salt; (2) [3-(3-Carboxy-2,2,3-trimethylcyclopentanecarboxamido)-2-methoxypropyl](hydrogen mercaptoacetato)mercury disodium salt. *CAS-21259-76-7; CAS-20223-84-1* [mercaptomerin]. USP XX; MI.

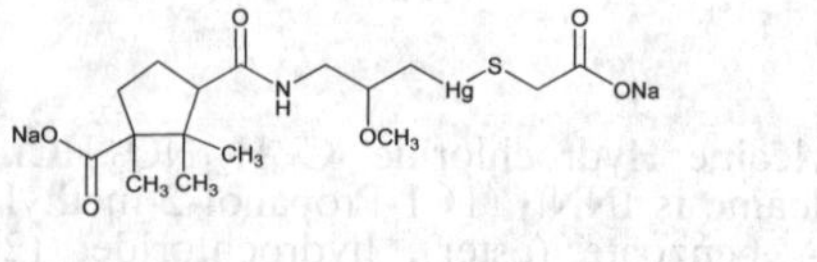

Mercaptopurine (mer kap″ toe pure′ een). USP. $C_5H_4N_4S.H_2O$. 170.19. (1) 6*H*-Purine-6-thione, 1,7-dihydro-, monohydrate; (2) Purine-6-thiol monohydrate. *UNII-E7WED276I5; UNII-PKK6MUZ20G* [mercaptopurine anhydrous]. *CAS-6112-76-1; CAS-50-44-2* [anhydrous]. INN; BAN; JAN. *Antineoplastic.* Purinethol (Teva) ◇*NSC-755*

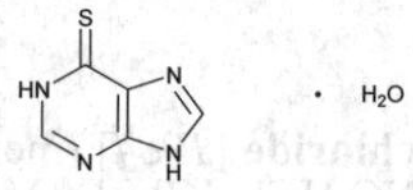

Mercuderamide. $C_{12}H_{15}HgNO_6$. 469.84. *o*-[[2-Hydroxy-3-(hydroxymercuri)propyl]carbamoyl]phenoxyacetic acid. *CAS-525-30-4.* INN; DCF.

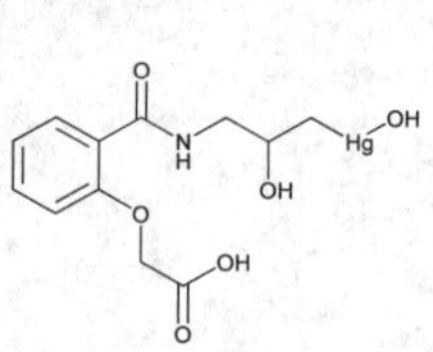

Mercufenol Chloride [*1980*] (mer″ kue fee′ nol klor′ ide). C_6H_5ClHgO. 329.15. (1) Mercury, chloro(2-hydroxyphenyl)-; (2) Chloro(*o*-hydroxyphenyl)mercury. *CAS-90-03-9.* *Anti-infective, topical.* ◇*U-7743*

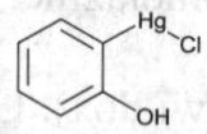

Mercumatilin Sodium. $C_{21}H_{21}HgN_4NaO_8.H_2O$. 699.01. A mixture of sodium salt of 8-[3-(hydroxymercuri)-2-methoxypropyl]-2-oxo-2*H*-1-benzopyran-3-carboxylic acid and theophylline. *CAS-60135-06-0; CAS-574-79-8* [replaced]; *CAS-43043-01-2* [mercumatilin]. INN; MI.

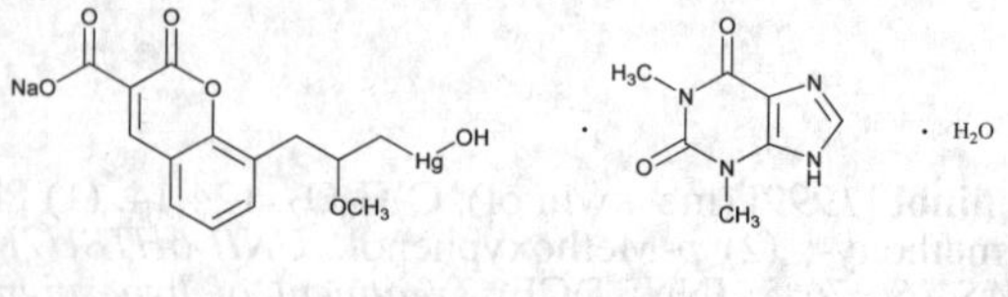

Mercuric Chloride. $HgCl_2$. 271.50. *CAS-7487-94-7.* JAN.

Mercuric Oxide, Yellow. *CAS-21908-53-2.* NF XIII; MI.

Mercuric Salicylate. *CAS-5970-32-1.* NF IX; MI.

Mercuric Succinimide. *CAS-584-43-0; CAS-123-56-8* [succinimide]. NF IX; MI.

Mercurobutol. $C_{10}H_{13}ClHgO$. 385.25. 4-*tert*-Butyl-2-chloro-mercuriphenol. *CAS-498-73-7*. INN; DCF. ◇*L 542*

Mercurochrome (JAN) — *See* Merbromin.

Mercurophylline. A mixture of sodium salt of 3-[3-(hydroxymercuri)-2-methoxypropyl]camphoramic acid ($C_{14}H_{24}HgNNaO_5$) and theophylline ($C_7H_8N_4O_2$). *CAS-8012-34-8*. NF XII; INN; BAN. *[Name previously used: Mercurophylline Sodium.]*

Mercurous Chloride — *See* Calomel.

Mercury, Ammoniated (mer′ kure e a moe′ nee ay″ ted). **USP**. $Hg(NH_2)Cl$. 252.07. (1) Mercury amide chloride; (2) Mercury amide chloride. *CAS-10124-48-8*. *Anti-infective, topical.*

Mercury Oleate. *CAS-1191-80-6*. NF XI.

Merethoxylline Procaine. NND 1964.

Mergocriptine. $C_{33}H_{43}N_5O_5$. 589.73. 2-Methyl-α-ergocryptine. *CAS-81968-16-3*. INN.

Meribendan. $C_{15}H_{14}N_6O$. 294.31. 4,5-Dihydro-5-methyl-6-(2-pyrazol-3-yl-5-benzimidazolyl)-3(2*H*)-pyridazinone. *CAS-119322-27-9*. INN.

Merimepodib [*2002*] (mer″ i mep′ oh dib). $C_{23}H_{24}N_4O_6$. 452.46. (1) Carbamic acid, [[3-[[[[3-methoxy-4-(5-oxazolyl)phenyl]amino]carbonyl]amino]phenyl]methyl]-, (3*S*)-tetrahydro-3-furanyl ester; (2) (*S*)-Tetrahydro-3-furyl [*m*-[3-[3-methoxy-4-(5-oxazolyl)phenyl]ureido]benzyl]carbamate. *UNII-2ZL2BA06FU*. *CAS-198821-22-6*. INN. *Inhibition of inosine monophosphate dehydrogenase (IMPDH),*

which has potential antiviral, antiproliferative, antiparasitic, and immunosuppressive activity. ◇*VX-497; VI-21,497*

Merisoprol Acetate Hg 197 [*1966*] (mer is′ oh prole as′ e tate). $C_5H_{10}{}^{197}HgO_3$. (1) Mercury-^{197}Hg, hydroxy(2-hydroxypropyl)-, acetate; (2) Hydroxy(2-hydroxypropyl)mercury-^{197}Hg, acetate. *CAS-24359-51-1*. INN. *Radioactive agent.*

Merisoprol Acetate Hg 203 [*1966*] (mer is′ oh prole as′ e tate). $C_5H_{10}{}^{203}HgO_3$. (1) Mercury-^{203}Hg, hydroxy(2-hydroxypropyl)-, acetate; (2) Hydroxy(2-hydroxypropyl)mercury-^{203}Hg, acetate. *CAS-24359-50-0. Radioactive agent.*

Merisoprol Hg 197 [*1965*] (mer is′ oh prole). $C_3H_8HgO_2$. 276.68. (1) Mercury-^{197}Hg, hydroxy(2-hydroxypropyl)-; (2) Hydroxy(2-hydroxypropyl)mercury-^{197}Hg. *CAS-5579-94-2. Diagnostic aid (renal function determination); radioactive agent.* Merprane (Bristol-Myers Squibb†)

Meropenem [*1992*] (mer″ oh pen′ em). **USP**. $C_{17}H_{25}N_3O_5S.3H_2O$. 437.51. (1) 1-Azabicyclo[3.2.0]hept-2-ene-2-carboxylic acid, 3-[[5-[(dimethylamino)carbonyl]-3-pyrrolidinyl]thio]-6-(1-hydroxyethyl)-4-methyl-7-oxo-, trihydrate, [4*R*-[3(3*S**,5*S**),4α,5β,6β(*R**)]]-; (2) (4*R*,5*S*,6*S*)-3-[[(3*S*,5*S*)-5-(Dimethylcarbamoyl)-3-pyrrolidinyl]thio]-6-[(1*R*)-1-hydroxyethyl]-4-methyl-7-oxo-1-azabicyclo[3.2.0]hept-2-ene-2-carboxylic acid, trihydrate. *UNII-FV9J3JU8B1*. *CAS-119478-56-7*; *CAS-96036-03-2* [anhydrous]. INN; BAN. *Antibacterial*. Merrem (AstraZeneca) ◇*ICI 194,660; SM-7338*

Mersalyl. $C_{13}H_{16}HgNNaO_6$. 505.85. Sodium salt of *o*-[(3-hydroxymercuri-2-methoxypropyl)carbamoyl]phenoxyacetic acid. *UNII-7RDI07K19U. CAS-492-18-2*. INN; DCF; MI. Salyrgan (Sterling Winthrop†)

Mersalyl Sodium — *See* Mersalyl.

---

† Brand name formerly used, and/or firm no longer concerned with this product.

Mertiatide. $C_8H_{13}N_3O_5S$. 263.27. *N*-[*N*-[*N*-(Mercaptoacetyl)glycyl]glycyl]glycine. *UNII-8NVY8268MY. CAS-66516-09-4.* INN.

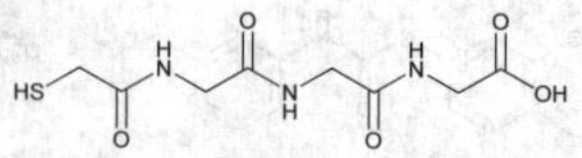

Mesabolone. $C_{26}H_{40}O_3$. 400.59. 17β-[(1-Methoxycyclohexyl)oxy]-5α-androst-1-en-3-one. *CAS-7483-09-2.* INN.

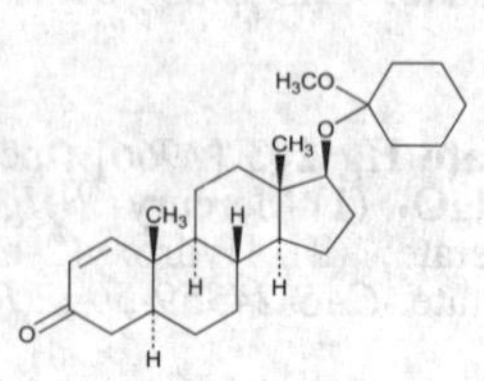

Mesalamine [*1986*] (me sal' a meen). **USP**. $C_7H_7NO_3$. 153.14. [Mesalazine is INN and BAN.] (1) Benzoic acid, 5-amino-2-hydroxy-; (2) 5-Aminosalicylic acid. *UNII-4Q81I59GXC. CAS-89-57-6. Anti-inflammatory*. Asacol (Procter & Gamble); Canasa (Axcan Scandipharm); Pentasa (Shire); Rowasa (Alaven)

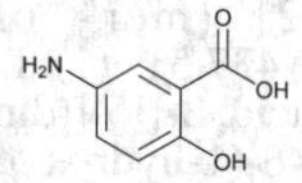

Mesalazine (INN, BAN) — *See* Mesalamine.

Meseclazone [*1976*] (me sek' la zone). $C_{11}H_{10}ClNO_3$. 239.66. (1) 2*H*,9*H*-Isoxazolo[3,2-*b*][1,3]benzoxacin-9-one, 7-chloro-3,3a-dihydro-2-methyl-; (2) 7-Chloro-3,3a-dihydro-2-methyl-2*H*,9*H*-isoxazolo[3,2-*b*][1,3]benzoxazin-9-one. *UNII-51KFT71THG. CAS-29053-27-8.* INN. *Anti-inflammatory*. ◇*W-2395*

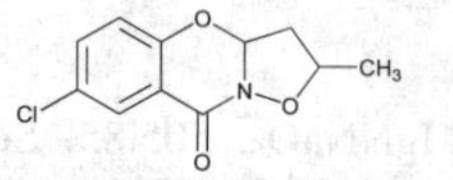

Mesifilcon A [*1980*] (me" si fil' kon). $(C_6H_9NO)_v$ $(C_6H_{10}O_3)_w(C_{16}H_{38}O_5Si_4)_x(C_7H_{10}O_2)_y(C_4H_5O$-$(C_2H_4O)_a(C_2$-$H_6OSi)_b(C_2H_4O)_c$-$O_2C_4H_5)_z$. (1) Siloxanes and silicones dimethyl, polymer with ethylene oxide, dimethacrylate, block, polymer with 1-vinyl-2-pyrrolidinone, 2-hydroxyethyl methacrylate, 3-[3,3,3-trimethyl-1,1-bis(trimethylsiloxy)disiloxanyl]propyl methacrylate and allyl methacrylate; (2) 1-Vinyl-2-pyrrolidinone polymer with 2-hydroxyethyl methacrylate, 3-[3,3,3-trimethyl-1,1-bis (trimethylsiloxy)-disiloxanyl]propyl methacrylate, allyl methacrylate and α-methacryloyl-ω-(methac-

ryloyloxy)poly[oxyethylene-*co*-oxy(dimethylsilylene)-*co*-oxyethylene]. *Contact lens material (hydrophilic)*. ◇*AO-PLUTO*

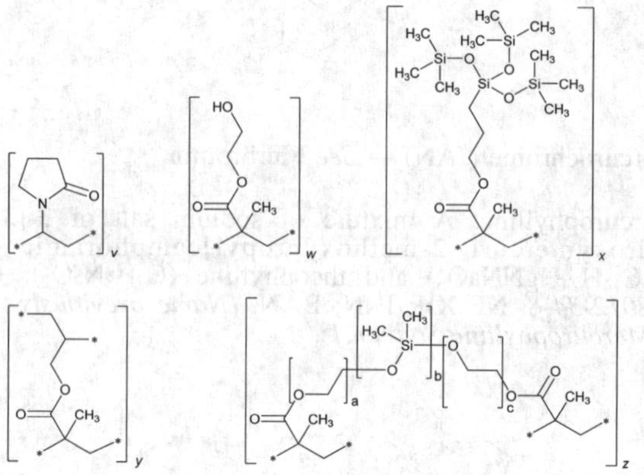

Mesna [*1990*] (mes' na). $C_2H_5NaO_3S_2$. 164.18. (1) Ethanesulfonic acid, 2-mercapto-, monosodium salt; (2) Sodium 2-mercaptoethanesulfonate. *UNII-NR7O1405Q9. CAS-19767-45-4; CAS-3375-50-6* [2-mercaptoethanesulfonic acid]. INN; BAN. *Detoxifying agent*. Mesnex (Baxter Healthcare) ◇*D 7093*

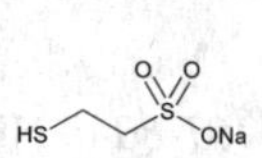

Mesocarb. $C_{18}H_{18}N_4O_2$. 322.36. 3-(α-Methylphenethyl)-*N*-(phenylcarbamoyl)sydnone imine. *CAS-34262-84-5.* INN.

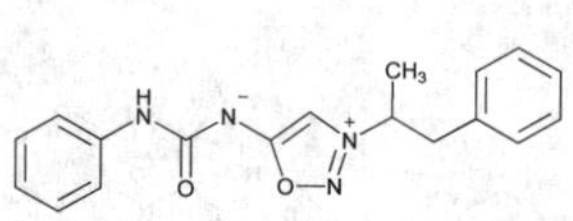

Meso-Inositol — *See* Inositol.

Meso-nordihydroguaiaretic Acid — *See* Masoprocol.

Mesoridazine [*1965*] (mes" oh rid' a zeen). $C_{21}H_{26}N_2OS_2$. 386.57. (1) 10*H*-Phenothiazine, 10-[2-(1-methyl-2-piperidinyl)ethyl]-2-(methylsulfinyl)-; (2) 10-[2(1-Methyl-2-piperidyl)ethyl]-2-(methylsulfinyl)-phenothiazine. *UNII-5XE4NWM740. CAS-5588-33-0.* INN; BAN. *Antipsychotic*. Lidanar (Novartis†) ◇*TPS-23; NC-123*

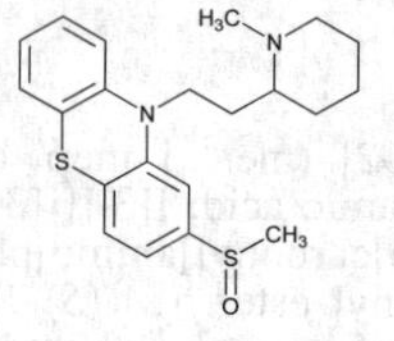

Mesoridazine Besylate (mes" oh rid' a zeen bes' i late). **USP**. $C_{21}H_{26}N_2OS_2 \cdot C_6H_6O_3S$. 544.75. (1) 10*H*-Phenothiazine, 10-[2-(1-methyl-2-piperidinyl)ethyl]-2-(methylsulfinyl)-, (±)-, monobenzenesulfonate; (2) (±)-10-[2-(1-Methyl-2-piperidyl)ethyl]-2-(methylsulfinyl)phenothiazine monobenzenesulfonate. *UNII-T4G2I958J2. CAS-32672-69-8; CAS-5588-33-0* [mesoridazine]. *Antipsychotic.* Serentil (Novartis)

Mespiperone C 11 [*1997*] (mes pi′ per one). **USP** [Injection]. $C_{23}^{11}CH_{28}FN_3O_2$. [Mespiperone (¹¹C) is INN.] 8-[3-(*p*-Fluorobenzoyl)propyl]-3-[¹¹C]methyl-1-phenyl-1,3,8-triazaspiro[4.5]decan-4-one. *CAS-94153-50-1. Diagnostic aid; radioactive agent. [Note—Because of the rapid decay rate of the radioactive isotope, the injectable form is not marketed but is produced near the patient's bedside for immediate administration.]*

Mespirenone. $C_{25}H_{30}O_4S$. 426.57. 15α,16α-Dihydro-17-hydroxy-7α-mercapto-3-oxo-3′*H*-cyclopropa[15,16]-17α-pregna-1,4,15-triene-21-carboxylic acid, γ-lactone, acetate. *CAS-87952-98-5.* INN.

Mestanolone. $C_{20}H_{32}O_2$. 304.47. 17β-Hydroxy-17-methyl-5α-androstan-3-one. *CAS-521-11-9.* INN; BAN; JAN; MI.

Mestenediol — *See* Methandriol.

Mesterolone [*1966*] (mes ter′ oh lone). $C_{20}H_{32}O_2$. 304.47. (1) Androstan-3-one, 17-hydroxy-1-methyl-, (1α,5α,17β)-; (2) 17β-Hydroxy-1α-methyl-5α-androstan-3-one. *CAS-1424-00-6.* INN; BAN. *Androgen.* ◇*SH 723; NSC-75054*

---

† Brand name formerly used, and/or firm no longer concerned with this product.

Mestranol [*1962*] (mes′ tra nol). **USP.** $C_{21}H_{26}O_2$. 310.43. (1) 19-Norpregna-1,3,5(10)-trien-20-yn-17-ol, 3-methoxy-, (17α)-; (2) 3-Methoxy-19-nor-17α-pregna-1,3,5(10)-trien-20-yn-17-ol. *UNII-B2V233XGE7. CAS-72-33-3.* INN; BAN; JAN. *Estrogen.* ◇*EE₃ME; 33355*

Mesudipine. $C_{19}H_{24}N_2O_4S$. 376.47. Diethyl 1′,4′-dihydro-2′,6′-dimethyl-2-(methylthio)[3,4′-bipyridine]-3′,5′-dicarboxylate. *UNII-DT27W93DFF. CAS-62658-88-2.* INN.

Mesulergine. $C_{18}H_{26}N_4O_2S$. 362.49. *N*′-(1,6-Dimethylergolin-8α-yl)-*N,N*-dimethylsulfamide. *CAS-64795-35-3.* INN; MI.

Mesulfamide. $C_7H_{10}N_2O_5S_2$. 266.29. (*p*-Sulfamoylanilino)-methanesulfonic acid. *UNII-Y19VNL22L0. CAS-122-89-4.* INN.

Mesulfen. $C_{14}H_{12}S_2$. 244.38. [Mesulphen is BAN.] 2,7-Dimethylthianthrene. *UNII-EG6V6W7WDD. CAS-135-58-0.* INN; DCF; MI.

Mesulphen (BAN) — *See* Mesulfen.

Mesuprine Hydrochloride [*1969*] (me′ su preen hye″ droe klor′ ide). $C_{19}H_{26}N_2O_5S$·HCl. 430.95. [Mesuprine is INN.] (1) Methanesulfonamide, *N*-[2-hydroxy-5-[1-hydroxy-2-[[2-(4-methoxyphenyl)ethyl]amino]propyl]phenyl]-, monohydrochloride; (2) 2′-Hydroxy-5′-[1-hydroxy-2-[*p*-methoxyphenethyl)amino]propyl]methanesulfonanilide monohydrochloride. *CAS-7660-71-1; CAS-7541-30-2* [mesuprine]. *Vasodilator; relaxant (smooth muscle).* ◇*MJ 1987*

Mesuximide (INN, BAN) — *See* Methsuximide.

Metabromsalan [*1966*] (met″ a brome′ sa lan). $C_{13}H_9Br_2NO_2$. 371.02. (1) Benzamide, 3,5-dibromo-2-hydroxy-*N*-phenyl-; (2) 3,5-Dibromosalicylanilide. *UNII-8Q21Y09R21. CAS-2577-72-2*. INN. *Disinfectant.* ◇*NSC-526280*

Metabutethamine Hydrochloride. $C_{13}H_{20}N_2O_2$.HCl. 272.77. 2-(Isobutylamino)ethanol *m*-aminobenzoate, hydrochloride. *CAS-553-58-2; CAS-4439-25-2* [metabutethamine]. NF XIII.

Metabutoxycaine Hydrochloride. $C_{17}H_{28}N_2O_2$.HCl. 328.88. 2-(Diethylamino)ethyl 3-amino-2-butoxybenzoate hydrochloride. *CAS-550-01-6; CAS-3624-87-1* [metabutoxycaine]. NF XII; MI.

Metacetamol. $C_8H_9NO_2$. 151.16. 3′-Hydroxyacetanilide. *UNII-V942ZCN81H. CAS-621-42-1*. INN; BAN. ◇*BS 749*

Metaclazepam. $C_{18}H_{18}BrClN_2O$. 393.71. 7-Bromo-5-(*o*-chlorophenyl)-2,3-dihydro-2-(methoxymethyl)-1-methyl-1*H*-1,4-benzodiazepine. *CAS-65517-27-3*. INN; MI.

Metacresol (met″ a kree′ sol). **USP.** C_7H_8O. 108.14. (1) 3-Methylphenol; (2) 3-Hydroxytoluene. *CAS-108-39-4*. BAN. *Antiseptic (topical); antifungal; antifungal (veterinary).*

Metacycline (INN) — *See* Methacycline.

Metaglycodol. $C_{11}H_{15}ClO_2$. 214.69. 2-(*m*-Chlorophenyl)-3-methyl-2,3-butanediol. *CAS-13980-94-4*. INN.

Metahexamide. $C_{14}H_{21}N_3O_3S$. 311.40. 1-(3-Amino-*p*-tolyl-sulfonyl)-3-cyclohexylurea. *CAS-565-33-3*. INN; BAN.

Metahexanamide — *See* Metahexamide.

Metalkonium Chloride. $C_{23}H_{41}ClN_2O$. 397.04. Benzyl[(dodecylcarbamoyl)methyl]dimethylammonium chloride. *CAS-100-95-8*. INN.

Metallibure (INN, BAN) — *See* Methallibure.

Metalol Hydrochloride [*1967*] (met′ a lol hye″ droe klor′ ide). $C_{11}H_{18}N_2O_3S$.HCl. 294.80. (1) Methanesulfonamide, *N*-[4-[1-hydroxy-2-(methylamino)propyl]phenyl]-, monohydrochloride; (2) 4′-[1-Hydroxy-2-(methylamino)propyl]-methanesulfonanilide monohydrochloride. *CAS-955-48-6; CAS-7701-65-7* [metalol]. *Anti-adrenergic (β-receptor).* ◇*MJ 1998*

Metamelfalan. $C_{13}H_{18}Cl_2N_2O_2$. 305.20. 3-[*m*-[Bis(2-chloroethyl)amino]phenyl]-L-alanine. *CAS-1088-80-8*. INN; BAN.

Metamfazone. $C_{11}H_{11}N_3O$. 201.22. 4-Amino-6-methyl-2-phenyl-3(2*H*)-pyridazinone. *UNII-6Q0YU79408. CAS-54063-49-9*. INN; BAN; DCF. *[Name previously used: Methamphazone.]* ◇*AGN 20*

Metamfepramone. $C_{11}H_{15}NO$. 177.24. 2-(Dimethylamino)-propiophenone. *CAS-15351-09-4*. INN; BAN; DCF; MI. ◇*MG 559*

Metamfetamine (INN) — *See* Methamphetamine Hydrochloride.

Metamizole Sodium (INN) — *See* Dipyrone.

Metampicillin. $C_{17}H_{19}N_3O_4S$. 361.42. [α-(Methyleneamino)benzyl]penicillin. *CAS-6489-97-0*. INN; DCF; MI.

Metandienone (INN) — *See* Methandrostenolone.

(*E*)-Metanicotine — *See* Rivanicline Galactarate.

trans-Metanicotine — *See* Rivanicline Galactarate.

Metanixin. $C_{14}H_{14}N_2O_2$. 242.27. 2-(2,6-Xylidino)nicotinic acid. *UNII-OWY6DMB1YX*. *CAS-4394-04-1*. INN.

Metaoxedrine Chloride — *See* Phenylephrine Hydrochloride.

Metapramine. $C_{16}H_{18}N_2$. 238.33. 10,11-Dihydro-5-methyl-10-(methylamino)-5*H*-dibenz[*b,f*]azepine. *CAS-21730-16-5*. INN; MI.

Metaproterenol Polistirex [*1989*] (met″ a proe ter′ e nol pol″ ee stye′ rex). [Orciprenaline is INN and BAN.] (1) Benzene, diethenyl-, polymer with ethenylbenzene, sulfonated, complex with 5-[1-hydroxy-2-[(1-methylethyl)amino]ethyl]-1,3-benzenediol; (2) Sulfonated styrene-divinylbenzene copolymer complex with 3,5-dihydroxy-α-[(isopropylamino)methyl]benzyl alcohol. *CAS-586-06-1* [metaproterenol]. *Bronchodilator.*

Metaproterenol Sulfate [*1964*] (met″ a proe ter′ e nol sul′ fate). USP. $(C_{11}H_{17}NO_3)_2.H_2SO_4$. 520.59. [Orciprenaline Sulfate is JAN.] (1) 1,3-Benzenediol, 5-[1-hydroxy-2-(1-methylethyl)amino]ethyl-, (±)-, sulfate (2:1) (salt); (2) (±)-3,5-Dihydroxy-α-[(isopropylamino)methyl]benzyl alcohol sulfate (2:1). *UNII-GJ20H50YF0*. *CAS-5874-97-5*. *Bronchodilator.* Alupent (Boehringer Ingelheim); Prometa (Muro) ◇*Th-152*

Metaradrine Bitartrate — *See* Metaraminol Bitartrate.

Metaraminol Bitartrate (met″ a ram′ i nol bye tar′ trate). USP. $C_9H_{13}NO_2.C_4H_6O_6$. 317.29. [Metaraminol is INN and BAN.] (1) Benzenemethanol, α-(1-aminoethyl)-3-hydroxy-, [*R*-(*R*,S**)]-, [*R*-(*R*,R**)]-2,3-dihydroxybutanedioate (1:1) (salt); (2) (-)-α-(1-Aminoethyl)-*m*-hydroxybenzyl alcohol tartrate (1:1) (salt). *UNII-ZC4202M9P3*; *UNII-818U2PZ2EH* [metaraminol]. *CAS-33402-03-8*; *CAS-17171-57-2* [replaced]; *CAS-54-49-9* [metaraminol]. JAN. *Adrenergic.* Aramine (Merck)

Metaterol. $C_{11}H_{17}NO_2$. 195.26. *m*-Hydroxy-α-[(isopropylamino)methyl]benzyl alcohol. *CAS-3571-71-9*. INN.

Metaxalone [*1962*] (me tax′ a lone). $C_{12}H_{15}NO_3$. 221.25. (1) 2-Oxazolidinone, 5-[(3,5-dimethylphenoxy)methyl]-; (2) 5-[(3,5-Xylyloxy)methyl]-2-oxazolidinone. *UNII-1NM-A9J598Y*. *CAS-1665-48-1*. INN; BAN. *Relaxant (skeletal muscle).* Skelaxin (Jones); Skelaxin (King) ◇*AHR-438*

---

† Brand name formerly used, and/or firm no longer concerned with this product.

Metazamide. $C_{11}H_{12}N_2O_2$. 204.23. 1-(*p*-Methoxyphenyl)-5-methyl-4-imidazolin-2-one. *UNII-T3Y0F5VOB8. CAS-14058-90-3.* INN. ◇*GPA-878*

Metazepium Iodide — *See* Buzepide Metiodide.

Metazide. $C_{13}H_{14}N_6O_2$. 286.29. Isonicotinic acid 2,2′-methylenedihydrazide. *UNII-NSL1M7IFYP. CAS-1707-15-9.* INN.

Metazocine. $C_{15}H_{21}NO$. 231.33. 2′-Hydroxy-2,5,9-trimethyl-6,7-benzomorphan. *CAS-3734-52-9.* INN; BAN; DCF; MI.

Metbufen. $C_{17}H_{16}O_3$. 268.31. 3-(4-Biphenylylcarbonyl)-2-methylpropionic acid. *CAS-63472-04-8.* INN.

Metcaraphen Hydrochloride. $C_{20}H_{31}NO_2 \cdot HCl$. 353.93. (1) Cyclopentanecarboxylic acid, 1-(3,4-xylyl)-, 2-diethylamino)ethyl ester, hydrochloride; (2) 2-(Diethylamino)ethyl 1-(3,4-dimethylphenyl)cyclopentanecarboxylate hydrochloride. *UNII-0W3C4GMZ2I. CAS-1950-31-8; CAS-561-79-5* [metcaraphen]. MI.

Metelimumab. Immunoglobulin G4, anti-(human transforming growth factor β1) (human monoclonal CAT-192 γ4-chain), disulfide with human monoclonal CAT-192 κ-chain, dimer. *CAS-272780-74-2.* INN.

Meteneprost [*1981*] (me teen′ prost). $C_{23}H_{38}O_4$. 378.55. (1) Prosta-5,13-dien-1-oic acid, 11,15-dihydroxy-16,16-dimethyl-9-methylene-, (5*Z*,11α,13*E*,15*R*)-; (2) (*Z*)-7-[(1*R*,2*R*,3*R*)-3-Hydroxy-2-[(*E*)-(3*R*)-3-hydroxy-4,4-dimethyl-1-octenyl]-5-methylenecyclopentyl]-5-heptenoic acid; (3) 9-Deoxo-16,16-dimethyl-9-methyleneprostaglandin E_2. *CAS-61263-35-2.* INN. *Oxytocic; prostaglandin.* ◇*U-46,785*

Metenkefalin. $C_{27}H_{35}N_5O_7S$. 573.66. L-Tyrosylglycylglycyl-L-phenylalanyl-L-methionine β-endorphin human-(1-5)-peptide. *CAS-58569-55-4.* INN.

Metenolone (INN, BAN) — *See* Methenolone Acetate.

Metenolone Acetate (JAN) — *See* Methenolone Acetate.

Metenolone Enanthate (JAN) — *See* Methenolone Enanthate.

Metergoline. $C_{25}H_{29}N_3O_2$. 403.52. (+)-*N*-(Carboxy)-1-methyl-9,10-dihydrolysergamine benzyl ester. *CAS-17692-51-2.* INN; BAN; MI. ◇*FI 6337; MCE*

Metergotamine. $C_{34}H_{37}N_5O_5$. 595.69. 1-Methylergotamine. *CAS-22336-84-1.* INN. ◇*MY-25 [as bitartrate]*

Metescufylline. $C_{25}H_{31}N_5O_8$. 529.54. 7-[2-(Diethylamino)ethyl]theophylline [(7-hydroxy-4-methyl-2-oxo-2*H*-1-benzopyran-6-yl)oxy]acetate. *UNII-I542T3H3T2. CAS-15518-82-8.* INN; DCF; MI.

Metesculetol. $C_{12}H_{10}O_6$. 250.20. [(7-Hydroxy-4-methyl-2-oxo-2*H*-1-benzopyran-6-yl)oxy]acetic acid. *UNII-HO6I89Z64J. CAS-52814-39-8.* INN.

Metesind Glucuronate [*1996*] (met′ e sind gloo″ kure on′ ate). $C_{23}H_{24}N_4O_3S \cdot C_6H_{10}O_7$. 630.67. [Metesind is INN.] (1) Morpholine, 4-[[4-[[(2-aminobenz[*cd*]indol-6-yl)methylamino]methyl]phenyl]sulfonyl]-, mono-D-glucuronate; (2)

4-[[α-[(2-Aminobenz[*cd*]indol-6-yl)methylamino]-*p*-tolyl]sulfonyl]morpholine mono-D-glucuronate. *CAS-157182-23-5; CAS-138384-68-6* [metesind]. *Antineoplastic (specific thymidylate synthase inhibitor).* ◇*AG331*

Metethoheptazine. $C_{17}H_{25}NO_2$. 275.39. Hexahydro-1,3-dimethyl-4-phenyl-azepinecarboxylic acid ethyl ester. *CAS-509-84-2.* INN.

Metetoin (INN, BAN) — *See* Methetoin.

Metformin [*1969*] (met for′ min). $C_4H_{11}N_5$. 129.16. (1) Imidodicarbonimidic diamide-, *N,N*-dimethyl-; (2) 1,1-Dimethylbiguanide. *UNII-9100L32L2N. CAS-657-24-9.* INN; BAN. *Antidiabetic.* ◇*LA-6023*

Metformin Hydrochloride [*1995*] (met for′ min hye″ droe klor′ ide). **USP**. $C_4H_{11}N_5$·HCl. 165.62. (1) Imidodicarbonimidic diamide, *N,N*-dimethyl-, monohydrochloride; (2) 1,1-Dimethylbiguanide monohydrochloride. *UNII-786Z46389E. CAS-1115-70-4.* JAN. *Antidiabetic.* Fortamet (Teva); Glucophage (Bristol-Myers Squibb); Glumetza (Depomed); Riomet (Ranbaxy) ◇*LA-6023*

Methacholine Bromide. $C_8H_{18}BrNO_2$. 240.14. *UNII-03V657ZD3V* [methacholine]. *CAS-333-31-3; CAS-55-92-5* [methacholine]. NF XIV.

Methacholine Chloride (meth″ a koe′ leen klor′ ide). **USP**. $C_8H_{18}ClNO_2$. 195.69. (1) 1-Propanaminium, 2-(acetyloxy)-*N,N,N*-trimethyl-, chloride, (±)-; (2) (±)-(2-Hydroxypropyl)trimethylammonium chloride acetate. *UNII-*

0W5ETF9M2K; UNII-03V657ZD3V [methacholine]. *CAS-62-51-1; CAS-55-92-5* [methacholine]. INN; BAN. *Cholinergic.* Provocholine (Methapharm)

Methacrylic Acid Copolymer (meth″ a kril′ ik as′ id koe pol′ i mer). **NF**. A fully polymerized copolymer of methacrylic acid and an acrylic or methacrylic ester. *Pharmaceutic aid (tablet coating agent).* Kollicoat MAE 300 (BASF)

Methacycline [*1962*] (meth″ a sye′ kleen). $C_{22}H_{22}N_2O_8$. 442.42. [Metacycline is INN.] (1) 2-Naphthacenecarboxamide, 4-(dimethylamino)-1,4,4a,5,5a,6,11,12a-octahydro-3,5,10,12,12a-pentahydroxy-6-methylene-1,11-dioxo-, [4*S*-(4α,4aα,5α,5aα,12aα)]-; (2) 4-(Dimethylamino)-1,4,4a,5,5a,6,11,12a-octahydro-3,5,10,12,12a-pentahydroxy-6-methylene-1,11-dioxo-2-naphthacenecarboxamide; (3) 6-Deoxy-6-demethyl-6-methylene-5-oxytetracycline. *UNII-IR235I7C5P. CAS-914-00-1.* BAN. *Antibacterial.* ◇*GS-2876*

Methacycline Hydrochloride (meth″ a sye′ kleen hye″ droe klor′ ide). **USP**. $C_{22}H_{22}N_2O_8$·HCl. 478.88. (1) 2-Naphthacenecarboxamide, 4-(dimethylamino)-1,4,4a,5,5a,6,11,12a-octahydro-3,5,10,12,12a-pentahydroxy-6-methylene-1,11-dioxo-, monohydrochloride, [4*S*-(4α,4aα,5α,5aα,12aα)]-; (2) 4-(Dimethylamino)-1,4,4a,5,5a,6,11,12a-octahydro-3,5,10,12,12a-pentahydroxy-6-methylene-1,11-dioxo-2-naphthacenecarboxamide monohydrochloride. *UNII-9GJ0N7ZAP0; UNII-IR235I7C5P* [methacycline]. *CAS-3963-95-9; CAS-914-00-1* [methacycline]. *Antibacterial.* Rondomycin (Medpointe)

Methadol — *See* Dimepheptanol.

Methadone Hydrochloride (meth′ a done hye″ droe klor′ ide). **USP**. $C_{21}H_{27}NO$·HCl. 345.91. [Methadone is INN and BAN.] (1) 3-Heptanone, 6-(dimethylamino)-4,4-diphenyl-, hydrochloride; (2) 6-(Dimethylamino)-4,4-diphenyl-3-heptanone hydrochloride. *UNII-229809935B; UNII-UC6VBE7V1Z* [methadone]. *CAS-1095-90-5; CAS-76-99-3* [methadone]. *Analgesic (narcotic).* Dolophine Hydrochloride (Xanodyne); Methadose (Mallinckrodt)

Methadonium Chloride — *See* Methadone Hydrochloride.

Methadyl Acetate [*1970*] (meth′ a dil as′ e tate). $C_{23}H_{31}NO_2$. 353.50. [Acetylmethadol is INN and BAN.] (1) Benzeneethanol, β-[2-(dimethylamino)propyl]-α-ethyl-β-phenyl-, acetate (ester); (2) 6-(Dimethylamino)-4,4-diphenyl-3-heptanol acetate (ester). *CAS-509-74-0. Analgesic (narcotic).*

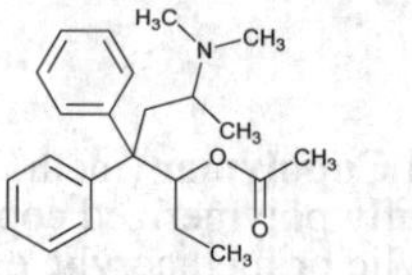

Methafilcon B [*1990*] (meth″ a fil′ kon). $(C_6H_{10}O_3)_w$ $(C_4H_6O_2)_x(C_{10}H_{14}O_4)_y(C_8H_{14}O_4)_z$. (1) 2-Propenoic acid, 2-methyl-, 2-hydroxyethyl ester, polymer with 2-methyl-2-propenoic acid, 1,2-ethanediyl bis(2-methyl-2-propenoate) and 2-(2-hydroxyethoxy)ethyl 2-methyl-2-propenoate; (2) 2-Hydroxyethyl methacrylate polymer with methacrylic acid, ethylene dimethacrylate and 2-(2-hydroxyethoxy) ethyl methacrylate. *CAS-115288-27-2. Contact lens material (hydrophilic).* Hydrasoft (CooperVision)

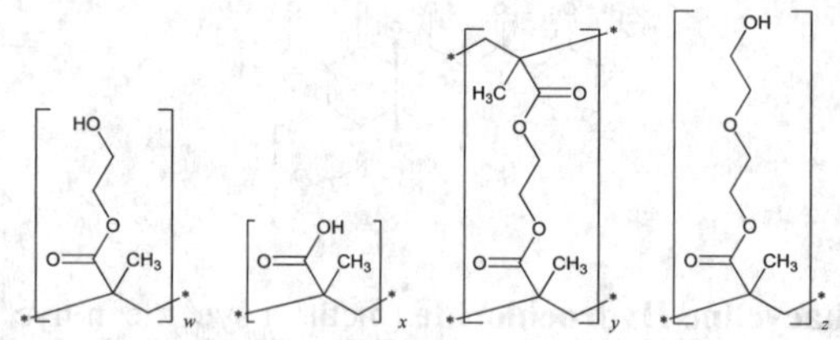

Methallenestril. $C_{18}H_{22}O_3$. 286.37. β-Ethyl-6-methoxy-α,α-dimethyl-2-naphthalenepropionic acid. *UNII-XL025389JS. CAS-517-18-0.* INN; BAN; MI.

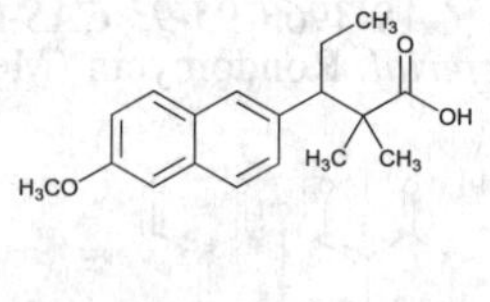

Methallenestrol — *See* Methallenestril.

Methallenoestril (previously used name) — *See* Methallenestril.

Methallibure [*1967*] (meth al′ i bure). $C_7H_{14}N_4S_2$. 218.34. [Metallibure is INN and BAN.] (1) 1,2-Hydrazinedicarbothioamide, N-methyl-N'-(1-methyl-2-propenyl)-; (2) 1-Methyl-6-(1-methylallyl)-2,5-dithiobiurea. *CAS-926-93-2. Anterior pituitary activator (for swine).* ◇*ICI-33,828; AY-61122; NSC-69536*

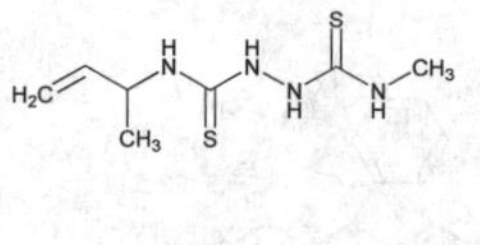

Methalthiazide [*1963*] (meth al thye′ a zide). $C_{12}H_{16}ClN_3O_4S_3$. 397.92. (1) 2H-1,2,4-Benzothiadiazine-7-sulfonamide, 6-chloro-3,4-dihydro-2-methyl-3-[(2-propenylthio)methyl]-, 1,1-dioxide; (2) 3-[(Allylthio)-

methyl]-6-chloro-3,4-dihydro-2-methyl-2H-1,2,4-benzothiadiazine-7-sulfonamide 1,1-dioxide. *CAS-5611-64-3. Diuretic; antihypertensive.* ◇*P-2530*

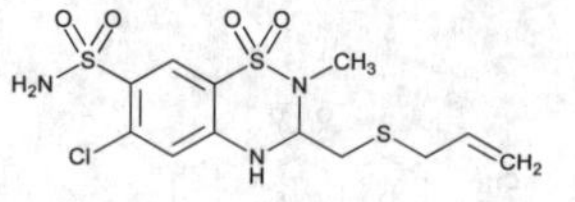

Methamoctol. Biochem. Pharmacol. 8: 12 (1961).

Methamphazone (previously used name) — *See* Metamfazone.

Methamphetamine Hydrochloride (meth″ am fet′ a meen hye″ droe klor′ ide). USP. $C_{10}H_{15}N \cdot HCl$. 185.69. [Metamfetamine is INN.] (1) Benzeneethanamine, N,α-dimethyl-, hydrochloride, (S)-; (2) (+)-(S)-N,α-Dimethylphenethylamine hydrochloride. *UNII-997F43Z9CV; UNII-44RAL3456C* [methamphetamine]. *CAS-51-57-0; CAS-537-46-2* [methamphetamine]. JAN. *Stimulant (central).* Desoxyn (Ovation)

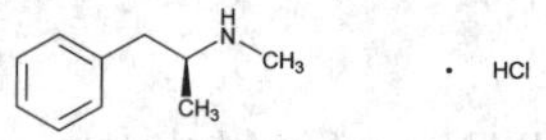

Methampyrone (previously used name) — *See* Dipyrone.

Methandienone (BAN) — *See* Methandrostenolone.

Methandriol. $C_{20}H_{32}O_2$. 304.47. 17α-Methylandrost-5-ene-3β,17β-diol. *CAS-521-10-8.* INN; MI. Methostan (Schering†)

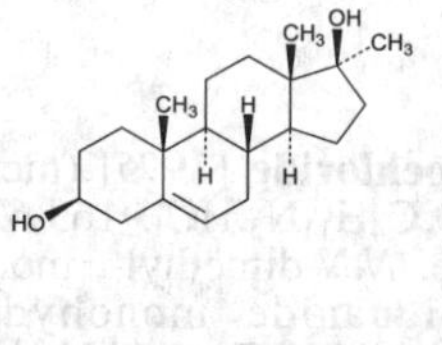

Methandrostenolone. $C_{20}H_{28}O_2$. 300.44. [Metandienone is INN; Methandienone is BAN.] (1) Androsta-1,4-diene-3-one, 17-hydroxy-17-methyl-, (17β)-; (2) 17β-Hydroxy-17-methylandrosta-1,4-dien-3-one. *CAS-72-63-9.* USP XX; MI. ◇*NSC-42722*

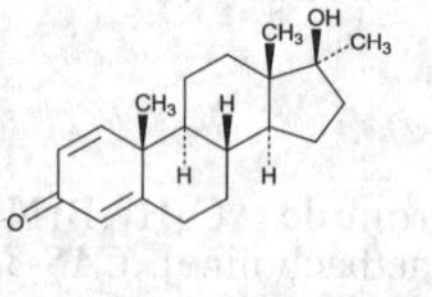

Methaniazide. $C_7H_9N_3O_4S$. 231.23. [Isoniazide Sodium Methanesulfonate is JAN.] Isonicotinic acid 2-(sulfomethyl)hydrazine. *UNII-GN8S7ZES0F. CAS-13447-95-5.* INN.

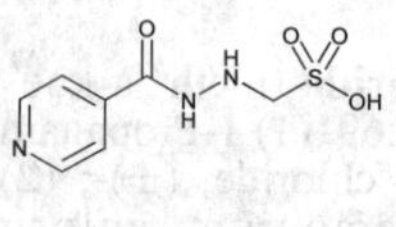

Methantheline Bromide. $C_{21}H_{26}BrNO_3$. 420.34. [Methanthelinium Bromide is INN and BAN.] (1) Ethanaminium, N,N-diethyl-N-methyl-2-[(9H-xanthen-9-ylcarbonyl)oxy]-, bromide; (2) Diethyl(2-hydroxyethyl)methylammonium bromide xanthene-9-carboxylate. *UNII-090519SAPF. CAS-53-46-3; CAS-5818-17-7* [methantheline]. USP XXII. Banthine (Shire)

Methanthelinium Bromide (INN, BAN, DCF) — *See* Methantheline Bromide.

Methaphenilene Hydrochloride. $C_{15}H_{20}N_2S.HCl$. 296.86. [Methaphenilene is INN and BAN.] *N,N*-Dimethyl-*N′*-(α-thenyl)-*N′*-phenethylenediamine hydrochloride. *UNII-DK0OIL461Z. CAS-7084-07-3; CAS-493-78-7* [methaphenilene]. NF X; MI.

Methapyrilene Fumarate. $(C_{14}H_{19}N_3S)_2.3C_4H_4O_4$. 870.99. [Methapyrilene is INN and BAN.] (1) 1,2-Ethanediamine, *N,N*-dimethyl-*N′*-2-pyridinyl-*N′*-(2-thienylmethyl)-, (*E*)-2-butenedioate (2:3); (2) 2-[[2-(Dimethylamino)ethyl]-2-thenylamino]pyridine fumarate (2:3). *UNII-A01LX40298* [methapyrilene]. *CAS-33032-12-1; CAS-91-80-5* [methapyrilene]. USP XX; MI.

Methapyrilene Hydrochloride. $C_{14}H_{19}N_3S.HCl$. 297.85. (1) 1,2-Ethanediamine, *N,N*-dimethyl-*N′*-2-pyridinyl-*N′*-(2-thienylmethyl)-, monohydrochloride; (2) 2-[[2-(Dimethylamino)ethyl]-2-thenylamino]pyridine monohydrochloride. *UNII-00S42N58OM. CAS-135-23-9; CAS-91-80-5* [methapyrilene]. USP XX; MI. Thenylene Hydrochloride (Abbott†)

Methaqualone [*1962*] (meth a′ kwa lone). $C_{16}H_{14}N_2O$. 250.30. (1) 4(3*H*)-Quinazolinone, 2-methyl-3-(2-methylphenyl)-; (2) 2-Methyl-3-*o*-tolyl-4(3*H*)-quinazolinone. *CAS-72-44-6.* USP XXI; INN; BAN. *Sedative-hypnotic.* ◇*CI-705; CN 38703; QZ-2; R-148; TR-495*

Methaqualone Hydrochloride. $C_{16}H_{14}N_2O.HCl$. 286.76. (1) 4(3*H*)-Quinazolinone, 2-methyl-3-(2-methylphenyl)-, monohydrochloride; (2) 2-Methyl-3-*o*-tolyl-4(3*H*)-quinazolinone monohydrochloride. *UNII-RJQ4G25ZRH. CAS-340-56-7; CAS-72-44-6* [methaqualone]. USP XX; MI. Optimil (Wallace†); Parest (Parke-Davis†)

____

† Brand name formerly used, and/or firm no longer concerned with this product.

Metharbital. $C_9H_{14}N_2O_3$. 198.22. (1) 2,4,6(1*H*,3*H*,5*H*)-Pyrimidinetrione, 5,5-diethyl-1-methyl-; (2) 5,5-Diethyl-1-methylbarbituric acid. *UNII-02OS7K758T. CAS-50-11-3.* USP XXII; INN; BAN; JAN. Gemonil (Abbott) *[Name previously used: Metharbitone.]*

Methastyridone. $C_{13}H_{15}NO_2$. 217.26. 2,2-Dimethyl-5-styryl-4-oxazolidinone. *CAS-721-19-7.* INN.

Methazolamide (meth″ a zoe′ la mide). **USP.** $C_5H_8N_4O_3S_2$. 236.27. (1) Acetamide, *N*-[5-(aminosulfonyl)-3-methyl-1,3,4-thiadiazol-2(3*H*)-ylidene]-; (2) *N*-(4-Methyl-2-sulfamoyl-Δ^2-1,3,4-thiadiazolin-5-ylidene)acetamide. *UNII-W733B0S9SD. CAS-554-57-4.* INN; BAN; JAN. *Carbonic anhydrase inhibitor.*

Methdilazine. $C_{18}H_{20}N_2S$. 296.43. (1) 10*H*-Phenothiazine, 10-[(1-methyl-3-pyrrolidinyl)methyl]-; (2) 10-[(1-Methyl-3-pyrrolidinyl)methyl]phenothiazine. *UNII-4Q13LY9Z8X. CAS-1982-37-2.* USP XXIII; INN; BAN. *Antipruritic.* Tacaryl (Westwood-Squibb)

Methdilazine Hydrochloride (meth dil′ a zeen hye″ droe klor′ ide). **USP.** $C_{18}H_{20}N_2S.HCl$. 332.89. (1) 10*H*-Phenothiazine, 10-[(1-methyl-3-pyrrolidinyl)methyl]-, monohydrochloride; (2) 10-[(1-Methyl-3-pyrrolidinyl)methyl]phenothiazine monohydrochloride. *UNII-T0GSO02UEZ; UNII-4Q13LY9Z8X* [methdilazine]. *CAS-1229-35-2; CAS-1982-37-2* [methdilazine]. *Antipruritic.* Tacaryl (Westwood-Squibb)

Methenamine (meth en′ a meen). **USP.** $C_6H_{12}N_4$. 140.19. [Hexamine is JAN.] (1) 1,3,5,7-Tetraazatricyclo[3.3.1.1^{3,7}]decane; (2) Hexamethylenetetramine. *UNII-J50OIX95QV. CAS-100-97-0.* INN. *Antibacterial (urinary).* Uritone (Parke-Davis†); Urotropin (Parke-Davis†) *[Name previously used: Hexamethylenamine.]*

Methenamine Hippurate [*1963*] (meth en′ a meen hip′ ure ate). **USP.** $C_6H_{12}N_4.C_9H_9NO_3$. 319.36. (1) Glycine, *N*-benzoyl, compd. with 1,3,5,7-tetraazatricyclo[3.3.1.1^{3,7}]-decane (1:1); (2) Hexamethylenetetramine monohippurate. *UNII-M329791L57. CAS-5714-73-8; CAS-100-97-0* [methenamine]. BAN. *Antibacterial (urinary)*. Hiprex (Sanofi Aventis); Urex (Vatring) *[Name previously used: Hexamine Hippurate.]*

Methenamine Mandelate (meth en′ a meen man′ de late). **USP**. $C_6H_{12}N_4 \cdot C_8H_8O_3$. 292.33. [Hexamine Mandelate is JAN.] (1) Benzeneacetic acid, α-hydroxy-, (±)-, compd. with 1,3,5,7-tetraazatricyclo[3.3.1.1^{3,7}]decane (1:1); (2) Hexamethylenetetramine mono-(±)-mandelate. *UNII-695N30CINR. CAS-587-23-5; CAS-100-97-0* [methenamine]. *Antibacterial (urinary)*. Mandelamine (Parke-Davis)

Methenolone Acetate [*1966*] (meth en′ oh lone as′ e tate). $C_{22}H_{32}O_3$. 344.49. [Metenolone is INN and BAN; Metenolone Acetate is JAN.] (1) Androst-1-en-3-one, 17-(acetyloxy)-1-methyl-, (5α,17β)-; (2) 17β-Hydroxy-1-methyl-5α-androst-1-en-3-one acetate. *CAS-434-05-9; CAS-153-00-4* [methenolone]. *Anabolic*. ◇*SH 567; SQ 16496; NSC-74226*

Methenolone Enanthate [*1964*] (e nan′ thate e nan′ thate). $C_{27}H_{42}O_3$. 414.62. [Metenolone Enanthate is JAN.] (1) Androst-1-en-3-one, 1-methyl-17-[(1-oxoheptyl)oxy]-, (5α,17β)-; (2) 17β-Hydroxy-1-methyl-5α-androst-1-en-3-one heptanoate. *CAS-303-42-4. Anabolic*. ◇*SH 601; SQ 16374; NSC-64967*

Metheptazine. $C_{16}H_{23}NO_2$. 261.36. Hexahydro-1,2-dimethyl-4-phenyl-4-azepinecarboxylic acid methyl ester. *CAS-469-78-3. INN*.

Methestrol. $C_{20}H_{26}O_2$. 298.42. 4,4′-(1,2-Diethylethylene)di-*o*-cresol. *CAS-130-73-4. INN; BAN; DCF; MI. [Name previously used: Promethoestrol.]*

Methetharimide — *See* Bemegride.

Methetoin [*1962*] (meth′ e toin; meth′ e toe in). $C_{12}H_{14}N_2O_2$. 218.25. [Metetoin is INN and BAN.] (1) 2,4-Imidazolidinedione, 5-ethyl-1-methyl-5-phenyl-; (2) 5-Ethyl-1-methyl-5-phenylhydantoin. *CAS-5696-06-0. Anticonvulsant*. Deltoin (Novartis†) ◇*N-3; NSC-524411*

Methicillin Sodium [*1962*] (meth″ i sil′ in soe′ dee um). $C_{17}H_{19}N_2NaO_6S \cdot H_2O$. 420.41. [Methicillin is BAN; Meticillin is INN; Meticillin Sodium is JAN.] (1) 4-Thia-1-azabicyclo[3.2.0]heptane-2-carboxylic acid, 6-[(2,6-dimethoxybenzoyl)amino]-3,3-dimethyl-7-oxo-, monosodium salt, monohydrate, [2S-(2α,5α,6β)]-; (2) Monosodium (2S,5R,6R)-6-(2,6-dimethoxybenzamido)-3,3-dimethyl-7-oxo-4-thia-1-azabicyclo[3.2.0]heptane-2-carboxylate monohydrate. *UNII-AO9YF4MN30; UNII-Q91FH1328A* [methicillin]. *CAS-7246-14-2; CAS-132-92-3* [anhydrous]; *CAS-61-32-5* [methicillin]. USP XXV. *Antibacterial*. Staphcillin (Apothecon) ◇*BRL-1241; SQ 16,123; X-1497*

Methimazole (meth im′ a zole). **USP**. $C_4H_6N_2S$. 114.17. [Thiamazole is INN, BAN and JAN.] (1) 2*H*-Imidazole-2-thione, 1,3-dihydro-1-methyl-; (2) 1-Methylimidazole-2-thiol. *UNII-554Z48XN5E. CAS-60-56-0. Thyroid inhibitor*. Tapazole (King)

Methindizate (previously used name) — *See* Metindizate.

Methiodal Sodium. CH_2INaO_3S. 243.98. (1) Methanesulfonic acid, iodo-, sodium salt; (2) Sodium iodomethanesulfonate. *CAS-126-31-8; CAS-143-47-5* [methiodal]. USP XXI; INN; BAN; MI. Skiodan Sodium (Sterling Winthrop†)

Methiomeprazine Hydrochloride. $C_{19}H_{24}N_2S_2 \cdot HCl$. 381.00. [Methiomeprazine is INN.] (±)-10-[3-(Dimethylamino)-2-methylpropyl]-2-(methylthio)phenothiazine monohydrochloride. *CAS-7009-43-0* [methiomeprazine].

Methionine [*1980*] (me thye′ oh neen). **USP**. $C_5H_{11}NO_2S$. 149.21. [L-Methionine is JAN.] (1) L-Methionine; (2) L-Methionine. *UNII-AE28F7PNPL. CAS-63-68-3. INN. Amino acid*.

L-Methionine (JAN) — *See* Methionine.

Methionine (NF XIV and previously used name) — *See* Racemethionine.

DL-Methionine (JAN) — *See* Racemethionine.

Methionine C 11. **USP** [Injection]. A sterile isotonic solution, of L[^{11}C] methionine, in which a portion of the molecules are labeled with radioactive ^{11}C. *Radioactive agent.*

Methiothepin — *See* Metitepine.

Methisazone [*1964*] (meth is' a zone). $C_{10}H_{10}N_4OS$. 234.28. [Metisazone is INN and BAN.] (1) Hydrazinecarbothioamide, 2-(1,2-dihydro-1-methyl-2-oxo-3*H*-indol-3-ylidene)-; (2) 1-Methylindole-2,3-dione 3-(thiosemicarbazone). *UNII-K3QML4J07E.* *CAS-1910-68-5. Antiviral.* ◇*BW 33-T-57; NSC-69811*

Methitural. $C_{12}H_{20}N_2O_2S_2$. 288.43. 5-(1-Methylbutyl)-5-[2-(methylthio)ethyl]-2-thiobarbituric acid. *CAS-467-43-6.* INN; MI.

Methixene Hydrochloride [*1964*] (me thix' een hye'' droe klor' ide). $C_{20}H_{23}NS.HCl.H_2O$. 363.94. [Metixene is INN and BAN; Metixene Hydrochloride is JAN.] (1) Piperidine, 1-methyl-3-(9*H*-thioxanthen-9-ylmethyl)-, hydrochloride, monohydrate; (2) 1-Methyl-3-(thioxanthen-9-ylmethyl)piperidine hydrochloride monohydrate. *UNII-84L8XK6N1G; UNII-32VY6L26ZW* [methixene]. *CAS-7081-40-5; CAS-1553-34-0* [anhydrous]; *CAS-4969-02-2* [methixene]. *Relaxant (smooth muscle).* Trest (Novartis) ◇*SJ 1977; NSC-78194*

Methocamphone Methylsulfate — *See* Trimethidinium Methosulfate.

Methocarbamol (meth'' oh kar' ba mol). **USP**. $C_{11}H_{15}NO_5$. 241.24. (1) 1,2-Propanediol, 3-(2-methoxyphenoxy)-, 1-carbamate, (±)-; (2) (±)-3-(*o*-Methoxyphenoxy)-1,2-pro-

panediol 1-carbamate. *UNII-125OD7737X. CAS-532-03-6.* INN; BAN; JAN. *Relaxant (skeletal muscle).* Robaxin (Schwarz Pharma)

Methocidin. Hydroxymethylgramicidin. *CAS-1407-05-2.* INN; DCF.

Methohexital (meth'' oh hex' i tal). **USP**. $C_{14}H_{18}N_2O_3$. 262.30. (1) 2,4,6(1*H*,3*H*,5*H*)-Pyrimidinetrione, 1-methyl-5-(1-methyl-2-pentynyl)-5-(2-propenyl)-, (±)-; (2) (±)-5-Allyl-1-methyl-5-(1-methyl-2-pentynyl)barbituric acid. *UNII-E5B8ND5IPE. CAS-18652-93-2.* INN; BAN. Pharmaceutic necessity for Methohexital Sodium for Injection. [*Name previously used: Methohexitone.*]

Methohexital Sodium (meth'' oh hex' i tal soe' dee um). **USP** [for Injection]. $C_{14}H_{17}N_2NaO_3$. 284.29. (1) 2,4,6(1*H*,3*H*,5*H*)-Pyrimidinetrione, 1-methyl-5-(1-methyl-2-pentynyl)-5-(2-propenyl)-, (±)-, monosodium salt; (2) Sodium 5-allyl-1-methyl-5-(1-methyl-2-pentynyl)barbiturate. *UNII-60200PNZ7Q. CAS-309-36-4; CAS-60634-69-7* [±]; *CAS-22151-68-4* [replaced]; *CAS-18652-93-2* [methohexital]. *Anesthetic (intravenous).* Brevital Sodium (King)

Methohexitone (previously used name) — *See* Methohexital.

Methoin (previously used name) — *See* Mephenytoin.

Methonaphthone — *See* Menbutone.

Methophedrine — *See* Methoxyphedrine.

Methophenazine — *See* Metofenazate.

Methopholine [*1963*] (meth oh' foe leen). $C_{20}H_{24}ClNO_2$. 345.86. [Metofoline is INN and BAN.] (1) Isoquinoline, 1-[2-(4-chlorophenyl)ethyl]-1,2,3,4-tetrahydro-6,7-dimethoxy-2-methyl-; (2) 1-(*p*-Chlorophenethyl)-1,2,3,4-tetrahydro-6,7-dimethoxy-2-methylisoquinoline. *CAS-2154-02-1. Analgesic.* ◇*ARC I-K-1; NIH 7672; Ro 4-1778/1*

Methoprene. $C_{19}H_{34}O_3$. 310.47. Isopropyl (2*E*,4*E*)-(7*S*)-11-methoxy-3,7,11-trimethyl-2,4-dodecadienoate. *UNII-8B830OJ2UX. CAS-40596-69-8.* INN; MI.

Methopromazine (INN, DCF) Maleate — *See* Methoxypromazine Maleate.

Methopyrimazole — *See* Epirizole.

Methoserpidine. $C_{33}H_{40}N_2O_9$. 608.68. 10-Methoxydeserpidine. *CAS-865-04-3.* INN; BAN; DCF.

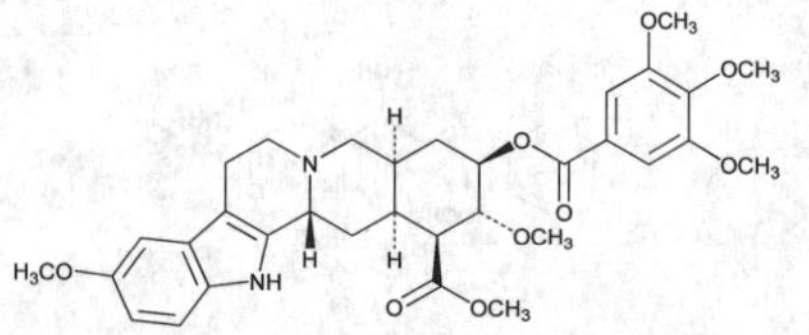

Methotrexate [*1961*] (meth″ oh trex′ ate). **USP.** $C_{20}H_{22}N_8O_5$. 454.44. (1) L-Glutamic acid, *N*-[4-[[(2,4-diamino-6-pteridinyl)methyl]methylamino]benzoyl]-; (2) L-(+)-*N*-[*p*-[[(2,4-Diamino-6-pteridinyl)methyl]methylamino]benzoyl]glutamic acid. *UNII-YL5FZ2Y5U1.* *CAS-59-05-2.* INN; BAN; JAN. *Antineoplastic.* Mexate (Bristol-Myers Oncology†); Rheumatrex (Wyeth-Ayerst) *[Name previously used: Amethopterin.]* ◇*CL 14377; NSC-740*

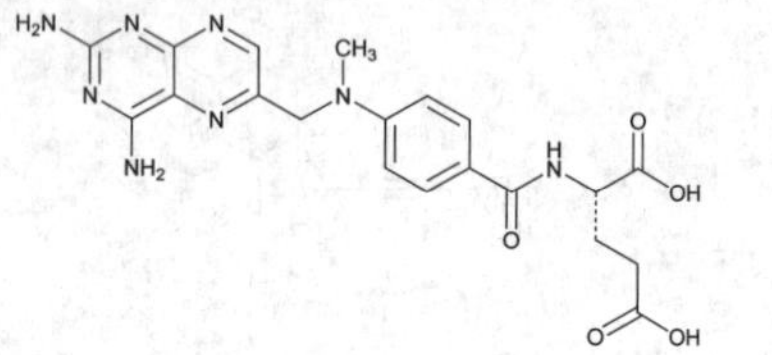

Methotrimeprazine (meth″ oh trye mep′ ra zeen). **USP.** $C_{19}H_{24}N_2OS$. 328.47. (1) 10*H*-Phenothiazine-10-propanamine, 2-methoxy-*N,N,β*-trimethyl-, (-)-; (2) (-)-10-[3-(Dimethylamino)-2-methylpropyl]-2-methoxyphenothiazine. *CAS-60-99-1.* *Analgesic.* Levoprome (Immunex) ◇*CL 36467; CL 39743; RP 7044; SK&F 5116*

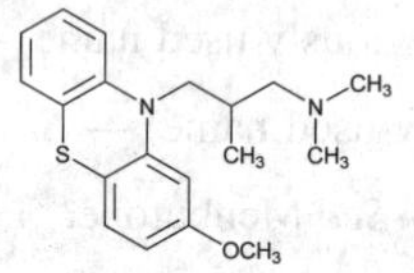

Methoxamine Hydrochloride. $C_{11}H_{17}NO_3 \cdot HCl$. 247.72. [Methoxamine is INN and BAN.] (1) Benzenemethanol, *α*-(1-aminoethyl)-2,5-dimethoxy-, hydrochloride; (2) (±)-*α*-(1-Aminoethyl)-2,5-dimethoxybenzyl alcohol hydrochloride. *UNII-8MB4MJ9R7L; UNII-HUQ1KC1YLI* [methoxamine]. *CAS-61-16-5; CAS-390-28-3* [methoxamine]. USP XXII; JAN. Vasoxyl (GlaxoSmithKline)

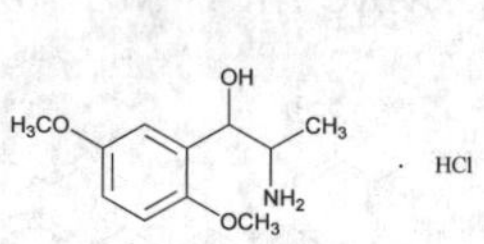

Methoxiflurane — *See* Methoxyflurane.

Methoxsalen (meth ox′ a len). **USP.** $C_{12}H_8O_4$. 216.19. (1) 7*H*-Furo[3,2-*g*][1]benzopyran-7-one, 9-methoxy-; (2) 9-Methoxy-7*H*-furo[3,2-*g*][1]benzopyran-7-one. *UNII-U4VJ29L7BQ.* *CAS-298-81-7.* BAN; JAN. *Pigmentation agent.* Oxsoralen (Valeant)

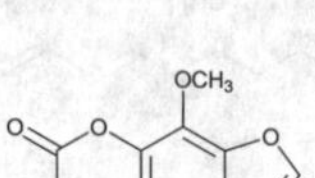

Methoxyfenoserpin — *See* Mefeserpine.

Methoxyflurane [*1962*] (meth ox″ ee floo′ rane). **USP.** $C_3H_4Cl_2F_2O$. 164.97. (1) Ethane, 2,2-dichloro-1,1-difluoro-1-methoxy-; (2) 2,2-Dichloro-1,1-difluoroethyl methyl ether. *UNII-30905R8O7B.* *CAS-76-38-0.* INN; BAN. *Anesthetic (inhalation).* Penthrane (Abbott) ◇*NSC-110432*

Methoxyphedrine. $C_{11}H_{15}NO_2$. 193.24. 1-*p*-Methoxyphenyl-2-methylaminopropan-1-one. *CAS-530-54-1.* INN; DCF.

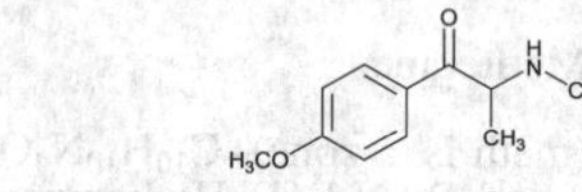

Methoxyphenamine Hydrochloride. $C_{11}H_{17}NO \cdot HCl$. 215.72. [Methoxyphenamine is INN and BAN.] (1) Benzeneethanamine, 2-methoxy-*N,α*-dimethyl-, hydrochloride; (2) *o*-Methoxy-*N,α*-dimethylphenethylamine hydrochloride. *CAS-5588-10-3; CAS-93-30-1* [methoxyphenamine]. USP XXI; JAN; MI.

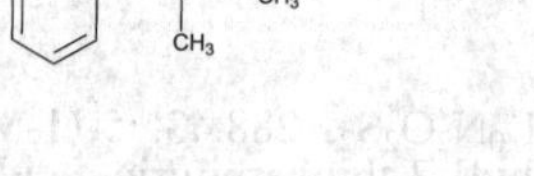

4-Methoxyphenol (previously used name) — *See* Mequinol.

Methoxypromazine Maleate. [Methopromazine is INN.] *UNII-OR0RPY2Y2V.* *CAS-3403-42-7; CAS-61-01-8* [methoxypromazine]. MI; NND 1962.

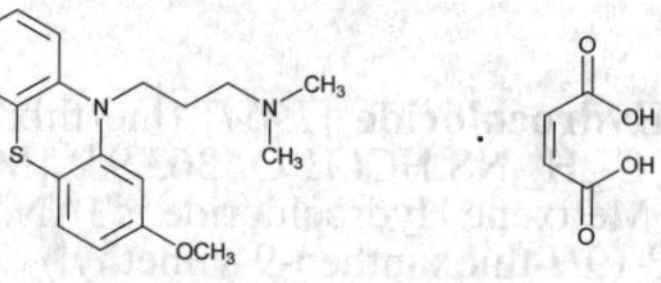

8-Methoxypsoralen — *See* Methoxsalen.

Methphenoxydiol — *See* Guaifenesin.

Methscopolamine Bromide (meth″ skoe pol′ a meen broe′ mide). **USP.** $C_{18}H_{24}BrNO_4$. 398.29. [Hyoscine Methobromide is BAN; *N*-Methylscopolamine Methylsulfate is JAN.] (1) 3-Oxa-9-azoniatricyclo[3.3.1.0^{2,4}]nonane, 7-(3-hydroxy-1-oxo-2-phenylpropoxy)-9,9-dimethyl-, bromide, [7(*S*)-(1*α*,2*β*,4*β*,5*α*,7*β*)]-; (2) 6*β*,7*β*-Epoxy-3*α*-hydroxy-8-methyl-1*α*H,5*α*H-tropanium bromide (-)-tropate. *UNII-RTN51LK7WL.* *CAS-155-41-9.* Pamine (Bradley)

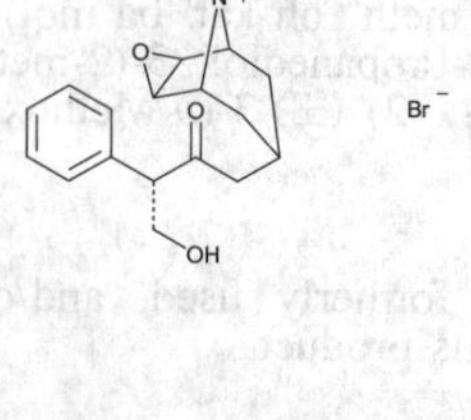

Methsuximide (meth sux′ i mide). **USP**. $C_{12}H_{13}NO_2$. 203.24. [Mesuximide is INN and BAN.] (1) 2,5-Pyrrolidine-dione,1,3-dimethyl-3-phenyl-, (±)-; (2) (±)-*N*,2-Dimethyl-2-phenylsuccinimide. *UNII-0G76K8X6C0. CAS-77-41-8. Anticonvulsant.* Celontin (Pfizer)

Methyclothiazide [*1963*] (meth″ i kloe thye′ a zide). **USP**. $C_9H_{11}Cl_2N_3O_4S_2$. 360.24. (1) 2*H*-1,2,4-Benzothiadiazine-7-sulfonamide, 6-chloro-3-(chloromethyl)-3,4-dihydro-2-methyl-, 1,1-dioxide, (±)-; (2) (±)-6-Chloro-3-(chloromethyl)-3,4-dihydro-2-methyl-2*H*-1,2,4-benzothiadiazine-7-sulfonamide 1,1-dioxide. *UNII-L3H46UAC61. CAS-135-07-9.* INN; BAN; JAN. *Diuretic; antihypertensive.* Aquatensen (Medpointe); Enduron (Abbott) ◇*NSC-110431*

Methydromorphine — *See* Methyldihydromorphine.

Methyl Alcohol (meth′ il al′ ka hol). **NF**. CH_4O. 32.04. (1) Methanol; (2) Methanol. *UNII-Y4S76JWI15. CAS-67-56-1. Pharmaceutic aid (solvent).*

Methyl Aminolevulinate Hydrochloride [*2002*] (meth′ il a mee″ noe lev″ ue lin′ ate hye″ droe klor′ ide). $C_6H_{11}NO_3 \cdot HCl$. 181.62. (1) Pentanoic acid, 5-amino-4-oxo-, methyl ester, hydrochloride; (2) Methyl 5-amino-4-oxopentanoate hydrochloride. *UNII-7S73606O1A. CAS-79416-27-6. Antineoplastic agent used in photodynamic therapy.* Metvixia (PhotoCure, Norway) ◇*P-1202*

Methyl Benzoquate (BAN) — *See* Nequinate.

Methyl Benzylidene Camphor (previously used name) — *See* Enzacamene.

Methyl Cysteine (previously used name) — *See* Mecysteine.

Methyl Isobutyl Ketone (meth′ il eye″ soe bue′ til kee′ tone). **NF**. $C_6H_{12}O$. 100.16. (1) 2-Pentanone, 4-methyl-; (2) 4-Methyl-2-pentanone. *CAS-108-10-1. Pharmaceutic aid (alcohol denaturant).*

Methyl Nicotinate [*1988*] (meth′ il nik″ oh tin′ ate). $C_7H_7NO_2$. 137.14. 3-Pyridinecarboxylic acid methyl ester. *UNII-7B1AVU9DJN.* Heat Spray (Whitehall-Robins†)

Methyl Palmoxirate [*1982*] (meth′ il pal mox′ ir ate). $C_{18}H_{34}O_3$. 298.46. (1) Oxiranecarboxylic acid, 2-tetradecyl-, methyl ester, (±)-; (2) Methyl (±)-2-tetradecylglycidate. *CAS-69207-52-9. Antidiabetic.* ◇*McN-3716*

Methyl Parahydroxybenzoate (JAN) — *See* Methylparaben.

Methyl Phthalate — *See* Dimethyl Phthalate.

Methyl Salicylate (meth′ il sa lis′ i late). **NF**. $C_8H_8O_3$. 152.15. (1) Benzoic acid, 2-hydroxy-, methyl ester; (2) Methyl salicylate. *UNII-LAV5U5022Y. CAS-119-36-8.* JAN. *Pharmaceutic aid (flavor).*

Methyl Violet — *See* Gentian Violet.

Methylaminopterin — *See* Methotrexate.

Methylandrostenediol — *See* Methandriol.

Methylatropine Nitrate [*1963*] (meth″ il at′ roe peen nye′ trate). $C_{18}H_{26}N_2O_6$. 366.41. [Atropine Methonitrate is INN, BAN and JAN.] (1) 8-Azoniabicyclo[3.2.1]octane, 3-(3-hydroxy-1-oxo-2-phenylpropoxy)-8,8-dimethyl-, *endo*-(±)-, nitrate (salt); (2) 3α-Hydroxy-8-methyl-1α*H*,5α*H*-tropanium bromide (±)-tropate; (3) Atropine methylnitrate. *CAS-52-88-0. Anticholinergic.* Ekomine (Hoechst-Roussel†); Eumydrin (Sterling Winthrop†)

Methylbenactyzium Bromide. $C_{21}H_{28}BrNO_3$. 422.36. Diethyl(2-hydroxyethyl)methylammonium bromide benzilate. *CAS-3166-62-9.* INN; JAN.

Methylbenzethonium Chloride (meth″ il ben″ ze thoe′ nee um klor′ ide). **USP**. $C_{28}H_{44}ClNO_2 \cdot H_2O$. 480.12. (1) Benzenemethanaminium, *N*,*N*-dimethyl-*N*-[2-[2-[methyl-4-(1,1,3,3-tetramethylbutyl)phenoxy]ethoxy]ethyl]-, chloride, monohydrate; (2) Benzyldimethyl[2-[2-[[4-(1,1,3,3-

---

† Brand name formerly used, and/or firm no longer concerned with this product.

tetramethylbutyl)tolyl]oxy]ethoxy]ethyl]ammonium chloride monohydrate. *CAS-1320-44-1; CAS-25155-18-4* [anhydrous]. INN; BAN. *Anti-infective, topical.* Delavan (Bayer†); Diaparene (Sterling Winthrop)

Methylcellulose (meth″ il sel′ ue lose). **USP.** (1) Cellulose, methyl ether; (2) Cellulose methyl ether. *CAS-9004-67-5.* INN; JAN. *Pharmaceutic aid (suspending agent).* Cologel (Lilly); Methocel A (Dow Chemical)

Methylcellulose, Propylene Glycol Ether of — *See* Hypromellose.

Methylchromone. $C_{10}H_8O_2$. 160.17. 3-Methyl-4(*H*)-chromen-4-one. *UNII-KJ0091KAAH. CAS-85-90-5.* INN; BAN.

Methyldesorphine. $C_{18}H_{21}NO_2$. 283.36. 6-Methyl-Δ^6-deoxy-morphine. *CAS-16008-36-9.* INN; BAN; DCF. ◇*MK 57*

Methyldigoxin — *See* Metildigoxin.

Methyldihydromorphine. $C_{18}H_{23}NO_3$. 301.38. 3,6-Dihydroxy-6,*N*-dimethyl-4,5-epoxymorphinan. *CAS-509-56-8.* INN; DCF.

Methyldihydromorphinone Hydrochloride — *See* Metopon Hydrochloride.

Methyldinitrobenzamide — *See* Dinitolmide.

Methyldioxatrine — *See* Meletimide.

Methyldopa [*1962*] (meth″ il doe′ pa). **USP.** $C_{10}H_{13}NO_4.1\frac{1}{2}$-$H_2O$. 238.24. (1) L-Tyrosine, 3-hydroxy-α-methyl-, sesquihydrate; (2) L-3-(3,4-Dihydroxyphenyl)-2-methylalanine sesquihydrate. *UNII-56LH93261Y. CAS-41372-08-1; CAS-555-30-6* [anhydrous]. INN; BAN; JAN. *Antihypertensive.* Aldomet (Merck) *[Name previously used: Alpha-Methyldopa.]* ◇*MK-351*

Methyldopate Hydrochloride [*1963*] (meth″ il doe′ pate hye″ droe klor′ ide). **USP.** $C_{12}H_{17}NO_4.HCl$. 275.73. [Methyldopate is BAN.] (1) L-Tyrosine, 3-hydroxy-α-

methyl-, ethyl ester, hydrochloride; (2) L-3-(3,4-Dihydroxyphenyl)-2-methylalanine ethyl ester hydrochloride. *UNII-7PX435DN5A; UNII-2579Z4P04J* [methyldopate]. *CAS-2508-79-4; CAS-5123-53-5* [replaced]; *CAS-2544-09-4* [methyldopate]. *Antihypertensive.* Aldomet (Merck)

Methylene Blue (meth′ i leen). **USP.** $C_{16}H_{18}ClN_3S.3H_2O$. 373.90. [Methylthioninium Chloride is INN and BAN.] (1) Phenothiazin-5-ium, 3,7-bis(dimethylamino)-, chloride, trihydrate; (2) C.I. Basic Blue 9 trihydrate. *UNII-T42P99266K. CAS-7220-79-3; CAS-61-73-4* [anhydrous]. *Antimethemoglobinemic; antidote (to cyanide poisoning).*

Methylene Chloride (meth′ i leen klor′ ide). **NF.** CH_2Cl_2. 84.93. (1) Methane, dichloro-; (2) Dichloromethane. *UNII-588X2YUY0A. CAS-75-09-2. Pharmaceutic aid (solvent).*

Methylenprednisolone — *See* Prednylidene.

Methylephedrine. $C_{11}H_{17}NO$. 179.26. [*dl*-Methylephedrine Hydrochloride, *l*-Methylephedrine Hydrochloride, and *dl*-Methylephedrine Saccharinate are JAN.] (1*RS*,2*RS*)-2-Dimethylamino-1-phenylpropan-1-ol. *CAS-552-79-4.* BAN.

dl-Methylephedrine Hydrochloride (JAN) — *See* Methylephedrine.

l-Methylephedrine Hydrochloride (JAN) — *See* Methylephedrine.

dl-Methylephedrine Saccharinate (JAN) — *See* Methylephedrine.

Methylergometrine (INN, BAN) — *See* Methylergonovine Maleate.

Methylergometrine Maleate (JAN) — *See* Methylergonovine Maleate.

Methylergonovine Maleate (meth″ il er″ goe noe′ veen mal′ ee ate). **USP.** $C_{20}H_{25}N_3O_2.C_4H_4O_4$. 455.50. [Methylergometrine is INN and BAN; Methylergometrine Maleate is JAN.] (1) Ergoline-8-carboxamide, 9,10-didehydro-*N*-[1-(hydroxymethyl)propyl]-6-methyl-, [8β(*S*)]-, (*Z*)-2-butenedioate (1:1) (salt); (2) 9,10-Didehydro-*N*-[(*S*)-1-(hydroxymethyl)propyl]-6-methylergoline-8β-carboxamide maleate (1:1) (salt). *UNII-IR84JPZ1RK; UNII-W53L6FE61V* [methylergonovine]. *CAS-57432-61-8; CAS-7054-07-1* [replaced]; *CAS-113-42-8* [methylergonovine]. *Oxytocic.* Methergine (Novartis)

Methylergonovinium Bimaleate — *See* Methylergonovine Maleate.

Methylestrenolone — *See* Normethandrone.

Methyl *p*-Hydroxybenzoate — *See* Methylparaben.

Methylmethionine Sulfonium Chloride. $C_6H_{14}ClNO_2S$. 199.70. (*S*)-(3-Amino-3-carboxypropyl)dimethylsulfonium chloride. *CAS-1115-84-0*. JAN.

Methylmorphine — *See* Codeine.

Methylnaltrexone Bromide [*2006*] (meth″ il nal trex′ one broe′ mide). $C_{21}H_{26}BrNO_4$. 436.34. (1) Morphinanium, 17-(cyclopropylmethyl)-4,5-epoxy-3,14-dihydroxy-17-methyl-6-oxo-, bromide, (5α)-; (2) (17*RS*)-17-(Cyclopropylmethyl)-4,5α-epoxy-3,14-dihydroxy-17-methyl-6-oxo-morphinanium bromide. *UNII-RFO6IL3D3M. CAS-73232-52-7*. INN. *Treatment of peripheral side effects of opioid therapy.* ◇*MRZ 2663BR*

Methylnortestosterone — *See* Normethandrone.

Methylparaben [*1986*] (meth″ il par′ a ben). **NF**. $C_8H_8O_3$. 152.15. [Methyl Parahydroxybenzoate is JAN.] (1) Benzoic acid, 4-hydroxy-, methyl ester; (2) Methyl *p*-hydroxy-benzoate. *UNII-A2I8C7HI9T. CAS-99-76-3. Pharmaceutic aid (antifungal agent).*

Methylparaben Sodium [*1986*] (meth″ il par′ a ben soe′ dee um). **NF**. $C_8H_7NaO_3$. 174.13. (1) Benzoic acid, 4-hydroxy-, methyl ester, sodium salt; (2) Methyl *p*-hydroxybenzoate, sodium salt. *UNII-CR6K9C2NHK. CAS-5026-62-0. Pharmaceutic aid (antimicrobial preservative).*

Methylparafynol — *See* Meparfynol.

Methylpentynol (INN, BAN, DCF) — *See* Meparfynol.

Methylperidol — *See* Moperone.

Methylphenidate [*2003*] (meth″ il fen′ i date). $C_{14}H_{19}NO_2$. 233.31. (1) 2-Piperidineacetic acid, α-phenyl-, methyl ester; (2) α-Phenyl-2-piperidineacetic acid methyl ester. *UNII-207ZZ9QZ49. CAS-113-45-1*. INN; BAN. *Stimulant (CNS).* Daytrana (Shire)

Methylphenidate Hydrochloride (meth″ il fen′ i date hye″ droe klor′ ide). **USP**. $C_{14}H_{19}NO_2 \cdot HCl$. 269.77. [Methylphenidate is INN and BAN.] (1) 2-Piperidineacetic acid, α-phenyl-, methyl ester, hydrochloride, (*R**,*R**)-(±)-; (2) Methyl α-phenyl-2-piperidineacetate hydrochloride. *UNII-*

4B3SC438HI. CAS-298-59-9; CAS-113-45-1 [methylphenidate]. JAN. *Stimulant (central).* Concerta (ALZA); Methylin (Mallinckrodt); ritalin (Novartis)

Methylphenobarbital (INN, BAN, DCF) — *See* Mephobarbital.

Methylphenobarbitone (previously used name) — *See* Mephobarbital.

Methylprednisolone (meth″ il pred nis′ oh lone). **USP**. $C_{22}H_{30}O_5$. 374.47. (1) Pregna-1,4-diene-3,20-dione, 11,17,21-trihydroxy-6-methyl-, (6α,11β)-; (2) 11β,17,21-Trihydroxy-6α-methylpregna-1,4-diene-3,20-dione. *UNII-X4W7ZR7023. CAS-83-43-2*. INN; BAN; JAN. *Glucocorticoid.* Medrol (Pfizer) ◇*U-67,590A; NSC-19987*

Methylprednisolone Aceponate. $C_{27}H_{36}O_7$. 472.57. 11β,17,21-Trihydroxy-6α-methylpregna-1,4-diene-3,20-dione, 21-acetate 17-propionate. *CAS-86401-95-8*. INN.

Methylprednisolone Acetate (meth″ il pred nis′ oh lone as′ e tate). **USP**. $C_{24}H_{32}O_6$. 416.51. (1) Pregna-1,4-diene-3,20-dione, 21-(acetyloxy)-11,17-dihydroxy-6-methyl-, (6α,11β)-; (2) 11β,17,21-Trihydroxy-6α-methylpregna-1,4-diene-3,20-dione 21-acetate. *UNII-43502P7F0P. CAS-53-36-1*. JAN. *Glucocorticoid.* Depo-medrol (Pfizer)

Methylprednisolone Hemisuccinate (meth″ il pred nis′ oh lone hem″ ee sux′ i nate). **USP**. $C_{26}H_{34}O_8$. 474.54. (1) Pregna-1,4-diene-3,20-dione, 21-(3-carboxy-1-oxopropoxy)-11,17-dihydroxy-6-methyl-, (6α,11β)-; (2) 11β,17,21-Trihydroxy-6α-methylpregna-1,4-diene-3,20-dione 21-(hydrogen succinate). *CAS-2921-57-5. Adrenocortical steroid.*

Methylprednisolone Sodium Phosphate [*1973*] (meth″ il pred nis′ oh lone soe′ dee um fos′ fate). $C_{22}H_{29}Na_2O_8P$. 498.41. (1) Pregna-1,4-diene-3,20-dione, 11,17-dihydroxy-6-methyl-21-(phosphonooxy)-, disodium salt (6α,11β)-; (2) 11β,17,21-Trihydroxy-6α-methylpregna-1,4-diene-

---

† Brand name formerly used, and/or firm no longer concerned with this product.

3,20-dione 21-(disodium phosphate). *CAS-5015-36-1; CAS-22252-38-6* [methylprednisolone 21-(dihydrogen phosphate)]. *Glucocorticoid.* ◇*U-12,019E*

Methylprednisolone Sodium Succinate (meth″ il pred nis′ oh lone soe′ dee um sux′ i nate). **USP.** $C_{26}H_{33}NaO_8$. 496.53. (1) Pregna-1,4-diene-3,20-dione, 21-(3-carboxy-1-oxopropoxy)-11,17-dihydroxy-6-methyl-, monosodium salt, (6α,11β)-; (2) 11β,17,21-Trihydroxy-6α-methylpregna-1,4-diene-3,20-dione 21-(sodium succinate). *UNII-LEC9GKY20K. CAS-2375-03-3; CAS-2921-57-5* [methylprednisolone 21-(hydrogen succinate)]. JAN. *Glucocorticoid.* Solu-medrol (Pfizer)

Methylprednisolone Suleptanate [*1987*] (meth″ il pred nis′ oh lone sul ep′ ta nate). $C_{33}H_{48}NNaO_{10}S$. 673.79. (1) Pregna-1,4-diene-3,20-dione, 11,17-dihydroxy-6-methyl-21-[[8-[methyl(2-sulfoethyl)amino]-1,8-dioxooctyl]oxy]-, monosodium salt, (6α,11β)-; (2) 7-[Methyl(2-sulfoethyl)-carbamoyl]heptanoic acid, *C*-21-ester with 11β,17,21-trihydroxy-6α-methylpregna-1,4-diene-3,20-dione, monosodium salt. *UNII-G6CS53NCVS. CAS-90350-40-6.* INN. *Anti-inflammatory.* ◇*U-67,590A*

Methylpromazine. *CAS-84-96-8.*

4-Methylpyrazole — *See* Fomepizole.

Methylrosaniline Chloride (previously used name) — *See* Gentian Violet.

Methylrosanilinium Chloride (INN, BAN, JAN) — *See* Gentian Violet.

Methylscopolamine Bromide — *See* Methscopolamine Bromide.

N-Methylscopolamine Methylsulfate (JAN) — *See* Methscopolamine Bromide.

Methyltestosterone (meth″ il tes tos′ ter one). **USP.** $C_{20}H_{30}O_2$. 302.45. (1) Androst-4-en-3-one, 17-hydroxy-17-methyl-, (17β)-; (2) 17β-Hydroxy-17-methylandrost-4-en-3-one. *UNII-V9EFU16ZIF. CAS-58-18-4.* INN; BAN; JAN. *Androgen.* Android (Valeant); Metandren (Novartis); Oreton (Schering); Testred (Valeant) ◇*NSC-9701*

Methyltheobromine — *See* Caffeine.

Methylthionine Chloride — *See* Methylene Blue.

Methylthionine Hydrochloride — *See* Methylene Blue.

Methylthioninium Chloride (INN; BAN) — *See* Methylene Blue.

Methylthiouracil. $C_5H_6N_2OS$. 142.18. (1) 4(1*H*)-Pyrimidinone, 2,3-dihydro-6-methyl-2-thioxo-; (2) 6-Methyl-2-thiouracil. *CAS-56-04-2.* USP XXI; INN; MI.

Methyltrienolone — *See* Metribolone.

Methynodiol Diacetate [*1972*] (meth″ in oh dye′ ol dye as′ e tate). $C_{25}H_{34}O_4$. 398.54. [Metynodiol is INN.] (1) 19-Norpregn-4-en-20-yne-3,17-diol, 11-methyl-, diacetate, (3β,11β,17α)-; (2) 11β-Methyl-19-nor-17α-pregn-4-en-20-yne-3β,17-diol diacetate. *CAS-23163-51-1; CAS-23163-42-0* [methynodiol]. *Progestin.* ◇*SC-19198*

Methyprylon. $C_{10}H_{17}NO_2$. 183.25. (1) 2,4-Piperidinedione, 3,3-diethyl-5-methyl-; (2) 3,3-Diethyl-5-methyl-2,4-piperidinedione. *UNII-CUT48I42ON. CAS-125-64-4.* USP XXII; INN; BAN. Noludar (Roche) [*Name previously used: Methyprylone.*]

Methyridine (BAN) — *See* Metyridine.

Methysergide [*1970*] (meth″ i ser′ jide). $C_{21}H_{27}N_3O_2$. 353.46. (1) Ergoline-8-carboxamide, 9,10-didehydro-*N*-[1-(hydroxymethyl)propyl]-1,6-dimethyl-, (8β)-; (2) (+)-9,10-Didehydro-*N*-[1-(hydroxymethyl)propyl]-1,6-dimethylergoline-8β-carboxamide; (3) (+)-*N*-[1-(Hydroxymethyl)propyl]-1-methyl-D-lysergamide. *UNII-XZA9HY6Z98. CAS-361-37-5.* INN; BAN. *Vasoconstrictor (specific in migraine).*

Methysergide Maleate (meth″ i ser′ jide mal′ ee ate). **USP.** $C_{21}H_{27}N_3O_2 \cdot C_4H_4O_4$. 469.53. (1) Ergoline-8-carboxamide, 9,10-didehydro-*N*-[1-(hydroxymethyl)propyl]-1,6-dimethyl-, (8β)-, (*Z*)-2-butenedioate (1:1) (salt); (2) 9,10-Didehydro-*N*-[1-(hydroxymethyl)propyl]-1,6-dimethylergoline-8β-carboxamide maleate (1:1) (salt). *UNII-

2U7H1466GH. CAS-129-49-7; CAS-361-37-5 [methysergide]. *Vasoconstrictor (specific in migraine)*. Sansert (Novartis)

Metiamide [*1973*] (me tye′ a mide). $C_9H_{16}N_4S_2$. 244.38. (1) Thiourea, *N*-methyl-*N*′-[2-[[(5-methyl-1*H*-imidazol-4-yl)methyl]thio]ethyl]-; (2) 1-Methyl-3-[2-[[(5-methylimidazol-4-yl)methyl]thio]ethyl]-2-thiourea. *CAS-34839-70-8.* INN; BAN. *Antagonist (to histamine H₂receptors).* ◇*SK&F 92058*

Metiapine [*1969*] (me tye′ a peen). $C_{19}H_{21}N_3S$. 323.46. (1) Dibenzo[*b,f*][1,4]thiazepine, 2-methyl-11-(4-methyl-1-piperazinyl)-; (2) 2-Methyl-11-(4-methyl-1-piperazinyl)dibenzo[*b,f*][1,4]thiazepine. *CAS-5800-19-1.* INN. *Antipsychotic.*

Metiazinic Acid. $C_{15}H_{13}NO_2S$. 271.33. 10-Methylphenothiazine-2-acetic acid. *CAS-13993-65-2.* INN; JAN; DCF; MI. ◇*RP 16091*

Metibride. $C_{18}H_{18}ClN_3O_2S_2$. 407.94. 2-Chloro-*N,N*-dimethyl-5-[3-methyl-2-(phenylimino)-4-thiazolin-4-yl]benzenesulfonamide. *UNII-OJF65U061Y. CAS-77989-60-7.* INN.

Meticillin (INN) — *See* Methicillin Sodium.

Meticillin Sodium (JAN) — *See* Methicillin Sodium.

Meticrane. $C_{10}H_{13}NO_4S_2$. 275.34. 6-Methylthiochroman-7-sulfonamide 1,1-dioxide. *UNII-I7EKN1924Q. CAS-1084-65-7.* INN; JAN; DCF; MI. ◇*SD 17102*

Metildigoxin. $C_{42}H_{66}O_{14}$. 794.97. 4‴-*O*-Methyldigoxin. *CAS-30685-43-9.* INN; BAN; JAN.

Metindizate. $C_{25}H_{31}NO_3$. 393.52. 2-(Hexahydro-1-methyl-3-indolinyl)ethyl benzilate. *CAS-15687-33-9.* INN; BAN. *[Name previously used: Methindizate.]*

Metioprim [*1980*] (me tye′ oh prim). $C_{14}H_{18}N_4O_2S$. 306.38. (1) 2,4-Pyrimidinediamine, 5-[[3,5-dimethoxy-4-(methylthio)phenyl]methyl]-; (2) 2,4-Diamino-5-[3,5-dimethoxy-4-(methylthio)benzyl]pyrimidine. *UNII-K29KWU39J0. CAS-68902-57-8.* INN; BAN. *Antibacterial.*

Metioxate. $C_{22}H_{27}N_3O_4S$. 429.53. 2-(4-Methylpiperidino)ethyl 6-ethyl-2,3,6,9-tetrahydro-3-methyl-2,9-dioxothiazolo[5,4-*f*]quinoline-8-carboxylate. *UNII-00V69U1QC7. CAS-42110-58-7.* INN.

Metipirox. $C_7H_9NO_2$. 139.15. 1-Hydroxy-4,6-dimethyl-2(1*H*)-pyridone. *UNII-IE9M6JG949. CAS-29342-02-7.* INN.

---

† Brand name formerly used, and/or firm no longer concerned with this product.

Metipranolol [*1990*] (met″ i pran′ oh lol). $C_{17}H_{27}NO_4$. 309.40. (1) Phenol, 4-[2-hydroxy-3-[(1-methylethyl)amino]propoxy]-2,3,6-trimethyl-, (±)-, 1-acetate; (2) (±)-1-(4-Hydroxy-2,3,5-trimethylphenoxy)-3-(isopropylamino)-2-propanol 4-acetate. *UNII-X39AL81KEB. CAS-22664-55-7.* INN; BAN. *Antihypertensive (β-blocker, ophthalmic).* OptiPranolol (Bausch & Lomb Pharmaceuticals) ◇*BM01.004; VUAB6453 (SPOFA)*

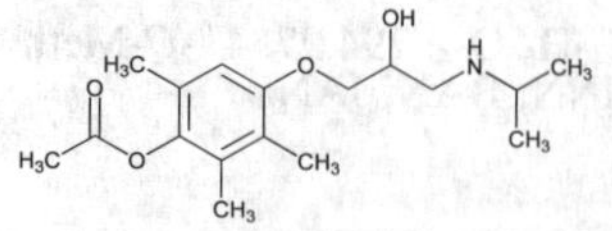

Metiprenaline. $C_{12}H_{19}NO_3$. 225.28. α-[(Isopropylamino)methyl]vanillyl alcohol. *CAS-1212-03-9.* INN.

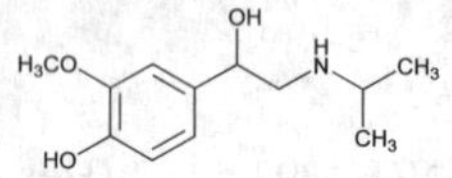

Metirosine (INN, BAN) — *See* Metyrosine.

Metisazone (INN, BAN) — *See* Methisazone.

Metitepine. $C_{20}H_{24}N_2S_2$. 356.55. 1-[10,11-Dihydro-8-(methylthio)dibenzo[*b,f*]thiepin-10-yl]-4-methylpiperazine. *CAS-20229-30-5.* INN.

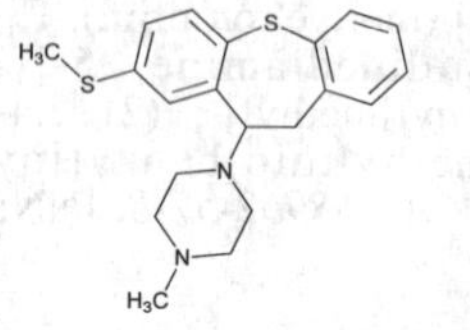

Metixene (INN, BAN) — *See* Methixene Hydrochloride.

Metixene Hydrochloride (JAN) — *See* Methixene Hydrochloride.

Metizoline Hydrochloride [*1969*] (me tiz′ oh leen hye″ droe klor′ ide). $C_{13}H_{14}N_2S.HCl$. 266.79. [Metizoline is INN and BAN.] (1) 1*H*-Imidazole, 4,5-dihydro-2-[(2-methylbenzo[*b*]thien-3-yl)methyl]-, monohydrochloride; (2) 2-[(2-Methylbenzo[*b*]thien-3-yl)methyl]-2-imidazoline monohydrochloride. *CAS-5090-37-9; CAS-17692-22-7* [metizoline]. *Adrenergic (vasoconstrictor).* Ellsyl (Marion Merrell Dow†) [*Name previously used: Metyzoline.*] ◇*EX 10-781; RMI 10,482A*

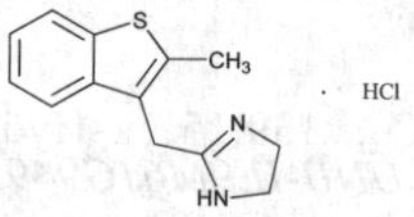

Metkefamide (INN) Acetate — *See* Metkephamid Acetate.

Metkephamid Acetate [*1980*] (met kef′ a mid as′ e tate). $C_{29}H_{40}N_6O_6S.C_2H_4O_2$. 660.78. [Metkefamide is INN.] (1) L-Methioninamide, L-tyrosyl-D-alanylglycyl-L-phenylalanyl-N^2-methyl-, monoacetate (salt); (2) L-Tyrosyl-D-alanylglycyl-L-phenylalanyl-N^2-methyl-L-methioninamide monoacetate (salt). *CAS-66960-35-8; CAS-66960-34-7* [metkephamid]. *Analgesic.* ◇*LY 127623*

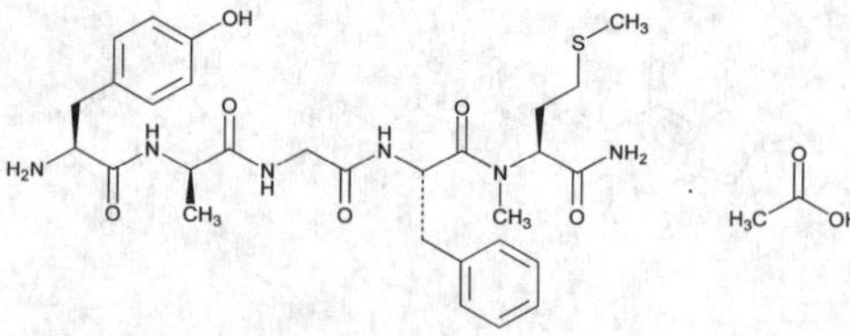

Metochalcone. $C_{18}H_{18}O_4$. 298.33. 2′,4,4′-Trimethoxychalcone. *UNII-1754ZE4075. CAS-18493-30-6.* INN; DCF; MI.

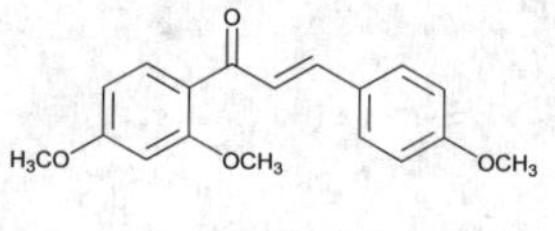

Metocinium Iodide. $C_{19}H_{24}INO_3$. 441.30. (2-Hydroxyethyl)trimethylammonium iodide benzilate. *UNII-R11SBP9F2B. CAS-2424-71-7.* INN.

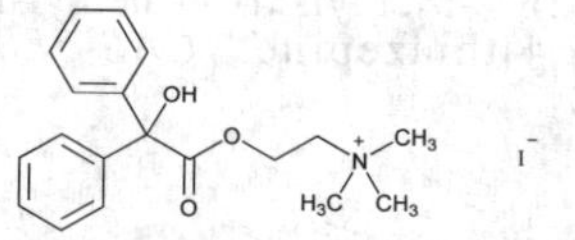

Metoclopramide Hydrochloride [*1964*] (met″ oh kloe′ pra mide hye″ droe klor′ ide). **USP.** $C_{14}H_{22}ClN_3O_2.HCl.H_2O$. 354.27. [Metoclopramide is INN, BAN, and JAN.] (1) Benzamide, 4-amino-5-chloro-*N*-[2-(diethylamino)ethyl]-2-methoxy-, monohydrochloride, monohydrate; (2) 4-Amino-5-chloro-*N*-[2-(diethylamino)ethyl]-*o*-anisamide monohydrochloride monohydrate. *UNII-W1792A2RVD; UNII-L4YEB44I46* [metoclopramide]. *CAS-54143-57-6; CAS-7232-21-5* [anhydrous]; *CAS-364-62-5* [metoclopramide]. JAN. *Anti-emetic.* Maxolon (King); Reglan (Schwarz Pharma) ◇*AHR-3070-C*

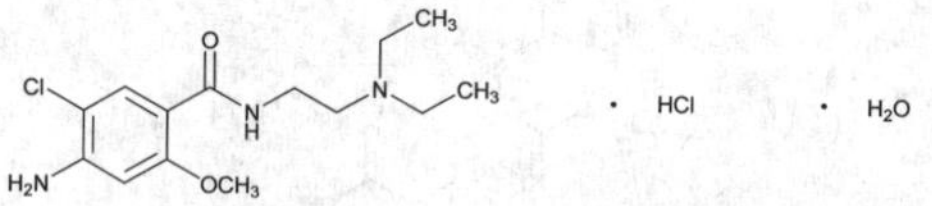

Metocurine Iodide [*1975*] (met″ oh kure′ een eye′ oh dide). $C_{40}H_{48}I_2N_2O_6$. 906.63. (1) Tubocuraranium, 6,6′,7′,12′-tetramethoxy-2,2,2′,2′-tetramethyl-, diiodide; (2) (+)-*O,O′*-Dimethylchondrocurarine diiodide. *UNII-O0U0E87X7F. CAS-7601-55-0.* USP XXIII. *Neuromuscular blocking agent.* Metubine Iodide (Lilly) [*Name previously used: Dimethyl Tubocurarine Iodide.*]

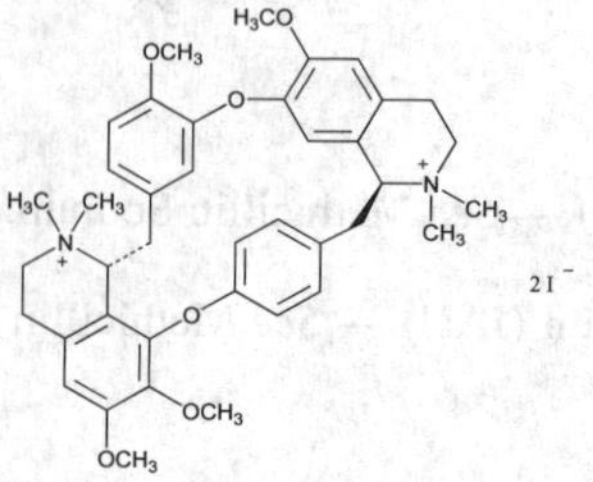

Metofenazate. $C_{31}H_{36}ClN_3O_5S$. 598.15. 2-[4-[3-(2-Chlorophenothiazin-10-yl)propyl]-1-piperazinyl]ethyl 3,4,5-trimethoxybenzoate. *UNII-27J5OW8OGT. CAS-388-51-2.* INN; MI.

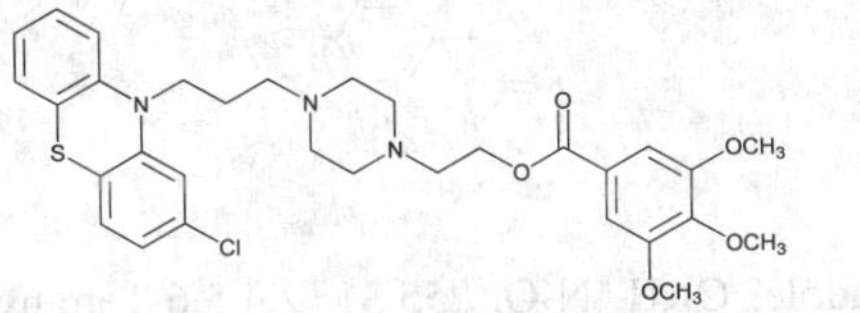

Metofoline (INN, BAN) — *See* Methopholine.

Metogest [*1975*] (met′ oh jest). $C_{20}H_{30}O_2$. 302.45. (1) Estr-4-en-3-one, 17-hydroxy, 16,16-dimethyl-, (17β)-; (2) 17β-Hydroxy-16,16-dimethylestr-4-en-3-one. *CAS-52279-58-0.* INN. *Hormone.* ◇*SC-14207*

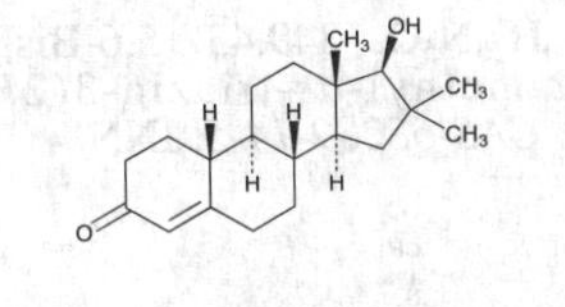

Metolazone [*1968*] (me tol′ a zone). **USP.** $C_{16}H_{16}ClN_3O_3S$. 365.83. (1) 6-Quinazolinesulfonamide, 7-chloro-1,2,3,4-tetrahydro-2-methyl-3-(2-methylphenyl)-4-oxo-; (2) 7-Chloro-1,2,3,4-tetrahydro-2-methyl-4-oxo-3-*o*-tolyl-6-quinazolinesulfonamide. *UNII-TZ7V40X7VX. CAS-17560-51-9.* INN; BAN; JAN. *Diuretic; antihypertensive.* Diulo (Pfizer); Mykrox (UCB); Zaroxolyn (UCB) ◇*SR 720-22*

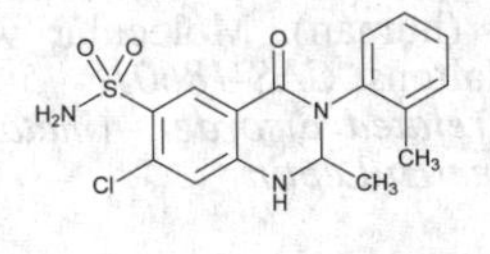

Metomidate. $C_{13}H_{14}N_2O_2$. 230.26. Methyl 1-(α-methylbenzyl)imidazole-5-carboxylate. *CAS-5377-20-8.* INN; BAN; MI.

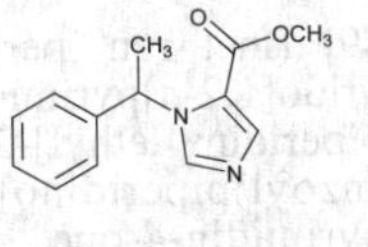

Metopimazine [*1967*] (met″ oh pim′ a zeen). $C_{22}H_{27}N_3O_3S_2$. 445.60. (1) 4-Piperidinecarboxamide, 1-[3-[2-(methylsulfonyl)-10*H*-phenothiazin-10-yl]propyl]-; (2) 1-[3-[2-(Methylsulfonyl)phenothiazin-10-yl]propyl]isonipecotamide. *UNII-238S75V9AV. CAS-14008-44-7.* INN; BAN. *Anti-emetic.* ◇*EXP 999*

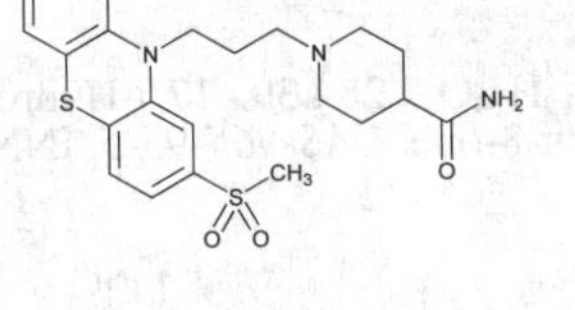

Metopon Hydrochloride. $C_{18}H_{21}NO_3 \cdot HCl$. 335.83. [Metopon is INN and BAN.] 5-Methyldihydromorphinone, hydrochloride. *CAS-124-92-5; CAS-143-52-2* [metopon]. MI; NND 1958.

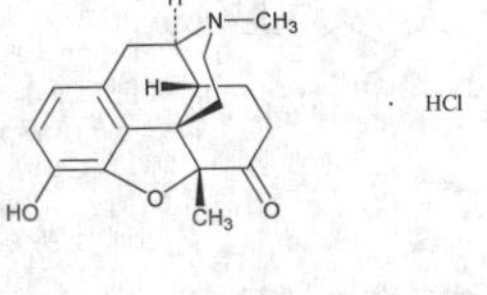

Metoprine [*1977*] (met′ oh preen). $C_{11}H_{10}Cl_2N_4$. 269.13. (1) 2,4-Pyrimidinediamine, 5-(3,4-dichlorophenyl)-6-methyl-; (2) 2,4-Diamino-5-(3,4-dichlorophenyl)-6-methylpyrimidine. *CAS-7761-45-7.* Antineoplastic.

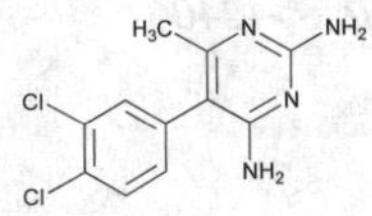

Metoprolol [*1976*] (met″ oh proe′ lol; me top′ roe lol). $C_{15}H_{25}NO_3$. 267.36. (1) 2-Propanol, 1-[4-(2-methoxyethyl)phenoxy]-3-[(1-methylethyl)amino]-; (2) 1-(Isopropylamino)-3-[*p*-(2-methoxyethyl)phenoxy]-2-propanol. *UNII-GEB06NHM23. CAS-37350-58-6; CAS-54163-88-1* [replaced]. INN; BAN. *Anti-adrenergic (β-receptor).*

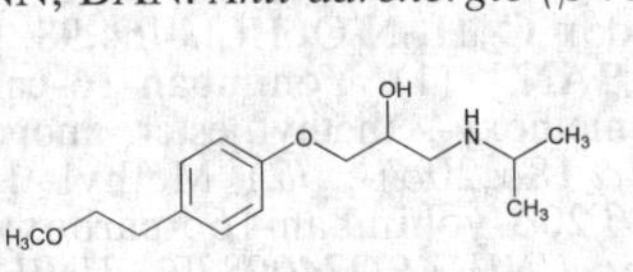

Metoprolol Fumarate [*1990*] (met″ oh proe′ lol fue′ ma rate; me top′ roe lol fue′ ma rate). **USP.** $(C_{15}H_{25}NO_3)_2 \cdot C_4H_4O_4$. 650.80. (1) 2-Propanol, 1-[4-(2-methoxyethyl)phenoxy]-3-[(1-methylethyl)amino]-, (±)-, (*E*)-2-butanedioate (2:1) (salt); (2) (±)-1-(Isopropylamino)-3-[*p*-(2-methoxyethyl)phenoxy]-2-propanol fumarate (2:1) (salt). *UNII-IO1C09Z674. CAS-119637-66-0.* Antihypertensive. Lopressor (Novartis) ◇*CGP 2175C*

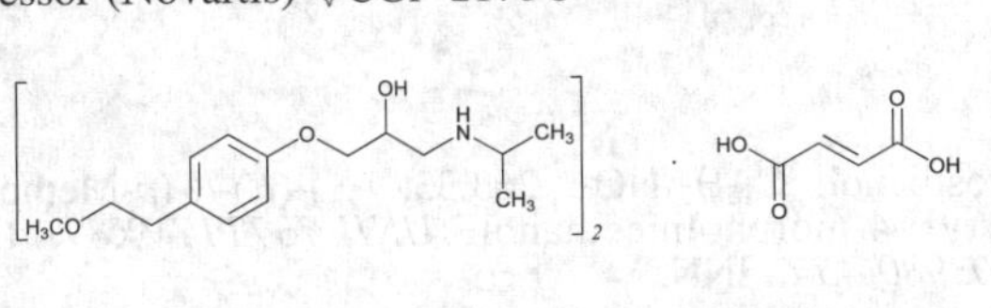

Metoprolol Succinate [*1991*] (met″ oh proe′ lol sux′ i nate; me top′ roe lol sux′ i nate). **USP.** $(C_{15}H_{25}NO_3)_2 \cdot C_4H_6O_4$. 652.82. (1) 2-Propanol, 1-[4-(2-methoxyethyl)phenoxy]-3-[(1-methylethyl)amino]-, (±)-, butanedioate (2:1) (salt); (2) (±)-1-(Isopropylamino)-3-[*p*-(2-methoxyethyl)phenoxy]-2-propanol succinate (2:1) (salt). *UNII-TH25PD4CCB. CAS-98418-47-4.* Anti-anginal; antihypertensive. Toprol (AstraZeneca) ◇*H 93/26 succinate*

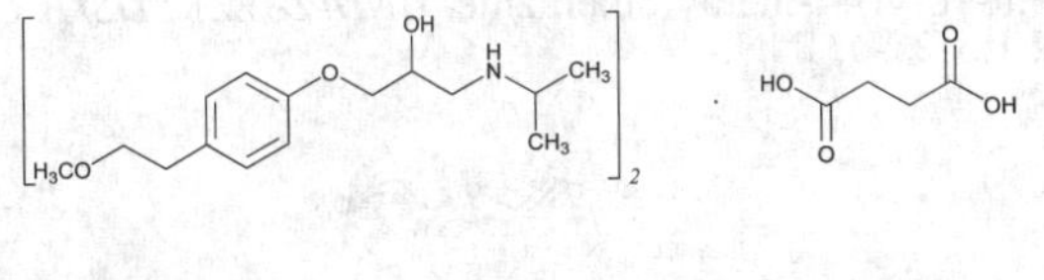

Metoprolol Tartrate [*1978*] (met″ oh proe′ lol tar′ trate; me top′ roe lol tar′ trate). **USP.** $(C_{15}H_{25}NO_3)_2 \cdot C_4H_6O_6$. 684.81. (1) 2-Propanol, 1-[4-(2-methoxyethyl)phenoxy]-3-[(1-methylethyl)amino]-, (±)-, [*R*-(*R**,*R**)]-2,3-dihydroxybutanedioate (2:1) (salt); (2) (±)-1-(Isopropylamino)-3-[*p*-(2-methoxyethyl)phenoxy]-2-propanol L-(+)-tartrate (2:1) (salt); (3) 1-Isopropylamino-3-[*p*-(2-methoxyethyl)phenoxy]-2-propanol (2:1) *dextro*-tartrate salt. *UNII-*

---

† Brand name formerly used, and/or firm no longer concerned with this product.

W5S57Y3A5L. CAS-56392-17-7; CAS-37350-58-6 [metroprolol]. *JAN. Anti-adrenergic (β-receptor).* Lopressor (Novartis) ◇*CGP-2175E*

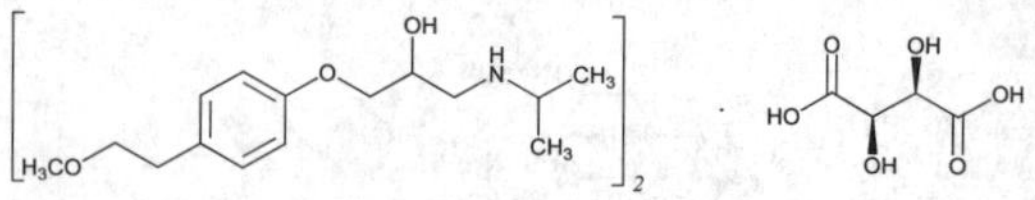

Metoquizine [*1966*] (met oh′ kwi zeen). $C_{22}H_{27}N_5O$. 377.48. (1) 1*H*-Pyrazole-1-carboxamide, 3,5-dimethyl-*N*-(4,6,6a,7,8,9,10,10a-octahydro-4,7-dimethylindolo[4,3-*fg*]quinolin-9-yl); (2) 3,5-Dimethyl-*N*-(4,6,6a,7,8,9,10,10a-octahydro-4,7-dimethylindolo[4,3-*fg*]quinolin-9-yl)pyrazole-1-carboxamide. *UNII-2DW6SEL94L. CAS-7125-67-9.* INN. *Anticholinergic.* ◇*42406*

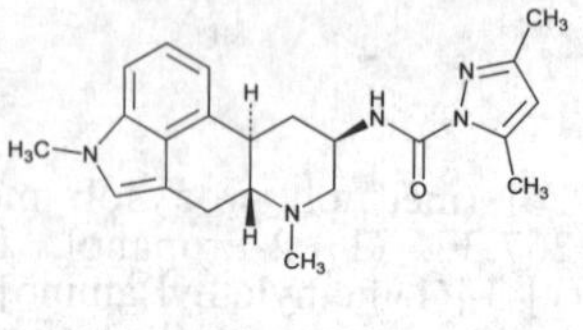

Metoserpate Hydrochloride [*1968*] (met″ oh ser′ pate hye″ droe klor′ ide). $C_{24}H_{32}N_2O_5 \cdot HCl$. 464.98. [Metoserpate is INN and BAN.] (1) Yohimban-16-carboxylic acid, 11,17,18-trimethoxy-, methyl ester, monohydrochloride, (3β,16β,17α,18α,20α)-; (2) Methyl 11,17α,18α-trimethoxy-3β,20α-yohimban-16β-carboxylate monohydrochloride. *UNII-KBO7409339; UNII-X3G4L02XQU* [metoserpate]. *CAS-1178-29-6; CAS-1178-28-5* [metoserpate]. *Sedative (veterinary).* ◇*Su-9064*

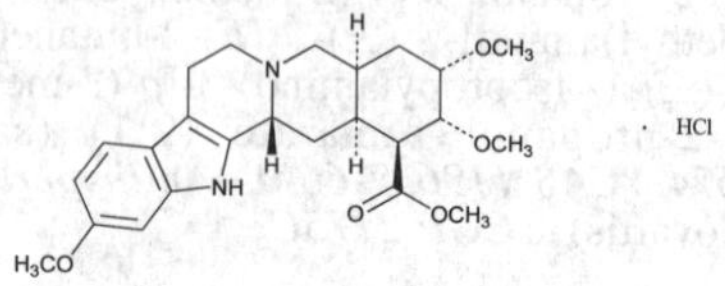

Metostilenol. $C_{15}H_{21}NO_3$. 263.33. (±)-(*E*)-α-(*p*-Methoxystyryl)-4-morpholineethanol. *UNII-737T1YVX89. CAS-103980-45-6.* INN.

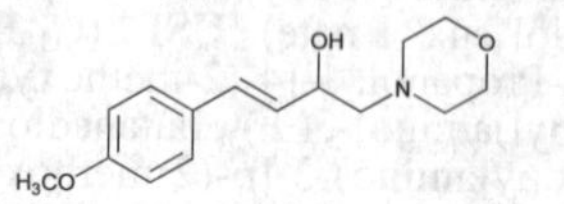

Metoxepin. $C_{20}H_{22}N_2O_2$. 322.40. 1-(8-Methoxydibenz[*b,f*]oxepin-10-yl)-4-methylpiperazine. *UNII-Z8EZK2DSIT. CAS-22013-23-6.* INN.

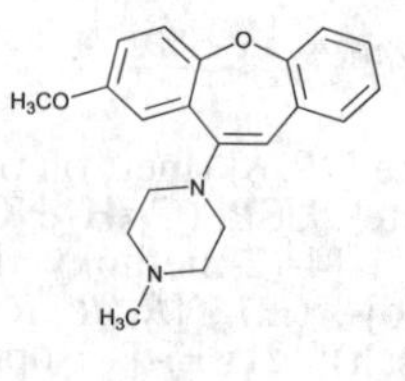

Metoxiestrol — *See* Moxestrol.

Metrafazoline. $C_{17}H_{22}N_2$. 254.37. 2-[(1,2,3,4-Tetrahydro-7-methyl-1,4-ethanonaphthalen-6-yl)methyl]-2-imidazoline. *UNII-89Q735AA4A. CAS-38349-38-1.* INN.

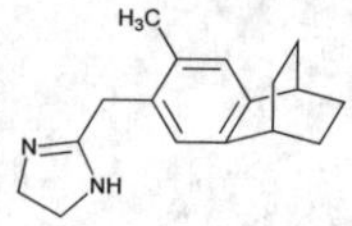

Metralindole. $C_{15}H_{17}N_3O$. 255.31. 2,4,5,6-Tetrahydro-9-methoxy-4-methyl-1*H*-3,4,6a-triazafluoranthene. *UNII-2QW3FL6OPA. CAS-54188-38-4.* INN; MI.

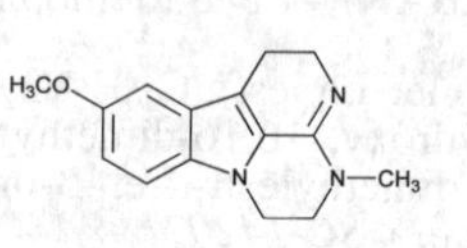

Metrazifone. $C_{20}H_{23}N_5O$. 349.43. 5,6-Bis[*p*-(dimethylamino)phenyl]-2-methyl-*as*-triazin-3(2*H*)-one. *UNII-1N1RL0G53P. CAS-68289-14-5.* INN.

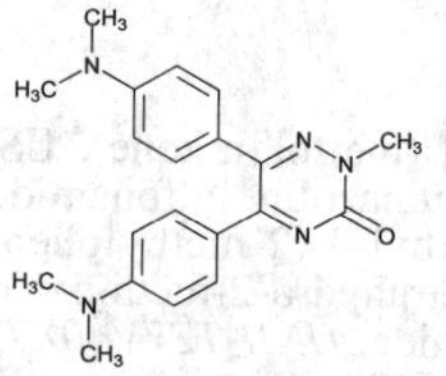

Metreleptin [*1999*] (met″ re lep′ tin). $C_{714}H_{1167}N_{191}O_{221}S_6$. *N*-Methionylleptin (human). Molecular weight is approximately 16,156 daltons. *CAS-186018-45-1.* INN. *Treatment of obesity and related disorders (metabolic homeostasis regulator).* ◇*r-metHuLeptin*

```
                                                      M
VPIQKVQDDT KTLIKTIVTR INDISHTQSV FIPGLHPILT LSKMDQTLAV
YQQILTSMPS ENLRDLLHVL AFSKSCHLPW ASGLETLDSL TEVVALSRLQ
GSLQDMLWQL DLSPGC
```

Metrenperone [*1989*] (met ren′ per one). $C_{24}H_{26}FN_3O_2$. 407.48. (1) 4*H*-Pyrido[1,2-*a*]pyrimidin-4-one, 3-[2-[4-(4-fluorobenzoyl)-1-piperidinyl]ethyl]-2,7-dimethyl-; (2) 3-[2-[4-(*p*-Fluorobenzoyl)piperidino]ethyl]-2,7-dimethyl-4*H*-pyrido[1,2-*a*]pyrimidin-4-one. *UNII-W1O4FV809G. CAS-81043-56-3.* INN; BAN. *Myopathic (veterinary).* ◇*R 50 970*

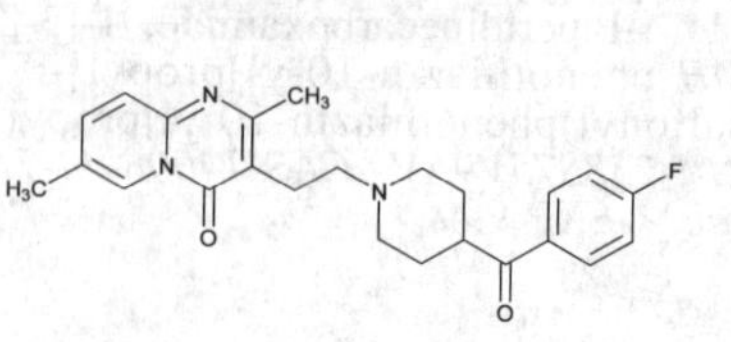

Metribolone. $C_{19}H_{24}O_2$. 284.39. 17β-Hydroxy-17-methylestra-4,9,11-trien-3-one. *CAS-965-93-5.* INN; DCF. ◇*R 1881*

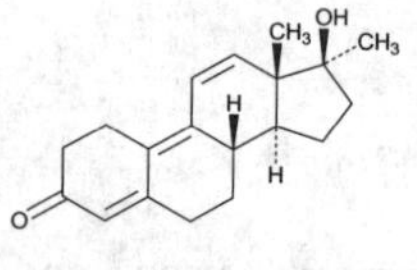

Metrifonate (met″ ri foe′ nate). **USP**. C₄H₈Cl₃O₄P. 257.44. (1) Phosphonic acid, (2,2,2-trichloro-1-hydroxyethyl)-, dimethyl ester; (2) Dimethyl (2,2,2-trichloro-1-hydroxyethyl)phosphonate. *CAS-52-68-6*. INN; BAN.

Metrifudil. C₁₈H₂₁N₅O₄. 371.39. 6-(*o*-Methylbenzylamino)-9-β-D-ribofuranosyl-9*H*-purine. *CAS-23707-33-7*. INN. ◇*Th 322*

Metriphonate (previously used name) — *See* Trichlorfon.

Metrizamide [*1975*] (me triz′ a mide). C₁₈H₂₂I₃N₃O₈. 789.10. (1) D-Glucose, 2-[[3-(acetylamino)-5-(acetylmethylamino)-2,4,6-triiodobenzoyl]amino]-2-deoxy-; (2) 2-[3-Acetamido-2,4,6-triiodo-5-(*N*-methylacetamido)benzamido]-2-deoxy-D-glucose; (3) 2-[3-Acetamido-2,4,6-triiodo-5-(*N*-methylacetamido)benzamido]-2-deoxy-D-glucopyranose. *UNII-RHH3W8F1CO*. *CAS-31112-62-6*. INN; BAN; JAN. *Diagnostic aid (radiopaque medium)*. Amipaque (GE Healthcare) ◇*Win 39103*

Metrizoate Sodium [*1965*] (met″ ri zoe′ ate soe′ dee um). C₁₂H₁₀I₃N₂NaO₄. 649.92. [Sodium Metrizoate is INN and BAN; Metrizoic Acid is JAN.] (1) Benzoic acid, 3-(acetylamino)-5-(acetylmethylamino)-2,4,6-triiodo-, monosodium salt; (2) Sodium 3-acetamido-2,4,6-triiodo-5-(*N*-methylacetamido)benzoate. *UNII-O65Q227UIC; UNII-CM1N99QR1M* [metrizoic acid]. *CAS-7225-61-8; CAS-1949-45-7* [metrizoic acid]. *Diagnostic aid (radiopaque medium)*. ◇*NSC-107431*

Metrizoic Acid (JAN) — *See* Metrizoate Sodium.

Metronidazole [*1962*] (met″ roe nye′ da zole). **USP**. C₆H₉N₃O₃. 171.15. (1) 1*H*-Imidazole-1-ethanol, 2-methyl-5-nitro-; (2) 2-Methyl-5-nitroimidazole-1-ethanol. *UNII-140QMO216E*. *CAS-443-48-1; CAS-13182-89-3* [benzoate]. INN; BAN; JAN. *Antiprotozoal (Trichomo-*

nas). Flagyl (Pfizer); Metrogel (Galderma); Noritate (Sanofi Aventis); Vandazole (Teva) ◇*Bayer 5360; RP 8823; NSC-50364*

Metronidazole Benzoate (met″ roe nye′ da zole ben′ zoe ate). **USP**. C₁₃H₁₃N₃O₄. 275.26. 2-(2-Methyl-5-nitroimidazol-1-yl)ethyl benzoate. *CAS-13182-89-3*. BAN.

Metronidazole Hydrochloride [*1980*] (met″ roe nye′ da zole hye″ droe klor′ ide). C₆H₉N₃O₃.HCl. 207.61. (1) 1*H*-Imidazole-1-ethanol, 2-methyl-5-nitro-, hydrochloride; (2) 2-Methyl-5-nitroimidazole-1-ethanol monohydrochloride. *UNII-76JC1633UF; UNII-140QMO216E* [metronidazole]. *CAS-69198-10-3; CAS-443-48-1* [metronidazole]. *Antibacterial*. Flagyl (Pfizer) ◇*SC-32642*

Metronidazole Phosphate [*1980*] (met″ roe nye′ da zole fos′ fate). C₆H₁₀N₃O₆P. 251.13. (1) 1*H*-Imidazole-1-ethanol, 2-methyl-5-nitro-, dihydrogen phosphate (ester); (2) 2-Methyl-5-nitroimidazole-1-ethanol dihydrogen phosphate (ester). *CAS-73334-05-1*. *Antibacterial; antiprotozoal*. ◇*U-54,555*

Metuclazepam — *See* Metaclazepam.

Meturedepa [*1962*] (met ure″ e de′ pa). C₁₁H₂₂N₃O₃P. 275.28. (1) Carbamic acid, [bis(2,2-dimethyl-1-aziridinyl)phosphinyl]-, ethyl ester; (2) Ethyl [bis(2,2-dimethyl-1-aziridinyl)phosphinyl]carbamate. *CAS-1661-29-6*. INN. *Antineoplastic*. ◇*AB-132; NSC-51325*

Metynodiol (INN) **Diacetate** — *See* Methynodiol Diacetate.

Metyrapone [*1963*] (me tir′ a pone). **USP**. C₁₄H₁₄N₂O. 226.27. (1) 1-Propanone, 2-methyl-1,2-di-3-pyridinyl-; (2) 2-Methyl-1,2-di-3-pyridyl-1-propanone. *UNII-ZS9KD92H6V*. *CAS-54-36-4*. INN; BAN; JAN. *Diagnostic aid (pituitary function determination)*. Metopirone (Novartis)

Metyrapone Tartrate [*1966*] (me tir′ a pone tar′ trate). C₁₄H₁₄N₂O.2C₄H₆O₆. 526.45. (1) 1-Propanone, 2-methyl-1,2-di-3-pyridinyl-, [*R*-(*R**,*R**)]-2,3-dihydroxybutanedioate (1:2); (2) 2-Methyl-1,2-di-3-pyridyl-1-propanone tartrate (1:2). *UNII-B6DRB5ZI7P; UNII-ZS9KD92H6V* [metyrapone]. *CAS-908-35-0; CAS-54-36-4* [metyrapone]. *Diagnostic aid (pituitary function determination)*. Metopirone Ditartrate (Ciba-Geigy†) ◇*Su-4885*

Metyridine. C₈H₁₁NO. 137.18. [Methyridine is BAN.] 2-(2-Methoxyethyl)pyridine. *UNII-08760H16R0*. *CAS-114-91-0*. INN; MI.

---

† Brand name formerly used, and/or firm no longer concerned with this product.

Metyrosine [*1976*] (me tye′ roe seen). **USP.** $C_{10}H_{13}NO_3$. 195.22. [Metirosine is INN and BAN.] (1) L-Tyrosine, α-methyl-, (-)-; (2) (-)-α-Methyl-L-tyrosine. *UNII-DOQ0J0TPF7. CAS-672-87-7. Antihypertensive.* Demser (Aton) ◇*MK-781; L-588357-0*

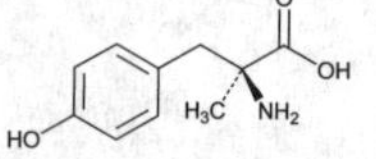

Metyzoline (previously used name) — *See* Metizoline Hydrochloride.

Mevastatin. $C_{23}H_{34}O_5$. 390.51. (1*S*,7*S*,8*S*,8a*R*)-1,2,3,7,8,8a-Hexahydro-7-methyl-8-[2-[(2*R*,4*R*)-tetrahydro-4-hydroxy-6-oxo-2*H*-pyran-2-yl]ethyl]-1-naphthyl (*S*)-2-methylbutyrate. *CAS-73573-88-3.* INN; MI.

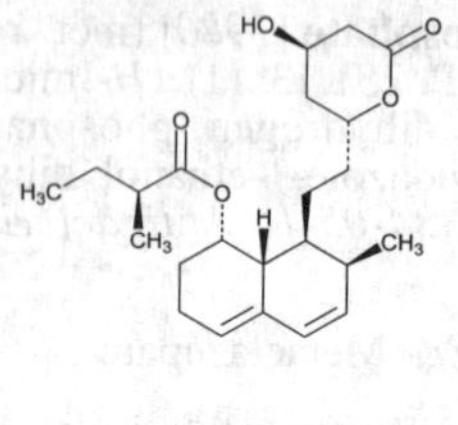

Mevinolin (previously used name) — *See* Lovastatin.

Mexafylline. $C_{14}H_{18}N_4O_2$. 274.32. 3-(3-Cyclohexen-1-yl-methyl)-1,8-dimethylxanthine. *CAS-80294-25-3.* INN.

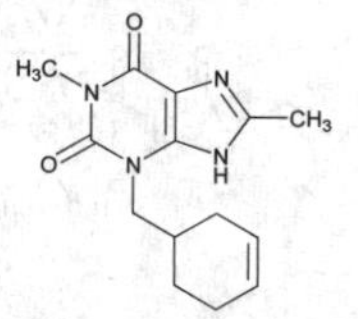

Mexazolam. $C_{18}H_{16}Cl_2N_2O_2$. 363.24. 10-Chloro-11b-(*o*-chlorophenyl)-2,3,7,11b-tetrahydro-3-methyloxazolo[3,2-*d*][1,4]benzodiazepin-6(5*H*)-one. *UNII-S5969B6237. CAS-31868-18-5.* INN; JAN; MI.

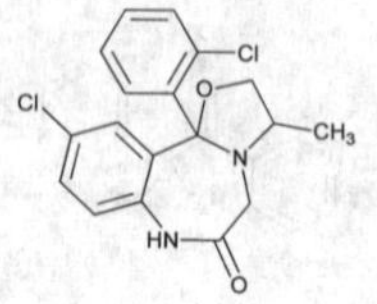

Mexenone. $C_{15}H_{14}O_3$. 242.27. 2-Hydroxy-4-methoxy-4′-methylbenzophenone. *UNII-ET1UGF4A0B. CAS-1641-17-4.* INN; BAN; MI.

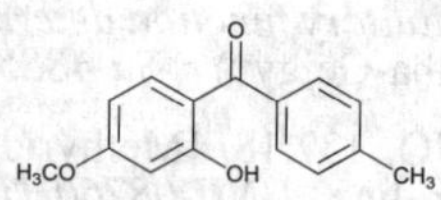

Mexiletine Hydrochloride [*1986*] (mex il′ e teen hye″ droe klor′ ide). **USP.** $C_{11}H_{17}NO·HCl$. 215.72. [Mexiletine is INN and BAN.] (1) 2-Propanamine, 1-(2,6-dimethylphenoxy)-, hydrochloride, (±)-; (2) (±)-1-Methyl-2-(2,6-xyloxy-y)ethylamine hydrochloride. *UNII-606D60IS38; UNII-*

1U511HHV4Z [mexiletine]. *CAS-5370-01-4; CAS-31828-71-4* [mexiletine]. JAN. *Cardiac depressant (anti-arrhythmic).* ◇*Ko 1173 Cl*

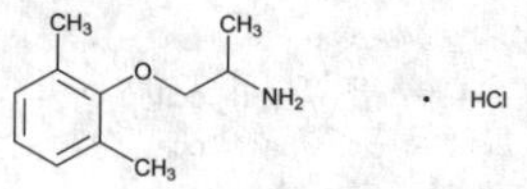

Mexiprostil. $C_{23}H_{40}O_6$. 412.56. Methyl (1*R*,2*R*,3*R*)-3-hydroxy-2-[(*E*)-(3*R*)-3-hydroxy-4-methoxy-4-methyloctyl]-5-oxocyclopentaneheptanoate. *UNII-L5U1X99Q9Z. CAS-88980-20-5.* INN.

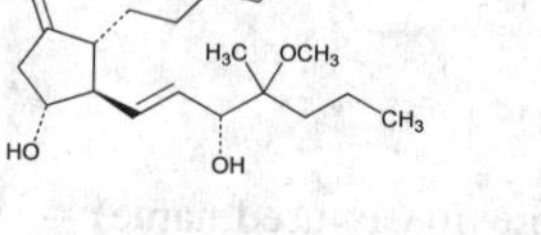

Mexoprofen. $C_{16}H_{22}O_2$. 246.34. *p*-(*trans*-2-Methylcyclohexyl)hydratropic acid. *CAS-37529-08-1.* INN; DCF.

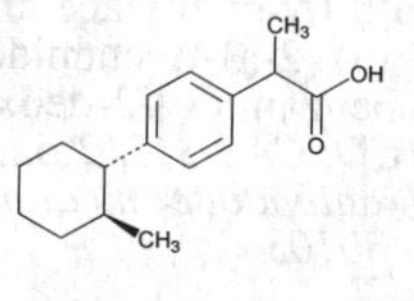

Mexrenoate Potassium [*1975*] (mex ren′ oh ate poe tas′ ee um). $C_{24}H_{33}KO_6·2H_2O$. 492.64. (1) Pregn-4-ene-7,21-dicarboxylic acid, 17-hydroxy-3-oxo-, 7-methyl ester, monopotassium salt, dihydrate, (7α,17α)-; (2) 7-Methyl 21-potassium 17-hydroxy-3-oxo-17α-pregn-4-ene-7α,21-dicarboxylate dihydrate. *CAS-43169-54-6; CAS-41020-67-1* [anhydrous]; *CAS-41020-68-2* [mexrenoic acid]. INN. *Aldosterone antagonist.* ◇*SC-26714*

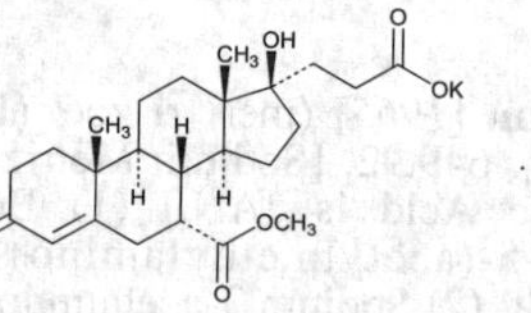

Mezacopride. $C_{16}H_{22}ClN_3O_2$. 323.82. (±)-5-Chloro-4-(methylamino)-*N*-3-quinuclidinyl-*o*-anisamide. *CAS-89613-77-4.* INN.

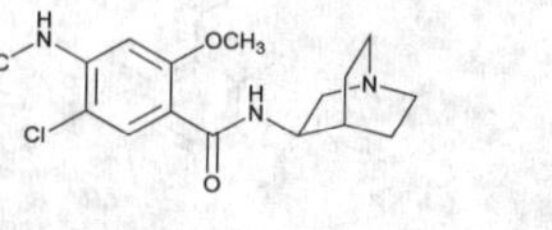

Mezepine. $C_{18}H_{22}N_2$. 266.38. 5,6-Dihydro-5-[3-(methylamino)propyl]-11*H*-dibenz[*b*,*e*]azepine. *UNII-P21N4Z6JHO. CAS-27432-00-4.* INN.

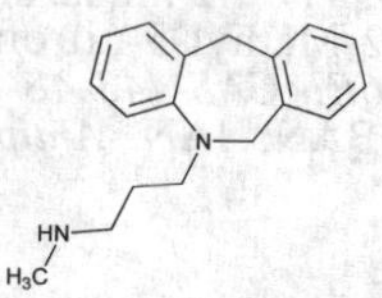

Mezilamine. $C_{11}H_{18}ClN_5S$. 287.81. 4-Chloro-2-(methylamino)-6-(4-methyl-1-piperazinyl)-5-(methylthio)pyrimidine. *UNII-V243ORA40X. CAS-50335-55-2.* INN.

Mezlocillin [*1976*] (mez″ loe sil′ in). $C_{21}H_{25}N_5O_8S_2$. 539.58. (1) 4-Thia-1-azabicyclo[3.2.0]heptane-2-carboxylic acid, 3,3-dimethyl-6-[[[[[3-(methylsulfonyl)-2-oxo-1-imidazolidinyl]carbonyl]amino]phenylacetyl]amino]-7-oxo-, [2S-[2α,5α,6β(S*)]]; (2) (2S,5R,6R)-3,3-Dimethyl-6-[(R)-2-[3-(methylsulfonyl)-2-oxo-1-imidazolidinecarboxamido]-2-phenylacetamido]-7-oxo-4-thia-1-azabicyclo[3.2.0]heptane-2-carboxylic acid. *UNII-OH2O403D1G. CAS-51481-65-3.* INN; BAN. *Antibacterial.* Multocillin (Bayer†)

Mezlocillin Sodium (mez″ loe sil′ in soe′ dee um). **USP**. $C_{21}H_{24}NaN_5O_8S_2$. 561.56. (1) 4-Thia-1-azabicyclo[3.2.0]-heptane-2-carboxylic acid, 3,3-dimethyl-6-[[[[[3-(methylsulfonyl)-2-oxo-1-imidazolidinyl]carbonyl]amino]phenylacetyl]amino]-7-oxo-, monosodium salt, [2S-[2α,5α,6β(S*)]]-; (2) Sodium (2S,5R,6R)-3,3-dimethyl-6-[(R)-2-[3-(methylsulfonyl)-2-oxo-1-imidazolidinecarboxamido]-2-phenylacetamido]-7-oxo-4-thia-1-azabicyclo[3.2.0]heptane-2-carboxylate. *CAS-59798-30-0.* JAN. *Antibacterial.* Mezlin (Bayer)

Mianserin Hydrochloride [*1968*] (mye an′ ser in hye″ droe klor′ ide). $C_{18}H_{20}N_2$·HCl. 300.83. [Mianserin is INN and BAN.] (1) Dibenzo[c,f]pyrazino[1,2-a]azepine, 1,2,3,4,10,14b-hexahydro-2-methyl-, monohydrochloride; (2) 1,2,3,4,10,14b-Hexahydro-2-methyldibenzo[c,f]-pyrazino[1,2-a]azepine monohydrochloride. *CAS-21535-47-7; CAS-24219-97-4* [mianserin]. JAN. *Serotonin inhibitor; antihistaminic.* ◇*Org GB 94*

Mibefradil Dihydrochloride [*1994*] (mye bef′ ra dil dye hye″ droe klor′ ide). $C_{29}H_{38}FN_3O_3$·2HCl. 568.55. [Mibefradil is INN and BAN.] (1) Acetic acid, methoxy-, 2-[2-[[3-(1H-benzimidazol-2-yl)propyl]methylamino]ethyl]-6-fluoro-1,2,3,4-tetrahydro-1-(1-methylethyl)-2-naphthalenyl ester, dihydrochloride, (1S-cis)-; (2) (1S,2S)-[2-[[3-(2-Benzimidazolyl)propyl]methylamino]ethyl]-6-fluoro-1,2,3,4-tetrahydro-1-isopropyl-2-naphthyl methoxyacetate, dihydrochloride. *CAS-116666-63-8; CAS-116644-53-2* [mibefradil]. *Vasodilator.* Posicor (Hoffmann-LaRoche) ◇*Ro 40-5967/001*

M^{131}IBG — *See* Iobenguane I 131.

M^{131}IBG — *See* Iobenguane Sulfate I 131.

MIBG-I-123 — *See* Iobenguane Sulfate I 123.

Mibolerone [*1972*] (mye bole′ er one). **USP**. $C_{20}H_{30}O_2$. 302.45. (1) Estr-4-en-3-one, 17-hydroxy-7,17-dimethyl-, (7α,17β)-; (2) 17β-Hydroxy-7α,17-dimethylestr-4-en-3-one. *UNII-9OGY4BOR8D. CAS-3704-09-4.* INN; BAN. *Anabolic; androgen.* ◇*U-10,997*

Miboplatin. $C_{11}H_{18}N_2O_4Pt$. 437.36. (-)-Cis-[(R)-2-(aminomethyl)pyrrolidine](1,1-cyclobutanedicarboxylato)platinum. *CAS-103775-75-3.* INN.

Micafungin Sodium [*2004*] (mye″ ka fun′ jin soe′ dee um). $C_{56}H_{70}N_9NaO_{23}S$. 1292.26. [Micafungin is INN.] (1) Pneumocandin A0, 1-[(4R,5R)-4,5-dihydroxy-N^2-[4-[5-[4-(pentyloxy)phenyl]-3-isoxazolyl]benzoyl]-L-ornithine]-4-[(4S)-4-hydroxy-4-[4-hydroxy-3-(sulfooxy)phenyl]-L-threonine]-, monosodium salt; (2) 5-[(1S,2S)-2-[(2R,6S,9S,11R,12R,14aS,15S,16S,20S,23S,25aS)-20-[(1R)-3-Amino-1-hydroxy-3-oxopropyl]-2,11,12,15-tetrahydroxy-6-[(1R)-1-hydroxyethyl]-16-methyl-5,8,14,19,22,25-hexaoxo-9-[[4-[5-[4-(pentyloxy)phenyl]isoxazol-3-yl]benzoyl]amino]tetracosahydro-1H-dipyrrolo[2,1-c:2′,1′-l][1,4,7,10,13,16]hexaazacyclohenicosin-23-yl]-1,2-dihydroxyethyl]-2-hydroxyphenyl sodium sulfate. *UNII-IS1UP79R56; UNII-R10H71BSWG* [micafungin].

---

† Brand name formerly used, and/or firm no longer concerned with this product.

CAS-208538-73-2; CAS-235114-32-6 [micafungin]. *Treatment of Aspergillus and Candida fungal infections.* Mycamine (Astellas) ◇*FK463*

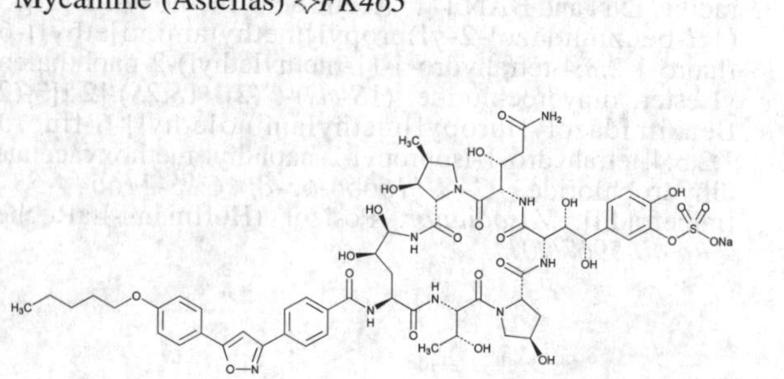

Micinicate. $C_{23}H_{27}NO_4$. 381.46. Nicotinic acid, ester with *cis*-3,3,5-trimethylcyclohexyl (±)-mandelate. *CAS-39537-99-0.* INN.

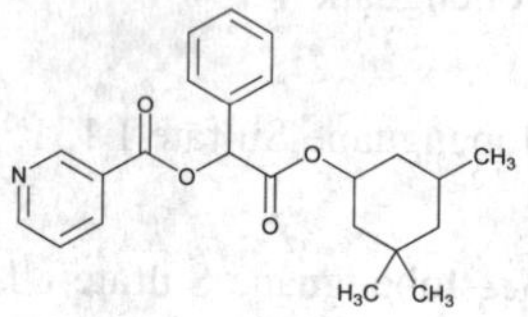

Miconazole (mye kon′ a zole). **USP.** $C_{18}H_{14}Cl_4N_2O$. 416.13. (1) 1*H*-Imidazole, 1-2-[(2,4-dichlorophenyl)-2-[(2,4-dichlorophenyl)]methoxy]ethyl]-, (±)-; (2) (±)-1-[2,4-Dichloro-β-[(2,4-dichlorobenzyl)oxy]phenethyl]imidazole. *UNII-7NNO0D7S5M. CAS-22916-47-8.* INN; BAN; JAN. *Antifungal.* Monistat (Johnson & Johnson)

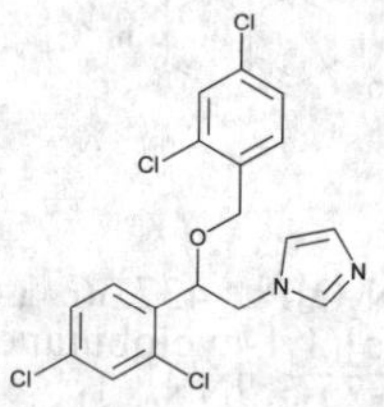

Miconazole Nitrate [*1970*] (mye kon′ a zole nye′ trate). **USP.** $C_{18}H_{14}Cl_4N_2O \cdot HNO_3$. 479.14. (1) 1*H*-Imidazole, 1-[2-(2,4-dichlorophenyl)-2-[(2,4-dichlorophenyl)methoxy]ethyl]-, mononitrate; (2) 1-[2,4-Dichloro-β-[(2,4-dichlorobenzyl)oxy]phenethyl]imidazole mononitrate. *UNII-VW4H1CYW1K; UNII-7NNO0D7S5M* [miconazole]. *CAS-22832-87-7; CAS-22916-47-8* [miconazole]. JAN. *Antifungal.* Monistat (Johnson & Johnson) ◇*R 14,889*

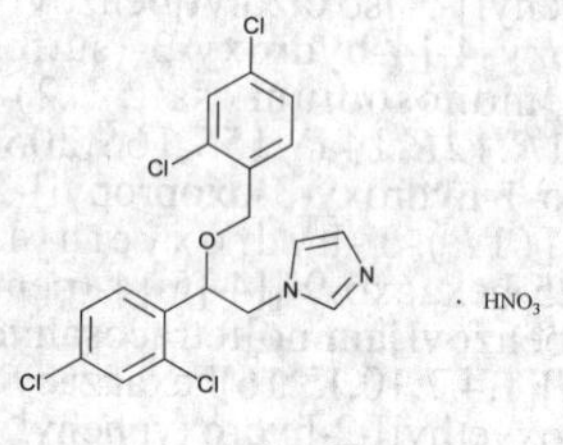

Micronomicin. $C_{20}H_{41}N_5O_7$. 463.57. [Micronomicin Sulfate is JAN.] *O*-2-Amino-2,3,4,6-tetradeoxy-6-(methylamino)-*a*-D-*erythro*-hexopyranosyl-(1→4)-*O*-[3-deoxy-4-*C*-methyl-3-(methylamino)-β-L-arabinopyranosyl-(1→6)]-2-deoxy-D-streptamine. *CAS-52093-21-7.* INN; MI.

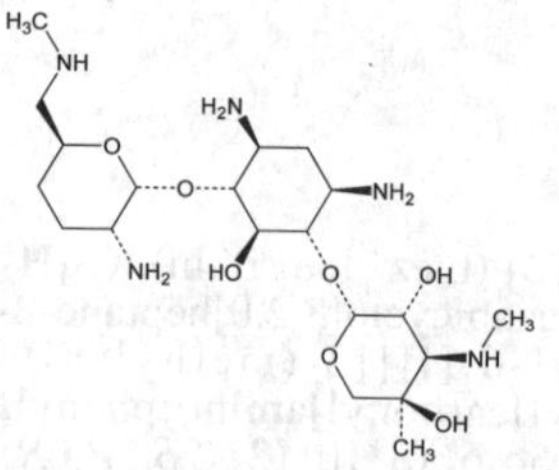

Midaflur [*1968*] (mye′ da flur). $C_7H_3F_{12}N_3$. 357.10. (1) 1*H*-Imidazol-4-amine, 2,5-dihydro-2,2,5,5-tetrakis(trifluoromethyl)-; (2) 4-Amino-2,2,5,5-tetrakis(trifluoromethyl)-3-imidazoline. *CAS-23757-42-8.* INN. *Sedative-hypnotic.* ◇*EXP 338*

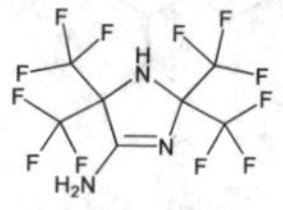

Midafotel. $C_8H_{15}N_2O_5P$. 250.19. (-)-(*R*)-4-[(*E*)-3-Phosphonoallyl]-2-piperazinecarboxylic acid. *CAS-117414-74-1.* INN.

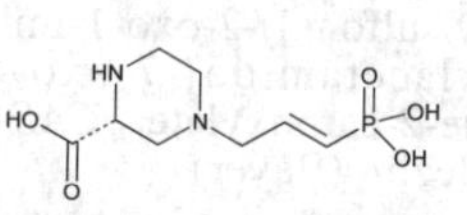

Midaglizole. $C_{16}H_{17}N_3$. 251.33. (±)-2-[α-(2-Imidazolin-2-ylmethyl)benzyl]pyridine. *UNII-44NWV6A237. CAS-66529-17-7.* INN.

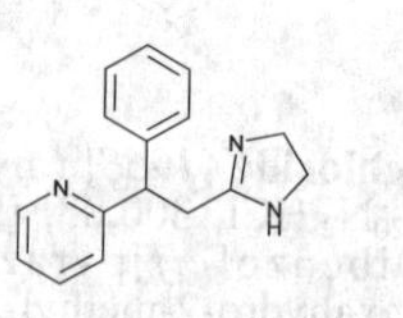

Midalcipran — *See* Milnacipran Hydrochloride.

Midamaline. $C_{18}H_{21}ClN_4$. 328.84. *N*-(5-Chloro-2-benzimidazolylmethyl)-*N*-phenyl-*N*′,*N*′-dimethylethylenediamine. *UNII-MK73KA425L. CAS-496-38-8; CAS-24360-03-0* [hydrochloride]. INN.

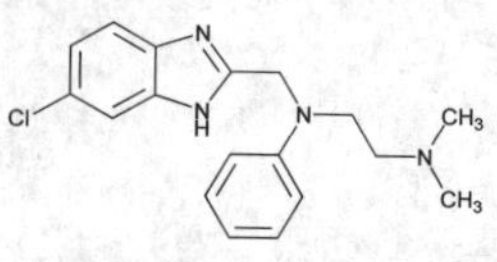

Midaxifylline. $C_{16}H_{25}N_5O_2$. 319.40. 8-(1-Aminocyclopentyl)-1,3-dipropylxanthine. *UNII-A937Z0MS6C. CAS-151159-23-8.* INN.

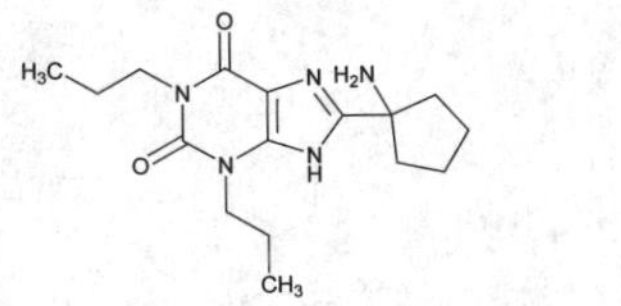

Midazogrel. $C_{18}H_{24}N_2O$. 284.40. (±)-1-[(*E*)-3-(Benzyloxy)-1-octenyl]imidazole. *UNII-04HCK0SD2O. CAS-80614-27-3.* INN.

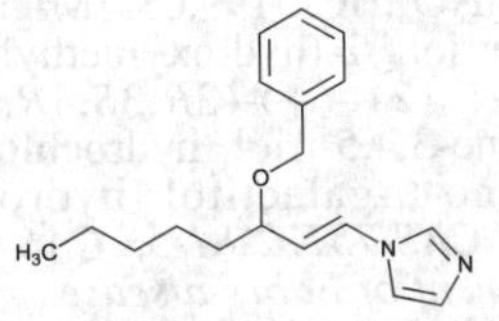

Midazolam Hydrochloride [*1981*] (mid ay′ oh lam hye″ droe klor′ ide). $C_{18}H_{13}ClFN_3 \cdot HCl$. 362.23. [Midazolam is INN, BAN, and JAN.] (1) 4*H*-Imidazo[1,5-*a*][1,4]benzodiazepine, 8-chloro-6-(2-fluorophenyl)-1-methyl-, monohydrochloride; (2) 8-Chloro-6-(*o*-fluorophenyl)-1-methyl-4*H*-imidazo[1,5-*a*][1,4]benzodiazepine monohydrochloride. *UNII-W7TTW573JJ. CAS-59467-96-8; CAS-59467-70-8* [midazolam]. *Anesthetic (injectable).* Versed (Roche) ◇*Ro 21-3981/003*

Midazolam Maleate [*1978*] (mid az′ oh lam mal′ ee ate). $C_{18}H_{13}ClFN_3 \cdot C_4H_4O_4$. 441.84. (1) 4*H*-Imidazo[1,5-*a*][1,4]benzodiazepine, 8-chloro-6-(2-fluorophenyl)-1-methyl-, (*Z*)-2-butenedioate (1:1); (2) 8-Chloro-6-(*o*-fluorophenyl)-1-methyl-4*H*-imidazo[1,5-*a*][1,4]benzodiazepine maleate (1:1). *UNII-R60L0SM5BC* [midazolam]. *CAS-59467-94-6; CAS-59467-70-8* [midazolam]. *Anesthetic (intravenous).* ◇*Ro 21-3981/001*

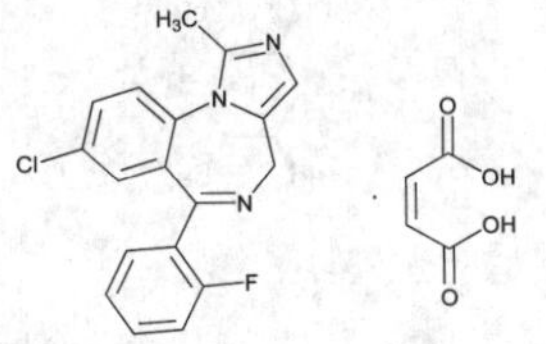

Midecamycin. $C_{41}H_{67}NO_{15}$. 813.97. [Midecamycin Acetate is JAN.] 7-(Formylmethyl)-4,10-dihydroxy-5-methoxy-9,16-dimethyl-2-oxooxacyclohexadeca-11,13-dien-6-yl 3,6-dideoxy-4-*O*-(2,6-dideoxy-3-*C*-methyl-α-L-*ribo*-hexopyranosyl)-3-(dimethylamino)-β-D-glucopyranoside 4′,4″-dipropionate (ester). *CAS-35457-80-8.* INN; JAN; DCF; MI.

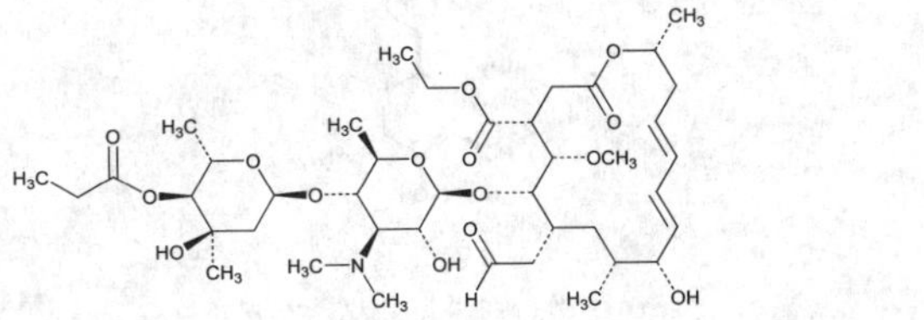

Mideplanin. $C_{93}H_{109}Cl_2N_{11}O_{32}$. 1963.82. A mixture of six substances of which 70% is: 34-[(2-acetamido-2-deoxy-β-D-glucopyranosyl)oxy]-15-amino-22,31-dichloro-56-[[2-deoxy-2-(8-methylnonanamido)-β-D-glucopyranosyl]oxy]-*N*-[3-(dimethylamino)propyl]-2,3,16,17,18,19,35,36,37,38,48,49,50,50a-tetradecahydro-6,11,40,44-tetrahydroxy-42-(α-D-mannopyranosyloxy)-2,16,36,50,51,59-hexaoxo-1*H*,15*H*,34*H*-20,23:30,33-dietheno-3,18:35,48-bis(iminomethano)-4,8:10,14:25,28:43,47-tetrametheno-28*H*-[1,14,6,22]dioxadiazacyclooctacosino[4,5-*m*][10,2,16]benzoxadiazacyclotetracosine-38-carboxamide. *CAS-122173-74-4.* INN.

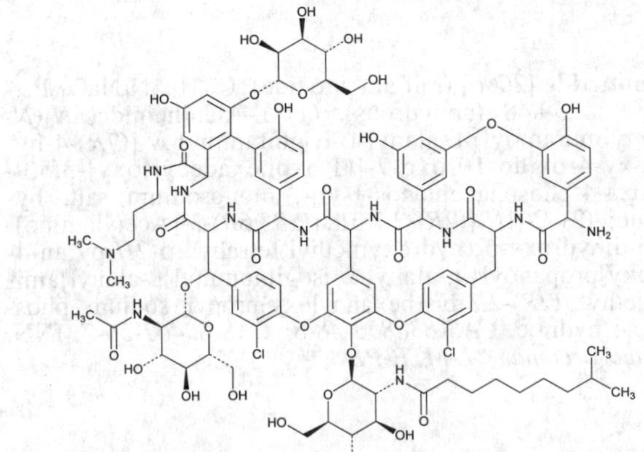

Midesteine. $C_{12}H_{13}NO_3S_3$. 315.43. 2-Thiophenecarbothioic acid, *S*-ester with (±)-2-mercapto-*N*-(tetrahydro-2-oxo-3-thienyl)propionamide. *CAS-94149-41-4.* INN.

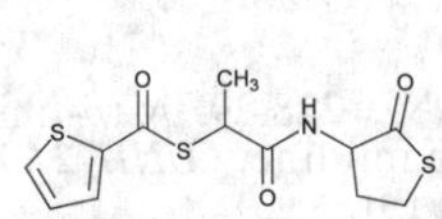

Midodrine Hydrochloride [*1983*] (mye′ doe dreen hye″ droe klor′ ide). $C_{12}H_{18}N_2O_4 \cdot HCl$. 290.74. [Midodrine is INN and BAN.] (1) Acetamide, 2-amino-*N*-[2-(2,5-dimethoxyphenyl)-2-hydroxyethyl]-, monohydrochloride, (±)-; (2) (±)-2-Amino-*N*-(β-hydroxy-2,5-dimethoxyphenethyl)acetamide monohydrochloride. *UNII-59JV96YTXV; UNII-6YE7PBM15H* [midodrine]. *CAS-3092-17-9; CAS-42794-76-3* [midodrine]. JAN. *Antihypotensive.* Orvaten (Upsher Smith); Proamatine (Shire) ◇*A-4020 Linz; St. Peter 224; St 1085 [as the base]*

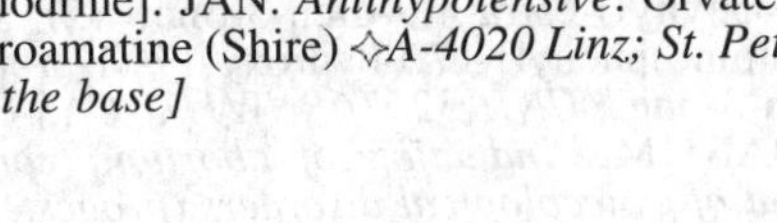

Midostaurin [*2004*] (mye″ doe staw′ rin). $C_{35}H_{30}N_4O_4$. 570.64. (1) Benzamide, *N*-[(9*S*,10*R*,11*R*,13*R*)-2,3,10,11,12,13-hexahydro-10-methoxy-9-methyl-1-oxo-9,13-epoxy-1*H*,9*H*-diindolo[1,2,3-*gh*:3′,2′,1′-*lm*]pyrrolo[3,4-*j*][1,7]benzodiazonin-11-yl]-*N*-methyl-; (2) *N*-[(9*S*,10*R*,11*R*,13*R*)-10-methoxy-9-methyl-1-oxo-2,3,10,11,12,13-hexahydro-9,13-epoxy-1*H*,9*H*-diindolo[1,2,3-*gh*:3′,2′,1′-*lm*]pyrrolo[3,4-*j*][1,7]benzodiazonin-

---

† Brand name formerly used, and/or firm no longer concerned with this product.

11-yl]-*N*-methylbenzamide. *CAS-120685-11-2.* INN. *Antineoplastic; protein kinase C inhibitor.* ◇*CGP 41251; PKC 412*

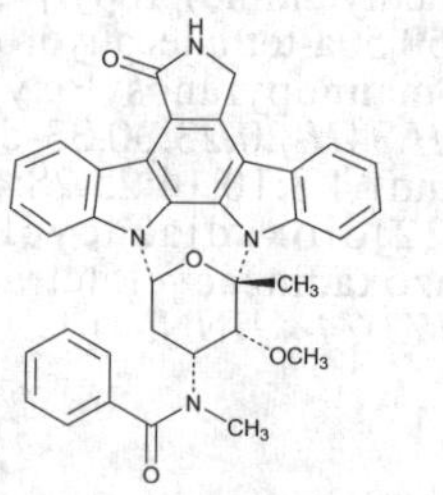

Mifamurtide [*2006*] (mif am′ ure tide). $C_{59}H_{108}N_6NaO_{19}P \cdot x\text{-}H_2O$. 1259.48 (anhydrous). (1) L-Alaninamide, *N*-(*N*-acetylmuramoyl)-L-alanyl-D-α-glutaminyl-*N*-[(7*R*)-4-hydroxy-4-oxido-10-oxo-7-[(1-oxohexadecyl)oxy]-3,5,9-trioxa-4-phosphapentacos-1-yl]-, monosodium salt, hydrate; (2) 2-[[*N*-[(2*R*)-2-[(3*R*,4*R*,5*S*,6*R*)-3-(Acetylamino)-2,5-dihydroxy-6-(hydroxymethyl)tetrahydro-2*H*-pyran-4-yloxy]propanoyl]-L-alanyl-D-isoglutaminyl-L-alanyl]amino]ethyl (2*R*)-2,3-bis(hexanoyloxy)propyl sodium phosphate hydrate. *CAS-838853-48-8; CAS-83461-56-7.* INN. *Osteosarcoma.* ◇*L-MTP-PE*

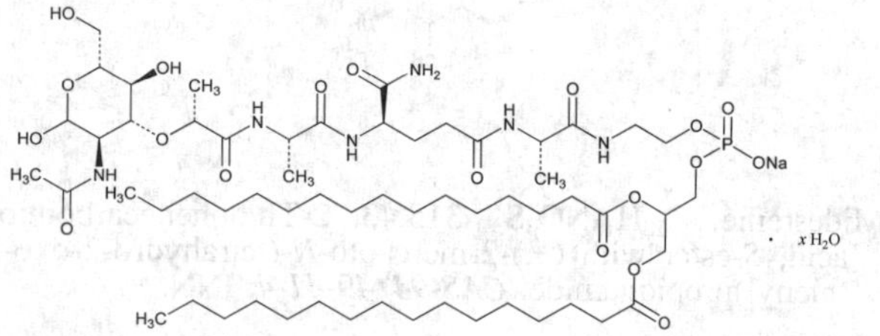

Mifentidine. $C_{13}H_{16}N_4$. 228.29. *N*-(*p*-Imidazol-4-ylphenyl)-*N*′-isopropylformamidine. *UNII-2F70KF5S0K. CAS-83184-43-4.* INN; MI.

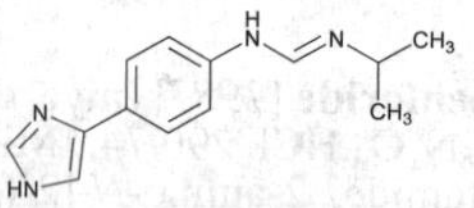

Mifepristone [*1998*] (mif″ e pris′ tone). $C_{29}H_{35}NO_2$. 429.59. (1) (11β,17β)-11-[4-(Dimethylamino)phenyl]-17-hydroxy-17-(1-propynyl)-estra-4,9-dien-3-one; (2) 11β-[*p*-(Dimethylamino)phenyl]-17β-hydroxy-17-(1-propynyl)estra-4,9-dien-3-one. *UNII-320T6RNW1F. CAS-84371-65-3.* INN; BAN; MI. *Induction of abortion; contraception; treatment of gynecological disorders (progesterone antagonist).* Mifeprex (Danco) [*Note—Mifepristone is marketed overseas as Mifegyne.*] ◇*RU 38486; RU 486*

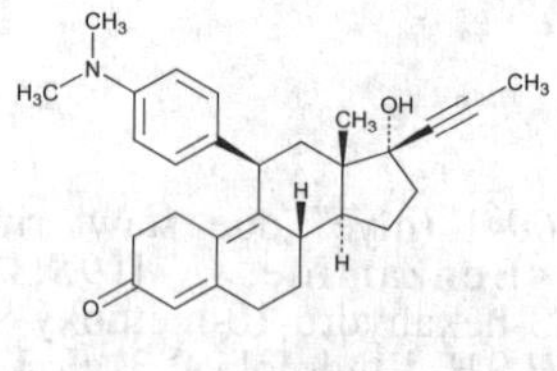

Mifobate [*1984*] (mif′ oh bate). $C_{11}H_{17}ClO_7P_2$. 358.65. (1) Phosphoric acid, (4-chlorophenyl)(dimethoxyphosphinyl)-methyl dimethyl ester; (2) Dimethyl (*p*-chloro-α-hydroxy-benzyl)phosphonate, dimethyl phosphate. *CAS-76541-72-5.* INN. *Anti-atherosclerotic.* Clenicor (Symphar S.A., Switzerland) ◇*SR-202*

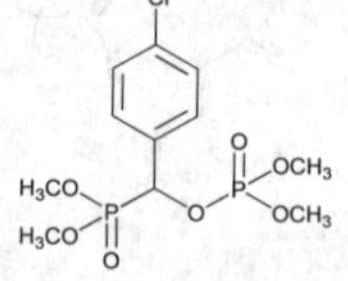

Migalastat Hydrochloride [*2005*] (mi gal′ a stat hye″ droe klor′ ide). $C_6H_{13}NO_4 \cdot HCl$. 199.63. [Migalastat is INN.] (1) 3,4,5-Piperidinetriol, 2-(hydroxymethyl)-, hydrochloride, (2*R*,3*S*,4*R*,5*S*)-; (2) (+)-(2*R*,3*S*,4*R*,5*S*)-2-(Hydroxymethyl)piperidine-3,4,5-triol hydrochloride; (3) 1,5-Dideoxy-1,5-imino-D-galactitol hydrochloride. *UNII-CLY7M0XD20. CAS-75172-81-5; CAS-108147-54-2* [migalastat]. *Treatment of Fabry disease.*

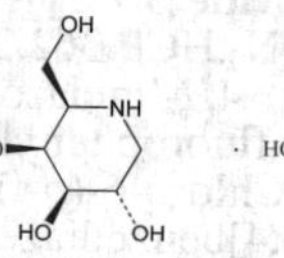

Miglitol [*1990*] (mig′ li tol). $C_8H_{17}NO_5$. 207.22. (1) 3,4,5-Piperidinetriol, 1-(2-hydroxyethyl)-2-(hydroxymethyl)-, [2*R*-(2α,3β,4α,5β)]-; (2) (2*R*,3*R*,4*R*,5*S*)-1-(2-Hydroxyethyl)-2-(hydroxymethyl)-3,4,5-piperidinetriol. *UNII-0V5436JAQW. CAS-72432-03-2.* INN; BAN. *Inhibitor (α-glucosidase).* Glyset (Pfizer) ◇*Bay m 1099*

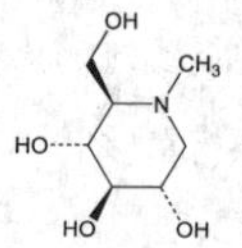

Miglustat [*2003*] (mi gloo′ stat). $C_{10}H_{21}NO_4$. 219.28. (1) 3,4,5-Piperidinetriol, 1-butyl-2-(hydroxymethyl)-, (2*R*,3*R*,4*R*,5*S*)-; (2) (2*R*,3*R*,4*R*,5*S*)-1-Butyl-2-(hydroxymethyl)piperidine-3,4,5-triol. *UNII-ADN3S497AZ. CAS-72599-27-0.* INN; BAN. *Treatment of glycolipid storage diseases.* Zavesca (Actelion) ◇*OGT 918*

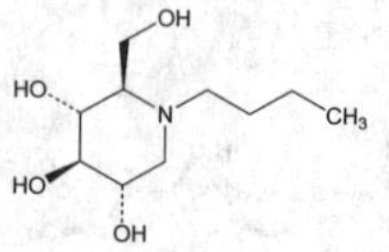

Migrenin. *CAS-8066-49-7.* JAN.

Mikamycin. Antibiotic produced by *Streptomyces mitakaensis,* or the same substance produced by any other means. *CAS-11006-76-1.* INN; BAN; DCF; MI.

Milacainide. $C_{19}H_{25}N_3O$. 311.42. (-)-(*R*)-2-Amino-*N*-[3-(3-pyridyl)propyl]-2′,6′-propionoxylidide. *UNII-7YB0YX4M89. CAS-141725-10-2.* INN.

Milacemide Hydrochloride [*1986*] (mil a′ se mide hye″ droe klor′ ide). $C_7H_{16}N_2O·HCl$. 180.68. [Milacemide is INN.] (1) Acetamide, 2-(pentylamino)-, monohydrochloride. (2) 2-(Pentylamino)acetamide monohydrochloride. *UNII-6XK4G40F6W. CAS-76990-85-7; CAS-76990-56-2* [milacemide]. *Anticonvulsant; antidepressant.* ◇*CP 1552 S*

Milameline Hydrochloride [*1996*] (mil a′ me leen hye″ droe klor′ ide). $C_8H_{14}N_2O·HCl$. 190.67. [Milameline is INN.] (1) 3-Pyridinecarboxaldehyde, 1,2,5,6-tetrahydro-1-methyl-, *O*-methyloxime, monohydrochloride, (*E*); (2) 1,2,5,6-Tetrahydro-1-methylnicotinaldehyde (*E*)-*O*-methyloxime monohydrochloride. *CAS-139886-04-7; CAS-139886-32-1* [milameline]. *Antidementia (partial muscarinic agonist).* ◇*CI-979; RU35926*

Milataxel. $C_{44}H_{55}NO_{16}$. 853.90. 1,10β-Dihydroxy-9-oxo-5β,20-epoxy-3ζ-tax-11-ene-2α,4,7β,13α-tetrayl 4-acetate 2-benzoate 13-[(2*R*,3*R*)-3-(*tert*-butoxycarbonylamino)-3-(furan-2-yl)-2-hydroxypropanoate] 7-propanoate. *CAS-393101-41-2.* INN.

Milatuzumab [*2007*] (mil″ a tooz′ oo mab). $C_{6518}H_{10066}N_{1758}O_{2020}S_{40}$. (1) Immunoglobulin G1, anti-(human class II antigen invariant chain) (human-mouse monoclonal hLL1 heavy chain), disulfide with human-mouse monoclonal hLL1 κ-chain, dimer; (2) Immunoglobulin G1, anti-(human HLA class II histocompatibility antigen γ chain (Ia antigen-associated invariant chain, CD74 antigen)) humanized mouse monoclonal hLL1 γ1 heavy chain (223-219′)-disulfide with humanized mouse monoclonal hLL1 κ light chain (229?229″:232?232″)-bisdisulfide dimer. Molecular weight is approximately 146,700 daltons. *CAS-899796-83-9.* INN. *Treatment of multiple myeloma and other hematological malignancies.* ◇*IMMU-115*

---

† Brand name formerly used, and/or firm no longer concerned with this product.

Milenperone [*1977*] (mil en′ per one). $C_{22}H_{23}ClFN_3O_2$. 415.89. (1) 2*H*-Benzimidazol-2-one, 5-chloro-1-[3-[4-(4-fluorobenzoyl)-1-piperidinyl]propyl]-1,3-dihydro-; (2) 5-Chloro-1-[3-[4-(*p*-fluorobenzoyl)piperidino]propyl]-2-benzimidazolinone. *UNII-9GC5JKP4BD. CAS-59831-64-0.* INN; BAN. *Antipsychotic.* ◇*R 34,009*

Milfasartan. $C_{30}H_{30}N_6O_3S$. 554.66. Methyl 2-[[4-butyl-2-methyl-6-oxo-5-[*p*-(*o*-1*H*-tetrazol-5-ylphenyl)benzyl]-1(6*H*)-pyrimidinyl]methyl]-3-thiophenecarboxylate. *UNII-8UAL5421CL. CAS-148564-47-0.* INN.

Milipertine [*1968*] (mil″ i per′ teen). $C_{24}H_{31}N_3O_3$. 409.52. (1) 1*H*-Indole, 5,6-dimethoxy-3-[2-[4-(2-methoxyphenyl)-1-piperazinyl]ethyl]-2-methyl-; (2) 5,6-Dimethoxy-3-[2-[4-(*o*-methoxyphenyl)-1-piperazinyl]ethyl]-2-methylindole. *CAS-24360-55-2.* INN. *Antipsychotic.* ◇*Win 18,935*

Milk Thistle. The dried ripe fruit of *Silybum marianum* (Linné) Gaertner (Fam. Asteraceae), the pappus having been removed. NF XXI.

Milnacipran Hydrochloride [*2007*] (mil na′ si pran hye″ droe klor′ ide). $C_{15}H_{22}N_2O·HCl$. 282.81. [Milnacipran is INN and BAN.] (1) Cyclopropanecarboxamide, 2-(aminomethyl)-*N*,*N*-diethyl-1-phenyl-, monohydrochloride, (1*R*,2*S*)-*rel*-; (2) (1*RS*,2*SR*)-2-(Aminomethyl)-*N*,*N*-diethyl-1-phenylcyclopropanecarboxamide hydrochloride; (3) *Z*-2 Aminomethyl-1-phenyl-*N*,*N*-diethylcyclopropane-carboxamide hydrochloride. *UNII-RNZ43O5WW5; UNII-G56VK1HF36* [milnacipran]. *CAS-101152-94-7; CAS-92623-85-3* [milnacipran]. *Treatment of fibromyalgia.*

Milodistim [*1996*] (mye loe′ di stim). $C_{1336}H_{2116}N_{362}O_{410}S_{13}$. 30,226.15. A glycoprotein expressed from *S. cerevisiae* as characterized using SDS polyacrylamide gel electrophoresis. The glycoprotein has a relative molecular weight of approximately 35,000 ±3,000 daltons due to glycosylation. The nucleotide sequence encoding the glycoprotein consists of an analog human granulocyte macrophage colony-stimulating factor (GM-CSF), an oligonucleotide linker, and an analog human interleukin 3 (IL-3) DNA sequence. (1) Colony-stimulating factor 2 (human clone pHG25 protein moiety reduced), 23-L-leucine-27-L-aspartic acid-39-L-glutamic acid-, (127→9′)-protein with 9-glycine-10-

glycine-11-glycine-12-glycine-13-L-serine-14-glycine-15-glycine-16-glycine-18-glycine-19-L-serine-34-L-aspartic acid-89-L-aspartic acid-9-152-interleukin 3 (human clone D11 precursor protein moiety reduced); (2) 23-L-Leucine-27-L-aspartic acid-39-L-glutamic acid-colony-stimulating factor 2 (human clone pHG25 protein moiety reduced), (127→9′)-protein with 9-glycine-10-glycine-11-glycine-12-glycine-13-L-serine-14-glycine-15-glycine-16-glycine-18-glycine-19-L-serine-34-L-aspartic acid-89-L-aspartic acid-9-152-interleukin 3 (human clone D11 precursor protein moiety reduced). *CAS-137463-76-4.* INN. *Hematopoietic stimulant; antineutropenic.* Pixykine (Immunex) ◇*PIXY321*

```
APARSPSPST QPWEHVNAIQ EALRLLDLSR DTAAEMNEEV EVISEMFDLQ
EPTCLQTRLE LYKQGLRGSL TKLKGPLTMM ASHYKQHCPP TPETSCATQI
ITFESFKENL KDFLLVIPFD CWEPVQEGGG GSGGGGGSAP MTQTTPLKTS
WVDCSNMIDE IITHLKQPPL PLLDFNNLNG EDQDILMENN LRRPNLEAFN
RAVKSLQDAS AIESILKNLL PCLPLATAAP TRHPIHIKDG DWNEFRRKLT
FYLKTLENAQ AQQTTLSLAI F
```

Miloxacin. $C_{12}H_9NO_6$. 263.20. 5,8-Dihydro-5-methoxy-8-oxo-1,3-dioxolo[4,5-g]quinoline-7-carboxylic acid. *UNII-VM4W7043SN. CAS-37065-29-5.* INN; MI.

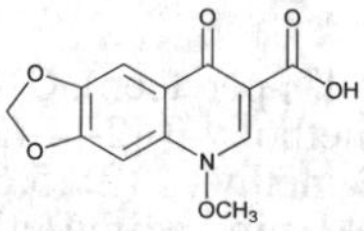

Milrinone [*1983*] (mil′ ri none). **USP.** $C_{12}H_9N_3O$. 211.22. (1) [3,4′-Bipyridine]-5-carbonitrile, 1,6-dihydro-2-methyl-6-oxo-; (2) 1,6-Dihydro-2-methyl-6-oxo[3,4′-bipyridine]-5-carbonitrile. *UNII-JU9YAX04C7. CAS-78415-72-2.* INN; BAN. *Cardiotonic.* Primacor (Sterling Winthrop) ◇*Win 47,203-2*

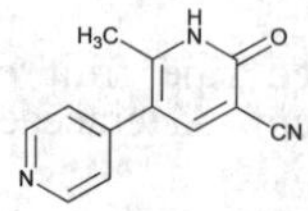

Miltefosine. $C_{21}H_{46}NO_4P$. 407.57. Choline hydroxide, hexadecyl hydrogen phosphate, inner salt. *UNII-53EY29-W7EC. CAS-58066-85-6.* INN; BAN. ◇*D-18506; HDPC*

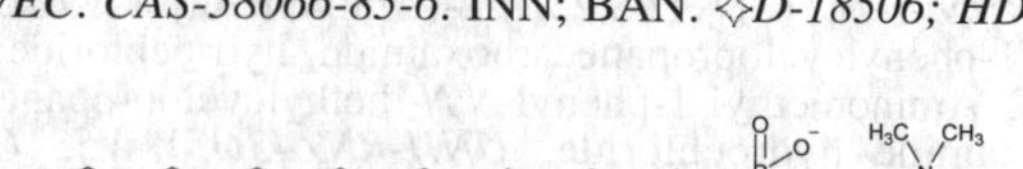

Milverine. $C_{20}H_{20}N_2$. 288.39. 4-[(3,3-Diphenylpropyl)amino]pyridine. *UNII-83B517YUVM. CAS-75437-14-8.* INN.

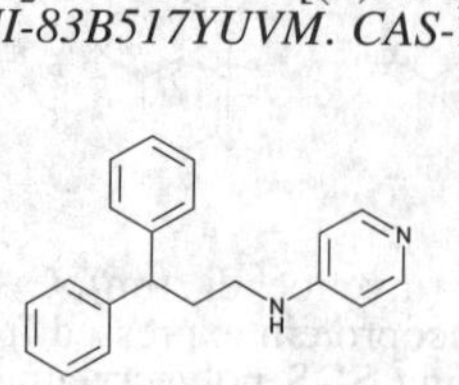

Milveterol Hydrochloride [*2006*] (mil ve′ ter ol hye″ droe klor′ ide). $C_{25}H_{29}N_3O_4$.HCl. 471.98. [Milveterol is INN.] (1) Formamide, N-[2-hydroxy-5-[(1R)-1-hydroxy-2-[[2-[4-[[(2R)-2-hydroxy-2-phenylethyl]amino]phenyl]ethyl]amino]ethyl]phenyl]-, monohydrochloride; (2) N-[2-Hydroxy-5-[(1R)-1-hydroxy-2-[[2-[4-[[(2R)-2-hydroxy-2-phenylethyl]amino]phenyl]ethyl]amino]ethyl]phenyl]formamide

monohydrochloride. *UNII-1D1MD355SJ. CAS-804518-03-4; CAS-652990-07-3* [milveterol]. *Asthma and chronic obstructive pulmonary disease.* ◇*GSK159797C*

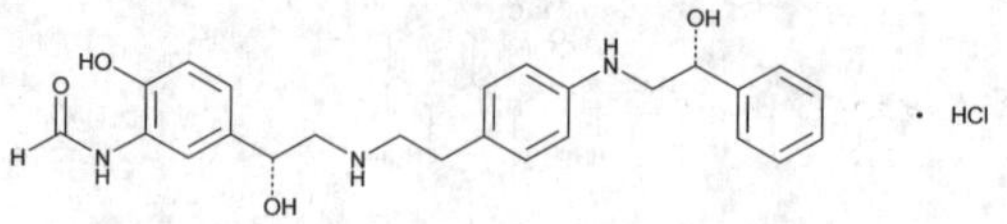

Mimbane Hydrochloride [*1963*] (mim′ bane hye″ droe klor′ ide). $C_{20}H_{26}N_2$.HCl. 330.89. [Mimbane is INN.] (1) Yohimban, 1-methyl-, monohydrochloride; (2) 1-Methylyohimbane monohydrochloride; (3) 1,2,3,4,4aβ,5,7,8,13,13bα,14,14aα-Dodecahydro-13-methylbenz[g]indolo[2,3-a]quinolizine monohydrochloride. *UNII-O9NUI7UT2S; UNII-J9XW583M0N* [mimbane]. *CAS-5560-73-6; CAS-3277-59-6* [mimbane]. *Analgesic.* ◇*W 2291A*

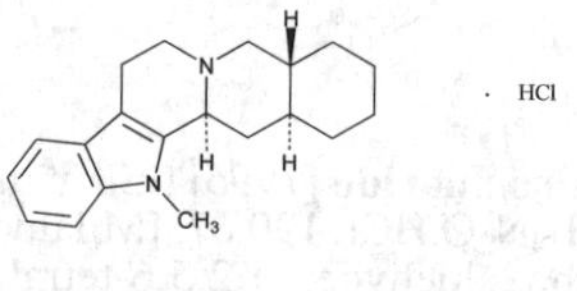

Mimopezil. $C_{23}H_{23}ClN_2O_3$. 410.89. (5R,9R)-5-{[(5-Chloro-2-hydroxy-3-methoxyphenyl)methylidene]amino}-11-[(E)-ethylidene]-7-methyl-5,6,9,10-tetrahydro-5,9-methanocycloocta[b]pyridin-2(1H)-one. *CAS-180694-97-7.* INN.

Minalrestat [*1996*] (min al′ re stat). $C_{19}H_{11}BrF_2N_2O_4$. 449.20. (1) Spiro[isoquinoline-4(1H),3′-pyrrolidine]-1,2′,3,5′(2H)-tetrone, 2-[(4-bromo-2-fluorophenyl)methyl]-6-fluoro-; (2) 2-(4-Bromo-2-fluorobenzyl)-6-fluorospiro[isoquinoline-4(1H),3′-pyrrolidine]-1,2′,3,5′(2H)-tetrone. *UNII-G44PE6QB31. CAS-129688-50-2.* INN. *Inhibitor (aldose reductase).* ◇*WAY-ARI-509*

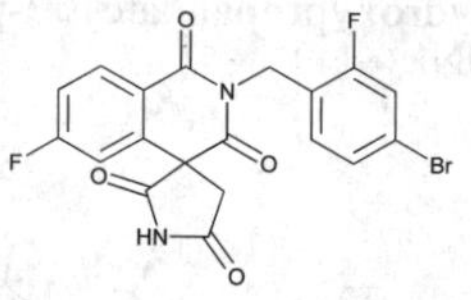

Minamestane. $C_{19}H_{23}NO_2$. 297.39. 4-Aminoandrosta-1,4,6-triene-3,17-dione. *CAS-105051-87-4.* INN.

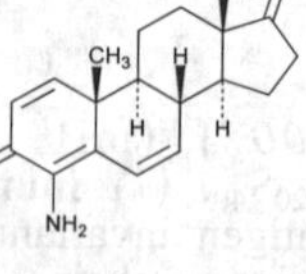

Minaprine [*1988*] (min′ a preen). $C_{17}H_{22}N_4O$. 298.38. (1) 4-Morpholineethanamine, N-(4-methyl-6-phenyl-3-pyridazinyl)-; (2) 4-[2-[(4-Methyl-6-phenyl-3-pyridazinyl)amino]ethyl]morpholine. *UNII-00U7GX0NLM. CAS-25905-77-5.* INN; BAN. *Psychotropic.* Cantor (Sanofi) ◇*CB-30038; AGR-1240*

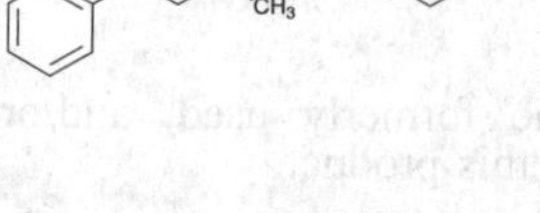

Minaprine Hydrochloride [*1986*] (min′ a preen hye″ droe klor′ ide). $C_{17}H_{22}N_4O·2HCl$. 371.30. (1) 4-Morpholineethanamine, *N*-(4-methyl-6-phenyl-3-pyridazinyl)-, dihydrochloride; (2) 4-[2-[(4-Methyl-6-phenyl-3-pyridazinyl)amino]ethyl]morpholine dihydrochloride. *UNII-82Y7NT6DFT; UNII-00U7GX0NLM* [minaprine]. *CAS-25953-17-7; CAS-25905-77-5* [minaprine]. *Antidepressant.* ◇*30038CB*

Minaxolone [*1979*] (min ax′ oh lone). $C_{25}H_{43}NO_3$. 405.61. (1) Pregnan-20-one, 11-(dimethylamino)-2-ethoxy-3-hydroxy-, $(2\beta,3\alpha,5\alpha,11\alpha)$-; (2) 11α-(Dimethylamino)-2β-ethoxy-3α-hydroxy-5α-pregnan-20-one. *CAS-62571-87-3.* INN; BAN. *Anesthetic.* ◇*C.C.I. 12923*

Mindodilol. $C_{23}H_{28}N_2O_3$. 380.48. $(\pm)$-α-[(Indol-4-yloxy)methyl]-4-(phenoxymethyl)-1-piperidineethanol. *UNII-5VI1D4HYXC. CAS-70260-53-6.* INN.

Mindolic Acid — *See* Clometacin.

Mindoperone. $C_{25}H_{29}FN_2O_2$. 408.51. 4′-Fluoro-4-[4-(6-methoxy-2-methylindol-3-yl)piperidino]butyrophenone. *UNII-556OP2G5M2. CAS-52157-83-2.* INN.

Minepentate. $C_{18}H_{27}NO_3$. 305.41. 2-[2-(Dimethylamino)ethoxy]ethyl 1-phenylcyclopentanecarboxylate. *UNII-2ZBF31C62F. CAS-13877-99-1.* INN; BAN. ◇*UCB 1549*

Mineral Oil (min′ er al). **USP.** [Liquid Paraffin is JAN.] A mixture of liquid hydrocarbons obtained from petroleum *CAS-8012-95-1. Laxative; pharmaceutic aid (solvent).* Balneol (Solvay Pharmaceuticals); Neo-Cultol (Fisons†); Nujol (Schering-Plough HealthCare†) *[Name previously used: Liquid Petrolatum.]*

Mineral Oil, Light (min′ er al). **NF.** A mixture of liquid hydrocarbons obtained from petroleum. *Pharmaceutic aid (tablet and/or capsule lubricant); pharmaceutic aid (vehicle). [Name previously used: Light Liquid Petrolatum.]*

---

† Brand name formerly used, and/or firm no longer concerned with this product.

Minocromil [*1985*] (min ok′ roe mil). $C_{18}H_{16}N_2O_6$. 356.33. (1) $4H$-Pyrano[3,2-*g*]quinoline-2,8-dicarboxylic acid, 6-(methylamino)-4-oxo-10-propyl-; (2) 6-(Methylamino)-4-oxo-10-propyl-$4H$-pyrano[3,2-*g*]quinoline-2,8-dicarboxylic acid. *UNII-F37A9VKY5Q. CAS-85118-44-1.* INN; BAN. *Anti-allergic (prophylactic).* ◇*FPL 59360*

Minocycline [*1966*] (min″ oh sye′ kleen). $C_{23}H_{27}N_3O_7$. 457.48. (1) 2-Naphthacenecarboxamide, 4,7-bis(dimethylamino)-1,4,4a,5,5a,6,11,12a-octahydro-3,10,12,12a-tetrahydroxy-1,11-dioxo-, [$4S$-($4\alpha,4a\alpha,5a\alpha,12a\alpha$)]-; (2) 4,7-Bis(dimethylamino)-1,4,4a,5,5a,6,11,12a-octahydro-3,10,12,12a-tetrahydroxy-1,11-dioxo-2-naphthacenecarboxamide. *UNII-FYY3R43WGO. CAS-10118-90-8.* INN; BAN. *Antibacterial.*

Minocycline Hydrochloride (min″ oh sye′ kleen hye″ droe klor′ ide). **USP.** $C_{23}H_{27}N_3O_7·HCl$. 493.94. (1) 2-Naphthacenecarboxamide, 4,7-bis(dimethylamino)-1,4,4a,5,5a,6,11,12a-octahydro-3,10,12,12a-tetrahydroxy-1,11-dioxo-, monohydrochloride, [$4S$-($4\alpha,4a\alpha,5a\alpha,12a\alpha$)]-; (2) 4,7-Bis(dimethylamino)-1,4,4a,5,5a,6,11,12a-octahydro-3,10,12,12a-tetrahydroxy-1,11-dioxo-2-naphthacenecarboxamide monohydrochloride. *UNII-0020414E5U. CAS-13614-98-7; CAS-10118-90-8* [minocycline]. JAN. *Antibacterial.* Dynacin (Medicis); Minocin (Triax); Solodyn (Medicis)

Minodronic Acid. $C_9H_{12}N_2O_7P_2$. 322.15. (1-Hydroxy-2-imidazo[1,2-*a*]pyridin-3-ylethylidene)diphosphonic acid. *UNII-40SGR63TGL. CAS-127657-42-5.* INN.

Minolteparin Sodium. Sodium salt of depolymerized heparin obtained by nitrous acid degradation of heparin from pork intestinal mucosa, the majority of the components have a 2-*O*-sulfo-α-L-idopyranosuronic acid structure at the non-reducing end and a 6-*O*-sulfo-2,5-anhydro-D-mannitol structure at the reducing end of their chain; the average relative molecular mass is between 1700 and 3300, 90% of which ranges between 1000 and 8000; the degree of sulfation is about 2.1 per disaccharide unit. INN.

Minopafant. $C_{46}H_{73}ClN_4O_9$. 861.55. (+)-1-Ethyl-2-[[N-[[(2R)-2-methoxy-3-[[(4-[(octadecylcarbamoyl)oxy]piperidino]carbonyl]oxy]propoxy]carbonyl]-o-anisamido]methyl]pyridinium chloride. *CAS-128420-61-1*. INN.

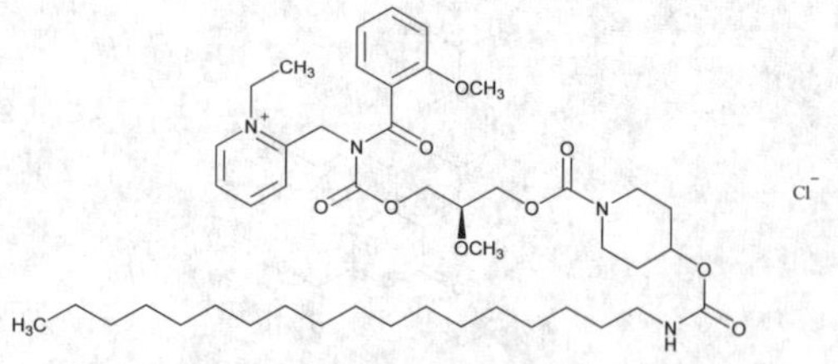

Minoxidil [*1970*] (min ox′ i dil). **USP.** $C_9H_{15}N_5O$. 209.25. (1) 2,4-Pyrimidinediamine, 6-(1-piperidinyl)-, 3-oxide; (2) 2,4-Diamino-6-piperidinopyrimidine 3-oxide. *UNII-5965120SH1. CAS-38304-91-5*. INN; BAN. *Antihypertensive; hair growth stimulant (topical).* Loniten (Pfizer); Rogaine (Johnson & Johnson) ◇*U-10,858*

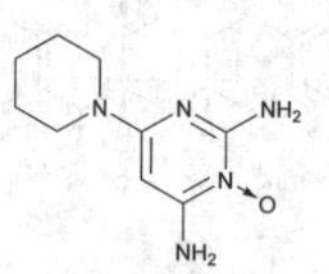

Minretumomab. Immunoglobulin G1 anti-(human tumor-associated glycoprotein 72) (mouse monoclonal Mab CC-49 λ1-chain), disulfide with mouse monoclonal Mab CC-49-chain, dimer. *CAS-195189-17-4*. INN.

Mioflazine Hydrochloride [*1984*] (mye oh′ fla zeen hye″ droe klor′ ide). $C_{29}H_{30}Cl_2F_2N_4O_2 \cdot 2HCl \cdot H_2O$. 666.41. [Mioflazine is INN and BAN.] (1) 1-Piperazineacetamide, 3-(aminocarbonyl)-4-[4,4-bis(4-fluorophenyl)butyl]-N-(2,6-dichlorophenyl)-, dihydrochloride, monohydrate; (2) 4-[4,4-Bis(p-fluorophenyl)butyl]-3-carbamoyl-2,6-dichloro-1-piperazineacetanilide dihydrochloride monohydrate. *CAS-79467-24-6; CAS-79467-23-5* [mioflazine]. *Vasodilator (coronary).* ◇*R-51,469*

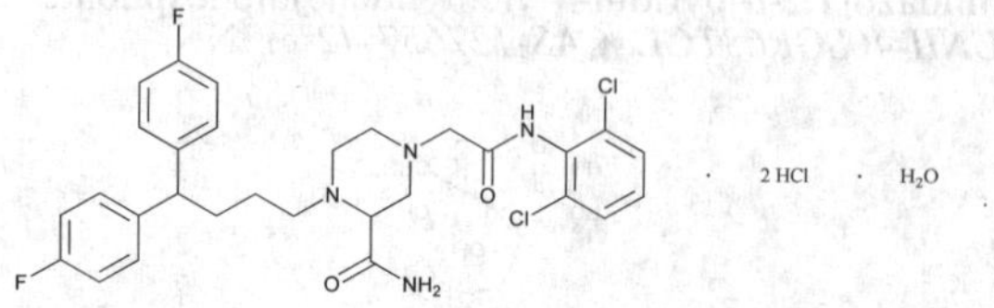

Mipafilcon A [*1993*] (mi″ pa fil′ kon). $(C_5H_9NO)_u$ $(C_6H_9NO)_v(C_5H_8O_2)_w(C_8H_{14}O_3)_x(C_{10}H_{14}O_4)_y(C_7H_{10}O_2)_z$. (1) 2-Propenamide, N,N-dimethyl-, polymer with 1-ethenyl-2-pyrrolidinone, methyl 2-methyl-2-propenoate, (±)-2-hydroxybutyl 2-methyl-2-propenoate, 1,2-ethanediyl bis(2-methyl-2-propenoate) and 2-propenyl 2-methyl-2-propenoate; (2) N,N-Dimethylacrylamide polymer with 1-vinyl-2-pyrrolidinone, methyl methacrylate, (±)-2-hydroxybutyl methacrylate, ethylene dimethacrylate and allyl methacrylate. *CAS-104868-24-8. Contact lens material (hydrophilic).* [Note—The water content of the contact lens material is 70% at 25°C.]

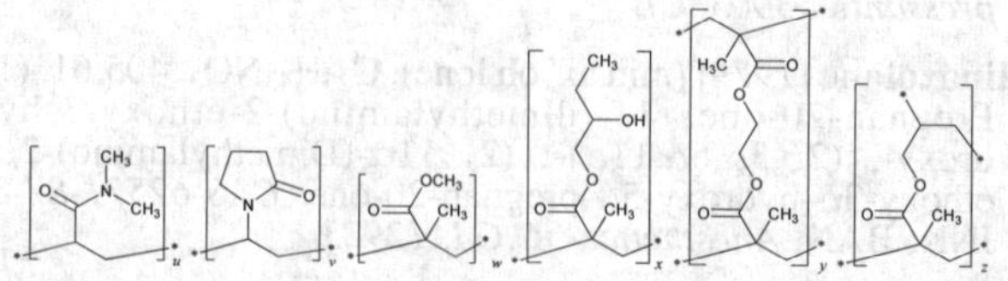

Mipimazole. $C_6H_{12}N_2S$. 144.24. 1-Isopropyl-2-imidazolidinethione. *UNII-UYN5I3I5YQ. CAS-20406-60-4*. INN.

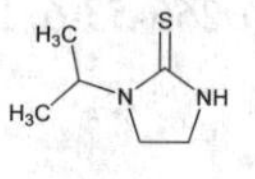

Mipitroban. $C_{19}H_{19}Cl_2N_3O_2$. 392.28. 6-Chloro-3-(p-chlorobenzyl)-β,β-dimethyl-3H-imidazo[4,5-b]pyridine-2-butyric acid. *UNII-2L6Q871829. CAS-136122-46-8*. INN.

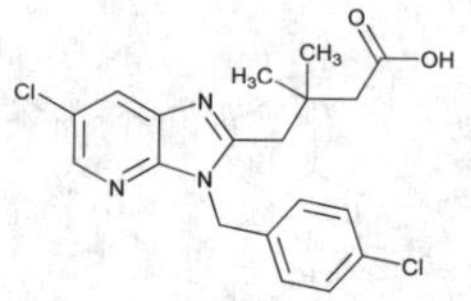

Mipomersen Sodium [*2007*] (mi″ poe mer′ sen soe′ dee um). $C_{230}H_{305}N_{67}Na_{19}O_{122}P_{19}S_{19}$. 7594.80. [Mipomersen is INN.] (1) DNA, d(P-thio)([2′-O-(2-methoxyethyl)]rG-[2′-O-(2-methoxyethyl)]m5rC-[2′-O-(2-methoxyethyl)]m5rC-[2′-O-(2-methoxyethyl)]m5rU-[2′-O-(2-methoxyethyl)]m5rC-A-G-T-m5C-T-G-m5C-T-T-m5C-[2′-O-(2-methoxyethyl)]rG-[2′-O-(2-methoxyethyl)]m5rC-[2′-O-(2-methoxyethyl)]rA-[2′-O-(2-methoxyethyl)]m5rC-[2′-O-(2-methoxyethyl)]m5rC), sodium salt; (2) 2′-O-(2-Methoxyethyl)-P-thioguanylyl-(3′→5′)-2′-O-(2-methoxyethyl)-5-methyl-P-thiocytidylyl-(3′→5′)-2′-O-(2-methoxyethyl)-5-methyl-P-thiocytidylyl-(3′→5′)-2′-O-(2-methoxyethyl)-5-methyl-P-thiouridylyl-(3′→5′)-2′-O-(2-methoxyethyl)-5-methyl-P-thiocytidylyl-(3′→5′)-2′-deoxy-P-thioadenylyl-(3′→5′)-2′-deoxy-P-thioguanylyl-(3′→5′)P-thiothymidylyl-(3′→5′)-2′-deoxy-5-methyl-P-thiocytidylyl-(3′→5′)-P-thiothymidylyl-(3′→5′)-2′-deoxy-P-thioguanylyl-(3′→5′)-2′-deoxy-5-methyl-P-thiocytidylyl-(3′→5′)-P-thiothymidylyl-(3′→5′)-P-thiothymidylyl-(3′→5′)-2′-deoxy-5-methyl-P-thiocytidylyl-(3′→5′)-2′-O-(2-methoxyethyl)-P-thioguanylyl-(3′→5′)-2′-O-(2-methoxyethyl)-5-methyl-P-thiocytidylyl-(3′→5′)-2′-O-(2-methoxyethyl)-P-thioadenylyl-(3′→5′)-2′-O-(2-methoxyethyl)-5-methyl-P-thiocytidylyl-(3′→5′)-2′-O-(2-methoxyethyl)-5-methylcytidine nonadecasodium salt. *CAS-629167-92-6; CAS-1000120-98-8* [mipomersen]. *Treatment of hypercholesterolemia.* ◇*ISIS 301012*

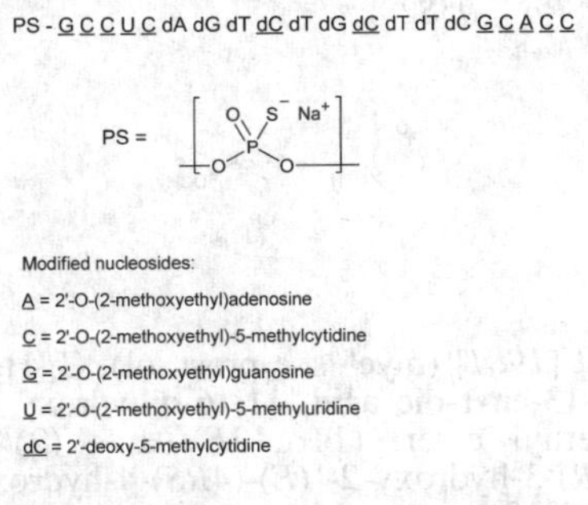

PS - $\underline{G}$ $\underline{C}$ $\underline{C}$ $\underline{U}$ $\underline{C}$ dA dG dT $\underline{dC}$ dT dG $\underline{dC}$ dT dT dC $\underline{G}$ $\underline{C}$ $\underline{A}$ $\underline{C}$ $\underline{C}$

Modified nucleosides:

A = 2'-O-(2-methoxyethyl)adenosine

C = 2'-O-(2-methoxyethyl)-5-methylcytidine

G = 2'-O-(2-methoxyethyl)guanosine

U = 2'-O-(2-methoxyethyl)-5-methyluridine

dC = 2'-deoxy-5-methylcytidine

Mipragoside. $C_{76}H_{137}N_3O_{31}$. 1588.90. *N*-(II³-*N*-Acetylneuraminosylgangliotetraosyl)ceramide, isopropyl ester. *CAS-131129-98-1*. INN.

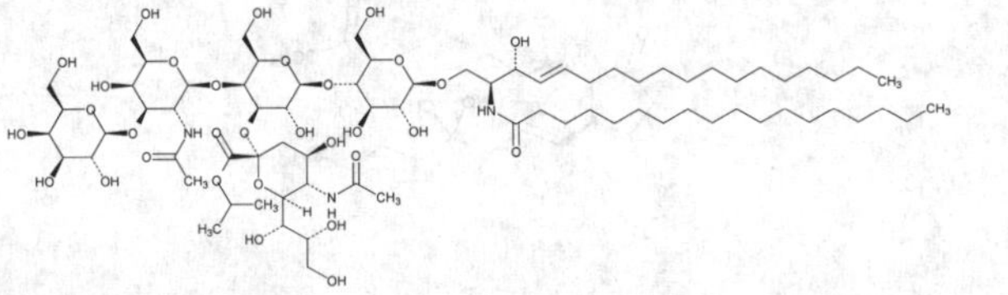

Miproxifene. $C_{29}H_{35}NO_2$. 429.59. (*Z*)-α-[*p*-[2-(Dimethylamino)ethoxy]phenyl]-α′-ethyl-4′-isopropyl-4-stilbenol. *UNII-BGJ4Z7930W. CAS-129612-87-9*. INN.

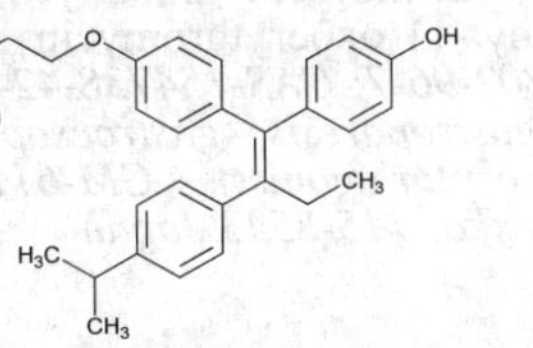

Mirabegron. $C_{21}H_{24}N_4O_2S$. 396.51. 2-(2-Amino-1,3-thiazol-4-yl)-*N*-[4-(2-{[(2*R*)-2-hydroxy-2-phenylethyl]amino}ethyl)phenyl]acetamide. *CAS-223673-61-8*. INN.

Mirfentanil Hydrochloride [*1990*] (mir fen′ ta nil hye″ droe klor′ ide). $C_{22}H_{24}N_4O_2$.HCl. 412.91. [Mirfentanil is INN.] (1) 2-Furancarboxamide, *N*-[1-(2-phenylethyl)-4-piperidinyl]-*N*-pyrazinyl-, monohydrochloride; (2) *N*-(1-Phenylethyl-4-piperidyl)-*N*-pyrazinyl-2-furamide monohydrochloride. *CAS-119413-53-5; CAS-117523-47-4* [mirfentanil]. *Analgesic.* ◇*A-3508.HCl*

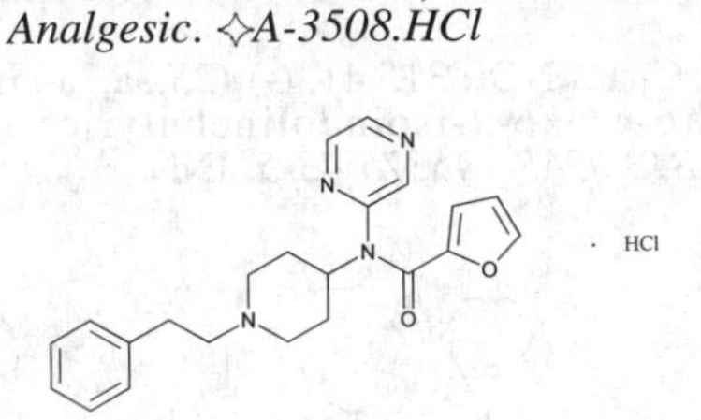

Mirimostim. $C_{1058}H_{1651}N_{277}O_{341}S_{14}$ (for non-glycosylated protein). 24,156.02. 1-214-Colony-stimulating factor 1 (human clone p3ACSF-69 protein moiety reduced), homodimer. *CAS-121547-04-4*. INN; JAN.

Mirincamycin Hydrochloride [*1974*] (mir in″ ka mye′ sin hye″ droe klor′ ide). $C_{19}H_{35}ClN_2O_5S$.HCl. 475.47. [Mirincamycin is INN.] (1) L-*threo*-α-D-*galacto*-Octopyranoside, methyl 7-chloro-6,7,8-trideoxy-6-[[(4-pentyl-2-pyrrolidinyl)carbonyl]amino]-1-thio-, monohydrochloride, (2*S-cis*)-mixture with methyl 7-chloro-6,7,8-trideoxy-6-[[(*trans*-4-pentyl-2(*S*)-pyrrolidinyl)carbonyl]amino]-1-thio-L-*threo*-α-D-*galacto*-octopyranoside monohydrochloride; (2) Methyl 7-chloro-6,7,8-trideoxy-6-(*cis*-4-pentyl-L-2-pyrrolidinecarboxamido)-1-thio-L-*threo*-α-D-*galacto*-octopyranoside monohydrochloride mixture with methyl 7-chloro-6,7,8-trideoxy-6-(*trans*-4-pentyl-L-2-pyrrolidinecarboxamido)-1-thio-L-*threo*-α-D-*galacto*-octopyranoside monohydrochloride. *CAS-8063-91-0; CAS-37217-18-8* [replaced]; *CAS-31101-25-4* [mirincamycin]. *Antibacterial; antimalarial.* ◇*U-24,729A*

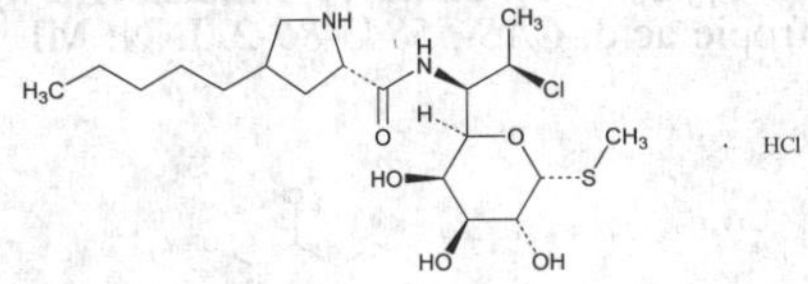

Miripirium Chloride. $C_{20}H_{36}ClN$. 325.96. 1-Tetradecyl-4-picolinium chloride. *CAS-2748-88-1*. INN.

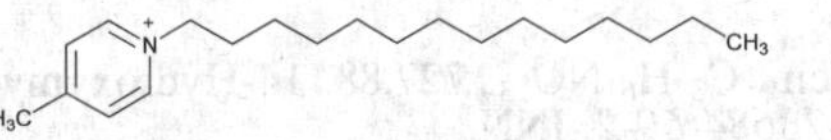

Miriplatin. $C_{34}H_{68}N_2O_4Pt$. 764.00. (*SP*-4-2)-[(1*R*,2*R*)-Cyclohexane-1,2-diamine-*N*,*N*′]bis(tetradecanoato-*O*)platinum. *CAS-141977-79-9*. INN.

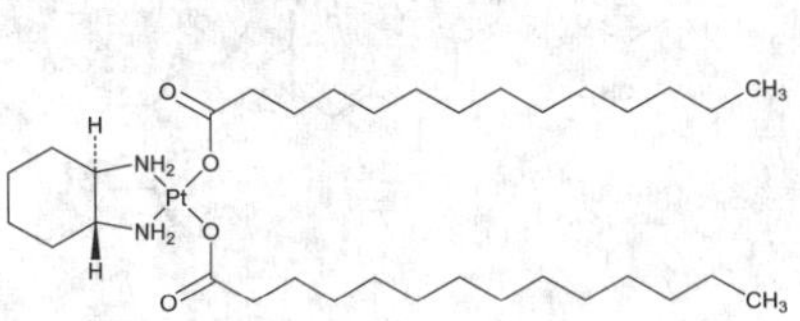

Mirisetron Maleate [*1994*] (mir eye′ se tron mal′ ee ate). $C_{24}H_{31}N_3O_2.C_4H_4O_4$. 509.59. [Mirisetron is INN.] (1) 3-Quinolinecarboxamide, 1-cyclohexyl-1,4-dihydro-*N*-(8-methyl-8-azabicyclo[3.2.1]oct-3-yl)-4-oxo-, *endo*-, (*Z*)-2-butenedioate (1:1); (2) 1-Cyclohexyl-1,4-dihydro-4-oxo-*N*-1αH,5αH-tropan-3α-yl-3-quinolinecarboxamide maleate (1:1). *CAS-148611-75-0; CAS-135905-89-4* [mirisetron]. *Anti-anxiety agent.* ◇*WAY-SEC-579*

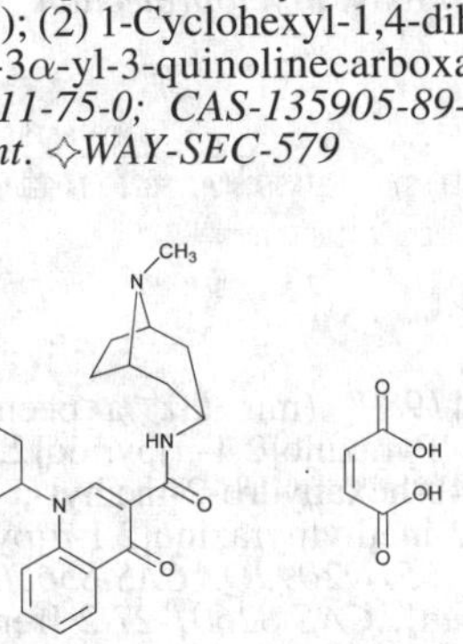

Miristalkonium Chloride. $C_{23}H_{42}ClN$. 368.04. Benzyldimethyltetradecylammonium chloride. *CAS-139-08-2*. INN; BAN.

---

† Brand name formerly used, and/or firm no longer concerned with this product.

Miroc60ept. $C_{1054}H_{1635}N_{293}O_{312}S_{16}$. (1) Myristoylated-peptidyl recombinant SCR1-3 of human complement receptor type 1; (2) Protein APT070 (synthetic human clone pET04-01 complement receptor type 1 short consensus repeat 1-3 fragment), (198→17′)-disulfide with *N*-(tetradecanoyl)glycyl-L-seryl-L-seryl-L-lysyl-L-seryl-L-prolyl-L-seryl-L-lysyl-L-lysyl-L-lysyl-L-lysyl-L-lysyl-L-lysyl-L-prolylglycyl-L-aspartyl-L-cysteinamide. *CAS-507453-82-9.* BAN; INN. ◇*APT 070*

Mirodenafil. $C_{26}H_{37}N_5O_5S$. 531.67. 5-Ethyl-2-(5-{[4-(2-hydroxyethyl)piperazin-1-yl]sulfonyl}-2-propoxyphenyl)-7-propyl-3,5-dihydro-4*H*-pyrrolo[3,2-*d*]pyrimidin-4-one. *CAS-862189-95-5.* INN.

Miroprofen. $C_{16}H_{14}N_2O_2$. 266.29. *p*-Imidazo[1,2-*a*]pyridin-2-ylhydratropic acid. *CAS-55843-86-2.* INN; MI.

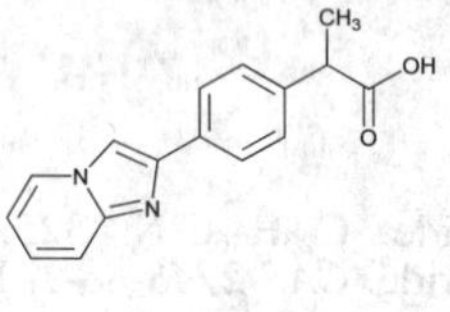

Mirosamicin. $C_{37}H_{61}NO_{13}$. 727.88. 14-Hydroxymycinamicin I. *CAS-73684-69-2.* INN.

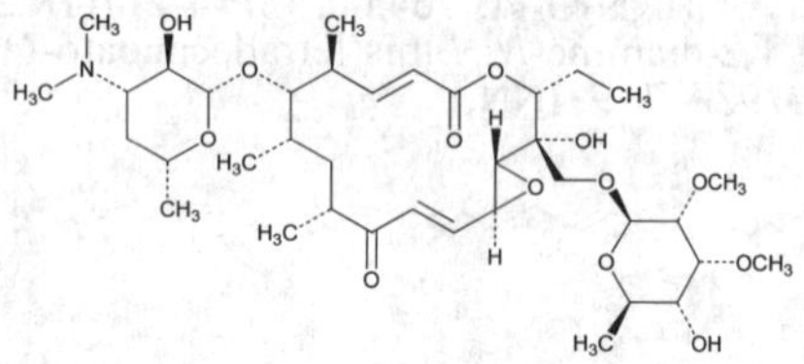

Mirostipen [*2000*] (mir oh stye′ pen). $C_{380}H_{612}N_{112}O_{112}S_9$. 8830.19 daltons. (1) 23-99-Myeloid progenitor inhibitory factor 1 [23-methionine] (human); (2) 23-L-Methionine-23-99-myeloid progenitor inhibitory factor 1 (human). *CAS-244130-01-6.* INN. *Myeloprotection.*

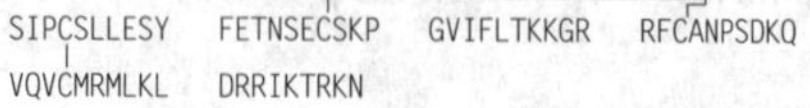

```
                            MDRFHATS  ADCCISYTPR
       SIPCSLLESY  FETNSECSKP  GVIFLTKKGR  RFCANPSDKQ
       VQVCMRMLKL  DRRIKTRKN
```

Mirtazapine [*1989*] (mir taz′ a peen). **USP.** $C_{17}H_{19}N_3$. 265.35. (1) Pyrazino[2,1-*a*]pyrido[2,3-*c*][2]benzazepine, 1,2,3,4,10,14b-hexahydro-2-methyl-; (2) 1,2,3,4,10,14b-Hexahydro-2-methylpyrazino[2,1-*a*]pyrido[2,3-*c*]benzazepine. *UNII-A051Q2099Q. CAS-85650-52-8; CAS-61337-67-5* [replaced]; *CAS-82601-27-2* [replaced]. INN; BAN. *Antidepressant.* Remeron (Organon) ◇*ORG 3770*

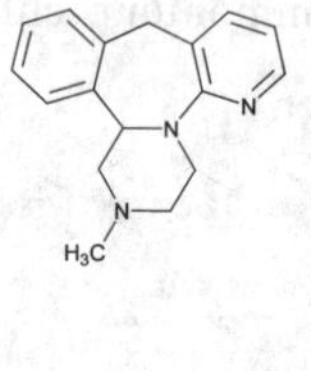

Misonidazole [*1978*] (mye″ soe nye′ da zole). $C_7H_{11}N_3O_4$. 201.18. (1) 1*H*-Imidazole-1-ethanol, α-(methoxymethyl)-2-nitro-; (2) α-(Methoxymethyl)-2-nitroimidazole-1-ethanol. *CAS-13551-87-6.* INN; BAN. *Antiprotozoal (Trichomonas).* ◇*Ro 7-0582*

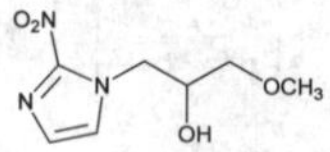

Misoprostol [*1981*] (mye″ soe prost′ ol). $C_{22}H_{38}O_5$. 382.53. (1) Prost-13-en-1-oic acid, 11,16-dihydroxy-16-methyl-9-oxo-, methyl ester, (11α,13*E*)-(±)-; (2) (±)-Methyl (1*R*,2*R*,3*R*)-3-hydroxy-2-[(*E*)-(4*RS*)-4-hydroxy-4-methyl-1-octenyl]-5-oxocyclopentaneheptanoate. *UNII-0E43V0BB57. CAS-59122-46-2.* INN; BAN; JAN. *Antiulcerative.* Cytotec (Pfizer) ◇*SC-29333*

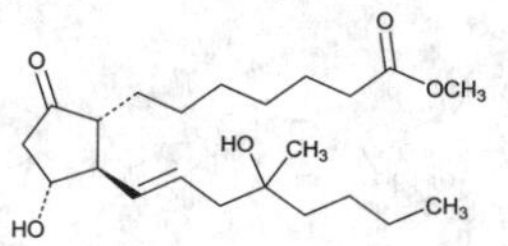

Mitemcinal Fumarate [*2002*] (mye tem′ sin al fue′ ma rate). $C_{40}H_{69}NO_{12}\cdot\frac{1}{2}(C_4H_4O_4)$. 814.01. [Mitemcinal is INN.] (1) Erythromycin, 8,9-didehydro-*N*-demethyl-9-deoxo-6,11-dideoxy-6,9-epoxy-12-*O*-methyl *N*-(1-methylethyl)-11-oxo-, (2*E*)-2-butenedioate (2:1); (2) 8,9-Didehydro-*N*-demethyl-9-deoxo-6,11-dideoxy-6,9-epoxy-*N*-isopropyl-12-*O*-methyl-11-oxoerythromycin fumarate (2:1) (salt). *CAS-154802-96-7; CAS-154738-42-8* [mitemcinal]. *Treatment of gastroparesis; gastroesophageal reflux disease (motilin receptor agonist).* ◇*GM-611; 5-1 Ukima 5 Chome; Kita-ku Toyko; 115-8543 Japan*

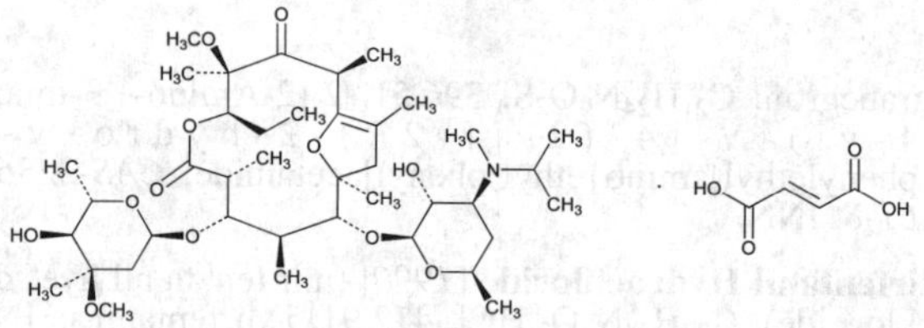

Mithramycin (previously used name) — *See* Plicamycin.

Mitiglinide. $C_{19}H_{25}NO_3$. 315.41. (-)-(2*S*,3a,7a-*cis*)-α-Benzylhexahydro-γ-oxo-2-isoindolinebutyric acid. *UNII-D86I0XLB13. CAS-145375-43-5.* INN.

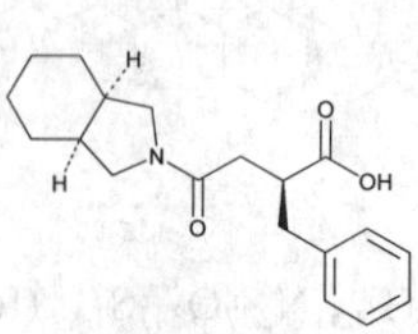

Mitindomide [*1983*] (mye tin′ doe mide). $C_{14}H_{12}N_2O_4$. 272.26. (1) 4,8-Ethenopyrrolo[3′,4′:3,4]cyclobut[1,2-*f*]isoindole-1,3,5,7(2*H*,6*H*)-tetrone, 3a,3b,4,4a,7a,8,8a,8b-octahydro-, (3aα,3bβ,4α,4aβ,7aβ,8α,8aβ,8bα)-; (2) (1*R**,2*S**,3*R**,4*S**,5*R**,6*S**,7*S**,8*R**)-Tricyclo[4.2.2.0^{2,5}]-

dec-9-ene-3,4,7,8-tetracarboxylic 3,4:7,8-diimide. *UNII-DK61ZER6T7. CAS-10403-51-7.* INN. *Antineoplastic.* ◇*NSC-284356*

Mitobronitol. $C_6H_{12}Br_2O_4$. 307.97. 1,6-Dibromo-1,6-dideoxy-D-mannitol. *CAS-488-41-5.* INN; BAN; JAN; DCF; MI. ◇*DBM*

Mitocarcin [*1970*] (mye″ toe kar′ sin). Antibiotic derived from *Streptomyces* species. (1) Mitocarcin; (2) Mitocarcin. *CAS-11056-14-7.* INN. *Antineoplastic.* ◇*24281*

Mitoclomine. $C_{16}H_{19}Cl_2NO$. 312.23. *N,N*-Bis(2-chloroethyl)-4-methoxy-3-methyl-1-naphthylamine. *UNII-02DQX562CR. CAS-17692-54-5.* INN; BAN.

Mitocromin [*1967*] (mye″ toe kroe′ min). Antibiotic produced by *Streptomyces viridochromogenes.* (1) Mitocromin; (2) Mitocromin. *CAS-11043-98-4. Antineoplastic.* ◇*B-35251; NSC-77471*

Mitoflaxone. $C_{17}H_{12}O_4$. 280.27. 4-Oxo-2-phenyl-4*H*-1-benzopyran-8-acetic acid. *CAS-87626-55-9.* INN.

Mitogillin [*1966*] (mye″ toe jil′ in). Antibiotic produced by *Aspergillus restrictus.* (1) Mitogillin; (2) Mitogillin. *CAS-1403-99-2.* INN. *Antineoplastic.* ◇*NSC-69529*

Mitoguazone. $C_5H_{12}N_8$. 184.20. 1,1′-[(Methylethanediylidene)dinitrilo]diguanidine. *CAS-459-86-9.* INN; DCF; MI.

Mitolactol. $C_6H_{12}Br_2O_4$. 307.97. 1,6-Dibromo-1,6-dideoxy-D-galactitol. *CAS-10318-26-0.* INN; MI.

Mitomalcin [*1967*] (mye″ toe mal′ sin). Antibiotic produced by *Streptomyces malayensis.* (1) Mitomalcin; (2) Mitomalcin. *CAS-11043-99-5.* INN. *Antineoplastic.* ◇*NSC-113233*

Mitomycin [*1972*] (mye″ toe mye′ sin). USP. $C_{15}H_{18}N_4O_5$. 334.33. [Mitomycin C is JAN.] (1) Azirino[2′,3′:3,4]pyrrolo[1,2-*a*]indole-4,7-dione, 6-amino-8-[[(aminocarbonyl)oxy]methyl]-1,1a,2,8,8a,8b-hexahydro-8a-methoxy-5-methyl-, [1a*S*-(1aα,8β,8aα,8bα)]-; (2) 6-Amino-1,1a,2,8,8a,8b-hexahydro-8-(hydroxymethyl)-8a-methoxy-5-methylazirino[2′,3′:3,4]pyrrolo[1,2-*a*]indole-4,7-dione carbamate (ester); (3) Mitomycin C. *UNII-50SG953SK6. CAS-50-07-7.* INN; BAN. *Antineoplastic.* Mutamycin (Bristol-Myers Squibb); Mytozytrex (SuperGen) ◇*NSC-26980*

Mitomycin C (JAN) — *See* Mitomycin.

Mitonafide. $C_{16}H_{15}N_3O_4$. 313.31. *N*-[2-(Dimethylamino)ethyl]-3-nitronaphthalimide. *UNII-06Q0V17SI9. CAS-54824-17-8.* INN.

Mitopodozide. $C_{24}H_{30}N_2O_8$. 474.50. Podophyllic acid 2-ethylhydrazide. *CAS-1508-45-8.* INN; BAN. ◇*SPI-77; NSC-72274*

Mitoquidone. $C_{20}H_{13}NO_2$. 299.32. 5,14-Dihydrobenz[5,6]isoindolo[2,1-*b*]isoquinoline-8,13-dione. *UNII-OWD9-JI448N. CAS-91753-07-0.* INN; BAN. ◇*GR 30921*

Mitosper [*1970*] (mye′ toe sper). Substance derived from *Aspergillus* of the *glaucus* group. (1) Mitosper; (2) Mitosper. *CAS-11056-15-8.* INN. *Antineoplastic.* ◇*31595C; NSC-117032*

---

† Brand name formerly used, and/or firm no longer concerned with this product.

Mitotane [*1968*] (mye′ toe tane). **USP**. $C_{14}H_{10}Cl_4$. 320.04. (1) Benzene, 1-chloro-2-[2,2-dichloro-1-(4-chlorophenyl)ethyl]-, (±)-; (2) (±)-1,1-Dichloro-2-(*o*-chlorophenyl)-2-(*p*-chlorophenyl)ethane. *UNII-78E4J5IB5J. CAS-53-19-0.* INN; JAN. *Antineoplastic.* Lysodren (Bristol-Myers Squibb) *[Name previously used: o,p′-DDD.]* ◇*CB 313; NSC-38721*

Mitotenamine. $C_{13}H_{15}BrClNS$. 332.69. 5-Bromo-*N*-(2-chloroethyl)-*N*-ethylbenzo[*b*]thiophene-3-methylamine. *UNII-2879S26V4P. CAS-7696-00-6.* INN; BAN.

Mitoxantrone Hydrochloride [*1980*] (mye tox′ an trone hye″ droe klor′ ide). **USP**. $C_{22}H_{28}N_4O_6$·2HCl. 517.40. [Mitoxantrone is INN and BAN.] (1) 9,10-Anthracenedione, 1,4-dihydroxy-5,8-bis[[2-[(2-hydroxyethyl)amino]ethyl]amino]-, dihydrochloride; (2) 1,4-Dihydroxy-5,8-bis[[2-[(2-hydroxyethyl)amino]ethyl]amino]anthraquinone dihydrochloride. *UNII-U6USW86RD0; UNII-BZ114NVM5P* [mitoxantrone]. *CAS-70476-82-3; CAS-65271-80-9* [mitoxantrone]. JAN. *Antineoplastic.* Novantrone (Serono) ◇*CL 232,315*

Mitozantrone (former BAN) — *See* Mitoxantrone Hydrochloride.

Mitozolomide. $C_7H_7ClN_6O_2$. 242.62. 3-(2-Chloroethyl)-3,4-dihydro-4-oxoimidazo[5,1-*d*]-*as*-tetrazine-8-carboxamide. *UNII-E3U7286V3W. CAS-85622-95-3.* INN; BAN.

Mitratapide [*2005*] (mye trat′ a pide). $C_{36}H_{41}ClN_8O_4S$. 717.28. (1) 3*H*-1,2,4-Triazol-3-one, 4-[4-[4-[4-[[(2*S*,4*R*)-2-(4-chlorophenyl)-2-[[(4-methyl-4*H*-1,2,4-triazol-3-yl)thio]methyl]-1,3-dioxolan-4-yl]methoxy]phenyl]-1-piperazinyl]phenyl]-2,4-dihydro-2-[(1*R*)-1-methylpropyl]-; (2) (-)-4-[4-[4-[4-[[(2*S*,4*R*)-2-(4-Chlorophenyl)-2-[[(4-methyl-4*H*-1,2,4-triazol-3-yl)sulfanyl]methyl]-1,3-dioxolan-4-yl]methoxy]phenyl]piperazin-1-yl]phenyl]-2-(1*R*)-1-methylpropyl]-2,4-dihydro-3*H*-1,2,4-triazol-3-one. *UNII-FVW7T75XP4. CAS-179602-65-4.* INN. *Management of obesity in dogs.* ◇*R103757*

Mitumomab [*1999*] (mye toom′ oh mab). (1) Immunoglobulin G2b, anti-(GD3 ganglioside) (mouse monoclonal γ2b-chain), disulfide with mouse monoclonal κ-chain, dimer; (2) Immunoglobulin G2b (mouse monoclonal BEC2 γ2b-chain anti-GD3 ganglioside), disulfide with mouse monoclonal BEC2 κ-chain, dimer. Molecular weight is approximately 170,000 daltons. *CAS-216503-58-1.* INN. *Antitumor monoclonal antibody (tumor cell expressing GD3 ganglioside).* ◇*BEC2*

Mitumprotimut-T [*2007*] (mye″ tum proe′ ti mut). Anti-lymphoma vaccine produced by conjugating recombinant patient-specific idiotype proteins to the immunostimulatory protein KLH (Keyhole Limpet Hemocyanin). Molecular weight is approximately 150,000 daltons. *Treatment of follicular B cell non-Hodgkins lymphoma.* Favid (Favrille) ◇*Id/KLH*

Mivacurium Chloride [*1990*] (mye″ va kue′ ree um klor′ ide; mye″ va kure′ ee um klor′ ide). $C_{58}H_{80}Cl_2N_2O_{14}$. 1100.17. (1) Isoquinolinium, 2,2′-[(1,8-dioxo-4-octene-1,8-diyl)bis(oxy-3,1-propanediyl)]bis[1,2,3,4-tetrahydro-6,7-dimethoxy-2-methyl-1-[(3,4,5-trimethoxyphenyl)methyl]-, dichloride, [*R*-[*R**,*R**-(*E*)]]-; (2) (*R*)-1,2,3,4-Tetrahydro-2-(3-hydroxypropyl)-6,7-dimethoxy-2-methyl-1-(3,4,5-trimethoxybenzyl)isoquinolinium chloride, (*E*)-4-octenedioate (2:1). *UNII-600ZG213C3. CAS-106861-44-3.* INN; BAN. *Neuromuscular blocking agent.* Mivacron (Abbott) ◇*BW B1090U dichloride*

Mivazerol. $C_{11}H_{11}N_3O_2$. 217.22. α-Imidazol-4-yl-2,3-cresotamide. *UNII-W5P1SSA8KD. CAS-125472-02-8.* INN.

Mivobulin Isethionate [*1997*] (mye″ voe bue′ lin). $C_{17}H_{19}N_5O_2 \cdot C_2H_6O_4S$. 451.50. [Mivobulin is INN.] (1) Carbamic acid, (5-amino-1,2-dihydro-2-methyl-3-phenylpyrido[3,4-*b*]pyrazin-7-yl) ethyl ester, (*S*)-, mono(2-hydroxyethanesulfonate); (2) Ethyl (*S*)-5-amino-1,2-dihydro-2-methyl-3-phenylpyrido[3,4-*b*]pyrazine-7-carbamate, mono(2-hydroxyethanesulfonate). *CAS-126268-81-3; CAS-122332-18-7* [mivobulin]. *Antineoplastic (microtubule inhibitor).* ◇*CI-980*

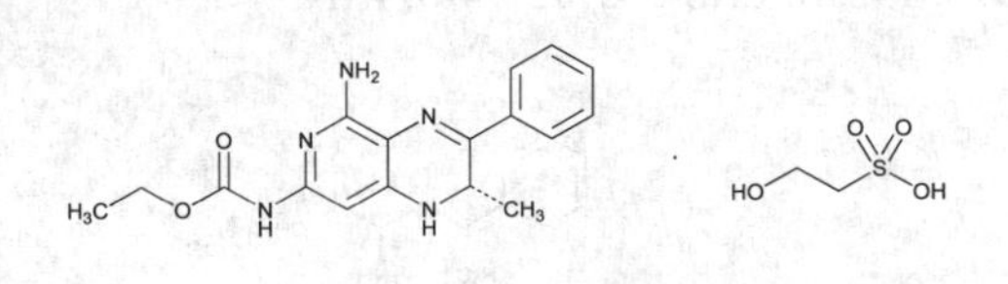

Mivotilate. $C_{12}H_{14}N_2O_3S_3$. 330.45. Isopropyl *N*-(4-methyl-2-thiazolyl)-1,3-dithietane-Δ^2,L-malonamate. *UNII-0789652QUL. CAS-130112-42-4.* INN.

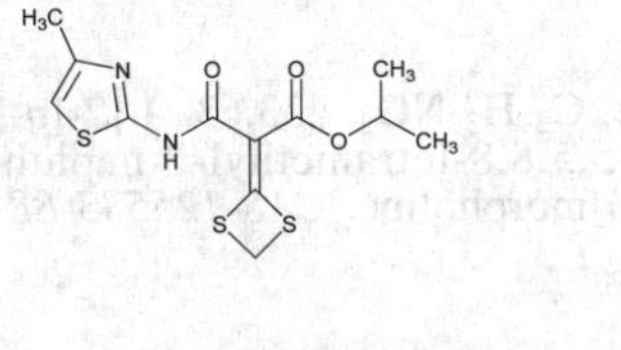

Mixidine [*1974*] (mix′ i deen). $C_{15}H_{22}N_2O_2$. 262.35. (1) Benzeneethanamine, 3,4-dimethoxy-*N*-(1-methyl-2-pyrrolidinylidene)-; (2) 2-[(3,4-Dimethoxyphenethyl)imino]-1-methylpyrrolidine. *CAS-27737-38-8; CAS-42540-38-5* [replaced]. INN. *Vasodilator (coronary).* ◇*McN-1589*

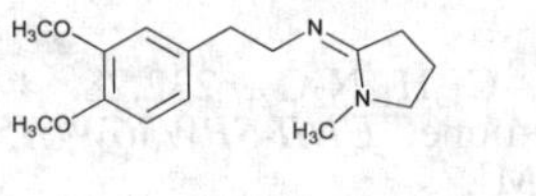

Mizolastine. $C_{24}H_{25}FN_6O$. 432.49. 2-[[1-[1-(*p*-Fluorobenzyl)-2-benzimidazolyl]-4-piperidyl]methylamino]-4(3*H*)-pyrimidinone. *UNII-244O1F90NA. CAS-108612-45-9.* INN; BAN.

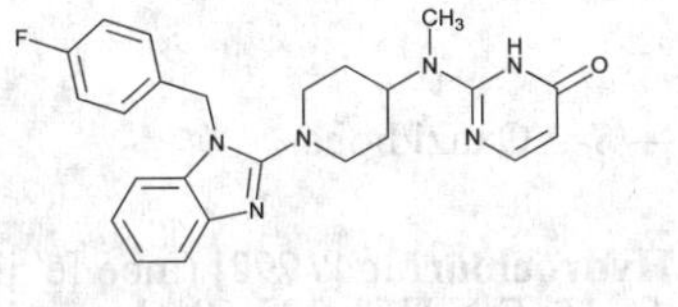

Mizoribine. $C_9H_{13}N_3O_6$. 259.22. 5-Hydroxy-1-β-D-ribofuranosylimidazole-4-carboxamide. *UNII-4JR41A10VP. CAS-50924-49-7.* INN; JAN; MI.

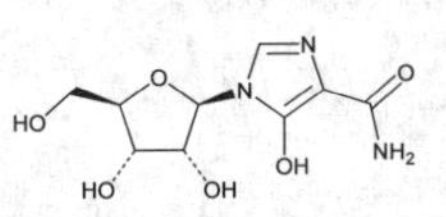

Mobecarb. $C_{14}H_{17}NO_4$. 263.29. Phenacyl 4-morpholineacetate. *UNII-46LG9K0Y24. CAS-15518-84-0.* INN.

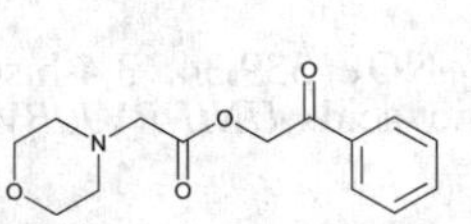

Mobenakin. $C_{773}H_{1219}N_{201}O_{238}S_7$. 17,360.62. 71-L-Serineinterleukin 1β (human clone pIL-1-14 reduced). *CAS-124146-64-1.* INN.

Mobenzoxamine. $C_{30}H_{35}FN_2O_3$. 490.61. 4′-Fluoro-4-[4-[2-[(*p*-methoxy-α-phenylbenzyl)oxy]ethyl]-1-piperazinyl]butyrophenone. *CAS-65329-79-5.* INN.

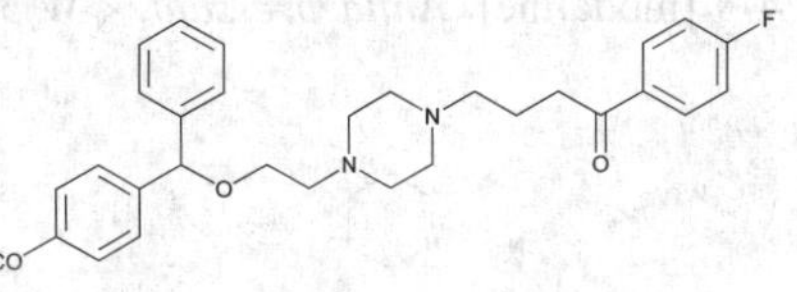

Mocetinostat Dihydrobromide [*2008*] (moe″ se tin′ oh stat dye hye″ droe broe′ mide). $C_{23}H_{20}N_6O.2HBr$. 558.27. (1) Benzamide, *N*-(2-aminophenyl)-4-[[[4-(3-pyridinyl)-2-pyrimidinyl]amino]methyl]-, hydrobromide (1:2); (2) *N*-(2-Aminophenyl)-4-({[4-(pyridin-3-yl)pyrimidin-2-yl]amino}methyl)benzamide dihydrobromide. *UNII-4V9P667Y2G. CAS-944537-89-7. Antineoplastic.*

Mocimycin. Antibiotic obtained from cultures of *Streptomyces ramocissimus* or the same substance obtained by any other means. *CAS-52212-85-8; CAS-50935-71-2* [trivial name]. INN; MI. ◇*MYC 8003*

Mociprazine. $C_{22}H_{32}N_2O_3$. 372.50. α-[[(1-Ethynylcyclohexyl)oxy]methyl]-4-(*o*-methoxyphenyl)-1-piperazineethanol. *CAS-56693-13-1.* INN.

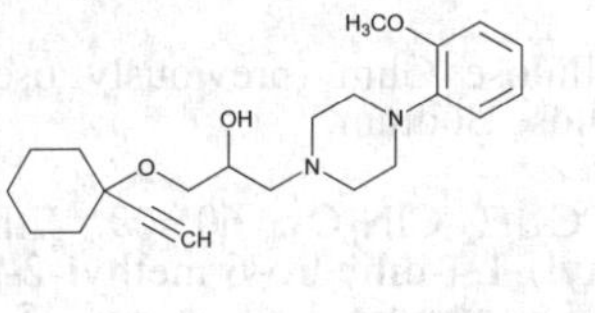

Moclobemide [*1987*] (moe kloe′ be mide). $C_{13}H_{17}ClN_2O_2$. 268.74. (1) Benzamide, 4-chloro-*N*-[2-(4-morpholinyl)ethyl]-; (2) *p*-Chloro-*N*-(2-morpholinoethyl)benzamide. *CAS-71320-77-9.* INN; BAN. *Antidepressant.* ◇*Ro 11-1163/000*

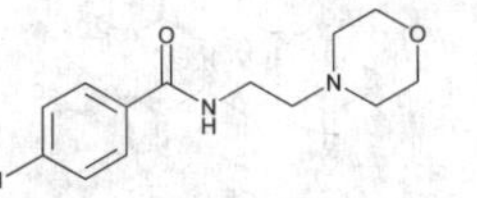

Moctamide. $C_{33}H_{47}NO$. 473.73. (-)-*N*-(*p*-Methyl-α-phenylphenethyl)linoleamide. *UNII-TN4C52M5ZT. CAS-29619-86-1.* INN.

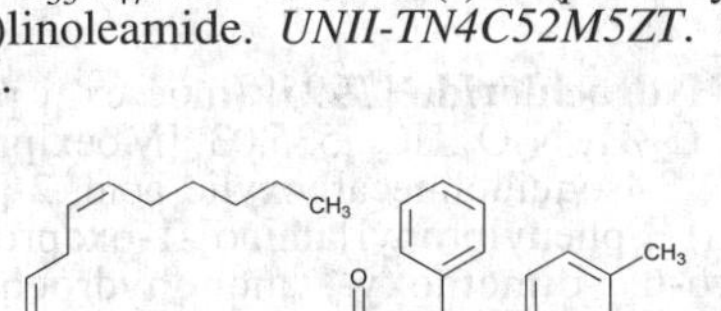

Modafinil [*1994*] (moe daf′ i nil). **USP.** $C_{15}H_{15}NO_2S$. 273.35. (1) Acetamide, 2-[(diphenylmethyl)sulfinyl]-; (2) 2-[(Diphenylmethyl)sulfinyl]acetamide. *UNII-R3UK8X3U3D. CAS-68693-11-8.* INN; BAN. *Analeptic (treatment of narcolepsy and hypersomnia).* Provigil (Cephalon) ◇*CRL 40476; CEP 1538*

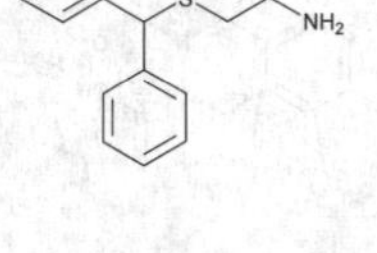

---

† Brand name formerly used, and/or firm no longer concerned with this product.

Modaline Sulfate [*1965*] (moe′ da leen sul′ fate). $C_{10}H_{15}N_3 \cdot H_2SO_4$. 275.32. [Modaline is INN.] (1) Pyrazine, 2-methyl-3-(1-piperidinyl)-, sulfate (1:1); (2) 2-Methyl-3-piperidinopyrazine sulfate (1:1). *CAS-2856-75-9; CAS-2856-74-8* [modaline]. *Antidepressant.* ◇*W 3207B; NSC-89277*

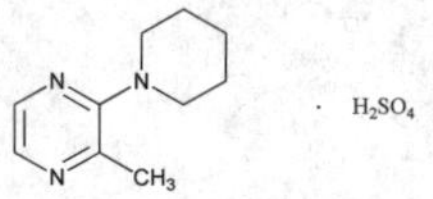

Modecainide [*1990*] (moe dek′ a nide). $C_{22}H_{28}N_2O_3$. 368.47. (1) Benzamide, 4-hydroxy-3-methoxy-*N*-[2-[2-(1-methyl-2-piperidinyl)ethyl]phenyl]-, (±)-; (2) (±)-2′-[2-(1-Methyl-2-piperidyl)ethyl]vanillanilide. *CAS-82522-70-1.* INN. *Cardiac depressant (anti-arrhythmic).* ◇*BMY-40327*

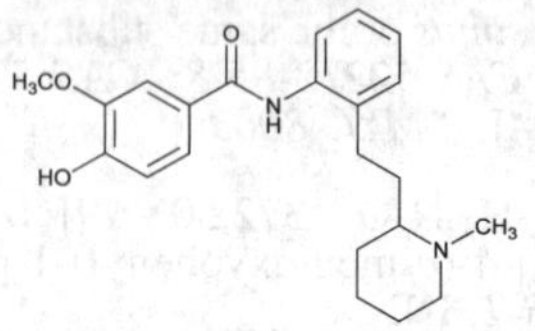

Modified Cellulose Gum (previously used name) — *See* Croscarmellose Sodium.

Modipafant. $C_{34}H_{29}ClN_6O_3$. 605.09. Ethyl (+)-(*R*)-4-(*o*-chlorophenyl)-1,4-dihydro-6-methyl-2-[*p*-(2-methyl-1*H*-imidazo[4,5-*c*]pyridin-1-yl)phenyl]-5-(2-pyridylcarbamoyl)nicotinate. *CAS-122957-06-6; CAS-122956-68-7* [racemate]. INN; BAN. ◇*UK-80067*

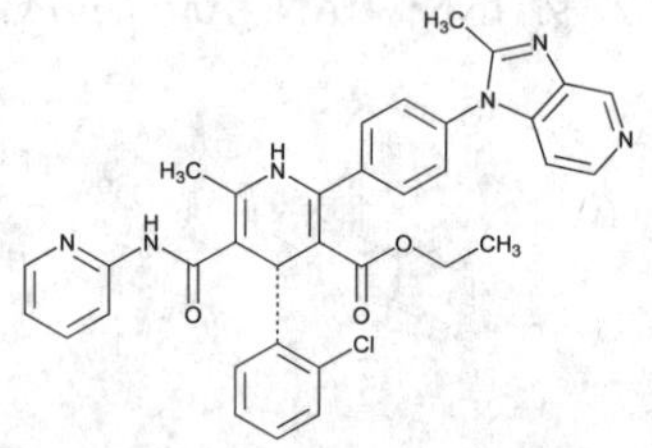

Moexipril Hydrochloride [*1995*] (moe ex′ i pril hye″ droe klor′ ide). $C_{27}H_{34}N_2O_7 \cdot HCl$. 535.03. [Moexipril is INN and BAN.] (1) 3-Isoquinolinecarboxylic acid, 2-[2-[[1-(ethoxycarbonyl)-3-phenylpropyl]amino]-1-oxopropyl]-1,2,3,4-tetrahydro-6,7-dimethoxy-, monohydrochloride, [3*S*-[2[*R**(*R**)],3*R**]]-; (2) (3*S*)-2-[(2*S*)-*N*-[(1*S*)-1-Carboxy-3-phenylpropyl]alanyl]-1,2,3,4-tetrahydro-6,7-dimethoxy-3-isoquinolinecarboxylic acid, 2-ethyl ester, monohydrochloride. *UNII-Q1UMG3UH45. CAS-82586-52-5; CAS-103775-10-6* [moexipril]. *Antihypertensive; enzyme inhibitor (angiotensin-converting).* Univasc (Schwarz Pharma) ◇*SPM 925; CI 925; RS-10085-197*

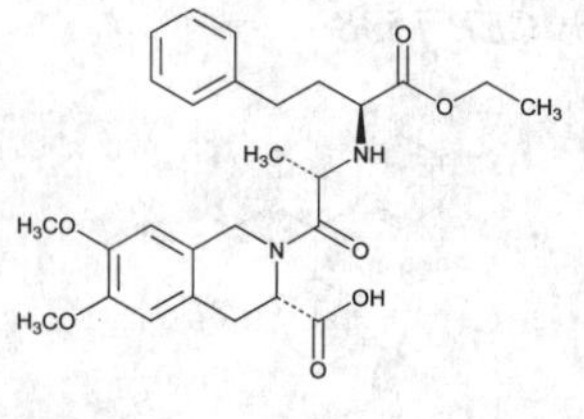

Moexiprilat. $C_{25}H_{30}N_2O_7$. 470.51. (3*S*)-2-[(2*S*)-*N*-[(1*S*)-1-Carboxy-3-phenylpropyl]alanyl]-1,2,3,4-tetrahydro-6,7-dimethoxy-3-isoquinolinecarboxylic acid. *UNII-H3753190JS. CAS-103775-14-0.* INN.

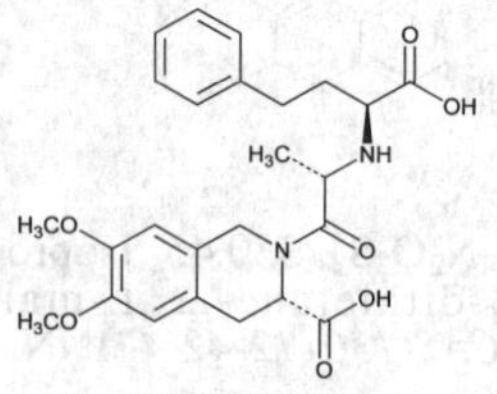

Mofarotene. $C_{29}H_{39}NO_2$. 433.63. 4-[2-[*p*-[(*E*)-2-(5,6,7,8-Tetrahydro-5,5,8,8-tetramethyl-2-naphthyl)propenyl]phenoxy]ethyl]morpholine. *CAS-125533-88-2.* INN.

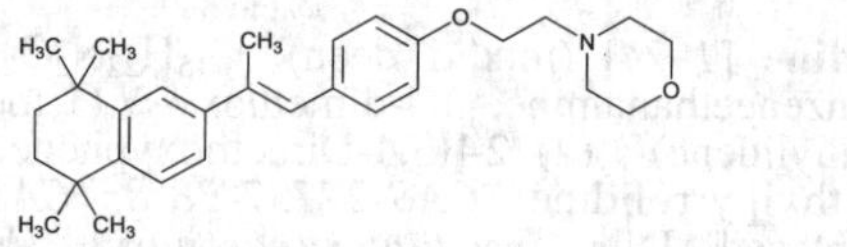

Mofebutazone. $C_{13}H_{16}N_2O_2$. 232.28. 4-Butyl-1-phenyl-3,5-pyrazolidinedione. *UNII-SPW36WUI5Z. CAS-2210-63-1.* INN; DCF; MI.

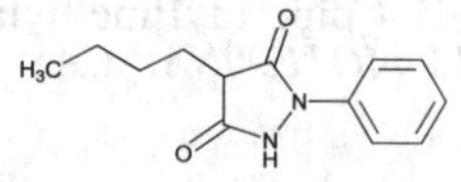

Mofedione — *See* Oxazidione.

Mofegiline Hydrochloride [*1992*] (moe fe′ ji leen hye″ droe klor′ ide). $C_{11}H_{13}F_2N \cdot HCl$. 233.69. [Mofegiline is INN.] (1) Benzenebutanamine, 4-fluoro-β-(fluoromethylene)-, hydrochloride, (*E*)-; (2) (*E*)-2-(Fluoromethylene)-4-(*p*-fluorophenyl)butylamine hydrochloride. *UNII-08331R10RY. CAS-120635-25-8; CAS-119386-96-8* [free base]. *Antiparkinsonian.* ◇*MDL 72,974A*

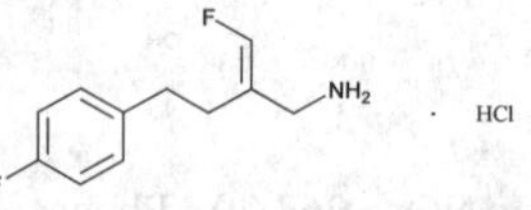

Mofezolac. $C_{19}H_{17}NO_5$. 339.34. 3,4-bis(*p*-Methoxyphenyl)-5-isoxazoleacetic acid. *UNII-RVJ0BV3H3Y. CAS-78967-07-4.* INN.

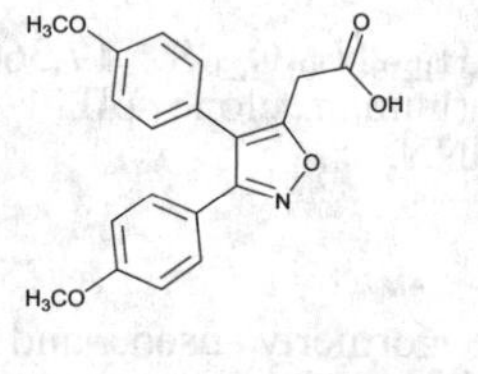

Mofloverine. $C_{16}H_{23}NO_6$. 325.36. 2,4,6-Trimethoxybenzoic acid, 2-morpholinoethyl ester. *UNII-L1G37N4EBS. CAS-54063-50-2.* INN; DCF.

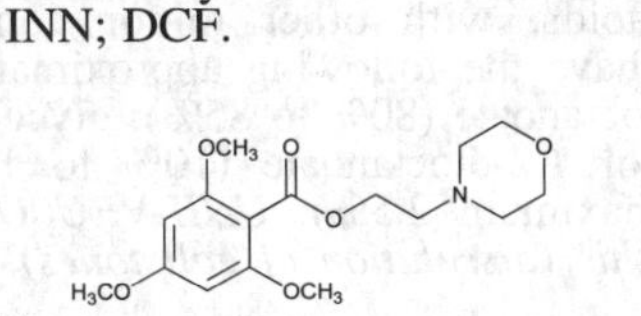

Mofoxime. $C_{14}H_{18}N_2O_4$. 278.30. 4-[(*p*-Acetylphenoxy)acetyl]morpholine *p*-oxime. *UNII-Q7FNA7HXLF. CAS-29936-79-6.* INN.

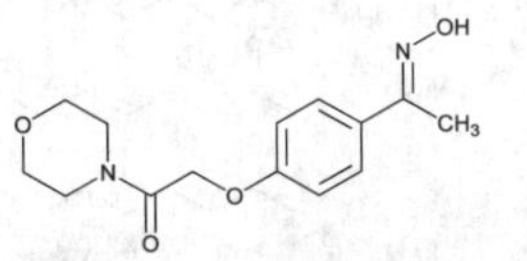

Moguisteine. $C_{16}H_{21}NO_5S$. 339.41. Ethyl (±)-2-[(*o*-methoxyphenoxy)methyl]-β-oxo-3-thiazolidinepropionate. *UNII-6Y556547YY. CAS-119637-67-1.* INN.

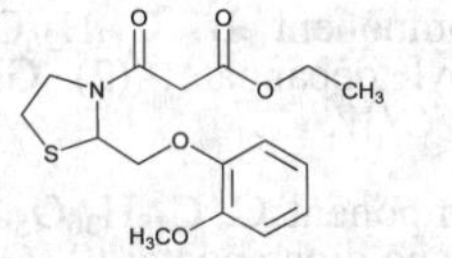

Molfarnate. $C_{31}H_{50}O_2$. 454.73. 3,7,11-Trimethyl-2,6,10-dodecatrienyl 4,8,12-trimethyl-3,7,11-tridecatrienoate. *UNII-5288I2K01S. CAS-83689-23-0.* INN.

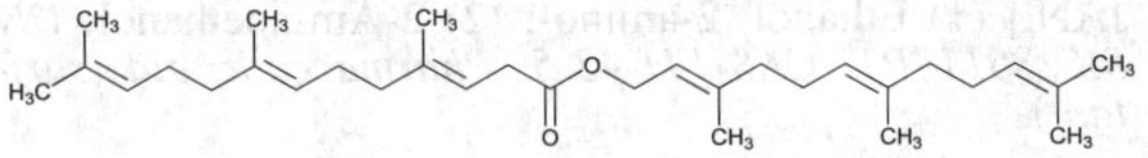

Molgramostim [*1992*] (mol gra′ moe stim). $C_{639}H_{1007}N_{171}O_{196}S_8$ (protein moiety). 14,477 daltons. (1) Colony-stimulating factor 2 (human clone pHG$_{25}$ protein moiety reduced); (2) Colony-stimulating factor 2 (human clone pHG$_{25}$ protein moiety reduced). *UNII-B321AL142J. CAS-99283-10-0.* INN; BAN. *Antineutropenic; hematopoietic stimulant.* ◇*Sch 39300*

```
APARSPSPST QPWEHVNAIQ EARRLLNLSR DTAAEMNGTV EVISEMFDLQ
EPTCLQTRLE LYKQGLRGSL TKLKGPLTMM ASHYKQHCPP TPETSCATQI
ITFESFKENL KDFLLVIPFN CWEPVQE
```

Molinazone [*1962*] (moe lin′ a zone). $C_{11}H_{12}N_4O_2$. 232.24. (1) 1,2,3-Benzotriazin-4(3*H*)-one, 3-(4-morpholinyl)-; (2) 3-Morpholino-1,2,3-benzotriazin-4(3*H*)-one. *UNII-NHQ2X2AKZO. CAS-5581-46-4.* INN. *Analgesic.*

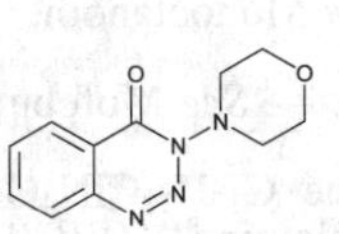

Molindone Hydrochloride [*1967*] (moe lin′ done hye″ droe klor′ ide). **USP.** $C_{16}H_{24}N_2O_2 \cdot HCl$. 312.83. [Molindone is INN and BAN.] (1) 4*H*-Indol-4-one, 3-ethyl-1,5,6,7-

tetrahydro-2-methyl-5-(4-morpholinylmethyl)-, monohydrochloride; (2) 3-Ethyl-6,7-dihydro-2-methyl-5-(morpholinomethyl)indol-4(5*H*)-one monohydrochloride. *UNII-1DWS68PNE6; UNII-RT3Y3QMF8N* [molindone]. *CAS-15622-65-8; CAS-7416-34-4* [molindone]. *Antipsychotic.* Moban (Endo) ◇*EN-1733A*

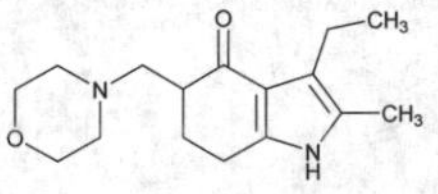

Molracetam. $C_{18}H_{25}N_3O_4$. 347.41. 4-[(4-*p*-Anisoyl-1-piperazinyl)acetyl]morpholine. *UNII-R47KMF9589. CAS-94746-78-8.* INN.

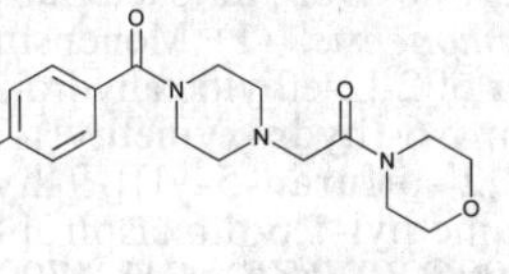

Molsidomine [*1980*] (mol si′ doe meen). $C_9H_{14}N_4O_4$. 242.23. (1) Sydnone imine, *N*-(ethoxycarbonyl)-3-(4-morpholinyl)-; (2) *N*-Carboxy-3-morpholinosydnone imine ethyl ester; (3) *N*-Ethoxycarbonyl-3-morpholinosydnonimine. *CAS-25717-80-0.* INN; BAN; JAN. *Anti-anginal; vasodilator (coronary).* Corvaton (Hoechst-Roussel†) ◇*CAS 276*

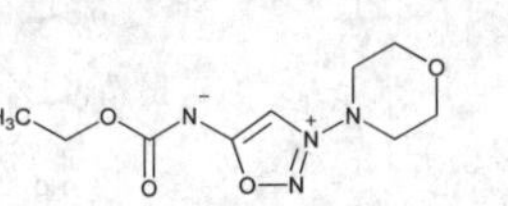

Mometasone Furoate [*1987*] (moe met′ a sone fure′ oh ate). **USP.** $C_{27}H_{30}Cl_2O_6$. 521.43. [Mometasone is INN and BAN.] (1) Pregna-1,4-diene-3,20-dione, 9,21-dichloro-17-[(2-furanylcarbonyl)oxy]-11-hydroxy-16-methyl-, (11β,16α)-; (2) 9,21-Dichloro-11β,17-dihydroxy-16α-methylpregna-1,4-diene-3,20-dione 17-(2-furoate). *UNII-04201GDN4R. CAS-83919-23-7.* JAN. *Steroid (topical).* Asmanex (Schering); Elocon (Schering) ◇*Sch 32088*

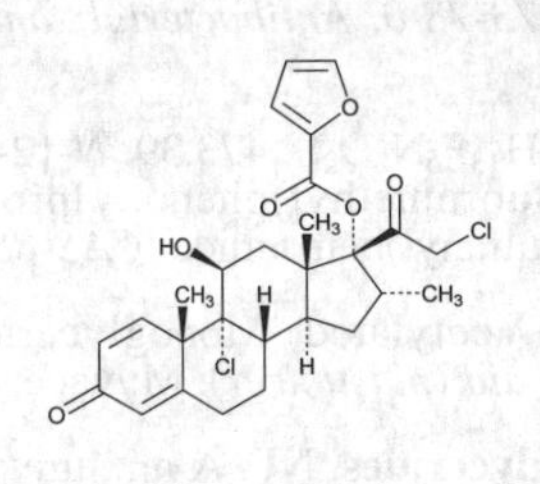

Monab B72.3-GYK-DTPA-^{111}In (previously used name) — *See* Indium In 111 Satumomab Pendetide.

Monalazone Disodium. $C_7H_4ClNNa_2O_4S$. 279.61. *p*-(Chlorosulfamoyl)benzoic acid disodium salt. *UNII-267GPF992J. CAS-61477-95-0.* INN.

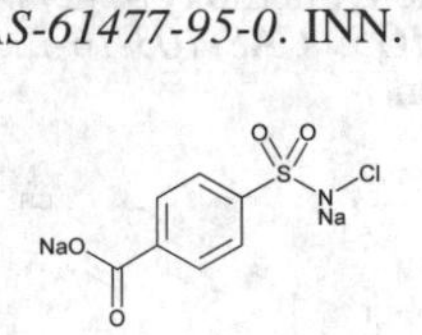

Monalium Hydrate — *See* Magaldrate.

Monatepil Maleate [*1995*] (moe na′ te pil mal′ ee ate). $C_{28}H_{30}FN_3OS \cdot C_4H_4O_4$. 591.69. [Monatepil is INN.] (1) 1-Piperazinebutanamide, *N*-(6,11-dihydrodibenzo[*b,e*]thiepin-11-yl)-4-(4-fluorophenyl)-, (±)-, (*Z*)-2-butenedioate

---

† Brand name formerly used, and/or firm no longer concerned with this product.

(1:1); (2) (±)-*N*-(6,11-Dihydrodibenzo[*b,e*]thiepin-11-yl)-4-(*p*-fluorophenyl)-1-piperazinebutyramide maleate (1:1). *UNII-W456I35SKD. CAS-132046-06-1; CAS-132019-54-6* [monatepil]. *Anti-anginal; antihypertensive.* ◇AJ-2615

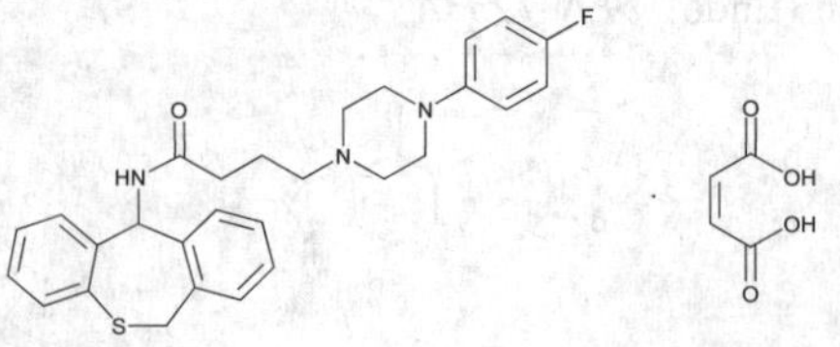

Monensin [*1968*] (moe nen′ sin). **USP.** $C_{36}H_{62}O_{11}$ (monensin A). 670.87; $C_{35}H_{60}O_{11}$ (monensin B). 656.84; $C_{37}H_{64}O_{11}$ (monensin C). 684.90. Antibacterial produced by *Streptomyces cinnamonensis.* (1) Monensin; (2) Monensin; (3) Stereoisomer of 2-[2-ethyloctahydro-3′-methyl-5′-[tetrahydro-6-hydroxy-6-(hydroxymethyl)-3,5-dimethyl-2*H*-pyran-2-yl][2,2′-bifuran-5-yl]]-9-hydroxy-*β*-methoxy-*α*,*γ*,2,8-tetramethyl-1,6-dioxaspiro[4.5]decan-7-butanoic acid. *UNII-906O0YJ6ZP. CAS-17090-79-8.* INN; BAN. *Antiprotozoal; antibacterial; antifungal.* Coban [as sodium salt] (Lilly); Rumensin [as sodium salt] (Lilly) ◇67314

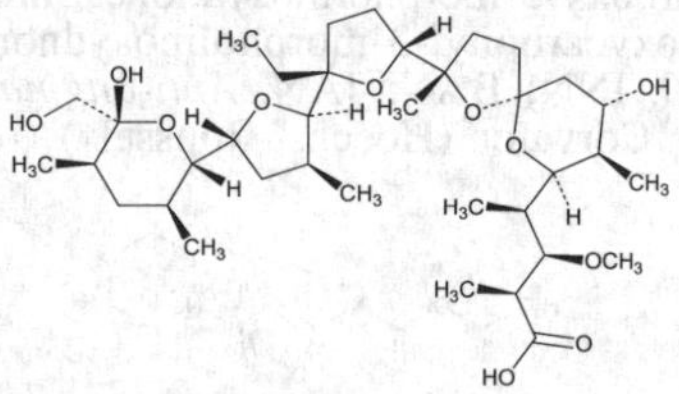

Monensin Sodium (moe nen′ sin soe′ dee um). **USP.** $C_{36}H_{61}NaO_{11}$ (monensin A sodium). 692.85; $C_{35}H_{59}NaO_{11}$ (monensin B sodium). 678.83; $C_{37}H_{63}NaO_{11}$ (monensin C sodium). 706.88. (1) Monensin, sodium salt; (2) Stereoisomer of 2-[2-ethyloctahydro-3′-methyl-5′-[tetrahydro-6-hydroxy-6-(hydroxymethyl)-3,5-dimethyl-2*H*-pyran-2-yl][2,2′-bifuran-5-yl]]-9-hydroxy-*β*-methoxy-*α*,*γ*,2,8-tetramethyl-1,6-dioxaspiro[4.5]decan-7-butanoic acid sodium salt. *CAS-22373-78-0. Antibacterial; antifungal; antiprotozoal.*

Monepantel. $C_{20}H_{13}F_6N_3O_2S.$ 473.39. *N*-{2-Cyano-1-[(2*S*)-5-cyano-2-(trifluoromethyl)phenoxy]propan-2-yl}-4-(trifluoromethylsulfanyl)benzamide. *CAS-887148-69-8.* INN.

Mono- and Di-acetylated Monoglycerides. NF XVIII. *Pharmaceutic aid (plasticizer).* Myvacet (Eastman†)

Mono- and Di-glycerides. NF. A mixture of glycerol mono- and di-esters, with minor amounts of tri-esters, of fatty acids from edible oils. *Pharmaceutic aid (emulsifying agent).* Myverol (Eastman†)

Monobenzone (mon oh ben′ zone). **USP.** $C_{13}H_{12}O_2.$ 200.23. (1) Phenol, 4-(phenylmethoxy)-; (2) *p*-(Benzyloxy)phenol. *UNII-9L2KA76MG5. CAS-103-16-2.* INN. *Depigmentor.* Benoquin (Valeant)

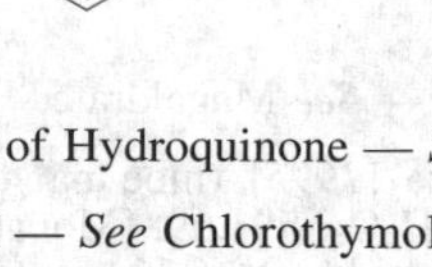

Monobenzyl Ether of Hydroquinone — *See* Monobenzone.

Monochlorothymol — *See* Chlorothymol.

Monochlorphenamide (DCF) — *See* Clofenamide.

Monoctanoin [*1992*] (mon ok′ ta noin). A semisynthetic mixture of mono- and diglycerides (of octanoic and decanoic acids, with other minor components. The glycerides have the following approximate composition: glycerol 1-octanoate (80% to 85%); glycerol 1-decanoate and glycerol 1,2-dioctanoate (10% to 15%); and free glycerol (maximum 2.5%). *UNII-VFU0OU98LO.* BAN. *Anticholelithic (dissolution of gallstones).* Moctanin (Ex-elixis)

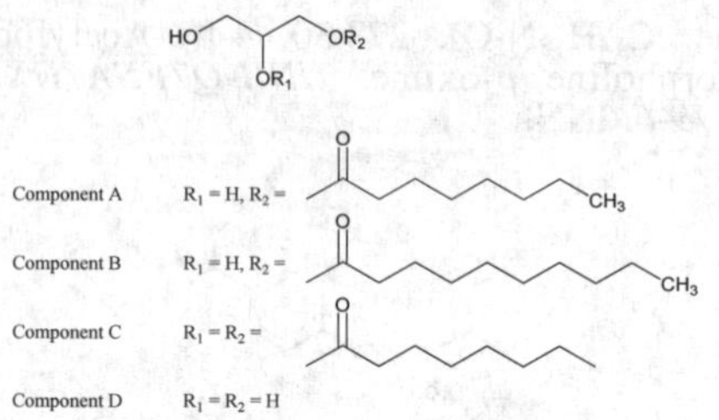

Monoctanoin Component A. $C_{11}H_{22}O_4.$ 218.29. (1) 2,3-Dihydroxypropyl octanoate; (2) Glycerol 1-octanoate. *UNII-TM2TZD4G4A.*

Monoctanoin Component B. $C_{13}H_{26}O_4.$ 246.34. (1) 2,3-Dihydroxypropyl decanoate; (2) Glycerol 1-decanoate. *UNII-197M6VFC1W.*

Monoctanoin Component C. $C_{19}H_{36}O_5.$ 344.49. (1) (Hydroxymethyl)ethylene dioctanoate; (2) Glycerol 1,2-dioctanoate. *UNII-SA9937IP23.*

Monoctanoin Component D. $C_3H_8O_3.$ 92.09. Glycerol.

Monoethanolamine (mon″ oh eth″ a nol′ a meen). **NF.** $C_2H_7NO.$ 61.08. [Monoethanolamine Oleate is INN and JAN.] (1) Ethanol, 2-amino-; (2) 2-Aminoethanol. *UNII-5KV86114PT. CAS-141-43-5. Pharmaceutic aid (surfactant).*

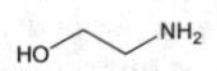

Monoglyceride Citrate. NF. Citric acid ester of glyceryl monooleate. *CAS-36291-32-4.*

Monometacrine. $C_{19}H_{24}N_2.$ 280.41. 9,9-Dimethyl-10-[3-(methylamino)propyl]acridan. *UNII-3FDC82890Y. CAS-4757-49-7.* INN.

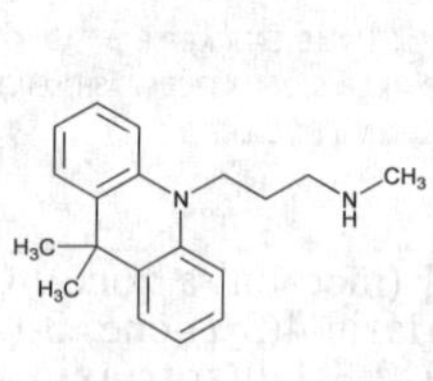

Monooctanoin — *See* Monoctanoin.

Monophenylbutazone — *See* Mofebutazone.

Monophosphothiamine. $C_{12}H_{18}ClN_4O_4PS.$ 380.79. Monophosphoric ester of thiamine. *UNII-P712T71Q3T. CAS-532-40-1.* INN; DCF.

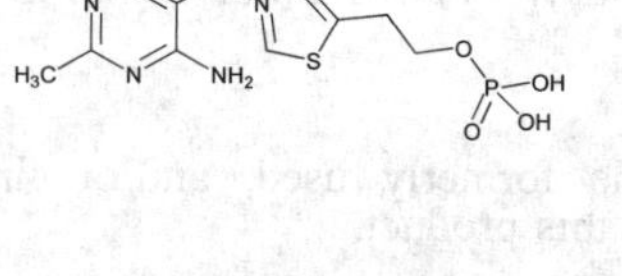

Monosodium Glutamate (mon″ oh soe′ dee um gloo′ ta mate). **NF**. $C_5H_8NNaO_4 \cdot H_2O$. 187.13. (1) L-Glutamic acid, sodium salt, hydrate; (2) Monosodium L-glutamate, hydrate. *Pharmaceutic aid (flavor); pharmaceutic aid (perfume)*.

Monosulfiram (previously used name) — *See* Sulfiram.

Monothioglycerol (mon″ oh thye″ oh glis′ er ol). **NF**. $C_3H_8O_2S$. 108.16. (1) 1,2-Propanediol, 3-mercapto-; (2) 3-Mercapto-1,2-propanediol. *CAS-96-27-5. Pharmaceutic aid (preservative)*.

Monoxerutin. $C_{29}H_{34}O_{17}$. 654.57. 3,3′,4′,5-Tetrahydroxy-7-(2-hydroxyethoxy)flavone 3-[6-O-(6-deoxy-α-L-mannopyranosyl)-β-D-glucopyranoside]. *UNII-EKF7043SBU. CAS-23869-24-1*. INN.

Montelukast Sodium [*1995*] (mon te loo′ kast soe′ dee um). $C_{35}H_{35}ClNNaO_3S$. 608.17. [Montelukast is INN and BAN.] (1) Cyclopropaneacetic acid, 1-[[[1-[3-[2-(7-chloro-2-quinolinyl)ethenyl]phenyl]-3-[2-(1-hydroxy-1-methylethyl)-phenyl]propyl]thio]methyl]-, sodium salt, [R-(E)]-; (2) Sodium 1-[[[(R)-m-[(E)-2-(7-chloro-2-quinolyl)vinyl]-α-[o-(1-hydroxy-1-methylethyl)phenethyl]benzyl]thio]methyl]cyclopropaneacetate. *UNII-U1O3J18SFL; UNII-MHM278SD3E* [montelukast]. *CAS-151767-02-1; CAS-158966-92-8* [montelukast]. *Anti-asthmatic (leukotriene antagonist)*. Singulair (Merck) ◇*MK-476*

Monteplase. $C_{2569}H_{3896}N_{746}O_{783}S_{39}$. 59,009.55. 84-L-Serine-plasminogen activator (human tissue-type 2-chain form), cyclic (6→36), (32′→48′), (34→43), (40′→109′), (51→73), (56→62), (75→83), (92→173), (113→155), (120′→264), (134′→209′), (144→168), (166′→182′), (180→261), (199′→227′), (201→243), (232→256)-heptadecakis(disulfide). *CAS-156616-23-8*. INN.

---

† Brand name formerly used, and/or firm no longer concerned with this product.

Montirelin. $C_{17}H_{24}N_6O_4S$. 408.48. N-[[(3R,6R)-6-Methyl-5-oxo-3-thiomorpholinyl]carbonyl]-L-histidyl-L-prolinamide. *UNII-30MUJ6YYUY. CAS-90243-66-6*. INN.

Moperone. $C_{22}H_{26}FNO_2$. 355.45. [Moperone Hydrochloride is JAN.] 4′-Fluoro-4-(4-hydroxy-4-p-tolylpiperidino)butyrophenone. *UNII-OU730881W5. CAS-1050-79-9*. INN; MI. ◇*R 1658*

Mopidamol. $C_{19}H_{31}N_7O_4$. 421.49. 2,2′,2″,2‴-[(4-Piperidinopyrimido[5,4-d]pyrimidine-2,6-diyl)dinitrilo]tetraethanol. *CAS-13665-88-8*. INN; BAN; MI.

Mopidralazine. $C_{14}H_{19}N_5O$. 273.33. 4-[6-[(2,5-Dimethylpyrrol-1-yl)amino]-3-pyridazinyl]morpholine. *UNII-96600S6GLK. CAS-75841-82-6*. INN.

Moprolol. $C_{13}H_{21}NO_3$. 239.31. 1-(Isopropylamino)-3-(o-methoxyphenoxy)-2-propanol. *CAS-5741-22-0*. INN; MI.

Moquizone. $C_{20}H_{21}N_3O_3$. 351.40. 2,3-Dihydro-1-(morpholinoacetyl)-3-phenyl-4(1H)-quinazolinone. *UNII-EG12MD1RMA. CAS-19395-58-5*. INN; MI.

Moracizine (INN, BAN) — *See* Moricizine.

Morantel Tartrate [*1969*] (moe ran' tel tar' trate). **USP.** $C_{12}H_{16}N_2S.C_4H_6O_6$. 370.42. [Morantel is INN and BAN.] (1) Pyrimidine, 1,4,5,6-tetrahydro-1-methyl-2-[2-(3-methyl-2-thienyl)ethenyl]-, (*E*)-,[*R*-(*R**,*R**)]-2,3-dihydroxybutanedioate (1:1); (2) (*E*)-1,4,5,6-Tetrahydro-1-methyl-2-[2-(3-methyl-2-thienyl)vinyl]pyrimidine tartrate (1:1). *UNII-5WF7E9QC3F; UNII-7NJ031HAX5* [morantel]. *CAS-26155-31-7; CAS-20574-50-9* [morantel]. *Anthelmintic.* ◇*CP-12,009-18*

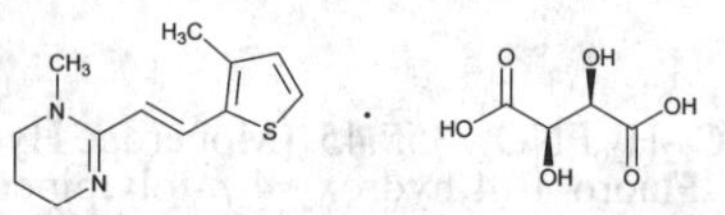

Morazone. $C_{23}H_{27}N_3O_2$. 377.48. 4-[(3-Methyl-2-phenylmorpholino)methyl]antipyrine. *UNII-870Q5BL2FN. CAS-6536-18-1.* INN; BAN; MI.

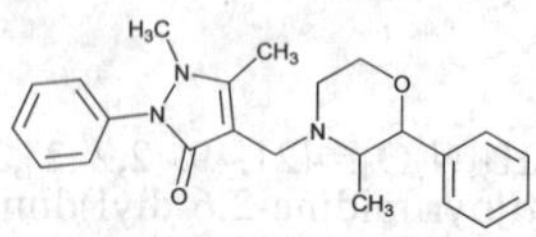

Morclofone. $C_{21}H_{24}ClNO_5$. 405.87. 4'-Chloro-3,5-dimethoxy-4-(2-morpholinoethoxy)benzophenone. *UNII-VY62TIB872. CAS-31848-01-8.* INN; MI.

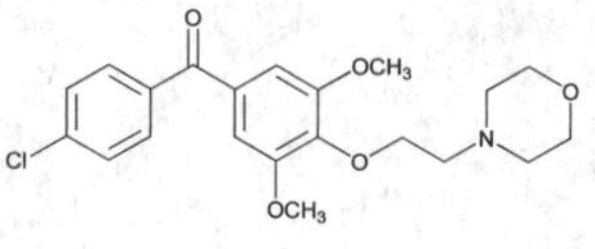

Morforex. $C_{15}H_{24}N_2O$. 248.36. 4-[2-[(α-Methylphenethyl)amino]ethyl]morpholine. *UNII-O9J6ITY8UX. CAS-41152-17-4.* INN; DCF.

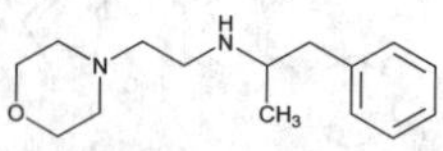

Moricizine [*1981*] (mor i' si zeen). $C_{22}H_{25}N_3O_4S$. 427.52. [Moracizine is INN and BAN.] (1) Carbamic acid, [10-[3-(4-morpholinyl)-1-oxopropyl]-10*H*-phenothiazin-2-yl]-, ethyl ester; (2) Ethyl 10-(3-morpholinopropionyl)phenothiazine-2-carbamate. *UNII-2GT1D0TMX1; UNII-71OK3Z1ESP* [moricizine hydrochloride]. *CAS-31883-05-3; CAS-29560-58-5* [moricizine hydrochloride]. *Cardiac depressant (anti-arrhythmic).* Ethmozine (Roberts Pharmaceutical) ◇*EN-313*

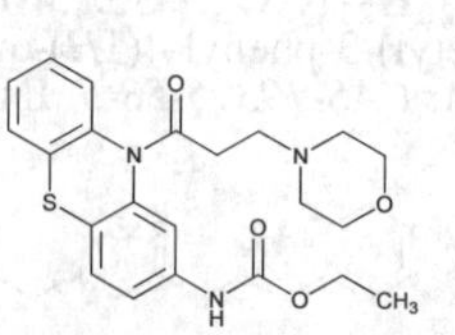

Moricizine Hydrochloride (mor i' si zeen hye" droe klor' ide). **USP.** $C_{22}H_{25}N_3O_4S.HCl$. 463.98. (1) Carbamic acid, [10-[3-(4-morpholinyl)-1-oxopropyl]-10*H*-phenothiazin-

2yl]-, ethyl ester, hydrochloride; (2) Ethyl 10-(3-morpholinopropionyl)phenothiazine-2-carbamate, hydrochloride. *UNII-71OK3Z1ESP. CAS-29560-58-5.* Ethmozine (Shire)

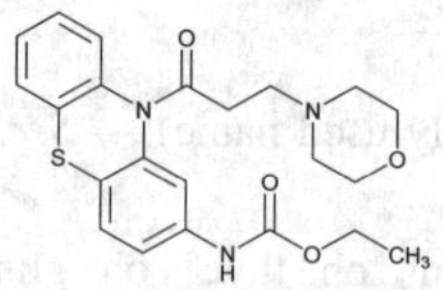

Morinamide. $C_{10}H_{14}N_4O_2$. 222.24. *N*-(Morpholinomethyl)-pyrazinecarboxamide. *UNII-8CFL28PA3W. CAS-952-54-5.* INN; DCF. ◇*B-2311*

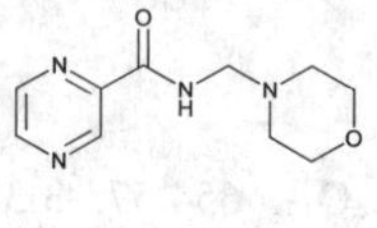

Morniflumate [*1978*] (mor ni floo' mate). $C_{19}H_{20}F_3N_3O_3$. 395.38. (1) 3-Pyridinecarboxylic acid, 2-[[3-(trifluoromethyl)phenyl]amino]-, 2-(4-morpholinylethyl) ester; (2) 2-Morpholinoethyl 2-(α,α,α-trifluoro-*m*-toluidino)nicotinate. *UNII-R133MWH7X1. CAS-65847-85-0.* INN. *Anti-inflammatory.* ◇*UP 164*

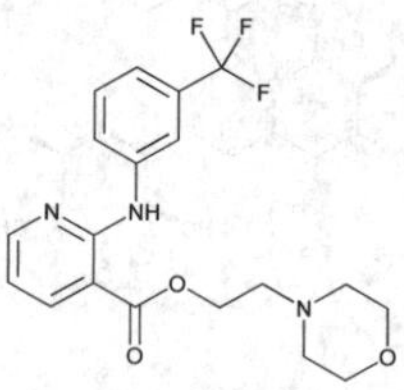

Morocromen. $C_{21}H_{27}N_3O_5$. 401.46. 4-Methyl-7-(4-morpholinecarboxamido)-3-(2-morpholinoethyl)coumarin. *UNII-762D3F7OY3. CAS-35843-07-3.* INN.

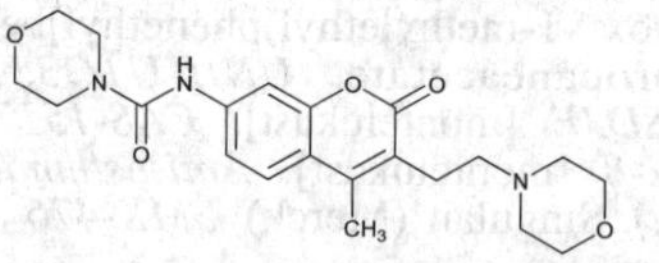

Moroctocog Alfa. $C_{3953}H_{6020}N_{1040}O_{1158}S_{29}$ + $C_{3553}H_{5412}N_{956}O_{1028}S_{33}$. 87,570.32. (1-742)-(1637-1648)-Blood-coagulation factor VIII (human reduced) complex with 1649-2332-blood-coagulation factor VIII (human reduced). INN; BAN.

Morolimumab. Human monoclonal IgG1 antibody against human Rhesus-D antigen. *CAS-202833-07-6.* INN.

Moroxydine. $C_6H_{13}N_5O$. 171.20. 4-Morpholinecarboximidoylguanidine. *UNII-O611591WAH. CAS-3731-59-7.* INN; BAN; DCF; MI. ◇*SKF 8898-A; ABOB*

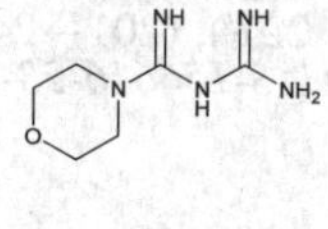

Morphazinamide — *See* Morinamide.

Morpheridine. $C_{20}H_{30}N_2O_3$. 346.46. 1-(2-Morpholinoethyl)-4-phenylpiperidine-4-carboxylic acid ethyl ester. *UNII-1854GKB41Y. CAS-469-81-8.* INN; BAN; DCF; MI.

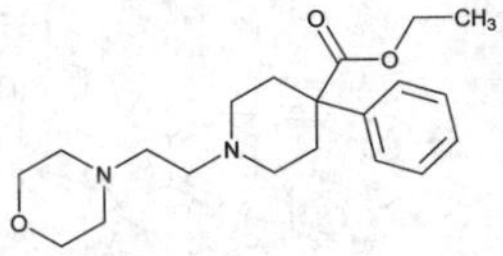

Morphine Glucuronide. $C_{23}H_{27}NO_9$. 461.46. 3-Hydroxy-17-methyl-4,5α-epoxymorphin-7-en-6α-yl β-D-glucopyranosiduronic acid. *CAS-20290-10-2.* INN.

Morphine Hydrochloride. *UNII-76I7G6D29C* [morphine]. *CAS-52-26-6; CAS-57-27-2* [morphine]. USP XV; JAN; MI.

Morphine Sulfate (mor′ feen sul′ fate). **USP**. $(C_{17}H_{19}NO_3)_2{\cdot}H_2SO_4{\cdot}5H_2O$. 758.83. [Morphine is BAN.] (1) Morphinan-3,6-diol, 7,8-didehydro-4,5-epoxy-17-methyl, (5α,6α)-, sulfate (2:1) (salt), pentahydrate; (2) 7,8-Didehydro-4,5α-epoxy-17-methylmorphinan-3,6α-diol sulfate (2:1) (salt) pentahydrate. *UNII-X3P646A2J0; UNII-76I7G6D29C* [morphine]. *CAS-6211-15-0; CAS-64-31-3* [anhydrous]; *CAS-57-27-2* [morphine]. JAN. *Analgesic (narcotic).* Duramorph (Baxter Healthcare); Kadian (Alpharma); Ms Contin (Purdue Frederick); Oramorph (Xanodyne)

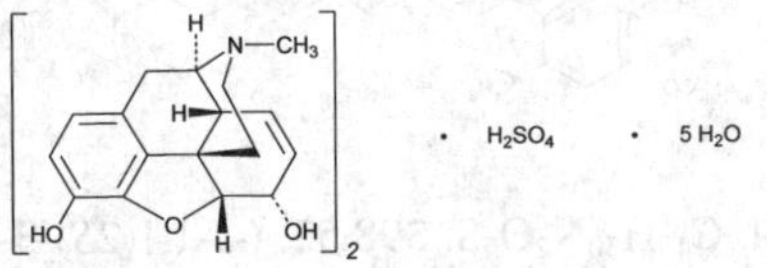

Morpholinyl Succinimide — *See* Morsuximide.

Morrhuate Sodium (mor′ ue ate soe′ dee um). **USP** [Injection]. [Sodium Morrhuate is INN.] A sterile solution of sodium salts of the fatty acids of cod liver oil. *CAS-8031-09-2. Sclerosing agent.*

Morsuximide. $C_{16}H_{20}N_2O_3$. 288.34. 2-Methyl-*N*-(morpholinomethyl)-2-phenylsuccinimide. *UNII-57G776P4EJ. CAS-3780-72-1.* INN. ◇S-210

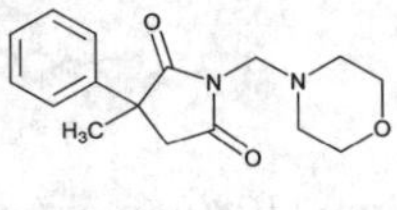

Morsydomine — *See* Molsidomine.

---

† Brand name formerly used, and/or firm no longer concerned with this product.

Mosapramine. $C_{28}H_{35}ClN_4O$. 479.06. [Mosapramine Hydrochloride is JAN.] ($\pm$)-1′-[3-(3-Chloro-10,11-dihydro-5*H*-dibenz[*b,f*]azepin-5-yl)propyl]hexahydrospiro[imidazo[1,2-*a*]pyridine-3(2*H*),4′-piperidin]-2-one. *UNII-04UZ-Q7O9SJ. CAS-89419-40-9.* INN.

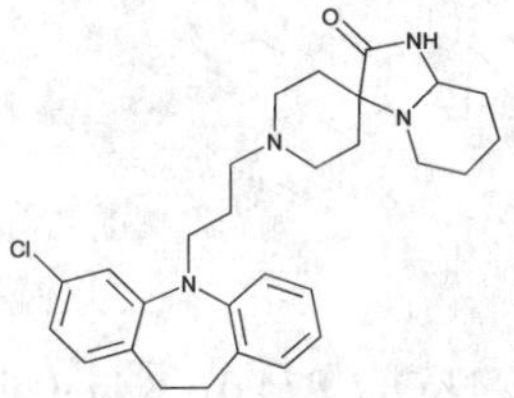

Mosapride. $C_{21}H_{25}ClFN_3O_3$. 421.89. ($\pm$)-4-Amino-5-chloro-2-ethoxy-*N*-[[4-(*p*-fluorobenzyl)-2-morpholinyl]methyl]-benzamide. *UNII-I8MFJ1C0BY. CAS-112885-41-3.* INN.

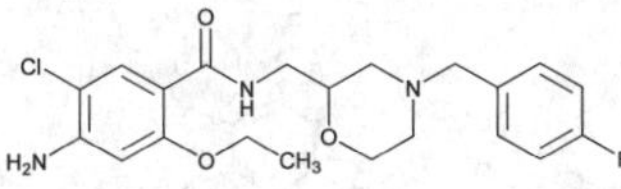

Motapizone. $C_{12}H_{12}N_4OS$. 260.31. ($\pm$)-4,5-Dihydro-6-(4-imidazol-1-yl-2-thienyl)-5-methyl-3(2*H*)-pyridazinone. *UNII-C4A61P8A37. CAS-90697-57-7.* INN.

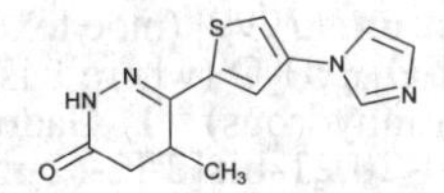

Motavizumab *[2005]* (moe″ ta viz′ oo mab). $C_{6476}H_{10014}N_{1706}O_{2008}S_{48}$. Immunoglobulin G1, anti-(respiratory syncytial virus glycoprotein F) (human-mouse monoclonal MEDI-524 γ1-chain), disulfide with human-mouse monoclonal MEDI-524κ-chain, dimer. Molecular weight is approximately 148,000 daltons. *CAS-677010-34-3.* INN. *Prevention of serious lower respiratory tract disease caused by respiratory syncytial virus (RSV) in pediatric patients at high risk of RSV disease.* ◇MEDI-524

MOTC — *See* Methacycline.

Motesanib *[2007]* (moe tes′ a nib). $C_{22}H_{23}N_5O$. 373.45. (1) 3-Pyridinecarboxamide, *N*-(2,3-dihydro-3,3-dimethyl-1*H*-indol-6-yl)-2-[(4-pyridinylmethyl)amino]-; (2) *N*-(3,3-Dimethyl-2,3-dihydro-1*H*-indol-6-yl)-2-[(pyridin-4-ylmethyl)amino]pyridine-3-carboxamide. *UNII-U1JK633AYI. CAS-453562-69-1.* INN. *Angiogenic agent.* ◇AMG 706

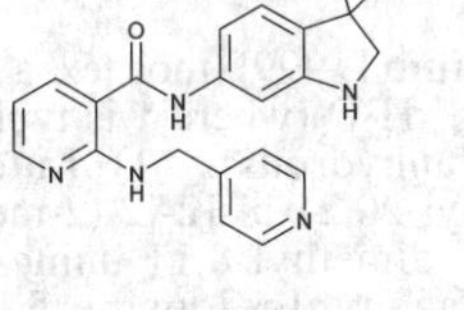

Motesanib Diphosphate *[2006]* (moe tes′ a nib dye fos′ fate). $C_{22}H_{23}N_5O{\cdot}2H_3O_4P$. 569.44. (1) 3-Pyridinecarboxamide, *N*-(2,3-dihydro-3,3-dimethyl-1*H*-indol-6-yl)-2-[(4-pyridinylmethyl)amino]-, phosphate (1:2); (2) *N*-(3,3-Dimethyl-2,3-dihydro-1*H*-indol-6-yl)-2-[(pyridin-4-ylmethyl)amino]pyridine-3-carboxamide phosphate (1:2). *UNII-T6Q3060U91. CAS-857876-30-3. Antiangiogenesis agent.* ◇*AMG 706*

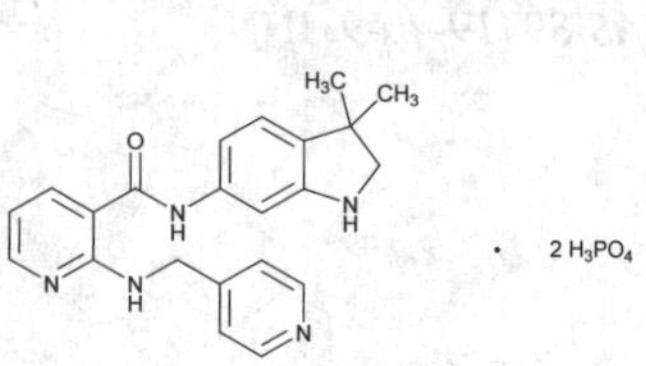

Motexafin. $C_{48}H_{67}N_5O_{10}$. 874.07. 8,11-Imino-3,6:16,13-dinitrilo-1,18-benzodiazacycloeicosine-5,14-dipropanol, 9,10-diethyl-20,21-bis[2-[2-(2-methoxyethoxy)ethoxy]ethoxy]-4,15-dimethyl-. *CAS-189752-49-6.* INN.

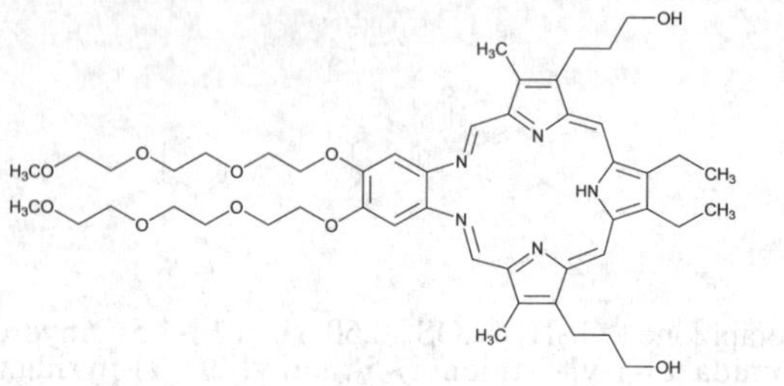

Motexafin Gadolinium [*1999*] (moe tex′ a fin gad″ oh lin′ ee um). $C_{52}H_{72}GdN_5O_{14} \cdot xH_2O$ (where *x* is typically between 0 and 2). 1148.40 (anhydrous). (1) Gadolinium, bis(acetato-*κO*)[9,10-diethyl-20,21-bis[2-[2-(2-methoxyethoxy)ethoxy]ethoxy]-4,15-dimethyl-8,11-imino-3,6:16,13-dinitrilo-1,18-benzodiazacycloeicosine-5,14-dipropanolato-*κN*^1,*κN*^18,*κN*^23,*κN*^24,*κN*^25]-hydrate, (*PB*-7-11-233′2′4)-; (2) Bis(acetato-*O*)[9,10-diethyl-20,21-bis[2-[2-(2-methoxy-ethoxy)ethoxy]ethoxy]-4,15-dimethyl-8,11-imino-3,6:16,13-dinitrilo-1,18-benzodiazacycloeicosine-5,14-dipropanolato-*N*^1,*N*^18,*N*^23,*N*^24,*N*^25]gadolinium hydrate. *CAS-156436-89-4. Antineoplastic.* Xcytrin (Pharmacyclics) ◇*PCI-0120; gadolinium texaphyrin; Gd texaphyrin; Gd-Tex; FP-GP1; API-GP3*

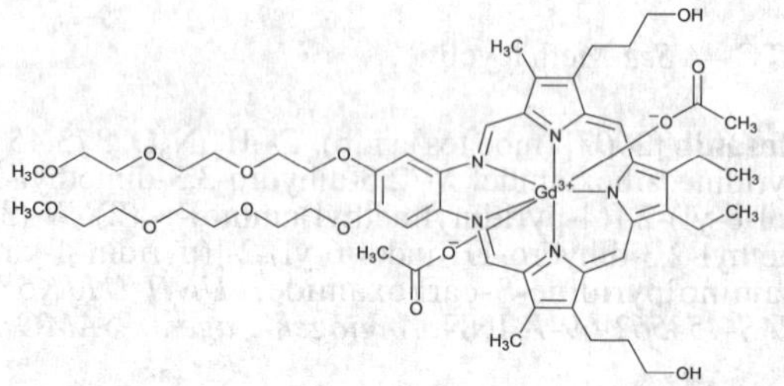

Motexafin Lutetium [*1999*] (moe tex′ a fin loo tee′ shee um). $C_{52}H_{72}LuN_5O_{14} \cdot xH_2O$ (where *x* is typically between 0 and 2). 1166.12 (anhydrous). (1) Lutetium, bis(acetato-*κO*)[9,10-diethyl-20,21-bis[2-[2-(2-methoxyethoxy)ethox-y]ethoxy]-4,15-dimethyl-8,11-imino-3,6:16,13-dinitrilo-1,18-benzodiazacycloeicosine-5,14-dipropanolato-*κN*^1,*κN*^18,*κN*^23,*κN*^24,*κN*^25]-, hydrate, (*PB*-7-11-233′2′4); (2) Bis(acetato-*O*)[9,10-diethyl-20,21-bis[2-[2-(2-methoxy-yethoxy)ethoxy]ethoxy]-4,15-dimethyl-8,11-imino-3,6:16,13-dinitrilo-1,18-benzodiazacycloeicosine-5,14-dipropanolato-*N*^1,*N*^18,*N*^23,*N*^24,*N*^25]-, hydrate, (*PB*-7-11-233′2′4). *CAS-156436-90-7. Antineoplastic/antiathero-*

sclerotic. Lutrin (Pharmacyclics); Antrin (Pharmacyclics); Optrin (Pharmacyclics) ◇*PCI-0123; lutetium texaphyrin; Lu texaphyrin; Lu-Tex; FP-LP1*

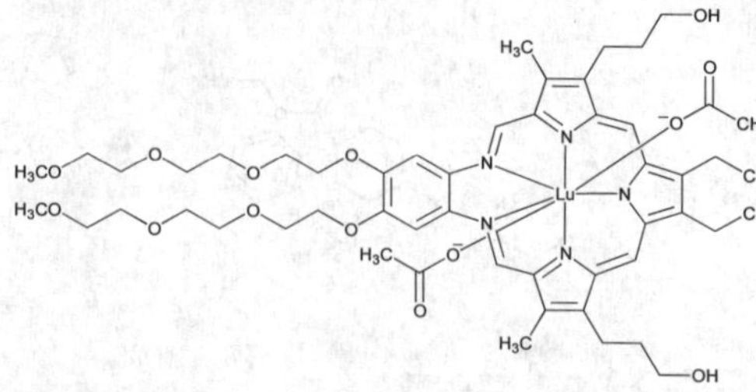

Motrazepam. $C_{17}H_{15}N_3O_4$. 325.32. 1,3-Dihydro-1-(methoxymethyl)-7-nitro-5-phenyl-2*H*-1,4-benzodiazepin-2-one. *UNII-36YG4ZMR69. CAS-29442-58-8.* INN.

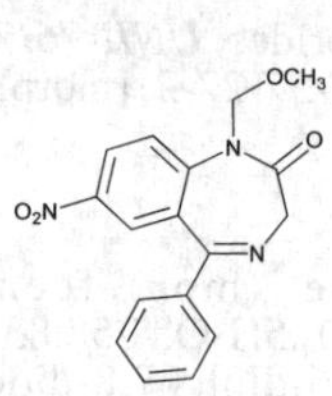

Motretinide [*1979*] (moe tret′ i nide). $C_{23}H_{31}NO_2$. 353.50. (1) 2,4,6,8-Nonatetraenamide, *N*-ethyl-9-(4-methoxy-2,3,6-tri-methylphenyl)-3,7-dimethyl-, (*all-E*)-; (2) *all-trans-N*-Ethyl-9-(4-methoxy-2,3,6-trimethylphenyl)-3,7-dimethyl-2,4,6,8-nonatetraenamide. *CAS-56281-36-8.* INN. *Keratolytic.* Tasmaderm (Hoffmann-LaRoche†) ◇*Ro 11-1430*

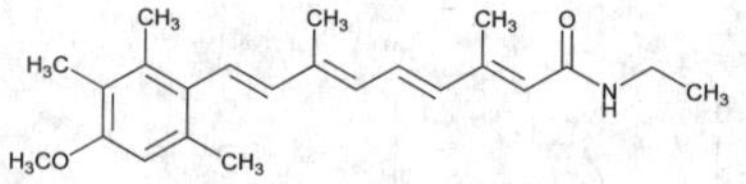

Moveltipril. $C_{19}H_{30}N_2O_5S$. 398.52. (-)-1-[(2*S*)-3-Mercapto-2-methylpropionyl]-L-proline, ester with *N*-(cyclohexylcarbonyl)thio-D-alanine. *CAS-85856-54-8.* INN; MI.

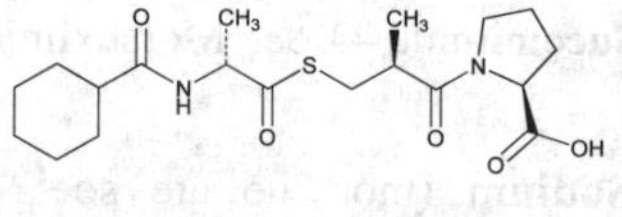

Moxadolen. $C_{11}H_{13}NO_4$. 223.23. Methylcarbamic acid, ester with (3*R**,3a*R**,4*S**,7*R**,7a*S**)-3a,4,7,7a-tetrahydro-3-hydroxy-4,7-methanoisobenzofuran-1(3*H*)-one. *CAS-75992-53-9.* INN.

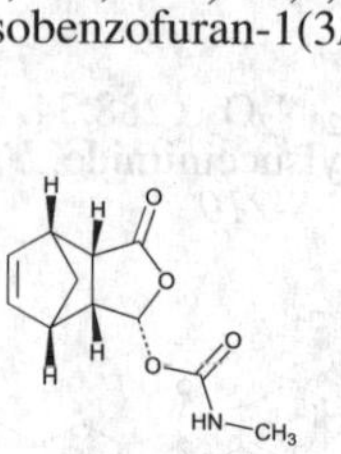

Moxalactam Disodium [*1980*] (mox″ a lak′ tam dye soe′ dee um). $C_{20}H_{18}N_6Na_2O_9S$. 564.44. [Latamoxef is INN and BAN; Latamoxef Sodium is JAN.] (1) 5-Oxa-1-azabicyclo[4.2.0]oct-2-ene-2-carboxylic acid, 7-[[carboxy(4-hydroxyphenyl)acetyl]amino]-7-methoxy-3-[[(1-methyl-1*H*-tetrazol-5-yl)thio]methyl]-8-oxo-, disodium salt; (2) *N*-[(6*R*,7*R*)-2-Carboxy-7-methoxy-3-[[(1-methyl-1*H*-tetra-zol-5-yl)thio]methyl]-8-oxo-5-oxa-1-azabicyclo[4.2.0]oct-2-en-7-yl]-2-(*p*-hydroxyphenyl)malonamic acid disodium salt. *UNII-5APW73W3QZ; UNII-VUF6C936Z3* [moxalactam]. *CAS-64953-12-4; CAS-64952-97-2* [moxalactam]. USP XXIII. *Anti-infective.* Moxam (Lilly) ◇*LY 127935*

Moxantrazole (previously used name) — *See* Teloxantrone Hydrochloride.

Moxaprindine. $C_{23}H_{32}N_2O$. 352.51. *N,N*-Diethyl-*N'*-(1-methoxy-2-indanyl)-*N'*-phenyl-1,3-propanediamine. *CAS-53076-26-9*. INN.

Moxastine. $C_{18}H_{23}NO$. 269.38. 2-(1,1-Diphenylethoxy)-*N,N*-dimethylethylamine. *UNII-ZSJ254W6SF. CAS-3572-74-5.* INN.

Moxaverine. $C_{20}H_{21}NO_2$. 307.39. 1-Benzyl-3-ethyl-6,7-dimethoxyisoquinoline. *UNII-P3P08Y1XJ4. CAS-10539-19-2.* INN; BAN; MI.

Moxazocine [*1977*] (mox az′ oh seen). $C_{18}H_{25}NO_2$. 287.40. (1) 2,6-Methano-3-benzazocin-8-ol, 3-(cyclopropylmethyl)-1,2,3,4,5,6-hexahydro-11-methoxy-6-methyl-, [2*R*-(2α,6α,11*R**)]-; (2) (-)-(2*R*,6*S*,11*R*)-3-(Cyclopropylmethyl)-1,2,3,4,5,6-hexahydro-11-methoxy-6-methyl-2,6-methano-3-benzazocin-8-ol. *CAS-58239-89-7.* INN. *Analgesic; antitussive.* ◇*levo-BL-4566*

Moxestrol. $C_{21}H_{26}O_3$. 326.43. 11β-Methoxy-19-nor-17α-pregna-1,3,5-(10)-trien-20-yne-3,17-diol. *CAS-34816-55-2; CAS-21375-12-2* [replaced]. INN; DCF; MI. ◇*R 2858*

Moxicoumone. $C_{22}H_{30}N_2O_6$. 418.48. 4-Methyl-5,7-bis(2-morpholinoethoxy)coumarin. *UNII-IG2442S013. CAS-17692-56-7.* INN.

Moxidectin [*1989*] (mox″ i dek′ tin). $C_{37}H_{53}NO_8$. 639.82. (1) Milbemycin B, 5-*O*-demethyl-28-deoxy-25-(1,3-dimethyl-1-butenyl)-6,28-epoxy-23-(methoxyimino)-, [6*R*,23*E*,25*S*(*E*)]-; (2) (6*R*,25*S*)-5-*O*-Demethyl-28-deoxy-25-[(*E*)-1,3-dimethyl-1-butenyl]-6,28-epoxy-23-oxomilbemycin B 23-(*E*)-(*O*-methyloxime); (3) (2a*E*,4*E*,5′*R*,6*R*,6′*S*,8*E*,11*R*,13*S*,15*S*,17a*R*,20*R*,20a*R*,20b*S*)-6′-[(*E*)-1,3-Dimethyl-1-butenyl]-5′,6,6′,7,10,11,14,15,17a,20,20a,20b-dodecahydro-20,20b-dihydroxy-5′,6,8,19-tetramethylspiro[11,15-methano-2*H*,13*H*,17*H*-furo[4,3,2-*pq*][2,6]benzodioxacyclooctadecin-13,2′-[2*H*]pyran]-4′,17(3′*H*)-dione 4′-(*E*)-(*O*-methyloxime). *UNII-NGU5-H31YO9. CAS-113507-06-5.* INN; BAN. *Antiparasitic (veterinary).* ◇*CL 301,423*

Moxifloxacin. $C_{21}H_{24}FN_3O_4$. 401.43. 1-Cyclopropyl-6-fluoro-1,4-dihydro-8-methoxy-7-[(4a*S*,7a*S*)-octahydro-6*H*-pyrrolo[3,4-*b*]pyridin-6-yl]-4-oxo-3-quinolinecarboxylic acid. *UNII-U188XYD42P. CAS-151096-09-2.* INN; BAN.

Moxifloxacin Hydrochloride [*1998*] (mox″ i flox′ a sin hye″ droe klor′ ide). $C_{21}H_{24}FN_3O_4 \cdot HCl$. 437.89. (1) (4a*S-cis*)-1-Cyclopropyl-6-fluoro-1,4-dihydro-8-methoxy-7-(octahydro-6*H*-pyrrolol[3,4-*b*]pyridin-6-yl)-4-oxo-3-quinolinecarboxylic acid, monohydrochloride; (2) 1-Cyclopropyl-6-fluoro-1,4-dihydro-8-methoxy-7-[(4a*S*,7a*S*)-octahydro-6*H*-pyrrolo[3,4-*b*]pyridin-6-yl]-4-oxo-3-quinolinecarboxylic acid, monohydrochloride. *UNII-C53598599T. CAS-186826-86-8. Antibacterial.* Avelox (Bayer); Vigamox (Alcon) ◇*BAY 12-8039*

---

† Brand name formerly used, and/or firm no longer concerned with this product.

Moxilubant Maleate [*1997*] (mox il′ ue bant mal′ ee ate). C$_{26}$H$_{37}$N$_3$O$_4$.C$_4$H$_4$O$_4$. 571.66. [Moxilubant is INN.] 4-[[5-(*p*-Amidinophenoxy)pentyl]oxy]-*N*,*N*-diisopropyl-3-methoxybenzamide maleate (1:1). *CAS-147398-01-4; CAS-146978-48-5* [moxilubant]. *Antirheumatic; anti-inflammatory (nonsteroidal); antipsoriatic.* ◇*CGS 25019C*

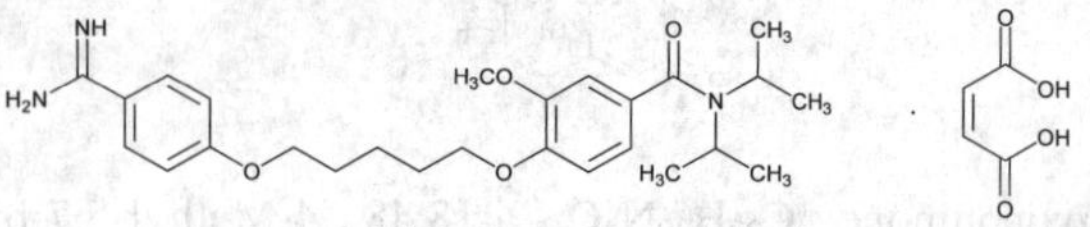

Moxipraquine. C$_{24}$H$_{38}$N$_4$O$_2$. 414.58. 4-[6-[(6-Methoxy-8-quinolyl)amino]hexyl]-α-methyl-1-piperazinepropanol. *CAS-23790-08-1.* INN; BAN. ◇*349 C59*

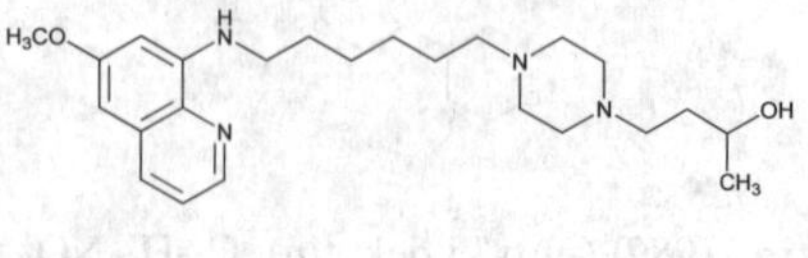

Moxiraprine. C$_{17}$H$_{22}$N$_4$O$_2$. 314.38. *p*-[5-Methyl-6-[(2-morpholinoethyl)amino]-3-pyridazinyl]phenol. *UNII-7ET381H9UA. CAS-82239-52-9.* INN.

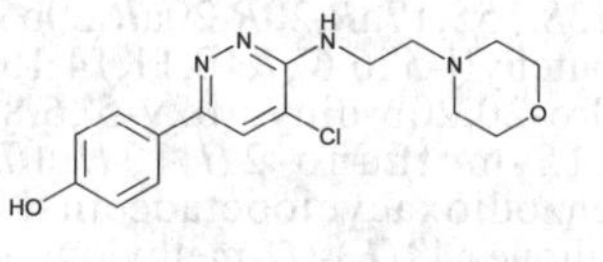

Moxisylyte. C$_{16}$H$_{25}$NO$_3$. 279.37. [Moxisylyte Hydrochloride is JAN.] [2-(4-Acetoxy-2-isopropyl-5-methylphenoxy)ethyl]dimethylamine. *CAS-54-32-0.* INN; BAN; DCF; MI.

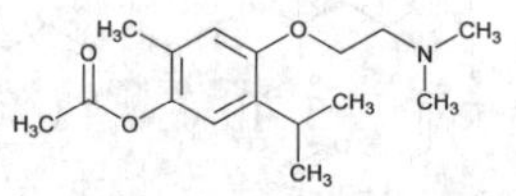

Moxnidazole [*1975*] (mox nye′ da zole). C$_{13}$H$_{18}$N$_6$O$_5$. 338.32. (1) 2-Oxazolidinone, 3-[[(1-methyl-5-nitro-1*H*-imidazol-2-yl)methylene]amino]-5-(4-morpholinyl-methyl)-; (2) 3-[[(1-Methyl-5-nitroimidazol-2-yl)methyl-ene]amino]-5-(morpholinomethyl)-2-oxazolidinone. *CAS-52279-59-1.* INN. *Antiprotozoal (Trichomonas).* ◇*SH 240*

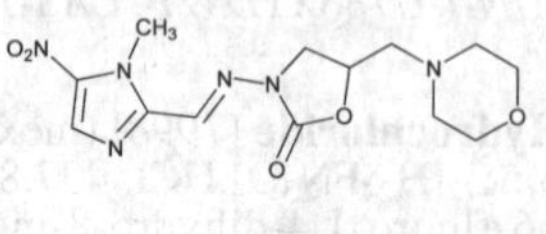

Moxonidine [*1998*] (mox oh′ ni deen). C$_9$H$_{12}$ClN$_5$O. 241.68. (1) 5-Pyrimidinamine, 4-chloro-*N*-(4,5-dihydro-1*H*-imidazol-2-yl)-6-methoxy-2-methyl-; (2) 4-Chloro-5-(2-imidazolidinyldeneamino)-6-methoxy-2-methylpyrimidine. *CAS-75438-57-2.* INN; BAN. *Antihypertensive; treatment of congestive heart failure; treatment of type 2 diabetes (centrally acting sympatholytic).* Cynt (Lilly); Nucynt (Lilly); Norcynt (Lilly) ◇*LY326869; BE5895; BDF5896*

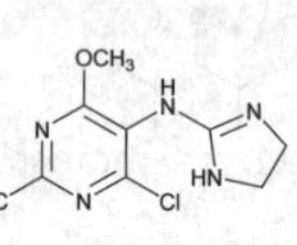

Mozavaptan. C$_{27}$H$_{29}$N$_2$O$_2$. 413.53. *N*-[4-[[(5*RS*)-5-(Dimethylamino)-2,3,4,5-tetrahydro-1*H*-1-benzazepin-1-yl]carbonyl]phenyl]-2-methylbenzamide. *UNII-17OJ42922Y. CAS-137975-06-5.* INN.

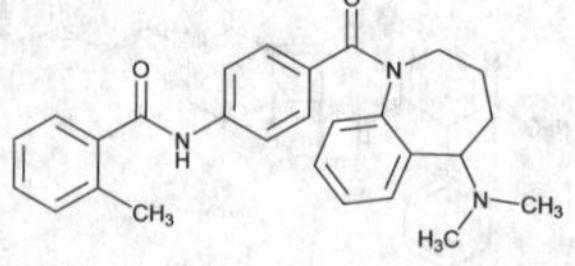

Mozenavir. C$_{33}$H$_{36}$N$_4$O$_3$. 536.66. (4*R*,5*S*,6*S*,7*R*)-1,3-Bis(3-aminobenzyl)-4,7-dibenzylhexahydro-5,6-dihydroxy-2*H*-1,3-diazepin-2-one. *UNII-64OO8946ER. CAS-174391-92-5.* INN.

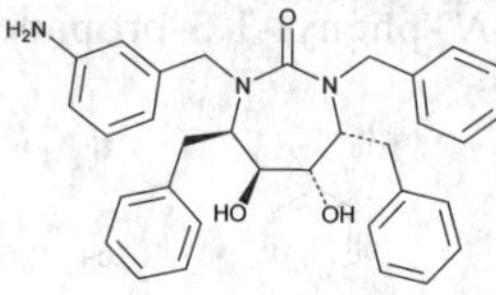

MP-537. Code designation for Iomethin I 125 and for Iomethin I 131.

mTHPC — *See* Temoporfin.

Mubritinib [*2003*] (mue bri′ ti nib). C$_{25}$H$_{23}$F$_3$N$_4$O$_2$. 468.47. (1) 1*H*-1,2,3-Triazole, 1-[4-[4-[[2-[(1*E*)-2-[4-(trifluoromethyl)phenyl]ethenyl]-4-oxazolyl]methoxy]phenyl]butyl]-; (2) 1-[4-[4-[[2-[(*E*)-2-[4-(Trifluoromethyl)phenyl]ethenyl]oxazol-4-yl]methoxy]phenyl]butyl]-1*H*-1,2,3-triazole. *UNII-V734AZP9BR. CAS-366017-09-6.* INN. *Treatment of cancer.* ◇*TAK-165*

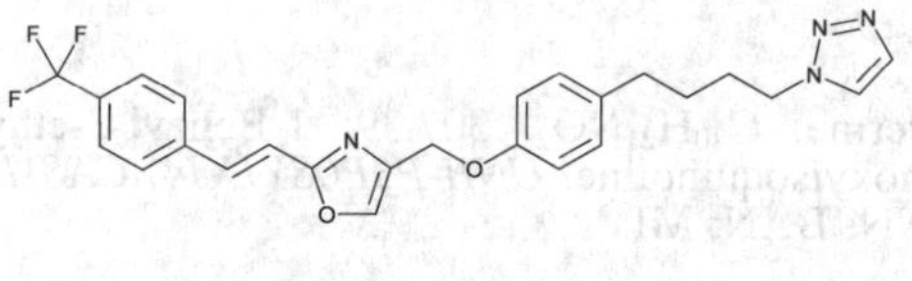

Mucopolysaccharide Polysulfate. JAN.

Mumps Skin Test Antigen. USP. A sterile suspension of formaldehyde-inactivated mumps virus prepared from the extra-embryonic fluids of the mumps virus-infected chicken embryo, concentrated and purified by differential centrifugation, and diluted with isotonic sodium chloride solution. *Diagnostic aid (dermal reactivity indicator).*

Mumps Virus Vaccine, Inactivated. [PHS: *Mumps Vaccine*]. NF XIV.

Mumps Virus Vaccine Live. USP. A bacterially sterile preparation of live virus derived from a strain of mumps virus tested for neurovirulence in monkeys, and for immunogenicity, free from all demonstrable viable microbial agents except unavoidable bacteriophage, and found suitable for human immunization. *Immunizing agent (active).* Mumpsvax (Merck)

Mupirocin [*1986*] (mue pir′ oh sin). USP. C$_{26}$H$_{44}$O$_9$. 500.62. (1) Nonanoic acid, 9-[[3-methyl-1-oxo-4-[tetrahydro-3,4-dihydroxy-5-[[3-(2-hydroxy-1-methylpropyl)oxiranyl]-methyl]-2*H*-pyran-2-yl]-2-butenyl]oxy]-, [2*S*-[2α(*E*),3β,4β,5α[2*R**,3*R**(1*R**,2*R**)]]]-; (2) (*E*)-(2*S*,3*R*,4*R*,5*S*)-5-[(2*S*,3*S*,4*S*,5*S*)-2,3-Epoxy-5-hydroxy-4-methylhexyl]tetrahydro-3,4-dihydroxy-β-methyl-2*H*-pyran-2-crotonic acid, ester with 9-hydroxynonanoic acid.

UNII-D0GX863OA5. CAS-12650-69-0. INN; BAN. *Antibacterial (topical).* Bactroban (GlaxoSmithKline); Centany (Johnson & Johnson) ◇*BRL 4910A*

Mupirocin Calcium [*1994*] (mue pir′ oh sin kal′ see um). **USP.** $C_{52}H_{86}CaO_{18}\cdot 2H_2O$. 1075.34. (1) Nonanoic acid, 9-[[3-methyl-1-oxo-4-[tetrahydro-3,4-dihydroxy-5-[[3-(2-hydroxy-1-methylpropyl)oxiranyl]methyl]-2*H*-pyran-2-yl]-2-butenyl]oxy]-, calcium salt (2:1), dihydrate, [2*S*-[2α(*E*),3β,4β,5α[2*R**,3*R**(1*R**,2*R**)]]]-; (2) (α*E*,2*S*,3*R*,4*R*,5*S*)-5-[(2*S*,3*S*,4*S*,5*S*)-2,3-Epoxy-5-hydroxy-4-methylhexyl]tetrahydro-3,4-dihydroxy-β-methyl-2*H*-pyran-2-crotonic acid, ester with 9-hydroxynonanoic acid, calcium salt (2:1), dihydrate. *UNII-RG38I2P540. CAS-115074-43-6; CAS-104486-81-9* [anhydrous]. *Antibacterial (topical).* Bactroban (GlaxoSmithKline) ◇*BRL 4910F*

Muplestim [*1996*] (mue′ ple stim). $C_{670}H_{1074}N_{186}O_{199}S_5$. 15,079.16. (1) Interleukin 3 (human); (2) Interleukin 3 (human). *CAS-148641-02-5.* INN. *Hematopoietic stimulant; antineutropenic.* Hemokine (Novartis) ◇*SDZ ILE 964*

```
APMTQTTSLK TSWVNCSNMI DEIITHLKQP PLPLLDFNNL NGEDQDILME
NNLRRPNLEA FNRAVKSLQN ASAIESILKN LLPCLPLATA APTRHPIHIK
DGDWNEFRRK LTFYLKTLEN AQAQQTTLSL AIF
```

Murabutide. $C_{23}H_{40}N_4O_{11}$. 548.58. 2-Acetamido-3-*O*-[(*R*)-1-[[(*S*)-1-[[(*R*)-3-carbamoyl-1-carboxypropyl]carbamoyl]-ethyl]carbamoyl]ethyl]-2-deoxy-D-glucopyranose, butyl ester. *CAS-74817-61-1.* INN.

Muraglitazar [*2003*] (mue″ ra gli′ ta zar). $C_{29}H_{28}N_2O_7$. 516.54. (1) Glycine, *N*-[(4-methoxyphenoxy)carbonyl]-*N*-[[4-[2-(5-methyl-2-phenyl-4-oxazolyl)ethoxy]phenyl]-methyl]-; (2) [[(4-Methoxyphenoxy)carbonyl][4-[2-(5-methyl-2-phenyloxazol-4-yl)ethoxy]benzyl]amino]acetic acid. *UNII-W1MKM70WQI. CAS-331741-94-7* [free acid]. INN. *Treatment of type-2 diabetes mellitus, mixed*

---

† Brand name formerly used, and/or firm no longer concerned with this product.

dyslipidemia, atherosclerosis, and metabolic syndrome (dual (alpha and gamma) peroxime proliferator activated (PPAR) agonist). ◇*BMS-298585*

Mureletecan. Poly[[*N*-(2-hydroxypropyl)methacrylamide]-*co*-[camptothecin ester with *N*-[6-(2-methacrylamidoacetamido)hexanoyl]glycine]-*co*-[*N*-[[(2-hydroxypropyl)carbamoyl]methyl]methacrylamide]]. *CAS-246527-99-1.* INN.

Murine Monoclonal Antibody — *See* Muromonab-CD3.

Murocainide. $C_{19}H_{27}N_3O_5$. 377.43. 1-[4,7-Dimethoxy-6-(2-piperidinoethoxy)-5-benzofuranyl]-3-methylurea. *UNII-U4THC4MHG7. CAS-66203-94-9.* INN.

Murodermin. $C_{257}H_{375}N_{73}O_{83}S_7$. 6039.62. Urogastrone (mouse salivary gland) or epidermal growth factor (mouse salivary gland). *CAS-54017-73-1.* INN.

```
NSYPGCPSSY DGYCLNGGVC MHIESLDSYT CNCVIGYSGD RCQTRDLRWW
ELR
```

Muromonab-CD3 [*1989*] (mue″ roe moe′ nab). A biochemically purified $IgG_{2\alpha}$ immunoglobulin consisting of a heavy chain of approximately 50,000 daltons and a light chain of approximately 25,000 daltons. It is manufactured by a process involving the fusion of mouse myeloma cells to lymphocytes from immunized animals to produce a hybridoma which secretes antigen-specific antibodies to the T3 antigen of human T-lymphocytes. INN; JAN. *Monoclonal antibody (immunosuppressant).* Orthoclone OKT3 (Ortho Pharmaceutical)

Mustard Oil — *See* Allyl Isothiocyanate.

Mustine (previously used name) — *See* Mechlorethamine Hydrochloride.

Muzolimine [*1977*] (mue zoe' li meen). $C_{11}H_{11}Cl_2N_3O$. 272.13. (1) 3*H*-Pyrazol-3-one, 5-amino-2-[1-(3,4-dichlorophenyl)ethyl]-2,4-dihydro-; (2) 3-Amino-1-(3,4-dichloro-α-methylbenzyl)-2-pyrazolin-5-one. *CAS-55294-15-0.* INN; BAN. *Diuretic; antihypertensive.* ◇*BAY g 2821*

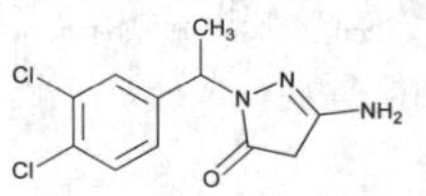

Mycophenolate Mofetil [*1990*] (mye" koe fen' oh late moe' fe til). $C_{23}H_{31}NO_7$. 433.49. (1) 4-Hexenoic acid, 6-(1,3-dihydro-4-hydroxy-6-methoxy-7-methyl-3-oxo-5-isobenzofuranyl)-4-methyl-, 2-(4-morpholinyl)ethyl ester, (*E*)-; (2) 2-Morpholinoethyl (*E*)-6-(4-hydroxy-6-methoxy-7-methyl-3-oxo-5-phthalanyl)-4-methyl-4-hexenoate. *UNII-9242ECW6R0. CAS-115007-34-6. Immunomodulator.* Cellcept (Roche) ◇*RS-61443*

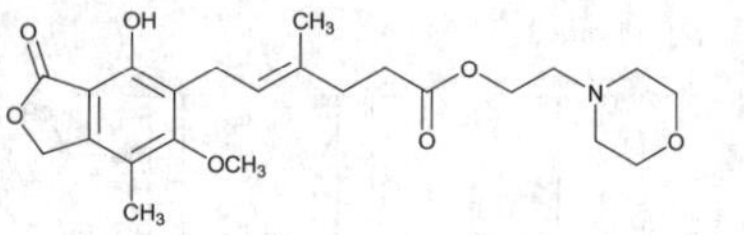

Mycophenolate Mofetil Hydrochloride [*1998*] (mye" koe fen' oh late moe' fe til hye" droe klor' ide). $C_{23}H_{31}NO_7 \cdot HCl$. 469.96. (1) 2-(4-Morpholinyl)ethyl ester (*E*)-6-(1,3-dihydro-4-hydroxy-6-methoxy-7-methyl-3-oxo-5-isobenzofuranyl)-4-methyl-4-hexenoic acid, hydrochloride; (2) 2-Morpholinoethyl (*E*)-6-(4-hydroxy-6-methoxy-7-methyl-3-oxo-5-phthalanyl)-4-methyl-4-hexenoate hydrochloride. *UNII-UXH81S8ZVB. CAS-116680-01-4. Transplantation (immunosuppressant).* Cellcept (Roche) ◇*RS-61443-190*

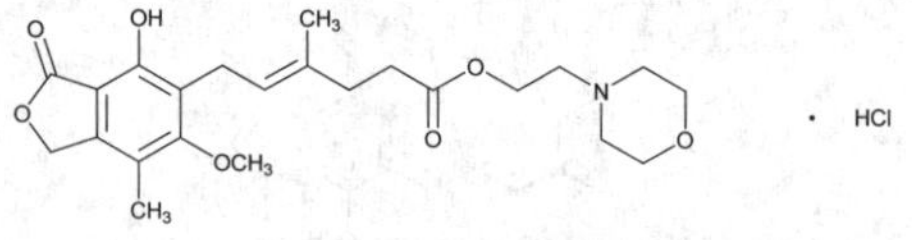

Mycophenolate Sodium [*2002*] (mye" koe fen' oh late soe' dee um). $C_{17}H_{19}NaO_6$. 342.32. (1) 4-Hexenoic acid, 6-(1,3-dihydro-4-hydroxy-6-methoxy-7-methyl-3-oxo-5-isobenzofuranyl)-4-methyl-, monosodium salt, (4*E*)-; (2) Sodium 4(*E*)-6-(4-hydroxy-6-methoxy-7-methyl-3-oxo-1,3-dihydroisobenzofuran-5-yl)-4-methylhex-4-enoate. *UNII-WX877SQI1G. CAS-37415-62-6. Transplantation (immunosuppressant).* ◇*ERL 080*

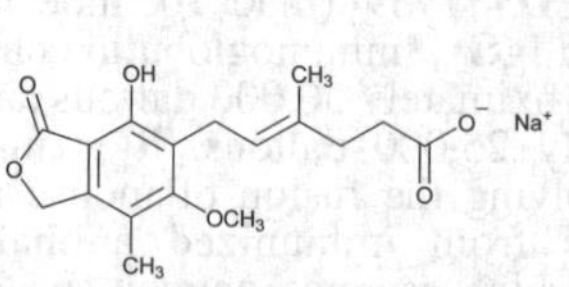

Mycophenolic Acid [*1970*] (mye" koe fe nole' ik as' id). $C_{17}H_{20}O_6$. 320.34. (1) 4-Hexenoic acid, 6-(1,3-dihydro-4-hydroxy-6-methoxy-7-methyl-3-oxo-5-isobenzofuranyl)-4-methyl-, (*E*)-; (2) (*E*)-6-(4-Hydroxy-6-methoxy-7-methyl-3-oxo-5-phthalanyl)-4-methyl-4-hexenoic acid. *UNII-*

HU9DX48N0T. CAS-24280-93-1. INN; BAN. *Antineoplastic.* Myfortic (Novartis) ◇*68618; RS-61443 [as mofetil]; NSC-129185*

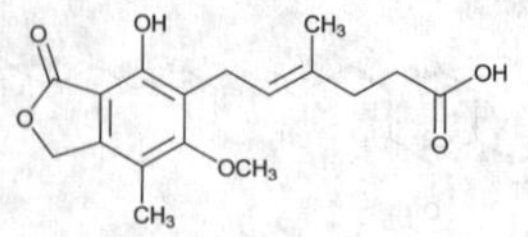

Mydeton — *See* Tolperisone.

Myelosan — *See* Busulfan.

Myfadol. $C_{21}H_{25}NO_2$. 323.43. 2-[3-(*m*-Hydroxyphenyl)-2,3-dimethylpiperidino]acetophenone. *CAS-4575-34-2.* INN.

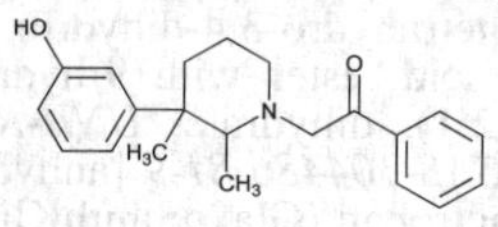

Myralact. $C_{19}H_{41}NO_4$. 347.53. 2-(Tetradecylamino)ethanol lactate. *CAS-15518-87-3.* INN; BAN.

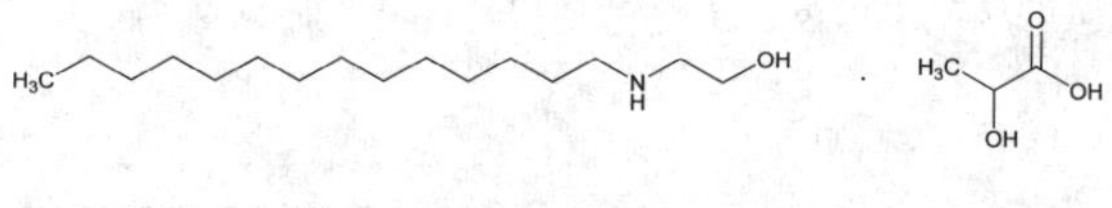

Myricodine — *See* Myrophine.

Myristic Acid. NF. $C_{14}H_{28}O_2$. 228.37. Tetradecanoic acid. *UNII-0I3V7S25AW. CAS-544-63-8.*

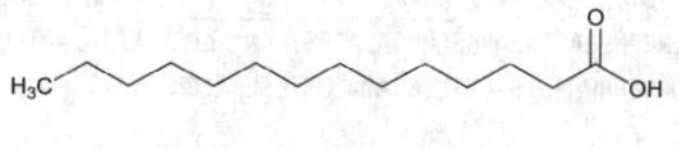

Myristica Oil — *See* Nutmeg Oil.

Myristyl Alcohol (mir is' til al' ka hol). NF. $C_{14}H_{30}O$. 214.39. Tetradecanol. *CAS-112-72-1. Pharmaceutic aid (stiffening agent).*

Myrophine. $C_{38}H_{51}NO_4$. 585.82. (1) Myristylbenzylmorphine; (2) 3-Benzyloxy-*N*-methyl-6-myristoyloxy-4,5-epoxymorphin-7-en. *CAS-467-18-5.* INN; BAN; DCF; MI.

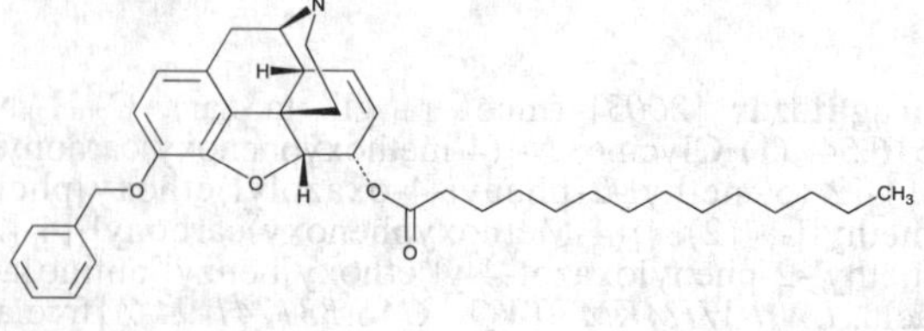

Myrrh (mur). **USP**. The oleo-gum resin obtained from stems and branches of *Commiphora molmol* Engler and other related species of *Commiphora* other than *Commiphora mukul* (Fam. Burseraceae). *UNII-JC71GJ1F3L.*

Myrtecaine. $C_{17}H_{31}NO$. 265.43. 2-[2-(6,6-Dimethyl-2-norpinen-2-yl)ethoxy]triethylamine. *CAS-7712-50-7.* INN; DCF; MI.

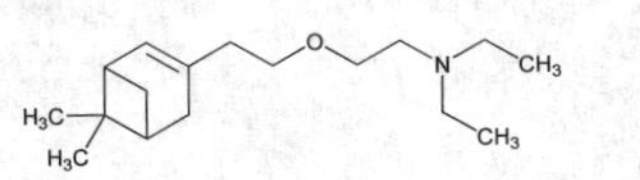

^{13}N — *See* Ammonia N 13.

^{22}Na — *See* Sodium Chloride Na 22.

Nabazenil [*1983*] (nab az′ e nil). $C_{35}H_{55}NO_3$. 537.82. (1) 1*H*-Azepine-1-butanoic acid, hexahydro-, 3-(1,2-dimethylheptyl)-7,8,9,10-tetrahydro-6,6,9-trimethyl-6*H*-dibenzo[*b,d*]pyran-1-yl ester; (2) 3-(1,2-Dimethylheptyl)-7,8,9,10-tetrahydro-6,6,9-trimethyl-6*H*-dibenzo[*b,d*]pyran-1-yl hexahydro-1*H*-azepine-1-butyrate. *CAS-58019-65-1.* INN. *Anticonvulsant.* ◇*SP-175*

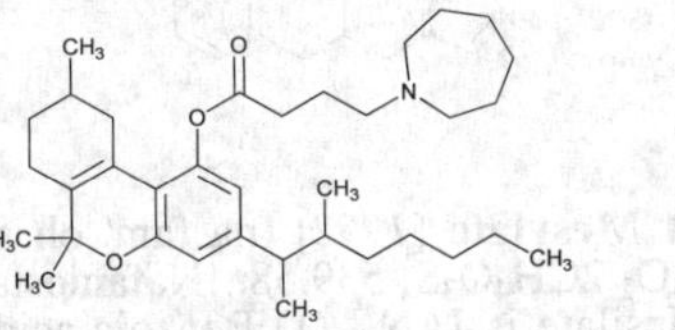

Nabilone [*1976*] (nab′ i lone). $C_{24}H_{36}O_3$. 372.54. (1) 9*H*-Dibenzo[*b,d*]pyran-9-one, 3-(1,1-dimethylheptyl)-6,6a,7,8,10,10a-hexahydro-1-hydroxy-6,6-dimethyl-, *trans-*, (±)-; (2) (±)-3-(1,1-Dimethylheptyl-6,6aβ,7,8,10,10aα-hexahydro-1-hydroxy-6,6-dimethyl-9*H*-dibenzo[*b,d*]pyran-9-one. *UNII-2N4O9L084N. CAS-51022-71-0.* INN; BAN. *Tranquilizer (minor).* Cesamet (Valeant) ◇*Cpd 109514*

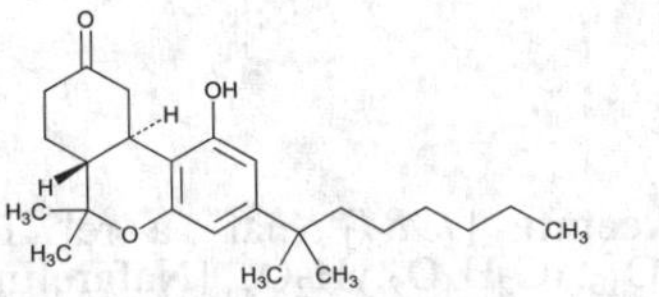

Nabitan Hydrochloride [*1979*] (nab′ i tan hye″ droe klor′ ide). $C_{35}H_{52}N_2O_3 \cdot HCl$. 585.26. [Nabitan is INN.] (1) 1-Piperidinebutanoic acid, 8-(1,2-dimethylheptyl)-1,3,4,5-tetrahydro-5,5-dimethyl-2-(2-propynyl)-2*H*-[1]benzopyrano[4,3-*c*]pyridin-10-yl ester monohydrochloride-; (2) 8-(1,2-Dimethylheptyl)-1,3,4,5-tetrahydro-5,5-dimethyl-2-(2-propynyl)-2*H*-[1]benzopyrano[4,3-*c*]pyridin-10-yl 1-piperidinebutyrate monohydrochloride. *CAS-49637-08-3; CAS-66556-74-9* [nabitan]. *Analgesic. [Name previously used: Nabutan Hydrochloride.]* ◇*SP-106; NIB*

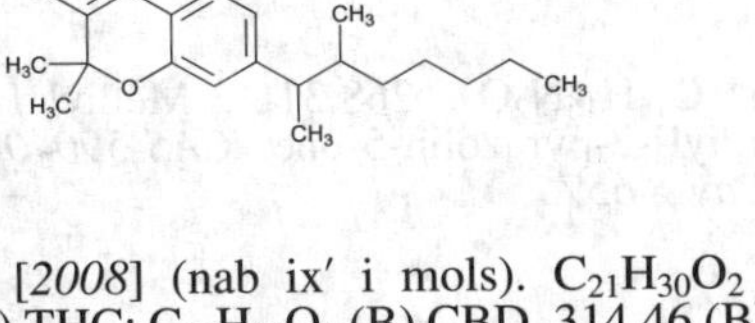

Nabiximols [*2008*] (nab ix′ i mols). $C_{21}H_{30}O_2$ (A) THC. 314.46 (A) THC; $C_{21}H_{30}O_2$ (B) CBD. 314.46 (B) CBD. (A) Delta-9-tetrahydrocannabinol (THC): (1) 6*H*-Dibenzo[*b,d*]pyran-1-ol, 6a,7,8,10a-tetrahydro-6,6,9-trimethyl-3-pentyl-, (6a*R*,10a*R*)-; (2) (6a*R*,10a*R*)-6,6,9-Trimethyl-3-pentyl-6a,7,8,10a-tetrahydro-6*H*-dibenzo[*b,d*]pyran-1-ol; (3) Highly characterized botanical extract of a defined chemotype of *Cannabis sativa* L. The major chemical constituent is the cannabinoid, delta-9-tetrahydrocannabinol (THC). Important minor constituents are related cannabinoids and non-cannabinoid components alpha- and trans-caryophyllenes. (B) Cannabidiol (CBD): (1) 1,3-Benzenediol, 2-[(1*R*,6*R*)-3-methyl-6-(1-methylethenyl)-2-cyclohexen-1-yl]-5-pentyl-; (2) 2-[(1*R*,6*R*)-3-Methyl-6-(1-methylethenyl)cyclohex-2-enyl]-5-pentylbenzene-1,3-diol; (3) Highly characterized botanical extract of a defined chemotype of *Cannabis sativa* L. The major chemical constituent is the cannabinoid cannabidiol (CBD). Important minor constituents are related cannabinoids and non-cannabinoid components alpha- and trans-caryophyllenes. *CAS-1972-08-3* [(A) THC]; *CAS-13956-29-1* [(A) CBD]. *Relief of pain in patients with advanced cancer, who experience inadequate analgesia during optimized chronic opioid therapy.* Sativex (GW Pharma Ltd) ◇*GW-1000*

Naboctate Hydrochloride [*1981*] (nab′ ok tate hye″ droe klor′ ide). $C_{33}H_{53}NO_3 \cdot HCl$. 548.24. [Naboctate is INN.] (1) Butanoic acid, 4-(diethylamino)-, 7,8,9,10-tetrahydro-6,6,9-trimethyl-3-(1-methyloctyl)-6*H*-dibenzo[*b,d*]pyran-1-yl ester, hydrochloride, (±)-; (2) (±)-7,8,9,10-Tetrahydro-6,6,9-trimethyl-3-(1-methyloctyl)6*H*-dibenzo[*b,d*]pyran-1-yl 4-(diethylamino)butyrate, hydrochloride. *CAS-73747-21-4. Antiglaucoma agent; antinauseant.* ◇*SP-325*

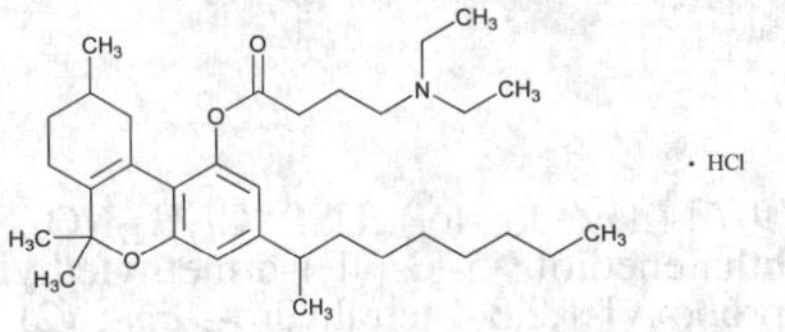

Nabumetone [*1986*] (nab ue′ me tone). USP. $C_{15}H_{16}O_2$. 228.29. (1) 2-Butanone, 4-(6-methoxy-2-naphthalenyl)-; (2) 4-(6-Methoxy-2-naphthyl)-2-butanone. *UNII-LW0TIW155Z. CAS-42924-53-8.* INN; BAN; JAN. *Anti-inflammatory.* Relafen (GlaxoSmithKline) ◇*BRL 14777*

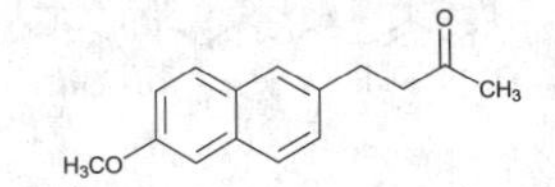

Nabutan Hydrochloride (previously used name) — *See* Nabitan Hydrochloride.

Nacartocin. $C_{46}H_{71}N_{11}O_{11}S$. 986.19. 1-(3-Mercaptopropionic acid)-2-[3-(*p*-ethylphenyl)-L-alanine]-6-(L-2-aminobutyric acid)oxytocin. *CAS-77727-10-7.* INN.

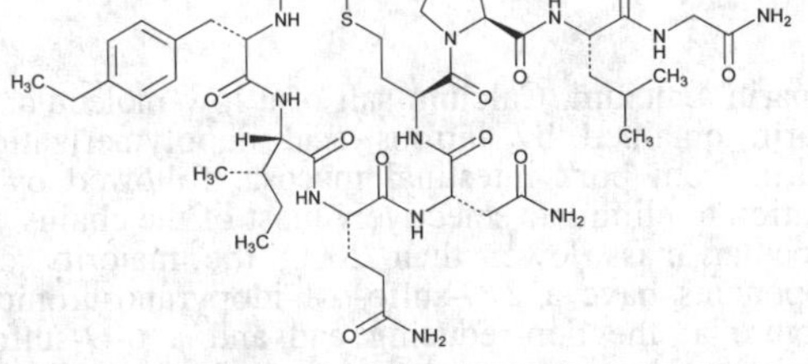

Nacolomab Tafenatox. Immunoglobulin G1, anti-(human colorectal tumor antigen C242) Fab fragment (mouse monoclonal r-C242Fab-SEA clone pkP941 γl-chain)

fusion protein with enterotoxin A (*Staphylococcus aureus*), disulfide with mouse monoclonal r-C242Fab-SEA clone pkP941 κ-chain. *CAS-150631-27-9.* INN.

Nadide [*1967*] (nay′ dide). $C_{21}H_{27}N_7O_{14}P_2$. 663.43. (1) Adenosine 5′-(trihydrogen diphosphate), 5′→5′-ester with 3-(aminocarbonyl)-1-β-D-ribofuranosylpyridinium, hydroxide, inner salt; (2) 3-Carbamoyl-1-β-D-ribofuranosyl-pyridinium hydroxide, 5′-ester with adenosine 5′-pyrophosphate, inner salt; (3) Codehydrogenase I. *CAS-53-84-9.* INN; BAN; JAN. *Antagonist (to alcohol and narcotics). [Names previously used: Diphosphopyridine Nucleotide; Nicotinamide Adenine Dinucleotide.]* ◇*DPN; CO-I; NAD; NSC-20272*

Nadifloxacin. $C_{19}H_{21}FN_2O_4$. 360.38. (±)-9-Fluoro-6,7-dihydro-8-(4-hydroxypiperidino)-5-methyl-1-oxo-1*H*,5*H*-benzo[*ij*]quinolizine-2-carboxylic acid. *CAS-124858-35-1.* INN; BAN; JAN. ◇*OPC-7251*

Nadolol [*1976*] (nay′ doe lol). **USP**. $C_{17}H_{27}NO_4$. 309.40. (1) 2,3-Naphthalenediol, 5-[3-[(1,1-dimethylethyl)amino]-2-hydroxypropoxy]-1,2,3,4-tetrahydro-, *cis*-; (2) 1-(*tert*-Butylamino)-3-[(5,6,7,8-tetrahydro-*cis*-6,7-dihydroxy-1-naphthyl)oxy]-2-propanol. *UNII-FEN504330V.* *CAS-42200-33-9.* INN; BAN; JAN. *Anti-adrenergic (β-receptor).* Corgard (King) ◇*SQ 11725*

Nadoxolol. $C_{14}H_{16}N_2O_3$. 260.29. 3-Hydroxy-4-(1-naphthyloxy)butyramidoxime. *CAS-54063-51-3.* INN; DCF; MI. ◇*LL 1530*

Nadroparin Calcium. Calcium salt of a low molecular mass heparin obtained by nitrous acid depolymerization of heparin from pork intestinal mucosa, followed by fractionation to eliminate selectively most of the chains with a molecular mass lower than 2000; the majority of the components have a 2-*O*-sulfo-α-L-idopyranosuronic acid structure at the non-reducing end and a 6-*O*-sulfo-2,5-anhydro-D-mannitol structure at the reducing end of their chain; the mass-average molecular mass ranges between 3600 and 5000 with a characteristic value of about 4300; the degree of sulfatation is about 2.1 per disaccharidic unit. INN; BAN. ◇*CY 216*

Naepaine Hydrochloride. $C_{14}H_{22}N_2O_2$.HCl. 286.80. (1) Benzoic acid, *p*-amino-, 2-(pentylamino)ethyl ester, hydrochloride; (2) 2-(Pentylamino)ethyl 4-aminobenzoate. *UNII-463O18JU8V.* *CAS-614-42-6; CAS-2188-67-2* [naepaine]. NF XI; MI.

Nafagrel. $C_{15}H_{16}N_2O_2$. 256.30. (±)-5,6,7,8-Tetrahydro-6-(imidazol-1-ylmethyl)-2-naphthoic acid. *UNII-98PDQ9OL4V.* *CAS-97901-21-8.* INN.

Nafamostat Mesylate [*1992*] (na fam′ oh stat mes′ i late). $C_{19}H_{17}N_5O_2$.2CH$_4$O$_3$S. 539.58. [Nafamostat is INN; Nafamostat Mesilate is JAN.] (1) Benzoic acid, 4-[(aminoiminomethyl)amino]-, 6-(aminoiminomethyl)-2-naphthalenyl ester, dimethanesulfonate; (2) 6-Amidino-2-naphthyl *p*-guanidinobenzoate, dimethanesulfonate. *CAS-82956-11-4; CAS-81525-10-2* [nafamostat]. *Anticoagulant; antifibrinolytic.* ◇*FUT-175*

Nafarelin Acetate [*1984*] (naf″ a rel′ in as′ e tate). $C_{66}H_{83}N_{17}O_{13}$.xC$_2$H$_4$O$_2$.yH$_2$O. [Nafarelin is INN and BAN.] (1) Luteinizing hormone-releasing factor (pig), 6-[3-(2-naphthalenyl)-D-alanine]-, acetate (salt), hydrate; (2) 5-Oxo-L-prolyl-L-histidyl-L-tryptophyl-L-seryl-L-tyrosyl-3-(2-naphthyl)-D-alanyl-L-leucyl-L-arginyl-L-prolylglycinamide acetate (salt) hydrate. *UNII-8ENZ0QJW4H; UNII-1X0094V6JV* [nafarelin]. *CAS-86220-42-0; CAS-76932-56-4* [nafarelin]. *LHRH agonist.* Synarel (Pfizer) ◇*RS-94991-298*

Nafazatrom. $C_{16}H_{16}N_2O_2$. 268.31. 3-Methyl-1-[2-(2-naphthyloxy)ethyl]-2-pyrazolin-5-one. *CAS-59040-30-1.* INN; BAN. ◇*Bay g 6575*

Nafcaproic Acid. $C_{16}H_{18}O_2$. 242.31. α,α-Diethyl-1-naphthaleneacetic acid. *UNII-0FI45II3D5. CAS-1085-91-2.* INN. ◇*DA-808*

Nafcillin Sodium [*1963*] (naf sil′ in soe′ dee um). **USP**. $C_{21}H_{21}N_2NaO_5S.H_2O$. 454.47. [Nafcillin is INN and BAN.] (1) 4-Thia-1-azabicyclo[3.2.0]heptane-2-carboxylic acid, 6-[[(2-ethoxy-1-naphthalenyl)carbonyl]amino]-3,3-dimethyl-7-oxo-, monosodium salt, monohydrate, [2S-(2α,5α,6β)]; (2) Monosodium (2S,5R,6R)-6-(2-ethoxy-1-naphthamido)-3,3-dimethyl-7-oxo-4-thia-1-azabicyclo[3.2.0]heptane-2-carboxylate monohydrate. *UNII-49G3001BCK; UNII-4CNZ27M7RV* [nafcillin]. *CAS-7177-50-6; CAS-985-16-0* [anhydrous]; *CAS-147-52-4* [nafcillin]. *Antibacterial.* Nallpen (GlaxoSmithKline); Unipen (Wyeth) ◇*Wy-3277*

Nafenodone. $C_{20}H_{23}NO$. 293.40. (±)-2-[2-(Dimethylamino)ethyl]-3,4-dihydro-2-phenyl-1(2H)-naphthalenone. *UNII-0O501R1CSQ. CAS-92615-20-8.* INN.

Nafenopin [*1970*] (na fen′ oh pin). $C_{20}H_{22}O_3$. 310.39. (1) Propanoic acid, 2-methyl-2-[4-(1,2,3,4-tetrahydro-1-naphthalenyl)phenoxy]-; (2) 2-Methyl-2-[p-(1,2,3,4-tetrahydro-1-naphthyl)phenoxy]propionic acid. *CAS-3771-19-5.* INN; BAN. *Antihyperlipoproteinemic.* ◇*Su-13437*

Nafetolol. $C_{19}H_{29}NO_3$. 319.44. 1-(*tert*-Butylamino)-3-[(1,2,3,4-tetrahydro-8-hydroxy-1,4-ethanonaphthalen-5-yl)oxy]-2-propanol. *CAS-42050-23-7.* INN.

Nafimidone Hydrochloride [*1983*] (naf im′ i done hye″ droe klor′ ide). $C_{15}H_{12}N_2O.HCl$. 272.73. [Nafimidone is INN.] (1) Ethanone, 2-(1H-imidazol-1-yl)-1-(2-naphthalenyl)-,

monohydrochloride; (2) 2-Imidazol-1-yl-2′-acetonaphthone monohydrochloride. *CAS-70891-37-1; CAS-64212-22-2* [nafimidone]. *Anticonvulsant.*

Nafiverine. $C_{34}H_{38}N_2O_4$. 538.68. 1,4-Piperazinediethanol α-methyl-1-naphthaleneacetate ester. *UNII-WLT400RC9Q. CAS-5061-22-3.* INN; MI. ◇*DA-914*

Naflocort [*1984*] (naf′ loe kort). $C_{29}H_{33}FO_4.H_2O$. 482.58. (1) 2′H-Naphtho[2′,3′:16,17]pregna-1,4-diene-3,20-dione, 9-fluoro-1′,4′-dihydro-11,21-dihydroxy-, monohydrate, (11β,16β)-; (2) 9-Fluoro-1′,4′-dihydro-11β,21-dihydroxy-2′βH-naphtho[2′,3′:16,17]pregna-1,4-diene-3,20-dione monohydrate. *CAS-80738-47-2; CAS-59497-39-1* [anhydrous]. INN. *Adrenocortical steroid (topical).* ◇*SQ 26490*

Nafomine Malate [*1970*] (naf′ oh meen mal′ ate). $C_{12}H_{13}NO.C_4H_6O_5$. 321.33. [Nafomine is INN.] (1) Butanedioic acid, hydroxy-, compd. with O-[(2-methyl-1-naphthalenyl)methyl]hydroxylamine (1:1); (2) Malic acid compound with O-[(2-methyl-1-naphthyl)methyl]hydroxylamine (1:1). *CAS-23247-36-1; CAS-46263-35-8* [nafomine]. *Relaxant (muscle).*

Nafoxadol. $C_{15}H_{15}NO_2$. 241.29. 5-(2-Naphthyl)-6,8-dioxa-3-azabicyclo[3.2.1]octane. *CAS-84145-90-4.* INN.

Nafoxidine Hydrochloride [*1965*] (naf ox′ i deen hye″ droe klor′ ide). $C_{29}H_{31}NO_2.HCl$. 462.02. (1) Pyrrolidine 1-[2-[4-(3,4-dihydro-6-methoxy-2-phenyl-1-naphthalenyl)phenoxy]ethyl]-, hydrochloride; (2) 1-[2-[p-(3,4-Dihydro-6-

methoxy-2-phenyl-1-naphthyl)phenoxy]ethyl]pyrrolidine hydrochloride. *CAS-1847-63-8; CAS-1845-11-0* [nafoxidine]. INN. *Anti-estrogen.* ◇*U-11100A; NSC-70735*

Nafronyl Oxalate [*1969*] (naf′ roe nil ox′ a late). $C_{24}H_{33}NO_3 \cdot C_2H_2O_4$. 473.56. [Naftidrofuryl is INN and BAN.] (1) 2-Furanpropanoic acid, tetrahydro-α-(1-naphthalenylmethyl)-, 2-(diethylamino)ethyl ester, ethanedioate (1:1); (2) 2-(Diethylamino)ethyl tetrahydro-α-(1-naphthylmethyl)-2-furanpropionate oxalate (1:1). *CAS-3200-06-4; CAS-31329-57-4* [nafronyl]. *Vasodilator.* Praxilene (Lipha, S.A., France) ◇*EU-1806; LS-121*

Naftalofos [*1972*] (naf tal′ oh fos). $C_{16}H_{16}NO_6P$. 349.28. (1) 1*H*-Benz[*de*]isoquinoline-1,3(2*H*)-dione, 2-[(diethoxyphosphinyl)oxy]-; (2) *N*-Hydroxynaphthalimide diethyl phosphate. *CAS-1491-41-4.* INN; BAN. *Anthelmintic (veterinary).* Maretin (Bayer Animal Health†) [*Name previously used: Naphthalophos.*] ◇*BAY 9002; E 9002; ENT-25567; S-940*

Naftazone. $C_{11}H_9N_3O_2$. 215.21. 1,2-Naphthoquinone 2-semicarbazone. *CAS-15687-37-3.* INN; BAN; DCF.

Naftidrofuryl (INN, BAN, DCF) — *See* Nafronyl Oxalate.

Naftifine Hydrochloride [*1981*] (naf′ ti feen hye″ droe klor′ ide). USP. $C_{21}H_{21}N \cdot HCl$. 323.86. [Naftifine is INN and BAN.] (1) 1-Naphthalenemethanamine, *N*-methyl-*N*-(3-phenyl-2-propenyl)-, hydrochloride, (*E*)-; (2) (*E*)-*N*-Cinnamyl-*N*-methyl-1-naphthalenemethylamine hydrochloride. *UNII-25UR9N9041; UNII-4FB1TON47A* [naftifine]. *CAS-65473-14-5; CAS-65472-88-0* [naftifine]. *Antifungal.* Naftin (Merz) ◇*AW 105-843*

Naftopidil. $C_{24}H_{28}N_2O_3$. 392.49. (±)-4-(*o*-Methoxyphenyl)-α-[(1-naphthyloxy)methyl]-1-piperazineethanol. *UNII-R9PHW59SFN. CAS-57149-07-2.* INN.

Naftoxate. $C_{19}H_{14}N_2OS_2$. 350.46. 2-Benzoxazolyl *N*-methyldithio-1-naphthalenecarbamate. *UNII-2781UEP67S. CAS-28820-28-2.* INN. ◇*K-F 224*

Naftypramide. $C_{19}H_{26}N_2O$. 298.42. α-Isopropyl-α-[2-(dimethylamino)ethyl]-1-naphthaleneacetamide. *CAS-1505-95-9.* INN. ◇*DA-992*

Naglivan. $C_{22}H_{46}N_4O_3S_2V$. 529.70. Bis[2-amino-3-mercapto-*N*-octylpropionamidato(1-)-*S*]oxovanadium. *CAS-122575-28-4.* INN.

Nagrestipen [*1997*] (na gres′ ti pen). $C_{338}H_{516}N_{88}O_{108}S_4$. 7668.50. 26-L-Alaninelymphokine MIP 1α (human clone pAT464 macrophage inflammatory). *CAS-166089-33-4.* INN; BAN. *Hematopoietic inhibitor.* ◇*BB-10010*

SLAADTPTAC CFSYTSRQIP QNFIAAYFET SSQCSLPGVI FLTKRSRQVC
ADPSEEWVQK YVSDLELSA

Nalazosulfamide — *See* Salazosulfamide.

Nalbuphine Hydrochloride [*1968*] (nal′ bue feen hye″ droe klor′ ide). $C_{21}H_{27}NO_4 \cdot HCl$. 393.90. [Nalbuphine is INN and BAN.] (1) Morphinan-3,6,14-triol, 17-(cyclobutylmethyl)-4,5-epoxy-, hydrochloride, (5α,6α)-; (2) 17-(Cyclobutylmethyl)-4,5α-epoxymorphinan-3,6α,14-triol hydrochloride. *UNII-ZU4275277R; UNII-L2T841QI2K* [nalbuphine]. *CAS-23277-43-2; CAS-20594-83-6* [nalbuphine]. *Analgesic; antagonist (to narcotics).* Nubain (Endo) ◇*EN-2234A*

Nalfurafine Hydrochloride [*2006*] (nal fure′ a feen hye″ droe klor′ ide). $C_{28}H_{32}N_2O_5 \cdot HCl$. 513.03. [Nalfurafine is INN.] (1) 2-Propenamide, N-[(5α,6β)-17-(cyclopropylmethyl)-4,5-epoxy-3,14-dihydroxymorphinan-6-yl]-3-(3-furanyl)-N-methyl-, monohydrochloride, (2E)-; (2) (E)-N-[17-(Cyclopropylmethyl)-4,5α-epoxy-3,14-dihydroxymorphinan-6β-yl]-3-(furan-3-yl)-N-methylprop-2-enamide monohydrochloride; (3) (-)-17-(Cyclopropylmethyl-3,14 β-dihydroxy-4,5 α-epoxy-6 β-[N-methyl-trans-3-(3-furyl)acrylamido]morphinan hydrochloride. *UNII-25CC4N0P8J. CAS-152658-17-8; CAS-152657-84-6* [nalfurafine]. JAN. *Treatment of uremic pruritus in hemodialysis patients.* ◇*TRK-820*

Nalidixane — *See* Nalidixic Acid.

Nalidixate Sodium [*1967*] (nal i dix′ ate soe′ dee um). $C_{12}H_{11}N_2NaO_3H_2O$. 272.23. (1) 1,8-Naphthyridine-3-carboxylic acid, 1-ethyl-1,4-dihydro-7-methyl-4-oxo-, sodium salt, monohydrate; (2) Sodium 1-ethyl-1,4-dihydro-7-methyl-4-oxo-1,8-naphthyridine-3-carboxylate monohydrate. *UNII-J17QL41ZAG; UNII-3B91HWA56M* [nalidixic acid]. *CAS-15769-77-4; CAS-3374-05-8* [anhydrous]; *CAS-389-08-2* [nalidixic acid]. *Antibacterial.* ◇*Win 18,320-3*

Nalidixic Acid [*1962*] (nal i dix′ ik as′ id). USP. $C_{12}H_{12}N_2O_3$. 232.24. (1) 1,8-Naphthyridine-3-carboxylic acid, 1-ethyl-1,4-dihydro-7-methyl-4-oxo-; (2) 1-Ethyl-1,4-dihydro-7-methyl-4-oxo-1,8-naphthyridine-3-carboxylic acid. *UNII-3B91HWA56M. CAS-389-08-2.* INN; BAN; JAN. *Antibacterial.* Neggram (Sanofi Aventis) ◇*Win 18,320; NSC-82174*

Nalmefene [*1981*] (nal′ me feen). $C_{21}H_{25}NO_3$. 339.43. (1) Morphinan-3,14-diol, 17-(cyclopropylmethyl)-4,5-epoxy-6-methylene-, (5α)-; (2) 17-(Cyclopropylmethyl)-4,5α-epoxy-6-methylenemorphinan-3,14-diol. *UNII-TOV02TD-*

P9I. CAS-55096-26-9. INN; BAN. *Antagonist (to narcotics). [Name previously used: Nalmetrene.]* ◇*JF-1; ORF 11676*

Nalmetrene (previously used name) — *See* Nalmefene.

Nalmexone Hydrochloride [*1967*] (nal mex′ one hye″ droe klor′ ide). $C_{21}H_{25}NO_4 \cdot HCl$. 391.89. [Nalmexone is INN.] (1) Morphinan-6-one, 4,5-epoxy-3,14-dihydroxy-17-(3-methyl-2-butenyl)-, hydrochloride, (5α)-; (2) 4,5α-Epoxy-3,14-dihydroxy-17-(3-methyl-2-butenyl)morphinan-6-one hydrochloride. *CAS-16676-27-0; CAS-16291-05-7* [replaced]; *CAS-16676-26-9* [nalmexone]. *Analgesic; antagonist (to narcotics).* ◇*EN-1620A*

Nalorphine Hydrochloride (nal or′ feen hye″ droe klor′ ide). USP. $C_{19}H_{21}NO_3 \cdot HCl$. 347.84. [Nalorphine is INN and BAN.] (1) Morphinan-3,6-diol, 7,8-didehydro-4,5-epoxy-17-(2-propenyl)-(5α,6α)-, hydrochloride; (2) 17-Allyl-7,8-didehydro-4,5α-epoxymorphinan-3,6α-diol hydrochloride. *UNII-9FPE56Z2TW. CAS-57-29-4; CAS-62-67-9* [nalorphine]. Nalline [Veterinary] (Merial)

Naloxiphane Tartrate — *See* Levallorphan Tartrate.

Naloxone Hydrochloride [*1963*] (nal ox′ one hye″ droe klor′ ide). USP. $C_{19}H_{21}NO_4 \cdot HCl$. 363.84. [Naloxone is INN and BAN.] (1) Morphinan-6-one, 4,5-epoxy-3,14-dihydroxy-17-(2-propenyl)-, hydrochloride, (5α)-; (2) 17-Allyl-4,5α-epoxy-3,14-dihydroxymorphinan-6-one hydrochloride; (3) (-)-N-Allyl-14-hydroxynordihydromorphinone hydrochloride. *UNII-F850569PQR; UNII-36B82AMQ7N* [naloxone]. *CAS-357-08-4; CAS-51481-60-8* [dihydrate]; *CAS-465-65-6* [naloxone]. JAN. *Antagonist (to narcotics).* Narcan (Bristol-Myers Squibb) ◇*EN-15304*

Naltrexone [*1973*] (nal trex′ one). $C_{20}H_{23}NO_4$. 341.40. (1) Morphinan-6-one, 17-(cyclopropylmethyl)-4,5-epoxy-3,14-dihydroxy-, (5α)-; (2) 17-(Cyclopropylmethyl)-4,5α-epoxy-3,14-dihydroxymorphinan-6-one. *UNII-*

---

† Brand name formerly used, and/or firm no longer concerned with this product.

5S6W795CQM. CAS-16590-41-3. INN; BAN. *Antagonist (to narcotics).* Vivitrol (Alkermes) ◇*EN-1639A [as hydrochloride]*

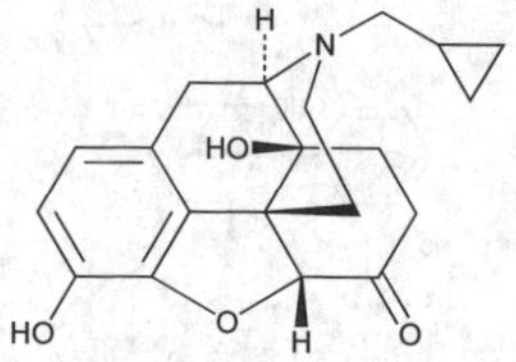

Naltrexone Hydrochloride (nal trex′ one hye″ droe klor′ ide). USP. $C_{20}H_{23}NO_4 \cdot HCl$. 377.86. (1) Morphinan-6-one, 17-(cyclopropylmethyl)-4,5-epoxy-3,14-dihydroxy-, hydrochloride, (5α)-; (2) 17-Cyclopropylmethyl-4,5α-epoxy-3,14-dihydroxymorphinan-6-one hydrochloride. *UNII-Z6375YW9SF. CAS-16676-29-2.* Revia (Duramed) ◇*EN-1639A*

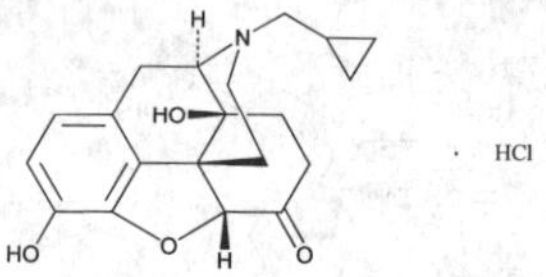

Naluzotan [*2008*] (nal″ ue zoe′ tan). $C_{23}H_{38}N_4O_3S$. 450.64. (1) Acetamide, *N*-[3-[4-[4-[[(cyclohexylmethyl)sulfonyl]amino]butyl]-1-piperazinyl]phenyl]-; (2) *N*-{3-[4-(4-{[(Cyclohexylmethyl)sulfonyl]amino}butyl)piperazin-1-yl]phenyl}acetamide. *UNII-LQ54E5B4EW. CAS-740873-06-7. Treatment of psychiatric disorders.* ◇*PRX-00023*

Naluzotan Hydrochloride [*2008*] (nal″ ue zoe′ tan hye″ droe klor′ ide). $C_{23}H_{38}N_4O_3S \cdot HCl$. 487.10. (1) Acetamide, *N*-[3-[4-[4-[[(cyclohexylmethyl)sulfonyl]amino]butyl]-1-piperazinyl]phenyl]-, monohydrochloride; (2) *N*-{3-[4-(4-{[(Cyclohexylmethyl)sulfonyl]amino}butyl)piperazin-1-yl]phenyl}acetamide hydrochloride. *UNII-7F2X95XC2A. CAS-740873-82-9. Treatment of depression and anxiety disorders.*

Naminidil [*2002*] (na min′ i dil). $C_{15}H_{19}N_5$. 269.34. (1) Guanidine, *N*-cyano-*N*′-(4-cyanophenyl)-*N*″-[(1*R*)-1,2,2-trimethylpropyl]-; (2) *N*-Cyano-*N*′-(4-cyanophenyl)-*N*″-[(1*R*)-1,2,2-trimethylpropyl] guanidine. *UNII-7K50VT05OD. CAS-220641-11-2.* INN. *Treatment of hair loss; an ATP-sensitive potassium channel vasodilator.* ◇*BMS-234303-01*

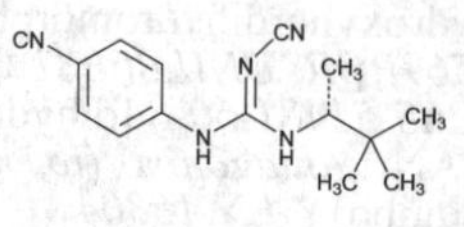

Naminterol. $C_{19}H_{26}N_2O_3$. 330.42. 5-Amino-α-[[(*p*-methoxy-α-methylphenethyl)amino]methyl]-*m*-xylene-α,α′-diol. *CAS-93047-40-6.* INN.

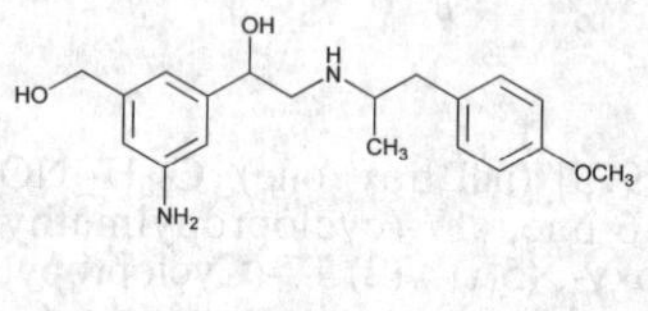

Namirotene. $C_{17}H_{18}O_2S$. 286.39. *p*-[(*E*)-2-(5-Isopropyl-2-thienyl)propenyl]benzoic acid. *CAS-101506-83-6.* INN.

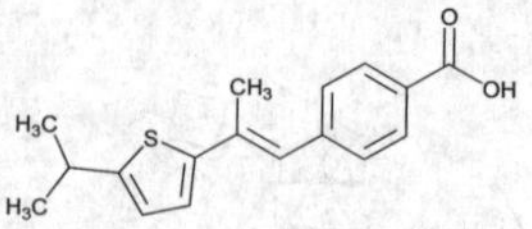

Namoxyrate [*1965*] (na mox′ i rate). $C_{16}H_{16}O_2 \cdot C_4H_{11}NO$. 329.43. (1) [1,1′-Biphenyl]-4-acetic acid, α-ethyl-, compd. with 2-(dimethylamino)ethanol (1:1); (2) α-Ethyl-4-biphenylacetic acid, compound with 2-dimethylaminoethanol (1:1). *CAS-1234-71-5.* INN. *Analgesic.* ◇*W 1760A*

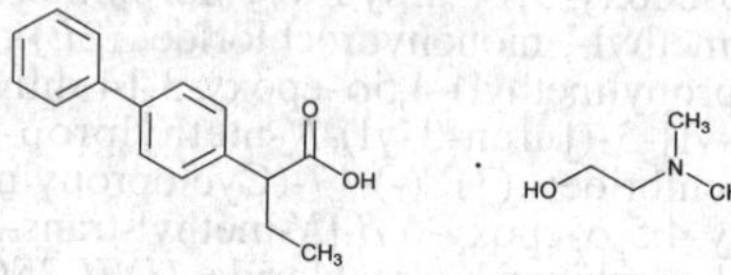

Nanafrocin. $C_{16}H_{14}O_6$. 302.28. (1*S*,3*R*)-3,4,5,10-Tetrahydro-9-hydroxy-1-methyl-5,10-dioxo-1*H*-naphtho-[2,3-*c*]pyran-3-acetic acid. *UNII-8XBV72641V. CAS-52934-83-5.* INN.

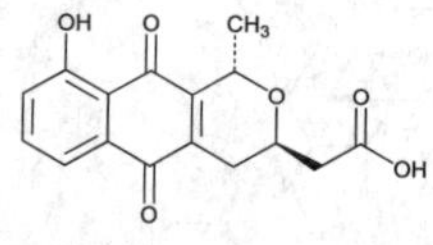

Nandrolone Cyclotate [*1972*] (nan′ droe lone sye′ kloe tate). $C_{28}H_{38}O_3$. 422.60. [Nandrolone is BAN; Nandrolone Cyclohexylpropionate is JAN.] (1) Estr-4-en-3-one, 17-[[(4-methylbicyclo[2.2.2]oct-2-en-1-yl)carbonyl]oxy]-, (17β)-; (2) 17β-Hydroxyestr-4-en-3-one 4-methylbicyclo[2.2.2]oct-2-ene-1-carboxylate. *CAS-22263-51-0. Anabolic.* ◇*RS-3268R*

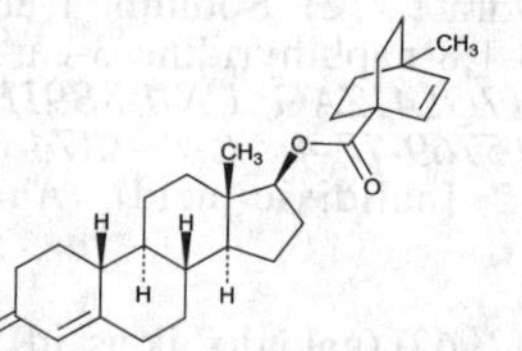

Nandrolone Decanoate [*1965*] (nan′ droe lone dek″ a noe′ ate). USP. $C_{28}H_{44}O_3$. 428.65. (1) Estr-4-en-3-one, 17-[(1-oxodecyl)oxy]-, (17β)-; (2) 17β-Hydroxyestr-4-en-3-one decanoate. *UNII-H45187T098. CAS-360-70-3.* JAN. *Androgen.* Durabolin (Organon)

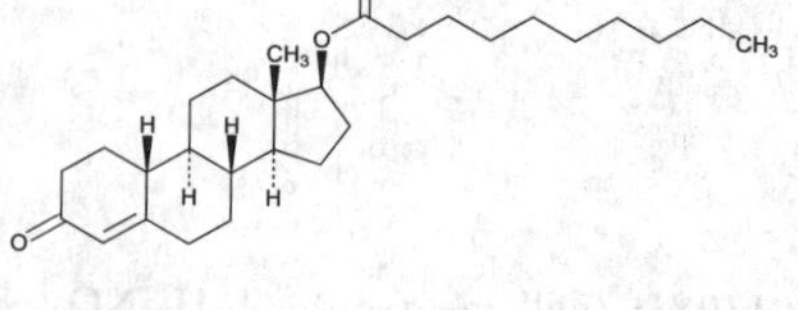

Nandrolone Phenpropionate (nan′ droe lone fen proe′ pee oh nate). USP. $C_{27}H_{34}O_3$. 406.56. [Nortestosterone Furanpropionate and Nandrolone Phenylpropionate are JAN.] (1) Estr-4-en-3-one, 17-(1-oxo-3-phenylpropoxy)-, (17β)-; (2) 17β-Hydroxyestr-4-en-3-one hydrocinnamate. *UNII-KF7Z9K2T3W. CAS-62-90-8. Androgen.* Durabolin (Organon) ◇*NSC-23162*

Naniopine — *See* Nanofin.

Nanofin. $C_7H_{15}N$. 113.20. 2,6-Lupetidine. *UNII-329I5805BP. CAS-504-03-0.* INN.

Nanterinone. $C_{15}H_{15}N_3O$. 253.30. 6-(2,4-Dimethylimidazol-1-yl)-8-methyl-2-quinolone. *UNII-1S169L7KAV. CAS-102791-47-9; CAS-102791-74-2* [mesylate]. INN; BAN. ◇*UK-61260-27*

Nantradol Hydrochloride [*1979*] (nan′ tra dol hye″ droe klor′ ide). $C_{27}H_{35}NO_4·HCl$. 474.03. [Nantradol is INN.] (1) 1,9-Phenanthridinediol, 5,6,6a,7,8,9,10,10a-octahydro-6-methyl-3-(1-methyl-4-phenylbutoxy)-, 1-acetate, hydrochloride; (2) (±)-5,6,6aβ,7,8,9α,10,10aα-Octahydro-6β-methyl-3-(1-methyl-4-phenylbutoxy)-1,9-phenanthridine-diol 1-acetate, hydrochloride. *UNII-CVN9D598JL. CAS-65511-42-4; CAS-65511-41-3* [nantradol]. *Analgesic.* ◇*CP-44,001-1*

Napactadine Hydrochloride [*1981*] (na pak′ ta deen hye″ droe klor′ ide). $C_{14}H_{16}N_2·HCl$. 248.75. [Napactadine is INN.] (1) 2-Naphthaleneethanimidamide, *N,N′*-dimethyl-, monohydrochloride; (2) *N,N′*-Dimethyl-2-naphthalene-acetamidine monohydrochloride. *CAS-57166-13-9. Anti-depressant.* ◇*DL-588*

Napamezole Hydrochloride [*1985*] (na pam′ e zole hye″ droe klor′ ide). $C_{14}H_{16}N_2·HCl$. 248.75. [Napamezole is INN.] (1) 1*H*-Imidazole, 2-[(3,4-dihydro-2-naphthalenyl)-methyl]-4,5-dihydro-, monohydrochloride; (2) 2-[(3,4-Di-hydro-2-naphthyl)methyl]-2-imidazoline monohydrochlor-ide. *UNII-DTN86H1ZWK. CAS-87495-33-8; CAS-91524-14-0* [napamezole]. *Antidepressant.* ◇*Win 51,181-2*

Naphazoline Hydrochloride (naf az′ oh leen hye″ droe klor′ ide). USP. $C_{14}H_{14}N_2·HCl$. 246.74. [Naphazoline is INN and BAN; Naphazoline Nitrate is JAN.] (1) 1*H*-Imidazole, 4,5-dihydro-2-(1-naphthalenylmethyl)-, monohydrochloride;

(2) 2-(1-Naphthylmethyl)-2-imidazoline monohydrochlor-ide. *UNII-MZ1131787D; UNII-H231GF11BV* [naphazo-line]. *CAS-550-99-2; CAS-835-31-4* [naphazoline]. JAN. *Adrenergic (vasoconstrictor).* Albalon (Allergan); Nafazair (Bausch & Lomb); Naphcon (Alcon); Vasocon (Novartis)

Naphthalophos (previously used name) — *See* Naftalofos.

Naphthonone. $C_{16}H_{16}O_2$. 240.30. 2-(2-Hydroxynaphth-1-yl)-cyclohexanone. *UNII-229YMD7GRO. CAS-7114-11-6.* INN; DCF.

Naphthypramide — *See* Naftypramide.

Naphuride — *See* Suramin Hexasodium.

Napirimus. $C_{17}H_{13}NO_3$. 279.29. 1-Methyl-4-(1-naphthoyl)-pyrrole-2-carboxylic acid. *UNII-45081SG6XT. CAS-70696-66-1.* INN.

Napitane Mesylate [*1996*] (na′ pi tane mes′ i late). $C_{22}H_{25}NO_2·CH_4O_3S$. 431.55. [Napitane is INN.] (1) Pyrrolidine, 3-phenyl-1-[(6,7,8,9-tetrahydronaphtho[1,2-*d*]-1,3-dioxol-6-yl)methyl]-, (*R**,*R**)-(±)-, methanesulfo-nate; (2) (±)-(3*R**)-3-Phenyl-1-[[(6*R**)-6,7,8,9-tetrahydro-naphtho[1,2-*d*]-1,3-dioxol-6-yl]methyl]pyrrolidine meth-anesulfonate. *CAS-149189-73-1; CAS-148152-63-0* [napi-tane]. *Antidepressant.* ◇*A-75200 mesylate*

Naprodoxime. $C_{13}H_{14}N_2O_2$. 230.26. 2-(1-Naphthyloxy)pro-pionamidoxime. *CAS-57925-64-1.* INN.

Naproxcinod [*2008*] (na prox′ sin od). $C_{18}H_{21}NO_6$. 347.36. (1) 2-Naphthaleneacetic acid, 6-methoxy-α-methyl-, 4-(nitrooxy)butyl ester, (α*S*)-; (2) 4-(Nitrooxy)butyl (2*S*)-2-

---

(6-methoxynaphthalen-2-yl)propanoate. *CAS-163133-43-5.* INN. *Osteoarthritis.* ◇*HCT 3012; AZD3582; AR-P900758XX*

Naproxen [*1970*] (na prox′ en). **USP**. $C_{14}H_{14}O_3$. 230.26. (1) 2-Naphthaleneacetic acid, 6-methoxy-α-methyl-, (*S*)-; (2) (+)-(*S*)-6-Methoxy-α-methyl-2-naphthaleneacetic acid. *UNII-57Y76R9ATQ. CAS-22204-53-1.* INN; BAN; JAN. *Anti-inflammatory; analgesic; antipyretic.* Naprosyn (Roche) ◇*RS-3540*

Naproxen Sodium [*1973*] (na prox′ en soe′ dee um). **USP**. $C_{14}H_{13}NaO_3$. 252.24. (1) 2-Naphthaleneacetic acid, 6-methoxy-α-methyl-, sodium salt, (*S*)-; (2) (-)-Sodium (*S*)-6-methoxy-α-methyl-2-naphthaleneacetate. *UNII-9TN87S3A3C; UNII-57Y76R9ATQ* [naproxen]. *CAS-26159-34-2; CAS-22204-53-1* [naproxen]. *Anti-inflammatory; analgesic; antipyretic.* Aleve (Bayer) ◇*RS-3650*

Naproxol [*1970*] (na prox′ ol). $C_{14}H_{16}O_2$. 216.28. (1) 2-Naphthaleneethanol, 6-methoxy-β-methyl-, (*S*)-; (2) (-)-(*S*)-6-Methoxy-β-methyl-2-naphthaleneethanol. *CAS-26159-36-4.* INN. *Anti-inflammatory; analgesic; antipyretic.* ◇*RS-4034*

Napsagatran [*1995*] (nap″ sa gat′ ran). $C_{26}H_{34}N_6O_6S.H_2O$. 576.67. (1) Glycine, *N*-[*N*-[[1-(aminoiminomethyl)-3-piperidinyl]methyl]-N^2-(2-naphthalenylsulfonyl)-L-asparaginyl]-*N*-cyclopropyl-, monohydrate, (*S*)-; (2) *N*-[N^4-[[(3*S*-1-Amidino-3-piperidyl]methyl]-N^2-(2-naphthylsulfonyl)-L-asparaginyl]-*N*-cyclopropylglycine monohydrate. *CAS-159668-20-9.* INN. *Antithrombotic.* ◇*Ro 46-6240/010*

Naptumomab Estafenatox. $C_{3255}H_{5025}N_{855}O_{1050}S_{18}$. Immunoglobulin fragment, anti-[trophoblast glycoprotein (TPBG, 5T4)] monoclonal 5T4 gamma1 heavy chain fragment fusion protein [*Mus musculus* VH (5T4V14: H41>P, S44>G, I69>T, V113>G)-IGHG1CH1)] - [Glycyl-Glycyl-Prolyl] - superantigen SEA/E-120 (synthetic), non-disulfide linked with monoclonal 5T4 kappa light chain [*Mus musculus* V-KAPPA (5T4V18: F10>S, T45>K, I63>S, F73>L, T77>S, L78>V, L83>A)-IGKC]. *CAS-676258-98-3.* INN.

Naranol Hydrochloride [*1971*] (nar′ a nol hye″ droe klor′ ide). $C_{18}H_{21}NO_2.HCl$. 319.83. [Naranol is INN.] (1) 7a*H*-Naphtho[1′,2′:5,6]pyrano[3,2-*c*]pyridin-7a-ol,

8,9,10,11,11a,12-hexahydro-8,10-dimethyl-, hydrochloride; (2) 8,9,10,11,11a,12-Hexahydro-8,10-dimethyl-7a*H*-naphtho[1′,2′:5:6]pyrano[3,2-*c*]pyridin-7a-ol hydrochloride. *CAS-34256-91-2; CAS-22292-91-7* [naranol]. *Antipsychotic.* ◇*W 5494A*

Narasin [*1976*] (nar′ a sin). **USP** [Granular]. $C_{43}H_{72}O_{11}$ (narasin A). 765.03; $C_{43}H_{71}O_{11}$ (narasin B). 764.02; $C_{44}H_{74}O_{11}$ (narasin D). 779.05; $C_{44}H_{74}O_{11}$ (narasin I). 779.05. (1) 2*H*-Pyran-2-acetic acid, α-ethyl-6-[5-[2-(5-ethyltetrahydro-5-hydroxy-6-methyl-2*H*-pyran-2-yl)-15-hydroxy-2,10,12-trimethyl-1,6,8-trioxadispiro[4.1.5.3]pentadec-13-en-9-yl]-2-hydroxy-1,3-dimethyl-4-oxoheptyl]tetrahydro-3,5-dimethyl-; (2) α-Ethyl-6-[5-[2-(5-ethyltetrahydro-5-hydroxy-6-methyl-2*H*-pyran-2-yl)-15-hydroxy-2,10,12-trimethyl-1,6,8-trioxadispiro[4.1.5.3]pentadec-13-en-9-yl]-2-hydroxy-1,3-dimethyl-4-oxoheptyl]tetrahydro-3,5-dimethyl-2*H*-pyran-2-acetic acid. *UNII-DZY9VU539P. CAS-55134-13-9.* INN; BAN. *Coccidiostat; growth stimulant (veterinary).* Monteban (Lilly) ◇*Compound 79891*

Naratriptan. $C_{17}H_{25}N_3O_2S$. 335.46. *N*-Methyl-2-[3-(1-methyl-piperiden-4-yl)indole-5-yl]ethanesulfonamide. *UNII-QX3KXL1ZA2. CAS-121679-13-8.* INN; BAN.

Naratriptan Hydrochloride [*1993*] (nar″ a trip′ tan hye″ droe klor′ ide). **USP**. $C_{17}H_{25}N_3O_2S.HCl$. 371.93. (1) 1*H*-Indole-5-ethanesulfonamide, *N*-methyl-3-(1-methyl-4-piperidinyl)-, monohydrochloride; (2) *N*-Methyl-3-(1-methyl-4-piperidyl)indole-5-ethanesulfonamide monohydrochloride. *UNII-10X8X4P12Z; UNII-QX3KXL1ZA2* [naratriptan]. *CAS-143388-64-1; CAS-121679-13-8* [naratriptan]. *Antimigraine.* Amerge (GlaxoSmithKline) ◇*GR 85548A*

Narcotine — *See* Noscapine.

Narcotine Hydrochloride — *See* Noscapine Hydrochloride.

Nardeterol. $C_{20}H_{24}FN_3O_2$. 357.42. (±)-α-[[[3-(1-Benzimidazolyl)-1,1-dimethylpropyl]amino]methyl]-2-fluoro-4-hydroxybenzyl alcohol. *UNII-70859437W3. CAS-73865-18-6.* INN.

Naroparcil. $C_{19}H_{17}NO_4S_2$. 387.47. *p*-[*p*-[(5-Thio-β-D-xylopyranosyl)thio]benzoyl]benzonitrile. *UNII-238M5105OY. CAS-120819-70-7.* INN.

Nartograstim. $C_{850}H_{1344}N_{226}O_{245}S_8$ (for non-glycosylated protein). 18,905.67. *N*-L-Methionyl-1-L-alanine-3-L-threonine-4-L-tyrosine-5-L-arginine-17-L-serinecolony-stimulating factor (human clone 1034). *CAS-134088-74-7.* INN; JAN.

Nasaruplase. $C_{2031}H_{3121}N_{585}O_{601}S_{31}$. 46,343.14. Prourokinase (enzyme-activating) (human clone pA3/pD2/pF1 protein moiety), glycosylated. *CAS-99821-44-0.* INN.

Nasaruplase Beta [*1999*] (na sar′ ue plase bay″ ta). $C_{2031}H_{3121}N_{585}O_{601}S_{31}$ (amino acid sequence). (1) Kinase (enzyme-activating), prouro-(human clone pUK4/pUK18); (2) Prourokinase (enzyme-activating)(human clone pUK4/pUK18 protein moiety), glycosylated. Molecular weight is approximately 49,500 daltons, including a carbohydrate moiety of approximately 3,000 daltons. *UNII-SYW4Z0B3KN. CAS-136653-69-5.* INN. *Treatment of acute ischemic stroke (fibrinolytic).* Prolyse (Abbott) ◇*Abbott-74187; ABT-187*

```
SNELHQVPSN   CDCLNGGTCV*  SNKYFSNIHW   CNCPKKFGGQ   HCEIDKSKTC

YEGNGHFYRG   KASTDTMGRP   CLPWNSATVL   QQTYHAHRSD   ALQLGLGKHN

YCRNPDNRRR   PWCYVQVGLK   PLVQECMVHD   CADGKKPSSP   PEELKFQCGQ

KTLRPRFKII   GGEFTTIENQ   PWFAAIYRRH   RGGSVTYVCG   GSLMSPCWVI

SATHCFIDYP   KKEDYIVYLG   RSRLNSNTQG   EMKFEVENLI   LHKDYSADTL

AHHNDIALLK   IRSKEGRCAQ   PSRTIQTICL   PSMYNDPQFG   TSCEITGFGK

ENSTDYLYPE*  QLKMTVVKLI   SHRECQQPHY   YGSEVTTKML   CAADPQWKTD

SCQGDSGGPL   VCSLQGRMTL   TGIVSWGRGC   ALKDKPGVYT   RVSHFLPWIR

SHTKEENGLA   L
```

* glycosylation sites

Natalizumab [*1998*] (na″ ta liz′ oo mab). Immunoglobulin G 4 (human-mouse monoclonal AN100226 4-chain anti-human integrin 4), disulfide with human-mouse monoclonal AN100226 light chain, dimer. *UNII-3JB47N2Q2P. CAS-189261-10-7.* INN.

Natamycin [*1977*] (na″ ta mye′ sin). **USP.** $C_{33}H_{47}NO_{13}$. 665.73. [Pimaricin is JAN.] (1) Pimaricin; (2) Stereoisomer of 22-[(3-amino-3,6-dideoxy-β-D-mannopyranosyl)oxy]-1,3,26-trihydroxy-12-methyl-10-oxo-6,11,28-trioxatricyclo[22.3.1.0⁵,⁷]octacosa-8,14,16,18,20-pentaene-25-carboxylic acid. *UNII-8O0C852CPO. CAS-7681-93-8.* INN; BAN. *Antibacterial (ophthalmic).* Natacyn (Alcon) ◇*CL 12,625; Antibiotic A-5283*

Nateglinide [*2000*] (na te glye′ nide). $C_{19}H_{27}NO_3$. 317.42. (1) D-Phenylalanine, *N*-[[*trans*-4-(1-methylethyl)cyclohexyl]carbonyl]-; (2) (-)-*N*-[(*trans*-4-Isopropylcyclohexyl)carbonyl]-D-phenylalanine. *UNII-41X3PWK4O2. CAS-105816-04-4.* INN; BAN. *Antidiabetic used in the treatment of Type II diabetes mellitus.* Starlix (Novartis) ◇*A-4166; AY4166; DJN 608; SDZ DJN 608*

Nateplase. A mixture of *N*-[*N*²-(*N*-Glycyl-L-alanyl)-L-arginyl]plasminogen activator (human tissue-type 1-chain form, protein moiety), glycoform β (major component) and plasminogen activator (human tissue-type 1-chain form, protein moiety), glycoform β. *CAS-159445-63-3.* INN.

Naveglitazar [*2004*] (nav″ e gli′ ta zar). $C_{25}H_{26}O_6$. 422.47. (1) Benzenepropanoic acid, α-methoxy-4-[3-(4-phenoxyphenoxy)propoxy]-, (α*S*)-; (2) (2*S*)-2-Methoxy-3-[4-[3-(4-phenoxyphenoxy)propoxy]phenyl]propanoic acid. *UNII-Y995M7GM0G. CAS-476436-68-7.* INN. *Treatment of Type II diabetes and associated cardiovascular indications.* ◇*LY9818; LY519818*

Navuridine. $C_9H_{11}N_5O_4$. 253.21. 3′-Azido-2′,3′-dideoxyuridine. *CAS-84472-85-5.* INN.

Naxagolide Hydrochloride [*1989*] (nax ag′ oh lide hye″ droe klor′ ide). $C_{15}H_{21}NO_2 \cdot HCl$. 283.79. [Naxagolide is INN.] (1) 2*H*-Naphth[1,2-*b*]-1,4-oxazin-9-ol, 3,4,4a,5,6,10b-hexahydro-4-propyl-, hydrochloride, (4a*R-trans*)-; (2) (+)-(4a*R*,10b*R*)-3,4,4a,5,6,10b-Hexahydro-4-propyl-2*H*-

---

† Brand name formerly used, and/or firm no longer concerned with this product.

naphth[1,2-*b*]-1,4-oxazin-9-ol hydrochloride. *CAS-99705-65-4; CAS-88058-88-2* [naxagolide]. *Antiparkinsonian; dopamine agonist.* ◇*MK-458; L-647,339*

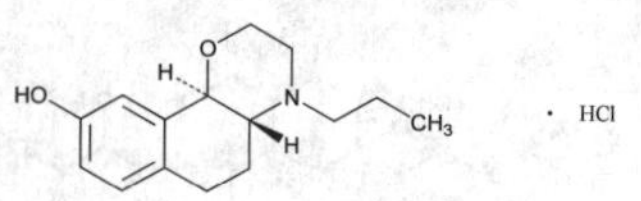

Naxaprostene. $C_{25}H_{32}O_4$. 396.52. α-[(2*E*,3a*S*,4*R*,5*R*,6a*S*)-4-[(1*E*,3*S*)-3-Cyclohexyl-3-hydroxypropenyl]hexahydro-5-hydroxy-2(1*H*)-pentalenylidene]-*m*-toluic acid. *CAS-87269-59-8.* INN.

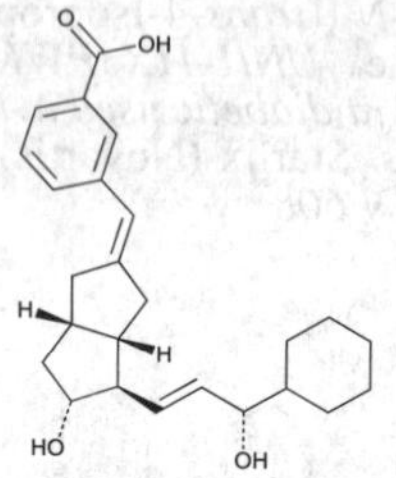

Naxifylline [*2002*] (nax if′ i lin). $C_{18}H_{24}N_4O_3$. 344.41. (1) 1*H*-Purine-2,6-dione, 3,7-dihydro-8-(3-oxatricyclo[3.2.1.0²,⁴]oct-6-yl)-1,3-dipropyl-, [1*S*-(1α,2β,4β,5α,6α)]-; (2) 8-[(2*S*,5,6-*exo*)-5,6-epoxy-2-norbonyl]-1,3-dipropylxanthine. *CAS-166374-49-8.* INN. *Treatment of edema associated with congestive heart failure.* ◇*BG9719; CVT-124*

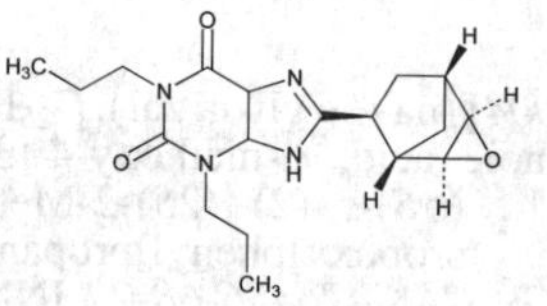

9-NC (previously used name) — *See* Rubitecan.

Nealbarbital. $C_{12}H_{18}N_2O_3$. 238.28. 5-Allyl-5-neopentylbarbituric acid. *UNII-25ATP958PA. CAS-561-83-1.* INN; BAN; MI. [*Name previously used: Nealbarbitone.*]

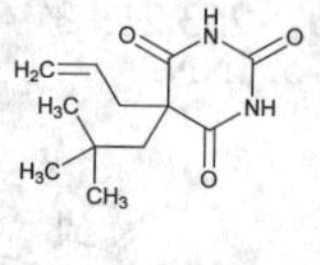

Nebacumab [*1993*] (ne bak′ ue mab). (1) Immunoglobulin M (human monoclonal HA-1A anti-endotoxin), disulfide with human monoclonal HA-1A κ-chain, pentameric dimer; (2) Immunoglobulin M (human monoclonal HA-1A anti-endotoxin), disulfide with human monoclonal HA-1A κ-chain, pentameric dimer. Molecular weight is approximately 1,000,000 daltons. *CAS-138661-01-5.* INN; BAN. *Monoclonal antibody (anti-endotoxin).* Centoxin (Centocor†) [*Name previously used: Septomonab*] ◇*HA-1A*

Nebentan. $C_{24}H_{21}N_5O_5S$. 491.52. (*E*)-*N*-[6-Methoxy-5-(2-methoxyphenoxy)-2,2′-bipyrimidin-4-yl]-2-phenylethene-sulfonamide. *UNII-IJ670B0H4A. CAS-403604-85-3.* INN.

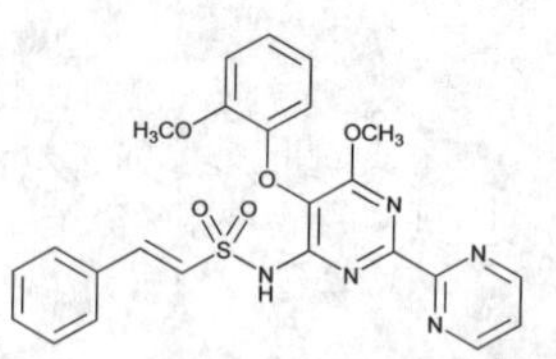

Nebicapone. $C_{14}H_{11}NO_5$. 273.24. 1-(3,4-Dihydroxy-5-nitrophenyl)-2-phenylethan-1-one. *CAS-274925-86-9.* INN.

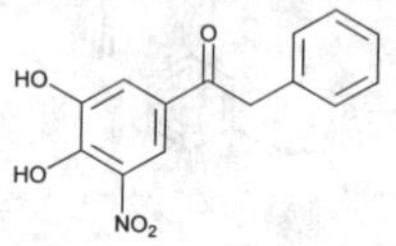

Nebidrazine. $C_9H_8Cl_2N_6$. 271.11. 2,6-Dichlorobenzaldehyde (4-amino-4*H*-1,2,4-triazol-3-yl)hydrazone. *CAS-55248-23-2.* INN.

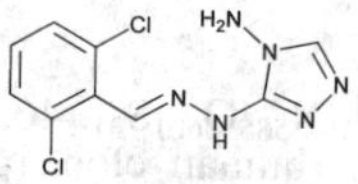

Nebivolol [*1988*] (ne biv′ oh lol). $C_{22}H_{25}F_2NO_4$. 405.44. (1) 2*H*-1-Benzopyran-2-methanol, α,α′-[iminobis(methylene)]bis[6-fluoro-3,4-dihydro-; (2) α,α′-(Iminodimethylene)bis[6-fluoro-2-chromanmethanol]. *UNII-030Y90569U. CAS-118457-14-0.* INN; BAN. *Antihypertensive (β-blocker).* ◇*R65,824*

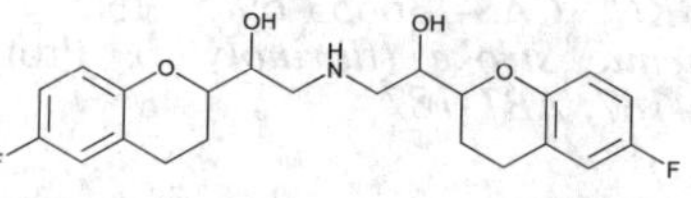

Nebivolol Hydrochloride [*2004*] (ne biv′ oh lol hye″ droe klor′ ide). $C_{22}H_{25}F_2NO_4$·HCl. 441.90. (1) 2*H*-1-Benzopyran-2-methanol, α,α′-[iminobis(methylene)]bis[6-fluoro-3,4-dihydro-, hydrochloride, (αR,α′*R*,2*R*,2′*S*)-*rel*-; (2) (1*RS*,1′*RS*)-1,1′-[(2*RS*,2′*SR*)-Bis(6-fluoro-3,4-dihydro-2*H*-1-benzopyran-2-yl)]-2,2′-iminodiethanol hydrochloride. *UNII-JGS34J7L9I. CAS-152520-56-4. Highly selective b1 antagonist with non-adrenergic vasodilating properties due to the release of nitric oxide from vascular endothelium, studied in the treatment of hypertension, congestive heart failure and other cardiovascular events.* ◇*R067555*

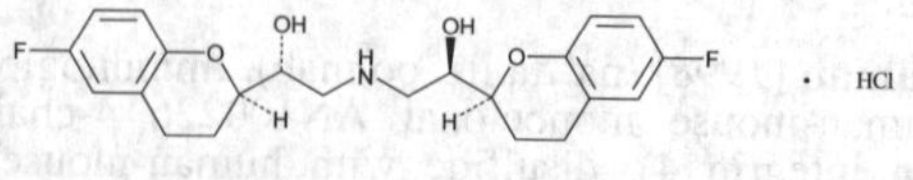

Neboglamine. $C_{13}H_{24}N_2O_3$. 256.34. (*S*)-4-Amino-*N*-(4,4-dimethylcyclohexyl)glutaramic acid. *UNII-12EA34U5B8. CAS-163000-63-3.* INN. [*Name previously used: Nebostinel.*]

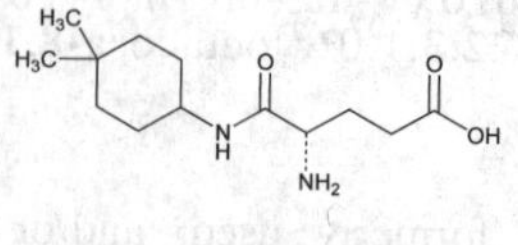

Nebracetam. $C_{12}H_{16}N_2O$. 204.27. (±)-4-(Aminomethyl)-1-benzyl-2-pyrrolidinone. *UNII-T30038QI8N. CAS-116041-13-5.* INN.

Nebramycin [*1968*] (ne″ bra mye′ sin). A complex of antibiotic substances produced by *Streptomyces tenebrarius.* (1) Nebramycin; (2) Nebramycin. *CAS-11048-13-8.* INN. *Antibacterial.* ◇*A-12253A*

Nebramycin Factor 6 — *See* Tobramycin.

Necopidem. $C_{23}H_{29}N_3O$. 363.50. *N*-[[2-(*p*-Ethylphenyl)-6-methylimidazo[1,2-*a*]pyridin-3-yl]methyl]-*N*,3-dimethyl-butyramide. *UNII-G4N2F166MN. CAS-103844-77-5.* INN.

Nedaplatin. $C_2H_8N_2O_3Pt$. 303.18. *cis*-Diammine(glycolato-O^1,O^2)platinum. *CAS-95734-82-0.* INN.

Nedocromil [*1985*] (ne dok′ roe′ mil). $C_{19}H_{17}NO_7$. 371.34. (1) 4*H*-Pyrano[3,2-*g*]quinoline-2,8-dicarboxylic acid, 9-ethyl-6,9-dihydro-4,6-dioxo-10-propyl-; (2) 9-Ethyl-6,9-dihydro-4,6-dioxo-10-propyl-4*H*-pyrano[3,2-*g*]quinoline-2,8-dicarboxylic acid. *UNII-0B535E0BN0. CAS-69049-73-6.* INN; BAN. *Anti-allergic (prophylactic).* ◇*FPL 59002*

Nedocromil Calcium [*1986*] (ne dok′ roe′ mil kal′ see um). $C_{19}H_{15}CaNO_7$. 409.40. (1) 4*H*-Pyrano[3,2-*g*]quinoline-2,8-dicarboxylic acid, 9-ethyl-6,9-dihydro-4,6-dioxo-10-propyl-, calcium salt (1:1); (2) Calcium 9-ethyl-6,9-dihydro-4,6-dioxo-10-propyl-4*H*-pyrano[3,2-*g*]quinoline-2,8-dicarboxylate (1:1). *CAS-101626-68-0. Anti-allergic (prophylactic).* ◇*FPL 59002KC*

Nedocromil Sodium [*1985*] (ne dok′ roe′ mil soe′ dee um). $C_{19}H_{15}NNa_2O_7$. 415.30. (1) 4*H*-Pyrano[3,2-*g*]quinoline-2,8-dicarboxylic acid, 9-ethyl-6,9-dihydro-4,6-dioxo-10-propyl-, disodium salt; (2) Disodium-9-ethyl-6,9-dihydro-4,6-dioxo-10-propyl-4*H*-pyrano[3,2-*g*]quinoline-2,8-dicarboxylate. *UNII-ET8IF4KS1T. CAS-69049-74-7. Anti-allergic (prophylactic).* Tilade (King) ◇*FPL 59002KP*

Nefazodone Hydrochloride [*1984*] (ne faz′ oh done hye″ droe klor′ ide). USP. $C_{25}H_{32}ClN_5O_2 \cdot HCl$. 506.47. [Nefazodone is INN and BAN.] (1) 3*H*-1,2,4-Triazol-3-one, 2-[3-[4-(3-chlorophenyl)-1-piperazinyl]]propyl]-5-ethyl-2,4-dihydro-4-(2-phenoxyethyl)-, monohydrochloride; (2) 1-[3-[4-(*m*-Chlorophenyl)-1-piperazinyl]propyl]-3-ethyl-4-(2-phenoxyethyl)-Δ^2-1,2,4-triazolin-5-one monohydrochloride. *UNII-27X63J94GR; UNII-59H4FCV1TF* [nefazodone]. *CAS-82752-99-6; CAS-83366-66-9* [nefazodone]. *Antidepressant.* Serzone (Bristol-Myers Squibb) ◇*MJ 13,754-1; BMY 13754*

Nefiracetam. $C_{14}H_{18}N_2O_2$. 246.30. 2-Oxo-1-pyrrolidineaceto-2′,6′-xylidide. *UNII-1JK12GX30N. CAS-77191-36-7.* INN.

Neflumozide Hydrochloride [*1986*] (ne floo′ moe zide hye″ droe klor′ ide). $C_{22}H_{23}FN_4O_2 \cdot HCl$. 430.90. [Neflumozide is INN.] (1) 2*H*-Benzimidazol-2-one, 1-[1-[3-(6-fluoro-1,2-benzisoxazol-3-yl)propyl]-4-piperidinyl]-1,3-dihydro-, monohydrochloride; (2) 1-[1-[3-(6-Fluoro-1,2-benzisoxazol-3-yl)propyl]-4-piperidyl]-2-benzimidazolinone monohydrochloride. *CAS-86015-38-5; CAS-86636-93-3* [neflumozide]. *Antipsychotic.* ◇*HRP 913; P79 3913*

Nefocon A [*1985*] (ne foe′ kon). $(C_5H_8O_2)_v(C_4H_6O_2)_w(C_{10}H_{14}O_4)_x(C_{16}H_{38}O_5Si_4)_y(C_9H_{15}NO_2)_z$. (1) 2-Propenoic acid, 2-methyl-, methyl ester, polymer with 2-methyl-2-propenoic acid, 1,2-ethanediyl bis(2-methyl-2-propenoate), 3-[3,3,3-trimethyl-1,1-bis[(trimethylsilyl)oxy]disiloxanyl]propyl 2-methyl-2-propenoate and *N*-(1,1-dimethyl-3-oxobutyl)-2-propenamide; (2) Methyl methacrylate polymer with methacrylic acid, ethylene dimethacrylate, 3-[3,3,3-trimethyl-1,1-bis(trimeth-

---

† Brand name formerly used, and/or firm no longer concerned with this product.

ylsiloxy)disiloxanyl]propylmethacrylate and *N*-(1,1-dimethyl-3-oxobutyl)acrylamide. *CAS-91524-13-9. Contact lens material (hydrophobic).*

Nefopam Hydrochloride [*1971*] (ne′ foe pam hye″ droe klor′ ide). $C_{17}H_{19}NO \cdot HCl$. 289.80. [Nefopam is INN and BAN.] (1) 1*H*-2,5-Benzoxazocine, 3,4,5,6-tetrahydro-5-methyl-1-phenyl-, hydrochloride; (2) 3,4,5,6-Tetrahydro-5-methyl-1-phenyl-1*H*-2,5-benzoxazocine hydrochloride. *CAS-23327-57-3; CAS-13669-70-0* [nefopam]. *Analgesic.* Acupan (3M Pharmaceuticals)

Nelarabine [*1998*] (nel ar′ a been). $C_{11}H_{15}N_5O_5$. 297.27. (1) 9-β-D-Arabinofuranosyl-6-methoxy-9*H*-purin-2-amine; (2) 2-Amino-9-β-D-arabinofuranosyl-6-methoxy-9*H*-purine. *UNII-60158CV180. CAS-121032-29-9. BAN. Antineoplastic used in the treatment of T-cell malignancies (including both T-cell and B-cell lymphomas).* Arranon (GlaxoSmithKline) ◇*MAY; 506U*

Neldazosin. $C_{18}H_{25}N_5O_4$. 375.42. (±)-1-(4-Amino-6,7-dimethoxy-2-quinazolinyl)-4-(3-hydroxybutyryl)piperazine. *UNII-G3E7RO42MB. CAS-109713-79-3. INN.*

Nelezaprine Maleate [*1988*] (nel ez′ a preen mal′ ee ate). $C_{18}H_{21}ClN_2 \cdot C_4H_4O_4$. 416.90. [Nelezaprine is INN.] (1) 1-Propanamine, 3-(9-chloro-5,6-dihydro-11*H*-pyrrolo[2,1-*b*][3]benzazepin-11-ylidene)-*N,N*-dimethyl-, (*E*)-, (*Z*)-2-butenedioate (1:1); (2) (*E*)-9-Chloro-11-[3-(dimethylamino)propylidene]-6,11-dihydro-5*H*-pyrrolo[2,1-*b*][3]benza-

zepine maleate (1:1). *UNII-3Q9L107XJB. CAS-107407-62-5; CAS-69624-60-8* [nelezaprine]. *Relaxant (muscle).* ◇*L-637,510*

Nelfilcon A [*1997*] (nel fil′ kon). Polymer of poly(vinyl alcohol) partially acetalized with *N*-(formylmethyl) acrylamide. *CAS-159073-29-7. Contact lens material (hydrophilic).* [Note—*The water content of the contact lens material is 69.4% at ambient temperature (23±2°C), the purity of modified poly vinyl alcohol is >95%, and the oxygen permeability is 26.8 × $10^{-11}(cm^2/sec)(ml\ O_2/ml ×\ mm\ Hg)$ at 35°C (Dk value).*]

Nelfinavir Mesylate [*1996*] (nel fin′ a vir mes′ i late). $C_{32}H_{45}N_3O_4S \cdot CH_4O_3S$. 663.89. [Nelfinavir is INN and BAN.] (1) 3-Isoquinolinecarboxamide, *N*-(1,1-dimethylethyl)decahydro-2-[2-hydroxy-3-[(3-hydroxy-2-methylbenzoyl)amino]-4-(phenylthio)butyl]-, [3*S*-[2(2*S**,3*S**),3α,4aβ,8aβ]]-, monomethanesulfonate (salt); (2) (3*S*,4a*S*,8a*S*)-*N-tert*-Butyl-2-[(2*R*,3*R*)-3-(3,2-cresotamido)-2-hydroxy-4-(phenylthio)butyl]decahydro-3-isoquinolinecarboxamide monomethanesulfonate (salt). *UNII-98D603VP8V; UNII-HO3OGH5D7I* [nelfinavir]. *CAS-159989-65-8; CAS-159989-64-7* [nelfinavir]. *Antiviral.* Viracept (Agouron) ◇*AG1343*

Nelivaptan. $C_{30}H_{32}ClN_3O_8S$. 630.11. (2*S*,4*R*)-1-{(3*R*)-5-Chloro-1-[(2,4-dimethoxybenzene)sulfonyl]-3-(2-methoxyphenyl)-2-oxo-2,3-dihydro-1*H*-indol-3-yl}-4-hydroxy-*N,N*-dimethylpyrrolidine-2-carboxamide. *CAS-439687-69-1. INN.*

Neltenexine. $C_{18}H_{20}Br_2N_2O_2S$. 488.24. 4′,6′-Dibromo-α-[(*trans*-4-hydroxycyclohexyl)amino]-2-thiophene-carboxy-*o*-toluidide. *CAS-99453-84-6. INN.*

Nelzarabine [*1997*] (nel zar′ a been). $C_{11}H_{15}N_5O_5$. 297.27. [Nelarabine is INN.] 2-Amino-9-β-D-arabinofuranosyl-6-methoxy-9*H*-purine. *UNII-60158CV180. CAS-121032-29-9. Antineoplastic.* ◇*MAY; 506U*

Nemadectin [*1989*] (ne″ ma dek′ tin). $C_{36}H_{52}O_8$. 612.79. (1) Milbemycin B, 5-*O*-demethyl-28-deoxy-25-(1,3-dimethyl-1-butenyl)-6,28-epoxy-23-hydroxy-, [6*R*,23*S*,25*S*(*E*)]-; (2) (6*R*,23*S*,25*S*)-5-*O*-Demethyl-28-deoxy-25-[(*E*)-1,3-di-methyl-1-butenyl]-6,28-epoxy-23-hydroxymilbemycin B; (3) (2a*E*,4*E*,4′*S*,5′*S*,6*R*,6′*S*,8*E*,11*R*,13*R*,15*S*,17a*R*,20-*R*,20a*R*,20b*S*)-6′-[(*E*)-1,3-Dimethyl-1-butenyl]-3′,4′,5′,6,6′,7,10,11,14,15,17a,20,20a,20b-tetradecahydro-4′,20,20b-trihydroxy-5′,6,8,19-tetramethylspiro[11,15-methano-2*H*,13*H*,17*H*-furo[4,3,2-*pq*][2,6]benzodioxacyclooctadecin-13,2′-[2*H*]pyran]-17-one. *CAS-102130-84-7. INN. Antiparasitic (veterinary).* ◇*F28249α; CL 287,088*

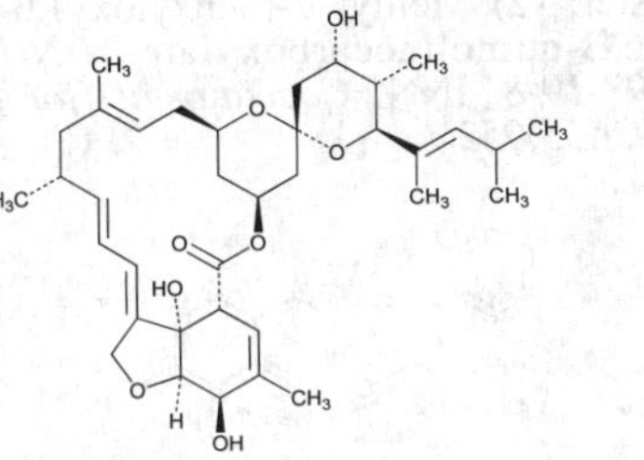

Nemazoline Hydrochloride [*1993*] (ne maz′ oh leen hye″ droe klor′ ide). $C_{10}H_{11}Cl_2N_3$.HCl. 280.58. [Nemazoline is INN.] (1) Benzenamine, 2,6-dichloro-4-[(4,5-dihydro-1*H*-imidazol-2-yl)methyl]-, monohydrochloride; (2) 2-(4-Amino-3,5-dichlorobenzyl)-2-imidazoline monohydrochloride. *CAS-111073-18-8; CAS-130759-56-7* [nemazoline]. *Nasal decongestant.* ◇*SCH 40054 HCl*

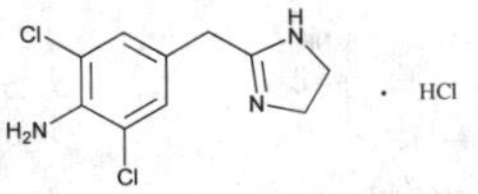

Nemifitide Ditriflutate [*2002*] (ne mif′ i tide dye trye floo′ tate). $C_{33}H_{43}FN_{10}O_6.2C_2HF_3O_2$. 922.80. [Nemifitide is INN.] (1) L-Tryptophanamide, 4-fluoro-L-phenylalanyl-(4*R*)-4-hydroxy-L-prolyl-L-arginylglycyl-bis(trifluoroacetate) (salt); (2) 4-Fluoro-L-phenylalanyl-*trans*-4-hydroxy-L-prolyl-L-arginylglycyl-L-tryptophanamide bis(trifluoroacetate) (salt). *CAS-204992-09-6; CAS-173240-15-9* [nemifitide]. *Antidepressant.* ◇*INN 00835*

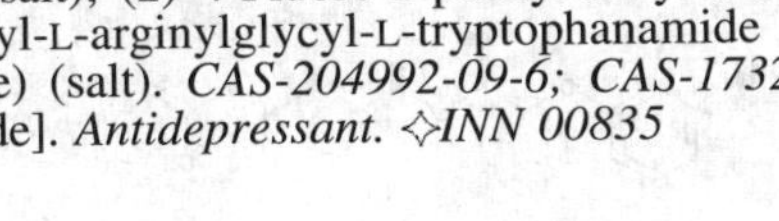

Nemonapride. $C_{21}H_{26}ClN_3O_2$. 387.90. (±)-*cis*-*N*-(1-Benzyl-2-methyl-3-pyrrolidinyl)-5-chloro-4-(methylamino)-*o*-anisamide. *UNII-Q88T5P3444. CAS-93664-94-9.* INN; JAN.

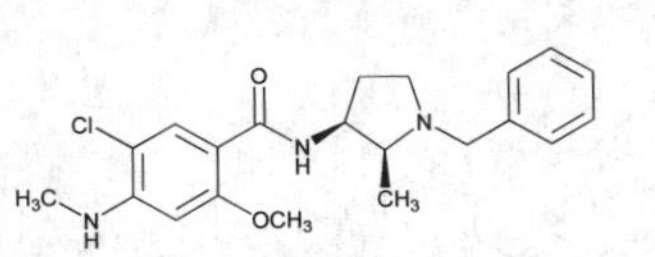

Nemonoxacin. $C_{20}H_{25}N_3O_4$. 371.43. 7-[(3*S*,5*S*)-3-Amino-5-methylpiperidin-1-yl]-1-cyclopropyl-8-methoxy-4-oxo-1,4-dihydroquinoline-3-carboxylic acid. *CAS-378746-64-6.* INN.

Nemorubicin. $C_{32}H_{37}NO_{13}$. 643.64. (1*S*,3*S*)-3-Glycoloyl-1,2,3,4,6,11-hexahydro-3,5,12-trihydroxy-10-methoxy-6,11-dioxo-1-naphthacenyl 2,3,6-trideoxy-3-[(*S*)-2-methoxymorpholino]-α-L-*lyxo*-hexopyranoside. *CAS-108852-90-0.* INN.

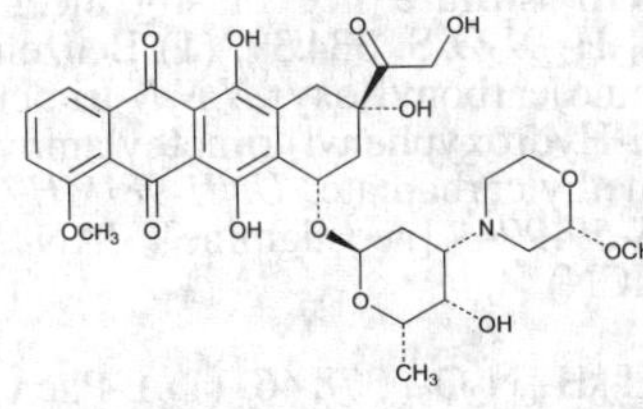

Neoarsphenamine. $C_{13}H_{13}As_2N_2NaO_4S$. 466.15. Sodium 3,3′-diamino-4,4′-dihydroxyarsenobenzene-*N*-formaldehyde-sulfoxylate. *CAS-457-60-3.* NF IX; INN; MI.

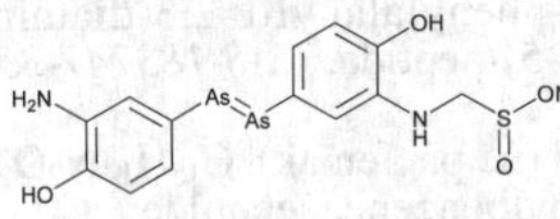

Neocarzinostatin (previously used name) — *See* Zinostatin.

Neocinchophen. $C_{19}H_{17}NO_2$. 291.34. Ethyl 6-methyl-2-phenyl-4-quinolinecarboxylate. *UNII-539M941Y9O. CAS-485-34-7.* NF XI; INN; BAN; MI.

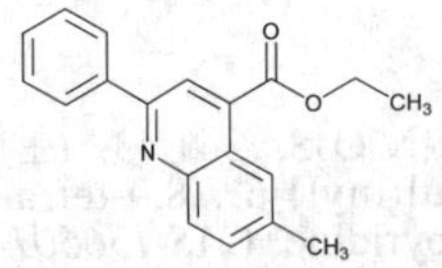

Neomycin B — *See* Framycetin.

Neomycin Palmitate [*1966*] (nee″ oh mye′ sin pal′ mi tate). [Neomycin is INN and BAN.] Palmitate salt of neomycin having a potency of not less than 180 γmg of neomycin base activity per mg. (1) Neomycin, palmitate; (2) Neomycin palmitate. *UNII-I16QD7X297* [neomycin]. *CAS-1405-12-5; CAS-1404-04-2* [neomycin]. *Antibacterial.*

Neomycin Sulfate (nee″ oh mye′ sin sul′ fate). **USP**. [Fradiomycin Sulfate is JAN.] (1) Neomycin sulfate; (2) Neomycins sulfate. *UNII-057Y626693; UNII-I16QD7X297* [neomycin]. *CAS-1405-10-3; CAS-1404-04-2* [neomycin]. *Antibacterial.* Mycifradin (Pfizer)

Neomycin Undecylenate [*1966*] (nee″ oh mye′ sin un de′ sil en ate). Undecylenate salt of neomycin having a potency of not less than 300 μg of neomycin base activity per mg. (1) Neomycin, undecenoate; (2) Neomycin undecylenate. *UNII-I16QD7X297* [neomycin]. *CAS-1406-04-8; CAS-1404-04-2* [neomycin]. *Antibacterial; antifungal.*

Neoquate — *See* Nequinate.

Neostigmine Bromide (nee″ oh stig′ meen broe′ mide). **USP**. $C_{12}H_{19}BrN_2O_2$. 303.20. [Neostigmine is BAN.] (1) Benzenaminium, 3-[[(dimethylamino)carbonyl]oxy]-*N*,*N*,*N*-trimethyl-, bromide; (2) (*m*-Hydroxyphenyl)trimethylammonium bromide dimethylcarbamate. *UNII-*

---

† Brand name formerly used, and/or firm no longer concerned with this product.

005SYP50G5; UNII-3982TWQ96G [neostigmine]. *CAS-114-80-7; CAS-59-99-4* [neostigmine]. INN; BAN; JAN. *Cholinergic.*

Neostigmine Methylsulfate (nee″ oh stig′ meen meth″ il sul′ fate). USP. $C_{13}H_{22}N_2O_6S$. 334.39. (1) Benzenaminium, 3-[[(dimethylamino)carbonyl]oxy]-*N,N,N*-trimethyl-, methyl sulfate; (2) (*m*-Hydroxyphenyl)trimethylammonium methyl sulfate dimethylcarbamate. *UNII-98IMH7M386. CAS-51-60-5; CAS-59-99-4* [neostigmine]. JAN. *Cholinergic.* Prostigmine (ICN)

Neotame. NF. $C_{20}H_{30}N_2O_5$. 378.46. (1) L-Phenylalanine, *N*-[*N*-(3,3-dimethylbutyl)-L-α-aspartyl]-1-methyl ester; (2) *N*-[*N*-(3,3-Dimethylbutyl)-L-α-aspartyl]-L-phenylalanine 1-methyl ester. *CAS-165450-17-9.*

Nepadutant. $C_{45}H_{58}N_{10}O_{13}$. 947.00. Cyclo[*N*-(2-acetamido-2-deoxy-β-D-glucopyranosyl)-L-asparaginyl-L-α-aspartyl-L-tryptophyl-L-phenylalanyl-L-2,3-diaminopropionyl-L-leucyl],cyclic(2-5)-peptide. *CAS-183747-35-5.* INN.

Nepafenac [*1997*] (ne pa′ fen ak). $C_{15}H_{14}N_2O_2$. 254.28. (1) 2-Amino-3-benzoylbenzeneacetamide; (2) 2-(2-Amino-3-benzoylphenyl)acetamide. *UNII-0J9L7J6V8C. CAS-78281-72-8.* INN; JAN. *Topical ocular anti-inflammatory and analgesic.* Nevanac (Alcon) ◇*AHR-9434; AL-6515*

Nepaprazole. $C_{18}H_{19}N_3O_2S$. 341.43. (±)-(9*R**)-9-[(*SS**)-2-Benzimidazolylsulfinyl]-6,7,8,9-tetrahydro-4-methoxy-5*H*-cyclohepta[*b*]pyridine. *CAS-156601-79-5.* INN.

Nepicastat Hydrochloride [*1997*] (ne pik′ a stat hye″ droe klor′ ide). $C_{14}H_{15}F_2N_3S.HCl.H_2O$. 349.83. [Nepicastat is INN.] (1) (*S*)-5-(Aminomethyl)-1-(5,7-difluoro-1,2,3,4-tetrahydro-2-naphthalenyl)-1,3-dihydro-2*H*-imidazole-2-thione monohydrochloride, monohydrate; (2) 5-(Aminomethyl)-1-[(*S*)-5,7-difluoro-1,2,3,4-tetrahydro-2-naphthyl]-4-imidazoline-2-thione monohydrochloride, monohydrate. *CAS-177645-08-8; CAS-173997-05-2* [nepicastat]. *Treatment of congestive heart failure (dopamine β-hydroxylase inhibitor).* ◇*RS-25560-197*

Nepidermin. $C_{270}H_{401}N_{73}O_{83}S_7$. 6221.97. Human epidermal growth factor, recombinant DNA origin. *CAS-62253-63-8.* INN.

Nepinalone. $C_{18}H_{25}NO$. 271.40. (±)-3,4-Dihydro-1-methyl-1-(2-piperidinoethyl)-2(1*H*)-naphthalenone. *UNII-L9806LPR7G. CAS-22443-11-4.* INN.

Neptamustine (INN) — *See* Pentamustine.

Nequinate [*1968*] (ne kwin′ ate). $C_{22}H_{23}NO_4$. 365.42. [Methyl Benzoquate is BAN.] (1) 3-Quinolinecarboxylic acid, 6-butyl-1,4-dihydro-4-oxo-7-(phenylmethoxy)-, methyl ester; (2) Methyl 7-(benzyloxy)-6-butyl-1,4-dihydro-4-oxo-3-quinolinecarboxylate. *UNII-91ZE013933. CAS-13997-19-8.* INN. *Coccidiostat (for poultry).* ◇*AY-20,385; ICI 55,052*

Neramexane Mesylate [*2003*] (ner a mex′ ane mes′ i late). $C_{11}H_{23}N.CH_4O_3S$. 265.41. [Neramexane is INN.] (1) Cyclohexanamine, 1,3,3,5,5-pentamethyl-, methanesulfonate; (2) 1,3,3,5,5-Pentamethylcyclohexanamine methanesulfonate. *UNII-9M85GXG84D; UNII-856DX0KJ84* [neramexane]. *CAS-457068-92-7; CAS-219810-59-0* [neramexane]. *Treatment of depression, Alzheimer's disease, and pain.*

Neraminol. $C_{20}H_{26}N_4O_2$. 354.45. (±)-1-(1*H*-Indazol-4-yloxy)-3-[[2-(2,6-xylidino)ethyl]amino]-2-propanol. *UNII-H5HKR8OEF3. CAS-86140-10-5.* INN.

Neratinib [*2006*] (ner a′ ti nib). $C_{30}H_{29}ClN_6O_3$. 557.04. (1) 2-Butenamide, *N*-[4-[[3-chloro-4-(2-pyridinylmethoxy)phenyl]amino]-3-cyano-7-ethoxy-6-quinolinyl]-4-(dimethylamino)-, (2*E*)-; (2) (2*E*)-*N*-[4-[[3-Chloro-4-[(pyridin-2-yl)methoxy]phenyl]amino]-3-cyano-7-ethoxyquinolin-6-yl]-4-(dimethylamino)but-2-enamide. *UNII-JJH94R3PWB. CAS-698387-09-6.* INN. *Treatment of cancer.* ◇*HKI-272*

Nerbacadol. $C_{10}H_{14}N_2O_2$. 194.23. 1-[(5-Methyl-4-isoxazolyl)carbonyl]piperidine. *UNII-A9W1Q28TT2. CAS-99803-72-2.* INN.

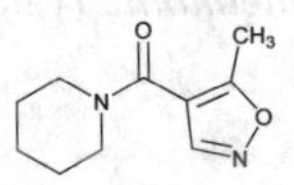

Nerelimomab [*1996*] (ner″ e lim′ oh mab). (1) Immunoglobulin G1 (mouse monoclonal BAYX1351 γ1-chain anti-human tumor necrosis factor α), disulfide with mouse monoclonal BAYX1351 light chain, dimer; (2) Immunoglobulin G1 (mouse monoclonal BAYX1351 γ1-chain anti-human tumor necrosis factor α), disulfide with mouse monoclonal BAYX1351 light chain, dimer. Molecular weight is approximately 150,000 daltons. *CAS-162774-06-3.* INN. *Monoclonal antibody.* ◇*TNF MAb; BAY X 1351*

Neridronic Acid. $C_6H_{17}NO_7P_2$. 277.15. (6-Amino-1-hydroxyhexylidene)diphosphonic acid. *UNII-8U27U3RIN4. CAS-79778-41-9.* INN.

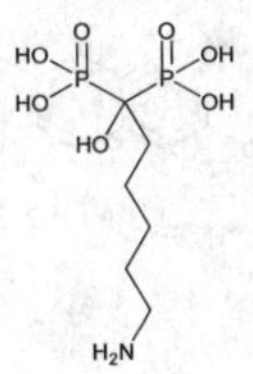

Nerisopam. $C_{18}H_{19}N_3O_2$. 309.36. 1-(*p*-Aminophenyl)-7,8-dimethoxy-4-methyl-5*H*-2,3-benzodiazepine. *UNII-18Q4O339AG. CAS-102771-12-0.* INN.

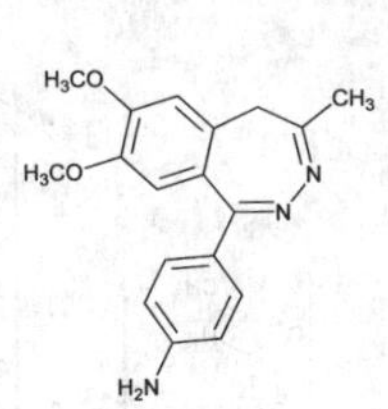

Nerispirdine. $C_{17}H_{18}FN_3$. 283.34. *N*-(3-Fluoropyridin-4-yl)-3-methyl-*N*-propyl-1*H*-indol-1-amine. *UNII-G7M7YWO6CG. CAS-119229-65-1.* INN.

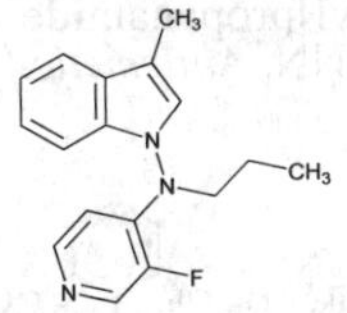

Nesapidil. $C_{23}H_{28}N_4O_4$. 424.49. (±)-1-[4-(*o*-Methoxyphenyl)-1-piperazinyl]-3-[*m*-(5-methyl-1,3,4-oxadiazol-2-yl)phenoxy]-2-propanol. *UNII-QRY8KPT3QI. CAS-90326-85-5.* INN.

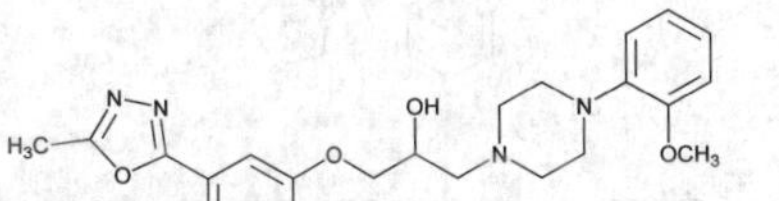

Nesbuvir [*2007*] (nes′ bue vir). $C_{22}H_{23}FN_2O_5S$. 446.49. (1) 3-Benzofurancarboxamide, 5-cyclopropyl-2-(4-fluorophenyl)-6-[(2-hydroxyethyl)(methylsulfonyl)amino]-*N*-methyl-; (2) 5-Cyclopropyl-2-(4-fluorophenyl)-6-[(2-hydroxyethyl)(methylsulfonyl)amino]-*N*-methyl-1-benzofuran-3-carboxamide. *UNII-EYK815W3Z8. CAS-691852-58-1.* INN. *Treatment of Hepatitis C.* ◇*HCV-796*

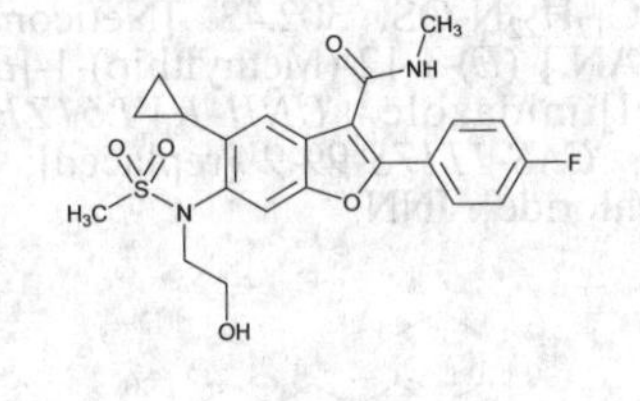

Nesiritide [*1998*] (ne sir′ i tide). $C_{143}H_{244}N_{50}O_{42}S_4$. 3464.04 g/mol. (1) Natriuretic factor-32 (human brain clone λhBNP57); (2) L-Seryl-L-prolyl-L-lysyl-L-methionyl-L-valyl-L-glutaminylglycyl-L-serylglycyl-L-cysteinyl-L-phenylalanylglycyl-L-arginyl-L-lysyl-L-methionyl-L-aspartyl-L-arginyl-L-isoleucyl-L-seryl-L-seryl-L-seryl-L-serylglycyl-L-leucylglycyl-L-cysteinyl-L-lysyl-L-valyl-L-leucyl-L-arginyl-L-arginyl-L-histidine cyclic (10→26)-disulfide. *UNII-P7WI8UL647. CAS-124584-08-3.* INN. *Treatment of congestive heart failure (renin-angiotensin system antagonist).* Natrecor (Biochemie, Austria)

SPKMVQGSGC FGRKMDRISS SSGLGCKVLR RH

Nesiritide Citrate [*1998*] (ne sir′ i tide sit′ rate). $C_{143}H_{244}N_{50}O_{42}S_4 \cdot xC_6H_8O_7$. (1) Natriuretic factor-32 (human brain clone λhBNP57), 2-hydroxy-1,2,3-propanetricarboxylate (salt); (2) L-Seryl-L-prolyl-L-lysyl-L-methionyl-L-valyl-L-glutaminylglycyl-L-serylglycyl-L-cys-teinyl-L-phenylalanylglycyl-L-arginyl-L-lysyl-L-methionyl-L-aspartyl-L-arginyl-L-isoleucyl-L-seryl-L-seryl-L-seryl-L-serylglycyl-L-leucylglycyl-L-cysteinyl-L-lysyl-L-valyl-L-leucyl-L-arginyl-L-arginyl-L-histidine cyclic(10→26) — disulfide citrate (salt). *CAS-189032-40-4. Treatment of congestive heart failure (renin-angiotensin system antagonist).* Natrecor (Biochemie, Austria)

SPKMVQGSGC FGRKMDRISS SSGLGCKVLR RH

---

† Brand name formerly used, and/or firm no longer concerned with this product.

Nesosteine. $C_{11}H_{11}NO_3S$. 237.27. *o*-(3-Thiazolidinylcarbonyl)benzoic acid. *UNII-445J9K442Z. CAS-84233-61-4.* INN.

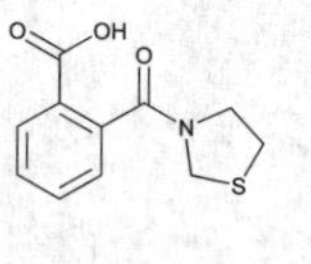

Nestifylline. $C_{11}H_{14}N_4O_2S_2$. 298.38. 7-(1,3-Dithiolan-2-ylmethyl)theophylline. *UNII-52915ASM3D. CAS-116763-36-1.* INN.

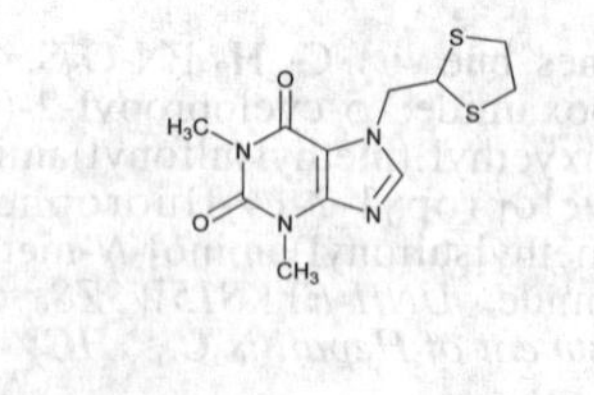

Nethalide — *See* Pronetalol.

Neticonazole. $C_{17}H_{22}N_2OS$. 302.43. [Neticonazole Hydrochloride is JAN.] (*E*)-1-[2-(Methylthio)-1-[*o*-(pentyloxy)-phenyl]vinyl]imidazole. *UNII-KVL61ZF9UO. CAS-130726-68-0; CAS-11178-99-9 [replaced]; CAS-130773-02-3 [hydrochloride].* INN.

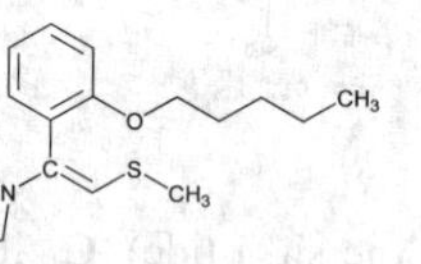

Netilmicin Sulfate [*1976*] (ne″ til mye′ sin sul′ fate). **USP**. $(C_{21}H_{41}N_5O_7)_2 \cdot 5H_2SO_4$. 1441.55. [Netilmicin is INN and BAN.] (1) D-Streptamine, *O*-3-deoxy-4-*C*-methyl-3-(methylamino)-β-L-arabinopyranosyl-(1→6)-*O*-[2,6-diamino-2,3,4,6-tetradeoxy-α-D-*glycero*-hex-4-enopyranosyl-(1→4)]-2-deoxy-N^1-ethyl-, sulfate (2:5) (salt); (2) *O*-3-Deoxy-4-*C*-methyl-3-(methylamino)-β-L-arabinopyranosyl-(1→4)-*O*-[2,6-diamino-2,3,4,6-tetradeoxy-α-D-*glycero*-hex-4-enopyranosyl-(1→6)]-2-deoxy-N^3-ethyl-L-streptamine sulfate (2:5) (salt). *UNII-S741ZJS97U; UNII-4O5J85GJJB [netilmicin]. CAS-56391-57-2; CAS-56391-56-1 [netilmicin].* JAN. *Antibacterial.* Netromycin (Schering) ◇*Sch 20569*

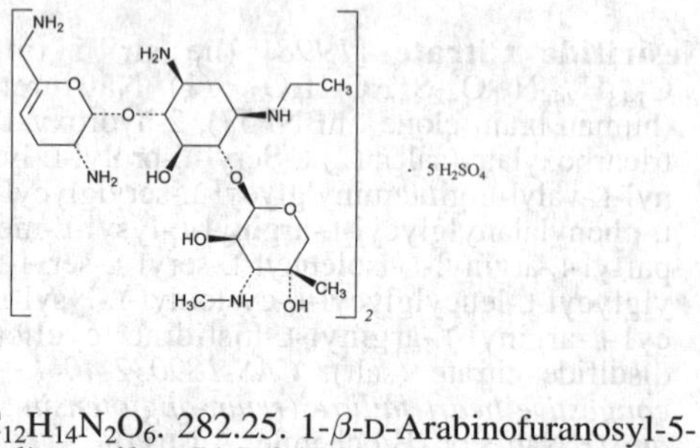

Netivudine. $C_{12}H_{14}N_2O_6$. 282.25. 1-β-D-Arabinofuranosyl-5-(1-propynyl)uracil. *CAS-84558-93-0.* INN; BAN. ◇*882C87*

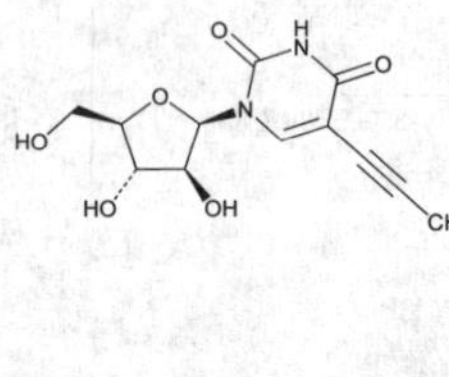

Netobimin [*1986*] (ne toe′ bi min). $C_{14}H_{20}N_4O_7S_2$. 420.46. (1) Ethanesulfonic acid, 2-[[[(methoxycarbonyl)amino][[2-nitro-5-(propylthio)phenyl]imino]methyl]amino]-; (2) Methyl [*N′*-[2-nitro-5-(propylthio)phenyl]-*N*-(2-sulfoethyl)amidino]carbamate. *UNII-U30C54N3MU. CAS-88255-01-0.* INN; BAN. *Anthelmintic (veterinary).* ◇*Sch 32481*

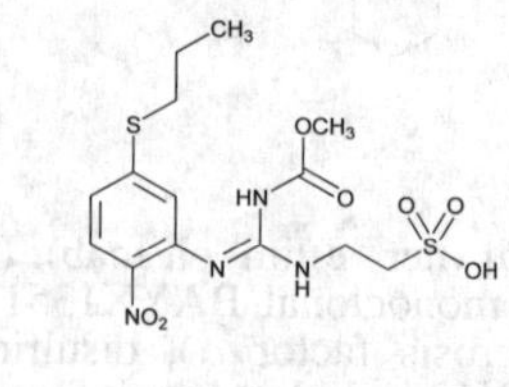

Netoglitazone [*2004*] (ne″ toe gli′ ta zone). $C_{21}H_{16}FNO_3S$. 381.42. (1) 2,4-Thiazolidinedione, 5-[[6-[(2-fluorophenyl)-methoxy]-2-naphthalenyl]methyl]-; (2) (5*RS*)-5-[[6-[(2-Fluorobenzyl)oxy]-2-naphthyl]methyl]thiazolidine-2,4-dione. *UNII-QOV2JZ647A. CAS-161600-01-7.* INN. *Antidiabetic; orally-administered insulin action enhancer to lower the plasma glucose in patients with non-insulin dependent diabetes mellitus (Type II).* ◇*MCC 555; RWJ-241947*

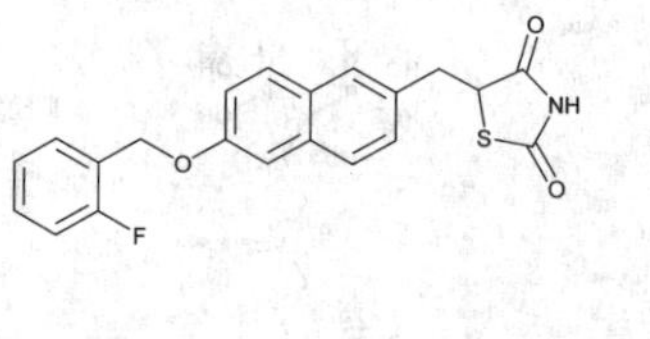

Netrafilcon A [*1990*] (ne″ tra fil′ kon). $(C_5H_8O_2)_x(C_5H_9NO)_y(C_{10}H_{14}O_4)_z$. (1) 2-Propenoic acid, 2-methyl-, methyl ester, polymer with *N,N*-dimethyl-2-propenamide and 1,2-ethanediyl bis(2-methyl-2-propenoate); (2) Methyl methacrylate polymer with *N,N*-dimethylacrylamide and ethylene dimethacrylate. *CAS-54116-21-1. Contact lens material (hydrophilic).*

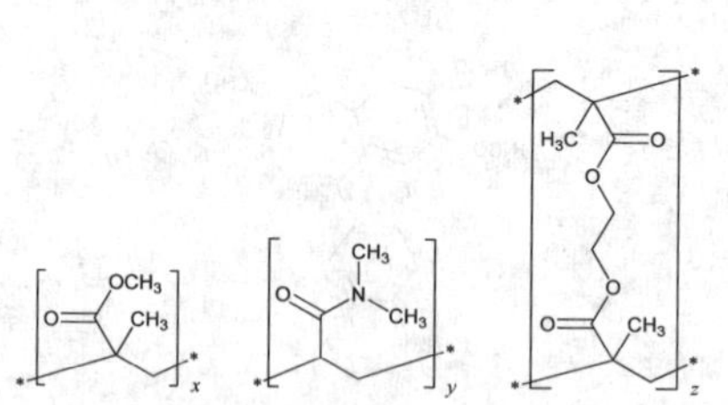

Netupitant [*2005*] (net ue′ pi tant). $C_{30}H_{32}F_6N_4O$. 578.59. (1) Benzeneacetamide, *N,α,α*-trimethyl-*N*-[4-(2-methylphenyl)-6-(4-methyl-1-piperazinyl)-3-pyridinyl]-3,5-bis(trifluoromethyl)-; (2) 2-[3,5-Bis(trifluoromethyl)phenyl]-*N,*2-dimethyl-*N*-[4-(2-methylphenyl)-6-(4-methylpiperazin-1-yl)pyridin-3-yl]propanamide. *UNII-7732P08TIR. CAS-290297-26-6.* INN. *Antiemetic.* ◇*Ro 67-3189/000*

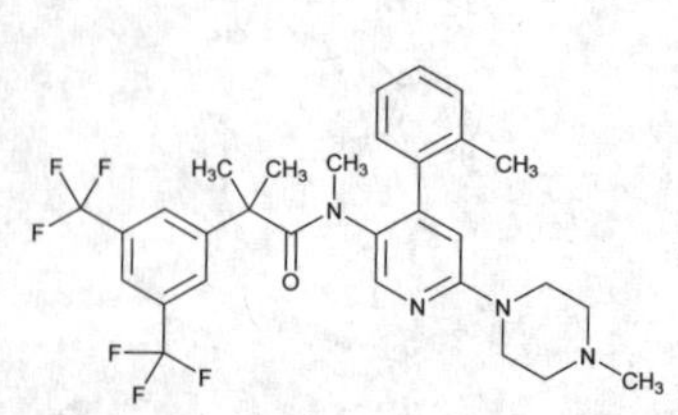

Neutramycin [*1964*] (nue″ tra mye′ sin). $C_{34}H_{54}O_{14}$. 686.78. Antibiotic produced by *Streptomyces rimosus.* (1) Neutramycin; (2) Neutramycin. *CAS-1404-08-6.* INN. *Antibacterial.* ◇*AE-705W; LL-705W*

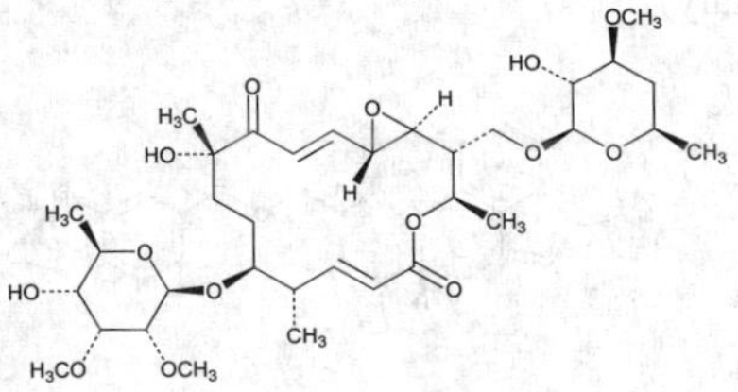

Nevirapine [*1991*] (ne vir′ a peen). **USP.** $C_{15}H_{14}N_4O$. 266.30. (1) 6*H*-Dipyrido[3,2-*b*:2′,3′-*e*][1,4]diazepin-6-one, 11-cyclopropyl-5,11-dihydro-4-methyl-; (2) 11-Cyclopropyl-5,11-dihydro-4-methyl-6*H*-dipyrido[3,2-*b*:2′,3′-*e*][1,4]diazepin-6-one. *UNII-99DK7FVK1H. CAS-129618-40-2.* INN; BAN. *Antiviral.* Viramune (Boehringer Ingelheim) ◇*BIRG 0587*

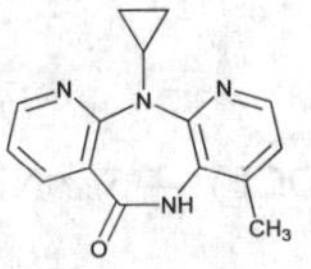

New-Estranol 1 — *See* Diethylstilbestrol.

Nexeridine Hydrochloride [*1976*] (nex er′ i deen hye″ droe klor′ ide). $C_{19}H_{29}NO_2$.HCl. 339.90. [Nexeridine is INN.] (1) Cyclohexanol, 1-[2-(dimethylamino)-1-methylethyl]-2-phenyl-, acetate (ester), hydrochloride; (2) 1-[2-(Dimethylamino)-1-methylethyl]-2-phenylcyclohexanol acetate (ester) hydrochloride. *CAS-53716-47-5; CAS-53716-48-6* [nexeridine]. *Analgesic.* ◇*673-082*

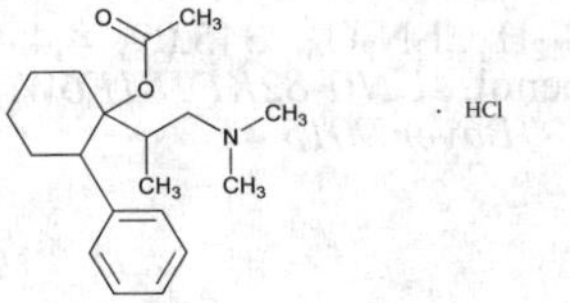

Nexopamil. $C_{24}H_{40}N_2O_3$. 404.59. (2*S*)-5-(Hexylmethylamino)-2-isopropyl-2-(3,4,5-trimethoxyphenyl)valeronitrile. *UNII-ECA0E1PO91. CAS-136033-49-3.* INN.

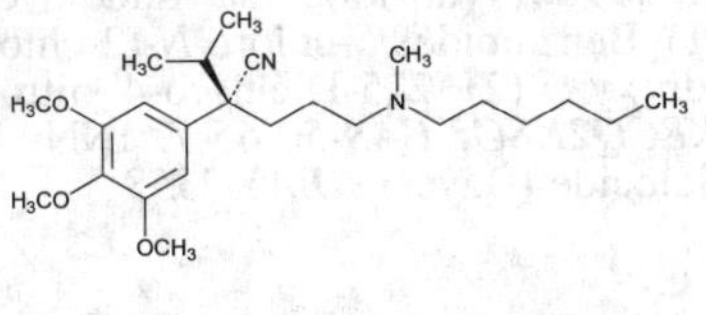

Niacin (nye′ a sin). **USP.** $C_6H_5NO_2$. 123.11. [Nicotinic Acid is INN and JAN.] (1) 3-Pyridinecarboxylic acid; (2) Nicotinic acid. *UNII-2679MF687A. CAS-59-67-6. Antihyperlipidemic; vitamin (enzyme co-factor).* Niacor (Upsher Smith); Niaspan (Abbott)

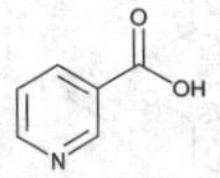

Niacinamide (nye″ a sin′ a mide). **USP.** $C_6H_6N_2O$. 122.12. [Nicotinamide is INN and JAN.] (1) 3-Pyridinecarboxamide; (2) Nicotinamide. *UNII-25X51I8RD4. CAS-98-92-0. Vitamin (enzyme co-factor).*

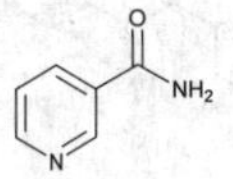

Nialamide. $C_{16}H_{18}N_4O_2$. 298.34. Isonicotinic acid 2-[(2-benzylcarbamoyl)ethyl]hydrazide. *CAS-51-12-7.* NF XIII; INN; BAN; MI.

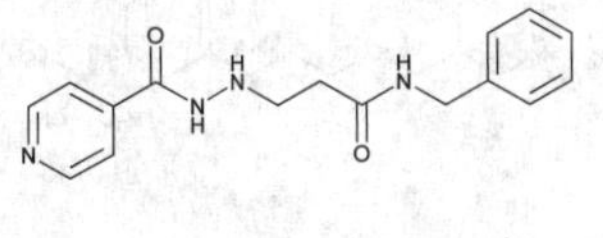

Niaprazine. $C_{20}H_{25}FN_4O$. 356.44. *N*-[3-[4-(*p*-Fluorophenyl)-1-piperazinyl]-1-methylpropyl]nicotinamide. *UNII-R2H3YN6E3L. CAS-27367-90-4.* INN; DCF; MI. ◇*1709 CERM*

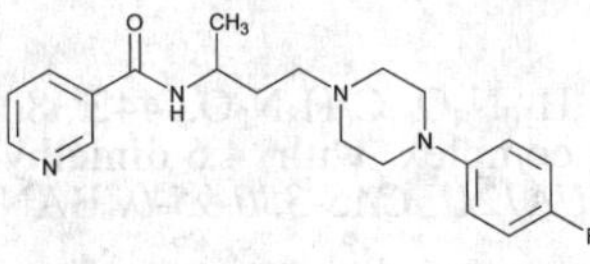

Nibroxane [*1976*] (nye brox′ ane). $C_5H_8BrNO_4$. 226.03. (1) 1,3-Dioxane, 5-bromo-2-methyl-5-nitro-; (2) 5-Bromo-2-methyl-5-nitro-*m*-dioxane. *CAS-53983-00-9.* INN. *Antimicrobial (topical).* ◇*Compound 85287*

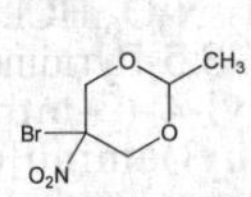

Nicafenine. $C_{24}H_{19}ClN_4O_3$. 446.89. *N*-(7-Chloro-4-quinolyl)anthranilic acid ester with *N*-(2-hydroxyethyl)nicotinamide. *UNII-F1DZD948G6. CAS-64039-88-9.* INN.

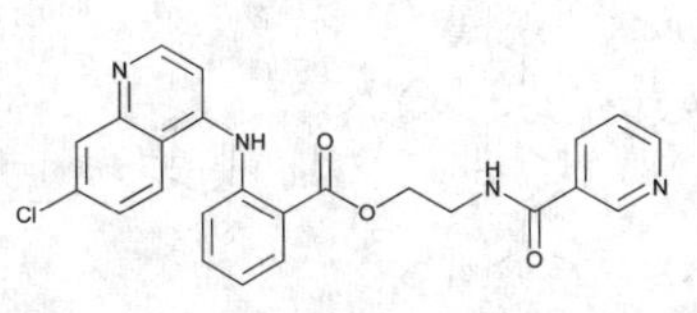

---

† Brand name formerly used, and/or firm no longer concerned with this product.

Nicainoprol. $C_{21}H_{27}N_3O_3$. 369.46. (±)-1,2,3,4-Tetrahydro-8-[2-hydroxy-3-(isopropylamino)propoxy]-1-nicotinoylquinoline. *UNII-1UA960P80H. CAS-76252-06-7.* INN.

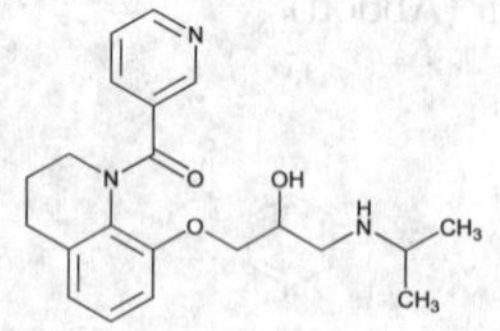

Nicametate. $C_{12}H_{18}N_2O_2$. 222.28. [Nicametate Citrate is JAN.] 2-(Diethylamino)ethyl nicotinate. *UNII-ML4O3-WYO2M. CAS-3099-52-3.* INN; BAN; DCF; MI.

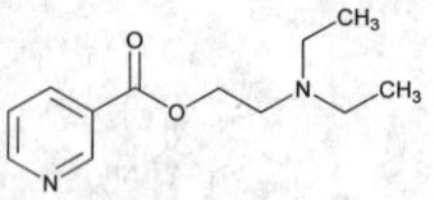

Nicanartine. $C_{23}H_{33}NO_2$. 355.51. 2,6-Di-*tert*-butyl-4-[3-(3-pyridylmethoxy)propyl]phenol. *UNII-85DV2PAF78. CAS-150443-71-3.* INN.

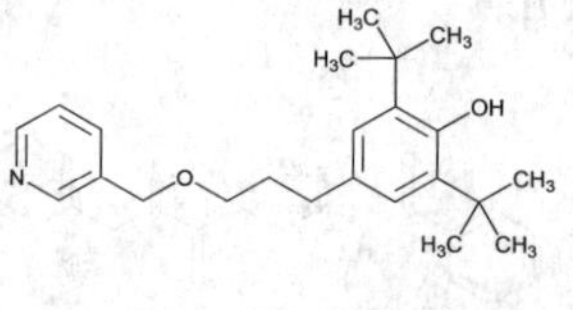

Nicaraven. $C_{15}H_{16}N_4O_2$. 284.31. (±)-*N,N'*-Propylenebis[nicotinamide]. *UNII-UD8PEV6JBD. CAS-79455-30-4.* INN.

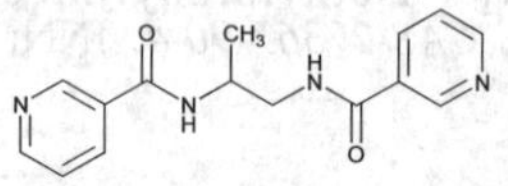

Nicarbazin. $C_{13}H_{10}N_4O_6 \cdot C_6H_8N_2O$. 442.38. 1,3-Bis(4-nitrophenyl)urea complex with 4,6-dimethylpyrimidin-2-ol. *UNII-11P9NUA12U. CAS-330-95-0.* BAN; MI.

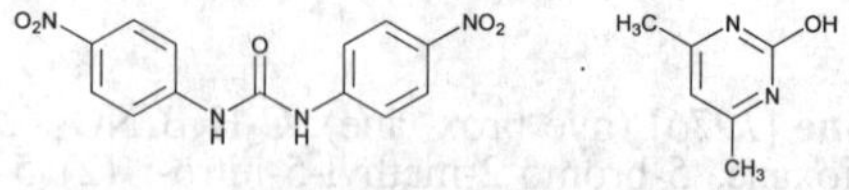

Nicardipine Hydrochloride [*1979*] (nye kar' di peen hye" droe klor' ide). $C_{26}H_{29}N_3O_6 \cdot HCl$. 515.99. [Nicardipine is INN and BAN.] (1) 3,5-Pyridinedicarboxylic acid, 1,4-dihydro-2,6-dimethyl-4-(3-nitrophenyl)-, methyl 2-[methyl(phenylmethyl)amino]ethyl ester, monohydrochloride; (2) 2-(Benzylmethylamino)ethyl methyl 1,4-dihydro-2,6-dimethyl-4-(*m*-nitrophenyl)-3,5-pyridinedicarboxylate monohydrochloride. *UNII-K5BC5011K3; UNII-CZ5312222S* [nicardipine]. *CAS-54527-84-3; CAS-55985-32-5* [nicardipine]. JAN. *Vasodilator*. Cardene (PDL Biopharma) ◇*YC-93; RS-69216; RS-69216-XX-07-0*

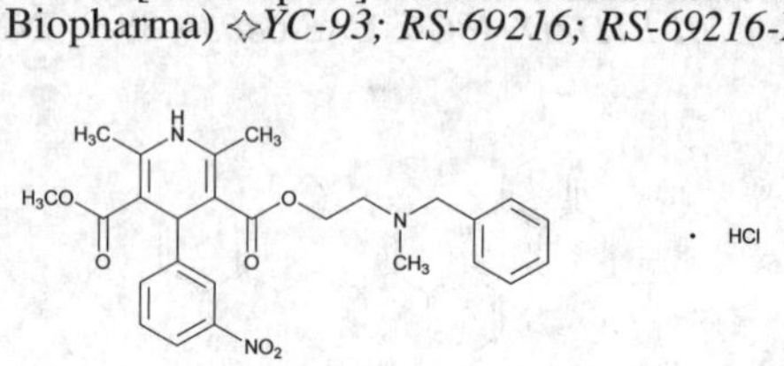

Nicergoline [*1976*] (nye ser' goe leen). $C_{24}H_{26}BrN_3O_3$. 484.39. (1) Ergoline-8-methanol, 10-methoxy-1,6-dimethyl-, (8β)-, 5-bromo-3-pyridinecarboxylate (ester); (2) 10-Methoxy-1,6-dimethylergoline-8β-methanol 5-bromonicotinate (ester). *CAS-27848-84-6.* INN; BAN; JAN. *Vasodilator*. Sermion (Farmitalia, Societa Farmaceutici Italia, Italy)

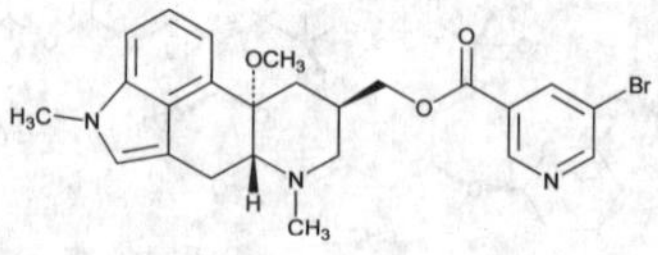

Niceritrol. $C_{29}H_{24}N_4O_8$. 556.52. Pentaerithritol tetranicotinate. *UNII-F54EHJ34MV. CAS-5868-05-3.* INN; BAN; JAN; MI; DCF.

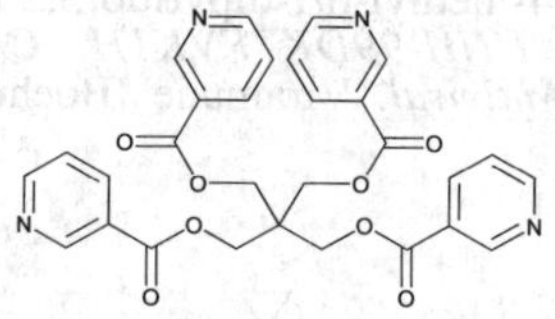

Nicethamide (BAN, DCF) — *See* Nikethamide.

Niceverine. $C_{30}H_{23}N_3O_6$. 521.52. 4-[(6,7-Dimethoxy-1-isoquinolyl)methyl]pyrocatechol dinicotinate. *UNII-U9YT4RM48N. CAS-2545-24-6.* INN; DCF. ◇*RC-167*

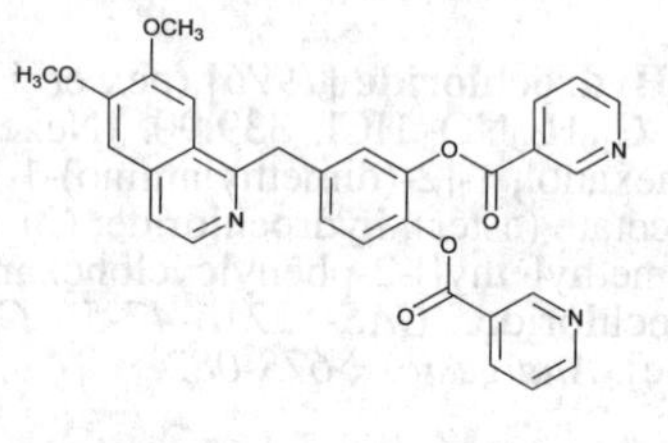

Niclofolan. $C_{12}H_6Cl_2N_2O_6$. 345.09. 4,4'-Dichloro-6,6'-dinitro-*o,o*-biphenol. *UNII-82KFT81F6W. CAS-10331-57-4.* INN; BAN. ◇*Bayer 9015*

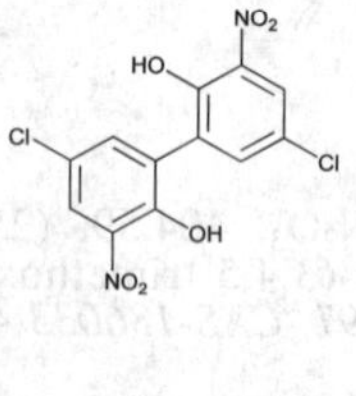

Niclosamide [*1966*] (ni kloe' sa mide). $C_{13}H_8Cl_2N_2O_4$. 327.12. (1) Benzamide, 5-chloro-*N*-(2-chloro-4-nitrophenyl)-2-hydroxy-; (2) 2',5-Dichloro-4'-nitrosalicylanilide. *UNII-8KK8CQ2K8G. CAS-50-65-7.* INN; BAN. *Anthelmintic*. Niclocide (Bayer) ◇*BAY 2353*

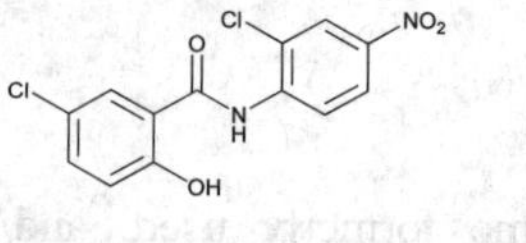

Nicoboxil. $C_{12}H_{17}NO_3$. 223.27. [β-Butoxyethyl Nicotinate is JAN.] 2-Butoxyethyl nicotinate. *CAS-13912-80-6*. INN.

Nicoclonate. $C_{16}H_{16}ClNO_2$. 289.76. *p*-Chloro-α-isopropyl-benzyl nicotinate. *UNII-9I4T8U1887*. *CAS-10571-59-2*. INN; DCF; MI.

Nicocodine. $C_{24}H_{24}N_2O_4$. 404.46. 6-Nicotinoylcodeine. *CAS-3688-66-2*. INN; BAN; DCF.

Nicocortonide. $C_{31}H_{37}NO_7$. 535.63. 11β,14,17,21-Tetra-hydroxypregn-4-ene-3,20-dione cyclic 14,17-acetal with crotonaldehyde, 21-isonicotinate. *CAS-65415-41-0*. INN.

Nicodicodine. $C_{24}H_{26}N_2O_4$. 406.47. 6-Nicotinoyl dihydro-codeine. *CAS-808-24-2*. INN; BAN; DCF.

Nicoduozide. Isonicotinic acid hydrazide mixture with nicotinaldehyde thiosemicarbazone. A mixture of Isoniazid with Nicothiazone.

Nicofibrate. $C_{16}H_{16}ClNO_3$. 305.76. 3-Pyridylmethyl 2-(*p*-chlorophenoxy)-2-methylpropionate. *UNII-4839MB71E7*. *CAS-31980-29-7*. INN; MI.

Nicofuranose. $C_{30}H_{24}N_4O_{10}$. 600.53. D-Fructofuranose 1,3,4,6-tetranicotinate. *CAS-15351-13-0*. INN; DCF; BAN; MI. ◇*ES 304*

Nicofurate. $C_{35}H_{28}N_4O_{11}$. 680.62. 2-Methyl-5-(D-*arabino*-1,2,3,4-tetrahydroxybutyl)-3-furoic acid methyl ester, tetranicotinate. *CAS-4397-91-5*. INN.

Nicogrelate. $C_{17}H_{21}N_3O_2$. 299.37. (±)-(*E*)-3-Imidazol-1-yl-1-pentylallyl nicotinate. *UNII-DW310SVK6Q*. *CAS-80614-21-7*. INN.

Nicomol. $C_{34}H_{32}N_4O_9$. 640.64. 2-Hydroxy-1,1,3,3-cyclohex-anetetramethanol 1,1,3,3-tetranicotinate. *CAS-27959-26-8*. INN; JAN; MI.

Nicomorphine. $C_{29}H_{25}N_3O_5$. 495.53. Morphine dinicotinate ester. *CAS-639-48-5*. INN; BAN; DCF; MI.

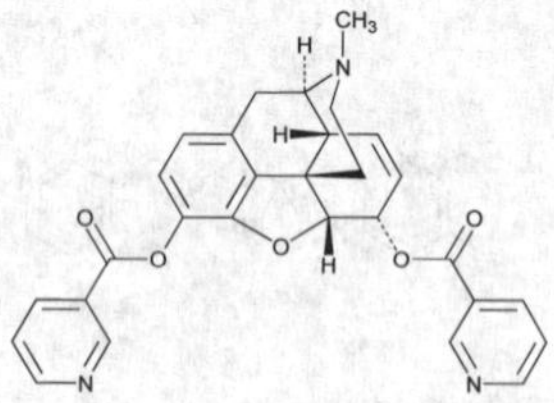

Nicopholine. $C_{10}H_{12}N_2O_2$. 192.21. 4-Nicotinoylmorpholine. *UNII-BT61K2O76Y. CAS-492-85-3*. INN; DCF.

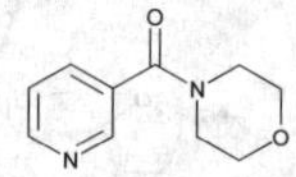

Nicoracetam. $C_{11}H_{12}N_2O_3$. 220.22. 1-(6-Methoxynicotinoyl)-2-pyrrolidinone. *UNII-8U10GC2V6Y. CAS-128326-80-7.* INN.

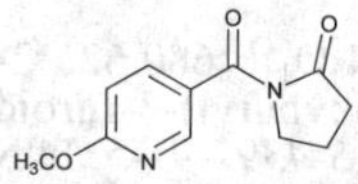

Nicorandil [*1981*] (ni kore′ an dil). $C_8H_9N_3O_4$. 211.17. (1) 3-Pyridinecarboxamide, *N*-[2-(nitroxy)ethyl]-; (2) *N*-(2-Hydroxyethyl)nicotinamide nitrate (ester). *CAS-65141-46-0.* INN; BAN; JAN. *Vasodilator (coronary).* ◇*SG-75*

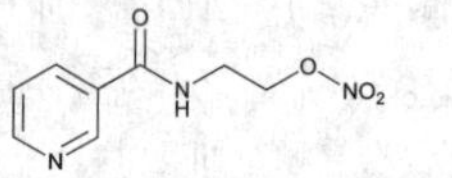

Nicothiazone. $C_7H_8N_4S$. 180.23. Nicotinaldehyde thiosemicarbazone. *CAS-555-90-8*. INN.

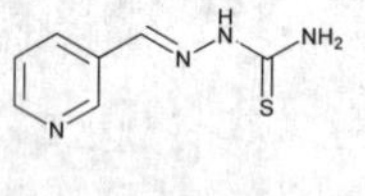

Nicotinaldehyde Thiosemicarbazone — *See* Nicothiazone.

Nicotinamide (INN, JAN) — *See* Niacinamide.

Nicotinamide Adenine Dinucleotide (previously used name) — *See* Nadide.

Nicotine (nik′ oh teen). **USP.** $C_{10}H_{14}N_2$. 162.23. (1) 3-(1-Methyl-2-pyrrolidinyl)pyridine; (2) *β*-Pyridyl-*α*-*N*-methyl pyrrolidine. *UNII-6M3C89ZY6R. CAS-54-11-5*. MI. *Smoking cessation adjunct*. Nicoderm (Sanofi Aventis); Nicotrol (Pfizer)

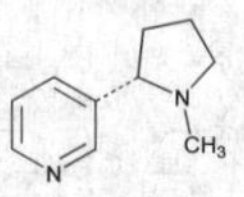

Nicotine Bitartrate [*2000*] (nik′ oh teen bye tar′ trate). $C_{10}H_{14}N_2 \cdot 2CH_4H_6O_6 \cdot 2H_2O$. 434.44. (1) Pyridine, 3-[(2*S*)-1-methyl-2-pyrrolidinyl]-, (2*R*,3*R*)-2,3-dihydroxybutane-

dioate (1:2), dihydrate; (2) Nicotine L-(+)-tartrate (1:2), dihydrate. *UNII-R7M676M8YV. CAS-65-31-6* [anhydrous]. *Treatment of smoking withdrawal syndrome.*

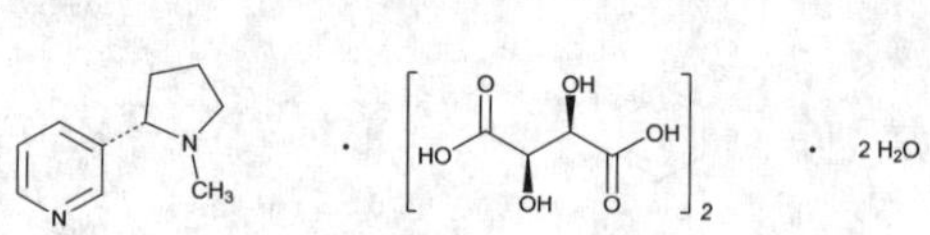

Nicotine Polacrilex [*1985*] (nik′ oh teen pol″ a kril′ ex). **USP.** $[(C_4H_6O_2)_x(C_{10}H_{10})_y](C_{10}H_{14}N_2)$. (1) 2-Propenoic acid, 2-methyl-, polymer with diethenylbenzene, complex with (*S*)-3-(1-methyl-2-pyrrolidinyl)pyridine; (2) Methacrylic acid polymer with divinylbenzene, complex with nicotine. *CAS-96055-45-7. Smoking cessation adjunct*. Commit (GlaxoSmithKline); Nicorette (GlaxoSmithKline)

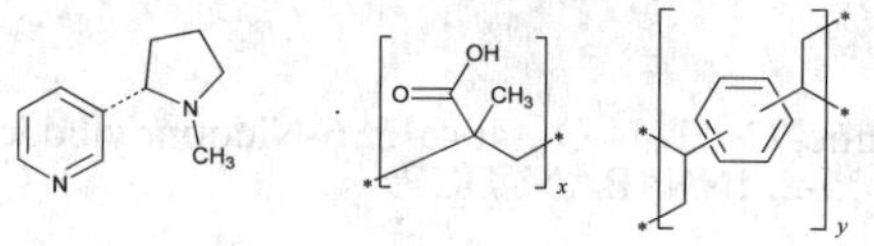

Nicotinic Acid (INN, JAN) — *See* Niacin.

Nicotinic Acid Amide — *See* Niacinamide.

Nicotinyl Alcohol [*1961*] (nik″ oh tin′ il al′ ka hol). C_6H_7NO. 109.13. [Nicotinyl Alcohol Tartrate is JAN.] (1) 3-Pyridinemethanol; (2) 3-Pyridinemethanol. *UNII-9TF312056Y. CAS-100-55-0.* BAN. *Vasodilator (peripheral).* Roniacol (Hoffmann-LaRoche†) ◇*NU-2121; RO 1-5155; NSC-526046*

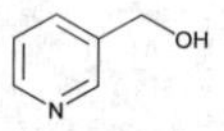

Nicotinyl Tartrate. 3-Pyridinemethanol tartrate (1:1) (salt). NND 1964; MI.

Nicotredole. $C_{16}H_{15}N_3O$. 265.31. *N*-(2-Indol-3-ylethyl)nicotinamide. *UNII-0F1T12OCLX. CAS-29876-14-0.* INN.

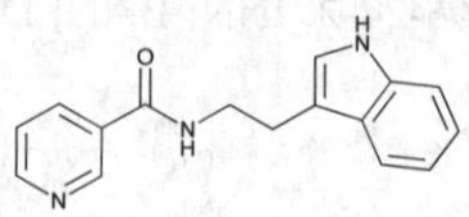

Nicotylamide — *See* Niacinamide.

Nicoumalone (former BAN) — *See* Acenocoumarol.

Nicoxamat. $C_6H_6N_2O_2$. 138.12. Nicotinohydroxamic acid. *UNII-Z3H2D4MF7A. CAS-5657-61-4.* INN.

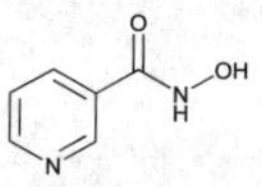

Nictiazem. $C_{26}H_{27}N_3O_4S$. 477.58. (+)-*cis*-5-[2-(Dimethyl-amino)ethyl]-2,3-dihydro-3-hydroxy-2-(*p*-methoxyphen-yl)-1,5-benzothiazepin-4(5*H*)-one nicotinate (ester). *CAS-95058-70-1.* INN.

Nictindole. $C_{17}H_{16}N_2O$. 264.32. 2-Isopropylindol-3-yl 3-pyridyl ketone. *UNII-EDK3Z2X1IV. CAS-36504-64-0.* INN. ◇*L 8027*

Nidroxyzone. $C_8H_{10}N_4O_5$. 242.19. 5-Nitro-2-furaldehyde 2-(2-hydroxyethyl)semicarbazone. *CAS-405-22-1.* INN; MI.

Nifedipine [*1973*] (nye fed′ i peen). **USP.** $C_{17}H_{18}N_2O_6$. 346.33. (1) 3,5-Pyridinedicarboxylic acid, 1,4-dihydro-2,6-dimethyl-4-(2-nitrophenyl)-, dimethyl ester; (2) Dimethyl 1,4-dihydro-2,6-dimethyl-4-(*o*-nitrophenyl)-3,5-pyridine-dicarboxylate. *UNII-I9ZF7L6G2L. CAS-21829-25-4.* INN; BAN; JAN. *Vasodilator (coronary).* Adalat (Bayer); Procardia (Pfizer) ◇*Bay a 1040*

Nifekalant. $C_{19}H_{27}N_5O_5$. 405.45. 6-[[2-[(2-Hydroxyethyl)[3-(*p*-nitrophenyl)propyl]amino]ethyl]amino]-1,3-dimethyluracil. *UNII-5VZ7GZM43E. CAS-130636-43-0.* INN.

Nifenalol. $C_{11}H_{16}N_2O_3$. 224.26. α-[(Isopropylamino)methyl]-*p*-nitrobenzyl alcohol. *UNII-D1DE63830P. CAS-7413-36-7.* INN; MI.

Nifenazone. $C_{17}H_{16}N_4O_2$. 308.33. *N*-Antipyrinylnicotina-mide. *UNII-8780F0K71U. CAS-2139-47-1.* INN; BAN; MI.

Niflumic Acid. $C_{13}H_9F_3N_2O_2$. 282.22. 2-[3-(Trifluoromethy-l)anilino]nicotinic acid. *UNII-4U5MP5IUD8. CAS-4394-00-7.* INN; DCF; MI. ◇*UP 83*

Nifluridide [*1980*] (nye flur′ i dide). $C_{10}H_6F_7N_3O_3$. 349.16. (1) Propanamide, *N*-[2-amino-3-nitro-5-(trifluoromethyl)-phenyl]-2,2,3,3-tetrafluoro-; (2) 6′-Amino-α,α,α,2,2,3,3-heptafluoro-5′-nitro-*m*-propionotoluidide. *UNII-849K45OH8R. CAS-61444-62-0. Ectoparasiticide.* ◇*Compound 109168*

Nifungin [*1970*] (nye fun′ jin). Substance derived from *Aspergillus giganteus.* (1) Nifungin; (2) Nifungin. *CAS-11056-16-9.* INN. ◇*18894*

Nifuradene [*1967*] (nye fure′ a deen). $C_8H_8N_4O_4$. 224.17. (1) 2-Imidazolidinone, 1-[[(5-nitro-2-furanyl)methylene]ami-no]-; (2) 1-[(5-Nitrofurfurylidene)amino]-2-imidazolidi-none. *CAS-555-84-0.* INN. *Antibacterial.* ◇*NF-246; NSC-6470*

Nifuralazine — *See* Furalazine.

Nifuraldezone [*1966*] (nye″ fure al′ de zone). $C_7H_6N_4O_5$. 226.15. (1) Acetic acid, aminooxo-, [(5-nitro-2-furanyl)methylene]hydrazide; (2) 5-Nitro-2-furaldehyde semioxamazone. *UNII-0180PBK4FC. CAS-3270-71-1.* INN. *Antibacterial.* ◇*NF-84; NSC-3184*

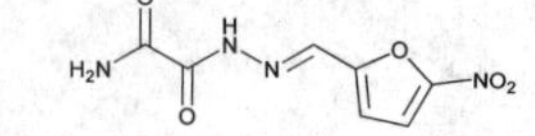

Nifuralide. $C_{14}H_{13}N_5O_4S$. 347.35. 2-(Allylamino)-4-thiazolecarboxylic acid [3-(5-nitro-2-furyl)allylidene]hydrazide. *CAS-54657-96-4.* INN.

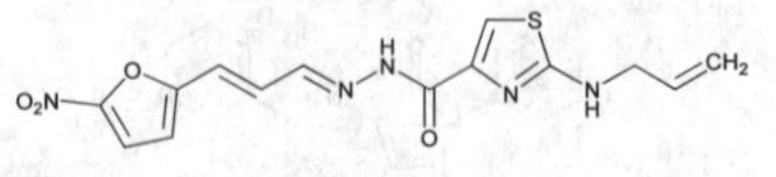

Nifuramizone — *See* Nifurethazone.

Nifuratel [*1967*] (nye fure′ a tel). $C_{10}H_{11}N_3O_5S$. 285.28. (1) 2-Oxazolidinone, 5-[(methylthio)methyl]-3-[[(5-nitro-2-furanyl)methylene]amino]-; (2) 5-[(Methylthio)methyl]-3-[(5-nitrofurfurylidene)amino]-2-oxazolidinone. *CAS-4936-47-4.* INN; BAN. *Antibacterial; antifungal; antiprotozoal (Trichomonas).* Macmiror (Polichimica Sap, Italy); Magmilor (Polichimica Sap, Italy); Polmiror (Polichimica Sap, Italy); Tydantil (Polichimica Sap, Italy)

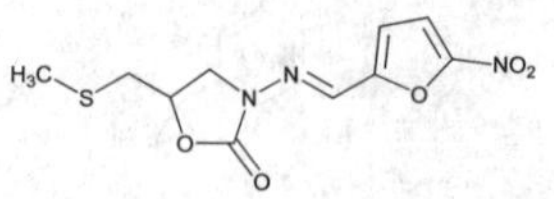

Nifuratrone [*1970*] (nye fure′ a trone). $C_7H_8N_2O_5$. 200.15. (1) Ethanol, 2-[[(5-nitro-2-furanyl)methylene]amino]-, *N*-oxide; (2) *N*-(2-Hydroxyethyl)-α-(5-nitro-2-furyl)nitrone. *CAS-19561-70-7.* INN. *Antibacterial.*

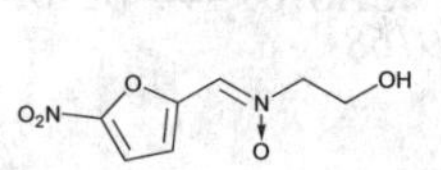

Nifurazolidone — *See* Furazolidone.

Nifurdazil [*1967*] (nye fure′ da zil). $C_{10}H_{12}N_4O_5$. 268.23. (1) 2-Imidazolidinone, 1-(2-hydroxyethyl)-3-[[(5-nitro-2-furanyl)methylene]amino]-; (2) 1-(2-Hydroxyethyl)-3-[(5-nitrofurfurylidene)amino]-2-imidazolidinone. *CAS-5036-03-3.* INN. *Antibacterial.* ◇*NF-1010*

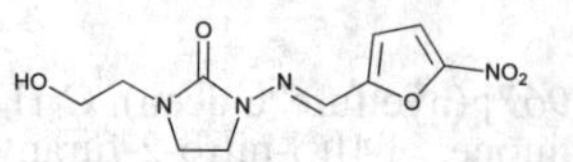

Nifurethazone. $C_{10}H_{15}N_5O_4$. 269.26. 5-Nitro-2-furaldehyde 2-(2-dimethylaminoethyl)semicarbazone. *CAS-5580-25-6.* INN.

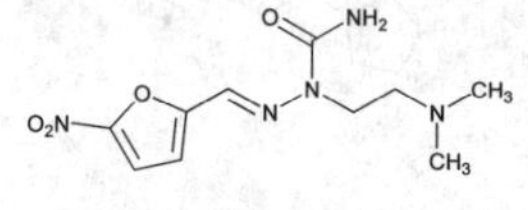

Nifurfoline. $C_{13}H_{15}N_5O_6$. 337.29. 3-(Morpholinomethyl)-1-[(5-nitrofurfurylidene)amino]hydantoin. *CAS-3363-58-4.* INN; MI.

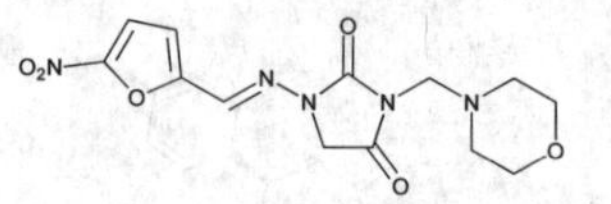

Nifurhydrazone — *See* Nihydrazone.

Nifurimide [*1967*] (nye fure′ i mide). $C_9H_{10}N_4O_4$. 238.20. (1) 2-Imidazolidinone, 4-methyl-1-[[(5-nitro-2-furanyl)methylene]amino]-, (±)-; (2) (±)-4-Methyl-1-[(5-nitrofurfurylidene)amino]-2-imidazolidinone. *CAS-15179-96-1.* INN. *Antibacterial.* ◇*NF-1120*

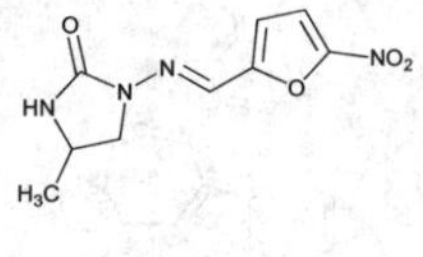

Nifurizone. $C_{12}H_{13}N_5O_5$. 307.26. 1-(Methylcarbamoyl)-3-[[3-(5-nitro-2-furyl)allylidene]amino]-2-imidazolidinone. *CAS-26350-39-0.* INN; DCF. ◇*CB 11380*

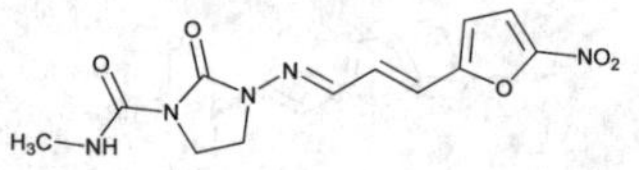

Nifurmazole. $C_{11}H_{10}N_4O_6$. 294.22. 3-(Hydroxymethyl)-1-[[3-(5-nitro-2-furyl)allylidene]amino]hydantoin. *CAS-18857-59-5.* INN; DCF. ◇*CB 10615*

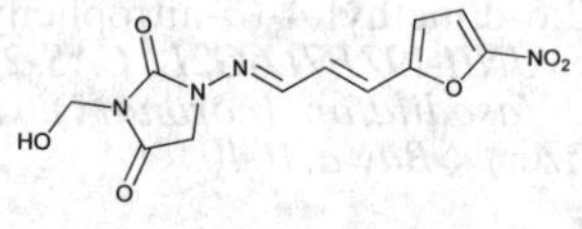

Nifurmerone [*1967*] (nye fure′ mer one). $C_6H_4ClNO_4$. 189.55. (1) Ethanone, 2-chloro-1-(5-nitro-2-furanyl)-; (2) Chloromethyl 5-nitro-2-furyl ketone. *UNII-F57Y390K2N. CAS-5579-95-3.* INN. *Antifungal.* ◇*NF-71*

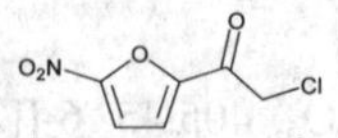

Nifuroquine. $C_{14}H_8N_2O_6$. 300.22. 4-(5-Nitro-2-furyl)quinaldic acid 1-oxide. *UNII-54T0T0F4O2. CAS-57474-29-0.* INN; BAN.

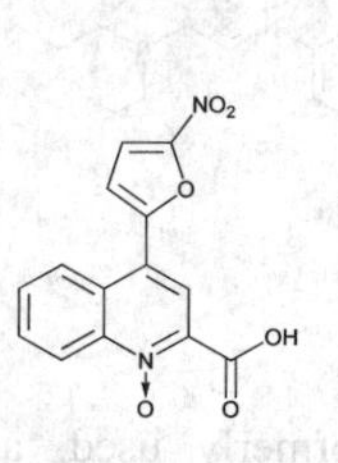

Nifuroxazide. $C_{12}H_9N_3O_5$. 275.22. *p*-Hydroxybenzoic acid 5-nitrofurfurylidene hydrazide. *CAS-965-52-6.* INN; DCF; MI. ◇*RC-27109*

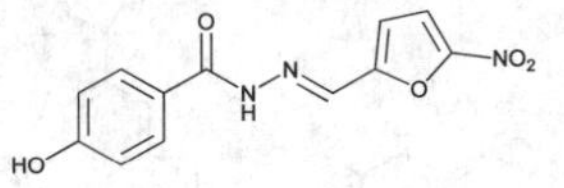

Nifuroxime. $C_5H_4N_2O_4$. 156.10. 5-Nitro-2-furaldehyde oxime. *UNII-465N7P5U85. CAS-6236-05-1.* NF XIII; INN; MI.

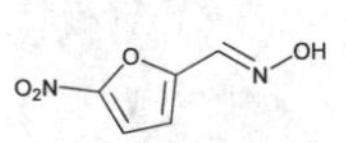

Nifurpipone. $C_{12}H_{17}N_5O_4$. 295.29. 4-Methyl-1-piperazine-acetic acid (5-nitrofurfurylidene)hydrazide. *CAS-24632-47-1.* INN. ◇*NP; Rec 15 0122*

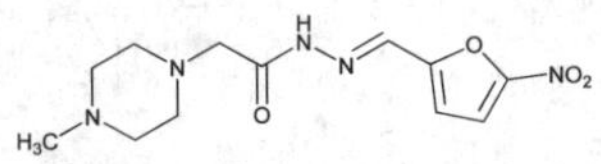

Nifurpirinol [*1973*] (nye″ fure pir′ i nol). $C_{12}H_{10}N_2O_4$. 246.22. (1) 2-Pyridinemethanol, 6-[2-(5-nitro-2-furanyl)ethenyl]-; (2) 6-[2-(5-Nitro-2-furyl)vinyl]-2-pyridine-methanol. *CAS-13411-16-0.* INN. *Antibacterial.* Furanace (Dainippon Pharmaceutical Co., Japan) ◇*P-7138*

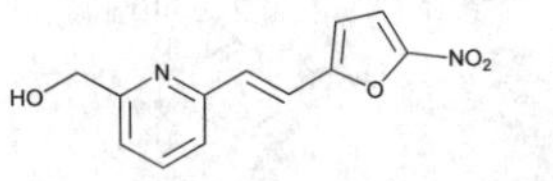

Nifurprazine. $C_{10}H_8N_4O_3$. 232.20. 3-Amino-6-[2-(5-nitro-2-furyl)vinyl]pyradizine. *CAS-1614-20-6.* INN; MI. ◇*HB 115*

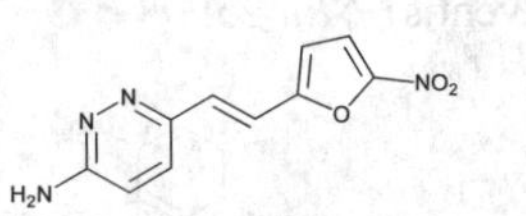

Nifurquinazol [*1967*] (nye″ fure kwin′ a zol). $C_{16}H_{16}N_4O_5$. 344.32. (1) Ethanol, 2,2′-[[2-(5-nitro-2-furanyl)-4-quinazo-linyl]imino]bis-; (2) 2,2′-[[2-(5-Nitro-2-furyl)-4-quinazoli-nyl]imino]diethanol. *CAS-5055-20-9.* INN. *Antibacterial.* ◇*NF-1088*

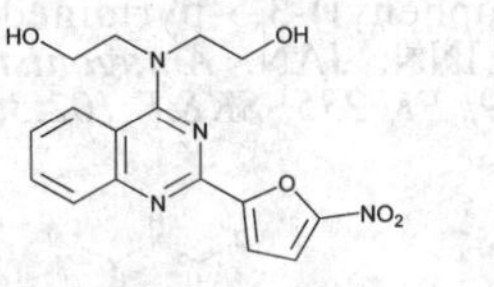

Nifursemizone [*1967*] (nye″ fure sem′ i zone). $C_8H_{10}N_4O_4$. 226.19. (1) Hydrazinecarboxamide, 1-ethyl-2-[(5-nitro-2-furanyl)methylene]-; (2) 5-Nitro-2-furaldehyde 2-ethylse-micarbazone. *UNII-BFE9UAV73M. CAS-5579-89-5.* INN. *Antiprotozoal (Histomonas, for poultry).* ◇*NF-161*

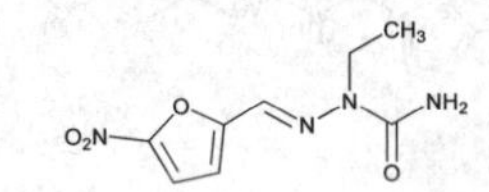

Nifursol [*1968*] (nye′ fure sol). $C_{12}H_7N_5O_9$. 365.21. (1) Benzoic acid, 2-hydroxy-3,5-dinitro-, [(5-nitro-2-furanyl)-methylene]hydrazide; (2) 3,5-Dinitrosalicylic acid (5-nitrofurfurylidene)hydrazide. *CAS-16915-70-1.* INN; BAN. *Antiprotozoal (Histomonas, for poultry).*

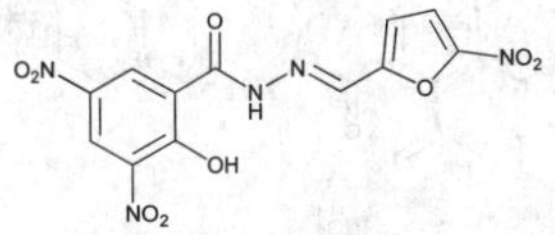

Nifurthiazole [*1964*] (nye″ fure thye′ a zole). $C_8H_6N_4O_4S$. 254.22. (1) Hydrazinecarboxaldehyde, 2-[4-(5-nitro-2-furanyl)-2-thiazolyl]-; (2) Formic acid 2-[4-(5-nitro-2-furyl)-2-thiazolyl]hydrazide. *CAS-3570-75-0.* INN. *Antibacterial.* ◇*AS-17665; NSC-525334*

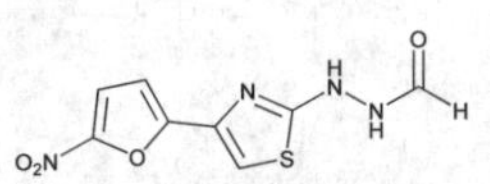

Nifurthiline — *See* Thiofuradene.

Nifurtimox. $C_{10}H_{13}N_3O_5S$. 287.29. 4-[(5-Nitrofurfuryl-idene)amino]-3-methylthiomorpholine 1,1-dioxide. *CAS-23256-30-6.* INN; BAN; MI. ◇*Bayer 2502*

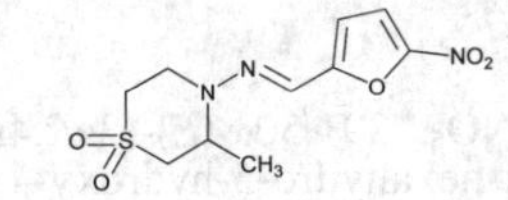

Nifurtoinol. $C_9H_8N_4O_6$. 268.18. 3-(Hydroxymethyl)-1-[(5-nitrofurfurylidene)amino]hydantoin. *CAS-1088-92-2.* INN; MI.

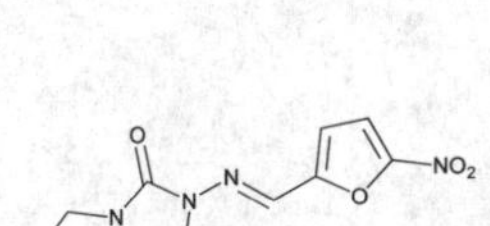

Nifurvidine. $C_{11}H_9N_3O_4$. 247.21. 2-Methyl-6-[2-(5-nitro-2-furyl)vinyl]-4-pyrimidinol. *CAS-1900-13-6.* INN.

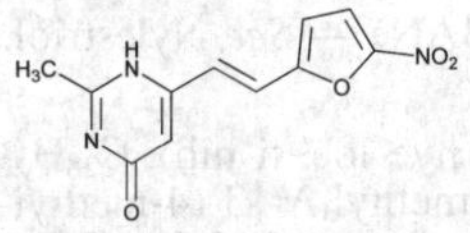

---

† Brand name formerly used, and/or firm no longer concerned with this product.

Nifurzide. $C_{12}H_8N_4O_6S$. 336.28. 5-Nitro-2-thiophenecarboxylic acid [3-(5-nitro-2-furyl)allylidene]hydrazide. *CAS-39978-42-2*. INN; MI.

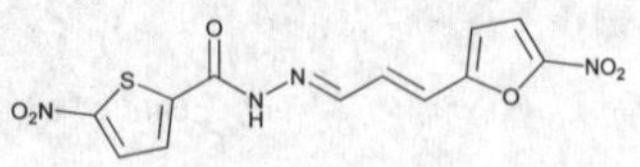

Niguldipine. $C_{36}H_{39}N_3O_6$. 609.71. (-)-(S)-3-(4,4-Diphenylpiperidino)propyl methyl 1,4-dihydro-2,6-dimethyl-4-(*m*-nitrophenyl)-3,5-pyridinedicarboxylate. *CAS-113165-32-5*. INN.

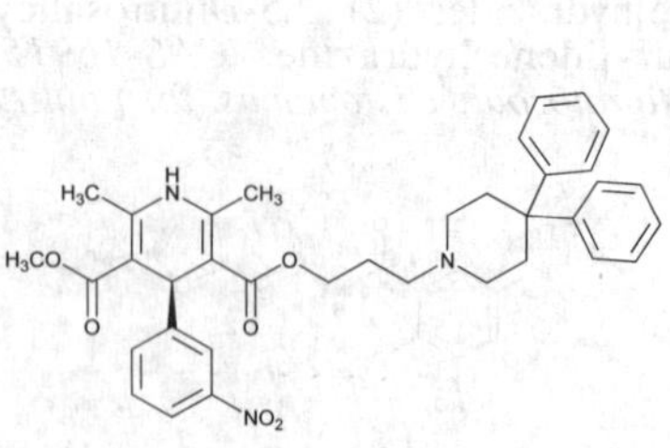

Nihydrazone. $C_7H_7N_3O_4$. 197.15. Acetic acid 5-nitrofurfurylidenehydrazide. *CAS-67-28-7*. INN; MI.

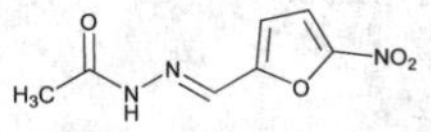

Nikethamide. $C_{10}H_{14}N_2O$. 178.23. *N,N*-Diethylnicotinamide. *UNII-368IVD6M32*. *CAS-59-26-7*. NF XIII; INN; BAN; MI. Coramine (Ciba-Geigy†); Nikethyl (Abbott†)

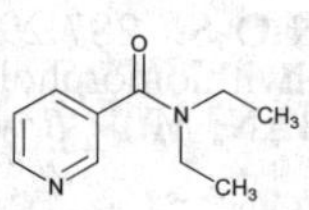

Nileprost. $C_{22}H_{33}NO_5$. 391.50. (*E*)-(3a*R*,4*R*,5*R*,6a*S*)-δ-Cyano-3,3a,4,5,6,6a-hexahydro-5-hydroxy-4-[(*E*)-(3*S*,4*RS*)-3-hydroxy-4-methyl-1-octenyl]-2*H*-cyclopenta[*b*]furan-$\Delta^{2,\Delta}$-valeric acid. *UNII-YGD81BG4SN*. *CAS-71097-83-1*. INN.

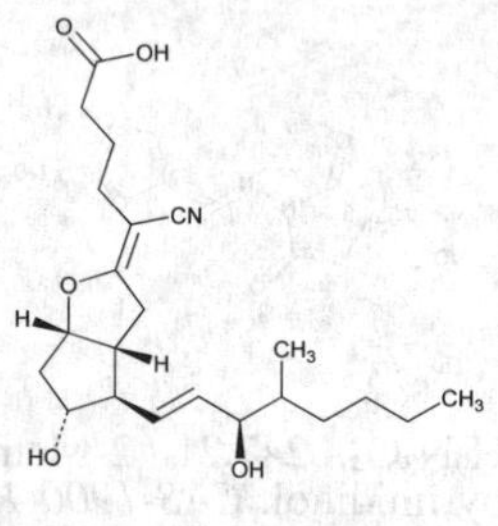

Nilestriol (INN, BAN) — *See* Nylestriol.

Nilotinib [*2006*] (nye loe′ ti nib). $C_{28}H_{22}F_3N_7O$. 529.52. (1) Benzamide, 4-methyl-*N*-[3-(4-methyl-1*H*-imidazol-1-yl)-5-(trifluoromethyl)phenyl]-3-[[4-(3-pyridinyl)-2-pyrimidinyl]amino; (2) 4-Methyl-*N*-[3-(4-methyl-1*H*-imidazol-1-yl)-5-(trifluoromethyl)phenyl]-3-{[4-(pyridin-3-yl)pyrimidin-2-yl]amino}benzamide. *UNII-F41401512X*. *CAS-641571-10-0*. INN. *Antineoplastic.* ◇*AMN 107*

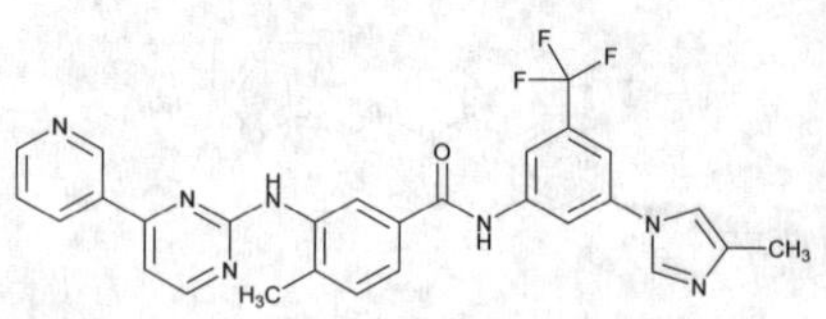

Nilprazole. $C_{26}H_{33}N_5O_2$. 447.57. 4-[[1-(2-Benzoylethyl)-2-benzimidazolyl]methyl]-*N*-isopropyl-1-piperazineacetamide. *UNII-AET4M101U3*. *CAS-60662-19-3*. INN; BAN.

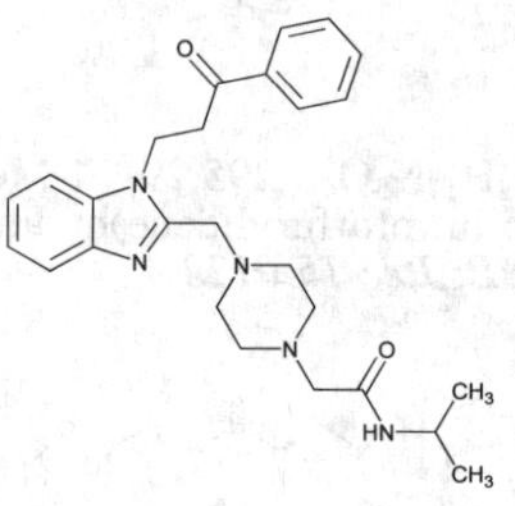

Niludipine. $C_{25}H_{34}N_2O_8$. 490.55. Bis(2-propoxyethyl) 1,4-dihydro-2,6-dimethyl-4-(*m*-nitrophenyl)-3,5-pyridinedicarboxylate. *UNII-9844OS3B0J*. *CAS-22609-73-0*. INN; BAN.

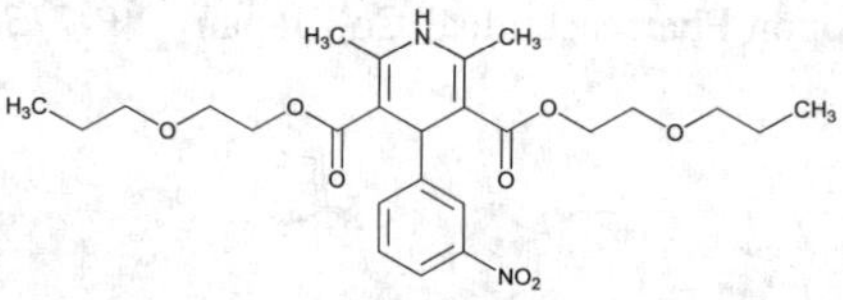

Nilutamide [*1995*] (nye loo′ ta mide). $C_{12}H_{10}F_3N_3O_4$. 317.22. (1) 2,4-Imidazolidinedione, 5,5-dimethyl-3-[4-nitro-3-(trifluoromethyl)phenyl]-; (2) 5,5-Dimethyl-3-(α,α,α-trifluoro-4-nitro-*m*-tolyl)hydantoin. *UNII-51G6I8B902*. *CAS-63612-50-0*. INN; BAN; MI. *Antineoplastic.* Nilandron (Sanofi Aventis) ◇*Ru 23908*

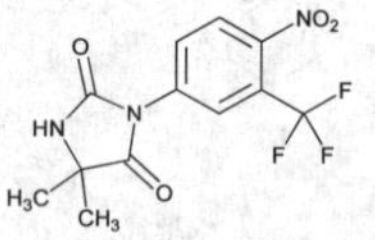

Nilvadipine [*1985*] (nil vad′ i peen). $C_{19}H_{19}N_3O_6$. 385.37. (1) 3,5-Pyridinedicarboxylic acid, 2-cyano-1,4-dihydro-6-methyl-4-(3-nitrophenyl)-, 3-methyl 5-(1-methylethyl) ester; (2) 5-Isopropyl 3-methyl 2-cyano-1,4-dihydro-6-methyl-4-(*m*-nitrophenyl)-3,5-pyridinedicarboxylate. *CAS-75530-68-6*. INN; JAN. *Antagonist (calcium channel).* ◇*CL 287,389; FK 235; SK&F 102,362*

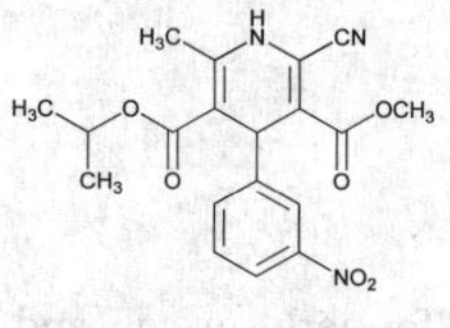

Nimazone [*1968*] (nim′ a zone). $C_{11}H_9ClN_4O$. 248.67. (1) 1-Imidazolidineacetonitrile, 3-(4-chlorophenyl)-4-imino-2-oxo-; (2) 3-(*p*-Chlorophenyl)-4-imino-2-oxo-1-imidazolidineacetonitrile. *UNII-N71M372MP4*. *CAS-17230-89-6*. INN. *Anti-inflammatory.* ◇*Win 25,347*

Nimesulide. $C_{13}H_{12}N_2O_5S$. 308.31. 4′-Nitro-2′-phenoxymethanesulfonanilide. *CAS-51803-78-2*. INN; BAN; MI. ◇*R 805*

Nimetazepam. $C_{16}H_{13}N_3O_3$. 295.29. 1,3-Dihydro-1-methyl-7-nitro-5-phenyl-2*H*-1,4-benzodiazepin-2-one. *UNII-4532264KW6*. *CAS-2011-67-8*. INN; JAN; MI. ◇*S 1530*

Nimidane [*1975*] (nim′ i dane). $C_9H_8ClNS_2$. 229.75. (1) Benzeneamine, 4-chloro-*N*-1,3-dithietan-2-ylidene-2-methyl-; (2) Cyclic methylene (4-chloro-*o*-tolyl)dithioimidocarbonate. *UNII-J3YYF867DV*. *CAS-50435-25-1*. INN. *Acaricide (veterinary).* ◇*CL 84,633; ENT 29,106*

Nimodipine [*1979*] (nye moe′ di peen). **USP**. $C_{21}H_{26}N_2O_7$. 418.44. (1) 3,5-Pyridinedicarboxylic acid, 1,4-dihydro-2,6-dimethyl-4-(3-nitrophenyl)-, 2-methoxyethyl 1-methylethyl ester; (2) Isopropyl 2-methoxyethyl 1,4-dihydro-2,6-dimethyl-4-(*m*-nitrophenyl)-3,5-pyridinedicarboxylate. *UNII-57WA9QZ5WH*. *CAS-66085-59-4*. INN; BAN. *Vasodilator.* Nimotop (Bayer) ◇*BAY e 9736*

Nimorazole. $C_9H_{14}N_4O_3$. 226.23. 4-[2-(5-Nitroimidazol-1-yl)ethyl]morpholine. *UNII-469ULX0H4G*. *CAS-6506-37-2*. INN; BAN; MI. ◇*K-1900*

Nimotuzumab. $C_{6566}H_{10082}N_{1746}O_{2056}S_{40}$. Immunoglobulin G1, anti-(humanized mouse monoclonal hR3 β1 chain anti-human epidermal growth factor receptor), disulfide with humanized mouse monoclonal hR3 K-chain, dimer. *CAS-828933-51-3*. INN.

Nimustine. $C_9H_{13}ClN_6O_2$. 272.69. [Nimustine Hydrochloride is JAN.] 3-[(4-Amino-2-methyl-5-pyrimidinyl)methyl]-1-(2-chloroethyl)-1-nitrosourea. *CAS-42471-28-3*. INN; MI.

Niometacin. $C_{18}H_{16}N_2O_4$. 324.33. 5-Methoxy-2-methyl-1-nicotinoylindole-3-acetic acid. *UNII-6EYW73T7SG*. *CAS-16426-83-8*. INN.

Niperotidine. $C_{20}H_{26}N_4O_5S$. 434.51. *N*-[2-[[5-[(Dimethylamino)methyl]furfuryl]thio]ethyl]-2-nitro-*N*′-piperonyl-1,1-ethenediamine. *CAS-84845-75-0*. INN.

Nipradilol. $C_{15}H_{22}N_2O_6$. 326.34. 8-[2-Hydroxy-3-(isopropylamino)propoxy]-3-chromanol, 3-nitrate. *UNII-FVM336I71Y*. *CAS-81486-22-8*. INN; JAN; MI.

Niprofazone. $C_{21}H_{25}N_5O_2$. 379.46. *N*-[(Antipyrinylisopropylamino)methyl]nicotinamide. *UNII-0A995E1KA6*. *CAS-15387-10-7*. INN.

---

† Brand name formerly used, and/or firm no longer concerned with this product.

Niravoline. C$_{22}$H$_{25}$N$_3$O$_3$. 379.45. *N*-Methyl-2-(*m*-nitrophenyl)-*N*-[(1*S*,2*S*)-2-(1-pyrrolidinyl)-1-indanyl]acetamide. *CAS-130610-93-4.* INN.

Niraxostat. C$_{16}$H$_{17}$N$_3$O$_3$. 299.32. 1-[3-Cyano-4-(2,2-dimethylpropoxy)phenyl]-1*H*-pyrazole-4-carboxylic acid. *CAS-206884-98-2.* INN. *[Name previously used: Piraxostat.]*

Niridazole [*1968*] (nye rid′ a zole). C$_6$H$_6$N$_4$O$_3$S. 214.20. (1) 2-Imidazolidinone, 1-(5-nitro-2-thiazolyl)-; (2) 1-(5-Nitro-2-thiazolyl)-2-imidazolidinone. *CAS-61-57-4.* INN; BAN. *Antischistosomal.* ◇*BA 32644; NSC-136947*

Nisbuterol Mesylate [*1977*] (nis bue′ ter ol mes′ i late). C$_{22}$H$_{27}$NO$_6$·CH$_4$O$_3$S. 497.56. [Nisbuterol is INN.] (1) Benzoic acid, 4-methoxy-, 2-(acetyloxy)-4-[2-[(1,1-dimethylethyl)amino]-1-hydroxyethyl]phenyl ester, methanesulfonate (salt), (±)-; (2) (±)-α-[(*tert*-Butylamino)methyl]-3,4-dihydroxybenzyl alcohol 3-acetate 4-*p*-anisate methanesulfonate (salt). *UNII-4ZSF6GBG5S. CAS-60734-88-5; CAS-60734-87-4* [nisbuterol]. *Bronchodilator.* ◇*Win 34886*

Nisobamate [*1969*] (nye″ soe bam′ ate). C$_{13}$H$_{26}$N$_2$O$_4$. 274.36. (1) Carbamic acid, (1-methylethyl)-, 2-[[(aminocarbonyl)oxy]methyl]-2,3-dimethylpentyl ester; (2) 2-(Hydroxymethyl)-2,3-dimethylpentyl isopropylcarbamate carbamate(ester). *CAS-25269-04-9.* INN. *Tranquilizer (minor); sedative-hypnotic.* ◇*W-1015*

Nisoldipine [*1981*] (nye sol′ di peen). C$_{20}$H$_{24}$N$_2$O$_6$. 388.41. (1) 3,5-Pyridinedicarboxylic acid, 1,4-dihydro-2,6-dimethyl-4-(2-nitrophenyl)-, methyl 2-methylpropyl ester, (±)-; (2) (±)-Isobutyl methyl 1,4-dihydro-2,6-dimethyl-4-(*o*-nitrophenyl)-3,5-pyridinedicarboxylate. *UNII-4I8HAB65SZ. CAS-63675-72-9.* INN; BAN; JAN. *Vasodilator (coronary).* Sular (Sciele) ◇*Bay k 5552*

Nisoxetine [*1975*] (nye sox′ e teen). C$_{17}$H$_{21}$NO$_2$. 271.35. (1) Benzenepropanamine, γ-(2-methoxyphenoxy)-*N*-methyl-, (±)-; (2) (±)-3-(*o*-Methoxyphenoxy)-*N*-methyl-3-phenylpropylamine. *UNII-17NV064B2D. CAS-53179-07-0.* INN. *Antidepressant.* ◇*Compound 89218*

Nisterime Acetate [*1977*] (nye ster′ eem as′ e tate). C$_{27}$H$_{35}$ClN$_2$O$_5$. 503.03. [Nisterime is INN.] (1) Androstan-3-one, 17-(acetyloxy)-2-chloro-, 3-[*O*-(4-nitrophenyl)oxime], (2α,5α,17β)-; (2) 2α-Chloro-17β-hydroxy-5α-androstan-3-one *O*-(*p*-nitrophenyl)oxime acetate (ester). *CAS-51354-31-5; CAS-51354-32-6* [nisterime]. *Androgen.* ◇*ORF 9326*

Nitarsone [*1966*] (nye tar′ sone). C$_6$H$_6$AsNO$_5$. 247.04. (1) Arsonic acid, (4-nitrophenyl)-; (2) *p*-Nitrobenzenearsonic acid. *UNII-JP2EN8WORU. CAS-98-72-6.* INN. *Antiprotozoal (Histomonas).* ◇*NSC-5085*

Nitazoxanide [*2003*] (nye″ ta zox′ a nide). C$_{12}$H$_9$N$_3$O$_5$S. 307.28. (1) Benzamide, 2-(acetyloxy)-*N*-(5-nitro-2-thiazolyl)-; (2) *N*-(5-Nitrothiazol-2-yl)salicylamide acetate ester. *UNII-SOA12P041N. CAS-55981-09-4.* INN; BAN. *Antiparasitic; treatment of Cryptosporidium parvum and Giardia lamblia.* Alinia (Romark) ◇*PH 5776*

Nitecapone. $C_{12}H_{11}NO_6$. 265.22. 3-(3,4-Dihydroxy-5-nitro-benzylidene)-2,4-pentanedione. *CAS-116313-94-1.* INN.

Nithiamide [*1976*] (nye thye′ a mide). $C_5H_5N_3O_3S$. 187.18. [Aminitrozole is INN and BAN.] (1) Acetamide, *N*-(5-nitro-2-thiazolyl)-; (2) *N*-(5-Nitro-2-thiazolyl)acetamide. *UNII-9CBM60191Z. CAS-140-40-9. Antibacterial (veterinary). [Name previously used: Acinitrazole.]* ◇*CL 5,279*

Nitisinone [*2002*] (nye tis′ i none). $C_{14}H_{10}F_3NO_5$. 329.23. (1) 1,3-Cyclohexanedione, 2-[2-nitro-4-(trifluoromethyl)benzoyl]-; (2) 2-(α,α,α-Trifluoro-2-nitro-*p*-tuluoyl)-1,3-cyclohexanedione. *UNII-K5BN214699. CAS-104206-65-7.* INN. *Treatment of hereditary tyrosinemia.* Orfadin (Swedish Orphan) ◇*SC-0735*

Nitracrine. $C_{18}H_{20}N_4O_2$. 324.38. 9-[[3-(Dimethylamino)propyl]amino]-1-nitroacridine. *UNII-712MLZ30SB. CAS-4533-39-5.* INN; MI.

Nitrafudam Hydrochloride [*1978*] (nye″ tra fue′ dam hye″ droe klor′ ide). $C_{11}H_9N_3O_3 \cdot HCl$. 267.67. [Nitrafudam is INN.] (1) 2-Furancarboximidamide, 5-(2-nitrophenyl)-, monohydrochloride; (2) 5-(*o*-Nitrophenyl)-2-furamidine monohydrochloride. *UNII-555ERF3D9O. CAS-57666-60-1; CAS-64743-09-5* [nitrafudam]. *Antidepressant.* ◇*F-853*

Nitralamine Hydrochloride [*1965*] (nye tral′ a meen hye″ droe klor′ ide). $C_{10}H_{13}ClN_2O_2S \cdot HCl$. 297.20. (1) Ethanamine, 2-[[1-(2-chlorophenyl)-2-nitroethyl]thio]-, monohydrochloride; (2) 2-[[*o*-Chloro-α-(nitromethyl) benzyl]thio]ethylamine monohydrochloride. *UNII-P5H9H0GK67. CAS-1432-75-3; CAS-71872-90-7* [nitralamine]. *Antifungal.* ◇*SC-12350*

Nitramisole Hydrochloride [*1976*] (nye tra′ mi sole hye″ droe klor′ ide). $C_{11}H_{11}N_3O_2S \cdot HCl$. 285.75. [Nitramisole is INN.] (1) Imidazo[2,1-*b*]thiazole, 2,3,5,6-tetrahydro-6-(3-nitrophenyl)-, monohydrochloride, (±)-; (2) (±)-2,3,5,6-Tetrahydro-6-(*m*-nitrophenyl)-imidazo[2,1-*b*]thiazole monohydrochloride. *CAS-56689-44-2; CAS-6363-02-6* [nitramisole]. *Anthelmintic.* ◇*R 29,860*

Nitraquazone. $C_{16}H_{13}N_3O_4$. 311.29. 3-Ethyl-1-(*m*-nitrophenyl)-2,4(1*H*,3*H*)-quinazolinedione. *UNII-1YF1KXP4QF. CAS-56739-21-0.* INN.

Nitrazepam [*1966*] (nye traz′ e pam). $C_{15}H_{11}N_3O_3$. 281.27. (1) 2*H*-1,4-Benzodiazepin-2-one, 1,3-dihydro-7-nitro-5-phenyl-; (2) 1,3-Dihydro-7-nitro-5-phenyl-2*H*-1,4-benzodiazepin-2-one. *CAS-146-22-5.* INN; BAN; JAN. *Anticonvulsant; sedative-hypnotic.* Mogadon (Hoffmann-LaRoche†) ◇*Ro 4-5360; Ro 5-3059; NSC-58775*

Nitre, Sweet Spirit of — *See* Ethyl Nitrite [Spirit].

Nitrefazole. $C_{10}H_8N_4O_4$. 248.19. 2-Methyl-4-nitro-1-(4-nitrophenyl)imidazole. *UNII-VFD629099M. CAS-21721-92-6.* INN; BAN; MI. ◇*EMD 15 700*

Nitrendipine [*1981*] (nye tren′ di peen). $C_{18}H_{20}N_2O_6$. 360.36. (1) 3,5-Pyridinedicarboxylic acid, 1,4-dihydro-2,6-dimethyl-4-(3-nitrophenyl)-, ethyl methyl ester, (±)-; (2) (±)-Ethyl methyl 1,4-dihydro-2,6-dimethyl-4-(*m*-nitrophenyl)-3,5-pyridinedicarboxylate. *CAS-39562-70-4*. INN; BAN; JAN. *Antihypertensive*. Baypress (Bayer) ◇*Bay e 5009*

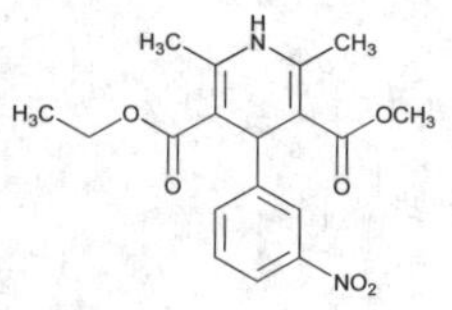

Nitric Acid (nye′ trik as′ id). **NF**. HNO_3. 63.01. (1) Nitric acid; (2) Nitric acid. *CAS-7697-37-2*. *Pharmaceutic aid (acidifying agent)*.

Nitric Oxide [*1998*] (nye′ trik ox′ ide). NO. 30.01. (1) Nitrogen oxide; (2) Nitrogen monoxide; (3) Nitric oxide. *UNII-31C4KY9ESH*. *CAS-10102-43-9*. *Endogenous vasodilator used in the treatment of hypoxic respiratory failure in the term and near-term neonate*. Inomax (Ino) ◇*OHM-11771*

Nitricholine Perchlorate. $C_5H_{13}ClN_2O_7$. 248.62. Nitrate ester of choline perchlorate. *UNII-79WCR09M2C*. *CAS-7009-91-8*. INN.

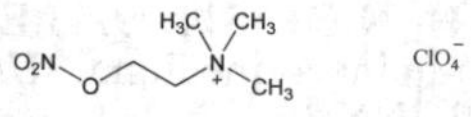

Nitroblue Tetrazolium Chloride. $C_{40}H_{30}Cl_2N_{10}O_6$. 817.64. 3,3′-[3,3′-Dimethoxy-(1,1′-biphenyl)-4,4′-dyl]bis[2-(*p*-nitrophenyl)-5-phenyl-2*H*-tetrazolium]dichloride. *UNII-X44P41F7ZK*. *CAS-38184-50-8*. JAN.

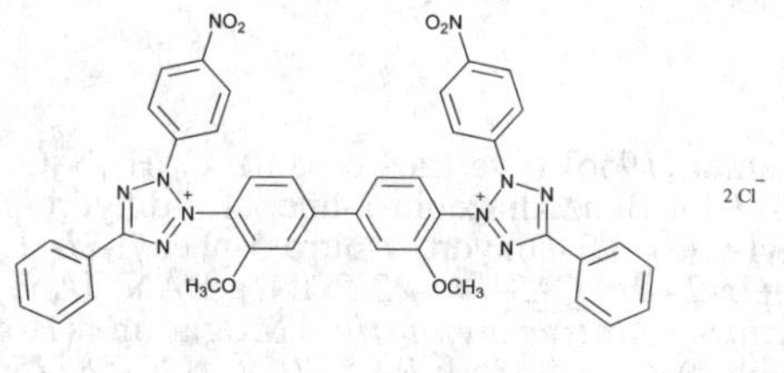

Nitrocefin. $C_{21}H_{16}N_4O_8S_2$. 516.50. (7*R*)-3-[(*E*)-2,4-Dinitrostyryl]-7-(2-thienylacetamido)-3-cephem-4-carboxylic acid. *UNII-EWP54G0J8F*. *CAS-41906-86-9*. BAN.

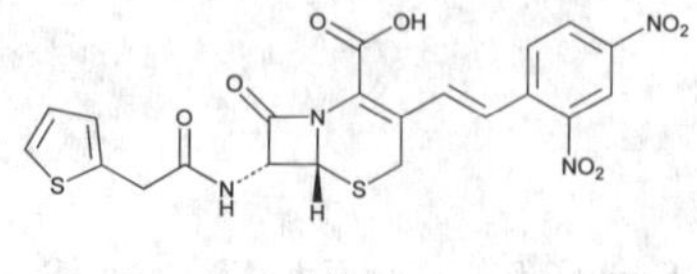

Nitroclofene. $C_{13}H_8Cl_2N_2O_6$. 359.12. 4,6′-Dichloro-4′,6-dinitro-2,2′-methylenediphenol. *UNII-NT0758136A*. *CAS-39224-48-1*. INN.

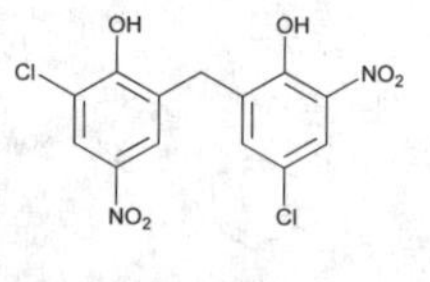

Nitrocycline [*1963*] (nye″ troe sye′ kleen). $C_{21}H_{21}N_3O_9$. 459.41. (1) 2-Naphthacenecarboxamide, 4-(dimethylamino)-1,4,4a,5,5a,6,11,12-octahydro-3,10,12,12a-tetrahydroxy-7-nitro-1,11-dioxo-, [4*S*-(4α,4aα,5aα,12aα)]-; (2) 4-(Dimethylamino)-1,4,4a,5,5a,6,11,12-octahydro-

3,10,12,12a-tetrahydroxy-7-nitro-1,11-dioxo-2-naphthacenecarboxamide. *UNII-2JH9LR1Y6S*. *CAS-5585-59-1*. INN. *Antibacterial*.

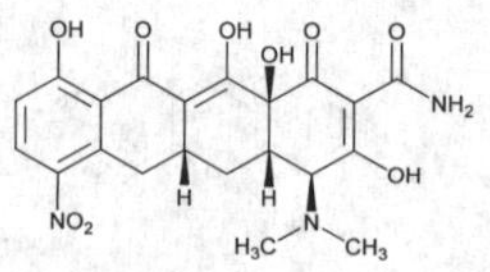

Nitrodan [*1964*] (nye′ troe dan). $C_{10}H_8N_4O_3S_2$. 296.33. (1) 4-Thiazolidinone, 3-methyl-5-[(4-nitrophenyl)azo]-2-thioxo-; (2) 3-Methyl-5-[(*p*-nitrophenyl)azo]rhodanine. *UNII-2STG09LA8F*. *CAS-962-02-7*. INN. *Anthelmintic*. ◇*CTR 6110*

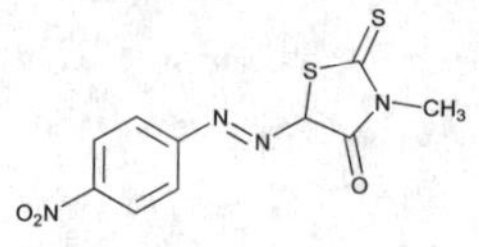

Nitroethanolamine — *See* Aminoethyl Nitrate.

Nitrofuradoxadone — *See* Furmethoxadone.

Nitrofural (INN and DCF) — *See* Nitrofurazone.

Nitrofurantoin (nye″ troe fure an′ toin; nye″ troe fure an′ toe in). **USP**. $C_8H_6N_4O_5$. 238.16. (1) 2,4-Imidazolidinedione, 1-[[(5-nitro-2-furanyl)methylene]amino]-; (2) 1-[(5-Nitrofurfurylidene)amino]hydantoin. *UNII-927AH8112L; UNII-E1QI2CQQ1I* [nitrofurantoin monohydrate]. *CAS-67-20-9; CAS-17140-81-7* [monohydrate]. INN; BAN; JAN. *Antibacterial (urinary)*. Furadantin (Sciele); Macrodantin (Procter & Gamble)

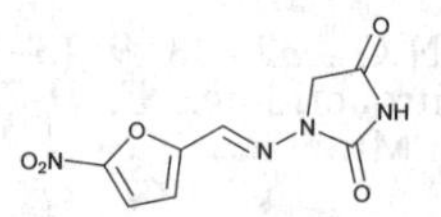

Nitrofurantoin Sodium. *UNII-MAL9M0T5LV*. *CAS-54-87-5; CAS-67-20-9* [nitrofurantoin].

Nitrofurazone (nye″ troe fure′ a zone). **USP**. $C_6H_6N_4O_4$. 198.14. [Nitrofural is INN.] (1) Hydrazinecarboxamide, 2-[(5-nitro-2-furanyl)methylene]-; (2) 5-Nitro-2-furaldehyde semicarbazone. *UNII-X8XI70B5Z6*. *CAS-59-87-0*. BAN. *Anti-infective, topical*. Actin-N (Sherwood); Furacin (Shire)

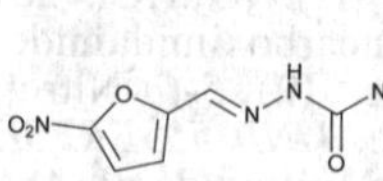

Nitrofurmethone — *See* Furaltadone.

Nitrofuroxizone — *See* Nidroxyzone.

Nitrogen (nye′ troe jen). **NF**. N_2. 28.01. (1) Nitrogen; (2) Nitrogen. *UNII-N762921K75*. *CAS-7727-37-9*. *Pharmaceutic aid (air displacement)*.

Nitrogen Monoxide — *See* Nitrous Oxide.

Nitrogen Mustard — *See* Mechlorethamine Hydrochloride.

Nitrogen Mustard *N*-Oxide Hydrochloride (JAN) — *See* Mechlorethamine Hydrochloride.

Nitroglycerin (nye″ troe glis′ er in). **USP** [Diluted]. $C_3H_5N_3O_9$. 227.09. (1) 1,2,3-Propanetriol, trinitrate; (2) Nitroglycerin. *UNII-G59M7S0WS3*. *CAS-55-63-0*. JAN.

Vasodilator (coronary). Minitran (Graceway); Nitro-bid (Sanofi Aventis); Nitro-dur (Key); Nitrostat (Pfizer) *[Name previously used: Glyceryl Trinitrate.]*

Nitrohydroxyquinoline — *See* Nitroxoline.

Nitromannitol — *See* Mannitol Hexanitrate.

Nitromersol (nye″ troe mer′ sol). **USP.** $C_7H_5HgNO_3$. 351.71. (1) 7-Oxa-8-mercurabicyclo[4.2.0]octa-1,3,5-triene, 5-methyl-2-nitro-; (2) 5-Methyl-2-nitro-7-oxa-8-mercurabicyclo[4.2.0]octa-1,3,5-triene. *CAS-133-58-4. Anti-infective, topical.*

Nitromide *[1966]* (nye′ troe mide). $C_7H_5N_3O_5$. 211.13. (1) Benzamide, 3,5-dinitro-; (2) 3,5-Dinitrobenzamide. *UNII-9DUJ3CMK8S. CAS-121-81-3. Coccidiostat (for poultry); antibacterial.* ◇*NSC-60719*

Nitromifene. $C_{27}H_{28}N_2O_4$. 444.52. 1-[2-[p-[α-(p-Methoxyphenyl)-β-nitrostyryl]phenoxy]ethyl]pyrrolidine. *CAS-10448-84-7.* INN.

Nitromifene Citrate *[1975]* (nye troe′ mi feen sit′ rate). $C_{27}H_{28}N_2O_4 \cdot C_6H_8O_7$. 636.65. (1) Pyrrolidine, 1-[2-[4-[1-(4-methoxyphenyl)-2-nitro-2-phenylethenyl]phenoxy]ethyl]-, 2-hydroxy-1,2,3-propanetricarboxylate (1:1); (2) 1-[2-[p-[α-(p-Methoxyphenyl)-β-nitrostyryl]phenoxy]ethyl]-pyrrolidine citrate (1:1). *CAS-5863-35-4; CAS-10448-84-7* [nitromifene]. *Anti-estrogen.*

---

† Brand name formerly used, and/or firm no longer concerned with this product.

p-Nitrophenyl-O-ethyl Ethylphosphonate. $C_{10}H_{14}NO_5P$. 259.20. Ethyl p-nitrophenyl ethylphosphonate. *CAS-546-71-4.* JAN.

Nitroscanate *[1976]* (nye troe skan′ ate). $C_{13}H_8N_2O_3S$. 272.28. (1) Benzene, 1-isothiocyanato-4-(4-nitrophenoxy)-; (2) p-(p-Nitrophenoxy)phenyl isothiocyanate. *UNII-P4IE5B6D6U. CAS-19881-18-6.* INN; BAN. *Anthelmintic (veterinary).* ◇*CGA-23654*

Nitrosulfathiazole (INN, DCF) — *See* Para-Nitrosulfathiazole.

Nitrous Oxide (nye′ trus ox′ ide). **USP.** N_2O. 44.01. (1) Nitrogen oxide (N_2O); (2) Nitrogen oxide (N_2O). *CAS-10024-97-2.* JAN. *Anesthetic (inhalation).*

Nitrovin. $C_{14}H_{12}N_6O_6$. 360.28. Bis[2-(5-nitro-2-furyl)vinyl]-methylenehydrazinoformamidine. *CAS-804-36-4.* BAN.

Nitroxinil. $C_7H_3IN_2O_3$. 290.01. 4-Hydroxy-3-iodo-5-nitrobenzonitrile. *UNII-9L0EXQ7125. CAS-1689-89-0.* INN; BAN; MI. *[Name previously used: Nitroxynil.]*

Nitroxoline. $C_9H_6N_2O_3$. 190.16. 5-Nitro-8-quinolinol. *UNII-A8M33244M6. CAS-4008-48-4.* INN; BAN; DCF; MI. ◇*A-82*

Nitroxynil (previously used name) — *See* Nitroxinil.

Nivacortol (INN) — *See* Nivazol.

Nivadipine — *See* Nilvadipine.

Nivazol *[1969]* (nye′ va zol). $C_{28}H_{31}FN_2O$. 430.56. [Nivacortol is INN.] (1) 2′H-Pregna-2,4-dien-20-yno[3,2-c]pyrazol-17-ol, 2′-(4-fluorophenyl)-, (17α)-; (2) 2′-(p-

Fluorophenyl)-2′*H*-17α-pregna-2,4-dien-20-yno[3,2-*c*]pyrazol-17-ol. *UNII-50U0Z120RS. CAS-24358-76-7. Glucocorticoid.* ◇*Win 27,914*

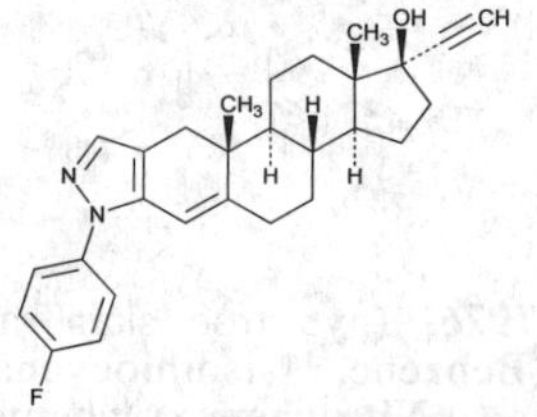

Nivimedone Sodium [*1977*] (nye vim′ e done soe′ dee um). $C_{11}H_8NNaO_4 \cdot H_2O$. 259.19. [Nivimedone is INN and BAN.] (1) 1*H*-Indene-1,3(2*H*)-dione, 5,6-dimethyl-2-nitro-, ion (1-), sodium, monohydrate; (2) 5,6-Dimethyl-2-*aci*-nitro-1,3-indandione sodium salt, monohydrate. *UNII-4953C873N2. CAS-62077-09-2; CAS-57441-90-4* [anhydrous]; *CAS-49561-92-4* [nivimedone]. *Anti-allergic.*

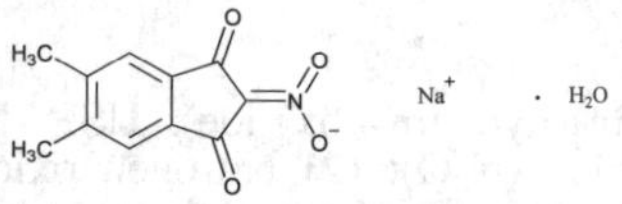

Nixylic Acid. $C_{14}H_{14}N_2O_2$. 242.27. 2-(2,3-Xylidino)nicotinic acid. *UNII-1ZI8H16Z5I. CAS-4394-05-2.* INN; DCF. ◇*UP 74*

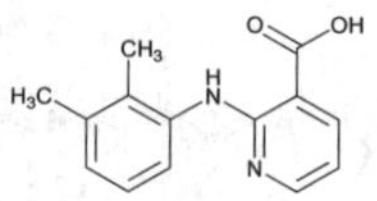

Nizatidine [*1983*] (nye za′ ti deen). **USP.** $C_{12}H_{21}N_5O_2S_2$. 331.46. (1) 1,1-Ethenediamine, *N*-[2-[[[2-[(dimethylamino)methyl]-4-thiazolyl]methyl]thio]ethyl]-*N*′-methyl-2-nitro-; (2) *N*-[2-[[[2-[(Dimethylamino)methyl]-4-thiazolyl]methyl]thio]ethyl]-*N*′-methyl-2-nitro-1,1-ethenediamine. *UNII-P41PML4GHR. CAS-76963-41-2.* INN; BAN; JAN. *Anti-ulcerative.* Axid (Reliant) ◇*LY 139037*

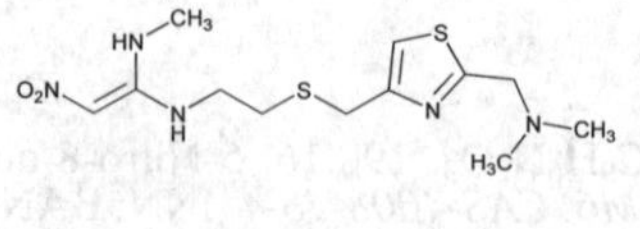

Nizofenone. $C_{21}H_{21}ClN_4O_3$. 412.87. [Nizofenone Fumarate is JAN.] 2′-Chloro-2-[2-[(diethylamino)methyl]imidazol-1-yl]-5-nitrobenzophenone. *UNII-7A2NOC3R88. CAS-54533-85-6.* INN; MI.

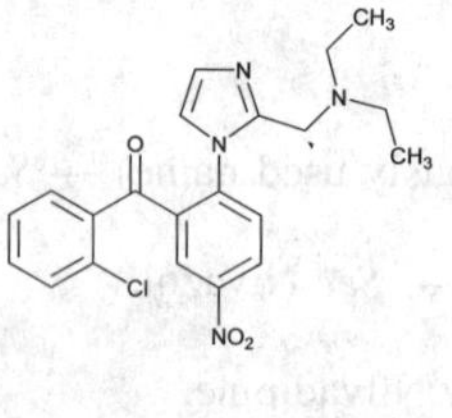

Noberastine [*1991*] (noe″ ber as′ teen). $C_{17}H_{21}N_5O$. 311.38. (1) 3*H*-Imidazo[4,5-*b*]pyridin-2-amine, 3-[(5-methyl-2-furanyl)methyl]-*N*-4-piperidinyl-; (2) 3-(5-Methylfurfur-

yl)-2-(4-piperidylamino)-3*H*-imidazo[4,5-*b*]pyridine. *UNII-9HPD98OUWN. CAS-110588-56-2.* INN; BAN. *Antihistaminic.* ◇*R 64947*

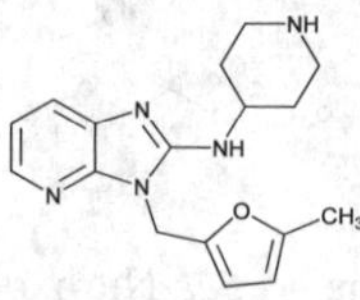

Nocloprost. $C_{22}H_{37}ClO_4$. 400.98. (*Z*)-7-[(1*R*,2*R*,3*R*,5*R*)-5-Chloro-3-hydroxy-2-[(*E*)-(3*R*)-3-hydroxy-4,4-dimethyl-1-octenyl]cyclopentyl]-5-heptenoic acid. *CAS-79360-43-3.* INN.

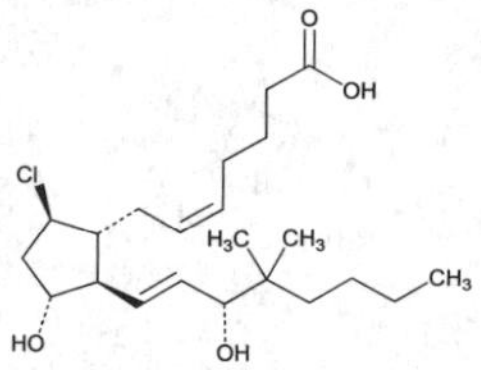

Nocodazole [*1976*] (noe koe′ da zole). $C_{14}H_{11}N_3O_3S$. 301.32. (1) Carbamic acid, [5-(2-thienylcarbonyl)-1*H*-benzimidazole-2-yl]-, methyl ester; (2) Methyl 5-(2-thenoyl)-2-benzimidazolecarbamate. *UNII-SH1WY3R615. CAS-31430-18-9.* INN. *Antineoplastic.* ◇*R 17,934*

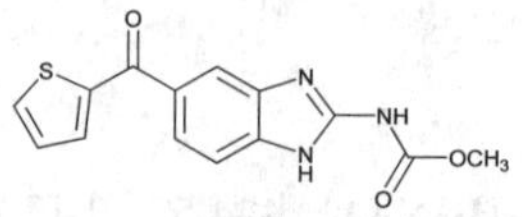

Nofecainide. $C_{20}H_{24}N_2O_3$. 340.42. 3-[2-Hydroxy-3-(isopropylamino)propoxy]-2-phenylphthalimidine. *UNII-07CJN646IN. CAS-50516-43-3.* INN.

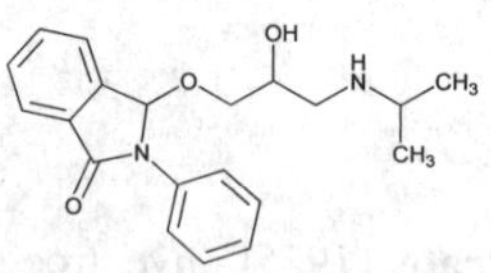

Nogalamycin [*1965*] (noe gal″ a mye′ sin). $C_{39}H_{49}NO_{16}$. 787.80. Antibiotic produced by *Streptomyces nogalater* variant. (1) Nogalamycin; (2) Nogalamycin. *CAS-1404-15-5.* INN. *Antineoplastic.* ◇*U-15167; NSC-70845*

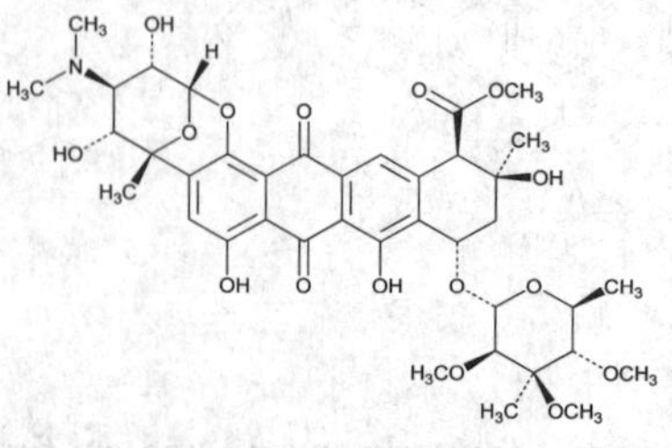

Nolatrexed. $C_{14}H_{12}N_4OS$. 284.34. 2-Amino-6-methyl-5-(4-pyridylthio)-4(3*H*)-quinazolinone. *CAS-147149-76-6*. INN.

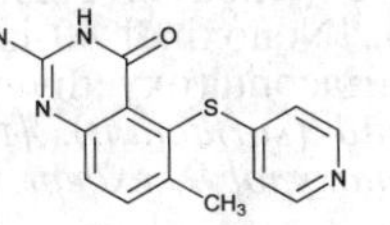

Nolinium Bromide [*1977*] (noe lin′ i um broe′ mide). $C_{15}H_{11}BrCl_2N_2$. 370.07. (1) Quinolizinium, 2-[(3,4-dichlorophenyl)amino]-, bromide; (2) 2-(3,4-Dichloroanilino)-quinolizinium bromide. *CAS-40759-33-9*. INN. *Antisecretory; anti-ulcerative.* ◇*EU-2972*

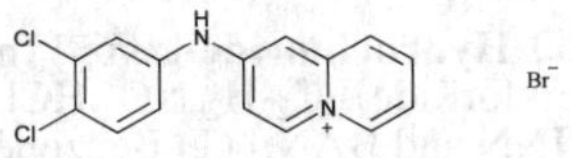

Nolomirole. $C_{19}H_{27}NO_4$. 333.42. (±)-5,6,7,8-Tetrahydro-6-(methylamino)-1,2-naphthylene diisobutyrate. *UNII-6EMF80C55F*. *CAS-90060-42-7*. INN.

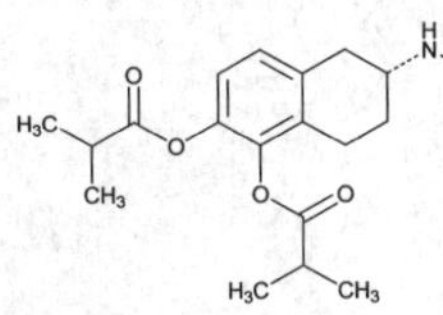

Nolpitantium Besilate. $C_{43}H_{50}Cl_2N_2O_5S$. 777.84. 1-[2-[(*S*)-3-(3,4-Dichlorophenyl)-1-[(*m*-isopropoxyphenyl)acetyl]-3-piperidyl]ethyl-4-phenylquinuclidinium benzenesulfonate. *CAS-155418-06-7*. INN.

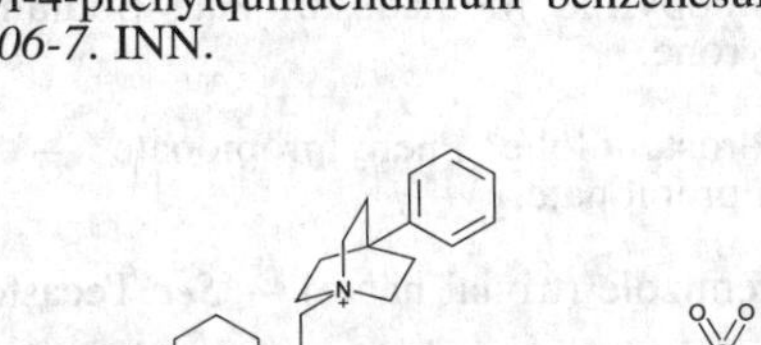

Nomegestrol Acetate [*2008*] (noe″ me jes′ trol as′ e tate). $C_{23}H_{30}O_4$. 370.48. [Nomegestrol is INN and BAN.] (1) 19-Norpregna-4,6-diene-3,20-dione, 17-(acetyloxy)-6-methyl-; (2) 6-Methyl-3,20-dioxo-19-norpregna-4,6-dien-17-yl acetate; (3) 17-Acetoxy-6-methyl-19-norpregn-4,6-dien-3,20-dione. *CAS-58652-20-3; CAS-58691-88-6* [nomegestrol]. *Prevention of pregnancy in women who elect to use a hormonal contraceptive as a method of contraception.* ◇*ORG 10486-0; TX 066*

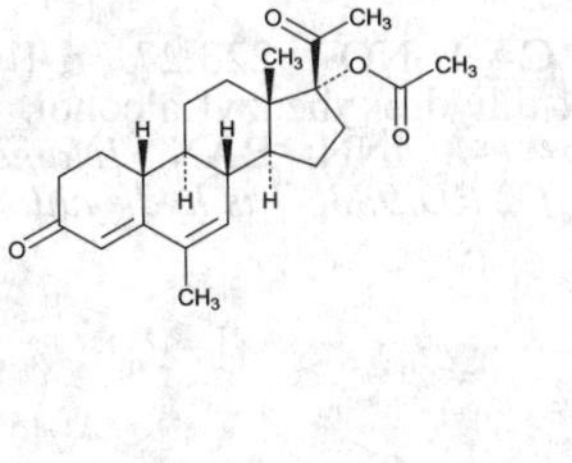

Nomelidine. $C_{15}H_{15}BrN_2$. 303.20. (*Z*)-3-[1-(*p*-Bromophenyl)-3-(methylamino)propenyl]pyridine. *UNII-FVL27C1DMG*. *CAS-60324-59-6*. INN.

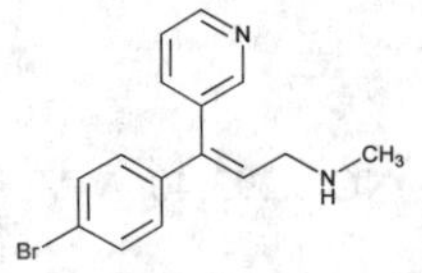

Nomifensine Maleate [*1975*] (noe″ mi fen′ seen mal′ ee ate). $C_{16}H_{18}N_2 \cdot C_4H_4O_4$. 354.40. [Nomifensine is INN and BAN.] (1) 8-Isoquinolinamine, 1,2,3,4-tetrahydro-2-methyl-4-phenyl-, (*Z*)-2-butenedioate (1:1); (2) 8-Amino-1,2,3,4-tetrahydro-2-methyl-4-phenylisoquinoline maleate (1:1). *UNII-76S8CUH5MR; UNII-1LGS5JRP31* [nomifensine]. *CAS-32795-47-4; CAS-24526-64-5* [nomifensine]. *Antidepressant.* Merital (Hoechst-Roussel†) ◇*HOE 984*

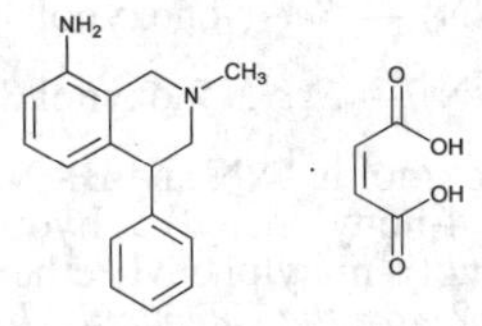

Nonabine. $C_{25}H_{33}NO_2$. 379.54. 7-(1,2-Dimethylheptyl)-2,2-dimethyl-4-(4-pyridyl)-2*H*-1-benzopyran-5-ol. *UNII-77DUK856J7*. *CAS-16985-03-8*. INN; BAN. ◇*BRL 4664*

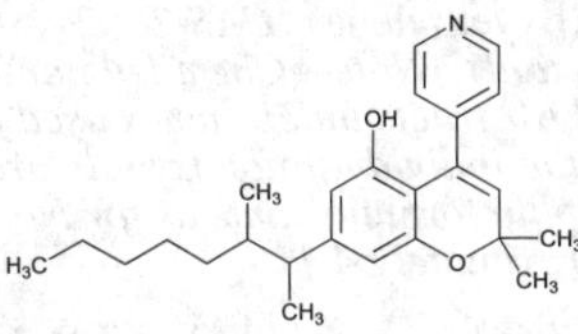

Nonachlazine (previously used name) — *See* Azaclorzine Hydrochloride.

Nonacog Alfa [*1996*] (noe′ na kog al′ fa). Blood-coagulation factor IX (synethic human). Molecular weight is approximately 66,000 daltons. *UNII-382L14738L*. *CAS-181054-95-5*. INN; BAN. *Correction of coagulation deficit.* BeneFix (Genetics Institute)

Nonaperone. $C_{18}H_{24}FNO$. 289.39. 4-(3-Azabicyclo[3.2.2]-non-3-yl)-4′-fluorobutyrophenone. *CAS-15997-76-9*. INN.

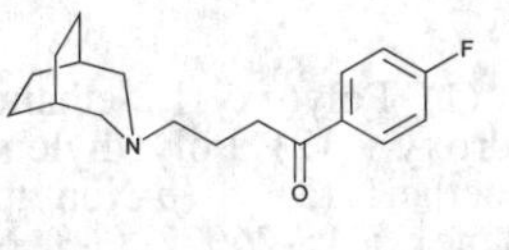

Nonapyrimine. $C_{15}H_{24}N_4$. 260.38. 4-(Nonylamino)-7*H*-pyrrolo[2,3-*d*]pyrimidine. *UNII-322D5Y3Q0G*. *CAS-5626-36-8*. INN.

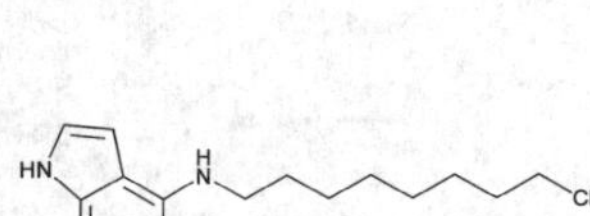

---

† Brand name formerly used, and/or firm no longer concerned with this product.

Nonathymulin. $C_{33}H_{54}N_{12}O_{15}$. 858.85. N^2-[N-[N-[N-[N^2-[N-[N^2-[N-(-5-Oxo-L-prolyl)-L-alanyl]-L-lysyl]-L-seryl]-L-glutaminyl]glycyl]glycyl]-L-seryl]-L-asparagine. *CAS-63958-90-7.* INN.

OXOPAKSQGGSD

Nonivamide. $C_{17}H_{27}NO_3$. 293.40. *N*-Vanillylnonamide. *CAS-2444-46-4.* INN.

Nonoxinol (INN, BAN) — *See* Nonoxynol.

Nonoxinol 4 (INN) — *See* Nonoxynol 4.

Nonoxinol 9 (INN) — *See* Nonoxynol 9.

Nonoxinol 15 (INN) — *See* Nonoxynol 15.

Nonoxinol 30 (INN) — *See* Nonoxynol 30.

Nonoxynol. [Nonoxinol is INN and BAN.] (1) Poly(oxy-1,2-ethanediyl), α-(4-nonylphenyl)-ω-hydroxy-; (2) Polyethylene glycol mono(*p*-nonylphenyl) ether. *[Note—Chemical names (1) and (2) are the Chemical Abstracts index names used for all nonoxynol compounds; the individual nonoxynols are not specifically indexed.]*

Nonoxynol 4 [*1967*] (non ox′ i nol). $C_{23}H_{40}O_5$ (Approximate). 396.56. [Nonoxinol 4 is INN.] (1) Poly(oxy-1,2-ethanediyl), α-(4-nonylphenyl)-ω-hydroxy; (2) Polyethylene glycol mono(*p*-nonylphenyl) ether; (3) α-(*p*-Nonylphenyl)-ω-hydroxytetra(oxyethylene). *CAS-26027-38-3.* *Pharmaceutic aid (surfactant). [Note—Chemical names (1) and (2) are the Chemical Abstracts index names used for all nonoxynol compounds; the individual nonoxynols are not specifically indexed. Graphic formula same as for Nonoxynol 9, except that n is approximately 4.]*

Nonoxynol 9 [*1966*] (non ox′ i nol). **USP.** $C_{15}H_{24}O(C_2H_4O)_n$ (n = approximately 9). [Nonoxinol 9 is INN.] (1) Poly(oxy-1,2-ethanediyl), α-(4-nonylphenyl)-ω-hydroxy-; (2) Polyethylene glycol mono(*p*-nonylphenyl) ether; (3) α-(*p*-Nonylphenyl)-ω-hydroxynona(oxyethylene). *CAS-26027-38-3. Pharmaceutic aid (wetting and/or solubilizing agent); spermaticide.* Conceptrol (Ortho Pharmaceutical); Emko (Schering-Plough HealthCare); Gynol II (Ortho Pharmaceutical); Intercept (Ortho Pharmaceutical); Semicid (Whitehall-Robins); Today Sponge (Whitehall-Robins†)

Nonoxynol 10. (1) Poly(oxy-1,2-ethanediyl), α-(4-nonylphenyl)-ω-hydroxy-; (2) Polyethylene glycol mono(*p*-nonylphenyl) ether; (3) α-(*p*-Nonylphenyl)-ω-hydroxydeca(oxyethylene). *CAS-26027-38-3.* NF XVIII. *Pharmaceutic aid (surfactant). [Note—Graphic formula same as for Nonoxynol 9, except that n is approximately 10.]*

Nonoxynol 15 [*1967*] (non ox′ i nol). $C_{45}H_{84}O_{16}$ (Approximate). 881.14. [Nonoxinol 15 is INN.] α-(*p*-Nonylphenyl)-ω-hydroxypentadeca(oxyethylene). *CAS-26027-38-3.*

Pharmaceutic aid (surfactant). [Note—Graphic formula same as for Nonoxynol 9, except that n is approximately 15.]

Nonoxynol 30 [*1967*] (non ox′ i nol). $C_{75}H_{144}O_{31}$ (Approximate). 1541.93. [Nonoxinol 30 is INN.] α-(*p*-Nonylphenyl)-ω-hydroxytriaconta(oxyethylene). *CAS-26027-38-3. Pharmaceutic aid (surfactant). [Note—Graphic formula same as for Nonoxynol 9, except that n is approximately 30.]*

Nonylphenoxypolyethoxyethanol — *See* Nonoxynol 15.

Nonylphenoxypolyethoxyethanol — *See* Nonoxynol 30.

Nonylphenoxypolyethoxyethanol — *See* Nonoxynol 4.

Nonylphenoxypolyethoxyethanol — *See* Nonoxynol 9.

Noracymethadol Hydrochloride [*1963*] (nor″ a sye meth′ a dol hye″ droe klor′ ide). $C_{22}H_{29}NO_2 \cdot HCl$. 375.93. [Noracymethadol is INN and BAN.] (1) Benzeneethanol, α-ethyl-β-[2-(methylamino)propyl]-β-phenyl-, acetate (ester), hydrochloride; (2) 6-(Methylamino)-4,4-diphenyl-3-heptanol acetate (ester) hydrochloride. *CAS-5633-25-0; CAS-1477-39-0 [noracymethadol]. Analgesic.* ◇NIH 7667; 30109

Noradrenaline (BAN) — *See* Norepinephrine Bitartrate.

Noradrenaline Bitartrate — *See* Norepinephrine Bitartrate.

Noramidopyrine Methanesulfonate Sodium (DCF) — *See* Dipyrone.

Norandrostenolone Phenylpropionate — *See* Nandrolone Phenpropionate.

Norastemizole (trivial name) — *See* Tecastemizole.

Norbolethone [*1964*] (nor bole′ e thone). $C_{21}H_{32}O_2$. 316.48. [Norboletone is INN.] (1) 18,19-Dinorpregn-4-en-3-one, 13-ethyl-17-hydroxy-, (17α)-, ($\pm$)-; (2) ($\pm$)-13-Ethyl-17-hydroxy-18,19-dinor-17α-pregn-4-en-3-one. *CAS-1235-15-0. Anabolic.* ◇Wy-3475

Norboletone (INN) — *See* Norbolethone.

Norbudrine. $C_{12}H_{17}NO_3$. 223.27. α-[(Cyclobutylamino)methyl]-3,4-dihydroxybenzyl alcohol. *UNII-8P6T83567P. CAS-15686-81-4.* INN; BAN. *[Name previously used: Norbutrine.]* ◇RD 9338 *[as hydrochloride]*

Norbutrine (previously used name) — *See* Norbudrine.

Norcholestenol Iodomethyl (^{131}I) [Injection]. $C_{27}H_{45}{}^{131}IO$. 6β-Iodo-^{131}I-methyl-19-norcholest-5(10)-en-3β-ol. *CAS-56897-09-7.* JAN.

Norclostebol. $C_{18}H_{25}ClO_2$. 308.84. 4-Chloro-17β-hydroxyestr-4-en-3-one. *UNII-VI1001O2DI. CAS-13583-21-6.* INN.

Norcodeine. $C_{17}H_{19}NO_3$. 285.34. *N*-Demethylcodeine. *CAS-467-15-2.* INN; BAN; MI.

Norcycline — *See* Sancycline.

Nordazepam. $C_{15}H_{11}ClN_2O$. 270.71. 7-Chloro-1,3-dihydro-5-phenyl-2*H*-1,4-benzodiazepin-2-one. *CAS-1088-11-5.* INN; MI.

Nordefrin Hydrochloride. $C_9H_{13}NO_3{\cdot}HCl$. 219.67. ($\pm$)-α-(1-Aminoethyl)-3,4-dihydroxybenzyl alcohol hydrochloride. *UNII-R81X549E70* [nordefrin]. *CAS-155-60-2; CAS-6539-57-7* [nordefrin]. NF XII; MI. Cobefrin (Sterling Winthrop)

Nordinone. $C_{20}H_{28}O_2$. 300.44. 11α-Hydroxy-17,17-dimethyl-18-norandrosta-4,13-dien-3-one. *CAS-33122-60-0.* INN.

Norelgestromin [*2000*] (nor el jes′ troe min). $C_{21}H_{29}NO_2$. 327.46. (1) 18,19-Dinorpregn-4-en-20-yn-3-one, 13-ethyl-17-hydroxy-, oxime, (17α)-; (2) 13-Ethyl-17-hydroxy-18,19-dinor-17α-pregn-4-en-20-yn-3-one oxime. *UNII-R0TAY3X631. CAS-53016-31-2.* INN; BAN. *Female contraceptive.* ORTHO EVRA (R. W. Johnson); EVRA (R. W. Johnson) [*Note—Norelgestromin has appeared in the literature as 17-deacylnorgestimate.*] ◇*RWJ-10553*

Norephedrine Hydrochloride — *See* Phenylpropanolamine Hydrochloride.

Norepinephrine Bitartrate [*1980*] (nor″ ep i nef′ rin bye tar′ trate). **USP.** $C_8H_{11}NO_3{\cdot}C_4H_6O_6{\cdot}H_2O$. 337.28. [Norepinephrine is INN; BAN and JAN; Norepinephrine Hydrochloride is JAN; Noradrenaline is BAN.] (1) 1,2-Benzenediol, 4-(2-amino-1-hydroxyethyl)-, (*R*)-[*R*-(*R*,R**)]-2,3-dihydroxybutanedioate (1:1) (salt), monohydrate; (2) (-)-α-(Aminomethyl)-3,4-dihydroxybenzyl alcohol tartrate (1:1) (salt) monohydrate. *UNII-IFY5PE3ZRW; UNII-X4W3ENH1CV* [norepinephrine]. *CAS-69815-49-2; CAS-51-40-1* [anhydrous]; *CAS-5794-08-1* [replaced]; *CAS-51-41-2* [norepinephrine]. *Adrenergic (vasoconstrictor).* Levophed (Hospira) [*Name previously used: Levarterenol Bitartrate.*]

Norethandrolone. $C_{20}H_{30}O_2$. 302.45. 17α-Ethyl-17β-hydroxyestr-4-en-3-one. *UNII-P7W01638W6. CAS-52-78-8.* NF XIII; INN; BAN; MI.

Norethindrone (nor eth′ in drone). **USP.** $C_{20}H_{26}O_2$. 298.42. [Norethisterone is INN, BAN, and JAN.] (1) 19-Norpregn-4-en-20-yn-3-one, 17-hydroxy-, (17α)-; (2) 17-Hydroxy-19-nor-17α-pregn-4-en-20-yn-3-one. *UNII-T18F433X4S. CAS-68-22-4. Progestin.* Micronor (Ortho-McNeil); Norlutin (Pfizer) ◇*NSC-9564*

Norethindrone Acetate (nor eth′ in drone as′ e tate). **USP.** $C_{22}H_{28}O_3$. 340.46. (1) 19-Norpregn-4-en-20-yn-3-one, 17-(acetyloxy)-, (17α); (2) 17-Hydroxy-19-nor-17α-pregn-4-en-20-yn-3-one acetate. *UNII-9S44LIC7OJ. CAS-51-98-9. Progestin.* Aygestin (Duramed); Norlutate (Pfizer)

Norethisterone (INN, BAN, JAN, DCF) — *See* Norethindrone.

---

† Brand name formerly used, and/or firm no longer concerned with this product.

Norethynodrel [*1962*] (nor″ e thye′ noe drel). **USP.** $C_{20}H_{26}O_2$. 298.42. [Noretynodrel is INN and BAN.] (1) 19-Norpregn-5(10)-en-20-yn-3-one, 17-hydroxy-, (17α)-; (2) 17-Hydroxy-19-nor-17α-pregn-5(10)-en-20-yn-3-one. *UNII-88181ACA0M. CAS-68-23-5. Progestin.* ◇*SC-4642; NSC-15432*

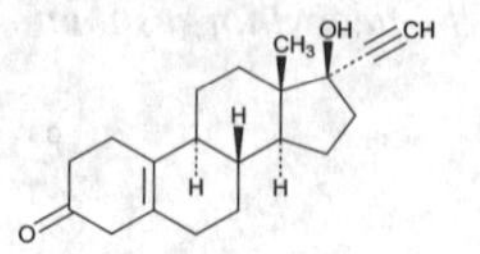

Noretynodrel (INN, BAN, DCF) — *See* Norethynodrel.

Noreximide. $C_9H_9NO_2$. 163.17. *cis-exo*-5-Norbornene-2,3-dicarboximide. *CAS-6319-06-8.* INN.

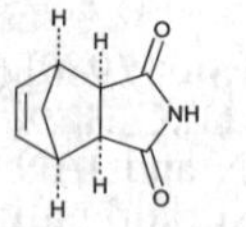

Norfenefrine. $C_8H_{11}NO_2$. 153.18. [Norfenefrine Hydrochloride is JAN.] α-(Aminomethyl)-*m*-hydroxybenzyl alcohol. *CAS-536-21-0.* INN; MI. ◇*WV 569 [as hydrochloride]*

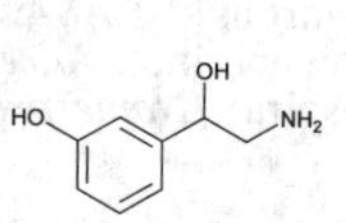

Norfloxacin [*1984*] (nor flox′ a sin). **USP.** $C_{16}H_{18}FN_3O_3$. 319.33. (1) 3-Quinolinecarboxylic acid, 1-ethyl-6-fluoro-1,4-dihydro-4-oxo-7-(1-piperazinyl)-; (2) 1-Ethyl-6-fluoro-1,4-dihydro-4-oxo-7-(1-piperazinyl)-3-quinolinecarboxylic acid. *UNII-N0F8P22L1P. CAS-70458-96-7.* INN; BAN; JAN. *Antibacterial.* Noroxin (Merck) ◇*MK-366*

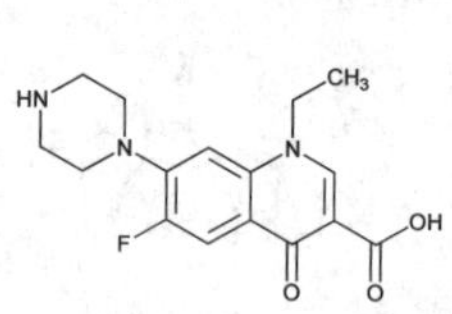

Norfloxacin Succinil. $C_{20}H_{22}FN_3O_6$. 419.40. 7-[4-(3-Carboxypropionyl)-1-piperazinyl]-1-ethyl-6-fluoro-1,4-dihydro-4-oxo-3-quinolinecarboxylic acid. *UNII-K40E7MO61Q. CAS-100587-52-8.* INN.

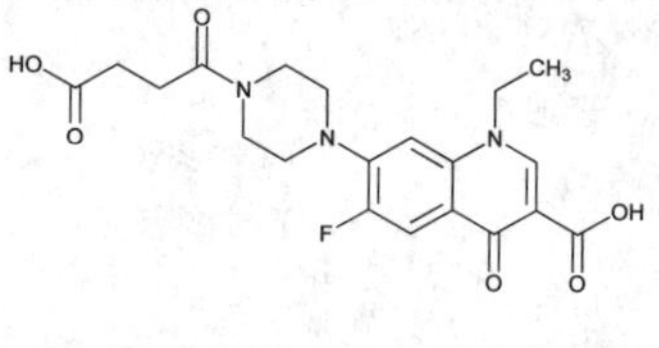

Norflurane [*1967*] (nor flur′ ane). $C_2H_2F_4$. 102.03. (1) Ethane, 1,1,1,2-tetrafluoro-; (2) 1,1,1,2-Tetrafluoroethane. *UNII-DH9E53K1Y8. CAS-811-97-2.* INN; BAN. *Anesthetic (inhalation).* ◇*HFA-134-a*

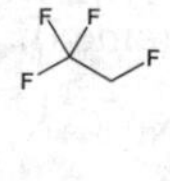

Norgesterone. $C_{20}H_{28}O_2$. 300.44. 17α-Vinyl-5(10)-estrene-17β-ol-3-one. *CAS-13563-60-5.* INN; MI.

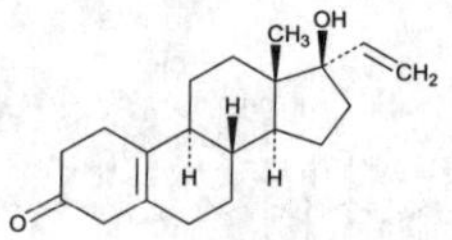

Norgestimate [*1975*] (nor jes′ ti mate). **USP.** $C_{23}H_{31}NO_3$. 369.50. (1) 18,19-Dinor-17-pregn-4-en-20-yn-3-one, 17-(acetyloxy)-13-ethyl-, oxime, (17α)-(+)-; (2) (+)-13-Ethyl-17-hydroxy-18,19-dinor-17α-pregn-4-en-20-yn-3-one oxime acetate (ester). *UNII-C291HFX4DY. CAS-35189-28-7.* INN; BAN. *Progestin. [Name previously used: Dexnorgestrel Acetime.]* ◇*ORF 10131; RWJ 10131*

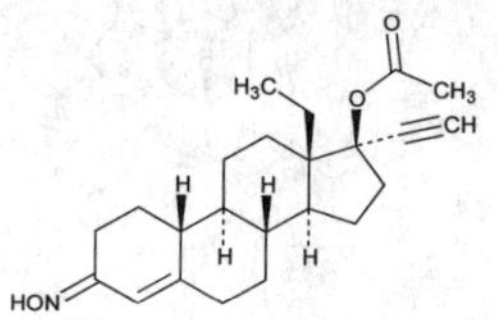

Norgestomet [*1974*] (nor jes′ toe met). $C_{23}H_{32}O_4$. 372.50. (1) 19-Norpregn-4-ene-3,20-dione, 17-(acetyloxy)-11-methyl-, (11β)-; (2) 17-Hydroxy-11β-methyl-19-norpregn-4-ene-3,20-dione acetate. *UNII-3L33UD42X4. CAS-25092-41-5.* INN; BAN. *Progestin.* ◇*SC-21009*

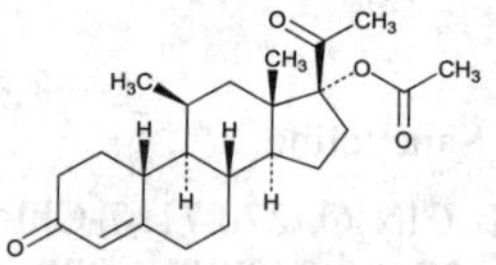

Norgestrel [*1966*] (nor jes′ trel). **USP.** $C_{21}H_{28}O_2$. 312.45. (1) 18,19-Dinorpregn-4-en-20-yn-3-one, 13-ethyl-17-hydroxy-, (17α)-(±)-; (2) (±)-13-Ethyl-17-hydroxy-18,19-dinor-17α-pregn-4-en-20-yn-3-one. *UNII-3J8Q1747Z2. CAS-6533-00-2.* INN; BAN; JAN. *Progestin.* Ovrette (Wyeth) ◇*Wy-3707*

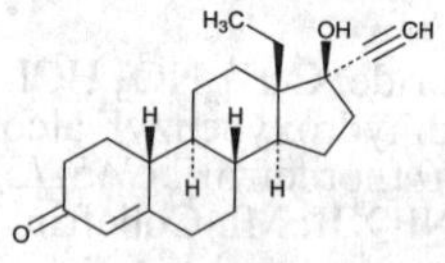

Norgestrienone. $C_{20}H_{22}O_2$. 294.39. 17-Hydroxy-19-nor-17α-pregna-4,9,11-trien-20-yn-3-one. *CAS-848-21-5.* INN; DCF; MI.

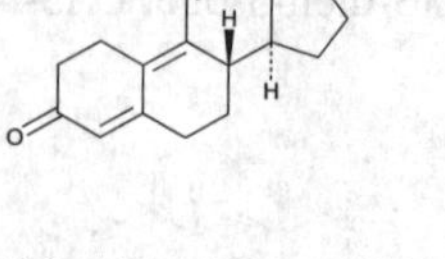

Norletimol. $C_{14}H_{13}NO$. 211.26. *o*-(*N*-Benzylformimidoyl)-phenol. *CAS-886-08-8.* INN; BAN.

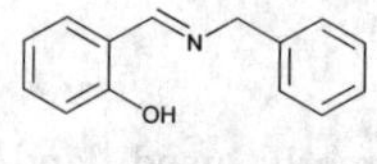

Norleusactide. $C_{142}H_{222}N_{42}O_{31}$. 3013.54. [Pentacosactride is BAN.] D-Seryl-L-tyrosyl-L-seryl-L-norleucyl-L-glutamyl-L-histadyl-L-phenylalanyl-L-arginyl-L-tryptophyl-glycyl-L-lysyl-L-propyl-L-valyl-glycyl-L-lysyl-L-lysyl-L-arginyl-L-arginyl-L-prolyl-L-valyl-L-lysyl-L-valyl-L-tyrosyl-L-prolyl-L-vallinamide. *CAS-17692-62-5.* INN; DCF. ◇*DW 75*

SYS-N1e-EHFRWG KPVGKKRRPV KVYPV —NH₂

Nle - norleucine

Norlevorphanol. $C_{16}H_{21}NO$. 243.34. (-)-3-Hydroxymorphinan. *CAS-1531-12-0.* INN; BAN; DCF; MI.

Normethadone. $C_{20}H_{25}NO$. 295.42. 6-Dimethylamino-4,4-diphenyl-3-hexanone. *UNII-KR2L2A68XL. CAS-467-85-6.* INN; BAN; DCF; MI. ◇*Hoechst 10582*

Normethandrolone — *See* Normethandrone.

Normethandrone. *CAS-514-61-4.* MI. ◇*NSC-10039*

Normethisterone — *See* Normethandrone.

Normorphine. $C_{16}H_{17}NO_3$. 271.31. 4,5-Epoxy-3,6-dihydroxy-morphin-7-ene. *CAS-466-97-7.* INN; BAN; DCF; MI.

Norpipanone. $C_{23}H_{29}NO$. 335.48. 4,4-Diphenyl-6-(1-piperidyl)-3-hexanone. *UNII-127X8DJ74M. CAS-561-48-8.* INN; BAN; DCF; MI. ◇*Hoechst 10495*

Nortestosterone Furanpropionate (JAN) — *See* Nandrolone Phenpropionate.

Nortestosterone Phenylpropionate — *See* Nandrolone Phenpropionate.

---

† Brand name formerly used, and/or firm no longer concerned with this product.

Nortetrazepam. $C_{15}H_{15}ClN_2O$. 274.75. 7-Chloro-5-(1-cyclohexen-1-yl)-1,3-dihydro-2*H*-1,4-benzodiazepin-2-one. *UNII-PWL441R6EQ. CAS-10379-11-0.* INN; DCF. ◇*CB 4260*

Nortopixantrone. $C_{20}H_{24}N_6O_2$. 380.44. 2-[2-[(2-Hydroxyethyl)amino]ethyl]-5-[[2-(methylamino)ethyl]amino]indazolo[4,3-*gh*]isoquinolin-6(2*H*)-one. *UNII-PH2639TAB4. CAS-156090-17-4.* INN; BAN. ◇*BBR 3438*

Nortriptyline Hydrochloride [*1963*] (nor trip′ ti leen hye″ droe klor′ ide). **USP**. $C_{19}H_{21}N \cdot HCl$. 299.84. [Nortriptyline is INN and BAN.] (1) 1-Propanamine, 3-(10,11-dihydro-5*H*-dibenzo[*a,d*]cyclohepten-5-ylidene)-*N*-methyl-, hydrochloride; (2) 10,11-Dihydro-*N*-methyl-5*H*-dibenzo[*a,d*]cycloheptene-$\Delta^{5,\gamma}$-propylamine hydrochloride. *UNII-00FN6IH15D; UNII-BL03SY4LXB* [nortriptyline]. *CAS-894-71-3; CAS-72-69-5* [nortriptyline]. JAN. *Antidepressant.* Aventyl Hydrochloride (Ranbaxy); Pamelor (Tyco) ◇*38489*

Norvinisterone. $C_{20}H_{28}O_2$. 300.44. 17β-Hydroxy-17α-vinyl-estr-4-en-3-one. *CAS-6795-60-4.* INN; MI.

Norvinodrel — *See* Norgesterone.

Nosantine. $C_{14}H_{22}N_4O_2$. 278.35. *erythro*-9-[1-(1-Hydroxyethyl)heptyl]hypoxanthine. *UNII-NYM432G79C. CAS-76600-30-1.* INN; BAN. ◇*NPT 15392*

Noscapine (nos′ ka peen). **USP**. $C_{22}H_{23}NO_7$. 413.42. (1) 1(3*H*)-Isobenzofuranone, 6,7-dimethoxy-3-(5,6,7,8-tetrahydro-4-methoxy-6-methyl-1,3-dioxolo[4,5-*g*]-isoquinolin-5-yl), [S-(R*,S*)]-; (2) Narcotine. *UNII-8V32U4AOQU. CAS-128-62-1.* INN; BAN; JAN. *Antitussive.* Tusscapine (Fisons†) ◇*NSC-5366*

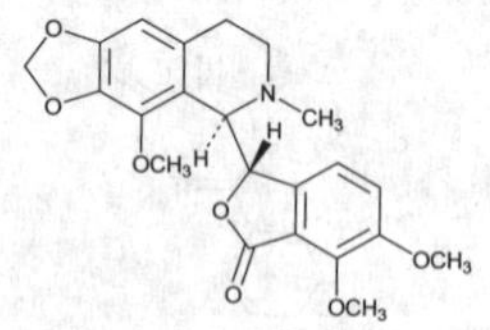

Noscapine Hydrochloride. *UNII-TTN62ITH9I. CAS-912-60-7; CAS-128-62-1* [noscapine]. NF XII; JAN; MI.

Nosiheptide [*1978*] (noe″ si hep′ tide). $C_{51}H_{43}N_{13}O_{12}S_6$. 1222.36. (1) Nosiheptide; (2) N-[1-(Aminocarbonyl)ethenyl]-2-[14-ethylidene-9,10,11,12,13,14,19,20,21,22,23,24,26,33,35,36-hexadecahydro-3,23-dihydroxy-11-(1-hydroxyethyl)-31-methyl-9,12,19,24,33,43-hexaoxo-30,32-imino-8,5:18,15:40,37-trinitrilo-21,36-([2,4]-*endo*-thiazolomethanimino)-5H,15H,37H-pyrido[3,2-w][2,11,21,27,31,7,14,17]ben-zoxatetrathiatriazacyclohexatriacontin-2-yl]-4-thiazolecarboxamide. *CAS-56377-79-8.* INN; BAN. *Growth stimulant (veterinary).* ◇*RP 9671*

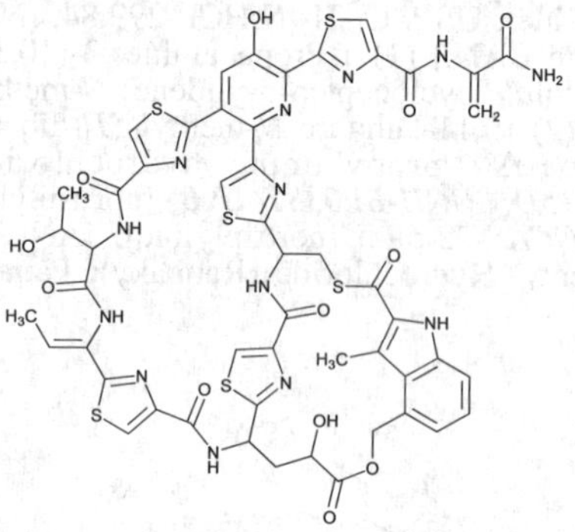

Novobiocin Calcium. $C_{62}H_{70}CaN_4O_{22}$. 1263.31. [Novobiocin is INN and BAN.] (1) Benzamide, N-[7-[[3-O-(aminocarbonyl)-6-deoxy-5-C-methyl-4-O-methyl-β-L-*lyxo*-hexopyranosyl]oxy]-4-hydroxy-8-methyl-2-oxo-2H-1-benzopyran-3-yl]-4-hydroxy-3-(3-methyl-2-butenyl)-, calcium salt (2:1); (2) Novobiocin, calcium salt. *UNII-RHW5BU180N; UNII-17EC19951N* [novobiocin]. *CAS-4309-70-0; CAS-303-81-1* [novobiocin]. USP XXII.

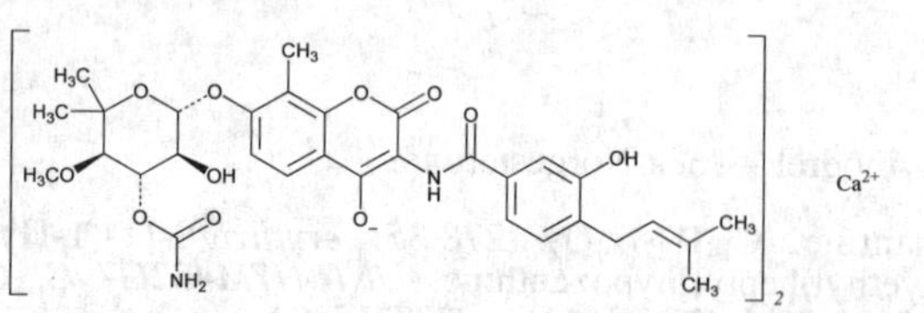

Novobiocin Sodium (noe″ voe bye′ oh sin soe′ dee um). **USP.** $C_{31}H_{35}N_2NaO_{11}$. 634.61. (1) Benzamide, N-[7-[[3-O-(aminocarbonyl)-6-deoxy-5-C-methyl-4-O-methyl-β-L-*lyxo*-hexopyranosyl]oxy]-4-hydroxy-8-methyl-2-oxo-2H-1-benzopyran-3-yl]-4-hydroxy-3-(3-methyl-2-butenyl-, monosodium salt; (2) Novobiocin, monosodium salt. *UNII-Q9S9NQ5YIY. CAS-1476-53-5. Antibacterial.* Albamycin (Pfizer)

Novo-Dermoquinona (previously used name) — *See* Mequinol.

Noxiptiline. $C_{19}H_{22}N_2O$. 294.39. 10,11-Dihydro-5H-dibenzo[a,d]cyclohepten-5-one O-[(2-dimethylamino)ethyl]oxime. *UNII-DF7D3NY7EL. CAS-3362-45-6.* INN; BAN; DCF; MI. *[Name previously used: Noxiptyline.]* ◇*BAY 1521*

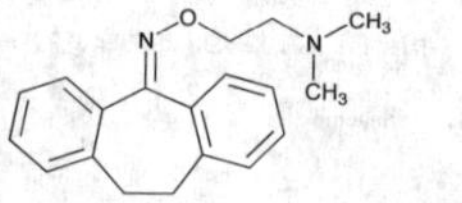

Noxiptyline (previously used name) — *See* Noxiptiline.

Noxythiolin (previously used name) — *See* Noxytiolin.

Noxytiolin. $C_3H_8N_2OS$. 120.17. 1-Hydroxymethyl-3-methyl-2-thiourea. *UNII-4DN3AF1FU6. CAS-15599-39-0.* INN; BAN; DCF; MI. *[Name previously used: Noxythiolin.]*

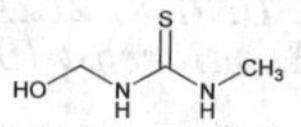

NSC [National Service Center, National Cancer Institute] Numbers—*See* Appendix II.

Nuclomedone. $C_{13}H_{11}ClN_2O_2S$. 294.76. (±)-6-(p-Chlorobenzyl)-2,3-dihydro-5H-thiazolo[3,2-a]pyrimidine-5,7(6H)-dione. *UNII-MR28U787Z2. CAS-75963-52-9.* INN.

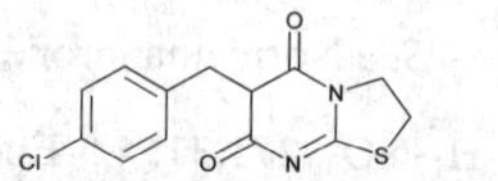

Nuclotixene. $C_{21}H_{20}ClNS$. 353.91. 3-[(2-Chlorothioxanthen-9-ylidene)methyl]quinuclidine. *CAS-36471-39-3.* INN.

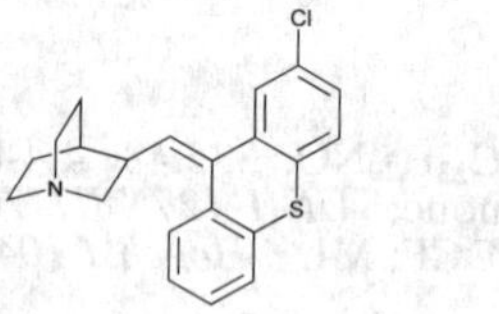

Nufenoxole [*1978*] (nue″ fen ox′ ole). $C_{25}H_{29}N_3O$. 387.52. (1) 2-Azabicyclo[2.2.2]octane, 2-[3-(5-methyl-1,3,4-oxadiazol-2-yl)-3,3-diphenylpropyl]-; (2) 2-[3-(5-Methyl-1,3,4-oxadiazol-2-yl)-3,3-diphenylpropyl]-2-azabicyclo[2.2.2]octane. *CAS-57726-65-5.* INN; BAN. *Antiperistaltic.* ◇*SC-27166*

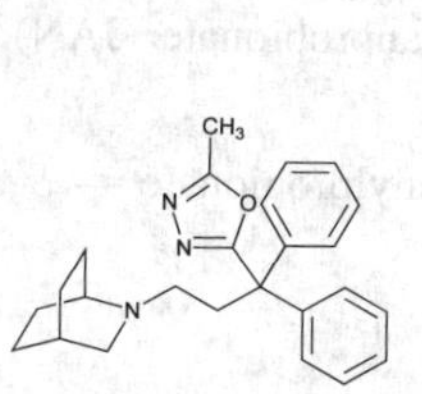

Nupafant. $C_{23}H_{32}N_4O_3S$. 444.59. N-[(S)-1-(Ethoxymethyl)-3-methylbutyl]-N-methyl-α-(2-methyl-1H-imidazo[4,5-c]pyridin-1-yl)-p-toluenesulfonamide. *UNII-02NKI0ARRJ. CAS-139133-27-0.* INN; BAN.

Nutmeg Oil. *CAS-8008-45-5.* NF XVI.

Nuvenzepine. $C_{19}H_{20}N_4O_2$. 336.39. 6,11-Dihydro-11-(1-methylisonipecotoyl)-5H-pyrido[2,3-b][1,5]benzodiazepin-5-one. *UNII-8OMO7K4W74. CAS-96487-37-5.* INN.

Nux Vomica Extract. An extract of the seed of *Strychnos nux-vomica* Linné (*Loganiaceae*). JAN.

Nylestriol [*1975*] (nye les′ tree ol). $C_{25}H_{32}O_3$. 380.52. [Nilestriol is INN and BAN.] (1) 19-Nor-17-pregna-1,3,5(10)-trien-20-yne-16,17-diol, 3-(cyclopentyloxy)-, (16α,17α)-; (2) 17α-Ethynylestra-1,3,5(10)-triene-3,16α,17β-triol 3-cyclopentyl ether. *CAS-39791-20-3. Estrogen.* ◇49825

Nylidrin Hydrochloride. $C_{19}H_{25}NO_2 \cdot HCl$. 335.87. [Buphenine is INN and BAN.] (1) Benzenemethanol, 4-hydroxy-α-[1-[(1-methyl-3-phenylpropyl)amino]ethyl]-, hydrochloride; (2) p-Hydroxy-α-[1-[(1-methyl-3-phenylpropyl)amino]ethyl]benzyl alcohol hydrochloride. *CAS-849-55-8; CAS-900-01-6* [replaced]; *CAS-447-41-6* [nylidrin]. USP XXII.

Nystatin (nye stat′ in). USP. $C_{47}H_{75}NO_{17}$. 926.09. (1) Nystatin A; (2) 14,39-Dioxabicyclo[33.3.1]nonatriaconta-19,21,25,27,29,31-hexaene-36-carboxylic acid, 33-[(3-amino-3,6-dideoxy-β-D-mannopyranosyl)oxy]-1,3,4,7,9,11,17,37-octahydroxy-15,16,18-trimethyl-13-oxo-, (1S,3R,4R,7R,9R,11R,15S,16R,17R,18S,19E,21E,25E,27E,29E,31E,33R,35S,36R,37S)-; (3) (1S,3R,4R,7R,9R,11R,15S,16R,17R,18S,19E,21E,25E,27E,29E,31E,33R,35S,36R,37S)-33-[(3-Amino-3,6-dideoxy-β-D-mannopyranosyl)oxy]-1,3,4,7,9,11,17,37-octahy-droxy-15,16,18-trimethyl-13-oxo-14,39-dioxabicyclo[33.3.1]nonatriaconta-19,21,25,27,29,31-hexaene-36-carboxylic acid. *UNII-BDF1O1C72E. CAS-1400-61-9.* INN; BAN; JAN. *Antifungal.* Mycostatin (Ranbaxy)

^{15}O — *See* Water O 15.

Obatoclax Mesylate [*2005*] (oh bat′ oh klax mes′ i late). $C_{20}H_{19}N_3O \cdot CH_4O_3S$. 413.49. [Obatoclax is INN.] (1) 1H-Indole, 2-[2-[(3,5-dimethyl-1H-pyrrol-2-yl)methylene]-3-methoxy-2H-pyrrol-5-yl]-, monomethanesulfonate; (2) 2-[2-[(3,5-Dimethyl-1H-pyrrol-2-yl)methylidene]-3-methox-y-2H-pyrrol-5-yl]-1H-indole monomethanesulfonate. *UNII-39200FJ43J; UNII-QN4128B52A* [obatoclax]. *CAS-803712-79-0; CAS-803712-67-6* [obatoclax]. *Treatment of chronic lymphocytic leukemia and solid tumor cancer.* (Gemin X Biotechnologies) ◇GX15-070MS

Oberadilol. $C_{25}H_{30}ClN_5O_3$. 483.99. ($\pm$)-4-Chloro-2-[3-[[1,1-dimethyl-2-[p-(1,4,5,6-tetrahydro-4-methyl-6-oxo-3-pyridazinyl)anilino]ethyl]amino]-2-hydroxypropoxy]benzonitrile. *UNII-7ZNX9ET039. CAS-114856-44-9.* INN.

Obeticholic Acid [*2008*] (oh bet″ i koe′ lik). $C_{26}H_{44}O_4$. 420.63. (1) Cholan-24-oic acid, 6-ethyl-3,7-dihydroxy-, (3α,5β,6α,7α)-; (2) 6α-Ethyl-3α,7α-dihydroxy-5β-cholan-24-oic acid. *CAS-459789-99-2. Treatment of primary biliary cirrhosis.* ◇INT-747

Obidoxime Chloride [*1971*] (oh″ bi dox′ eem klor′ ide). $C_{14}H_{16}Cl_2N_4O_3$. 359.21. (1) Pyridinium, 1,1′-[oxybis(methylene)]bis[4-(hydroxyimino)methyl]-, dichloride; (2) 1,1′-(Oxydimethylene)bis[4-formylpyridinium] dichloride dioxime. *UNII-3HXR312Z9M. CAS-114-90-9.* INN. *Cholinesterase reactivator.*

Obinepitide. $C_{185}H_{288}N_{54}O_{55}S_2$. 4212.73. [34-L-Glutamine]-pancreatic hormone (human). *CAS-348119-84-6.* INN.

Oblimersen Sodium [*2002*] (oh″ bli mer′ sen soe′ dee um). $C_{172}H_{204}N_{62}Na_{17}O_{91}P_{17}S_{17}$. 6058.31. [Oblimersen is INN.] (1) DNA, d(P-thio)(T-C-T-C-C-C-A-G-C-G-T-G-C-G-C-C-A-T); (2) P-Thiothymidylyl-(3′→5′)-2′-deoxy-P-thiocytidylyl-(3′→5′)-P-thiothymidylyl-(3′→5′)-2′-deoxy-P-thiocytidylyl-(3′→5′)-2′-deoxy-P-thiocytidylyl-(3′→5′)-2′-

---

† Brand name formerly used, and/or firm no longer concerned with this product.

deoxy-*P*-thiocytidylyl-(3′→5′)-2′-deoxy-*P*-thioadenylyl-(3′→5′)-2′-deoxy-*P*-thioguanylyl-(3′→5′)-2′-deoxy-*P*-thiocytidylyl-(3′→5′)-2′-deoxy-*P*-thioguanylyl-(3′→5′)-*P*-thiothymidylyl-(3′→5′)-2′-deoxy-*P*-thioguanylyl-(3′→5′)-2′-deoxy-*P*-thiocytidylyl-(3′→5′)-2′-deoxy-*P*-thioguany-lyl-(3′→5′)-2′-deoxy-*P*-thiocytidylyl-(3′→5′)-2′-deoxy-*P*-thiocytidylyl-(3′→5′)-2′-deoxy-*P*-thioadenylyl-(3′→5′)-thymidine heptadecasodium salt. *UNII-SH55B0RQ9K. CAS-190977-41-4. Treatment of cancer and rheumatological diseases (an antisense oligonucleotide).* Genasense (Genta) ◇*G3139*

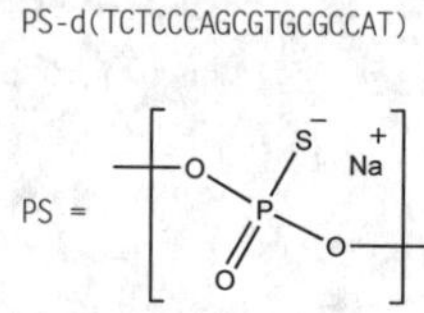

PS-d(TCTCCCAGCGTGCGCCAT)

PS =

Ocaperidone [*1993*] (oh″ ka per′ i done). $C_{24}H_{25}FN_4O_2$. 420.48. (1) 4*H*-Pyrido[1,2-*a*]pyrimidin-4-one, 3-[2-[4-(6-fluoro-1,2-benzisoxazol-3-yl)-1-piperidinyl]ethyl]-2,9-dimethyl-; (2) 3-[2-[4-(6-Fluoro-1,2-benzisoxazol-3-yl)piperidino]ethyl]-2,9-dimethyl-4*H*-pyrido[1,2-*a*]pyrimidin-4-one. *UNII-26HUS7139V. CAS-129029-23-8.* INN; BAN. *Antipsychotic.* ◇*R 79598*

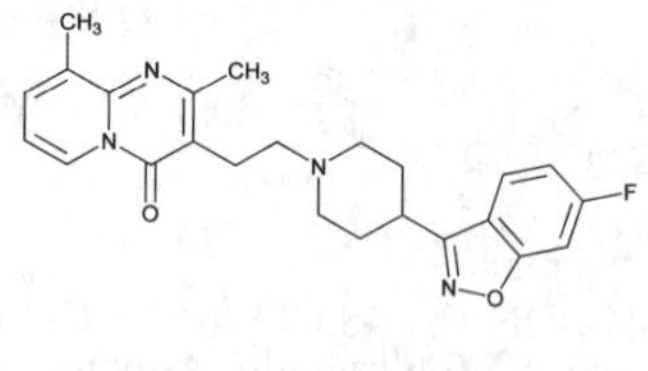

Ocfentanil Hydrochloride [*1989*] (ok fen′ ta nil hye″ droe klor′ ide). $C_{22}H_{27}FN_2O_2 \cdot HCl$. 406.92. [Ocfentanil is INN.] (1) Acetamide, *N*-(2-fluorophenyl)-2-methoxy-*N*-[1-(2-phenylethyl)-4-piperidinyl]-, monohydrochloride; (2) 2′-Fluoro-2-methoxy-*N*-(1-phenethyl)-4-piperidyl)acetanilide monohydrochloride. *UNII-Z8T88FVW9V. CAS-112964-97-3; CAS-101343-69-5* [ocfentanil]. *Analgesic (narcotic).* ◇*A-3217*

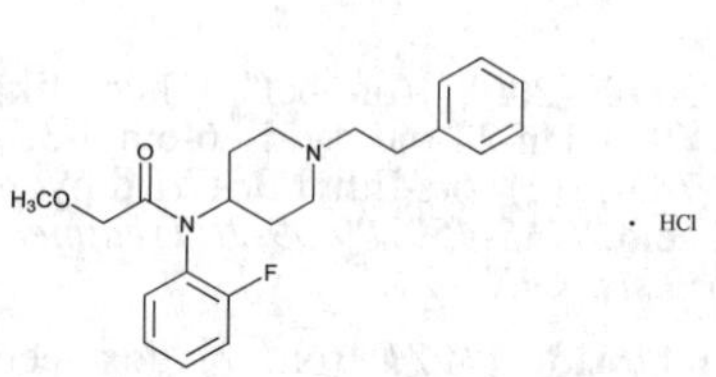

Ociltide. $C_{31}H_{40}N_6O_7S$. 640.75. L-Tyrosyl-*N*ᵋ-formyl-D-lysyl-glycylphenyl-*N*-(tetrahydro-2-oxo-3-thienyl)-L-alaninamide. *CAS-78410-57-8.* INN.

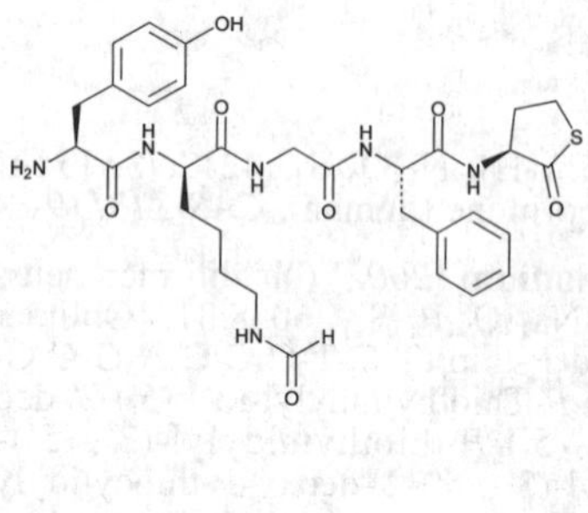

Ocinaplon [*1994*] (oh sin′ a plon). $C_{17}H_{11}N_5O$. 301.30. (1) Methanone, 2-pyridinyl[7-(4-pyridinyl)pyrazolo[1,5-*a*]pyrimidin-3-yl]-; (2) 2-Pyridyl 7-(4-pyridyl)pyrazolo-[1,5-*a*]pyrimidin-3-yl ketone. *CAS-96604-21-6.* INN. *Anti-anxiety agent.* ◇*CL 273,547*

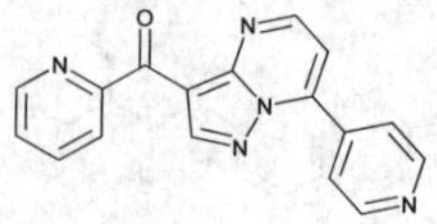

Ocrase. Fibrinolytic enzyme derived from *Aspergillus ochraceus.CAS-51899-01-5.* INN.

Ocrelizumab [*2005*] (ok″ re liz′ oo mab). $C_{6494}H_{9978}N_{1718}O_{2014}S_{46}$. 148,000 daltons. Immunoglobulin G1, anti-(human CD20 (antigen)) (human-mouse monoclonal 2H7 γ1-chain), disulfide with human-mouse monoclonal 2H7 κ-chain, dimer. *UNII-A10SJL62JY. CAS-637334-45-3.* INN. *Treatment of rheumatoid arthritis.* ◇*PR070769*

Ocrilate (INN) — *See* Ocrylate.

Ocrylate [*1969*] (ok′ ri late). $C_{12}H_{19}NO_2$. 209.28. [Ocrilate is INN.] (1) 2-Propenoic acid, 2-cyano-, octyl ester; (2) Octyl-2-cyanoacrylate. *CAS-6701-17-3. Surgical aid (tissue adhesive).*

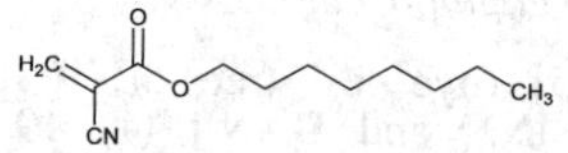

Octabenzone [*1967*] (ok″ ta ben′ zone). $C_{21}H_{26}O_3$. 326.43. (1) Methanone, [2-hydroxy-4-(octyloxy)phenyl]phenyl-; (2) 2-Hydroxy-4-(octyloxy)benzophenone. *UNII-73P3618V2E. CAS-1843-05-6.* INN. *Ultraviolet screen.*

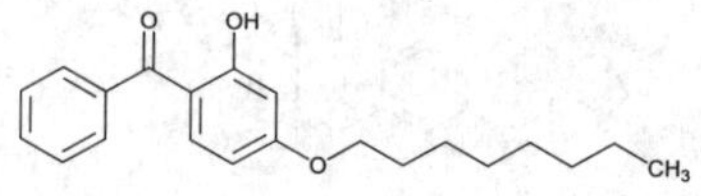

Octacaine. $C_{14}H_{22}N_2O$. 234.34. 3-Diethylaminobutyranilide. *UNII-5BZF8S8IL5. CAS-13912-77-1.* INN; MI.

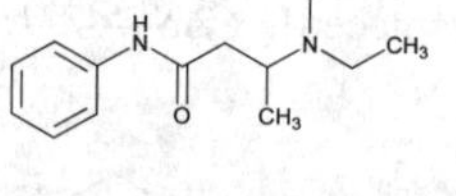

Octacosactrin (previously used name) — *See* Tosactide.

Octafonium Chloride. $C_{27}H_{42}ClNO$. 432.08. Benzyldiethyl[2-[4-(1,1,3,3-tetramethylbutyl)phenoxy]ethyl]ammonium chloride. *CAS-78-05-7.* INN; BAN. *[Name previously used: Octaphonium Chloride.]*

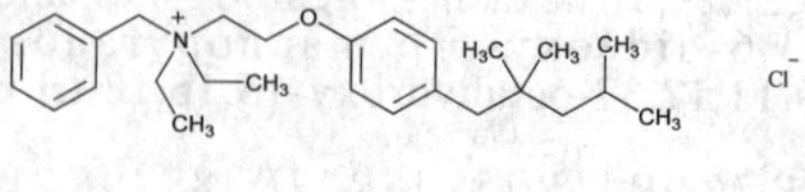

Octamoxin. $C_8H_{20}N_2$. 144.26. (1-Methylheptyl)hydrazine. *UNII-0HXY3M6S54. CAS-4684-87-1.* INN; DCF; MI.

Octamylamine. $C_{13}H_{29}N$. 199.38. *N*-Isopentyl-1,5-dimethyl-hexylamine. *CAS-502-59-0.* INN; DCF; MI.

Octanoic Acid [*1983*] (ok″ ta noe′ ik as′ id). $C_8H_{16}O_2$. 144.21. (1) Octanoic acid; (2) Octanoic acid. *UNII-OBL58JN025. CAS-124-07-2.* INN. *Antifungal.*

Octaphonium Chloride (previously used name) — *See* Octafonium Chloride.

Octapinol. $C_{15}H_{31}NO$. 241.41. 4-(2-Propylpentyl)-1-piperidineethanol. *CAS-71138-71-1.* INN.

Octastine. $C_{23}H_{30}ClNO$. 371.94. 1-[2-[(*p*-Chloro-α-methyl-α-phenylbenzyl)oxy]ethyl]octahydroazocine. *CAS-59767-12-3.* INN.

Octatropine Methylbromide (INN, BAN) — *See* Anisotropine Methylbromide.

Octatropone Bromide — *See* Anisotropine Methylbromide.

Octaverine. $C_{23}H_{27}NO_5$. 397.46. 6,7-Dimethoxy-1-(3,4,5-triethoxyphenyl)isoquinoline. *CAS-549-68-8.* INN; BAN; DCF; MI.

Octazamide [*1976*] (ok taz′ a mide). $C_{13}H_{15}NO_2$. 217.26. (1) 1*H*-Furo[3,4-*c*]pyrrole, 5-benzoylhexahydro-; (2) 5-Benzoylhexahydro-1*H*-furo[3,4-*c*]pyrrole. *CAS-56391-55-0.* INN. *Analgesic.* ◇*ICI-U.S. 457*

Octenidine Hydrochloride [*1979*] (ok ten′ ni deen hye″ droe klor′ ide). $C_{36}H_{62}N_4$.2HCl. 623.83. [Octenidine is INN and BAN.] (1) 1-Octanamine, *N,N′*-(1,10-decanediyldi-1(4*H*)-

pyridinyl-4-ylidene)bis-, dihydrochloride; (2) 1,1′-Decamethylenebis[1,4-dihydro-4-(octylimino)pyridine] dihydrochloride. *CAS-70775-75-6; CAS-71251-02-0* [octenidine]. *Anti-infective, topical.* ◇*Win 41464-2*

Octenidine Saccharin [*1984*] (ok ten′ ni deen sak′ a rin). $C_{36}H_{62}N_4$.2($C_7H_5NO_3S$). 917.27. (1) 1-Octanamine, *N,N′*-(1,10-decanediyldi-1(4*H*)-pyridinyl-4-ylidene)bis-, compound with 1,2-benzisothiazol-3(2*H*)-one 1,1-dioxide (1:2); (2) 1,1′-Decamethylenebis[1,4-dihydro-4-(octylimino)pyridine] compound with 1,2-benzisothiazolin-3-one 1,1-dioxide (1:2). *UNII-R337868TDW. CAS-86767-75-1. Dental plaque inhibitor.* ◇*Win 41,464-6*

Octicizer [*1967*] (ok″ ti sye′ zer). $C_{20}H_{27}O_4P$. 362.40. (1) Phosphoric acid, 2-ethylhexyl diphenyl ester; (2) 2-Ethylhexyl diphenyl phosphate. *CAS-1241-94-7. Pharmaceutic aid (plasticizer).*

Octimibate. $C_{29}H_{30}N_2O_3$. 454.56. 8-[(1,4,5-Triphenylimidazol-2-yl)oxy]octanoic acid. *CAS-89838-96-0.* INN.

Octinoxate [*1999*] (ok″ tin ox′ ate). **USP.** $C_{18}H_{26}O_3$. 290.40. (1) 2-Propenoic acid, 3-(4-methoxyphenyl)-, 2-ethylhexyl ester; (2) 2-Ethylhexyl *p*-methoxycinnamate. *UNII-4Y5P7MUD51. CAS-5466-77-3.* INN. *Sunscreen (ultraviolet B absorber).* Parsol (Roche); Neo Heliopan (H & R Florasynth); Escalol (ISP Van Dyk) *[Name previously used: Octyl Methoxycinnamate.] [Note—The International Cosmetic Ingredient (INCI) name for octinoxate is octyl methoxycinnamate.]*

Octisalate [*1999*] (ok″ ti sal′ ate). **USP.** $C_{15}H_{22}O_3$. 250.33. (1) Benzoic acid, 2-hydroxy-, 2-ethylhexyl ester; (2) 2-Ethylhexyl salicylate. *CAS-118-60-5.* INN. *Sunscreen*

---

† Brand name formerly used, and/or firm no longer concerned with this product.

(ultraviolet absorber). Escalol (ISP Van Dyk); Neo Heliopan (Haarmann & Reimer, Germany); Uvinul (BASF) *[Name previously used: Octyl Salicylate.] [Note—The International Cosmetic Ingredient (INCI) name for octisalate is octyl salicylate.]*

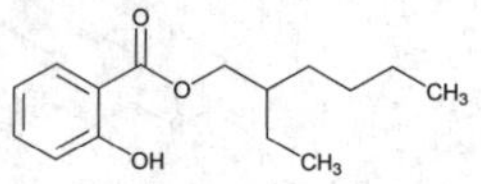

Octisamyl — *See* Octamylamine.

Octoclothepine — *See* Clorotepine.

Octocog Alfa (BAN) — *See* Factor VIII (rDNA).

Octocog Alfa. Blood-coagulation factor VIII (human), glycoform α. *UNII-P89DR4NY54. CAS-139076-62-3.* INN; BAN.

Octocrilene (INN) — *See* Octocrylene.

Octocrylene [*1979*] (ok′ toe kril″ een). **USP.** $C_{24}H_{27}NO_2$. 361.48. [Octocrilene is INN.] (1) 2-Propenoic acid, 2-cyano-3,3-diphenyl-, 2-ethylhexyl ester; (2) 2-Ethylhexyl 2-cyano-3,3-diphenylacrylate. *CAS-6197-30-4. Ultraviolet screen.*

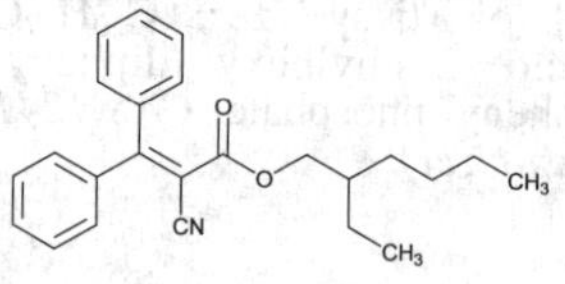

Octodecactide (DCF) — *See* Codactide.

Octodrine [*1967*] (ok′ toe dreen). $C_8H_{19}N$. 129.24. (1) Hexylamine, 1,5-dimethyl-; (2) 1,5-Dimethylhexylamine. *UNII-3GQ9E911BI. CAS-543-82-8.* INN. *Adrenergic (vasoconstrictor); anesthetic (local).* ◇*SK&F 51*

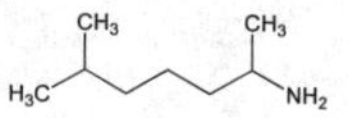

Octopamine. $C_8H_{11}NO_2$. 153.18. α-(Aminomethyl)-*p*-hydroxybenzyl alcohol. *UNII-14O50WS8JD. CAS-104-14-3.* INN; MI. ◇*ND 50*

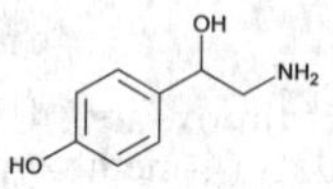

Octotiamine. $C_{23}H_{36}N_4O_5S_3$. 544.75. 8-[[2-[*N*-[(4-Amino-2-methyl-5-pyrimidinyl)methyl]formamido]-1-(2-hydroxyethyl)propenyl]dithio]-6-mercaptooctanoic acid, methyl ester acetate. *CAS-137-86-0.* INN; JAN; MI.

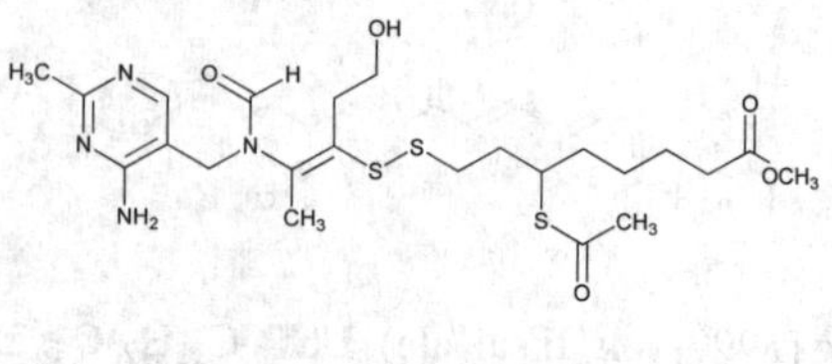

Octoxinol (INN, BAN) — *See* Octoxynol 9.

Octoxynol 9 [*1975*] (ok tox′ i nol). **NF.** [Octoxinol is INN and BAN.] (1) Poly(oxy-1,2-ethanediyl), α-(octylphenyl)-ω-hydroxy-; (2) Polyethylene glycol mono(octylphenyl) ether. *CAS-9002-93-1. Pharmaceutic aid (surfactant).* Triton X-100 (Union Carbide)

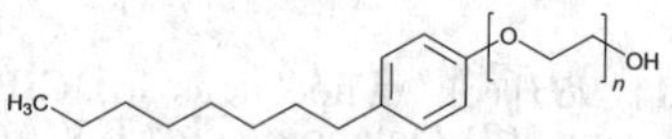

Octreotide [*1987*] (ok tree′ oh tide). $C_{49}H_{66}N_{10}O_{10}S_2$. 1019.24. (1) L-Cysteinamide, D-phenylalanyl-L-cysteinyl-L-phenylalanyl-D-tryptophyl-L-lysyl-L-threonyl-*N*-[2-hydroxy-1-(hydroxymethyl)propyl]-, cyclic (2→7)-disulfide, [*R*-(*R**,*R**)]-; (2) D-Phenylalanyl-L-cysteinyl-L-phenylalanyl-D-tryptophyl-L-lysyl-L-threonyl-*N*-[(1*R*,2*R*)-2-hydroxy-1-(hydroxymethyl)propyl]-L-cysteinamide cyclic (2→7)-disulfide; (3) D-Phenylalanyl-L-cysteinyl-L-phenylalanyl-D-tryptophyl-L-lysyl-L-threonyl-L-cysteinyl-L-threoninol cyclic (2→7)-disulfide. *UNII-RWM8CCW8GP. CAS-83150-76-9.* INN; BAN. *Antisecretory (gastric).* Sandostatin (Novartis) ◇*SMS-201-995*

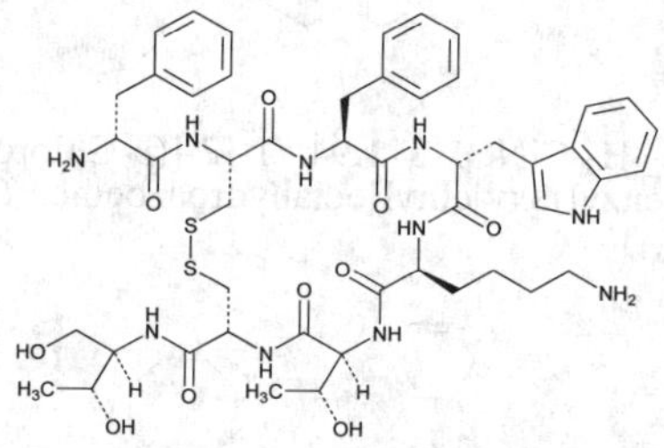

Octreotide Acetate [*1990*] (ok tree′ oh tide as′ e tate). $C_{49}H_{66}N_{10}O_{10}S_2 \cdot xC_2H_4O_2$. (1) L-Cysteinamide, D-phenylalanyl-L-cysteinyl-L-phenylalanyl-D-tryptophyl-L-lysyl-L-threonyl-*N*-[2-hydroxy-1-(hydroxymethyl)propyl]-, cyclic (2→7)-disulfide, [*R*-(*R**,*R**)]-, acetate (salt); (2) D-Phenylalanyl-L-cysteinyl-L-phenylalanyl-D-tryptophyl-L-lysyl-L-threonyl-*N*-[(1*R*,2*R*)-2-hydroxy-1-(hydroxymethyl)propyl]-L-cysteinamide cyclic (2→7)-disulfide acetate (salt); (3) D-Phenylalanyl-L-hemicystyl-L-phenylalanyl-D-tryptophyl-L-lysyl-L-threonyl-L-hemicystyl-L-threoninol cyclic (2→7)-disulfide acetate (salt). *UNII-75R0U2568I. CAS-79517-01-4.* JAN. *Antisecretory (gastric).* Sandostatin (Novartis) ◇*SMS 201-995 ac*

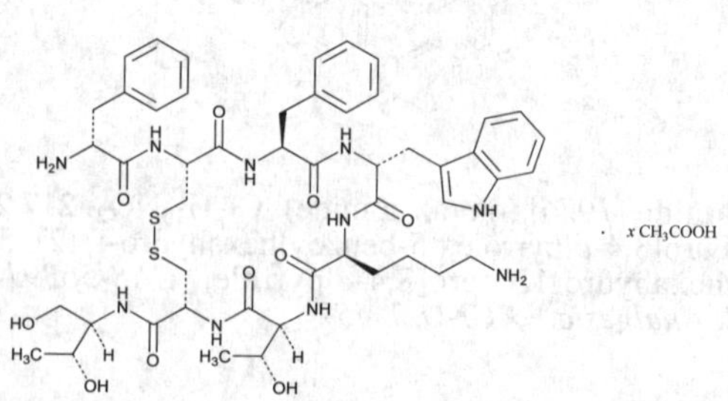

Octreotide Pamoate [*1997*] (ok tree′ oh tide pam′ oh ate). $C_{49}H_{66}N_{10}O_{10}S_2 \cdot C_{23}H_{16}O_6$. 1407.61. (1) L-Cysteinamide, D-phenylalanyl-L-cysteinyl-L-phenylalanyl-D-tryptophyl-L-lysyl-L-threonyl-*N*-[2-hydroxy-1-(hydroxymethyl)propyl]-, cyclic (2→7)-disulfide [*R*-(*R**,*R**)]-, 4,4′-methylenebis[3-hydroxy-2-naphthalenecarboxylate] (1:1) (salt); (2) D-Phenylalanyl-L-cysteinyl-L-phenylalanyl-D-tryptophyl-L-lysyl-L-threonyl-*N*-[(1*R*,2*R*)-2-hydroxy-1-(hydroxymethyl)propyl]-L-cysteinamide cyclic (2→7)-disulfide 4,4′-methylenebis[3-hydroxy-2-naphthoate] (1:1) (salt); (3) D-Phenylalanyl-L-cysteinyl-L-phenylalanyl-D-tryptophyl-

L-lysyl-L-threonyl-L-cysteinyl-L-threoninol cyclic (2→7)-disulfide pamoate (1:1) (salt). *CAS-135467-16-2. Antineoplastic.* ◇*SMS 201-995 pa; SMS pa*

Octriptyline Phosphate [*1975*] (ok trip′ ti leen fos′ fate). $C_{20}H_{21}N \cdot H_3PO_4$. 373.38. [Octriptyline is INN.] (1) 1-Propanamine, 3-(1a,10b-dihydrodibenzo[*a,e*]cyclopropa[*c*]cyclohepten-6(1*H*)-ylidene)-*N*-methyl-, phosphate (1:1); (2) 1a,10b-Dihydro-*N*-methyldibenzo[*a,e*]cyclopropa[*c*]cycloheptene-$\Delta^{6(1H),\gamma}$-propylamine phosphate (1:1). *CAS-51481-67-5; CAS-47166-67-6* [octriptyline]. *Antidepressant.* ◇*SC-27123*

Octrizole [*1979*] (ok′ tri zole). $C_{20}H_{25}N_3O$. 323.43. (1) Phenol, 2-(2*H*-benzotriazol-2-yl)-4-(1,1,3,3-tetramethylbutyl)-; (2) 2-(2*H*-Benzotriazol-2-yl)-4-(1,1,3,3-tetramethylbutyl)phenol. *UNII-R775Y233N3. CAS-3147-75-9.* INN. *Ultraviolet screen.*

Octyl Methoxycinnamate (previously used name) — *See* Octinoxate.

Octyl Salicylate (previously used name) — *See* Octisalate.

Octyldodecanol (ok″ til doe dek′ a nol). **NF.** $C_{20}H_{42}O$. 298.55. (1) Decanol, 2-octyl; (2) Icosan-9-ol. *Pharmaceutic aid (vehicle, oleaginous).*

Ocufilcon A [*1977*] (ok″ ue fil′ kon). $(C_6H_{10}O_3)_x(C_4H_6O_2)_y(C_{10}H_{14}O_4)_z$. (1) 2-Propenoic acid, 2-methyl-, 2-hydroxyethyl ester, polymer with 2-methyl-2-propenoic acid and 1,2-ethanediyl bis(2-methyl-2-propenoate); (2) 2-Hydroxy-

ethyl methacrylate polymer with methacrylic acid and ethylene dimethacrylate. *CAS-33410-59-2. Contact lens material (hydrophilic).*

Ocufilcon B [*1978*] (ok″ ue fil′ kon). $(C_6H_{10}O_3)_x(C_4H_6O_2)_y(C_{10}H_{14}O_4)_z$. (1) 2-Propenoic acid, 2-methyl-, 2-hydroxyethyl ester, polymer with 2-methyl-2-propenoic acid and 1,2-ethanediyl bis(2-methyl-2-propenoate); (2) 2-Hydroxyethyl methacrylate polymer with methacrylic acid and ethylene dimethacrylate. *CAS-33410-59-2. Contact lens material (hydrophilic). [Note—Graphic formula same as for Ocufilcon A.]*

Ocufilcon C [*1981*] (ok″ ue fil′ kon). $(C_6H_{10}O_3)_x(C_4H_6O_2)_y(C_{10}H_{14}O_4)_z$. (1) 2-Propenoic acid, 2-methyl-, 2-hydroxyethyl, ester, polymer with 2-methyl-2-propenoic acid and 1,2-ethanediyl bis(2-methyl-2-propenoate); (2) 2-Hydroxyethyl methacrylate polymer with methacrylic acid and ethylene dimethacrylate. *CAS-33410-59-2. Contact lens material (hydrophilic). [Note—Graphic formula same as for Ocufilcon A.]*

Ocufilcon D [*1989*] (ok″ ue fil′ kon). $(C_6H_{10}O_3)_x(C_4H_6O_2)_y(C_{10}H_{14}O_4)_z$. (1) 2-Propenoic acid, 2-methyl-, 2-hydroxyethyl ester, polymer with 2-methyl-2-propenoic acid and 1,2-ethanediyl bis(2-methyl-2-propenoate); (2) 2-Hydroxyethyl methacrylate polymer with methacrylic acid and ethylene dimethacrylate. *CAS-33410-59-2. Contact lens material (hydrophilic). [Note—Graphic formula same as for Ocufilcon A.]*

Ocufilcon E [*1991*] (ok″ ue fil′ kon). $(C_6H_{10}O_3)_x(C_4H_6O_2)_y(C_{10}H_{14}O_4)_z$. (1) 2-Propenoic acid, 2-methyl-, 2-hydroxyethyl ester, polymer with 2-methyl-2-propenoic acid and 1,2-ethanediyl bis(2-methyl-2-propenoate); (2) 2-Hydroxyethyl methacrylate, polymer with methacrylic acid and ethylene dimethacrylate. *CAS-33410-59-2. Contact lens material (hydrophilic). [Note—Ocufilcon E has a reported water content of 65%. Graphic formula same as for Ocufilcon A.]*

Ocufilcon F [*1999*] (ok″ ue fil′ kon). $(C_6H_{10}O_3)_x(C_4H_6O_2)_y(C_{10}H_{14}O_4)_z$. (1) 2-Propenoic acid, 2-methyl-, 2-hydroxyethyl ester, polymer with 2-methyl-2-propenoic acid and 1,2-ethanediyl bis(2-methyl-2-propenoate); (2) 2-Hydroxyethyl methacrylate, polymer with methacrylic acid and ethylene dimethacrylate. *CAS-33410-59-2. Contact lens material (hydrophilic). [Notes—The water content of the contact lens material is 60.0% ($\pm2\%$) at ambient temperature ($23\pm2°C$), the purity of 2-hydroxyethyl methacrylate (HEMA) is 98.5%, and the oxygen permeability is 25.3 (±1.6) $\times 10^{-11}(cm^2/sec)(ml\ O_2/ml \times mm\ Hg)$ at $35°C$ (Dk value). Graphic formula same as for Ocufilcon A.]*

Odalprofen. $C_{20}H_{20}N_2O_2$. 320.39. Methyl ($\pm$)-*m*-(α-imidazol-1-ylbenzyl)hydratropate. *CAS-137460-88-9.* INN.

Odanacatib [*2007*] (oh dan″ a ka′ tib). C$_{25}$H$_{27}$F$_4$N$_3$O$_3$S. 525.56. (1) Pentanamide, *N*-(1-cyanocyclopropyl)-4-fluoro-4-methyl-2-[[(1*S*)-2,2,2-trifluoro-1-[4′-(methylsulfonyl)[1,1′-biphenyl]-4-yl]ethyl]amino]-, (2*S*)-; (2) (2*S*)-*N*-(1-Cyanocyclopropyl)-4-fluoro-4-methyl-2-({(1*S*)-2,2,2-trifluoro-1-[4′-(methylsulfonyl)[1,1′-biphenyl]-4-yl]ethyl}amino)pentanamide. *UNII-N673F6W2VH. CAS-603139-19-1.* INN. *Bone resorption inhibitor.*

Odapipam. C$_{19}$H$_{20}$ClNO$_2$. 329.82. (+)-(*S*)-8-Chloro-5-(2,3-dihydro-7-benzofuranyl)-2,3,4,5-tetrahydro-3-methyl-1*H*-3-benzazepin-7-ol. *CAS-131796-63-9.* INN.

Odiparcil. C$_{15}$H$_{16}$O$_6$S. 324.35. 4-Methyl-7-(5-thio-β-D-xylo-pyranosyloxy)-2*H*-chromen-2-one. *CAS-137215-12-4.* INN.

Odulimomab. Immunoglobulin G1, anti-(human CD11 (antigen) α-chain) (mouse monoclonal 25.3 γ1-chain), disulfide with mouse monoclonal 25.3 light chain, dimer. *CAS-159445-64-4.* INN.

Oestradiol (previously used name) — *See* Estradiol.

Oestradiol Benzoate (previously used name) — *See* Estradiol Benzoate.

Oestradiol Valerate (previously used name) — *See* Estradiol Valerate.

Oestriol (previously used name) — *See* Estriol.

Oestrone (previously used name) — *See* Estrone.

Ofatumumab. C$_{6480}$N$_{10022}$N$_{1742}$O$_{2020}$S$_{44}$. Immunoglobulin G1, anti-(human CD20 (antigen))(human monoclonal HuMax-CD20 heavy chain), disulfide with human monoclonal HuMax-CD20 κ-chain, dimer. *CAS-679818-59-8.* INN.

Ofloxacin [*1984*] (oh flox′ a sin). **USP.** C$_{18}$H$_{20}$FN$_3$O$_4$. 361.37. (1) 7*H*-Pyrido[1,2,3-*de*]-1,4-benzoxazine-6-carboxylic acid, 9-fluoro-2,3-dihydro-3-methyl-10-(4-methyl-1-piperazinyl)-7-oxo-, (±)-; (2) (±)-9-Fluoro-2,3-dihydro-3-methyl-10-(4-methyl-1-piperazinyl)-7-oxo-7*H*-pyrido[1,2,3-*de*]-1,4-benzoxazine-6-carboxylic acid. *UNII-*

A4P49JAZ9H. CAS-82419-36-1. INN; BAN; JAN. *Antibacterial.* Floxin (Ortho-McNeil); Ocuflox (Allergan) ◇*DL-8280; HOE 280*

Ofornine [*1984*] (oh for′ neen). C$_{17}$H$_{19}$N$_3$O. 281.35. (1) Piperidine, 1-[2-(4-pyridinylamino)benzoyl]-; (2) 1-(*N*-4-Pyridylanthraniloyl)piperidine. *UNII-WK1LBP1F3L. CAS-87784-12-1.* INN. *Antihypertensive.* ◇*Win 48,049*

Oftasceine. C$_{30}$H$_{26}$N$_2$O$_{13}$. 622.53. 2′,7′-Bis[[bis(carboxymethyl)amino]methyl]fluorescein. *CAS-1461-15-0.* INN.

Oglemilast. C$_{20}$H$_{13}$Cl$_2$F$_2$N$_3$O$_5$S. 516.30. *N*-(3,5-Dichloropyridin-4-yl)-4-(difluoromethoxy)-8-[(methylsulfonyl)amino]dibenzo[*b,d*]furan-1-carboxamide. *CAS-778576-62-8.* INN.

Oglufanide Disodium [*2002*] (oh gloo′ fa nide dye soe′ dee um). C$_{16}$H$_{17}$N$_3$Na$_2$O$_5$. 377.30. [Oglufanide is INN.] (1) L-Tryptophan, L-α-glutamyl-, disodium salt; (2) L-α-Glutamyl-L-tryptophan, disodium salt. *UNII-Q60AU1LLNU. CAS-237068-57-4; CAS-38101-59-6* [oglufanide]. *Treatment of Kaposi's sarcoma and solid tumor cancers (angiogenesis inhibitor); immunomodulator.[Name previously used: Glufanide Disodium.] [Note—Marketed in the former USSR as Thymogen.]* ◇*IM862*

Olaflur [*1973*] (oh′ la flur). C$_{27}$H$_{58}$N$_2$O$_3$.2HF. 498.77. (1) Ethanol, 2,2′-[[3-[(2-hydroxyethyl)octadecylamino]propyl]imino]bis-, dihydrofluoride; (2) 2,2′-[[3-[(2-Hydroxyethyl)octadecylamino]propyl]imino]diethanol dihydrofluoride. *CAS-6818-37-7; CAS-17671-49-1* [olaflur base]. INN; BAN. *Dental caries prophylactic.* ◇*SK&F 38095*

Olamufloxacin. $C_{20}H_{23}FN_4O_3$. 386.42. (-)-5-Amino-7-[(*S*)-7-amino-5-azaspiro[2,4]hept-5-yl]-1-cyclopropyl-6-fluoro-1,4-dihydro-8-methyl-4-oxo-3-quinolinecarboxylic acid. *CAS-167887-97-0*. INN.

Olanexidine. $C_{17}H_{27}Cl_2N_5$. 372.34. 1-(3,4-Dichlorobenzyl)-5-octylbiguanide. *CAS-146510-36-3*. INN.

Olanexidine Hydrochloride [*1999*] (oh″ lan ex′ i deen hye″ droe klor′ ide). $C_{17}H_{27}Cl_2N_5 \cdot HCl \cdot \frac{1}{2}H_2O$. 417.80. (1) Imidodicarbonimidic diamide, *N*-[(3,4-dichlorophenyl)methyl]-*N'*-octyl-, monohydrochloride, hydrate (2:1); (2) 1-(3,4-Dichlorobenzyl)-5-octylbiguanide monohydrochloride hemihydrate. *CAS-218282-71-4*. *Topical antimicrobial for pathogenic microorganisms, particularly those causing nosocomial or wound infection.* ◇*OPB-2045*

Olanzapine [*1992*] (oh lan′ za peen). $C_{17}H_{20}N_4S$. 312.43. (1) 10*H*-Thieno[2,3-*b*][1,5]benzodiazepine, 2-methyl-4-(4-methyl-1-piperazinyl)-; (2) 2-Methyl-4-(4-methyl-1-piperazinyl)-10*H*-thieno[2,3-*b*][1,5]benzodiazepine. *UNII-N7U69T4SZR. CAS-132539-06-1*. INN; BAN. *Antipsychotic.* Zyprexa (Lilly) ◇*LY170053*

Olanzapine Pamoate [*2004*] (oh lan′ za peen pam′ oh ate). $C_{23}H_{16}O_6 \cdot C_{17}H_{20}N_4S \cdot H_2O$. 718.82. (1) 2-Naphthalenecarboxylic acid, 4,4′-methylenebis[3-hydroxy-, compound with 2-methyl-4-(4-methyl-1-piperazinyl)-10*H*-thieno[2,3-*b*][1,5]benzodiazepine (1:1), monohydrate; (2) 10*H*-Thieno[2,3-*b*][1,5]benzodiazepine, 2-methyl-4-(4-methyl-1-piperazinyl)-, 4,4′-methlenebis[3-hydroxy-2-naphthalenecarboxylate] (1:1), monohydrate; (3) 2-Methyl-4-(4-methyl-1-piperazinyl)-10*H*-thieno[2,3-*b*][1,5]benzodiazepine pamoate monohydrate. *UNII-X7S6Q4MHCB. CAS-221373-18-8. Treatment of schizophrenia (selective monoaminergic antagonist).*

Olaparib. $C_{24}H_{23}FN_4O_3$. 434.46. 4-[(3-{[4-(Cyclopropylcarbonyl)piperazin-1-yl]carbonyl}-4-fluorophenyl)methyl]phthalazin-1(2*H*)-one. *CAS-763113-22-0*. INN.

Olaquindox. $C_{12}H_{13}N_3O_4$. 263.25. *N*-(2-Hydroxyethyl)-3-methyl-2-quinoxalinecarboxamide 1,4-dioxide. *CAS-23696-28-8*. INN; BAN; MI. ◇*BAY Va 9391*

Olcegepant. $C_{38}H_{47}Br_2N_9O_5$. 869.65. *N*-[(1*R*)-2-[[(1*S*)-5-Amino-1-[[4-(pyridin-4-yl)piperazin-1-yl]carbonyl]pentyl]amino]-1-(3,5-dibromo-4-hydroxybenzyl)-2-oxoethyl]-4-(2-oxo-1,4-dihydroquinazolin-3(2*H*)-yl)piperidine-1-carboxamide. *CAS-204697-65-4*. INN.

---

† Brand name formerly used, and/or firm no longer concerned with this product.

Oleandomycin Phosphate. $C_{35}H_{61}NO_{12} \cdot H_3PO_4$. 785.85. [Oleandomycin is INN and BAN.] Oleandomycin phosphate (1:1). *UNII-8681H0C27P; UNII-P8ZQ646136* [oleandomycin]. *CAS-7060-74-4; CAS-3922-90-5* [oleandomycin]. NF XIII; JAN; MI. Matromycin (Pfizer)

Oleic Acid (oh lay′ ik as′ id). **NF.** $C_{18}H_{34}O_2$. 282.46. (1) 9-Octadecenoic acid, (Z)-; (2) Oleic acid. *CAS-112-80-1. Pharmaceutic aid (emulsion adjunct).*

Oleic Acid I 125 [*1963*] (oh lay′ ik as′ id). (1) 9-Octadecenoic acid (Z), labeled with iodine-125; (2) Oleic acid, labeled with iodine-125. *Radioactive agent.* Oleotope I-125 (Bristol-Myers Squibb†)

Oleic Acid I 131 [*1963*] (oh lay′ ik as′ id). (1) 9-Octadecenoic acid (Z), labeled with iodine-131; (2) Oleic acid, labeled with iodine-131. *Radioactive agent.* Oleotope (Bristol-Myers Squibb†); Oleotope Diagnostic (Bristol-Myers Squibb†); Raoleic Acid-131 (Abbott†)

Oleovitamin A (previously used name) — *See* Vitamin A.

Oleovitamin A and D (oh″ lee oh vye′ ta min). **USP.** A solution of vitamin A and vitamin D in fish liver oil or in an edible vegetable oil. *Vitamins A and D, source of.*

Oleovitamin D, Synthetic (previously used name) — *See* Ergocalciferol.

Oleoyl Polyoxylglycerides. **NF.** Mixtures of monoesters, diesters, and triesters of glycerol and monoesters and diesters of polyethylene glycols with a mean relative molecular weight between 300 and 400.

Olesoxime. $C_{27}H_{45}NO$. 399.65. (*EZ*)-*N*-(Cholest-4-en-3-ylidene)hydroxylamine. *CAS-22033-87-0.* INN.

Olethytan 20 — *See* Polysorbate 80.

Oletimol. $C_{15}H_{15}NO$. 225.29. *o*-(*N*-Benzylacetimidoyl)phenol. *CAS-5879-67-4.* INN; BAN.

Oleum Caryophylii — *See* Clove Oil.

Oleum Gossypii Seminis — *See* Cottonseed Oil.

Oleum Maydis — *See* Corn Oil.

Oleum Ricini — *See* Castor Oil.

Oleyl Alcohol (oh lay′ il al′ ka hol). **NF.** $C_{18}H_{36}O$. 268.48. (1) 9-Octadecen-1-ol, (Z)-; (2) (Z)-9-Octadecen-1-ol. *UNII-172F2WN8DV. CAS-143-28-2. Pharmaceutic aid (emulsifying agent); pharmaceutic aid (emollient).* Witcohol 85 (Witco); Witcohol 90 (Witco)

Oleyl Oleate (oh lay′ il oh′ lee ate). **NF.** $C_{36}H_{68}O_2$. 532.92. (1) 9-Octadecenoic acid, (Z)-, oleyl ester; (2) Oleyl oleate. *CAS-3687-45-4.*

Olive Oil (ol′ iv). **NF.** The fixed oil obtained from the ripe fruit of *Olea europaea* Linné (Fam. Oleaceae). *CAS-8001-25-0.* JAN. *Pharmaceutic aid.*

Olivomycin. Antibiotic obtained from cultures of *Actinomyces olivoreticuli,* or the same substance obtained by any other means. *CAS-11006-70-5.* INN; MI.

Olmesartan [*2002*] (ol″ me sar′ tan). $C_{24}H_{26}N_6O_3$. 446.50. 1*H*-Imidazole-5-carboxylic acid, 4-(1-hydroxy-1-methylethyl)-2-propyl-1-[[2′-(1*H*-tetrazol-5-yl) [1,1′-biphenyl]-4-yl]methyl]-. *UNII-8W1IQP3U10. CAS-144689-24-7.* BAN; INN. *Treatment of hypertension (novel angiotensin (Ang II) antagonist).* ◇RNH-6270

Olmesartan Medoxomil [*2002*] (ol″ me sar′ tan me dox′ oh mil). $C_{29}H_{30}N_6O_6$. 558.59. 1*H*-Imidazole-5-carboxylic acid, 4-(1-hydroxy-1-methylethyl)-2-propyl-1-[[2′-(1*H*-tetrazol-5-yl) [1,1′-biphenyl]-4-yl]methyl]-, (5-methyl-2-oxo-1,3-dioxol-4-yl) methyl ester. *UNII-6M97XTV3HD. CAS-144689-63-4.* INN; BAN. *Treatment of hypertension (novel angiotensin (Ang II) antagonist).* Benicar (Sankyo) ◇CS-866

Olmidine. $C_9H_{10}N_2O_3$. 194.19. 3,4-(Methylenedioxy)mandelamidine. *CAS-22693-65-8.* INN; DCF.

Olopatadine Hydrochloride [*1995*] (oh″ loe pa′ ta deen hye″ droe klor′ ide). $C_{21}H_{23}NO_3 \cdot HCl$. 373.87. [Olopatadine is INN and BAN.] (1) Dibenz[*b,e*]oxepin-2-acetic acid, 11-[3-(dimethylamino)propylidene]-6,11-dihydro-, hydrochloride, (Z)-; (2) 11-[(Z)-3-(Dimethylamino)propylidene]-6,11-dihydrodibenz[*b,e*]oxepin-2-acetic acid, hydrochloride. *UNII-2XG66W44KF; UNII-D27V6190PM* [olopatadine]. *CAS-140462-76-6; CAS-113806-05-6* [olopatadine]. *Anti-allergic.* Patanol (Alcon) ◇KW4679; ALO4943A

Olpadronic Acid. $C_5H_{15}NO_7P_2$. 263.12. [3-(Dimethylamino)-1-hydroxypropylidene]diphosphonic acid. *UNII-874HHB2V3S. CAS-63132-39-8.* INN.

Olpimedone. $C_7H_{10}N_2OS$. 170.23. ($\pm$)-2,3,6,7-Tetrahydro-7-methyl-5*H*-thiazolo[3,2-*a*]pyrimidin-5-one. *CAS-39567-20-9.* INN.

Olprinone. $C_{14}H_{10}N_4O$. 250.26. 1,2-Dihydro-5-imidazo[1,2-α]pyridin-6-yl-6-methyl-2-oxonicotinonitrile. *CAS-106730-54-5.* INN.

Olradipine. $C_{22}H_{28}Cl_2N_2O_6$. 487.37. 3-Ethyl 5-methyl ($\pm$)-2-[[2-(2-aminoethoxy)ethoxy]methyl]-4-(2,3-dichlorophenyl)-1,4-dihydro-6-methyl-3,5-pyridinedicarboxylate. *CAS-115972-78-6.* INN.

Olsalazine Sodium [*1987*] (ol sal′ a zeen soe′ dee um). $C_{14}H_8N_2Na_2O_6$. 346.20. [Olsalazine is INN and BAN.] (1) Benzoic acid, 3,3′-azobis[6-hydroxy-, disodium salt; (2) C. I. Mordant Yellow 5, disodium salt; (3) Disodium 5,5′-azodisalicylate. *UNII-Y7JEW0XG7I; UNII-ULS5I8J03O* [olsalazine]. *CAS-6054-98-4; CAS-15722-48-2* [olsalazine]. *Anti-inflammatory (gastrointestinal).* Dipentum (UCB) *[Names previously used: Sodium Azodisalicylate; Azodisal Sodium.]* ◇*CJ 91B*

Oltipraz. $C_8H_6N_2S_3$. 226.34. 4-Methyl-5-(pyrazinyl)-3*H*-1,2-dithiole-3-thione. *UNII-6N510JUL1Y. CAS-64224-21-1.* INN.

Olvanil [*1986*] (ol′ va nil). $C_{26}H_{43}NO_3$. 417.62. (1) 9-Octadecenamide, *N*-[(4-hydroxy-3-methoxyphenyl)-methyl]-, (*Z*)-; (2) *N*-Vanillyloleamide. *CAS-58493-49-5.* INN. *Analgesic.* ◇*NE-19550*

Omacetaxine Mepesuccinate [*2007*] (oh″ ma se tax′ een mep″ e sux′ i nate). $C_{29}H_{39}NO_9$. 545.62. (1) Cephalotaxine, 4-methyl (2*R*)-2-hydroxy-2-(4-hydroxy-4-methylpentyl)-butanedioate (ester); (2) 1-[(1*S*,3a*R*,14b*S*)-2-Methoxy-1,5,6,8,9,14b-hexahydro-4*H*-cyclopenta[*a*][1,3]dioxolo[4,5-*h*]pyrrolo[2,1-*b*][3]benzazepin-1-yl] 4-methyl (2*R*)-2-hydroxy-2-(4-hydroxy-4-methylpentyl)butanedioate *UNII-6FG8041S5B. CAS-26833-87-4.* INN. *Treatment of chronic myeloid leukemia, acute myeloid leukemia and myelodysplasia.* ◇*CGX-635; Homoharringtonine*

Omaciclovir [*2000*] (oh″ ma sye′ kloe vir). $C_{10}H_{15}N_5O_3$. 253.26. (1) 6*H*-Purin-6-one, 2-amino-1,9-dihydro-9-[4-hydroxy-2-(hydroxymethyl)butyl]- (*R*)-; (2) 9-[(*R*)-4-Hydroxy-2-(hydroxymethyl)butyl]guanine. *CAS-124265-89-0.* INN. *Treatment of herpes zoster (inhibitor of DNA polymerase).* ◇*ABT-091; A-182091.0; H2G; 2-HMHBG*

Omafilcon A [*1995*] (oh″ ma fil′ kon). $(C_6H_{10}O_3)_x(C_{11}H_{22}NO_6P)_y(C_{10}H_{14}O_4)_z$. (1) 2-Hydroxyethyl 2-methyl-2-propenoate polymer with 4-hydroxy-*N,N,N*,10-tetramethyl-9-oxo-3,5,8-trioxa-4-phosphaundec-10-en-1-aminium inner salt 4-oxide and 1,2-ethanediyl bis(2-methyl-2-propenoate); (2) 2-Hydroxyethyl methacrylate polymer with choline hydroxide, 2-hydroxyethyl hydrogen phosphate, inner salt, methacrylate and ethylene dimethacrylate. *CAS-144056-32-6. Contact lens material (hydrophilic).* Proclear (Biocompatibles) *[Note—The water content of the contact*

---

† Brand name formerly used, and/or firm no longer concerned with this product.

lens material is 59±1% at ambient temperature (23±2°C), and the oxygen permeability is 25 ± 1 × 10⁻¹¹(cm²/sec)(ml O₂/ml × mm Hg) at 35°C (Dk value).]

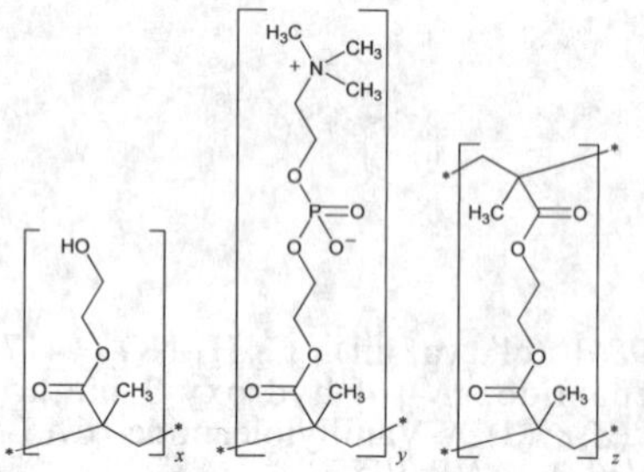

Omalizumab [*2002*] (oh″ ma liz′ oo mab). (1) Immunoglobulin G, anti-(human immunoglobulin E Fc region) (human-mouse monoclonal E25 clone pSVIE26 γ-chain), disulfide with human-mouse monoclonal E25 clone pSVIE26 κ-chain, dimer; (2) Immunoglobulin G (human-mouse monoclonal E25 clone pSVIE26 γ-chain anti-human immunoglobulin E Fc region), disulfide with human-mouse monoclonal E25 clone pSVIE126 κ-chain, dimer. Molecular weight is approximately 150,000 daltons. *CAS-242138-07-4.* INN; BAN. *Treatment of atopic disease (asthma; rhinitis) (monoclonal antibody).* Xolair (Genentech) ◇*rhuMab-E25*

Omapatrilat [*1997*] (oh″ ma pa′ tril at). $C_{19}H_{24}N_2O_4S_2$. 408.53. (1) [4S-[4α(R*),7α,10aβ]]-Octahydro-4-[(2-mercapto-1-oxo-3-phenylpropyl)amino]-5-oxo-7*H*-pyrido[2,1-*b*][1,3]thiazepine-7-carboxylic acid; (2) (4S,7S,10aS)-Octahydro-4-[(*S*)-α-mercaptohydrocinnamamido]-5-oxo-7*H*-pyrido[2,1-*b*][1,3]thiazepine-7-carboxylic acid. *CAS-167305-00-2.* INN; BAN. *Treatment of hypertension and congestive heart failure (neutral endopeptidase and angiotensin converting enzyme inhibitor).* ◇*BMS-186716; BMS-186716-01*

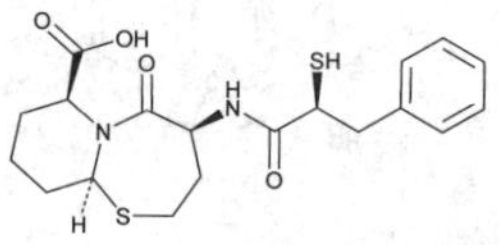

Ombrabulin. $C_{21}H_{26}N_2O_6$. 402.44. (2S)-2-Amino-3-hydroxy-*N*-{2-methoxy-5-[(1Z)-2-(3,4,5-trimethoxyphenyl)ethenyl]phenyl}propanamide. *CAS-181816-48-8.* INN.

Omega-3-acid Ethyl Esters [*2002*] (oh may′ ga as′ id eth′ il es′ ters). $C_{22}H_{34}O_2$ (EPA ethyl ester). 330.50 (EPA ethyl ester); $C_{24}H_{36}O_2$ (DHA ethyl ester). 356.54 (DHA ethyl ester). [Omega-3 Marine Triglycerides is BAN; Doconexent (DHA ethyl ester) and Icosapent (EPA ethyl ester) are INN.] EPA ethyl ester: (1) 5,8,11,14,17-Eicosapentaenoic acid, ethyl ester, (all-*Z*)-; (2) Ethyl (5Z,8Z,11Z,14Z,17Z)-eicosa-5,8,11,14,17-pentaenoate. DHA ethyl ester: (1) 4,7,10,13,16,19-Docosahexaenoic acid, ethyl ester, (all-*Z*)-; (2) Ethyl (4Z,7Z,10Z,13Z,16Z,19Z)-docosa-4,7,10,13,16,19-hexaenoate. *UNII-D87YGH4Z0Q.* CAS-86227-47-6 [EPA ethyl ester]; *CAS-81926-94-5* [DHA ethyl ester]. *Hypolipidemic.* Lovaza (Reliant) ◇*K85*

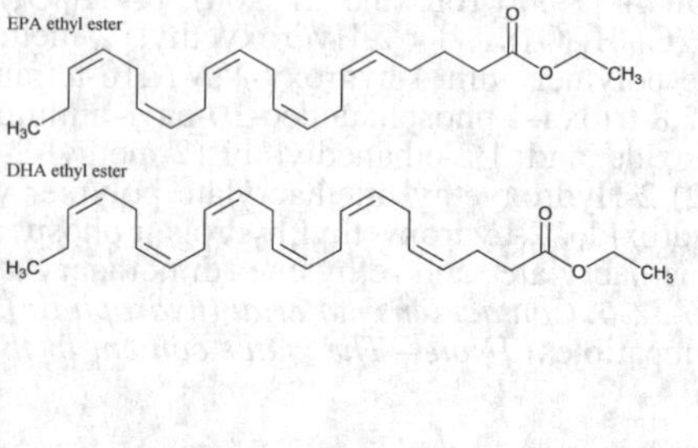

EPA ethyl ester

DHA ethyl ester

Omeprazole [*1986*] (oh mep′ ra zole). USP. $C_{17}H_{19}N_3O_3S$. 345.42. (1) 1*H*-Benzimidazole, 5-methoxy-2-[[(4-methoxy-3,5-dimethyl-2-pyridinyl)methyl]sulfinyl]-; (2) 5-Methoxy-2-[[(4-methoxy-3,5-dimethyl-2-pyridyl)methyl]sulfinyl]benzimidazole. *UNII-KG60484QX9. CAS-73590-58-6.* INN; BAN; JAN. *Depressant (gastric acid secretory).* Prilosec (AstraZeneca) ◇*H 168/68*

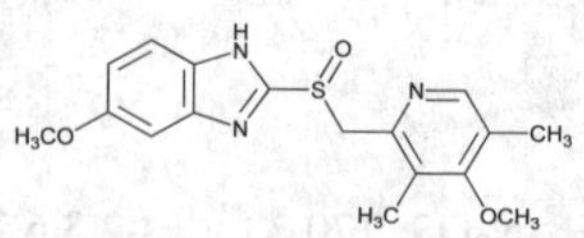

Omeprazole Magnesium [*2000*] (oh mep′ ra zole mag nee′ zee um). $C_{34}H_{36}MgN_6O_6S_2$. 713.12. (1) 5-Methoxy-2-[[(4-methoxy-3,5-dimethyl-2-pyridinyl)methyl]sulfinyl]-1*H*-benzimidazole, magnesium salt (2:1); (2) 5-Methoxy-2-[[(4-methoxy-3,5-dimethyl-2-pyridyl)methyl]sulfinyl]benzimidazole, magnesium salt (2:1). *UNII-426QFE7XLK. CAS-95382-33-5. Gastric acid secretory depressant.* Prilosec (AstraZeneca) ◇*H 168/68 magnesium*

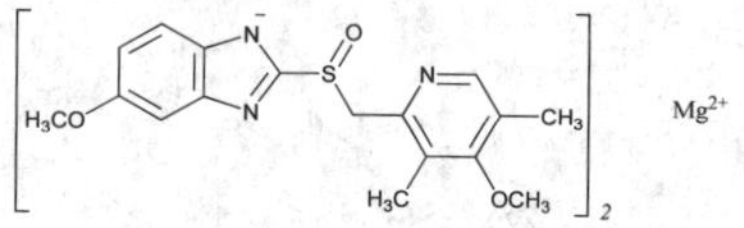

Omeprazole Sodium [*1993*] (oh mep′ ra zole soe′ dee um). $C_{17}H_{18}N_3NaO_3S$. 367.40. (1) 1*H*-Benzimidazole, 5-methoxy-2-[[(4-methoxy-3,5-dimethyl-2-pyridinyl)methyl]sulfinyl]-, sodium salt; (2) 5-Methoxy-2-[[(4-methoxy-3,5-dimethyl-2-pyridyl)methyl]sulfinyl]benzimidazole, sodium salt. *UNII-KV03YZ6QLW. CAS-95510-70-6. Antisecretory (gastric).* Losec Sodium (Astra Pharmaceutical Production AB, Sweden) ◇*H 168/68 sodium*

Omidoline. $C_{22}H_{27}N_3O_2$. 365.47. 2-Methyl-3-(β-piperidino-*p*-phenetidino)phthalimidine. *CAS-21590-91-0.* INN.

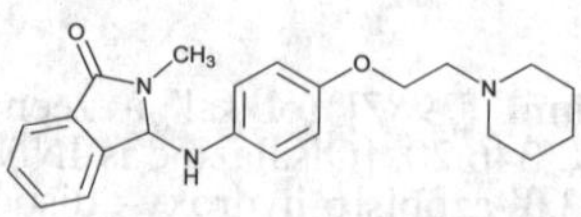

Omiganan Pentahydrochloride [*2003*] (oh″ mi gan′ an pen″ ta hye″ droe klor′ ide). $C_{90}H_{127}N_{27}O_{12}$.5HCl. 1961.45. [Omiganan is INN.] (1) L-Lysinamide, L-isoleucyl-L-leucyl-L-arginyl-L-tryptophyl-L-prolyl-L-tryptophyl-L-tryptophyl-L-prolyl-L-tryptophyl-L-arginyl-L-arginyl-, pentahydrochloride; (2) L-Isoleucyl-L-leucyl-L-arginyl-L-tryptophyl-L-prolyl-L-tryptophyl-L-tryptophyl-L-prolyl-L-tryptophyl-L-arginyl-L-arginyl-L-lysinamide pentahydrochloride. *CAS-269062-93-3; CAS-204248-78-2* [omiganan]. *Anti-microbial agent.*

ILRWPWWPWRRK——NH₂ · 5HCl

Omigapil. $C_{19}H_{17}NO$. 275.34. *N*-(Dibenzo[*b,f*]oxepin-10-ylmethyl)-*N*-methylprop-2-yn-1-amine. *CAS-181296-84-4*. INN.

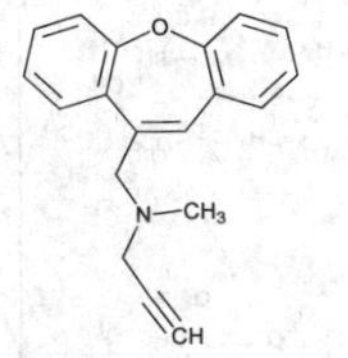

Omiloxetine. $C_{27}H_{25}F_2NO_4$. 465.49. 4′-Fluoro-2-[*trans*-4-(*p*-fluorophenyl)-3-[[3,4-(methylenedioxy)phenoxy]-methyl]piperidino]acetophenone. *CAS-176894-09-0*. INN.

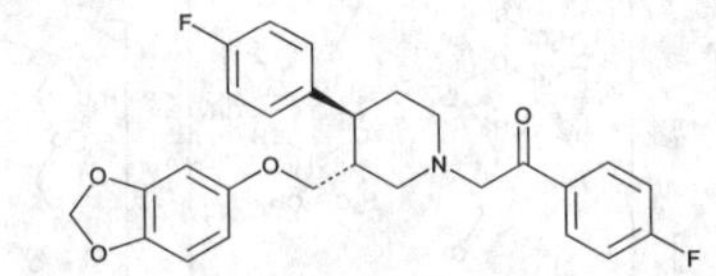

Omocianine. $C_{32}H_{38}N_2O_{12}S_4$. 770.91. Trihydrogen 2-{(1*E*,3*E*,5*E*)-7-[(2*E*)-3,3-dimethyl-5-sulfonato-1-(2-sulfonatoethyl)-1,3-dihydro-2*H*-indol-2-ylidene]-4-methylhepta-1,3,5-trienyl}-3,3-dimethyl-1-(2-sulfonatoethyl)-3*H*-indolium-5-sulfonate. *CAS-154082-13-0*. INN.

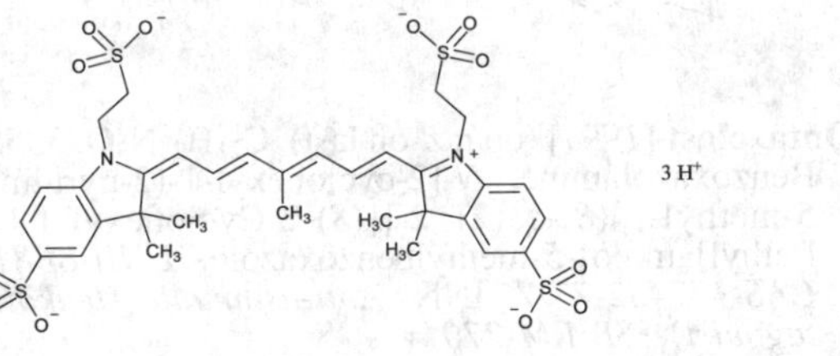

Omoconazole Nitrate [*1996*] (oh″ moe kon′ a zole nye′ trate). $C_{20}H_{17}Cl_3N_2O_2.HNO_3$. 486.73. [Omoconazole is INN.] (1) 1*H*-Imidazole, 1-[2-[2-(4-chlorophenoxy) ethoxy]-2-(2,4-dichlorophenyl)-1-methylethenyl]-, (*Z*)-, mononitrate; (2) (*Z*)-1-[2,4-Dichloro-β-[2-(*p*-chlorophenoxy)ethoxy]-α-methylstyryl]imidazole mononitrate. *UNII-15LTY5STY6; UNII-GQ8ADD54E1* [omoconazole]. *CAS-83621-06-1; CAS-74512-12-2* [omoconazole]. *Antifungal.* ✧*10 80 07*

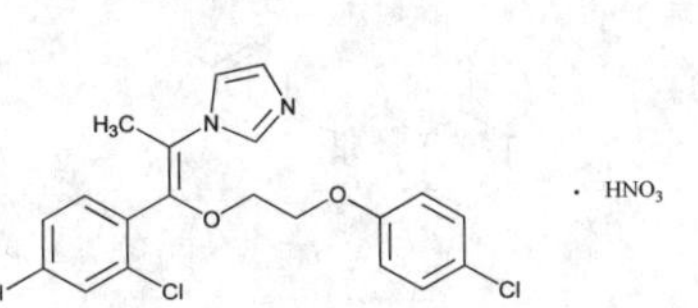

Omonasteine. $C_5H_9NO_2S$. 147.20. Tetrahydro-2*H*-1,3-thiazine-4-carboxylic acid. *CAS-60175-95-3*. INN.

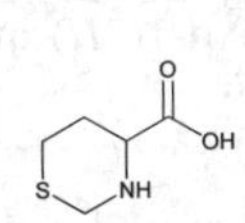

Omtriptolide Sodium [*2006*] (om trip′ toe lide soe′ dee um). $C_{24}H_{27}NaO_9$. 482.46. [Omtriptolide is INN.] (1) Butanedioic acid, mono[(3b*S*,4a*S*,5a*R*,6*R*,6a*S*,7a*S*,7b*S*,8a*S*,8b*S*)-1,3,3b,4,4a,6,6a,7a,7b,8b,9,10-dodecahydro-8b-methyl-6a-(1-methylethyl)-1-oxotrisoxireno[4b,5:6,7:8a,9]phenanthro[1,2-*c*]furan-6-yl] ester, sodium salt; (2) Sodium 4-[(3b*S*,4a*S*,5a*R*,6*R*,6a*S*,7a*S*,7b*S*,8a*S*,8b*S*)-8b-methyl-6a-(1-methylethyl)-1-oxo-1,3,3b,4,4a,6,6a,7a,7b,8b,9,10-dodecahydrotrisoxireno[4b,5:6,7:8a,9]phenanthro[1,2-*c*]furan-6-yl]-4-oxobutanoate. *UNII-PVH9FQC04V. CAS-195883-09-1; CAS-195883-06-8* [omtriptolide]. *Anti-neoplastic.* ✧*PG490-88Na*

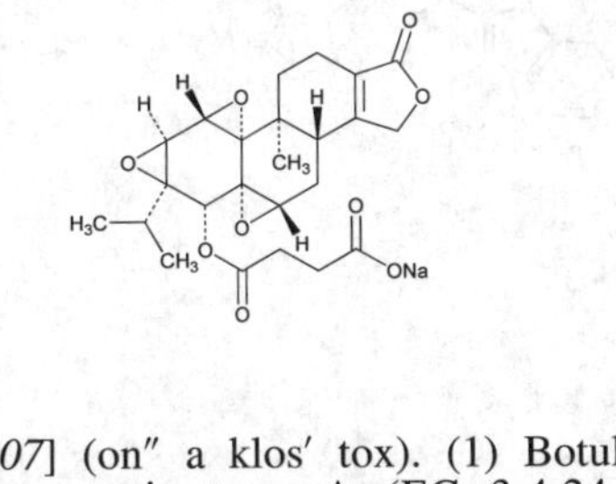

Onaclostox [*2007*] (on″ a klos′ tox). (1) Botulin A; (2) Botulinum neurotoxin type A (EC 3.4.24.69) from *Clostridium botulinum*; (3) *Clostridium botulinum* Type A-1 neurotoxin complex (Allergan strain-900,000 Daltons). Molecular weight is approximately 900,000 daltons. *CAS-93384-43-1. Treatment of blepharospasm, strabismus, cervical dystonia, severe primary axillary hyperhidrosis, glabellar lines.* Botox (Allergan); Botox Cosmetic (Allergan)

Onamelatucel-L [*2005*] (on″ a mel″ a too′ sel - el). Product is a specific active immunotherapeutic composed of approximately equal numbers of viable, gamma-irradiated, replication-incompetent whole cells derived from three (3) human melanoma cell lines designated as M10-VACC, M24-VACC, and M101-VACC. *Treatment of cancer, primarily melanoma.* Canvaxin (Cancervax)

Onapristone. $C_{29}H_{39}NO_3$. 449.62. 11β-[*p*-(Dimethylamino)-phenyl]-17α-hydroxy-17-(3-hydroxypropyl)-13α-estra-4,9-dien-3-one. *CAS-96346-61-1*. INN.

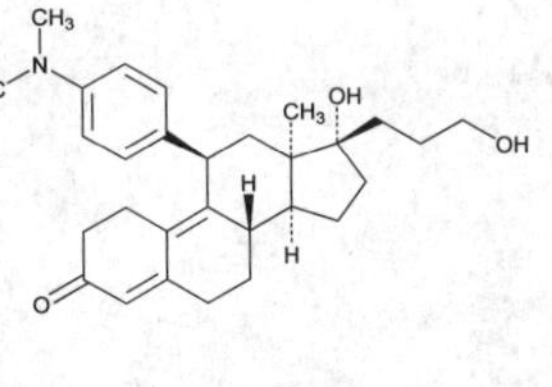

Ondansetron (on dan′ se tron). **USP**. $C_{18}H_{19}N_3O$. 293.36. (1) 4*H*-Carbazol-4-one, 1,2,3,9-tetrahydro-9-methyl-3-[(2-methyl-1*H*-imidazol-1-yl)methyl]- (±)-; (2) (±)-2,3-Dihydro-9-methyl-3-[(2-methylimidazol-1-yl)methyl]carbazol-4(1*H*)-one. *UNII-4AF302ESOS. CAS-99614-02-5; CAS-108303-49-1* [replaced]; *CAS-116002-70-1* [replaced]. INN; BAN. Zofran (GlaxoSmithKline)

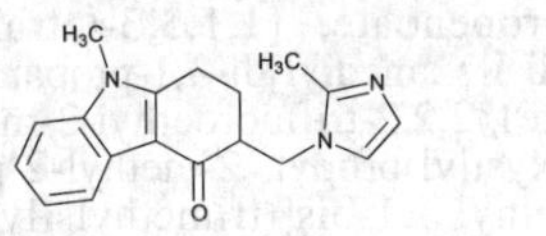

Ondansetron Hydrochloride [*1989*] (on dan′ se tron hye″ droe klor′ ide). **USP**. $C_{18}H_{19}N_3O.HCl.2H_2O$. 365.85. (1) 4*H*-Carbazol-4-one, 1,2,3,9-tetrahydro-9-methyl-3-[(2-methyl-1*H*-imidazol-1-yl)methyl]-, monohydrochloride, (±)-, dihydrate; (2) (±)-2,3-Dihydro-9-methyl-3-[(2-methylimidazol-1-yl)methyl]carbazol-4(1*H*)-one monohy-

† Brand name formerly used, and/or firm no longer concerned with this product.

drochloride dihydrate. *UNII-NMH84OZK2B. CAS-103639-04-9.* JAN. *Anti-anxiety agent; anti-emetic; antischizophrenic.* Zofran (GlaxoSmithKline) ◇*GR 38032F*

Onercept [*2001*] (on′ er sept). $C_{753}H_{1156}N_{228}O_{247}S_{25}$. Glycoprotein TNF-BP (tumor necrosis factor-binding protein) (human disulfide variant 1). Molecular weight is approximately 18,000 daltons. *CAS-199685-57-9.* INN. *Anti-TNF (tumor necrosis factor) activity.* ◇*r-hTBP-1*

```
DSVCPQGKYI HPQNNSICCT KCHKGTYLYN DCPGPGQDTD CRECESGSFT

ASENHLRHCL SCSKCRKEMG QVEISSCTVD RDTVCGCRKN QYRHYWSENL

FQCFNCSLCL NGTVHLSCQE KQNTVCTCHA GFFLRENECV SCSNCKKSLE

CTKLCLPQIE N
```

* glycosylation sites

Onsifocon A [*2002*] (on″ si foe′ kon). $(C_6H_7F_3O_2)_s$ $(C_{16}H_{38}O_5Si_4)_t(C_{10}H_{20}O_5Si)_u(C_4H_6O_2)_v(C_{26}H_{58}O_9Si_6)_w(C_{10}$ $H_{14}O_4)_x(C_6H_{10}O_3)_y(C_6H_9NO)_z$. (1) 2-Propenoic acid, 2-methyl-, polymer with 1,2-ethanediyl bis(2-methyl-2-propenoate), 1-ethenyl-2-pyrrolidinone, 2-hydroxyethyl 2-methyl-2-propenoate, [1,1,3,3-tetrakis[(trimethylsilyl)oxy]-1,3-disiloxanediyl]di-3,1-propanediyl bis(2-methyl-2-propenoate), 2,2,2-trifluoroethyl 2-methyl-2-propenoate, 3-(trimethoxysilyl)propyl 2-methyl-2-propenoate and 3-[3,3,3-trimethyl-1,1-bis[(trimethylsilyl)oxy]disiloxanyl]-propyl 2-methyl-2-propenoate; (2) Trifluoroethyl methacrylate polymer with tris(trimethylsiloxy)methacryloxypropylsilane 3-trimethoxysilylpropyl methacrylate methacrylic acid 1,3-bis(3-methacryloxypropyl)tetrakis (trimethylsiloxy)disiloxane ethylene glycol dimethacrylate 2-hydroxyethyl methacrylate *N*-vinylpyrrolidone. *CAS-311330-20-8. Contact lens material (hydrophobic).*[-*Note—The water content of the contact lens material is <*

0.2% at ambient temperature (23±2°C), and the oxygen permeability is 57 × 10^{-11}(cm²/sec)(ml O₂/ml × mm Hg) at 35°C (Dk value).]

Ontazolast [*1994*] (on taz′ oh last). $C_{21}H_{25}N_3O$. 335.44. (1) 2-Benzoxazolamine, *N*-[2-cyclohexyl-1-(2-pyridinyl)ethyl]-5-methyl-, (*S*)-; (2) 2-[[(*S*)-2-Cyclohexyl-1-(2-pyridyl)ethyl]amino]-5-methylbenzoxazole. *UNII-8P8TW6B25I. CAS-147432-77-7.* INN. *Anti-asthmatic (leukotriene antagonist).* ◇*BIRM-270*

Ontianil. $C_{13}H_{12}ClNO_2S$. 281.76. 4′-Chloro-2,6-dioxocyclohexanecarbothioanilide. *CAS-35727-72-1.* INN; MI.

Opanixil. $C_{19}H_{21}F_3N_6O_2$. 422.40. 4-Amino-2-(4,4-dimethyl-2-oxo-1-imidazolidinyl)-*N*-ethyl-α,α,α-trifluoro-5-pyrimidinecarboxy-*m*-toluidide. *CAS-152939-42-9.* INN.

Opaviraline. $C_{14}H_{17}FN_2O_3$. 280.29. Isopropyl (*S*)-2-ethyl-7-fluoro-3,4-dihydro-3-oxo-1(2*H*)-quinoxalinecarboxylate. *CAS-178040-94-3.* INN.

Opebacan [*1999*] (oh pe′ bay kan). (1) 1-193-Bactericidal/permeability-increasing protein [132-alanine] (human); (2) 132-L-Alanine-1-193-bactericidal/permeability-increasing protein (human). Molecular weight is approximately 21,000 daltons. *CAS-206254-79-7.* INN; BAN. *Antimicrobial for gram negative bacterial infections.* ◇rBPI-21

```
VNPGVVVRIS   QKGLDYASQQ   GTAALQKELK   RIKIPDYSDS
FKIKHLGKGH   YSFYSMDIRE   FQLPSSQISM   VPNVGLKFSI
SNANIKISGK   WKAQKRFLKM   SGNFDLSIEG   MSISADLKLG
SNPTSGKPTI   TASSCSSHIN   SVHVHISKSK   VGWLIQLFHK
KIESALRNKM   NSQVCEKVTN   SVSSELQPYF   QTL
```

Opiniazide. $C_{16}H_{15}N_3O_5$. 329.31. 5,6-Dimethoxyphthalaldehydic acid isonicotinoyl hydrazone. *CAS-2779-55-7.* INN; MI.

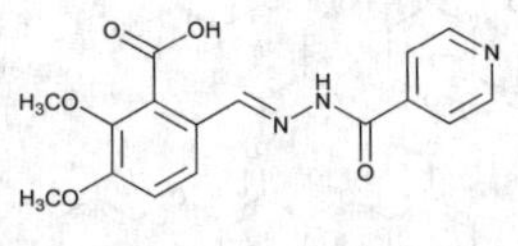

Opipramol Hydrochloride [*1964*] (oh pip′ ra mol hye″ droe klor′ ide). $C_{23}H_{29}N_3O.2HCl$. 436.42. [Opipramol is INN and BAN.] (1) 1-Piperazineethanol, 4-[3-(5*H*-dibenz[*b,f*]azepin-5-yl)propyl]-, dihydrochloride; (2) 4-[3-(5*H*-Dibenz[*b,f*]azepin-5-yl)propyl]-1-piperazineethanol dihydrochloride. *CAS-909-39-7; CAS-315-72-0* [opipramol]. *Antidepressant; antipsychotic.* ◇G-33040

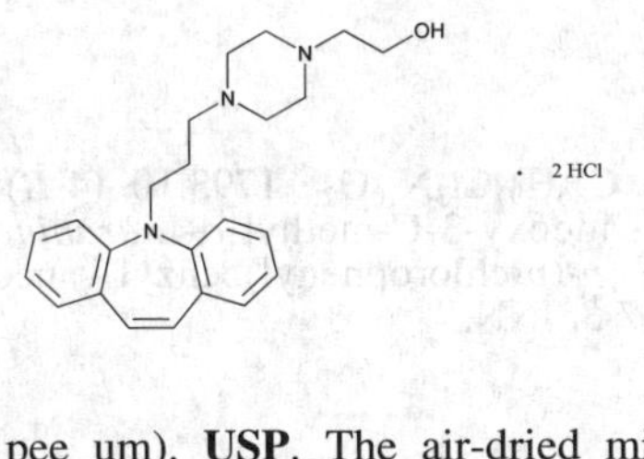

Opium (oh′ pee um). **USP**. The air-dried milky exudate obtained by incising the unripe capsules of *Papaver somniferum* Linné or its variety *album* De Candolle (Fam. Papaveraceae). Pharmaceutic necessity for Powdered Opium.

Opratonium Iodide. $C_{17}H_{35}IN_2O$. 410.38. Trimethyl[3-(10-undecenamido)propyl]ammonium iodide. *CAS-210419-36-6.* INN.

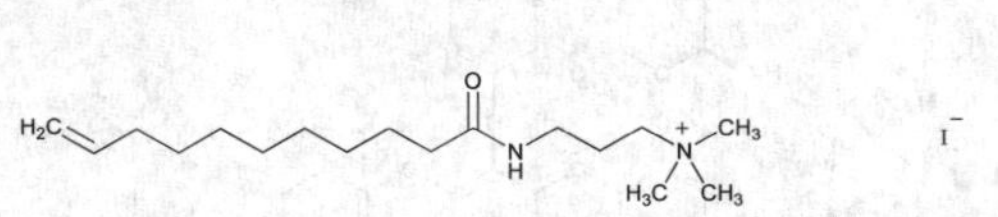

Oprelvekin [*1996*] (oh prel′ ve kin″). $C_{854}H_{1411}N_{253}O_{235}S_2$. 19,047.04. (1) 2-178-Interleukin 11 (human clone pXM/IL-11); (2) 2-178-Interleukin 11 (human clone pXM/IL-11). *UNII-HM5641GA6F. CAS-145941-26-0.* INN. *Hematopoietic stimulant.* Neumega (Genetics Institute)

```
GPPPGPPRVS PDPRAELDST VLLTRSLLAD TRQLAAQLRD KFPADGDHNL
DSLPTLAMSA GALGALQLPG VLTRLRADLL SYLRHVQWLR RAGGSSLKTL
EPELGTLQAR LDRLLRRLQL LMSRLALPQP PPDPPAPPLA PPSSAWGGIR
AAHAILGGLH LTLDWAVRGL LLLKTRL
```

Orange Flower Oil. NF XVII.

Orange Flower Water. NF XVI.

Orange Oil (or′ enj). **NF.** The volatile oil obtained by expression from the fresh peel of the ripe fruit of *Citrus sinensis* L. Osbeck (Fam. Rutaceae). *Pharmaceutic aid (flavor).*

Orange Peel, Bitter. JAN.

Orange Peel Tincture, Sweet (or′ enj). **NF.** Prepared from sweet orange peel, which is the outer rind of the non-artifically colored, fresh, ripe fruit of *Citrus sinesis* (L.) Osbeck (Fam. Rutaceae).

Orazamide. $C_4H_6N_4O.C_5H_4N_2O_4.2H_2O$. 318.24. 5-Aminoimidazole-4-carboxamide orotate. *UNII-CLY9MRR8FV. CAS-60104-30-5.* INN; DCF; MI. ◇AICA

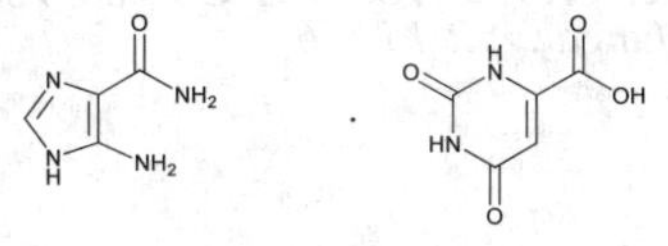

Orazipone. $C_{13}H_{14}O_4S$. 266.31. 3-[*p*-(Methylsulfonyl)benzylidene]-2,4-pentanedione. *CAS-137109-78-5.* INN.

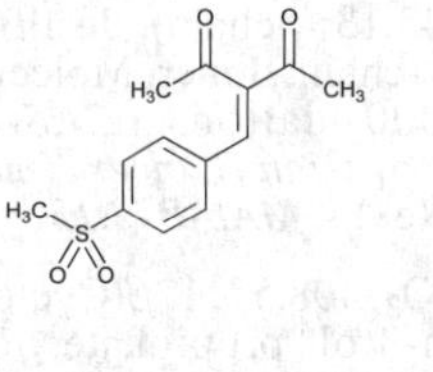

Orbifloxacin. $C_{19}H_{20}F_3N_3O_3$. 395.38. 1-Cyclopropyl-7-(*cis*-3,5-dimethyl-1-piperazinyl)-5,6,8-trifluoro-1,4-dihydro-4-oxo-3-quinolinecarboxylic acid. *UNII-660932TPY6. CAS-113617-63-3.* INN. Orbax (Schering-Plough Animal Health)

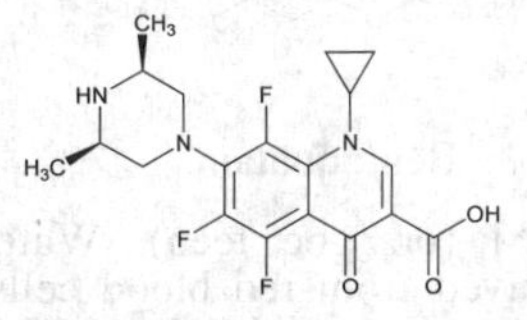

Orbofiban Acetate [*1996*] (or″ boe fye′ ban as′ e tate). $C_{17}H_{23}N_5O_4.C_2H_4O_2.H_2O$. 425.95. [Orbofiban is INN.] (1) β-Alanine, *N*-[[[1-[4-(aminoiminomethyl)phenyl]-2-oxo-3-pyrrolidinyl]amino]carbonyl]-, ethyl ester (*S*)-, monoacetate, hydrate (4:1); (2) *N*-[[(3*S*)-1-(*p*-Amidinophenyl)-2-oxo-3-pyrrolidinyl]carbamoyl]-β-alanine, ethyl ester, monoacetate quadrantihydrate. *CAS-165800-05-5; CAS-163250-90-6* [orbofiban]. *Antithrombotic; platelet aggregation inhibitor.* ◇SC-57099B

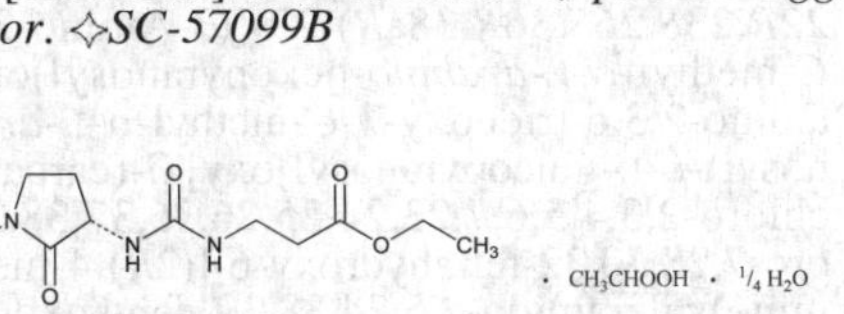

Orbutopril. $C_{20}H_{34}N_2O_5$. 382.49. (2S,3aS,7aS)-1-[(S)-N-[(S)-1-Carboxypentyl]alanyl]hexahydro-2-indolinecarboxylic acid, 1-ethyl ester. *CAS-108391-88-4*. INN.

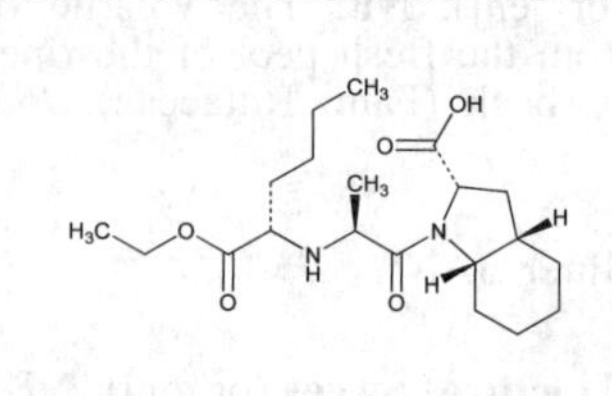

Orciprenaline (INN, BAN) — *See* Metaproterenol Polistirex.

Orciprenaline Sulfate (JAN) — *See* Metaproterenol Sulfate.

Orconazole Nitrate [*1978*] (or kon′ a zole nye′ trate). $C_{18}H_{15}Cl_3N_2O.HNO_3$. 444.70. [Orconazole is INN.] (1) 1*H*-Imidazole, 1-[2-(4-chlorophenyl)-2-[(2,6-dichlorophenyl)methoxy]ethyl]-, mononitrate, (±)-; (2) (±)-1[*p*-Chloro-*β*-[(2,6-dichlorobenzyl)oxy]phenethyl]imidazole mononitrate. *CAS-66778-38-9; CAS-66778-37-8* [orconazole]. *Antifungal.* ◇*R 15,556*

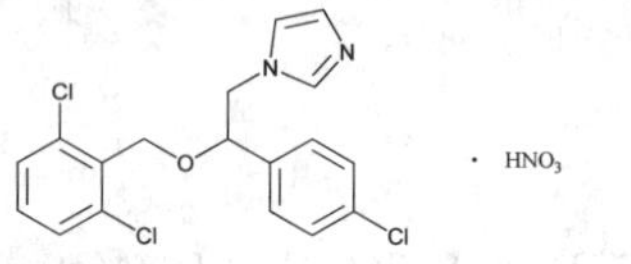

Oregovomab [*2002*] (or″ e goe′ voe mab). Immunoglobulin G1, anti-(human CA125 (carbohydrate antigen)) (mouse monoclonal B43.13γ_1-chain), disulfide with mouse monoclonal B43.13κ-chain, dimer. Molecular weight is approximately 150,000 daltons. *CAS-213327-37-8*. INN. *Treatment of ovarian cancer (monoclonal antibody).* OvaRex (AltaRex) ◇*MAb-B43.13*

Orestrate. $C_{27}H_{36}O_3$. 408.57. 17*β*(Cyclohexen-1-yloxy)-estra-1,3,5(10)-trien-3-ol propionate. *UNII-G9VC23W7W0. CAS-13885-31-9*. INN.

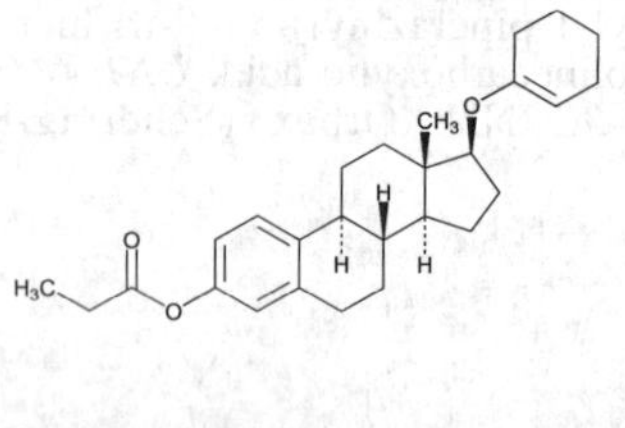

Organoclay — *See* Bentoquatam.

Orgotein [*1968*] (or′ goe teen). Water-soluble protein congeners derived from red blood cells, liver, and other tissues, of molecular weight about 33,000 with compact conformation maintained by about 4 gram-atoms of divalent metal. Produced from beef liver as Cu-Zn mixed chelate having superoxide dismutase activity. (1) Orgotein; (2) Orgotein. *CAS-9016-01-7*. INN; BAN. *Anti-inflammatory; antirheumatic.* Palosein [Veterinary] (Oxis)

Orientiparcin. $C_{73}H_{89}ClN_{10}O_{26}$ (Orienticine A). 1557.99 (Orienticine A); $C_{74}H_{91}ClN_{10}O_{26}$ (Orienticine D). 1572.02 (Orienticine D). A mixture of Orienticine A and Orienticine D. Orienticine A (major component): (-) (3S,6R,7R,22R,23S,26S,36R,38aR)-22-[(3-Amino-2,3,6-trideoxy-3-*C*-methyl-α-L-*arabino*-hexopyranosyl)oxy]-44-[[2-*O*-(3-amino-2,3,6-trideoxy-3-*C*-methyl-α-L-*arabino*-hexopyranosyl)-*β*-D-glucopyranosyl]oxy]-3-(carbamoylmethyl)-19-chloro-2,3,4,5,6,7,23,24,25,26,36,37,38,38a-tetradecahydro-7,28,30,32-tetrahydroxy-6-[(2R)-4-methyl-2-(methylamino)valeramido]-2,5,24,38,39-pentaoxo-22*H*-8,11:18,21-dietheno-23,36-(iminomethano)-13,16:31,35-dimetheno-1*H*,16*H*-[1,6,9]oxadiazacyclohexadecino[4,5-*m*][10,2,16]benzoxadiazacyclotetracosine-26-carboxylic

acid; Orienticine D (minor component): (-)-(3S,6R,7R,22R,23S,26S,36R,38aR)-22-[(3-Amino-2,3,6-trideoxy-3-*C*-methyl-α-L-*arabino*-hexopyranosyl)oxy]-44-[[2-*O*-(3-amino-2,3,6-trideoxy-3-*C*-methyl-α-L-*arabino*-hexopyranosyl)-*β*-D-glucopyranosyl]oxy]-3-(carbamoyl-methyl)-19-chloro-6-[(2R)-2-(dimethylamino)-4-methyl-valeramido]-2,3,4,5,6,7,23,24,25,26,36,37,38,38a-tetradecahydro-7,28,30,32-tetrahydroxy-2,5,24,38,39-pentaoxo-22*H*-8,11:18,21-dietheno-23,36-(iminomethano)-13,16:31,35-dimetheno-1*H*,16*H*-[1,6,9]oxadiazacyclohexadecino[4,5-*m*][10,2,16]benzoxadiazacyclotetracosine-26-carboxylic acid. *CAS-159445-62-2; CAS-111073-20-2* [Orienticine A]; *CAS-112848-46-1* [Orienticine D]. INN.

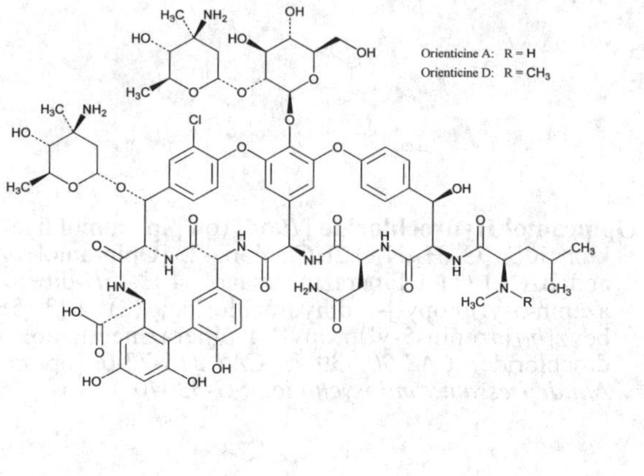

Oritavancin. $C_{86}H_{97}Cl_3N_{10}O_{26}$. 1793.10. (4″*R*)-22-*O*-(3-Amino-2,3,6-trideoxy-3-*C*-methyl-α-L-*arabino*-hexopyranosyl)-*N*$^{3″}$-[*p*-(*p*-chlorophenyl)benzyl]vancomycin. *CAS-171099-57-3*. INN.

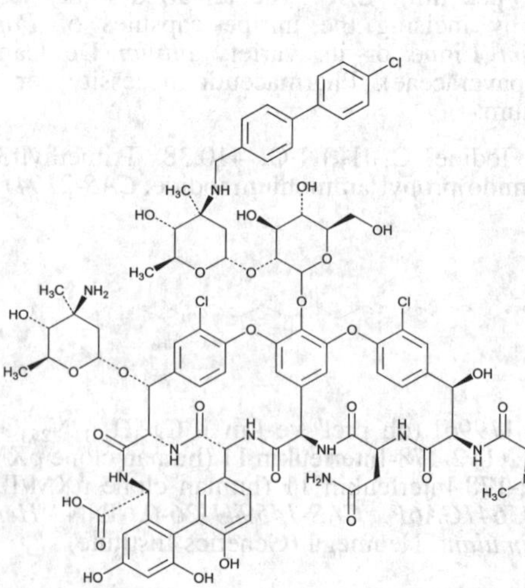

Oritavancin Diphosphate [*1999*] (or it″ a van′ sin dye fos′ fate). $C_{86}H_{97}Cl_3N_{10}O_{26}.2H_3PO_4$. 1989.09. (1) (4″*R*)-22-*O*-(3-Amino-2,3,6-trideoxy-3-*C*-methyl-α-L-*arabino*-hexo-pyranosyl)-*N*$^{3″}$-[(4′-chloro[1,1′-biphenyl]-4-yl)methyl]vancomycin phosphate (1:2) (salt); (2) (4″*R*)-22-*O*-(3-Amino-2,3,6-trideoxy-3-*C*-methyl-α-L-*arabino*-hexopyra-nosyl)-*N*$^{3″}$-[*p*-(*p*-chlorophenyl)benzyl]vancomycin phosphate (1:2) (salt). *CAS-192564-14-0. Antibacterial (peptidoglycan synthesis inhibitor).* ◇*LY333328 diphosphate*

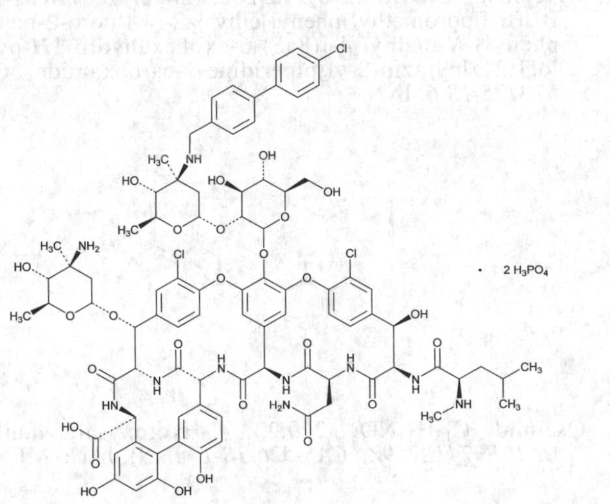

Orlipastat — *See* Orlistat.

Orlistat [*1991*] (or′ li stat). $C_{29}H_{53}NO_5$. 495.73. (1) L-Leucine, *N*-formyl-, 1-[(3-hexyl-4-oxo-2-oxetanyl)-methyl]dodecyl ester, [2*S*-[2α(*R**),3β]]-; (2) *N*-Formyl-L-leucine, ester with (3*S*,4*S*)-3-hexyl-4-[(2*S*)-2-hydroxytridecyl]-2-oxetanone. *UNII-95M8R751W8. CAS-96829-58-2.* INN; BAN. *Inhibitor (pancreatic lipase).* Xenical (Roche) ◇*Ro 18-0647/002*

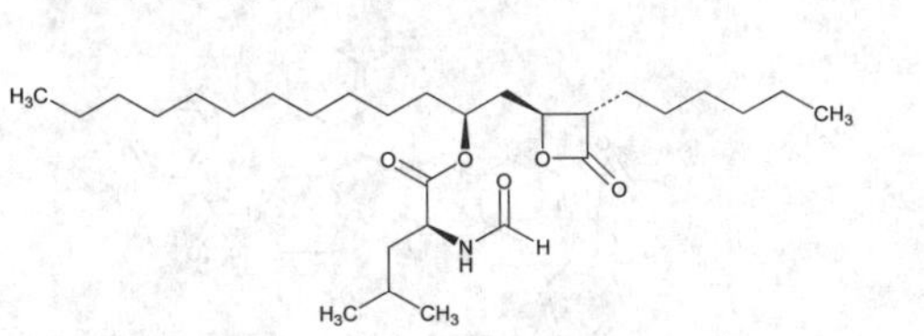

Ormaplatin [*1990*] (or″ ma pla′ tin). $C_6H_{14}Cl_4N_2Pt$. 451.08. (1) Platinum, tetrachloro(1,2-cyclohexanediamine-*N*,*N*′)-, [*OC*-6-22-(*trans*)]-; (2) (±)-*trans*-Tetrachloro(1,2-cyclohexanediamine)platinum. *CAS-62816-98-2.* INN. *Antineoplastic.* ◇*U-77,233*

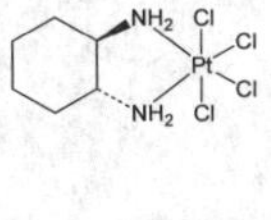

Ormeloxifene. $C_{30}H_{35}NO_3$. 457.60. (±)-1-[2-[*p*-(*trans*-7-Methoxy-2,2-dimethyl-3-phenyl-4-chromanyl)phenoxy]-ethyl]pyrrolidine. *CAS-78994-24-8.* INN.

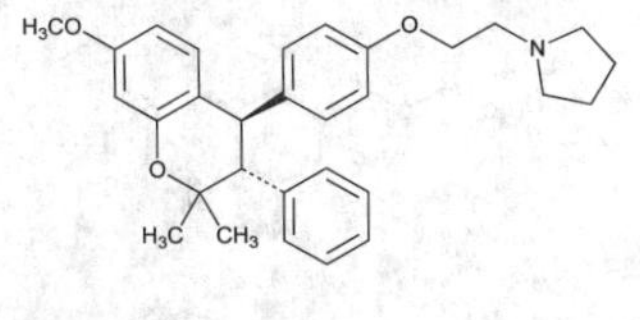

Ormetoprim [*1969*] (or met′ oh prim). $C_{14}H_{18}N_4O_2$. 274.32. (1) 2,4-Pyrimidinediamine, 5-[(4,5-dimethoxy-2-methyl-phenyl)methyl]-; (2) 2,4-Diamino-5-(6-methylveratryl)-pyrimidine. *UNII-M3EFS94984. CAS-6981-18-6.* INN. *Antibacterial.* ◇*Ro 5-9754; NSC-95072*

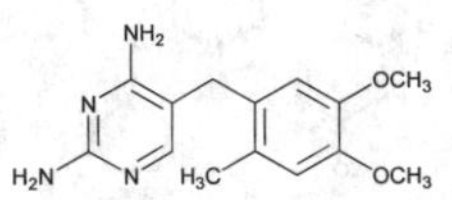

Ornidazole [*1977*] (or nye′ da zole). $C_7H_{10}ClN_3O_3$. 219.63. (1) 1*H*-Imidazole-1-ethanol, α-(chloromethyl)-2-methyl-5-nitro-; (2) α-(Chloromethyl)-2-methyl-5-nitroimidazole-1-ethanol. *CAS-16773-42-5.* INN. *Anti-infective.* ◇*Ro 7-0207*

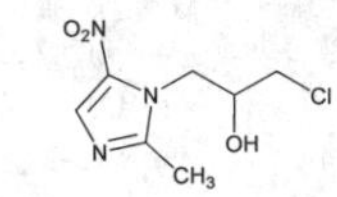

Ornipressin. $C_{45}H_{63}N_{13}O_{12}S_2$. 1042.19. 8-Ornithinevasopressin. *CAS-3397-23-7.* INN; MI. ◇*POR 8*

Ornithine. $C_5H_{12}N_2O_2$. 132.16. L-Ornithine. *UNII-E524N2IXA3. CAS-70-26-8.* INN; MI.

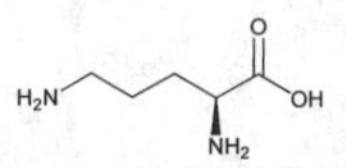

Ornithine Vasopressin — *See* Ornipressin.

Ornoprostil. $C_{23}H_{38}O_6$. 410.54. Methyl (-)-(1*R*,2*R*,3*R*)-3-hydroxy-2-[(*E*)-(3*S*,5*S*)-3-hydroxy-5-methyl-1-nonenyl]-ε,5-dioxocyclopentaneheptanoate. *CAS-70667-26-4.* INN; JAN; MI.

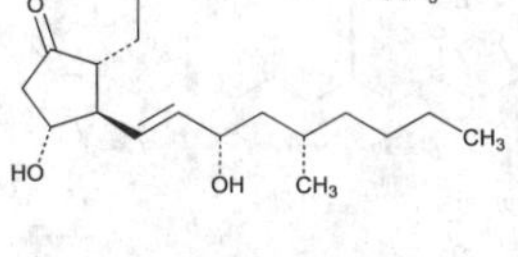

Orotic Acid. $C_5H_4N_2O_4$. 156.10. (1) 1,2,3,4-Tetrahydro-2,6-dioxopyrimidine-4-carboxylic acid; (2) Orotic acid. *UNII-61H4T033E5. CAS-65-86-1.* INN; BAN; JAN; MI.

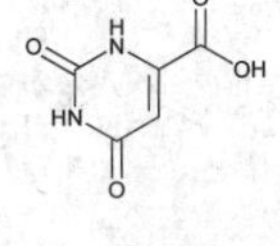

---

† Brand name formerly used, and/or firm no longer concerned with this product.

Orotirelin. $C_{16}H_{19}N_7O_5$. 389.37. *N*-[(1,2,3,6-Tetrahydro-2,6-dioxo-4-pyrimidinyl)carbonyl]-L-histidyl-L-prolinamide. *CAS-62305-86-6*. INN.

Orpanoxin [*1977*] (or″ pa nox′ in). $C_{13}H_{11}ClO_4$. 266.68. (1) 2-Furanpropanoic acid, 5-(4-chlorophenyl)-β-hydroxy-; (2) 5-(*p*-Chlorophenyl)-2-furanhydracrylic acid. *CAS-60653-25-0*. INN. *Anti-inflammatory.* ◇*F-776*

Orphenadine Citrate — *See* Orphenadrine Citrate.

Orphenadrine Citrate (or fen′ a dreen sit′ rate). **USP**. $C_{18}H_{23}NO.C_6H_8O_7$. 461.50. [Orphenadrine is INN and BAN.] (1) Ethanamine, *N,N*-dimethyl-2-[(2-methylphenyl)phenylmethoxy]-, (±)-, 2-hydroxy-1,2,3-propanetricarboxylate (1:1); (2) (±)-*N,N*-Dimethyl-2-[(*o*-methyl-α-phenylbenzyl)oxy]ethylamine citrate (1:1). *UNII-X0A40N8I4S; UNII-AL805O9OG9* [orphenadrine]. *CAS-4682-36-4; CAS-83-98-7* [orphenadrine]. *Relaxant (skeletal muscle); antihistaminic.* Norflex (3M Pharmaceuticals)

Orpressin — *See* Ornipressin.

Ortataxel. $C_{44}H_{57}NO_{17}$. 871.92. (3a*S*,4*R*,5*E*,7*R*,8a*S*,9-*S*,10a*R*,12a*S*,12b*R*,13*S*,13a*S*)-7,12a-Bis(acetyloxy)-13-(benzoyloxy)-9-hydroxy-5,8a,14,14-tetramethyl-2,8-dioxo-3a,4,7,8,8a,9,10,10a,12,12a,12b,13-dodecahydro-6,13a-methano-13a*H*-oxeto[2″,3″:5′,6′]benzo[1′,2′:4,5]cyclodeca[1,2-*d*]-1,3-dioxol-4-yl(2*R*,3*S*)-3-[[(1,1-dimethylethoxy)carbonyl]amino]-2-hydroxy-5-methylhexanoate. *CAS-186348-23-2*. INN.

Ortetamine. $C_{10}H_{15}N$. 149.23. *o,α*-Dimethylphenethylamine. *UNII-VF4N11KKKR. CAS-5580-32-5*. INN.

Orthocresol. *CAS-95-48-7*. NF V.

Orthotolidine. *CAS-119-93-7*.

Orvepitant. $C_{31}H_{35}F_7N_4O_2$. 628.62. (2*R*,4*S*)-*N*-{(1*R*)-1-[3,5-Bis(trifluoromethyl)phenyl]ethyl}-2-(4-fluoro-2-methylphenyl)-*N*-methyl-4-[(8a*S*)-6-oxohexahydro-1*H*-pyrrolo[1,2-*a*]pyrazin-2-yl]piperidine-1-carboxamide. *CAS-579475-18-6*. INN.

Osalmid. $C_{13}H_{11}NO_3$. 229.23. 4′-Hydroxysalicylanilide. *UNII-89741L759Z. CAS-526-18-1*. INN; JAN; MI. ◇*L-1718*

Osanetant. $C_{35}H_{41}Cl_2N_3O_2$. 606.62. *N*-[1-[3-[(*R*)-1-Benzoyl-3-(3,4-dichlorophenyl)-3-piperidyl]propyl]-4-phenyl-4-piperidyl]-*N*-methylacetamide. *CAS-160492-56-8*. INN.

Osaterone. $C_{20}H_{25}ClO_4$. 364.86. (+)-6-Chloro-17-hydroxy-2-oxapregna-4,6-diene-3,20-dione. *CAS-105149-04-0*. INN.

Oseltamivir. $C_{16}H_{28}N_2O_4$. 312.40. Ethyl (3*R*,4*R*,5*S*)-4-acetamido-5-amino-3-(1-ethylpropoxy)-1-cyclohexene-1-carboxylate. *UNII-20O93L6F9H. CAS-196618-13-0*. INN; BAN. ◇*RO 640796*

Oseltamivir Phosphate [*1998*] (oh″ sel tam′ i vir fos′ fate). $C_{16}H_{28}N_2O_4.H_3PO_4$. 410.40. (1) [3*R*-(3$\alpha$,4$\beta$,5$\alpha$)]-Ethyl 4-(acetylamino)-5-amino-3-(1-ethylpropoxy)-1-cyclohexene-1-carboxylate phosphate (1:1); (2) Ethyl (3*R*,4*R*,5*S*)-4-acetamido-5-amino-3-(1-ethylpropoxy)-1-cyclohexene-1-

carboxylate, phosphate (1:1). *UNII-4A3O49NGEZ. CAS-204255-11-8. Antiviral (neuraminidase inhibitor).* Tamiflu (Roche) ◇*Ro 64-0796/002*

Osemozotan. $C_{19}H_{21}NO_5$. 343.37. 3-(1,3-Benzodioxol-5-yloxy)-*N*-[[(2*S*)-2,3-dihydro-1,4-benzodioxin-2-yl]-methyl]propan-1-amine. *CAS-137275-81-1.* INN.

Osmadizone. $C_{23}H_{22}N_2O_4S$. 422.50. [2-(Phenylsulfinyl)ethyl]malonic acid mono(1,2-diphenylhydrazide). *CAS-27450-21-1.* INN.

Ospemifene [*2006*] (os pem′ i feen). $C_{24}H_{23}ClO_2$. 378.89. (1) Ethanol, 2-[4-[(1*Z*)-4-chloro-1,2-diphenyl-1-butenyl]phenoxy]-; (2) 2-[*p*-[(*Z*)-4-Chloro-1,2-diphenyl-1-butenyl]-phenoxy]ethanol. *UNII-B0P231ILBK. CAS-128607-22-7.* INN; BAN. *Treatment of vaginal atrophy, osteoporosis, and vasomotor symptoms.* ◇*FC-1271a; Fc-1271*

Ostreogrycin. Antibiotic substances derived from cultures of *Streptomyces osteogriseus*, or the same substance produced by any other means. *CAS-11006-76-1.* INN; BAN.

Osutidine. $C_{19}H_{28}N_4O_5S_2$. 456.58. (±)-*N*-[(*E*)-[(*p*,β-Dihydroxyphenethyl)amino][[2-[[5-[(methylamino)methyl]furfuryl]thio]ethyl]amino]methylene]methanesulfonamide. *CAS-140695-21-2.* INN.

Otamixaban. $C_{25}H_{26}N_4O_4$. 446.50. Methyl (2*R*,3*R*)-2-(3-carbamimidoylbenzyl)-3-[[4-(1-oxidopyridin-4-yl)benzoyl]amino]butanoate. *CAS-193153-04-7.* INN.

Otelixizumab [*2007*] (oh″ te lix iz′ oo mab). $C_{6448}H_{9954}N_{1718}O_{2016}S_{42}$. (1) Immunoglobulin G1, anti-(human CD3 (antigen)) (human-rat monoclonal heavy chain), disulfide with human-rat monoclonal λ-chain, dimer; (2) Unglycosylated immunoglobulin G1, anti-(human CD3 epsilon chain) humanized rat monoclonal YTH12.5; gamma 1 heavy chain [humanized VH (*Homo sapiens* FR/*Rattus norvegicus* CDR)-[297-alanine] *Homo sapiens* IGHG1] (222-214)-disulfide with chimeric lambda light chain [*Rattus norvegicus* VL/*Homo sapiens* IGLC2]; (228-228″:231-231″)-bisdisulfide dimer. Molecular weight is approximately 145,100 daltons. *CAS-881191-44-2.* INN. *Type 1 diabetes and psoriasis.* ◇*TRX4; ChAglyCD3*

Otenabant [*2007*] (oh ten′ a bant). $C_{25}H_{25}Cl_2N_7O$. 510.42. (1) 4-Piperidinecarboxamide, 1-[8-(2-chlorophenyl)-9-(4-chlorophenyl)-9*H*-purin-6-yl]-4-(ethylamino)-; (2) 1-[8-(2-Chlorophenyl)-9-(4-chlorophenyl)-9*H*-purin-6-yl]-4-(ethylamino)piperidine-4-carboxamide. *CAS-686344-29-6.* INN. *Treatment of obesity.* ◇*CP-945,598*

Otenabant Hydrochloride [*2007*] (oh ten′ a bant hye″ droe klor′ ide). $C_{25}H_{25}Cl_2N_7O·HCl$. 546.88. (1) 4-Piperidinecarboxamide, 1-[8-(2-chlorophenyl)-9-(4-chlorophenyl)-9*H*-purin-6-yl]-4-(ethylamino)-, monohydrochloride; (2) 1-[8-(2-Chlorophenyl)-9-(4-chlorophenyl)-9*H*-purin-6-yl]-4-(ethylamino)piperidine-4-carboxamide monohydrochloride. *CAS-686347-12-6. Treatment of obesity.* ◇*CP-945,598*

Otenzepad. $C_{24}H_{31}N_5O_2$. 421.54. (±)-11-[[2-[(Diethylamino)methyl]piperidino]acetyl]-5,11-dihydro-6*H*-pyrido[2,3-*b*][1,4]benzodiazepin-6-one. *UNII-OM7J0XAL0S. CAS-100158-38-1*. INN.

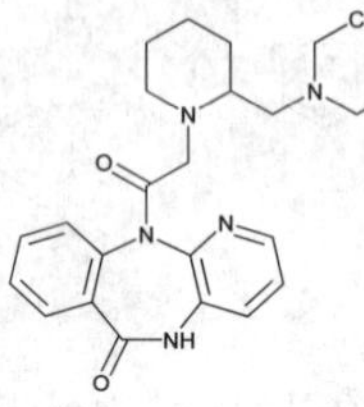

Oteracil. $C_4H_3N_3O_4$. 157.08. 1,4,5,6-Tetrahydro-4,6-dioxo-*s*-triazine-2-carboxylic acid. *UNII-5VT6420TIG. CAS-937-13-3*. INN.

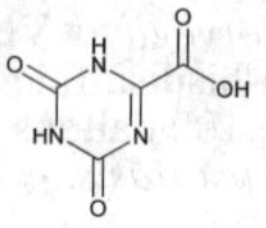

Otilonium Bromide. $C_{29}H_{43}BrN_2O_4$. 563.57. Diethyl(2-hydroxyethyl)methylammonium bromide *p*-[*o*-(octyloxy)-benzamido]-benzoate. *CAS-26095-59-0*. INN; BAN. ⋄*SP63*

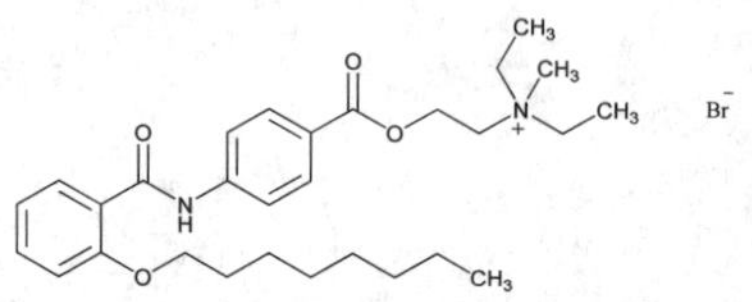

Otimerate Sodium. $C_{10}H_8HgNNaO_3S$. 445.82. Ethyl(hydrogen 2-mercapto-5-benzoxazolecarboxylato)mercury, sodium salt. *CAS-16509-11-8*. INN.

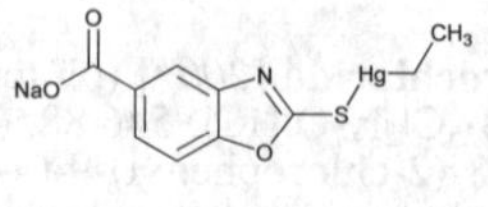

Ouabain. $C_{29}H_{44}O_{12} \cdot 8H_2O$. 728.77. [G-Strophanthin is JAN.] (1) Card-20(22)-enolide, 3-[(6-deoxy-α-L-mannopyranosyl)oxy]-1,5,11,14,19-pentahydroxy-, octahydrate, (1β,3β,5β,11α)-; (2) Ouabain octahydrate. *CAS-11018-89-6; CAS-630-60-4* [anhydrous]. USP XX; MI.

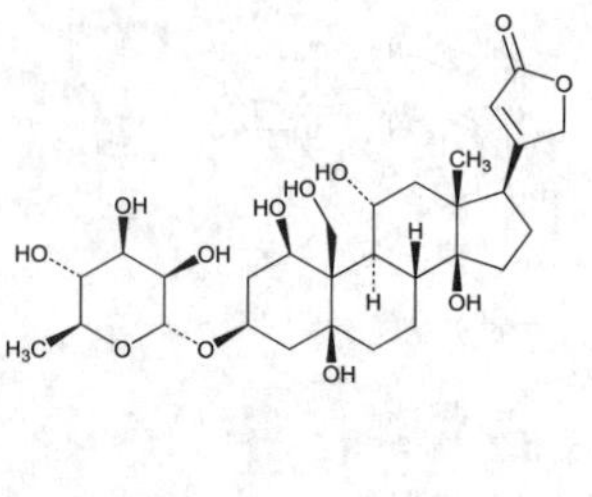

Ovandrotone Albumin. 3-[(3,17-Dioxoandrost-4-en-7α-yl)thio]propionic acid, serum albumin conjugate. INN; BAN. ⋄*GR 33207*

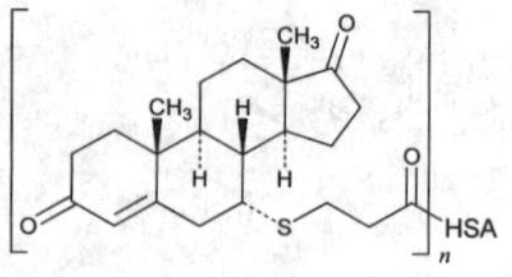

HSA = Human Serum Albumin

Ovemotide [*2005*] (oh vem′ oh tide). $C_{46}H_{71}N_9O_{14}$. 974.11. (1) L-Valine, L-tyrosyl-L-leucyl-L-α-glutamyl-L-prolylglycyl-L-prolyl-L-valyl-L-threonyl-; (2) [264-L-Valine]melanocyte protein Pmel 17 (human melanoma-associated ME20 antigen)-(256-264)-peptide. *CAS-181477-91-8*. INN. *Melanoma peptide vaccine.* ⋄*MPS-21*

Y L E P G P V T V

Ox Bile. An alcoholic extract of ox bile reduced by evaporation and containing bile salts. BAN.

Oxabolone Cipionate. $C_{26}H_{38}O_4$. 414.58. 4,17β-Dihydroxyestr-4-en-3-one 17-cyclopentanepropionate. *UNII-5RXY50Q01N. CAS-1254-35-9*. INN. ⋄*FI 5852*

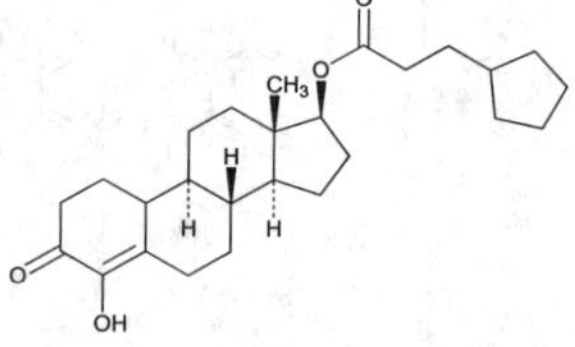

Oxabrexine. $C_{18}H_{25}Br_2NO_3$. 463.20. Ethyl[[4,6-dibromo-α-(cyclohexylmethylamino)-*o*-tolyl]oxy]acetate. *CAS-65415-42-1*. INN.

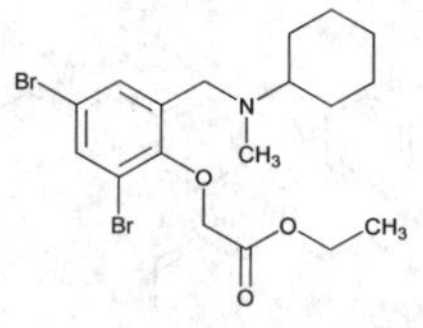

22-Oxacalcitriol (previously used name) — *See* Maxacalcitol.

Oxaceprol. $C_7H_{11}NO_4$. 173.17. (-)-1-Acetyl-4-hydroxy-L-proline. *CAS-33996-33-7*. INN; MI.

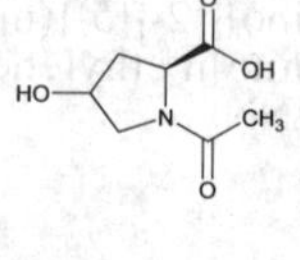

Oxacillin Sodium [*1962*] (ox″ a sil′ in soe′ dee um). **USP.** $C_{19}H_{18}N_3NaO_5S \cdot H_2O$. 441.43. [Oxacillin is INN and BAN.] (1) 4-Thia-1-azabicyclo[3.2.0]heptane-2-carboxylic acid, 3,3-dimethyl-6-[[(5-methyl-3-phenyl-4-isoxazolyl)carbonyl]amino]-7-oxo-, monosodium salt, monohydrate, [2*S*-(2α,5α,6β)]-; (2) Monosodium (2*S*,5*R*,6*R*)-3,3-dimethyl-6-(5-methyl-3-phenyl-4-isoxazolecarboxamido)-7-oxo-4-thia-1-azabicyclo[3.2.0]heptane-2-carboxylate monohydrate. *UNII-G0V6C994Q5; UNII-UH95VD7V76* [oxacillin]. *CAS-7240-38-2; CAS-1173-88-2* [anhydrous];

CAS-66-79-5 [oxacillin].   JAN.   *Antibacterial*.   Bactocill (GlaxoSmithKline); Prostaphlin (Apothecon) ◇*P-12; SQ 16,423*

Oxadimedine Hydrochloride. C$_{18}$H$_{21}$N$_3$O.HCl. 331.84. [Oxadimedine is INN.] *N*-(Benzoxazolyl)-*N*-benzyl-*N,N*-dimethylethylenediamine hydrochloride. *CAS-6314-69-8; CAS-16485-05-5* [oxadimedine].

Oxaflozane. C$_{14}$H$_{18}$F$_3$NO. 273.29. 4-Isopropyl-2-(α,α,α-trifluoro-*m*-tolyl)morpholine. *UNII-V4WLW77V5Q. CAS-26629-87-8*. INN; DCF; MI.

Oxaflumazine. C$_{26}$H$_{32}$F$_3$N$_3$O$_2$S. 507.61. 10-[3-[4-(2-*m*-Dioxanylethyl)-1-piperazinyl]propyl]-2-(trifluoromethyl) phenothiazine. *CAS-16498-21-8*. INN; DCF; MI. ◇*SD 270-31 [as disuccinate]*

Oxafuradene — *See* Nifuradene.

Oxagrelate [*1981*] (ox ag′ re late). C$_{14}$H$_{16}$N$_2$O$_4$. 276.29. (1) 6-Phthalazinecarboxylic acid, 3,4-dihydro-1-(hydroxymethyl)-5,7-dimethyl-4-oxo-, ethyl ester; (2) Ethyl 3,4-dihydro-1-(hydroxymethyl)-5,7-dimethyl-4-oxo-6-phthalazinecarboxylate. *UNII-V17MYO89WO. CAS-56611-65-5*. INN. *Platelet aggregation inhibitor*. ◇*SC-32840*

---

† Brand name formerly used, and/or firm no longer concerned with this product.

Oxalinast. C$_{14}$H$_{13}$NO$_4$. 259.26. ($\pm$)-(6,7,8,8a-Tetrahydro-2-oxo-3-acenaphthenyl)oxamic acid. *CAS-70009-66-4*. INN.

Oxaliplatin [*1998*] (ox al″ i pla′ tin). C$_8$H$_{14}$N$_2$O$_4$Pt. 397.29. (1) [*SP*-4-2-(1*R*-trans)]-(1,2-cyclohexanediamine-*N,N′*)[ethanedioato(2-)-*O,O′*]platinum; (2) *cis*-[(1*R*,2*R*)-1,2-Cyclohexanediamine-*N,N′*][oxalato(2-)-*O,O′*]platinum. *UNII-04ZR38536J. CAS-61825-94-3*. INN; BAN. *Antineoplastic (DNA adduct alkylating agent)*. Eloxatin (Sanofi Aventis) ◇*SR-96669; l-OHP; RP-54780; JM-83; NSC-266046*

Oxamarin Hydrochloride [*1981*] (ox am′ a rin hye″ droe klor′ ide). C$_{22}$H$_{34}$N$_2$O$_4$.2HCl. 463.44. [Oxamarin is INN.] (1) 2*H*-1-Benzopyran-2-one, 6,7-bis[2-(diethylamino)ethoxy]-4-methyl-, dihydrochloride; (2) 6,7-Bis[2-(diethylamino)ethoxy]-4-methylcoumarin dihydrochloride. *CAS-6830-17-7* [dihydrochloride]; *CAS-15301-80-1* [oxamarin]. *Hemostatic*. Idro P$_3$ (Maggioni Farmaceutici S.p.A., Italy) ◇*M.G. 652*

Oxametacin. C$_{19}$H$_{17}$ClN$_2$O$_4$. 372.80. 1-(*p*-Chlorobenzoyl)-5-methoxy-2-methylindole-3-acetohydroxamic acid. *UNII-8G02RSW5CM. CAS-27035-30-9*. INN; MI.

Oxamisole Hydrochloride [*1988*] (ox am′ i sole hye″ droe klor′ ide). C$_{15}$H$_{20}$N$_2$O$_2$.HCl. 296.79. [Oxamisole is INN.] (1) Imidazo[1,2-*a*]pyridine, 2,3,5,6,7,8-hexahydro-8,8-dimethoxy-2-phenyl-, monohydrochloride, ($\pm$)-; (2) ($\pm$)-2,3,6,7-Tetrahydro-2-phenylimidazo[1,2-*a*]pyridin-8(5*H*)-one, dimethyl acetal, monohydrochloride. *CAS-99258-55-6; CAS-99258-56-7* [oxamisole]. *Immunoregulator*. ◇*PR 879-317A*

Oxamniquine [*1975*] (ox am′ ni kwin). C$_{14}$H$_{21}$N$_3$O$_3$. 279.33. (1) 6-Quinolinemethanol, 1,2,3,4-tetrahydro-2-[[(1-methylethyl)amino]methyl]-7-nitro-; (2) 1,2,3,4-Tetrahydro-2-

[(isopropylamino)methyl]-7-nitro-6-quinolinemethanol. *UNII-0O977R722D. CAS-21738-42-1.* USP XXIII; INN; BAN. *Antischistosomal.* Vansil (Pfizer) ◇*UK-4271*

Oxamphetamine Hydrobromide — *See* Hydroxyamphetamine Hydrobromide.

Oxanamide. $C_8H_{15}NO_2$. 157.21. 2,3-Epoxy-2-ethylhexanamide. *CAS-126-93-2.* INN; MI.

Oxandrolone [*1962*] (ox an′ droe lone). USP. $C_{19}H_{30}O_3$. 306.44. (1) 2-Oxaandrostan-3-one, 17-hydroxy-17-methyl-, (5α,17β)-; (2) 17β-Hydroxy-17-methyl-2-oxa-5α-androstan-3-one. *UNII-7H6TM3CT4L. CAS-53-39-4.* INN; BAN; JAN. *Androgen.* Oxandrin (Savient) ◇*SC 11585; NSC-67068*

Oxantel Pamoate [*1974*] (ox′ an tel pam′ oh ate). $C_{13}H_{16}N_2O.C_{23}H_{16}O_6$. 604.65. [Oxantel is INN and BAN.] (1) Phenol, 3-[2-(1,4,5,6-tetrahydro-1-methyl-2-pyrimidinyl)ethenyl], (*E*)-, 4,4′-methylenebis[3-hydroxy-2-naphthalenecarboxylate] (1:1) (salt); (2) (*E*)-*m*-[2-(1,4,5,6-Tetrahydro-1-methyl-2-pyrimidinyl)vinyl]phenol 4,4′-methylenebis[3-hydroxy-2-naphthoate] (1:1) (salt). *CAS-68813-55-8; CAS-36531-26-7* [oxantel]. *Anthelmintic.* Telopar (Pfizer) ◇*CP-14,445-16*

Oxapadol. $C_{17}H_{14}N_2O_2$. 278.31. 4,5-Dihydro-1-phenyl-1,4-epoxy-1*H*,3*H*-[1,4]oxazepino[4,3-*a*]benzimidazole. *CAS-56969-22-3.* INN.

Oxapium Iodide. $C_{22}H_{34}INO_2$. 471.42. 1-[(2-Cyclohexyl-2-phenyl-1,3-dioxolan-4-yl)methyl]-1-methylpiperidinium iodide. *CAS-6577-41-9.* INN; JAN. ◇*SH 100*

Oxaprazine. 10-[3-[4-(2-*m*-Dioxan-2-ylethyl)-1-piperazinyl]propyl]phenothiazine. DCF. ◇*SD 270-07 [as succinate]*

Oxapropanium Iodide. $C_7H_{16}INO_2$. 273.11. (1,3-Dioxolan-4-ylmethyl)trimethylammonium iodide. *CAS-541-66-2; CAS-5818-18-8* [oxapropanium]. INN; MI.

Oxaprotiline Hydrochloride [*1981*] (ox″ a proe′ ti leen hye″ droe klor′ ide). $C_{20}H_{23}NO.HCl$. 329.86. [Oxaprotiline is INN.] (1) 9,10-Ethanoanthracene-9(10*H*)-ethanol, α-[(methylamino)methyl]-, hydrochloride, (±)-; (2) (±)-α-[(Methylamino)methyl]-9,10-ethanoanthracene-9(10*H*)-ethanol hydrochloride. *CAS-39022-39-4; CAS-56433-44-4* [oxaprotiline]. *Antidepressant.* ◇*C-49802B-Ba*

Oxaprozin [*1973*] (ox″ a proe′ zin). USP. $C_{18}H_{15}NO_3$. 293.32. (1) 2-Oxazolepropanoic acid, 4,5-diphenyl-; (2) 4,5-Diphenyl-2-oxazolepropionic acid. *UNII-MHJ80W9LRB. CAS-21256-18-8.* INN; BAN; JAN. *Anti-inflammatory.* Daypro (Pfizer) ◇*WY-21,743*

Oxarbazole [*1977*] (ox ar′ ba zole). $C_{21}H_{19}NO_4$. 349.38. (1) 1*H*-Carbazole-3-carboxylic acid, 9-benzoyl-2,3,4,9-tetrahydro-6-methoxy-; (2) 9-Benzoyl-1,2,3,4-tetrahydro-6-methoxycarbazole-3-carboxylic acid. *UNII-A34YCH7N8A. CAS-35578-20-2.* INN. *Anti-asthmatic.* ◇*Win 34284*

Oxarutine — *See* Ethoxazorutoside.

Oxatomide [*1977*] (ox at′ oh mide). $C_{27}H_{30}N_4O$. 426.55. (1) 2*H*-Benzimidazol-2-one, 1-[3-[4-(diphenylmethyl)-1-piperazinyl]propyl]-1,3-dihydro-; (2) 1-[3-[4-(Diphenylmethyl)-1-piperazinyl]propyl]-2-benzimidazolinone. *UNII-J31IL9Z2EE. CAS-60607-34-3.* INN; BAN; JAN. *Anti-allergic; anti-asthmatic.* ◇*R 35,443*

Oxazafone. $C_{19}H_{21}ClN_2O_3$. 360.83. 2′-Benzoyl-4′-chloro-2-[(2-hydroxyethyl)methylamino]-*N*-methylacetanilide. *CAS-70541-17-2.* INN.

Oxazepam [*1965*] (ox az′ e pam). **USP.** $C_{15}H_{11}ClN_2O_2$. 286.71. (1) 2*H*-1,4-Benzodiazepin-2-one, 7-chloro-1,3-dihydro-3-hydroxy-5-phenyl-, (±)-; (2) (±)-7-Chloro-1,3-dihydro-3-hydroxy-5-phenyl-2*H*-1,4-benzodiazepin-2-one. *UNII-6GOW6DWN2A. CAS-604-75-1.* INN; BAN; JAN. *Tranquilizer (minor).* Serax (Alpharma); Zaxopam (Quantum Pharmics) ◇*Wy-3498*

Oxazidione. $C_{20}H_{19}NO_3$. 321.37. 2-(Morpholinomethyl)-2-phenyl-1,3-indanedione. *UNII-OPC1BN901Y. CAS-27591-42-0.* INN; DCF; MI.

Oxazolam. $C_{18}H_{17}ClN_2O_2$. 328.79. 10-Chloro-2,3,7,11b-tetrahydro-2-methyl-11b-phenyloxazolo[3,2-*d*][1,4]benzodiazepin-6(5*H*)-one. *CAS-24143-17-7.* INN; JAN; MI.

Oxazolidin — *See* Oxyphenbutazone.

---

† Brand name formerly used, and/or firm no longer concerned with this product.

Oxazorone. $C_{14}H_{15}NO_4$. 261.27. 7-Hydroxy-4-(morpholino-methyl)coumarin. *UNII-77243B845F. CAS-25392-50-1.* INN; DCF.

Oxcarbazepine [*2002*] (ox″ kar baz′ e peen). $C_{15}H_{12}N_2O_2$. 252.27. (1) 5*H*-Dibenz[*b,f*]azepine-5-carboxamide, 10,11-dihydro-10-oxo-; (2) 10,11-Dihydro-10-oxo-5*H*-dibenz[*b,-f*]azepine-5-carboxamide. *UNII-VZI5B1W380. CAS-28721-07-5.* INN; BAN. *Anticonvulsant; antiepileptic.* Trileptal (Novartis) ◇*GP-47680; KIN-493*

Oxdralazine. $C_8H_{15}N_5O_2$. 213.24. 2,2′-[(6-Hydrazino-3-pyridazinyl)imino]diethanol. *UNII-K6SU81C9V1. CAS-17259-75-5.* INN.

Oxeclosporin. $C_{64}H_{115}N_{11}O_{14}$. 1262.66. Cyclo[[(2*S*,3*R*,4*R*,6*E*)-3-hydroxy-4-methyl-2-(methylamino)-6-octenoyl]-L-2-aminobutyryl-*N*-methylglycyl-*N*-methyl-L-leucyl-L-valyl-*N*-methyl-L-leucyl-L-alanyl-*O*-(2-hydroxyethyl)-D-seryl-*N*-methyl-L-leucyl-*N*-methyl-L-leucyl-*N*-methyl-L-valyl]. *CAS-135548-15-1.* INN.

Oxedrine. $C_9H_{13}NO_2$. 167.21. (*RS*)-1-(4-Hydroxyphenyl)-2-(methylamino)ethanol. *CAS-94-07-5.* BAN.

Oxeglitazar. $C_{19}H_{22}O_4$. 314.38. (2*E*,4*E*)-5-(7-Methoxy-3,3-dimethyl-2,3-dihydro-1-benzoxepin-5-yl)-3-methylpenta-2,4-dienoic acid. *UNII-LKX634SL5X. CAS-280585-34-4.* INN.

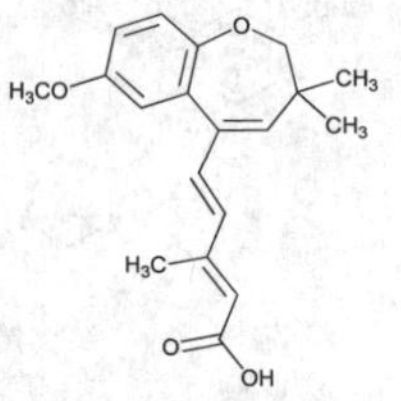

Oxeladin. $C_{20}H_{33}NO_3$. 335.48. [Oxeladin Citrate and Oxeladin Tannate are JAN.] 2-(2-Diethylaminoethoxy)ethyl 2-ethyl-2-phenylbutyrate. *CAS-468-61-1.* INN; BAN; DCF; MI.

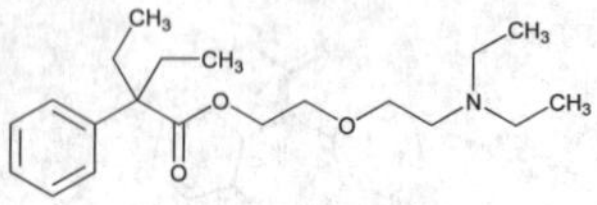

Oxendolone [*1987*] (ox en′ doe lone). $C_{20}H_{30}O_2$. 302.45. (1) Estr-4-en-3-one, 16-ethyl-17-hydroxy-, (16β,17β)-; (2) 16β-Ethyl-17β-hydroxyestr-4-en-3-one. *CAS-33765-68-3.* INN; JAN. *Anti-androgen (benign prostatic hypertrophy).* ◇*TSAA-291*

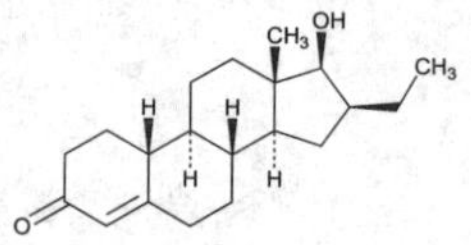

Oxepinac. $C_{16}H_{12}O_4$. 268.26. 6,11-Dihydro-11-oxodibenz [*b,e*]oxepin-3-acetic acid. *UNII-PF3750D8AE. CAS-55689-65-1.* INN.

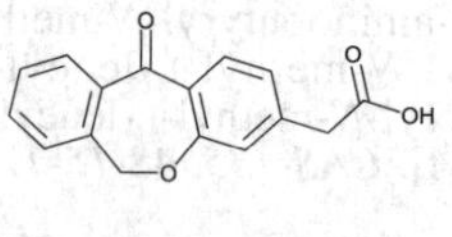

Oxerutins. A mixture of 5 different O-(β-hydroxyethyl) rutosides, not less than 45% of which is troxerutin. BAN.

Oxetacaine (INN, BAN, DCF) — *See* Oxethazaine.

Oxetacillin. $C_{19}H_{23}N_3O_5S$. 405.47. (2*S*,5*R*,6*R*)-6-[(*R*)-4-(*p*-Hydroxyphenyl)-2,2-dimethyl-5-oxo-1-imidazolidinyl]]-3,3-dimethyl-7-oxo-4-thia-1-azabicyclo[3.2.0]heptane-2-carboxylic acid. *UNII-47UDJ8GA54. CAS-53861-02-2.* INN.

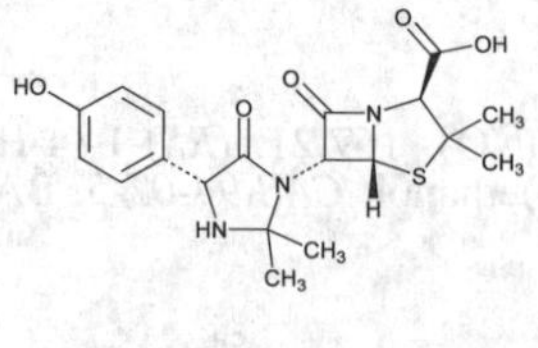

Oxethazaine [*1962*] (ox eth′ a zane). $C_{28}H_{41}N_3O_3$. 467.64. [Oxetacaine is INN and BAN.] (1) Acetamide, 2,2′-[(2-hydroxyethyl)imino]bis[*N*-(1,1-dimethyl-2-phenylethyl)-*N*-methyl-; (2) 2,2′-[(2-Hydroxyethyl)imino]bis[*N*-(α,α-dimethylphenethyl)-*N*-methylacetamide]. *UNII-IP8QT76V17. CAS-126-27-2.* JAN. *Anesthetic (topical).* ◇*Wy-806*

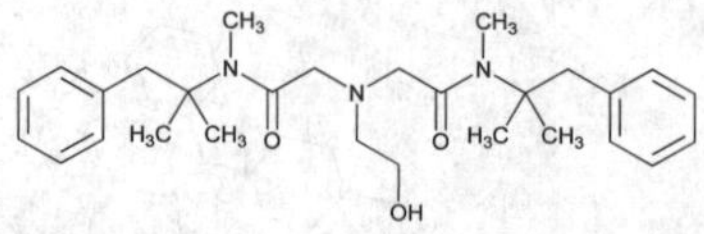

Oxetorone Fumarate [*1978*] (ox et′ oh rone fue′ ma rate). $C_{21}H_{21}NO_2.C_4H_4O_4$. 435.47. [Oxetorone is INN.] (1) 1-Propanamine, 3-benzofuro[3,2-*c*][1]benzoxepin-6(12*H*)-ylidene-*N,N*-dimethyl-, (*E*)-2-butenedioate (1:1); (2) *N,N*-Dimethylbenzofuro[3,2-*c*][1]benzoxepin-$\Delta^{6(12H),\gamma}$-propylamine fumarate (1:1). *UNII-5SYZ8I05SH. CAS-34522-46-8; CAS-26020-55-3* [oxetorone]. *Analgesic (specific in migraine).* Nocertone (Labaz S.A., France) ◇*L-6257*

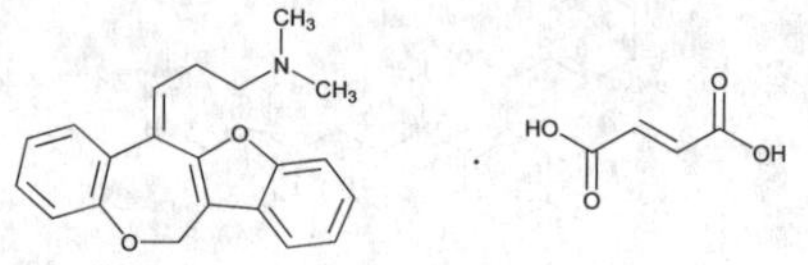

Oxfenamide — *See* Oxiramide.

Oxfendazole [*1976*] (ox fen′ da zole). USP. $C_{15}H_{13}N_3O_3S$. 315.35. (1) Carbamic acid, 5-(phenylsulfinyl)-1*H*-benzimidazol-2-yl-, methyl ester; (2) Methyl 5-(phenylsulfinyl)-2-benzimidazolecarbamate. *UNII-OMP2H17F9E. CAS-53716-50-0.* INN; BAN. *Anthelmintic.* Synanthic [Veterinary] (Syntex) ◇*RS-8858*

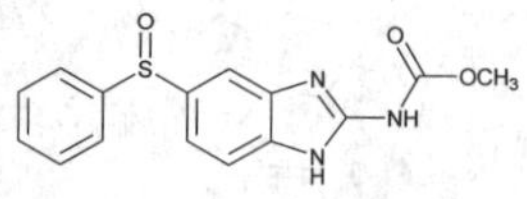

Oxfenicine [*1979*] (ox fen′ i seen). $C_8H_9NO_3$. 167.16. (1) Benzeneacetic acid, α-amino-4-hydroxy-, (*S*)-; (2) L-2-(*p*-Hydroxyphenyl)glycine. *CAS-32462-30-9.* INN; BAN. *Vasodilator.* ◇*UK-25,842*

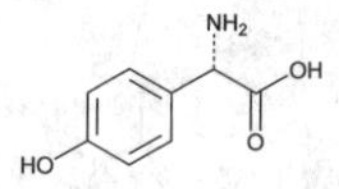

Oxibendazole [*1973*] (ox″ i ben′ da zole). $C_{12}H_{15}N_3O_3$. 249.27. (1) Carbamic acid, (5-propoxy-1*H*-benzimidazol-2-yl)-, methyl ester; (2) Methyl 5-propoxy-2-benzimidazolecarbamate. *UNII-022N12KJ0X. CAS-20559-55-1.* INN; BAN. *Anthelmintic.* Anthelcide EQ (SmithKline Beecham Animal Health); Filaribits Plus (SmithKline Beecham Animal Health) ◇*SK&F 30310*

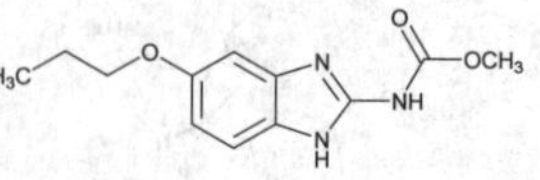

Oxibetaine. $C_6H_{13}NO_3$. 147.17. (Carboxymethyl)dimethyl(2-hydroxyethyl)ammonium hydroxide inner salt. *UNII-Y0WVV18VUI. CAS-7002-65-5.* INN; DCF.

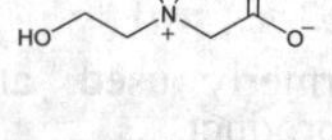

Oxibuprocaine Chloride — *See* Benoxinate Hydrochloride.

Oxichlorochine Sulfate — *See* Hydroxychloroquine Sulfate.

Oxicinchophen — *See* Oxycinchophen.

Oxiconazole Nitrate [*1987*] (ox″ i kon′ a zole nye′ trate). $C_{18}H_{13}Cl_4N_3O \cdot HNO_3$. 492.14. [Oxiconazole is INN and BAN.] (1) Ethanone, 1-(2,4-dichlorophenyl)-2-(1*H*-imidazol-1-yl)-, *O*-[(2,4-dichlorophenyl)methyl]oxime, (*Z*)-, mononitrate; (2) 2′,4′-Dichloro-2-imidazol-1-ylacetophenone (*Z*)-[*O*-(2,4-dichlorobenzyl)oxime], mononitrate. *UNII-RQ8UL4C17S; UNII-C668Q9I33J* [oxiconazole]. *CAS-64211-46-7; CAS-64211-45-6* [oxiconazole]. JAN. *Antifungal.* Oxistat (Altana) ◇*SGD 301-76; Ro 13-8996; ST-813*

Oxicone — *See* Oxycodone.

Oxidopamine [*1977*] (ox″ i doe′ pa meen). $C_8H_{11}NO_3$. 169.18. (1) 1,2,4-Benzenetriol, 5-(2-aminoethyl)-; (2) 5-(2-Aminoethyl)-1,2,4-benzenetriol. *CAS-1199-18-4*. INN. *Adrenergic (ophthalmic).*

Oxidronic Acid [*1979*] (ox″ i dron′ ik as′ id). $CH_6O_7P_2$. 192.00. (1) Phosphonic acid, (hydroxymethylene)bis-; (2) (Hydroxymethylene)diphosphonic acid. *CAS-15468-10-7*. INN; BAN. *Regulator (calcium).* ◇*HMDP*

Oxifenamate — *See* Hydroxyphenamate.

Oxifentorex. $C_{17}H_{21}NO$. 255.35. *N*-Benzyl-*N*,α-dimethylphenethylamine *N*-oxide. *CAS-4075-88-1*. INN; DCF.

Oxifungin Hydrochloride [*1978*] (ox″ i fun′ jin hye″ droe klor′ ide). $C_{13}H_{12}N_4O \cdot HCl$. 276.72. [Oxifungin is INN.] (1) Pyrido[3,4-*e*]-1,2,4-triazine, 1,2-dihydro-3-(phenoxymethyl)-, monohydrochloride; (2) 1,2-Dihydro-3-(phenoxymethyl)pyrido[3,4-*e*]*as*-triazine monohydrochloride.

____

† Brand name formerly used, and/or firm no longer concerned with this product.

UNII-34711907NJ; UNII-F14V3I66R3 [oxifungin]. *CAS-55242-74-5; CAS-64057-48-3* [oxifungin]. *Antifungal.* ◇*EU-3421*

Oxiglutatione. $C_{20}H_{32}N_6O_{12}S_2$. 612.63. *N,N′*-[Dithiobis[(*R*)-1-[(carboxymethyl)carbamoyl]ethylene]]di-L-glutamine. *CAS-27025-41-8*. INN.

Oxilofrine. $C_{10}H_{15}NO_2$. 181.23. *erythro-p*-Hydroxy-α-[1-(methylamino)ethyl]benzyl alcohol. *UNII-F49638UBDR*. *CAS-365-26-4*. INN.

Oxilorphan [*1974*] (ox″ il or′ fan). $C_{20}H_{27}NO_2$. 313.43. (1) Morphinan-3,14-diol, 17-(cyclopropylmethyl)-; (2) (-)-17-(Cyclopropylmethyl)morphinan-3,14-diol. *CAS-42281-59-4*. INN. *Antagonist (to narcotics).* ◇*levo-BC-2605*

Oximetazoline Hydrochloride — *See* Oxymetazoline Hydrochloride.

Oximetholone — *See* Oxymetholone.

Oximonam [*1985*] (ox″ i moe′ nam). $C_{12}H_{15}N_5O_6S$. 357.34. (1) Acetic acid, [[3-[[(2-amino-4-thiazolyl)(methoxyimino)acetyl]amino]-2-methyl-4-oxo-1-azetidinyl]oxy]-, [2*S*-[2α,3β(*Z*)]]-; (2) [[(2*S*,3*S*)-3-[(2-Amino-4-thiazolyl)glyoxylamido]-2-methyl-4-oxo-1-azetidinyl]oxy]acetic acid, 3²-(*Z*)-(*O*-methyloxime). *UNII-482M43SL0K*. *CAS-90898-90-1*. INN. *Antibacterial.* ◇*SQ 82291*

Oximonam Sodium [*1985*] (ox″ i moe′ nam soe′ dee um). $C_{12}H_{14}N_5NaO_6S$. 379.32. (1) Acetic acid, [[3-[[(2-amino-4-thiazolyl)(methoxyimino)acetyl]amino]-2-methyl-4-oxo-1-azetidinyl]oxy]-, monosodium salt, [2*S*-[2α,3β(*Z*)]]-; (2) Sodium [[(2*S*,3*S*)-3-[(2-amino-4-thiazolyl)glyoxylamido]-

2-methyl-4-oxo-1-azetidinyl]oxy]acetate, 3^2-(Z)-(O-methyloxime). *UNII-G274R51QFV. CAS-90849-08-4. Antibacterial.* ◇*SQ 82629*

Oxindanac. $C_{17}H_{14}O_4$. 282.29. (±)-5-Benzoyl-6-hydroxy-1-indancarboxylic acid. *UNII-ZY400R3BNT. CAS-68548-99-2.* INN.

Oxiniacic Acid. $C_6H_5NO_3$. 139.11. Nicotinic acid 1-oxide. *UNII-YY03Q39E6L. CAS-2398-81-4.* INN; DCF; MI.

Oxiperomide [*1973*] (ox″ i per′ oh mide). $C_{20}H_{23}N_3O_2$. 337.42. (1) 2*H*-Benzimidazol-2-one, 1,3-dihydro-1-[1-(2-phenoxyethyl)-4-piperidinyl]-; (2) 1-[1-(2-Phenoxyethyl)-4-piperidyl]-2-benzimidazolinone. *UNII-WRO75M6RW2. CAS-5322-53-2.* INN. *Antipsychotic.* ◇*R 4714*

Oxipertine — *See* Oxypertine.

Oxipethidine — *See* Hydroxypethidine.

Oxiphenbutazone — *See* Oxyphenbutazone.

Oxiphencyclimine Chloride — *See* Oxyphencyclimine Hydrochloride.

Oxiprocaine — *See* Hydroxyprocaine.

Oxiprogesterone Caproate — *See* Hydroxyprogesterone Caproate.

Oxipurinol (INN, BAN) — *See* Oxypurinol.

Oxiracetam. $C_6H_{10}N_2O_3$. 158.16. 4-Hydroxy-2-oxo-1-pyrrolidineacetamide. *UNII-P7U817352G. CAS-62613-82-5.* INN; BAN; MI. ◇*CGP 21690E*

Oxiramide [*1975*] (ox ir′ a mide). $C_{25}H_{34}N_2O_2$. 394.55. (1) Benzeneacetamide, *N*-[4-(2,6-dimethyl-1-piperidinyl)butyl]-α-phenoxy-, *cis*-(±)-; (2) *N*-[4-(2,6-Dimethylpiperidino)butyl]-2-phenoxy-2-phenylacetamide. *CAS-13958-40-2.* INN. *Cardiac depressant (anti-arrhythmic).* ◇*Cl-661*

Oxisopred. $C_{21}H_{28}O_6$. 376.44. 11β,17,21-Trihydroxy-*B*-homo-*A*-norpregn-1-ene-3,6,20-trione. *UNII-0C39YBM73T. CAS-18118-80-4.* INN.

Oxistilbamidine Isethionate — *See* Hydroxystilbamidine Isethionate.

Oxisuran [*1971*] (ox″ i sur′ an). $C_8H_9NO_2S$. 183.23. (1) Ethanone, 2-(methylsulfinyl)-1-(2-pyridinyl)-; (2) (Methylsulfinyl)methyl 2-pyridyl ketone. *CAS-27302-90-5.* INN. *Antineoplastic.* ◇*W 6495*

Oxitefonium Bromide. $C_{19}H_{26}BrNO_3S$. 428.38. Diethyl(2-hydroxyethyl)methylammonium bromide α-phenyl-2-thiopheneglycolate. *CAS-17692-63-6.* INN.

Oxitetracaine — *See* Hydroxytetracaine.

Oxitetracycline — *See* Oxytetracycline.

Oxitriptan. $C_{11}H_{12}N_2O_3$. 220.22. 5-Hydroxy-L-tryptophan. *UNII-C1LJO185Q9. CAS-4350-09-8.* INN.

Oxitriptyline. $C_{19}H_{21}NO_2$. 295.38. 2-[(10,11-Dihydro-5*H*-dibenzo[*a,d*]cyclohepten-5-yl)oxy]-*N,N*-dimethylacetamide. *UNII-5YGV817KFT. CAS-29541-85-3.* INN.

Oxitropium Bromide. $C_{19}H_{26}BrNO_4$. 412.32. (8*r*)-6β,7β-Epoxy-8-ethyl-3α-hydroxy-1αH,5αH-tropanium bromide (-)-tropate. *UNII-SF4NW7NH7C. CAS-30286-75-0.* INN; BAN; JAN; MI. Oxivent (Boehringer Ingelheim)

Oxmetidine Hydrochloride [*1980*] (ox me′ ti deen hye″ droe klor′ ide). $C_{19}H_{21}N_5O_3S.2HCl$. 472.39. [Oxmetidine is INN and BAN.] (1) 4(1*H*)-Pyrimidinone, 5-(1,3-benzodioxol-5-ylmethyl)-2-[[2-[[(5-methyl-1*H*-imidazol-4-yl)-methyl]thio]ethyl]amino]-, dihydrochloride; (2) 2-[[2-[[(5-Methylimidazol-4-yl)methyl]thio]ethyl]amino]-5-piperonyl-4(1*H*)-pyrimidinone dihydrochloride. *CAS-63204-23-9; CAS-72830-39-8* [oxmetidine]. *Antagonist (to histamine H₂receptors).* ◇*SK&F 92994-A₂*

Oxmetidine Mesylate [*1983*] (ox me′ ti deen mes′ i late). $C_{19}H_{21}N_5O_3S.2CH_4O_3S$. 591.68. (1) 4(1*H*)-Pyrimidinone, 5-(1,3-benzodioxol-5-ylmethyl)-2-[[2-[[(5-methyl-1*H*-imidazol-4-yl)methyl]thio]ethyl]amino]-, dimethanesulfonate; (2) 2-[[2-[[(5-Methylimidazol-4-yl)methyl]thio]ethyl]amino]-5-piperonyl-4(1*H*)-pyrimidinone dimethanesulfonate. *CAS-84455-52-7. Antagonist (to histamine H₂receptors).* ◇*SK&F 92994-J₂*

trans-π-Oxocamphor (JAN) — *See* Camphor.

Oxodipine. $C_{19}H_{21}NO_6$. 359.37. Ethyl methyl 1,4-dihydro-2,6-dimethyl-4-[2,3-(methylenedioxy)phenyl]-3,5-pyridinedicarboxylate. *CAS-90729-41-2.* INN.

Oxogestone Phenpropionate [*1968*] (ox″ oh jes′ tone fen proe′ pee oh nate). $C_{29}H_{38}O_3$. 434.61. [Oxogestone is INN.] (1) 19-Norpregn-4-en-3-one, 20-(1-oxo-3-phenylpropoxy)-, (20*R*)-; (2) 20β-Hydroxy-19-norpregn-4-en-3-one hydrocinnamate. *CAS-16915-80-3; CAS-3643-00-3* [oxogestone]. *Progestin.*

Oxolamine. $C_{14}H_{19}N_3O$. 245.32. 5-[2-(Diethylamino)ethyl]-3-phenyl-1,2,4-oxadiazole. *UNII-90BEA145GY. CAS-959-14-8.* INN; DCF; MI. ◇*SKF 9976 [as citrate]; AF-438 [as citrate]*

Oxolinic Acid [*1968*] (ox″ oh lin′ ik as′ id). $C_{13}H_{11}NO_5$. 261.23. (1) 1,3-Dioxolo[4,5-*g*]quinoline-7-carboxylic acid, 5-ethyl-5,8-dihydro-8-oxo-; (2) 5-Ethyl-5,8-dihydro-8-oxo-1,3-dioxolo[4,5-*g*]quinoline-7-carboxylic acid. *UNII-L0A22B22FT. CAS-14698-29-4.* INN; BAN. *Antibacterial.* Utibid (Parke-Davis†) ◇*W 4565; NSC-110364*

Oxomemazine. $C_{18}H_{22}N_2O_2S$. 330.44. 10-[3-(Dimethylamino)-2-methylpropyl]phenothiazine 5,5-dioxide. *UNII-305MB38V1C. CAS-3689-50-7.* INN; DCF; MI. ◇*RP 6847*

Oxonazine. $C_9H_{14}N_6O$. 222.25. N^2,N^2-Diallylmelamine N^2-oxide. *UNII-0Q3H898100. CAS-5580-22-3.* INN.

Oxophenarsine Hydrochloride. $C_6H_6AsNO_2.HCl$. 235.50. [Oxophenarsine is INN.] 2-Amino-4-arsenosophenol hydrochloride. *CAS-538-03-4; CAS-306-12-7* [oxophenarsine]. USP XVII; MI. Mapharsen (Parke-Davis†)

Oxoprostol. $C_{22}H_{32}O_4$. 360.49. (±)-*trans*-2-(7-Hydroxyheptyl)-3-(3-oxo-4-phenoxybutyl)cyclopentanone. *UNII-53C97244OY. CAS-69648-40-4.* INN; BAN. ◇*M&B 33153*

Oxozepam — *See* Oxazepam.

Oxpentifylline (BAN) — *See* Pentoxifylline.

Oxpheneridine. $C_{22}H_{27}NO_3$. 353.45. 1-(β-Hydroxyphenethyl)-4-phenylpiperidine-4-carboxylic acid ethyl ester. *UNII-5OO7RKH9WL. CAS-546-32-7.* INN; DCF.

Oxprenoate Potassium. $C_{25}H_{37}KO_4$. 440.66. Potassium 17-hydroxy-3-oxo-7α-propyl-17α-pregn-4-ene-21-carboxylate. *UNII-167NDD8MTE. CAS-76676-34-1.* INN.

Oxprenolol Hydrochloride [*1968*] (ox pren' oh lol hye" droe klor' ide). **USP**. $C_{15}H_{23}NO_3 \cdot HCl$. 301.81. [Oxprenolol is INN and BAN.] (1) 2-Propanol, 1-(*o*-allyloxyphenoxy)-3-isopropylamino-, hydrochloride; (2) 1-(*o*-Allyloxyphenoxy)-3-isopropylamino-2-propanol hydrochloride. *UNII-F4XSI7SNIU; UNII-519MXN9YZR* [oxprenolol]. *CAS-6452-73-9; CAS-6452-71-7* [oxprenolol]. JAN. *Vasodilator (coronary).* Trasicor (Novartis) ✧*Ba-39,089*

Oxtriphylline (ox trif' i lin). **USP**. $C_{12}H_{21}N_5O_3$. 283.33. [Choline Theophyllinate is INN and BAN; Choline Theophylline is JAN.] (1) Ethanaminium, 2-hydroxy-*N,N,N*-trimethyl-, salt with 3,7-dihydro-1,3-dimethyl-1*H*-purine-2,6-dione; (2) Choline salt with theophylline (1:1). *UNII-3K045XR58X. CAS-4499-40-5; CAS-13930-27-3* [replaced]. *Bronchodilator.* Choledyl (Warner Chilcott)

Oxybenzone [*1965*] (ox" i ben' zone). **USP**. $C_{14}H_{12}O_3$. 228.24. (1) Methanone, (2-hydroxy-4-methoxyphenyl)phenyl-; (2) 2-Hydroxy-4-methoxybenzophenone. *UNII-95OOS7VE0Y. CAS-131-57-7.* INN. *Ultraviolet screen.* Uvinul M40 (BASF) ✧*NSC-7778*

Oxybuprocaine (INN, BAN) — *See* Benoxinate Hydrochloride.

Oxybuprocaine Hydrochloride (JAN) — *See* Benoxinate Hydrochloride.

Oxybutynin [*2001*] (ox" i bue' ti nin). $C_{22}H_{31}NO_3$. 357.49. (1) Benzeneacetic acid, α-cyclohexyl-α-hydroxy-, 4-(diethylamino)-2-butynyl ester; (2) 4-(Diethylamino)-2-butynyl

α-phenylcyclohexaneglycolic acid ester. *UNII-K9P6MC7092. CAS-5633-20-5.* INN; BAN. *Anticholinergic.* Oxytrol (Watson)

Oxybutynin Chloride [*1962*] (ox" i bue' ti nin klor' ide). **USP**. $C_{22}H_{31}NO_3 \cdot HCl$. 393.95. [Oxybutynin Hydrochloride is JAN.] (1) Benzeneacetic acid, α-cyclohexyl-α-hydroxy-, 4-(diethylamino)-2-butynyl ester hydrochloride, ($\pm$)-; (2) 4-(Diethylamino)-2-butynyl ($\pm$)-α-phenylcyclohexaneglycolate hydrochloride. *UNII-L9F3D9RENQ. CAS-1508-65-2. Anticholinergic.* Ditropan (ALZA) ✧*MJ 4309-1; 5058*

Oxychlorosene [*1962*] (ox" i klor' oh seen). The hypochlorous acid complex of a mixture of the phenyl sulfonate derivatives of aliphatic hydrocarbons. (1) Oxychlorosene; (2) Oxychlorosene. *CAS-8031-14-9. Anti-infective, topical.*

Oxychlorosene Sodium [*1962*] (ox" i klor' oh seen soe' dee um). (1) Oxychlorosene sodium; (2) Oxychlorosene sodium. *CAS-52906-84-0; CAS-8031-14-9* [oxychlorosene]. *Anti-infective, topical.* Clorpactin WCS-90 (Guardian Laboratories)

Oxycinchophen. $C_{16}H_{11}NO_3$. 265.26. 3-Hydroxy-2-phenyl-4-quinolinecarboxylic acid. *UNII-UK6392GD5W. CAS-485-89-2.* INN; BAN; MI.

Oxyclipine (INN) Hydrochloride — *See* Propenzolate Hydrochloride.

Oxyclozanide. $C_{13}H_6Cl_5NO_3$. 401.46. 3,3',5,5',6-Pentachloro-2'-hydroxysalicylanilide. *UNII-1QS9G4876X. CAS-2277-92-1.* INN; BAN; MI. ✧*ICI 46683*

Oxycodone [*1963*] (ox" i koe' done). $C_{18}H_{21}NO_4$. 315.36. (1) Morphinan-6-one, 4,5-epoxy-14-hydroxy-3-methoxy-17-methyl-, (5α)-; (2) 4,5α-Epoxy-14-hydroxy-3-methoxy-17-methylmorphinan-6-one; (3) (-)-14-Hydroxydihydrocodeinone. *UNII-CD35PMG570. CAS-76-42-6.* INN; BAN. *Analgesic (narcotic).* OxyContin (Purdue Frederick) ✧*NSC-19043*

Oxycodone Hydrochloride [*1966*] (ox" i koe' done hye" droe klor' ide). **USP**. $C_{18}H_{21}NO_4 \cdot HCl$. 351.82. (1) Morphinan-6-one, 4,5-epoxy-14-hydroxy-3-methoxy-17-methyl-, hydrochloride, (5α)-; (2) 4,5α-Epoxy-14-hydroxy-3-methoxy-

17-methylmorphinan-6-one hydrochloride. *UNII-C1EN-J2TE6C; UNII-CD35PMG570* [oxycodone]. *CAS-124-90-3; CAS-76-42-6* [oxycodone]. JAN. *Analgesic (narcotic).* Oxycontin (Purdue); Roxicodone (Roxane)

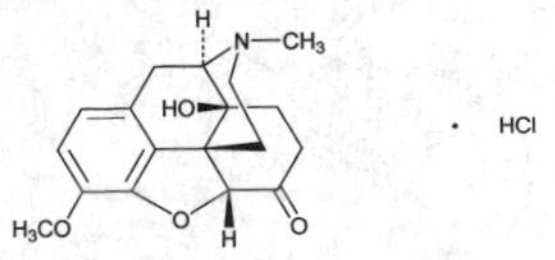

Oxycodone Terephthalate (ox″ i koe′ done ter″ e thal′ ate). **USP.** $(C_{18}H_{21}NO_4)_2.C_8H_6O_4$. 796.86. (1) Morphinan-6-one, 4,5-epoxy-14-hydroxy-3-methoxy-17-methyl-, 1,4-benzenedicarboxylate (2:1 salt), (5α); (2) 4,5α-Epoxy-14-hydroxy-3-methoxy-17-methylmorphinan-6-one 1,4-benzenedicarboxylate (2:1 salt). *UNII-M04XWV43UF. CAS-64336-55-6. Analgesic (narcotic).*

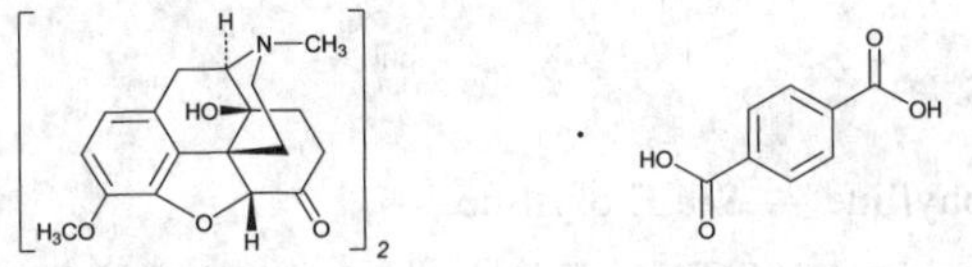

Oxydipentonium Chloride. $C_{16}H_{38}Cl_2N_2O$. 345.39. [Oxybis(pentamethylene)]bis(trimethylammonium chloride). *UNII-VV0B5MP6VI. CAS-7174-23-4.* INN.

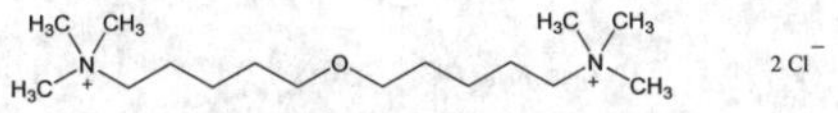

Oxydol (JAN) — *See* Hydrogen Peroxide.

Oxyethyltheophylline — *See* Etofylline.

Oxyfedrine. $C_{19}H_{23}NO_3$. 313.39. [Oxyfedrine Hydrochloride is JAN.] 3-[[(αS,βR)-β-Hydroxy-α-methylphenethyl]amino]-3′-methoxypropiophenone. *UNII-DWL616XF1K. CAS-15687-41-9.* INN; BAN; DCF; MI.

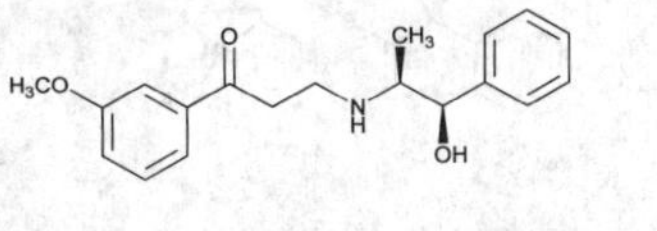

Oxyfenamate (INN and DCF) — *See* Hydroxyphenamate.

Oxyfilcon A [*1981*] (ox″ i fil′ kon). $[[(C_2H_6OSi)_v]_3C_3H_7 OSi]_w(C_4H_6O_2)_x(C_6H_9NO)_y(C_5H_8O_2)_z$. (1) Siloxane, dimethyl, 3-hydroxypropyl-terminated, polymer with 2-methyl-2-propenoic acid, 1-ethenyl-2-pyrrolidinone and methyl 2-methyl-2-propenoate; (2) 3-Hydroxypropyl-terminated dimethyl siloxane, polymer with methacrylic acid, 1-vinyl-2-pyrrolidinone and methyl methacrylate. *Contact lens material (hydrophilic).* ◇*AL-T150*

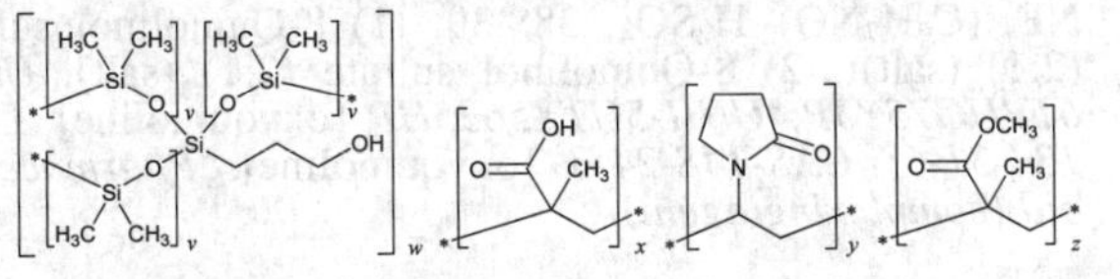

Oxygen (ox′ i jen). **USP.** O_2. 32.00. (1) Oxygen; (2) Oxygen. *CAS-7782-44-7. Gas, medicinal.*

Oxygen 93 Percent (ox′ i jen). **USP.** Contains 93 ± 3.0%, by volume, of O_2, the remainder consisting mostly of argon and nitrogen. *Gas, medicinal.*

Oxymesterone. $C_{20}H_{30}O_3$. 318.45. 4,17β-Dihydroxy-17-methylandrost-4-en-3-one. *UNII-4R73K9MRMX. CAS-145-12-0.* INN; BAN; DCF; MI.

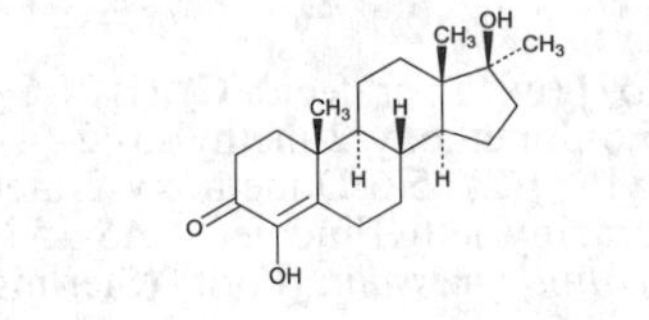

Oxymetazoline Hydrochloride [*1963*] (ox″ i me taz′ oh leen hye″ droe klor′ ide). **USP.** $C_{16}H_{24}N_2O.HCl$. 296.84. [Oxymetazoline is INN and BAN.] (1) Phenol, 3-[(4,5-dihydro-1H-imidazol-2-yl)methyl]-6-(1,1-dimethylethyl)-2,4-dimethyl-, monohydrochloride; (2) 6-*tert*-Butyl-3-(2-imidazolin-2-ylmethyl)-2,4-dimethylphenol monohydrochloride. *UNII-K89MJ0S5VY; UNII-8VLN5B44ZY* [oxymetazoline]. *CAS-2315-02-8; CAS-1491-59-4* [oxymetazoline]. JAN. *Adrenergic (vasoconstrictor).* Ocuclear (Schering-Plough); Visine (Pfizer) ◇*Sch 9384*

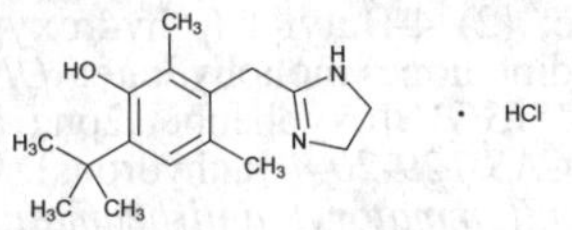

Oxymetebanol (JAN) — *See* Drotebanol.

Oxymetholone [*1963*] (ox″ i meth′ oh lone). **USP.** $C_{21}H_{32}O_3$. 332.48. (1) Androstan-3-one, 17-hydroxy-2-(hydroxymethylene)-17-methyl-, (5α,17β)-; (2) 17β-Hydroxy-2-(hydroxymethylene)-17-methyl-5α-androstan-3-one. *UNII-L76T0ZCA8K. CAS-434-07-1.* INN; BAN; JAN. *Androgen.* Anadrol (Alaven) ◇*CI-406; HMD*

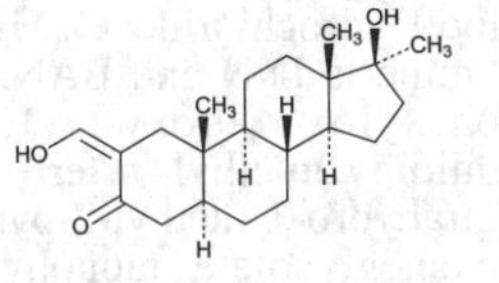

Oxymethylene Urea — *See* Polynoxylin.

Oxymorphone Hydrochloride (ox″ i mor′ fone hye″ droe klor′ ide). **USP.** $C_{17}H_{19}NO_4.HCl$. 337.80. [Oxymorphone is INN and BAN.] (1) Morphinan-6-one, 4,5-epoxy-3,14-dihydroxy-17-methyl-, hydrochloride, (5α)-; (2) 4,5α-Epoxy-3,14-dihydroxy-17-methylmorphinan-6-one hydrochloride. *UNII-5Y2EI94NBC; UNII-9VXA968E0C* [oxymorphone]. *CAS-357-07-3; CAS-76-41-5* [oxymorphone]. *Analgesic (narcotic).* Numorphan (Endo); Opana (Endo)

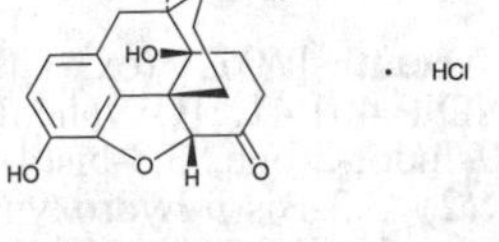

---

† Brand name formerly used, and/or firm no longer concerned with this product.

Oxypendyl. $C_{20}H_{26}N_4OS$. 370.51. 4-[3-(10*H*-Pyrido[3,2-*b*][1,4]benzothiazin-10-yl)-propyl]piperazin-1-ylethanol. *UNII-Q76F3HAE5V. CAS-5585-93-3.* INN; MI.

Oxypertine [*1967*] (ox″ i per′ teen). $C_{23}H_{29}N_3O_2$. 379.50. (1) 1*H*-Indole, 5,6-dimethoxy-2-methyl-3-[2-(4-phenyl-1-piperazinyl)ethyl]-; (2) 5,6-Dimethoxy-2-methyl-3-[2-(4-phenyl-1-piperazinyl)ethyl]indole. *CAS-153-87-7.* INN; BAN; JAN. *Antidepressant.* Forit (Sterling Winthrop) ◇*Win 18,501-2*

Oxyphenbutazone. $C_{19}H_{20}N_2O_3 \cdot H_2O$. 342.39. (1) 3,5-Pyrazolidinedione, 4-butyl-1-(4-hydroxyphenyl)-2-phenyl-, monohydrate; (2) 4-Butyl-1-(*p*-hydroxyphenyl)-2-phenyl-3,5-pyrazolidinedione monohydrate. *UNII-H806S4B3NS; UNII-A7D84513GV* [oxyphenbutazone anhydrous]. *CAS-7081-38-1; CAS-129-20-4* [anhydrous]. USP XXIII; INN; BAN. *Anti-inflammatory; antirheumatic.* Tandearil (Novartis)

Oxyphencyclimine Hydrochloride. $C_{20}H_{28}N_2O_3 \cdot HCl$. 380.91. [Oxyphencyclimine is INN and BAN.] (1) Benzeneacetic acid, α-cyclohexyl-α-hydroxy-, (1,4,5,6-tetrahydro-1-methyl-2-pyrimidinyl)methyl ester monohydrochloride; (2) (1,4,5,6-Tetrahydro-1-methyl-2-pyrimidinyl)methyl α-phenylcyclohexaneglycolate monohydrochloride. *UNII-GWO1432WOU; UNII-4V44H1O8XI* [oxyphencyclimine]. *CAS-125-52-0; CAS-125-53-1* [oxyphencyclimine]. USP XXII; JAN. Daricon (Pfizer)

Oxyphenhydrazine — *See* Carsalam.

Oxyphenisatin Acetate [*1962*] (ox″ i fen eye′ sa tin as′ e tate). $C_{24}H_{19}NO_5$. 401.41. [Oxyphenisatine is INN and BAN.] (1) 2*H*-Indol-2-one, 3,3-bis[4-(acetyloxy)phenyl]-1,3-dihydro-; (2) 3,3-Bis(*p*-hydroxyphenyl)-2-indolinone diacetate (ester). *UNII-3BT0VQG2GQ* [oxyphenisatine].

CAS-115-33-3; CAS-125-13-3 [oxyphenisatine]. *Laxative.* Isocrin (Parke-Davis†); Lavema (Sterling Winthrop†) ◇*NSC-59687*

Oxyphenonium Bromide. $C_{21}H_{34}BrNO_3$. 428.40. Diethyl(2-hydroxyethyl)methylammonium bromide α-phenylcyclohexaneglycolate. *UNII-S9421HWB3Z. CAS-50-10-2; CAS-14214-84-7* [oxyphenonium]. INN; BAN; MI. Antrenyl (Novartis)

Oxyphylline — *See* Etofylline.

Oxypurinol [*1967*] (ox″ i pure′ i nol). $C_5H_4N_4O_2$. 152.11. [Oxipurinol is INN and BAN.] (1) 1*H*-Pyrazolo[3,4-*d*]pyrimidine,4,6(5*H*,7*H*)-dione; (2) 1*H*-Pyrazolo[3,4-*d*]pyrimidine-4,6-diol. *CAS-2465-59-0. Xanthine oxidase inhibitor.* ◇*NSC-76239*

Oxypyrronium Bromide. $C_{21}H_{32}BrNO_3$. 426.39. 2-(2-Hydroxymethyl)-1,1-dimethyl)pyrrolidinium bromide α-phenylcyclohexaneglycolate. *UNII-1D79RM7Q04. CAS-561-43-3.* INN. ◇*LD 3055*

Oxyquinoline [*1978*] (ox″ i kwin′ oh leen). C_9H_7NO. 145.16. (1) 8-Quinolinol; (2) 8-Quinolinol. *UNII-5UTX5635HP. CAS-148-24-3. Disinfectant.*

Oxyquinoline Benzoate — *See* Benzoxiquine.

Oxyquinoline Sulfate [*1980*] (ox″ i kwin′ oh leen sul′ fate). **NF.** $(C_9H_7NO)_2 \cdot H_2SO_4$. 388.39. (1) 8-Quinolinol sulfate (2:1) (salt); (2) 8-Quinolinol sulfate (2:1) (salt). *UNII-61VUG75Y3P; UNII-5UTX5635HP* [oxyquinoline]. *CAS-134-31-6; CAS-148-24-3* [oxyquinoline]. *Pharmaceutic aid (complexing agent).*

Oxyridazine. $C_{21}H_{26}N_2OS$. 354.51. 2-Methoxy-10-[2-(1-methyl-2-piperidyl)ethyl]phenothiazine. *UNII-OCW5XQ-Q13I. CAS-14759-04-7.* INN. ◇*KS 33*

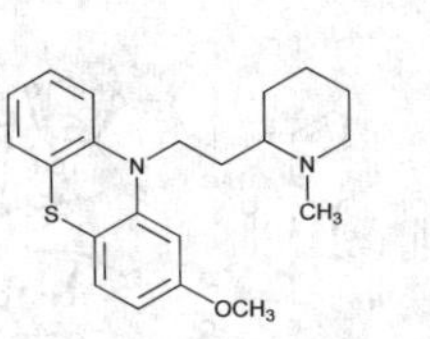

Oxysonium Iodide. $C_{18}H_{27}IO_3S$. 450.37. (2-Hydroxyethyl)dimethylsulfoniumiodide α-phenylcyclohexane glycolate. *UNII-A5Q7SNC216. CAS-3569-58-2.* INN.

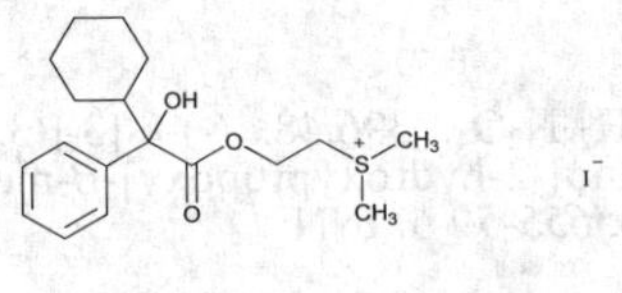

Oxytetracycline (ox″ i tet″ ra sye′ kleen). **USP**. $C_{22}H_{24}N_2O_9 \cdot 2H_2O$. 496.46. (1) 2-Naphthacenecarboxamide, 4-(dimethylamino)-1,4,4a,5,5a,6,11,12a-octahydro-3,5,6,10,12,12a-hexahydroxy-6-methyl-1,11-dioxo-, [4S-(4α,4aα,5α,5aα,6β,12aα)]-, dihydrate; (2) 4-(Dimethylamino)-1,4,4a,5,5a,6,11,12a-octahydro-3,5,6,10,12,12a-hexahydroxy-6-methyl-1,11-dioxo-2-naphthacenecarboxamide dihydrate. *UNII-X20I9EN955; UNII-SLF0D9077S* [oxytetracycline anhydrous]. *CAS-6153-64-6; CAS-79-57-2* [anhydrous]. INN; BAN; JAN. *Antibacterial.* Terramycin (Pfizer)

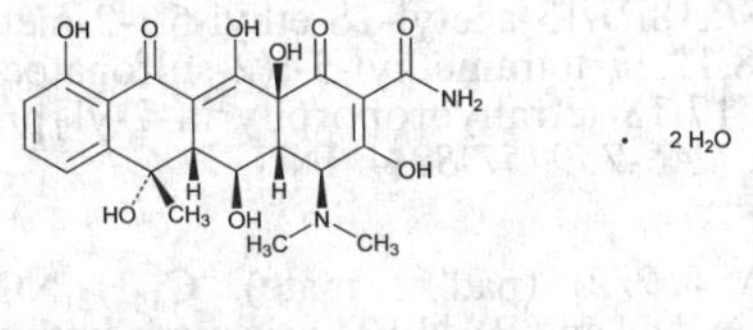

Oxytetracycline Calcium (ox″ i tet″ ra sye′ kleen kal′ see um). **USP**. $C_{44}H_{46}CaN_4O_{18}$. 958.93. (1) 2-Naphthacenecarboxamide, 4-(dimethylamino)-1,4,4a,5,5a,6,11,12a-octahydro-3,5,6,10,12,12a-hexahydroxy-6-methyl-1,11-dioxo-, calcium salt, [4S-(4α,4aα,5α,5aα,6β,12aα)]-; (2) 4-(Dimethylamino)-1,4,4a,5,5a,6,11,12a-octahydro-3,5,6,10,12,12a-hexahydroxy-6-methyl-1,11-dioxo-2-naphthacenecarboxamide calcium salt. *UNII-C8MRZ07FDV. CAS-15251-48-6; CAS-79-57-2* [oxytetracycline]. *Antibacterial.* Terramycin (Pfizer)

Oxytetracycline Hydrochloride (ox″ i tet″ ra sye′ kleen hye″ droe klor′ ide). **USP**. $C_{22}H_{24}N_2O_9 \cdot HCl$. 496.89. (1) 2-Naphthacenecarboxamide, 4-(dimethylamino)-1,4,4a,5,5a,6,11,12a-octahydro-3,5,6,10,12,12a-hexahydroxy-6-methyl-1,11-dioxo-, monohydrochloride, [4S-(4α,4aα,5α,5aα,6β,12aα)]-; (2) 4-(Dimethylamino)-1,4,4a,5,5a,6,11,12a-octahydro-3,5,6,10,12,12a-hexahydroxy-6-methyl-1,11-dioxo-2-naphthacenecarboxamide monohydrochloride. *UNII-4U7K4N52ZM; UNII-X20I9EN955* [oxytetracycline]. *CAS-2058-46-0; CAS-79-57-2* [oxytetracycline]. JAN. *Antibacterial; antirickettsial.* Terramycin (Pfizer)

Oxytocin (ox″ i toe′ sin). **USP**. $C_{43}H_{66}N_{12}O_{12}S_2$. 1007.19. (1) Oxytocin; (2) Oxytocin. *UNII-1JQS135EYN. CAS-50-56-6.* INN; BAN; JAN. *Oxytocic.* Pitocin (King); Syntocinon (Novartis)

Ozagrel. $C_{13}H_{12}N_2O_2$. 228.25. [Ozagrel Sodium is JAN.] (*E*)-*p*-(Imidazol-1-ylmethyl)cinnamic acid. *UNII-L256JB984D. CAS-82571-53-7.* INN; MI.

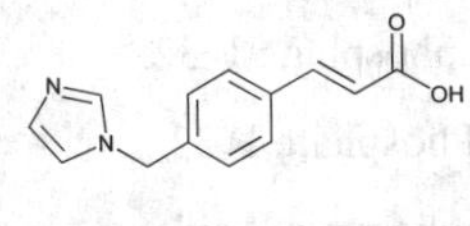

Ozarelix. $C_{72}H_{96}ClN_{17}O_{14}$. 1459.09. *N*-Acetyl-3-(naphthalen-2-yl)-D-alanyl-4-chloro-D-phenylalanyl-3-(pyridin-3-yl)-D-alanyl-L-seryl-*N*-methyl-L-tyrosyl-N^6-carbamoyl-D-lysyl-L-2-aminohexanoyl-L-arginyl-L-prolyl-D-alaninamide. *CAS-295350-45-7.* INN.

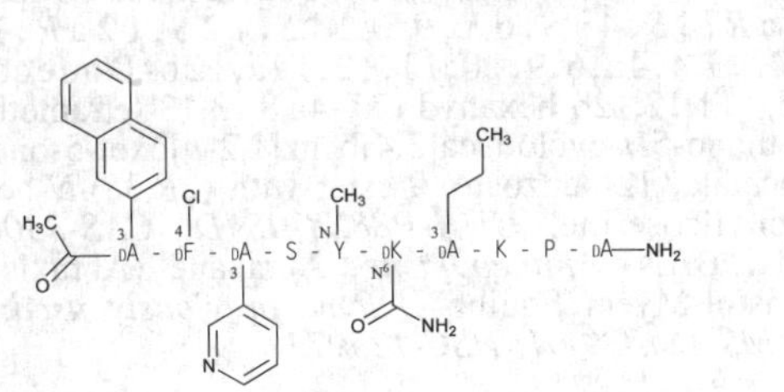

Ozenoxacin. $C_{21}H_{21}N_3O_3$. 363.41. 1-Cyclopropyl-8-methyl-7-[5-methyl-6-(methylamino)pyridin-3-yl]-4-oxo-1,4-dihydroquinoline-3-carboxylic acid. *CAS-245765-41-7.* INN.

Ozogamicin. $C_{73}H_{97}IN_6O_{25}S_3$. 1681.68. Methyl (1*R*,4*Z*,8*S*,13*E*)-13-[2-[[2-[[[*p*-(3-carbamoylpropoxy)-α-methylbenzylidene]hydrazino]carbonyl]-1,1-dimethylethyl]dithio]ethylidene]-8-[[4,6-dideoxy-4-[[[2,6-dideoxy-4-*S*-[4-[(6-deoxy-3-*O*-methyl-α-L-mannopyranosyl)oxy]-3-iodo-5,6-dimethoxy-*o*-toluoyl]-4-thio-β-D-*ribo*-hexopyranosyl]oxy]amino]-2-*O*-[2,4-dideoxy-4-(*N*-ethylacetamido)-3-*O*-methyl-α-L-*threo*-pentopyranosyl]-β-D-glucopyranosyl]oxy]-1-hydroxy-11-oxobicyclo[7.3.1]trideca-4,9-diene-2,6-diyne-10-carbamate. *CAS-400046-53-9.* INN.

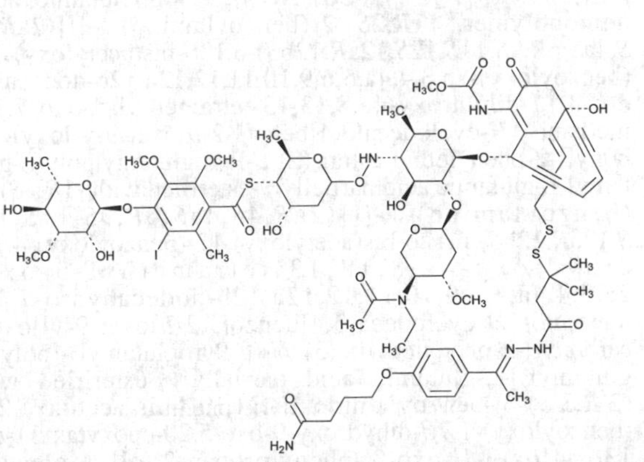

---

† Brand name formerly used, and/or firm no longer concerned with this product.

Ozolinone [*1978*] (oh zoe′ li none). $C_{11}H_{16}N_2O_3S$. 256.32. (1) Acetic acid, [3-methyl-4-oxo-5-(1-piperidinyl)-2-thiazolidinylidene]-, (Z)-; (2) (Z)-3-Methyl-4-oxo-5-piperidino-$\Delta^{2,\alpha}$-thiazolidineacetic acid. *UNII-55TIT7J81D. CAS-56784-39-5*. INN. *Diuretic.* ◊*Goedecke 3282*

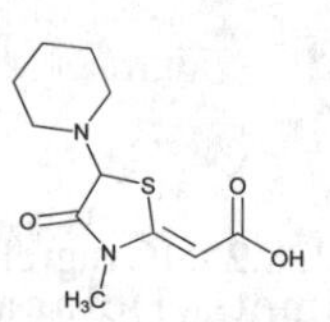

^{32}P — *See* Chromic Phosphate P 32.

^{32}P — *See* Polymetaphosphate P 32.

^{32}P — *See* Sodium Phosphate P 32.

PABA — *See* Aminobenzoic Acid.

Paclitaxel [*1993*] (pak″ li tax′ el). **USP.** $C_{47}H_{51}NO_{14}$. 853.91. (1) Benzenepropanoic acid, β-(benzoylamino)-α-hydroxy-, 6,12b-bis(acetyloxy)-12-(benzoyloxy)-2a,3,4,4a,5,6,9,10,11,12,12a,12b-dodecahydro-4,11-dihydroxy-4a,8,13,13-tetramethyl-5-oxo-7,11-methano-1*H*-cyclodeca[3,4]benz[1,2-b]oxet-9-yl ester, [2a*R*-[2aα,4β,4aβ,6β,9α(α*R**,β*S**),11α,12α,12aα,12bα]]-; (2) (2a*R*,4*S*,4a*S*,6*R*,9*S*,11*S*,12*S*,12a*R*,12b*S*)-1,2a,3,4,4a,6,9,10,11,12,12a,12b-Dodecahydro-4,6,9,11,12,12b-hexahydroxy-4a,8,13,13-tetramethyl-7,11-methano-5*H*-cyclodeca[3,4]benz[1,2-*b*]oxet-5-one 6,12b-diacetate, 12-benzoate, 9-ester with (2*R*,3*S*)-*N*-benzoyl-3-phenylisoserine. *UNII-P88XT4IS4D. CAS-33069-62-4.* INN; BAN. *Antineoplastic.* Abraxane (Abraxis); Taxol (Bristol-Myers Squibb) [*Name previously used: Taxol.*] ◊*BMS-181339-01; NSC-125973*

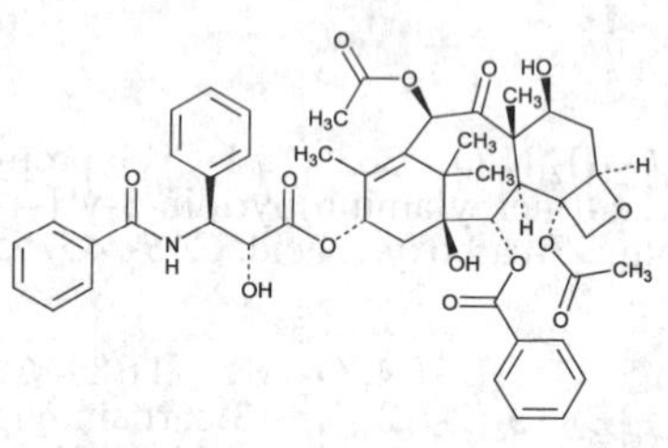

Paclitaxel Ceribate. $C_{51}H_{57}NO_{18}$. 971.99. 7β-[(2*RS*)-2,3-Dihydroxypropoxycarbonyloxy]-1-hydroxy-9-oxo-5β,20-epoxytax-11-ene-2α,4,10β,13α-tetrayl 4,10-diacetate 2-benzoate 13-[(2*R*,3*S*)-3-benzamido-2-hydroxy-3-phenylpropanoate]. *CAS-186040-50-6.* INN.

Paclitaxel Poliglumex [*2004*] (pak″ li tax′ el pol″ ee gloo′ mex). $(C_{52}H_{56}N_2O_{16})_n·(C_5H_7NO_3)_x$. (1) L-Glutamic acid, homopolymer, (1*R*,2*S*)-2-(benzoylamino)-1-[[[(2a*R*,4*S*,4a*S*,6*R*,9*S*,11*S*,12*S*,12a*R*,12b*S*)-6,12b-bis(acetyloxy)-12-(benzoyloxy)-2a,3,4,4a,5,6,9,10,11,12,12a,12b-dodecahydro-4,11-dihydroxy-4a,8,13,13-tetramethyl-5-oxo-7,11-methano-1*H*-cyclodeca[3,4]benz[1,2-*b*]oxet-9-yl]oxy]carbonyl]-2-phenylethyl ester; (2) L-Pyroglutamylpoly-L-glutamyl-L-glutamic acid partially γ-esterified with (1*R*,2*S*)-2-(benzoylamino)-1-[[[(2a*R*,4*S*,4a*S*,6*R*,9*S*,11*S*,12-*S*,12a*R*,12b*S*)-6,12b-bis(acetyloxy)-12-dihydroxy-4a,8,13,13-tetramethyl-5-oxo-2a,3,4,4a,5,6,9,10,11,12,12a,12b-dodecahydro-7,11-methano-1*H*-cyclodeca[3,4]benzo[1,2-*b*]oxet-9-yl]oxy]-carbonyl]-2-phenylethyl; (3) *N*-(L-Pyroglutamyl)-[poly(L-glutamyl)]-L-glutamic acid partially γ-esterified with (2′*R*,3′*S*)-3′-benzoylamido-1′-[[4,10β-bis(acetoxy)-2α-(benzoyloxy)-1,7β-dihydroxy-9-oxo-5,20-epoxytax-11-en-13α-yl]oxy]-1′-oxo-3′-phenylpropan-2′-ol. Molecular weight is approximately 45,000 daltons. *CAS-263351-82-*

2. INN. *Anticancer therapy as a single agent or in combination with other anticancer therapies.* Xyotax (Amcis) ◊*CT-2103*

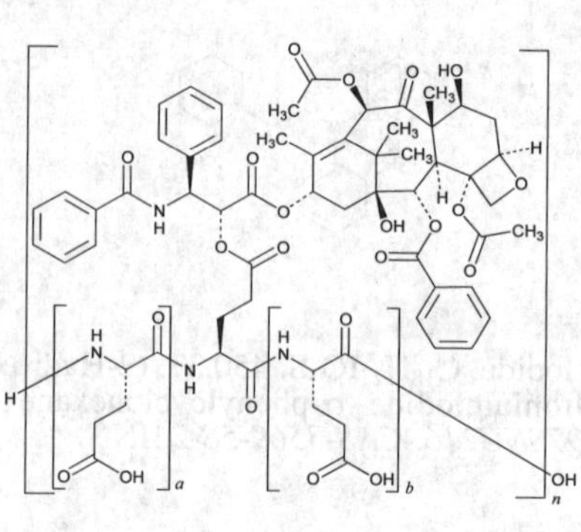

Pacrinolol. $C_{23}H_{28}N_2O_4$. 396.48. (-)-*p*-[3-[(3,4-Dimethoxyphenetyl)amino]-2-hydroxypropoxy]-β-methylcinnamonitrile. *CAS-65655-59-6.* INN.

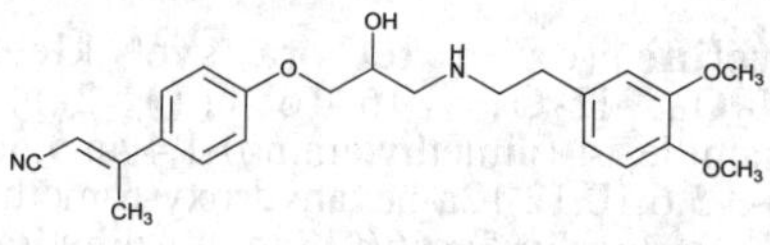

Pactimibe. $C_{25}H_{40}N_2O_3$. 416.60. [7-(2,2-Dimethylpropanamido)-4,6-dimethyl-1-octylindolin-5-yl]acetic acid. *UNII-D874R9PZ9T. CAS-189198-30-9.* INN; BAN.

Padeliporfin. $C_{37}H_{43}N_5O_9PdS$. 840.25. Dihydrogen (3-{(7*S*,8*S*,17*R*,18*R*)-13-acetyl-18-ethyl-5-(-2-methoxy-2-oxoethyl)-2,8,12,17-tetramethyl-3-[(2-sulfonatoethyl)carbamoyl]-7,8,17,18-tetrahydroporphyrin-7-yl}propanoato)-palladium. *CAS-759457-82-4.* INN.

Padimate A [*1972*] (pad′ i mate). $C_{14}H_{21}NO_2$. 235.32. [Padimate is INN and BAN.] This is made with commercial amyl alcohol consisting of approximately 67% of *n*-pentanol and a mixture of 2-methyl and 3-methyl butanols. (1) Benzoic acid, 4-(dimethylamino)-, pentyl ester; (2) Pentyl *p*-(dimethylamino)benzoate. *CAS-14779-78-3. Ultraviolet screen.*

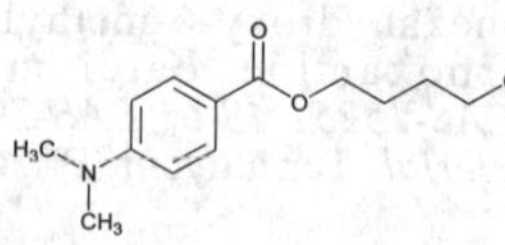

Padimate O [*1974*] (pad′ i mate). **USP.** $C_{17}H_{27}NO_2$. 277.40. (1) Benzoic acid, 4-(dimethylamino)-, 2-ethylhexyl ester; (2) 2-Ethylhexyl *p*-(dimethylamino)benzoate. *CAS-21245-02-3. Ultraviolet screen.* Arlatone UVB (ICI Americas†); Escalol 507 (ISP Van Dyk)

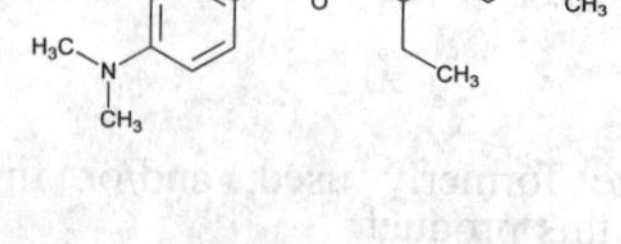

Padoporfin. $C_{35}H_{38}N_4O_6Pd$. 717.12. {Hydrogen 3-[(2²*R*,7*R*,8*R*,17*S*,18*S*)-12-acetyl-7-ethyl-2²-(methoxycarbonyl)-3,8,13,17-tetramethyl-2¹-oxo-2¹,2²,7,8,17,18-hexahydrocyclopenta[*at*]porphyrin-18-yl]propanoato-κ4N²¹,N²²,N²³,N²⁴}palladium. *CAS-274679-00-4*. INN.

Pafenolol. $C_{18}H_{31}N_3O_3$. 337.46. (±)-1-[*p*-[2-Hydroxy-3-(isopropylamino)propoxy]phenethyl]-3-isopropylurea. *UNII-5AEP5YJ9MZ. CAS-75949-61-0*. INN.

Paflufocon A [*1987*] (pa″ floo foe′ kon). $(C_6H_7F_3O_2)_i$ $(C_{26}H_{58}O_9Si_6)_u(C_5H_8O_2)_v(C_4H_6,O_2)_w(C_{13}H_{30}O_5Si_3)_x(C_{16}H_{38}O_5Si_4)_y(C_{10}H_{14}O_4)_z$. [Oxygen permeability at 35°C is (Dk) 92 × 10⁻¹¹ (cm²/sec)(ml O₂/ml × mm Hg)] (1) 2-Propenoic acid, 2-methyl-, 2,2,2-trifluoroethyl ester, polymer with [1,1,3,3-tetrakis[(trimethylsilyl)oxy]-1,3-disiloxanediyl]di-3,1-propanediyl bis(2-methyl-2-propenoate), methyl 2-methyl-2-propenoate, 2-methyl-2-propenoic acid, 3-[1-hydroxy-3,3,3-trimethyl-1-[(trimethylsilyl)oxy]disiloxanyl]propyl 2-methyl-2-propenoate, 3-[3,3,3-trimethyl-1,1-bis[(trimethylsilyl)oxy]disiloxanyl]propyl 2-methyl-2-propenoate and 1,2-ethanediyl bis(2-methyl-2-propenoate); (2) 2,2,2-Trifluoroethyl methacrylate polymer with [1,1,3,3-tetrakis(trimethylsiloxy)disiloxanylene]bis(trimethylene) dimethacrylate, methyl methacrylate, methacrylic acid, 3-[1-hydroxy-3,3,3-trimethyl-1-(trimethylsiloxy)disiloxanyl]propyl metacrylate, 3-[3,3,3-trimethyl-1,1-bis(trimethylsiloxy)disiloxanyl]propyl methacrylate and ethylene dimethacrylate. *CAS-109550-08-5. Contact lens material (hydrophobic)*. Fluoroperm 92 (Paragon)

Paflufocon B [*1987*] (pa″ floo foe′ kon). [Oxygen permeability at 35°C is (Dk) 62 × 10⁻¹¹ (cm²/sec)(ml O₂/ml × mm Hg).] *Contact lens material (hydrophobic)*. Fluoroperm 62 (Paragon) *[Note—The chemical names, structural and molecular formula, manufacturer and CAS Registry Number are identical to Paflufocon A.]*

Paflufocon C [*1987*] (pa″ floo foe′ kon). [Oxygen permeability at 35°C is (Dk) 32 × 10⁻¹¹ (cm²/sec)(ml O₂/ml × mm Hg).] *Contact lens material (hydrophobic)*. Fluoroperm 32 (Paragon) *[Note—The chemical names, structural and molecular formula, manufacturer and CAS Registry Number are identical to Paflufocon A.]*

Paflufocon D [*1990*] (pa″ floo foe′ kon). [Oxygen permeability at 35°C is (Dk) 151 × 10⁻¹¹ (cm²/sec)(ml O₂/ml × mm Hg).] *Contact lens material (hydrophobic)*. Fluoroperm 151 (Paragon) *[Note—The chemical names, structural and molecular formula, manufacturer and CAS Registry Number are identical to Paflufocon A.]*

Paflufocon D-HEM-Iberfilcon A [*2005*] (pa″ floo foe′ kon eye″ ber fil′ kon). $(C_6H_7F_3O_2)_t$ $(C_{26}H_{58}O_8Si_6)_u$ $(C_5H_8O_2)_v$ $(C_4H_6O_2)_w$ $(C_{13}H_{30}O_5Si_3)_x$ $(C_{16}H_{38}O_5Si_4)_y$ $(C_{10}H_{14}O_4)_z$ (Component A: paflufocon D) $(C_{18}H_{26}O_6)_w$ $(C_{12}H_{16}O_3)_x$ $(C_7H_{12}O_3)_y$, $(C_6H_{10}O_3)_z$ (Component B: iberfilcon A). A hybrid contact lens material composed of: Component A (paflufocon D), 2-Propenoic acid, 2-methyl-, 2,2,2-trifluoroethyl ester, polymer with [1,1,3,3-tetrakis[(trimethylsilyl)oxy]-1,3-disiloxanediyl]di-3,1-propanediyl bis(2-methyl-2-propenoate), methyl 2-methyl-2-propenoate, 2-methyl-2-propenoic acid, 3-[1-hydroxy-3,3,3-trimethyl-1-[(trimethylsilyl)oxy]disiloxanyl]propyl 2-methyl-2-propenoate, 3-[3,3,3-trimethyl-1,1-bis[(trimethylsilyl)oxy]disiloxanyl]propyl 2-methyl-2-propenoate and 1,2-ethanediyl bis(2-methyl-2-propenoate); Component B: (iberfilcon A), 2-Propenoic acid, 2-methyl-, 2-ethyl-2-[[(2-methyl-1-oxo-2-propenyl)oxy]methyl]-1,3-propanediyl ester, polymer with 2,2-diethoxy-1-phenylethanone, 2-hydroxyethyl 2-methyl-2-propenoate and 2-methoxyethyl 2-methyl-2-propenoate. *CAS-109550-08-5* (paflufocon D); *CAS-847923-13-1* (iberfilcon A). *Contact lens material (hybrid)*. Synergeyes (Synergeyes) *[Note—The water content of the component A (paflufocon D) is <1% at ambient temperature (23±2°C), and the oxygen permeability is 145 × 10⁻¹¹(cm²/sec)(ml O₂/ml × mm Hg) at 35°C (Dk value). The water content of the component B (iberfilcon A) is 27% at ambient temperature (23±2°C), and the oxygen permeability is 145 × 10⁻¹¹(cm²/sec)(ml O₂/ml × mm Hg) at 35°C (Dk value).*

Paflufocon E [*1998*] (pa″ floo foe′ kon). [The water content of the contact lens material is less than 0.1% at ambient temperature (23±2°C), and the oxygen permeability is 66.4 ± 2.2 × 10⁻¹¹ (cm²/sec)(ml O₂/ml × mm Hg) at 35°C (Dk value).] *Contact lens material (hydrophobic)*. PVS Basics (Paragon) *[Note—The chemical names, structural and molecular formula, manufacturer and CAS Registry Number are identical to Paflufocon A.]*

Pafuramidine Maleate [*2006*] (paf″ ue ram′ i deen mal′ ee ate). $C_{20}H_{20}N_4O_3 \cdot C_4H_4O_4$. 480.47. [Pafuramidine is INN.] (1) Benzenecarboximidamide, 4,4′-(2,5-furandiyl)bis[*N*-methoxy-, (2*Z*)]-2-butenedioate (1:1); (2) 4,4′-(Furan-2,5-diyl)bis(*N*-methoxybenzenecarboximidamide) (2*Z*)-2-butenedioate (1:1); (3) 2,5-Bis[4-(*N*-methoxyamidino)phenyl] furan monomaleate salt. *UNII-K27F04K3A9. CAS-837369-26-3; CAS-186953-56-0* [pafuramidine]. *Treatment of malaria, African sleeping sickness, and pneumocystis pneumonia.* ◇DB289

Pagibaximab [*2004*] (pag″ i bax′ i mab). $C_{6462}H_{9996}N_{1728}O_{2028}S_{54}$. (10 Immunoglobulin G1, anti-(*Staphylococcus epidermidis* lipoteichoic acid) (human-mouse monoclonal heavy chain), disulfide with human-mouse monoclonal κ-chain, dimer; (2) Immunoglobulin G1, anti-(*Staphylococcus epidermidis* lipoteichoic acid)

---

† Brand name formerly used, and/or firm no longer concerned with this product.

(human–mouse monoclonal HU96-110 heavy chain), disulfide with human–mouse monoclonal HU96-110 κ-chain, dimer. *CAS-595566-61-3.* INN. *Prevention of staphylococcal sepsis in premature neonates.* ◇*A110*

Pagoclone [*1995*] (pag′ oh klone). $C_{23}H_{22}ClN_3O_2$. 407.89. (1) 1*H*-Isoindol-1-one, 2-(7-chloro-1,8-naphthyridin-2-yl)-2,3-dihydro-3-(5-methyl-2-oxohexyl)-, (+)-; (2) (+)-2-(7-Chloro-1,8-naphthyridin-2-yl)-3-(5-methyl-2-oxohexyl)phthalimidine. *CAS-133737-32-3.* INN. *Anti-anxiety agent.* Bextra (Interneuron) ◇*IP 456; RP 62955*

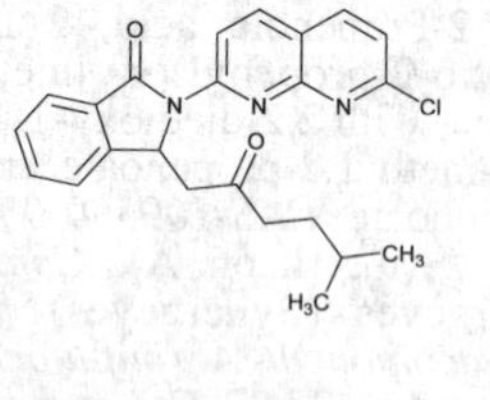

PAHA — *See* Aminohippuric Acid.

Palatrigine. $C_{12}H_{13}Cl_2N_5$. 298.17. 5-Amino-6-(2,3-dichlorophenyl)-2,3-dihydro-3-imino-2-isopropyl-*as*-triazine. *CAS-98410-36-7.* INN; BAN. ◇*BW A256C*

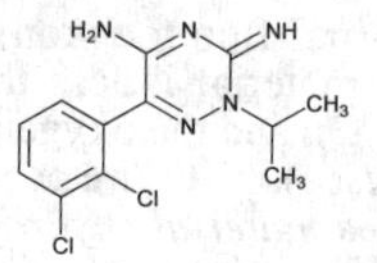

Paldimycin [*1987*] (pal″ di mye′ sin). Antibiotic produced by *Streptomyces* organism; a mixture of Paldimycin A and Paldimycin B, in approximately a 1:1 ratio. *CAS-102426-96-0.* INN. *Antibacterial.* ◇*U-70138*

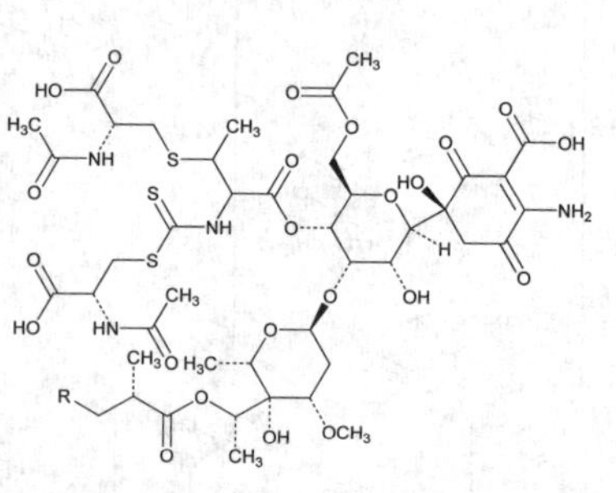

Paldimycin A   R = —CH₃
Paldimycin B   R = —H

Paldimycin A. $C_{44}H_{64}N_4O_{23}S_3$. 1113.19. (1) L-Cysteine, *N*-acetyl-, [2-[[2-(acetylamino)-2-carboxyethyl]thio]-1-carboxypropyl]carbamodithioate(ester), 4′-ester with 5-[6-*O*-acetyl-3-*O*-[2,6-dideoxy-3-*O*-methyl-4-*C*-[1-(2-methyl-1-oxobutoxy)ethyl]-α-L-*lyxo*-hexopyranosyl]-β-D-allopyranosyl]-2-amino-5-hydroxy-3,6-dioxo-1-cyclohexene-1-carboxylic acid; (2) 2-Amino-5-[3-*O*-[2,6-dideoxy-4-*C*-[(1*S*)-1-hydroxyethyl]-3-*O*-methyl-α-L-*lyxo*-hexopyranosyl]-β-D-allopyranosyl]-5-hydroxy-3,6-dioxo-1-cyclohexene-1-carboxylic acid, 4′-[3-[[(2*R*)-2-acetamido-2-carboxyethyl]thio]-2-[(dithiocarboxy)amino]butyrate], 6′-acetate, 4″-*C*-[(2*S*)-2-methylbutyrate], *S*-ester with *N*-acetyl-L-cysteine. *CAS-101411-70-5.*

Paldimycin B. $C_{43}H_{62}N_4O_{23}S_3$. 1099.16. (1) L-Cysteine, *N*-acetyl-, [2-[[2-(acetylamino)-2-carboxyethyl]thio]-1-carboxypropyl]carbamodithioate (ester), 4′-ester with 5-[6-*O*-acetyl-3-*O*-[2,6-dideoxy-3-*O*-methyl-4-*C*-[1-(2-methyl-1-oxopropoxy)ethyl]-α-L-*lyxo*-hexopyranosyl]-β-D-allopyranosyl]-2-amino-5-hydroxy-3,6-dioxo-1-cyclohexene-1-carboxylic acid; (2) 2-Amino-5-[3-*O*-[2,6-dideoxy-4-*C*-[(1*S*)-1-hydroxyethyl]-3-*O*-methyl-α-L-*lyxo*-hexopyra-

nosyl]-β-D-allopyranosyl]-5-hydroxy-3,6-dioxo-1-cyclohexene-1-carboxylic acid, 4′-[3-[[(2*R*)-2-acetamido-2-carboxyethyl]thio]-2-[(dithiocarboxy)amino]butyrate], 6′-acetate, 4″-*C*-isobutyrate, *S*-ester with *N*-acetyl-L-cysteine. *CAS-101411-71-6.*

Palestrol — *See* Diethylstilbestrol.

Palifermin [*2002*] (pal″ ee fer′ min). $C_{729}H_{1156}N_{204}O_{207}S_{10}$. 24-163 fibroblast growth factor 7 (human). Molecular weight is approximately 16,300 daltons. *UNII-QMS40680K6.* *CAS-162394-19-6.* INN. *Treatment of mucositis; KGF (keratinocyte growth factor).*

MSYDYMEGGD	IRVRRLFCRT	QWYLRIDKRG	KVKGTQEMKN	NYNIMEIRTV
AVGIVAIKGV	ESEFYLAMNK	EGKLYAKKEC	NEDCNFKELI	LENHYNTYAS
AKWTHNGGEM	FVALNQKGIP	VRGKKTKKEQ	KTAHFLPMAI	T

Palifosfamide [*2008*] (pal″ i fos′ fa mide). $C_4H_{11}Cl_2N_2O_2P$. 221.02. (1) Phosphorodiamidic acid, *N,N′*-bis(2-chloroethyl)-; (2) *N,N′*-Bis(2-chloroethyl)phosphorodiamidic acid. *CAS-31645-39-3.* INN. *Antineoplastic.* ◇*IPM; ZIO-201*

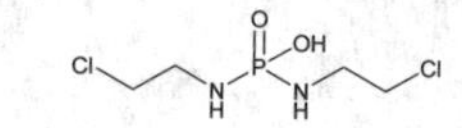

Palinavir [*1995*] (pa lin′ a vir). $C_{41}H_{52}N_6O_5$. 708.89. (1) 2-Quinolinecarboxamide, *N*-[1-[[[3-[2-[[(1,1-dimethylethyl)amino]carbonyl]-4-(4-pyridinylmethoxy)-1-piperidinyl]-2-hydroxy-1-(phenylmethyl)propyl]amino]carbonyl]-2-methylpropyl]-[2*S*-[1[1*R**(*R**),2*S**],2α,4α]]-; (2) *N*-[(1*S*)-1-[[(1*S*,2*R*)-1-Benzyl-3-[(2*S*,4*R*)-2-(*tert*-butylcarbamoyl)-4-(4-pyridylmethoxy)piperidino]-2-hydroxypropyl]carbamoyl]-2-methylpropyl]quinaldamide. *UNII-632S1WU9Z2.* *CAS-154612-39-2.* INN. *Antiviral.* ◇*BILA 2011 BS*

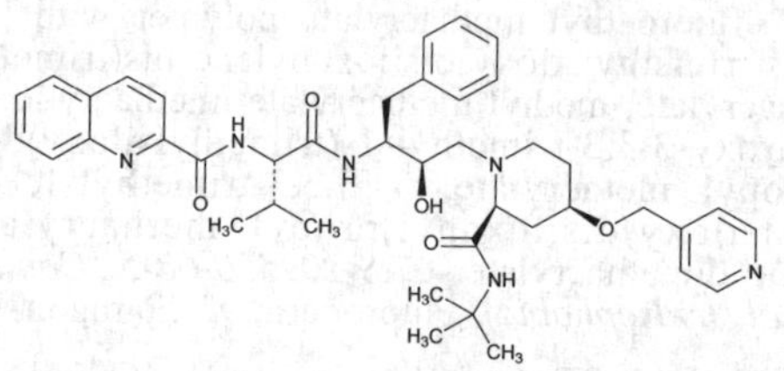

Palindore Fumarate (previously used name) — *See* Aplindore Fumarate.

Paliperidone [*2004*] (pal″ ee per′ i done). $C_{23}H_{27}FN_4O_3$. 426.48. (1) 4*H*-Pyrido[1,2-*a*]pyrimidin-4-one, 3-[2-[4-(6-fluoro-1,2-benzisoxazol-3-yl)-1-piperidinyl]ethyl]-6,7,8,9-tetrahydro-9-hydroxy-2-methyl-; (2) (9*RS*)-3-[2-[4-(6-Fluoro-1,2-benzisoxazol-3-yl)piperidin-1-yl]]ethyl]-9-hydroxy-2-methyl-6,7,8,9-tetrahydro-4*H*-pyrido[1,2-*a*]pyrimidin-4-one. *UNII-838F01T721.* *CAS-144598-75-4.* INN; JAN. *Treatment of schizophrenia.* Invega (Janssen) ◇*RO76477*

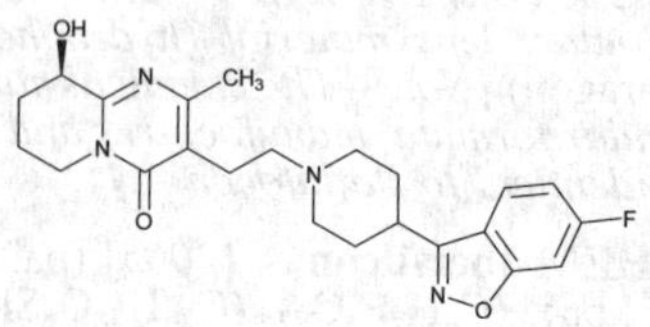

Paliperidone Palmitate [*2004*] (pal″ ee per′ i done pal′ mi tate). $C_{39}H_{57}FN_4O_4$. 664.89. (1) Hexadecanoic acid, 3-[2-[4-(6-fluoro-1,2-benzisoxazol-3-yl)-1-piperidinyl]ethyl]-6,7,8,9-tetrahydro-2-methyl-4-oxo-4*H*-pyrido[1,2-*a*]pyrimidin-9-yl ester; (2) (9*RS*)-3-[2-[4-(6-Fluoro-1,2-benzisox-azol-3-yl)piperidin-1-yl]ethyl]-2-methyl-4-oxo-6,7,8,9-tet-rahydro-4*H*-pyrido[1,2-*a*]pyrimidin-9-yl hexadecanoate. *CAS-199739-10-1. Treatment of schizophrenia.* ✧*RO92670*

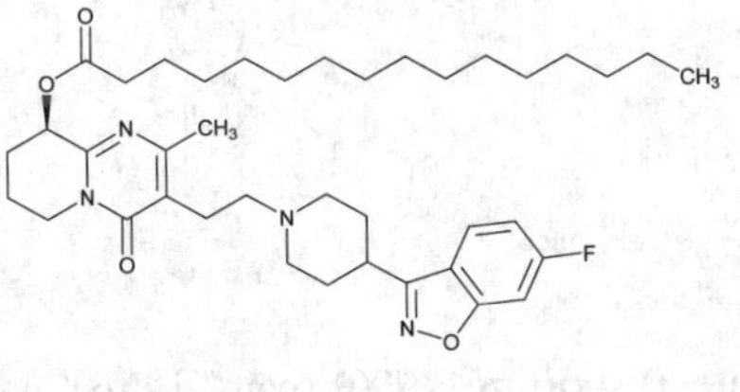

Paliroden. $C_{26}H_{24}F_3N$. 407.47. 1-[2-(Biphenyl-4-yl)ethyl]-4-[3-(trifluoromethyl)phenyl]-1,2,3,6-tetrahydropyridine. *UNII-17VJ76L90T. CAS-188396-77-2. INN.*

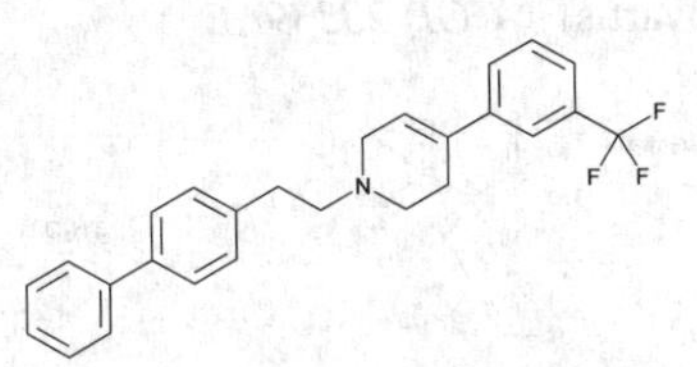

Palivizumab [*1997*] (pal″ i viz′ oo mab). Immunoglobulin G 1 (human-mouse monoclonal MEDI-493γ1-chain antire-spiratory syncytial virus protein F), disulfide with human-mouse monoclonal MEDI-493κ1-chain, dimer. *UNII-DQ448MW7KS. CAS-188039-54-5.* BAN; INN.

Palm Kernel Oil. **NF.** *Elaeis guineensis* seed oil. *CAS-8023-79-8.*

Palmidrol. $C_{18}H_{37}NO_2$. 299.49. *N*-(2-Hydroxyethyl)palmita-mide. *UNII-6R8T1UDM3V. CAS-544-31-0. INN; MI.*

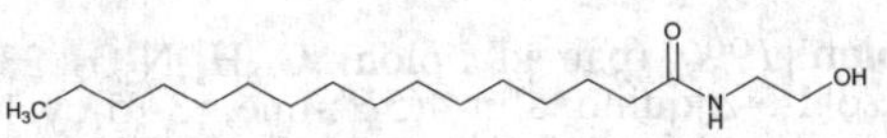

Palmitic Acid [*2000*] (pal mit′ ik as′ id). **NF.** $C_{16}H_{32}O_2$. 256.42. Hexadecanoic acid. *UNII-2V16EO95H1. CAS-57-10-3. Ingredient in a diagnostic aid (ultrasound contrast medium).[Note—The International Nomenclature Cosmetic Ingredient (INCI) name assigned to this substance by the Cosmetic, Toiletry, and Fragrance Association is palmitic acid.]*

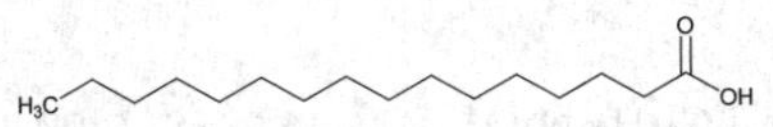

Palmoxirate Sodium [*1982*] (pal mox′ i rate soe′ dee um). $C_{17}H_{31}NaO_3.2H_2O$. 342.45. [Palmoxiric Acid is INN.] (1) Oxiranecarboxylic acid, 2-tetradecyl-, sodium salt, dihy-drate, (±)-; (2) Sodium (±)-2-tetradecylglycidate dihy-drate. *UNII-P5P95SB639; UNII-R326X4TRBY* [palmoxiric

acid]. *CAS-79069-97-9; CAS-68170-97-8* [palmoxiric acid]. *Antidiabetic.* ✧*McN-3802-21-98; McN-3802 [anhy-drous free acid]*

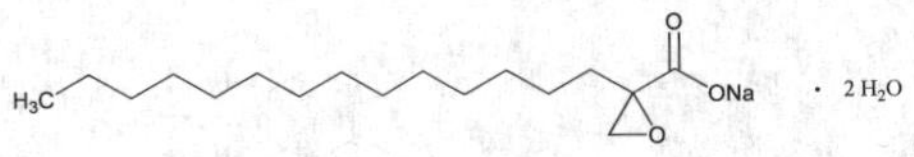

Palmoxiric Acid (INN) — *See* Palmoxirate Sodium.

Palonidipine. $C_{29}H_{34}FN_3O_6$. 539.60. (±)-3-(Benzylmethyla-mino)-2,2-dimethylpropyl methyl 4-(2-fluoro-5-nitrophe-nyl)-1,4-dihydro-2,6-dimethyl-3,5-pyridinedicarboxylate. *UNII-FMS4X67Q96. CAS-96515-73-0. INN.*

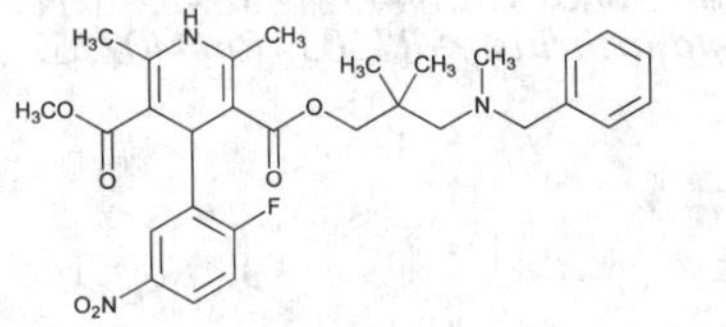

Palonosetron Hydrochloride [*1995*] (pal″ oh noe′ se tron hye″ droe klor′ ide). $C_{19}H_{24}N_2O.HCl$. 332.87. [Palonose-tron is INN.] (3a*S*)-2,3,3a,4,5,6-Hexahydro-2-[(3*S*)-3-qui-nuclidinyl]-1*H*-benz[*de*]isoquinolin-1-one monohy-drochloride. *UNII-23310D4I19; UNII-5D06587D6R* [palonosetron]. *CAS-135729-62-3; CAS-135729-56-5* [pa-lonosetron]. JAN. *Anti-emetic; antinauseant.* Aloxi (Hel-sinn) ✧*RS-25259-197*

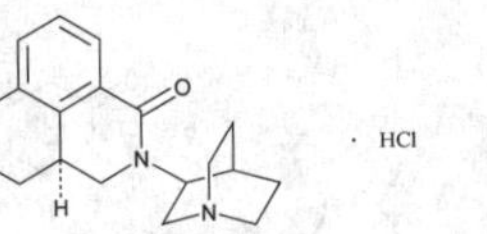

Palosuran. $C_{25}H_{30}N_4O_2$. 418.53. 1-[2-(4-Benzyl-4-hydroxypi-peridin-1-yl)ethyl]-3-(2-methylquinolin-4-yl)urea. *UNII-ULD9ZKE457. CAS-540769-28-6. INN.*

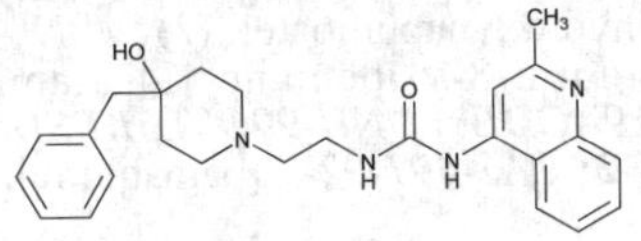

Palovarotene [*2008*] (pal″ oh var′ oh teen). $C_{27}H_{30}N_2O_2$. 414.54. (1) Benzoic acid, 4-[(1*E*)-2-[5,6,7,8-tetrahydro-5,5,8,8-tetramethyl-3-(1*H*-pyrazol-1-ylmethyl)-2-naphtha-lenyl]ethenyl]-; (2) 4-{(1*E*)-2-[5,5,8,8-Tetramethyl-3-(1*H*-pyrazol-1-ylmethyl)-5,6,7,8-tetrahydronaphthalen-2-yl]ethenyl}benzoic acid. *UNII-28K6I5M16G. CAS-410528-02-8. INN. Treatment of emphysema.* ✧*RO3300074*

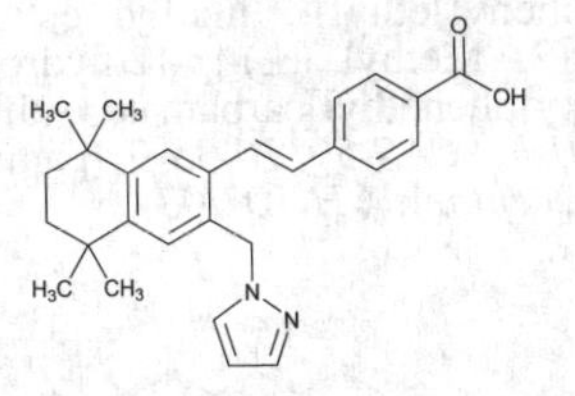

Pamabrom [*1988*] (pam′ a brom). **USP.** $C_{11}H_{18}BrN_5O_3$. 348.20. (1) 8-Bromo-3,7-dihydro-1,3-dimethyl-1*H*-purine-2,6-dione compound with 2-amino-2-methyl-1-propanol

---

(1:1); (2) 8-Bromotheophylline compound with 2-amino-2-methyl-1-propanol (1:1). *UNII-UA8U0KJM72. CAS-606-04-2.*

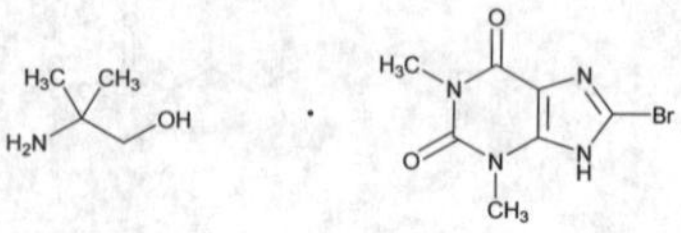

Pamapimod [*2007*] (pa map′ i mod). $C_{19}H_{20}F_2N_4O_4$. 406.38. (1) Pyrido[2,3-*d*]pyrimidin-7(8*H*)-one, 6-(2,4-difluorophenoxy)-2-[[3-hydroxy-1-(2-hydroxyethyl)propyl]amino]-8-methyl-; (2) 6-(2,4-Difluorophenoxy)-2-{[3-hydroxy-1-(2-hydroxyethyl)propyl]amino}-8-methylpyrido[2,3-*d*]pyrimidin-7(8*H*)-one. *CAS-449811-01-2.* INN. *Treatment of rheumatoid arthritis.* ◇*R1503; Ro 4402257*

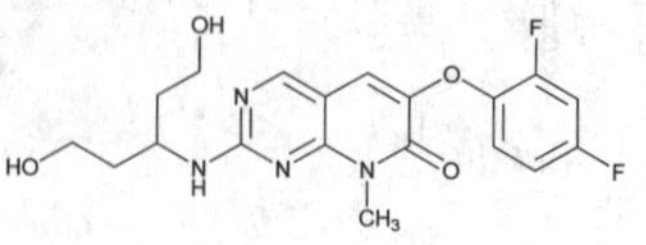

Pamaqueside [*1995*] (pam a′ kwe side). $C_{39}H_{62}O_{14}$. 754.90. (1) Spirostan-11-one, 3-[(4-*O*-β-D-glucopyranosyl-β-D-glucopyranosyl)oxy]-, (3β,5α,25*R*)-; (2) 11-Oxo-(25*R*)-5α-spirostan-3β-yl 4-*O*-β-D-glucopyranosyl-β-D-glucopyranoside. *CAS-150332-35-7.* INN. *Anti-atherosclerotic; hypocholesterolemic.* ◇*CP-148,623*

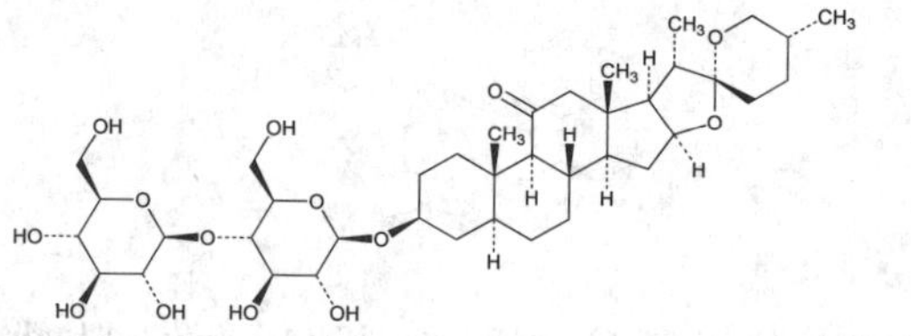

Pamaquine Naphthoate. $C_{42}H_{45}N_3O_7$. 703.82. (1) Quinoline, 6-methoxy-8-(1-methyl-4-diethylamino)butylamino, methylene-bis-β-hydroxynaphthoate; (2) N^1,N^1-Diethyl-N^4-(6-methoxyquinolin-8-yl)pentane-1,4-diamine pamoate. *UNII-96Y4A9AODB; UNII-99QVL5KPSU* [pamaquine]. *CAS-635-05-2; CAS-491-92-9* [pamaquine]. NF IX; MI.

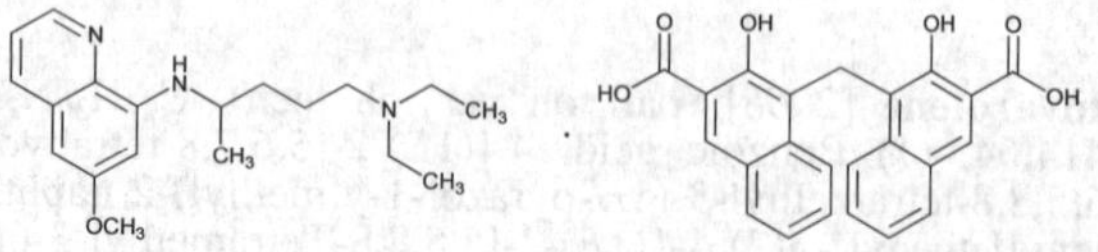

Pamatolol Sulfate [*1977*] (pam a′ toe lol sul′ fate). $(C_{16}H_{26}N_2O_4)_2{\cdot}H_2SO_4$. 718.86. [Pamatolol is INN.] (1) Carbamic acid, [2-[4-[2-hydroxy-3-[(1-methylethyl)amino]propoxy]phenyl]ethyl]-, methyl ester, (±)-, sulfate (salt) (2:1); (2) Methyl (±)-[*p*-[2-hydroxy-3-(isopropylamino)propoxy]phenethyl]carbamate sulfate (salt) (2:1). *CAS-59954-01-7; CAS-59110-35-9* [pamatolol]. *Anti-adrenergic (β-receptor).* ◇*H 104/08*

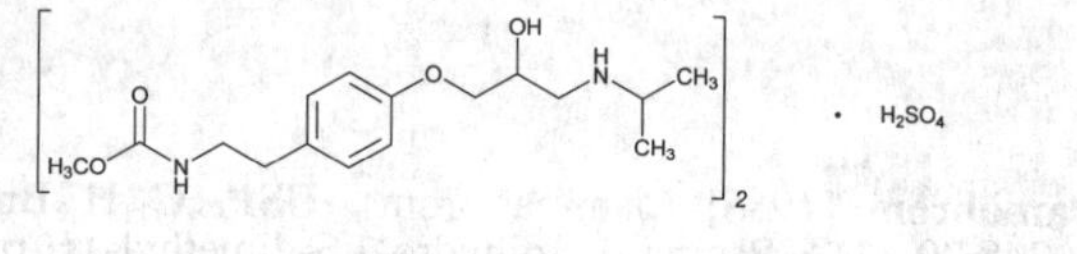

Pamicogrel. $C_{25}H_{24}N_2O_4S$. 448.53. Ethyl 2-[4,5-bis(*p*-methoxyphenyl)-2-thiazolyl]pyrrole-1-acetate. *UNII-398FD8EDAL. CAS-101001-34-7.* INN.

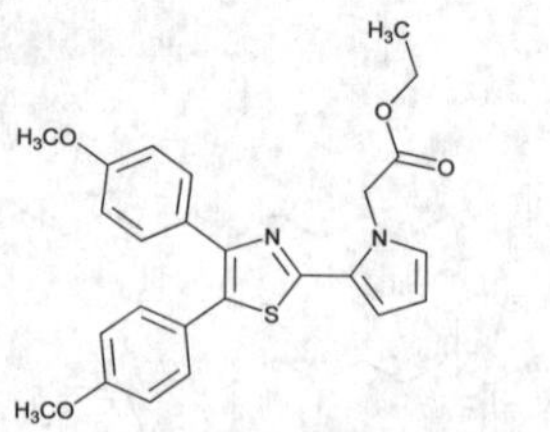

Pamidronate Disodium [*1990*] (pam″ i droe′ nate dye soe′ dee um). USP. $C_3H_9NNa_2O_7P_2{\cdot}5H_2O$. 369.11. (1) Phosphonic acid, (3-amino-1-hydroxypropylidene)bis-, disodium salt, pentahydrate; (2) Disodium dihydrogen (3-amino-1-hydroxypropylidene)diphosphonate, pentahydrate. *UNII-8742T8ZQZA. CAS-109552-15-0; CAS-57248-88-1* [anhydrous]. JAN. *Bone resorption inhibitor.* Aredia (Novartis) ◇*CGP 23339AE*

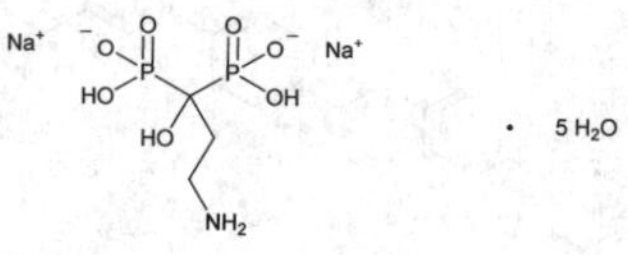

Pamidronic Acid. $C_3H_{11}NO_7P_2$. 235.07. (3-Amino-1-hydroxypropylidene)diphosphonic acid. *UNII-OYY3447OMC. CAS-40391-99-9.* INN; BAN; MI.

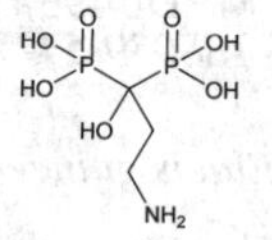

Pamiteplase. $C_{2172}H_{3309}N_{627}O_{658}S_{34}$. 49,822.59. 275-L-Glutamic acid-(1-91)-(174-527)-plasminogen activator (human tissue-type protein moiety). *CAS-151912-42-4.* INN.

Panadiplon [*1990*] (pan ad′ i plon). $C_{18}H_{17}N_5O_2$. 335.36. (1) Imidazo[1,5-*a*]quinoxalin-4(5*H*)-one, 3-(5-cyclopropyl-1,2,4-oxadiazol-3-yl)-5-(1-methylethyl)-; (2) 3-(5-Cyclopropyl-1,2,4-oxadiazol-3-yl)-5-isopropylimidazo[1,5-*a*]quinoxalin-4(5*H*)-one. *UNII-V4PW0S7ZP7. CAS-124423-84-3.* INN. *Anti-anxiety agent.* ◇*U-78875; FG-10571*

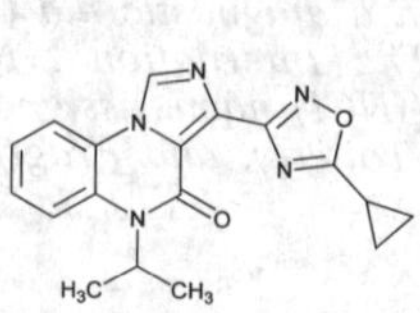

Panamesine. $C_{23}H_{26}N_2O_6$. 426.46. (5*S*)-5-[[4-Hydroxy-4-[3,4-(methylenedioxy)phenyl]piperidino]methyl]-3-(*p*-methoxyphenyl)-2-oxazolidinone. *UNII-023D9E916L. CAS-139225-22-2.* INN.

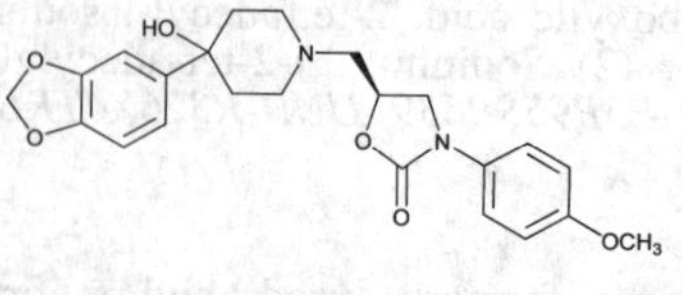

Pancopride [*1990*] (pan′ koe pride). $C_{18}H_{24}ClN_3O_2$. 349.86. (1) Benzamide, 4-amino-*N*-1-azabicyclo[2.2.2]oct-3-yl-5-chloro-2-(cyclopropylmethoxy)-, (±)-; (2) (±)-4-Amino-5-chloro-α-cyclopropyl-*N*-3-quinuclidinyl-*o*-anisamide. *CAS-121243-20-7* [nonstereospecific]; *CAS-121650-80-4* [±]. INN. *Anti-anxiety agent; anti-emetic; stimulant (peristaltic).* ◇*LAS 30451*

Pancreatin (pan′ kree a tin). **USP.** (1) Pancreatin; (2) Pancreatin. *CAS-8049-47-6.* BAN; JAN. *Enzyme (digestant adjunct).* Panteric (Parke-Davis†)

Pancrelipase [*1963*] (pan″ kree lye′ pase). **USP.** A concentrate of pancreatic enzymes standardized for lipase content. (1) Lipase, triacylglycerol; (2) Lipase of pancreas. *CAS-53608-75-6. Enzyme (digestant adjunct).* Accelerase (Organon†); Cotazym (Organon); Cotazym-S (Organon); Creon (Solvay Pharmaceuticals); Entolase (Robins†); Ilozyme (Savage); Ku-zyme HP (Schwarz Pharma); Pancrease (Ortho-McNeil); Viokase (Robins); Zymase (Organon)

Pancreozymin. A polypeptide hormone obtained from duodenal mucosa cholecystokinin. BAN.

Pancuronium Bromide [*1971*] (pan kure oh′ nee um broe′ mide). **USP.** $C_{35}H_{60}Br_2N_2O_4$. 732.67. (1) Piperidinium, 1,1′-[(2β,3α,5α,16β,17β)-3,17-bis(acetyloxy)androstane-2,16-diyl]bis[1-methyl]-, dibromide; (2) 1,1′-(3α,17β-Dihydroxy-5α-androstan-2β,16β-ylene)bis[1-methylpiperidinium] dibromide diacetate; (3) 2β,16β-Dipiperidino-5α-androstane-3α,17β-diol diacetate dimethobromide. *UNII-U9LY9Y75X2. CAS-15500-66-0.* INN; BAN; JAN. *Neuromuscular blocking agent.* Pavulon (Organon) ◇*Org NA 97*

Panidazole. $C_{11}H_{12}N_4O_2$. 232.24. 4-[2-(2-Methyl-5-nitroimidazol-1-yl)ethyl]pyridine. *UNII-08AHL2YV5K. CAS-13752-33-5.* INN; BAN.

Panipenem. $C_{15}H_{21}N_3O_4S$. 339.41. (+)-(5*R*,6*S*)-3-[[(*S*)-1-acetimidoyl-3-pyrrolidinyl]thio]-6-[(*R*)-1-hydroxyethyl]-7-oxo-1-azabicyclo[3.2.0]hept-2-ene-2-carboxylic acid. *UNII-W9769W09JF. CAS-87726-17-8.* INN; JAN.

Panitumumab [*2004*] (pan″ i toom′ ue mab). $C_{6398}H_{9878}N_{1694}O_{2016}S_{48}$. [Panitumumab (genetical recombination) is JAN.] (1) Immunoglobulin, anti-(human epidermal growth factor receptor) (human monoclonal ABX-EGF heavy chain), disulfide with human monoclonal ABX-EGF light chain, dimer; (2) Immunoglobulin, human (anti-human epidermal growth factor receptor) monoclonal antibody (ABX-EGF). Molecular weight is approximately 144,324 daltons. *UNII-6A901E312A. CAS-339177-26-3.* INN. *Antineoplastic.* ◇*ABX-EGF*

Panobinostat. $C_{21}H_{23}N_3O_2$. 349.43. (2*E*)-*N*-Hydroxy-3-[4-({[2-(2-methyl-1*H*-indol-3-yl)ethyl]amino}methyl)phenyl]prop-2-enamide. *CAS-404950-80-7.* INN.

Panomifene. $C_{25}H_{24}F_3NO_2$. 427.46. (*E*)-2-[[2-[*p*-(3,3,3-Trifluoro-1,2-diphenylpropenyl)phenoxy]ethyl]amino]ethanol. *UNII-GCW5E728OC. CAS-77599-17-8.* INN.

Pantenicate. $C_{62}H_{78}N_8O_{20}S_2$. 1319.45. [*R*-(*R**,*R**)]-3-Pyridylmethyl hydrogen succinate, tetraester with *N*,*N*′-[dithiobis(ethyleneiminocarbonylethylene)]bis[2,4-dihydroxy-3,3-dimethylbutyramide]. *CAS-96922-80-4.* INN.

Pantethine. $C_{22}H_{42}N_4O_8S_2$. 554.72. D-Bis(*N*-pantothenyl-2-aminoethyl)-disulfide. *CAS-16816-67-4.* JAN.

D-**Panthenol** — *See* Dexpanthenol.

(+)-**Panthenol** — *See* Dexpanthenol.

Panthenol [*1964*] (pan′ the nol). **USP.** $C_9H_{19}NO_4$. 205.25. (1) Butanamide, 2,4-dihydroxy-*N*-(3-hydroxypropyl)-3,3-dimethyl-, (±)-; (2) (±)-2,4-Dihydroxy-*N*-(3-hydroxypropyl)-3,3-dimethylbutyramide; (3) (±)-Pantothenyl alcohol. *CAS-16485-10-2.* INN; BAN; JAN. *Vitamin.*

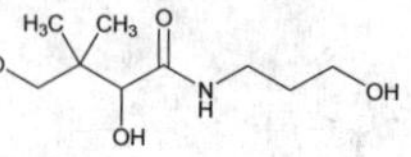

Pantoprazole [*1991*] (pan toe′ pra zole). $C_{16}H_{15}F_2N_3O_4S$. 383.37. (1) 1*H*-Benzimidazole, 5-(difluoromethoxy)-2-[[(3,4-dimethoxy-2-pyridinyl)methyl]sulfinyl]-; (2) 5-(Difluoromethoxy)-2-[[(3,4-dimethoxy-2-pyridyl)methyl]sulfinyl]benzimidazole. *UNII-D8TST4O562. CAS-102625-70-7.* INN; BAN. *Anti-ulcerative.* ◇SK&F 96022; BY 1023

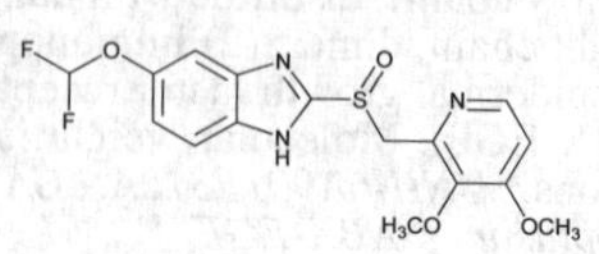

Pantoprazole Sodium [*1999*] (pan toe′ pra zole soe′ dee um). $C_{16}H_{14}F_2N_3NaO_4S.1.5H_2O$. 432.37. (1) 1*H*-Benzimidazole, 5-(difluoromethoxy)-2-[[(3,4-dimethoxy-2-pyridinyl)-methyl]sulfinyl]-, sodium salt, hydrate (2:3); (2) 5-(Difluoromethoxy)-2-[[(3,4-dimethoxy-2-pyridyl)methyl]-sulfinyl]benzimidazole, sodium salt, sesquihydrate. *UNII-6871619Q5X. CAS-164579-32-2. Treatment of various acid-related gastrointestinal diseases, including acute erosive esophagitis healing and maintenance, treatment of hypersecretory conditions, Zollinger-Ellison Syndrome (ZES), and eradication of Helicobacter pylori infection.* Protonix (Wyeth)

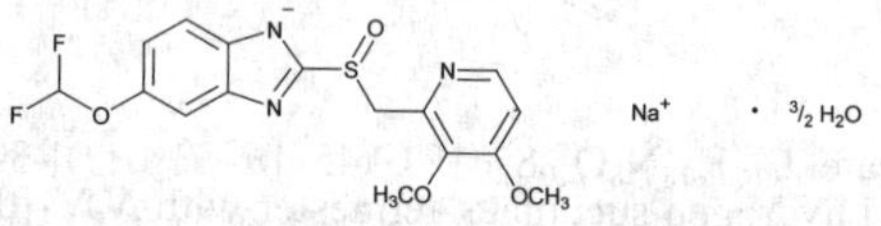

Pantothenic Acid (BAN) — *See* Calcium Pantothenate.

Pantothenol — *See* Dexpanthenol.

D-Pantothenyl Alcohol — *See* Dexpanthenol.

Panuramine. $C_{24}H_{25}N_3O_2$. 387.47. 1-Benzoyl-3-[1-(2-naphthylmethyl)-4-piperidyl]urea. *UNII-1UWS3T8EAB. CAS-80349-58-2.* INN; BAN.

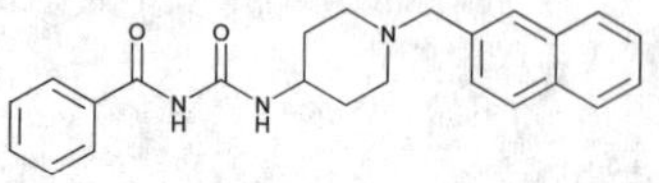

Papain (pa pay′ in). **USP.** (1) Papain; (2) Papain. *CAS-9001-73-4. Enzyme (proteolytic).* Caroid (Sterling Winthrop†)

Papaveretum. A mixture of 253 parts of morphine hydrochloride, 23 parts of papaverine hydrochloride and 20 parts of codeine hydrochloride. *CAS-8002-76-4.* BAN.

Papaverine Hydrochloride (pa pav′ er een hye″ droe klor′ ide). **USP.** $C_{20}H_{21}NO_4.HCl$. 375.85. [Papaverine is BAN.] (1) Isoquinoline, 1-[(3,4-dimethoxyphenyl)methyl]-6,7-dimethoxy-, hydrochloride; (2) 6,7-Dimethoxy-1-veratrylisoquinoline hydrochloride. *UNII-23473EC6BQ; UNII-*

DAA13NKG2Q [papaverine]. *CAS-61-25-6; CAS-58-74-2* [papaverine]. JAN. *Relaxant (smooth muscle).* Pavabid (Hoechst Marion Roussel)

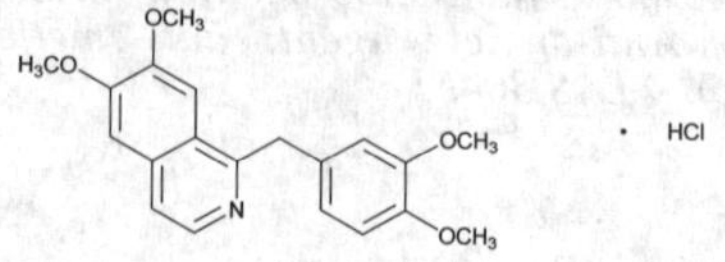

Papaveroline. $C_{16}H_{13}NO_4$. 283.28. 1-(3,4-Dihydroxybenzyl)-6,7-isoquinolinediol. *UNII-A0CR5J8X17. CAS-574-77-6.* INN; BAN.

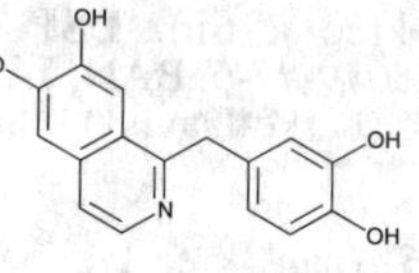

Paquinimod. $C_{21}H_{22}N_2O_3$. 350.41. *N*,5-Diethyl-4-hydroxy-1-methyl-2-oxo-*N*-phenyl-1,2-dihydroquinoline-3-carboxamide. *CAS-248282-01-1.* INN.

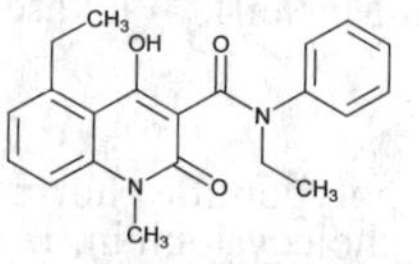

Para-Aminobenzoic Acid (previously used name) — *See* Aminobenzoic Acid.

Para-Aminohippurate Sodium [Injection] — *See* Aminohippurate Sodium.

Para-Aminohippuric Acid — *See* Aminohippuric Acid.

Para-Aminosalicylic Acid — *See* Aminosalicylic Acid.

Parabromdylamine Maleate — *See* Brompheniramine Maleate.

Paracetaldehyde — *See* Paraldehyde.

Paracetamol (INN, BAN, DCF) — *See* Acetaminophen.

Parachlorophenol (par″ a klor″ oh fee′ nol). **USP.** C_6H_5ClO. 128.56. (1) Phenol, 4-chloro-; (2) *p*-Chlorophenol. *CAS-106-48-9. Antibacterial (topical).*

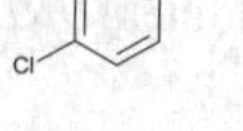

Paraffin (par′ a fin). **NF.** A purified mixture of solid hydrocarbons obtained from petroleum. *CAS-8002-74-2.* JAN. *Pharmaceutic aid (stiffening agent).*

Paraffin, Liquid (JAN) — *See* Mineral Oil.

Paraffin, Synthetic (par′ a fin). **NF.** Synthesized by the Fischer-Tropsch process from carbon monoxide and hydrogen, which are catalytically converted to a mixture of paraffin hydrocarbons. *Pharmaceutic aid (stiffening agent).*

Paraflutizide. $C_{14}H_{13}ClFN_3O_4S_2$. 405.85. 6-Chloro-3,4-dihydro-3-(*p*-fluorobenzyl)-2*H*-1,2,4-benzothiadiazine-7-sulfonamide 1,1-dioxide. *UNII-53A5V9FGN9. CAS-1580-83-2.* INN; DCF; MI. ◇*LD 3612*

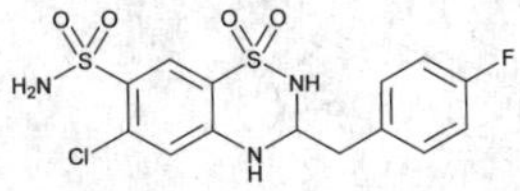

Paraformaldehyde. Poly(oxymethylene). *CAS-30525-89-4.* USP X; JAN; MI.

Parahydrecin (previously used name) — *See* Isomerol.

Paraldehyde (par al′ de hyde). **USP.** $C_6H_{12}O_3$. 132.16. (1) 1,3,5-Trioxane, 2,4,6-trimethyl-; (2) 2,4,6-Trimethyl-*s*-trioxane. *CAS-123-63-7. Sedative-hypnotic.* Paral (Forest)

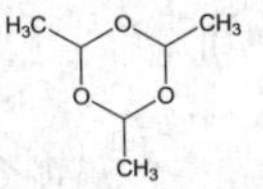

Paramethadione. $C_7H_{11}NO_3$. 157.17. (1) 2,4-Oxazolidinedione, 5-ethyl-3,5-dimethyl-; (2) 5-Ethyl-3,5-dimethyl-2,4-oxazolidinedione. *UNII-Z615FRW64N. CAS-115-67-3.* USP XXII; INN; BAN. Paradione (Abbott)

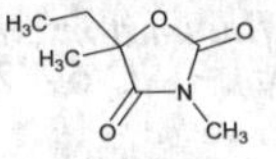

Paramethasone Acetate [*1962*] (par″ a meth′ a sone as′ e tate). **USP.** $C_{24}H_{31}FO_6$. 434.50. [Paramethasone is INN and BAN.] (1) Pregna-1,4-diene-3,20-dione, 21-(acetyloxy)-6-fluoro-11,17-dihydroxy-16-methyl-, (6α,11β,16α)-; (2) 6α-Fluoro-11β,17,21-trihydroxy-16α-methylpregna-1,4-diene-3,20-dione 21-acetate. *UNII-8X50N88ZDP; UNII-VFC6ZX3584* [paramethasone]. *CAS-1597-82-6; CAS-53-33-8* [paramethasone]. JAN. *Glucocorticoid.* Haldrone (Lilly)

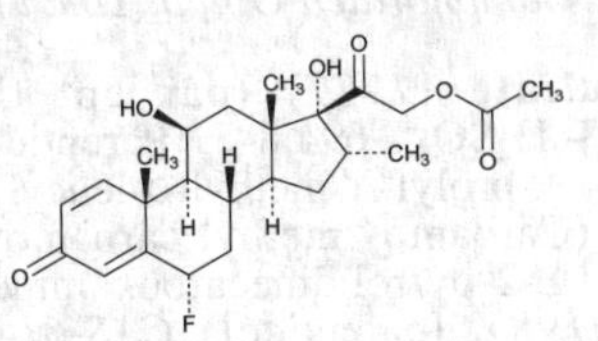

Para-Nitrosulfathiazole. $C_9H_7N_3O_4S_2$. 285.30. [Nitrosulfathiazole is INN.] *p*-Nitro-*N*-2-thiazolylbenzenesulfonamide. *CAS-473-42-7.* NF XI. Nisulfazole (Sterling Winthrop†)

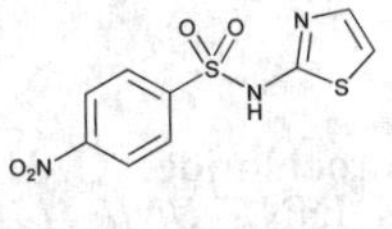

Paranyline Hydrochloride [*1962*] (par″ a nye′ leen hye″ droe klor′ ide). $C_{21}H_{16}N_2$.HCl. 332.83. [Renyfoline is INN.] (1) Benzenecarboximidamide, 4-(9*H*)-fluoren-9-ylidenemethyl)-, monohydrochloride; (2) α-Fluoren-9-ylidene-*p*-toluamidine monohydrochloride. *UNII-3QW5SNZ81H; UNII-O2ILF29K8B* [paranyline]. *CAS-5585-60-4; CAS-1729-61-9* [paranyline]. *Anti-inflammatory.*

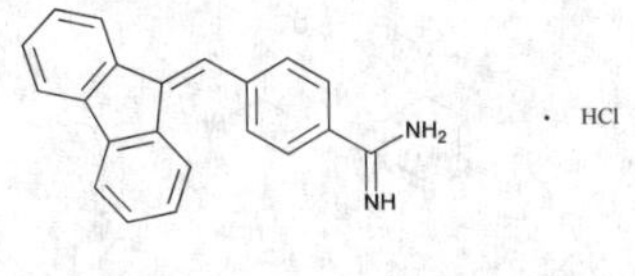

Parapenzolate Bromide [*1963*] (par″ a pen′ zoe late broe′ mide). $C_{21}H_{26}BrNO_3$. 420.34. (1) Piperidinium, 4-[(hydroxydiphenylacetyl)oxy]-1,1-dimethyl-, bromide; (2) 4-Hydroxy-1,1-dimethylpiperidinium bromide benzilate. *UNII-K2A047674O. CAS-5634-41-3.* INN. *Anticholinergic.* ◇*Sch 3444*

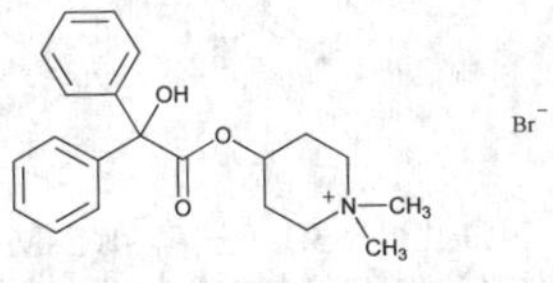

Parapropamol. $C_9H_{11}NO_2$. 165.19. 4′-Hydroxypropionanilid. *UNII-I729P6N0P7. CAS-1693-37-4.* INN; DCF.

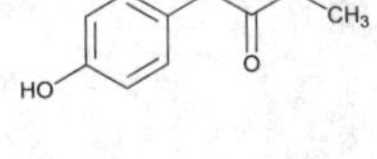

Pararosaniline Embonate (INN) — *See* Pararosaniline Pamoate.

Pararosaniline Pamoate [*1964*] (par″ a roe zan′ i lin pam′ oh ate). $[(C_{19}H_{18}N_3)_2.C_{23}H_{14}O_6].2H_2O$. 999.12. [Pararosaniline Embonate is INN.] (1) 2-Naphthalenecarboxylic acid, 4,4′-methylenebis[3-hydroxy-, compd. with 4-[(4-aminophenyl)(4-imino-2,5-cyclohexadien-1-ylidene)methyl]benzenamine (1:2) dihydrate; (2) α-(*p*-Aminophenyl)-α-(4-imino-2,5-cyclohexadien-1-ylidene)-*p*-toluidine 4,4′-methylenebis(3-hydroxy-2-naphthoate) (2:1) dihydrate. *CAS-7232-51-1; CAS-569-61-9* [pararosaniline]. *Antischistosomal.* ◇*CI 403A; CN-15,573-23A; PS-1286; NSC-107529*

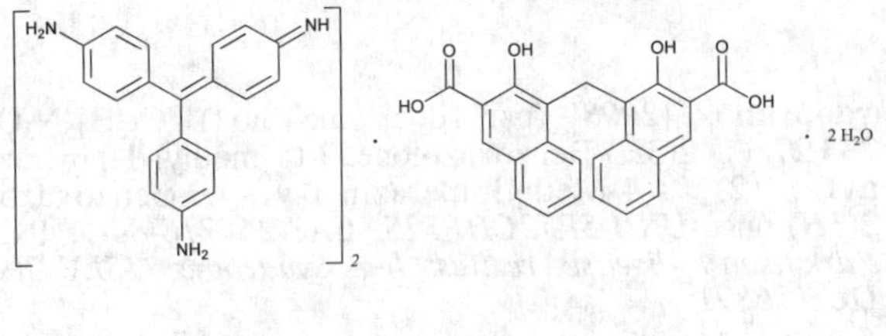

Parathiazine (INN) — *See* Pyrathiazine Hydrochloride.

Parathyroid Hormone [*2003*] (par″ a thye′ roid hor′ mone). $C_{408}H_{674}N_{126}O_{126}S_2$. Parathormone (human recombinant). Molecular weight is 9414 daltons. *CAS-68893-82-3* [human]; *CAS-345663-45-8* [human recombinant]; *CAS-9002-64-6* [parathyroid]. USP XXI; INN; BAN; MI. *Treatment of osteoporosis, as an antiosteoporotic, in the treatment of bone and mineral disease and disorders, bone metabolism regulator, blood calcium regulator, and as a diagnostic aid (pseudohypoparathyroidism; hypocalcemia).* Paroidin (Parke-Davis†) ◇*ALX1-11*

---

† Brand name formerly used, and/or firm no longer concerned with this product.

Paraxazone. $C_{10}H_{10}N_2O_3$. 206.20. 2,3-Dihydro-3-oxo-4*H*-1,4-benzoxazine-4-acetamide. *UNII-2H6ON8WA7L*. *CAS-26513-79-1*. INN.

Parbendazole [*1968*] (par ben′ da zole). $C_{13}H_{17}N_3O_2$. 247.29. (1) Carbamic acid, (5-butyl-1*H*-benzimidazol-2-yl)-, methyl ester; (2) Methyl 5-butyl-2-benzimidazolecarbamate. *CAS-14255-87-9*. INN; BAN. *Anthelmintic.* ◇*SK&F 29044*

Parcetasal. $C_{17}H_{15}NO_5$. 313.30. (±)-4′-[(2-Methyl-4-oxo-1,3-benzodioxan-2-yl)oxy]acetanilide. *UNII-3LSZ7869T2*. *CAS-87549-36-8*. INN.

Parconazole Hydrochloride [*1978*] (par kon′ a zole hye″ droe klor′ ide). $C_{17}H_{16}Cl_2N_2O_3{\cdot}HCl$. 403.69. [Parconazole is INN.] (1) 1*H*-Imidazole, 1-[[2-(2,4-dichlorophenyl)-4-[(2-propynyloxy)methyl]-1,3-dioxolan-2-yl]methyl]-, monohydrochloride, *cis*-; (2) *cis*-1-[[2-(2,4-Dichlorophenyl)-4-[(2-propynyloxy)methyl]-1,3-dioxolan-2-yl]methyl]imidazole monohydrochloride. *UNII-8IF7HES548*; *UNII-8Z2Z19C8Z1* [parconazole]. *CAS-62973-77-7*; *CAS-61400-59-7* [parconazole]. *Antifungal.* ◇*R 39,500*

Pardoprunox [*2008*] (par″ doe prue′ nox). $C_{12}H_{15}N_3O_2$. 233.27. (1) 2(3*H*)-Benzoxazolone, 7-(4-methyl-1-piperazinyl)-; (2) 7-(4-Methylpiperazin-1-yl)-1,3-benzoxazol-2(3*H*)-one. *UNII-5R72CHP32S*. *CAS-269718-84-5*. INN. *Parkinson's disease, restless legs syndrome.* ◇*SLV 308; DU 126891*

Pardoprunox Hydrochloride [*2008*] (par″ doe prue′ nox hye″ droe klor′ ide). $C_{12}H_{15}N_3O_2{\cdot}HCl$. 269.73. (1) 2(3*H*)-Benzoxazolone, 7-(4-methyl-1-piperazinyl)-, hydrochloride (1:1); (2) 7-(4-Methylpiperazin-1-yl)-1,3-benzoxazol-

2(3*H*)-one monohydrochloride. *UNII-U40903X6V8*. *CAS-269718-83-4*. *Parkinson's disease, restless legs syndrome.* ◇*SLV 308 hydrochloride; DU 126891 hydrochloride*

Parecoxib [*2000*] (par″ e kox′ ib). $C_{19}H_{18}N_2O_4S$. 370.42. (1) Propanamide, *N*-[[4-(5-methyl-3-phenyl-4-isoxazolyl)phenyl]sulfonyl]-; (2) *N*-[[*p*-(5-methyl-3-phenyl-4-isoxazolyl)phenyl]sulfonyl]propionamide. *UNII-9TUW81Y3CE*. *CAS-198470-84-7*. INN; BAN. *Anti-inflammatory; analgesic (cyclooxygenase [COX]-2 inhibitor).* ◇*SC-69124*

Parecoxib Sodium [*1998*] (par″ e kox′ ib soe′ dee um). $C_{19}H_{17}N_2NaO_4S$. 392.40. (1) *N*-[[4-(5-Methyl-3-phenyl-4-isoxazolyl)phenyl]sulfonyl]propanamide, sodium salt; (2) *N*-[[*p*-(5-Methyl-3-phenyl-4-isoxazolyl)phenyl]sulfonyl]-propanamide, sodium salt. *UNII-EB87433V6F*. *CAS-197502-82-2*. *Anti-inflammatory; analgesic (cyclooxygenase [COX]-2 inhibitor).* ◇*SC-69124A*

Paregoric (par″ e gor′ ik). **USP**. Consists of powdered opium, suitable essential oil(s), benzoic acid, diluted alcohol and glycerin. *CAS-8029-99-0*. *Antiperistaltic.* [*Name previously used: Camphorated Opium Tincture.*]

Pareptide Sulfate [*1977*] (par ep′ tide sul′ fate). $[C_{14}H_{26}N_4O_3]_2{\cdot}H_2SO_4$. 694.84. [Pareptide is INN.] (1) Glycinamide, L-prolyl-*N*-methyl-D-leucyl-, sulfate (2:1); (2) *N*-[D-1-[(Carbamoylmethyl)carbamoyl]-3-methylbutyl]-*N*-methyl-L-2-pyrrolidinecarboxamide sulfate (2:1). *UNII-4743XI19RY* [pareptide]. *CAS-61484-39-7*; *CAS-61484-38-6* [pareptide]. *Antiparkinsonian.* ◇*AY-24,856*

Parethoxycaine Hydrochloride. $C_{15}H_{23}NO_3{\cdot}HCl$. 301.81. [Parethoxycaine is INN.] *UNII-414P5USJ7F*. *CAS-136-46-9*; *CAS-94-23-5* [parethoxycaine]. MI. Intracaine Hydrochloride (Bristol-Myers Squibb†)

Pargeverine. $C_{21}H_{23}NO_3$. 337.41. 2-(Dimethylamino)ethyl diphenyl(2-propynyloxy)acetate. *UNII-UC61HM8FX0. CAS-13479-13-5.* INN.

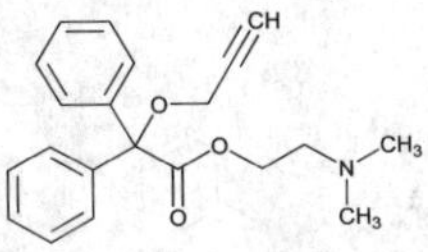

Pargolol. $C_{16}H_{23}NO_3$. 277.36. 1-(*tert*-Butylamino)-3-[*o*-(2-propynyloxy)phenoxy]-2-propanol. *UNII-5OPO851W5L. CAS-47082-97-3.* INN.

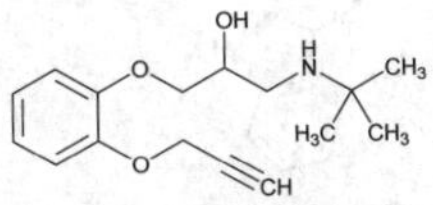

Pargyline Hydrochloride [*1962*] (par′ ji leen hye″ droe klor′ ide). $C_{11}H_{13}N \cdot HCl$. 195.69. [Pargyline is INN and BAN.] (1) Benzenemethanamine, *N*-methyl-*N*-2-propynyl-, hydrochloride; (2) *N*-Methyl-*N*-2-propynylbenzylamine hydrochloride. *UNII-W70V6I2OMY; UNII-9MV14S8G3E* [pargyline]. *CAS-306-07-0; CAS-555-57-7* [pargyline]. USP XXII. *Antihypertensive.* Eutonyl (Abbott) ◇*A-19120; MO-911; NSC-43798*

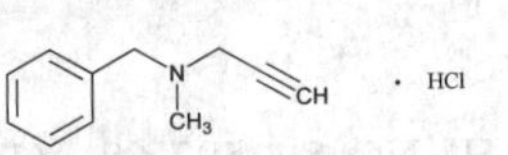

Paricalcitol [*1997*] (par″ i kal′ si tol). **USP.** $C_{27}H_{44}O_3$. 416.64. (1) 19-Nor-1-α,25-dihydroxyvitamin D_2; (2) (1α,3β,7E,22E)-19-Nor-9,10-secoergosta-5,7,22-triene-1,3,25-triol; (3) (7E,22E)-19-Nor-9,10-secoergosta-5,7,22-triene-1α,3β,25-triol. *UNII-6702D36OG5. CAS-131918-61-1.* INN. *Treatment of osteodystrophy (for the reduction of parathyroid hormone levels).* Zemplar (Abbott) ◇*Compound 49510*

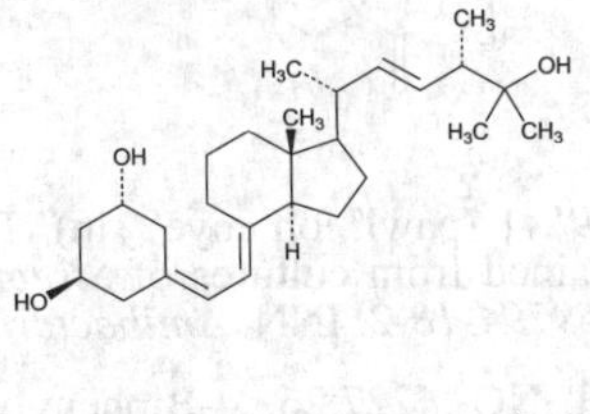

Paridocaine. $C_{17}H_{26}N_2O_2$. 290.40. 1-Methyl-4-piperidinol *p*-butylaminobenzoate. *UNII-795182TM5G. CAS-7162-37-0.* INN.

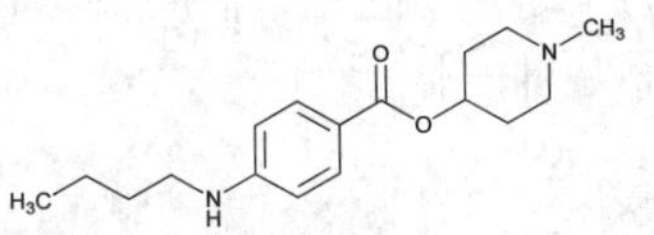

Parnaparin Sodium. Sodium salt of a low molecular mass heparin that is obtained by radical-catalyzed depolymerization, with hydrogen peroxide and with a cupric salt, of heparin from bovine or pork intestinal mucosa; the majority of the components have a 2-*O*-sulfo-α-L-idopyranosuronic acid structure at the non-reducing end and a 2-*N*,6-*O*-disulfo-D-glucosamine structure at the reducing end of their chain; the mass-average molecular mass ranges between 4000 and 6000 with a characteristic value of about 5000; the degree of sulfatation is 2.0 to 2.6 per disaccharidic unit. INN; BAN. ◇*OP 21-23*

Parodilol. $C_{23}H_{27}N_3O_2$. 377.48. (±)-1-[(2-Indol-3-yl-1,1-dimethylethyl)amino]-3-(indol-4-yloxy)-2-propanol. *UNII-0Q1O6G98Q8. CAS-103238-56-8.* INN.

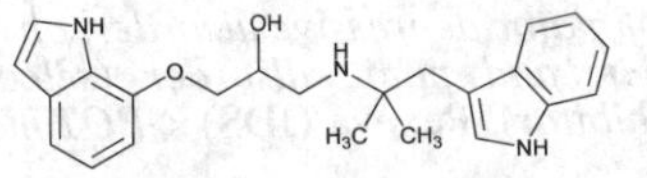

Parogrelil. $C_{19}H_{18}BrClN_4O_2$. 449.73. 4-Bromo-6-[3-(4-chlorophenyl)propoxy]-5-[(pyridin-3-ylmethyl)amino]pyridazin-3(2*H*)-one. *CAS-139145-27-0.* INN.

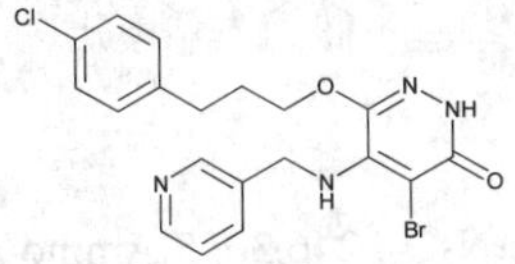

Paromomycin Sulfate (par oh″ moe mye′ sin sul′ fate). **USP.** $C_{23}H_{45}N_5O_{14} \cdot xH_2SO_4$. 615.63 (base). [Paromomycin is INN and BAN.] (1) D-Streptamine, *O*-2-amino-2-deoxy-α-D-glucopyranosyl-(1→4)-*O*-[*O*-2,6-diamino-2,6-dideoxy-β-L-idopyranosyl-(1→3)-β-D-ribofuranosyl-(1→5)]-2-deoxy-, sulfate (salt); (2) *O*-2,6-Diamino-2,6-dideoxy-β-L-idopyranosyl-(1→3)-*O*-β-D-ribofuranosyl-(1→5)-*O*-[2-amino-2-deoxy-α-D-glucopyranosyl-(1→4)]-2-deoxy-streptamine sulfate (salt). *UNII-845NU6GJPS; UNII-61JJC8N5ZK* [paromomycin]. *CAS-1263-89-4; CAS-7542-37-2* [paromomycin]; *CAS-59-04-1* [paromomycin, replaced]. JAN. *Anti-amebic.* Humatin (King)

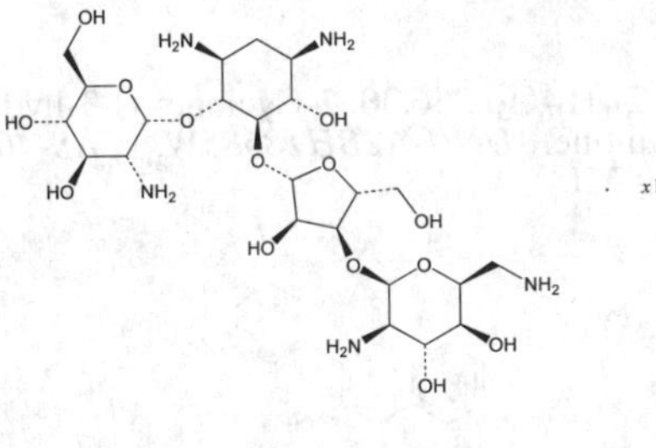

Paroxetine [*1989*] (par ox′ e teen). $C_{19}H_{20}FNO_3$. 329.37. (1) Piperidine, 3-[(1,3-benzodioxol-5-yloxy)methyl]-4-(4-fluorophenyl)-, (3*S-trans*)-; (2) (-)-(3*S*,4*R*)-4-(*p*-Fluorophenyl)-3-[(3,4-methylenedioxy)phenoxy]methyl]piperidine. *UNII-41VRH5220H. CAS-61869-08-7.* INN; BAN. *Antidepressant.* Paxil [as hydrochloride] (SmithKline Beecham) ◇*BRL 29060*

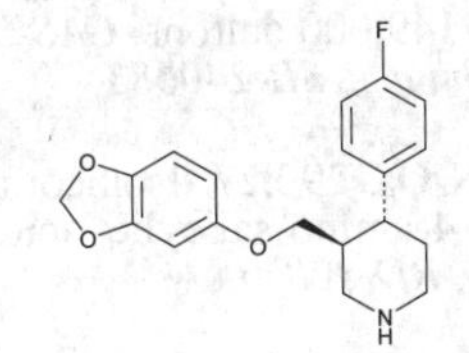

Paroxetine Hydrochloride (par ox′ e teen hye″ droe klor′ ide). **USP.** $C_{19}H_{20}FNO_3 \cdot HCl$. 365.83. (1) Piperidine, 3-[[(1,3-benzodioxol-5-yloxy)methyl]-4-(4-fluorophenyl)-, hydrochloride, (3*S-trans*)-; (2) (-)-(3*S*,4*R*)-4-(*p*-Fluorophe-

---

† Brand name formerly used, and/or firm no longer concerned with this product.

nyl)-3-[(3,4-methylenedioxy)phenoxy]-methyl]piperidine hydrochloride. *UNII-3I3T11UD2S. CAS-78246-49-8.* Paxil (GlaxoSmithKline)

Paroxetine Mesylate [*2003*] (par ox′ e teen mes′ i late). $C_{19}H_{20}FNO_3 \cdot CH_4O_4S$. 441.47. (1) Piperidine, 3-[(1,3-benzodioxol-5-yloxy)methyl]-4-(4-fluorophenyl)-, (3S,4R)-, methanesulfonate; (2) (-)-*trans*-4R-(4′-Fluorophenyl)-3S-[(3′,4′-methylenedioxyphenoxy)methyl]piperidine, mesylate. *UNII-M711N184JE. CAS-217797-14-3. Treatment of major depressive disorder, obsessive compulsive disorder, and panic disorder (selective serotonin reuptake inhibitor).* Pexeva (JDS) ◇*POT.mes*

Paroxypropione. $C_9H_{10}O_2$. 150.17. 4′-Hydroxypropiophenone. *CAS-70-70-2.* INN; DCF; MI. ◇*B-360; H 365; NSC-2834*

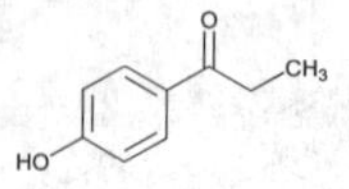

Parsalmide. $C_{14}H_{18}N_2O_2$. 246.30. 5-Amino-*N*-butyl-2-(2-propynyloxy)benzamide. *UNII-YQH5093J7C. CAS-30653-83-9.* INN; DCF; MI.

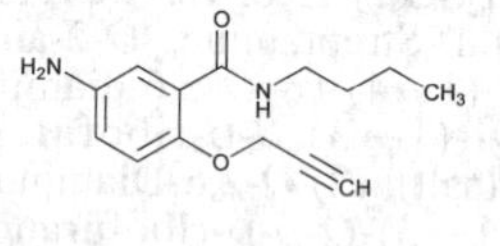

Partricin [*1971*] (par trye′ sin). A mixture in a constant ratio (about 1:1) of two polyene (heptaene) substances having very similar structures (not yet fully elucidated) and very similar biological properties. (1) Partricin; (2) Partricin. *CAS-11096-49-4.* INN. *Antifungal; antiprotozoal.* ◇*SPA-S-132*

Parvaquone. $C_{16}H_{16}O_3$. 256.30. 2-Cyclohexyl-3-hydroxy-1,4-naphthoquinone. *UNII-A2BH18685W. CAS-4042-30-2.* INN; BAN; MI.

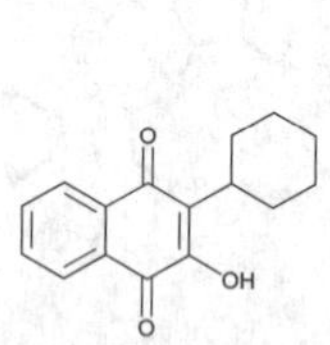

PAS — *See* Aminosalicylic Acid.

Pascolizumab [*2002*] (pas″ koe liz′ oo mab). Immunoglobulin G1, anti-(human interleukin 4) (human-mouse monoclonal SB-240683 γ1-chain), disulfide with human-mouse monoclonal SB-240683 κ-chain, dimer. Molecular weight is approximately 149,000 daltons. *CAS-331243-22-2.* INN. *Treatment of asthma.* ◇*SB-240683*

Pasiniazid. $C_{13}H_{14}N_4O_4$. 290.27. Isonicotinic acid hydrazide compound with 4-amino-salicylic acid. *CAS-2066-89-9.* INN; DCF; MI. ◇*RD 328*

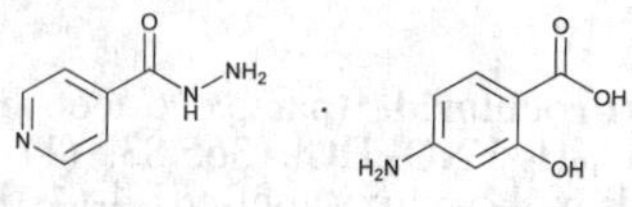

Pasireotide. $C_{58}H_{66}N_{10}O_9$. 1047.21. Cyclo[(4R)-4-(2-aminoethylcarbamoyloxy)-L-prolyl-L-phenylglycyl-D-tryptophyl-L-lysyl-4-*O*-benzyl-L-tyrosyl-L-phenylalanyl-]. *UNII-98H1T17066. CAS-396091-73-9.* INN.

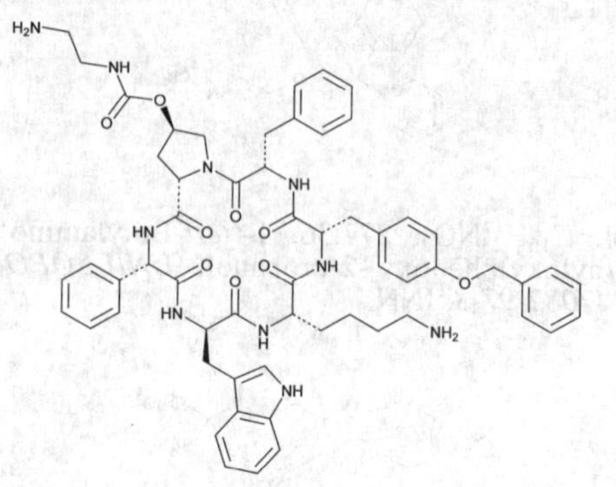

Patamostat. $C_{20}H_{20}N_4O_4S$. 412.46. *p*-[(2-Succinimidoethyl)thio]phenyl *p*-guanidinobenzoate. *UNII-2T7W4EA51W. CAS-114568-26-2.* INN.

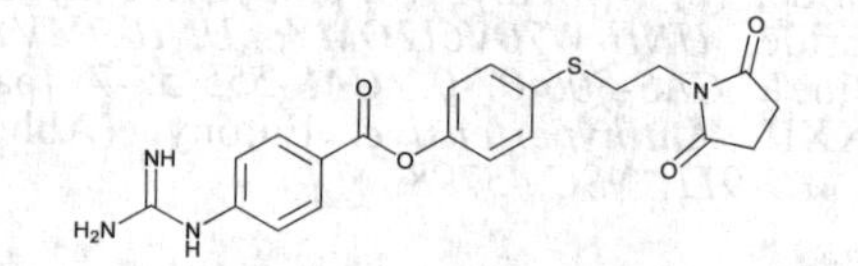

Patupilone. $C_{27}H_{41}NO_6S$. 507.68. (1S,3S,7S,10R,11S,12S,16R)-7,11-Dihydroxy-8,8,10,12,16-pentamethyl-3-[(1E)-1-(2-methyl-1,3-thiazol-4-yl)prop-1-en-2-yl]-4,17-dioxabicyclo[14.1.0]heptadecane-5,9-dione. *CAS-152044-54-7.* INN.

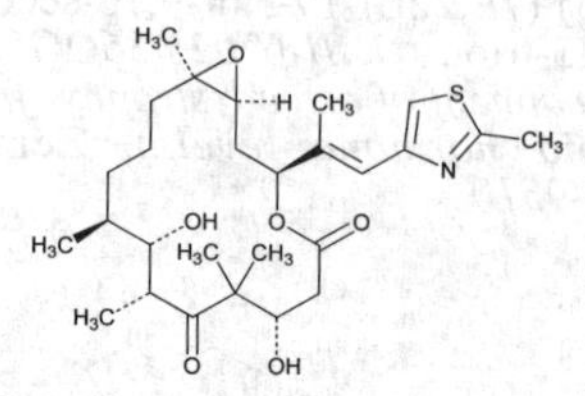

Paulomycin [*1984*] (pawl″ oh mye′ sin). Paulomycin. An antibiotic obtained from cultures of *Streptomyces paulus, variant.CAS-59794-18-2.* INN. *Antibacterial.* ◇*U-43,120*

Paxamate. $C_{14}H_{13}NO_2$. 227.26. 4-Biphenylyl methylcarbamate. *UNII-27P0WQO4ZB. CAS-5579-05-5.* INN.

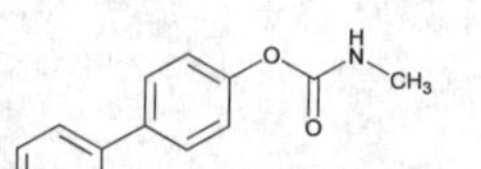

Pazelliptine. $C_{22}H_{27}N_5$. 361.48. 10-[[3-(Diethylamino)propyl]amino]-6-methyl-5*H*-pyrido[3′,4′:4,5]pyrrolo[2,3-*g*]isoquinoline. *UNII-2CSP4U82HK. CAS-65222-35-7.* INN.

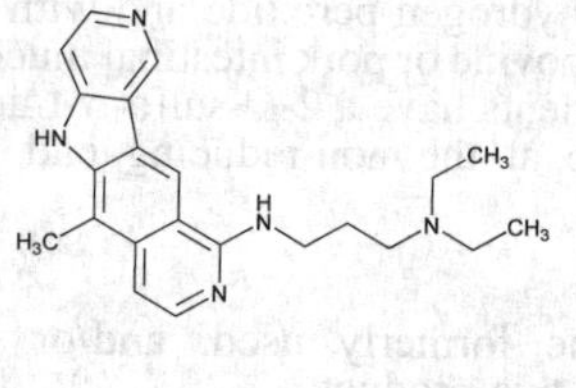

Pazinaclone [*1994*] (pa zin′ a klone). $C_{25}H_{23}ClN_4O_4$. 478.93. (1) 1,4-Dioxa-8-azaspiro[4.5]decane, 8-[[2-(7-chloro-1,8-naphthyridin-2-yl)-2,3-dihydro-3-oxo-1*H*-isoindol-1-yl]-acetyl]-, (±)-; (2) (±)-8-[[2-(7-Chloro-1,8-naphthyridin-2-yl)-3-oxo-1-isoindolinyl]acetyl]-1,4-dioxa-8-azaspiro-[4.5]decane; (3) (±)-2-(7-Chloro-1,8-naphthyridin-2-yl)-3-[[(1,4-dioxa-8-azaspiro[4.5]dec-8-yl)carbonyl]methyl]-1-isoindolinone. *CAS-103255-66-9*. INN. *Anti-anxiety agent.* *✧A-77000; DN-2327*

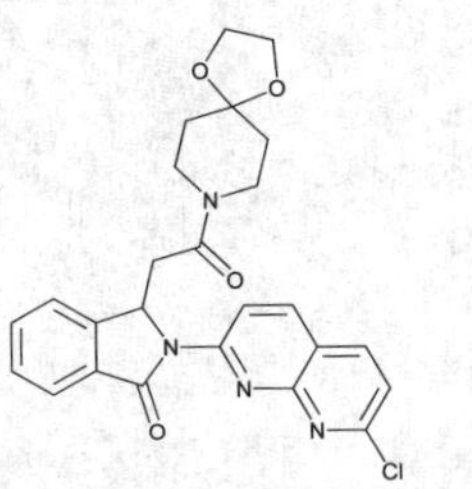

Pazopanib Hydrochloride [*2005*] (paz oh′ pa nib hye″ droe klor′ ide). $C_{21}H_{23}N_7O_2S.HCl$. 473.98. [Pazopanib is INN.] (1) Benzenesulfonamide, 5-[[4-[(2,3-dimethyl-2*H*-indazol-6-yl)methylamino]-2-pyrimidinyl]amino]-2-methyl-, monohydrochloride; (2) 5-[[4-[(2,3-Dimethyl-2*H*-indazol-6-yl)methylamino]pyrimidin-2-yl]amino]-2-methylbenzenesulfonamide monohydrochloride. *UNII-33Y9ANM545; UNII-7RN5DR86CK* [pazopanib]. *CAS-635702-64-6; CAS-444731-52-6* [pazopanib]. *Antineoplastic agent, a potent and selective inhibitor of VEGFR-1, -2 and -3 tyrosine kinases, blocking angiogenesis.* *✧GW786034B*

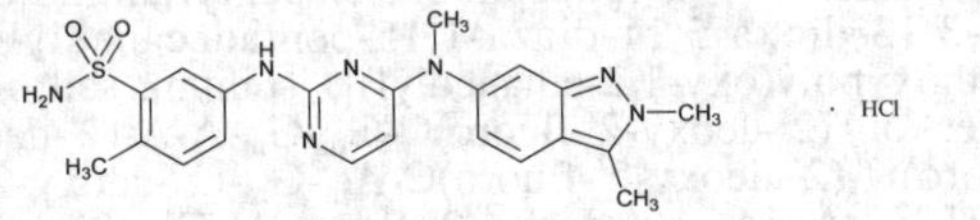

Pazoxide [*1974*] (pa zox′ ide). $C_{12}H_{10}Cl_2N_2O_2S$. 317.19. (1) 2*H*-1,2,4-Benzothiadiazine, 6,7-dichloro-3-(3-cyclopenten-1-yl)-, 1,1-dioxide; (2) 6,7-Dichloro-3-(3-cyclopenten-1-yl)-2*H*-1,2,4-benzothiadiazine 1,1-dioxide. *UNII-QZE8T5D680*. *CAS-21132-59-2*. INN. *Antihypertensive.* *✧Sch 12149*

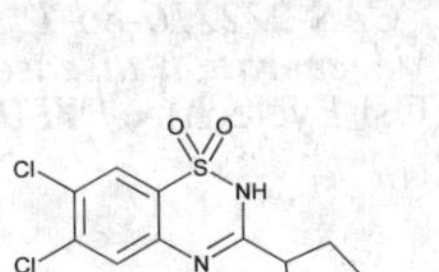

Pazufloxacin. $C_{16}H_{15}FN_2O_4$. 318.30. (-)-(3*S*)-10-(1-Aminocyclopropyl)-9-fluoro-2,3-dihydro-3-methyl-7-oxo-7*H*-pyrido[1,2,3-*de*]-1,4-benzoxazine-6-carboxylic acid. *UNII-4CZ1R38NDI*. *CAS-127045-41-4*. INN.

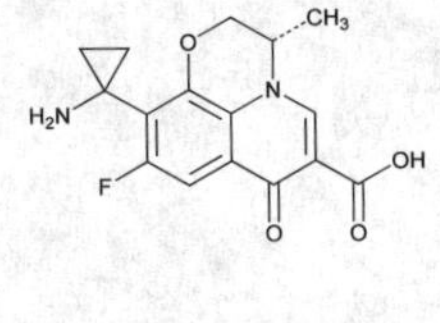

PCP — *See* Phencyclidine Hydrochloride.

† Brand name formerly used, and/or firm no longer concerned with this product.

Peanut Oil (pee′ nut). **NF**. The fully-refined oil obtained from the seed kernels of one or more of the cultivated varieties of *Arachis hypogaea* Linné (Fam. Leguminosae). *UNII-5TL50QU0W4*. *CAS-8002-03-7*. JAN. *Pharmaceutic aid (solvent).*

Pecazine (INN, BAN) — *See* Mepazine Acetate.

Pecilocin. $C_{17}H_{25}NO_3$. 291.39. [Variotin is JAN.] 2-Pyrrolidinone, 1-(8-hydroxy-6-methyl-2,4,6-dodecatrienoyl)-, (*E,E,E*)-(*R*)-. *UNII-TSA7W27MF8*. *CAS-19504-77-9*. INN; BAN; MI.

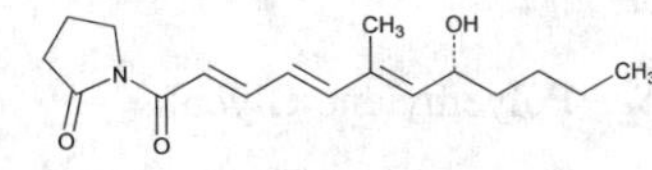

Pecocycline. $C_{29}H_{35}N_3O_{10}$. 585.60. *N*-[[4-(Dimethylamino)-1,4,4a,5,5a,6,11,12a-octahydro-3,6,10,12,12a-pentahydroxy-6-methyl-1,11-dioxo-2-naphthacene carboxamido]-methyl]nipecotic acid. *UNII-0CG6O25ZC4*. *CAS-15301-82-3*. INN.

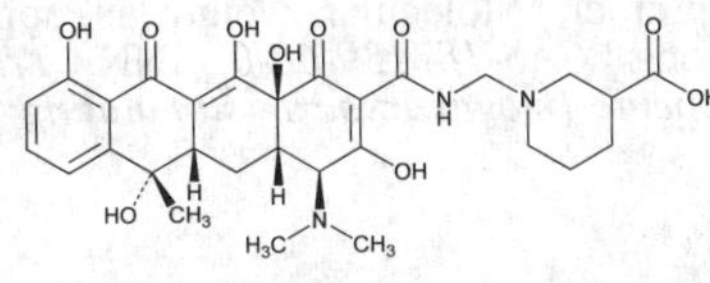

Pectin (pek′ tin). **USP**. (1) Pectin; (2) Pectin. *CAS-9000-69-5*. *Pharmaceutic aid (suspending agent); protectant.*

Pefloxacin [*1981*] (pe flox′ a sin). $C_{17}H_{20}FN_3O_3$. 333.36. (1) 3-Quinolinecarboxylic acid, 1-ethyl-6-fluoro-1,4-dihydro-7-(4-methyl-1-piperazinyl)-4-oxo; (2) 1-Ethyl-6-fluoro-1,4-dihydro-7-(4-methyl-1-piperazinyl)-4-oxo-3-quinolinecarboxylic acid. *UNII-2H52Z9F2Q5*. *CAS-70458-92-3*. INN; BAN. *Antibacterial.* *✧EU-5306; 1589 RB*

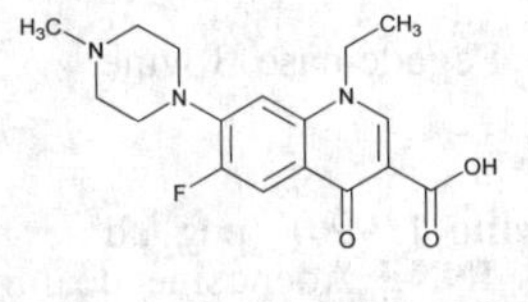

Pefloxacin Mesylate [*1987*] (pe flox′ a sin mes′ i late). $C_{17}H_{20}FN_3O_3.CH_4O_3S$. 429.46. (1) 3-Quinolinecarboxylic acid, 1-ethyl-6-fluoro-1,4-dihydro-7-(4-methyl-1-piperazinyl)-4-oxo-, monomethanesulfonate; (2) 1-Ethyl-6-fluoro-1,4-dihydro-7-(4-methyl-1-piperazinyl)-4-oxo-3-quinolinecarboxylic acid, monomethanesulfonate. *UNII-5IA-D0UV3FH*. *CAS-70458-95-6*. *Antibacterial.* *✧41 982 RP*

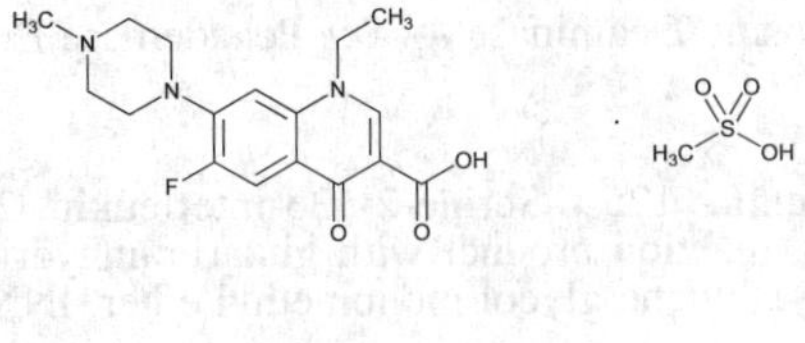

Peforelin. $C_{59}H_{74}N_{18}O_{14}$. 1259.33. 5-Oxo-L-prolyl-L-histidyl-L-tryptophyl-L-seryl-L-histidyl-L-α-asparagyl-L-tryptophyl-L-lysyl-L-prolylglycinamide. *CAS-147859-97-0.* INN.

HWSHDWLPG—NH₂

PEG (PEN) — *See* Polyethylene Glycol.

Pegacaristim [*1998*] (peg″ a kar′ i stim). CH_3-$(OCH_2CH_2)_n$ $OCH_2CH_2CH_2$-$C_{781}H_{1288}N_{220}O_{220}S_7$. (1) *N*-(3-Hydroxypropyl)-1-163-thrombopoietin (human), monoether with α-methyl-ω-hydroxypoly(oxy-1,2-ethanediyl); (2) *N*-(3-Hydroxypropyl)-1-163-megakaryocyte growth and development factor (human), monoether with polyethylene glycol monomethyl ether. Molecular weight is approximately 37,505 daltons. *CAS-187139-68-0.* INN. *Treatment of thrombocytopenia (megakaryocyte stimulating factor).*

```
*SPAPPACDLR   VLSKLLRDSH   VLHSKLSQCP   EVHPLPTPVL   LPAVDFSLGE
WKTQMEETKA   QDILGAVTLL   LEGVMAARGQ   LGPTCLSSLL   GQLSEQVRLL
LGALQSLLGT   QLPPQGRTTA   HKDPNAIFLS   FQHLLRGKVR   FLMLVGGSTL
CVRRAPPTTA   VPS
```

* pegylation site

H₃C—[O—]ₙ—O——pegacaristim

PEG-ADA — *See* Pegademase Bovine.

Pegademase Bovine [*1990*] (peg ad′ e mase boe′ vine). [Pegademase is INN.] Adenosine deaminase is obtained from calf intestine. (1) Deaminase, adenosine, cattle, reaction product with succinic anhydride, esters with polyethylene glycol mono-Me ether; (2) Adenosine deaminase, cattle, reaction product with succinic anhydride, esters with polyethylene glycol monomethyl ether. *UNII-HW3H7D91F6.* *Replacement therapy (adenosine deaminase deficiency).* Adagen (Enzon)

PEG-Adenosine Deaminase — *See* Pegademase Bovine.

Pegaldesleukin. 125-L-Serine-2-133-interleukin 2 (human reduced), reaction product with glutaric anhydride, esters with polyethylene glycol monomethyl ether. INN.

Pegamotecan [*2004*] (peg am″ oh tee′ kan). $C_{50}H_{44}N_6O_{13}$ $[C_2H_4O]_n$. (1) L-Alanine, (4*S*)-4-ethyl-3,4,12,14-tetrahydro-3,14-dioxo-1H-pyrano[3′,4′:6,7]indolizino [1,2-b]quinolin-4-yl ester, mono(trifluoroacetate), reaction products with polyethylene glycol bis (carboxymethyl) ether; (2) Derivative of camptothecin and polyethylene glycol produced by amide formation between [(4*S*)-4-ethyl-3,14-dioxo-3,4,12,14-tetrahydro-1*H*-pyrano[3′,4′:6,7]indolizino[1,2-*b*]quinolin-4-yl] (2*S*)-2-aminopropanoate (camptothecin L-alaninate) and α-(carboxymethyl)-ω-

(carboxymethoxy)poly(oxyethylene). *CAS-581079-18-7.* INN. *Treatment of gastric and gastroesophageal junction adenocarcinoma.* Prothecan (Enzon) ◇*EZ-246*

Pegaptanib Sodium [*2002*] (peg ap′ ta nib soe′ dee um). $C_{294}H_{342}F_{13}N_{107}Na_{28}O_{188}P_{28}[C_2H_4O]_n$. [Pegaptanib is INN and BAN.] (1) RNA, ((2′-Deoxy-2′-fluoro)C-G$_m$-G$_m$-A-A-(2′-deoxy-2′-fluoro)U-(2′-deoxy-2′-fluoro)C-A$_m$-G$_m$-(2′-deoxy-2′-fluoro)U-G$_m$-A$_m$-A$_m$-(2′-deoxy-2′-fluoro)U-G$_m$-(2′-deoxy-2′-fluoro)C-(2′-deoxy-2′-fluoro)U-(2′-deoxy-2′-fluoro)U-A$_m$-(2′-deoxy-2′-fluoro)U-A$_m$-(2′-deoxy-2′-fluoro)C-A$_m$-(2′-deoxy-2′-fluoro)U-(2′-deoxy-2′-fluoro)C-(2′-deoxy-2′-fluoro)C-G$_m$-(3→3′)-dT), 5′-ester with α,α'-[4,12-dioxo-6-[[[5-(phosphoonoxy)pentyl]amino]carbonyl]-3,13-dioxa-5,11-diaza-1,15-pentadecanediyl]bis[ω-methoxypoly(oxy-1,2-ethanediyl)], sodium salt; (2) 5′-Ester of (2′-deoxy-2′-fluoro)C-G$_m$-G$_m$-A-A-(2′-deoxy-2′-fluoro)U-(2′-deoxy-2′-fluoro)C-A$_m$-G$_m$-(2′-deoxy-2′-fluoro)U-G$_m$-A$_m$-A$_m$-(2′-deoxy-2′-fluoro)U-G$_m$-(2′-deoxy-2′-fluoro)C-(2′-deoxy-2′-fluoro)U-(2′-deoxy-2′-fluoro)U-A$_m$-(2′-deoxy-2′-fluoro)U-A$_m$-(2′-deoxy-2′-fluoro)C-A$_m$-(2′-deoxy-2′-fluoro)U-(2′-deoxy-2′-fluoro)C-(2′-deoxy-2′-fluoro)C-G$_m$-(3′→3′)-dT with α,α'-[[(1*S*)-1-[[5-(phosphonooxy)pentyl]carbamoyl]pentane-1,5-diyl]bis(iminocarbonyl)]bis[ω-methoxypoly(oxyethane-1,2-diyl)] sodium salt. Molecular weight is approximately 50,000 daltons. *CAS-222716-86-1.* *Treatment of age-related macular degeneration disease (anti-VEGF apatamer).* Macugen (Osi Eyetech) ◇*EYE001; NX1838*

C$_f$G$_m$G$_m$AAU$_f$C$_f$A$_m$G$_m$U$_f$G$_m$A$_m$A$_m$U$_f$G$_m$C$_f$U$_f$U$_f$A$_m$U$_f$A$_{ra}$C$_f$A$_m$U$_f$C$_f$C$_f$G$_m$T

A	- adenosine
A$_m$	- 2′-O-methyladenosine
C$_f$	- 2′-deoxy-2′-fluorocytidine
G$_m$	- 2′-O-methylguanosine
U$_f$	- 2′-deoxy-2′-fluorouracil
T	- thymidine

Pegaspargase [*1990*] (peg as′ par jase). (1) Pegaspargase; (2) Asparaginase, reaction product with succinic anhydride, esters with polyethylene glycol, monomethyl ether; (3) (Monomethoxypolyethylene glycol succinimidyl)$_{74}$-L-asparaginase. *UNII-7D96IR0PPM.* *CAS-130167-69-0.* INN. *Antineoplastic.* Oncaspar (Enzon)

Pegfilgrastim. $C_{849}H_{1347}N_{223}O_{244}S_9 \cdot (C_2H_4O)_n$. *N*-(3-Hydroxypropyl)methionylcolony-stimulating factor (human), 1-ether with α-methyl-ω-hydroxypoly(oxyethylene). *UNII-3A58010674. CAS-208265-92-3.* INN; BAN.

TPLGPASSLP	QSFLLKCLEQ	VRKIQGDGAA	LQEKLCATYK
LCHPEELVLL	GHSLGIPWAP	LSSCPSQALQ	LAGCLSQLHS
GLFLYQGLLQ	ALEGISPELG	PTLDTLQLDV	ADFATTIWQQ
MEELGMAPAL	QPTQGAMPAF	ASAFQRRAGG	VLVASHLQSF
LEVSYRVLRH	LAQP		

Peginterferon Alfa-2a [*2003*] (peg in″ ter feer′ on al′ fa). (1) Interferon αA (human leukocyte), mono(N^2,N^6-dicarboxyl-L-lysyl) derivative, diester with α-methyl-ω-hydroxypoly(oxy-1,2-ethanediyl); (2) Interferon αA (human leukocyte), mono(N^2,N^6-dicarboxyl-L-lysyl) derivative, diester with polyethylene glycol monomethyl ether. *UNII-Q46947FE7K. CAS-198153-51-4.* INN; BAN. *Treatment of hepatitis C.* Pegasys (Hoffmann-LaRoche) ◇*Ro 25-8310/000*

CDLPQTHSLG	SRRTLMLLAQ	MRKISLFSCL	*KDRHDFGFPQ
EEFGNQFQKA	ETIPVLHEMI	QQIFNLFSTK	DSSAAWDETL
LDKFYTELYQ	QLNDLEACVI	QGVGVTETPL	MKEDSILAVR
*KYFQRITLYL	*KE*KKYSPCAW	EVVRAEIMRS	FSLSTNLQES
LRSKE			

* pegylation sites

Peginterferon Alfa-2b. (1) Monocarboxyinterferon alfa-2b, diesters with polyethylene glycol monomethyl ether. The molecular mass of the pegylated part may be indicated in the name by adding a number, for example: peginterferon alfa-2b (12KD); (2) Pegylated, recombinant interferon alfa-2b. *UNII-G8RGG88B68. CAS-215647-85-1.* INN; BAN.

*CDLPQTHSLG	SRRTLMLLAQ	MRRISLFSCL	KDRHDFGFPQ
EEFGNQFQKA	ETIPVLHEMI	QQIFNLFSTK	DSSAAWDETL
LDKFYTELYQ	QLNDLEACVI	QGVGVTETPL	MKEDSILAVR
*KYFQRITLYL	KEKKYSPCAW	EVVRAEIMRS	FSLSTNLQES
LRSKE			

* pegylation sites

Peglicol 5 Oleate [*1974*] (pe glye′ kol oh′ lee ate). Product obtained by the alcoholysis of natural vegetable oils in the presence of polyethylene glycols of molecular weights between 200 and 400. It consists of a mixture of partial mixed esters of glycerin and these polyethylene glycols.

The average number of ethylene glycol units is 5. *Pharmaceutic aid (emulsifying agent).* Labrafil M1944CS (Gattefosse Etablissements, France)

Pegloticase [*2007*] (peg loe′ ti kase). $C_{1549}H_{2430}N_{408}O_{448}S_8$ (peptide monomer). (1) Oxidase, urate (synthetic *Sus scrofa* variant pigKS-ΔN subunit), homotetramer, amide with α-carboxy-ω-methoxypoly(oxy-1,2-ethanediyl); (2) Des-(1-6)-[7-threonine,46-threonine,291-lysine,301-serine]uricase (EC 1.7.3.3, urate oxidase) *Sus scrofa* (pig) tetramer, non acetylated, carbamates with α-carboxy-ω-methoxypoly(oxyethylene). Molecular weight is approximately 497,000 daltons (polymer-modifeid tetramer). *CAS-885051-90-1.* INN. *Treatment failure gout.* Puricase (Savient)

Pegmusirudin. $(C_2H_4O)_n(C_2H_4O)_nC_{302}H_{451}N_{85}O_{112}S_6$. L-Valyl-L-valyl-L-tyrosyl-L-threonyl-L-α-aspartyl-L-cysteinyl-L-threonyl-L-α-glutamyl-L-serylglycyl-L-glutaminyl-L-asparaginyl-L-leucyl-L-cysteinyl-L-leucyl-L-cysteinyl-L-α-glutamylglycyl-L-seryl-L-asparaginyl-L-valyl-L-cysteinylglycyl-L-glutamylglycyl-L-asparaginyl-N^6-carboxy-L-lysyl-L-cysteinyl-L-isoleucyl-L-leucylglycyl-L-seryl-N^6-carboxy-L-lysylglycyl-L-α-glutamyl-L-arginyl-L-asparaginyl-L-glutaminyl-L-cysteinyl-L-valyl-L-threonylglycyl-L-α-glutamylglycyl-L-threonyl-L-prolyl-L-arginyl-L-prolyl-L-glutaminyl-L-seryl-L-histidyl-L-asparaginyl-L-α-aspartylglycyl-L-α-aspartyl-L-phenylalanyl-L-α-glutamyl-L-α-glutamyl-L-isoleucyl-L-prolyl-L-α-glutamyl-L-α-glutamyl-L-tyrosyl-L-leucyl-L-glutamine cyclic (6→14), (16→28), (22→39)-tris(disulfide), 27,33-diester with polyethylene glycol monoethyl ether. *CAS-186638-10-8.* INN.

Pegnartograstim [*1998*] (peg nar″ toe gra′ stim). (1) Pegnartograstim; (2) *N*-L-Methionyl-1-L-alanine-3-L-threonine-4-L-tyrosine-5-L-arginine-17-L-serinecolony-stimulating factor (human clone 1034), reaction product with succinic anhydride, esters with polyethylene glycol monomethyl ether. Molecular weight is approximately 20,000 daltons. *CAS-204565-76-4.* INN. *1) Parenteral adjuvant to anticancer chemotherapy; 2) Immunomodulator.* ◇*Ro-25-8315/000*

Pegorgotein [*1994*] (peg ore′ go teen). (1) Pegorgotein; (2) Superoxide dismutase, reaction product with succinic anhydride, esters with polyethylene glycol monomethyl ether. Molecular weight is $88,352 \pm 17,039$ daltons. *CAS-155773-57-2.* INN. *Free oxygen radical scavenger.* Dismutec (Sterling Winthrop) ◇*WIN 22118; PEG-SOD*

Pegoterate [*1974*] (peg oh′ te rate). $(C_{10}H_8O_4)_n$, in which $n = 20$ to 100. Condensation polymer between terephthalic acid and ethylene glycol as microcrystals of colloidal dimensions, having a molecular weight range of 5000 ± 2000. (1) Poly(oxy-1,2-ethanediyloxycarbonyl-1,4-phenylenecarbonyl); (2) Poly(oxyethyleneoxyterephthaloyl). *CAS-9003-68-3.* INN. *Pharmaceutic aid (suspending agent).*

Pegoxol 7 Stearate [*1974*] (peg ox′ ol steer′ ate). A mixture of mono- and distearic esters of ethylene glycol and of polyoxyethylene glycol, the latter having an average molecular weight of 450. The average number of ethylene glycol units is 7. *Pharmaceutic aid (emulsifying agent).*

Pegsunercept [*2002*] (peg soon′ er sept). $C_{502}H_{758}N_{154}O_{165}S_{16}$. (1) 1-105-Tumor necrosis factor receptor p55 [methionyl] (human), 30-kilodalton pegylated; (2) Pegylated (30 kilodaltons) L-methionyl-1-105-tumor necrosis factor receptor p55 (human). Molecular weight is approximately 42,000 daltons. *CAS-330988-75-5.* INN. *Treatment of inflammatory and autoimmune condi-*

---

† Brand name formerly used, and/or firm no longer concerned with this product.

tions (*e.g. rheumatoid arthritis, Crohn's disease*) (*binds and thereby inhibits the inflammatory activity of tumor necrosis factor*).[*Note—The molecular formula and amino acid sequence represents the unpegylated moiety.*] ◇*sTNF-RI*

```
DSVCPQGKYI  HPQNNSICCT  KCHKGTYLYN  DCPGPGQDTD  CRECESGSFT
ASENHLRHCL  SCSKCRKEMG  QVEISSCTVD  RDTVCGCRKN  QYRHYWSENL
FQCFN
```

Pegvisomant [*1999*] (peg vi′ soe mant). (1) Pegwisomant; (2) 18-L-Aspartic acid-21-L-asparagine-120-L-lysine-167-L-asparagine-168-L-alanine-171-L-serine-172-L-arginine-174-serine-179-L-threonine growth hormone (human), reaction product with polyethylene glycol. Molecular weight is approximately 50,000 daltons. *UNII-N824AOU5XV*. INN. *Treatment of acromegaly (competitive inhibition of peripheral growth hormone receptors to block IFG-I production)*. Somavert (Pfizer) [*Note—The FDA has designated pegvisomant (B2036-PEG) as an Orphan Drug for the treatment of acromegaly.*] ◇*B2036-PEG*

Pelanserin Hydrochloride [*1987*] (pel an′ ser in hye″ droe klor′ ide). $C_{21}H_{24}N_4O_2$·HCl. 400.90. [Pelanserin is INN.] (1) 2,4(1*H*,3*H*)-Quinazolinedione, 3-[3-(4-phenyl-1-piperazinyl)propyl]-, monohydrochloride; (2) 3-[3-(4-Phenyl-1-piperazinyl)propyl]-2,4(1*H*,3*H*)-quinazolinedione monohydrochloride. *UNII-4J8I18ZP0A; UNII-6SNR96E409* [pelanserin]. *CAS-42877-18-9; CAS-2208-51-7* [pelanserin]. *Antihypertensive; vasodilator (serotonin S₂and α₁adrener-c receptor blocker)*. ◇*TR-2515*

Peldesine [*1995*] (pel′ de seen). $C_{12}H_{11}N_5O$. 241.25. (1) 4*H*-Pyrrolo[3,2-*d*]pyrimidin-4-one, 2-amino-3,5-dihydro-7-(3-pyridinylmethyl)-; (2) 2-Amino-3,5-dihydro-7-(3-pyridyl-methyl)-4*H*-pyrrolo[3,2-*d*]pyrimidin-4-one. *CAS-133432-71-0*. INN. *Antineoplastic; antipsoriatic*. ◇*BCX-34*

Peliglitazar [*2005*] (pel″ i gli′ ta zar). $C_{30}H_{30}N_2O_7$. 530.57. (1) Glycine, *N*-[(4-methoxyphenoxy)carbonyl]-*N*-[(1*S*)-1-[4-[2-(5-methyl-2-phenyl-4-oxazolyl)ethoxy]phenyl]ethyl]-; (2) [[(4-Methoxyphenoxy)carbonyl][(1*S*)-1-[4-[2-(5-methyl-2-phenyloxazol-4-yl)ethoxy]phenyl]ethyl]amino]acetic acid. *CAS-331744-64-0*. INN. *Treatment of Type II diabetes mellitus, mixed dyslipidemia, atherosclerosis, and metabolic syndrome*. ◇*BMS-426707-1*

Peliomycin [*1964*] (pel″ i oh mye′ sin). $C_{46}H_{76}O_{14}$. 853,09. Antibiotic produced by *Streptomyces luteogriseus* n. sp. (1) Peliomycin; (2) Peliomycin. *CAS-1404-20-2*. INN. *Antineoplastic*. ◇*NSC-76455*

Pelitinib [*2004*] (pel i′ ti nib). $C_{24}H_{23}ClFN_5O_2$. 467.92. (1) 2-Butenamide, *N*-[4-[(3-chloro-4-fluorophenyl)amino]-3-cy-ano-7-ethoxy-6-quinolinyl]-4-(dimethylamino)-, (2*E*)-; (2) (2*E*)-*N*-[4-[(3-Chloro-4-fluorophenyl)amino]-3-cyano-7-ethoxyquinolin-6-yl]-4-(dimethylamino)but-2-enamide. *UNII-X5DWL380Z6. CAS-257933-82-7*. INN. *Treatment of cancer*. ◇*EKB-569*

Pelitrexol [*2004*] (pel″ i trex′ ol). $C_{20}H_{25}N_5O_6S$. 463.51. (1) L-Glutamic acid, *N*-[[5-[2-[(6*S*)-2-amino-1,4,5,6,7,8-hexahy-dro-4-oxopyrido[2,3-*d*]pyrimidin-6-yl]ethyl]-4-methyl-2-thienyl]carbonyl]-; (2) (2*S*)-2-[[[5-[2-[(6*S*)-2-Amino-4-oxo-1,4,5,6,7,8-hexahydropyrido[2,3-*d*]pyrimidin-6-yl]ethyl]-4-methylthiophen-2-yl]carbonyl]amino]pentane-dioic acid. *UNII-DHT6E8M4KP. CAS-446022-33-9*. INN. *Antineoplastic (glycinamide ribonucleotide formyltransfer-ase (GARFT) inhibitor)*. ◇*AG2037*

Pelretin [*1989*] (pel′ re tin). $C_{23}H_{28}O_2$. 336.47. (1) Benzoic acid, 4-[4-methyl-6-(2,6,6-trimethyl-1-cyclohexen-1-yl)-1,3,5-hexatrienyl]-, (*E,E,E*)-; (2) (*E,E,E*)-*p*-[4-Methyl-6-(2,6,6-trimethyl-1-cyclohexen-1-yl)-1,3,5-hexatrienyl]ben-zoic acid. *CAS-91587-01-8*. INN. *Antikeratinizing agent*. ◇*ORF 18704; RWJ 18704; BASF 43915*

Pelrinone Hydrochloride [*1985*] (pel′ ri none hye″ droe klor′ ide). $C_{12}H_{11}N_5O$·HCl. 277.71. [Pelrinone is INN.] (1) 5-Pyrimidinecarbonitrile, 1,4-dihydro-2-methyl-4-oxo-6-[(3-pyridinylmethyl)amino]-, monohydrochloride; (2) 1,4-Di-hydro-2-methyl-4-oxo-6-[(3-pyridylmethyl)amino]-5-pyri-midinecarbonitrile monohydrochloride. *CAS-89232-84-8; CAS-94386-65-9* [pelrinone]. *Cardiotonic*. Myotrope (Wyeth-Ayerst) ◇*AY-28,768*

Pelubiprofen. $C_{16}H_{18}O_3$. 258.31. (±)-*p*-[[(*E*)-2-Oxocyclohex-ylidene]methyl]hydratropic acid. *UNII-1619C79FVJ. CAS-69956-77-0*. INN.

Pemaglitazar. $C_{18}H_{17}F_3O_3S$. 370.39. (2*S*)-4-[(2-Methylphenyl)sulfanyl]-2-[4-(trifluoromethyl)phenoxy]butanoic acid. *CAS-496050-39-6.* INN.

Pemedolac [*1987*] (pem ed′ oh lak). $C_{22}H_{23}NO_3$. 349.42. (1) Pyrano[3,4-*b*]indole-1-acetic acid, 1-ethyl-1,3,4,9-tetrahydro-4-(phenylmethyl)-, *cis*-(±)-; (2) (±)-*cis*-4-Benzyl-1-ethyl-1,3,4,9-tetrahydropyrano[3,4-*b*]indole-1-acetic acid. *CAS-114716-16-4.* INN. *Analgesic.* ◇*AY-30,715*

Pemerid Nitrate [*1971*] (pem′ e rid nye′ trate). $C_{15}H_{32}N_2O\cdot2HNO_3$. 382.45. [Pemerid is INN.] (1) Piperidine, 4-[3-(dimethylamino)propoxy]-1,2,2,6,6-pentamethyl-, dinitrate; (2) 4-[3-(Dimethylamino)propoxy]-1,2,2,6,6-pentamethylpiperidine dinitrate. *UNII-9ABL5H8Y29.* *CAS-34114-01-7; CAS-50432-78-5* [pemerid]. *Antitussive.* ◇*W 2394A*

Pemetrexed Disodium [*2004*] (pem″ e trex′ ed dye soe′ dee um). $C_{20}H_{19}N_5Na_2O_6$. 471.37. [Pemetrexed is INN and BAN.] (1) L-Glutamic acid, *N*-[4-[2-(2-amino-4,7-dihydro-4-oxo-1*H*-pyrrolo[2,3-*d*]pyrimidin-5-yl)ethyl]benzoyl]-, disodium salt; (2) Disodium *N*-[*p*-[2-(2-amino-4,7-dihydro-4-oxo-1*H*-pyrrolo[2,3-*d*]pyrimidin-5-yl)ethyl]benzoyl]-L-glutamate. *UNII-2PKU919BA9; UNII-04Q9AIZ7NO* [pemetrexed]. *CAS-150399-23-8; CAS-137281-23-3* [pemetrexed]. *Antineoplastic (specific thymidylate synthase inhibitor).* Alimta (Lilly) ◇*LY231514*

Pemirolast Potassium [*1989*] (pem ir′ oh last poe tas′ ee um). $C_{10}H_7KN_6O$. 266.30. [Pemirolast is INN.] (1) 4*H*-Pyrido[1,2-*a*]pyrimidin-4-one, 9-methyl-3-(1*H*-tetrazol-5-yl)-, potassium salt; (2) 9-Methyl-3-(1*H*-tetrazol-5-yl)-4*H*-pyrido[1,2-*a*]pyrimidin-4-one, potassium salt. *UNII-497A17OUUE; UNII-2C09NV773M* [pemirolast]. *CAS-*

---

† Brand name formerly used, and/or firm no longer concerned with this product.

100299-08-9; CAS-69372-19-6 [pemirolast]. JAN. *Antiallergic; inhibitor (mediator release).* Alamast (Sanofi Winthrop) ◇*BMY-26517*

Pemoline [*1966*] (pem′ oh leen). $C_9H_8N_2O_2$. 176.17. (1) 4(5*H*)-Oxazolone, 2-amino-5-phenyl-; (2) 2-Imino-5-phenyl-4-oxazolidinone. *UNII-7GAQ2332NK.* *CAS-2152-34-3.* INN; BAN; JAN. *Stimulant (central).* Cylert (Abbott) ◇*NSC-25159*

Pempidine. $C_{10}H_{21}N$. 155.28. 1,2,2,6,6-Pentamethylpiperidine. *UNII-N5I18JI9D6.* *CAS-79-55-0.* INN; BAN; MI.

Penamecillin [*1987*] (pen″ am e sil′ in). $C_{19}H_{22}N_2O_6S$. 406.45. (1) 4-Thia-1-azabicyclo[3.2.0]heptane-2-carboxylic acid, 3,3-dimethyl-7-oxo-6-[(phenylacetyl)amino]-[2*S*-(2α,5α,6β)]-, (acetyloxy)methyl ester; (2) Hydroxymethyl (2*S*,5*R*,6*R*)-3,3-dimethyl-7-oxo-6-(2-phenylacetamido)-4-thia-1-azabicyclo[3.2.0]heptane-2-carboxylate, acetate (ester). *CAS-983-85-7.* INN; BAN. *Antibacterial.* ◇*WY-20,788*

Penbutolol Sulfate [*1977*] (pen bue′ toe lol sul′ fate). **USP.** $(C_{18}H_{29}NO_2)_2\cdot H_2SO_4$. 680.94. [Penbutolol is INN and BAN.] (1) 2-Propanol, 1-(2-cyclopentylphenoxy)-3-[(1,1-dimethylethyl)amino]-, (*S*)-, sulfate (2:1) (salt); (2) (*S*)-1-(*tert*-Butylamino)-3-(*o*-cyclopentylphenoxy)-2-propanol sulfate (2:1) (salt). *UNII-US71433228; UNII-78W62V43DY* [penbutolol]. *CAS-38363-32-5; CAS-38363-40-5* [penbutolol]. JAN. *Anti-adrenergic (β-receptor).* Levatol (Schwarz Pharma) ◇*HOE 893d; HOE 39-893d*

Penciclovir [*1992*] (pen sye′ kloe vir). $C_{10}H_{15}N_5O_3$. 253.26. (1) 6*H*-Purin-6-one, 2-amino-1,9-dihydro-9-[4-hydroxy-3-(hydroxymethyl)butyl]-; (2) 9-[4-Hydroxy-3-(hydroxymethyl)butyl]guanine. *UNII-359HUE8FJC. CAS-39809-25-1*. INN; BAN. *Antiviral*. Denavir (SmithKline Beecham) ◇*BRL-39123*

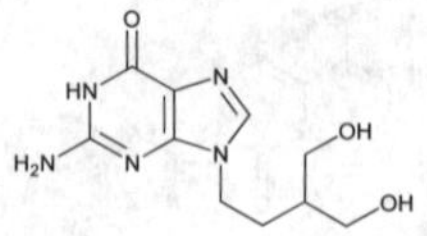

Penciclovir Sodium [*1998*] (pen sye′ kloe vir soe′ dee um). $C_{10}H_{14}N_5NaO_3$. 275.24. (1) 2-Amino-1,9-dihydro-9-[4-hydroxy-3-(hydroxymethyl)butyl]-6*H*-purin-6-one monosodium salt; (2) 9-[4-Hydroxy-3-(hydroxymethyl)butyl]-guanine monosodium salt. *UNII-P06226385L. CAS-97845-62-0. Antiviral (treatment of herpes virus infections)*. Denavir (Novartis) ◇*BRL-39123-D*

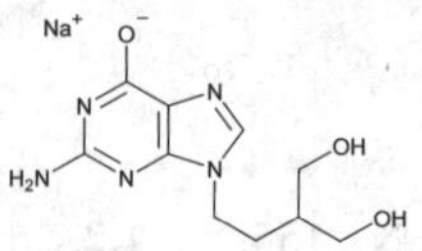

Pendecamaine. $C_{23}H_{46}N_2O_3$. 398.62. (Carboxymethyl)dimethyl(3-palmitamidopropyl)ammonium hydroxide inner salt. *UNII-WP8C6WF33S. CAS-32954-43-1*. INN; BAN.

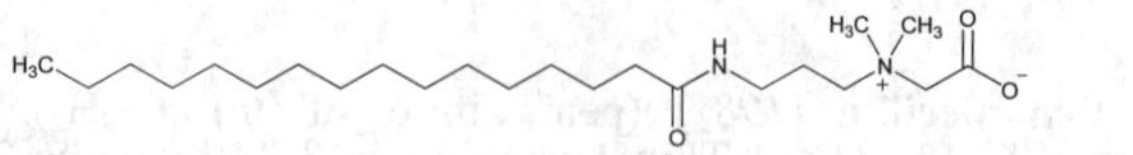

Pendetide. $C_{31}H_{47}N_7O_{14}$. 741.74. Glycyl-L-tyrosyl-N^6-[*N*-(2-{2-[bis(carboxymethyl)amino]ethyl(carboxymethyl)amino}ethyl)-*N*-(carboxymethyl)glycyl]-L-lysine. BAN. *[Note—Pendetide is the recommended radical name for this entry.]*

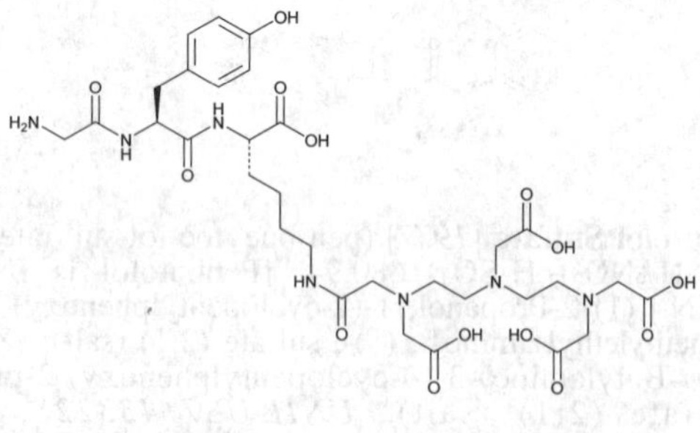

Penethamate Hydriodide. $C_{22}H_{31}N_3O_4S \cdot HI$. 561.48. [Penethamate is BAN.] 2-Diethylaminoethyl (6*R*)-6-(2-phenylacetamido)penicillanate hydriodide. *CAS-808-71-9*.

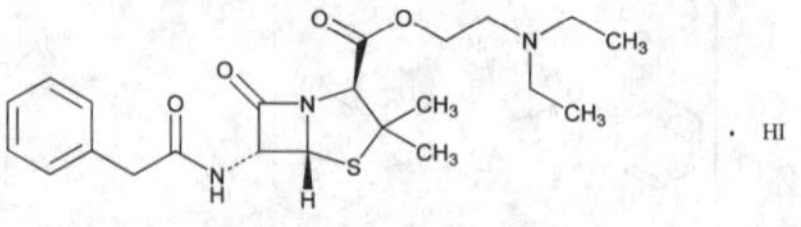

Penfluridol [*1971*] (pen flur′ i dol). $C_{28}H_{27}ClF_5NO$. 523.97. (1) 4-Piperidinol, 1-[4,4-bis(4-fluorophenyl)butyl]-4-[4-chloro-3-(trifluoromethyl)phenyl]-; (2) 1-[4,4-Bis(*p*-fluo-rophenyl)butyl]-4-(4-chloro-α,α,α-trifluoro-*m*-tolyl)-4-piperidinol. *CAS-26864-56-2*. INN; BAN. *Antipsychotic*. Semap (Ortho-McNeil†) ◇*McN-JR-16,341; R 16,341*

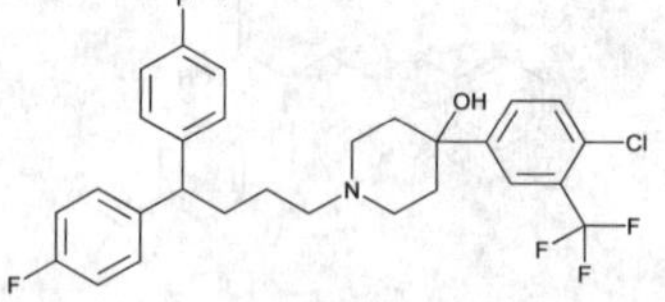

Penflutizide. $C_{13}H_{18}F_3N_3O_4S_2$. 401.42. 3,4-Dihydro-3-pentyl-6-(trifluoromethyl)-2*H*-1,2,4-benzothiadiazine-7-sulfonamide 1,1-dioxide. *UNII-91NGD0O6FZ. CAS-1766-91-2*. INN; JAN.

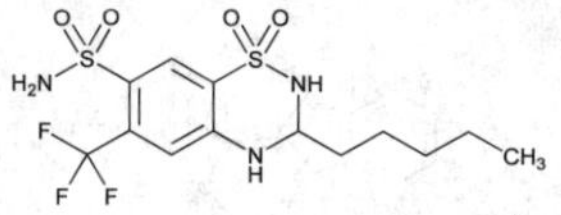

Pengitoxin. $C_{51}H_{74}O_{19}$. 991.12. Gitoxin pentaacetate. *CAS-7242-04-8*. INN.

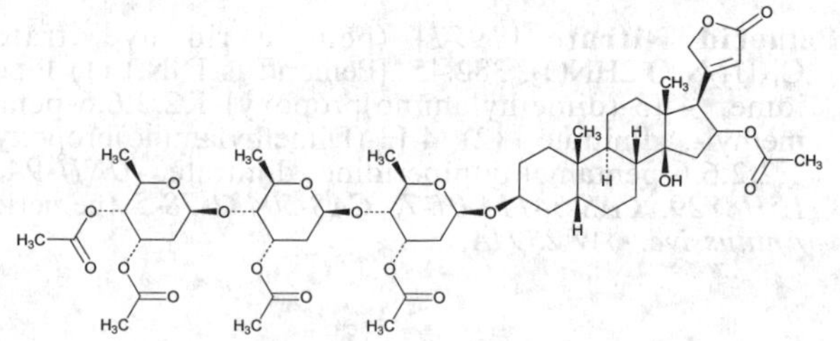

Penicillamine [*1963*] (pen″ i sil′ a meen). **USP.** $C_5H_{11}NO_2S$. 149.21. (1) D-Valine, 3-mercapto-; (2) D-3-Mercaptovaline. *UNII-GNN1DV99GX. CAS-52-67-5*. INN; BAN; JAN. *Chelating agent*. Cuprimine (Merck); Depen (Medpointe)

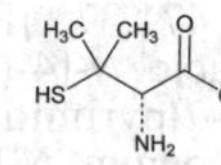

Penicillin-152 Potassium — *See* Phenethicillin Potassium.

Penicillin Aluminum. *CAS-1406-06-0*. NND 1962.

Penicillin Benzathine Phenoxymethyl (previously used name) — *See* Penicillin V Benzathine.

Penicillin Calcium. Calcium 3,3-dimethyl-7-oxo-6-(2-phenylacetamido)-4-thia-1-azabicyclo[3.2.0]heptane-2-carboxylate. *UNII-Q42T66VG0C* [penicillin g]. *CAS-1406-07-1; CAS-61-33-6* [penicillin G]. USP XIII.

Penicillin G Benzathine (pen″ i sil′ in ben′ za theen). **USP.** $(C_{16}H_{18}N_2O_4S)_2 \cdot C_{16}H_{20}N_2 \cdot 4H_2O$. 981.18. [Benzathine Benzylpenicillin is INN and BAN; Benzathine Penicillin is BAN; Benzylpenicillin Benzathine is JAN.] (1) 4-Thia-1-azabicyclo[3.2.0]heptane-2-carboxylic acid, 3,3-dimethyl-7-oxo-6-[(phenylacetyl)amino]-, [2*S*-(2α,5α,6β)]-, compd. with *N,N*′-bis(phenylmethyl)-1,2-ethanediamine (2:1), tetrahydrate; (2) (2*S*,5*R*,6*R*)-3,3-Dimethyl-7-oxo-6-(2-phenylacetamido)-4-thia-1-azabicyclo[3.2.0]heptane-2-carboxylic acid compound with *N,N*′-dibenzylethylenediamine (2:1), tetrahydrate. *UNII-RIT82F58GK; UNII-Q42T66VG0C* [penicillin g]. *CAS-41372-02-5; CAS-*

1538-09-6 [anhydrous]; *CAS-61-33-6* [penicillin G]. *Antibacterial*. Bicillin (King); Permapen (Pfizer) *[Name previously used: Benzathine Penicillin.]*

Penicillin G Hydrabamine. *UNII-Q42T66VG0C* [penicillin g]. *CAS-3344-16-9; CAS-61-33-6* [penicillin G]. MI; NNR 1957.

Penicillin G Potassium (pen″ i sil′ in poe tas′ ee um). **USP**. $C_{16}H_{17}KN_2O_4S$. 372.48. [Benzylpenicillin Potassium is BAN and JAN.] (1) 4-Thia-1-azabicyclo[3.2.0]heptane-2-carboxylic acid, 3,3-dimethyl-7-oxo-6-[(phenylacetyl)amino]-, monopotassium salt, [2S-(2α,5α,6β)]-; (2) Monopotassium (2S,5R,6R)-3,3-dimethyl-7-oxo-6-(2-phenylacetamido)-4-thia-1-azabicyclo[3.2.0]heptane-2-carboxylate. *UNII-VL775ZTH4C. CAS-113-98-4; CAS-61-33-6* [penicillin G]. *Antibacterial*. Pentids (Apothecon)

Penicillin G Procaine (pen″ i sil′ in proe′ kane). **USP**. $C_{16}H_{18}N_2O_4S.C_{13}H_{20}N_2O_2.H_2O$. 588.72. [Procaine Benzylpenicillin is BAN.] (1) 4-Thia-1-azabicyclo[3.2.0]heptane-2-carboxylic acid, 3,3-dimethyl-7-oxo-6-[(phenylacetyl)amino]-, [2S-(2α,5α,6β)]-, compd. with 2-(diethylamino)ethyl 4-aminobenzoate (1:1) monohydrate; (2) (2S,5R,6R)-3,3-Dimethyl-7-oxo-6-(2-phenylacetamido)-4-thia-1-azabicyclo[3.2.0]heptane-2-carboxylic acid compound with 2-(diethylamino)ethyl p-aminobenzoate (1:1) monohydrate. *UNII-Q42T66VG0C* [penicillin g]. *CAS-6130-64-9; CAS-54-35-3* [anhydrous]; *CAS-61-33-6* [penicillin G]. *Antibacterial*. Duracillin (Lilly); Pfizerpen (Pfizer)

Penicillin G Sodium (pen″ i sil′ in soe′ dee um). **USP**. $C_{16}H_{17}N_2NaO_4S$. 356.37. (1) 4-Thia-1-azabicyclo[3.2.0]-heptane-2-carboxylic acid, 3,3-dimethyl-7-oxo-6-[(phenylacetyl)amino]-, [2S-(2α,5α,6β)]-, monosodium salt; (2) Monosodium (2S,5R,6R)-3,3-dimethyl-7-oxo-6-(2-phenylacetamido)-4-thia-1-azabicyclo[3.2.0]heptane-2-carboxylate. *UNII-YS5LY7JF4N. CAS-69-57-8; CAS-61-33-6* [penicillin G]. *Antibacterial*.

Penicillin G Sodium, Crystalline — *See* Penicillin G Sodium.

Penicillin Hydrabamine Phenoxymethyl (previously used name) — *See* Penicillin V Hydrabamine.

Penicillin N — *See* Adicillin.

Penicillin O — *See* Almecillin.

Penicillin O Chloroprocaine. *CAS-575-52-0*. MI; NND 1963.

Penicillin O Potassium. *CAS-897-61-0; CAS-87-09-2* [penicillin O]. MI.

Penicillin O Sodium. *CAS-7177-54-0; CAS-87-09-2* [penicillin O]. MI; NND 1963.

Penicillin Phenoxymethyl (previously used name) — *See* Penicillin V.

Penicillin Potassium G, Crystalline — *See* Penicillin G Potassium.

Penicillin Potassium Phenoxymethyl (previously used name) — *See* Penicillin V Potassium.

Penicillin V [*1975*] (pen″ i sil′ in). **USP**. $C_{16}H_{18}N_2O_5S$. 350.39. [Phenoxymethylpenicillin is INN and BAN.] (1) 4-Thia-1-azabicyclo[3.2.0]heptane-2-carboxylic acid, 3,3-dimethyl-7-oxo-6-[(phenoxyacetyl)amino]-, [2S-(2α,5α,6β)]-; (2) (2S,5R,6R)-3,3-Dimethyl-7-oxo-6-(2-phenoxyacetamido)-4-thia-1-azabicyclo[3.2.0]heptane-2-carboxylic acid. *UNII-Z61I075U2W. CAS-87-08-1*. *Antibacterial*. V-Cillin (Lilly) *[Name previously used: Penicillin Phenoxymethyl.]*

Penicillin V Benzathine [*1975*] (pen″ i sil′ in ben′ za theen). **USP**. $(C_{16}H_{18}N_2O_5S)_2.C_{16}H_{20}N_2$. 941.12. (1) 4-Thia-1-azabicyclo[3.2.0]heptane-2-carboxylic acid, 3,3-dimethyl-7-oxo-6-[(2-phenoxyacetyl)amino]-, [2S-(2α,5α,6β)]-, compd. with N,N′-bis(phenylmethyl)-1,2-ethanediamine (2:1); (2) (2S,5R,6R)-3,3-Dimethyl-7-oxo-6-(2-phenoxyacetamido)-4-thia-1-azabicyclo[3.2.0]heptane-2-carboxylic acid compound with N,N′-dibenzylethylenediamine (2:1). *UNII-Z61I075U2W* [penicillin v]. *CAS-5928-84-7; CAS-63690-57-3* [tetrahydrate]; *CAS-87-08-1* [penicillin V]. *Antibacterial*. *[Name previously used: Penicillin Benzathine Phenoxymethyl.]*

Penicillin V Hydrabamine [*1975*] (pen″ i sil′ in hye″ dra bam′ een). $(C_{16}H_{18}N_2O_5S)_2.C_{42}H_{64}N_2$. 1297.75. (1) 4-Thia-1-azabicyclo[3.2.0]heptane-2-carboxylic acid, 3,3-dimethyl-7-oxo-6-[(phenoxyacetyl)amino]-, [2S-(2α,5α,6β)]-, compd. with [1R-[1α(1R*,4aS*,10aR*), 4aβ,10aα]]-N,N′-bis-[(1,2,3,4,4a,9,10,10a-octahydro-1,4a-dimethyl-7-(1-methylethyl)-1-phenanthrenyl]methyl-1,2-ethanediamine (2:1) (principal component); (2) 3,3-Dimethyl-7-oxo-6-(2-phenoxyacetamido)-4-thia-1-azabicyclo[3.2.0]heptane-2-carboxylic acid compound with N,N′-bis[(1α,2,3,4,4aβ,9,10,10aα-octahydro-7-isopropyl-1,4a-dimethyl-1-phenanthryl)methyl]ethylenediamine (2:1) (principal component). *UNII-Z61I075U2W* [penicil-

---

† Brand name formerly used, and/or firm no longer concerned with this product.

lin v]. *CAS-6591-72-6; CAS-87-08-1* [penicillin V]. USP XX. *Antibacterial. [Name previously used: Penicillin Hydrabamine Phenoxymethyl.]*

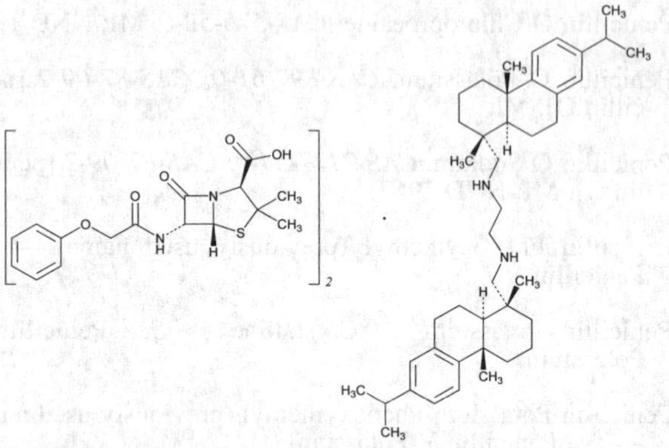

Penicillin V Potassium [*1975*] (pen″ i sil′ in poe tas′ ee um). **USP.** $C_{16}H_{17}KN_2O_5S$. 388.48. [Phenoxymethylpenicillin Potassium is JAN.] (1) 4-Thia-1-azabicyclo[3.2.0]heptane-2-carboxylic acid, 3,3-dimethyl-7-oxo-6-[(phenoxyacetyl)amino]-, monopotassium salt, [2*S*-(2α,5α,6β)]-; (2) Monopotassium (2*S*,5*R*,6*R*)-3,3-dimethyl-7-oxo-6-(2-phenoxyacetamido)-4-thia-1-azabicyclo[3.2.0]heptane-2-carboxylate. *UNII-146T0TU1JB. CAS-132-98-9; CAS-87-08-1* [penicillin V]. *Antibacterial.* Beepen-vk (Glaxo SmithKline); Betapen-vk (Apothecon); Pen-vee K (Wyeth); Pfizerpen Vk (Pfizer); V-cillin K (Lilly); Veetids (Apothecon) *[Name previously used: Penicillin Potassium Phenoxymethyl.]*

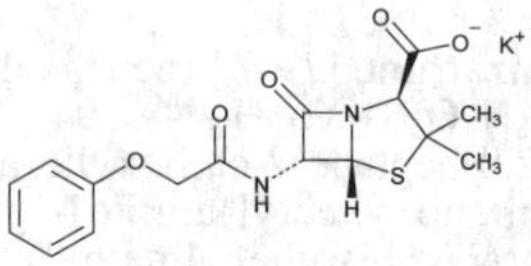

Penicillinase. Enzyme obtained by fermentation from cultures of *Bacillus cereus. CAS-9001-74-5.* INN; BAN; AMA-DE 1973. Neutrapen (3M Pharmaceuticals†)

Penicillinphenyrazine — *See* Phenyracillin.

Penimepicycline. $C_{45}H_{56}N_6O_{14}S$. 937.02. 4-(Dimethyl-amino)-1,4,4a,5,5a,6,11,12a-octahydro-3,6,10,12,12a-pentahydroxy-*N*-[[4-(2-hydroxyethyl)-1-piperazinyl]methyl]-6-methyl-1,11-dioxo-2-naphthacenecarboxamide salt with phenoxymethylpenicillin. *CAS-4599-60-4.* INN; DCF; MI.

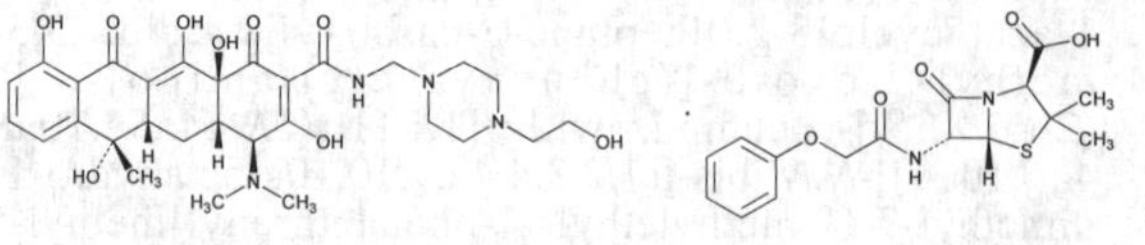

Penimocycline. $C_{39}H_{43}N_5O_{12}S$. 805.85. 6-[2-[[[4-(Dimethyl-amino)-1,4,4a,5,5a,6,11,12a-octahydro-3,6,10,12,12a-pentahydroxy-6-methyl-1,11-dioxo-2-naphthacenecarbox-

amido]methyl]amino]-2-phenylacetamido]-3,3-dimethyl-7-oxo-4-thia-1-azabicyclo[3.2.0]heptane-2-carboxylic acid. *CAS-16259-34-0.* INN; DCF.

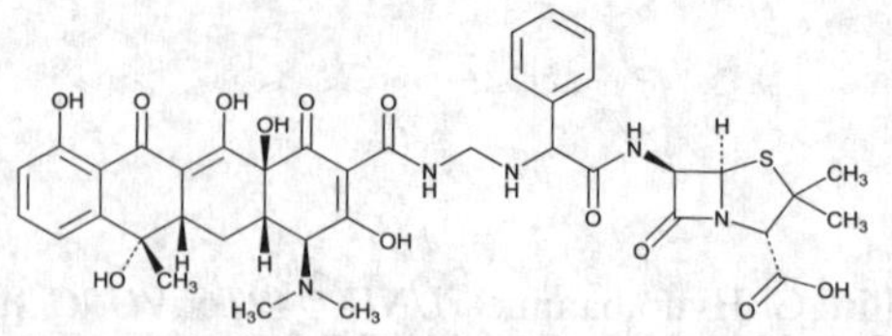

Penirolol. $C_{15}H_{22}N_2O_2$. 262.35. *o*-[2-Hydroxy-3-(*tert*-penty-lamino)propoxy]benzonitrile. *UNII-BT9Y6D2DR0. CAS-58503-83-6.* INN.

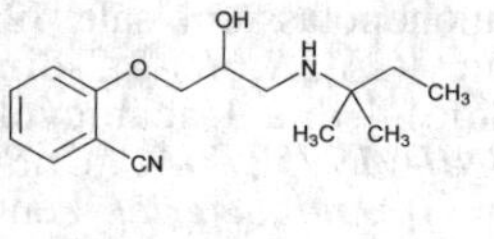

Penmesterol. $C_{25}H_{38}O_2$. 370.57. 3-(Cyclopentyloxy)-17-methyl-androsta-3,5-dien-17β-ol. *CAS-67-81-2.* INN; DCF. ◇*RP 12222*

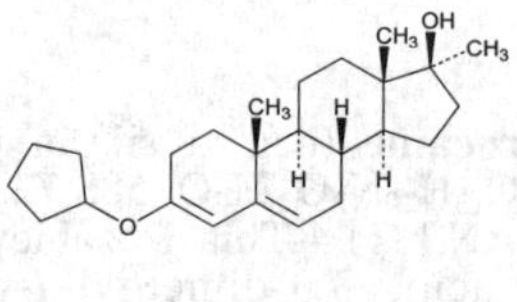

Penoctonium Bromide. $C_{26}H_{50}BrNO_2$. 488.58. Diethyl(2-hydroxyethyl)octyl ammonium bromide dicyclopentylac-etate. *UNII-HF11NTT6MZ. CAS-17088-72-1.* INN.

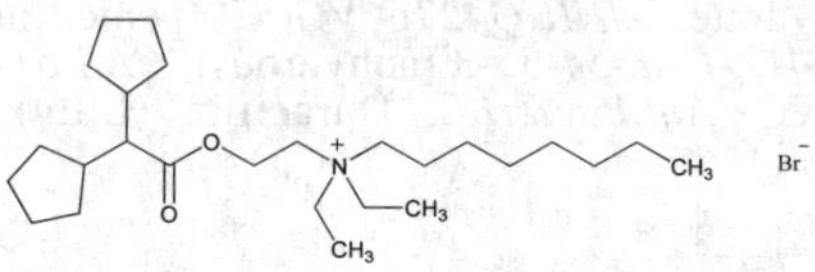

Penprostene. $C_{21}H_{32}O_5$. 364.48. (±)-(*Z*)-7-[(1*R**,2*R**)-2-[(*E*)-3*R**-5-Ethoxy-3-hydroxy-4,4-dimethyl-1-pentenyl]-5-oxo-3-cyclopenten-1-yl]-5-heptenoic acid. *CAS-61557-12-8.* INN.

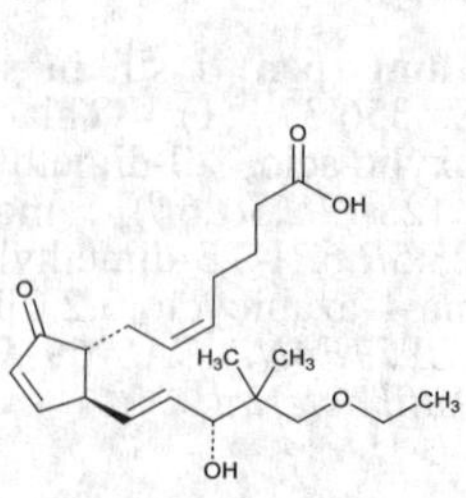

Pentabamate [*1963*] (pen″ ta bam′ ate). $C_8H_{16}N_2O_4$. 204.22. (1) 2,4-Pentanediol, 3-methyl-, dicarbamate; (2) 3-Methyl-2,4-pentanediol dicarbamate. *UNII-8871ZB4UGC. CAS-5667-70-9.* INN. *Tranquilizer (minor).*

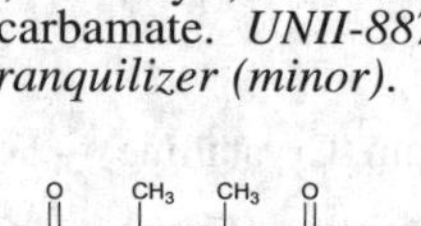

Pentacosactride (BAN) — *See* Norleusactide.

Pentacynium Chloride. $C_{27}H_{39}Cl_2N_3O$. 492.52. [Pentacynium Metilsulfate is BAN.] N-[N'-(5-Cyano-5,5-diphenylpentyl)-N'-dimethylammoniummethyl]-N-methylmorpholinium dichloride. *UNII-B08O4ROE04. CAS-77-12-3.* INN. [*Name previously used: Pentacynium Methylsulphate.*]

Pentacyone Chloride — *See* Pentacynium Chloride.

Pentaerythritol Tetranitrate. $C_5H_8N_4O_{12}$. 316.14. [Pentaerithrityl Tetranitrate is INN and BAN.] (1) 1,3-Propanediol, 2,2-bis[(nitrooxy)methyl]-, dinitrate (ester); (2) 2,2-Bis(hydroxymethyl)-1,3-propanediol tetranitrate. *UNII-10L39TRG1Z. CAS-78-11-5.* USP XXIII; JAN. *Vasodilator.* Pentritol Tempules (Rhone-Poulenc Rorer†); Peritrate (Parke-Davis†)

Pentafilcon A [*1983*] (pen″ ta fil′ kon). $(C_6H_{10}O_3)_v(C_9H_{15}NO_2)_w(C_4H_6O_2)_x(C_5H_8O_2)_y(C_{10}H_{14}O_4)_z$. (1) 2-Propenoic acid, 2-hydroxyethyl 2-methyl-, polymer with N-(1,1-dimethyl-3-oxobutyl)-2-propenamide, 2-methyl-2-propenoic acid, methyl 2-methyl-2-propenoate and 1,2-ethanediyl bis(2-methyl-2-propenoate); (2) 2-Hydroxyethyl methacrylate polymer with N-(1,1-dimethyl-3-oxobutyl)-acrylamide, methacrylic acid, methyl methacrylate and ethylene dimethacrylate. *CAS-82571-55-9. Contact lens material (hydrophilic).* E-40 (Lombart); E-50 (Lombart); E-60 (Lombart) ◇*E-52*

Pentafluranol. $C_{17}H_{15}F_5O_2$. 346.29. 4,4′-[(1R,2S)-1-Methyl-2-(2,2,2-trifluoroethyl)ethylene]bis(2-fluorophenol). *UNII-95RFZ48151. CAS-65634-39-1.* INN; BAN.

Pentafuside (trivial name) — *See* Enfuvirtide.

Pentagastrin [*1967*] (pen″ ta gas′ trin). $C_{37}H_{49}N_7O_9S$. 767.89. (1) L-Phenylalaninamide, N-[(1,1-dimethylethoxy)carbonyl]-β-alanyl-L-tryptophyl-L-methionyl-L-α-aspartyl-; (2) N-Carboxy-β-alanyl-L-tryptophyl-L-methionyl-L-aspartyl-phenyl-L-alaninamide N-*tert*-butyl ester. *UNII-*

EF0NX91490. CAS-5534-95-2. INN; BAN; JAN. *Diagnostic aid (gastric secretion indicator).* Peptavlon (Wyeth) ◇*ICI 50,123; AY-6608*

Pentagestrone. $C_{26}H_{38}O_3$. 398.58. 3-(Cyclopentyloxy)-17-hydroxypregna-3,5-dien-20-one. *CAS-7001-56-1.* INN; MI.

Pentalamide. $C_{12}H_{17}NO_2$. 207.27. *o*-(Pentyloxy)benzamide. *UNII-6SK5U4T3II. CAS-5579-06-6.* INN; BAN.

Pentalyte [*1981*] (pen′ ta lite). A combination of the following components in amounts that yield a descending order of concentration in the finished product: sodium chloride, USP; potassium chloride, USP; magnesium sulfate, USP; sodium phosphate dibasic, USP; potassium phosphate monobasic, NF. This combination of electrolytes is used to prepare a physiologic irrigation solution intended for use on wounds and open tissue surfaces. *Electrolyte combination.* Tis-U-Sol (Baxter Healthcare)

Pentamethazene — *See* Azamethonium Bromide.

Pentamethonium Bromide. $C_{11}H_{28}Br_2N_2$. 348.16. Pentamethylenebis(trimethylammonium bromide). *UNII-0UX03A6JJC. CAS-541-20-8; CAS-2365-25-5* [pentamethonium]. INN; BAN; MI.

Pentamethonium Iodide. $C_{11}H_{28}I_2N_2$. 442.16. N,N'-Pentamethylenebis(trimethylammonium) di-iodide. *CAS-5282-80-4.* BAN.

Pentamethylenetetrazol — *See* Pentylenetetrazol.

Pentamidine. $C_{19}H_{24}N_4O_2$. 340.42. [Pentamidine Isetionate is JAN.] 4,4′-(Pentamethylenedioxy)dibenzamidine. *UNII-673LC5J4LQ. CAS-100-33-4.* INN; BAN; DCF; MI. Nebupent [as isethionate] (Fujisawa); Pentacarinat [as isethionate] (Rhone-Poulenc Rorer); Pentam 300 [as isethionate] (Fujisawa) ◇*MB 800 [as isethionate]; RP 2512 [as isethionate]*

Pentamidine Isethionate [*2007*] (pen tam′ i deen eye″ se thye′ oh nate). $C_{23}H_{36}N_4O_{10}S_2$. 592.68. (1) Ethanesulfonic acid, 2-hydroxy-, compd. with 4,4′-[1,5-pentanediylbis(oxy)]bis [benzenecarboximidamide]; (2) 4,4′-(Pentane-1,5-diylbis(oxy))dibenzimidamide bis(2-hydroxyethanesulfonate). *UNII-V2P3K60DA2. CAS-140-64-7. Prevention and treatment of pneumonia.* Nebupent (Abraxis); Pentam (Abraxis)

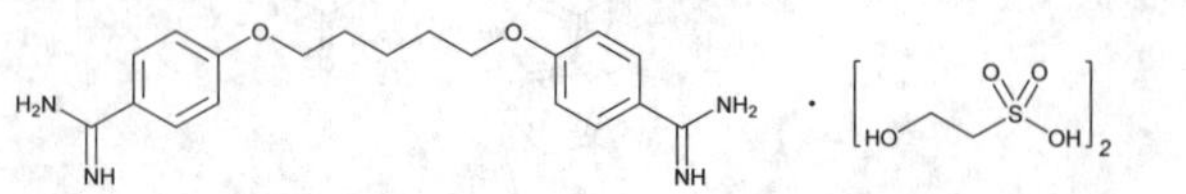

Pentamidine Isetionate (JAN) — *See* Pentamidine.

Pentamorphone [*1989*] (pen″ ta mor′ fone). $C_{22}H_{28}N_2O_3$. 368.47. (1) Morphinan-6-one, 7,8-didehydro-4,5-epoxy-3-hydroxy-17-methyl-14-(pentylamino)-, (5α)-; (2) 7,8-Didehydro-4,5α-epoxy-3-hydroxy-17-methyl-14-(pentylamino)morphinan-6-one. *CAS-68616-83-1.* INN. *Analgesic (narcotic).* ◇RX77989; A-4492

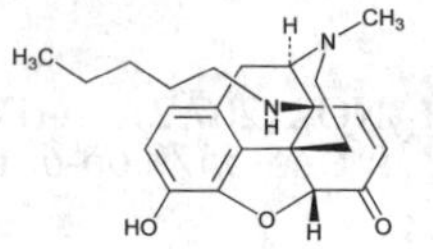

Pentamoxane Hydrochloride. $C_{14}H_{21}NO_2$.HCl. 271.78. [Pentamoxane is INN.] *CAS-4729-93-5; CAS-4730-07-8* [pentamoxane].

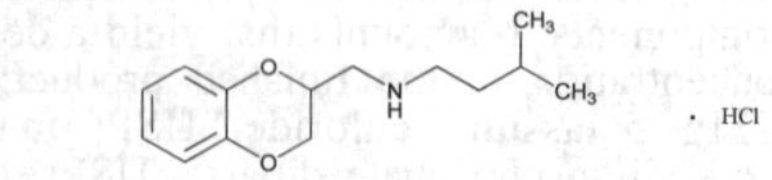

Pentamustine [*1980*] (pen″ ta mus′ teen). $C_8H_{16}ClN_3O_2$. 221.68. [Neptamustine is INN.] (1) Urea, *N*-(2-chloroethyl)-*N′*-(2,2-dimethylpropyl)-*N*-nitroso-; (2) 1-(2-Chloroethyl)-3-neopentyl-1-nitrosourea. *UNII-VB67O9FBGM. CAS-73105-03-0. Antineoplastic.* Salisburystin (National Foundation for Cancer Research) ◇NCNU

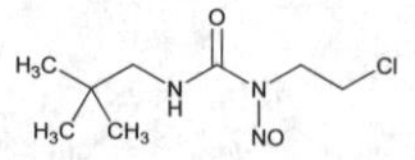

Pentanitrol — *See* Pentaerythritol Tetranitrate.

Pentaphonate. *CAS-24360-58-5.* JAMA 155: 1581 (1954).

Pentapiperide. $C_{18}H_{27}NO_2$. 289.41. 1-Methyl-4-piperidyl 3-methyl-2-phenylvalerate ester. *CAS-7009-54-3.* INN; BAN; MI.

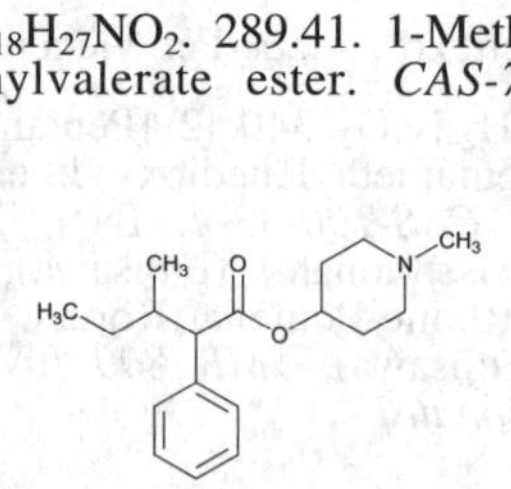

Pentapiperium Methylsulfate [*1971*] (pen″ ta pye per′ ee um meth″ il sul′ fate). $C_{20}H_{33}NO_6S$. 415.54. [Pentapiperium Metilsulfate is INN.] (1) Piperidinium, 1,1-dimethyl-4-[(3-methyl-1-oxo-2-phenylpentyl)oxy]-, methyl sulfate; (2) 4-Hydroxy-1,1-dimethylpiperidinium methyl sulfate 3-methyl-2-phenylvalerate. *CAS-7681-80-3; CAS-26372-86-1* [pentapiperium]. *Anticholinergic.*

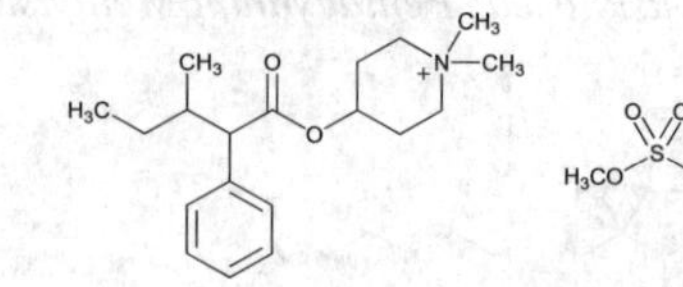

Pentapiperium Metilsulfate (INN) — *See* Pentapiperium Methylsulfate.

Pentaquine Phosphate. $C_{18}H_{27}N_3O$.H_3PO_4. 399.42. [Pentaquine is INN and BAN.] 8-(5-Isopropylaminoamylamino)-6-methoxy quinoline phosphate. *CAS-5428-64-8; CAS-86-78-2* [pentaquine]. USP XIV.

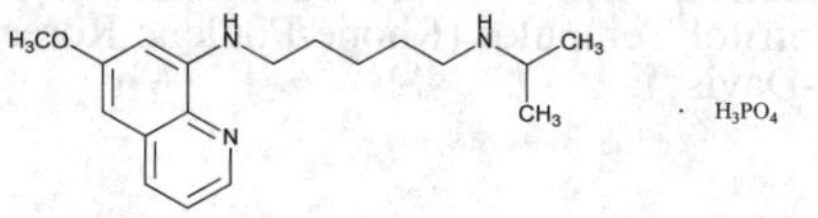

Pentastarch [*1987*] (pen′ ta starch). A starch composed of more than 90% amylopectin that has been etherified to the extent that an average of 4 to 5 of the OH groups present in every 10 D-glucopyranose units of the starch polymer have been converted to OCH$_2$CH$_2$OH groups. Starch 2-hydroxyethyl ether. *CAS-9005-27-0.* BAN. *Leukopheresis adjunct (red cell sedimenting agent).* Pentaspan (DuPont Merck) ◇ASL-607

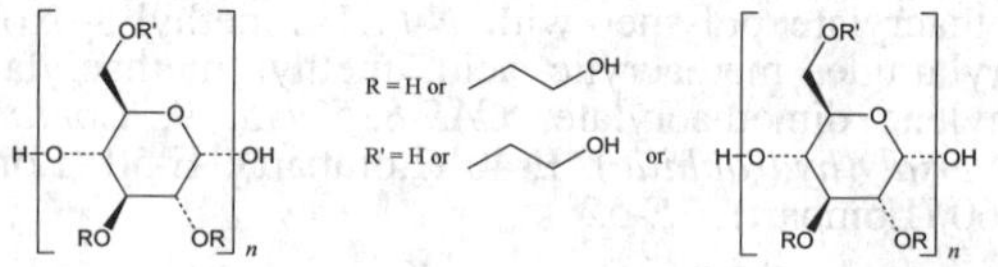

Pentazocine [*1963*] (pen taz′ oh seen). USP. $C_{19}H_{27}NO$. 285.42. (1) 2,6-Methano-3-benzazocin-8-ol, 1,2,3,4,5,6-hexahydro-6,11-dimethyl-3-(3-methyl-2-butenyl)-, (2α,6α,11*R**)-; (2) (2*R**,6*R**,11*R**)-1,2,3,4,5,6-Hexahydro-6,11-dimethyl-3-(3-methyl-2-butenyl)-2,6-methano-3-benzazocin-8-ol. *UNII-RP4A60D26L. CAS-359-83-1.* INN; BAN; JAN. *Analgesic.* Fortral (Sterling Winthrop); Talwin (Sterling Winthrop) ◇Win 20,228; NSC-107430

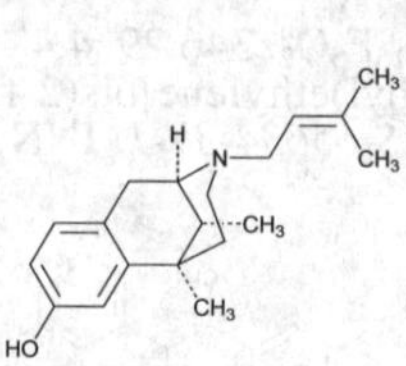

Pentazocine Hydrochloride [*1969*] (pen taz′ oh seen hye″ droe klor′ ide). USP. $C_{19}H_{27}NO$.HCl. 321.88. (1) 2,6-Methano-3-benzazocin-8-ol, 1,2,3,4,5,6-hexahydro-6,11-dimethyl-3-(3-methyl-2-butenyl)-, hydrochloride, (2α,6α,11*R**)-; (2) (2*R**,6*R**,11*R**)-1,2,3,4,5,6-Hexahydro-6,11-dimethyl-3-(3-methyl-2-butenyl)-2,6-methano-3-benzazocin-8-ol hydrochloride. *UNII-A36BXO4PPX. CAS-64024-15-3; CAS-359-83-1* [pentazocine]. *Analgesic.* Talwin (Sanofi Aventis)

Pentazocine Lactate [*1969*] (pen taz′ oh seen lak′ tate). $C_{19}H_{27}NO$.$C_3H_6O_3$. 375.50. (1) 2,6-Methano-3-benzazocin-8-ol, 1,2,3,4,5,6-hexahydro-6,11-dimethyl-3-(3-methyl-2-butenyl)-, (2α,6α,11*R**)-, compd. with 2-hydroxypropanoic acid (1:1); (2) (2*R**,6*R**,11*R**)-

1,2,3,4,5,6-Hexahydro-6,11-dimethyl-3-(3-methyl-2-butenyl)-2,6-methano-3-benzazocin-8-ol lactate (salt). *UNII-1P2XIB510O. CAS-17146-95-1; CAS-359-83-1* [pentazocine]. *Analgesic.* Talwin (Hospira)

Pentetate Calcium Trisodium [*1964*] (pen′ te tate kal′ see um trye soe′ dee um). $C_{14}H_{18}CaN_3Na_3O_{10}$. 497.35. [Calcium Trisodium Pentetate is INN and BAN.] (1) Calciate(3-), [*N,N*-bis[2-[bis(carboxymethyl)amino]ethyl]-glycinato(5-)]-, trisodium; (2) Trisodium [*N,N*-bis[2-[bis(carboxymethyl)amino]ethyl]glycinato(5-)]calciate(3-). *UNII-G79YN26H5B; UNII-7A314HQM0I* [pentetic acid]. *CAS-12111-24-9; CAS-67-43-6* [pentetic acid]. *Chelating agent (plutonium).* ◇*NSC-34249*

Pentetate Calcium Trisodium Yb 169 [*1971*] (pen′ te tate kal′ see um trye soe′ dee um). (1) Calciate(3-), [*N,N*-bis[2-[bis(carboxymethyl)amino]ethyl]glycinato(5-)]-, trisodium, labeled with ytterbium-169; (2) Trisodium [*N,N*-bis[2-[bis(carboxymethyl)amino]ethyl]glycinato(5-)]calciate(3-), labeled with ytterbium-169. *Radioactive agent.* ◇*Material A; Compound 24266; MRP-10*

Pentetate Indium Disodium In 111 [*1979*] (pen′ te tate in′ dee um dye soe′ dee um). $C_{14}H_{18}{}^{111}InN_3Na_2O_{10}$. (1) Indate(2-)-$^{111}In$-, [*N,N*-bis[2-[bis(carboxymethyl)amino]ethyl]glycinato(5-)]-, disodium; (2) Disodium [*N,N*-bis[2-[bis(carboxymethyl)amino]ethyl]glycinato(5-)]indate(2-)-^{111}In. *CAS-60662-14-8. Diagnostic aid; radioactive agent.*

Pentethylcyclanone — *See* Cyclexanone.

Pentetic Acid [*1977*] (pen tet′ ik as′ id). USP. $C_{14}H_{23}N_3O_{10}$. 393.35. (1) Glycine, *N,N*-bis[2-[bis(carboxymethyl)amino]ethyl]-; (2) Diethylenetriaminepentaacetic acid. [Note—The sodium salts are named as follows: pentetate monosodium (1 Na ion); pentetate disodium (2 Na ions); pentetate trisodium (3 Na ions); pentetate tetrasodium (4 Na ions); pentetate pentasodium (5 Na ions).] *UNII-7A314HQM0I. CAS-67-43-6.* INN; BAN. *Diagnostic aid.* ◇*DTPA*

Pentetrazol (INN, BAN, DCF) — *See* Pentylenetetrazol.

Pentetreotide. $C_{63}H_{87}N_{13}O_{19}S_2$. 1394.57. *N*-[2-[[2-[Bis(carboxymethyl)amino]ethyl](carboxymethyl)amino]ethyl]-*N*-(carboxymethyl)glycyl-D-phenylalanyl-L-cysteinyl-L-phenylalanyl-D-tryptophyl-L-lysyl-L-threonyl-*N*-[(1*R*,2*R*)-2-hydroxy-1-(hydroxymethyl)propyl]-L-cysteinamide cyclic (3→8)-disulfide. *UNII-G083B71P98. CAS-138661-02-6.* INN; BAN. ◇*SDZ 215-811; SDZ 215-811s; DTPA-SMS*

Penthienate Bromide. $C_{18}H_{30}BrNO_3S$. 420.40. [Penthienate is BAN.] (1) Diethyl(2-hydroxyethyl)methylammonium bromide α-cyclopentyl-2-thiopheneglycolate; (2) 2-(2-Cyclopentyl-2-hydroxy-2-(thiophen-2-yl)acetoxy)-*N,N*-diethyl-*N*-methylethanaminium bromide. *CAS-60-44-6; CAS-22064-27-3* [penthienate]. NF XIII; MI. Monodral Bromide (Sterling Winthrop)

Penthrichloral. $C_7H_{11}Cl_3O_4$. 265.52. 5,5-Di(hydroxymethyl)-2-trichloromethyl-1,3-dioxan. *UNII-ADN850L91I. CAS-5684-90-2.* INN; BAN; DCF.

Pentiapine Maleate [*1987*] (pen tye′ a peen mal′ ee ate). $C_{15}H_{17}N_5S \cdot C_4H_4O_4$. 415.47. [Pentiapine is INN.] (1) Imidazo[2,1-*b*][1,3,5]benzothiadiazepine, 5-(4-methyl-1-piperazinyl)-, (*Z*)-2-butenedioate(1:1); (2) 5-(4-Methyl-1-piperazinyl)imidazo[2,1-*b*][1,3,5]benzothiadiazepine maleate (1:1). *CAS-81382-52-7. Antipsychotic.* ◇*CGS 10746B*

Penticide — *See* Chlorophenothane.

Pentifylline. $C_{13}H_{20}N_4O_2$. 264.32. 1-Hexyltheobromine. *UNII-MBM1C4K26S. CAS-1028-33-7.* INN; DCF; BAN; MI.

---

† Brand name formerly used, and/or firm no longer concerned with this product.

Pentigetide [*1988*] (pen tye′ je tide). $C_{22}H_{36}N_8O_{11}$. 588.57. (1) L-Arginine, N^2-[1-[N-(N-L-α-aspartyl-L-seryl)-L-α-aspartyl]-L-prolyl]-; (2) N^2-[1-[N-(N-L-α-Aspartyl-L-seryl)-L-α-aspartyl]-L-prolyl]-L-arginine. *CAS-62087-72-3*. INN. *Anti-allergic*. Pentyde (Immunetech) ◇*HEPP; Pentapeptide DSDPR; IgE Pentapeptide*

Pentisomicin [*1979*] (pen tis″ oh mye′ sin). $C_{19}H_{37}N_5O_7$. 447.53. (1) D-*myo*-Inositol, O-3-deoxy-4-C-methyl-3-(methylamino)-β-L-arabinopyranosyl-(1→1)-O-[2,6-diamino-2,3,4,6-tetradeoxy-α-D-*glycero*-hex-4-enopyranosyl-(1→3)]-4,6-diamino-4,5,6-trideoxy-; (2) O-3-Deoxy-4-C-methyl-3-(methylamino)-β-L-arabinopyranosyl-(1→1)-O-[2,6-diamino-2,3,4,6-tetradeoxy-α-D-*glycero*-hex-4-enopyranosyl-(1→3)]-4,6-diamino-4,5,6-trideoxy-D-*myo*-inositol. *CAS-55870-64-9*. INN. *Anti-infective*. ◇*Sch 22591*

Pentisomide. $C_{19}H_{33}N_3O$. 319.48. (±)-α-[2-(Diisopropylamino)ethyl]-α-isobutyl-2-pyridineacetamide. *CAS-96513-83-6*. INN.

Pentizidone Sodium [*1977*] (pen ti′ zi done soe′ dee um). $C_8H_{11}N_2NaO_3 \cdot \frac{1}{2}H_2O$. 215.18. [Pentizidone is INN.] (1) 3-Isoxazolidinone, 4-[(1-methyl-3-oxo-1-butenyl)amino]-, monosodium salt, hemihydrate, (R)-; (2) (R)-4-[(1-Methyl-3-oxo-1-butenyl)amino]-3-isoxazolidinone monosodium salt hemihydrate. *CAS-59831-62-8; CAS-55694-83-2* [pentizidone]. *Antibacterial*.

Pentobarbital (pen″ toe bar′ bi tal). **USP.** $C_{11}H_{18}N_2O_3$. 226.27. [Pentobarbital Calcium is JAN.] (1) 2,4,6(1H,3H,5H)-Pyrimidinetrione, 5-ethyl-5-(1-methylbutyl)-, (±)-; (2) (±)-5-Ethyl-5-(1-methylbutyl)barbituric

acid. *UNII-I4744080IR*. *CAS-76-74-4*. INN; BAN. *Sedative-hypnotic*. Nembutal (Ovation) [*Name previously used: Pentobarbitone.*]

Pentobarbital Sodium (pen″ toe bar′ bi tal soe′ dee um). **USP.** $C_{11}H_{17}N_2NaO_3$. 248.25. (1) 2,4,6(1H,3H,5H)-Pyrimidinetrione, 5-ethyl-5-(1-methylbutyl), monosodium salt; (2) Sodium 5-ethyl-5-(1-methylbutyl)barbiturate. *UNII-NJJ0475N0S; UNII-I4744080IR* [pentobarbital]. *CAS-57-33-0; CAS-76-74-4* [pentobarbital]. JAN. *Sedative-hypnotic*. Nembutal Sodium (Ovation)

Pentolinium Tartrate. $C_{23}H_{42}N_2O_{12}$. 538.59. [Pentolonium Tartrate is INN and BAN.] Pyrrolidinium 1,1′-(1,5-pentanediyl)bis-[1-methyl-, [R-(R^*,R^*)]-2,3-dihydroxybutanedioate. *UNII-953357GACY*. *CAS-52-62-0; CAS-144-44-5* [pentolinium]. NF XIV; MI. Ansolysen (Wyeth)

Pentolonium Tartrate (INN, BAN) — *See* Pentolinium Tartrate.

Pentolonum Bitartrate — *See* Pentolinium Tartrate.

Pentomone [*1979*] (pen′ toe mone). $C_{24}H_{26}O_5$. 394.46. (1) 5aH,13H-[1]Benzopyrano[3,2-b]xanthen-13-one, 6,6a,12,12a,13a,14-hexahydro-4,8-dimethoxy-6,6-dimethyl-, (5aα,6aα,12aα,13aα)-; (2) 6,6aα,12,12aα,13aα,14-Hexahydro-4,8-dimethoxy-6,6-dimethyl-5aαH,13H-[1]benzopyrano[3,2-b]xanthen-13-one. *CAS-67102-87-8*. INN. *Prostate growth inhibitor*. ◇*Compound 113935*

Pentopril [*1985*] (pen′ toe pril). $C_{18}H_{23}NO_5$. 333.38. (1) 1H-Indole-1-pentanoic acid, 2-carboxy-2,3-dihydro-α,γ-dimethyl-δ-oxo-, ethyl ester, [2S-[1(αS^*,γS^*),2R^*]]-; (2) Ethyl (αR,γR,2S)-2-carboxy-α,γ-dimethyl-δ-oxo-1-indolinevalerate. *UNII-Z99269057A*. *CAS-82924-03-6*. INN. *Enzyme inhibitor (angiotensin-converting)*. ◇*CGS 13945*

Pentorex. $C_{11}H_{17}N$. 163.26. α,α,β-Trimethylphenethylamine. *UNII-K97CJK0FXR*. *CAS-434-43-5*. INN; DCF.

Pentosalen. 9-(3-Methylbut-2-enyloxy)furo[3,2-*g*]chromen-7-one. *CAS-482-44-0.* BAN.

Pentosan Polysulfate Sodium [*1988*] (pen′ toe san pol″ ee sul′ fate soe′ dee um). $[C_5H_6Na_2O_{10}S_2]_n$ (*n* = 6 to 12). (1) 4-*O*-Methyl-α-D-glucurono-β-D-xylan, hydrogen sulfate, sodium salt; (2) (4-*O*-Methyl-α-D-glucurono)-(1→2)-(1→4)-β-D-xylopyranan, hydrogen sulfate, sodium salt. *UNII-914032762Y. CAS-140207-93-8; CAS-116001-96-8* [replaced]. INN; BAN. *Anti-inflammatory (interstitial cystitis).* Elmiron (Ortho-McNeil) *[Name previously used: Pentosan Polysulphate Sodium.]* ◇SP54; PZ68

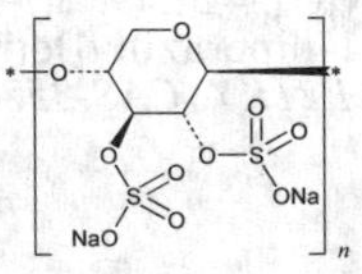

Pentostatin [*1977*] (pen″ toe stat′ in). $C_{11}H_{16}N_4O_4$. 268.27. (1) Imidazo[4,5-*d*][1,3]diazepin-8-ol, 3-(2-deoxy-β-D-*erythro*-pentofuranosyl)-3,6,7,8-tetrahydro-, (*R*)-; (2) (*R*)-3-(2-Deoxy-β-D-*erythro*-pentofuranosyl)-3,6,7,8-tetrahydroimidazo[4,5-*d*][1,3]diazepin-8-ol. *UNII-395575MZO7. CAS-53910-25-1.* INN; BAN; JAN. *Potentiator.* Nipent (Hospira) ◇CI-825; PD 81565; NSC-218321

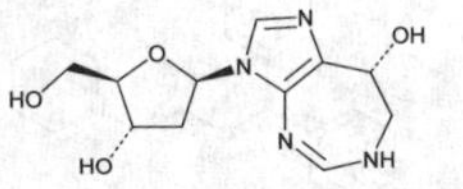

Pentoxifylline [*1976*] (pen″ tox if′ i lin). **USP.** $C_{13}H_{18}N_4O_3$. 278.31. [Oxpentifylline is BAN.] (1) 1*H*-Purine-2,6-dione, 3,7-dihydro-3,7-dimethyl-1-(5-oxohexyl)-; (2) 1-(5-Oxohexyl)theobromine. *UNII-SD6QCT3TSU. CAS-6493-05-6.* INN; BAN; JAN. *Vasodilator.* Pentoxil (Upsher Smith); Trental (Sanofi Aventis) ◇BL 191

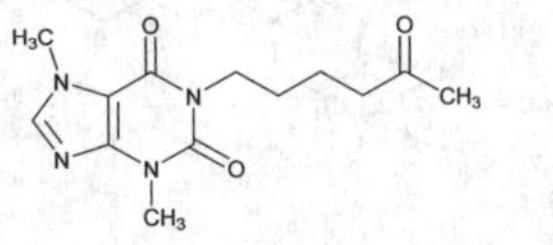

Pentoxyverine (INN, BAN, DCF) — *See* Carbetapentane Citrate.

Pentoxyverine Citrate (JAN) — *See* Carbetapentane Citrate.

Pentrinitrol [*1973*] (pen″ trye nye′ trol). $C_5H_9N_3O_{10}$. 271.14. (1) 1,3-Propanediol, 2,2-bis[(nitrooxy)methyl]-, mononitrate (ester); (2) Pentaerythritol trinitrate. *CAS-1607-17-6.* INN. *Vasodilator (coronary).* Petrin (Parke-Davis†) ◇W 2197

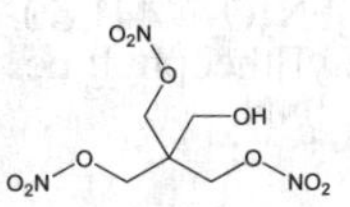

Pentylenetetrazol. $C_6H_{10}N_4$. 138.17. [Pentetrazol is INN and BAN.] 6,7,8,9-Tetrahydro-5*H*-tetrazoloazepine. *CAS-54-95-5.* NF XIII; MI. Cardiazol (Knoll†)

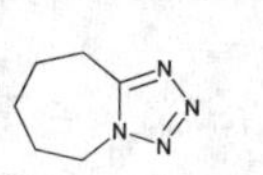

Pentymal — *See* Amobarbital.

Pepleomycin — *See* Peplomycin Sulfate.

Peplomycin Sulfate [*1981*] (pep″ loe mye′ sin sul′ fate). $C_{61}H_{88}N_{18}O_{21}S_2 \cdot H_2SO_4$. 1571.67. [Peplomycin is INN.] (1) Bleomycinamide, N^1-[3-[(1-phenylethyl)amino]propyl]-, (*S*)-, sulfate (1:1) (salt); (2) N^1-[3-[[(*S*)-(α-Methylbenzyl)]amino]propyl]bleomycinamide sulfate (1:1) (salt). *CAS-70384-29-1* [sulfate salt, 1:1]; *CAS-68247-85-8* [peplomycin]. JAN. *Antineoplastic.* ◇NK-631

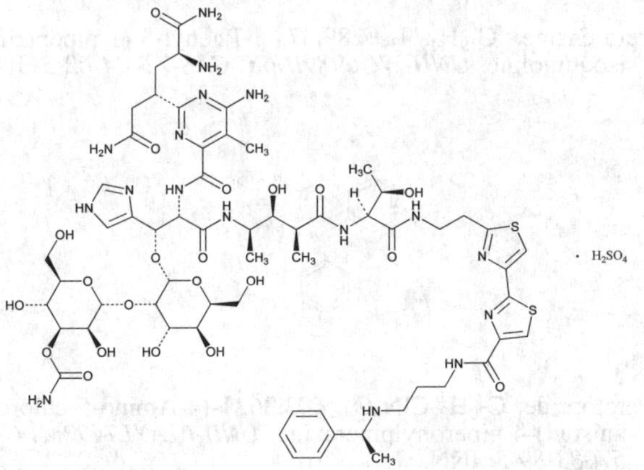

Peppermint (pep′ er mint). **NF.** The dried leaf and flowering top of *Mentha piperita* Linné (Fam. Labiatae). *UNII-V95R5KMY2B. Pharmaceutic aid (flavor); pharmaceutic aid (perfume).*

Peppermint Oil (pep′ er mint). **NF.** The volatile oil distilled with steam from the fresh overground parts of the flowering plant of *Mentha piperita* Linné (Fam. Labiatae), rectified by distillation and neither partially nor wholly dementholized. *CAS-8006-90-4. Pharmaceutic aid (flavor).*

Pepstatin [*1972*] (pep stat′ in). $C_{34}H_{63}N_5O_9$. 685.89. (1) Pepstatin A; (2) *N*-(3-Methyl-1-oxobutyl)-L-valyl-L-valyl-4-amino-3-hydroxy-6-methylheptanoyl-L-alanyl-4-amino-3-hydroxy-6-methylheptanoic acid. *CAS-26305-03-3; CAS-39324-30-6* [nonspecific]. INN. *Enzyme inhibitor (pepsin).*

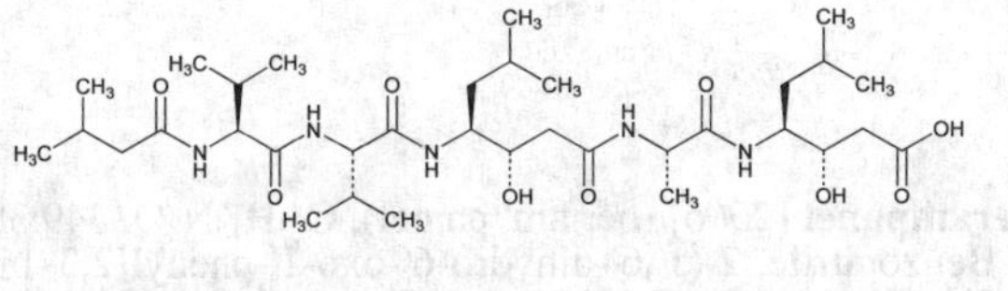

---

† Brand name formerly used, and/or firm no longer concerned with this product.

Peraclopone. $C_{20}H_{23}Cl_2N_3O_2$. 408.32. *p*-Chlorobenzaldehyde (±)-(*E*)-*O*-[3-[4-(*o*-chlorophenyl)-1-piperazinyl]-2-hydroxypropyl]oxime. *UNII-231HZQ66PD. CAS-96164-19-1.* INN.

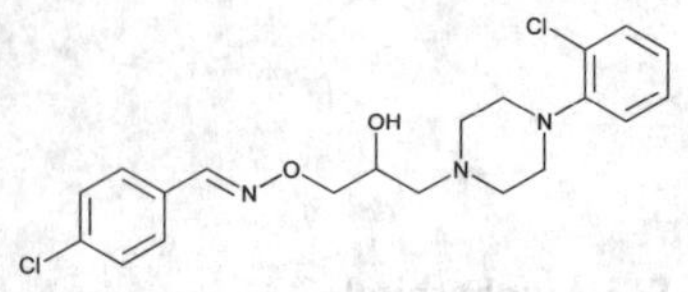

Peradoxime. $C_{22}H_{29}N_3O_4$. 399.48. *m*-Anisaldehyde *O*-[2-hydroxy-3-[4-(*o*-methoxyphenyl)-1-piperazinyl]propyl] oxime. *UNII-7A977PW795. CAS-67254-81-3.* INN.

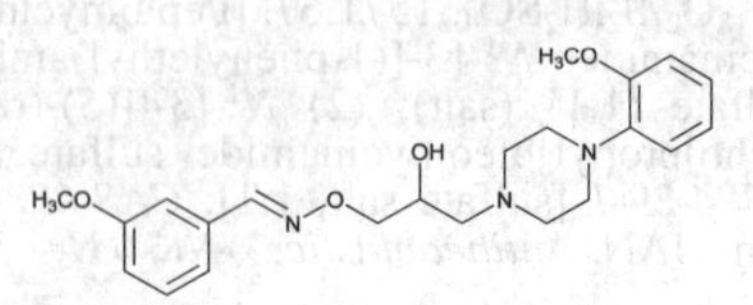

Perafensine. $C_{19}H_{19}N_3$. 289.37. 1-Phenyl-3-(1-piperazinyl) isoquinoline. *UNII-WU6989IN6X. CAS-72444-62-3.* INN.

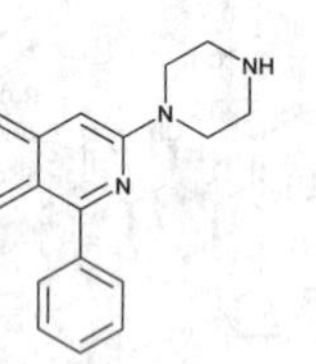

Peralopride. $C_{20}H_{22}ClN_3O_4$. 403.86. 1-(4-Amino-5-chloro-*o*-anisoyl)-4-piperonylpiperazine. *UNII-61AYL7492M. CAS-57083-89-3.* INN.

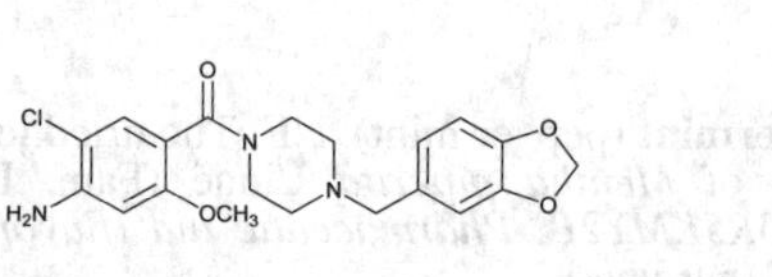

Peramivir [*2002*] (per am′ i vir). $C_{15}H_{28}N_4O_4.3H_2O$. 382.45. (1) Cyclopentanecarboxylic acid, 3-[(1*S*)-1-(acetylamino)-2-ethylbutyl]-4-[(aminoiminomethyl)amino]-2-hydroxy-, trihydrate (1*S*,2*S*,3*R*,4*R*); (2) (1*S*,2*S*,3*R*,4*R*)-3-[(1*S*)-1-Acetylamino-2-ethylbutyl]-4-[(aminoiminomethyl)amino]-2-hydroxycyclopentanecarboxylic acid, trihydrate. *UNII-QW7Y7ZR15U. CAS-229614-55-5* (monohydrate). INN. *Treatment and prevention of influenza A and B viruses (neuroaminidase inhibitor).* ◇*RWJ-270201*

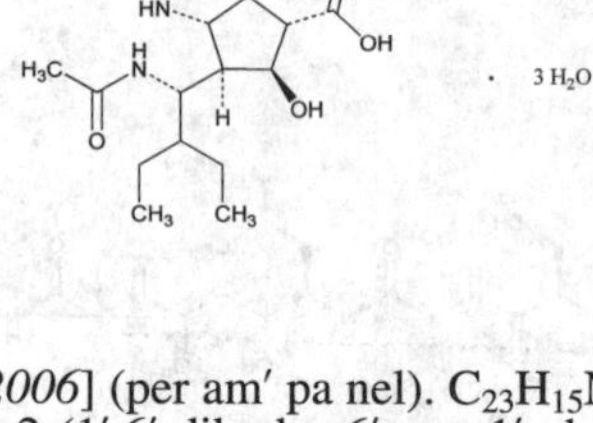

Perampanel [*2006*] (per am′ pa nel). $C_{23}H_{15}N_3O$. 349.38. (1) Benzonitrile, 2-(1′,6′-dihydro-6′-oxo-1′-phenyl[2,3′-bipyridin]-5′-yl)-; (2) 5′-(2-Cyanophenyl)-1′-phenyl-2,3′-bipyridinyl-6′(1′*H*)-one. *UNII-H821664NPK. CAS-380917-97-5.* INN. *AMPA-type glutamate receptor antagonist.* ◇*E2007; ER-155055-90*

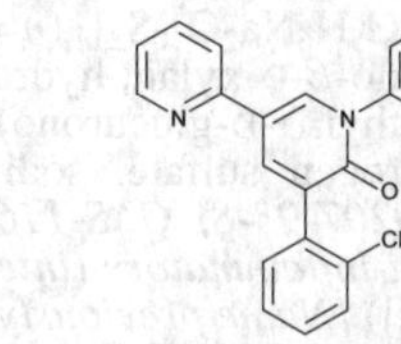

Peraquinsin. $C_{23}H_{28}N_4O_4$. 424.49. 6,7-Dimethoxy-2-[2-[4-(*o*-methoxyphenyl)-1-piperazinyl]ethyl]-4(3*H*)-quinazolinone. *UNII-5726CF21KY. CAS-35265-50-0.* INN.

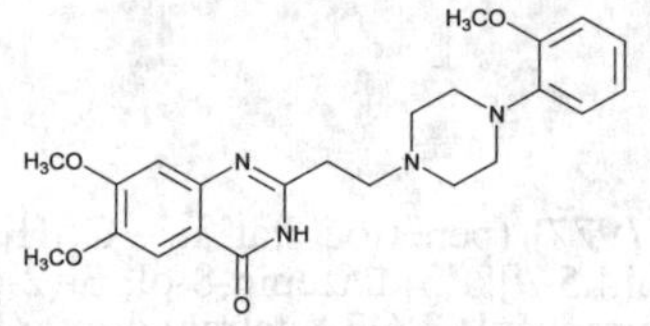

Perastine. $C_{20}H_{25}NO$. 295.42. 1-[2-(Diphenylmethoxy)ethyl]-piperidine. *UNII-BJ563H8V4W. CAS-4960-10-5.* INN.

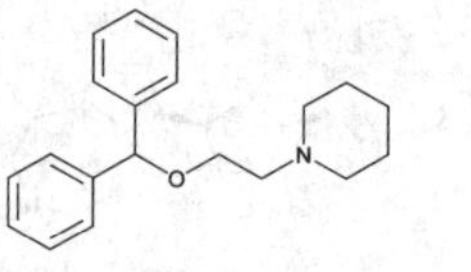

Peratizole. $C_{17}H_{26}N_4S_2$. 350.55. 1-[4-(2,4-Dimethyl-5-thiazolyl)butyl]-4-(4-methyl-2-thiazolyl)piperazine. *UNII-17071G0W3C. CAS-29952-13-4.* INN; BAN. ◇*EMD 19698 [as hydrogen maleate]*

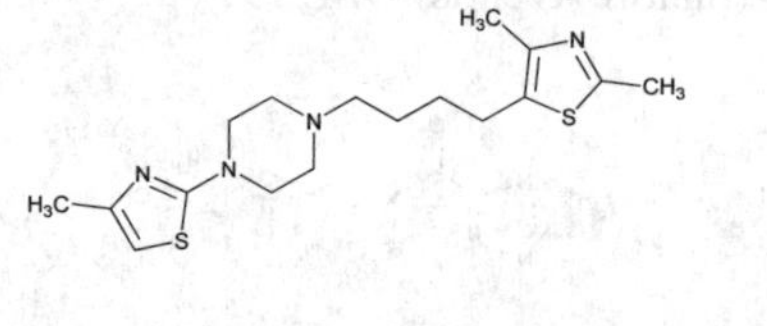

Perazine Fendizoate. $C_{20}H_{25}N_3S.2C_{20}H_{14}O_4$. 976.14. [Perazine Maleate is JAN.] 10-[3-(4-Methylpiperazin-1-yl)propyl]phenothiazine difendizoate. *UNII-8915147A2B* [perazine]. *CAS-84-97-9* [perazine]; *CAS-14516-56-4* [perazine maleate]. JAN.

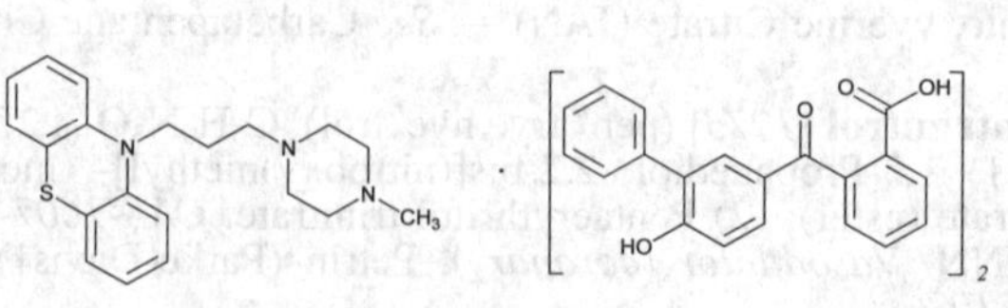

Perbufylline. $C_{23}H_{28}FN_5O_3$. 441.50. 7-[4-[4-(*p*-Fluorobenzoyl)piperidino]butyl]theophylline. *UNII-M69H5TDQ1K. CAS-110390-84-6.* INN.

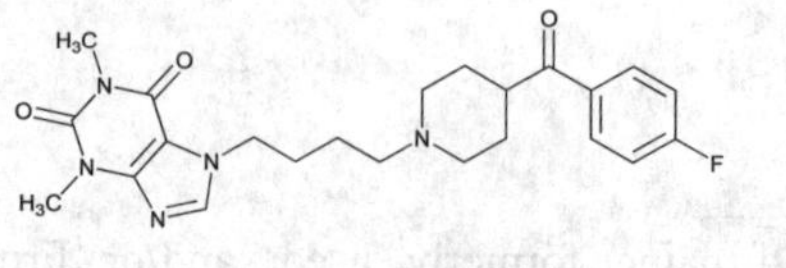

Peretinoin. C₂₀H₃₀O₂. 302.45. (2*E*,4*E*,6*E*,10*E*)-3,7,11,15-Tetramethylhexadeca-2,4,6,10,14-pentaenoic acid. *CAS-81485-25-8.* INN.

Perfilcon A [*1978*] (per fil′ kon). (C₆H₁₀O₃)ₓ(C₆H₉NO)ᵧ(C₄H₆O₂)ᵤ. (1) 2-Propenoic acid, 2-methyl-, 2-hydroxyethyl ester polymer with 1-ethenyl-2-pyrrolidinone and 2-methyl-2-propenoic acid; (2) 2-Hydroxyethyl methacrylate polymer with 1-vinyl-2-pyrrolidinone and methacrylic acid. *CAS-37017-46-2.* *Contact lens material (hydrophilic).* Permalens (CooperVision)

Perflenapent [*1996*] (per flen′ a pent). C₅F₁₂. 288.03. (1) Pentane, dodecafluoro-; (2) Dodecafluoropentane. *CAS-678-26-2.* INN. *Diagnostic aid.* [*Note—The trademark EchoGen Emulsion has been selected for the mixture of Perflenapent and Perflisopent in a ratio of 85:15, respectively.*] ◇*FC41-12 (Perflenapent/Perflisopent mixture)*

Perflexane [*1999*] (per flex′ ane). C₆F₁₄. 338.04. (1) Hexane, tetradecafluoro-; (2) Tetradecafluorohexane. *UNII-FX3WJ41CMX.* CAS-355-42-0. INN. *(1) Diagnostic aid. [Note—Perflexane is a component of Imagent (AF0150), an echopharmaceutical for contrast enhancement during ultrasound studies.]* ◇*AF0150*

Perflisobutane. C₄F₁₀. 238.03. 1,1,1,2,3,3,3-Heptafluoro-2-(trifluoromethyl)propane. *UNII-7W4TAI502Z.* *CAS-354-92-7.* INN.

Perflisopent [*1996*] (per flye′ soe pent). C₅F₁₂. 288.03. (1) Butane, 1,1,1,2,2,3,4,4,4-nonafluoro-3-(trifluoromethyl)-; (2) Nonafluoro-2-(trifluoromethyl)butane. *CAS-594-91-2.* INN. *Diagnostic aid. [Note—The trademark EchoGen Emulsion has been selected for the mixture of Perflenapent and Perflisopent in a ratio of 85:15, respectively.]* ◇*FC41-12 (Perflenapent/Perflisopent mixture)*

Perfluamine. C₉F₂₁N. 521.07. Heneicosafluorotripropylamine. *CAS-338-83-0.* INN; BAN.

Perflubrodec [*2001*] (per floo′ broe dek). C₁₀BrF₂₁. 598.98. (1) Decane, 1-bromo-1,1,2,2,,3,3,4,4,5,5,6,6,7,7,8,8,9,9,10,10,10-heneicosafluoro-; (2) 1-Bromoheneicosafluorodecane. *UNII-4818HEA280.* CAS-307-43-7. INN. *Treatment of acute anemia (component of an intravascular temporary oxygen carrier that is intended to enhance oxygen transport).* Component of Oxygent (Atofina) ◇*AF0144*

Perflubron [*1991*] (per floo′ bron). **USP.** C₈BrF₁₇. 498.96. (1) Octane, 1-bromo-1,1,2,2,3,3,4,4,5,5,6,6,7,7,8,8,8-heptadecafluoro-; (2) 1-Bromoheptadecafluorooctane; (3) Perfluorooctyl bromide. *UNII-Q1D0Q7R4D9.* CAS-423-55-2. INN. *Blood substitute.* Imagent (Alliance)

Perflubutane [*2005*] (per floo′ bue tane). C₄F₁₀. 238.03. (1) Butane, decafluoro-; (2) Decafluorobutane. *UNII-SE4TWR0K2C.* CAS-355-25-9. INN. *Ultrasound contrast agent intended for assessing myocardial perfusion in patients with coronary artery disease.* ◇*AI-700*

Perflunafene. C₁₀F₁₈. 462.08. Octadecafluorodecahydronaphthalene. *CAS-306-94-5.* INN; BAN.

Perfluorooctylbromide — *See* Perflubron.

Perflutren [*1999*] (per floo′ tren). C₃F₈. 188.02. (1) Propane, octafluoro-; (2) Octafluoropropane. *UNII-CK0N3WH0SR.* CAS-76-19-7. INN. *Ultrasound contrast imaging in cardiology and radiology (diagnostic).* Definity (Bristol-Myers Squibb) ◇*DMP 115; FS069; MRX-115*

Perflutren Protein-Type A Microspheres (per floo′ tren proe′ teen mye′ kroe sfeerz″). **USP** [Injectable Suspension]. A sterile, nonpyrogenic suspension of microspheres produced by dispersing perflutren (octafluoropropane) gas in an aqueous solution of diluted sterile albumin human.

---

† Brand name formerly used, and/or firm no longer concerned with this product.

Perfomedil. $C_{19}H_{29}NO_4$. 335.44. (±)-2′,4′,6′-Trimethoxy-4-(3-methylpiperidino)butyrophenone. *UNII-8A8NY1Z12E. CAS-92268-40-1.* INN.

Perfosfamide [*1991*] (per fos′ fa mide). $C_7H_{15}Cl_2N_2O_4P$. 293.08. (1) Hydroperoxide, 2-[bis(2-chloroethyl)amino]-tetrahydro-2*H*-1,3,2-oxazaphosphorin-4-yl, *P*-oxide, *cis*-(±)-; (2) (±)-*cis*-2-[Bis(2-chloroethyl)amino]tetrahydro-2*H*-1,3,2-oxazaphosphorin-4-yl hydroperoxide, *P*-oxide. *CAS-62435-42-1.* INN. *Antineoplastic.* Pergamid (Scios Nova) ◇*4-HC; NSC-181815*

Pergolide Mesylate [*1979*] (per′ goe lide mes′ i late). **USP.** $C_{19}H_{26}N_2S \cdot CH_4O_3S$. 410.59. [Pergolide is INN and BAN.] (1) Ergoline, 8-[(methylthio)methyl]-6-propyl-, monomethanesulfonate, (8β)-; (2) 8β-[(Methylthio)methyl]-6-propylergoline monomethanesulfonate. *UNII-55B9HQY616; UNII-24MJ822NZ9* [pergolide]. *CAS-66104-23-2; CAS-66104-22-1* [pergolide]. *Dopamine agonist.* Permax (Valeant) ◇*LY 127809*

Perhexiline Maleate [*1966*] (per hex′ i leen mal′ ee ate). $C_{19}H_{35}N \cdot C_4H_4O_4$. 393.56. [Perhexiline is INN and BAN.] (1) Piperidine, 2-(2,2-dicyclohexylethyl)-, (*Z*)-2-butenedioate (1:1); (2) 2-(2,2-Dicyclohexylethyl)piperidine maleate (1:1). *CAS-6724-53-4; CAS-6621-47-2* [perhexiline]. *Vasodilator (coronary).* Pexid (Marion Merrell Dow†)

Periciazine. $C_{21}H_{23}N_3OS$. 365.49. [Periciazine is BAN; Propericiazine is JAN.] 10-[3-(4-Hydroxypiperidino)propyl]phenothiazine-2-carbonitrile. *UNII-3405M6FD73. CAS-2622-26-6.* INN; MI. ◇*RP 8909; SKF 20716*

Pericyazine (BAN) — *See* Periciazine.

Perifosine. $C_{25}H_{52}NO_4P$. 461.66. 1,1-Dimethylpiperidinium-4-yl octadecyl phosphate, inner salt. *UNII-2GWV496552. CAS-157716-52-4.* INN.

Perimetazine. $C_{22}H_{28}N_2O_2S$. 384.53. 1-[3-(2-Methoxyphenothiazin-10-yl)-2-methylpropyl]-4-piperidinol. *UNII-2R880S54IS. CAS-13093-88-4.* INN; DCF; MI. ◇*AN 1317; RP 9159*

Perindopril [*1988*] (per in′ doe pril). $C_{19}H_{32}N_2O_5$. 368.47. (1) 1*H*-Indole-2-carboxylic acid, 1-[2-[[1-(ethoxycarbonyl)butyl]amino]-1-oxopropyl]octahydro-, [2*S*-[1[*R**(*R**)],2α,3aβ,7aβ]]-; (2) (2*S*,3a*S*,7a*S*)-1-[(*S*)-*N*-[(*S*)-1-Carboxybutyl]alanyl]hexahydro-2-indolinecarboxylic acid, 1-ethyl ester. *UNII-Y5GMK36KGY. CAS-82834-16-0.* INN; BAN. *Enzyme inhibitor (angiotensin-converting).* ◇*S-9490; McN-A-2833*

Perindopril Erbumine [*1989*] (per in′ doe pril er′ bue meen). $C_{19}H_{32}N_2O_5 \cdot C_4H_{11}N$. 441.60. (1) 1*H*-Indole-2-carboxylic acid, 1-[2-[[1-(ethoxycarbonyl)butyl]amino]-1-oxopropyl]octahydro-, [2*S*-[1[*R**(*R**)],2α,3aβ,7aβ]]-, compd. with 2-methyl-2-propanamine (1:1); (2) (2*S*,3a*S*,7a*S*)-1-[(*S*)-*N*-[(*S*)-1-Carboxybutyl]alanyl]hexahydro-2-indolinecarboxylic acid, 1-ethyl ester, compound with *tert*-butylamine (1:1). *UNII-1964X464OJ. CAS-107133-36-8.* *Antihypertensive.* Aceon (Solvay Pharmaceuticals) ◇*S-9490-3; McN-A-2833-109*

Perindoprilat. $C_{17}H_{28}N_2O_5$. 340.41. (2*S*,3a*S*,7a*S*)-1-[(*S*)-*N*-[(*S*)-1-Carboxybutyl]alanyl]hexahydro-2-indolinecarboxylic acid. *UNII-2UV6ZNQ92K. CAS-95153-31-4.* INN; BAN. ◇*S-9780*

Perisoxal. $C_{16}H_{20}N_2O_2$. 272.34. [Perisoxal Citrate is JAN.] α-(5-Phenyl-3-isoxazolyl)-1-piperidineethanol. *CAS-2055-44-9*. INN; MI.

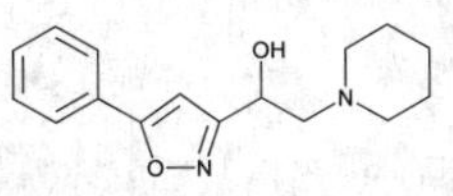

Perlapine [*1970*] (per′ la peen). $C_{19}H_{21}N_3$. 291.39. (1) 11*H*-Dibenz[*b,e*]azepine, 6-(4-methyl-1-piperazinyl)-; (2) 6-(4-Methyl-1-piperazinyl)morphanthridine. *UNII-4N8UJ-J27IM*. *CAS-1977-11-3*. INN; BAN; JAN. *Sedative-hypnotic.* ◇*AW 14′2333*

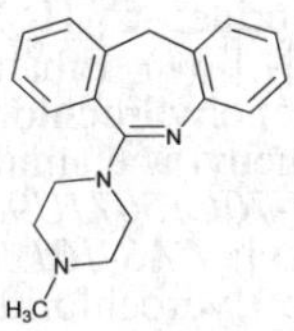

Permethrin [*1987*] (per meth′ rin). $C_{21}H_{20}Cl_2O_3$. 391.29. (1) Cyclopropanecarboxylic acid, 3-(2,2-dichloroethenyl)-2,2-dimethyl-, (3-phenoxyphenyl)methyl ester; (2) *m*-Phenoxybenzyl (±)-3-(2,2-dichlorovinyl)-2,2-dimethylcyclopropanecarboxylate; (3) (±)-3-Phenoxybenzyl 3-(2,2-dichlorovinyl)-2,2-dimethylcyclopropanecarboxylate. *UNII-509F88P9SZ*. *CAS-52645-53-1*. INN; BAN. *Ectoparasiticide.* Elimite (Allergan); Nix (Insight)

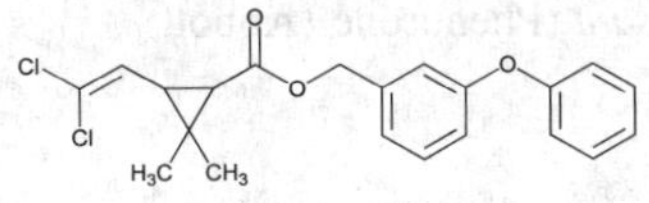

Perospirone. $C_{23}H_{30}N_4O_2S$. 426.57. *cis-N*-[4-[4-(1,2-Benzisothiazol-3-yl)-1-piperazinyl]butyl]-1,2-cyclohexanedicarboximide. *UNII-N303OK87DT*. *CAS-150915-41-6*. INN.

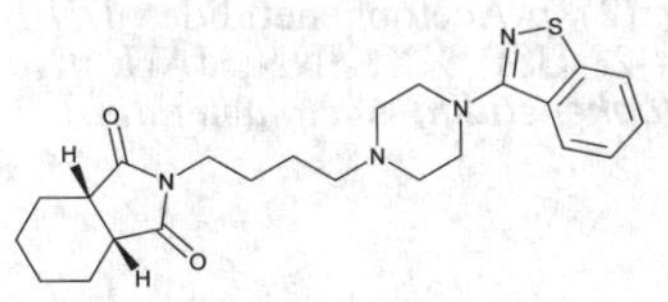

Perphenazine (per fen′ a zeen). **USP**. $C_{21}H_{26}ClN_3OS$. 403.97. [Perphenazine Fendizoate and Perphenazine Maleate are JAN.] (1) Piperazineethanol, 4-[3-(2-chloro-10*H*-phenothiazin-10-yl)propyl]-; (2) 4-[3-(2-Chlorophenothiazin-10-yl)propyl]-1-piperazineethanol. *UNII-FTA7XXY4EZ*. *CAS-58-39-9*. INN; BAN; JAN. *Antipsychotic.* Trilafon (Schering)

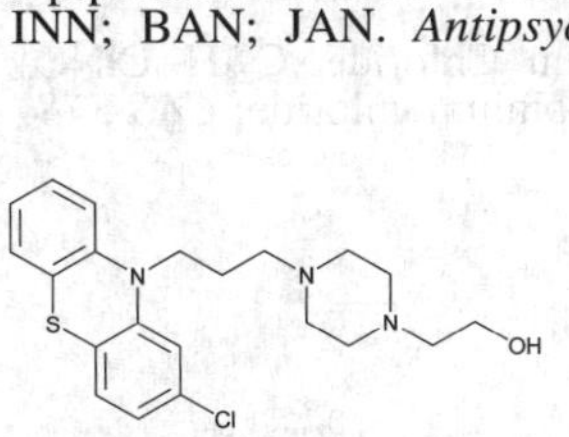

Persic Oil. *CAS-8002-78-6*. NF XVII.

---

† Brand name formerly used, and/or firm no longer concerned with this product.

Persilic Acid. $C_6H_6O_8S_2$. 270.24. 2,5-Dihydroxy-*p*-benzenedisulfonic acid. *UNII-35VER614H0*. *CAS-4444-23-9*. INN.

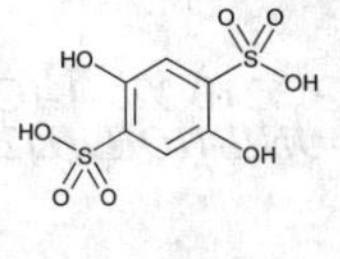

Pertussis Immune Globulin (per tus′ is i mune′ glob′ ue lin). **USP**. A sterile, nonpyrogenic solution of globulins derived from blood plasma of adult human donors who have been immunized with pertussis vaccine. *Immunizing agent (passive).* [*Name previously used: Pertussis Immune Human Globulin.*]

Pertussis Immune Human Globulin (previously used name) — *See* Pertussis Immune Globulin.

Pertussis Vaccine. USP XXVI. *Immunizing agent (active).*

Pertussis Vaccine Adsorbed. USP XXVI. *Immunizing agent (active).*

Pertuzumab [*2003*] (per tooz′ oo mab). Immunoglobulin G1, anti-(human neu (receptor)) (human-mouse monoclonal 2C4 heavy chain), disulfide with human-mouse monoclonal 2C4 κ-chain, dimer. *UNII-K16AIQ8CTM*. *CAS-380610-27-5*. INN; BAN. *Anti-neoplastic.* ◇*rhuMab 2C4*

Peruvian Balsam. *CAS-8007-00-9*. NF XIII.

Perzinfotel [*2004*] (per zin′ foe tel). $C_9H_{13}N_2O_5P$. 260.18. (1) Phosphonic acid, [2-(8,9-dioxo-2,6-diazabicyclo[5.2.0]non-1(7)-en-2-yl)ethyl]-; (2) [2-(8,9-Dioxo-2,6-diazabicyclo[5.2.0]non-1(7)-en-2-yl)ethyl]phosphonic acid. *UNII-FX5AUU7Z8T*. *CAS-144912-63-0*. INN. *Treatment of neuropathic pain (NMDA receptor antagonist).* ◇*EAA-090*

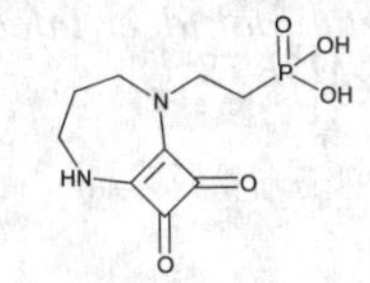

Pethidine (INN, BAN) — *See* Meperidine Hydrochloride.

Pethidine Hydrochloride (JAN) — *See* Meperidine Hydrochloride.

Petrichloral. $C_{13}H_{16}Cl_{12}O_8$. 725.70. 1,1′,1″,1‴-(Neopentanetetryltetraoxy)tetrakis(2,2,2-trichloroethanol). *CAS-78-12-6*. INN.

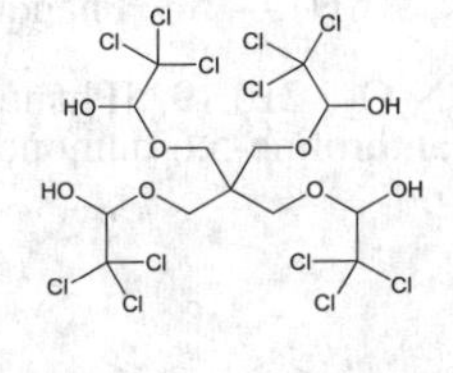

Petrolatum (pet″ roe lay′ tum). **USP**. [Yellow Petrolatum is JAN.] A purified mixture of semisolid hydrocarbons obtained from petroleum. *CAS-8009-03-8*. *Pharmaceutic aid (ointment base).*

Petrolatum, White (pet″ roe lay′ tum). **USP**. A purified mixture of semisolid hydrocarbons obtained from petroleum, and wholly or nearly decolorized. *UNII-4T6H12BN9U*. JAN. *Pharmaceutic aid (ointment base, oleaginous); protectant (topical).* Moroline (Schering-Plough HealthCare†)

Petroleum Jelly — *See* Petrolatum.

Pexacerfont. $C_{18}H_{24}N_6O$. 340.42. N-[(2R)-Butan-2-yl]-8-(6-methoxy-2-methylpyridin-3-yl)-2,7-dimethylpyrazolo[1,5-a][1,3,5]triazin-4-amine. *UNII-LF1VBG4ZUK. CAS-459856-18-9.* INN.

Pexantel. $C_{12}H_{22}N_2O$. 210.32. 1-(Cyclohexylcarbonyl)-4-methylpiperazine. *UNII-HOH9HJ2737. CAS-10001-13-5.* INN.

Pexelizumab [*2000*] (pex″ e liz′ oo mab). (1) Immunoglobulin, anti-(human complement C5 α-chain) (human-mouse monoclonal 5G1.1-SC single chain); (2) Immunoglobulin (human-mouse monoclonal 5G1.1-SC single chain anti-human complement C5 α-chain). Molecular weight is approximately 26,500 daltons. *CAS-219685-93-5.* INN; BAN. *Complement inhibitor used to reduce the impact of complement-mediated injuries sustained during cardiopulmonary bypass (humanized monoclonal antibody).* (Alexion) ◇*h5G1.1 scFv; h5G1.1 scFv (CDR)*

Pexiganan. $C_{122}H_{210}N_{32}O_{22}$. 2477.17. Glycyl-L-isoleucylglycyl-L-lysyl-L-phenylalanyl-L-leucyl-L-lysyl-L-lysyl-L-alanyl-L-lysyl-L-lysyl-L-phenylalanylglycyl-L-lysyl-L-alanyl-L-phenylalanyl-L-valyl-L-lysyl-L-isoleucyl-L-leucyl-L-lysyl-L-lysinamide. *CAS-147664-63-9.* INN.

Pexiganan Acetate [*1998*] (pex″ i gan′ an as′ e tate). $C_{122}H_{210}N_{32}O_{22} \cdot xC_2H_4O_2$. 2477.17 (free base). Glycyl-L-isoleucylglycyl-L-lysyl-L-phenylalanyl-L-leucyl-L-lysyl-L-lysyl-L-alanyl-L-lysyl-L-lysyl-L-phenylalanylglycyl-L-lysyl-L-alanyl-L-phenylalanyl-L-valyl-L-lysyl-L-isoleucyl-L-leucyl-L-lysyl-L-lysinamide acetate. *CAS-172820-23-4. Treatment of diabetic foot ulcer infections (antibacterial).* Cytolex (Abbott) ◇*MSI-78*

GIGKFLKKAK KFGKAFVKIL KK —NH₂   *x* CH₃COOH

PFOB — *See* Perflubron.

PGE₁ (previously used name) — *See* Alprostadil.

PGI₂ (previously used name) — *See* Epoprostenol.

PGX (previously used name) — *See* Epoprostenol.

Phanchinone — *See* Phanquone.

Phanquinone (INN, BAN) — *See* Phanquone.

Phanquone. $C_{12}H_6N_2O_2$. 210.19. [Phanquinone is INN and BAN.] 4,7-Phenanthroline-5,6-quinone. *CAS-84-12-8.* ◇*C-11925*

Phebutazine — *See* Febuverine.

Phebutyrazine — *See* Febuverine.

Phemfilcon A [*1977*] (fem fil′ kon). $(C_6H_{10}O_3)_x(C_8H_{14}O_3)_y$. (1) 2-Propenoic acid, 2-methyl-, 2-hydroxyethyl ester, polymer with 2-ethoxyethyl 2-methyl-2-propenoate; (2) 2-Hydroxyethyl methacrylate polymer with 2-ethoxyethyl

methacrylate. *CAS-29403-23-4. Contact lens material (hydrophilic).* DuraSoft 2 (Wesley-Jessen); DuraSoft 3 (Wesley-Jessen); Fresh Look (Wesley-Jessen)

Phenacaine Hydrochloride. $C_{18}H_{22}N_2O_2 \cdot HCl \cdot H_2O$. 352.86. [Phenacaine is INN.] (1) Ethanimidamide, N,N'-bis(4-ethoxyphenyl)-, monohydrochloride, monohydrate; (2) N,N'-Bis(p-ethoxyphenyl)acetamidine monohydrochloride monohydrate. *UNII-70C1507JU9. CAS-6153-19-1; CAS-620-99-5* [anhydrous]; *CAS-101-93-9* [phenacaine]. USP XXI; MI. Holocaine Hydrochloride (Abbott†)

Phenacemide. $C_9H_{10}N_2O_2$. 178.19. (1) Benzeneacetamide, N-(aminocarbonyl)-; (2) (Phenylacetyl)urea. *UNII-PAI7J52V09. CAS-63-98-9.* USP XXIII; INN; BAN. *Anticonvulsant.* Phenurone (Abbott)

Phenacetin. $C_{10}H_{13}NO_2$. 179.22. (1) Acetamide, N-(4-ethoxyphenol)-; (2) p-Acetophenetidide. *UNII-ER0CTH01H9. CAS-62-44-2.* USP XX; INN; JAN. [*Names previously used: Acetophenetidin; Acetphenetidin.*]

Phenacon — *See* Fenaclon.

Phenactropinium Chloride. $C_{24}H_{28}ClNO_4$. 429.94. N-Phenacylhomatropinium chloride. *CAS-3784-89-2.* INN; BAN; MI.

Phenadoxone. $C_{23}H_{29}NO_2$. 351.48. 6-Morpholino-4,4-diphenyl-3-heptanone. *UNII-375W3TA42N. CAS-467-84-5.* INN; BAN; DCF; MI. ◇*CB 11 [as hydrochloride]*

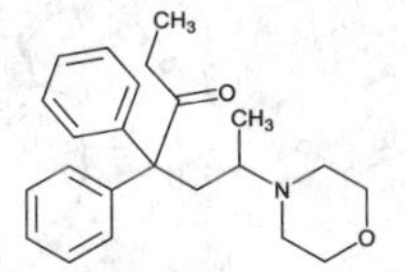

Phenaglycodol. $C_{11}H_{15}ClO_2$. 214.69. 2-(*p*-Chlorophenyl)-3-methyl-2,3-butanediol. *CAS-79-93-6.* INN; BAN; AMA-DE 1973; MI.

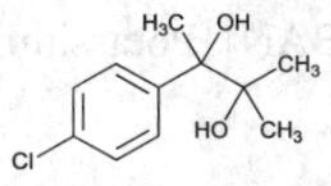

Phenamazoline Hydrochloride. $C_{10}H_{13}N_3$.HCl. 211.69. [Phenamazoline is INN.] *N*-((4,5-Dihydro-1*H*-imidazol-2-yl)methyl)aniline hydrochloride. *UNII-090O8Q78KU; UNII-09L091X49E [phenamazoline]. CAS-24359-77-1; CAS-501-62-2 [phenamazoline].*

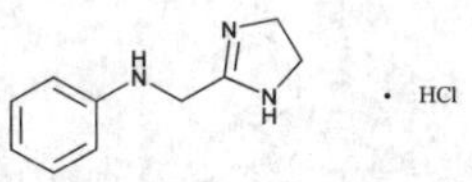

Phenampromide. $C_{17}H_{26}N_2O$. 274.40. *N*-(1-Methyl-2-piperidinoethyl)propionanilide. *UNII-0600L2M6EZ. CAS-129-83-9.* INN; BAN; MI.

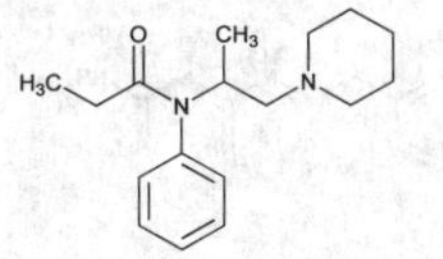

Phenaphthazine. *UNII-4U1WVN6KUX. CAS-5423-07-4.* Nitrazine Paper (Apothecon)

Phenarbutal — *See* Phetharbital.

Phenarsone Sulfoxylate. $C_7H_8AsNNa_2O_6S$. 355.11. 4-Hydroxy-*m*-arsanilic acid, compound with sodium formaldehydesulfoxylate. *CAS-535-51-3.* INN; MI. Aldarsone (Abbott†)

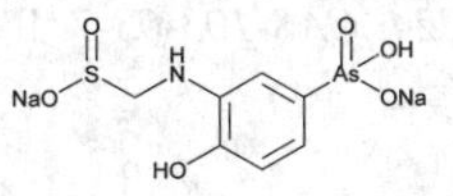

Phenazocine Hydrobromide. $C_{22}H_{27}NO$.HBr. 402.37. [Phenazocine is INN and BAN.] 2′-Hydroxy-5,9-dimethyl-2-phenethyl-6,7-benzomorphan. *CAS-1239-04-9; CAS-127-35-5 [phenazocine].* MI; ND 1966. Prinadol (SmithKline Beecham†)

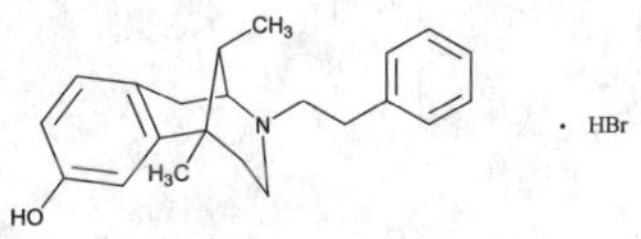

Phenazone (INN, BAN, DCF) — *See* Antipyrine.

Phenazopyridine Hydrochloride [*1961*] (fen ay″ zoe pir′ i deen hye″ droe klor′ ide). **USP.** $C_{11}H_{11}N_5$.HCl. 249.70. [Phenazopyridine is INN and BAN.] (1) 2,6-Pyridinediamine, 3-(phenylazo)-, monohydrochloride; (2) 2,6-Diamino-3-(phenylazo)pyridine monohydrochloride. *UNII-0EWG668W17; UNII-K2J09EMJ52 [phenazopyridine]. CAS-136-40-3; CAS-94-78-0 [phenazopyridine]. Analgesic (urinary tract).* Pyridium (Warner Chilcott) ◇*NC 150; W 1655; NSC-1879*

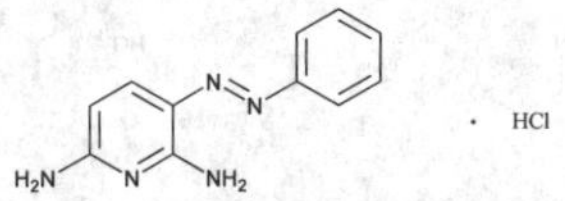

Phenbenicillin (previously used name) — *See* Fenbenicillin.

Phenbutazone Sodium Glycerate [*1971*] (fen bue′ ta zone soe′ dee um glis′ er ate). $C_{19}H_{19}N_2NaO_2$.$C_3H_8O_3$. 422.45. (1) 3*H*-Pyrazol-3-one, 4-butyl-1,2-dihydro-5-hydroxy-1,2-diphenyl sodium salt, compd. with 1,2,3-propanetriol; (2) 4-Butyl-3-hydroxy-1,2-diphenyl-3-pyrazolin-5-one sodium salt compound with glycerol (1:1). *UNII-RKC4AOX590; UNII-GN5P7K3T8S [phenylbutazone]. CAS-34214-49-8; CAS-28013-70-9 [replaced]; CAS-50-33-9 [phenylbutazone]. Anti-inflammatory.* ◇*G 26,872*

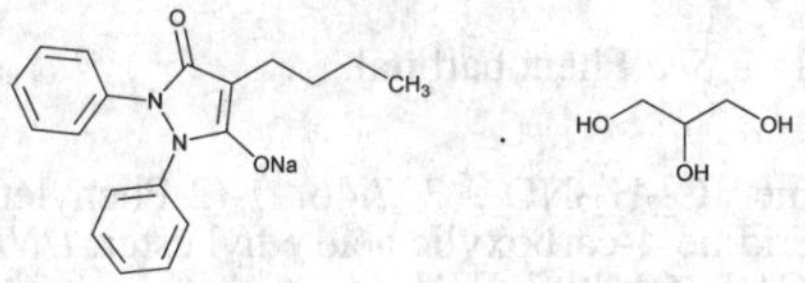

Phenbutrazate (previously used name) — *See* Fenbutrazate.

Phencarbamide [*1962*] (fen kar′ ba mide). $C_{19}H_{24}N_2OS$. 328.47. [Fencarbamide is INN.] (1) Carbamothioic acid, diphenyl-, *S*-[2-(diethylamino)ethyl] ester; (2) *S*-[2-(Diethylamino)ethyl] diphenylthiocarbamate. *UNII-59H17J9F1B. CAS-3735-90-8. Anticholinergic.* Escorpal (Farbenfabriken Bayer A.G., Germany)

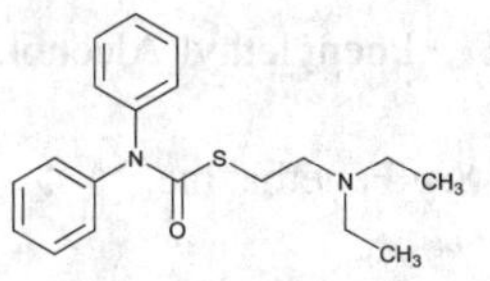

Phencyclidine Hydrochloride [*1963*] (fen sye′ kli deen hye″ droe klor′ ide). $C_{17}H_{25}N$.HCl. 279.85. [Phencyclidine is INN and BAN.] (1) Piperidine, 1-(1-phenylcyclohexyl)-, hydrochloride; (2) 1-(1-Phenylcyclohexyl)piperidine hydrochloride. *UNII-V1JZQ7GDTX; UNII-J1DOI7UV76*

---

† Brand name formerly used, and/or firm no longer concerned with this product.

[phencyclidine]. *CAS-956-90-1; CAS-77-10-1* [phencyclidine]. *Anesthetic.* Sernylan (Parke-Davis†) ◇*CI-395; CN-25,253-2; GP-121; NSC-40902*

Phendimetrazine Tartrate (fen″ dye met′ ra zeen tar′ trate). **USP.** $C_{12}H_{17}NO.C_4H_6O_6$. 341.36. [Phendimetrazine is INN and BAN.] (1) Morpholine, 3,4-dimethyl-2-phenyl-, (2*S-trans*)-, [*R*-(*R*,R**)]-2,3-dihydroxybutanedioate (1:1); (2) (2*S*,3*S*)-3,4-Dimethyl-2-phenylmorpholine L-(+)-tartrate (1:1). *UNII-6985IP0T80; UNII-AB2794W8KV* [phendimetrazine]. *CAS-50-58-8; CAS-21102-82-9* [replaced]; *CAS-634-03-7* [phendimetrazine]. *Appetite suppressant (systemic).* Bontril (Mallinckrodt); plegine (Wyeth); X-trozine (Shire Richwood)

Phenelzine Sulfate (fen′ el zeen sul′ fate). **USP.** $C_8H_{12}N_2.H_2SO_4$. 234.27. [Phenelzine is INN and BAN.] (1) Hydrazine, (2-phenylethyl)-, sulfate (1:1); (2) Phenethylhydrazine sulfate (1:1). *UNII-2681D7P965; UNII-O408N561GF* [phenelzine]. *CAS-156-51-4; CAS-51-71-8* [phenelzine]. *Antidepressant.* Nardil (Pfizer)

Phenemal — *See* Phenobarbital.

Pheneridine. $C_{22}H_{27}NO_2$. 337.46. 1-(2-Phenylethyl)-4-phenylpiperidine-4-carboxylic acid ethyl ester. *UNII-2UG271-VI0Z. CAS-469-80-7.* INN.

Phenethanol — *See* Phenylethyl Alcohol.

Phenethazine — *See* Fenethazine.

Phenethicillin Potassium. $C_{17}H_{19}KN_2O_5S$. 402.51. [Pheneticillin is INN and BAN.] (1) 4-Thia-1-azabicyclo[3.2.0]-heptane-2-carboxylic acid, 3,3-dimethyl-7-oxo-6-[(1-oxo-2-phenoxypropyl)amino]-, [2*S*-(2α,5α,6β)]-, monopotassium salt; (2) Monopotassium (2*S*,5*R*,6*R*)-3,3-dimethyl-7-oxo-6-(2-phenoxypropionamido)-4-thia-1-azabicyclo[3.2.0]heptane-2-carboxylate. *CAS-132-93-4; CAS-147-*

55-7 [phenethicillin]. USP XX; JAN; MI. Chemipen (Bristol-Myers Squibb†); Syncillin (Bristol-Myers Squibb†) *[Name previously used: Phenethicillin.]*

Phenethyl Alcohol (BAN) — *See* Phenylethyl Alcohol.

Phenethylazocine Bromide — *See* Phenazocine Hydrobromide.

Pheneticillin (INN, BAN) Potassium — *See* Phenethicillin Potassium.

Phenetsal — *See* Acetaminosalol.

Pheneturide. $C_{11}H_{14}N_2O_2$. 206.24. [Acetylpheneturide is JAN.] 2-Phenylbutyrylurea. *UNII-878CEJ4HGX. CAS-90-49-3.* INN; BAN; MI.

Phenformin Hydrochloride. $C_{10}H_{15}N_5.HCl$. 241.72. [Phenformin is INN and BAN.] Imidodicarbonimidic diamide, *N*-(2-phenylethyl)-, monohydrochloride. *UNII-91XC93EU03. CAS-834-28-6; CAS-114-86-3* [phenformin]. USP XIX; MI. DBI (Ciba-Geigy†)

Phenglutarimide. $C_{17}H_{24}N_2O_2$. 288.38. 2,2-Diethyl-aminoethyl-2-phenylglutarimide. *CAS-1156-05-4.* INN; BAN; DCF; MI.

Phenicarbazide. $C_7H_9N_3O$. 151.17. 1-Phenylsemicarbazide. *UNII-1LR2578324. CAS-103-03-7.* INN; DCF; MI.

Phenidiemal — *See* Phetharbital.

Phenindamine Tartrate [*1988*] (fen in′ da meen tar′ trate). $C_{19}H_{19}N.C_4H_6O_6$. 411.45. [Phenindamine is INN and BAN.] 2,3,4,9-Tetrahydro-2-methyl-9-phenyl-1*H*-indeno[2,1-*c*]pyridine. *CAS-569-59-5; CAS-82-88-2* [phenindamine]. Thephorin (Hoffmann-LaRoche†)

Phenindione. $C_{15}H_{10}O_2$. 222.24. (1) 1*H*-Indene-1,3(2*H*)-dione, 2-phenyl-; (2) 2-Phenyl-1,3-indandione. *UNII-5M7Y6274ZE. CAS-83-12-5.* USP XXII; INN; BAN. Hedulin (Sanofi Aventis)

Pheniodol Sodium (INN) — *See* Iodoalphionic Acid.

Pheniprazine Hydrochloride. $C_9H_{14}N_2$. 150.22. [Pheniprazine is INN and BAN.] *UNII-5B3OM8452C. CAS-66-05-7; CAS-55-52-7* [pheniprazine]. MI. Catron Hydrochloride (Marion Merrell Dow†)

Pheniramine Maleate [*1988*] (fen ir′ a meen mal′ ee ate). **USP.** $C_{16}H_{20}N_2.C_4H_4O_4$. 356.42. [Pheniramine is INN and BAN.] (1) 2-[α-[2-Dimethylaminoethyl]benzyl]pyridine bimaleate; (2) *N,N*-Dimethyl-3-phenyl-3-(2-pyridyl)propylamine hydrogen maleate. *UNII-NYW905655B; UNII-134FM9ZZ6M* [pheniramine]. *CAS-132-20-7; CAS-86-21-5* [pheniramine].

Phenisonone Hydrobromide. *CAS-530-10-9; CAS-28227-96-5* [phenisonone].

Phenmetraline Hydrochloride — *See* Phenmetrazine Hydrochloride.

Phenmetrazine Hydrochloride (fen met′ ra zeen hye″ droe klor′ ide). **USP.** $C_{11}H_{15}NO.HCl$. 213.70. [Phenmetrazine is INN and BAN.] (1) Morpholine, 3-methyl-2-phenyl-, hydrochloride; (2) 3-Methyl-2-phenylmorpholine hydro-

chloride. *UNII-6U85YRT588; UNII-XA501VL3VR* [phenmetrazine]. *CAS-1707-14-8; CAS-134-49-6* [phenmetrazine]. *Anorexic.* Preludin (Boehringer Ingelheim)

Phenobamate — *See* Febarbamate.

Phenobarbital (fee″ noe bar′ bi tal). **USP.** $C_{12}H_{12}N_2O_3$. 232.24. (1) 2,4,6(1*H*,3*H*,5*H*)-Pyrimidinetrione, 5-ethyl-5-phenyl-; (2) 5-Ethyl-5-phenylbarbituric acid. *UNII-YQE403BP4D. CAS-50-06-6.* INN; BAN; JAN. *Anticonvulsant; sedative-hypnotic.* Eskabarb (SmithKline Beecham†); Luminal (Sterling Winthrop); Solfoton (ECR†); Talpheno (Marion Merrell Dow†) [*Name previously used: Phenobarbitone.*]

Phenobarbital Sodium (fee″ noe bar′ bi tal soe′ dee um). **USP.** $C_{12}H_{11}N_2NaO_3$. 254.22. (1) 2,4,6(1*H*,3*H*,5*H*)-Pyrimidinetrione, 5-ethyl-5-phenyl-, monosodium salt; (2) Sodium 5-ethyl-5-phenylbarbiturate. *UNII-SW9M9BB5K3. CAS-57-30-7; CAS-50-06-6* [phenobarbital]. INN; JAN. *Anticonvulsant; sedative-hypnotic.* Luminal Sodium (Sterling Winthrop)

Phenobutiodil. $C_{10}H_9I_3O_3$. 557.89. 2-(2,4,6-Triiodophenoxy)butyric acid. *CAS-554-24-5.* INN; BAN; MI.

Phenododecinium Bromide (DCF) — *See* Domiphen Bromide.

Phenol (fee′ nol). **USP.** C_6H_6O. 94.11. (1) Phenol; (2) Phenol. *UNII-339NCG44TV. CAS-108-95-2.* JAN. *Pharmaceutic aid (preservative).* [*Note—Depicted as C_6H_5OH.*]

Phenol Red — *See* Phenolsulfonphthalein.

Phenolate Sodium [*1978*] (fee′ noe late soe′ dee um). C_6H_5NaO. 116.09. (1) Phenol, sodium salt; (2) Sodium phenolate. *CAS-139-02-6. Disinfectant.*

Phenolphthalein. $C_{20}H_{14}O_4$. 318.32. (1) 1(3*H*)-Isobenzofuranone, 3,3-bis(4-hydroxyphenyl)-; (2) 3,3-Bis(*p*-hydroxyphenyl)phthalide. *UNII-6QK969R2IF. CAS-77-09-8.* USP

---

† Brand name formerly used, and/or firm no longer concerned with this product.

XXIII; INN; BAN. *Laxative.* Evac-Q-Tabs (Savage†); Ex-Lax (Novartis); Modane (Savage†); Prulet (Mission Pharmacal†)

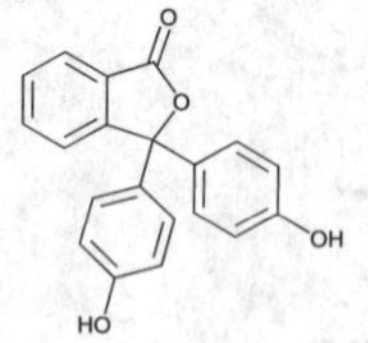

Phenolphthalein, Yellow. USP XXIII. *Laxative.* Feen-a-Mint Gum (Schering-Plough HealthCare†)

Phenolsulfonic Acid (JAN) — *See* Zinc Phenolsulfonate.

Phenolsulfonphthalein (fee″ nol sul″ fon thal′ een). **NF.** $C_{19}H_{14}O_5S$. 354.38. [Phenolsulphonphthalein is BAN.] (1) Phenol Red; (2) Phenol, 4,4′-($3H$-2,1-benzoxathiol-3-ylidene)bis-, (S,S-dioxide); (3) 3,3-Bis(4-hydroxyphenyl)-$3H$-2,1-benzoxathiole 1,1-dioxide. *UNII-I6G9Y0J1OJ. CAS-143-74-8.* JAN; MI.

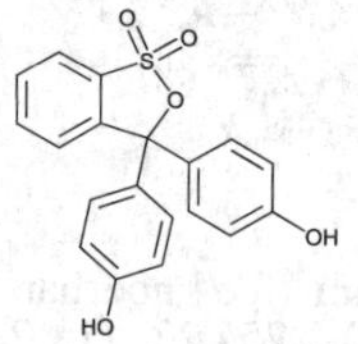

Phenolsulphonate Sodium. $C_6H_5NaO_4S.2H_2O$. 232.19. Sodium 4-hydroxybenzenesulfonate, dihydrate. *CAS-10580-19-5.* USP IX.

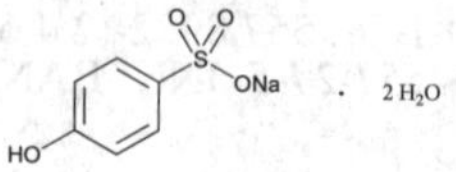

Phenolsulphonphthalein (BAN) — *See* Phenolsulfonphthalein.

Phenomorphan. $C_{24}H_{29}NO$. 347.49. 3-Hydroxy-N-phenethyl-morphinan. *CAS-468-07-5.* INN; BAN; DCF; MI.

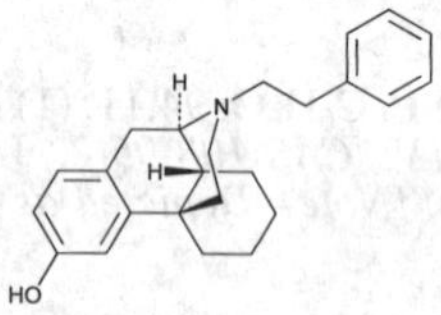

Phenomycilline — *See* Penicillin V.

Phenoperidine. $C_{23}H_{29}NO_3$. 367.48. 1-(3-Hydroxy-3-phenyl-propyl)-4-phenylpiperidine-4-carboxylic acid ethyl ester. *UNII-G9BH09J4JW. CAS-562-26-5.* INN; BAN; DCF; MI. ◇*R 1406*

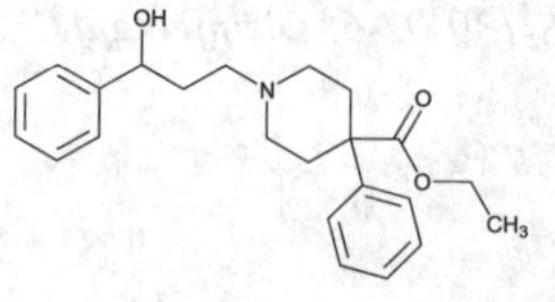

Phenopryldiasulfone Sodium (DCF) — *See* Solasulfone.

Phenosulfophthalein — *See* Phenolsulfonphthalein.

Phenothiazine. $C_{12}H_9NS$. 199.27. Thiodiphenylamine. *UNII-GS9EX7QNU6. CAS-92-84-2.* NF XII; INN; MI. Nemazine (Parke-Davis†)

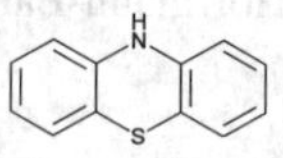

Phenothrin. $C_{23}H_{26}O_3$. 350.45. *m*-Phenoxybenzyl (±)-*cis, trans*-2,2-dimethyl-3-(2-methylpropenyl)cyclopropanecarboxylate. *CAS-26002-80-2.* INN; BAN; MI. ◇*S-2539F*

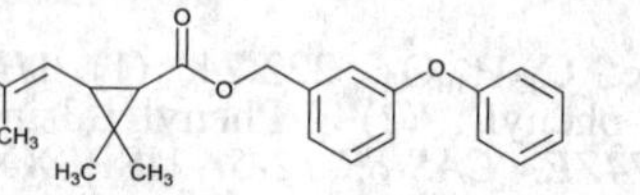

Phenovalin. A mixture of isovalerylphenolphthalein and acetylphenolphthalein (1:1). JAN.

Phenoxazoline Hydrochloride — *See* Fenoxazoline Hydrochloride.

Phenoxodiol (trivial name) — *See* Idronoxil.

Phenoxybenzamine Hydrochloride (fen ox″ ee ben′ za meen hye″ droe klor′ ide). **USP.** $C_{18}H_{22}ClNO.HCl$. 340.29. [Phenoxybenzamine is INN and BAN.] (1) Benzenemethanamine, N-(2-chloroethyl)-N-(1-methyl-2-phenoxyethyl)-, hydrochloride; (2) N-(2-Chloroethyl)-N-(1-methyl-2-phenoxyethyl)benzylamine hydrochloride. *UNII-X11E-G24OHL; UNII-0TTZ664R7Z* [phenoxybenzamine]. *CAS-63-92-3; CAS-59-96-1* [phenoxybenzamine]. *Antihypertensive.* Dibenzyline (WellSpring)

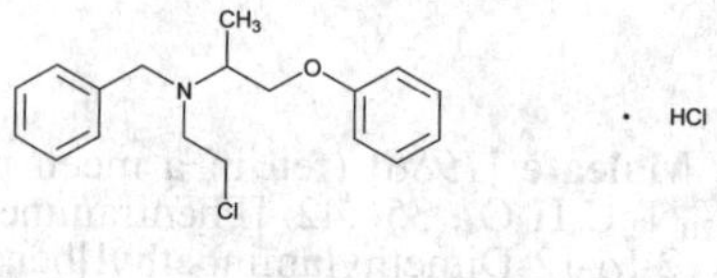

Phenoxyethanol. NF. $C_8H_{10}O_2$. 138.16. (1) 2-Phenoxyethanol; (2) 2-Phenoxyethyl alcohol; (3) Ethylene glycol, 2-monophenyl ether. *UNII-HIE492ZZ3T. CAS-122-99-6.*

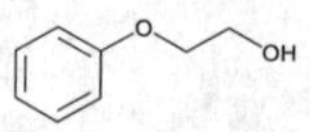

Phenoxymethylpenicillin (INN, BAN) — *See* Penicillin V.

Phenoxymethylpenicillin Potassium (JAN) — *See* Penicillin V Potassium.

Phenoxypropazine. $C_9H_{14}N_2O$. 166.22. [Fenoxypropazine is INN and BAN.] (1-Methyl-2-phenoxyethyl)hydrazine. *UNII-8E92V52324. CAS-3818-37-9.* MI.

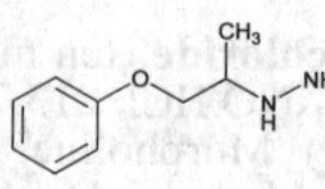

Phenoxypropylpenicillin — *See* Propicillin.

Phenozolone — *See* Fenozolone.

Phenprobamate. $C_{10}H_{13}NO_2$. 179.22. 3-Phenyl-1-propanol carbamate. *CAS-673-31-4*. INN; BAN; JAN; DCF; MI. *✧MH-532*

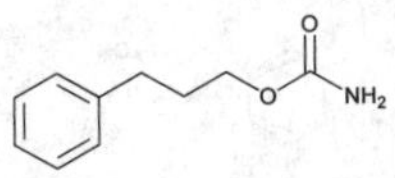

Phenprocoumon [*1961*] (fen″ proe koo′ mon). $C_{18}H_{16}O_3$. 280.32. (1) 2*H*-1-Benzopyran-2-one, 4-hydroxy-3-(1-phenylpropyl)-; (2) 3-(α-Ethylbenzyl)-4-hydroxycoumarin. *UNII-Q08SIO485D*. *CAS-435-97-2*. USP XXII; INN; BAN. *Anticoagulant*. Liquamar (Organon)

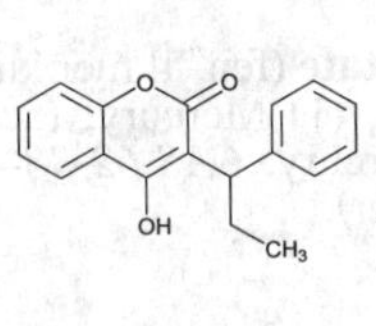

Phenprocumone — *See* Phenprocoumon.

Phenpromethadrine — *See* Phenpromethamine.

Phenpromethamine. $C_{10}H_{15}N$. 149.23. *N,β*-Dimethylphenethylamine. *CAS-93-88-9*. INN; DCF. Vonedrine (Marion Merrell Dow†)

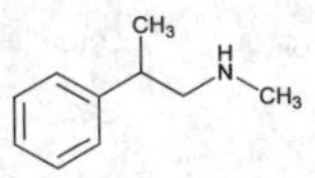

Phenpropamine Citrate — *See* Alverine Citrate.

Phensuximide (fen sux′ i mide). **USP**. $C_{11}H_{11}NO_2$. 189.21. (1) 2,5-Pyrrolidinedione, 1-methyl-3-phenyl-, (±)-; (2) (±)-*N*-Methyl-2-phenylsuccinimide. *UNII-6WVL9C355G*. *CAS-86-34-0*. INN; BAN. *Anticonvulsant*. Milontin (Pfizer)

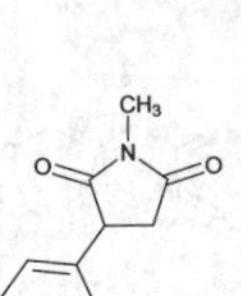

Phentermine [*1962*] (fen′ ter meen). $C_{10}H_{15}N$. 149.23. (1) Benzeneethanamine, α,α-dimethyl-; (2) α,α-Dimethylphenethylamine. *UNII-C045TQL4WP*. *CAS-122-09-8*. INN; BAN. *Anorexic*. Ionamin (Fisons)

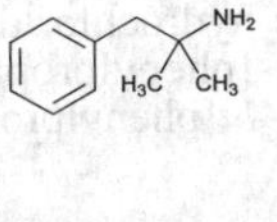

Phentermine Hydrochloride (fen′ ter meen hye″ droe klor′ ide). **USP**. $C_{10}H_{15}N.HCl$. 185.69. (1) Benzeneethanamine, α,α-dimethyl-, hydrochloride; (2) α,α-Dimethylphenethylamine hydrochloride. *UNII-0K2I505OTV; UNII-C045TQL4WP* [phentermine]. *CAS-1197-21-3; CAS-122-09-8* [phentermine]. *Appetite suppressant (systemic)*. Fastin (GlaxoSmithKline)

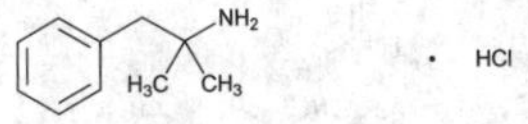

Phenthiazine — *See* Phenothiazine.

Phentolamine Hydrochloride. $C_{17}H_{19}N_3O.HCl$. 317.81. [Phentolamine is INN and BAN.] (1) Phenol, 3-[[(4,5-dihydro-1*H*-imidazol-2-yl)methyl](4-methylphenyl)amino], monohydrochloride; (2) *m*-[*N*-(2-Imidazolin-2-ylmethyl)-*p*-toluidino]phenol monohydrochloride. *UNII-86DRW83R1H; UNII-Z468598HBV* [phentolamine]. *CAS-73-05-2; CAS-50-60-2* [phentolamine]. USP XX; MI. Regitine Hydrochloride (Ciba-Geigy†)

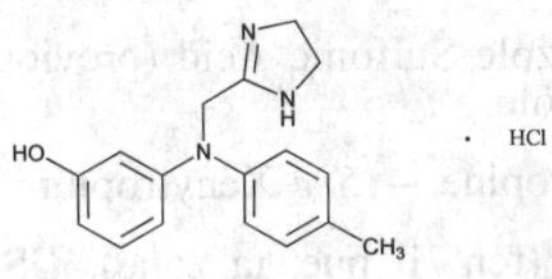

Phentolamine Mesylate (fen tol′ a meen mes′ i late). **USP**. $C_{17}H_{19}N_3O.CH_4O_3S$. 377.46. [Phentolamine Mesilate is INN and JAN.] (1) Phenol, 3-[[(4,5-dihydro-1*H*-imidazol-2-yl)methyl](4-methylphenyl)amino]-, monomethanesulfonate (salt); (2) *m*-[*N*-(2-Imidazolin-2-ylmethyl)-*p*-toluidino]phenol monomethanesulfonate (salt). *UNII-Y7543E5K9T; UNII-Z468598HBV* [phentolamine]. *CAS-65-28-1; CAS-50-60-2* [phentolamine]. *Anti-adrenergic*. Regitine (Novartis) *[Name previously used: Phentolamine Methanesulfonate.]*

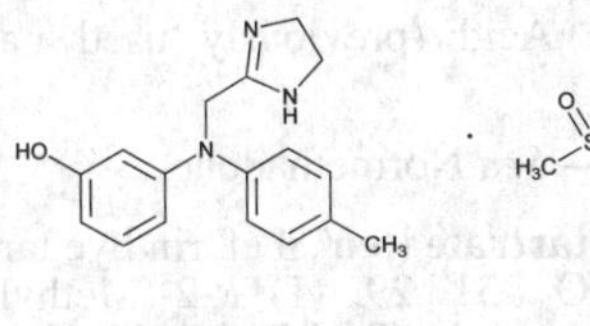

Phentolamine Methanesulfonate (previously used name) — *See* Phentolamine Mesylate.

Phentydrone. *UNII-GF6SPR73DW*. *CAS-634-19-5*. MI.

Phenyl Aminosalicylate [*1964*] (fen′ il a mee″ noe sa lis′ i late). $C_{13}H_{11}NO_3$. 229.23. [Fenamisal is INN and BAN.] (1) Benzoic acid, 4-amino-2-hydroxy-, phenyl ester; (2) Phenyl 4-aminosalicylate. *UNII-52936SIP7V*. *CAS-133-11-9*. *Antibacterial (tuberculostatic)*. Pheny-Pas-Tebamin (Purdue Frederick) *✧NSC-40144*

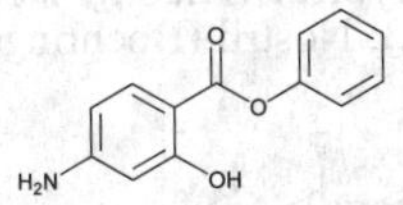

Phenyl Salicylate. *UNII-28A37T47QO*. *CAS-118-55-8*. NF XI; MI.

† Brand name formerly used, and/or firm no longer concerned with this product.

Phenylacetylglycine Dimethylamide. $C_{12}H_{16}N_2O_2$. 220.27. *N*-Phenyl-*N*-acetylglycine dimethylamide. *UNII-7TUY98X69L. CAS-3738-06-5.* JAN.

Phenylalanine [*1980*] (fen″ il al′ a neen). **USP.** $C_9H_{11}NO_2$. 165.19. [L-Phenylalanine is JAN.] (1) L-Phenylalanine; (2) L-Phenylalanine. *UNII-47E5O17Y3R. CAS-63-91-2.* INN; JAN. *Amino acid.*

Phenylalanine Mustard — *See* Melphalan.

Phenylbenzimidazole Sulfonic Acid (previously used name) — *See* Ensulizole.

Phenylbenzyl Atropine — *See* Xenytropium Bromide.

Phenylbutazone (fen″ il bue′ ta zone). **USP.** $C_{19}H_{20}N_2O_2$. 308.37. (1) 3,5-Pyrazolidinedione, 4-butyl-1,2-diphenyl-; (2) 4-Butyl-1,2-diphenyl-3,5-pyrazolidinedione. *UNII-GN5P7K3T8S. CAS-50-33-9.* INN; BAN; JAN. *Antirheumatic.* Azolid (Sanofi Aventis); Butazolidin (Novartis)

Phenylcarbinol — *See* Benzyl Alcohol.

Phenylcinchoninic Acid (previously used name) — *See* Cinchophen.

Phenyldimazone — *See* Normethadone.

Phenylephrine Bitartrate (fen″ il ef′ rin bye tar′ trate). **USP.** $C_9H_{13}NO_2 \cdot C_4H_6O_6$. 317.29. (1) *R*-2-(Methylamino)-1-(3-hydroxyphenyl)ethanol-, (2*R*,3*R*)-2,3-dihydroxybutanedioate (1:1) (salt); (2) (-)-1-(3-Hydroxyphenyl)-2-methylaminoethanol, hydrogen tartrate; (3) (-)-3 Hydroxy-α-[(methylamino)methyl]benzenemethanol, hydrogen tartrate; (4) 1-*m*-Hydroxy-α-[(methylamino)methyl]benzyl alcohol, hydrogen tartrate. *UNII-27O3Q5ML57. CAS-17162-39-9.*

Phenylephrine Hydrochloride (fen″ il ef′ rin hye″ droe klor′ ide). **USP.** $C_9H_{13}NO_2 \cdot HCl$. 203.67. [Phenylephrine is INN and BAN.] (1) Benzenemethanol, 3-hydroxy-α-[(methylamino)methyl]-, hydrochloride (*R*)-; (2) (-)-*m*-Hydroxy-α-[(methylamino)methyl]benzyl alcohol hydrochloride. *UNII-04JA59TNSJ. CAS-61-76-7; CAS-59-42-7* [phenylephrine]. JAN. *Adrenergic (ophthalmic).* Afrin 4 Hour Nasal Spray (Schering-Plough HealthCare); Biomydrin (Parke-Davis†); Mydfrin (Alcon); Neo-Synephrine (Sterling Health U.S.A.); Nostril (Boehringer Ingelheim†)

Phenylethanol — *See* Phenylethyl Alcohol.

Phenylethyl Alcohol (fen″ il eth′ il al′ ka hol). **USP.** $C_8H_{10}O$. 122.16. [Phenethyl Alcohol is BAN.] (1) Benzeneethanol; (2) Phenethyl alcohol. *CAS-60-12-8. Pharmaceutic aid (antimicrobial agent).*

Phenylethylmalonylurea — *See* Phenobarbital.

Phenylindanedione — *See* Phenindione.

Phenyliodoundecynoate. $C_{17}H_{21}IO_2$. 384.25. 11-Iodoundecynoic acid phenyl ester. *UNII-VXD0H11TQ7. CAS-2020-25-9.* JAN.

Phenylmercuric Acetate (fen″ il mer kure′ ik as′ e tate). **NF.** $C_8H_8HgO_2$. 336.74. (1) Mercury, (acetato-*O*)phenyl-; (2) (Acetato)phenylmercury. *CAS-62-38-4. Pharmaceutic aid (antimicrobial agent).*

Phenylmercuric Borate. $C_6H_7BHgO_3 \cdot C_6H_6HgO$. 633.22. Equimolecular compound of phenylmercury borate and phenylmercuric hydroxide. *CAS-8017-88-7.* INN.

Phenylmercuric Chloride. Chlorophenylmercury. *CAS-100-56-1.* NF IX; MI.

Phenylmercuric Nitrate (fen″ il mer kure′ ik nye′ trate). **NF.** (1) Mercury, (nitrato-*O*)phenyl-; (2) Nitratophenylmercury. *CAS-55-68-5. Pharmaceutic aid (antimicrobial agent).* Phenmerzyl Nitrate (Marion Merrell Dow†)

Phenylpropanol. $C_9H_{12}O$. 136.19. 1-Phenylpropanol. *CAS-93-54-9.* JAN.

Phenylpropanolamine Bitartrate (fen″ il proe″ pa nol′ a meen bye tar′ trate). **USP.** $C_9H_{13}NO \cdot C_4H_6O_6$. 301.29. (*R*,S**)-(±)-α-(1-Aminoethyl)benzenemethanol bitartrate. *CAS-67244-90-0.*

Phenylpropanolamine Hydrochloride (fen″ il proe″ pa nol′ a meen hye″ droe klor′ ide). **USP.** $C_9H_{13}NO \cdot HCl$. 187.67. [Phenylpropanolamine is INN and BAN.] (1) Benzenemethanol, α-(1-aminoethyl)-, hydrochloride, (*R*,S**)-, (±); (2) (±)-Norephedrine hydrochloride. *UNII-8D5I63UE1Q; UNII-33RU150WUN* [phenylpropanolamine]. *CAS-154-41-6; CAS-14838-15-4* [phenylpropanolamine]. *Adrenergic (vasoconstrictor).*

Phenylpropanolamine Polistirex [*1987*] (fen″ il proe″ pa nol′ a meen pol″ ee stye′ rex). (1) Benzene, diethenyl-, polymer with ethenylbenzene, sulfonated, complex with

(±)-(*R*,S**)-α-(1-aminoethyl)benzenemethanol; (2) Sulfonated styrene-divinylbenzene copolymer complex with (±)-norephedrine. *Adrenergic (vasoconstrictor)*.

Phenylthilone. $C_{12}H_{13}NO_2S$. 235.30. [Phenythilone is INN.] 2-Ethyl-2-phenyl-3,5-thiamorpholinedione. *UNII-V8350F4A37. CAS-115-55-9.*

Phenyltoloxamine. $C_{17}H_{21}NO$. 255.35. *N,N*-Dimethyl-2-(α-phenyl-*o*-tolyloxy)ethylamine. *UNII-K65LB6598J. CAS-92-12-6; CAS-1176-08-5* [citrate]. INN; BAN; MI.

Phenyltoloxamine Citrate. **USP**. $C_{17}H_{21}NO.C_6H_8O_7$. 447.48. (1) *N,N*-Dimethyl-2-(α-phenyl-*o*-tolyloxy)ethylamine, citrate (1:1) salt; (2) 2-(2-Dimethylaminoethoxy)-diphenylmethane, citrate (1:1) salt; (3) Phenyltoloxamine dihydrogen citrate. *CAS-1176-08-5.*

Phenyracillin. $(C_{16}H_{18}N_2O_4S)_2.C_{16}H_{18}N_2$. 907.11. 2,5-Diphenylpiperazine salt of benzylpenicillin. *UNII-3V721R4XYY. CAS-7009-88-3.* INN; DCF.

Phenyramidol Hydrochloride [*1961*] (fen″ i ram′ i dol hye″ droe klor′ ide). $C_{13}H_{14}N_2O.HCl$. 250.72. [Fenyramidol is INN and BAN.] (1) Benzenemethanol, α-[(2-pyridinylamino)methyl]-, monohydrochloride; (2) α-[(2-Pyridyl-amino)methyl]benzyl alcohol monohydrochloride. *CAS-326-43-2; CAS-553-69-5* [phenyramidol]. *Analgesic; relaxant (skeletal muscle)*. ◇*IN 511; MJ 505; NSC-17777*

Phenythilone (INN) — *See* Phenylthilone.

Phenytoin [*1975*] (fen′ i toin; fen′ i toe in). **USP**. $C_{15}H_{12}N_2O_2$. 252.27. (1) 2,4-Imidazolidinedione, 5,5-diphenyl-; (2) 5,5-Diphenylhydantoin. *UNII-6158TKW0C5. CAS-57-41-0.* INN; BAN; JAN. *Anticonvulsant*. Dilantin (Pfizer) [*Name previously used: Diphenylhydantoin.*]

Phenytoin Sodium (fen′ i toin soe′ dee um; fen′ i toe in soe′ dee um). **USP**. $C_{15}H_{11}N_2NaO_2$. 274.25. (1) 2,4-Imidazolidinedione, 5,5-diphenyl-, monosodium salt; (2) 5,5-Diphenylhydantoin sodium salt. *UNII-4182431BJH. CAS-630-93-3; CAS-57-41-0* [phenytoin]. JAN [for Injection]. *Anticonvulsant*. Dilantin (Parke-Davis) [*Name previously used: Diphenylhydantoin Sodium.*]

Phetharbital. $C_{14}H_{16}N_2O_3$. 260.29. 5,5-Diethyl-1-phenyl-barbituric acid. *CAS-357-67-5.* INN.

Phezathion — *See* Fezatione.

Phloroglucinol. $C_6H_6O_3$. 126.11. Benzene-1,3,5-triol. *CAS-108-73-6.* BAN.

Phloropropiophenone — *See* Flopropione.

Pholcodine. $C_{23}H_{30}N_2O_4$. 398.50. Morpholinylethylmorphine. *CAS-509-67-1.* INN; BAN; MI. Ethnine Simplex (Purdue Frederick†)

Pholedrine. $C_{10}H_{15}NO$. 165.23. *p*-(2-Methylaminopropyl)-phenol. *UNII-AY28O44JGD. CAS-370-14-9.* INN; BAN; DCF; MI.

Pholescutol — *See* Folescutol.

Phoscolic Acid — *See* Foscolic Acid.

---

† Brand name formerly used, and/or firm no longer concerned with this product.

Phosmet. $C_{11}H_{12}NO_4PS_2$. 317.32. *O,O*-Dimethyl phthalimidomethyl phosphorodithioate. *UNII-VN04LI540Y. CAS-732-11-6.* BAN.

Phosphate Salt of Tricyclic Nucleoside (previously used name) — *See* Triciribine Phosphate.

Phosphoric Acid (fos for′ ik as′ id). **NF**. H_3PO_4. 98.00. (1) Phosphoric acid; (2) Phosphoric acid. *UNII-E4GA8884NN. CAS-7664-38-2. Pharmaceutic aid (solvent).*

Phosphothiamine — *See* Monophosphothiamine.

Phoxim. $C_{12}H_{15}N_2O_3PS$. 298.30. Phenylglyoxylnitrile oxime *O,O*-diethyl phosphorothioate. *UNII-6F5V775VPO. CAS-14816-18-3.* INN; BAN; MI. ◇*Bayer 9053*

Phthalofyne [*1966*] (thal′ oh fine). $C_{14}H_{14}O_4$. 246.26. [Ftalofyne is INN.] (1) 1,2-Benzenedicarboxylic acid, mono(1-ethyl-1-methyl-2-propynyl) ester; (2) Mono(1-ethyl-1-methyl-2-propynyl) phthalate; (3) 3-Methyl-1-pentyn-3-yl acid phthalate. *UNII-TA9XO4D05J. CAS-131-67-9. Anthelmintic (veterinary).* ◇*NSC-25614*

Phthalylsulfacetamide. $C_{16}H_{14}N_2O_6S$. 362.36. 4′-(Acetylsulfamoyl)phthalanilic acid. *UNII-24PUW23GRX. CAS-131-69-1.* NF XIII; BAN; MI. Talsigel (Bristol-Myers Squibb†); Thalamyd (Schering†) *[Name previously used: Phthalylsulphacetamide.]*

Phthalylsulfamethizole. $C_{17}H_{14}N_4O_5S_2$. 418.45. 4′-[(5-Methyl-1,3,4-thiadiazol-2-yl)sulfamoyl]phthalanilic acid. *UNII-TAY5ZBM0MO. CAS-485-24-5.* INN; DCF.

Phthalylsulfathiazole. $C_{17}H_{13}N_3O_5S_2$. 403.43. (1) Benzoic acid, 2-[[[4-[(2-thiazolylamino)sulfonyl]phenyl]amino]-carbonyl]-; (2) 4′-(2-Thiazolylsulfamoyl)phthalanilic acid. *UNII-6875L5852V. CAS-85-73-4.* USP XX; INN; BAN. *[Name previously used: Phthalylsulphathiazole.]*

Phthalylsulphacetamide (previously used name) — *See* Phthalylsulfacetamide.

Phthalylsulphathiazole (previously used name) — *See* Phthalylsulfathiazole.

Physostigmine (fye″ soe stig′ meen). **USP**. $C_{15}H_{21}N_3O_2$. 275.35. (1) Pyrrolo[2,3-*b*]indol-5-ol, 1,2,3,3a,8,8a-hexahydro-1,3a,8-trimethyl-, methylcarbamate (ester), (3a*S-cis*); (2) Physostigmine; (3) 1,2,3,3aβ,8aβ-Hexahydro-1,3a,8-trimethylpyrrolo[2,3-*b*]-indol-5-yl methylcarbamate. *UNII-9U1VM840SP. CAS-57-47-6.* BAN. *Cholinergic (ophthalmic).*

Physostigmine Salicylate (fye″ soe stig′ meen sa lis′ i late). **USP**. $C_{15}H_{21}N_3O_2 \cdot C_7H_6O_3$. 413.47. (1) Pyrrolo[2,3-*b*]indol-5-ol, 1,2,3,3a,8,8a-hexahydro-1,3a,8-trimethyl-, methylcarbamate (ester), (3a*S-cis*)-, mono(2-hydroxybenzoate); (2) Physostigmine monosalicylate. *UNII-2046ZRO9VU; UNII-9U1VM840SP* [physostigmine]. *CAS-57-64-7; CAS-57-47-6* [physostigmine]. JAN. *Cholinergic (ophthalmic).* Antilirium (Forest); Isopto Eserine (Alcon†)

Physostigmine Sulfate (fye″ soe stig′ meen sul′ fate). **USP**. $(C_{15}H_{21}N_3O_2)_2 \cdot H_2SO_4$. 648.77. (1) Pyrrolo[2,3-*b*]indol-5-ol, 1,2,3,3a,8,8a-hexahydro-1,3a,8-trimethyl-, methylcarbamate (ester), (3a*S-cis*)-, sulfate (2:1); (2) Physostigmine sulfate (2:1). *UNII-G63V2J2N71; UNII-9U1VM840SP* [physostigmine]. *CAS-64-47-1; CAS-57-47-6* [physostigmine]. *Cholinergic (ophthalmic).* Eserine Sulfate (Ciba Vision, US Ophthalmics)

Phytate Persodium [*1977*] (fye′ tate per soe′ dee um). $C_6H_6Na_{12}O_{24}P_6$. 923.82. (1) Inositol hexakis(dihydrogen phosphate), dodecasodium salt, *myo*-; (2) *myo*-Inositol hexakis(disodium phosphate). *CAS-17211-15-3. Pharmaceutic aid.*

Phytate Sodium [*1962*] (fye′ tate soe′ dee um). $C_6H_9Na_9O_{24}P_6$. 857.87. (1) *myo*-Inositol, hexakis(dihydrogen phosphate), nonasodium salt; (2) Sodium cyclohexanehexyl (hexaphosphate). *CAS-7205-52-9. Chelating agent (calcium).* Rencal (Bristol-Myers Squibb†) ◇*SQ 9343*

Phytic Acid. $C_6H_{18}O_{24}P_6$. 660.04. [Fytic Acid is INN.] Phytic acid. *CAS-83-86-3.* MI.

Phytomenadione (INN, BAN, DCF) — *See* Phytonadione.

Phytonadiol Sodium Diphosphate. $C_{31}H_{48}Na_2O_8P_2$. 656.64. 2-Methyl-3-phytyl-1,4-naphthalenediol disodium diphosphate. *CAS-5988-22-7.* INN.

Phytonadione (fye toe″ na dye′ one). **USP.** $C_{31}H_{46}O_2$. 450.70. [Phytomenadione is INN and BAN.] (1) 1,4-Naphthalenedione, 2-methyl-3-(3,7,11,15-tetramethyl-2-hexadecenyl)-, [*R*-[*R**,*R**-(*E*)]]-; (2) Phylloquinone. *UNII-A034SE7857. CAS-84-80-0.* JAN. *Vitamin (prothrombogenic).* Aquamephyton (Merck); Konakion (Roche); Vitamin K1 (Hospira)

Pibaxizine. $C_{24}H_{29}NO_4$. 395.49. [2-[2-[4-(Diphenylmethylene)piperidino]ethoxy]ethoxy]acetic acid. *UNII-224TL37A39. CAS-82227-39-2.* INN.

Pibecarb. $C_{13}H_{16}O_3$. 220.26. Phenacylpivalate. *UNII-MOA3-SO592J. CAS-2522-81-8.* INN.

Piberaline. $C_{17}H_{19}N_3O$. 281.35. 1-Benzyl-4-picolinoylpiperazine. *UNII-8M09P36809. CAS-39640-15-8.* INN; MI.

Piboserod Hydrochloride [*1999*] (pi boe′ ser od hye″ droe klor′ ide). $C_{22}H_{31}N_3O_2$·HCl. 405.96. [Piboserod is BAN.] (1) 2*H*-[1,3]Oxazino[3,2-*a*]indole-10-carboxamide, *N*-[(1-butyl-4-piperidinyl)methyl]-3,4-dihydro-, monohydrochloride; (2) *N*-[(1-Butyl-4-piperidyl)methyl]-3,4-dihydro-2*H*-[1,3]oxazino[3,2-*a*]indole-10-carboxamide monohydrochloride. *UNII-61Z0VMM0AJ; UNII-4UQ3S81B25* [piboserod]. *CAS-178273-87-5; CAS-152811-62-6* [piboserod]. *Treatment of irritable bowel syndrome (selective 5HT₄receptor antagonist).* ◇*SB-207266-A*

Pibrozelesin. $C_{32}H_{36}BrN_5O_8$. 698.56. Methyl (*S*)-8-(bromomethyl)-3,6,7,8-tetrahydro-4-hydroxy-2-methyl-6-[(5,6,7-trimethoxyindol-2-yl)carbonyl]benzo[1,2-*b*:4,3-*b′*]dipyrrole-1-carboxylate, 4-methyl-1-piperazinecarboxylate (ester). *UNII-IHK933KCIC. CAS-154889-68-6.* INN.

Pibrozelesin Hydrobromide [*1998*] (pi″ broe zel′ e sin hye″ droe broe′ mide). $C_{32}H_{36}BrN_5O_8$·HBr. 779.47. (1) 8-(Bromomethyl)-3,6,7,8-tetrahydro-2-methyl-4-[[(4-methyl-1-piperazinyl)carbonyl]oxy]-6-[(1,6,7-trimethoxy-1*H*-indol-2-yl)carbonyl]benzo[1,2-*b*:4,3-*b′*]dipyrrole-1-carboxylic acid, methyl ester, monohydrobromide; (2) Methyl (*S*)-8-(bromomethyl)-3,6,7,8-tetrahydro-4-hydroxy-2-methyl-6-[(5,6,7-trimethoxyindol-2-yl)carbonyl]benzo[1,2-*b*:4,3-*b′*]dipyrrole-1-carboxylate, 4-methyl-1-piperazinecarboxylate (ester), monohydrobromide. *UNII-0481JCC90T. CAS-148778-32-9. Antineoplastic.* ◇*KW-2189*

---

† Brand name formerly used, and/or firm no longer concerned with this product.

Pibutidine. $C_{19}H_{24}N_4O_3$. 356.42. 3-Amino-4-[[(*Z*)-4-[[4-(piperidinomethyl)-2-pyridyl]oxy]-2-butenyl]amino]-3-cyclobutene-1,2-dione. *UNII-4XRL9PL02Y. CAS-103922-33-4.* INN.

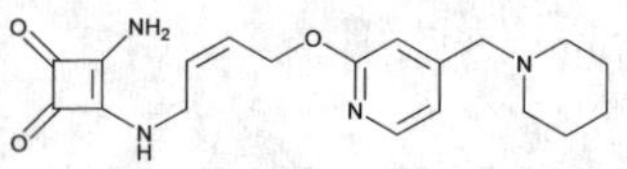

Picafibrate. $C_{18}H_{19}ClN_2O_4$. 362.81. 2-(*p*-Chlorophenoxy)-2-methylpropionic acid ester with *N*-(2-hydroxyethyl)nicotinamide. *UNII-12L83YI68T. CAS-57548-79-5.* INN.

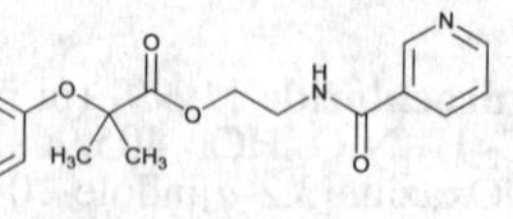

Picartamide. $C_{11}H_{14}N_2S_2$. 238.37. (±)-Tetrahydro-*N*-methyl-2-(2-pyridyl)thio-2-thiophenecarboxamide. *UNII-7JZ930H2M6. CAS-76732-75-7.* INN.

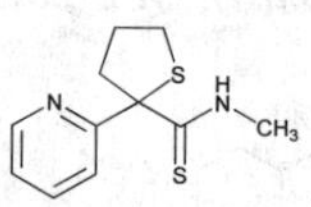

Picenadol Hydrochloride [*1981*] (pi sen′ a dol hye″ droe klor′ ide). $C_{16}H_{25}NO·HCl$. 283.84. [Picenadol is INN.] (1) Phenol, 3-(1,3-dimethyl-4-propyl-4-piperidinyl)-, hydrochloride, (±)-*trans*-; (2) (±)-*trans*-*m*-(1,3-Dimethyl-4-propyl-4-piperidyl)phenol hydrochloride. *UNII-29610N9WR1. CAS-74685-16-8; CAS-79201-85-7* [picenadol]. *Analgesic.* ◇*LY 150720*

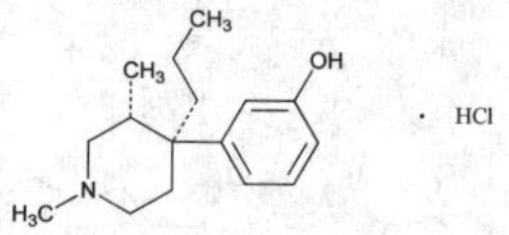

Picilorex. $C_{14}H_{18}ClN$. 235.75. 3-(*p*-Chlorophenyl)-5-cyclopropyl-2-methylpyrrolidine. *UNII-S8K2JDR3NZ. CAS-62510-56-9.* INN; MI.

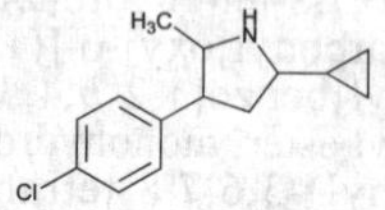

Piclamilast [*1996*] (pi kla′ mi last). $C_{18}H_{18}Cl_2N_2O_3$. 381.25. (1) Benzamide, 3-(cyclopentyloxy)-*N*-(3,5-dichloro-4-pyridinyl)-4-methoxy-; (2) 3-(Cyclopentyloxy)-*N*-(3,5-dichloro-4-pyridyl)-*p*-anisamide. *CAS-144035-83-6.* INN. *Antiasthmatic (type IV phosphodiesterase inhibitor).* ◇*RP 73401*

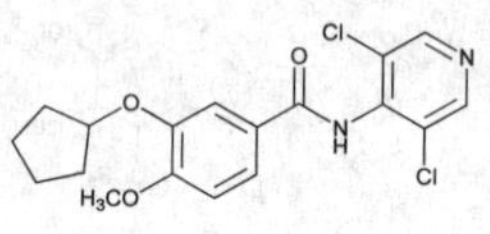

Piclonidine. $C_{14}H_{17}Cl_2N_3O$. 314.21. (±)-2-[2,6-Dichloro-*N*-(tetrahydro-2*H*-pyran-2-yl)anilino-2-imidazoline. *UNII-R7P4D56J1Z. CAS-72467-44-8.* INN.

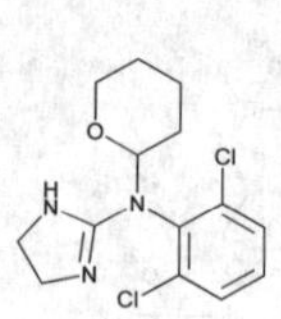

Piclopastine. $C_{20}H_{26}ClN_3O_2$. 375.89. 2-[2-[4-(*p*-Chloro-α-2-pyridylbenzyl)-1-piperazinyl]ethoxy]ethanol. *UNII-0939APN2IR. CAS-55837-13-3.* INN; DCF.

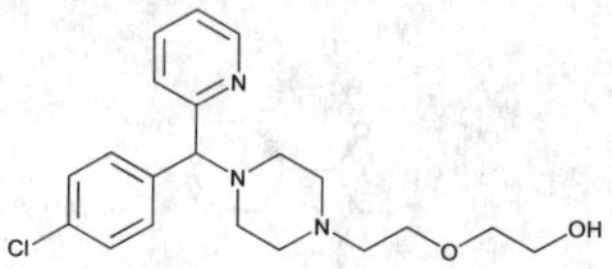

Picloxydine. $C_{20}H_{24}Cl_2N_{10}$. 475.38. 1,1′-[1,4-Piperazinediylbis(imidocarbonyl)]bis[3-(*p*-chlorophenyl)guanidine]. *UNII-4YC2PY3AEU. CAS-5636-92-0.* INN; BAN; DCF; MI.

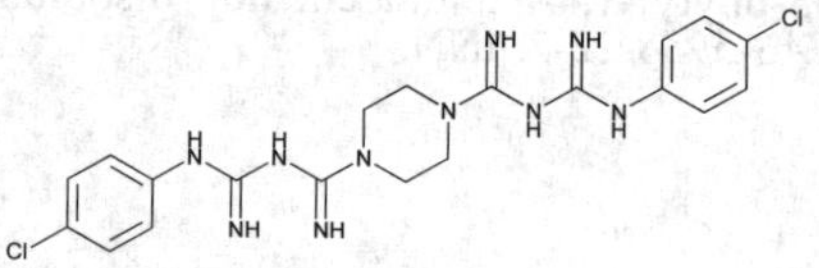

Piclozotan. $C_{23}H_{24}ClN_3O_2$. 409.91. 3-Chloro-4-[4-(1′,2′,3′,6′-tetrahydro-[2,4′-bipyridin]-1′-yl)butyl]-1,4-benzoxazepin-5(4*H*)-one. *CAS-182415-09-4.* INN.

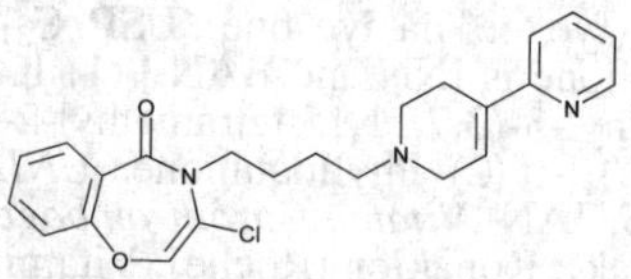

Picobenzide. $C_{15}H_{16}N_2O$. 240.30. 3,5-Dimethyl-*N*-(4-pyridylmethyl)benzamide. *UNII-C46317G8F0. CAS-51832-87-2.* INN.

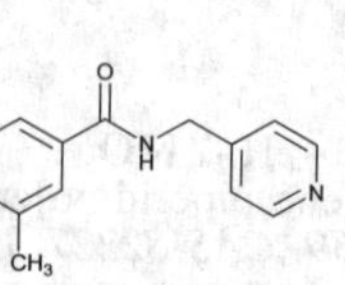

Picodralazine. $C_{14}H_{13}N_5$. 251.29. 1-Hydrazino-4-(4-pyridylmethyl)phthalazine. *UNII-O9D004V63I. CAS-17692-43-2.* INN; DCF.

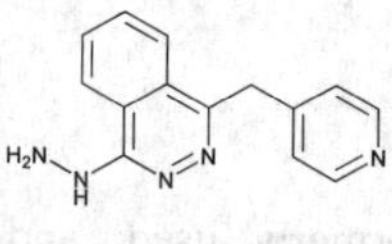

Picolamine. $C_6H_8N_2$. 108.14. 3-(Aminomethyl)pyridine. *UNII-31LA41942J. CAS-3731-52-0*. INN; DCF.

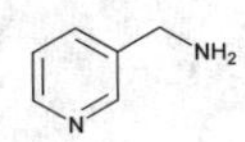

Piconol. C_6H_7NO. 109.13. 2-Pyridinemethanol. *UNII-7HQ8UT1TPS. CAS-586-98-1*. INN.

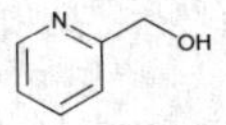

Picoperine. $C_{19}H_{25}N_3$. 295.42. 1-[2-[N-(2-Pyridylmethyl)anilino]ethyl]piperidine. *UNII-YK3XA0K1O1. CAS-21755-66-8*. INN; MI. ◇*TAT-3*

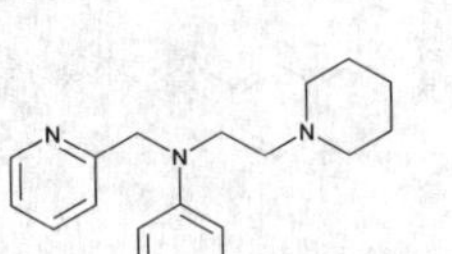

Picoplatin [*2006*] (pi″ koe pla′ tin). $C_6H_{10}Cl_2N_2Pt$. 376.15. (1) Platinum, amminedichloro(2-methylpyridine)-, (*SP*-4-3)-; (2) (*SP*-4-3)-Amminedichloro(2-methylpyridine)platinium. *CAS-181630-15-9*. INN; BAN. *Treatment of cancer.* ◇*NX 473; ZD0473; AMD473*

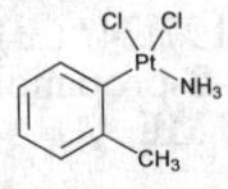

Picoprazole. $C_{17}H_{17}N_3O_3S$. 343.40. Methyl 6-methyl-2-[[(3-methyl-2-pyridyl)methyl]sulfinyl]-5-benzimidazolecarboxylate. *CAS-78090-11-6*. INN.

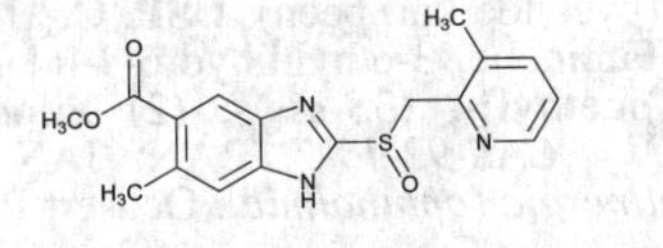

Picotamide. $C_{21}H_{20}N_4O_3$. 376.41. *N,N′*-Bis(3-pyridylmethyl)-4-methoxyisophthalamide. *UNII-654G2VCI4Q. CAS-32828-81-2*. BAN.

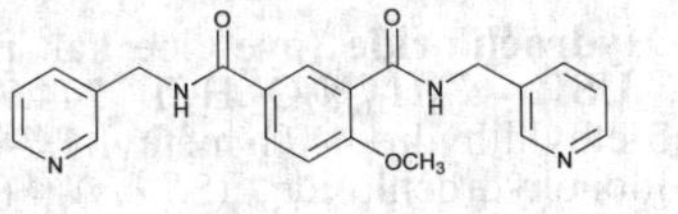

Picotrin Diolamine [*1978*] (pi′ koe trin dye ole′ a meen). $C_{25}H_{19}NO_2 \cdot C_4H_{11}NO_2$. 470.56. [Picotrin is INN.] (1) 2-Pyridinecarboxylic acid, 5-(triphenylmethyl)-, compound with 2,2′-iminobis[ethanol] (1:1); (2) 5-Tritylpicolinic acid compound with 2,2′-iminodiethanol (1:1). *CAS-64063-83-8; CAS-64063-57-6* [picotrin]. *Keratolytic.* ◇*Sch 19741*

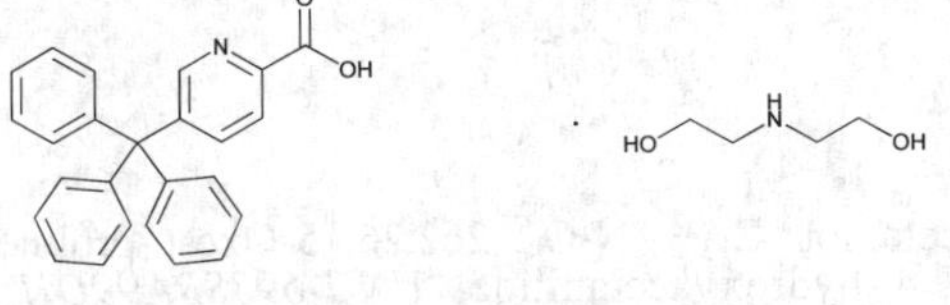

Picric Acid — *See* Trinitrophenol.

Picrotoxin. $C_{15}H_{18}O_7 \cdot C_{15}H_{16}O_6$. 602.58. (1) 3,6-Methano-8*H*-1,5,7-trioxacyclopenta(*ij*)cycloprop(*a*)azulene-4,8(3*H*)-dione, hexahydro-2a-hydroxy-9-(1-hydroxy-1-methylethyl)-8b-methyl-, (1a*R*-(1aα,2aβ,3β,6β,6aβ,8aS*,8bβ,9S*))-, compound with (1aR-(1aα,2aβ,3β,6β,6aβ,8aS*,8bβ,9R*))-hexahydro-2a-hydroxy-8b-methyl-9-(1-methylethenyl)-3,6-methano-8*H*-1,5,7-trioxacyclopenta(*ij*)cycloprop(*a*)azulene-4,8(3*H*)-dione; (2) (1*R*,2*S*,5*S*,7*R*,9*R*,10*S*,13*S*,14*R*)-3,6,12-Trioxapentacyclo[8.2.1.1^{2,5}.0^{5,7}.0^{9,14}]-4,11-dioxo-9-hydroxy-13-(2-hydroxypropan-2-yl)-1,4-methyltetradecane compound with (1*R*,2*S*,5*S*,7*R*,9*R*,10*S*,13*R*,14*R*)-3,6,12-Trioxapentacyclo[8.2.1.1^{2,5}.0^{5,7}.0^{9,14}]-4,11-dioxo-9-hydroxy-13-(propen-2-yl)-1,4-methyltetradecane. *CAS-124-87-8*. NF XIII; MI.

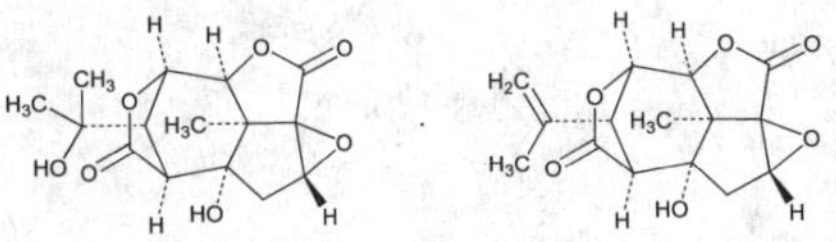

Picumast. $C_{25}H_{29}ClN_2O_3$. 440.96. 7-[3-[4-(*p*-Chlorobenzyl)-1-piperazinyl]propoxy]-3,4-dimethylcoumarin. *UNII-125267OAUF. CAS-39577-19-0*. INN; BAN.

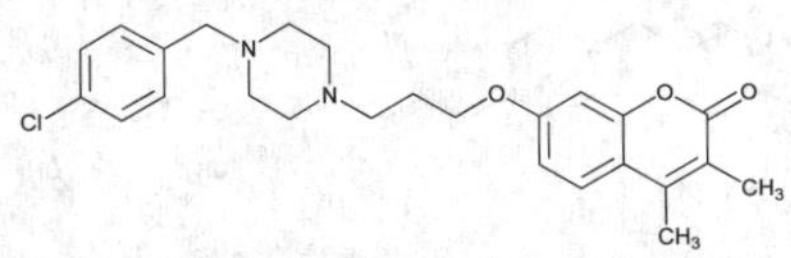

Picumeterol Fumarate [*1991*] (pi″ kue me′ ter ol fue′ ma rate). $(C_{21}H_{29}Cl_2N_3O_2)_2 \cdot C_4H_4O_4$. 968.83. [Picumeterol is INN and BAN.] (1) Benzenemethanol, 4-amino-3,5-dichloro-α-[[[6-[2-(2-pyridinyl)ethoxy]hexyl]amino]methyl]-, (*R*)-, (*E*)-2-butenedioate (2:1) (salt); (2) (-)-(*R*)-4-Amino-3,5-dichloro-α-[[[6-[2-(2-pyridyl)ethoxy]hexyl]amino]methyl]benzyl alcohol, fumarate (2:1) (salt). *UNII-0SUN4UF93Y; UNII-86WEQ311WF* [picumeterol]. *CAS-130641-37-1; CAS-130641-36-0* [picumeterol]. *Bronchodilator.* ◇*GR 114297A; GR 114297X* [picumeterol]

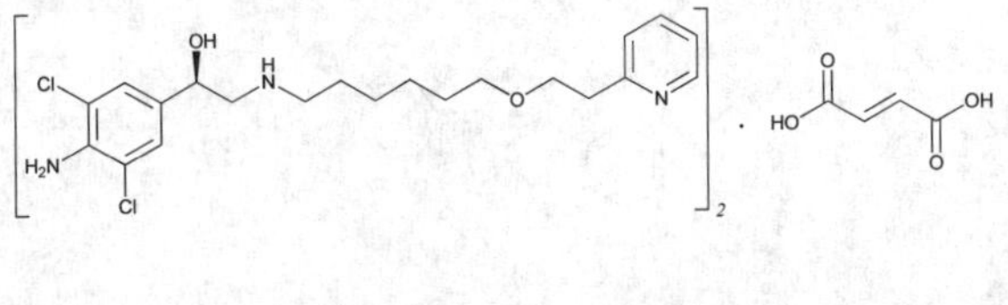

---

† Brand name formerly used, and/or firm no longer concerned with this product.

Pidobenzone. $C_{11}H_{11}NO_4$. 221.21. 5-Oxo-L-proline,*p*-hydroxyphenyl ester. *UNII-X7D2GSX1C1. CAS-138506-45-3.* INN.

Pidolacetamol. $C_{13}H_{14}N_2O_4$. 262.26. 5-Oxo-L-proline, ester with 4′-hydroxyacetanilide. *UNII-693SRA99OH. CAS-114485-92-6.* INN.

Pidolic Acid. $C_5H_7NO_3$. 129.11. 5-Oxoproline. *CAS-98-79-3.* INN; BAN.

Pidotimod. $C_9H_{12}N_2O_4S$. 244.27. (*R*)-3-[(*S*)-5-Oxoprolyl]-4-thiazolidinecarboxylic acid. *UNII-785363R681. CAS-121808-62-6.* INN.

Pifarnine [*1977*] (pi far′ neen). $C_{27}H_{40}N_2O_2$. 424.62. (1) Piperazine, 1-(1,3-benzodioxol-5-ylmethyl)-4-(3,7,11-trimethyl-2,6,10-dodecatrienyl)-; (2) 1-Piperonyl-4-(3,7,11-trimethyl-2,6,10-dodecatrienyl)piperazine. *UNII-3W85193GZ4. CAS-56208-01-6.* INN. *Anti-ulcerative (gastric).*

Pifenate. $C_{22}H_{27}NO_2$. 337.46. Ethyl α,α-diphenyl-2-piperidinepropionate. *UNII-STW31V60ZL. CAS-15686-87-0.* INN; BAN.

Pifexole. $C_{13}H_8ClN_3O$. 257.68. 4-[5-(*o*-Chlorophenyl)-1,2,4-oxadiazol-3-yl]pyridine. *UNII-36DL76CZNI. CAS-27199-40-2.* INN. ◇RI-64

Piflutixol. $C_{24}H_{25}F_4NOS$. 451.52. 1-[3-[6-Fluoro-2-(trifluoromethyl)thioxanthen-9-ylidene]propyl]-4-piperidineethanol. *CAS-54341-02-5.* INN.

Pifonakin. 36-L-Aspartic acid-141-L-serineinterleukin 1α (human clone p10A). *CAS-112721-39-8.* INN.

Pifoxime. $C_{15}H_{20}N_2O_3$. 276.33. 1-[(*p*-Acetylphenoxy)-acetyl]piperidine *p*-oxime. *CAS-31224-92-7.* INN; MI.

Piketoprofen. $C_{22}H_{20}N_2O_2$. 344.41. *m*-Benzoyl-*N*-(4-methyl-2-pyridyl)hydratropamide. *UNII-362QBC4NL0. CAS-60576-13-8.* INN; MI.

Pildralazine. $C_8H_{15}N_5O$. 197.24. ($\pm$)-1-[(6-Hydrazino-3-pyridazinyl)methylamino]-2-propanol. *UNII-FU2BGC781U. CAS-64000-73-3.* INN; MI.

Pilocarpine (pye″ loe kar′ peen). **USP.** $C_{11}H_{16}N_2O_2$. 208.26. (1) 2(3*H*)-Furanone, 3-ethyldihydro-4-[(1-methyl-1*H*-imidazol-5-yl)methyl]-, (3*S-cis*)-; (2) Pilocarpine. *UNII-01MI4Q9DI3. CAS-92-13-7.* BAN; JAN. *Antiglaucoma agent; cholinergic (ophthalmic).* Ocusert Pilo (Akorn)

Pilocarpine Hydrochloride (pye″ loe kar′ peen hye″ droe klor′ ide). **USP.** $C_{11}H_{16}N_2O_2 \cdot HCl$. 244.72. (1) 2(3*H*)-Furanone, 3-ethyldihydro-4-[(1-methyl-1*H*-imidazol-5-yl)methyl]-, monohydrochloride, (3*S-cis*)-; (2) Pilocarpine monohydrochloride. *UNII-0WW6D218XJ. CAS-54-71-7; CAS-92-13-7* [pilocarpine]. JAN. *Cholinergic (ophthalmic).* Pilopine (Alcon); Salagen (MGI Pharma)

Pilocarpine Nitrate (pye″ loe kar′ peen nye′ trate). **USP.** $C_{11}H_{16}N_2O_2 \cdot HNO_3$. 271.27. (1) 2(3*H*)-Furanone, 3-ethyldihydro-4-[(1-methyl-1*H*-imidazol-5-yl)methyl]-, (3*S-cis*)-, mononitrate; (2) Pilocarpine mononitrate. *UNII-01MI4Q9-DI3* [pilocarpine]. *CAS-148-72-1; CAS-92-13-7* [pilocarpine]. *Cholinergic (ophthalmic).* Pilagan (Allergan)

Pilsicainide. $C_{17}H_{24}N_2O$. 272.39. [Pilsicainide Hydrochloride is JAN.] Tetrahydro-1*H*-pyrrolizine-7a(5*H*)-aceto-2′,6′-xylidide. *UNII-AV0X7V6CSE. CAS-88069-67-4.* INN.

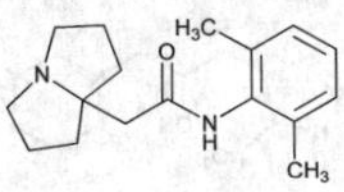

Pimagedine Hydrochloride [*1993*] (pim a′ je deen hye″ droe klor′ ide). $CH_6N_4.HCl$. 110.55. [Pimagedine is INN.] (1) Hydrazinecarboximidamide, monohydrochloride; (2) Aminoguanidine monohydrochloride. *UNII-A2Z7G2RGAH. CAS-1937-19-5; CAS-79-17-4* [pimagedine]. *Inhibitor (advanced glycosylation end-product formation). ✧GER-11*

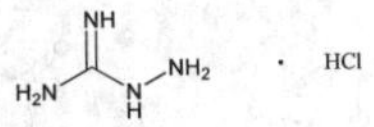

Pimaricin (JAN) — *See* Natamycin.

Pimavanserin Tartrate [*2006*] (pim″ a van′ ser in). $(C_{25}H_{34}FN_3O_2)_2.C_4H_6O_6$. 1005.20. [Pimavanserin is INN.] (1) Urea, *N*-[(4-fluorophenyl)methyl]-*N*-(1-methyl-4-piperidinyl)-*N′*-[[4-(2-methylpropoxy)phenyl]methyl]-, (2*R*,3*R*)-2,3-dihydroxybutanedioate (2:1); (2) Bis[1-(4-fluorobenzyl)-1-(1-methylpiperidin-4-yl)-3-[4-(2-methylpropoxy)benzyl]urea] (2*R*,3*R*)-2,3-dihydroxybutanedioate. *UNII-NA83F1SJSR; UNII-JZ963P0DIK* [pimavanserin]. *CAS-706782-28-7; CAS-706779-91-1* [pimavanserin]. *Treatment of psychosis in Parkinson's disease patients and in schizophrenia patients. ✧ACP-103*

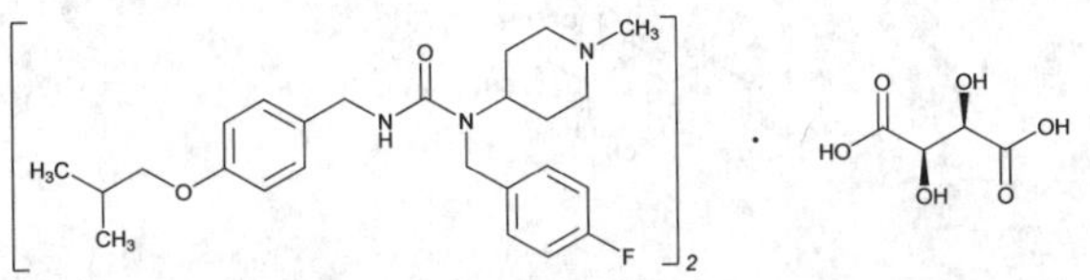

Pimeclone. $C_{12}H_{21}NO$. 195.30. 2-(Piperidinomethyl)cyclohexanone. *UNII-F0PVL84ZWR. CAS-534-84-9.* INN; DCF; MI. *✧NA-66*

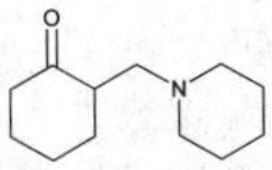

Pimecrolimus [*2000*] (pim″ e kroe′ li mus). $C_{43}H_{68}ClNO_{11}$. 810.45. (1) 15,19-Epoxy-3*H*-pyrido[2,1-*c*][1,4]oxaazacyclotricosine-1,17,20,21(4*H*,23*H*)-tetrone, 3-[(1*E*)-2-[(1*R*,3*R*,4*S*)-4-chloro-3-methoxycyclohexyl]-1-methylethenyl]-8-ethyl-5,6,8,11,12,13,14,15,16,17,18,19,24,26,26a-hexadecahydro-5,19-dihydroxy-14,16-dimethoxy-4,10,12,18-tetramethyl-, (3*S*,4*R*,5*S*,8*R*,9*E*,12*S*,14*S*,15*R*,16*S*,18*R*,19*R*,26a*S*)-; (2) (3*S*,4*R*,5*S*,8*R*,9*E*,12*S*,14*S*,15*R*,16*S*,18*R*,19*R*,26a*S*)-3-[(*E*)-2-[(1*R*,3*R*,4*S*)-4-chloro-3-methoxycyclohexyl]-1-methylvinyl]-8-ethyl-5,6,8,11,12,13,14,15,16,17,18,19,24,26,26a-hexadecahydro-5,19-epoxy-3H-pyrido[2,1-*c*][1,4]oxaazacyclotricosine-1,17,20,21(4*H*,23*H*)-tetrone. *UNII-7KYV510875. CAS-137071-32-0.* INN; BAN. *Treatment of inflammatory skin disease (immunosuppressant).* Elidel (Novartis) *✧SDZ ASM 981*

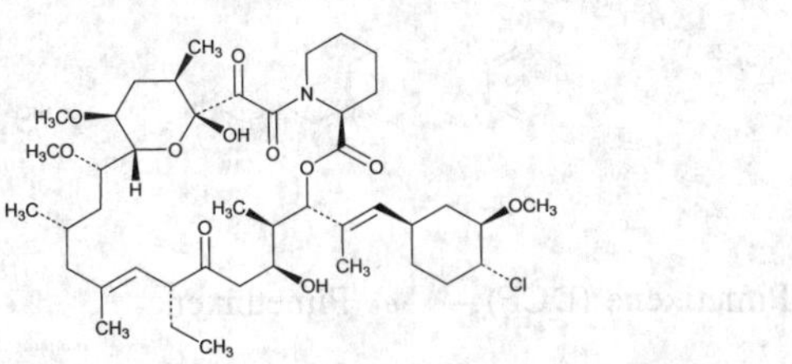

Pimefylline. $C_{15}H_{18}N_6O_2$. 314.34. 7-[2-[(3-Pyridylmethyl)amino]ethyl]theophylline. *UNII-8680B5Y37A. CAS-10001-43-1.* INN; MI.

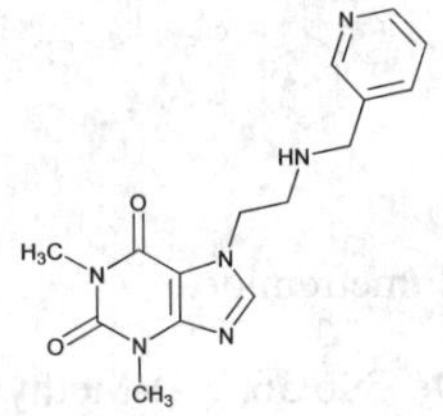

Pimelautide. $C_{29}H_{52}N_6O_9$. 628.76. *threo*-6-Carbamoyl-N^2-[*N*-(*N*-lauroyl-L-alanyl)-D-γ-glutamyl]-N^6-glycyl-DL-lysine. *UNII-O9643CJL3T. CAS-78512-63-7.* INN.

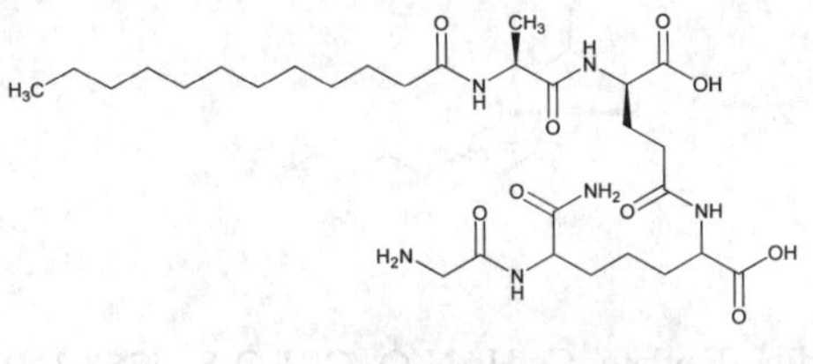

Pimetacin. $C_{25}H_{21}ClN_2O_3S$. 464.96. 1-(*p*-Chlorobenzoyl)-5-methoxy-2-methyl-3-indoleacetic acid 3-pyridylmethyl thioester. *UNII-Z6RX3C7B5V. CAS-79992-71-5.* INN.

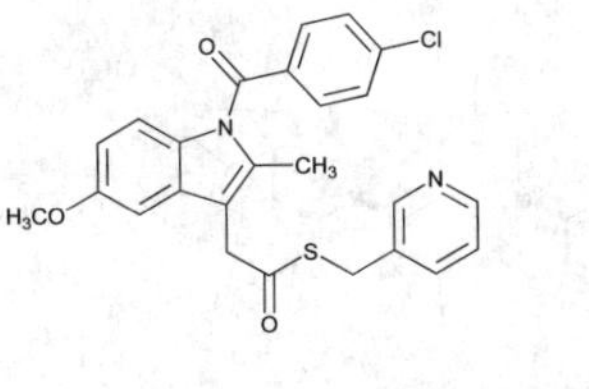

Pimethixene. $C_{19}H_{19}NS$. 293.43. 1-Methyl-4-(thioxanthen-9-ylidene)piperidine. *CAS-314-03-4.* INN. *✧BP 400*

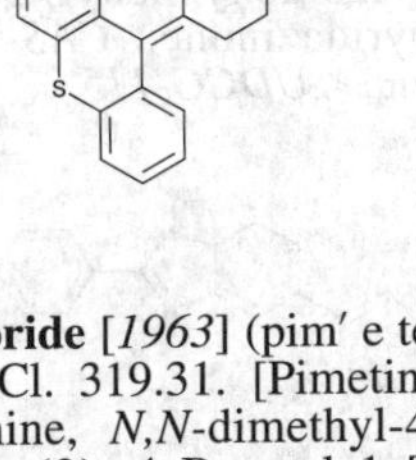

Pimetine Hydrochloride [*1963*] (pim′ e teen hye″ droe klor′ ide). $C_{16}H_{26}N_2.2HCl$. 319.31. [Pimetine is INN.] (1) 1-Piperidineethanamine, *N*,*N*-dimethyl-4-(phenylmethyl)-, dihydrochloride; (2) 4-Benzyl-1-[2-(dimethylami-

† Brand name formerly used, and/or firm no longer concerned with this product.

no)ethyl]piperidine dihydrochloride. *CAS-4991-68-8; CAS-3565-03-5* [pimetine]. *Antihyperlipoproteinemic.* ◇*IN 379; NSC-528880*

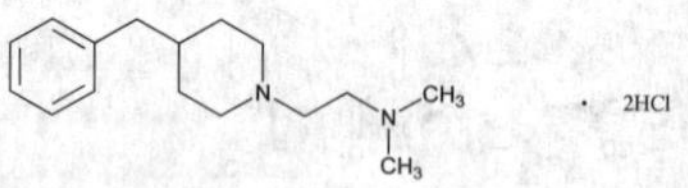

Pimetixene (DCF) — *See* Pimethixene.

Pimetremide. $C_{16}H_{18}N_2O_2$. 270.33. *N*-Methyl-2-phenyl-*N*-3-pyridylmethylhydracrylamide. *UNII-3VY58MWL7J. CAS-578-89-2.* INN.

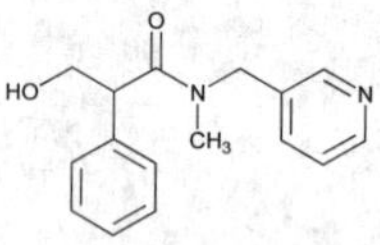

Pimeverine — *See* Pimetremide.

Pimilprost. $C_{23}H_{40}O_5$. 396.56. (+)-Methyl [2-[(2*R*,3a*S*,4*R*,5-*R*,6a*S*)-octahydro-5-hydroxy-4-[(1*E*,3*S*,5*S*)-3-hydroxy-5-methyl-1-nonenyl]-2-pentalenyl]ethoxy]acetate. *UNII-O316O1ZGEG. CAS-139403-31-9.* INN.

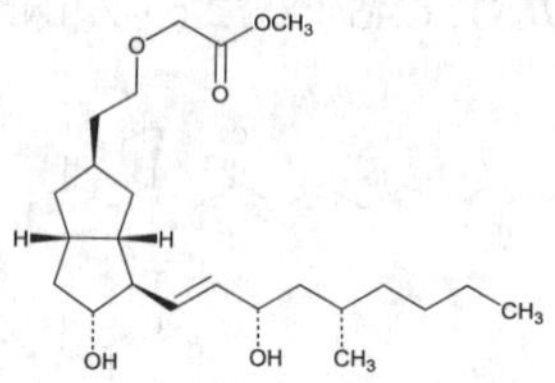

Piminodine Esylate. $C_{23}H_{30}N_2O_2 \cdot C_2H_6O_3S$. 476.63. [Piminodine is INN and BAN.] 4-Piperidinecarboxylic acid, 4-phenyl-1-[3-(phenylamino)propyl]-, ethyl ester, monoethanesulfonate. *UNII-2C29WCQ951. CAS-7081-52-9; CAS-13495-09-5* [piminodine]. NF XIV; MI. Alvodine Ethanesulfonate (Sterling Winthrop†)

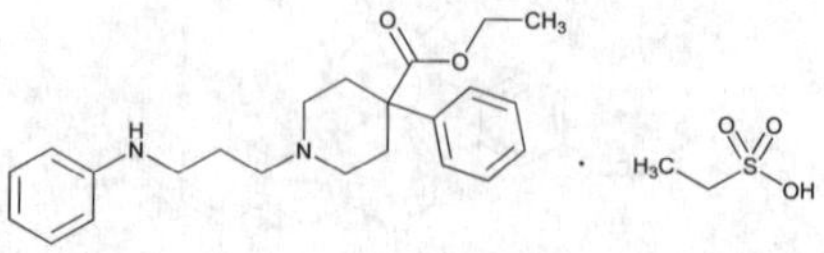

Piminodine Ethanesulfonate — *See* Piminodine Esylate.

Pimobendan [*1990*] (pim″ oh ben′ dan). $C_{19}H_{18}N_4O_2$. 334.37. (1) 3(2*H*)-Pyridazinone, 4,5-dihydro-6-[2-(4-methoxyphenyl)-1*H*-benzimidazol-5-yl]-5-methyl-, (±)-; (2) (±)-4,5-Dihydro-6-[2-(*p*-methoxyphenyl)-5-benzimidazolyl]-5-methyl-3(2*H*)-pyridazinone. *CAS-118428-36-7.* INN; BAN. *Cardiotonic.* ◇*UDCG-115*

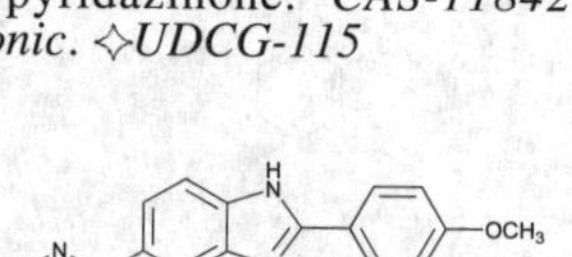

Pimonidazole. $C_{11}H_{18}N_4O_3$. 254.29. (±)-α-[(2-Nitroimidazol-1-yl)methyl]-1-piperidineethanol. *CAS-70132-50-2.* INN; BAN. ◇*Ro 03-8799*

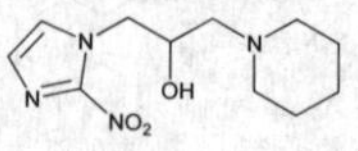

Pimozide [*1967*] (pim′ oh zide). **USP**. $C_{28}H_{29}F_2N_3O$. 461.55. (1) 2*H*-Benzimidazol-2-one, 1-[1-[4,4-bis(4-fluorophenyl)-butyl]-4-piperidinyl]-1,3-dihydro-; (2) 1-[1-[4,4-Bis(*p*-fluorophenyl)butyl]-4-piperidyl]-2-benzimidazolinone. *UNII-1HIZ4DL86F. CAS-2062-78-4.* INN; BAN; JAN. *Antipsychotic.* Orap (Teva) ◇*McN-JR-6238; R 6238*

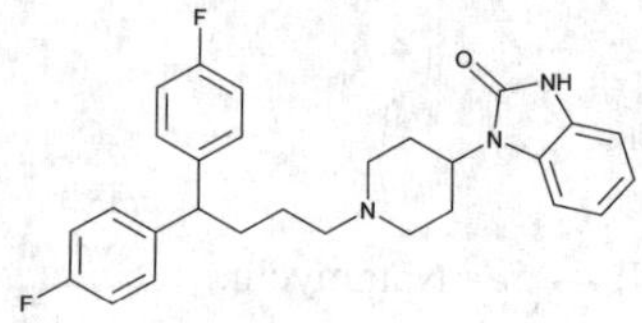

Pinacidil [*1984*] (pin a′ si dil). $C_{13}H_{19}N_5 \cdot H_2O$. 263.34. (1) Guanidine, *N″*-cyano-*N*-4-pyridinyl-*N′*-(1,2,2-trimethylpropyl)-, monohydrate, (±)-; (2) (±)-2-Cyano-1-(4-pyridyl)-3-(1,2,2-trimethylpropyl)guanidine monohydrate; (3) Guanidine, *N*-cyano-*N′*-4-pyridinyl-*N″*-(1,2,2-trimethylpropyl)-, monohydrate, (±)-. *UNII-7B0ZZH8P2W. CAS-85371-64-8; CAS-60560-33-0* [anhydrous]. INN. *Antihypertensive.* Pindac (Leo)

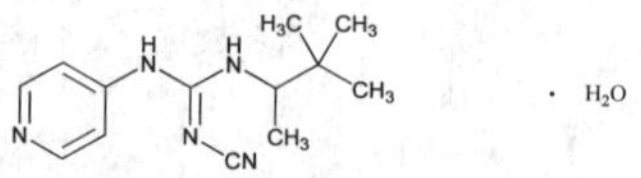

Pinadoline [*1984*] (pin ad′ oh leen). $C_{19}H_{19}Cl_2N_3O_3$. 408.28. (1) Dibenz[*b,f*][1,4]oxazepine-10(11*H*)-carboxylic acid, 8-chloro-, 2-(5-chloro-1-oxopentyl)hydrazide; (2) 1-[(8-Chlorodibenz[*b,f*][1,4]oxazepin-10(11*H*-yl)carbonyl]-2-(5-chlorovaleryl)hydrazine. *CAS-38955-22-5.* INN. *Analgesic.* ◇*SC-25469*

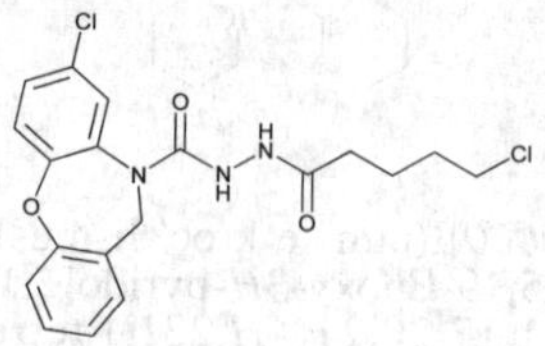

Pinafide. $C_{18}H_{17}N_3O_4$. 339.35. 3-Nitro-*N*-[2-(1-pyrrolidinyl)ethyl]naphthalimide. *UNII-1OZ94FI615. CAS-54824-20-3.* INN.

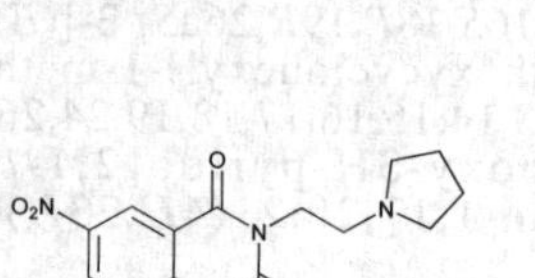

Pinaverium Bromide. $C_{26}H_{41}Br_2NO_4$. 591.42. 4-(6-Bromo-veratryl)-4-[2-[2-(6,6-dimethyl-2-norpinyl)ethoxy]ethyl]-morpholinium bromide. *CAS-53251-94-8; CAS-59995-65-2* [pinaverium]. INN; MI.

Pinazepam. $C_{18}H_{13}ClN_2O$. 308.76. 7-Chloro-1,3-dihydro-5-phenyl-1-(2-propynyl)-2*H*-1,4-benzodiazepin-2-one. *UNII-5286RBZ882. CAS-52463-83-9*. INN; MI.

Pincainide. $C_{16}H_{24}N_2O$. 260.37. 2,3,4,5,6,7-Hexahydro-1*H*-azepine-1-aceto-2′,6′-xylidide. *UNII-66803GMO3G. CAS-83471-41-4*. INN.

Pindolol [*1970*] (pin′ doe lol). **USP.** $C_{14}H_{20}N_2O_2$. 248.32. (1) 2-Propanol, 1-(1*H*-indol-4-yloxy)-3-(1-methylethyl)ami-no-; (2) 1-(Indol-4-yloxy)-3-(isopropylamino)-2-propanol. *UNII-BJ4HF6IU1D. CAS-13523-86-9*. INN; BAN; JAN. *Vasodilator*. Visken (Novartis) ◇*LB-46*

Pine Needle Oil. *CAS-8016-46-4*. NF XVI.

Pine Tar. USP XXI; JAN.

Pinokalant. $C_{41}H_{48}N_2O_9$. 712.83. (±)-3,4-Dihydro-6,7-di-methoxy-α-phenyl-*N,N*-bis(2,3,4-trimethoxyphenethyl)-1-isoquinolineacetamide. *UNII-7J9ZZ971AO. CAS-149759-26-2*. INN.

---

† Brand name formerly used, and/or firm no longer concerned with this product.

Pinolcaine. $C_{23}H_{29}NO_2$. 351.48. D-(+)-1-Methyl-1-(1-meth-yl-2-piperidyl)ethyl diphenylacetate. *UNII-S0U059XF2E. CAS-28240-18-8*. INN.

Pinoxepin Hydrochloride [*1967*] (pin ox′ e pin hye″ droe klor′ ide). $C_{23}H_{27}ClN_2O_2$.2HCl. 471.85. [Pinoxepin is INN.] (1) 1-Piperazineethanol, 4-[3-(2-chlorodibenz[*b,e*]oxepin-11(6*H*)-ylidene)propyl]-, dihydrochloride, (*Z*)-; (2) (*Z*)-4-[3-(2-Chlorodibenz[*b,e*]oxepin-11-(6*H*)-yli-dene)propyl]-1-piperazineethanol dihydrochloride. *UNII-7KE5R66TSY. CAS-14008-46-9; CAS-14008-66-3* [pinox-epin]. *Antipsychotic*. ◇*P-5227*

Pioglitazone Hydrochloride [*1989*] (pye″ oh gli′ ta zone hye″ droe klor′ ide). $C_{19}H_{20}N_2O_3S$.HCl. 392.90. [Pioglita-zone is INN and BAN.] (1) 2,4-Thiazolidinedione, 5-[[4-[2-(5-ethyl-2-pyridinyl)ethoxy]phenyl]methyl]-, monohy-drochloride, (±)-; (2) (±)-5-[*p*-[2-(5-Ethyl-2-pyridy-l)ethoxy]benzyl]-2,4-thiazolidinedione monohydrochlor-ide. *UNII-JQT35NPK6C; UNII-X4OV71U42S* [pioglitazone]. *CAS-112529-15-4; CAS-111025-46-8* [pio-glitazone]. *Antidiabetic*. Actos (Takeda) ◇*U-72107A*

Pipacycline. $C_{29}H_{38}N_4O_9$. 586.63. 4-Dimethylamino-1,4,4a,5,5a,6,11,12a-octahydro-3,6,10,12,12a-pentahy-droxy-*N*-[[4-(2-hydroxyethyl)-1-piperazinyl]methyl]-6-methyl-1,11-dioxo-2-naphthacenecarboxamide. *UNII-PQ3P6082I5. CAS-1110-80-1*. INN; MI.

Pipamazine. $C_{21}H_{24}ClN_3OS$. 401.95. 10-[3-(4-Carbamoylpi-peridino)propyl]-2-chlorophenothiazine. *UNII-653552FHIN. CAS-84-04-8*. INN; BAN; MI.

Pipamperone [*1967*] (pi pam′ per one). $C_{21}H_{30}FN_3O_2$. 375.48. [Pipamperone Hydrochloride is JAN.] (1) [1,4′-Bipiperidine]-4′-carboxamide, 1′-[4-(4-fluorophenyl)-4-

oxobutyl]-; (2) 1'-[3-(*p*-Fluorobenzoyl)propyl]-[1,4'-bipiperidine]-4'-carboxamide. *UNII-5402501F0W. CAS-1893-33-0.* INN; BAN. *Antipsychotic. [Name previously used: Floropipamide.]* ◇*R 3345*

Pipaneperone — *See* Pipamperone.

Pipazetate (INN, BAN, DCF) — *See* Pipazethate.

Pipazethate [*1963*] (pi paz' e thate). C$_{21}$H$_{25}$N$_3$O$_3$S. 399.51. [Pipazetate is INN and BAN.] (1) 10*H*-Pyrido[3,2-*b*][1,4]benzothiazine-10-carboxylic acid, 2-[2-(1-piperidinyl)ethoxy]ethyl ester; (2) 2-(2-Piperidinoethoxy)ethyl 10*H*-pyrido[3,2-*b*][1,4]benzothiazine-10-carboxylate. *CAS-2167-85-3. Antitussive.* ◇*D-254; SK&F 70230-A; SQ 15,874*

Pipebuzone. C$_{25}$H$_{32}$N$_4$O$_2$. 420.55. 4-Butyl-4-[(4-methyl-1-piperazinyl)methyl]-1,2-diphenyl-3,5-pyrazolidinedione. *UNII-2B2ZV6F5HG. CAS-27315-91-9.* INN; DCF; MI. ◇*LD 4644*

Pipecuronium Bromide [*1987*] (pi″ pe kure oh′ nee um broe′ mide). C$_{35}$H$_{62}$Br$_2$N$_4$O$_4$. 762.70. (1) Piperazinium, 4,4'-[(2β,3α,5α,16β,17β)-3,17-bis(acetyloxy)androstane-2,16-diyl]bis[1,1-dimethyl-, dibromide; (2) 4,4'-(3α,17β-Dihydroxy-5α-androstan-2β,16β-ylene)bis[1,1-dimethylpiperazinium]dibromide, diacetate (ester). *UNII-R6ZTY81RE1. CAS-52212-02-9.* INN; BAN. *Neuromuscular blocking agent.* Arduan (Organon) ◇*RGH 1106*

Pipemidic Acid. C$_{14}$H$_{17}$N$_5$O$_3$. 303.32. [Pipemidic Acid Trihydrate is JAN.] 8-Ethyl-5,8-dihydro-5-oxo-2-(1-piperazinyl)pyrido[2,3-*d*]pyrimidine-6-carboxylic acid. *UNII-LT12J5HVR8. CAS-51940-44-4.* INN; BAN; DCF; MI.

Pipendoxifene. C$_{29}$H$_{32}$N$_2$O$_3$. 456.58. 2-(*p*-Hydroxyphenyl)-3-methyl-1-[*p*-(2-piperidinoethoxy)benzyl]indol-5-ol. *UNII-TPC5Q8496G. CAS-198480-55-6.* INN.

Pipenzolate Bromide. C$_{22}$H$_{28}$BrNO$_3$. 434.37. 1-Ethyl-3-hydroxy-1-methylpiperidinium bromide benzilate. *CAS-125-51-9; CAS-13473-38-6* [pipenzolate]. INN; BAN; MI. Piptal (Marion Merrell Dow†)

Pipenzolate Methylbromide — *See* Pipenzolate Bromide.

Pipenzolone Bromide — *See* Pipenzolate Bromide.

Pipequaline. C$_{22}$H$_{24}$N$_2$. 316.44. 2-Phenyl-4-[2-(4-piperidyl)ethyl]quinoline. *UNII-J3S205V4I2. CAS-77472-98-1.* INN.

Piperacetazine [*1962*] (pi″ per a seet′ a zeen). C$_{24}$H$_{30}$N$_2$O$_2$S. 410.57. (1) Ethanone, 1-[10-[3-[4-(2-hydroxyethyl)-1-piperidinyl]propyl]-10*H*-phenothiazin-2-yl]-; (2) 10-[3-[4-(2-Hydroxyethyl)piperidino]propyl]phenothiazin-2-yl methyl ketone. *UNII-KL6248WNW4. CAS-3819-00-9.* USP XXII; INN. *Antipsychotic.* Quide (Dow Chemical) ◇*PC-1421*

Piperacillin (pi″ per a sil′ in). **USP.** $C_{23}H_{27}N_5O_7S.H_2O$. 535.57. (1) 4-Thia-1-azabicyclo[3.2.0]heptane-2-carboxylic acid, 6-[[[[(4-ethyl-2,3-dioxo-1-piperazinyl)carbonyl]amino]phenylacetyl]amino]-3,3-dimethyl-7-oxo-, monohydrate, [2S-[2α,5α,6β(S*)]]; (2) (2S,5R,6R)-6-[(R)-2-(4-Ethyl-2,3-dioxo-1-piperazinecarboxamido)-2-phenylacetamido]-3,3-dimethyl-7-oxo-4-thia-1-azabicyclo[3.2.0]heptane-2-carboxylic acid monohydrate. *UNII-X00B0D5O0E. CAS-66258-76-2; CAS-61477-96-1* [anhydrous]. INN; BAN. *Antibacterial.*

Piperacillin Sodium [*1977*] (pi″ per a sil′ in soe′ dee um). **USP.** $C_{23}H_{26}N_5NaO_7S$. 539.54. (1) 4-Thia-1-azabicyclo[3.2.0]heptane-2-carboxylic acid, 6-[[[[(4-ethyl-2,3-dioxo-1-piperazinyl)carbonyl]amino]phenylacetyl]amino]-3,3-dimethyl-7-oxo-, monosodium salt, [2S-[2α,5α,6β(S*)]]; (2) Sodium (2S,5R,6R)-6-[(R)-2-(4-ethyl-2,3-dioxo-1-piperazinecarboxamido)-2-phenylacetamido]-3,3-dimethyl-7-oxo-4-thia-1-azabicyclo[3.2.0]heptane-2-carboxylate. *UNII-M98T69Q7HP. CAS-59703-84-3.* JAN. *Antibacterial.* Pipracil (Wyeth) ◇T-1220; CL 227,193

Piperamide Maleate [*1964*] (pi per′ a mide mal′ ee ate). $C_{17}H_{28}N_4O.2C_4H_4O_4$. 536.57. [Piperamide is INN.] (1) Acetamide, N-[4-[4-[3-(dimethylamino)propyl]-1-piperazinyl]phenyl]-, (Z)-2-butenedioate (1:2); (2) 4′-{4-[3-(Dimethylamino)propyl]-1-piperazinyl}acetanilide maleate (1:2). *UNII-7T952LZM7T; UNII-83B7UZO20C* [piperamide]. *CAS-1252-69-3; CAS-299-48-9* [piperamide]. *Anthelmintic.* ◇CL 54131

Piperamine — *See* Bamipine.

Piperazine (pi per′ a zeen). **USP.** $C_4H_{10}N_2$. 86.14. (1) Piperazine; (2) Piperazine. *UNII-1RTM4PAL0V. CAS-110-85-0. Anthelmintic.*

Piperazine Adipate (JAN) — *See* Piperazine Edetate Calcium.

Piperazine Calcium Edetate (INN, BAN) — *See* Piperazine Edetate Calcium.

Piperazine Citrate (pi per′ a zeen sit′ rate). **USP.** $(C_4H_{10}N_2)_3.2C_6H_8O_7.xH_2O$. 642.65 (anhydrous). (1) Piperazine, 2-hydroxy-1,2,3-propanetricarboxylate (3:2), hydrate; (2) Piperazine citrate (3:2) hydrate. *UNII-63KP7FXF2I. CAS-41372-10-5; CAS-144-29-6* [anhydrous]; *CAS-110-85-0* [piperazine]. *Anthelmintic.* Antepar (GlaxoSmithKline); Bryrel (Sanofi Aventis)

Piperazine Edetate Calcium [*1964*] (pi per′ a zeen e′ de tate kal′ see um). $C_{14}H_{24}CaN_4O_8$. 416.44. [Piperazine Calcium Edetate is INN and BAN; Piperazine Adipate is JAN.] (1) Calcium, (T-4)-[[N,N′-1,2-ethanediylbis[N-(carboxymethyl)glycinato]](2-)-N,N′,O,O′]-, compd. with piperazine (1:1); (2) Dihydrogen [(ethylenedinitrilo)tetraacetato]calciate(2-) compound with piperazine (1:1). *UNII-1RTM4PAL0V* [piperazine]. *CAS-12002-30-1; CAS-50322-15-1* [dihydrate]; *CAS-110-85-0* [piperazine]; *CAS-60-00-4* [edetic acid]. *Anthelmintic.*

Piperazine Estrone Sulfate (previously used name) — *See* Estropipate.

Piperazine Phosphate. $C_4H_{10}N_2.H_3PO_4.H_2O$. 202.15. (1) Piperazine phosphate (1:1), monohydrate; (2) Piperazine phosphate (1:1) monohydrate. *UNII-8TIF7T48FP. CAS-18534-18-4; CAS-14538-56-8* [anhydrous]; *CAS-110-85-0* [piperazine]. USP XX; JAN; MI. Pincets (Marion Merrell Dow†); Pinsirup (Marion Merrell Dow†)

Piperazine Theophylline Ethanoate — *See* Acefylline Piperazine.

Piperidine Phosphate. $C_5H_{11}N.H_3PO_4$. 183.14. *CAS-767-21-5; CAS-110-89-4* [piperidine]. MI. Cypentil (Abbott†)

Piperidolate Hydrochloride. $C_{21}H_{25}NO_2.HCl$. 359.89. [Piperidolate is INN and BAN.] (1) Benzeneacetic acid, α-phenyl-, 1-ethyl-3-piperidinyl ester, hydrochloride; (2) 1-Ethyl-3-piperidyl diphenylacetate hydrochloride. *CAS-129-77-1; CAS-82-98-4* [piperidolate]. USP XX; JAN; MI. Dactil (Marion Merrell Dow†)

---

† Brand name formerly used, and/or firm no longer concerned with this product.

Piperilate. $C_{21}H_{25}NO_3$. 339.43. [Pipethanate is INN; Pipethanate Ethobromide and Pipethanate Hydrochloride are JAN.] α-Hydroxy-α-phenylbenzeneacetic acid 2-(1-piperidinyl)ethyl ester. *UNII-P32MG14U83. CAS-4546-39-8; CAS-4544-15-4* [hydrochloride]. MI.

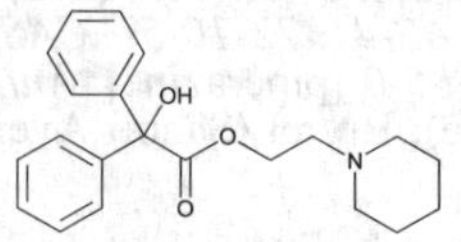

Piperine. $C_{17}H_{19}NO_3$. 285.34. (1) Piperidine, 1-(5-(1,3-benzodioxol-5-yl)-1-oxo-2,4-pentadienyl)-, (*E,E*)-; (2) (2*E*,4*E*)-5-(Benzo[*d*][1,3]dioxol-5-yl)-1-(piperidin-1-yl)-penta-2,4-dien-1-one. *UNII-U71XL721QK. CAS-94-62-2.* USP VIII; MI.

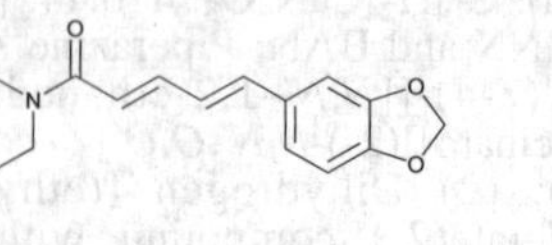

Piperocaine Hydrochloride. $C_{16}H_{23}NO_2 \cdot HCl$. 297.82. [Piperocaine is INN and BAN.] 3-(2-Methylpiperidino)propyl benzoate hydrochloride. *CAS-533-28-8; CAS-136-82-3* [piperocaine]. USP XVI; MI. Metycaine Hydrochloride (Lilly†)

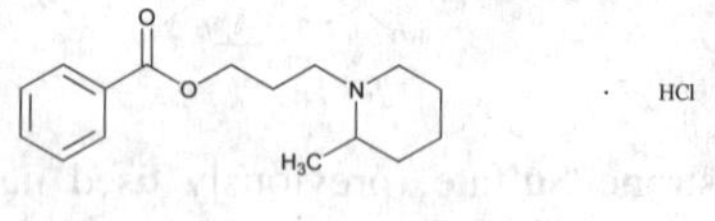

Piperonyl Butoxide. $C_{19}H_{30}O_5$. 338.44. 5-[2-(2-Butoxyethoxy)ethoxymethyl]-6-propyl-1,3-benzodioxole. *UNII-LWK91TU9AH. CAS-51-03-6.* BAN.

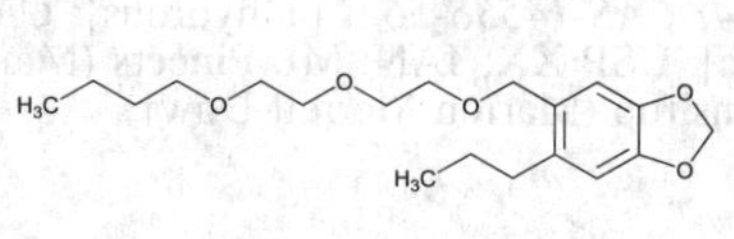

Piperoxan. $C_{14}H_{19}NO_2$. 233.31. 2-Piperidinomethyl-1,4-benzodioxan. *UNII-9ZCS27634Y. CAS-59-39-2; CAS-135-87-5* [hydrochloride]. INN; BAN; MI.

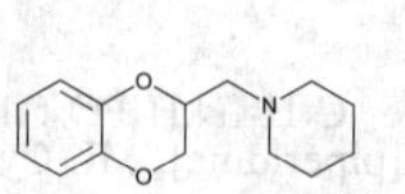

Piperphenidol Hydrochloride. *UNII-407JU2B9IS. CAS-6091-56-1; CAS-90-23-3* [piperphenidol].

Piperylone. $C_{17}H_{23}N_3O$. 285.38. 4-Ethyl-1-(1-methyl-4-piperidyl)-3-phenyl-3-pyrazolin-5-one. *UNII-XWH5VH1L2F. CAS-2531-04-6.* INN; MI.

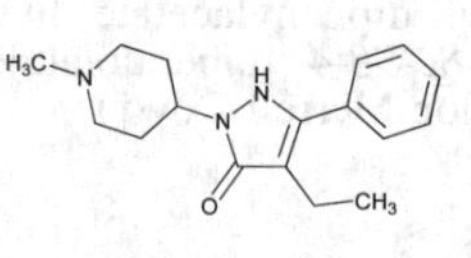

Pipethanate (INN) — *See* Piperilate.

Pipethanate Ethobromide (JAN) — *See* Piperilate.

Pipethanate Hydrochloride (JAN) — *See* Piperilate.

Pipobroman [*1965*] (pi″ poe broe′ man). $C_{10}H_{16}Br_2N_2O_2$. 356.05. (1) Piperazine, 1,4-bis(3-bromo-1-oxopropyl)-; (2) 1,4-Bis(3-bromopropionyl)piperazine. *UNII-6Q99RDT97R. CAS-54-91-1.* USP XXII; INN. *Antineoplastic.* Vercyte (Abbott) ◇*A-8103; NSC-25154*

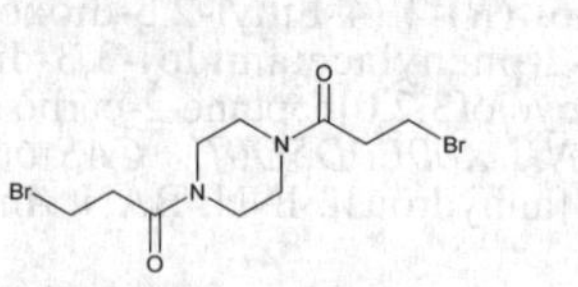

Pipoctanone. $C_{22}H_{35}NO$. 329.52. 4′-Octyl-3-piperidinopropiophenone. *UNII-24N16QE4S0. CAS-18841-58-2.* INN.

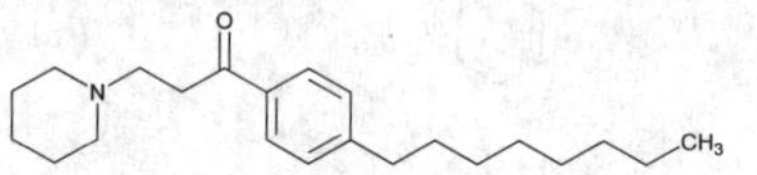

Pipofezine. $C_{16}H_{19}N_5O$. 297.35. 5-Methyl-3-(4-methyl-1-piperazinyl)-5*H*-pyridazino[3,4-*b*][1,4]benzoxazine. *UNII-P8T739L1FA. CAS-24886-52-0.* INN.

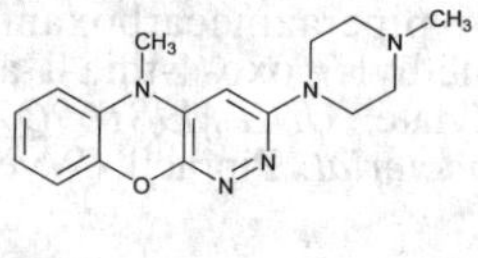

Piposulfan [*1965*] (pi″ poe sul′ fan). $C_{12}H_{22}N_2O_8S_2$. 386.44. (1) Piperazine, 1,4-bis[3-[(methylsulfonyl)oxy]-1-oxopropyl]-; (2) 1,4-Dihydracryloylpiperazine dimethanesulfonate (ester). *CAS-2608-24-4.* INN. *Antineoplastic.* Ancyte (Abbott†) ◇*A-20968; NSC-47774*

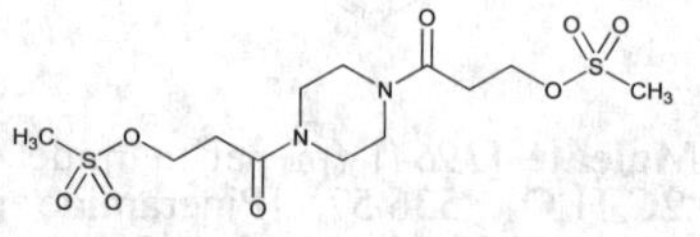

Pipotiazine Palmitate [*1973*] (pi″ poe tye′ a zeen pal′ mi tate). $C_{40}H_{63}N_3O_4S_2$. 714.08. [Pipotiazine is INN and BAN.] (1) Hexadecanoic acid, 2-[1-[3-[2-[(dimethylamino)sulfonyl]-10*H*-phenothiazin-10-yl]propyl]-4-piperidinyl]ethyl ester; (2) 10-[3-[4-(2-Hydroxyethyl)piperidino]propyl]-*N,N*-dimethylphenothiazine-2-sulfonamide palmitate (ester). *CAS-37517-26-3; CAS-39860-99-6* [pipotiazine]. *Antipsychotic. [Name previously used: Pipothiazine.]* ◇*RP 19552; IL-19552*

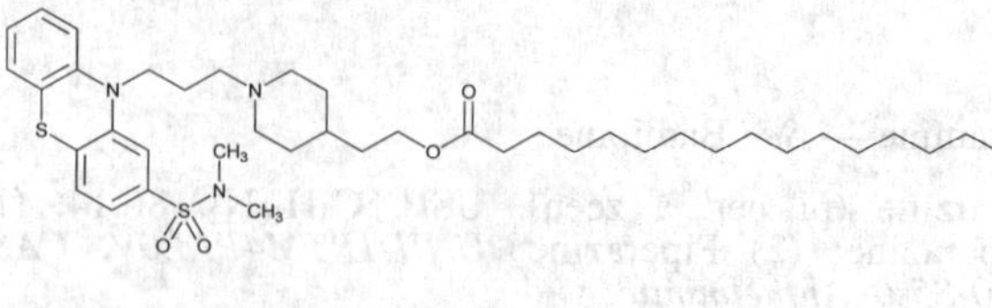

Pipoxizine. $C_{24}H_{31}NO_3$. 381.51. 2-[2-[2-[4-(Diphenylmethylene)piperidino]ethoxy]exothy]ethanol. *UNII-B9A98D632Z. CAS-55837-21-3.* INN.

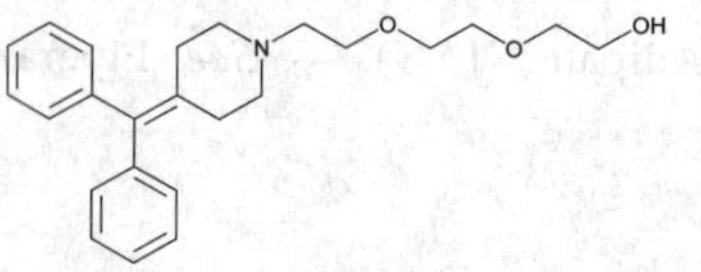

Pipoxolan Hydrochloride [*1970*] (pi pox′ oh lan hye″ droe klor′ ide). $C_{22}H_{25}NO_3.HCl$. 387.90. [Pipoxolan is INN and BAN.] (1) 1,3-Dioxolan-4-one, 5,5-diphenyl-2-[2-(1-piperidinyl)ethyl]-, hydrochloride; (2) 5,5-Diphenyl-2-(2-piperidinoethyl)-1,3-dioxolan-4-one hydrochloride. *CAS-18174-58-8; CAS-23744-24-3* [pipoxolan]. *Relaxant (muscle).* Rowapraxin (Rowa Ltd., Ireland)

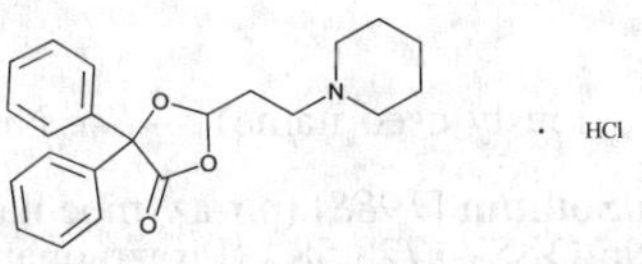

Pipradimadol. $C_{24}H_{37}ClN_2O_2$. 421.02. 1-(*o*-Chlorophenethyl)-*N*-cyclohexyl-4-hydroxy-*N*,α,α-trimethyl-4-piperidineacetamide. *UNII-CBI6614BOL. CAS-68797-29-5.* INN.

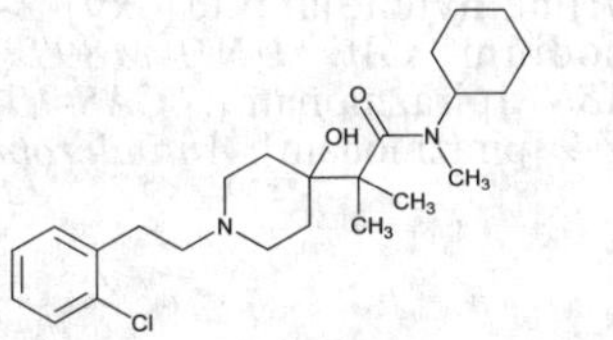

Pipradrol Hydrochloride. $C_{18}H_{21}NO.HCl$. 303.83. [Pipradrol is INN and BAN.] α,α-Diphenyl-2-piperidinemethanol hydrochloride. *CAS-71-78-3; CAS-467-60-7* [pipradrol]. NF XII; JAN; MI. Meratran (Marion Merrell Dow†)

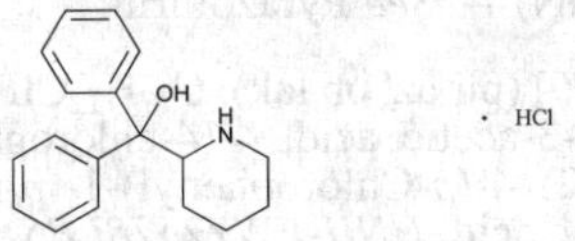

Pipramadol. $C_{23}H_{35}ClN_2O_2$. 406.99. (±)-1-(*o*-Chlorophenethyl)-*N*-cyclohexyl-4-hydroxy-*N*,α-dimethyl-4-piperidineacetamide. *UNII-6QR1645G9S. CAS-55313-67-2.* INN.

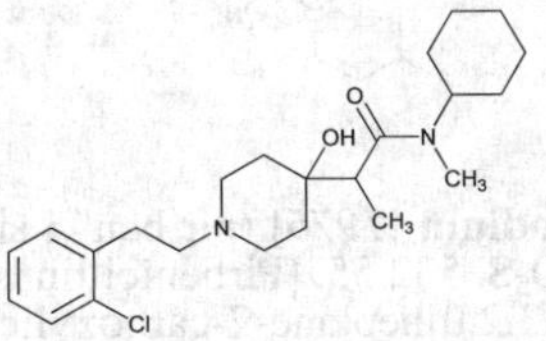

Pipratecol. $C_{19}H_{24}N_2O_4$. 344.40. α-(3,4-Dihydroxyphenyl)-4-(2-methoxyphenyl)-1-piperazineethanol. *UNII-E33L6C08A5. CAS-15534-05-1.* INN; DCF. *◇711 SE*

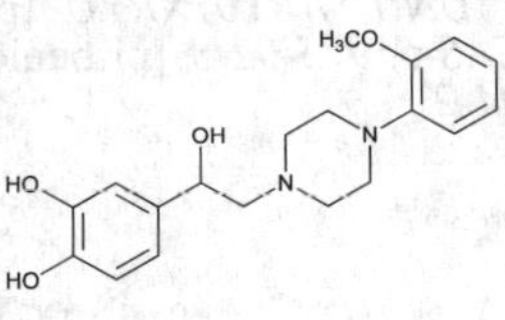

† Brand name formerly used, and/or firm no longer concerned with this product.

Piprinhydrinate. $C_{19}H_{23}NO.C_7H_7ClN_4O_2$. 496.00. 4-Diphenylmethoxy-1-methylpiperidine compound of 8-chlorotheophylline. *UNII-SI78RFJ7XI. CAS-606-90-6.* INN; BAN; MI.

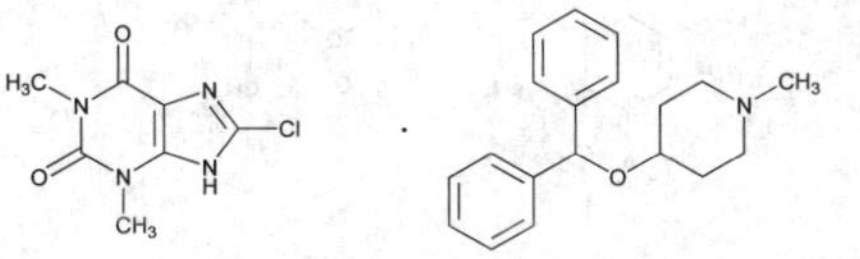

Piprocurarium Iodide. $C_{23}H_{40}I_2N_2O_3$. 646.38. 1-α-Carboxybenzyl-1-methylpiperidinium iodide diethyl[2-(2-hydroxyethoxy)ethyl]methylammonium iodide ester. *CAS-3562-55-8.* INN. *◇LD 2480*

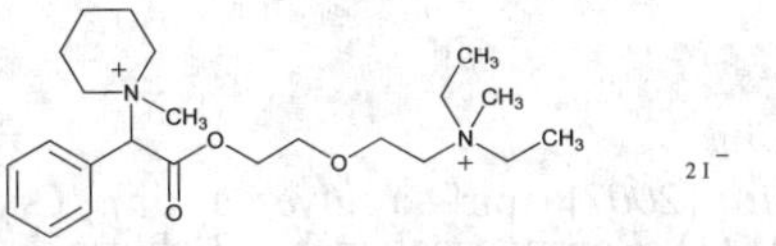

Piprofurol. $C_{26}H_{33}NO_6$. 455.54. α-(*p*-Hydroxyphenethyl)-4,7-dimethoxy-6-(2-piperidineethoxy)-5-benzofuranmethanol. *UNII-3745QN167A. CAS-40680-87-3.* INN.

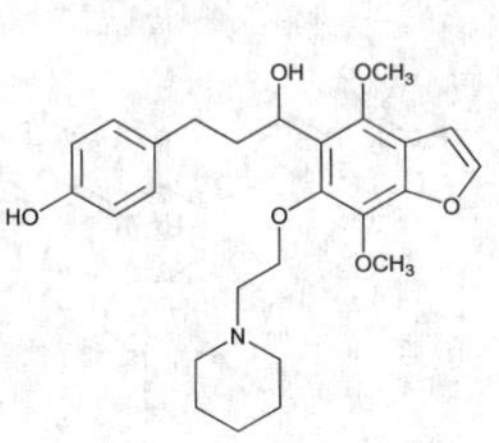

Piprozolin [*1968*] (pi″ proe zoe′ lin). $C_{14}H_{22}N_2O_3S$. 298.40. (1) Acetic acid, [3-ethyl-4-oxo-5-(1-piperidinyl)-2-thiazolidinylidene]-, ethyl ester; (2) Ethyl 3-ethyl-4-oxo-5-piperidino-$\Delta^{2,\alpha}$-thiazolidineacetate. *CAS-17243-64-0.* INN. *Choleretic.* Probkin (Parke-Davis) *◇W 3699; Go 919*

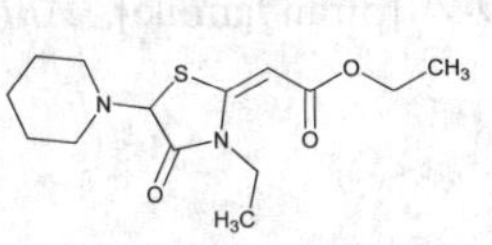

Piquindone Hydrochloride [*1984*] (pi′ kwin done hye″ droe klor′ ide). $C_{15}H_{22}N_2O.HCl.2H_2O$. 318.84. [Piquindone is INN.] (1) 4*H*-Pyrrolo[2,3-*g*]isoquinolin-4-one, 3-ethyl-1,4a,5,6,7,8,8a,9-octahydro-2,6-dimethyl-, monohydrochloride, dihydrate, *trans*-(±)-; (2) (±)-*trans*-3-Ethyl-1,4a,5,6,7,8,8a,9-octahydro-2,6-dimethyl-4*H*-pyrrolo[2,3-*g*]isoquinolin-4-one monohydrochloride dihydrate. *CAS-83784-19-4; CAS-78541-97-6* [piquindone]. *Antipsychotic. ◇Ro 22-1319/003*

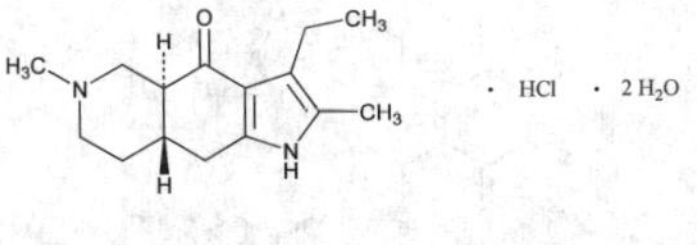

Piquizil Hydrochloride [*1969*] (pi′ kwi zil hye″ droe klor′ ide). $C_{19}H_{26}N_4O_4.HCl$. 410.90. [Piquizil is INN.] (1) 1-Piperazinecarboxylic acid, 4-(6,7-dimethoxy-4-quinazolinyl)-, 2-methylpropyl ester, monohydrochloride; (2) Isobutyl 4-(6,7-dimethoxy-4-quinazolinyl)-1-piperazine-carboxylate monohydrochloride. *CAS-23256-26-0; CAS-21560-58-7* [piquizil]. *Bronchodilator.* ◇*CP-12,521-1*

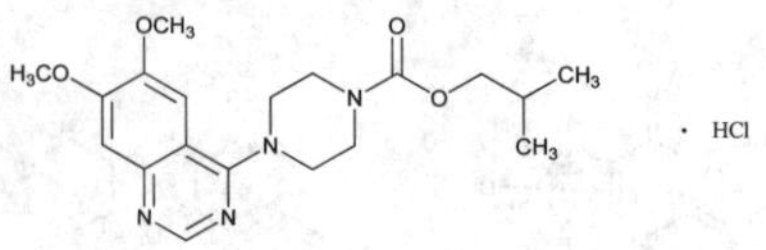

Piracetam [*1980*] (pir a′ se tam). $C_6H_{10}N_2O_2$. 142.16. (1) 1-Pyrrolidineacetamide, 2-oxo-; (2) 2-Oxo-1-pyrrolidineacetamide. *UNII-ZH516LNZ10. CAS-7491-74-9.* INN; BAN. *Cognition adjuvant.* ◇*Cl-871*

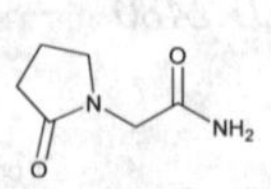

Piragliatin [*2007*] (pir″ a glye′ a tin). $C_{19}H_{20}ClN_3O_4S$. 421.90. (1) Benzeneacetamide, 3-chloro-4-(methylsulfonyl)-α-[[(1R)-3-oxocyclopentyl]methyl]-N-pyrazinyl-, (αR)-; (2) (2R)-2-[3-Chloro-4-(methylsulfonyl)phenyl]-3-[(1R)-3-oxocyclopentyl]-N-pyrazinylpropanamide. *UNII-BM1HR7IP1L. CAS-625114-41-2.* INN. *Treatment of type 2 diabetes.* ◇*RO4389620-R1440*

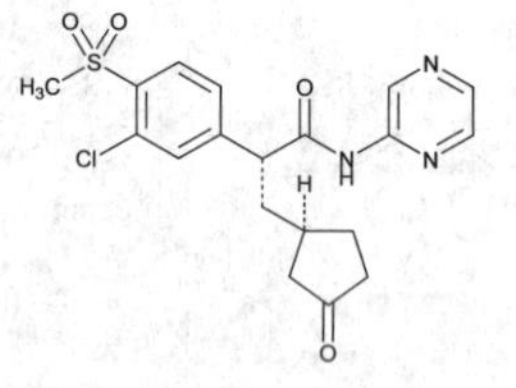

Pirandamine Hydrochloride [*1974*] (pir an′ da meen hye″ droe klor′ ide). $C_{17}H_{23}NO.HCl$. 293.83. [Pirandamine is INN.] (1) Indeno[2,1-c]pyran-1-ethanamine, 1,3,4,9-tetrahydro-N,N,1-trimethyl-, hydrochloride; (2) 1,3,4,9-Tetrahydro-N,N,1-trimethylindeno[2,1-c]pyran-1-ethylamine hydrochloride. *UNII-Y4F9MIF6M1. CAS-42408-78-6; CAS-42408-79-7* [pirandamine]. *Antidepressant.* ◇*AY-23,713*

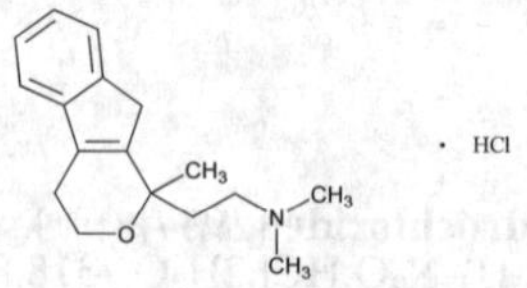

Pirarubicin. $C_{32}H_{37}NO_{12}$. 627.64. (8S,10S)-10-[[3-Amino-2,3,6-trideoxy-4-O-(2R-tetrahydro-2H-pyran-2-yl)-α-L-lyxo-hexopyranosyl]oxy]-8-glycoloyl-7,8,9,10-tetrahydro-6,8,11-trihydroxy-1-methoxy-5,12-naphthacenedione. *CAS-72496-41-4.* INN; JAN; MI.

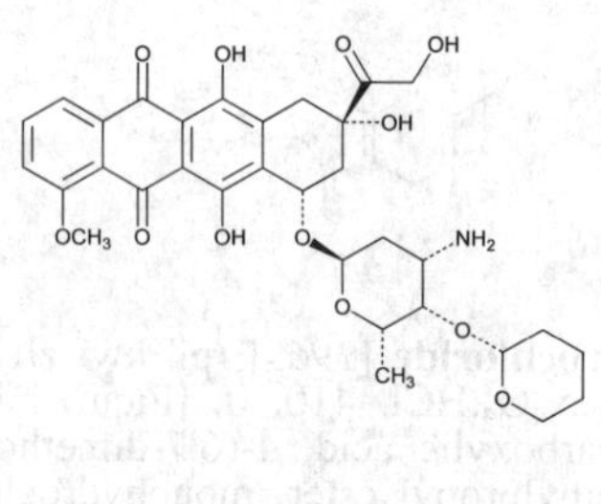

Piraxelate. $C_{15}H_{25}NO_3$. 267.36. 3,3,5-Trimethylcyclohexyl-2-oxo-1-pyrrolidineacetate. *UNII-Y1P25NQI7X. CAS-82209-39-0.* INN.

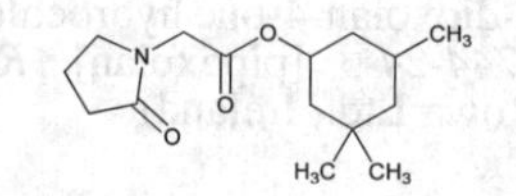

Piraxostat (previously used name) — *See* Niraxostat.

Pirazmonam Sodium [*1988*] (pir az′ moe nam soe′ dee um). $C_{22}H_{22}N_{10}Na_2O_{12}S_2$. 728.58. [Pirazmonam is INN.] (1) Propanoic acid, 2-[[[1-(2-amino-4-thiazolyl)-2-[1-[[[[3-[[(1,4-dihydro-5-hydroxy-4-oxo-2-pyridinyl)carbonyl]amino]-2-oxo-1-imidazolidinyl]sulfonyl]amino]carbonyl]-2-oxo-3-azetidinyl]amino]-2-oxoethylidene]amino]oxy]-2-methyldisodium salt; (2) 2-[[[(2-Amino-4-thiazolyl)[[1-[[[3-(1,4-dihydro-5-hydroxy-4-oxopicolinamido)-2-oxo-1-imidazolidinyl]sulfonyl]carbamoyl]-2-oxo-3-azetidinyl]-carbamoyl]methylene]amino]oxy]-2-methylpropionic acid, disodium salt. *UNII-M89TPX4O2C; UNII-1S3Z442A8N* [pirazmonam]. *CAS-104393-00-2; CAS-108319-07-9* [pirazmonam]. *Antimicrobial.* ◇*SQ 83360*

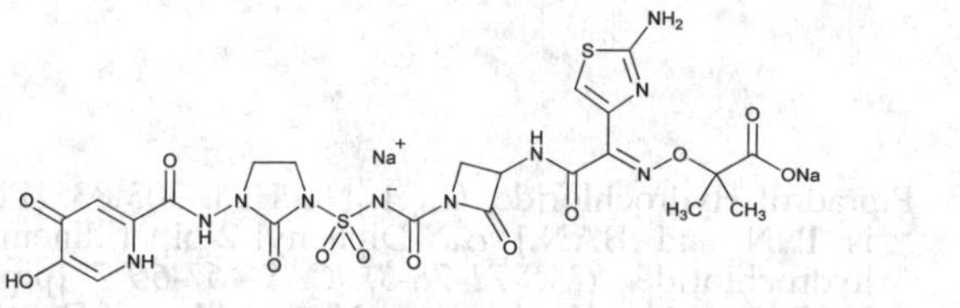

Pirazofurin (INN) — *See* Pyrazofurin.

Pirazolac [*1980*] (pir az′ oh lak). $C_{17}H_{12}ClFN_2O_2$. 330.74. (1) 1H-Pyrazole-3-acetic acid, 4-(4-chlorophenyl)-1-(4-fluorophenyl)-; (2) 4-(p-Chlorophenyl)-1-(p-fluorophenyl)pyrazole-3-acetic acid. *UNII-FWY2578LP5. CAS-71002-09-0.* INN; BAN. *Antirheumatic.* ◇*ZK 76 604*

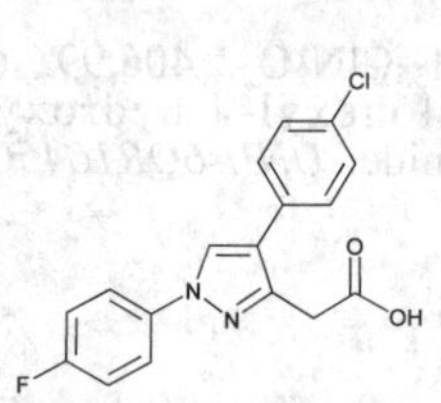

Pirbenicillin Sodium [*1976*] (pir ben″ i sil′ in soe′ dee um). $C_{24}H_{25}N_6NaO_5S$. 532.55. [Pirbenicillin is INN.] (1) 4-Thia-1-azabicyclo[3.2.0]heptane-2-carboxylic acid, 6-[[[[[(imino-4-pyridinylmethyl)amino]acetyl]amino]phenylacetyl]amino]-3,3-dimethyl-7-oxo-, monosodium salt, [2S-[2α,5α,6β(S*)]]-; (2) Sodium (2S,5R,6R)-6-[(R)-2-[2-(isonicotinimidoylamino)acetamido]-2-phenylacetamido]-3,3-dimethyl-7-oxo-4-thia-1-azabicyclo[3.2.0]heptane-2-carboxylate. *UNII-638D8M316Y; UNII-8ARY01XRYU* [pirbenicillin]. *CAS-55162-26-0; CAS-55975-92-3* [pirbenicillin]. *Antibacterial.* ◇*CP-33,994-2*

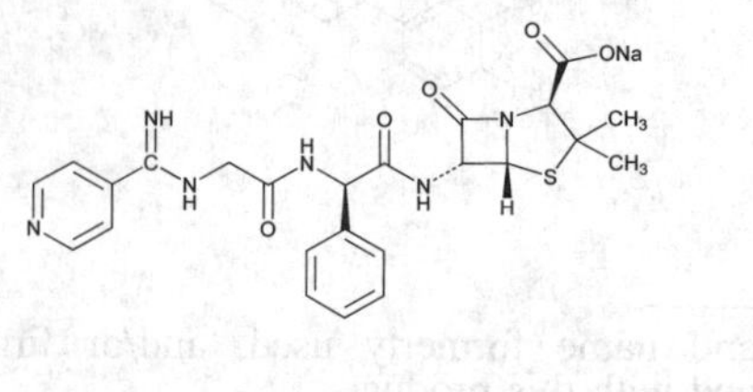

Pirbuterol Acetate [*1978*] (pir bue′ ter ol as′ e tate). $C_{12}H_{20}N_2O_3 \cdot C_2H_4O_2$. 300.35. [Pirbuterol is INN and BAN.] (1) 2,6-Pyridinedimethanol, α^6-[[(1,1-dimethylethyl)amino]methyl]-3-hydroxy-, monoacetate (salt); (2) α^6-[(*tert*-Butylamino)methyl]-3-hydroxy-2,6-pyridinedimethanol monoacetate (salt). *UNII-1EH73XKR9N; UNII-OG645J8RVW* [pirbuterol]. *CAS-65652-44-0; CAS-38677-81-5* [pirbuterol]. *Bronchodilator.* Maxair (Graceway) ◇*CP-24,314-14*

Pirbuterol Hydrochloride [*1973*] (pir bue′ ter ol hye″ droe klor′ ide). $C_{12}H_{20}N_2O_3 \cdot 2HCl$. 313.22. (1) 2,6-Pyridinedimethanol, α^6-[[(1,1-dimethylethyl)amino]methyl]-3-hydroxy-, dihydrochloride; (2) α^6[(*tert*-Butylamino)methyl]-3-hydroxy-2,6-pyridinedimethanol dihydrochloride. *UNII-J6793T658K. CAS-38029-10-6; CAS-38677-81-5* [pirbuterol]. JAN. *Bronchodilator.* ◇*CP-24,314-1*

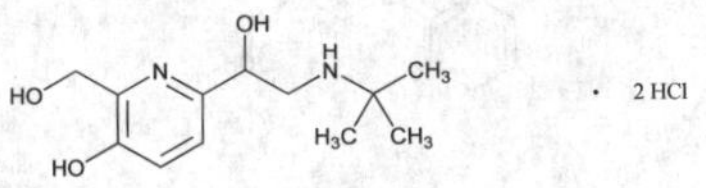

Pirdonium Bromide. $C_{22}H_{30}BrNO$. 404.38. 1,1-Dimethyl-2-[[(*p*-methyl-α-phenylbenzyl)oxy]methyl]piperidinium bromide. *UNII-5123Q291S5. CAS-35620-67-8.* INN.

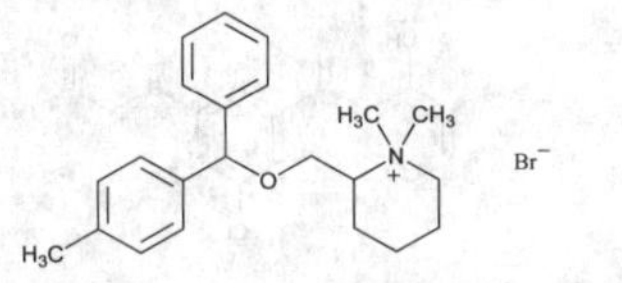

Pirenoxine. $C_{16}H_8N_2O_5$. 308.25. 1-Hydroxy-5-oxo-5*H*-pyrido[3,2-*a*]phenoxazine-3-carboxylic acid. *UNII-27L0EP6IZK. CAS-1043-21-6.* INN; JAN; MI.

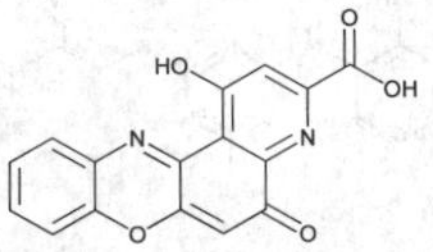

Pirenperone [*1981*] (pir en′ per one). $C_{23}H_{24}FN_3O_2$. 393.45. (1) 4*H*-Pyrido[1,2-*a*]pyrimidin-4-one, 3-[2-[4-(4-fluorobenzoyl)-1-piperidinyl]ethyl]-2-methyl-; (2) 3-[2-[4-(*p*-Fluorobenzoyl)piperidino]ethyl]-2-methyl-4*H*-pyrido[1,2-*a*]pyrimidin-4-one. *UNII-Y9FMC4513X. CAS-75444-65-4.* INN; BAN. *Tranquilizer.* ◇*R-47,465*

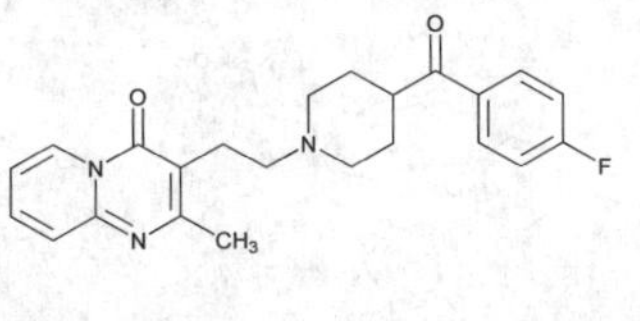

Pirenzepine Hydrochloride [*1986*] (pir en′ ze peen hye″ droe klor′ ide). $C_{19}H_{21}N_5O_2 \cdot 2HCl$. 424.32. [Pirenzepine is INN and BAN.] (1) 6*H*-Pyrido[2,3-*b*][1,4]benzodiazepin-6-one, 5,11-dihydro-11-[(4-methyl-1-piperazinyl)acetyl]-, dihydrochloride; (2) 5,11-Dihydro-11-[(4-methyl-1-piperazinyl)acetyl]-6*H*-pyrido[2,3-*b*][1,4]benzodiazepin-6-one dihydrochloride. *UNII-10YM403FLS; UNII-*

---

† Brand name formerly used, and/or firm no longer concerned with this product.

3G0285N20N [pirenzepine]. *CAS-29868-97-1; CAS-28797-61-7* [pirenzepine]. JAN. *Anti-ulcerative.* ◇*LS 519 Cl2*

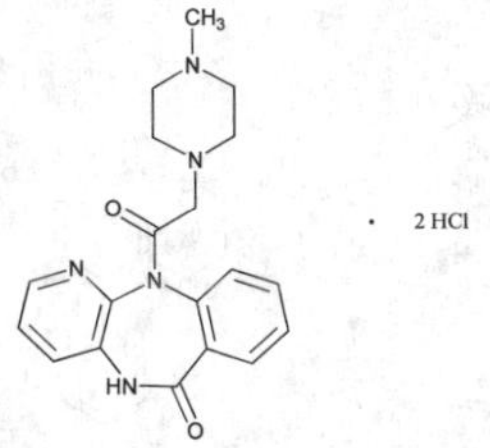

Pirepolol. $C_{21}H_{32}N_4O_5$. 420.50. ($\pm$)-6-[[2-[[3-(*p*-Butoxyphenoxy)-2-hydroxypropyl]amino]ethyl]amino]-1,3-dimethyluracil. *UNII-V1J0B4P41O. CAS-69479-26-1.* INN.

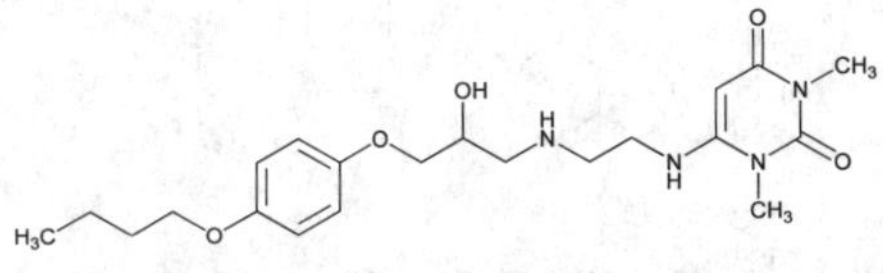

Piretanide [*1978*] (pir et′ a nide). $C_{17}H_{18}N_2O_5S$. 362.40. (1) Benzoic acid, 3-(aminosulfonyl)-4-phenoxy-5-(1-pyrrolidinyl)-; (2) 4-Phenoxy-3-(1-pyrrolidinyl)-5-sulfamoylbenzoic acid. *UNII-DQ6KK6GV93. CAS-55837-27-9.* INN; BAN; JAN. *Diuretic.* Arlix (Hoechst-Roussel†) ◇*HOE 118; S 73 4118*

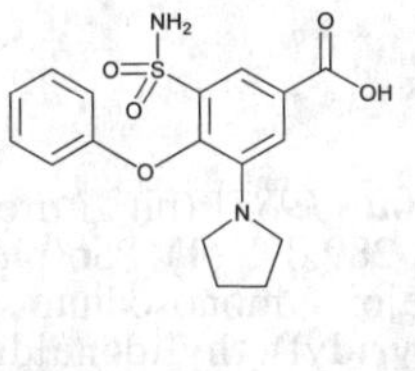

Pirfenidone [*1975*] (pir fen′ i done). $C_{12}H_{11}NO$. 185.22. (1) 2(1*H*)-Pyridinone, 5-methyl-1-phenyl-; (2) 5-Methyl-1-phenyl-2(1*H*)-pyridone. *CAS-53179-13-8.* INN. *Analgesic; anti-inflammatory; antipyretic.* ◇*AMR-69*

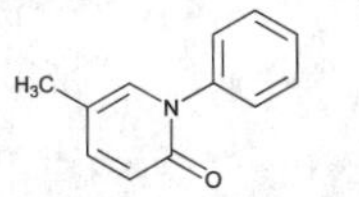

Piribedil. $C_{16}H_{18}N_4O_2$. 298.34. 2-(4-Piperonyl-1-piperazinyl)-pyrimidine. *UNII-DO22K1PRDJ. CAS-3605-01-4.* INN; DCF; MI. ◇*EU-4200; ET-495*

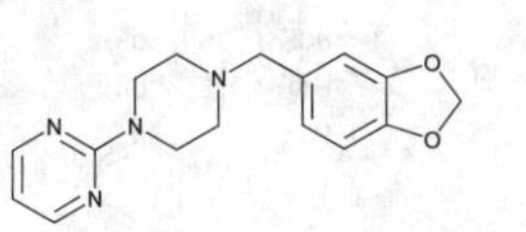

Piribenzyl Methylsulfate — *See* Bevonium Metilsulfate.

Piridicillin Sodium [*1979*] (pir i″ di sil′ in soe′ dee um). $C_{32}H_{34}N_5NaO_{11}S_2$. 751.76. [Piridicillin is INN.] (1) 4-Thia-1-azabicyclo[3.2.0]heptane-2-carboxylic acid, 6-[[[[[6-[4-[[bis(2-hydroxyethyl)amino]sulfonyl]phenyl]-1,2-dihydro-2-oxo-3-pyridinyl]carbonyl]amino](4-hydroxyphenyl)acetyl]amino]-3,3-dimethyl-7-oxo-, sodium salt [2*S*-[2α,5α,6β(*S**)]]-; (2) Sodium (2*S*,5*R*,6*R*)-6-[(*R*)-2-[6-[*p*-[bis(2-hydroxyethyl)sulfamoyl]phenyl]-1,2-dihydro-2-oxonicotinamido]-2-(*p*-hydroxyphenyl)acetamido]-3,3-dimethyl-7-oxo-4-thia-1-azabicyclo[3.2.0]heptane-2-carboxylate. *UNII-1Q728MH9P9; UNII-6502ONO3L0* [piridicillin]. *CAS-69402-03-5; CAS-69414-41-1* [piridicillin]. *Antibacterial.* ◇CL-867

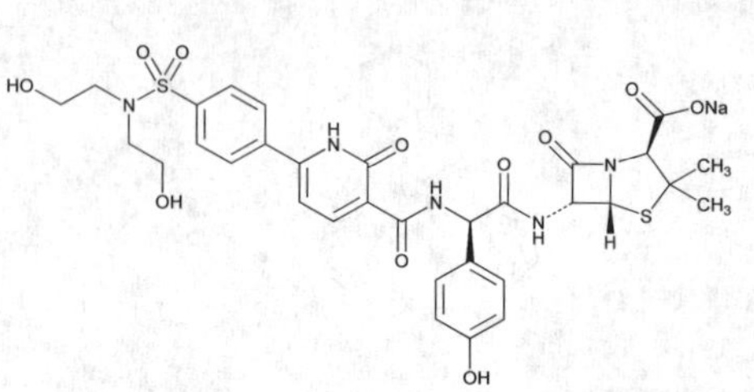

Piridocaine Hydrochloride. $C_{14}H_{20}N_2O_2$.HCl. 284.78. [Piridocaine is INN.] *CAS-87-21-8* [piridocaine]. MI.

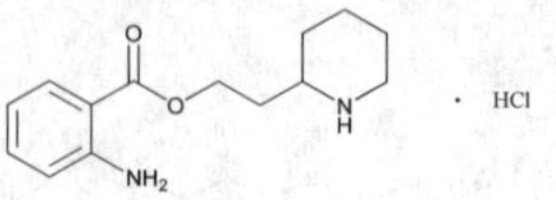

Piridoxilate. $C_{10}H_{13}NO_6.C_{10}H_{13}NO_6$. 486.43. [[5-Hydroxy-4-(hydroxymethyl)-6-methyl-3-pyridyl]methoxy]glycolic acid compound with [[4,5-bis(hydroxymethyl)-2-methyl-3-pyridyl]oxy]glycolic acid (1:1). *UNII-13X224L936. CAS-24340-35-0.* INN; BAN; DCF.

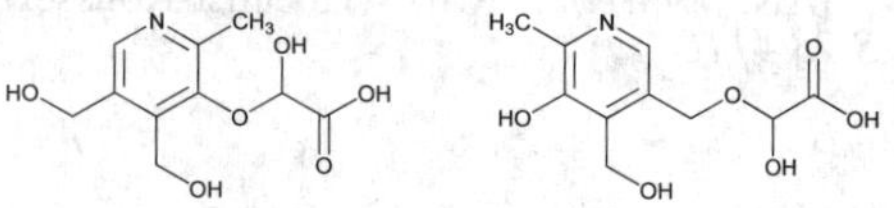

Piridronate Sodium [*1987*] (pir″ i droe′ nate soe′ dee um). $C_7H_{10}NNaO_6P_2$. 289.09. (1) Phosphonic acid, [2-(2-pyridinyl)ethylidene]bis-, monosodium salt; (2) Sodium trihydrogen [2-(2-pyridyl)ethylidene]diphosphonate. *CAS-100188-33-8. Regulator (calcium).* ◇NE 97221

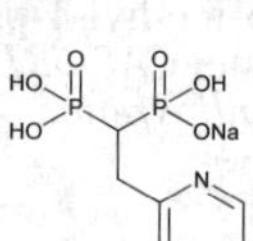

Piridronic Acid. $C_7H_{11}NO_6P_2$. 267.11. (1) Phosphonic acid, [2-(2-pyridinyl)ethylidene]bis-; (2) [2-(2-Pyridyl)ethylidene]diphosphonic acid. *UNII-ADD4H8T3K9. CAS-75755-07-6.* INN.

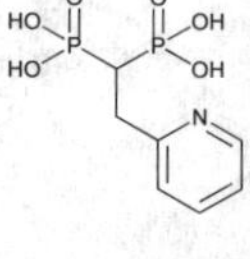

Pirifibrate. $C_{17}H_{18}ClNO_4$. 335.78. [6-(Hydroxymethyl)-2-pyridyl]methyl 2-(p-chlorophenoxy)-2-methylpropionate. *UNII-E82B3Z65BN. CAS-55285-45-5.* INN; MI.

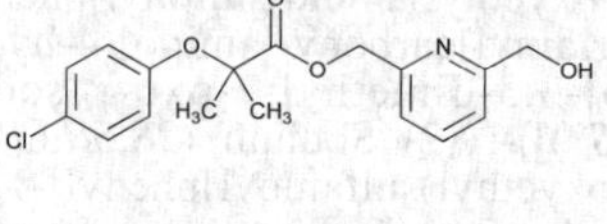

Pirimiphos-ethyl. $C_{13}H_{24}N_3O_3PS$. 333.39. *O*-(2-Diethylamino-6-methylpyrimidin-4-yl) *O,O*-diethyl phosphorothioate. *UNII-3L26N84757. CAS-23505-41-1.* BAN.

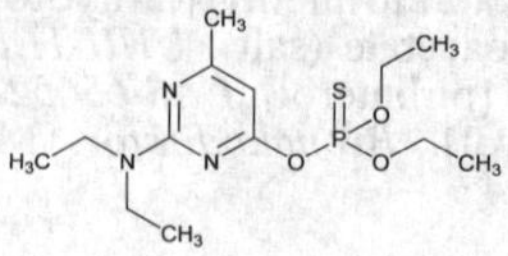

Pirinidazole. $C_{10}H_{10}N_4O_2S$. 250.28. 2-[[(1-Methyl-5-nitroimidazol-2-yl)methyl]thio]pyridine. *UNII-YLO2E256HT. CAS-55432-15-0.* INN.

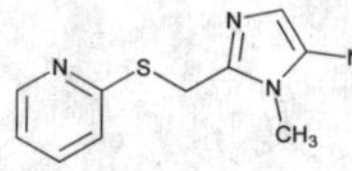

Pirinitramide — *See* Piritramide.

Pirinixic Acid. $C_{14}H_{14}ClN_3O_2S$. 323.80. [[4-Chloro-6-(2,3-xylidino)-2-pyrimidinyl]thio]acetic acid. *UNII-86C4MRT55A. CAS-50892-23-4.* INN.

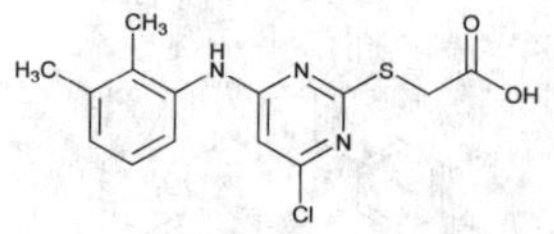

Pirinixil. $C_{16}H_{19}ClN_4O_2S$. 366.87. 2-[[4-Chloro-6-(2,3-xylidino)-2-pyrimidinyl]thio]-*N*-(2-hydroxyethyl)acetamide. *UNII-969LVT6GJ2. CAS-65089-17-0.* INN.

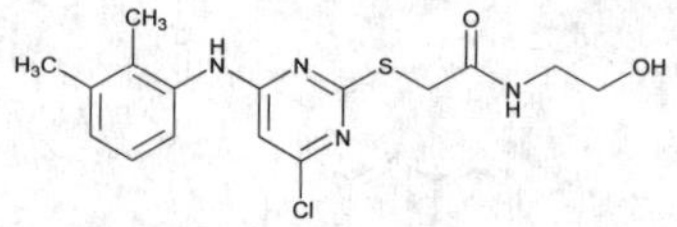

Piriprost [*1984*] (pir′ i prost). $C_{26}H_{35}NO_4$. 425.56. (1) Cyclopenta[*b*]pyrrole-2-pentanoic acid, 1,4,5,6-tetrahydro-5-hydroxy-4-(3-hydroxy-1-octenyl)-1-phenyl-, [4*R*-[4α(1*E*,3*S**),5β]]-; (2) (4*R*,5*R*)-1,4,5,6-Tetrahydro-5-hydroxy-4-[(*E*)-(3*S*)-3-hydroxy-1-octenyl]-1-phenylcyclopenta[*b*]pyrrole-2-valeric acid. *UNII-R802O5NILK. CAS-79672-88-1.* INN. *Anti-asthmatic.* ◇U-60,257

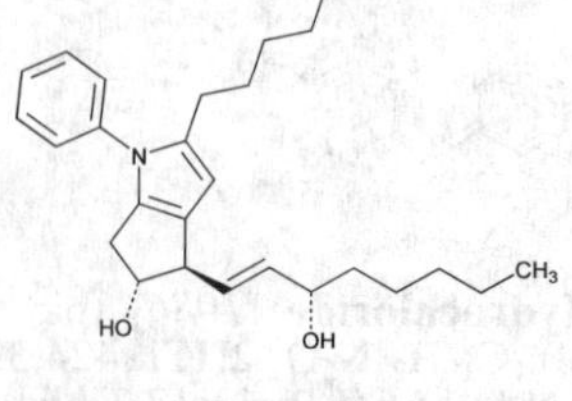

Piriprost Potassium [*1984*] (pir′ i prost poe tas′ ee um). $C_{26}H_{34}KNO_4$. 463.65. (1) Cyclopenta[*b*]pyrrole-2-pentanoic acid, 1,4,5,6-tetrahydro-5-hydroxy-4-(3-hydroxy-1-octenyl)-1-phenyl-, monopotassium salt, [4*R*-[4α(1*E*,3*S**),5β]]-; (2) Potassium (4*R*,5*R*)-1,4,5,6-tetrahydro-5-hydroxy-4-[(*E*)-(3*S*)-3-hydroxy-1-octenyl]-1-phenylcyclopenta[*b*]pyrrole-2-valerate. *UNII-2ZYM2BH34M. CAS-88851-62-1. Anti-asthmatic.* ◇U-60,257B

Piriqualone. $C_{22}H_{17}N_3O$. 339.39. 2-[2-(2-Pyridyl)vinyl]-3-*o*-tolyl-4(3*H*)-quinazolinone. *UNII-9O52U70AP4. CAS-1897-89-8.* INN.

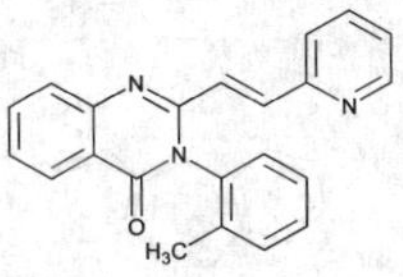

Pirisudanol. $C_{16}H_{24}N_2O_6$. 340.37. 2-(Dimethylamino)ethyl[5-hydroxy-4-(hydroxymethyl)-6-methyl-3-pyridyl]methyl succinate. *UNII-W618Z2SMVL. CAS-33605-94-6.* INN.

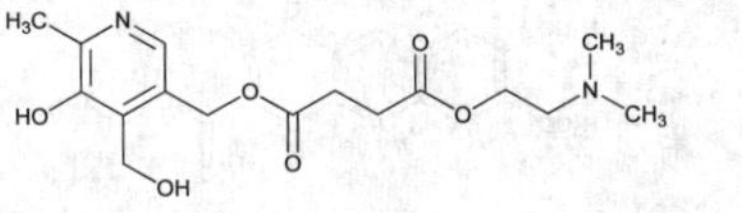

Piritramide. $C_{27}H_{34}N_4O$. 430.59. 1'-(3-Cyano-3,3-diphenyl-propyl)-[1,4'-bipiperidine]-4'-carboxamide. *CAS-302-41-0.* INN; BAN; DCF; MI. ◇*R 3365*

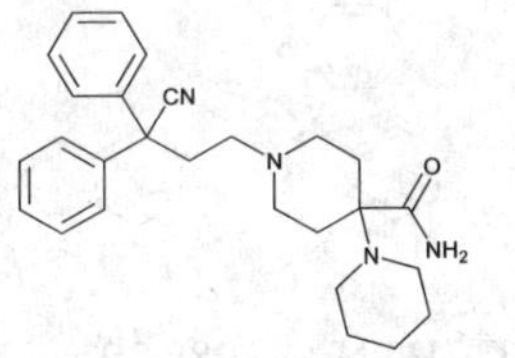

Piritrexim Isethionate [*1986*] (pir″ i trex′ im). $C_{17}H_{19}N_5O_2$. $C_2H_6O_4S$. 451.50. [Piritrexim is INN.] (1) Pyrido[2,3-*d*]pyrimidine-2,4-diamine, 6-[(2,5-dimethoxyphenyl)-methyl]-5-methyl-, mono(2-hydroxyethanesulfonate); (2) 2,4-Diamino-6-(2,5-dimethoxybenzyl)-5-methylpyri-do[2,3-*d*]pyrimidine mono(2-hydroxyethanesulfonate). *CAS-79483-69-5; CAS-72732-56-0* [piritrexim]. *Antiproli-ferative agent.* ◇*BW 301U isethionate*

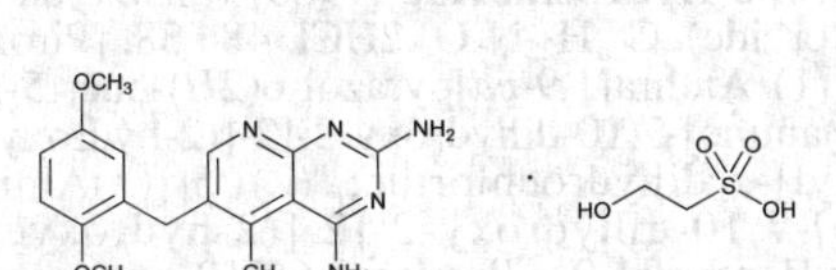

Pirlimycin Hydrochloride [*1982*] (pir″ li mye′ sin hye″ droe klor′ ide). $C_{17}H_{31}ClN_2O_5S.HCl.H_2O$. 465.43. [Pirlimycin is INN.] (1) L-*threo*-α-D-*galacto*-Octopyranoside, methyl 7-chloro-6,7,8-trideoxy-6-[[(4-ethyl-2-piperidinyl)carbony-l]amino]-1-thio-, monohydrochloride, monohydrate, (2*S-cis*)-; (2) Methyl 7-chloro-6,7,8-trideoxy-6-*cis*-4-ethyl-L-pipecolamido)-1-thio-L-*threo*-α-D-*galacto*-octopyranoside

---

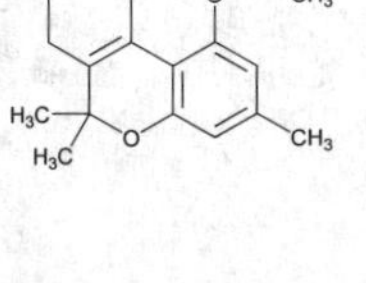

† Brand name formerly used, and/or firm no longer concerned with this product.

monohydrochloride monohydrate. *UNII-8S09O559AQ. CAS-77495-92-2* [monohydrate]. *Antibacterial.* ◇*U-57,930E*

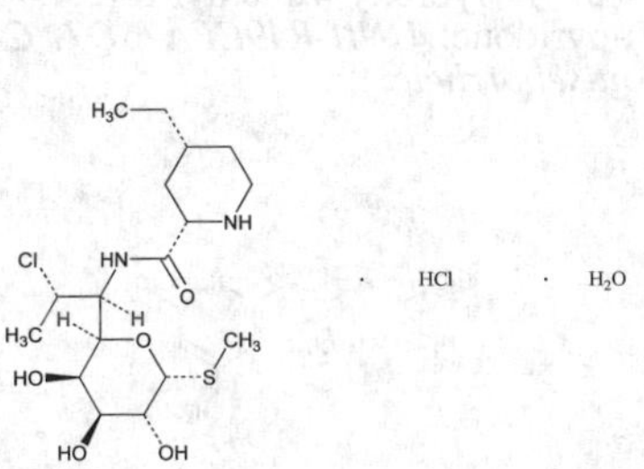

Pirlindole. $C_{15}H_{18}N_2$. 226.32. 2,3,3a,4,5,6-Hexahydro-8-methyl-1*H*-pyrazino[3,2,1-*jk*]carbazole. *UNII-V39YPH45FZ. CAS-60762-57-4.* INN.

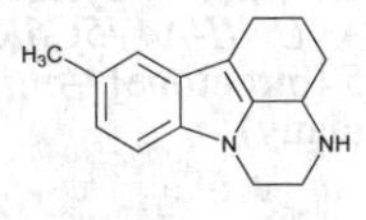

Pirmagrel [*1985*] (pir′ ma grel). $C_{13}H_{16}N_2O_2$. 232.28. (1) Imidazo[1,5-*a*]pyridine-5-hexanoic acid; (2) Imidazo[1,5-*a*]pyridine-5-hexanoic acid. *CAS-85691-74-3.* INN. *Inhib-itor (thromboxane synthetase).* ◇*CGS 13080*

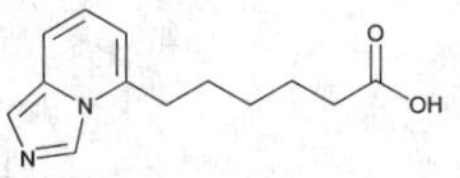

Pirmenol Hydrochloride [*1979*] (pir′ me nol hye″ droe klor′ ide). $C_{22}H_{30}N_2O.HCl$. 374.95. [Pirmenol is INN.] (1) 2-Pyridinemethanol, α-[3-(2,6-dimethyl-1-piperidinyl)pro-pyl]-α-phenyl-, monohydrochloride, *cis*-, (±)-; (2) (±)-*cis*-2,6-Dimethyl-α-phenyl-α-2-pyridyl-1-piperidinebuta-nol monohydrochloride. *UNII-JA79OMG4QT. CAS-61477-94-9; CAS-68252-19-7* [pirmenol]. *Cardiac depres-sant (anti-arrhythmic).* Pirmavar (Parke-Davis) ◇*CI-845*

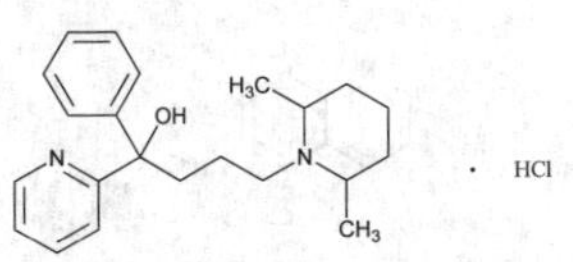

Pirnabin (INN) — *See* Pirnabine.

Pirnabine [*1979*] (pir′ na been). $C_{19}H_{24}O_3$. 300.39. [Pirnabin is INN.] (1) 6*H*-Dibenzo[*b,d*]pyran-1-ol, 7,8,9,10-tetrahy-dro-3,6,6,9-tetramethyl-, acetate, (±)-; (2) (±)-7,8,9,10-Tetrahydro-3,6,6,9-tetramethyl-6*H*-dibenzo[*b,d*]pyran-1-ol acetate. *CAS-19825-63-9; CAS-68298-00-0* [(±)-pirna-bine]. *Antiglaucoma agent.* ◇*SP-304*

Piroctone [*1979*] (pir ok′ tone). C$_{14}$H$_{23}$NO$_2$. 237.34. (1) 2(1*H*)-Pyridinone, 1-hydroxy-4-methyl-6-(2,4,4-trimethylpentyl)-; (2) 1-Hydroxy-4-methyl-6-(2,4,4-trimethylpentyl)-2(1*H*)-pyridone. *UNII-R49EFA73Q7. CAS-50650-76-5.* INN. *Antiseborrheic.*

Piroctone Olamine [*1979*] (pir ok′ tone ole′ a meen). C$_{14}$H$_{23}$NO$_2$.C$_2$H$_7$NO. 298.42. (1) 2(1*H*)-Pyridinone, 1-hydroxy-4-methyl-6-(2,4,4-trimethylpentyl)-, compound with 2-aminoethanol (1:1); (2) 1-Hydroxy-4-methyl-6-(2,4,4-trimethylpentyl)-2(1*H*)-pyridone compound with 2-aminoethanol (1:1). *UNII-A4V5C6R9FB. CAS-68890-66-4; CAS-50650-76-5* [piroctone]. *Antiseborrheic.* Octopirox (Hoechst AG, Germany)

Pirodavir [*1993*] (pir oh′ da vir). C$_{21}$H$_{27}$N$_3$O$_3$. 369.46. (1) Benzoic acid, 4-[2-[1-(6-methyl-3-pyridazinyl)-4-piperidinyl]ethoxy]-, ethyl ester; (2) Ethyl *p*-[2-[1-(6-methyl-3-pyridazinyl)-4-piperidyl]ethoxy]benzoate. *CAS-124436-59-5.* INN; BAN. *Antiviral.* ◇*R 77975*

Pirodomast. C$_{18}$H$_{17}$N$_3$O$_2$. 307.35. 4-Hydroxy-1-phenyl-3-(1-pyrrolidinyl)-1,8-naphthyridin-2(1*H*)-one. *CAS-108310-20-9.* INN.

Pirogliride Tartrate [*1978*] (pir oh′ glir ide tar′ trate). C$_{16}$H$_{22}$N$_4$.C$_4$H$_6$O$_6$. 420.46. [Pirogliride is INN.] (1) 1-Pyrrolidinecarboximidamide, *N*-(1-methyl-2-pyrrolidinylidene)-*N*′-phenyl-[*R*-(*R**,*R**)]-2,3-dihydroxybutanedioate (1:1); (2) *N*-(1-Methyl-2-pyrrolidinylidene)-*N*′-phenyl-1-pyrrolidinecarboxamidine L-(+)-tartrate (1:1). *CAS-62625-19-8; CAS-62625-18-7* [pirogliride]. *Antidiabetic.* ◇*McN-3495*

Piroheptine. C$_{22}$H$_{25}$N. 303.44. [Piroheptine Hydrochloride is JAN.] 3-(10,11-Dihydro-5*H*-dibenzo[*a,d*]cyclohepten-5-ylidene)-1-ethyl-2-methylpyrrolidine. *UNII-AR6Y753ARL. CAS-16378-21-5.* INN; MI.

Pirolate [*1977*] (pir′ oh late). C$_{16}$H$_{15}$N$_3$O$_5$. 329.31. (1) Pyrimido[4,5-*b*]quinoline-2-carboxylic acid, 1,4-dihydro-7,8-dimethoxy-4-oxo-, ethyl ester; (2) Ethyl 1,4-dihydro-7,8-dimethoxy-4-oxopyrimido[4,5-*b*]quinoline-2-carboxylate. *CAS-55149-05-8.* INN. *Anti-asthmatic.* ◇*CP-32,387*

Pirolazamide [*1975*] (pir″ oh laz′ a mide). C$_{23}$H$_{29}$N$_3$O. 363.50. (1) Pyrrolo[1,2-*a*]pyrazine-2(1*H*)-butanamide, hexahydro-α,α-diphenyl-; (2) Hexahydro-α,α-diphenylpyrrolo[1,2-*a*]pyrazine-2(1*H*)-butyramide. *UNII-GQN5BVM24W. CAS-39186-49-7.* INN. *Cardiac depressant (anti-arrhythmic).* ◇*SC-26438*

Piromidic Acid. C$_{14}$H$_{16}$N$_4$O$_3$. 288.30. 8-Ethyl-5,8-dihydro-5-oxo-2-(1-pyrrolidinyl)pyrido[2,3-*d*]pyrimidine-6-carboxylic acid. *UNII-3I12WH4EWF. CAS-19562-30-2.* INN; JAN; MI. ◇*PD-93*

Piroxantrone Hydrochloride [*1988*] (pir ox′ an trone hye″ droe klor′ ide). C$_{21}$H$_{25}$N$_5$O$_4$.2HCl. 484.38. [Piroxantrone is INN.] (1) Anthra[1,9-*cd*]pyrazol-6(2*H*)-one, 5-[(3-aminopropyl)amino]-7,10-dihydroxy-2-[2-[(2-hydroxyethyl)amino]ethyl]-, dihydrochloride; (2) 5-[(3-Aminopropyl)amino]-7,10-dihydroxy-2-[2-[(2-hydroxyethyl)amino]ethyl]anthra[1,9-*cd*]pyrazol-6(2*H*)-one dihydrochloride. *UNII-PS51OZG63Z. CAS-105118-12-5; CAS-91441-23-5* [piroxantrone]. *Antineoplastic.* ◇*CI-942*

Piroxicam [*1974*] (pir ox′ i kam). **USP.** C$_{15}$H$_{13}$N$_3$O$_4$S. 331.35. (1) 2*H*-1,2-Benzothiazine-3-carboxamide, 4-hydroxy-2-methyl-*N*-2-pyridinyl-, 1,1-dioxide; (2) 4-Hydroxy-2-methyl-*N*-2-pyridyl-2*H*-1,2-benzothiazine-3-carboxamide 1,1-dioxide. *UNII-13T4O6VMAM. CAS-36322-90-4.* INN; BAN; JAN. *Anti-inflammatory.* Feldene (Pfizer) ◇*CP-16,171*

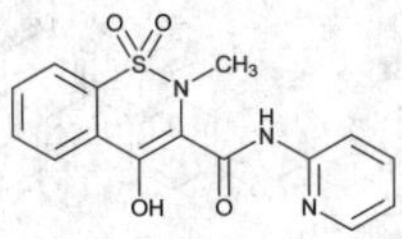

Piroxicam Betadex [*1996*] (pir ox′ i kam bay′ ta dex). $(C_{15}H_{13}N_3O_4S)_2.(C_{42}H_{70}O_{35})_5.$ 6337.61. (1) 2*H*-1,2-Benzothiazine-3-carboxamide, 4-hydroxy-2-methyl-*N*-2-pyridinyl-, 1,1-dioxide compound with β-cyclodextrin (2:5); (2) 4-Hydroxy-2-methyl-*N*-2-pyridyl-2*H*-1,2-benzothiazine-3-carboxamide 1,1-dioxide, compound with β-cyclodextrin (2:5). *CAS-96684-40-1. Analgesic; anti-inflammatory; antirheumatic.*

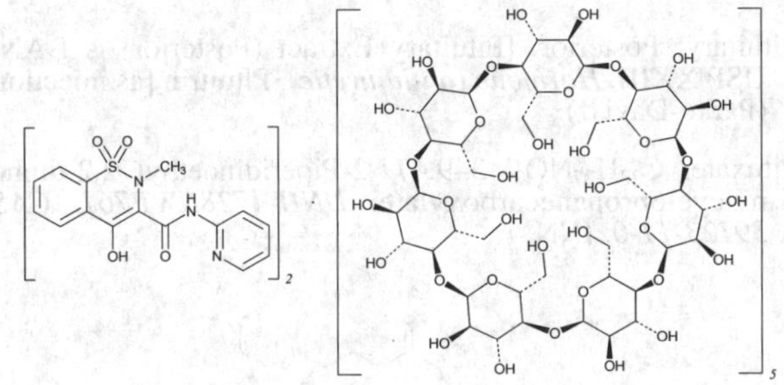

Piroxicam Cinnamate [*1987*] (pir ox′ i kam sin′ a mate). $C_{24}H_{19}N_3O_5S.$ 461.49. (1) 2-Propenoic acid, 3-phenyl-, 2-methyl-3-[(2-pyridinylamino)carbonyl]-2*H*-1,2-benzothiazin-4-yl ester, *S,S*-dioxide; (2) 4-Hydroxy-2-methyl-*N*-2-pyridyl-2*H*-1,2-benzothiazine-3-carboxamide 1,1-dioxide, cinnamate (ester). *UNII-7E8Q32N75N. CAS-87234-24-0. Anti-inflammatory.* ◇*SPA-S-510*

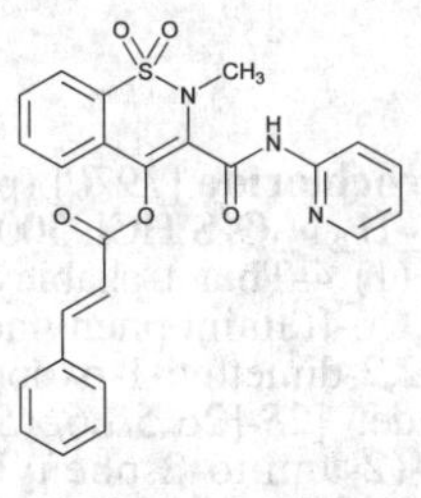

Piroxicam Olamine [*1984*] (pir ox′ i kam ole′ a meen). $C_{15}H_{13}N_3O_4S.C_2H_7NO.$ 392.43. (1) 2*H*-1,2-Benzothiazine-3-carboxamide, 4-hydroxy-2-methyl-*N*-2-pyridinyl-, 1,1-dioxide, compound with 2-aminoethanol (1:1); (2) 4-Hydroxy-2-methyl-*N*-2-pyridyl-2*H*-1,2-benzothiazine-3-carboxamide 1,1-dioxide, compound with 2-aminoethanol (1:1). *UNII-T4O2MP4507. CAS-85056-47-9. Analgesic; anti-inflammatory.* ◇*CP-16,171-85*

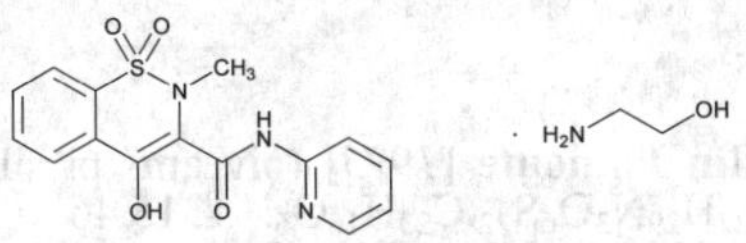

Piroxicillin. $C_{27}H_{28}N_8O_9S_2.$ 672.69. (2*S*,5*R*,6*R*)-6-[(*R*)-2-(*p*-Hydroxyphenyl)-2-[3-[4-hydroxy-2-(*p*-sulfamoylanilino)-5-pyrimidinyl]ureido]acetamido]-3,3-dimethyl-7-oxo-4-thia-1-azabicyclo[3.2.0]heptane-2-carboxylic acid. *UNII-HPI5A94GD9. CAS-82509-56-6.* INN.

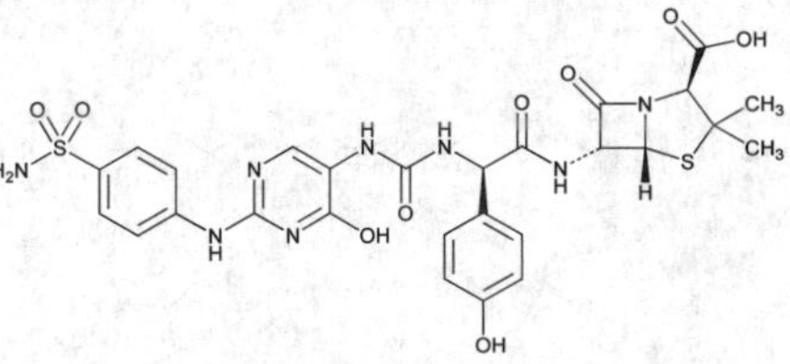

Piroximone [*1985*] (pir ox′ i mone). $C_{11}H_{11}N_3O_2.$ 217.22. (1) 2*H*-Imidazol-2-one, 4-ethyl-1,3-dihydro-5-(4-pyridinylcarbonyl)-; (2) 4-Ethyl-5-isonicotinoyl-4-imidazolin-2-one. *CAS-84490-12-0.* INN; BAN. *Cardiotonic.* ◇*MDL 19,205*

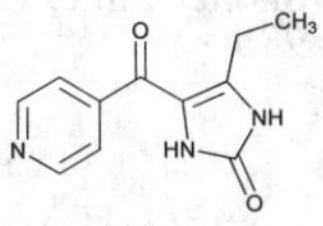

Pirozadil. $C_{27}H_{29}NO_{10}.$ 527.52. 2,6-Pyridinediyldimethylenebis(3,4,5-trimethoxybenzoate). *UNII-54978VNA4T. CAS-54110-25-7.* INN; MI.

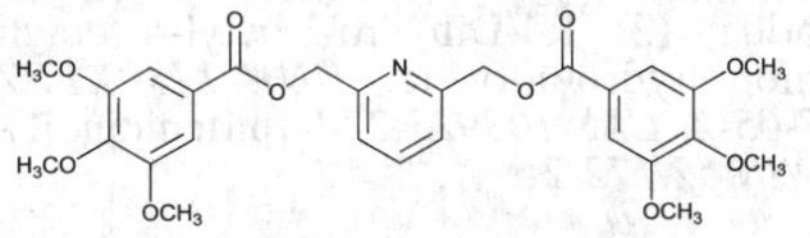

Pirprofen [*1974*] (pir proe′ fen). $C_{13}H_{14}ClNO_2.$ 251.71. (1) Benzeneacetic acid, 3-chloro-4-(2,5-dihydro-1*H*-pyrrol-1-yl)-α-methyl-; (2) 3-Chloro-4-(3-pyrrolin-1-yl)hydratropic acid. *CAS-31793-07-4.* INN; BAN. *Anti-inflammatory.* ◇*Su 21524*

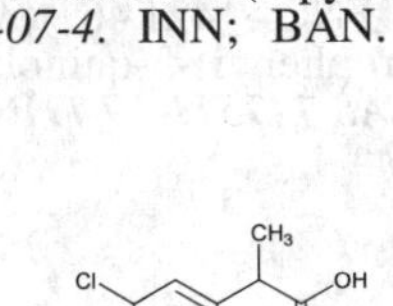

Pirquinozol [*1979*] (pir kwin′ oh zol). $C_{11}H_9N_3O_2.$ 215.21. (1) Pyrazolo[1,5-*c*]quinazolin-5(6*H*)-one, 2-(hydroxymethyl)-; (2) 2-(Hydroxymethyl)pyrazolo[1,5-*c*]quinazolin-5(6*H*)-one. *CAS-65950-99-4.* INN; BAN. *Anti-allergic.* ◇*SQ 13847*

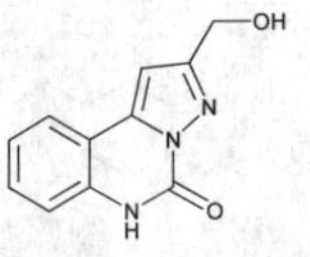

---

† Brand name formerly used, and/or firm no longer concerned with this product.

Pirralkonium Bromide. $C_{35}H_{72}BrN_3$. 614.87. Bis[3-(2,5-dimethyl-1-pyrrolidinyl)propyl]hexadecylmethylammonium bromide. *UNII-6WVM5HPV4T. CAS-17243-65-1.* INN.

Pirroksan (previously used name) — *See* Proroxan Hydrochloride.

Pirsidomine [*1993*] (pir sid′ oh meen). $C_{17}H_{22}N_4O_3$. 330.38. (1) Sydnone imine, 3-(2,6-dimethyl-1-piperidinyl)-*N*-(4-methoxybenzoyl)-, *cis*-; (2) *N-p*-Anisoyl-3-(*cis*-2,6-dimethylpiperidino)sydnone imine. *CAS-132722-74-8.* INN. *Vasodilator.* ◇*CAS 936*

Pirtenidine Hydrochloride [*1986*] (pir ten′ i deen hye″ droe klor′ ide). $C_{21}H_{38}N_2$.HCl. 355.00. [Pirtenidine is INN.] (1) *N*-(1-Octyl-4(1*H*)-pyridinylidene-1-octanamine monohydrochloride; (2) 1,4-Dihydro-1-octyl-4-(octylimino)pyridine monohydrochloride. *UNII-1J30XTP76F. CAS-100227-05-2; CAS-103923-27-9* [pirtenidine]. *Antigingivitus.* ◇*WIN 52,172-2*

Pitavastatin. $C_{25}H_{24}FNO_4$. 421.46. (3*R*,5*S*,6*E*)-7-[2-Cyclopropyl-4-(*p*-fluorophenyl)-3-quinolyl]-3,5-dihydroxy-6-heptenoic acid. *CAS-147511-69-1.* INN. [*Name previously used: Itavastatin]*

Pitenodil. $C_{17}H_{27}N_3O_3S$. 353.48. 2-[4-[3-(2-Thenoyl)propyl]-1-piperazinyl]ethyl dimethylcarbamate. *UNII-ZIB93J9J6L. CAS-59840-71-0.* INN.

Pitofenone. $C_{22}H_{25}NO_4$. 367.44. Methyl *o*-[*p*-(2-piperidinoethoxy)benzoyl]benzoate. *UNII-M09N8K7YJY. CAS-54063-52-4.* INN; DCF.

Pitrakinra. $C_{651}H_{1054}N_{190}O_{200}S_8$. L-Methionyl-[121-aspartic acid,124-aspartic acid]interleukin-4. INN.

```
                                                   M
HKCDITLQEI   IKTLNSLTEQ   KTLCTELTVT   DIFAASKNTT
EKETFCRAAT   VLRQFYSHHE   KDTRCLGATA   QQFHRHKQLI
RFLKRLDRNL   WGLAGLNSCP   VKEANQSTLE   NFLERLKTIM
DEKDSKCSS
```

Pituitary, Posterior. [Pituitary Extract (Posterior) is BAN.] USP XXIII. *Hormone (antidiuretic).* Pituitrin [as injection] (Parke-Davis†)

Pituxate. $C_{23}H_{27}NO_2$. 349.47. 2-Piperidinoethyl 2,2-diphenylcyclopropanecarboxylate. *UNII-4728AWF76J. CAS-39123-11-0.* INN.

Pivagabine. $C_9H_{17}NO_3$. 187.24. 4-Pivalamidobutyric acid. *UNII-C53SV0WO4V. CAS-69542-93-4.* INN.

Pivampicillin Hydrochloride [*1970*] (piv am″ pi sil′ in hye″ droe klor′ ide). $C_{22}H_{29}N_3O_6S$.HCl. 500.01. [Pivampicillin is INN and BAN.] (1) 4-Thia-1-azabicyclo[3.2.0]heptane-2-carboxylic acid, 6-[(aminophenylacetyl)amino]-3,3-dimethyl-7-oxo-, (2,2-dimethyl-1-oxopropoxy)methyl ester, monohydrochloride, [2*S*-[2α,5α,6β(*S**)]]-; (2) Hydroxymethyl D-(-)-6-(2-amino-2-phenylacetamido)-3,3-dimethyl-7-oxo-4-thia-1-azabicyclo[3.2.0]heptane-2-carboxylate pivalate (ester) monohydrochloride. *UNII-V9HOC53L7L. CAS-26309-95-5; CAS-33817-20-8* [pivampicillin]. *Antibacterial.*

Pivampicillin Pamoate [*1973*] (piv am″ pi sil′ in pam′ oh ate). $(C_{22}H_{29}N_3O_6S)_2$.$C_{23}H_{16}O_6$. 1315.46. (1) 4-Thia-1-azabicyclo[3.2.0]heptane-2-carboxylic acid, 6-[(aminophenylacetyl)amino]-3,3-dimethyl-7-oxo-, (2,2-dimethyl-1-oxopropoxy)methyl ester, [2*S*-[(2α,5α, 6β(*S**)])]-, 4,4′-methylenebis[3-hydroxy-2-naphthalenecarboxylate] (2:1); (2) Hydroxymethyl D-(-)-6-(2-amino-2-phenylacetamido)-3,3-dimethyl-7-oxo-4-thia-1-azabicyclo[3.2.0]heptane-2-carboxylate pivalate (ester) compound with 4,4′-methylenebis[3-hydroxy-2-naphthoic acid] (2:1). *UNII-5Z5TRG74EY. CAS-39030-72-3; CAS-59549-62-1* [replaced]; *CAS-33817-20-8* [pivampicillin]. *Antibacterial.*

Pivampicillin Probenate [*1973*] (piv am″ pi sil′ in proe′ be nate). $C_{22}H_{29}N_3O_6S.C_{13}H_{19}NO_4S$. 748.91. (1) 4-Thia-1-azabicyclo[3.2.0]heptane-2-carboxylic acid, 6-[(aminophenylacetyl)amino]-3,3-dimethyl-7-oxo-, (2,2-dimethyl-1-oxopropoxy)methyl ester, [2*S*-[2α,5α,6β(*S**)]]-, mono[4-[(dipropylamino)sulfonyl]benzoate] (1:1); (2) Hydroxymethyl D-(-)-6-(2-amino-2-phenylacetamido)-3,3-dimethyl-7-oxo-4-thia-1-azabicyclo[3.2.0]heptane-2-carboxylate pivalate (ester) compound with *p*-(dipropylsulfamoyl)benzoic acid (1:1). *UNII-M3MYK6R22U. CAS-42190-91-0; CAS-39030-71-2* [replaced]; *CAS-33817-20-8* [pivampicillin]. *Antibacterial.*

Pivenfrine. $C_{14}H_{21}NO_3$. 251.32. (±)-*m*-[1-Hydroxy-2-(methylamino)ethyl]phenyl pivalate. *UNII-RB4XQ0T71U. CAS-67577-23-5.* INN.

Pivhydrazine. $C_{12}H_{18}N_2O$. 206.28. 2′-Benzylpivalohydrazide. *CAS-306-19-4.* BAN.

Pivmecillinam (INN, BAN) — *See* Amdinocillin Pivoxil.

Pivmecillinam Hydrochloride (JAN) — *See* Amdinocillin Pivoxil.

Pivopril [*1985*] (piv′ oh pril). $C_{16}H_{27}NO_4S$. 329.45. (1) Glycine, *N*-cyclopentyl-*N*-[3-[(2,2-dimethyl-1-oxopropyl)thio]-2-methyl-1-oxopropyl]-, (*S*)-(-)-; (2) 2,2-Dimethylthiopropionic acid, *S*-ester with (-)-(*S*)-*N*-cyclopentyl-*N*-(3-mercapto-2-methylpropionyl)glycine. *UNII-3V6I5962EM. CAS-81045-50-3.* INN. *Antihypertensive.* ◇*REV 3659-(S); RHC 3659-(S); USV 3659-(S)*

Pivoxazepam. $C_{20}H_{19}ClN_2O_3$. 370.83. 7-Chloro-1,3-dihydro-3-hydroxy-5-phenyl-2*H*-1,4-benzodiazepin-2-one pivalate (ester). *UNII-F4ER8Z6Q3U. CAS-55299-10-0.* INN.

Pivsulbactam (BAN) — *See* Sulbactam Pivoxil.

Pix Pini — *See* Pine Tar.

---

† Brand name formerly used, and/or firm no longer concerned with this product.

Pixantrone [*2003*] (pix′ an trone). $C_{17}H_{19}N_5O_2$. 325.37. (1) Benz[*g*]isoquinoline-5,10-dione, 6,9-bis[(2-aminoethyl)amino]-; (2) 6,9-Bis[(2-aminoethyl)amino]benzo[*g*]isoquinoline-5,10-dione. *UNII-F5SXN2KNMR. CAS-144510-96-3.* INN; BAN. *Anti-neoplastic.* ◇*BBR 2778*

Pizotifen (INN and BAN) — *See* Pizotyline.

Pizotyline [*1970*] (pi zoe′ ti leen). $C_{19}H_{21}NS$. 295.44. [Pizotifen is INN and BAN.] (1) Piperidine, 4-(9,10-dihydro-4*H*-benzo[4,5]cyclohepta[1,2-*b*]thien-4-ylidene)-1-methyl-; (2) 4-(9,10-Dihydro-4*H*-benzo[4,5]cyclohepta[1,2-*b*]thien-4-ylidene)-1-methylpiperidine. *CAS-15574-96-6. Anabolic; antidepressant; serotonin inhibitor (specific in migraine).* Sandomigran (Novartis†) ◇*BC-105*

Plafibride. $C_{16}H_{22}ClN_3O_4$. 355.82. 1-[2-(*p*-Chlorophenoxy)-2-methylpropionyl]-3-(morpholinomethyl)urea. *UNII-5J7C4JZ564. CAS-63394-05-8.* INN; MI.

Plague Vaccine. USP XXVI. *Immunizing agent (active).*

Plantago Seed (plan tay′ goe). **USP.** The cleaned, dried, ripe seed of *Plantago psyllium* Linné, or of *Plantago indica* Linné (*Plantago arenaria* Waldstein et Kitaibel), known in commerce as Spanish or French Psyllium Seed; or of *Plantago ovata* Forskal, known in commerce as Blond Psyllium or Indian Plantago Seed (Fam. Plantaginaceae). *UNII-9C60Y73166. Laxative.*

Plantain Seed — *See* Plantago Seed.

Plasma, Antihemophilic Human. [PHS: *Antihemophilic Plasma (Human)*]. USP XVIII.

Plasma Concentrate Factor IX — *See* Factor IX Complex.

Plasma Protein Fraction. USP. A sterile preparation of serum albumin and globulin obtained by fractionating material (source blood, plasma, or serum) from healthy human donors, the source material being tested for the absence of hepatitis B surface antigen. *Blood volume supporter.* Plasmanate (Bayer); Plasma Plex (Centeon); Plasmatein (Alpha Therapeutic); Protenate (Hyland) *[Name previously used: Plasma Protein Fraction, Human.]*

Plasma Protein Fraction, Human (previously used name) — *See* Plasma Protein Fraction.

Plasmin (previously used name) — *See* Fibrinolysin, Human.

Plasminogen. The specific substance derived from plasma that, when activated, has the property of lysing fibrinogen, fibrin and some other proteins. BAN.

Platelet Concentrate. **USP**. Contains the platelets taken from plasma obtained by whole blood collection, by plasma pheresis, or by platelet pheresis, from a single suitable donor of whole blood; or from a plasma pheresis donor; or from a platelet pheresis donor who meets the criteria described in the product license application. *Replenisher (platelets).*

Platelets. **USP**. The portion of blood that contains platelet cells.

cis-Platinum II (previously used name) — *See* Cisplatin.

Platonin. $C_{38}H_{61}I_2N_3S_3$. 909.91. 2,2′-[3-[(3-Heptyl-4-methyl-2(3*H*)-thiazolylidene)ethylidene]-1-propene-1,3-diyl]-bis[3-heptyl-4-methylthiazolium]diiodide. *UNII-0X9JDS6MF1. CAS-3571-88-8.* JAN.

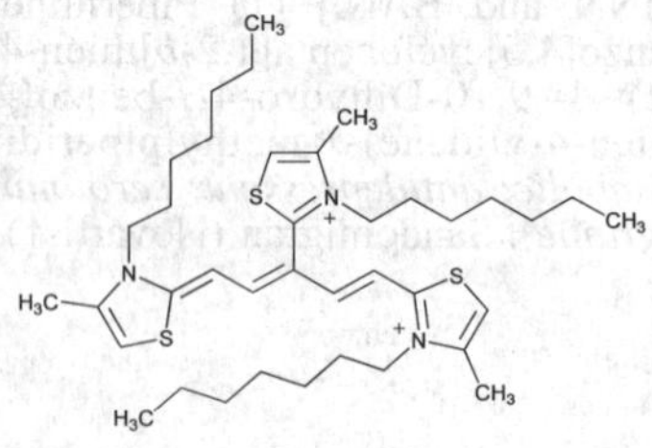

Plaunotol. $C_{20}H_{34}O_2$. 306.48. (2*Z*,6*E*)-2-[(3*E*)-4,8-Dimethyl-3,7-nonadienyl]-6-methyl-2,6-octadiene-1,8-diol. *UNII-MV715X4634. CAS-64218-02-6.* INN; JAN; MI.

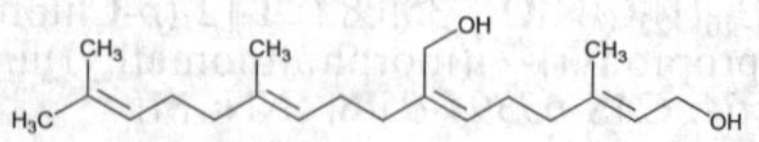

Plauracin [*1977*] (plaw′ ra sin). $C_{26}H_{35}N_3O_7$(ML)+$C_{45}H_{53}N_7O_{11}$(D). Antibiotic complex produced by *Actinoplanes auranticolor* (ATCC No. 31011). A mixture of two major components, a macrocyclic lactone (ML) and a depsipeptide (D), the structures of which are not fully confirmed. (1) Plauracin; (2) Plauracin. *CAS-62107-94-2.* INN. *Growth stimulant (veterinary).* ◇*CP-38,754*

Pleconaril [*1997*] (ple kon′ a ril). $C_{18}H_{18}F_3N_3O_3$. 381.35. 3-[4-[3-(3-Methyl-5-isoxazolyl)propoxy]-3,5-xylyl]-5-trifluoromethyl-1,2,4-oxadizole. *UNII-9H4570Q89D. CAS-153168-05-9.* INN. *Antiviral.* ◇*VP 63843; WIN 63843*

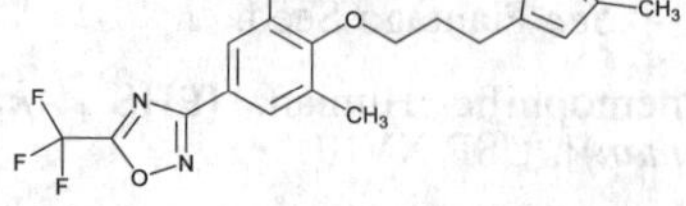

Plerixafor [*2004*] (pler ix′ a fore). $C_{28}H_{54}N_8$. 502.78. (1) 1,4,8,11-Tetraazacyclotetradecane, 1,1′-[1,4-phenylene-bis(methylene)]bis-; (2) 1,1′-(1,4-Phenylenebismethylene)-bis(1,4,8,11-tetraazacyclotetradecane). *UNII-S915P5499N. CAS-110078-46-1.* INN. *Stem cell mobilization (CXCR4 receptor antagonist).* ◇*AMD3100*

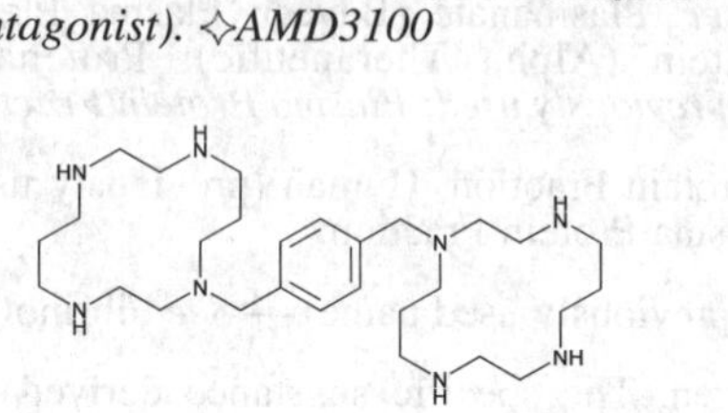

Pleuromulin. $C_{22}H_{34}O_5$. 378.50. Glycolic acid 8-ester with octahydro-5,8-dihydroxy-4,6,9,10-tetramethyl-6-vinyl-3a,9-propano-3a*H*-cyclopentacycloocten-1(4*H*)-one. *CAS-125-65-5.* INN.

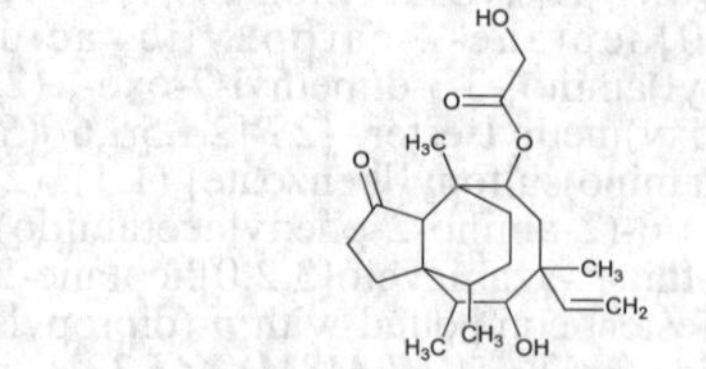

Plevitrexed. $C_{26}H_{25}FN_8O_4$. 532.53. (2*S*)-2-[[4-[[(2,7-Di-methyl-4-oxo-1,4-dihydroquinazolin-6-yl)methyl](prop-2-ynyl)amino]-2-fluorobenzoyl]amino]-4-(1*H*-tetrazol-5-yl)-butanoic acid. *UNII-L9P2881C3H. CAS-153537-73-6.* INN; BAN. ◇*ZD9331*

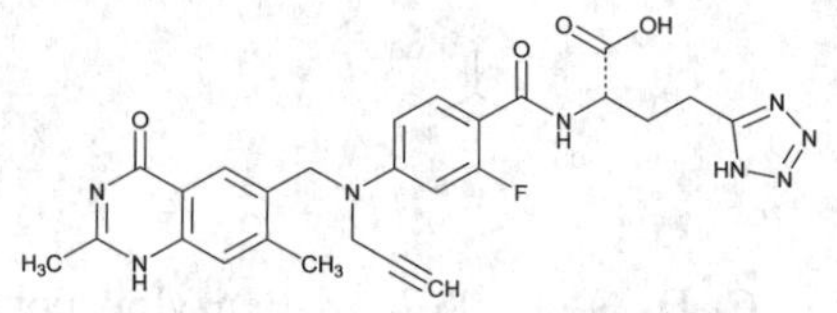

Plicamycin [*1965*] (plye″ ka mye′ sin). **USP**. $C_{52}H_{76}O_{24}$. 1085.15. Antibiotic produced by *Streptomyces argillaceus* n. sp., *Streptomyces tanashiensis*, and *Streptomyces plicatus*. (1) Plicamycin; (2) Plicamycin; (3) [2*S*-[2α,3β(1*R**,3*R**,4*S**)]]-6-[[2,6-Dideoxy-3-*O*-(2,6-di-deoxy-β-D-*arabino*-hexopyranosyl)-β-D-*arabino*-hexopyr-anosyl]oxy]-2-[(*O*-2,6-dideoxy-3-*C*-methyl-β-D-*ribo*-hex-opyranosyl-(1→4)-*O*-2,6-dideoxy-α-D-*lyxo*-hexopyrano-syl-(1→3)-2,6-dideoxy-β-D-*arabino*-hexopyranosyl)oxy]-3-(3,4-dihydroxy-1-methyl-2-oxopentyl)-3,4-dihydro-8,9-dihydroxy-7-methyl-1(2*H*)-anthracenone. *UNII-NIJ123W41V. CAS-18378-89-7.* INN; BAN. *Antineoplastic.* Mithracin (Pfizer) *[Name previously used: Mithramycin.]* ◇*PA-144; A-2371; NSC-24559*

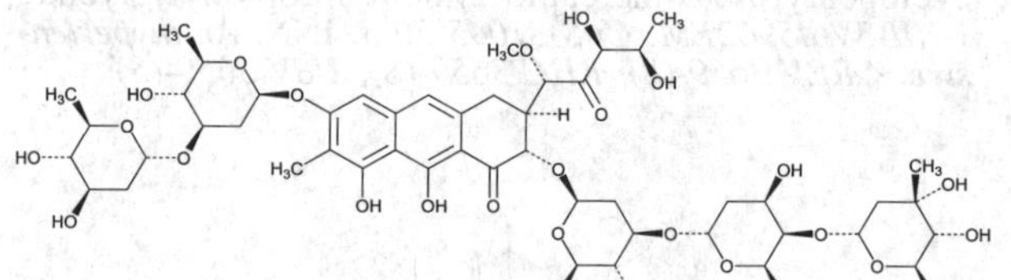

Plitidepsin. $C_{57}H_{87}N_7O_{15}$. 1110.34. 3,6-Anhydro(*N*-{(2*S*,4*S*)-4-[(3*S*,4*R*,5*S*)-3-hydroxy-4-{[*N*-(2-oxopropanoyl)-L-pro-lyl-*N*-methyl-D-leucyl-L-threonyl]amino}-5-methylhepta-noyloxy]-2,5-dimethyl-3-oxohexanoyl}-L-leucyl-L-prolyl-*N*,*O*-dimethyl-L-tyrosine). *CAS-137219-37-5.* INN; BAN.

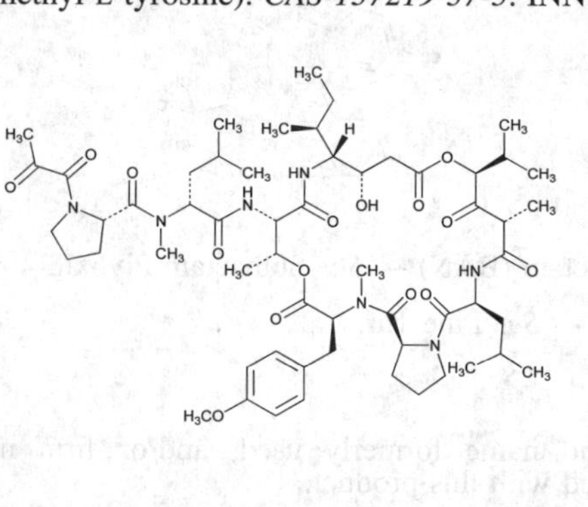

Plomestane [*1991*] (ploe mes′ tane). $C_{21}H_{26}O_2$. 310.43. (1) Estr-4-ene-3,17-dione, 10-(2-propynyl)-; (2) 10-(2-Propynyl)estr-4-ene-3,17-dione. *CAS-77016-85-4*. INN. *Antineoplastic.* ◇*MDL 18,962*

Plusonermin. A mixture of tumor necrosis factor proteins (human): 1-157-tumor necrosis factor, 3-157-tumor necrosis factor (major component), and 5-157-tumor necrosis factor. INN.

Pobilukast Edamine [*1994*] (poe″ bi loo′ kast ed′ a meen). $C_{26}H_{34}O_5S.C_2H_8N_2.H_2O$. 536.72. [Pobilukast is INN.] (1) Benzenepropanoic acid, β-[(2-carboxyethyl)thio]-α-hydroxy-2-(8-phenyloctyl)-, [R-(R^*,S^*)]-, compd. with 1,2-ethanediamine (1:1), monohydrate; (2) ($2S,3R$)-3-[(2-Carboxyethyl)thio]-3-[o-(8-phenyloctyl)phenyl]lactic acid, compound with ethylenediamine (1:1), monohydrate. *CAS-137232-03-2; CAS-107023-41-6* [pobilukast]. *Anti-asthmatic (leukotriene antagonist).* ◇*SK&F 104353-Q*

Podilfen. $C_{18}H_{23}N_3O_2S$. 345.46. 1-[α-Methyl-3,4-(methylenedioxy)phenethyl]-4-(4-methyl-2-thiazolyl)piperazine. *UNII-LI81FMI713. CAS-13409-53-5*. INN.

Podofilox [*1989*] (poe dof′ il lox). $C_{22}H_{22}O_8$. 414.41. [Podophyllotoxin is BAN.] (1) Furo[3′,4′:6,7]naphtho[2,3-d]-1,3-dioxol-6(5aH)-one, 5,8,8a,9-tetrahydro-9-hydroxy-5-(3,4,5-trimethoxyphenyl)-, [$5R$-($5\alpha,5a\beta,8a\alpha,9\alpha$)]-; (2) Podophyllotoxin; (3) ($5R,5aR,8aR,9R$)-5,8,8a,9-Tetrahydro-9-hydroxy-5-(3,4,5-trimethoxyphenyl)furo[3′,4′:6,7]-naphtho[2,3-d]-1,3-dioxol-6(5aH)-one. *UNII-L36H50F353. CAS-518-28-5. Antimitotic.* Condylox (Oclassen)

Podophyllotoxin (BAN) — *See* Podofilox.

Podophyllum (pode oh fil′ um; po dof′ il um). **USP**. Pharmaceutic necessity for Podophyllum Resin. *UNII-2S713A4VP3. Pharmaceutic necessity.*

Poison Ivy Extract, Alum Precipitated [*1962*]. A repository form of a pyridine extract of poison ivy (*Toxicodendron radicans*). *Ivy poisoning counteractant.* Aqua Ivy, AP (Bayer†); Rhus Tox Antigen (Lemmon†)

Poison Oak Extract [*1963*]. A sterile extract prepared from *Toxicodendron quercifolium*. *UNII-UD3030V43F. Antiallergic.*

Polacrilin [*1969*] (pol″ a kril′ in). A synthetic ion-exchange resin, supplied in the hydrogen or free acid form. (1) 2-Propenoic acid, 2-methyl-, polymer with diethenylbenzene; (2) Methacrylic acid polymer with divinylbenzene. *CAS-50602-21-6; CAS-9017-36-1* [replaced]. INN. *Pharmaceutic aid.*

Polacrilin Potassium [*1969*] (pol″ a kril′ in poe tas′ ee um). **NF**. (1) 2-Propenoic acid, 2-methyl-, potassium salt, polymer with diethenylbenzene; (2) Potassium methacrylate-divinylbenzene, copolymer. *CAS-65405-55-2; CAS-54182-62-6* [replaced]; *CAS-50602-21-6* [polacrilin]. *Pharmaceutic aid (tablet disintegrant).* Amberlite IRP88 Resin (Rohm and Haas)

Polaprezinc. $(C_9H_{12}N_4O_3Zn)_n$. *catena*-Poly[zinc-μ-[β-alanyl-L-histidinato(2-)-$N,N^N,O:N^\tau$]]. *CAS-107667-60-7*. INN.

Poldine Methylsulfate [*1962*] (pol′ deen meth″ il sul′ fate). $C_{22}H_{29}NO_7S$. 451.53. [Poldine Metilsulfate is INN and BAN.] (1) Pyrrolidinium 2-[[(hydroxydiphenylacetyl)oxy]methyl]-1,1-dimethyl-, methyl sulfate; (2) 2-(Hydroxymethyl)-1,1-dimethylpyrrolidinium methyl sulfate benzilate. *CAS-545-80-2; CAS-596-50-9* [poldine]. USP XX. *Anticholinergic.* Nacton (Ortho-McNeil†) *[Name previously used: Poldine Methylsulphate.]* ◇*I.S. 499; McN-R-726-47*

Policapram [*1974*] (pol″ i ka′ pram). $(C_6H_{11}NO)_n$. Linear polymer of caprolactam (ϵ-aminocaproic lactam) as microcrystals of colloidal dimensions. (1) Poly[imino(1-oxo-1,6-hexanediyl)]; (2) Poly(iminocarbonylpentamethylene). *CAS-25038-54-4*. INN. *Pharmaceutic aid (tablet binder).*

Policresulen. $(C_8H_9O_4S)(C_8H_8O_4S)_n(C_7H_7O_4S)$. 2-Hydroxy-*p*-toluenesulfonic acid, polymer with formaldehyde. *CAS-101418-00-2.* INN.

Polidexide Sulfate. [Polidexide is BAN.] Dextran 2-(diethyl-amino)ethyl 2-[[2-(diethylamino)ethyl]diethylammo-nio]ethyl ether sulfate, epichlorohydrin crosslinked. *CAS-63494-82-6; CAS-56227-39-5 [polidexide].* INN.

Polidocanol. Polyethylene glycol monododecyl ether (aver-age polymer, n = 9; nonaethylene glycol monododecyl ether). *CAS-3055-99-0.* INN; JAN; MI; DCF.

Polidronium Chloride. $(C_6H_{12}ClN)_n \cdot C_{16}H_{36}Cl_2N_2O_6$. α-[(*E*)-4-[Tris(2-hydroxyethyl)ammonio]-2-butenyl-ω-[tris(2-hy-droxyethyl)ammonio]poly[(dimethyliminio)[(*E*)-2-buten-ylene]chloride]dichloride. *CAS-75345-27-6.* INN; BAN.

Polifeprosan 20 [*1991*] (pol″ ee fep′ roe san). $(C_{17}H_{16}O_6)_m$ $(C_{10}H_{18}O_4)_n$. 20,000–200,000. [Polifeprosan is INN.] The numerical value 20 represents the weight percent of the 4,4′-(trimethylenedioxy)dibenzoic acid monomer (mono-mer *m*) present in the polymer. (1) Benzoic acid, 4,4′-[1,3-propanediylbis(oxy)]bis-, polymer with decanedioic acid; (2) 4,4′-(Trimethylenedioxy)dibenzoic acid, polymer with sebacic acid. *CAS-90409-78-2. Pharmaceutic aid.*

Poligeenan [*1969*] (pol″ ee gee′ nan). $[C_{12}H_{16}M_2O_{15}S_2]n$ (Nominal, the value of *n* is 30 to 60). Polysaccharide derived from extensive acid hydrolysis of carrageenan from red algae. (1) Poligeenan; (2) 3,6-Anhydro-4-*O*-β-D-galactopyranosyl-α-D-galactopyranose 2,4′-bis(potassium/sodium sulfate)-(1→3′)-polysaccharide. *CAS-53973-98-1.* INN. *Pharmaceutic aid (dispersing agent).*

Poliglecaprone 25 [*1991*] (pol″ ee glek′ a prone). $(C_6H_{10}O_2)_m(C_4H_4O_4)_n$. 70,000 (wt. avg.). [Poliglecaprone is BAN.] (1) 2-Oxepanone, polymer with 1,4-dioxane-2,5-dione; (2) 2-Oxepanone polymer with *p*-dioxane-2,5-dione. *CAS-41706-81-4.* INN. *Surgical aid (surgical suture material, absorbable).*

Poliglecaprone 90 [*1991*] (pol″ ee glek′ a prone). $(C_6H_{10}O_2)_m(C_4H_4O_4)_n$. 5,000–15,000 (wt. avg.). (1) 2-Oxepanone, polymer with 1,4-dioxane-2,5-dione; (2) 2-Oxepanone polymer with *p*-dioxane-2,5-dione. *CAS-41706-81-4.* INN. *Surgical aid (surgical suture coating, absorbable).*

Poliglusam [*1991*] (pol″ ee gloo′ sam). Linear homopolymer of partially acetylated glucosamine. (1) Chitosan; (2) Chitosan. *CAS-9012-76-4.* INN. *Antihemorrhagic.*

Polignate Sodium [*1970*] (poe lig′ nate soe′ dee um). The sulfonated form of a polymer similar to the sub-unit of coniferyl alcohol polymer derived from coniferous wood. (The individual polymer units are considered to be three-dimensional structures with molecular weights in the range of several thousand.) (1) Lignosulfonic acid, sodium salt; (2) Sodium lignosulfonate. *CAS-8061-51-6; CAS-7061-51-6 [sodium lignosulfonate]. Enzyme inhibitor (pepsin).* ◇AHR-2438B

Polihexanide. $(C_8H_{17}N_5 \cdot HCl)_n$. Poly(iminoimidocarbonyl-iminoimidocarbonylimino hexamethylene monohydrochloride). *CAS-32289-58-0; CAS-28757-48-4* [replaced]. INN; BAN. [*Name previously used: Polyhexanide.*]

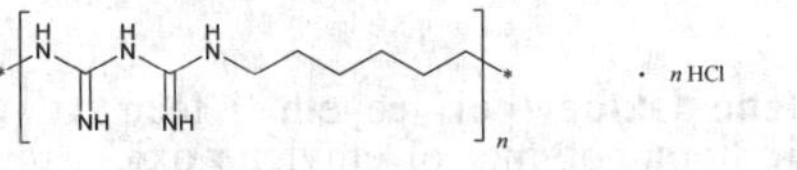

Poliomyelitis Vaccine (previously used name) — *See* Poliovirus Vaccine Inactivated.

Poliovirus Vaccine Inactivated (poe″ lee oh vye′ rus vax′ een in ak′ ti vay″ ted). **USP**. A sterile aqueous suspension of inactivated poliomyelitis virus of Types 1, 2, and 3. *Immunizing agent (active).* [*Name previously used: Poliomyelitis Vaccine.*]

Poliovirus Vaccine Live Oral. USP XXVI. *Immunizing agent (active).* Orimune (Lederle)

Polipropene 25 [*1974*] (pol″ ee proe′ peen). $(C_3H_6)_n$. (1) 1-Propene homopolymer; (2) Polypropene. *CAS-9003-07-0. Pharmaceutic aid (tablet excipient).*

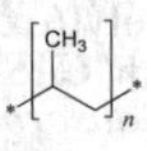

Polisaponin. A mixture of all the steroid saponins isolated from the rhizome of *Dioscorea polystachya.CAS-8063-80-7.* INN.

Politef (INN) — *See* Polytef.

Polixetonium Chloride [*1993*] (poe″ lix e toe′ nee um klor′ ide). $(C_{10}H_{24}Cl_2N_2O)_n$. (1) Poly[oxy-1,2-ethanediyl(dimethyliminio)-1,2-ethanediyl(dimethyliminio)-1,2-ethanediyl dichloride]; (2) Poly[oxyethylene(dimethyliminio) ethylene(dimethyliminio)ethylene dichloride]. *CAS-31512-74-0.* INN. *Pharmaceutic aid (preservative).*

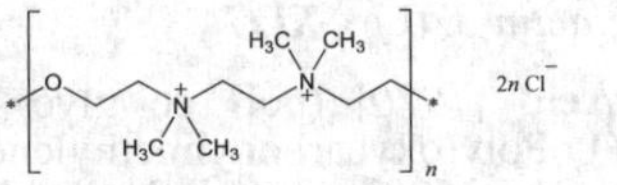

Poloxalene [*1965*] (pol ox′ a leen). **USP**. Liquid nonionic surfactant polymer of the polyethylene-polypropylene glycol type, having a molecular weight of approximately 3000. (In the graphic formula, average values are: $a = 12$; $b = 34$; $c = 12$.) (1) Oxirane, methyl-, polymer with oxirane; (2) Polyethylene-polypropylene glycol. *CAS-9003-11-6.* INN; BAN. *Pharmaceutic aid (surfactant).* Bloat Guard (SmithKline Beecham Animal Health); Therabloat (SmithKline Beecham Animal Health) ◇*SK&F 18,667*

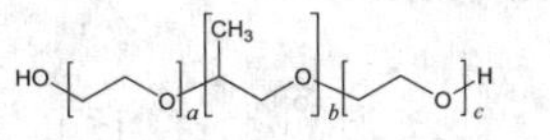

Poloxamer [*1971*] (pol ox′ a mer). **NF**. $HO(C_2H_4O)_a(C_3H_6O)_b(C_2H_4O)_aH$. [Poloxamer-188 is JAN.] (1) Oxirane, methyl-, polymer with oxirane; (2) α-Hydro-ω-hydroxy-poly(oxyethylene)$_a$-poly(oxopropylene)$_b$-poly(oxyethyle-ne)$_a$ block copolymer; (3) Polyethylene-polypropylene glycol. [*Note—Poloxamer* (*used in conjunction with a numeric suffix for individual unique identification*) *is the nonproprietary name that applies to products for which a food, drug, or cosmetic use is likely. These copolymers may function as surfactants, emulsifiers, solubilizers, or stabilizers.*] *CAS-9003-11-6; CAS-106392-12-5* [block copolymer]. INN; BAN. *Pharmaceutic aid (ointment base); pharmaceutic aid (suppository base); pharmaceutic aid (surfactant); pharmaceutic aid (tablet binder and emulsifying agent); pharmaceutic aid (tablet coating agent).* Lutrol F (BASF); Pluracare (BASF); Pluronic (BASF)

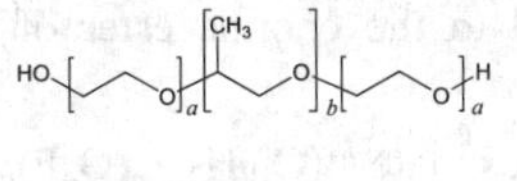

Poloxyl Lanolin. A polyoxyethylene condensation product of anhydrous lanolin. BAN.

Polyamine-Methylene Resin. Phenol condensation product with polyamines. MI. Resinat (Marion Merrell Dow†)

Polybenzarsol. A mixture of polymers formed by reacting formaldehyde with 4-hydroxybenzenearsonic acid. *CAS-54531-52-1; CAS-9006-68-2* [replaced]. INN; MI. Benzocal (Marion Merrell Dow†)

Polybutester [*1985*] (pol″ ee bue′ tes ter). $[(C_4H_8O)xH_2O]_m(C_8H_6O_4)_n(C_4H_{10}O_2)_o$. (1) Poly(oxy-1,4-butanediyl), α-hydro-ω-hydroxy-, polymer with 1,4-benzenedicarboxylic acid and 1,4-butanediol; (2) Polytetramethylene glycol, polymer with terephthalic acid and 1,4-butanediol. *CAS-37282-12-5. Surgical aid (surgical suture material).* Novafil (Davis & Geck) ◇*XM-72*

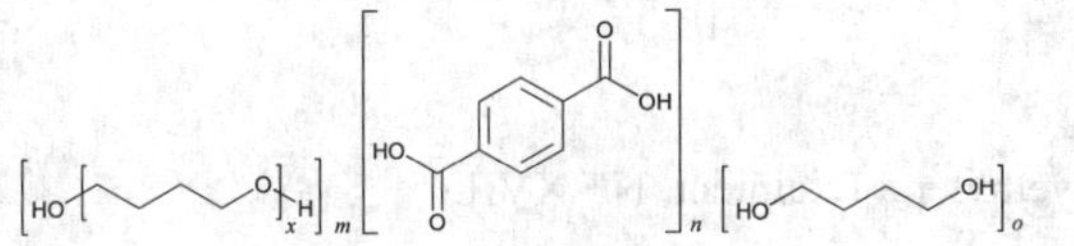

Polybutilate [*1976*] (pol″ ee bue′ ti late). $(C_{10}H_{16}O_4)_n$. (1) Poly[oxy-1,4-butanediyloxy(1,6-dioxo-1,6-hexanediyl)]; (2) Poly(oxytetramethyleneoxyadipoyl). *CAS-24936-97-8. Surgical aid (surgical suture coating).*

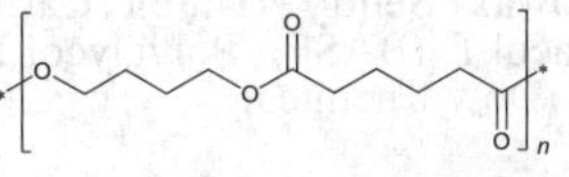

Polycarbokane — *See* Polycarbophil.

Polycarbophil (pol″ ee kar′ boe fil). **USP**. (1) Polycarbophil; (2) Polycarbophil. *CAS-9003-97-8.* INN; BAN. *Laxative.* Noveon AA-1 (Goodrich)

Polydextrose [*1979*] (pol″ ee dex′ trose). **NF**. A randomly bonded glucose polymer with some sorbitol end-groups, and with citric acid residues attached to the polymer by mono- or diester bonds. The $1\rightarrow6$ bond predominates, but all possible bonds are present in the molecule. Molecular weight: average of 1500, with upper limit of 20,000. (1) Polydextrose; (2) D-Glucose polymer, reaction product with citric acid and sorbitol. *CAS-68424-04-4. Food additive.* ◇*CP-31,081*

---

† Brand name formerly used, and/or firm no longer concerned with this product.

Polydioxanone [*1978*] (pol″ ee dye ox′ a none). $(C_4H_6O_3)_n$. (1) Poly[oxy(1-oxo-1,2-ethanediyl)oxy-1,2-ethanediyl]; (2) Poly(oxycarbonylmethyleneoxyethylene). *CAS-31621-87-1.* BAN. *Surgical aid (surgical suture material, absorbable).* PDS II (Ethicon)

Polyelectrolyte 211 — *See* Sodium Alginate.

Polyenephosphatidyl Choline. A mixture of the diglyceride of polyene, linked to the choline ester of phosphoric acid. JAN.

Polyestradiol Phosphate. $(C_{18}H_{22})_m(O_4P)_n$ (Approximate). Estradiol phosphate polymer. *CAS-28014-46-2.* INN; BAN; MI. Estradurin (Wyeth) ◇*Leo 114*

Polyetadene (INN) — *See* Polyethadene.

Polyethadene [*1964*] (pol″ ee eth′ a deen). $(C_4H_6O_2)_m(C_2H_5N)_n$. [Polyetadene is INN.] (1) 2,2′-Biox-irane polymer with aziridine; (2) 1,2:3,4-Diepoxybutane polymer with ethylenimine. *CAS-9003-23-0. Antacid.* ◇*30639*

Polyethylene Excipient. NF XVII.

Polyethylene Glycol (pol″ ee eth′ i leen glye′ kol). **NF.** $H(OCH_2CH_2)_nOH$. [Macrogol is BAN and JAN; PEG is PEN.] (1) Poly(oxy-1,2-ethanediyl, α-hydro-ω-hydroxy-; (2) Polyethylene glycol. *CAS-25322-68-3; CAS-9002-90-8* [macrogol]. *Pharmaceutic aid (ointment base); pharmaceutic aid (suppository base); pharmaceutic aid (solvent); pharmaceutic aid (tablet excipient); pharmaceutic aid (tablet and/or capsule lubricant).* Atpeg 300 (ICI Americas†); Carbowax Sentry (Union Carbide); Lutrol E (BASF); Pluracol E (BASF); Polyglycol E 300, E 400, E 1450, E 8000 (Dow Chemical)

Polyethylene Glycol 1540. NF XIV.

Polyethylene Glycol 4000. [Macrogol 4000 is INN.] USP XIX; MI. Atpeg 4000 (ICI Americas†) *[Note—A number of forms of polyethylene glycol are consolidated under a composite monograph, Polyethylene Glycol, in NF.]*

Polyethylene Glycol 6000. USP XIX; MI. *[Note—A number of forms of polyethylene glycol are consolidated under a composite monograph, Polyethylene Glycol, in NF.]*

Polyethylene Glycol Monomethyl Ether (pol″ ee eth′ i leen glye′ kol mon″ oh meth′ il ee′ ther). **NF.** (1) Poly(oxy-1,2-ethanediyl), α-methyl-ω-hydroxy-; (2) Methoxy polyethy-

lene glycol. *CAS-9004-74-4. Pharmaceutic aid (excipient).* Carbowax Sentry Methoxypolyethylene Glycol (Union Carbide)

Polyethylene Oxide (pol″ ee eth′ i leen ox′ ide). **NF.** A nonionic homopolymer of ethylene oxide, represented by the formula $(OCH_2CH_2)_n$, in which *n* represents the average number of oxyethylene groups. *Pharmaceutic aid (suspending and/or viscosity agent); pharmaceutic aid (tablet binder).* Sentry Polyox WSR (Union Carbide)

Polyferose [*1962*] (pol″ ee fer′ ose). A chelate complex of iron and a polymerized derivative of sucrose. (1) β-D-Fructofuranosyl α-D-glucopyranoside deriv., polymer, iron complex; (2) Carbohydrates, compounds, iron complex. *CAS-9009-29-4. Hematinic.* Jefron (Marion Merrell Dow†)

Polygeline. Polymer of urea and polypeptides derived from denatured gelatin. *CAS-9015-56-9.* INN; BAN.

Polyglactin 370 [*1978*] (pol″ ee glak′ tin). $(C_6H_8O_4)_m (C_4H_4O_4)_n$. [Polyglactin is BAN.] (1) 1,4-Dioxane-2,5-dione, 3,6-dimethyl-, polymer with 1,4-dioxane-2,5-dione; (2) 3,6-Dimethyl-*p*-dioxane-2,5-dione polymer with *p*-dioxane-2,5-dione; (3) Poly[(oxycarbonylmethylene)$_m$-co-(oxycarbonylethylidene)$_n$]. *CAS-26780-50-7. Surgical aid (surgical suture coating, absorbable).*

Polyglactin 910 [*1972*] (pol″ ee glak′ tin). $(C_6H_8O_4)_m (C_4H_4O_4)_n$. (1) 1,4-Dioxane-2,5-dione, 3,6-dimethyl-, polymer with 1,4-dioxane-2,5-dione; (2) 3,6-Dimethyl-*p*-dioxane-2,5-dione polymer with *p*-dioxane-2,5-dione; (3) Poly[(oxycarbonylmethylene)$_m$-co-(oxycarbonylethylidene)$_n$]. Molecular weight is approximately 80,000. *CAS-26780-50-7. Surgical aid (surgical suture material, absorbable).* Vicryl (Ethicon) *[Note—Graphic formula same as for Polyglactin 370.]* ◇*XLG*

Polyglycolic Acid [*1970*] (pol″ ee glye kol′ ik as′ id). $(C_2H_2O_2)_n$. (1) Poly(oxycarbonylmethylene); (2) Poly(glycolic acid). *CAS-26009-03-0.* INN; BAN. *Surgical aid (surgical suture material).* Dexon (Davis & Geck)

Polyglyconate [*1983*] (pol″ ee glye′ koe nate). $(C_4H_4O_4)_m (C_4H_6O_3)_n$. (1) 1,4-Dioxane-2,5-dione polymer with 1,3-dioxan-2-one; (2) *p*-Dioxane-2,5-dione polymer with cyclic trimethylene carbonate. *CAS-75734-93-9.* BAN. *Surgical aid (surgical suture material, absorbable).* Maxon (Davis & Geck) ◇*MAS-1*

Polyhexanide (previously used name) — *See* Polihexanide.

Polyisobutylene (pol″ ee eye″ soe bue′ ti leen). **NF.** A synthetic polymer produced by the low-temperature polymerization of isobutylene in liquid ethylene, methylene chloride, or hexane, using an aluminum-chloride or boron-trifluoride catalyst. *CAS-9003-27-4.*

Polymacon [*1971*] (pol″ ee may′ kon). $(C_6H_{10}O_3)_n$. (The material is loosely cross-linked as a result of the combination of a small amount of ethyleneglycol dimethacrylate with the hydroxyethyl methacrylate monomer. The result is a cross-link every few hundred monomer units. See graphic formula.) (1) 2-Propenoic acid, 2-methyl-, 1,2-ethanediyl ester, polymer with 2-hydroxyethyl 2-methyl-2-propenoate; (2) Poly(2-hydroxyethyl methacrylate). *CAS-25053-81-0. Contact lens material (hydrophilic).* BENZ 38 (Benz Research and Development); Cooper Thin (CooperVision); Criterion Ultra DW (Bausch & Lomb†); Criterion Ultra FW (Bausch & Lomb†); Criterion Ultra SP (Bausch & Lomb†); Criterion XLT (Bausch & Lomb†); LL-38 (Lombart); Medalist (Bausch & Lomb); Occasions Multifocal (Bausch & Lomb); Occasions Single Use (Bausch & Lomb); Optima 38 (Bausch & Lomb); Optima 38/SP (Bausch & Lomb); Optima FW (Bausch & Lomb); Plano T (Bausch & Lomb); SeeQuence (Bausch & Lomb); SeeQuence 2 (Bausch & Lomb†); Soflens (Bausch & Lomb); Sofspin (Bausch & Lomb)

Polymanoacetate (previously used name) — *See* Acemannan.

Polymetaphosphate P 32 [*1966*] (pol″ ee met″ a fos′ fate). *Radioactive agent.*

Polymixin E — *See* Colistin Sulfate.

Polymonine. Formaldehyde reaction product with *p*-methoxy-*N*-methylphenethylamine. JAMA 155: 158 (1954).

Polymyxin B Sulfate (pol″ ee mix′ in sul′ fate). **USP.** [Polymyxin B is INN and BAN.] (1) Polymyxin B, sulfate; (2) Polymyxin B sulfate. *UNII-19371312D4; UNII-J2VZ07J96K [polymyxin b]. CAS-1405-20-5; CAS-1404-26-8 [polymyxin B].* JAN. *Antibacterial.* Aerosporin (GlaxoSmithKline)

Polynoxylin. Poly[methi[bis(hydroxymethyl)]ureylene]amer. *CAS-9011-05-6.* INN; BAN; MI.

Polyoxyethylene 50 Stearate (previously used name) — *See* Polyoxyl 50 Stearate.

Polyoxyl 8 Stearate [*1964*] (pol″ ee ox′ il steer′ ate). $C_{34}H_{68}O_{10}$ (Approximate). 636.90. [Macrogol Ester 400 is INN; Macrogol 8 Stearate is BAN.] (1) Poly(oxy-1,2-ethanediyl), α-hydro-ω-hydroxy-, octadecanoate; (2) Polyethylene glycol 8 monostearate. [Compound usually contains also associated fatty acids.] *CAS-9004-99-3. Pharmaceutic aid (surfactant).*

Polyoxyl 10 Oleyl Ether (pol″ ee ox′ il oh lay′ il ee′ ther). **NF.** (1) Polyoxy-1,2-ethanediyl, α-[(Z)-9-octadecenyl-ω-hydroxy-; (2) Polyethylene glycol monooleyl ether. *CAS-9004-98-2. Pharmaceutic aid (surfactant).* Brij 96 (ICI Americas†); Brij 97 (ICI Americas)

Polyoxyl 20 Cetostearyl Ether (pol″ ee ox′ il see″ toe steer′ il ee′ ther). **NF.** A mixture of monocetostearyl (mixed hexadecyl and octadecyl) ethers of mixed polyoxyethylene diols, the average polymer length being 21.1 ± 3.9 oxyethylene units. *Pharmaceutic aid (surfactant).*

Polyoxyl 35 Castor Oil (pol″ ee ox′ il kas′ tor). **NF.** Contains mainly the tri-ricinoleate ester of ethoxylated glycerol, with smaller amounts of polyethylene glycol ricinoleate and the corresponding free glycols. *Pharmaceutic aid (emulsifying agent); pharmaceutic aid (surfactant).* Cremophor EL (BASF); Cremophor ELP (BASF)

Polyoxyl 40 Hydrogenated Castor Oil (pol″ ee ox′ il hye droj′ en ay″ ted kas′ tor). **NF.** Contains mainly the tri-hydroxystearate ester of ethoxylated glycerol, with smaller amounts of polyethylene glycol tri-hydroxystearate and of the corresponding free glycols. *Pharmaceutic aid (emulsifying agent); pharmaceutic aid (surfactant).* Cremophor RH40 (BASF)

Polyoxyl 40 Stearate [*1964*] (pol″ ee ox′ il steer′ ate). **NF.** [Macrogol Ester 2000 is INN; Macrogol 40 Stearate is BAN.] (1) Poly(oxy-1,2-ethanediyl), α-hydro-ω-hydroxy-, octadecanoate; (2) Polyethylene glycol monostearate. *CAS-9004-99-3.* JAN. *Pharmaceutic aid (surfactant).* Myrj 52 (ICI Americas)

Polyoxyl 50 Stearate. (1) Poly(oxy-1,2-ethanediyl), α-(1-oxooctadecyl)-ω-hydroxy-; (2) Polyethylene glycol monostearate. *CAS-9004-99-3.* NF XVIII. *Pharmaceutic aid (surfactant); pharmaceutic aid (emulsifying agent).* Myrj 53 (ICI Americas) [*Name previously used: Polyoxyethylene 50 Stearate.*]

Polyoxyl Lauryl Ether (pol″ ee ox′ il lawr′ il ee′ ther). **NF.** Polyethylene glycol monolauryl ether. *CAS-9002-92-0.*

Polyoxyl Oleate (pol″ ee ox′ il oh′ lee ate). **NF.** Polyethylene glycol monooleate. *CAS-9004-96-0.*

Polyoxyl Stearyl Ether (pol″ ee ox′ il steer′ il ee′ ther). **NF.** Polyethylene glycol monostearyl ether. *CAS-9005-00-9.*

Polyoxypropylene 15 Stearyl Ether [*1981*] (pol″ ee ox″ ee proe′ pi leen steer′ il ee′ ther). Stearyl Ether is the polypropylene glycol ether of stearyl alcohol represented predominantly by the graphic formula shown below, in which the average value of *n* is 15. It has an iodine value of less than 4, an acid value of less than 2, and a Karl Fischer moisture content of less than 0.7%. (1) Poly[oxy(methyl-1,2-ethanediyl)]-, α-octadecyl-ω-hydroxy-; (2) Polypropylene glycol monooctadecyl ether. *CAS-25231-21-4.* CID. *Pharmaceutic aid (solvent).* Arlamol E (ICI Americas) [*Name previously used: PPG-15 Stearyl Ether.*]

Polypropylene Glycol. NF XVI.

Polysorbate 20 [*1964*] (pol″ ee sor′ bate). **NF.** $C_{58}H_{114}O_{26}$ (Approximate). 1227.51. (1) Sorbitan, monododecanoate, poly(oxy-1,2-ethanediyl) derivs.; (2) Polyoxyethylene 20 sorbitan monolaurate. [Compound usually contains also

---

associated fatty acids.] *UNII-7T1F30V5YH. CAS-9005-64-5.* INN; BAN. *Pharmaceutic aid (surfactant).* Tween 20 (ICI Americas)

Polysorbate 40 [*1964*] (pol″ ee sor′ bate). **NF.** $C_{62}H_{122}O_{26}$ (Approximate). 1283.62. (1) Sorbitan, monohexadecanoate, poly(oxy-1,2-ethanediyl) derivs.; (2) Polyoxyethylene 20 sorbitan monopalmitate. [Compound usually contains also associated fatty acids.] *CAS-9005-66-7.* INN; BAN. *Pharmaceutic aid (surfactant).* Tween 40 (ICI Americas) *[Note—Graphic formula same as for Polysorbate 20, except that R is $(C_{15}H_{31})COO$.]*

Polysorbate 60 [*1964*] (pol″ ee sor′ bate). **NF.** $C_{64}H_{126}O_{26}$ (Approximate). 1311.67. (1) Sorbitan, monooctadecanoate, poly(oxy-1,2-ethanediyl) derivs.; (2) Polyoxyethylene 20 sorbitan monostearate. [Compound usually contains also associated fatty acids.] *CAS-9005-67-8.* INN; BAN. *Pharmaceutic aid (surfactant).* Tween 60 (ICI Americas) *[Note—Graphic formula same as for Polysorbate 20, except that R is $(C_{17}H_{35})COO$.]*

Polysorbate 65 [*1964*] (pol″ ee sor′ bate). $C_{100}H_{194}O_{28}$ (Approximate). 1844.59. (1) Sorbitan, trioctadecanoate, poly(oxy-1,2-ethanediyl) derivs.; (2) Polyoxyethylene 20 sorbitan tristearate. [Compound usually contains also associated fatty acids.] *CAS-9005-71-4.* INN; BAN. *Pharmaceutic aid (surfactant).* Tween 65 (ICI Americas)

Polysorbate 80 [*1964*] (pol″ ee sor′ bate). **NF.** (1) Sorbitan, mono-9-octadecenoate, poly(oxy-1,2-ethanediyl) derivs., (Z)-; (2) Polyoxyethylene 20 sorbitan monooleate. *UNII-6OZP39ZG8H. CAS-9005-65-6.* INN; BAN; JAN. *Pharmaceutic aid (surfactant).* Sorlate (Abbott†); Tween 80 (ICI Americas) *[Note—Graphic formula same as for Polysorbate 20, except that R is $(C_{17}H_{33})COO$.]*

Polysorbate 85 [*1964*] (pol″ ee sor′ bate). $C_{100}H_{188}O_{28}$ (Approximate). 1838.55. (1) Sorbitan, tri-9-octadecenoate, poly(oxy-1,2-ethanediyl) derivs., (Z,Z,Z)-; (2) Polyoxyethylene 20 sorbitan trioleate. [Compound usually contains also associated fatty acids.] *CAS-9005-70-3.* INN; BAN. *Pharmaceutic aid (surfactant).* Tween 85 (ICI Americas) *[Note—Graphic formula same as for Polysorbate 65, except that R is $(C_{17}H_{33})COO$.]*

Polytef [*1969*] (pol′ ee tef). $(C_2F_4)_n$. [Politef is INN.] (1) Ethene, tetrafluoro, homopolymer; (2) Poly(tetrafluoroethylene). *CAS-9002-84-0.*

Polythiazide [*1961*] (pol″ ee thye′ a zide). $C_{11}H_{13}ClF_3N_3O_4S_3$. 439.88. (1) 2*H*-1,2,4-Benzothiadiazine-7-sulfonamide, 6-chloro-3,4-dihydro-2-methyl-3-[[(2,2,2-trifluoroethyl)thio]methyl]-, 1,1-dioxide; (2) 6-Chloro-3,4-dihydro-2-methyl-3-[[(2,2,2-trifluoroethyl)thio]methyl]-2*H*-1,2,4-benzothiadiazine-7-sulfonamide 1,1-dioxide. *UNII-36780APV5N. CAS-346-18-9.* USP XXIII; INN; BAN; JAN. *Diuretic; antihypertensive.* Renese (Pfizer) ◇*P-2525; NSC-108161*

Polyurethane Foam [*1961*] (pol″ ee ure′ e thane). Product resulting from the combination of the contents of two separately packaged ingredients that polymerize upon being mixed to yield a rigid, porous mass. (1) Urethane polymers; (2) Urethane polymers. *CAS-9009-54-5. Prosthetic aid (internal bone splint).* Ostamer (Marion Merrell Dow†)

Polyvidone (previously used name) — *See* Povidone.

Polyvinox. Poly(1-butoxyethylene). BAN.

Polyvinyl Acetate Phthalate (pol″ ee vye′ nil as′ e tate thal′ ate). **NF.** A reaction product of phthalic anhydride and a partially hydrolyzed polyvinyl acetate. *Pharmaceutic aid (coating agent).*

Polyvinyl Alcohol (pol″ ee vye′ nil al′ ka hol). **USP.** $(C_2H_4O)_n$. [Polyvinyl Alcohol Iodine Solution is JAN.] (1) Ethenol, homopolymer; (2) Vinyl alcohol polymer. *CAS-9002-89-5. Pharmaceutic aid (viscosity-increasing agent).* Liquifilm Tears (Allergan)

Polyvinylpyrrolidone (previously used name) — *See* Povidone.

Polyvinylpyrrolidone [K25, K30, K90] (JAN) — *See* Povidone.

Pomalidomide [*2006*] (poe″ ma lid′ oh mide). $C_{13}H_{11}N_3O_4$. 273.24. (1) 1*H*-Isoindole-1,3(2*H*)-dione, 4-amino-2-(2,6-dioxo-3-piperidinyl)-; (2) 4-Amino-2-[(3*RS*)-2,6-dioxopiperidin-3-yl]-1*H*-isoindole-1,3(2*H*)-dione. *UNII-D2UX06XLB5. CAS-19171-19-8.* INN. *Treatment of cancer.* ◇*CC-4047; IMiD 3*

Pomisartan. $C_{31}H_{30}N_4O_2$. 490.60. 4′-[[2-Ethyl-4-methyl-6-(5,6,7,8-tetrahydroimidazo[1,2-*a*]pyridin-2-yl)-1-benzimidazolyl]methyl]-2-biphenylcarboxylic acid. *UNII-7539319JYI. CAS-144702-17-0.* INN.

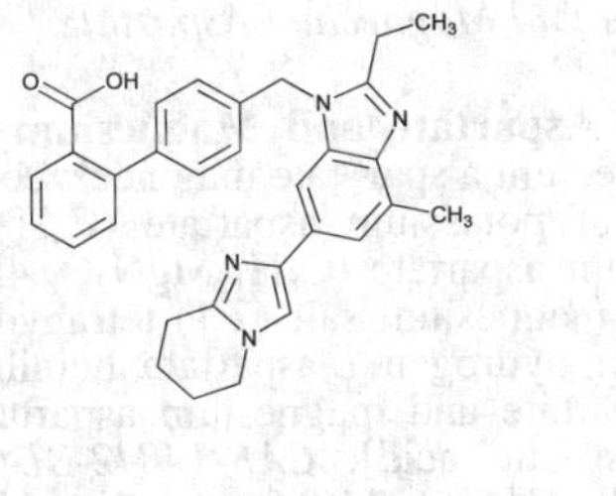

Ponalrestat [*1988*] (poe nal′ re stat). $C_{17}H_{12}BrFN_2O_3$. 391.19. (1) 1-Phthalazineacetic acid, 3-[(4-bromo-2-fluorophenyl)methyl]-3,4-dihydro-4-oxo-; (2) 3-(4-Bromo-2-fluorobenzyl)-3,4-dihydro-4-oxo-1-phthalazineacetic acid. *CAS-72702-95-5.* INN; BAN. *Inhibitor (aldose reductase).* ◇*ICI 128,436*

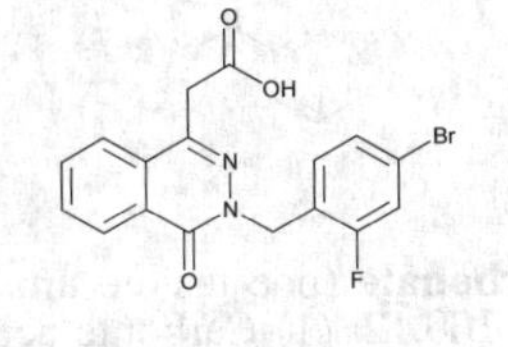

Ponazuril. $C_{18}H_{14}F_3N_3O_6S$. 457.38. 1-Methyl-3-[4-[*p*-[(trifluoromethyl)sulfonyl]phenoxy]-*m*-tolyl]-*s*-triazine-2,4,6(1*H*,3*H*,5*H*)-trione. *UNII-JPW84AS66U. CAS-69004-04-2.* INN.

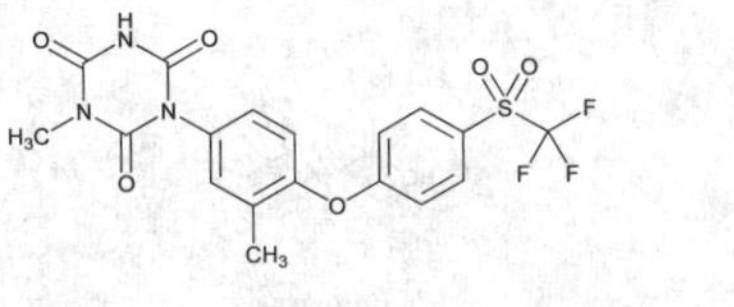

Ponfibrate. $C_{18}H_{16}Cl_2O_4$. 367.22. Ethyl *trans*-2,10-dichloro-12-methyl-12*H*-dibenzo[*d,g*][1,3]dioxocin-6-carboxylate. *UNII-0ARR2L0V0A. CAS-53341-49-4.* INN.

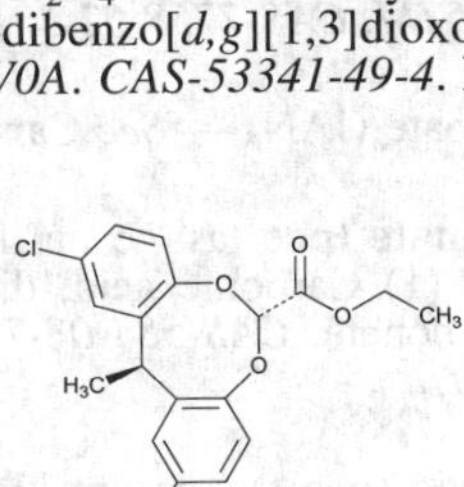

Poractant Alfa. An extract of porcine lung containing not less than 90% of phospholipids, about 1% of hydrophobic proteins (SP-B and SP-C) and about 9% of other lipids. *UNII-KE3U2023NP. CAS-129069-19-8.* BAN. Curosurf (Dey)

Porfimer Sodium [*1990*] (por′ fi mer soe′ dee um). Polyporphrin oligomer containing ester and ether linkage. (1) Photofrin II; (2) Photofrin II. *UNII-Y3834SIK5F. CAS-87806-31-3.* INN; BAN. *Antineoplastic.* Photofrin (Axcan Scandipharm) ◇*CL 184,116*

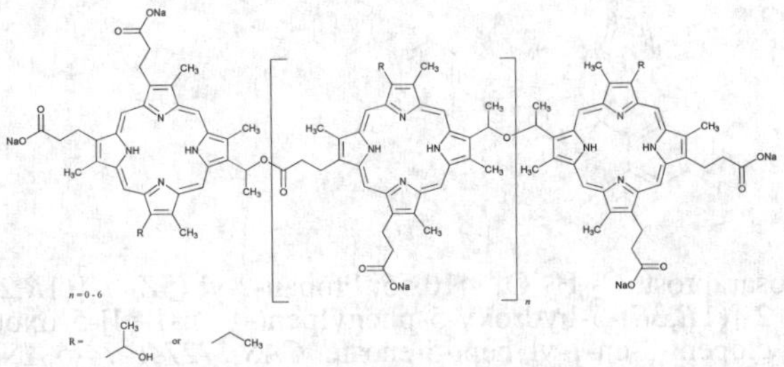

Porfiromycin [*1965*] (por fir″ oh mye′ sin). $C_{16}H_{20}N_4O_5$. 348.35. (1) Azirino[2′,3′:3,4]pyrrolo[1,2-*a*]-indole-4,7-dione, 6-amino-8-[[(aminocarbonyl)oxy]methyl]-1,1a,2,8,8a,8b-hexahydro-8a-methoxy-1,5-dimethyl-; (2) 6-Amino-1,1a,2,8,8a,8b-hexahydro-8-(hydroxymethyl)-8a-methoxy-1,5-dimethylazirino[2′,3′:3,4]pyrrolo[1,2-*a*]indole-4,7-dione carbamate (ester). *CAS-801-52-5.* INN; BAN. *Antibacterial; antineoplastic.* ◇*U-14,743; NSC-56410*

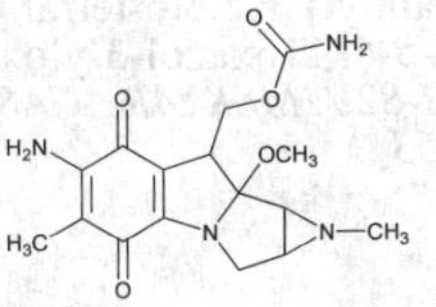

Porofocon A [*1977*] (por″ oh foe′ kon). $(C_{32}H_{48}O_{16})_n$. (1) Cellulose, acetate, dibutanoate; (2) Cellulose acetate dibutyrate. *CAS-60840-55-3. Contact lens material (hydrophobic).*

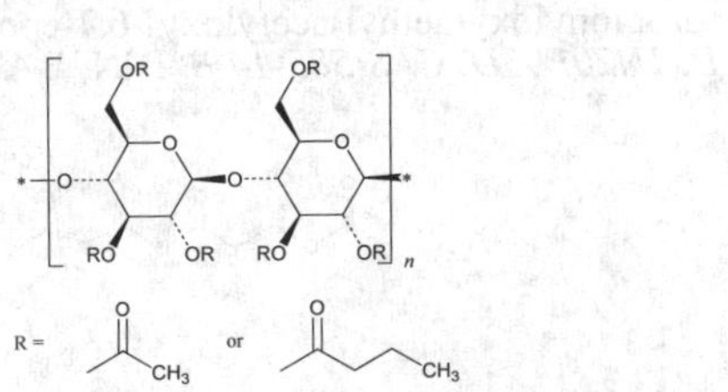

Porofocon B [*1977*] (por″ oh foe′ kon). $(C_{32}H_{48}O_{16})_n$. (1) Cellulose, acetate, dibutanoate; (2) Cellulose acetate dibutyrate. *CAS-60840-55-3. Contact lens material (hydrophobic). [Note—Graphic formula same as for Porofocon A.]* ◇*Continuous Curve-CAB Contact Lens*

Posaconazole [*1999*] (poe″ sa kon′ a zole). $C_{37}H_{42}F_2N_8O_4$. 700.78. (1) 3*H*-1,2,4-Triazol-3-one, 4-[4-[4-[4-[[5-(2,4-difluorophenyl)tetrahydro-5-(1*H*-1,2,4-triazol-1-ylmethyl)-3-furanyl]methoxy]phenyl]-1-piperazinyl]phenyl]-2-(1-ethyl-2-hydroxypropyl)-2,4-dihydro-, [3*R*-[3α(1*S**,2*S**),5α]]-; (2) 4-[*p*-[4-[*p*-[[(3*R*,5*R*)-5-(2,4-Difluorophenyl)tetrahydro-5-(1*H*-1,2,4-triazol-1-ylmethyl)-3-furyl]methoxy]phenyl]-1-piperazinyl]phenyl]-1-[(1*S*,2*S*)-1-ethyl-2-hydroxypropyl]-Δ^2-1,2,4-triazolin-5-

---

one. *UNII-6TK1G07BHZ. CAS-171228-49-2.* INN; BAN. *Antifungal (α-demethylase fungal P450 cytochrome system inhibitor).* Noxafil (Schering) ◇*SCH 56592*

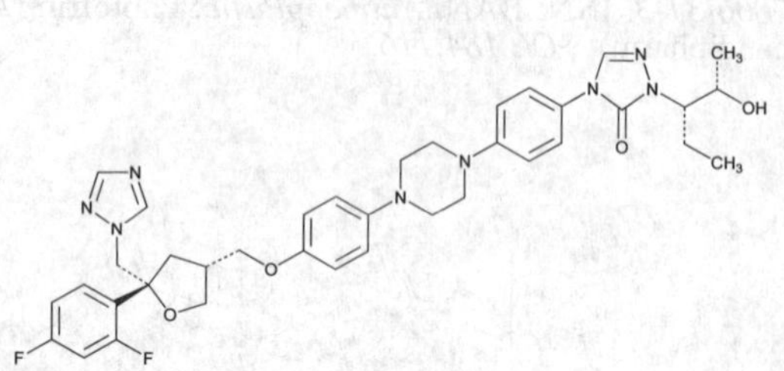

Posaraprost. $C_{26}H_{34}O_4$. 410.55. Propan-2-yl (5*Z*)-7-{(1*R*,2*S*)-2-[(1*E*,3*S*)-3-hydroxy-5-phenylpent-1-en-1-yl]-5-oxocyclopent-3-en-1-yl}hept-5-enoate. *CAS-172740-14-6.* INN.

Posatirelin. $C_{17}H_{28}N_4O_4$. 352.43. (2*S*)-*N*[(1*S*)-1-[[(2*S*)-2-Carbamoyl-1-pyrrolidinyl]carbonyl]-3-methylbutyl]-6-oxopipecolamide. *UNII-78U6302ARL. CAS-78664-73-0.* INN.

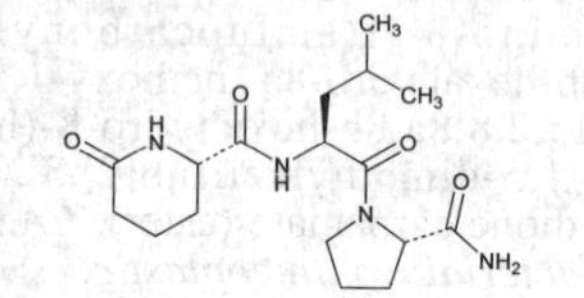

Posizolid. $C_{21}H_{21}F_2N_3O_7$. 465.40. (5*R*)-3-(4-{1-[(2*S*)-2,3-Dihydroxypropanoyl]-1,2,3,6-tetrahydro-4-pyridyl}-3,5-difluorophenyl)-5-(1,2-oxazol-3-yloxymethyl)-1,3-oxazolan-2-one. *UNII-82V2M8K24R. CAS-252260-06-3.* INN; BAN. ◇*AZD2563*

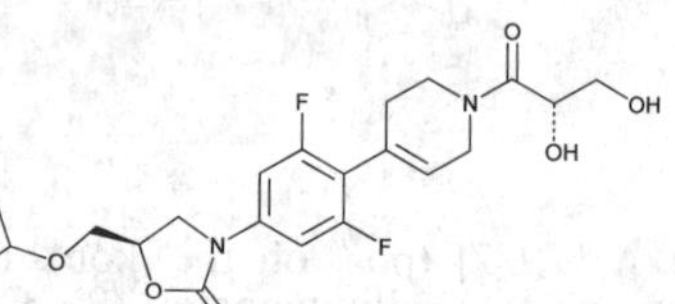

Poskine. $C_{20}H_{25}NO_5$. 359.42. 3-[2-Phenyl-2-(propionyloxymethyl)acetyloxy]-6,7-epoxytropane. *UNII-DJ1N20F93D. CAS-585-14-8.* INN; BAN.

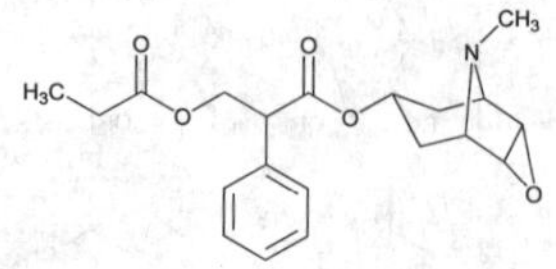

Potash, Sulfurated (pot′ ash sul′ fur ay″ ted). **USP.** (1) Thiosulfuric acid, dipotassium salt, mixt. with potassium sulfide (K_2S_x); (2) Dipotassium thiosulfate mixture with potassium sulfide (K_2S_x). *CAS-39365-88-3. Sulfide, source of.*

Potassic Saline [Injection], Lactated. NF XIII.

Potassium Acetate (poe tas′ ee um as′ e tate). **USP.** $C_2H_3KO_2$. 98.14. (1) Acetic acid, potassium salt; (2) Potassium acetate. *UNII-M911911U02. CAS-127-08-2.* JAN. *Replenisher (electrolyte).*

Potassium Alginate (poe tas′ ee um al′ ji nate). **NF.** (1) Alginic acid, potassium salt; (2) Potassium alginate. *CAS-9005-36-1.*

Potassium Aspartate. $C_4H_6KNO_4.\frac{1}{2}H_2O$. 180.20. [L-Aspartate Potassium is JAN.] *[See also the entry for Potassium Aspartate and Magnesium Aspartate.]*

Potassium Aspartate and Magnesium Aspartate [*1963*] (poe tas′ ee um a spar′ tate mag nee′ zee um a spar′ tate). A mixture of potassium aspartate ($C_4H_6KNO_4.\frac{1}{2}H_2O$) and magnesium aspartate ($C_8H_{12}MgN_2O_8.4H_2O$). (1) Aspartic acid, L-, magnesium salt (2:1) tetrahydrate, mixture with potassium hydrogen L-aspartate hemihydrate; (2) Potassium aspartate and magnesium aspartate. *UNII-30KYC7-MIAI* [aspartic acid]. *CAS-14842-81-0; CAS-8000-90-6* [replaced]; *CAS-56-84-8* [L-aspartic acid]. JAN. *Nutrient.* ◇*Wy-2837; Wy-2838*

Potassium Benzoate (poe tas′ ee um ben′ zoe ate). **NF.** $C_7H_5KO_2$. 160.21. (1) Benzoic acid, potassium salt; (2) Potassium benzoate. *CAS-582-25-2. Pharmaceutic aid (preservative).*

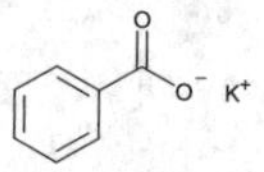

Potassium Bicarbonate (poe tas′ ee um bye kar′ bo nate). **USP.** $KHCO_3$. 100.12. (1) Carbonic acid, monopotassium salt; (2) Monopotassium carbonate. *CAS-298-14-6. Pharmaceutic necessity.*

Potassium Bitartrate [*1988*] (poe tas′ ee um bye tar′ trate). **USP.** $C_4H_5KO_6$. 188.18. [Potassium Hydrogen Tartrate is JAN.] (1) Butanedioic acid 2,3-dihydroxy-, [*R*-(*R**,*R**)]-, monopotassium salt; (2) Potassium hydrogen tartrate. *CAS-868-14-4.*

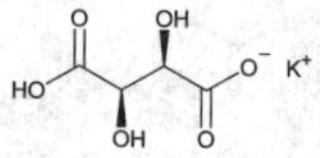

Potassium Bromide (poe tas′ ee um broe′ mide). **USP.** KBr. 119.00. (1) Potassium bromide; (2) Potassium bromide. *UNII-OSD78555ZM. CAS-7758-02-3.* JAN.

Potassium Canrenoate (JAN) — *See* Canrenoate Potassium.

Potassium Carbonate (poe tas′ ee um kar′ bo nate). **USP.** K_2CO_3. 138.21. (1) Carbonic acid, dipotassium salt; (2) Dipotassium carbonate. *CAS-584-08-7. Pharmaceutic aid (alkalizing agent).*

Potassium Chloride (poe tas′ ee um klor′ ide). **USP.** KCl. 74.55. (1) Potassium chloride; (2) Potassium chloride. *UNII-660YQ98I10. CAS-7447-40-7.* JAN. *Replenisher (electrolyte).* K-dur (Key); Kaon Cl (Savage); Klor-con (Upsher Smith); Klotrix (Apothecon); Micro-k (KV Pharmaceutical)

Potassium Chloride K 42 [*1963*] (poe tas′ ee um klor′ ide). ^{42}KCl. (1) Potassium chloride (^{42}KCl); (2) Potassium chloride (^{42}KCl). *Radioactive agent.*

Potassium Citrate (poe tas′ ee um sit′ rate). **USP.** $C_6H_5K_3O_7.H_2O$. 324.41. (1) 1,2,3-Propanetricarboxylic acid, 2-hydroxy-, tripotassium salt, monohydrate; (2)

Tripotassium citrate monohydrate. *UNII-EE90ONI6FF. CAS-6100-05-6; CAS-866-84-2* [anhydrous]. *Alkalizer.* Urocit-K (Mission)

Potassium Glucaldrate [*1963*] (poe tas′ ee um gloo kal′ drate). $C_6H_{16}AlKO_{11}$. 330.26. (1) Aluminate(1-), diaqua[gluconato(2-)-O^1,O^2]dihydroxy-, potassium, (*OC*-6-44); (2) Potassium diaqua[gluconato(2-)]dihydroxyaluminate(1-). *CAS-23835-15-6; CAS-1317-30-2* [replaced]. INN. *Antacid.* Aciquel (Ortho-McNeil†) ◇*McN-R-1162-22*

Potassium Gluconate (poe tas′ ee um gloo′ koe nate). **USP**. $C_6H_{11}KO_7$. 234.25. (1) D-Gluconic acid, monopotassium salt; (2) Monopotassium D-gluconate. *UNII-12H3K5QKN9. CAS-299-27-4; CAS-35398-15-3* [monohydrate]; *CAS-526-95-4* [D-gluconic acid]. JAN. *Replenisher (electrolyte).* Kaon (Savage†)

Potassium Guaiacolsulfonate (poe tas′ ee um gwye″ a kol sul′ foe nate). **USP**. $C_7H_7KO_5S.\frac{1}{2}H_2O$. 251.30. [Sulfogaiacol is INN.] (1) Benzenesulfonic acid, hydroxymethoxy-, monopotassium salt, hemihydrate; (2) Potassium hydroxymethoxybenzenesulfonate hemihydrate. *CAS-78247-49-1*. JAN. *Expectorant.*

Potassium Hydrogen Tartrate (JAN) — *See* Potassium Bitartrate.

Potassium Hydroxide (poe tas′ ee um hye drox′ ide). **NF**. KOH. 56.11. (1) Potassium hydroxide; (2) Potassium hydroxide. *CAS-1310-58-3*. JAN. *Pharmaceutic aid (alkalizing agent).*

Potassium Iodide (poe tas′ ee um eye′ oh dide). **USP**. KI. 166.00. (1) Potassium iodide; (2) Potassium iodide. *UNII-1C4QK22F9J. CAS-7681-11-0*. JAN. *Antifungal; expectorant; supplement (iodine).* Iosat (Anbex); Thyro-Block (Medpointe); Thyrosafe (R R Registrations); Thyroshield (Fleming)

Potassium Menaphthosulphate (previously used name) — *See* Menadiol Sodium Sulfate.

Potassium Mercuric Iodide. *CAS-7783-33-7*. NF X.

---

† Brand name formerly used, and/or firm no longer concerned with this product.

Potassium Metabisulfite (poe tas′ ee um met″ a bye sul′ fite). **NF**. $K_2S_2O_5$. 222.32. (1) Disulfurous acid, dipotassium salt; (2) Dipotassium pyrosulfite. *CAS-16731-55-8. Pharmaceutic aid (antioxidant).*

Potassium Metaphosphate (poe tas′ ee um met″ a fos′ fate). **NF**. KPO_3. 118.07. (1) Metaphosphoric acid (HPO_3), potassium salt; (2) Potassium metaphosphate. *CAS-7790-53-6. Pharmaceutic aid (buffering agent).*

Potassium Nitrate (poe tas′ ee um nye′ trate). **USP**. KNO_3. 101.10. (1) Potassium nitrate; (2) Potassium nitrate. *CAS-7757-79-1*. JAN.

Potassium Nitrazepate. $C_{16}H_{10}KN_3O_5$. 363.37. Potassium 2,3-dihydro-7-nitro-2-oxo-5-phenyl-1*H*-1,4-benzodiazepine-3-carboxylate. *UNII-3D69H48U8Q. CAS-5571-84-6*. INN.

Potassium Perchlorate (poe tas′ ee um per klor′ ate). **USP**. $KClO_4$. 138.55. Potassium perchlorate. *UNII-42255P5X4D. CAS-7778-74-7*. Perchloracap (Mallinckrodt)

Potassium Permanganate (poe tas′ ee um per man′ ga nate). **USP**. $KMnO_4$. 158.03. (1) Permanganic acid ($HMnO_4$), potassium salt; (2) Potassium permanganate ($KMnO_4$). *UNII-00OT1QX5U4. CAS-7722-64-7*. JAN. *Anti-infective, topical.*

Potassium Phosphate, Dibasic (poe tas′ ee um fos′ fate dye bay′ sik). **USP**. K_2HPO_4. 174.18. (1) Phosphoric acid, dipotassium salt; (2) Dipotassium hydrogen phosphate. *UNII-CI71S98N1Z. CAS-7758-11-4*. JAN. *Regulator (calcium).* Isolyte (McGaw)

Potassium Phosphate, Monobasic (poe tas′ ee um fos′ fate mon″ oh bay′ sik). **NF**. KH_2PO_4. 136.09. (1) Phosphoric acid, monopotassium salt; (2) Monopotassium phosphate. *CAS-7778-77-0. Pharmaceutic aid (buffering agent).*

Potassium Sodium Tartrate (poe tas′ ee um soe′ dee um tar′ trate). **USP**. $C_4H_4KNaO_6.4H_2O$. 282.22. (1) Butanedioic acid, 2,3-dihydroxy-, [*R*-(*R**,*R**)]-, monopotassium monosodium salt, tetrahydrate; (2) Monopotassium monosodium tartrate tetrahydrate. *CAS-6381-59-5; CAS-304-59-6* [anhydrous]; *CAS-6100-16-9* [replaced]. *Laxative.*

Potassium Sorbate (poe tas′ ee um sor′ bate). **NF**. $C_6H_7KO_2$. 150.22. (1) 2,4-Hexadienoic acid, (*E,E′*)-, potassium salt; 2,4-Hexadienoic acid, potassium salt; (2) Potassium (*E,E′*)-sorbate; Potassium sorbate. *UNII-1VPU26JZZ4. CAS-590-00-1; CAS-24634-61-5* [*E,E*]; *CAS-110-44-1* [sorbic acid]; *CAS-22500-92-1* [(*E,E*)-sorbic acid]. *Pharmaceutic aid (antimicrobial agent).*

Potassium Sulfate. K_2SO_4. 174.26. *CAS-7778-80-5*. JAN.

Potassium Thiocyanate. *CAS-333-20-0*. NF X; MI.

Potato Starch (JAN) — *See* Starch.

Povidone [*1968*] (poe′ vi done). **USP.** ($C_6H_9NO)_n$. [Polyvinylpyrrolidone (K25, K30, K90) is JAN.] (1) 2-Pyrrolidinone, 1-ethenyl-, homopolymer; (2) 1-Vinyl-2-pyrrolidinone polymer. *UNII-FZ989GH94E. CAS-9003-39-8.* INN; BAN. *Pharmaceutic aid (dispersing and suspending agent).* Kollidon 25, 30, 12PF, 17PF, 90F (BASF); Plasdone (International Specialty Products); Vinisil (Abbott†) [*Name previously used: Polyvidone; Polyvinylpyrrolidone.*]

Povidone I 125 [*1964*] (poe′ vi done). (1) 2-Pyrrolidinone, 1-ethenyl-, homopolymer, labeled with iodine-125; (2) 1-Vinyl-2-pyrrolidinone polymer, labeled with iodine-125. *Radioactive agent.*

Povidone I 131 [*1964*] (poe′ vi done). (1) 2-Pyrrolidinone, 1-ethenyl-, homopolymer, labeled with iodine-131; (2) 1-Vinyl-2-pyrrolidinone polymer, labeled with iodine-131. *Radioactive agent.*

Povidone-Iodine. **USP.** ($C_6H_9NO)_n$·*x*I. (1) 2-Pyrrolidinone, 1-ethenyl-, homopolymer, compd. with iodine; (2) 1-Vinyl-2-pyrrolidinone polymer, compound with iodine. *UNII-85H0HZU99M. CAS-25655-41-8.* BAN; JAN. *Anti-infective, topical.* Betadine (Alcon); E-z Scrub (Becton Dickinson Microbiology)

Pozanicline [*2008*] (poe zan′ i kleen). $C_{11}H_{16}N_2O$. 192.26. (1) Pyridine, 2-methyl-3-[(2*S*)-2-pyrrolidinylmethoxy]-; (2) 2-Methyl-3-{[(2*S*)-pyrrolidin-2-yl]methoxy}pyridine. *UNII-CL2002R563. CAS-161417-03-4. Attention deficit/hyperactivity disorder, Alzheimer's type dementia.* ◇A-87089.0; ABT-089

Pozanicline Tartrate [*2008*] (poe zan′ i kleen tar′ trate). $C_{11}H_{16}N_2O \cdot C_4H_4O_6$. 340.33. (1) Pyridine, 2-methyl-3-[(2*S*)-2-pyrrolidinylmethoxy]-, (2*R*,3*R*)-2,3-dihydroxybutanedioate (1:1); (2) 2-Methyl-3-{[(2*S*)-pyrrolidin-2-yl]methoxy}pyridine (2*R*,3*R*)-2,3-dihydroxybutanedioate. *UNII-8CY265YM5K. CAS-945405-37-8. Attention deficit/ hyperactivity disorder (ADHD); dementia of the Alzheimer's type (AD).* ◇A-87089.74

PPG-15 Stearyl Ether (previously used name) — *See* Polyoxypropylene 15 Stearyl Ether.

Practolol [*1969*] (prak′ toe lol). $C_{14}H_{22}N_2O_3$. 266.34. (1) Acetamide, *N*-[4-[2-hydroxy-3-[(1-methylethyl) amino]propoxy]phenyl]-; (2) 4′-[2-Hydroxy-3-

(isopropylamino)propoxy]acetanilide. *UNII-SUG9176GRW. CAS-6673-35-4.* INN; BAN. *Anti-adrenergic (β-receptor).* ◇AY-21,011; I.C.I. 50,172

Pradefovir Mesylate [*2005*] (pra def′ oh vir mes′ i late). $C_{17}H_{19}ClN_5O_4P \cdot CH_4O_3S$. 519.90. [Pradefovir is INN.] (1) 9*H*-Purin-6-amine, 9-[2-[[(2*R*,4*S*)-4-(3-chlorophenyl)-2-oxido-1,3,2-dioxaphosphorinan-2-yl]methoxy]ethyl]-, monomethanesulfonate; (2) (2*R*,4*S*)-2-[[2-(6-Amino-9*H*-purin-9-yl)ethoxy]methyl]-4-(3-chlorophenyl)-1,3,2λ^5-dioxaphosphinan-2-one monomethanesulfonate. *UNII-0D5204ZSIX; UNII-GZE85Q9Q61* [pradefovir]. *CAS-625095-61-6; CAS-625095-60-5* [pradefovir]. *Antiviral.*

Pradofloxacin. $C_{21}H_{21}FN_4O_3$. 396.41. 8-Cyano-1-cyclopropyl-6-fluoro-7-[(4a*S*,7a*S*)-octahydro-6*H*-pyrrolo[3,4-*b*]pyridin-6-yl]-4-oxo-1,4-dihydroquinoline-3-carboxylic acid. *UNII-6O0T5E048I. CAS-195532-12-8.* INN.

Prajmalium Bitartrate. $C_{27}H_{38}N_2O_8$. 518.60. *N*-Propylajmalinium tartrate. *CAS-2589-47-1; CAS-35080-11-6* [prajmalium]. INN; BAN; MI. ◇NPAP

Pralatrexate [*2004*] (pral″ a trex′ ate). $C_{23}H_{23}N_7O_5$. 477.47. (1) L-Glutamic acid, *N*-[4-[1-[(2,4-diamino-6-pteridinyl)-methyl]-3-butynyl]benzoyl]-; (2) (2*S*)-2-[[4-[(1*RS*)-1-[(2,4-Diaminopteridin-6-yl)methyl]but-3-ynyl]benzoyl]amino]pentanedioic acid. *UNII-A8Q8I19Q20. CAS-146464-95-1.* INN. *Treatment of malignancies.* ◇PDX

Pralidoxime Chloride [*1962*] (pral″ i dox′ eem klor′ ide). **USP.** $C_7H_9ClN_2O$. 172.61. [Pralidoxime is INN and BAN.] (1) Pyridinium, 2-[(hydroxyimino)methyl]-1-methyl-, chloride; (2) 2-Formyl-1-methylpyridinium chloride oxime. *UNII-38X7XS076H. CAS-51-15-0. Cholinesterase reactivator.* Protopam Chloride (Wyeth) ◇*2-PAM; 2-PAM Chloride*

Pralidoxime Iodide [*1966*] (pral″ i dox′ eem eye′ oh dide). $C_7H_9IN_2O$. 264.06. (1) Pyridinium, 2-[(hydroxyimino)-methyl]-1-methyl-, iodide; (2) 2-Formyl-1-methylpyridinium iodide oxime. *UNII-7H254VC0NT. CAS-94-63-3.* INN; JAN. *Cholinesterase reactivator.* ◇*NSC-7760*

Pralidoxime Mesylate [*1966*] (pral″ i dox′ eem mes′ i late). $C_8H_{12}N_2O_4S$. 232.26. (1) Pyridinium, 2-[(hydroxyimino)-methyl]-1-methyl-, methanesulfonate; (2) 2-Formyl-1-methylpyridinium methanesulfonate oxime. *UNII-45CO7XIN2K. CAS-154-97-2. Cholinesterase reactivator.*

Pralmorelin Dihydrochloride [*1997*] (pral″ moe rel′ in dye hye″ droe klor′ ide). $C_{45}H_{55}N_9O_6$.2HCl. 890.90. [Pralmorelin is INN.] (1) L-Lysinamide, D-alanyl-3-(2-naphthalenyl)-D-alanyl-L-alanyl-L-tryptophyl-D-phenylalanyl-, dihydrochloride; (2) D-Alanyl-3-(2-naphthyl)-D-alanyl-L-alanyl-L-tryptophyl-D-phenylalanyl-L-lysinamide dihydrochloride. *UNII-R4AVR27MM8. CAS-158827-34-0; CAS-158861-67-7* [pralmorelin]. *Growth hormone releasing factor.* ◇*WAY-GPA-748*

Pralnacasan [*2000*] (pral na′ ka san). $C_{26}H_{29}N_5O_7$. 523.54. 6*H*-Pyridazino [1,2-*a*][1,2]diazepine-1-carboxamide, *N*-[(2*R*,3*S*)-2-ethoxytetrahydro-5-oxo-3-furanyl]octahydro-9-[(1-isoquinolinylcarbonyl)amino]-6,10-dioxo-, (1*S*,9*S*)-. *UNII-N986NI319S. CAS-192755-52-5.* INN. *Treatment of rheumatoid arthritis; (interleukin-1β converting enzyme (also known as caspase-1) inhibitor).* (Aventis); (Vertex) ◇*VX-740; HMR3480; HMR3480/VX-740*

Pramiconazole [*2006*] (pram″ i kon′ a zole). $C_{35}H_{39}F_2N_7O_4$. 659.73. (1) 2-Imidazolidinone, 1-[4-[4-[4-[[(2*S*,4*R*)-4-(2,4-difluorophenyl)-4-(1*H*-1,2,4-triazol-1-ylmethyl)-1,3-dioxolan-2-yl]methoxy]phenyl]-1-piperazinyl]phenyl]-3-(1-methylethyl)-; (2) 1-[4-[4-[4-[[(2*S*,4*R*)-4-(2,4-Difluorophenyl)-4-(1*H*-1,2,4-triazol-1-ylmethyl)-1,3-dioxolan-2-yl]-

methoxy]phenyl]piperazin-1-yl]phenyl]-3-(1-methylethyl)imidazolidin-2-one. *UNII-4SYH0R661F. CAS-219923-85-0.* INN. *Antifungal agent.* ◇*R126638*

Pramipexole [*1995*] (pram″ i pex′ ole). $C_{10}H_{17}N_3S$. 211.33. (1) 2,6-Benzothiazolediamine, 4,5,6,7-tetrahydro-*N*⁶-propyl-, (*S*)-; (2) (*S*)-2-Amino-4,5,6,7-tetrahydro-6-(propylamino)benzothiazole. *UNII-83619PEU5T. CAS-104632-26-0.* INN; BAN. *Antidepressant; antiparkinsonian; antischizophrenic; dopamine agonist.* ◇*U-98528E; SUD919CL2Y*

Pramipexole Dihydrochloride [*1997*] (pram″ i pex′ ole dye hye″ droe klor′ ide). $C_{10}H_{17}N_3S$.2HCl.H_2O. 302.26. (*S*)-2-Amino-4,5,6,7-tetrahydro-6-(propylamino)benzothiazole dihydrochloride monohydrate. *UNII-3D867NP06J. CAS-191217-81-9. Antidepressant; antiparkinsonian; antischizophrenic; dopamine agonist.* Mirapex (Boehringer Ingelheim) ◇*PNU-98528E; SND919CL2Y*

Pramiracetam Hydrochloride [*1981*] (pram″ i ra′ se tam hye″ droe klor′ ide). $C_{14}H_{27}N_3O_2$.HCl. 305.84. [Pramiracetam is INN.] (1) 1-Pyrrolidineacetamide, *N*-[2-[bis(1-methylethyl)amino]ethyl]-2-oxo-, monohydrochloride; (2) *N*-[2-(Diisopropylamino)ethyl]-2-oxo-1-pyrrolidineacetamide monohydrochloride. *UNII-WIU553VC0S. CAS-75733-50-5; CAS-68497-62-1* [pramiracetam]. *Cognition adjuvant.* Remen (Parke-Davis†) [*Name previously used: Amacetam Hydrochloride.*] ◇*CI-879*

Pramiracetam Sulfate [*1981*] (pram″ i ra′ se tam sul′ fate). $C_{14}H_{27}N_3O_2$.H_2SO_4. 367.46. (1) 1-Pyrrolidineacetamide, *N*-[2-[bis(1-methylethyl)amino]ethyl]-2-oxo-, sulfate (1:1); (2) *N*-[2-(Diisopropylamino)ethyl]-2-oxo-1-pyrrolidineacetamide sulfate (1:1). *CAS-72869-16-0; CAS-68497-62-1* [pramiracetam]. *Cognition adjuvant.* [*Name previously used: Amacetam Sulfate.*] ◇*CI-879 [sulfate]*

Pramiverine. $C_{21}H_{27}N$. 293.45. 4,4-Diphenyl-*N*-isopropylcyclohexylamine *UNII-157NY06G9T. CAS-14334-40-8.* INN; BAN; MI. ◇*HSP 2986; EMD 9806*

Pramlintide [*1996*] (pram′ lin tide). $C_{171}H_{267}N_{51}O_{53}S_2$. 3949.39. (1) L-Tyrosinamide, L-lysyl-L-cysteinyl-L-asparaginyl-L-threonyl-L-alanyl-L-threonyl-L-cysteinyl-L-alanyl-L-threonyl-L-glutaminyl-L-arginyl-L-leucyl-L-alanyl-L-asparaginyl-L-phenylalanyl-L-leucyl-L-valyl-L-histidyl-L-

---

† Brand name formerly used, and/or firm no longer concerned with this product.

seryl-L-seryl-L-asparaginyl-L-asparaginyl-L-phenylalanyl-glycyl-L-prolyl-L-isoleucyl-L-leucyl-L-prolyl-L-prolyl-L-threonyl-L-asparaginyl-L-valylglycyl-L-seryl-L-asparaginyl-L-threonyl-, cyclic (2→7)-disulfide; (2) L-Lysyl-L-cysteinyl-L-asparaginyl-L-threonyl-L-alanyl-L-threonyl-L-cysteinyl-L-alanyl-L-threonyl-L-glutaminyl-L-arginyl-L-leucyl-L-alanyl-L-asparaginyl-L-phenylalanyl-L-leucyl-L-valyl-L-histidyl-L-seryl-L-seryl-L-asparaginyl-L-asparaginyl-L-phenylalanylglycyl-L-prolyl-L-isoleucyl-L-leucyl-L-prolyl-L-prolyl-L-threonyl-L-asparaginyl-L-valylglycyl-L-seryl-L-asparaginyl-L-threonyl-L-tyrosinamide, cyclic (2→7)-disulfide. *UNII-D3FM8FA78T. CAS-151126-32-8.* INN; BAN. *Antidiabetic.* ◇*AC0137*

Pramlintide Acetate [*1997*] (pram′ lin tide as′ e tate). $C_{171}H_{267}N_{51}O_{53}S_2 \cdot xC_2H_4O_2 \cdot yH_2O$ (x and y are variable). 3949.39. (1) 25-L-Proline-28-L-proline-29-L-prolineamylin (human) acetate (salt), hydrate; (2) L-Lysyl-L-cysteinyl-L-asparaginyl-L-threonyl-L-alanyl-L-threonyl-L-cysteinyl-L-alanyl-L-threonyl-L-glutaminyl-L-arginyl-L-leucyl-L-alanyl-L-asparaginyl-L-phenylalanyl-L-leucyl-L-valyl-L-histidyl-L-seryl-L-seryl-L-asparaginyl-L-asparaginyl-L-phenylalanylglycyl-L-prolyl-L-isoleucyl-L-leucyl-L-prolyl-L-prolyl-L-threonyl-L-asparaginyl-L-valylglycyl-L-seryl-L-asparaginyl-L-threonyl-L-tyrosinamide, cyclic (2→7)-disulfide, acetate (salt), hydrate. *UNII-726I6TE06G. CAS-196078-30-5. Treatment of metabolic disorders, antidiabetic.* Symlin (Amylin) ◇*AC0137*

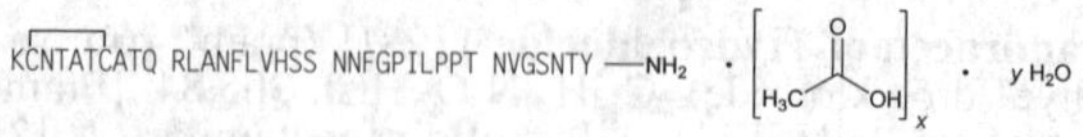

Pramocaine (INN, BAN) Hydrochloride — *See* Pramoxine Hydrochloride.

Pramoxine Hydrochloride (pram ox′ een hye″ droe klor′ ide). **USP.** $C_{17}H_{27}NO_3 \cdot HCl$. 329.86. [Pramocaine is INN and BAN.] (1) Morpholine, 4-[3-(4-butoxyphenoxy)propyl]-, hydrochloride; (2) 4-[3-(*p*-Butoxyphenoxy)propyl]-morpholine hydrochloride. *UNII-88AYB867L5; UNII-068X84E056* [pramoxine]. *CAS-637-58-1; CAS-140-65-8* [pramoxine]. *Anesthetic (topical).* Tronolane (Ross); Tronothane (Abbott)

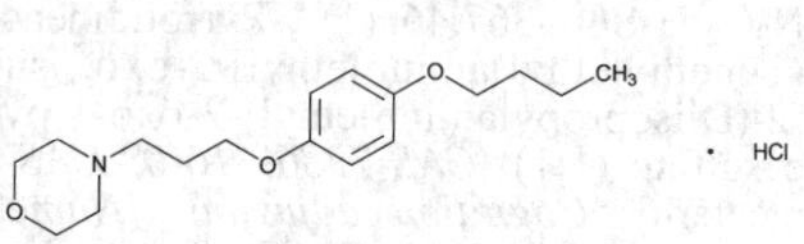

Prampine. $C_{20}H_{27}NO_4$. 345.43. Atropine propionate. *UNII-B4XTR3PC33. CAS-7009-65-6.* INN; BAN. ◇*PAMN [as methonitrate]*

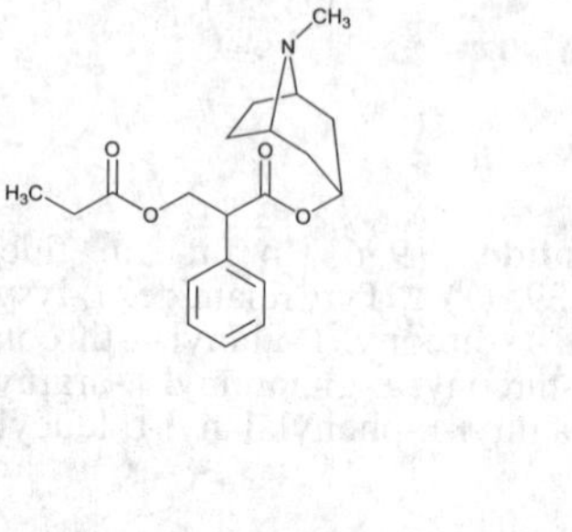

Pranazepide. $C_{26}H_{19}FN_4O_2$. 438.45. (-)-*N*-[(*S*)-1-(*o*-Fluorophenyl)-3,4,6,7-tetrahydro-4-oxopyrrolo[3,2,1-*jk*][1,4]benzodiazepin-3-yl]indole-2-carboxamide. *UNII-10TO0RP68C. CAS-150408-73-4.* INN.

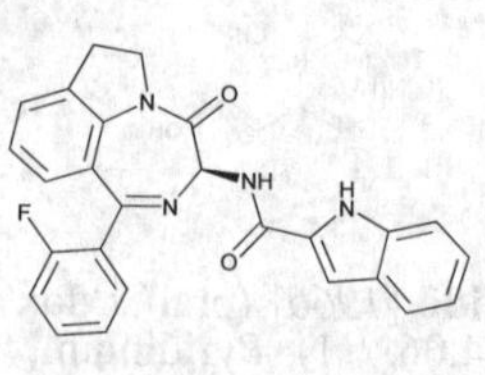

Pranidipine. $C_{25}H_{24}N_2O_6$. 448.47. (*E*)-Cinnamyl methyl (±)-1,4-dihydro-2,6-dimethyl-4-(*m*-nitrophenyl)-3,5-pyridinedicarboxylate. *UNII-9DES9QVH58. CAS-99522-79-9.* INN.

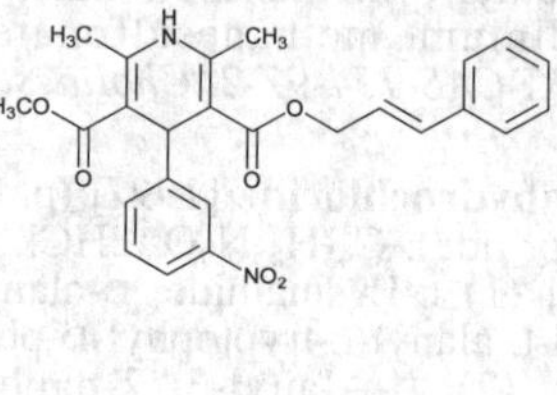

Pranlukast. $C_{27}H_{23}N_5O_4$. 481.50. *N*-[4-Oxo-2-(1*H*-tetrazol-5-yl)-4*H*-1-benzopyran-8-yl]-*p*-(4-phenylbutoxy)benzamide. *CAS-103177-37-3.* INN; BAN. ◇*ONO-1078; SB 205312*

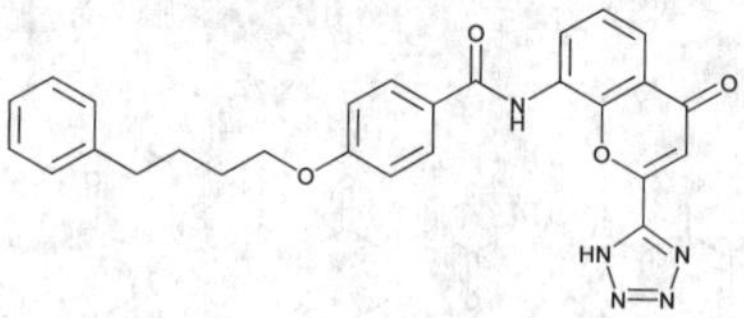

Pranolium Chloride [*1974*] (pran oh′ le um klor′ ide). $C_{18}H_{26}ClNO_2$. 323.86. (1) 1-Propanaminium, 2-hydroxy-*N,N*-dimethyl-*N*-(1-methylethyl)-3-(1-naphthalenyloxy)-, chloride; (2) [2-Hydroxy-3-(1-naphthyloxy)propyl]isopropyldimethylammonium chloride. *CAS-42879-47-0.* INN. *Cardiac depressant (anti-arrhythmic).* ◇*SC-27761*

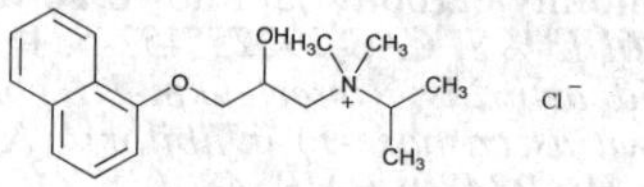

Pranoprofen. $C_{15}H_{13}NO_3$. 255.27. *α*-Methyl-5*H*-[1]benzopyrano[2,3-*b*]pyridine-7-acetic acid. *UNII-2R7O1ET613. CAS-52549-17-4.* INN; JAN; MI.

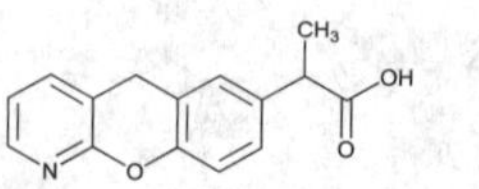

Pranosal. $C_{16}H_{23}NO_3$. 277.36. 2,5-Dimethyl-1-pyrrolidine-propanol salicylate (ester). *UNII-4JB9426X1H. CAS-17716-89-1.* INN; DCF.

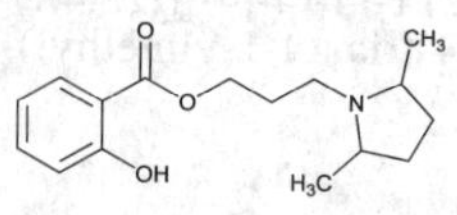

Prasterone. $C_{19}H_{28}O_2$. 288.42. 3β-Hydroxyandrost-5-en-17-one. *CAS-53-43-0*. INN; MI.

Prasugrel Hydrochloride [*2004*] (pra′ soo grel hye″ droe klor′ ide). $C_{20}H_{20}FNO_3S\cdot HCl$. 409.90. [Prasugrel is INN.] (1) Ethanone, 2-[2-(acetyloxy)-6,7-dihydrothieno[3,2-*c*]pyridin-5(4*H*)-yl]-1-cyclopropyl-2-(2-fluorophenyl)-, hydrochloride; (2) 5-[(1*RS*)-2-Cyclopropyl-1-(2-fluorophenyl)-2-oxoethyl]-4,5,6,7-tetrahydrothieno[3,2-*c*]pyridin-2-yl acetate hydrochloride. *UNII-G89JQ59I13*. *CAS-389574-19-0; CAS-150322-43-3* [prasugrel]. *Inhibits platelet aggregation (platelet ADPP 2Y12 antagonist).* ◇LY640315

Pratosartan. $C_{25}H_{26}N_6O$. 426.51. 2-Propyl-3-[[2′-(1*H*-tetrazol-5-yl)biphenyl-4-yl]methyl]-5,6,7,8-tetrahydrocycloheptaimidazol-4(3*H*)-one. *UNII-66VLQ6E6DL*. *CAS-153804-05-8*. INN.

Pravadoline Maleate [*1989*] (prav ad′ oh leen mal′ ee ate). $C_{23}H_{26}N_2O_3\cdot C_4H_4O_4$. 494.54. [Pravadoline is INN.] (1) Methanone, (4-methoxyphenyl)[2-methyl-1-[2-(4-morpholinyl)ethyl]-1*H*-indol-3-yl]-, (*Z*)-2-butenedioate (1:1); (2) *p*-Methoxyphenyl 2-methyl-1-(2-morpholinoethyl)indol-3-yl ketone maleate (1:1). *UNII-2DH4X8278M*. *CAS-92623-84-2; CAS-92623-83-1* [pravadoline]. *Analgesic.* ◇Win 48,098-6

Pravastatin Sodium [*1988*] (pra″ va stat′ in soe′ dee um). USP. $C_{23}H_{35}NaO_7$. 446.51. [Pravastatin is INN and BAN.] (1) 1-Naphthaleneheptanoic acid, 1,2,6,7,8,8a-hexahydro-β,δ,6-trihydroxy-2-methyl-8-(2-methyl-1-oxobutoxy)-, monosodium salt, [1*S*-[1α(βS^*,δS^*),2α,6α,8β(R^*),8aα]]-; (2) Sodium (+)-($\beta R,\delta R$,1*S*,2*S*,6*S*,8*S*,8a*R*)-1,2,6,7,8,8a-hexahydro-β,δ,6,8-tetrahydroxy-2-methyl-1-naphthaleneheptanoate, 8-[(2*S*)-2-methylbutyrate]. *UNII-3M8608UQ61;*

UNII-KXO2KT9N0G [pravastatin]. *CAS-81131-70-6; CAS-81093-37-0* [pravastatin]. JAN. *Antihyperlipidemic.* Pravachol (Bristol-Myers Squibb) ◇CS-514; SQ-31,000

Praxadine. $C_4H_6N_4$. 110.12. Pyrazole-1-carboxamidine. *UNII-12L58GX4AS*. *CAS-4023-00-1*. INN; DCF.

Prazarelix. $C_{80}H_{102}ClN_{23}O_{12}$. 1613.27. *N*-Acetyl-3-(2-naphthyl)-D-alanyl-*p*-chloro-D-phenylalanyl-3-(3-pyridyl)-D-alanyl-L-seryl-*p*-[(5-amino-*s*-triazol-3-yl)amino]-L-phenylalanyl-*p*-[(5-amino-*s*-triazol-3-yl)amino]-D-phenyl-alanyl-L-leucyl-N^6-isopropyl-L-lysyl-L-prolyl-D-alanin-amide. *CAS-134457-28-6*. INN.

Prazarelix Acetate [*1998*] (praz″ a rel′ ix as′ e tate). $C_{80}H_{102}ClN_{23}O_{12}\cdot C_2H_4O_2$. 1673.32. (1) *N*-Acetyl-3-(2-naphthalenyl)-D-alanyl-4-chloro-D-phenylalanyl-3-(3-pyridinyl)-D-alanyl-L-seryl-4-[(5-amino-1*H*-1,2,4-triazol-3-yl)amino]-L-phenylalanyl-4-[(5-amino-1*H*-1,2,4-triazol-3-yl)amino]-D-phenylalanyl-L-leucyl-N^6-(1-methylethyl)-L-lysyl-L-prolyl-D-alaninamide acetate (salt); (2) *N*-Acetyl-3-(2-naphthyl)-D-alanyl-*p*-chloro-D-phenylalanyl-3-(3-pyridyl)-D-alanyl-L-seryl-*p*-[(5-amino-*s*-triazol-3-yl)amino]-L-phenylalanyl-*p*-[5-amino-*s*-triazol-3-yl)amino]-D-phenylalanyl-L-leucyl-N^6-isopropyl-L-lysyl-L-prolyl-D-alaninamide acetate (salt). *CAS-134485-10-2. Treatment of uterine fibroids, endometriosis, and prostate cancer (gonadotropin-releasing hormone antagonist).[Previously used name: Azaline B.]* ◇RWJ 47428

Prazepam [*1968*] (praz′ e pam). $C_{19}H_{17}ClN_2O$. 324.80. (1) 2*H*-1,4-Benzodiazepin-2-one, 7-chloro-1-(cyclopropyl-methyl)-1,3-dihydro-5-phenyl-; (2) 7-Chloro-1-(cyclopropylmethyl)-1,3-dihydro-5-phenyl-2*H*-1,4-benzodiazepin-

---

† Brand name formerly used, and/or firm no longer concerned with this product.

2-one. *UNII-Q30VCC064M. CAS-2955-38-6.* USP XXIII; INN; BAN; JAN. *Sedative-hypnotic.* Centrax (Pfizer) ◇*W 4020*

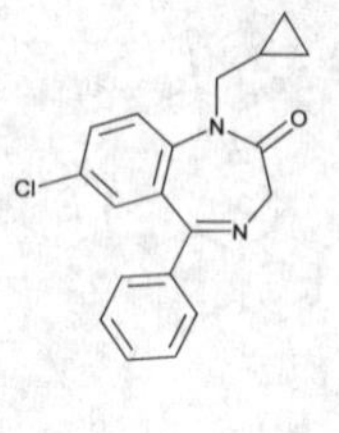

Prazepine. $C_{19}H_{24}N_2$. 280.41. 5,6-Dihydro-*N*-[3-(dimethylamino)propyl]-11*H*-dibenz[*b,e*]azepine. *UNII-72O4809PU1. CAS-73-07-4.* INN.

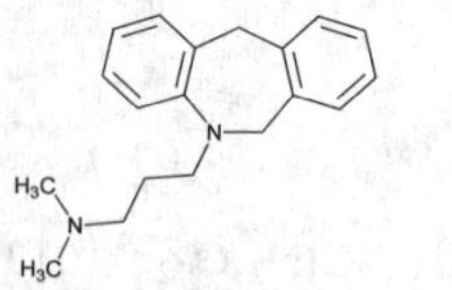

Praziquantel [*1978*] (praz″ i kwon′ tel). **USP.** $C_{19}H_{24}N_2O_2$. 312.41. (1) 4*H*-Pyrazino[2,1-*a*]isoquinolin-4-one, 2-(cyclohexylcarbonyl)-1,2,3,6,7,11b-hexahydro-; (2) 2-(Cyclohexylcarbonyl)-1,2,3,6,7,11b-hexahydro-4*H*-pyrazino[2,1-*a*]isoquinolin-4-one. *UNII-6490C9U457. CAS-55268-74-1.* INN; BAN; JAN. *Anthelmintic (veterinary).* Biltricide (Bayer) ◇*EMBAY 8440*

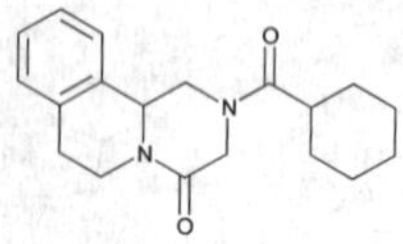

Prazitone. $C_{16}H_{19}N_3O_3$. 301.34. 5-Phenyl-5-(2-piperidylmethyl)barbituric acid. *UNII-6DZB018428. CAS-2409-26-9.* INN; BAN. ◇*AGN 511 [as hydrochloride]*

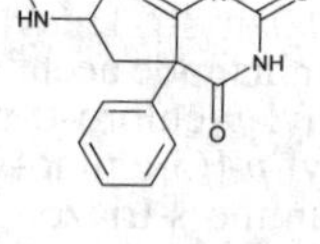

Prazocillin. $C_{19}H_{18}Cl_2N_4O_4S$. 469.34. 6-[1-(2,6-Dichlorophenyl)-4-methylpyrazole-5-carboxamido]-3,3-dimethyl-7-oxo-4-thia-1-azabicyclo[3.2.0]heptane-2-carboxylic acid. *UNII-IRZ1462XXF. CAS-15949-72-1.* INN.

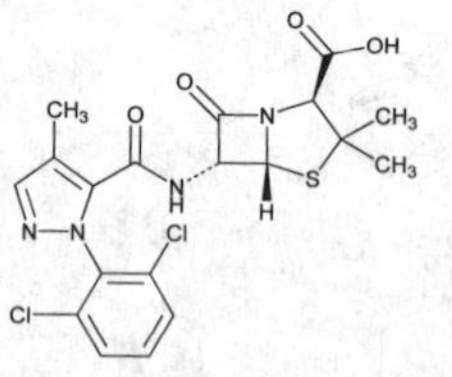

Prazosin Hydrochloride [*1968*] (praz′ oh sin hye″ droe klor′ ide). **USP.** $C_{19}H_{21}N_5O_4 \cdot HCl$. 419.86. [Prazosin is INN and BAN.] (1) Piperazine, 1-(4-amino-6,7-dimethoxy-2-quinazolinyl)-4-(2-furanylcarbonyl)-, monohydrochloride; (2) 1-(4-Amino-6,7-dimethoxy-2-quinazolinyl)-4-(2-furoyl)piperazine monohydrochloride. *UNII-X0Z7454B90; UNII-*

XM03YJ541D [prazosin]. *CAS-19237-84-4; CAS-19216-56-9* [prazosin]. JAN. *Antihypertensive.* Minipress (Pfizer) ◇*CP-12,299-1*

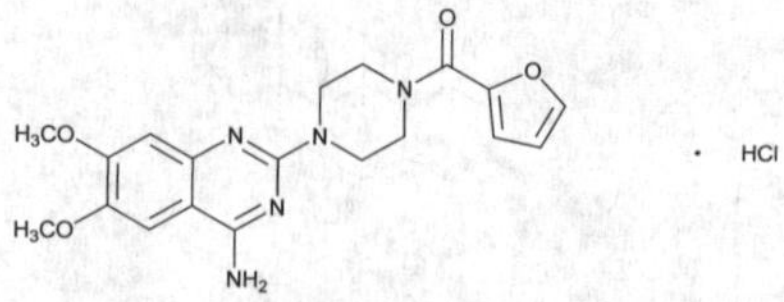

Preclamol. $C_{14}H_{21}NO$. 219.32. (-)-(*S*)-*m*-(1-Propyl-3-piperidyl)phenol. *CAS-85966-89-8.* INN.

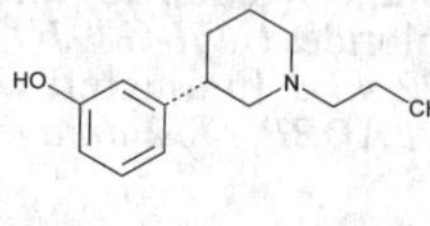

Prednazate [*1965*] (pred′ na zate). $C_{25}H_{32}O_8 \cdot C_{21}H_{26}ClN_3OS$. 864.49. (1) Pregna-1,4-diene-3,20-dione, 21-(3-carboxy-1-oxopropoxy)-11,17-dihydroxy-, (11β)-, compd. with 4-[3-(2-chloro-10*H*-phenothiazin-10-yl)propyl]-1-piperazineethanol (1:1); (2) 11β,17,21-Trihydroxypregna-1,4-diene-3,20-dione, 21-(hydrogen succinate), compound with 4-[3-(2-chlorophenothiazin-10-yl)propyl]-1-piperazine-ethanol (1:1). *CAS-5714-75-0.* INN. *Anti-inflammatory.* ◇*Sch 6620*

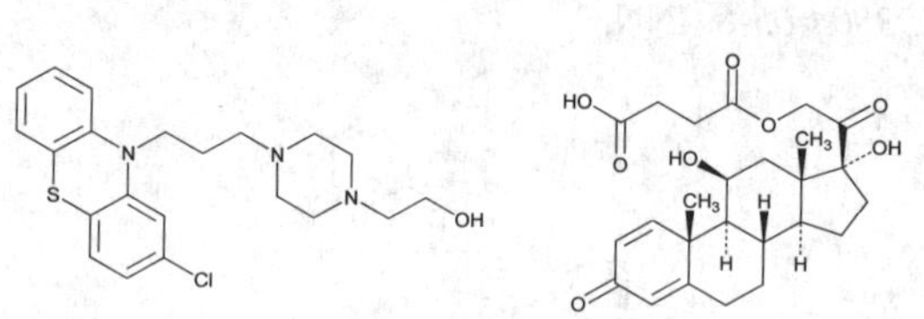

Prednazoline. $C_{22}H_{29}O_8P \cdot C_{13}H_{18}N_2O$. 670.73. 11β,17,21-Trihydroxypregna-1,4-diene-3,20-dione 21-(di-H phosphate) compound with 2-[(2-isopropylphenoxy)methyl]-2-imidazoline. *CAS-6693-90-9.* INN; DCF.

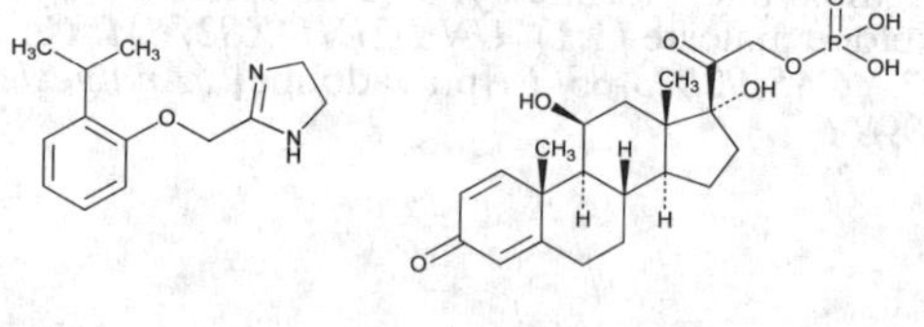

Prednicarbate [*1983*] (pred″ ni kar′ bate). **USP.** $C_{27}H_{36}O_8$. 488.57. (1) Pregna-1,4-diene-3,20-dione, 17-[(ethoxycarbonyl)oxy]-11-hydroxy-21-(1-oxopropoxy)-, (11β)-; (2) 11β,17,21-Trihydroxypregna-1,4-diene-3,20-dione 17-(ethyl carbonate) 21-propionate. *UNII-V901LV1K7D. CAS-73771-04-7.* INN; BAN. *Glucocorticoid.* Dermatop (Sanofi Aventis) ◇*HOE 777; S 77 0777*

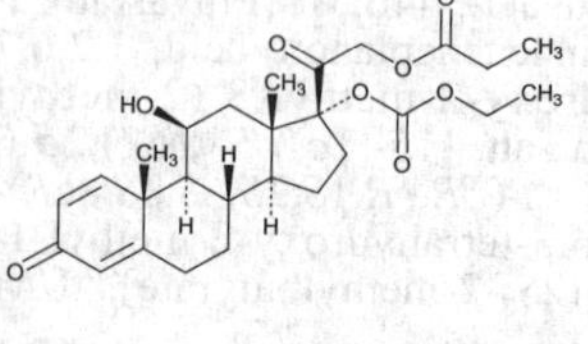

Prednimustine [*1979*] (pred″ ni mus′ teen). $C_{35}H_{45}Cl_2NO_6$. 646.64. (1) Pregna-1,4-diene-3,20-dione, 21-[4-[4-[bis(2-chloroethyl)amino]phenyl]-1-oxobutoxy]-11,17-dihydroxy-, (11*β*)-; (2) 11*β*,17,21-Trihydroxypregna-1,4-diene-3,20-dione 21-[4-[*p*-[bis(2-chloroethyl)amino]phenyl]butyrate]. *CAS-29069-24-7*. INN. *Antineoplastic*.

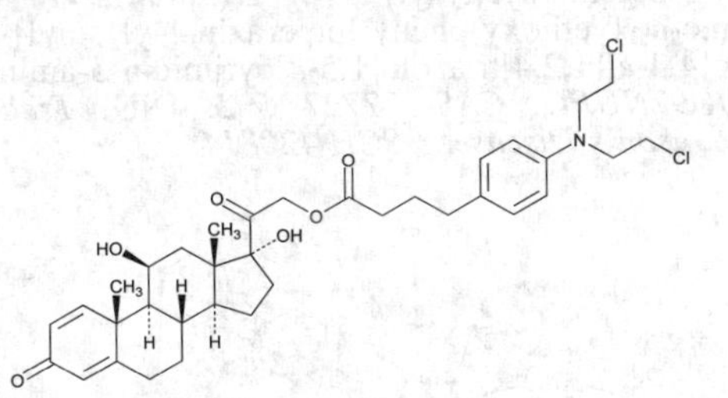

Prednisolamate. $C_{27}H_{39}NO_6$. 473.60. 11*β*,17,21-Trihydroxypregna-1,4-diene-3,20-dione 21-*N,N*-diethylglycine ester. *CAS-5626-34-6*. INN; BAN.

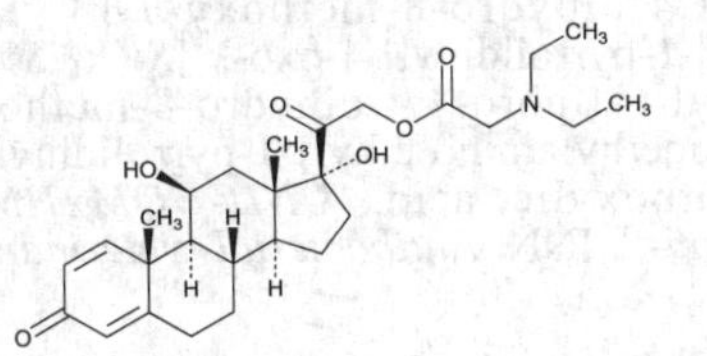

Prednisolone (pred nis′ oh lone). **USP**. $C_{21}H_{28}O_5$. 360.44. (1) Pregna-1,4-diene-3,20-dione, 11,17,21-trihydroxy-, (11*β*)-; (2) 11*β*,17,21-Trihydroxypregna-1,4-diene-3,20-dione. *UNII-9PHQ9Y1OLM*. *CAS-50-24-8* [anhydrous]; *CAS-52438-85-4* [sesquihydrate]. INN; BAN; JAN. *Glucocorticoid*. Delta-cortef (Pfizer); Meti-derm (Schering); Sterane (Pfizer) ✧*NSC-9120*

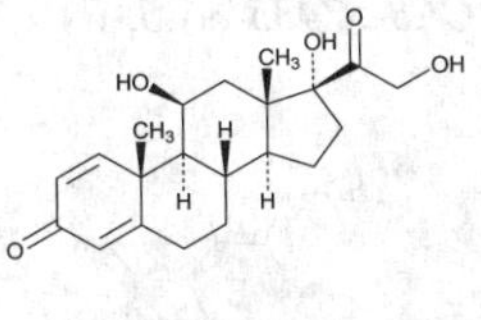

Prednisolone Acetate (pred nis′ oh lone as′ e tate). **USP**. $C_{23}H_{30}O_6$. 402.48. (1) Pregna-1,4-diene-3,20-dione, 21-(acetyloxy)-11,17-dihydroxy-, (11*β*)-; (2) 11*β*,17,21-Trihydroxypregna-1,4-diene-3,20-dione 21-acetate. *UNII-8B2807733D*. *CAS-52-21-1*. JAN. *Glucocorticoid*. Meticortelone (Schering); Omnipred (Alcon); Sterane (Pfizer)

Prednisolone Butylacetate (JAN) — *See* Prednisolone Tebutate.

Prednisolone Hemisuccinate (pred nis′ oh lone hem″ ee sux′ i nate). **USP**. $C_{25}H_{32}O_8$. 460.52. [Prednisolone Succinate is JAN.] (1) Pregna-1,4-diene-3,20-dione,21-(3-carboxy-1-oxopropoxy)-11,17-dihydroxy-, (11*β*)-; (2) 11*β*,17,21-Trihydroxypregna-1,4-diene-3,20-dione 21-(hydrogen succinate). *CAS-2920-86-7*. *Glucocorticoid*.

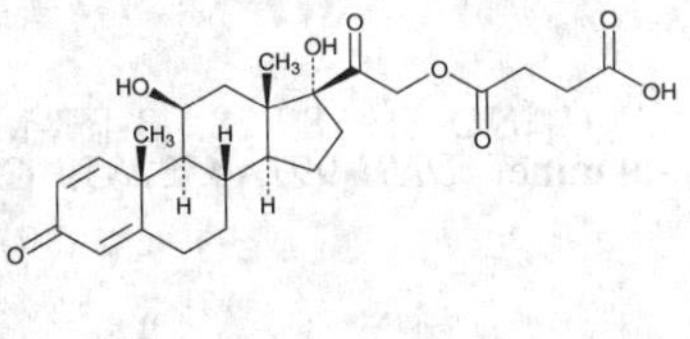

† Brand name formerly used, and/or firm no longer concerned with this product.

Prednisolone Sodium Phosphate (pred nis′ oh lone soe′ dee um fos′ fate). **USP**. $C_{21}H_{27}Na_2O_8P$. 484.39. (1) Pregna-1,4-diene-3,20-dione, 11,17-dihydroxy-21-(phosphonooxy)-, disodium salt, (11*β*)-; (2) 11*β*,17,21-Trihydroxypregna-1,4-diene-3,20-dione 21-(disodium phosphate). *UNII-IV021NXA9J*. *CAS-125-02-0; CAS-302-25-0* [prednisolone 21-(dihydrogen phosphate)]. JAN. *Glucocorticoid*. Hydeltrasol (Merck); Metreton (Schering); Orapred (Medicis); Pediapred (UCB)

Prednisolone Sodium Succinate (pred nis′ oh lone soe′ dee um sux′ i nate). **USP** [for Injection]. $C_{25}H_{31}NaO_8$. 482.50. (1) Pregna-1,4-diene-3,20-dione, 21-(3-carboxyl-1-oxopropoxy)-11,17-dihydroxy-, monosodium salt, (11*β*)-; (2) 11*β*,17,21-Trihydroxypregna-1,4-diene-3,20-dione 21-(sodium succinate). *UNII-8223RR9DWF*. *CAS-1715-33-9; CAS-2920-86-7* [prednisolone 21-(hydrogen succinate)]. JAN. *Glucocorticoid*.

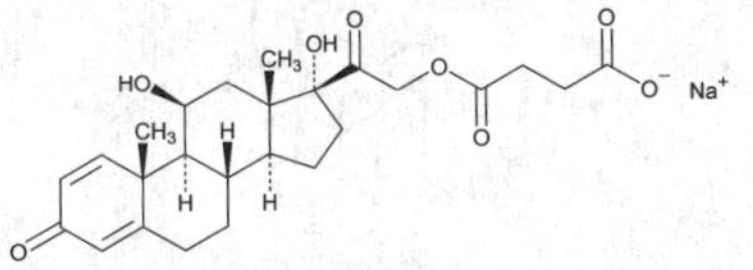

Prednisolone Steaglate. $C_{41}H_{64}O_8$. 684.94. Stearate ester of 11*β*,17,21-trihydroxypregna-1,4-diene-3,20-dione-21-glycolate. *UNII-OZQ2XN817F*. *CAS-5060-55-9*. INN; BAN; MI.

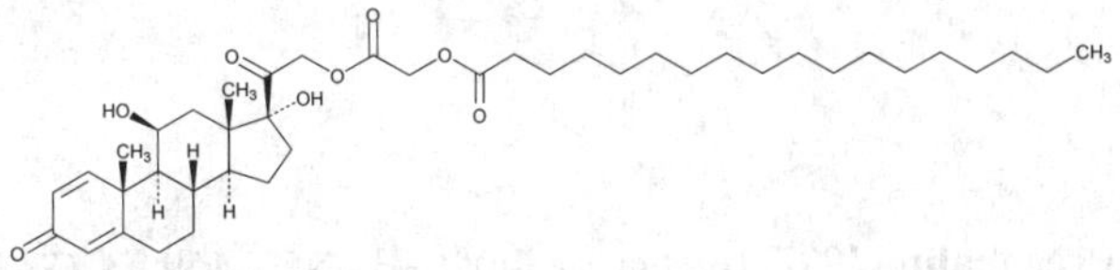

Prednisolone Tebutate (pred nis′ oh lone teb′ ue tate). **USP**. $C_{27}H_{38}O_6$. 458.59. [Prednisolone Butylacetate is JAN.] (1) Pregna-1,4-diene-3,20-dione, 11,17-dihydroxy-21-[(3,3-dimethyl-1-oxobutyl)oxy]-, (11*β*)-; (2) 11*β*,17,21-Trihydroxypregna-1,4-diene-3,20-dione 21-(3,3-dimethylbutyrate). *UNII-1V7A1U282K*. *CAS-7681-14-3*. *Glucocorticoid*. Hydeltra-TBA (Merck)

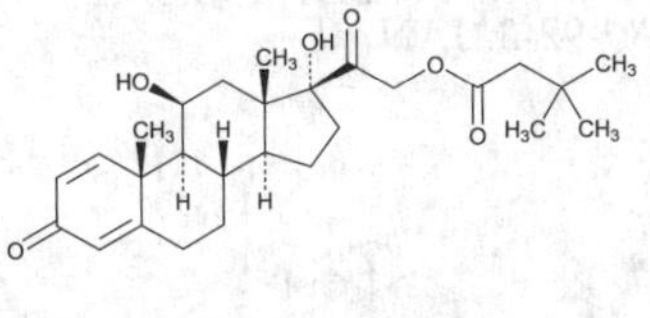

Prednisolone Valerate Acetate. $C_{28}H_{38}O_7$. 486.60. 11*β*,17*α*,21-Trihydroxy-1,4-pregnadiene-3,20-dione 21-acetate 17-valerate. *UNII-2JB27QJW3D*. *CAS-72064-79-0*. JAN.

Prednisone (pred′ ni sone). **USP**. $C_{21}H_{26}O_5.H_2O$. 376.44. (1) Pregna-1,4-diene-3,11,20-trione monohydrate, 17,21-dihydroxy-; (2) 17,21-Dihydroxypregna-1,4-diene-3,11,20-trione monohydrate. *UNII-VB0R961HZT*. *CAS-53-03-2*. INN; BAN. *Glucocorticoid*. Delta-dome (Bayer); Deltasone (Pfizer); Meticorten (Schering); Orasone (Solvay Pharmaceuticals) ✧*NSC-10023*

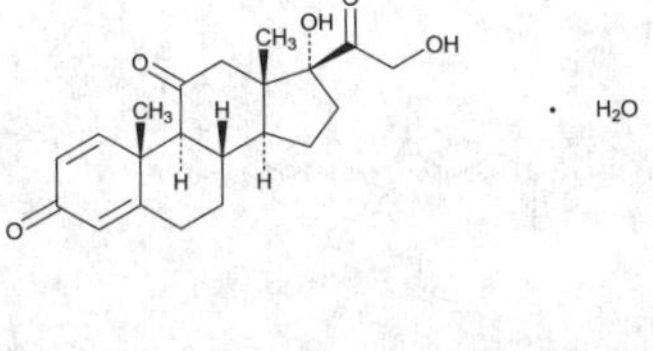

Prednival [*1967*] (pred′ ni val). $C_{26}H_{36}O_6$. 444.56. (1) Pregna-1,4-diene-3,20-dione, 11,21-dihydroxy-17-[(1-oxopentyl)oxy]-, (11β)-; (2) 11β,17,21-Trihydroxypregna-1,4-diene-3,20-dione 17-valerate. *CAS-15180-00-4. Glucocorticoid.* ◇*W 4869*

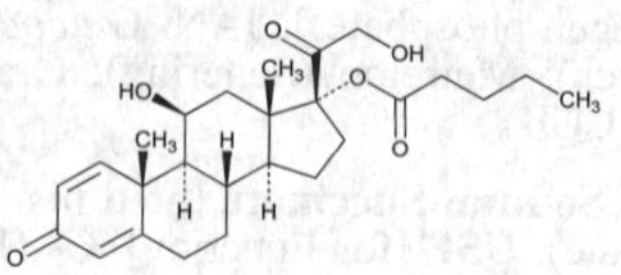

Prednylidene. $C_{22}H_{28}O_5$. 372.45. 11β,17,21-Trihydroxy-16-methylenepregna-1,4-diene-3,20-dione. *CAS-599-33-7.* INN; BAN; DCF; MI.

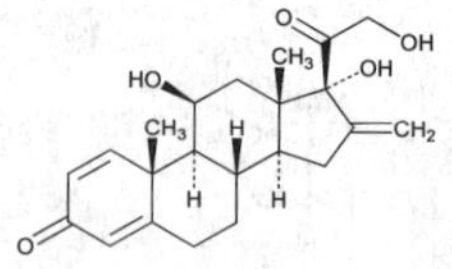

Prefenamate. $C_{19}H_{18}F_3NO_2$. 349.35. 3-Methyl-2-butenyl *N*-(α,α,α-trifluoro-*m*-tolyl)anthranilate. *UNII-G1SCZ6N70K. CAS-57775-28-7.* INN.

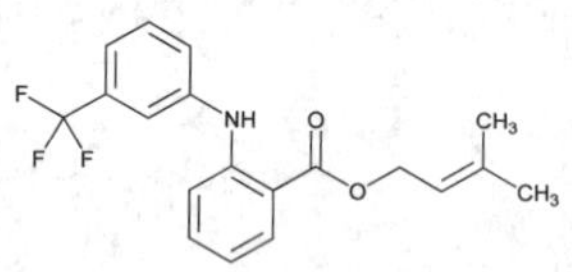

Pregabalin [*1997*] (pre ga′ ba lin). $C_8H_{17}NO_2$. 159.23. (*S*)-3-(Aminomethyl)-5-methylhexanoic acid. *UNII-55JG375S6M. CAS-148553-50-9.* INN; BAN; JAN. *Anticonvulsant.* Lyrica (Pfizer) ◇*CI-1008*

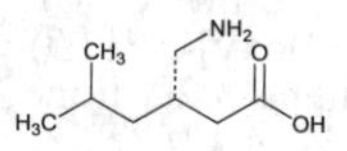

Pregnandiol. $C_{21}H_{36}O_2$. 320.51. (3α,5β,20α)-Pregnane-3,20-diol. *CAS-80-92-2.* JAN.

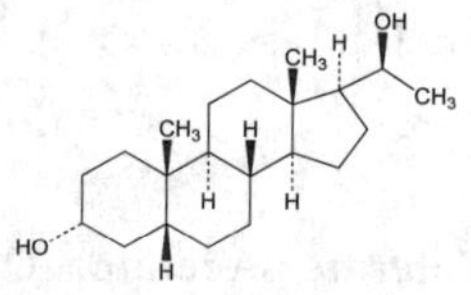

Pregneninolone — *See* Ethisterone.

Pregnenolone Succinate [*1961*] (preg nen′ oh lone sux′ i nate). $C_{25}H_{36}O_5$. 416.55. [Pregnenolone is INN and BAN.] (1) Pregn-5-en-20-one, 3-(3-carboxy-1-oxopropoxy)-, (3β)-; (2) 3β-Hydroxypregn-5-en-20-one hydrogen succinate. *CAS-4598-67-8; CAS-145-13-1* [pregnenolone]. *Nonhormonal sterol derivative.* Formula 405 (Doak)

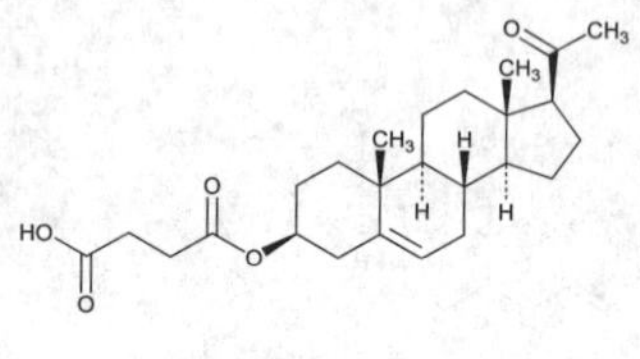

Preladenant [*2007*] (prel a′ de nant). $C_{25}H_{29}N_9O_3$. 503.56. (1) 7*H*-Pyrazolo[4,3-*e*][1,2,4]triazolo[1,5-*c*]pyrimidin-5-amine, 2-(2-furanyl)-7-[2-[4-[4-(2-methoxyethoxy)phenyl]-1-piperazinyl]ethyl]-; (2) 2-(Furan-2-yl)-7-[2-[4-[4-(2-methoxyethoxy)phenyl]piperazin-1-yl]ethyl]-7*H*-pyrazolo[4,3-*e*][1,2,4]triazolo[1,5-*c*]pyrimidin-5-amine. *UNII-950O97NUPO. CAS-377727-87-2.* INN. *Treatment of Parkinson's Disease.* ◇*SCH 420814*

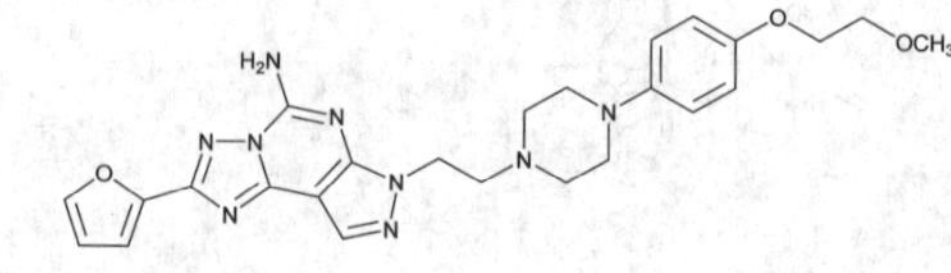

Premafloxacin [*1995*] (prem″ a flox′ a sin). $C_{21}H_{26}FN_3O_4$. 403.45. (1) 3-Quinolinecarboxylic acid, 1-cyclopropyl-6-fluoro-1,4-dihydro-8-methoxy-7-[3-[1-(methylamino)ethyl]-1-pyrrolidinyl]-4-oxo-, [*S*-(*R**,*S**)]-; (2) 1-Cyclopropyl-6-fluoro-1,4-dihydro-8-methoxy-7-[(3*R*)-3-[(1*S*)-1-(methylamino)ethyl]-1-pyrrolidinyl]-4-oxo-3-quinolinecarboxylic acid. *UNII-UOM2HMO524. CAS-143383-65-7.* INN. *Antibacterial (veterinary).* ◇*U-95376*

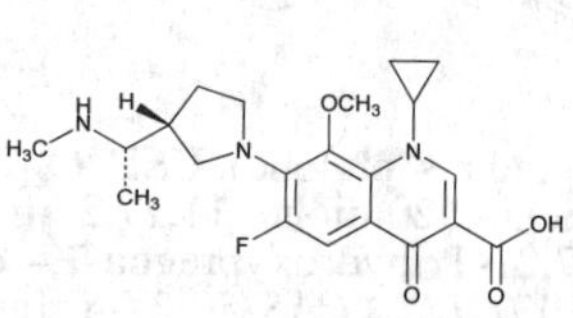

Premazepam. $C_{15}H_{15}N_3O$. 253.30. 3,7-Dihydro-6,7-dimethyl-5-phenylpyrrolo[3,4-*e*]-1,4-diazepin-2(1*H*)-one. *UNII-OI7443PDLB. CAS-57435-86-6.* INN; BAN.

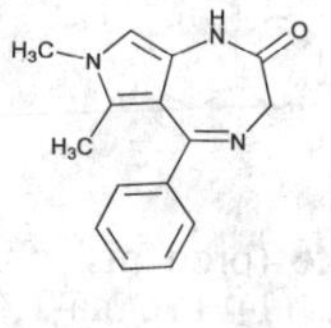

Prenalterol Hydrochloride [*1980*] (pre nal′ ter ol hye″ droe klor′ ide). $C_{12}H_{19}NO_3 \cdot HCl$. 261.75. [Prenalterol is INN and BAN.] (1) Phenol, 4-[2-hydroxy-3-[(1-methylethyl)amino]propoxy]-, hydrochloride, (*S*)-; (2) (-)-(*S*)-1-(*p*-Hydroxyphenoxy)-3-(isopropylamino)-2-propanol hydrochloride. *CAS-61260-05-7; CAS-57526-81-5* [prenalterol]. *Adrenergic.* ◇*H 133/22; CGP 7760B*

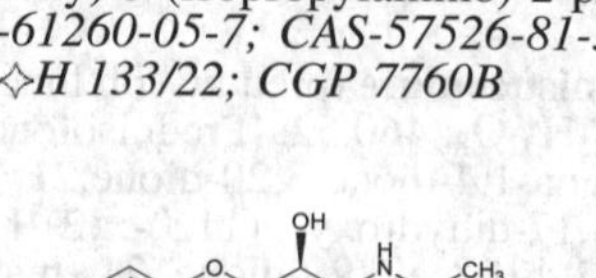

Prenisteine. $C_8H_{15}NO_2S$. 189.28. 3-[(3-Methyl-2-butenyl)thio]-L-alanine. *UNII-99TA452185. CAS-5287-46-7.* INN.

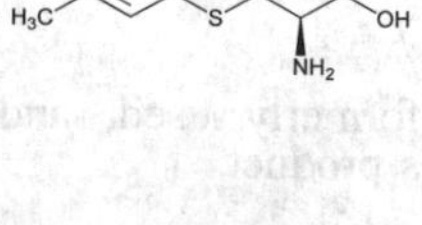

Prenoverine. $C_{25}H_{29}NO_2$. 375.50. ($\pm$)-2′-(Diphenylmethoxy)-*N*,1-dimethyl-2-phenoxydiethylamine. *UNII-PK3852O88V. CAS-65236-29-5.* INN.

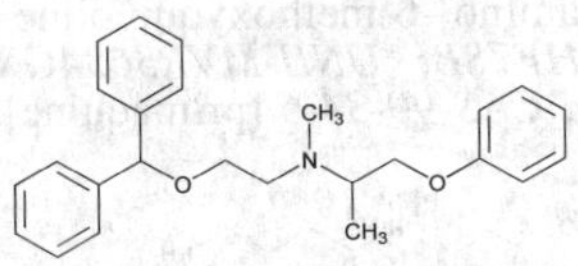

Prenoxdiazine. $C_{23}H_{27}N_3O$. 361.48. 1-[2-[3-(2,2-Diphenylethyl)-1,2,4-oxadiazol-5-yl]ethyl]piperidine. *UNII-S491HH391H. CAS-47543-65-7.* INN; MI.

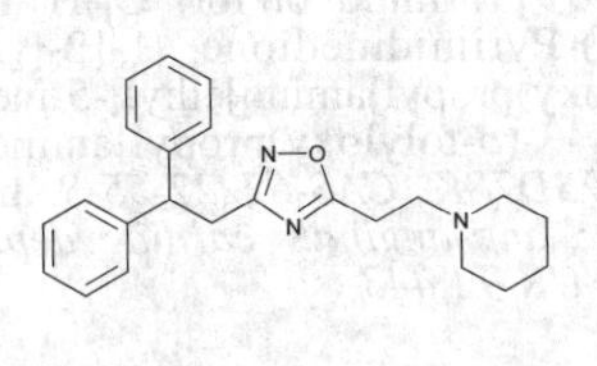

Prenylamine [*1962*] (pre nil′ a meen). $C_{24}H_{27}N$. 329.48. [Prenylamine Lactate is JAN.] (1) Benzenepropanamine, *N*-(1-methyl-2-phenylethyl)-γ-phenyl-; (2) *N*-(3,3-Diphenylpropyl)-α-methylphenethylamine. *CAS-390-64-7; CAS-69-43-2* [prenylamine lactate]. INN; BAN. *Vasodilator (coronary).* ◇*B-436*

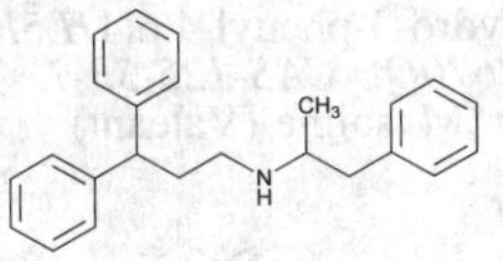

Pretamazium Iodide. $C_{29}H_{29}IN_2S$. 564.52. 4-(4-Biphenylyl)-3-ethyl-2-(*p*-1-pyrrolidinylstyryl)thiazolium iodide. *UNII-7Z32Z641H2. CAS-24840-59-3.* INN; BAN. ◇*66-269*

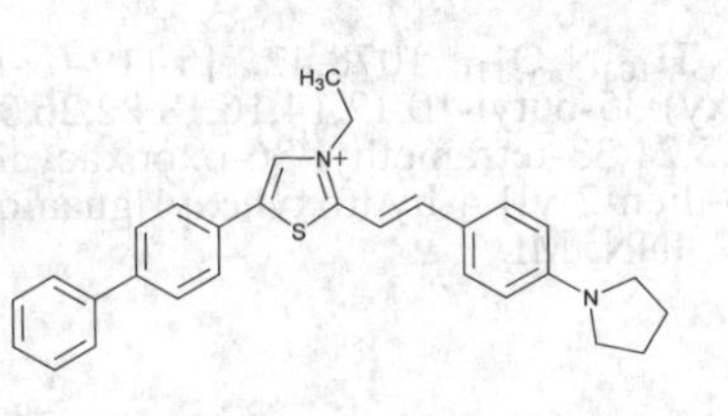

Prethcamide. *UNII-41A1FCW148. CAS-8015-51-8.*

Pretiadil. $C_{26}H_{31}N_3O_2S$. 449.61. 6,11-Dihydro-6-methyl-11-[3-[methyl(α-methylphenethyl)amino]propyl]dibenzo[1,2,5]thiadiazepine 5,5-dioxide. *UNII-9MG4L920HS. CAS-30840-27-8.* INN; DCF.

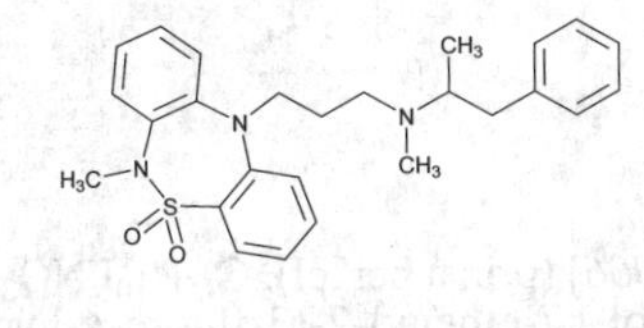

Prezatide Copper Acetate [*1993*] (prez′ a tide kop′ er as′ e tate). $C_{28}H_{46}CuN_{12}O_8 \cdot 2C_2H_4O_2$. 862.39. (1) Cuprate (1-), [*N*^{2}-(*N*-glycyl-L-histidyl)-L-lysinato][*N*^{2}-(*N*-glycyl-L-histidyl)-L-lysinato(2-)]-, hydrogen, diacetate; (2) Hydrogen [*N*^{2}-(*N*-glycyl-L-histidyl)-L-lysinato)][*N*^{2}-(*N*-glycyl-L-his-

tidyl)-L-lysinato(2-)]cuprate(1-), diacetate. *CAS-130120-57-9.* INN. *Immunomodulator.* Iamin (ProCyte) ◇*PC1020 acetate*

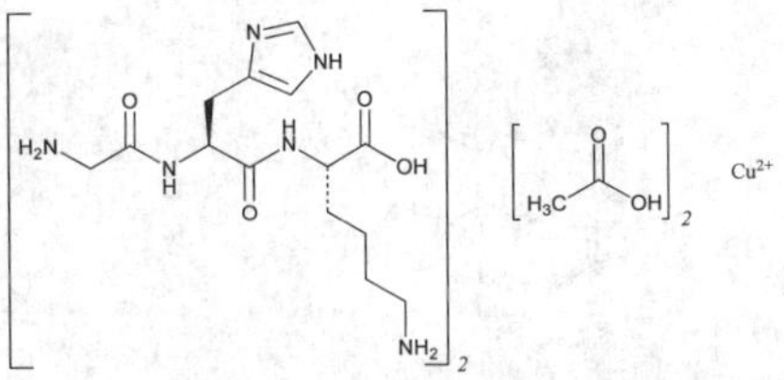

Pribecaine. $C_{16}H_{23}NO_3$. 277.36. 3-Piperidinopropyl *m*-anisate. *UNII-382TLA8X28. CAS-55837-22-4.* INN.

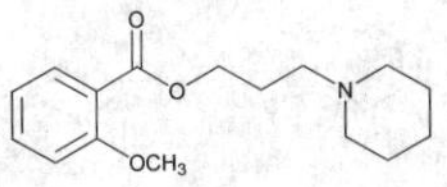

Pridefine Hydrochloride [*1979*] (pri′ de feen hye″ droe klor′ ide). $C_{19}H_{21}N \cdot HCl$. 299.84. [Pridefine is INN.] Pyrrolidine, 3-(diphenylmethylene)-1-ethyl-, hydrochloride. *CAS-23239-78-3; CAS-5370-41-2* [pridefine]. *Antidepressant.* ◇*AHR-1118*

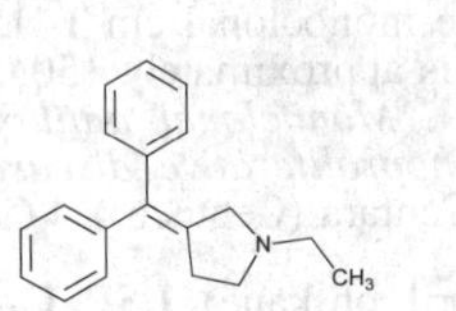

Prideperone. $C_{23}H_{24}FN_3O_3$. 409.45. 5-Cyano-*N*-[2-[4-(*p*-fluorobenzoyl)piperidino]ethyl]-*o*-anisamide. *UNII-78W508SA0Q. CAS-95374-52-0.* INN.

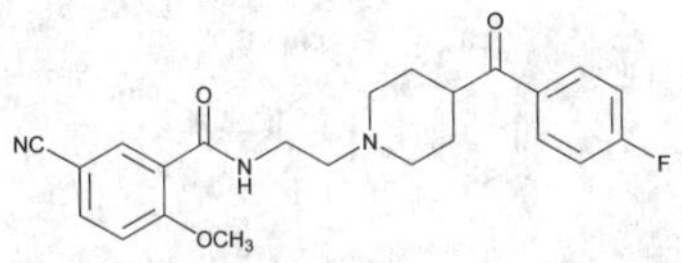

Pridinol. $C_{20}H_{25}NO$. 295.42. [Pridinol Mesilate is JAN.] α,α-Diphenyl-1-piperidinepropanol. *UNII-9E75Q6SUUB. CAS-511-45-5.* INN; DCF; MI. ◇*C-238*

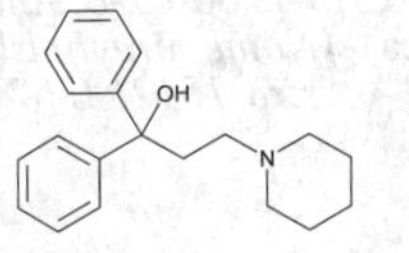

Prifelone [*1988*] (pri′ fe lone). $C_{19}H_{24}O_2S$. 316.46. (1) Methanone, [3,5-bis(1,1-dimethylethyl)-4-hydroxyphenyl]-2-thienyl-; (2) 3,5-Di-*tert*-butyl-4-hydroxyphenyl 2-thienyl ketone. *UNII-0414BW860U. CAS-69425-13-4.* INN. *Anti-inflammatory (dermatologic).* ◇*R-830; R-830T; S-16820*

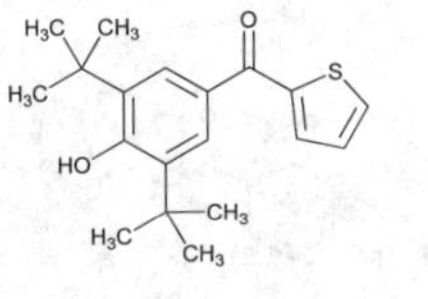

---

† Brand name formerly used, and/or firm no longer concerned with this product.

Prifinium Bromide. C$_{22}$H$_{28}$BrN. 386.37. 3-(Diphenylmethylene)-1,1-diethyl-2-methylpyrrolidinium bromide. *UNII-3B7O9ZC520. CAS-4630-95-9; CAS-10236-81-4* [prifinium]. INN; JAN; MI. ◇*PDB*

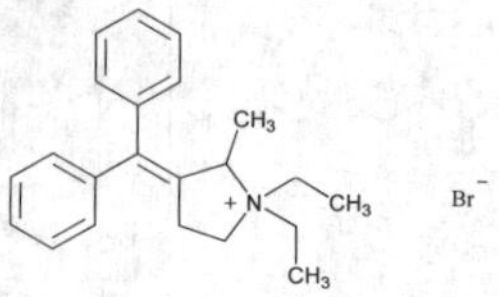

Prifuroline. C$_{14}$H$_{16}$N$_2$O. 228.29. 4-(2-Benzofuranyl)-2-(dimethylamino)-1-pyrroline. *UNII-OP2V3XRV2Y. CAS-70833-07-7.* INN.

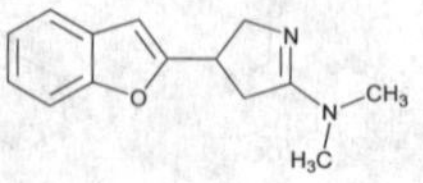

Priliximab [*1996*] (pri lix′ i mab). (1) Immunoglobulin G 1 (human-mouse monoclonal cm-T412 anti-human antigen CD 4), disulfide with human-mouse monoclonal cm-T412 κ-chain, dimer; (2) Immunoglobulin G 1 (human-mouse monoclonal cm-T412 anti-human antigen CD 4), disulfide with human-mouse monoclonal cm-T412 κ-chain, dimer. Molecular weight is approximately 150,000 daltons. *CAS-147191-91-1.* INN. *Monoclonal antibody (treatment of autoimmune lymphoproliferative diseases and in organ transplantation).* Centara (Centocor) ◇*CEN 000029*

Prilocaine [*1996*] (pril′ oh kane). **USP.** C$_{13}$H$_{20}$N$_2$O. 220.31. (1) Propanamide, *N*-(2-methylphenyl)-2-(propylamino)-; (2) 2-(Propylamino)-*o*-propionotoluidide; (3) (*RS*)-*N*-(2-Methylphenyl)-2-(propylamino)propanamide. *UNII-046O35D44R. CAS-721-50-6.* INN; BAN. *Anesthetic (local).*

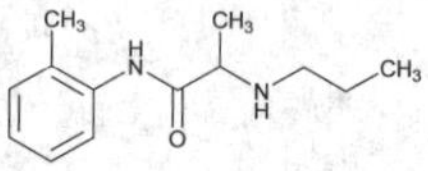

Prilocaine Hydrochloride [*1966*] (pril′ oh kane hye″ droe klor′ ide). **USP.** C$_{13}$H$_{20}$N$_2$O.HCl. 256.77. [Propitocaine Hydrochloride is JAN.] (1) Propanamide, *N*-(2-methylphenyl)-2-(propylamino)-, monohydrochloride; (2) 2-(Propylamino)-*o*-propionotoluidide monohydrochloride. *UNII-MJW015BAPH. CAS-1786-81-8. Anesthetic (local).* Citanest (AstraZeneca) *[Name previously used: Propitocaine Hydrochloride.]* ◇*Astra 1512; L-67*

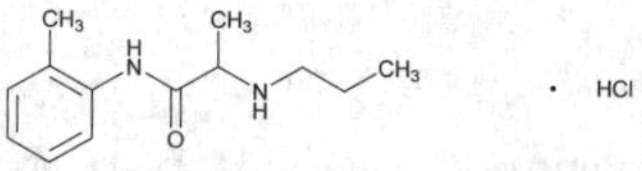

Primachine Phosphate — *See* Primaquine Phosphate.

Primaperone. C$_{15}$H$_{20}$FNO. 249.32. 4′-Fluoro-4-piperidinobutyrophenone. *UNII-BR551134L6. CAS-1219-35-8.* INN; DCF; MI.

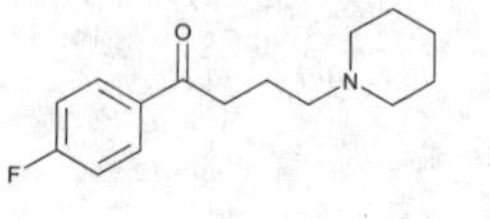

Primaquine Phosphate (prim′ a kwin fos′ fate). **USP.** C$_{15}$H$_{21}$N$_3$O.2H$_3$PO$_4$. 455.34. [Primaquine is INN and BAN.] (1) 1,4-Pentanediamine, *N*^{4}-(6-methoxy-8-quinolinyl)-, (±)-, phosphate (1:2); (2) (±)-8-[(4-Amino-1-methylbutyl)amino]-6-methoxyquinoline phosphate (1:2). *UNII-H0982HF78B; UNII-MVR3634GX1* [primaquine]. *CAS-63-45-6; CAS-90-34-6* [primaquine]. *Antimalarial.*

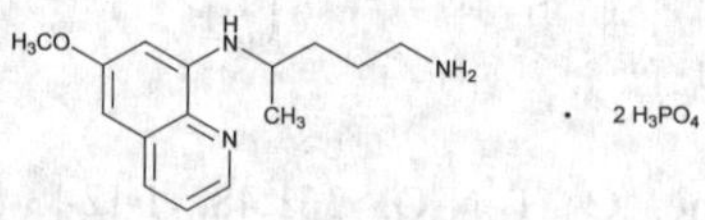

Primidolol [*1979*] (prim id′ oh lol). C$_{17}$H$_{23}$N$_3$O$_4$. 333.38. (1) 2,4-(1*H*,3*H*)-Pyrimidinedione, 1-[2-[[2-hydroxy-3-(2-methylphenoxy)propyl]amino]ethyl]-5-methyl-; (2) 1-[2-[[2-Hydroxy-3-(*o*-tolyloxy)propyl]amino]ethyl]thymine. *UNII-56QH73D78K. CAS-67227-55-8.* INN; BAN. *Antihypertensive; anti-anginal; cardiac depressant (anti-arrhythmic).* ◇*UK-11,443*

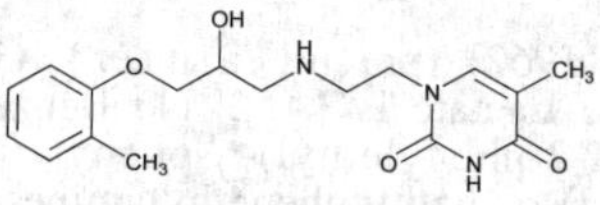

Primidone (prim′ i done). **USP.** C$_{12}$H$_{14}$N$_2$O$_2$. 218.25. (1) 4,6(1*H*,5*H*)-Pyrimidinedione, 5-ethyldihydro-5-phenyl-; (2) 5-Ethyldihydro-5-phenyl-4,6(1*H*,5*H*)-pyrimidinedione. *UNII-13AFD7670Q. CAS-125-33-7.* INN; BAN; JAN. *Anticonvulsant.* Mysoline (Valeant)

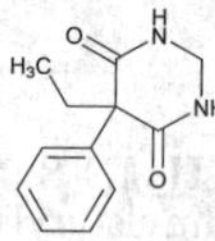

Primycin. C$_{55}$H$_{103}$N$_3$O$_{17}$. 1078.42. [5-[19-(α-D-Arabinofuranosyloxy)-35-butyl-10,12,14,16,18,22,26,30,34-nonahydroxy-3,5,21,33-tetramethyl-36-oxooxacyclohexatriaconta-4,20-dien-2-yl]-4-hydroxyhexyl]guanidine. *CAS-47917-41-9.* INN; MI.

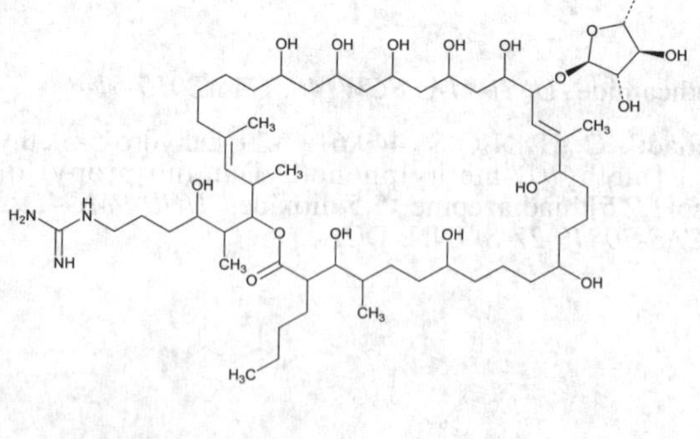

Prinaberel [*2006*] (prin a ber′ el). C$_{15}$H$_{10}$FNO$_3$. 271.24. (1) 5-Benzoxazolol, 7-ethenyl-2-(3-fluoro-4-hydroxyphenyl)-; (2) 7-Ethenyl-2-(3-fluoro-4-hydroxyphenyl)benzoxazol-5-ol. *UNII-A9C8MNF7CA. CAS-524684-52-4.* INN. *Treatment of arthritis.* ◇*ERB-041*

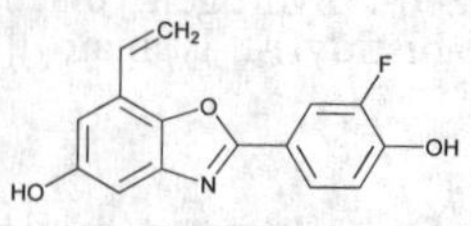

Prinodolol — *See* Pindolol.

Prinomastat [*1999*] (prin oh′ ma stat). $C_{18}H_{21}N_3$ O_5S_2. 423.51. (1) 3-Thiomorpholinecarboxamide, *N*-hydroxy-2,2-dimethyl-4-[[4-(4-pyridinyloxy)phenyl]sulfonyl]-, (*S*)-; (2) (*S*)-2,2-Dimethyl-4-[[*p*-(4-pyridyloxy)phenyl]sulfonyl]-3-thiomorpholinecarbohydroxamic acid. *CAS-192329-42-3.* INN. *Antineoplastic; antiangiogenic; treatment for retinal and subfoveal choroidal neovascularization (matrix metalloproteinase inhibitor).* ◇*AG3340*

Prinomide Tromethamine [*1988*] (prin′ oh mide troe meth′ a meen). $C_{15}H_{13}N_3O_2 \cdot C_4H_{11}NO_3$. 388.42. [Prinomide is INN.] (1) 1*H*-Pyrrole-2-propanamide, α-cyano-1-methyl-β-oxo-*N*-phenyl-, compound with 2-amino-2-hydroxymethyl)-1,3-propanediol (1:1); (2) α-Cyano-1-methyl-β-oxopyrrole-2-propionanilide compound with 2-amino-2-(hydroxymethyl)-1,3-propanediol (1:1). *UNII-33S1GFG04E; UNII-6NHC09L02I* [prinomide]. *CAS-109636-76-2; CAS-77639-66-8* [prinomide]. *Antirheumatic.* ◇*CGS 10787D*

Prinoxodan [*1990*] (prin ox′ oh dan). $C_{13}H_{14}N_4O_2$. 258.28. (1) 2(1*H*)-Quinazolinone, 3,4-dihydro-3-methyl-6-(1,4,5,6-tetrahydro-6-oxo-3-pyridazinyl)-; (2) 3,4-Dihydro-3-methyl-6-(1,4,5,6-tetrahydro-6-oxo-3-pyridazinyl)-2(1*H*)-quinazolinone. *UNII-W4VMH2E80M. CAS-111786-07-3.* INN. *Cardiotonic.* ◇*RGW-2938*

Prisotinol. $C_{11}H_{18}N_2O$. 194.27. (±)-6-[2-(Isopropylamino)-propyl]-3-pyridinol. *UNII-ZPO6B92P5Y. CAS-78997-40-7.* INN.

Pristinamycin. Antibiotic produced by *Streptomyces pristina spiralis,* or the same substance produced by any other means. *CAS-11006-76-1.* INN; BAN; DCF; MI. ◇*RP 7293*

Pritumumab. $C_{6440}H_{9968}N_{1708}O_{2016}S_{42}$. Immunoglobulin G, anti-(human vimentin) (human monoclonal CLN G11 γ1-chain), disulfide with human monoclonal CLN G11 κ-chain, dimer. *CAS-499212-74-7.* INN.

Prizidilol Hydrochloride [*1980*] (pri zye′ dil ol hye″ droe klor′ ide). $C_{17}H_{25}N_5O_2 \cdot 2HCl \cdot H_2O$. 422.35. [Prizidilol is INN and BAN.] (1) 2-Propanol, 1-[[(1,1-dimethylethyl)a-mino]-3-[2-(6-hydrazino-3-pyridazinyl)phenoxy]-, dihydrochloride monohydrate; (2) 1-(*tert*-Butylamino)-3-[*o*-(6-hydrazino-3-pyridazinyl)phenoxy]-2-propanol dihydrochloride monohydrate. *UNII-1Q4C0XA9H4; UNII-U6QG1RWA7B* [prizidilol hydrochloride anhydrous]. *CAS-73398-12-6; CAS-63642-19-3* [anhydrous]; *CAS-59010-44-5* [prizidilol]. *Antihypertensive.* ◇*SK&F 92657-A_2*

Proadifen Hydrochloride [*1964*] (proe ad′ i fen hye″ droe klor′ ide). $C_{23}H_{31}NO_2 \cdot HCl$. 389.96. [Proadifen is INN.] (1) Benzeneacetic acid, α-phenyl-α-propyl-, 2-(diethylamino)ethyl ester hydrochloride; (2) 2-(Diethylamino)ethyl 2,2-diphenylvalerate hydrochloride. *UNII-30624AA6X2. CAS-62-68-0; CAS-302-33-0* [proadifen]. *Synergist (nonspecific).* ◇*SK&F 525-A; RP 5171; NSC-39690*

Probarbital Sodium. $C_9H_{13}N_2NaO_3$. 220.20. Sodium derivative of 5-ethyl-5-isopropylbarbituric acid. *UNII-YDA0W423G6. CAS-143-82-8; CAS-76-76-6* [probarbital]. NF X; INN; MI. Ipral Sodium (Bristol-Myers Squibb†)

Probenecid (proe ben′ e sid). **USP.** $C_{13}H_{19}NO_4S$. 285.36. (1) Benzoic acid, 4-[(dipropylamino)sulfonyl]-; (2) *p*-(Dipropylsulfamoyl)benzoic acid. *UNII-PO572Z7917. CAS-57-66-9.* INN; BAN; JAN. *Uricosuric.* Benemid (Merck)

Probicromil Calcium [*1981*] (proe bik′ roe mil kal′ see um). $C_{17}H_{10}CaO_8$. 382.33. [Ambicromil is INN and BAN.] (1) 4*H*,6*H*-Benzo[1,2-*b*:5,4-*b*′]dipyran-2,8-dicarboxylic acid, 4,6-dioxo-10-propyl-, calcium salt (1:1); (2) Calcium 4,6-dioxo-10-propyl-4*H*,6*H*-benzo[1,2-*b*:5,4-*b*′]dipyran-2,8-dicarboxylate (1:1). *UNII-0U434950BU. CAS-71144-97-3* [Ca salt (1:1)]; *CAS-58805-38-2* [probicromil]. *Antiallergic (prophylactic).* ◇*FPL 58668KC*

Probucol [*1970*] (proe′ bue kol). **USP.** C$_{31}$H$_{48}$O$_2$S$_2$. 516.84. (1) Phenol, 4,4′-[(1-methylethylidene)bis(thio)]bis[2,6-bis(1,1-dimethylethyl)-; (2) Acetone bis(3,5-di-*tert*-butyl-4-hydroxyphenyl) mercaptole. *UNII-P3CTH044XJ. CAS-23288-49-5.* INN; BAN; JAN. *Antihyperlipidemic.* Lorelco (Sanofi Aventis) ◇*DH-581*

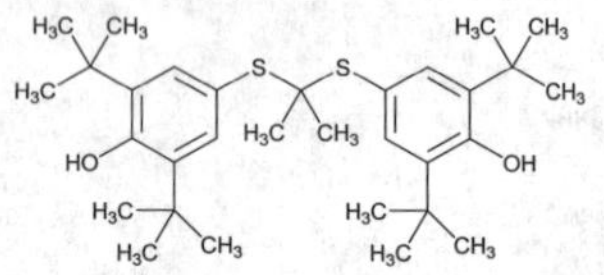

Procainamide Hydrochloride (proe kane′ a mide hye″ droe klor′ ide). **USP.** C$_{13}$H$_{21}$N$_3$O.HCl. 271.79. [Procainamide is INN and BAN.] (1) Benzamide, 4-amino-*N*-[2-(diethylamino)ethyl]-, monohydrochloride; (2) *p*-Amino-*N*-[2-(diethylamino)ethyl]benzamide monohydrochloride. *UNII-SI4064OOLX; UNII-L39WTC366D* [procainamide]. *CAS-614-39-1; CAS-51-06-9* [procainamide]. JAN. *Cardiac depressant (anti-arrhythmic).* Procan (Pfizer); Pronestyl (Apothecon)

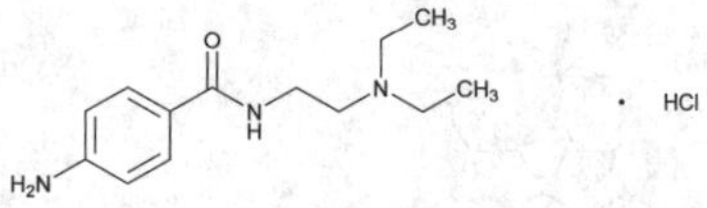

Procaine Borate. C$_{13}$H$_{25}$B$_5$N$_2$O$_{12}$. 455.40. [Procaine is INN and BAN.] 2-(Diethylamino)ethyl *p*-aminobenzoate borate (1:5). *UNII-4Z8Y51M438* [procaine]. *CAS-149-13-3; CAS-59-46-1* [procaine]. NF IX; MI.

Procaine Hydrochloride (proe′ kane hye″ droe klor′ ide). **USP.** C$_{13}$H$_{20}$N$_2$O$_2$.HCl. 272.77. (1) Benzoic acid, 4-amino-, 2-(diethylamino)ethyl ester, monohydrochloride; (2) 2-(Diethylamino)ethyl *p*-aminobenzoate monohydrochloride. *UNII-95URV01IDQ. CAS-51-05-8; CAS-59-46-1* [procaine]. JAN. *Anesthetic (local).* Novocain (Hospira)

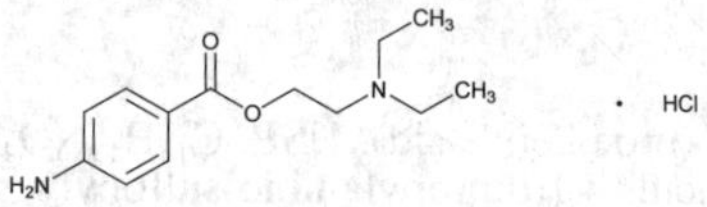

Procaine Penicillin (former BAN) — *See* Penicillin G Procaine.

Procarbazine Hydrochloride [*1967*] (proe kar′ ba zeen hye″ droe klor′ ide). **USP.** C$_{12}$H$_{19}$N$_3$O.HCl. 257.76. [Procarbazine is INN and BAN.] (1) Benzamide, *N*-(1-methylethyl)-4-[(2-methylhydrazino)methyl]-, monohydrochloride; (2) *N*-Isopropyl-α-(2-methylhydrazino)-*p*-toluamide monohydrochloride. *UNII-XH0NPH5ZX8; UNII-35S93Y190K* [procarbazine]. *CAS-366-70-1; CAS-671-16-9* [procarbazine]. JAN. *Antineoplastic.* Matulane (Sigma-Tau) ◇*Ro 4-6467/1; NSC-77213*

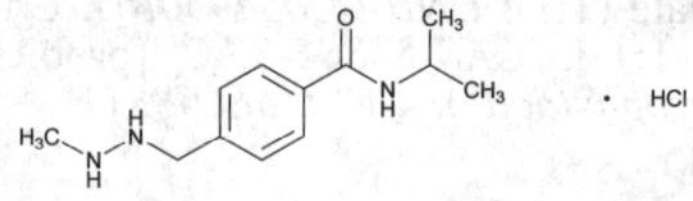

Procaterol Hydrochloride [*1980*] (proe ka′ ter ol hye″ droe klor′ ide). C$_{16}$H$_{22}$N$_2$O$_3$.HCl. 326.82. [Procaterol is INN and BAN.] (1) 2(1*H*)-Quinolinone, 8-hydroxy-5-[1-hydroxy-2-[(1-methylethyl)amino]butyl]-, monohydrochloride, (*R**,*S**)-, (±)-; (2) (±)-*erythro*-8-Hydroxy-5-[1-hydroxy-2-(isopropylamino)butyl]carbostyril monohydrochloride.

CAS-59828-07-8; CAS-72332-33-3 [procaterol]; *CAS-60443-17-6* [replaced]. JAN. *Bronchodilator.* Pro-Air (Parke-Davis†) ◇*CI-888*

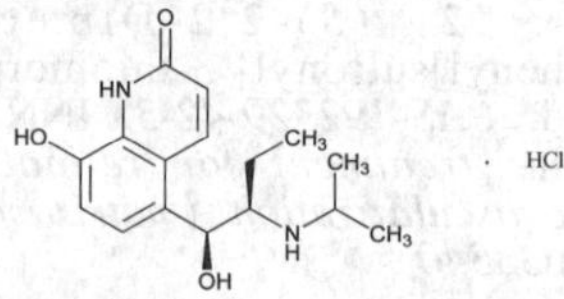

Prochlorperazine (proe″ klor per′ a zeen). **USP.** C$_{20}$H$_{24}$ClN$_3$S. 373.94. [Prochlorperazine Mesilate is JAN.] (1) 10*H*-Phenothiazine, 2-chloro-10-[3-(4-methyl-1-piperazinyl)propyl]-; (2) 2-Chloro-10-[3-(4-methyl-1-piperazinyl)propyl]phenothiazine. *UNII-YHP6YLT61T. CAS-58-38-8.* INN; BAN; JAN. *Anti-emetic.* Compazine (GlaxoSmithKline)

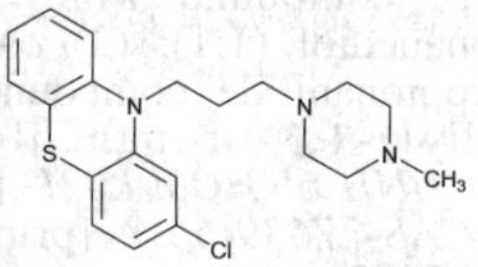

Prochlorperazine Edisylate (proe″ klor per′ a zeen e dis′ i late). **USP.** C$_{20}$H$_{24}$ClN$_3$S.C$_2$H$_6$O$_6$S$_2$. 564.14. (1) 10*H*-Phenothiazine, 2-chloro-10-[3-(4-methyl-1-piperazinyl)-propyl]-, 1,2-ethanedisulfonate (1:1); (2) 2-Chloro-10-[3-(4-methyl-1-piperazinyl)propyl]phenothiazine 1,2-ethanedisulfonate (1:1). *UNII-PG20W5VQZS. CAS-1257-78-9; CAS-58-38-8* [prochlorperazine]. *Anti-emetic; antipsychotic.* Compazine (GlaxoSmithKline)

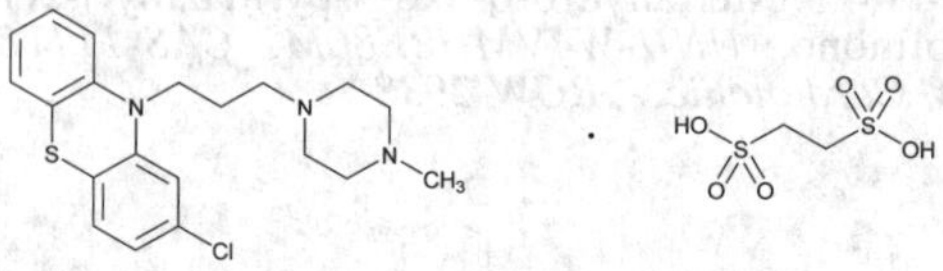

Prochlorperazine Ethanedisulfonate — *See* Prochlorperazine Edisylate.

Prochlorperazine Maleate (proe″ klor per′ a zeen mal′ ee ate). **USP.** C$_{20}$H$_{24}$ClN$_3$S.2C$_4$H$_4$O$_4$. 606.09. (1) 10*H*-Phenothiazine, 2-chloro-10-[3-(4-methyl-1-piperazinyl)pro-pyl]-, (*Z*)-2-butenedioate (1:2); (2) 2-Chloro-10-[3-(4-methyl-1-piperazinyl)propyl]phenothiazine maleate (1:2). *UNII-I1T8O1JTL6. CAS-84-02-6; CAS-58-38-8* [prochlorperazine]. JAN. *Anti-emetic; antipsychotic.* Compazine (GlaxoSmithKline)

Procinolol. C$_{15}$H$_{23}$NO$_2$. 249.35. 1-(*o*-Cyclopropylphenoxy)-3-(isopropylamino)-2-propanol. *UNII-SLJ0HIL21J. CAS-27325-36-6.* INN; DCF. ◇*SD 2124-01*

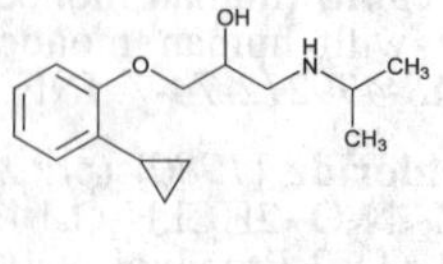

Procinonide [*1977*] (proe sin′ oh nide). C$_{27}$H$_{34}$F$_2$O$_7$. 508.55. (1) Pregna-1,4-diene-3,20-dione, 6,9-difluoro-11-hydroxy-16,17-[(1-methylethylidene)bis(oxy)]-21-(1-oxopropoxy)-, (6α,11β,16α)-; (2) 6α,9-Difluoro-11β,16α,17,21-tetrahydroxypregna-1,4-diene-3,20-dione cyclic 16,17-acetal with acetone, 21-propionate. *CAS-58497-00-0.* INN. *Adrenocortical steroid.* ◇*RS-2362*

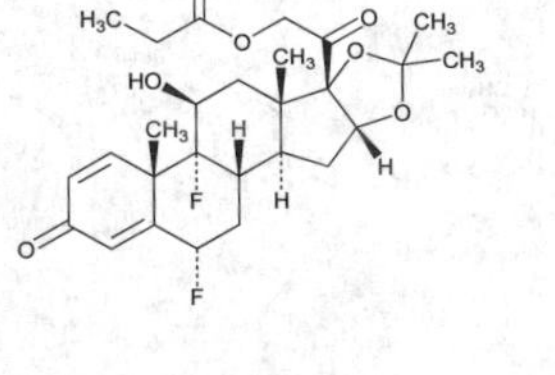

Proclonol [*1967*] (proe′ klo nol). $C_{16}H_{14}Cl_2O$. 293.19. (1) Benzenemethanol, 4-chloro-α-(4-chlorophenyl)-α-cyclopropyl-; (2) Bis(*p*-chlorophenyl)cyclopropylmethanol. *CAS-14088-71-2.* INN; BAN. *Anthelmintic; antifungal.* ◇*R 8284*

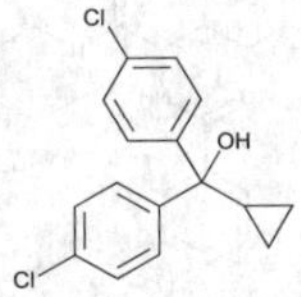

Procodazole. $C_{10}H_{10}N_2O_2$. 190.20. 2-Benzimidazolepropionic acid. *UNII-SG5IU7FD3R. CAS-23249-97-0.* INN; MI.

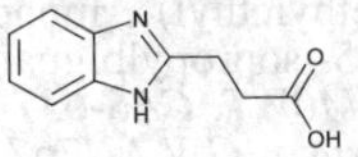

Procromil. $C_{17}H_{18}O_4$. 286.32. 6,7,8,9-Tetrahydro-4-oxo-10-propyl-4*H*-benzo[*g*]chromene-2-carboxylic acid. *CAS-60400-86-4.* BAN.

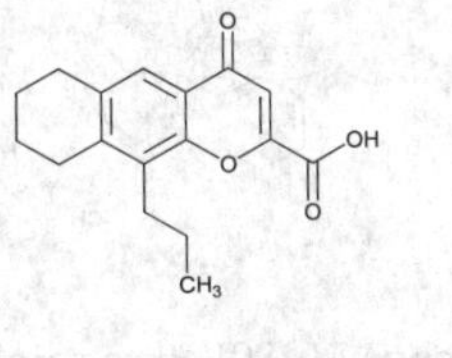

Procyclidine Hydrochloride (proe sye′ kli deen hye″ droe klor′ ide). **USP.** $C_{19}H_{29}NO.HCl$. 323.90. [Procyclidine is INN and BAN.] (1) 1-Pyrrolidinepropanol, α-cyclohexyl-α-phenyl-, hydrochloride; (2) α-Cyclohexyl-α-phenyl-1-pyrrolidinepropanol hydrochloride. *UNII-CQC932Z7YW; UNII-C6QE1Q1TKR* [procyclidine]. *CAS-1508-76-5; CAS-77-37-2* [procyclidine]. *Antiparkinsonian; relaxant (skeletal muscle).* Kemadrin (King)

Procymate. $C_{10}H_{19}NO_2$. 185.26. 1-Cyclohexylpropyl carbamate. *UNII-308EUN932K. CAS-13931-64-1.* INN; DCF; MI.

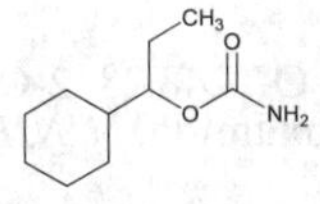

Prodeconium Bromide. $C_{28}H_{58}Br_2N_2O_6$. 678.58. Dipropyl ester of [decamethylenebis(oxymethylene)]bis[(carboxymethyl)dimethylammonium bromide]. *UNII-I38846JP2L. CAS-3690-61-7.* INN. ◇*G-25178*

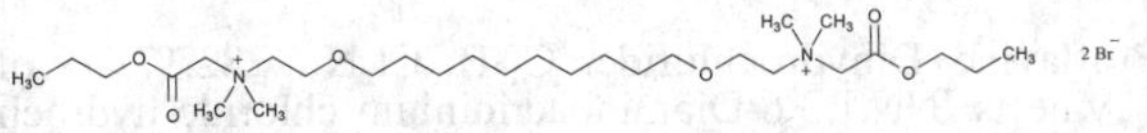

Prodilidine Hydrochloride [*1962*] (proe dil′ i deen hye″ droe klor′ ide). $C_{15}H_{21}NO_2.HCl$. 283.79. [Prodilidine is INN.] (1) 3-Pyrrolidinol, 1,2-dimethyl-3-phenyl-, propanoate (ester), hydrochloride; (2) 1,2-Dimethyl-3-phenyl-3-pyrrolidinol propionate (ester) hydrochloride. *CAS-3734-16-5; CAS-3734-17-6* [prodilidine]. *Analgesic.* ◇*A-1981-12; CI 427; 5054*

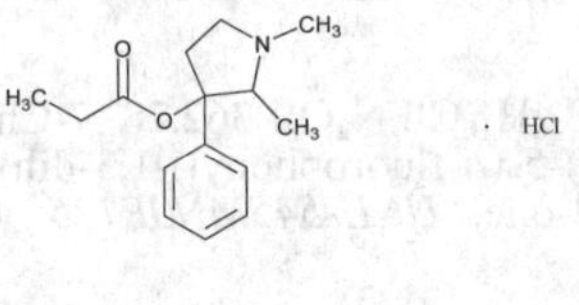

Prodipine. $C_{20}H_{25}N$. 279.42. 1-Isopropyl-4,4-diphenylpiperidine. *UNII-51567MYG7V. CAS-31314-38-2.* INN; MI.

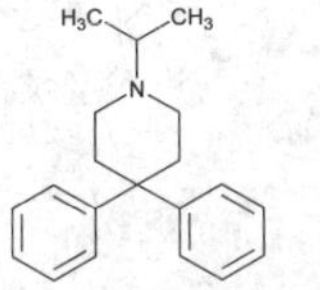

Prodolic Acid [*1973*] (proe doe′ lik as′ id). $C_{16}H_{19}NO_3$. 273.33. (1) Pyrano[3,4-*b*]indole-1-acetic acid, 1,3,4,9-tetrahydro-1-propyl-; (2) 1,3,4,9-Tetrahydro-1-propylpyrano[3,4-*b*]indole-1-acetic acid. *CAS-36505-82-5.* INN. *Anti-inflammatory.* ◇*AY-23,289*

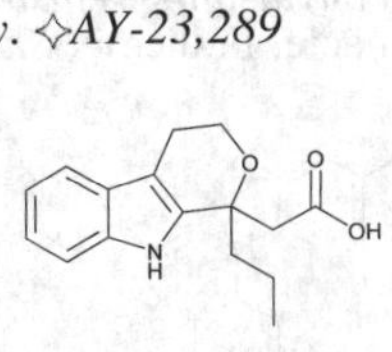

Profadol Hydrochloride [*1971*] (proe′ fa dol hye″ droe klor′ ide). $C_{14}H_{21}NO.HCl$. 255.78. [Profadol is INN and BAN.] (1) Phenol, 3-(1-methyl-3-propyl-3-pyrrolidinyl)-, hydrochloride; (2) *m*-(1-Methyl-3-propyl-3-pyrrolidinyl)phenol hydrochloride. *CAS-2324-94-9; CAS-428-37-5* [profadol]. *Analgesic.* Centrac (Parke-Davis†) ◇*CI-572; A-2205*

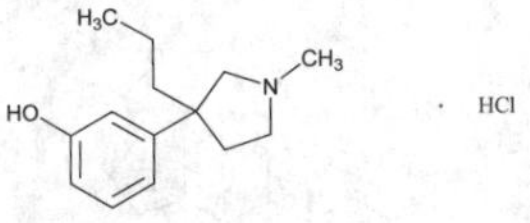

Profenamine (INN, BAN, DCF) — *See* Ethopropazine Hydrochloride.

---

† Brand name formerly used, and/or firm no longer concerned with this product.

Profenamine Hibenzate (JAN) — *See* Ethopropazine Hydrochloride.

Profenamine Hydrochloride (JAN) — *See* Ethopropazine Hydrochloride.

Profexalone. $C_{13}H_{16}N_2O_3$. 248.28. 2-Oxo-5-phenyl-*N*-propyl-3-oxazolidinecarboxamide. *UNII-3T29053XGS*. *CAS-34740-13-1*. INN.

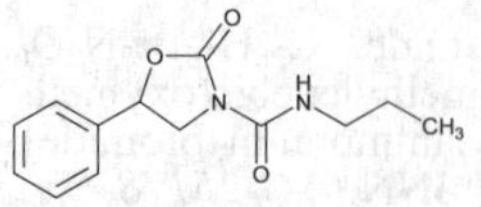

Proflavine Dihydrochloride. $C_{13}H_{13}Cl_2N_3$. 282.17. [Proflavine is INN.] 3,6-Diaminoacridinium chloride hydrochloride. *UNII-CY3RNB3K4T* [proflavine]. *CAS-531-73-7; CAS-92-62-6* [proflavine]. NF IX; MI.

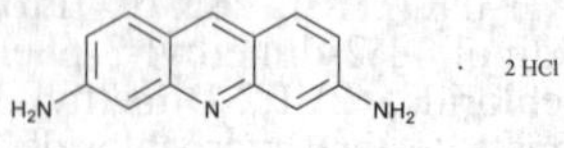

Proflavine Sulfate. *UNII-2961Y60ATP; UNII-CY3RNB3K4T* [proflavine]. *CAS-553-30-0; CAS-92-62-6* [proflavine]. NF IX; MI.

Proflazepam. $C_{18}H_{16}ClFN_2O_3$. 362.78. 7-Chloro-1-(2,3-dihydroxypropyl)-5-(*o*-fluorophenyl)-1,3-dihydro-2*H*-1,4-benzodiazepin-2-one. *UNII-545MN0F125*. *CAS-52829-30-8*. INN.

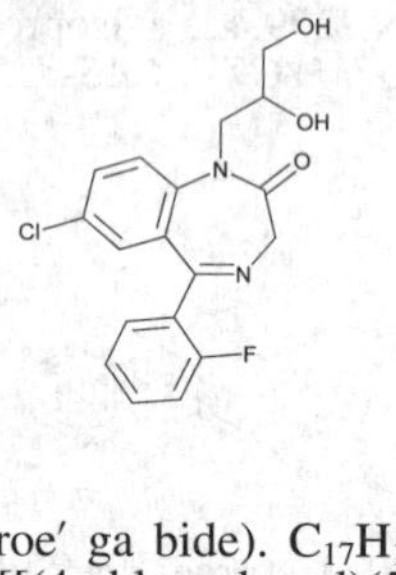

Progabide [*1984*] (proe′ ga bide). $C_{17}H_{16}ClFN_2O_2$. 334.77. (1) Butanamide, 4-[[(4-chlorophenyl)(5-fluoro-2-hydroxyphenyl)methylene]amino]-; (2) 4-[[α-(*p*-Chlorophenyl)-5-fluorosalicylidene]amino]butyramide. *CAS-62666-20-0*. INN; BAN. *Anticonvulsant; relaxant (muscle)*. Gabren (Synthelabo Pharmacie, France) ✧*SL 76 002*

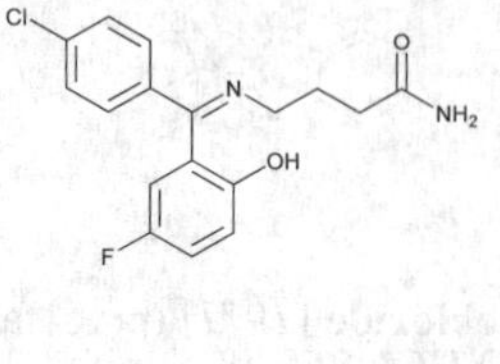

Progesterone (proe jes′ ter one). **USP**. $C_{21}H_{30}O_2$. 314.46. (1) Pregn-4-ene-3,20-dione; (2) Progesterone. *UNII-4G7DS2Q64Y*. *CAS-57-83-0*. INN; BAN; JAN. *Progestin*. Crinone (Columbia); Endometrin (Ferring Pharmaceuticals); Prometrium (Unimed) ✧*NSC-9704*

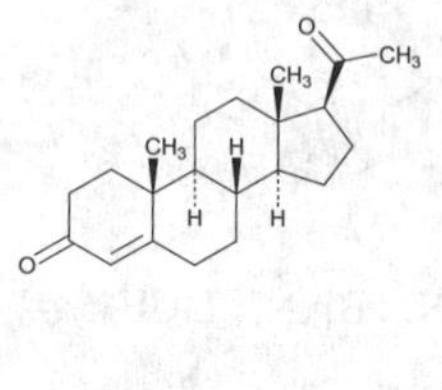

Proglumetacin. $C_{46}H_{58}ClN_5O_8$. 844.43. [Proglumetacin Maleate is JAN.] 3-[4-(2-Hydroxyethyl)-1-piperazinyl]propyl DL-4-benzamido-*N,N*-dipropylglutaramate 1-(*p*-chlorobenzoyl)-5-methoxy-2-methylindole-3-acetate (ester). *CAS-57132-53-3*. INN; BAN; MI.

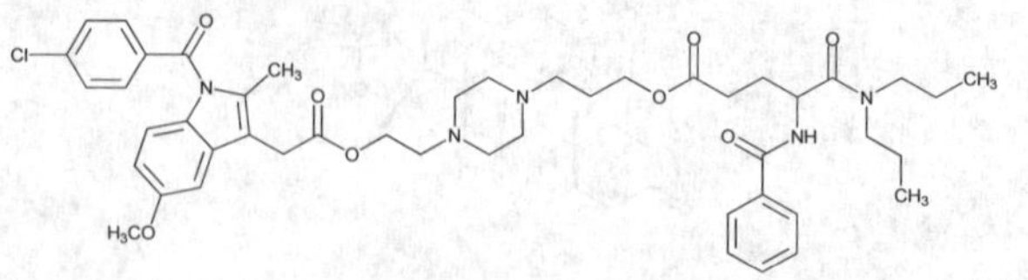

Proglumide [*1969*] (proe gloo′ mide). $C_{18}H_{26}N_2O_4$. 334.41. (1) Pentanoic acid, 4-(benzoylamino)-5-(dipropylamino)-5-oxo-, (±)-; (2) (±)-4-Benzamido-*N,N*-dipropylglutaramic acid. *CAS-6620-60-6*. INN; BAN; JAN. *Anticholinergic*. Nulsa (Wallace†) ✧*W-5219*

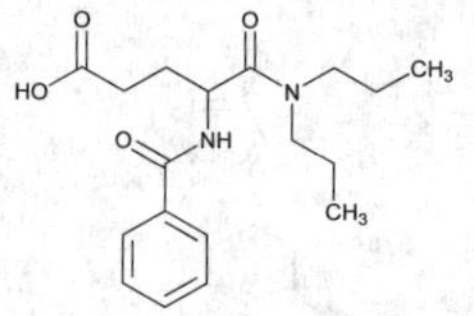

Proguanil (INN, BAN, DCF) — *See* Chloroguanide Hydrochloride.

Proguanil Hydrochloride [*2000*] (proe gwahn′ il hye″ droe klor′ ide). (1) Imidodicarbonimidic diamide, *N*-(4-chlorophenyl)-*N′*-(1-methylethyl)-, monohydrochloride; (2) 1-(*p*-Chlorophenyl)-5-isopropylbiguanide monohydrochloride. *UNII-R71Y86M0WT*. *CAS-637-32-1*. *Prophylaxis and treatment of malaria*. ✧*GW AH7673A; 336U50*

Proheptazine. $C_{17}H_{25}NO_2$. 275.39. 1,3-Dimethyl-4-phenyl-4-propionyloxyazacycloheptane. *UNII-S23189WW7E*. *CAS-77-14-5*. INN; BAN; MI.

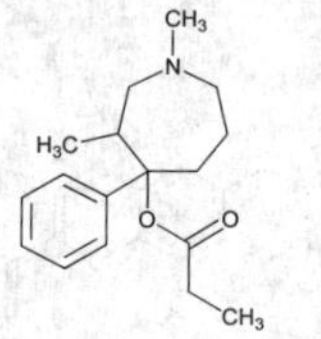

Proinsulin Human [*1989*] (proe in′ su lin hue′ man). $C_{410}H_{638}N_{114}O_{127}S_6$. 9388.53. (1) Proinsulin (pig), 30-L-threonine-36-L-aspartic acid-37-L-leucine-39-L-valine-41-L-glutamine-48-L-proline-49a-*endo*-L-alanine-50a-*endo*-L-serine-53-L-proline-59-L-serine-60-L-leucine-; (2) Proinsulin (human). *CAS-67422-14-4*. *Antidiabetic*. ✧*LY167005*

FVNQHLCGSH LVEALYLVCG ERGFFYTPKT RREAEDLQVG QVELGGGPGA
GSLQPLALEG SLQKRGIVEQ CCTSICSLYQ LENYCN

Proligestone. $C_{24}H_{34}O_4$. 386.52. 14,17-Dihydroxypregn-4-ene-3,20-dione, cyclic acetal with propionaldehyde. *UNII-55772LJ01V*. *CAS-23873-85-0*. INN; BAN.

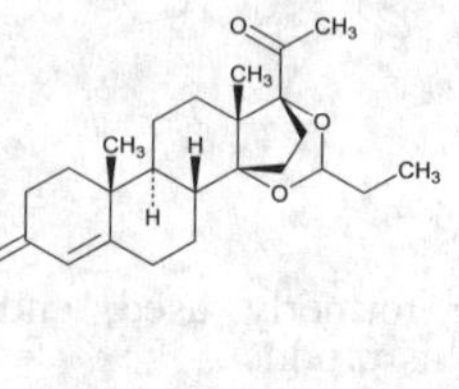

Proline [*1979*] (proe′ leen). **USP**. $C_5H_9NO_2$. 115.13. (1) L-Proline; (2) L-Proline. *UNII-9DLQ4CIU6V. CAS-147-85-3* [L]. INN. *Amino acid.*

Prolintane Hydrochloride [*1966*] (proe lin′ tane hye″ droe klor′ ide). $C_{15}H_{23}N.HCl$. 253.81. [Prolintane is INN and BAN.] (1) Pyrrolidine, 1-[1-(phenylmethyl)butyl]-, hydrochloride; (2) 1-(α-Propylphenethyl)pyrrolidine hydrochloride. *CAS-1211-28-5; CAS-493-92-5* [prolintane]. *Antidepressant.*

Prolonium Iodide. $C_9H_{24}I_2N_2O$. 430.11. (2-Hydroxytrimethylene)bis(trimethylammonium iodide). *UNII-VKH95UNQ6N. CAS-123-47-7.* INN; MI. Entodon (Sterling Winthrop†)

Promazine Hydrochloride (proe′ ma zeen hye″ droe klor′ ide). **USP**. $C_{17}H_{20}N_2S.HCl$. 320.88. [Promazine is INN and BAN.] (1) 10-*H*-Phenothiazine-10-propanamine, *N,N*-dimethyl-, monohydrochloride; (2) 10-[3-(Dimethylamino)propyl]phenothiazine monohydrochloride. *UNII-U16EOR79U4; UNII-O9M39HTM5W* [promazine]. *CAS-53-60-1; CAS-58-40-2* [promazine]. *Antipsychotic.* Sparine (Wyeth)

Promegestone. $C_{22}H_{30}O_2$. 326.47. 17α-Methyl-17-propionylestra-4,9-dien-3-one. *UNII-9XE0V2SQYX. CAS-34184-77-5.* INN; MI.

Promelase. [Semi-alkaline Proteinase is JAN.] *Aspergillus melleus* alkaline proteinase. INN.

Promestriene. $C_{22}H_{32}O_2$. 328.49. 17β-Methoxy-3-propoxyestra-1,3,5(10)-triene. *UNII-GXM4PER6WZ. CAS-39219-28-8.* INN; DCF.

Promethazine Hydrochloride (proe meth′ a zeen hye″ droe klor′ ide). **USP**. $C_{17}H_{20}N_2S.HCl$. 320.88. [Promethazine is INN and BAN.] (1) 10*H*-Phenothiazine-10-ethanamine, *N,N*,α-trimethyl-, monohydrochloride, (±)-; (2) (±)-10-[2-(Dimethylamino)propyl]phenothiazine monohydrochloride. *UNII-R61ZEH7I1I; UNII-FF28EJQ494* [promethazine]. *CAS-58-33-3; CAS-60-87-7* [promethazine]. JAN. *Anti-emetic; antihistaminic.* Phenergan (Wyeth); Remsed (Bristol-Myers Squibb)

Promethazine Teoclate. $C_{17}H_{20}N_2S.C_7H_7ClN_4O_2$. 499.03. 10-(2-Dimethylaminopropyl)phenothiazine compound of 8-chlorotheophylline. *UNII-S5PUP23U26. CAS-17693-51-5.* INN; BAN; JAN. *[Name previously used: Promethazine Theoclate.]*

Promethestrol — *See* Methestrol.

Promethoestrol (previously used name) — *See* Methestrol.

Promolate. $C_{16}H_{23}NO_4$. 293.36. 2-Morpholinoethyl 2-methyl-2-phenoxypropionate. *UNII-5WGM277OKR. CAS-3615-74-5.* INN.

Promoxolane. $C_{10}H_{20}O_3$. 188.26. 2,2-Diisopropyl-1,3-dioxolane-4-methanol. *CAS-470-43-9.* INN; BAN; MI. Dimethylane (Marion Merrell Dow†) *[Name previously used: Promoxolan.]*

Pronase. Proteolytic enzyme obtained from *Streptomyces griseus.* JAN.

Pronetalol. $C_{15}H_{19}NO$. 229.32. 2-Isopropylamino-1-(naphth-2-yl)ethanol. *CAS-54-80-8*. INN; BAN. *[Name previously used: Pronethalol.]* ⟡*ICI 38174 [as hydrochloride]; AY 6204 [as hydrochloride]*

Pronethalol (previously used name) — *See* Pronetalol.

Propacetamol. $C_{14}H_{20}N_2O_3$. 264.32. *N,N*-Diethylglycine, ester with 4′-hydroxyacetanilide. *UNII-5CHW4JMR82. CAS-66532-85-2*. INN; BAN; MI.

Propafenone Hydrochloride [*1988*] (proe pa′ fen one hye″ droe klor′ ide). **USP**. $C_{21}H_{27}NO_3 \cdot HCl$. 377.90. [Propafenone is INN and BAN.] (1) 1-Propanone, 1-[2-[2-hydroxy-3-(propylamino)propoxy]phenyl]-3-phenyl-, hydrochloride; (2) 2′-[2-Hydroxy-3-(propylamino)propoxy]-3-phenylpropiophenone hydrochloride. *UNII-33XCH0HOCD; UNII-68IQX3T69U [propafenone]. CAS-34183-22-7; CAS-54063-53-5 [propafenone]*. JAN. *Cardiac depressant (anti-arrhythmic)*. Rythmol (Reliant)

Propagermanium. $(C_3H_5GeO_{3.5})_n$. Polymer obtained from 3-(trihydroxygermyl)propionic acid. INN.

Propamidine. $C_{17}H_{20}N_4O_2$. 312.37. 4,4′-(Trimethylenedioxy)dibenzamidine. *CAS-104-32-5*. INN; BAN; DCF; MI. ⟡*M&B 782 [as isethionate]*

Propaminodiphen — *See* Pramiverine.

Propane (proe′ pane). **NF**. C_3H_8. 44.10. Propane. *UNII-T75W9911L6. CAS-74-98-6. Aerosol propellant.*

Propanidid [*1963*] (proe pan′ i did). $C_{18}H_{27}NO_5$. 337.41. (1) Benzeneacetic acid, 4-[2-(diethylamino)-2-oxoethoxy]-3-methoxy-, propyl ester; (2) Propyl {4-[(diethylcarbamoyl)methoxy]-3-methoxyphenyl}acetate. *CAS-1421-14-3.*

INN; BAN. *Anesthetic (intravenous)*. Epontol (Farbenfabriken Bayer A.G., Germany) ⟡*FBA 1420; Bayer 1420; WH 5668; TH-2180*

Propanocaine. $C_{20}H_{25}NO_2$. 311.42. α-(2-Diethylaminoethyl)-benzyl benzoate. *UNII-99LL28NYJ2. CAS-493-76-5*. INN; DCF; MI.

Propantheline Bromide (proe pan′ the leen broe′ mide). **USP**. $C_{23}H_{30}BrNO_3$. 448.39. (1) 2-Propanaminium, *N*-methyl-*N*-(1-methylethyl)-*N*-[2-[(9*H*-xanthen-9-ylcarbonyl)oxy]ethyl]-, bromide; (2) (2-Hydroxyethyl)diisopropylmethylammonium bromide xanthene-9-carboxylate. *UNII-UX9Z118X9F. CAS-50-34-0; CAS-298-50-0 [propantheline]*. INN; BAN; JAN. *Anticholinergic*. Probanthine (Shire)

Proparacaine Hydrochloride (proe par′ a kane hye″ droe klor′ ide). **USP**. $C_{16}H_{26}N_2O_3 \cdot HCl$. 330.85. [Proxymetacaine is INN and BAN.] (1) Benzoic acid, 3-amino-4-propoxy-, 2-(diethylamino)ethyl ester, monohydrochloride; (2) 2-(Diethylamino)ethyl 3-amino-4-propoxybenzoate monohydrochloride. *UNII-U96OL57GOY; UNII-B4OB0JHI1X [proparacaine]. CAS-5875-06-9; CAS-499-67-2 [proparacaine]*. *Anesthetic (topical, ophthalmic)*. Alcaine (Alcon); Ophthaine (Apothecon); Ophthetic (Allergan); Paracaine (Optopics)

Propatyl Nitrate [*1963*] (proe′ pa til nye′ trate). $C_6H_{11}N_3O_9$. 269.17. [Propatylnitrate is INN and BAN.] (1) 1,3-Propanediol, 2-ethyl-2-[(nitrooxy)methyl]-, dinitrate (ester); (2) 2-Ethyl-2-(hydroxymethyl)-1,3-propanediol trinitrate. *UNII-AJT2YN495R. CAS-2921-92-8*. *Vasodilator (coronary)*. Etrynit (Sterling Winthrop†) ⟡*ETTN; Win 9317*

Propazolamide. $C_5H_8N_4O_3S_2$. 236.27. 5-Propionamido-1,3,4-thiadiazole-2-sulfonamide. *CAS-98-75-9.* INN.

Propenidazole. $C_{11}H_{13}N_3O_5$. 267.24. Ethyl *trans*-α-acetyl-1-methyl-5-nitroimidazole-2-acrylate. *UNII-F0O89MB7QE. CAS-76448-31-2.* INN.

Propentofylline. $C_{15}H_{22}N_4O_3$. 306.36. 3-Methyl-1-(5-oxohexyl)-7-propylxanthine. *CAS-55242-55-2.* INN; BAN; JAN; MI. ◇*HWA 285*

Propenzolate Hydrochloride [*1962*] (proe pen′ zoe late hye″ droe klor′ ide). $C_{20}H_{29}NO_3$.HCl. 367.91. [Oxyclipine is INN.] (1) Benzeneacetic acid, α-cyclohexyl-α-hydroxy-, ($\pm$)-, (+)-1-methyl-3-piperidinyl ester, hydrochloride; (2) (+)-1-Methyl-3-piperidyl ($\pm$)-α-phenylcyclohexaneglycolate hydrochloride. *CAS-1420-03-7; CAS-4354-45-4* [propenzolate]. *Anticholinergic.* Delinal (Marion Merrell Dow†) ◇*NDR 263*

Propericiazine (JAN, DCF) — *See* Periciazine.

Properidine. $C_{16}H_{23}NO_2$. 261.36. 1-Methyl-4-phenylpiperidine-4-carboxylic acid isopropyl ester. *UNII-R1493W1CJ0. CAS-561-76-2.* INN; BAN; DCF; MI.

Propetamide. $C_{14}H_{22}N_2O_2$. 250.34. 2-*p*-Phenetidino-*N*-propylpropionamide. *UNII-U9R24EH050. CAS-730-07-4.* INN.

Propetamphos. $C_{10}H_{20}NO_4PS$. 281.31. Isopropyl (*E*)-3-[(ethylamino)(methoxy)phosphino-thioyloxy]but-2-enoate. *UNII-G4A07F635U. CAS-31218-83-4.* BAN.

Propetandrol. $C_{23}H_{36}O_3$. 360.53. 19-Nor-17α-pregn-4-ene-3β,17-diol 3-propionate. *CAS-3638-82-2.* INN; DCF. ◇*SC-7294*

Prophenamine Hydrochloride — *See* Ethopropazine Hydrochloride.

Propicillin. $C_{18}H_{22}N_2O_5S$. 378.44. [Propicillin Potassium is JAN.] (1-Phenoxypropyl)penicillin. *UNII-8X1R260V33. CAS-551-27-9.* INN; BAN; DCF; MI.

Propikacin [*1980*] (proe″ pi kay′ sin). $C_{21}H_{43}N_5O_{12}$. 557.59. (1) D-Streptamine, *O*-3-amino-3-deoxy-α-D-glucopyranosyl(1→6)-*O*-[2,6-diamino-2,6-dideoxy-α-D-glucopyranosyl(1→4)]-2-deoxy-N^1-[2-hydroxy-1-(hydroxymethyl)ethyl]-; (2) *O*-3-Amino-3-deoxy-α-D-glucopyranosyl(1→4)-*O*-[2,6-diamino-2,6-dideoxy-α-D-glucopyranosyl(1→6)]-2-deoxy-N^3-[2-hydroxy-1-(hydroxymethyl)ethyl]-L-streptamine. *UNII-9X6F5H479X. CAS-66887-96-5.* INN. *Antibacterial.* ◇*UK-31,214*

Propinetidine. $C_{19}H_{25}NO_2$. 299.41. 1-Phenethyl-4-(2-propynyl)-4-piperidinol propionate. *UNII-70QV580PA4. CAS-3811-53-8.* INN.

---

† Brand name formerly used, and/or firm no longer concerned with this product.

Propiodal — *See* Prolonium Iodide.

Propiolactone [*1964*] (proe″ pee oh lak′ tone). $C_3H_4O_2$. 72.06. (1) 2-Oxetanone; (2) β-Propiolactone. *UNII-6RC3ZT4HB0. CAS-57-57-8.* INN; BAN. *Disinfectant.* Betaprone (Forest) ◇*NSC-21626*

Propiomazine [*1962*] (proe″ pee oh′ ma zeen). $C_{20}H_{24}N_2OS$. 340.48. (1) 1-Propanone, 1-[10-[2-(dimethylamino)propyl]-10*H*-phenothiazin-2-yl]-; (2) 1-[10-[2-(Dimethylamino)propyl]phenothiazin-2-yl]-1-propanone. *UNII-242Z0PM79Y. CAS-362-29-8.* INN; BAN. *Sedative (preanesthetic).* ◇*CB 1678; Wy-1359*

Propiomazine Hydrochloride. $C_{20}H_{24}N_2OS{\cdot}HCl$. 376.94. (1) 1-Propanone, 1-[10-[2-(dimethylamino)propyl]-10*H*-phenothiazin-2-yl]-, monohydrochloride; (2) 1-[10-[2-(Dimethylamino)propyl]phenothiazin-2-yl]-1-propanone monohydrochloride. *UNII-70BO17YR03; UNII-242Z0PM79Y* [propiomazine]. *CAS-1240-15-9; CAS-362-29-8* [propiomazine]. USP XXII. Largon (Baxter Healthcare)

Propionic Acid (proe″ pee on′ ik as′ id). **NF.** $C_3H_6O_2$. 74.08. (1) Propanoic acid; (2) Propionic acid. *UNII-JHU490R-VYR. CAS-79-09-4. Antimicrobial; pharmaceutic aid (acidifying agent).*

Propionyl Erythromycin Lauryl Sulfate — *See* Erythromycin Estolate.

Propipocaine. $C_{17}H_{25}NO_2$. 275.39. 3-Piperidino-4′-propoxy-propiophenone. *UNII-U09698V56W. CAS-3670-68-6.* INN; MI.

Propiram Fumarate [*1967*] (proe′ pi ram fue′ ma rate). $C_{16}H_{25}N_3O{\cdot}C_4H_4O_4$. 391.46. [Propiram is INN and BAN.] (1) Propanamide, *N*-[1-methyl-2-(1-piperidinyl)ethyl]-*N*-2-pyridinyl-, (*E*)-2-butenedioate (1:1); (2) *N*-(1-Methyl-2-piperidinoethyl)-*N*-2-pyridylpropionamide fumarate (1:1). *UNII-AVG0GBV8AP. CAS-13717-04-9; CAS-15686-91-6* [propiram]. *Analgesic.* Dirame (Bayer†) ◇*BAY 4503*

Propisergide. $C_{20}H_{25}N_3O_2$. 339.43. 9,10-Didehydro-*N*-[(*S*)-2-hydroxy-1-methylethyl]-1,6-dimethylergoline-8β-carboxamide. *UNII-1Q1AWW2JET. CAS-5793-04-4.* INN.

Propitocaine Hydrochloride (JAN and previously used name) — *See* Prilocaine Hydrochloride.

Propiverine. $C_{23}H_{29}NO_3$. 367.48. [Propiverine Hydrochloride is JAN.] 1-Methyl-4-piperidyl diphenylpropoxyacetate. *UNII-468GE2241L. CAS-60569-19-9; CAS-54556-98-8* [hydrochloride]. INN; BAN.

Propizepine. $C_{17}H_{20}N_4O$. 296.37. 6,11-Dihydro-6-[2-(dimethylamino)-2-methylethyl]-5*H*-pyrido[2,3-*b*][1,5]benzodiazepin-5-one. *UNII-09B57945V9. CAS-10321-12-7.* INN; DCF; MI. ◇*UP 106*

Propofol [*1984*] (proe′ poe fol). **USP.** $C_{12}H_{18}O$. 178.27. (1) Phenol, 2,6-bis(1-methylethyl); (2) 2,6-Diisopropylphenol. *UNII-YI7VU623SF. CAS-2078-54-8.* INN; BAN. *Anesthetic (intravenous).* Diprivan (Abraxis) ◇*ICI 35,868*

Propoxate. $C_{15}H_{18}N_2O_2$. 258.32. (±)-Propyl 1-(α-methylbenzyl)imidazole-5-carboxylate. *UNII-M42D353K88. CAS-7036-58-0.* INN. ◇*R 7464*

Propoxur. $C_{11}H_{15}NO_3$. 209.24. 2-Isopropoxyphenyl methylcarbamate. *CAS-114-26-1.* BAN.

Propoxycaine Hydrochloride (proe pox′ i kane hye″ droe klor′ ide). **USP.** $C_{16}H_{26}N_2O_3{\cdot}HCl$. 330.85. [Propoxycaine is INN.] (1) Benzoic acid, 4-amino-2-propoxy-, 2-(diethylamino)ethyl ester, monohydrochloride; (2) 2-(Diethylamino)ethyl 4-amino-2-propoxybenzoate monohydrochloride. *UNII-K490D39G46; UNII-EPD1EH7F53* [propoxycaine]. *CAS-550-83-4; CAS-86-43-1* [propoxycaine]. *Anesthetic (local).* Blockain Hydrochloride (Sterling Winthrop†); Ravocaine Hydrochloride (Cook-Waite)

Propoxyphene Hydrochloride [*1964*] (proe pox′ i feen hye″ droe klor′ ide). **USP.** C$_{22}$H$_{29}$NO$_2$.HCl. 375.93. [Dextropropoxyphene is INN and BAN.] (1) Benzeneethanol, α-[2-(dimethylamino)-1-methylethyl]-α-phenyl-, propanoate (ester), hydrochloride, [S-(R*,S*)]-; (2) (2S,3R)-(+)-4-(Dimethylamino)-3-methyl-1,2-diphenyl-2-butanol propionate (ester) hydrochloride. *UNII-CB2TL9PS0T. CAS-1639-60-7; CAS-469-62-5* [propoxyphene]. *Analgesic.* Darvon (Xanodyne)

Propoxyphene Napsylate [*1969*] (proe pox′ i feen nap′ si late). **USP.** C$_{22}$H$_{29}$NO$_2$.C$_{10}$H$_8$O$_3$S.H$_2$O. 565.72. (1) Benzeneethanol, α-[2-(dimethylamino)-1-methylethyl]-α-phenyl-, propanoate (ester), [S-(R*,S*)]-, compd. with 2-naphthalenesulfonic acid (1:1), monohydrate; (2) (αS,1R)-α-[2-(Dimethylamino)-1-methylethyl]-α-phenylphenethyl propionate compound with 2-naphthalenesulfonic acid (1:1) monohydrate. *UNII-38M219L1OJ. CAS-26570-10-5; CAS-17140-78-2* [anhydrous]; *CAS-23239-43-2* [replaced]; *CAS-469-62-5* [propoxyphene]. *Analgesic.* Darvon-N (Xanodyne)

Propranolol Hydrochloride [*1965*] (proe pran′ oh lol hye″ droe klor′ ide). **USP.** C$_{16}$H$_{21}$NO$_2$.HCl. 295.80. [Propranolol is INN and BAN.] (1) 2-Propanol, 1-[(1-methylethyl)amino]-3-(1-naphthalenyloxy)-, hydrochloride, ($\pm$)-; (2) ($\pm$)-1-(Isopropylamino)-3-(1-naphthyloxy)-2-propanol hydrochloride. *UNII-F8A3652H1V; UNII-9Y8NXQ24VQ* [propranolol]. *CAS-318-98-9; CAS-525-66-6* [propranolol]. JAN. *Cardiac depressant (anti-arrhythmic); anti-adrenergic (β-receptor).* Inderal (Wyeth); Innopran (Reliant) ◇AY 64043; ICI 45520; NSC-91523

---

† Brand name formerly used, and/or firm no longer concerned with this product.

Propyl Docetrizoate. C$_{14}$H$_{14}$I$_3$NO$_4$. 640.98. Propyl 3-diacetylamino-2,4,6-triiodobenzoate. *UNII-0B62S0B44U. CAS-5579-08-8.* INN; BAN; MI.

Propyl Gallate (proe′ pil gal′ ate). **NF.** C$_{10}$H$_{12}$O$_5$. 212.20. (1) Benzoic acid, 3,4,5-trihydroxy-, propyl ester; (2) Propyl gallate. *UNII-8D4SNN7V92. CAS-121-79-9. Pharmaceutic aid (antioxidant).*

Propyl Parahydroxybenzoate (JAN) — *See* Propylparaben.

Propylene Carbonate (proe′ pi leen kar′ bo nate). **NF.** C$_4$H$_6$O$_3$. 102.09. (1) 4-Methyl-1,3-dioxolan-2-one; (2) Cyclic propylene carbonate. *UNII-8D08K3S51E. CAS-108-32-7. Pharmaceutic aid (gelling agent).*

Propylene Glycol (proe′ pi leen glye′ kol). **USP.** C$_3$H$_8$O$_2$. 76.09. [Propylene Glycol Cefatrizine is JAN.] (1) 1,2-Propanediol; (2) 1,2-Propanediol. *UNII-6DC9Q167V3. CAS-57-55-6.* JAN. *Pharmaceutic aid (humectant); pharmaceutic aid (solvent); pharmaceutic aid (suspending agent).* Sentry Propylene Glycol (Union Carbide†); Sirlene (Dow Chemical)

Propylene Glycol Alginate (proe′ pi leen glye′ kol al′ ji nate). **NF.** A propylene glycol ester of alginic acid. *Pharmaceutic aid (suspending agent); pharmaceutic aid (viscosity-increasing agent).*

Propylene Glycol Cefatrizine (JAN) — *See* Propylene Glycol.

Propylene Glycol Diacetate. C$_7$H$_{12}$O$_4$. 160.17. *UNII-5Z492UNF9O.* NF XVIII. *Pharmaceutic aid (solvent).*

Propylene Glycol Dilaurate (proe′ pi leen glye′ kol). **NF.** (1) Dodecanoic acid, monoester wih 1,2-propanediol; (2) Lauric acid, monoester with propane-1,2-diol; (3) Propylene dilaurate.

Propylene Glycol Ether of Methylcellulose — *See* Hypromellose.

Propylene Glycol Monolaurate (proe′ pi leen glye′ kol mon″ oh lawr′ ate). **NF.** (1) Dodecanoic acid, monoester wih 1,2-propanediol; (2) Lauric acid, monoester with propane-1,2-diol. *UNII-M4AW13H75T.*

Propylene Glycol Monostearate (proe′ pi leen glye′ kol mon″ oh steer′ ate). **NF.** (1) Octadecanoic acid, monoester with 1,2-propanediol; (2) 1,2-Propanediol monostearate. *UNII-F76354LMGR. CAS-1323-39-3. Pharmaceutic aid (emulsifying agent).*

Propylhexedrine (proe″ pil hex′ e dreen). **USP**. $C_{10}H_{21}N$. 155.28. (1) Cyclohexaneethanamine, N,α-dimethyl-, (±)-; (2) (±)-N,α-Dimethylcyclohexaneethylamine. *UNII-LQU92IU8LL. CAS-101-40-6*. INN; BAN. *Adrenergic (vasoconstrictor).* Dristan Inhaler (Whitehall-Robins†)

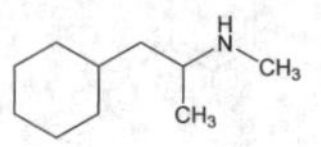

Propyliodone (proe″ pil eye′ oh done). **USP**. $C_{10}H_{11}I_2NO_3$. 447.01. (1) 1(4*H*)-Pyridineacetic acid, 3,5-diiodo-4-oxo-, propyl ester; (2) Propyl 3,5-diiodo-4-oxo-1(4*H*) pyridine-acetate. *UNII-5NPJ6BPX36. CAS-587-61-1*. INN; BAN; JAN. *Diagnostic aid (radiopaque medium).* Dionosil (GlaxoSmithKline)

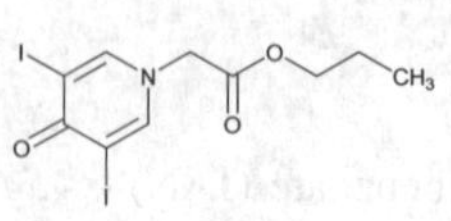

Propylorvinol — *See* Etorphine.

Propylparaben [*1986*] (proe″ pil par′ a ben). **NF**. $C_{10}H_{12}O_3$. 180.20. [Propyl Parahydroxybenzoate is JAN.] (1) Benzoic acid, 4-hydroxy-, propyl ester; (2) Propyl *p*-hydroxybenzo-ate. *UNII-Z8IX2SC1OH. CAS-94-13-3. Pharmaceutic aid (antifungal agent).*

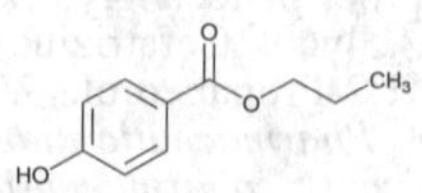

Propylparaben Sodium [*1986*] (proe″ pil par′ a ben soe′ dee um). **NF**. $C_{10}H_{11}NaO_3$. 202.18. (1) Benzoic acid, 4-hydroxy-, propyl ester, sodium salt; (2) Propyl *p*-hydroxybenzoate, sodium salt. *CAS-35285-69-9. Pharmaceutic aid (antimicrobial preservative).*

Propylthiouracil (proe″ pil thye″ oh ure′ a sil). **USP**. $C_7H_{10}N_2OS$. 170.23. (1) 4(1*H*)-Pyrimidinone, 2,3-dihydro-6-propyl-2-thioxo-; (2) 6-Propyl-2-thiouracil. *UNII-721M9407IY. CAS-51-52-5*. INN; BAN; JAN. *Thyroid inhibitor.*

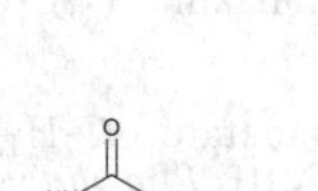

Propyperone. $C_{23}H_{33}FN_2O_2$. 388.52. 4′-Fluoro-4-(4-piperidi-no-4-propionylpiperidino)butyrophenone. *UNII-HG22108KQK. CAS-3781-28-0*. INN. ◇*R 4082*

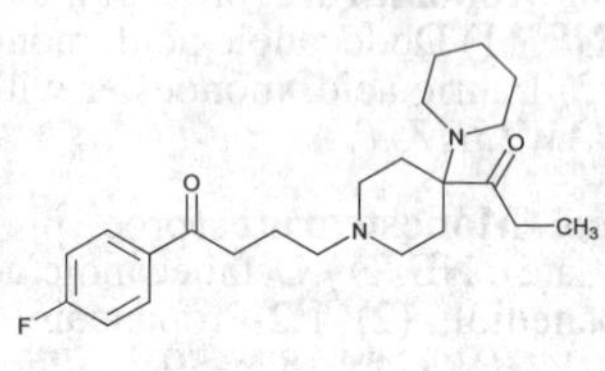

Propyphenazone. $C_{14}H_{18}N_2O$. 230.31. [Isopropylantipyrine is JAN.] 4-Isopropyl-2,3-dimethyl-1-phenyl-3-pyrazolin-5-one. *UNII-OED8FV75PY. CAS-479-92-5*. INN; BAN; DCF; MI.

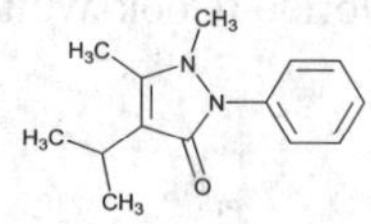

Propyromazine Bromide. $C_{20}H_{23}BrN_2OS$. 419.38. 1-Methyl-1-(1-phenothiazin-10-ylcarbonylethyl)pyrrolidinium bro-mide. *UNII-G69033J83V. CAS-145-54-0*. INN. ◇*LD 335*

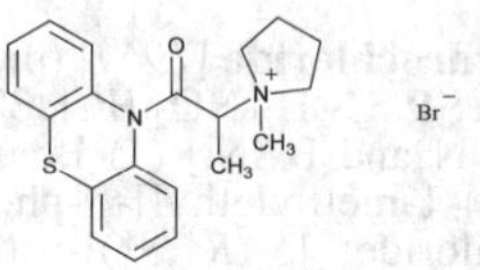

Proquamezine (previously used name) — *See* Aminoproma-zine.

Proquazone [*1971*] (proe′ kwa zone). $C_{18}H_{18}N_2O$. 278.35. (1) 2(1*H*)-Quinazolinone, 7-methyl-1-(1-methylethyl)-4-phe-nyl-; (2) 1-Isopropyl-7-methyl-4-phenyl-2(1*H*)-quinazoli-none. *UNII-42VPJ2980S. CAS-22760-18-5*. INN; BAN. *Anti-inflammatory.* Arthrex (Novartis) ◇*43-715*

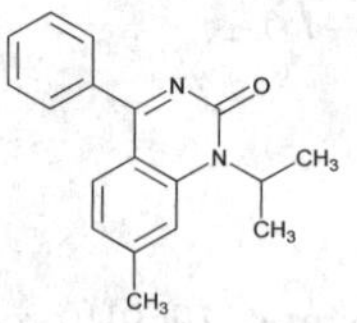

Proquinolate [*1967*] (proe kwin′ oh late). $C_{17}H_{21}NO_5$. 319.35. (1) 3-Quinolinecarboxylic acid, 4-hydroxy-6,7-bis(1-methylethoxy)-, methyl ester; (2) Methyl 4-hydroxy-6,7-diisopropoxy-3-quinolinecarboxylate. *CAS-1698-95-9*. INN. *Coccidiostat (for poultry).* ◇*EU-1063*

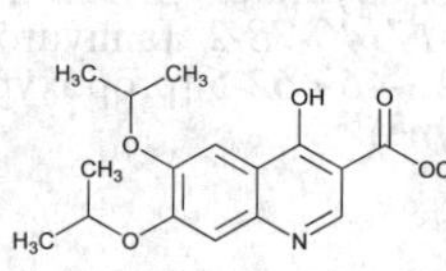

Prorenoate Potassium [*1974*] (proe ren′ oh ate poe tas′ ee um). $C_{23}H_{31}KO_4$. 410.59. (1) 3′*H*-Cyclopropa[6,7]pregna-4,6-diene-21-carboxylic acid, 6,7-dihydro-17-hydroxy-3-oxo-, ($6\alpha,7\alpha,17\alpha$)-, monopotassium salt; (2) Potassium 6,7-dihydro-17-hydroxy-3-oxo-3′*H*-cyclopropa[6,7]-17α-pregna-4,6-diene-21-carboxylate. *CAS-49847-97-4*. INN; BAN. *Aldosterone antagonist.* ◇*SC-23992*

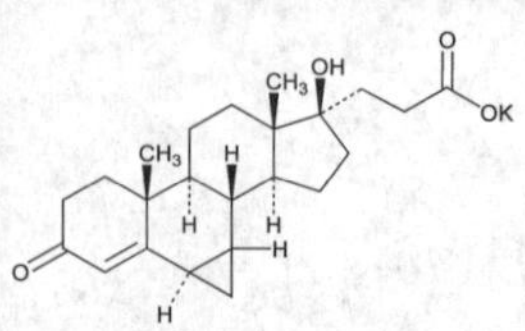

Proroxan Hydrochloride [*1978*] (proe rox′ an hye″ droe klor′ ide). $C_{21}H_{23}NO_3 \cdot HCl$. 373.87. [Proroxan is INN.] (1) 1-Propanone, 1-(2,3-dihydro-1,4-benzodioxin-6-yl)-3-(3-phenyl-1-pyrrolidinyl)-, hydrochloride; (2) 1-(1,4-Benzo-dioxan-6-yl)-3-(3-phenyl-1-pyrrolidinyl)-1-propanone hydrochloride. *CAS-33025-33-1; CAS-33743-96-3* [prorox-an]. *Anti-adrenergic (α-receptor). [Names previously used: Pyrroxane; Pirroksan.]* ◇*AY-24,269*

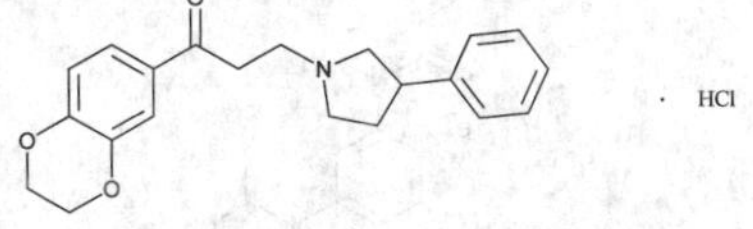

Proscillaridin [*1967*] (proe″ si lar′ i din). $C_{30}H_{42}O_8$. 530.65. (1) Bufa-4,20,22-trienolide, 3-[(6-deoxy-α-L-mannopyra-nosyl)oxy]-14-hydroxy-, (3β)-; (2) Proscillaridin A; (3) [(6-Deoxy-α-L-mannopyranosyl)oxy]-14-hydroxybufa-4,20,22-trienolide. *CAS-466-06-8.* INN; BAN; JAN. *Cardiotonic.* Tradenal (Knoll†) ◇*A-32686; 2936*

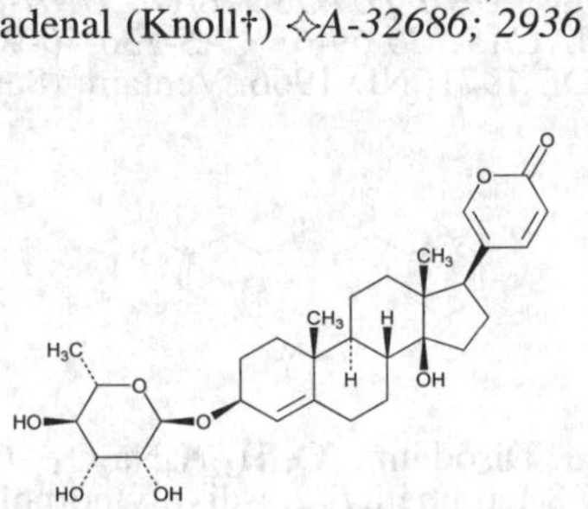

Prospidium Chloride. $C_{18}H_{36}Cl_4N_4O_2$. 482.32. 3,12-Bis(3-chloro-2-hydroxypropyl)-3,12-diaza-6,9-diazoniadispir-o[5.2.5.2]hexadecane dichloride. *UNII-7G733H6RES. CAS-23476-83-7.* INN.

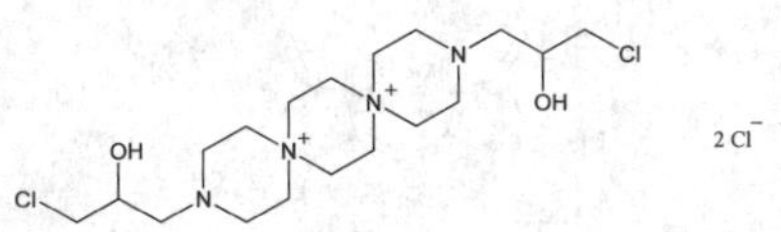

Prostacyclin (previously used name) — *See* Epoprostenol.

Prostaglandin E₁ (previously used name) — *See* Alprostadil.

Prostaglandin I₂ (previously used name) — *See* Epoprostenol.

Prostaglandin X (previously used name) — *See* Epoprostenol.

Prostalene [*1976*] (prost′ a leen). $C_{22}H_{36}O_5$. 380.52. (1) Prosta-4,5,13-trien-1-oic acid, 9,11,15-trihydroxy-15-methyl-, methyl ester, (9α,11α,13E)-, (±)-; (2) (±)-Methyl 7-[(1R*,2R*,3R*,5S*)-3,5-dihydroxy-2-[(E)-3-hydroxy-3-methyl-1-octenyl]cyclopentyl]-4,5-heptadienoate. *UNII-OO2SWY8981. CAS-54120-61-5.* INN; BAN. *Prostaglandin.* Synchrocept [Veterinary] (Syntex) ◇*RS-9390*

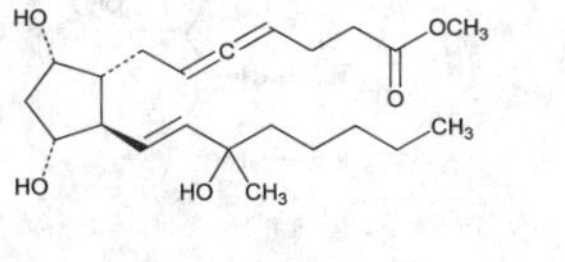

Prosulpride. $C_{16}H_{25}N_3O_4S$. 355.45. *N*-[(1-Propyl-2-pyrrolidi-nyl)methyl]-5-sulfamoyl-*o*-anisamide. *UNII-H9JT455SZ7. CAS-68556-59-2.* INN.

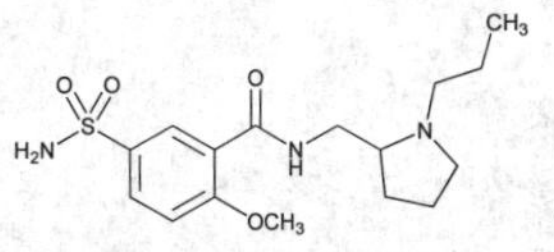

Prosultiamine. $C_{15}H_{24}N_4O_2S_2$. 356.51. *N*-[(4-Amino-2-methyl-5-pyrimidinyl)methyl]-*N*-[4-hydroxy-1-methyl-2-(propyldithio)-1-butenyl]formamide. *CAS-59-58-5.* INN; JAN; DCF; MI.

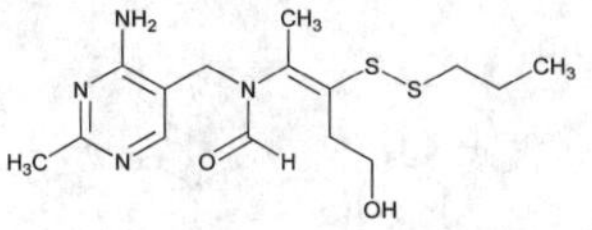

Protamine Hydrochloride. BAN.

Protamine Sulfate (proe′ ta meen sul′ fate). **USP.** [Protamine Sulphate is BAN.] A purified mixture of simple protein principles obtained from the sperm or testes of suitable species of fish, which has the property of neutralizing heparin. *CAS-9009-65-8.* INN; JAN. *Antidote (to heparin).*

Protargin, Mild — *See* Silver Protein, Mild.

Protein Hydrolysate (proe′ teen hye drol′ i sate). **USP** [Injection]. A sterile solution of amino acids and short-chain peptides, which represent the approximate nutritive equivalent of the casein, lact-albumin, plasma, fibrin, or other suitable protein from which it is derived by acid, enzymatic, or other methods of hydrolysis. *CAS-9015-54-7. Replenisher (fluid and nutrient).* Aminosol (Abbott); Hyprotigen (B Braun)

Proterguride. $C_{22}H_{32}N_4O$. 368.52. 1,1-Diethyl-3-(6-propyler-golin-8α-yl)urea. *UNII-10661OD4VE. CAS-77650-95-4.* INN.

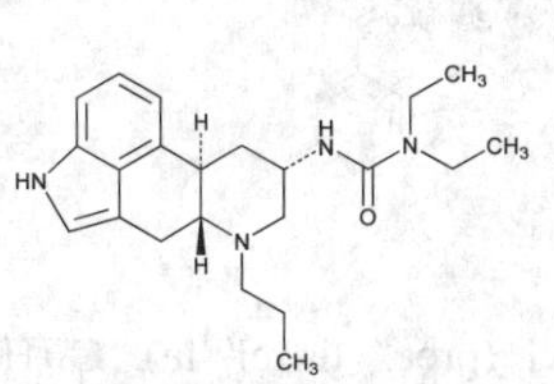

Protheobromine. $C_{10}H_{14}N_4O_3$. 238.24. 1-(2-Hydroxypro-pyl)theobromine. *UNII-8067S1388X. CAS-50-39-5.* INN; MI.

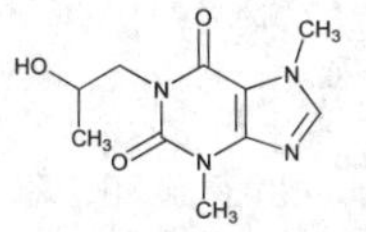

Prothionamide (JAN) — *See* Protionamide.

---

† Brand name formerly used, and/or firm no longer concerned with this product.

Prothipendyl Hydrochloride. $C_{16}H_{19}N_3S \cdot HCl$. 321.87. [Prothipendyl is INN and BAN.] *N,N*-Dimethyl-10*H*-pyrido[3,2-*b*][1,4]benzothiazine-10-propanamine, monohydrochloride. *UNII-7610629RVH. CAS-1225-65-6; CAS-303-69-5* [prothipendyl]. MI.

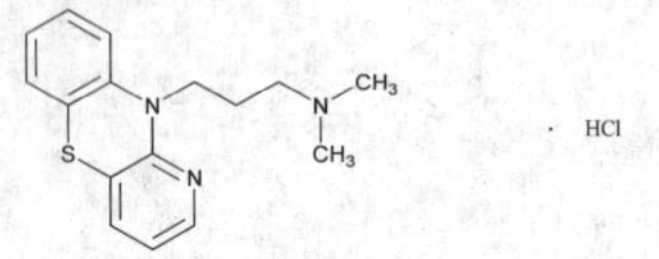

Prothixene. $C_{18}H_{19}NS$. 281.42. *N,N*-Dimethylthioxanthene-$\Delta^{9,\gamma}$-propylamine. *UNII-2HX2OJH78L. CAS-2622-24-4.* INN.

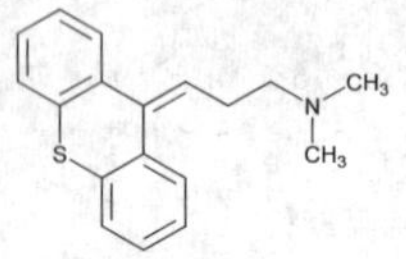

Prothrombin Complex, Activated. A preparation from human plasma containing factor VIII inhibitor by-passing activity. BAN.

Protiofate. $C_{12}H_{16}O_6S$. 288.32. Dipropyl 3,4-dihydroxy-2,5-thiophenedicarboxylate. *UNII-FIP88CI9Y3. CAS-58416-00-5.* INN; MI.

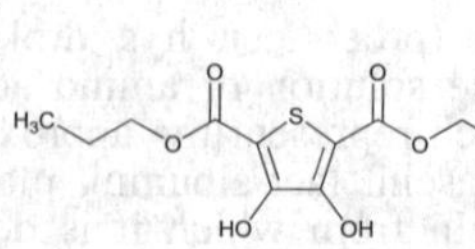

Protionamide. $C_9H_{12}N_2S$. 180.27. [Prothionamide is JAN.] 2-Propylthioisonicotinamide. *UNII-76YOO33643. CAS-14222-60-7.* INN; BAN; DCF; MI. ◇*TH-1321; RP 9778*

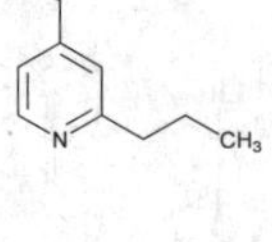

Protirelin [*1974*] (proe″ ti rel′ in). $C_{16}H_{22}N_6O_4$. 362.38. [Protirelin Tartrate is JAN.] (1) L-Prolinamide, 5-oxo-L-prolyl-L-histidyl-; (2) 5-Oxo-L-prolyl-L-histidyl-L-prolinamide. *UNII-5Y5F15120W. CAS-24305-27-9.* INN; BAN; JAN. *Prothyrotropin.* Thypinone (Abbott); Thyrel Trh (Ferring Pharmaceuticals) [*Name previously used: Lopremone.*] ◇*Abbott-38579; Synthetic TRH*

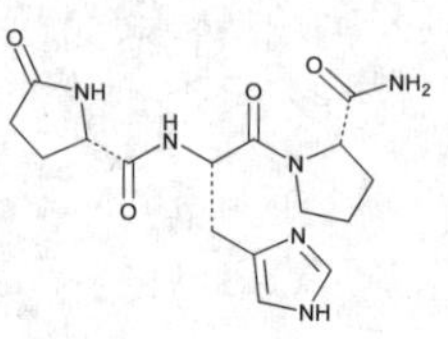

Protizinic Acid. $C_{17}H_{17}NO_3S$. 315.39. 7-Methoxy-α,10-dimethylphenothiazine-2-acetic acid. *UNII-N40195UTPI. CAS-13799-03-6.* INN; JAN; DCF; MI.

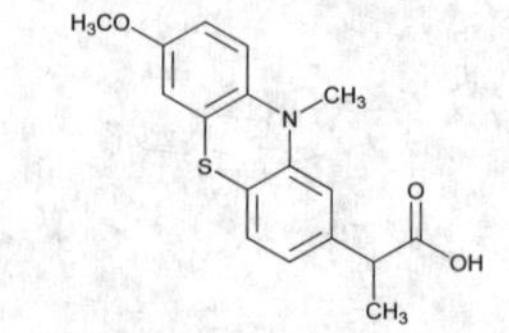

Protokylol Hydrochloride. $C_{18}H_{21}NO_5 \cdot HCl$. 367.82. [Protokylol is BAN.] α-[[(α-Methyl-3,4-methylenedioxyphenethyl)amino]methyl]protocatechuyl alcohol, hydrochloride. *UNII-7U7O8Q48IO; UNII-8Y5Y4EEO2V* [protokylol]. *CAS-136-69-6; CAS-136-70-9* [protokylol]. MI; AMA-DE 1971; ND 1966. Ventaire (Sanofi Aventis)

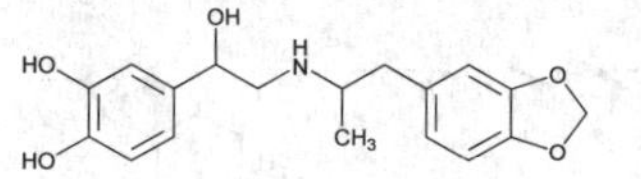

Protoporphyrin Disodium. $C_{34}H_{32}N_4Na_2O_4$. 606.62. Disodium 1,3,5,8-tetramethyl-2,4-divinylporphine-6,7-dipropionate. *UNII-54N4UY1C7C. CAS-50865-01-5.* JAN.

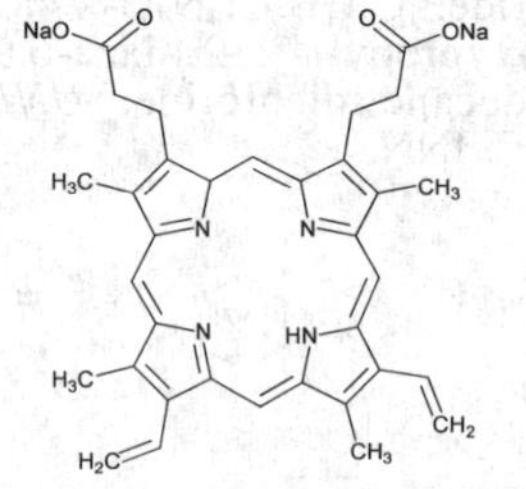

Protoveratrine A. $C_{41}H_{63}NO_{14}$. 793.94. (1) [3β(S),4α,6α,7α,15α(R),16β]-4,9-Epoxycevane-3,4,6,7,14,15,16,20-octol 6,7-diacetate 3-(2-hydroxy-2-methylbutanoate) 15-(2-methylbutanoate); (2) (3S,4S,4aR,5R,6S,6aS,6bS,7S,8R,8aR,9S,9aS,12-S,15aS,15bS,16aR,16bS)-5,6-Bis(acetyloxy)-4,6b,8,9-tetrahydroxy-9,12,16b-trimethyl-7-{[(2R)-2-methylbutanoyl]oxy}docosahydro-2H-4,16a-epoxybenzo[4,5]indeno[1,2-*h*]pyrido[1,2-*b*]isoquinolin-3-yl (2S)-2-hydroxy-2-methyl butanoate. *UNII-XP343X1HJU. CAS-143-57-7.* MI. Protalba (Marion Merrell Dow†)

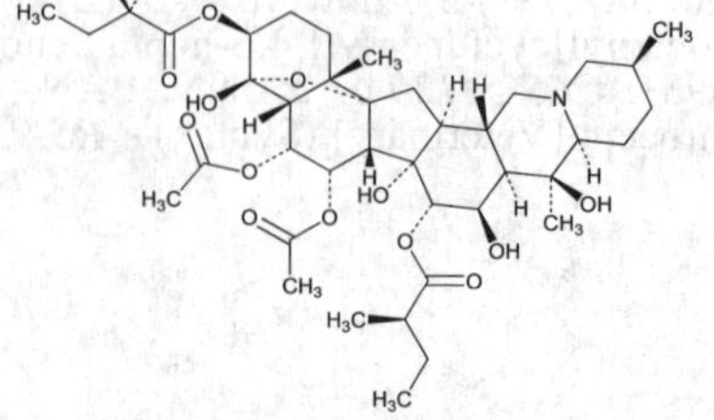

Protriptyline Hydrochloride [*1963*] (proe trip′ ti leen hye″ droe klor′ ide). **USP.** $C_{19}H_{21}N \cdot HCl$. 299.84. [Protriptyline is INN and BAN.] (1) 5*H*-Dibenzo[*a,d*]cycloheptene-5-propanamine, *N*-methyl-, hydrochloride; (2) *N*-Methyl-5*H*-dibenzo[*a,d*]cycloheptene-5-propylamine hydrochloride.

UNII-44665V00O8; UNII-4NDU154T12 [protriptyline]. *CAS-1225-55-4; CAS-438-60-8* [protriptyline]. *Antidepressant.* Vivactil (Odyssey) ✧*MK-240*

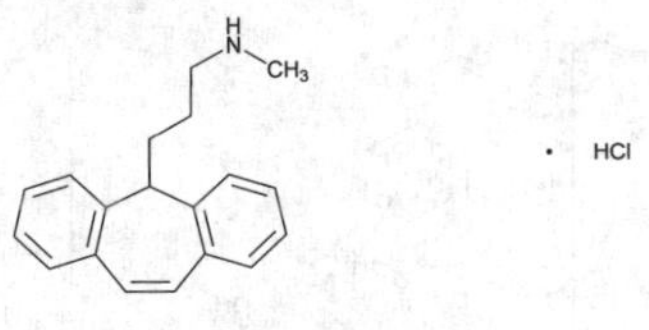

Proxazole [*1965*] (prox′ a zole). $C_{17}H_{25}N_3O$. 287.40. (1) 1,2,4-Oxadiazole-5-ethanamine, *N,N*-diethyl-3-(1-phenylpropyl)-; (2) 5-[2-(Diethylamino)ethyl]-3-(α-ethylbenzyl)-1,2,4-oxadiazole. *UNII-FD72T13M0K. CAS-5696-09-3.* INN. *Relaxant (smooth muscle); analgesic; anti-inflammatory.* Aerbron (Angelini Francesco, Italy)

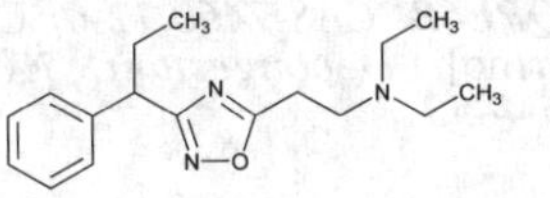

Proxazole Citrate [*1966*] (prox′ a zole sit′ rate). $C_{17}H_{25}N_3O.C_6H_8O_7$. 479.52. (1) 1,2,4-Oxadiazole-5-ethanamine, *N,N*-diethyl-3-(1-phenylpropyl)-, 2-hydroxy-1,2,3-propanetricarboxylate (1:1); (2) 5-[2-(Diethylamino)ethyl]-3-(α-ethylbenzyl)-1,2,4-oxadiazole citrate (1:1). *UNII-FD72T13M0K* [proxazole]. *CAS-132-35-4; CAS-5696-09-3* [proxazole]. *Relaxant (smooth muscle); analgesic; anti-inflammatory.* Toness (Angelini Francesco, Italy) ✧*AF-634*

Proxibarbal. $C_{10}H_{14}N_2O_4$. 226.23. 5-Allyl-5-(2-hydroxypropyl)barbituric acid. *UNII-F97OMS297F. CAS-2537-29-3.* INN; MI.

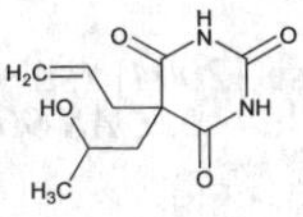

Proxibutene. $C_{22}H_{27}NO_2$. 337.46. 3-[(Dimethylamino)-methyl]-1,2-diphenyl-3-buten-2-ol propionate (ester). *UNII-7F228A0THI. CAS-14089-84-0.* INN. ✧*Ba-40088*

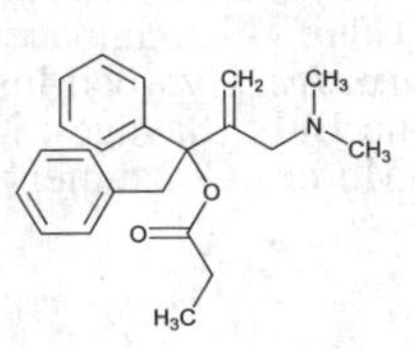

Proxicromil [*1980*] (prox ik′ roe mil). $C_{17}H_{18}O_5$. 302.32. (1) 4*H*-Naphtho[2,3-*b*]pyran-2-carboxylic acid, 6,7,8,9-tetrahydro-5-hydroxy-4-oxo-10-propyl-; (2) 6,7,8,9-Tetrahydro-5-hydroxy-4-oxo-10-propyl-4*H*-naphtho[2,3-*b*]pyran-2-carboxylic acid. *UNII-8WWZ0E633P. CAS-60400-92-2.* INN; BAN. *Anti-allergic.*

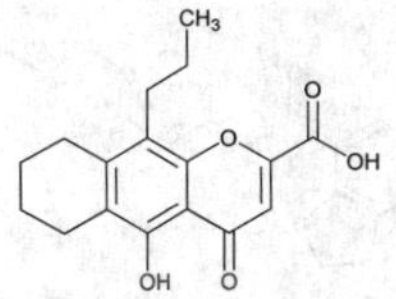

Proxifezone. $C_{22}H_{29}NO_2.C_{19}H_{20}N_2O_2$. 647.85. (+)-4-(Dimethylamino)-3-methyl-1,2-diphenyl-2-butanol propionate (ester) compound with 4-butyl-1,2-diphenyl-3,5-pyrazolidinedione (1:1). *UNII-005MKH0F6D. CAS-34427-79-7.* INN; DCF.

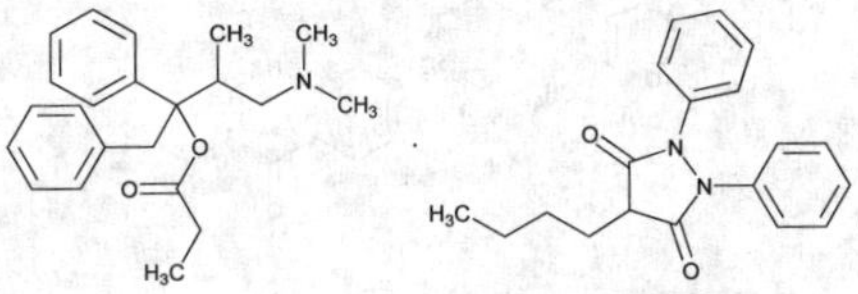

Proxorphan Tartrate [*1980*] (prox′ or fan tar′ trate). $(C_{19}H_{25}NO_2)_2.C_4H_6O_6$. 748.90. [Proxorphan is INN.] (1) 6-Oxamorphinan-3-ol, 17-(cyclopropylmethyl)-, [*S*-(*R**,*R**)]-2,3-dihydroxybutanedioate (2:1) (salt); (2) (-)-(4a*R*,5*R*,10b*S*)-13-(Cyclopropylmethyl)-4,4a,5,6-tetrahydro-3*H*-5,10b-(iminoethano)-1*H*-naphtho[1,2-*c*]-pyran-9-ol D-(-)-tartrate (2:1) (salt). *UNII-T32BM3AM71. CAS-69815-39-0; CAS-69815-38-9* [proxorphan]. *Analgesic; antitussive.* ✧*BL-5572M*

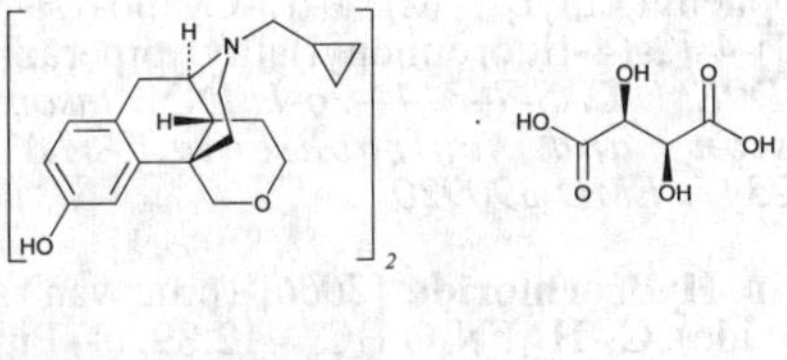

Proxymetacaine (INN, BAN, DCF) — *See* Proparacaine Hydrochloride.

Proxyphylline. $C_{10}H_{14}N_4O_3$. 238.24. 7-(2-Hydroxypropyl)-theophylline. *CAS-603-00-9.* INN; BAN; JAN; MI.

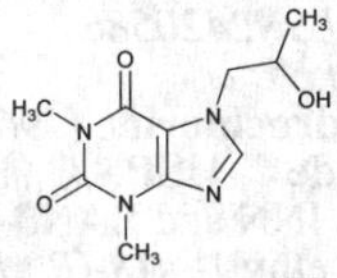

Prozapine. $C_{21}H_{27}N$. 293.45. 1-(3,3-Diphenylpropyl)cyclohexamethyleneimine. *UNII-E9503DM633. CAS-3426-08-2.* INN; MI.

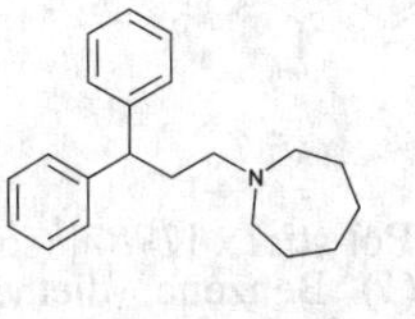

† Brand name formerly used, and/or firm no longer concerned with this product.

Prucalopride. $C_{18}H_{26}ClN_3O_3$. 367.87. 4-Amino-5-chloro-2,3-dihydro-N-[1-(3-methoxypropyl)-4-piperidyl]-7-benzofurancarboxamide. *UNII-0A09IUW5TP. CAS-179474-81-8.* INN; BAN.

Prulifloxacin. $C_{21}H_{20}FN_3O_6S$. 461.46. ($\pm$)-7-[4-[(Z)-2,3-Dihydroxy-2-butenyl]-1-piperazinyl]-6-fluoro-1-methyl-4-oxo-$1H,4H$-[1,3]thiazeto[3,2-a]quinoline-3-carboxylic acid, cyclic carbonate. *UNII-J42298IESW. CAS-123447-62-1.* INN.

Prussian Blue Insoluble [*2005*] (prush' un). $C_{18}Fe_7N_{18}$. 859.23. (1) Ferrate(4-), hexakis(cyano-κC)-, iron(3+) (3:4) (OC-6-11)-; (2) Ferric hexacyanoferrate (II). *UNII-TLE294X33A. CAS-14038-43-8. Antidote indicated in the treatment of patients with known or suspected internal contamination with radioactive cesium and/or non-radioactive thallium to increase their rates of elimination.* Antidotum-Thallii-Heyl (Heyl, Germany); Radiogardase-Cs (Heyl, Germany)

Pruvanserin [*2006*] (prue van' ser in). $C_{22}H_{21}FN_4O$. 376.43. (1) Piperazine, 1-[(3-cyano-$1H$-indol-7-yl)carbonyl]-4-[2-(4-fluorophenyl)ethyl]-; (2) 1-[(3-Cyano-$1H$-indol-7-yl)-carbonyl]-4-[2-(4-fluorophenyl)ethyl]piperazine. *UNII-UL09X1D9EM. CAS-443144-26-1.* INN. *Insomnia, major depression, and schizophrenia.* ◇*LY2420586; LSN2422347; EMD 390920*

Pruvanserin Hydrochloride [*2006*] (prue van' ser in hye" droe klor' ide). $C_{22}H_{21}FN_4O \cdot HCl$. 412.89. (1) Piperazine, 1-[(3-cyano-$1H$-indol-7-yl)carbonyl]-4-[2-(4-fluorophenyl)ethyl]-, monohydrochloride; (2) 7-{4-[2-(4-fluorophenyl)ethyl]piperazine-1-carbonyl}-$1H$-indole-3-carbonitrile, monohydrochloride; (3) 7-{4-[2-(4-fluorophenyl)ethyl]piperazine-1-ylcarbonyl}-$1H$-indole-3-carbonitrile hydrochloride. *UNII-AWA682DH9Z; UNII-UL09X1D9EM* [pruvanserin]. *CAS-443144-27-2; CAS-443144-26-1* [pruvanserin]. *Insomnia, major depression, and schizophrenia.* ◇*LY2422347 HCl; LSN2420586*

Pseudoephedrine Hydrochloride [*1963*] (soo" doe e fed' rin hye" droe klor' ide). **USP.** $C_{10}H_{15}NO \cdot HCl$. 201.69. [Pseudoephedrine is INN and BAN.] (1) Benzenemethanol, α-[1-(methylamino)ethyl]-, [S-(R^*,R^*)]-, hydrochloride; (2) (+)-Pseudoephedrine hydrochloride. *UNII-6V9V2RYJ8N; UNII-7CUC9DDI9F* [pseudoephedrine]. *CAS-345-78-8; CAS-90-82-4* [pseudoephedrine]. *Adrenergic (vasoconstrictor).* Sudafed (McNeil)

Pseudoephedrine Polistirex [*1987*] (soo" doe e fed' rin pol" ee stye' rex). (1) Benzene, diethenyl-, polymer with ethenylbenzene, sulfonated, complex with [S-(R^*,R^*)]-α-[1-(methylamino)ethyl]benzenemethanol; (2) Sulfonated styrene-divinylbenzene copolymer complex with (+)-pseudoephedrine. *Nasal decongestant.* Pseudo (UCB)

Pseudoephedrine Sulfate [*1978*] (soo" doe e fed' rin sul' fate). **USP.** $(C_{10}H_{15}NO)_2 \cdot H_2SO_4$. 428.54. (1) Benzenemethanol, α-[1-(methylamino)ethyl]-, [S-(R^*,R^*)]-, sulfate (2:1) (salt); (2) (+)-Pseudoephedrine sulfate (2:1) (salt). *UNII-Y9DL7QPE6B. CAS-7460-12-0; CAS-90-82-4* [(+)-pseudoephedrine]. *Decongestant.* Afrinol (Schering-Plough) ◇*Sch 4855*

Pseudomonic Acid — *See* Mupirocin.

Psilocybine. $C_{12}H_{17}N_2O_4P$. 284.25. 3-(2-Dimethylaminoethyl)indol-4-yl dihydrogen phosphate. *CAS-520-52-5.* INN; BAN; DCF; MI. ◇*CY 39*

Psyllium Hemicellulose [*2004*] (sil' ee um hem" ee sel' ue lose). **USP.** Hemicellulose. *CAS-9034-32-6. Laxation and cholesterol lowering.*

Psyllium Husk (sil' ee um). **USP.** The cleaned, dried seed coat (epidermis) separated by winnowing and thrashing from the seeds of *Plantago ovata* Forskal, known in commerce as Blond Psyllium or Indian Psyllium or Ispaghula, or from *Plantago arenaria* Waldstein et Kitaibel (Plantago psyllium L.) known in commerce as Spanish or French Psyllium (Fam. Plantaginaceae), in whole or in powdered form. *Laxative.* Hydrocil Instant (Solvay Pharmaceuticals); Modane Bulk (Savage); Mylanta Fiber (Johnson & Johnson-Merck Consumer†); Syllact (Carter-Wallace)

Psyllium Seed — *See* Plantago Seed.

Pteroylglutamic Acid — *See* Folic Acid.

Pumactant. A mixture of 7 parts by weight of 1,2-dipalmitoyl-sn-glycero(3)phosphocholine (DPPC) and 3 parts by weight of 2-oleoyl-1-palmitoyl-sn-glycero(3)phospho(1)-sn-glycerol (PG). BAN.

Pumafentrine. $C_{29}H_{39}N_3O_3$. 477.64. (-)-*p*-[(4a*R**,10b*S**)-9-Ethoxy-1,2,3,4,4a,10b-hexahydro-8-methoxy-2-methyl-benzo[*c*][1,6]naphthyridin-6-yl]-*N*,*N*-diisopropylbenza-mide. *UNII-063D2YI19E. CAS-207993-12-2.* INN.

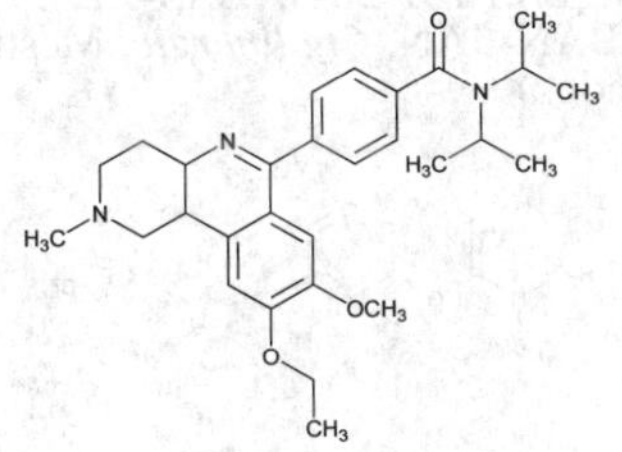

Pumaprazole. $C_{19}H_{22}N_4O_2$. 338.40. Methyl 2-[[(2,3-dimethy-limidazo[1,2-*a*]pyridin-8-yl)amino]methyl]-3-methylcar-banilate. *UNII-DK95Z519WL. CAS-158364-59-1.* INN.

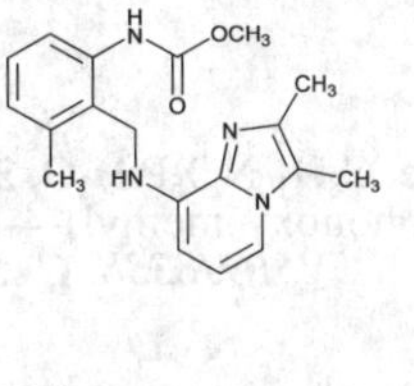

Pumice (pum′ is). **USP.** A substance of volcanic origin, consisting of complex silicates of aluminum, potassium, and sodium. *Abrasive (dental).*

Pumitepa. $C_{12}H_{19}N_8OP$. 322.31. *P*,*P*-Bis(1-aziridinyl)-*N*-[2-(dimethylamino)-7-methylpurin-6-yl]phosphinic amide. *UNII-7AYY495RE0. CAS-42061-52-9.* INN.

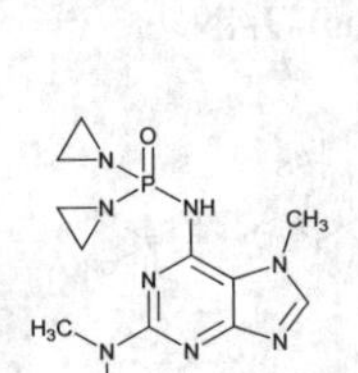

Pumosetrag. $C_{15}H_{17}N_3O_2S$. 303.38. *N*-[(3*R*)-1-Azabicy-clo[2.2.2]oct-3-yl]-7-oxo-4,7-dihydrothieno[3,2-*b*]pyri-dine-6-carboxamide. *CAS-153062-94-3.* INN.

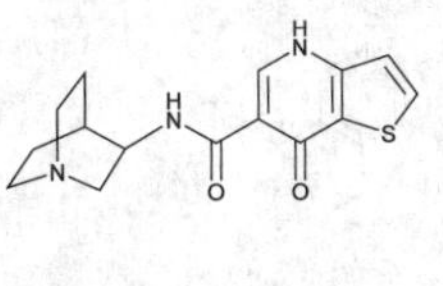

Puromycin [*1965*] (pure″ oh mye′ sin). $C_{22}H_{29}N_7O_5$. 471.51. (1) Adenosine, 3′-[(2-amino-3-(4-methoxyphenyl)-1-oxo-propyl]amino]-3′-deoxy-*N*,*N*-dimethyl-, (*S*)-; (2) 3′-(L-α-Amino-*p*-methoxyhydrocinnamamido)-3′-deoxy-*N*,*N*-di-

methyladenosine. *CAS-53-79-2.* INN; BAN. *Antineoplas-tic; antiprotozoal (Trypanosoma).* ◇*P-638; CL 13,900; 3123L*

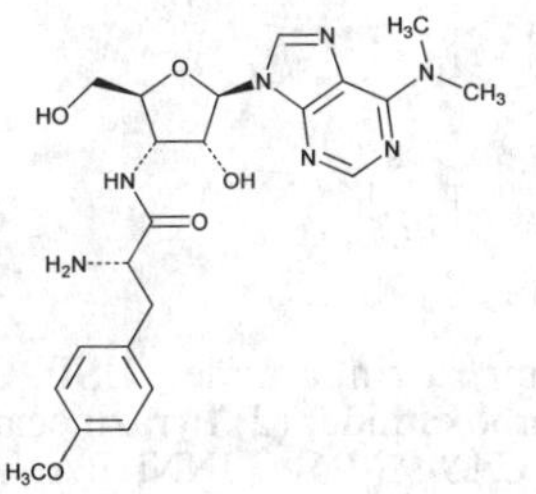

Puromycin Hydrochloride [*1968*] (pure″ oh mye′ sin hye″ droe klor′ ide). $C_{22}H_{29}N_7O_5 \cdot 2HCl$. 544.43. (1) Adenosine, 3′-[(2-amino-3-(4-methoxyphenyl)-1-oxopropyl]amino]-3′-deoxy-*N*,*N*-dimethyl-, dihydrochloride, (*S*)-; (2) 3′-(L-α-Amino-*p*-methoxyhydrocinnamamido)-3′-deoxy-*N*,*N*-di-methyladenosine dihydrochloride. *UNII-PGN54228S5. CAS-58-58-2; CAS-53-79-2* [puromycin]. *Antineoplastic; antiprotozoal (Trypanosoma).* ◇*CL 16,536; NSC-3055*

Pyrabrom [*1970*] (pir′ a brom). $C_{24}H_{30}BrN_7O_3$. 544.44. (1) 1*H*-Purine-2,6-dione, 8-bromo-3,7-dihydro-1,3-dimethyl, compd. with *N*-[(4-methoxyphenyl)methyl]-*N*′,*N*′-di-methyl-*N*-2-pyridinyl-1,2-ethanediamine (1:1); (2) 8-Bro-motheophylline compound with 2-[[2-(dimethylamino)ethyl](*p*-methoxybenzyl)amino]pyridine (1:1). *CAS-606-05-3. Antihistaminic.* ◇*SMP 68-40; NSC-14279*

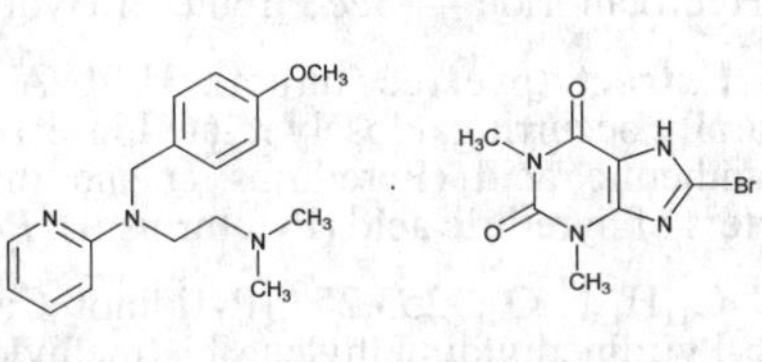

Pyrantel Pamoate [*1969*] (pi ran′ tel pam′ oh ate). **USP.** $C_{11}H_{14}N_2S \cdot C_{23}H_{16}O_6$. 594.68. [Pyrantel is INN and BAN.] (1) Pyrimidine, 1,4,5,6-tetrahydro-1-methyl-2-[2-(2-thie-nyl)ethenyl]-, (*E*)-, compd. with 4,4′-methylenebis[3-hy-droxy-2-naphthalenecarboxylic acid] (1:1); (2) (*E*)-1,4,5,6-Tetrahydro-1-methyl-2-[2-(2-thienyl)vinyl]pyrimidine 4,4′-methylenebis[3-hydroxy-2-naphthoate] (1:1). *UNII-81BK194Z5M. CAS-22204-24-6; CAS-15686-83-6* [pyran-tel]. JAN. *Anthelmintic.* Antiminth (Roerig); Combantrin (Pfizer) ◇*CP-10,423-16*

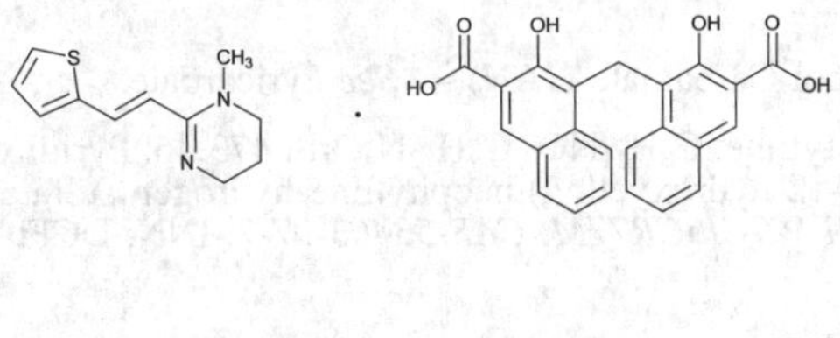

Pyrantel Tartrate [*1966*] (pi ran′ tel tar′ trate). $C_{11}H_{14}N_2S \cdot C_4H_6O_6$. 356.39. (1) Pyrimidine, 1,4,5,6-tetra-hydro-1-methyl-2-[2-(2-thienyl)ethenyl]-, (*E*)-, [*R*-(*R**,*R**)]-2,3-dihydroxybutanedioate (1:1); (2) (*E*)-1,4,5,6-Tetrahydro-1-methyl-2-[2-(2-thienyl)vinyl]pyrimidine tar-trate (1:1). *UNII-4QIH0N49E7* [pyrantel]. *CAS-33401-94-4; CAS-15686-83-6* [pyrantel]. *Anthelmintic.* Banminth (Pfizer) ◇*CP-10,423-18*

---

† Brand name formerly used, and/or firm no longer concerned with this product.

Pyrathiazine Hydrochloride. $C_{18}H_{20}N_2S.HCl$. 332.89. [Parathiazine is INN.] 10-[2-(1-Pyrrolidinyl)ethyl]phenothiazine hydrochloride. *UNII-X0SMC42Q5O. CAS-522-25-8; CAS-84-08-2.* MI.

Pyrazinamide (pir″ a zin′ a mide). **USP.** $C_5H_5N_3O$. 123.11. (1) Pyrazinecarboxamide; (2) Pyrazinecarboxamide. *UNII-2KNI5N06TI. CAS-98-96-4.* INN; BAN; JAN. *Antibacterial (tuberculostatic).*

Pyrazinecarboxamide — *See* Pyrazinamide.

Pyrazofurin [*1974*] (pir az″ oh fure′ in). $C_9H_{13}N_3O_6$. 259.22. [Pirazofurin is INN.] (1) 1*H*-Pyrazole-5-carboxamide, 4-hydroxy-3-β-D-ribofuranosyl-; (2) 4-Hydroxy-3-β-D-ribofuranosylpyrazole-5-carboxamide. *CAS-30868-30-5.* *Antineoplastic.* ◇47599

Pyrbuterol Hydrochloride — *See* Pirbuterol Hydrochloride.

Pyrethrum Extract (pye ree′ thrum). **USP.** A mixture of three naturally occurring, closely related insecticidal esters of chrysanthemic acid (Pyrethrins I) and three closely related esters of pyrethric acid (Pyrethrins II). *Pediculicide.*

Pyricarbate. $C_{11}H_{15}N_3O_4$. 253.25. [Pyridinol Carbamate is JAN.] 2,6-Pyridinediyldimethylene bis(methylcarbamate). *CAS-1882-26-4.* INN.

Pyridarone. $C_{13}H_9NO$. 195.22. 2-(4-Pyridyl)benzofuran. *UNII-83L91231V7. CAS-7035-04-3.* INN. ◇L-4269

Pyridinol Carbamate (JAN) — *See* Pyricarbate.

Pyridofylline. $C_8H_{11}NO_3.C_9H_{12}N_4O_6S$. 473.46. Pyridoxol salt of 7-(2-hydroxyethyl)theophylline hydrogen sulfate ester. *UNII-W9CI6CR77M. CAS-53403-97-7.* INN; DCF; MI.

Pyridoglutethimide — *See* Rogletimide.

Pyridostigmine Bromide (pir id″ oh stig′ meen broe′ mide). **USP.** $C_9H_{13}BrN_2O_2$. 261.12. (1) Pyridinium, 3-[[(dimethylamino)carbonyl]oxy]-1-methyl-, bromide; (2) 3-Hydroxy-1-methylpyridinium bromide dimethylcarbamate. *UNII-KVI30INA53. CAS-101-26-8; CAS-155-97-5* [pyridostigmine]. INN; BAN; JAN. *Cholinergic.* Mestinon (Valeant); Regonol (Sandoz)

Pyridoxal Calcium Phosphate. $C_8H_8CaNO_6P.3H_2O$. 339.25. 2-Methyl-3-hydroxy-4-formyl-5-hydroxymethylpyridine-5-calcium phosphate trihydrate. *CAS-54-47-7.* JAN.

Pyridoxal Phosphate. $C_8H_{10}NO_6P.H_2O$. 265.16. 3-Hydroxy-2-methyl-5-[(phosphonoxy)methyl]-4-pyridinecarboxaldehyde hydrate. *UNII-5V5IOJ8338. CAS-41468-25-1.* JAN.

Pyridoxamine Phosphate. $C_8H_{13}N_2O_5P.2H_2O$. 284.20. 4-Aminomethyl-3-hydroxy-2-methyl-5-[(phosphonooxy)methyl]pyridine dihydrate. *UNII-QWW7V29814. CAS-529-96-4* (anhydrous). JAN.

Pyridoxine Hydrochloride (pir″ i dox′ een hye″ droe klor′ ide). **USP.** $C_8H_{11}NO_3.HCl$. 205.64. [Pyridoxine is INN and BAN.] (1) 3,4-Pyridinedimethanol, 5-hydroxy-6-methyl-, hydrochloride; (2) Pyridoxol hydrochloride. *UNII-68Y4CF58BV; UNII-KV2JZ1BI6Z* [pyridoxine]. *CAS-58-56-0; CAS-65-23-6* [pyridoxine]. JAN. *Vitamin (enzyme co-factor).* Hexa-Betalin (Lilly)

Pyridylcarbinol — *See* Nicotinyl Alcohol.

Pyridylmethanol — *See* Nicotinyl Alcohol.

Pyrilamine Maleate (pir il′ a meen mal′ ee ate). **USP.** $C_{17}H_{23}N_3O.C_4H_4O_4$. 401.46. [Mepyramine is INN and BAN.] (1) 1,2-Ethanediamine, *N*-[(4-methoxyphenyl)methyl]-*N′,N′*-dimethyl-*N*-2-pyridinyl-, (*Z*)-2-butenedioate (1:1); (2) 2-[[2-(Dimethylamino)ethyl](*p*-methoxybenzyl)amino]pyridine maleate (1:1). *UNII-R35D29L3ZA; UNII-HPE317O9TL* [pyrilamine]. *CAS-59-33-6; CAS-91-84-9* [pyrilamine]. *Antihistaminic.*

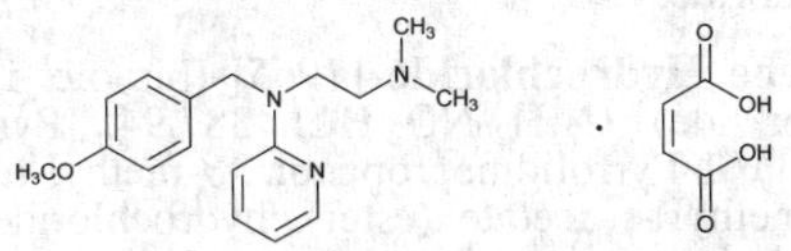

Pyrimethamine (pir″ i meth′ a meen). **USP.** $C_{12}H_{13}ClN_4$. 248.71. (1) 2,4-Pyrimidinediamine, 5-(4-chlorophenyl)-6-ethyl-; (2) 2,4-Diamino-5-(*p*-chlorophenyl)-6-ethylpyrimidine. *UNII-Z3614QOX8W. CAS-58-14-0.* INN; BAN; JAN. *Antimalarial.* Daraprim (GlaxoSmithKline)

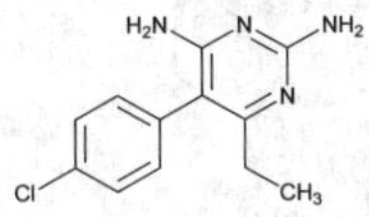

Pyrimitate. $C_{11}H_{20}N_3O_3PS$. 305.33. *O,O*-Diethyl *O*-(2-dimethylamino-6-methyl-4-pyrimidinyl) phosphorothioate. *UNII-6U704SC0N2. CAS-5221-49-8.* INN; BAN. ◇*ICI 29661*

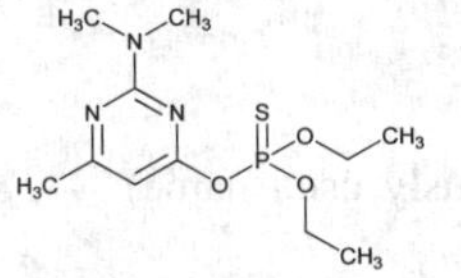

Pyrimithate — *See* Pyrimitate.

Pyrinoline [*1965*] (pir in′ oh leen). $C_{27}H_{20}N_4O$. 416.47. (1) 2-Pyridinemethanol, α-[3-(di-2-pyridinylmethylene)-1,4-cyclopentadien-1-yl]-α-2-pyridinyl-; (2) 3-(Di-2-pyridylmethylene)-α,α-di-2-pyridyl-1,4-cyclopentadiene-1-methanol. *UNII-14PEC3LEVH. CAS-1740-22-3.* INN. *Cardiac depressant (anti-arrhythmic).* Surexin (Ortho-McNeil†) ◇*McN-1210*

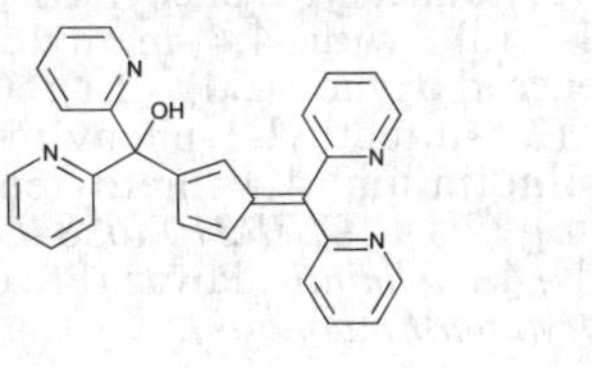

Pyrithidium Bromide (previously used name) — *See* Pyritidium Bromide.

Pyrithione Sodium [*1989*] (pir″ i thye′ one soe′ dee um). C_5H_4NNaOS. 149.15. (1) 2(1*H*)-Pyridinethione, 1-hydroxy-, sodium salt; (2) 1-Hydroxy-2(1*H*)-pyridinethione, sodium salt. *UNII-6L3991491R. CAS-15922-78-8. Antimicrobial (topical).* Sodium Omadine (Olin) ◇*AL02725*

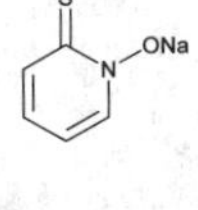

---

† Brand name formerly used, and/or firm no longer concerned with this product.

Pyrithione Zinc [*1966*] (pir″ i thye′ one zink). $C_{10}H_8N_2O_2S_2Zn$. 317.69. (1) Zinc, bis(1-hydroxy-2(1*H*)-pyridinethionato-*O,S*)-(T-4)-; (2) Bis[1-hydroxy-2(1*H*)-pyridinethionato]zinc. *UNII-R953O2RHZ5. CAS-13463-41-7.* INN. *Antibacterial; antifungal; antiseborrheic.* Head & Shoulders Conditioner (Procter & Gamble)

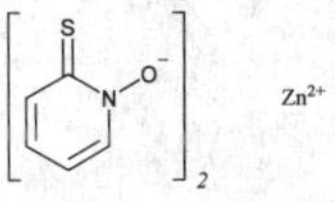

Pyrithioxine (JAN) — *See* Pyritinol.

Pyrithioxine Hydrochloride (JAN) — *See* Pyritinol.

Pyrithyldione. $C_9H_{13}NO_2$. 167.21. 3,3-Diethyl-2,4(1*H*,3*H*)-pyridinedione. *CAS-77-04-3.* INN; MI.

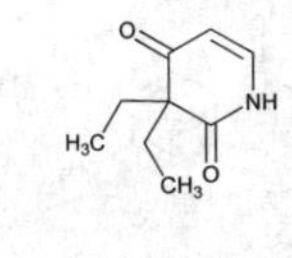

Pyritidium Bromide. $C_{26}H_{27}Br_2N_7$. 597.35. 3-Amino-8-[(2-amino-6-methyl-4-pyrimidinyl)amino]-6-(*p*-aminophenyl)-5-methylphenanthridinium bromide 1′-methobromide. *UNII-3K01419ADP. CAS-14222-46-9; CAS-3616-05-5* [pyritidium]. INN. *[Name previously used: Pyrithidium Bromide.]* ◇*RD 2801*

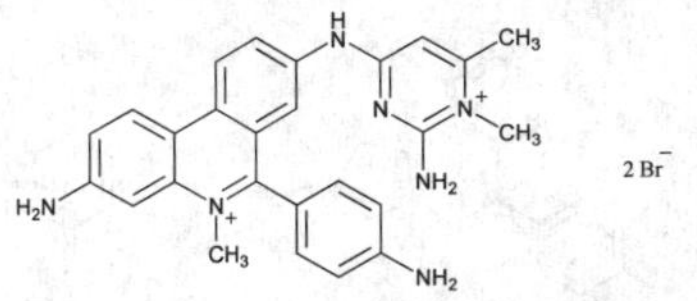

Pyritinol. $C_{16}H_{20}N_2O_4S_2$. 368.47. [Pyrithioxine and Pyrithioxine Hydrochloride are JAN.] 3,3′-(Dithiodimethylene)-bis(5-hydroxy-6-methyl-4-pyridinemethanol). *UNII-AK5Q5FZH2R. CAS-1098-97-1.* INN; BAN; DCF; MI.

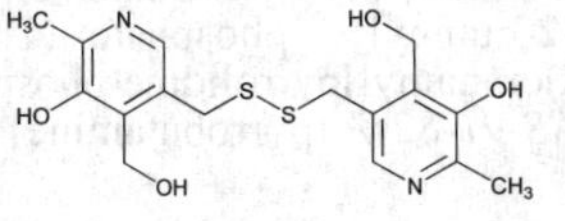

Pyrodifenium Bromide — *See* Prifinium Bromide.

Pyrogallic Acid — *See* Pyrogallol.

Pyrogallol. $C_6H_6O_3$. 126.11. 1,2,3-Trihydroxybenzene. *CAS-87-66-1.* NF X; MI.

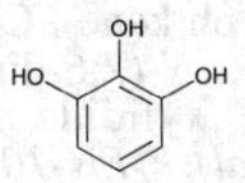

Pyronaridine. $C_{29}H_{32}ClN_5O_2$. 518.05. 4-[(7-Chloro-2-methoxybenzo[*b*][1,5]naphthyridin-10-yl)amino]-2,6-bis[(pyrrolidin-1-yl)methyl]phenol. *CAS-74847-35-1.* INN.

Pyrophendane (INN) — *See* Pyrophenindane.

Pyrophenindane. $C_{21}H_{25}N$. 291.43. [Pyrophendane is INN.] 1-Methyl-3-(3-phenyl-1-indanylmethyl)pyrrolidine. *UNII-TYG45UE07V. CAS-7009-69-0.*

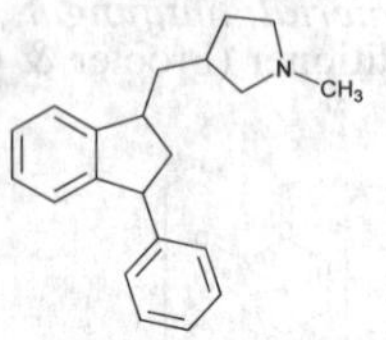

Pyrovalerone Hydrochloride [*1964*] (pir″ oh val′ er one hye″ droe klor′ ide). $C_{16}H_{23}NO.HCl$. 281.82. [Pyrovalerone is INN.] (1) 1-Pentanone, 1-(4-methylphenyl)-2-(1-pyrrolidinyl)-, hydrochloride; (2) 4′-Methyl-2-(1-pyrrolidinyl)valerophenone hydrochloride. *UNII-Z95Z9C2201. CAS-1147-62-2; CAS-3563-49-3* [pyrovalerone]. *Stimulant (central).* ◇*F 1983*

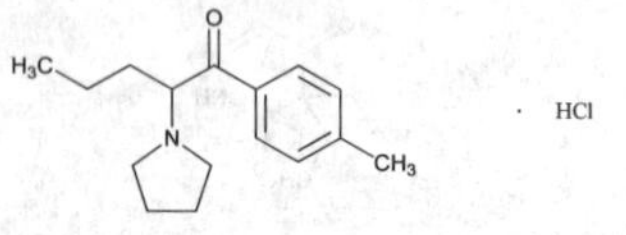

Pyroxamine Maleate [*1963*] (pir ox′ a meen mal′ ee ate). $C_{18}H_{20}ClNO.C_4H_4O_4$. 417.88. [Pyroxamine is INN.] (1) Pyrrolidine, 3-[(4-chlorophenyl)phenylmethoxy]-1-methyl-, (Z)-2-butenedioate (1:1); (2) 3-[(*p*-Chloro-α-phenylbenzyl)oxy]-1-methylpyrrolidine maleate (1:1). *UNII-T38B9T1F30. CAS-5560-75-8; CAS-7009-68-9* [pyroxamine]. *Antihistaminic.* ◇*AHR-224; NSC-64540*

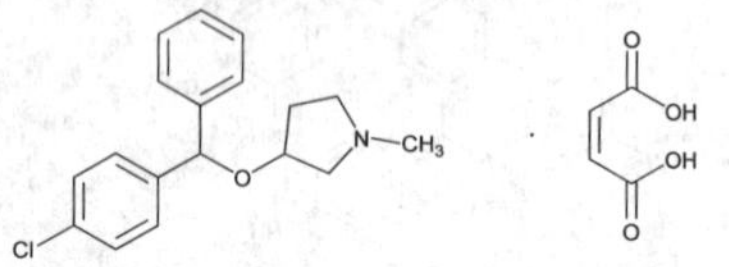

Pyroxylin (pye rox′ i lin). **USP.** (1) Cellulose, nitrate; (2) Pyroxylin. *CAS-9004-70-0.* INN; JAN. Pharmaceutic necessity for Collodion.

Pyrrobutamine Phosphate. $C_{20}H_{22}ClN.2H_3PO_4$. 507.84. [Pyrrobutamine is BAN.] (1) Pyrrolidine, 1-[4-(4-chlorophenyl)-3-phenyl-2-butenyl]-, phosphate (1:2); (2) 1-[γ-(*p*-Chlorobenzyl)cinnamyl]pyrrolidine phosphate (1:2). *CAS-135-31-9; CAS-91-82-7* [pyrrobutamine]. USP XXI. Pyronil (Lilly†)

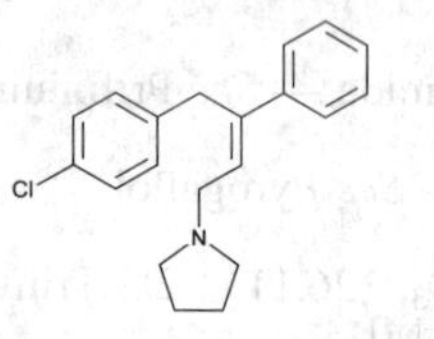

Pyrrocaine [*1962*] (pir′ oh kane). $C_{14}H_{20}N_2O$. 232.32. (1) 1-Pyrrolidineacetamide, *N*-(2,6-dimethylphenyl)-; (2) 1-Pyrrolidineaceto-2′,6′-xylidide. *CAS-2210-77-7.* INN; BAN. *Anesthetic (local).* ◇*EN-1010; NSC-52644*

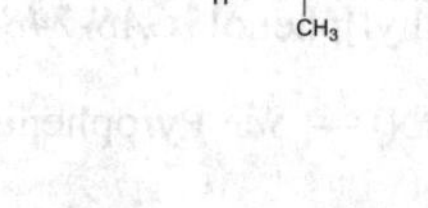

Pyrrocaine Hydrochloride. *CAS-2210-64-2; CAS-2210-77-7* [pyrrocaine]. NF XIV; MI.

Pyrrolifene (INN) Hydrochloride — *See* Pyrroliphene Hydrochloride.

Pyrroliphene Hydrochloride [*1965*] (pir ole′ i feen hye″ droe klor′ ide). $C_{23}H_{29}NO_2.HCl$. 387.94. [Pyrrolifene is INN.] (1) 1-Pyrrolidinepropanol, β-methyl-α-phenyl-α-(phenylmethyl)-, acetate (ester), hydrochloride; (2) (+)-α-Benzyl-β-methyl-α-phenyl-1-pyrrolidinepropanol acetate (ester) hydrochloride. *CAS-5591-44-6; CAS-15686-97-2* [pyrroliphene]. *Analgesic.* ◇*31518*

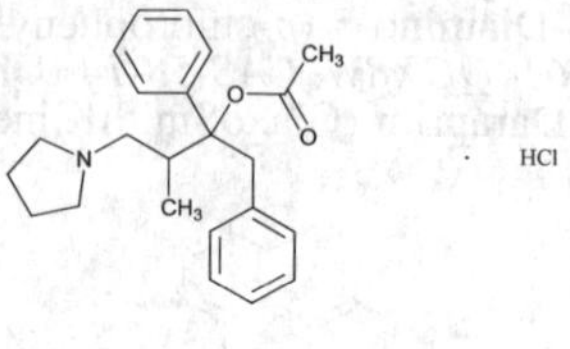

Pyrrolnitrin [*1968*] (pir″ ole nye′ trin). $C_{10}H_6Cl_2N_2O_2$. 257.07. (1) 1*H*-Pyrrole, 3-chloro-4-(3-chloro-2-nitrophenyl)-; (2) 3-Chloro-4-(3-chloro-2-nitrophenyl)pyrrole. *CAS-1018-71-9.* INN; JAN. *Antifungal.* ◇*52230; NSC-107654*

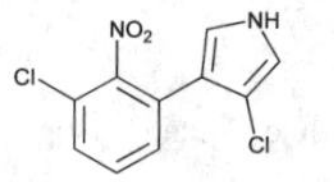

Pyrroxane (previously used name) — *See* Proroxan Hydrochloride.

Pyruvic Acid Calcium Isoniazid. $C_9H_8CaN_3O_3$. 246.26. Pyruvic acid calcium isoniazid heptahydrate. *CAS-3428-05-5* [anhydrous]. JAN.

Pyrvinium Chloride. $C_{26}H_{28}ClN_3$. 417.97. 6-Dimethylamino-2′-[2-(2,5-dimethyl-1-phenyl-3-pyrrolyl)vinyl]-1-methylquinolinium chloride. *CAS-548-84-5.* INN; MI.

Pyrvinium Embonate (DCF) — *See* Pyrvinium Pamoate.

Pyrvinium Pamoate (pir vin′ ee um pam′ oh ate). **USP.** $C_{75}H_{70}N_6O_6$. 1151.39. (1) Quinolinium, 6-(dimethylamino)-2-[2-(2,5-dimethyl-1-phenyl-1*H*-pyrrol-3-yl)ethenyl]-1-methyl-, salt with 4,4′-methylenebis[3-hydroxy-2-naphthalenecarboxylic acid] (2:1); (2) 6-(Dimethylamino)-2-[2-(2,5-dimethyl-1-phenylpyrrol-3-yl)vinyl]-1-methylquinolinium 4,4′-methylenebis[3-hydroxy-2-naphthoate] (2:1). *UNII-310X6S84LW. CAS-3546-41-6.* BAN; JAN. *Anthelmintic.* Povan (Pfizer) *[Name previously used: Viprynium Embonate.]*

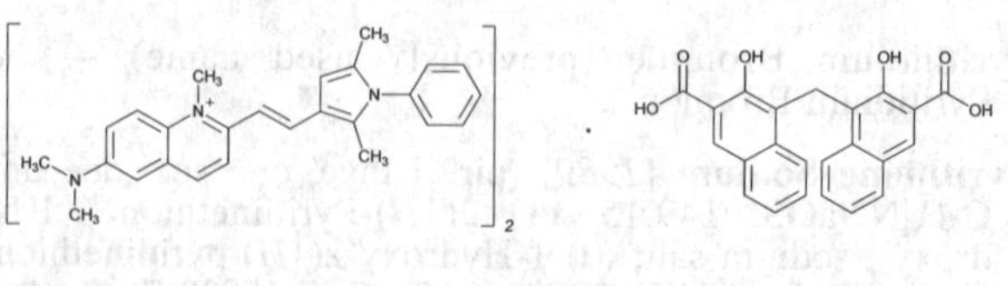

Pytamine. $C_{20}H_{28}N_2O$. 312.45. 2-[α-[2-(Dimethylamino)ethoxy]-2,6-diethylbenzyl]pyridine. *UNII-B8414665Y7. CAS-15301-88-9.* INN. ◇*BS 7161 D [as hydrochloride]*

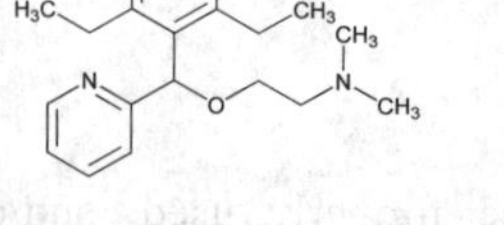

Quadazocine Mesylate [*1985*] (kwad az' oh seen mes' i late). $C_{25}H_{37}NO_2 \cdot CH_4O_3S$. 479.67. [Quadazocine is INN and BAN.] (1) 3-Pentanone, 1-cyclopentyl-5-(1,2,3,4,5,6-hexahydro-8-hydroxy-3,6,11-trimethyl-2,6-methano-3-benzazocin-11-yl)-, [2*R*-(2α,6α,11*S**)]-, methanesulfonate (salt); (2) (-)-(2*R*,6*S*,11*S*)-1-Cyclopentyl-5-(1,2,3,4,5,6-hexahydro-8-hydroxy-3,6,11-trimethyl-2,6-methano-3-benzazocin-11-yl)-3-pentanone methanesulfonate (salt). *CAS-71276-44-3; CAS-71276-43-2* [quadazocine]. *Antagonist (opioid).* ◇*Win 44,441-3*

Quadrosilan. $C_{18}H_{28}O_4Si_4$. 420.75. *cis*-2,2,4,6,6,8-Hexamethyl-4,8-diphenylcyclotetrasiloxane. *UNII-C5KT601WPM. CAS-33204-76-1.* INN; BAN.

Quarfloxin [*2007*] (kwar flox' in). $C_{35}H_{33}FN_6O_3$. 604.67. (1) 3*H*-Benzo[*b*]pyrido[3,2,1-*kl*]phenoxazine-2-carboxamide, 5-fluoro-*N*-[2-[(2*S*)-1-methyl-2-pyrrolidinyl]ethyl]-3-oxo-6-(3-pyrazinyl-1-pyrrolidinyl)-; (2) 5-Fluoro-*N*-[2-[(2*S*)-1-methylpyrrolidin-2-yl]ethyl]-3-oxo-6-[3-(pyrazin-2-yl)-pyrrolidin-1-yl]-3*H*-benzo[*b*]pyrido[3,2,1-*kl*]phenoxazine-2-carboxamide. *CAS-865311-47-3.* INN. *Antineoplastic.* ◇*CX-3543*

Quatacaine. $C_{14}H_{22}N_2O$. 234.34. 2-Methyl-2-(propylamino)-*o*-propionotoluidide. *UNII-49BR7256ZY. CAS-17692-45-4.* INN. ◇*LA-012 [as hydrochloride]*

Quaternium-18 bentonite (CTFA) — *See* Bentoquatam.

Quazepam [*1976*] (kwaz' e pam). **USP.** $C_{17}H_{11}ClF_4N_2S$. 386.79. (1) 2*H*-1,4-Benzodiazepine-2-thione, 7-chloro-5-(2-fluorophenyl)-1,3-dihydro-1-(2,2,2-trifluoroethyl)-; (2) 7-Chloro-5-(*o*-fluorophenyl)-1,3-dihydro-1-(2,2,2-trifluoroethyl)-2*H*-1,4-benzodiazepine-2-thione. *UNII-JF8V0828ZI. CAS-36735-22-5.* INN; BAN. *Sedative-hypnotic.* Doral (Questcor) ◇*Sch 16134*

Quazinone [*1985*] (kwaz' i none). $C_{11}H_{10}ClN_3O$. 235.67. (1) Imidazo[2,1-*b*]quinazolin-2(3*H*)-one, 6-chloro-1,5-dihydro-3-methyl-, (*R*)-; (2) (*R*)-6-Chloro-1,5-dihydro-3-methylimidazo[2,1-*b*]quinazolin-2(3*H*)-one. *UNII-D1Q7F6C2FP. CAS-70018-51-8.* INN. *Cardiotonic.* ◇*Ro 13-6438/006*

Quazodine [*1968*] (kwaz' oh deen). $C_{12}H_{14}N_2O_2$. 218.25. (1) Quinazoline, 4-ethyl-6,7-dimethoxy-; (2) 4-Ethyl-6,7-dimethoxyquinazoline. *CAS-4015-32-1.* INN. *Cardiotonic; bronchodilator.* ◇*MJ 1988*

Quazolast [*1986*] (kwaz' oh last). $C_{12}H_7ClN_2O_3$. 262.65. (1) Oxazolo[4,5-*h*]quinoline-2-carboxylic acid, 5-chloro-, methyl ester; (2) Methyl 5-chlorooxazolo[4,5-*h*]quinoline-2-carboxylate. *CAS-86048-40-0.* INN. *Anti-asthmatic; inhibitor (mediator release).* ◇*RHC 3988*

Quercus stenophylla Extract. JAN.

Quetiapine Fumarate [*1996*] (kwe tye' a peen fue' ma rate). $(C_{21}H_{25}N_3O_2S)_2 \cdot C_4H_4O_4$. 883.09. [Quetiapine is INN and BAN.] (1) Ethanol, 2-[2-(4-dibenzo[*b*,*f*][1,4]thiazepin-11-yl-1-piperazinyl)ethoxy]-, (*E*)-2-butenedioate (2:1) (salt); (2) 2-[2-[2-(4-Dibenzo[*b*,*f*][1,4]thiazepin-11-yl-1-piperaziny-l)ethoxy]ethanol fumarate (2:1) (salt). *UNII-2S3PL1B6UJ;*

---

† Brand name formerly used, and/or firm no longer concerned with this product.

UNII-BGL0JSY5SI [quetiapine]. *CAS-111974-72-2; CAS-111974-69-7* [quetiapine]. *Antipsychotic.* Seroquel (Astra-Zeneca) ◇*ICI 204,636; ZD5077; ZM 204,636*

Quifenadine. $C_{20}H_{23}NO$. 293.40. α,α-Diphenyl-3-quinuclidi-nemethanol. *UNII-W9A18RJ49B. CAS-10447-39-9.* INN.

Quiflapon Sodium [*1995*] (kwi′ flap on soe′ dee um). $C_{34}H_{34}ClN_2NaO_3S$. 609.15. [Quiflapon is INN.] (1) 1*H*-Indole-2-propanoic acid, 1-[(4-chlorophenyl)methyl]-3-[(1,1-dimethylethyl)thio]-α,α-dimethyl-5-(2-quinolinyl-methoxy)-, sodium salt; (2) Sodium 3-(*tert*-butylthio)-1-(*p*-chlorobenzyl)-α,α-dimethyl-5-(2-quinolylmethoxy)in-dole-2-propionate. *UNII-321US0I5R6. CAS-147030-01-1; CAS-136668-42-3* [quiflapon]. *Anti-asthmatic; suppressant (inflammatory bowel disease).* ◇*MK-591*

Quillifoline. $C_{21}H_{24}ClNO_2$. 357.87. 2-(*p*-Chlorophenyl)-1,3,4,6,7,11b-hexahydro-9,10-dimethoxy-2*H*-benzo[*a*]qui-nolizine. *UNII-8JD13PH39Q. CAS-15301-89-0.* INN.

Quilostigmine [*1996*] (kwil″ oh stig′ meen). $C_{23}H_{27}N_3O_2$. 377.48. (1) 2(1*H*)-Isoquinolinecarboxylic acid, 3,4-dihy-dro-, 1,2,3,3a,8,8a-hexahydro-1,3a,8-trimethylpyrrolo[2,3-*b*]indol-5-yl ester, (3a*S*-cis); (2) (3a*S*,8a*R*)-1,2,3,3a,8,8a-Hexahydro-1,3a,8-trimethylpyrrolo[2,3-*b*]indol-5-yl 3,4-dihydro-2(1*H*)-isoquinolinecarboxylate. *CAS-139314-01-5.* INN. *Cholinergic.* ◇*HP 290; NXX-066*

Quinacainol. $C_{21}H_{30}N_2O$. 326.48. (±)-2-*tert*-Butyl-α-[2-(4-piperidyl)ethyl]-4-quinolinemethanol. *CAS-86024-64-8.* INN.

Quinacillin. $C_{18}H_{16}N_4O_6S$. 416.41. (3-Carboxy-2-quinoxali-nyl)penicillin. *UNII-83NB50X92M. CAS-1596-63-0.* INN; BAN; MI.

Quinacrine Hydrochloride. $C_{23}H_{30}ClN_3O.2HCl.2H_2O$. 508.91. [Mepacrine is INN and BAN.] (1) 1,4-Pentanedia-mine, N^4-(6-chloro-2-methoxy-9-acridinyl)-N^1,N^1-diethyl-, dihydrochloride, dihydrate; (2) 6-Chloro-9-[[4-(diethyl-amino)-1-methylbutyl]amino]-2-methoxyacridine dihy-drochloride dihydrate. *CAS-6151-30-0; CAS-69-05-6* [an-hydrous]; *CAS-83-89-6* [quinacrine]. USP XXII. Atabrine Hydrochloride (Sterling Winthrop)

Quinagolide. $C_{20}H_{33}N_3O_3S$. 395.56. (±)-*N,N*-Diethyl-*N*′-[(3*R**,4a*R**,10a*S**)-1,2,3,4,4a,5,10,10a-octahydro-6-hy-droxy-1-propylbenzo[*g*]quinolin-3-yl]sulfamide. *UNII-80Q9QWN15M. CAS-87056-78-8; CAS-94424-50-7* [hy-drochloride]. INN; BAN.

Quinalbarbitone Sodium (previously used name) — *See* Secobarbital Sodium.

Quinaldine Blue [*1966*] (kwin′ al deen). $C_{25}H_{25}ClN_2$. 388.93. (1) Quinolinium, 1-ethyl-2-[3-(1-ethyl-2(1*H*)-quinolinyli-dene)-1-propenyl]-, chloride; (2) 1-Ethyl-2-[3-(1-ethyl-2(1*H*)quinolylidene)propenyl]quinolinium chloride. *UNII-91SZ6DGY86. CAS-2768-90-3.* INN. *Diagnostic aid (ob-stetrics).* ◇*NSC-56808*

Quinapril (kwin′ a pril). **USP** [Tablets]. $C_{25}H_{30}N_2O_5$. 438.52. (3*S*)-2-{*N*-[(*S*)-1-Ethoxycarbonyl-3-phenylpropyl]-L-alanyl}-1,2,3,4-tetrahydroisoquinoline-3-carboxylic acid. *UNII-RJ84Y44811. CAS-85441-61-8.* INN; BAN.

Quinapril Hydrochloride [*1985*] (kwin′ a pril hye″ droe klor′ ide). **USP**. $C_{25}H_{30}N_2O_5 \cdot HCl$. 474.98. (1) 3-Isoquinolinecarboxylic acid, 2-[2-[[1-(ethoxycarbonyl)-3-phenylpropyl]amino]-1-oxopropyl]-1,2,3,4-tetrahydro-, monohydrochloride, [3*S*-[2[*R**(*R**)],3*R**]]; (2) (*S*)-2-[(*S*)-*N*-[(*S*)-1-Carboxy-3-phenylpropyl]alanyl]-1,2,3,4-tetrahydro-3-isoquinolinecarboxylic acid, 1-ethyl ester, monohydrochloride. *UNII-33067B3N2M; UNII-RJ84Y44811* [quinapril]. *CAS-82586-55-8; CAS-85441-61-8* [quinapril]. *Antihypertensive; enzyme inhibitor (angiotensin-converting).* Accupril (Pfizer) ◇*CI-906*

Quinaprilat [*1988*] (kwin′ a pril at″). $C_{23}H_{26}N_2O_5$. 410.46. (1) 3-Isoquinolinecarboxylic acid, 2-[2-[(1-carboxy-3-phenylpropyl)amino]-1-oxopropyl]-1,2,3,4-tetrahydro-, [3*S*-[2[*R**(*R**)],3*R**]]-; (2) (3*S*)-2-[(*S*)-*N*-[(*S*)-1-Carboxy-3-phenylpropyl]alanyl]-1,2,3,4-tetrahydro-3-isoquinolinecarboxylic acid. *CAS-85441-60-7.* INN. *Antihypertensive; enzyme inhibitor (angiotensin-converting).* ◇*CI-928*

Quinazosin Hydrochloride [*1966*] (kwin az′ oh sin hye″ droe klor′ ide). $C_{17}H_{23}N_5O_2 \cdot 2HCl$. 402.32. [Quinazosin is INN.] (1) 4-Quinazolinamine, 6,7-dimethoxy-2-[4-(2-propenyl)-1-piperazinyl]-, dihydrochloride; (2) 2-(4-Allyl-1-piperazinyl)-4-amino-6,7-dimethoxyquinazoline dihydrochloride. *UNII-2N2LI66RRO; UNII-436XK6QFMR* [quinazosin]. *CAS-7262-00-2; CAS-15793-38-1* [quinazosin]. *Antihypertensive.* ◇*CP-11,332-1*

Quinbolone [*1964*] (kwin′ boe lone). $C_{24}H_{32}O_2$. 352.51. (1) Androsta-1,4-dien-3-one, 17-(1-cyclopenten-1-yloxy)-, (17β); (2) 17β-(1-Cyclopenten-1-yloxy)androsta-1,4-dien-3-one. *CAS-2487-63-0.* INN. *Anabolic.*

Quincarbate. $C_{17}H_{18}ClNO_6$. 367.78. Ethyl 10-chloro-3-(ethoxymethyl)-2,3,6,9-tetrahydro-9-oxo-*p*-dioxino[2,3-g]quinoline-8-carboxylate. *UNII-U40Q9GE876. CAS-54340-59-9.* INN. ◇*DU-23187*

Quindecamine Acetate [*1965*] (kwin dek′ a meen as′ e tate). $C_{30}H_{38}N_4 \cdot 2C_2H_4O_2 \cdot 2H_2O$. 610.78. [Quindecamine is INN.] (1) 1,10-Decanediamine, *N*,*N*′-bis(2-methyl-4-quinolinyl)-, diacetate dihydrate; (2) 4,4′-(Decamethylenediimino)diquinaldine diacetate dihydrate. *CAS-5714-05-6; CAS-19146-62-4* [anhydrous]; *CAS-19056-26-9* [quindecamine]. *Antibacterial.* ◇*RMI 8090DJ*

Quindonium Bromide [*1964*] (kwin doe′ nee um broe′ mide). $C_{16}H_{20}BrNO$. 322.24. (1) 1*H*-Benzo[*a*]cyclopenta[*f*]quinolizinium, 2,3,3*a*,5,6,11,12,12*a*-octahydro-8-hydroxy-, bromide; (2) 2,3,3*a*,5,6,11,12,12*a*-Octahydro-8-hydroxy-1*H*-benzo[*a*]cyclopenta[*f*]quinolizinium bromide. *CAS-130-81-4.* INN. *Cardiac depressant (antiarrhythmic).* ◇*W 3366A*

Quindoxin. $C_8H_6N_2O_2$. 162.15. Quinoxaline 1,4-dioxide. *UNII-AMX8J6YS1H. CAS-2423-66-7.* INN; BAN. ◇*ICI 8173*

Quinelorane Hydrochloride [*1989*] (kwin el′ oh rane hye″ droe klor′ ide). $C_{14}H_{22}N_4 \cdot 2HCl$. 319.27. [Quinelorane is INN and BAN.] (1) Pyrido[2,3-g]quinazolin-2-amine, 5,5a,6,7,8,9,9a,10-octahydro-6-propyl-, dihydrochloride, (5a*R*-*trans*)-; (2) (-)-(5a*R*,9a*R*)-2-Amino-5,5a,6,7,8,9,9a,10-octahydro-6-propylpyrido[2,3-g]quinazoline dihydrochloride. *CAS-97548-97-5; CAS-97466-90-5* [quinelorane]. *Antihypertensive; antiparkinsonian.* ◇*LY163502*

---

† Brand name formerly used, and/or firm no longer concerned with this product.

Quinestradol. $C_{23}H_{32}O_3$. 356.50. 3-(Cyclopentyloxy)estra-1,3,5(10)-triene-16α,17β-diol. *UNII-422L8173W8. CAS-1169-79-5.* INN; BAN; MI.

Quinestrol [*1963*] (kwin es' trol). $C_{25}H_{32}O_2$. 364.52. (1) 19-Norpregna-1,3,5(10)-trien-20-yn-17-ol, 3-(cyclopenty-loxy)-, (17α)-; (2) 3-(Cyclopentyloxy)-19-nor-17α-preg-na-1,3,5(10)-trien-20-yn-17-ol. *UNII-JR0N7XD5GZ. CAS-152-43-2.* USP XXII; INN; BAN. *Estrogen.* Estrovis (Pfizer) ◇*W 3566*

Quinetalate (INN) — *See* Quinetolate.

Quinethazone. $C_{10}H_{12}ClN_3O_3S$. 289.74. (1) 6-Quinazoline-sulfonamide, 7-chloro-2-ethyl-1,2,3,4-tetrahydro-4-oxo-; (2) 7-Chloro-2-ethyl-1,2,3,4-tetrahydro-4-oxo-6-quinazoli-nesulfonamide. *UNII-455E0S048W. CAS-73-49-4.* USP XXII; INN; BAN; JAN.

Quinetolate [*1965*] (kwin et' oh late). $C_{14}H_{19}N_3O.2C_{12}H_{19}NO_3$. 695.89. [Quinetalate is INN.] (1) 3-Cyclohexene-1-carboxylic acid, 6-[(diethylamino)carbonyl]-, compd. with N'-(6-methoxy-4-quinolinyl)-N,N-dimethyl-1,2-ethane-diamine (2:1); (2) 6-(Diethylcarbamoyl)-3-cyclohexene-1-carboxylic acid compound with 4-[[2-(dimethylamino)-ethyl]amino]-6-methoxyquinoline (2:1). *CAS-5714-76-1.* *Relaxant (smooth muscle).*

Quinezamide. $C_{13}H_{12}N_4O$. 240.26. N-(5-Methylpyrazolo[1,5-c]quinazolin-1-yl)acetamide. *UNII-005MIM19QV. CAS-77197-48-9.* INN.

Quinfamide [*1978*] (kwin' fa mide). $C_{16}H_{13}Cl_2NO_4$. 354.18. (1) 2-Furancarboxylic acid, 1-(dichloroacetyl)-1,2,3,4-tet-rahydro-6-quinolinyl ester; (2) 2-Furoic acid ester with 1-(dichloroacetyl)-1,2,3,4-tetrahydro-6-quinolinol. *UNII-O1ZB1046R1. CAS-62265-68-3.* INN. *Anti-amebic.* Ame-nide (Sterling Winthrop) ◇*Win 40014*

Quingestanol Acetate [*1967*] (kwin jes' ta nol as' e tate). $C_{27}H_{36}O_3$. 408.57. [Quingestanol is INN and BAN.] (1) 19-Norpregna-3,5-dien-20-yn-17-ol, 3-(cyclopentyloxy)-, ace-tate, (17α)-; (2) 3-(Cyclopentyloxy)-19-nor-17α-pregna-3,5-dien-20-yn-17-ol acetate. *CAS-3000-39-3; CAS-10592-65-1* [quingestanol]. *Progestin.* ◇*W 4540*

Quingestrone [*1963*] (kwin jes' trone). $C_{26}H_{38}O_2$. 382.58. (1) Pregna-3,5-dien-20-one, 3-(cyclopentyloxy)-; (2) 3-(Cy-clopentyloxy)pregna-3,5-dien-20-one. *CAS-67-95-8.* INN. *Progestin.* ◇*W 3399*

Quinidine. $C_{20}H_{24}N_2O_2$. 324.42. (8R,9S)-6'-Methoxycincho-nan-9-ol. *UNII-ITX08688JL. CAS-56-54-2.* NF V; BAN; MI.

Quinidine Gluconate (kwin' i deen gloo' koe nate). **USP**. $C_{20}H_{24}N_2O_2.C_6H_{12}O_7$. 520.57. (1) Cinchonan-9-ol, 6'-methoxy-, (9S)-, mono-D-gluconate (salt); (2) Quinidine mono-D-gluconate (salt). *UNII-R6875N380F. CAS-7054-25-3; CAS-56-54-2* [quinidine]. *Cardiac depressant (anti-arrhythmic).* Duraquin (Warner Chilcott); Quinaglute (Bayer)

Quinidine Sulfate (kwin' i deen sul' fate). **USP**. $(C_{20}H_{24}N_2O_2)_2.H_2SO_4.2H_2O$. 782.94. (1) Cinchonan-9-ol, 6'-methoxy-, (9S)-, sulfate (2:1) (salt), dihydrate; (2) Quinidine sulfate (2:1) (salt) dihydrate. *UNII-J13S2394HE. CAS-6591-63-5; CAS-50-54-4* [anhydrous]; *CAS-56-54-2* [quinidine]. JAN. *Cardiac depressant (anti-arrhythmic).* Cin-quin (Solvay Pharmaceuticals); Quinidex (Wyeth); Quinora (Schering)

Quinine. $C_{20}H_{24}N_2O_2$. 324.42. (8S,9R)-6'-Methoxycincho-nan-9-ol. *UNII-A7V27PHC7A. CAS-130-95-0.* NF X; BAN; MI.

Quinine Ascorbate [*1980*] (kwye' nine a skor' bate). $C_{20}H_{24}N_2O_2.2C_6H_8O_6$. 676.67. (1) L-Ascorbic acid, com-pound with (8α,9R)-6'-methoxycinchonan-9-ol (2:1); (2) L-

Ascorbic acid, compound with quinine (2:1). *CAS-146-40-7. Deterrent (smoking). [Name previously used: Quinine Biascorbate.]*

Quinine Biascorbate (previously used name) — *See* Quinine Ascorbate.

Quinine Bisulfate. *UNII-A7V27PHC7A* [quinine]. *CAS-549-56-4; CAS-130-95-0* [quinine]. NF XI; MI.

Quinine Dihydrochloride. *UNII-A7V27PHC7A* [quinine]. *CAS-60-93-5; CAS-130-95-0* [quinine]. NF XIII; MI.

Quinine Ethylcarbonate. *CAS-83-75-0.* NF VIII; JAN; MI.

Quinine Glycerophosphate. Quinine compound with glycerol phosphate. *UNII-ZP61X8C21F.* NF IV.

Quinine Hydrobromide. Quinine monohydrobromide. NF IX; MI.

Quinine Hydrochloride. Quinine monohydrochloride. *UNII-711S8Y0T33. CAS-6119-47-7.* NF XI; JAN; MI.

Quinine Hypophosphite. Quinine phosphinate (1:1) (salt). NF IV.

Quinine Phosphate. Quinine phosphate (3:2) (salt). NF XI.

Quinine Salicylate. Quinine monosalicylate (salt). *UNII-A7V27PHC7A* [quinine]. *CAS-750-90-3; CAS-130-95-0* [quinine]. NF VIII; MI.

Quinine Sulfate (kwye′ nine sul′ fate). **USP**. $(C_{20}H_{24}N_2O_2)_2 \cdot H_2SO_4 \cdot 2H_2O.$ 782.94. (1) Cinchonan-9-ol, 6′-methoxy-, $(8\alpha,9R)$-, sulfate (2:1) (salt), dihydrate; (2) Quinine sulfate (2:1) (salt) dihydrate. *UNII-KF7Z0E0Q2B. CAS-6119-70-6; CAS-804-63-7* [anhydrous]; *CAS-130-95-0* [quinine]. JAN. *Antimalarial.*

Quinine Tannate. Quinine tannate. *UNII-A7V27PHC7A* [quinine]. *CAS-1407-83-6; CAS-130-95-0* [quinine]. USP X; MI.

Quinisocaine (INN) — *See* Dimethisoquin Hydrochloride.

Quinocide. $C_{15}H_{21}N_3O.$ 259.35. 8-[(4-Aminopentyl)amino]-6-methoxyquinoline. *UNII-CNG7995Y4B. CAS-525-61-1.* INN; MI.

Quinotolast. $C_{17}H_{12}N_6O_3.$ 348.32. 4-Oxo-1-phenoxy-*N*-1*H*-tetrazol-5-yl-4*H*-quinolizine-3-carboxamide. *UNII-SU-C3551A8U. CAS-101193-40-2.* INN.

Quinpirole Hydrochloride [*1984*] (kwin′ pir ole hye″ droe klor′ ide). $C_{13}H_{21}N_3 \cdot HCl.$ 255.79. [Quinpirole is INN.] (1) 1*H*-Pyrazolo[3,4-*g*]quinoline, 4,4a,5,6,7,8,8a,9-octahydro-5-propyl-, monohydrochloride, (4a*R*-*trans*)-; (2) (-)-(4a*R*,8a*R*)-4,4a,5,6,7,8,8a,9-Octahydro-5-propyl-1*H*-pyrazolo[3,4-*g*]quinoline monohydrochloride. *CAS-85798-08-9; CAS-85760-74-3* [quinpirole]. *Antihypertensive.* ◇*LY171555*

Quinprenaline (INN) Sulfate — *See* Quinterenol Sulfate.

Quinterenol Sulfate [*1967*] (kwin ter′ e nol sul′ fate). $(C_{14}H_{18}N_2O_2)_2 \cdot H_2SO_4.$ 590.69. [Quinprenaline is INN.] (1) 5-Quinolinemethanol, 8-hydroxy-α-[[(1-methylethyl)amino]methyl]-, sulfate (2:1); (2) 8-Hydroxy-α-[(isopropylamino)methyl]-5-quinolinemethanol sulfate (2:1). *CAS-13758-23-1; CAS-13757-97-6* [quinterenol]. *Bronchodilator.* ◇*CP-10,303-8*

Quintiofos. $C_{17}H_{16}NO_2PS.$ 329.35. *O*-Ethyl *O*-(8-quinolyl) phenylphosphonothioate. *UNII-X50ZS5010Z. CAS-1776-83-6.* INN; BAN. ◇*Bayer 9037*

Quinuclium Bromide [*1978*] (kwin ue′ klee um broe′ mide). $C_{14}H_{18}BrNO \cdot \tfrac{1}{2}H_2O.$ 305.21. (1) 1-Azoniabicyclo[2.2.2]octane, 1-methyl-3-oxo-4-phenyl-, bromide, hemihydrate; (2) 1-Methyl-3-oxo-4-phenylquinuclidinium bromide hemihydrate. *UNII-502H53WMM0. CAS-64755-06-2; CAS-35425-83-3* [anhydrous]. INN. *Antihypertensive.* ◇*MA-540*

Quinupramine. $C_{21}H_{24}N_2$. 304.43. 10,11-Dihydro-5-(3-quinuclidinyl)-5H-dibenz[b,f]azepine. *CAS-31721-17-2.* INN; DCF; MI.

Quinupristin [*1993*] (kwin″ ue pris′ tin). $C_{53}H_{67}N_9O_{10}S$. 1022.22. (1) Virginiamycin S_1, 4-[4-(dimethylamino)-N-methyl-L-phenylalanine]-5-[5-[(1-azabicyclo[2.2.2]oct-3-ylthio)methyl]-4-oxo-L-2-piperidinecarboxylic acid]-, (S)-; (2) N-[(6R,9S,10R,13S,15aS,18R,22S,24aS)-22-[p-(Dimethylamino)benzyl]-6-ethyldocosahydro-10,23-dimethyl-5,8,12,15,17,21,24-heptaoxo-13-phenyl-18-[[(3S)-3-quinuclidinylthio]methyl]-12H-pyrido[2,1-f]pyrrolo[2,1-l][1,4,7,10,13,16]oxapentaazacyclononadecin-9-yl]-3-hydroxypicolinamide. *UNII-23OW28RS7P. CAS-120138-50-3.* INN; BAN. *Antibacterial.* ◇*RP 57669*

Quipazine Maleate [*1966*] (kwip′ a zeen mal′ ee ate). $C_{13}H_{15}N_3 \cdot C_4H_4O_4$. 329.35. [Quipazine is INN.] (1) Quinoline, 2-(1-piperazinyl)-, (Z)-2-butenedioate (1:1); (2) 2-(1-Piperazinyl)quinoline maleate (1:1). *UNII-JY444CK9IG; UNII-4WCY05C0SJ* [quipazine]. *CAS-5786-68-5; CAS-4774-24-7* [quipazine]. *Antidepressant; oxytocic.* ◇*MA 1291*

Quisultazine. $C_{21}H_{25}N_3O_2S_2$. 415.57. N,N-Dimethyl-10-(3-quinuclidinyl)phenothiazine-2-sulfonamide. *UNII-60J29WG4Q6. CAS-64099-44-1.* INN.

Quisultidine — *See* Quisultazine.

Rabeprazole Sodium [*1995*] (ra bep′ ra zole soe′ dee um). $C_{18}H_{20}N_3NaO_3S$. 381.42. [Rabeprazole is INN and BAN.] (1) 1H-Benzimidazole, 2-[[[4-(3-methoxypropoxy)-3-methyl-2-pyridinyl]methyl]sulfinyl]-, sodium salt; (2) 2-[[[4-(3-Methoxypropoxy)-3-methyl-2-pyridyl]methyl]sulfinyl]benzimidazole sodium salt. *UNII-3L36P16U4R.*

CAS-117976-90-6; CAS-117976-89-3 [rabeprazole]. *Antiulcerative; gastric acid pump inhibitor.* Aciphex (Eisai Medical Research) ◇*LY307640 sodium; E-3810*

Rabeximod. $C_{22}H_{24}ClN_5O$. 409.91. 2-(9-Chloro-2,3-dimethyl-6H-indolo[2,3-b]quinoxalin-6-yl)-N-[2-(dimethylamino)ethyl]acetamide. *CAS-872178-65-9.* INN.

Rabies Immune Globulin (ray′ beez i mune′ glob′ ue lin). **USP.** A sterile, nonpyrogenic, slightly opalescent solution consisting of globulins derived from blood plasma or serum that has been tested for the absence of hepatitis B surface antigen, derived from selected adult human donors who have been immunized with rabies vaccine and have developed high titers of rabies antibody. *Immunizing agent (passive).* BayRab (Bayer)

Rabies Vaccine (ray′ beez vax′ een). **USP.** A sterile preparation, in dried or liquid form, of inactivated rabies virus harvested from inoculated diploid cell cultures. *Immunizing agent (active).*

Racecadotril. $C_{21}H_{23}NO_4S$. 385.48. ($\pm$)-N-[α-(Mercaptomethyl)hydrocinnamoyl]glycine, benzyl ester, acetate (ester). *UNII-76K53XP4TO. CAS-81110-73-8.* INN.

Racefemine. $C_{18}H_{23}NO$. 269.38. ($\pm$)-α-Methyl-N-(1-methyl-2-phenoxyethyl)phenethylamine. *UNII-GFK50B8Y78. CAS-22232-57-1; CAS-15686-98-3* [replaced]. INN; DCF; MI. ◇*CB 3697*

Racefenicol (INN) — *See* Racephenicol.

Racementhol. $C_{10}H_{20}O$. 156.27. ($\pm$)-(1R*,3R*,4S*)-Menthol. *UNII-YS08XHA860. CAS-15356-70-4.* INN; BAN.

Racemethadol — *See* Dimepheptanol.

Racemethionine [*1980*] (rayse″ e me thye′ oh neen). $C_5H_{11}NO_2S$. 149.21. [Methionine is INN; DL-Methionine is JAN.] (1) Methionine, DL-; (2) DL-2-Amino-4-

(methylthio)-butyric acid. *CAS-59-51-8.* USP XXI. *Acidifier (urinary).* Pedameth (Forest) *[Name previously used: Methionine (NF XIV).]*

Racemethorphan. $C_{18}H_{25}NO$. 271.40. (±)-3-Methoxy-*N*-methylmorphinan. *CAS-510-53-2.* INN; BAN; DCF; MI.

Racemetirosine. $C_{10}H_{13}NO_3$. 195.22. (±)-α-Methyl-DL-tyrosine. *UNII-X88TTO174Z. CAS-620-30-4.* INN.

Racemoramide. $C_{25}H_{32}N_2O_2$. 392.53. (±)-4-[2-Methyl-4-oxo-3,3-diphenyl-4-(1-pyrrolidinyl)butyl]morpholine. *UNII-L3J8QT828G. CAS-545-59-5.* INN; BAN; DCF. ◇*R 610*

Racemorphan. $C_{17}H_{23}NO$. 257.37. (±)-3-Hydroxy-*N*-methylmorphinan. *CAS-297-90-5.* INN; BAN.

Racephedrine Hydrochloride [*1988*] (rayse″ e fed′ rin hye″ droe klor′ ide). $C_{10}H_{15}NO.HCl$. 201.69. [Racephedrine is INN and BAN.] *dl*-α[1-(Methylamino)ethyl]benzyl alcohol hydrochloride. *UNII-43SK4LAO7D. CAS-134-71-4; CAS-90-81-3* [racephedrine].

Racephenicol [*1968*] (rayse fen′ i kol). $C_{12}H_{15}Cl_2NO_5S$. 356.22. [Racefenicol is INN.] (1) Acetamide, 2,2-dichloro-*N*-[2-hydroxy-1-(hydroxymethyl)-2-[4-(methylsulfonyl)-phenyl]ethyl]-, (*R*,R**)-(±)-; (2) (±)-*threo*-2,2-Dichloro-*N*-[β-hydroxy-α-(hydroxymethyl)-*p*-

(methylsulfonyl)phenethyl]acetamide. *UNII-283383NO13. CAS-847-25-6. Antibacterial.* Dexawin (Sterling Winthrop†) ◇*Win 5063*

Racepinefrine (INN) — *See* Racepinephrine.

Racepinephrine (rayse ep″ i nef′ rin). USP. $C_9H_{13}NO_3$. 183.20. [Racepinefrine is INN.] (1) 1,2-Benzenediol, 4-[1-hydroxy-2-(methylamino)ethyl]-, (±)-; (2) (±)-3,4-Dihydroxy-α-[(methylamino)methyl]benzyl alcohol. *UNII-GR0L9S3J0F. CAS-329-65-7. Bronchodilator.* Vaponefrin (Fisons†)

Racepinephrine Hydrochloride (rayse ep″ i nef′ rin hye″ droe klor′ ide). USP. $C_9H_{13}NO_3.HCl$. 219.67. (1) 1,2-Benzenediol, 4-[1-hydroxy-2-(methylamino)ethyl]-, hydrochloride (±)-; (2) (±)-3,4-Dihydroxy-α-[(methylamino)methyl]benzyl alcohol, hydrochloride. *UNII-336096P2WE. CAS-329-63-5; CAS-329-65-7* [racepinephrine]. *Bronchodilator.*

Raclopride C 11 [*1997*] (rak′ loe pride). USP [Injection]. $C_{14}{}^{11}CH_{20}Cl_2N_2O_3$. [Raclopride is INN and BAN.] (1) Benzamide, 3,5-dichloro-*N*-[(1-ethyl-2-pyrrolidinyl)methyl]-2-hydroxy-6-(methoxy-^{11}C)-, (*S*)-; (2) (*S*)-3,5-Dichloro-*N*-[(1-ethyl-2-pyrrolidinyl)methyl]-6-hydroxy-[α-^{11}C]-*o*-anisamide. *CAS-97849-54-2; CAS-84225-95-6* [raclopride]. *Radioactive agent.*

Ractopamine Hydrochloride [*1987*] (rak toe′ pa meen hye″ droe klor′ ide). $C_{18}H_{23}NO_3.HCl$. 337.84. [Ractopamine is INN.] (1) Benzenemethanol, 4-hydroxy-α-[[[3-(4-hydroxyphenyl)-1-methylpropyl]amino]methyl]-, hydrochloride; (2) (±)-*all-rac-p*-Hydroxy-α-[[[3-(*p*-hydroxyphenyl)-1-methylpropyl]amino]methyl]benzyl alcohol, hydrochloride. *CAS-90274-24-1; CAS-97825-25-7* [ractopamine]. *Growth stimulant (veterinary).* ◇*LYO31537; EL737*

Radafaxine Hydrochloride [*2004*] (rad″ a fax′ een hye″ droe klor′ ide). $C_{13}H_{18}ClNO_2.HCl$. 292.20. [Radafaxine is INN.] (1) 2-Morpholinol, 2-(3-chlorophenyl)-3,5,5-trimethyl-, hydrochloride, (2*S*,3*S*)-; (2) (+)-(2*S*,3*S*)-2-(3-Chlorophe-

---

† Brand name formerly used, and/or firm no longer concerned with this product.

nyl)-3,5,5-trimethylmorpholin-2-ol hydrochloride. *UNII-SYD411HZ3S. CAS-106083-71-0; CAS-192374-14-4* [radafaxine]. *Antidepressant; antianxiety.* ◇*GW353162A*

Radezolid [*2008*] (ra dez' oh lid). $C_{22}H_{23}FN_6O_3$. 438.45. (1) Acetamide, *N*-[[(5*S*)-3-[2-fluoro-4'-[[(1*H*-1,2,3-triazol-5-ylmethyl)amino]methyl][1,1'-biphenyl]-4-yl]-2-oxo-5-oxazolidinyl]methyl]-; (2) *N*-{[(5*S*)-3-(2-Fluoro-4'-{[(1*H*-1,2,3-triazol-5-ylmethyl)amino]methyl}biphenyl-4-yl)-2-oxo-1,3-oxazolidin-5-yl]methyl}acetamide. *UNII-53PC6LO35W. CAS-869884-78-6.* INN. *Antibacterial.* ◇*RX-103; RX-1741; RX-01667*

Radezolid Hydrochloride [*2008*] (ra dez' oh lid hye″ droe klor′ ide). $C_{22}H_{23}FN_6O_3$·HCl. 474.92. (1) Acetamide, *N*-[[(5*S*)-3-[2-fluoro-4'-[[(1*H*-1,2,3-triazol-5-ylmethyl)amino]methyl][1,1'-biphenyl]-4-yl]-2-oxo-5-oxazolidinyl]-methyl]-, hydrochloride; (2) *N*-{[(5*S*)-3-(2-Fluoro-4'-{[(1*H*-1,2,3-triazol-5-ylmethyl)amino]methyl}biphenyl-4-yl)-2-oxo-1,3-oxazolidin-5-yl]methyl}acetamide hydrochloride. *UNII-37CW568NXL. CAS-869884-77-5. Antibacterial.* ◇*RX-103; RX-1741; RX-01667*

Radiomerisoprol 197 Hg — *See* Merisoprol Hg 197.

Radioselenomethionine 75 Se — *See* Selenomethionine Se 75.

Radiotolpovidone I 131 (INN) — *See* Tolpovidone I 131.

Radiprodil. $C_{21}H_{20}FN_3O_4$. 397.40. 2-{4-[(4-Fluorophenyl)-methyl]piperidin-1-yl}-2-oxo-*N*-(2-oxo-2,3-dihydro-1,3-benzoxazol-6-yl)acetamide. *CAS-496054-87-6.* INN.

Radolmidine (previously used name) — *See* Fadolmidine.

Radolmidine Hydrochloride (previously used name) — *See* Fadolmidine Hydrochloride.

Radotermin. $C_{1184}H_{1844}N_{330}O_{350}S_{22}$. Growth differentiation factor 5 (human), homodimer. *CAS-575458-75-2.* INN.

Rafabegron. $C_{21}H_{23}ClN_2O_4$. 402.87. (3-{(2*R*)-2-[(2*R*)-2-(3-Chlorophenyl)-2-hydroxyethylamino]propyl}-1*H*-indol-7-yloxy)acetic acid. *CAS-244081-42-3.* INN.

Rafivirumab. $C_{6462}H_{9942}N_{1714}O_{2036}S_{46}$. Immunoglobulin G1, anti-[rabies virus glycoprotein], *Homo sapiens* monoclonal antibody, CR57; gamma1 heavy chain (1-456) [*Homo sapiens* VH (IGHV1-69-(IGHD)-IGHJ5*02) [8.8.20] (1-127) - IGHG1*03, CH3 K130>del (128-456)], (230-217')-disulfide with lambda light chain (1'-218') [*Homo sapiens* V-LAMBDA (IGLV2-11-IGLJ2*01) [9.3.12] (1'-112') - IGLC2*01 (113'-218')]; (236-236″:239-239″)-bisdisulfide dimer. *CAS-944548-37-2.* INN.

Rafoxanide [*1970*] (ra fox′ a nide). $C_{19}H_{11}Cl_2I_2NO_3$. 626.01. (1) Benzamide, *N*-[3-chloro-4-(4-chlorophenoxy)phenyl]-2-hydroxy-3,5-diiodo-; (2) 3′-Chloro-4′-(*p*-chlorophenoxy)-3,5-diiodosalicylanilide. *CAS-22662-39-1.* INN; BAN. *Anthelmintic.*

Ragaglitazar. $C_{25}H_{25}NO_5$. 419.47. (-)-(2*S*)-2-Ethoxy-3-[4-[2-(10*H*-phenoxazin-10-yl)ethoxy]phenyl]propanoic acid. *UNII-Q5ELR5A7Y5. CAS-222834-30-2.* INN.

Ralfinamide. $C_{17}H_{19}FN_2O_2$. 302.34. (2*S*)-2-[4-(2-Fluorobenzyloxy)benzylamino]propanamide. *UNII-3LPF0S0GVV. CAS-133865-88-0.* INN.

Ralitoline [*1991*] (ra lit′ oh leen). $C_{13}H_{13}ClN_2O_2S$. 296.77. (1) Acetamide, *N*-(2-chloro-6-methylphenyl)-2-(3-methyl-4-oxo-2-thiazolidinylidene)-, (*Z*)-; (2) (*Z*)-6′-Chloro-3-methyl-4-oxo-$\Delta^{2,\alpha}$-thiazolidineaceto-*o*-toluide. *UNII-Q4MW9RM93A. CAS-93738-40-0.* INN. *Anticonvulsant.* ◇*CI-946*

Raloxifene Hydrochloride [*1988*] (ral ox′ i feen hye″ droe klor′ ide). $C_{28}H_{27}NO_4S$·HCl. 510.04. [Raloxifene is INN and BAN.] (1) Methanone, [6-hydroxy-2-(4-hydroxyphenyl)benzo[*b*]thien-3-yl][4-[2-(1-piperidinyl)ethoxy]phenyl]-, hydrochloride; (2) 6-Hydroxy-2-(*p*-hydroxyphenyl)benzo[*b*]thien-3-yl-*p*-(2-piperidinoethoxy)phenyl ketone, hydrochloride. *UNII-4F86W47BR6; UNII-YX9162EO3I* [raloxifene]. *CAS-82640-04-8; CAS-84449-90-1* [raloxifene]. *Anti-estrogen.* Evista (Lilly) [*Name previously used: Keoxifene Hydrochloride.*] ◇*LY156758*

Raltegravir Potassium [*2007*] (ral teg′ ra vir poe tas′ ee um). $C_{20}H_{20}FKN_6O_5$. 482.51. [Raltegravir is INN.] (1) 4-Pyrimidinecarboxamide, *N*-[(4-fluorophenyl)methyl]-1,6-dihydro-5-hydroxy-1-methyl-2-[1-methyl-1-[[(5-methyl-1,3,4-oxadiazol-2-yl)carbonyl]amino]ethyl]-6-oxo-, monopotassium salt; (2) Potassium 4-[(4-fluorobenzyl)carbamoyl]-1-methyl-2-[1-methyl-1-[[(5-methyl-1,3,4-oxadia-zol-2-yl)carbonyl]amino]ethyl]-6-oxo-1,6-dihydropyrimi-din-5-olate. *UNII-43Y000U234; UNII-22VKV8053U* [raltegravir]. *CAS-871038-72-1; CAS-518048-05-0* [ralte-gravir]. JAN. *Antiviral.* ◇*MK-0518*

Raltitrexed [*1996*] (ral″ ti trex′ ed). $C_{21}H_{22}N_4O_6S$. 458.49. (1) L-Glutamic acid, *N*-[[5-[[(1,4-dihydro-2-methyl-4-oxo-6-quinazolinyl)methyl]methylamino]-2-thienyl]carbonyl]-; (2) *N*-[5-[[(3,4-Dihydro-2-methyl-4-oxo-6-quinazolinyl)-methyl]methylamino]-2-thenoyl]-L-glutamic acid. *CAS-112887-68-0*. INN; BAN. *Advanced colorectal cancer treatment (thymidylate synthase inhibitor).* Tomudex (Zeneca) ◇*ZD1694*

Raluridine [*1996*] (ral ure′ i deen). $C_9H_{10}ClFN_2O_4$. 264.64. (1) Uridine, 5-chloro-2′,3′-dideoxy-3′-fluoro-; (2) 5-Chloro-2′,3′-dideoxy-3′-fluorouridine. *CAS-119644-22-3*. *Antiviral.* ◇*935U83*

Ramatroban. $C_{21}H_{21}FN_2O_4S$. 416.47. (+)-(3*R*)-3-(*p*-Fluoro-benzenesulfonamido)-1,2,3,4-tetrahydrocarbazole-9-propi-onic acid. *UNII-P1ALI72U6C*. *CAS-116649-85-5*. INN; BAN. ◇*BAY u 3405; EN 137774*

Rambufaside — *See* Meproscillarin.

Ramciclane. $C_{21}H_{33}NO$. 315.49. 2-[(2-Benzyl-2-bornyl)oxy]-*N,N*-dimethylethylamine. *UNII-I8AB3P944K*. *CAS-96743-96-3*. INN.

Ramelteon [*2004*] (ra mel′ tee on). $C_{16}H_{21}NO_2$. 259.34. (1) Propanamide, *N*-[2-[(8*S*)-1,6,7,8-tetrahydro-2*H*-inde-no[5,4-*b*]furan-8-yl]ethyl]-; (2) (-)-*N*-[2-([(8*S*)-1,6,7,8-Tet-rahydro-2*H*-indeno[5,4-*b*]furan-8-yl]ethyl]propanamide. *UNII-901AS54I69*. *CAS-196597-26-9*. INN; BAN; JAN. *Treatment of sleep disorders.* Rozerem (Takeda) ◇*TAK-375*

Ramifenazone. $C_{14}H_{19}N_3O$. 245.32. 4-(Isopropylamino)-2,3-dimethyl-1-phenyl-3-pyrazolin-5-one. *UNII-GKH2KOV2RF*. *CAS-3615-24-5*. INN; MI.

Ramipril [*1986*] (ra′ mi pril). USP. $C_{23}H_{32}N_2O_5$. 416.51. (1) Cyclopenta[*b*]pyrrole-2-carboxylic acid, 1-[2-[[1-(ethoxy-carbonyl)-3-phenylpropyl]amino]-1-oxopropyl]octahy-dro-, [2*S*-[1[*R**(*R**)],2α,3aβ,6aβ]]-; (2) (2*S*,3a*S*,6a*S*)-1-[(*S*)-*N*-[(*S*)-1-Carboxy-3-phenylpropyl]alanyl]octahydro-cyclopenta[*b*]pyrrole-2-carboxylic acid, 1-ethyl ester. *UNII-L35JN3I7SJ*. *CAS-87333-19-5*. INN; BAN. *Antihy-pertensive; enzyme inhibitor (angiotensin-converting).* Altace (King) ◇*HOE 498*

Ramiprilat. $C_{21}H_{28}N_2O_5$. 388.46. (2*S*,3a*S*,6a*S*)-1-[(*S*)-*N*-[(*S*)-1-Carboxy-3-phenylpropyl]alanyl]octahydrocyclopen-ta[*b*]pyrrole-2-carboxylic acid. *UNII-6N5U4QFC3G*. *CAS-87269-97-4*. INN.

Ramixotidine. $C_{16}H_{21}N_3O_3S$. 335.42. *N*-[2-[[5-[(Dimethyla-mino)methyl]furfuryl]thio]ethyl]nicotinamide 1-oxide. *UNII-957W618927*. *CAS-84071-15-8*. INN.

---

† Brand name formerly used, and/or firm no longer concerned with this product.

Ramnodigin. $C_{29}H_{44}O_6$. 488.66. 14-Hydroxy-3β-[(2,3,6-trideoxy-α-L-*erythro*-hexopyranosyl)oxy]-5β-card-20(22)-enolide. *UNII-Z8SRY7BR30. CAS-33156-28-4.* INN.

Ramoplanin [*1992*] (ra″ moe plan′ in). Glycolipodepsi peptide antibiotic produced by *actinoplanes* species ATCC33076. Ramoplanin is a complex antibiotic consisting of a main component designated as ramoplanin A_2 and a small amount of related substances, ramoplanin A_1, A'_1, A'_2, A_3, and A'_3. *CAS-76168-82-6.* INN. *Antibacterial.* ◇*MDL 62,198*

Ramoplanin A_1. $C_{118}H_{152}ClN_{21}O_{40}$. 2540.04. (1) Ramoplanin A 1 (peptide moiety), 11-[L-2-[4-[(2-O-α-D-mannopyranosyl-α-D-mannopyranosyl)oxy]phenyl]glycine]-; (2) (S)-2-(3-Chloro-4-hydroxyphenyl)-N-[N^2-[(2Z,4E)-2,4-octadienoyl]-(S)-asparaginyl-(2S,3S)-3-hydroxyasparaginyl-(R)-2-(p-hydroxyphenyl)glycyl-(R)-ornithyl-(2R,3R)-allothreonyl-2-(p-hydroxyphenyl)glycyl-2-(p-hydroxyphenyl)glycyl-(2S,3S)-allothreonyl-(S)-phenylalanyl-(R)-ornithyl-(S)-2-[p-[(2-O-α-D-mannopyranosyl-α-D-mannopyranosyl)oxy]phenyl]glycyl-(2R,3R)-allothreonyl-(S)-2-(p-hydroxyphenyl)glycylglycyl-(S)-leucyl-(R)-alanyl]glycine ψ_1-lactone. *CAS-81988-87-6.*

Ramoplanin A'_1. $C_{112}H_{142}ClN_{21}O_{35}$. 2377.90. (1) Ramoplanin A 1 (peptide moiety), 11-[L-2-[4-[(α-D-mannopyranosyloxy)phenyl]glycine]-; (2) (S)-2-(3-Chloro-4-hydroxyphenyl)-N-[N^2-[(2Z,4E)-2,4-octadienoyl]-(S)-asparaginyl-(2S,3S)-3-hydroxyasparaginyl-(R)-2-(p-hydroxyphenyl)-glycyl-(R)-ornithyl-(2R,3R)-allothreonyl-2-(p-hydroxyphenyl)glycyl-2-(p-hydroxyphenyl)glycyl-(2S,3S)-allothreonyl-(S)-phenylalanyl-(R)-ornithyl-(S)-2-[p-(α-D-mannopyranosyloxy)phenyl]glycyl-(2R,3R)-allothreonyl-(S)-2-(p-hydroxyphenyl)glycylglycyl-(S)-leucyl-(R)-alanyl]-glycine ψ_1-lactone. *CAS-124884-28-2.*

Ramoplanin A_2 (Main Component). $C_{119}H_{154}ClN_{21}O_{40}$. 2554.07. (1) Ramoplanin A 1 (peptide moiety), 1-[N^2-(7-methyl-1-oxo-2,4-octadienyl)-L-asparagine]-11-[L-2-[4-[(2-O-α-D-mannopyranosyl-α-D-mannopyranosyl)oxy]-phenyl]glycine]-,(Z,E)-; (2) (S)-2-(3-Chloro-4-hydroxyphenyl)-N-[N^2-[(2Z,4E)-7-methyl-2,4-octadienoyl]-(S)-asparaginyl-(2S,3S)-3-hydroxyasparaginyl-(R)-2-(p-hydro-

xyphenyl)glycyl-(R)-ornithyl-(2R,3R)-allothreonyl-2-(p-hydroxyphenyl)glycyl-2-(p-hydroxyphenyl)glycyl-(2S,3S)-allothreonyl-(S)-phenylalanyl-(R)-ornithyl-(S)-2-[p-[(2-O-α-D-mannopyranosyl-α-D-mannopyranosyl)oxy]phenyl]glycyl-(2R,3R)-allothreonyl-(S)-2-(p-(hydroxyphenyl)glycylglycyl-(S)-leucyl-(R)-alanyl]glycine ψ_1-lactone. *CAS-81988-88-7.*

Ramoplanin A'_2. $C_{113}H_{144}ClN_{21}O_{35}$. 2391.93. (1) Ramoplanin A 1 (peptide moiety), 1-[N^2-(7-methyl-1-oxo-2,4-octadienyl)-L-asparagine]-11-[L-2-[4-(α-D-mannopyranosyloxy)-phenyl]glycine]-, (Z,E)-; (2) (S)-2-(3-Chloro-4-hydroxyphenyl)-N-[N^2-[(2Z,4E)-7-methyl-2,4-octadienoyl]-(S)-asparaginyl-(2S,3S)-3-hydroxyasparaginyl-(R)-2-(p-hydroxyphenyl)glycyl-(R)-ornithyl-(2R,3R)-allothreonyl-2-(p-hydroxyphenyl)glycyl-2-(p-hydroxyphenyl)glycyl-(2S,3S)-allothreonyl-(S)-phenylalanyl-(R)-ornithyl-(S)-2-[p-(α-D-mannopyranosyloxy)phenyl]glycyl-(2R,3R)-allothreonyl-(S)-2-(p-hydroxyphenyl)glycylglycyl-(S)-leucyl-(R)-alanyl]glycine ψ_1-lactone. *CAS-124884-29-3.*

Ramoplanin A_3. $C_{120}H_{156}ClN_{21}O_{40}$. 2568.09. (1) Ramoplanin A 1 (peptide moiety), 1-[N^2-methyl-1-oxo-2,4-nonadienyl)-L-asparagine]-11-[L-2-[4-[(2-O-α-D-mannopyranosyl-α-D-mannopyranosyl)oxy]phenyl]glycine]-, (Z,E)-; (2) (S)-2-(3-Chloro-4-hydroxyphenyl)-N-[N^2-[(2Z,4E)-8-methyl-2,4-nonadienoyl]-(S)-asparaginyl-(2S,3S)-3-hydroxyasparaginyl-(R)-2-(p-hydroxyphenyl)glycyl-(R)-ornithyl-(2R,3R)-allothreonyl-2-(p-hydroxyphenyl)glycyl-2-(p-hydroxyphenyl)glycyl-(2S,3S)-allothreonyl-(S)-phenylalanyl-(R)-ornithyl-(S)-2-[p-[(2-O-α-D-mannopyranosyl-α-D-mannopyranosyl)oxy]phenyl]glycyl-(2R,3R)-allothreonyl-(S)-2-(p-hydroxyphenyl)glycylglycyl-(S)-leucyl-(R)-alanyl]glycine ψ_1-lactone. *CAS-81988-89-8.*

Ramoplanin A'_3. $C_{114}H_{146}ClN_{21}O_{35}$. 2405.95. (1) Ramoplanin A 1 (peptide moiety), 1-[N^2-(8-methyl-1-oxo-2,4-nonadienyl)-L-asparagine]-11-[L-2-[4-(α-D-mannopyranosyloxy)phenyl]glycine]-, (Z,E)-; (2) (S)-2-(3-Chloro-4-hydroxyphenyl)-N-[N^2-[(2Z,4E)-8-methyl-2,4-nonadienoyl]-(S)-asparaginyl-(2S,3S)-3-hydroxyasparaginyl-(R)-2-(p-hydroxyphenyl)glycyl-(R)-ornithyl-(2R,3R)-allothreonyl-2-(p-hydroxyphenyl)glycyl-2-(p-hydroxyphenyl)glycyl-(2S,3S)-allothreonyl-(S)-phenylalanyl-(R)-ornithyl-(S)-2-[p-(α-D-mannopyranosyloxy)phenyl]glycyl-(2R,3R)-allothreonyl-(S)-2-(p-hydroxyphenyl)glycylglycyl-(S)-leucyl-(R)-alanyl]glycine ψ_1-lactone. *CAS-124884-30-6.*

Ramorelix. $C_{74}H_{95}ClN_{16}O_{18}$. 1532.10. 1-[$N$-Acetyl-3-(2-naphthyl)-D-alanyl-p-chloro-D-phenylalanyl-D-tryptophyl-L-seryl-L-tyrosyl-O-(6-deoxy-α-L-mannopyranosyl)-D-seryl-L-leucyl-L-arginyl-L-prolyl]semicarbazide. *CAS-127932-90-5.* INN.

Ramosetron. $C_{17}H_{17}N_3O$. 279.34. (-)-(R)-1-Methylindol-3-yl-4,5,6,7-tetrahydro-5-benzimidazolyl ketone. *UNII-7ZROOSC54Y. CAS-132036-88-5.* INN.

Ramucirumab [*2008*] (ra″ mue sir′ ue mab). $C_{6374}H_{9864}N_{1692}O_{1996}S_{46}$. (1) Immunoglobulin G1, anti-(human vascular endothelial growth factor receptor type VEGFR-2 extracellular domain) (human monoclonal IMC-1121B γ-chain), disulfide with human monoclonal IMC-1121B κ-chain, dimer; (2) Immunoglobulin G1, anti-(vascular endothelial growth factor receptor 2 (EC 2.7.10.1 or protein-tyrosine kinase receptor Flk-1 or CD309 antigen) extracellular domain); human monoclonal IMC-1121B γ1 heavy chain (219-214′)-disulfide with human monoclonal IMC-1121B κ light chain (225-225″:228-228″)-bisdisulfide dimer. Molecular weight is approximately 143,600 daltons. *CAS-947687-13-0. Antineoplastic, treatment of solid tumors.* ◇*IMC-1121B*

Ran4 (trivial name) — *See* Ranolazine.

Ran D (trivial name) — *See* Ranolazine.

Ranagengliotucel-T [*2007*] (ran″ a jen glye″ oh too′ sel - el). Autologous vaccine cocktail of TGF-β blocked, whole brain cancer tumor cells. *Cell therapy treatment for brain cancer.* Glionix (NovaRx)

Ranelic Acid. $C_{12}H_{10}N_2O_8S$. 342.28. 5-[Bis(carboxymethyl)amino]-2-carboxy-4-cyano-3-thiopheneacetic acid. *UNII-K9CCS0RIBT. CAS-135459-90-4.* INN.

Ranibizumab [*2002*] (ra″ ni biz′ oo mab). $C_{2158}H_{3282}N_{562}O_{681}S_{12}$. Immunoglobulin G1, anti-(human vascular endothelial growth factor) Fab fragment (human-mouse monoclonal rhuFAB V2 γ1-chain), disulfide with human-mouse monoclonal rhuFAB V2 light chain. Molecular weight is approximately 48,000 daltons. *UNII-ZL1R02VT79. CAS-347396-82-1.* INN; BAN; JAN. *Treatment of age-related macular degeneration.*

Ranimustine. $C_{10}H_{18}ClN_3O_7$. 327.72. Methyl 6-[3-(2-chloroethyl)-3-nitrosoureido]-6-deoxy-α-D-glucopyranoside. *UNII-RYH2T97J77. CAS-58994-96-0.* INN; JAN; MI.

Ranimycin [*1968*] (ra″ ni mye′ sin). $C_{12}H_{18}O_6$. 258.27. Antibiotic derived from *Streptomyces lincolnensis* variant. (1) Ranimycin; (2) Ranimycin. *CAS-11056-09-0.* INN. *Antibacterial.* ◇*U-25,873*

---

† Brand name formerly used, and/or firm no longer concerned with this product.

Ranirestat. $C_{17}H_{11}BrFN_3O_4$. 420.19. (3*R*)-2′-(4-Bromo-2-fluorobenzyl)spiro[pyrrolidine-3,4′(1′*H*)-pyrrolo[1,2-*a*]pyrazine]-1′,2,3′,5(2′*H*)-tetrone. *CAS-147254-64-6.* INN.

Ranitidine [*1979*] (ra ni′ ti deen). $C_{13}H_{22}N_4O_3S$. 314.40. (1) 1,1-Ethenediamine, *N*-[2-[[[5-[(dimethylamino)methyl]-2-furanyl]methyl]thio]ethyl]-*N*′-methyl-2-nitro-; (2) *N*-[2-[[5-[(Dimethylamino)methyl]furfuryl]thio]ethyl]-*N*′-methyl-2-nitro-1,1-ethenediamine. *UNII-884KT10YB7. CAS-66357-35-5.* INN; BAN. *Antagonist (to histamine H_2receptors).*

Ranitidine Bismuth Citrate [*1993*] (ra ni′ ti deen biz′ muth sit′ rate). $C_{13}H_{22}N_4O_3S \cdot C_6H_5BiO_7$. 712.48. (1) 1,2,3-Propanetricarboxylic acid, 2-hydroxy-, bismuth(3+) salt (1:1), compd. with *N*-[2-[[[5-[(dimethylamino)methyl]-2-furanyl]methyl]thio]ethyl]-*N*′-methyl-2-nitro-1,1-ethenediamine (1:1); (2) *N*-[2-[[5-[(Dimethylamino)methyl]furfuryl]thio]ethyl]-*N*′-methyl-2-nitro-1,1-ethenediamine, compound with bismuth(3+) citrate (1:1). *UNII-7AJ51I17KG. CAS-128345-62-0.* BAN. *Antagonist (to histamine H_2receptors).* Tritec (GlaxoSmithKline) *[BAN name previously used: Ranitidine Bismutrex.]* ◇*GR 122311X*

Ranitidine Bismutrex (BAN previously used name) — *See* Ranitidine Bismuth Citrate.

Ranitidine Hydrochloride (ra ni′ ti deen hye″ droe klor′ ide). USP. $C_{13}H_{22}N_4O_3S \cdot HCl$. 350.86. (1) 1,1-Ethenediamine, *N*-[2-[[[5-[(dimethylamino)methyl]-2-furanyl]methyl]thio]ethyl]-*N*′-methyl-2-nitro-, monohydrochloride; (2) *N*-[2-[[[5-[(Dimethylamino)methyl]-2-furanyl]methyl]thio]ethyl]-*N*′-methyl-2-nitro-1,1-ethenediamine, hydrochloride. *UNII-BK764651HM. CAS-66357-59-3.* JAN. *Antagonist (to histamine H_2receptors).* Zantac (GlaxoSmithKline) ◇*AH 19065*

Ranolazine [*2004*] (ra noe′ la zeen). $C_{24}H_{33}N_3O_4$. 427.54. (1) 1-Piperazineacetamide, *N*-(2,6-dimethylphenyl)-4-[2-hydroxy-3-(2-methoxyphenoxy)propyl]-; (2) (±)-*N*-(2,6-Dimethylphenyl)-4-[2-hydroxy-3-(2-methoxyphenoxy)propyl]-1-piperazineacetamide; (3) 1-Piperazineacetamide, *N*-(2,6-dimethylphenyl)-4-[2-hydroxy-3-(2-methoxyphenoxy)propyl]-, (±)-. *UNII-A6IEZ5M406. CAS-95635-55-5.*

INN. *Anti-anginal; anti-ischemic.* Ranexa (Sensus) [*Note—The trivial names, Ran D and Ran4, have appeared in literature.*] ◇*RS-43285-003; CVT-303*

Ranolazine Hydrochloride [*1988*] (ra noe′ la zeen hye″ droe klor′ ide). $C_{24}H_{33}N_3O_4 \cdot 2HCl$. 500.46. (1) 1-Piperazineacetamide, *N*-(2,6-dimethylphenyl)-4-[2-hydroxy-3-(2-methoxyphenoxy)propyl]-, dihydrochloride, (±)-; (2) (±)-4-[2-Hydroxy-3-(*o*-methoxyphenoxy)propyl]-1-piperazineaceto-2′,6′-xylidide dihydrochloride. *UNII-F71253DJUN; UNII-A6IEZ5M406* [ranolazine]. *CAS-95635-56-6; CAS-95635-55-5* [ranolazine]. *Anti-anginal.* ◇*RS-43285*

Ranpirnase [*1998*] (ran′ pir nase). $C_{520}H_{810}N_{142}O_{155}S_9$. 11,819.44 daltons. Ribonuclease (*Rana pipiens*). *CAS-196488-72-9.* INN. *Antineoplastic for the treatment of solid tumors.* Onconase (Alfacell) ◇*P-30 Protein*

```
oxoPDWLTFQKKH ITNTRDVDCD NIMSTNLFHC KDKNTFIYSR PEPVKAICKG
IIASKNVLTT SEFYLSDCNV TSRPCKYKLK KSTNKFCVTC ENQAPVHFVG
VGSC
```

Rapacuronium Bromide [*1997*] (ra″ pa kure oh′ nee um broe′ mide). $C_{37}H_{61}BrN_2O_4$. 677.80. 1-Allyl-1-(3α,17β-dihydroxy-2β-piperidino-5α-androstan-16β-yl)piperidinium bromide, 3-acetate 17-propionate. *UNII-65Q4QDG4KC. CAS-156137-99-4.* INN; BAN. *Neuromuscular blocking agent.* Raplon (Organon) ◇*Org 9487*

Rapamycin (previously used name) — *See* Sirolimus.

Rapeseed Oil, Fully Hydrogenated. **NF**. The product obtained by refining and hydrogenating oil obtained from the seeds of *Brassica napus* and *Brassica campestris* (Fam. Cruciferae). The product is a mixture of triglycerides in which the fatty acid composition is a mixture of saturated fatty acids. *CAS-84681-71-0.*

Rapeseed Oil, Fully Hydrogenated Superglycerinated. **NF**. The product obtained by refining, hydrogenating, and glycerinating oil obtained from the seeds of *Brassica napus* and *Brassica campestris* (Fam. Cruciferae). The product is a mixture of mono-, di-, and triglycerides, with triglycerides as a minor component.

Rasagiline Mesylate [*1995*] (ra sa′ ji leen mes′ i late). $C_{12}H_{13}N \cdot CH_4O_3S$. 267.34. [Rasagiline is INN.] (1) 1*H*-Inden-1-amine, 2,3-dihydro-*N*-2-propynyl-, (*R*)-, methanesulfonate; (2) (*R*)-*N*-2-Propynyl-1-indanamine methanesul-fonate. *UNII-LH8C2JI290; UNII-003N66TS6T* [rasagiline]. *CAS-161735-79-1; CAS-136236-51-6* [rasagiline]. *Antiparkinsonian.* Azilect (Teva) ◇*TVP-1012*

Rasburicase [*2000*] (ras bure′ i kase). $C_{1523}H_{2383}N_{417}O_{462}S_7$ (monomer). (1) Oxidase, urate (*Aspergillus flavus* clone 9C/9A reduced); (2) Urate oxydase (tetramer of the *N*-acetylpolypeptide of 301 amino acids). Molecular weight is approximately 34,151.65 daltons (monomer). *UNII-08GY9K1EUO. CAS-134774-45-1.* INN; BAN; JAN. *Treatment of malignancy-associated or chemotherapy-induced hyperuricemia.* ◇*SR29142*

Raspberry Syrup. *CAS-8027-62-1.* USP XVIII; MI.

Rathyronine. $C_{15}H_{12}I_3NO_4$. 650.97. DL-3-[4-(4-Hydroxy-3-iodophenoxy)-3,5-diiodophenyl]alanine. *CAS-3130-96-9.* INN; DCF.

Rauwolfia Serpentina (row wool′ fee a ser″ pen teen′ a). **USP**. [Rauwolfia Alkaloids is JAN.] The dried root of *Rauwolfia* (Linné) Bentham ex Kurz (Fam. Apocynaceae), sometimes having fragments of rhizome and aerial stem bases attached. *Antihypertensive.* Raudixin (Apothecon)

Ravuconazole. $C_{22}H_{17}F_2N_5OS$. 437.47. *p*-[2-[(α*R*,β*R*)-2,4-Difluoro-β-hydroxy-α-methyl-β-(1*H*-1,2,4-triazol-1-yl-methyl)phenethyl]-4-thiazolyl]benzonitrile. *CAS-182760-06-1.* INN.

Raxibacumab [*2004*] (rax″ i bak′ ue mab). $C_{6320}H_{9794}N_{1702}O_{1998}S_{42}$. 142,900 daltons. Immunoglobulin G1, anti-(anthrax protective antigen) (human monoclonal PA heavy chain), disulfide with human monoclonal PAλ-chain, dimer. *CAS-565451-13-0.* INN. *Treatment of anthrax infection.* ABthrax (Human Genome Sciences)

Raxofelast. $C_{15}H_{18}O_5$. 278.30. (±)-2,3-Dihydro-5-hydroxy-4,6,7-trimethyl-2-benzofuranacetic acid, acetate. *UNII-TC0T0O9VYO. CAS-128232-14-4.* INN.

Rayon, Purified [*1968*] (ray′ on). **USP**. A fibrous form of regenerated cellulose, manufactured by the viscose process, desulfured, washed, and bleached. *Surgical aid.*

Razaxaban Hydrochloride [*2003*] (ra zax′ a ban hye″ droe klor′ ide). $C_{24}H_{20}F_4N_8O_2 \cdot HCl$. 564.92. [Razaxaban is INN.] (1) 1*H*-Pyrazole-5-carboxamide, 1-(3-amino-1,2-benzisoxazol-5-yl)-*N*-[4-[2-[(dimethylamino)methyl]-1*H*-imidazol-

1-yl]-2-fluorophenyl]-3-[trifluoromethyl)-, monohydrochloride; (2) 1-(3-Amino-1,2-benzisoxazol-5-yl)-*N*-[4-[2-[(dimethylamino)methyl]-1*H*-imidazol-1-yl]-2-fluorophenyl]-3-(trifluoromethyl)-1*H*-pyrazole-5-carboxamide monohydrochloride. *UNII-7CLJ1MEZ8V. CAS-405940-76-3; CAS-218298-21-6 [razaxaban]. Anticoagulant; antithrombotic (Factor Xa inhibitor).* ◇*BMS-561389*

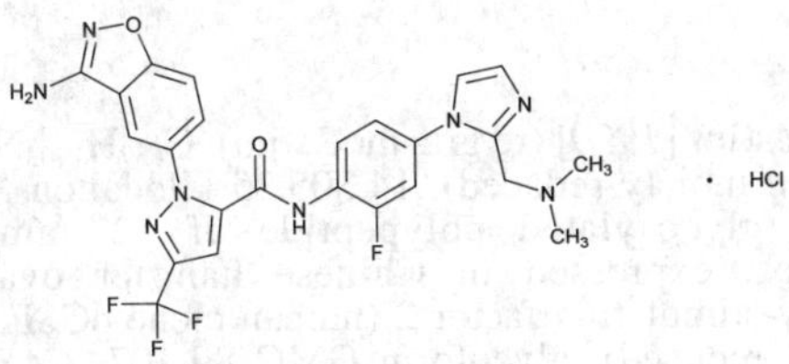

Razinodil. C$_{27}$H$_{34}$N$_4$O$_{10}$. 574.58. 3,4,5-Trimethoxybenzoic acid ester with 3-(2-hydroxy-3-morpholinopropyl)-6,7,8-trimethoxy-1,2,3-benzotriazin-4(3*H*)-one. *UNII-UJ1O5LVT0G. CAS-30271-85-3.* INN.

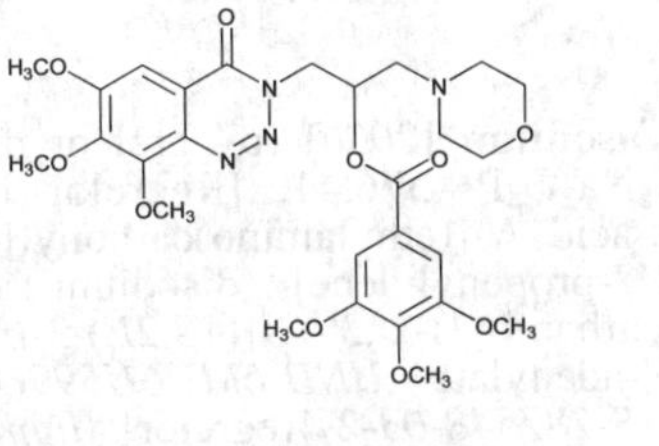

Razobazam. C$_{14}$H$_{14}$N$_4$O$_2$. 270.29. 4,8-Dihydro-3,8-dimethyl-4-phenylpyrazolo[3,4-*b*][1,4]diazepine-5,7(1*H*,6*H*)-dione. *UNII-LZ84VWN0U4. CAS-78466-98-5.* INN.

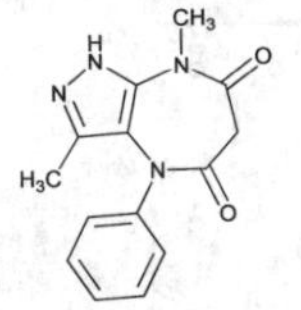

Razoxane. C$_{11}$H$_{16}$N$_4$O$_4$. 268.27. (±)-4,4′-Propylenedi-2,6-piperazinedione. *UNII-5AR83PR647. CAS-21416-87-5; CAS-21416-67-1 [replaced].* INN; BAN; MI. ◇*ICI 59118; ICRF 159*

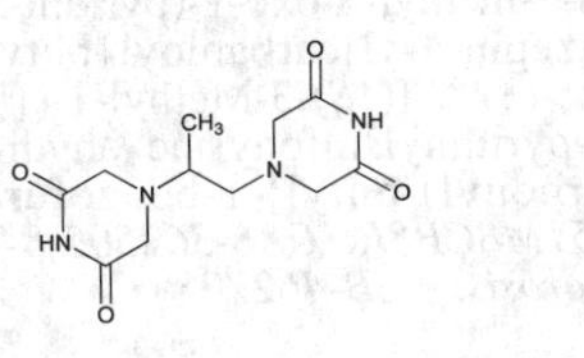

^{82}RbCl — *See* Rubidium Chloride Rb 82.

^{86}RbCl — *See* Rubidium Chloride Rb 86.

^{81}RbOH — *See* Rubidium Hydroxide (^{81}Rb) [Injection].

---

† Brand name formerly used, and/or firm no longer concerned with this product.

Rebamipide. C$_{19}$H$_{15}$ClN$_2$O$_4$. 370.79. (±)-α-(*p*-Chlorobenzamido)-1,2-dihydro-2-oxo-4-quinolinepropionic acid. *CAS-111911-87-6.* INN; JAN.

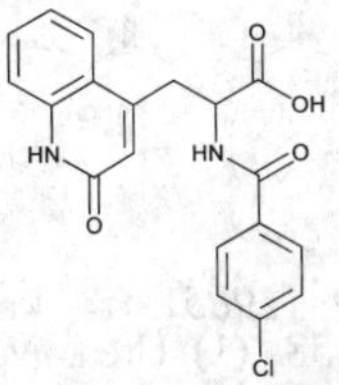

Rebimastat [*2003*] (re bim′ a stat). C$_{23}$H$_{41}$N$_5$O$_5$S. 499.67. (1) L-Valinamide, *N*-[(2*S*)-2-mercapto-1-oxo-4-(3,4,4-trimethyl-2,5-dioxo-1-imidazolidinyl)butyl]-L-leucyl-*N*,3-dimethyl-; (2) (2*S*)-*N*-[(1*S*)-2,2-dimethyl-1-(methylcarbamoyl)propyl]-4-methyl-2-[[(2*S*)-2-sulfanyl-4-(3,4,4-trimethyl-2,5-dioxoimidazolidin-1-yl)butanoyl]amino]pentanamide. *UNII-1B47R6ZX4K. CAS-259188-38-0.* INN. *Antineoplastic (matrix metalloproteinase inhibitor).* ◇*BMS 275291-01; D2163*

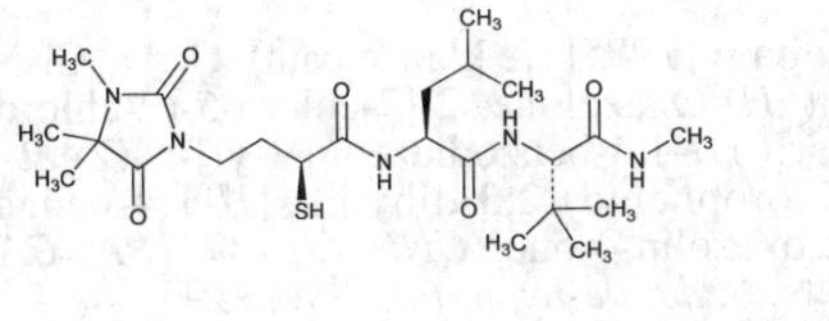

Reboxetine. C$_{19}$H$_{23}$NO$_3$. 313.39. (±)-(2*R**)-2-[(α*R**)-α-(*o*-Ethoxyphenoxy)benzyl]morpholine. *UNII-947S0YZ36I. CAS-98769-81-4.* INN; BAN.

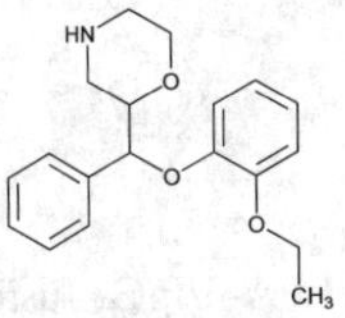

Reboxetine Mesylate [*1997*] (re box′ e teen mes′ i late). C$_{19}$H$_{23}$NO$_3$.CH$_4$O$_3$S. 409.50. (1) (±)-(*R**,*S**)-2-[(2-Ethoxyphenoxy)phenylmethyl]morpholine methanesulfonate; (2) (±)-(2*R**)-2-[(α*S**)-α-(*o*-Ethoxyphenoxy)benzyl]morpholine methanesulfonate. *CAS-98769-84-7. Antidepressant (selective noradrenaline reuptake inhibitor).* Edronax (Pharmacia & Upjohn) ◇*PNU-155950E; FCE 20124*

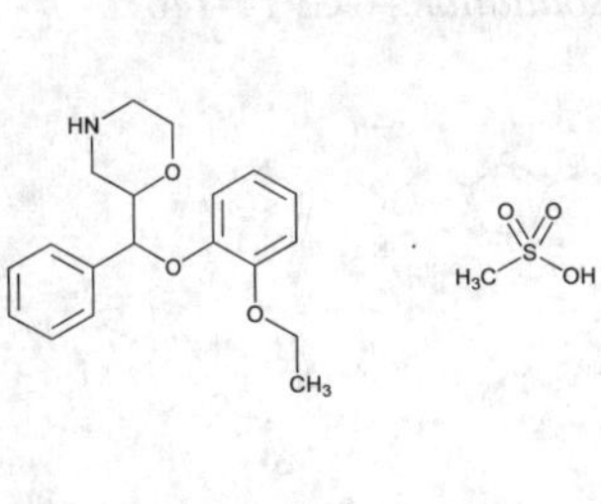

Recainam Hydrochloride [*1985*] (re kane′ am hye″ droe klor′ ide). C$_{15}$H$_{25}$N$_3$O.HCl. 299.84. [Recainam is INN and BAN.] (1) Urea, *N*-(2,6-dimethylphenyl)-*N*′-[3-[(1-methylethyl)amino]propyl]-, monohydrochloride; (2) 1-[3-(Isopropylamino)propyl]-3-(2,6-xylyl)urea monohydrochloride. *CAS-74752-07-1; CAS-74738-24-2* [recainam]. *Cardiac depressant (anti-arrhythmic).* Vanorm (Wyeth-Ayerst) ◇*WY-42,362 HCl*

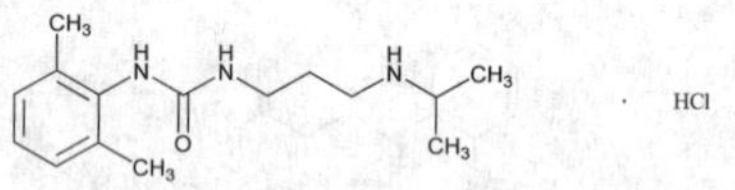

Recainam Tosylate [*1985*] (re kane′ am tos′ i late). $C_{22}H_{33}N_3O_4S$. 435.58. (1) Urea, *N*-(2,6-dimethylphenyl)-*N′*-[3-[(1-methylethyl)amino]propyl]-, mono(4-methylbenzenesulfonate); (2) 1-[3-(Isopropylamino)propyl]-3-(2,6-xylyl)urea mono-*p*-toluenesulfonate. *CAS-74752-08-2. Cardiac depressant (anti-arrhythmic).* ◇*WY-42,362 tosylate*

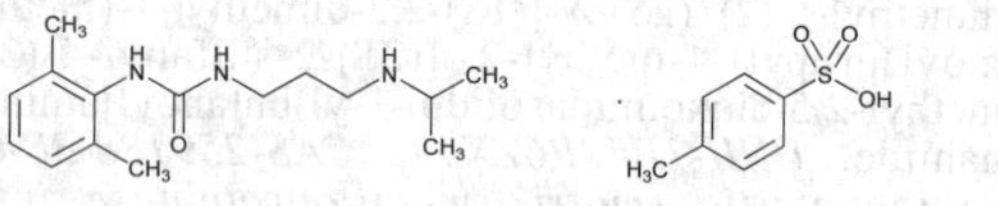

Recanescin — *See* Deserpidine.

Reclazepam [*1985*] (re klaz′ e pam). $C_{18}H_{13}Cl_2N_3O_2$. 374.22. (1) 4(5*H*)-Oxazolone, 2-[7-chloro-5-(2-chlorophenyl)-2,3-dihydro-1*H*-1,4-benzodiazepin-1-yl]-; (2) 2-[7-Chloro-5-(*o*-chlorophenyl)-2,3-dihydro-1*H*-1,4-benzodiazepin-1-yl]-2-oxazolin-4-one. *UNII-YJL42911RA. CAS-76053-16-2.* INN. *Sedative-hypnotic.* ◇*SC-33963*

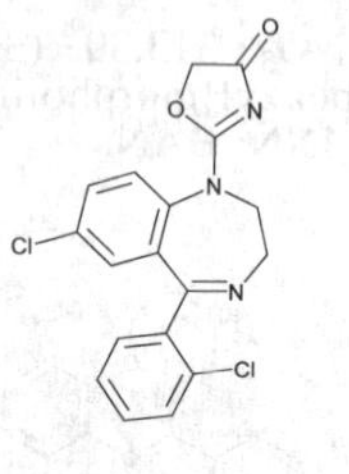

Recombinant human LFA-3/IgG₁ fusion protein (previously used name) — *See* Alefacept.

Regadenoson [*2006*] (re″ ga den′ oh son). $C_{15}H_{18}N_8O_5 \cdot H_2O$. 408.37. (1) Adenosine, 2-[4-[(methylamino)carbonyl]-1*H*-pyrazol-1-yl]-, monohydrate; (2) 1-(6-Amino-9-*β*-D-ribofuranosyl-9*H*-purin-2-yl)-*N*-methyl-1*H*-pyrazole-4-carboxamide, monohydrate. *UNII-2XLN4Y044H. CAS-875148-45-1; CAS-313348-27-5* [anhydrous]. INN; BAN. *Intravenous use in radionuclide myocardial perfusion imaging as a pharmacologic stress agent to produce coronary vasodilation.* ◇*CVT-3146*

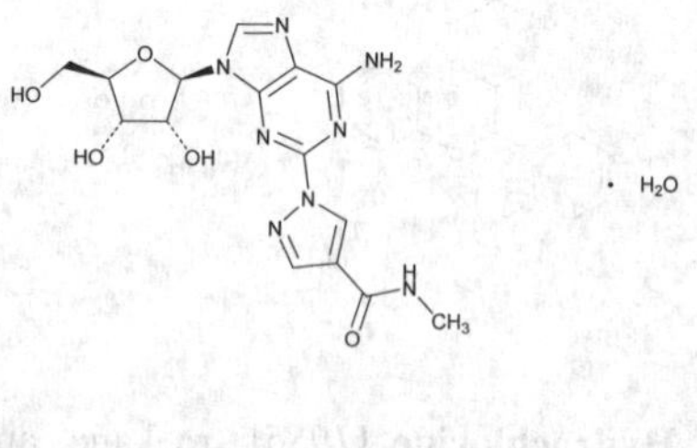

Regavirumab. Immunoglobulin G1, anti-(human herpesvirus 5 glycoprotein B) (human monoclonal γl-chain), disulfide with human monoclonal κ-chain, dimer. *CAS-153101-26-9.* INN.

Reglitazar. $C_{22}H_{20}N_2O_5$. 392.40. (4*RS*)-4-[4-[2-(5-Methyl-2-phenyl-4-oxazolyl)ethoxy]benzyl]-3,5-isoxazolidinedione. *CAS-170861-63-9.* INN.

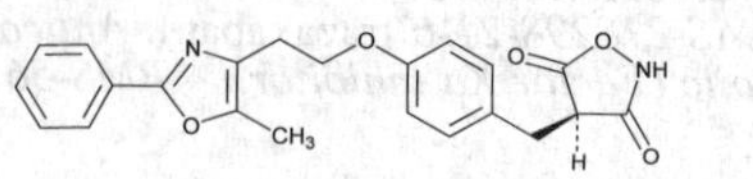

Regramostim [*1990*] (re gra′ moe stim). $C_{637}H_{1003}N_{171}O_{187}S_8$ (protein moiety reduced). 14,305.35 kilodaltons. A single chain, glycosylated polypeptide of 127 amino acid residues, expressed in Chinese hamster ovary cells. Colony-stimulating factor 2 (human clone pCSF-1 protein moiety reduced), glycoform GMC 89-107. *CAS-127757-91-9.* INN. *Antineutropenic; hematopoietic stimulant.* ◇*GMC 89-107; GM-CSF; rhGm-CSF*

APARSPSPST QPWEHVNAIQ EARRLLNLSR DTAAEMNETV EVISEMFDLQ
EPTCLQTRLE LYKQGLRGSL TKLKGPLTMM ASHYKQHCPP TPETSCATQT
ITFESFKENL KDFLLVIPFD CWEPVQE

Regrelor Disodium [*2006*] (re′ grel or dye soe′ dee um). $C_{22}H_{23}N_6Na_2O_8P$. 576.41. [Regrelor is INN.] (1) 5′-Adenylic acid, *N*-[(ethylamino)carbonyl]-2′,3′-*O*-[(1*S*,2*E*)-3-phenyl-2-propenylidene]-, disodium salt; (2) Disodium *N*-(ethylcarbamoyl)-2′,3′-*O*-[(1*S*,2*E*)-3-phenyl-2-propenylidene]-5′-adenylate. *UNII-6MU6U599QZ. CAS-676251-22-2; CAS-787548-03-2* [regrelor]. *Inhibition of platelet aggregation to prevent thrombosis and resulting complications.* ◇*INS50589*

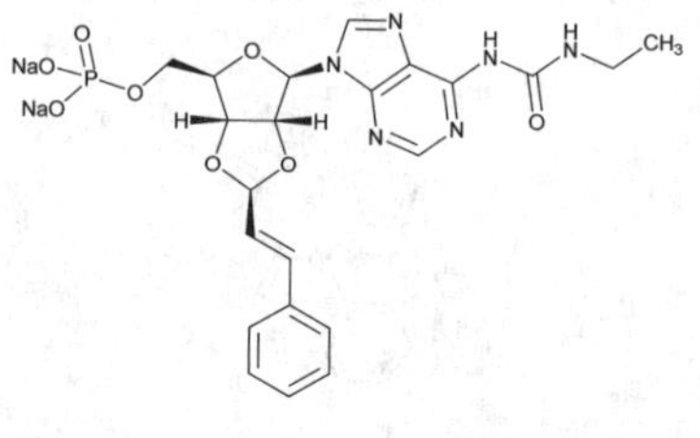

Relacatib [*2006*] (rel″ a ka′ tib). $C_{27}H_{32}N_4O_6S$. 540.63. (1) 2-Benzofurancarboxamide, *N*-[(1*S*)-1-({[(4*S*,7*R*)-hexahydro-7-methyl-3-oxo-1-(2-pyridinylsulfonyl)-1*H*-azepin-4-yl]amino}carbonyl)-3-methylbutyl]-; (2) *N*-[(1*S*)-3-Methyl-1-{[(4*S*,7*R*)-7-methyl-3-oxo-1-(pyridin-2-ylsulfonyl)hexahydro-1*H*-azepin-4-yl]carbamoyl}butyl]benzofuran-2-carboxamide; (3) *N*-[(1*S*)-3-Methyl-1-({[(4*S*,7*R*)-7-methyl-3-oxo-1-(2-pyridinylsulfonyl)hexahydro-1*H*-azepin-4-yl]amino}carbonyl)-butyl]-1-benzofuran-2-carboxamide. *UNII-BL51M8CB8R. CAS-362505-84-8.* INN. *Treatment of osteoporosis.* ◇*SB-462795*

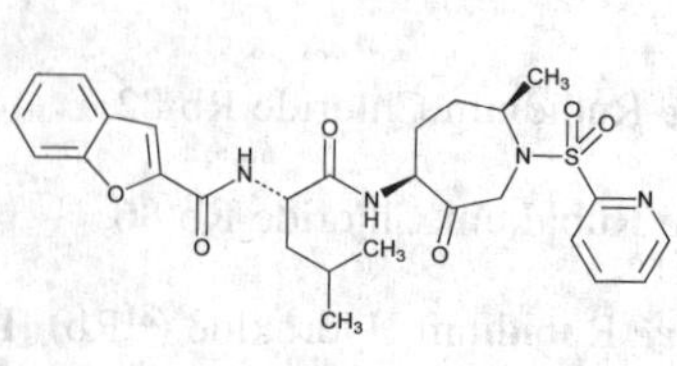

Relaxin. MI. Cervilaxin (Marion Merrell Dow†); Releasin (Parke-Davis†)

Relcovaptan. $C_{28}H_{27}Cl_2N_3O_7S$. 620.50. (2*S*)-1-[[(2*R*,3*S*)-5-Chloro-3-(*o*-chlorophenyl)-1-[(3,4-dimethoxyphenyl)sulfonyl]-3-hydroxy-2-indolinyl]carbonyl]-2-pyrrolidinecarboxamide. *CAS-150375-75-0*. INN.

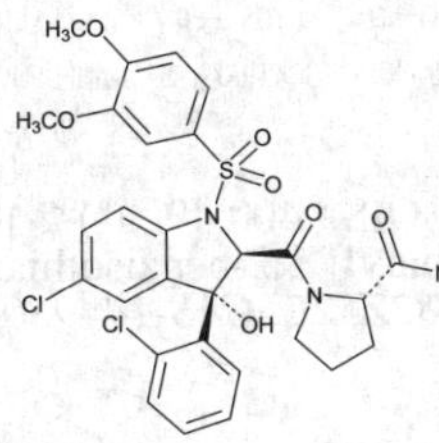

Relomycin [*1964*] (rel″ oh mye′ sin). Antibiotic produced by *Streptomyces hygroscopicus.* (1) Relomycin; (2) Relomycin. *UNII-E70CPL81IY*. *CAS-1404-48-4*. INN. *Antibacterial.* ◇*AM-684-Beta*

Remacemide Hydrochloride [*1990*] (rem a′ se mide hye″ droe klor′ ide). $C_{17}H_{20}N_2O.HCl$. 304.81. [Remacemide is INN.] (1) Acetamide, 2-amino-*N*-(1-methyl-1,2-diphenylethyl)-, monohydrochloride, (±)-; (2) (±)-2-Amino-*N*-(1-methyl-1,2-diphenylethyl)acetamide monohydrochloride. *CAS-111686-79-4; CAS-128298-28-2* [remacemide]. *Anticonvulsant (neuroprotective).* ◇*FPL 12924AA; PR 934-423A*

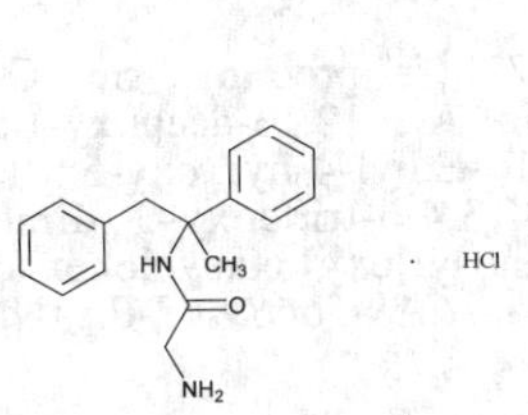

Remifentanil Hydrochloride [*1992*] (rem″ i fen′ ta nil hye″ droe klor′ ide). $C_{20}H_{28}N_2O_5.HCl$. 412.91. [Remifentanil is INN and BAN.] (1) 1-Piperidinepropanoic acid, 4-(methoxycarbonyl)-4-[(1-oxopropyl)phenylamino]-, methyl ester, monohydrochloride; (2) 4-Carboxy-4-(*N*-phenylpropionamido)-1-piperidine propionic acid, dimethyl ester, monohydrochloride. *UNII-5V444H5WIC; UNII-P10582JYYK* [remifentanil]. *CAS-132539-07-2; CAS-132875-61-7* [remifentanil]. *Analgesic.* Ultiva (Abbott) ◇*GI 87084B*

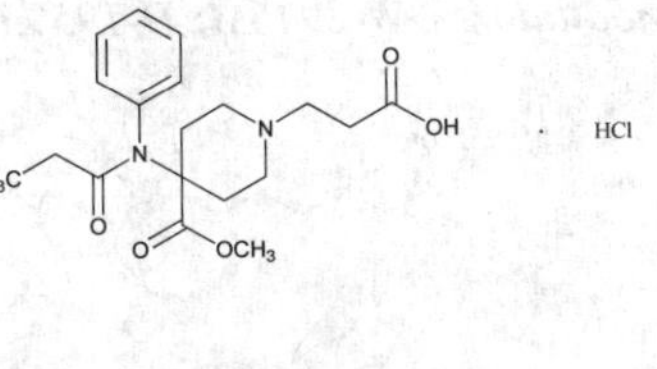

Remikiren. $C_{33}H_{50}N_4O_6S$. 630.84. (α*S*)-α-[(α*S*)-α-[(*tert*-Butylsulfonyl)methyl]hydrocinnamamido]-*N*-[(1*S*,2*R*,3*S*)-1-(cyclohexylmethyl)-3-cyclopropyl-2,3-dihydroxypropyl]imidazole-4-propionamide. *UNII-LC7FBL96A4*. *CAS-126222-34-2*. INN.

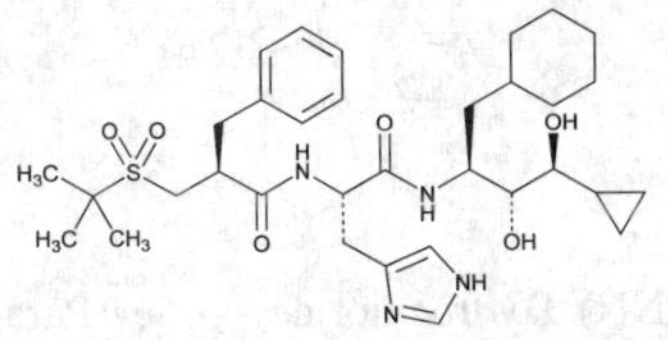

Reminertant (previously used name) — *See* Meclinertant.

Remiprostol [*1993*] (rem″ i prost′ ol). $C_{25}H_{36}O_5$. 416.55. (1) 4-Heptenoic acid, 7-[2-[6-(1-cyclopenten-1-yl)-4-hydroxy-4-methyl-1,5-hexadienyl]-3-hydroxy-5-oxocyclopentyl]-, methyl ester; (2) (±)-Methyl (*Z*)-7-[(1*R*,2*R*,3*R*)-2-[(1*E*,5*E*)-(4*RS*)-6-(1-cyclopenten-1-yl)-4-hydroxy-4-methyl-1,5-hexadienyl]-3-hydroxy-5-oxocyclopentyl]-4-heptenoate. *CAS-110845-89-1*. INN. *Anti-ulcerative.* ◇*SC-48834*

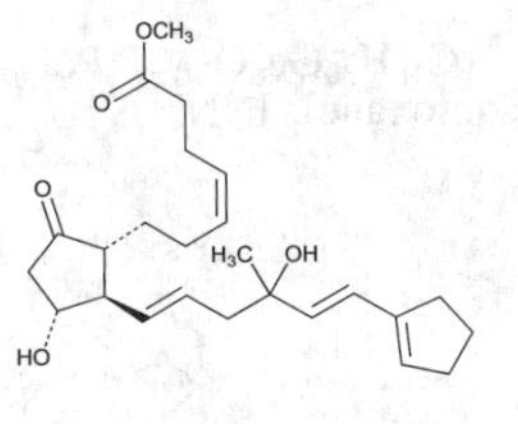

Remogliflozin Etabonate. $C_{26}H_{38}N_2O_9$. 522.59. 5-Methyl-1-(propan-2-yl)-4-({4-[(propan-2-yl)oxy]phenyl}methyl)-1*H*-pyrazol-3-yl 6-*O*-(ethoxycarbonyl)-β-D-glucopyranoside. *UNII-TR0QT6QSUL*. *CAS-442201-24-3*. INN.

Remoxipride [*1985*] (rem ox′ i pride). $C_{16}H_{23}BrN_2O_3$. 371.27. (1) Benzamide, 3-bromo-*N*-[(1-ethyl-2-pyrrolidinyl)methyl]-2,6-dimethoxy-, (*S*)-; (2) (-)-(*S*)-3-Bromo-*N*-[(1-ethyl-2-pyrrolidinyl)methyl]-2,6-dimethoxybenzamide. *UNII-0223RD59PE*. *CAS-80125-14-0*. INN; BAN. *Antipsychotic.* ◇*A 33547; FLA 731*

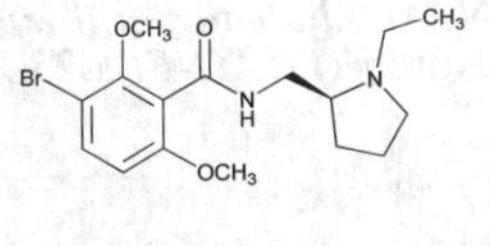

Remoxipride Hydrochloride [*1993*] (rem ox′ i pride hye″ droe klor′ ide). $C_{16}H_{23}BrN_2O_3.HCl.H_2O$. 425.75. (1) Benzamide, 3-bromo-*N*-[(1-ethyl-2-pyrrolidinyl)methyl]-2,6-dimethoxy-, monohydrochloride, monohydrate, (*S*)-; (2) (-)-(*S*)-3-Bromo-*N*-[(1-ethyl-2-pyrrolidinyl)methyl]-2,6-dimethoxybenzamide monohydrochloride, monohydrate. *UNII-MH4OU8RWCW*. *CAS-117591-79-4*. *Antipsychotic.* ◇*A 33547.HCl.H₂O; FLA 731(-)*

Renanolone. $C_{21}H_{32}O_3$. 332.48. 3α-Hydroxy-5β-pregnane-11,20-dione. *UNII-D8Z6E4IR2J*. *CAS-565-99-1*. INN.

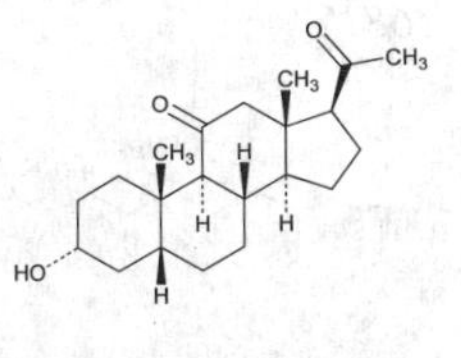

† Brand name formerly used, and/or firm no longer concerned with this product.

Rentiapril. $C_{13}H_{15}NO_4S_2$. 313.39. (2*R*,4*R*)-2-(*o*-Hydroxyphenyl)-3-(3-mercaptopropionyl)-4-thiazolidinecarboxylic acid. *UNII-D0TAM1017B. CAS-80830-42-8.* INN.

Renytoline (INN) **Hydrochloride** — *See* Paranyline Hydrochloride.

Renzapride. $C_{16}H_{22}ClN_3O_2$. 323.82. [(±)-*endo*]-4-Amino-*N*-(1-azabicyclo[3.3.1]non-4-yl)-5-chloroanisamide. *CAS-88721-77-1.* INN; BAN.

Repagermanium. $(C_{18}H_{30}Ge_6O_{21})_n$. Poly-*trans*-[(2-carboxyethyl)germasesquioxane]. INN.

Repaglinide [*1998*] (re pag′ li nide). **USP.** $C_{27}H_{36}N_2O_4$. 452.59. (1) (*S*)-2-Ethoxy-4-[2-{methyl-1-[2-(1-piperidinyl)phenyl]butylamino}-2-oxoethyl]-benzoic acid; (2) (+)-2-Ethoxy-α-[[(*S*)-α-isobutyl-*o*-piperidinobenzyl]carbamoyl]-*p*-toluic acid. *UNII-668Z8C33LU. CAS-135062-02-1.* INN; BAN. *Antidiabetic (oral hypoglycemic agent).* Prandin (Novo Nordisk) ◇*AG-EE 623 ZW*

Reparixin [*2005*] (re″ pa rix′ in). $C_{14}H_{21}NO_3S$. 283.39. (1) Benzeneacetamide, α-methyl-4-(2-methylpropyl)-*N*-(methylsulfonyl)- (α*R*)-; (2) (-)-(2*R*)-2-[4-(2-Methylpropyl)phenyl]-*N*-(methylsulfonyl)propanamide. *UNII-U604E1NB3K. CAS-266359-83-5.* INN. *Prevention of delayed graft function in solid organ transplant (CXCL8 inhibitor).* ◇*DF 1681Y*

Repifermin [*1999*] (re″ pi fer′ min). $C_{723}H_{1131}N_{209}O_{204}S_5$. 33-172-Keratinocyte growth factor 2 (human). Molecular weight is approximately 16,175 daltons. *CAS-219527-63-6.* INN. *Treatment of mucositis and to promote wound healing.* ◇*KGF-2*

```
SYNHLQGDVR   WRKLFSFTKY   FLKIEKNGKV   SGTKKENCPY   SILEITSVEI
GVVAVKAINS   NYYLAMNKKG   KLYGSKEFNN   DCKLKERIEE   NGYNTYASFN
WQHNGRQMYV   ALNGKGAPRR   GQKTRRKNTS   AHFLPMVVHS
```

Repinotan. $C_{21}H_{24}N_2O_4S$. 400.49. (-)-2-[4-[[(*R*)-2-Chromanylmethyl]amino]butyl]-1,2-benzisothiazolin-3-one 1,1-dioxide. *UNII-05PB82Z52L. CAS-144980-29-0.* INN.

Repirinast [*1990*] (re pir′ i nast). $C_{20}H_{21}NO_5$. 355.38. (1) 4*H*-Pyrano[3,2-*c*]quinoline-2-carboxylic acid, 5,6-dihydro-7,8-dimethyl-4,5-dioxo-, 3-methylbutyl ester; (2) Isopentyl 5,6-dihydro-7,8-dimethyl-4,5-dioxo-4*H*-pyrano[3,2-*c*]quinoline-2-carboxylate. *UNII-4K8KA8B61G. CAS-73080-51-0.* INN; JAN; MI. *Anti-allergic; anti-asthmatic.* ◇*MY-5116*

Repromicin [*1977*] (re″ proe mye′ sin). $C_{31}H_{51}NO_8$. 565.74. (1) Cirramycin A_1, 12,13-deepoxy-12,13-didehydro-4′-deoxy-; (2) 16-Ethyl-4-hydroxy-5,9,13,15-tetramethyl-2,10-dioxo-6-[[3,4,6-trideoxy-3-(dimethylamino)-β-D-*xylo*-hexopyranosyl]oxy]oxacyclohexadeca-11,13-diene-7-acetaldehyde. *CAS-56689-42-0.* INN. *Antibacterial.* ◇*Sch 16524*

Reproterol Hydrochloride [*1977*] (re proe′ ter ol hye″ droe klor′ ide). $C_{18}H_{23}N_5O_5$·HCl. 425.87. [Reproterol is INN and BAN.] (1) 1*H*-Purine-2,6-dione, 7-[3-[[2-(3,5-dihydroxyphenyl)-2-hydroxyethyl]amino]propyl]-3,7-dihydro-1,3-dimethyl-, monohydrochloride; (2) 7-[3-[(β,3,5-Trihydroxyphenethyl)amino]propyl]theophylline monohydrochloride. *CAS-13055-82-8; CAS-54063-54-6* [reproterol]. *Bronchodilator.* ◇*W-2946M; D-1959.HCl*

Resatorvid. $C_{15}H_{17}ClFNO_4S$. 361.82. Ethyl (6*R*)-6-[(2-chloro-4-fluorophenyl)sulfamoyl]cyclohex-1-ene-1-carboxylate. *CAS-243984-11-4.* INN.

Rescimetol. $C_{33}H_{38}N_2O_8$. 590.66. Methyl 18β-hydroxy-11,17α-dimethoxy-3β,20α-yohimban-16β-carboxylate (*E*)-4-hydroxy-3-methoxycinnamate (ester). *UNII-25YF317R6S. CAS-73573-42-9*. INN; JAN; MI.

Rescinnamine. $C_{35}H_{42}N_2O_9$. 634.72. Methyl 18β-hydroxy-11,17α-dimethoxy-3β,20α-yohimban-16β-carboxylate. *UNII-Q6W1F7DJ2D. CAS-24815-24-5*. NF XIII; INN; JAN; BAN; MI. Moderil (Pfizer)

Resequinil. $C_{18}H_{14}N_4O_3$. 334.33. 5-(3-Methoxyphenyl)-3-(5-methyl-1,2,4-oxadiazol-3-yl)-1,6-naphthyridin-2(1*H*)-one. *UNII-2G222T03EY. CAS-219846-31-8*. INN.

Reserpine (re ser′ peen). **USP**. $C_{33}H_{40}N_2O_9$. 608.68. (1) Yohimban-16-carboxylic acid, 11,17-dimethoxy-18-[(3,4,5-trimethoxybenzoyl)oxy]-, methyl ester, (3β,16β,17α,18β,20α)-; (2) Methyl 18β-hydroxy-11,17α-dimethoxy-3β,20α-yohimban-16β-carboxylate 3,4,5-trimethoxybenzoate (ester). *UNII-8B1QWR724A. CAS-50-55-5*. INN; BAN; JAN. *Antihypertensive*. Rau-Sed (Bristol-Myers Squibb); Sandril (Lilly); Serpasil (Novartis)

Resiquimod. $C_{17}H_{22}N_4O_2$. 314.38. 4-Amino-2-(ethoxymethyl)-α,α-dimethyl-1*H*-imidazo[4,5-*c*]quinoline-1-ethanol. *UNII-V3DMU7PVXF. CAS-144875-48-9*. INN.

Reslizumab [*2000*] (res liz ′ oo mab). (1) Immunoglobulin G4, anti-(human interleukin 5) (human-rat monoclonal SCH 55700 γ4-chain), disulfide with human-rat monoclonal SCH 55700 light chain, dimer; (2) Immunoglobulin G4 (human-rat monoclonal SCH 55700 γ4-chain anti-human interleukin 5), disulfide with human-rat monoclonal SCH 55770 light chain, dimer. Molecular weight is approximately 150,000 daltons. *CAS-241473-69-8*. INN. *Treatment of bronchial asthma as well as a pharmacological tool to elucidate the role of IL-5 in human eosinophilic diseases*. (Schering-Plough) ◇*SCH 55700*

Resocortol Butyrate [*1995*] (re soe′ kor tol bue′ ti rate). $C_{26}H_{38}O_5$. 430.58. [Resocortol is INN.] (1) Androst-4-en-3-one, 11β-hydroxy-17α-(1-oxobutoxy)-17-(1-oxopropyl)-; (2) 11β,17α-Dihydroxy-17-propionylandrost-4-en-3-one 17-butyrate. *CAS-76738-96-0; CAS-76675-97-3* [resocortol]. *Anti-inflammatory (topical)*. ◇*ALO 2184; ORG7417*

Resorantel. $C_{13}H_{10}BrNO_3$. 308.13. 4′-Bromo-γ-resorcylanilide. *UNII-2I8V5Q9A78. CAS-20788-07-2*. INN; MI. ◇*Hoe 296 V*

Resorcin (JAN) — *See* Resorcinol.

Resorcin Acetate — *See* Resorcinol Monoacetate.

Resorcin Brown. C. I. Acid Orange 24 monosodium salt. NF IX.

Resorcinol (re sor′ si nol). **USP**. $C_6H_6O_2$. 110.11. [Resorcin is JAN.] (1) 1,3-Benzenediol; (2) Resorcinol. *UNII-YUL4-LO94HK. CAS-108-46-3. Keratolytic*.

Resorcinol Monoacetate (re sor′ si nol mon″ oh as′ e tate). **USP**. $C_8H_8O_3$. 152.15. (1) 1,3-Benzenediol, monoacetate; (2) Resorcinol monoacetate. *CAS-102-29-4. Antiseborrheic; keratolytic*. Euresol (Knoll†)

Retapamulin [*2004*] (re″ te pam′ ue lin). $C_{30}H_{47}NO_4S$. 517.76. (1) Acetic acid, [[(3-*exo*)-8-methyl-8-azabicyclo[3.2.1]oct-3-yl]thio]-, (3a*S*,4*R*,5*S*,6*S*,8*R*,9*R*,9a*R*,10*R*)-6-ethenyldecahydro-5-hydroxy-4,6,9,10-tetramethyl-1-oxo-3a,9-propano-3a*H*-cyclopentacycloocten-8-yl ester; (2) (3a*S*,4*R*,5*S*,6*S*,8*R*,9*R*,9a*R*,10*R*)-6-ethenyl-5-hydroxy-

---

† Brand name formerly used, and/or firm no longer concerned with this product.

4,6,9,10-tetramethyl-1-oxodecahydro-3a,9-propano-3a*H*-cyclopenta[8]annulen-8-yl [[(1*R*,3*s*,5*S*)-8-methyl-8-azabicyclo[3.2.1]oct-3-yl]sulfanyl]acetate. *UNII-4MG6O8991R. CAS-224452-66-8.* INN. *Topical antibiotic for secondarily infected traumatic lesions (SITL) and secondarily infected dermatoses (SID) or impetigo.* Altabax (GlaxoSmithKline) ◇*SB-275833*

Retaspimycin [*2008*] (ret″ asp i mye′ sin). $C_{31}H_{45}N_3O_8$. 587.70. (1) Geldanamycin, 18,21-didehydro-17-demethoxy-18,21-dideoxo-18,21-dihydroxy-17-(2-propenylamino)-; (2) (4*E*,6*Z*,8*S*,9*S*,10*E*,12*S*,13*R*,14*S*,16*R*)-13,20,22-Trihydroxy-8,14-dimethoxy-4,10,12,16-tetramethyl-3-oxo-19-(prop-2-enylamino)-2-azabicyclo[16.3.1]docosa-1(21),4,6,10,18(22),19-hexen-9-yl carbamate. *UNII-BZF2ZM0I5Z. CAS-857402-23-4.* INN. *Treatment of patients with metastatic and/or unresectable gastrointestinal stromal tumors (GIST); treatment of patients with relapsed and/or refractory stage IIIb (with pleural or pericardial effusions) or IV NSCLC..* ◇*IPI-504*

Retaspimycin Hydrochloride [*2008*] (ret″ asp i mye′ sin). $C_{31}H_{45}N_3O_8$·HCl. 624.17. (1) Geldanamycin, 18,21-didehydro-17-demethoxy-18,21-dideoxo-18,21-dihydroxy-17-(2-propenylamino)-, monohydrochloride; (2) (4*E*,6*Z*,8*S*,9*S*,10*E*,12*S*,13*R*,14*S*,16*R*)-13,20,22-Trihydroxy-8,14-dimethoxy-4,10,12,16-tetramethyl-3-oxo-19-(prop-2-enylamino)-2-azabicyclo[16.3.1]docosa-1(21),4,6,10,18(22),19-hexen-9-yl carbamate hydrochloride. *UNII-928Q33Q049. CAS-857402-63-2. Antineoplastic, Hsp 90 inhibitor.* ◇*IPI-504*

Retelliptine. $C_{25}H_{32}N_4O$. 404.55. 1-[[3-(Diethylamino)propyl]amino]-9-methoxy-5,11-dimethyl-6*H*-pyrido[4,3-*b*]carbazole. *UNII-SZ0F94M68J. CAS-72238-02-9.* INN.

Reteplase [*1997*] (re′ te plase). $C_{1736}H_{2653}N_{499}O_{522}S_{22}$·39,571.14. (1) 173-527-Plasminogen activator (human tissue-type), 173-L-serine-174-L-tyrosine-175-L-glutamine-; (2) 173-L-Serine-174-L-tyrosine-175-L-glutamine-173-527-plasminogen activator (mutant of human tissue-type). *CAS-133652-38-7.* INN; BAN. *Myocardial infarction therapy; plasminogen activator.* ◇*BM 06.022*

SYQGNSDCYF	GNGSAYRGTH	SLTESGASCL	PWNSMILIGK	VYTAQNPSAQ
ALGLGKHNYC	RNPDGDAKPW	CHVLKNRRLT	WEYCDVPSCS	TCGLRQYSQP
QFRIKGGLFA	DIASHPWQAA	IFAKHRRSPG	ERFLCGGILI	SSCWILSAAH
CFQERFPPHH	LTVILGRTYR	VVPGEEEQKF	EVEKYIVHKE	FDDDTYDNDI
ALLQLKSDSS	RCAQESSVVR	TVCLPPADLQ	LPDWTECELS	GYGKHEALSP
FYSERLKEAH	VRLYPSSRCT	SQHLLNRTVT	DNMLCAGDTR	SGGPQANLHD
ACQGDSGGPL	VCLNDGRMTL	VGIISWGLGC	GQKDVPGVYT	KVTNYLDWIR
DNMRP				

Retigabine [*2006*] (re tig′ a been). $C_{16}H_{18}FN_3O_2$. 303.33. (1) Carbamic acid, [2-amino-4-[[(4-fluoro-phenyl)methyl]amino]phenyl]-ethyl ester; (2) *N*-[2-Amino-4-(4-fluorobenzylamino)-phenyl]carbamic acid ethyl ester. *UNII-12G01I6BBU. CAS-150812-12-7.* INN. *Antiepileptic, adjunctive therapy for partial onset seizures.* ◇*D-23129*

Retinol. $C_{20}H_{30}O$. 286.45. [Retinol Acetate and Retinol Palmitate are JAN.] 3,7-Dimethyl-9-(2,6,6-trimethyl-1-cyclohexen-1-yl)-2,4,6,8-nonate-traen-1-ol. *UNII-G2SH0XKK91. CAS-68-26-8.* INN; BAN.

Retosiban [*2007*] (re toe′ si ban). $C_{27}H_{34}N_4O_5$. 494.58. (1) Morpholine, 4-[(2*R*)-[(3*R*,6*R*)-3-(2,3-dihydro-1*H*-inden-2-yl)-6-[(1*S*)-1-methylpropyl]-2,5-dioxo-1-piperazinyl](2-methyl-4-oxazolyl)acetyl]-; (2) (3*R*,6*R*)-6-[(2*S*)-Butan-2-yl]-3-(2,3-dihydro-1*H*-inden-2-yl)-1-[(1*R*)-1-(2-methyl-1,3-oxazol-4-yl)-2-(morpholin-4-yl)-2-oxoethyl]piperazine-2,5-dione. *UNII-GIE06H28OX. CAS-820957-38-8.* INN. *Oxytocin receptor antagonist for delaying preterm birth.* ◇*GSK221149A*

Revaprazan Hydrochloride [*2003*] (re va′ pra zan hye″ droe klor′ ide). $C_{22}H_{23}FN_4$·HCl. 398.90. [Revaprazan is INN.] (1) 2-Pyrimidinamine, 4-(3,4-dihydro-1-methyl-2(1*H*)-isoquinolinyl)-*N*-(4-fluorophenyl)-5,6-dimethyl-, monohydrochloride; (2) *N*-(4-Fluorophenyl)-5,6-dimethyl-4-[(1*RS*)-1-methyl-3,4-dihydroisoquinolin-2(1*H*)-yl]pyrimidin-2-amine monohydrochloride. *UNII-4DQ6T10R64; UNII-5P184180P5* [revaprazan]. *CAS-178307-42-1; CAS-*

199463-33-7 [revaprazan]. *Treatment of peptic ulcer, gastric ulcer, duodenal ulcer, and GERD (acid pump antagonist).* ◇*YH1885*

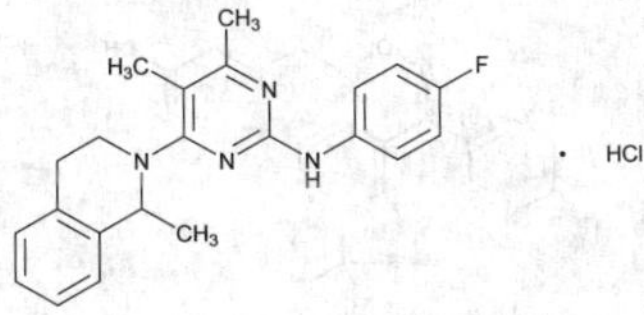

Revatropate. $C_{19}H_{27}NO_4S$. 365.49. (*R*)-3-Quinuclidinyl (*S*)-β-hydroxy-α-[2-(*R*)-methylsulfinyl]ethyl]hydratropate. *UNII-3W7L15V40W. CAS-149926-91-0.* INN; BAN. ◇*UK-112,166; UK-112,166-04 [as hydrobromide]*

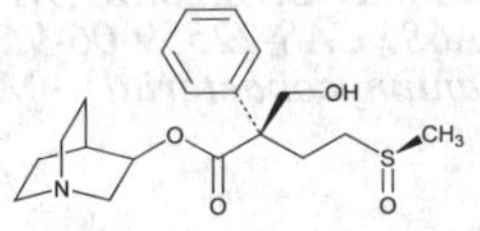

Revenast. $C_{27}H_{29}N_5O$. 439.55. 2,3-Diphenyl-1-[3-[4-(2-pyridyl)-1-piperazinyl]propyl]-3-pyrazolin-5-one. *UNII-24G45TQO8A. CAS-85673-87-6.* INN.

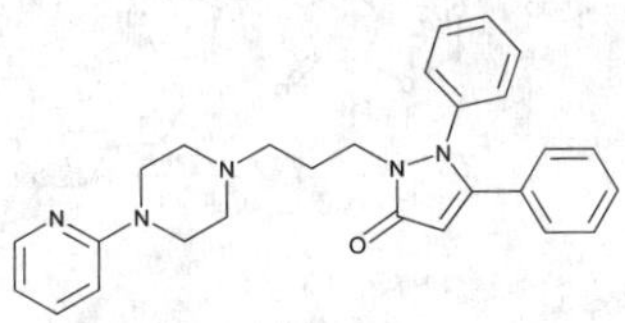

Reviparin Sodium. Sodium salt of a low molecular mass heparin that is obtained by nitrous acid depolymerization of heparin from porcine intestinal mucosa; the majority of the components have a 2-*O*-sulfo-α-L-idopyranosuronic acid structure at the non-reducing end and a 6-*O*-sulfo-2,5-anhydro-D-mannitol structure at the reducing end of their chain; the mass-average molecular mass ranges between 3150 and 5150, with a characteristic value of about 4150; the degree of sulfatation is about 2.1 per disaccharidic unit. INN; BAN.

Revizinone. $C_{26}H_{29}N_5O_3$. 459.54. (*E*)-*N*-Cyclohexyl-*N*-methyl-2-[[[α-(1,2,3,5-tetrahydro-2-oxoimidazo[2,1-*b*]quinazolin-7-yl)benzylidene]amino]oxy]acetamide. *UNII-6208ZO6MLG. CAS-133718-29-3.* INN.

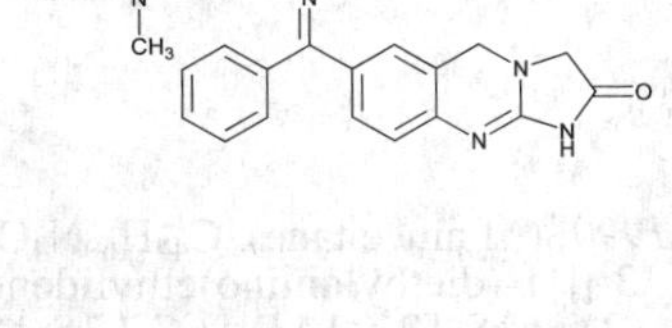

---

† Brand name formerly used, and/or firm no longer concerned with this product.

Revospirone. $C_{18}H_{21}N_5O_3S$. 387.46. 2-[3-[4-(2-Pyrimidinyl)-1-piperazinyl]propyl]-1,2-benzisothiazolin-3-one 1,1-dioxide. *UNII-6X8764TW2J. CAS-95847-87-3.* INN; BAN.

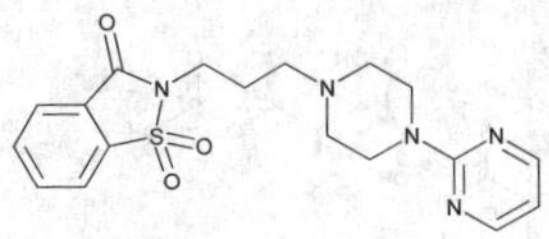

Rh₀(D) Immune Globulin. USP. A sterile, nonpyrogenic solution of globulins derived from human blood plasma containing antibody to the erythrocyte factor Rh₀ (D). *Immunizing agent (passive).* BayRho-D (Bayer); Gamulin Rh (Centeon); MICRhoGAM (Ortho Diagnostic); Mini-Gamulin Rh (Centeon); RhoGAM (Ortho Diagnostic) *[Name previously used: Rh₀(D) Immune Human Globulin.]*

Rh₀ (D) Immune Human Globulin (previously used name) — *See* Rh₀ (D) Immune Globulin.

Rhamnus Purshiana — *See* Cascara Sagrada.

Rhetinic Acid — *See* Enoxolone.

rhIGF-1 — *See* Mecasermin.

rhM-CSF (previously used name) — *See* Cilmostim.

Ribaminol [*1967*] (rye ba′ mi nol). (1) Ribonucleic acids, transfer, 2-(diethylamino)ethanol complex; (2) Ribonucleic acid compound with 2-(diethylamino)ethanol. *CAS-8063-28-3.* INN. *Memory adjuvant.* ◇*ICN-542*

Ribavirin [*1974*] (rye″ ba vir′ in). **USP.** $C_8H_{12}N_4O_5$. 244.20. (1) 1*H*-1,2,4-Triazole-3-carboxamide, 1-β-D-ribofuranosyl-; (2) 1-β-D-Ribofuranosyl-1*H*-1,2,4-triazole-3-carboxamide. *UNII-49717AWG6K. CAS-36791-04-5.* INN; BAN. *Antiviral.* Copegus (Roche); Rebetol (Schering-Plough); Ribasphere (Three Rivers); Virazole (Valeant)

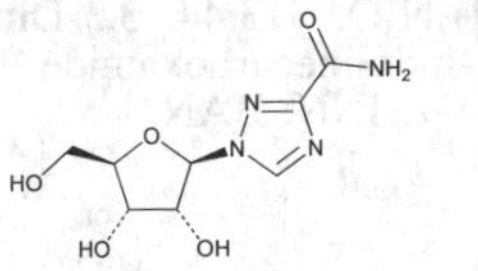

Riboflavin (rye′ boe flay vin). **USP.** $C_{17}H_{20}N_4O_6$. 376.36. [Riboflavin Tetrabutyrate is JAN.] (1) Riboflavine; (2) Riboflavine. *UNII-TLM2976OFR. CAS-83-88-5.* INN; BAN. *Vitamin (enzyme co-factor).* Flavaxin (Sterling Winthrop†) *[Name previously used: Riboflavine.]*

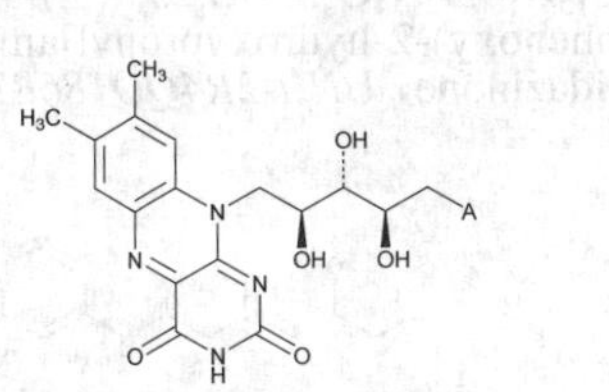

Riboflavin 5′-Phosphate Sodium (rye′ boe flay vin fos′ fate soe′ dee um). **USP.** $C_{17}H_{20}N_4NaO_9P.2H_2O$. 514.36. [Riboflavin Sodium Phosphate is JAN.] (1) Riboflavin 5′-

(dihydrogen phosphate), monosodium salt, dihydrate; (2) Riboflavine 5′-(sodium hydrogen phosphate), dihydrate. *CAS-130-40-5* [anhydrous]. *Vitamin.*

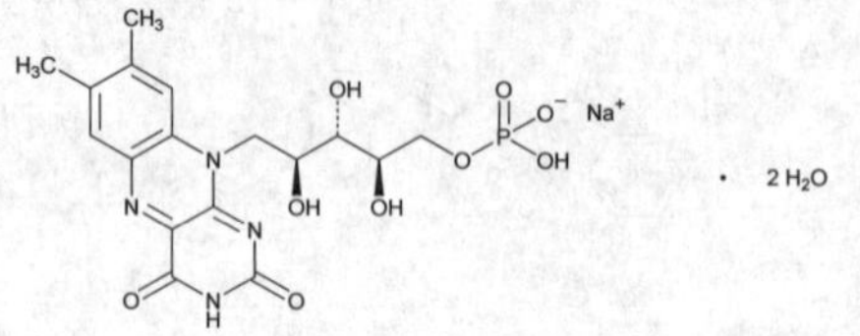

Riboflavin Sodium Phosphate (JAN) — *See* Riboflavin 5′-Phosphate Sodium.

Riboprine [*1968*] (rye′ boe preen). $C_{15}H_{21}N_5O_4$. 335.36. (1) Adenosine, *N*-(3-methyl-2-butenyl)-; (2) *N*-(3-Methyl-2-butenyl)adenosine; (3) 6-*N*-[(3-Methyl-2-butenyl)amino]-9-β-D-ribofuranosyl-9*H*-purine. *CAS-7724-76-7.* INN. *Antineoplastic.* ◇*IPA; NSC-105546*

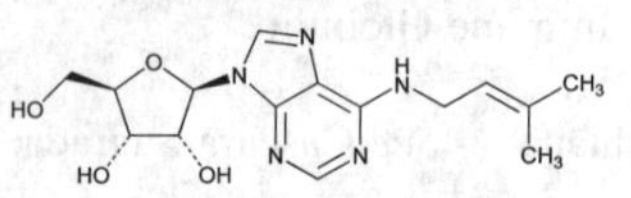

Ribostamycin. $C_{17}H_{34}N_4O_{10}$. 454.47. [Ribostamycin Sulfate is JAN.] *O*-2,6-Diamino-2,6-dideoxy-α-D-glucopyranosyl-(1→4)-*O*-[β-D-ribofuranosyl-(1→5)]-2-deoxystreptamine. *CAS-25546-65-0.* INN; BAN; MI.

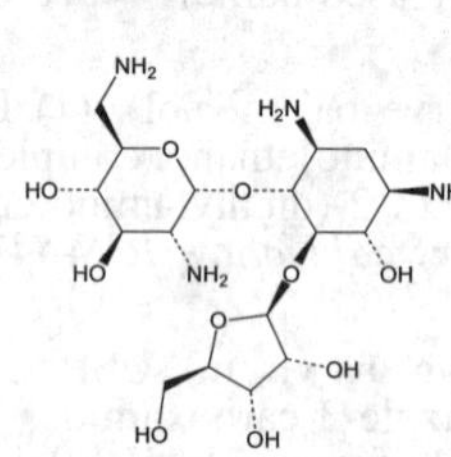

Riboxamide — *See* Tiazofurin.

Ricainide — *See* Indecainide Hydrochloride.

Ricasetron. $C_{19}H_{27}N_3O$. 313.44. 3,3-Dimethyl-*N*-1α*H*,5α*H*-tropan-3α-yl-1-indolinecarboxamide. *UNII-R92JB88O88. CAS-117086-68-7.* INN; BAN.

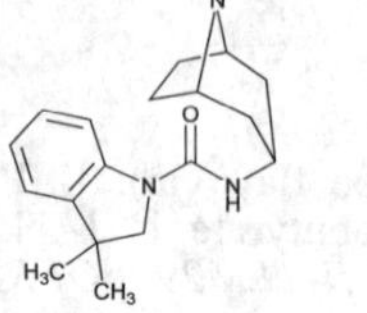

Ridazolol. $C_{15}H_{18}Cl_2N_4O_3$. 373.23. (±)-4-Chloro-5-[[2-[[3-(*o*-chlorophenoxy)-2-hydroxypropyl]amino]ethyl]amino]-3(2*H*)-pyridazinone. *UNII-2R4QO1868Y. CAS-83395-21-5.* INN.

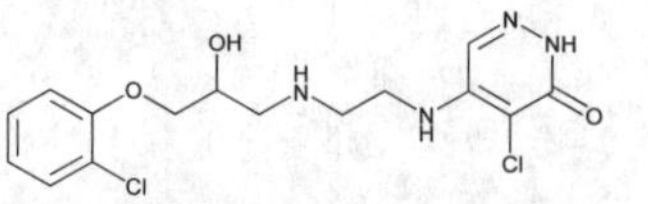

Ridogrel [*1991*] (rye′ doe grel). $C_{18}H_{17}F_3N_2O_3$. 366.33. (1) Pentanoic acid, 5-[[[3-pyridinyl[3-(trifluoromethyl)phen-yl]methylene]amino]oxy]-, (*E*)-; (2) (*E*)-5-[[[α-3-Pyridyl-

m-(trifluoromethyl)benzylidene]amino]oxy]valeric acid. *CAS-110140-89-1.* INN; BAN. *Inhibitor (thromboxane synthetase).* ◇*R 68070*

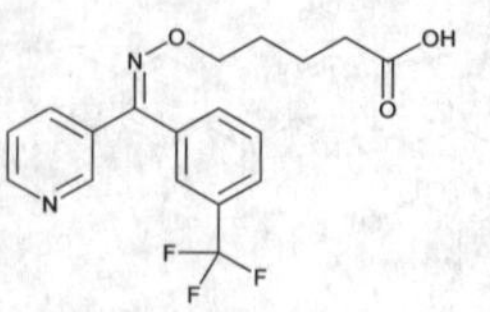

Rifabutin [*1993*] (rif″ a bue′ tin). **USP.** $C_{46}H_{62}N_4O_{11}$. 847.00. (9*S*,12*E*,14*S*,15*R*,16*S*,17*R*,18*R*,19*R*,20*S*,21*S*,22*E*,24*Z*)-6-16,18,20-Tetrahydroxy-1′-isobutyl-14-methoxy-7,9,15,17,19,21,25-heptamethylspiro[9,4-(epoxypentadeca[1,11,13]trienimino)-2*H*-furo[2′,3′:7,8]naphth[1,2-*d*]imidazole-2,4′-piperidine]-5,10,26(3*H*,9*H*)-trione,16-acetate. *UNII-1W306TDA6S. CAS-72559-06-9.* INN; BAN; JAN. *Antibacterial (antimycobacterial).* Mycobutin (Pfizer) ◇*LM-427*

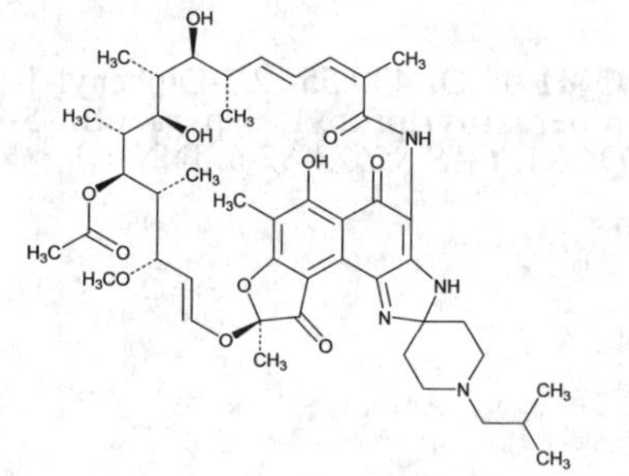

Rifalazil [*1997*] (rif al′ a zil). $C_{51}H_{64}N_4O_{13}$. 941.07. (2*S*,16*Z*,18*E*,20*S*,21*S*,22*R*,23*R*,24*R*,25*S*,26*R*,27*S*,28*E*)-5,12,21,23,25-Pentahydroxy-10-(4-isobutyl-1-piperazinyl)-27-methoxy-2,4,16,20,22,24,26-heptamethyl-2,7-(epoxypentadeca[1,11,13]trienimino)-6*H*-benzofuro[4,5-*a*]phenoxazine-1(2*H*),6,15-trione 25-acetate. *CAS-129791-92-0.* INN. *Antibacterial (antimycobacterial).* ◇*KRM-1648*

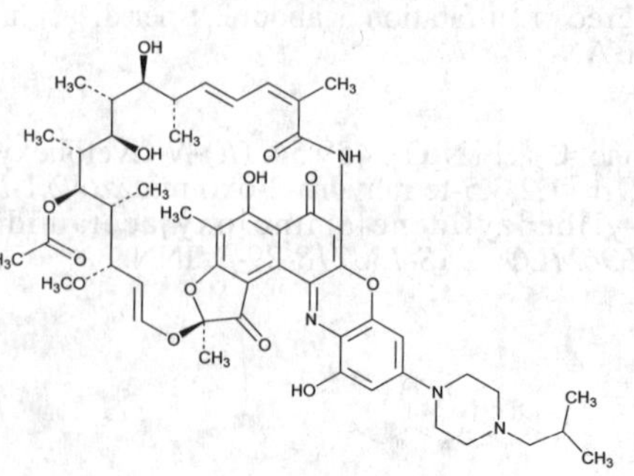

Rifametane [*1990*] (rif am′ e tane). $C_{44}H_{60}N_4O_{12}$. 836.97. (1) Rifamycin, 3-[[[1-(diethylamino)ethylidene]hydrazono]-methyl]-; (2) (2*S*,12*Z*,14*E*,16*S*,17*S*,18*R*,19*R*,20*R*,21*S*,22*S*,23*S*,24*E*)-1,2-Dihydro-5,6,9,17,19,21-hexahy-droxy-23-methoxy-2,4,12,16,18,20,22-heptamethyl-1,11-dioxo-2,7-(epoxypentadeca[1,11,13]trienimino)-

naphtho[2,1-*b*]furan-8-carboxyaldehyde, 8-azine with *N,N*-diethylacetamide, 21-acetate. *CAS-94168-98-6*. INN. *Antibacterial. ◇SPA-S-565*

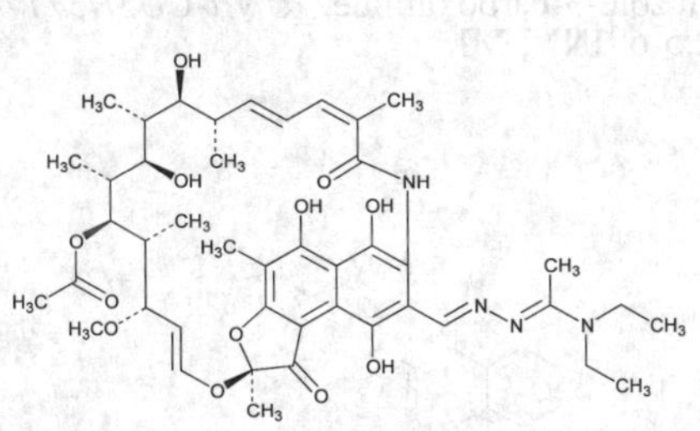

Rifamexil [*1992*] (rif″ a mex′ il). $C_{42}H_{55}N_3O_{11}S$. 809.96. (1) Rifamycin P, 2′-(diethylamino)-; (2) (9*S*,12*E*,14*S*,15*S*,16*S*,17*R*,18*R*,19*R*,20*S*,21*S*,22*E*,24*Z*)-2-(Diethylamino)-5,6,16,18,20-pentahydroxy-14-methoxy-7,9,15,17,19,21,25-heptamethyl-9,4-(epoxypentadeca[1,11,13]trienimino)furo[2′,3′:7,8]naphtho[1,2-*d*]thiazole-10,26(9*H*)-dione, 16-acetate. *CAS-113102-19-5*. INN. *Antibacterial. ◇MDL 62,769*

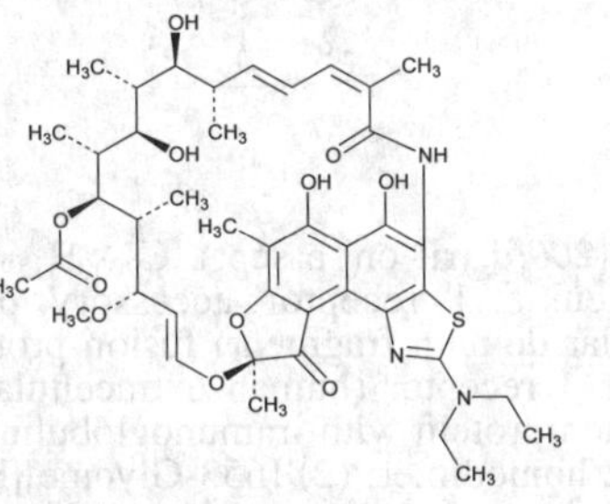

Rifamide [*1966*] (rif′ a mide). $C_{43}H_{58}N_2O_{13}$. 810.93. (1) Rifamycin, 4-*O*-[2-(diethylamino)-2-oxoethyl]-; (2) Stereoisomer of *N,N*-Diethyl-2-[(1,2-dihydro-5,6,17,19,21-pentahydroxy-23-methoxy-2,4,12,16,18,20,22-heptamethyl-1,11-dioxo-2,7-(epoxypentadeca[1,11,13]trienimino)naphtho[2,1-*b*]furan-9-yl)oxy]acetamide 21-acetate; (3) Rifamycin B *N,N*-diethylamide. *CAS-2750-76-7*. INN; BAN. *Antibacterial. ◇Rifamycin M-14; NSC-133099*

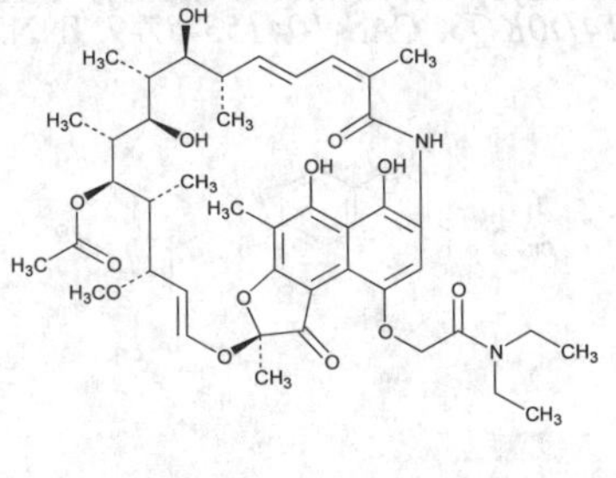

Rifampicin (INN, BAN, JAN) — *See* Rifampin.

Rifampin [*1968*] (rif am′ pin). **USP**. $C_{43}H_{58}N_4O_{12}$. 822.94. [Rifampicin is INN, BAN, and JAN.] (1) Rifamycin, 3-[[(4-methyl-1-piperazinyl)imino]methyl]-; (2) 5,6,9,17,19,21-Hexahydroxy-23-methoxy-2,4,12,16,18,20,22-heptamethyl-8-[*N*-(4-methyl-1-piperazinyl)formimidoyl]-2,7-(epoxypentadeca[1,11,13]trienimino)naphtho[2,1-*b*]furan-1,11(2*H*)-dione 21-acetate. *UNII-VJT6J7R4TR. CAS-13292-46-1*. *Antibacterial.* Rifadin (Sanofi Aventis); Rimactane (Actavis) *◇L-5103 Lepetit; Ba 41166/E; NSC-113926*

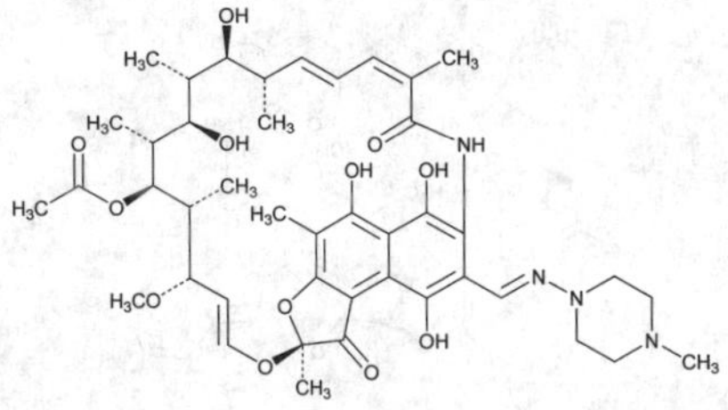

Rifamycin. $C_{37}H_{47}NO_{12}$. 697.77. Rifamycin SV, an antibiotic produced by certain strains of *Streptomyces mediterranei*, or the same substance produced by any other means. *CAS-6998-60-3*. INN; BAN; DCF; MI. *◇M-14*

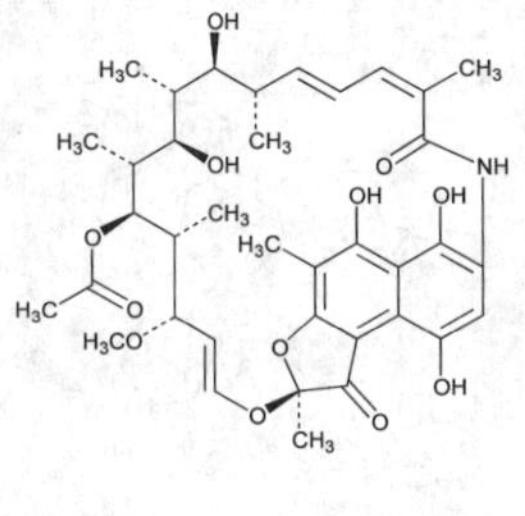

Rifamycin Diethylamide — *See* Rifamide.

Rifapentine [*1985*] (rif″ a pen′ teen). $C_{47}H_{64}N_4O_{12}$. 877.03. (1) Rifamycin, 3-[[(4-cyclopentyl-1-piperazinyl)imino]methyl]-; (2) 3-[*N*-(4-Cyclopentyl-1-piperazinyl)formimidoyl]rifamycin. *UNII-XJM390A33U. CAS-61379-65-5*. INN; BAN. *Antibacterial.* Priftin (Sanofi Aventis) *◇MDL 473*

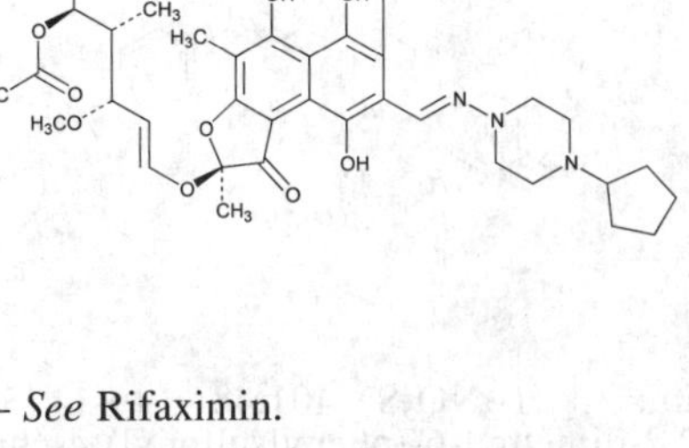

Rifaxidin — *See* Rifaximin.

Rifaximin [*1992*] (rif ax′ i min). $C_{43}H_{51}N_3O_{11}$. 785.88. (1) 2,7-(Epoxypentadeca[1,11,13]trienimino)benzofuro[4,5-*e*]pyrido[1,2-*a*]benzimidazole-1,15(2*H*)-dione, 25-(acetyloxy)-5,6,21,23-tetrahydroxy-27-methoxy-2,4,11,16,20,22,24,26-octamethyl-, [2*S*-(2*R**, 16*Z*,18*E*,20*R**,21*R**,22*S**,23*S**,24*S**,25*R**,26*S**,27*R**,28-*E*)]-; (2) (2*S*,16*Z*,18*E*,20*S*,21*S*,22*R*,23*R*,24*R*,25*S*,26*S*,27*S*,28*E*)-5,6,21,23,25 Pentahydroxy-27-methoxy-2,4,11,16,20,22,24,26-octamethyl-2,7-(epoxypentadeca[1,11,13]trienimino)benzofuro[4,5-*e*]pyrido[1,2-*a*]ben-

† Brand name formerly used, and/or firm no longer concerned with this product.

zimidazole-1,15(2*H*)-dione, 25-acetate. *UNII-L36O5T016N. CAS-80621-81-4.* INN; MI. *Antibacterial.* Xifaxan (Salix)

Rifomycin — *See* Rifamycin.

Rilapine. $C_{22}H_{20}ClN_3$. 361.87. (*Z*)-2-Chloro-10-(4-methyl-1-piperazinyl)-5*H*-dibenzo[*a,d*]cycloheptene-$\Delta^{5,\alpha}$-acetonitrile. *UNII-7QCG0RP106. CAS-79781-95-6.* INN.

Rilapladib [*2005*] (ril ap′ la dib). $C_{40}H_{38}F_5N_3O_3S$. 735.81. (1) 1(4*H*)-Quinolineacetamide, 2-[[(2,3-difluorophenyl)-methyl]thio]-*N*-[1-(2-methoxyethyl)-4-piperidinyl]-4-oxo-*N*-[[4′-(trifluoromethyl)[1,1′-biphenyl]-4-yl]methyl]-; (2) 2-[2-[(2,3-Difluorobenzyl)sulfanyl]-4-oxoquinolin-1(4*H*)-yl]-*N*-[1-(2-methoxyethyl)piperidin-4-yl]-*N*-[[4′-(trifluoromethyl)biphenyl-4-yl]methyl]acetamide. *UNII-O14CWE893Z. CAS-412950-08-4.* INN. *Treatment of atherosclerosis.* ◇SB-659032

Rilmakalim. $C_{21}H_{23}NO_5S$. 401.48. (+)-1-[(3*S*,4*R*)-3-hydroxy-2,2-dimethyl-6-(phenylsulfonyl)-4-chromanyl]-2-pyrrolidinone. *UNII-47Y56T6LEI. CAS-132014-21-2.* INN.

Rilmazafone. $C_{21}H_{20}Cl_2N_6O_3$. 475.33. [Rilmazafone Hydrochloride is JAN.] 5-[(2-Aminoacetamido)methyl]-1-[4-chloro-2-(*o*-chlorobenzoyl)phenyl]-*N*,*N*-dimethyl-1*H*-1,2,4-triazole-3-carboxamide. *UNII-CU3H37T766. CAS-99593-25-6.* INN; MI.

Rilmenidine. $C_{10}H_{16}N_2O$. 180.25. 2-[(Dicyclopropylmethyl)amino]-2-oxazoline. *UNII-P67IM25ID8. CAS-54187-04-1.* INN; MI.

Rilonacept [*2006*] (ril on′ a sept). $C_{9030}H_{13932}N_{2400}O_{2670}S_{74}$. (1) Interleukin 1 receptor accessory protein (human extracellular domain fragment) fusion protein with type I interleukin 1 receptor (human extracellular domain fragment) fusion protein with immunoglobulin G1 (human Fc fragment), homodimer; (2) [653-Glycine][human interleukin-1 receptor accessory protein-(1-339)-peptide (extracellular domain fragment) fusion protein with human type I interleukin-1 receptor-(5-316)-peptide (extracellular domain fragment) fusion protein with human immunoglobulin G1-(229 *C*-terminal residues)-peptide (Fc fragment)] dimer. Molecular weight is approximately 201,210 daltons. *CAS-501081-76-1.* INN. *Treatment of rheumatoid arthritis, autoinflammatory diseases, and osteoarthritis.* ◇IL-1 Trap; *Interleukin-1 Trap*

Rilopirox. $C_{19}H_{16}ClNO_4$. 357.79. 6-[[*p*-(*p*-Chlorophenoxy)phenoxy]methyl]-1-hydroxy-4-methyl-2(1*H*)-pyridone. *UNII-595T4D0KQ3. CAS-104153-37-9.* INN.

Rilozarone. $C_{32}H_{36}BrClN_2O_2$. 596.00. 1-Bromo-2-phenyl-3-indolizinyl 3-chloro-4-[3-(dibutylamino)propoxy]phenyl ketone. *UNII-E521I6380L. CAS-79282-39-6.* INN.

Rilpivirine. $C_{22}H_{18}N_6$. 366.42. 4-{[4-({4-[(1*E*)-2-Cyanoethenyl]-2,6-dimethylphenyl}amino)pyrimidin-2-yl]amino}-benzonitrile. *UNII-FI96A8X663. CAS-500287-72-9.* INN.

Riluzole [*1995*] (ril′ ue zole). $C_8H_5F_3N_2OS$. 234.20. (1) 2-Benzothiazolamine, 6-(trifluoromethoxy)-; (2) 2-Amino-6-(trifluoromethoxy)benzothiazole. *UNII-7LJ087RS6F. CAS-1744-22-5.* INN; BAN. *Amyotrophic lateral sclerosis treatment.* Rilutek (Sanofi Aventis) ◇*RP 54274*

Rimacalib. $C_{22}H_{23}FN_4O_2$. 394.44. *N*-{3-[(1*S*)-1-(2-Fluorobiphenyl-4-yl)ethyl]-1,2-oxazol-5-yl}morpholine-4-carboximidamide. *CAS-215174-50-8.* INN.

Rimantadine Hydrochloride [*1966*] (ri man′ ta deen hye″ droe klor′ ide). **USP.** $C_{12}H_{21}N{\cdot}HCl$. 215.76. [Rimantadine is INN and BAN.] (1) Tricyclo[3.3.1.1^{3,7}]-decane-1-methanamine, α-methyl-, hydrochloride; (2) α-Methyl-1-adamantanemethylamine hydrochloride. *UNII-JEIO7OOS8Y; UNII-0T2EF4JQTU* [rimantadine]. *CAS-1501-84-4; CAS-13392-28-4* [rimantadine]. *Antiviral.* Flumadine (Forest) ◇*EXP 126*

Rimazolium Metilsulfate. $C_{14}H_{22}N_2O_7S$. 362.40. 3-(Ethoxycarbonyl)-6,7,8,9-tetrahydro-1,6-dimethyl-4-oxo-4*H*-pyrido[1,2-*a*]pyrimidinium methyl sulfate. *UNII-99YI50276I. CAS-28610-84-6; CAS-35615-72-6* [rimazolium]. INN; MI. ◇*MZ-144*

Rimcazole Hydrochloride [*1986*] (rim′ ka zole hye″ droe klor′ ide). $C_{21}H_{27}N_3{\cdot}2HCl$. 394.38. [Rimcazole is INN.] (1) 9*H*-Carbazole, 9-[3-(3,5-dimethyl-1-piperazinyl)propyl]-, dihydrochloride, *cis*-; (2) 9-[3-(*cis*-3,5-Dimethyl-1-piper-

azinyl)propyl]carbazole dihydrochloride. *CAS-75859-03-9; CAS-75859-04-0* [rimcazole]. *Antipsychotic.* ◇*BW 234U dihydrochloride*

Rimeporide. $C_{11}H_{15}N_3O_5S_2$. 333.38. *N*-(Aminoiminomethyl)-4,5-bis(methanesulfonyl)-2-methylbenzamide. *CAS-187870-78-6.* INN.

Rimexolone [*1990*] (ri mex′ oh lone). **USP.** $C_{24}H_{34}O_3$. 370.52. (1) Androsta-1,4-dien-3-one, 11-hydroxy-16,17-dimethyl-17-(1-oxopropyl)-, (11β,16α,17β)-; (2) 11β-Hydroxy-16α,17α-dimethyl-17-propionylandrosta-1,4-dien-3-one. *UNII-O7M2E4264D. CAS-49697-38-3.* INN; BAN. *Anti-inflammatory.* Vexol (Alcon) ◇*Org 6216*

Rimiterol Hydrobromide [*1971*] (ri mi′ ter ol hye″ droe broe′ mide). $C_{12}H_{17}NO_3{\cdot}HBr$. 304.18. [Rimiterol is INN and BAN.] (1) 2-Piperidinemethanol, α-(3,4-dihydroxyphenyl)-, (*R**,*S**)-, hydrobromide; (2) *erythro*-α-(3,4-Dihydroxyphenyl)-2-piperidinemethanol hydrobromide. *UNII-I29DRR8S3R. CAS-31842-61-2; CAS-31931-97-2* [nonstereospecific]; *CAS-32953-89-2* [rimiterol]. *Bronchodilator.* ◇*WG-253; R 798*

Rimonabant [*2005*] (ri mone′ a bant). $C_{22}H_{21}Cl_3N_4O$. 463.79. (1) 5-(*p*-Chlorophenyl)-1-(2,4-dichlorophenyl)-4-methyl-*N*-piperidinopyrazole-3-carboxamide; (2) 1*H*-Pyrazole-3-carboxamide, 5-(4-chlorophenyl)-1-(2,4-dichlorophenyl)-4-methyl-*N*-piperidinyl. *UNII-RML78EN3XE. CAS-168273-06-1.* INN. *Smoking cessation; treatment of obesity.* Acomplia (Sanofi-Synthelabo) ◇*SR141716*

---

† Brand name formerly used, and/or firm no longer concerned with this product.

Rimoprogin. $C_8H_7IN_2OS$. 306.12. 5-[(3-Iodo-2-propynyl)oxy]-2-(methylthio)pyrimidine. *UNII-QG8198SR7M. CAS-37750-83-7.* INN.

Rinfabate [*2006*] (rin′ fa bate). (1) Insulin-like growth factor-binding protein-3 (human); (2) Recombinant human insulin-like growth factor-binding protein 3. Molecular weight is approximately 28,732 daltons. *CAS-405341-12-0. Anti-cancer agent.* ◇*rhIGFBP-3*

```
GASSAGLGPV VRCEPCDARA LAQCAPPPAV CAELVREPGC GCCLTCALSE
GQPCGIYTER CGSGLRCQPS PDEARPLQAL LDGRGLCVNA SAVSRLRAYL
LPAPPAPGNA SESEEDRSAG SVESPSVSST HRVSDPKFHP LHSKIIIKK
GHAKDSQRYK VDYESQSTDT QNFSSESKRE TEYGPCRREM EDTLNHLKFL
NVLSPRGVHI PNCDKKGFYK KKQCRPSKGR KRGFCWCVDK YGQPLPGYTT
KGKEDVHCYS MQSK
```

Ringer's Injection. **USP**. [Compound Solution of Sodium Chloride is INN.] A sterile solution of sodium chloride, potassium chloride and calcium chloride in water. *Replenisher (fluid); replenisher (electrolyte)*.

Riociguat. $C_{20}H_{19}FN_8O_2$. 422.42. Methyl *N*-(4,6-diamino-2-{1-[(2-fluorophenyl)methyl]-1*H*-pyrazolo[3,4-*b*]pyridin-3-yl}pyrimidin-5-yl)-*N*-methylcarbamate. *CAS-625115-55-1.* INN.

Riodipine. $C_{18}H_{19}F_2NO_5$. 367.34. Dimethyl 4-[*o*-(difluoromethoxy)phenyl]-1,4-dihydro-2,6-dimethyl-3,5-pyridinedicarboxylate. *UNII-W12VDB26LB. CAS-71653-63-9.* INN.

Rioprostil [*1983*] (rye″ oh prost′ il). $C_{21}H_{38}O_4$. 354.52. (1) Prost-13-en-9-one, 1,11,16-trihydroxy-16-methyl-, (11α,13*E*)-; (2) (2*R*,3*R*,4*R*)-4-Hydroxy-2-(7-hydroxyheptyl)-3-[(*E*)-(4*RS*)-(4-hydroxy-4-methyl-1-octenyl)]cyclopentanone. *CAS-77287-05-9.* INN; BAN. *Antisecretory (gastric).* ◇*TR-4698; ORF 15927; RWJ 15927*

Ripazepam [*1976*] (ri paz′ e pam). $C_{15}H_{16}N_4O$. 268.31. (1) Pyrazolo[4,3-*e*][1,4]diazepin-5(1*H*)-one, 1-ethyl-4,6-dihydro-3-methyl-8-phenyl-; (2) 1-Ethyl-4,6-dihydro-3-methyl-8-phenylpyrazolo[4,3-*e*][1,4]diazepin-5(1*H*)-one. *CAS-26308-28-1.* INN. *Tranquilizer (minor).* ◇*Cl-683*

Ripisartan. $C_{23}H_{22}N_8O$. 426.47. 5-Methyl-7-propyl-8-[*p*-(*o*-1*H*-tetrazol-5-ylphenyl)benzyl]-*s*-triazolo[1,5-*c*]pyrimidin-2(3*H*)-one. *CAS-148504-51-2.* INN.

Risarestat. $C_{16}H_{21}NO_4S$. 323.41. ($\pm$)-5-[3-Ethoxy-4-(pentyloxy)phenyl]-2,4-thiazolidinedione. *CAS-79714-31-1.* INN.

Risedronate Sodium [*1990*] (ris″ e droe′ nate soe′ dee um). $C_7H_{10}NNaO_7P_2$. 305.09. (1) Phosphonic acid, [1-hydroxy-2-(3-pyridinyl)ethylidene]bis-, monosodium salt; (2) Sodium trihydrogen [1-hydroxy-2-(3-pyridyl)ethylidene]diphosphonate. *UNII-OFG5EXG60L. CAS-115436-72-1. Regulator (calcium).* Actonel (Procter & Gamble) ◇*NE-58095*

Risedronic Acid. $C_7H_{11}NO_7P_2$. 283.11. [1-Hydroxy-2-(3-pyridyl)ethylidene]diphosphonic acid. *UNII-KM2Z91756Z. CAS-105462-24-6.* INN; BAN.

Rismorelin Porcine [*1995*] (ris″ moe rel′ in por′ sine). $C_{379}H_{623}N_{127}O_{118}$. 8846.78. [Rismorelin is INN.] (1) Prosomatoliberin (pig), 1-[*N*-(4-methylbenzoyl)glycine]-9-L-asparagine-12-L-arginine-15-L-threonine-21-L-arginine-27-L-leucine-51-L-leucine-56-L-arginine-58-L-leucine-; (2) 1-(*p*-Methylhippuric acid)-9-L-asparagine-12-L-arginine-15-L-threonine-21-L-arginine-27-L-leucine-51-L-leucine-56-L-arginine-58-L-leucineprosomatoliberin (pig). *CAS-146706-68-5. Growth hormone-releasing hormone.* ◇*LY293404*

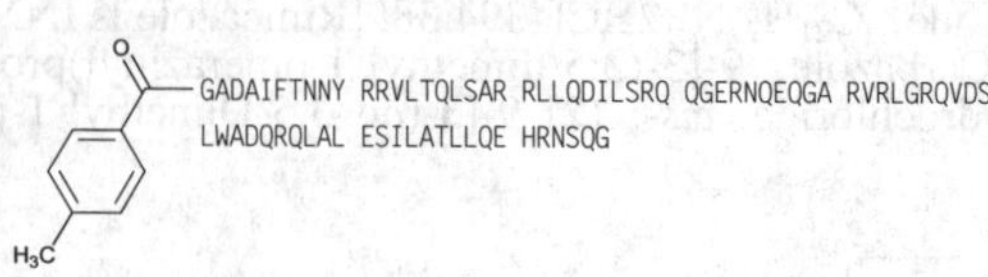

Risocaine [*1971*] (ris′ oh kane). $C_{10}H_{13}NO_2$. 179.22. (1) Benzoic acid, 4-amino-, propyl ester; (2) Propyl *p*-aminobenzoate. *CAS-94-12-2*. INN. *Anesthetic (local)*. ◇*NSC-23516*

Risotilide Hydrochloride [*1990*] (ris ote′ i lide hye″ droe klor′ ide). $C_{15}H_{27}N_3O_4S_2$.HCl. 413.98. [Risotilide is INN.] (1) Benzenesulfonamide, *N*-(1-methylethyl)-*N*-[2-[(1-methylethyl)amino]ethyl]-4-[(methylsulfonyl)amino]-, monohydrochloride; (2) 4′-[Isopropyl[2-(isopropylamino)ethyl]sulfamoyl]methanesulfonanilide monohydrochloride. *CAS-116907-13-2; CAS-120688-08-6* [risotilide]. *Cardiac depressant (anti-arrhythmic)*. ◇*WY-48986*

Rispenzepine. $C_{19}H_{20}N_4O_2$. 336.39. (±)-6,11-Dihydro-11-(1-methylnipecotoyl)-5*H*-pyrido[2,3-*b*][1,5]benzodiazepin-5-one. *UNII-W99LLM73R7. CAS-96449-05-7*. INN.

Risperidone [*1989*] (ris per′ i done). **USP.** $C_{23}H_{27}FN_4O_2$. 410.48. (1) 4*H*-Pyrido[1,2-*a*]pyrimidin-4-one, 3-[2-[4-(6-fluoro-1,2-benzisoxazol-3-yl)-1-piperidinyl]ethyl]-6,7,8,9-tetrahydro-2-methyl-; (2) 3-[2-[4-(6-Fluoro-1,2-benzisoxazol-3-yl)piperidino]ethyl]-6,7,8,9-tetrahydro-2-methyl-4*H*-pyrido[1,2-*a*]pyrimidin-4-one. *UNII-L6UH7ZF8HC. CAS-106266-06-2*. INN; BAN. *Neuroleptic*. Risperdal (Janssen) ◇*R 64 766*

Ristianol Phosphate [*1984*] (ris tye′ a nol fos′ fate). $C_8H_{11}NOS.H_3PO_4$. 267.24. [Ristianol is INN and BAN.] (1) Ethanol, 2-[(4-pyridinylmethyl)thio]-, phosphate (1:1) (salt); (2) 2-(4-Pyridylmethyl)thioethanol phosphate (1:1) (salt). *CAS-78092-66-7*. *Immunoregulator*. ◇*CP-48,867-9*

Ristocetin. Antibiotic obtained from cultures of *Nocardia lurida*, or the same substance produced by any other means. *CAS-1404-55-3*. USP XVII; INN; BAN; MI. Spontin (Abbott†)

Ritanserin [*1985*] (ri tan′ ser in). $C_{27}H_{25}F_2N_3OS$. 477.57. (1) 5*H*-Thiazolo[3,2-*a*]pyrimidin-5-one, 6-[2-[4-bis(4-fluorophenyl)methylene]-1-piperidinyl]ethyl]-7-methyl-; (2) 6-[2-[4-[Bis(*p*-fluorophenyl)methylene]-piperidino]ethyl]-7-methyl-5*H*-thiazolo-[3,2-*a*]pyrimidin-5-one. *CAS-87051-43-2*. INN; BAN. *Serotonin antagonist*. Tiserton (Janssen) ◇*R 55,667*

Ritiometan. $C_7H_{10}O_6S_3$. 286.35. (Methylidynetrithio)triacetic acid. *UNII-J89LM8QVEE. CAS-34914-39-1*. INN.

Ritipenem. $C_{10}H_{12}N_2O_6S$. 288.28. (5*R*,6*S*)-3-(Carbamoyloxymethyl)-6-((*R*)-1-hydroxyethyl)-7-oxo-4-thia-1-azabicyclo[3.2.0]hept-2-ene-2-carboxylic acid. *UNII-D4SL77931L. CAS-84845-57-8*. INN.

Ritobegron. $C_{21}H_{27}NO_5$. 373.44. [4-(2-{[(1*R*,2*S*)-1-Hydroxy-1-(4-hydroxyphenyl)propan-2-yl]amino}ethyl)-2,5-dimethylphenoxy]acetic acid. *CAS-255734-04-4*. INN.

Ritodrine [*1969*] (rit′ oh dreen). $C_{17}H_{21}NO_3$. 287.35. (1) Benzenemethanol, 4-hydroxy-α-[1-[[2-(4-hydroxyphenyl)ethyl]amino]ethyl]-, (*R**,*S**)-; (2) *erythro-p*-Hydroxy-α-[1-[(*p*-hydroxyphenethyl)amino]ethyl]benzyl alcohol. *UNII-I0Q6O6740J. CAS-26652-09-5*. INN; BAN. *Relaxant (smooth muscle)*. ◇*DU-21220*

Ritodrine Hydrochloride [*1981*] (rit′ oh dreen hye″ droe klor′ ide). **USP.** $C_{17}H_{21}NO_3$.HCl. 323.81. (1) Benzenemethanol, 4-hydroxy-α-[1-[[2-(4-hydroxyphenyl)ethyl]amino]ethyl]-, hydrochloride, (*R**,*S**)-; (2) *erythro-p*-Hydroxy-α-[1-[(*p*-hydroxyphenethyl)amino]ethyl]benzyl

---

† Brand name formerly used, and/or firm no longer concerned with this product.

alcohol hydrochloride. *UNII-ESJ56Q60GC. CAS-23239-51-2.* JAN. *Relaxant (smooth muscle).* Yutopar (AstraZeneca)

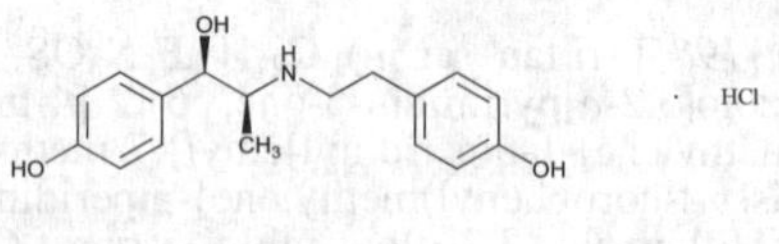

Ritolukast [*1990*] (rit″ oh loo′ kast). C$_{17}$H$_{13}$F$_3$N$_2$O$_3$S. 382.36. (1) Methanesulfonamide, 1,1,1-trifluoro-*N*-[3-(2-quinolinylmethoxy)phenyl]-; (2) 1,1,1-Trifluoro-α-2-quinolylmethanesulfon-*m*-anisidide. *UNII-0E8R4GDE2Q. CAS-111974-60-8.* INN. *Anti-asthmatic (leukotriene antagonist).* ◇*WY-48252*

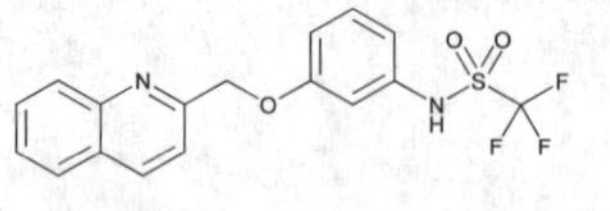

Ritonavir [*1995*] (rit oh′ na vir). USP. C$_{37}$H$_{48}$N$_6$O$_5$S$_2$. 720.94. (1) 2,4,7,12-Tetraazatridecan-13-oic acid, 10-hydroxy-2-methyl-5-(1-methylethyl)-1-[2-(1-methylethyl)-4-thiazolyl]-3,6-dioxo-8,11-bis(phenylmethyl)-5-thiazolylmethyl ester [5*S*-(5*R**,8*R**,10*R**,11*R**)]-; (2) 5-Thiazolylmethyl [(α*S*)-α-[(1*S*,3*S*)-1-hydroxy-3-[(2*S*)-2-[3-[(2-isopropyl-4-thiazolyl)methyl]-3-methylureido]-3-methylbutyramido]-4-phenylbutyl]phenethyl]carbamate. *UNII-O3J8G9O825. CAS-155213-67-5.* INN; BAN. *Antiviral.* Norvir (Abbott) ◇*Abbott-84538*

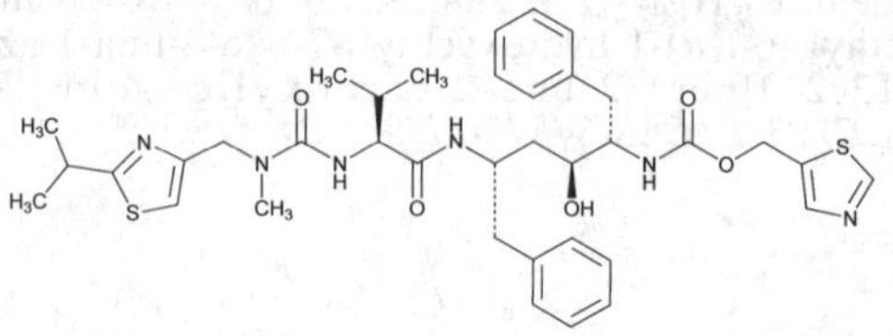

Ritropirronium Bromide. C$_{19}$H$_{28}$BrNO$_3$. 398.33. *erythro*-3-Hydroxy-1,1-dimethylpyrrolidinium bromide α-cyclopentylmandelate. *CAS-53808-86-9.* INN.

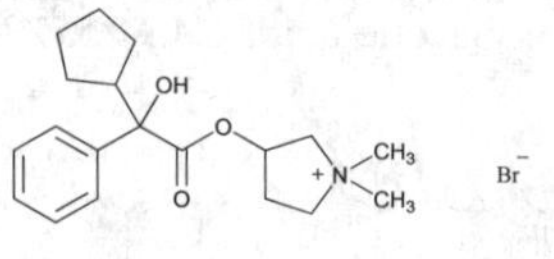

Ritrosulfan. C$_{10}$H$_{24}$N$_2$O$_8$S$_2$. 364.44. 1,4-Dideoxy-1,4-bis[(2-hydroxyethyl)amino]erythritol 1,4-dimethanesulfonate (ester). *UNII-YIY0662KX9. CAS-4148-16-7.* INN.

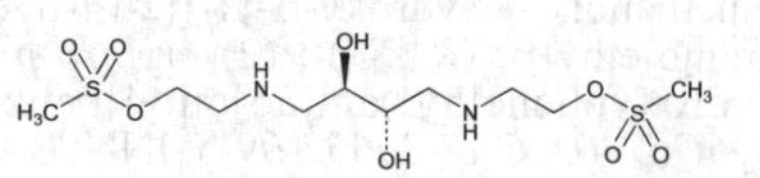

Rituximab [*1997*] (ri tux′ i mab). (1) Immunoglobulin G 1 (human-mouse monoclonal IDEC-C2B8 γ1-chain anti-human antigen CD 20), disulfide with human-mouse monoclonal IDEC-C2B8 κ-chain, dimer; (2) Immunoglobulin G 1 (human-mouse monoclonal IDEC-C2B8 γ1-chain anti-human antigen CD 20), disulfide with human-mouse monoclonal IDEC-C2B8 κ-chain, dimer. Molecular weight is approximately 144,187 daltons. *UNII-4F4X42SYQ6. CAS-174722-31-7.* INN; BAN. *Antineoplastic (microtubule inhibitor); monoclonal antibody.* Rituxan (IDEC) ◇*IDEC-C2B8; IDEC-102*

Rivanicline Galactarate [*2004*] (riv an′ i kleen gal ak′ tar ate). (C$_{10}$H$_{14}$N$_2$)$_2$.C$_6$H$_{10}$O$_8$. 534.60. [Rivanicline is INN.] (1) Galactaric acid, compound with *N*-methyl-4-(3-pyridinyl)-(3*E*)-3-buten-1-amine (1:2); (2) Bis[(3*E*)-*N*-methyl-4-(pyridin-3-yl)but-3-en-1-amine] galactarate. *UNII-VAS2-V13A9H; UNII-6H35LF645A* [rivanicline]. *CAS-675132-86-2; CAS-15585-43-0* [rivanicline]. *Treatment of ulcerative colitis (nicotinic receptor agonist).[Note—Rivanicline has appeared in the literature as (E)-metanicotine and trans-metanicotine.]* ◇*TC-02403-12*

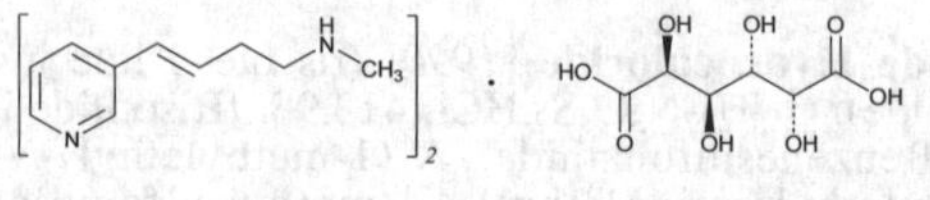

Rivaroxaban [*2006*] (riv″ a rox′ a ban). C$_{19}$H$_{18}$ClN$_3$O$_5$S. 435.88. (1) 2-Thiophenecarboxamide, 5-chloro-*N*-[[(5*S*)-2-oxo-3-[4-(3-oxo-4-morpholinyl)phenyl]-5-oxazolidinyl]methyl]-; (2) 5-Chloro-*N*-({(5*S*)-2-oxo-3-[4-(3-oxomorpholin-4-yl)phenyl]-1,3-oxazolidin-5-yl}methyl)thiophene-2-carboxamide. *UNII-9NDF7JZ4M3. CAS-366789-02-8.* INN; JAN. *Prophylaxis of venous thromboembolism.* ◇*BAY 59-7939*

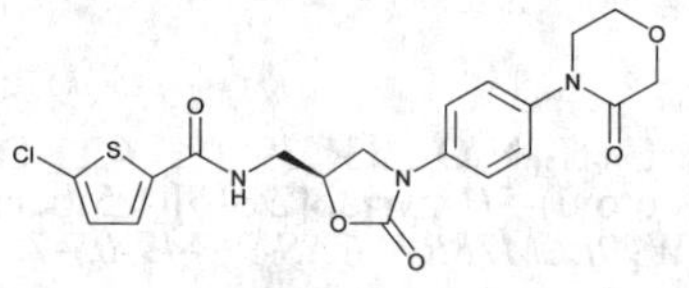

Rivastigmine [*1997*] (riv″ a stig′ meen). C$_{14}$H$_{22}$N$_2$O$_2$. 250.34. (1) (*S*)-3-[1-(Dimethylamino)ethyl]phenyl ethylmethylcarbamate; (2) *m*-[(*S*)-1-(Dimethylamino)ethyl]phenyl ethylmethylcarbamate. *UNII-PKI06M3IW0. CAS-123441-03-2.* INN; BAN. *Treatment of Alzheimer's disease (acetylcholinesterase inhibitor).* Exelon (Novartis) ◇*SDZ-ENA-713; SDZ-212-713; ENA-713*

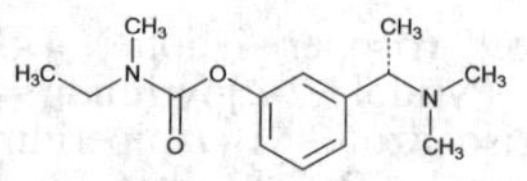

Rivenprost. C$_{24}$H$_{34}$O$_6$S. 450.59. Methyl 4-({2-[(1*R*,2*R*,3*R*)-3-hydroxy-2-{(1*E*,3*S*)-3-hydroxy-4-[3-(methoxymethyl)phenyl]but-1-en-1-yl}-5-oxocyclopentyl]ethyl}sulfanyl)butanoate. *CAS-256382-08-8.* INN.

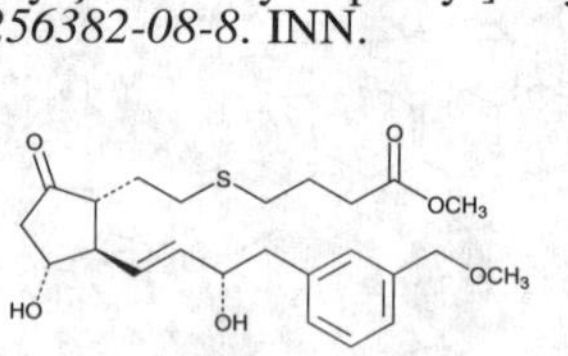

Rivoglitazone [*2000*] (riv″ oh gli′ ta zone). C$_{20}$H$_{19}$N$_3$O$_4$S. 397.45. (1) 2,4-Thiazolidinedione, 5-[[4-[(6-methoxy-1-methyl-1*H*-benzimidazol-2-yl)methoxy]phenyl]methyl]-; (2) (±)-5-[*p*-[(6-Methoxy-1-methyl-2-benzimidazolyl)methoxy]benzyl]-2,4-thiazolidinedione. *UNII-3A3N0634Q6. CAS-185428-18-6.* INN. *Treatment of type II diabetes mellitus.* ◇*R-106056*

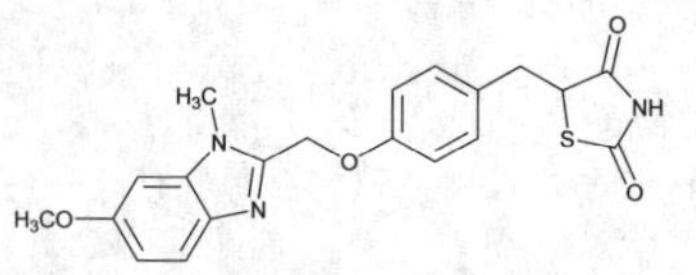

Rizatriptan Benzoate [*1996*] (rye″ za trip′ tan ben′ zoe ate). $C_{15}H_{19}N_5 \cdot C_7H_6O_2$. 391.47. [Rizatriptan is INN and BAN.] (1) 1*H*-Indole-3-ethanamine, *N,N*-dimethyl-5-(1*H*-1,2,4-triazol-1-ylmethyl)-, monobenzoate; (2) 3-[2-(Dimethylamino)ethyl]-5-(1*H*-1,2,4-triazol-1-ylmethyl)indole monobenzoate. *UNII-WR978S7QHH; UNII-51086HBW8G* [rizatriptan]. *CAS-145202-66-0; CAS-144034-80-0* [rizatriptan]. *Antimigraine*. Maxalt (Merck) ◇*MK-0462*

Rizatriptan Sulfate [*1996*] (rye″ za trip′ tan sul′ fate). $(C_{15}H_{19}N_5)_2 \cdot H_2SO_4 \cdot H_2O$. 654.78. (1) 1*H*-Indole-3-ethanamine, *N,N*-dimethyl-5-(1*H*-1,2,4-triazol-1-ylmethyl)-, sulfate (2:1), monohydrate; (2) 3-[2-(Dimethylamino)ethyl]-5-(1*H*-1,2,4-triazol-1-ylmethyl)indole sulfate (2:1), monohydrate. *UNII-13RRH2218G. CAS-159776-67-7; CAS-144034-80-0* [rizatriptan]. *Antimigraine.* ◇*MK-A462*

Rizolipase. Lipase of *Rhizopus arrhizus* var. *Delemar. CAS-9001-62-1*. INN; DCF.

Robalzotan. $C_{18}H_{23}FN_2O_2$. 318.39. (*R*)-3-(Dicyclobutylamino)-8-fluoro-5-chromancarboxamide. *UNII-I18M56OGME. CAS-169758-66-1*. INN; BAN.

Robenacoxib. $C_{16}H_{13}F_4NO_2$. 327.27. {5-Ethyl-2-[(2,3,5,6-tetrafluorophenyl)amino]phenyl}acetic acid. *UNII-Z588009C7C. CAS-220991-32-2*. INN.

Robenidine Hydrochloride [*1971*] (roe ben′ i deen hye″ droe klor′ ide). $C_{15}H_{13}Cl_2N_5 \cdot HCl$. 370.66. [Robenidine is INN and BAN.] (1) Carbonimidic dihydrazide, bis[(4-chlorophenyl)methylene]-, monohydrochloride; (2) 1,3-Bis[(*p*-chlorobenzylidene)amino]guanidine monohydrochloride.

---

† Brand name formerly used, and/or firm no longer concerned with this product.

UNII-8STT15Y392; UNII-4888ME6C4E [robenidine]. *CAS-25875-50-7; CAS-25875-51-8* [robenidine]. *Coccidiostat (for poultry)*.

Rocastine Hydrochloride [*1987*] (roe kas′ teen hye″ droe klor′ ide). $C_{13}H_{19}N_3OS \cdot HCl \cdot H_2O$. 319.85. [Rocastine is INN.] (1) Pyrido[3,2-*f*]-1,4-oxazepine-5(2*H*)-thione, 2-[2-(dimethylamino)ethyl]-3,4-dihydro-4-methyl-, monohydrochloride, monohydrate; (2) (±)-2-[2-(Dimethylamino)ethyl]-3,4-dihydro-4-methylpyrido[3,2-*f*]-1,4-oxazepine-5(2*H*)-thione monohydrochloride monohydrate. *CAS-99617-35-3; CAS-91833-77-1* [rocastine]. *Antihistaminic.* ◇*AHR-11325-D*

Rocepafant. $C_{26}H_{23}ClN_6OS_2$. 535.08. 6-(*o*-Chlorophenyl)-7,10-dihydro-1-methylthio-4*H*-pyrido[4′,3′:4,5]thieno[3,2-*f*]-*s*-triazolo[4,3-*a*][1,4]diazepine-9(8*H*)-carboxy-*p*-anisidide. *UNII-4KGX1STY2N. CAS-132418-36-1*. INN.

Rochelle Salt — *See* Potassium Sodium Tartrate.

Rociclovir. $C_{15}H_{25}N_5O_3$. 323.39. 2-Amino-9-[[2-isopropoxy-1-(isopropoxymethyl)ethoxy]methyl]purine. *UNII-6DF29U51Y7. CAS-108436-80-2*. INN.

Rociverine. $C_{20}H_{37}NO_3$. 339.51. 2-(Diethylamino)-1-methylethyl *cis*-1-hydroxy[bicyclohexyl]-2-carboxylate. *CAS-53716-44-2*. INN; MI.

Rocky Mountain Spotted Fever Vaccine. USP XX.

Rocuronium Bromide [*1993*] (roe″ kure oh′ nee um broe′ mide). $C_{32}H_{53}BrN_2O_4$. 609.68. (1) Pyrrolidinium, 1-[(2β,3α,5α,16β,17β)-17-(acetyloxy)-3-hydroxy-2-(4-morpholinyl)androstan-16-yl]-1-(2-propenyl)-, bromide; (2) 1-Allyl-1-(3α,17β-dihydroxy-2β-morpholino-5α-androstan-16β-yl)pyrrolidinium bromide, 17-acetate. *UNII-I65MW4OFHZ. CAS-119302-91-9.* INN; BAN. *Neuromuscular blocking agent.* Zemuron (Organon) ◇*ORG 9426*

Rodocaine [*1972*] (roe′ doe kane). $C_{18}H_{25}ClN_2O$. 320.86. (1) 1*H*-Pyridine-1-propanamide, *N*-(2-chloro-6-methylphenyl)octahydro- *trans*-; (2) *trans*-6′-Chloro-2,3,4,4a,5,6,7,7a-octahydro-1*H*-1-pyrindine-1-propiono-*o*-toluidide. *UNII-9W0Z08C70V. CAS-38821-80-6.* INN. *Anesthetic (local).* ◇*R 19,317; R 22,700 [as hydrochloride]*

Rodorubicin. $C_{48}H_{64}N_2O_{17}$. 941.02. (1*S*,3*R*,4*R*)-3-Ethyl-1,2,3,4,6,11-hexahydro-3,5,10,12-tetrahydroxy-6,11-dioxo-4-[[2,3,6-trideoxy-3-(dimethylamino)-α-L-*lyxo*-hexopyranosyl]oxy]-1-naphthacenyl *O*-3,6-dideoxy-α-L-*erythro*-hexopyranos-4-ulosyl-(1→4)-*O*-2,6-dideoxy-α-L-*lyxo*-hexopyranosyl-(1→4)-2,3,6-trideoxy-3-(dimethylamino)-α-L-*lyxo*-hexopyranoside, 2″,3′-anhydride. *CAS-96497-67-5.* INN.

Rofecoxib [*1998*] (roe″ fe kox′ ib). $C_{17}H_{14}O_4S$. 314.36. (1) 4-[4-(Methylsulfonyl)phenyl]-3-phenyl-2(5*H*)-furanone; (2) 4-[*p*-(Methylsulfonyl)phenyl]-3-phenyl-2(5*H*)-furanone. *UNII-0QTW8Z7MCR. CAS-162011-90-7.* INN; BAN. *Antiinflammatory; analgesic (cyclooxygenase-2 [COX-2] inhibitor).* Vioxx (Merck) ◇*MK-0966*

Rofelodine. $C_{13}H_{14}N_2O$. 214.26. (±)-2,6,7,8-Tetrahydro-7-phenylpyrrolo[1,2-*a*]pyrimidin-4(3*H*)-one. *UNII-146D7G2I94. CAS-76696-97-4.* INN.

Rofleponide. $C_{25}H_{34}F_2O_6$. 468.53. 6α,9-Difluoro-11β,16α,17,21-tetrahydroxypregn-4-ene-3,20-dione, cyclic (*R*)-16,17-acetal with butyraldehyde. *UNII-R9IQ7GVL3E. CAS-144459-70-1.* INN.

Roflumilast [*2002*] (roe flue′ mi last). $C_{17}H_{14}Cl_2F_2N_2O_3$. 403.21. (1) Benzamide, 3-(cyclopropylmethoxy)-*N*-(3,5-dichloro-4-pyridinyl)-4-(difluoromethoxy)-; (2) 3-Cyclopropylmethoxy-*N*-(3,5-dichloropyridin-4-yl)-4-(difluoromethoxy)benzamide. *UNII-0P6C6ZOP5U. CAS-162401-32-3.* INN. *Treatment of bronchial asthma and chronic obstructive pulmonary disease.* ◇*BY217; B9302-107; BYK20869*

Roflurane [*1962*] (roe flur′ ane). $C_3H_4BrF_3O$. 192.96. (1) Ethane, 2-bromo-1,1,2-trifluoro-1-methoxy-; (2) 2-Bromo-1,1,2-trifluoro-ethyl methyl ether. *CAS-679-90-3.* INN. *Anesthetic (inhalation).* ◇*DA-893*

Rogletimide [*1991*] (roe glet′ i mide). $C_{12}H_{14}N_2O_2$. 218.25. (1) 2,6-Piperidinedione, 3-ethyl-3-(4-pyridinyl)-, (±)-; (2) (±)-2-Ethyl-2-(4-pyridyl)glutarimide. *CAS-121840-95-7.* INN; BAN. *Antineoplastic.*

Rokitamycin. $C_{42}H_{69}NO_{15}$. 827.99. [(4*R*,5*S*,6*S*,7*R*,9*R*,10*R*,11*E*,13*E*,16*R*)-7-(Formylmethyl)-4,10-dihydroxy-5-methoxy-9,16-dimethyl-2-oxooxacyclohexadeca-11,13-dien-6-yl]-3,6-dideoxy-4-*O*-(2,6-dideoxy-3-*C*-methyl-α-L-

ribo-hexopyranosyl)-3-(dimethyl-amino)-β-D-glucopyra-noside 4″-butyrate 3″-propionate. *CAS-74014-51-0.* INN; JAN; MI.

Rolafagrel. $C_{14}H_{12}N_2O_2$. 240.26. 5,6-Dihydro-7-imidazol-1-yl-2-naphthoic acid. *CAS-89781-55-5.* INN.

Rolapitant Hydrochloride [*2006*] (roe la′ pi tant hye″ droe klor′ ide). $C_{25}H_{26}F_6N_2O_2 \cdot HCl \cdot H_2O$. 554.95. [Rolapitant is INN.] (1) 1,7-Diazaspiro[4.5]decan-2-one, 8-[[(1*R*)-1-[3,5-bis(trifluoromethyl)phenyl]ethoxy]methyl]-8-phenyl-, monohydrochloride, monohydrate, (5*S*,8*S*)-; (2) (5*S*,8*S*)-8-[[(1*R*)-1-[3,5-Bis(trifluoromethyl)phenyl]ethoxy]methyl]-8-phenyl-1,7-diazaspiro[4.5]decan-2-one monohy-drochloride monohydrate. *UNII-57O5S1QSAQ. CAS-914462-92-3; CAS-552292-08-7* [rolapitant]. *Prevention of nausea and vomiting.* ◇*SCH619734*

Roletamide [*1967*] (roe let′ a mide). $C_{16}H_{19}NO_4$. 289.33. (1) 2-Propen-1-one, 3-(2,5-dihydro-1*H*-pyrrol-1-yl)-1-(3,4,5-trimethoxyphenyl)-; (2) 3′,4′,5′-Trimethoxy-3-(3-pyrrolin-1-yl)acrylophenone. *CAS-10078-46-3.* INN. *Sedative-hypnotic.* ◇*CL 59112*

Rolgamidine [*1987*] (role gam′ i deen). $C_9H_{16}N_4O$. 196.25. (1) 1*H*-Pyrrole-1-acetamide, *N*-(diaminomethylene)-2,5-dihydro-2,5-dimethyl-, *trans*-; (2) *trans-N*-(Diamino-methylene)-2,5-dimethyl-3-pyrroline-1-acetamide. *UNII-2M3NG13839. CAS-66608-04-6.* INN; BAN. *Antidiarrhe-al.* ◇*WY-25,021*

---

† Brand name formerly used, and/or firm no longer concerned with this product.

Rolicyclidine. $C_{16}H_{23}N$. 229.36. 1-(1-Phenylcyclohexyl)pyr-rolidine. *UNII-183O9O9JE3. CAS-2201-39-0.* INN.

Rolicyprine [*1963*] (roe″ li sye′ preen). $C_{14}H_{16}N_2O_2$. 244.29. (1) 2-Pyrrolidinecarboxamide, 5-oxo-*N*-(2-phenylcyclo-propyl)-; (2) L-*trans*-(+)-5-Oxo-*N*-(2-phenylcyclopropyl)-2-pyrrolidinecarboxamide. *CAS-2829-19-8.* INN; BAN. *Antidepressant.* Cypromin (Schering†) [*Name previously used: Rolicypram.*] ◇*Ex 4883; RMI 83,027*

Rolipoltide. $C_{561}H_{887}N_{169}O_{136}S_4$. Protein derived from two major allergens of *Cryptomeria japonica* pollen: Sugi basic protein (Cry j 1) and the polygalacturonase (Cry j 2): (Cry j 1-(213-225)-peptidyl)-L-arginyl-L-arginyl(Cry j 1-(108-120)-peptidyl)-L-arginyl-L-arginyl(Cry j 2-(191-209)-pep-tidyl)-L-arginyl-L-arginyl(Cry j 2-(88-107)-peptidyl)-L-ar-ginyl-L-arginyl(Cry j 1-(80-95)-peptidyl)-L-arginyl(Cry j 2-(75-89)-peptide). *CAS-698389-00-3.* INN.

```
MKVTVAFNQF GPNRRVFIKR VSNVIIHGRR IDIFASKNFH LQKNTIGTGR
RWKNNRIWLQ FAKLTGFTLM GRRLKMPMYI AGYKTFDGRR VDGIIAAYQN
PASWK
```

Rolipram [*1980*] (roe′ li pram). $C_{16}H_{21}NO_3$. 275.34. (1) 2-Pyrrolidinone, 4-[3-(cyclopentyloxy)-4-methoxyphenyl]-; (2) 4-[3-(Cyclopentyloxy)-4-methoxyphenyl]-2-pyrrolidi-none. *UNII-K676NL63N7. CAS-61413-54-5.* INN. *Tran-quilizer.* ◇*ZK 62 711*

Rolitetracycline [*1963*] (roe″ li tet″ ra sye′ kleen). $C_{27}H_{33}N_3O_8$. 527.57. (1) 2-Naphthacenecarboxamide, 4-(dimethylamino)-1,4,4a,5,5a,6,11,12a-octahydro-3,6,10,12,12a-pentahydroxy-6-methyl-1,11-dioxo-*N*-(1-pyrrolidinylmethyl)-, [4*S*-(4α,4aα,5aα,6β,12aα)]-; (2) 4-(Dimethylamino)-1,4,4a,5,5a,6,11,12a-octahydro-3,6,10,12,12a-pentahydroxy-6-methyl-1,11-dioxo-*N*-(1-pyrrolidinylmethyl)-2-naphthacenecarboxamide. *UNII-GH9IW85221. CAS-751-97-3.* USP XXII; INN; BAN; JAN. *Antibacterial.* Syntetrin (Bristol-Myers Squibb†) ◇*SQ 15,659*

Rolitetracycline Nitrate [*1965*] (roe″ li tet″ ra sye′ kleen nye′ trate). $C_{27}H_{33}N_3O_8 \cdot HNO_3 \cdot 1\frac{1}{2}H_2O$. 617.60. (1) 2-Naphtha-cenecarboxamide, 4-(dimethylamino)-1,4,4a,5,5a,6,11,12a-octahydro-3,6,10,12,12a-pentahydroxy-6-meth-yl-1,11-dioxo-*N*-(1-pyrrolidinylmethyl)-, [4*S*-(4α,4aα,5aα,6β,12aα)]-, mononitrate (salt), sesquihydrate; (2) 4-(Dimethylamino)-1,4,4a,5,5a,6,11,12a-octahydro-

3,6,10,12,12a-pentahydroxy-6-methyl-1,11-dioxo-*N*-(1-pyrrolidinylmethyl)-2-naphthacenecarboxamide nitrate sesquihydrate. *CAS-26657-13-6; CAS-7681-32-5* [anhydrous]; *CAS-751-97-3* [rolitetracycline]. JAN. *Antibacterial.*

Rolodine [*1964*] (roe′ loe deen). $C_{14}H_{14}N_4$. 238.29. (1) 7*H*-Pyrrolo[2,3-*d*]pyrimidin-4-amine, 2-methyl-*N*-(phenylmethyl)-; (2) 4-(Benzylamino)-2-methyl-7*H*-pyrrolo[2,3-*d*]pyrimidine. *CAS-1866-43-9.* INN. *Relaxant (skeletal muscle).* ◇*BW 58-271; NSC-106570*

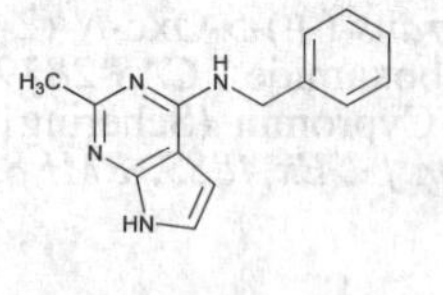

Rolofylline [*2007*] (roe lof′ i lin). $C_{20}H_{28}N_4O_2$. 356.46. (1) 1*H*-Purine-2,6-dione, 8-(hexahydro-2,5-methanopentalen-3a(1*H*)-yl)-3,7-dihydro-1,3-dipropyl-; (2) 1,3-Dipropyl-8-(tricyclo[3.3.1.0^{3,7}]non-3-yl)-3,7-dihydro-1*H*-purine-2,6-dione; (3) 3,7-Dihydro-1,3-dipropyl-8-(3-tricyclo[3.3.1.0^{3,7}]nonyl)-1*H*-purine-2,6-dione. *CAS-136199-02-5.* INN. *Treatment of heart failure in patients with renal impairment undergoing diuresis.* ◇*KW-3902*

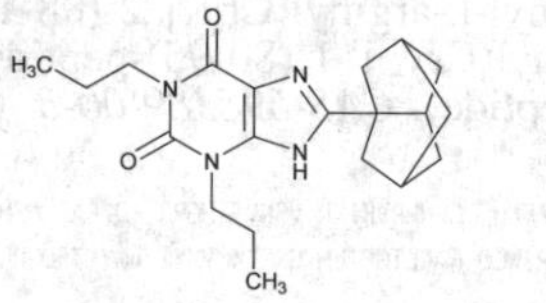

Rolziracetam. $C_7H_9NO_2$. 139.15. Dihydro-1*H*-pyrrolizine-3,5(2*H*,6*H*)-dione. *UNII-RES9I0LGG5. CAS-18356-28-0.* INN; BAN. ◇*CI-911*

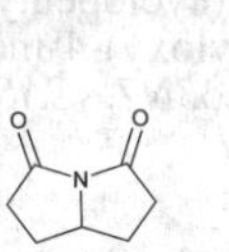

Romazarit [*1990*] (roe maz′ a rit). $C_{15}H_{16}ClNO_4$. 309.74. (1) Propanoic acid, 2-[[2-(4-chlorophenyl)-4-methyl-5-oxazolyl]methoxy]-2-methyl-; (2) 2-[[2-(*p*-Chlorophenyl)-4-methyl-5-oxazolyl]methoxy]-2-methylpropionic acid. *UNII-CN68E94R2X. CAS-109543-76-2.* INN; BAN. *Antiinflammatory; antirheumatic.* ◇*Ro 31-3948/000*

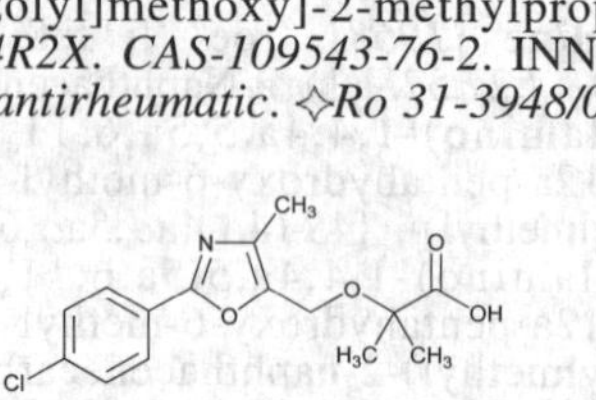

Romergoline. $C_{20}H_{22}N_4O_2$. 350.41. 4-[(9,10-Didehydro-6-methylergolin-8β-yl)methyl]-2,6-piperazinedione. *CAS-107052-56-2.* INN.

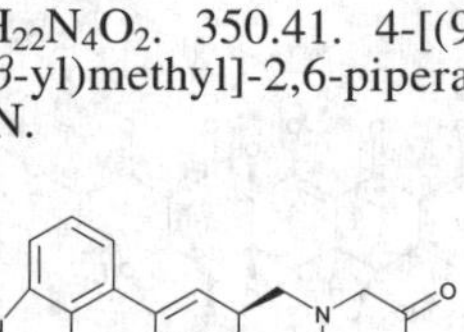

Romidepsin [*2006*] (roe″ mi dep′ sin). $C_{24}H_{36}N_4O_6S_2$. 540.70. (1) Cyclo[(2*Z*)-2-amino-2-butenoyl-L-valyl-(3*S*,4*E*)-3-hydroxy-7-mercapto-4-heptenoyl-D-valyl-D-cysteinyl], cyclic (3→5)-disulfide; (2) (1*S*,4*S*,7*Z*,10*S*,16*E*,21*R*)-7-Ethylidene-4,21-bis(1-methylethyl)-2-oxa-12,13-dithia-

5,8,20,23-tetraazabicyclo[8.7.6]tricos-16-ene-3,6,9,19,22-pentone. *CAS-128517-07-7.* INN. *Antitumor/anticancer drug.* Chromadax (Gloucester) ◇*FR901228; FK228*

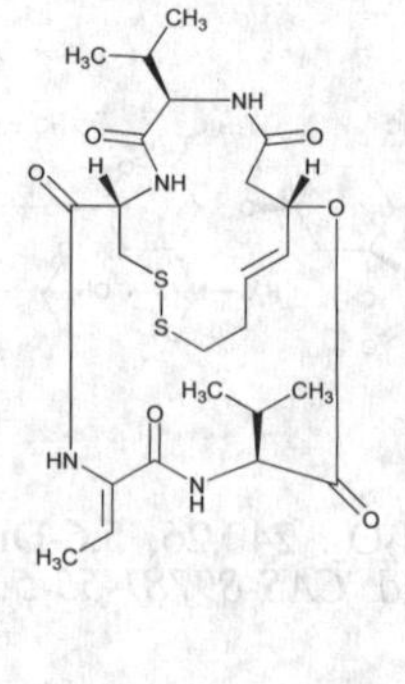

Romifenone. $C_{13}H_{17}NO_3$. 235.28. 2′-Hydroxy-3-morpholinopropiophenone. *UNII-672T0ES47P. CAS-38373-83-0.* INN.

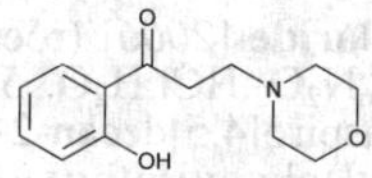

Romifidine. $C_9H_9BrFN_3$. 258.09. 2-(2-Bromo-6-fluoroanilino)-2-imidazoline. *UNII-876351L05K. CAS-65896-16-4; CAS-65896-14-2* [hydrochloride]. INN; BAN.

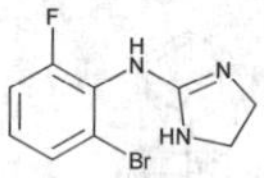

Romiplostim [*2006*] (roe mip′ loe stim). $C_{1317}H_{2043}N_{361}O_{395}S_9$ (monomer). 29,542 (monomer). Methionyl, 227 amino acid C-terminal Immunoglobulin G1 (human Fc fragment) fusion protein with 41 amino acid peptide, dimer. *UNII-GN5XU2DXKV. CAS-267639-76-9.* INN. *Treatment of immune thrombocytopenic purpura (ITP).*

Romurtide. $C_{43}H_{78}N_6O_{13}$. 887.11. 2-Acetamido-3-*O*-[(*R*)-1-[[(*S*)-1-[[(*R*)-1-carbamoyl-3-[[(*S*)-1-carboxy-5-stearamidopentyl]carbamoyl]propyl]carbamoyl]ethyl]carbamoyl]-ethyl]-2-deoxy-D-glucopyranose. *CAS-78113-36-7.* INN; JAN.

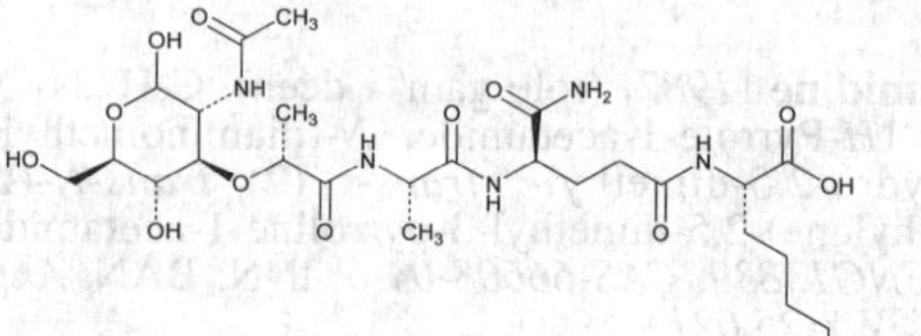

Ronacaleret Hydrochloride [*2007*] (roe″ na kal′ er et hye″ droe klor′ ide). $C_{25}H_{31}F_2NO_4 \cdot HCl$. 483.98. [Ronacaleret is INN.] (1) Benzenepropanoic acid, 3-[(2*R*)-3-[[2-(2,3-dihydro-1*H*-inden-2-yl)-1,1-dimethylethyl]amino]-2-hydroxypropoxy]-4,5-difluoro-, hydrochloride; (2) 3-[3-[(2*R*)-3-[[2-(2,3-dihydro-1*H*-inden-2-yl)-1,1-dimethylethyl]amino]-2-hydroxypropoxy]-4,5-difluorophenyl]propanoic acid hydrochloride. *UNII-LZM2DSH251. CAS-702686-96-2; CAS-753449-67-1* [ronacaleret]. *Treatment of osteoporosis.* ◇*SB-751689-A*

Ronactolol. $C_{20}H_{26}N_2O_4$. 358.43. (±)-4′-[2-Hydroxy-3-(iso-propylamino)propoxy]-*p*-anisanilide. *UNII-PJ691WQY08. CAS-90895-85-5.* INN.

Ronidazole [*1967*] (roe nye′ da zole). $C_6H_8N_4O_4$. 200.15. (1) 1*H*-Imidazole-2-methanol, 1-methyl-5-nitro-, carbamate (ester); (2) 1-Methyl-5-nitroimidazole-2-methanol carbamate ester. *CAS-7681-76-7.* INN; BAN. *Antiprotozoal.*

Ronifibrate. $C_{19}H_{20}ClNO_5$. 377.82. 3-Hydroxypropyl nicotinate, 2-(*p*-chlorophenoxy)-2-methylpropionate (ester). *UNII-W86I18X716. CAS-42597-57-9.* INN; MI.

Ronipamil. $C_{32}H_{48}N_2$. 460.74. (±)-2-[3-(Methylphenethylamino)propyl]-2-phenyltetradecanenitrile. *UNII-BP76593251. CAS-85247-77-4.* INN.

Ronnel [*1973*] (ron′ el). $C_8H_8Cl_3O_3PS$. 321.55. [Fenclofos is INN; Fenclorfos is BAN.] (1) Phosphorothioic acid, *O,O*-dimethyl *O*-(2,4,5-trichlorophenyl) ester; (2) *O,O*-Dimethyl *O*-(2,4,5-trichlorophenyl) phosphorothioate. *UNII-89RAG7SB3B. CAS-299-84-3. Insecticide (systemic).* [*Name previously used: Fenchlorphos.*]

Ropidoxuridine [*2007*] (roe pye″ dox ure′ i deen). $C_9H_{11}IN_2O_4$. 338.10. (1) 2(1*H*)-Pyrimidinone, 1-(2-deoxy-*β*-D-*erythro*-pentofuranosyl)-5-iodo-; (2) 1-(2-Deoxy-*β*-D-*erythro*-pentofuranosyl)-5-iodopyrimidin-2(1*H*)-one. *UNII-3HX21A3SQF. CAS-93265-81-7.* INN. *Treatment of cancer.* ◇*IPdR*

Ropinirole [*2007*] (roe pin′ i role″). $C_{16}H_{24}N_2O$. 260.37. (1) 2*H*-Indol-2-one, 4-[2-(dipropylamino)ethyl]-1,3-dihydro-; (2) 4-[2-(Dipropylamino)ethyl]-1,3-dihydro-2*H*-indol-2-one. *UNII-030PYR8953. CAS-91374-21-9. Parkinson's disease and Restless Leg Syndrome (RLS).* Requip (GlaxoSmithKline) ◇*SK&F 101468*

Ropinirole Hydrochloride [*1993*] (roe pin′ i role″ hye″ droe klor′ ide). $C_{16}H_{24}N_2O.HCl$. 296.84. [Ropinirole is INN and BAN.] (1) 2*H*-Indol-2-one, 4-[2-(dipropylamino)ethyl]-1,3-dihydro-, monohydrochloride; (2) 4-[2-(Dipropylamino)ethyl]-2-indolinone monohydrochloride. *UNII-D7ZD41RZI9. CAS-91374-20-8; CAS-91374-21-9* [ropinirole]. *Antiparkinsonian (D₂ receptor agonist).* Requip (GlaxoSmithKline) ◇*SK&F 101468-A*

Ropitoin Hydrochloride [*1978*] (roe′ pi toin; roe′ pi toe in hye″ droe klor′ ide). $C_{30}H_{33}N_3O_3.HCl$. 520.06. [Ropitoin is INN.] (1) 2,4-Imidazolidinedione, 5-(4-methoxyphenyl)-5-phenyl-3-[3-(4-phenyl-1-piperidinyl)propyl]-, monohydrochloride; (2) 5-(*p*-Methoxyphenyl)-5-phenyl-3-[3-(4-phenylpiperidino)propyl]hydantoin monohydrochloride. *CAS-56079-80-2; CAS-56079-81-3* [ropitoin]. *Cardiac depressant (anti-arrhythmic).* ◇*TR-2985*

Ropivacaine Hydrochloride (roe piv′ a kane hye″ droe klor′ ide). USP. $C_{17}H_{26}N_2O.HCl.H_2O$. 328.88. [Ropivacaine is INN and BAN.] (1) (*S*)-(-)-1-Propylpiperidine-2-carboxylic acid (2,6-dimethylphenyl)amide hydrochloride monohydrate; (2) (*S*)-(-)-1-Propyl-2′,6′-pipecoloxylidide hydrochloride monohydrate. *UNII-7IO5LYA57N* [ropivacaine]. *CAS-132112-35-7; CAS-84057-95-4* [ropivacaine]. Narapin (Astra)

Ropizine [*1976*] (roe′ pi zeen). $C_{24}H_{26}N_4$. 370.49. (1) 1-Piperazinamine, 4-(diphenylmethyl)-*N*-[(6-methyl-2-pyridinyl)methylene]-; (2) 1-(Diphenylmethyl)-4-[[(6-methyl-

---

† Brand name formerly used, and/or firm no longer concerned with this product.

2-pyridyl)methylene]amino]piperazine. *UNII-Q5128GW9D4*. *CAS-3601-19-2*. INN. *Anticonvulsant.* ◇*SC-13504*

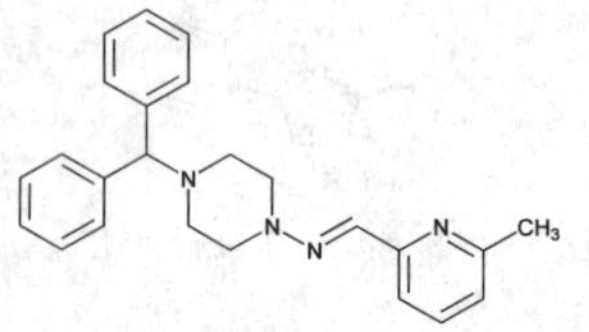

Roquinimex [*1995*] (roe kwin′ i mex). $C_{18}H_{16}N_2O_3$. 308.33. (1) 3-Quinolinecarboxamide, 1,2-dihydro-4-hydroxy-*N*,1-dimethyl-2-oxo-*N*-phenyl; (2) 1,2-Dihydro-4-hydroxy-*N*,1-dimethyl-2-oxo-3-quinolinecarboxanilide. *CAS-84088-42-6*. INN. *Biological response modifier; immunomodulator.* ◇*LS 2616; FCF 89*

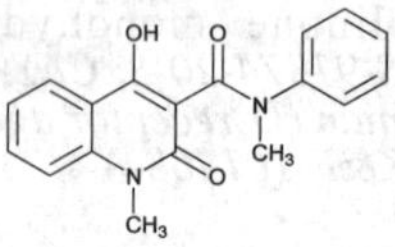

Rosabulin [*2006*] (roe″ za bue′ lin). $C_{22}H_{16}N_4O_2S$. 400.45. (1) 1-Indolizineacetamide, 3-[(4-cyanophenyl)methyl]-*N*-(3-methyl-5-isothiazolyl)-α-oxo-; (2) 2-[3-(4-Cyanobenzyl)indolizin-1-yl]-*N*-(3-methylisothiazol-5-yl)-2-oxoacetamide. *UNII-6Z674O12T6*. *CAS-501948-05-6*. INN. *Treatment of therapeutic resistant cancers.* ◇*STA-5312*

Rosamicin (previously used name) — *See* Rosaramicin.

Rosamicin Butyrate (previously used name) — *See* Rosaramicin Butyrate.

Rosamicin Propionate (previously used name) — *See* Rosaramicin Propionate.

Rosamicin Sodium Phosphate (previously used name) — *See* Rosaramicin Sodium Phosphate.

Rosamicin Stearate (previously used name) — *See* Rosaramicin Stearate.

Rosaprostol. $C_{18}H_{34}O_3$. 298.46. (1*RS*,2*SR*,5*RS*)-2-Hexyl-5-hydrocyclopentaneheptanoic acid, mixture with (1*RS*,2*SR*,5*SR*)-2-hexyl-5-hydroxycyclopentaneheptanoic acid. *CAS-56695-65-9*. INN; MI.

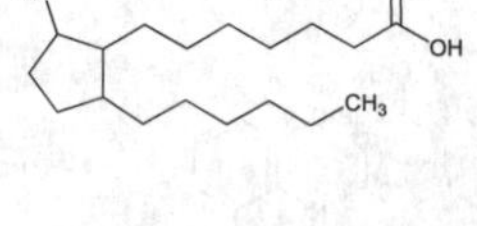

Rosaramicin [*1973*] (roe sar″ a mye′ sin). $C_{31}H_{51}NO_9$. 581.74. Antibiotic derived from *Micromonospora rosaria*. (1) Cirramycin A₁, 4′-deoxy-; (2) Rosamicin; (3) Stereoisomer of 3-ethyl-7-hydroxy-2,8,12,16-tetramethyl-5,13-dioxo-9-[[3,4,6-trideoxy-3-(dimethylamino)-β-D-*xylo*-hexopyranosyl]oxy]-4,17-dioxabicyclo[14.1.0]heptadec-14-

ene-10-acetaldehyde. *CAS-35834-26-5*. INN; BAN. *Antibacterial.* [*Name previously used: Rosamicin.*] ◇*Sch 14947*

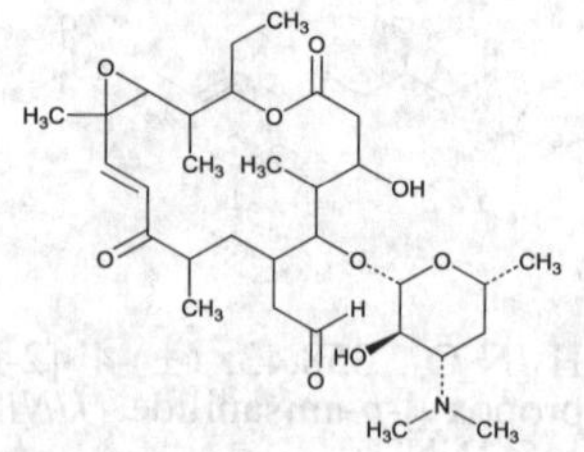

Rosaramicin Butyrate [*1976*] (roe sar″ a mye′ sin bue′ ti rate). $C_{35}H_{57}NO_{10}$. 651.83. (1) Cirramycin A₁, 4′-deoxy-, 2′-butanoate; (2) Rosamicin 2′-butanoate; (3) 3-Ethyl-7-hydroxy-2,8,12,16-tetramethyl-5,13-dioxo-9-[[3,4,6-trideoxy-3-(dimethylamino)-β-D-*xylo*-hexopyranosyl]oxy]-4,17-dioxabicyclo[14.1.0]heptadec-14-ene-10-acetaldehyde 2′-butyrate. *CAS-55103-30-5; CAS-35834-26-5* [rosaramicin]. *Antibacterial.* [*Name previously used: Rosamicin Butyrate.*] ◇*Sch 18667*

Rosaramicin Propionate [*1974*] (roe sar″ a mye′ sin proe′ pee oh nate). $C_{34}H_{55}NO_{10}$. 637.80. (1) Cirramycin A₁, 4′-deoxy-, 2′-propanoate; (2) Rosamicin 2′-propanoate; (3) 3-Ethyl-7-hydroxy-2,8,12,16-tetramethyl-5,13-dioxo-9-[[3,4,6-trideoxy-3-(dimethylamino)-β-D-*xylo*-hexopyranosyl]oxy]-4,17-dioxabicyclo[14.1.0]heptadec-14-ene-10-acetaldehyde 2′-propionate. *CAS-51481-64-2; CAS-35834-26-5* [rosaramicin]. *Antibacterial.* [*Name previously used: Rosamicin Propionate.*] ◇*Sch 17894*

Rosaramicin Sodium Phosphate [*1977*] (roe sar″ a mye′ sin soe′ dee um fos′ fate). $C_{31}H_{51}NO_9 \cdot NaH_2PO_4$. 701.71. (1) Cirramycin A₁, 4′-deoxy-, compd. with sodium dihydrogen phosphate; (2) Rosamicin compound with sodium dihydrogen phosphate (1:1); (3) Stereoisomer of 3-ethyl-7-hydroxy-2,8,12,16-tetramethyl-5,13-dioxo-9-[[3,4,6-trideoxy-3-(dimethylamino)-β-D-*xylo*-hexopyranosyl]oxy]-4,17-dioxabicyclo[14.1.0]heptadec-14-ene-10-acetaldehyde, compound with sodium dihydrogen phosphate (1:1). *CAS-60802-40-6; CAS-35834-26-5* [rosaramicin]. *Antibacterial.* [*Name previously used: Rosamicin Sodium Phosphate.*] ◇*Sch 14947.NaH₂PO₄*

Rosaramicin Stearate [*1974*] (roe sar″ a mye′ sin steer′ ate). $C_{31}H_{51}NO_9 \cdot C_{18}H_{36}O_2$. 866.22. (1) Cirramycin A₁, 4′-deoxy-, octadecanoate (salt); (2) Rosamicin octadecanoate (salt); (3) 3-Ethyl-7-hydroxy-2,8,12,16-tetramethyl-5,13-dioxo-9-[[3,4,6-trideoxy-3-(dimethylamino)-β-D-*xylo*-hexopyranosyl]oxy]-4,17-dioxabicyclo[14.1.0]heptadec-14-ene-10-acetaldehyde stearate (salt). *CAS-51547-64-9; CAS-35834-26-5* [rosaramicin]. *Antibacterial.* [*Name previously used: Rosamicin Stearate.*] ◇*Sch 14947 Stearate*

Rose Bengal Sodium I 125 [*1966*] (roze ben′ gal soe′ dee um). $C_{20}H_2Cl_4{}^{125}I_4Na_2O_5$. (1) Spiro[isobenzofuran-1(3*H*),9′-[9*H*]-xanthene]-3-one, 4,5,6,7-tetrachloro-3′,6′-dihydroxy-2′,4′,5′,7′-tetraiodo-, disodium salt, labeled with iodine-125; (2) 4,5,6,7-Tetrachloro-2′,4′,5′,7′-tetraiodofluorescein-^{125}*I*, disodium salt. *Radioactive agent.* Robengatope I-125 (Bristol-Myers Squibb†)

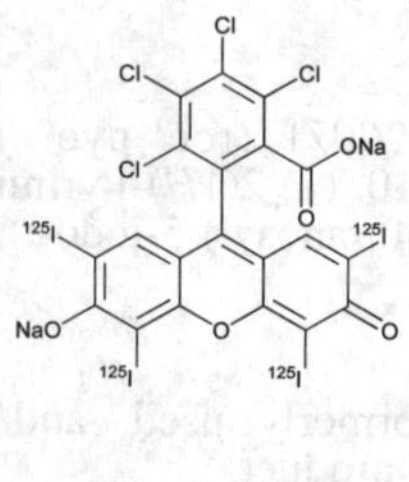

Rose Bengal Sodium I 131 [*1966*] (roze ben′ gal soe′ dee um). **USP** [Injection]. $C_{20}H_2Cl_4{}^{131}I_4Na_2O_5$. [Rose Bengal Sodium ($^{131}I$) is INN.] (1) Spiro[isobenzofuran-1(3*H*),9′-[9*H*]-xanthene]-3-one, 4,5,6,7-tetrachloro-3′,6′-dihydroxy-2′,4′,5′,7′-tetraiodo-, disodium salt, labeled with iodine-131; (2) 4,5,6,7-Tetrachloro-2′,4′,5′,7′-tetraiodofluorescein-^{131}I, disodium salt. *UNII-24I7KUI7MK. CAS-50291-21-9* [closed form]; *CAS-24916-55-0* [open form]. *Diagnostic aid (hepatic function determination); radioactive agent.* Robengatope I-131 (Bristol-Myers Squibb†)

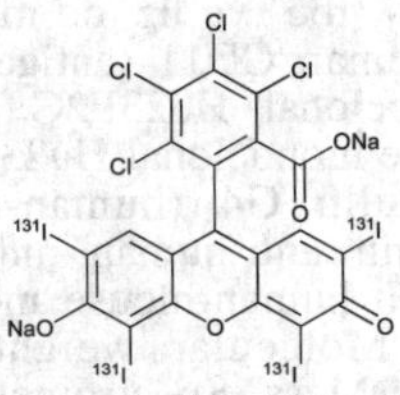

Rose Oil (roze). **NF**. Volatile oil distilled with steam from the fresh flowers of *Rosa gallica* Linné, *Rosa damascena* Miller, *Rosa alba* Linné, *Rosa centifolia* Linné, and varieties of these species (Fam. Rosaceae). *UNII-WU-B68Y35M7. CAS-8007-01-0. Pharmaceutic aid (perfume).*

Rose Water, Stronger (roze wa′ ter). **NF**. A saturated solution of the odoriferous principles of the flowers of *Rosa centifolia* Linné (Fam. Rosaceae). *CAS-8030-26-0. Pharmaceutic aid (perfume).*

Rosiglitazone Maleate [*1997*] (roe″ si gli′ ta zone mal′ ee ate). $C_{18}H_{19}N_3O_3S.C_4H_4O_4$. 473.50. [Rosiglitazone is INN and BAN.] (±)-5-[*p*-[2-(Methyl-2-pyridylamino)ethoxy]-benzyl]-2,4-thiazolidinedione maleate (1:1). *UNII-KX2339DP44; UNII-05V02F2KDG* [rosiglitazone]. *CAS-155141-29-0; CAS-122320-73-4* [rosiglitazone]. *Antidiabetic.* Avandia (GlaxoSmithKline) ✧*BRL-49653-C*

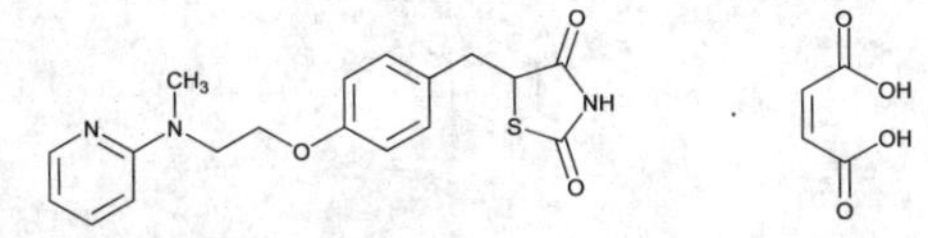

Rosin. *CAS-8050-09-7*. USP XXI.

Rosonabant. $C_{21}H_{21}Cl_3N_4O$. 451.78. (5*RS*)-5-(4-Chlorophenyl)-1-(2,4-dichlorophenyl)-*N*-(piperidin-1-yl)-4,5-dihydro-1*H*-pyrazole-3-carboxamide. *CAS-861151-12-4*. INN.

Rosoxacin [*1976*] (roe sox′ a sin). $C_{17}H_{14}N_2O_3$. 294.30. [Acrosoxacin is BAN.] (1) 3-Quinolinecarboxylic acid, 1-ethyl-1,4-dihydro-4-oxo-7-(4-pyridinyl)-; (2) 1-Ethyl-1,4-dihydro-4-oxo-7-(4-pyridyl)-3-quinolinecarboxylic acid. *UNII-3Y1OT3J4NW. CAS-40034-42-2*. INN; BAN. *Antibacterial.* Roxadyl (Sterling Winthrop) ✧*Win 35,213*

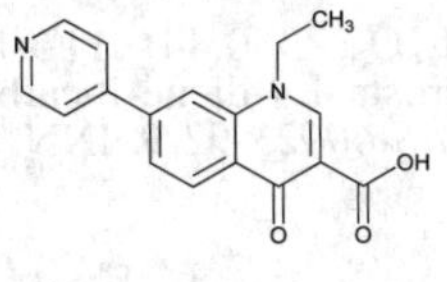

Rostafuroxin. $C_{23}H_{34}O_4$. 374.51. 21,23-Epoxy-24-nor-14*β*,5*β*-chola-20,21-diene-3*β*,14,17*α*-triol. *CAS-156722-18-8*. INN.

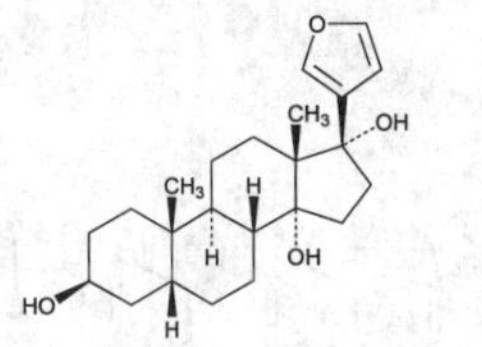

Rostaporfin [*1999*] (roe″ sta por′ fin). $C_{37}H_{42}Cl_2N_4O_2Sn$. 764.37. (1) Tin, dichloro[*rel*-ethyl(18*R*,19*S*)-3,4,20,21-tetradehydro-4,9,14,19-tetraethyl-18,19-dihydro-3,8,13,18-tetramethyl-20-phorbinecarboxylato(2-)-*κ*-N^{23},-*κ*-N^{24},-*κ*-N^{25},-*κ*-N^{26}]-, (*OC*-6-13)-; (2) (*OC*-6-13)-Dichloro[*rel*-ethyl(18*R*,19*S*)-3,4,20,21-tetradehydro-4,9,14,19-tetraethyl-18,19-dihydro-3,8,13,18-tetramethyl-20-phorbinecarboxylato(2-)-*κ*N^{23}, *κ*N^{24}, *κ*N^{25}, *κ*N^{26}]tin. *CAS-284041-10-7*. INN. *Age related macular degeneration and other ophthalmic indications.* ✧*SnET2*

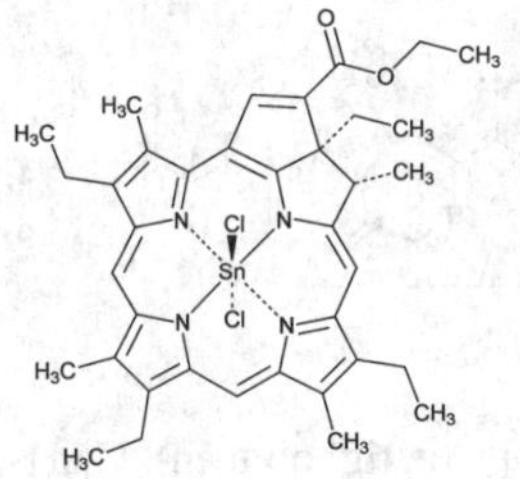

Rosterolone. $C_{23}H_{38}O_2$. 346.55. 17*β*-Hydroxy-1*α*-methyl-17-propyl-5*α*-androstan-3-one. *UNII-3L5C5C8ZNG. CAS-79243-67-7*. INN.

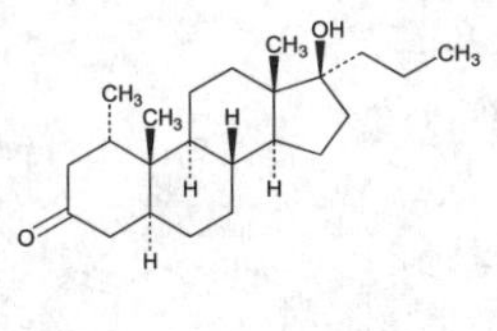

Rosuvastatin Calcium [*2000*] (roe soo″ va stat′ in kal′ see um). $2C_{22}H_{27}FN_3O_6S.Ca$. 1001.14. [Rosuvastatin is INN and BAN.] (1) 6-Heptenoic acid, 7-[4-(4-fluorophenyl)-6-(1-methylethyl)-2-[methyl(methylsulfonyl)amino]-5-pyrimidinyl]-3,5-dihydroxy-, calcium salt (2:1), (3*R*,5*S*,6*E*)-; (2) [*S*-[*R**,*S**-(*E*)]]-7-[4-(4-Fluorophenyl)-6-(1-methylethyl)-2-[methyl(methylsulfonyl)amino]-5-pyrimidinyl]-3,5-dihydroxy-6-heptenoic acid, calcium salt (2:1). *UNII-83MVU38M7Q; UNII-413KH5ZJ73* [rosuvastatin]. *CAS-147098-20-2; CAS-287714-41-4* [rosuvastatin]. *Antihyperlipidemic (HMGCoA reductase inhibitor).* Crestor (AstraZeneca) ✧*ZD4522 (calcium salt); S-4522*

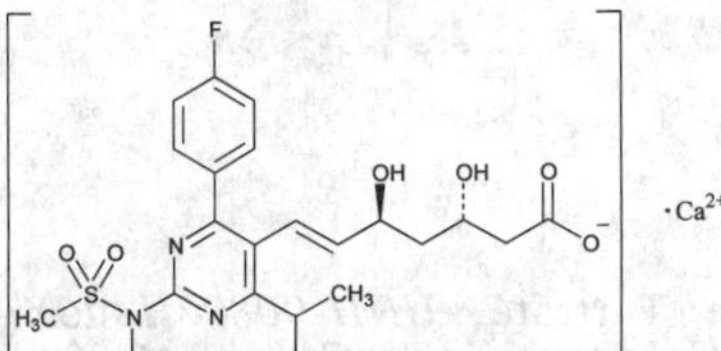

† Brand name formerly used, and/or firm no longer concerned with this product.

Rotamicillin. $C_{28}H_{31}N_5O_5S$. 549.64. (2*S*,5*R*,6*R*)-3,3-Dimethyl-7-oxo-6-[(*R*)-2-phenyl-2-[2-[*p*-(1,4,5,6-tetrahydro-2-pyrimidinyl)phenyl]acetamido]acetamido]-4-thia-1-azabicyclo[3.2.0]heptane-2-carboxylic acid. *CAS-55530-41-1*. INN.

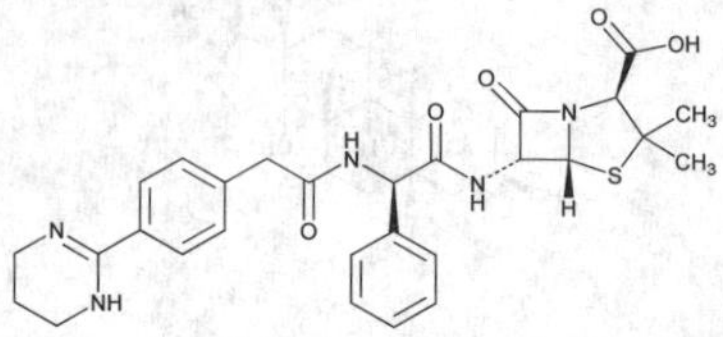

Rotigaptide [*2005*] (roe″ ti gap′ tide). $C_{28}H_{39}N_7O_9$. 617.65. (1) Glycinamide, *N*-acetyl-D-tyrosyl-D-prolyl-(4*S*)-4-hydroxy-D-prolylglycyl-D-alanyl-; (2) *N*-Acetyl-D-tyrosyl-D-prolyl-(4*S*)-4-hydroxy-D-prolylglycyl-D-alanylglycinamide. *CAS-355151-12-1*. INN. *Treatment of ventricular tachycardia or ventricular fibrillation.* ◇*GAP (Wyeth); ZP-123 (Zealand)*

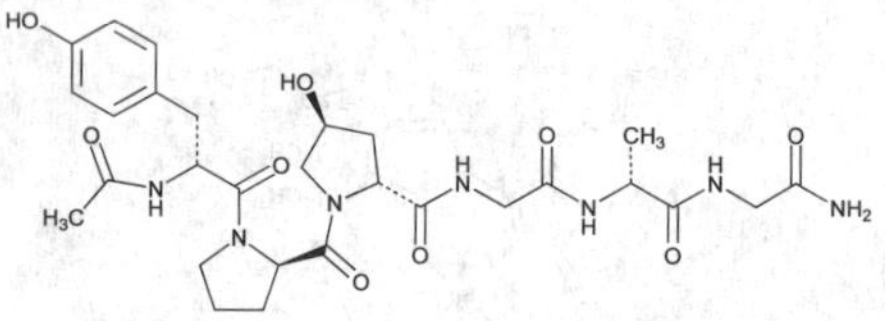

Rotigotine [*2004*] (roe tig′ oh teen). $C_{19}H_{25}NOS$. 315.47. (1) 1-Naphthalenol, 5,6,7,8-tetrahydro-6-[propyl [2-(2-thienyl)ethyl]amino-(6*S*)-; (2) (-)-(*S*)-5,6,7,8-Tetrahydro-6-[propyl[2-(2-thienyl)ethyl]amino]-1-naphthol; (3) (6*S*)-6-[Propyl(2-(2-thienyl)ethyl)amino]-5,6,7,8-tetrahydro-1-naphthalenol. *UNII-87T4T8BO2E*. *CAS-99755-59-6*. INN. *Treatment of early and advanced Parkinson's disease and restless leg syndrome.* Neupro (Schwarz Pharma) ◇*SPM 962*

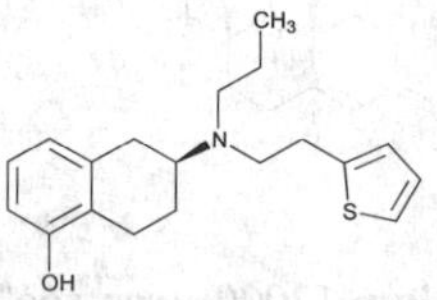

Rotoxamine [*1963*] (roe tox′ a meen). $C_{16}H_{19}ClN_2O$. 290.79. (1) Ethanamine, 2-[(4-chlorophenyl)(2-pyridinyl)-methoxy]-*N*,*N*-dimethyl-, (-)-; (2) (-)-2-[*p*-Chloro-α-[2-(dimethylamino)ethoxy]benzyl]pyridine. *UNII-VE-D9E376NC*. *CAS-5560-77-0*. INN. *Antihistaminic.* ◇*McN-R-73-Z*

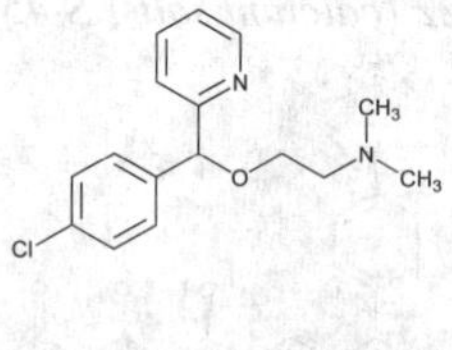

Rotoxamine Tartrate. *UNII-90897H496X; UNII-VE-D9E376NC* [rotoxamine]. *CAS-49746-00-1; CAS-5560-77-0* [rotoxamine]. NF XIV. Twiston (Ortho-McNeil†); Twiston R-A (Ortho-McNeil†)

Rotraxate. $C_{17}H_{23}NO_3$. 289.37. *p*-[[*trans*-4-(Aminomethyl)-cyclohexyl]carbonyl]hydrocinnamic acid. *UNII-KRN50N3Y2T*. *CAS-92071-51-7*. INN; MI.

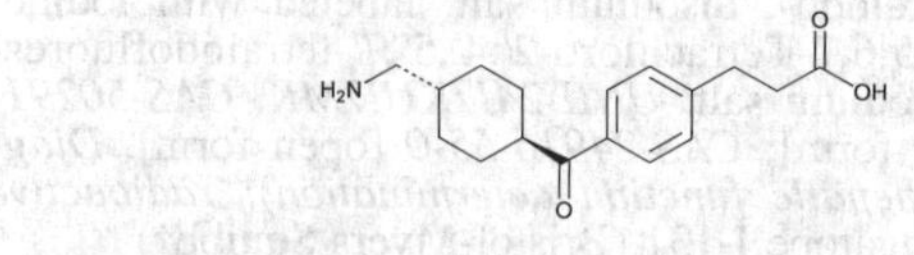

Rovelizumab [*1998*] (roe″ ve liz′ oo mab). (1) Immunoglobulin G4, anti-(human CD11 (antigen)/integrin β2) (human-mouse monoclonal Hu23F2G γ4-chain), disulfide with human-mouse monoclonal Hu23F2G κ-chain, dimer; (2) Immunoglobulin G4 (human-mouse monoclonal Hu23F2G γ4-chain anti-human antigen CD11/integrin β2), disulfide with human-mouse monoclonal Hu23F2G κ-chain, dimer. Molecular weight is approximately 148,100 daltons (Mass Spectrometry analysis). *CAS-197099-66-4*. INN. Leukarrest (ICOS) ◇*Hu23F2G*

Roxadimate [*1990*] (rox ad′ i mate). $C_{15}H_{23}NO_4$. 281.35. (1) Benzoic acid, 4-[bis(2-hydroxypropyl)amino]-, ethyl ester; (2) Ethyl (±)-*p*-[bis(2-hydroxypropyl)amino]benzoate. *CAS-58882-17-0*. INN. *Sunscreen.*

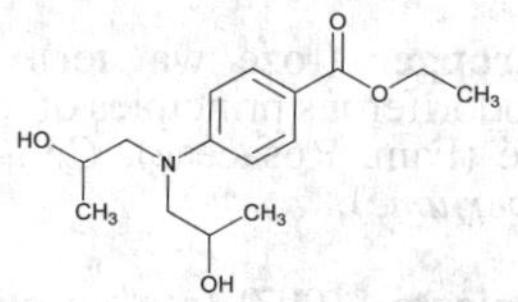

Roxarsone [*1966*] (rox ar′ sone). **USP**. $C_6H_6AsNO_6$. 263.04. (1) Arsonic acid, (4-hydroxy-3-nitrophenyl)-; (2) 4-Hydroxy-3-nitrobenzenearsonic acid. *UNII-H5GU9YQL7L*. *CAS-121-19-7*. INN; BAN. *Antibacterial.* ◇*NSC-2101*

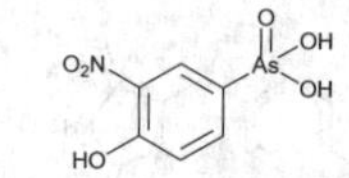

Roxatidine Acetate Hydrochloride [*1989*] (rox a′ ti deen as′ e tate hye″ droe klor′ ide). $C_{19}H_{28}N_2O_4 \cdot HCl$. 384.90. [Roxatidine is INN and BAN; Roxatidine Acetate is INN and BAN.] (1) Acetamide, 2-(acetyloxy)-*N*-[3-[3-(1-piperidinylmethyl)phenoxy]propyl-, monohydrochloride; (2) *N*-[3-[(α-Piperidino-*m*-tolyl)oxy]propyl]glycolamide acetate (ester), monohydrochloride. *CAS-93793-83-0; CAS-78273-80-0* [roxatidine]; *CAS-78628-28-1* [roxatidine acetate]. JAN. *Anti-ulcerative.* ◇*HOE 760; HOE 062 [Roxatidine]*

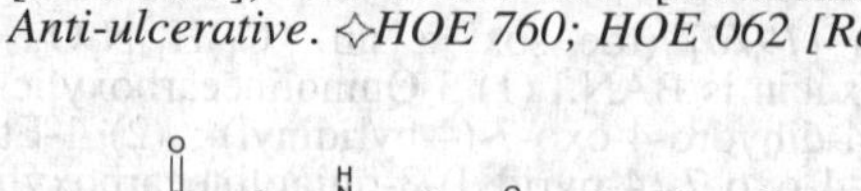

Roxibolone. $C_{21}H_{28}O_5$. 360.44. 11β,17β-Dihydroxy-17-methyl-3-oxoandrosta-1,4-diene-2-carboxylic acid. *UNII-3R7NLP419C*. *CAS-60023-92-9*. INN.

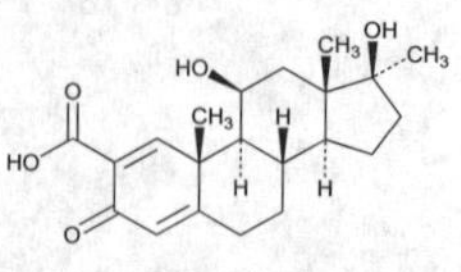

Roxifiban Acetate [*1997*] (rox″ i fye′ ban as′ e tate). $C_{21}H_{29}N_5O_6 \cdot C_2H_4O_2$. 507.54. [Roxifiban is INN.] (1) L-Alanine, 3-[[[3-[4-(aminoiminomethyl]phenyl]-4,5-dihydro-5-isoxazolyl]acetyl]amino]-*N*-(butoxycarbonyl)-, methyl ester, (*R*)-, monoacetate; (2) (2*S*)-3-[2-[(5*R*)-3-(*p*-Amidinophenyl)-2-isoxazolin-5-yl]acetamido]-2-(carboxyamino)propionic acid, 2-butyl methyl ester, monoacetate. *CAS-176022-59-6; CAS-170902-47-3* [roxifiban]. *Antithrombotic; fibrinogen receptor antagonist.* ◇*DMP 754*

Roxindole. $C_{23}H_{26}N_2O$. 346.47. 3-[4-(3,6-Dihydro-4-phenyl-1(2*H*)-pyridylbutyl]indol-5-ol. *CAS-112192-04-8.* INN.

Roxithromycin [*1986*] (rox ith″ roe mye′ sin). $C_{41}H_{76}N_2O_{15}$. 837.05. (1) Erythromycin, 9-[*O*-[(2-methoxyethoxy)methyl]oxime]; (2) Erythromycin 9-[*O*-[(2-methoxyethoxy)methyl]oxime]. *CAS-80214-83-1.* INN; JAN. *Antibacterial.* Rulide (Hoechst-Roussel†) ◇*RU 965; RU 28965*

Roxolonium Metilsulfate. $C_{38}H_{63}NO_8S$. 693.97. 2-(Hydroxymethyl)-1,1-dimethylpyrrolidinium methyl sulfate 3β-hydroxy-11-oxoolean-12-en-30-oate. *CAS-53862-80-9.* INN.

Roxoperone. $C_{19}H_{23}FN_2O_3$. 346.40. 8-[3-(*p*-Fluorobenzoyl)propyl]-2-methyl-2,8-diazaspiro[4.5]decane-1,3-dione. *UNII-5RS1CY853F. CAS-2804-00-4.* INN.

Rubella Virus Vaccine Live (roo bel′ a). **USP**. A bacterially sterile preparation of live virus derived from a strain of rubella virus that has been tested for neurovirulence in monkeys, and for immunogenicity, that is free from all demonstrable viable microbial agents except unavoidable bacteriophage, and that has been found suitable for human immunization. *Immunizing agent (active).* Meruvax (Merck)

Rubidium Chloride Rb 82 [*1993*] (roo bid′ e um klor′ ide). **USP** [Injection]. $Cl^{82}Rb$. (1) Rubidium chloride ($^{82}RbCl$); (2) Rubidium chloride ($^{82}RbCl$). *UNII-F0Z746KRKQ. CAS-132486-03-4. Diagnostic aid (radioactive, cardiac disease); radioactive agent.* Cardiogen (Bristol-Myers Squibb†) [*Note—Rubidium Chloride Rb 82 is the drug product eluted from Cardiogen-82 (rubidium 82 generator).*]

Rubidium Chloride Rb 86 [*1963*] (roo bid′ e um klor′ ide). $^{86}RbCl$. (1) Rubidium chloride ($^{86}RbCl$); (2) Rubidium chloride ($^{86}RbCl$). *CAS-21031-72-1. Radioactive agent.*

Rubidium Hydroxide (^{81}Rb) [Injection]. $^{81}RbOH$. *CAS-1310-82-3* [rubidium hydroxide]. JAN.

Rubitecan [*1999*] (roo″ bi tee′ kan). $C_{20}H_{15}N_3O_6$. 393.35. (1) 1*H*-Pyrano[3′,4′:6,7]indolizino[1,2-*b*]quinoline-3,14(4*H*,12*H*)-dione, 4-ethyl-4-hydroxy-10-nitro-, (4*S*)-; (2) 9-Nitrocamptothecin; (3) 9-Nitro-20(*S*)-camptothecin. *CAS-91421-42-0.* INN. *Antineoplastic (topoisomerase I inhibitor).[Name previously used: 9-NC.]* ◇*RFS 2000*

Ruboxistaurin. $C_{28}H_{28}N_4O_3$. 468.55. (9*S*)-9-[(Dimethylamino)methyl]-6,7,10,11-tetrahydro-9*H*,19*H*-5,21:12,17-dimethenodibenzo[*e,k*]pyrrolo[3,4-*h*][1,4,13]oxadiazacyclohexadecene-18,20-dione. *UNII-721809WQCP. CAS-169939-94-0.* INN.

Rufinamide [*2000*] (roo fin′ a mide). $C_{10}H_8F_2N_4O$. 238.19. (1) 1*H*-1,2,3-Triazole-4-carboxamide, 1-[(2,6-difluorophenyl)methyl]-; (2) 1-(2,6-Difluorobenzyl)-1*H*-1,2,3-triazole-4-carboxamide. *UNII-WFW942PR79. CAS-106308-*

44-5. INN; BAN. *Treatment of partial-onset seizures and seizures in Lennox-Gastaut syndrome.* ◇*CGP 33101; RUF 331; E2080; 60231/4*

Rufloxacin. $C_{17}H_{18}FN_3O_3S$. 363.41. 9-Fluoro-2,3-dihydro-10-(4-methyl-1-piperazinyl)-7-oxo-7*H*-pyrido[1,2,3-*de*]-1,4-benzothiazine-6-carboxylic acid. *UNII-Y521XM2900. CAS-101363-10-4.* INN; BAN. ◇*MF 934*

Rufocromomycin (INN, BAN, DCF) — *See* Streptonigrin.

Rupatadine. $C_{26}H_{26}ClN_3$. 415.96. 8-Chloro-6,11-dihydro-11-[1-[(5-methyl-3-pyridyl)methyl]-4-piperidylidene]-5*H*-benzo[5,6]cyclohepta[1,2-*b*]pyridine. *UNII-2AE8M83G3E. CAS-158876-82-5.* INN.

Rupintrivir [*2002*] (roo pin′ tri vir). $C_{31}H_{39}FN_4O_7$. 598.66. (1) 2-Pentenoic acid, 4-[[(2*R*,5*S*)-2-[(4-fluorophenyl) methyl]-6-methyl-5-[[(5-methyl-3-isoxazolyl)carbonyl]amino]-1,4-dioxoheptyl]amino]-5-[(3*S*)-2-oxo-3-pyrrolidinyl]-, ethylester, (2*E*,4*S*)-; (2) Ethyl (2*E*,4*S*)-4-[[(2*R*,5*S*)-2-(4-fluorobenzyl)-6-methyl-5-[[(5-methylisoxazol-3-yl)carbonyl]amino]-4-oxoheptanoyl]amino]-5-[(3*S*)-2-oxopyrrolidin-3-yl]pent-2-enoate. *CAS-223537-30-2.* INN. *Antiviral intended for use in the treatment of the common cold (human rhinovirus 3C protease inhibitor).* ◇*AG7088*

Ruplizumab [*1999*] (roo pliz′ oo mab). (1) Immunoglobulin G1, (anti-human CD40 ligand) (human-mouse monoclonal 5c8 γ_1-chain), disulfide with human-mouse monoclonal 5c8 κ-chain, dimer; (2) Immunoglobulin G1 (human-mouse monoclonal 5c8 γ1-chain anti-human CD40 ligand), disulfide with human-mouse monoclonal 5c8 κ-chain, dimer. Molecular weight is approximately 145,448 daltons (with two additional N-linked glycans consisting of several glycoform species with an average molecular weight of approximately 1500 daltons). *CAS-220651-94-5.* INN. *Treatment of immune thrombocytopenic purpura and systemic lupus erythematosus (humanized monoclonal antibody).* ◇*BG9588; hu5c8*

Rusalatide Acetate [*2006*] (roo sal′ a tide as′ e tate). $(C_{97}H_{147}N_{29}O_{35}S)_3 \cdot (C_2H_4O_2)_2$. 7054.43. [Rusalatide is INN.] (1) L-Valinamide, L-alanylglycyl-L-tyrosyl-L-lysyl-L-prolyl-L-α-aspartyl-L-α-glutamylglycyl-L-lysyl-L-arginylglycyl-L-α-aspartyl-L-alanyl-L-cysteinyl-L-α-glutamylglycyl-L-α-aspartyl-L-serylglycylglycyl-L-prolyl-L-phenylalanyl-, acetate (3:2) (salt); (2) L-Alanylglycyl-L-tyrosyl-L-lysyl-L-prolyl-L-α-aspartyl-L-α-glutamylglycyl-L-lysyl-L-arginylglycyl-L-α-aspartyl-L-alanyl-L-cysteinyl-L-α-glutamylglycyl-L-α-aspartyl-L-serylglycylglycyl-L-prolyl-L-phenylalanyl-L-valinamide, acetate (3:2) salt. *CAS-875455-82-6; CAS-497221-38-2* [rusalatide]. *Promotes healing of bone, skin wounds, cartilage, cardiovascular tissue and ligaments/tendons.* Chrysalin (OrthoLogic) ◇*TP 508; TRAP-508*

Rutamycin [*1963*] (roo″ ta mye′ sin). Antibiotic produced by *Streptomyces rutgersensis.* (1) Rutamycin (Oligomycin D); (2) Rutamycin. *CAS-1404-59-7.* INN. *Antifungal.* ◇*A-272; RR No. 32705*

Rutin. $C_{27}H_{30}O_{16} \cdot 3H_2O$. 664.56. [Rutoside is INN and BAN.] (1) 3-Rhamnoglucoside of 5,7,3′,4′-tetrahydroxyflavonol; (2) 2-(3,4-Dihydroxyphenyl)-5,7-dihydroxy-4*H*-chromen-4-one-3-yl 6-*O*-α-L-rhamnopyranosyl-β-D-glucoside. *CAS-153-18-4.* NF XI; JAN; MI.

Rutoside (INN, BAN, DCF) — *See* Rutin.

Ruvazone. $C_{12}H_{14}N_2O_4$. 250.25. *o*-Ethoxybenzoic acid (1-carboxyethylidene)hydrazide. *CAS-20228-27-7.* INN.

Ruzadolane. $C_{18}H_{19}F_2N_5S$. 375.44. 3-[[2-[4-(2,4-Difluoro-phenyl)-1-piperazinyl]ethyl]thio]-*S*-triazolo[4,3-*a*]pyridine. *UNII-ZKV3GT35TR. CAS-115762-17-9.* INN.

s1^{11}In — *See* Indium In 111 Pentetate.

^{35}S — *See* Sodium Sulfate S 35.

Sabarubicin. $C_{32}H_{37}NO_{13}$. 643.64. (7*S*,9*S*)-7-{[4-*O*-(3-Amino-2,3,6-trideoxy-α-L-*lyxo*-hexopyranosyl)-2,6-dideoxy-α-L-*lyxo*-hexopyranosyl]oxy}-6,9,11-trihydroxy-9-(hydroxyacetyl)-7,8,9,10-tetrahydrotetracene-5,12-dione. *CAS-211100-13-9.* INN.

Sabcomeline Hydrochloride [*1997*] (sab koe′ me leen hye″ droe klor′ ide). $C_{10}H_{15}N_3O \cdot HCl$. 229.71. [Sabcomeline is INN and BAN.] (*R*)-3-Quinuclidineglyoxylonitrile (*Z*)-*O*-methyloxime, monohydrochloride. *CAS-159912-58-0; CAS-159912-53-5* [sabcomeline]. *Alzheimer's disease treatment (adjunct).* ◇SB-202026-A

Sabeluzole [*1988*] (sa bel′ ue zole). $C_{22}H_{26}FN_3O_2S$. 415.52. (1) 1-Piperidineethanol, 4-(2-benzothiazolylmethylamino)-α-[(4-fluorophenoxy)methyl]-, (±)-; (2) (±)-4-(2-Benzothiazolylmethylamino)-α-[(*p*-fluorophenoxy)methyl]-1-piperidineethanol. *CAS-104383-17-7.* INN; BAN. *Anticonvulsant; antihypoxic.* ◇R 58735

Sabiporide. $C_{18}H_{19}F_3N_6O_2$. 408.38. *N*-Carbamimidoyl-4-[4-(1*H*-pyrrol-2-ylcarbonyl)piperazin-1-yl]-3-(trifluoromethyl)benzamide. *UNII-U52APA00X7. CAS-324758-66-9.* INN.

Saccharated Ferric Oxide (JAN) — *See* Iron Sucrose.

Saccharated Iron (previously used name) — *See* Iron Sucrose.

Saccharated Iron Oxide (previously used name) — *See* Iron Sucrose.

Saccharated Pepsin. A mixture of pepsin obtained from the gastric mucosa of hogs or cattle and lactose. It is an enzyme drug having a proteolytic activity. *CAS-9001-75-6.* JAN.

Saccharin (sak′ a rin). **NF.** $C_7H_5NO_3S$. 183.18. (1) 1,2-Benzisothiazol-3(2*H*)-one, 1,1-dioxide; (2) 1,2-Benzisothiazolin-3-one 1,1-dioxide. *UNII-FST467XS7D. CAS-81-07-2. Pharmaceutic aid (flavor).* Sweeta (Bristol-Myers Squibb†)

Saccharin Calcium (sak′ a rin kal′ see um). **USP.** $C_{14}H_8CaN_2O_6S_2 \cdot 3\frac{1}{2}H_2O$. 467.48. (1) 1,2-Benzisothiazol-3(2*H*)-one, 1,1-dioxide, calcium salt, hydrate (2:7); (2) 1,2-Benzisothiazolin-3-one 1,1-dioxide calcium salt hydrate (2:7). *UNII-FST467XS7D* [saccharin]. *CAS-6381-91-5; CAS-6485-34-3* [anhydrous]; *CAS-81-07-2* [saccharin]. *Sweetener (non-nutritive).*

Saccharin Sodium (sak′ a rin soe′ dee um). **USP.** $C_7H_4NNaO_3S \cdot 2H_2O$. 241.20. (1) 1,2-Benzisothiazol-3(2*H*)-one, 1,1-dioxide, sodium salt, dihydrate; (2) 1,2-Benzisothiazolin-3-one 1,1-dioxide sodium salt dihydrate. *UNII-SB8ZUX40TY. CAS-6155-57-3; CAS-128-44-9* [anhydrous]; *CAS-81-07-2* [saccharin]. JAN. *Sweetener (non-nutritive).* Sucaryl (Ross†)

Sacrosidase [*1997*] (sak roe′ si dase). β-Fructofuranosidase (*Saccharomyces cerevisiae* clone FI4 protein moiety reduced). Molecular weight is approximately 140,000

---

† Brand name formerly used, and/or firm no longer concerned with this product.

daltons. *UNII-8A7F670F2Y. CAS-85897-35-4. Treatment of congenital sucrase-isomaltase deficiency (enzyme replacement).* Sucraid (QOL)

```
SMTNETSDRP LVHFTPNKGW MNDPNGLWYD EKDAKWHLYF QYNPNDTVWG
TPLFWGHATS DDLTNWEDQP IAIAPKRNDS GAFSGSMVVD YNNTSGFFND
TIDPRQRCVA IWTYNTPESE EQYISYSLDG GYTFTEYQKN PVLAANSTQF
RDPKVFWYEP SQKWIMTAAK SQDYKIEIYS SDDLKSWKLE SAFANEGFLG
YQYECPGLIE VPTEQDPSKS YWVMFISINP GAPAGGSFNQ YFVGSFNGTH
FEAFDNQSRV VDFGKDYYAL QTFFNTDPTY GSALGIAWAS NWEYSAFVPT
NPWRSSMSLV RKFSLNTEYQ ANPETELINL KAEPILNISN AGPWSRFATN
TTLTKANSYN VDLSNSTGTL EFELVYAVNT TQTISKSVFA DLSLWFKGLE
DPEEYLRMGF EVSASSFFLD RGNSKVKFVK ENPYFTNRMS VNNQPFKSEN
DLSYYKVYGL LDQNILELYF NDGDVVSTNT YFMTTGNALG SVNMTTGVDN
LFYIDKFQVR EVK
```

Safflower Oil (saf' low er). **USP**. The refined fixed oil obtained from the seed of *Carthamus tinctorius* Linné (Fam. Compositae). *UNII-65UEH262IS. Pharmaceutic aid (vehicle, oleaginous).* Liposyn (Abbott)

Safinamide. $C_{17}H_{19}FN_2O_2$. 302.34. (+)-(*S*)-2-[[*p*-[(*m*-Fluorobenzyl)oxy]benzyl]amino]propionamide. *UNII-90ENL74SIG. CAS-133865-89-1.* INN.

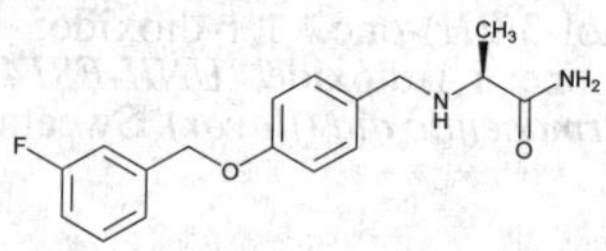

Safingol [*1994*] (sa fin' gol). $C_{18}H_{39}NO_2$. 301.51. (1) 1,3-Octadecanediol, 2-amino-, [*S*-(*R**,*R**)]-; (2) (2*S*,3*S*)-2-Amino-1,3-octadecanediol. *CAS-15639-50-6.* INN. *Antineoplastic (adjunct); antipsoriatic.* ◇*SPC-100270*

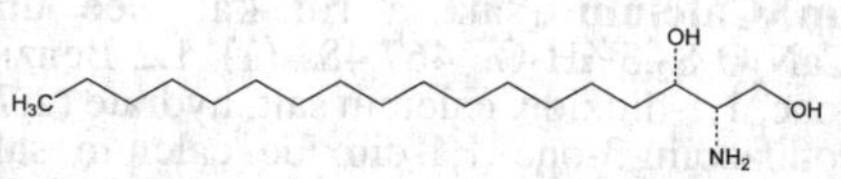

Safingol Hydrochloride [*1994*] (sa fin' gol hye" droe klor' ide). $C_{18}H_{39}NO_2 \cdot HCl$. 337.97. (1) 1,3-Octadecanediol, 2-amino-, hydrochloride, [*S*-(*R**,*R**)]-; (2) (2*S*,3*S*)-2-Amino-1,3-octadecanediol hydrochloride. *CAS-139755-79-6. Antineoplastic (adjunct); antipsoriatic.* ◇*SPC-100271*

Safironil. $C_{15}H_{23}N_3O_4$. 309.36. *N,N′*-Bis(3-methoxypropyl)-2,4-pyridinedicarboxamide. *UNII-CK4M8AX1LN. CAS-134377-69-8.* INN.

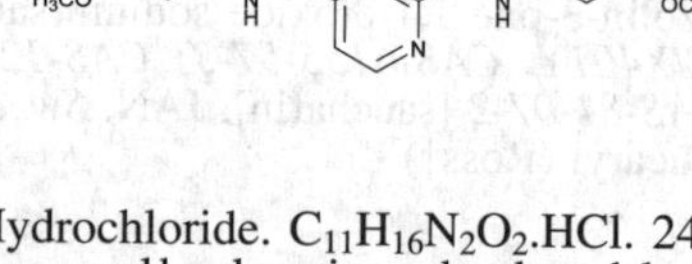

Safrazine Hydrochloride. $C_{11}H_{16}N_2O_2 \cdot HCl$. 244.72. β-Piperonylisopropylhydrazine hydrochloride. *UNII-5985O24GLM. CAS-7296-30-2; CAS-33419-68-0* [safrazine]. JAN.

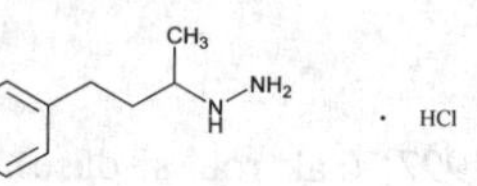

Safrole. $C_{10}H_{10}O_2$. 162.19. 4-Allyl-1,2-(methylenedioxy)benzene. USP VIII; MI.

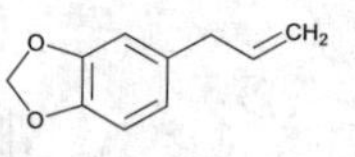

Sagandipine. $C_{27}H_{31}FN_2O_5$. 482.54. Methyl (5-piperidinomethyl)furfuryl 4-(*o*-fluorophenyl)-1,4-dihydro-2,6-dimethyl-3,5-pyridinedicarboxylate. *UNII-20O65J0B72. CAS-126294-30-2.* INN.

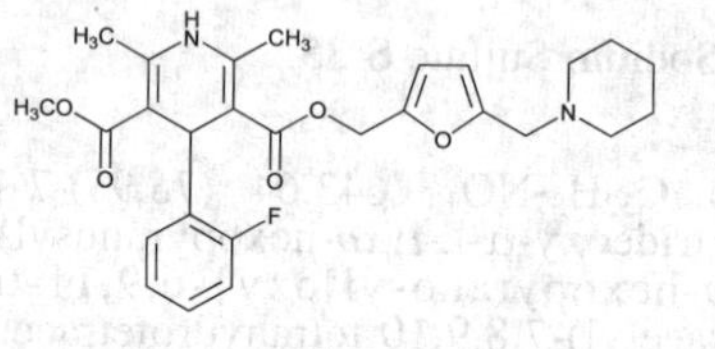

Sagopilone. $C_{30}H_{41}NO_6S$. 543.71. (1*S*,3*S*,7*S*,10*R*,11*S*,12*S*,16*R*)-7,11-Dihydroxy-8,8,12,16-tetramethyl-3-(2-methyl-1,3-benzothiazol-5-yl)-10-(prop-2-enyl)-4,17-dioxabicyclo[14.1.0]heptadecane-5,9-dione. *CAS-305841-29-6.* INN.

Salacetamide. $C_9H_9NO_3$. 179.17. *N*-Acetylsalicylamide. *UNII-7G29CRR596. CAS-487-48-9.* INN; DCF; MI. ◇*L-749*

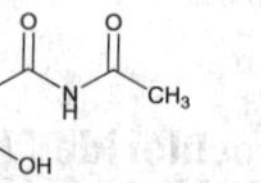

Salafibrate. $C_{32}H_{32}Cl_2O_{10}$. 647.50. 2-Hydroxy-1-(hydroxymethyl)ethyl salicylate 2-acetate bis[2-(*p*-chlorophenoxy)-2-methylpropionate]. *UNII-HJ57229JPX. CAS-64496-66-8.* INN.

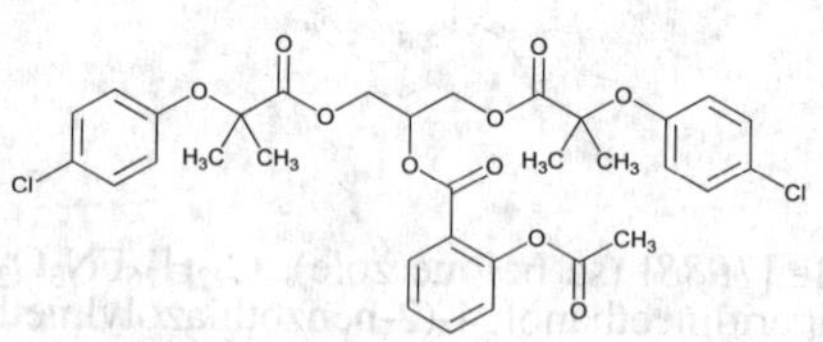

Salantel [*1973*] (sal an' tel). $C_{20}H_{11}Cl_2I_2NO_3$. 638.02. (1) Benzamide, *N*-[3-chloro-4-(4-chlorobenzoyl)phenyl]-2-hydroxy-3,5-diiodo-; (2) 3′-Chloro-4′-(*p*-chlorobenzoyl)-3,5-diiodosalicylanilide. *UNII-BIY8B0682Q. CAS-36093-47-7.* INN. *Anthelmintic (veterinary).* ◇*R 23,050*

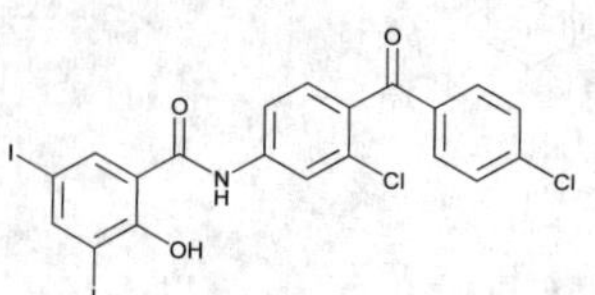

Salazodine. $C_{18}H_{15}N_5O_6S$. 429.41. 5-[[*p*-[(6-Methoxy-3-pyridazinyl)sulfamoyl]phenyl]azo]salicylic acid. *UNII-4L219Q1D16*. *CAS-22933-72-8*. INN.

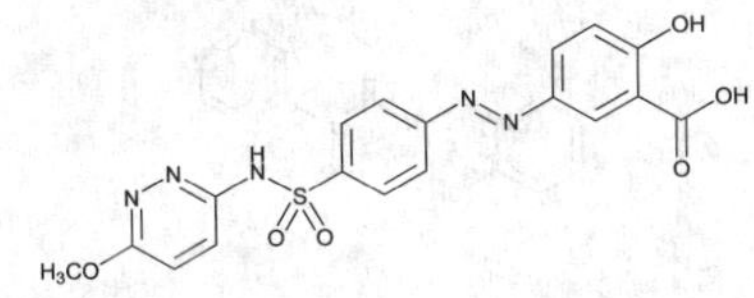

Salazosulfadimidine. $C_{19}H_{17}N_5O_5S$. 427.43. 5-[*p*-[(4,6-Dimethyl-2-pyrimidinyl)sulfamoyl]phenylazo]salicylic acid. *UNII-W33009B02O*. *CAS-2315-08-4*. INN; BAN; MI. *[Name previously used: Salazosulphadimidine.]*

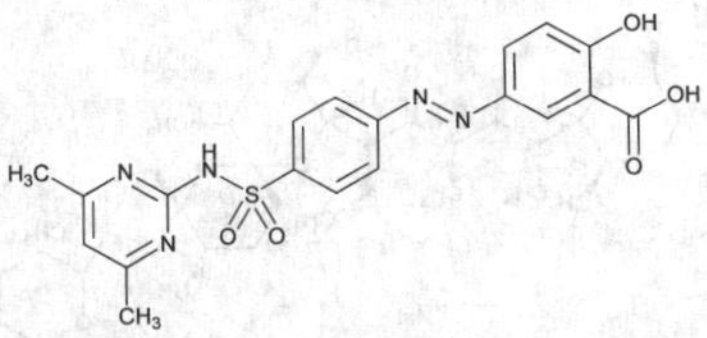

Salazosulfamide. $C_{13}H_{11}N_3O_5S$. 321.31. 5-(*p*-Sulfamoylphenylazo)salicylic acid. *UNII-B6831ORH7W*. *CAS-139-56-0*. INN; DCF.

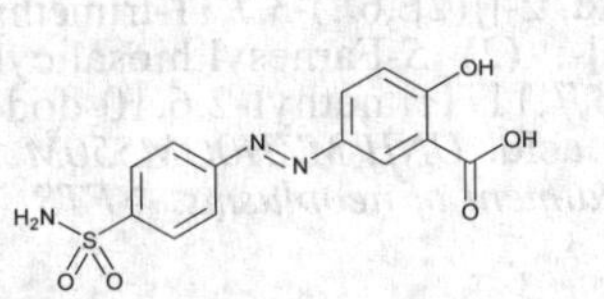

Salazosulfapyridine (JAN) — *See* Sulfasalazine.

Salazosulfathiazole. $C_{16}H_{12}N_4O_5S_2$. 404.42. 5-[*p*-(2-Thiazolylsulfamoyl)phenylazo]salicylic acid. *UNII-56PE10-F2EA*. *CAS-515-58-2*. INN; DCF.

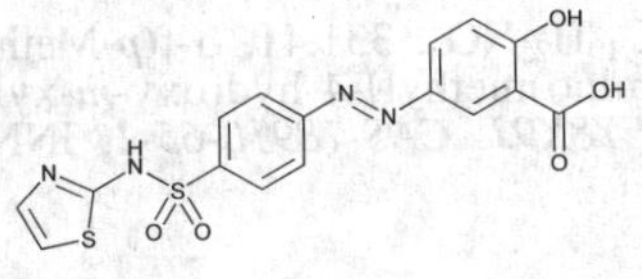

Salazosulphadimidine (previously used name) — *See* Salazosulfadimidine.

Salbutamol (INN, BAN, DCF) — *See* Albuterol.

Salbutamol Sulfate (JAN) — *See* Albuterol Sulfate.

Salcaprozate Sodium [*2002*] (sal kap′ roe zate soe′ dee um). $C_{15}H_{20}NNaO_4$. 301.31. (1) Octanoic acid, 8-[(2-hydroxybenzoyl)amino]-, monosodium salt; (2) Sodium 8-[(2-hydroxybenzoyl)amino]octanoate. *UNII-1YTW0422YU*. *CAS-203787-91-1*. *Oral absorption promoter*. *✧E414; SNAC*

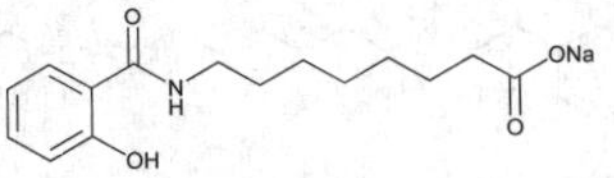

† Brand name formerly used, and/or firm no longer concerned with this product.

Salcaprozic Acid. $C_{15}H_{21}NO_4$. 279.33. 8-(2-Hydroxybenzamido)octanoic acid. *UNII-X88E147FCU*. *CAS-183990-46-7*. INN.

Salcatonin (MI) — *See* Calcitonin.

Salclobuzate Sodium [*2004*] (sal kloe′ bue zate soe′ dee um). $C_{11}H_{11}ClNNaO_4$. 279.65. (1) Butanoic acid, 4-[(4-chloro-2-hydroxybenzoyl)amino]-, monosodium salt; (2) Sodium 4-[(4-chloro-2-hydroxybenzoyl)amino]butanoate. *UNII-7V49F22020*. *CAS-387825-07-2*. *Oral absorption promoter*. (Emisphere Technologies) *✧4-CNAB*

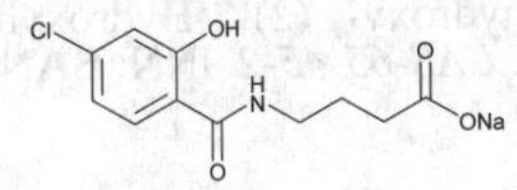

Salclobuzic Acid. $C_{11}H_{12}ClNO_4$. 257.67. 4-(4-Chloro-2-hydroxybenzamido)butanoic acid. *CAS-387825-03-8*. INN.

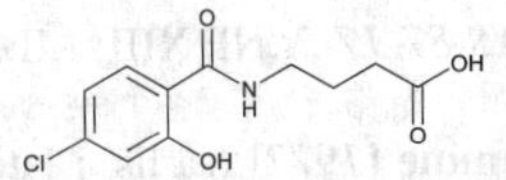

Salcolex [*1969*] (sal′ koe lex). $[C_{12}H_{19}NO_4]_2.MgSO_4.4H_2O$. 675.00. (1) Ethanaminium, 2-hydroxy-*N,N,N*-trimethyl-, 2-hydroxybenzoate (salt), compd. with magnesium sulfate (2:1), tetrahydrate; (2) Choline salicylate (salt) compound with magnesium sulfate (2:1) tetrahydrate. *CAS-28038-04-2*; *CAS-54194-00-2* [anhydrous]. INN. *Analgesic; anti-inflammatory; antipyretic*.

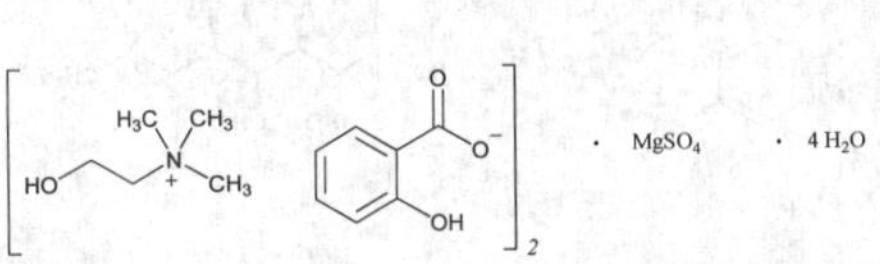

Saletamide (INN) Maleate — *See* Salethamide Maleate.

Salethamide Maleate [*1968*] (sal eth′ a mide mal′ ee ate). $C_{13}H_{20}N_2O_2.C_4H_4O_4$. 352.38. [Saletamide is INN.] (1) Benzamide, *N*-[2-(diethylamino)ethyl]-2-hydroxy-, (*Z*)-2-butenedioate (1:1) (salt); (2) *N*-[2-(Diethylamino)ethyl] salicylamide maleate (1:1) (salt). *CAS-24381-55-3*; *CAS-46803-81-0* [salethamide]. *Analgesic*. *✧MA-593*

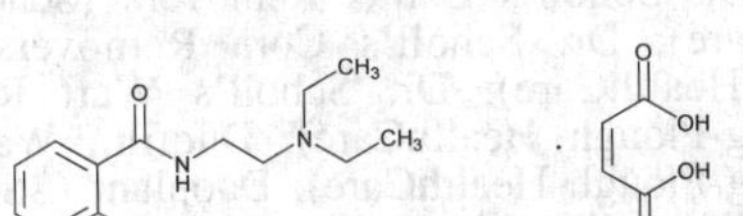

Salfluverine. $C_{14}H_{10}F_3NO_2$. 281.23. α,α,α-Trifluoro-*m*-salicylotoluidide. *UNII-GAK955D9Q5*. *CAS-587-49-5*. INN; DCF.

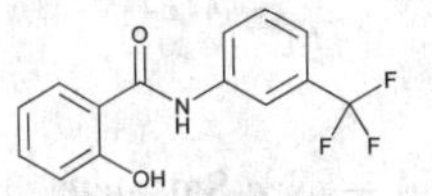

Salicain (previously used name) — *See* Salicyl Alcohol.

Salicin. *CAS-138-52-3*. USP IX; MI.

Salicyl Alcohol [*1979*] (sal′ i sil al′ ka hol). $C_7H_8O_2$. 124.14. (1) Benzenemethanol, 2-hydroxy-; (2) *o*-Hydroxybenzyl alcohol. *UNII-FA1N0842KB. CAS-90-01-7. Anesthetic (local). [Names previously used: Saligenin, Saligenol, Salicain]*

Salicylamide (sal″ i sil′ a mide). **USP.** $C_7H_7NO_2$. 137.14. (1) Benzamide, 2-hydroxy-; (2) 2-Hydroxybenzamide. *UNII-EM8BM710ZC. CAS-65-45-2.* INN; BAN; JAN. *Analgesic.*

Salicylanilide. *CAS-87-17-2.* NF XIII; MI.

Salicylate Meglumine [*1972*] (sa lis′ i late me′ gloo meen). $C_7H_{17}NO_5.C_7H_6O_3$. 333.33. (1) Benzoic acid, 2-hydroxy-, compd. with 1-deoxy-1-(methylamino)-D-glucitol; (2) Salicylic acid compound with 1-deoxy-1-(methylamino)-D-glucitol (1:1); (3) *N*-Methylglucamine salicylate. *UNII-6HG8UB2MUY* [meglumine]. *CAS-23277-50-1; CAS-6284-40-8* [meglumine]. *Antirheumatic; analgesic.* ◇*PFA-186*

Salicylazosulfapyridine (previously used name) — *See* Sulfasalazine.

Salicylic Acid (sal″ i sil′ ik as′ id). **USP.** $C_7H_6O_3$. 138.12. (1) Benzoic acid, 2-hydroxy-; (2) Salicylic acid. *UNII-O414PZ4LPZ. CAS-69-72-7.* JAN. *Keratolytic.* Advanced Pain Relief Callus Removers (Schering-Plough HealthCare); Advanced Pain Relief Corn Removers (Schering-Plough HealthCare); Clear Away Wart Remover (Schering-Plough HealthCare); Compound W (Whitehall-Robins†); Dr. Scholl's Callus Removers (Schering-Plough HealthCare); Dr. Scholl's Corn Removers (Schering-Plough HealthCare); Dr. Scholl's Wart Remover Kit (Schering-Plough HealthCare); Duofilm Wart Remover (Schering-Plough HealthCare); Duoplant (Stiefel†); Freezone (Whitehall-Robins†); Ionil (Galderma†); Ionil-Plus (Galderma†); Salicylic Acid Soap (Stiefel); Saligel (Stiefel†); Stri-Dex (Sterling Health U.S.A.)

Salicylsalicylic Acid — *See* Salsalate.

Saligenin (previously used name) — *See* Salicyl Alcohol.

Saligenol (previously used name) — *See* Salicyl Alcohol.

Salinazid. $C_{13}H_{11}N_3O_2$. 241.25. 1-Isonicotinoyl-2-salicylidenehydrazine. *CAS-495-84-1.* INN; BAN; MI. Salizid (Parke-Davis†)

Saliniazid — *See* Salinazid.

Salinomycin. $C_{42}H_{70}O_{11}$. 751.00. Salinomycin. *UNII-62UXS86T64. CAS-53003-10-4.* INN; BAN; MI.

Salirasib [*2006*] (sal ir′ a sib). $C_{22}H_{30}O_2S$. 358.54. (1) Benzoic acid, 2-[[(2*E*,6*E*)-3,7,11-trimethyl-2,6,10-dodecatrienyl]thio]-; (2) *S*-Farnesylthiosalicylic acid; (3) 2-[[(2*E*,6*E*)-3,7,11-Trimethyl-2,6,10-dodecatrienyl]sulfanyl]benzoic acid. *UNII-MZH0OM550M. CAS-162520-00-5.* INN. *Treatment of neoplasms.* ◇*FTS*

Salmaterol — *See* Salmeterol.

Salmefamol. $C_{19}H_{25}NO_4$. 331.41. α-[(*p*-Methoxy-α-methylphenethylamino)methyl]-4-hydroxy-*m*-xylene-α,α′-diol. *UNII-Q56SEY8X9J. CAS-18910-65-1.* INN; BAN. ◇*AH 3923*

Salmeterol [*1985*] (sal me′ ter ol). $C_{25}H_{37}NO_4$. 415.57. (1) 1,3-Benzenedimethanol, 4-hydroxy-α¹-[[[6-(4-phenylbutoxy)hexyl]amino]methyl-, (±)-; (2) (±)-4-Hydroxy-α′-[[[6-(4-phenylbutoxy)hexyl]amino]methyl]-*m*-xylene-α,α′-diol. *UNII-2I4BC502BT. CAS-89365-50-4.* INN; BAN. *Bronchodilator.* ◇*GR 33343 X*

Salmeterol Xinafoate [*1990*] (sal me′ ter ol zye naf′ oh ate). $C_{25}H_{37}NO_4.C_{11}H_8O_3$. 603.75. (1) 1,3-Benzenedimethanol, 4-hydroxy-α¹-[[[6-(4-phenylbutoxy)hexyl]amino]methyl]-, (±)-, 1-hydroxy-2-naphthalenecarboxylate (salt); (2) (±)-4-Hydroxy-α¹-[[[6-(4-phenylbutoxy)hexyl]amino]-

methyl]-*m*-xylene-α,α′-diol 1-hydroxy-2-naphthoate (salt). *UNII-6EW8Q962A5. CAS-94749-08-3. Bronchodilator.* Serevent (GlaxoSmithKline) ◇*GR 33343 G*

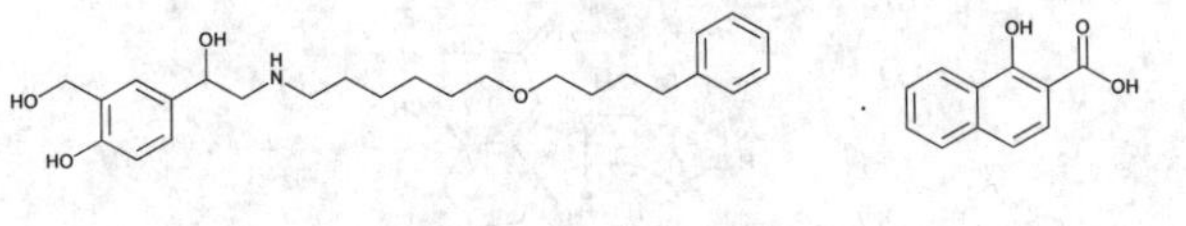

Salmisteine. $C_{14}H_{15}NO_6S$. 325.34. *N*-Acetyl-L-cysteine salicylate (ester), acetate (ester). *CAS-89767-59-9.* INN.

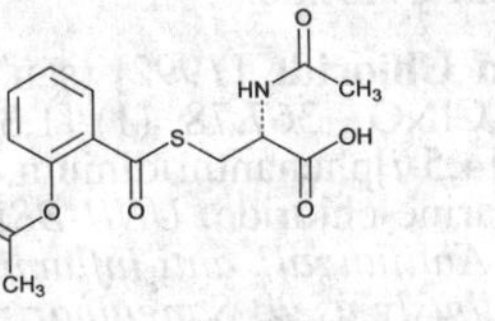

Salmotin — *See* Adicillin.

Salnacedin [*1995*] (sal na′ se din). $C_{12}H_{13}NO_5S$. 283.30. (1) L-Cysteine, *N*-acetyl-, 2-hydroxybenzoate (ester); (2) *N*-Acetyl-L-cysteine salicylate (ester). *CAS-87573-01-1.* INN. *Anti-inflammatory (topical).* ◇*G-201,SCY*

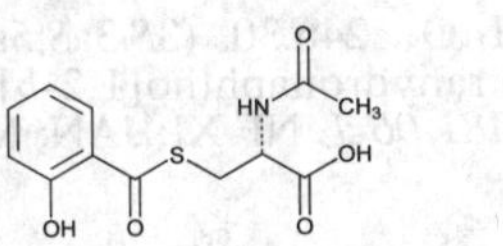

Salol — *See* Phenyl Salicylate.

Salprotoside. $C_{25}H_{30}O_{10}$. 490.50. Ethyl 3-*O*-propyl-D-glucofuranoside 5,6-disalicylate. *CAS-33779-37-2.* INN.

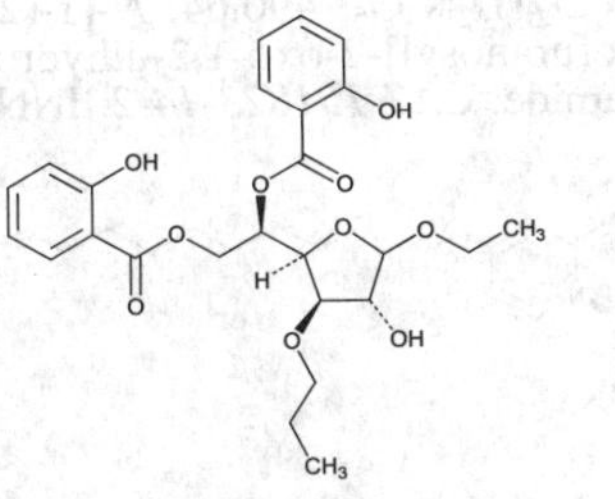

Salsalate [*1972*] (sal′ sa late). **USP.** $C_{14}H_{10}O_5$. 258.23. [Sasapyrine is JAN.] (1) Benzoic acid, 2-hydroxy-, 2-carboxyphenyl ester; (2) Disalicylic acid; (3) Salicylic acid, bimolecular ester; (4) Salicylsalicylic acid. *CAS-552-94-3.* INN; BAN. *Analgesic; anti-inflammatory.* Disalcid (3M Pharmaceuticals) ◇*NSC-49171*

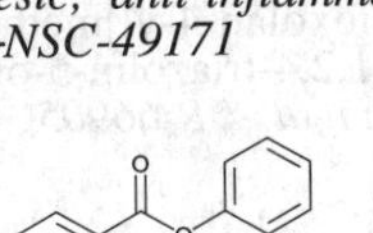

Salts, Rehydration. **USP** [Oral]. A dry mixture of sodium chloride, potassium chloride, sodium bicarbonate, and dextrose (anhydrous). *Electrolyte combination.*

Saluzide — *See* Opiniazide.

---

† Brand name formerly used, and/or firm no longer concerned with this product.

Salverine. $C_{19}H_{24}N_2O_2$. 312.41. 2-[2-(Diethylamino)ethoxy]-benzanilide. *UNII-BA484813BO. CAS-6376-26-7.* INN; MI. ◇*M-811*

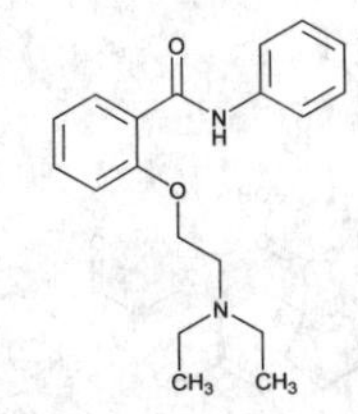

Samarium Sm 153 Lexidronam (sa mar′ ee um lex id′ roe nam). **USP** [Injection]. $C_6H_{12}N_2O_{12}P_4{}^{153}Sm$. 586.02. (1) Samarate(5-)-153Sm, [[[1,2-ethanediylbis[nitrilobis(-methylene)]]tetrakis [phosphonato]](8-)-*N,N′,OP,OP′,O-P²,OP*;p2²]-, (OC-6-21)-; (2) (OC-6-21)-[[[ethylenebis(nitrilodimethylene)]tetraphosphonato](8-)-*N,N′,OP,OP′,OP²,OP′²*]samarate (5-)-153Sm. *CAS-154427-83-5.* INN.

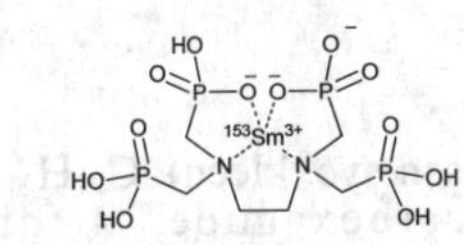

Samarium Sm 153 Lexidronam Pentasodium [*1995*] (sa mar′ ee um lex id′ roe nam pen″ ta soe′ dee um). $C_6H_{12}N_2Na_5O_{12}P_4{}^{153}Sm$. 696.01. (1) Samarate(5-)-^{153}Sm, [[[1,2-ethanediylbis[nitrilobis(methylene)]]tetrakis[phosphonato]](8-)-*N,N′,OP,OP′,OP″,OP‴*]-, pentasodium, (OC-6-21)-; (2) Pentasodium (OC-6-21)-[[[ethylenebis(nitrilodimethylene)]tetraphosphonato](8-)-*N,N′,OP,OP′,O-P″,OP‴*]samarate(5-)-^{153}Sm. *CAS-160369-78-8; CAS-154427-83-5* [samarium (^{153}Sm) lexidronam]. *Antineoplastic; radioactive agent.* Quadramet (Cytogen) ◇*CYT-424*

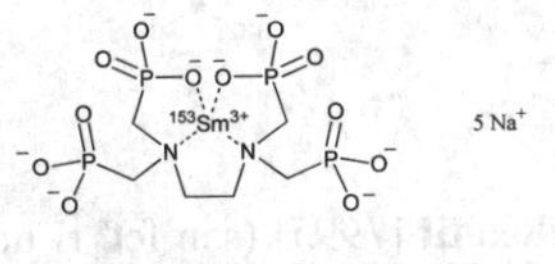

Sameridine. $C_{21}H_{34}N_2O$. 330.51. *N*-Ethyl-1-hexyl-*N*-methyl-4-phenylisonipecotamide. *UNII-NQP2Y50Y6B. CAS-143257-97-0.* INN.

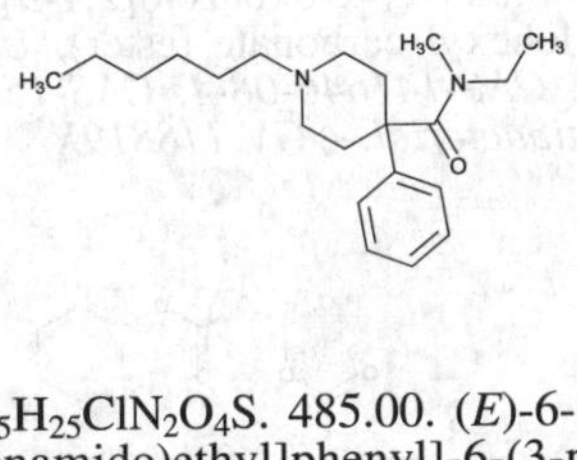

Samixogrel. $C_{25}H_{25}ClN_2O_4S$. 485.00. (*E*)-6-[*p*-[2-(*p*-Chlorobenzenesulfonamido)ethyl]phenyl]-6-(3-pyridyl)-5-hexenoic acid. *UNII-5MB73H1ADH. CAS-133276-80-9.* INN.

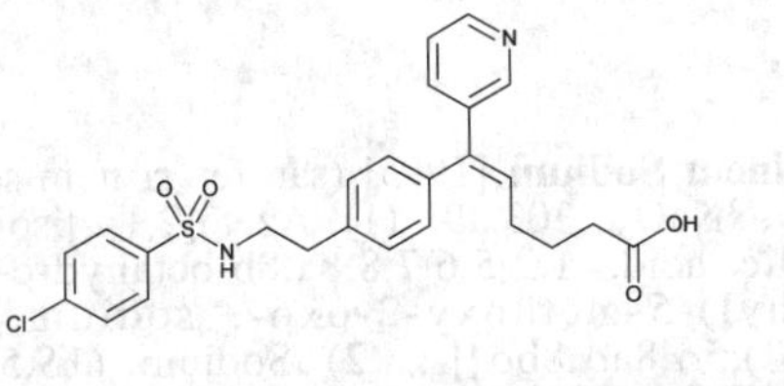

Sampatrilat. $C_{26}H_{40}N_4O_9S$. 584.68. *N*-[[1-[(*S*)-3-[(*S*)-6-Amino-2-methanesulfonamidohexanamido]-2-carboxypropyl]-cyclopentyl]carbonyl]-L-tyrosine. *CAS-129981-36-8*. INN; BAN. ◇*UK-81,252*

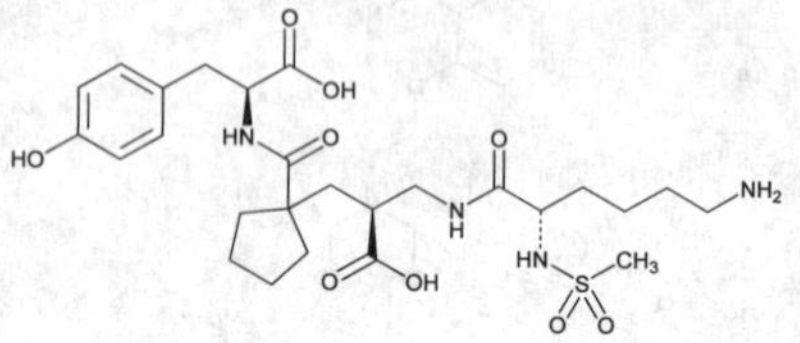

Sampirtine. $C_{12}H_{12}FN_3$. 217.24. 2,6-Diamino-3-(*p*-fluorobenzyl)pyridine *UNII-9684V5J83L. CAS-115911-28-9*. INN.

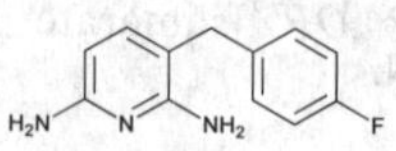

Sancycline [*1964*] (san sye′ kleen). $C_{21}H_{22}N_2O_7$. 414.41. (1) 2-Naphthacenecarboxamide, 4-(dimethylamino)-1,4,4a,5,5a,6,11,12a-octahydro-3,10,12,12a-tetrahydroxy-1,11-dioxo-, [4*S*-(4α,4aα,5aα,12aα)]-; (2) 4-(Dimethylamino)-1,4,4a,5,5a,6,11,12a-octahydro-3,10,12,12a-tetrahydroxy-1,11-dioxo-2-naphthacenecarboxamide; (3) 6-Demethyl-6-deoxytetracycline. *CAS-808-26-4*. INN. *Antibacterial.* Bonomycin (Pfizer) ◇*GS 2147; NSC-51812 [as hydrochloride]*

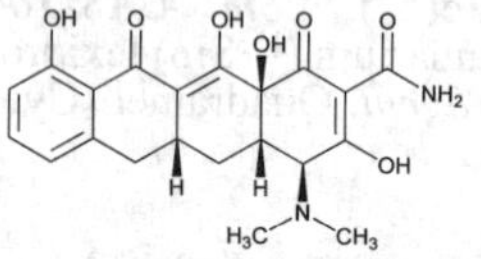

Sanfetrinem Cilexetil [*1995*] (san fet′ ri nem sye lex′ e til). $C_{23}H_{33}NO_8$. 451.51. [Sanfetrinem is INN and BAN.] (1) Azeto[2,1-*a*]isoindole-4-carboxylic acid, 1,2,5,6,7,8,8a,8b-octahydro-1-(1-hydroxyethyl)-5-methoxy-2-oxo-, 1-[[(cyclohexyloxy)carbonyl]oxy]ethyl ester; (2) 1-Hydroxyethyl (1*S*,5*S*,8a*S*,8b*R*)-1,2,5,6,7,8,8a,8b-octahydro-1-[(*R*)-1-hydroxyethyl]-5-methoxy-2-oxoazeto[2,1-*a*]isoindole-4-carboxylate, cyclohexyl carbonate (ester). *UNII-0S36458I44* [sanfetrinem]. *CAS-141646-08-4; CAS-156769-21-0* [sanfetrinem]. *Antibacterial.* ◇*GV 118819X*

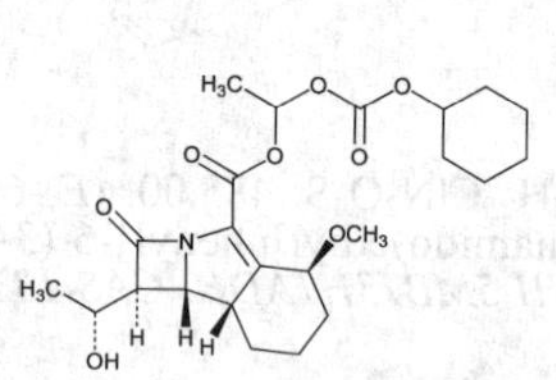

Sanfetrinem Sodium [*1995*] (san fet′ ri nem soe′ dee um). $C_{14}H_{18}NNaO_5$. 303.29. (1) Azeto[2,1-*a*]isoindole-4-carboxylic acid, 1,2,5,6,7,8,8a,8b-octahydro-1-(1-hydroxyethyl)-5-methoxy-2-oxo-, sodium salt, [1*S*-[1α(*S**),5α,8aα,8bα]]-; (2) Sodium (1*S*,5*S*,8a*S*,8b*R*)-1,2,5,6,7,8,8a,8b-octahydro-1-[(*R*)-1-hydroxyethyl]-5-me-

thoxy-2-oxoazeto[2,1-*a*]isoindole-4-carboxylate. *UNII-R0OS2S9G4U. CAS-141611-76-9. Antibacterial.* ◇*GV 104326B*

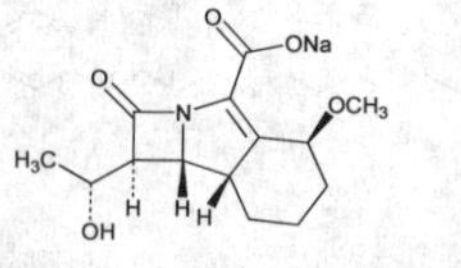

Sanguinarine Chloride (previously used name) — *See* Sanguinarium Chloride.

Sanguinarium Chloride [*1992*] (san″ gwi nar′ ee um klor′ ide). $C_{20}H_{14}ClNO_4$. 367.78. (1) [1,3]Benzodioxolo[5,6-*c*]-1,3-dioxolo[4,5-*i*]phenanthridinium, 13-methyl-, chloride; (2) Sanguinarine chloride. *UNII-B8Z8J4400H. CAS-5578-73-4*. INN. *Antifungal; anti-inflammatory; antimicrobial. [Name previously used: Sanguinarine Chloride.]*

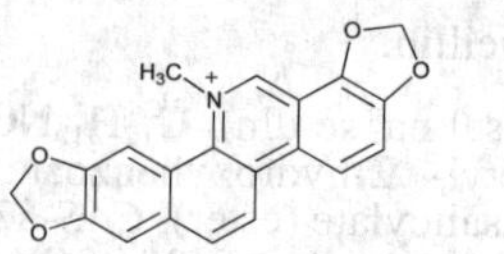

Santonin. $C_{15}H_{18}O_3$. 246.30. (3*S*,3a*S*,5a*S*)-3,5a,9-Trimethyl-3a,4,5,5a-tetrahydronaphtho[1,2-*b*]furan-2,8(3*H*,9b*H*)-dione. *CAS-481-06-1*. NF XI; JAN; MI.

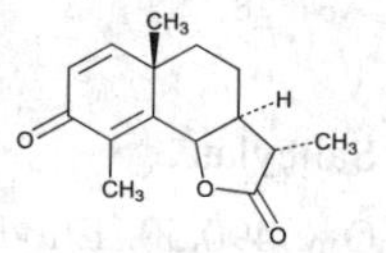

Sapacitabine. $C_{26}H_{42}N_4O_5$. 490.64. *N*-[1-(2-Cyano-2-deoxy-β-D-arabinofuranosyl]-2-oxo-1,2-dihydropyrimidin-4-yl}-hexadecanamide. *CAS-151823-14-2*. INN.

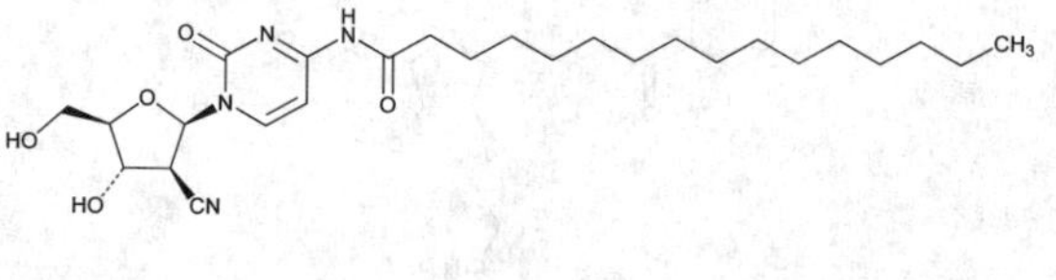

Saperconazole [*1991*] (sa″ per kon′ a zole). $C_{35}H_{38}F_2N_8O_4$. 672.72. (1) 3*H*-1,2,4-Triazol-3-one, 4-[4-[4-[4-[[2-(2,4-difluorophenyl)-2-(1*H*-1,2,4-triazol-1-ylmethyl)-1,3-dioxolan-4-yl]methoxy]phenyl]-1-piperazinyl]phenyl]-2,4-dihydro-2-(1-methylpropyl)-; (2) (±)-1-*sec*-Butyl-4-[*p*-[4-[*p*-[[(2*R**,4*S**)-2-(2,4-difluorophenyl)-2-(1*H*-1,2,4-triazol-1-ylmethyl)-1,3-dioxolan-4-yl]methoxy]phenyl]-1-piperazinyl]phenyl]-Δ²-1,2,4-triazolin-5-one. *CAS-110588-57-3*. INN; BAN. *Antifungal.* ◇*R 66905*

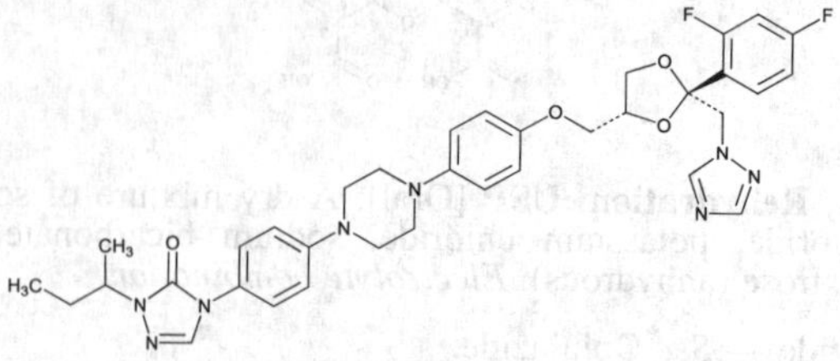

Saprisartan Potassium [*1995*] (sap″ ri sar′ tan poe tas′ ee um). $C_{25}H_{21}BrF_3KN_4O_4S$. 649.52. [Saprisartan is INN and BAN.] (1) 1*H*-Imidazole-5-carboxamide, 1-[[3-bromo-2-

[2-[[(trifluoromethyl)sulfonyl]amino]phenyl-5-benzofuranyl]methyl]-4-cyclopropyl-2-ethyl-, monopotassium salt; (2) 1-[[3-Bromo-2-[*o*-(1,1,1-(trifluoromethanesulfonamido)phenyl]-5-benzofuranyl]methyl]-4-cyclopropyl-2-ethylimidazole-5-carboxamide, monopotassium salt. *CAS-146613-90-3; CAS-146623-69-0* [saprisartan]. *Antihypertensive.* ◇*GR 138950C*

Sapropterin Dihydrochloride [*2005*] (sap″ roe ter′ in dye hye″ droe klor′ ide). $C_9H_{15}N_5O_3$·2HCl. 314.17. [Sapropterin is INN.] (1) 4(1*H*)-Pteridinone, 2-amino-6-[(1*R*,2*S*)-1,2-dihydroxypropyl]-5,6,7,8-tetrahydro-, dihydrochloride, (6*R*)-; (2) (6*R*)-2-Amino-6-[(1*R*,2*S*)-1,2-dihydroxypropyl]-5,6,7,8-tetrahydro-4(1*H*)-pteridinone dihydrochloride. *UNII-RG277LF5B3. CAS-69056-38-8; CAS-62989-33-7* [sapropterin]. *Treatment of mild-to-moderate phenylketonuria (PKU).* ◇*T1401 (BioMarin); SUN-0588 (Shiratori)*

Saquinavir [*1997*] (sa kwin′ a vir). **USP** [Capsules]. $C_{38}H_{50}N_6O_5$. 670.84. (1) [3*S*-[2[1*R**(*R**),2*S**], 3I,4aϑ,8aϑ]]-*N*¹-[3-[3-[[(1,1-Dimethylethyl)amino]carbonyl]octahydro-2(1*H*)-isoquinolinyl]-2-hydroxy-1-(phenylmethyl)propyl]-2-[(2-quinolinylcarbonyl)amino]butanediamide; (2) (*S*)-*N*-[(I*S*)-I-[(1*R*)-2-[(3*S*,4a*S*,8a*S*)-3-(*tert*-Butylcarbamoyl)octahydro-2(1*H*)-isoquinolyl]-1-hydroxyethyl]phenethyl]-2-quinaldamidosuccinamide. *UNII-L3JE09KZ2F. CAS-127779-20-8. INN; BAN. Antiviral (HIV protease inhibitor).* Fortovase (Roche) ◇*Ro 31-8959/000*

Saquinavir Mesylate [*1994*] (sa kwin′ a vir mes′ i late). **USP**. $C_{38}H_{50}N_6O_5$·CH₄O₃S. 766.95. (1) Butanediamide, *N*¹-[3-[3-[[(1,1-dimethylethyl)amino]carbonyl]octahydro-2(1*H*)-isoquinolinyl]-2-hydroxy-1-(phenylmethyl)propyl]-2-[(2-quinolinylcarbonyl)amino]-, [3*S*-[2[1*R**(*R**),2*S**], 3α,4aβ,8aβ]]-, monomethanesulfonate (salt); (2) (*S*)-*N*-[(α*S*)-α-[(1*R*)-2-[(3*S*,4a*S*,8a*S*)-3-(*tert*-Butylcarbamoyl)octahydro-2(1*H*)-isoquinolyl]-1-hydroxyethyl]phenethyl]-2-

quinaldamidosuccinamide monomethanesulfonate (salt). *UNII-UHB9Z3841A. CAS-149845-06-7. Antiviral.* Invirase (Roche) ◇*Ro 31-8959/003*

Saracatinib. $C_{27}H_{32}ClN_5O_5$. 542.03. *N*-(5-Chloro-1,3-benzodioxol-4-yl)-7-[2-(4-methylpiperazin-1-yl)ethoxy]-5-[(oxan-4-yl)oxy]quinazolin-4-amine. *CAS-379231-04-6.* INN.

Sarafloxacin Hydrochloride [*1990*] (sar″ a flox′ a sin hye″ droe klor′ ide). $C_{20}H_{17}F_2N_3O_3$·HCl. 421.83. [Sarafloxacin is INN and BAN.] (1) 3-Quinolinecarboxylic acid, 6-fluoro-1-(4-fluorophenyl)-1,4-dihydro-4-oxo-7-(1-piperazinyl)-, monohydrochloride; (2) 6-Fluoro-1-(*p*-fluorophenyl)-1,4-dihydro-4-oxo-7-(1-piperazinyl)-3-quinolinecarboxylic acid monohydrochloride. *UNII-I36JP4Q9DF. CAS-91296-87-6; CAS-98105-99-8* [sarafloxacin]. *Anti-infective (DNA gyrase inhibitor).* SaraFlox Injectable (Abbott); SaraFlox WSP (Abbott) ◇*Abbott-56620; Abbott-57135* [*sarafloxacin*]

Sarakalim. $C_{20}H_{19}F_3N_2O_4$. 408.37. *N*-[[2,2-Dimethyl-4-(2-oxo-1(2*H*)-pyridyl)-6-(trifluoromethyl)-2*H*-1-benzopyran-3-yl]methyl]acetohydroxamic acid. *UNII-2BY2U8GO3M. CAS-148430-28-8.* INN.

Saralasin Acetate [*1973*] (sar al′ a sin as′ e tate). $C_{42}H_{65}N_{13}O_{10}·xC_2H_4O_2·xH_2O$. 912.05 (base). [Saralasin is INN and BAN.] (1) Angiotensin II, 1-(*N*-methylglycine)-5-L-valine-8-L-alanine-, acetate (salt) hydrate; (2) *N*-[1-[*N*-[*N*-[*N*-[*N*-[*N*²-(*N*-Methylglycyl-L-arginyl]-L-valyl]-L-tyrosyl]-L-valyl]-L-histidyl]-L-prolyl]-L-alanine acetate (salt) hydrate. *UNII-FO21Z580M4; UNII-H2AFV2HE66* [saralasin]. *CAS-39698-78-7; CAS-54194-01-3* [anhydrous]; *CAS-34273-10-4* [saralasin]. *Antihypertensive.* Sarenin (Procter & Gamble) ◇*P-113*

$$H_3C\text{—— GRVYVHPA} \quad \cdot x\,CH_3COOH \quad \cdot x\,H_2O$$

L-Sarcolysin — *See* Melphalan.

---

† Brand name formerly used, and/or firm no longer concerned with this product.

Sarcolysin. $C_{13}H_{18}Cl_2N_2O_2$. 305.20. DL-3-[*p*-[Bis(2-chloroethyl)amino]phenyl]alanine. *UNII-A960M0G5TP. CAS-531-76-0.* INN.

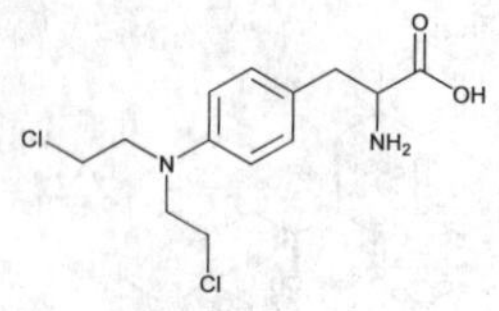

Sardomozide. $C_{11}H_{14}N_6$. 230.27. Urea azine with 1-oxo-4-indancarboxamidine. *CAS-149400-88-4.* INN.

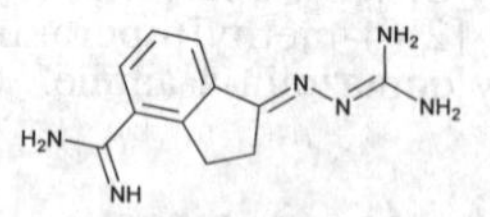

Saredutant. $C_{31}H_{35}Cl_2N_3O_2$. 552.53. *N*-[(*S*)-β-[2-(4-Acetamido-4-phenylpiperidino)ethyl]-3,4-dichlorophenethyl]-*N*-methylbenzamide. *CAS-142001-63-6.* INN.

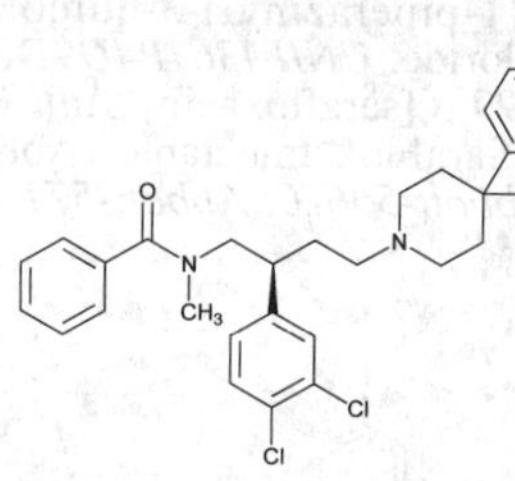

Sargramostim [*1992*] (sar gra' moe stim). **USP.** $C_{639}H_{1002}N_{168}O_{196}S_8$ (protein moiety). 14,414. A single chain, glycosylated polypeptide of 127 amino acid residues expressed from *Saccharomyces cerevisiae*. The glycoprotein is represented by three molecular species having relative molecular weights of approximately 19,500, 16,800 and 15,500 due to different levels of glycosylation. (1) Colony-stimulating factor 2 (human clone pHG$_{25}$ protein moiety), 23-L-leucine-; (2) 23-L-Leucinecolony-stimulating factor 2 (human clone pHG$_{25}$ protein moiety). *UNII-5TAA004E22. CAS-123774-72-1.* INN; BAN; JAN. *Antineutropenic; hematopoietic stimulant.* Leukine (Immunex) ◇*B1 61.012; rhu GM-CSF*

```
APARSPSPST QPWEHVNAIQ EALRLLNLSR DTAAEMNETV EVISEMFDLQ
EPTCLQTRLE LYKQGLRGSL TKLKGPLTMM ASHYKQHCPP TPETSCATQI
ITFESFKENL KDFLLVIPFD CWEPVQE
```

Saripidem. $C_{19}H_{20}ClN_3O$. 341.83. *N*-[[2-(*p*-Chlorophenyl)imidazo[1,2-*a*]pyridin-3-yl]methyl]-*N*-methylbutyramide. *UNII-0J6174G60N. CAS-103844-86-6.* INN.

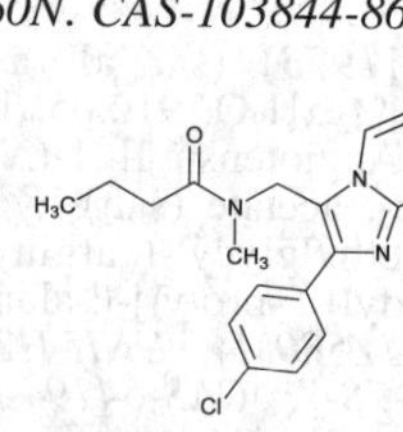

Sarizotan Hydrochloride [*2005*] (sar″ i zoe′ tan hye″ droe klor′ ide). $C_{22}H_{21}FN_2O \cdot HCl$. 384.87. [Sarizotan is INN.] (1) 3-Pyridinemethanamine, *N*-[[(2*R*)-3,4-dihydro-2*H*-1-benzopyran-2-yl]methyl]-5-(4-fluorophenyl)-, monohydrochloride; (2) (-)-*N*-[[(2*R*)-3,4-Dihydro-2*H*-1-benzopyran-2-yl)methyl]-5-(4-fluorophenyl)pyridine-3-

yl]methanamine monohydrochloride. *UNII-5P71E6YO9H; UNII-467LU0UCUW* [sarizotan]. *CAS-195068-07-6; CAS-351862-32-3* [sarizotan]; *CAS-177975-08-5* [sarizotan, replaced]. *Treatment—associated dyskinesia in Parkinson's disease.* ◇*EMD 128130*

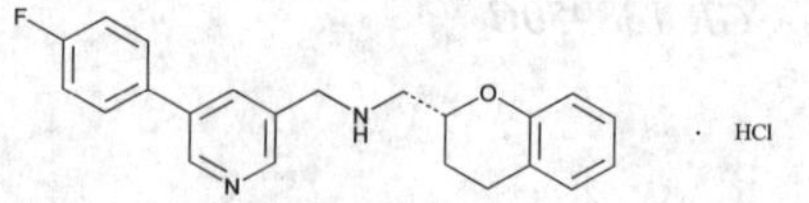

Sarmazenil. $C_{15}H_{14}ClN_3O_3$. 319.74. Ethyl 7-chloro-5,6-dihydro-5-methyl-6-oxo-4*H*-imidazo-[1,5-*a*][1,4]benzodiazepine-3-carboxylate. *UNII-F84AE7X24P. CAS-78771-13-8.* INN.

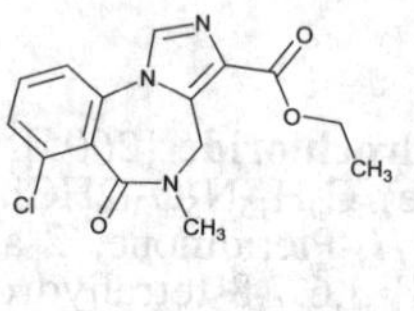

Sarmoxicillin [*1979*] (sar mox″ i sil′ in). $C_{21}H_{27}N_3O_6S$. 449.52. (1) 4-Thia-1-azabicyclo[3.2.0]heptane-2-carboxylic acid, 6-[4-(4-hydroxyphenyl)-2,2-dimethyl-5-oxo-1-imidazolidinyl]-3,3-dimethyl-7-oxo-, methoxymethyl ester, [2*S*-(2α,5α,6β)]-, (2) Methoxymethyl (2*S*,5*R*,6*R*)-6-[4-(*p*-hydroxyphenyl)-2,2-dimethyl-5-oxo-1-imidazolidinyl]-3,3-dimethyl-7-oxo-4-thia-1-azabicyclo[3.2.0]heptane-2-carboxylate. *CAS-67337-44-4.* INN. *Antibacterial.* ◇*BL-P1780*

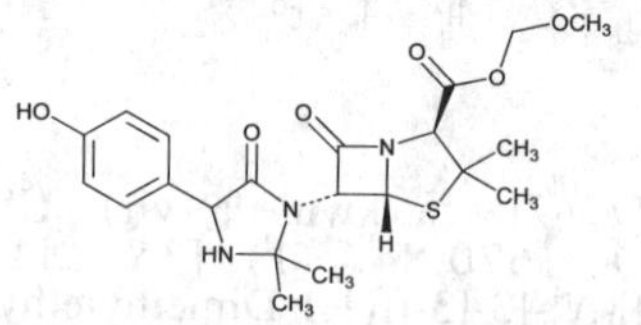

Sarpicillin [*1976*] (sar″ pi sil′ in). $C_{21}H_{27}N_3O_5S$. 433.52. (1) 4-Thia-1-azabicyclo[3.2.0]heptane-2-carboxylic acid, 6-(2,2-dimethyl-5-oxo-4-phenyl-1-imidazolidinyl)-3,3-dimethyl-7-oxo-, [2*S*-(2α,5α,6β)]-, methoxymethyl ester; (2) Methoxymethyl (2*S*,5*R*,6*R*)-6-(2,2-dimethyl-5-oxo-4-phenyl-1-imidazolidinyl)-3,3-dimethyl-7-oxo-4-thia-1-azabicyclo[3.2.0]heptane-2-carboxylate. *CAS-40966-79-8.* INN. *Antibacterial.* ◇*BL-P1761*

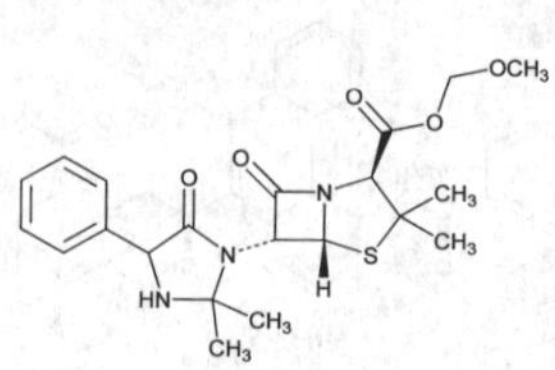

Sarpogrelate. $C_{24}H_{31}NO_6$. 429.51. [Sarpogrelate Hydrochloride is JAN.] (±)-2-(Dimethylamino)-1-[[*o*-(*m*-methoxyphenethyl)phenoxy]methyl]ethyl hydrogen succinate. *UNII-19P708E787. CAS-125926-17-2.* INN.

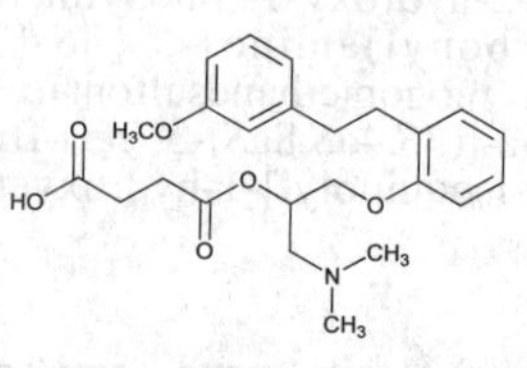

Saruplase. $C_{2031}H_{3121}N_{585}O_{601}S_{31}$. Prourokinase (enzyme activating) (human clone pUK4/pUK18), nonglycosylated. *CAS-99149-95-8.* INN; BAN.

Sasapyrine (JAN) — *See* Salsalate.

Satavaptan. $C_{33}H_{45}N_3O_8S$. 643.79. N-*tert*-Butyl-4-({cis-5′-ethoxy-4-[2-(morpholin-4-yl)ethoxy)]-2′-oxo-1′,2′-dihydrospiro[cyclohexane-1:3′-indole]-1′-yl}sulfonyl)-3-methoxybenzamide. *UNII-AJS8S3P31H. CAS-185913-78-4.* INN.

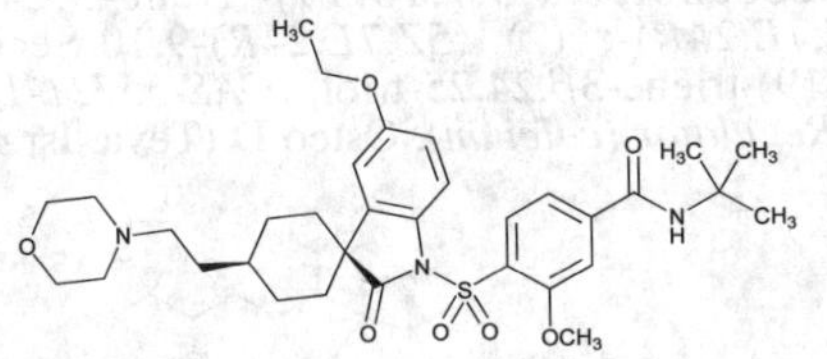

Saterinone. $C_{27}H_{30}N_4O_4$. 474.55. (±)-1,2-Dihydro-5-[*p*-[2-hydroxy-3-[4-(*o*-methoxyphenyl)-1-piperazinyl]propoxy]-phenyl]-6-methyl-2-oxonicotinonitrile. *UNII-W4P85FO7GS. CAS-102669-89-6.* INN.

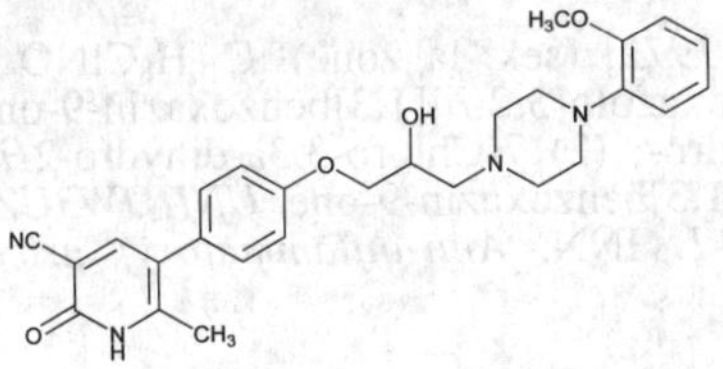

Satigrel. $C_{20}H_{19}NO_4$. 337.37. 4-Cyano-5,5-bis(*p*-methoxyphenyl)-4-pentenoic acid. *UNII-XPV71VQL72. CAS-111753-73-2.* INN.

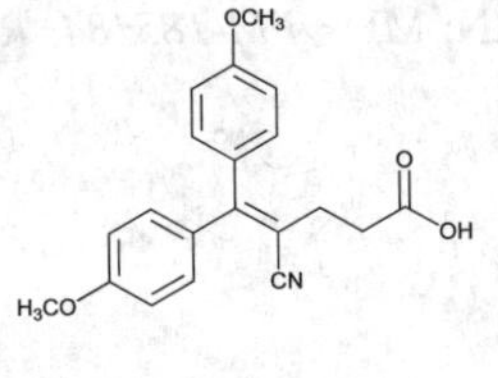

Satranidazole. $C_8H_{11}N_5O_5S$. 289.27. 1-(1-Methyl-5-nitroimidazol-2-yl)-3-(methylsulfonyl)-2-imidazolidinone. *UNII-4N7G8A6439. CAS-56302-13-7.* INN.

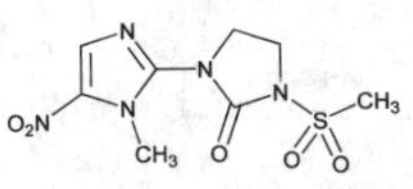

Satraplatin [*1998*] (sat″ ra pla′ tin). $C_{10}H_{22}Cl_2N_2O_4Pt$. 500.28. (1) (*OC*-6-43)-Bis(acetato-*O*)amminedichloro(cyclohexanamine)platinum; (2) (*OC*-6-43)-Bis(ac-etato)amminedichloro(cyclohexylamine)platinum. *CAS-129580-63-8.* INN. *Antineoplastic.* ◇BMS-182751; JM-216; BMY-45594

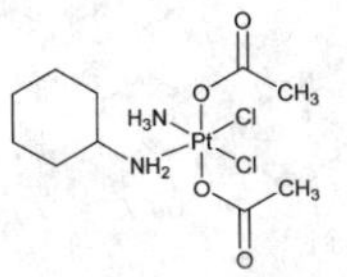

Satumomab (INN, BAN) — *See* Indium In 111 Satumomab Pendetide.

Satumomab Pendetide — *See* Indium In 111 Satumomab Pendetide.

Saviprazole. $C_{15}H_{10}F_7N_3O_2S_2$. 461.38. 2-[[[4-(2,2,3,3,4,4,4-Heptafluorobutoxy)-2-pyridyl]methyl]sulfinyl]-1*H*-thieno[3,4-*d*]imidazole. *CAS-121617-11-6.* INN.

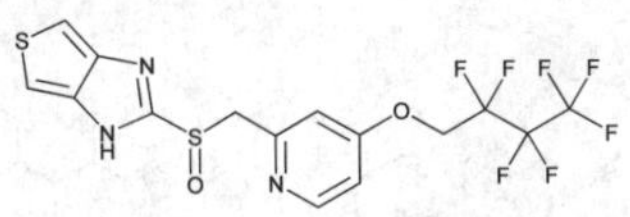

Savoxepin. $C_{25}H_{26}N_2O$. 370.49. 3-(Cyclopentylmethyl)-2,3,4,5-tetrahydro-1*H*-dibenz[2,3:6,7]oxepino[4,5-*d*]azepine-7-carbonitrile. *CAS-79262-46-7.* INN.

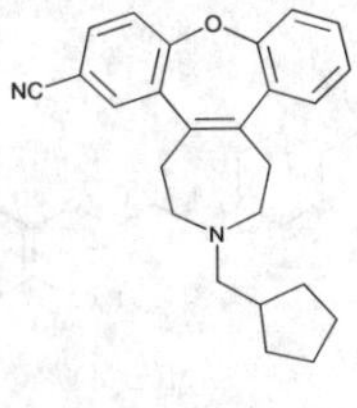

Saw Palmetto. Saw Palmetto consists of partially dried, ripe fruit of *Serenoa repens* (Bartram) Small (Fam. Arecaceae) [*Serenoa serrulatum* Schultes; *Sabal serrulata* (Michaux) Nichols]. NF XXI.

Saxagliptin [*2004*] (sax″ a glip′ tin). $C_{18}H_{27}N_3O_3$. 333.43. (1) 2-Azabicyclo[3.1.0]hexane-3-carbonitrile, 2-[(2*S*)-amino(3-hydroxytricyclo[3.3.1.1^{3,7}]dec-1-yl)acetyl]-, hydrate (1:1), (1*S*,3*S*,5*S*)-; (2) (1*S*,3*S*,5*S*)-2-[(2*S*)-Amino(3-hydroxytricyclo[3.3.1.1^{3,7}]dec-1-yl)acetyl]-2-azabicyclo[3.1.0]-hexane-3-carbonitrile monohydrate. *UNII-9GB927LAJW. CAS-945667-22-1; CAS-361442-04-8* [anhydrous]. INN. *Treatment of Type II diabetes mellitus and metabolic syndrome.* ◇BMS-477118-11

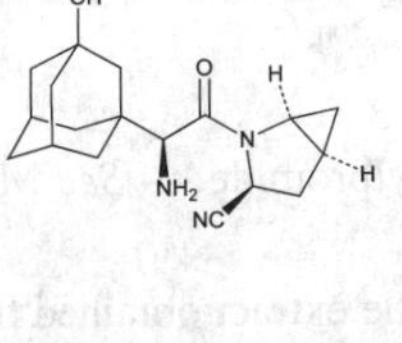

Scarlet Fever Streptococcus Toxin. AMA-DE 1973.

---

† Brand name formerly used, and/or firm no longer concerned with this product.

Scarlet Red. $C_{24}H_{20}N_4O$. 380.44. *o*-Tolylazo-*o*-tolylazo-β-naphthol. *CAS-85-83-6.* NF X; MI.

Schick Test Control. USP XXX. *Diagnostic aid (dermal reactivity indicator). [Name previously used: Diphtheria Toxin, Inactivated Diagnostic.]*

Scopafungin [*1970*] (skoe″ pa fun′ jin). $C_{59}H_{103}N_3O_{18}$·1142.46. Antibiotic derived from *Streptomyces hygroscopicus* variant. (1) Scopafungin; (2) Scopafungin. *CAS-11056-18-1. Antifungal; antibacterial.* ◇*U-29,479; NSC-107041*

Scopinast. $C_{31}H_{31}F_2NO_5$. 535.58. 7-[3-[4-[Bis(*p*-fluorophenyl)hydroxymethyl]piperidino]propoxy]-6-methoxycoumarin. *UNII-LZ9041E1BO. CAS-145574-90-9.* INN.

Scopolamine Hydrobromide (skoe pol′ a meen hye″ droe broe′ mide). USP. $C_{17}H_{21}NO_4 \cdot HBr \cdot 3H_2O$. 438.31. [Hyoscine is BAN.] (1) Benzeneacetic acid, α-(hydroxymethyl)-, 9-methyl-3-oxa-9-azatricyclo[3.3.1.0^{2,4}]non-7-yl ester, hydrobromide, trihydrate, [7(*S*)-(1α,2β,4β,5α,7β)]-; (2) 6β,7β-Epoxy-1αH,5αH-tropan-3α-ol (-)-tropate (ester) hydrobromide trihydrate. *UNII-451IFR0GXB; UNII-DL48G20X8X* [scopolamine]. *CAS-6533-68-2; CAS-114-49-8* [anhydrous]; *CAS-51-34-3* [scopolamine]. JAN. *Anticholinergic (ophthalmic).* Isopto Hyoscine (Alcon); Transderm-Scop (Ciba-Geigy†) *[Name previously used: Hyoscine Hydrobromide.]*

Scopolamine Methylbromide — *See* Methscopolamine Bromide.

Scopolia Extract. The extract obtained from the rhizome and/or root of *Scopolia japonica* Maximowicz or other species of the same genus *Solanaceae.* JAN.

^{75}Se — *See* Selenomethionine Se 75.

Sebriplatin. $C_{11}H_{20}N_2O_4Pt$. 439.37. (+)-*cis*-(1,1-Cyclobutanedicarboxylato)[(2*R*)-2-methyl-1,4-butanediamine-*N,N′*]platinum. *CAS-110172-45-7.* INN.

Secalciferol [*1989*] (se″ kal sif′ er ol). $C_{27}H_{44}O_3$. 416.64. (1) 9,10-Secocholesta-5,7,10(19)-triene-3,24,25-triol, (3β,5*Z*,7*E*,24*R*)-; (2) (5*Z*,7*E*,24*R*)-9,10-Secocholesta-5,7,10(19)-triene-3β,24,25-triol. *CAS-55721-11-4.* INN; BAN. *Regulator (calcium).* Osteo D (Teva, Israel)

Secbutabarbital (INN) **Sodium** — *See* Butabarbital Sodium.

Secbutobarbitone (previously used name) — *See* Butabarbital.

Seclazone [*1972*] (sek′ la zone). $C_{10}H_8ClNO_3$. 225.63. (1) 2*H*,9*H*-Isoxazolo[3,2-*b*][1,3]benzoxazin-9-one, 7-chloro-3,3a-dihydro-; (2) 7-Chloro-3,3a-dihydro-2*H*,9*H*-isoxazolo[3,2-*b*][1,3]benzoxazin-9-one. *UNII-JW3UZ4I1A8. CAS-29050-11-1.* INN. *Anti-inflammatory; uricosuric.* ◇*W-2354*

Secnidazole. $C_7H_{11}N_3O_3$. 185.18. α,2-Dimethyl-5-nitroimidazole-1-ethanol. *UNII-R3459K699K. CAS-3366-95-8.* INN; DCF; BAN; MI. ◇*PM-185184; RP 14539*

Secobarbital (see″ koe bar′ bi tal). USP. $C_{12}H_{18}N_2O_3$. 238.28. (1) 2,4,6(1*H*,3*H*,5*H*)-Pyrimidinetrione, 5-(1-methylbutyl)-5-(2-propenyl)-; (2) 5-Allyl-5-(1-methylbutyl)barbituric acid. *UNII-1P7H87IN75. CAS-76-73-3.* INN. *Sedative-hypnotic.* Seconal (Lilly†)

Secobarbital Sodium (see″ koe bar′ bi tal soe′ dee um). USP. $C_{12}H_{17}N_2NaO_3$. 260.26. (1) 2,4,6(1*H*,3*H*,5*H*)-Pyrimidinetrione, 5-(1-methylbutyl)-5-(2-propenyl)-, monosodium salt; (2) Sodium 5-allyl-5-(1-methylbutyl)barbiturate. *UNII-XBP604F6UM. CAS-309-43-3; CAS-76-73-3* [secobarbital]. BAN; JAN. *Sedative-hypnotic.* Seconal Sodium (Ranbaxy) *[Name previously used: Quinalbarbitone Sodium.]*

Secoverine. $C_{22}H_{35}NO_2$. 345.52. 1-Cyclohexyl-4-[ethyl(*p*-methoxy-α-methylphenethyl)amino]-1-butanone. *CAS-57558-44-8.* INN.

Secretin [*2004*] (se kree′ tin). $C_{130}H_{220}N_{44}O_{40}$ (human). 3039.41 (human); $C_{130}H_{220}N_{44}O_{41}$ (porcine). 3055.41 (porcine). CHEMICAL NAMES (human): (1) Secretin (porcine), 15-L-glutamic acid-16-glycine-; (2) L-Histidyl-L-seryl-L-α-aspartylglycyl-L-threonyl-L-phenylalanyl-L-threonyl-L-seryl-L-α-glutamyl-L-leucyl-L-seryl-L-arginyl-L-leucyl-L-arginyl-L-α-glutamylglycyl-L-alanyl-L-arginyl-L-leucyl-L-glutaminyl-L-arginyl-L-leucyl-L-leucyl-L-glutaminylglycyl-L-leucyl-L-valinamide. CHEMICAL NAMES (porcine): (1) Secretin (porcine): (2) L-Histidyl-L-seryl-L-α-aspartylglycyl-L-threonyl-L-phenylalanyl-L-threonyl-L-seryl-L-α-glutamyl-L-leucyl-L-seryl-L-arginyl-L-leucyl-L-arginyl-L-α-aspartyl-L-seryl-L-alanyl-L-arginyl-L-leucyl-L-glutaminyl-L-arginyl-L-leucyl-L-leucyl-L-glutaminylglycyl-L-leucyl-L-valinamide. *UNII-88C55N56UU. CAS-108153-74-8* [human]; *CAS-17034-35-4* [porcine]; *CAS-1393-25-5.* INN; BAN; JAN; DCF; MI. *Stimulates pancreatic and gastric secretions to aid in the diagnosis of pancreatic exocrine dysfunction and the diagnosis of gastrinoma.* Secretin-Kabi (KabiVitrum, Sweden) *[NOTE—The source of the product (human, porcine, etc.) must be indicated in the labeling.]*

HSDGTFTSEL SRLREGARLQ RLLQGLV

Securinine. $C_{13}H_{15}NO_2$. 217.26. (6*S*,11a*R*,11b*S*)-9,10,11,11a-Tetrahydro-8*H*-6,11b-methanofuro[2,3-*c*]pyrido[1,2-*a*]azepin-2(6*H*)-one. *UNII-G4VS580P5E. CAS-5610-40-2.* INN; MI.

Sedecamycin [*1987*] (se dek″ a mye′ sin). $C_{27}H_{35}NO_8$. 501.57. (1) Propanamide, *N*-[13-(acetyloxy)-7-hydroxy-1,4,10,19-tetramethyl-17,18-dioxo-16-oxabicyclo[13.2.2]nonadeca-3,5,9,11-tetraen-2-yl]-2-oxo-, [1*S*-(1*R**,2*S**,3*E*,5*E*,7*R**,9*E*,11*E*,13*R**,15*S**,19*S**)]-; (2) (-)-*N*-[(1*S*,2*R*,3*E*,5*E*,7*S*,9*E*,11*E*,13*S*,15*R*,19*R*)-7,13-Dihydroxy-1,4,10,19-tetramethyl-17,18-dioxo-16-oxabicyclo[13.2.2]nonadeca-3,5,9,11-tetraen-2-yl]pyruvamide 13-

acetate. *UNII-WLK252Z51F. CAS-23477-98-7.* INN. *Antibacterial (veterinary). [Name previously used: Bundlin.]* ◇*Ro 23-0731/000; T-2636; T-2636A*

Sedoxantrone Trihydrochloride [*1996*] (se dox′ an trone trye hye″ droe klor′ ide). $C_{21}H_{27}N_5OS.3HCl$. 506.92. (1) 2*H*-[1]Benzothiopyrano[4,3,2-*cd*]indazol-8-ol, 5-[(2-aminoethyl)amino]-2-[2-(diethylamino)ethyl]-, trihydrochloride; (2) 5-[(2-Aminoethyl)amino]-2-[2-(diethylamino)ethyl]-2*H*-[1]benzothiopyrano[4,3,2-*cd*]indazol-8-ol trihydrochloride. *CAS-119221-49-7. Antineoplastic (DNA topoisomerase II inhibitor).* ◇*CI-958*

Seganserin. $C_{29}H_{27}F_2N_3O$. 471.54. 3-[2-[4-[Bis(*p*-fluorophenyl)methylene]piperidino]ethyl]-2-methyl-4*H*-pyrido[1,2-*a*]pyrimidin-4-one. *UNII-197HL4EZCC. CAS-87729-89-3.* INN; BAN.

Segesterone. $C_{21}H_{28}O_3$. 328.45. 17-Hydroxy-16-methylene-19-norpregn-4-ene-3,20-dione. *UNII-09Q5UV3747. CAS-7690-08-6.* INN.

---

† Brand name formerly used, and/or firm no longer concerned with this product.

Seglitide Acetate [*1987*] (seg′ li tide as′ e tate). $C_{44}H_{56}N_8O_7$. $C_2H_4O_2$. 869.02. [Seglitide is INN.] Cyclo(*N*-methyl-L-alanyl-L-tyrosyl-D-tryptophyl-L-lysyl-L-valyl-L-phenylalanyl) monoacetate (salt). *CAS-99248-33-6; CAS-81377-02-8* [seglitide]. *Antidiabetic*. ◇*MK-678*

Selamectin [*1998*] (sel″ a mek′ tin). $C_{43}H_{63}NO_{11}$. 769.96. (1) 25-Cyclohexyl-4′-*O*-de(2,6-dideoxy-3-*O*-methyl-α-L-arabino-hexopyranosyl)-5-demethoxy-25-de(1-methylpropyl)-22,23-dihydro-5-(hydroxyimino)-avermectin A1a; (2) (2a*E*,4*E*,5′*S*,6*S*,6′*S*,7*S*,8*E*,11*R*,13*R*,15*S*,17a*R*,20a*R*,20b*S*)-6′-cyclohexyl-7-[(2,6-dideoxy-3-*O*-methyl-α-L-*arabino*-hexopyranosyl)oxy]-3′,4′,5′,6,6′,7,10,11,14,15,20a,20b-dodecahydro-20b-hydroxy-5′,6,8,19-tetramethylspiro[11,15-methano-2*H*,13*H*,17*H*-furo[4,3,2-*pq*][2,6]benzodioxacyclooctadecin-13,2′-[2*H*]pyran]-17,20(17a*H*)-dione 20-oxime. *UNII-A2669OWX9N*. *CAS-165108-07-6*. INN. *Antiparasitic (veterinary)*. ◇*UK-124,114*

Selegiline [*2004*] (se lej′ i leen). $C_{13}H_{17}N$. 187.28. (1) Benzeneethanamine, *N*,α-methyl-*N*-2-propynyl-, (α*R*)-; (2) (-)-(*N*)-Methyl-*N*-[(1*R*)-1-methyl-2-phenylethyl]prop-2-yn-1-amine. *UNII-2K1V7GP655*. *CAS-14611-51-9*. *Antidepressant (MAO inhibitor)*. Emsam (Somerset)

Selegiline Hydrochloride [*1992*] (se le′ ji leen hye″ droe klor′ ide). **USP**. $C_{13}H_{17}N$.HCl. 223.74. [Selegiline is INN and BAN.] (1) Benzeneethanamine, *N*,α-dimethyl-*N*-2-propynyl-, hydrochloride, (*R*)-; (2) (-)-(*R*)-*N*,α-Dimethyl-*N*-2-propynylphenethylamine hydrochloride. *UNII-6W731X367Q*. *CAS-14611-52-0; CAS-14611-51-9* [selegiline]. *Antidyskinetic; antiparkinsonian (in combination with levodopa/carbidopa)*. Eldepryl (Somerset); Zelapar (Valeant); Ensam (Somerset)

Selenious Acid (se lee′ nee us as′ id). **USP**. H_2SeO_3. 128.97. (1) Selenium dioxide, monohydrated; (2) Selenious acid. *CAS-7783-00-8*. *Supplement (trace mineral)*.

Selenium Sulfide (se lee′ nee um sul′ fide). **USP**. SeS_2. 143.09. (1) Selenium sulfide (SeS_2); (2) Selenium sulfide (SeS_2). *UNII-Z69D9E381Q*. *CAS-7488-56-4*. *Antifungal; antiseborrheic*. Selsun (Chattem)

Selenomethionine (se lee″ noe me thye′ oh neen). $C_5H_{11}NO_2Se$. 196.11. (1) Butanoic acid, 2-amino-4-(methylseleno)-, (*S*)-; (2) (*S*)-2-Amino-4-(methylselenyl)-butyric acid. *CAS-1464-42-2*.

Selenomethionine Se 75 [*1964*] (se lee″ noe me thye′ oh neen). $C_5H_{11}NO_2{}^{75}Se$. [Selenomethionine (75 Se) is INN; Selenomethionine (^{75}Se) Injection is JAN.] (1) Butanoic acid, 2-amino-4-(methylseleno-^{75}Se)-, (*S*)-; (2) (*S*)-2-Amino-4-(methylselenyl-^{75}Se)butyric acid. *UNII-P6708E7555*. *CAS-1187-56-0*. USP XXII. *Diagnostic aid (pancreas function determination); radioactive agent*. Sethotope (Bristol-Myers Squibb†)

Seletracetam [*2005*] (sel″ e tra′ se tam). $C_{10}H_{14}F_2N_2O_2$. 232.23. (1) 1-Pyrrolidineacetamide, 4-(2,2-difluoroethenyl)-α-ethyl-2-oxo-, (α*S*,4*S*)-; (2) (2*S*)-2-[(4*S*)-4-(2,2-Difluoroethenyl)-2-oxopyrrolidin-1-yl]butanamide. *UNII-RFR2CH3QZK*. *CAS-357336-74-4*. INN. *Treatment of epilepsy, hyperkinetic movement disorders*. ◇*ucb 44212*

Selfotel [*1993*] (sel′ fo tel). $C_7H_{14}NO_5P$. 223.16. (1) 2-Piperidinecarboxylic acid, 4-(phosphonomethyl)-, *cis*-; (2) *cis*-4-(Phosphonomethyl)pipecolic acid. *CAS-110347-85-8*. INN. *NMDA antagonist*. ◇*CGS 19755*

Seliciclib. $C_{19}H_{26}N_6O$. 354.45. (2*R*)-2-{[6-Benzylamino-9-(propan-2-yl)-9*H*-purin-2-yl]amino}butan-1-ol. *CAS-186692-46-6*. INN.

Selodenoson [*2004*] (sel″ oh den′ oh son). $C_{17}H_{24}N_6O_4$. 376.41. (1) β-D-Ribofuranuronamide, 1-[6-(cyclopentylamino)-9*H*-purin-9-yl]-1-deoxy-*N*-ethyl-; (2) 1-[6-(Cyclopentylamino)-9*H*-purin-9-yl]-1-deoxy-*N*-ethyl-β-D-ribofuranuronamide. *UNII-103G5E953K. CAS-110299-05-3. INN. Management of atrial fibrillation and atrial flutter.* ◇*DTI-0009*

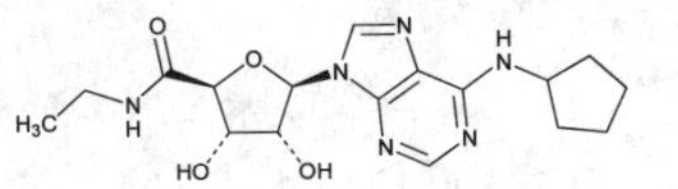

Selprazine. $C_{24}H_{31}N_3O_3$. 409.52. 6-[3-[4-(*o*-Ethoxyphenyl)-1-piperazinyl]propoxy]-3,4-dihydrocarbostyril. *UNII-VA472258QN. CAS-103997-59-7.* INN.

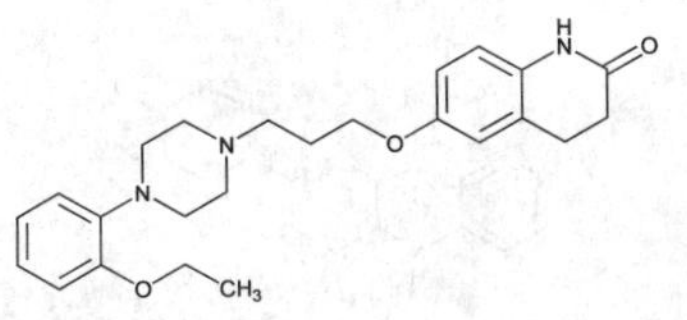

Semagacestat [*2007*] (sem″ a gas′ e stat). $C_{19}H_{27}N_3O_4$. 361.44. (1) Butanamide, 2-hydroxy-3-methyl-*N*-[(1*S*)-1-methyl-2-oxo-2-[[(1*S*)-2,3,4,5-tetrahydro-3-methyl-2-oxo-1*H*-3-benzazepin-1-yl]amino]ethyl]-, (2*S*)-; (2) (2*S*)-2-Hydroxy-3-methyl-*N*-[(2*S*)-1-{[(1*S*)-3-methyl-2-oxo-2,3,4,5-tetrahydro-1*H*-3-benzazepin-1-yl]amino}-1-oxopropan-2-yl]butanamide; (3) N^2-[(2*S*)-2-Hydroxy-3-methylbutanoyl]-N^1-[(1*S*)-3-methyl-2-oxo-2,3,4,5-tetrahydro-1*H*-3-benzazepin-1-yl]-L-alaninamide; (4) (*N*)-((*S*)-2-Hydroxy-3-methyl-butyryl)-1-(*L*-alaninyl)-(*S*)-1-amino-3-methyl-2,3,4,5-tetrahydro-1*H*-3-benzazepin-2-one. *UNII-3YN0602W4W. CAS-425386-60-3.* INN. *Treatment of Alzheimer's disease.* ◇*LY450139*

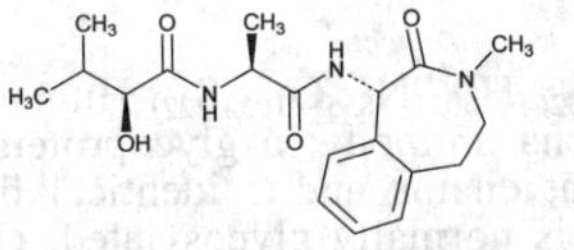

Semapimod. $C_{34}H_{52}N_{18}O_2$. 744.90. *N,N*′-Bis{3,5-bis[1-(carbamimidoylhydrazono)ethyl]phenyl}decanediamide. *CAS-352513-83-8.* INN.

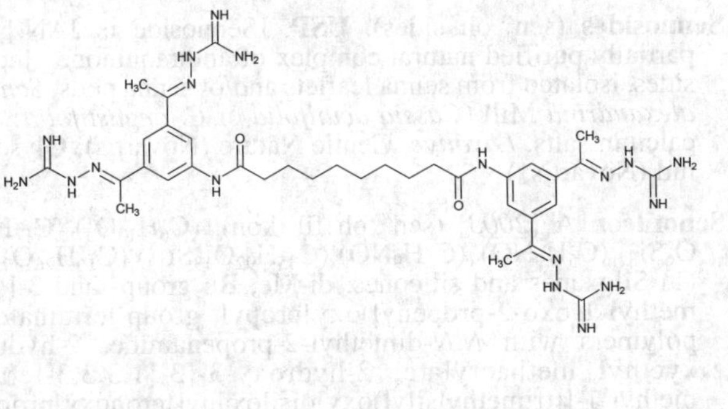

Sematilide Hydrochloride [*1988*] (se mayt′ i lide hye″ droe klor′ ide). $C_{14}H_{23}N_3O_3S \cdot HCl$. 349.88. [Sematilide is INN.] (1) Benzamide, *N*-[2-(diethylamino)ethyl]-4-[(methylsulfonyl)amino]-, monohydrochloride; (2) *N*-[2-(Diethylamino)ethyl]-*p*-methanesulfonamidobenzamide monohy-

drochloride. *CAS-101526-62-9; CAS-101526-83-4* [sematilide]. *Cardiac depressant (anti-arrhythmic).* ◇*CK-1752A*

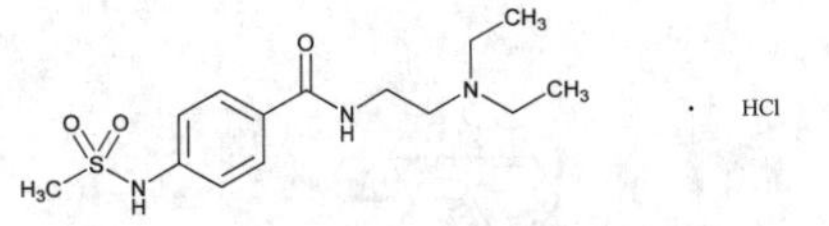

Semaxanib [*2000*] (se max′ a nib). $C_{15}H_{14}N_2O$. 238.28. (1) 2*H*-Indol-2-one, 3-[3,5-dimethyl-1*H*-pyrrol-2-yl)methylene]- 1,3-dihydro-, (*Z*)-; (2) 3-[(*Z*)-(3,5-Dimethylpyrrol-2-yl)methylene]-2-indolinone. *UNII-71IA9S35AJ. CAS-194413-58-6.* INN. *Antineoplastic (anti-angiogenic by selective inhibition of vascular endothelial growth factor-mediated Flk-1 signaling).* ◇*SU5416*

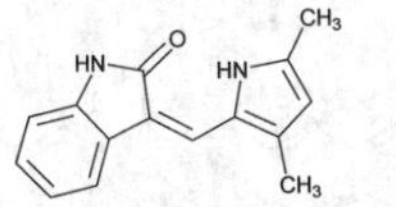

Semduramicin [*1989*] (sem dur″ a mye′ sin). $C_{45}H_{76}O_{16}$. 873.08. (1) Lonomycin A, 23,27-didemethoxy-2,6,22-tridemethyl-5,11-di-*O*-demethyl-6-methoxy-22-[(tetrahydro-5-methoxy-6-methyl-2*H*-pyran-2-yl)oxy]-, [3*R*,4*S*,5*S*,6*R*,7*S*,22*S*(2*S*,5*S*,6*R*)]-; (2) (3*R*,4*S*,5*S*,6*R*,7*S*,22*S*)-23,27-Didemethoxy-2,6,22-tridemethyl-5,11-di-*O*-demethyl-6-methoxy-22-[[(2*S*,5*S*,6*R*)-tetrahydro-5-methoxy-6-methyl-2*H*-pyran-2-yl]oxy]lonomycin A; (3) (2*R*,3*S*,4*S*,5*R*,6*S*)-Tetrahydro-2,4-dihydroxy-6-[(1*R*)-1-[(2*S*,5*R*,7*S*,8*R*,9*S*)-9-hydroxy-2,8-dimethyl-2-[(2*R*,5*S*)-tetrahydro-5-methyl-5-[(2*R*,3*S*,5*R*)-tetrahydro-5-[(2*S*,3*S*,5*R*,6*S*)-tetrahydro-6-hydroxy-3,5,6-trimethyl-2*H*-pyran-2-yl]-3-[[(2*S*,5*S*,6*R*)-tetrahydro-5-methoxy-6-methyl-2*H*-pyran-2-yl]oxy]-2-furyl]-2-furyl]-1,6-dioxaspiro[4.5]dec-7-yl]ethyl]-5-methoxy-3-methyl-2*H*-pyran-2-acetic acid. *UNII-P6VXL377WL. CAS-113378-31-7.* INN; BAN. *Coccidiostat.* ◇*UK-61,689*

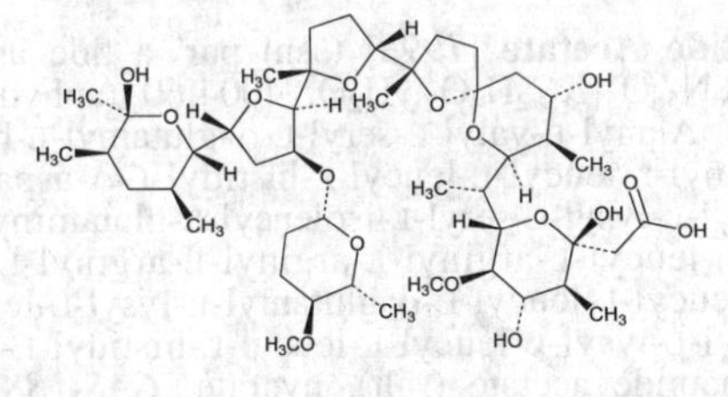

Semduramicin Sodium [*1989*] (sem dur″ a mye′ sin soe′ dee um). $C_{45}H_{75}NaO_{16}$. 895.06. (1) Lonomycin A, 23,27-didemethoxy-2,6,22-tridemethyl-5,11-di-*O*-demethyl-6-methoxy-22-[(tetrahydro-5-methoxy-6-methyl-2*H*-pyran-2-yl)oxy]-, monosodium salt, [3*R*,4*S*,5*S*,6*R*,7*S*,22*S*(2*S*,5*S*,6*R*)]-; (2) (3*R*,4*S*,5*S*,6*R*,7*S*,22*S*)-23,27-Didemethoxy-2,6,22-tridemethyl-5,11-di-*O*-demethyl-6-methoxy-22-[[(2*S*,5*S*,6*R*)-tetrahydro-5-methoxy-6-methyl-2*H*-pyran-2-yl]oxy]lonomycin A, monosodium salt; (3) Sodium (2*R*,3*S*,4*S*,5*R*,6*S*)-tetrahydro-2,4-dihydroxy-6-[(1*R*)-1-[(2*S*,5*R*,7*S*,8*R*,9*S*)-9-hydroxy-2,8-dimethyl-2-[(2*R*,5*S*)-tetrahydro-5-methyl-5-[(2*R*,3*S*,5*R*)-tetrahydro-5-[(2*S*,3*S*,5*R*,6*S*)-tetrahydro-6-hydroxy-3,5,6-trimethyl-2*H*-pyran-2-yl]-3-[[(2*S*,5*S*,6*R*)-tetrahydro-5-methoxy-6-methyl-2*H*-pyran-2-yl]oxy]-2-furyl]-2-furyl]-1,6-dioxaspiro[4.5]dec-7-yl]ethyl]-5-methoxy-3-methyl-2*H*-pyran-2-acetate. *UNII-8B50X0IVEC. CAS-119068-77-8. Coccidiostat.* ◇*UK-61,689-2*

Semi-alkaline Proteinase (JAN) — *See* Promelase.

Semisodium Valproate (BAN) — *See* Divalproex Sodium.

---

† Brand name formerly used, and/or firm no longer concerned with this product.

Semorphone. $C_{19}H_{23}NO_5$. 345.39. (-)-4,5α-Epoxy-3,14-dihydroxy-17-(2-methoxyethyl)morphinan-6-one. *UNII-2HD556171I2. CAS-88939-40-6.* INN.

Semotiadil. $C_{29}H_{32}N_2O_6S$. 536.64. (+-(R)-2-[5-Methoxy-2-[3-[methyl[2-[3,4-(methylenedioxy)phenoxy]ethyl]amino]propoxy]phenyl]-4-methyl-2H-1,4-benzothiazin-3(4H)-one. *UNII-DGN08QZ30G. CAS-116476-13-2.* INN.

Semparatide. $C_{175}H_{300}N_{56}O_{51}$. 4004.60. L-Alanyl-L-valyl-L-seryl-L-α-glutamyl-L-histidyl-L-glutaminyl-L-leucyl-L-leucyl-L-histidyl-L-α-aspartyl-L-lysylglycyl-L-lysyl-L-seryl-L-isoleucyl-L-glutaminyl-L-α-aspartyl-L-leucyl-L-arginyl-L-arginyl-L-arginyl-L-α-glutamyl-L-leucyl-L-leucyl-L-α-glutamyl-L-lysyl-L-leucyl-L-leucyl-L-α-glutamyl-L-lysyl-L-leucyl-L-histidyl-L-threonyl-L-alaninamide. *CAS-154906-40-8.* INN.

AVSEHQLLHD KGKSIQDLRR RELLEKLLEK LHTA—NH2

Semparatide Acetate [*1998*] (sem par' a tide as' e tate). $C_{175}H_{300}N_{56}O_{51} \cdot xC_2H_4O_2 \cdot yH_2O$. 4004.60 (anhydrous free base). L-Alanyl-L-valyl-L-seryl-L-α-glutamyl-L-histidyl-L-glutaminyl-L-leucyl-L-leucyl-L-histidyl-L-α-aspartyl-L-lysylglycyl-L-lysyl-L-seryl-L-isoleucyl-L-glutaminyl-L-α-aspartyl-L-leucyl-L-arginyl-L-arginyl-L-arginyl-L-α-glutamyl-L-leucyl-L-leucyl-L-α-glutamyl-L-lysyl-L-leucyl-L-α-glutamyl-L-lysyl-L-leucyl-L-leucyl-L-histidyl-L-threonyl-L-alaninamide acetate (salt), hydrate. *CAS-188106-30-1. Shorten time for fracture healing (parathyroid-hormone-related peptide).* ⬦*RS-66271-297; Ro 70-0001/001; Ro 106-6271/297*

AVSEHQLLHD KGKSIQDLRR RELLEKLLEK LHTA—NH2 · xCH3COOH · yH2O

Semuloparin Sodium. Sodium salt of a low molecular mass heparin that is obtained by phosphazene promoted depolymerization of heparin from porcine intestinal mucosa; the majority of the components have a 4-deoxy-2-O-sulfo-α-L-*threo*-hex-4-enopyranosuronic acid structure at the non-reducing end and a 2-deoxy-6-O-sulfo-2-(sulfoamino)-D-glucopyranose structure at the reducing end of their chain; the molecular mass is defined by a repartition, no more than 40% is inferior to 1600 and no more than 11% is superior to 4500 Daltons, and by a mass-average value comprised between 2000 and 3000 Daltons; the degree of sulfation is about 2.0 per disaccharidic unit. *CAS-9041-08-1.* INN.

Semustine [*1972*] (se mus' teen). $C_{10}H_{18}ClN_3O_2$. 247.72. (1) Urea, N-(2-chloroethyl)-N'-(4-methylcyclohexyl)-N-nitroso-; (2) 1-(2-Chloroethyl)-3-(4-methylcyclohexyl)-1-nitrosourea. *CAS-13909-09-6.* INN. *Antineoplastic.* ⬦*Methyl-CCNU; NSC-95441*

Senazodan. $C_{15}H_{14}N_4O$. 266.30. 6-[4-(Pyridin-4-ylamino)phenyl]-4,5-dihydropyridazin-3(2H)-one. *UNII-427L2I2KIM. CAS-98326-32-0.* INN.

Senega Syrup. JAN.

Senicapoc [*2006*] (sen" i kay' pok). $C_{20}H_{15}F_2NO$. 323.34. (1) Benzeneacetamide, 4-fluoro-α-(4-fluorophenyl)-α-phenyl-; (2) 2,2-Bis(4-fluorophenyl)-2-phenylacetamide. *UNII-TS6G201A6Q. CAS-289656-45-7.* INN. *Treatment of disorders mediated by a calcium activated intermediate conductance potassium ion channel antagonist.* ⬦*ICA-17043*

Senlizumab. $C_{3261}H_{5027}N_{855}O_{1034}S_{22}$. Humanised monoclonal anti-TNF alpha antibody; a glycoprotein consisting of 2 identical light chains and 2 identical heavy chains; the heavy chain is normally glycosylated. *CAS-336128-48-4.* BAN. ⬦*CDP571*

Senna (sen' a). **USP.** [Senna Extract is JAN.] The dried leaflet of *Senna alexandrina* Mill also known as *Cassia acutifolia* Delile (Alexandrian senna) or *C. angustifolia* Vahl (Tinnevelly senna) (Fam. Fabaceae). *Laxative.* Senokot (Purdue Frederick)

Sennosides (sen' oh sides). **USP.** [Sennoside is JAN.] A partially purified natural complex of anthraquinone glucosides, isolated from senna leaflets and/or senna pods, *Senna alexandrina* Mill (*Cassia acutifolia* or *C. angustifolia*), as calcium salts. *Laxative.* Gentle Nature (Novartis); Glysennid (Novartis†)

Senofilcon A [*2003*] (sen" oh fil' kon). $(C_6H_{10}O_3)_u(C_{17}H_{38}O_6Si_3)_v(C_5H_9NO)_w(C_6H_9NO)_x(C_{35}H_{92}O_{13}Si_{12})_y(C_{16}H_{26}O_7)_z$. (1) Siloxanes and silicones, di-Me, Bu group- and 3-[(2-methyl-1-oxo-2-propenyl)oxy]propyl group-terminated, polymers with N,N-dimethyl-2-propenamide, 2-hydroxyethyl methacrylate, 2-hydroxy-3-[3-[1,3,3,3-tetramethyl-1-[(trimethylsilyl)oxy]disiloxanyl]propoxy]propyl methacrylate, tetraethylene glycol dimethacrylate and vinylpyrrolidone; (2) Copolymer of 3-(23-butyltetracosamethyldodecasiloxanyl)propyl 2-methylprop-2-enoate (n=11), N,N-dimethylprop-2-enamide, 1-ethenylpyrrolidin-2-one, 2-hydroxyethyl 2-methylprop-2-enoate, (2RS)-2-hydroxy-3-[3-[1,3,3,3-tetramethyl-1-[(trimethylsilyl)oxy]disiloxanyl]propoxy]propyl 2-methylprop-2-enoate and oxybis(ethyleneoxyethylene) bis(2-methylprop-2-enoate). *CAS-478799-92-7. Contact lens material (hydrophilic).[-Note—The water content of the contact lens material is*

38% at ambient temperature (23±2°C), and the oxygen permeability is $103 \times 10^{-11}(cm^2/sec)(ml\ O_2/ml \times mm\ Hg)$ at 35°C (Dk value).]

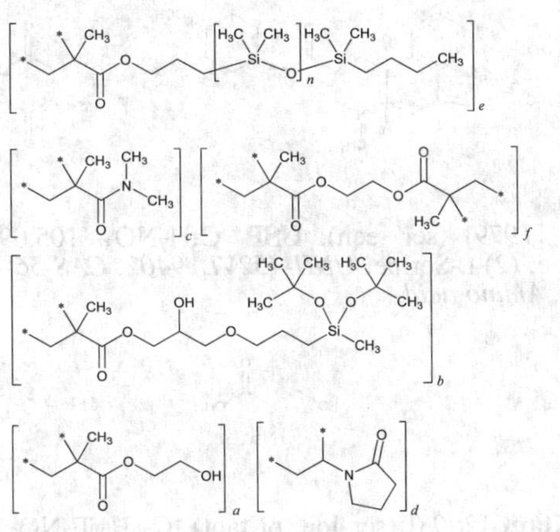

Seocalcitol. $C_{30}H_{46}O_3$. 454.68. (5Z,7E,22E,24E)-24a,26a,27a-Trihomo-9,10-secocholesta-5,7,10(19),22,24-pentaene-1α,3β,25-triol. *CAS-134404-52-7.* INN; BAN.

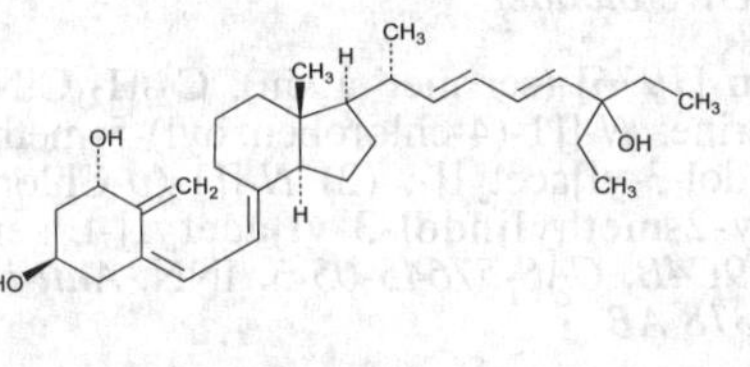

Sepazonium Chloride [*1976*] (sep a zoe′ nee um klor′ ide). $C_{26}H_{23}Cl_5N_2O$. 556.74. (1) 1*H*-Imidazolium, 1-[2-(2,4-dichlorophenyl)-2-[(2,4-dichlorophenyl)methoxy]ethyl]-3-(2-phenylethyl)-, chloride; (2) 1-[2,4-Dichloro-β-[(2,4-dichlorobenzyl)oxy]phenethyl]-3-phenethylimidazolium chloride. *UNII-54473012UK. CAS-54143-54-3.* INN; BAN. *Anti-infective, topical.* ◇R 27,500

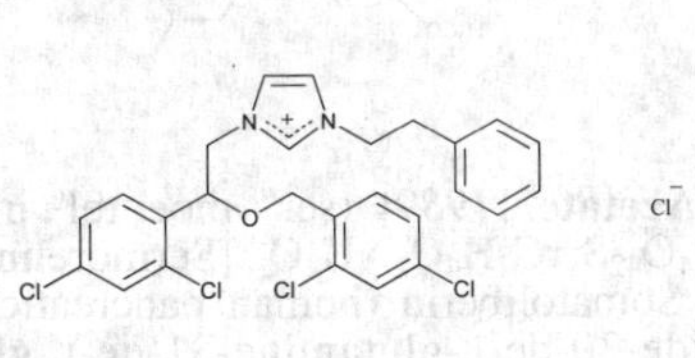

Seperidol Hydrochloride [*1968*] (se per′ i dol hye″ droe klor′ ide). $C_{22}H_{22}ClF_4NO_2.HCl$. 480.32. [Clofluperol is INN and BAN.] (1) 1-Butanone, 4-[4-[4-chloro-3-(trifluoromethyl)-phenyl]-4-hydroxy-1-piperidinyl]-1-(4-fluorophenyl)-, hydrochloride; (2) 4-[4-(4-Chloro-α,α,α-trifluoro-*m*-tolyl)-4-hydroxypiperidino]-4′-fluorobutyrophenone hydrochloride. *CAS-17230-87-4; CAS-10457-91-7* [seperidol]. *Antipsychotic.* ◇R 9298

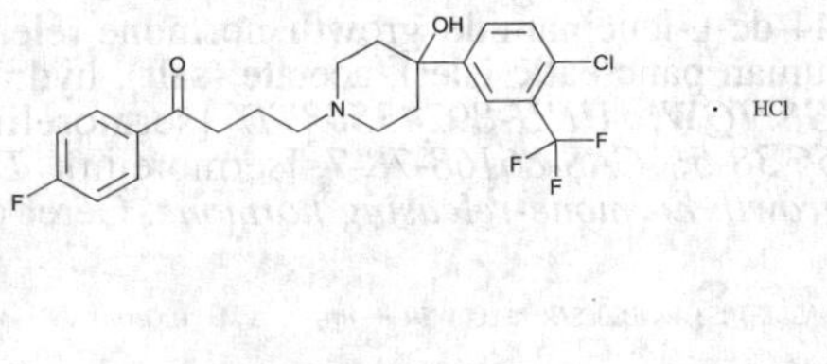

Sepimostat. $C_{21}H_{19}N_5O_2$. 373.41. 6-Amidino-2-naphthyl *p*-(2-imidazolin-2-ylamino)benzoate. *UNII-5ZFR16F4QQ. CAS-103926-64-3.* INN.

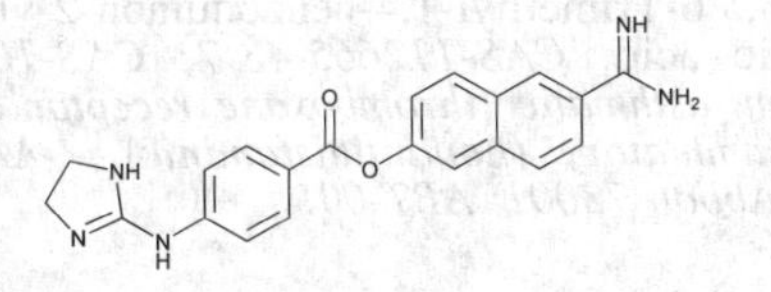

Seprilose [*1994*] (sep′ ri lose). $C_{16}H_{30}O_6$. 318.41. (1) α-D-Glucofuranose, 3-*O*-heptyl-1,2-*O*-(1-methylethylidene)-; (2) 3-*O*-Heptyl-1,2-*O*-isopropylidene-α-D-glucofuranose. *CAS-133692-55-4.* INN. *Antirheumatic.* ◇GW-80126

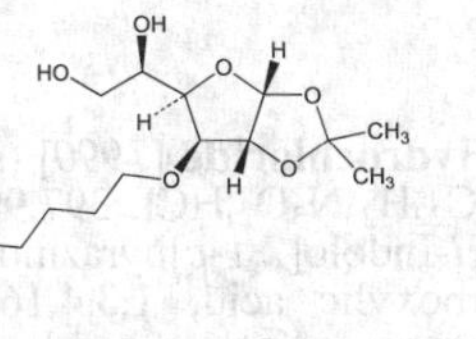

Seproxetine Hydrochloride [*1991*] (se prox′ e teen hye″ droe klor′ ide). $C_{16}H_{16}F_3NO.HCl$. 331.76. [Seproxetine is INN.] (1) Benzenepropanamine, γ-[4-(trifluoromethyl)phenoxy]-, hydrochloride, (*S*)-; (2) (*S*)-3-Phenyl-3-[(α,α,α-trifluoro-*p*-tolyl)oxy]propylamine hydrochloride. *UNII-K4QYN23H2N; UNII-25CO3X0R31* [seproxetine]. *CAS-127685-30-7; CAS-126924-38-7* [seproxetine]. *Antidepressant.* ◇LY215229 hydrochloride

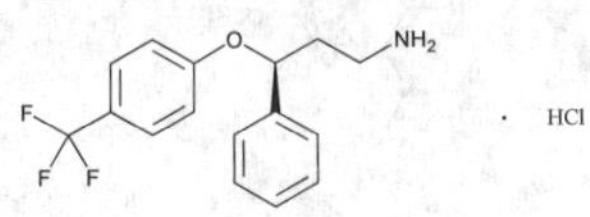

Septomonab (previously used name) — *See* Nebacumab.

Sequifenadine. $C_{22}H_{27}NO$. 321.46. α,α-Di-*o*-tolyl-3-quinu-clidinemethanol. *UNII-C7Q3TBR3FP. CAS-57734-69-7.* INN.

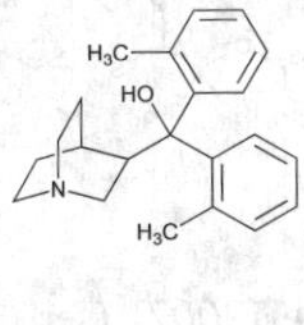

Seractide Acetate [*1974*] (ser ak′ tide as′ e tate). $C_{207}H_{308}N_{56}O_{58}S.(C_2H_4O_2)_x.xH_2O$. 4541.07 (base). [Seractide is INN and BAN.] (1) α^{1-39}-Corticotropin (pig), 25-L-aspartic acid-26-L-alanine-27-glycine-30-L-glutamine-31-L-serine-, acetate (salt) hydrate; (2) L-Seryl-L-tyrosyl-L-seryl-L-methionyl-L-α-glutamyl-L-histidyl-L-phenylala-nyl-L-arginyl-L-tryptophylglycyl-L-lysyl-L-prolyl-L-valyl-glycyl-L-lysyl-L-lysyl-L-arginyl-L-arginyl-L-prolyl-L-va-lyl-L-lysyl-L-valyl-L-tyrosyl-L-prolyl-L-α-aspartyl-L-ala-nylglycyl-L-α-glutamyl-L-α-aspartyl-L-glutaminyl-L-ser-yl-L-alanyl-L-α-glutamyl-L-alanyl-L-phenylalanyl-L-pro-lyl-L-leucyl-L-α-glutamyl-L-phenylalanine acetate (salt) hydrate. *UNII-DI9132OQ3R; UNII-IGM44CEY2I* [serac-tide]. *CAS-39295-97-1; CAS-39294-79-6* [anhydrous]; *CAS-63304-56-3* [seractide]. *Hormone (adrenocorticotropic).* Acthar Gel-Synthetic (Armour)

SYSMEHFRWG KPVGKKRRPV KVYPDAGEDQ SAEAFPLEF · CH_3COOH · xH_2O

---

† Brand name formerly used, and/or firm no longer concerned with this product.

Seratrodast [*1995*] (ser a′ troe dast). $C_{22}H_{26}O_4$. 354.44. (1) Benzeneheptanoic acid, ζ-(2,4,5-trimethyl-3,6-dioxo-1,4-cyclohexadien-1-yl)-, (±)-; (2) (±)-2,4,5-Trimethyl-3,6-dioxo-ζ-phenyl-1,4-cyclohexadiene-1-heptanoic acid; (3) (±)-7-(3,5,6-Trimethyl-1,4-benzoquinon-2-yl)-7-phenyl-heptanoic acid. *CAS-112665-43-7; CAS-103186-19-2.* INN. *Anti-asthmatic (thromboxane receptor antagonist); anti-inflammatory (nonantihistaminic).* ◇*AA-2414; A-73001; Abbott-73001; ABT-001*

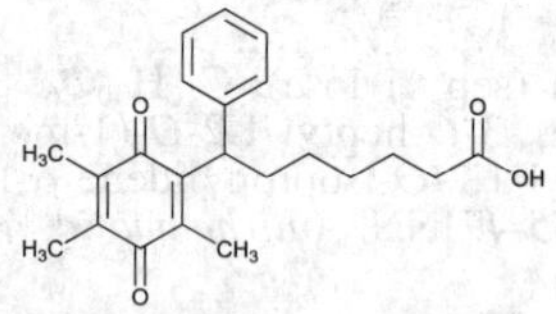

Serazapine Hydrochloride [*1990*] (ser az′ a peen hye″ droe klor′ ide). $C_{22}H_{23}N_3O_2.HCl$. 397.90. [Serazapine is INN.] (1) 2*H*,10*H*-Indolo[2,1-*c*]pyrazino[1,2-*a*][1,4]benzodiazepine-16-carboxylic acid, 1,3,4,16b-tetrahydro-2-methyl-, methyl ester, monohydrochloride; (2) (±)-Methyl 1,3,4,16b-tetrahydro-2-methyl-2*H*,10*H*-indolo[2,1-*c*]pyrazino[1,2-*a*][1,4]benzodiazepine-16-carboxylate, monohydrochloride. *CAS-117581-05-2; CAS-115313-22-9* [serazapine]. *Anti-anxiety agent.* ◇*CGS 15040A*

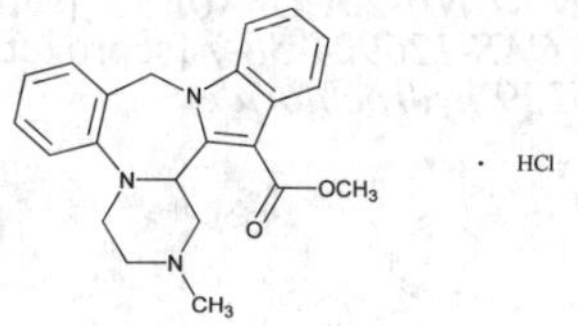

Serfibrate. $C_{16}H_{20}ClNO_5S$. 373.85. 2-Acetamido-4-mercaptobutyric acid 2-(*p*-chlorophenoxy)-2-methylpropionate (ester). *UNII-910906N64M. CAS-54657-98-6.* INN.

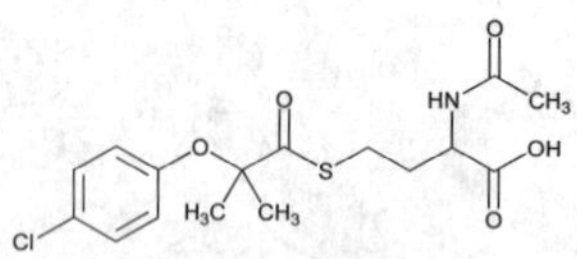

Sergliflozin Etabonate [*2007*] (ser″ gli floe′ zin et″ a boe′ nate). $C_{23}H_{28}O_9$. 448.46. (1) β-D-Glucopyranoside, 2-[(4-methoxyphenyl)methyl]phenyl, 6-(ethyl carbonate); (2) 2-(4-Methoxybenzyl)phenyl 6-*O*-(ethoxycarbonyl)-β-D-glucopyranoside. *CAS-408504-26-7.* INN. *Treatment of type 2 diabetes.* ◇*GW869682X*

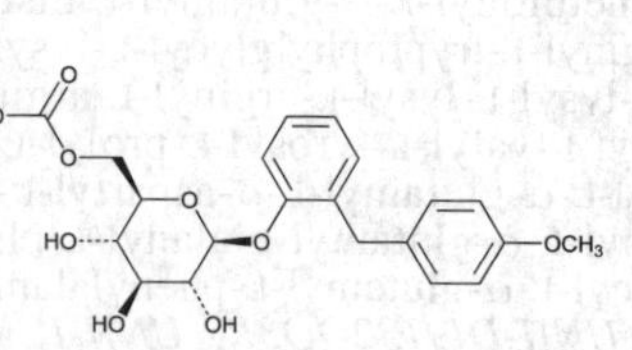

Sergolexole Maleate [*1989*] (ser″ goe lex′ ole mal′ ee ate). $C_{26}H_{36}N_2O_3.C_4H_4O_4$. 540.65. [Sergolexole is INN.] (1) Ergoline-8-carboxylic acid, 6-methyl-1-(1-methylethyl)-, 4-methoxycyclohexyl ester, [8β(*trans*)]-, (*Z*)-2-butenedioate (1:1); (2) *trans*-4-Methoxycyclohexyl 1-isopropyl-6-

methylergoline-8β-carboxylate, maleate (1:1). *CAS-108674-87-9; CAS-108674-86-8* [sergolexole]. *Antimigraine.* ◇*LY281067*

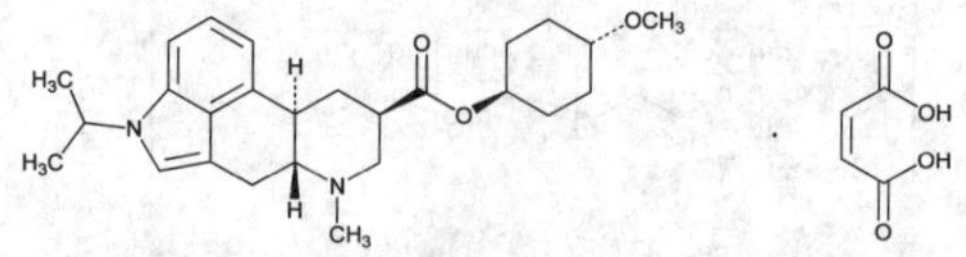

Serine [*1979*] (ser′ een). **USP.** $C_3H_7NO_3$. 105.09. (1) L-Serine; (2) L-Serine. *UNII-452VLY9402. CAS-56-45-1* [L]. INN. *Amino acid.*

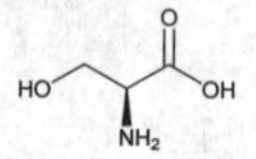

Serlopitant [*2008*] (ser loe′ pi tant). $C_{29}H_{28}F_7NO_2$. 555.53. (1) 2-Cyclopenten-1-one, 3-[(3a*R*,4*R*,5*S*,7a*S*)-5-[(1*R*)-1-[3,5-bis(trifluoromethyl)phenyl]ethoxy]-4-(4-fluorophenyl)octahydro-2*H*-isoindol-2-yl]-; (2) 3-[(3a*R*,4*R*,5*S*,7a*S*)-5-{(1*R*)-1-[3,5-bis(trifluoromethyl)phenyl]ethoxy}-4-(4-fluorophenyl)octahydro-2*H*-isoindol-2-yl]cyclopent-2-en-1-one. *UNII-277V92K32B. CAS-860642-69-9. Treatment of overactive bladder.*

Sermetacin [*1976*] (ser met′ a sin). $C_{22}H_{21}ClN_2O_6$. 444.86. (1) L-Serine, *N*-[[1-(4-chlorobenzoyl)-5-methoxy-2-methyl-1*H*-indol-3-yl]acetyl]-; (2) *N*-[[1-(*p*-Chlorobenzoyl)-5-methoxy-2-methylindol-3-yl]acetyl]-L-serine. *UNII-04O7H69C4B. CAS-57645-05-3.* INN. *Anti-inflammatory.* ◇*SH G 318 AB*

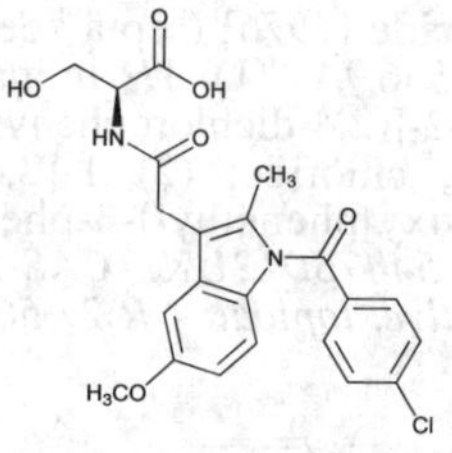

Sermorelin Acetate [*1989*] (ser″ moe rel′ in as′ e tate). $C_{149}H_{246}N_{44}O_{42}S.xC_2H_4O_2.yH_2O$. [Sermorelin is INN and BAN.] (1) Somatoliberin (human pancreatic islet), 29-L-argininamide-30-de-L-glutamine-31-de-L-glutamine-32-deglycine-33-de-L-glutamic acid-34-de-L-serine-35-de-L-asparagine-36-de-L-glutamine-37-de-L-glutamic acid-38-de-L-arginine-39-deglycine-40-de-L-alanine-41-de-L-arginine-42-de-L-alanine-43-de-L-arginine-44-de-L-leucinamide-, acetate (salt), hydrate; (2) Growth hormone-releasing factor (human)-(1-29)-peptide amide, acetate (salt), hydrate; (3) 29-L-Argininamide-30-de-L-glutamine-31-de-L-glutamine-32-deglycine-33-de-L-glutamic acid-34-de-L-serine-35-de-L-asparagine-36-de-L-glutamine-37-de-L-glutamic acid-38-de-L-arginine-39-deglycine-40-de-L-alanine-41-de-L-arginine-42-de-L-alanine-43-de-L-arginine-44-de-L-leucinamide growth hormone-releasing factor (human pancreatic islet), acetate (salt), hydrate. *UNII-00IBG87IQW; UNII-89243S03TE* [sermorelin]. *CAS-114466-38-5; CAS-86168-78-7* [sermorelin]. *Diagnostic aid; growth hormone-releasing hormone.* Geref (Serono)

YADAIFTNSY RKVLGQLSAR KLLQDIMSR —NH₂   · x CH₃COOH   · y H₂O

Serrapeptase. A proteolytic enzyme derived from *Serratia sp.*E15. *CAS-37312-62-2.* INN; JAN; DCF.

Sertaconazole. $C_{20}H_{15}Cl_3N_2OS$. 437.77. ($\pm$)-1-[2,4-Dichloro-β-[(7-chlorobenzo[*b*]thien-3-yl)methoxy]phenethyl]imidazole. *UNII-72W71I16EG. CAS-99592-32-2.* INN; BAN.

Sertindole [*1992*] (ser tin′ dole). $C_{24}H_{26}ClFN_4O$. 440.94. (1) 2-Imidazolidinone, 1-[2-[4-[5-chloro-1-(4-fluorophenyl)-1*H*-indol-3-yl]-1-piperidinyl]ethyl]-; (2) 1-[2-[4-[5-Chloro-1-(*p*-fluorophenyl)indol-3-yl]piperidino]ethyl]-2-imidazolidinone. *UNII-GVV4Z879SP. CAS-106516-24-9.* INN; BAN. *Antipsychotic; neuroleptic.* SerLect (Abbott) ◇*Lu 23-174*

Sertraline Hydrochloride [*1983*] (ser′ tra leen hye″ droe klor′ ide). $C_{17}H_{17}Cl_2N\cdot HCl$. 342.69. [Sertraline is INN and BAN.] (1) 1-Naphthalenamine, 4-(3,4-dichlorophenyl)-1,2,3,4-tetrahydro-*N*-methyl-, hydrochloride, (1*S-cis*)-; (2) (1*S,4S*)-4-(3,4-Dichlorophenyl)-1,2,3,4-tetrahydro-*N*-methyl-1-naphthylamine hydrochloride. *UNII-UTI8907Y6X; UNII-QUC7NX6WMB* [sertraline]. *CAS-79559-97-0; CAS-79617-96-2* [sertraline]. *Antidepressant.* Zoloft (Pfizer) ◇*Cp-51,974-1*

Serum Albumin, Iodinated (^{125}I) Human (INN) — *See* Albumin, Iodinated I 125 Serum.

Sesame Oil (ses′ a me). **NF**. The refined fixed oil obtained from the seed of one or more cultivated varieties of *Sesamum indicum* Linné (Fam. Pedaliaceae). *UNII-QX10HYY4QV. CAS-8008-74-0.* JAN. *Pharmaceutic aid (solvent); pharmaceutic aid (vehicle, oleaginous).*

Setastine. $C_{22}H_{28}ClNO$. 357.92. 1-[2-[(*p*-Chloro-α-methyl-α-phenylbenzyl)oxy]ethyl]hexahydro-1*H*-azepine. *UNII-6G3OCF528J. CAS-64294-95-7.* INN; MI.

Setazindol. $C_{15}H_{16}ClNO$. 261.75. 4′-Chloro-2-[(methylamino)methyl]benzhydrol. *UNII-92D9H0A3WN. CAS-56481-43-7.* INN; BAN.

Setipafant. $C_{26}H_{23}ClN_6O_2S$. 519.02. 6-(*o*-Chlorophenyl)-7,10-dihydro-1-methyl-4*H*-pyrido[4′,3′:4,5]thieno[3,2-*f*]-*s*-triazolo[4,3-*a*][1,4]diazepine-9(8*H*)-carbox-*p*-anisidide. *UNII-UFN2Q54HS6. CAS-132418-35-0.* INN.

Setiptiline. $C_{19}H_{19}N$. 261.36. [Setiptiline Maleate is JAN.] 2,3,4,9-Tetrahydro-2-methyl-1*H*-dibenzo[3,4:6,7]cyclohepta[1,2-*c*]pyridine. *UNII-7L38105Z6E. CAS-57262-94-9.* INN.

Setoperone [*1985*] (se toe′ per one). $C_{21}H_{24}FN_3O_2S$. 401.50. (1) 5*H*-Thiazolo[3,2-*a*]pyrimidin-5-one, 6-[2-[4-(4-fluorobenzoyl)-1-piperidinyl]ethyl]-2,3-dihydro-7-methyl-; (2) 6-[2-[4-(*p*-Fluorobenzoyl)piperidino]ethyl]-2,3-dihydro-7-methyl-5*H*-thiazolo[3,2-α]pyrimidin-5-one. *UNII-BQ67CS3Q3E. CAS-86487-64-1.* INN. *Antipsychotic.* ◇*R 52,245*

Sevelamer Carbonate [*2006*] (se vel′ a mer kar′ bo nate). $[(C_3H_7N)_m(C_3H_5ClO)_n]\cdot xCH_2O_3$. (1) Carbonic acid, compound with (chloromethyl)oxirane polymer with 2-propen-1-amine; (2) Prop-2-en-1-amine polymer with (chloromethyl)oxirane carbonate. *UNII-9YCX42I8IU. CAS-845273-93-0. Control of serum phosphorus in patients with chronic kidney disease (phosphate binder).* ◇*GT335-012*

Sevelamer Hydrochloride [*1997*] (se vel′ a mer hye″ droe klor′ ide). $(C_3H_7N)_m(C_3H_5ClO)_n\cdot xHCl$. [Sevelamer is INN and BAN.] (1) 2-Propen-1-amine polymer with (chloromethyl)oxirane, hydrochloride; (2) Allylamine polymer with 1-chloro-2,3-epoxypropane, hydrochloride. *UNII-*

---

† Brand name formerly used, and/or firm no longer concerned with this product.

GLS2PGI8QG. CAS-182683-00-7; CAS-52757-95-6 [seve-lamer]. *Antihyperphosphatemic.* Renagel (Genzyme) ◇*GT16-026A*

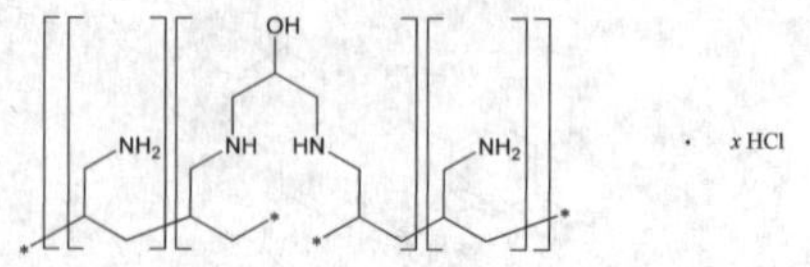

Sevirumab [*1993*] (se vir′ ue mab). (1) Immunoglobulin G 1 (human monoclonal EV2-7 anti-cytomegalovirus), disulfide with human monoclonal EV2-7 κ-chain, dimer; (2) Immunoglobulin G 1 (human monoclonal EV2-7 anti-cytomegalovirus), disulfide with human monoclonal EV2-7 κ-chain, dimer. Molecular weight is approximately 150,000 daltons. *CAS-138660-96-5.* INN. *Monoclonal antibody (antiviral).* ◇*EV2-7; SDZ MSL 109*

Sevitropium Mesilate. $C_{24}H_{29}NO_5S_2$. 475.62. (±)-3α-[(6,11-Dihydrodibenzo[*b,e*]thiepin-11-yl)oxy]-6β,7β-epoxy-8-methyl-1αH,5αH-tropanium methanesulfonate. *CAS-88199-75-1.* INN.

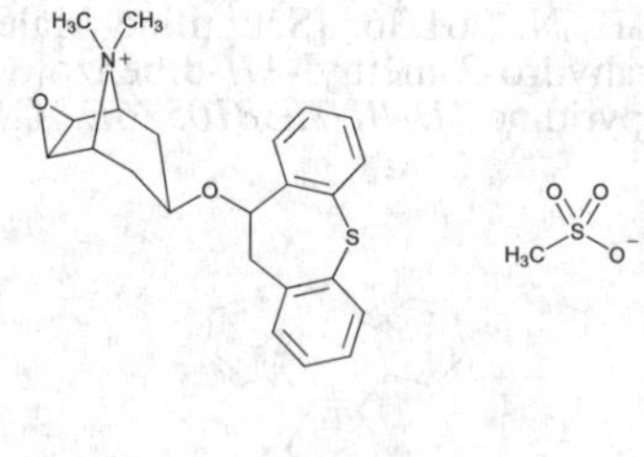

Sevoflurane [*1971*] (see″ voe floo′ rane). $C_4H_3F_7O$. 200.05. (1) Propane, 1,1,1,3,3,3-hexafluoro-2-(fluoromethoxy)-; (2) Fluoromethyl 2,2,2-trifluoro-1-(trifluoromethyl)ethyl ether. *UNII-38LVP0K73A. CAS-28523-86-6.* INN; BAN; JAN. *Anesthetic (inhalation).* Ultane (Abbott) ◇*MR6S4*

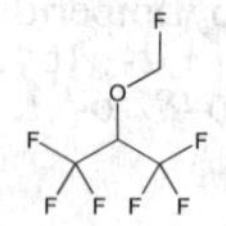

Sevopramide. $C_{29}H_{43}N_3O_3$. 481.67. (±)-α-Benzamido-*p*-[3-(diethylamino)propoxyl]-*N,N*-dipropylhydrocinnamamide. *UNII-18USM69UB1. CAS-57227-17-5.* INN.

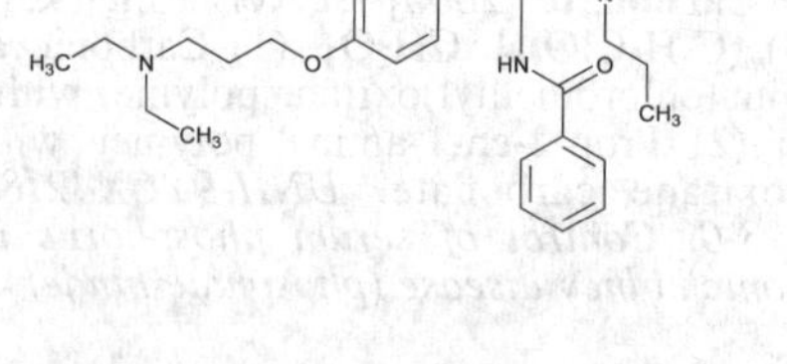

Sezolamide Hydrochloride [*1990*] (se zoe′ la mide hye″ droe klor′ ide). $C_{11}H_{18}N_2O_4S_3$.HCl. 374.93. [Sezolamide is INN.] (1) 4*H*-Thieno[2,3-*b*]thiopyran-2-sulfonamide, 5,6-dihydro-4-[(2-methylpropyl)amino]-, 7,7-dioxide, mono-hydrochloride, (*S*)-; (2) (+)-(*S*)-5,6-Dihydro-4-(isobutyla-mino)-4*H*-thieno[2,3-*b*]thiopyran-2-sulfonamide, 7,7-

dioxide, monohydrochloride. *CAS-119271-78-2; CAS-123308-22-5* [sezolamide]. *Carbonic anhydrase inhibitor.* ◇*MK-417*

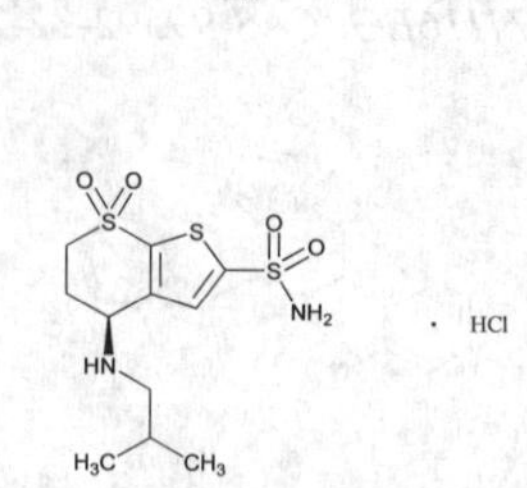

Sfericase. Alkaline *Bacillus sphaericus* proteinase. *CAS-63551-77-9.* INN.

Shellac (she lak′). **NF.** Obtained by the purification of Lac, the resinous secretion of the insect *Laccifer Lacca Kerr* (Fam. Coccidae). *Pharmaceutic aid (tablet coating agent).*

Siagoside. $C_{73}H_{129}N_3O_{30}$. 1528.81. *N*-(ll³-*N*-Acetylneurami-nosylgangliotetraosyl)ceramide, intramolecular ester. *CAS-100345-64-0.* INN.

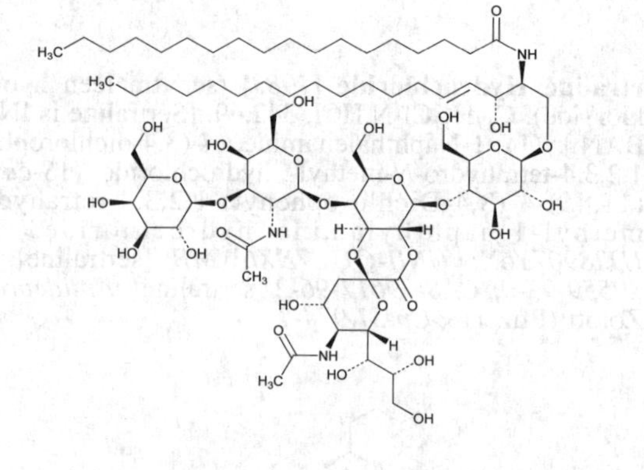

Sibenadet Hydrochloride [*2002*] (si ben′ a det hye″ droe klor′ ide). $C_{22}H_{28}N_2O_5S_2$.HCl. 501.06. [Sibenadet is INN and BAN.] (1) 2 (3*H*)-Benzothiazolone, 4-hydroxy-7-[2-[[2-[[3-(2-phenylethoxy)propyl]sulfonyl]ethyl]ami-no]ethyl]-, monohydrochloride; (2) 4-Hydroxy-7-[2-[2-[3-phenylethoxy-propane-1-sulfonyl]-ethylamino]ethyl]-3*H*-benzothiazol-2-one, hydrochloride; (3) 4-Hydroxy-7-[2-[[2-[[3-(2-phenylethoxy)propyl]sulfonyl]ethyl]ami-no]ethyl]-1,3-benzothiazol-2(3*H*)-one, hydrochloride. *UNII-659OIV373Y; UNII-N32934RHGW* [sibenadet]. *CAS-154189-24-9; CAS-154189-40-0* [sibenadet]. *Treatment of symptoms of Chronic Obstructive Pulmonary Disease.* Viozan (AstraZeneca) ◇*AR-C68397AA*

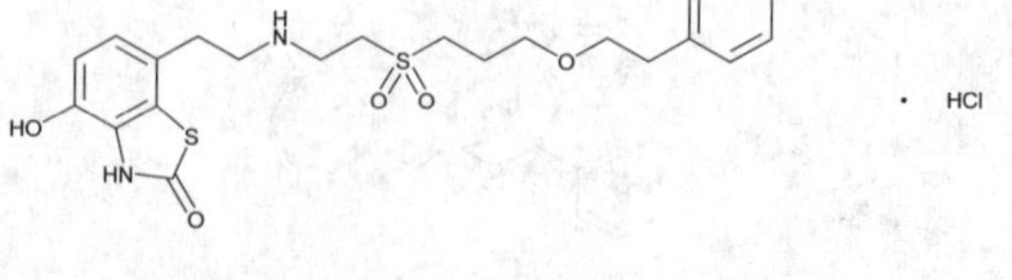

Sibopirdine [*1993*] (si boe′ pir deen). $C_{23}H_{18}N_4$.H_2O. 368.43. (1) 5*H*-Cyclopenta[2,1-*b*:3,4-*b*′]dipyridine, 5,5-bis(4-pyri-dinylmethyl)-, monohydrate; (2) 5,5-Bis(4-pyridylmethyl)-5*H*-cyclopenta[2,1-*b*:3,4-*b*′]dipyridine monohydrate.

UNII-RAG2185DR1. CAS-139781-09-2. INN. *Alzheimer's disease treatment (cognition enhancer); nootropic.* ◇*DuP 921*

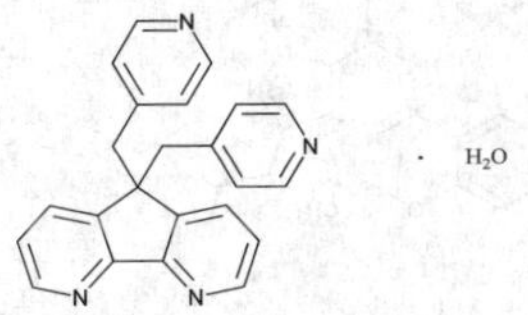

Sibrafiban [*1997*] (si″ bra fye′ ban). $C_{20}H_{28}N_4O_6$. 420.46. (1) Acetic acid, [[1-[2-[[4-[amino(hydroxyimino)methyl]benzoyl]amino]-1-oxopropyl]-4-piperidinyl]oxy]-, ethyl ester, [*S*-(*Z*)]-; (2) Ethyl (*Z*)-[[1-[*N*-[(*p*-hydroxyamidino)benzoyl]-L-alanyl]-4-piperidyl]oxy]acetate. *CAS-172927-65-0.* INN; BAN. *Antithrombotic; fibrinogen receptor antagonist; platelet aggregation inhibitor.* ◇*Ro 48-3657/001*

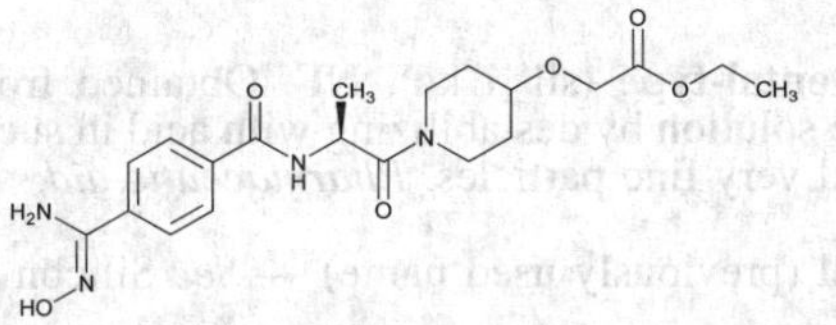

Sibrotuzumab. Immunoglobulin G1, anti-(human FAP (fibroblast activation protein)) (human-mouse monoclonal BIBH1 γ1-chain), disulfide with human-mouse monoclonal BIBH1 κ-chain, dimer. *CAS-216669-97-5.* INN.

Sibutramine Hydrochloride [*1990*] (si bue′ tra meen hye″ droe klor′ ide). $C_{17}H_{26}ClN.HCl.H_2O$. 334.32. [Sibutramine is INN and BAN.] (1) Cyclobutanemethanamine, 1-(4-chlorophenyl)-*N,N*-dimethyl-α-(2-methylpropyl)-, hydrochloride, monohydrate, ($\pm$)-; (2) ($\pm$)-1-(*p*-Chlorophenyl)-α-isobutyl-*N,N*-dimethylcyclobutanemethylamine hydrochloride monohydrate. *UNII-OGM0YHD1WF. CAS-125494-59-9* [monohydrate]; *CAS-84485-00-7* [anhydrous]; *CAS-106650-56-0* [sibutramine]. JAN. *Anorexic; antidepressant.* Meridia (Abbott) ◇*BTS 54524*

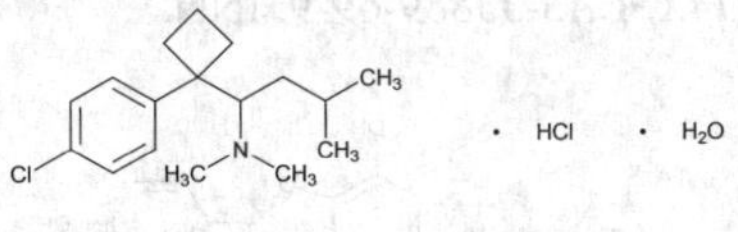

Siccanin. $C_{22}H_{30}O_3$. 342.47. (13a*S*)-1,2,3,4,4aβ,5,6,6a,11bβ,13bβ-Decahydro-4,4,6aβ,9-tetramethyl-13*H*-benzo[*a*]furo[2,3,4-*mn*]xanthen-11-ol. *UNII-L702S858Z6. CAS-22733-60-4.* INN; JAN; MI.

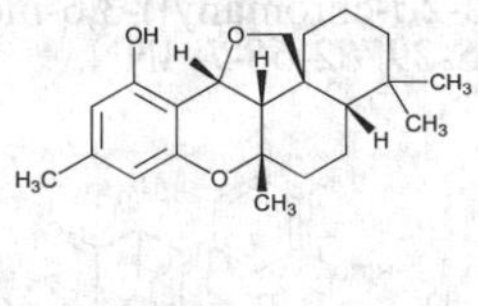

Sifaprazine. $C_{18}H_{22}N_2$. 266.38. 1-Methyl-4-(α-phenyl-*o*-tolyl)piperazine. *UNII-372MWC170E. CAS-131635-06-8.* INN.

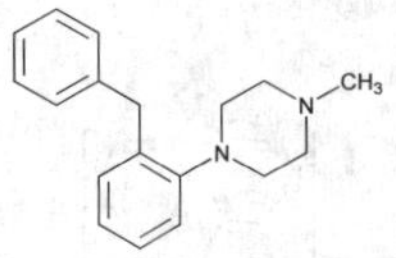

Sifilcon A [*2006*] (sye fil′ kon). $(C_{103}H_{217}N_3F_{36}O_{49}Si_{27})_a(C_{5-103}H_{217}N_3F_{36}O_{49}Si_{27})_a(C_5H_9NO)_b(C_{16}H_{38}O_5Si_4)_c(C_8H_8)_d$. 2-Propenoic acid, 2-methyl-, 2-isocyanatoethyl ester, polymers with *N,N*-dimethyl-2-propenamide, α-[[3-(2-hydroxyethoxy)propyl]dimethylsilyl]-ω-[[[3-(2-hydroxyethoxy)-propyl]dimethylsilyl]oxy]poly [oxy(dimethylsilylene)], 5-isocyanato-1-(isocyanatomethyl)-1,3,3-trimethylcyclohexane, reduced Me esters of reduced polymd. Oxidized tetrafluoroethylene, styrene and 3-[3,3,3-trimethyl-1,1-bis[(trimethylsilyl)oxy]disiloxanyl]propyl methacrylate. *CAS-867217-46-7. Contact lens material (hydrophilic).[-Note—The water content of the contact lens material is 32.0±2% at ambient temperature (23±2°C), and the oxygen permeability is 82 ± 1 barrers at 35°C (Dk value).]*

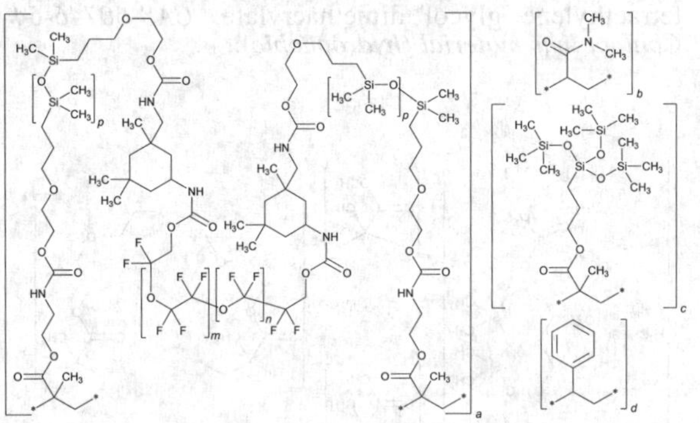

Siflufocon A [*1987*] (si″ floo foe′ kon). $(C_{16}H_{38}O_5Si_4)_w$ $(C_6H_7F_3O_2)_x(C_4H_6O_2)_y(C_{26}H_{58}O_9Si_6)_z$. (1) 3-[3,3,3-Trimethyl-1,1-bis[(trimethylsilyl)oxy]disiloxanyl]propyl 2-methyl-2-propenoate polymer with 2,2,2-trifluoroethyl 2-methyl-2-propenoate, 2-methyl-2-propenoic acid and [1,1,3,3-tetrakis[(trimethylsilyl)oxy]-1,3-disiloxanediyl]di-3,1-propanediyl bis(2-methyl-2-propenoate); (2) 3-[3,3,3-Trimethyl-1,1-bis(trimethylsiloxy)disiloxanyl]propyl methacrylate polymer with 2,2,2-trifluoroethyl methacrylate, methacrylic acid and [1,1,3,3-tetrakis(trimethylsiloxy)disiloxanylene]bis(trimethylene) dimethacrylate. *Contact lens material (hydrophobic).*

Siguazodan. $C_{14}H_{16}N_6O$. 284.32. 2-Cyano-1-methyl-3-[4-(4-methyl-6-oxo-1,4,5,6-tetrahydropyridazin-3-yl)phenyl]guanidine. *UNII-5E4UI00UQJ. CAS-115344-47-3.* INN; BAN. ◇*SK&F 94836*

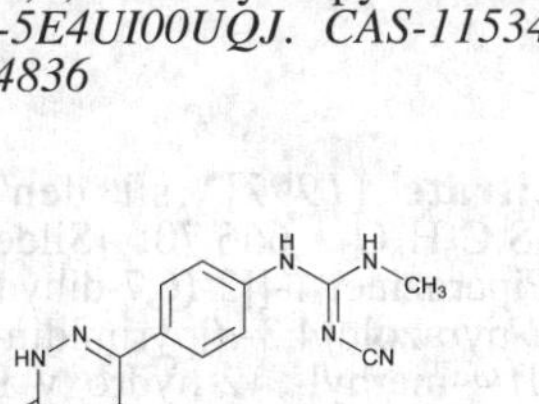

---

† Brand name formerly used, and/or firm no longer concerned with this product.

Silafilcon A [*1980*] (sil″ a fil′ kon). $(C_2H_6OSi)_a$ $(C_{12}H_{10}OSi)_b(C_3H_6OSi)_c(C_6H_5O_{3/2}Si)_d(C_2H_7O_{1/2}Si)_e$. (1) Silafilcon A; (2) Poly(dimethyl diphenyl methylvinyl phenyl hydrodimethyl siloxane). *Contact lens material (hydrophilic).*

Silafocon A [*1978*] (sil″ a foe′ kon). $(C_{22}H_{56}O_8Si_7)_w$ $(C_5H_8O_2)_x(C_4H_6O_2)_y(C_{16}H_{26}O_7)_z$. (1) 2-Propenoic acid, 2-methyl-, 3-[3,3,5,5,5-pentamethyl-1,1-bis[(pentamethyldisiloxanyl)oxy]trisiloxanyl]propyl ester, polymer with 2-methyl-2-propenoate, 2-methyl-2-propenoic acid and oxybis(2,1-ethanediyloxy-2,1-ethanediyl)bis(2-methyl-2-propenoate); (2) 3-[3,3,5,5,5-Pentamethyl-1,1-bis[(pentamethyldisiloxanyl)oxy]trisiloxanyl]propyl methacrylate polymer with methyl methacrylate, methacrylic acid and tetraethylene glycol dimethacrylate. *CAS-60746-64-7. Contact lens material (hydrophobic).*

Silandrone [*1967*] (sil′ an drone). $C_{22}H_{36}O_2Si$. 360.61. (1) Androst-4-en-3-one, 17-[(trimethylsilyl)oxy]-, (17β)-; (2) 17β-(Trimethylsiloxy)androst-4-en-3-one. *CAS-5055-42-5. INN. Androgen.* ◇SC-16148; NSC-95147

Sildenafil Citrate [*1997*] (sil den′ a fil sit′ rate). $C_{22}H_{30}N_6O_4S.C_6H_8O_7$. 666.70. [Sildenafil is INN and BAN.] (1) Piperazine, 1-[[3-(6,7-dihydro-1-methyl-7-oxo-3-propyl-1*H*-pyrazolo[4,3-*d*]pyrimidin-5-yl)-4-ethoxyphenyl]sulfonyl]-4-methyl-, 2-hydroxy-1,2,3-propanetricarboxylate (1:1); (2) 1-[[3-(6,7-Dihydro-1-methyl-7-oxo-3-propyl-1*H*-pyrazolo[4,3-*d*]pyrimidin-5-yl)-4-ethoxyphenyl]sulfonyl]-4-methylpiperazine citrate (1:1). *UNII-BW9B0ZE037; UNII-3M7OB98Y7H* [sildenafil]. *CAS-171599-83-0; CAS-139755-83-2* [sildenafil]. *Impotence therapy.* Viagra (Pfizer) ◇UK-92,480-10

Silibinin. $C_{25}H_{22}O_{10}$. 482.44. 3,5,7-Trihydroxy-2-[3-(4-hydroxy-3-methoxyphenyl)-2-(hydroxymethyl)-1,4-benzodioxan-6-yl]-4-chromanone. *CAS-22888-70-6. INN.*

Silica, Dental-type (sil′ i ka). **NF.** Obtained from sodium silicate solution by destabilizing with acid in such a way as to yield very fine particles. *Pharmaceutic aid.*

Silica Gel (previously used name) — *See* Silicon Dioxide.

Siliceous Earth, Purified (si lish′ us). **NF.** A form of silica (SiO_2) consisting of the frustules and fragments of diatoms, purified by calcining. *CAS-7631-86-9. Pharmaceutic aid (filtering medium).*

Silicon Dioxide (sil′ i kon dye ox′ ide). **NF.** SiO_2xH_2O. 60.08 (anhydrous). Obtained by insolubilizing the dissolved silica in sodium silicate solution. *Pharmaceutic aid (dispersing and suspending agent). [Name previously used: Silica Gel.]*

Silicon Dioxide, Colloidal (sil′ i kon dye ox′ ide koe loid′ al). **NF.** SiO_2. 60.08. (1) Silica; (2) Silica. *CAS-7631-86-9. Pharmaceutic aid (suspending agent); pharmaceutic aid (tablet and capsule diluent); pharmaceutic aid (thickening agent). [The CAS Registry Number for Silicon Dioxide, Colloidal is the same as that for Siliceous Earth, Purified.]*

Silicristin. $C_{25}H_{22}O_{10}$. 482.44. 2-[2,3-Dihydro-7-hydroxy-2-(4-hydroxy-3-methoxyphenyl)-3-(hydroxymethyl)-5-benzofuranyl]-3,5,7-trihydroxy-4-chromanone. *UNII-LK279ER14X. CAS-33889-69-9. INN.*

Silidianin. $C_{25}H_{22}O_{10}$. 482.44. (+)-2,3α,3aα,7a-Tetrahydro-7aα-hydroxy-8-(4-hydroxy-3-methoxyphenyl)-4-(3α,5,7-trihydroxy-4-oxo-2β-chromanyl)-3,6-methanobenzofuran-7(6αH)-one. *CAS-29782-68-1. INN.*

Silodosin. $C_{25}H_{32}F_3N_3O_4$. 495.53. (-)-1-(3-Hydroxypropyl)-5-[(2*R*)-2-[[2-[2-(2,2,2-trifluoroethoxy)phenoxy]ethyl]amino]propyl]-2,3-dihydro-1*H*-indole-7-carboxamide. *UNII-CUZ39LUY82. CAS-160970-54-7.* INN.

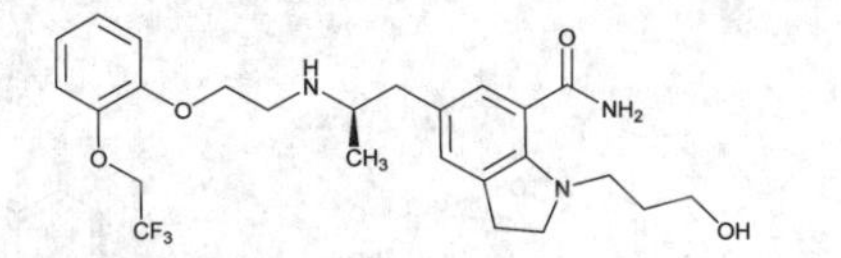

Silodrate [*1964*] (sil′ oh drate). $Al_2Mg_2O_{11}Si_3 \cdot xH_2O$. 362.82 (anhydrous). [Magnesium Aluminometasilicate is JAN; Simaldrate is INN.] (1) Aluminosilicic acid ($H_4Al_2Si_3O_{11}$), magnesium salt (1:2) hydrate; (2) Aluminosilicic acid ($H_4Al_2Si_3O_{11}$), magnesium salt (1:2) hydrate. *CAS-12408-47-8. Antacid.* ◇*MP-1051*

Silperisone. $C_{15}H_{24}FNSi$. 265.44. 1-[[(*p*-Fluorobenzyl)dimethylsilyl]methyl]piperidine. *UNII-R16SK8726X. CAS-140944-31-6.* INN.

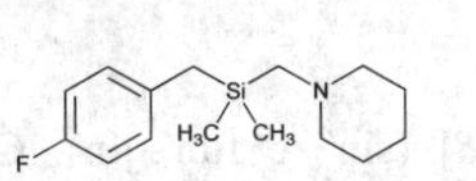

Siltenzepine. $C_{19}H_{20}ClN_3O_4$. 389.83. 5-[*N,N*-Bis(2-hydroxyethyl)glycyl]-8-chloro-5,10-dihydro-11*H*-dibenzo[*b,e*][1,4]diazepin-11-one. *UNII-DJF293UV6K. CAS-98374-54-0.* INN.

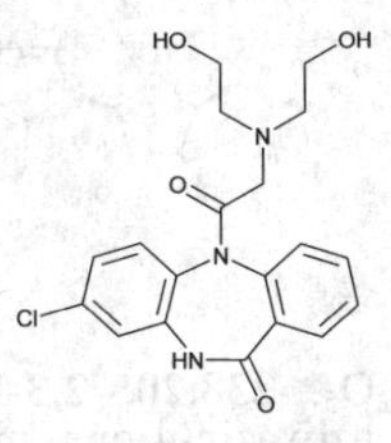

Silteplase. $C_{2580}H_{3948}N_{752}O_{784}S_{40}$ (non-glycosylated protein). 59,326.19. *N*-[*N*²-(*N*-glycyl-*L*-alanyl)-*L*-arginyl]plasminogen activator (human tissue-type protein moiety reduced), glycoform. *CAS-131081-40-8.* INN; JAN.

Silver Diammine Fluoride. $[Ag(NH_3)_2]F$. 160.93. Silver diammine fluoride. *CAS-34445-07-3.* JAN.

Silver Nitrate (sil′ ver nye′ trate). **USP**. $AgNO_3$. 169.87. (1) Nitric acid silver(1+) salt; (2) Silver(1+) nitrate. *UNII-95IT3W8JZE. CAS-7761-88-8.* JAN. *Anti-infective, topical.*

Silver Nitrate, Toughened (sil′ ver nye′ trate). **USP**. Contains not less than 94.5% of $AgNO_3$, the remainder consisting of silver chloride (AgCl). *CAS-8007-31-6. Caustic.*

Silver Protein, Mild. [Silver Protein is JAN.] *CAS-9015-51-4.* NF XIII; MI.

Simaldrate (INN) — *See* Silodrate.

---

† Brand name formerly used, and/or firm no longer concerned with this product.

Simendan. $C_{14}H_{12}N_6O$. 280.28. Mesoxalonitrile (±)-[*p*-(1,4,5,6-tetrahydro-4-methyl-6-oxo-3-pyridazinyl)phenyl]hydrazone. *CAS-131741-08-7.* INN.

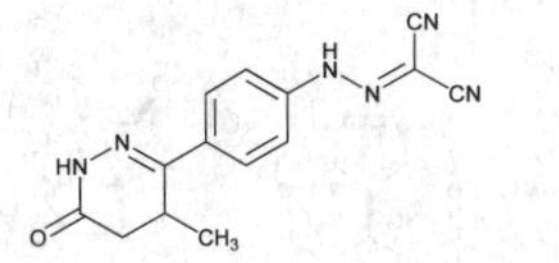

Simethicone [*1963*] (sye meth′ i kone). **USP**. A mixture of poly(dimethylsiloxane) (in the graphic formula, the calculated average value of *n* is 200 to 350) and silicon dioxide. (1) Simethicone; (2) α-(Trimethylsilyl)-ω-methylpoly[oxy(dimethylsilylene)], mixture with silicon dioxide. *CAS-8050-81-5. Antiflatulent.* Gas-X (Novartis); Mylanta Gas Relief (Johnson & Johnson-Merck Consumer); Mylicon Infant's Drops (Johnson & Johnson-Merck Consumer); Sentry Simethicone (Witco); Sentry Simethicone Emulsion (Witco) ◇*Antifoam A; Antifoam AF*

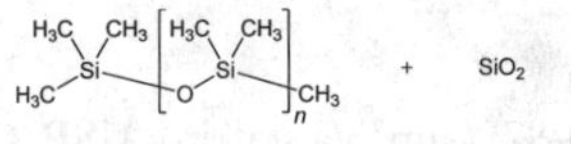

Simeticone. α-(Trimethylsilyl)-ω-methylpoly[oxy(dimethylsilylene)], mixture with silicon dioxide. *CAS-8050-81-5.* INN; BAN.

Simetride. $C_{28}H_{38}N_2O_6$. 498.61. 1,4-Bis[(2-methoxy-4-propylphenoxy)acetyl]piperazine. *UNII-QU6P2P8XLW. CAS-154-82-5.* INN; JAN; MI.

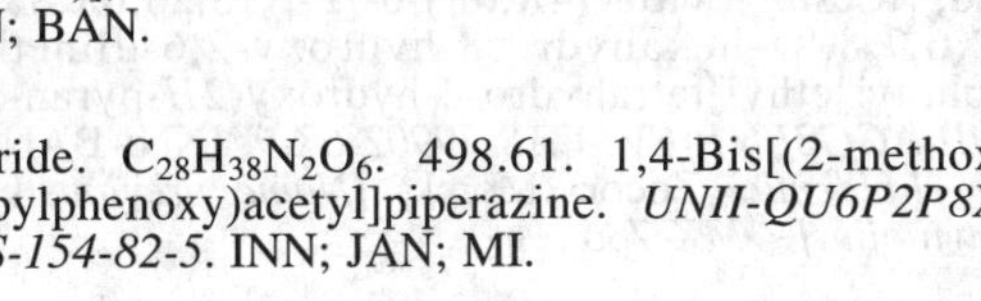

Simfibrate. $C_{23}H_{26}Cl_2O_6$. 469.35. 2-(*p*-Chlorophenoxy)-2-methylpropionic acid trimethylene ester. *UNII-L2R75RQX26. CAS-14929-11-4.* INN; JAN; MI. ◇*CLY-503*

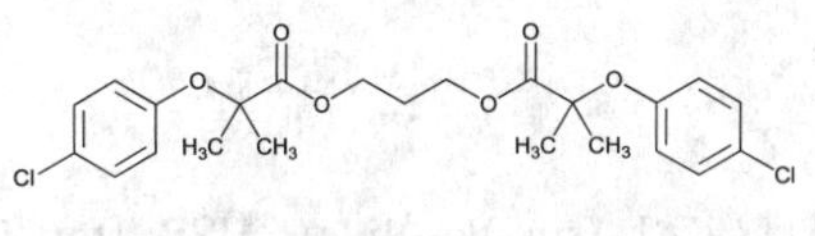

Simotaxel [*2005*] (sim″ oh tax′ el). $C_{46}H_{57}NO_{15}S$. 896.01. (1) 2-Thiophenepropanoic acid, α-hydroxy-β-[[(1-methylethoxy)carbonyl]amino]-, (2a*R*,4*S*,4a*S*,6*R*,9*S*,11*S*,12*S*,12a*R*,12b*S*)-12b-(acetyloxy)-12-(benzoyloxy)-6-[(cyclopentylcarbonyl)oxy]-2a,3,4,4a,5,6,9,10,11,12,12a,12b-dodecahydro-4,11-dihydroxy-4a,8,13,13-tetramethyl-5-oxo-7,11-methano-1*H*-cyclodeca[3,4]benz[1,2-*b*]oxet-9-yl ester, (α*R*,β*R*)-; (2) (2a*R*,4*S*,4a*S*,6*R*,9*S*,11*S*,12*S*,12a*R*,12b*S*)-4,11-Dihydroxy-4a,8,13,13-tetramethyl-5-oxo-2a,3,4,4a,5,6,9,10,11,12,12a,12b-dodecahydro-7,11-methano-1*H*-cyclodeca[3,4]benz[1,2-*b*]oxete-6,9,12,12b-tetrayl 12b-acetate 12-benzoate 6-cyclopentanecarboxylate 9-[(2*R*,3*R*)-2-hydroxy-3-[[(1-methylethoxy)carbonyl]amino]-3-(thiophen-2-yl)propanoate]. *CAS-791635-59-1*. INN. *Second-line treatment of NSCLC and metastatic breast cancer.* ◇*MST-997*

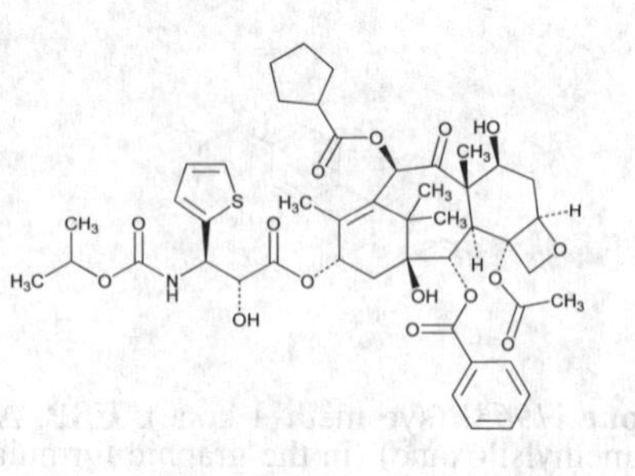

Simtrazene [*1964*] (sim′ tra zeen). $C_{14}H_{16}N_4$. 240.30. (1) 2-Tetrazene, 1,4-dimethyl-1,4-diphenyl-; (2) 1,4-Dimethyl-1,4-diphenyl-2-tetrazene. *UNII-HSD1XP51CR. CAS-5579-27-1*. INN. *Antineoplastic.* ◇*CL 26193; NSC-83799*

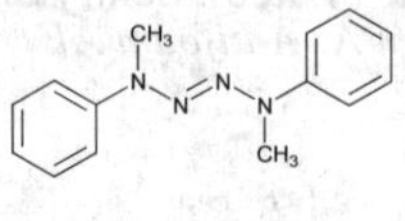

Simvastatin [*1987*] (sim″ va stat′ in). **USP.** $C_{25}H_{38}O_5$. 418.57. (1) Butanoic acid, 2,2-dimethyl-, 1,2,3,7,8,8a-hexahydro-3,7-dimethyl-8-[2-(tetrahydro-4-hydroxy-6-oxo-2*H*-pyran-2-yl)ethyl]-1-naphthalenyl ester, [1*S*-[1α,3α,7β,8β(2*S**,4*S**),8aβ]]-; (2) 2,2-Dimethylbutyric acid, 8-ester with (4*R*,6*R*)-6-[2-[(1*S*,2*S*,6*R*,8*S*,8a*R*)-1,2,6,7,8,8a-hexahydro-8-hydroxy-2,6-dimethyl-1-naphthyl]ethyl]tetrahydro-4-hydroxy-2*H*-pyran-2-one. *UNII-AGG2FN16EV. CAS-79902-63-9*. INN; BAN. *Antihyperlipidemic.* Zocor (Merck) *[Name previously used: Synvinolin.]* ◇*MK-733*

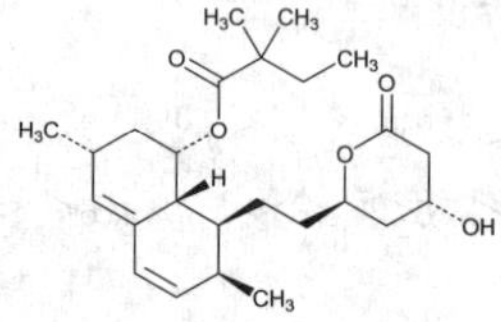

Sinapultide [*1997*] (sin″ a pul′ tide). $C_{126}H_{238}N_{26}O_{22}$. 2469.40. L-Lysyl-L-leucyl-L-leucyl-L-leucyl-L-leucyl-L-lysyl-L-leucyl-L-leucyl-L-leucyl-L-leucyl-L-lysyl-L-leucyl-L-leucyl-L-leucyl-L-leucyl-L-lysyl-L-leucyl-L-leucyl-L-leucyl-L-leucyl-L-leucyl-L-lysine. *CAS-138531-07-4*. INN. *Pulmonary surfactant.* ◇*ATI 01*

KLLLLKLLLL KLLLLKLLLL K

Sincalide [*1974*] (sin′ ka lide). **USP** [for Injection]. $C_{49}H_{62}N_{10}O_{16}S_3$. 1143.27. (1) Caerulein, 1-de(5-oxo-L-proline)-2-de-L-glutamine-5-L-methionine-; (2) L-Aspartyl-L-tyrosyl-L-methionylglycyl-L-tryptophyl-L-methionyl-L-aspartylphenyl-L-alaninamide hydrogen sulfate (ester); (3) L-α-Aspartyl-*O*-sulfo-L-tyrosyl-L-methionylglycyl-L-tryptophyl-L-methionyl-L-α-aspartyl-L-phenylalaninamide. *UNII-M03GIQ7Z6P. CAS-25126-32-3*. INN; BAN. *Choleretic.* Kinevac (Bracco) ◇*SQ 19844*

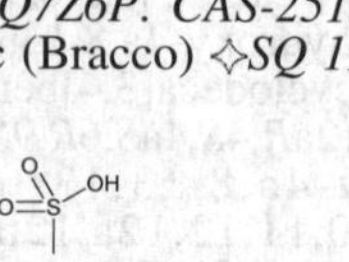

D Y M G W M D F —NH₂

Sinecatechins [*2006*] (sin″ e kat′ e kins). (1) Tea (*Camellia sinensis*), ext; (2) Major chemical constituents are (-)-Epicatechin, (-)-Epigallocatechin with their corresponding 3-gallate esters, and their corresponding epimers. *UNII-W2ZU1RY8B0. CAS-811420-59-4. Treatment of external genital and perianal warts.* Veregen (Medigene)

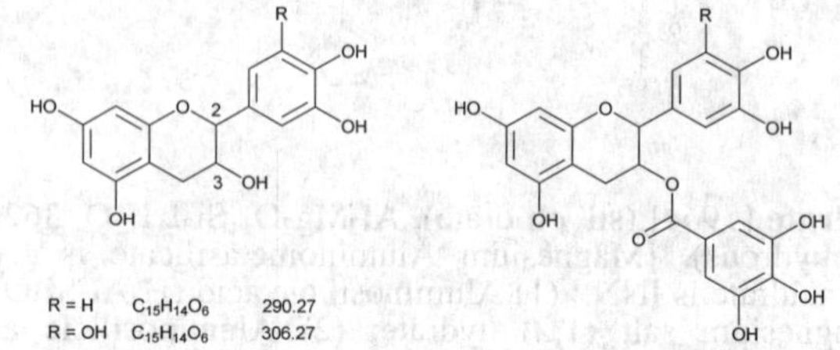

| R = H | $C_{15}H_{14}O_6$ | 290.27 |
| R = OH | $C_{15}H_{14}O_6$ | 306.27 |

| R = H | $C_{22}H_{18}O_{10}$ | 442.37 |
| R = OH | $C_{22}H_{18}O_{11}$ | 458.37 |

R = H	(-)-Epicatechin	[*cis*-; 2*R*,3*R*]
R = OH	(-)-Epigallocatechin	[*cis*-; 2*R*,3*R*]
R = H	(+)-Catechin	[*trans*-; 2*R*,3*S*]
R = H	(-)-Catechin	[*trans*-; 2*S*,3*R*]
R = OH	(+)-Gallocatechin	[*trans*-; 2*R*,3*S*]
R = OH	(-)-Gallocatechin	[*trans*-; 2*S*,3*R*]

R = H	(-)-Epicatechin gallate	[*cis*-; 2*R*,3*R*]
R = OH	(-)-Epigallocatechin gallate	[*cis*-; 2*R*,3*R*]
R = H	(-)-Catechin gallate	[*trans*-; 2*S*,3*R*]
R = OH	(-)-Gallocatechin gallate	[*trans*-; 2*S*,3*R*]

Sinefungin [*1978*] (sin″ e fun′ jin). $C_{15}H_{23}N_7O_5$. 381.39. *Antibiotic derived from Streptomyces griseolus.* (1) Decofuranuronic acid, 6,9-diamino-1-(6-amino-9*H*-purin-9-yl)-1,5,6,7,8,9-hexadeoxy-, (β-D-*ribo*)-; (2) 6,9-Diamino-1-(6-amino-9*H*-purin-9-yl)-1,5,6,7,8,9-hexadeoxy-β-D-*ribo*-decofuranuronic acid. *UNII-W2U467CIIL. CAS-58944-73-3*. INN. *Antifungal.* ◇*Compound 57926*

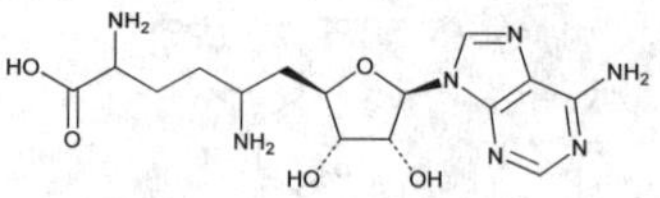

Sinitrodil. $C_{10}H_{10}N_2O_5$. 238.20. 2,3-Dihydro-3-(2-hydroxyethyl)-4*H*-1,3-benzoxazin-4-one nitrate (ester). *UNII-Y3FJ2C4H75. CAS-143248-63-9*. INN.

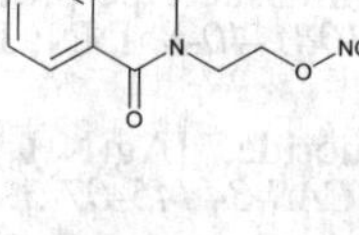

Sinorphan — *See* Ecadotril.

Sintropium Bromide. $C_{19}H_{36}BrNO_2$. 390.40. (8*r*)-3α-Hydroxy-8-isopropyl-1α*H*,5α*H*-tropanium bromide 2-propylvalerate. *CAS-79467-19-9*. INN.

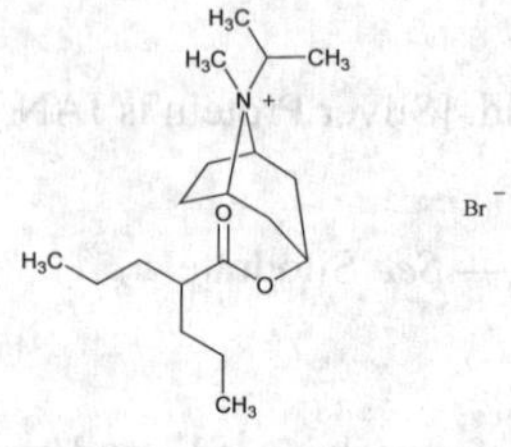

Sipatrigine. $C_{15}H_{16}Cl_3N_5$. 372.68. 4-Amino-2-(4-methyl-1-piperazinyl)-5-(2,3,5-trichlorophenyl)pyrimidine. *CAS-130800-90-7*. INN; BAN. ◊*619C89*

Siplizumab [*2002*] (si pliz' oo mab). Immunoglobulin G1, anti-[human CD2 (antigen)] (human-rat monoclonal MEDI-507 γ1-chain), disulfide with human-rat monoclonal MEDI-507 light chain, dimer. Molecular weight is approximately 150,000 daltons. *CAS-288392-69-8*. INN. *Treatment of auto-immune diseases/immune disorders.* ◊*MEDI-507*

Sipoglitazar. $C_{25}H_{25}N_3O_4S$. 463.55. 3-(3-Ethoxy-1-{4-[(2-phenyl-1,3-thiazol-4-yl)methoxy]benzyl}-1*H*-pyrazol-4-yl)propanoic acid. *CAS-342026-92-0*. INN.

Sipuleucel-T [*2005*] (si″ pu loo' sel - tee). Product is a specific active immunotherapeutic composed of antigen-loaded autologous antigen presenting cells designed to stimulate a T cell immune response specific for the tumor-associated antigen prostatic acid phosphatase (PAP). *Treatment of prostate cancer.* Provenge (Dendreon) ◊*APC8015*

Siramesine. $C_{30}H_{31}FN_2O$. 454.58. 1′-[4-[1-(*p*-Fluorophenyl)indol-3-yl]butyl]spiro[phthalan-1,4′-piperidine]. *UNII-3IX8CWR24V*. *CAS-147817-50-3*. INN.

Siratiazem. $C_{24}H_{30}N_2O_4S$. 442.57. (+)-(2*S*,3*S*)-2,3-Dihydro-3-hydroxy-5-[2-(isopropylmethylamino)ethyl]-2-(*p*-methoxyphenyl)-1,5-benzothiazepin-4(5*H*)-one acetate (ester). *CAS-138778-28-6*. INN.

Sirolimus [*1993*] (sir oh' li mus). $C_{51}H_{79}NO_{13}$. 914.17. (1) Rapamycin; (2) (3*S*,6*R*,7*E*,9*R*,10*R*,12*R*,14*S*,15*E*,17*E*,19*E*,21*S*,23*S*,26*R*,27*R*,34a*S*)-9,10,12,13,14,21,22,23,24,25,26,27,32,33,34,34a-Hexadecahydro-9,27-dihydroxy-3-[(1*R*)-2-[(1*S*,3*R*,4*R*)-4-hydroxy-3-methoxycyclohexyl]-1-methylethyl]-10,21-dimethoxy-6,8,12,14,20,26-hexamethyl-23,27-epoxy-3*H*-pyrido[2,1-*c*][1,4]oxaazacyclohentriacontine-1,5,11,28,29(4*H*,6*H*,31*H*)-pentone. *UNII-W36ZG6FT64*. *CAS-53123-88-9*. INN; BAN. *Immunosuppressant.* Rapamune (Wyeth) [*Name previously used: rapamycin.*] ◊*AY-22989; WY-090217*

Sisomicin [*1972*] (sis″ oh mye' sin). $C_{19}H_{37}N_5O_7$. 447.53. Antibiotic produced by *Micromonospora inyoensis.* (1) (2*S-cis*)-4-*O*-[3-Amino-6-(aminomethyl)-3,4-dihydro-2*H*-pyran-2-yl]-2-deoxy-6-*O*-[3-deoxy-4-*C*-methyl-3-(methylamino)-β-L-arabinopyranosyl]-D-streptamine; (2) *O*-3-Deoxy-4-*C*-methyl-3-(methylamino)-β-L-arabinopyranosyl-(1→4)-*O*-[2,6-diamino-2,3,4,6-tetradeoxy-α-D-*glycero*-hex-4-enopyranosyl-(1→6)]-2-deoxy-L-streptamine. *UNII-X55XSL74YQ*. *CAS-32385-11-8*. INN. *Antibacterial.* [*Note—This antibiotic is closely related to gentamicin C_{1A}, one of the components of the gentamicin complex.*]

Sisomicin Sulfate [*1975*] (sis″ oh mye' sin sul' fate). **USP**. $(C_{19}H_{37}N_5O_7)_2·5H_2SO_4$. 1385.45. [Sissomicin is BAN.] (1) D-Streptamine, (2*S-cis*)-4-*O*-[3-amino-6-(aminomethyl)-3,4-dihydro-2*H*-pyran-2-yl]-2-deoxy-6-*O*-[3-deoxy-4-*C*-methyl-3-(methylamino)-β-L-arabinopyranosyl]-, sulfate (2:5) (salt); (2) *O*-3-Deoxy-4-*C*-methyl-3-(methylamino)-β-L-arabinopyranosyl-(1→4)-*O*-[2,6-diamino-2,3,4,6-tetradeoxy-α-D-*glycero*-hex-4-enopyranosyl-(1→6)]-2-deoxy-L-streptamine sulfate (2:5) (salt). *UNII-X55XSL74YQ* [sisomicin]. *CAS-53179-09-2; CAS-32385-11-8* [sisomicin]. JAN. *Antibacterial.* Siseptin (Schering†) ◊*Sch 13475 sulfate*

Sissomicin (BAN) — *See* Sisomicin.

Sissomicin (BAN) — *See* Sisomicin Sulfate.

Sitafloxacin [*1999*] (sye″ ta flox' a sin). $C_{19}H_{18}ClF_2N_3O_3·1½H_2O$. 436.84. (1) 3-Quinolinecarboxylic acid, 7-(7-amino-5-azaspiro[2.4]hept-5-yl)-8-chloro-6-fluoro-1-(2-fluorocyclopropyl)-1,4-dihydro-4-oxo-, hydrate (2:3), [1*R*-[1α(*S**),

---

2α]]-; (2) (-)-7-[(7*S*)-7-Amino-5-azaspiro[2.4]hept-5-yl]-8-chloro-6-fluoro-1-[(1*R*,2*S*)-2-fluorocyclopropyl]-1,4-dihydro-4-oxo-3-quinolinecarboxylic acid, sesquihydrate. *UNII-9TD681796G; UNII-3GJC60U4Q8* [sitafloxacin anhydrous]. *CAS-163253-35-8; CAS-127254-12-0* [anhydrous]. INN. *Antibacterial (DNA-gyrase inhibitor).* ◇*DU-6859a*

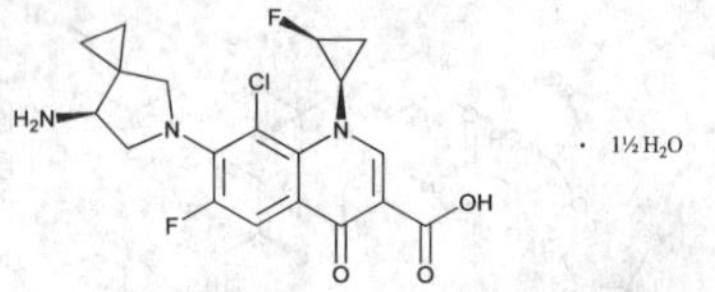

Sitagliptin Phosphate [*2005*] (sye″ ta glip′ tin fos′ fate). $C_{16}H_{15}F_6N_5O \cdot H_3O_4P \cdot H_2O$. 523.32. [Sitagliptin is INN; Sitagliptin Phosphate Hydrate is JAN.] (1) 1,2,4-Triazolo[4,3-*a*]pyrazine, 7-[(3*R*)-3-amino-1-oxo-4-(2,4,5-trifluorophenyl)butyl]-5,6,7,8-tetrahydro-3-(trifluoromethyl)-, phosphate (1:1) monohydrate; (2) 7-[(3*R*)-3-Amino-4-(2,4,5-trifluorophenyl)butanoyl]-3-(trifluoromethyl)-5,6,7,8-tetrahydro-1,2,4-triazolo[4,3-*a*]pyrazine-monophosphate monohydrate. *UNII-TS63EW8X6F; UNII-QFP0P1DV7Z* [sitagliptin]. *CAS-654671-77-9; CAS-486460-32-6* [sitagliptin]. *Treatment of type 2 diabetes mellitus and related disorders.* Januvia (Merck)

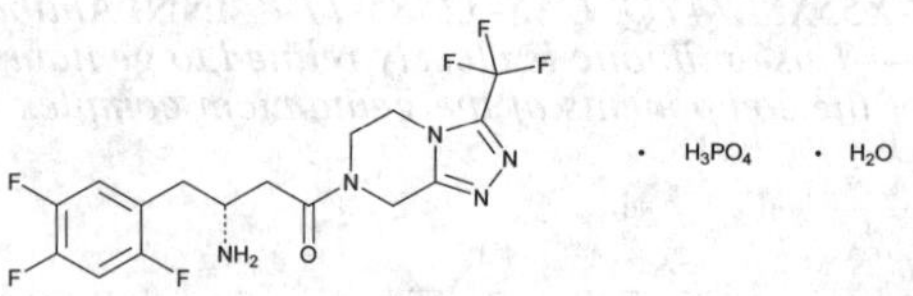

Sitalidone. $C_{23}H_{29}ClN_2O_5S$. 481.00. (±)-2-Chloro-4′-hydroxy-5-(2-hydroxy-1-methyl-5-oxo-2-pyrrolidinyl)-3′,5′-diisopropylbenzenesulfonanilide. *UNII-06H9KWB6IB*. *CAS-108894-39-9*. INN.

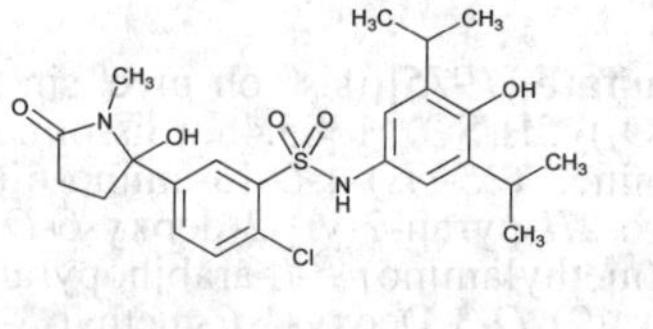

Sitamaquine. $C_{21}H_{33}N_3O$. 343.51. *N,N*-Diethyl-*N*′-(6-methoxy-4-methyl-8-quinolyl)-hexane-1,6-diamine. *UNII-5AIJ4TGC6B*. *CAS-57695-04-2*. INN; BAN. ◇*WR 6026*

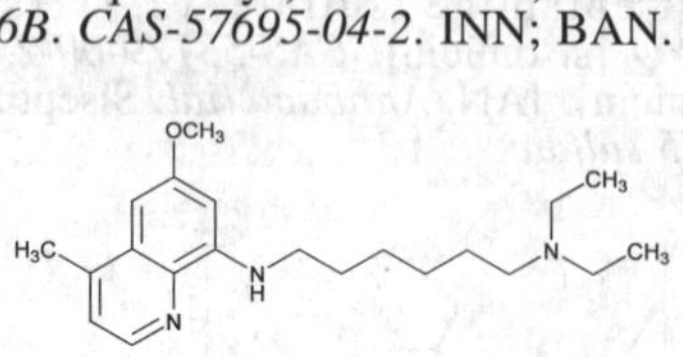

Sitaxentan. $C_{18}H_{15}ClN_2O_6S_2$. 454.90. *N*-(4-Chloro-3-methyl-5-isoxazolyl)-2-[[4,5-(methylenedioxy)-*o*-tolyl]acetyl]-3-thiophenesulfonamide. *UNII-J9QH779MEM*. *CAS-184036-34-8*. INN.

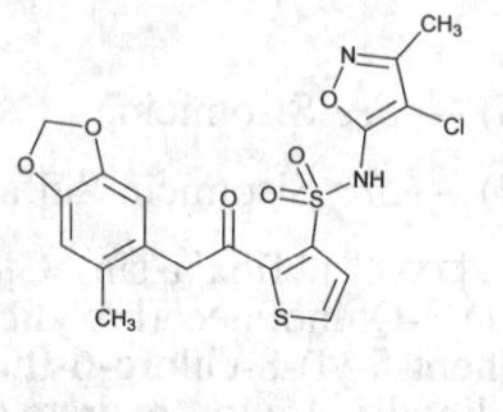

Sitimagene Ceradenovec. (Recombinant) replication restricted adenovirus (type 5) vector, E1 and E3 deleted, containing/expressing the *Herpes simplex virus* thymidine kinase (HSV-tk) gene. *CAS-898830-54-1*. INN.

Sitofibrate. $C_{39}H_{59}ClO_3$. 611.34. Stigmast-5-en-3β-ol 2-(*p*-chlorophenoxy)-2-methylpropionate. *CAS-55902-94-8*. INN.

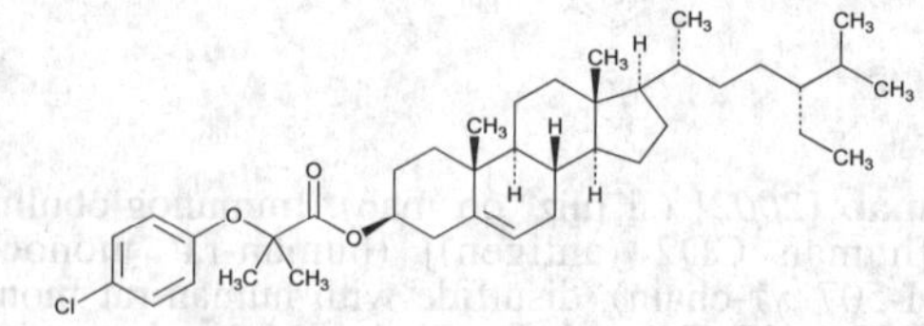

Sitogluside [*1980*] (si″ toe gloo′ side). $C_{35}H_{60}O_6$. 576.85. (1) β-D-Glucopyranoside, (3β)-stigmast-5-en-3-yl; (2) 3β-(β-D-Glucopyranosyloxy)stigmast-5-ene. *CAS-474-58-8*. INN. *Antiprostatic hypertrophy.* ◇*BSSG; EU-4906; AW 10; WA 184*

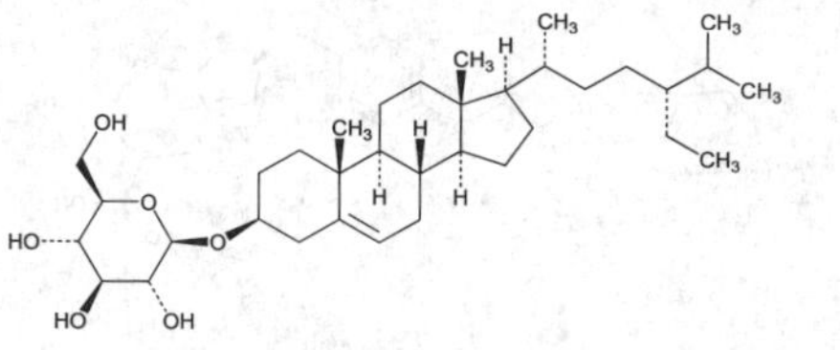

Sitosterols. NF XIII. Cytellin (Lilly†)

Sivelestat [*2002*] (si vel′ e stat). $C_{20}H_{22}N_2O_7S$. 434.46. (1) Glycine, *N*-[2-[[[4-(2,2-dimethyl-1-oxopropoxy)phenyl]sulfonyl]amino]benzoyl]-; (2) *o*-(*p*-Hydroxybenzenesulfonamido)hippuric acid, pivalate (ester). *UNII-DWI62G0P59*. *CAS-127373-66-4*. INN. *Treatment of acute lung injury; acute respiratory distress syndrome (elastase inhibitor).* ◇*LY544349; ONO-5046*

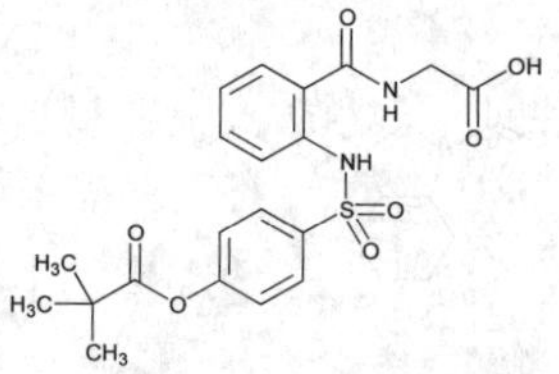

Sivelestat Sodium [*2002*] (si vel′ e stat soe′ dee um). $C_{20}H_{21}N_2NaO_7S \cdot 4H_2O$. 528.51. (1) Glycine, *N*-[2-[[[4-(2,2-dimethyl-1-oxopropoxy)phenyl]sulfonyl]amino]benzoyl]-, monosodium salt, tetrahydrate; (2) Sodium [[2-[[[4-[(2,2-dimethylpropanoyl)oxy]phenyl]sulfonyl]amino]benzoyl]amino]acetate tetrahydrate. *UNII-737RR8Y409*. *CAS-201677-61-4*. *Treatment of acute lung injury; acute respiratory distress syndrome (elastase inhibitor).* ◇*LY544349 Sodium Hydrate; ONO-5046.Na*

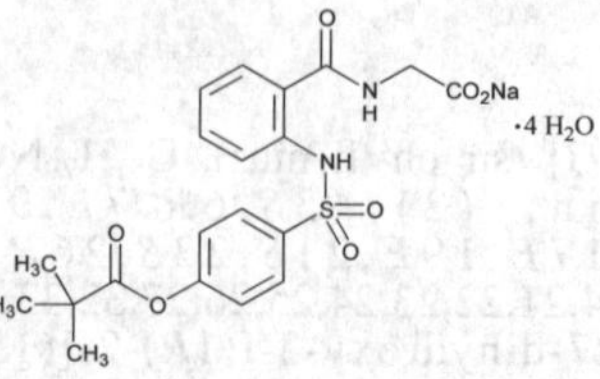

Sivifene [*2007*] (siv′ i feen). $C_{19}H_{14}N_4O_6$. 394.34. (1) Methanone, bis(4-hydroxyphenyl)-, (2,4-dinitrophenyl)hydrazone; (2) 4,4′-[[2-(2,4-Dinitrophenyl)hydrazinylidene]-

methylene]diphenol. *CAS-2675-35-6*. INN. *Treatment of high-grade squamous intraepithelial lesions of the cervix and other neoplasms.* ◇*A-007*

Sizofiran. $(C_{24}H_{40}O_{20})_n$. Poly[3→(O-β-D-glucopyranosyl-(1→3)-O-[β-D-glucopyranosyl-(1→6)]-O-β-D-glucopyranosyl-(1→3)-O-β-D-glucopyranosyl→1]. *CAS-9050-67-3*. INN; JAN; MI.

Skin, Sterile Freeze-dried Porcine Dermal. JAN.

Skin, Sterile Freeze-dried Porcine Epidermal. JAN.

Skin Substitute, Human Fibroblast-Derived Temporary. **USP**. A nonliving monolayer skin substitute derived from neonatal foreskins. It is composed of fibroblasts, an extracellular matrix, and a nylon mesh bonded to a transparent, semi-permeable silicone membrane.

[153]Sm — *See* Samarium Sm 153 Lexidronam Pentasodium.

Smallpox Vaccine (smawl′ pox vax′ een). **USP**. A suspension or solid containing the living virus of vaccinia of a strain of approved origin and manipulation, that has been grown in the skin of a vaccinated bovine calf. *Immunizing agent (active).*

Soap, Green. **USP**. A potassium soap made by the saponification of suitable vegetable oils, excluding coconut oil and palm kernel oil, without the removal of glycerin. *Detergent.*

Sobetirome [*2008*] (soe″ be tye′ rome). $C_{20}H_{24}O_4$. 328.40. (1) Acetic acid, 2-[4-[[4-hydroxy-3-(1-methylethyl)phenyl]methyl]-3,5-dimethylphenoxy]-; (2) (4-{[4-Hydroxy-3-(1-methylethyl)phenyl]methyl}-3,5-dimethylphenoxy)acetic acid. *UNII-XQ31741E9Q. CAS-211110-63-3. Treatment of hypercholestemia, obesity, and thyroid proliferative disorders.* ◇*GC-1; QRX-431*

---

† Brand name formerly used, and/or firm no longer concerned with this product.

Soblidotin. $C_{39}H_{67}N_5O_6$. 701.98. N^2-(*N,N*-Dimethyl-L-valyl)-N^1-[(1*S*,2*R*)-2-methoxy-4-[(2*S*)-2-[(1*R*,2*R*)-1-methoxy-2-methyl-3-oxo-3-[(2-phenylethyl)amino]propyl]-1-pyrrolidinyl]-1-[(1*S*)-1-methylpropyl]-4-oxobutyl]-N^1-methyl-L-valinamide. *CAS-149606-27-9*. INN.

Sobuzoxane. $C_{22}H_{34}N_4O_{10}$. 514.53. 4,4′-Ethylenebis[1-(hydroxymethyl)-2,6-piperazinedione] bis(isobutyl carbonate) (ester). *UNII-R1308VH37P. CAS-98631-95-9*. INN; JAN.

SOD — *See* Orgotein.

Soda Lime (soe′ da lyme). **NF**. A mixture of calcium hydroxide and sodium or potassium hydroxide or both. *CAS-8006-28-8. Carbon dioxide absorbant.* Sodasorb (Grace)

Sodelglitazar [*2006*] (soe″ del gli′ ta zar). $C_{23}H_{21}F_4NO_3S_2$. 499.54. (1) Propanoic acid, 2-[4-[[[2-[2-fluoro-4-(trifluoromethyl)phenyl]-4-methyl-5-thiazolyl]methyl]thio]-2-methylphenoxy]-2-methyl-; (2) 2-[4-[[[2-[2-Fluoro-4-(trifluoromethyl)phenyl]-4-methyl-1,3-thiazol-5-yl]methyl]-sulfanyl]-2-methylphenoxy]-2-methylpropanoic acid. *UNII-6G973E04VI. CAS-447406-78-2.* INN. *Treatment of type 2 diabetes.* (GlaxoSmithKline) ◇*GW677954*

Sodium Acetate (soe′ dee um as′ e tate). **USP**. $C_2H_3NaO_2$.3-H_2O. 136.08. (1) Acetic acid, sodium salt, trihydrate; (2) Sodium acetate trihydrate. *UNII-4550K0SC9B. CAS-6131-90-4; CAS-127-09-3* [anhydrous]. JAN. *Pharmaceutic aid (in dialysis solutions).*

Sodium Acetate C 11 (soe′ dee um as′ e tate). **USP** [Injection]. A sterile solution of sodium acetate in which a portion of the carboxyl molecules are labeled with radioactive [11]C. *Radioactive agent.*

Sodium Alginate (soe′ dee um al′ ji nate). **NF**. (1) Alginic acid, sodium salt; (2) Sodium alginate. *CAS-9005-38-3; CAS-9005-32-7* [alginic acid]. *Pharmaceutic aid (suspending agent).*

Sodium Amidotrizoate (INN, BAN) — *See* Diatrizoate Sodium.

Sodium Aminobenzoate. *UNII-75UI7QUZ5J. CAS-555-06-6; CAS-150-13-0* [4-Aminobenzoic acid].

Sodium Amylosulfate [*1964*] (soe′ dee um am″ i loe sul′ fate). Sodium salt of the sulfated form of amylopectin [derived from potatoes (tubers of *Solanum tuberosum*)]. (1) Amylopectin, sulfate, sodium salt; (2) Sodium amylopectin sulfate. *CAS-9010-01-9. Enzyme inhibitor.* ◇*SN-263*

Sodium Anoxynaphthonate (BAN) — *See* Anazolene Sodium.

Sodium Antimonylgluconate. $C_6H_8NaO_7Sb$. 336.87. Sodium salt of a trivalent antimony derivative of gluconic acid. *CAS-12550-17-3.* BAN.

Sodium Apolate (INN, BAN) — *See* Lyapolate Sodium.

Sodium Arsenate As 74 [*1963*] (soe′ dee um ar′ se nate). (1) Arsenic acid ($H_3^{74}AsO_4$), sodium salt; (2) Sodium arsenate-^{74}As. *Radioactive agent.*

Sodium Arsenate, Exsiccated. *CAS-7778-43-0.* NF VIII.

Sodium Ascorbate (soe′ dee um a skor′ bate). **USP**. $C_6H_7NaO_6$. 198.11. (1) L-Ascorbic acid, monosodium salt; (2) Monosodium L-ascorbate. *UNII-PQ6CK8PD0R* [ascorbic acid]. *CAS-134-03-2; CAS-50-81-7* [ascorbic acid]. INN. *Vitamin (antiscorbutic).* Ascorbin (Marion Merrell Dow†); Cevalin (Lilly)

Sodium Aurothiomalate (INN, JAN) — *See* Gold Sodium Thiomalate.

Sodium Aurotiosulfate (INN) — *See* Gold Sodium Thiosulfate.

Sodium Azodisalicylate (previously used name) — *See* Olsalazine Sodium.

Sodium Benzoate [*1989*] (soe′ dee um ben′ zoe ate). **NF**. $C_7H_5NaO_2$. 144.10. (1) Benzoic acid, sodium salt; (2) Sodium benzoate. *UNII-OJ245FE5EU. CAS-532-32-1.* JAN. *Antihyperammonemic; pharmaceutic aid (antifungal agent).*

Sodium Bicarbonate (soe′ dee um bye kar′ bo nate). **USP**. $NaHCO_3$. 84.01. (1) Carbonic acid monosodium salt; (2) Monosodium carbonate. *UNII-8MDF5V39QO. CAS-144-55-8.* JAN. *Replenisher (electrolyte); alkalizer (systemic).*

Sodium Bisulfite. (1) Sulfurous acid, monosodium salt; (2) Monosodium sulfite. *UNII-TZX5469Z6I. CAS-7631-90-5.* NF XV; JAN; MI.

Sodium Bitionolate (INN) — *See* Bithionolate Sodium.

Sodium Borate (soe′ dee um bore′ ate). **NF**. $Na_2B_4O_7 \cdot 10H_2O$. 381.37. (1) Borax; (2) Borax. *UNII-91MBZ8H3QO. CAS-1303-96-4; CAS-1330-43-4* [anhydrous]. JAN. *Pharmaceutic aid (alkalizing agent).*

Sodium Borocaptate (^{10}B) (INN) — *See* Borocaptate Sodium B 10.

Sodium Bromide (soe′ dee um broe′ mide). **USP**. NaBr. 102.89. (1) Sodium bromide; (2) Sodium bromide. *CAS-7647-15-6.* JAN.

Sodium Butyrate (soe′ dee um bue′ ti rate). **USP**. $C_4H_7NaO_2$. 110.09. (1) Butyric acid sodium salt; (2) Sodium butyrate. *CAS-156-54-7.*

Sodium Cacodylate. *CAS-124-65-2; CAS-75-60-5* [cacodylic acid]. NF X; MI.

Sodium Calcium Edetate (INN, BAN, JAN) — *See* Edetate Calcium Disodium.

Sodium Calciumedetate (previously used name) — *See* Edetate Calcium Disodium.

Sodium Caprylate (soe′ dee um kap′ ri late). **NF**. $C_8H_{15}NaO_2$. 166.19. Sodium octanoate. *UNII-9XTM81VK2B. CAS-1984-06-1; CAS-142-62-1* [caproic acid]. NND 1963.

Sodium Carbonate (soe′ dee um kar′ bo nate). **NF**. Na_2CO_3. 105.99. (1) Carbonic acid, disodium salt; (2) Disodium carbonate. *UNII-45P3261C7T. CAS-497-19-8; CAS-5968-11-6* [monohydrate]. *Pharmaceutic aid (alkalizing agent).*

Sodium Cefapirin (JAN) — *See* Cephapirin Sodium.

Sodium Cetostearyl Sulfate (soe′ dee um see″ toe steer′ il sul′ fate). **NF**. A mixture of sodium cetyl sulfate and sodium stearyl sulfate.

Sodium Chloride (soe′ dee um klor′ ide). **USP**. NaCl. 58.44. [10% Sodium Chloride Injection and Sodium Chloride Solution, Isotonic are also JAN.] (1) Sodium chloride; (2) Sodium chloride. *UNII-451W47IQ8X. CAS-7647-14-5.* JAN. *Pharmaceutic aid (tonicity agent).*

Sodium Chloride, Compound Solution of (INN) — *See* Ringer's Injection.

Sodium Chloride Na 22 [*1963*] (soe′ dee um klor′ ide). $^{22}NaCl$. (1) Sodium chloride ($^{22}NaCl$); (2) Sodium chloride ($^{22}NaCl$). *CAS-17112-21-9. Radioactive agent.* Natritope Chloride (Bristol-Myers Squibb†)

Sodium Chromate Cr 51 [*1963*] (soe′ dee um kroe′ mate). **USP** [Injection]. $Na_2^{51}CrO_4$. [Sodium Chromate (^{51}Cr) is INN; Sodium Chromate (^{51}Cr) Injection is JAN.] (1) Chromic acid ($H_2^{51}CrO_4$), disodium salt; (2) Disodium chromate ($Na_2^{51}CrO_4$). *CAS-7775-11-3. Diagnostic aid (blood volume determination); radioactive agent.* Chromitope Sodium (Bristol-Myers Squibb†); Rachromate (Abbott†)

Sodium Citrate (soe′ dee um sit′ rate). **USP**. $C_6H_5Na_3O_7$. 258.07 (anhydrous). (1) 1,2,3-Propanetricarboxylic acid, 2-hydroxy-, trisodium salt; (2) Trisodium citrate; (3) Trisodium citrate dihydrate. *UNII-1Q73Q2JULR. CAS-6132-04-3; CAS-68-04-2* [anhydrous]. JAN. *Alkalizer (systemic).*

Sodium Cromoglicate (JAN) — *See* Cromolyn Sodium.

Sodium Cyclamate. $C_6H_{12}NNaO_3S$. 201.22. Sodium cyclohexanesulfamate. *CAS-139-05-9.* NF XIII; INN; BAN; MI.

Sodium Dehydroacetate (soe′ dee um dee hye″ droe as′ e tate). **NF**. $C_8H_7NaO_4$. 190.13. 2*H*-Pyran-2,4(3*H*)-dione, 3-acetyl-6-methyl-, monosodium salt. *CAS-4418-26-2. Pharmaceutic aid (antimicrobial preservative).*

Sodium Dehydrocholate (INN) — *See* Dehydrocholate Sodium.

Sodium Diatrizoate (previously used name) — *See* Diatrizoate Sodium.

Sodium Dibunate. $C_{18}H_{23}NaO_3S$. 342.43. Sodium 2,6-di-*tert*-butyl-1(or 3)-naphthalenesulfonate. *UNII-FRS4SO3K8D. CAS-14992-59-7.* INN; BAN. ◇*L-1633*

Sodium Dichloroacetate [*1999*] (soe′ dee um dye klor″ oh as′ e tate). $C_2HCl_2NaO_2$. 150.92. (1) Dichloroacetic acid, sodium salt; (2) Sodium dichloroacetate. *UNII-42932X67B5. CAS-2156-56-1. Treatment of neurologic injury (pyruvate dehydrogenase activator).* Ceresine (Cypros) ◇*CPC-211; DCA*

Sodium Dioctyl Sulfosuccinate (INN) — *See* Docusate Sodium.

Sodium Diprotrizoate (BAN) — *See* Diprotrizoate Sodium.

Sodium Etasulfate (INN) — *See* Sodium Ethasulfate.

Sodium Ethasulfate [*1962*] (soe′ dee um eth″ a sul′ fate). $C_8H_{17}NaO_4S$. 232.27. [Sodium Etasulfate is INN.] (1) Hexanol, 2-ethyl-, hydrogen sulfate, sodium salt; (2) Mono(2-ethylhexyl) sulfate sodium salt. *CAS-126-92-1; CAS-5254-16-0* [mono(2-ethylhexyl)sulfate]. *Detergent.*

Sodium Feredetate. $C_{10}H_{12}FeN_2NaO_8$. 367.05. Iron chelate of the monosodium salt of (ethylenedinitrilo)tetraacetic acid. *UNII-403J23EMFA. CAS-15708-41-5.* INN; BAN; DCF. *[Name previously used: Sodium Ironedetate.]*

Sodium Ferric Gluconate Complex [*2002*] (soe′ dee um fer′ ik gloo′ koe nate). $[NaFe_2O_3(C_6H_{11}O_7)(C_{12}H_{22}O_{11})_5]_x$ (where x is approximately $_{200}$). D-Gluconic acid, iron (3+) sodium salt. Molecular weight is approximately 350,000 daltons ±23,000. *UNII-CC9149U2QX. CAS-34089-81-1. Hematinic used in the management of iron deficiency in hemodialysis patients for whom oral iron is insufficient.* Ferrlecit (Watson)

---

† Brand name formerly used, and/or firm no longer concerned with this product.

Sodium Ferrous Citrate. $C_{12}H_{10}FeNa_4O_{14}$. 526.00. Tetrasodium biscitrato iron (II). *CAS-50717-86-7.* JAN.

Sodium Fluoride (soe′ dee um floor′ ide). **USP**. NaF. 41.99. (1) Sodium fluoride; (2) Sodium fluoride. *UNII-8ZYQ1474W7. CAS-7681-49-4.* JAN. *Dental caries prophylactic.* Fluorinse (Oral-B); Minute-Gel (Oral-B); Neutra Care (Oral-B); Pediaflor (Ross)

Sodium Fluoride F 18 (soe′ dee um floor′ ide). **USP** [Injection]. A sterile solution of sodium fluoride in sodium chloride in which a portion of the molecules are labeled with radioactive ^{18}F. *CAS-22554-99-0. Radioactive agent.*

Sodium Formaldehyde Sulfoxylate (soe′ dee um for mal′ de hyde sul fox′ il ate). **NF**. CH_3NaO_3S. 118.09. (1) Methanesulfinic acid, hydroxy-, monosodium salt; (2) Monosodium hydroxymethanesulfinate. *UNII-X4ZGP7K714. CAS-6035-47-8; CAS-149-44-0* [anhydrous]; *CAS-79-25-4* [hydroxymethanesulfinic acid]. *Pharmaceutic aid (preservative).*

Sodium Fusidate (JAN) — *See* Fusidate Sodium.

Sodium Gentisate. $C_7H_5NaO_4$. 176.10. Sodium 2,5-dihydroxybenzoate. *UNII-VP36V95O3T* [gentisic acid]. *CAS-4955-90-2; CAS-490-79-9* [gentisic acid]. INN.

Sodium Glucaldrate. Sodium diaquagluconato(2-)-O^1,O^2-dihydroxoaluminate. BAN.

Sodium Glucaspaldrate. $C_{42}H_{54}Al_2Na_8O_{38}$·$2H_2O$. 1440.77. Sodium bis(acetato)tetrakis[gluconato(2-)]bis[salicylato(2-)] dialuminate dihydrate. *CAS-12214-50-5.* INN; BAN.

Sodium Gluconate (soe′ dee um gloo′ koe nate). **USP**. $C_6H_{11}NaO_7$. 218.14. (1) D-Gluconic acid, monosodium salt; (2) Monosodium D-gluconate. *UNII-R6Q3791S76. CAS-527-07-1. Replenisher (electrolyte).*

Sodium Glucosulfone. *CAS-554-18-7.* USP XVIII.

Sodium Glucuronate. $C_6H_9NaO_7$·H_2O. 234.14. Sodium glucuronate. *CAS-14984-34-0.* JAN.

Sodium Glutamate. [Glutamate Sodium is JAN.] *UNII-3KX376GY7L* [glutamic acid]. *CAS-142-47-2; CAS-56-86-0* [L-glutamic acid]. AMA-DE 1973.

Sodium Glycerophosphate. *CAS-55073-41-1; CAS-1334-74-3* [anhydrous]; *CAS-27082-31-1* [glycerophosphoric acid]. NF X; MI.

Sodium Gualenate. $C_{15}H_{17}NaO_3S$. 300.35. [Azulene Sulfonate Sodium is JAN.] Sodium 5-isopropyl-3,8-dimethyl-1-azulene sulfonate. *UNII-19WSH095WP. CAS-6223-35-4; CAS-16915-32-5* [gualenic acid]. INN.

Sodium Hydroxide (soe′ dee um hye drox′ ide). **NF**. NaOH. 40.00. (1) Sodium hydroxide; (2) Sodium hydroxide. *UNII-55X04QC32I. CAS-1310-73-2. Pharmaceutic aid (alkalizing agent).*

Sodium Hypochlorite (soe′ dee um hye″ poe klor′ ite). **USP** [Solution]. NaClO. 74.44. (1) Hypochlorous acid, sodium salt; (2) Sodium hypochlorite. *UNII-DY38VHM5OD. CAS-7681-52-9.* JAN. *Disinfectant.*

Sodium Hypochlorite [Solution, Diluted]. [Dental Antiformin is JAN.] *CAS-8007-59-8.* NF; MI.

Sodium Hypophosphite. *CAS-7681-53-0.* NF X; MI.

Sodium Iodide (soe′ dee um eye′ oh dide). **USP**. NaI. 149.89. (1) Sodium iodide; (2) Sodium iodide. *UNII-F5WR8N145C. CAS-7681-82-5.* JAN. *Supplement (iodine).*

Sodium Iodide I 123 (soe′ dee um eye′ oh dide). **USP**. [Sodium Iodide (^{123}I) Capsules is JAN.] (1) Sodium iodide (Na^{123}I); (2) Sodium iodide (Na^{123}I). *UNII-29UKX3A616. CAS-41927-88-2. Diagnostic aid (thyroid function determination); radioactive agent.*

Sodium Iodide I 125 [*1963*] (soe′ dee um eye′ oh dide). Na^{125}I. [Sodium Iodide (^{125}I) is INN.] (1) Sodium iodide (Na^{125}I); (2) Sodium iodide (Na^{125}I). *UNII-HII3IK0W0I. CAS-24359-64-6.* USP XXII. *Diagnostic aid (thyroid function determination); radioactive agent.* Iodotope I-125 (Bristol-Myers Squibb†)

Sodium Iodide I 131 [*1963*] (soe′ dee um eye′ oh dide). **USP**. Na^{131}I. [Sodium Iodide (^{131}I) Capsules is JAN.] (1) Sodium iodide (Na^{131}I); (2) Sodium iodide (Na^{131}I). *UNII-29VCO8-ACHH. CAS-7790-26-3.* INN. *Antineoplastic; diagnostic aid (thyroid function determination); radioactive agent.* Iodotope I-131 (Bristol-Myers Squibb†); Iodotope Therapeutic (Bristol-Myers Squibb†); Oriodide (Abbott†); Radiocaps-131 (Abbott†); Theriodide (Abbott†); Tracervial-131 (Abbott†)

Sodium Iodohippurate (^{131}I) (INN) — *See* Iodohippurate Sodium I 131.

Sodium Iodohippurate (^{131}I) Injection (JAN) — *See* Iodohippurate Sodium I 131.

Sodium Iopodate (INN, BAN, JAN) — *See* Ipodate Sodium.

Sodium Iotalamate (^{125}I) (INN) — *See* Iothalamate Sodium I 125.

Sodium Iotalamate (^{131}I) (INN) — *See* Iothalamate Sodium I 131.

Sodium Iotalamate Injection (JAN) — *See* Iothalamate Sodium.

Sodium Iothalamate (BAN) — *See* Iothalamate Sodium I 125.

Sodium Ioxaglate (BAN) — *See* Ioxaglate Sodium.

Sodium Ipodate (previously used name) — *See* Ipodate Sodium.

Sodium Ironedetate (previously used name) — *See* Sodium Feredetate.

Sodium Lactate (soe′ dee um lak′ tate). **USP** [Injection]. $C_3H_5NaO_3$. 112.06. (1) Propanoic acid, 2-hydroxy-, monosodium salt; (2) Sodium lactate. *UNII-TU7HW0W0QT. CAS-72-17-3.* JAN. *Replenisher (electrolyte).*

Sodium Lauryl Sulfate (soe′ dee um lawr′ il sul′ fate). **NF**. (1) Sulfuric acid monododecyl ester sodium salt; (2) Sodium monododecyl sulfate. *UNII-368GB5141J. CAS-151-21-3; CAS-151-41-7* [monododecyl hydrogen sulfate]. JAN. *Pharmaceutic aid (surfactant).*

Sodium Metabisulfite (soe′ dee um met″ a bye sul′ fite). **NF**. $Na_2S_2O_5$. 190.11. (1) Disulfurous acid, disodium salt; (2) Disodium pyrosulfite. *CAS-7681-57-4. Pharmaceutic aid (antioxidant).*

Sodium Metrizoate (INN, BAN) — *See* Metrizoate Sodium.

Sodium Monofluorophosphate (soe′ dee um mon″ oh floor″ oh fos′ fate). **USP**. Na_2PFO_3. 143.95. (1) Phosphorofluoridic acid, disodium salt; (2) Disodium phosphorofluoridate. *UNII-C810JCZ56Q. CAS-10163-15-2. Dental caries prophylactic.* [Note—Depicted as $FPO(ONa)_2$.]

Sodium Morrhuate (INN) — *See* Morrhuate Sodium.

Sodium Nitrite (soe′ dee um nye′ trite). **USP**. $NaNO_2$. 69.00. (1) Nitrous acid, sodium salt; (2) Sodium nitrite. *CAS-7632-00-0. Antidote (to cyanide poisoning).*

Sodium Nitroferricyanide — *See* Sodium Nitroprusside.

Sodium Nitroprusside (soe′ dee um nye″ troe prus′ ide). **USP**. $Na_2[Fe(CN)_5NO].2H_2O$. 297.95. (1) Ferrate(2-), pentakis(cyano-*C*)nitrosyl-, disodium, dihydrate, (*OC*-6-22)-; (2) Disodium pentacyanonitrosylferrate(2-) dihydrate; (3) Sodium nitroferricyanide dihydrate. *UNII-EAO03PE1TC. CAS-13755-38-9; CAS-14402-89-2* [anhydrous]. *Antihypertensive.* Nitropress (Hospira)

Sodium Oxybate [*1966*] (soe′ dee um ox′ i bate). $C_4H_7NaO_3$. 126.09. (1) Butanoic acid, 4-hydroxy-, sodium salt; (2) Sodium 4-hydroxybutyrate. *UNII-7G33012534. CAS-502-85-2; CAS-591-81-1* [4-hydroxybutanoic acid]. *Anesthesia, adjunct to.* Xyrem (Jazz) ◇*Wy-3478; NSC-84223*

Sodium Perborate Monohydrate [*1988*] (soe′ dee um per bore′ ate mon″ oh hye′ drate). $NaBO_3.H_2O$. 99.81.

Sodium Pertechnetate Tc 99m [*1966*] (soe′ dee um per tek′ ne tate). **USP** [Injection]. Na^{99m}TcO$_4$. [Sodium Pertechnetium (^{99m}Tc) Injection is JAN.] (1) Pertechnetic acid (H^{99m}TcO$_4$), sodium salt; (2) Sodium pertechnetate (Na^{99m}TcO$_4$). *CAS-23288-60-0. Radioactive agent.* Tc 99m Generator (Medi-Physics); Pertscan-99m (Abbott†); Ultra-Technekow FM (Mallinckrodt)

Sodium Pertechnetium (^{99m}Tc) Injection (JAN) — *See* Sodium Pertechnetate Tc 99m.

Sodium Phenylacetate [*1989*] (soe′ dee um fen″ il as′ e tate). $C_8H_7NaO_2$. 158.13. (1) Benzeneacetic acid, sodium salt; (2) Sodium phenylacetate. *UNII-48N6U1781G. CAS-114-70-5. Antihyperammonemic.*

Sodium Phenylbutyrate [*1995*] (soe′ dee um fen″ il bue′ ti rate). $C_{10}H_{11}NaO_2$. 186.18. (1) Benzenebutanoic acid, sodium salt; (2) Sodium 4-phenylbutyrate. *UNII-NT6K61736T. CAS-1716-12-7.* BAN. *Antihyperammonemic.* Buphenyl (Medicis)

Sodium Phosphate, Dibasic (soe′ dee um fos′ fate dye bay′ sik). **USP**. $Na_2HPO_4.xH_2O$. 141.96 (anhydrous). (1) Phosphoric acid, disodium salt, dodecahydrate; (2) Disodium hydrogen phosphate, dodecahydrate; (3) Phosphoric acid, disodium salt, heptahydrate; (4) Disodium hydrogen phosphate heptahydrate; (5) Phosphoric acid, disodium salt, dihydrate; (6) Disodium hydrogen phosphate, dihydrate; (7) Phosphoric acid, sodium salt, monohydrate; (8) Disodium hydrogen phosphate, monohydrate; (9) Phosphoric acid, disodium salt, hydrate; (10) Disodium hydrogen phosphate hydrate. *CAS-10140-65-5; CAS-10039-32-4* [dodecahydrate]; *CAS-7782-85-6* [heptahydrate]; *CAS-10028-24-7* [dihydrate]; *CAS-118830-14-1* [monohydrate]; *CAS-7558-79-4* [anhydrous]. *Laxative.*

Sodium Phosphate, Monobasic (soe′ dee um fos′ fate mon″ oh bay′ sik). **USP**. $NaH_2PO_4.xH_2O$. 119.98 (anhydrous). (1) Phosphoric acid, monosodium salt, monohydrate; (2) Monosodium phosphate monohydrate. (1) Phosphoric acid, monosodium salt, dihydrate; (2) Monosodium phosphate dihydrate. *CAS-7558-80-7* [anhydrous]; *CAS-10049-21-5* [monohydrate]; *CAS-13472-35-0* [dihydrate].

Sodium Phosphate P 32 [*1963*] (soe′ dee um fos′ fate). **USP** [Solution]. [Sodium Phosphate (^{32}P) is INN.] (1) Phosphoric-^{32}P acid, disodium salt; (2) Dibasic sodium phosphate-^{32}P. *CAS-7635-46-3. Antineoplastic; antipolycythemic; diagnostic aid (neoplasm); radioactive agent.* Phosphotope (Bristol-Myers Squibb†)

Sodium Phosphate, Tribasic (soe′ dee um fos′ fate trye bay′ sik). **NF**. Na_3PO_4. 163.94 (anhydrous). (1) Phosphoric acid, trisodium salt, dodecahydrate; (2) Trisodium phosphate, dodecahydrate; (3) Trisodium phosphate, monohydrate. *CAS-7601-54-9* [anhydrous]; *CAS-10101-89-0* [dodecahydrate].

Sodium Picofosfate. $C_{18}H_{13}NNa_4O_8P_2$. 525.20. 4,4′-(2-Pyridylmethylene)diphenol bis(dihydrogen phosphate) tetrasodium salt. *UNII-9164VT6ANB. CAS-36175-05-0.* INN.

Sodium Picosulfate. $C_{18}H_{13}NNa_2O_8S_2$. 481.41. 4,4′-(2-Pyridylmethylene)diphenol bis(hydrogen sulfate) disodium salt. *UNII-LR57574HN8. CAS-10040-45-6; CAS-10040-34-3* [picosulfuric acid]. INN; BAN; JAN. *[Name previously used: Sodium Picosulphate.]* ◇*LA 391; DA 1773*

Sodium Polyethylenesulfonate (JAN) — *See* Lyapolate Sodium.

Sodium Polyphosphate [*1977*] (soe′ dee um pol″ ee fos′ fate). $(NaPO_3)_n$. (1) Polyphosphoric acid, sodium salt; (2) Sodium polyphosphate. (In the graphic formula, *n* is 12 to 20.) *Pharmaceutic aid.*

Sodium Polystyrene Sulfonate (soe′ dee um pol″ ee stye′ reen sul′ foe nate). **USP**. (1) Benzene, diethenyl-, polymer with ethenylbenzene, sulfonated, sodium salt; (2) Divinylbenzene copolymer with styrene, sulfonated, sodium salt. *UNII-1699G8679Z.* JAN. *Ion-exchange resin (potassium).* Kayexalate (Sanofi Aventis)

Sodium Prasterone Sulfate. $C_{19}H_{27}NaO_5S.2H_2O$. 426.50. 3β-Hydroxy-5-androsten-17-one sodium sulfate dihydrate. *UNII-E1CR8487EN. CAS-1099-87-2.* JAN.

Sodium Propionate (soe′ dee um proe′ pee oh nate). **NF**. $C_3H_5NaO_2.xH_2O$. 96.06 (anhydrous). (1) Propanoic acid, sodium salt, hydrate; (2) Sodium propionate hydrate. *CAS-6700-17-0; CAS-137-40-6* [anhydrous]. *Pharmaceutic aid (preservative).*

Sodium Psylliate [Injection]. *CAS-8021-76-9.* NF XI.

Sodium Pyrophosphate [*1977*] (soe′ dee um pye″ roe fos′ fate). $Na_4P_2O_7$. 265.90. (1) Diphosphoric acid, tetrasodium salt; (2) Tetrasodium pyrophosphate. *UNII-O352864B8Z. CAS-7722-88-5. Pharmaceutic aid.*

Sodium Radiochromate — *See* Sodium Chromate Cr 51.

Sodium Rhodanate — *See* Thiocyanate Sodium.

Sodium Salicylate (soe′ dee um sa lis′ i late). **USP**. $C_7H_5NaO_3$. 160.10. (1) Benzoic acid, 2-hydroxy-, monosodium salt; (2) Monosodium salicylate. *UNII-WIQ1H85SYP. CAS-54-21-7.* JAN. *Analgesic.* Alysine (Marion Merrell Dow†)

Sodium Starch Glycolate (soe′ dee um stahrch glye′ koe late). **NF**. Starch carboxymethyl ether, sodium salt. *Pharmaceutic aid (tablet excipient).*

Sodium Stearate (soe′ dee um steer′ ate). **NF**. (1) Octadecanoic acid, sodium salt; (2) Sodium stearate. *UNII-QU7E2XA9TG. CAS-822-16-2. Pharmaceutic aid (emulsifying and stiffening agent).*

Sodium Stearyl Fumarate (soe′ dee um steer′ il fue′ ma rate). **NF**. 2-Butenedioic acid (2*E*)-, monooctadecyl ester, sodium salt. *CAS-4070-80-8. Pharmaceutic aid (tablet and/ or capsule lubricant).*

Sodium Stibocaptate. $C_{12}H_6Na_6O_{12}S_6Sb_2$. 916.02. Hexasodium salt of the *S,S*-diester of the cyclic thioantimonate(III) of 2,3-dimercaptosuccinic acid. *CAS-3064-61-7; CAS-1986-66-9* [stibocaptate]. INN; BAN. *[Name previously used: Stibocaptate.]* ◇*TWSB; Ro 4-1544-6*

Sodium Stibogluconate. Antimony (V) derivative of sodium gluconate. *CAS-16037-91-5.* INN; BAN; DCF.

Sodium Sulfate (soe′ dee um sul′ fate). **USP**. $Na_2SO_4.10H_2O$. 322.19. [Sodium Sulfate, Dried is JAN.] (1) Sulfuric acid disodium salt, decahydrate; (2) Disodium sulfate decahydrate. *UNII-0YPR65R21J. CAS-7727-73-3; CAS-7757-82-6* [anhydrous]. *Regulator (calcium).*

Sodium Sulfate S 35 [*1963*] (soe′ dee um sul′ fate). $Na_2{}^{35}SO_4$. (1) Sulfuric-^{35}S acid, disodium salt; (2) Disodium sulfate-^{35}S.*CAS-14262-80-7. Radioactive agent.*

Sodium Sulfide (soe′ dee um sul′ fide). **USP**. $Na_2S.9H_2O$. 240.18. (1) Sodium sulfide nonahydrate; (2) Disodium sulfide nonahydrate. *CAS-1313-84-4.*

Sodium Sulfite (soe′ dee um sul′ fite). **NF**. Na_2SO_3. 126.04. (1) Sulfurous acid, sodium salt; (2) Sulfurous acid, disodium salt. *UNII-VTK01UQK3G. CAS-7757-83-7.*

Sodium Sulfocyanate — *See* Thiocyanate Sodium.

Sodium Tartrate (soe′ dee um tar′ trate). **NF**. $C_4H_4Na_2O_6.2$-H_2O. 230.08. (1) Disodium L-tartrate; (2) Disodium (+)-2,3-dihydroxybutanedioic acid. *UNII-QTO9JB4MDD. CAS-868-18-8.*

Sodium Tetradecyl Sulfate. $C_{14}H_{29}NaO_4S$. 316.43. Sodium 7-ethyl-2-methyl-4-undecanol sulfate. *UNII-Q1SUG5KBD6. CAS-139-88-8; CAS-4754-44-3* [1-tetradecanol hydrogen sulfate]. INN; MI. Sotradecol (Bioniche)

Sodium Thiosulfate (soe′ dee um thye″ oh sul′ fate). **USP**. $Na_2S_2O_3.5H_2O$. 248.18. (1) Thiosulfuric acid, disodium salt, pentahydrate; (2) Disodium thiosulfate pentahydrate. *UNII-HX1032V43M. CAS-10102-17-7; CAS-7772-98-7* [anhydrous]. JAN. *Antidote (to cyanide poisoning).*

Sodium Timerfonate (INN, BAN) — *See* Thimerfonate Sodium.

Sodium Trimetaphosphate [*1977*] (soe′ dee um trye met″ a fos′ fate). $Na_3P_3O_9$. 305.89. (1) Metaphosphoric acid $(H_3P_3O_9)$, trisodium salt; (2) Sodium trimetaphosphate. *UNII-3IH6169RL0. CAS-7785-84-4. Pharmaceutic aid.*

Sodium Tyropanoate (INN, BAN, JAN) — *See* Tyropanoate Sodium.

Sodium Valproate (JAN) — *See* Valproate Sodium.

Sodium *o*-Iodo-^{123}I-Hippurate (JAN) — *See* Iodohippurate Sodium I 123.

Sofalcone. $C_{27}H_{30}O_6$. 450.52. [5-[(3-Methyl-2-butenyl)oxy]-2-[*p*-[(3-methyl-2-butenyl)oxy]cinnamoyl]phenoxy]acetic acid. *CAS-64506-49-6.* INN; JAN; MI.

Sofigatran. $C_{24}H_{44}N_4O_4S$. 484.70. Propyl {(1*S*)-1-{(2*S*)-2-[(*trans*-4-aminocyclohexylmethyl)carbamoyl]pyrrolidine-1-carbonyl}-2-methyl-2-[(propan-2-yl)sulfanyl]propyl}-carbamate. *CAS-187602-11-5.* INN.

Sofinicline [*2008*] (soe fin′ i kleen). $C_{10}H_{11}Cl_2N_3$. 244.12. (1) 3,6-Diazabicyclo[3.2.0]heptane, 3-(5,6-dichloro-3-pyridinyl)-, (1*S*,5*S*)-; (2) (-)-(1*S*,5*S*)-3-(5,6-Dichloropyridin-3-yl)-3,6-diazabicyclo[3.2.0]heptane. *CAS-799279-80-4. Attention deficit/hyperactivity disorder, neuropathic pain, Alzheimer's type dementia.* ◇*A-422894.0; ABT-894*

Sofinicline Benzenesulfonate [*2008*] (soe fin′ i kleen ben″ zeen sul′ foe nate). $C_{10}H_{11}Cl_2N_3.C_6H_6O_3S$. 402.30. (1) 3,6-Diazabicyclo[3.2.0]heptane, 3-(5,6-dichloro-3-pyridinyl)-, (1*S*,5*S*)-, monobenzenesulfonate; (2) (-)-(1*S*,5*S*)-3-(5,6-Dichloropyridin-3-yl)-3,6-diazabicyclo[3.2.0]heptane monobenzenesulfonate. *CAS-876170-44-4. Diabetic neuropathic pain, attention deficit/hyperactivity disorder (ADHD), dementia of the Alzheimer's type (AD).* ◇*A-422894.112*

Solabegron Hydrochloride [*2003*] (soe la beg′ ron hye″ droe klor′ ide). $C_{23}H_{23}ClN_2O_3.HCl$. 447.35. [Solabegron is INN.] (1) [1,1′-Biphenyl]-3-carboxylic acid, 3′-[[2-[[(2*R*)-2-(3-chlorophenyl)-2-hydroxyethyl]amino]ethyl]amino]-, hydrochloride; (2) 3′-[[2-[[(2*R*)-2-(3-Chlorophenyl)-2-hydroxyethyl]amino]ethyl]amino]biphenyl-3-carboxylic acid hydrochloride. *CAS-451470-34-1; CAS-252920-94-8* [solabegron]. *Antidiabetic (β3 adrenoreceptor agonist).* ◇*GW427353B*

Solapsone (BAN) — *See* Solasulfone.

Solasulfone. $C_{30}H_{28}N_2Na_4O_{14}S_5$. 892.83. [Solapsone is BAN.] Tetrasodium salt of 1,1′-[sulfonylbis(*p*-phenylimino)]bis-(3-phenyl-1,3-propanedisulfonic acid). *CAS-133-65-3.* INN; MI.

Solifenacin Succinate [*2001*] (soe″ li fen′ a sin sux′ i nate). $C_{23}H_{26}N_2O_2.C_4H_6O_4$. 480.55. [Solifenacin is INN and BAN.] Butanedioic acid, cmpd. with (1*S*)-(3*R*)-1-azabicyclo[2.2.2]oct-3-yl 3,4-dihydro-1-phenyl-2(1*H*)-isoquinolinecarboxylate (1:1). *UNII-KKA5DLD701; UNII-A8910SQJ1U* [solifenacin]. *CAS-242478-38-2; CAS-242478-37-1* [solifenacin]. *Treatment for relief of symptoms of urinary frequency, urinary urgency, or urge urinary incontinence (UUI) associated with an overactive bladder (muscarinic M3 receptor antagonist).* Vesicare (Astellas) ◇*YM905; YM-67905; YM67905*

Solimastat. $C_{20}H_{32}N_4O_5$. 408.49. (2*S*,3*R*)-3-[(1*S*)-(2,2-Dimethyl-1-(2-pyridylcarbamoyl)propyl)carbamoyl]-2-methoxy-5-methylhexanohydroxamic acid. *CAS-226072-63-5.* BAN, INN. *Matrix Metalloproteinase Inhibitor.* ◇*BB-3644*

Solpecainol. $C_{18}H_{23}NO_3$. 301.38. (1*R**,2*S**)-2-[[(*S**)-1-Methyl-2-phenoxyethyl]amino]-1-phenyl-1,3-propanediol. *CAS-68567-30-6.* INN.

Solypertine Tartrate [*1963*] (soe″ li per′ teen tar′ trate). $C_{22}H_{25}N_3O_3.C_4H_6O_6$. 529.54. [Solypertine is INN.] (1) 5*H*-1,3-Dioxolo[4,5-*f*]indole, 7-[2-[4-(2-methoxyphenyl)-1-piperazinyl]ethyl]-, [*R*-(*R**,*R**)]-2,3-dihydroxybutanedioate (1:1); (2) 7-[2-[4-(*o*-Methoxyphenyl)-1-piperazinyl]ethyl]-5*H*-1,3-dioxolo-[4,5-*f*]-indole tartrate (1:1). *CAS-5591-43-5; CAS-4448-96-8* [solypertine]. *Anti-adrenergic.* ◇*Win 18,413-2*

Somagrebove [*1990*] (soe ma′ gre bove). $C_{987}H_{1550}N_{268}O_{291}S_9$. 22,115.09. (1) Somatotropin (ox reduced), 1-[*N²*-L-methionyl-L-α-aspartyl]-L-glutamine]-; (2) 1-[*N²*-(*N*-L-Methionyl-L-α-aspartyl)-L-glutamine]growth hormone (ox reduced). *CAS-96353-48-9.* INN. *Galactopoietic agent (veterinary).* ◇*CL 291,894*

```
                                               MD
QFPAMSLSGL FANAVLRAQH LHQLAADTFK EFERTYIPEG QRYSIQNTQV
AFCFSETIPA PTGKNEAQQK SDLELLRISL LLIQSWLGPL QFLSRVFTNS
LVFGTSDRVY EKLKDLEEGI LALMRELEDG TPRAGQILKQ TYDKFDTNMR
SDDALLKNYG LLSCFRKDLH KTETYLRVMK CRRFGEASCA F
```

Somalapor [*1990*] (soe ma′ la pore). $C_{977}H_{1527}N_{265}O_{287}S_7$. 21,801.65 gm/mole. (1) Somatotropin (pig clone pPGH-1 reduced), *N*-L-alanyl-; (2) *N*-L-Alanylgrowth hormone (pig reduced). *CAS-106282-98-8.* INN; BAN. *Hormone (growth, porcine).*

```
AFPAMPLSSL FANAVLRAQH LHQLAADTYK EFERAYIPEG QRYSIQNAQA
AFCFSETIPA PTGKNEAQQR SDVELLRFSL LLIQSWLGPV QFLSRVFTNS
LVFGTSDRVY EKLKDLEEGI QALMRELEDG SPRAGQILKQ TYDKFDTNLR
SDDALLKNYG LLSCFKKDLH KAETYLRVMK CRRFVESSCA F
```

Somantadine Hydrochloride [*1984*] (soe man′ ta deen hye″ droe klor′ ide). $C_{14}H_{25}N.HCl$. 243.82. [Somantadine is INN.] (1) Tricyclo[3.3.1.^{3,7}] decane-1-ethanamine, α,α-dimethyl-, hydrochloride; (2) α,α-Dimethyl-1-adamantaneethylamine hydrochloride. *CAS-68693-30-1; CAS-79594-24-4* [somantadine]. *Antiviral.* ◇*PR-741-976A*

Somatomedin-C — *See* Mecasermin.

Somatorelin. $C_{215}H_{358}N_{72}O_{66}S$. 5039.65. [Somatorelin Acetate is JAN.] Growth hormone-releasing factor (human). *CAS-83930-13-6.* INN.

Somatosalm. $C_{952}H_{1524}N_{266}O_{290}S_8$. 21,592.43. Somatotropin (Oncorhyncus mykiss clone ptGH-II isoform II reduced). *CAS-123212-08-8.* INN.

Somatostatin. $C_{76}H_{104}N_{18}O_{19}S_2$. 1637.88. Growth hormone-release inhibiting factor: L-alanylglycyl-L-cysteinyl-L-lysyl-L-asparaginyl-L-phenylalanyl-L-phenylalanyl-L-trypto-

---

† Brand name formerly used, and/or firm no longer concerned with this product.

phyl-L-lysyl-L-threonyl-L-phenylalanyl-L-threonyl-L-seryl-L-cysteine cyclic (3→14) disulfide. *CAS-38916-34-6.* INN; BAN; MI.

```
                AGCKNFFWKT FTSC
```

Somatrem [*1984*] (soe′ ma trem). $C_{995}H_{1537}N_{263}O_{301}S_8$. 22,255.97. (1) Somatotropin (human), *N*-L-methionyl-; (2) *N*-L-Methionylgrowth hormone (human). *UNII-CU8-D464EDW. CAS-82030-87-3.* INN; BAN; JAN. *Hormone (growth).* Protropin (Genentech)

```
                                                       M
     FPTIPLSRLF   DNAMLRAHRL   HQLAFDTYQE   FEEAYIPKEQ   KYSFLQNPQT
     SLCFSESIPT   PSNREETQQK   SNLELLRISL   LLIQSWLEPV   QFLRSVFANS
     LVYGASDSNV   YDLLKDLEEG   IQTLMGRLED   GSPRTGQIFK   QTYSKFDTNS
     HNDDALLKNY   GLLYCFRKDM   DKVETFLRIV   QCRSVEGSCG   F
```

Somatropin [*1977*] (soe″ ma troe′ pin). **USP.** $C_{990}H_{1528}N_{262}O_{300}S_7$. 22,124.77. [Human Growth Hormone is JAN.] A single polypeptide chain of 191 amino acids having the normal structure of the principal growth stimulating hormone obtained from the anterior lobe of the human pituitary gland. (1) Growth hormone (human); (2) Somatotropin (human). *UNII-NQX9KB6PCL. CAS-12629-01-5.* INN; BAN; JAN. *Hormone (growth).* Genotropin (Pfizer); Humatrope (Lilly); Nutropin (Genentech); Saizen (Serono); Serostim (Serono) ◇*CB-311; LY137998*

```
     FPTIPLSRLF   DNAMLRAHRL   HQLAFDTYQE   FEEAYIPKEQ   KYSFLQNPQT
     SLCFSESIPT   PSNREETQQK   SNLELLRISL   LLIQSWLEPV   QFLRSVFANS
     LVYGASDSNV   YDLLKDLEEG   IQTLMGRLED   GSPRTGQIFK   QTYSKFDTNS
     HNDDALLKNY   GLLYCFRKDM   DKVETFLRIV   QCRSVEGSCG   F
```

Somavubove [*1990*] (soe ma′ vue bove). $C_{976}H_{1533}N_{265}O_{286}S_8$. 21,811.76. (1) Somatotropin (ox), 127-L-leucine-; (2) 127-L-leucine growth hormone (ox). *CAS-126752-39-4.* INN. *Galactopoietic agent (veterinary). [Note—One of four naturally occurring molecular variants in bovine pituitary somatotropin.]*

```
     AFPAMSLSGL   FANAVLRAQH   LHQLAADTFK   EFERTYIPEG   QRYSIQNTQV
     AFCFSETIPA   PTGKNEAQQK   SDLELLRISL   LLIQSWLGPL   QFLRSVFTNS
     LVFGTSDRVY   EKLKDLEEGI   LALMRELEDG   TPRAGQILKQ   TYDKFDTNMR
     SDDALLKNYG   LLSCFRKDLH   KTETYLRVMK   CRRFGEASCA   F
```

Somenopor [*1990*] (soe me′ noe pore). $C_{938}H_{1469}N_{255}O_{275}S_7$. 20,942.72. (1) Somatotropin (pig clone pPGH-1 reduced), *N*-L-alanyl-32-de-L-glutamic acid-33-de-L-arginine-34-de-L-alanine-35-de-L-tyrosine-36-de-L-isoleucine-37-de-L-proline-38-de-L-glutamic acid-; (2) *N*-L-Alanyl-32-de-L-glutamic acid-33-de-L-arginine-34-de-L-alanine-35-de-L-tyrosine-36-de-L-isoleucine-37-de-L-proline-38-de-L-glutamic acidgrowth hormone (pig clone pPGH-1 reduced). *CAS-119693-74-2.* INN; BAN. *Hormone (growth, porcine).*

```
     AFPAMPLSSL   FANAVLRAQH   LHQLAADTYK   EFGQRYSIQN   AQAAFCFSET
     IPAPTGKDEA   QQRSDVELLR   FSLLLIQSWL   GPVQFLSRVF   TNSLVFGTSD
     RVYEKLKDLE   EGIQALMREL   EDGSPRAGQI   LKQTYDKFDT   NLRSDDALLK
     NYGLLSCFKK   DLHKAETYLR   VMKCRRFVES   SCAF
```

Sometribove [*1989*] (soe me′ tri bove). $C_{978}H_{1537}N_{265}O_{286}S_9$. 21,871.88. (1) Somatotropin (ox), 1-L-methionine-127-L-leucine-; (2) 1-L-Methionine-127-L-leucinegrowth hormone (ox). *CAS-102744-97-8.* INN; BAN. *Growth stimulant (veterinary).* Posilac (Monsanto)

```
     MFPAMSLSGL   FANAVLRAQH   LHQLAADTFK   EFERTYIPEG   QRYSIQNTQV
     AFCFSETIPA   PTGKNEAQQK   SDLELLRISL   LLIQSWLGPL   QFLSRVFTNS
     LVFGTSDRVY   EKLKDLEEGI   LALMRELEDG   TPRAGQILKQ   TYDKFDTNMR
     SDDALLKNYG   LLSCFRKDLH   KTETYLRVMK   CRRFGEASCA   F
```

Sometripor [*1989*] (soe me′ tri pore). $C_{979}H_{1527}N_{265}O_{287}S_8$. 21,857.74. (1) Somatotropin (pig), *N*-L-methionyl-; (2) *N*-L-Methionylgrowth hormone (pig). *CAS-102733-72-2.* INN; BAN. *Growth stimulant (veterinary).*

```
     MFPAMPLSSL   FANAVLRAQH   LHQLAADTYK   EFERAYIPEG   QRYSIQNAQA
     AFCFSETIPA   PTGKNEAQQR   SDVELLRFSL   LLIQSWLGPV   QFLSRVFTNS
     LVFGTSDRVY   EKLKDLEEGI   QALMRELEDG   SPRAGQILKQ   TYDKFDTNLR
     SDDALLKNYG   LLSCFKKDLH   KAETYLRVMK   CRRFVESSCA   F
```

Somfasepor [*1991*] (sohm fas′ e pore). $C_{938}H_{1465}N_{257}O_{278}S_6$. 20,982.63. (1) 8-190-Somatotropin (pig clone pPGH-1); (2) 8-190-Growth hormone (pig). *CAS-129566-95-6.* INN. *Growth stimulant (veterinary).* Grolene (Pitman-Moore); Leanstar (Pitman-Moore) ◇*P-3232; P-3895*

```
     SLFANAVLRA   QHLHQLAADT   YKEFERAYIP   EGQRYSIQNA   QAAFCFSETI
     PAPTGKNEAQ   QRSDVELLRF   SLLLIQSWLG   PVQFLSRVFT   NSLVFGTSDR
     VYEKLKDLEE   GIQALMRELE   DGSPRAGQIL   KQTYDKFDTN   LRSDDALLKN
     YGLLSCFKKD   LHKAETYLRV   MKCRRFVESS   CAF
```

Somidobove [*1989*] (soe mi′ doe bove). $C_{1020}H_{1596}N_{274}O_{302}S_9$. 22,817.85. (1) Somatotropin (ox), 1-[N^2-[*N*-[*N*-[*N*-[*N*-[*N*-[1-(*N*-L-methionyl-L-phenylalanyl)-L-prolyl]-L-leucyl]-L-α-aspartyl]-L-α-aspartyl]-L-α-aspartyl]-L-α-aspartyl]-L-lysine]-; (2) 1-[N^2-[*N*-[*N*-[*N*-[*N*-[*N*-[1-(*N*-L-Methionyl-L-phenylalanyl)-L-prolyl]-L-leucyl]-L-aspartyl]-L-aspartyl]-L-aspartyl]-L-aspartyl]-L-lysine]growth hormone (ox). *CAS-89383-13-1.* INN; BAN. *Hormone (growth, synthetic bovine).* Optiflex (Lilly) ◇*LY177837; EL349*

```
     MFPLDDDDKF   PAMSLSGLFA   NAVLRAQHLH   QLAADTFKEF   ERTYIPEGQR
     YSIQNTQVAF   CFSETIPAPT   GKNEAQQKSD   LELLRISLLL   IQSWLGPLQF
     LSRVFTNSLV   FGTSDRVYEK   LKDLEEGILA   LMRELEDGTP   RAGQILKQTY
     DKFDTNMRSD   DALLKNYGLL   SCFRKDLHKT   ETYLRVMKCR   RFGEASCAF
```

Soneclosan. $C_{12}H_8Cl_2O_2$. 255.10. 5-Chloro-2-(*p*-chlorophenoxy)phenol. *CAS-3380-30-1.* INN.

Sonedenoson [*2007*] (son″ e den′ oh son). $C_{18}H_{20}ClN_5O_5$. 421.83. (1) Adenosine, 2-[2-(4-chlorophenyl)ethoxy]-; (2) 9-β-D-Ribofuranosyl-2-[2-(4-chlorophenyl)ethoxy]-9*H*-purin-6-amine. *CAS-131865-88-8. Wound healing; Adenosine A_{2A}Receptor agonist.* ✧*MRE0094*

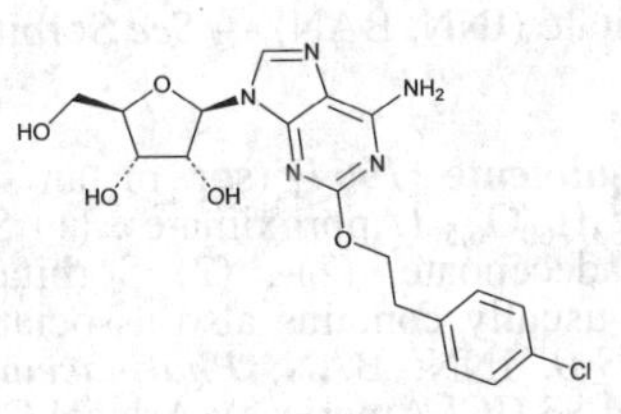

Sonepiprazole. $C_{21}H_{27}N_3O_3S$. 401.52. (-)-*p*-[4-[2-[(*S*)-1-Isochromanyl]ethyl]-1-piperazinyl]benzenesulfonamide. *UNII-O609V24217. CAS-170858-33-0.* INN.

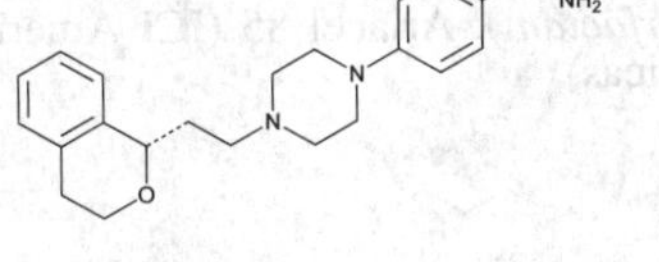

Sonepiprazole Mesylate [*1998*] (soe″ ne pi′ pra zole mes′ i late). $C_{21}H_{27}N_3O_3S.CH_4O_3S$. 497.63. (1) (*S*)-4-[4-[2-(3,4-Dihydro-1*H*-2-benzopyran-1-yl)ethyl]-1-piperazinyl]benzenesulfonamide monomethanesulfonate; (2) (-)-*p*-[4-[2-[(*S*)-1-Isochromanyl]ethyl]-1-piperazinyl]benzenesulfonamide monomethanesulfonate. *CAS-170858-34-1. Antipsychotic (dopamine D_4antagonist).* ✧*PNU-101387G*

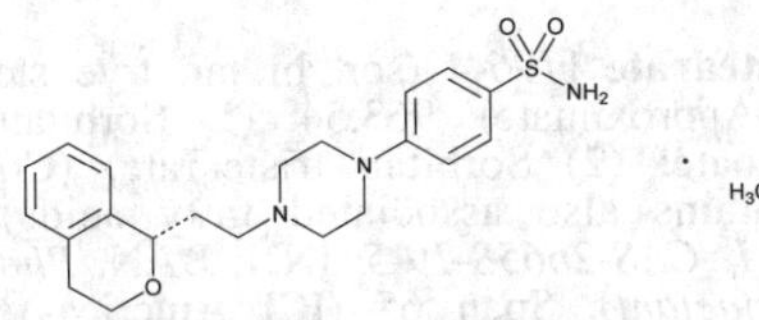

Sonermin. $C_{767}H_{1204}N_{210}O_{229}S_2$. 17,095.18. 3-157-Tumor necrosis factor (human). *CAS-144916-42-7.* INN.

Sontuzumab. Immunoglobulin G1, anti-(human episialin) (mouse monoclonal HMFG-1 γ1-chain), disulfide with mouse monoclonal HMFG-1, dimer. *CAS-372075-37-1.* INN.

Sopecainol — *See* Solpecainol.

Sopitazine. $C_{20}H_{23}N_3OS$. 353.48. 10-[(4-Isopropyl-1-piperazinyl)carbonyl]phenothiazine. *UNII-QI0U3D4X3M. CAS-23492-69-5.* INN.

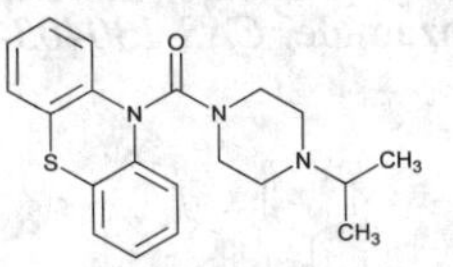

Sopromidine. $C_{14}H_{23}N_7S$. 321.44. (-)-1-[(*R*)-2-Imidazol-4-yl-1-methylethyl]-3-[2-[[(5-methylimidazol-4-yl)-methyl]thio]ethyl]guanidine. *CAS-79313-75-0.* INN.

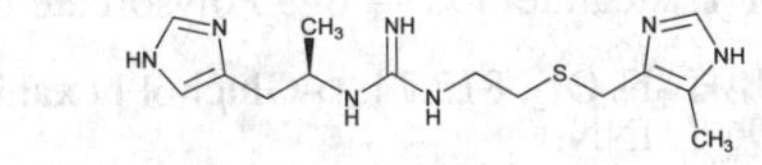

Soquinolol. $C_{17}H_{26}N_2O_3$. 306.40. 5-[3-(*tert*-Butylamino)-2-hydroxypropoxy]-3,4-dihydro-2(1*H*)-isoquinolinecarboxaldehyde. *UNII-15CC9BOH7Q. CAS-61563-18-6.* INN.

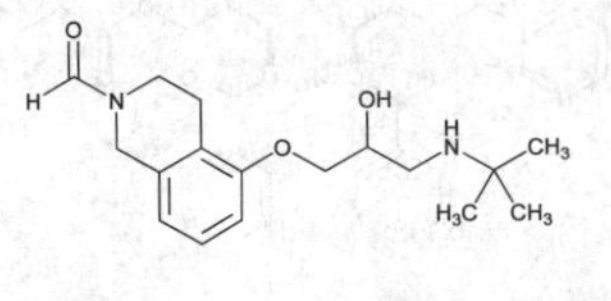

Sorafenib [*2006*] (soe raf′ e nib). $C_{21}H_{16}ClF_3N_4O_3$. 464.82. (1) 2-Pyridinecarboxamide, 4-[4-[[[[4-chloro-3-trifluoromethyl)phenyl]amino]carbonyl]amino]phenoxy]-*N*-methyl-; (2) 4-(4{3-[4 Chloro-3-(trifluoromethyl)phenyl]ureido}phenoxy)-*N*2-methylpyridine-2-carboxamide. *UNII-9ZOQ3TZI87. CAS-284461-73-0.* INN. *Treatment of cancer.* Nexavar (Bayer HealthCare); Xarelto (Bayer HealthCare) ✧*BAY 43-9006*

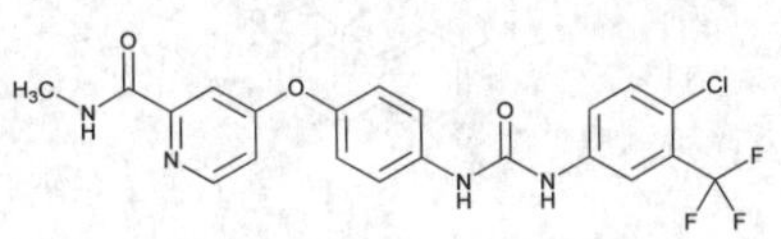

Sorafenib Tosylate [*2006*] (soe raf′ e nib tos′ i late). $C_{21}H_{16}ClF_3N_4O_3.C_7H_8O_3S$. 637.03. (1) 2-Pyridinecarboxamide, 4-[4-[[[[4-chloro-3-(trifluoromethyl)phenyl]amino]carbonyl]amino]phenoxy]-*N*-methyl-, mono(4-methylbenzenesulfonate); (2) 1-[4-Chloro-3-(trifluoromethyl)phenyl]-3-[4-[[2-(methylcarbamoyl)pyridin-4-yl]oxy]phenyl]urea mono(4-methylbenzenesulfonate); (3) 4-(4-{3-[4-Chloro-3-(trifluoromethyl)phenyl]ureido}phenoxy)-*N*2-methylpyridine-2-carboxamide mono (4-methylbenzenesulfonate). *UNII-5T62Q3B36J. CAS-475207-59-1. Treatment of cancer.* Nexavar (Bayer) ✧*BAY 54-9085*

Soraprazan. $C_{21}H_{25}N_3O_3$. 367.44. (7*R*,8*R*,9*R*)-7-(2-Methoxyethoxy)-2,3-dimethyl-9-phenyl-7,8,9,10-tetrahydroimidazo[1,2-*h*][1,7]naphtyridin-8-ol. *CAS-261944-46-1.* INN.

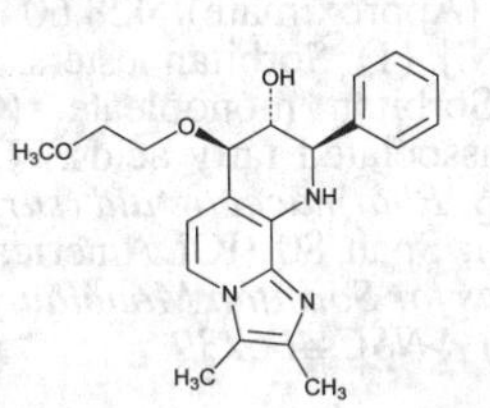

Sorbic Acid (sor′ bik as′ id). **NF**. $C_6H_8O_2$. 112.13. (1) 2,4-Hexadienoic acid, (*E,E*)-; 2,4-Hexadienoic acid. (2) (*E,E*)-Sorbic acid; Sorbic acid. *CAS-110-44-1; CAS-22500-92-1 [E,E]. Pharmaceutic aid (antimicrobial agent).*

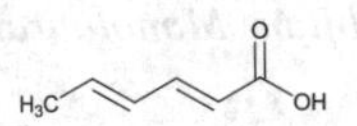

Sorbide Nitrate — *See* Isosorbide Dinitrate.

Sorbimacrogol Laurate 300 — *See* Polysorbate 20.

Sorbimacrogol Oleate 300 — *See* Polysorbate 80.

† Brand name formerly used, and/or firm no longer concerned with this product.

Sorbimacrogol Palmitate 300 — *See* Polysorbate 40.

Sorbimacrogol Stearate — *See* Polysorbate 60.

Sorbimacrogol Tristearate 300 — *See* Polysorbate 65.

Sorbinicate. $C_{42}H_{32}N_6O_{12}$. 812.74. D-Glucitol hexanicotinate. *CAS-6184-06-1.* INN.

Sorbinil [*1979*] (sor′ bi nil). $C_{11}H_9FN_2O_3$. 236.20. (1) Spiro[4*H*-1-benzopyran-4,4′-imidazolidine]-2′,5′-dione, 6-fluoro-2,3-dihydro-, (*S*)-; (2) (*S*)-6-Fluorospiro[chroman-4,4′-imidazolidine]-2′,5′-dione. *CAS-68367-52-2.* INN; BAN. *Enzyme inhibitor (aldose reductase).* ◇*CP-45,634*

Sorbitan Laurate (INN, BAN) — *See* Sorbitan Monolaurate.

Sorbitan Monolaurate [*1964*] (sor′ bi tan mon″ oh lawr′ ate). **NF.** $C_{18}H_{34}O_6$. 346.46. [Sorbitan Laurate is INN and BAN.] (1) Sorbitan, esters, monododecanoate; (2) Sorbitan monolaurate. (Compound usually contains also associated fatty acids.) *UNII-6W9PS8B71J. CAS-1338-39-2. Pharmaceutic aid (surfactant).* Span 20 (ICI Americas)

Sorbitan Monooleate [*1964*] (sor′ bi tan mon″ oh oh′ lee ate). **NF.** $C_{24}H_{44}O_6$ (Approximate). 428.60. [Sorbitan Oleate is INN and BAN.] (1) Sorbitan esters, mono(*Z*)-9-octadecenoate; (2) Sorbitan monooleate. (Compound usually contains also associated fatty acids.) *UNII-06XEA2VD56. CAS-1338-43-8. Pharmaceutic aid (surfactant).* Arlacel 80 (ICI Americas); Span 80 (ICI Americas) *[Note—Graphic formula same as for Sorbitan Monolaurate, except that R is $(C_{17}H_{33})COO$.]* ◇*NSC-406239*

Sorbitan Monopalmitate [*1964*] (sor′ bi tan mon″ oh pal′ mi tate). **NF.** $C_{22}H_{42}O_6$ (Approximate). 402.57. [Sorbitan Palmitate is INN and BAN.] (1) Sorbitan, esters, monohexadecanoate; (2) Sorbitan monopalmitate. (Compound usually contains also associated fatty acids.) *UNII-77K6Z421KU. CAS-26266-57-9. Pharmaceutic aid (surfactant).* Span 40 (ICI Americas) *[Note—Graphic formula same as for Sorbitan Monolaurate, except that R is $(C_{15}H_{31})COO$.]*

Sorbitan Monostearate [*1964*] (sor′ bi tan mon″ oh steer′ ate). **NF.** $C_{24}H_{46}O_6$ (Approximate). 430.62. [Sorbitan Stearate is INN and BAN.] (1) Sorbitan, esters, monooctadecanoate; (2) Sorbitan monostearate. (Compound usually contains also associated fatty acids.) *UNII-NVZ4I0H58X. CAS-1338-41-6. Pharmaceutic aid (surfac-*

tant). Span 60 (ICI Americas) *[Note—Graphic formula same as for Sorbitan Monolaurate, except that R is $(C_{17}H_{35})COO$.]*

Sorbitan Oleate (INN, BAN) — *See* Sorbitan Monooleate.

Sorbitan Palmitate (INN, BAN) — *See* Sorbitan Monopalmitate.

Sorbitan Sesquioleate [*1964*] (sor′ bi tan ses″ kwi oh′ lee ate). **NF.** $C_{33}H_{60}O_{6.5}$ (Approximate). (1) Sorbitan, esters, sesqui-9-octadecenoate, (*Z*)-; (2) Sorbitan sesquioleate. (Compound usually contains also associated fatty acids.) *CAS-8007-43-0.* INN; BAN. *Pharmaceutic aid (surfactant).* Arlacel 83 (ICI Americas); Arlacel C (ICI Americas)

Sorbitan Stearate (INN, BAN) — *See* Sorbitan Monostearate.

Sorbitan Trioleate [*1964*] (sor′ bi tan trye oh′ lee ate). **NF.** $C_{60}H_{108}O_8$ (Approximate). 957.49. (1) Sorbitan, esters, tri-9-octadecenoate, (*Z,Z,Z*)-; (2) Sorbitan trioleate. (Compound usually contains also associated fatty acids.) *UNII-QE6F49RPJ1. CAS-26266-58-0.* INN; BAN. *Pharmaceutic aid (surfactant).* Arlacel 85 (ICI Americas†); Span 85 (ICI Americas)

Sorbitan Tristearate [*1964*] (sor′ bi tan trye steer′ ate). $C_{60}H_{114}O_8$ (Approximate). 963.54. (1) Sorbitan, esters, trioctadecanoate; (2) Sorbitan tristearate. (Compound usually contains also associated fatty acids). *UNII-6LUM696811. CAS-26658-19-5.* INN; BAN. *Pharmaceutic aid (surfactant).* Span 65 (ICI Americas) *[Note—Graphic formula same as for Sorbitan Trioleate, except that R is $(C_{17}H_{35})COO$.]*

Sorbitol (sor′ bi tol). **NF, USP (Solution).** $C_6H_{14}O_6$. 182.17. [D-Sorbitol is JAN.] (1) D-Glucitol; (2) D-Glucitol. *UNII-506T60A25R. CAS-50-70-4. Pharmaceutic aid (flavor); pharmaceutic aid (tablet excipient).*

D-Sorbitol (JAN) — *See* Sorbitol.

Soretolide. $C_{13}H_{14}N_2O_2$. 230.26. 2,6-Dimethyl-*N*-(5-methyl-3-isoxazolyl)benzamide. *CAS-130403-08-6.* INN.

Sorivudine [*1992*] (soe riv′ ue deen). $C_{11}H_{13}BrN_2O_6$. 349.13. (1) 2,4(1*H*,3*H*)-Pyrimidinedione, 1-β-D-arabinofuranosyl-5-(2-bromoethenyl)-, (*E*)-; (2) (+)-1-β-D-Arabinofuranosyl-5-[(*E*)-2-bromovinyl]uracil. *CAS-77181-69-2.* INN; BAN; JAN. *Antiviral.* Bravavir (Bristol-Myers Squibb) ◇*SQ 32,756; YN-72*

Sornidipine. C$_{22}$H$_{24}$N$_2$O$_9$. 460.43. (+)-1,4-Dihydro-2,6-dimethyl-4-(*o*-nitrophenyl)-3,5-pyridinedicarboxylic acid, methyl ester, 5-ester with 1,4:3,6-dianhydro-D-glucitol. *UNII-Z82YP691V7. CAS-95105-77-4.* INN.

Sotalol Hydrochloride [*1967*] (soe′ ta lol hye″ droe klor′ ide). **USP.** C$_{12}$H$_{20}$N$_2$O$_3$S.HCl. 308.82. [Sotalol is INN and BAN.] (1) Methanesulfonamide, *N*-[4-[1-hydroxy-2-[(1-methylethyl)amino]ethyl]phenyl]-, monohydrochloride; (2) 4′-[1-Hydroxy-2-(isopropylamino)ethyl]methanesulfonanilide monohydrochloride. *UNII-HEC37C70XX; UNII-A6D97U294I* [sotalol]. *CAS-959-24-0; CAS-3930-20-9* [sotalol]. *Anti-adrenergic (β-receptor).* Betapace (Bayer); Sorine (Upsher Smith) ◇*MJ 1999*

Soterenol Hydrochloride [*1968*] (soe ter′ e nol hye″ droe klor′ ide). C$_{12}$H$_{20}$N$_2$O$_4$S.HCl. 324.82. [Soterenol is INN.] (1) Methanesulfonamide, *N*-[2-hydroxy-5-[1-hydroxy-2-[(1-methylethyl)amino]ethyl]phenyl]-, monohydrochloride; (2) 2′-Hydroxy-5′-[1-hydroxy-2-(isopropylamino)ethyl]methanesulfonamide monohydrochloride. *CAS-14816-67-2; CAS-13642-52-9* [soterenol]. *Bronchodilator.* ◇*MJ 1992*

Sotirimod [*2005*] (soe tir′ i mod). C$_{14}$H$_{17}$N$_5$. 255.32. (1) 1*H*-Imidazo[4,5-*c*][1,5]naphthyridin-4-amine, 2-methyl-1-(2-methylpropyl)-; (2) 2-Methyl-1-(2-methylpropyl)-1*H*-imidazo[4,5-*c*][1,5]naphthyridin-4-amine. *UNII-*

X04FQM7J4M. CAS-227318-75-4. INN. *Treatment of dermatologic diseases, including actinic keratosis, infections, cancer.* ◇*R-850; S-30594*

Sotrastaurin Acetate [*2008*] (soe″ tra staw′ rin as′ e tate). C$_{25}$H$_{22}$N$_6$O$_2$.C$_2$H$_4$O$_2$. 498.53. [Sotrastaurin is INN.] (1) 1*H*-Pyrrole-2,5-dione, 3-(1*H*-indol-3-yl)-4-[2-(4-methyl-1-piperazinyl)-4-quinazolinyl]-, acetate; (2) 3-(1*H*-Indol-3-yl)-4-[2-(4-methylpiperazin-1-yl)quinazolin-4-yl]-1*H*-pyrrole-2,5-dione acetate. *UNII-R1SIA15KZ1. CAS-908351-31-5; CAS-425637-18-9* [sotrastaurin]. *Transplantation, T-cell mediated acute or chronic inflammatory diseases.* ◇*AEB071*

Soybean Oil (soi′ been). **USP.** The refined fixed oil obtained from the seeds of the soya plant *Glycine max* Merr. (Fabaceae). *UNII-241ATL177A.* JAN. *Pharmaceutic necessity.* Intralipid (Fresenius); Liposyn (Hospira); Nutrilipid (B Braun)

Soybean Oil, Hydrogenated (soi′ been hye droj′ en ay″ ted). **NF.** The product obtained by refining, bleaching, hydrogenation, and deordorization of oil obtained from seeds of the soya plant *Glycine max* Merr. (Fabaceae). *CAS-8016-70-4.*

Soybean Phospholipids. A mixture of the diglycerides of stearic, palmitic, and oleic acids, linked to the choline ester of phosphoric acid. JAN.

Soysterol. Unsaponifiable matter of soybean oil. JAN.

Spaglumic Acid. C$_{11}$H$_{16}$N$_2$O$_8$. 304.25. *N*-(*N*-Acetyl-L-β-aspartyl)-L-glutamic acid. *UNII-X81L78B3RB. CAS-4910-46-7.* INN.

Sparfloxacin [*1991*] (spar flox′ a sin). C$_{19}$H$_{22}$F$_2$N$_4$O$_3$. 392.40. (1) 3-Quinolinecarboxylic acid, 5-amino-1-cyclopropyl-7-(3,5-dimethyl-1-piperazinyl)-6,8-difluoro-1,4-dihydro-4-oxo-, *cis*-; (2) 5-Amino-1-cyclopropyl-7-(*cis*-3,5-dimethyl-1-piperazinyl)-6,8-difluoro-1,4-dihydro-4-oxo-3-quinoli-

---

† Brand name formerly used, and/or firm no longer concerned with this product.

necarboxylic acid. *UNII-Q90AGA787L. CAS-110871-86-8.* INN; BAN; JAN. *Antibacterial.* Zagam (Mylan) ◇*CI-978; AT-4140*

Sparfosate Sodium [*1981*] (spar fos′ ate soe′ dee um). $C_6H_8NNa_2O_8P$. 299.08. [Sparfosic Acid is INN.] (1) L-Aspartic acid, *N*-(phosphonoacetyl)-, disodium salt; (2) *N*-(phosphonoacetyl)-L-aspartic acid, disodium salt. *CAS-66569-27-5* [disodium salt]; *CAS-51321-79-0* [sparfosic acid]. *Antineoplastic.* ◇*CI-882*

Sparfosic Acid (INN) — *See* Sparfosate Sodium.

Sparsomycin [*1962*] (spar″ soe mye′ sin). $C_{13}H_{19}N_3O_5S_2$. 361.44. Antibiotic produced by *Streptomyces sparsogenes* variant. (1) 2-Propenamide, *N*-[1-(hydroxymethyl)-2-[[(methylthio)methyl]sulfinyl]ethyl]-3-(1,2,3,4-tetrahydro-6-methyl-2,4-dioxo-5-pyrimidinyl)-, [*S*-(*E*)]-; (2) Sparsomycin. *CAS-1404-64-4.* INN. *Antineoplastic.* ◇*U-19183; NSC-59729*

Sparteine Sulfate [*1962*] (spar′ teen sul′ fate). $C_{15}H_{26}N_2 \cdot H_2SO_4 \cdot 5H_2O$. 422.54. [Sparteine is INN.] (1) 7,14-Methano-2*H*,6*H*-dipyrido[1,2-*a*:1′,2′-*e*][1,5]diazocine, dodecahydro-, [7*S*-(7α,7aα,14α,14aβ)]-, sulfate (1:1), pentahydrate; (2) Sparteine sulfate (1:1) pentahydrate. *CAS-6160-12-9; CAS-299-39-8* [anhydrous]; *CAS-90-39-1* [sparteine]. JAN. *Oxytocic.*

Spearmint. NF XVI.

Spearmint Oil. *CAS-8008-79-5.* NF XVI.

Spectinomycin Hydrochloride [*1962*] (spek″ tin oh mye′ sin hye″ droe klor′ ide). **USP.** $C_{14}H_{24}N_2O_7 \cdot 2HCl \cdot 5H_2O$. 495.35. [Spectinomycin is INN and BAN.] (1) 4*H*-Pyrano[2,3-*b*][1,4]benzodioxin-4-one, decahydro-4a,7,9-trihydroxy-2-methyl-6,8-bis(methylamino)-, dihydrochloride, pentahydrate; (2) Decahydro-4a,7,9-trihydroxy-2-methyl-6,8-bis(-methylamino)-4*H*-pyrano[2,3-*b*][1,4]benzodioxin-4-one dihydrochloride pentahydrate. *UNII-HWT06H303Z; UNII-93AKI1U6QF* [spectinomycin]. *CAS-22189-32-8; CAS-*

21736-83-4 [anhydrous]; *CAS-1695-77-8* [spectinomycin]. JAN. *Antibacterial.* Trobicin (Pfizer) ◇*M-141; U-18,409AE*

Spermaceti, Synthetic — *See* Cetyl Esters Wax.

Spiclamine. $C_{20}H_{25}ClN_2O$. 344.88. (-)-(1*R*,2*R*,3*S*,4*S*)-3-(*p*-Chlorophenyl)-2′-morpholinospiro[norbornane-2,5′-[1]pyrroline]. *CAS-90243-97-3.* INN.

Spiclomazine. $C_{22}H_{24}ClN_3OS_2$. 446.03. 8-[3-(2-Chloro-10-phenothiazinyl)propyl]-1-thia-4,8-diazaspiro[4,5]decan-3-one. *UNII-G2V8248111. CAS-24527-27-3.* INN.

Spinosad [*2008*] (spin′ oh sad). $C_{41}H_{65}NO_{10}$ (factor A). 731.46; $C_{42}H_{67}NO_{10}$ (factor D). 745.48. (1) Factor A: 1*H*-*as*-Indaceno[3,2-*d*]oxacyclododecin-7,15-dione, 2-[(6-deoxy-2,3,4-tri-*O*-methyl-α-L-mannopyranosyl)oxy]-13-[[(2*R*,5*S*,6*R*)-5-(dimethylamino)tetrahydro-6-methyl-2*H*-pyran-2-yl]oxy]-9-ethyl-2,3,3a,5a,5b,6,9,10,11,12,13,14, 16a,16b-tetradecahydro-14-methyl-, (2*R*,3a*S*,5a*R*,5b*S*,9*S*,13*S*,14*R*,16a*S*,16b*R*)-, Factor D: 1*H*-*as*-Indaceno[3,2-*d*]oxacyclododecin-7,15-dione, 2-[(6-deoxy-2,3,4-tri-*O*-methyl-α-L-mannopyranosyl)oxy]-13-[[(2*R*,5*S*,6*R*)-5-(dimethylamino)tetrahydro-6-methyl-2*H*-pyran-2-yl]oxy]-9-ethyl-2,3,3a,5a,5b,6,9,10,11,12,13,14, 16a,16b-tetradecahydro-4,14-dimethyl-, (2*S*,3a*R*,5a-*S*,5b*S*,9*S*,13*S*,14*R*,16a*S*,16b*S*)-; (2) Factor A: (2*R*,3a*S*,5a*R*,5b*S*,9*S*,13*S*,14*R*,16a*S*,16b*R*)-2-[(6-Deoxy-2,3,4-tri-*O*-methyl-α-L-mannopyranosyl)oxy]-13-[[(2*R*,5*S*,6*R*)-5-(dimethylamino)tetrahydro-6-methyl-2*H*-pyran-2-yl]oxy]-9-ethyl-14-methyl-2,3,3a,5a,5b,6,9,10,11,12,13,14,16a,16b-tetradecahydro-1*H*-*as*-indaceno[3,2-*d*]oxacyclododecin-7,15-dione, Factor D: (2*R*,3a*S*,5a*R*,5b*S*,9*S*,13*S*,14*R*,16a*S*,16b*R*)-2-[(6-Deoxy-2,3,4-tri-*O*-methyl-α-L-mannopyranosyl)oxy]-13-[[(2*R*,5*S*,6*R*)-5-(dimethylamino)tetrahydro-6-methyl-2*H*-pyran-2-yl]oxy]-9-ethyl-4,14-dimethyl-2,3,3a,5a,5b,6,9,10,11,12,13,14,16a,16b-tetradecahydro-1*H*-*as*-indaceno[3,2-*d*]oxacyclododecin-7,15-dione. *CAS-131929-60-7* [factor A]; *CAS-131929-63-0* [factor D]. *Pediculicide.* ◇*XDE-105; LY-232105; PP-105*

Spiperone [*1966*] (spye′ per one). $C_{23}H_{26}FN_3O_2$. 395.47. (1) 1,3,8-Triazaspiro[4.5]decan-4-one, 8-[4-(4-fluorophenyl)-4-oxobutyl]-1-phenyl-; (2) 8-[3-(*p*-Fluorobenzoyl)propyl]-1-phenyl-1,3,8-triazaspiro[4.5]decan-4-one. *UNII-*

4X6E73CJ0Q. CAS-749-02-0. INN; BAN; JAN. *Antipsychotic.* Spiropitan (Janssen Pharmaceutica, Belgium) ◊*R 5147*

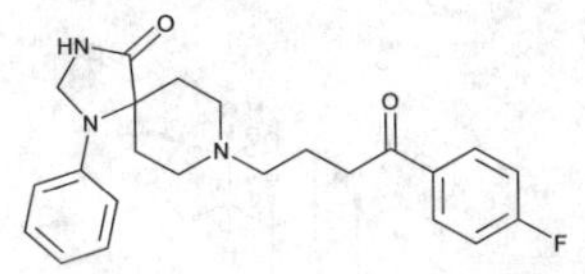

Spiradoline Mesylate [*1989*] (spir ad' oh leen mes' i late). $C_{22}H_{30}Cl_2N_2O_2 \cdot CH_4O_3S$. 521.50. [Spiradoline is INN.] (1) Benzeneacetamide, 3,4-dichloro-*N*-methyl-*N*-[7-(1-pyrrolidinyl)-1-oxaspiro[4.5]dec-8-yl]-, (5α,7α,8β)-(±)-, monomethanesulfonate; (2) (±)-2-(3,4-Dichlorophenyl)-*N*-methyl-*N*-[(5*R**,7*S**,8*S**)-7-(1-pyrrolidinyl)-1-oxaspiro[4.5]dec-8-yl]acetamide monomethanesulfonate. *CAS-87173-97-5; CAS-87151-85-7* [spiradoline]. *Analgesic.* ◊*U-62066E*

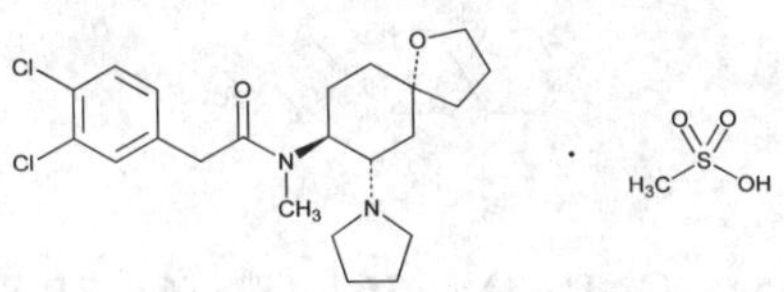

Spiramide. $C_{22}H_{26}FN_3O_2$. 383.46. 8-[3-(4-Fluorophenoxy)propyl]-1-phenyl-1,3,8-triazaspiro[4.5]decan-4-one. *UNII-471LF4O004. CAS-510-74-7.* INN. ◊*R 5808*

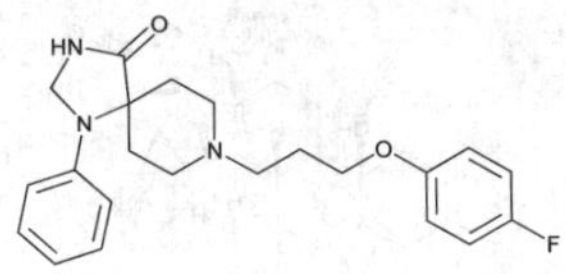

Spiramycin [*1962*] (spir" a mye' sin). $C_{43}H_{74}N_2O_{14}$. 843.05. [Acetylspiramycin is JAN.] Antibiotic produced by *Streptomyces ambofaciens.* (1) Leucomycin; (2) Leucomycin. *CAS-8025-81-8.* INN; BAN. *Antibacterial.* Rovamycin (Rhone-Poulenc Rorer) ◊*IL 5902; RP 5337; NSC-55926; NSC-64393 [as hydrochloride]*

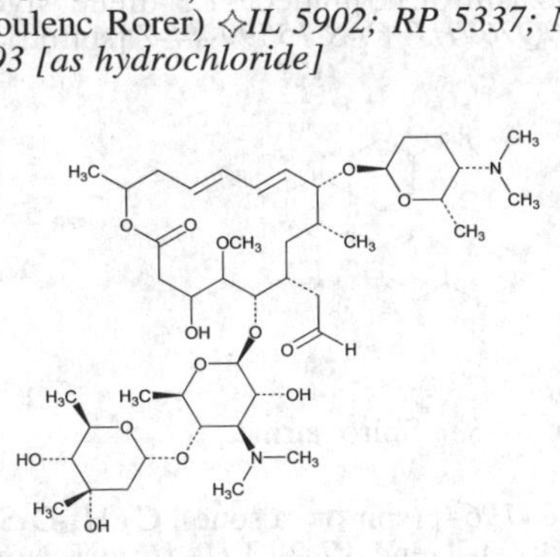

Spirapril Hydrochloride [*1987*] (spir' a pril hye" droe klor' ide). $C_{22}H_{30}N_2O_5S_2 \cdot HCl$. 503.07. [Spirapril is INN and BAN.] (1) 1,4-Dithia-7-azaspiro[4.4]nonane-8-carboxylic acid, 7-[2-[[1-(ethoxycarbonyl)-3-phenylpropyl]amino]-1-oxopropyl]-, monohydrochloride, [8*S*-[7[*R**(*R**)],8*R**]]-; (2) (8*S*)-7-[(*S*)-*N*-[(*S*)-1-Carboxy-3-phenylpropyl]alanyl]-1,4-dithia-7-azaspiro[4.4]nonane-8-carboxylic acid, 1-ethyl ester, monohydrochloride. *UNII-OCC25LM897;*

---

† Brand name formerly used, and/or firm no longer concerned with this product.

UNII-96U2K78I3V [spirapril]. *CAS-94841-17-5; CAS-83647-97-6* [spirapril]. *Enzyme inhibitor (angiotensin-converting).* Renormax (Schering) ◊*Sch 33844*

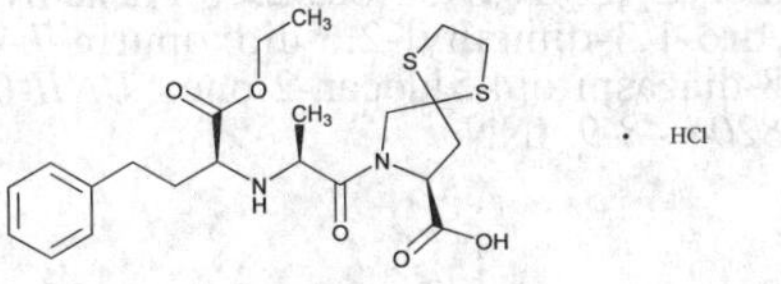

Spiraprilat [*1988*] (spir' a pril at"). $C_{20}H_{26}N_2O_5S_2$. 438.56. (1) 1,4-Dithia-7-azaspiro[4.4]nonane-8-carboxylic acid, 7-[2-[(1-carboxy-3-phenylpropyl)amino]-1-oxopropyl]-, [8*S*-[7[*R**(*R**)],8*R**]]-; (2) (8*S*)-7-[(*S*)-*N*-[(*S*)-1-Carboxy-3-phenylpropyl]alanyl]-1,4-dithia-7-azaspiro[4.4]nonane-8-carboxylic acid. *CAS-83602-05-5.* INN. *Enzyme inhibitor (angiotensin-converting).* ◊*Sch 33861*

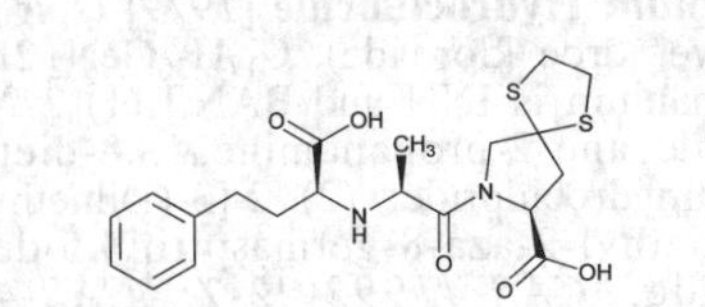

Spirazine (INN) Hydrochloride — *See* Spirotriazine Hydrochloride.

Spirendolol. $C_{21}H_{31}NO_3$. 345.48. (±)-4'-[3-(*tert*-Butylamino)-2-hydroxypropoxy]spiro[cyclohexane-1,2'-indan]-1'-one. *UNII-96789094BR. CAS-65429-87-0.* INN.

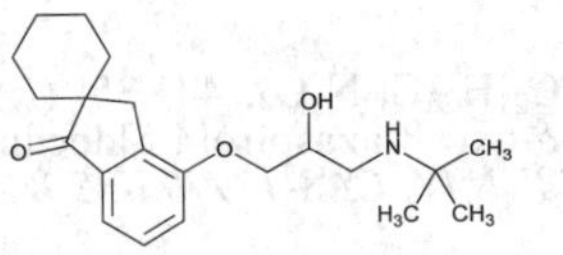

Spirgetine. $C_{10}H_{20}N_4$. 196.29. [2-(6-Azaspiro[2.5]oct-6-yl)ethyl]guanidine. *UNII-8J8O0MK4JG. CAS-144-45-6.* INN; DCF.

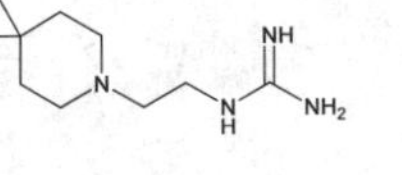

Spirilene. $C_{24}H_{28}FN_3O$. 393.50. 8-[4-(*p*-Fluorophenyl)-3-pentenyl]-1-phenyl-1,3,8-triazaspiro[4,5]decan-4-one. *CAS-357-66-4.* INN; BAN; MI. ◊*R 6109*

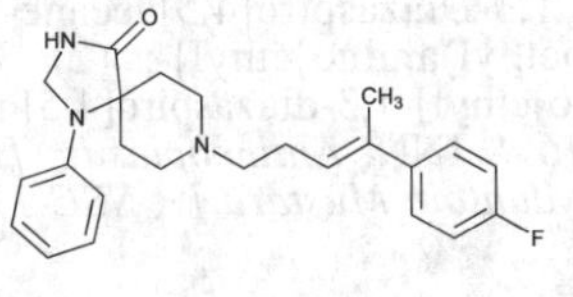

Spiriprostil. $C_{20}H_{34}N_2O_4$. 366.49. (±)-(5*R**,6*S**,7*R**)-7-Hexyl-2,4-dioxo-1,3-diazaspiro[4,4]nonane-6-heptanoic acid. *UNII-Q2LN8K1MS7. CAS-122946-42-3.* INN.

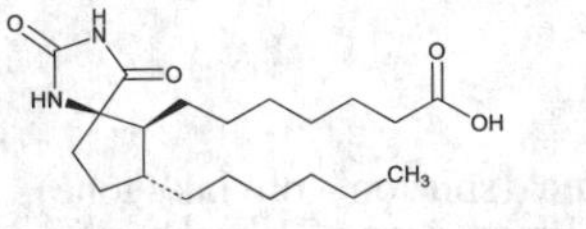

Spirit of Nitrous Ether — *See* Ethyl Nitrite [Spirit].

Spirobarbital Sodium. *CAS-12262-77-0; CAS-72035-36-0* [spirobarbital].

Spirofylline. $C_{24}H_{28}N_6O_5$. 480.52. 8-Phenethyl-3-[(1,2,3,6-tetrahydro-1,3-dimethyl-2,6-dioxopurin-7-yl)acetyl]-1-oxa-3,8-diazaspiro[4,5]decan-2-one. *UNII-000F949089. CAS-98204-48-9.* INN.

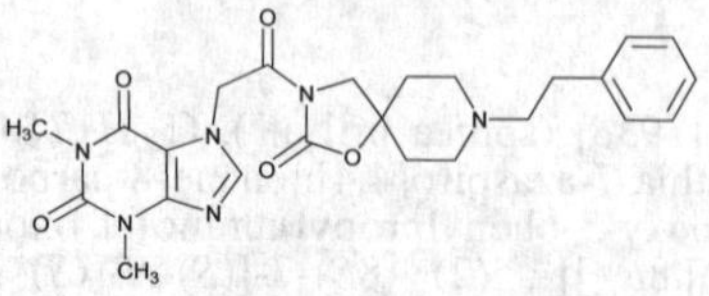

Spirogermanium Hydrochloride [*1979*] (spir″ oh jer may′ nee um hye″ droe klor′ ide). $C_{17}H_{36}GeN_2.2HCl$. 414.04. [Spirogermanium is INN and BAN.] (1) 2-Aza-8-germaspiro[4.5]decane-2-propanamine, 8,8-diethyl-*N*,*N*-dimethyl-, dihydrochloride; (2) 2-[3-(Dimethylamino)propyl]-8,8-diethyl-2-aza-8-germaspiro[4.5]decane dihydrochloride. *CAS-41992-22-7; CAS-41992-23-8* [spirogermanium]. *Antineoplastic.* Spiro-32 (Unimed) ◇*NSC-192965*

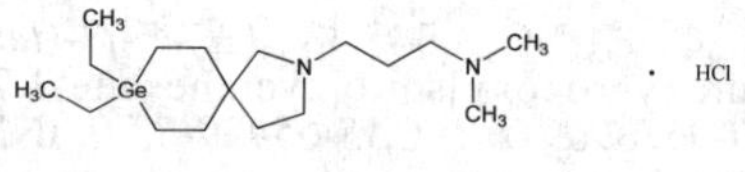

Spiroglumide. $C_{21}H_{26}Cl_2N_2O_4$. 441.35. (*R*)-γ-(3,5-Dichlorobenzamido)-δ-oxo-8-azaspiro[4.5]decane-8-valeric acid. *UNII-EZS5V8UN4Y. CAS-137795-35-8.* INN.

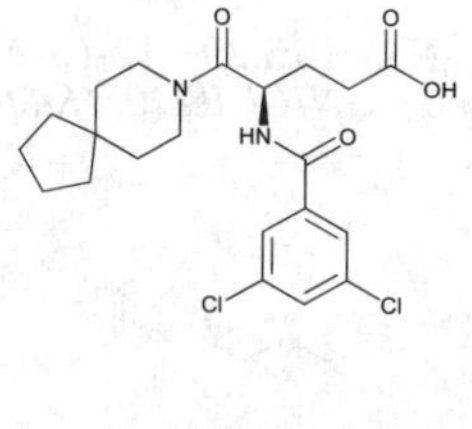

Spirohydantoin Mustard (previously used name) — *See* Spiromustine.

Spiromustine [*1981*] (spir″ oh mus′ teen). $C_{14}H_{23}Cl_2N_3O_2$. 336.26. (1) 1,3-Diazaspiro[4.5]decane-2,4-dione, 3-[2-[bis(2-chloroethyl)amino]ethyl]-; (2) 3-[2-[Bis(2-chloroethyl)amino]ethyl]-1,3-diazaspiro[4.5]decane-2,4-dione. *CAS-56605-16-4.* INN. *Antineoplastic.* [*Name previously used: Spirohydantoin Mustard.*] ◇*NSC-172112*

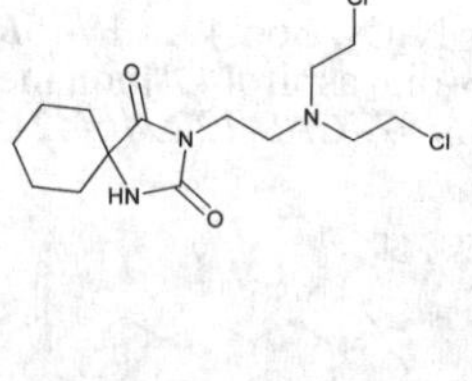

Spironolactone (spir on″ oh lak′ tone). **USP.** $C_{24}H_{32}O_4S$. 416.57. (1) Pregn-4-ene-21-carboxylic acid, 7-(acetylthio)-17-hydroxy-3-oxo-, γ-lactone, (7α,17α)-; (2) 17-Hydroxy-7α-mercapto-3-oxo-17α-pregn-4-ene-21-carboxylic acid,

γ-lactone acetate. *UNII-27O7W4T232. CAS-52-01-7.* INN; BAN; JAN. *Diuretic; aldosterone antagonist.* Aldactone (Pfizer)

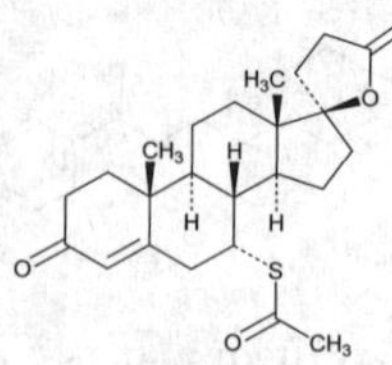

Spiroplatin [*1983*] (spir″ oh pla′ tin). $C_8H_{18}N_2O_4PtS$. 433.39. (1) Platinum, (1,1-cyclohexanedimethanamine-*N*,*N*′)[sulfato(2-)-*O*,*O*′]-, (*SP*-4-2)-; (2) *cis*-[1,1-Cyclohexanebis(methylamine)](sulfato)platinum. *CAS-74790-08-2.* INN; BAN. *Antineoplastic.* ◇*TNO-6; NSC-311056*

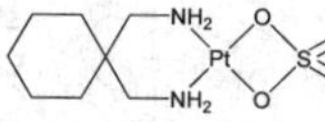

Spirorenone. $C_{24}H_{28}O_3$. 364.48. (6*R*,7*R*,8*R*,9*S*,10*R*,13*S*,14*R*,15*S*,16*S*,17*S*)-3′,4′,6,7,8,9,11,12,13,14,15,16,20,21-Tetradecahydro-10,13-dimethylspiro[17*H*-dicyclopropa[6,7:15,16]cyclopenta[*a*]phenanthrene-17,2′(5′*H*)-furan]-3(10*H*),5′-dione. *CAS-74220-07-8.* INN.

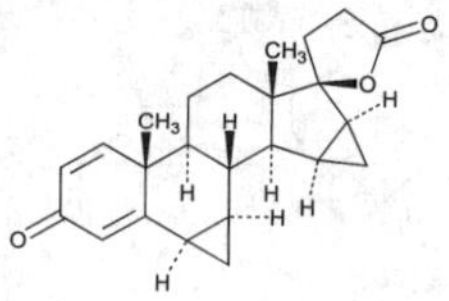

Spirotriazine Hydrochloride. $C_{15}H_{20}ClN_5.HCl$. 342.27. [Spirazine is INN.] 2,4-Diamino-5-(*p*-chlorophenyl)-9-methyl-1,3,5-triazaspiro[5.5]undeca-1,3-diene hydrochloride. *UNII-I4I0Q76VHJ. CAS-15599-44-7* [spirotriazine].

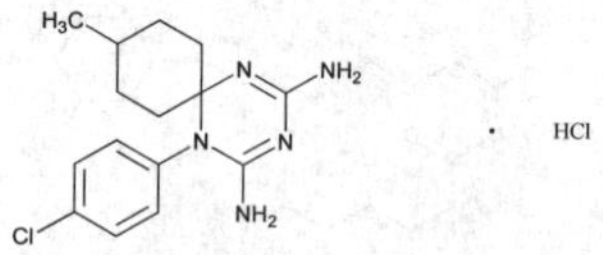

Spiroxamide — *See* Spiroxatrine.

Spiroxasone [*1964*] (spir ox′ a sone). $C_{24}H_{34}O_3S$. 402.59. (1) Spiro[androst-4-ene-17,2′(3′*H*)-furan]-3-one, 2-(acetylthio)-4′,5′-dihydro-, (7α,17β)-; (2) 4′,5′-Dihydro-7α-mercaptospiro[androst-4-ene-17,2′-(3′*H*)-furan]-3-one acetate. *CAS-6673-97-8.* INN. *Diuretic.*

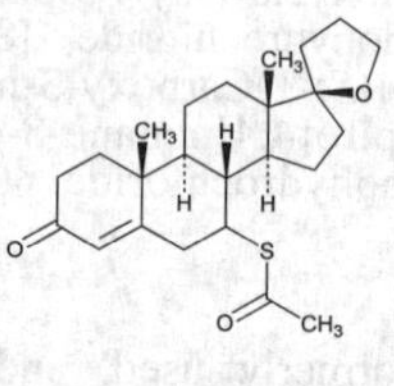

Spiroxatrine. $C_{22}H_{25}N_3O_3$. 379.45. 8-(1,4-Benzodioxan-2-ylmethyl)-1-phenyl-1,3,8-trianaspiro[4,5]decane-4-one. *UNII-DR0QR50ALL. CAS-1054-88-2.* INN. ◇*R 5188*

Spiroxepin. $C_{19}H_{21}NO_3$. 311.37. *N,N*-Dimethylspiro[dibenz[-*b,e*]oxepin-11(6*H*),2'-[1,3]dioxolane]-4'-methylamine. *UNII-80O018LGCI. CAS-47254-05-7.* INN.

Spizofurone. $C_{12}H_{10}O_3$. 202.21. 5-Acetylspiro[benzofuran-2(3*H*),1'-cyclopropan]-3-one. *UNII-94F21T5G3C. CAS-72492-12-7.* INN; JAN; MI.

Sprodiamide [*1994*] (sproe dye′ a mide). $C_{16}H_{26}DyN_5O_8$. 578.91 (anhydrous). (1) Dysprosium, [5,8-bis(carboxymethyl)-11-[2-(methylamino)-2-oxoethyl]-3-oxo-2,5,8,11-tetraazatridecan-13-oato(3-)]-; (2) [*N,N*-Bis[2-[(carboxymethyl)[(methylcarbamoyl)methyl]amino]ethyl]glycinato(3-)]dysprosium. *UNII-0E6DA2DHBE* [anhydrous]. *CAS-128470-17-7* [anhydrous]. INN. *Diagnostic aid (paramagnetic).* ◇*DyDTPA-BMA; S-043*

Squalamine Lactate [*2002*] (skwah′ la meen lak′ tate). $C_{34}H_{65}N_3O_5S.xC_3H_6O_3.yH_2O$. 627.96. [Squalamine is INN.] Cholestane-7,24-diol, 3-[[3-[(4-aminobutyl)amino]propyl]amino]-, 24-(hydrogen sulfate), (3β,5α,7α,24*R*)-, (2*S*)-2-hydroxypropanoate (salt). *CAS-32072-47-1; CAS-*

148717-90-2 [squalamine]. *Antineoplastic used in the treatment of advanced malignancies (angiogenesis inhibitor).* ◇*MSI-1256F*

Squalane (skwah′ lane). **NF**. $C_{30}H_{62}$. 422.81. (1) Tetracosane, 2,6,10,15,19,23-hexamethyl-; (2) 2,6,10,15,19,23-Hexamethyltetracosane. *UNII-GW89575KF9. CAS-111-01-3. Pharmaceutic aid (vehicle, oleaginous).*

^{85}Sr — *See* Strontium Chloride Sr 85.

^{85}Sr — *See* Strontium Nitrate Sr 85.

^{85}Sr — *See* Strontium Sr 85.

^{89}Sr — *See* Strontium Chloride Sr 89.

St. John's Wort. St. John's Wort consists of the dried flowering tops or aerial parts of *Hypericum perforatum* Linné (Fam. Hypericaceae), gathered shortly before or during flowering. *UNII-UFH8805FKA*. NF XXI.

Stacofylline. $C_{20}H_{33}N_7O_3$. 419.52. *N,N*-Diethyl-4-[3-(1,2,3,6-tetrahydro-1,3,7-trimethyl-2,6-dioxopurin-8-yl)propyl]-1-piperazinecarboxamide. *UNII-C7K8PK4Q0E. CAS-98833-92-2.* INN.

Stallimycin Hydrochloride [*1976*] (stal″ i mye′ sin hye″ droe klor′ ide). $C_{22}H_{27}N_9O_4.HCl$. 517.97. [Stallimycin is INN.] (1) 1*H*-Pyrrole-2-carboxamide, *N*-[5-[[(3-amino-3-iminopropyl)amino]carbonyl]-1-methyl-1*H*-pyrrol-3-yl]-4-[[[4-(formylamino)-1-methyl-1*H*-pyrrol-2-yl]carbonyl]amino]-1-methyl-, monohydrochloride; (2) *N‴*-(2-Amidinoethyl)-4-formamido-1,1′,1″-trimethyl-*N,4′:N′,4″*-ter[pyrrole-2-carboxamide] monohydrochloride. *UNII-80O63P88IS* [stallimycin]. *CAS-6576-51-8; CAS-636-47-5* [stallimycin]. *Antibacterial.* Herperal (Farmitalia, Societa Farmaceutici Italia, Italy) ◇*F.I. 6426*

Stamulumab [*2005*] (sta mul′ ue mab). $C_{6330}H_{9748}N_{1672}O_{1998}S_{48}$. Immunoglobulin G1, anti-(human growth differentiation factor 8) (human MYO-029 heavy chain), disulfide with human MYO-029 λ-chain, dimer. *CAS-705287-60-1.* INN. *Treatment of muscular dystrophy and age-related sarcopenia or frailty.* ◇*MYO-029*

---

† Brand name formerly used, and/or firm no longer concerned with this product.

Stannous Chloride [*1977*] (stan′ us klor′ ide). $SnCl_2.2H_2O$. 225.65. (1) Tin chloride ($SnCl_2$) dihydrate; (2) Tin chloride ($SnCl_2$) dihydrate. *UNII-1BQV3749L5. CAS-10025-69-1; CAS-7772-99-8* [anhydrous]. *Pharmaceutic aid.*

Stannous Fluoride (stan′ us floor′ ide). **USP.** SnF_2. 156.71. (1) Tin fluoride (SnF_2); (2) Tin fluoride (SnF_2). *UNII-3FTR44B32Q. CAS-7783-47-3. Dental caries prophylactic.* Stop (Oral-B)

Stannous Pyrophosphate [*1974*] (stan′ us pye″ roe fos′ fate). $Sn_2P_2O_7$. 411.36. (1) Diphosphoric acid, ditin(2+) salt; (2) Ditin(2+) pyrophosphate (4-). *CAS-15578-26-4. Diagnostic aid (skeletal imaging).* TechneScan PYP (Mallinckrodt) ◇*MP 4018*

Stannous Sulfur Colloid [*1976*] (stan′ us sul′ fur kol′ oid). A sulfur colloid containing stannous ions formed by reacting sodium thiosulfate with hydrochloric acid, then adding stannous ions. *Diagnostic aid (bone, liver, and spleen imaging)* [when combined with Technetium Tc 99m]. TechneScan S.S.C. (Mallinckrodt†) ◇*MP 7010*

Stannsoporfin [*1997*] (stan″ soe pore′ fin). $C_{34}H_{36}Cl_2N_4O_4Sn$. 754.29. (1) (*OC*-6-13)-Dihydrogen dichloro[7,12-diethyl-3,8,13,17-tetramethyl-21*H*,23*H*-porphine-2,18-dipropanoato(4-)-*N*^{21},*N*^{22},*N*^{23},*N*^{24}]stannate(2-); (2) Dihydrogen (*OC*-6-13)-dichloro[7,12-diethyl-3,8,13,17-tetramethylporphyrin-2,18-dipropionato(4-)-*N*^{21},*N*^{22},*N*^{23},*N*^{24}]stannate(2-). *CAS-106344-20-1.* INN. *Control of hyperbilirubinemia in preterm and term newborns (inhibitor of bilirubin).* Stanate (Torcan) ◇*B992*

Stanolone. $C_{19}H_{30}O_2$. 290.44. [Androstanolone is INN and BAN.] 17β-Hydroxy-5α-androstan-3-one. *UNII-08J2K08A3Y. CAS-521-18-6.* MI. Neodrol (Pfizer)

Stanozolol [*1962*] (stan oh′ zoe lol). **USP.** $C_{21}H_{32}N_2O$. 328.49. (1) 2′*H*-Androst-2-eno[3,2-*c*]pyrazol-17-ol, 17-methyl-, (5α,17β)-; (2) 17-Methyl-2′*H*-5α-androst-2-eno[3,2-*c*]pyrazol-17β-ol. *UNII-4R1VB9P8V3. CAS-10418-03-8.* INN; BAN; JAN. *Androgen.* Winstrol (Ovation) ◇*Win 14833; NSC-43193*

Starch. [Corn Starch, Potato Starch, and Wheat Starch are JAN.] (1) Starch; (2) Starch. *CAS-9005-25-8.* NF XXIII. *Dusting powder; pharmaceutic aid.*

Starch, Corn (stahrch korn). **NF.** Consists of the starch granules separated from the mature grain of corn [*Zea mays* Linné (Fam. Gramineae)].

Starch Glycerite. *CAS-8050-68-8.* NF XV.

Starch, Modified (stahrch). **NF.** Starch modified by chemical means.

Starch, Potato (stahrch). **NF.** Obtained from the tuber of *Solanum tuberosum* L.

Starch, Pregelatinized (stahrch pree jel at′ i nized). **NF.** Starch that has been chemically and/or mechanically processed to rupture all or part of the granules in the presence of water and subsequently dried. *Pharmaceutic aid (tablet excipient).*

Starch, Pregelatinized Modified (stahrch pree jel at′ i nized). **NF.** Modified Starch that has been chemically or mechanically processed, or both, to rupture all or part of the granules to produce a product that swells in cold water.

Starch, Rice. *CAS-9005-25-8* [starch]. JAN.

Starch, Tapioca (stahrch). **NF.** Consists of the starch granules separated from the tubers of tapioca (cassava) [*Manihot utilissima* Pohl (Fam. Euphorbiaceae)].

Starch, Topical (stahrch). **USP.** Consists of the granules separated from the mature grain of corn [*Zea mays* Linné (Fam. Gramineae)]. *Dusting powder.*

Starch, Wheat (stahrch). **NF.** Obtained from the caryopsis of *Triticum aestivum* L. (*T. vulgare Vill.*).

Statolon [*1967*] (stat′ oh lon). [Vistatolon is INN.] Substance derived from *Penicillium stoloniferum* (1) Statolon; (2) Statolon. *CAS-11006-77-2. Antiviral.* ◇*NSC-71901*

Stavudine [*1991*] (stav′ ue deen). **USP.** $C_{10}H_{12}N_2O_4$. 224.21. (1) Thymidine, 2′,3′-didehydro-3′-deoxy-; (2) 1-(2,3-Dideoxy-β-D-*glycero*-pent-2-enofuranosyl)thymine. *UNII-BO9LE4QFZF. CAS-3056-17-5.* INN; BAN. *Antiviral.* Zerit (Bristol-Myers Squibb) ◇*BMY-27857; d4T*

Stearethate 40 — *See* Polyoxyl 40 Stearate.

Stearic Acid (steer′ ik as′ id). **NF.** (1) Octadecanoic acid; (2) Stearic acid. *CAS-57-11-4.* JAN. *Pharmaceutic aid (emulsion adjunct); pharmaceutic aid (tablet and/or capsule lubricant).* Hystrene 5016 (Witco)

Stearoyl Polyoxylglcerides. **NF.** Mixtures of monoesters, diesters, and triesters of glycerol and monoesters and diesters of polyethylene glycols with a nominal mean relative molecular weight between 300 and 4000.

Stearyl Alcohol (steer′ il al′ ka hol). **NF.** (1) 1-Octadecanol; (2) 1-Octadecanol. *UNII-2KR89I4H1Y. CAS-112-92-5.* JAN. *Pharmaceutic aid (emulsion adjunct).*

Stearylsulfamide. $C_{24}H_{42}N_2O_3S$. 438.67. *N*-Sulfanilylstearamide. *UNII-CH8C36F1MO. CAS-498-78-2.* INN; DCF.

Steffimycin [*1968*] (stef″ fi mye′ sin). Antibiotic produced by *Streptomyces steffisburgensis* var. *steffisburgensis* n.sp. (1) Steffimycin; (2) Steffimycin. *CAS-11033-34-4.* INN. *Antibacterial; antiviral.* ◇*U-20,661*

Stenbolone Acetate [*1967*] (sten′ boe lone as′ e tate). $C_{22}H_{32}O_3$. 344.49. [Stenbolone is INN.] (1) Androst-1-en-3-one, 17-(acetyloxy)-2-methyl-, (5α,17β)-; (2) 17β-Hydroxy-2-methyl-5α-androst-1-en-3-one acetate. *CAS-1242-56-4; CAS-5197-58-0* [stenbolone]. *Anabolic.*

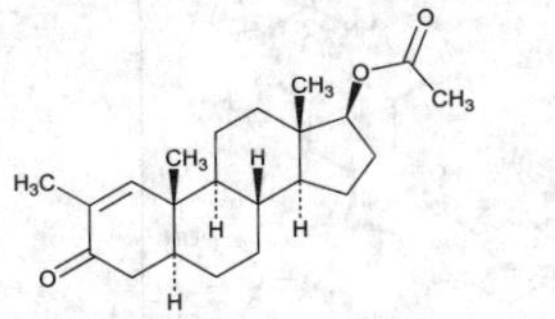

Stepronin. $C_{10}H_{11}NO_4S_2$. 273.33. *N*-(2-Mercaptopropionyl)-glycine 2-thiophenecarboxylate (ester). *UNII-0NOY894QRB. CAS-72324-18-6.* INN; MI.

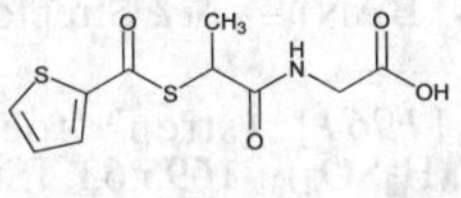

Stercuronium Iodide. $C_{26}H_{43}IN_2$. 510.54. (Cona-4,6-dienin-3β-yl)dimethylethylammonium iodide. *CAS-30033-10-4.* INN.

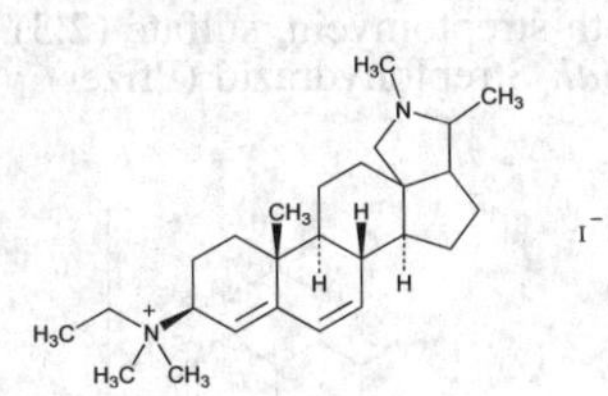

Stevaladil. $C_{27}H_{45}NO_4$. 447.65. 3β-(Dimethylamino)-5α-pregnane-18,20α-diol diacetate (ester). *CAS-6535-03-1.* INN.

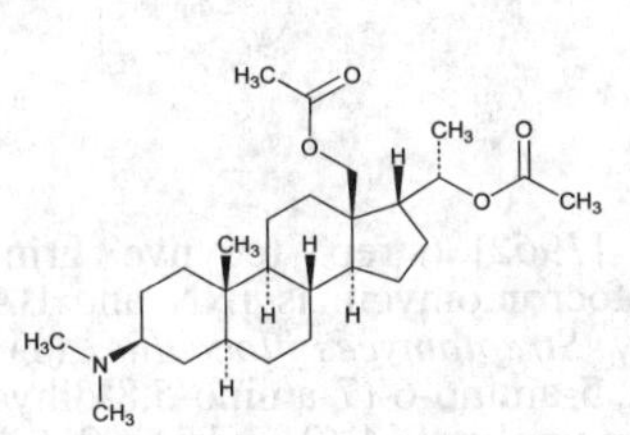

Stibamine Glucoside. $C_{36}H_{49}N_3NaO_{22}Sb_3$. 1264.05. *N*-Glucoside of sodium 4-aminobenzenestibonate. *CAS-1344-34-9.* INN; BAN.

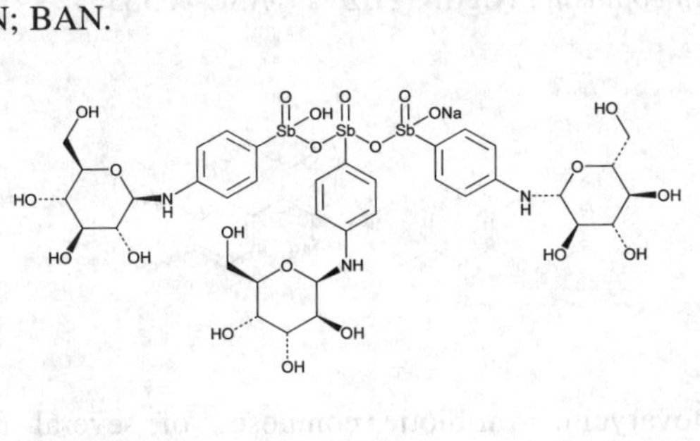

Stibocaptate (previously used name) — *See* Sodium Stibocaptate.

Stibophen. $C_{12}H_4Na_5O_{16}S_4Sb.7H_2O$. 895.23. (1) Antimonate(5-), bis[4,5-dihydroxy-1,3-benzenedisulfonato(4-)-O^4,O^5]-, pentasodium heptahydrate; (2) Pentasodium bis[4,5-dihydroxy-*m*-benzenedisulfonato(4-)]antimonate(5-) heptahydrate. *CAS-15489-16-4; CAS-23940-36-5* [anhydrous]; *CAS-16028-21-0* [replaced]. NF XIV; MI. Fuadin (Sterling Winthrop)

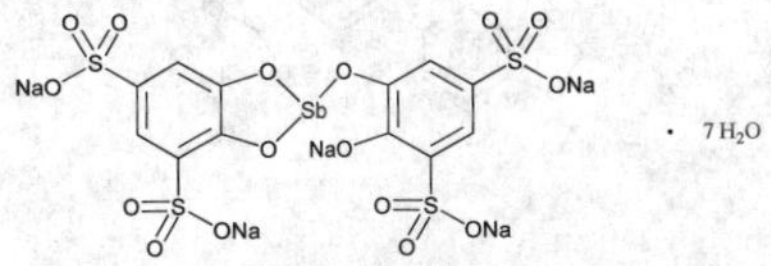

Stibosamine (INN, DCF) — *See* Ethylstibamine.

Stilbamidine Isethionate. $C_{20}H_{28}N_4O_8S_2$. 516.59. [Stilbamidine Isetionate is INN; Stilbamidine is BAN.] 4,4′-Stilbenedicarboxamidine bis(2-hydroxyethanesulfonate). *CAS-140-59-0; CAS-122-06-5* [stilbamidine]. MI.

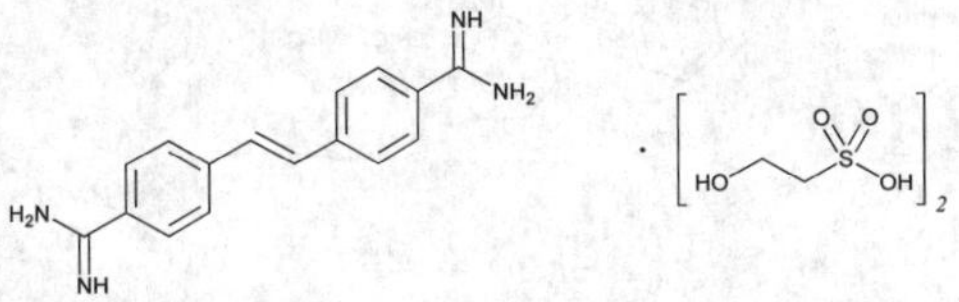

Stilbazium Iodide [*1963*] (stil baz′ ee um eye′ oh dide). $C_{31}H_{36}IN_3$. 577.54. (1) Pyridinium, 1-ethyl-2,6-bis[2-[4-(1-pyrrolidinyl)phenyl]ethenyl]-, iodide; (2) 1-Ethyl-2,6-bis-(*p*-pyrrolidinylstyryl)pyridinium iodide. *CAS-3784-99-4.* INN; BAN. *Anthelmintic.* ◇BW-61-32

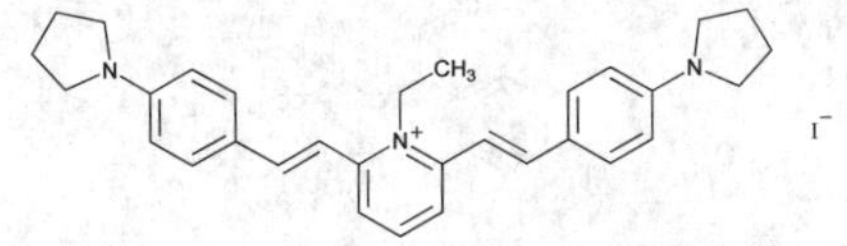

Stilbestroform — *See* Diethylstilbestrol.

Stilbestrol — *See* Diethylstilbestrol.

Stilboestrol — *See* Diethylstilbestrol.

Stilonium Iodide [*1981*] (stil oh′ nee um eye′ oh dide). $C_{22}H_{30}INO$. 451.38. (1) Ethanaminium, *N,N,N*-triethyl-2-[4-(2-phenylethenyl)phenoxy]-, iodide, (*E*)-; (2) Triethyl[2-[(*E*)-(*p*-styrylphenoxy)]ethyl]ammonium iodide. *UNII-19B3530KQ6. CAS-77257-42-2.* INN. *Antispasmodic.* Elvetil (Maggioni Farmaceutici S.p.A., Italy) ◇M.G. 624

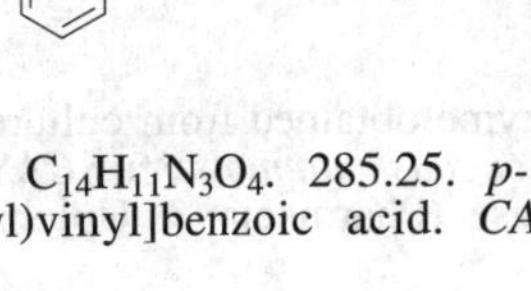

Stirimazole. $C_{14}H_{11}N_3O_4$. 285.25. *p*-[2-(5-Nitro-1-vinyl-2-imidazolyl)vinyl]benzoic acid. *CAS-30529-16-9.* INN; BAN.

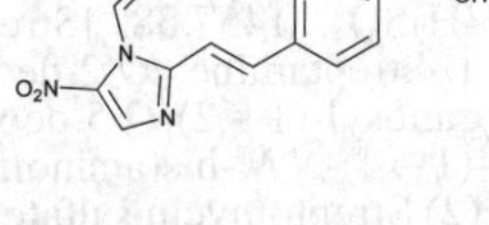

---

† Brand name formerly used, and/or firm no longer concerned with this product.

Stiripentol [*1979*] (stir″ i pen′ tol). $C_{14}H_{18}O_3$. 234.29. (1) 1-Penten-3-ol, 1-(1,3-benzodioxol-5-yl)-4,4-dimethyl-; (2) 4,4-Dimethyl-1-[(3,4-methylenedioxy)phenyl]-1-penten-3-ol. *CAS-49763-96-4*. INN. *Anticonvulsant.* ◇*BCX 2600*

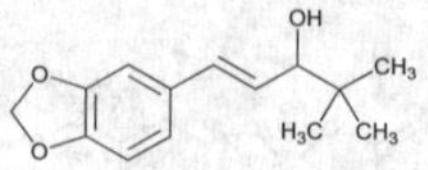

Stirocainide. $C_{22}H_{34}N_2O$. 342.52. (*E*)-2-Benzylidenecyclo-heptanone(*E*)-*O*-[2-(diisopropylamino)ethyl]oxime. *UNII-LXD20TIK6Y*. *CAS-78372-27-7*. INN.

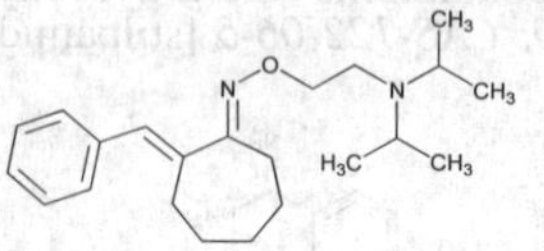

Stirofos [*1972*] (stir′ oh fos). $C_{10}H_9Cl_4O_4P$. 365.96. (1) Phosphoric acid, 2-chloro-1-(2,4,5-trichlorophenyl)ethenyl dimethyl ester, (*Z*)-; (2) 2-Chloro-1-(2,4,5-trichlorophenyl)vinyl dimethyl phosphate. *CAS-22248-79-9*. *Insecticide (veterinary).*

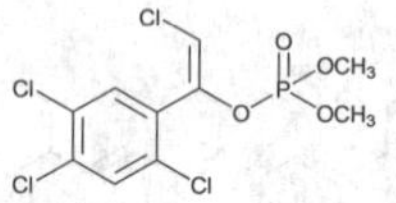

Storax (stor′ ax). **USP.** A balsam obtained from the trunk of *Liquidambar orientalis* Miller, known in commerce as Levant Storax, or of *Liquidambar styraciflua* Linné, known in commerce as American Storax (Fam. Hamamelidaceae). Component of Benzoin [Tincture, Compound].

Streptodornase. Enzyme obtained from cultures of various strains of *Streptococcus haemolyticus.* *CAS-37340-82-2*. INN; BAN; DCF; NND 1964.

Streptoduocin. Dihydrostreptomycin sulfate (2:3) (salt) mixture with streptomycin sulfate (2:3). USP XVI; BAN. Combistrep (Pfizer); Distrycin (Bristol-Myers Squibb†)

Streptokinase. Co-enzyme obtained from cultures of various strains of *Streptococcus haemolyticus.* *CAS-9002-01-1*. INN; MI. Kabikinase (Pharmacia & Upjohn); Streptase (Astra)

Streptomycin Sulfate (strep″ toe mye′ sin sul′ fate). **USP.** $(C_{21}H_{39}N_7O_{12})_2 \cdot 3H_2SO_4$. 1457.38. [Streptomycin is INN and BAN.] (1) D-Streptamine, *O*-2-deoxy-2-(methylamino)-α-L-glucopyranosyl-(1→2)-*O*-5-deoxy-3-*C*-formyl-α-L-lyxofuranosyl-(1→4)-*N,N′*-bis(aminoiminomethyl)-, sulfate (2:3) (salt); (2) Streptomycin sulfate (2:3) (salt). *UNII-*

CW25IKJ202; UNII-Y45QSO73OB [streptomycin]. *CAS-3810-74-0; CAS-57-92-1* [streptomycin]. JAN. *Antibacterial (tuberculostatic).*

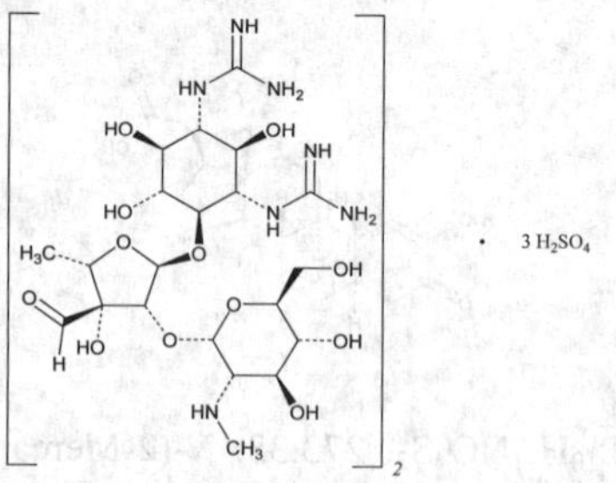

Streptoniazid (INN, BAN) — *See* Streptonicozid.

Streptonicozid [*1961*] (strep″ toe nye′ koe zid). $(C_{27}H_{44}N_{10}O_{12})_2 \cdot (H_2SO_4)_3$. 1695.63. [Streptoniazid is INN and BAN.] (1) 4-Pyridinecarboxylic acid hydrazide, hydrazone with *O*-2-deoxy-2-(methylamino)-α-L-glucopyranosyl-(1→2)-*O*-5-deoxy-3-*C*-formyl-α-L-lyxofuranosyl-(1→4)-*N,N′*-bis(aminoiminomethyl)-D-streptamine sulfate (2:3) (salt); (2) Isonicotinic acid hydrazide, hydrazone with streptomycin, sulfate (2:3). *CAS-5667-71-0*. *Antibacterial.* Streptohydrazid (Pfizer)

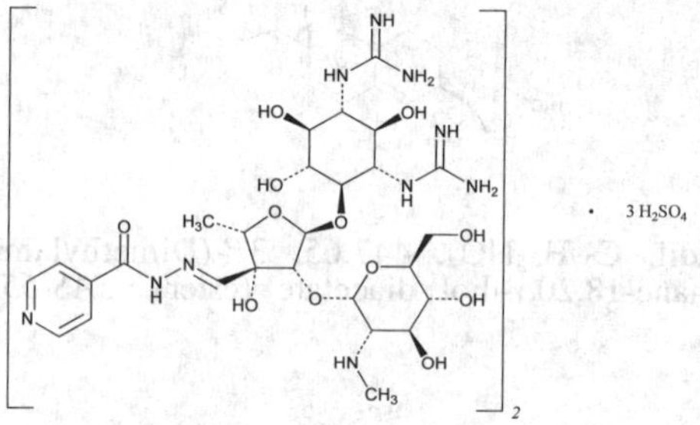

Streptonigrin [*1962*] (strep″ toe nye′ grin). $C_{25}H_{22}N_4O_8$. 506.46. [Rufocromomycin is INN and BAN.] Antibiotic produced by *Streptomyces flocculus*. (1) 2-Pyridinecarboxylic acid, 5-amino-6-(7-amino-5,8-dihydro-6-methoxy-5,8-dioxo-2-quinolinyl)-4-(2-hydroxy-3,4-dimethoxyphenyl)-3-methyl-; (2) 5-Amino-6-(7-amino-5,8-dihydro-6-methoxy-5,8-dioxo-2-quinolyl)-4-(2-hydroxy-3,4-dimethoxyphenyl)-3-methylpicolinic acid. *CAS-3930-19-6*. *Antineoplastic.* Nigrin (Pfizer) ◇*NSC-45383*

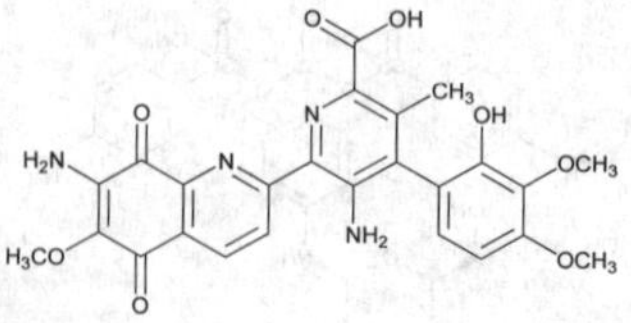

Streptovarycin. Antibiotic composed of several related components obtained from cultures of *Streptomyces variabilis. CAS-1404-74-6*. INN; MI. ◇*U-7750*

Streptozocin [*1975*] (strep″ toe zoe′ sin). $C_8H_{15}N_3O_7$. 265.22. (1) D-Glucopyranose, 2-deoxy-2-[[(methylnitrosoamino)-carbonyl]amino]-; (2) 2-Deoxy-2-(3-methyl-3-nitrosoureido)-D-glucopyranose; (3) 2-Deoxy-2-(3-methyl-3-

nitrosoureido)-α(and β)-D-glucopyranose. *UNII-5W494URQ81. CAS-18883-66-4.* INN. *Antineoplastic.* Zanosar (Teva) ◇*U-9889; NSC-85998*

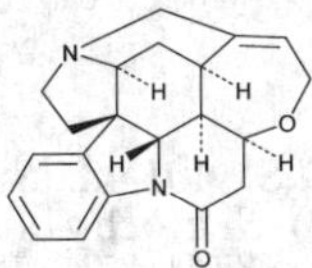

Streptozotocin — *See* Streptozocin.

Strinoline. $C_{10}H_6N_4$. 182.18. *as*-Triazino[5,6-*c*]quinoline. *UNII-K356C79875. CAS-39862-58-3.* INN.

Strong Co-Danthramer — *See* Co-danthramer.

Strontium Chloride Sr 85 [*1966*] (stron′ shee um klor′ ide). $^{85}SrCl_2$. (1) Strontium chloride ($^{85}SrCl_2$); (2) Strontium chloride ($^{85}SrCl_2$). *CAS-24359-46-4. Radioactive agent.* Stronscan-85 (Abbott†)

Strontium Chloride Sr 89 [*1993*] (stron′ shee um klor′ ide). **USP** [Injection]. $^{89}SrCl_2$. 159.90. (1) Strontium chloride ($^{89}SrCl_2$); (2) Strontium chloride ($^{89}SrCl_2$). *UNII-5R78837D4A. CAS-38270-90-5. Antineoplastic; radioactive agent.* Metastron (Nycomed Amersham) ◇*Sms2PA*

Strontium Nitrate Sr 85 [*1963*] (stron′ shee um nye′ trate). $^{85}Sr(NO_3)_2$. (1) Nitric acid, strontium-^{85}Sr salt; (2) Strontium-^{85}Sr nitrate. *CAS-24381-59-7. Radioactive agent.* Strotope (Bristol-Myers Squibb†)

Strontium Salicylate. Strontium salicylate. NF IX.

Strontium Sr 85. *CAS-13967-73-2.* USP XIX.

Strychnine. $C_{21}H_{22}N_2O_2$. 334.41. (1) Strychnidin-10-one; (2) (4b*R*,7a*S*,8a*R*,13*S*,13a*R*,13b*S*)-5,6,7a,8,8a,11,13a,13b-octahydro-13*H*-13,14-ethano-7,9-methanooxepino[3,4-*a*]pyrrolo[2,3-*d*]carbazol-15-one. *CAS-57-24-9.* NF X; MI.

Strychnine Glycerophosphate. Strychnine compound with glycerol phosphate (2:1). NF IV; MI.

Strychnine Nitrate. *CAS-66-32-0; CAS-57-24-9* [strychnine]. NF X; MI.

Strychnine Phosphate. NF XI; MI.

Strychnine Sulfate. *CAS-60-41-3; CAS-57-24-9* [strychnine]. NF XI; MI.

Strychnine Valerate. Valeric acid compound with strychnine (1:1). *CAS-6101-07-1; CAS-57-24-9* [strychnine]. NF IV.

Stutgin — *See* Cinnarizine.

---

† Brand name formerly used, and/or firm no longer concerned with this product.

Styramate. $C_9H_{11}NO_3$. 181.19. β-Hydroxyphenethyl carbamate. *CAS-94-35-9.* INN; BAN; MI.

Styronate Resins. *CAS-8053-19-8.*

Subathizone. $C_{10}H_{13}N_3O_2S_2$. 271.36. *p*-Ethylsulfonylbenzaldehyde thiosemicarbazone. *UNII-BSC36V44TK. CAS-121-55-1.* INN; DCF; MI.

Subendazole. $C_{10}H_5Cl_3N_4S_3$. 383.73. 4,5,7-Trichloro-2-[[3-(methylthio)-1,2,4-thiadiazol-5-yl]-thio]benzimidazole. *UNII-YT3IDN1WR0. CAS-54340-66-8.* INN; DCF. ◇*CB 12592*

Substance F — *See* Demecolcine.

Succimer [*1978*] (sux′ i mer). $C_4H_6O_4S_2$. 182.22. (1) Butanedioic acid, 2,3-dimercapto-, (*R**,*S**)-; (2) *meso*-2,3-Dimercaptosuccinic acid. *UNII-DX1U2629QE. CAS-304-55-2.* INN; BAN. *Diagnostic aid.* Chemet (Ovation) ◇*DMSA; DIM-SA*

Succinchlorimide. *N*-Chlorosuccinimide. *CAS-128-09-6.* NF IX.

Succinic Acid. NF. $C_4H_6O_4$. 118.09. Butanedioic acid. *UNII-AB6MNQ6J6L. CAS-110-15-6.*

Succinobucol [*2006*] (sux″ in oh bue′ kol). $C_{35}H_{52}O_5S_2$. 616.91. (1) Butanedioic acid, mono[4-[[1-[[3,5-bis(1,1-dimethylethyl)-4-hydroxyphenyl]thio]-1-methylethyl]thio]-2,6-bis(1,1-dimethylethyl)phenyl] ester; (2) 4-[4-[[1-[[3,5-Bis(1,1-dimethylethyl)-4-hydroxyphenyl]sulfanyl]-1-methylethyl]sulfanyl]-2,6-bis(1,1-dimethylethyl)phenoxy]-4-oxobutanoic acid. *UNII-J1J54V24R4. CAS-216167-82-7.* INN. *Reduction of cardiovascular events.* ◇*AGI-1067*

Succinylcholine Chloride (sux″ i nil koe′ leen klor′ ide). **USP.** $C_{14}H_{30}Cl_2N_2O_4$. 361.31. [Suxamethonium Chloride is INN, BAN, and JAN.] (1) Ethanaminium, 2,2′-[(1,4-dioxo-1,4-butanediyl)bis(oxy)]bis[*N,N,N*-trimethyl-], dichloride;

(2) Choline chloride succinate (2:1). *UNII-I9L0DDD30I. CAS-71-27-2; CAS-6101-15-1* [dihydrate]. *Neuromuscular blocking agent*. Anectine (Sandoz); Quelicin (Hospira)

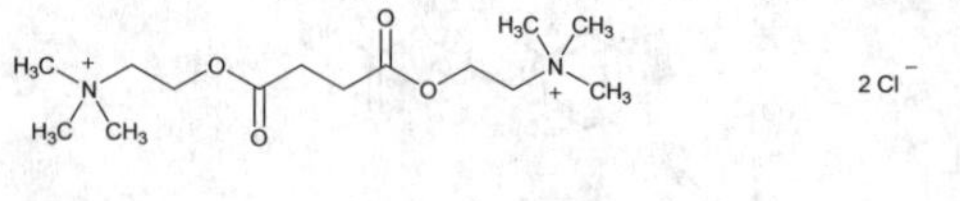

Succinyldapsone — *See* Succisulfone.

Succinylsulfathiazole. $C_{13}H_{13}N_3O_5S_2.H_2O$. 373.40. 4′-(2-Thiazolylsulfamoyl)succinanilic acid. *CAS-116-43-8*. USP XVIII; INN; BAN; MI.

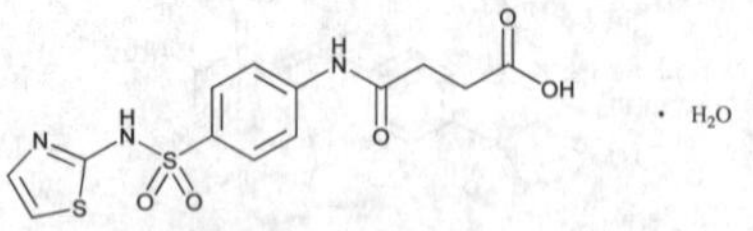

Succisulfone. $C_{16}H_{16}N_2O_5S$. 348.37. 4′-Sulfanilylsuccinanilic acid. *UNII-0Z4EEC962O. CAS-5934-14-5*. INN; DCF; MI. ◇*F 1500*

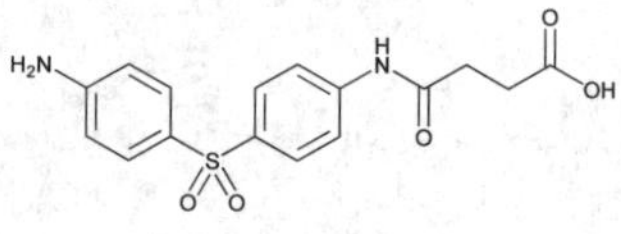

Suclofenide. $C_{16}H_{13}ClN_2O_4S$. 364.80. 3-Chloro-4-(phenyl-succinimido)benzenesulfonamide. *UNII-3V0537Z59Q. CAS-30279-49-3*. INN; BAN; MI.

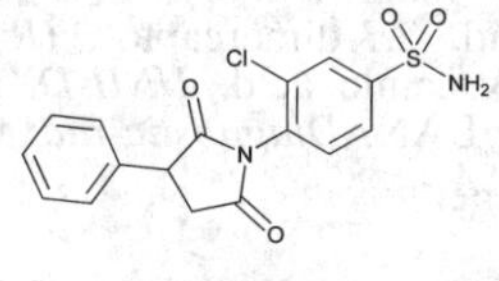

Sucralfate [*1976*] (soo kral′ fate). **USP.** $Al_8(OH)_{16}(C_{12}H_{14}O_{35}S_8)[Al(OH)_3]_x[H_2O]_y$ in which $x = 8$ to 10, and $y = 22$ to 31. (1) α-D-Glucopyranoside, β-D-fructofurano-syl-, octakis(hydrogen sulfate), aluminum complex; (2) Sucrose octakis(hydrogen sulfate) aluminum complex. *CAS-54182-58-0*. INN; BAN; JAN. *Anti-ulcerative (gastrointestinal)*. Carafate (Axcan Scandipharm)

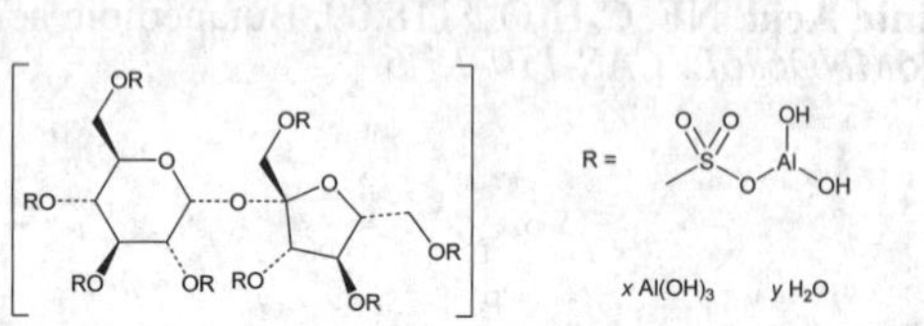

Sucralose (soo′ kra lose). **NF.** $C_{12}H_{19}Cl_3O_8$. 397.63. (1) 1,6-Dichloro-1,6-dideoxy-β-D-fructofuranosyl-4-chloro-4-deoxy-α-D-galactopyranoside; (2) 1′,4,6′-Trichlorogalac-tosucrose. *UNII-96K6UQ3ZD4. CAS-56038-13-2*. BAN; MI.

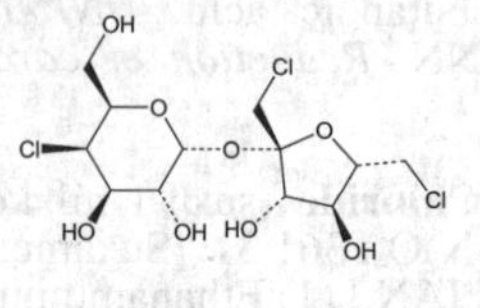

Sucralox. Sucrose complex with aluminum hydroxide. *CAS-12040-73-2*. INN; BAN.

Sucrose (soo′ krose). **NF.** $C_{12}H_{22}O_{11}$. 342.30. (1) α-D-Glucopyranoside, β-D-fructofuranosyl-; (2) Sucrose. *UNII-C151H8M554. CAS-57-50-1*. JAN. *Pharmaceutic aid (flavor); pharmaceutic aid (tablet excipient)*.

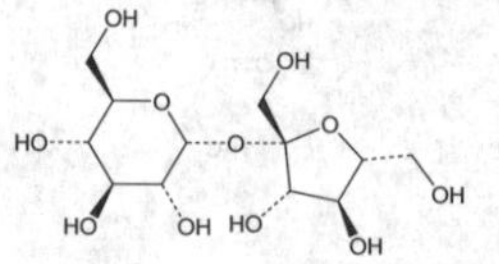

Sucrose Octaacetate (soo′ krose ok″ ta as′ e tate). **NF.** $C_{28}H_{38}O_{19}$. 678.59. (1) α-D-Glucopyranoside, 1,3,4,6-tetra-*O*-acetyl-β-D-fructofuranosyl, tetraacetate; (2) Sucrose octaacetate. *CAS-126-14-7. Pharmaceutic aid (alcohol denaturant)*.

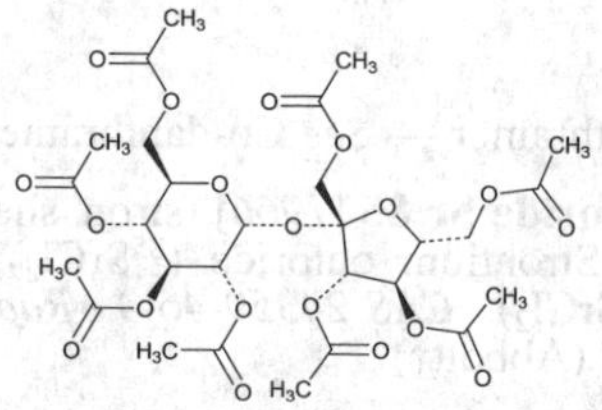

Sucrosofate Potassium [*1990*] (soo kroe′ soe fate poe tas′ ee um). $C_{12}H_{14}K_8O_{35}S_8.7H_2O$. 1413.63. [Sucrosofate is INN.] (1) α-D-Glucopyranoside, 1,3,4,6-tetra-*O*-sulfo-β-D-fruc-tofuranosyl, tetrakis(hydrogen sulfate), octapotassium salt, heptahydrate; (2) Sucrose octakis(potassium sulfate), heptahydrate. *CAS-76578-81-9; CAS-57680-56-5* [sucrosofate]. *Anti-ulcerative*. ◇*Agent M-01*

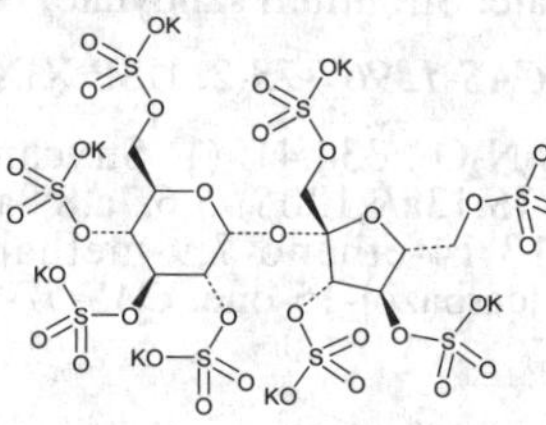

Sudexanox. $C_{21}H_{23}NO_5S$. 401.48. *S*-(7-Carboxy-4-hexyl-9-oxoxanthen-2-yl)-*S*-methylsulfoximine. *UNII-H6C0F5AD7D. CAS-58761-87-8*. INN.

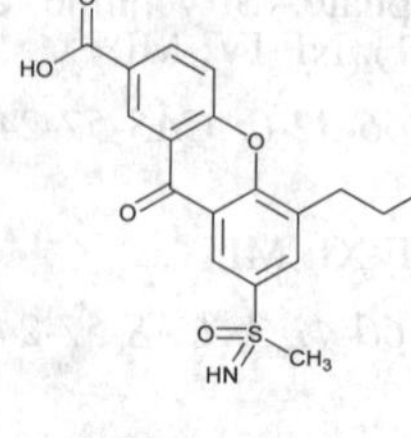

Sudismase. $C_{681}H_{1087}N_{203}O_{225}S_4$. 15,846.41. *N*-Acetylsuper-oxide dismutase (human clone pS 61-10 copper-zinc subunit protein moiety reduced). *CAS-110294-55-8*. INN.

Sudoxicam [*1972*] (soo dox′ i kam). $C_{13}H_{11}N_3O_4S_2$. 337.37. (1) 2*H*-1,2-Benzothiazine-3-carboxamide, 4-hydroxy-2-methyl-*N*-2-thiazolyl-, 1,1-dioxide; (2) 4-Hydroxy-2-methyl-*N*-2-thiazolyl-2*H*-1,2-benzothiazine-3-carboxamide 1,1-dioxide. *CAS-34042-85-8*. INN; BAN. *Anti-inflammatory.* ✧*CP-15,973*

Sufentanil [*1976*] (soo fen′ ta nil). $C_{22}H_{30}N_2O_2S$. 386.55. (1) Propanamide, *N*-[4-(methoxymethyl)-1-[2-(2-thienyl)ethyl]-4-piperidinyl]-*N*-phenyl-; (2) *N*-[4-(Methoxymethyl)-1-[2-(2-thienyl)ethyl]-4-piperidyl]propionanilide. *UNII-AFE2YW0IIZ. CAS-56030-54-7.* INN; BAN. *Analgesic.* ✧*R 30,730*

Sufentanil Citrate [*1984*] (soo fen′ ta nil sit′ rate). **USP.** $C_{22}H_{30}N_2O_2S.C_6H_8O_7$. 578.67. (1) Propanamide, *N*-[4-(methoxymethyl)-1-[2-(thienyl)ethyl]-4-piperidinyl]-*N*-phenyl-, 2-hydroxy-1,2,3-propanetricarboxylate (1:1); (2) *N*-[4-(Methoxymethyl)-1-[2-(2-thienyl)ethyl]-4-piperidyl]-propionanilide citrate (1:1). *UNII-S9ZFX8403R. CAS-60561-17-3. Analgesic (narcotic).* Sufenta (Akorn) ✧*R 33800*

Sufosfamide. $C_8H_{18}ClN_2O_5PS$. 320.73. 2-[[3-(2-Chloroethyl)tetrahydro-2*H*-1,3,2-oxazaphosphorin-2-yl]amino]ethanol methanesulfonate (ester) *P*-oxide. *UNII-2208Y59985. CAS-37753-10-9.* INN.

Sufotidine [*1987*] (soo foe′ ti deen). $C_{20}H_{31}N_5O_3S$. 421.56. (1) 1*H*-1,2,4-Triazol-5-amine, 1-methyl-3-[(methylsulfonyl)methyl]-*N*-[3-[3-(1-piperidinylmethyl)phenoxy]propyl]-; (2) 1-[*m*-[3-[[1-Methyl-3-[(methylsulfonyl)methyl]-1*H*-1,2,4-triazol-5-yl]amino]propoxy]benzyl]piperidine. *UNII-56B0591Y76. CAS-80343-63-1.* INN; BAN. *Antagonist (to histamine H$_2$receptors).* ✧*AH 25352X*

Sufugolix. $C_{36}H_{31}F_2N_5O_4S$. 667.72. 5-{[Benzyl(methyl)amino]methyl}-1-(2,6-difluorobenzyl)-6-[4-(3-methoxyureido)phenyl]-3-phenylthieno[2,3-*d*]pyrimidine-2,4(1*H*,3*H*)-dione. *CAS-308831-61-0.* INN; BAN.

Sugammadex Sodium [*2004*] (soo gam′ ma dex soe′ dee um). $C_{72}H_{104}Na_8O_{48}S_8$. 2178.01. [Sugammadex is INN.] (1) γ-Cyclodextrin, 6A,6B,6C,6D,6E,7F,6G,6H-octakis-*S*-(2-carboxyethyl)-6A,6B,6C,6D,6E,7F,6G,6H-octathio-, octasodium salt; (2) Octasodium 6,6′,6″,6‴,6⁗,6″‴,6‴‴,6⁗‴-octakis-*S*-(2-carboxylatoethyl)-6,6′,6″,6‴,6⁗,6″‴,6‴‴,6⁗‴-octathiocyclo-α-(1→4)-D-octaglucopyranoside. *UNII-ERJ6X2MXV7. CAS-343306-79-6; CAS-343306-71-8* [sugammadex]. JAN. *Reversal agent for neuromuscular blocking agents.* ✧*Org 25969*

Sugar, Compressible (shug er). **NF.** Sugar previously dried at 105° for 4 hours, containing 96.5 ± 1.5% sucrose ($C_{12}H_{22}O_{11}$). *Pharmaceutic aid (flavor); pharmaceutic aid (tablet excipient).*

Sugar, Confectioner's (shug er). **NF.** Sucrose ground together with corn starch to a fine powder. *Pharmaceutic aid (flavor); pharmaceutic aid (tablet excipient).*

Sugar, Invert (shug er). **USP** [Injection]. A sterile solution of a mixture of equal amounts of dextrose and fructose in water, or an equivalent sterile solution produced by the hydrolysis of sucrose, in water. *Replenisher (fluid and nutrient).*

Sugar Spheres (shug er). **NF.** Contains 77.0 ± 15.5% sucrose ($C_{12}H_{22}O_{11}$), calculated on the dried basis, the remainder consisting chiefly of starch. *Pharmaceutic aid (vehicle, solid carrier).*

Sulamserod Hydrochloride [*1999*] (sul am′ se rod hye″ droe klor′ ide). $C_{19}H_{28}ClN_3O_5S.HCl$. 482.42. [Sulamserod is INN.] (1) *N*-[2-[4-[3-(8-Amino-7-chloro-2,3-dihydro-1,4-benzodioxin-5-yl)-3-oxopropyl]-1-piperidinyl]ethyl]-methanesulfonamide monohydrochloride; (2) *N*-[2-[4-[2-

[(8-Amino-7-chloro-1,4-benzodioxan-5-yl)carbony-l]ethyl]piperidino]ethyl]methanesulfonamide monohydrochloride. *CAS-184159-40-8; CAS-219757-90-1* [sulamserod]. INN. *Treatment of urge incontinence; atrial fibrillations (selective 5-HT$_4$receptor antagonist).* ◇*RS-100302-190*

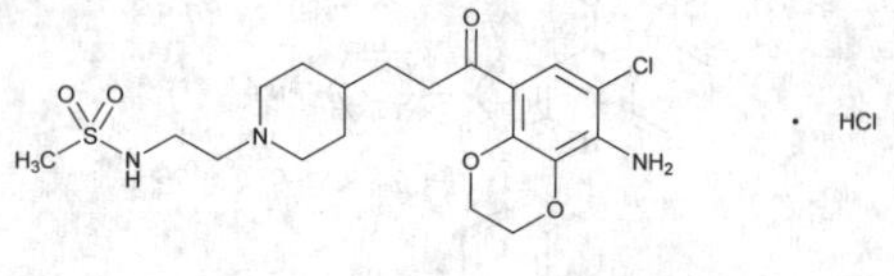

Sulazepam [*1968*] (sul az′ e pam). C$_{16}$H$_{13}$ClN$_2$S. 300.81. (1) 2*H*-1,4-Benzodiazepine-2-thione, 7-chloro-1,3-dihydro-1-methyl-5-phenyl-; (2) 7-Chloro-1,3-dihydro-1-methyl-5-phenyl-2*H*-1,4-benzodiazepine-2-thione. *UNII-NZ779Q5S0W. CAS-2898-13-7.* INN. *Tranquilizer (minor).* ◇*W 3676*

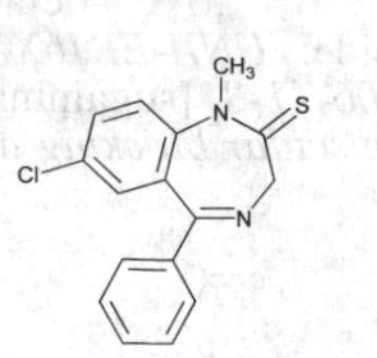

Sulazuril. C$_{17}$H$_{15}$Cl$_2$N$_3$O$_5$S. 444.29. 2-[3,5-Dichloro-4-[*p*-(methylsulfonyl)phenoxy]phenyl]dihydro-1-methyl-*as*-triazine-3,5(2*H*,4*H*)-dione. *UNII-2136B7T7KE. CAS-108258-89-5.* INN.

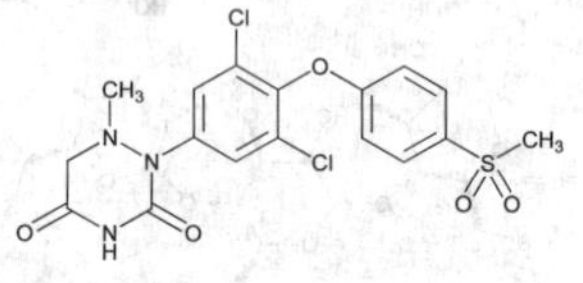

Sulbactam Benzathine [*1984*] (sul bak′ tam ben′ za theen). (C$_8$H$_{11}$NO$_5$S)$_2$.C$_{16}$H$_{20}$N$_2$. 706.83. [Sulbactam is INN and BAN.] (1) 4-Thia-1-azabicyclo[3.2.0]heptane-2-carboxylic acid, 3,3-dimethyl-7-oxo-, 4,4-dioxide, (2*S-cis*)-, compound with *N,N′*-bis(phenylmethyl)-1,2-ethanediamine (2:1); (2) (2*S*,5*R*)-3,3-Dimethyl-7-oxo-4-thia-1-azabicyclo[3.2.0]heptane-2-carboxylic acid, 4,4-dioxide, compound with *N,N′*-dibenzylethylenediamine (2:1). *UNII-S4TF6I2330* [sulbactam]. *CAS-83031-43-0; CAS-68373-14-8* [sulbactam]. *Inhibitor (β-lactamase); synergist (penicillin/cephalosporin).* ◇*CP-45,899-99*

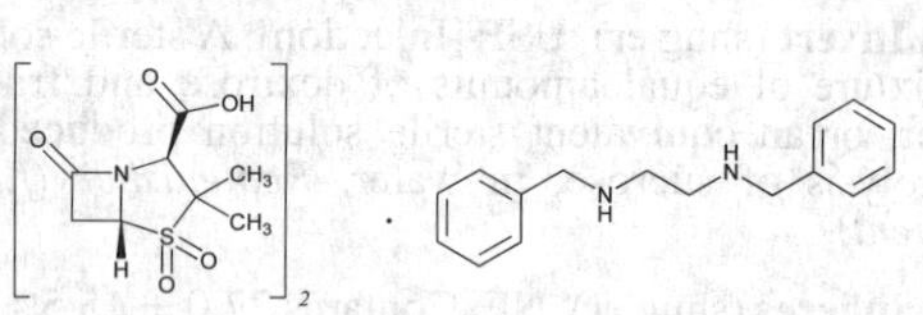

Sulbactam Pivoxil [*1980*] (sul bak′ tam piv ox′ il). C$_{14}$H$_{21}$NO$_7$S. 347.38. [Pivsulbactam is BAN.] (1) 4-Thia-1-azabicyclo[3.2.0]heptane-2-carboxylic acid, 3,3-dimethyl-7-oxo-, 4,4-dioxide, (2,2-dimethyl-1-oxopropoxy)-methyl ester, (2*S-cis*)-; (2) Hydroxymethyl (2*S*,5*R*)-3,3-dimethyl-7-oxo-4-thia-1-azabicyclo[3.2.0]heptane-2-car-

boxylate pivalate (ester), 4,4-dioxide. *CAS-69388-79-0. Inhibitor (β-lactamase); synergist (penicillin/cephalosporin).* ◇*CP-47,904*

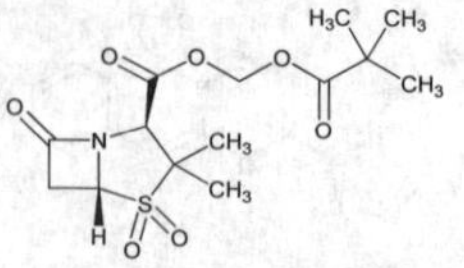

Sulbactam Sodium [*1980*] (sul bak′ tam soe′ dee um). **USP**. C$_8$H$_{10}$NNaO$_5$S. 255.22. (1) 4-Thia-1-azabicyclo[3.2.0]heptane-2-carboxylic acid, 3,3-dimethyl-7-oxo-, 4,4-dioxide, sodium salt, (2*S-cis*)-; (2) Sodium (2*S*,5*R*)-3,3-dimethyl-7-oxo-4-thia-1-azabicyclo[3.2.0]heptane-2-carboxylate 4,4-dioxide. *UNII-DKQ4T82YE6. CAS-69388-84-7; CAS-68373-14-8* [sulbactam]. JAN. *Inhibitor (β-lactamase); synergist (penicillin/cephalosporin).* ◇*CP-45,899-2*

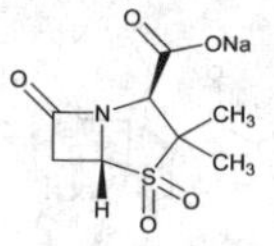

Sulbenicillin. C$_{16}$H$_{18}$N$_2$O$_7$S$_2$. 414.45. [Sulbenicillin Sodium is JAN.] 3,3-Dimethyl-7-oxo-6-(2-phenyl-2-sulfoacetamido)-4-thia-1-azabicyclo[3.2.0]heptane-2-carboxylic acid. *CAS-34779-28-7.* INN; MI.

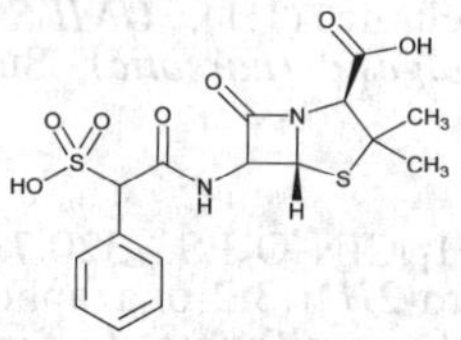

Sulbenox [*1977*] (sul′ ben ox). C$_9$H$_{10}$N$_2$O$_2$S. 210.25. (1) Urea, (4,5,6,7-tetrahydro-7-oxobenzo[*b*]thien-4-yl)-; (2) (4,5,6,7-Tetrahydro-7-oxobenzo[*b*]thien-4-yl)urea. *UNII-6J4L7U7I9D. CAS-58095-31-1.* INN. *Growth stimulant (veterinary).* ◇*CL 206,576*

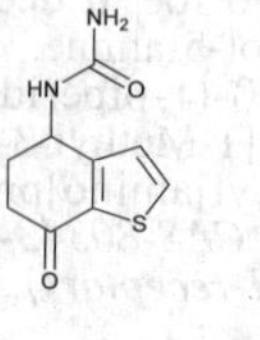

Sulbentine. C$_{17}$H$_{18}$N$_2$S$_2$. 314.47. 3,5-Dibenzyltetrahydro-2*H*-1,3,5-thiadiazine-2-thione. *UNII-D0NR12WK9J. CAS-350-12-9.* INN; MI. ◇*D 47*

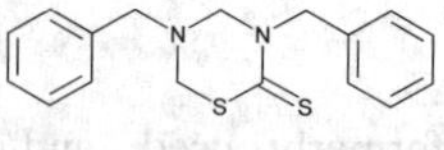

Sulbutiamine. $C_{32}H_{46}N_8O_6S_2$. 702.89. [Bisibuthiamine is JAN.] *N,N'*-[Dithiobis[2-(2-hydroxyethyl)-1-methylvinyl-ene]]bis[*N*-[(4-amino-2-methyl-5-pyrimidinyl)methyl]formamide] diisobutyrate (ester). *CAS-3286-46-2.* INN.

Sulclamide. $C_7H_7ClN_2O_3S$. 234.66. 4-Chloro-3-sulfamoyl-benzamide. *UNII-7GHI2O527Q.* *CAS-2455-92-7.* INN; DCF. ◇*SD 14112*

Sulconazole Nitrate [*1977*] (sul kon' a zole nye' trate). **USP**. $C_{18}H_{15}Cl_3N_2S.HNO_3$. 460.76. [Sulconazole is INN and BAN.] (1) 1*H*-Imidazole, 1-[2-[[(4-chlorophenyl)-methyl]thio]-2-(2,4-dichlorophenyl)ethyl]-, mononitrate, (±)-; (2) (±)-1-[2,4-Dichloro-*β*-[(*p*-chlorobenzyl)thio]-phenethyl]imidazole mononitrate. *UNII-1T89100D5U;* *UNII-5D9HAA5Q5S* [sulconazole]. *CAS-61318-91-0;* *CAS-61318-90-9* [sulconazole]. JAN. *Antifungal.* Exel-derm (Ranbaxy) ◇*RS-44872; RS-44872-00-10-3*

Suleparoid Sodium. $(C_{14}H_{18}NO_{17}S_2Na_3)_n$. Heparitin sulfate, sodium salt. *CAS-57459-72-0.* INN.

Sulergine — *See* Disulergine.

Sulesomab [*1996*] (soo les' oh mab). (1) Immunoglobulin G1 (mouse monoclonal IMMU-MN3 Fab' fragment *γ*-chain anti-human NCA-90 granulocyte cell antigen), disulfide with mouse monoclonal IMMU-MN3 light chain; (2) Immunoglobulin G1 (mouse monoclonal IMMU-MN3 Fab' fragment *γ*-chain anti-human NCA-90 granulocyte cell antigen), disulfide with mouse monoclonal IMMU-MN3 light chain. Molecular weight is approximately 50,000 daltons. *CAS-167747-19-5.* INN. *Monoclonal anti-body (diagnostic for the detection of infectious lesions).* LeukoScan (Immunomedics) *[Note—The marketed prod-uct will be labeled with technetium Tc 99m at the clinical site; the nonproprietary name for the radiodiagnostic is technetium Tc 99m sulesomab.]* ◇*IMMU-MN3*

Sulfa, Triple — *See* Triple Sulfa.

---

† Brand name formerly used, and/or firm no longer concerned with this product.

Sulfabenz [*1966*] (sul' fa benz). $C_{12}H_{12}N_2O_2S$. 248.30. (1) Benzenesulfonamide, 4-amino-*N*-phenyl-; (2) Sulfanilani-lide. *CAS-127-77-5.* INN. *Antibacterial; coccidiostat (for poultry).* ◇*NSC-2619*

Sulfabenzamide [*1971*] (sul″ fa benz′ a mide). **USP**. $C_{13}H_{12}N_2O_3S$. 276.31. (1) Benzamide, *N*-[(4-aminophen-yl)sulfonyl]-; (2) *N*-Sulfanilylbenzamide. *CAS-127-71-9.* INN; BAN. *Antibacterial.*

Sulfabromomethazine Sodium. $C_{12}H_{12}BrN_4NaO_2S.H_2O$. 397.22. Sodium N^1-(5-bromo-4,6-dimethyl-2-pyrimidi-nyl)sulfanilamide, monohydrate. *UNII-PQK2N461KJ* [sul-f a b r o m o m e t h a z i n e]. *C A S - 1 1 6 - 4 5 - 0* [sulfabromomethazine]. NF XII; MI.

Sulfacarbamide. $C_7H_9N_3O_3S$. 215.23. Sulfanilylurea. *CAS-547-44-4.* INN; BAN; DCF. *[Name previously used: Sulphaurea.]*

Sulfacecole. $C_{14}H_{17}N_3O_5S$. 339.37. 2-Ethoxy-4′-[(5-methyl-3-isoxazolyl)sulfamoyl]acetanilide. *UNII-AP3C1V2UPV.* *CAS-21662-79-3.* INN.

Sulfacetamide (sul″ fa seet′ a mide). **USP**. $C_8H_{10}N_2O_3S$. 214.24. (1) Acetamide, *N*-[(4-aminophenyl)sulfonyl]-; (2) *N*-Sulfanilylacetamide. *UNII-4965G3J0F5.* *CAS-144-80-9.* INN; BAN. *Antibacterial. [Name previously used: Sulph-acetamide.]*

Sulfacetamide Sodium (sul″ fa seet′ a mide soe′ dee um). **USP**. $C_8H_9N_2NaO_3S.H_2O$. 254.24. (1) Acetamide, *N*-[(4-aminophenyl)sulfonyl]-, monosodium salt, monohydrate; (2) *N*-Sulfanilylacetamide monosodium salt monohydrate. *UNII-4NRT660KJQ.* *CAS-6209-17-2;* *CAS-127-56-0* [an-hydrous]; *CAS-144-80-9* [sulfacetamide]. *Antibacterial.*

Bleph (Allergan); Cetamide (Alcon); Klaron (Sanofi Aventis); Ocusulf (MIZA); Sodium Sulamyd (Schering); Sulfacel (Optopics)

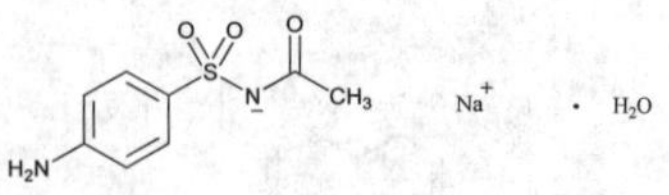

Sulfachlorpyridazine (sul″ fa klor″ pir id′ a zeen). **USP**. $C_{10}H_9ClN_4O_2S$. 284.72. N^1-(6-Chloro-3-pyridazinyl)sulfanilamide. *UNII-P78D9P90C0. CAS-80-32-0*. INN; BAN; MI. *Antibacterial (veterinary)*. Nefrosul (3M Pharmaceuticals†); Sonilyn (Carter-Wallace†); Vetisulid [Veterinary] (Fort Dodge Animal Health) *[Name previously used: Sulphachlorpyridazine.]*

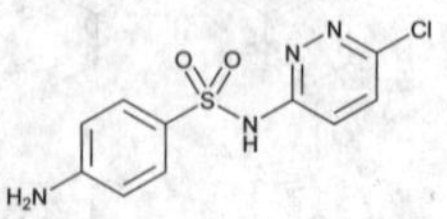

Sulfachrysoidine. $C_{13}H_{13}N_5O_4S$. 335.34. 3,5-Diamino-2-(*p*-sulfamoylphenylazo)benzoic acid. *UNII-39O1389K38. CAS-485-41-6*. INN; DCF; MI.

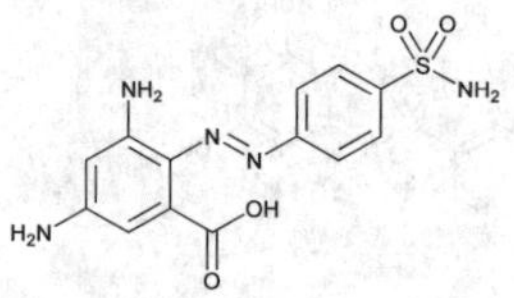

Sulfacitine (INN) — *See* Sulfacytine.

Sulfaclomide. $C_{12}H_{13}ClN_4O_2S$. 312.78. N^1-(5-Chloro-2,6-dimethyl-4-pyrimidinyl)sulfanilamide. *UNII-AXA8-K5U95M. CAS-4015-18-3*. INN.

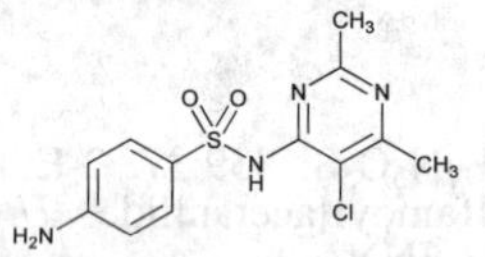

Sulfaclorazole. $C_{16}H_{15}ClN_4O_2S$. 362.83. N^1-[1-(*m*-Chlorophenyl)-3-methyl-5-pyrazolyl]sulfanilamide. *UNII-13HX5F227D. CAS-54063-55-7*. INN.

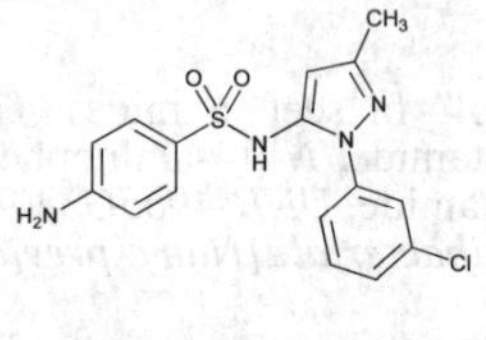

Sulfaclozine. $C_{10}H_9ClN_4O_2S$. 284.72. N^1-(6-Chloropyrazinyl)sulfanilamide. *UNII-69YP7Z48CW. CAS-27890-59-1*. INN.

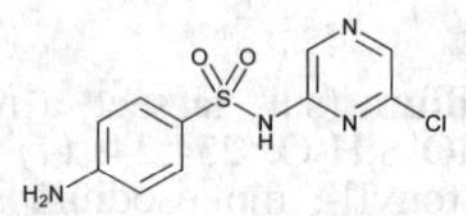

Sulfacombin — *See* Sulfadiazine.

Sulfacytine [*1972*] (sul″ fa sye′ teen). $C_{12}H_{14}N_4O_3S$. 294.33. [Sulfacitine is INN.] (1) Benzenesulfonamide, 4-amino-*N*-(1-ethyl-1,2-dihydro-2-oxo-4-pyrimidinyl)-; (2) N^1-(1-Ethyl-1,2-dihydro-2-oxo-4-pyrimidinyl)sulfanilamide; (3) 1-Ethyl-*N*-sulfanilylcytosine. *UNII-T795873AJP. CAS-17784-12-2*. BAN. *Antibacterial*. Renoquid (Glenwood) ◇*CI-636*

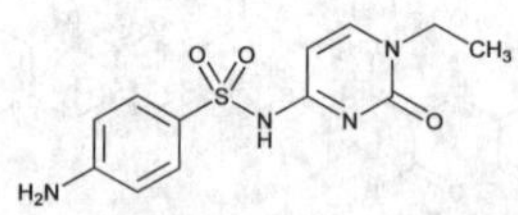

Sulfadiasulfone Sodium (INN) — *See* Acetosulfone Sodium.

Sulfadiazine (sul″ fa dye′ a zeen). **USP**. $C_{10}H_{10}N_4O_2S$. 250.28. (1) Benzenesulfonamide, 4-amino-*N*-2-pyrimidinyl-; (2) N^1-2-Pyrimidinylsulfanilamide. *UNII-0N7609K889. CAS-68-35-9*. INN; BAN; JAN. *Antibacterial*. Coco-diazine (Lilly) *[Name previously used: Sulphadiazine.]*

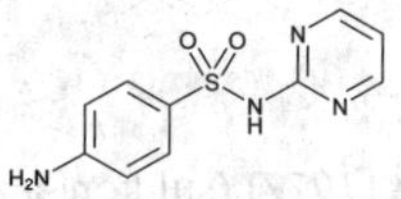

Sulfadiazine, Silver [*1975*] (sul″ fa dye′ a zeen sil′ ver). **USP**. $C_{10}H_9AgN_4O_2S$. 357.14. [Sulfadiazine Silver is JAN.] (1) Benzenesulfonamide, 4-amino-*N*-2-pyrimidinyl-, monosilver(1+) salt; (2) N^1-2-Pyrimidinylsulfanilamide monosilver(1+) salt. *UNII-0N7609K889* [sulfadiazine]. *CAS-22199-08-2; CAS-68-35-9* [sulfadiazine]. *Anti-infective, topical*. Silvadene (Hoechst Marion Roussel)

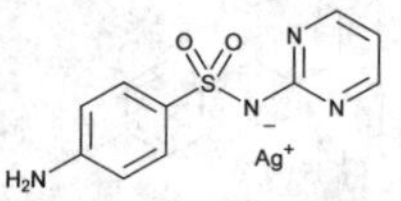

Sulfadiazine Sodium (sul″ fa dye′ a zeen soe′ dee um). **USP**. $C_{10}H_9N_4NaO_2S$. 272.26. (1) Benzenesulfonamide, 4-amino-*N*-2-pyrimidinyl-, monosodium salt; (2) N^1-2-Pyrimidinylsulfanilamide monosodium salt. *UNII-84CS1P306F. CAS-547-32-0; CAS-68-35-9* [sulfadiazine]. INN. *Antibacterial*.

Sulfadicramide. $C_{11}H_{14}N_2O_3S$. 254.31. N'-(3,3-Dimethylacroyl)sulfanilamide. *CAS-115-68-4*. INN; DCF; MI.

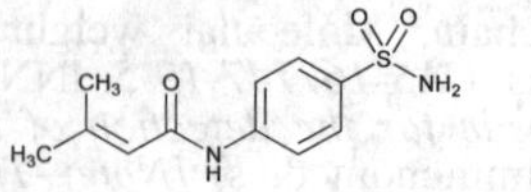

Sulfadicrolamide — *See* Sulfadicramide.

Sulfadimethoxine (sul″ fa dye″ meth ox′ een). **USP**. $C_{12}H_{14}N_4O_4S$. 310.33. (1) Benzenesulfonamide, 4-amino-*N*-(2,6-dimethoxy-4-pyrimidinyl)-; (2) N^1-(2,6-Dimethoxy-4-pyrimidinyl)sulfanilamide. *UNII-30CPC5LDEX. CAS-122-11-2*. NF XIV; BAN; JAN; MI.

Agribon [Veterinary] (Hoffmann-LaRoche); Albon [Veterinary] (Hoffmann-LaRoche); Madribon (Hoffmann-LaRoche†) *[Name previously used: Sulphadimethoxine.]*

Sulfadimethoxine Sodium (sul″ fa dye″ meth ox′ een soe′ dee um). **USP**. $C_{12}H_{13}N_4NaO_4S$. 332.31. (1) Benzenesulfonamide, 4-amino-*N*-(2,6-dimethoxy-4-pyrimidinyl)-, monosodium salt; (2) N^1-(2,6-Dimethoxy-4-pyrimidinyl)-sulfanilamide monosodium salt. *UNII-49DG2B481W*. *CAS-1037-50-9.*

Sulfadimidine (INN, BAN) — *See* Sulfamethazine.

Sulfadoxine [*1968*] (sul″ fa dox′ een). **USP**. $C_{12}H_{14}N_4O_4S$. 310.33. (1) Benzenesulfonamide, 4-amino-*N*-(5,6-dimethoxy-4-pyrimidinyl)-; (2) N^1-(5,6-Dimethoxy-4-pyrimidinyl)sulfanilamide. *UNII-88463U4SM5*. *CAS-2447-57-6.* INN; BAN; JAN. *Antibacterial.* Fanasil (Hoffmann-LaRoche-International); Fanzil (Hoffmann-LaRoche†) ◇*Ro 4-4393*

Sulfaethidole. $C_{10}H_{12}N_4O_2S_2$. 284.36. (1) Benzenesulfonamide, 4-amino-*N*-(5-ethyl-1,3,4-thiadiazol-2-yl)-; (2) N^1-(5-Ethyl-1,3,4-thiadiazol-2-yl)sulfanilamide. *CAS-94-19-9.* NF XIV; INN; BAN; MI. *[Name previously used: Sulphaethidole.]*

Sulfafurazole (INN, BAN) — *See* Sulfisoxazole.

Sulfaguanidine. $C_7H_{10}N_4O_2S$. 214.24. (1) Benzenesulfonamide, 4-amino-*N*-(diaminomethylene)-; (2) N^1-(Diaminomethylene)sulfanilamide. *UNII-15XQ8043FN*. *CAS-57-67-0.* NF XI; INN; BAN; MI. *[Name previously used: Sulphaguanidine.]*

Sulfaguanole. $C_{12}H_{15}N_5O_3S$. 309.34. N^1-[(4,5-Dimethyl-2-oxazolyl)amidino]sulfanilamide. *UNII-0X9P7B60UD*. *CAS-27031-08-9.* INN; MI.

Sulfaisodimidine — *See* Sulfisomidine.

Sulfalene [*1965*] (sul′ fa leen). $C_{11}H_{12}N_4O_3S$. 280.30. [Sulfametopyrazine is BAN; Sulfamethopyrazine is JAN.] (1) Benzenesulfonamide, 4-amino-*N*-(3-methoxypyrazinyl)-; (2) N^1-(3-Methoxypyrazinyl)sulfanilamide. *UNII-T6BL4ZC15G*. *CAS-152-47-6.* INN. *Antibacterial.* Kelfizina (Abbott†) ◇*NSC-110433*

Sulfaloxic Acid. $C_{16}H_{15}N_3O_7S$. 393.37. 4′-[[(Hydroxymethyl)carbamoyl]sulfamoyl]phthalanilic acid. *UNII-4YSI0ZY4W9*. *CAS-14376-16-0.* INN; BAN; MI. *[Name previously used: Sulphaloxic Acid.]*

Sulfamazone. $C_{23}H_{24}N_6O_7S_2$. 560.60. α-[*p*-[(6-Methoxy-3-pyridazinyl)sulfamoyl]anilino]-2,3-dimethyl-5-oxo-1-phenyl-3-pyrazoline-4-methanesulfonic acid. *UNII-D7B8U8-VA9J*. *CAS-65761-24-2.* INN.

Sulfamerazine. $C_{11}H_{12}N_4O_2S$. 264.30. (1) Benzenesulfonamide, 4-amino-*N*-(4-methyl-2-pyrimidinyl)-; (2) N^1-(4-Methyl-2-pyrimidinyl)sulfanilamide. *UNII-UR1SAB295F*. *CAS-127-79-7.* USP XXIII; INN; BAN. *Antibacterial.*

Sulfamerazine Sodium [Injection]. $C_{11}H_{11}N_4NaO_2S$. 286.29. *UNII-JOV4UJY07O; UNII-UR1SAB295F* [sulfamerazine]. *CAS-127-58-2; CAS-127-79-7* [sulfamerazine]. NF XII; INN.

Sulfameter [*1967*] (sul″ fa mee′ ter). $C_{11}H_{12}N_4O_3S$. 280.30. [Sulfametoxydiazine is INN and BAN.] (1) Benzenesulfonamide, 4-amino-*N*-(5-methoxy-2-pyrimidinyl)-; (2) N^1-(5-Methoxy-2-pyrimidinyl)sulfanilamide. *UNII-*

3L179F09D6. CAS-651-06-9. Antibacterial. Sulla (Bayer) *[Name previously used: Sulphamethoxydiazine.]* ◇*AHR-857*

Sulfamethazine (sul″ fa meth′ a zeen). **USP.** C$_{12}$H$_{14}$N$_4$O$_2$S. 278.33. [Sulfadimidine is INN and BAN.] (1) Benzenesulfonamide, 4-amino-*N*-(4,6-dimethyl-2-pyrimidinyl)-; (2) *N*^{1}-(4,6-Dimethyl-2-pyrimidinyl)sulfanilamide. *UNII-48U51W007F. CAS-57-68-1. Antibacterial.* Calfspan Tablets [Veterinary] (Fort Dodge Animal Health); Sulka S Boluses [Veterinary] (Fort Dodge Animal Health); Sulfa-SURE SR Bolus [Veterinary] (Boehringer Ingelheim Animal Health)

Sulfamethizole (sul″ fa meth′ i zole). **USP.** C$_9$H$_{10}$N$_4$O$_2$S$_2$. 270.33. (1) Benzenesulfonamide, 4-amino-*N*-(5-methyl-1,3,4-thiadiazol-2-yl)-; (2) *N*^{1}-(5-Methyl-1,3,4-thiadiazol-2-yl)sulfanilamide. *UNII-25W8454H16. CAS-144-82-1.* INN; BAN; JAN. *Antibacterial.* Thiosulfil (Wyeth) *[Name previously used: Sulphamethizole.]*

Sulfamethopyrazine (JAN) — *See* Sulfalene.

Sulfamethoxazole [*1962*] (sul″ fa meth ox′ a zole). **USP.** C$_{10}$H$_{11}$N$_3$O$_3$S. 253.28. [Acetylsulfamethoxazole and Sulfamethoxazole Sodium are JAN.] (1) Benzenesulfonamide, 4-amino-*N*-(5-methyl-3-isoxazolyl)-; (2) *N*^{1}-(5-Methyl-3-isoxazolyl)sulfanilamide. *UNII-JE42381TNV. CAS-723-46-6.* INN; BAN; JAN. *Antibacterial.* Gantanol (Roche) *[Name previously used: Sulphamethoxazole.]* ◇*Ro 4-2130*

Sulfamethoxypyridazine. C$_{11}$H$_{12}$N$_4$O$_3$S. 280.30. *N*^{1}-(6-Methoxy-3-pyridazinyl)sulfanilamide. *UNII-T034E4NS2Z. CAS-80-35-3.* USP XVII; INN; BAN; MI. Midicel (Parke-Davis†) *[Name previously used: Sulphamethoxypyridazine.]*

Sulfamethoxypyridazine Acetyl. *UNII-T034E4NS2Z* [sulfamethoxypyridazine]. *CAS-3568-43-2; CAS-80-35-3* [sulfamethoxypyridazine]. ND 1966. Midicel Acetyl (Parke-Davis†)

Sulfametin — *See* Sulfameter.

Sulfametomidine. C$_{12}$H$_{14}$N$_4$O$_3$S. 294.33. *N*^{1}-(6-Methoxy-2-methyl-4-pyrimidinyl)sulfanilamide. *UNII-940ZL3AHKB. CAS-3772-76-7.* INN; DCF.

Sulfametopyrazine (BAN, DCF) — *See* Sulfalene.

Sulfametoxydiazine (INN, BAN, DCF) — *See* Sulfameter.

Sulfametrole. C$_9$H$_{10}$N$_4$O$_3$S$_2$. 286.33. *N*^{1}-(4-Methoxy-1,2,5-thiadiazol-3-yl)sulfanilamide. *UNII-F5AK41IPQG. CAS-32909-92-5.* INN; BAN; MI.

Sulfamidothiodiazol — *See* Glybuzole.

Sulfamonomethoxine [*1963*] (sul″ fa mon″ oh meth ox′ een). C$_{11}$H$_{12}$N$_4$O$_3$S. 280.30. (1) Benzenesulfonamide, 4-amino-*N*-(6-methoxy-4-pyrimidinyl)-; (2) *N*^{1}-(6-Methoxy-4-pyrimidinyl)sulfanilamide. *UNII-U700P169W2. CAS-1220-83-3.* INN; BAN; JAN. *Antibacterial.*

Sulfamoprine (BAN) — *See* Sulphamoprine.

Sulfamoxole [*1968*] (sul″ fa mox′ ole). C$_{11}$H$_{13}$N$_3$O$_3$S. 267.30. (1) Benzenesulfonamide, 4-amino-*N*-(4,5-dimethyl-2-oxazolyl)-; (2) *N*^{1}-(4,5-Dimethyl-2-oxazolyl)sulfanilamide. *CAS-729-99-7.* INN; BAN. *Antibacterial.*

Sulfanilamide. C$_6$H$_8$N$_2$O$_2$S. 172.20. *p*-Aminobenzenesulfonamide. *UNII-21240MF57M. CAS-63-74-1.* NF XI; INN; DCF; MI.

Sulfanilate Zinc [*1970*] (sul fan′ i late zink). C$_{12}$H$_{12}$N$_2$O$_6$S$_2$Zn.4H$_2$O. 481.80. (1) Benzenesulfonic acid, 4-amino-, zinc salt (2:1), tetrahydrate; (2) Zinc sulfanilate tetrahydrate. *CAS-31884-76-1; CAS-22484-64-6* [anhydrous]; *CAS-121-57-3* [sulfanilic acid]. *Antibacterial.* Nizin (Broemmel†)

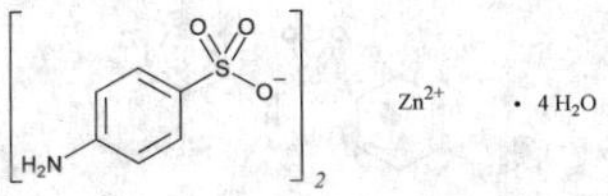

Sulfanitran [*1964*] (sul″ fa nye′ tran). $C_{14}H_{13}N_3O_5S$. 335.34. (1) Acetamide, *N*-[4-[[(4-nitrophenyl)amino]sulfonyl]phenyl]-; (2) 4′-[(*p*-Nitrophenyl)sulfamoyl]acetanilide. *UNII-QT35T5T35Q. CAS-122-16-7.* INN; BAN. *Antibacterial; coccidiostat (for poultry).* ◇*NSC-77120*

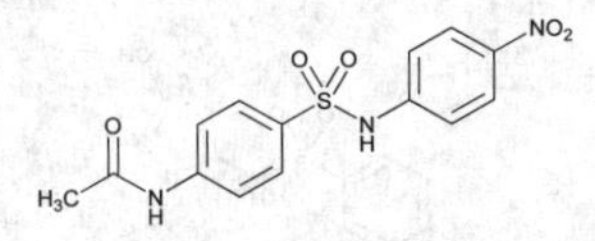

Sulfaperin. $C_{11}H_{12}N_4O_2S$. 264.30. *N*[1]-(5-Methyl-2-pyrimidinyl)sulfanilamide. *UNII-W5E840UV9P. CAS-599-88-2.* INN; MI.

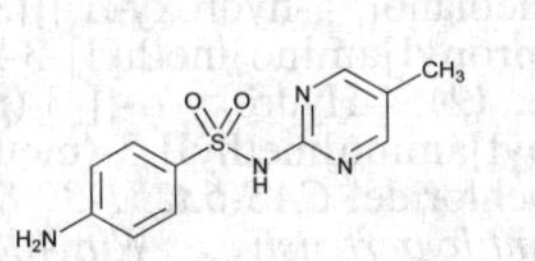

Sulfaphenazole. $C_{15}H_{14}N_4O_2S$. 314.36. *N*[1]-(1-Phenylpyrazol-5-yl)sulfanilamide. *UNII-0J8L4V3F81. CAS-526-08-9.* INN; BAN; JAN; MI. Sulfabid (Purdue Frederick) *[Name previously used: Sulphaphenazole.]*

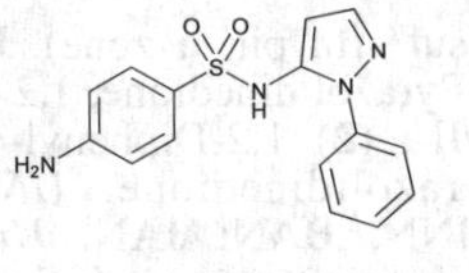

Sulfaphtalylthiazol — *See* Phthalylsulfathiazole.

Sulfaproxyline. $C_{16}H_{18}N_2O_4S$. 334.39. *N*[1]-(4-Isopropoxybenzoyl)sulfanilamide. *UNII-YR841R53VW. CAS-116-42-7.* INN; BAN; MI. *[Name previously used: Sulphaproxyline.]*

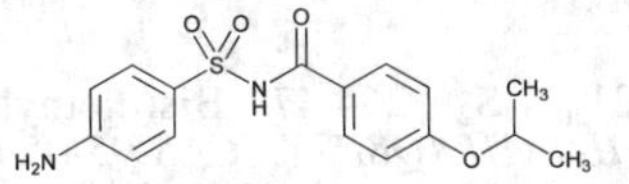

Sulfapyrazole (INN, BAN) — *See* Sulfazamet.

---

† Brand name formerly used, and/or firm no longer concerned with this product.

Sulfapyridine (sul″ fa pir′ i deen). **USP.** $C_{11}H_{11}N_3O_2S$. 249.29. (1) Benzenesulfonamide, 4-amino-*N*-2-pyridinyl-; (2) *N*[1]-2-Pyridylsulfanilamide. *UNII-Y5V2N1KE8U. CAS-144-83-2.* INN; BAN. *Suppressant (dermatitis herpetiformis). [Name previously used: Sulphapyridine.]*

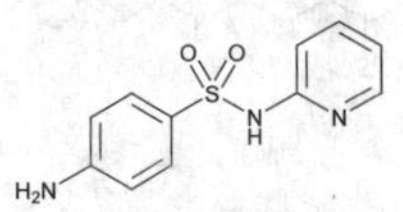

Sulfapyridine Sodium. *UNII-H3SKB3662O. CAS-127-57-1; CAS-144-83-2* [sulfapyridine]. NF X; MI.

Sulfaquinoxaline (sul″ fa kwin ox′ a leen). **USP.** $C_{14}H_{12}N_4O_2S$. 300.34. *N*[1]-2-Quinoxalinylsulfanilamide. *UNII-WNW8115TM9. CAS-59-40-5.* INN; BAN; MI. *Coccidiostat (veterinary).*

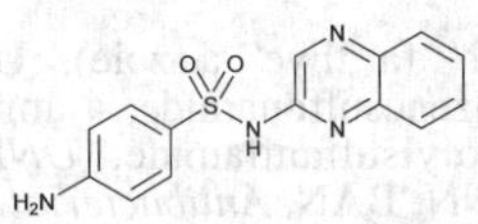

Sulfarsphenamine. $C_{14}H_{14}As_2N_2Na_2O_8S_2$. 598.22. Disodium [arsenobis[(6-hydroxy-*m*-phenylene)imino]]dimethanesulfonate. *CAS-618-82-6.* NF IX; INN; MI.

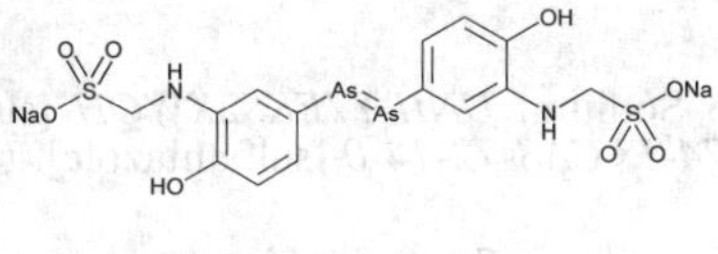

Sulfasalazine [*1975*] (sul″ fa sal′ a zeen). **USP.** $C_{18}H_{14}N_4O_5S$. 398.39. [Salazosulfapyridine is JAN.] (1) Benzoic acid, 2-hydroxy-5-[[4-[(2-pyridinylamino)sulfonyl]phenyl]azo]-; (2) 5-[[*p*-(2-Pyridylsulfamoyl)phenyl]azo]salicylic acid. *UNII-3XC8GUZ6CB. CAS-599-79-1.* INN; BAN. *Antibacterial.* Azulfidine (Pfizer); S.a.s. (Solvay Pharmaceuticals) *[Names previously used: Salicylazosulfapyridine; Sulphasalazine.]*

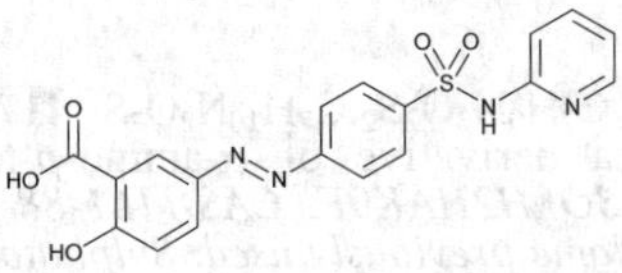

Sulfasomizole [*1962*] (sul″ fa soe′ mi zole). $C_{10}H_{11}N_3O_2S_2$. 269.34. (1) Benzenesulfonamide, 4-amino-*N*-(3-methyl-5-isothiazolyl)-; (2) *N*[1]-(3-Methyl-5-isothiazolyl)sulfanilamide. *UNII-U3227B174V. CAS-632-00-8.* INN; BAN. *Antibacterial. [Name previously used: Sulphasomizole.]* ◇*NSC-139593*

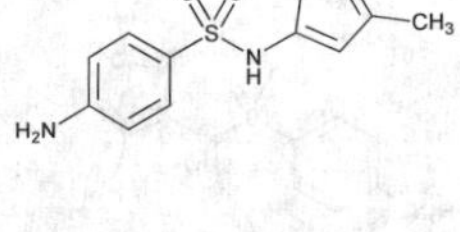

Sulfastearyl — *See* Stearylsulfamide.

Sulfasuccinamide. $C_{10}H_{12}N_2O_5S$. 272.28. 4'-Sulfamoylsuccinanilic acid. *UNII-8286I9062N. CAS-3563-14-2.* INN.

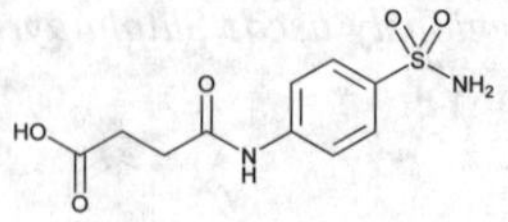

Sulfasymazine. $C_{13}H_{17}N_5O_2S$. 307.37. N^1-(4,6-Biethyl-*s*-triazin-2-yl)sulfanilamide. *CAS-1984-94-7.* INN; MI.

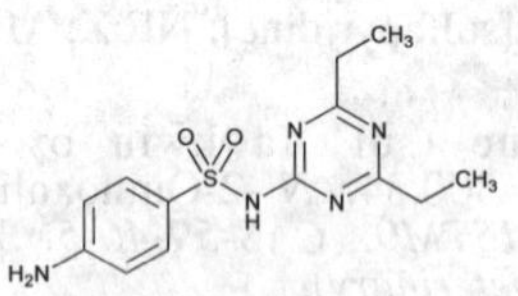

Sulfathiazole (sul″ fa thye′ a zole). **USP.** $C_9H_9N_3O_2S_2$. 255.32. (1) Benzenesulfonamide, 4-amino-*N*-2-thiazolyl-; (2) N^1-2-Thiazolylsulfanilamide. *UNII-Y7FKS2XWQH. CAS-72-14-0.* INN; BAN. *Antibacterial. [Name previously used: Sulphathiazole.]*

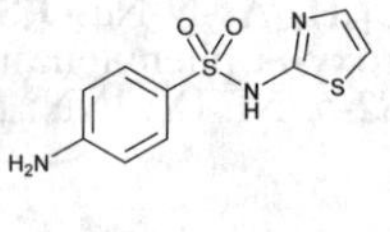

Sulfathiazole Sodium. *UNII-Y7FKS2XWQH* [sulfathiazole]. *CAS-144-74-1; CAS-72-14-0* [sulfathiazole]. NF XI; MI.

Sulfathiocarbamide — *See* Sulfathiourea.

Sulfathiourea. $C_7H_9N_3O_2S_2$. 231.30. 1-Sulfanilyl-2-thiourea. *UNII-MXF9G4I1V5. CAS-515-49-1.* INN; BAN; DCF; MI. *[Name previously used: Sulphathiourea.]*

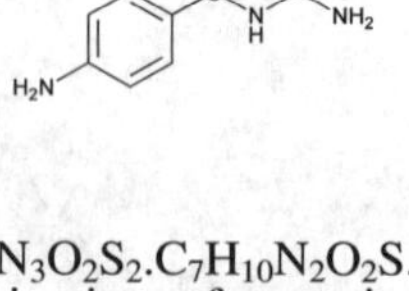

Sulfatolamide. $C_7H_9N_3O_2S_2 \cdot C_7H_{10}N_2O_2S$. 417.53. 1-Sulfanilyl-2-thiourea derivative of α-amino-*p*-toluenesulfonamide. *UNII-3OLH2HAK9F. CAS-1161-88-2.* INN; BAN; JAN; MI. *[Name previously used: Sulphatolamide.]*

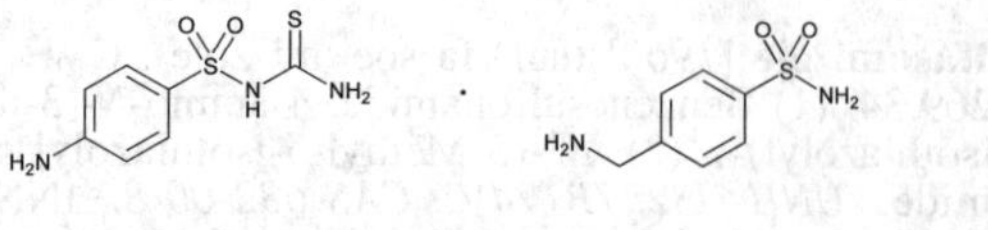

Sulfatroxazole. $C_{11}H_{13}N_3O_3S$. 267.30. N^1-(4,5-Dimethyl-3-isoxazolyl)sulfanilamide. *CAS-23256-23-7.* INN; BAN.

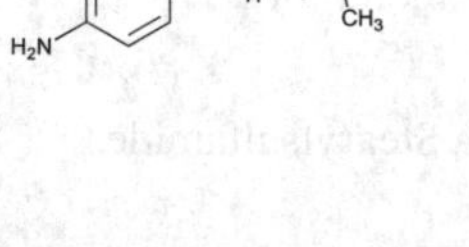

Sulfatrozole. $C_{10}H_{12}N_4O_3S_2$. 300.36. N^1-(4-Ethoxy-1,2,5-thiadiazol-3-yl)sulfanilamide. *UNII-G91KDP4M35. CAS-13369-07-8.* INN.

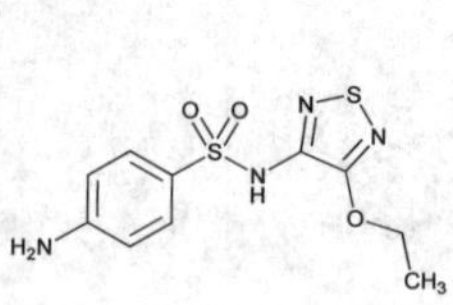

Sulfazamet [*1969*] (sul faz′ a met). $C_{16}H_{16}N_4O_2S$. 328.39. [Sulfapyrazole is INN and BAN.] (1) Benzenesulfonamide, 4-amino-*N*-(3-methyl-1-phenyl-1*H*-pyrazol-5-yl)-; (2) N^1-(3-Methyl-1-phenylpyrazol-5-yl)sulfanilamide. *CAS-852-19-7. Antibacterial.*

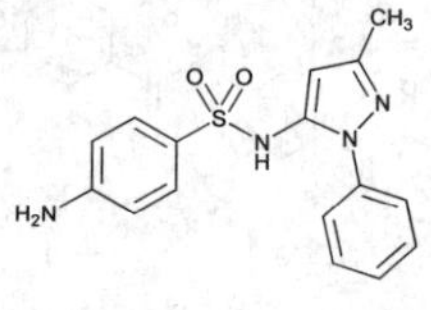

Sulfinalol Hydrochloride [*1979*] (sul fin′ a lol hye″ droe klor′ ide). $C_{20}H_{27}NO_4S \cdot HCl$. 413.96. [Sulfinalol is INN.] (1) Benzenemethanol, 4-hydroxy-α-[[[3-(4-methoxyphenyl)-1-methylpropyl]amino]methyl]-3-(methylsulfinyl)-, hydrochloride; (2) 4-Hydroxy-α-[[[3-(*p*-methoxyphenyl)-1-methylpropyl]amino]methyl]-3-(methylsulfinyl)benzyl alcohol hydrochloride. *CAS-63251-39-8; CAS-66264-77-5* [sulfinalol]. *Antihypertensive.* ◇Win 40808-7

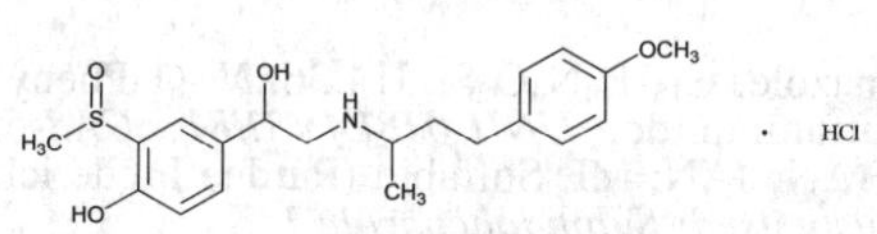

Sulfinpyrazone (sul″ fin pir′ a zone). **USP.** $C_{23}H_{20}N_2O_3S$. 404.48. (1) 3,5-Pyrazolidinedione, 1,2-diphenyl-4-[2-(phenylsulfinyl)ethyl]-; (2) 1,2-Diphenyl-4-[2-(phenylsulfinyl)ethyl]-3,5-pyrazolidinedione. *UNII-V6OFU47K3W. CAS-57-96-5.* INN; BAN; JAN. *Uricosuric.* Anturane (Novartis) *[Name previously used: Sulphinpyrazone.]*

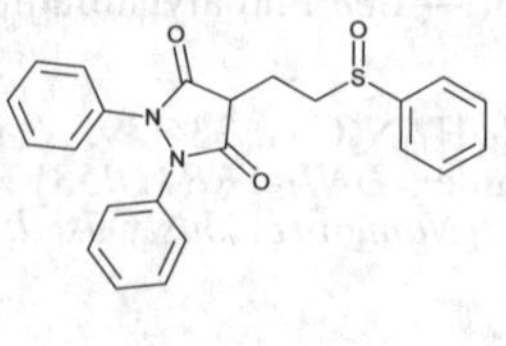

Sulfiram. $C_{10}H_{20}N_2S_3$. 264.47. Bis(diethylthiocarbamoyl) sulfide. *UNII-1XHL4Q8P7Y. CAS-95-05-6.* INN; BAN; MI. *[Name previously used: Monosulfiram.]*

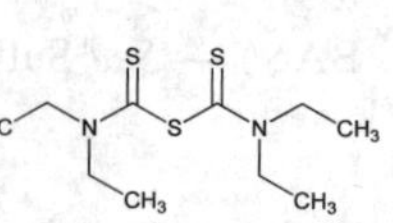

Sulfisomidine. $C_{12}H_{14}N_4O_2S$. 278.33. [Sulfisomidine Sodium is JAN.] N^1-(2,6-Dimethyl-4-pyrimidinyl)sulfanilamide. *CAS-515-64-0.* JAN; BAN; MI. *[Name previously used: Sulphasomidine.]*

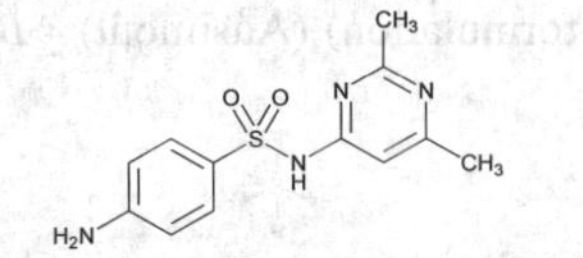

Sulfisoxazole (sul″ fi sox′ a zole). **USP.** $C_{11}H_{13}N_3O_3S$. 267.30. [Sulfafurazole is INN and BAN.] (1) Benzenesulfonamide, 4-amino-*N*-(3,4-dimethyl-5-isoxazolyl)-; (2) N^1-(3,4-Dimethyl-5-isoxazolyl)sulfanilamide. *UNII-740T4C525W.* CAS-127-69-5. JAN. *Antibacterial.* Gantrisin (Roche) *[Name previously used: Sulphafurazole.]*

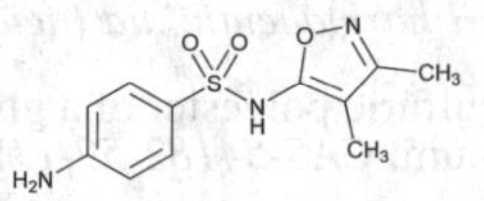

Sulfisoxazole Acetyl (sul″ fi sox′ a zole). **USP.** $C_{13}H_{15}N_3O_4S$. 309.34. [Acetylsulfisoxazole is JAN.] (1) Acetamide, *N*-[(4-aminophenyl)sulfonyl]-*N*-(3,4-dimethyl-5-isoxazolyl)-; (2) *N*-(3,4-Dimethyl-5-isoxazolyl)-*N*-sulfanilylacetamide. *UNII-WBT5QH3KED.* CAS-80-74-0. *Antibacterial.* Gantrisin (Roche)

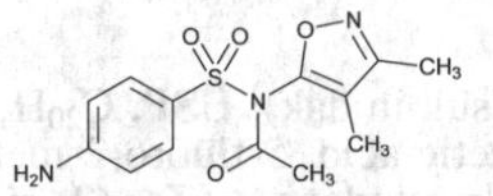

Sulfisoxazole Diolamine *[1966]* (sul″ fi sox′ a zole dye ole′ a meen). $C_{11}H_{13}N_3O_3S.C_4H_{11}NO_2$. 372.44. (1) Benzenesulfonamide, 4-amino-*N*-(3,4-dimethyl-5-isoxazolyl)-, compd. with 2,2′-iminobis[ethanol] (1:1); (2) N^1-(3,4-Dimethyl-5-isoxazolyl)sulfanilamide compound with 2,2′-iminodiethanol (1:1). *UNII-30S4B46J8B.* CAS-4299-60-9; *CAS-127-69-5* [sulfisoxazole]. USP XXIII. *Antibacterial.* Gantrisin (Roche) ◇*NU-445*

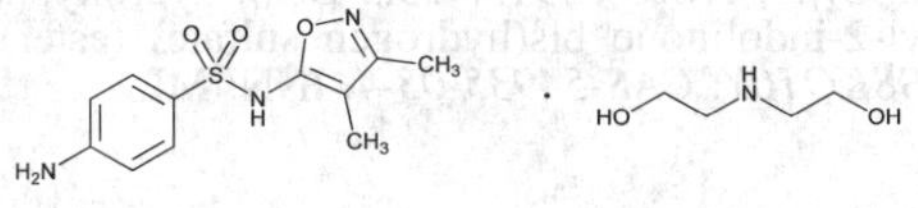

Sulfobenzylpenicillin — *See* Sulbenicillin.

Sulfobromophthalein Sodium. $C_{20}H_8Br_4Na_2O_{10}S_2$. 838.00. [Sulphobromophthalein is BAN.] (1) Benzenesulfonic acid, 3,3′-(4,5,6,7-tetrabromo-3-oxo-1(3*H*)-isobenzofuranylide-ne)bis[6-hydroxy-, disodium salt; (2) 4,5,6,7-Tetrabromo-3′,3″-disulfophenolphthalein disodium salt. *CAS-71-67-0; CAS-297-83-6* [sulfobromophthalein]. USP XXII; JAN.

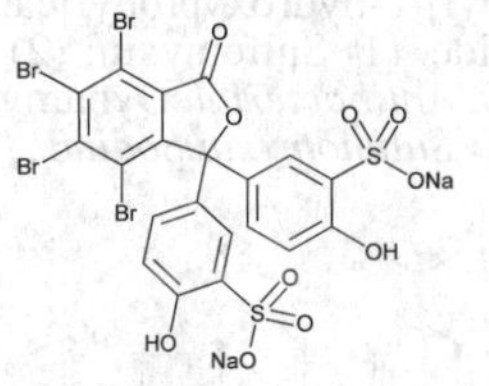

Sulfobromphthalein Sodium — *See* Sulfobromophthalein Sodium.

Sulfocon B *[2002]* (sul foe′ kon). $(C_5H_8O_2)_n$ $(C_{10}H_{16}O_2)_m(C_{19}H_{50}O_8Si_7)_x(C_{14}H_{22}O_6)_y(C_6H_9NO)_z(C_{16}H_{14}F_{17}NO_4S)_g(C_4H_6O_2)_q$. (1) Methyl 2-methyl-2-propenoate polymer with cyclohexyl 2-methyl-2-propenoate, 3-[1-[(dimethylsily)oxy]-3,3,5,5,7,7-hexamethyl-1-[(1,1,3,3-tetramethyldisiloxanyl)oxy]-tetrasiloxanyl]propyl-2-methyl-2-propenoate, 1,2-ethanediylbis(oxy-2,1-ethanediyl) bis(2-methyl-2-propenoate), 1-ethenyl-2-pyrrolidinone, 2-[ethyl[(heptadecafluorooctyl)sulfonyl]amino]ethyl 2-methyl-2-propenoate and 2-methyl-2-propenoic acid; (2) Methyl methacrylate polymer with cyclohexyl methacrylate, 3-[1-(dimethylsiloxy)-3,3,5,5,7,7-hexamethyl-1-(1,1,3,3-tetramethyldisiloxanoxy)tetrasiloxanyl]propyl methacrylate, triethylene glycol dimethacrylate, 1-vinyl-2-pyrrolidinone, 2-(*N*-ethyl-1,1,2,2,3,3,4,4,5,5,6,6,7,7,8,8,8-heptadecafluoro-1-octanesulfonamido)ethyl methacrylate and methacrylic acid. *Contact lens material (hydrophobic).* The Alberta Lens SM2 (Progressive Optical) *[Note—The water content of the contact lens material is <0.2% at ambient temperature (23±2°C), and the oxygen permeability is 45 × 10^{-11}(cm²/sec)(ml O₂/ml × mm Hg) at 35°C (Dk value).]*

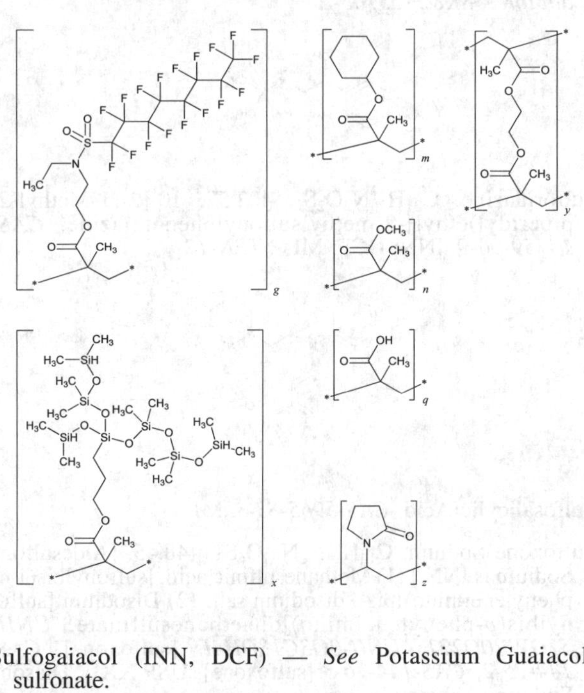

Sulfogaiacol (INN, DCF) — *See* Potassium Guaiacolsulfonate.

Sulfomyxin *[1966]* (sul″ foe mix′ in). $C_{61}H_{103}N_{16}Na_5O_{28}S_5$ (major component). 1783.83. [Sulfomyxin Sodium is BAN.] A mixture consisting mainly of the pentasodium salt of the pentakis(*N*-sulfomethyl) derivative of polymyxin B_1 with a lesser amount of the corresponding salt derived from polymyxin B_2 and a trace of the corresponding salt derived from polymyxin B_3. Major component: The pentasodium salt of the pentakis(*N*-sulfomethyl) derivative

---

of a specific stereoisomer of *N*-(3-amino-1-[[1-[[3-amino-1-[[6,9,18-tris-(2-aminoethyl)-15-benzyl-3-(1-hydroxyethyl)-12-isobutyl-2,5,8,11,14,17-20-heptaoxo-1,4,7,10,13,16,19-heptaazacyclotricos-21-yl]carbamoyl]propyl]carbamoyl]-2-hydroxypropyl]carbamoyl]propyl]-6-methyloctanamide. (1) Sulfomyxin; (2) Sulfomyxin. *CAS-1405-52-3*. INN. *Antibacterial.* Dynamyxin (Pfizer) *[Name previously used: Sulphomyxin Sodium.]* ◇*GS-6742*

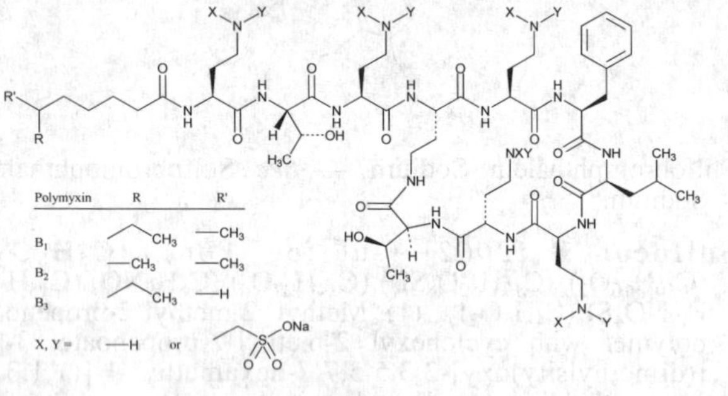

Sulfonal — *See* Sulfonmethane.

Sulfonethylmethane. *UNII-217727W28W. CAS-76-20-0.* NF VIII; MI.

Sulfonmethane. *CAS-115-24-2.* NF VIII; MI.

Sulfonterol Hydrochloride [*1975*] (sul fon′ ter ol hye″ droe klor′ ide). $C_{14}H_{23}NO_4S \cdot HCl$. 337.86. [Sulfonterol is INN.] (1) Benzenemethanol, α-[[(1,1-dimethylethyl)amino]methyl]-4-hydroxy-3-[(methylsulfonyl)methyl]-, hydrochloride; (2) α-[(*tert*-Butylamino)methyl]-4-hydroxy-3-[(methylsulfonyl)methyl]benzyl alcohol hydrochloride. *UNII-AJ14S16J7N; UNII-Z540ZT2MI6* [sulfonterol]. *CAS-42461-78-9; CAS-42461-79-0* [sulfonterol]. *Bronchodilator.* ◇*SK&F 53705-A*

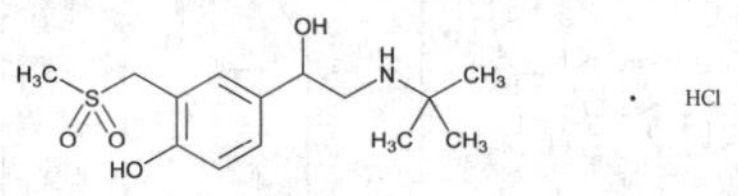

Sulforidazine. $C_{21}H_{26}N_2O_2S_2$. 402.57. 10-[2-(1-Methyl-2-piperidyl)ethyl]-2-methylsulfonylphenothiazine. *CAS-14759-06-9.* INN; DCF; MI. ◇*TPN-12*

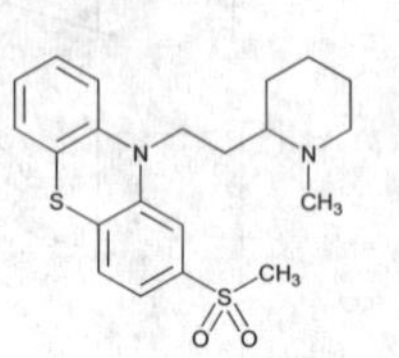

Sulfosalicylic Acid. *CAS-5965-83-3.* MI.

Sulfoxone Sodium. $C_{14}H_{14}N_2Na_2O_6S_3$. 448.45. [Aldesulfone Sodium is INN.] (1) Methanesulfinic acid, [sulfonylbis(1,4-phenyleneimino)]bis-, disodium salt; (2) Disodium [sulfonylbis(*p*-phenyleneimino)]dimethanesulfinate. *UNII-57OWB0Q221; UNII-0G3C18OH4D* [sulfoxone]. *CAS-144-75-2; CAS-144-76-3* [sulfoxone]. USP XXII. Diasone Sodium (Abbott)

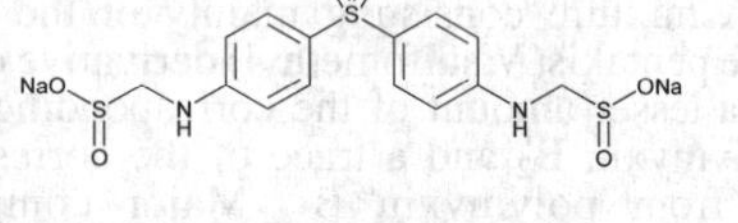

Sulfur Dioxide (sul′ fur dye ox′ ide). **NF.** SO_2. 64.06. (1) Sulfur dioxide; (2) Sulfur dioxide. *CAS-7446-09-5. Pharmaceutic aid (antioxidant).*

Sulfur Hexafluoride [*1999*] (sul′ fur hex″ a floor′ ide). SF_6. 146.06. (1) Sulfur fluoride (SF_6); (2) Sulfur hexafluoride. *CAS-2551-62-4. Diagnostic (ultrasound).* SonoVue (for the microbubble formulation) (Ausimont) ◇*BRI*

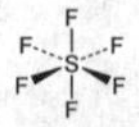

Sulfur, Precipitated (sul′ fur pre sip′ i tay″ ted). **USP.** S. 32.07. [Sulfur is JAN.] (1) Sulfur; (2) Sulfur. *CAS-7704-34-9. Scabicide.* Liquamat (Galderma†); Sastid (Stiefel); Sulfur Soap (Stiefel)

Sulfur, Sublimed (sul′ fur sub lymed′). **USP.** S. 32.07. (1) Sulfur; (2) Sulfur. *CAS-7704-34-9. Scabicide.*

Sulfuric Acid (sul fure′ ik as′ id). **NF.** H_2SO_4. 98.08. (1) Sulfuric acid; (2) Sulfuric acid. *UNII-O40UQP6WCF. CAS-7664-93-9. Pharmaceutic aid (acidifying agent).*

Sulglicotide. The sulfuric polyester of a glycopeptide isolated from pig duodenum. *CAS-54182-59-1.* INN; BAN.

Sulglycotide (previously used name) — *See* Sulglicotide.

Sulicrinat. $C_{15}H_{10}Cl_3NO_6S$. 438.67. [2,3-Dichloro-4-(4-chloro-3-sulfamoylbenzoyl)phenoxy]acetic acid. *UNII-DJH1LFU42E. CAS-90207-12-8.* INN.

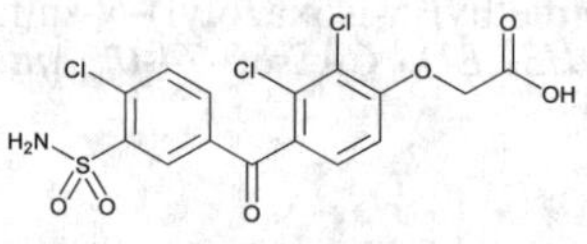

Sulindac [*1975*] (sul′ in dak). **USP.** $C_{20}H_{17}FO_3S$. 356.41. (1) 1*H*-Indene-3-acetic acid, 5-fluoro-2-methyl-1-[[4-(methylsulfinyl)phenyl]methylene]-, (*Z*)-; (2) *cis*-5-Fluoro-2-methyl-1-[(*p*-methylsulfinyl)benzylidene]indene-3-acetic acid. *UNII-184SNS8VUH. CAS-38194-50-2.* INN; BAN; JAN. *Anti-inflammatory.* Clinoril (Merck)

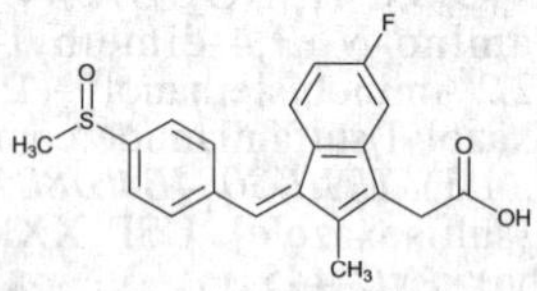

Sulisatin. $C_{21}H_{17}NO_9S_2$. 491.49. 3,3-Bis(*p*-hydroxyphenyl)-7-methyl-2-indolinone bis(hydrogen sulfate) (ester). *UNII-5EOG8KQT0Y. CAS-54935-03-4.* INN; MI.

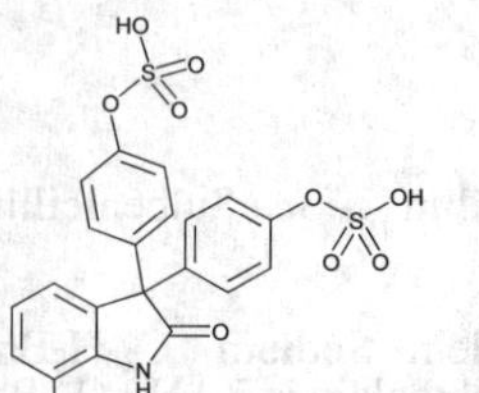

Sulisobenzone [*1966*] (sul″ i soe ben′ zone). **USP.** $C_{14}H_{12}O_6S$. 308.31. (1) Benzenesulfonic acid, 5-benzoyl-4-hydroxy-2-methoxy-; (2) 5-Benzoyl-4-hydroxy-2-methoxybenzenesulfonic acid. *UNII-1W6L629B4K. CAS-4065-45-6.* INN. *Ultraviolet screen.* Sungard (Bayer†) ◇*NSC-60584*

Sulmarin [*1981*] (sul′ ma rin). $C_{10}H_8O_{10}S_2$. 352.29. (1) 2*H*-1-Benzopyran-2-one, 4-methyl-6,7-bis(sulfooxy)-; (2) 6,7-Dihydroxy-4-methylcoumarin bis(hydrogen sulfate). *UNII-73W96524XT. CAS-29334-07-4.* INN. *Hemostatic.* Idro P_2 (Maggioni Farmaceutici S.p.A., Italy) ◇*M.G. 143*

Sulmazole. $C_{14}H_{13}N_3O_2S$. 287.34. 2-[2-Methoxy-4-(methylsulfinyl)phenyl]-3*H*-imidazo[4,5-*b*]pyridine. *CAS-73384-60-8.* INN; MI.

Sulmepride. $C_{14}H_{21}N_3O_4S$. 327.40. *N*-[(1-Methyl-2-pyrrolidinyl)methyl]-5-sulfamoyl-*o*-anisamide. *UNII-DX60O-V32AE. CAS-57479-88-6.* INN; MI.

Sulnidazole [*1975*] (sul nye′ da zole). $C_9H_{14}N_4O_3S$. 258.30. (1) Carbamothioic acid, [2-(2-ethyl-5-nitro-1*H*-imidazol-1-yl)ethyl]-, *O*-methyl ester; (2) *O*-Methyl [2-(2-ethyl-5-nitroimidazol-1-yl)ethyl]thiocarbamate. *UNII-504LR309YV. CAS-51022-76-5.* INN. *Antiprotozoal (Trichomonas).* ◇*R 26,412*

Sulocarbilate. $C_9H_{12}N_2O_5S$. 260.27. 2-Hydroxyethyl *p*-sulfamoylcarbanilate. *UNII-5VZ26183XG. CAS-121-64-2.* INN.

Suloctidil [*1978*] (sul ok′ ti dil). $C_{20}H_{35}NOS$. 337.56. (1) Benzenemethanol, 4-[(1-methylethyl)thio]-α-[1-(octylamino)ethyl]-, (*R**,*S**)-; (2) *erythro-p*-(Isopropylthio)-α-[1-(octylamino)ethyl]benzyl alcohol. *CAS-54063-56-8.* INN; BAN. *Vasodilator (peripheral).* ◇*MJF 12637; CP-556S*

Sulodexide. Glucorono-2-amino-2-deoxyglucoglucan sulfate. *CAS-57821-29-1.* INN.

Sulofenur [*1990*] (sul″ oh fen′ ur). $C_{16}H_{15}ClN_2O_3S$. 350.82. (1) 1*H*-Indene-5-sulfonamide, *N*-[[(4-chlorophenyl)amino]carbonyl]-2,3-dihydro-; (2) 1-(*p*-Chlorophenyl)-3-(5-indanylsulfonyl)urea. *CAS-110311-27-8.* INN; BAN. *Antineoplastic.* ◇*LY186641*

Sulopenem [*1992*] (sul″ oh pen′ em). $C_{12}H_{15}NO_5S_3$. 349.45. (1) 4-Thia-1-azabicyclo[3.2.0]hept-2-ene-2-carboxylic acid, 6-(1-hydroxyethyl)-7-oxo-3-[(tetrahydro-3-thienyl)thio]-, *S*-oxide, [5*R*-[3(1*R**,3*S**),5α,6α(*R**)]]-; (2) (5*R*,6*S*)-6-[(1*R*)-1-Hydroxyethyl]-7-oxo-3-[[(3*S*)-tetrahydro-3-thienyl]thio]-4-thia-1-azabicyclo[3.2.0]hept-2-ene-2-carboxylic acid, (*R*)-*S*-oxide. *CAS-120788-07-0.* INN. *Antibacterial.* ◇*CP-70,429*

Sulosemide. $C_{17}H_{16}N_2O_7S_2$. 424.45. 2-(Furfurylamino)-4-phenoxy-5-sulfamoylbenzenesulfonic acid. *UNII-CY351D07GJ. CAS-82666-62-4.* INN.

Sulotroban [*1989*] (sul″ oh troe′ ban). $C_{16}H_{17}NO_5S$. 335.37. (1) Acetic acid, [4-[2-[(phenylsulfonyl)amino]ethyl]phenoxy]-; (2) [*p*-(2-Benzenesulfonamidoethyl)phenoxy] acetic acid. *CAS-72131-33-0.* INN; BAN. *Glomerulonephritis treatment.* ◇*BM 13.177; SK&F 95587*

Suloxifen Oxalate [*1973*] (sul ox′ i fen ox′ a late). $C_{18}H_{24}N_2OS.C_2H_2O_4$. 406.50. [Suloxifen is INN.] (1) Sulfoximine, *N*-[2-(diethylamino)ethyl]-*S*,*S*-diphenyl-, ethanedioate (1:1); (2) *N*-[2-(Diethylamino)ethyl]-*S*,*S*-diphenylsulfoximine oxalate (1:1). *UNII-C0HG40P7PY;*

UNII-LD18TA6Q06 [suloxifen]. *CAS-25827-13-8; CAS-25827-12-7* [suloxifen]. *Bronchodilator.* ◇*Go 1733; W 6439A*

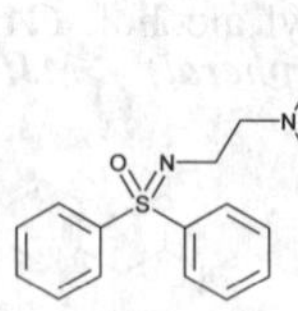

Sulphabutin — *See* Busulfan.

Sulphacetamide (previously used name) — *See* Sulfacetamide.

Sulphachlorpyridazine (previously used name) — *See* Sulfachlorpyridazine.

Sulphadiazine (previously used name) — *See* Sulfadiazine.

Sulphadimethoxine (previously used name) — *See* Sulfadimethoxine.

Sulphaethidole (previously used name) — *See* Sulfaethidole.

Sulphafurazole (previously used name) — *See* Sulfisoxazole.

Sulphaguanidine (previously used name) — *See* Sulfaguanidine.

Sulphaloxic Acid (previously used name) — *See* Sulfaloxic Acid.

Sulphamethizole (previously used name) — *See* Sulfamethizole.

Sulphamethoxazole (previously used name) — *See* Sulfamethoxazole.

Sulphamethoxydiazine (previously used name) — *See* Sulfameter.

Sulphamethoxypyridazine (previously used name) — *See* Sulfamethoxypyridazine.

Sulphamoprine. $C_{12}H_{14}N_4O_4S$. 310.33. [Sulfamoprine is BAN.] N^1-(4,6-Dimethoxypyrimidin-2-yl)sulphanilamide. *UNII-E7C6PMZ54M. CAS-155-91-9.*

Sulphamoxole (previously used name) — *See* Sulfamoxole.

Sulphan Blue (BAN) — *See* Isosulfan Blue.

Sulphaphenazole (previously used name) — *See* Sulfaphenazole.

Sulphaproxyline (previously used name) — *See* Sulfaproxyline.

Sulphapyridine (previously used name) — *See* Sulfapyridine.

Sulphasalazine (previously used name) — *See* Sulfasalazine.

Sulphasomidine (previously used name) — *See* Sulfisomidine.

Sulphasomizole (previously used name) — *See* Sulfasomizole.

Sulphathiazole (previously used name) — *See* Sulfathiazole.

Sulphathiourea (previously used name) — *See* Sulfathiourea.

Sulphatolamide (previously used name) — *See* Sulfatolamide.

Sulphaurea (previously used name) — *See* Sulfacarbamide.

Sulphinpyrazone (previously used name) — *See* Sulfinpyrazone.

Sulphobromophthalein (BAN) — *See* Sulfobromophthalein Sodium.

Sulphocarbolate Sodium — *See* Phenolsulphonate Sodium.

Sulphomyxin Sodium (previously used name) — *See* Sulfomyxin.

Sulphonal — *See* Sulfonmethane.

Sulpiride [*1968*] (sul′ pir ide). $C_{15}H_{23}N_3O_4S$. 341.43. (1) Benzamide, 5-(aminosulfonyl)-*N*-[(1-ethyl-2-pyrrolidinyl)methyl]-2-methoxy-; (2) *N*-[(1-Ethyl-2-pyrrolidinyl)methyl]-5-sulfamoyl-*o*-anisamide. *CAS-15676-16-1.* INN; BAN; JAN. *Antidepressant.* Dogmatyl (Laboratoires Delagrange, France)

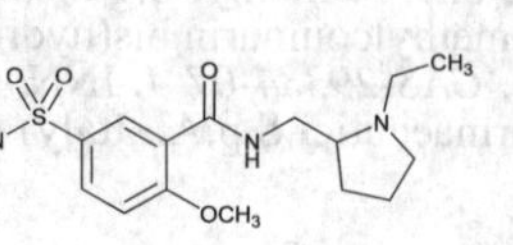

Sulprosal. $C_{10}H_{12}O_6S$. 260.26. Salicylic acid ester with 3-hydroxy-1-propanesulfonic acid. *UNII-85LCU5151G. CAS-58703-77-8.* INN.

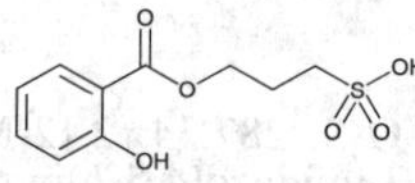

Sulprostone [*1977*] (sul prost′ one). $C_{23}H_{31}NO_7S$. 465.56. (1) 5-Heptenamide, 7-[3-hydroxy-2-(3-hydroxy-4-phenoxy-1-butenyl)-5-oxocyclopentyl]-*N*-(methylsulfonyl)-, [1*R*-[1α(*Z*),2β(1*E*,3*R**),3α]]-; (2) (*Z*)-7-[(1*R*,2*R*,3*R*)-3-Hydroxy-2-[(*E*)-(3*R*)-(3-hydroxy-4-phenoxy-1-butenyl)]-5-oxocyclopentyl]-*N*-(methylsulfonyl)-5-heptenamide. *CAS-60325-46-4.* INN. *Prostaglandin.* ◇*ZK 57 671; CP-34,089*

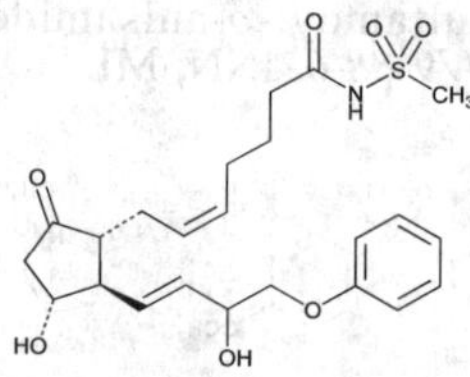

Sulpyrine (JAN) — *See* Dipyrone.

Sultamicillin [*1982*] (sul tam″ i sil′ in). $C_{25}H_{30}N_4O_9S_2$. 594.66. [Sultamicillin Tosilate is JAN.] (1) 4-Thia-1-azabicyclo[3.2.0]heptane-2-carboxylic acid, 6-[(aminophenylacetyl)amino]-3,3-dimethyl-7-oxo-, [[(3,3-dimethyl-7-oxo-4-thia-1-azabicyclo[3.2.0]hept-2-yl)carbonyl]oxy]methyl ester, *S*,*S*-dioxide, [2*S*-[2α(2*R**,5*S**),5α,6β(*S**)]]-; (2) Hydroxymethyl (2*S*,5*R*,6*R*)-6-[(*R*)-(2-amino-2-phenylacetamido)]-3,3-dimethyl-7-oxo-4-thia-1-azabicyclo[3.2.0]heptane-2-carboxylate, (2*S*,5*R*)-3,3-dimethyl-7-oxo-4-thia-1-azabicyclo[3.2.0]heptane-2-carboxylate (ester) *S*,*S*-dioxide. *CAS-76497-13-7.* INN; BAN. *Antibacterial.* ◇*CP-49,952*

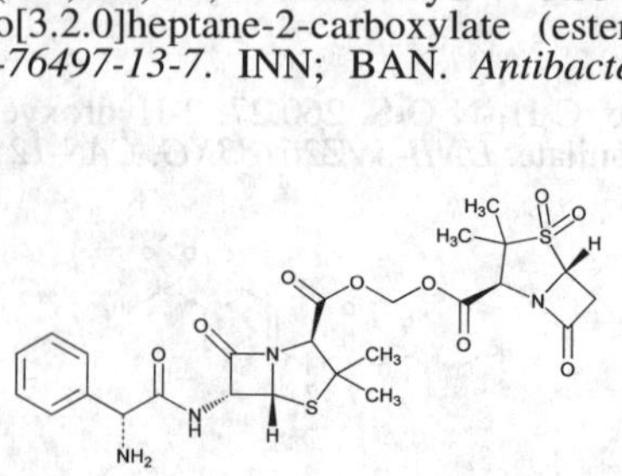

Sulthiame [*1962*] (sul thye′ ame). $C_{10}H_{14}N_2O_4S_2$. 290.36. [Sultiame is INN and JAN.] (1) Benzenesulfonamide, 4-(tetrahydro-2*H*-1,2-thiazin-2-yl)-, *S*,*S*-dioxide; (2) *p*-(Tetrahydro-2*H*-1,2-thiazin-2-yl)benzenesulfonamide, *S*,*S*-dioxide. *CAS-61-56-3*. BAN. *Anticonvulsant*. Conadil (3M Pharmaceuticals†); Trolone (3M Pharmaceuticals†) ◇*Riker 594*

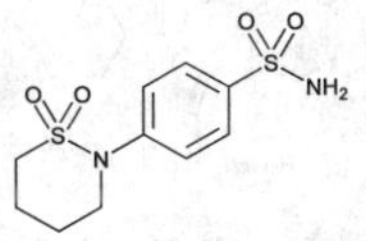

Sultiame (INN, JAN, DCF) — *See* Sulthiame.

Sultopride. $C_{17}H_{26}N_2O_4S$. 354.46. [Sultopride Hydrochloride is JAN.] *N*-[(1-Ethyl-2-pyrrolidinyl)methyl]-5-(ethylsulfonyl)-*o*-anisamide. *UNII-AA0G3TW31W*. *CAS-53583-79-2*. INN; DCF; MI.

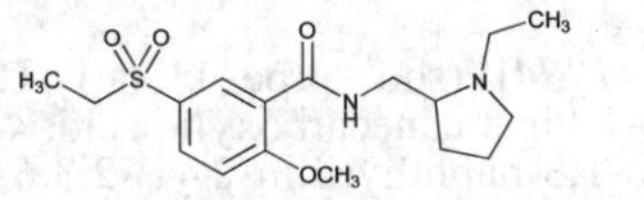

Sultosilic Acid. $C_{13}H_{12}O_7S_2$. 344.36. 2,5-Dihydroxybenzenesulfonic acid 5-*p*-toluenesulfonate. *UNII-62734PD6SM*. *CAS-57775-26-5*. INN; MI.

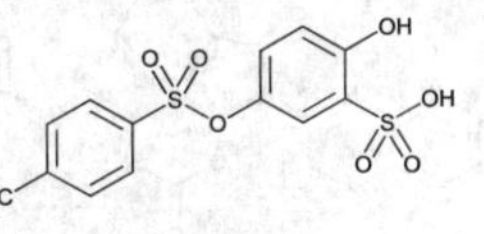

Sultroponium. $C_{20}H_{29}NO_6S$. 411.51. 8-(3-Sulfopropyl)atropinium hydroxide inner salt. *UNII-8WNY0897ER*. *CAS-15130-91-3*. INN; DCF; MI. ◇*A-118*

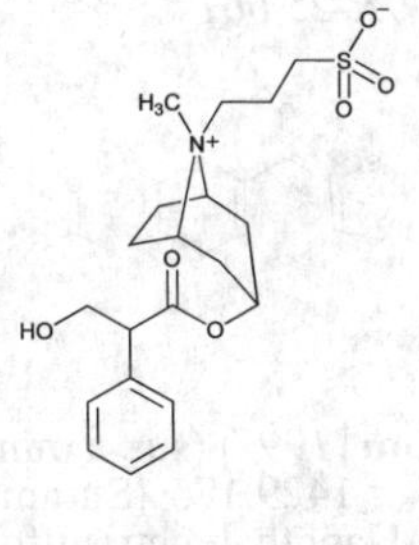

Sulukast [*1990*] (soo loo′ kast). $C_{25}H_{36}N_4O_3S$. 472.64. (1) Propanoic acid, 3-[[1-[hydroxy[3-(1*H*-tetrazol-5-yl)phenyl]methyl]-2,4-tetradecadienyl]thio]-, [*R*-[*R**,*S**-(*E*,*Z*)]]-; (2) 3-[[(1*R*,2*E*,4*Z*)-1-[(α*S*)-α-Hydroxy-*m*-1*H*-tetrazol-5-ylbenzyl]-2,4-tetradecadienyl]thio]propionic acid. *UNII-M652A5186T*. *CAS-98116-53-1*. INN. *Anti-asthmatic (leukotriene antagonist)*. ◇*LY170680*

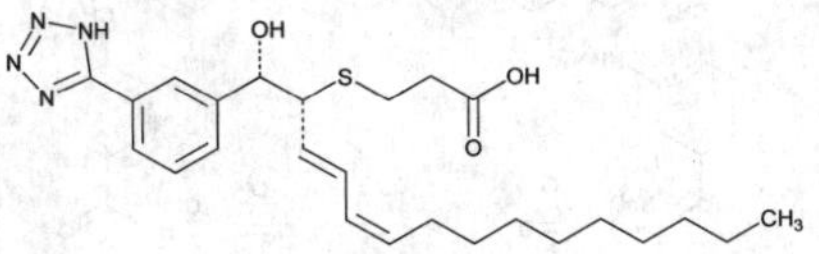

Sulverapride. $C_{16}H_{25}N_3O_5S$. 371.45. *N*-[(1-Methyl-2-pyrrolidinyl)methyl]-5-(methylsulfamoyl)-*o*-veratramide. *UNII-87C4V63NWI*. *CAS-73747-20-3*. INN.

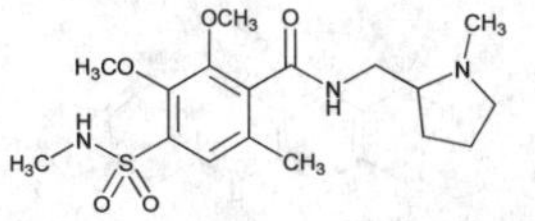

Sumacetamol. $C_{15}H_{20}N_2O_4S$. 324.40. *N*-Acetyl-DL-methionine, ester with 4′-hydroxyacetanilide. *UNII-A0BK6FM64M*. *CAS-69217-67-0*. INN; BAN. ◇*SUR 2647*

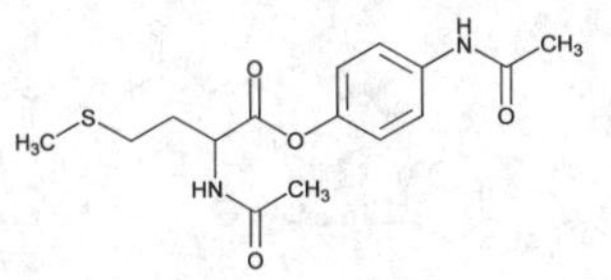

Sumanirole. $C_{11}H_{13}N_3O$. 203.24. (*R*)-5,6-Dihydro-5-(methylamino)-4*H*-imidazo[4,5,1-*ij*]quinolin-2(1*H*)-one. *UNII-3E93IV1U45*. *CAS-179386-43-7*. INN.

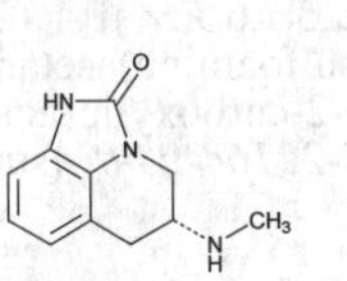

Sumarotene [*1990*] (soo mar′ oh teen). $C_{24}H_{30}O_2S$. 382.56. (1) Naphthalene, 1,2,3,4-tetrahydro-1,1,4,4-tetramethyl-6-[1-methyl-2-[4-(methylsulfonyl)phenyl]ethenyl]-, (*E*)-; (2) 1,2,3,4-Tetrahydro-1,1,4,4-tetramethyl-6-[(*E*)-α-methyl-*p*-(methylsulfonyl)styryl]naphthalene. *UNII-8896RX4S4J*. *CAS-105687-93-2*. INN. *Keratolytic*. ◇*Ro 14-9706/000*

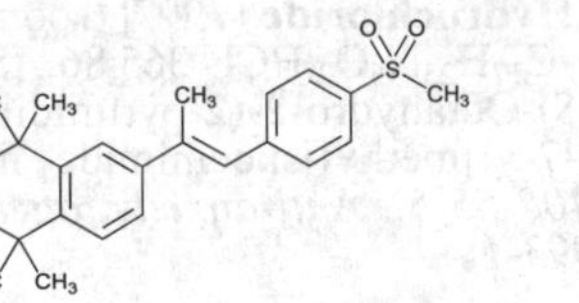

Sumatriptan (soo″ ma trip′ tan). **USP**. $C_{14}H_{21}N_3O_2S$. 295.40. (1) 1*H*-Indole-5-methanesulfonamide, 3-[2-(dimethylamino)ethyl]-*N*-methyl-; (2) 3-[2-(Dimethylamino)ethyl]-*N*-methy-1*H*-indole-5-methanesulfonamide. *UNII-8R78F6L9VO*. *CAS-103628-46-2*. INN; BAN. Imitrex (GlaxoSmithKline)

Sumatriptan Succinate [*1989*] (soo″ ma trip′ tan sux′ i nate). $C_{14}H_{21}N_3O_2S.C_4H_6O_4$. 413.49. (1) 1*H*-Indole-5-methanesulfonamide, 3-[2-(dimethylamino)ethyl]-*N*-methyl-, butanedioate (1:1); (2) 3-[2-(Dimethylamino)ethyl]-*N*-methylindole-5-methanesulfonamide succinate (1:1). *UNII-J8BDZ68989*. *CAS-103628-48-4; CAS-103628-46-2* [sumatriptan]. *Antimigraine*. Imitrex (GlaxoSmithKline) ◇*GR 43175C*

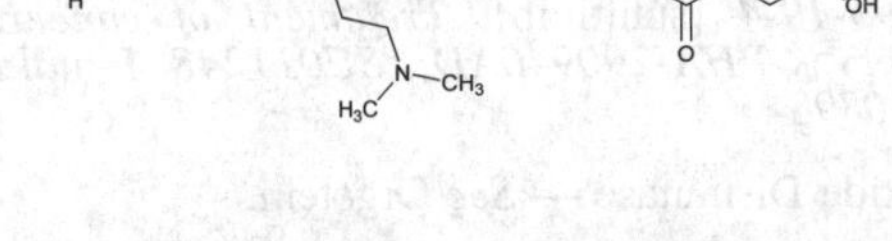

---

† Brand name formerly used, and/or firm no longer concerned with this product.

Sumetizide. $C_{12}H_{13}ClN_4O_6S_2$. 408.84. 6-Chloro-3,4-dihydro-3-succinimidomethyl-2*H*-1,2,4-benzothiadiazine-7-sulfonamide 1,1-dioxide. *UNII-LWP0997QUF. CAS-32059-27-1.* INN; DCF.

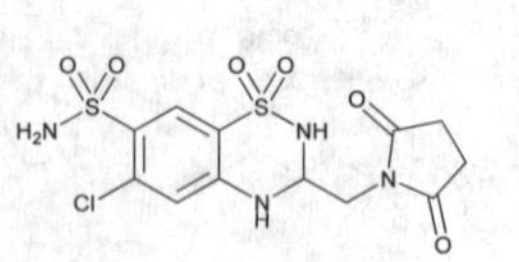

Sunagrel. $C_{25}H_{32}N_2O_2S$. 424.60. *erythro*-4-Cinnamoyl-α-[*p*-(isopropylthio)phenyl]-β-methyl-1-piperazineethanol. *CAS-85418-85-5.* INN.

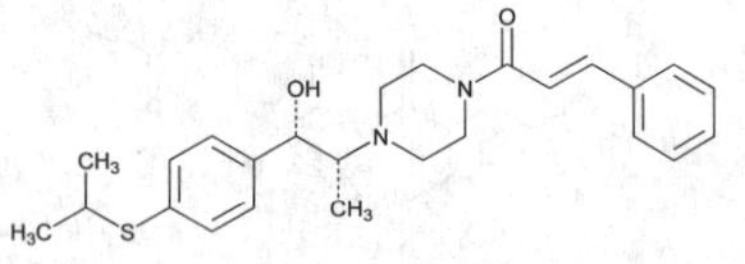

Suncillin Sodium [*1971*] (sun sil′ in soe′ dee um). $C_{16}H_{17}N_3Na_2O_7S_2$. 473.43. [Suncillin is INN.] (1) 4-Thia-1-azabicyclo[3.2.0]heptane-2-carboxylic acid, 3,3-dimethyl-7-oxo-6-[(phenylsulfaminoacetyl)amino]-, disodium salt, [2*S*-[2α,5α,6β(*S**)]]-; (2) 3,3-Dimethyl-7-oxo-6-[2-phenyl-D-2-(sulfoamino)acetamido]-4-thia-1-azabicyclo-[3.2.0]heptane-2-carboxylic acid disodium salt. *CAS-23444-86-2; CAS-22164-94-9* [suncillin]. *Antibacterial.* ◇*BL-P 1462*

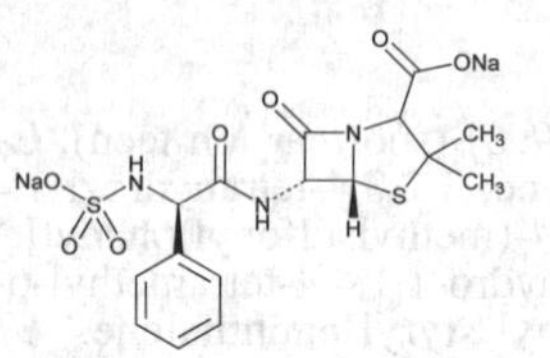

Sunepitron Hydrochloride [*1997*] (soo ne′ pi tron hye″ droe klor′ ide). $C_{17}H_{23}N_5O_2$.HCl. 365.86. [Sunepitron is INN.] *N*-[[(7*S*,9a*S*)-Octahydro-2-(2-pyrimidinyl)-2*H*-pyrido[1,2-*a*]pyrazin-7-yl]methyl]succinimide monohydrochloride. *CAS-148408-65-5.* *Anti-anxiety agent; antidepressant.* ◇*CP-93,393-1*

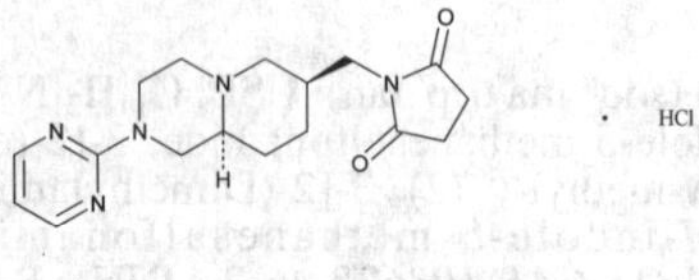

Sunflower Oil. NF. A refined fixed oil obtained from the seeds of the sunflower plant *Helianthus annuus* Linné (Fam, Asteraceae alt. Compositae). *UNII-3W1JG795YI.*

Sunitinib Malate [*2006*] (soo ni′ ti nib mal′ ate). $C_{22}H_{27}FN_4O_2$.$C_4H_6O_5$. 532.56. [Sunitinib is INN.] (1) Butanedioic acid, hydroxy-, (2*S*)-, compound with *N*-[2-(diethylamino)ethyl]-5-[(*Z*)-(5-fluoro-1,2-dihydro-2-oxo-3*H*-indol-3-ylidine)methyl]-2,4-dimethyl-1*H*-pyrrole-3-carboxamide (1:1); (2) *N*-[2-Diethylamino)ethyl]-5-[(*Z*)-(5-fluoro-2-oxo-1,2-dihydro-3*H*-indol-3-ylidene)methyl]-2,4-dimethyl-1*H*-pyrrole-3-carboxamide (2*S*)-2-hydroxybutanedioate. *UNII-LVX8N1UT73; UNII-V99T50803M* [sunitinib]. *CAS-341031-54-7; CAS-557795-19-4* [sunitinib]. *Treatment of cancer.* Sutent (Pfizer) ◇*PHA-290940AD; SU011248 L-malate salt; SU010398*

Superoxide Dismutase — *See* Orgotein.

Supidimide. $C_{12}H_{12}N_2O_4S$. 280.30. 2-(2-Oxo-3-piperidyl)-1,2-benzisothiazolin-3-one 1,1-dioxide. *UNII-L2GWR3US1G. CAS-49785-74-2.* INN.

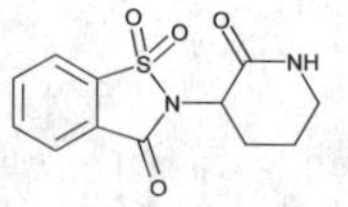

Suplatast Tosilate. $C_{23}H_{33}NO_7S_2$. 499.64. ($\pm$)-[2-[[*p*-(3-Ethoxy-2-hydroxypropoxy)phenyl]carbamoyl]ethyl]dimethylsulfonium *p*-toluenesulfonate. *CAS-94055-76-2.* INN.

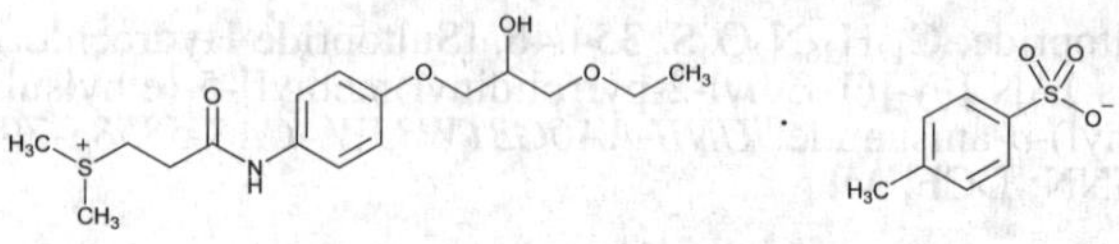

Suproclone [*1984*] (soo′ proe klone). $C_{22}H_{22}ClN_5O_4S_2$. 520.02. (1) 1-Piperazinecarboxylic acid, 4-(1-oxopropyl)-, 6-(7-chloro-1,8-naphthyridin-2-yl)-2,3,6,7-tetrahydro-7-oxo-5*H*-1,4-dithiino[2,3-*c*]pyrrol-5-yl ester, ($\pm$)-; (2) 4-Propionyl-1-piperazinecarboxylic acid, ester with ($\pm$)-6-(7-chloro-1,8-naphthyridin-2-yl)-2,3,6,7-tetrahydro-7-hydroxy-5*H*-*p*-dithiino[2,3-*c*]pyrrol-5-one. *CAS-77590-92-2.* INN. *Sedative-hypnotic.* ◇*37 162 R.P.*

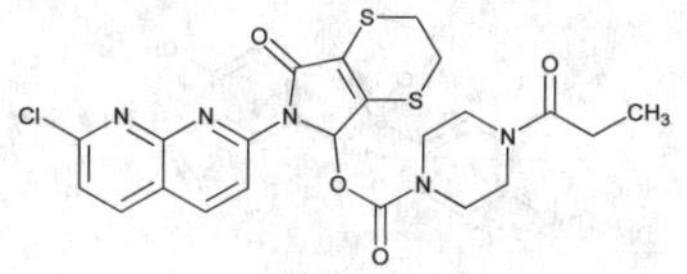

Suprofen [*1974*] (soo proe′ fen). **USP.** $C_{14}H_{12}O_3S$. 260.31. (1) Benzeneacetic acid, α-methyl-4-(2-thienylcarbonyl)-; (2) *p*-2-Thenoylhydratropic acid. *UNII-988GU2F9PE. CAS-40828-46-4.* INN; BAN; JAN. *Anti-inflammatory.* Profenal (Alcon) ◇*R-25,061*

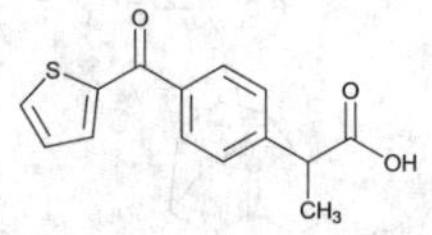

Suramin Hexasodium [*1997*] (sur′ a min hex″ a soe′ dee um). $C_{51}H_{34}N_6Na_6O_{23}S_6$. 1429.17. [Suramin Sodium is USP XVII.] (1) 1,3,5-Naphthalenetrisulfonic acid, 8,8′-[carbonylbis[imino-3,1-phenylenecarbonylimino(4-methyl-3,1-phenylene)carbonylimino]]bis-, hexasodium salt; (2) Hexasodium 8,8′-[ureylenebis[*m*-phenylenecarbonylimino(4-methyl-*m*-phenylene)carbonylimino]]di-1,3,5-naphthalenetrisulfonate. *CAS-129-46-4; CAS-145-63-1* [suramin]. *Antineoplastic.* ◇*CI-1003*

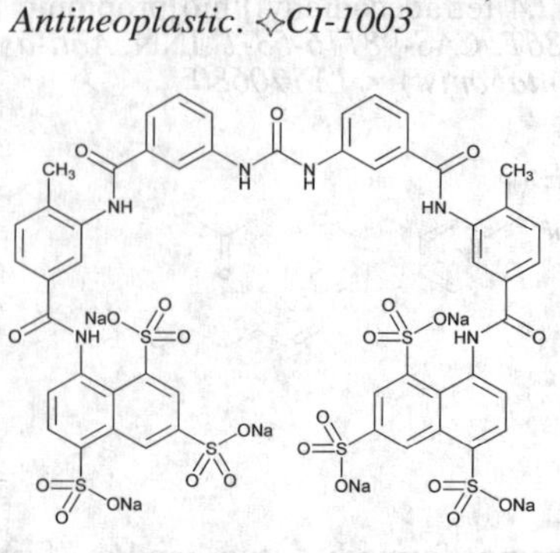

Surfactant TA — *See* Beractant.

Surfilcon A [*1985*] (sur fil′ kon). $(C_6H_9NO)_x(C_5H_8O_2)_y$ $(C_7H_{10}O_2)_z$. (1) 2-Pyrrolidinone, 1-ethenyl-, polymer with methyl 2-methyl-2-propenoate and 2-propenyl 2-methyl-2-propenoate; (2) 1-Vinyl-2-pyrrolidinone polymer with methyl methacrylate and allyl methacrylate. *CAS-38809-73-3*. *Contact lens material (hydrophilic)*. Permaflex Naturals (CooperVision)

Surfomer [*1980*] (surf′ o mer). $(C_{22}H_{40}O_4)_n$. (1) Poly(1,2-dicarboxy-3-hexadecyl-1,4-butanediyl); (2) Poly(1,2-dicarboxy-3-hexadecyltetramethylene). *CAS-71251-04-2*. INN. *Hypolipidemic*. ◇*AOMA*

Surgibone [*1963*] (sur′ ji bone). Sterile, specially processed mature bovine bone. *Prosthetic aid (internal bone splint)*. Unilab Surgibone (Unilab)

Suricainide Maleate [*1986*] (sur i′ ka nide mal′ ee ate). $C_{18}H_{31}N_3O_3S.C_4H_4O_4$. 485.59. [Suricainide is INN.] (1) Urea, *N*′-[2-(diethylamino)ethyl]-*N*-(1-methylethyl)-*N*-[2-(phenylsulfonyl)ethyl]-, (*Z*)-2-butenedioate (1:1); (2) 3-[2-(Diethylamino)ethyl]-1-isopropyl-1-[2-(phenylsulfonyl)ethyl]urea maleate (1:1). *CAS-85053-47-0; CAS-85053-46-9* [suricainide]. INN. *Cardiac depressant (anti-arrhythmic)*. ◇*AHR-10718*

Suriclone. $C_{20}H_{20}ClN_5O_3S_2$. 477.99. 4-Methyl-1-piperazinecarboxylic acid ester with (±)-6-(7-chloro-1,8-naphthyridin-2-yl)-2,3,6,7-tetrahydro-7-hydroxy-5*H*-*p*-dithiino[2,3-*c*]pyrrol-5-one. *CAS-53813-83-5*. INN; BAN; MI. ◇*RP 31264*

Surinabant. $C_{23}H_{23}BrCl_2N_4O$. 522.26. 5-(4-Bromophenyl)-1-(2,4-dichlorophenyl)-4-ethyl-*N*-(piperidin-1-yl)-1*H*-pyrazole-3-carboxamide. *CAS-288104-79-0*. INN.

Suritozole [*1993*] (sur it′ oh zole). $C_{10}H_{10}FN_3S$. 223.27. (1) 3*H*-1,2,4-Triazole-3-thione, 5-(3-fluorophenyl)-2,4-dihydro-2,4-dimethyl-; (2) 3-(*m*-Fluorophenyl-1,4-dimethyl-Δ^2-1,2,4-triazoline-5-thione. *CAS-110623-33-1*. INN. *Antidepressant*. ◇*MDL 26,479*

Suronacrine Maleate [*1989*] (sur one′ a kreen mal′ ee ate). $C_{20}H_{20}N_2O.C_4H_4O_4$. 420.46. [Suronacrine is INN.] (1) 1-Acridinol, 1,2,3,4-tetrahydro-9-[(phenylmethyl)amino]-, (±)-(*Z*)-2-butenedioate (1:1) (salt); (2) (±)-9-(Benzylamino)-1,2,3,4-tetrahydro-1-acridinol maleate (1:1) (salt). *CAS-113108-86-4; CAS-104675-35-6* [suronacrine]. *Inhibitor (cholinesterase)*. ◇*HP 128*

Susalimod. $C_{21}H_{16}N_2O_5S$. 408.43. 5-[[*p*-[(3-Methyl-2-pyridyl)sulfamoyl]phenyl]ethynyl]salicylic acid. *UNII-I5MPG6F043. CAS-149556-49-0*. INN.

Sutilains [*1967*] (soo′ ti lains). Proteolytic enzymes derived from *Bacillus subtilis*. (1) Sutilains; (2) Sutilains. *CAS-12211-28-8*. USP XXIII; INN; BAN. *Enzyme (proteolytic)*. Travase (Abbott) ◇*BAX 1515*

Sutoprofen — *See* Suprofen.

Suture, Absorbable Surgical (soo′ chur). **USP**. A sterile, flexible strand prepared from collagen derives from healthy mammals, or from synthetic polymer. It is capable of being absorbed by living mammalian tissue. *Surgical aid*.

Suture, Nonabsorbable Surgical (soo′ chur). **USP**. A flexible strand of material that is suitably resistant to the action of living mammalian tissue. *Surgical aid*. Ethibond (Ethicon); Ethiflex (Ethicon†); Ethilon (Ethicon); Mersilene (Ethicon); Nurolon (Ethicon); Prolene (Ethicon)

Suxamethone — *See* Succinylcholine Chloride.

---

† Brand name formerly used, and/or firm no longer concerned with this product.

Suxamethonium Bromide. $C_{14}H_{30}Br_2N_2O_4$. 450.21. 2,2′-Succinyldioxybis(ethyltrimethylammonium) dibromide. *UNII-1MBL83KX8J. CAS-55-94-7.* BAN.

Suxamethonium Chloride (INN, BAN, JAN, DCF) — *See* Succinylcholine Chloride.

Suxemerid Sulfate [*1971*] (sux em′ e rid sul′ fate). $C_{24}H_{44}N_2O_4 \cdot 2H_2SO_4$. 620.77. [Suxemerid is INN.] (1) Butanedioic acid, bis(1,2,2,6,6-pentamethyl-4-piperidinyl) ester, sulfate (1:2); (2) Bis(1,2,2,6,6-pentamethyl-4-piperidyl) succinate sulfate (1:2). *UNII-9JP0YSJ4IC. CAS-34144-82-6; CAS-47662-15-7* [suxemerid]. *Antitussive.* ✧*W 2180*

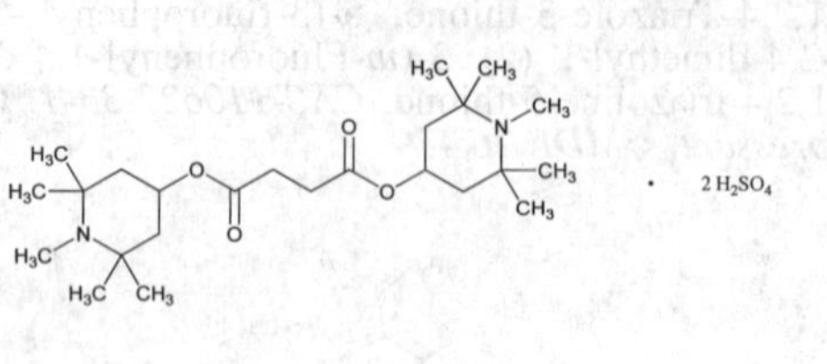

Suxethonium Chloride. $C_{16}H_{34}Cl_2N_2O_4$. 389.36. [Suxethonium Bromide is BAN.] Ethyl(2-hydroxyethyl)dimethyl-lammonium chloride succinate. *UNII-U5026H7S5S. CAS-54063-57-9.* INN.

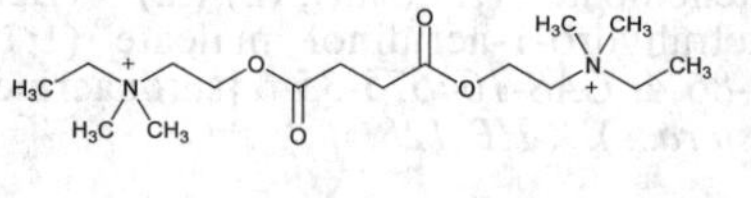

Suxibuzone. $C_{24}H_{26}N_2O_6$. 438.47. 4-Butyl-4-(hydroxymethyl)-1,2-diphenyl-3,5-pyrazolidinedione hydrogen succinate (ester). *UNII-86TDZ5WP2B. CAS-27470-51-5.* INN; BAN; JAN; MI.

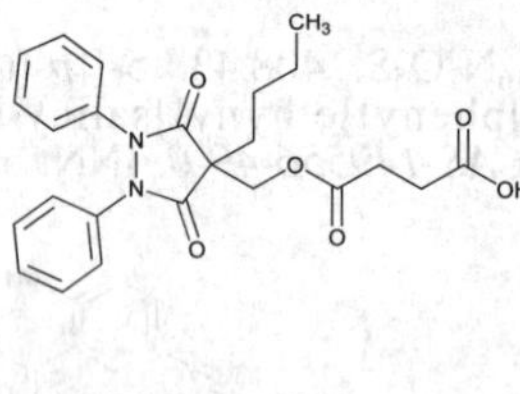

Sweet Birch Oil — *See* Methyl Salicylate.

Swertia Herb. JAN.

Symclosene [*1964*] (sim′ kloe seen). $C_3Cl_3N_3O_3$. 232.41. (1) 1,3,5-Triazine, 2,4,6(1*H*,3*H*,5*H*)-trione, 1,3,5-trichloro-; (2) 1,3,5-Trichloro-*s*-triazine-2,4,6(1*H*,3*H*,5*H*)-trione; (3) Trichloroisocyanuric acid. *UNII-RL3HK1I66B. CAS-87-90-1.* INN. *Anti-infective, topical.* ✧*NSC-405124*

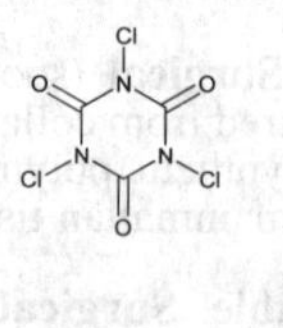

Symetine Hydrochloride [*1962*] (sim′ e teen hye″ droe klor′ ide). $C_{30}H_{48}N_2O_2 \cdot 2HCl$. 541.64. [Symetine is INN.] (1) Benzenemethanamine, 4,4′-[1,2-ethanediylbis(oxy)]bis[*N*-hexyl-*N*-methyl-, dihydrochloride; (2) 4,4′-(Ethylenedioxy)bis[*N*-hexyl-*N*-methylbenzylamine] dihydrochloride. *UNII-S175C652YS; UNII-UZ8WTY8051* [symetine]. *CAS-5585-62-6; CAS-15599-45-8* [symetine]. *Anti-amebic.* ✧*16726*

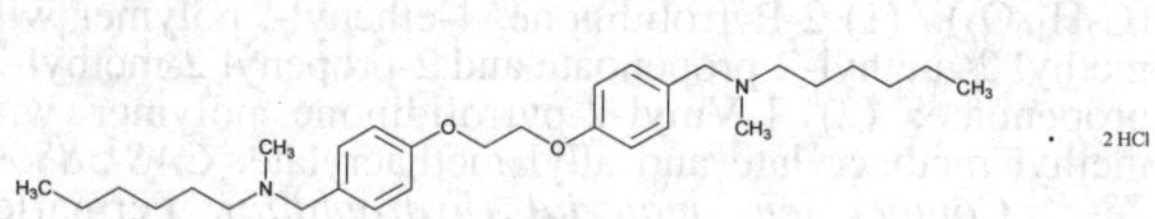

Synestrin — *See* Diethylstilbestrol.

Synnematin B — *See* Adicillin.

Synthestrin — *See* Diethylstilbestrol.

Synthetic Conjugated Estrogens, B [*2003*] (kon′ joo gay″ ted es′ troe jens). Synthetic conjugated estrogens, B, contains the sodium sulfate forms of estrone, equilin, 17α-estradiol, 17α-dihydroequilin, 17β-dihydroequilin, 17α-dihydroequilenin, 17β-dihydroequilenin, equilenin, 17β-estradiol, and $\Delta^{8,9}$-dehydroestrone. The total percent label claim for the sum of estrone and equilin, is 79.5% - 88.0%. The individual levels for each component are: estrone 52.5% - 61.5%, equilin 22.5% - 30.5%, 17α-estradiol 2.5% - 9.5%, 17α-dihydroequilin 13.5% - 19.5%, 17β-dihydroequilin 0.5% - 4.0%, 17α-dihydroequilenin 0.2% - 3.25%, 17β-dihydroequilenin 0.2% - 2.75%, equilenin 0.2% - 5.5%, 17β-estradiol 0.2% - 2.25%, and $\Delta^{8,9}$-dehydroestrone 0.2% - 6.25%. *Estrogen therapy.* ✧*CE-10*

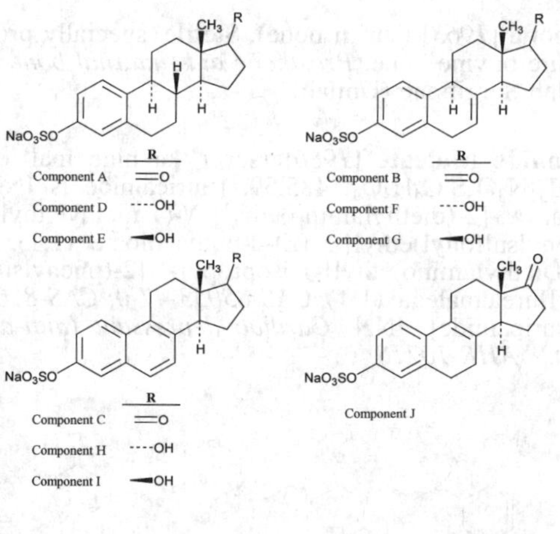

Synthetic Spermaceti (previously used name) — *See* Cetyl Esters Wax.

Synvinolin (previously used name) — *See* Simvastatin.

Syrosingopine. $C_{35}H_{42}N_2O_{11}$. 666.71. Methyl 18β-hydroxy-11,17α-dimethoxy-3β,20α-yohimban-16β-carboxylate 4-hydroxy. *CAS-84-36-6.* NF XIII; INN; BAN; JAN; MI.

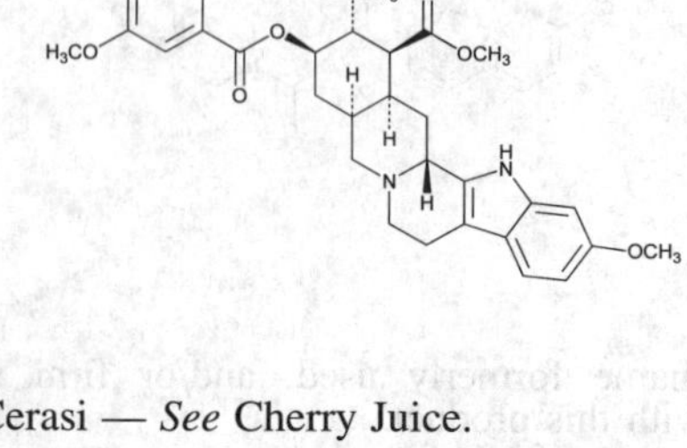

Syrupus Cerasi — *See* Cherry Juice.

Tabilautide. $C_{27}H_{49}N_5O_8$. 571.71. *threo*-6-Carbamoyl-N^2-[N-(N-lauroyl-L-alanyl)-D-γ-glutamyl]-L-lysine. *UNII-EZ61NB05TG. CAS-78088-46-7.* INN.

Tabimorelin. $C_{32}H_{40}N_4O_3$. 528.69. (R)-α-[(E)-5-Amino-N,5-dimethyl-2-hexenamido]-N-methyl-N-[(R)-α-(methylcarbamoyl)phenethyl]-2-naphthalenepropionamide. *UNII-L51CBE03KF. CAS-193079-69-5.* INN.

Tacalcitol. $C_{27}H_{44}O_3$. 416.64. (+)-(5Z,7E,24R)-9,10-Secocholesta-5,7,10(19)-triene-1α,3β,24-triol. *CAS-57333-96-7.* INN; BAN; JAN.

Tacapenem. $C_{14}H_{18}N_2O_5S$. 326.37. (+)-(4R,5S,6S)-6-[(1R)-1-Hydroxyethyl]-4-methyl-7-oxo-3-[[(3R)-5-oxopyrrolidin-3-yl]sulfanyl]-1-azabicyclo[3.2.0]hept-2-ene-2-carboxylic acid. *UNII-5216EI628Q. CAS-193811-33-5.* INN.

Tacedinaline [*2002*] (ta see dye′ na leen). $C_{15}H_{15}N_3O_2$. 269.30. (1) Benzamide, 4-(acetylamino)-N-(2-aminophenyl)-; (2) 4-(Acetylamino)-N-(2-aminophenyl)benzamide. *UNII-UMF554N5FG. CAS-112522-64-2.* INN. *Combination therapy for selected tumors including non-small cell lung, pancreatic, breast, and colorectal cancers.* ◇*CI-994; PD 123654; GOE 5549*

Taclamine Hydrochloride [*1972*] (tak′ la meen hye″ droe klor′ ide). $C_{21}H_{23}N$.HCl. 325.87. [Taclamine is INN.] (1) 1H-Benzo[6,7]cyclohepta[1,2,3-*de*]pyrido[2,1-*a*]isoquinoline, 2,3,4,4a,8,9,13b,14-octahydro-, hydrochloride; (2) 2,3,4,4a,8,9,13b,14-Octahydro-1H-benzo[6,7]cyclohepta[1,2,3-*de*]pyrido[2,1-*a*]isoquinoline hydrochloride. *CAS-34061-34-2; CAS-34061-33-1* [taclamine]. *Tranquilizer (minor).* ◇*AY-22,214*

Tacrine Hydrochloride [*1988*] (tak reen hye″ droe klor′ ide). **USP.** $C_{13}H_{14}N_2$.HCl.H_2O. 252.74. [Tacrine is INN and BAN.] (1) 9-Acridinamine, 1,2,3,4-tetrahydro-, monohydrochloride; (2) 9-Amino-1,2,3,4-tetrahydroacridine monohydrochloride. *UNII-4966RNG0BU; UNII-4VX7YNB537* [tacrine]. *CAS-1684-40-8; CAS-321-64-2* [tacrine]. *Cognition adjuvant; dementia symptoms treatment adjunct.* Cognex (Sciele) ◇*CI-970*

Tacrolimus [*1992*] (ta kroe′ li mus). $C_{44}H_{69}NO_{12}$.H_2O. 822.03. [Tacrolimus Hydrate is JAN.] (1) 15,19-Epoxy-3H-pyrido[2,1-*c*][1,4]oxaazacyclotricosine-1,7,20,21(4H,23H)-tetrone, 5,6,8,11,12,13,14,15,16,17,18,19,24,25,26,26a-hexadecahydro-5,19-dihydroxy-3-[2-(4-hydroxy-3-methoxycyclohexyl)-1-methylethenyl]-14,16-dimethoxy-4,10,12,18-tetramethyl-8-(2-propenyl)-, monohydrate, [3S-[3R*,[E(1S*,3S*,4S*)],4S*,5R*,8-S*,9E,12R*,14R*,15S*,16R*,18S*,19S*,26aR*]]-; (2) (-)-(3S,4R,5S,8R,9E,12S,14S,15R,16S,18R,19R,26aS)-8-allyl-5,6,8,11,12,13,14,15,16,17,18,19,24,25,26,26a-Hexadecahydro-5,19-dihydroxy-3-[(E)-2-[(1R,3R,4R)-4-hydroxy-3-methoxycyclohexyl]-1-methylvinyl]-14,16-dimethoxy-4,10,12,18-tetramethyl-15-epoxy-3H-pyrido[2,1-*c*][1,4]oxaazacyclotricosine-1,7,20,21(4H,23H)-tetrone)monohydrate. *UNII-WM0HAQ4WNM. CAS-109581-93-3; CAS-104987-11-3* [anhydrous]. INN; BAN. *Immunosuppressant.* Prograf (Astellas); Protopic (Astellas) ◇*FK 506; FR900506*

Tadalafil [*2001*] (ta dal′ a fil). $C_{22}H_{19}N_3O_4$. 389.40. (1) Pyrazino[1′,2′:1,6]pyrido[3,4-*b*]indole-1,4-dione, 6-(1,3-benzodioxol-5-yl)-2,3,6,7,12,12a-hexahydro-2-methyl-, (6R-12aR)-; (2) (6R,12aR)-2,3,6,7,12,12a-Hexahydro-2-methyl-6-[3,4-(methylenedioxy)phenyl] pyrazino[1′,2′:1,6]pyrido[3,4-*b*]indole-1,4-dione; (3) (6R-*trans*)-6-(1,3-Benzodioxol-5-yl)-2,3,6,7,12,12a-hexahydro-2-methyl-pyrazino[1′,2′:1,6]pyrido[3,4-*b*]indole-1,4-dione.

---

† Brand name formerly used, and/or firm no longer concerned with this product.

872 **TADEK–TALAC**   *USP Dictionary of USAN and International Drug Names*

UNII-742SXX0ICT. CAS-171596-29-5. INN; BAN. *Treatment of male erectile and female sexual dysfunction.* Cialis (Lilly) ◇*IC351*

Tadekinig Alfa. $C_{781}H_{1230}N_{216}O_{237}S_6$ (protein). Interleukin-18 binding protein (human gene IL18BP isoform a precursor). *CAS-220712-29-8.* INN.

Tadocizumab [*2005*] (tad″ oh siz′ oo mab). $C_{2107}H_{3252}N_{562}O_{673}S_{12}$. Immunoglobulin G1, anti-(human integrin αIIbβ3) Fab fragment (human-mouse monoclonal C4G1 γ1-chain), disulfide with human-mouse monoclonal C4G1 κ-chain. *CAS-339086-80-5.* INN. *Treatment of patients undergoing percutaneous coronary interventions.* ◇*YM337*

```
DIQMTQTPST LSASVGDRVT      QVQLVQSGAE VKKPGSSVKV
ISCRASQDIN NYLNWYQQKP      SCKASGYAFT NYLIEWVRQA
GKAPKLLIYY TSTLHSGVPS      PGQGLEWIGV IYPGSGGTNY
RFSGSGSGTD YTLTISSLQP      NEKFKGRVTL TVDESTNTAY
DDFATYFCQQ GNTLPWTFGQ      MELSSLRSED TAVYFCARRD
GTKVEVKRTV AAPSVFIFPP      GNYGWFAYWG QGTLVTVSSA
SDEQLKSGTA SVVCLLNNFY      STKGPSVFPL APSSKSTSGG
PREAKVQWKV DNALQSGNSQ      TAALGCLVKD YFPEPVTVSW
ESVTEQDSKD STYSLSSTLT      NSGALTSGVH TFPAVLQSSG
LSKADYEKHK VYACEVTHQG      LYSLSSVVTV PSSSLGTQTY
LSSPVTKSFN RGEC           ICNVNHKPSN TKVDKKVEPK
                          SCDKTH
```

Tafenoquine. $C_{24}H_{28}F_3N_3O_3$. 463.49. (*RS*)-N^4-(2,6-Dimethoxy-4-methyl-5-(3-trifluoro-methylphenoxy)quinolin-8-yl)pentane-1,4-diamine. *UNII-262P8GS9L9. CAS-106635-80-7.* BAN, INN. ◇*WR 238605*

Tafluposide. $C_{45}H_{35}F_{10}O_{20}P$. 1116.71. 4-[(5*R*,5a*R*,8a*R*,9*S*)-9-[[4,6-*O*-[(1*R*)-Ethylidene]-2,3-bis*O*-[(pentafluorophenoxy)acetyl]-β-D-glucopyranosyl]oxy]-6-oxo-5,5a,6,8,8a,9-hexahydrofuro[3′,4′:6,7]naphtho[2,3-*d*]-1,3-dioxol-5-yl]-2,6-dimethoxyphenyle dihydrogen phosphate. *CAS-179067-42-6.* INN.

Tafluprost. $C_{25}H_{34}F_2O_5$. 452.53. Isopropyl (5*Z*)-7-{(1*R*,2*R*,3*R*,5*S*)-2-[(1*E*)-3,3-difluoro-4-phenoxybut-1-enyl]-3,5-dihydroxycyclopentyl}hept-5-enoate. *CAS-209860-87-7.* INN.

Tagatose. NF. $C_6H_{12}O_6$. 180.16. (1) D-Tagatose; (2) D-*lyxo*-Hexulose. *CAS-87-81-0.*

Taglutimide. $C_{14}H_{16}N_2O_4$. 276.29. *cis-endo-N*-(2,6-Dioxo-3-piperidyl)-2,3-norbornanedicarboximide. *CAS-14166-26-8.* INN; MI.

Tagorizine. $C_{30}H_{36}N_4O$. 468.63. (*E*)-*N*-[4-[4-(Diphenyl-methyl)-1-piperazinyl]butyl]-6-methyl-3-pyridineac-rylamide. *UNII-668QM8QJFS. CAS-118420-47-6.* INN.

Talabostat [*2005*] (tal ab′ oh stat). $C_9H_{19}BN_2O_3$. 214.07. (1) Boronic acid, [(2*R*)-1-[(2*S*)-2-amino-3-methyl-1-oxobutyl]-2-pyrrolidinyl]-; (2) [(2*R*)-1-[(2*S*)-2-Amino-3-methyl-butanoyl]pyrrolidin-2-yl]boronic acid. *UNII-KZ1O2SH88Z. CAS-149682-77-9.* INN. *Treatment of cancer; hematopoietic stimulant.* ◇*PT-100*

Talabostat Mesylate [*2005*] (tal ab′ oh stat mes′ i late). $C_9H_{19}BN_2O_3 \cdot CH_4O_3S$. 310.18. (1) Boronic acid, [(2*R*)-1-[(2*S*)-2-amino-3-methyl-1-oxobutyl]-2-pyrrolidinyl]-monomethanesulfonate; (2) [(2*R*)-1-[(2*S*)-2-Amino-3-methylbutanoyl]pyrrolidin-2-yl]boronic acid methanesul-fonate. *UNII-V8ZG4Y1B51. CAS-150080-09-4. Treatment of cancer; hematopoetic stimulant.* ◇*PT-100*

Talactoferrin Alfa [*2004*] (ta lak″ toe fer′ in al′ fa). $C_{3345}H_{5215}N_{963}O_{1015}S_{37}$ (protein). (1) Lactoferrin (recombinant human LF00); (2) [11-L-Threonine,29-L-arginine]lactoferrin(human) produced by *Aspergillus niger* var. *awamori*. Molecular weight is approximately 80,000 daltons (glycosylated). *CAS-308240-58-6.* INN. *Recombi-*

nant human lactoferrin (rhLF), intended for use as an anti-infective (anti-microbial and antiviral); anti-inflammatory, and antineoplastic. ◇LF00

```
GRRRRSVQWC TVSQPEATKC FQWQRNMRRV RGPPVSCIKR DSPIQCIQAI
AENRADAVTL DGGFIYEAGL APYKLRPVAA EVYGTERQPR THYYAVAVVK
KGGSFQLNEL QGLKSCHTGL RRTAGWNVPI GTLRPFLNWT GPPEPIEAAV
ARFFSASCVP GADKGQFPNL CRLCAGTGEN KCAFSSQEPY FSYSGAFKCL
RDGAGDVAFI RESTVFEDLS DEAERDEYEL LCPDNTRKPV DKFKDCHLAR
VPSHAVVARS VNGKEDAIWN LLRQAQEKFG KDKSPKFQLF GSPSGQKDLL
FKDSAIGFSR VPPRIDSGLY LGSGYFTAIQ NLRKSEEEVA ARRARVVWCA
VGEQELRKCN QWSGLSEGSV TCSSASTTED CIALVLKGEA DAMSLDGGYV
YTAGKCGLVP VLAENYKSQQ SSDPDPNCVD RPVEGYLAVA VVRRSDTSLT
WNSVKGKKSC HTAVDRTAGW NIPMGLLFNQ TGSCKFDEYF SQSCAPGSDP
RSNLCALCIG DEQGENKCVP NSNERYYGYT GAFRCLAENA GDVAFVKDVT
VLQNTDGNNN EAWAKDLKLA DFALLCLDGK RKPVTEARSC HLAMAPNHAV
VSRMDKVERL KQVLLHQQAK FGRNGSDCPD KFCLFQSETK NLLFNDNTEC
LARLHGKTTY EKYLGPQYVA GITNLKKCST SPLLEACEFL RK
```

N* - glycosylation site

Talaglumetad Hydrochloride [*2004*] (ta″ la gloo′ me tad hye″ droe klor′ ide). $C_{11}H_{16}N_2O_5$·HCl. 292.72. [Talaglumetad is INN.] (1) Bicyclo[3.1.0]hexane-2,6-dicarboxylic acid, 2-[[(2*S*)-2-amino-1-oxopropyl]amino]-, monohydrochloride, (1*S*,2*S*,5*R*,6*S*)-; (2) (1*S*,2*S*,5*R*,6*S*)-2-[[(2*S*)-2-Aminopropanoyl]amino]bicyclo[3.1.0]hexane-2,6-dicarboxylic acid hydrochloride. *UNII-X30300EU7I. CAS-441765-97-5; CAS-441765-98-6* [talaglumetad]. *Treatment of anxiety and stress disorders (metabotropic glutamate (mGlu) agonist).* (Lilly) ◇LY544344 hydrochloride

Talampanel. $C_{19}H_{19}N_3O_3$. 337.37. (*R*)-7-Acetyl-5-(*p*-aminophenyl)-8,9-dihydro-8-methyl-7*H*-1,3-dioxolo[4,5-*h*][2,3]benzodiazepine. *CAS-161832-65-1.* INN.

Talampicillin Hydrochloride [*1974*] (tal am″ pi sil′ in hye″ droe klor′ ide). $C_{24}H_{23}N_3O_6S$·HCl. 517.98. [Talampicillin is INN and BAN.] (1) 4-Thia-1-azabicyclo[3.2.0]heptane-2-carboxylic acid, 6-[(aminophenylacetyl)amino]-3,3-dimethyl-7-oxo-, 1,3-dihydro-3-oxo-1-isobenzofuranyl ester, monohydrochloride, [2*S*-[2α,5α,6β(*S**)]]-; (2) (2*S*,5*R*,6*R*)-6-[(*R*)-2-Amino-2-phenylacetamido]-3,3-dimethyl-7-oxo-4-thia-1-azabicyclo[3.2.0]heptane-2-carboxylic acid ester

with 3-hydroxyphthalide, monohydrochloride. *CAS-39878-70-1; CAS-47747-56-8* [talampicillin]. JAN. *Antibacterial.* ◇*BRL 8988 Hydrochloride*

Talaporfin Sodium [*2002*] (tal a pore′ fin soe′ dee um). $C_{38}H_{41}N_5Na_4O_9$. 803.72. [Talaporfin is INN.] (1) L-Aspartic acid, *N*-[[(7*S*,8*S*,)-3-carboxy-7-(2-carboxyethyl)-13-ethenyl-18-ethyl-7,8-dihydro-2,8,12,17-tetramethyl-21*H*,23*H*-porphin-5-yl]acetyl]-, tetrasodium salt; (2) Tetrasodium (2*S*)-2-[[[(7*S*,8*S*)-3-carboxylato-7-(2-carboxylatoethyl)-13-ethenyl-18-ethyl-2,8,12,17-tetramethyl-7,8-dihydroporphyrin-5-yl]acetyl]amino]butanedioate. *CAS-220201-34-3; CAS-110230-98-3* [talaporfin]. *Photosensitizer for use in photodynamic therapy to destroy tumor tissue.* ◇LS-11

Talarozole [*2007*] (ta lar′ oh zole). $C_{21}H_{23}N_5S$. 377.51. (1) 2-Benzothiazolamine, *N*-[4-[2-ethyl-1-(1*H*-1,2,4-triazol-1-yl)butyl]phenyl]-; (2) *N*-[4-[(1*RS*)-2-Ethyl-1-(1*H*-1,2,4-triazol-1-yl)butyl]phenyl]benzothiazol-2-amine. *CAS-201410-53-9.* INN. *Treatment of keratinization disorders; acne and psoriasis.* Rambazole (Barrier) ◇*R115866*

Talastine. $C_{19}H_{21}N_3O$. 307.39. 2-[2-(Dimethylamino)ethyl]-4-benzyl-1(2*H*)phthalazinone. *UNII-49AB2PA48B. CAS-16188-61-7.* INN; MI.

---

† Brand name formerly used, and/or firm no longer concerned with this product.

Talbutal. $C_{11}H_{16}N_2O_3$. 224.26. (1) 2,4,6($1H,3H,5H$)-Pyrimidinetrione, 5-(1-methypropyl)-5-(2-propenyl)-; (2) 5-Allyl-5-*sec*-butylbarbituric acid. *UNII-4YIR8202AX. CAS-115-44-6.* USP XXII; INN. Lotusate (Sanofi Aventis)

Talc (talk). **USP.** A powdered, selected, natural, hydrated magnesium silicate. *UNII-7SEV7J4R1U. CAS-14807-96-6.* JAN. *Dusting powder; pharmaceutic aid (tablet and/or capsule lubricant).* Sclerosol (Bryan)

Taleranol [*1975*] (tal er′ a nol). $C_{18}H_{26}O_5$. 322.40. (1) $1H$-2-Benzoxacyclotetradecin-1-one, 3,4,5,6,7,8,9,10,11,12-decahydro-7,14,16-trihydroxy-3-methyl-, [$3S$-($3R^*,7R^*$)]; (2) ($3S,7S$)-3,4,5,6,7,8,9,10,11,12-Decahydro-7,14,16-trihydroxy-3-methyl-$1H$-2-benzoxacyclotetradecin-1-one; (3) ($6S,10S$)-6-(6,10-Dihydroxyundecyl)-β-resorcyclic acid μ-lactone. *UNII-HUN219N434. CAS-42422-68-4.* INN. *Enzyme inhibitor (gonadotropin).* ◇*P-1560*

Talibegron Hydrochloride [*2002*] (tal″ ee beg′ ron hye″ droe klor′ ide). $C_{18}H_{21}NO_4 \cdot HCl$. 351.82. [Talibegron is INN.] Benzeneacetic acid, 4-[2-[[($2R$)-2-hydroxy-2-phenylethyl]amino]ethoxy]-, hydrochloride. *UNII-N251Q608VU. CAS-178600-17-4; CAS-146376-58-1* [talibegron]. *Treatment of obesity in dogs and cats (β-3 adrenoreceptor agonist).* ◇*SCH 417849; ZD2079; ICID2079*

Talinolol. $C_{20}H_{33}N_3O_3$. 363.49. ($\pm$)-1-[p-[3-(*tert*-Butylamino)-2-hydroxypropoxy]phenyl]-3-cyclohexylurea. *UNII-3S82268BKG. CAS-57460-41-0.* INN; MI.

Talipexole. $C_{10}H_{15}N_3S$. 209.31. 6-Allyl-2-amino-5,6,7,8-tetrahydro-$4H$-thiazolo[4,5-d]azepine. *CAS-101626-70-4.* INN.

Talisomycin [*1978*] (tal″ i soe mye′ sin). $C_{68}H_{110}N_{22}O_{27}S_2$. 1731.86. Antibiotic produced by *Streptoalloteichus hindustanus* strain E 465-94. (1) Bleomycinamide, N^1-[4-amino-6-[[3-[(4-aminobutyl)amino]propyl]amino]-6-oxohexyl]-13-[(4-amino-4,6-dideoxy-α-L-talopyranosyl)oxy]-19-demethyl-12-hydroxy-; (2) N^1-[4-Amino-5-[[3-[(4-aminobutyl)amino]propyl]carbamoyl]pentyl]-13-[(4-amino-4,6-dideoxy-α-L-talopyranosyl)oxy]-19-demethyl-12-hy-droxybleomycinamide. *CAS-65057-90-1.* INN. *Antineoplastic.* [*Name previously used: Tallysomycin A.*] ◇*BU-2231A*

Talizumab [*2003*] (ta liz′ oo mab). $C_{6518}H_{10020}N_{1728}O_{2036}S_{42}$. Immunoglobulin G, anti-(human immunoglobulin E Fc region) (human-mouse monoclonal Hu901 γ-chain), disulfide with human-mouse monoclonal Hu901 κ-chain, dimer. Molecular weight is approximately 146,348 daltons. *CAS-380610-22-0.* INN; BAN. *Treatment to increase the threshold for peanut-induced anaphylaxis from unintended ingestion by those with peanut allergy.* ◇*TNX-901*

Tallimustine. $C_{32}H_{38}Cl_2N_{10}O_4$. 697.61. N''-(2-Amidinoethyl)-4-[p-[bis(2-chloroethyl)amino]benzamido]-1,1′,1″-trimethyl-$N,4'$:$N',4''$-ter[pyrrole-2-carboxamide]. *UNII-71193OXG6S. CAS-115308-98-0.* INN.

Tallysomycin A (previously used name) — *See* Talisomycin.

Talmapimod [*2007*] (tal map′ i mod). $C_{27}H_{30}ClFN_4O_3$. 513.00. (1) $1H$-Indole-3-acetamide, 6-chloro-5-[[($2R,5S$)-4-[(4-fluorophenyl)methyl]-2,5-dimethyl-1-piperazinyl]carbonyl]-N,N,1-trimethyl-α-oxo-; (2) 2-[6-Chloro-5-[[($2R,5S$)-4-(4-fluorobenzyl)-2,5-dimethylpiperazin-1-yl]carbonyl]-1-methyl-$1H$-indol-3-yl]-N,N-dimethyl-2-oxoacetamide. *UNII-B1E00KQ6NT. CAS-309913-83-5.* INN. *Immunomodulator.* ◇*SCIO 469*

Talmetacin [*1981*] (tal met′ a sin). $C_{27}H_{20}ClNO_6$. 489.90. (1) $1H$-Indole-3-acetic acid, 1-(4-chlorobenzoyl)-5-methoxy-2-methyl-, 1,3-dihydro-3-oxo-1-isobenzofuranyl ester, ($\pm$)-; (2) ($\pm$)-Phthalidyl 1-(p-chlorobenzoyl)-5-methoxy-2-methylindole-3-acetate. *UNII-6FY017I6S7. CAS-67489-39-8.* INN. *Analgesic; anti-inflammatory; antipyretic.* ◇*BA 7605-06*

Talmetoprim. C$_{22}$H$_{20}$N$_4$O$_5$. 420.42. *N*-[4-Amino-5-(3,4,5-trimethoxybenzyl)-2-pyrimidinyl]phthalimide. *UNII-X8W4CW0QHK. CAS-66093-35-4.* INN.

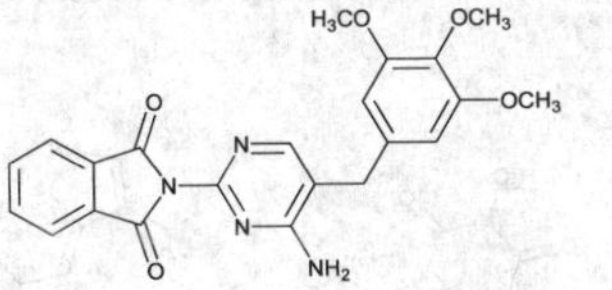

Talnetant. C$_{25}$H$_{22}$N$_2$O$_2$. 382.45. *N*-[(*S*)-α-Ethylbenzyl]-3-hydroxy-2-phenylcinchoninamide. *UNII-CZ3T9T146K. CAS-174636-32-9.* INN.

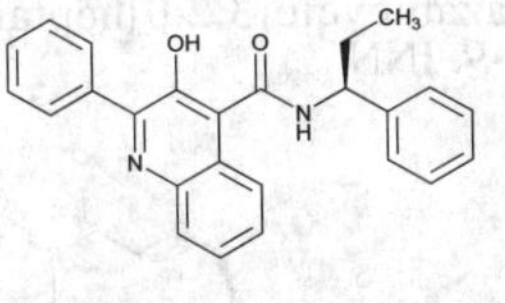

Talnetant Hydrochloride [*1998*] (tal′ ne tant hye″ droe klor′ ide). C$_{25}$H$_{22}$N$_2$O$_2$.HCl. 418.92. (1) (*S*)-3-Hydroxy-2-phenyl-*N*-(1-phenylpropyl)-4-quinolinecarboxamide monohydrochloride; (2) *N*-[(*S*)-α-Ethylbenzyl]-3-hydroxy-2-phenylcinchoninamide monohydrochloride. *CAS-204519-66-4. Treatment of symptoms associated with bladder dysfunction (SABD), including urinary urgency, frequency and/or urinary incontinence (NK-3 receptor antagonist).* ◇*SB-223412-A*

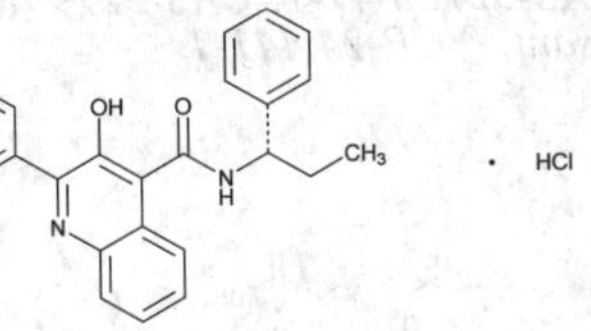

Talniflumate [*1979*] (tal nye′ floo mate). C$_{21}$H$_{13}$F$_3$N$_2$O$_4$. 414.33. (1) 3-Pyridinecarboxylic acid, 2-[[3-(trifluoromethyl)phenyl]amino]-, 1,3-dihydro-3-oxo-1-isobenzofuranyl ester; (2) Phthalidyl 2-(α,α,α,-trifluoro-*m*-toluidino)nicotinate. *UNII-JFK78S0U9S. CAS-66898-62-2.* INN. *Anti-inflammatory; analgesic.* Somalgen (Laboratorio Bago, S.A., Argentina) ◇*BA 7602-06*

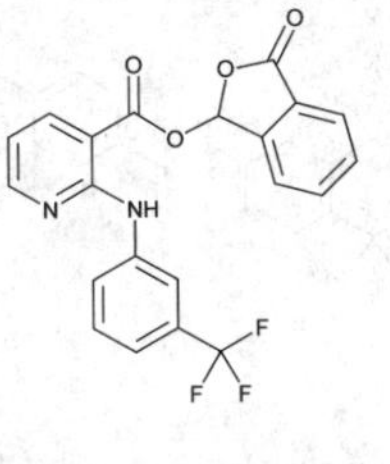

Talopram Hydrochloride [*1973*] (tal′ oh pram hye″ droe klor′ ide). C$_{20}$H$_{25}$NO.HCl. 331.88. [Talopram is INN.] (1) 1-Isobenzofuranpropanamine, 1,3-dihydro-*N*,3,3-trimethyl-1-phenyl-, hydrochloride; (2) *N*,3,3-Trimethyl-1-phenyl-1-phthalanpropylamine hydrochloride. *UNII-*

0X97008FCC. CAS-7013-41-4; CAS-7182-51-6 [talopram]. *Potentiator (catecholamine).* ◇*AY-21,554; LU3-010*

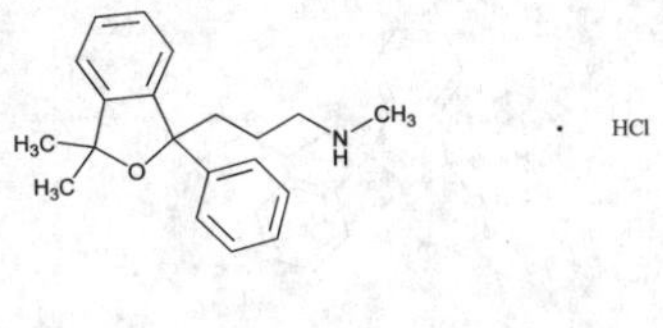

Talosalate [*1979*] (tal″ oh sal′ ate). C$_{17}$H$_{12}$O$_6$. 312.27. (1) Benzoic acid, 2-(acetyloxy)-, 1,3-dihydro-3-oxo-1-isobenzofuranyl ester; (2) Phthalidyl salicylate, acetate; (3) Salicylic acid acetate, ester with 3-hydroxyphthalide. *UNII-1356SD6O2G. CAS-66898-60-0.* INN. *Analgesic; anti-inflammatory.* ◇*BA 7604-02*

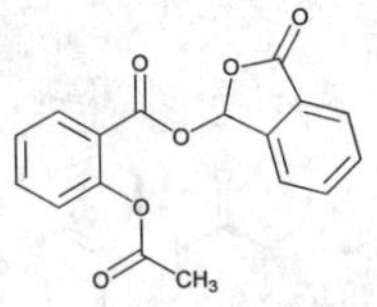

Talotrexin Ammonium [*2005*] (tal″ oh trex′ in a moe′ nee um). C$_{27}$H$_{27}$N$_9$O$_6$.H$_3$N. 590.59. [Talotrexin is INN.] (1) Benzoic acid, 2-[[[(4*S*)-4-carboxy-4-[[4-[[(2,4-diamino-6-pteridinyl)methyl]amino]benzoyl]amino]butyl]amino]carbonyl]-, monoammonium salt; (2) 2-[[(4*S*)-4-Carboxy-4-[[4-[[(2,4-diaminopteridin-6-yl)methyl]amino]benzoyl]amino]butyl]carbamoyl]benzoic acid monoammonium salt. *UNII-686WJT9102. CAS-648420-92-2; CAS-113857-87-7* [talotrexin]. *Antineoplastic.* ◇*PT-523; PT523; NSC-712783*

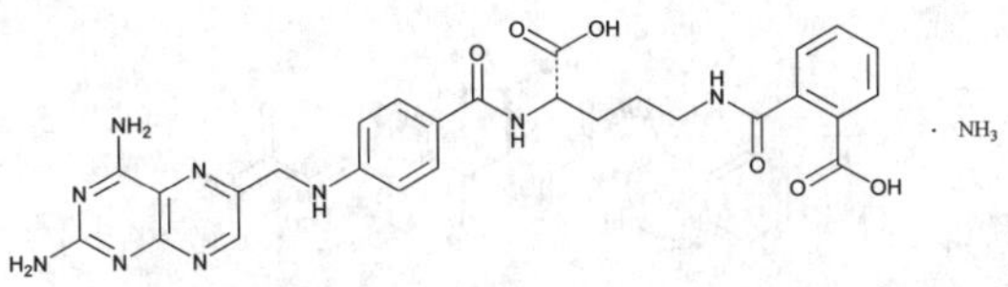

Taloximine. C$_{12}$H$_{16}$N$_4$O$_2$. 248.28. 4-[2-(Dimethylamino)ethoxy]-1(2*H*)phthalazinone oxime. *CAS-17243-68-4.* INN; BAN.

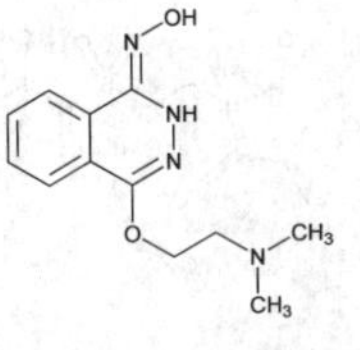

Talsaclidine Fumarate [*1995*] (tal sa′ kli deen fue′ ma rate). C$_{10}$H$_{15}$NO.C$_4$H$_4$O$_4$. 281.30. [Talsaclidine is INN.] (1) 3-(2-Propynyloxy)-1-azabicyclo[2.2.2]octane, (*R*)-, (*E*)-2-butenedioate (1:1); (2) (*R*)-3-(2-Propynyloxy)quinuclidine fumarate (1:1). *CAS-147025-54-5; CAS-147025-53-4* [talsaclidine]. *Alzheimer's disease treatment (muscarinic M$_1$-agonist).* ◇*WAL 2014 FU*

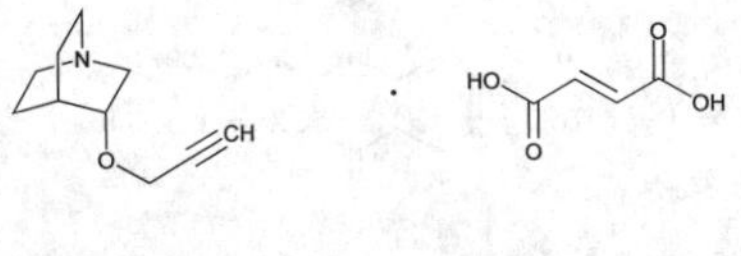

---

† Brand name formerly used, and/or firm no longer concerned with this product.

Talsupram. $C_{20}H_{25}NS$. 311.48. 1,3-Dihydro-*N*,3,3-trimethyl-1-phenylbenzo(*c*)thiophene-1-propylamine. *UNII-C6Z73MW6CR. CAS-21489-20-3.* INN.

Taltibride — *See* Metibride.

Taltirelin. $C_{17}H_{23}N_7O_5$. 405.41. (-)-*N*-[[(*S*)-Hexahydro-1-methyl-2,6-dioxo-4-pyrimidinyl]carbonyl]-L-histidyl-L-prolinamide. *UNII-DOZ62MV6A5. CAS-103300-74-9.* INN.

Taltobulin [*2004*] (tal″ toe bue′ lin). $C_{27}H_{43}N_3O_4$. 473.65. (1) L-Valinamide, *N*,β,β-trimethyl-L-phenylalanine-*N*-[(1*S*,2*E*)-3-carboxy-1-(1-methylethyl)-2-butenyl]-*N*,3-dimethyl-; (2) (4*S*)-4-[[(2*S*)-3,3-Dimethyl-2-[[(2*S*)-3-methyl-2-(methylamino)-3-phenylbutanoyl]amino]butanoyl]methylamino]-2,5-dimethylhex-2-enoic acid. *UNII-J6D6912BXS. CAS-228266-40-8.* INN. *Treatment of solid tumors.* ◇HTI-286

Taltrimide. $C_{13}H_{16}N_2O_4S$. 296.34. *N*-Isopropyl-1,3-dioxo-2-isoindolineethanesulfonamide. *UNII-NQ74U9QR5D. CAS-81428-04-8.* INN.

Taludipine Hydrochloride (previously used USAN) — *See* Teludipine Hydrochloride.

Talviraline. $C_{15}H_{20}N_2O_3S_2$. 340.46. Isopropyl (2*S*)-3,4-dihydro-7-methoxy-2-[(methylthio)methyl]-3-thioxo-1(2*H*)-quinoxalinecarboxylate. *CAS-169312-27-0.* INN.

Tameridone [*1989*] (ta mer′ i done). $C_{22}H_{26}N_6O_2$. 406.48. (1) 1*H*-Purine-2,6-dione, 3,7-dihydro-7-[2-[4-(1*H*-indol-3-yl)-1-piperidinyl]ethyl]-1,3-dimethyl-; (2) 7-[2-(4-Indol-3-yl-piperidino)ethyl]theophylline. *UNII-74ATQ0K1LA. CAS-102144-78-5.* INN; BAN. *Sedative (veterinary).* ◇R 51 163

Tameticillin. $C_{23}H_{33}N_3O_6S$. 479.59. 2-(Diethylamino)ethyl (2*S*,5*R*,6*R*)-6-(2,6-dimethoxybenzamido)-3,3-dimethyl-7-oxo-4-thia-1-azabicyclo[3.2.0]heptane-2-carboxylate. *CAS-56211-43-9.* INN.

Tametraline Hydrochloride [*1981*] (ta me′ tra leen hye″ droe klor′ ide). $C_{17}H_{19}N \cdot HCl$. 273.80. [Tametraline is INN.] (1) 1-Naphthalenamine, 1,2,3,4-tetrahydro-*N*-methyl-4-phenyl-, hydrochloride, (1*R-trans*)-; (2) (1*R*,4*S*)-1,2,3,4-Tetrahydro-*N*-methyl-4-phenyl-1-naphthylamine hydrochloride. *CAS-52760-47-1; CAS-52795-02-5* [tametraline]. *Antidepressant.* ◇CP-24,441-1

Tamibarotene. $C_{22}H_{25}NO_3$. 351.44. *N*-(5,6,7,8-Tetrahydro-5,5,8,8-tetramethyl-2-naphthyl)terephthalamic acid. *UNII-08V52GZ3H9. CAS-94497-51-5.* INN.

Tamitinol. $C_{11}H_{18}N_2OS$. 226.34. 4-[(Ethylamino)methyl]-2-methyl-5-[(methylthio)methyl]-3-pyridinol. *UNII-9H440NF95E. CAS-59429-50-4.* INN; BAN.

Tamolarizine. $C_{27}H_{32}N_2O_3$. 432.55. $(\pm)$-α-(3,4-Dimethoxyphenyl)-4-(diphenylmethyl)-1-piperazineethanol. *UNII-0PG3PMK9YA. CAS-128229-52-7*. INN.

Tamoxifen Citrate [*1976*] (ta mox′ i fen sit′ rate). **USP**. $C_{26}H_{29}NO.C_6H_8O_7$. 563.64. [Tamoxifen is INN and BAN.] (1) Ethanamine, 2-[4-(1,2-diphenyl-1-butenyl)phenoxy]-*N,N*-dimethyl, (*Z*)-, 2-hydroxy-1,2,3-propanetricarboxylate (1:1); (2) (*Z*)-2-[*p*-(1,2-Diphenyl-1-butenyl)phenoxy]-*N,N*-dimethylethylamine citrate (1:1). *UNII-7FRV7310N6; UNII-094ZI81Y45* [tamoxifen]. *CAS-54965-24-1; CAS-10540-29-1* [tamoxifen]. JAN. *Anti-estrogen.* Nolvadex (AstraZeneca); Soltamox (Rosemont) ◇*ICI 46,474*

Tampramine Fumarate [*1986*] (tamp′ ra meen fue′ ma rate). $C_{23}H_{24}N_4.C_4H_4O_4$. 472.54. [Tampramine is INN.] (1) 11*H*-Pyrido[2,3-*b*][1,4]benzodiazepine-11-propanamine, *N,N*-dimethyl-6-phenyl-, (*E*)-2-butenedioate (1:1); (2) 11-[3-(Dimethylamino)propyl]-6-phenyl-11*H*-pyrido[2,3-*b*][1,4]benzodiazepine fumarate (1:1). *CAS-83166-18-1; CAS-83166-17-0* [tampramine]. *Antidepressant.* ◇*AHR-9377*

Tamsulosin Hydrochloride [*1993*] (tam soo′ loe sin hye″ droe klor′ ide). $C_{20}H_{28}N_2O_5S.HCl$. 444.97. [Tamsulosin is INN and BAN.] (1) Benzenesulfonamide, 5-[2-[[2-(2-ethoxyphenoxy)ethyl]amino]propyl]-2-methoxy-, monohydrochloride, (*R*)-; (2) (-)-(*R*)-5-[2-[[2-(*o*-Ethoxyphenoxy)ethyl]amino]propyl]-2-methoxybenzenesulfonamide monohydrochloride. *UNII-11SV1951MR; UNII-G3P28OML5I* [tamsulosin]. *CAS-106463-17-6; CAS-106133-20-4* [tamsulosin]. JAN. *Benign prostatic hyperplasia therapy agent.* Flomax (Boehringer Ingelheim) ◇*LY253351; R-(-)-YM-12617; YM-12617-1; YM617*

Tanaproget [*2004*] (tan ap′ roe jet). $C_{16}H_{15}N_3OS$. 297.37. (1) 1*H*-Pyrrole-2-carbonitrile, 5-(1,4-dihydro-4,4-dimethyl-2-thioxo-2*H*-3,1-benzoxazin-6-yl)-1-methyl-; (2) 5-(4,4-Dimethyl-2-thioxo-1,4-dihydro-2*H*-3,1-benzoxazin-6-yl)-1-methyl-1*H*-pyrrole-2-carbonitrile. *UNII-W9F9H8GXWR. CAS-304853-42-7*. INN. *Oral contraception; nonsteroidal ligand for the progesterone receptor.* ◇*NSP-989*

Tandamine Hydrochloride [*1974*] (tan′ da meen hye″ droe klor′ ide). $C_{18}H_{26}N_2S.HCl$. 338.94. [Tandamine is INN.] (1) Thiopyrano[3,4-*b*]indole-1-ethanamine, 9-ethyl-1,3,4,9-tetrahydro-*N,N*,1-trimethyl-, monohydrochloride; (2) 1-[2-(Dimethylamino)ethyl]-9-ethyl-1,3,4,9-tetrahydro-1-methylthiopyrano[3,4-*b*]indole monohydrochloride. *CAS-58167-78-5; CAS-42408-80-0* [tandamine]. *Antidepressant.* ◇*AY-23,946*

Tandospirone Citrate [*1990*] (tan″ doe spye′ rone sit′ rate). $C_{21}H_{29}N_5O_2.C_6H_8O_7$. 575.61. [Tandospirone is INN and BAN.] (1) 4,7-Methano-1*H*-isoindole-1,3(2*H*)-dione, hexahydro-2-[4-[4-(2-pyrimidinyl)-1-piperazinyl]butyl]-, $(3a\alpha,4\beta,7\beta,7a\alpha)$-, 2-hydroxy-1,2,3-propanetricarboxylate (1:1); (2) (1*R**,2*S**,3*R**,4*S**)-*N*-[4-[4-(2-Pyrimidinyl)-1-piperazinyl]butyl]-2,3-norbornanedicarboximide citrate (1:1). *UNII-0R8E9BWM4J. CAS-112457-95-1; CAS-87760-53-0* [tandospirone]. *Anti-anxiety agent.* ◇*SM-3997*

Tandutinib [*2004*] (tan doo′ ti nib). $C_{31}H_{42}N_6O_4$. 562.70. (1) 1-Piperazinecarboxamide, 4-[6-methoxy-7-[3-(1-piperidinyl)propoxy]-4-quinazolinyl]-*N*-[4-(1-methylethoxy)phenyl]-; (2) 4-[6-Methoxy-7-[3-(piperidin-1-yl)propoxy]quinazolin-4-yl]-*N*-[4-(1-methylethoxy)phenyl]piperazine-1-carboxamide. *UNII-E11O3ICJ9A. CAS-387867-13-2*. INN. *Treatment of cardiovascular diseases, fibrotic diseases and acute myelogenous leukemia (tyrosine kinase inhibitor).* ◇*CT 53518*

Taneptacogin Alfa. $O^{344},N^{T.193}$- Cyclic hemiacetal obtained by the action of L-phenylalanyl L-phenylalanyl-L-arginine chloromethane on the blood coagulation factor VII (eptacog alfa) activated. *CAS-465540-87-8*. INN.

Tanespimycin [*2006*] (tan es″ pi mye′ sin). $C_{31}H_{43}N_3O_8$. 585.69. (1) Geldanamycin, 17-demethoxy-17-(2-propenylamino)-; (2) (4*E*,6*Z*,8*S*,9*S*,10*E*,12*S*,13*R*,14*S*,16*R*)-13-Hy-

---

† Brand name formerly used, and/or firm no longer concerned with this product.

droxy-8,14-dimethoxy-4,10,12,16-tetramethyl-3,20,22-trioxo-19-(prop-2-enylamino)-2-azabicyclo[16.3.1]docosa-1(21),4,6,10,18-pentaen-9-yl carbamate. *UNII-4GY0AVT3L4. CAS-75747-14-7.* INN. *Treatment of solid and hematological tumors.* ◇*KOS-953; 17-AAG*

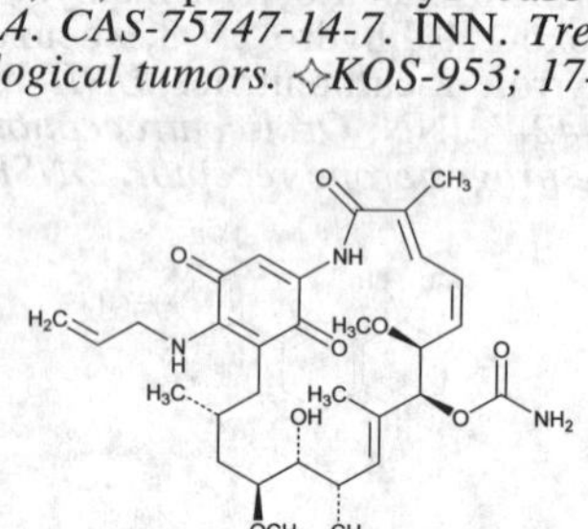

Tanezumab [*2007*] (tan ez' oo mab). $C_{6464}H_{9942}N_{1706}O_{2026}S_{46}$. (1) Immunoglobulin G2, anti-(human nerve growth factor) (human-mouse monoclonal RN624 heavy chain), disulfide with human-mouse monoclonal RN624 light chain, dimer; (2) Immunoglobulin G2, anti-(human nerve growth factor) h u m a n i z e d   m o u s e   m o n o c l o n a l   R N 6 2 4 [Lys^{71},Ser^{330},Ser^{331}]γ2 heavy chain (135-214')-disulfide with κ light chain (223-223":224-224":227-227":230-230")-tetrakisdisulfide dimer. Molecular weight is approximately 145,400 daltons. *CAS-880266-57-9.* INN. *Treatment of pain.* ◇*RN624; PF-4383119*

Taniplon. $C_{14}H_{15}N_5O_2$. 285.30. 6,7,8,9-Tetrahydro-5-methoxy-2-(5-methyl-1,2,4-oxadiazol-3-yl)imidazo-[1,2-*a*]-quinazoline. *UNII-OKS0I0BBLP. CAS-106073-01-2.* INN.

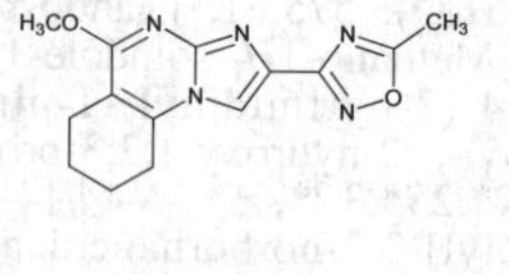

Tannic Acid (tan' ik as' id). **USP.** (1) Tannin. (2) Tannic acid; Tannin. *UNII-28F9E0DJY6. CAS-1401-55-4.* JAN. *Astringent.*

Tannyl Acetate — *See* Acetyltannic Acid.

Tanogitran. $C_{25}H_{31}N_7O_3$. 477.56. *N*-[(2*R*)-2-{2-[(4-Carbamimidoylanilino)methyl]-1-methyl-1*H*-benzimidazol-5-yl}-1-oxo-1-(pyrrolidin-1-yl)propan-2-yl]glycine. *CAS-637328-69-9.* INN.

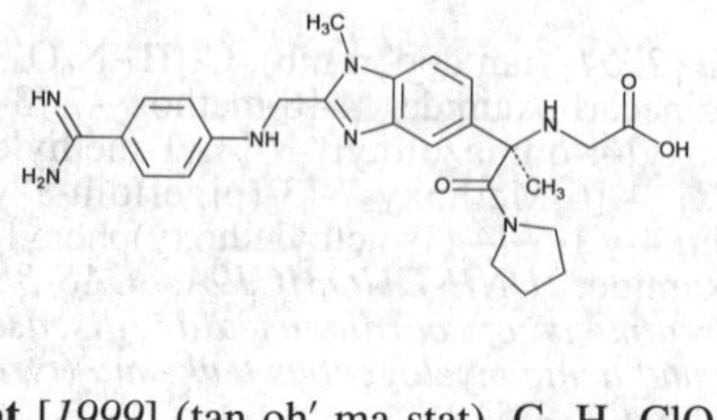

Tanomastat [*1999*] (tan oh' ma stat). $C_{23}H_{19}ClO_3S$. 410.91. (1) (*S*)-4'-Chloro-γ-oxo-α-[(phenylthio)methyl][1,1'-biphenyl]-4-butanoic acid; (2) (*S*)-3-[(4'-Chloro-4-biphenylyl)carbonyl]-2-[(phenylthio)methyl]propionic acid. *CAS-179545-77-8.* INN. *Treatment of osteoarthritis and in oncology (matrix metalloproteinase inhibitor).* ◇*BAY 12-9566*

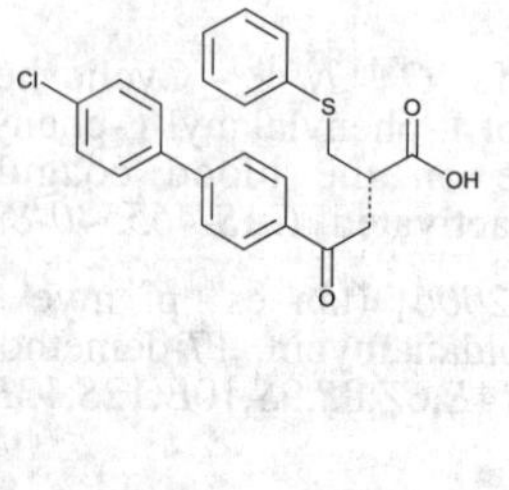

Tape, Adhesive (tape). **USP.** Consists of fabric and/or film evenly coated on one side with a pressure-sensitive, adhesive mixture. *Surgical aid.*

Tapentadol [*2005*] (ta pen' ta dol). $C_{14}H_{23}NO$. 221.34. (1) Phenol, 3-[(1*R*,2*R*)-3-(dimethylamino)-1-ethyl-2-methylpropyl]-; (2) 3-[(1*R*,2*R*)-3-(Dimethylamino)-1-ethyl-2-methylpropyl]phenol. *UNII-H8A007M585. CAS-175591-23-8.* INN. *Analgesic (μ-agonist).* ◇*CG5503 (base); BN 200 (base)*

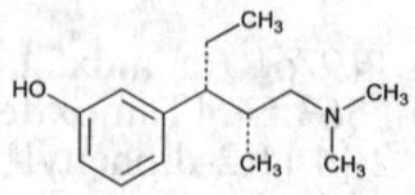

Taplitumomab Paptox. Immunoglobulin G1, anti-(human antigen CD19) (mouse monoclonal B43 γ1-chain), disulfide with mouse monoclonal B43 κ-chain, dimer, disulfide with protein PAP (pokeweed antiviral). *CAS-235428-87-2.* INN.

Taprizosin. $C_{25}H_{26}N_6O_4S$. 506.58. *N*-{2-[4-Amino-6,7-dimethoxy-5-(2-pyridyl)quinazolin-2-yl]-1,2,3,4-tetrahydro-5-isoquinolyl}methanesulfonamide. *UNII-EQ8YV2D86Y. CAS-210538-44-6.* INN; BAN. ◇*UK-338,003*

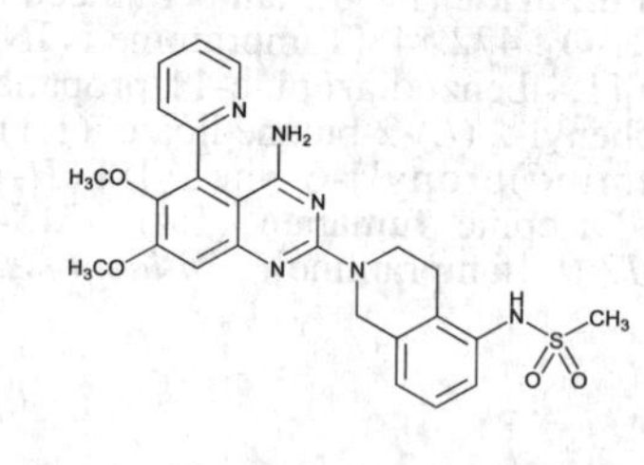

Taprostene. $C_{24}H_{30}O_5$. 398.49. α-[(2*Z*,3a*R*,4*R*,5*R*,6a*S*)-4-[(1*E*,3*S*)-3-cyclohexyl-3-hydroxypropenyl]hexahydro-5-hydroxy-2*H*-cyclopenta[*b*]furan-2-ylidene]-*m*-toluic acid. *UNII-7MS1HEY2IZ. CAS-108945-35-3.* INN.

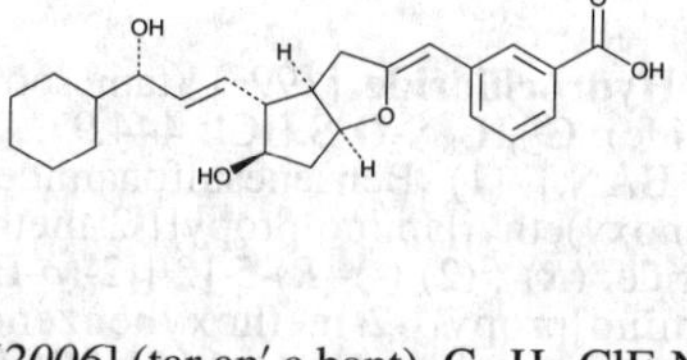

Taranabant [*2006*] (tar an' a bant). $C_{27}H_{25}ClF_3N_3O_2$. 515.95. (1) Propanamide, *N*-[(1*S*,2*S*)-3-(4-chlorophenyl)-2-(3-cyanophenyl)-1-methylpropyl]-2-methyl-2-[[5-(trifluoromethyl)-2-pyridinyl]oxy]-; (2) *N*-[(1*S*,2*S*)-3-(4-Chlorophenyl)-2-(3-cyanophenyl)-1-methylpropyl]-2-methyl-2-[[5-(trifluoromethyl)pyridin-2-yl]oxy]propanamide. *UNII-X9U622S114. CAS-701977-09-5.* INN. *Treatment of obesity.*

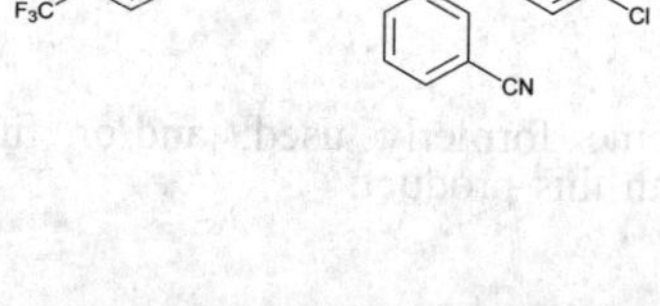

Tarazepide. $C_{28}H_{24}N_4O_2$. 448.52. (-)-*N*-[(*S*)-2,3-Dihydro-1-methyl-2-oxo-5-phenyl-1*H*-1,4-benzodiazepin-3-yl]-5,6-dihydro-4*H*-pyrrolo[3,2,1-*ij*]quinoline-2-carboxamide. *UNII-RK2972YZ2U. CAS-141374-81-4.* INN.

Tarenflurbil [*2006*] (tar″ en flur′ bil). $C_{15}H_{13}FO_2$. 244.26. (1) [1,1′-Biphenyl]-4-acetic acid, 2-fluoro-α-methyl-, (α*R*)-; (2) (-)-(2*R*)-2-(2-Fluorobiphenyl-4-yl)propanoic acid. *UNII-501W0OOOWA. CAS-51543-40-9.* INN. *Treatment of Alzheimer's disease.* Flurizan (Myriad) ◇*MPC-7869; E-7869*

Targinine (previously used name) — *See* Tilarginine Acetate.

Taribavirin Hydrochloride [*2005*] (ta″ rye ba vir′ in hye″ droe klor′ ide). $C_8H_{13}N_5O_4$·HCl. 279.68. [Taribavirin is INN.] (1) 1*H*-1,2,4-Triazole-3-carboximidamide, 1-β-D-ribofuranosyl-, monohydrochloride; (2) 1-β-D-Ribofuranosyl-1*H*-1,2,4-triazole-3-carboximidamide monohydrochloride. *UNII-R3B1994K2E* [taribavirin]. *CAS-40372-00-7; CAS-119567-79-2* [taribavirin]. *Antiviral.* Viramidine (Valeant)

Tariquidar [*2002*] (tar i′ kwi dar). $C_{38}H_{38}N_4O_6$. 646.73. (1) 3-Quinolinecarboxamide,*N*-[2-[[[4-[2-(3,4-dihydro-6,7-dimethoxy-2(1*H*)-isoquinolinyl)ethyl]phenyl]amino]carbonyl]-4,5-dimethoxyphenyl]-; (2) *N*-[2-[[4-[2-(6,7-Dimethoxy-3,4-dihydroisoquinolin-2(1*H*)-yl)ethyl]phenyl]carbamoyl]-4,5-dimethoxyphenyl]quinoline-3-carboxamide. *UNII-J58862DTVD. CAS-206873-63-4.* INN; BAN. *Adjunct to cytotoxic chemotherapies in oncology, P-glycoprotein pump inhibitor.* ◇*XR9576*

Tartar Emetic — *See* Antimony Potassium Tartrate.

Tartaric Acid (tar tar′ ik as′ id). **NF.** $C_4H_6O_6$. 150.09. (1) Butanedioic acid, 2,3-dihydroxy-; Butanedioic acid, 2,3-dihydroxy-, [*R*-(*R**,*R**)]-; (2) Tartaric acid; L-(+)-Tartaric acid. *UNII-W48881119H. CAS-87-69-4; CAS-526-83-0.* JAN. *Pharmaceutic aid (buffering agent).*

Tasidotin Hydrochloride [*2005*] (tas″ i doe′ tin hye″ droe klor′ ide). $C_{32}H_{58}N_6O_5$·HCl. 643.30. [Tasidotin is INN.] (1) L-Prolinamide, *N*,*N*-dimethyl-L-valyl-L-valyl-*N*-methyl-L-valyl-L-prolyl-*N*-(1,1-dimethylethyl)-, monohydrochloride; (2) *N*,*N*-Dimethyl-L-valyl-L-valyl-*N*-methyl-L-valyl-L-prolyl-*N*-(1,1-dimethylethyl)-L-prolinamide monohydrochloride. *UNII-05G07285DK* [tasidotin]. *CAS-623174-*

20-9; CAS-192658-64-3 [tasidotin]. *Treatment of patients with advanced, refractory neoplasms (microtubule stabilizing agent).* ◇*ILX651*

Tasimelteon [*2007*] (tas″ i mel′ tee on). $C_{15}H_{19}NO_2$. 245.32. (1) Propanamide, *N*-[[(1*R*,2*R*)-2-(2,3-dihydro-4-benzofuranyl)cyclopropyl]methyl]-; (2) *N*-[[(1*R*,2*R*)-2-(2,3-Dihydro-1-benzofuran-4-yl)cyclopropyl]methyl]propanamide. *CAS-609799-22-6.* INN. *Sleep disorders.* ◇*VEC-162; BMS-214778*

Tasisulam Sodium [*2007*] (tas″ i soo′ lam). $C_{11}H_5BrCl_2NO_3S_2Na$. 437.09. [Tasisulam is INN.] (1) Benzamide, *N*-[(5-bromo-2-thienyl)sulfonyl]-2,4-dichloro-, sodium salt; (2) Sodium *N*-[(5-bromothiophen-2-yl)sulfonyl]-2,4-dichlorobenzamide. *CAS-519055-63-1; CAS-519055-62-0* [tasisulam]. *Antineoplastic.* ◇*LY-573636.Na*

Tasonermin. $C_{778}H_{1225}N_{215}O_{231}S_2$. 17,350.49. 1-157-Tumor necrosis factor alfa-1a (human). *CAS-94948-59-1.* INN; BAN.

```
VRSSSRTPSD KPVAHVVANP QAEGQLQWLN RRANALLANG VELRDNQLVV
PSEGLYLIYS QVLFKGQGCP STHVLLTHTI SRIAVSYQTK VNLLSAIKSP
CQRETPEGAE AKPWYEPIYL GGVFQLEKGD RLSAEINRPD YLDFAESGQV
YFGIIAL
```

Tasosartan [*1995*] (tas″ oh sar′ tan). $C_{23}H_{21}N_7O$. 411.46. (1) Pyrido[2,3-*d*]pyrimidin-7(6*H*)-one, 5,8-dihydro-2,4-dimethyl-8-[[2′-(1*H*-tetrazol-5-yl)[1,1′-biphenyl]-4-yl]methyl]-; (2) 5,8-Dihydro-2,4-dimethyl-8-[*p*-(*o*-1*H*-tetrazol-5-ylphenyl)benzyl]pyrido[2,3-*d*]pyrimidin-7(6*H*)-one. *CAS-145733-36-4.* INN; BAN. *Antihypertensive.* ◇*WAY-ANA-756*

Taspoglutide. $C_{152}H_{232}N_{40}O_{45}$. 3339.71. [8-(2-Amino-2-methylpropanoic acid),35-(2-amino-2-methylpropanoic acid)]human glucagon-like peptide 1 (GLP-1)-(7-36)-peptidamide L-histidyl-2-methyl-L-alanyl-L-glutamylglycyl-L-threonyl-L-phenylalanyl-L-threonyl-L-seryl-L-aspartyl-L-valyl-L-seryl-L-seryl-L-tyrosyl-L-leucyl-L-glutamylglycyl-L-glutaminyl-L-alanyl-L-lysyl-L-glutamyl-L-phenylalanyl-L-isoleucyl-L-alanyl-L-tryptophyl-L-leucyl-L-valyl-L-lysyl-2-methyl-L-alanyl-L-arginamide. *CAS-275371-94-3.* INN.

---

† Brand name formerly used, and/or firm no longer concerned with this product.

Tasquinimod. $C_{20}H_{17}F_3N_2O_4$. 406.36. 4-Hydroxy-5-methoxy-*N*,1-dimethyl-2-oxo-*N*-[4-(trifluoromethyl)phenyl]-1,2-dihydroquinoline-3-carboxamide. *CAS-254964-60-8*. INN.

Tasuldine. $C_{10}H_9N_3S$. 203.26. 2-[(3-Pyridylmethyl)thio]pyrimidine. *UNII-S4ZCE64Q3O*. *CAS-88579-39-9*. INN.

Taurine (taw′ reen). **USP**. $C_2H_7NO_3S$. 125.15. [Aminoethylsulfonic Acid is JAN.] Taurine. *UNII-1EQV5MLY3D*. *CAS-107-35-7*. INN; MI.

Taurolidine. $C_7H_{16}N_4O_4S_2$. 284.36. 4,4′-Methylenebis(tetrahydro-1,2,4-thiadiazine 1,1-dioxide). *CAS-19388-87-5*. INN; BAN.

Tauromustine. $C_7H_{15}ClN_4O_4S$. 286.74. 1-(2-Chloroethyl)-3-[2-(dimethylsulfamoyl)ethyl]-1-nitrosourea. *CAS-85977-49-7*. INN.

Tauroselcholic Acid. $C_{26}H_{45}NO_7SSe$. 594.66. *N*-[[[(20*S*)-3α,7α,12α-Trihydroxy-20-methyl-5β-pregnan-21-yl]selenyl]acetyl]taurine. *CAS-75018-71-2*. INN; BAN. ◇*SeHCAT*

Taurosteine. $C_7H_9NO_4S_2$. 235.28. *N*-2-Thenoyltaurine. *UNII-43A07PH183*. *CAS-124066-33-7*. INN.

Taurultam. $C_3H_8N_2O_2S$. 136.17. Tetrahydro-2*H*-1,2,4-thiadiazine 1,1-dioxide. *UNII-LIX7OM008P*. *CAS-38668-01-8*. INN; BAN.

Taxol (previously used name) — *See* Paclitaxel.

Tazadolene Succinate [*1985*] (taz″ a doe′ leen sux′ i nate). $C_{16}H_{21}N.C_4H_6O_4$. 345.43. [Tazadolene is INN.] (1) Azetidine, 1-[2-(phenylmethylene)cyclohexyl]-, (*E*)-(±)-, butanedioate (1:1); (2) (±)-1-[(*E*)-2-Benzylidenecyclohexyl] azetidine succinate (1:1). *CAS-87936-82-1; CAS-87936-75-2* [tazadolene]. *Analgesic*. ◇*U-53,996H*

Tazanolast. $C_{13}H_{15}N_5O_3$. 289.29. Butyl 3′-(1*H*-tetrazol-5-yl)oxanilate. *UNII-T0248823H1*. *CAS-82989-25-1*. INN; JAN.

Tazarotene [*1994*] (taz ar′ oh teen). $C_{21}H_{21}NO_2S$. 351.46. (1) 3-Pyridinecarboxylic acid, 6-[(3,4-dihydro-4,4-dimethyl-2*H*-1-benzothiopyran-6-yl)ethynyl]-, ethyl ester; (2) Ethyl 6-[(4,4-dimethylthiochroman-6-yl)ethynyl]nicotinate. *UNII-81BDR9Y8PS*. *CAS-118292-40-3*. INN; BAN. *Keratolytic*. Avage (Allergan); Tazorac (Allergan) ◇*AGN 190168*

Tazasubrate. $C_{18}H_{17}NO_3S_2$. 359.46. (±)-α-[(6-Ethoxy-2-benzothiazolyl)thio]hydratropic acid. *UNII-6SGF1AP698*. *CAS-79071-15-1*. INN; BAN.

Tazeprofen. $C_{16}H_{13}NO_2S$. 283.34. (±)-α-Methyl-2-phenyl-6-benzothiazoleacetic acid. *UNII-S05RV1R3LZ*. *CAS-85702-89-2*. INN.

Tazifylline Hydrochloride [*1985*] (taz if′ i lin hye″ droe klor′ ide). $C_{23}H_{32}N_6O_3S \cdot 2HCl$. 545.53. [Tazifylline is INN.] (1) 1*H*-Purine-2,6-dione, 3,7-dihydro-7-[2-hydroxy-3-[4-[3-(phenylthio)propyl]-1-piperazinyl]propyl]-1,3-dimethyl-, dihydrochloride, (±)-; (2) (±)-7-[2-Hydroxy-3-[4-[3-(phenylthio)propyl]-1-piperazinyl]propyl]theophylline dihydrochloride. *CAS-79712-53-1; CAS-79712-55-3* [tazifylline]. *Antihistaminic.* ◇RS-49014

Taziprinone. $C_{22}H_{31}N_3O_3$. 385.50. (±)-*N*-[(4*R**,4a*R**,9b*S**)-1,2,3,4,4a,9b-Hexahydro-8,9b-dimethyl-3-oxo-4-dibenzofuranyl]-4-methyl-1-piperazinepropionamide. *UNII-MVC7EI41TU. CAS-79253-92-2.* INN; MI.

Tazobactam [*1989*] (taz″ oh bak′ tam). USP. $C_{10}H_{12}N_4O_5S$. 300.29. (1) 4-Thia-1-azabicyclo[3.2.0]heptane-2-carboxylic acid, 3-methyl-7-oxo-3-(1*H*-1,2,3-triazol-1-ylmethyl)-, 4,4-dioxide, [2*S*-(2α,3β,5α)]-; (2) (2*S*,3*S*,5*R*)-3-Methyl-7-oxo-3-(1*H*-1,2,3-triazol-1-ylmethyl)-4-thia-1-azabicyclo[3.2.0]heptane-2-carboxylic acid, 4,4-dioxide. *UNII-SE10G96M8W. CAS-89786-04-9.* INN; BAN. *Inhibitor (β-lactamase).* ◇CL 298,741; YTR-830H

Tazobactam Sodium [*1989*] (taz″ oh bak′ tam soe′ dee um). $C_{10}H_{11}N_4NaO_5S$. 322.27. (1) 4-Thia-1-azabicyclo[3.2.0]-heptane-2-carboxylic acid, 3-methyl-7-oxo-3-(1*H*-1,2,3-triazol-1-ylmethyl)-, 4,4-dioxide, sodium salt, [2*S*-(2α,3β,5α)]-; (2) Sodium (2*S*,3*S*,5*R*)-3-methyl-7-oxo-3-(1*H*-1,2,3-triazol-1-ylmethyl)-4-thia-1-azabicyclo[3.2.0]-heptane-2-carboxylate, 4,4-dioxide. *UNII-UXA545ABTT. CAS-89785-84-2. Inhibitor (β-lactamase).* ◇CL 307,579

Tazofelone [*1994*] (taz oh′ fe lone). $C_{18}H_{27}NO_2S$. 321.48. (1) 4-Thiazolidinone, 5-[[3,5-bis(1,1-dimethylethyl)-4-hydroxyphenyl]methyl]-, (±)-; (2) (±)-5-(3,5-Di-*tert*-butyl-4-hydroxybenzyl)-4-thiazolidinone. *UNII-VH2I1JN8Q1. CAS-136433-51-7.* INN. *Suppressant (inflammatory bowel disease).* ◇LY213829

Tazolol Hydrochloride [*1974*] (taz′ oh lol hye″ droe klor′ ide). $C_9H_{16}N_2O_2S \cdot HCl$. 252.76. [Tazolol is INN.] (1) 2-Propanol, 1-[(1-methylethyl)amino]-3-(2-thiazolyloxy)-, monohydrochloride, (±)-; (2) (±)-1-(Isopropylamino)-3-(2-thiazolyloxy)-2-propanol monohydrochloride. *CAS-38241-39-3; CAS-39832-48-9* [tazolol]. *Cardiotonic.* ◇RS-6245

Tazomeline Citrate [*1997*] (taz oh′ me leen sit′ rate). $C_{14}H_{23}N_3S_2 \cdot C_6H_8O_7$. 489.61. [Tazomeline is INN.] (1) Pyridine, 3-[4-(hexylthio)-1,2,5-thiadiazol-3-yl]-1,2,5,6-tetrahydro-1-methyl-, 2-hydroxy-1,2,3-propanetricarboxylate (1:1); (2) 3-[4-(Hexylthio)-1,2,5-thiadiazol-3-yl]-1,2,5,6-tetrahydro-1-methylpyridine citrate (1:1). *UNII-O494QX2F4D. CAS-175615-45-9; CAS-131987-54-7* [tazomeline]. *Alzheimer's disease treatment (cholinergic agonist).* ◇LY287041

⁹⁹ᵐTc — *See* Bectumomab.

⁹⁹ᵐTc — *See* Biciromab.

⁹⁹ᵐTc — *See* Macrosalb (⁹⁹ᵐTc).

⁹⁹ᵐTc — *See* Sodium Pertechnetate Tc 99m.

⁹⁹ᵐTc — *See* Sulesomab.

⁹⁹ᵐTc — *See* Technetium (⁹⁹ᵐTc) Human Serum Albumin [Injection].

⁹⁹ᵐTc — *See* Technetium (⁹⁹ᵐTc) Phytate [Injection].

⁹⁹ᵐTc — *See* Technetium Tc 99m (Pyro- and trimeta-) Phosphates.

⁹⁹ᵐTc — *See* Technetium Tc 99m Albumin.

⁹⁹ᵐTc — *See* Technetium Tc 99m Albumin Aggregated.

⁹⁹ᵐTc — *See* Technetium Tc 99m Albumin Colloid.

⁹⁹ᵐTc — *See* Technetium Tc 99m Albumin Microaggregated.

⁹⁹ᵐTc — *See* Technetium Tc 99m Antimony Trisulfide Colloid.

⁹⁹ᵐTc — *See* Technetium Tc 99m Arcitumomab.

⁹⁹ᵐTc — *See* Technetium Tc 99m Bicisate.

⁹⁹ᵐTc — *See* Technetium Tc 99m Depreotide.

⁹⁹ᵐTc — *See* Technetium Tc 99m Disofenin.

⁹⁹ᵐTc — *See* Technetium Tc 99m Etidronate.

⁹⁹ᵐTc — *See* Technetium Tc 99m Exametazime.

---

† Brand name formerly used, and/or firm no longer concerned with this product.

⁹⁹ᵐTc — *See* Technetium Tc 99m Ferpentetate.

⁹⁹ᵐTc — *See* Technetium Tc 99m Furifosmin.

⁹⁹ᵐTc — *See* Technetium Tc 99m Gluceptate.

⁹⁹ᵐTc — *See* Technetium Tc 99m Lidofenin.

⁹⁹ᵐTc — *See* Technetium Tc 99m Mebrofenin.

⁹⁹ᵐTc — *See* Technetium Tc 99m Medronate.

⁹⁹ᵐTc — *See* Technetium Tc 99m Medronate Disodium.

⁹⁹ᵐTc — *See* Technetium Tc 99m Mertiatide.

⁹⁹ᵐTc — *See* Technetium Tc 99m Oxidronate.

⁹⁹ᵐTc — *See* Technetium Tc 99m Pentetate.

⁹⁹ᵐTc — *See* Technetium Tc 99m Pentetate Calcium Trisodium.

⁹⁹ᵐTc — *See* Technetium Tc 99m Pyrophosphate.

⁹⁹ᵐTc — *See* Technetium Tc 99m Red Blood Cells.

⁹⁹ᵐTc — *See* Technetium Tc 99m Sestamibi.

⁹⁹ᵐTc — *See* Technetium Tc 99m Siboroxime.

⁹⁹ᵐTc — *See* Technetium Tc 99m Succimer.

⁹⁹ᵐTc — *See* Technetium Tc 99m Sulfur Colloid.

⁹⁹ᵐTc — *See* Technetium Tc 99m Teboroxime.

⁹⁹ᵐTc — *See* Technetium Tc 99m Tetrofosmin.

⁹⁹ᵐTc — *See* Technetium Tc 99m Tiatide.

Teaberry Oil — *See* Methyl Salicylate.

Tebanicline Tosylate [*2001*] (te ban′ i kleen tos′ i late). $C_9H_{11}ClN_2O.C_7H_{19}O_3S$. 381.94. [Tebanicline is INN.] (1) Pyridine, 5-[(2*R*)-2-azetidinylmethoxy]-2-chloro-, mono(4-methylbenzenesulfonate); (2) 5-[[(*R*)-2-Azetidnyl]methoxy]-2-chloropyridine mono-*p*-toluenesulfonate. *UNII-CP1A26546Z. CAS-198283-74-8; CAS-198283-73-7* [tebanicline]. *Analgesic (cholinergic channel modulator).[- Name previously used: Ebanicline Tosylate.]* ◇*A-166594.47; ABT-594; A-165594*

Tebatizole. $C_{12}H_{21}N_3S$. 239.38. 1-(4-*tert*-Butyl-2-thiazolyl)-4-methylpiperazine. *UNII-P0S37156TW. CAS-54147-28-3.* INN.

Tebipenem Pivoxil. $C_{22}H_{31}N_3O_6S_2$. 497.63. (4*R*,5*S*,6*S*)-3-[[1-(4,5-Dihydro-2-thiazolyl)-3-azetidinyl]thio]-6-[(1*R*)-1-hydroxyethyl]-4-methyl-7-oxo-1-azabicyclo[3.2.0]hept-2-ene-2-carboxylic acid (2,2-dimethyl-1-oxopropoxy) methyl ester. *UNII-95AK1A52I8. CAS-161715-24-8.* INN.

Tebufelone [*1990*] (te bue′ fe lone). $C_{20}H_{28}O_2$. 300.44. (1) 5-Hexyn-1-one, 1-[3,5-bis(1,1-dimethylethyl)-4-hydroxyphenyl]-; (2) 3′,5′-Di-*tert*-butyl-4′-hydroxy-5-hexynophenone. *CAS-112018-00-5.* INN. *Analgesic; anti-inflammatory.* ◇*NE 11740*

Tebuquine [*1983*] (te′ bue kwin). $C_{26}H_{25}Cl_2N_3O$. 466.40. (1) [1,1′-Biphenyl]-2-ol, 4′-chloro-5-[(7-chloro-4-quinolinyl)amino]-3-[[(1,1-dimethylethyl)amino]methyl]-; (2) 3-[(*tert*-Butylamino)methyl]-4′-chloro-5-[(7-chloro-4-quinolyl)amino]-2-biphenylol. *UNII-699Q1XT4EN. CAS-74129-03-6.* INN. *Antimalarial.* ◇*CI-897; WR-228,258*

Tecadenoson [*2002*] (tek″ a den′ o son). $C_{14}H_{19}N_5O_5$. 337.33. (1) Adenosine, *N*-[3*R*]-tetrahydro-3-furanyl]-; (2) (2*R*,3*R*,4*S*,5*R*)-2-Hydroxymethyl)-5-[6-[(3*R*)-(tetrahydrofuran-3-ylamino]-9*H*-purin-9-yl]tetrahydrofuran-3,4-diol; (3) 2-(6-[((3*R*)Oxolan-3-yl)amino]purin-9-yl](2*R*,4*S*,3*R*,5*R*)-5-(hydroxymethyl)oxolane-3,4-diol. *UNII-GZ1X96601Z. CAS-204512-90-3.* INN. *Treatment of paroxysmal supraventricular tachycardia and rate control in atrial fibrillation and atrial flutter.* ◇*CVT-510*

Tecalcet Hydrochloride [*2002*] (tek′ al set hye″ droe klor′ ide). $C_{18}H_{22}ClNO.HCl$. 340.29. [Tecalcet is INN.] (1) Benzenepropanamine, 2-chloro-*N*-[(1*R*)-1-(3-methoxyphenyl)ethyl]-, hydrochloride; (2) 3-(2-Chlorophenyl)-*N*-[(1*R*)-1-(3-methoxyphenyl)ethyl]propan-1-amine hydrochloride. *UNII-3HP28R98LC; UNII-8I16YLE4US* [tecalcet]. *CAS-177172-49-5; CAS-148717-54-8* [tecalcet]. *Treatment of hyperparathyroidism and related disorders, such as hypercalcemia (reduction of PTH secretion* *through modulation of calcium ion receptors on parathyroid cells).* Norcalcin (Amgen) ◇*NPS R-568; R-568; KRN-568*

Tecastemizole [*2002*] (tek″ a stem′ i zole). $C_{19}H_{21}FN_4$. 324.40. (1) 1*H*-Benzimidazol-2-amine, 1-[(4-fluorophenyl)methyl]-*N*-4-piperidinyl-; (2) 1-(-Fluorobenzyl)-*N*-(piperidin-4-yl)-1*H*-benzimidazol-2-amine. *UNII-W5DCO14M05. CAS-75970-99-9.* INN. *Antihistamine used in the treatment of allergic rhinitis.[Note—The trivial name, norastemizole, has appeared in literature.]* ◇*R-43512*

Teceleukin [*1987*] (tek″ e loo′ kin). $C_{698}H_{1127}N_{179}O_{204}S_8$. 15,547.03. (1) Interleukin 2 (human), *N*-L-methionyl-; (2) *N*-L-Methionylinterleukin 2 (human). *CAS-136279-32-8; CAS-94218-75-4* [reduced protein moiety]. INN; BAN. *Immunostimulant.* ◇*Ro 23-6019; BG 8301*

```
                                                      M
APTSSSTKKT QLQLEHLLLD LQMILNGINN YKNPKLTRML TFKFYMPKKA
TELKHLQCLE EELKPLEEVL NLAQSKNFHL RPRDLISNIN VIVLELKGSE
TTFMCEYADE TATIVEFLNR WITFCQSIIS TLT
```

Technetium (^{99m}Tc) Dimercaptosuccinic Acid for Injection (JAN) — *See* Technetium Tc 99m Succimer.

Technetium (^{99m}Tc) Human Serum Albumin [Injection]. JAN.

Technetium (^{99m}TC) Labelled Macroaggregated Human Serum Albumin Injection (JAN) — *See* Macrosalb (^{99m}Tc).

Technetium (^{99m}Tc) Methylenediphosphonate for Injection (JAN) — *See* Technetium Tc 99m Medronate.

Technetium (^{99m}Tc) Phytate [Injection]. JAN.

Technetium (^{99m}Tc) Pintumomab. Immunoglobulin G1, anti-(human adenocarcinoma antigen) (mouse monoclonal 170 γ1-chain), disulfide with mouse monoclonal 170 κ-chain, dimer, technetium [^{99m}Tc] salt. *CAS-157476-76-1.* INN.

Technetium Tc 99m Albumin (tek nee′ shee um al bue′ min). **USP** [Injection]. A sterile, aqueous solution of albumin human that is labeled with ^{99m}Tc. *Radioactive agent.* Technetium Tc 99m HSA (Medi-Physics)

Technetium Tc 99m Albumin Aggregated [*1974*] (tek nee′ shee um al bue′ min ag′ re gay″ ted). **USP** [Injection]. Albumins, blood serum, metastable technetium-99 labeled. *Diagnostic aid (lung imaging); radioactive agent.* AN-MAA (CL Pharma AG, Austria†); Macrotec (Bracco Diagnostics); Pulmolite (DuPont Merck); TechneScan MAA (Mallinckrodt); Technetium Tc 99m MAA (Medi-Physics) ◇*Tc99m-MP 4006*

---

† Brand name formerly used, and/or firm no longer concerned with this product.

Technetium Tc 99m Albumin Colloid [*1974*] (tek nee′ shee um al bue′ min kol′ oid). **USP** [Injection]. A sterile, pyrogen-free, aqueous suspension of albumin human that has been denatured to produce colloids of controlled particle size and that are labeled with ^{99m}Tc. *Radioactive agent.* Microlite (DuPont Merck)

Technetium Tc 99m Albumin Microaggregated [*1985*] (tek nee′ shee um al bue′ min mye″ kroe ag′ re gay″ ted). *Radioactive agent.* Microloid (Bristol-Myers Squibb†)

Technetium Tc 99m Antimony Trisulfide Colloid [*1974*] (tek nee′ shee um an′ ti moe″ nee trye sul′ fide kol′ oid). *Radioactive agent.*

Technetium Tc 99m Apcitide [*1997*] (tek nee′ shee um ap′ si tide). **USP** [Injection]. $C_{51}H_{73}N_{17}NaO_{20}S_5{}^{99m}$Tc. [Technetium (^{99m} Tc) Apcitide is INN.] Sodium hydrogen [*N*-(mercaptoacetyl)-D-tyrosyl-*S*-(3-aminopropyl)-L-cysteinylglycyl-L-α-aspartyl-L-cysteinylglycylglycyl-*S*-(acetamidomethyl)-L-cysteinylglycyl-*S*-(acetamidomethyl)-L-cysteinylglycylglycyl-L-cysteinamide cyclic (1→5)-sulfidato(5-)-$N^{11},N^{12},N^{13},S^{13}$]oxo[^{99m}Tc]technetate(V). *UNII-IV7T84QA4T. CAS-178959-14-3. Diagnostic aid (radioactive, vascular disorders). [Note—Technetium Tc 99m apcitide is the technetium complex that is formed when bibapcitide is combined with sodium pertechnetate.]* ◇*[99mTc]-P246*

Technetium Tc 99m Arcitumomab (tek nee′ shee um ar″ si toom′ oh mab). **USP** [Injection]. A sterile, nonpyrogenic preparation of the 50,000-dalton Fab′ fragment generated from the murine IgG monoclonal antibody Immu-4 that is labeled with ^{99m}Tc. *Radioactive agent.*

Technetium Tc 99m Bectumomab — *See* Bectumomab.

Technetium Tc 99m Biciromab — *See* Biciromab.

Technetium Tc 99m Bicisate [*1990*] (tek nee′ shee um bye sis′ ate). **USP** [Injection]. $C_{12}H_{21}N_2O_5S_2{}^{99m}$Tc. (1) Technetium-^{99m}*Tc*, [[diethyl *N*,*N*′-1,2-ethanediylbis[L-cysteinato]](3-)-*N*,*N*′,*S*,*S*′]oxo-, (*SP*-5-35)-; (2) [*N*,*N*′-Ethylenedi-L-cysteinato(3-)]oxo[^{99m}Tc]technetium(V), diethyl ester. *CAS-121281-41-2.* INN; BAN. *Diagnostic aid (brain imaging); radioactive agent.* Neurolite (DuPont Merck)

Technetium Tc 99m Depreotide (tek nee′ shee um de pree′ oh tide). **USP** [Injection]. A sterile, aqueous solution that contains ^{99m}Tc in the form of a depreotide complex. *Radioactive agent.*

Technetium Tc 99m Disofenin (tek nee′ shee um dye″ soe fen′ in). **USP** [Injection]. A sterile, aqueous solution of disofenin that is labeled with ^{99m}Tc. *Diagnostic aid (hepatobiliary function determination); radioactive agent.* Hepatolite (DuPont Merck)

Technetium Tc 99m Etidronate (tek nee′ shee um e ti droe′ nate). **USP** [Injection]. A sterile, clear, colorless solution of radioactive technetium (^{99m}Tc) in the form of a chelate of etidronate sodium. *Radioactive agent.*

Technetium Tc 99m Exametazime [*1989*] (tek nee′ shee um ex″ a met′ a zeem). **USP** [Injection]. (1) 2-Butanone, 3,3′-[(2,2-dimethyl-1,3-propanediyl)diimino]bis-dioxime-^{99m}Tc; (2) d,1-Hexamethylpropylene amine oxime-^{99m}Tc. *UNII-G29272NCKL. CAS-105613-48-7. Radioactive agent.* Ceretec (Nycomed Amersham)

Technetium Tc 99m Fanolesomab [*2002*] (tek nee′ shee um fan″ oh les′ oh mab). **USP** [Injection]. (1) Immunoglobulin M, anti-(human CD15 (antigen)) (mouse monoclonal RB5 μ-chain), disulfide with mouse monoclonal RB5 light chain, pentamer, technetium-^{99m}Tc salt; (2) Immunoglobulin M (mouse monoclonal RB5 μ-chain anti-human antigen CD 15), disulfide with mouse monoclonal RB5 light chain, pentamer, [^{99m}Tc]technetium salt. The molecular weight is approximately 670,000 Daltons (measured by size exclusion HPLC, other methods yield different results). *CAS-225239-31-6.* INN. *In vivo diagnostic for imaging sites of infection associated with polymorphonuclear neutrophil (PMN) accumulation.* Leutech (Palatin) ◇*RB5 IgM; anti-SSEA-1; Tc 99m anti-SSEA-1; Tc99m RB5 IgM*

Technetium Tc 99m Ferpentetate. (1) Iron, ascorbic acid and *N,N*-bis[2-[bis(carboxymethyl)amino]-ethyl]glycine complex, metastable technetium-99 labeled; (2) Iron, ascorbic acid and *N,N*-bis[2-[bis(carboxymethyl)amino]-ethyl]glycine complex, metastable technetium-99 labeled. USP XXII. *[Name previously used: Technetium Tc 99m Iron Ascorbate Pentetic Acid Complex.]*

Technetium Tc 99m Furifosmin [*1994*] (tek nee′ shee um fure″ i fos′ min). $C_{44}H_{84}ClN_2O_{10}P_2{}^{99m}$Tc. (1) Technetium(1+)-^{99m}*Tc*, [[4,4′-[1,2-ethanediylbis(nitrilomethylidyne)]bis[dihydro-2,2,5,5-tetramethyl-3(2*H*)-furanonato]](2-)-*N*^{4},*N*$^{4'}$,*O*^{3},*O*$^{3'}$]bis[tris(3-methoxypropyl)phosphine-*P*]-, chloride, (*OC*-6-13)-; (2) (*OC*-6-13)-[[4,4′-[Ethylenebis(nitrilomethylidyne)]bis[dihydro-2,2,5,5-tetramethyl-3(2*H*)-furanonato]](2-)-*N*,*N*′,*O*^{3},*O*$^{3'}$]bis[tris(3-methoxypropyl)phosphine-*P*][^{99m}Tc]technetium(1+) chloride. *CAS-142481-95-6.* INN. *Diagnostic aid (radioactive, cardiac disease); radioactive agent.* TechneScan Q-12 (Mallinckrodt) ◇*MP-1554; Q-12*

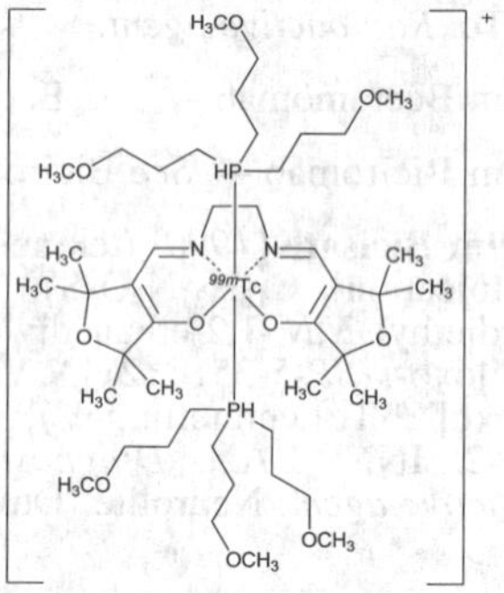

Technetium Tc 99m Gluceptate (tek nee′ shee um gloo sep′ tate). **USP** [Injection]. (1) D-*glycero*-D-*gulo*-Heptonic acid, technetium-^{99m}*Tc* complex; (2) Technetium-^{99m}Tc D-*glycero*-D-*gulo*-heptonate complex. *Radioactive agent.* Glucoscan (DuPont Merck); TechneScan Gluceptate (Mallinckrodt) *[Name previously used: Technetium Tc 99m Sodium Gluceptate.]*

Technetium Tc 99m Iron Ascorbate Pentetic Acid Complex (previously used name) — *See* Technetium Tc 99m Ferpentetate.

Technetium Tc 99m Lidofenin [*1988*] (tek nee′ shee um lye″ doe fen′ in). **USP** [Injection]. A sterile, clear, colorless solution of lidofenin complexed to radioactive technetium (^{99m}Tc) in the form of a chelate. *Radioactive agent.* TechneScan HIDA (Mallinckrodt)

Technetium Tc 99m Mebrofenin [*1984*] (tek nee′ shee um me″ broe fen′ in). **USP** [Injection]. A sterile, aqueous solution of stannous fluoride and mebrofenin labeled with radioactive technetium ^{99m}Tc. *Radioactive agent.* Choletec (Bracco Diagnostics)

Technetium Tc 99m Medronate (tek nee′ shee um me′ droe nate). **USP** [Injection]. [Technetium (^{99m}Tc) Methylenediphosphonate for Injection is JAN.] A sterile, aqueous solution of sodium medronate and stannous chloride or stannous fluoride that is labeled with radioactive technetium (^{99m}Tc). *Diagnostic aid (skeletal imaging); radioac-*

tive agent. AN-MDP (CL Pharma AG, Austria); MDP-Bracco (Bracco Diagnostics); MDP Kit (Medi-Physics); Osteolite (DuPont Merck); TechneScan MDP (Mallinckrodt)

Technetium Tc 99m Medronate Disodium [*1984*] (tek nee′ shee um me′ droe nate dye soe′ dee um). *Radioactive agent.* Amerscan MDP (Nycomed Amersham†)

Technetium Tc 99m Mertiatide [*1990*] (tek nee′ shee um mer tye′ a tide). **USP** [Injection]. $C_8H_8N_3Na_2O_6S^{99m}$Tc. (1) Technetate(2-)-^{99m}*Tc*, [*N*-[*N*-[*N*-(mercaptoacetyl)glycyl]glycyl]glycinato(5-)-*N*,*N*′,*N*″,*S*]-oxo-, disodium, (*SP*-5-25)-; (2) Disodium [*N*-[*N*-[*N*-(mercaptoacetyl)glycyl]glycyl]glycinato(5-)-*N*,*N*′,*N*″,*S*]-oxo[^{99m}Tc]technetate(V). *CAS-125224-05-7. Diagnostic aid (renal function determination); radioactive agent.* TechneScan MAG3 (Mallinckrodt) ◇*Tc-MAG₃*

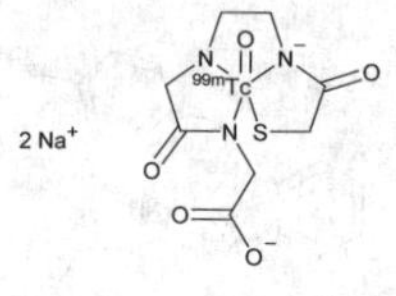

Technetium Tc 99m Nitridocade [*2003*] (tek nee′ shee um nye trid′ oh kade). $C_{10}H_{20}N_3O_2S_4{}^{99}$Tc. 441.50. (1) Technetium-^{99}*Tc*, bis(ethoxyethylcarbamodithioato-κS,κS′)nitrido-, (*SP*-5-21)-; (2) (*SP*-5-21)-Bis(ethoxyethyl-carbamodithioato-κS,κS′)nitrido[^{99m}Tc]technetium. *CAS-131608-78-1.* INN. *For in-vivo diagnosis of coronary artery disease.* Cisnoet (Berlex) ◇^{99m}*TcN-NOET*

Technetium Tc 99m Nofetumomab Merpentan (tek nee′ shee um noe″ fe toom′ oh mab mer pen′ tan). **USP** [Injection]. Immunoglobulin G2b anti-(human tumor) Fab fragment (mouse monoclonal NR-LU-10 γ2b-chain), disulfide with mouse monoclonal NR-LU-10 κ-chain, oxo[[*N*,*N*′-[1-(3-oxopropyl)-1,2-ethanediyl]bis[2-mercaptoacetamidato]](4-)-*N*,*N*′,*S*,*S*′]technetate(1-)-[^{99m}Tc] conjugate. *CAS-165942-79-0.* INN. Verluma (DuPont Merck)

Technetium Tc 99m Oxidronate (tek nee′ shee um ox″ i droe′ nate). **USP** [Injection]. A sterile, clear, colorless solution of radioactive technetium (^{99m}Tc) in the form of a chelate of oxidronate sodium. *Diagnostic aid (skeletal imaging); radioactive agent.* TechneScan HDP (Mallinckrodt)

Technetium Tc 99m Pentetate (tek nee′ shee um pen′ te tate). **USP** [Injection]. $C_{14}H_{18}N_3NaO_{10}{}^{99m}$Tc. [Human Serum Albumin Diethylenetriaminepentaacetic Acid Technetium (^{99m}Tc) Injection is JAN.] (1) Technetate (1-)-^{99m}*Tc*, [*N*,*N*-bis[2-bis(carboxymethyl)amino]ethyl]glycinato(5-)]-, sodium; (2) Sodium [*N*,*N*-bis[2-bis(carboxymethyl)amino]ethyl]glycinato(5-)]-technetate(1-)-^{99m}Tc. *CAS-65454-61-7. Radioactive agent.* AN-DTPA (CL Pharma AG, Austria); Tc 99m DTPA Kit (chelate) (Medi-Physics); Techneplex (Bracco Diagnostics) *[Name previously used: Technetium Tc 99m Pentetate Sodium.]*

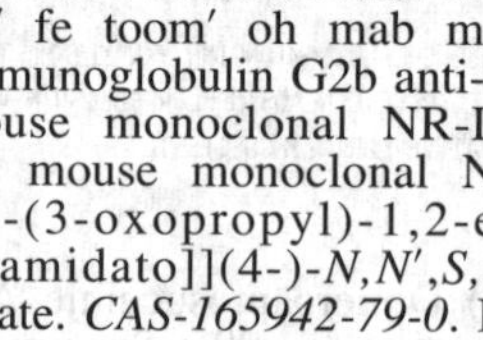

Technetium Tc 99m Pentetate Calcium Trisodium [*1990*] (tek nee′ shee um pen′ te tate kal′ see um trye soe′ dee um). *Radioactive agent.*

Technetium Tc 99m Pentetate Sodium (previously used name) — *See* Technetium Tc 99m Pentetate.

Technetium Tc 99m (Pyro- and trimeta-) Phosphates (tek nee′ shee um pye″ roe and trye met″ a fos′ fates). **USP** [Injection]. A sterile, aqueous solution of sodium pyrophosphate, sodium trimetaphosphate, and stannous chloride labeled with radioactive technetium ^{99m}Tc. *Radioactive agent.* Pyrolite (DuPont Merck)

Technetium Tc 99m Pyrophosphate (tek nee′ shee um pye″ roe fos′ fate). **USP** [Injection]. A sterile, aqueous solution of pyrophosphate that is labeled with ^{99m}Tc. JAN. *Radioactive agent.* CIS-PYRO (CL Pharma AG, Austria); Pyrophosphate Kit (Medi-Physics); Phosphotec (Bracco Diagnostics); TechneScan PYP Kit (Mallinckrodt)

Technetium Tc 99m Red Blood Cells [*1986*] (tek nee′ shee um red blud sels). **USP** [Injection]. A preparation of anticoagulated whole blood that is labeled with ^{99m}Tc. *Radioactive agent.* UltraTag RBC (Mallinckrodt)

Technetium Tc 99m Sestamibi [*1990*] (tek nee′ shee um ses″ ta mib′ ee). **USP** [Injection]. $C_{36}H_{66}N_6O_6^{99m}$Tc. (1) Technetium(1+)-^{99m}Tc, hexakis(1-isocyano-2-methoxy-2-methylpropane)-, (*OC*-6-11)-; (2) Hexakis(2-methoxy-2-methylpropyl isocyanide)[^{99m}Tc]technetium(1+). *CAS-109581-73-9.* INN; BAN. *Diagnostic aid (radiopaque medium, cardiac perfusion); radioactive agent.* Cardiolite (DuPont Merck) ◇*Tc99m RP-30A*

Technetium Tc 99m Siboroxime [*1990*] (tek nee′ shee um sye″ boe rox′ eem). $C_{16}H_{29}BClN_6O_6^{99m}$Tc. (1) Technetium-$^{99m}Tc$, [bis[(2,3-butanedione dioximato)(1-)-*O*][(2,3-butanedione dioximato)(2-)-*O*](2-methylpropyl)borato(2-)-*N,N′,N″,N‴,N⁗,N⁗′*]chloro-, (*TPS*-7-1-232′4′54)-; (2) [Bis[(2,3-butanedione dioximato)(1-)-*O*][(2,3-butanedione dioximato)(2-)-*O*]isobutylborato(2-)-*N,N′, N″,N‴,N⁗,N⁗′*]chloro[^{99m}Tc]technetium(III). *CAS-106417-28-1.* INN. *Diagnostic aid (brain imaging); radioactive agent.* ◇*SQ 32,097*

Technetium Tc 99m Sodium Gluceptate (previously used name) — *See* Technetium Tc 99m Gluceptate.

Technetium Tc 99m Succimer (tek nee′ shee um sux′ i mer). **USP** [Injection]. [Technetium (^{99m}Tc) Dimercaptosuccinic Acid for Injection is JAN.] meso-2,3-Dimercaptosuccinic acid, ^{99m}Tc complex. *Diagnostic aid (renal function determination); radioactive agent.* DMSA Kidney Reagent (Medi-Physics)

Technetium Tc 99m Sulesomab — *See* Sulesomab.

Technetium Tc 99m Sulfur Colloid [*1967*] (tek nee′ shee um sul′ fur kol′ oid). **USP** [Injection]. Sulfur, colloidal, metastable technetium-99 labeled. *CAS-7704-34-9.* *Radioactive agent.* AN-Sulfur Colloid Kit (CL Pharma AG, Austria); TechneColl (Mallinckrodt†); TechneScan Sulfur Colloid (Mallinckrodt); Technetium Tc 99m TSC (Medi-Physics); Tesuloid (Bristol-Myers Squibb†)

Technetium Tc 99m Teboroxime [*1990*] (tek nee′ shee um te″ boe rox′ eem). $C_{19}H_{29}BClN_6O_6^{99m}$Tc. (1) Technetium-$^{99m}Tc$, [bis[(1,2-cyclohexanedione dioximato)(1-)-*O*][(1,2-cyclohexanedione dioximato)(2-)-*O*]methylborato(2-)-*N,N′,N″,N‴,N⁗,N⁗′*]chloro-, (*TPS*-7-1-232′4′54)-; (2) Bis[(1,2-cyclohexanedione dioximato)(1-)-*O*][(1,2-cyclohexanedione dioximato)(2-)-*O*]methylborato(2-)-*N,N′,N″,N‴,N⁗,N⁗′*]chloro[^{99m}Tc]technetium (III). *CAS-104716-22-5.* INN; BAN. *Diagnostic aid (radiopaque medium, cardiac perfusion); radioactive agent.* Cardiotec (Bracco Diagnostics) ◇*SQ 30217*

Technetium Tc 99m Tetrofosmin (tek nee′ shee um te″ troe fos′ min). **USP** [Injection]. A sterile, aqueous solution that contains ^{99m}Tc in the form of a complex of tetrofosmin. *Radioactive agent.* Myoview (Nycomed Amersham)

Technetium Tc 99m Tiatide. $C_{16}H_{16}N_6Na_2O_{12}S_2Tc_2$. 790.44. Disodium [*N*-(mercaptoacetyl)glycylglycylglycinato(2-)-*N,N′,N″,S*]oxotechnetate(2-). *CAS-104348-91-6* [anion]. BAN.

Teclothiazide. $C_8H_7Cl_4N_3O_4S_2$. 415.10. 6-Chloro-3,4-dihydro-3-(trichloromethyl)-2*H*-1,2,4-benzothiadiazine-7-sulfonamide 1,1-dioxide. *UNII-M69O7IV78O. CAS-4267-05-4.* INN; BAN; DCF.

Teclozan [*1963*] (tek′ loe zan). $C_{20}H_{28}Cl_4N_2O_4$. 502.26. (1) Acetamide, *N,N′*-[1,4-phenylenebis(methylene)]bis[2,2-dichloro-*N*-(2-ethoxyethyl)-; (2) *N,N′*-(*p*-Phenylenedimethylene)bis[2,2-dichloro-*N*-(2-ethoxyethyl)acetamide]. *CAS-5560-78-1.* INN. *Anti-amebic.* Falmonox (Sterling Winthrop) ◇*Win 13,146; NSC-107433*

Tecogalan Sodium [*1994*] (tek oh′ ga lan soe′ dee um). (1) Fermentation product of *Arthrobacter* sp. AT-25, and composed of sulfated polysaccharide and small amounts of peptidoglycan and phosphorus. The polysaccharide is composed primarily of galactose and glucose (molar ratio of approximately 5:1) which could contain approximately one sulfate group (as sodium salt) per sugar unit on the average. The peptidoglycan contains glucosamine, mura-

---

mic acid, alanine, glutamic acid, glycine and diaminopimelic acid. (2) CA General Subject Indexes description: Polysaccharides sulfated, peptidoglycan complexes, of *Arthrobacter* species AT-25. Molecular weight is ca. 29,000 by GPC method using dextrans as standard. *CAS-134633-29-7. Antineoplastic (adjunct).* ◊*DS-4152*

Tecovirimat [*2008*] (tek″ oh vir′ i mat). $C_{19}H_{15}F_3N_2O_3$. 376.33. (1) Benzamide, *N*-[(3a*R*,4*R*,4a*R*,5a*S*,6*S*,6a*S*)-3,3a,4,4a,5,5a,6,6a-octahydro-1,3-dioxo-4,6-ethenocycloprop[*f*]isoindol-2(1*H*)-yl]-4-(trifluoromethyl)-, rel-; (2) *N*-[(3a*R*,4*R*,4a*R*,5a*S*,6*S*,6a*S*)-1,3-dioxo-3,3a,4,4a,5,5a,6,6a-octahydro-4,6-ethenocyclopropa[*f*]isoindol-2(1*H*)-yl]-4-(trifluoromethyl)benzamide. *UNII-F925RR824R. CAS-869572-92-9.* INN. *Treatment of small pox.* ◊*siga-246*

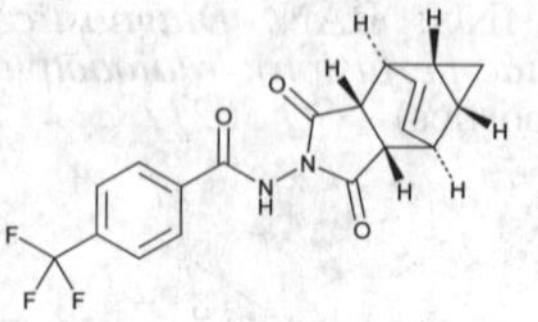

Tedisamil [*2005*] (te dis′ a mil). $C_{19}H_{32}N_2$. 288.47. (1) Spiro[cyclopentane-1,9′-[3,7]diazabicyclo[3.3.1]nonane], 3′,7′-bis(cyclopropylmethyl)-; (2) 3′,7′-Bis(cyclopropylmethyl)spiro[cyclopentane-1,9′-[3,7]diazabicyclo[3.3.1]nonane]. *UNII-A5VAY2U3R8. CAS-90961-53-8.* INN. *Antiarrhythmic agent (K⁺channel blocker).* ◊*KC8857*

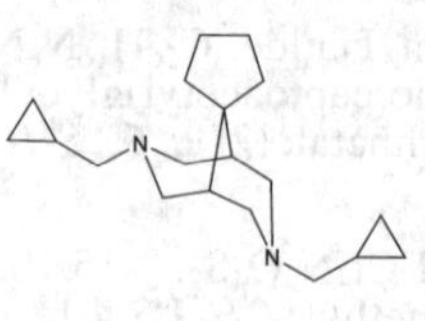

Tedisamil Sesquifumarate [*2005*] (te dis′ a mil ses″ kwi fue′ ma rate). $2C_{19}H_{32}N_2.3C_4H_4O_4$. 925.16. (1) Spiro[cyclopentane-1,9′-[3,7]diazabicyclo[3.3.1]nonane], 3′,7′-bis(cyclopropylmethyl)-, (2*E*)-2-butenedioate (2:3); (2) Bis[3′,7′-bis(cyclopropylmethyl)spiro[cyclopentane-1,9′-[3,7]diazabicyclo[3.3.1]nonane]] dihydrogen tris[(2*E*-but-2-enedioate]. *UNII-Y4HRG433UU. CAS-150501-62-5. Antiarrhythmic agent (K⁺channel blocker);.* ◊*KC8857*

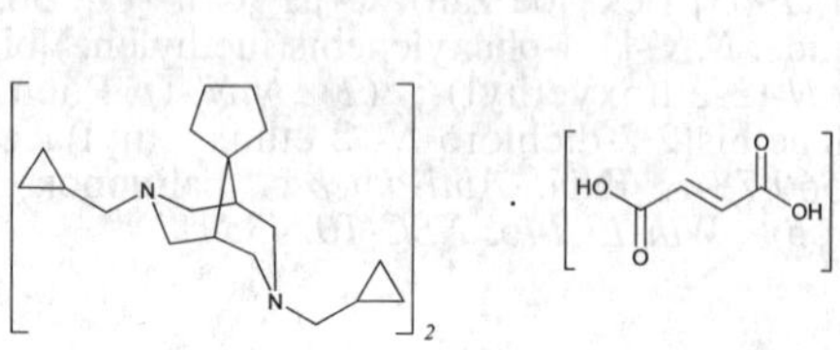

Teduglutide [*2004*] (te″ due gloo′ tide). $C_{164}H_{252}N_{44}O_{55}S$. 3752.08. (1) ALX 0600 (2-glycine-1-33-glucagon-like peptide II (human)); (2) [2-Glycine]-1-33-glucagon-like peptide II (human). *UNII-7M19191IKG. CAS-287714-30-1.* INN; BAN. *Treatment of intestinal diseases characterized by chemical or surgical damage of the intestinal epithelium such as Short Bowel Syndrome (SBS) or damage to the intestinal epithelium due to disease (glucagon-like peptide-2 (GLP-2) analog).* ◊*ALX 0600*

HGDGSFSDEM NTILDNLAAR DFINWLIQTK ITD

Tefazoline. $C_{14}H_{18}N_2$. 214.31. 2-[(5,6,7,8-Tetrahydro-1-naphthyl)methyl]-2-imidazoline. *UNII-9738II2CCH. CAS-1082-56-0.* INN; DCF.

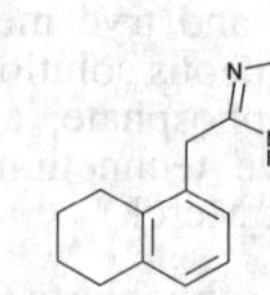

Tefenperate. $C_{29}H_{37}Cl_2NO_4$. 534.51. 2-(2,2,6,6-Tetramethyl-piperidino)ethyl *o*-chloro-α-(*o*-chlorobenzyl)-α-hydroxyhydrocinnamate acetate (ester). *UNII-W5P145L26T. CAS-77342-26-8.* INN.

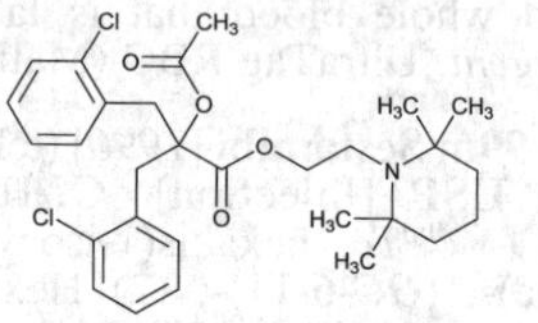

Tefibazumab [*2004*] (te″ fi baz′ oo mab). $C_{6548}H_{10122}N_{1730}O_{2034}S_{44}$. Immunoglobulin G1, anti-(*Staphylococcus aureus* protein ClfA (clumping factor A)) (human-Mus musculus monoclonal Aurexis heavy chain), disulfide with human-Mus musculus monoclonal Aurexis κ-chain, dimer. Molecular weight is approximately 147,590 daltons. *CAS-521079-87-8.* INN. *Treatment of Staphylococcus aureus infections.* Aurexis (Avid Bioservices) ◊*INH-H2002*

Tefilcon A [*1981*] (te fil′ kon). $(C_6H_{10}O_3)_v(C_4H_6O_2)_w(C_8H_{14}O_2)_x(C_8H_{15}NO_2)_y(C_{10}H_{14}O_4)_z$. (1) 2-Hydroxethyl 2-methyl-2-propenoate polymer with 2-methyl-2-propenoic acid, butyl 2-methyl-2-propenoate, 2-(dimethylamino)-ethyl 2-methyl-propenoate and 1,2-ethanediyl bis(2-methyl-2-propenoate); (2) 2-Hydroxyethyl methacrylate polymer with methacrylic acid, butyl methacrylate, 2-(dimethylamino)ethyl methacrylate and ethylene dimethacrylate. *CAS-78372-26-6. Contact lens material (hydrophilic).* Weicon 60 (Titmus Eurocon Kontaktlinsen GmbH & Co. KG, Germany)

Tefludazine. $C_{22}H_{24}F_4N_2O$. 408.43. *trans*-4-[3-(*p*-Fluorophenyl)-6-(trifluoromethyl)-1-indanyl]-1-piperazineethanol. *CAS-80680-06-4.* INN.

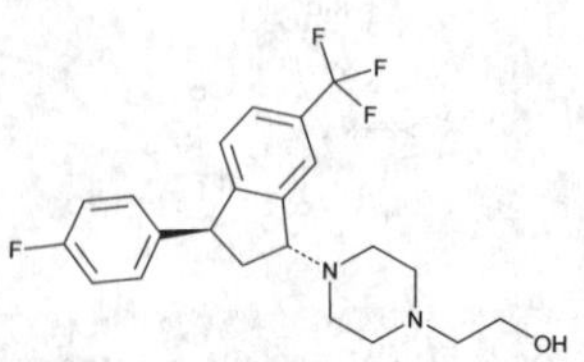

Teflurane [*1965*] (te flur′ ane). C_2HBrF_4. 180.93. (1) Ethane, 2-bromo-1,1,1,2-tetrafluoro-; (2) 2-Bromo-1,1,1,2-tetrafluoroethane. *CAS-124-72-1.* INN. *Anesthetic (inhalation).* ◊*Abbott-16900; DA-708*

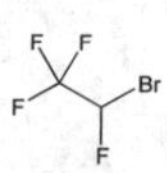

Teflutixol. $C_{23}H_{26}F_4N_2OS$. 454.52. 4-[3-[6-Fluoro-2-(trifluoromethyl)thioxanthen-9-yl]propyl]-1-piperazineethanol. *UNII-1O8A15G935. CAS-55837-23-5.* INN.

Tegafur [*1979*] (teg′ a fur). $C_8H_9FN_2O_3$. 200.17. (1) 2,4(1*H*,3*H*)Pyrimidinedione, 5-fluoro-1-(tetrahydro-2-furanyl)-; (2) 5-Fluoro-1-(tetrahydro-2-furyl)uracil. *CAS-17902-23-7.* INN; BAN; JAN. *Antineoplastic.* ◇*MJF-12264; NSC-148958*

Tegaserod [*1999*] (teg″ a ser′ od). $C_{16}H_{23}N_5O$. 301.39. (1) Hydrazinecarboximidamide, 2-[(5-methoxy-1*H*-indol-3-yl)methylene]-*N*-pentyl-; (2) 1-[[(5-Methoxyindol-3-yl)methylene]amino]-3-pentylguanidine. *UNII-458VC51857. CAS-145158-71-0.* INN; BAN. *Treatment of gastrointestinal motility disorders (selective serotonin 5HT4antagonist).* Zelmac (Novartis) ◇*HTF 919; SDZ-HTF-919*

Tegaserod Maleate [*2002*] (teg″ a ser′ od mal′ ee ate). $C_{16}H_{23}N_5O \cdot C_4H_4O_4$. 417.46. (1) Hydrazinecarboximidamide, 2-[(5-methoxy-1*H*-indol-3-yl)methylene]-*N*-pentyl-, (2*Z*)-2-butenedioate (1:1); (2) 3-(5-Methoxy-1*H*-indol-3-ylmethylene)-*N*-pentylcarbazimidamide hydrogen maleate. *UNII-E5XNT3RF5A. CAS-189188-57-6. Treatment of gastrointestinal motility disorders (selective serotonin 5HT4antagonist).* Zelnorm (Novartis) ◇*HTF 919*

Teglicar. $C_{22}H_{45}N_3O_3$. 399.61. (3*R*)-3-[(Tetradecylaminocarbonyl)amino]-4-(trimethylazaniumyl)butanoate. *CAS-250694-07-6.* INN.

TEIB — *See* Triaziquone.

Teicoplanin [*1986*] (tye″ koe plan′ in). $C_{72-89}H_{68-99}Cl_2N_{8-9}O_{28-33}$. 1564.27-1893.71. Antibiotic obtained from cultures of *Actinoplanes teichomyceticus*, or the same substance produced by other means. (1) Teicoplanin; (2) Teicoplanin. *CAS-61036-62-2.* INN; BAN. *Antibacterial.* Targocid (Hoechst Marion Roussel) *[Note—See below for chemical names of components and structural formulas.]* ◇*MDL 507*

Teicoplanin A2-1. $C_{88}H_{95}Cl_2N_9O_{33}$. 1877.64. (1) (*Z*)-34-*O*-[2-(Acetylamino)-2-deoxy-β-D-glucopyranosyl]-22,31-dichloro-7-demethyl-64-*O*-demethyl-19-deoxy-56-*O*-[2-deoxy-2-[(1-oxo-4-decenyl)amino]-β-D-glucopyranosyl]42-*O*-α-D-mannopyranosylristomycin A aglycone; (2) (3*S*,15*R*,18*R*,34*R*,35*S*,38*S*,48*R*,50a*R*)-34-[(2-Acetamido-2-deoxy-β-D-glucopyranosyl)oxy]-15-amino-22,31-dichloro-56-[[2-(*Z*)-4-decenamido-2-deoxy-β-D-glucopyranosyl]oxy]-2,3,16,17,18,19,35,36,37,38,48,49,50,50a-tetradecahydro-6,11,40,44-tetrahydroxy-42-(α-D-mannopyranosyloxy)-2,16,36,50,51,59-hexaoxo-1*H*,15*H*,34*H*-20,23:30,33-dietheno-3,18:35,48-bis(iminomethano)-4,8:10,14:25,28:43,47-tetratheno-28*H*-[1,14,6,22]dioxadiazacyclooctacosino[4,5-*m*][10,2,16]benzoxadiazacyclotetracosine-38-carboxylic acid. *CAS-91032-34-7.*

Teicoplanin A2-2. $C_{88}H_{97}Cl_2N_9O_{33}$. 1879.66. (1) 34-*O*-[2-(Acetylamino)-2-deoxy-β-D-glucopyranosyl]-22,31-dichloro-7-demethyl-64-*O*-demethyl-19-deoxy-56-*O*-[2-deoxy-2-[(8-methyl-1-oxononyl)amino]-β-D-glucopyranosyl]-42-*O*-α-D-mannopyranosylristomycin A aglycone; (2) (3*S*,15*R*,18*R*,34*R*,35*S*,38*S*,48*R*,50a*R*)-34-[(2-Acetamido-2-deoxy-β-D-glucopyranosyl)oxy]-15-amino-22,31-dichloro-56-[[2-deoxy-2-(8-methylnonanamido)-β-D-glucopyranosyl]oxy]-2,3,16,17,18,19,35,36,37,38,48,49,50,50a-tetradecahydro-6,11,40,44-tetrahydroxy-42-(α-D-mannopyranosyloxy)-2,16,36,50,51,59-hexaoxo-1*H*,15*H*,34*H*-20,23:30,33-dietheno-3,18:35,48-bis(iminomethano)-4,8:10,14:25,28:43,47-tetratheno-28*H*-[1,14,6,22]dioxadiazacyclooctacosino[4,5-*m*][10,2,16]benzoxadiazacyclotetracosine-38-carboxylic acid. *CAS-91032-26-7.*

Teicoplanin A₂₋₃. C₈₈H₉₇Cl₂N₉O₃₃. 1879.66. (1) 34-*O*-[2-(Acetylamino)-2-deoxy-β-D-glucopyranosyl]-22,31-dichloro-7-demethyl-64-*O*-demethyl-19-deoxy-56-*O*-[2-deoxy-2-[(1-oxodecyl)amino]-β-D-glucopyranosyl]-42-*O*-α-D-mannopyranosylristomycin A aglycone; (2) (3*S*,15*R*,18*R*,34*R*,35*S*,38*S*,48*R*,50a*R*)-34-[(2-Acetamido-2-deoxy-β-D-glucopyranosyl)oxy]-15-amino-22,31-dichloro-56-[(2-decanamido-2-deoxy-β-D-glucopyranosyl)oxy]-2,3,16,17,18,19,35,36,37,38,48,49,50,50a-tetradecahydro-6,11,40,44-tetrahydroxy-42-(α-D-mannopyranosyloxy)-2,16,36,50,51,59-hexaoxo-1*H*,15*H*,34*H*-20,23:30,33-dietheno-3,18:35,48-bis(iminomethano)-4,8:10,14:25,28:43,47-tetrametheno-28*H*-[1,14,6,22]dioxadiazacyclooctacosino[4,5-*m*][10,2,16]benzoxadiazacyclotetracosine-38-carboxylic acid. *CAS-91032-36-9.*

Teicoplanin A₂₋₄. C₈₉H₉₉Cl₂N₉O₃₃. 1893.68. (1) 34-*O*-[2-(Acetylamino)-2-deoxy-β-D-glucopyranosyl]-22,31-dichloro-7-demethyl-64-*O*-demethyl-19-deoxy-56-*O*-[2-deoxy-2-[(8-methyl-1-oxodecyl)amino]-β-D-glucopyranosyl]-42-*O*-α-D-mannopyranosylristomycin A aglycone; (2) (3*S*,15*R*,18*R*,34*R*,35*S*,38*S*,48*R*,50a*R*)-34-[(2-Acetamido-2-deoxy-β-D-glucopyranosyl)oxy]-15-amino-22,31-dichloro-56-[[2-deoxy-2-(8-methyldecanamido)-β-D-glucopyranosyl]oxy]-2,3,16,17,18,19,35,36,37,38,48,49,50,50a-tetradecahydro-6,11,40,44-tetrahydroxy-42-(α-D-mannopyranosyloxy)-2,16,36,50,51,59-hexaoxo-1*H*,15*H*,34*H*-20,23:30,33-dietheno-3,18:35,48-bis(iminomethano)-4,8:10,14:25,28:43,47-tetrametheno-28*H*-[1,14,6,22]dioxadiazacyclooctacosino[4,5-*m*][10,2,16]benzoxadiazacyclotetracosine-38-carboxylic acid. *CAS-91032-37-0.*

Teicoplanin A₂₋₅. C₈₉H₉₉Cl₂N₉O₃₃. 1893.68. (1) 34-*O*-[2-(Acetylamino)-2-deoxy-β-D-glucopyranosyl]-22,31-dichloro-7-demethyl-64-*O*-demethyl-19-deoxy-56-*O*-[2-deoxy-2-[(9-methyl-1-oxodecyl)amino]-β-D-glucopyranosyl]-42-*O*-α-D-mannopyranosylristomycin A aglycone; (2) (3*S*,15*R*,18*R*,34*R*,35*S*,38*S*,48*R*,50a*R*)-34-[(2-Acetamido-2-deoxy-β-D-glucopyranosyl)oxy]-15-amino-22,31-dichloro-56-[[2-deoxy-2-(9-methyldecanamido)-β-D-glucopyranosyl]oxy]-2,3,16,17,18,19,35,36,37,38,48,49,50,50a-tetradecahydro-6,11,40,44-tetrahydroxy-42-(α-D-mannopyranosyloxy)-2,16,36,50,51,59-hexaoxo-1*H*,15*H*,34*H*-20,23:30,33-dietheno-3,18:35,48-bis(iminomethano)-4,8:10,14:25,28:43,47-tetrametheno-28*H*-[1,14,6,22]dioxadiazacyclooctacosino[4,5-*m*][10,2,16]benzoxadiazacyclotetracosine-38-carboxylic acid. *CAS-91032-38-1.*

Teicoplanin A₃₋₁. C₇₂H₆₈Cl₂N₈O₂₈. 1564.25. (1) 34-*O*-[2-(Acetylamino)-2-deoxy-β-D-glucopyranosyl]-22,31-dichloro-7-demethyl-64-*O*-demethyl-19-deoxy-42-*O*-α-D-mannopyranosylristomycin A aglycone; (2) (3*S*,15*R*,18*R*,34*R*,35*S*,38*S*,48*R*,50a*R*)-34-[(2-Acetamido-2-deoxy-β-D-glucopyranosyl)oxy]-15-amino-22,31-dichloro-2,3,16,17,18,19,35,36,37,38,48,49,50,50a-tetradecahydro-6,11,40,44,56-pentahydroxy-42-(α-D-mannopyranosyloxy)-2,16,36,50,51,59-hexaoxo-1*H*,15*H*,34*H*-20,23:30,33-dietheno-3,18:35,48-bis(iminomethano)-4,8:10,14:25,28:43,47-tetrametheno-28*H*-[1,14,6,22]dioxadiazacyclooctacosino[4,5-*m*][10,2,16]benzoxadiazacyclotetracosine-38-carboxylic acid. *CAS-93616-27-4.*

Telaprevir [*2006*] (tel a′ pre vir). C₃₆H₅₃N₇O₆. 679.85. (1) Cyclopenta[*c*]pyrrole-1-carboxamide, (2*S*)-2-cyclohexyl-*N*-(pyrazinylcarbonyl)glycyl-3-methyl-L-valyl-*N*-[(1*S*)-1-[(cyclopropylamino)oxoacetyl]butyl]octahydro-, (1*S*,3a*R*,6a*S*)-; (2) (1*S*,3a*R*,6a*S*)-2-[(2*S*)-2-[[(2*S*)-Cyclohexyl[(pyrazinylcarbonyl)amino]acetyl]amino]-3,3-dimethylbutanoyl]-*N*-[(1*S*)-1-[(cyclopropylamino)oxoacetyl]butyl] octahydrocyclopenta[*c*]pyrrole-1-carboxamide.

UNII-655M5O3W0U. CAS-402957-28-2. INN. *Treatment of hepatitis C viral infection.* ◇*VX-950; LY-570310; VRT-111950; MP-424*

Telatinib. C₂₀H₁₆ClN₅O₃. 409.83. 4-[({4-[(4-Chlorophenyl)amino]furo[2,3-*d*]pyridazin-7-yl}oxy)methyl]-*N*-methylpyridine-2-carboxamide. *CAS-332012-40-5.* INN.

Telavancin Hydrochloride [*2004*] (tel″ a van′ sin hye″ droe klor′ ide). C₈₀H₁₀₆Cl₂N₁₁O₂₇P.HCl. 1792.10. [Telavancin is INN.] (1) Vancomycin, *N*³″-[2-(decylamino)ethyl]-29-[[(phosphonomethyl)amino]methyl]-, monohydrochloride; (2) (3*S*,6*R*,7*R*,22*R*,23*S*,26*S*,36*R*,38a*R*)-3-(2-Amino-2-oxoethyl)-10,19-dichloro-44-[[2-*O*-[3-[[2-(decylamino)ethyl]amino]-3-*C*-methyl-2,3,6-trideoxy-α-L-*lyxo*-hexopyranosyl]-β-D-glucopyranosyl]oxy]-7,22,28,30,32-pentahydroxy-6-[[(2*R*)-4-methyl-2-(methylamino)pentanoyl]amino]-2,5,24,38,39-pentaoxo-29-[[(phosphonomethyl)amino]methyl]-2,3,4,5,6,7,23,24,25,26,36,37,38,38a-tetradecahydro-8,11:18,21-dietheno-23,36-(iminomethano)-22*H*-13,16:31,35-dimetheno-1*H*,13*H*-[1,6,9]oxadiazacyclohexadecino[4,5-*m*][10,2,16]benzoxadiazacyclotetracosine-26-carboxylic acid monohydrochloride. *CAS-560130-42-9; CAS-372151-71-8 [telavancin]. Antibacterial agent active against gram-positive pathogens.* ◇*Td-6424*

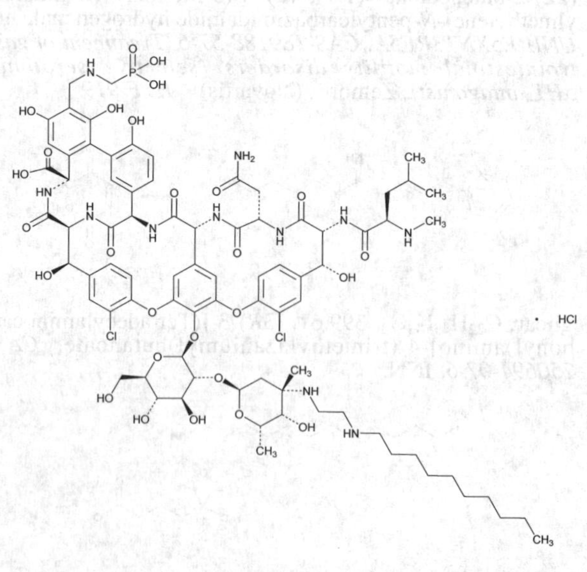

Telbermin [*2000*] (tel ber′ min). C₁₆₁₂H₂₅₆₈N₅₀₀O₄₉₈S₄₄. 38,200 daltons. (1) Vascular endothelial growth factor; (2) Vascular endothelial growth factor (human), dimer.

CAS-205887-54-3. INN. *Angiogenesis, vascular reactivity (recombinant human endothelial growth factor).* ◇*rhVEGF*

APMAEGGGQN HHEVVKFMDV YQRSYCHPIE TLVDIFQEYP DEIEYIFKPS
CVPLMRCGGC CNDEGLECVP TEESNITMQI MRIKPHQGQH IGEMSFLQHN
KCECRPKKDR ARQENPCGPC SERRKHLFVQ DPQTCKCSCK NTDSRCKARQ
LELNERTCRC DKPRR

↳ disulfide

Telbivudine [*2002*] (tel biv′ ue deen). $C_{10}H_{14}N_2O_5$. 242.23. (1) 2,4(1*H*,3*H*)-Pyrimidinedione, 1-(2-deoxy-β-L-*erythro*-pentofuranosyl)-5-methyl-; (2) 2′-Deoxy-L-thymidine. *UNII-2OC4HKD3SF. CAS-3424-98-4.* INN; BAN. *Antiviral (treatment of hepatitis B infection).* Tyzeka (Idenix) ◇*NV-02B*

Telcagepant [*2008*] (tel ka′ je pant). $C_{26}H_{27}F_5N_6O_3$. 566.52. (1) 1-Piperidinecarboxamide, *N*-[(3*R*,6*S*)-6-(2,3-difluoro-phenyl)hexahydro-2-oxo-1-(2,2,2-trifluoroethyl)-1*H*-aze-pin-3-yl]-4-(2,3-dihydro-2-oxo-1*H*-imidazo[4,5-*b*]pyridin-1-yl)-; (2) *N*-[(3*R*,6*S*)-6-(2,3-Difluorophenyl)-2-oxo-1-(2,2,2-trifluoroethyl)hexahydro-1*H*-azepin-3-yl]-4-(2-oxo-2,3-dihydro-1*H*-imidazo[4,5-*b*]pyridin-1-yl)piperidine-1-carboxamide. *UNII-D42O649ALL. CAS-781649-09-0. Treatment of migraine.*

Telcagepant Potassium [*2008*] (tel ka′ je pant poe tas′ ee um). $C_{26}H_{26}F_5KN_6O_3 \cdot C_2H_6O$. 650.68. (1) 1-Piperidinecar-boxamide, *N*-[(3*R*,6*S*)-6-(2,3-difluorophenyl)hexahydro-2-oxo-1-(2,2,2-trifluoroethyl)-1*H*-azepin-3-yl]-4-(2,3-dihy-dro-2-oxo-1*H*-imidazo[4,5-*b*]pyridin-1-yl)-, compd. with ethanol, potassium salt (1:1:1); (2) Potassium 1-(1-{[(3*R*,6*S*)-6-(2,3-difluorophenyl)-2-oxo-1-(2,2,2-trifluor-oethyl)hexahydro-1*H*-azepin-3-yl]carbamoyl}piperidin-4-yl)-1*H*-imidazo[4,5-*b*]pyridin-2-olate compound with etha-nol (1:1). *CAS-953077-35-5. Treatment of migraine.*

Telenzepine. $C_{19}H_{22}N_4O_2S$. 370.47. 4,9-Dihydro-3-methyl-4-[(4-methyl-1-piperazinyl)acetyl]-10*H*-thieno[3,4-*b*][1,5]benzodiazepin-10-one. *UNII-0990EG3K10. CAS-80880-90-6.* INN.

Telimomab Aritox. Ricin A chain-antibody T 101 Fab fragment immunotoxin. *CAS-117305-33-6.* INN.

Telinavir [*1995*] (tel in′ a vir). $C_{33}H_{44}N_6O_5$. 604.74. (1) Butanediamide, N^1-[3-[[[(1,1-dimethylethyl)amino]carbo-nyl](2-methylpropyl)amino]-2-hydroxy-1-(phenylmethyl)-propyl]-2-[(2-quinolinylcarbonyl)amino]-, [1*S*-

[1*R**(*R**),2*S**]]-; (2) (2*S*)-*N*-[(1*S*,2*R*)-1-Benzyl-3-(3-*tert*-butyl-1-isobutylureido)-2-hydroxypropyl]-2-quinaldami-dosuccinamide. *UNII-IZF55EH3CG. CAS-143224-34-4.* INN. *Antiviral.* ◇*SC-52151*

Telithromycin [*2004*] (tel ith″ roe mye′ sin). $C_{43}H_{65}N_5O_{10}$. 812.00. (1) Erythromycin, 3-de[(2,6-dideoxy-3-*C*-methyl-3-*O*-methyl-α-L-*ribo*-hexopyranosyl)oxy]-11,12-dideoxy-6-*O*-methyl-3-oxo-12,11-[oxycarbonyl[[4-[4-(3-pyridi-nyl)-1*H*-imidazol-1-yl]butyl]imino]-; (2) (3a*S*,4*R*,7*R*,9*R*,10*R*,11*R*,13*R*,15*R*,15a*R*)-4-Ethyl-11-me-thoxy-3a,7,9,11,13,15-hexamethyl-1-[4-[4-(pyridin-3-yl)-1*H*-imidazol-1-yl]butyl]-10-[[3,4,6-trideoxy-3-(dimethyla-mino)-β-D-*xylo*-hexopyranosyl]oxy]octahydro-2*H*-oxac-yclotetradecino[4,3-*d*]oxazole-2,6,8,14(1*H*,7*H*,9*H*)-te-trone. *UNII-KI8H7H19WL. CAS-191114-48-4; CAS-173838-31-8.* INN; BAN. *Antimicrobial (via inhibition of bacterial protein synthesis).* Ketek (Sanofi Aventis) ◇*HMR 3647*

Telmesteine. $C_7H_{11}NO_4S$. 205.23. (-)-3-Ethyl hydrogen (*R*)-3,4-thiazolidinedicarboxylate. *UNII-124I3FE35T. CAS-122946-43-4.* INN.

Telmisartan [*1997*] (tel″ mi sar′ tan). $C_{33}H_{30}N_4O_2$. 514.62. (1) [1,1′-Biphenyl]-2-carboxylic acid, 4′-[[1,4′-dimethyl-2′-propyl[2,6′-bi-1*H*-benzimidazol]-1′-yl)methyl]-; (2) 4′-[[4-Methyl-6-(1-methyl-2-benzimidazolyl)-2-propyl-1-benzimidazolyl]methyl]-2-biphenylcarboxylic acid. *UNII-*

---

† Brand name formerly used, and/or firm no longer concerned with this product.

U5SYW473RQ. CAS-144701-48-4. INN; BAN. *Antagonist (angiotensin II receptor); antihypertensive.* Micardis (Boehringer Ingelheim) ◇*BIBR 277 SE*

Teloxantrone Hydrochloride [*1992*] (tel ox′ an trone hye″ droe klor′ ide). $C_{21}H_{25}N_5O_4 \cdot 2HCl \cdot H_2O$. 502.39. [Teloxantrone is INN.](1) Anthra[1,9-*cd*]pyrazol-6(2*H*)-one, 7,10-dihydroxy-2-[2-[(2-hydroxyethyl)amino]ethyl]-5-[[2-(methylamino)ethyl]amino]-, dihydrochloride, monohydrate; (2) 7,10-Dihydroxy-2-[2-[(2-hydroxyethyl)amino]ethyl]-5-[[2-(methylamino)ethyl]amino]anthra[1,9-*cd*]pyrazol-6(2*H*)-one, dihydrochloride, monohydrate. *UNII-7ZQK8VIO6V; UNII-96521WL61B* [teloxantrone]. *CAS-132937-88-3; CAS-91441-48-4* [teloxantrone]. *Antineoplastic. [Name previously used: Moxantrazole.]* ◇*DUP 937; NSC-355644*

Teludipine Hydrochloride [*1991*] (tel oo′ di peen hye″ droe klor′ ide). $C_{28}H_{38}N_2O_6 \cdot HCl$. 535.07. [Teludipine is INN and BAN.](1) 3,5-Pyridinedicarboxylic acid, 2-[(dimethylamino)methyl]-4-[2-[3-(1,1-dimethylethoxy)-3-oxo-1-propenyl]phenyl]-1,4-dihydro-6-methyl-, diethyl ester, monohydrochloride, (*E*)-; (2) 4-[*o*-[(*E*)-2-Carboxyvinyl]phenyl]-2-[(dimethylamino)methyl]-1,4-dihydro-6-methyl-3,5-pyridinedicarboxylic acid, 4-*tert*-butyl diethyl ester, monohydrochloride. *UNII-7P6B96QLKN. CAS-108700-03-4; CAS-108687-08-7* [teludipine]. *Antagonist (calcium channel); antihypertensive. [USAN previously used: Taludipine Hydrochloride.]* ◇*GR 53992B (GX 1296B)*

Temafloxacin Hydrochloride [*1988*] (tem″ a flox′ a sin hye″ droe klor′ ide). $C_{21}H_{18}F_3N_3O_3 \cdot HCl$. 453.84. [Temafloxacin is INN and BAN.] (1) 3-Quinolinecarboxylic acid, 1-(2,4-difluorophenyl)-6-fluoro-1,4-dihydro-7-(3-methyl-1-piperazinyl)-4-oxo-, monohydrochloride, (±)-; (2) (±)-1-(2,4-Difluorophenyl)-6-fluoro-1,4-dihydro-7-(3-methyl-1-piperazinyl)-4-oxo-3-quinolinecarboxylic acid, monohydrochloride. *UNII-OC5IGJ7J6I. CAS-105784-61-0; CAS-*

108319-06-8 [temafloxacin]. *Antibacterial (microbial DNA topoisomerase inhibitor).* Omniflox (Abbott†) ◇*Abbott-62254*

Temarotene. $C_{23}H_{28}$. 304.47. 1,2,3,4-Tetrahydro-1,1,4,4-tetramethyl-6-[(*E*)-α-methylstyryl]naphthalene. *UNII-A28G39IJ7K. CAS-75078-91-0.* INN.

Tematropium Methylsulfate [*1990*] (tem″ a troe′ pee um meth″ il sul′ fate). $C_{21}H_{31}NO_8S$. 457.54. [Tematropium Metilsulfate is INN.] (1) 8-Azoniabicyclo[3.2.1]octane, 3-(3-ethoxy-1,3-dioxo-2-phenylpropoxy)-8,8-dimethyl-, *endo*-(±)-, methyl sulfate; (2) 3α-Hydroxy-8-methyl-1αH,5αH-tropanium methyl sulfate (salt), (±)-ethyl hydrogen phenylmalonate. *CAS-113932-41-5. Anticholinergic.* ◇*HGP-6; CDDD 3602*

Temazepam [*1969*] (tem az′ e pam). **USP**. $C_{16}H_{13}ClN_2O_2$. 300.74. (1) 2*H*-1,4-Benzodiazepin-2-one, 7-chloro-1,3-dihydro-3-hydroxy-1-methyl-5-phenyl-; (2) 7-Chloro-1,3-dihydro-3-hydroxy-1-methyl-5-phenyl-2*H*-1,4-benzodiazepin-2-one. *UNII-CHB1QD2QSS. CAS-846-50-4.* INN; BAN. *Tranquilizer (minor).* Restoril (Tyco) ◇*Wy-3917*

Temefos [*1974*] (tem′ e fos). $C_{16}H_{20}O_6P_2S_3$. 466.47. (1) Phosphorothioic acid, *O,O′*-(thiodi-4,1-phenylene) *O,O,O′,O′*-tetramethyl ester; (2) *O,O′*-(Thiodi-*p*-phenylene) *O,O,O′,O′*-tetramethyl bis(phosphorothioate). *UNII-ONP3ME32DL. CAS-3383-96-8.* INN. *Ectoparasiticide (veterinary).* ◇*27165*

Temelastine [*1986*] (tem″ e las′ teen). $C_{21}H_{24}BrN_5O$. 442.35. (1) 4(1*H*)-Pyrimidinone, 2-[[4-(5-bromo-3-methyl-2-pyridinyl)butyl]amino]-5-[(6-methyl-3-pyridinyl)methyl]-; (2)

2-[[4-(5-Bromo-3-methyl-2-pyridyl)butyl]amino]-5-[(6-methyl-3-pyridyl)methyl]-4(1*H*)-pyrimidinone. *UNII-BF6IGI53XH. CAS-86181-42-2.* INN; BAN. *Antihistaminic.* ◇*SK&F 93944*

Temiverine. $C_{24}H_{35}NO_3$. 385.54. 4-(Diethylamino)-1,1-dimethyl-2-butynyl ($\pm$)-α-phenylcyclohexaneglycolate. *CAS-173324-94-2.* INN.

Temocapril Hydrochloride [*1993*] (tem oh′ ka pril hye″ droe klor′ ide). $C_{23}H_{28}N_2O_5S_2$·HCl. 513.07. [Temocapril is INN and BAN.] (1) 1,4-Thiazepine-4-(5*H*)-acetic acid, 6-[[1-(ethoxycarbonyl)-3-phenylpropyl]amino]tetrahydro-5-oxo-2-(2-thienyl)-, monohydrochloride, [2*S*-[2α,6β(*R**)]]-; (2) (+)-(2*S*,6*R*)-6-[[(1*S*)-1-Carboxy-3-phenylpropyl]amino]tetrahydro-5-oxo-2-(2-thienyl)-1,4-thiazepine-4(5*H*)-acetic acid, 6-ethyl ester, monohydrochloride. *CAS-110221-44-8; CAS-111902-57-9* [temocapril]. JAN. *Antihypertensive.* ◇*CS-622*

Temocaprilat. $C_{21}H_{24}N_2O_5S_2$. 448.56. (+)-(2*S*,6*R*)-6-[[(1*S*)-1-carboxy-3-phenylpropyl]amino]tetrahydro-5-oxo-2-(2-thienyl)-1,4-thiazepine-4(5*H*)-acetic acid. *UNII-2D6A12Q12R. CAS-110221-53-9.* INN; BAN. ◇*RNH-5139*

Temocillin [*1985*] (tem″ oh sil′ in). $C_{16}H_{18}N_2O_7S_2$. 414.45. (1) 4-Thia-1-azabicyclo[3.2.0]heptane-2-carboxylic acid, 6-[(carboxy-3-thienylacetyl)amino]-6-methoxy-3,3-dimethyl-7-oxo-, [2*S*-(2α,5α,6α)]-; (2) *N*-[(2*S*,5*R*,6*S*)-2-Carboxy-6-methoxy-3,3-dimethyl-7-oxo-4-thia-1-azabicyclo[3.2.0]hept-6-yl]-3-thiophenemalonamic acid. *UNII-03QB156W6I. CAS-66148-78-5; CAS-61545-06-0* [temocillin sodium]. INN; BAN. *Antibacterial.* ◇*BRL 17421 [as sodium]*

Temodox [*1975*] (tem′ oh dox). $C_{12}H_{12}N_2O_5$. 264.23. (1) 2-Quinoxalinecarboxylic acid, 3-methyl-, 2-hydroxyethyl ester, 1,4-dioxide; (2) 2-Hydroxyethyl 3-methyl-2-quinoxalinecarboxylate 1,4-dioxide. *UNII-5P41KX11BT. CAS-34499-96-2.* INN. *Growth stimulant (veterinary).* ◇*CP-22,341*

Temoporfin [*1995*] (tem″ oh pore′ fin). $C_{44}H_{32}N_4O_4$. 680.75. (1) Phenol, 3,3′,3″,3‴-(7,8-dihydro-21*H*,23*H*-porphine-5,10,15,20-tetrayl)tetrakis-; (2) 3,3′,3″,3‴-(7,8-Dihydroporphyrin-5,10,15,20-tetrayl)tetraphenol. *CAS-122341-38-2.* INN; BAN. *Antineoplastic.* ◇*EF9*

Temozolomide [*1999*] (tem″ oh zoe′ loe mide). $C_6H_6N_6O_2$. 194.15. (1) Imidazo[5,1-*d*]-1,2,3,5-tetrazine-8-carboxamide, 3,4-dihydro-3-methyl-4-oxo-; (2) 3,4-Dihydro-3-methyl-4-oxoimidazo[5,1-*d*]-*as*-tetrazine-8-carboxamide. *UNII-YF1K15M17Y. CAS-85622-93-1.* INN; BAN. *Treatment of recurrent high-grade gliomas and advanced metastatic melanoma (alkylating agent).* Temodar (Schering) ◇*SCH 52365; M&B 39831; CCRG-81045; NSC-362856*

Temsirolimus [*2004*] (tem″ sir oh′ li mus). $C_{56}H_{87}NO_{16}$. 1030.29. (1) Rapamycin, 42-[3-hydroxy-2-(hydroxymethyl)-2-methylpropanoate]; (2) (3*S*,6*R*,7*E*,9-*R*,10*R*,12*R*,14*S*,15*E*,17*E*,19*E*,21*S*,23*S*,26*R*,27*R*,34a*S*)-9,10,12,13,14,21,22,23,24,25,26,27,32,33,34,34a-Hexadecahydro-9,27-dihydroxy-3-[(1*R*)-2-[(1*S*,3*R*,4*R*)-4-hydroxy-3-methoxycyclohexyl]-1-methylethyl]-10,21-dimethoxy-6,8,12,14,20,26-hexamethyl-23,27-epoxy-3*H*-pyrido[2,1-*c*][1,4]oxaazacyclohentriacontine-1,5,11,28,29(4*H*,6*H*,31*H*)-pentone 4′-[2,2-bis(hydroxymethyl)propionate]; (3) Rapamycin 42-[2,2-bis(hydroxy-methyl)propionate]. *CAS-162635-04-3.* INN; BAN; JAN. *Antineoplastic (mTOR inhibitor).* ◇*CCI-779*

Temurtide [*1989*] (tem′ ure tide). $C_{20}H_{34}N_4O_{12}$. 522.50. (1) D-α-Glutamine, N^2-[*N*-(*N*-acetylmuramoyl)-L-threonyl]-; (2) 2-Acetamido-3-*O*-[[(1*R*)-1-[(1*S*,2*R*)-1-[[(1*R*)-1-carba-moyl-3-carboxypropyl]carbamoyl]-2-hydroxypropyl]car-bamoyl]ethyl]-2-deoxy-D-glucopyranose. *CAS-66112-59-2.* INN; BAN. *Vaccine adjuvant.* ◇*RS-37449*

Tenamfetamine. $C_{10}H_{13}NO_2$. 179.22. (±)-α-Methyl-3,4-(methylenedioxy)phenethylamine. *CAS-51497-09-7.* INN.

Tenatoprazole. $C_{16}H_{18}N_4O_3S$. 346.40. (±)-5-Methoxy-2-[[(4-methoxy-3,5-dimethyl-2-pyridyl)methyl]sulfinyl]-1*H*-imi-dazo[4,5-*b*]pyridine. *CAS-113712-98-4.* INN.

Tenatumomab. Immunoglobulin G2b, anti-[human tenascin C (TNC, hexabrachion, HBX) *Mus musculus*] monoclonal antibody ST2146; gamma2b heavy chain (*Mus musculus* VH [8.8.13]-IGHG2B*02 from clone ST2146) (135-219′)-disulfide with kappa light chain (*Mus musculus* V-KAPPA [11.3.9]-IGKC*01 from clone ST 2146); (229-229″:232-232″:235-235″:238-238″)-tetradisulfide dimer. *CAS-592557-43-2* [light chain]; *CAS-592557-41-0* [heavy chain]. INN.

Tendamistat. An α-amylase inhibiting polypeptide obtained from cultures of *Streptomyces tendae.* INN.

Tenecteplase [*1997*] (ten ek′ te plase). $C_{2558}H_{3872}N_{738}O_{781}S_{40}\cdot$103-L-Asparagine-117-L-glutamine-296-L-alanine-297-L-alanine-298-L-alanine-299-L-alanineplasminogen activator (human tissue type). Molecular weight is approximately

58,742 daltons (polypeptide portion only). *UNII-WGD229O42W. CAS-191588-94-0.* INN; BAN. *Treatment of acute thrombotic disorders.* ◇*TNK-tPA*

```
SYQVICRDEK TQMIYQQHQS WLRPVLRSNR VEYCWCNSGR AQCHSVPVKS
CSEPRCFNGG TCQQALYFSD FVCQCPEGFA GKCCEIDTRA TCYEDQGISY
RGNWSTAESG AECTNWQSSA LAQKPYSGRR PDAIRLGLGN HNYCRNPDRD
SKPWCYVFKA GKYSSEFCST PACSEGNSDC YFGNGSAYRG THSLTESGAS
CLPWNSMILI GKVYTAQNPS AQALGLGKHN YCRNPDGDAK PWCHVLKNRR
LTWEYCDVPS CSTCGLRQYS QPQFRIKGGL FADIASHPWQ AAIFAAAAAS
PGERFLCGGI LISSCWILSA AHCFQERFPP HHLTVILGRT YRVVPGEEEQ
KFEVEKYIVH KEFDDDTYDN DIALLQLKSD SSRCAQESSV VRTVCLPPAD
LQLPDWTECE LSGYGKHEAL SPFYSERLKE AHVRLYPSSR CTSQHLLNRT
VTDNMLCAGD TRSGGPQANL HDACQGDSGG PLVCLNDGRM TLVGIISWGL
GCGQKDVPGV YTKVTNYLDW IRDNMRP
```

Tenegliptin. **C22H30N6OS**. {(2*S*,4*S*)-4-[4-(3-Methyl-1-phenyl-1*H*-pyrazol-5-yl)piperazin-1-yl]pyrrolidin-2-yl}(1,3-thiazolidin-3-yl)methanone. *CAS-760937-92-6.* INN.

Teneliximab [*2002*] (ten″ e lix′ i mab). Immunoglobulin G1, anti-[human CD40 (antigen)] (human-mouse monoclonal chi220 γ1-chain), disulfide with human-mouse monoclonal chi220 light chain, dimer. Molecular weight is approxi-mately 73,046 daltons. *CAS-299423-37-3.* INN. *Treatment of auto-immune diseases and prevention of organ trans-plant rejection.* ◇*BMS-224819*

Tenidap [*1990*] (ten′ i dap). $C_{14}H_9ClN_2O_3S$. 320.75. (1) 1*H*-Indole-1-carboxamide, 5-chloro-2,3-dihydro-3-(hydroxy-2-thienylmethylene)-2-oxo-, (*Z*)-; (2) (*Z*)-5-Chloro-3-(α-hydroxy-2-thenylidene)-2-oxo-1-indolinecarboxamide. *CAS-120210-48-2.* INN; BAN. *Anti-inflammatory (os-teoarthritis and rheumatoid arthritis).* ◇*CP-66,248*

Tenidap Sodium [*1990*] (ten′ i dap soe′ dee um). $C_{14}H_8ClN_2NaO_3S$. 342.73. (1) 1*H*-Indole-1-carboxamide, 5-chloro-2,3-dihydro-3-(hydroxy-2-thienylmethylene)-2-oxo-, monosodium salt, (*Z*)-; (2) (*Z*)-5-Chloro-3-(α-hy-droxy-2-thenylidene)-2-oxo-1-indolinecarboxamide, monosodium salt. *UNII-DCV1328NH2. CAS-119784-94-0.* *Anti-inflammatory (osteoarthritis and rheumatoid arthri-tis).* ◇*CP-66,248-2*

Tenilapine. $C_{17}H_{16}N_4S_2$. 340.47. (*E*)-5-(4-Methyl-1-piperazi-nyl)-9*H*-dithieno[3,4-*b*:3′,4′-*e*]-azepine-$\Delta^{9,\alpha}$-acetonitrile. *UNII-D0U312O2BE. CAS-82650-83-7.* INN.

Teniloxazine. $C_{16}H_{19}NO_2S$. 289.39. (±)-2-[[(α-2-Thienyl-*o*-tolyl)oxy]methyl]morpholine. *UNII-95Q6WNP25P*. *CAS-62473-79-4*. INN; MI.

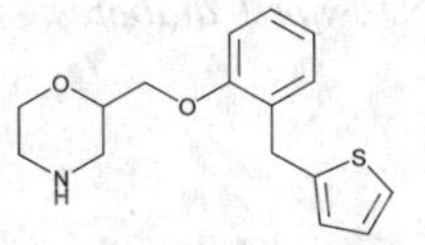

Tenilsetam. $C_8H_{10}N_2OS$. 182.24. (±)-3-(2-Thienyl)-2-piperazinone. *UNII-O4Q7XM74N6*. *CAS-86696-86-8*. INN.

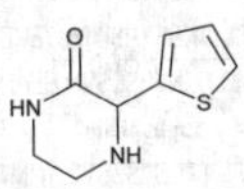

Teniposide [*1978*] (ten″ i poe′ side). $C_{32}H_{32}O_{13}S$. 656.65. (1) Furo[3′,4′:6,7]naphtho[2,3-*d*]-1,3-dioxol-6(5a*H*)-one, 5,8,8a,9-tetrahydro-5-(4-hydroxy-3,5-dimethoxyphenyl)-9-[[4,6-*O*-(2-thienylmethylene)-β-D-glucopyranosyl]-oxy]-, [5*R*-[5α,5aβ,8aα,9β(*R**)]]-; (2) 4′-Demethylepipodophyllotoxin 9-[4,6-*O*-(*R*)-2-thenylidene-β-D-glucopyranoside]. *UNII-957E6438QA*. *CAS-29767-20-2*. INN; BAN. *Antineoplastic*. Vumon (Bristol-Myers Squibb) ✧*VM-26*

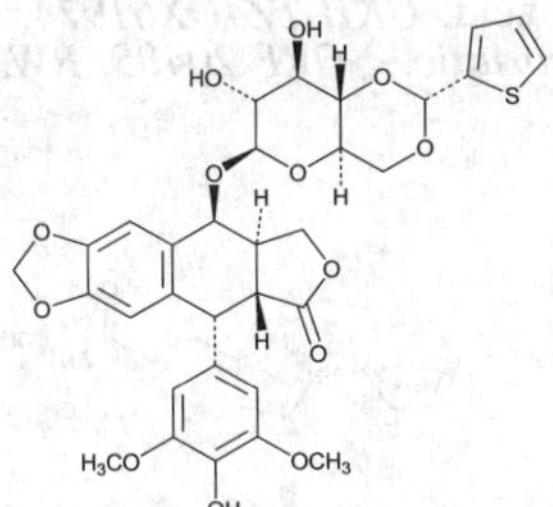

Tenivastatin Calcium [*2002*] (ten i″ va stat′ in kal′ see um). $C_{50}H_{78}CaO_{12}$. 911.23 (anhydrous). [Tenivastatin is INN.] (1) 1-Naphthaleneheptanoic acid, 8-(2,2-dimethyl-1-oxobutoxy)-1,2,6,7,8,8a-hexahydro-β,δ-dihydroxy-2,6-dimethyl-, calcium salt, (2:1), (βR,δR,1*S*,2*S*,6*R*,8*S*,8a*R*)-; (2) Calcium (3*R*,5*R*)-7-[(1*S*,2*S*,6*R*,8*S*,8a*R*)-8-(2,2-dimethylbutyryloxy)-2,6-dimethyl-1,2,6,7,8,8a-hexahydronaphthalen-1-yl]-3,5-dihydroxyheptanoate (1:2). *UNII-YNO268EI8T*. *CAS-151006-18-7* [anhydrous]; *CAS-121009-77-6* [tenivastatin]. *Antihyperlipidemic (HMG-CoA reductase inhibitor)*.

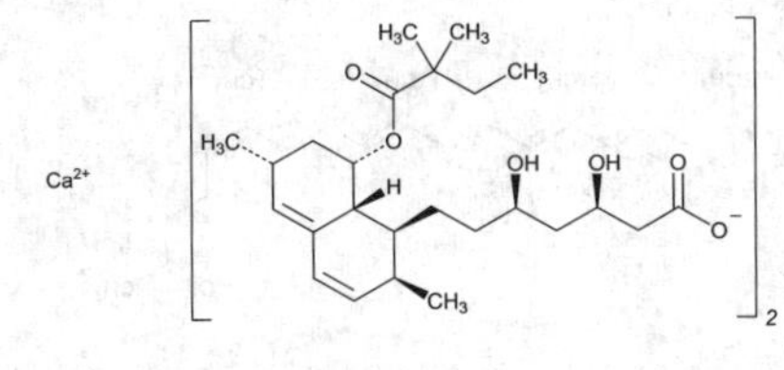

Tenocyclidine. $C_{15}H_{23}NS$. 249.41. 1-[1-(2-Thienyl)cyclohexyl]piperidine. *CAS-21500-98-1*. INN.

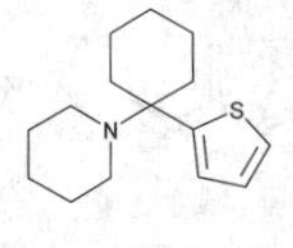

Tenofovir [*1999*] (ten of′ oh vir). $C_9H_{14}N_5O_4P.H_2O$. 305.23. (1) (*R*)-[[2-(6-Amino-9*H*-purin-9-yl)-1-methylethoxy]-methyl]phosphonic acid monohydrate; (2) [[(*R*)-2-(6-Amino-9*H*-purin-9-yl)-1-methylethoxy]methyl]phosphonic acid, monohydrate; (3) 9-[(*R*)-2-(Phosphonomethoxy)propyl]adenine monohydrate. *UNII-99YXE507IL*. *CAS-147127-20-6*. INN; BAN. *Antiviral (reverse transcriptase inhibitor)*. ✧*GS-1278; PMPA*

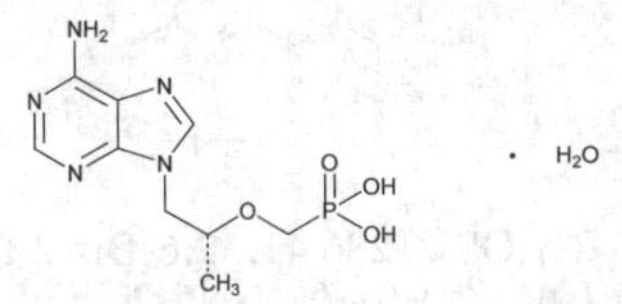

Tenofovir Disoproxil Fumarate [*1999*] (ten of′ oh vir dye″ soe prox′ il fue′ ma rate). $C_{19}H_{30}N_5O_{10}P.C_4H_4O_4$. 635.51. (1) (*R*)-5-[[2-(6-Amino-9*H*-purin-9-yl)-1-methylethoxy]-methyl]-2,4,6,8-tetraoxa-5-phosphanonanedioic acid, bis(1-methylethyl) ester, 5-oxide, (*E*)-2-butenedioate (1:1); (2) Bis(hydroxymethyl) [[(*R*)-2-(6-amino-9*H*-purin-9-yl)-1-methylethoxy]methyl]phosphonate, bis(isopropyl carbonate) (ester), fumarate (1:1); (3) 9-[(*R*)-2-[[Bis[[(isopropoxycarbonyl)oxy]methoxy]phosphinyl]methoxy]propyl]adenine fumarate (1:1). *UNII-OTT9J7900I*. *CAS-202138-50-9*. *Antiviral (reverse transcriptase inhibitor)*. Viread (Gilead Sciences) ✧*GS-4331-05; PMPA Prodrug*

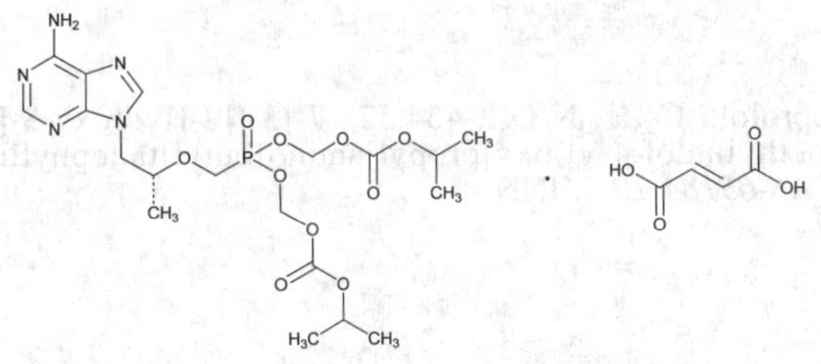

Tenonitrozole. $C_8H_5N_3O_3S_2$. 255.27. *N*-(5-Nitro-2-thiazolyl)-2-thiophenecarboxamide. *CAS-3810-35-3*. INN; MI.

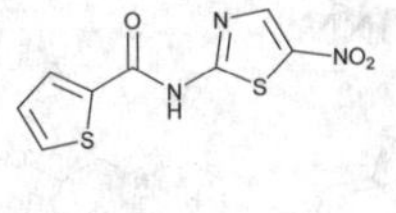

Tenosal. $C_{12}H_8O_4S$. 248.25. 2-Thiophenecarboxylic acid, ester with salicylic acid. *UNII-EEK88K197T*. *CAS-95232-68-1*. INN.

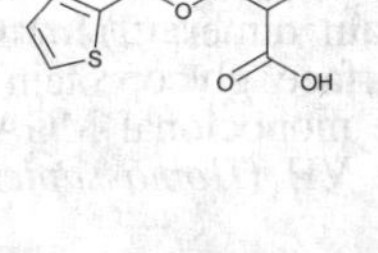

† Brand name formerly used, and/or firm no longer concerned with this product.

894 **TENOS–TEPRO** *USP Dictionary of USAN and International Drug Names*

Tenosiprol. $C_{10}H_{11}NO_4S$. 241.26. (*R*)-4-Hydroxy-L-proline 2-thiophenecarboxylate (ester). *UNII-3E44064G8N. CAS-129336-81-8.* INN.

Tenoxicam [*1987*] (ten ox' i kam). $C_{13}H_{11}N_3O_4S_2$. 337.37. (1) 2*H*-Thieno[2,3-*e*]-1,2-thiazine-3-carboxamide, 4-hydroxy-2-methyl-*N*-2-pyridinyl-, 1,1-dioxide; (2) 4-Hydroxy-2-methyl-*N*-2-pyridyl-2*H*-thieno[2,3-*e*]-1,2-thiazine-3-carboxamide 1,1-dioxide. *UNII-Z1R9N0A399. CAS-59804-37-4.* INN; BAN; JAN. *Anti-inflammatory.* ◇*Ro 12-0068/000*

Tenylidone. $C_{16}H_{14}OS_2$. 286.41. 2,6-Bis(2-thenylidene)cyclohexanone. *CAS-893-01-6.* INN; DCF.

Teopranitol. $C_{16}H_{22}N_6O_7$. 410.38. 1,4:3,6-Dianhydro-2-deoxy-2-[[3-(1,2,3,6-tetrahydro-1,3-dimethyl-2,6-dioxopurin-7-yl)propyl]amino]-L-iditol 5-nitrate. *UNII-631R1KON85. CAS-81792-35-0.* INN.

Teoprolol. $C_{23}H_{30}N_6O_4$. 454.52. 7-[3-[[2-Hydroxy-3-[(2-methylindol-4-yl)oxy]propyl]amino]butyl]theophylline. *CAS-65184-10-3.* INN.

Tepirindole. $C_{16}H_{19}ClN_2$. 274.79. 5-Chloro-3-(1,2,3,6-tetrahydro-1-propyl-4-pyridyl)indole. *UNII-X235XX30GK. CAS-72808-81-2.* INN.

Teplizumab [*2006*] (tep liz' oo mab). $C_{6462}H_{9938}N_{1738}O_{2022}S_{46}$. (1) Immunoglobulin G1, anti-(human CD3 (antigen) ε-chain) (human-mouse monoclonal MGA031 heavy chain), disulfide with human-mouse monoclonal MGA031 light-chain, dimer; (2) Immunoglobulin G1, anti-(human T-cell surface glycoprotein CD3 epsilon chain) humanized mouse monoclonal MGA031; gamma1 heavy chain [humanized VH (*Homo sapiens* FR/*Mus musculus* CDR)-[117-alanine,118-alanine]*Homo sapiens* IGHG1] (222-213')-disulfide with kappa light chain [humanized V-KAPPA (*Homo sapiens* FR/*Mus musculus* CDR)-*Homo sapiens* IGKC]; (228-228″:231-231″)-bisdisulfide dimer. Molecular weight is approximately 145,800 daltons. *CAS-876387-05-2.* INN. *Type 1 diabetes.* ◇*MGA031*

Heavy chain

```
QVQLVQSGGG VVQPGRSLRL SCKASGYTFT RYTMHWVRQA PGKGLEWIGY
INPSRGYTNY NQKVKDRFTI SRDNSKNTAF LQMDSLRPED TGVYFCARYY
DDHYCLDYWG QGTPVTVSSA STKGPSVFPL APSSKSTSGG TAALGCLVKD
YFPEPVTVSW NSGALTSGVH TFPAVLQSSG LYSLSSVVTV PSSSLGTQTY
ICNVNHKPSN TKVDKKVEPK SCDKTHTCPP CPAPEAAGGP SVFLFPPKPK
DTLMISRTPE VTCVVVDVSH EDPEVKFNWY VDGVEVHNAK TKPREEQYNS
TYRVVSVLTV LHQDWLNGKE YKCKVSNKAL PAPIEKTISK AKGQPREPQV
YTLPPSRDEL TKNQVSLTCL VKGFYPSDIA VEWESNGQPE NNYKTTPPVL
DSDGSFFLYS KLTVDKSRWQ QGNVFSCSVM HEALHNHYTQ KSLSLSPGK
```
2

Light chain

```
DIQMTQSPSS LSASVGDRVT ITCSASSSVS YMNWYQQTPG KAPKRWIYDT
SKLASGVPSR FSGSGSGTDY TFTISSLQPE DIATYYCQQW SSNPFTFGQG
TKLQITRTVA APSVFIFPPS DEQLKSGTAS VVCLLNNFYP REAKVQWKVD
NALQSGNSQE SVTEQDSKDS TYSLSSTLTL SKADYEKHKV YACEVTHQGL
SSPVTKSFNR GEC
```
2

Tepoxalin [*1987*] (te pox' a lin). $C_{20}H_{20}ClN_3O_3$. 385.84. (1) 1*H*-Pyrazole-3-propanamide, 5-(4-chlorophenyl)-*N*-hydroxy-1-(4-methoxyphenyl)-*N*-methyl-; (2) 5-(*p*-Chlorophenyl)-1-(*p*-methoxyphenyl)-*N*-methylpyrazole-3-propionohydroxamic acid. *UNII-TZ4OX61974. CAS-103475-41-8.* INN. *Antipsoriatic.* ◇*ORF 20485; RWJ 20485*

Teprenone. $C_{23}H_{38}O$. 330.55. 6,10,14,18-Tetramethyl-5,9,13,17-nonadecatetraen-2-one, mixture of (5*E*,9*E*,13*E*) and (5*Z*,9*E*,13*E*) isomers. *UNII-S8S8451A4O.* INN; JAN; MI.

5E : 5Z = 3 : 2

Teprotide [*1976*] (tep' roe tide). $C_{53}H_{76}N_{14}O_{12}$. 1101.26. (1) Bradykinin potentiator B, 2-L-tryptophan-3-de-L-leucine-4-de-L-proline-8-L-glutamine-; (2) 5-Oxo-L-prolyl-L-tryptophyl-L-prolyl-L-arginyl-L-prolyl-L-glutaminyl-L-isoleucyl-L-prolyl-L-proline. *CAS-35115-60-7.* INN; BAN. *Enzyme inhibitor (angiotensin-converting).* ◇*SQ 20881*

Terameprocol [*2006*] (ter am″ e proe′ kol). $C_{22}H_{30}O_4$. 358.47. (1) Benzene, 1,1′-(2,3-dimethyl-1,4-butanediyl)-bis[3,4-dimethoxy-, (*R**,*S**)-; (2) 1,1′-[(2*R**,3*S**)-2,3-Dimethylbutane-1,4-diyl)bis[3,4-dimethoxybenzene]. *CAS-24150-24-1.* INN. *Treatment of human neoplasms.* ◇*EM-1421*

Terazosin Hydrochloride [*1980*] (ter az′ oh sin hye″ droe klor′ ide). **USP.** $C_{19}H_{25}N_5O_4 \cdot HCl \cdot 2H_2O$. 459.92. [Terazosin is INN and BAN.] (1) Piperazine, 1-(4-amino-6,7-dimethoxy-2-quinazolinyl)-4-[(tetrahydro-2-furanyl)carbonyl]-, monohydrochloride, dihydrate; (2) 1-(4-Amino-6,7-dimethoxy-2-quinazolinyl)-4-(tetrahydro-2-furoyl)piperazine monohydrochloride dihydrate. *UNII-D32S14F082; UNII-8L5014XET7* [terazosin]. *CAS-70024-40-7; CAS-63074-08-8* [anhydrous]; *CAS-63590-64-7* [terazosin]. JAN. *Antihypertensive.* Hytrin (Abbott) ◇*Abbott-45975*

Terbequinil. $C_{15}H_{18}N_2O_3$. 274.32. 1,4-Dihydro-1-(methoxymethyl)-4-oxo-*N*-propyl-3-quinolinecarboxamide. *UNII-0DH9WUS03O. CAS-113079-82-6.* INN.

Terbinafine [*1987*] (ter′ bin a feen). $C_{21}H_{25}N$. 291.43. [Terbinafine Hydrochloride is JAN.] (1) 1-Naphthalenemethanamine, *N*-(6,6-dimethyl-2-hepten-4-ynyl)-*N*-methyl-, (*E*)-; (2) (*E*)-*N*-(6,6-Dimethyl-2-hepten-4-ynyl)-*N*-methyl-1-naphthalenemethylamine. *UNII-G7RIW8S0XP;*

---

† Brand name formerly used, and/or firm no longer concerned with this product.

UNII-012C11ZU6G [terbinafine hydrochloride]. *CAS-91161-71-6; CAS-78628-80-5* [hydrochloride]. INN; BAN. *Antifungal.* Lamisil (Novartis) ◇*SF 86-327*

Terbogrel [*1998*] (ter′ boe grel). $C_{23}H_{27}N_5O_2$. 405.49. (1) (*E*)-6-[3-[[(Cyanoamino)[(1,1-dimethylethyl)amino]methylene]amino]phenyl]-6-(3-pyridinyl)-5-hexenoic acid; (2) (5*E*)-6-[*m*-(3-*tert*-Butyl-2-cyanoguanidino)phenyl]-6-(3-pyridyl)-5-hexenoic acid. *CAS-149979-74-8.* INN. *Platelet aggregation inhibitor.* ◇*BIBV 308 SE*

Terbucromil. $C_{18}H_{22}O_4$. 302.36. 6,8-Di-*tert*-butyl-4-oxo-4*H*-1-benzopyran-2-carboxylic acid. *CAS-37456-21-6.* INN; BAN.

Terbufibrol. $C_{20}H_{24}O_5$. 344.40. *p*-[3-(*p*-*tert*-Butylphenoxy)-2-hydroxypropoxy]benzoic acid. *CAS-56488-59-6.* INN.

Terbuficin. $C_{30}H_{44}O_4$. 468.67. Bis(3,5-di-*tert*-butyl-4-hydroxyphenyl)acetic acid. *UNII-470XML6G45. CAS-15534-92-6.* INN.

Terbuprol. $C_8H_{18}O_3$. 162.23. 1-*tert*-Butoxy-3-methoxy-2-propanol. *CAS-13021-53-9.* INN.

Terbutaline Sulfate [*1970*] (ter bue′ ta leen sul′ fate). **USP.** $(C_{12}H_{19}NO_3)_2 \cdot H_2SO_4$. 548.65. [Terbutaline is INN and BAN.] (1) 1,3-Benzenediol, 5-[2-[(1,1-dimethylethyl)amino]-1-hydroxyethyl]-, sulfate (2:1) (salt); (2) (±)-α-[(*tert*-Butylamino)methyl]-3,5-dihydroxybenzyl alcohol sulfate (2:1) (salt). *UNII-576PU70Y8E; UNII-N8ONU3L3PG* [terbutaline]. *CAS-23031-32-5; CAS-23031-25-6* [terbutaline]. JAN. *Bronchodilator*. Brethaire (Novartis); Brethine (Aaipharma) ◇*KWD 2019*

Terciprazine. $C_{22}H_{29}F_3N_2O_2$. 410.47. (±)-α-[[(1-Ethynylcyclohexyl)oxy]methyl]-4-(α,α,α-trifluoro-*m*-tolyl)-1-piperazineethanol. *CAS-56693-15-3*. INN.

Terconazole [*1980*] (ter kon′ a zole). $C_{26}H_{31}Cl_2N_5O_3$. 532.46. (1) Piperazine, 1-[4-[[2-(2,4-dichlorophenyl)-2-(1*H*-1,2,4-triazol-1-ylmethyl)-1,3-dioxolan-4-yl]methoxy]phenyl]-4-(1-methylethyl)-, *cis*-; (2) *cis*-1-[*p*-[[2-(2,4-Dichlorophenyl)-2-(1*H*-1,2,4-triazol-1-ylmethyl)-1,3-dioxolan-4-yl]methoxy]phenyl]-4-isopropylpiperazine. *UNII-0KJ2VE664U*. *CAS-67915-31-5*. INN; BAN. *Antifungal*. Terazol (Ortho-McNeil) [*Name previously used: Triaconazole.*] ◇*R-42,470*

Terdecamycin. $C_{31}H_{43}N_3O_8$. 585.69. 4-Methyl-1-piperazinecarboxylic acid, 7-ester with (-)-*N*-[(1*S*,2*R*,3*E*,5*E*,7-*S*,9*E*,11*E*,13*S*,15*R*,19*R*)-7,13-dihydroxy-1,4,10,19-tetramethyl-17,18-dioxo-16-oxabicyclo[13.2.2]nonadeca-3,5,9,11-tetraen-2-yl]pyruvamide. *CAS-113167-61-6*. INN.

Terestigmine. $C_{21}H_{33}N_3O_3$. 375.51. (4a*S*,9a*S*)-2,3,4,4a,9,9a-Hexahydro-2,4a,9-trimethyl-1,2-oxazino[6,5-*b*]indol-6-yl heptylcarbamate. *CAS-147650-57-5*. INN.

Terfenadine [*1975*] (ter fen′ a deen). $C_{32}H_{41}NO_2$. 471.67. (1) 1-Piperidinebutanol, α-[4-(1,1-dimethylethyl)phenyl]-4-(hydroxydiphenylmethyl)-; (2) α-(*p-tert*-Butylphenyl)-4-(hydroxydiphenylmethyl)-1-piperidinebutanol. *UNII-7BA5G9Y06Q*. *CAS-50679-08-8*. USP XXIII; INN; BAN; JAN. *Antihistaminic*. Seldane (Merrell) ◇*RMI 9918*

Terflavoxate. $C_{26}H_{29}NO_4$. 419.51. 1,1-Dimethyl-2-piperidinoethyl 3-methyl-4-oxo-2-phenyl-4*H*-1-benzopyran-8-carboxylate. *UNII-NKF031O02G*. *CAS-86433-40-1*. INN.

Terfluranol. $C_{17}H_{17}F_3O_2$. 310.31. 4,4′-[(1*R*,2*S*)-1-Methyl-2-(2,2,2-trifluoroethyl)ethylene]diphenol. *UNII-WUF1DL156G*. *CAS-64396-09-4*. INN; BAN.

Terguride. $C_{20}H_{28}N_4O$. 340.46. 1,1-Diethyl-3-(6-methylergolin-8α-yl)urea. *CAS-37686-84-3*. INN; MI.

Teriflunomide. $C_{12}H_9F_3N_2O_2$. 270.21. (*Z*)-2-Cyano-α,α,α-trifluoro-3-hydroxy-*p*-crotonotoluidide. *UNII-1C058IKG3B*. *CAS-108605-62-5*. INN.

Terikalant. $C_{24}H_{31}NO_3$. 381.51. (-)-(*S*)-1-[2-(4-Chromanyl)ethyl]-4-(3,4-dimethoxyphenyl)piperidine. *UNII-G8ZMP77RGJ*. *CAS-121277-96-1*. INN.

Teriparatide [*1996*] (ter″ i par′ a tide). $C_{181}H_{291}N_{55}O_{51}S_2$. 4117.72. (1) L-Phenylalanine, L-seryl-L-valyl-L-seryl-L-α-glutamyl-L-isoleucyl-L-glutaminyl-L-leucyl-L-methionyl-L-histidyl-L-asparaginyl-L-leucylglycyl-L-lysyl-L-histidyl-L-leucyl-L-asparaginyl-L-seryl-L-methionyl-L-α-glutamyl-L-arginyl-L-valyl-L-α-glutamyl-L-triptophyl-L-leucyl-L-arginyl-L-lysyl-L-lysyl-L-leucyl-L-glutaminyl-L-α-aspartyl-L-valyl-L-histidyl-L-asparaginyl-; (2) L-Seryl-L-valyl-L-seryl-L-α-glutamyl-L-isoleucyl-L-glutaminyl-L-leucyl-L-methionyl-L-histidyl-L-asparaginyl-L-leucylglycyl-L-lysyl-L-histidyl-L-leucyl-L-asparaginyl-L-seryl-L-methionyl-L-α-glutamyl-L-arginyl-L-valyl-L-α-glutamyl-L-tryptophyl-L-leucyl-L-arginyl-L-lysyl-L-lysyl-L-leucyl-L-glutaminyl-L-α-aspartyl-L-valyl-L-histidyl-L-asparaginyl-L-phenylalanine. *UNII-10T9CSU89I. CAS-52232-67-4.* INN; JAN. *Bone resorption inhibitor; osteoporosis therapy adjunct.* ◇*LY 333334*

SVSEIQLMHN LGKHLNSMER VEWLRKKLQD VHNF——OH

Teriparatide Acetate [*1986*] (ter″ i par′ a tide as′ e tate). $C_{181}H_{291}N_{55}O_{51}S_2.xH_2O.yC_2H_4O_2$. (1) L-Phenylalanine, L-seryl-L-valyl-L-seryl-L-α-glutamyl-L-isoleucyl-L-glutaminyl-L-leucyl-L-methionyl-L-histidyl-L-asparaginyl-L-leucylglycyl-L-lysyl-L-histidyl-L-leucyl-L-asparaginyl-L-seryl-L-methionyl-L-α-glutamyl-L-arginyl-L-valyl-L-α-glutamyl-L-tryptophyl-L-leucyl-L-arginyl-L-lysyl-L-lysyl-L-leucyl-L-glutaminyl-L-α-aspartyl-L-valyl-L-histidyl-L-asparaginyl-, acetate (salt) hydrate; (2) L-Seryl-L-valyl-L-seryl-L-α-glutamyl-L-isoleucyl-L-glutaminyl-L-leucyl-L-methionyl-L-histidyl-L-asparaginyl-L-leucylglycyl-L-lysyl-L-histidyl-L-leucyl-L-asparaginyl-L-seryl-L-methionyl-L-α-glutamyl-L-arginyl-L-valyl-L-α-glutamyl-L-tryptophyl-L-leucyl-L-arginyl-L-lysyl-L-lysyl-L-leucyl-L-glutaminyl-L-α-aspartyl-L-valyl-L-histidyl-L-asparaginyl-L-phenylalanine acetate (salt) hydrate. *UNII-9959P4V12N. CAS-99294-94-7.* JAN. *Diagnostic aid (hypocalcemia).* Parathar (Sanofi Aventis) ◇*hPTH 1-34 (acetate salt)*

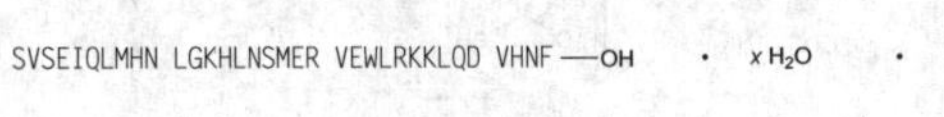

SVSEIQLMHN LGKHLNSMER VEWLRKKLQD VHNF——OH   ·   x H₂O   ·   [H₃C—CO—OH]y

Terizidone. $C_{14}H_{14}N_4O_4$. 302.29. 4,4′-[*p*-Phenylenebis-(methyleneamino)]di-(isoxazolidin-3-one). *CAS-25683-71-0.* INN.

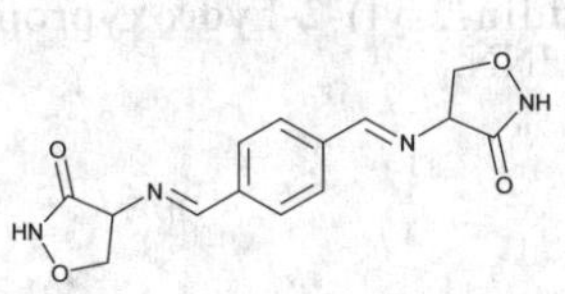

Terlakiren [*1991*] (ter la kye′ ren). $C_{31}H_{48}N_4O_7S$. 620.80. (1) L-Cysteinamide, *N*-(4-morpholinylcarbonyl)-L-phenylalanyl-*N*-[1-(cyclohexylmethyl)-2-hydroxy-3-(1-methylethoxy)-3-oxopropyl]-*S*-methyl-, [*R*-(*R**,*S**)]-; (2) Isopropyl ($\alpha R,\beta S$)-α-hydroxy-β-[(*R*)-3-(methylthio)-2-[(*S*)-α-4-morpholinecarboxamidohydrocinnamamido]propionamido]cyclohexanebutyrate. *CAS-119625-78-4.* INN. *Antihypertensive.* ◇*CP-80,794*

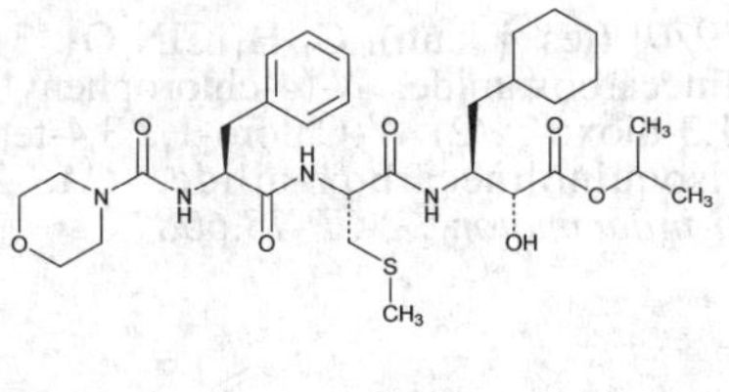

Terlipressin [*2006*] (ter″ li pres′ in). $C_{52}H_{74}N_{16}O_{15}S_2$. 1227.37. (1) *N*-[*N*-(*N*-Glycylglycyl)glycyl]-8-L-lysinevasopressin; (2) Glycylglycylglycyl[8-L-lysine]vasopressin. *UNII-7Z5X49W53P. CAS-14636-12-5.* INN; BAN; MI. *Vasoconstrictor (vasopressin derivative).*

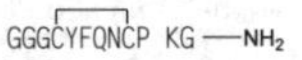

GGGCYFQNCP KG——NH₂

Ternidazole. $C_7H_{11}N_3O_3$. 185.18. 2-Methyl-5-nitroimidazole-1-propanol. *UNII-4N8R018QB0. CAS-1077-93-6.* INN.

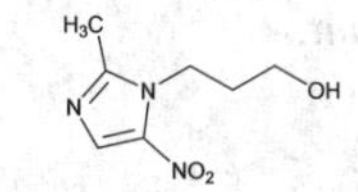

Terodiline Hydrochloride [*1966*] (ter oh′ dil een hye″ droe klor′ ide). $C_{20}H_{27}N.HCl$. 317.90. [Terodiline is INN, BAN, and JAN.] (1) Benzenepropanamine, *N*-(1,1-dimethylethyl)-α-methyl-γ-phenyl-, hydrochloride; (2) *N*-*tert*-Butyl-1-methyl-3,3-diphenylpropylamine hydrochloride. *CAS-7082-21-5; CAS-15793-40-5* [terodiline]. *Vasodilator (coronary).*

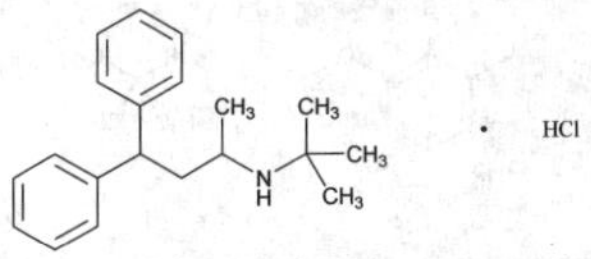

Terofenamate. $C_{17}H_{17}Cl_2NO_3$. 354.23. Ethoxymethyl *N*-(2,6-dichloro-*m*-tolyl)anthranilate. *UNII-A53154FC4N. CAS-29098-15-5.* INN; MI.

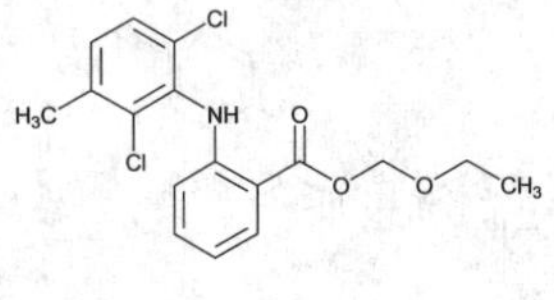

Teroxalene Hydrochloride [*1966*] (ter ox′ a leen hye″ droe klor′ ide). $C_{28}H_{41}ClN_2O.HCl$. 493.55. [Teroxalene is INN.] (1) Piperazine, 1-(3-chloro-4-methylphenyl)-4-[6-[4-(1,1-dimethylpropyl)phenoxy]hexyl]-, monohydrochloride; (2) 1-(3-Chloro-*p*-tolyl)-4-[6-(*p*-*tert*-pentylphenoxy)hexyl]piperazine monohydrochloride. *CAS-3845-22-5; CAS-14728-33-7* [teroxalene]. *Antischistosomal.* ◇*A-16612; PR-3847*

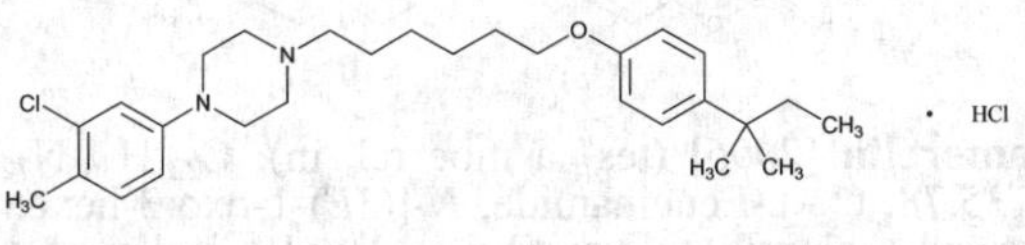

Teroxirone [*1981*] (ter ox′ i rone). $C_{12}H_{15}N_3O_6$. 297.26. (1) 1,3,5-Triazine-2,4,6(1*H*,3*H*,5*H*)-trione, 1,3,5-tris(oxiranylmethyl)-, [1(*R**),3(*R**),5(*S**)]-($\pm$)-; (2) (*RS,RS,SR*)-1,3,5-

---

† Brand name formerly used, and/or firm no longer concerned with this product.

Tris(2,3-epoxypropyl)-*s*-triazine-2,4,6(1*H*,3*H*,5*H*)-trione; (3) α-Triglycidyl isocyanurate. *UNII-456V4159SL. CAS-59653-73-5.* INN. *Antineoplastic.* ◇αTGI; NSC-296934

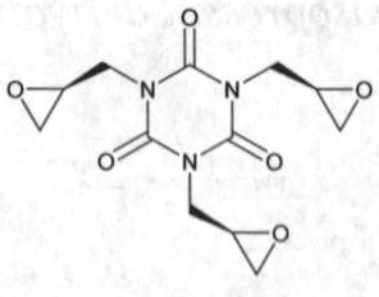

Terpin Hydrate (ter′ pin hye′ drate). **USP.** $C_{10}H_{20}O_2 \cdot H_2O$. 190.28. [Terpin is BAN.] (1) Cyclohexanemethanol, 4-hydroxy-α,α,4-trimethyl-, monohydrate; (2) *p*-Menthane-1,8-diol monohydrate. *CAS-2451-01-6; CAS-80-53-5* [anhydrous]. *Expectorant.*

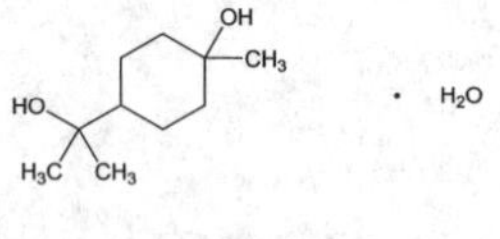

Terpinol — *See* Terpin Hydrate.

Terrafungine — *See* Oxytetracycline.

Tertatolol. $C_{16}H_{25}NO_2S$. 295.44. (±)-1-(*tert*-Butylamino)-3-(thiochroman-8-yloxy)-2-propanol. *CAS-34784-64-0.* INN; BAN; MI. ◇S-2395

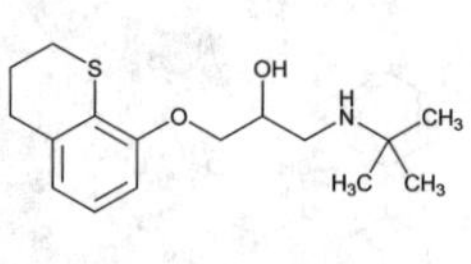

Tertomotide. $C_{85}H_{146}N_{26}O_{21}$. 1868.23. Human telomerase reverse transcriptase (EC 2.7.7.49)-(611-626)-peptide (telomerase catalytic subunit fragment). *CAS-915019-08-8.* INN.

Terutroban. $C_{20}H_{22}ClNO_4S$. 407.91. 3-[(6*R*)-6-(4-Chlorobenzenesulfonamido)-2-methyl-5,6,7,8-tetrahydronaphthalen-1-yl]propanoic acid. *CAS-165538-40-9.* INN.

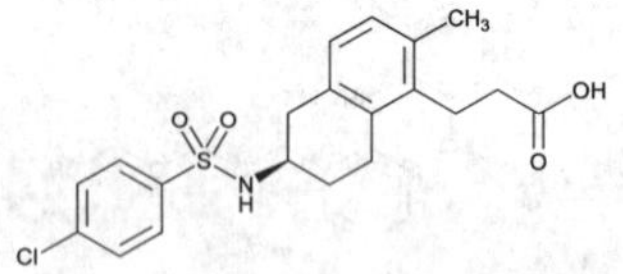

Tesaglitazar [*2004*] (tes″ a gli′ ta zar). $C_{20}H_{24}O_7S$. 408.47. (1) Benzenepropanoic acid, α-ethoxy-4-[2-[4-[(methylsulfonyl)oxy]phenyl]ethoxy]-, (α*S*)-; (2) (2*S*)-2-Ethoxy-3-[4-[2-[4-[(methylsulfonyl)oxy]phenyl]ethoxy]phenyl]propanoic acid. *UNII-6734037O3L. CAS-251565-85-2.* INN. *Treatment of type 2 diabetes and insulin resistance syndrome.* Galida (AstraZeneca) ◇AR-H039242XX

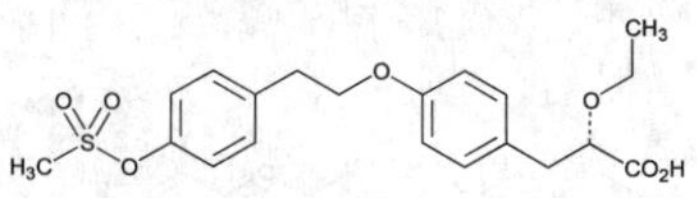

Tesamorelin [*2006*] (tes″ a moe rel′ in). $C_{221}H_{366}N_{72}O_{67}S$. 5135.78. (1) L-Leucinamide, *N*-[(3*E*)-1-oxo-3-hexenyl]-L-tyrosyl-L-alanyl-L-α-aspartyl-L-alanyl-L-isoleucyl-L-phenylalanyl-L-threonyl-L-asparaginyl-L-seryl-L-tyrosyl-L-arginyl-L-lysyl-L-valyl-L-leucylglycyl-L-glutaminyl-L-leucyl-L-seryl-L-alanyl-L-arginyl-L-lysyl-L-leucyl-L-leucyl-L-glutaminyl-L-α-aspartyl-L-isoleucyl-L-methionyl-L-seryl-L-arginyl-L-glutaminyl-L-glutaminylglycyl-L-α-glutamyl-

L-seryl-L-asparaginyl-L-glutaminyl-L-α-glutamyl-L-arginylglycyl-L-alanyl-L-arginyl-L-alanyl-L-arginyl-; (2) (3*E*)-Hex-3-enoylsomatoliberin (human). *UNII-MQG94M5EEO. CAS-218949-48-5.* INN. *Reduction of visceral adipose tissue in patients receiving antiretroviral therapy.* ◇TH9507

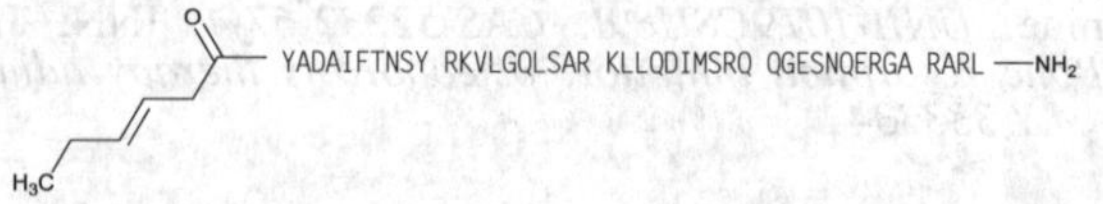

Tesamorelin Acetate [*2007*] (tes″ a moe rel′ in as′ e tate). $C_{221}H_{366}N_{72}O_{67}S \cdot xC_2H_4O_2$. (1) L-Leucinamide, *N*-[(3*E*)-1-oxo-3-hexenyl]-L-tyrosyl-L-alanyl-L-α-aspartyl-L-alanyl-L-isoleucyl-L-phenylalanyl-L-threonyl-L-asparaginyl-L-seryl-L-tyrosyl-L-arginyl-L-lysyl-L-valyl-L-leucylglycyl-L-glutaminyl-L-leucyl-L-seryl-L-alanyl-L-arginyl-L-lysyl-L-leucyl-L-leucyl-L-glutaminyl-L-α-aspartyl-L-isoleucyl-L-methionyl-L-seryl-L-arginyl-L-glutaminyl-L-glutaminyl-glycyl-L-α-glutamyl-L-seryl-L-asparaginyl-L-glutaminyl-L-α-glutamyl-L-arginylglycyl-L-alanyl-L-arginyl-L-alanyl-L-arginyl-, acetate (salt); (2) (3*E*)-Hex-3-enoylsomatoliberin (human) acetate (salt). *CAS-901758-09-6. Reduction of visceral adipose tissue in patients receiving antiretroviral therapy.* ◇TH9507

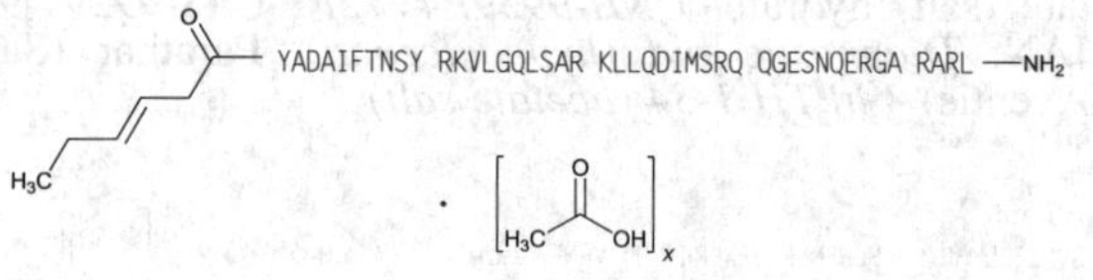

Tesetaxel. $C_{46}H_{60}FN_3O_{13}$. 881.98. 2′-[(Dimethylamino)methyl]-1-hydroxy-5β,20-epoxy-9α,10α-dihydro[1,3]-dioxolo[4′,5′:9,10]tax-11-ene-2α,4,13α-triyl 4-acetate 2-benzoate 13-{(2*R*,3*S*)-3-[(*tert*-butoxycarbonyl)amino]-3-(3-fluoropyridin-2-yl)-2-hydroxypropanoate}. *CAS-333754-36-2.* INN.

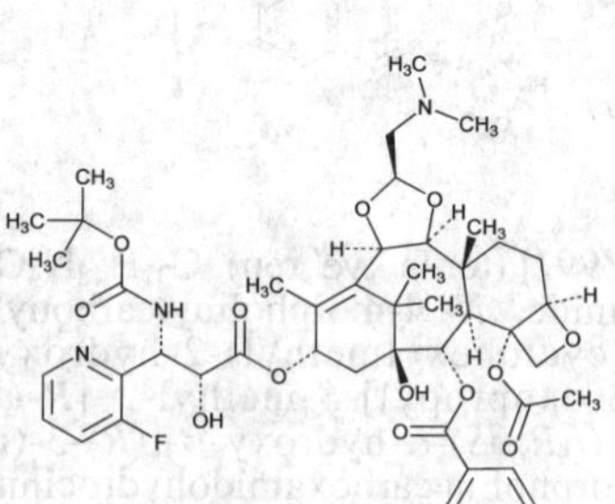

Tesicam [*1970*] (tes′ i kam). $C_{16}H_{11}ClN_2O_3$. 314.72. (1) 4-Isoquinolinecarboxamide, *N*-(4-chlorophenyl)-1,2,3,4-tetrahydro-1,3-dioxo-; (2) 4′-Chloro-1,2,3,4-tetrahydro-1,3-dioxo-4-isoquinolinecarboxanilide. *CAS-21925-88-2.* INN. *Anti-inflammatory.* ◇CP-13,608

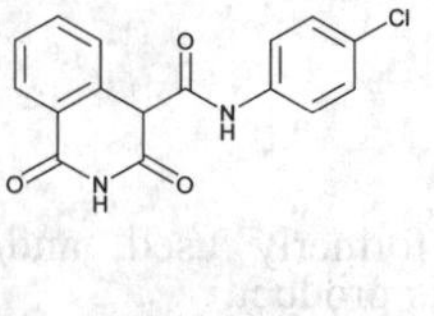

Tesimide [*1974*] (tes' i mide). $C_{16}H_{15}NO_2$. 253.30. (1) 1,3(2*H*,4*H*)-Isoquinolinedione, 5,6,7,8-tetrahydro-4-(phenylmethylene)-; (2) 4-Benzylidene-5,6,7,8-tetrahydro-1,3(2*H*,4*H*)-isoquinolinedione. *CAS-35423-09-7*. INN. *Anti-inflammatory*.

Tesmilifene. $C_{19}H_{25}NO$. 283.41. 2-[(α-Phenyl-*p*-tolyl)oxy]-triethylamine. *UNII-I43T3ID6G2*. *CAS-98774-23-3*. INN.

Tesmilifene Hydrochloride [*1998*] (tes mil' i feen hye″ droe klor' ide). $C_{19}H_{25}NO.HCl$. 319.87. (1) Ethanamine, *N*,*N*-diethyl-2-[4-(phenylmethyl)phenoxy]-, hydrochloride; (2) 2-[(α-Phenyl-*p*-tolyl)oxy]triethylamine hydrochloride. *UNII-1U4B477260*. *CAS-92981-78-7*. *Chemopotentiator used in the treatment of patients with malignant solid tumors (antihistamine)*. ◇*BMS-217380-01; BMY-33419; DPPE*

Tesofensine. $C_{17}H_{23}Cl_2NO$. 328.28. (1*R*,2*R*,3*S*,5*S*)-3-(3,4-Dichlorophenyl)-2-(ethoxymethyl)-8-methyl-8-azabicyclo[3.2.1]octane. *UNII-BLH9UKX9V1*. *CAS-195875-84-4*. INN.

Testolactone [*1964*] (tes″ toe lak' tone). **USP**. $C_{19}H_{24}O_3$. 300.39. (1) D-Homo-17a-oxaandrosta-1,4-diene-3,17-dione; (2) 13-Hydroxy-3-oxo-13,17-secoandrosta-1,4-dien-17-oic acid δ-lactone. *UNII-6J9BLA949Q*. *CAS-968-93-4*. INN. *Antineoplastic*. Teslac (Bristol-Myers Squibb) ◇*SQ 9538; NSC-23759*

Testosterone (tes tos' ter one). **USP**. $C_{19}H_{28}O_2$. 288.42. (1) Androst-4-en-3-one, 17-hydroxy-, (17β)-; (2) 17β-Hydroxyandrost-4-en-3-one. *UNII-3XMK78S47O*. *CAS-58-22-0*. INN; BAN. *Androgen*. Androderm (Watson); Androgel (Unimed); Testim (Auxilium)

Testosterone Cyclopentylpropionate — *See* Testosterone Cypionate.

Testosterone Cypionate (tes tos' ter one sip' ee oh nate). **USP**. $C_{27}H_{40}O_3$. 412.60. (1) Androst-4-en-3-one, 17-(3-cyclopentyl-1-oxopropoxy)-, (17β)-; (2) Testosterone cyclopentanepropionate. *UNII-M0XW1UBI14*. *CAS-58-20-8*. *Androgen*. Depo-testosterone (Pfizer); Testosterone (Pfizer)

Testosterone Enanthate (tes tos' ter one e nan' thate). **USP**. $C_{26}H_{40}O_3$. 400.59. (1) Androst-4-en-3-one, 17-(1-oxoheptyl)oxy-, (17β)-; (2) Testosterone heptanoate. *UNII-7Z6522T8N9*. *CAS-315-37-7*. JAN. *Androgen*. Delatestryl (Indevus) ◇*NSC-17591*

Testosterone Heptanoate — *See* Testosterone Enanthate.

Testosterone Ketolaurate [*1965*] (tes tos' ter one kee″ toe lawr' ate). $C_{31}H_{48}O_4$. 484.71. (1) Androst-4-en-3-one, 17-[(1,3-dioxododecyl)oxy]-, (17β)-; (2) Testosterone 3-oxododecanoate. *CAS-5874-98-6*. INN. *Androgen*.

Testosterone Phenylacetate [*1965*] (tes tos' ter one fen″ il as' e tate). $C_{27}H_{34}O_3$. 406.56. (1) Androst-4-en-3-one, 17-[(phenylacetyl)oxy]-; (2) Testosterone phenylacetate. *CAS-5704-03-0*. *Androgen*.

Testosterone Propionate (tes tos' ter one proe' pee oh nate). **USP**. $C_{22}H_{32}O_3$. 344.49. (1) Androst-4-en-3-one, 17-(1-oxopropoxy)-, (17β)-; (2) Testosterone propionate. *UNII-WI93Z9138A*. *CAS-57-85-2*. JAN. *Androgen*. ◇*NSC-9166*

Testosterone Undecanoate [*2003*] (tes tos' ter one un dek″ a noe' ate). $C_{30}H_{48}O_3$. 456.70. (1) 3-Oxoandrost-4-en-17β-yl undecanoate; (2) Androst-4-en-3-one, 17-[(1-oxoundecyl)oxy]-(17β). *UNII-H16A5VCT9C*. *CAS-5949-44-0*. *In males: testosterone replacement therapy for primary or*

---

† Brand name formerly used, and/or firm no longer concerned with this product.

secondary hypogonadal disorders. In female-to-male transsexuals: masculinization. Moreover, in men, testosterone therapy may be indicated in osteoporosis caused by androgen deficiency. Andriol (Diosynth B.V., Netherlands); Andriol (Organon) ◇*Org 538*

Tetanus and Gas Gangrene Antitoxins. [*PHS: Tetanus and Gas Gangrene Polyvalent Antitoxin*]. NF XIV.

Tetanus Antitoxin. USP XXVI. *Immunizing agent (passive).*

Tetanus Immune Globulin (tet′ a nus i mune′ glob′ ue lin). **USP.** A sterile, nonpyrogenic solution of globulins derived from the blood plasma of adult human donors who have been immunized with tetanus toxoid. *Immunizing agent (passive).* BayTet (Bayer); Homo-Tet (Savage†); Immu-Tetanus (Parke-Davis†) *[Name previously used: Tetanus Immune Human Globulin.]*

Tetanus Immune Human Globulin (previously used name) — *See* Tetanus Immune Globulin.

Tetanus Toxoid (tet′ a nus). **USP.** A sterile solution of the formaldehyde-treated products of growth of the tetanus bacillus (*Clostridium tetani*). *Immunizing agent (active).*

Tetanus Toxoid Adsorbed (tet′ a nus). **USP.** A sterile preparation of plain tetanus toxoid that meets all the requirements for the product with the exception of those for potency, and that has been precipitated or absorbed by alum, aluminum hydroxide, or aluminum phosphate adjuvants. *Immunizing agent (active).*

Tetiothalein Sodium — *See* Iodophthalein Sodium.

Tetnicoran — *See* Nicofurate.

Tetomilast. $C_{19}H_{18}N_2O_4S$. 370.42. 6-[2-(3,4-Diethoxyphenyl)-1,3-thiazol-4-yl]pyridine-2-carboxylic acid. *CAS-145739-56-6.* INN.

Tetrabarbital. $C_{12}H_{20}N_2O_3$. 240.30. 5-Ethyl-5-(1-ethylbutyl)-barbituric acid. *UNII-3K441526FO. CAS-76-23-3.* INN; DCF; MI.

Tetrabenazine. $C_{19}H_{27}NO_3$. 317.42. 1,3,4,6,7,11b-Hexahydro-3-isobutyl-9,10-dimethoxy-2*H*-benzo[*a*]quinolizin-2-one. *UNII-Z9O08YRN8O. CAS-58-46-8.* INN; BAN; MI. ◇*Ro 1-9569*

Tetracaine (te′ tra kane). **USP.** $C_{15}H_{24}N_2O_2$. 264.36. (1) Benzoic acid, 4-(butylamino)-, 2-(dimethylamino)ethyl ester; (2) 2-(Dimethylamino)ethyl *p*-(butylamino)benzoate. *UNII-0619F35CGV. CAS-94-24-6.* INN; BAN. *Anesthetic*

(topical). Medihaler-Tetracaine (3M Pharmaceuticals†); Metraspray (3M Pharmaceuticals†); Pontocaine (Sterling Winthrop)

Tetracaine Hydrochloride (te′ tra kane hye″ droe klor′ ide). **USP.** $C_{15}H_{24}N_2O_2$·HCl. 300.82. (1) Benzoic acid, 4-(butylamino)-, 2-(dimethylamino)ethyl ester, monohydrochloride; (2) 2-(Dimethylamino)ethyl *p*-(butylamino)benzoate monohydrochloride. *UNII-5NF5D4OPCI. CAS-136-47-0; CAS-94-24-6* [tetracaine]. JAN. *Anesthetic (local).* Pontocaine Hydrochloride (Sterling Winthrop)

Tetrachloroethylene. C_2Cl_4. 165.83. (1) Ethene, tetrachloro-; (2) Tetrachloroethylene. *UNII-TJ904HH8SN. CAS-127-18-4.* USP XXI; MI.

Tetracosactide (INN, BAN) — *See* Cosyntropin.

Tetracosactrin (previously used name) — *See* Cosyntropin.

Tetracycline (tet″ ra sye′ kleen). **USP.** $C_{22}H_{24}N_2O_8$. 444.43. (1) 2-Naphthacenecarboxamide, 4-(dimethylamino)-1,4,4a,5,5a,6,11,12a-octahydro-3,6,10,12,12a-pentahydroxy-6-methyl-1,11-dioxo-, [4*S*-(4α,4aα,5aα,6β,12aα)]-; (2) (4*S*,4a*S*,5a*S*,12a*S*)-4-(Dimethylamino)-1,4,4a,5,5a,6,11,12a-octahydro-3,6,10,12,12a-pentahydroxy-6-methyl-1,11-dioxo-2-naphthacenecarboxamide. *UNII-F8VB5M810T. CAS-60-54-8; CAS-6416-04-2* [trihydrate]. INN; BAN; JAN. *Anti-amebic; antibacterial; antirickettsial.* Liquamycin [Veterinary] (Pfizer)

Tetracycline Hydrochloride (tet″ ra sye′ kleen hye″ droe klor′ ide). **USP.** $C_{22}H_{24}N_2O_8$·HCl. 480.90. (1) 2-Naphthacenecarboxamide, 4-(dimethylamino)-1,4,4a,5,5a,6,11,12a-octahydro-3,6,10,12,12a-pentahydroxy-6-methyl-1,11-dioxo-, monohydrochloride, [4*S*-(4α,4aα,5aα,6β,12aα)]-; (2) (4*S*,4a*S*,5a*S*,6*S*,12a*S*)-4-(Dimethylamino)-1,4,4a,5,5a,6,11,12a-octahydro-3,6,10,12,12a-pentahydroxy-6-methyl-1,11-dioxo-2-naphthacenecarboxamide monohydrochloride. *UNII-P6R62377KV. CAS-64-75-5; CAS-60-54-8* [tetracycline]. JAN. *Anti-amebic; antibacterial; antirickettsial.* Achromycin (Lederle); Bristacycline (Bristol-Myers Squibb); Cyclopar (Warner Chilcott); Panmycin (Pfizer); Sumycin (Par); Tetracyn (Pfizer)

Tetracycline Metaphosphate (JAN) — *See* Tetracycline Phosphate Complex.

Tetracycline Phosphate Complex. [Tetracycline Metaphosphate is JAN.] (1) 2-Naphthacenecarboxamide, 4-(dimethylamino)-1,4,4a,5,5a,6,11,12a-octahydro-3,6,10,12,12a-pentahydroxy-6-methyl-1,11-dioxo, [4*S*-(4α,4aα,5aα,6β,12aα)]-, phosphate complex; (2) (4*S*,4a*S*,5a*S*,6*S*,12a*S*)-4-(Dimethylamino)-1,4,4a,5,5a,6,11,12a-octahydro-3,6,10,12,12a-pentahydroxy-6-methyl-1,11-dioxo-2-naphthacenecarboxamide phosphate complex. *UNII-F8VB5M810T* [tetracycline]. *CAS-1336-20-5; CAS-60-54-8* [tetracycline]. USP XXIII; BAN. *Antibacterial.* Tetrex (Bristol-Myers Squibb)

Tetradonium Bromide. $C_{17}H_{38}BrN$. 336.39. Trimethyltetradecylammonium bromide. *UNII-8483H94W1E. CAS-1119-97-7.* INN.

Tetraethylammonium Chloride. *CAS-56-34-8.* MI.

Tetrafilcon A [*1976*] (te″ tra fil′ kon). $(C_6H_{10}O_3)_w(C_{10}H_{10})_x$ $(C_5H_8O_2)_y(C_6H_9NO)_z$. (1) 2-Propenoic acid, 2-methyl-, 2-hydroxyethyl ester, polymer with diethenylbenzene, 1-ethenyl-2-pyrrolidinone and methyl 2-methyl-2-propenoate; (2) 2-Hydroxyethyl methacrylate polymer with divinylbenzene, methyl methacrylate and 1-vinyl-2-pyrrolidinone. *CAS-53626-53-2. Contact lens material (hydrophilic).* Alliance (CooperVision); Cooper Clear (CooperVision); Cooper Toric (CooperVision); Preference (CooperVision); Preference Standard (CooperVision); Preference Toric (CooperVision); Vantage (CooperVision); Vantage Thin (CooperVision)

Tetragastrin. $C_{37}H_{42}N_6O_8S$. 730.83. L-Triptophyl-L-methyionyl-L-α-aspartyl-L-phenylalaninamide. *CAS-1947-37-1.* JAN.

Tetrahydrolipstatin — *See* Orlistat.

Tetrahydrozoline Hydrochloride (tet″ ra hye droz′ oh leen hye″ droe klor′ ide). **USP.** $C_{13}H_{16}N_2.HCl$. 236.74. [Tetryzoline is INN and BAN; Tetryzoline Hydrochloride is JAN; Tetrahydrozoline Nitrate is JAN.] (1) 1*H*-Imidazole, 4,5-dihydro-2-(1,2,3,4-tetrahydro-1-naphthalenyl)-, monohydrochloride; (2) 2-(1,2,3,4-Tetrahydro-1-naphthyl)-2-imidazoline monohydrochloride. *UNII-0YZT43HS7D; UNII-S9U025Y077* [tetrahydrozoline]. *CAS-522-48-5; CAS-84-22-0* [tetrahydrozoline]. *Adrenergic (vasoconstrictor).* Tyzine (Kenwood)

Tetraiodophenolphthalein Sodium — *See* Iodophthalein Sodium.

Tetrallobarbital — *See* Butalbital.

Tetramal — *See* Tetrabarbital.

Tetrameprozine — *See* Aminopromazine.

Tetramethrin. $C_{19}H_{25}NO_4$. 331.41. (1) 2,2-Dimethyl-3-(2-methylpropenyl)cyclopropanecarboxylic acid, ester with *N*-(hydroxymethyl)-1-cyclohexene-1,2-dicarboximide; (2)

1-cyclohexene-1,2-dicarboximidomethyl 2,2-dimethyl-3-(2-methylpropenyl)cyclopropanecarboxylate. *UNII-Z72930Q46K. CAS-7696-12-0.* INN; MI.

Tetramisole Hydrochloride [*1966*] (te tram′ i sole hye″ droe klor′ ide). $C_{11}H_{12}N_2S.HCl$. 240.75. [Tetramisole is INN and BAN.] (1) Imidazo[2,1-*b*]thiazole, 2,3,5,6-tetrahydro-6-phenyl-, monohydrochloride, (±)-; (2) (±)-2,3,5,6-Tetrahydro-6-phenylimidazo[2,1-*b*]thiazole monohydrochloride. *CAS-5086-74-8; CAS-5036-02-2* [tetramisole]. *Anthelmintic.* Anthelvet (Ortho-McNeil†) ◇*R 8299; McN-JR-8299-11*

Tetranitrol — *See* Erythrityl Tetranitrate.

Tetrantoin. *UNII-3NM8B9838N. CAS-52094-70-9.* MI.

Tetraxetan [*2004*] (te trax′ e tan). $C_{16}H_{28}N_4O_8$. 404.42. (1) 1,4,7,10-Tetraazacyclododecane-1,4,7,10-tetraacetic acid; (2) 2,2′,2″,2‴-(1,4,7,10-Tetraazacyclododecane-1,4,7,10-tetryl)tetraacetic acid. *UNII-1HTE449DGZ. CAS-60239-18-1. Radical designation for a chelating agent.[Note— Tetraxetan has been used in conjunction with yttrium Y 90 epratuzumab tetraxetan (N04/58) and yttrium Y 90 labetuzumab tetraxetan (N04/59).]* ◇*DOTA*

Tetrazepam. $C_{16}H_{17}ClN_2O$. 288.77. 7-Chloro-5-(cyclohexen-1-yl)-1,3-dihydro-1-methyl-2*H*-1,4-benzodiazepin-2-one. *UNII-FO92091VP8. CAS-10379-14-3.* INN; BAN; DCF; MI. ◇*CB 4261*

Tetrazolast Meglumine [*1992*] (te traz′ oh last me′ gloo meen). $C_{10}H_6N_8.C_7H_{17}NO_5.H_2O$. 451.44. [Tetrazolast is INN.] (1) Tetrazolo[1,5-*a*]quinoline, 4-(1*H*-tetrazol-5-yl)-compd. with 1-deoxy-1-(methylamino)-D-glucitol, (1:1), monohydrate; (2) 4-(1*H*-Tetrazol-5-yl)tetrazolo[1,5-*a*]quinoline compound with 1-deoxy-1-(methylamino)-D-glucitol (1:1), monohydrate. *UNII-2IY97B405I. CAS-133008-33-0; CAS-121762-69-4* [anhydrous]; *CAS-95104-27-1* [tetrazolast]. *Anti-allergic; anti-asthmatic.* ◇*MDL 26,024G0*

Tetridamine (INN) — *See* Tetrydamine.

Tetriprofen. $C_{15}H_{18}O_2$. 230.30. *p*-1-Cyclohexen-1-ylhydratropic acid. *CAS-28168-10-7*. INN. ◇*47-210 [as sodium]*

Tetrofosmin [*1992*] (te″ troe fos′ min). $C_{18}H_{40}O_4P_2$. 382.46. (1) 3,12-Dioxa-6,9-diphosphatetradecane, 6,9-bis(2-ethoxyethyl)-; (2) Ethylenebis[bis(2-ethoxyethyl)phosphine]. *UNII-3J0KPB596Q*. *CAS-127502-06-1*. INN; BAN; JAN. *Diagnostic aid.* ◇*P53*

Tetronasin. $C_{35}H_{54}O_8$. 602.80. 4-Hydroxy-3-[(2*S*)-2-[(1*S*,2*S*,6*R*)-2-[(1*E*)-3-hydroxy-2-[(2*R*,3*R*,6*S*)-tetrahydro-3-methyl-6-[(1*E*,3*S*)-3-[(2*R*,3*S*,5*R*)-tetrahydro-5-[(1*S*)-1-methoxyethyl]-3-methyl-2-furyl]-1-butenyl]-2*H*-pyran-2-yl]propenyl]-6-methylcyclohexyl]propionyl]-2(5*H*)-furanone. *UNII-BZ5N591H97*. *CAS-75139-06-9*. MI.

Tetronasin Sodium [*1986*] (te troe′ na sin soe′ dee um). $C_{35}H_{53}NaO_8$. 624.78. [Tetronasin is INN and BAN.] (1) Antibiotic M 139603; (2) 4-Hydroxy-3-[(2*S*)-2-[(1*S*,2*S*,6*R*)-2-[(1*E*)-3-hydroxy-2-[(2*R*,3*R*,6*S*)-tetrahydro-3-methyl-6-[(1*E*,3*S*)-3-[(2*R*,3*S*,5*R*)-tetrahydro-5-[(1*S*)-1-methoxyethyl]-3-methyl-2-furyl]-1-butenyl]-2*H*-pyran-2-yl]propenyl]-6-methylcyclohexyl]propionyl]-2-(5*H*)-furanone, monosodium salt. *UNII-IH245EI7CP*. *CAS-75139-05-8*. *Growth promoter (veterinary).* ◇*ICI 139603; CH690001*

Tetroquinone [*1966*] (te″ troe kwin′ one). $C_6H_4O_6$. 172.09. (1) 2,5-Cyclohexadiene-1,4-dione, 2,3,5,6-tetrahydroxy-; (2) Tetrahydroxy-*p*-benzoquinone. *CAS-319-89-1*. INN. *Keratolytic (systemic).* ◇*HPEK-1; THQ; NSC-112931*

Tetroxoprim [*1978*] (te trox′ oh prim). $C_{16}H_{22}N_4O_4$. 334.37. (1) 2,4-Pyrimidinediamine, 5-[[3,5-dimethoxy-4-(2-methoxyethoxy)phenyl]methyl]-; (2) 2,4-Diamino-5-[3,5-dimethoxy-4-(2-methoxyethoxy)benzyl]pyrimidine. *UNII-5R6712AY0K*. *CAS-53808-87-0*. INN; BAN. *Antibacterial.*

Tetrydamine [*1968*] (te trid′ a meen). $C_9H_{15}N_3$. 165.24. [Tetridamine is INN.] (1) 2*H*-Indazol-3-amine, 4,5,6,7-tetrahydro-*N*,2-dimethyl-; (2) 4,5,6,7-Tetrahydro-2-methyl-3-(methylamino)-2*H*-indazole. *CAS-17289-49-5*. *Analgesic; anti-inflammatory.* ◇*POLI 67*

Tetrylammonium Bromide. $C_8H_{20}BrN$. 210.16. Tetraethylammonium bromide. *CAS-71-91-0*. INN. ◇*TEAB*

Tetryzoline (INN, BAN, DCF) — *See* Tetrahydrozoline Hydrochloride.

Tetryzoline Hydrochloride (JAN) — *See* Tetrahydrozoline Hydrochloride.

Teverelix. $C_{74}H_{100}ClN_{15}O_{14}$. 1459.13. *N*-Acetyl-3-(2-naphthyl)-D-alanyl-*p*-chloro-D-phenylalanyl-3-(3-pyridyl)-D-alanyl-L-seryl-L-tyrosyl-*N*[6]-carbamoyl-D-lysyl-L-leucyl-*N*[6]-isopropyl-L-lysyl-L-prolyl-D-alaninamide. *CAS-144743-92-0*. INN.

Texacromil. $C_{14}H_{14}O_6S$. 310.32. (±)-5-[2-Hydroxy-3-(methylthio)propoxy]-4-oxo-4*H*-1-benzopyran-2-carboxylic acid. *UNII-2B562K7K56*. *CAS-77005-28-8*. INN.

Tezacitabine [*2000*] (te″ za sye′ ta been). $C_{10}H_{12}FN_3O_4$·H_2O. 275.23. [Tezacitabine, anhydrous, is INN.] (1) Cytidine, 2′-deoxy-2′-(fluoromethylene)-, monohydrate, (2′*E*)-; (2) 2′-

Deoxy-2'-[(*E*)-fluoromethylene]cytidine monohydrate. *CAS-171176-43-5; CAS-130306-02-4* [anhydrous]. INN. *Antineoplastic.* ◇*FMdC; MDL 101,731*

Tezampanel [*2006*] (tez am′ pa nel). $C_{13}H_{21}N_5O_2.H_2O$. 297.35. (1) 3-Isoquinolinecarboxylic acid, decahydro-6-[2-(1*H*-tetrazol-5-yl)ethyl]-, monohydrate, (3*S*,4a*R*,6-*R*,8a*R*)-; (2) (3*S*,4a*R*,6*R*,8a*R*)-6-[2-(1*H*-Tetrazol-5-yl)ethyl]decahydroisoquinoline-3-carboxylic acid monohydrate. *UNII-6XN50U405Y. CAS-317819-68-4; CAS-154652-83-2* [anhydrous]. INN. *Treatment of migraine, neuropathic pain.* ◇*LY293558; NGX424*

Tezosentan. $C_{27}H_{27}N_9O_6S$. 605.62. *N*-[6-(2-Hydroxyethoxy)-5-(*o*-methoxyphenoxy)-2-[2-(1*H*-tetrazol-5-yl)-4-pyridyl]-4-pyrimidinyl]-5-isopropyl-2-pyridinesulfonamide. *CAS-180384-57-0.* INN; BAN.

Thalidomide [*1961*] (tha lid′ oh mide). **USP.** $C_{13}H_{10}N_2O_4$. 258.23. (1) 1*H*-Isoindole-1,3(2*H*)-dione, 2-(2,6-dioxo-3-piperidinyl)-, (±)-; (2) (±)-*N*-(2,6-Dioxo-3-piperidyl)phthalimide; (3) α-(*N*-Phthalimido)glutarimide. *UNII-4Z8R6ORS6L. CAS-50-35-1.* INN; BAN; JAN. *Sedative-hypnotic.* Thalomid (Celgene) ◇*K-17; NSC-66847*

Thallium Chloride (²⁰¹Tl) Injection (JAN) — *See* Thallous Chloride Tl 201.

Thallous Chloride Tl 201 [*1977*] (thal′ us klor′ ide). **USP** [Injection]. ²⁰¹TlCl. [Thallium Chloride (²⁰¹Tl) Injection is JAN.] (1) Thallium chloride (²⁰¹TlCl); (2) Thallium chloride (²⁰¹TlCl). *UNII-3I8Y076A0E. CAS-55172-29-7. Diagnostic aid (radiopaque medium); radioactive agent.*

Thaumatin. A mixture in the ratio 2:1 of two polypeptides, thaumatin I and II, each consisting of 207 amino acid residues and having a molecular weight of about 22,000, extracted from the aril of the tropical fruit *Thaumatococcus daniellii. CAS-53850-34-3.* BAN; MI.

Thebacon. $C_{20}H_{23}NO_4$. 341.40. Acetyldihydrocodeinone. *CAS-466-90-0.* INN; BAN; DCF.

Theine — *See* Caffeine.

Thenalidine. $C_{17}H_{22}N_2S$. 286.43. 1-Methyl-4-*N*-2-thenylanilinopiperidine. *CAS-86-12-4.* INN; BAN; MI.

Thenium Closylate [*1962*] (then′ ee um kloe′ si late). $C_{21}H_{24}ClNO_4S_2$. 454.00. [Thenium Closilate is INN and BAN.] (1) 2-Thiophenemethanaminium, *N,N*-dimethyl-*N*-(2-phenoxyethyl)-, salt with 4-chlorobenzenesulfonic acid (1:1); (2) Dimethyl(2-phenoxyethyl)-2-thenylammonium *p*-chlorobenzenesulfonate. *CAS-4304-40-9. Anthelmintic (veterinary).* ◇*611 C 65; NSC-106569*

Thenyldiamine. $C_{14}H_{19}N_3S$. 261.39. 2-[[2-(Dimethylamino)ethyl]-3-thenylamino]pyridine. *CAS-91-79-2; CAS-958-93-0* [hydrochloride]. INN; BAN; MI.

Thenylpyramine Hydrochloride — *See* Methapyrilene Hydrochloride.

Theobromine. *CAS-83-67-0.* NF XII; BAN; MI.

Theobromine Calcium Salicylate. [Theosalicin is JAN.] Theobromine calcium salt mixture with calcium salicylate. NF XI; MI. Theocalcin (Knoll†)

Theobromine Sodium Acetate. *CAS-8002-88-8; CAS-83-67-0* [theobromine]. NF XI; MI.

Theobromine Sodium Salicylate. *CAS-8048-31-5; CAS-83-67-0* [theobromine]. NF XI; JAN; MI.

Theodrenaline. $C_{17}H_{21}N_5O_5$. 375.38. 7-[2-[2-(3,4-Dihydroxyphenyl)-2-hydroxyethylamino]ethyl]theophylline. *CAS-13460-98-5.* INN; BAN.

---

† Brand name formerly used, and/or firm no longer concerned with this product.

Theofibrate [*1981*] (thee″ oh fye′ brate). $C_{19}H_{21}ClN_4O_5$. 420.85. [Etofylline Clofibrate is INN.] (1) Propanoic acid, 2-(4-chlorophenoxy)-2-methyl-, 2-(1,2,3,6-tetrahydro-1,3-dimethyl-2,6-dioxo-7*H*-purin-7-yl)ethyl ester; (2) 2-(*p*-Chlorophenoxy)-2-methylpropionic acid, ester with 7-(2-hydroxyethyl)theophylline. *CAS-54504-70-0. Antihyperlipoproteinemic.* Duolip (L. Merckle, Germany) ◇*ML-1024*

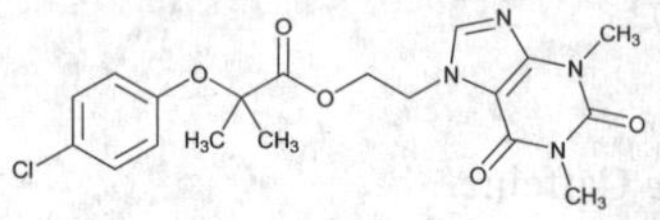

Theophyllamine — *See* Aminophylline.

Theophylline (thee of′ i lin). **USP.** $C_7H_8N_4O_2 \cdot H_2O$. 198.18. (1) 1*H*-Purine-2,6-dione, 3,7-dihydro-1,3-dimethyl-, monohydrate; (2) Theophylline monohydrate. *UNII-C137DTR5RG. CAS-5967-84-0; CAS-58-55-9* [anhydrous]. BAN; JAN. *Bronchodilator* Pharmaceutic necessity for Aminophylline Injection. Elixophyllin (Forest); Theo-24 (UCB); Theochron (Inwood); Theolair-sr (Graceway); Uniphyl (Purdue Frederick)

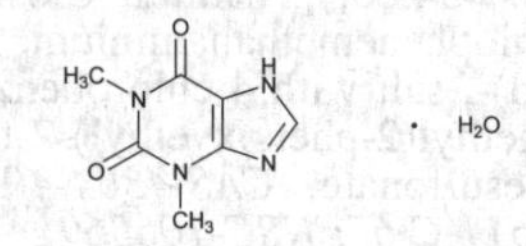

Theophylline Ethylenediamine (previously used name) — *See* Aminophylline.

Theophylline Olamine. $C_7H_8N_4O_2 \cdot C_2H_7NO$. 241.25. (1) 1*H*-Purine-2,6-dione, 3,7-dihydro-1,3-dimethyl-, compd. with 2-aminoethanol (1:1); (2) Theophylline compound with 2-aminoethanol (1:1). *UNII-C137DTR5RG* [theophylline]. *CAS-573-41-1; CAS-58-55-9* [theophylline]. USP XX.

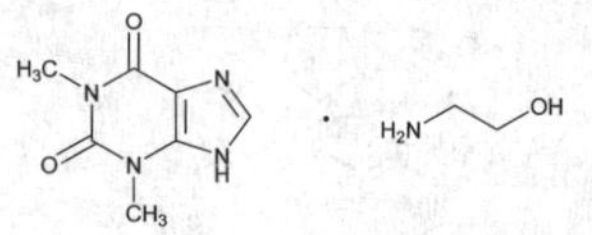

Theophylline Sodium Acetate. *UNII-88AO1K4HJ3.* NF XIII; MI. Theocin (Sterling Winthrop†)

Theophylline Sodium Glycinate (thee of′ i lin soe′ dee um glye′ sin ate). **USP.** (1) Glycine, mixt. with 3,7-dihydro-1,3-dimethyl-1*H*-purine-2,6-dione, monosodium salt; (2) Theophylline sodium mixture with glycine. *UNII-C137DTR5RG* [theophylline]. *CAS-8000-10-0; CAS-58-55-9* [theophylline]. *Relaxant (smooth muscle).* Asbron (Novartis)

Theosalicin (JAN) — *See* Theobromine Calcium Salicylate.

Thiabendazole [*1962*] (thye″ a ben′ da zole). **USP.** $C_{10}H_7N_3S$. 201.25. [Tiabendazole is INN, BAN and JAN.] (1) 1*H*-Benzimidazole, 2-(4-thiazolyl)-; (2) 2-(4-Thiazolyl)benzimidazole. *UNII-N1Q45E87DT. CAS-148-79-8. Anthelmintic.* Mintezol (Merck) ◇*MK-360*

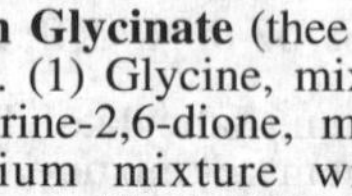

Thiabutazide — *See* Buthiazide.

Thiacetarsamide. $C_{11}H_{12}AsNO_5S_2$. 377.27. [Thiacetarsamide is INN and DCF.] (1) Benzamide, *p*-bis(carboxymethyl-mercapto)arsino-; (2) 4-Carbamylphenyl biscarboxymethylthioarsenite. *UNII-VMF4ELY9TZ. CAS-531-72-6.* USP XXVII.

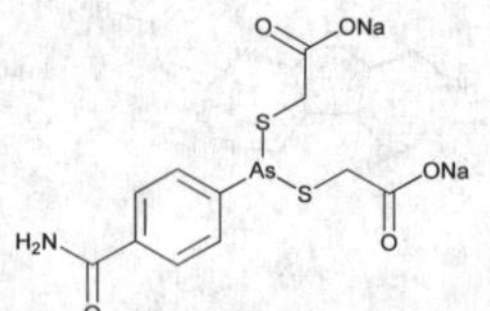

Thiacetazone (previously used name) — *See* Amithiozone.

Thialbarbital. $C_{13}H_{16}N_2O_2S$. 264.34. 5-Allyl-5-(2-cyclohexen-1-yl)-2-thiobarbituric acid. *UNII-ENV72C33QD. CAS-467-36-7.* INN; BAN; DCF; MI. *[Name previously used: Thialbarbitone.]*

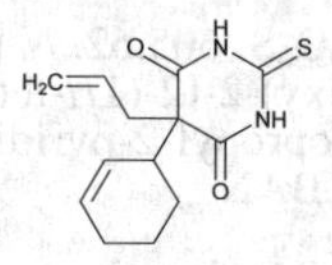

Thialisobumal Sodium — *See* Buthalital Sodium.

Thiamazole (INN, BAN, JAN, DCF) — *See* Methimazole.

Thiambutosine. $C_{19}H_{25}N_3OS$. 343.49. 1-(*p*-Butoxyphenyl)-3-(*p*-dimethylaminophenyl)-2-thiourea. *UNII-X92J960C7P. CAS-500-89-0.* INN; BAN. ◇*CIBA 1906*

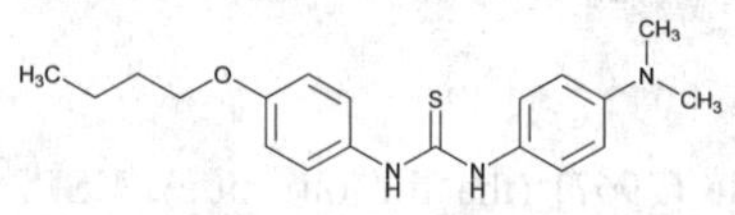

Thiamine Cobalt Chlorophyllin Complex. $C_{46}H_{55}CoN_8O_{10}S$. 970.97. Complex consisting of thiamine, cobalt (1+), and chlorophyllin. JAN.

Thiamine Hydrochloride (thye′ a min hye″ droe klor′ ide). **USP.** $C_{12}H_{17}ClN_4OS \cdot HCl$. 337.27. [Thiamine is INN and BAN; Thiamine Disulfide is JAN.] (1) Thiazolium, 3-[(4-amino-2-methyl-5-pyrimidinyl)methyl]-5-(2-hydroxyethyl)-4-methyl-, chloride, monohydrochloride; (2) Thiamine monohydrochloride. *UNII-M572600E5P; UNII-X66NSO3N35* [thiamine]. *CAS-67-03-8; CAS-59-43-8* [thiamine]. JAN. *Vitamin (enzyme co-factor).* Betalin S (Lilly)

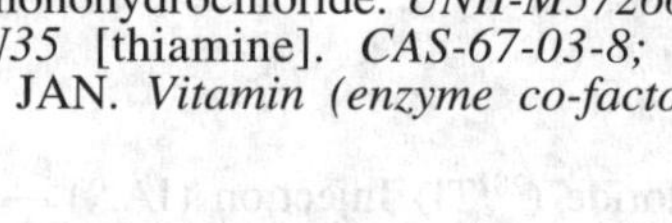

Thiamine Mononitrate (thye′ a min mon″ oh nye′ trate). **USP.** $C_{12}H_{17}N_5O_4S$. 327.36. [Thiamine Nitrate is JAN.] (1) Thiazolium, 3-[(4-amino-2-methyl-5-pyrimidinyl)methyl]-5-(2-hydroxyethyl)-4-methyl-, nitrate (salt); (2) Thiamine nitrate (salt). *UNII-X66NSO3N35* [thiamine]. *CAS-532-43-4; CAS-59-43-8* [thiamine]. *Vitamin (enzyme co-factor).*

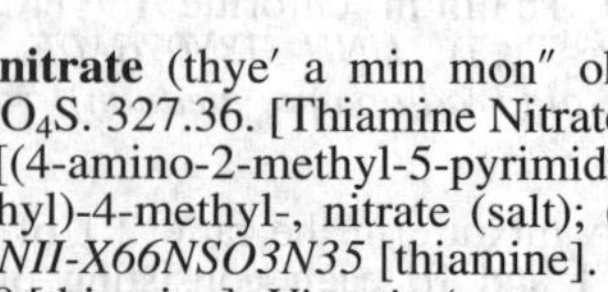

Thiamine Nitrate (JAN) — *See* Thiamine Mononitrate.

Thiamine Propyl Disulfide — *See* Prosultiamine.

Thiamiprine [*1964*] (thye am′ i preen). $C_9H_8N_8O_2S$. 292.28. [Tiamiprine is INN.] (1) 1*H*-Purin-2-amine, 6-[(1-methyl-4-nitro-1*H*-imidazol-5-yl)thio]-; (2) 2-Amino-6-[(1-methyl-4-nitroimidazol-5-yl)thio]purine. *UNII-E2EV7ZDD1M. CAS-5581-52-2. Antineoplastic.* ◇BW 57-323; NSC-38887

Thiamphenicol [*1968*] (thye″ am fen′ i kol). $C_{12}H_{15}Cl_2NO_5S$. 356.22. [Thiamphenicol Aminoacetate Hydrochloride is JAN.] (1) Acetamide, 2,2-dichloro-*N*-[2-hydroxy-1-(hydroxymethyl)-2-[4-(methylsulfonyl)phenyl]ethyl]-, [*R*-(*R**,*R**)]-; (2) D-(+)-*threo*-2,2-Dichloro-*N*-[β-hydroxy-α-(hydroxymethyl)-*p*-(methylsulfonyl)phenethyl]acetamide. *UNII-FLQ7571NPM. CAS-15318-45-3.* INN; BAN; JAN. *Antibacterial.* Thiocymetin (Sterling Winthrop†) ◇Win 5063-2

Thiamylal. $C_{12}H_{18}N_2O_2S$. 254.35. (1) Dihydro-5-(1-methylbutyl)-5-(2-propenyl)-2-thioxo-4,6-(1*H*,5*H*)-pyrimidinedione; (2) 5-Allyl-5-(1-methylbutyl)-2-thiobarbituric acid. *UNII-01T23W89FR. CAS-77-27-0.* USP XXIII. *Anesthetic (intravenous).*

Thiamylal Sodium. $C_{12}H_{17}N_2NaO_2S$. 276.33. (1) 4,6-(1*H*,5*H*)-Pyrimidinedione, dihydro-5-(1-methylbutyl)-5-(2-propenyl)-2-thioxo-, monosodium salt; (2) Sodium 5-allyl-5-(1-methylbutyl)-2-thiobarbiturate. *UNII-T4L2P3KH7K. CAS-337-47-3.* USP XXIII; JAN. *Anesthetic (intravenous).* Surital (Parkdale)

Thianthol. A mixture of dimethylthianthrene and ditoluenedisulfide. JAN.

Thiazesim Hydrochloride [*1966*] (thye az′ e sim hye″ droe klor′ ide). $C_{19}H_{22}N_2OS \cdot HCl$. 362.92. [Tiazesim is INN and BAN.] (1) 1,5-Benzothiazepin-4(5*H*)-one, 5-[2-(dimethyl-

amino)ethyl]-2,3-dihydro-2-phenyl-, monohydrochloride; (2) 5-[2-(Dimethylamino)ethyl]-2,3-dihydro-2-phenyl-1,5-benzothiazepin-4(5*H*)-one monohydrochloride. *CAS-3122-01-8; CAS-5845-26-1* [thiazesim]. *Antidepressant.* Altinil (Bristol-Myers Squibb†) ◇SQ 10,496

Thiazinamium Chloride [*1978*] (thye a zin′ a mee um klor′ ide). $C_{18}H_{23}ClN_2S$. 334.91. (1) 10*H*-Phenothiazine-10-ethanaminium, *N*,*N*,*N*,α-tetramethyl-, chloride; (2) Trimethyl(1-methyl-2-phenothiazin-10-ylethyl)-ammonium chloride. *CAS-4320-13-2; CAS-2338-21-8* [thiazinamium]. *Anti-allergic.* ◇WY-460E

Thiazinamium Metilsulfate. $C_{19}H_{26}N_2O_4S_2$. 410.55. Trimethyl(1-methyl-2-phenothiazin-10-ylethyl)ammonium methyl sulfate. *UNII-IA16WBX317. CAS-58-34-4; CAS-2338-21-8* [thiazinamium]. INN; MI.

Thiazolsulfone (previously used name) — *See* Thiazosulfone.

Thiazosulfone. $C_9H_9N_3O_2S_2$. 255.32. 2-Amino-5-sulfanilylthiazole. *CAS-473-30-3.* INN. Promizole (Parke-Davis†) [*Name previously used: Thiazolsulfone.*]

Thiazothielite — *See* Antienite.

Thiazothienol — *See* Antazonite.

Thiethylperazine [*1969*] (thye eth″ il per′ a zeen). $C_{22}H_{29}N_3S_2$. 399.62. (1) 10*H*-Phenothiazine, 2-(ethylthio)-10-[3-(4-methyl-1-piperazinyl)propyl]-; (2) 2-(Ethylthio)-10-[3-(4-methyl-1-piperazinyl)propyl]phenothiazine. *UNII-8ETK1WAF6R. CAS-1420-55-9.* INN; BAN. *Anti-emetic.*

Thiethylperazine Malate. $C_{22}H_{29}N_3S_2 \cdot 2C_4H_6O_5$. 667.79. [Thietylperazine Malate is JAN.] (1) 10*H*-Phenothiazine, 2-(ethylthio)-10-[3-(4-methyl-1-piperazinyl)propyl]-, 2-hydroxy-1,4-butanedioate (1:2); (2) 2-(Ethylthio)-10-[3-(4-methyl-1-piperazinyl)propyl]phenothiazine malate (1:2). *UNII-HP46XK89XB. CAS-52239-63-1; CAS-1420-55-9* [thiethylperazine]. USP XXIII. *Anti-emetic.* Torecan (Novartis)

---

† Brand name formerly used, and/or firm no longer concerned with this product.

Thiethylperazine Maleate [*1962*] (thye eth″ il per′ a zeen mal′ ee ate). **USP.** $C_{22}H_{29}N_3S_2 \cdot 2C_4H_4O_4$. 631.76. [Thietylperazine Maleate is JAN.] (1) 10*H*-Phenothiazine, 2-(ethylthio)-10-[3-(4-methyl-1-piperazinyl)propyl]-, (*Z*)-2-butenedioate (1:2); (2) 2-(Ethylthio)-10-[3-(4-methyl-1-piperazinyl)propyl]phenothiazine maleate (1:2). *UNII-RUK64CF26E. CAS-1179-69-7; CAS-1420-55-9* [thiethylperazine]. *Anti-emetic.* Torecan (Novartis) ◇*GS-95; NSC-130044*

Thietylperazine Malate (JAN) — *See* Thiethylperazine Malate.

Thietylperazine Maleate (JAN) — *See* Thiethylperazine Maleate.

Thihexinol Methylbromide. $C_{18}H_{26}BrNOS_2$. 416.44. [4-(Hydroxydi-2-thienylmethyl)cyclohexyl]trimethylammonium bromide. *UNII-03CPZ5439O. CAS-7219-91-2.* NF XIII; INN; MI.

Thimerfonate Sodium [*1963*] (thye mer′ foe nate soe′ dee um). $C_8H_9HgNaO_3S_2$. 440.87. [Sodium Timerfonate is INN and BAN.] (1) Mercury, ethyl(4-mercaptobenzenesulfonato-*S*⁴)- sodium salt; (2) Ethyl(hydrogen *p*-mercaptobenzenesulfonato)mercury sodium salt; (3) Sodium *p*-[(ethylmercuri)thio]benzenesulfonate. *CAS-5964-24-9; CAS-33305-56-5* [thimerfonate]. *Anti-infective, topical.*

Thimerosal (thye mer′ oh sal). **USP.** $C_9H_9HgNaO_2S$. 404.81. [Thiomersal is INN and BAN.] (1) Mercury, ethyl (2-mercaptobenzoato-*S*)-, sodium salt; (2) Ethyl (sodium *o*-mercaptobenzoato)mercury. *UNII-2225PI3MOV. CAS-54-64-8.* JAN. *Anti-infective, topical; pharmaceutic aid (preservative).* Merthiolate (Lilly)

Thioacetazone (INN, BAN, DCF) — *See* Amithiozone.

Thiocarbanidin. *UNII-370694U45W. CAS-92-97-7.* MI. Thioban (Parke-Davis†)

Thiocarlide (previously used name) — *See* Tiocarlide.

Thiocolchicine Glycoside — *See* Thiocolchicoside.

Thiocolchicoside. $C_{27}H_{33}NO_{10}S$. 563.62. 2-10-Di(demethoxy)-2-glucosyloxy-10-methylthiocolchicine. *CAS-602-41-5.* INN; DCF.

Thioctic Acid. $C_8H_{14}O_2S_2$. 206.33. 1,2-Dithiolane-3-valeric acid. *CAS-62-46-4.* BAN; JAN.

Thioctic Acid Amide. $C_8H_{15}NOS_2$. 205.34. 1,2-Dithiolane-3-pentanamide. JAN.

Thiocyanate Sodium. *CAS-540-72-7.* NF X; MI.

Thiodiglycol. $C_4H_{10}O_2S$. 122.19. 2,2′-Thiodiethanol. *UNII-9BW5T43J04. CAS-111-48-8.* INN; MI.

Thiodiphenylamine — *See* Phenothiazine.

Thiofuradene. $C_8H_8N_4O_3S$. 240.24. 1-(5-Nitrofurfurylideneamino)-2-imidazolidinethione. *CAS-2240-21-3.* INN.

Thioguanine [*1965*] (thye″ oh gwa′ neen). **USP.** $C_5H_5N_5S \cdot xH_2O$. 167.19 (anhydrous). [Tioguanine is INN and BAN.] (1) 6*H*-Purine-6-thione, 2-amino-1,7-dihydro-; (2) 2-Aminopurine-6(1*H*)-thione. *UNII-FTK8U1GZNX. CAS-154-42-7; CAS-5580-03-0* [hemihydrate]. *Antineoplastic.* ◇*NSC-752*

Thiohexallymal — *See* Thialbarbital.

Thiohexamide. $C_{14}H_{20}N_2O_3S_2$. 328.45. 1-Cyclohexyl-3-[*p*-(methylthio)phenylsulfonyl]urea. *UNII-6M8CV4TKXL. CAS-3692-44-2.* INN.

Thioinosine. $C_{10}H_{12}N_4O_4S$. 284.29. 9-*β*-D-Ribofuranosyl-6-mercaptopurine. *CAS-574-25-4.* JAN.

Thiomebumal Sodium — *See* Thiopental Sodium.

Thiomersal (INN, BAN) — *See* Thimerosal.

Thiomesterone (previously used name) — *See* Tiomesterone.

Thiopental Sodium (thye″ oh pen′ tal soe′ dee um). **USP.** $C_{11}H_{17}N_2NaO_2S$. 264.32. [Thiopental is BAN.] (1) 4,6(1*H*,5*H*)-Pyrimidinedione, 5-ethyldihydro-5-(1-methylbutyl)-2-thioxo-, monosodium salt, (±)-; (2) Sodium (±)-

5-ethyl-5-(1-methylbutyl)-2-thiobarbiturate. *UNII-49Y44QZL70; UNII-JI8Z5M7NA3* [thiopental]. *CAS-71-73-8; CAS-76-75-5* [thiopental]. INN; JAN. *Anesthetic (intravenous); anticonvulsant.* Pentothal (Abbott) *[Name previously used: Thiopentone.]*

Thiophanate. $C_{14}H_{18}N_4O_4S_2$. 370.45. 4,4′-*o*-Phenylenebis(ethyl 3-thioallophanate). *UNII-5Q0Y96D5I8. CAS-23564-06-9.* BAN; MI.

Thiopropazate Hydrochloride. $C_{23}H_{28}ClN_3O_2S.2HCl$. 518.93. [Thiopropazate is INN and BAN.] 4-[3-(2-Chlorophenothiazin-10-yl)propyl]-1-piperazineethanol acetate dihydrochloride. *CAS-84-06-0* [thiopropazate]. NF XIII; MI.

Thioproperazine Dimethanesulfonate (JAN) — *See* Thioproperazine Mesylate.

Thioproperazine Mesylate. $C_{22}H_{30}N_4O_2S_2.2CH_4O_3S$. 638.84. [Thioproperazine is INN and BAN; Thioproperazine Dimethanesulfonate is JAN.] *N,N*-Dimethyl-10-(3-(4-methylpiperazin-1-yl)propyl)-10*H*-phenothiazine-2-sulfonamide, dimethanesulfonate. *UNII-71P630M192; UNII-YJ050AQ56X* [thioproperazine]. *CAS-2347-80-0; CAS-316-81-4* [thioproperazine]. MI. Vontil (SmithKline Beecham†)

Thioproperazine Methanesulfonate — *See* Thioproperazine Mesylate.

Thioridazine [*1962*] (thye″ oh rid′ a zeen). **USP.** $C_{21}H_{26}N_2S_2$. 370.57. (1) 10*H*-Phenothiazine, 10-[2-(1-methyl-2-piperidinyl)ethyl]-2-(methylthio)-; (2) 10-[2-(1-Methyl-2-piper-

idyl)ethyl]-2-(methylthio)phenothiazine. *UNII-N3D6TG58NI. CAS-50-52-2.* INN; BAN. *Antipsychotic; sedative-hypnotic.* Mellaril (Novartis) ◇*TP-21*

Thioridazine Hydrochloride (thye″ oh rid′ a zeen hye″ droe klor′ ide). **USP.** $C_{21}H_{26}N_2S_2.HCl$. 407.04. (1) 10*H*-Phenothiazine, 10-[2-(1-methyl-2-piperidinyl)ethyl]-2-(methylthio)-, monohydrochloride; (2) 10-[2-(1-Methyl-2-piperidyl)ethyl]-2-(methylthio)phenothiazine monohydrochloride. *UNII-4WCI67NK8M. CAS-130-61-0; CAS-50-52-2* [thioridazine]. JAN. *Antipsychotic; sedative-hypnotic.* Mellaril (Novartis)

Thiosalan [*1967*] (thye oh′ sa lan). $C_{13}H_8Br_3NOS$. 465.99. [Tiosalan is INN.] (1) Benzamide, 3,5-dibromo-*N*-(4-bromophenyl)-2-mercapto-; (2) 3,4′,5-Tribromo-2-mercaptobenzanilide. *CAS-15686-78-9. Disinfectant.*

Thiostrepton (thye″ oh strep′ ton). **USP.** $C_{72}H_{85}N_{19}O_{18}S_5$. 1664.89. An antibacterial substance produced by the growth of strains of *Streptomyces azureus* (Fam. Streptomycetaceae). *CAS-1393-48-2. Antibacterial (veterinary).*

Thiotepa (thye″ oh tep′ a). **USP.** $C_6H_{12}N_3PS$. 189.22. (1) Aziridine,1,1′,1″-phosphinothioylidynetris-; (2) Tris(1-aziridinyl)phosphine sulfide. *UNII-905Z5W3GKH. CAS-52-24-4.* INN; BAN; JAN. *Antineoplastic.* Thioplex (Immunex) ◇*NSC-6396*

---

† Brand name formerly used, and/or firm no longer concerned with this product.

Thiotetrabarbital. $C_{12}H_{20}N_2O_2S$. 256.36. 5-Ethyl-5-(1-ethyl-butyl)-2-thiobarbituric acid. *UNII-1P93TO196Z. CAS-467-38-9.* INN.

Thiothixene [*1965*] (thye″ oh thix′ een). **USP.** $C_{23}H_{29}N_3O_2S_2$. 443.63. [Tiotixene is INN, BAN and JAN.] (1) 9*H*-Thioxanthene-2-sulfonamide, *N,N*-dimethyl-9-[3-(4-methyl-1-piperazinyl)propylidene]-, (*Z*)-; (2) *N,N*-Dimethyl-9-[3-(4-methyl-1-piperazinyl)propylidene]thioxanthene-2-sulfonamide. *UNII-7318FJ13YJ. CAS-5591-45-7; CAS-3313-26-6* [*Z*]. *Antipsychotic.* Navane (Pfizer) ◇*P-4657 B; NSC-108165*

Thiothixene Hydrochloride [*1969*] (thye″ oh thix′ een hye″ droe klor′ ide). **USP.** $C_{23}H_{29}N_3O_2S_2 \cdot 2HCl \cdot 2H_2O$. 552.58. (1) 9*H*-Thioxanthene-2-sulfonamide, *N,N*-dimethyl-9-[3-(4-methyl-1-piperazinyl)propylidene]-, dihydrochloride, dihydrate (*Z*)-; (2) *N,N*-Dimethyl-9-[3-(4-methyl-1-piper-azinyl)propylidene]thioxanthene-2-sulfonamide dihy-drochloride dihydrate. *UNII-B3CRJ1EWJU. CAS-22189-31-7; CAS-49746-09-0* [*Z*]; *CAS-58513-59-0* [anhydrous]; *CAS-49746-04-5* [anhydrous (*Z*)]; *CAS-5591-45-7* [base]. *Antipsychotic.* Navane (Pfizer) ◇*CP-12,252-1*

Thiouracil. *CAS-141-90-2.*

Thioxolone (previously used name) — *See* Tioxolone.

Thiphenamil Hydrochloride [*1962*] (thye fen′ a mil hye″ droe klor′ ide). $C_{20}H_{25}NOS \cdot HCl$. 363.94. [Tifenamil is INN.] (1) Benzeneethanethioic acid, α-phenyl-, *S*-[2-(diethylamino)ethyl] ester hydrochloride; (2) *S*-[2-(Diethylamino)ethyl] diphenylthioacetate hydrochloride. *CAS-548-68-5; CAS-82-99-5* [thiphenamil]. *Relaxant (smooth muscle).*

Thiphencillin Potassium [*1962*] (thye″ fen sil′ in poe tas′ ee um). $C_{16}H_{17}KN_2O_4S_2$. 404.55. [Tifencillin is INN.] (1) 4-Thia-1-azabicyclo[3.2.0]heptane-2-carboxylic acid, 3,3-di-methyl-7-oxo-6-[[(phenylthio)acetyl]amino]-, monopotas-sium salt, [2*S*-(2α,5α,6β)]-; (2) Potassium 3,3-dimethyl-7-oxo-6-[2-(phenylthio)acetamido]-4-thia-1-azabicy-clo[3.2.0]heptane-2-carboxylate. *UNII-OCS3IA7WA0; UNII-Z4T2YRI005* [thiphencillin]. *CAS-4803-45-6; CAS-26552-51-2* [thiphencillin]. *Antibacterial.* ◇*26383*

Thiram [*1962*] (thye′ ram). $C_6H_{12}N_2S_4$. 240.43. (1) Thioper-oxydicarbonic diamide, tetramethyl-; (2) Bis(dimethylthio-carbamoyl) disulfide. *UNII-0D771ISOFH. CAS-137-26-8.* INN. *Antifungal.* Rezifilm (Bristol-Myers Squibb†) ◇*SQ 1489; NSC-1771*

Thonzonium Bromide [*1963*] (thon zoe′ nee um broe′ mide). $C_{32}H_{55}BrN_4O$. 591.71. [Tonzonium Bromide is INN.] (1) 1-Hexadecanaminium, *N*-[2-[[(4-methoxyphenyl)methyl]-2-pyrimidinylamino]ethyl]-*N,N*-dimethyl-, bromide; (2) Hexadecyl[2-[(*p*-methoxybenzyl)-2-pyrimidinylami-no]ethyl]dimethylammonium bromide. *UNII-JI2B19CR0R. CAS-553-08-2.* USP XXII. *Detergent.* Thon-zide (Parke-Davis†) ◇*NC 1264; NSC-5648*

Thonzylamine Hydrochloride [*1988*] (thon zil′ a meen hye″ droe klor′ ide). $C_{16}H_{22}N_4O \cdot HCl$. 322.83. [Thonzylamine is INN and BAN.] 2-{[2-(Dimethylamino)ethyl](*p*-methoxy-benzyl)amino}pyrimidine hydrochloride. *CAS-63-56-9; CAS-91-85-0* [thonzylamine]. Super Anahist (Parke-Davis)

Thozalinone [*1963*] (thoe zal′ i none). $C_{11}H_{12}N_2O_2$. 204.23. [Tozalinone is INN.] (1) 4(5*H*)-Oxazolone, 2-(dimethyl-amino)-5-phenyl-; (2) 2-(Dimethylamino)-5-phenyl-2-ox-azolin-4-one. *CAS-655-05-0. Antidepressant.* ◇*CL 39808*

Threonine [*1979*] (three′ oh neen). **USP.** $C_4H_9NO_3$. 119.12. [L-Threonine is JAN.] (1) L-Threonine; (2) L-Threonine. *UNII-2ZD004190S. CAS-72-19-5* [L]. INN. *Amino acid.*

L-Threonine (JAN) — *See* Threonine.

Thrombin (throm′ bin). **USP.** A sterile, freeze-dried powder derived from bovine plasma containing the protein substance prepared from prothrombin through interaction with added thromboplastin in the presence of calcium INN; JAN. *Hemostatic (local).* Thrombostat (Parke-Davis)

Thrombin Alfa [*2007*] (throm′ bin al′ fa). $C_{1511}H_{2342}N_{418}O_{436}S_{15}$. (1) Thrombin (synthetic human); (2) Human thrombin (recombinant, glycosylated). Molecular weight is approximately 33,820 daltons. *UNII-SCK81AMR7R. CAS-869858-13-9.* INN. *Topical surgical hemastat.*

Light chain
TFGSGEADCG LRPLFEKKSL EDKTERELLE SYIDGR

Heavy chain
                                         IVEG SDAEIGMSPW
QVMLFRKSPQ ELLCGASLIS DRWVLTAAHC LLYPPWDKNF TENDLLVRIG
KHSRTRYERN IEKISMLEKI YIHPRYNWRE NLDRDIALMK LKKPVAFSDY
IHPVCLPDRE TAASLLQAGY KGRVTGWGNL KETWTANVGK GQPSVLQVVN
LPIVERPVCK DSTRIRITDN MFCAGYKPDE GKRGDACEGD SGGPFVMKSP
FNNRWYQMGI VSWGEGCDRD GKYGFYTHVF RLKKWIQKVI DQFGE

* glycosylation site

Thrombomodulin Alfa. $C_{2230}H_{3357}N_{633}O_{718}S_{50}$. 1-498-Thrombomodulin (human clone TMP26/TMJ1 protein moiety reduced). *CAS-120313-91-9.* INN.

Thromboplastin. *CAS-9002-05-5.* USP XVIII; MI.

Thurfyl Nicotinate. $C_{11}H_{13}NO_3$. 207.23. Tetrahydrofurfuryl nicotinate. *CAS-70-19-9.* BAN.

Thymalfasin [*1995*] (thye mal′ fa sin). $C_{129}H_{215}N_{33}O_{55}$. 3108.28. (1) Thymosin α1 (ox); (2) *N*-Acetyl-L-seryl-L-α-aspartyl-L-alanyl-L-alanyl-L-valyl-L-α-aspartyl-L-threonyl-L-seryl-L-seryl-L-α-glutamyl-L-isoleucyl-L-threonyl-L-threonyl-L-lysyl-L-α-aspartyl-L-leucyl-L-lysyl-L-α-glutamyl-L-lysyl-L-lysyl-L-α-glutamyl-L-valyl-L-valyl-L-α-glutamyl-L-α-glutamyl-L-alanyl-L-α-glutamyl-L-asparagine. *CAS-62304-98-7.* INN. *Antineoplastic; hepatitis treatment; infectious disease treatment; vaccine enhancement.* Zadaxin (SciClone) [*Name previously used: Thymosin α1.*]

SDAAVDTSSE ITTKDLKEKK EVVEEAEN

Thymocartin. $C_{21}H_{40}N_8O_7$. 516.59. *N*-[*N*-(N^2-L-Arginyl-L-lysyl)-L-α-aspartyl]-L-valine. *CAS-85466-18-8.* INN.

Thymoctonan. $C_{43}H_{67}N_9O_{13}$. 918.04. *N*-[*N*-[N^2-[1-[*N*-[*N*-(*N*-L-Leucyl-L-α-glutamyl)-L-α-aspartyl]glycyl]-L-prolyl]-L-lysyl]-L-phenylalanyl]-L-leucine. *CAS-107489-37-2.* INN.

Thymol (thye′ mol). **NF.** $C_{10}H_{14}O$. 150.22. (1) Phenol, 5-methyl-2-(1-methylethyl)-; (2) Thymol; (3) *p*-Cymen-3-ol. *UNII-3J50XA376E. CAS-89-83-8.* JAN. *Pharmaceutic aid (stabilizer).*

Thymol Iodide. *CAS-552-22-7.* NF X; MI.

Thymopentin [*1981*] (thye″ moe pen′ tin). $C_{30}H_{49}N_9O_9$. 679.76. L-Tyrosine, *N*-[*N*-[*N*-(N^2-L-arginyl-L-lysyl)-L-α-aspartyl]-L-valyl]-. *CAS-69558-55-0.* INN; BAN. *Immunoregulator.* [*Name previously used: Thymopoietin 32-36.*] ◇ORF 15244; TP-5

Thymopoietin 32-36 (previously used name) — *See* Thymopentin.

Thymosin α1 (previously used name) — *See* Thymalfasin.

Thymostimulin. Polypeptide immunostimulant factor extracted from thymus of mammalian species. The source of the product should be indicated, e.g. thymostimulin (calf). INN.

Thymotrinan. $C_{16}H_{31}N_7O_6$. 417.46. *N*-(N^2-L-Arginyl-L-lysyl)-L-aspartic acid. *UNII-29OE04A6C9. CAS-85465-82-3.* INN.

Thymoxamine (former BAN) — *See* Moxisylyte.

Thyroglobulin [*1971*] (thye″ roe glob′ ue lin). Substance obtained by the fractionation of thyroid glands from the hog, *Sus scrofa* Linné var. *domesticus* Gray (Fam. *Suidae*),

---

† Brand name formerly used, and/or firm no longer concerned with this product.

containing not less than 0.7% of total iodine (I). (1) Thyroglobulin; (2) Thyroglobulin. *CAS-9010-34-8*. USP XXII; INN. *Thyroid hormone*. Proloid (Pfizer)

Thyroid (thye′ roid). **USP**. [Dried Thyroid is JAN.] The cleaned, dried, and powdered thyroid gland previously deprived of connective tissue and fat, obtained from domesticated animals that are used for food by humans. *Thyroid hormone*. ◇*NSC-26492*

Thyromedan Hydrochloride [*1964*] (thye roe′ me dan hye″ droe klor′ ide). $C_{21}H_{24}I_3NO_4 \cdot HCl$. 771.59. [Tyromedan is INN.] (1) Benzeneacetic acid, 3,5-diiodo-4-(3-iodo-4-methoxyphenoxy)-, 2-(diethylamino)ethyl ester, hydrochloride; (2) 2-(Diethylamino)ethyl [3,5-diiodo-4-(3-iodo-4-methoxyphenoxy)phenyl]acetate hydrochloride. *CAS-57-65-8; CAS-15301-96-9* [thyromedan]. *Thyromimetic.* ◇*SK&F 13364-A*

Thyropropic Acid. $C_{15}H_{11}I_3O_4$. 635.96. 4-(4-Hydroxy-3-iodophenoxy)-3,5-diiodohydrocinnamic acid. *CAS-51-26-3*. INN; MI.

Thyrotropin. [Thyrotrophin is INN and BAN.] Thyrotrophic hormone. *CAS-9002-71-5*. Thytropar (Sanofi Aventis)

Thyrotropin Alfa [*1997*] (thye″ roe troe′ pin al′ fa). $C_{1039}H_{1602}N_{274}O_{307}S_{27}$. 23,709.28; $C_{437}H_{682}N_{122}O_{134}S_{13}$ (α-subunit). 10,205.69 (α-subunit); $C_{602}H_{920}N_{152}O_{173}S_{14}$ (β-subunit). 13,503.59 (β-subunit). Recombinant form of human, thyroid stimulating hormone (rhTSH). RhTSH is produced by mammalian cell culture technology using a Chinese Hamster Ovary (CHO) cell line. A CHO cell line was co-transfected with two recombinant plasmids containing respectively the DNA coding sequences of the alpha and beta subunits of TSH. Thyrotropin (human β-subunit protein moiety), complex with chorionic gonadotropin (human α-subunit protein moiety). *UNII-AVX3D5A4LM*. *CAS-194100-83-9*. INN; BAN. *Thyroid hormone*. Thyrogen (Genzyme) *[Note—The observed type of glycosylation in the recombinant hTSH differs slightly from that of the pituitary protein. Due to this fact and the fact that the glycosylation is variable and heterogeneous, the molecular formula and weight provided here represent the theoretical protein backbone only.]*

Thyroxine (former BAN) — *See* Levothyroxine Sodium.

Thyroxine I 125 [*1964*] (thye rox′ een). $C_{15}H_{11}{}^{125}I_4NO_4$. (1) Tyrosine, *O*-(4-hydroxy-3,5-diiodophenyl)-3,5-diiodo-, labeled with iodine-125; (2) Thyroxine, labeled with iodine-125. *CAS-24486-40-6*. *Radioactive agent*. Tetramet (Abbott†)

Thyroxine I 131 [*1963*] (thye rox′ een). $C_{15}H_{11}{}^{131}I_4NO_4$. (1) Tyrosine, *O*-(4-hydroxy-3,5-diiodophenyl)-3,5-diiodo-, labeled with iodine-131; (2) Thyroxine, labeled with iodine-131. *CAS-7019-69-4*. *Radioactive agent*.

Tiabendazole (INN, BAN, JAN) — *See* Thiabendazole.

Tiacrilast [*1984*] (tye ak′ ri last). $C_{12}H_{10}N_2O_3S$. 262.28. (1) 2-Propenoic acid, 3-[6-(methylthio)-4-oxo-3(4*H*)-quinazolinyl]-, (*E*)-; (2) (*E*)-6-(Methylthio)-4-oxo-3(4*H*)-quinazolineacrylic acid. *UNII-74L3DXN051*. *CAS-78299-53-3*. INN. *Anti-allergic*. ◇*Ro 22-3747/000*

Tiacrilast Sodium [*1988*] (tye ak′ ri last soe′ dee um). $C_{12}H_9N_2NaO_3S \cdot H_2O$. 302.28. (1) 2-Propenoic acid, 3-[6-(methylthio)-4-oxo-3(4*H*)-quinazolinyl]-, sodium salt, monohydrate; (2) Sodium (*E*)-6-(methylthio)-4-oxo-3(4*H*)-quinazolineacrylate, monohydrate. *UNII-4PG8A6UTDX*. *CAS-111868-63-4*. *Anti-allergic*. ◇*Ro 22-3747/007*

Tiadenol. $C_{14}H_{30}O_2S_2$. 294.52. 2,2′-(Decamethylenedithio)diethanol. *CAS-6964-20-1*. INN; DCF; MI.

Tiafibrate. $C_{34}H_{48}Cl_2O_6S_2$. 687.78. 2-(*p*-Chlorophenoxy)-2-methylpropionic acid diester with 2,2′-(decamethylenedithio)diethanol. *CAS-55837-28-0*. INN.

Tiagabine Hydrochloride [*1996*] (tye ag′ a been hye″ droe klor′ ide). **USP**. $C_{20}H_{25}NO_2S_2 \cdot HCl$. 412.01. [Tiagabine is INN and BAN.] (1) 3-Piperidinecarboxylic acid, 1-[4,4-bis(3-methyl-2-thienyl)-3-butenyl]-, hydrochloride, (*R*)-; (2) (-)-(*R*)-1-[4,4-Bis(3-methyl-2-thienyl)-3-butenyl]nipecotic acid, hydrochloride. *UNII-DQH6T6D8OY; UNII-Z80I64HMNP* [tiagabine]. *CAS-145821-59-6; CAS-115103-54-3* [tiagabine]. *Anticonvulsant*. Gabitril (Cephalon) ◇*Abbott-70569.1; Abbott-70569.HCl; ABT-569; NO-05-0328; NNC-05-0328*

Tiamenidine [*1989*] (tye″ a men′ i deen). $C_8H_{10}ClN_3S$. 215.70. (1) 1*H*-Imidazol-2-amine, *N*-(2-chloro-4-methyl-3-thienyl)-4,5-dihydro-; (2) 2-[(2-Chloro-4-methyl-3-thienyl)amino]-2-imidazoline. *UNII-195V08O55G*. *CAS-31428-61-2*. INN; BAN. *Antihypertensive*. Symcor Base TTS (Hoechst-Roussel†) ◇*HOE 440*

Tiamenidine Hydrochloride [*1977*] (tye″ a men′ i deen hye″ droe klor′ ide). $C_8H_{10}ClN_3S.HCl$. 252.16. (1) 1*H*-Imidazol-2-amine, *N*-(2-chloro-4-methyl-3-thienyl)-4,5-dihydro-, monohydrochloride; (2) 2-[(2-Chloro-4-methyl-3-thienyl)amino]-2-imidazoline monohydrochloride. *UNII-9SE2T8DW90. CAS-51274-83-0. Antihypertensive.* Symcor (Hoechst-Roussel†) ◇*HOE 42-440*

Tiametonium Iodide. $C_{12}H_{30}I_2N_2S$. 488.25. (Thiodiethylene)-bis(ethyldimethylammonium iodide). *UNII-Z0OMD60978. CAS-10433-71-3.* INN.

Tiamiprine (INN) — *See* Thiamiprine.

Tiamizide (INN) — *See* Diapamide.

Tiamulin [*1979*] (tye″ a mue′ lin). **USP.** $C_{28}H_{47}NO_4S$. 493.74. (1) Acetic acid, [[2-(diethylamino)ethyl]thio]-, 6-ethenyl-decahydro-5-hydroxy-4,6,9,10-tetramethyl-1-oxo-3a,9-propano-3a*H*-cyclopentacycloocten-8-yl ester [3a*S*-(3aα, 4β,5α,6α,8β,9α,9aβ,10*S**)]-; (2) [[2-(Diethylamino)ethyl]thio]acetic acid 8-ester with (3a*S*,4*R*,5*S*,6*S*,8*R*,9-*R*,9a*R*,10*R*)-octahydro-5,8-dihydroxy-4,6,9,10)-tetramethyl-6-vinyl-3a,9-propano-3a*H*-cyclopentacycloocten-1(4*H*)-one. *CAS-55297-95-5; CAS-56142-71-3* [replaced]. INN; BAN. *Antibacterial (veterinary).* Denagard (Boehringer Ingelheim Animal Health) ◇*SQ 14055*

Tiamulin Fumarate [*1979*] (tye″ a mue′ lin fue′ ma rate). **USP.** $C_{28}H_{47}NO_4S.C_4H_4O_4$. 609.81. (1) Tiamulin Hydrogen Fumarate; (2) Acetic acid, [[2-(diethylamino)ethyl]thio]-, 6-ethenyldecahydro-5-hydroxy-4,6,9,10-tetramethyl-1-oxo-3a,9-propano-3a*H*-cyclopentacycloocten-8-yl ester [3a*S*-(3aα,4β,5α,6α,8β,9α,9aβ,10*S**)]-, (*E*)-2-butenedioate (1:1) (salt); (3) [[2-(Diethylamino)ethyl]thio]acetic acid 8-ester with (3a*S*,4*R*,5*S*,6*S*,8*R*,9*R*,9a*R*,10*R*)-octahydro-5,8-dihydroxy-4,6,9,10-tetramethyl-6-vinyl-3a,9-propano-3a*H*-cyclopentacycloocten-1(4*H*)-one fumarate (1:1) (salt). *CAS-55297-96-6; CAS-55297-95-5* [tiamulin]. *Antibacterial (veterinary).* Dynamutilin (Bristol-Myers Squibb†) ◇*SQ 22947*

Tianafac. $C_{11}H_9ClO_2S$. 240.71. 5-Chloro-3-methylbenzo[*b*]thiophene-2-acetic acid. *UNII-P0T3ZRK3XV. CAS-51527-19-6.* INN.

Tianeptine. $C_{21}H_{25}ClN_2O_4S$. 436.95. 7-[(3-Chloro-6,11-dihydro-6-methyldibenzo[*c*,*f*][1,2]thiazepin-11-yl)amino]heptanoic acid *S*,*S*-dioxide. *CAS-66981-73-5.* INN; MI.

Tiapamil Hydrochloride [*1984*] (tye ap′ a mil hye″ droe klor′ ide). $C_{26}H_{37}NO_8S.HCl.H_2O$. 578.12. [Tiapamil is INN and BAN.] (1) 1,3-Dithiane-2-propanamine, 2-(3,4-dimethoxyphenyl)-*N*-[2-(3,4-dimethoxyphenyl)ethyl]-*N*-methyl-, 1,1,3,3-tetraoxide, hydrochloride, monohydrate; (2) *N*-(3,4-Dimethoxyphenethyl)-2-(3,4-dimethoxyphenyl)-*N*-methyl-*m*-dithiane-2-propylamine 1,1,3,3-tetraoxide hydrochloride monohydrate. *CAS-87434-83-1; CAS-57010-31-8* [tiapamil]. *Antagonist (to calcium).* ◇*Ro 11-1781/023*

Tiapirinol. $C_{12}H_{16}N_2O_4S$. 284.33. Tetrahydro-2-[3-hydroxy-5-(hydroxymethyl)-2-methyl-4-pyridyl]-2*H*-1,3-thiazine-4-carboxylic acid. *CAS-14785-50-3.* INN.

Tiapride. $C_{15}H_{24}N_2O_4S$. 328.43. [Tiapride Hydrochloride is JAN.] *N*-[2-(Diethylamino)ethyl]-5-(methylsulfonyl)-*o*-anisamide. *CAS-51012-32-9.* INN; BAN; DCF; MI.

Tiaprofenic Acid. $C_{14}H_{12}O_3S$. 260.31. 5-Benzoyl-α-methyl-2-thiopheneacetic acid. *CAS-33005-95-7.* INN; BAN; JAN; DCF; MI. ◇*RU 15060*

Tiaprost. $C_{20}H_{28}O_6S$. 396.50. (±)-(Z)-7-[(1R*,2R*,3R*,5S*)-3,5-Dihydroxy-2-[(E)-(3R*S*)-3-hydroxy-4-(3-thienyloxy)-1-butenyl]cyclopentyl]-5-heptenoic acid. *CAS-71116-82-0.* INN; BAN; MI.

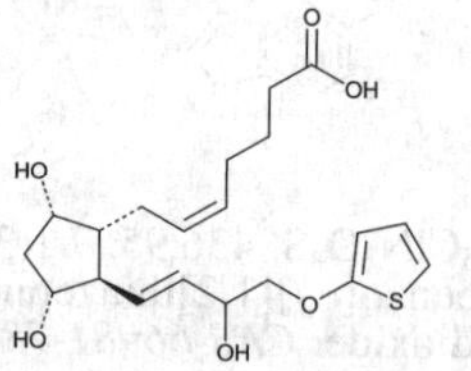

Tiaramide Hydrochloride [*1981*] (tye ar′ a mide hye″ droe klor′ ide). $C_{15}H_{18}ClN_3O_3S$·HCl. 392.30. [Tiaramide is INN and BAN.] (1) 1-Piperazineethanol, 4-[(5-chloro-2-oxo-3(2H)-benzothiazolyl)acetyl]-, monohydrochloride; (2) 4-[(5-Chloro-2-oxo-3-benzothiazolinyl)acetyl]-1-piperazineethanol monohydrochloride. *CAS-35941-71-0* [monohydrochloride]; *CAS-32527-55-2* [tiaramide]. JAN. *Antiasthmatic.*

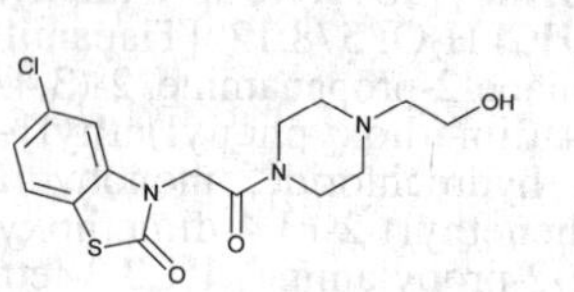

Tiazesim (INN, BAN) Hydrochloride — *See* Thiazesim Hydrochloride.

Tiazofurin [*1982*] (tye az″ oh fure′ in). $C_9H_{12}N_2O_5S$. 260.27. [Tiazofurine is INN.] (1) 4-Thiazolecarboxamide, 2-β-D-ribofuranosyl-; (2) 2-β-D-Ribofuranosyl-4-thiazolecarboxamide. *CAS-60084-10-8. Antineoplastic.* ◊CI-909; NSC-286193

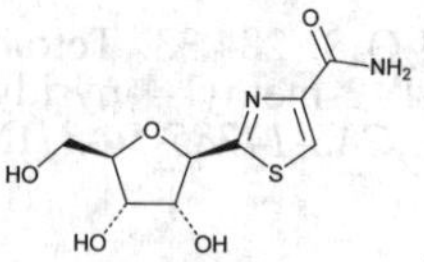

Tiazuril [*1972*] (tye az′ ue ril; tye az′ ure il). $C_{17}H_{14}ClN_3O_2S$. 359.83. (1) 1,2,4-Triazine-3,5(2H,4H)-dione, 2-[4-[(4-chlorophenyl)thio]-3,5-dimethylphenyl]-; (2) 2-[4-[(p-Chlorophenyl)thio]-3,5-xylyl]-as-triazine-3,5-(2H,4H)-dione. *UNII-14LS8QHX0U. CAS-35319-70-1.* INN. *Coccidiostat (for poultry).* ◊CP-25,673

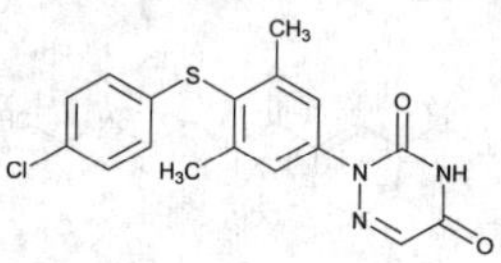

Tibalosin. $C_{21}H_{27}NOS$. 341.51. (±)-erythro-2,3-Dihydro-α-[1-[(4-phenylbutyl)amino]ethyl]benzo[b]thiophene-5-methanol. *CAS-63996-84-9.* INN.

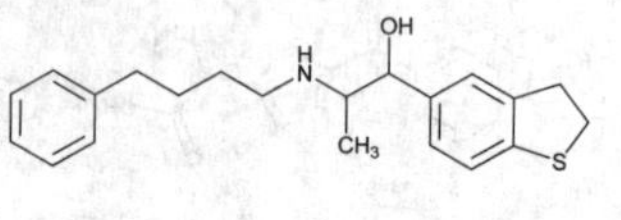

Tibeglisene. $C_{18}H_{15}ClO_4S$. 362.83. (±)-5-(p-Chlorophenyl)-2-(p-tolylsulfonyl)-4-pentynoic acid. *CAS-129731-11-9.* INN.

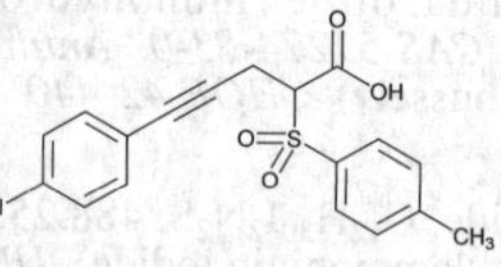

Tibenelast Sodium [*1987*] (tye ben′ e last soe′ dee um). $C_{13}H_{13}NaO_4S$. 288.29. [Tibenelast is INN.] (1) Benzo[b]thiophene-2-carboxylic acid, 5,6-diethoxy-, sodium salt; (2) Sodium 5,6-diethoxybenzo[b]thiophene-2-carboxylate. *UNII-V58CN2SY21. CAS-105102-18-9. Anti-asthmatic; bronchodilator.* ◊LY 186655

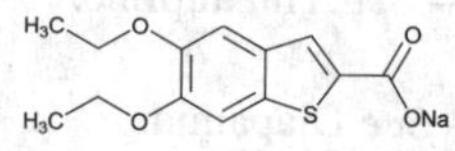

Tibenzate. $C_{14}H_{12}OS$. 228.31. S-Benzyl thiobenzoate. *UNII-0I93JSA6L6. CAS-13402-51-2.* INN.

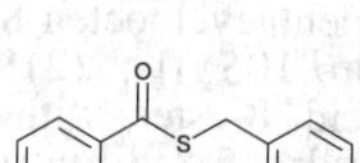

Tibezonium Iodide. $C_{28}H_{32}IN_3S_2$. 601.61. Diethylmethyl[2-[[4-[p-(phenylthio)phenyl]-3H-1,5-benzodiazepin-2-yl]thio]ethyl]ammonium iodide. *UNII-E9P274AJEW. CAS-54663-47-7.* INN; MI.

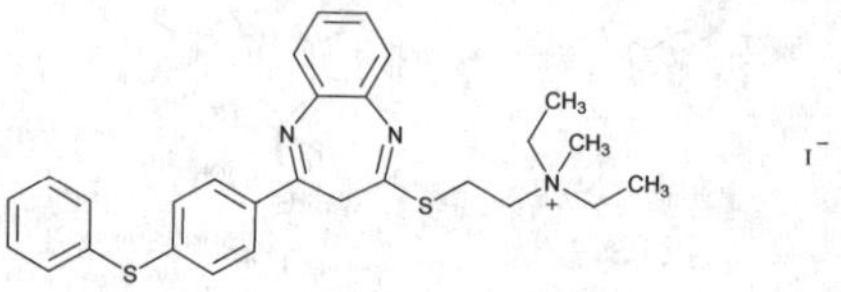

Tibolone [*1969*] (tye′ boe lone). $C_{21}H_{28}O_2$. 312.45. (1) 19-Norpregn-5(10)-en-20-yn-3-one, 17-hydroxy-7-methyl-, (7α,17α)-; (2) 17-Hydroxy-7α-methyl-19-nor-17α-pregn-5(10)-en-20-yn-3-one. *CAS-5630-53-5.* INN; BAN. *Menopausal symptoms suppressant.* ◊Org OD 14

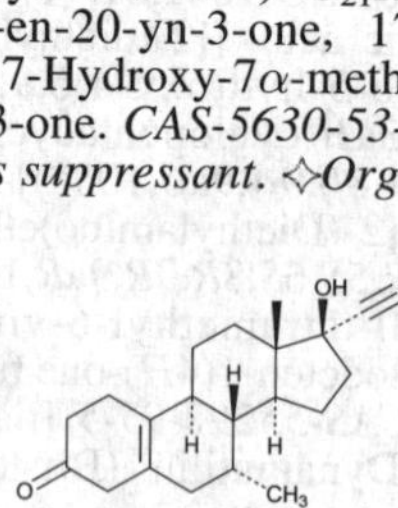

Tibric Acid [*1973*] (tye′ brik as′ id). $C_{14}H_{18}ClNO_4S$. 331.82. (1) Benzoic acid, 2-chloro-5-[(3,5-dimethyl-1-piperidinyl)sulfonyl]-, (cis)-; (2) 2-Chloro-5-[(cis-3,5-dimethylpiperidino)sulfonyl]benzoic acid. *CAS-37087-94-8; CAS-24358-29-0* [nonstereospecific]. INN; BAN. *Antihyperlipoproteinemic.* ◊CP-18,524

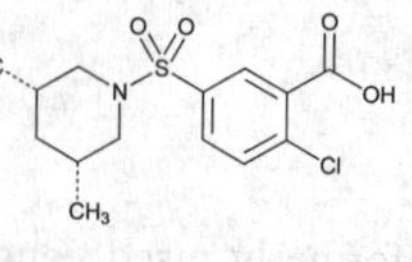

Tibrofan [*1967*] (tye′ broe fan). C₁₁H₆Br₃NOS. 439.95. (1) 2-Thiophenecarboxamide, 4,5-dibromo-*N*-(4-bromophenyl)-; (2) 4,4′,5-Tribromo-2-thiophenecarboxanilide. *CAS-15686-72-3.* INN. *Disinfectant.*

Ticabesone Propionate [*1983*] (tye ka′ be sone proe′ pee oh nate). C₂₅H₃₂F₂O₅S. 482.58. [Ticabesone is INN.] (1) Androsta-1,4-diene-17-carbothioic acid, 6,9-difluoro-11-hydroxy-16-methyl-3-oxo-17-(1-oxopropoxy)-, *S*-methyl ester, (6α,11β,16α,17α)-; (2) *S*-Methyl 6α,9-difluoro-11β,17-dihydroxy-16α-methyl-3-oxoandrosta-1,4-diene-17β-carbothioate, 17-propionate. *CAS-73205-13-7; CAS-74131-77-4* [ticabesone]. *Glucocorticoid.* ◇*RS-35909-00-00-0*

Ticagrelor [*2007*] (tye ka′ grel or). C₂₃H₂₈F₂N₆O₄S. 522.57. (1) 1,2-Cyclopentanediol, 3-[7-[[(1*R*,2*S*)-2-(3,4-difluorophenyl)cyclopropyl]amino]-5-(propylthio)-3*H*-1,2,3-triazolo[4,5-*d*]pyrimidin-3-yl]-5-(2-hydroxyethoxy)-, (1*S*,2*S*,3*R*,5*S*)-; (2) (1*S*,2*S*,3*R*,5*S*)-3-(7-((1*R*,2*S*)-2-(3,4-Difluorophenyl)cyclopropylamino)-5-(propylthio)-3*H*-[1,2,3]triazolo[4,5-*d*]pyrimidin-3-yl)-5-(2-hydroxyethoxy)cyclopentane-1,2-diol. *UNII-GLH0314RVC. CAS-274693-27-5.* INN. *Prevention of thromboembolic events in patients with acute coronary syndrome.* ◇*AZD6140; AR-C126532XX*

Ticalopride. C₁₄H₂₀ClN₃O₃. 313.78. 4-Amino-5-chloro-*N*-[(3*S*,4*R*)-3-methoxy-4-piperidyl]-*o*-anisamide. *UNII-QNG273A81O. CAS-202590-69-0.* INN.

Ticarbodine [*1971*] (tye kar′ boe deen). C₁₅H₁₉F₃N₂S. 316.38. (1) 1-Piperidinecarbothioamide, 2,6-dimethyl-*N*-[3-(trifluoromethyl)phenyl]-; (2) α,α,α-Trifluoro-2,6-dimethylthio-1-piperidinecarboxy-*m*-toluidide. *UNII-J4CLF34O60. CAS-31932-09-9.* INN; BAN. *Anthelmintic.* ◇*EL-974*

Ticarcillin Cresyl Sodium [*1976*] (tye″ kar sil′ in kres′ il soe′ dee um). C₂₂H₂₁N₂NaO₆S₂. 496.53. (1) 4-Thia-1-azabicyclo[3.2.0]heptane-2-carboxylic acid, 3,3-dimethyl-6-[[3-(4-methylphenoxy)-1,3-dioxo-2-(3-thienyl)propyl]amino]-7-oxo-, monosodium salt, [2*S*-[2α,5α,6β(*S**)]]-; (2) *p*-Tolyl (*R*)-*N*-[(2*S*,5*R*,6*R*)-(2-carboxy-3,3-dimethyl-7-oxo-4-thia-1-azabicyclo[3.2.0]hept-6-yl)]-3-thiophenemalonamate sodium salt. *CAS-59070-06-3; CAS-59070-07-4* [ticarcillin cresyl]. *Antibacterial.* ◇*BRL 12594*

Ticarcillin Disodium [*1973*] (tye″ kar sil′ in dye soe′ dee um). USP. C₁₅H₁₄N₂Na₂O₆S₂. 428.39. [Ticarcillin is INN and BAN; Ticarcillin Sodium is JAN.] (1) 4-Thia-1-azabicyclo[3.2.0]heptane-2-carboxylic acid, 6-[(carboxy-3-thienylacetyl)amino]-3,3-dimethyl-7-oxo-, disodium salt, [2*S*-[2α,5α,6β(*S**)]]-; (2) *N*-(2-Carboxy-3,3-dimethyl-7-oxo-4-thia-1-azabicyclo[3.2.0]hept-6-yl)-3-thiophenemalonamic acid disodium salt. *UNII-G8TVV6DSYG; UNII-F93UJX4SWT* [ticarcillin]. *CAS-4697-14-7; CAS-34787-01-4* [ticarcillin]. *Antibacterial.* Ticar (GlaxoSmithKline) ◇*BRL 2288*

Ticarcillin Monosodium (tye″ kar sil′ in mon″ oh soe′ dee um). USP. C₁₅H₁₅N₂NaO₆S₂.H₂O. 424.42. (1) 4-Thia-1-azabicyclo[3.2.0]heptane-2-carboxylic acid, 6-[(carboxy-3-thienylacetyl)amino]-3,3-dimethyl-7-oxo, monosodium salt, [2*S*-[2α,5α,6β(*S**)]]-, monohydrate; (2) (*R*)-*N*-[(2*S*,5*R*,6*R*)-2-Carboxy-3,4-dimethyl-7-oxo-4-thia-1-azabicyclo[3.2.0]hept-6-yl]-3-thiophenemalonamic acid monosodium salt. *CAS-74682-62-5* [anhydrous]. *Antibacterial.*

Ticilimumab (previously used name) — *See* Tremelimumab.

Ticlatone [*1970*] (tye′ kla tone). C₇H₄ClNOS. 185.63. (1) 1,2-Benzisothiazol-3(2*H*)-one, 6-chloro-; (2) 6-Chloro-1,2-benzisothiazolin-3-one. *CAS-70-10-0.* INN. *Antibacterial; antifungal.* ◇*FER-1443*

Ticlopidine Hydrochloride [*1978*] (tye kloe′ pi deen hye″ droe klor′ ide). C₁₄H₁₄ClNS.HCl. 300.25. [Ticlopidine is INN and BAN.] (1) Thieno[3,2-*c*]pyridine, 5-[(2-chloro-

---

† Brand name formerly used, and/or firm no longer concerned with this product.

phenyl)methyl]-4,5,6,7-tetrahydro-, hydrochloride; (2) 5-(*o*-Chlorobenzyl)-4,5,6,7-tetrahydrothieno-[3,2-*c*]pyridine hydrochloride. *UNII-A1L4914FMF; UNII-OM90ZUW7M1* [ticlopidine]. *CAS-53885-35-1; CAS-55142-85-3* [ticlopidine]. JAN. *Inhibitor (platelet).* Ticlid (Roche) ◇*53-32C; 4-C-32*

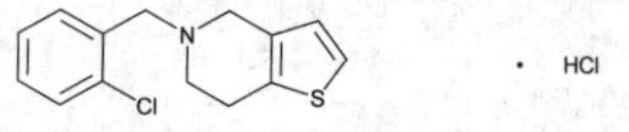

Ticolubant [*1996*] (tye kol′ ue bant). $C_{23}H_{19}Cl_2NO_3S$. 460.37. (1) 2-Propenoic acid, 3-[6[[(2,6-dichlorophenyl)thio]-methyl]-3-(2-phenylethoxy)-2-pyridinyl]-, (*E*)-; (2) (*E*)-6-[[(2,6-Dichlorophenyl)thio]methyl]-3-(phenethyloxy)-2-pyridineacrylic acid. *CAS-154413-61-3*. INN. *Antipsoriatic.* ◇*SB-209247*

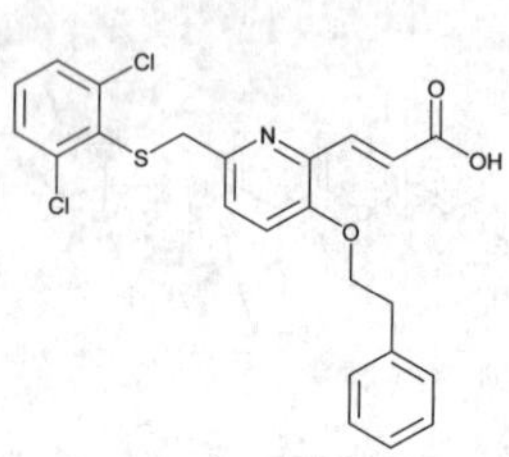

Ticrynafen [*1975*] (tye krin′ a fen). $C_{13}H_8Cl_2O_4S$. 331.17. [Tienilic Acid is INN and BAN.] (1) Acetic acid, [[2,3-dichloro-4-(2-thienylcarbonyl)phenoxy]-; (2) [2,3-Dichloro-4-(2-thenoyl)phenoxy]acetic acid. *CAS-40180-04-9. Diuretic; uricosuric; antihypertensive.* Selacryn (SmithKline Beecham†) ◇*SK&F 62698*

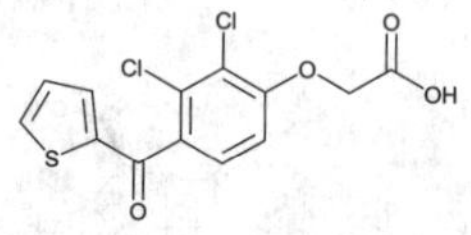

Tidembersat [*2000*] (tye dem′ ber sat). $C_{20}H_{19}F_2NO_4$. 375.37. (1) Benzamide, *N*-(6-acetyl-3,4-dihydro-3-hydroxy-2,2-di-methyl-2*H*-1-benzopyran-4-yl)-3,5-difluoro-, (3*R*-*trans*)-; (2) *N*-[(3*R*,4*S*)-6-Acetyl-3-hydroxy-2,2-dimethyl-4-chromanyl]-3,5-difluorobenzamide. *CAS-175013-73-7.* INN. *Antimigraine.* ◇*SB-218842*

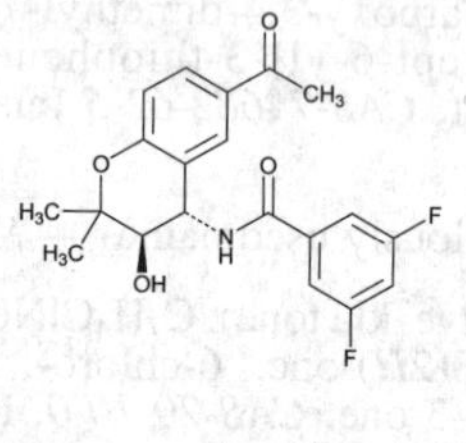

Tidiacic. $C_5H_7NO_4S$. 177.18. 2,4-Thiazolidinedicarboxylic acid. *UNII-F39KSS6R80. CAS-30097-06-4.* INN; DCF.

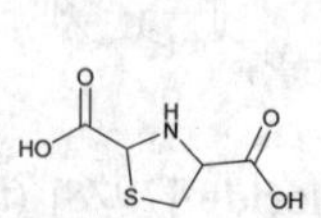

Tiemonium Iodide. $C_{18}H_{24}INO_2S$. 445.36. 4-[3-Hydroxy-3-phenyl-3-(2-thienyl)propyl]-4-methyl-morpholinium iodide. *UNII-FZ2LZ7U304. CAS-144-12-7; CAS-6252-92-2* [tiemonium]. INN; BAN; JAN; MI. ◇*TE 114*

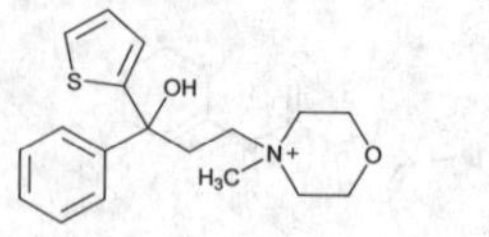

Tienilic Acid (INN, BAN, DCF) — *See* Ticrynafen.

Tienocarbine. $C_{15}H_{16}N_2S$. 256.37. 7,8,9,10-Tetrahydro-1,9-dimethyl-6*H*-pyrido[4,3-*b*]thieno[3,2-*e*]indole. *UNII-B255B0J51N. CAS-75458-65-0.* INN.

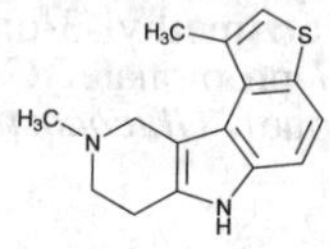

Tienopramine. $C_{17}H_{20}N_2S$. 284.42. 4-[3-(Dimethylamino)-propyl]-4*H*-thieno[3,2-*b*][1]benzazepine. *UNII-36L0QUK8SY. CAS-37967-98-9.* INN.

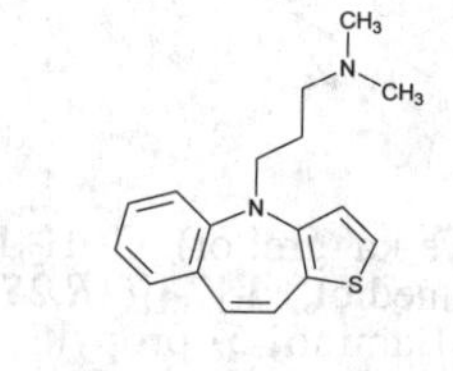

Tienoxolol. $C_{21}H_{28}N_2O_5S$. 420.52. (±)-Ethyl 2-[3-(*tert*-butylamino)-2-hydroxypropoxy]-5-(2-thiophenecarboxamido)benzoate. *CAS-90055-97-3.* INN.

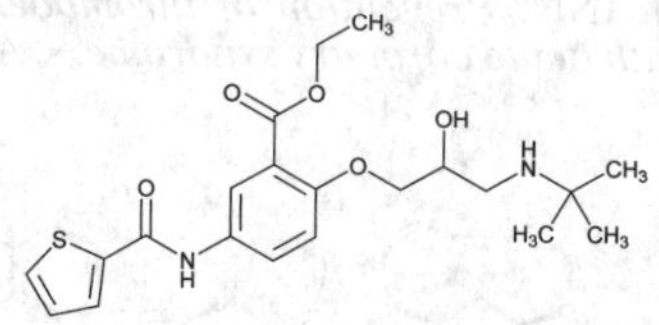

Tifacogin [*1997*] (tye″ fa ko′ gin). $C_{1400}H_{2167}N_{395}O_{422}S_{23}$. 32,021.11. *N*-L-Alanylblood-coagulation factor LACI (human clone λ P9 protein moiety reduced). *CAS-148883-56-1.* INN. *Anticoagulant (lipoprotein associated coagulation inhibitor).* ◇*SC-59735; LACI*

```
ADSEEDEEHT IITDTELPPL KLMHSFCAFK ADDGPCKAIM KRFFFNIFTR
QCEEFIYGGC EGNQNRFESL EECKKMCTRD NANRIIKTTL QQEKPDFCFL
EEDPGICRGY ITRYFYNNQT KQCERFKYGG CLGNMNNFET LEECKNICED
GPNGFQVDNY GTQLNAVNNS LTPQSTKVPS LFEFHGPSWC LTPADRGLCR
ANENRFYYNS VIGKCRPFKY SGCGGNENNF TSKQECLRAC KKGFIQRISK
GGLIKTKRKR KKQRVKIAYE EIFVKNM
```

Tifemoxone. $C_{11}H_{13}NO_2S$. 223.29. Tetrahydro-6-(phenoxy-methyl)-2*H*-1,3-oxazine-2-thione. *UNII-09I93HJ3Y4. CAS-39754-64-8.* INN.

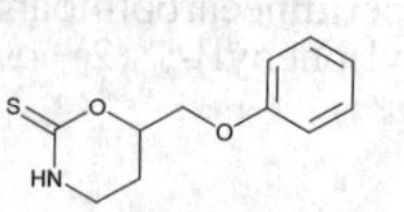

Tifenamil (INN) Hydrochloride — *See* Thiphenamil Hydrochloride.

Tifenazoxide. $C_9H_{10}ClN_3O_2S_2$. 291.78. 6-Chloro-*N*-(1-methylcyclopropyl)-1,1-dioxo-1,4-dihydro-1λ^6-thieno[3,2-*e*][1,2,4]thiadiazin-3-amine. *CAS-279215-43-9*. INN.

Tifencillin (INN) Potassium — *See* Thiphencillin Potassium.

Tiflamizole. $C_{17}H_{10}F_6N_2O_2S$. 420.33. 4,5-Bis(*p*-fluorophenyl)-2-[(1,1,2,2-tetrafluoroethyl)sulfonyl]imidazole. *CAS-62894-89-7*. INN.

Tiflorex. $C_{12}H_{16}F_3NS$. 263.32. (+)-*N*-Ethyl-α-methyl-*m*-[(trifluoromethyl)thio]phenethylamine. *UNII-EG3B69DFQ5*. *CAS-53993-67-2*. INN.

Tifluadom. $C_{22}H_{20}FN_3OS$. 393.48. (±)-*N*-[[5-(*o*-Fluorophenyl)-2,3-dihydro-1-methyl-1*H*-1,4-benzodiazepin-2-yl]methyl]-3-thiophenecarboxamide. *CAS-81656-30-6*. INN.

Tiflucarbine. $C_{16}H_{17}FN_2S$. 288.38. 9-Ethyl-4-fluoro-7,8,9,10-tetrahydro-1-methyl-6*H*-pyrido[4,3-*b*]thieno[3,2-*e*]indole. *UNII-M2108NUY0C*. *CAS-89875-86-5*. INN.

Tiformin. $C_5H_{12}N_4O$. 144.17. 4-Guanidinobutyramide. *CAS-4210-97-3*. INN; BAN; MI. *[Name previously used: Tyformin.]* ◇*HL 523 [as hydrochloride]*

Tifurac Sodium [*1987*] (tye′ fure ak soe′ dee um). $C_{18}H_{13}NaO_4S.xH_2O$. 348.35 (anhydrous). [Tifurac is INN.] (1) 5-Benzofuranacetic acid, 7-[4-(methylthio)benzoyl]-, sodium salt, hydrate; (2) Sodium 7-[*p*-(methylthio)benzoyl]-5-benzofuranacetate, hydrate. *UNII-S5TJ79BX74*. *CAS-102488-97-1*; *CAS-97483-17-5* [tifurac]. *Analgesic*. ◇*RS-82917-030*

Tifuvirtide. $C_{235}H_{341}N_{57}O_{67}$. 5036.56. *N*-Acetyl-L-tryptophyl-L-glutaminyl-L-glutamyl-L-tryptophyl-L-glutamyl-L-glutaminyl-L-lysyl-L-isoleucyl-L-threonyl-L-alanyl-L-leucyl-L-leucyl-L-glutamyl-L-glutaminyl-L-alanyl-L-glutaminyl-L-isoleucyl-L-glutaminyl-L-glutaminyl-L-glutamyl-L-lysyl-L-asparagyl-L-glutamyl-L-tyrosyl-L-glutamyl-L-leucyl-L-glutaminyl-L-lysyl-L-leucyl-L-aspartyl-L-lysyl-L-tryptophyl-L-alanyl-L-seryl-L-leucyl-L-tryptophyl-L-glutamyl-L-tryptophyl-L-phenylalaninamide. *CAS-251562-00-2*. INN.

Tigapotide Triflutate [*2006*] (tye gap′ oh tide trye floo′ tate). $C_{82}H_{119}N_{21}O_{34}S_3.C_2HF_3O_2$. 2153.16. [Tigapotide is INN.] (1) L-Threonine, L-α-glutamyl-L-tryptophyl-L-glutaminyl-L-threonyl-L-α-aspartyl-L-asparaginyl-*S*-[(acetylamino)methyl]-L-cysteinyl-L-α-glutamyl-L-threonyl-*S*-[(acetylamino)methyl]-L-cysteinyl-L-threonyl-*S*-[(acetylamino)methyl]-L-cysteinyl-L-tyrosyl-L-α-glutamyl-, mono(trifluoroacetate); (2) L-α-Glutamyl-L-tryptophyl-L-glutaminyl-L-threonyl-L-α-aspartyl-L-asparaginyl-*S*-[(acetylamino)methyl]-L-cysteinyl-L-α-glutamyl-L-threonyl-*S*-[(acetylamino)methyl]-L-cysteinyl-L-threonyl-*S*-[(acetylamino)methyl]-L-cysteinyl-L-tyrosyl-L-α-glutamyl-L-threonine mono(trifluoroacetate). *CAS-848084-84-4*; *CAS-848084-83-3* [tigapotide]. *Treatment of metastatic hormone refractory prostate cancer*. ◇*PCK3145*

Tigatuzumab. $C_{6406}H_{9924}N_{1716}O_{2012}S_{46}$. Immunoglobulin G1, anti-[*Homo sapiens* TNFRSF10B (tumor necrosis factor receptor superfamily member 10b, DR5, TRAIL-R2, CD262)] humanized monoclonal TRA-8 (or CS-1008); gamma1 heavy chain [humanized VH (*Homo sapiens* FR/*Mus musculus* CDR) [8.8.12]-*Homo sapiens* IGHG1*03] (222-213′)-disulfide with kappa light chain [humanized V-KAPPA (*Homo sapiens* FR/*Mus musculus* CDR) [6.3.8]-*Homo sapiens* IGKC*01]; (228-228″:231-231″)-bisdisulfide dimer. *CAS-918127-53-4*. INN.

Tigecycline [*2002*] (tye″ ge sye′ kleen). $C_{29}H_{39}N_5O_8$. 585.65. (1) 2-Naphthacenecarboxamide, 4,7-bis(dimethylamino)-9-[[[(1,1-dimethylethyl)amino]acetyl]amino]-1,4,4a,5,5a,6,11,12a-octahydro-3,10,12,12a-tetrahydroxy-1,11-dioxo-, (4*S*,4a*S*,5a*R*,12a*S*)-; (2) (4*S*,4a*S*,5a*R*,12a*S*)-9-[2-(*tert*-butylamino)acetamido]-4,7-bis(dimethylamino)-1,4,4a,5,5a,6,11,12a-octahydro-3,10,12,12a-tetrahydroxy-1,11-dioxo-2-naphthacenecarboxamide. *UNII-70JE2N95KR*. *CAS-220620-09-7*. INN. *Antibacterial (bacterial protein synthesis inhibitor)*. Tygacil (Wyeth) ◇*WAY-GAR-936*

---

† Brand name formerly used, and/or firm no longer concerned with this product.

Tigemonam Dicholine [*1987*] (tye″ ge moe′ nam dye koe′ leen). $C_{12}H_{13}N_5O_9S_2$.2($C_5H_{14}NO$). 643.73. [Tigemonam is INN.] (1) Ethanaminium, 2-hydroxy-*N,N,N*-trimethyl-, salt with [*S(Z)*]-[[[1-(2-amino-4-thiazolyl)-2-[[2,2-dimethyl-4-oxo-1-sulfooxy)-3-azetidinyl]amino]-2-oxoethylidene]amino]oxylacetic acid (2:1); (2) Choline, salt with [[[(Z)-(2-amino-4-thiazolyl)[[(3*S*)-1-hydroxy-2,2-dimethyl-4-oxo-3-azetidinyl]carbamoyl]methylene]amino]oxy]acetic acid hydrogen sulfate (ester) (2:1). *CAS-102916-21-2; CAS-102507-71-1* [tigemonam]. *Antimicrobial.* Tigemen (Bristol-Myers Squibb†) ◇*SQ 30836*

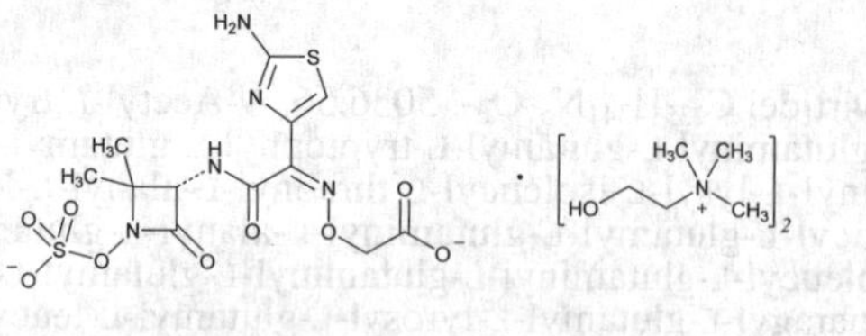

Tigestol [*1968*] (tye jes′ tol). $C_{20}H_{28}O$. 284.44. (1) 19-Norpregn-5(10)-en-20-yn-17-ol, (17α)-; (2) 19-Nor-17α-pregn-5(10)-en-20-yn-17-ol. *CAS-896-71-9.* INN. *Progestin.*

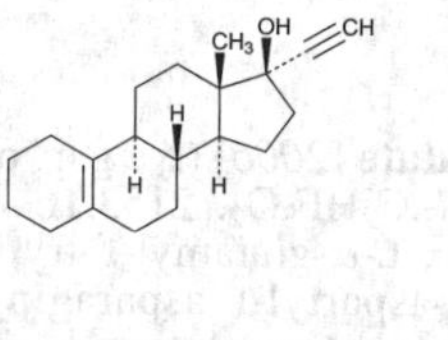

Tigloidine. $C_{13}H_{21}NO_2$. 223.31. Tiglyl*pseudo*tropine. *CAS-495-83-0.* INN; BAN; MI.

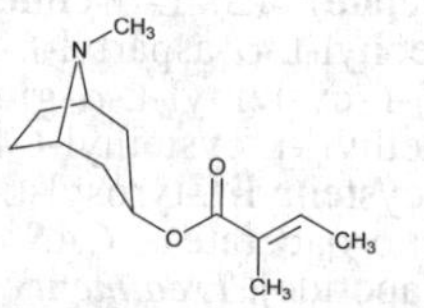

Tiglyltropeine — *See* Tropigline.

Tilactase. [Galactosidase is JAN.] β-D-Galactosidase. *CAS-9031-11-2.* INN; JAN.

Tilarginine Acetate [*2004*] (til ar′ ji neen as′ e tate). $C_7H_{16}N_4O_2$.$C_2H_4O_2$. 248.28. [Tilarginine is INN; Targinine is BAN.] (1) L-Ornithine, N^5-[imino(methylamino)-methyl]-, monoacetate; (2) (2*S*)-2-Amino-5-[(methylcarbamimidoyl)amino]pentanoic acid monoacetate. *CAS-53308-83-1; CAS-17035-90-4* [tilarginine]. *Treatment of cardiogenic shock complicating acute myocardial infarction (MI).* (Ferro Pfanstiehl) [*Name previously used: Targinine.*] ◇*ANO-1020*

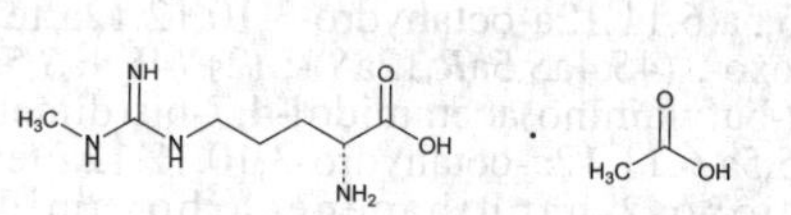

Tilbroquinol. $C_{10}H_8BrNO$. 238.08. 7-Bromo-5-methyl-8-quinolinol. *UNII-P6SB125NHA. CAS-7175-09-9.* INN.

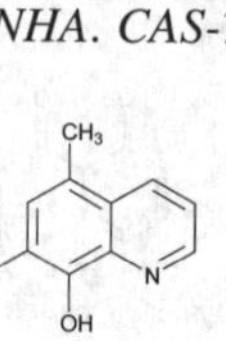

Tildipirosin. $C_{41}H_{71}N_3O_8$. 734.02. (4*R*,5*S*,6*S*,7*R*,9*R*,11*E*,13*E*,15*R*,16*R*-6-{[3,6-Dideoxy-3-(dimethylamino)-β-D-glucopyranosyl]oxy}-16-ethyl-4-hydroxy-5,9,13-trimethyl-7-[2-(piperidin-1-yl)ethyl]-15-[(piperidin-1-yl)methyl]oxacyclohexadeca-11,13-diene-2,10-dione. *CAS-328898-40-4.* INN.

Tiletamine Hydrochloride [*1970*] (tye let′ a meen hye″ droe klor′ ide). **USP.** $C_{12}H_{17}NOS$.HCl. 259.80. [Tiletamine is INN and BAN.] (1) Cyclohexanone, 2-(ethylamino)-2-(2-thienyl)-, hydrochloride; (2) 2-(Ethylamino)-2-(2-thienyl)-cyclohexanone hydrochloride. *CAS-14176-50-2; CAS-14176-49-9* [tiletamine]. *Anesthetic; anticonvulsant.* ◇*CI-634; CL 399; CN-54521-2*

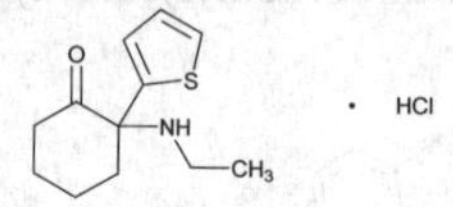

Tilidate (BAN) — *See* Tilidine Hydrochloride.

Tilidine Hydrochloride [*1969*] (tye′ li deen hye″ droe klor′ ide). $C_{17}H_{23}NO_2$.HCl. 309.83. [Tilidine is INN; Tilidate is BAN.] (1) 3-Cyclohexene-1-carboxylic acid, 2-(dimethylamino)-1-phenyl-, ethyl ester, hydrochloride (*trans*)-(±)-; (2) (±)-Ethyl *trans*-2-(dimethylamino)-1-phenyl-3-cyclohexene-1-carboxylate hydrochloride. *CAS-27107-79-5* [(±)-*trans*-]; *CAS-24357-97-9* [(+)-*trans*-]; *CAS-20380-58-9* [(±)-*trans*-tilidine]. *Analgesic.* Valoron (Parke-Davis†) ◇*W 5759A*

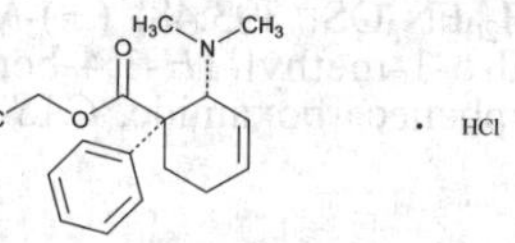

Tiliquinatine (previously used name) — *See* Intiquinatine.

Tiliquinol. $C_{10}H_9NO$. 159.18. 5-Methyl-8-quinolinol. *UNII-813OG1OGVG. CAS-5541-67-3.* INN.

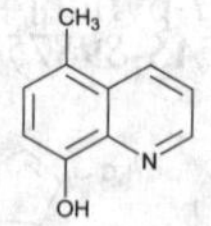

Tilisolol. $C_{17}H_{24}N_2O_3$. 304.38. (±)-4-[3-(*tert*-Butylamino)-2-hydroxypropoxy]-2-methylisocarbostyril. *UNII-QUF41MF56G. CAS-85136-71-6.* INN.

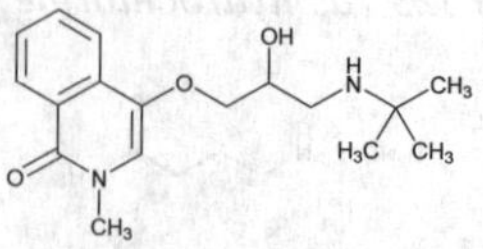

Tilmacoxib [*2002*] (til″ ma kox′ ib). $C_{16}H_{19}FN_2O_3S$. 338.40. (1) Benzenesulfonamide, 4-(4-cyclohexyl-2-methyl-5-oxazolyl)-2-fluoro-; (2) 4-(4-Cyclohexyl-2-methyloxazol-5-yl)-2-fluorobenzenesulfonamide. *UNII-G6VI5P84SX.*

CAS-180200-68-4. INN. Treatment of osteoarthritis and rheumatoid arthritis (COX-2 inhibitor). ◇*JTE-522; JTP-19605; RWJ-57504*

Tilmicosin [*1988*] (til″ mi koe′ sin). **USP.** $C_{46}H_{80}N_2O_{13}$. 869.13. (1) Tylosin, 4^A-*O*-de(2,6-dideoxy-3-*C*-methyl-α-L-*ribo*-hexopyranosyl)-20-deoxo-20-(3,5-dimethyl-1-piperidinyl)-, 20(*cis*)-; (2) 4^A-*O*-de(2,6-Dideoxy-3-*C*-methyl-α-L-*ribo*-hexopyranosyl)-20-deoxo-20-(*cis*-3,5-dimethylpiperidino)tylosin. *CAS-108050-54-0. INN; BAN. Antibacterial (veterinary).* Micotil (Lilly) ◇*LY177370; EL870*

Tilmicosin Phosphate [*1993*] (til″ mi koe′ sin fos′ fate). $C_{46}H_{80}N_2O_{13}$·H_3O_4P. 967.13. (1) Tylosin, 4^A-*O*-de(2,6-dideoxy-3-*C*-methyl-α-L-*ribo*-hexopyranosyl)-20-deoxo-20-(3,5-dimethyl-1-piperidinyl)-, [20(*cis*)]-, phosphate (1:1) (salt); (2) 4^A-*O*-de(2,6-Dideoxy-3-*C*-methyl-α-L-*ribo*-hexopyranosyl)-20-deoxo-20-(*cis*-3,5-dimethylpiperidino)tylosin phosphate (1:1) (salt). *CAS-137330-13-3. Antibacterial (veterinary).* ◇*LY177370 phosphate*

Tilnoprofen Arbamel. $C_{20}H_{22}N_2O_4$. 354.40. (±)-α,2-Dimethyl-5*H*-[1]-benzopyrano[2,3-*b*]pyridine-7-acetic acid, ester with *N,N*-dimethylglycolamide. *UNII-HY45T0EF6G. CAS-159098-79-0. INN.*

Tilomisole [*1987*] (tye loe′ mi sole). $C_{17}H_{11}ClN_2O_2S$. 342.80. (1) Thiazolo[3,2-*a*]benzimidazole-2-acetic acid, 3-(4-chlorophenyl); (2) 3-(*p*-Chlorophenyl)thiazolo[3,2-*a*]benzimidazole-2-acetic acid. *CAS-58433-11-7. INN. Immunoregulator.* ◇*WY-18,251*

Tilorone Hydrochloride [*1970*] (tye′ lor one hye″ droe klor′ ide). $C_{25}H_{34}N_2O_3$·2HCl. 483.47. [Tilorone is INN.] (1) 9*H*-Fluoren-9-one, 2,7-bis[2-(diethylamino)ethoxy]-, dihydrochloride; (2) 2,7-Bis[2-(diethylamino)ethoxy]fluoren-

9-one dihydrochloride. *UNII-BJ507J4LKY; UNII-O6W7VEW6KS* [tilorone]. *CAS-27591-69-1; CAS-27591-97-5* [tilorone]. *Antiviral.* ◇*NSC-143969*

Tilozepine. $C_{17}H_{18}ClN_3S$. 331.86. 7-Chloro-4-(4-methyl-1-piperazinyl)-10*H*-thieno[3,2-*c*][1]benzazepine. *UNII-3RG8Q831DX. CAS-42239-60-1. INN.*

Tilsuprost. $C_{20}H_{33}NO_4S$. 383.55. Methyl (±)-4-[[(3a*R**,4*R**,5*R**,6a*S**)-3,3a,4,5,6,6a-hexahydro-5-hydroxy-4-[(*E*)-(3*S**)-3-hydroxy-1-octenyl]cyclopenta[*b*]pyrrol-2-yl]thio]butyrate. *UNII-C23W8PF2D4. CAS-80225-28-1. INN.*

Tiludronate Disodium [*1994*] (tye″ loo droe′ nate dye soe′ dee um). $C_7H_7ClNa_2O_6P_2S$. 362.57. (1) Phosphonic acid, [[(4-chlorophenyl)thio]methylene]bis-, disodium salt; (2) Disodium dihydrogen [[(*p*-chlorophenyl)thio]methylene]diphosphonate. *UNII-BH6M93CIA0. CAS-149845-07-8. Paget's disease treatment; osteoporosis treatment and prevention.* Skelid (Sanofi Aventis) ◇*SR 41319B*

Tiludronic Acid. $C_7H_9ClO_6P_2S$. 318.61. [[(*p*-Chlorophenyl)thio]methylene]diphosphonic acid. *UNII-6PNS59HP4Y. CAS-89987-06-4. INN; BAN.* ◇*SR 41319*

---

† Brand name formerly used, and/or firm no longer concerned with this product.

Timcodar. $C_{43}H_{45}ClN_4O_6$. 749.29. (S)-N-Benzyl-p-chloro-α-[N-methyl-2-(3,4,5-trimethoxyphenyl)glyoxylamido]-N-[3-(4-pyridyl)-1-[2-(4-pyridyl)ethyl]propyl]hydrocinnamamide. *UNII-U141W322WZ. CAS-179033-51-3.* INN.

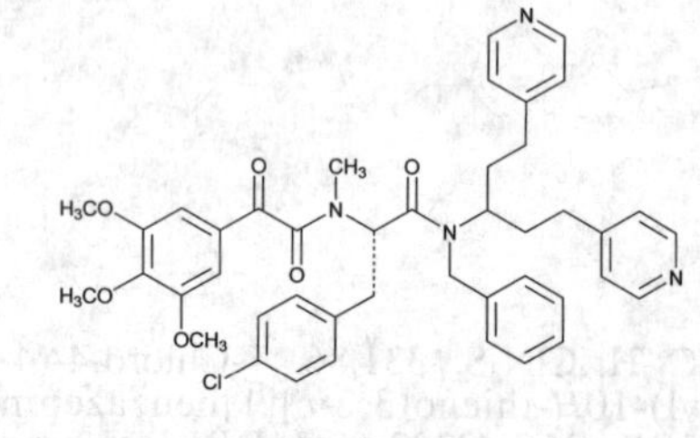

Timcodar Dimesylate [*1998*] (tim′ koe dar dye mes′ i late). $C_{43}H_{45}ClN_4O_6$·$2CH_4O_3S$. 941.50. (1) (S)-4-Chloro-α-[methyl[oxo(3,4,5-trimethoxyphenyl)acetyl]amino]-N-(phenylmethyl)-N-[3-(4-pyridinyl)-1-[2-(4-pyridinyl)ethyl]propyl]benzenepropanamide dimethanesulfonate; (2) (S)-N-Benzyl-p-chloro-α-[methyl[oxo(3,4,5-trimethoxyphenyl)glyoxylamido]-N-[3-(4-pyridyl)-1-[2-(4-pyridyl)ethyl]propyl]hydrocinnamide dimethanesulfonate. *UNII-44277I316G. CAS-183313-30-6. Used in adjuvant chemotherapy regimens to treat or prevent emergence of multidrug resistant cancers (multidrug resistance inhibitor).* ◇VX-853-2

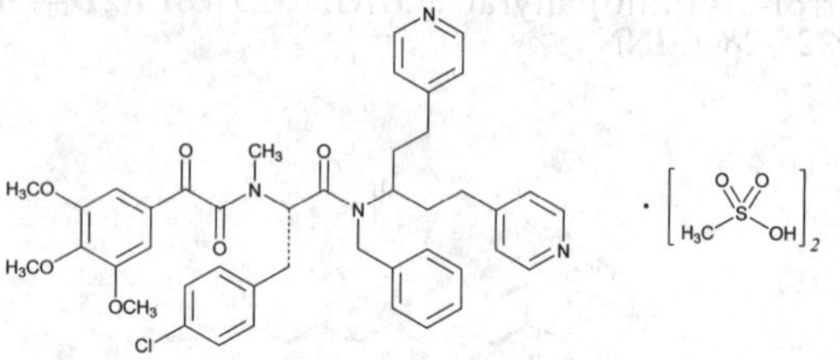

Timefurone [*1984*] (tye″ me fure′ one). $C_{15}H_{14}O_5S$. 306.33. (1) 5H-Furo[3,2-g][1]benzopyran-5-one, 4,9-dimethoxy-7-[(methylthio)methyl]-; (2) 4,9-Dimethoxy-7-[(methylthio)methyl]-5H-furo[3,2-g][1]benzopyran-5-one. *CAS-76301-19-4.* INN. *Anti-atherosclerotic.* ◇U-56,321

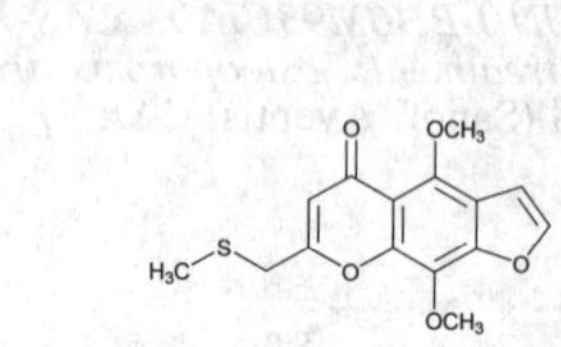

Timegadine. $C_{20}H_{23}N_5S$. 365.50. 1-Cyclohexyl-2-(2-methyl-4-quinolyl)-3-(2-thiazolyl)guanidine. *CAS-71079-19-1.* INN.

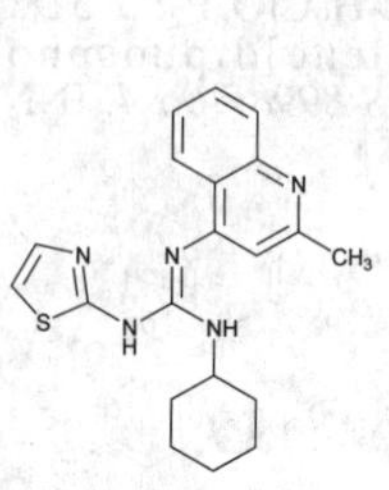

Timelotem. $C_{17}H_{18}FN_3S$. 315.41. (±)-10-Fluoro-1,2,3,4,4a,5-hexahydro-3-methyl-7-(2-thienyl)pyrazino[1,2-a][1,4]benzodiazepine. *UNII-090DE9CRP1. CAS-96306-34-2.* INN.

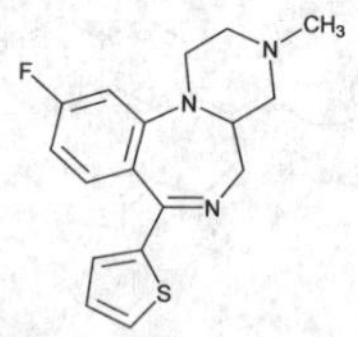

Timepidium Bromide. $C_{17}H_{22}BrNOS_2$. 400.40. 3-(Di-2-thienylmethylene)-5-methoxy-1,1-dimethyl-piperidinium bromide. *UNII-8R9E4766V4. CAS-35035-05-3.* INN; JAN; MI.

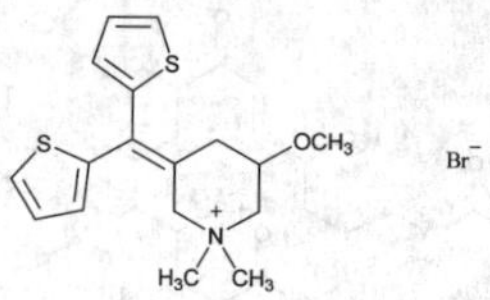

Timiperone. $C_{22}H_{24}FN_3OS$. 397.51. 4-Fluoro-4-[4-(2-thioxo-1-benzimidazolinyl)piperidino]butyrophenone. *UNII-626DQ7N19L. CAS-57648-21-2.* INN; JAN; MI.

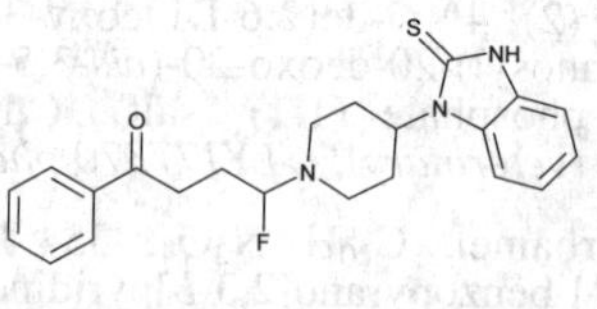

Timirdine. $C_9H_{10}ClN_3S$. 227.71. 3-(2-Amino-4-chlorophenyl)-2-iminothiazolidine. *UNII-313H31VAS6. CAS-100417-09-2.* INN.

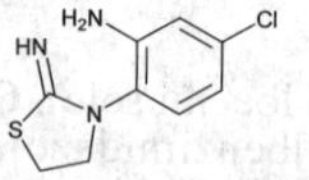

Timobesone Acetate [*1984*] (tye moe′ be sone as′ e tate). $C_{24}H_{31}FO_5S$. 450.56. [Timobesone is INN.] (1) Androsta-1,4-diene-17-carbothioic acid, 17-(acetyloxy)-9-fluoro-11-hydroxy-16-methyl-3-oxo-, S-methyl ester, (11β,16β,17α)-; (2) S-Methyl 9-fluoro-11β,17-dihydroxy-16β-methyl-3-oxoandrosta-1,4-diene-17β-carbothioate, 17-acetate. *CAS-79578-14-6; CAS-87116-72-1* [timobesone]. *Adrenocortical steroid (topical).* ◇RS-85446-007

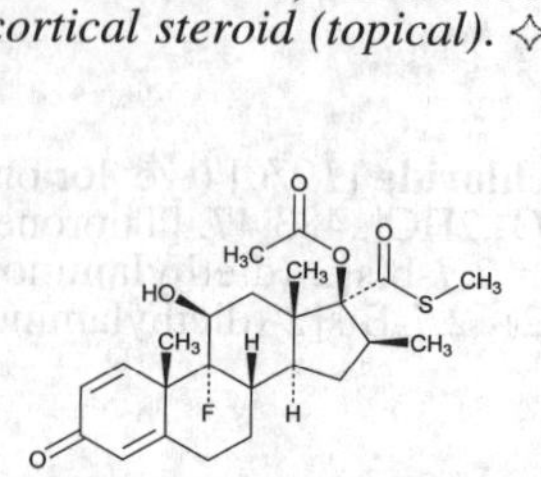

Timofibrate. C$_{14}$H$_{16}$ClNO$_4$S. 329.80. 3-[2-(*p*-Chlorophenoxy)-2-methylpropionyl]-4-thiazolidinecarboxylic acid. *UNII-85P20FW39R*. *CAS-64179-54-0*. INN.

Timolol [*1985*] (tim′ oh lol). C$_{13}$H$_{24}$N$_4$O$_3$S.½H$_2$O. 325.43. (1) 2-Propanol, 1-[(1,1-dimethylethyl)amino]-3-[[4-(4-morpholinyl)-1,2,5-thiadiazol-3-yl]oxy]-, hemihydrate, (*S*)-; (2) (*S*)-1-(*tert*-Butylamino)-3-[(4-morpholino-1,2,5-thiadiazol-3-yl)oxy]-2-propanol hemihydrate. *UNII-817W3C6175*. *CAS-91524-16-2*. INN; BAN. *Anti-adrenergic (β-receptor)*. Betimol (Sanofi Winthrop)

Timolol Maleate [*1973*] (tim′ oh lol mal′ ee ate). **USP.** C$_{13}$H$_{24}$N$_4$O$_3$S.C$_4$H$_4$O$_4$. 432.49. (1) 2-Propanol, 1-[(1,1-dimethylethyl)amino]-3-[[4-(4-morpholinyl)-1,2,5-thiadiazol-3-yl]oxy]-, (*S*)-, (*Z*)-2-butenedioate (1:1) (salt); (2) (-)-1-(*tert*-Butylamino)-3-[(4-morpholino-1,2,5-thiadiazol-3-yl)oxy]-2-propanol maleate (1:1) (salt). *UNII-P8Y54F701R*. *CAS-26921-17-5*. JAN. *Anti-adrenergic (β-receptor)*. Blocadren (Merck); Istalol (Ista); Timoptic (Merck)

Timonacic. C$_4$H$_7$NO$_2$S. 133.17. 4-Thiazolidinecarboxylic acid. *CAS-444-27-9*. INN; MI.

Timoprazole. C$_{13}$H$_{11}$N$_3$OS. 257.31. 2-[(2-Pyridylmethyl)sulfinyl]benzimidazole. *UNII-95H6S1X9CC*. *CAS-57237-97-5*. INN.

Tinabinol [*1983*] (tye nab′ i nol). C$_{23}$H$_{34}$O$_2$S. 374.58. (1) Thiopyrano[2,3-*c*][1]benzopyran-10-ol, 8-(1,2-dimethylheptyl)-1,2,3,5-tetrahydro-5,5-dimethyl-; (2) 8-(1,2-Dimethylheptyl)-1,2,3,5-tetrahydro-5,5-dimethylthiopyrano[2,3-*c*]-[1]benzopyran-10-ol. *UNII-455Y914AKK*. *CAS-50708-95-7*. INN. *Antihypertensive*. ◇*SP-119*

Tinazoline. C$_{11}$H$_{11}$N$_3$S. 217.29. 3-(2-Imidazolin-2-ylthio)indole. *UNII-88174AK70T*. *CAS-62882-99-9*. INN.

Tinidazole [*1970*] (tye nye′ da zole). **USP.** C$_8$H$_{13}$N$_3$O$_4$S. 247.27. (1) 1*H*-Imidazole, 1-[2-(ethylsulfonyl)ethyl]-2-methyl-5-nitro-; (2) 1-[2-(Ethylsulfonyl)ethyl]-2-methyl-5-nitroimidazole. *UNII-033KF7V46H*. *CAS-19387-91-8*. INN; BAN; JAN. *Antiprotozoal*. Tindamax (Mission) ◇*CP-12,574*

Tinisulpride. C$_{20}$H$_{29}$N$_3$O$_4$S. 407.53. 5-[(1,1-Dimethyl-2-propynyl)sulfamoyl]-*N*-[(1-ethyl-2-pyrrolidinyl)methyl]-*o*-anisamide. *UNII-037S03TJ5M*. *CAS-69387-87-7*. INN.

Tinofedrine. C$_{20}$H$_{21}$NOS$_2$. 355.52. (+)-(*R*)-α-[(*S*)-1-[(3,3-Di-3-thienylallyl)amino]ethyl]benzyl alcohol. *CAS-66788-41-8*. INN; MI.

Tinoridine. C$_{17}$H$_{20}$N$_2$O$_2$S. 316.42. [Tinoridine Hydrochloride is JAN.] Ethyl 2-amino-6-benzyl-4,5,6,7-tetrahydrothieno[2,3-*c*]pyridine-3-carboxylate. *UNII-C9Z9ICZ7YR*. *CAS-24237-54-5*. INN; MI. ◇*Y 3642*

Tinzaparin Sodium [*1993*] (tin zap′ a rin soe′ dee um; tin″ za par′ in soe′ dee um). Sodium salt of depolymerized heparin obtained by heparinase from *Flavobacteriumheparinum* (heparin lyase: EC 4.2.2.7) degradation of heparin from pork intestinal mucosa. The majority of the components

---

† Brand name formerly used, and/or firm no longer concerned with this product.

have a 2-*O*-sulfo-4-enepyranosuronic acid structure at the non-reducing end and a 2-*N*:6-*O*-disulfo-D-glucosamine structure at the reducing end of their chain. The relative molecular mass is 4500 ± 1500, 70% of which ranges between 1500 and 10,000. The degree of sulfation is 2 to 2.5 per disaccharide unit. *UNII-3S182ET3UA. CAS-9041-08-1.* INN; BAN. *Anticoagulant; antithrombotic.* Innohep (Pharmion)

Tiocarlide. $C_{23}H_{32}N_2O_2S$. 400.58. 4,4′-Bis(isopentyloxy)thiocarbanilide. *CAS-910-86-1.* INN; BAN; DCF; MI. ◇*DATC*

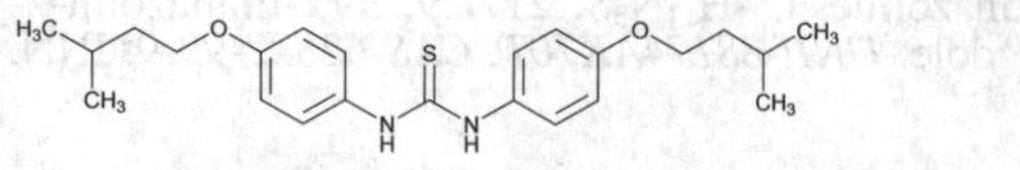

Tioclomarol. $C_{22}H_{16}Cl_2O_4S$. 447.33. 3-[5-Chloro-α-(*p*-chloro-β-hydroxyphenethyl)-2-thenyl]-4-hydroxycoumarin. *UNII-E5B7C16LFK. CAS-22619-35-8.* INN; DCF; MI.

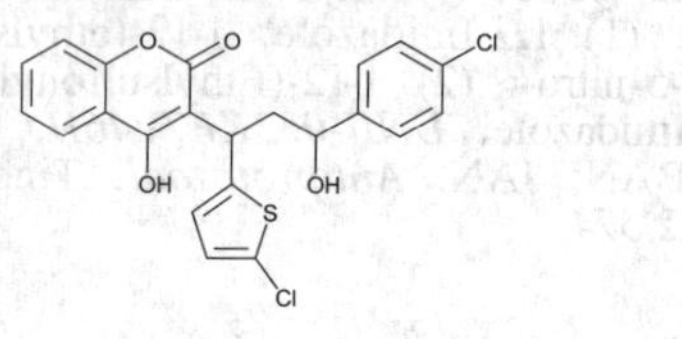

Tioconazole [*1978*] (tye″ oh kon′ a zole). **USP.** $C_{16}H_{13}Cl_3N_2OS$. 387.71. (1) 1*H*-Imidazole, 1-[2-[(2-chloro-3-thienyl)methoxy]-2-(2,4-dichlorophenyl)ethyl]-; (2) 1-[2,4-Dichloro-[β-(2-chloro-3-thenyl)oxy]phenethyl]imidazole. *UNII-S57Y5X1117. CAS-65899-73-2.* INN; BAN; JAN. *Antifungal.* Vagistat (Novartis) ◇*UK-20,349*

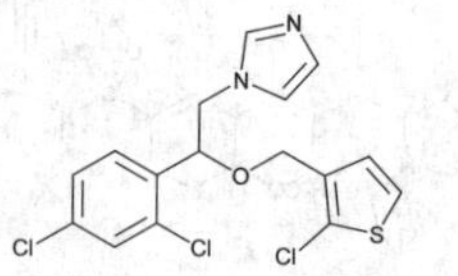

Tioctilate. $C_{15}H_{22}OS$. 250.40. *S*-Octyl thiobenzoate. *UNII-7JEE2JF5OB. CAS-10489-23-3.* INN.

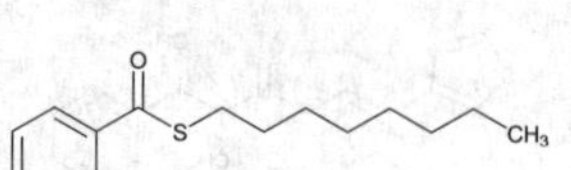

Tiodazosin [*1979*] (tye″ oh daz′ oh sin). $C_{18}H_{21}N_7O_4S$. 431.47. (1) Piperazine, 1-(4-amino-6,7-dimethoxy-2-quinazolinyl)-4-[[5-(methylthio)-1,3,4-oxadiazol-2-yl]carbonyl]-; (2) 1-(4-Amino-6,7-dimethoxy-2-quinazolinyl)-4-[[5-(methylthio)-1,3,4-oxadiazol-2-yl]carbonyl]-piperazine. *UNII-FQI0PYJ799. CAS-66969-81-1.* INN. *Antihypertensive.* ◇*BL-5111*

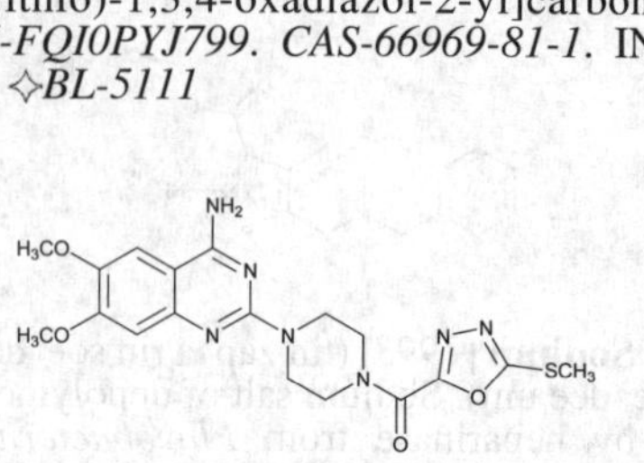

Tiodonium Chloride [*1976*] (tye″ oh doe′ nee um klor′ ide). $C_{10}H_7Cl_2IS$. 357.04. (1) Iodonium, (4-chlorophenyl)-2-thienyl-, chloride; (2) (*p*-Chlorophenyl)-2-thienyliodonium chloride. *CAS-38070-41-6.* INN. *Antibacterial.* ◇*DL-164*

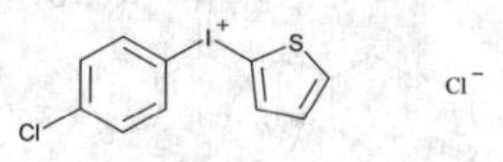

Tiofacic — *See* Stepronin.

Tioguanine (INN, BAN) — *See* Thioguanine.

Tiomergine. $C_{21}H_{21}N_3S$. 347.48. 9,10-Didehydro-6-methyl-8β-[(2-pyridylthio)methyl]ergoline. *CAS-57935-49-6.* INN.

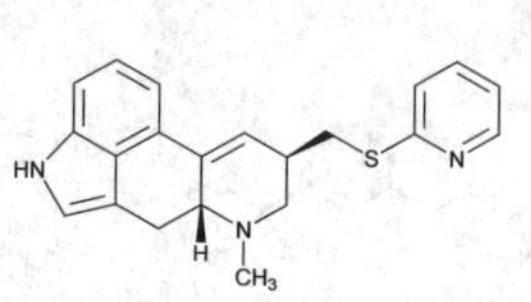

Tiomesterone. $C_{24}H_{34}O_4S_2$. 450.65. 1α,7α-Diacetylthio 17β-hydroxy-17-methylandrost-4-en-3-one. *UNII-W5K3712F4H. CAS-2205-73-4.* INN; BAN; MI. ◇*STA-307*

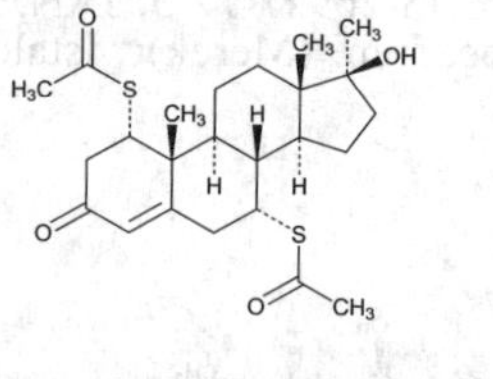

Tioperidone Hydrochloride [*1977*] (tye″ oh per′ i done hye″ droe klor′ ide). $C_{25}H_{32}N_4O_2S$·HCl. 489.07. [Tioperidone is INN.] (1) 2,4(1*H*,3*H*)-Quinazolinedione, 3-[4-[4-[2-(propylthio)phenyl]-1-piperazinyl]butyl]-, monohydrochloride; (2) 3-[4-[4-[*o*-(Propylthio)phenyl]-1-piperazinyl]butyl]-2,4(1*H*,3*H*)-quinazolinedione monohydrochloride. *CAS-52618-68-5; CAS-52618-67-4* [tioperidone]. *Antipsychotic.* ◇*CI 787*

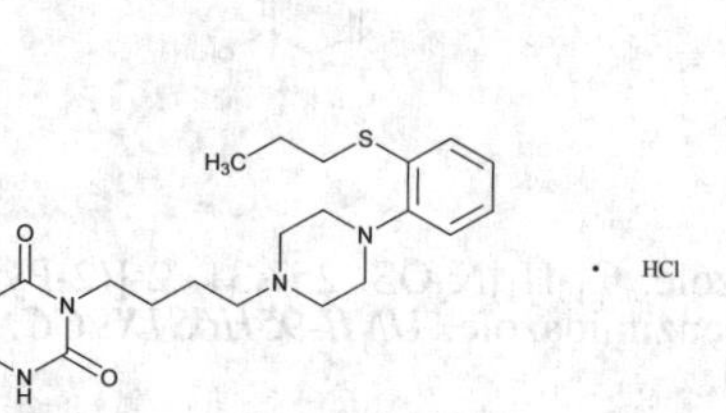

Tiopinac [*1978*] (tye oh′ pi nak). $C_{16}H_{12}O_3S$. 284.33. (1) Dibenzo[*b,e*]thiepin-3-acetic acid, 6,11-dihydro-11-oxo-; (2) 6,11-Dihydro-11-oxodibenzo[*b,e*]thiepin-3-acetic acid. *CAS-61220-69-7.* INN; BAN. *Anti-inflammatory; analgesic; antipyretic.* ◇*RS-40974-00-00-0*

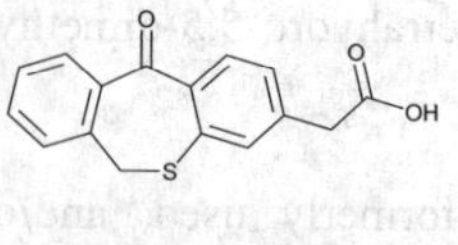

Tiopronin. $C_5H_9NO_3S$. 163.19. *N*-(2-Mercaptopropionyl)glycine. *UNII-C5W04GO61S*. *CAS-1953-02-2*. INN; JAN; DCF; MI.

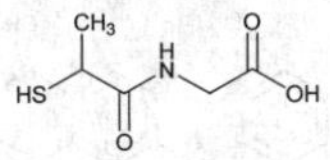

Tiopropamine. $C_{24}H_{27}NS$. 361.54. 3,3-Diphenyl-3′-(phenylthio)dipropylamine. *UNII-E9584TMZ4M*. *CAS-39516-21-7*. INN.

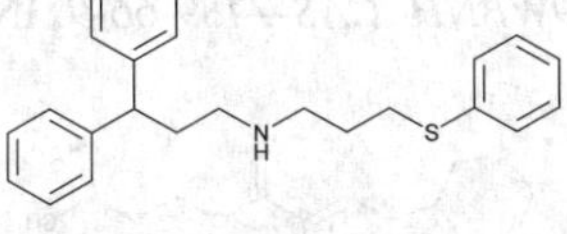

Tiosalan (INN) — *See* Thiosalan.

Tiosinamine — *See* Allylthiourea.

Tiospirone Hydrochloride [*1987*] (tye″ oh spye′ rone hye″ droe klor′ ide). $C_{24}H_{32}N_4O_2S$·HCl. 477.06. [Tiospirone is INN.] (1) 8-Azaspiro[4.5]decane-7,9-dione, 8-[4-[4-(1,2-benzisothiazol-3-yl)-1-piperazinyl]butyl]-, monohydrochloride; (2) *N*-[4-[4-(1,2-Benzisothiazol-3-yl)-1-piperazinyl]butyl]-1,1-cyclopentanediacetimide monohydrochloride. *UNII-45Q1DF53NN*; *UNII-35C6UMO5SR* [tiospirone]. *CAS-87691-92-7*; *CAS-87691-91-6* [tiospirone]. *Antipsychotic*. ◇*BMY 13859-1*

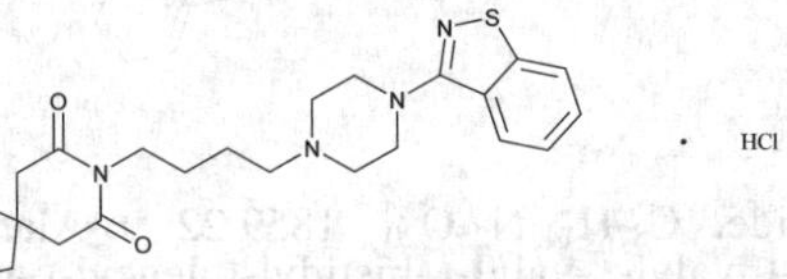

Tiotidine [*1980*] (tye oh′ ti deen). $C_{10}H_{16}N_8S_2$. 312.42. (1) Guanidine, *N″*-cyano-*N*-[2-[[[2-[(diaminomethylene)amino]-4-thiazolyl]methyl]thio]ethyl]-*N′*-methyl-; (2) 2-Cyano-1-[2-[[[2-[(diaminomethylene)amino]-4-thiazolyl]methyl]thio]ethyl]-3-methylguanidine. *CAS-69014-14-8*. INN. *Antagonist (to histamine H_2receptors)*. ◇*ICI 125,211*

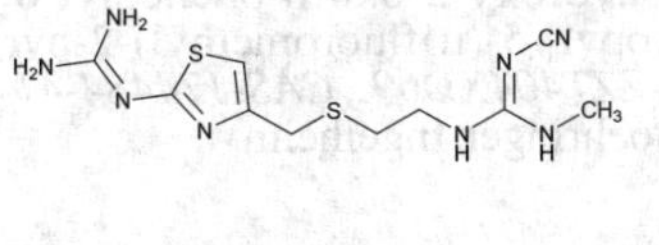

Tiotixene (INN, BAN, JAN, DCF) — *See* Thiothixene.

Tiotropium Bromide [*2000*] (tye″ oh troe′ pee um broe′ mide). $C_{19}H_{22}BrNO_4S_2$. 472.42. (1) 3-Oxa-9-azoniatricyclo[3.3.1.02,4]nonane, 7-[(hydroxydi-2-thienacetyl)oxy]-9,9-dimethyl-, bromide, $(1\alpha,2\beta,4\beta,5\alpha,7\beta)$-; (2) $6\beta,7\beta$-Epoxy-3β-hydroxy-8-methyl-1αH,5αH-tropanium bromide, di-2-thienylglycolate. *UNII-XX112XZP0J*. *CAS-136310-93-5*; *CAS-139404-48-1* [hydrate]. INN; BAN.

Anticholinergic used in the treatment of chronic obstructive disease (COPD). Spiriva (Boehringer Ingelheim KG, Germany) ◇*BA 679 BR*

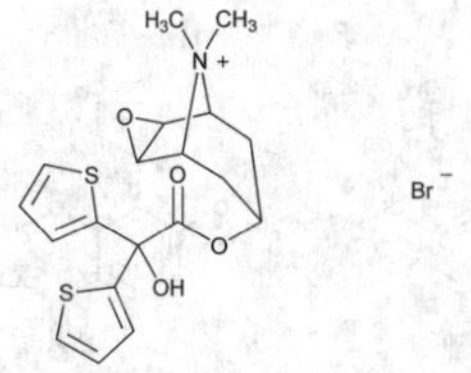

Tioxacin. $C_{14}H_{12}N_2O_4S$. 304.32. 6-Ethyl-2,3,6,9-tetrahydro-3-methyl-2,9-dioxothiazolo[5,4-*f*]quinoline-8-carboxylic acid. *UNII-0K40CNM74K*. *CAS-34976-39-1*. INN.

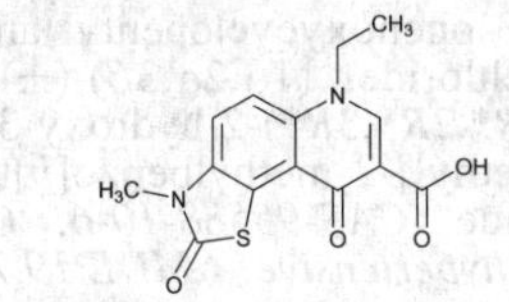

Tioxamast. $C_{14}H_{14}N_2O_4S$. 306.34. Ethyl [4-(*p*-methoxyphenyl)-2-thiazolyl]oxamate. *UNII-HQ7F53TO3L*. *CAS-74531-88-7*. INN.

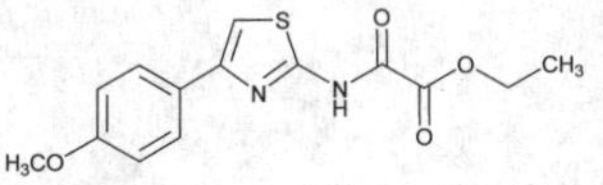

Tioxaprofen. $C_{18}H_{13}Cl_2NO_3S$. 394.27. 2-[[4,5-Bis(*p*-chlorophenyl)-2-oxazolyl]thio]propionic acid. *UNII-RA6D4LW87K*. *CAS-40198-53-6*. INN; BAN.

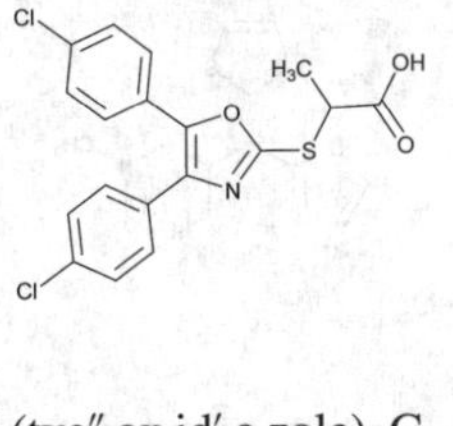

Tioxidazole [*1978*] (tye″ ox id′ a zole). $C_{12}H_{14}N_2O_3S$. 266.32. (1) Carbamic acid, (6-propoxy-2-benzothiazolyl)-, methyl ester; (2) Methyl 6-propoxy-2-benzothiazolecarbamate. *UNII-NZW046NI85*. *CAS-61570-90-9*. INN. *Anthelmintic*. Tiox [Veterinary] (Schering-Plough Animal Health†) ◇*Sch 21480*

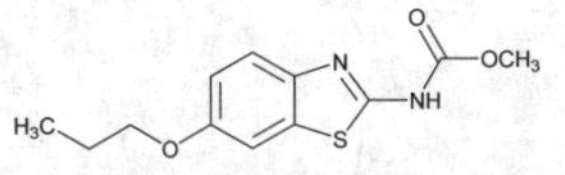

Tioxolone. $C_7H_4O_3S$. 168.17. 6-Hydroxy-1,3-benzoxathiol-2-one. *UNII-S0FAJ1R9CD*. *CAS-4991-65-5*. INN; BAN; DCF; MI.

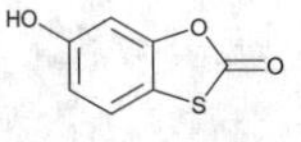

Tipelukast [*2006*] (tye″ pe loo′ kast). $C_{29}H_{38}O_7S$. 530.67. (1) Butanoic acid, 4-[6-acetyl-3-[3-[(4-acetyl-3-hydroxy-2-propylphenyl)thio]propoxy]-2-propylphenoxy]-; (2) 4-[6-Acetyl-3-[3-[(4-acetyl-3-hydroxy-2-propylphenyl)sulfa-

---

† Brand name formerly used, and/or firm no longer concerned with this product.

nyl]propoxy]-2-propylphenoxy]butanoic acid. *UNII-08379P260O. CAS-125961-82-2.* INN. *Treatment of asthma and interstitial cystitis.* ◇*KCA-757; MN-001*

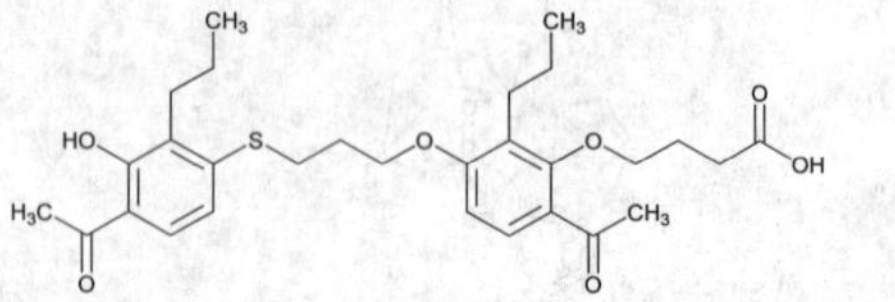

Tipentosin Hydrochloride [*1986*] (tye pen′ toe sin hye″ droe klor′ ide). $C_{21}H_{25}NO_3S \cdot HCl$. 407.95. [Tipentosin is INN and BAN.] (1) Benzo[*b*]thiophen-4(5*H*)-one, 6,7-dihydro-5-[[(2-hydroxy-3-phenoxycyclopentyl)amino]methyl]-2-methyl-, hydrochloride, (1α,2α,3β)-(±)-; (2) (±)-6,7-Dihydro-5-[[[(1*R**,2*R**,3*R**)-2-hydroxy-3-phenoxycyclopentyl]amino]methyl]-2-methylbenzo[*b*]thiophen-4(5*H*)-one hydrochloride. *CAS-95588-10-6; CAS-95588-08-2* [tipentosin]. *Antihypertensive.* ◇*MDL 19,744*

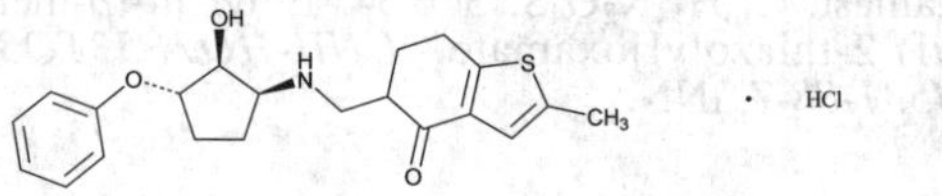

Tipepidine. $C_{15}H_{17}NS_2$. 275.43. [Tipepidine Hibenzate is JAN.] 3-(Di-2-thienylmethylene)-1-methylpiperidine. *UNII-2260ZP67IT. CAS-5169-78-8.* INN; DCF; MI. ◇*AT 327; CR/662*

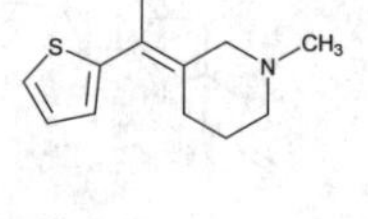

Tipetropium Bromide. $C_{25}H_{32}BrNOS$. 474.50. 3α-[(6,11-Dihydrodibenzo[*b,e*]thiepin-11-yl)oxy]-8*r*-propyl-1α*H*,5α*H*-tropanium bromide. *UNII-5F8F2A90IA. CAS-54376-91-9.* INN.

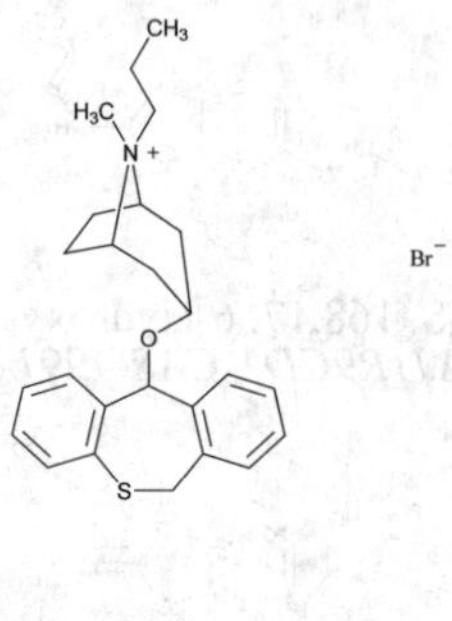

Tipifarnib [*2002*] (tip″ i far′ nib). $C_{27}H_{22}Cl_2N_4O$. 489.40. (1) 2 (1*H*)-Quinolinone,6-[amino(4-chlorophenyl)(1-methyl-1*H*-imidazol-5-yl)methyl]-4-(3-chlorophenyl)-1-methyl-, (+)-; (2) (*R*)-6-[Amino(4-chlorophenyl)(1-methyl-1*H*-imidazol-5-yl)methyl]-4-(3-chlorophenyl)-1-methyl-2(1*H*)-

quinolinone. *UNII-MAT637500A. CAS-192185-72-1.* INN. *Treatment of advanced pancreatic cancer, colorectal cancer, and non-small cell lung cancer.* ◇*R115777*

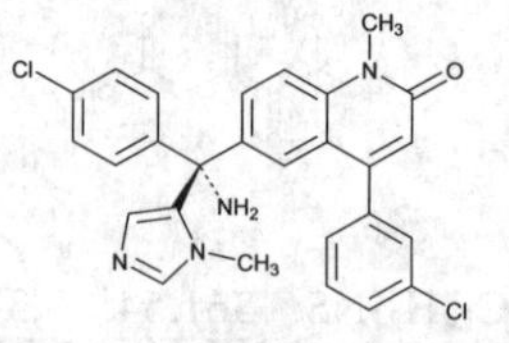

Tipindole. $C_{16}H_{20}N_2O_2S$. 304.41. 2-(Dimethylamino)ethyl 1,3,4,5-tetrahydrothiopyrano[4,3-*b*]indole-8-carboxylate. *UNII-US65H9WBNH. CAS-7489-66-9.* INN.

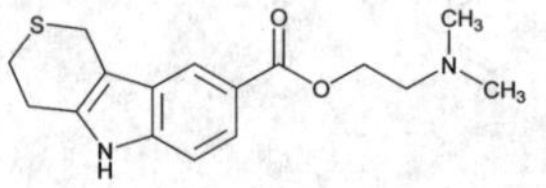

Tiplasinin [*2005*] (tye plas′ in in). $C_{24}H_{16}F_3NO_4$. 439.38. (1) 1*H*-Indole-3-acetic acid, α-oxo-1-(phenylmethyl)-5-[4-(trifluoromethoxy)phenyl]-; (2) [1-Benzyl-5-[4-(trifluoromethoxy)phenyl]-1*H*-indol-3-yl]oxoacetic acid. *UNII-L396QIB983. CAS-393105-53-8.* INN. *Treatment of fibrinolytic impairment diseases.* ◇*PAI-039*

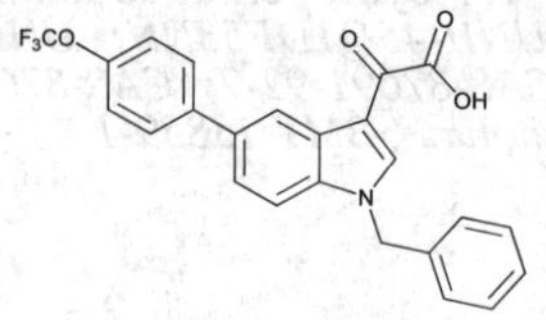

Tiplimotide. $C_{87}H_{143}N_{25}O_{20}$. 1859.22. D-Alanyl-L-lysyl-L-prolyl-L-valyl-L-valyl-L-histidyl-L-leucyl-L-phenylalanyl-L-alanyl-L-asparaginyl-L-isoleucyl-L-valyl-L-threonyl-L-prolyl-L-arginyl-L-threonyl-L-prolinamide. *CAS-178823-49-9.* INN.

DAKPVVHLFAN IVTPRTP —NH₂

Tipranavir. $C_{31}H_{33}F_3N_2O_5S$. 602.66. 3′-[(1*R*)-1-[(6*R*)-5,6-Dihydro-4-hydroxy-2-oxo-6-phenethyl-6-propyl-2*H*-pyran-3-yl]propyl]-5-(trifluoromethyl)-2-pyridinesulfonanilide. *UNII-ZZT404XD09. CAS-174484-41-4.* INN; BAN. Aptivus (Boehringer Ingelheim)

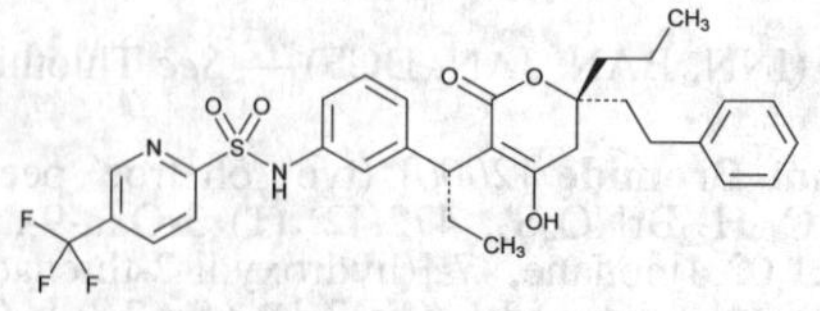

Tipranavir Disodium [*1998*] (tye pran′ a vir dye soe′ dee um). $C_{31}H_{31}F_3N_2Na_2O_5S$. 646.63. (1) [*R*-(*R**,*R**)]-*N*-[3-[1-[5,6-Dihydro-4-hydroxy-2-oxo-6-(2-phenylethyl)-6-propyl-2*H*-pyran-3-yl]propyl]phenyl]-5-(trifluoromethyl)-2-pyridinesulfonamide disodium salt; (2) 3′-[(1*R*)-1-[(6*R*)-5,6-Dihydro-4-hydroxy-2-oxo-6-phenethyl-6-propyl-2*H*-

pyran-3-yl]propyl]-5-(trifluoromethyl)-2-pyridinesulfona-nilide, disodium salt. *UNII-9BAN2XG1ZW. CAS-191150-83-1. Antiviral (protease inhibitor).* ◇*PNU-140690E*

Tipredane [*1986*] (tye pred′ ane). $C_{22}H_{31}FO_2S_2$. 410.61. (1) Androsta-1,4-dien-3-one, 17-(ethylthio)-9-fluoro-11-hy-droxy-17-(methylthio)-, (11β,17α)-; (2) 9-Fluoro-11β-hydroxyandrosta-1,4-diene-3,17-dione (17R)-17-(ethyl methyl mercaptole). *CAS-85197-77-9.* INN; BAN. *Adren-ocortical steroid (topical).* ◇*SQ 27,239*

Tiprenolol Hydrochloride [*1970*] (tye pren′ oh lol hye″ droe klor′ ide). $C_{13}H_{21}NO_2S.HCl$. 291.84. [Tiprenolol is INN and BAN.] (1) Propanol, 1-[(1-methylethyl)amino]-3-[2-(methylthio)phenoxy]-, hydrochloride, (±)-; (2) (±)-1-(Isopropylamino)-3-[o-(methylthio)phenoxy]-2-propanol hydrochloride. *CAS-39832-43-4; CAS-26481-51-6* [tipren-olol]. *Anti-adrenergic (β-receptor).* ◇*DU-21445*

Tiprinast Meglumine [*1983*] (tye′ pri nast me′ gloo meen). $C_{12}H_{14}N_2O_3S.C_7H_{17}NO_5$. 461.53. [Tiprinast is INN.] (1) Thieno[2,3-*d*]pyrimidine-2-carboxylic acid, 3,4-dihydro-5-methyl-6-(2-methylpropyl)-4-oxo, compound with 1-deoxy-1-(methylamino)-D-glucitol (1:1); (2) 3,4-Dihydro-6-isobutyl-5-methyl-4-oxothieno[2,3-*d*]pyrimidine-2-car-boxylic acid, compound with 1-deoxy-1-(methylamino)-D-glucitol (1:1). *UNII-7GWN8D7165. CAS-83198-90-7; CAS-83153-39-3* [tiprinast]. *Anti-allergic.* ◇*MJ 12,175-170*

Tiprolisant. $C_{17}H_{26}ClNO$. 295.85. 1-{3-[3-(4-Chlorophenyl)-propoxy]propyl}piperidine. *CAS-362665-56-3.* INN.

Tipropidil Hydrochloride [*1980*] (tye proe′ pi dil hye″ droe klor′ ide). $C_{20}H_{35}NO_2S.HCl$. 390.02. [Tipropidil is INN.] (1) 2-Propanol, 1-[4-[(1-methylethyl)thio]phenoxy]-3-(oc-tylamino)-, hydrochloride; (2) 1-[*p*-(Isopropylthio)phe-noxy]-3-(octylamino)-2-propanol hydrochloride. *UNII-34K00NS0TZ. CAS-70895-39-5; CAS-70895-45-3* [tipropi-dil]. *Vasodilator.* ◇*MJ 12,880-1*

Tiprostanide. $C_{33}H_{45}NO_6S$. 583.78. (1S,2R,3R)-3-Hydroxy-2-[(2-hydroxy-2-methylheptyl)thio]-5-oxocyclopentanehep-tanoic acid, ester with 4′-hydroxybenzanilide. *CAS-67040-53-3.* INN; BAN.

Tiprotimod. $C_{10}H_{13}NO_4S_2$. 275.34. 2-[(3-Carboxypro-pyl)thio]-4-methyl-5-thiazoleacetic acid. *UNII-FZ7ZH245CO. CAS-105523-37-3.* INN.

Tiqueside [*1992*] (tye′ kwe side). $C_{39}H_{64}O_{13}$. 740.92. (1) β-D-Glucopyranoside, (3β,5α,25R)-spirostan-3-yl 4-*O*-β-D-glucopyranosyl-; (2) (25R)-5α-Spirostan-3β-yl 4-*O*-β-D-glucopyranosyl-β-D-glucopyranoside. *CAS-99759-19-0.* INN. *Antihyperlipidemic.* ◇*CP-88,818*

Tiquinamide Hydrochloride [*1976*] (tye kwin′ a mide hye″ droe klor′ ide). $C_{11}H_{14}N_2S.HCl$. 242.77. [Tiquinamide is INN and BAN.] (1) 8-Quinolinecarbothioamide, 5,6,7,8-tetrahydro-3-methyl-, monohydrochloride; (2) 5,6,7,8-Tet-rahydro-3-methylthio-8-quinolinecarboxamide monohy-drochloride. *CAS-53400-68-3; CAS-53400-67-2* [tiquinamide]. *Anticholinergic (gastric).* ◇*WY-24,081 HCl*

Tiquizium Bromide. $C_{19}H_{24}BrNS_2$. 410.43. *trans*-3-(Di-2-thienylmethylene)octahydro-5-methyl-2*H*-quinolizinium bromide. *CAS-71731-58-3*. INN; JAN; MI.

Tiracizine. $C_{21}H_{25}N_3O_3$. 367.44. Ethyl 5-(*N*,*N*-dimethylgly-cyl)-10,11-dihydro-5*H*-dibenz[*b*,*f*]azepine-3-carbamate. *UNII-9UUO2T61K7*. *CAS-83275-56-3*. INN.

Tirapazamine [*1992*] (tye″ ra paz′ a meen). $C_7H_6N_4O_2$. 178.15. (1) 1,2,4-Benzotriazin-3-amine, 1,4-dioxide; (2) 3-Amino-1,2,4-benzotriazine 1,4-dioxide. *UNII-1UD32YR59G*. *CAS-27314-97-2*. INN. *Antineoplastic*. ◇*WIN 59075*

Tiratricol. $C_{14}H_9I_3O_4$. 621.93. [4-(4-Hydroxy-3-iodophe-noxy)-3,5-diiodophenyl]acetic acid. *UNII-29OQ9EU4R1*. *CAS-51-24-1*. INN; MI.

Tirilazad Mesylate [*1993*] (tye ril′ a zad mes′ i late). $C_{38}H_{52}N_6O_2 \cdot CH_4O_3S \cdot xH_2O$. 720.96 (anhydrous). [Tirilazad is INN and BAN.] (1) Pregna-1,4,9(11)-triene-3,20-dione, 21-[4-(2,6-di-1-pyrrolidinyl-4-pyrimidinyl)-1-piperazi-nyl]-16-methyl-, (16α)-, monomethanesulfonate, hydrate (1:1:?); (2) 21-[4-(2,6-Di-1-pyrrolidinyl-4-pyrimidinyl)-1-piperazinyl]-16α-methylpregna-1,4,9(11)-triene-3,20-dione monomethanesulfonate, hydrate. *CAS-149042-61-5; CAS-110101-66-1* [tirilazad]. *Inhibitor (lipid peroxida-tion)*. ◇*U-74006F*

Tirofiban Hydrochloride [*1994*] (tye″ roe fye′ ban hye″ droe klor′ ide). $C_{22}H_{36}N_2O_5S \cdot HCl \cdot H_2O$. 495.07. [Tirofiban is INN and BAN.] (1) L-Tyrosine, *N*-(butylsulfonyl)-*O*-[4-(4-piperidinyl)butyl]-, monohydrochloride, monohydrate; (2) *N*-(Butylsulfonyl)-4-[4-(4-piperidyl)butoxy]-L-phenylala-nine monohydrochloride monohydrate. *UNII-6H925F8O5J; UNII-GGX234SI5H* [tirofiban]. *CAS-*

150915-40-5; CAS-142373-60-2 [anhydrous]; *CAS-144494-65-5* [tirofiban]. *Treatment of unstable angina.* Aggrastat (Medicure) ◇*MK-383; L-700,462*

Tiropramide. $C_{28}H_{41}N_3O_3$. 467.64. DL-α-Benzamido-*p*-[2-(diethylamino)ethoxy]-*N*,*N*-dipropylhydrocinnamamide. *CAS-55837-29-1*. INN; MI.

Tisartan (previously used name) — *See* Abitesartan.

Tisilfocon A [*1992*] (tye″ sil foe′ kon). $(C_{17}H_{34}O_3Si_4)_u$ $(C_7H_6F_6O_2)_v(C_6H_9NO)_w(C_4H_6O_2)_x(C_{10}H_{14}O_4)_y(C_{13}H_{14}O_2)_z$. (1) Trisiloxane, 3-(4-ethenylphenyl)-1,1,1,5,5,5-hexa-methyl-3-[(trimethylsilyl)oxy]-, polymer with 2,2,2-tri-fluoro-1-(trifluoromethyl)ethyl 2-methyl-2-propenoate, 1-ethenyl-2-pyrrolidinone, 2-methyl-2-propenoic acid, 1,2-ethanediyl bis(2-methyl-2-propenoate) and (4-ethenylphe-nyl)methyl 2-methyl-2-propenoate; (2) 1,1,1,5,5,5-Hexam-ethyl-3-(trimethylsiloxy)-3-(*p*-vinylphenyl)trisiloxane polymer with 2,2,2-trifluoro-1-(trifluoromethyl)ethyl methacrylate, 1-vinyl-2-pyrrolidinone, methacrylic acid, ethylene dimethacrylate and *p*-vinylbenzyl methacrylate. *CAS-132978-98-4*. *Contact lens material (hydrophobic)*.

Tisocalcitate [*2004*] (tye″ soe kal′ si tate). $C_{31}H_{48}O_5$. 500.71. (1) 9,10-Secocholesta-5,7,10(19), 22-tetraene-25-car-boxylic acid, 1,3,24-trihydroxy-, 1-methylethyl ester, (1α, 3β, 5Z,7E,22E,24R)-; (2) 1-Methylethyl (5Z,7E,22E,24R)-1α,3β,24-trihydroxy-9,10-secocholesta-5,7,10(19),22-tetraene-25-carboxylate. *UNII-8O4QYK6G4Y. CAS-156965-06-9.* INN. *Topical treatment for plaque type psoriasis (vitamin D analogue).* ◇ZK 156942

Tisocromide. $C_{19}H_{30}N_2O_6S$. 414.52. *N*-[3-(Dimethylamino)-1,3-dimethylbutyl]-6,7-dimethoxy-2,1-benzoxathian-3-carboxamide 1,1-dioxide. *CAS-35423-51-9.* INN.

Tisokinase. $C_{2569}H_{3894}N_{746}O_{781}S_{40}$. 59,007.61. Glycoprotein (molecular weight: ca. 63,000; one chain form >80%) consisting of 527 amino acid residues, produced in diploid fibroblast cells derived from human lung. JAN.

Tisopurine. $C_5H_4N_4S$. 152.18. 1*H*-Pyrazolo[3,4-*d*]pyrimidine-4-thiol. *CAS-5334-23-6.* INN.

Tisoquone. $C_{17}H_{17}NS$. 267.39. 4-Ethyl-3,4-dihydro-4-phenylthioisocarbostyril. *CAS-40692-37-3.* INN.

Tissue Plasminogen Activator — *See* Alteplase.

Titanium Dioxide (tye tay′ nee um dye ox′ ide). **USP.** TiO_2. 79.87. (1) Titanium oxide (TiO_2); (2) Titanium oxide (TiO_2). *UNII-15FIX9V2JP. CAS-13463-67-7. Protectant (topical).*

Tivanidazole. $C_{11}H_{13}N_5O_2S$. 279.32. (*E*)-2-Ethyl-5-[1-methyl-2-(1-methyl-5-nitroimidazol-2-yl)vinyl]-1,3,4-thiadiazole. *UNII-7E136TJT00. CAS-80680-05-3.* INN.

Tiviciclovir. $C_9H_{13}N_5O_3$. 239.23. 2-Amino-9-[3-hydroxy-2-(hydroxymethyl)propyl]-1,9-dihydro-6*H*-purin-6-one. *UNII-JBP1N46HPN. CAS-103024-93-7.* INN.

Tivirapine. $C_{16}H_{20}ClN_3S$. 321.87. (*S*)-8-Chloro-4,5,6,7-tetrahydro-5-methyl-6-(3-methyl-2-butenyl)imidazo[4,5,1-*jk*][1,4]benzodiazepine-2(1*H*)-thione. *UNII-7WP69N3Y3Y. CAS-137332-54-8.* INN.

Tixadil. $C_{24}H_{25}NS$. 359.53. *N*-(α-Methylphenethyl)thioxanthene-9-ethylamine. *UNII-4F4L1E450W. CAS-2949-95-3.* INN. ◇B.S. 7561 [as hydrochloride]

Tixanox [*1976*] (tix′ a nox). $C_{15}H_{10}O_5S$. 302.30. (1) 9*H*-Xanthene-2-carboxylic acid, 7-(methylsulfinyl)-9-oxo-; (2) 7-(Methylsulfinyl)-9-oxoxanthene-2-carboxylic acid. *UNII-KQT9O2462E. CAS-40691-50-7.* INN. *Anti-allergic.* ◇RS-7337

Tixanoxum (INN) — *See* Tixanox.

Tixocortol Pivalate [*1987*] (tix″ oh kor′ tol piv′ a late). $C_{26}H_{38}O_5S$. 462.64. [Tixocortol is INN and BAN.] (1) Pregn-4-ene-3,20-dione, 21-[(2,2-dimethyl-1-oxopropyl)thio]-11,17-dihydroxy-, (11β)-; (2) 11β,17-Dihydroxy-21-mercaptopregn-4-ene-3,20-dione 21-pivalate. *CAS-55560-96-8; CAS-61951-99-3* [tixocortol]. *Anti-inflammatory (topical).*

Tizabrin. C₈H₁₅NO₃S. 205.27. (1*R*,3*S*,5*R*)-2,2,5-Trimethyl-3-thiomorpholinecarboxylic acid, 1-oxide. *CAS-83573-53-9.* INN.

Tizanidine Hydrochloride [*1993*] (tye zan′ i deen hye″ droe klor′ ide). **USP.** C₉H₈ClN₅S.HCl. 290.17. [Tizanidine is INN and BAN.] (1) 2,1,3-Benzothiadiazol-4-amine, 5-chloro-*N*-(4,5-dihydro-1*H*-imidazol-2-yl)-, monohydrochloride; (2) 5-Chloro-4-(2-imidazolin-2-ylamino)-2,1,3-benzothiadiazole monohydrochloride. *UNII-B53E3NMY5C; UNII-6AI06C00GW* [tizanidine]. *CAS-64461-82-1; CAS-51322-75-9* [tizanidine]. JAN. *Antispasmodic.* Zanaflex (Acorda) ◇*AN021; DS 103-282*

Tizolemide. C₁₁H₁₄ClN₃O₃S₂. 335.83. 2-Chloro-5-[4-hydroxy-3-methyl-2-(methylimino)-4-thiazolidinyl]benzenesulfonamide. *CAS-56488-58-5.* INN; BAN.

Tizoprolic Acid. C₇H₉NO₂S. 171.22. 2-Propyl-5-thiazolecarboxylic acid. *UNII-VGT0G37N5M. CAS-30709-69-4.* INN.

²⁰¹Tl — *See* Thallous Chloride Tl 201.

Tobicillin. C₂₇H₃₀N₂O₆S. 510.60. (+)-α-Hydroxy-*m*-tolyl(2*S*,5*R*,6*R*)-3,3-dimethyl-7-oxo-6-(2-phenylacetamido)-4-thia-1-azabicyclo[3.2.0]heptane-2-carboxylate, isobutyrate (ester). *UNII-2P43Z53ESB. CAS-151287-22-8.* INN.

Toborinone [*1997*] (toe boe′ ri none). C₂₁H₂₄N₂O₅. 384.43. (±)-6-[2-Hydroxy-3-(veratrylamino)propoxy]carbostyril. *CAS-143343-83-3.* INN. *Cardiotonic.* ◇*OPC-18790*

Tobramycin [*1972*] (toe″ bra mye′ sin). **USP.** C₁₈H₃₇N₅O₉. 467.51. Antibiotic produced by *Streptomyces tenebrarius.* (1) D-Streptamine, *O*-3-amino-3-deoxy-α-D-glucopyrano-syl-(1→6)-*O*-[2,6-diamino-2,3,6-trideoxy-α-D-*ribo*-hexopyranosyl-(1→4)]-2-deoxy-; (2) *O*-3-Amino-3-deoxy-α-D-glucopyranosyl-(1→4)-*O*-[2,6-diamino-2,3,6-trideoxy-α-D-*ribo*-hexopyranosyl-(1→6)]-2-deoxy-L-streptamine. *UNII-VZ8RRZ51VK. CAS-32986-56-4.* INN; BAN; JAN. *Antibacterial.* Aktob (Akorn); Tobi (Novartis); Tobrex (Alcon) ◇*47663*

Tobramycin Sulfate (toe″ bra mye′ sin sul′ fate). **USP.** (C₁₈H₃₇N₅O₉)₂.5H₂SO₄. 1425.42. (1) D-Streptamine, *O*-3-amino-3-deoxy-α-D-glucopyranosyl-(1→6)-*O*-[2,6-diamino-2,3,6-trideoxy-α-D-*ribo*-hexopyranosyl-(1→4)]-2-deoxy-, sulfate (2:5) (salt); (2) *O*-3-Amino-3-deoxy-α-D-glucopyranosyl-(1→4)-*O*-[2,6-diamino-2,3,6-trideoxy-α-D-*ribo*-hexopyranosyl-(1→6)]-2-deoxy-L-streptamine, sulfate (2:5) (salt); (3) Tobramycin sulfate (2:5) (salt). *UNII-HJT0RXD7JK. CAS-79645-27-5. Antibacterial.* Nebcin (Lilly)

Tobuterol. C₂₈H₃₁NO₅. 461.55. (±)-5-[2-(*tert*-Butylamino)-1-hydroxyethyl]-*m*-phenylene di-*p*-toluate. *UNII-17B9PXO2SW. CAS-75626-99-2.* INN.

Tocainide [*1976*] (toe′ ka nide). C₁₁H₁₆N₂O. 192.26. (1) Propanamide, 2-amino-*N*-(2,6-dimethylphenyl)-; (2) 2-Amino-2′,6′-propionoxylidide. *UNII-27DXO59SAN. CAS-41708-72-9.* INN; BAN. *Cardiac depressant (anti-arrhythmic).* ◇*W-36095*

Tocainide Hydrochloride (toe′ ka nide hye″ droe klor′ ide). **USP.** C₁₁H₁₆N₂O.HCl. 228.72. (1) Propanamide, 2-amino-*N*-(2,6-dimethylphenyl)-, hydrochloride, (±)-; (2) (±)-Amino-2′,6′-propionoxylidide hydrochloride. *UNII-2K7I38CKN5. CAS-35891-93-1. Cardiac depressant (anti-arrhythmic).* Tonocard (AstraZeneca)

Tocamphyl [*1964*] (toe kam′ fil). C₁₉H₂₆O₄.C₄H₁₁NO₂. 423.54. (1) 1,3-Cyclopentanedicarboxylic acid, 1,2,2-trimethyl-, 1-[1-(4-methylphenyl)ethyl] ester, compd. with 2,2′-iminobis[ethanol] (1:1); (2) 1-(*p*,α-Dimethylbenzyl) camphorate compound with 2,2′-iminodiethanol (1:1); (3)

Diethanolamine salt of the mono-(+)-camphoric acid ester of *p*-tolylmethylcarbinol. *CAS-5634-42-4.* INN. *Choleretic.*

Toceranib [*2008*] (toe ser′ a nib). $C_{22}H_{25}FN_4O_2$. 396.46. (1) 1*H*-Pyrrole-3-carboxamide, 5-[(*Z*)-(5-fluoro-1,2-dihydro-2-oxo-3*H*-indol-3-ylidene)methyl]-2,4-dimethyl-*N*-[2-(1-pyrrolidinyl)ethyl]-; (2) 5-[(*Z*)-(5-Fluoro-2-oxo-1,2-dihydro-3*H*-indol-3-ylidene)methyl]-2,4-dimethyl-*N*-[2-(pyrrolidin-1-yl)ethyl]-1*H*-pyrrole-3-carboxamide; (3) (*Z*)-5-[(5-Fluoro-2-oxo-1,2-dihydro-3*H*-indol-3-ylidene)methyl]-2,4-dimethyl-*N*-(2-pyrrolidin-1-ylethyl)-1*H*-pyrrole-3-carboxamide. *UNII-59L7Y0530C. CAS-356068-94-5. Treatment of mast cell tumors in dogs.* ◇PHA-291639

Toceranib Phosphate [*2008*] (toe ser′ a nib). $C_{22}H_{25}FN_4O_2$.H_3O_4P. 494.45. (1) 1*H*-Pyrrole-3-carboxamide, 5-[(*Z*)-(5-fluoro-1,2-dihydro-2-oxo-3*H*-indol-3-ylidene)methyl]-2,4-dimethyl-*N*-[2-(1-pyrrolidinyl)ethyl]-, phosphate (1:1); (2) 5-[(*Z*)-(5-Fluoro-2-oxo-1,2-dihydro-3*H*-indol-3-ylidene)-methyl]-2,4-dimethyl-*N*-[2-(pyrrolidin-1-yl)ethyl]-1*H*-pyrrole-3-carboxamide phosphate (1:1); (3) (*Z*)-5-[(5-Fluoro-2-oxo-1,2-dihydro-3*H*-indol-3-ylidene)methyl]-2,4-dimethyl-*N*-(2-pyrrolidin-1-ylethyl)-1*H*-pyrrole-3-carboxamide phosphate. *UNII-24F9PF7J3R. CAS-874819-74-6. Treatment of mast cell tumors in dogs.* ◇PHA-291639E

Tocilizumab [*2004*] (toe″ si liz′ oo mab). $C_{6428}H_{9976}N_{1720}O_{2018}S_{42}$. Immunoglobulin G1, anti-(human interleukin 6 receptor) (human-mouse monoclonal MRA heavy chain), disulfide with human-mouse monoclonal MRA κ-chain, dimer. Molecular weight is approximately 144,986 daltons. *CAS-375823-41-9.* INN. *Treatment of Castelman's disease; treatment of multiple myeloma; treatment of systemic lupus erythematosus; treatment of Crohn's disease; treatment of rheumatoid arthritis; treatment of systemic juvenile idiopathic arthritis.* ◇MRA

Tocladesine [*1999*] (toe kla′ de seen). $C_{10}H_{11}ClN_5O_6P$. 363.65. (1) Adenosine, 8-chloro-, cyclic 3′,5′-(hydrogen phosphate); (2) 8-Chloroadenosine 3′,5′-cyclic phosphate. *CAS-41941-56-4.* INN; BAN. *Antineoplastic.[Name previously used: Adenazole.]* ◇ICN-1256; 8-Cl-cAMP; NSC-614491

Tocofenoxate. $C_{37}H_{55}ClO_4$. 599.28. *all-rac*-2,5,7,8-Tetramethyl-2-(4,8,12-trimethyltridecyl)-6-chromanyl (*p*-chlorophenoxy)acetate. *CAS-61343-44-0.* INN.

Tocofersolan (INN) — *See* Tocophersolan.

Tocofibrate. $C_{39}H_{59}ClO_4$. 627.34. 2,5,7,8-Tetramethyl-2-(4,8,12-trimethyltridecyl)-6-chromanyl 2-(*p*-chlorophenoxy)-2-methylpropionate. *CAS-50465-39-9.* INN.

Tocopherol (JAN) — *See* Vitamin E.

Tocopherols Excipient (toe kof′ er ols ex sip′ ee ent). **NF.** A vegetable oil solution containing not less than 50.0% of total tocopherols, of which not less than 80.0% consists of varying amounts of beta, gamma, and delta tocopherols. *Pharmaceutic aid (antioxidant).*

Tocophersolan [*1963*] (toe″ koe fer′ soe lan). $C_{33}H_{54}O_5(C_2H_4O)_n$ (*n* = approximately 22). [Tocofersolan is INN.] (1) Poly(oxy-1,2-ethanediyl), α-[4-[[3,4-dihydro-2,5,7,8-tetramethyl-2-(4,8,12-trimethyltridecyl)-2*H*-1-benzopyran-6-yl]oxy]-1,4-dioxobutyl-ω-hydroxy-; (2) Mono-[2,5,7,8-tetramethyl-2-(4,8,12-trimethyltridecyl)-6-chromanyl] succinate polyethylene glycol monoester; (3) (+)-α-Tocopheryl polyethylene glycol 1000 succinate. *CAS-30999-06-5. Vitamin E supplement.* "EASTMAN" Vitamin E TPGS (Eastman) ◇TPGS

Tocopheryl Acetate, *d*-Alpha — *See* Vitamin E.

Tocopheryl Acetate, *dl*-Alpha — *See* Vitamin E.

Tocopheryl Acid Succinate, *d*-Alpha — *See* Vitamin E.

Todralazine. $C_{11}H_{12}N_4O_2$. 232.24. [Todralazine Hydrochloride is JAN.] Ethyl 3-(1-phthalazinyl)carbazate. *UNII-WEN3K83YKD. CAS-14679-73-3.* INN; BAN; MI. ◇CEPH [*as hydrochloride*]; BT 621 [*as hydrochloride*]

Tofenacin Hydrochloride [*1968*] (toe fen′ a sin hye″ droe klor′ ide). $C_{17}H_{21}NO.HCl$. 291.82. [Tofenacin is INN and BAN.] (1) Ethanamine, *N*-methyl-2-[(2-methylphenyl)phenylmethoxy]-, hydrochloride; (2) *N*-Methyl-2-[(*o*-methyl-α-phenylbenzyl)oxy]ethylamine hydrochloride. *UNII-3A10ND4DWR; UNII-C4A112M10H* [tofenacin]. *CAS-10488-36-5; CAS-15301-93-6* [tofenacin]. *Anticholinergic.*

---

† Brand name formerly used, and/or firm no longer concerned with this product.

Tofetridine. C₁₅H₂₁NO. 231.33. (-)-1,2,3,4,4a,5,6,10b-Octa-hydro-9-methoxy-10b-methylphenanthridine. *CAS-40173-75-9.* INN.

Tofimilast [*2000*] (toe fim′ i last). C₁₈H₂₁N₅S. 339.46. (1) 5*H*-Pyrazolo[3,4-*c*]-1,2,4-triazolo[4,3-*a*]pyridine, 9-cyclopen-tyl-7-ethyl-6,9-dihydro-3-(2-thienyl)-; (2) 9-Cyclopentyl-7-ethyl-6,9-dihydro-3-(2-thienyl)-5*H*-pyrazolo[3,4-*c*]-1,2,4-triazolo[4,3-*a*]pyridine. *UNII-5D7022962A.* *CAS-185954-27-2.* INN. *Treatment of asthma and chronic obstructive disease (phosphodiesterase isoenzyme 4) (PDE4 inhibitor).* (Pfizer) ◇*CP-325,366*

Tofisoline. C₂₂H₂₆N₂O₄. 382.45. 1-(3,4-Dimethoxyphenyl)-4-ethyl-6,7-dimethoxy-3-methylisoquinoline 2-imide. *UNII-2AV3RNM4HV.* *CAS-29726-99-6.*

Tofisopam. C₂₂H₂₆N₂O₄. 382.45. 1-(3,4-Dimethoxyphenyl)-5-ethyl-7,8-dimethoxy-4-methyl-5*H*-2,3-benzodiazepine. *CAS-22345-47-7.* INN; JAN; DCF; MI.

Tolafentrine. C₂₈H₃₁N₃O₄S. 505.63. (-)-4′-(*cis*-1,2,3,4,4a,10b-Hexahydro-8,9-dimethoxy-2-methylben-zo[*c*][1,6]naphthyridin-6-yl)-*p*-toluenesulfonanilide. *CAS-139308-65-9.* INN.

Tolamolol [*1973*] (tol am′ oh lol). C₁₉H₂₄N₂O₄. 344.40. (1) Benzamide, 4-[2-[[2-hydroxy-3-(2-methylphenoxy)propy-l]amino]ethoxy]-; (2) *p*-[2-[[2-Hydroxy-3-(*o*-tolyloxy)pro-

pyl]amino]ethoxy]benzamide. *CAS-38103-61-6.* INN; BAN. *Vasodilator (coronary); cardiac depressant (anti-arrhythmic); anti-adrenergic (β-receptor).*

Tolazamide [*1964*] (tol az′ a mide). **USP.** C₁₄H₂₁N₃O₃S. 311.40. (1) Benzenesulfonamide, *N*-[[(hexahydro-1*H*-aze-pin-1-yl)amino]carbonyl]-4-methyl-; (2) 1-(Hexahydro-1*H*-azepin-1-yl)-3-(*p*-tolylsulfonyl)urea. *UNII-9LT1BRO48Q.* *CAS-1156-19-0.* INN; BAN; JAN. *Antidi-abetic.* Tolinase (Pfizer) ◇*U-17835; NSC-70762*

Tolazoline Hydrochloride (tol az′ oh leen hye″ droe klor′ ide). **USP.** C₁₀H₁₂N₂.HCl. 196.68. [Tolazoline is INN and BAN.] (1) 1*H*-Imidazole, 4,5-dihydro-2-(phenylmethyl)-, monohydrochloride; (2) 2-Benzyl-2-imidazoline monohy-drochloride. *UNII-E669Z6S1JG; UNII-CHH9H12AQ3* [to-lazoline]. *CAS-59-97-2; CAS-59-98-3* [tolazoline]. JAN. *Vasodilator (peripheral).* Priscoline (Novartis)

Tolboxane. C₁₄H₂₁BO₂. 232.13. 5-Methyl-5-propyl-2-*p*-tolyl-1,3,2-dioxaborinane. *UNII-33P8JV23L7.* *CAS-2430-46-8.* INN; DCF; MI.

Tolbutamide (tol bue′ ta mide). **USP.** C₁₂H₁₈N₂O₃S. 270.35. (1) Benzenesulfonamide, *N*-[(butylamino)carbonyl]-4-methyl-; (2) 1-Butyl-3-(*p*-tolylsulfonyl)urea. *UNII-982XCM1FOI.* *CAS-64-77-7.* INN; BAN; JAN. *Antidia-betic.* Orinase (Pfizer)

Tolbutamide Sodium, Sterile. C₁₂H₁₇N₂NaO₃S. 292.33. (1) Benzenesulfonamide, *N*-[(butylamino)carbonyl]-4-meth-yl-, monosodium salt; (2) 1-Butyl-3-(*p*-tolylsulfonyl)urea monosodium salt. *UNII-982XCM1FOI* [tolbutamide]. *CAS-473-41-6; CAS-64-77-7* [tolbutamide]. USP XXIII. *Diag-nostic aid (diabetes).* Orinase Diagnostic (Pharmacia & Upjohn)

Tolcapone [*1993*] (tole′ ka pone). **USP.** $C_{14}H_{11}NO_5$. 273.24. (1) Methanone, (3,4-dihydroxy-5-nitrophenyl)(4-methylphenyl)-; (2) 3,4-Dihydroxy-4′-methyl-5-nitrobenzophenone. *UNII-CIF6334OLY. CAS-134308-13-7.* INN; BAN. *Antiparkinsonian.* Tasmar (Valeant) ◇*Ro 40-7592*

Tolciclate [*1976*] (tole sye′ klate). $C_{20}H_{21}NOS$. 323.45. (1) Carbamothioic acid, methyl(3-methylphenyl)-, *O*-(1,2,3,4-tetrahydro-1,4-methanonaphthalen-6-yl) ester; (2) *O*-(1,2,3,4-Tetrahydro-1,4-methanonaphthalen-6-yl) *m,N*-dimethylthiocarbanilate. *CAS-50838-36-3.* INN; JAN. *Antifungal.* ◇*K 9147*

Tolclotide — *See* Disulfamide.

Toldimfos. $C_9H_{14}NO_2P$. 199.19. [4-(Dimethylamino)-*o*-tolyl]phosphinic acid. *CAS-57808-64-7.* INN; BAN; MI.

Tolevamer Potassium Sodium [*2005*] (tole ev′ a mer poe tas′ ee um soe′ dee um). $(C_8H_7O_3S)_n \cdot K_{(n-a)}Na_a$. (1) Benzenesulfonic acid, 4-ethenyl-, homopolymer, potassium sodium salt; (2) Poly[1-(4-sulfophenyl)ethylene], potassium sodium salt. Molecular weight is greater than 400,000 daltons. *CAS-1011713-07-7; CAS-81998-90-5. Treatment of Clostridium difficle associated diarrhea.* ◇*GT267-004*

Tolevamer Sodium [*2002*] (tole ev′ a mer soe′ dee um). $(C_8H_7NaO_3S)_n$. [Tolevamer is INN.] (1) Benzenesulfonic acid, 4-ethenyl-, homopolymer, sodium salt; (2) Poly[1-(4-sulfophenyl)ethylene], sodium salt. Molecular weight is greater than 400,000 daltons. *CAS-28038-50-8; CAS-*

28210-41-5 [tolevamer]. *Treatment and prevention of Clostridium difficile (C.difficile) associated diarrheal disease (toxin binder).* ◇*GT160-246*

Tolfamide [*1980*] (tol′ fa mide). $C_8H_{12}N_3O_2P$. 213.17. (1) Benzamide, *N*-(diaminophosphinyl)-2-methyl-; (2) *N*-(Diaminophosphinyl)-*o*-toluamide. *UNII-7TJT8X832U. CAS-70788-29-3.* INN. *Enzyme inhibitor (urease).* ◇*EU-4584*

Tolfenamic Acid. $C_{14}H_{12}ClNO_2$. 261.70. *N*-(3-Chloro-*o*-tolyl)anthranilic acid. *CAS-13710-19-5.* INN; BAN; JAN; MI.

Tolgabide [*1987*] (tole′ ga bide). $C_{18}H_{18}Cl_2N_2O_2$. 365.25. (1) Butanamide, 4-[[(5-chloro-2-hydroxy-3-methylphenyl)(4-chlorophenyl)methylene]amino]-, (*E*)-; (2) (*E*)-4-[[5-Chloro-α-(*p*-chlorophenyl)-3-methylsalicylidene]amino]-butyramide. *UNII-0L55QF645F. CAS-86914-11-6.* INN; BAN. *Anti-epileptic (control of abnormal movements).* ◇*SL 81.0142-00*

Tolhexamide — *See* Glycyclamide.

Tolimidone [*1978*] (tole i′ mi done). $C_{11}H_{10}N_2O_2$. 202.21. (1) 2(1*H*)-Pyrimidinone, 5-(3-methylphenoxy)-; (2) 5-(*m*-Tolyloxy)-2(1*H*)-pyrimidinone. *CAS-41964-07-2.* INN. *Antiulcerative.* ◇*CP-26,154*

Tolindate [*1972*] (tole in′ date). $C_{18}H_{19}NOS$. 297.41. (1) Carbamothioic acid, methyl(3-methylphenyl)-, *O*-(2,3-dihydro-1*H*-inden-5-yl) ester; (2) *O*-5-Indanyl *m,N*-dimethylthiocarbanilate. *CAS-27877-51-6.* INN. *Antifungal.*

---

† Brand name formerly used, and/or firm no longer concerned with this product.

Toliodium Chloride [*1976*] (tole″ i oh′ di um klor′ ide). $C_{14}H_{14}ClI$. 344.62. (1) Iodonium, bis(4-methylphenyl)-, chloride; (2) Di-*p*-tolyliodonium chloride. *UNII-QV3QF1EF2P. CAS-19028-28-5.* INN. *Food additive (veterinary).* ◇*SK&F 15601A*

Toliprolol. $C_{13}H_{21}NO_2$. 223.31. 1-(Isopropylamino)-3-(*m*-tolyloxy)-2-propanol. *CAS-2933-94-0.* INN; MI. ◇*ICI 45763 [as hydrochloride]; Ko 592 [as hydrochloride]*

Tolmesoxide. $C_{10}H_{14}O_3S$. 214.28. 4,5-Dimethoxy-2-(methyl-sulfinyl)toluene. *CAS-38452-29-8.* INN; BAN.

Tolmetin [*1971*] (tol′ met in). $C_{15}H_{15}NO_3$. 257.28. (1) 1*H*-Pyrrole-2-acetic acid, 1-methyl-5-(4-methylbenzoyl)-; (2) 1-Methyl-5-*p*-toluoylpyrrole-2-acetic acid. *UNII-D8K2JPN18B. CAS-26171-23-3.* INN; BAN. *Anti-inflam-matory.* ◇*McN-2559*

Tolmetin Sodium [*1976*] (tol′ met in soe′ dee um). **USP**. $C_{15}H_{14}NNaO_3 \cdot 2H_2O$. 315.30. (1) 1*H*-Pyrrole-2-acetic acid, 1-methyl-5-(4-methylbenzoyl)-, sodium salt, dihydrate; (2) Sodium 1-methyl-5-*p*-toluoylpyrrole-2-acetate dihydrate. *UNII-02N1TZF99F. CAS-64490-92-2; CAS-35711-34-3* [anhydrous]. JAN. *Anti-inflammatory.* Tolectin (Ortho-McNeil) ◇*McN-2559-21-98*

Tolnaftate [*1963*] (tol naf′ tate). **USP**. $C_{19}H_{17}NOS$. 307.41. (1) Carbamothioic acid, methyl(3-methylphenyl)-, *O*-2-naphthalenyl ester; (2) *O*-2-Naphthyl *m,N*-dimethylthio-carbanilate. *UNII-06KB629TKV. CAS-2398-96-1.* INN; BAN; JAN. *Antifungal.* Aftate (Schering-Plough Health-Care); Dr. Scholl's Athlete's Foot Spray (Schering-Plough HealthCare); Tinactin (Schering-Plough HealthCare); Tritin (Schering-Plough HealthCare†) ◇*Sch 10144*

Tolnapersine. $C_{21}H_{26}N_2O$. 322.44. 5,6,7,8-Tetrahydro-6-(4-*o*-tolyl-1-piperazinyl)-2-naphthol. *CAS-70312-00-4.* INN.

Tolnidamine. $C_{16}H_{13}ClN_2O_2$. 300.74. 1-(4-Chloro-2-methyl-benzyl)-1*H*-indazole-3-carboxylic acid. *UNII-Z5M7SC6D5P. CAS-50454-68-7.* INN.

Toloconium Metilsulfate. $C_{23}H_{43}NO_4S$. 429.66. Trimethyl(1-*p*-tolyldodecyl)ammonium methylsulfate. *CAS-552-92-1.* INN.

Tolofocon A [*1987*] (tole″ oh foe′ kon). $(C_{16}H_{38}O_5Si_4)_v$ $(C_6H_7F_3O_2)_w(C_5H_8O_2)_x(C_4H_6O_2)_y(C_{10}H_{14}O_4)_z$. (1) 2-Prope-noic acid, 2-methyl-, 3-[3,3,3-trimethyl-1,1-bis[(trimethyl-silyl)oxy]disiloxanyl]propyl ester, polymer with 2,2,2-trifluoroethyl 2-methyl-2-propenoate, methyl 2-methyl-2-propenoate, 2-methyl-2-propenoic acid and 1,2-ethanediyl bis(2-methyl-2-propenoate); (2) 3-[3,3,3-Trimethyl-1,1-bis(trimethylsiloxy)disiloxanyl]propyl methacrylate poly-mer with 2,2,2-trifluoroethyl methacrylate, methyl meth-acrylate, methacrylic acid and ethylene dimethacrylate. *CAS-105581-52-0. Contact lens material (hydrophobic).*

Tolonidine. $C_{10}H_{12}ClN_3$. 209.68. 2-(2-Chloro-*p*-toluidino)-2-imidazoline. *UNII-I4O795Q03O. CAS-4201-22-3.* INN; DCF; MI. ◇*ST 375*

Tolonium Chloride. $C_{15}H_{16}ClN_3S$. 305.83. 3-Amino-7-dimethylamino-2-methylphenazathionium. *CAS-92-31-9*. MI; INN. Blutene (Abbott†)

Toloxatone. $C_{11}H_{13}NO_3$. 207.23. 5-(Hydroxymethyl)-3-*m*-tolyl-2-oxazolidinone. *CAS-29218-27-7*. INN; MI.

Toloxichloral — *See* Toloxychlorinol.

Toloxychlorinol. $C_{14}H_{16}Cl_6O_5$. 476.99. 1,1′-(3-*o*-Tolyloxypropylenedioxy)-bis(2,2,2-trichloroethanol). *CAS-6055-48-7*. INN; MI.

Tolpadol. $C_{28}H_{26}N_4O_2$. 450.53. *N,N′*-(1,2-Di-4-pyridylethylene)bis[*o*-toluamide]. *CAS-77502-27-3*. INN.

Tolpentamide. $C_{13}H_{18}N_2O_3S$. 282.36. 1-Cyclopentyl-3-*p*-tolylsulfonylurea. *UNII-4G278XM8KC*. *CAS-1027-87-8*. INN; BAN.

Tolperisone. $C_{16}H_{23}NO$. 245.36. [Tolperisone Hydrochloride is JAN.] 2,4′-Dimethyl-3-piperidinopropiophenone. *CAS-728-88-1*. INN; BAN; MI. ◇*N-553 [as hydrochloride]*

Tolpiprazole. $C_{17}H_{24}N_4$. 284.40. 1-[2-(5-Methylpyrazol-3-yl)ethyl]-4-*m*-tolylpiperazine. *UNII-8XP74P4HO3*. *CAS-20326-13-0*. INN; BAN. ◇*H 4170*

Tolpovidone I 131 [*1962*] (tole poe′ vi done). (1) Poly[1-(2-oxo-1-pyrrolidinyl)-1,2-ethanediyl], α-hydro-ω-[[4-(iodo-^{131}I)phenyl]methyl]-; (2) α-Hydro-ω-(*p*-iodobenzyl)-poly[1-(2-oxo-1-pyrrolidinyl)ethylene]-^{131}I. (A small part of the iodine is the radioactive isotope, ^{131}I.) *CAS-9015-62-7*. INN. *Diagnostic aid (hypoalbuminemia); radioactive agent.*

Tolpronine. $C_{15}H_{21}NO_2$. 247.33. 3,6-Dihydro-α-(*o*-toloxymethyl)-1(2*H*)-pyridenethanol. *CAS-97-57-4*. INN; BAN; MI.

Tolpropamine. $C_{18}H_{23}N$. 253.38. *N,N*-Dimethyl-3-phenyl-3-*p*-tolylpropylamine. *CAS-5632-44-0*. INN; BAN; MI.

Tolpyrramide [*1965*] (tol pir′ a mide). $C_{12}H_{16}N_2O_3S$. 268.33. (1) 1-Pyrrolidinecarboxamide, *N*-[(4-methylphenyl)sulfonyl]-; (2) *N-p*-Tolylsulfonyl-1-pyrrolidinecarboxamide. *UNII-W68DD2C7VG*. *CAS-5588-38-5*. INN. *Antidiabetic.* ◇*NSC-106572*

Tolquinzole. $C_{16}H_{23}NO$. 245.36. 2-Ethyl-1,3,4,6,7,11b-hexahydro-10-methyl-2*H*-benzo[*a*]quinolizin-2-ol. *CAS-6187-50-4*. INN.

Tolrestat [*1984*] (tol′ re stat). $C_{16}H_{14}F_3NO_3S$. 357.35. (1) Glycine, *N*-[6-methoxy-5-(trifluoromethyl)-1-naphthalenyl]thioxomethyl]-*N*-methyl-; (2) *N*-[6-Methoxythio-5-(trifluoromethyl)-1-naphthoyl]sarcosine. *CAS-82964-04-3.* INN; BAN. *Inhibitor (aldose reductase).* Alredase (Wyeth-Ayerst) ◇*AY-27,773*

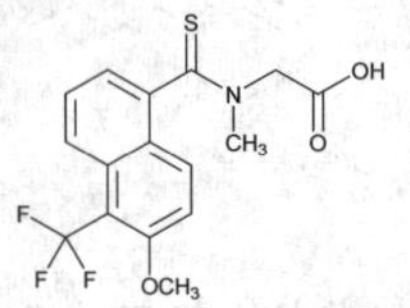

Tolterodine [*1997*] (tol ter′ oh deen). $C_{22}H_{31}NO$. 325.49. (+)-(*R*)-2-[α-[2-(Diisopropylamino)ethyl]benzyl]-*p*-cresol. *UNII-WHE7A56U7K. CAS-124937-51-5.* INN; BAN. *Anticholinergic.* ◇*Kabi 2234*

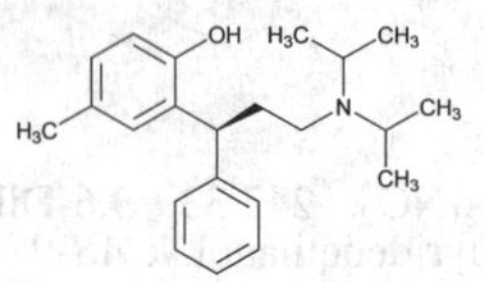

Tolterodine Tartrate [*1997*] (tol ter′ oh deen tar′ trate). $C_{22}H_{31}NO.C_4H_6O_6$. 475.57. (1) (*R*)-2-[3-[Bis(1-methylethyl)amino]-1-phenylpropyl]-4-methylphenol [*R*-(*R*,R**)]-2,3-dihydroxybutanedioate (1:1) (salt); (2) (+)-(*R*)-2-[I-[2-(Diisopropylamino)ethyl]benzyl]-*p*-cresol L-tartrate (1:1) (salt). *UNII-5T619TQR3R. CAS-124937-52-6. Treatment of urinary incontinence (muscarinic receptor antagonist).* Detrol (Pfizer) ◇*PNU-200583E*

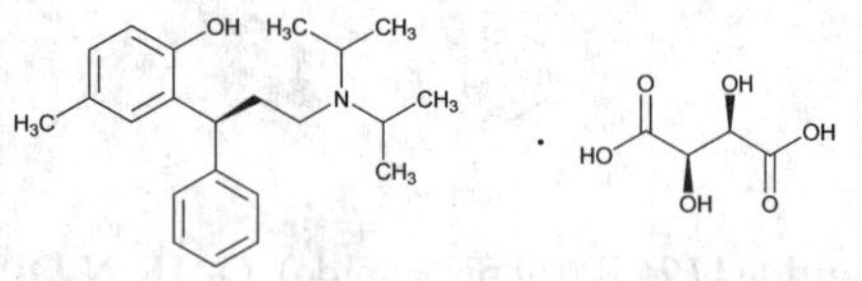

Toltrazuril [*1988*] (tole traz′ ure il). $C_{18}H_{14}F_3N_3O_4S$. 425.38. (1) 1,3,5-Triazine-2,4,6(1*H*,3*H*,5*H*)-trione, 1-methyl-3-[3-methyl-4-[4-[(trifluoromethyl)thio]phenoxy]phenyl]-; (2) 1-Methyl-3-[4-[*p*-[(trifluoromethyl)thio]phenoxy]-*m*-tolyl]-*s*-triazine-2,4,6(1*H*,3*H*,5*H*)-trione. *UNII-QVZ3IAR3JS. CAS-69004-03-1.* INN; BAN. *Coccidiostat (veterinary).* ◇*Bay Vi 9142*

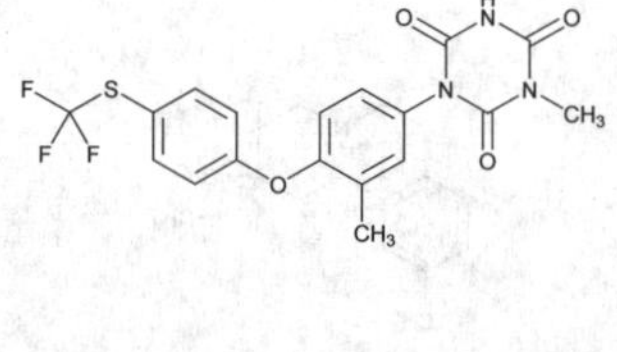

Tolu Balsam (toe loo′ bawl′ sam). **USP.** A balsam obtained from *Myroxylon balsamum* (Linné) Harms (Fam. Leguminosae). *CAS-8017-09-2.* NF XVII. *Pharmaceutic aid.*

Tolufazepam. $C_{24}H_{20}Cl_2N_2O_3S$. 487.40. 7-Chloro-5-(*o*-chlorophenyl)-1,3-dihydro-1-[2-(*p*-tolylsulfonyl)ethyl]-2*H*-1,4-benzodiazepin-2-one. *UNII-98SR74X50D. CAS-86273-92-9.* INN.

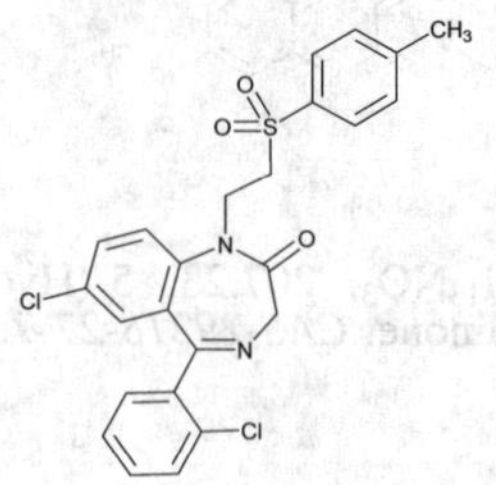

Toluidine Blue O — *See* Tolonium Chloride.

Tolvaptan [*1999*] (tol vap′ tan). $C_{26}H_{25}ClN_2O_3$. 448.94. (1) Benzamide, *N*-[4-[(7-chloro-2,3,4,5-tetrahydro-5-hydroxy-1*H*-1-benzazepin-1-yl)carbonyl]-3-methylphenyl]-2-methyl-; (2) (±)-4′-[(7-Chloro-2,3,4,5-tetrahydro-5-hydroxy-1*H*-1-benzazepin-1-yl) carbonyl]-*o*-tolu-*m*-toluidide. *UNII-21G72T1950. CAS-150683-30-0.* INN. *Treatment of congestive heart failure and hyponatremia (vasopressin V2 receptor antagonist).* ◇*OPC-41061*

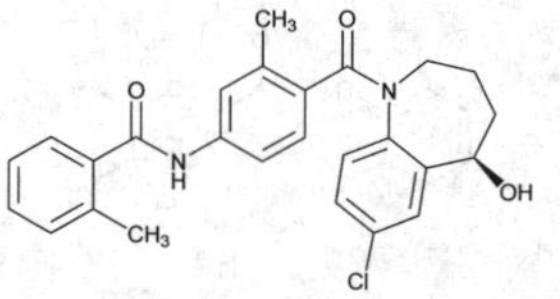

Tolycaine. $C_{15}H_{22}N_2O_3$. 278.35. [Tolycaine Hydrochloride is JAN.] Methyl 2-[2-(diethylamino)acetamido]-*m*-toluate. *UNII-12R8659YM6. CAS-3686-58-6.* INN; BAN; MI.

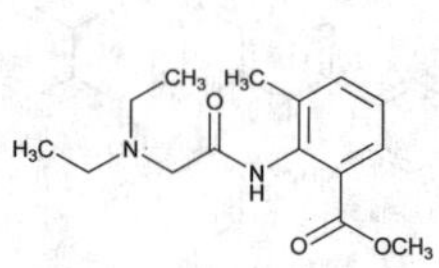

Tomeglovir. $C_{23}H_{27}N_3O_4S$. 441.54. *N*-[4-[[[5-(Dimethylamino)-1-naphthyl]sulfonyl]amino]phenyl]-3-hydroxy-2,2-dimethylpropionamide. *CAS-233254-24-5.* INN.

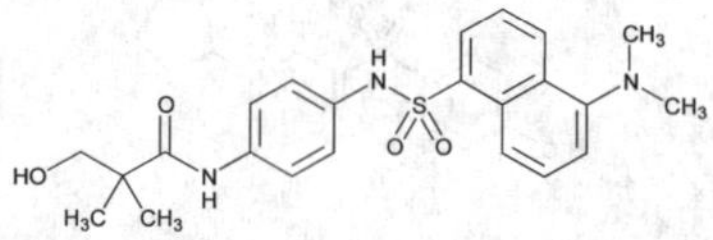

Tomelukast [*1988*] (toe″ me loo′ kast). $C_{16}H_{22}N_4O_3$. 318.37. (1) Ethanone, 1-[2-hydroxy-3-propyl-4-[4-(1*H*-tetrazol-5-yl)butoxy]phenyl]-; (2) 2′-Hydroxy-3′-propyl-4′-[4-(1*H*-tetrazol-5-yl)butoxy]acetophenone. *UNII-59762X5CLS. CAS-88107-10-2.* INN. *Anti-asthmatic (leukotriene antagonist).* ◇*LY171883*

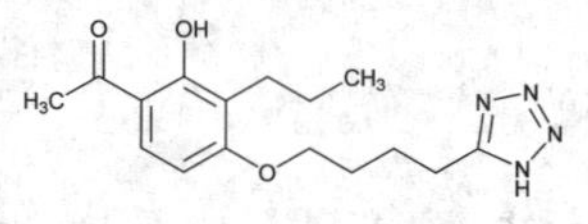

Tomoglumide. $C_{24}H_{38}N_2O_4$. 418.57. (±)-4-(3,4-Dimethyl-benzamido)-N,N-dipentylglutaramic acid. *UNII-4AO6I17SLB. CAS-97964-54-0.* INN.

Tomopenem [*2007*] (toe″ moe pen′ em). $C_{23}H_{35}N_7O_6S$. 537.63. (1) 1-Azabicyclo[3.2.0]hept-2-ene-2-carboxylic acid, 3-[[(3S,5S)-5-[[(3S)-3-[[[(aminoiminomethyl)amino]acetyl]amino]-1-pyrrolidinyl]carbonyl]-1-methyl-3-pyrrolidinyl]thio]-6-[(1R)-1-hydroxyethyl]-4-methyl-7-oxo-, (4R,5S,6S)-; (2) (4R,5S,6S)-3-({(3S,5S)-5-[(3S)-3-(Carbamimidamidoac-etamido)pyrrolidine-1-carbonyl]-1-methylpyrrolidin-3-yl}sulfanyl)-6-[(1R)-1-hydroxyethyl]-4-methyl-7-oxo-1-azabicyclo[3.2.0]hept-2-ene-2-carboxylic acid (3) (4R,5S,6S)-3-{[(3S,5S)-5-({(3S)-3-[(2-Guanidinoac-etyl)amino]pyrrolidin-1-yl}carbonyl)-1-methylpyrrolidin-3-yl]sulfanyl}-6-[(1R)-1-hydroxyethyl]-4-methyl-7-oxo-1-azabicyclo[3.2.0]hept-2-ene-2-carboxylic acid. *UNII-1654W9611T. CAS-222400-20-6.* INN. *Antibiotic.* ◇*RO4908463; CS-023; R-115685; R-1558*

Tomoxetine Hydrochloride (previously used name) — *See* Atomoxetine Hydrochloride.

Tomoxiprole. $C_{21}H_{20}N_2O$. 316.40. 3-Isopropyl-2-(p-methoxyphenyl)-3H-naphth[1,2-d]imidazole. *UNII-EZ948T2878. CAS-76145-76-1.* INN.

Tonabersat. $C_{20}H_{19}ClFNO_4$. 391.82. N-[(3S,4S)-6-Acetyl-3-hydroxy-2,2-dimethylchroman-4-yl]-3-chloro-4-fluoro-benzamide. *CAS-175013-84-0.* BAN, INN. ◇*SB-220453*

Tonazocine Mesylate [*1981*] (toe naz′ oh seen mes′ i late). $C_{23}H_{35}NO_2 \cdot CH_4O_3S$. 453.64. [Tonazocine is INN.] (1) 3-Octanone, 1-(1,2,3,4,5,6-hexahydro-8-hydroxy-3,6,11-tri-methyl-2,6-methano-3-benzazocin-11-yl)-, methanesulfo-nate (salt), (2$α$,6$α$,11S*)-(±)-; (2) (±)-1-[(2R*,6S*,11S*)-1,2,3,4,5,6-Hexahydro-8-hydroxy-3,6,11-trimethyl-2,6-methano-3-benzazocin-11-yl)-3-octanone methanesulfonate (salt). *UNII-2F5K551CB4. CAS-73789-00-1; CAS-71461-18-2* [tonazocine]. *Analgesic.* ◇*Win 42156-2*

Tonzonium Bromide (INN) — *See* Thonzonium Bromide.

Topilutamide. $C_{13}H_{11}F_6N_3O_5$. 403.23. (2RS)-2-Hydroxy-2-methyl-N-[4-nitro-3-(trifluoromethyl)phenyl]-3-[(trifluoroacetyl)amino]propanamide. *UNII-A8EU2FXY13. CAS-260980-89-0.* INN.

Topiramate [*1987*] (toe pir′ a mate). **USP**. $C_{12}H_{21}NO_8S$. 339.36. (1) $β$-D-Fructopyranose, 2,3:4,5-bis-O-(1-methyl-ethylidene)-, sulfamate; (2) 2,3:4,5-Di-O-isopropylidene-$β$-D-fructopyranose sulfamate. *UNII-0H73WJJ391. CAS-97240-79-4.* INN; BAN. *Anticonvulsant.* Topamax (Ortho-McNeil) ◇*McN-4853; RWJ-17021*

Topixantrone [*2003*] (toe pix′ an trone). $C_{21}H_{26}N_6O_2$. 394.47. (1) Indazolo[4,3-gh]isoquinolin-6(2H)-one, 5-[[2-(di-methylamino)ethyl]amino]-2-[2-[(2-hydroxyethyl)ami-no]ethyl]-; (2) 5-[[2-(Dimethylamino)ethyl]amino]-2-[2-[(2-hydroxyethyl)amino]ethyl]indazolo[4,3-gh]isoquino-lin-6(2H)-one. *UNII-R40RXC296C. CAS-156090-18-5.* INN; BAN. *Anti-neoplastic.* ◇*BBR 3576 (dihydrochloride)*

Topotecan Hydrochloride [*1990*] (toe″ poe tee′ kan hye″ droe klor′ ide). $C_{23}H_{23}N_3O_5 \cdot HCl$. 457.91. [Topotecan is INN and BAN.] (1) 1H-Pyrano[3′,4′:6,7]indolizino[1,2-b]quinoline-3,14(4H,12H)-dione, 10-[(dimethylamino)-methyl]-4-ethyl-4,9-dihydroxy-, monohydrochloride, (S)-; (2) (S)-10-[(Dimethylamino)methyl]-4-ethyl-4,9-dihy-droxy-1H-pyrano[3′,4′:6,7]indolizino[1,2-b]quinoline-3,14(4H,12H)-dione monohydrochloride. *UNII-956S425ZCY; UNII-7M7YKX2N15* [topotecan]. *CAS-*

---

† Brand name formerly used, and/or firm no longer concerned with this product.

119413-54-6; CAS-123948-87-8 [topotecan]. *Antineoplastic (DNA topoisomerase I inhibitor).* Hycamtin (Glaxo SmithKline) ◇*SK&F S-104864-A*

Toprilidine. $C_{19}H_{25}N_3O$. 311.42. 1-[3-(2-Pyridyloxy)propyl]-4-*o*-tolylpiperazine. *UNII-E66RIC936T. CAS-54063-58-0.* INN.

Topterone [*1977*] (top′ te rone). $C_{22}H_{34}O_2$. 330.50. (1) Androst-4-en-3-one, 17-hydroxy-17-propyl-, (17β)-; (2) 17β-Hydroxy-17-propylandrost-4-en-3-one. *UNII-77WPB17ZK1. CAS-60607-35-4.* INN. *Anti-androgen.* ◇*Win 17665*

Toquizine [*1966*] (toe′ kwi zeen). $C_{23}H_{29}N_5O$. 391.51. (1) 1H-Pyrazole-1-carboxamide, N-(4-ethyl-4,6,6a,7,8,9,10,10a-octahydro-7-methylindolo[4,3-*fg*]quinolin-9-yl)-3,5-dimethyl-; (2) N-(4-Ethyl-4,6,6a,7,8,9,10,10a-octahydro-7-methylindolo[4,3-*g*]quinolin-9-yl)-3,5-dimethylpyrazole-1-carboxamide. *CAS-7125-71-5.* INN. *Anticholinergic.* ◇*44106*

Toralizumab [*2002*] (tore″ a liz′ oo mab). Immunoglobulin G1, anti-(human CD40 ligand) (human-mouse monoclonal IDEC-131 γ1 chain), disulfide with human-mouse monoclonal IDEC-131 κ-chain, dimer. Molecular weight is approximately 148,426 daltons. *CAS-252662-47-8.* INN. *Treatment of antibody-mediated disorders (immune thrombocytopenic purpura, lupus nephritis, rheumatoid arthritis), T-cell-mediated diseases (multiple sclerosis, Crohn's disease, and transplantation such as solid organ transplantation, pancreatic islet cell transplantation, and corneal transplantation), and B-cell malignancies (such as CLL/small lymphocytic lymphoma, follicular cell lymphoma grade I or II, marginal zone lymphoma, mantle cell lymphoma, MALT lymphoma, Waldenstrom's macroglobulinemia, monocytoid B-cell lymphoma; relapsed/refractory Hodgkin's disease) (monoclonal antibody).* ◇*anti-gp39; anti-CD40L; anti-CD154*

Torapsel [*2004*] (tore ap′ sel). $C_{2726}H_{4186}N_{710}O_{846}S_{20}$ (peptidic part). 61,083 (peptidic part). 42-89-Glycoprotein (human clone PMT21:PL85 P-selectin glycoprotein ligand 1) fusion protein with immunoglobulin (human constant region). *CAS-204658-47-9.* INN. *P-selectin antagonist.* ◇*WAY 164339*

```
QATEYEYLDY DFLPETEPPE MLRNSTDTTP LTGPGTPEST TVEPAARPHT
CPPCPAPEAL GAPSVFLFPP KPKDTLMISR TPEVTCVVVD VSHEDPEVKF
NWYVDGVEVH NAKTKPREEQ YNSTYRVVSV LTVLHQDWLN GKEYKCKVSN
KALPVPIEKT ISKAKGQPRE PQVYTLPPSR EEMTKNQVSL TCLVKGFYPS
DIAVEWESNG QPENNYKTTP PVLDSDGSFF LYSKLTVDKS RWQQGNVFSC
SVMHEALHNH YTQKSLSLSP GK
```
2

Torasemide (INN, BAN) — *See* Torsemide.

Torbafylline. $C_{16}H_{26}N_4O_4$. 338.40. 7-(Ethoxymethyl)-1-(5-hydroxy-5-methylhexyl)-3-methylxanthine. *CAS-105102-21-4.* INN.

Torcetrapib [*2002*] (tore set′ ra pib). $C_{26}H_{25}F_9N_2O_4$. 600.47. (1) 1(2H)-Quinolinecarboxylic acid, 4-[[[3,5-bis(trifluoromethyl)phenyl]methyl] (methoxycarbonyl)amino]-2-ethyl-3,4-dihydro-6-(trifluoromethyl)-, ethyl ester, (2R,4S)-; (2) Ethyl (2R,4S)-4-[[3,5-bis(trifluoromethyl)benzyl](methoxycarbonyl)amino]-2-ethyl-6-(trifluoromethyl)-3,4-dihydroquinoline-1(2H)-carboxylate. *CAS-262352-17-0.* INN. *Treatment of atherosclerosis; heart disease (cholesteryl ester transfer protein inhibitor).* ◇*CP-529,414*

Torcitabine [*2002*] (tore sye′ ta been). $C_9H_{13}N_3O_4$. 227.22. (1) 2(1H)-Pyrimidinone, 4-amino-1-(2-deoxy-β-L-*erythro*-pentofuranosyl)-; (2) 4-Amino-1-(2-deoxy-β-L-*erythro*-pentofuranosyl)pyrimidin-2(1H)-one. *UNII-6BZN07BMW3. CAS-40093-94-5.* INN. *Treatment of hepatitis B infection (polymerase inhibitor).* ◇*NV-02C*

Toremifene Citrate [*1988*] (tore em′ i feen sit′ rate). $C_{26}H_{28}ClNO \cdot C_6H_8O_7$. 598.08. [Toremifene is INN and BAN.] (1) Ethanamine, 2-[4-(4-chloro-1,2-diphenyl-1-butenyl)phenoxy]-N,N-dimethyl-, (Z)-, 2-hydroxy-1,2,3-propanetricarboxylate (1:1); (2) 2-[*p*-[(Z)-4-Chloro-1,2-diphenyl-1-butenyl]phenoxy]-N,N-dimethylethylamine citrate (1:1). *UNII-2498Y783QT; UNII-7NFE54O27T* [toremifene]. *CAS-89778-27-8; CAS-89778-26-7* [toremifene]. *Anti-estrogen; antineoplastic.* Fareston (GTX) ◇*FC-1157a*

Toripristone. $C_{31}H_{39}NO_2$. 457.65. 17β-Hydroxy-11β-[*p*-(isopropylmethylamino)phenyl]-17-(1-propynyl)estra-4,9-dien-3-one. *CAS-91935-26-1.* INN.

Torsemide [*1989*] (tore′ se mide). **USP.** $C_{16}H_{20}N_4O_3S$. 348.42. [Torasemide is INN and BAN.] (1) 3-Pyridinesulfonamide, *N*-[[(1-methylethyl)amino]carbonyl]-4-[(3-methylphenyl)amino]-; (2) 1-Isopropyl-3-[(4-*m*-toluidino-3-pyridyl)sulfonyl]urea. *UNII-W31X2H97FB. CAS-56211-40-6. Diuretic.* Demadex (Roche) ◇*BM02.015; AC4464*

Tosactide. $C_{150}H_{230}N_{44}O_{38}S$. 3289.77. α^{1-28}-Corticotropin (human). *CAS-47931-80-6.* INN; BAN. *[Name previously used: Octacosactrin.]*

SYSMEHFRWG KPVGKKRRPV KVYPDAGE

Tosagestin [*2002*] (toe″ sa jes′ tin). $C_{21}H_{24}O_2$. 308.41. (1) 19-Norpregna-4,15-dien-20-yn-3-one, 17-hydroxy-11-methylene-, (17α)-; (2) 17-Hydroxy-11-methylene-19-nor-17α-pregna-4,15-dien-20-yn-3-one; (3) 11-Methylene-Δ-15-norethisterone. *UNII-YS7Z529O22. CAS-110072-15-6.* INN. *Hormonal contraception; hormone replacement therapy.[Name previously used: Letogestin.]* ◇*Org 30659*

Tosedostat. $C_{21}H_{30}N_2O_6$. 406.47. Cyclopentyl (2*S*)-2-{(2*R*)-2-[(1*S*)-1-hydroxy-2-(hydroxyamino)-2-oxoethyl]-4-methylpentanamido}-2-phenylacetate. *CAS-238750-77-1.* INN.

---

† Brand name formerly used, and/or firm no longer concerned with this product.

Tosifen [*1976*] (toe′ si fen). $C_{17}H_{20}N_2O_3S$. 332.42. (1) Benzenesulfonamide, 4-methyl-*N*-[[(1-methyl-2-phenylethyl)amino]carbonyl]-, (*S*)-; (2) (*S*)-1-(α-Methylphenethyl)-3-(*p*-tolylsulfonyl)urea. *CAS-32295-18-4.* INN. *Anti-anginal.* ◇*Sch 11973*

Tositumomab. Immunoglobulin G2a anti-(human antigen CD 20) (mouse monoclonal clone B1R1 γ2a-chain), disulfide with mouse monoclonal clone B1R1 λ_x-chain, dimer. *UNII-0343IGH41U. CAS-192391-48-3.* INN.

Tosufloxacin [*1989*] (toe″ soo flox′ a sin). $C_{19}H_{15}F_3N_4O_3$. 404.34. [Tosufloxacin Tosilate is JAN.] (1) 1,8-Naphthyridine-3-carboxylic acid, 7-(3-amino-1-pyrrolidinyl)-1-(2,4-difluorophenyl)-6-fluoro-1,4-dihydro-4-oxo-, (±)-; (2) (±)-7-(3-Amino-1-pyrrolidinyl)-1-(2,4-difluorophenyl)-6-fluoro-1,4-dihydro-4-oxo-1,8-naphthyridine-3-carboxylic acid. *UNII-6239812J7L* [tosufloxacin monohydrate]. *CAS-108138-46-1* [anhydrous (±)]; *CAS-107097-79-0* [monohydrate]. INN. *Antibacterial.* ◇*Abbott-61827*

Tosulur. $C_{11}H_{15}NO_5S$. 273.31. 2-Methoxyethyl (*p*-tolylsulfonyl)carbamate. *UNII-I04MF82GW9. CAS-87051-13-6.* INN.

Tosylchloramide Sodium (INN, BAN) — *See* Chloramine-T.

Totrombopag Choline [*2006*] (toe trom′ boe pag koe′ leen). $C_{25}H_{21}N_8O_2 \cdot C_5H_{14}NO$. 569.66. [Totrombopag is INN.] (1) Ethanaminium, 2-hydroxy-*N,N,N*-trimethyl-, salt with 2-(3,4-dimethylphenyl)-2,4-dihydro-4-[[2-hydroxy-3′-(1*H*-tetrazol-5-yl)[1,1′-biphenyl]-3-yl]azo]-5-methyl-3*H*-pyrazol-3-one (1:1); (2) 2-Hydroxy-*N,N,N*-trimethylethanaminium 5-[3′-[(2*Z*)-2-[1-(3,4-dimethylphenyl)-3-methyl-5-oxo-1,5-dihydro-4*H*-pyrazol-4-ylidene]diazanyl]-2′-hydroxybiphenyl-3-yl]tetrazolide. *UNII-IRH58115R1. CAS-851606-62-7; CAS-376592-42-6* [totrombopag]. *Treatment of chemotherapy-induced thrombocytopenia, treatment of thrombocytopenia-associated liver diseases, and idiopathic thrombocytopenic purpura.* ◇*SB-559448-AAA*

Tozalinone (INN) — *See* Thozalinone.

Tozasertib [*2008*] (toe″ za ser′ tib). $C_{23}H_{28}N_8OS$. 464.59. (1) Cyclopropanecarboxamide, *N*-[4-[[4-(4-methyl-1-piperazinyl)-6-[(5-methyl-1*H*-pyrazol-3-yl)amino]-2-pyrimidinyl]thio]phenyl]-; (2) *N*-[4-({4-(4-methylpiperazin-1-yl)-6-[(5-methyl-1*H*-pyrazol-3-yl)amino]pyrimidin-2-yl}sulfanyl)phenyl]cyclopropanecarboxamide. *UNII-234335M86K. CAS-639089-54-6. Antineoplastic.*

Tozasertib Lactate [*2008*] (toe″ za ser′ tib lak′ tate). $C_{23}H_{28}N_8OS.xC_3H_6O_3$. 464.59 (base). (1) Propanoic acid, 2-hydroxy-, (2*S*)-, compd. with *N*-[4-[[4-(4-methyl-1-piperazinyl)-6-[(5-methyl-1*H*-pyrazol-3-yl)amino]-2-pyrimidinyl]thio]phenyl]cyclopropanecarboxamide; (2) *N*-[4-[[4-(4-Methylpiperazin-1-yl)-6-[(5-methyl-1*H*-pyrazol-3-yl)amino]pyrimidin-2-yl]sulfanyl]phenyl]cyclopropanecarboxamide (2*S*)-2-hydroxypropanoate. *UNII-CN8EF9N084. CAS-899827-04-4. Antineoplastic.* ◊*MK-0457; VX-680*

Trabectedin [*2004*] (tra bek′ te din). $C_{39}H_{43}N_3O_{11}S$. 761.84. (1) Spiro[6,16-(epithiopropanoxymethano)-7,13-imino-12*H*-1,3-dioxolo[7,8]isoquino[3,2-*b*][3]benzazocine-20,1′(2′*H*)-isoquinolin]-19-one, 5-(acetyloxy)-3′,4′,6,6a,7,13,14,16-octahydro-6′,8,14-trihydroxy-7′,9-dimethoxy-4,10,23-trimethyl-, (1′*R*,6*R*,6a*R*,7*R*,13*S*,14*S*,16*R*)-; (2) (1′*R*,6*R*,6a*R*,7*R*,13*S*,14*S*,16*R*)-6′,8,14-Trihydroxy-7′,9-dimethoxy-4,10,23-trimethyl-19-oxo-3′,4′,6,7,12,13,14,16-octahydrospiro[6,16-(epithiopropanooxymethano)-7,13-imino-6a*H*-1,3-dioxolo[7,8]isoquino[3,2-*b*][3]benzazocine-20,1′(2′*H*)-isoquinolin]-5-yl acetate. *UNII-ID0YZQ2TCP. CAS-114899-77-3. INN. Anticancer, antineoplastic and antitumoral.* Yondelis (Pharma Mar) ◊*ET-743*

Trabedersen. $C_{177}H_{225}N_{60}O_{94}P_{17}S_{17}$. 5768.68. 2′-Deoxy-*P*-thiocytidylyl-(3′→5′)-2′-deoxy-*P*-thioguanylyl-(3′→5′)-2′-deoxy-*P*-thioguanylyl-(3′→5′)-2′-deoxy-*P*-thiocytidylyl-(3′→5′)-2′-deoxy-*P*-thioadenylyl-(3′→5′)-*P*-thiothymidylyl-(3′→5′)-2′-deoxy-*P*-thioguanylyl-(3′→5′)-*P*-thiothymidylyl-(3′→5′)-2′-deoxy-*P*-thiocytidylyl-(3′→5′)-*P*-thiothymidylyl-(3′→5′)-2′-deoxy-*P*-thioadenylyl-(3′→5′)-*P*-thiothymidylyl-(3′→5′)-*P*-thiothymidylyl-(3′→5′)-*P*-

thiothymidylyl-(3′→5′)-*P*-thiothymidylyl-(3′→5′)-2′-deoxy-*P*-thioguanylyl-(3′→5′)-*P*-thiothymidylyl-(3′→5′)-2′-deoxyadenosine. *CAS-925681-61-4.* INN.

Traboxopine. $C_{19}H_{23}ClN_2O_2$. 346.85. (±)-2-Chloro-12-[3-(dimethylamino)-2-methylpropyl]-12*H*-dibenzo[*d,g*][1,3,6]-dioxazocine. *UNII-NRU90S9ANF. CAS-103624-59-5.* INN.

Tracazolate [*1980*] (trak az′ oh late). $C_{16}H_{24}N_4O_2$. 304.39. (1) 1*H*-Pyrazolo[3,4-*b*]pyridine-5-carboxylic acid, 4-(butylamino)-1-ethyl-6-methyl-, ethyl ester; (2) Ethyl 4-(butylamino)-1-ethyl-6-methyl-1*H*-pyrazolo[3,4-*b*]pyridine-5-carboxylate. *CAS-41094-88-6. INN; BAN. Sedative-hypnotic.* ◊*ICI 136,753*

Tradecamide. $C_{15}H_{31}NO_2$. 257.41. 13-Hydroxy-*N,N*-dimethyltridecanamide. *UNII-127M91LHX5. CAS-132787-19-0.* INN.

Trafermin [*1997*] (tra fer′ min). $C_{764}H_{1201}N_{217}O_{219}S_6$. 17,122.44. 2-155-Basic fibroblast growth factor (human clone λKB7/λHFL1 precursor reduced). *CAS-131094-16-1. INN. Stroke treatment; fibroblast growth factor.* Fiblast (Scios Nova) ◊*CAB-2001*

Tragacanth (traj′ a kanth). **NF.** The dried gummy exudation from *Astragalus gummifer* Labillardière, or other species of *Astragalus* (Fam. Leguminosae). *Pharmaceutic aid (suspending agent).*

Tralonide [*1972*] (tral′ oh nide). $C_{24}H_{28}Cl_2F_2O_4$. 489.38. (1) Pregna-1,4-diene-3,20-dione, 9,11-dichloro-6,21-difluoro-16,17-[(1-methylethylidene)bis(oxy)](6α,11β,16α)-; (2) 9,11β-Dichloro-6α,21-difluoro-16α,17-dihydroxypregna-1,4-diene-3,20-dione cyclic acetal with acetone. *CAS-21365-49-1. INN. Glucocorticoid.*

Tramadol Hydrochloride [*1969*] (tram′ a dol hye″ droe klor′ ide). $C_{16}H_{25}NO_2.HCl$. 299.84. [Tramadol is INN and BAN.] (1) (±)-*cis*-2-[(Dimethylamino)methyl]-1-(3-methoxyphenyl)cyclohexanol hydrochloride; (2) (±)-*cis*-2-[(Dimethylamino)methyl]-1-(*m*-methoxyphenyl)cyclohexanol hydrochloride. *UNII-9N7R477WCK; UNII-39J1LGJ30J* [tramadol]. *CAS-36282-47-0; CAS-27203-92-5* [tramadol]. JAN. *Analgesic.* Ultram (Ortho-McNeil) ◇*U-26,225A; CG-315E*

Tramazoline Hydrochloride [*1970*] (tra maz' oh leen hye" droe klor' ide). $C_{13}H_{17}N_3$.HCl. 251.76. [Tramazoline is INN and BAN.] (1) 1*H*-Imidazol-2-amine, 4,5-dihydro-*N*-(5,6,7,8-tetrahydro-1-naphthalenyl)-, monohydrochloride; (2) 2-[(5,6,7,8-Tetrahydro-1-naphthyl)amino]-2-imidazoline monohydrochloride. *CAS-3715-90-0; CAS-1082-57-1* [tramazoline]. JAN. *Adrenergic.*

Tramiprosate [*2005*] (tram ip' roe sate). $C_3H_9NO_3S$. 139.17. (1) 1-Propanesulfonic acid, 3-amino-; (2) 3-Aminopropane-1-sulfonic acid. *UNII-5K8EAX0G53. CAS-3687-18-1.* INN. *Treatment of mild-to-moderate Alzheimer's disease, treatment of cerebral amyloid angiopathy.* ◇*NC-758*

Trandolapril. $C_{24}H_{34}N_2O_5$. 430.54. (2*S*,3a*R*,7a*S*)-1-[(*S*)-*N*-[(*S*)-1-Carboxy-3-phenylpropyl]alanyl]hexahydro-2-indolinecarboxylic acid, 1-ethyl ester. *UNII-1T0N3G9CRC. CAS-87679-37-6.* INN; BAN. Mavik (Abbott) ◇*RU 44570*

Trandolaprilat. $C_{22}H_{30}N_2O_5$. 402.48. (2*S*,3a*R*,7a*S*)-1-[(*S*)-*N*-[(*S*)-1-Carboxy-3-phenylpropyl]alanyl]hexahydro-2-indolinecarboxylic acid. *UNII-RR6866VL0O. CAS-87679-71-8.* INN.

Tranexamic Acid [*1967*] (tran" ex am' ik as' id). $C_8H_{15}NO_2$. 157.21. (1) Cyclohexanecarboxylic acid, 4-(aminomethyl)-, *trans*-; (2) *trans*-4-(Aminomethyl)cyclohexanecarboxylic

acid. *UNII-6T84R30KC1. CAS-1197-18-8.* INN; BAN; JAN. *Hemostatic.* Cyklokapron (Pfizer) ◇*Trans AMCHA; CL 65336*

Tranilast [*1985*] (tran' i last). $C_{18}H_{17}NO_5$. 327.33. (1) Benzoic acid, 2-[[3-(3,4-dimethoxyphenyl)-1-oxo-2-propenyl]amino]-; (2) *N*-(3,4-Dimethoxycinnamoyl)anthranilic acid. *CAS-53902-12-8.* INN; JAN. *Anti-asthmatic.* ◇*MK-341*

Transcainide [*1985*] (trans' ka nide). $C_{22}H_{35}N_3O_2$. 373.53. (1) 4-Piperidinecarboxamide, 4-(dimethylamino)-*N*-(2,6-dimethylphenyl)-1-(2-hydroxycyclohexyl)-, *trans*-(±)-; (2) (±)-*trans*-4-(Dimethylamino)-1-(2-hydroxycyclohexyl)-2',6'-isonipectoxylidide. *CAS-88296-62-2.* INN. *Cardiac depressant (anti-arrhythmic).* ◇*R 54,718*

Transclomiphene (previously used name) — *See* Zuclomiphene.

Transferrin Aldifitox. $C_{5992}H_{9317}N_{1641}O_{1834}S_{63}$. A conjugate of the precursor of human serotransferrin (siderophillin) with a primary amine group used to form an amidine with (4-iminobutane-1,4-diyl)sulfanediyl[(3RS)-2,5-dioxopyrrolidine-1,3-diyl]-1,3-phenylenecarbonyl and forming an *N*-

---

† Brand name formerly used, and/or firm no longer concerned with this product.

benzoyl derivative of a primary amine group of diphtheria [550-L-phenylalanine]toxin from *Corynebacterium diphtheriae*-(26-560)-peptide. *CAS-721946-42-5.* INN.

Transferrin

MRLAVGALLV CAVLGLCLAV PDKTVRWCAV SEHEATKCQS FRDHMKSVIP
SDGPSVACVK KASYLDCIRA IAANEADAVT LDAGLVYDAY LAPNNLKPVV
AEFYGSKEDP QTFYYAVAVV KKDSGFQMNQ LRGKKSCHTG LGRSAGWNIP
IGLLYCDLPE PRKPLEKAVA NFFSGSCAPC ADGTDFPQLC QLCPGCGCST
LNQYFGYSGA FKCLKDGAGD VAFVKHSTIF ENLANKADRD QYELLCLDNT
RKPVDEYKDC HLAQVPSHTV VARSMGGKED LIWELLNQAQ EHFGKDKSKE
FQLFSSPHGK DLLFKDSAHG FLKVPPRMDA KMYLGYEYVT AIRNLREGTC
PEAPTDECKP VKWCALSHHE RLKCDEWSVN SVGKIECVSA ETTEDCIAKI
MNGEADAMSL DGGFVYIAGK CGLVPVLAEN YNKSDNCEDT PEAGYFAVAV
VKKSASDLTW DNLKGKKSCH TAVGRTAGWN IPMGLLYNKI NHCRFDEFFS
EGCAPGSKKD SSLCKLCMGS GLNLCEPNNK EGYYGYTGAF RCLVEKGDVA
FVKHQTVPQN TGGKNPDPWA KNLNEKDYEL LCLDGTRKPV EEYANCHLAR
APNHAVVTRK DKEACVHKIL RQQQHLFGSN VTDCSGNFCL FRSETKDLLF
RDDTVCLAKL HDRNTYEKYL GEEYVKAVGN LRKCSTSSLL EACTFRRP

* glycosylation sites

CRM107

GADDVVDSSK SFVMENFSSY HGTKPGYVDS IQKGIQKPKS GTQGNYDDDW
KGFYSTDNKY DAAGYSVDNE NPLSGKAGGV VKVTYPGLTK VLALKVDNAE
TIKKELGLSL TEPLMEQVGT EEFIKRFGDG ASRVVLSLPF AEGSSSVEYI
NNWEQAKALS VELEINFETR GKRGQDAMYE YMAQACAGNR VRRSVGSSLS
CINLDWDVIR DKTKTKIESL KEHGPIKNKM SESPNKTVSE EKAKQYLEEF
HQTALEHPEL SELKTVTGTN PVFAGANYAA WAVNVAQVID SETADNLEKT
TAALSILPGI GSVMGIADGA VHHNTEEIVA QSIALSSLMV AQAIPLVGEL
VDIGFAAYNF VESIINLFQV VHNSYNRPAY SPGHKTQPFL HDGYAVSWNT
VEDSIIRTGF QGESGHDIKI TAENTPLPIA GVLLPTIPGK LDVNKSKTHI
SVNGRKIRMR CRAIDGDVTF CRPKSPVYVG NGVHANLHVA FHRSSSEKIH
SNEISSDSIG VLGYQKTVDH TKVNFKLSLF FEIKS

Trantelinium Bromide. $C_{23}H_{26}BrNO_3$. 444.36. 8-Methyltropinium bromide xanthene-9-carboxylate. *CAS-4047-34-1.* INN.

Tranylcypromine Sulfate. $(C_9H_{11}N)_2.H_2SO_4$. 364.46. [Tranylcypromine is INN and BAN.] (1) Cyclopropanamine, 2-phenyl-, *trans*-(±)-, sulfate (2:1); (2) (±)-*trans*-2-Phenylcyclopropylamine sulfate (2:1). *UNII-7ZAT6ES870; UNII-3E3V44J4Z9* [tranylcypromine]. *CAS-13492-01-8; CAS-7081-36-9* [replaced]; *CAS-155-09-9* [tranylcypromine]. USP XXI; MI. Parnate (GlaxoSmithKline)

Trapencaine. $C_{22}H_{34}N_2O_3$. 374.52. (±)-*trans*-2-(1-Pyrrolidinyl)cyclohexyl *m*-(pentyloxy)carbanilate. *UNII-6H10WF5D0H. CAS-104485-01-0.* INN.

Trapidil. $C_{10}H_{15}N_5$. 205.26. 7-(Diethylamino)-5-methyl-*s*-triazolo[1,5-*a*]pyrimidine. *UNII-EYG5Y6355E. CAS-15421-84-8.* INN; BAN; JAN; MI. ◇*AR 12008*

Trapymin — *See* Trapidil.

Trastuzumab [*1997*] (tras tooz′ oo mab). Immunoglobulin G 1 (human-mouse monoclonal rhuMab HER2$_{\gamma 1}$-chain anti-human p185$^{c-erbB2}$ receptor), disulfide with human-mouse monoclonal rhuMab HER2 light chain, dimer. *UNII-P188ANX8CK. CAS-180288-69-1.* INN; BAN.

Travoprost [*1998*] (trav′ oh prost). $C_{26}H_{35}F_3O_6$. 500.55. (1) [1*R*-[1α(*Z*),2β(1*E*,3*R**),3α,5α]]-7-[3,5-Dihydroxy-2-[3-hydroxy-4-[3-(trifluoromethyl)phenoxy]-1-butenyl]cyclopentyl]-5-heptenoic acid, 1-methylethyl ester; (2) (*Z*)-7-[(1*R*,2*R*,3*R*,5*S*)-3,5-Dihydroxy-2-[(1*E*,3*R*)-3-hydroxy-4-[(α,α,α-trifluoro-*m*-isopropyl-tolyl)oxy]-1-butenyl]cyclopentyl]-5-heptenoate. *UNII-WJ68R08KX9. CAS-157283-68-6.* INN; BAN. *Treatment of elevated intraocular pressure associated with glaucoma (prostaglandin FP-receptor agonist).* Travatan (Alcon) ◇*AL-6221*

Traxanox. $C_{13}H_6ClN_5O_2$. 299.67. 9-Chloro-7-(1*H*-tetrazol-5-yl)-5*H*-[1]benzopyrano[2,3-*b*]pyridine-5-one. *UNII-HDU53A8A4S. CAS-58712-69-9.* INN; MI.

Traxoprodil Mesylate [*2000*] (trax oh′ pro dil mes′ i late). $C_{20}H_{25}NO_3.CH_4O_3S.3H_2O$. 477.57. [Traxoprodil is INN.] (1) 1-Piperidineethanol, 4-hydroxy-α-(4-hydroxyphenyl)-β-methyl-4-phenyl-, [*S*-(*R**,*R**)]-, methanesulfonate (salt), trihydrate; (2) (α*S*,β*S*)-4-Hydroxy-α-(*p*-hydroxyphenyl)-β-methyl-4-phenyl-1-piperidineethanol methanesulfonate (salt), trihydrate. *UNII-BD2A56I30W. CAS-189894-57-3;*

CAS-134234-12-1 [traxoprodil]. INN. *Treatment of traumatic brain injury (highly selective NR21 NMDA receptor antagonist).* ◇*CP-101,606-27*

Trazitiline. $C_{21}H_{24}N_2$. 304.43. 1-(9,10-Dihydro-9,10-ethano-9-anthryl)-4-methylpiperazine. *UNII-7I6MS3VHQE. CAS-26070-23-5.* INN; DCF. ◇*SD 1223-01*

Trazium Esilate. $C_{19}H_{18}ClN_3O_4S$. 419.88. 1-(*p*-Chlorophenyl)-1,2-dihydro-1-hydroxy-*as*-triazino[6,1-*a*]isoquinolin-5-ium ethanesulfonate. *UNII-1PO9LWW5IN. CAS-97110-59-3.* INN.

Trazodone Hydrochloride [*1970*] (traz′ oh done hye″ droe klor′ ide). **USP.** $C_{19}H_{22}ClN_5O\cdot HCl$. 408.32. [Trazodone is INN and BAN.] (1) 1,2,4-Triazolo[4,3-*a*]pyridin-3(2*H*)-one, 2-[3-[4-(3-chlorophenyl)-1-piperazinyl]propyl]-, monohydrochloride; (2) 2-[3-[4-(*m*-Chlorophenyl)-1-piperazinyl]propyl]-*s*-triazolo[4,3-*a*]pyridin-3(2*H*)-one monohydrochloride. *UNII-6E8ZO8LRNM; UNII-YBK48BXK30* [trazodone]. *CAS-25332-39-2; CAS-19794-93-5* [trazodone]. JAN. *Antidepressant.* Desyrel (Apothecon) ◇*AF-1161*

Trazolopride. $C_{20}H_{23}N_5O_2$. 365.43. *N*-(1-Benzyl-4-piperidyl)-6-methoxy-1*H*-benzotriazole-5-carboxamide. *UNII-MF4NR5U03L. CAS-86365-92-6.* INN.

Trebenzomine Hydrochloride [*1975*] (tre ben′ zoe meen hye″ droe klor′ ide). $C_{12}H_{17}NO\cdot HCl$. 227.73. [Trebenzomine is INN.] (1) 2*H*-1-Benzopyran-3-amine, 3,4-dihydro-*N,N*,2-trimethyl-, hydrochloride, (*cis* or *trans*)-(±)-; (2) (±)-(*cis* or *trans*)-*N,N*,2-Trimethyl-3-chromanamine hydrochloride. *CAS-23915-74-4; CAS-23915-73-3* [trebenzomine]. *Antidepressant.* ◇*CI-686.HCl*

Trecadrine. $C_{27}H_{29}NO$. 383.53. (1*R*,2*S*)-α-[1-[[2-(10,11-Dihydro-5*H*-dibenzo[*a,d*]cyclohepten-5-ylidene)ethyl]methylamino]ethyl]benzyl alcohol. *UNII-34H206R8A5. CAS-90845-56-0.* INN.

Trecetilide. $C_{21}H_{37}FN_2O_3S$. 416.59. (-)-4′-[(*S*)-4-[Ethyl(6-fluoro-6-methylheptyl)amino]-1-hydroxybutyl]methanesulfonanilide. *CAS-180918-68-7.* INN.

Trecetilide Fumarate [*1997*] (tre set′ i lide fue′ ma rate). $(C_{21}H_{37}FN_2O_3S)_2\cdot C_4H_4O_4$. 949.26. (1) (*S*)-*N*-[4-[4-[Ethyl(6-fluoro-6-methylheptyl)amino]-1-hydroxybutyl]phenyl] methanesulfonamide (*E*)-2-butenedioate (2:1) (salt); (2) (-)-4′-[(*S*)-4-[Ethyl(6-fluoro-6-methylheptyl)amino]-1-hydroxybutyl] methanesulfonanilide fumarate (2:1) (salt). *CAS-191349-60-7. Antiarrythmic (Class III).* ◇*U-108342E*

Trecovirsen Sodium [*1997*] (tre″ koe vir′ sen soe′ dee um). $C_{237}H_{286}N_{72}Na_{24}O_{131}P_{24}S_{24}$. 8303.90. [Trecovirsen is INN.] (1) Deoxyribonucleic acid d(*P*-thio)(T-C-T-T-C-C-T-C-T-C-T-C-T-A-C-C-C-A-C-G-C-T-C-T-C), tetracosasodium salt; (2) *P*-Thiothymidylyl-(5′→3′)-2′-deoxy-*P*-thiocytidylyl-(5′→3′)-*P*-thiothymidylyl-(5′→3′)-*P*-thiothymidylyl-(5′→3′)-2′-deoxy-*P*-thiocytidylyl-(5′→3′)-2′-deoxy-*P*-thiocytidylyl-(5′→3′)-*P*-thiothymidylyl-(5′→3′)-2′-deoxy-*P*-thiocytidylyl-(5′→3′)-*P*-thiothymidylyl-(5′→3′)-2′-deoxy-*P*-thiocytidylyl-(5′→3′)-*P*-thiothymidylyl-(5′→3′)-2′-deoxy-*P*-thiocytidylyl-(5′→3′)-*P*-thiothymidylyl-(5′→3′)-2′-deoxy-*P*-thioadenylyl-(5′→3′)-2′-deoxy-*P*-thiocytidylyl-(5′→3′)-2′-deoxy-*P*-thiocytidylyl-(5′→3′)-2′-deoxy-*P*-thiocytidylyl-(5′→3′)-2′-deoxy-*P*-thioadenylyl-(5′→3′)-2′-deoxy-*P*-thiocytidylyl-(5′→3′)-2′-deoxy-*P*-thioguanylyl-(5′→3′)-2′-deoxy-*P*-thiocytidylyl-(5′→3′)-*P*-thiothymidylyl-(5′→3′)-2′-deoxy-*P*-thiocytidylyl-(5′→3′)-

P-thiothymidylyl-(5′→3′)-2′-deoxycytosine, tetracosasodium salt. *CAS-170274-79-0; CAS-148998-94-1* [trecovirsen]. *Antiviral.* Gem 91 (Hybridon)

PS-d(TCTTCCTCTCTCTACCCACGCTCTC)

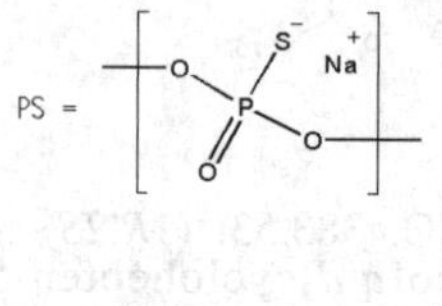

PS =

Trefentanil Hydrochloride [*1992*] (tre fen′ ta nil hye″ droe klor′ ide). $C_{25}H_{31}FN_6O_2$.HCl. 503.01. [Trefentanil is INN.] (1) Propanamide, *N*-[1-[2-(4-ethyl- 4,5-dihydro-5-oxo-1*H*-tetrazol-1-yl)ethyl]-4-phenyl-4-piperidinyl]-*N*-(2-fluorophenyl)-, monohydrochloride; (2) *N*-[1-[2-(4-Ethyl-5-oxo-Δ^2-tetrazolin-1-yl)ethyl]-4-phenyl-4-piperidyl]-2′-fluoropropionanilide monohydrochloride. *CAS-120656-93-1; CAS-120656-74-8* [trefentanil]. *Analgesic.* ◇A-3665.HCl

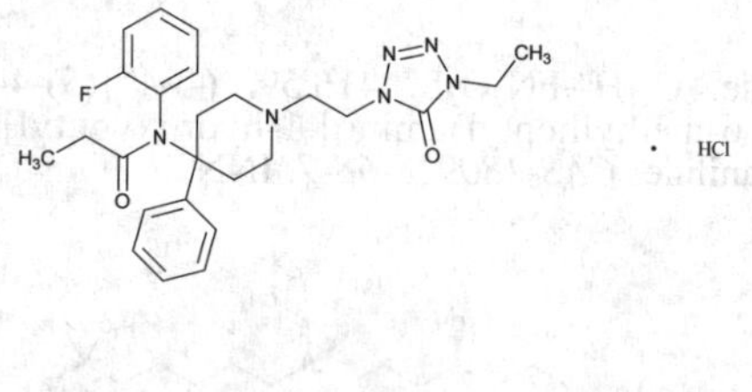

Trelanserin. $C_{24}H_{24}FN_5O_2S$. 465.54. 2-(7-Fluoro-2-oxo-4-{2-[4-(thieno[3,2-*c*]pyridin-4-yl)piperazin-1-yl]ethyl}-1,2-dihydroquinolin-1-yl)acetamide. *CAS-189003-92-7.* INN.

Trelnarizine. $C_{28}H_{30}F_2N_2O_2$. 464.55. (*E*)-1-[Bis(*p*-fluorophenyl)methyl]-4-(3,4-dimethoxycinnamyl)piperazine. *UNII-SE8X571K4C. CAS-123205-52-7.* INN.

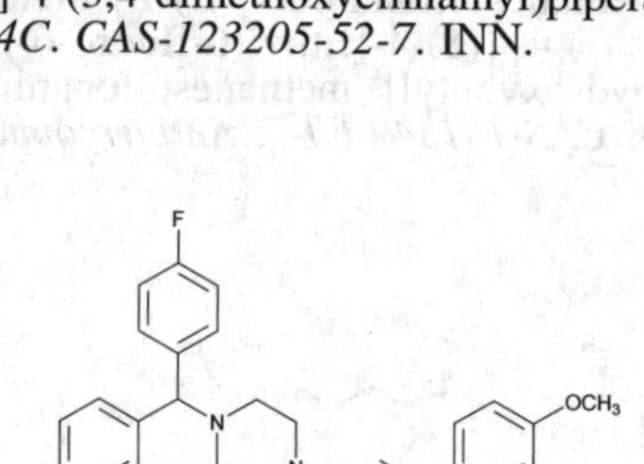

Treloxinate [*1971*] (tre lox′ i nate). $C_{16}H_{12}Cl_2O_4$. 339.17. (1) 12*H*-Dibenzo[*d,g*][1,3]dioxocin-6-carboxylic acid, 2,10-dichloro-, methyl ester; (2) Methyl 2,10-dichloro-12*H*-dibenzo[*d,g*][1,3]dioxocin-6-carboxylate. *UNII-7YA71J-CD50. CAS-30910-27-1.* INN. *Antihyperlipoproteinemic.*

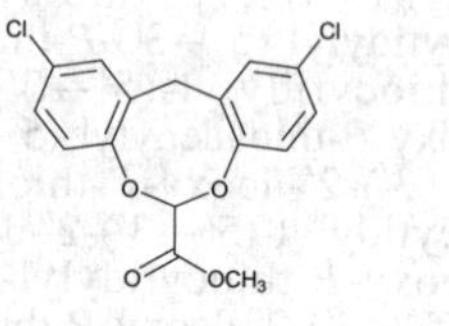

Tremacamra [*1997*] (tre ma kam′ ra). 1-453-Glycoprotein ICAM-1 (human reduced). Molecular weight is approximately 82,000 daltons (SDS-Page). *CAS-155576-45-7.* INN. *Antiviral (inhibitor of viral attachment to host cells).* ◇BIRR004

```
QTSVSPSKVI LPRGGSVLVT CSTSCDQPKL LGIETPLPKK ELLLPGNNRK
VYELSNVQED SQPMCYSNCP DGQSTAKTFL TVYWTPERVE LAPLPSWQPV
GKNLTLRCQV EGGAPRANLT VVLLRGEKEL KREPAVGEPA EVTTTVLVRR
DHHGANFSCR TELDLRPQGL ELFENTSAPY QLQTFVLPAT PPQLVSPRVL
EVDTQGTVVC SLDGLFPVSE AQVHLALGDQ RLNPTVTYGN DSFSAKASVS
VTAEDEGTQR LTCAVILGNQ SQETLQTVTI YSFPAPNVIL TKPEVSEGTE
VTVKCEAHPR AKVTLNGVPA QPLGPRAQLL LKATPEDNGR SFSCSATLEV
AGQLIHKNQT RELRVLYGPR LDERDCPGNW TWPENSQQTP MCQAWGNPLP
ELKCLKDGTF PLPIGESVTV TRDLEGTYLC RARSTQGEVT REVTVNVLSP
RYE
```

Tremelimumab [*2006*] (tre″ me lim′ ue mab). $C_{6500}H_{9974}N_{1726}O_{2026}S_{52}$. (1) Immunoglobulin G2, anti-(human CTLA-4 (antigen)) (human monoclonal CP-675206 clone 11.2.1 heavy chain) disulfide with human monoclonal CP-675206 clone 11.2.1 light chain, dimer; (2) Immunoglobulin G2, anti-(human Cytotoxic T-lymphocyte protein 4 (CD 152 antigen)) (human monoclonal CP-675206 clone 11.2.1 heavy chain) disulfide with human monoclonal CP-675206 clone 11.2.1 light chain, dimer. Molecular weight is approximately 150,000 daltons. *CAS-745013-59-6.* INN. *Treatment of cancer.[Name previously used: Ticilimumab.]* ◇CP-675,206

```
DIQMTQSPSS LSASVGDRVT ITCRASQSIN SYLDWYQQKP GKAPKLLIYA
ASSLQSGVPS RFSGSGSGTD FTLTISSLQP EDFATYYCQQ YYSTPFTFGP
GTKVEIKRTV AAPSVFIFPP SDEQLKSGTA SVVCLLNNFY PREAKVQWKV
DNALQSGNSQ ESVTEQDSKD STYSLSSTLT LSKADYEKHK VYACEVTHQG
LSSPVTKSFN RGEC

QVQLVESGGG VVQPGRSLRL SCAASGFTFS SYGMHWVRQA PGKGLEWVAV
IWYDGSNKYY ADSVKGRFTI SRDNSKNTLY LQMNSLRAED TAVYYCARDP
RGATLYYYYY GMDVWGQGTT VRVSSASTKG PSVFPLAPCS RSTSESTALL
GCLVKDYFPE PVTVSWNSGA LTSGVHTFPA VLQSSGLYSL SSVVTVPSSN
FGTQTYTCNV DHKPSNTKVD KTVERKCCVE CPPCPAPPVA GPSVFLFPPK
PKDTLMISRT PEVTCVVVDV SHEDPEVQFN WYVDGVEVHN AKTKPREEQF
NSTFRVVSVL TVVHQDWLNG KEYKCKVSNK GLPAPIEKTI SKTKGQPREP
QVYTLPPSRE EMTKNQVSLT CLVKGFYPSD IAVEWESNGQ PENNYKTTPP
MLDSDGSFFL YSKLTVDKSR WQQGNVFSCS VMHEALHNHY TQKSLSLSPG
K
```
$_2$

Trenbolone Acetate [*1984*] (tren′ boe lone as′ e tate). **USP**. $C_{20}H_{24}O_3$. 312.40. [Trenbolone is INN and BAN.] (1) Estra-4,9,11-trien-3-one, 17-(acetyloxy)-, (17*β*)-; (2) 17*β*-Hydroxyestra-4,9,11-trien-3-one, acetate. *UNII-RU-D5Y4SV0S. CAS-10161-34-9; CAS-10161-33-8* [trenbolone]. *Anabolic (veterinary).* Finaplix (Roussel-UCLAF, France) ◇RU-1697

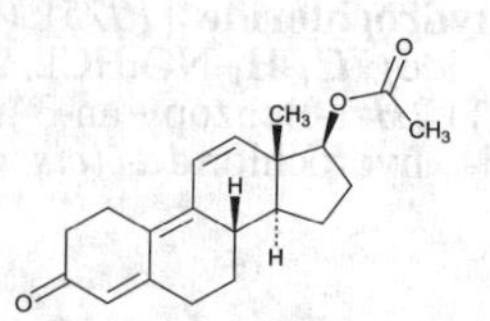

Trengestone. $C_{21}H_{25}ClO_2$. 344.88. 6-Chloro-9β,10α-pregna-1,4,6-triene-3,20-dione. *UNII-VY6S496SVX. CAS-5192-84-7*. INN; DCF; MI. ◇*Ro 48347*

Trenizine. $C_{31}H_{40}N_2O$. 456.66. ($\pm$)-α-(*p-tert*-Butylphenyl)-4-(diphenylmethyl)-1-piperazinebutanol. *UNII-1WPQ720NCK. CAS-82190-93-0*. INN.

Treosulfan. $C_6H_{14}O_8S_2$. 278.30. L-Threitol 1,4-dimethanesulfonate. *CAS-299-75-2*. INN; BAN.

Trepibutone. $C_{16}H_{22}O_6$. 310.34. 3-(2,4,5-Triethoxybenzoyl)-propionic acid. *UNII-H1187LU49Q. CAS-41826-92-0*. INN; JAN; MI.

Trepipam Maleate [*1979*] (tre′ pi pam mal′ ee ate). $C_{19}H_{23}NO_2 \cdot C_4H_4O_4$. 413.46. [Trepipam is INN.] (1) 1*H*-3-Benzazepine, 2,3,4,5-tetrahydro-7,8-dimethoxy-3-methyl-1-phenyl-, (+)-, (*Z*)-2-butenedioate (1:1); (2) (+)-2,3,4,5-Tetrahydro-7,8-dimethoxy-3-methyl-1-phenyl-1*H*-3-benzazepine maleate (1:1). *CAS-39624-66-3; CAS-56030-50-3* [trepipam]. *Sedative-hypnotic. [Name previously used: Trimopam Maleate.]* ◇*Sch 12679*

Trepirium Iodide. $C_{12}H_{26}I_2N_2O_2$. 484.16. 2-Carboxy-1,1-dimethylpyrrolidinium iodide, ester with (2-hydroxyethyl)trimethylammonium iodide. *UNII-7GGP8DTV34. CAS-1018-34-4*. INN.

Treprostinil [*2002*] (tre prost′ i nil). $C_{23}H_{34}O_5$. 390.51. (1) Acetic acid, [[(1*R*,2*R*,3a*S*,9a*S*)-2,3,3a,4,9,9a-hexahydro-2-hydroxy-1-[(3*S*)-3-hydroxyoctyl]-1*H*-benz[*f*]inden-5-yl]oxy]-; (2) [(1*R*,2*R*,3a*S*,9a*S*)-2-Hydroxy-1-((3*S*)-3-hydroxyoctyl)-2,3,3a,4,9,9a-hexahydro-1*H*-cyclopent[*b*]naphthalen-5-yl]oxy]acetate. *UNII-RUM6K67ESG. CAS-81846-19-7*. INN. *Treatment of pulmonary arterial hypertension and peripheral arterial occlusive disease.* Remodulin (United Therapeutics) ◇*UT-15; LRX-15; 15AU81*

Treptilamine. $C_{20}H_{27}NO$. 297.43. 2-[(α-Tricyclo[2.2.1.0^{2,6}]-hept-3-ylidenebenzyl)oxy]triethylamine. *UNII-1URW272384. CAS-58313-74-9*. INN.

Trequinsin. $C_{24}H_{27}N_3O_3$. 405.49. 2,3,6,7-Tetrahydro-2-(mesitylimino)-9,10-dimethoxy-3-methyl-4*H*-pyrimido[6,1-*a*]isoquinolin-4-one. *CAS-79855-88-2*. INN.

Tresperimus. $C_{17}H_{37}N_7O_3$. 387.52. [4-[(3-Aminopropyl)amino]butyl]carbamic acid, ester with *N*-(6-guanidinohexyl)glycolamide. *UNII-286F595V8H. CAS-160677-67-8*. INN; BAN. ◇*LF 08-0299*

Trestolone Acetate [*1971*] (tres′ toe lone as′ e tate). $C_{21}H_{30}O_3$. 330.46. [Trestolone is INN.] (1) Estr-4-en-3-one, 17-(acetyloxy)-7-methyl-, (7α,17β)-; (2) 17β-Hydroxy-7α-methylestr-4-en-3-one acetate. *CAS-6157-87-5; CAS-3764-87-2* [trestolone]. *Antineoplastic; androgen.* ✧*U-15,614; NSC-69948*

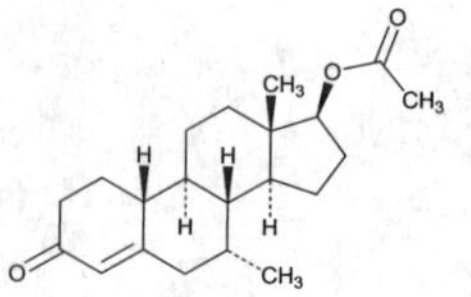

Tretamine (INN, BAN, and DCF) — *See* Triethylenemelamine.

Tretazicar. $C_9H_8N_4O_5$. 252.18. 5-(Aziridin-1-yl)-2,4-dinitrobenzamide. *UNII-7865D5D01M. CAS-21919-05-1.* INN.

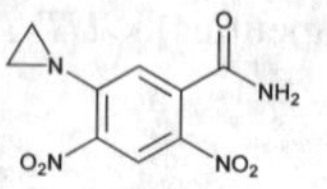

Trethinium Tosilate. $C_{19}H_{25}NO_3S$. 347.47. 2-Ethyl-1,2,3,4-tetrahydro-2-methylisoquinolinium *p*-toluenesulfonate. *UNII-3HA6AVV4EI. CAS-1748-43-2.* INN; BAN. *[Name previously used: Trethinium Tosylate.]*

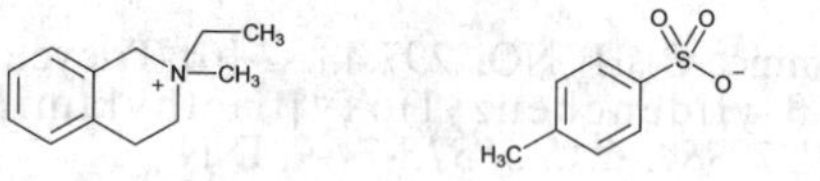

Trethocanic Acid (INN) — *See* Trethocanoic Acid.

Trethocanoic Acid. $C_{15}H_{30}O_3$. 258.40. [Trethocanic Acid is INN.] 3-Hydroxy-3,7,11-trimethyldodecanoic acid. *CAS-7007-81-0.*

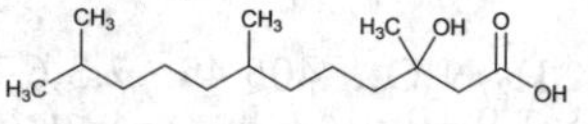

Tretinoin [*1970*] (tret′ i noin). **USP.** $C_{20}H_{28}O_2$. 300.44. (1) Retinoic acid; (2) all-*trans*-Retinoic acid. *UNII-5688UTC01R. CAS-302-79-4.* INN; BAN. *Keratolytic.* Avita (Mylan Bertek); Renova (Johnson & Johnson); Retin-A (Johnson & Johnson); Vesanoid (Roche) ✧*NSC-122758*

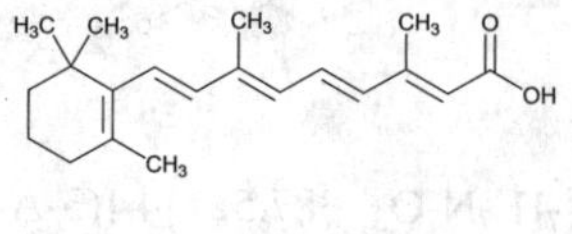

Tretinoin Tocoferil. $C_{49}H_{76}O_3$. 713.13. (±)-(2R*)-2,5,7,8-Tetramethyl-2-[(4R*,8R*)-4,8,12-trimethyltridecyl]-6-chromanyl retinoate. *UNII-CTD060B1SS. CAS-40516-48-1.* INN.

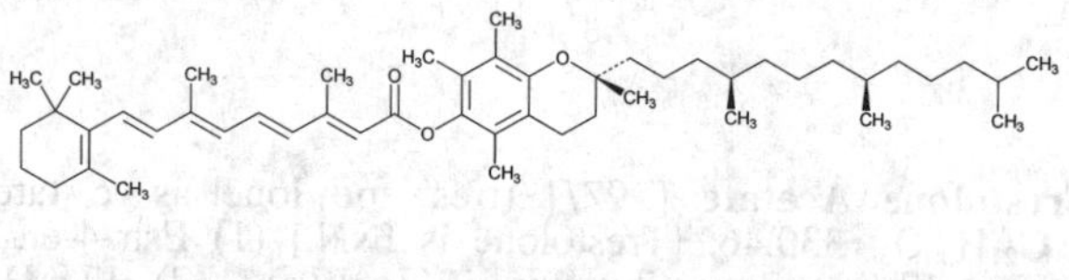

Tretoquinol. $C_{19}H_{23}NO_5$. 345.39. [Trimetoquinol Hydrochloride is JAN.] 1,2,3,4-Tetrahydro-1-(3,4,5-trimethoxybenzyl)-6,7-isoquinolinediol. *UNII-JIO3275WGI. CAS-30418-38-3.* INN; MI. ✧*AQ-110*

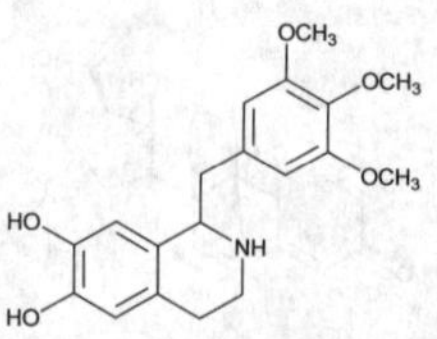

Triacetin (trye as′ e tin). **USP.** $C_9H_{14}O_6$. 218.20. (1) 1,2,3-Propanetriol triacetate; (2) Triacetin; (3) Glyceryl triacetate. *CAS-102-76-1.* INN; BAN. *Antifungal.* "EASTMAN" Triacetin (Eastman); Enzactin (Whitehall-Robins†) *[Name previously used: Glyceryl Triacetate.]*

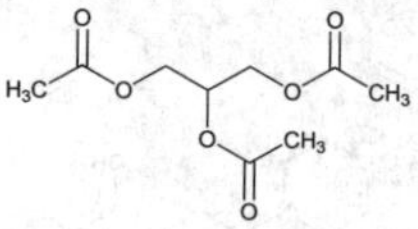

Triacetyloleandomycin (JAN and previously used name) — *See* Troleandomycin.

Triaconazole (previously used name) — *See* Terconazole.

Triafungin [*1978*] (trye a fun′ jin). $C_{13}H_{10}N_4$. 222.25. (1) Pyrido[3,4-*e*]-1,2,4-triazine, 3-(phenylmethyl)-; (2) 3-Benzylpyrido[3,4-*c*]-*as*-triazine. *UNII-E51A927SNR. CAS-55242-77-8.* INN. *Antifungal.* ✧*EU-3325*

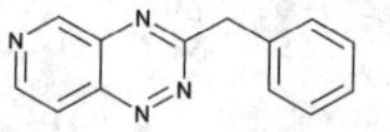

Triamcinolone (trye″ am sin′ oh lone). **USP.** $C_{21}H_{27}FO_6$. 394.43. (1) Pregna-1,4-diene-3,20-dione, 9-fluoro-11,16,17,21-tetrahydroxy-, (11β,16α); (2) 9-Fluoro-11β,16α,17,21-tetrahydroxypregna-1,4-diene-3,20-dione. *UNII-1ZK20VI6TY. CAS-124-94-7.* INN; BAN; JAN. *Glucocorticoid.* Aristocort (Astellas); Kenacort (Bristol-Myers Squibb)

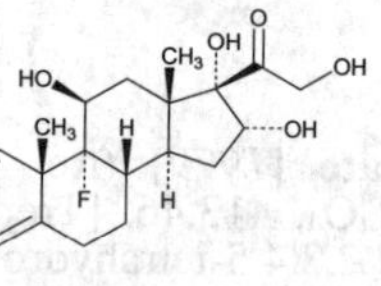

Triamcinolone Acetonide (trye″ am sin′ oh lone a seet′ oh nide). **USP.** $C_{24}H_{31}FO_6$. 434.50. (1) Pregna-1,4-diene-3,20-dione, 9-fluoro-11,21-dihydroxy-16,17-[(1-methylethylidene)bis(oxy)]-, (11β,16α)-; (2) 9-Fluoro-11β,16α,17,21-tetrahydroxypregna-1,4-diene-3,20-dione cyclic 16,17-acetal with acetone. *UNII-F446C597KA. CAS-76-25-5.* BAN; JAN. *Glucocorticoid.* Aristocort (Astellas); Azmacort (Abbott); Kenalog (Apothecon); Nasacort (Sanofi Aventis); Oralone (Taro); Triacet (Teva); Triderm (Del Ray)

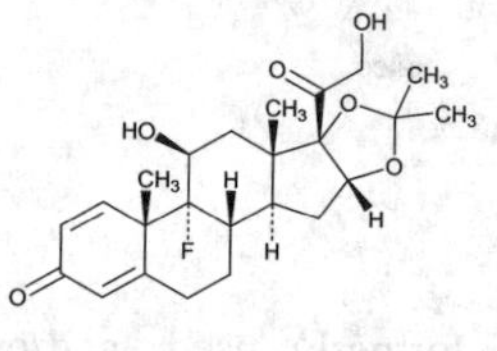

Triamcinolone Acetonide Sodium Phosphate [*1963*] (trye″ am sin′ oh lone a seet′ oh nide soe′ dee um fos′ fate). $C_{24}H_{30}FNa_2O_9P$. 558.44. (1) Pregna-1,4-diene-3,20-dione, 9-fluoro-11-hydroxy-16,17-[(1-methylethylidene)-bis(oxy)]-21-(phosphonooxy)-, disodium salt, (11β,16α)-; (2) 9-Fluoro-11β,16α,17,21-tetrahydroxypregna-1,4-diene-3,20-dione cyclic 16,17-acetal with ace-tone 21-(dihydrogen phosphate) disodium salt. *CAS-1997-15-5; CAS-989-96-8* [triamcinolone acetonide 21-(dihydrogen phosphate)]. *Glucocorticoid.* ◇*CL 61965; CL 106359*

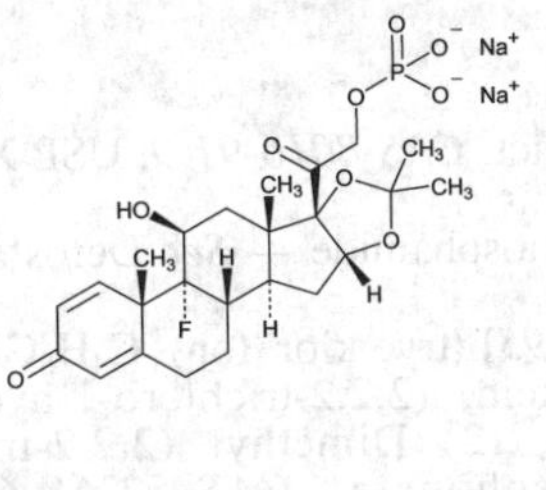

Triamcinolone Benetonide. $C_{35}H_{42}FNO_8$. 623.71. 9-Fluoro-11β,16α,17,21-tetrahydroxypregna-1,4-diene-3,20-dione cyclic 16,17-acetal with acetone 21-ester with *N*-benzoyl-2-methyl-β-alanine. *CAS-31002-79-6.* INN; MI.

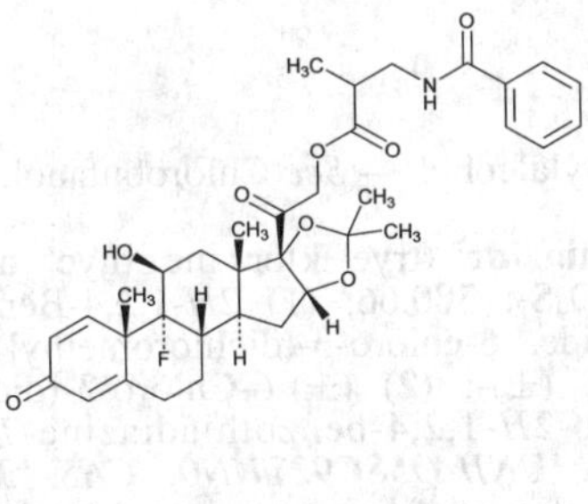

Triamcinolone Diacetate (trye″ am sin′ oh lone dye as′ e tate). USP. $C_{25}H_{31}FO_8$. 478.51. (1) Pregna-1,4-diene-3,20-dione, 16,21-bis(acetyloxy)-9-fluoro-11,17-dihydroxy-, (11β,16α)-; (2) 9-Fluoro-11β,16α,17,21-tetrahydroxy-pregna-1,4-diene-3,20-dione 16,21-diacetate. *UNII-A73MM2Q32P. CAS-67-78-7.* JAN. *Glucocorticoid.* Aristocort (Astellas); Kenacort (Bristol-Myers Squibb)

Triamcinolone Furetonide. $C_{33}H_{35}FO_8$. 578.62. 9-Fluoro-11β,16α,17,21-tetrahydroxypregna-1,4-diene-3,20-dione cyclic 16,17-acetal with acetone, 21-(2-benzofurancarbox-ylate). *UNII-O49NOC9ROC. CAS-4989-94-0.* INN.

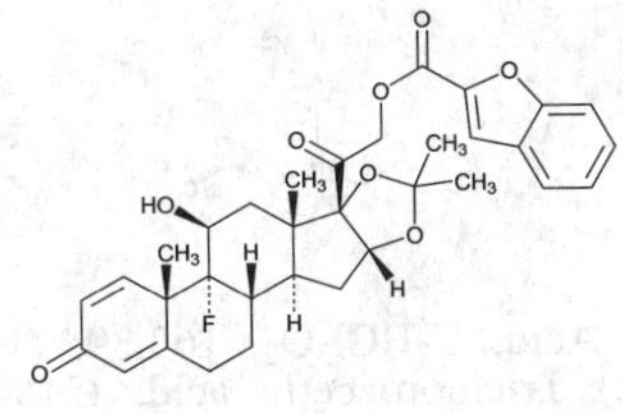

Triamcinolone Hexacetonide [*1964*] (trye″ am sin′ oh lone hex″ a seet′ oh nide). USP. $C_{30}H_{41}FO_7$. 532.64. (1) Pregna-1,4-diene-3,20-dione, 21-(3,3-dimethyl-1-oxobutoxy)-9-fluoro-11-hydroxy-16,17-[(1-methylethylidene)bis(oxy)]-, (11β,16α)-; (2) 9-Fluoro-11β,16α,17,21-tetrahydroxy-pregna-1,4-diene-3,20-dione cyclic 16,17-acetal with acet-

one 21-(3,3-dimethylbutyrate). *UNII-I7GT1U99Y9. CAS-5611-51-8.* INN; BAN. *Glucocorticoid.* Aristospan (Sandoz) ◇*CL 34433; TATBA*

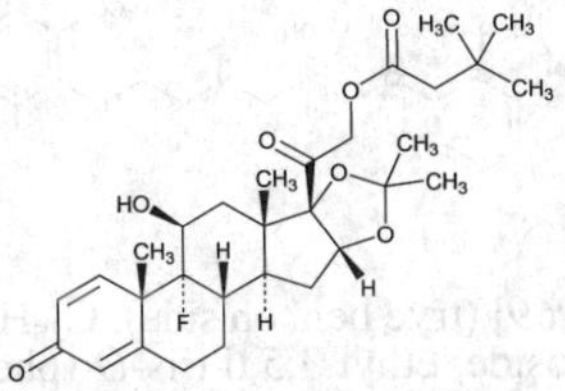

Triampyzine Sulfate [*1966*] (trye am′ pi zeen sul′ fate). $C_9H_{15}N_3 \cdot H_2SO_4$. 263.31. [Triampyzine is INN.] (1) 2-Pyrazinamine, *N,N*,3,5,6-pentamethyl-, sulfate (1:1); (2) (Dimethylamino)trimethylpyrazine sulfate (1:1). *UNII-05835HKX9S. CAS-7082-30-6; CAS-6503-95-3* [triampyzine]. *Anticholinergic.* ◇*W 3976B*

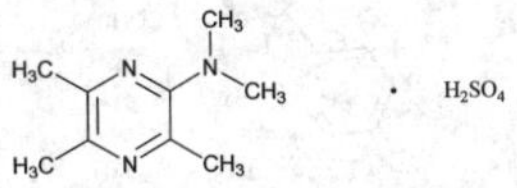

Triamterene [*1963*] (trye am′ ter een). USP. $C_{12}H_{11}N_7$. 253.26. (1) 2,4,7-Pteridinetriamine, 6-phenyl-; (2) 2,4,7-Triamino-6-phenylpteridine. *UNII-WS821Z52LQ. CAS-396-01-0.* INN; BAN; JAN. *Diuretic.* Dyrenium (Well-Spring) ◇*SK&F 8542; NSC-77625*

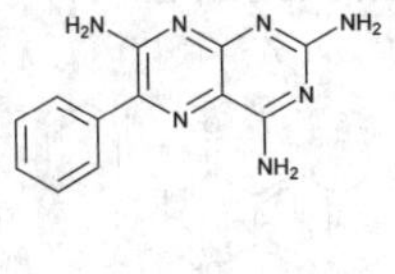

Trianisestrol — *See* Chlorotrianisene.

Triaziquone. $C_{12}H_{13}N_3O_2$. 231.25. Tris(1-aziridinyl)-*p*-benzoquinone. *CAS-68-76-8.* INN; BAN; MI. ◇*Bayer 3231; Riker 601; NSC-29215*

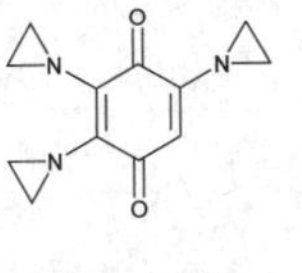

Triazolam [*1973*] (trye az′ oh lam). USP. $C_{17}H_{12}Cl_2N_4$. 343.21. (1) 4*H*-[1,2,4]Triazolo[4,3-*a*][1,4]benzodiazepine, 8-chloro-6-(2-chlorophenyl)-1-methyl-; (2) 8-Chloro-6-(*o*-chlorophenyl)-1-methyl-4*H*-*s*-triazolo[4,3-*a*][1,4]benzo-diazepine. *UNII-1HM943223R. CAS-28911-01-5.* INN; BAN; JAN. *Sedative-hypnotic.* Halcion (Pfizer) ◇*U-33,030*

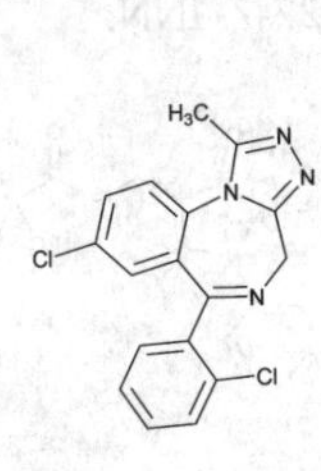

Tribavirin (BAN) — *See* Ribavirin.

---

† Brand name formerly used, and/or firm no longer concerned with this product.

Tribendilol. $C_{18}H_{22}N_4O_4$. 358.39. (±)-1-(1*H*-Benzotriazol-4-yloxy)-3-[[2-(*o*-methoxyphenoxy)ethyl]amino]-2-propanol. *UNII-K0744Q5ALP. CAS-96258-13-8.* INN.

Tribenoside [*1969*] (trye ben′ oh side). $C_{29}H_{34}O_6$. 478.58. (1) D-Glucofuranoside, ethyl 3,5,6-tris-*O*-(phenylmethyl)-; (2) Ethyl 3,5,6-tri-*O*-benzyl-D-glucofuranoside. *CAS-10310-32-4.* INN; BAN; JAN. *Sclerosing agent.* ◇*21401-Ba*

Tribromoethanol. *CAS-75-80-9.* NF XIII; MI. Avertin (Sterling Winthrop†)

Tribromsalan [*1963*] (trye brome′ sa lan). $C_{13}H_8Br_3NO_2$. 449.92. (1) Benzamide, 3,5-dibromo-*N*-(4-bromophenyl)-2-hydroxy-; (2) 3,4′,5-Tribromosalicylanilide. *UNII-6MCE3VTF0O. CAS-87-10-5.* INN; BAN. *Disinfectant.* Tuasol 100 (Marion Merrell Dow†) ◇*ET-394; NSC-20526*

Tributyl Citrate (trye bue′ til sit′ rate). **NF.** $C_{18}H_{32}O_7$. 360.44. (1) 1,2,3-Propanetricarboxylic acid, 2-hydroxy-, 1,2,3-tributyl ester; (2) 1,2,3-Propanetricarboxylic acid, 2-hydroxy-, tributyl ester. *CAS-77-94-1.*

Tribuzone. $C_{22}H_{24}N_2O_3$. 364.44. 4-(4,4-Dimethyl-3-oxopentyl)-1,2-diphenyl-3,5-pyrazolidinedione. *UNII-DUU9G-VA746. CAS-13221-27-7.* INN.

Tricaprilin. $C_{27}H_{50}O_6$. 470.68. Propane-1,2,3-triyl trioctanoate. *UNII-6P92858988. CAS-538-23-8.* JAN.

Tricetamide [*1963*] (trye set′ a mide). $C_{16}H_{24}N_2O_5$. 324.37. (1) Benzamide, *N*-[2-(diethylamino)-2-oxoethyl]-3,4,5-trimethoxy-; (2) *N*-[(Diethylcarbamoyl)methyl]-3,4,5-trimethoxybenzamide. *UNII-V6X0RFU7AF. CAS-363-20-2. Sedative-hypnotic.* ◇*R-548*

Trichinella Extract. *CAS-8016-91-9.* USP XIX.

Trichlorethoxyphosphamide — *See* Defosfamide.

Trichlorfon [*1995*] (trye klor′ fon). $C_4H_8Cl_3O_4P$. 257.44. (1) Phosphonic acid, (2,2,2-trichloro-1-hydroxyethyl)-, dimethyl ester; (2) Dimethyl (2,2,2-trichloro-1-hydroxyethyl)phosphonate. *CAS-52-68-6. Anthelmintic (veterinary). [Name previously used: Metriphonate.]* ◇*Bayer L 1359; DETF*

Trichlorisobutylalcohol — *See* Chlorobutanol.

Trichlormethiazide (trye klor me thye′ a zide). **USP.** $C_8H_8Cl_3N_3O_4S_2$. 380.66. (1) 2*H*-1,2,4-Benzothiadiazine-7-sulfonamide, 6-chloro-3-(dichloromethyl)-3,4-dihydro-, 1,1-dioxide, (±)-; (2) (±)-6-Chloro-3-(dichloromethyl)-3,4-dihydro-2*H*-1,2,4-benzothiadiazine-7-sulfonamide 1,1-dioxide. *UNII-Q58C92TUN0. CAS-133-67-5.* INN; JAN. *Diuretic; antihypertensive.* Metahydrin (Sanofi Aventis); Naqua (Schering)

Trichlormethine. $C_6H_{12}Cl_3N$. 204.53. 2,2′,2″-Trichlorotriethylamine. *UNII-66WBM7N0NM. CAS-555-77-1.* INN; BAN. *[Name previously used: Trimustine.]*

Trichloroacetic Acid. $C_2HCl_3O_2$. 163.39. (1) Acetic acid, trichloro-; (2) Trichloroacetic acid. *CAS-76-03-9.* USP XXI; MI.

Trichloroethyl Phosphate Sodium — *See* Triclofos Sodium.

Trichloroethylene. C_2HCl_3. 131.39. Ethene, trichloro-. *UNII-290YE8AR51. CAS-79-01-6.* NF XIV; INN; MI. Chlorylen (Schering†)

Trichloromonofluoromethane (trye klor″ oh mon″ oh floor″ oh meth′ ane). **NF**. CCl$_3$F. 137.37. (1) Methane, trichloro-fluoro-; (2) Trichlorofluoromethane. *UNII-990TYB331R*. *CAS-75-69-4*. *Pharmaceutic aid (aerosol propellant)*. Freon 11 (DuPont Merck†)

Trichomycin (JAN) — *See* Hachimycin.

Triciribine Phosphate [*1981*] (trye sir′ i been fos′ fate). C$_{13}$H$_{17}$N$_6$O$_7$P. 400.28. [Triciribine is INN.] (1) 1,4,5,6,8-Pentaazaacenaphthylen-3-amine, 1,5-dihydro-5-methyl-1-(5-*O*-phosphono-β-D-ribofuranosyl)-; (2) 3-Amino-1,5-dihydro-5-methyl-1-β-D-ribofuranosyl-1,4,5,6,8-pentaazaacenaphthylene 5′-(dihydrogen phosphate). *UNII-5L5GE3DV88*. *CAS-61966-08-3*. *Antineoplastic*. [*Name previously used: Phosphate Salt of Tricyclic Nucleoside.*] ◇*NSC-280594*

Tricitrates (trye sit′ rates). **USP** [Oral Solution]. A solution of Sodium Citrate, Potassium Citrate, and Citric Acid. *Alkalizer (systemic); alkalizer (urinary); anti-urolithic (cystine calculi); anti-urolithic (uric acid calculi); buffer (neutralizing)*.

Triclabendazole. C$_{14}$H$_9$Cl$_3$N$_2$OS. 359.66. 5-Chloro-6-(2,3-dichlorophenoxy)-2-(methylthio)benzimidazole. *UNII-4784C8E03O*. *CAS-68786-66-3*. INN; BAN; MI.

Triclacetamol. C$_8$H$_6$Cl$_3$NO$_2$. 254.50. 2,2,2-Trichloro-4′-hydroxyacetanilide. *UNII-L56P3532KI*. *CAS-6340-87-0*. INN; DCF.

Triclazate. C$_{20}$H$_{23}$NO$_3$. 325.40. 1-Methyl-3-pyrrolidine-methanol benzilate ester. *UNII-4661WA7OCU*. *CAS-7009-76-9*. INN.

Triclobisonium Chloride. C$_{36}$H$_{74}$Cl$_2$N$_2$. 605.89. Hexamethyl-enebis[dimethyl[1-methyl-3-(2,2,6-trimethylcyclohexyl)-propyl]ammonium] dichloride. *CAS-79-90-3*. NF XIII; INN; MI.

Triclocarban [*1965*] (trye″ kloe kar′ ban). C$_{13}$H$_9$Cl$_3$N$_2$O. 315.58. (1) Urea, *N*-(4-chlorophenyl)-*N*′-(3,4-dichlorophe-nyl)-; (2) 3,4,4′-Trichlorocarbanilide. *UNII-BGG1Y1ED0Y*. *CAS-101-20-2*. INN. *Disinfectant*. TCC Soap (Monsanto†) ◇*TCC; NSC-72005*

Triclodazol. C$_{17}$H$_{15}$Cl$_3$N$_2$O$_2$. 385.67. 3-(2,2,2-Trichloro-1-hydroxyethyl)-5,5-diphenyl-4-imidazolidinone. *UNII-0757XV4DZR*. *CAS-56-28-0*. INN; DCF; MI.

Triclofenol Piperazine [*1963*] (trye″ kloe fee′ nol pi per′ a zeen). C$_4$H$_{10}$N$_2$,2C$_6$H$_3$Cl$_3$O. 481.03. (1) Phenol, 2,4,5-trichloro-, compd. with piperazine (2:1); (2) Piperazine compound (1:2) with 2,4,5-trichlorophenol. *CAS-5714-82-9*. INN; BAN. *Anthelmintic*. Ranestol (Parke-Davis†) ◇*CI-416; CN-5834-5931B; IN 29-5931B; NSC-77747*

Triclofos Sodium [*1963*] (trye′ kloe fos soe′ dee um). C$_2$H$_3$Cl$_3$NaO$_4$P. 251.37. [Triclofos is INN and BAN.] (1) Ethanol, 2,2,2-trichloro-, dihydrogen phosphate monosodium salt; (2) 2,2,2-Trichloroethanol dihydrogen phosphate monosodium salt. *UNII-9F90KA5Q8U*. *CAS-7246-20-0; CAS-306-52-5* [triclofos]. JAN. *Sedative-hypnotic*. Triclos (Sanofi Aventis) ◇*Sch 10159*

Triclofylline. C$_{11}$H$_{13}$Cl$_3$N$_4$O$_4$. 371.60. 7-[2-(2,2,2-Trichloro-1-hydroxyethoxy)ethyl]theophylline. *UNII-2T7T4YO42R*. *CAS-17243-70-8*. INN; DCF.

Triclonide [*1973*] (trye′ kloe nide). C$_{24}$H$_{28}$Cl$_3$FO$_4$. 505.83. (1) Pregna-1,4-diene-3,20-dione, 9,11,21-trichloro-6-fluoro-16,17-[(1-methylethylidene)bis(oxy)]-, (6α,11β,16α)-; (2) 9,11β,21-Trichloro-6α-fluoro-16α,17-

---

dihydroxypregna-1,4-diene-3,20-dione cyclic acetal with acetone. *UNII-PSM3RT117Z. CAS-26849-57-0.* INN. *Anti-inflammatory.* ◇*RS-4464*

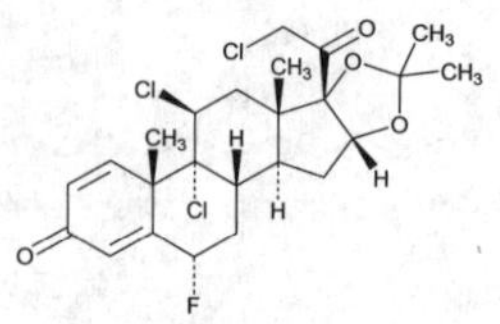

Triclosan [*1972*] (trye' kloe san). **USP.** $C_{12}H_7Cl_3O_2$. 289.54. (1) Phenol, 5-chloro-2-(2,4-dichlorophenoxy)-; (2) 2,4,4'-Trichloro-2'-hydroxydiphenyl ether. *UNII-4NM5039Y5X. CAS-3380-34-5.* INN; BAN. *Disinfectant.* Stri-Dex Cleansing Bar (Sterling Health U.S.A.); Stri-Dex Face Wash (Sterling Health U.S.A.) ◇*CH 3565*

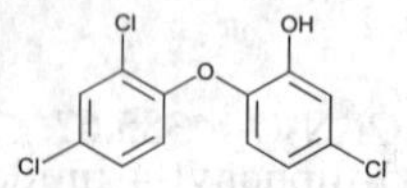

Tricosactide. $C_{131}H_{204}N_{40}O_{29}S$. 2835.34. 23-L-Tyrosinamide-$\alpha^{1\text{-}23}$-corticotropin. *CAS-20282-58-0.* INN.

SYSMEHFRWG KPVGKKRRPV KVY ——NH₂

Tricyclamol Chloride. $C_{20}H_{32}ClNO$. 337.93. (±)-1-(3-Cyclohexyl-3-hydroxy-3-phenylpropyl)-1-methylpyrrolidinium chloride. *CAS-3818-88-0.* INN; BAN.

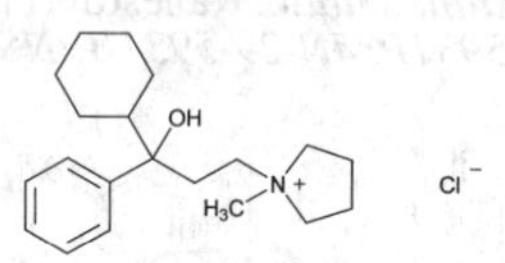

Tridecactide. $C_{75}H_{106}N_{20}O_{19}S$. 1623.83. Alpha-1-13-corticotropin, human L-seryl-L-tyrosyl-L-seryl-L-methionyl-L-glutamyl-L-histidyl-L-phenylalanyl-L-arginyl-L-tryptophyl-glycyl-L-lysyl-L-prolyl-L-valine. *CAS-22006-64-0.* INN.

Tridihexethyl Chloride. $C_{21}H_{36}ClNO$. 353.97. (1) Benzenepropanaminium, γ-cyclohexyl-*N,N,N*-triethyl-γ-hydroxy-, chloride; (2) (3-Cyclohexyl-3-hydroxy-3-phenylpropyl)-triethylammonium chloride. *UNII-25YK75CYMX. CAS-4310-35-4; CAS-60-49-1* [tridihexethyl]. USP XXII; BAN. Pathilon (Lederle)

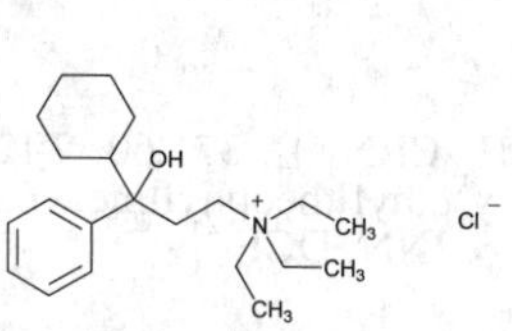

Tridihexethyl Iodide. $C_{21}H_{36}INO$. 445.42. (3-Cyclohexyl-3-hydroxy-3-phenylpropyl)triethylammonium iodide. *CAS-125-99-5.* INN; MI.

Tridolgosir Hydrochloride [*2000*] (trye dol' goe sir hye" droe klor' ide). $C_8H_{15}NO_3\cdot HCl$. 209.67. [Tridolgosir is INN.] (1) 1,2,8-Indolizinetriol, octahydro-, hydrochloride, [1*S*-(1α,2α,8β,8aβ)]-; (2) (1*S*,2*R*,8*R*,8a*R*)-Octahydro-

1,2,8-indolizinetriol hydrochloride. *CAS-214462-68-7; CAS-72741-87-8* [tridolgosir]. INN. *Treatment of solid tumor cancers; chemoprotectant.* ◇*GD0039*

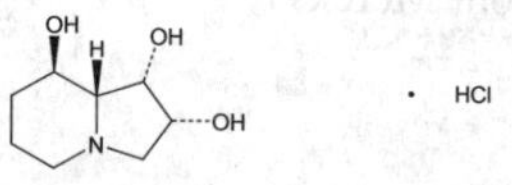

Trientine Hydrochloride [*1984*] (trye' en teen hye" droe klor' ide). **USP.** $C_6H_{18}N_4\cdot 2HCl$. 219.16. [Trientine is INN; Trientine Dihydrochloride is BAN.] (1) 1,2-Ethanediamine, *N,N'*-bis(2-aminoethyl)-, dihydrochloride; (2) Triethylenetetramine dihydrochloride. *UNII-HC3NX54582; UNII-SJ76Y07H5F* [trientine]. *CAS-38260-01-4; CAS-112-24-3* [trientine]. *Chelating agent.* Syprine (Aton) ◇*MK-0681*

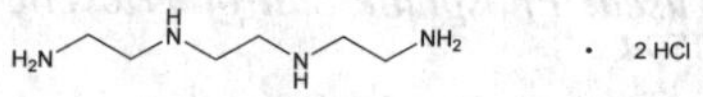

Triethanolamine (previously used name) — *See* Trolamine.

Triethyl Citrate (trye eth' il sit' rate). **NF.** $C_{12}H_{20}O_7$. 276.28. (1) 1,2,3-Propanetricarboxylic acid, 2-hydroxy-, 1,2,3-triethyl ester; (2) 1,2,3-Propanetricarboxylic acid, 2-hydroxy-, triethyl ester. *UNII-8Z96QXD6UM. CAS-77-93-0. Pharmaceutic aid (plasticizer).*

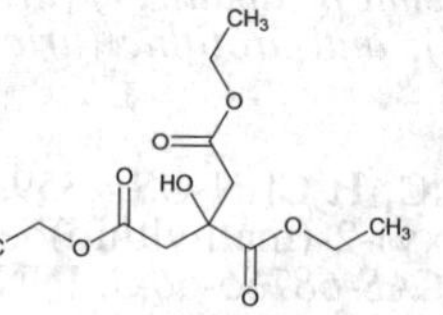

Triethyleneiminobenzoquinone — *See* Triaziquone.

Triethylenemelamine. $C_9H_{12}N_6$. 204.23. [Tretamine is INN and BAN.] 1,3,5-Triazine, 2,4,6-tris(1-aziridinyl)-. *CAS-51-18-3.* NF XIV; MI. ◇*NSC-9706*

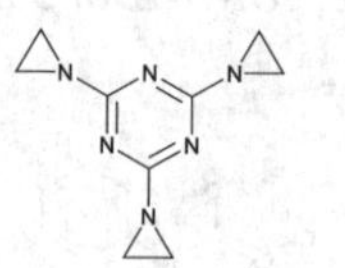

Trifenagrel [*1985*] (trye fen' a grel). $C_{25}H_{25}N_3O$. 383.49. (1) Ethanamine, 2-[2-[2-(4,5-diphenyl-1*H*-imidazol-2-yl)phenoxy]-*N,N*-dimethyl-; (2) 2-[*o*-[2-(Dimethylamino)ethoxy]phenyl]-4,5-diphenylimidazole. *UNII-59X5ME2O06. CAS-84203-09-8.* INN. *Antithrombotic.* ◇*BW 325U*

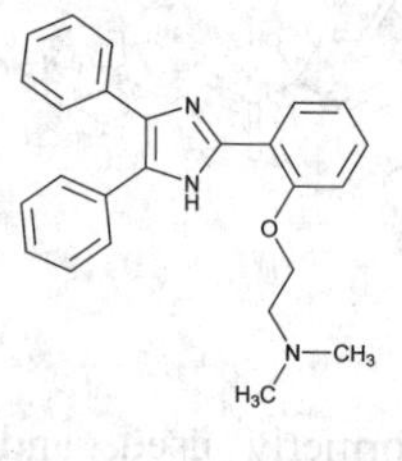

Trifezolac. $C_{23}H_{18}N_2O_2$. 354.40. 1,3,5-Triphenylpyrazole-4-acetic acid. *UNII-XJ3W180C22. CAS-32710-91-1.* INN.

Triflocin [*1969*] (trye floe′ sin). $C_{13}H_9F_3N_2O_2$. 282.22. (1) 3-Pyridinecarboxylic acid, 4-[[3-(trifluoromethyl)phenyl]amino]-; (2) 4-(α,α,α-Trifluoro-*m*-toluidino)nicotinic acid. *UNII-S01B3A38SK. CAS-13422-16-7.* INN. *Diuretic.* ◇CL 65,562

Triflubazam [*1973*] (trye floo′ ba zam). $C_{17}H_{13}F_3N_2O_2$. 334.29. (1) 1*H*-1,5-Benzodiazepine-2,4(3*H*,5*H*)-dione, 1-methyl-5-phenyl-7-(trifluoromethyl)-; (2) 1-Methyl-5-phenyl-7-(trifluoromethyl-1*H*-1,5-benzodiazepine-2,4(3*H*,5*H*)-dione. *CAS-22365-40-8.* INN. *Tranquilizer (minor).* ◇WE352; ORF-8063

Triflumidate [*1969*] (trye floo′ mi date). $C_{17}H_{14}F_3NO_5S$. 401.36. (1) Carbamic acid, (3-benzoylphenyl)[(trifluoromethyl)sulfonyl]-, ethyl ester; (2) Ethyl *m*-benzoyl-*N*-[(trifluoromethyl)sulfonyl]carbanilate. *UNII-V6G94Z48FK. CAS-24243-89-8.* INN. *Anti-inflammatory.* ◇BA 4223; MBR 4223

Trifluomeprazine. $C_{19}H_{21}F_3N_2S$. 366.44. 10-[3-(Dimethylamino)-2-methylpropyl]-2-(trifluoromethyl)phenothiazine. *UNII-OF4T2241HQ. CAS-2622-37-9.* INN; BAN; MI.

Trifluoperazine Hydrochloride (trye″ floo oh per′ a zeen hye″ droe klor′ ide). **USP.** $C_{21}H_{24}F_3N_3S.2HCl$. 480.42. [Trifluoperazine is INN and BAN; Trifluoperazine Maleate is JAN.] (1) 10*H*-Phenothiazine, 10-[3-(4-methyl-1-piperazinyl)propyl]-2-(trifluoromethyl)-, dihydrochloride; (2) 10-[3-(4-Methyl-1-piperazinyl)propyl]-2-(trifluoromethyl)phenothiazine dihydrochloride. *UNII-6P1Y2SNF5V; UNII-214IZI85K3* [trifluoperazine]. *CAS-440-17-5; CAS-117-89-5* [trifluoperazine]. JAN. *Antipsychotic; sedative-hypnotic.* Stelazine (GlaxoSmithKline)

Trifluperidol [*1965*] (trye″ floo per′ i dol). $C_{22}H_{23}F_4NO_2$. 409.42. (1) 1-Butanone, 1-(4-fluorophenyl)-4-[4-hydroxy-4-[3-(trifluoromethyl)phenyl]-1-piperidinyl]-; (2) 4′-Fluoro-4-[4-hydroxy-4-(α,α,α-trifluoro-*m*-tolyl)piperidino]butyrophenone. *UNII-R8869Q7R8I. CAS-749-13-3.* INN; BAN. *Antipsychotic.* Triperidol (Ortho-McNeil†) ◇McN-JR-2498; R-2498

Triflupromazine (trye″ floo proe′ ma zeen). **USP.** $C_{18}H_{19}F_3N_2S$. 352.42. (1) 10*H*-Phenothiazine-10-propanamine, *N,N*-dimethyl-2-(trifluoromethyl)-; (2) 10-3-(Dimethylamino)propyl-2-(trifluoromethyl)phenothiazine. *UNII-RO16TQF95Y. CAS-146-54-3.* INN; BAN. *Antipsychotic.* Vesprin (Apothecon) *[Name previously used: Fluopromazine.]*

Triflupromazine Hydrochloride (trye″ floo proe′ ma zeen hye″ droe klor′ ide). **USP.** $C_{18}H_{19}F_3N_2S.HCl$. 388.88. (1) 10*H*-Phenothiazine-10-propanamine, *N,N*-dimethyl-2-(trifluoromethyl)-, monohydrochloride; (2) 10-[3-(Dimethylamino)propyl]-2-(trifluoromethyl)phenothiazine monohydrochloride. *UNII-9E75N4A5HM. CAS-1098-60-8; CAS-146-54-3* [triflupromazine]. JAN. *Antipsychotic.* Vesprin (Apothecon)

Trifluridine [*1977*] (trye flur′ i deen). **USP.** $C_{10}H_{11}F_3N_2O_5$. 296.20. (1) Thymidine, α,α,α-trifluoro-; (2) 2′-Deoxy-5-(trifluoromethyl)uridine. *UNII-RMW9V5RW38. CAS-70-00-8.* INN. *Antiviral (ophthalmic).* Viroptic (King)

---

† Brand name formerly used, and/or firm no longer concerned with this product.

Triflusal. $C_{10}H_7F_3O_4$. 248.16. α,α,α-Trifluoro-2,4-cresotic acid acetate. *UNII-1Z0YFI05OO. CAS-322-79-2.* INN; BAN; MI.

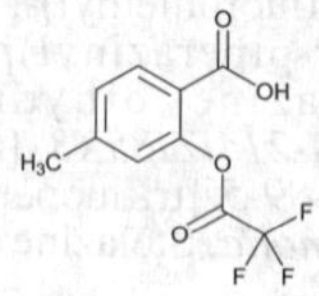

Trifosmin. $C_{12}H_{27}O_3P$. 250.31. Tris(3-methoxypropyl)phosphine. *UNII-38HR17LI0U. CAS-83622-85-9.* INN; BAN.

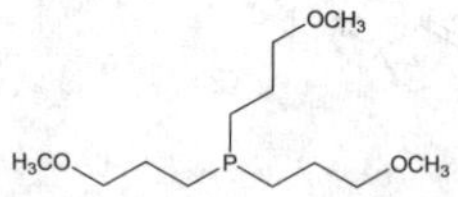

Trigevolol. $C_{21}H_{28}N_2O_7$. 420.46. ($\pm$)-5-[2-[[2-Hydroxy-3-[*p*-(2-methoxyethoxy)phenoxy]propyl]amino]ethoxy]salicylamide. *CAS-76812-98-1.* INN.

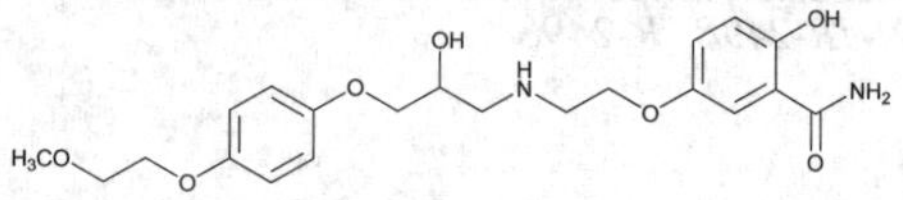

Triglycerides, Medium-Chain (trye glis′ er ides). **NF.** (1) Glycerides, mixed decanoyl and octanoyl; (2) Caprylic and capric triglycerides.

Trihexyphenidyl Hydrochloride (trye hex″ ee fen′ i dil hye″ droe klor′ ide). **USP.** $C_{20}H_{31}NO.HCl$. 337.93. [Trihexyphenidyl is INN and BAN; Benzhexol is BAN.] (1) 1-Piperidinepropanol, α-cyclohexyl-α-phenyl-, hydrochloride, ($\pm$)-; (2) ($\pm$)-α-Cyclohexyl-α-phenyl-1-piperidinepropanol hydrochloride. *UNII-AO61G82577; UNII-6RC5V8B7PO* [trihexyphenidyl]. *CAS-52-49-3; CAS-144-11-6* [trihexyphenidyl]. JAN. *Anticholinergic; antiparkinsonian.* Artane (Lederle); Tremin (Schering)

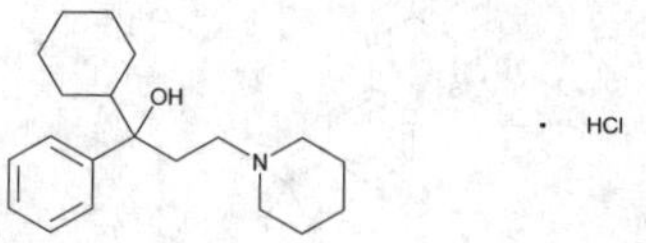

Triiodothyronine Sodium, Levo — *See* Liothyronine Sodium.

Trikates (trye′ kates). **USP** [Oral Solution]. A solution of Potassium Acetate, Potassium Bicarbonate, and Potassium Citrate. *Replenisher (electrolyte).*

Triletide. $C_{27}H_{31}N_5O_5$. 505.57. *N*-[*N*-(*N*-Acetyl-3-phenyl-L-alanyl)-3-phenyl-L-alanyl]-L-histidine, methyl ester. *CAS-62087-96-1.* INN.

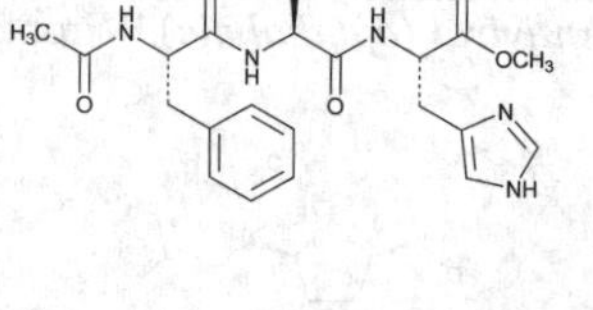

Trilostane [*1976*] (trye′ loe stane). $C_{20}H_{27}NO_3$. 329.43. (1) Androst-2-ene-2-carbonitrile, 4,5-epoxy-3,17-dihydroxy-, ($4\alpha,5\alpha,17\beta$)-; (2) $4\alpha,5$-Epoxy-3,17β-dihydroxy-5α-androst-2-ene-2-carbonitrile. *UNII-L0FPV48Q5R. CAS-13647-35-3.* INN; BAN; JAN. *Adrenocortical suppressant.* Modrastane (Bioenvision) ◇*Win 24,540*

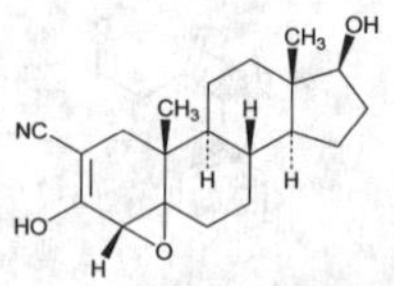

Trimazosin Hydrochloride [*1974*] (trye maz′ oh sin hye″ droe klor′ ide). $C_{20}H_{29}N_5O_6.HCl.H_2O$. 489.95. [Trimazosin is INN and BAN.] (1) 1-Piperazinecarboxylic acid, 4-(4-amino-6,7,8-trimethoxy-2-quinazolinyl)-, 2-hydroxy-2-methylpropyl ester, monohydrochloride, monohydrate; (2) 2-Hydroxy-2-methylpropyl 4-(4-amino-6,7,8-trimethoxy-2-quinazolinyl)-1-piperazinecarboxylate monohydrochloride monohydrate. *UNII-827T79ILE7; UNII-31L760807H* [trimazosin]. *CAS-53746-46-6; CAS-35795-17-6* [anhydrous]; *CAS-35795-16-5* [trimazosin]. *Antihypertensive.* ◇*CP-19,106-1*

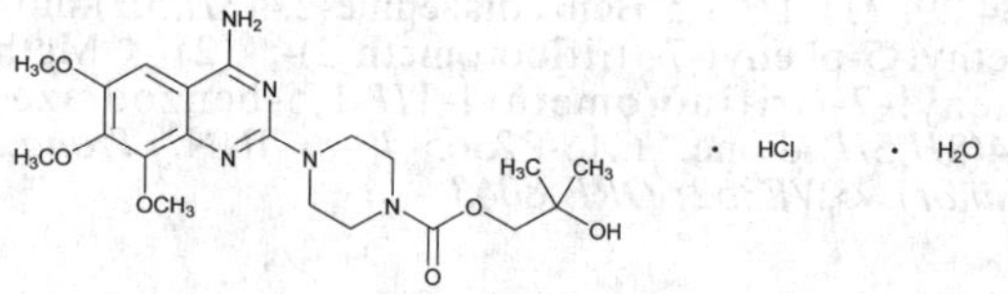

Trimebutine. $C_{22}H_{29}NO_5$. 387.47. [Trimebutine Maleate is JAN.] β-(Dimethylamino)-β-ethylphenethyl alcohol 3,4,5-trimethoxybenzoate (ester). *CAS-39133-31-8.* INN; BAN; DCF; MI.

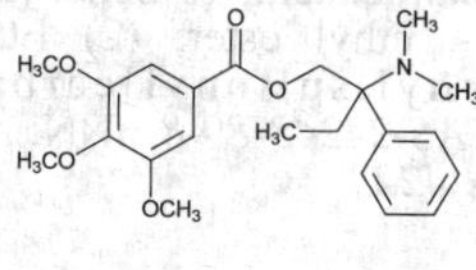

Trimecaine. $C_{15}H_{24}N_2O$. 248.36. 2-Diethylamino-2′,4′,6′-trimethylacetanilide. *UNII-IN1233R0JO. CAS-616-68-2.* INN; MI.

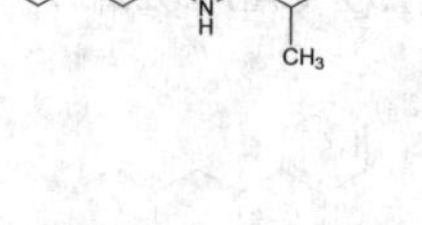

Trimedoxime Bromide. $C_{15}H_{18}Br_2N_4O_2$. 446.14. 1,1′-Trimethylenebis(4-formylpyridinium bromide)dioxime. *CAS-56-97-3.* INN. ◇*TMB-4; C-434*

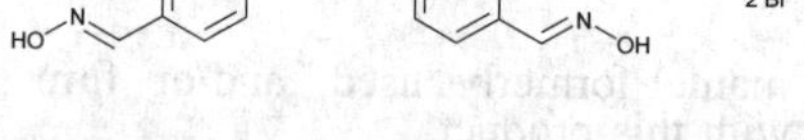

Trimegestone [*1996*] (trye me jes' tone). $C_{22}H_{30}O_3$. 342.47. (1) Estra-4,9-dien-3-one, 17-(2-hydroxy-1-oxopropyl)-17-methyl-, [17β(S)]-; (2) 17β-(S)-Lactoyl-17-methylestra-4,9-dien-3-one. *CAS-74513-62-5*. INN; BAN. *Progestin.* ◇RU 27987

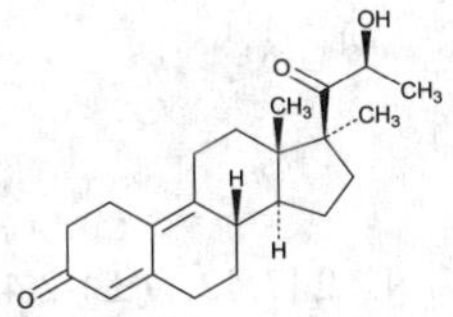

Trimeperidine. $C_{17}H_{25}NO_2$. 275.39. 1,2,5-Trimethyl-4-phenyl-4-propionyloxypiperidine. *UNII-1M2IB31DTS. CAS-64-39-1*. INN; BAN; DCF.

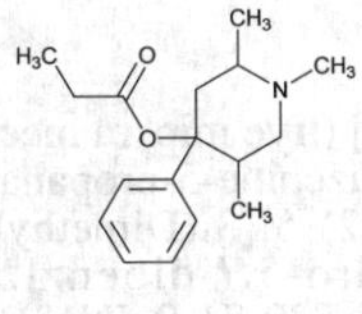

Trimeprazine Tartrate (trye mep' ra zeen tar' trate). **USP**. $(C_{18}H_{22}N_2S)_2 \cdot C_4H_6O_6$. 746.98. [Alimemazine is INN and BAN; Alimemazine Tartrate is JAN.] (1) 10*H*-Phenothiazine-10-propanamine N,N,β-trimethyl-, [R-(R*,R*)]-2,3-dihydroxybutanedioate (2:1); (2) 10-[3-(Dimethylamino)-2-methylpropyl]phenothiazine tartrate (2:1). *UNII-362NW1LD6Z; UNII-76H78MJJ52* [trimeprazine]. *CAS-4330-99-8; CAS-41375-66-0* [replaced]; *CAS-84-96-8* [trimeprazine]. *Antipruritic.* Temaril (Allergan)

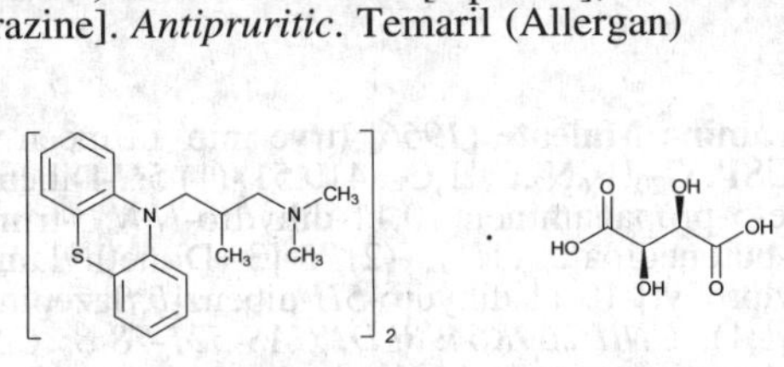

Trimeproprimine — *See* Trimipramine.

Trimetamide (INN) — *See* Trimethamide.

Trimetaphan Camsilate (INN, BAN, JAN, DCF) — *See* Trimethaphan Camsylate.

Trimetaphan Camsylate (previously used name) — *See* Trimethaphan Camsylate.

Trimetazidine. $C_{14}H_{22}N_2O_3$. 266.34. [Trimetazidine Hydrochloride is JAN.] 1-(2,3,4-Trimethoxybenzyl)piperazine. *UNII-N9A0A0R9S8. CAS-5011-34-7*. INN; BAN; DCF; MI. ◇40045

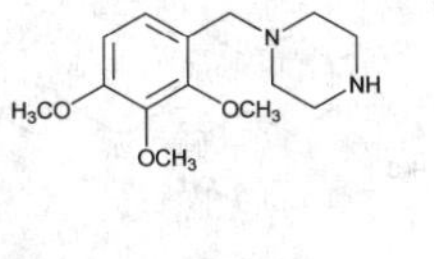

Trimethadione. $C_6H_9NO_3$. 143.14. (1) 2,4-Oxazolidinedione, 3,5,5-trimethyl-; (2) 3,5,5-Trimethyl-2,4-oxazolidinedione. *UNII-R7GV3H6FQ4. CAS-127-48-0*. USP XXIII; INN; BAN; JAN. *Anticonvulsant.* Tridione (Abbott) [*Name previously used: Troxidone.*]

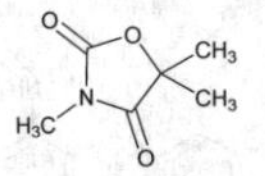

Trimethamide. $C_{17}H_{21}N_3O_4$. 331.37. [Trimetamide is INN.] N-[(2-Amino-6-methyl-3-pyridyl)methyl]-3,4,5-trimethoxybenzamide. *UNII-839184U8NM. CAS-5789-72-0*.

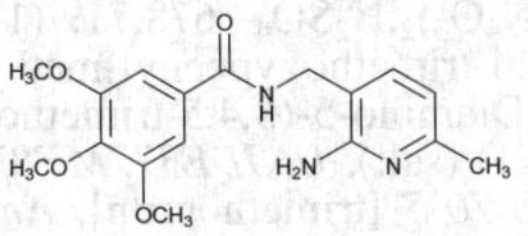

Trimethaphan Camphorsulfonate — *See* Trimethaphan Camsylate.

Trimethaphan Camsylate. $C_{32}H_{40}N_2O_5S_2$. 596.80. [Trimetaphan Camsilate is INN, BAN and JAN.] (1) Thieno[1',2':1,2]thieno[3,4-*d*]imidazol-5-ium, decahydro-2-oxo-1,3-bis(phenylmethyl)-, salt with (+)-7,7-dimethyl-2-oxobicyclo[2.2.1]heptane-1-methanesulfonic acid (1:1); (2) (+)-1,3-Dibenzyldecahydro-2-oxoimidazo[4,5-*c*]thieno[1,2-*a*]-thiolium 2-oxo-10-bornanesulfonate (1:1). *UNII-8W556014K9. CAS-68-91-7*. USP XXIII. *Antihypertensive.* Arfonad (Roche) [*Name previously used: Trimetaphan Camsylate.*]

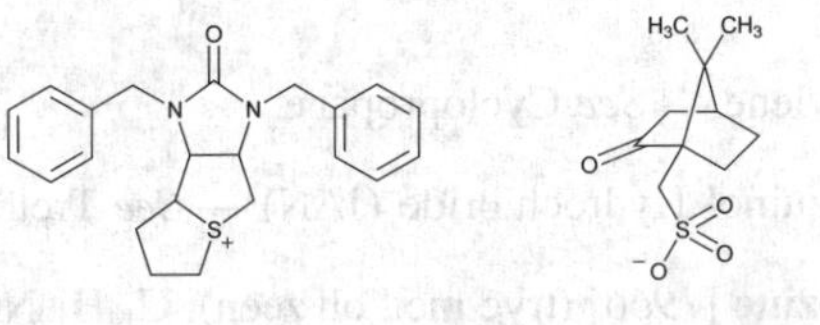

Trimethidinium Methosulfate. $C_{19}H_{42}N_2O_8S_2$. 490.68. [Trimethidinium Methosulphate is BAN.] 1,3,8,8-Tetramethyl-3-[3-(trimethylammonio)propyl]-3-azoniabicyclo[3.2.1]octane bis(methyl sulfate). *CAS-14149-43-0; CAS-2624-50-2* [trimethidinium]. NF XIII; INN; MI.

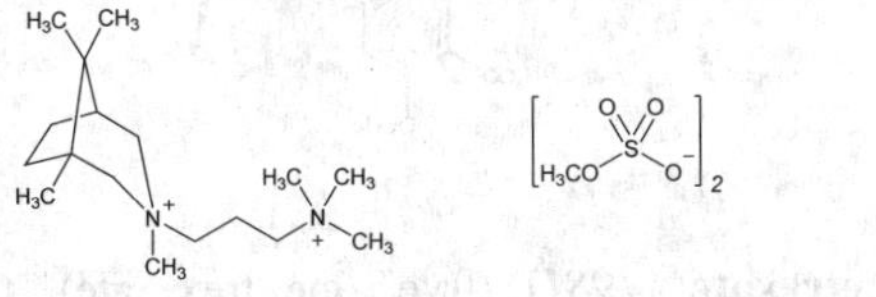

Trimethobenzamide Hydrochloride (trye meth" oh benz' a mide hye" droe klor' ide). **USP**. $C_{21}H_{28}N_2O_5 \cdot HCl$. 424.92. [Trimethobenzamide is INN.] (1) Benzamide, N-[[4-[2-(dimethylamino)ethoxy]phenyl]methyl]-3,4,5-trimethoxy-, monohydrochloride; (2) N-[*p*-[2-(Dimethylamino)ethoxy]benzyl]-3,4,5-trimethoxybenzamide monohydrochloride. *UNII-WDQ5P1SX7Q; UNII-W2X096QY97* [trimethobenzamide]. *CAS-554-92-7; CAS-138-56-7* [trimethobenzamide]. *Anti-emetic.* Tigan (King)

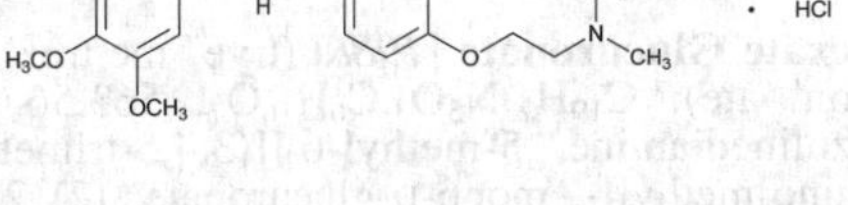

---

† Brand name formerly used, and/or firm no longer concerned with this product.

Trimethoprim [*1964*] (trye meth′ oh prim). **USP**. $C_{14}H_{18}N_4O_3$. 290.32. (1) 2,4-Pyrimidinediamine, 5-[(3,4,5-trimethoxyphenyl)methyl]-; (2) 2,4-Diamino-5-(3,4,5-trimethoxybenzyl)pyrimidine. *UNII-AN164J8Y0X*. *CAS-738-70-5*. INN; BAN; JAN. *Antibacterial*. Proloprim (King); Trimpex (Roche) ◇*BW 56-72; NSC-106568*

Trimethoprim Sulfate [*1984*] (trye meth′ oh prim sul′ fate). **USP**. $(C_{14}H_{18}N_4O_3)_2.H_2SO_4$. 678.71. (1) 2,4-Pyrimidinediamine, 5-[(3,4-trimethoxyphenyl)methyl]-, sulfate (2:1) (salt); (2) 2,4-Diamino-5-(3,4,5-trimethoxybenzyl)pyrimidine sulfate (2:1) (salt). *UNII-E377MF8EQ8*. *CAS-56585-33-2; CAS-738-70-5* [trimethoprim]. *Antibacterial*. ◇*BW 72U*

Trimethoquinol — *See* Tretoquinol.

Trimethylcetylammonium Pentachlorophenate. $C_{19}H_{42}N.C_6Cl_5O$. 549.87. *N,N,N*-Trimethyl-1-hexadecanaminium salt with pentachlorophenol (1:1). *CAS-87-76-3*. JAN.

Trimethylene — *See* Cyclopropane.

Trimetoquinol Hydrochloride (JAN) — *See* Tretoquinol.

Trimetozine [*1966*] (trye met′ oh zeen). $C_{14}H_{19}NO_5$. 281.30. (1) Morpholine, 4-(3,4,5-trimethoxybenzoyl)-; (2) 4-(3,4,5-Trimethoxybenzoyl)morpholine. *UNII-31EPT7G9PL*. *CAS-635-41-6*. INN. *Sedative-hypnotic*. ◇*Abbott-22370; PS 2383; NSC-62939*

Trimetrexate [*1981*] (trye″ me trex′ ate). $C_{19}H_{23}N_5O_3$. 369.42. (1) 2,4-Quinazolinediamine, 5-methyl-6-[[(3,4,5-trimethoxyphenyl)amino]methyl]-; (2) 2,4-Diamino-5-methyl-6-[(3,4,5-trimethoxyanilino)methyl]quinazoline. *UNII-UPN4ITI8T4*. *CAS-52128-35-5*. INN; BAN. *Antineoplastic*. ◇*CI-898*

Trimetrexate Glucuronate [*1988*] (trye″ me trex′ ate gloo″ kure on′ ate). $C_{19}H_{23}N_5O_3.C_6H_{10}O_7$. 563.56. (1) 2,4-Quinazolinediamine, 5-methyl-6-[[(3,4,5-trimethoxyphenyl)amino]methyl]-, mono-D-glucuronate; (2) 2,4-Diami-no-5-methyl-6-[(3,4,5-trimethoxyanilino)methyl]quinazoline mono-D-glucuronate. *UNII-L137U4A79K*. *CAS-82952-64-5*. *Antineoplastic*. Neutrexin (MedImmune)

Trimexiline. $C_{17}H_{29}N$. 247.42. (±)-2,4,6-Trimethyl-*N*-(1-methylhexyl)benzylamine. *UNII-HUH663DN8F*. *CAS-58757-61-2*. INN.

Trimipramine [*1966*] (trye mip′ ra meen). $C_{20}H_{26}N_2$. 294.43. (1) 5*H*-Dibenz[*b,f*]azepine-5-propanamine, 10,11-dihydro-*N,N,β*-trimethyl-; (2) 5-[3-(Dimethylamino)-2-methylpropyl]-10,11-dihydro-5*H*-dibenz[*b,f*]azepine. *UNII-6S082C9NDT*. *CAS-739-71-9*. INN; BAN. *Antidepressant*. Surmontil (Wyeth-Ayerst) ◇*IL 6001; 7162 RP*

Trimipramine Maleate [*1966*] (trye mip′ ra meen mal′ ee ate). **USP**. $C_{20}H_{26}N_2.C_4H_4O_4$. 410.51. (1) 5*H*-Dibenz[*b,f*]azepine-5-propanamine, 10,11-dihydro-*N,N,β*-trimethyl-, (*Z*)-2-butenedioate (1:1); (2) 5-[3-(Dimethylamino)-2-methylpropyl]-10,11-dihydro-5*H*-dibenz[*b,f*]azepine maleate (1:1). *UNII-269K6498LD*. *CAS-521-78-8; CAS-739-71-9* [trimipramine]. JAN. *Antidepressant*. Surmontil (Odyssey)

Trimolide — *See* Trimetozine.

Trimopam Maleate (previously used name) — *See* Trepipam Maleate.

Trimoprostil [*1983*] (trye″ moe prost′ il). $C_{23}H_{38}O_4$. 378.55. (1) Prosta-5,13-dien-1-oic acid, 15-hydroxy-11,16,16-trimethyl-9-oxo-, (5Z,11α,13E,15R)-; (2) (*Z*)-7-[(1*R*,2*R*,3*R*)-2-[(*E*)-(3*R*)-3-Hydroxy-4,4-dimethyl-1-octenyl]-3-methyl-5-oxocyclopentyl]-5-heptenoic acid. *CAS-69900-72-7*. INN. *Antisecretory (gastric)*. ◇*Ro 21-6937/000*

Trimoxamine Hydrochloride [*1966*] (trye mox′ a meen hye″ droe klor′ ide). $C_{15}H_{23}NO_3.HCl$. 301.81. [Trimoxamine is INN.] (1) Benzeneethanamine, 3,4,5-trimethoxy-*N*-methyl-α-2-propenyl-, hydrochloride; (2) α-Allyl-3,4,5-trimethoxy-*N*-methylphenethylamine hydrochloride. *CAS-7082-27-1; CAS-15686-23-4* [trimoxamine]. *Antihypertensive.* ◇*NAT-327; NDR-5523A*

Trimustine (previously used name) — *See* Trichlormethine.

Trinecol (pullus) [*1999*] (trye′ ne kol pool′ us). Trinecol (pullus) consists of purified, native, truncated (telopeptides largely removed) triple stranded monomers of type II collagen from chicken sternal cartilage solubilized in 0.1 M acetic acid. The first 15 residues on the N terminus of each chain are removed and the last 21, 22, or 24 residues of the C terminus of each chain are cleaved. Glycosylation can occur on hydroxylysine residues. The substance contains a heterogeneous mixture of α-D-glucopyranosyl-$(1\rightarrow2)$-β-D-galactopyranosyl-5-hydroxylysine and β-D-galactopyranosyl-5-hydroxylysine, and non-glycosylated hydroxylysines. Trinecol (pullus). Molecular weight is approximately 300,000 daltons. *CAS-212115-71-4. To reduce the signs and symptoms of rheumatoid arthritis (''oral tolerance therapy''*). Colloral (AutoImmune)

Trinitrin Tablets — *See* Nitroglycerin.

Trinitrophenol. Picric acid. NF IX.

Triolein I 125 [*1964*] (trye′ oh leen). (1) 9-Octadecenoic acid (*Z*), 1,2,3-propanetriyl ester, labeled with iodine-125; (2) Triolein, labeled with iodine-125. *Radioactive agent.*

Triolein I 131 [*1963*] (trye′ oh leen). (1) 9-Octadecenoic acid (*Z*), 1,2,3-propanetriyl ester, labeled with iodine-131; (2) Triolein, labeled with iodine-131. *Radioactive agent.* Raolein (Abbott†); Trioleotope (Bristol-Myers Squibb†)

Trional — *See* Sulfonethylmethane.

Trioxifene Mesylate [*1979*] (trye ox′ i feen mes′ i late). $C_{30}H_{31}NO_3.CH_4O_3S$. 549.68. [Trioxifene is INN.] (1) Methanone, [3,4-dihydro-2-(4-methoxyphenyl)-1-naphthalenyl][4-[2-(1-pyrrolidinyl)ethoxy]phenyl]-, methanesulfonate; (2) 3,4-Dihydro-2-(*p*-methoxyphenyl)-1-naphthyl *p*-[2-(1-pyrrolidinyl)ethoxy]phenyl ketone methanesulfonate. *CAS-68307-81-3; CAS-63619-84-1* [trioxifene]. *Anti-estrogen.* ◇*Compound 133314*

Trioxsalen [*1965*] (trye ox′ sa len). **USP.** $C_{14}H_{12}O_3$. 228.24. [Trioxysalen is INN and JAN.] (1) 7*H*-Furo[3,2-*g*][1]benzopyran-7-one, 2,5,9-trimethyl-; (2) 2,5,9-Trimethyl-7*H*-furo[3,2-*g*][1]benzopyran-7-one. *UNII-Y6UY8OV51T. CAS-3902-71-4. Pigmentation agent.* Trisoralen (Valeant) ◇*NSC-71047*

Trioxyethylrutin — *See* Troxerutin.

Trioxymethylene — *See* Paraformaldehyde.

Trioxysalen (INN, JAN) — *See* Trioxsalen.

Tripalmitin. $C_{51}H_{98}O_6$. 807.32. Tripalmitin *or* 1,2,3-propanetriyl trihexadecanoate. *UNII-D133ZRF50U. CAS-555-44-2.* INN.

Tripamide [*1981*] (trip′ a mide). $C_{16}H_{20}ClN_3O_3S$. 369.87. (1) Benzamide, 3-(aminosulfonyl)-4-chloro-*N*-(octahydro-4,7-methano-2*H*-isoindol-2-yl)-, (3aα,4α,7α,7aα)-; (2) 4-Chloro-*N*-(*endo*-hexahydro-4,7-methanoisoindolin-2-yl)-3-sulfamoylbenzamide. *CAS-73803-48-2.* INN; JAN. *Antihypertensive; diuretic.* ◇*ADR-033; E-614*

Triparanol. $C_{27}H_{32}ClNO_2$. 438.00. 2-*p*-Chlorophenyl-1-[*p*-(2-diethylaminoethoxy)phenyl]-1-*p*-tolylethanol. *CAS-78-41-1.* INN; BAN; MI.

Tripelennamine Citrate. $C_{16}H_{21}N_3.C_6H_8O_7$. 447.48. [Tripelennamine is INN and BAN.] (1) 1,2-Ethanediamine, *N,N*-dimethyl-*N*′-(phenylmethyl)-*N*′-2-pyridinyl-, 2-hydroxy-1,2,3-propanetricarboxylate (1:1); (2) 2-[Benzyl[2-(dimethylamino)ethyl]amino]pyridine citrate (1:1). *UNII-30OC46A3J9. CAS-6138-56-3; CAS-91-81-6* [tripelennamine]. USP XXIII. *Antihistaminic.* PBZ (Novartis)

Tripelennamine Hydrochloride (trip″ el en′ a meen hye″ droe klor′ ide). **USP.** $C_{16}H_{21}N_3.HCl$. 291.82. (1) 1,2-Ethanediamine, *N,N*-dimethyl-*N*′-(phenylmethyl)-*N*′-2-pyridinyl-, monohydrochloride; (2) 2-[Benzyl[2-(dimethy-

---

† Brand name formerly used, and/or firm no longer concerned with this product.

lamino)ethyl]amino]pyridine monohydrochloride. *UNII-FWV8GJ56ZN*. *CAS-154-69-8; CAS-91-81-6* [tripelennamine]. *Antihistaminic*. PBZ (Novartis)

Triplatin Tetranitrate. $C_{12}H_{50}Cl_2N_{14}O_{12}Pt_3$. 1238.77. *(SP-4-1)*-Diamminebis[*(SP-4-2)*-diamminechloroplatinum(II)(μ-hexane-1,6-diamine)]platinum tetranitrate. *CAS-172903-00-3*. INN; BAN. ◇*BBR 3464*

Triple Sulfa (trip′ el sul′ fa). **USP**. A mixture of sulfathiazole, sulfacetamide, and sulfabenzamide.

Tripro-amylin — *See* Pramlintide.

Triprolidine Hydrochloride (trye proe′ li deen hye″ droe klor′ ide). **USP**. $C_{19}H_{22}N_2 \cdot HCl \cdot H_2O$. 332.87. [Triprolidine is INN and BAN.] (1) Pyridine, 2-[1-(4-methylphenyl)-3-(1-pyrrolidinyl)-1-propenyl]-, monohydrochloride, monohydrate, (*E*)-; (2) (*E*)-2-[3-(1-Pyrrolidinyl)-1-*p*-tolylpropenyl]pyridine monohydrochloride monohydrate. *UNII-YAN7R5L890; UNII-2L8T9S52QM* [triprolidine]. *CAS-6138-79-0; CAS-550-70-9* [anhydrous]; *CAS-486-12-4* [triprolidine]. JAN. *Antihistaminic*. Actidil (GlaxoSmithKline); Myidyl (USl)

Triptorelin [*1987*] (trip″ toe rel′ in). $C_{64}H_{82}N_{18}O_{13}$. 1311.45. (1) Luteinizing hormone-releasing factor (pig), 6-D-tryptophan; (2) 5-Oxo-L-prolyl-L-histidyl-L-tryptophyl-L-seryl-L-tyrosyl-D-tryptophyl-L-leucyl-L-arginyl-L-prolylglycinamide. *UNII-9081Y98W2V*. *CAS-57773-63-4*. INN; BAN. *Antineoplastic*. ◇*CL 118,532*

Triptorelin Pamoate [*2000*] (trip″ toe rel′ in pam′ oh ate). $C_{64}H_{82}N_{18}O_{13} \cdot C_{23}H_{16}O_6$. 1699.82. (1) Luteinizing hormone-releasing factor (swine), 6-D-tryptophan-, 4,4′-methylenebis[3-hydroxy-2-naphthalenecarboxylate] (salt); (2) 5-Oxo-L-prolyl-L-histidyl-L-tryptophyl-L-seryl-L-tyrosyl-D-tryptophyl-L-leucyl-L-arginyl-L-prolylglycine amide, 4,4′-methylenebis[3-hydroxy-2-naphthoate] (salt). *UNII-08AN7WA2G0*. *CAS-124508-66-3*. *Antineoplastic (GnRH agonist, inhibitor of gonadotropin secretion)*. Trelstar (Watson)

Trisulfapyrimidines (trye sul″ fa pir i′ mi deens). **USP**. A mixture of Sulfadiazine, Sulfamerazine, and Sulfamethazine. *Antibacterial*. Metha-Meridiazine (Ortho-McNeil†);

Neotrizine (Lilly†); Sulfatryl (Wallace†); Sulfonsol (Marion Merrell Dow†); Terfonyl (Bristol-Myers Squibb†); Thi-Di-Mer (Marion Merrell Dow†); Truozine (Abbott†)

Tritiated Water — *See* Water, Tritiated.

Tritiozine. $C_{14}H_{19}NO_4S$. 297.37. 4-(3,4,5-Trimethoxythiobenzoyl)morpholine. *CAS-35619-65-9*. INN; MI.

Tritoqualine. $C_{26}H_{32}N_2O_8$. 500.54. 7-Amino-4,5,6-triethoxy-3-(5,6,7,8-tetrahydro-4-methoxy-6-methyl-1,3-dioxolo[4,5-*g*]isoquinolin-5-yl)phthalide. *UNII-F4MW5166YH*. *CAS-14504-73-5*. INN; DCF; MI. ◇*L-554*

Trixolane. $C_{18}H_{27}NO_6$. 353.41. 4-[[2-Methyl-2-(3,4,5-trimethoxyphenyl)-1,3-dioxolan-4-yl]methyl]morpholine. *CAS-47420-28-0*. INN.

Trizoxime. $C_{16}H_{15}N_5O_2$. 309.32. 5-Benzyl-4,5-dihydro-4-oxo-1*H*-1,2,5-benzotriazepine-3-carboxamidoxime. *CAS-35710-57-7*. INN; DCF.

Trocimine. $C_{17}H_{25}NO_4$. 307.38. Octahydro-1-(3,4,5-trimethoxybenzoyl)azocine. *CAS-14368-24-2*. INN.

Troclosene Potassium [*1964*] (troe′ kloe seen poe tas′ ee um). $C_3Cl_2KN_3O_3$. 236.05. (1) 1,3,5-Triazine-2,4,6(1*H*,3*H*,5*H*)-trione, 1,3-dichloro-, potassium salt; (2)

1,3-Dichloro-*s*-triazine-2,4,6(1*H*,3*H*,5*H*)trione potassium salt; (3) Potassium dichloroisocyanurate. *CAS-2244-21-5; CAS-2782-57-2* [troclosene]. INN. *Anti-infective, topical.*

Trodusquemine [*2004*] (troe doo′ skwe meen). $C_{37}H_{72}N_4O_5S$. 685.06. (1) Cholestane-7,24-diol, 3-[[3-[[4-[(3-aminopropyl)amino]butyl]amino]propyl]amino]-, 24-(hydrogen sulfate), (3β,5α,7α,24R)-; (2) (24R)-3β-[[3-[[4-[(3-aminopropyl)amino]butyl]amino]propyl]amino]-7α-hydroxy-5α-cholestan-24-yl hydrogen sulfate. *CAS-186139-09-3*. INN. *Treatment of medically significant obesity.* ◇*MSI-1436*

Trofosfamide. $C_9H_{18}Cl_3N_2O_2P$. 323.58. 3-(2-Chloroethyl)-2-[bis(2-chloroethyl)amino]tetrahydro-2*H*-1,3,2-oxazaphosphorin 2-oxide. *CAS-22089-22-1*. INN; MI. ◇*A-4828; Z-4828*

Troglitazone [*1995*] (troe gli′ ta zone). $C_{24}H_{27}NO_5S$. 441.54. (1) 2,4-Thiazolidinedione, 5-[[4-[(3,4-dihydro-6-hydroxy-2,5,7,8-tetramethyl-2*H*-1-benzopyran-2-yl)methoxy]phenyl]methyl]-; (2) (±)-*all-rac*-5-[*p*-[(6-Hydroxy-2,5,7,8-tetramethyl-2-chromanyl)methoxy]benzyl]-2,4-thiazolidinedione. *UNII-I66ZZ0ZN0E*. *CAS-97322-87-7*. INN; BAN. *Antidiabetic.* Prelay (Sankyo); Rezulin (Pfizer) ◇*CS-045; CI-991; GR92132X*

Trolamine (troe′ la meen). **NF.** $C_6H_{15}NO_3$. 149.19. (1) Ethanol, 2,2′,2″-nitrilotris-; (2) 2,2′,2″-Nitrilotriethanol. *CAS-102-71-6. Pharmaceutic aid (alkalizing agent); analgesic.* Mobisyl [as salicylate] (Ascher) *[Name previously used: Triethanolamine.]*

───────

† Brand name formerly used, and/or firm no longer concerned with this product.

Trolamine Salicylate (troe′ la meen sa lis′ i late). **USP.** $C_{13}H_{21}NO_6$. 287.31. Triethanolamine salicylate. *CAS-2174-16-5.*

Troleandomycin [*1968*] (troe″ lee an″ doe mye′ sin). **USP.** $C_{41}H_{67}NO_{15}$. 813.97. [Triacetyloleandomycin is JAN.] (1) Oleandomycin, triacetate (ester); (2) Triacetyloleandomycin. *UNII-C4DZ64560D. CAS-2751-09-9.* INN; BAN. *Antibacterial.* Tao (Pfizer) *[Name previously used: Triacetyloleandomycin.]* ◇*NSC-108166*

Trolnitrate Phosphate. $C_6H_{18}N_4O_{17}P_2$. 480.17. [Trolnitrate is INN.] 2,2′,2″-Nitrilotrisethanol trinitrate (ester) phosphate (1:2) (salt). *CAS-588-42-1; CAS-7077-34-1* [trolnitrate]. BAN; MI. Nitretamin (Bristol-Myers Squibb†)

Tromantadine. $C_{16}H_{28}N_2O_2$. 280.41. *N*-1-Adamantyl-2-[2-(dimethylamino)ethoxy]acetamide. *UNII-H191JFG8WA. CAS-53783-83-8.* INN; DCF; MI.

Trometamol (INN, BAN) — *See* Tromethamine.

Tromethamine [*1962*] (troe meth′ a meen). **USP.** $C_4H_{11}NO_3$. 121.14. [Trometamol is INN and BAN.] (1) 1,3-Propanediol, 2-amino-2-(hydroxymethyl)-; (2) 2-Amino-2-(hydroxymethyl)-1,3-propanediol. *UNII-023C2WHX2V. CAS-77-86-1. Alkalizer.* Tham (Hospira) ◇*NSC-6365*

Tropabazate. $C_{15}H_{19}N_3O_4$. 305.33. Phenyl 3α-hydroxy-8-azabicyclo[3.2.1]octane-8-carboxylate carbazate (ester). *CAS-64294-94-6.* INN.

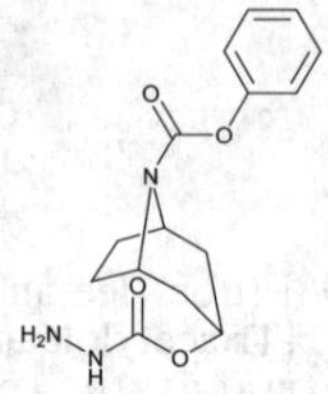

Tropanserin Hydrochloride [*1986*] (troe pan′ ser in hye″ droe klor′ ide). $C_{17}H_{23}NO_2 \cdot HCl$. 309.83. [Tropanserin is INN and BAN.] (1) Benzoic acid, 3,5-dimethyl-, 8-methyl-8-azabicyclo[3.2.1]oct-3-yl ester, hydrochloride, *endo-*; (2) 1αH,5αH-Tropan-3α-yl 3,5-dimethylbenzoate, hydrochloride. *CAS-85181-38-0; CAS-85181-40-4* [tropanserin]. *Serotonin receptor antagonist (specific in migraine).* ◇*MDL 72,422*

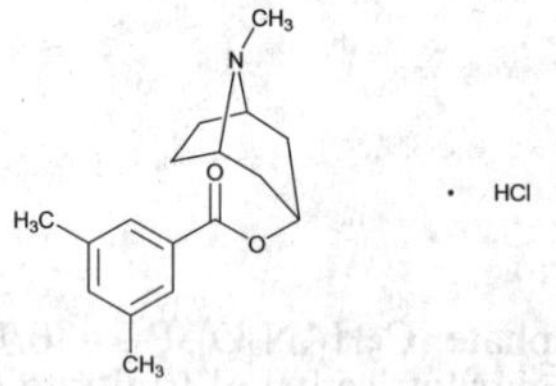

Tropantiol [*2006*] (troe″ pan tye′ ol). $C_{21}H_{34}ClN_3S_2$. 428.10. (1) Ethanethiol, 2-[[2-[[[(1*R*,2*R*,3*S*,5*S*)-3-(4-chlorophenyl)-8-methyl-8-azabicyclo[3.2.1]oct-2-yl]methyl](2-mercaptoethyl)amino]ethyl]amino]-; (2) 2-[[[(1*R*,2*R*,3*S*,5*S*)-3-(4-Chlorophenyl)-8-methyl-8-azabicyclo[3.2.1]oct-2-yl]methyl][2-[(2-sulfanylethyl)amino]ethyl]amino]ethanethiol. *UNII-7844H41L5Z. CAS-189950-11-6.* INN. *Diagnosis or exclusion of Parkinsonian syndrome with or without dopaminergic deficit.* ◇*NC100697*

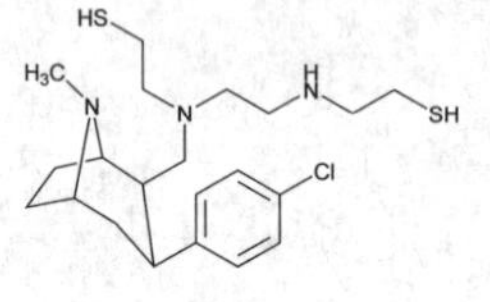

Tropapride. $C_{23}H_{28}N_2O_3$. 380.48. *N*-(8-Benzyl-1αH,5αH-nortropan-3β-yl)-*o*-veratramide. *CAS-76352-13-1.* INN.

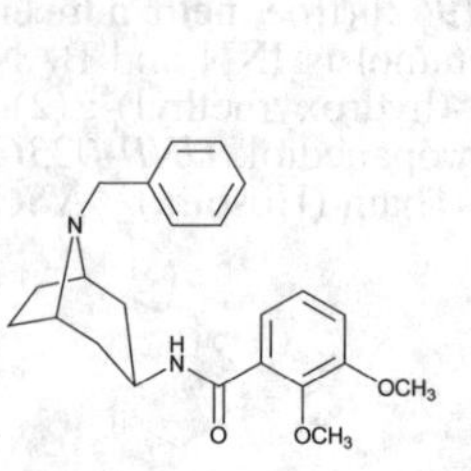

Tropatepine. $C_{22}H_{23}NS$. 333.49. 3-Dibenzo[*b,e*]thiepin-11(6*H*)-ylidene-1αH,5αH-tropane. *CAS-27574-24-9.* INN; DCF. ◇*SD 1248-17 [as hydrochloride]*

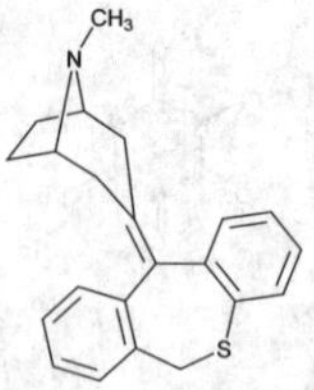

Tropenziline Bromide. $C_{24}H_{30}BrNO_4$. 476.40. 7-Methoxy-8-methyltropinium bromide benzilate. *CAS-143-92-0.* INN. ◇*MTS 263*

Trophosphamide — *See* Trofosfamide.

Tropicamide [*1962*] (troe pik′ a mide). **USP.** $C_{17}H_{20}N_2O_2$. 284.35. (1) Benzeneacetamide, *N*-ethyl-α-(hydroxymethyl)-*N*-(4-pyridinylmethyl)-, (±)-; (2) (±)-*N*-Ethyl-2-phenyl-*N*-(4-pyridylmethyl)hydracrylamide. *UNII-N0A3Z5XTC6. CAS-1508-75-4.* INN; BAN; JAN. *Anticholinergic (ophthalmic).* Mydriacyl (Alcon); Tropicacyl (Akorn)

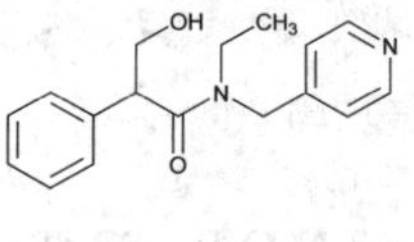

Tropigline. $C_{13}H_{21}NO_2$. 223.31. Tropyl 2,3-dimethylacrylate. *CAS-533-08-4.* INN; BAN.

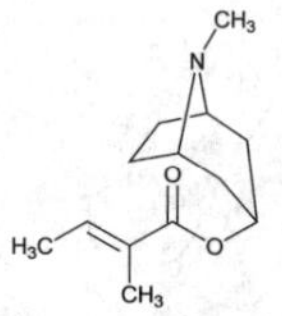

Tropirine. $C_{22}H_{24}N_2O$. 332.44. 3α-[(5*H*-Benzo[4,5]cyclohepta[1,2-*b*]pyridyl)-5-oxy]tropane. *CAS-19410-02-7.* INN. ◇*BS 7723 [as maleate]*

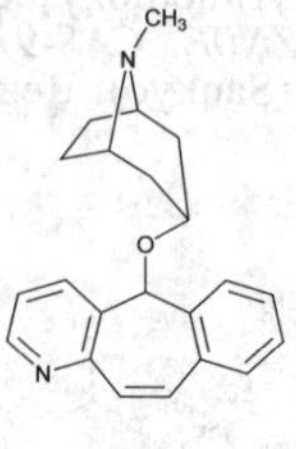

Tropisetron. $C_{17}H_{20}N_2O_2$. 284.35. 1αH,5αH-Tropan-3α-yl indole-3-carboxylate. *CAS-89565-68-4.* INN; BAN.

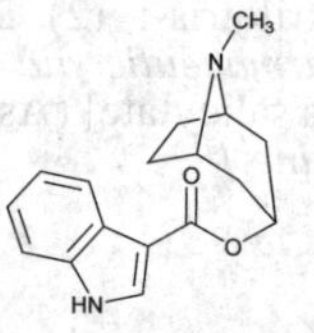

Troplasminogen Alfa. $C_{3875}H_{5917}N_{1107}O_{1190}S_{58}$. Thrombin-activable plasminogen: endo-[(558a(*559*)-558h(*365*))-human coagulation factor XI-(363-370)-peptide]-des-(559-562)-[606(*610*)-lysine,623(*627*)-lysine]human plasminogen, glycoform α. *CAS-931101-84-7*. INN.

Tropodifene. $C_{25}H_{29}NO_4$. 407.50. Tropine 3-(*p*-hydroxyphenyl-2-phenylpropionate (ester) acetate (ester). *CAS-15790-02-0*. INN.

Troquidazole. $C_{14}H_{15}N_5O_3$. 301.30. *N*′-(3-Nitro-4-quinolyl)-4-morpholinecarboxamidine. *UNII-41X4FOR202*. *CAS-108001-60-1*. INN.

Trospectomycin Sulfate [*1985*] (troe spek″ toe mye′ sin sul′ fate). $C_{17}H_{30}N_2O_7.H_2SO_4.5H_2O$. 562.58. [Trospectomycin is INN and BAN.] (1) 4*H*-Pyrano[2,3-*b*][1,4]benzodioxin-4-one, 2-butyldecahydro-4a,7,9-trihydroxy-6,8-bis(methylamino)-, [2*R*-(2α,4aβ,5aβ,6β,7β,8β,9α,9aα,10aβ)]-, sulfate (1:1) (salt), pentahydrate; (2) (2*R*,4a*R*,5a*R*,6*S*,7*S*,8*R*,9*S*,9a*R*,10a*S*)-2-Butyldecahydro-4a,7,9-trihydroxy-6,8-bis(methylamino)-4*H*-pyrano[2,3-*b*][1,4]benzodioxin-4-one sulfate (1:1) (salt), pentahydrate. *CAS-88851-61-0; CAS-88669-04-9* [trospectomycin]. *Antibacterial*. ◇*U-63,366F*

Trospium Chloride [*2001*] (trose′ pee um klor′ ide). $C_{25}H_{30}ClNO_3$. 427.96. (1) Spiro [8-azoniabicyclo[3.2.1]octane-8,1′-pyrrolidinium], 3-[(hydroxydiphenylacetyl)oxy]-, chloride, (1α, 3β, 5α); (2) 3α-Hydroxyspiro[1αH,5αH-nortropane-8,1′-pyrrolidinium] chloride benzilate. *UNII-1E6682427E*. *CAS-10405-02-4*. INN; BAN; JAN; MI. *Treatment of urinary incontinence*. Sanctura (Indevus) ◇*IP631*

Trovafloxacin Mesylate [*1995*] (troe″ va flox′ a sin mes′ i late). $C_{20}H_{15}F_3N_4O_3.CH_4O_3S$. 512.46. [Trovafloxacin is INN.] (1) 1,8-Naphthyridine-3-carboxylic acid, 7-(6-amino-3-azabicyclo[3.1.0]hex-3-yl)-1-(2,4-difluorophenyl)-6-fluoro-1,4-dihydro-4-oxo-(1α,5α,6α)-, monomethanesulfonate; (2) 7-[(1*R*,5*S*,6*s*)-6-Amino-3-azabicyclo[3.1.0]hex-3-yl]-1-(2,4-difluorophenyl)-6-fluoro-1,4-dihydro-4-oxo-1,8-naphthyridine-3-carboxylic acid, monomethanesulfonate. *UNII-0P1LKO80WN; UNII-9F388J00UK* [trovafloxacin]. *CAS-147059-75-4; CAS-147059-72-1* [trovafloxacin]. *Antibacterial*. Trovan (Pfizer) ◇*CP-99,219-27*

Trovirdine. $C_{13}H_{13}BrN_4S$. 337.24. 1-(5-Bromo-2-pyridyl)-3-[2-(2-pyridyl)ethyl]-2-thiourea. *UNII-ZE3K6J8614*. *CAS-149488-17-5*. INN.

Troxacitabine [*1998*] (trox″ a sye′ ta been). $C_8H_{11}N_3O_4$. 213.19. (1) (2*S*-*cis*)-4-Amino-1-[2-(hydroxymethyl)-1,3-dioxolan-4-yl]-2(1*H*)-pyrimidinone; (2) (-)-1-[(2*S*,4*S*)-2-(Hydroxymethyl)-1,3-dioxolan-4-yl]cytosine. *CAS-145918-75-8*. INN. *Antineoplastic used in the treatment of leukemias and solid tumors*. ◇*BCH-4556; (-)-OddC*

Troxerutin. $C_{33}H_{42}O_{19}$. 742.68. 3′,4′,7-Tris(hydroxyethyl)rutin. *UNII-7Y4N11PXO8*. *CAS-7085-55-4*. INN; BAN; DCF; MI. ◇*Z 6000; THR*

Troxidone (previously used name) — *See* Trimethadione.

Troxipide. $C_{15}H_{22}N_2O_4$. 294.35. (±)-3,4,5-Trimethoxy-*N*-3-piperidylbenzamide. *CAS-30751-05-4*. INN; JAN; MI.

---

† Brand name formerly used, and/or firm no longer concerned with this product.

Troxolamide. $C_{13}H_{25}N_2O_5$. 289.35. 3-[[2,3-Dihydroxy-1-(hydroxymethyl)propyl]carbamoyl]-2,2,5,5-tetramethyl-1-pyrrolidinyloxy. *CAS-97546-74-2.* INN.

Troxonium Tosilate. $C_{25}H_{37}NO_8S$. 511.63. Triethyl(2-hydroxyethyl)ammonium *p*-toluenesulfonate 3,4,5-trimethoxybenzoate. *CAS-391-70-8; CAS-4386-76-9* [troxonium]. INN; BAN. *[Name previously used: Troxonium Tosylate.]* ◇*FWH 399*

Troxypyrrolium Tosilate. $C_{25}H_{35}NO_8S$. 509.61. 1-Ethyl-1-(2-hydroxyethyl)pyrrolidinium *p*-toluenesulfonate 3,4,5-trimethoxybenzoate. *CAS-3612-98-4.* INN; BAN. *[Name previously used: Troxypyrrolium Tosylate.]*

Truxicurium Iodide. $C_{34}H_{52}I_2N_2O_4$. 806.60. Diethyl(3-hydroxypropyl)methylammonium iodide α-2,4-diphenyl-1,3-cyclobutanedicarboxylate. *CAS-4304-01-2.* INN.

Truxipicurium Iodide. $C_{38}H_{56}I_2N_2O_4$. 858.67. 1-Ethyl-1-(3-hydroxypropyl)piperidinium iodide α-2,4-diphenyl-1,3-cyclobutanedicarboxylate. *CAS-35515-77-6.* INN.

Tryparsamide. $C_8H_{10}AsN_2NaO_4.\frac{1}{2}H_2O$. 305.10. Monosodium *N*-(carbamoylmethyl)arsanilate. *UNII-4NN21HAX16. CAS-554-72-3.* USP XVII; INN; MI.

Trypsin, Crystallized (trip′ sin). **USP.** [Trypsin is BAN and JAN.] Proteolytic enzyme crystallized from an extract of the pancreas gland of the ox, *Bos taurus* Linné (Fam. Bovidae). *Enzyme (proteolytic).* Parenzyme (Marion Merrell Dow†)

Tryptophan [*1979*] (trip′ toe fan). **USP.** $C_{11}H_{12}N_2O_2$. 204.23. [L-Tryptophan is JAN.] (1) L-Tryptophan; (2) L-Tryptophan. *UNII-8DUH1N11BX. CAS-73-22-3* [L]. INN. *Amino acid.*

L-Tryptophan (JAN) — *See* Tryptophan.

Tuaminoheptane. $C_7H_{17}N$. 115.22. (1) 2-Heptanamine; (2) 1-Methylhexylamine. *CAS-123-82-0.* USP XXII; INN; BAN.

Tuaminoheptane Sulfate. $(C_7H_{17}N)_2.H_2SO_4$. 328.51. (1) 2-Heptanamine, sulfate (2:1); (2) 1-Methylhexylamine sulfate. *CAS-6411-75-2; CAS-123-82-0* [tuaminoheptane]. USP XX. Tuamine Sulfate (Lilly†)

Tuberculin (too ber′ kue lin). **USP.** A sterile solution derived from the concentrated, soluble products of growth of the tubercle bacillus (*Mycobacterium tuberculosis* or *Mycobacterium bovis*) prepared in a special medium. *Diagnostic aid (dermal reactivity indicator).* Aplisol (Parke-Davis); Aplitest (Parke-Davis†); Tine Test (Lederle); Tine Test PPD (Lederle)

Tuberculin, Old — *See* Tuberculin.

Tuberculin, Purified Protein Derivative of — *See* Tuberculin.

Tuberculosis Vaccine — *See* BCG Vaccine.

Tubocurarine Chloride (too″ boe kure ar′ een klor′ ide). **USP.** $C_{37}H_{41}ClN_2O_6.HCl.5H_2O$. 771.72. (1) Tubocuraranium, 7′,12′-dihydroxy-6,6′-dimethoxy-2,2′,2′-trimethyl-, chloride, hydrochloride, pentahydrate; (2) (+)-Tubocurarine chloride hydrochloride pentahydrate. *UNII-900961Z8VR. CAS-6989-98-6; CAS-57-94-3* [anhydrous]; *CAS-41354-45-4* [replaced]; *CAS-57-95-4* [tubocurarine]. INN; BAN; JAN. *Neuromuscular blocking agent.*

Tubulozole Hydrochloride [*1985*] (too bue′ loe zole hye″ droe klor′ ide). $C_{23}H_{23}Cl_2N_3O_4S.HCl$. 544.88. [Tubulozole is INN.] (1) Carbamic acid, [4-[[[2-(2,4-dichlorophenyl)-2-(1*H*-imidazol-1-ylmethyl)-1,3-dioxolan-4-yl]methyl]thio]phenyl]-, ethyl ester, monohydrochloride, *cis*-(±)-; (2) Ethyl (±)-*cis-p*-[[[2-(2,4-dichlorophenyl)-2-(imidazol-1-ylmethyl)-1,3-dioxolan-4-yl]methyl]thio]carbanilate, monohydrochloride. *CAS-83529-08-2; CAS-84697-22-3* [free base]. INN. *Antineoplastic (microtubule inhibitor).* ◇*R 46,846*

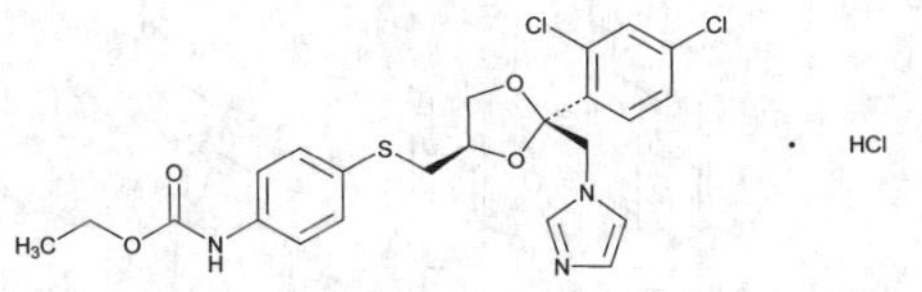

Tucaresol. $C_{15}H_{12}O_5$. 272.25. α-(2-Formyl-3-hydroxyphenoxy)-*p*-toluic acid. *CAS-84290-27-7.* INN; BAN. ◇*589C*

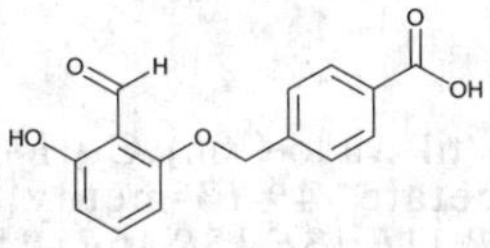

Tuclazepam. $C_{17}H_{16}Cl_2N_2O$. 335.23. 7-Chloro-5-(*o*-chlorophenyl)-2,3-dihydro-1-methyl-1*H*-1,4-benzodiazepine-2-methanol. *CAS-51037-88-8.* INN.

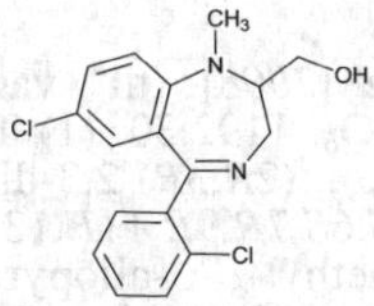

Tucotuzumab Celmoleukin [*2005*] (too″ koe tooz′ oo mab sel″ moe loo′ kin). $C_{7812}H_{12114}N_{2042}O_{2406}S_{60}$. Immunoglobulin G1, anti-(human antigen 17-1A) (human-mouse monoclonal huKS-IL2 heavy chain) fusion protein with interleukin 2 (human), disulfide with human-mouse monoclonal huKS-IL2 light chain, dimer. *CAS-339986-90-2.* INN. ◇*EMD 273066*

Tulathromycin [*2002*] (too lath″ roe mye′ sin). $C_{41}H_{79}N_3O_{12}$ (components A & B). 806.08. Component A: (1) 1-Oxa-6-azacyclopentadecan-15-one, 13-[(2,6-dideoxy-3-*C*-methyl-3-*O*-methyl-4-*C*-[(propylamino)methyl]-α-L-*ribo*-hexopyranosyl)oxy]-2-ethyl-3,4,10-trihydroxy-3,5,8,10,12,14-hexamethyl-11-[[3,4,6-trideoxy-3-(dimethylamino)-β-D-*xylo*-hexopyranosyl]oxy]-, (2*R*,3*S*,4*R*,5*R*,8*R*,10*R*,11*R*,12*S*,13*S*,14*R*)-; (2) (2*R*,3*S*,4*R*,5*R*,8*R*,10*R*,11*R*,12*S*,13*S*,14*R*)-13-[(2,6-Dideoxy-3-*C*-methyl-3-*O*-methyl-4-*C*-[(propylamino)methyl]-α-L-*ribo*-hexopyranosyl]oxy]-2-ethyl-3,4,10-trihydroxy-3,5,8,10,12,14-hexamethyl-11-[[3,4,6-trideoxy-3-(dimethylamino)-β-D-*xylo*-hexopyranosyl]oxy]-1-oxa-6-azacyclopentadecan-15-one. Component B: (1) 1-Oxa-4-azacyclotridecan-13-one, 11-[(2,6-dideoxy-3-*C*-methyl-3-*O*-methyl-4-*C*-[(propylamino)methyl]-α-L-*ribo*-hexopyranosyl)oxy]-2-(1,2-dihydroxy-1-methylbutyl)-8-hydroxy-3,6,8,10,12-pentamethyl-9-[[3,4,6-trideoxy-3-(dimethyl-amino)-β-D-*xylo*-hexopyranosyl]oxy]-, (2*S*,3*S*,6*R*,8*R*,9*R*,10*S*,11*S*,12*R*)-; (2) (2*R*,3*R*,6*R*,8*R*,9*R*,10*S*,11*S*,12*R*)-11-[(2,6-Dideoxy-3-*C*-methyl-3-*O*-methyl-4-*C*-[(propylamino)methyl]-α-L-*ribo*-hexopyranosyl]oxy]-2-[(1*S*,2*R*)-1,2-dihydroxy-1-methylbutyl]-8-hydroxy-3,6,8,10,12-pentamethyl-9-[[3,4,6-trideoxy-3-(dimethylamino)-β-D-*xylo*-hexopyranosyl]oxy]-

1-oxa-4-azacyclotridecan-13-one. *CAS-217500-96-4* (component A); *CAS-280755-12-6* (component B). INN. *Veterinary antibacterial.* ◇*CP-472,295; CP-547,272*

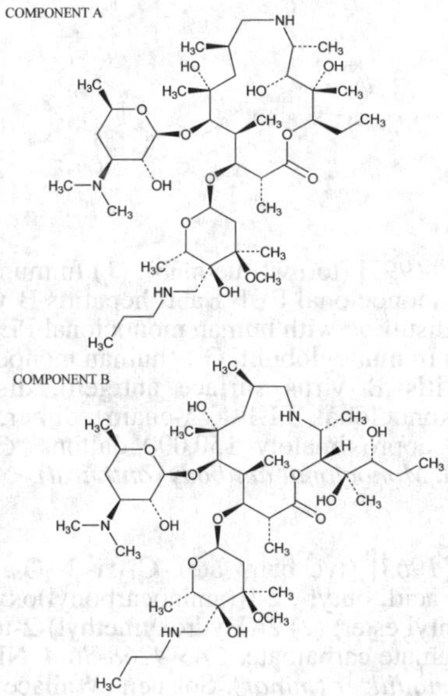

Tulobuterol. $C_{12}H_{18}ClNO$. 227.73. [Tulobuterol Hydrochloride is JAN.] α-[(*tert*-Butylamino)methyl]-*o*-chlorobenzyl alcohol. *CAS-41570-61-0.* INN; BAN; JAN; MI.

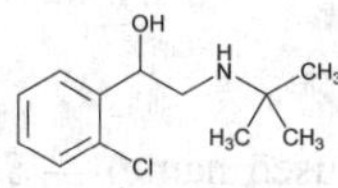

Tulopafant. $C_{25}H_{19}N_3O_2S$. 425.50. (+)-3′-Benzoyl-3-(3-pyridyl)-1*H*,3*H*-pyrrolo[1,2-*c*]thiazole-7-carboxanilide. *CAS-116289-53-3.* INN.

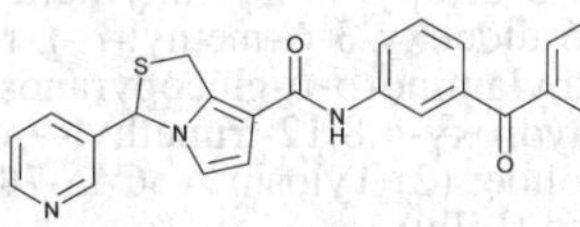

Turofexorate Isopropyl [*2008*] (tur″ oh fex′ oh rate). $C_{25}H_{24}F_2N_2O_3$. 438.47. (1) Azepino[4,5-*b*]indole-5-carboxylic acid, 3-(3,4-difluorobenzoyl)-1,2,3,6-tetrahydro-1,1-dimethyl-,1-methylethyl ester; (2) Isopropyl 3-(3,4-difluorobenzoyl)-1,1-dimethyl-1,2,3,6-tetrahydroazepino[4,5-*b*]indole-5-carboxylate. *UNII-S6KDM312I5. CAS-629664-81-9. Treatment of lipid disorders including hypertriglyceridemia and hypercholesterolemia.* ◇*FXR-450; WAY-362450*

Turosteride. $C_{27}H_{45}N_3O_3$. 459.66. 1,3-Diisopropyl-1-[(4-methyl-3-oxo-4-aza-5α-androstan-17β-yl)carbonyl]urea. *CAS-137099-09-3.* INN.

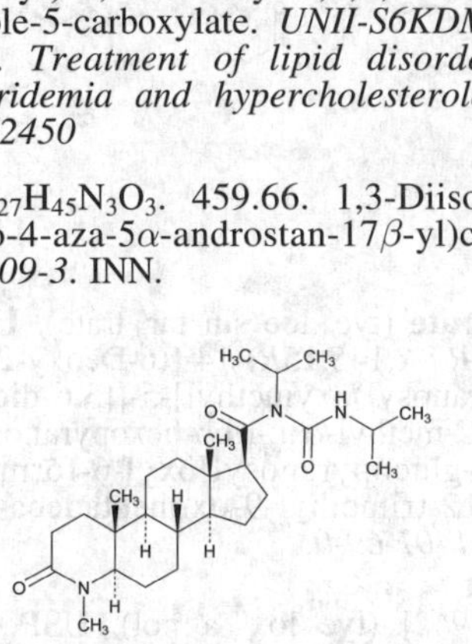

---

† Brand name formerly used, and/or firm no longer concerned with this product.

Tuvatidine. $C_{10}H_{17}N_9O_2S_3$. 391.50. [4-[[[2-[(5-Amino-4-methyl-4H-1,24,6-thriatriazin-3-yl)amino]ethyl]thio]methyl]-2-thiazolyl]guanidine S'',S''-dioxide. *UNII-TWN203TLYT. CAS-91257-14-6*. INN.

Tuvirumab [*1993*] (too vir' ue mab). (1) Immunoglobulin G 1 (human monoclonal PE1-1 anti-hepatitis B virus surface antigen), disulfide with human monoclonal PE1-1 λ-chain, dimer; (2) Immunoglobulin G 1 (human monoclonal PE1-1 anti-hepatitis B virus surface antigen), disulfide with human monoclonal PE1-1 λ-chain, dimer. Molecular weight is approximately 150,000 daltons. *CAS-138660-97-6*. INN. *Monoclonal antibody (antiviral).* ◇*PE1-1; SDZ OST 577*

Tybamate [*1963*] (tye bam' ate). $C_{13}H_{26}N_2O_4$. 274.36. (1) Carbamic acid, butyl-, 2-[[(aminocarbonyl)oxy]methyl]-2-methylpentyl ester; (2) 2-(Hydroxymethyl)-2-methylpentyl butylcarbamate carbamate. *CAS-4268-36-4*. NF XIII; INN; BAN. *Tranquilizer (minor).* Solacen (Wallace†) ◇*W 713*

Tyformin (previously used name) — *See* Tiformin.

Tylemalum — *See* Carbubarb.

Tylosin (tye' loe sin). **USP.** $C_{46}H_{77}NO_{17}$. 916.10. (1) (10E,12E)-(3R,4S,5S,6R,8R,14S,15R)-14-[(6-deoxy-2,3-di-O-methyl-β-D-allopyranosyl)oxymethyl]-5-[[3,6-dideoxy-4-O-(2,6-dideoxy-3-C-methyl-α-L-ribo-hexopyranosyl)-3-dimethylamino-β-D-glucopyranosyl]oxy]-6-formylmethyl-3-hydroxy-4,8,12-trimethyl-9-oxoheptadeca-10,12-dien-15-olide; (2) Tylosin A. *CAS-1401-69-0*. INN; BAN; MI. Tylan (Lilly)

Tylosin Tartrate (tye' loe sin tar' trate). **USP.** (10E,12E)-(3R,4S,5S,6R,8R,14S,15R)-14-[(6-Deoxy-2,3-di-O-methyl-β-D-allopyranosyl)oxymethyl]-5-[[3,6-dideoxy-4-O-(2,6-dideoxy-3-C-methyl-α-L-ribo-hexopyranosyl)-3-dimethyl-amino-β-D-glucopyranosyl]oxy]-6-formylmethyl-3-hydroxy-4,8,12-trimethyl-9-oxoheptadeca-10,12-dien-15-olide. *CAS-1401-69-0*.

Tyloxapol [*1962*] (tye lox' a pol). **USP.** (1) Phenol, 4-(1,1,3,3-tetramethylbutyl)-, polymer with formaldehyde and oxirane; (2) p-(1,1,3,3-Tetramethylbutyl)phenol poly-

mer with ethylene oxide and formaldehyde. *CAS-25301-02-4*. INN; BAN. *Detergent.* Superinone (Sterling Winthrop)

Tylvalosin [*2008*] (til'' va loe' sin). $C_{53}H_{87}NO_{19}$. 1042.25. (1) Tylosin, 3-acetate 4^B-(3-methylbutanoate); (2) (4R,5S,6S,7R,9R,11E,13E,15R,16R)-15-{[(6-Deoxy-2,3-di-O-methyl-β-D-allopyranosyl)oxy]methyl}-6-({3,6-dideoxy-4-O-[2,6-dideoxy-3-C-methyl-4-O-(3-methylbutanoyl)-α-L-*ribo*-hexopyranosyl]-3-(dimethylamino)-β-D-glucopyranosyl}oxy)-16-ethyl-5,9,13-trimethyl-2,10-dioxo-7-(2-oxoethyl)oxacyclohexadeca-11,13-dien-4-yl acetate. *CAS-63409-12-1*. INN. *Veterinary antibacterial.* Aivlosin (ECO Animal Health)

Tylvalosin Tartrate [*2008*] (til'' va loe' sin tar' trate). $C_{53}H_{87}NO_{19}.xC_4H_6O_6$. 1192.30. (1) Tylosin, 3-acetate 4^B-(3-methylbutanoate), (2R,3R)-2,3-dihydroxybutanedioate (salt); (2) (4R,5S,6S,7R,9R,11E,13E,15R,16R)-15-{[(6-Deoxy-2,3-di-O-methyl-β-D-allopyranosyl)oxy]methyl}-6-({3,6-dideoxy-4-O-[2,6-dideoxy-3-C-methyl-4-O-(3-methylbutanoyl)-α-L-*ribo*-hexopyranosyl]-3-(dimethylamino)-gb-D-glucopyranosyl}oxy)-16-ethyl-5,9,13-trimethyl-2,10-dioxo-7-(2-oxoethyl)oxacyclohexadeca-11,13-dien-4-yl acetate (2R,3R)-2,3-dihydroxybutanedioate. *CAS-63428-13-7*. *Control of swine enzootic pneumonia caused by Mycoplasma hyopneumoniae, swine dysentery caused by Brachyspira hyodysenteriae, and porcine proliferative enteropathy caused by Lawsonia intracellularis.* Aiviosin (ECO Animal Health)

Tymazoline. $C_{14}H_{20}N_2O$. 232.32. 2-(2-Isopropyl-5-methylphenoxymethyl)-2-imidazoline. *CAS-24243-97-8*. BAN.

Typhoid Vaccine. USP XXVI. *Immunizing agent (active).*

Typhus Vaccine. USP XX.

Tyromedan (INN) **Hydrochloride** — *See* Thyromedan Hydrochloride.

Tyropanoate Sodium [*1962*] (tye'' roe pa noe' ate soe' dee um). $C_{15}H_{17}I_3NNaO_3$. 663.00. [Sodium Tyropanoate is INN, BAN, and JAN.] (1) Benzenepropanoic acid, α-ethyl-2,4,6-triiodo-3-[(1-oxobutyl)amino]-, monosodium salt; (2) Sodium 3-butyramido-α-ethyl-2,4,6-triiodohydrocinnamate. *UNII-XRJ0P5FAYO; UNII-4F05V145YR* [tyropanic acid]. *CAS-7246-21-1; CAS-27293-82-9* [tyropanic acid]. USP XXIII. *Diagnostic aid (radiopaque medium, cholecystographic).* Bilopaque (GE Healthcare) ◇*Win 8851-2; NSC-107434*

Tyrosine [*1979*] (tye′ roe seen). **USP**. $C_9H_{11}NO_3$. 181.19. (1) L-Tyrosine; (2) L-Tyrosine. *UNII-42HK56048U. CAS-60-18-4* [L]. INN. *Amino acid.*

L-Tyrosine Ethylester Monohydrochloride. $C_{11}H_{15}NO_3 \cdot HCl$. 245.70. L-Tyrosine ethylester monohydrochloride. JAN.

Tyrothricin (tye″ roe thrye′ sin). **USP**. An antibacterial substance produced by the growth of *Bacillus brevis* Dubos (Fam. *Bacteriaceae*). *CAS-1404-88-2*. INN; BAN. *Antibacterial.* Bactratycin (Wallace†)

Ubenimex. $C_{16}H_{24}N_2O_4$. 308.37. (-)-*N*-[(2*S*,3*R*)-3-Amino-2-hydroxy-4-phenylbutyryl]-L-leucine. *CAS-58970-76-6*. INN; JAN; MI.

Ubidecarenone. $C_{59}H_{90}O_4$. 863.34. (1) 2,5-Cyclohexadiene-1,4-dione, 2-[(2*E*,6*E*,10*E*,14*E*,18*E*,22*E*,26*E*,30*E*,34*E*)-3,7,11,15,19,23,27,31,35,39-decamethyl-2,6,10,14,18,22,26,30,34,38-tetracontadecaenyl]-5,6-dimethoxy-3-methyl; (2) 2-[(*all-E*)-3,7,11,15,19,23,27,31,35,39-Decamethyl-2,6,10,14,18,22,26,30,34,38-tetracontadecaenyl)-5,6-dimethoxy-3-methyl-*p*-benzoquinone. *CAS-303-98-0*. NF XXI; INN; BAN; JAN.

Ubisindine. $C_{20}H_{24}N_2O$. 308.42. 2-[2-(Diethylamino)ethyl]-3-phenylphthalimidine. *UNII-FV251T245M. CAS-26070-78-0*. INN; BAN.

Udenafil. $C_{25}H_{36}N_6O_4S$. 516.66. 3-(1-Methyl-7-oxo-3-propyl-4,7-dihydro-1*H*-pyrazolo[4,3-*d*]pyrimidin-5-yl)-*N*-{2-[(2*RS*)-1-methylpyrrolidin-2-yl]ethyl}-4-propoxybenzenesulfonamide. *CAS-268203-93-6*. INN.

Ufenamate. $C_{18}H_{18}F_3NO_2$. 337.34. Butyl *N*-(α,α,α-trifluoro-*m*-tolyl)anthranilate. *CAS-67330-25-0*. INN; JAN.

Ufiprazole. $C_{17}H_{19}N_3O_2S$. 329.42. 5-Methoxy-2-[[(4-methoxy-3,5-dimethyl-2-pyridyl)methyl]thio]benzimidazole. *UNII-6FFV1V867C. CAS-73590-85-9*. INN.

Ularitide. $C_{145}H_{234}N_{52}O_{44}S_3$. 3505.93. L-Threonyl-L-alanyl-L-prolyl-L-arginyl-L-seryl-L-leucyl-L-arginyl-L-arginyl-L-seryl-L-seryl-L-cysteinyl-L-phenylalanylglycylglycyl-L-arginyl-L-methionyl-L-aspartyl-L-arginyl-L-isoleucylglycyl-L-alanyl-L-glutaminyl-L-serylglycyl-L-leucylglycyl-L-cysteinyl-L-asparaginyl-L-seryl-L-phenylalanyl-L-arginyl-L-tyrosine cyclic (11→27)-disulfide. *CAS-118812-69-4*. INN.

TAPRSLRRSS CFGGRMDRIG AQSGLGCNSF RY

Uldazepam [*1974*] (ul daz′ e pam). $C_{18}H_{15}Cl_2N_3O$. 360.24. (1) 3*H*-1,4-Benzodiazepin-2-amine, 7-chloro-5-(2-chlorophenyl)-*N*-(2-propenyloxy)-; (2) 2-[(Allyloxy)amino]-7-chloro-5-(*o*-chlorophenyl)-3*H*-1,4-benzodiazepine. *CAS-28546-58-9*. INN. *Sedative-hypnotic.* ◇*U-31,920*

Ulifloxacin. $C_{16}H_{16}FN_3O_3S$. 349.38. (1*RS*)-6-Fluoro-1-methyl-4-oxo-7-(piperazin-1-yl)-4*H*-[1,3]thiazeto[3,2-*a*]quinoline-3-carboxylic acid. *UNII-C38638H76Y. CAS-112984-60-8*. INN.

---

† Brand name formerly used, and/or firm no longer concerned with this product.

Ulinastatin. A glycoprotein of molecular weight about 67,000 isolated from human urine, inhibiting mainly proteolytic enzymes. INN; JAN.

Ulipristal. $C_{28}H_{35}NO_3$. 433.58. 11β-[4-(Dimethylamino)phenyl]-17-hydroxy-19-norpregna-4,9-diene-3,20-dione. *CAS-159811-51-5*. INN.

Ulobetasol (INN) — *See* Halobetasol Propionate.

Umespirone. $C_{28}H_{40}N_4O_5$. 512.64. *N*-Butyl-*N'*-[4-[4-(*o*-methoxyphenyl)-1-piperazinyl]butyl]-2,2-dimethyl-1,1,3,3-propanetetracarboxylic 1,3:1,3-diimide. *CAS-107736-98-1*. INN.

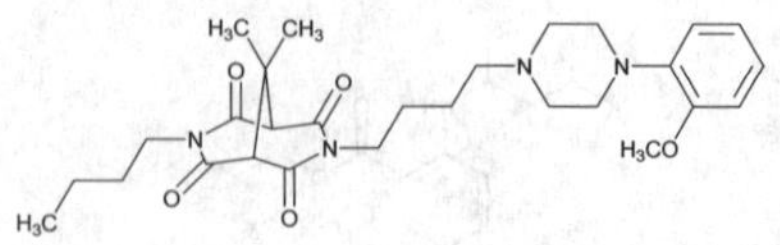

Undecoylium Chloride-Iodine. *CAS-1338-54-1*. MI; ND 1966.

Undecylenic Acid (un″ de sil en′ ik as′ id). USP. $C_{11}H_{20}O_2$. 184.28. (1) 10-Undecenoic acid; (2) 10-Undecenoic acid. *UNII-K3D86KJ24N*. *CAS-112-38-9*. JAN. *Antifungal*.

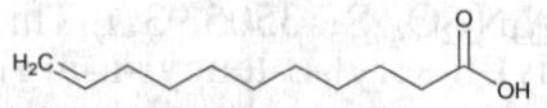

Unifocon A [*1990*] (ue″ ni foe′ kon). $(C_{16}H_{38}O_5Si_4)_v$ $(C_5H_8O_2)_w(C_8H_8F_6O_2)_x(C_4H_6O_2)_y(C_{16}H_{26}O_7)_z$. (1) 2-Propenoic acid, 2-methyl-, 3-[3,3,3-trimethyl-1,1-bis[(trimethylsilyl)oxy]disiloxanyl]propyl ester, polymer with methyl 2-methyl-2-propenoate, 2,2,3,4,4,4-hexafluorobutyl 2-methyl-2-propenoate, 2-methyl-2-propenoic acid and oxybis(2,1-ethanediyloxy-2,1-ethanediyl) bis(2-methyl-2-propenoate); (2) 3-[3,3,3-Trimethyl-1,1-bis(trimethylsiloxy)disiloxanyl]propyl methacrylate polymer with methyl methacrylate, 2,2,3,4,4,4-hexafluorobutyl methacrylate, methacrylic acid and tetraethylene glycol dimethacrylate. *CAS-126871-95-2*. *Contact lens material (hydrophobic)*. SGP 3 (Permeable Technologies) ◇*SGP 3*

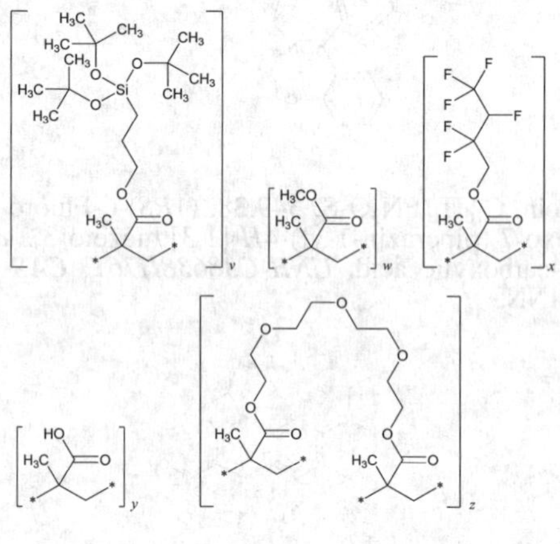

Unoprostone. $C_{22}H_{38}O_5$. 382.53. (+)-(*Z*)-7-[(1*R*,2*R*,3*R*,5*S*)-3,5-Dihydroxy-2-(3-oxodecyl)cyclopentyl]-5-heptenoic acid. *UNII-6X4F561V3W*. *CAS-120373-36-6*. INN.

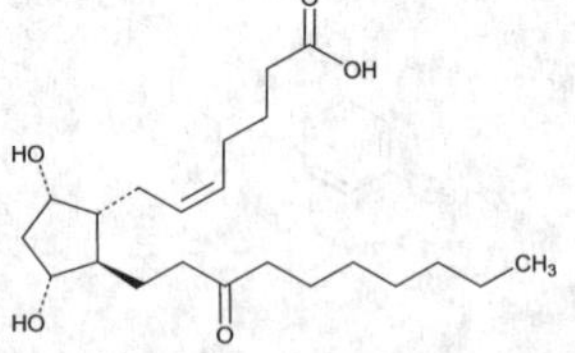

Upenazime. $C_{14}H_{30}N_4O_2$. 286.41. 3,3′-(Tetramethylenediimino)bis[3-methyl-2-butanone]dioxime. *CAS-95268-62-5*. INN; BAN. ◇*HL91*

Upidosin. $C_{31}H_{33}N_3O_4$. 511.61. *N*-[3-[4-(*o*-Methoxyphenyl)-1-piperazinyl]propyl]-3-methyl-4-oxo-2-phenyl-4*H*-1-benzopyran-8-carboxamide. *UNII-TXG28R7G4Y*. *CAS-152735-23-4*. INN.

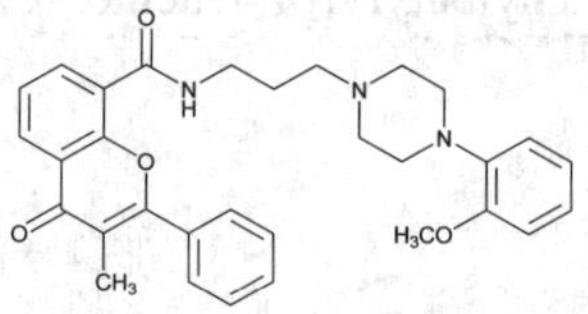

Uracil [*1997*] (ue′ ra sil; ure′ a sil). $C_4H_4N_2O_2$. 112.09. 2,4(1*H*,3*H*)-Pyrimidinedione. *CAS-66-22-8*. JAN. *Antineoplastic (adjunct)*. ◇*BMS-205603-01; SQ-6201; SQ-7726; SQ-8493*

Uracil Mustard [*1962*] (ue′ ra sil; ure′ a sil mus′ tard). $C_8H_{11}Cl_2N_3O_2$. 252.10. [Uramustine is INN and BAN.] (1) 2,4(1*H*,3*H*)-Pyrimidinedione, 5-[bis(2-chloroethyl)amino]-; (2) 5-[Bis(2-chloroethyl)amino]uracil. *UNII-W7KQ46GJ8U*. *CAS-66-75-1*. USP XXII. *Antineoplastic*. ◇*U-8344; NSC-34462*

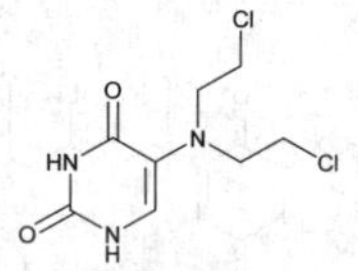

Uralenic Acid — *See* Enoxolone.

Uramustine (INN, BAN) — *See* Uracil Mustard.

Uranin — *See* Fluorescein Sodium.

Urapidil. $C_{20}H_{29}N_5O_3$. 387.48. 6-[[3-[4-(*o*-Methoxyphenyl)-1-piperazinyl]propyl]amino]-1,3-dimethyluracil. *CAS-34661-75-1*. INN; BAN; JAN; MI.

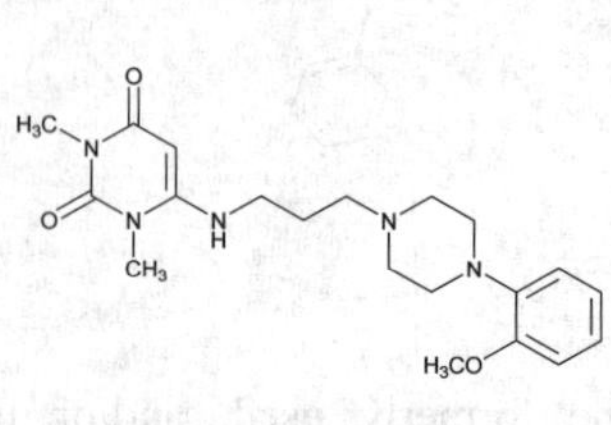

Urea (ue ree′ a; ure ee′ a). **USP.** CH_4N_2O. 60.06. (1) Urea; (2) Carbamide. *UNII-8W8T17847W. CAS-57-13-6.* JAN. *Diuretic.* Ureaphil (Hospira)

Urea C 13. USP. $^{13}CH_4N_2O$. 61.05. Urea [^{13}C]. *CAS-58069-82-2.*

Urea C 14. USP [Capsules]. $^{14}CH_4N_2O$. 62.05. Urea [^{14}C].

Uredepa [*1962*] (ure″ e dee′ pa). $C_7H_{14}N_3O_3P$. 219.18. (1) Carbamic acid, [bis(1-aziridinyl)phosphinyl]-, ethyl ester; (2) Ethyl [bis(1-aziridinyl)phosphinyl]carbamate. *CAS-302-49-8.* INN. *Antineoplastic.* ◇*AB-100; NSC-37095*

Uredofos [*1977*] (ue red′ oh fos; ure e′ doe fos). $C_{19}H_{25}N_4O_6PS_2$. 500.53. (1) Phosphoramidic acid, [[[2-[[[[(4-methylphenyl)sulfonyl]amino]carbonyl]amino]phenyl]amino]thioxomethyl]-, diethyl ester; (2) Diethyl [thio[*o*-3-(*p*-tolylsulfonyl)ureido]phenyl]carbamoyl]phosphoramidate. *UNII-P8W25X9B3K. CAS-52406-01-6.* INN; BAN. *Anthelmintic (veterinary).* ◇*RH-32,565; RH-565*

Urefibrate. $C_{15}H_{12}Cl_2N_2O_4$. 355.17. Glyoxyloylurea *aldehydo*-[bis(*p*-chlorophenyl)acetal]. *UNII-K0T77AAY7G. CAS-38647-79-9.* INN.

Urethan (NF XIII) — *See* Urethane.

---

† Brand name formerly used, and/or firm no longer concerned with this product.

Urethane. $C_3H_7NO_2$. 89.09. *UNII-3IN71E75Z5. CAS-51-79-6.* INN; DCF. *[Name previously used: Ethyl Carbamate.]* ◇*NSC-746*

Urofollitropin [*1987*] (ure″ oh fol″ i troe″ pin). A preparation of purified extract of human post-menopausal urine containing follicle-stimulating hormone (FSH). (1) Urofollitropin; (2) Urofollitropin. *UNII-W9BB98U6HP. CAS-97048-13-0.* INN; BAN. *Hormone (follicle-stimulating).* Bravelle (Ferring Pharmaceuticals); Fertinex (Serono); Metrodin (Serono) *[Name previously used: Urofollitrophin.]*

Urogastrone. An inhibitory factor of gastric secretion derived from human urine. *CAS-9010-53-1.* JAN.

Urokinase [*1965*] (ure″ oh kye′ nase). A plasminogen activator isolated from human sources. (1) Kinase (enzyme-activating), uro-; (2) Urokinase. *UNII-83G67E21XI. CAS-9039-53-6.* INN; BAN; JAN. *Plasminogen activator.* Abbokinase (Imarx)

Urokinase Alfa [*1997*] (ure″ oh kye′ nase al′ fa). Urokinase (enzyme-activating) (human clone pA3/pD2/pF1 high-molecular-weight isoenzyme protein moiety). Molecular weight is approximately 54,000 daltons (SDS gels). *CAS-99821-47-3.* INN. *Thrombolytic; plasminogen activator.* r-UK (Abbott) ◇*Abbott-76120; ABT-120*

Ursodeoxycholic Acid (INN, BAN) — *See* Ursodiol.

Ursodesoxycholic Acid (JAN) — *See* Ursodiol.

Ursodiol [*1988*] (ur″ soe dye′ ol). **USP.** $C_{24}H_{40}O_4$. 392.57. [Ursodeoxycholic Acid is INN and BAN; Ursodesoxycholic Acid is JAN.] (1) Cholan-24-oic acid, 3,7-dihydroxy-, ($3\alpha,5\beta,7\beta$)-; (2) $3\alpha,7\beta$-Dihydroxy-5β-cholan-24-oic acid. *UNII-724L30Y2QR. CAS-128-13-2. Anticholelithogenic.* Actigall (Watson); Urso (Axcan Scandipharm)

Ursulcholic Acid. $C_{24}H_{40}O_{10}S_2$. 552.70. $3\alpha,7\beta$-Dihydroxy-5β-cholan-24-oic acid bis(hydrogen sulfate). *CAS-88426-32-8.* INN.

Urtoxazumab. $C_{6414}H_{9934}N_{1718}O_{2010}S_{40}$. Immunogobulin anti-(*Escherichia coli* Shiga-like toxin II B subunit)(human-mouse hybridoma HuVTm1.1 γ-chain V-D-J region), disulfur with human-mouse hybridoma HuVTm1.1 κ-chain V-J region, dimer. *CAS-502496-16-4.* INN.

Ustekinumab [*2007*] (us″ te kin′ ue mab). $C_{6482}H_{10004}N_{1712}O_{2016}S_{46}$. (1) Immunoglobulin G1, anti-(human interleukin 12 p40 subunit) (human monoclonal CNTO 1275 γ1-chain), disulfide with human monoclonal CNTO 1275 κ-chain, dimer; (2) Immunoglobulin G1, anti-(human interleukin-12 subunit beta (IL-12B, CLMF p40,

NKSF2)) (human monoclonal CNTO 1275 γ1-chain), disulfide with human monoclonal CNTO 1275 κ-chain, dimer. Molecular weight is approximately 145,650 daltons. *CAS-815610-63-0.* INN. *Treatment of immunologically mediated inflammatory disorders.* ◇CNTO 1275

Utibapril. $C_{22}H_{31}N_3O_5S$. 449.56. (*S*)-2-*tert*-Butyl-4-[(*S*)-*N*-[(*S*)-1-carboxy-3-phenylpropyl]alanyl]-Δ²-1,3,4-thiadiazoline-5-carboxylic acid, 4-ethyl ester. *CAS-109683-61-6.* INN; BAN.

Utibaprilat. $C_{20}H_{27}N_3O_5S$. 421.51. (*S*)-2-*tert*-Butyl-4-[(*S*)-*N*-[(*S*)-1-carboxy-3-phenylpropyl]alanyl-Δ²-1,3,4-thiadiazoline-5-carboxylic acid. *UNII-KN82541NHV. CAS-109683-79-6.* INN; BAN.

Uva Ursi Fluidextract. The fluidextract obtained from bearberry leaf [the leaf of *Arctostaphylos uva-ursi* (Linné) Sprengel (*Ericaceae*)]. JAN.

Vabicaserin Hydrochloride [*2006*] (va″ bi ka′ ser in hye″ droe klor′ ide). $C_{15}H_{20}N_2$.HCl. 264.79. [Vabicaserin is INN.] (1) Cyclopenta[4,5]pyrido[3,2,1-*jk*][1,4]benzodiazepine, 4,5,6,7,9,9a,10,11,12,12a-decahydro-, monohydrochloride, (9a*R*,12a*S*)-rel-(-)-; (2) (-)-(9a*R**,12a*S**)-4,5,6,7,9,9a,10,11,12,12a-Decahydrocyclopenta[4,5]pyrido[3,2,1-*jk*][1,4]benzodiazepine monohydrochloride. *CAS-620948-34-7; CAS-620948-93-8* [vabicaserin]. *Treatment of schizophrenia.* ◇SCA-136

Vaccinia Immune Globulin (vax in′ ee a i mune′ glob′ ue lin). **USP.** A sterile, nonpyrogenic solution of globulins derived from the blood plasma of adult human donors who have been immunized with vaccinia virus (Smallpox Vaccine). *Immunizing agent (passive). [Name previously used: Vaccinia Immune Human Globulin.]*

Vaccinia Immune Human Globulin (previously used name) — *See* Vaccinia Immune Globulin.

Vadimezan. $C_{17}H_{14}O_4$. 282.29. 2-(5,6-Dimethyl-9-oxo-9*H*-xanthen-4-yl)acetic acid. *CAS-117570-53-3.* INN.

Vadocaine. $C_{18}H_{28}N_2O_2$. 304.43. (±)-6′-Methoxy-2-methyl-1-piperidinepropiono-2′,4′-xylidide. *UNII-OKA45SU1Q4. CAS-72005-58-4.* INN.

Valaciclovir (INN) — *See* Valacyclovir Hydrochloride.

Valacyclovir Hydrochloride [*1993*] (val″ ay sye′ kloe vir hye″ droe klor′ ide). $C_{13}H_{20}N_6O_4$.HCl. 360.80. [Valaciclovir is INN and BAN.] (1) L-Valine, 2-[(2-amino-1,6-dihydro-6-oxo-9*H*-purin-9-yl)methoxy]ethyl ester, mono-

hydrochloride; (2) L-Valine, ester with 9-[(2-hydroxyethoxy)methyl]guanine, monohydrochloride. *UNII-G447S0T1VC. CAS-124832-27-5; CAS-124832-26-4* [valacyclovir]. *Antiviral.* Valtrex (GlaxoSmithKline) ◇256U87 hydrochloride

Valategrast Hydrochloride [*2005*] (val a′ te grast hye″ droe klor′ ide). $C_{30}H_{32}Cl_3N_3O_4$.HCl. 641.41. [Valategrast is INN.] (1) L-Phenylalanine, *N*-(2-chloro-6-methylbenzoyl)-4-[(2,6-dichlorobenzoyl)amino-, 2-(diethylamino)ethyl ester, monohydrochloride; (2) 2-(Diethylamino)ethyl (2*S*)-2-[(2-chloro-6-methylbenzoyl)amino]-3-[4-[(2,6-dichlorobenzoyl)amino]phenyl]propanoate hydrochloride. *UNII-XN95730F0N. CAS-828271-96-1; CAS-220847-86-9* [valategrast]. *Treatment of asthma (dual α4β1/α4β7 integrin antagonist).* ◇R-411; Ro27-2441/002; Ro0272441/002

Valconazole. $C_{16}H_{18}Cl_2N_2O_2$. 341.23. (±)-2-(2,4-Dichlorophenoxy)-1-imidazol-1-yl-4,4-dimethyl-3-pentanone. *UNII-3EVI8KD2BC. CAS-56097-80-4.* INN; BAN.

Valdecoxib [*1998*] (val″ de kox′ ib). $C_{16}H_{14}N_2O_3S$. 314.36. (1) 4-(5-Methyl-3-phenyl-4-isoxazolyl)benzenesulfonamide; (2) *p*-(5-Methyl-3-phenyl-4-isoxazolyl)benzenesulfonamide. *UNII-2919279Q3W. CAS-181695-72-7.* INN; BAN. *Anti-inflammatory; analgesic (cyclooxygenase [COX]-2 inhibitor).* Bextra (Pfizer) ◇SC-65872

Valdetamide. $C_9H_{17}NO$. 155.24. 2,2-Diethyl-4-pentenamide. *UNII-1X50HHA8FY. CAS-512-48-1.* INN.

Valdipromide. $C_{11}H_{23}NO$. 185.31. 2,2-Dipropylvaleramide. *UNII-8JAK753213. CAS-52061-73-1.* INN.

Valepotriate — *See* Valtrate.

Valerian. Valerian consists of the subterranean parts of *Valeriana officinalis* Linné (Fam. Valerianaceae) including the rhizome, roots, and stolons. *UNII-JWF5YAW3QW.* NF XXI.

Valerian Extract, Powdered. NF XXI.

Valethamate Bromide. $C_{19}H_{32}BrNO_2$. 386.37. *N,N*-Diethyl-*N*-methyl-2-(3-methyl-2-phenylvaleryloxy)ethylammonium bromide. *CAS-90-22-2.* NF XIII; JAN; MI.

Valganciclovir Hydrochloride [*1997*] (val″ gan sye′ kloe vir hye″ droe klor′ ide). $C_{14}H_{22}N_6O_5 \cdot HCl$. 390.82. [Valganciclovir is INN and BAN.] L-Valine, ester with 9-[[2-hydroxy-1-(hydroxymethyl)ethoxy]methyl]guanine, monohydrochloride. *UNII-4P3T9QF9NZ; UNII-GCU97FKN3R* [valganciclovir]. *CAS-175865-59-5; CAS-175865-60-8* [valganciclovir]. *Antiviral.* Valcyte (Roche) ⟐*Ro107-9070/194; RS-079070-194*

Valine [*1979*] (val′ een). **USP.** $C_5H_{11}NO_2$. 117.15. [L-Valine is JAN.] (1) L-Valine; (2) L-Valine. *UNII-HG18B9YRS7. CAS-72-18-4* [L]. INN. *Amino acid.*

L-**Valine (JAN)** — *See* Valine.

Valnemulin. $C_{31}H_{52}N_2O_5S$. 564.82. [[2-[(*R*)-2-Amino-3-methylbutyramido]-1,1-dimethylethyl]thio]acetic acid, 8-ester with (3a*S*,4*R*,5*S*,6*S*,8*R*,9*R*,9a*R*,10*R*)-octahydro-5,8-dihydroxy-4,6,9,10-tetramethyl-6-vinyl-3a,9-propano-3a*H*-cyclopentacycloocten-1(4*H*)-one. *UNII-2AHC415BQG. CAS-101312-92-9.* INN; BAN.

Valnoctamide [*1963*] (val nok′ ta mide). $C_8H_{17}NO$. 143.23. (1) Pentanamide, 2-ethyl-3-methyl-; (2) 2-Ethyl-3-methyl-valeramide. *CAS-4171-13-5.* INN. *Tranquilizer.* Axiquel (Ortho-McNeil†) ⟐*McN-X-181; NSC-32363*

Valofane. $C_{10}H_{14}N_2O_4$. 226.23. (3-Allyltetrahydro-5-methyl-2-oxo-3-furoyl)urea. *UNII-X71N6E5IPO. CAS-3258-51-3.* INN.

Valomaciclovir. $C_{15}H_{24}N_6O_4$. 352.39. L-Valine, 4-ester with 9-[(*R*)-4-hydroxy-2-(hydroxymethyl)butyl]guanine. *CAS-195157-34-7.* INN.

Valomaciclovir Stearate [*2000*] (val oh ma sye′ kloe vir steer′ ate). $C_{33}H_{58}N_6O_5$. 618.85. (1) L-Valine, (3*R*)-3-[(2-amino-1,6-dihydro-6-oxo-9*H*-purin-9-yl)methyl]-4-[(1-oxooctadecyl)oxy]butyl ester; (2) L-Valine, 4-ester with 9-[(*R*)-4-hydroxy-2-(hydroxymethyl)butyl]guanine, stearate (ester). *CAS-195156-77-5. Treatment of herpes zoster (inhibitor of DNA polymerase).* ⟐*ABT-606; A-174606.0; MIV 606*

Valopicitabine Dihydrochloride [*2004*] (val oh″ pi sye′ ta been dye hye″ droe klor′ ide). $C_{15}H_{24}N_4O_6 \cdot 2HCl$. 429.30. [Valopicitabine is INN.] (1) L-Valine, 3′-ester with 2′-*C*-methylcytidine, dihydrochloride; (2) 4-Amino-1-[3-*O*-[(2*S*)-2-amino-3-methylbutanoyl]-2-*C*-methyl-β-D-ribofuranosyl]pyrimidin-2(1*H*)-one dihydrochloride; (3) Dihydrochloride of (2*R*,3*R*,4*R*,5*R*)-2-(4-amino-2-oxopyrimidin-1(2*H*)-yl)-3-hydroxy-5-(hydroxymethyl)-3-methyltetrahydrofuran-4-yl (2*S*)-2-amino-3-methylbutanoate. *UNII-7KNU786IT4; UNII-I2T0B5G94M* [valopicitabine]. *CAS-640725-71-9; CAS-640281-90-9* [valopicitabine]. *Treatment of chronic hepatitis C (HCV RNA polymerase inhibitor).* ⟐*NM283*

---

† Brand name formerly used, and/or firm no longer concerned with this product.

Valperinol. $C_{16}H_{27}NO_4$. 297.39. ($2R*,4R*,4aS*,5R*,7-S*,7aR*,8R*$)-Hexahydro-4-methoxy-8-methyl-7a(piperidinomethyl)-2,5-methanocyclopenta-*m*-dioxin-7-ol. *CAS-64860-67-9.* INN.

Valproate Pivoxil. $C_{14}H_{26}O_4$. 258.35. Hydroxymethyl 2-propylvalerate, pivalate. *UNII-9F5A05A29T. CAS-77372-61-3.* INN.

Valproate Semisodium (INN) — *See* Divalproex Sodium.

Valproate Sodium [*1975*] (val′ proe ate soe′ dee um). $C_8H_{15}NaO_2$. 166.19. [Sodium Valproate is JAN.] (1) Pentanoic acid, 2-propyl-, sodium salt; (2) Sodium 2-propylvalerate. *UNII-5VOM6GYJ0D; UNII-614OI1Z5WI* [valproic acid]. *CAS-1069-66-5; CAS-99-66-1* [valproic acid]. *Anticonvulsant.* Depacon (Abbott) ◇*Abbott 44090*

Valproic Acid [*1978*] (val proe′ ik as′ id). **USP.** $C_8H_{16}O_2$. 144.21. (1) Pentanoic acid, 2-propyl-; (2) Propylvaleric acid. *UNII-614OI1Z5WI. CAS-99-66-1.* INN; BAN. *Anticonvulsant.* Depakene (Abbott) ◇*44089*

Valpromide. $C_8H_{17}NO$. 143.23. 2-Propylvaleramide. *CAS-2430-27-5.* INN; MI.

Valrocemide [*2004*] (val roe′ se mide). $C_{10}H_{20}N_2O_2$. 200.28. (1) Pentanamide, *N*-(2-amino-2-oxoethyl)-2-propyl-; (2) *N*-(Carbamoylmethyl)-2-propylvaleramide; (3) *N*-(2-Amino-2-oxoethyl)-2-propylpentanamide. *UNII-1C7GO6OW7L. CAS-92262-58-3.* INN. *Antiepileptic; anticonvulsant.* ◇*TV-1901*

Valrubicin [*1997*] (val roo′ bi sin). **USP.** $C_{34}H_{36}F_3NO_{13}$. 723.64. (1) (*2S-cis*)-2-[1,2,3,4,6,11-Hexahydro-2,5,12-trihydroxy-7-methoxy-6,11-dioxo-4-[[2,3,6-trideoxy-3-[(trifluoroacetyl)amino]-α-L-*lyxo*-hexopyranosyl]oxy]-2-naphthacenyl]-2-oxoethyl pentanoate; (2) (8*S*,10*S*)-8-Glycoloyl-7,8,9,10-tetrahydro-6,8,11-trihydroxy-1-methoxy-10-[[2,3,6-trideoxy-3-(2,2,2-trifluoroacetamido)-α-L-*lyxo*-hexopyranosyl]oxy]-5,12-naphthacenedione 8^2-valerate. *UNII-2C6NUM6878. CAS-56124-62-0.* INN. *Antineoplastic.* Valstar (Indevus) ◇*AD 32; NSC-246131*

Valsartan [*1995*] (val sar′ tan). **USP.** $C_{24}H_{29}N_5O_3$. 435.52. (1) L-Valine, *N*-(1-oxopentyl)-*N*-[[2′-(1*H*-tetrazol-5-yl)[1,1′-biphenyl]-4-yl]methyl]-; (2) *N*-[*p*-(*o*-1*H*-Tetrazol-5-ylphenyl)benzyl]-*N*-valeryl-L-valine. *UNII-80M03YXJ7I. CAS-137862-53-4.* INN; BAN. *Antihypertensive.* Diovan (Novartis) ◇*CGP 48933*

Valspodar [*2000*] (val′ spoe dar). $C_{63}H_{111}N_{11}O_{12}$. 1214.62. (1) Cyclosporin D, 6-[(2*S*,4*R*,6*E*)-4-methyl-2-methylamino)-3-oxo-6-octenoic acid]-; (2) Cyclo[[(2*S*,4*R*,6*E*)-4-methyl-2-(methylamino)-3-oxo-6-octenoyl]-L-valyl-*N*-methylglycyl-*N*-methyl-L-leucyl-L-valyl-*N*-methyl-L-leucyl-L-alanyl-D-alanyl-*N*-methyl-L-leucyl-*N*-methyl-L-leucyl-*N*-methyl-L-valyl]. *CAS-121584-18-7.* INN; BAN. *Antineoplastic; multidrug resistance inhibitor.* Amdray (Novartis) ◇*SDZ PSC 833*

Valtorcitabine Dihydrochloride [*2003*] (val tor sye′ ta been dye hye″ droe klor′ ide). $C_{14}H_{22}N_4O_5$.2HCl. 399.27. [Valtorcitabine is INN.] (1) L-Valine, 3′-ester with β-L-2′-deoxycytidine, dihydrochloride; (2) 4-Amino-1-[3-*O*-[(2*S*)-2-amino-3-methylbutanoyl]-2-deoxy-β-L-*erythro*-pentofuranosyl]pyrimidin-2(1*H*)-one dihydrochloride. *UNII-5816OWJ81W. CAS-359689-54-6; CAS-380886-95-3* [valtorcitabine]. *Antiviral; treatment of Hepatitis B.* ◇*NM-147*

Valtrate. $C_{22}H_{30}O_8$. 422.47. 1,7a-Dihydro-1,6-dihydroxyspiro[cyclopenta[*c*]pyran-7-(6*H*),2′-oxirane]-4-methanol 4-acetate 1,6-diisovalerate. *CAS-18296-44-1.* INN.

Vamicamide. $C_{18}H_{23}N_3O$. 297.39. (±)-(*R**)-α-[(*R**)-2-(Dimethylamino)propyl]-α-phenyl-2-pyridineacetamide. *UNII-RU10K34QRU. CAS-132373-81-0.* INN.

Vancomycin (van″ koe mye′ sin). **USP.** $C_{66}H_{75}Cl_2N_9O_{24}$. 1449.25. (1) Vancomycin; (2) Vancomycin; (3) (S_a)-(3*S*,6*R*,7*R*,22*R*,23*S*,26*S*,36*R*,38a*R*)-44-[[2-*O*-(3-Amino-2,3,6-trideoxy-3-*C*-methyl-α-L-*lyxo*-hexopyranosyl)-β-D-glucopyranosyl]oxy]-3-(carbamoylmethyl)-10,19-dichloro-2,3,4,5,6,7,23,24,25,26,36,37,38,38a-tetradecahydro-7,22,28,30,32-pentahydroxy-6-[(2*R*)-4-methyl-2-(methylamino)valeramido]-2,5,24,38,39-pentaoxo-22*H*-8,11:18,21-dietheno-23,36-(iminomethano)-13,16:31,35-dimetheno-1*H*,16*H*-[1,6,9]oxadiazacyclohexadecino[4,5-*m*][10,2,16]benzoxadiazacyclotetracosine-26-carboxylic acid; (4) [3*S*-[3*R**,6*S**(*S**),7*S**,22*S**,23*R**,26*R**,36*S**,38a*S**]]-3-(2-Amino-2-oxoethyl)-44-[[2-*O*-(3-amino-2,3,6-trideoxy-3-*C*-methyl-α-L-*lyxo*-hexopyranosyl)-β-D-glucopyranosyl]oxy]-10,19-dichloro-2,3,4,5,6,7,23,24,25,26,36,37,38,38a-tetradecahydro-7,22,28,30,32-pentahydroxy-6-[[4-methyl-2-(methylamino)-1-oxopentyl]amino]-2,5,24,38,39-pentaoxo-22*H*-8,11:18,21-dietheno-23,36-(iminomethano)-13,16:31,35-dimetheno-1*H*,16*H*-[1,6,9]oxadiazacyclohexadecino[4,5-*m*][10,2,16]benzoxadiazacyclotetracosine-26-carboxylic acid. *UNII-6Q205EH1VU. CAS-1404-90-6.* BAN. *Antibacterial.*

Vancomycin Hydrochloride (van″ koe mye′ sin hye″ droe klor′ ide). **USP.** $C_{66}H_{75}Cl_2N_9O_{24}$.HCl. 1485.71. [Vancomycin is INN and BAN.] (1) Vancomycin, monohydrochloride; (2) Vancomycin monohydrochloride; (3) (S_a)-(3*S*,6*R*,7*R*,22*R*,23*S*,26*S*,36*R*,38a*R*)-44-[[2-*O*-(3-Amino-2,3,6-trideoxy-3-*C*-methyl-α-L-*lyxo*-hexopyranosyl)-β-D-glucopyranosyl]oxy]-3-(carbamoylmethyl)-10,19-dichloro-2,3,4,5,6,7,23,24,25,26,36,37,38,38a-tetradecahydro-7,22,28,30,32-pentahydroxy-6-[(2*R*)-4-methyl-2-(methylamino)valeramido]-2,5,24,38,39-pentaoxo-22*H*-8,11:18,21-dietheno-23,36-(iminomethano)-13,16:31,35-dimetheno-1*H*,16*H*-[1,6,9]oxadiazacyclohexadecino[4,5-*m*][10,2,16]benzoxadiazacyclotetracosine-26-carboxylic acid, monohydrochloride; (4) [3*S*-[3*R**,6*S** (*S**),7*S**,22*S**,23*R**,26*R**,36*S**,38a*S**]]-3-(2-Amino-2-oxoethyl)-44-[[2-*O*-(3-amino-2,3,6-trideoxy-3-*C*-methyl-α-L-*lyxo*-hexopyranosyl)-β-D-glucopyranosyl]oxy]-10,19-dichloro-2,3,4,5,6,7,23,24,25,26,36,37,38,38a-tetradecahydro-7,22,28,30,32-pentahydroxy-6-[[4-methyl-2-(methylamino)-1-oxopentyl]amino]-2,5,24,38,39-pentaoxo-22*H*-8,11:18,21-dietheno-23,36-(iminomethano)-13,16:31,35-dimetheno-1*H*,16*H*-[1,6,9]oxadiazacyclohexadecino[4,5-*m*][10,2,16]benzoxadiazacyclotetracosine-26-carboxylic acid, monohydrochloride. *UNII-71WO621TJD. CAS-1404-93-9; CAS-1404-90-6* [vancomycin]. JAN. *Antibacterial.* Vancocin Hydrochloride (ViroPharma)

Vandetanib [*2006*] (van det′ a nib). $C_{22}H_{24}BrFN_4O_2$. 475.35. (1) 4-Quinazolinamine, *N*-(4-bromo-2-fluorophenyl)-6-methoxy-7-[(1-methyl-4- piperidinyl)methoxy]-; (2) *N*-(4-Bromo-2-fluorophenyl)-6-methoxy-7-[(1-methylpiperidin-4-yl)methoxy]quinazolin-4-amine. *UNII-YO460OQ37K. CAS-443913-73-3; CAS-338992-00-0* [replaced]. INN; BAN; JAN. *Treatment of non-small cell lung cancer and other solid tumors.* Zactima (AstraZeneca) ◇ZD6474

Vaneprim. $C_{23}H_{28}N_4O_8S$. 520.56. (±)-α-[[4-Amino-5-(3,4,5-trimethoxybenzyl)-2-pyrimidinyl]amino]-3-ethoxy-4-hydroxy-α-toluenesulfonic acid. *UNII-M3EKF65MHG. CAS-81523-49-1.* INN.

Vangatalcite. $Al_2Mg_4(OH)_{12}CO_3 \cdot 3H_2O$. 469.33. Dialuminum tetramagnesium carbonate dodecahydroxide trihydrate. INN.

Vanilla (va nil′ a). **NF.** The cured, full-grown, unripe fruit of *Vanilla planifolia* Jacks., known in commerce as Mexican, Bourbon, or Madagascar vanilla, or of *Vanilla tahitensis* J.W. Moore, known in commerce as Tahitian vanilla (Fam. Orchidaceae). *Pharmaceutic aid (flavor).*

Vanillin (va nil′ in). **NF.** $C_8H_8O_3$. 152.15. (1) Benzaldehyde, 4-hydroxy-3-methoxy-; (2) Vanillin. *UNII-CHI530446X. CAS-121-33-5. Pharmaceutic aid (flavor).*

---

† Brand name formerly used, and/or firm no longer concerned with this product.

Vanitiolide. $C_{12}H_{15}NO_3S$. 253.32. 4-(Thiovanilloyl)morpholine. *UNII-26Y8H6WPAW. CAS-17692-71-6.* INN; DCF; MI.

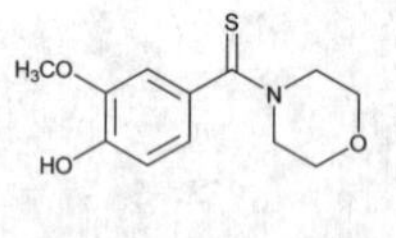

Vanoxerine. $C_{28}H_{32}F_2N_2O$. 450.56. 1-[2-[Bis(*p*-fluorophenyl)methoxy]ethyl]-4-(3-phenylpropyl)piperazine. *UNII-90X28IKH43. CAS-67469-69-6.* INN.

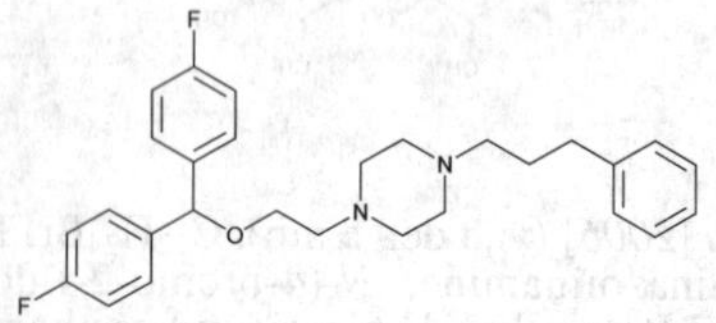

Vanyldisulfamide. $C_{20}H_{22}N_4O_6S_2$. 478.54. $N^4,N^{4'}$-Vanillylidenebis(sulfanilamide). *UNII-541ZDL2E7U. CAS-119-85-7.* INN; DCF.

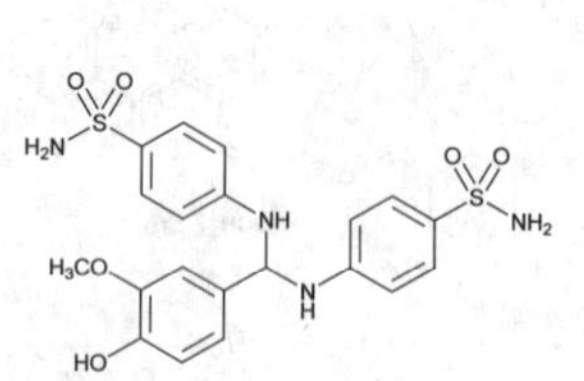

Vapaliximab. Immunoglobulin G2, anti-(human vascular adhesion protein VAP-1) (human-mouse monoclonal 2D10 γ2-chain), disulfide with human-mouse monoclonal 2D10 κ-chain, dimer. *CAS-336801-86-6.* INN.

Vapiprost Hydrochloride [*1989*] (va′ pi prost hye″ droe klor′ ide). $C_{30}H_{39}NO_4$·HCl. 514.10. [Vapiprost is INN and BAN.] (1) 4-Heptenoic acid, 7-[5-([1,1′-biphenyl]-4-ylmethoxy)-3-hydroxy-2-(1-piperidinyl)cyclopentyl]-, hydrochloride, [1*R*-[1α(*Z*),2β,3β,5α]]-; (2) (+)-(4*Z*)-7-[(1*R*,2*R*,3*S*,5*S*)-5-(4-Biphenylmethoxy)-3-hydroxy-2-piperidinocyclopentyl]-4-heptenoic acid, hydrochloride. *UNII-292V8Q1MXQ; UNII-H84XT1COAU* [vapiprost]. *CAS-87248-13-3; CAS-85505-64-2* [vapiprost]. *Antagonist (thromboxane A_2). ◇GR 32191B; GR 32191* [vapiprost]

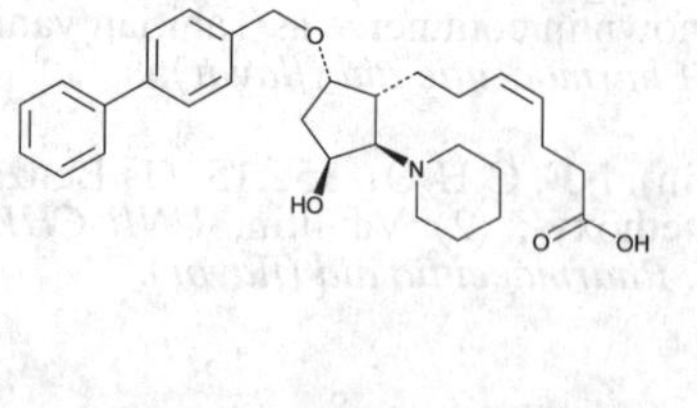

Vapitadine Dihydrochloride [*2006*] (va pi′ ta deen dye hye″ droe klor′ ide). $C_{17}H_{20}N_4O$·2HCl. 369.29. [Vapitadine is INN.] (1) Spiro[11*H*-imidazo[2,1-*b*][3]benzazepine-11,4′-piperidine]-3-carboxamide, 5,6-dihydro-, dihydrochloride; (2) 5,6-Dihydrospiro[11*H*-imidazo[2,1-*b*][3]benzazepine-11,4′-piperidine]-3-carboxamide dihydrochloride. *UNII-R612XR8A9F. CAS-279253-83-7; CAS-793655-64-8* [vapitadine]. *Treatment of atopic dermatitis. ◇R129160*

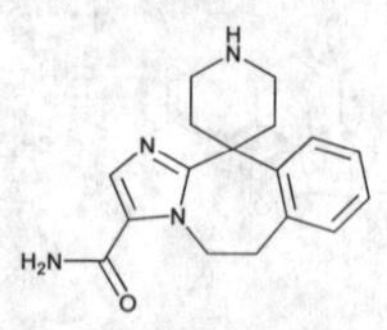

Vapreotide [*1989*] (va pree′ oh tide). $C_{57}H_{70}N_{12}O_9S_2$. 1131.37. (1) L-Tryptophanamide, D-phenylalanyl-L-cysteinyl-L-tyrosyl-D-tryptophyl-L-lysyl-L-valyl-L-cysteinyl-, cyclic (2→7)-disulfide; (2) D-Phenylalanyl-L-cysteinyl-L-tyrosyl-D-tryptophyl-L-lysyl-L-valyl-L-cysteinyl-L-tryptophanamide cyclic (2→7)-disulfide. *CAS-103222-11-3.* INN; BAN. *Antineoplastic. ◇RC-160; BMY-41606*

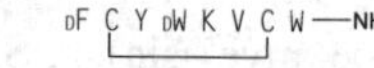

Vardenafil. $C_{23}H_{32}N_6O_4S$. 488.60. 1-[[3-(3,4-Dihydro-5-methyl-4-oxo-7-propylimidazo[5,1-*f*]-*as*-triazin-2-yl)-4-ethoxyphenyl]sulfonyl]-4-ethylpiperazine. *UNII-UCE6F4125H. CAS-224785-90-4.* INN; BAN.

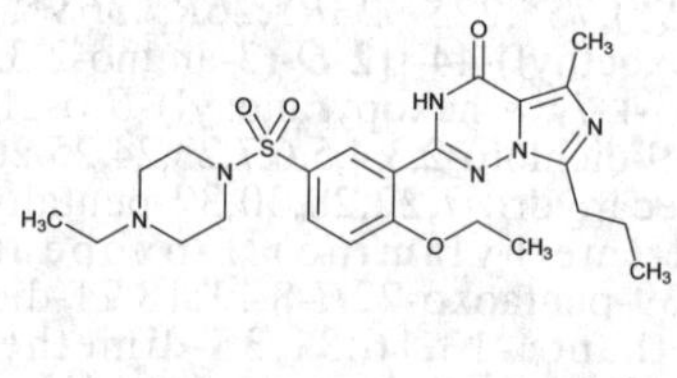

Vardenafil Dihydrochloride [*2001*] (var den′ a fil dye hye″ droe klor′ ide). $C_{23}H_{32}N_6O_4S$·2HCl. 561.52. Piperazine, 1-[[3-(1,4-dihydro-5-methyl-4-oxo-7-propylimidazo[5,1-*f*][1,2,4]triazin-2-yl)-4-ethoxyphenyl]sulfonyl]-4-ethyl-, dihydrochloride. *UNII-5O8R96XMH7. CAS-224789-15-5. Treatment of erectile dysfunction (PDE 5 inhibitor).*

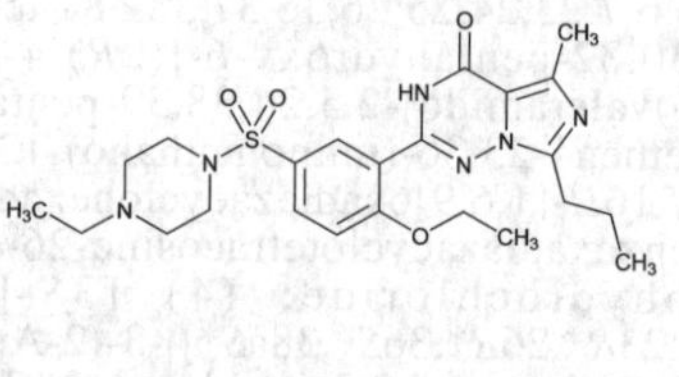

Varenicline Tartrate [*2003*] (var en′ i kleen tar′ trate). $C_{13}H_{13}N_3$·$C_4H_6O_6$. 361.35. [Varenicline is INN and BAN.] (1) 6,10-Methano-6*H*-pyrazino[2,3-*h*][3]benzazepine, 7,8,9,10-tetrahydro-, (2*R*,3*R*)-2,3-dihydroxybutanedioate (1:1); (2) 7,8,9,10-Tetrahydro-6,10-methano-6*H*-pyrazino[2,3-*h*][3]benzazepine (2*R*,3*R*)-2,3-dihydroxybutanedioate. *UNII-82269ASB48; UNII-W6HS99O8ZO* [varenicline]. *CAS-375815-87-5; CAS-249296-44-4* [varenicline]. *Smoking cessation (selective nicotinic receptor modulator).* Chantix (Pfizer) *◇CP-526,555-18*

Varespladib [*2008*] (var esp′ la dib). $C_{21}H_{20}N_2O_5$. 380.39. (1) Acetic acid, 2-[[3-(2-amino-2-oxoacetyl)-2-ethyl-1-(phenylmethyl)-1*H*-indol-4-yl]oxy]-; (2) {[3-(Aminooxoacetyl)-1-benzyl-2-ethyl-1*H*-indol-4-yl]oxy}acetic acid. *CAS-172732-68-2*. INN. *Treatment of dyslipidemia.*

Varespladib Methyl [*2008*] (var esp′ la dib meth′ il). $C_{22}H_{22}N_2O_5$. 394.42. (1) Acetic acid, [[3-(aminooxoacetyl)-2-ethyl-1-(phenylmethyl)-1*H*-indol-4-yl]oxy]-, methyl; ester; (2) Methyl {[3-(aminooxoacetyl)-1-benzyl-2-ethyl-1*H*-indol-4-yl]oxy}acetate. *UNII-0NB98NBX3D*. *CAS-172733-08-3*. *Treatment of dyslipidemia.* ◇*A-002; LY333013; S-3013*

Varespladib Sodium [*2002*] (var esp′ la dib soe′ dee um). $C_{21}H_{19}N_2NaO_5$. 402.38. [Varepladib is INN.] (1) Acetic acid, [[3-(aminooxoacetyl)-2-ethyl-1-(phenylmethyl)-1*H*-indol-4-yl]oxy]-, monosodium salt; (2) Sodium [[3-(aminooxoacetyl)-1-benzyl-2-ethyl-1*H*-indol-4-yl]oxy]acetate. *UNII-F6M52CDT0W*. *CAS-172733-42-5; CAS-172732-68-2* [varespladib]. *Treatment of sepsis (sPLA₂inhibitor)*. ◇*LY315920-Na⁺*

Varicella-Zoster Immune Globulin (var″ i sel′ a zos′ ter i mune′ glob′ ue lin). USP. A sterile $16.5 \pm 1.5\%$ solution of pH 7.0 containing the globulin fraction of human plasma consisting of not less than 99% of immunoglobulin G with traces of immunoglobulin A and immunoglobulin M, in 0.3 M glycine as a stabilizer and 1:10,000 thimerosal as a preservative. *Immunizing agent (passive).*

Variotin (JAN) — *See* Pecilocin.

Vasopressin (vay″ soe pres′ in). USP. $C_{46}H_{65}N_{15}O_{12}S_2$. 1084.23 (arginine form); $C_{46}H_{65}N_{13}O_{12}S_2$. 1056.22 (lysine form). (1) Vasopressin, 8-L-arginine-; (2) Vasopressin, 8-L-lysine-. *UNII-Y49070O6MFD* [arginine form]; *UNII-*

7CZF3L922Y [lysine form]. *CAS-113-79-1* [arginine form]; *CAS-50-57-7* [lysine form]. INN; JAN. *Hormone (antidiuretic).* Pitressin (Parke-Davis)

* in pig vasopressin, R is K

Vasopressin Tannate. A mixture of 8-L-arginine vasopressin tannate and 8-L-lysine vasopressin tannate. JAN. Pitressin Tannate (King)

Vasurfilcon A [*1987*] (vay″ sur fil′ kon). $(C_{18}H_{18}ClN_3O)_w(C_6H_9NO)_x(C_5H_8O_2)_y(C_7H_{10}O_2)_z$. 1-Vinyl-2-pyrrolidinone polymer with methyl methacrylate, allyl methacrylate and 2-(3′-*t*-butyl-2′-hydroxy-5′-vinylphenyl)-5-chlorobenzotriazole. *Contact lens material (hydrophilic).* Permaflex UV Naturals 74 (CooperVision)

Vatalanib [*2004*] (va tal′ a nib). $C_{20}H_{15}ClN_4$. 346.81. (1) 1-Phtalazinamine, *N*-(4-chlorophenyl)-4-(4-pyridinylmethyl)-; (2) *N*-(4-chlorophenyl)-4-(pyridin-4-ylmethyl)phtalazin-1-amine. *UNII-5DX9U76296*. *CAS-212141-54-3*. INN. *Treatment of tumors.* ◇*PTK787*

Vatanidipine. $C_{41}H_{42}N_4O_6$. 686.80. (±)-*p*-[4-(Diphenylmethyl)-1-piperazinyl]phenethyl]methyl 1,4-dihydro-2,6-dimethyl-4-(*m*-nitrophenyl)-3,5-pyridinedicarboxylate. *CAS-116308-55-5*. INN.

Vatreptacog Alfa (activated). $C_{1981}H_{3051}N_{561}O_{620}S_{27}$. [158-Aspartic acid, 296-valine, 298-glutamine]human coagulation factor VII activated, recombinant DNA origin. *CAS-897936-89-9*. INN.

Vebufloxacin. $C_{19}H_{22}FN_3O_3$. 359.39. (±)-9-Fluoro-6,7-dihydro-5-methyl-8-(4-methyl-1-piperazinyl)-1-oxo-1*H*,5*H*-benzo[*ij*]quinolizine-2-carboxylic acid. *CAS-79644-90-9*. INN.

Vecuronium Bromide [*1984*] (vek″ ue roe′ nee um broe′ mide; vek′ ure oh″ nee um broe′ mide). USP. $C_{34}H_{57}BrN_2O_4$. 637.73. (1) Piperidinium, 1-[(2β,3α,5α,16β,17β)-3,17-bis(acetyloxy)-2-(1-piperidinyl)androstan-16-yl]-1-methyl-, bromide; (2) 1-(3α,17β-Dihydroxy-2β-piperidino-5α-androstan-16β,5α-yl)-1-methylpiperidinium bromide, diacetate. *UNII-7E4PHP5N1D*. *CAS-50700-72-6*. INN; BAN; JAN. *Neuromuscular blocking agent.* Norcuron (Organon) ◇*ORG NC 45*

---

† Brand name formerly used, and/or firm no longer concerned with this product.

Vedaclidine. C$_{13}$H$_{21}$N$_3$S$_2$. 283.46. (*S*)-3-[4-(Butylthio)-1,2,5-thiadiazol-3-yl]quinuclidine. *UNII-98IW5HAV1N. CAS-141575-50-0.* INN.

Vedaprofen [*1994*] (ved″ a proe′ fen). C$_{19}$H$_{22}$O$_2$. 282.38. (1) 1-Naphthaleneacetic acid, 4-cyclohexyl-α-methyl-, (±)-; (2) (±)-4-Cyclohexyl-α-methyl-1-naphthaleneacetic acid. *UNII-OKX88EO7OI. CAS-71109-09-6.* INN; BAN. *Anti-inflammatory (veterinary).* ◇*CERM 10202; PM 150*

Vedolizumab [*2008*] (ve″ doe liz′ oo mab). C$_{6528}$H$_{10072}$N$_{1732}$O$_{2042}$S$_{42}$. Immunoglobulin G1, anti-(human integrin LPAM-1 (lymphocyte Peyer's patch adhesion molecule 1)) (human-*Mus musculus* heavy chain), disulfide with human-*Mus musculus* κ-chain, dimer. Molecular weight is approximately 146,800 daltons. *CAS-943609-66-3. Treatment of ulcerative colitis and Crohn's disease.* ◇*MLN0002; MLN02; LDP02*

Vegetable Oil, Hydrogenated (vej′ ta bul). **NF**. A mixture of triglycerides of fatty acids. *Pharmaceutic aid (tablet and/or capsule lubricant).*

Velafermin [*2005*] (vel″ a fer′ min). C$_{1047}$H$_{1632}$N$_{306}$O$_{302}$S$_5$. Fibroblast growth factor-20 (human recombinant CG53135). Molecular weight is approximately 23,500 daltons. *CAS-697766-75-9.* INN. *Treatment and/or prevention of mucositis.* ◇*CG53135-05*

```
MAPLAEVGGF LGGLEGLGQQ VGSHFLLPPA GERPPLLGER RSAAERSARG
GPGAAQLAHL HGILRRRQLY CRTGFHLQIL PDGSVQGTRQ DHSLFGILEF
ISVAVGLVSI RGVDSGLYLG MNDKGELYGS EKLTSECIFR EQFEENWYNT
YSSNIYKHGD TGRRYFVALN KDGTPRDGAR SKRHQKFTHF LPRPVDPERV
PELYKDLLMY T
```

Velaglucerase Alfa [*2007*] (vel″ a gloo′ ser ase al′ fa). C$_{2532}$H$_{3850}$N$_{672}$O$_{711}$S$_{16}$. (1) Ceramidase, glucosyl-(human HT-1080 cell); (2) Human glucosylceramidase (EC 3.2.1.45 or Beta-glucocerebrosidase), glycoform α. Molecular weight is approximately 55,600 daltons (protein). *CAS-884604-91-5.* INN. *Treatment of patients with Gaucher disease.* ◇*EC 3.2.1.45*

```
          *
ARPCIPKSFG YSSVVCVCNA TYCDSFDPPT FPALGTFSRY ESTRSGRRME
     *
LSMGPIQANH TGTGLLLTLQ PEQKFQKVKG FGGAMTDAAA LNILALSPPA
QNLLLKSYFS EEGIGYNIIR VPMASCDFSI RTYTYADTPD DFQLHNFSLP
EEDTKLKIPL IHRALQLAQR PVSLLASPWT SPTWLKTNGA VNGKGSLKGQ
PGDIYHQTWA RYFVKFLDAY AEHKLQFWAV TAENEPSAGL LSGYPFQCLG
FTPEHQRDFI ARDLGPTLAN STHHNVRLLM LDDQRLLLPH WAKVVLTDPE
AAKYVHGIAV HWYLDFLAPA KATLGETHRL FPNTMLFASE ACVGSKFWEQ
SVRLGSWDRG MQYSHSIITN LLYHVVGWTD WNLALNPEGG PNWVRNFVDS
PIIVDITKDT FYKQPMFYHL GHFSKFIPEG SQRVGLVASQ KNDLDAVALM
HPDGSAVVVV LNRSSKDVPL TIKDPAVGFL ETISPGYSIH TYLWRRQ
```

* - glycosylation site

Velaresol. C$_{12}$H$_{14}$O$_5$. 238.24. 5-(2-Formyl-3-hydroxyphenoxy)valeric acid. *CAS-77858-21-0.* INN; BAN. ◇*12C*

Veliflapon [*2006*] (vel″ i flap′ on). C$_{23}$H$_{23}$NO$_3$. 361.43. (1) Benzeneacetic acid, α-cyclopentyl-4-(2-quinolinyl-methoxy)-, (αR)-; (2) (+)-(2R)-Cyclopentyl(quinolin-2-ylmethoxy)acetic acid. *CAS-128253-31-6.* INN. *Prevention of acute cardiovascular events.* ◇*DG-031; Bay x 1005*

Velimogene Aliplasmid [*2006*] (ve lim′ oh jeen″ al″ i plas′ mid). (1) DNA (plasmid VCL-1005); (2) VCL-1005 plasmid DNA formulated with a lipid-based system, DMRIE/DOPE [(±)-*N*-(2-hydroxyethyl)-*N*,*N*-dimethyl-2,3-bis(tetradecyloxy)-1-propanaminium bromide/dioleoylphosphatidylethanolamine]. *CAS-296251-72-4.* INN. *Treatment of cancer.* Allovectin (Vical)

Velnacrine Maleate [*1989*] (vel′ na kreen mal′ ee ate). C$_{13}$H$_{14}$N$_2$O.C$_4$H$_4$O$_4$. 330.34. [Velnacrine is INN and BAN.] (1) 1-Acridinol, 9-amino-1,2,3,4-tetrahydro-, (±)-, (Z)-2-butenedioate (1:1) (salt); (2) (±)-9-Amino-1,2,3,4-tetrahydro-1-acridinol maleate (1:1) (salt). *CAS-118909-22-1; CAS-104675-29-8 [velnacrine]. Inhibitor (cholinesterase).* Mentane (Hoechst-Roussel†) ◇*HP 029; P83 6029A*

Velneperit [*2008*] (vel nep′ er it). C$_{17}$H$_{24}$F$_3$N$_3$O$_3$S. 407.45. (1) Cyclohexanecarboxamide, 4-[[(1,1-dimethylethyl)sulfonyl]amino]-*N*-[5-(trifluoromethyl)-2-pyridinyl]-, *trans*-; (2) *trans*-4-[[(1,1-Dimethylethyl)sulfonyl]amino]-*N*-[5-(trifluoromethyl)pyridin-2-yl]cyclohexanecarboxamide. *CAS-342577-38-2.* INN. *Treatment of clinical obesity.* ◇*S-2367*

Veltuzumab [*2007*] (vel tooz′ oo mab). C$_{6458}$H$_{9918}$N$_{1706}$O$_{2026}$S$_{46}$. (1) Immunoglobulin G1, anti-(human CD20 (antigen)) (human-mouse monoclonal hA20 heavy chain), disulfide with human-mouse monoclonal hA20 κ-chain, dimer; (2) Immunoglobulin G1, anti-(human B-lymphocyte antigen CD20 (Membrane-spanning 4-domains subfamily A member 1, Leu-16, Bp35)); [218-arginine,360-glutamic acid,362-methionine]humanized mouse monoclonal hA20 γ1 heavy chain (224-213′)-disulfide with humanized mouse monoclonal hA20 κ light chain (230-230″:233-233″)-bisdisulfide dimer. Molecular weight is approximately 145,300 daltons. *CAS-728917-18-8.* INN. *Treatment of non-Hodgkin's lymphoma.* ◇*IMMU-106*

Venlafaxine Hydrochloride [*1989*] (ven″ la fax′ een hye″ droe klor′ ide). C$_{17}$H$_{27}$NO$_2$.HCl. 313.86. [Venlafaxine is INN and BAN.] (1) Cyclohexanol, 1-[2-(dimethylamino)-1-(4-methoxyphenyl)ethyl]-, hydrochloride; (2) (±)-1-[α-[(Dimethylamino)methyl]-*p*-methoxybenzyl]cyclohexanol hydrochloride. *UNII-7D7RX5A8MO; UNII-*

GRZ5RCB1QG [venlafaxine]. *CAS-99300-78-4; CAS-93413-69-5* [venlafaxine]. *Antidepressant.* Effexor (Wyeth) ◇*WY-45,030*

Venritidine. $C_{18}H_{26}N_4O_3S$. 378.49. (±)-(*Z*)-*N*-Methyl-2-nitro-*N'*-[2-[[5-[(tricyclo[2.2.1.O^{2,6}]hept-3-ylamino)methyl]-furfuryl]thio]ethyl]-1,1-ethenediamine. *CAS-93064-63-2.* INN.

Vepalimomab. Immunoglobulin M (mouse monoclonal 1B2 *μ*-chain anti-human vascular adhesion protein VAP-1), disulfide with mouse monoclonal 1B2 light chain, dimer. *CAS-195158-85-1.* INN.

Veradoline Hydrochloride [*1981*] (ver ad′ oh leen hye″ droe klor′ ide). $C_{20}H_{26}N_2O_2$.2HCl. 399.35. [Veradoline is INN.] (1) Benzenamine, 4-[2-(3,4-dihydro-6,7-dimethoxy-1-methyl-2(1*H*)-isoquinolinyl)ethyl]-, dihydrochloride, (±)-; (2) (±)-2-(*p*-Aminophenethyl)-1,2,3,4-tetrahydro-6,7-dimethoxy-1-methylisoquinoline dihydrochloride. *CAS-76448-47-0; CAS-79201-80-2* [veradoline]. *Analgesic.* ◇*PR-870-714A*

Veralipride. $C_{17}H_{25}N_3O_5S$. 383.46. *N*-[(1-Allyl-2-pyrrolidinyl)methyl]-5-sulfamoyl-*o*-veratramide. *CAS-66644-81-3.* INN; MI.

Verapamil [*1968*] (ver ap′ a mil). $C_{27}H_{38}N_2O_4$. 454.60. (1) Benzeneacetonitrile, *α*-[3-[[2-(3,4-dimethoxyphenyl)ethyl]methylamino]propyl]-3,4-dimethoxy-*α*-(1-methylethyl)-; (2) 5-[(3,4-Dimethoxyphenethyl)methylamino]-2-(3,4-dimethoxyphenyl)-2-isopropylvaleronitrile. *UNII-CJ0O37KU29. CAS-52-53-9.* INN; BAN. *Vasodilator (coronary).* ◇*D-365; CP-16,533-1*

---

† Brand name formerly used, and/or firm no longer concerned with this product.

Verapamil Hydrochloride [*1981*] (ver ap′ a mil hye″ droe klor′ ide). **USP.** $C_{27}H_{38}N_2O_4$.HCl. 491.06. (1) Benzeneacetonitrile, *α*-[3-[[2-(3,4-dimethoxyphenyl)ethyl]methylamino]propyl]-3,4-dimethoxy-*α*-(1-methylethyl)-, monohydrochloride, (±)-; (2) (±)-5-[(3,4-Dimethoxyphenethyl)methylamino]-2-(3,4-dimethoxyphenyl)-2-isopropylvaleronitrile monohydrochloride. *UNII-V3888OEY5R. CAS-152-11-4.* JAN. *Anti-anginal; cardiac depressant (anti-arrhythmic).* Calan (Pfizer); Covera (Pfizer); Isoptin (Ranbaxy); Verelan (Elan)

Veratrylidene-Isoniazid — *See* Verazide.

Verazide. $C_{15}H_{15}N_3O_3$. 285.30. 1-Isonicotinoyl-2-veratrylidenehydrazine. *CAS-93-47-0.* INN; BAN; MI.

Verilopam Hydrochloride [*1979*] (ver il′ oh pam hye″ droe klor′ ide). $C_{20}H_{26}N_2O_2$.2HCl. 399.35. [Verilopam is INN.] (1) Benzenamine, 4-[2-(1,2,4,5-tetrahydro-7,8-dimethoxy-3*H*-3-benzazepin-3-yl)ethyl]-, dihydrochloride; (2) 3-(*p*-Aminophenethyl)-2,3,4,5-tetrahydro-7,8-dimethoxy-1*H*-3-benzazepine dihydrochloride. *UNII-7SJF09406G. CAS-67394-31-4; CAS-68318-20-7* [verilopam]. *Analgesic.* ◇*PR-0818-156A*

Verlukast [*1990*] (ver loo′ kast). $C_{26}H_{27}ClN_2O_3S_2$. 515.09. (1) Propanoic acid, 3-[[[3-[2-(7-chloro-2-quinolinyl)ethenyl]phenyl][[3-(dimethylamino)-3-oxopropyl]thio]methyl]thio]-, [*R*-(*E*)]-; (2) 3-[[(*αR*)-*m*-[(*E*)-2-(7-Chloro-2-quinolyl)vinyl]-*α*-[[2-(dimethylcarbamoyl)ethyl]thio]benzyl]thio]propionic acid. *CAS-120443-16-5.* INN. *Anti-asthmatic (leukotriene antagonist).* ◇*MK-679; L-668,019*

Vernakalant Hydrochloride [*2006*] (ver nak′ a lant hye″ droe klor′ ide). $C_{20}H_{31}NO_4$.HCl. 385.93. [Vernakalant is INN.] (1) 3-Pyrrolidinol, 1-[(1*R*,2*R*)-2-[2-(3,4-dimethoxyphenyl)ethoxy]cyclohexyl]-, hydrochloride, (3*R*)-; (2) (3*R*)-1-[(1*R*,2*R*)-2-[2-(3,4-dimethoxyphenyl)ethoxy]cyclohexyl]pyrrolidin-3-ol hydrochloride. *CAS-748810-28-8; CAS-794466-70-9* [vernakalant]. *Treatment of patients with atrial fibrillation and atrial flutter.* ◇*RSD1235*

Verofylline [*1979*] (ver of′ i lin). $C_{12}H_{18}N_4O_2$. 250.30. (1) 1*H*-Purine-2,6-dione, 3,7-dihydro-1,8-dimethyl-3-(2-methylbutyl)-, (±)-; (2) (±)-1,8-Dimethyl-3-(2-methybutyl)xanthine. *CAS-66172-75-6.* INN. *Bronchodilator; anti-asthmatic.* ◇*CK-0383*

Verpasep Caltespen [*2005*] (ver′ pa sep kal tes′ pen). $C_{2959}H_{4860}N_{810}O_{965}S_{16}$ (reduced peptide). Heat-shock protein HSP 65 (*Mycobacterium bovis* strain BCG) fusion protein with transcription factor E7 (human papillomavirus 16). *CAS-295371-00-5.* INN. *Treatment of diseases caused by human papillomavirus.* ◇*HspE7; BCG65-E7*

```
AKTIAYDEEA RRGLERGLNA LADAVKVTLG PKGRNVVLEK KWGAPTITND
GVSIAKEIEL EDPYEKIGAE LVKEVAKKTD DVAGDGTTTA TVLAQALVRE
GLRNVAAGAN PLGLKRGIEK AVEKVTETLL KGAKEVETKE QIAATAAISA
GDQSIGDLIA EAMDKVGNEG VITVEESNTF GLQLELTEGM RFDKGYISGY
FVTDPERQEA VLEDPYILLV SSKVSTVKDL LPLLEKVIGA GKPLLIIAED
VEGEALSTLV VNKIRGTFKS VAVKAPGFGD RRKAMLQDMA ILTGGQVISE
EVGLTLENAD LSLLGKARKV VVTKDETTIV EGAGDTDAIA GRVAQIRQEI
ENSDSDYDRE KLQERLAKLA GGVAVIKAGA ATEVELKERK HRIEDAVRNA
KAAVEEGIVA GGGVTLLQAA PTLDELKLEG DEATGANIVK VALEAPLKQI
AFNSGLEPGV VAEKVRNLPA GHGLNAQTGV YEDLLAAGVA DPVKVTRSAL
QNAASIAGLF LTTEAVVADK PEKEKASVPG GGDMGGMDFH MHGDTPTLHE
YMLDLQPETT DLYCYEQLND SSEEEDEIDG PAGQAEPDRA HYNIVTFCCK
CDSTLRLCVQ STHVDIRTLE DLLMGTLGIV CPICSQKP
```

Versetamide [*1994*] (ver set′ a mide). $C_{20}H_{37}N_5O_{10}$. 507.54. (1) 2-Oxa-5,8,11,14-tetraazahexadecan-16-oic acid, 8,11-bis(carboxymethyl)-14-[2-[(2-methoxyethyl)amino]-2-oxoethyl]-6-oxo-; (2) *N,N*-Bis[2-[(carboxymethyl)[[(2-methoxyethyl)carbamoyl]methyl]amino]ethyl]glycine. *UNII-N78PI4C683.* *CAS-129009-83-2.* INN. *Pharmaceutic aid.* [*Note—Versetamide is used as a carrier for the diagnostic aid, gadoversetamide.*] ◇*MP-1196*

Verteporfin [*1993*] (ver″ te pore′ fin). **USP.** $C_{41}H_{42}N_4O_8$. 718.79. (1) 23*H*,25*H*-Benzo[*b*]porphine-9,13-dipropanoic acid, 18-ethenyl-4,4a-dihydro-3,4-bis(methoxycarbonyl)-4a,8,14,19-tetramethyl-, monomethyl ester, *trans-*; (2) (±)-*trans*-3,4-Dicarboxy-4,4a-dihydro-4a,8,14,19-tetramethyl-18-vinyl-23*H*,25*H*-benzo[*b*]porphine-9,13-dipropionic acid, 3,4,9-trimethyl ester mixture with (±)-*trans*-3,4-dicarboxy-4,4a-dihydro-4a,8,14,19-tetramethyl-18-vinyl-23*H*,25*H*-benzo[*b*]porphine-9,13-dipropionic acid,

3,4,13-trimethyl ester. *UNII-0X9PA28K43.* *CAS-129497-78-5.* INN; BAN. *Antineoplastic.* Visudyne (QLT) ◇*CL 318,952*

Vesnarinone [*1988*] (ves na′ ri none). $C_{22}H_{25}N_3O_4$. 395.45. (1) Piperazine, 1-(3,4-dimethoxybenzoyl)-4-(1,2,3,4-tetrahydro-2-oxo-6-quinolinyl)-; (2) 1-(1,2,3,4-Tetrahydro-2-oxo-6-quinolyl)-4-veratroylpiperazine; (3) 6-[4-(3,4-Dimethoxybenzoyl)-1-piperazinyl]-3,4-dihydro-2(1*H*)-quinolone. *UNII-5COW40EV8M.* *CAS-81840-15-5.* INN; JAN. *Cardiotonic.* Arkin (Otsuka America) ◇*OPC-8212*

Vestipitant Mesylate [*2004*] (ves tee′ pi tant mes′ i late). $C_{23}H_{24}F_7N_3O·CH_4O_3S$. 587.55. [Vestipitant is INN.] (1) 1-Piperazinecarboxamide, *N*-[(1*R*)-1-[3,5-bis(trifluoromethyl)phenyl]ethyl]-2-(4-fluoro-2-methylphenyl)-*N*-methyl-, (2*S*)-, monomethanesulfonate; (2) (+)-(2*S*)-*N*-[(1*R*)-1-[3,5-bis(trifluoromethyl)phenyl]ethyl]-2-(4-fluoro-2-methylphenyl)-*N*-methylpiperazine-1-carboxamide methanesulfonate. *CAS-334476-64-1; CAS-334476-46-9* [vestipitant]. *Antidepressant/anti-anxiety; prevention of nausea and vomiting; used in the treatment of functional dyspepsia, irritable bowel syndrome and GERD.* ◇*GW597588B*

Vetrabutine. $C_{20}H_{27}NO_2$. 313.43. *N,N*-Dimethyl-α-(3-phenylpropyl)veratrylamine. *UNII-I3E2J32F37.* *CAS-3735-45-3.* INN; BAN; MI.

Vicotrope — *See* Cosyntropin.

Vicriviroc Maleate [*2005*] (vi″ kri vir′ ok mal′ ee ate). $C_{28}H_{38}F_3N_5O_2·C_4H_4O_4$. 649.70. [Vicriviroc is INN.] (1) Piperidine, 1-[(4,6-dimethyl-5-pyrimidinyl)carbonyl]-4-[(3*S*)-4-[(1*R*)-2-methoxy-1-[4-(trifluoromethyl)phenyl]ethyl]-3-methyl-1-piperazinyl]-4-methyl-, (2*Z*)-2-butene-dioate (1:1); (2) 1-[(4,6-Dimethylpyrimidin-5-yl)carbonyl]-4-[(3*S*)-4-[(1*R*)-2-methoxy-1-[4-(trifluoromethyl)phenyl]ethyl]-3-methylpiperazin-1-yl]-4-methylpiperidine-(2*Z*)-but-2-enedioate. *UNII-EP3QG127N9; UNII-TL515DW4QS* [vicriviroc]. *CAS-599179-03-0; CAS-306296-47-9* [vicriviroc]. *Antiviral, CCR5 antagonist, treatment of autoimmune conditions.* ◇*SCH 417690*

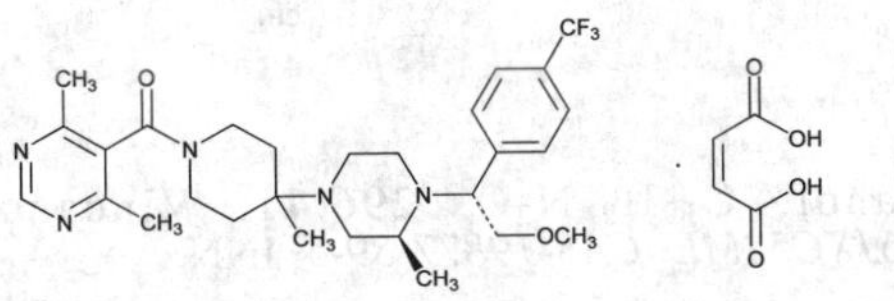

Vidarabine [*1974*] (vye dar′ a been). **USP**. $C_{10}H_{13}N_5O_4.H_2O$. 285.26. (1) 9*H*-Purin-6-amine, 9-β-D-arabinofuranosyl-, monohydrate; (2) 9-β-D-Arabinofuranosyladenine monohydrate. *UNII-FA2DM6879K. CAS-24356-66-9; CAS-5536-17-4* [anhydrous]. INN; BAN; JAN. *Antiviral.* Vira-A (Parkdale) ◇*ara-A; CI 673*

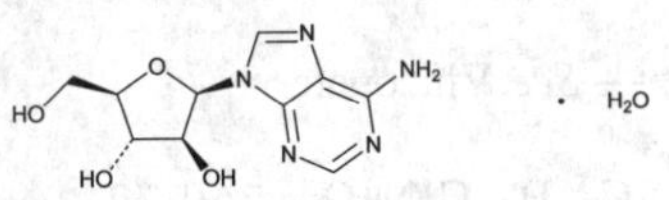

Vidarabine Phosphate [*1979*] (vye dar′ a been fos′ fate). $C_{10}H_{14}N_5O_7P$. 347.22. (1) 9*H*-Purin-6-amine, 9-(5-*O*-phosphono-β-D-arabinofuranosyl)-; (2) 9-β-D-Arabinofuranosyladenine 5′-(dihydrogen phosphate). *UNII-FA2DM6879K* [vidarabine]. *CAS-29984-33-6; CAS-5536-17-4* [vidarabine]. *Antiviral.* ◇*Cl-808*

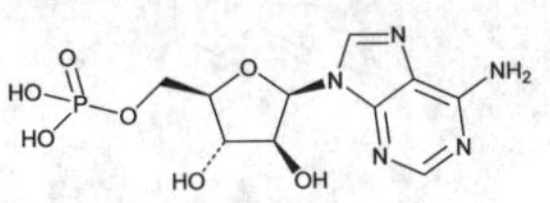

Vidarabine Sodium Phosphate [*1979*] (vye dar′ a been soe′ dee um fos′ fate). $C_{10}H_{12}N_5Na_2O_7P$. 391.18. (1) 9*H*-Purin-6-amine, 9-(5-*O*-phosphono-β-D-arabinofuranosyl)-, disodium salt; (2) 9-β-D-Arabinofuranosyladenine 5′-(dihydrogen phosphate), disodium salt. *UNII-FA2DM6879K* [vidarabine]. *CAS-71002-10-3; CAS-29984-33-6* [vidarabine phosphate]; *CAS-5536-17-4* [vidarabine]. *Antiviral.* ◇*Cl-808 sodium*

Vifilcon A [*1974*] (vye fil′ kon). $(C_4H_6O_2)_w(C_{10}H_{14}O_4)_x$ $(C_6H_{10}O_3)_y(C_6H_9NO)_z$. (1) 2-Propenoic acid, 2-methyl-, polymer with 1,2-ethanediyl bis(2-methyl-2-propenoate), 1-ethenyl-2-pyrrolidinone and 2-hydroxyethyl 2-methyl-2-propenoate; (2) Methacrylic acid polymer with ethylene dimethacrylate, 2-hydroxyethyl methacrylate and 1-vinyl-2-pyrrolidinone. *CAS-35528-20-2. Contact lens material (hydrophilic).* ◇*W 10168*

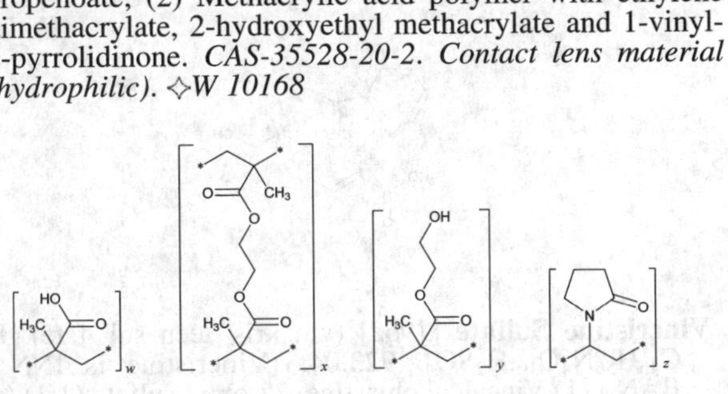

Vifilcon B [*1987*] (vye fil′ kon). $(C_4H_6O_2)_w(C_{10}H_{14}O_4)_x$ $(C_6H_{10}O_3)_y(C_6H_9NO)_z$. (1) 2-Propenoic acid, 2-methyl-, polymer with 1,2-ethanediyl bis(2-methyl-2-propenoate), 2-hydroxyethyl 2-methyl-2-propenoate and 1-ethenyl-2-pyrrolidinone; (2) Methacrylic acid polymer with ethylene dimethacrylate, 2-hydroxyethyl methacrylate and 1-vinyl-2-pyrrolidinone. *CAS-35528-20-2. Contact lens material (hydrophilic).* [*Note—Graphic formula same as for Vifilcon A.*]

Vigabatrin [*1985*] (vye ga′ ba trin). $C_6H_{11}NO_2$. 129.16. (1) 5-Hexenoic acid, 4-amino-; (2) 4-Amino-5-hexenoic acid. *CAS-60643-86-9.* INN; BAN. *Anticonvulsant (tardive dyskinesia).* Sabril (Hoechst Marion Roussel) ◇*MDL 71,754*

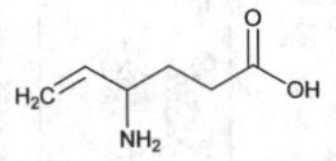

Vilazodone. $C_{26}H_{27}N_5O_2$. 441.52. 5-[4-[4-(5-Cyanoindol-3-yl)butyl]-1-piperazinyl]-2-benzofurancarboxamide. *CAS-163521-12-8.* INN.

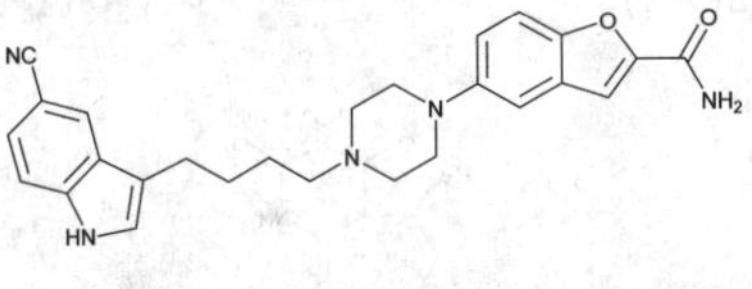

Vildagliptin [*2005*] (vil″ da glip′ tin). $C_{17}H_{25}N_3O_2$. 303.40. (1) 2-Pyrrolidinecarbonitrile, 1-[[(3-hydroxytricyclo[3.3.1.1^{3,7}]dec-1-yl)amino)acetyl]-, 2(*S*)-; (2) (-)-(2*S*)-1-[[(3-Hydroxytricyclo[3.3.1.1^{3,7}]dec-1-yl)amino]acetyl]pyrrolidine-2-carbonitrile. *UNII-I6B4B2U96P. CAS-274901-16-5.* INN; JAN. *Antidiabetic.* ◇*LAF237*

Viloxazine Hydrochloride [*1976*] (vye lox′ a zeen hye″ droe klor′ ide). $C_{13}H_{19}NO_3.HCl$. 273.76. [Viloxazine is INN and BAN.] (1) Morpholine, 2-[(2-ethoxyphenoxy)methyl]-, hydrochloride; (2) 2-[(*o*-Ethoxyphenoxy)methyl]morpholine hydrochloride. *CAS-35604-67-2; CAS-46817-91-8* [viloxazine]. *Antidepressant.* ◇*ICI 58,834*

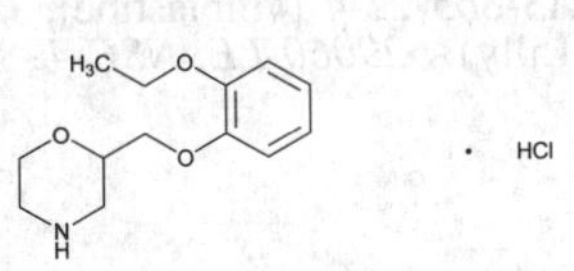

Viminol. $C_{21}H_{31}ClN_2O$. 362.94. 1-(*o*-Chlorobenzyl)-α-[(di-*sec*-butylamino)methyl]pyrrole-2-methanol. *CAS-21363-18-8.* INN; MI. ◇*Z 424*

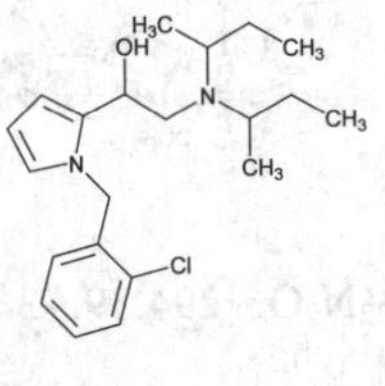

Vinafocon A [*1983*] (vin″ a foe′ kon). $[[(C_2H_6OSi)_u]_3C_3H_7$ $OSi]_v(C_4H_6O_2)_w[C_8H_{10}O_3(C_2H_4O)_n]_x(C_5H_9NO)_y(C_5H_8O_2)_z$, (*n* = 1, 2, or 3). (1) Siloxanes and silicones, dimethyl, 3-hydroxypropyl-terminated, polymer with 2-methyl-2-propenoic acid, α-(2-methyl-1-oxo-2-propenyl-ω-[(2-methyl-1-oxo-2-propenyl)oxy]poly(oxy-1,2-ethanediyl), *N*,*N*-dimethyl-2-propenamide and methyl 2-methyl-2-propenoate; (2) 3-Hydroxypropyl-terminated dimethyl siloxane, poly-

---

mer with methacrylic acid, polyethylene glycol dimethacrylate, *N,N*-dimethylacrylamide and methyl methacrylate. *Contact lens material (hydrophobic).* ◇*AL-T30*

Vinbarbital. $C_{11}H_{16}N_2O_3$. 224.26. 5-Ethyl-5-(1-methyl-1-butenyl)barbituric acid. *UNII-7NZH2C1T6O. CAS-125-42-8.* NF XIII; INN; BAN; DCF. *[Name previously used: Vinbarbitone.]*

Vinbarbital Sodium [Injection]. *UNII-7NZH2C1T6O* [vinbarbital]. NF XIII; MI.

Vinbarbitone (previously used name) — *See* Vinbarbital.

Vinblastine Sulfate *[1962]* (vin blas′ teen sul′ fate). **USP**. $C_{46}H_{58}N_4O_9 \cdot H_2SO_4$. 909.05. [Vinblastine is INN and BAN.] (1) Vincaleukoblastine, sulfate (1:1) (salt); (2) Vincaleukoblastine sulfate (1:1) (salt). *UNII-N00W22YO2B; UNII-5V9KLZ54CY* [vinblastine]. *CAS-143-67-9; CAS-865-21-4* [vinblastine]. JAN. *Antineoplastic.* Velban (Lilly) ◇*29060-LE; NSC-49842*

Vinburnine. $C_{19}H_{22}N_2O$. 294.39. 3α,16α-Eburnamonine. *CAS-4880-88-0.* INN.

Vincamine. $C_{21}H_{26}N_2O_3$. 354.44. Alkaloid obtained from *Vinca minor. CAS-1617-90-9.* INN; BAN; DCF; MI.

Vincanol. $C_{19}H_{24}N_2O$. 296.41. Vincanol. *UNII-6H6JXC52ME. CAS-19877-89-5.* INN.

Vincantenate — *See* Vinconate.

Vincantril. $C_{14}H_{13}ClN_2O$. 260.72. (±)-10-Chloro-1,2,3,3a,4,5-hexahydro-6*H*-indolo[3,2,1-*de*][1,5]naphthyridin-6-one. *UNII-S0KXB0NKWN. CAS-65285-58-7.* INN.

Vincofos *[1972]* (vin′ koe fos). $C_{11}H_{21}Cl_2O_4P$. 319.16. (1) Phosphoric acid, 2,3-dichloroethenyl methyl octyl ester; (2) 2,2-Dichlorovinyl methyl octyl phosphate. *CAS-17196-88-2.* INN. *Anthelmintic.* ◇*SD 15803*

Vinconate. $C_{18}H_{20}N_2O_2$. 296.36. (±)-Methyl 3-ethyl-2,3,3a,4-tetrahydro-1*H*-indolo[3,2,1-*de*][1,5]naphthyridine-6-carboxylate. *UNII-807MP0MJ61. CAS-70704-03-9.* INN.

Vincristine Sulfate *[1962]* (vin kris′ teen sul′ fate). **USP**. $C_{46}H_{56}N_4O_{10} \cdot H_2SO_4$. 923.04. [Vincristine is INN and BAN.] (1) Vincaleukoblastine, 22-oxo-, sulfate (1:1) (salt); (2) Leurocristine sulfate (1:1) (salt). *UNII-T5IRO3534A; UNII-5J49Q6B70F* [vincristine]. *CAS-2068-78-2; CAS-57-22-7* [vincristine]. JAN. *Antineoplastic.* Oncovin (Lilly); Vincrex (Bristol-Myers Squibb) *[Note—Graphic formula same as for Vinblastine Sulfate, except that R is CHO.]* ◇*37231; NSC-67574*

Vindeburnol. $C_{17}H_{20}N_2O$. 268.35. (±)-20,21-Dinor-16α-eburnamine. *CAS-74709-54-9*. INN.

Vindesine [*1976*] (vin′ de seen). $C_{43}H_{55}N_5O_7$. 753.93. (1) Vincaleukoblastine, 23-amino-O^4-deacetyl-23-demethoxy-; (2) 3-Carbamoyl-4-deacetyl-3-de(methoxycarbonyl)vincaleukoblastine. *CAS-53643-48-4*. INN; BAN. *Antineoplastic.* ◇*Compound 112531*

Vindesine Sulfate [*1980*] (vin′ de seen sul′ fate). $C_{43}H_{55}N_5O_7.H_2SO_4$. 852.00. (1) Vincaleukoblastine, 3-(aminocarbonyl)-O^4-deacetyl-3-de(methoxycarbonyl)sulfate (1:1) (salt); (2) 3-Carbamoyl-4-deacetyl-3-de(methoxycarbonyl)vincaleukoblastine sulfate (1:1) (salt). *CAS-59917-39-4; CAS-53643-48-4* [vindesine]. JAN. *Antineoplastic.* Eldisine (Lilly) ◇*LY099094; NSC-245467*

Vinepidine Sulfate [*1983*] (vin ep′ i deen sul′ fate). $C_{46}H_{56}N_4O_9.H_2SO_4$. 907.04. [Vinepidine is INN.] (1) Vincaleukoblastine, 4′-deoxy-22-oxo-, (4′α)-, sulfate (1:1); (2) (4′S)-4′-Deoxyleurocristine sulfate (1:1). *CAS-83200-11-7; CAS-68170-69-4* [vinepidine]. *Antineoplastic.* ◇*LY 119863*

Vinflunine. $C_{45}H_{54}F_2N_4O_8$. 816.93. 4′-Deoxy-20′,20′-difluoro-8′-norvincaleukoblastine. *UNII-5BF646324K. CAS-162652-95-1*. INN.

Vinflunine Ditartrate [*2007*] (vin′ floo neen dye tar′ trate). $C_{45}H_{54}F_2N_4O_8.2C_4H_6O_6$. 1117.10. [Vinflunine is INN.] (1) Aspidospermidine-3-carboxylic acid, 4-(acetyloxy)-6,7-didehydro-15-[(2R,4R,6S,8S)-4-(1,1-difluoroethyl)-1,3,4,5,6,7,8,9-octahydro-8-(methoxycarbonyl)-2,6-methano-2H-azecino[4,3-b]indol-8-yl]-3-hydroxy-16-methoxy-1-methyl-, methyl ester, (2β,3β,4β,5,12R,19.alpha.)-, (2R,3R)-2,3-dihydroxybutanedioate (1:2); (2) 4′-Deoxy-20′,20′-difluoro-8′-norvincaleucoblastine ditartrate. *UNII-33MG53C7XW; UNII-5BF646324K* [vinflunine]. *CAS-194468-36-5; CAS-162652-95-1* [vinflunine]. *Treatment of cancer.* Javlor (Middlebrook) ◇*BMS-710485; F-12158*

Vinformide. $C_{46}H_{54}N_4O_{10}$. 822.94. N-Demethyl-N-formyl-leurosine. *CAS-54022-49-0*. INN.

Vinfosiltine. $C_{51}H_{72}N_5O_{10}P$. 946.12. [23(*S*)]-4-Deacetyl-3-de(methoxycarbonyl)-3-[(2-methyl-1-phosphonopropyl)carbamoyl]vincaleukoblastine, diethyl ester. *CAS-123286-00-0.* INN.

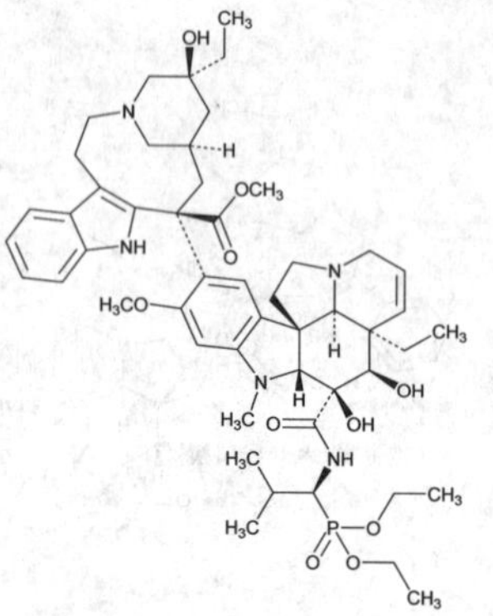

Vinglycinate Sulfate [*1965*] (vin glye′ sin ate sul′ fate). $C_{48}H_{63}N_5O_9 \cdot 1\frac{1}{2}H_2SO_4$. 1001.16. [Vinglycinate is INN.] (1) Vincaleukoblastine, 26-(dimethylamino)-, sulfate (2:3) (salt); (2) 4-Deacetylvincaleukoblastine 4-(*N,N*-dimethylglycinate) (ester) sulfate (2:3) (salt). *CAS-7281-31-4; CAS-865-24-7* [vinglycinate]. *Antineoplastic.* [*Note—Graphic formula for the free alkaloid is same as that for Vinblastine, except that the $OCOCH_3$ group at locus 4 is $OCOCH_2N(CH_3)_2$. See Vinblastine Sulfate.*] ◇49040

Vinleucinol. $C_{51}H_{69}N_5O_9$. 896.12. [23(1*S*,2*S*)]-4-Deacetyl-3-[(1-carboxy-2-methylbutyl)carbamoyl]-3-de(methoxycarbonyl)vincaleukoblastine, ethyl ester. *CAS-81571-28-0.* INN.

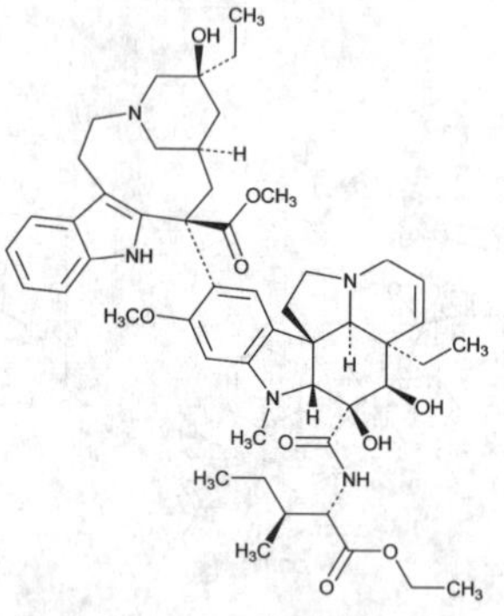

Vinleurosine Sulfate [*1962*] (vin loor′ oh seen sul′ fate). [Vinleurosine is INN.] A sulfate salt of an alkaloid derived from *Vinca rosea* Linné. (1) Vinleurosine sulfate; (2) Vinleurosine sulfate. *CAS-1404-95-1; CAS-23360-92-1* [vinleurosine]. *Antineoplastic.* ◇32645; NSC-528004

Vinmegallate. $C_{30}H_{32}N_2O_5$. 500.59. 17,18-Didehydro-3α,16α-eburnamenine-14-methanol 3,4,5-trimethoxybenzoate (ester). *CAS-83482-77-3.* INN.

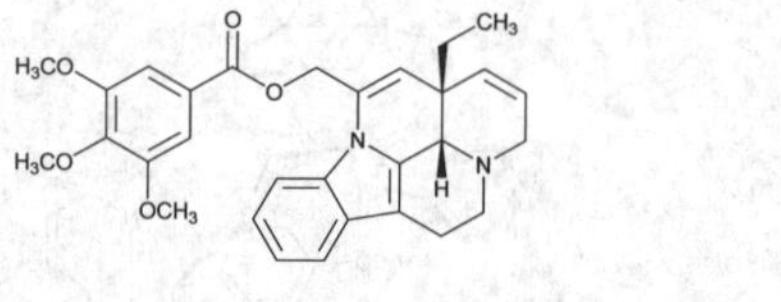

Vinorelbine Tartrate [*1993*] (vin or′ el been tar′ trate). **USP**. $C_{45}H_{54}N_4O_8 \cdot 2C_4H_6O_6$. 1079.11. [Vinorelbine is INN and BAN.] (1) *C*′-Norvincaleukoblastine, 3′,4′-didehydro-4′-deoxy-, [*R*-(*R**,*R**)]-2,3-dihydroxybutanedioate (1:2) (salt); (2) 3′,4′-Didehydro-4′-deoxy-8′-norvincaleukoblastine L-(+)-tartrate (1:2) (salt). *UNII-253GQW851Q; UNII-Q6C979R91Y* [vinorelbine]. *CAS-125317-39-7; CAS-71486-22-1* [vinorelbine]. *Antineoplastic.* Navelbine (Pierre)

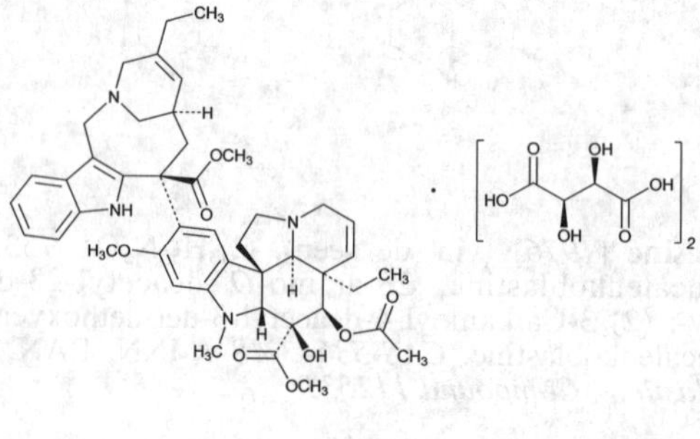

Vinpocetine [*1981*] (vin poe′ se teen). $C_{22}H_{26}N_2O_2$. 350.45. (1) Eburnamenine-14-carboxylic acid, ethyl ester, (3α, 16α)-; (2) Ethyl apovincamin-22-oate. *CAS-42971-09-5.* INN; JAN. ◇AY-27,255

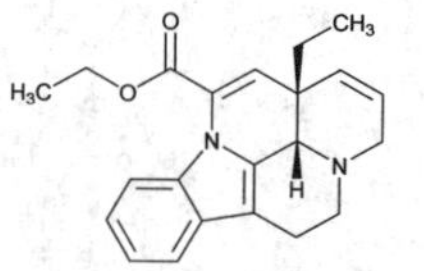

Vinpoline. $C_{23}H_{30}N_2O_3$. 382.50. 2-Hydroxypropyl 14-deoxyvincaminate. *CAS-57694-27-6.* INN.

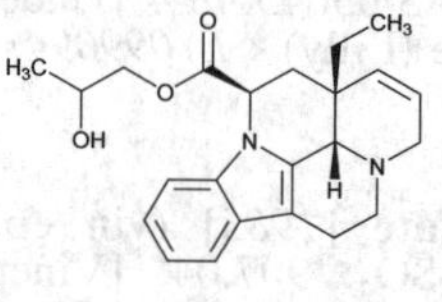

Vinrosidine Sulfate [*1962*] (vin roe′ zi deen sul′ fate). $C_{46}H_{58}N_4O_9 \cdot xH_2SO_4$. [Vinrosidine is INN.] A sulfate salt of an alkaloid derived from *Vinca rosea* Linné. (1) Vincaleukoblastine, 4′-deoxy-3′-hydroxy-, sulfate (salt); (2) Vinrosidine sulfate. *CAS-18556-44-0; CAS-15228-71-4* [vinrosidine]. *Antineoplastic.* ◇36781

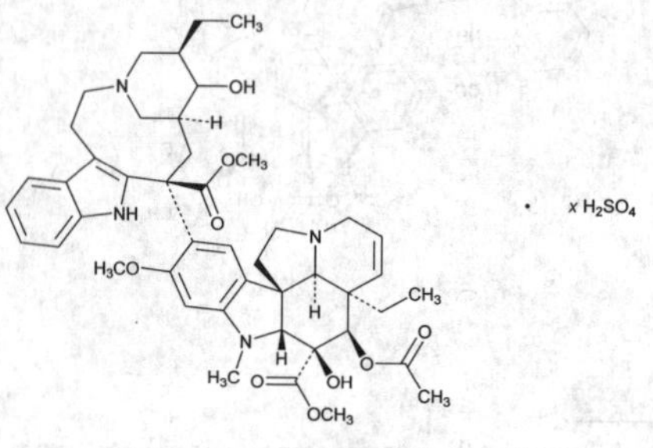

Vintiamol. $C_{21}H_{24}N_4O_3S$. 412.51. *N*-[(4-Amino-2-methyl-5-pyrimidinyl)methyl]-*N*-[2-[(2-benzoylvinyl)thio]-4-hydroxy-1-methyl-1-butenyl]formamide. *CAS-26242-33-1*. INN; MI.

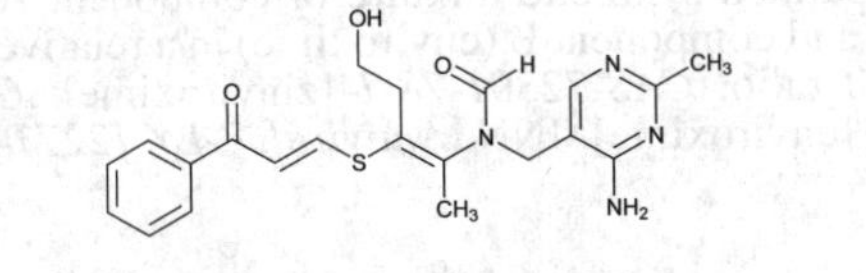

Vintoperol. $C_{18}H_{24}N_2O$. 284.40. (-)-(1*S*,12b*S*)-1-Ethyl-1,2,3,4,6,7,12,12b-octahydroindolo[2,3-*a*]quinolizine-1-methanol. *UNII-IS7C3GTW01*. *CAS-106498-99-1*. INN.

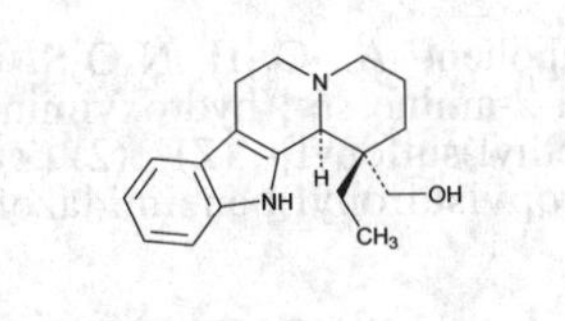

Vintriptol. $C_{56}H_{68}N_6O_9$. 969.17. [23(*S*)]-4-Deacetyl-3-[(1-carboxy-2-indol-3-ylethyl)carbamoyl]-3-de(methoxycarbonyl)vincaleukoblastine, ethyl ester. *CAS-81600-06-8*. INN.

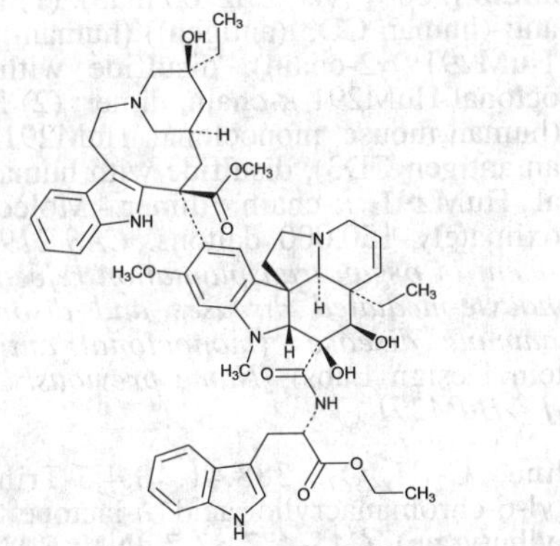

Vinyl Ether. C_4H_6O. 70.09. (1) Ethene, 1,1′-oxybis-; (2) Vinyl ether. *CAS-109-93-3*. USP XXI; MI.

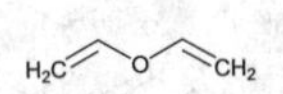

Vinyl Gamma-aminobutyric Acid — *See* Vigabatrin.

Vinylbital. $C_{11}H_{16}N_2O_3$. 224.26. 5-(1-Methylbutyl)-5-vinyl-barbituric acid. *UNII-3W58ITX06Q*. *CAS-2430-49-1*. INN; BAN; DCF; MI. *[Name previously used: Vinylbitone.]* ◇*JD-96*

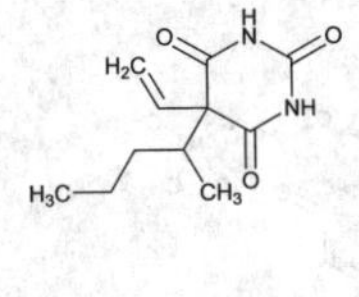

Vinylestrenolone — *See* Norgesterone.

Vinymal — *See* Vinylbital.

---

† Brand name formerly used, and/or firm no longer concerned with this product.

Vinzolidine Sulfate [*1981*] (vin zol′ i deen sul′ fate). $C_{48}H_{58}ClN_5O_9 \cdot H_2SO_4$. 982.53. [Vinzolidine is INN.] (1) 2*H*-3,7-Methanoazacycloundecino[5,4-*b*]indole-9-carboxylic acid, 9-[(2β,3β,4β,5α,12β,19α)-4-(acetyloxy)-3′-(2-chloroethyl)-6,7-didehydro-16-methoxy-1-methyl-2′,4′-dioxospiro[aspidospermidine-3,5′-oxazolidin]-15-yl]-5-ethyl-1,4,5,6,7,8,9,10-octahydro-5-hydroxy-, methyl ester, [3*R*-(3*R**,5*S**,7*R**,9*S**)]-, sulfate (1:1) (salt); (2) Methyl (3*R*,5*S*,7*R*,9*S*)-9-[3′-(2-chloroethyl)-6,7-didehydro-4β-hydroxy-16-methoxy-1-methyl-2′,4′-dioxo-2β,3β,5α,12β,19α-spiro[aspidospermidine-3,5′-oxazolidin]-15-yl]-5-ethyl-1,4,5,6,7,8,9,10-octahydro-5-hydroxy-2*H*-3,7-methanoazacycloundecino[5,4-*b*]indole-9-carboxylate 4′-acetate (ester) sulfate (1:1) (salt). *CAS-67699-41-6*. *Antineoplastic.* ◇*LY104208*

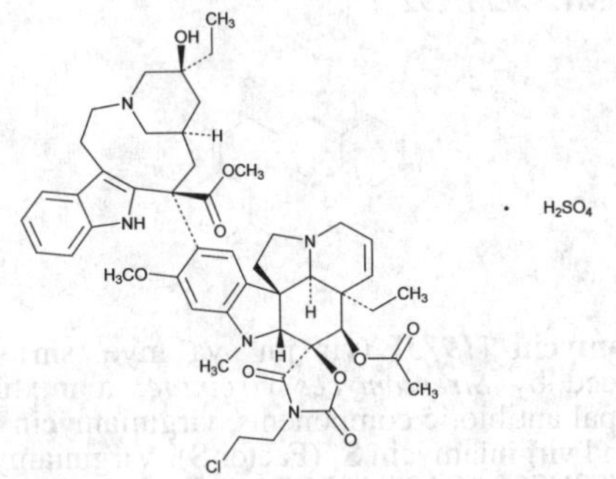

Viomycin Sulfate. [Viomycin is INN and BAN.] *UNII-LKO141R05V; UNII-YVU35998K5* [viomycin]. *CAS-37883-00-4; CAS-32988-50-4* [viomycin]. USP XX; MI. Viocin Sulfate (Pfizer)

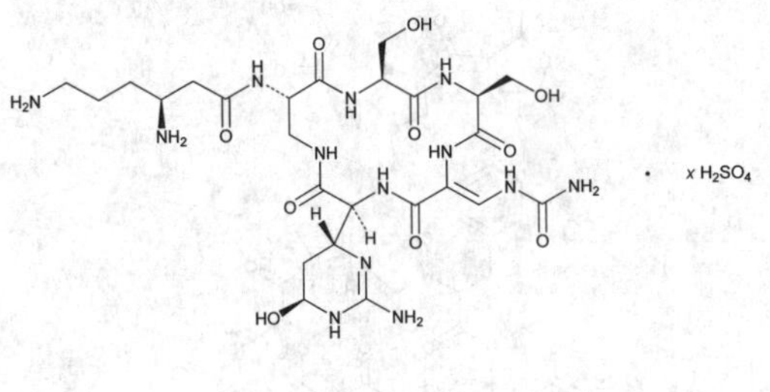

Viosterol in Oil — *See* Ergocalciferol.

Viprostol [*1985*] (vye prost′ ol). $C_{23}H_{36}O_5$. 392.53. (1) Prosta-5,13-dien-1-oic acid, 16-ethenyl-11,16-dihydroxy-9-oxo-, methyl ester, (5Z,11α,13E)-(±)-; (2) (±)-Methyl (Z)-7-[(1*R*,2*R*,3*R*)-2-[(*E*)-(4*RS*)-4-butyl-4-hydroxy-1,5-hexadienyl]-3-hydroxy-5-oxocyclopentyl]-5-heptenoate. *CAS-73647-73-1*. INN; BAN. *Hypotensive; vasodilator.* ◇*CL 115,347*

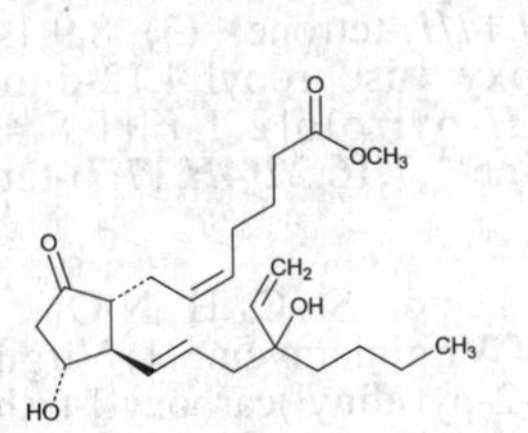

Viprynium Embonate (previously used name) — *See* Pyrvinium Pamoate.

Viqualine. $C_{20}H_{26}N_2O$. 310.43. 6-Methoxy-4-[3-[(3*R*,4*R*)-3-vinyl-4-piperidyl]propyl]quinoline. *CAS-72714-74-0.* INN.

Viquidacin. $C_{25}H_{29}FN_2O_4S_2$. 504.64. (3*R*,4*R*)-4-{(3*S*)-3-[3-Fluoro-6-methoxyquinolin-4-yl]-3-hydroxypropyl}-1-{2-[(thiophen-2-yl)sulfanyl]ethyl}piperidine-3-carboxylic acid. *CAS-904302-98-3.* INN.

Viquidil. $C_{20}H_{24}N_2O_2$. 324.42. 1-(6-Methoxy-4-quinolyl)-3-(3-vinyl-4-piperidyl)-1-propanone. *CAS-84-55-9.* INN; DCF; MI. ◇*LM 192*

Virginiamycin [*1973*] (vir jin″ ya mye′ sin). Antibiotic produced by *Streptomyces virginiae;* a mixture of two principal antibiotic components, virginiamycin M_1 (Factor M_1) and virginiamycin S_1 (Factor S). Virginiamycin. *UNII-C49WS9N75L. CAS-11006-76-1.* INN; BAN. *Antibacterial; food additive (veterinary).* Stafac (SmithKline Beecham Animal Health) ◇*SK&F 7988*

Virginiamycin Factor M_1. $C_{28}H_{35}N_3O_7$. 525.59. Antibiotic component of Virginiamycin. (1) Virginiamycin M_1; (2) 8,9,14,15,24,25-Hexahydro-14-hydroxy-4,12-dimethyl-3-(1-methylethyl)-3*H*-21,18-nitrilo-1*H*,22*H*-pyrrolo[2,1-*c*][1,8,4,19]dioxadiazacyclotetracosine-1,7,16,22(4*H*,17*H*)-tetrone; (3) 8,9,14,15,24,25-Hexahydro-14-hydroxy-3-isopropyl-4,12-dimethyl-3*H*-21,18-nitrilo-1*H*,22*H*-pyrrolo[2,1-*c*][1,8,4,19]dioxadiazacyclotetracosine-1,7,16,22(4*H*,17*H*)-tetrone. *CAS-21411-53-0.* MI.

Virginiamycin Factor S. $C_{43}H_{49}N_7O_{10}$. 823.89. Antibiotic component of Virginiamycin. (1) Virginiamycin S_1; (2) *N*-[(3-Hydroxy-2-pyridinyl)carbonyl]-L-threonyl-D-α-aminobutyryl-L-prolyl-*N*-methyl-L-phenylalanyl-4-oxo-L-pipecoloyl-L-2-phenylglycine ρ-lactone; (3) *N*-(3-Hydroxypicolinoyl)-L-threonyl-D-α-aminobutyryl-L-prolyl-*N*-methyl-L-phenylalanyl-4-oxo-L-pipecoloyl-L-2-phenylglycine ρ-lactone. *CAS-23152-29-6.* MI.

Viridofulvin [*1966*] (vir id″ oh ful′ vin). Antibiotic derived from *Streptomyces viridogriseus.* (1) Viridofulvin; (2) Viridofulvin. *CAS-1405-00-1.* INN. *Antifungal.*

Viroxime [*1983*] (vir ox′ eem). $C_{17}H_{18}N_4O_3S$. 358.41. An unseparated synthetic mixture of component A (zinviroxime) and component B (enviroxime) in a relatively constant 50-50 ratio. *CAS-72301-78-1* [zinviroxime]; *CAS-72301-79-2* [enviroxime]. INN. *Antiviral.* ◇*LY 12271-72*

Viroxime Component A. $C_{17}H_{18}N_4O_3S$. 358.41. (1) 1*H*-Benzimidazol-2-amine, 6-[(hydroxyimino)phenylmethyl]-1-[(1-methylethyl)sulfonyl]-, (*Z*)-; (2) (*Z*)-2-Amino-6-benzoyl-1-(isopropylsulfonyl)benzimidazole oxime. *CAS-72301-78-1.*

Viroxime Component B. $C_{17}H_{18}N_4O_3S$. 358.41. (1) 1*H*-Benzimidazol-2-amine, 6-[(hydroxyimino)phenylmethyl]-1-[(1-methylethyl)sulfonyl]-, (*E*)-; (2) (*E*)-2-Amino-6-benzoyl-1-(isopropylsulfonyl)benzimidazole oxime. *CAS-72301-79-2.*

Visilizumab [*2000*] (vis″ i liz′ oo mab). (1) Immunoglobulin G2, anti-(human CD3 (antigen)) (human-mouse monoclonal HuM291 γ2-chain), disulfide with human-mouse monoclonal HuM291 κ-chain, dimer; (2) Immunoglobulin G2 (human-mouse monoclonal HuM291 γ2-chain anti-human antigen CD3), disulfide with human-mouse monoclonal HuM291 κ-chain, dimer. Molecular weight is approximately 150,000 daltons. *CAS-219716-33-3.* INN. *Treatment of organ transplantation rejection and other T lymphocyte-mediated diseases and disorders, including autoimmune diseases (monoclonal antibody).* Nuvion (Protein Design Labs) [*Name previously used: Visiluzumab.*] ◇*HuM291*

Visnadine. $C_{21}H_{24}O_7$. 388.41. 3,4,5-Trihydroxy-2,2-dimethyl-6-chromanacrylic acid δ-lactone 4-acetate 3-(2-methylbutyrate). *CAS-477-32-7.* INN; BAN; MI.

Visnafylline. $C_{25}H_{29}N_5O_7$. 511.53. [2-[(9-Methoxy-7-methyl-5-oxo-5*H*-furo[3,2-*g*][1]benzopyran-4-yl)oxy]ethyl]trimethylammonium theophylline derivative. *UNII-GB901PL1KW. CAS-17243-56-0.* INN.

Vistatolon (INN) — *See* Statolon.

Vitamin A (vye′ ta min). **USP.** [Vitamin A Oil is JAN.] Contains a suitable form of retinol ($C_{20}H_{30}O$; vitamin A alcohol). It may consist of retinol or esters of retinol formed from edible fatty acids, principally acetic and palmitic acids. *Vitamin (anti-xerophthalmic).* Aquasol A (AstraZeneca) *[Name previously used: Oleovitamin A.]*

Vitamin B_1 — *See* Thiamine Hydrochloride.

Vitamin B_1 Mononitrate — *See* Thiamine Mononitrate.

Vitamin B_2 — *See* Riboflavin.

Vitamin B_6 — *See* Pyridoxine Hydrochloride.

Vitamin B_8 — *See* Adenosine Phosphate.

Vitamin B_{12} (previously used name) — *See* Cyanocobalamin.

Vitamin B Complex. Becotin (Lilly); Becozym (Hoffmann-LaRoche-International); Betalin Complex (Lilly); Betalin Compound (Lilly)

Vitamin C — *See* Ascorbic Acid.

Vitamin D — *See* Cholecalciferol.

Vitamin D_1 — *See* Dihydrotachysterol.

Vitamin D_2 — *See* Ergocalciferol.

Vitamin E (vye′ ta min). **USP**. [Tocopherol, Tocopherol Acetate, Tocopherol Calcium Succinate, and Tocopherol Nicotinate are JAN.] It may consist of *d*- or *dl*-alpha tocopherol ($C_{29}H_{50}O_2$), *d*- or *dl*-alpha tocopheryl acetate ($C_{31}H_{52}O_3$), *d*- or *dl*-alpha tocopheryl acid succinate ($C_{33}H_{54}O_5$), mixed tocopherols concentrate, or *d*-alpha tocopheryl acetate concentrate. *Vitamin E supplement.* Aquasol E (Astra); Eprolin (Lilly†); Natopherol (Abbott†)

Vitamin E Polyethylene Glycol Succinate (vye′ ta min pol″ ee eth′ i leen glye′ kol sux′ i nate). **NF**. A mixture formed by the esterification of *d*-alpha tocopheryl acid succinate and polyethylene glycol.

Vitamin G — *See* Riboflavin.

Vitamin K_1 — *See* Phytonadione.

Vitamin P_4 — *See* Troxerutin.

Vitespen [*2006*] (vye tes′ pen). $C_{3970}H_{6275}N_{1047}O_{1302}S_{21}$. (1) gp96; (2) Glucose regulated protein 94 (grp 94); (2) Endoplasmin (human tumor rejection antigen 1). Molecular weight is approximately 90,100 daltons *CAS-492448-75-6. Autologous heat shock protein immuno-stimulant for the treatment of cancer.* Oncophage (Antigenics) *✧HSPPC-96*

Voclosporin [*2006*] (voe″ kloe spor′ in). $C_{63}H_{111}N_{11}O_{12}$. 1214.62. (1) Cyclosporin A, 6-[(2*S*,3*R*,4*R*,6*E*)-3-hydroxy-4-methyl-2-(methylamino)-6,8-nonadienoic acid]-; (2) Cyclo[L-alanyl-D-alanyl-*N*-methyl-L-leucyl-*N*-methyl-L-leucyl-*N*-methyl-L-valyl-[(2*S*,3*R*,4*R*,6*E*)-3-hydroxy-4-methyl-2-(methylamino)nona-6,8-dienoyl]-(2*S*)-2-aminobutanoyl-*N*-methylglycyl-*N*-methyl-L-leucyl-L-valyl-*N*-methyl-L-leucyl]. *CAS-515814-01-4.* INN. *Immunosuppressant. ✧ISATX247; ISA247*

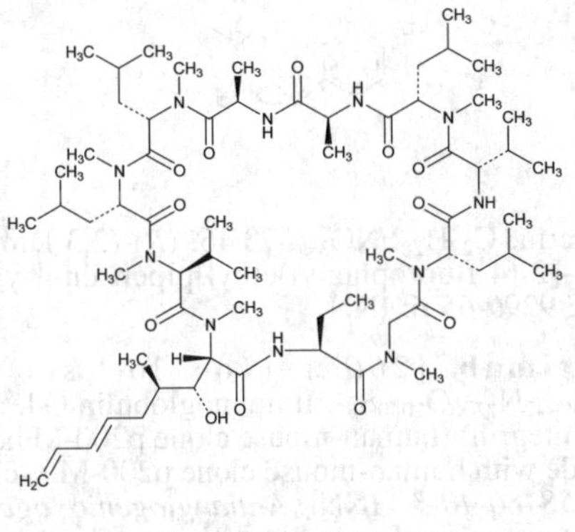

Vofopitant. $C_{21}H_{23}F_3N_6O$. 432.44. (2*S*,3*S*)-3-[[2-Methoxy-5-[5-(trifluoromethyl)-1*H*-tetrazol-1-yl]benzyl]amino]-2-phenylpiperidine. *UNII-K08BK043YS. CAS-168266-90-8.* INN.

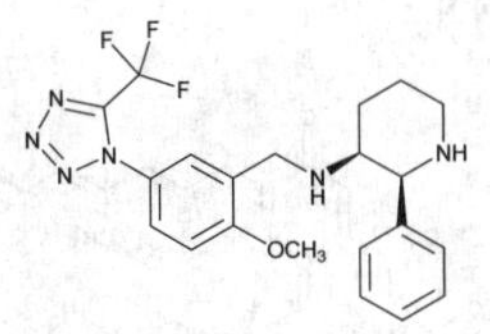

Vofopitant Dihydrochloride [*1999*] (voe foe′ pi tant dye hye″ droe klor′ ide). $C_{21}H_{23}F_3N_6O.2HCl$. 505.36. (1) 3-Piperidinamine, *N*-[[2-methoxy-5-[5-(trifluoromethyl)-1*H*-tetrazol-1-yl]phenyl]methyl]-2-phenyl-, dihydrochloride, (2*S*-*cis*)-; (2) (2*S*,3*S*)-3-[[2-Methoxy-5-[5-(trifluoromethyl)-1*H*-tetrazol-1-yl]benzyl]amino]-2-phenylpiperidine dihydrochloride. *CAS-168266-51-1. Antiemetic (tachykinin NK_1receptor antagonist). ✧GR205171A*

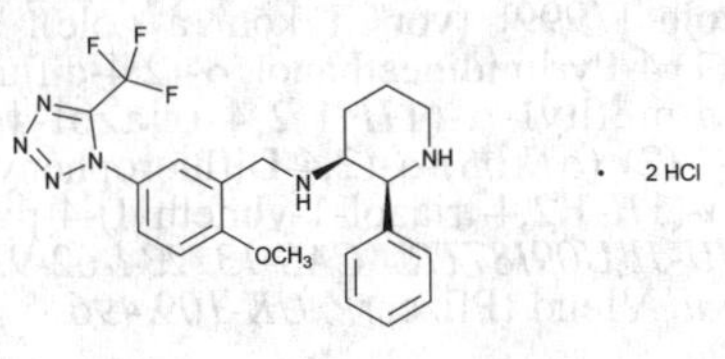

Voglibose [*1997*] (voe glye′ bose). $C_{10}H_{21}NO_7$. 267.28. 3,4-Dideoxy-4-[[2-hydroxy-1-(hydroxymethyl)ethyl]amino]-2-*C*-(hydroxymethyl)-*D*-epi-inositol. *CAS-83480-29-9.* INN. *Antidiabetic (α-glucosidase inhibitor).* Basen (Takeda); Glustat (Takeda) *✧AO-128; A-71100*

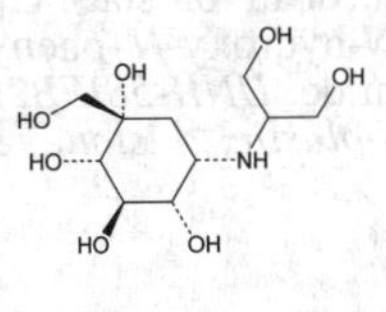

Volazocine [*1967*] (voe laz′ oh seen). $C_{18}H_{25}N$. 255.40. (1) 2,6-Methano-3-benzazocine, 3-(cyclopropylmethyl)-1,2,3,4,5,6-hexahydro-6,11-dimethyl-, *cis*-; (2) 3-(Cyclo-

† Brand name formerly used, and/or firm no longer concerned with this product.

propylmethyl)-1,2,3,4,5,6-hexahydro-*cis*-6,11-dimethyl-2,6-methano-3-benzazocine. *CAS-15686-68-7*. INN. *Analgesic.* ⋄*Win 23,200*

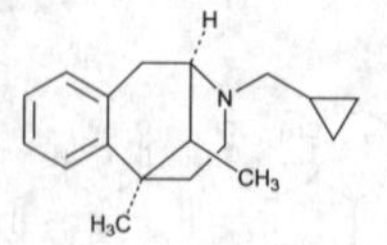

Volinanserin. $C_{22}H_{28}FNO_3$. 373.46. (*R*)-(2,3-Dimethoxyphenyl){1-[2-(4-fluorophenyl)ethyl]piperidin-4-yl}methanol. *CAS-139290-65-6.* INN.

Volociximab [*2005*] (voe loe six′ i mab). $C_{6434}H_{9942}N_{1706}O_{2040}S_{52}$. Immunoglobulin G4, anti-(human $\alpha5\beta1$ integrin) (human-mouse clone p200-M heavy chain), disulfide with human-mouse clone p200-M κ-chain, dimer. *CAS-558480-40-3.* INN. *Antiangiogenic agent to treat solid tumors and age-related macular degeneration.* ⋄*M200*

Volpristin. $C_{28}H_{37}N_3O_7$. 527.61. (3*R*,4*R*,5*E*,10*E*,12*E*,14-*S*,26a*R*)-8,9,14,15,24,25,26,26a-Octahydro-14-hydroxy-3-isopropyl-4,12-dimethyl-3*H*-21,18-nitrilo-1*H*,22*H*-pyrrolo[2,1-*c*][1,8,4,19]dioxadiazacyclotetracosine-1,7,16,22(4*H*,17*H*)-tetrone. *UNII-18UAN5144E.* *CAS-21102-49-8.* INN.

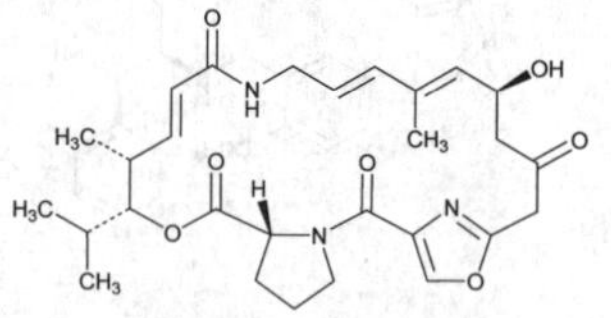

Voreloxin [*2008*] (vor″ e lox′ in). $C_{18}H_{19}N_5O_4S$. 401.44. (1) 1,8-Naphthyridine-3-carboxylic acid, 1,4-dihydro-7-[(3*S*,4*S*)-3-methoxy-4-(methylamino)-1-pyrrolidinyl]-4-oxo-1-(2-thiazolyl)-; (2) (+)-7-[(3*S*,4*S*)-3-Methoxy-4-(methylamino)pyrrolidin-1-yl]-4-oxo-1-(thiazol-2-yl)-1,4-dihydro-1,8-naphthyridine-3-carboxylic acid. *UNII-K6A90IIZ19.* *CAS-175414-77-4.* *Antineoplastic.* ⋄*SNS-595*

Voriconazole [*1999*] (vor″ i kon′ a zole). $C_{16}H_{14}F_3N_5O$. 349.31. (1) 4-Pyrimidineethanol, α-(2,4-difluorophenyl)-5-fluoro-β-methyl-α-(1*H*-1,2,4-triazol-1-ylmethyl)-, ($\alpha R,\beta S$)-; (2) ($\alpha R,\beta S$)-α-(2,4-Difluorophenyl)-5-fluoro-β-methyl-α-(1*H*-1,2,4-triazol-1-ylmethyl)-4-pyrimidineethanol. *UNII-JFU09I87TR.* *CAS-137234-62-9.* INN; BAN. *Antifungal.* Vfend (Pfizer) ⋄*UK-109,496*

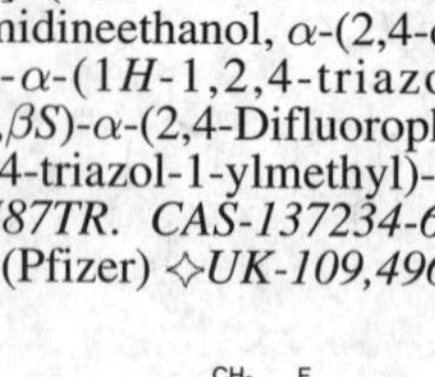

Vorinostat [*2005*] (vor in′ oh stat). $C_{14}H_{20}N_2O_3$. 264.32. (1) Octanediamide, *N*-hydroxy-*N*′-phenyl-; (2) *N*-Hydroxy-*N*′-phenyloctanediamide. *UNII-58IFB293JI.* *CAS-149647-78-9.* INN. *Antineoplastic, histone deacetylase inhibitor.* Zolinza (Merck)

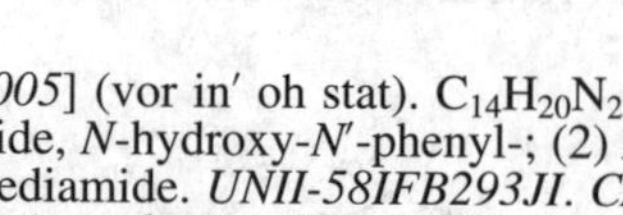

Vorozole [*1993*] (vor′ oh zole). $C_{16}H_{13}ClN_6$. 324.77. (1) 1*H*-Benzotriazole, 6-[(4-chlorophenyl)-1*H*-1,2,4-triazol-1-yl-methyl]-1-methyl-, (*S*)-; (2) (+)-(*S*)-6-(*p*-Chloro-α-1*H*-1,2,4-triazol-1-ylbenzyl)-1-methyl-1*H*-benzotriazole. *CAS-129731-10-8.* INN; BAN. *Antineoplastic.* Rivizor (Janssen) ⋄*R 83842*

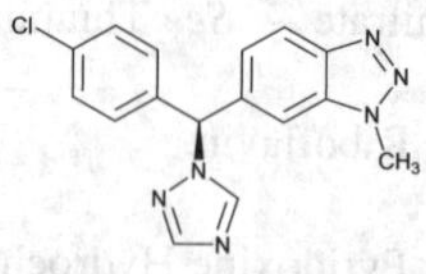

Votucalis. $C_{858}H_{1259}N_{221}O_{289}S_{10}$. Methionyl[145-leucine]FS-HBP2 (*Rhipicephalus appendiculatus* (Brown ear tick) Female-Specific Histamine-Bending Protein 2). *CAS-872525-61-6.* INN.

Votumumab [*1994*] (voe toom′ ue mab). (1) Immunoglobulin G 3 (human monoclonal 88BV59 heavy chain anti-human carcinoma-associated antigen), disulfide with human monoclonal 88BV59 κ-chain, dimer; (2) Immunoglobulin G 3 (human monoclonal 88BV59 heavy chain anti-human carcinoma-associated antigen), disulfide with human monoclonal 88BV59 κ-chain, dimer. Molecular weight is approximately 170,000 daltons. *CAS-148189-70-2.* INN; BAN. *Monoclonal antibody.* HumaSPECT (Intracel) ⋄*88BV59H21-2V67-66*

Voxergolide. $C_{16}H_{20}N_2OS$. 288.41. ($\pm$)-(6a*R*,9*R*,10a*R*)-4,6a,7,8,9,10a-Hexahydro-7-methyl-9-[(methylthio)-methyl]-6*H*-indolo[3,4-*gh*][1,4]benzoxazine. *UNII-PP012U645Q.* *CAS-89651-00-3.* INN.

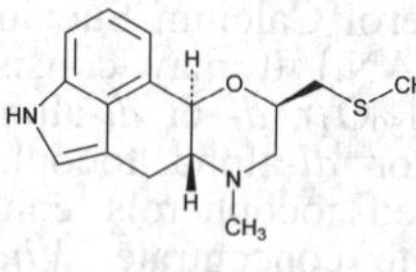

Warfarin Potassium. $C_{19}H_{15}KO_4$. 346.42. [Warfarin is INN and BAN.] (1) 2*H*-1-Benzopyran-2-one, 4-hydroxy-3-(3-oxo-1-phenylbutyl)-, potassium salt; (2) 3-(α-Acetonylbenzyl)-4-hydroxycoumarin potassium salt. *UNII-147IU4-FOCO.* *CAS-2610-86-8;* *CAS-81-81-2* [warfarin]. USP XXI; JAN; MI. Athrombin-K (Purdue Frederick)

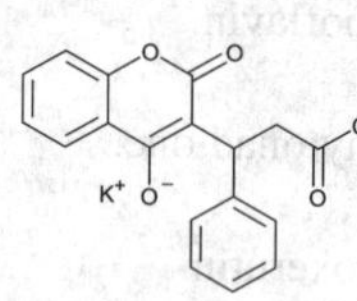

Warfarin Sodium (war′ far in soe′ dee um). **USP.** $C_{19}H_{15}NaO_4$. 330.31. (1) 2*H*-1-Benzopyran-2-one, 4-hydroxy-3-(3-oxo-1-phenylbutyl)-, sodium salt; (2) 3-(α-Acetonylbenzyl)-4-hydroxycoumarin sodium salt. *UNII-6153CWM0CL.* *CAS-129-06-6;* *CAS-81-81-2* [warfarin]. *Anticoagulant.* Athrombin (Purdue Frederick); Coumadin (Bristol-Myers Squibb); Jantoven (USl)

Water O 15 [*1992*] (wa′ ter). **USP** [Injection]. $H_2{}^{15}O$. (1) Water-${}^{15}O$; (2) [${}^{15}O$]Water. *UNII-63M8RYN44N.* *CAS-24286-21-3.* *Diagnostic aid (radioactive, vascular disorders); radioactive agent.* [*Note—This radiopharmaceutical, labeled with a cyclotron-generated radionuclide, is prepared in individual nuclear medical centers.*]

Water, Tritiated [*1963*] (wa′ ter trit′ ee ay″ ted). (1) Water, tritium cont′g.; (2) Water, tritium cont′g. *Radioactive agent.* Tritiotope (Bristol-Myers Squibb†)

Wax, Carnauba (wax kar noe′ ba). **NF**. Obtained from the leaves of *Copernicia cerifera* Mart. (Fam. Palmae). *Pharmaceutic aid (tablet coating agent).*

Wax, Emulsifying (wax ee mul″ si fye′ ing). **NF**. A waxy solid prepared from Cetostearyl Alcohol containing a polyoxyethylene derivative of a fatty acid ester of sorbitan. *Pharmaceutic aid (emulsifying agent); pharmaceutic aid (stiffening agent).*

Wax, Microcrystalline (wax mye″ kroe kris′ ta lin). **NF**. A mixture of straight-chain, branched-chain, and cyclic hydrocarbons, obtained by solvent fractionation of the still bottom fraction of petroleum by suitable dewaxing or deoiling means. *Pharmaceutic aid (stiffening agent); pharmaceutic aid (tablet coating agent).*

Wax, White (wax). **NF**. [White Beeswax is JAN.] Produced by bleaching and purifying Yellow Wax. *Pharmaceutic aid (stiffening agent).*

Wax, Yellow (wax yel′ oh). **NF**. [Yellow Beeswax is JAN.] The purified wax from the honeycomb of the bee [*Apis mellifera* Linné (Fam. Apidae)]. *CAS-8012-89-3. Pharmaceutic aid (stiffening agent).*

Wheat Bran. USP. Wheat Bran is the outer fraction of the cereal grain, comprising the pericarp, seed coat (testa), nucellar epidermis, and aleuronic layer, and is derived from *Triticum aestivum* Linné, *T, compactum* Host, *T. durum* Desf., and other common einkorn and emmer wheat cultivars. It is obtained by the milling and processing of the whole wheat grain meeting U.S. Standards for Number 1 wheat (7 CFR 810.2201).

Wheat Germ Oil—*Seed*l-Alpha Tocopherol, under Vitamin E.

Wheat Starch (JAN) — *See* Starch.

Widow Spider Species Antivenin (Latrodectus mactans) (previously used name) — *See* Antivenin (Latrodectus mactans).

Wild Cherry Syrup. USP XVIII; MI.

Wintergreen Oil — *See* Methyl Salicylate.

Witch Hazel (wich′ hay′ zel). **USP**. A clear, odorless distillate prepared from recently cut and partially dried dormant twigs of *Hamamelis virginiana* Linné. *Astringent.* Dickinson's Witch Hazel Formula (Dickinson)

Witepsol. A mixture of mono-, di- and triglyceride of saturated fatty acids. JAN.

Woolley's Antiserotonin — *See* Benanserin Hydrochloride.

Wound Matrix, Small Intestinal Submucosa. USP. A biologically derived, collagen-based wound care product, translucent and off-white in color, obtained from the small intestinal submucosa layer of the domestic pig (*Sus scrofa* L.).

Xaliproden [*1999*] (zal ip′ roe den). C$_{24}$H$_{22}$F$_3$N. 381.43. (1) Pyridine, 1,2,3,6-tetrahydro-1-[2-(2-naphthalenyl)ethyl]-4-[3-(trifluoromethyl)phenyl]-; (2) 1,2,3,6-Tetrahydro-1-[2-(2-naphthyl)ethyl]-4-(α,α,α-trifluoro-*m*-tolyl)pyridine. *CAS-135354-02-8.* INN; BAN. *Nootrope (5HT$_{1A}$agonist; potentiator of the action and endogenous synthesis of neurotrophins).* ◇SR 57746

Xamoterol [*1984*] (zam oh′ ter ol). C$_{16}$H$_{25}$N$_3$O$_5$. 339.39. (1) 4-Morpholinecarboxamide, *N*-[2-[[2-hydroxy-3-(4-hydroxyphenoxy)propyl]amino]ethyl]-, (±)-; (2) (±)-*N*-[2-

[[2-Hydroxy-3-(*p*-hydroxyphenoxy)propyl]amino]ethyl]-4-morpholinecarboxamide. *CAS-81801-12-9.* INN; BAN. *Stimulant (cardiac).*

Xamoterol Fumarate [*1992*] (zam oh′ ter ol fue′ ma rate). C$_{36}$H$_{54}$N$_6$O$_{14}$. 794.85. (1) 4-Morpholinecarboxamide, *N*-[2-[[2-hydroxy-3-(4-hydroxyphenoxy)propyl]amino]ethyl]-, (±)-, (*E*)-2-butenedioate (2:1) (salt); (2) (±)-*N*-[2-[[2-Hydroxy-3-(*p*-hydroxyphenoxy)propyl]amino]ethyl]-4-morpholinecarboxamide fumarate (2:1) (salt). *CAS-90730-93-1. Stimulant (cardiac).* ◇ICI 118,587

X-Andron — *See* Cioteronel.

Xanomeline [*1994*] (zan oh′ me leen). C$_{14}$H$_{23}$N$_3$OS. 281.42. (1) Pyridine, 3-[4-(hexyloxy)-1,2,5-thiadiazol-3-yl]-1,2,5,6-tetrahydro-1-methyl-; (2) 3-[4-(Hexyloxy)-1,2,5-thiadiazol-3-yl]-1,2,5,6-tetrahydro-1-methylpyridine. *CAS-131986-45-3.* INN. *Alzheimer's disease treatment (cholinergic agonist).* ◇LY246708

Xanomeline Tartrate [*1994*] (zan oh′ me leen tar′ trate). C$_{14}$H$_{23}$N$_3$OS.C$_4$H$_6$O$_6$. 431.50. (1) Pyridine, 3-[4-(hexyloxy)-1,2,5-thiadiazol-3-yl]-1,2,5,6-tetrahydro-1-methyl-, [*R*-(*R**,*R**)]-2,3-dihydroxybutanedioate (1:1); (2) 3-[4-(Hexyloxy)-1,2,5-thiadiazol-3-yl]-1,2,5,6-tetrahydro-1-methylpyridine L-(+)-tartrate (1:1). *CAS-152854-19-8. Alzheimer's disease treatment (cholinergic agonist).* ◇LY246708 tartrate

Xanoxate Sodium [*1975*] (zan ox′ ate soe′ dee um). C$_{17}$H$_{13}$NaO$_5$. 320.27. (1) 9*H*-Xanthene-2-carboxylic acid, 7-(1-methylethoxy)-9-oxo-, sodium salt; (2) Sodium 7-isopropoxy-9-oxoxanthene-2-carboxylate. *UNII-WA-S1IG4146. CAS-41147-04-0; CAS-33459-27-7* [xanoxic acid]. *Bronchodilator.* ◇RS-6818

Xanoxic Acid. $C_{17}H_{14}O_5$. 298.29. 7-Isopropoxy-9-oxoxanthene-2-carboxylic acid. *UNII-S6V5I726MH. CAS-33459-27-7.* INN.

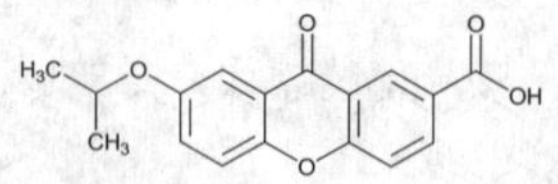

Xanthan Gum (zan′ than gum). **NF**. A high molecular weight polysaccharide gum produced by a pure-culture fermentation of a carbohydrate with *Xanthomonas Campestris*, then purified by recovery with Isopropyl Alcohol, dried, and milled. *Pharmaceutic aid (suspending agent).* Rhodigel (Vanderbilt)

Xanthinol Niacinate [*1963*] (zan′ thi nol nye′ a sin ate). $C_{13}H_{21}N_5O_4 \cdot C_6H_5NO_2$. 434.45. [Xantinol Nicotinate is INN and BAN.] (1) 3-Pyridinecarboxylic acid compd. with 3,7-dihydro-7-[2-hydroxy-3-[(2-hydroxyethyl)methylamino]-propyl]-1,3-dimethyl-1*H*-purine-2,6-dione (1:1); (2) 7-{2-Hydroxy-3-[(2-hydroxyethyl)methylamino]propyl}theophylline, compound with nicotinic acid (1:1). *CAS-437-74-1. Vasodilator (peripheral).* Complamin (3M Pharmaceuticals†)

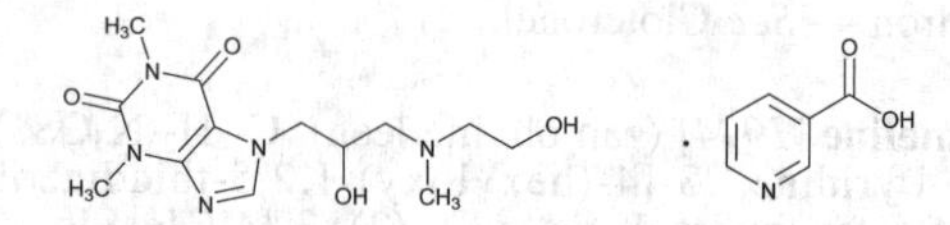

Xanthiol Hydrochloride. $C_{23}H_{31}Cl_3N_2OS$. 489.93. [Xanthiol is INN.] *CAS-17162-32-2; CAS-14008-71-0* [xanthiol]. Daxid (Roerig)

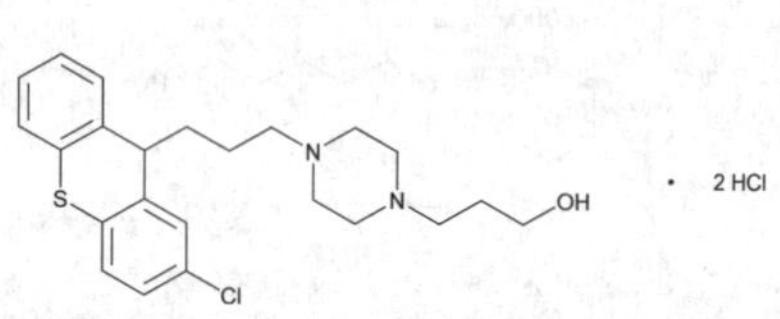

Xanthocillin (previously used name) — *See* Xantocillin.

Xanthotoxin — *See* Methoxsalen.

Xantifibrate. $C_{13}H_{21}N_5O_4 \cdot C_{10}H_{11}ClO_3$. 525.98. 7-[2-Hydroxy-3-[(2-hydroxyethyl)methylamino]propyl]theophylline compound with 2-(*p*-chlorophenoxy)-2-methylpropionic acid (1:1). *UNII-9FEN3M88VP. CAS-36921-54-7; CAS-882-09-7* [clofibric acid]. INN.

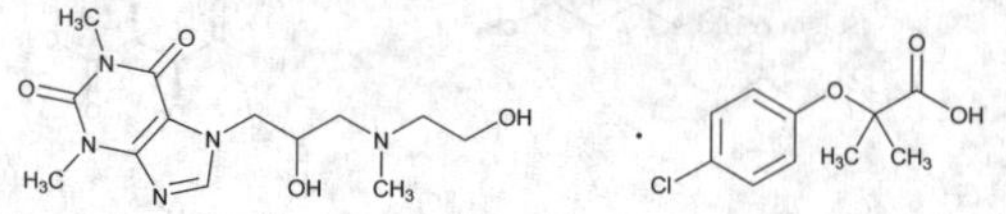

Xantinol Nicotinate (INN, BAN, DCF) — *See* Xanthinol Niacinate.

Xantocillin. Antibiotic obtained from cultures of *Penicillium notatum* or the same substance produced by any other means. *UNII-EX637I77PC. CAS-580-74-5.* INN; BAN.

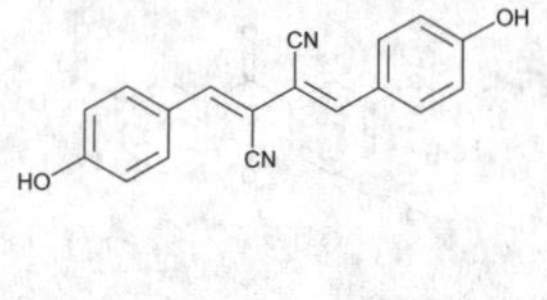

Xantofyl Palmitate. $C_{72}H_{116}O_4$. 1045.69. [Helenien is JAN.] β-Carotene-4,4′-diol dipalmitate. *UNII-V2W1791D7V. CAS-547-17-1.* INN.

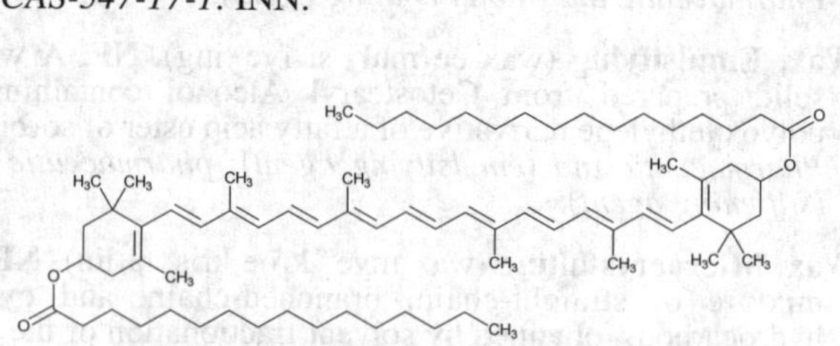

^{127}Xe — *See* Xenon Xe 127.

^{133}Xe — *See* Xenon Xe 133.

Xemilofiban Hydrochloride [*1995*] (ze mil″ oh fye′ ban hye″ droe klor′ ide). $C_{18}H_{22}N_4O_4 \cdot HCl$. 394.85. [Xemilofiban is INN.] (1) 4-Pentynoic acid, 3-[[4-[[4-(aminoiminomethyl)-phenyl]amino]-1,4-dioxobutyl]amino]-, ethyl ester, monohydrochloride, (*S*)-; (2) Ethyl (3*S*)-3-[3-[(*p*-amidinophenyl)carbamoyl]propionamido]-4-pentynoate, monohydrochloride. *CAS-156586-91-3; CAS-149820-74-6* [xemilofiban]. *Prevention of post-recanalization reocclusion of coronary vessels; treatment of unstable angina.* ◇*SC-54684A*

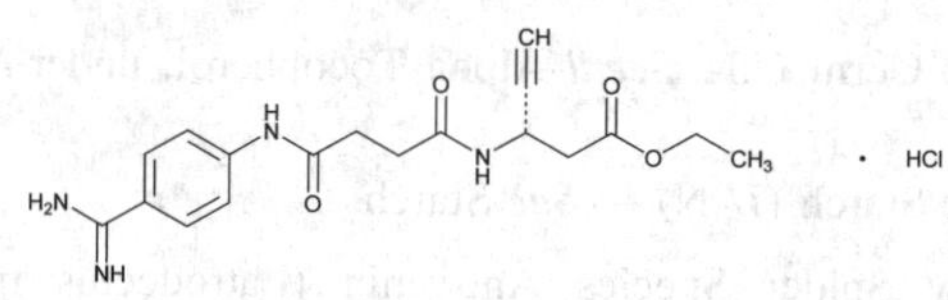

Xenalamine — *See* Xenazoic Acid.

Xenaldial — *See* Xenygloxal.

Xenalipin [*1989*] (zen″ a li′ pin). $C_{14}H_9F_3O_2$. 266.22. (1) [1,1′-Biphenyl]-2-carboxylic acid, 4′-(trifluoromethyl)-; (2) 4′-(Trifluoromethyl)-2-biphenylcarboxylic acid. *CAS-84392-17-6.* INN. *Hypolipidemic.* ◇*BW 207U*

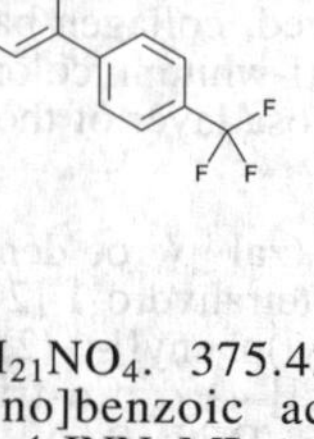

Xenazoic Acid. $C_{23}H_{21}NO_4$. 375.42. *p*-[(α-Ethoxy-*p*-phenylphenacyl)amino]benzoic acid. *UNII-KDU8V-H09O8. CAS-1174-11-4.* INN; MI. ◇*CV 58903; SKF-8318*

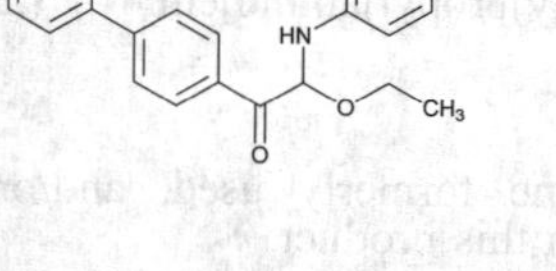

Xenbucin [*1981*] (zen bue′ sin). $C_{16}H_{16}O_2$. 240.30. (1) [1,1′-Biphenyl]-4-acetic acid, α-ethyl-, (±)-; (2) (±)-α-Ethyl-4-biphenylacetic acid. *UNII-R3U09W4H4I. CAS-959-10-4.* INN. *Antihyperlipidemic.* Liosol (Maggioni Farmaceutici S.p.A., Italy) ◇*M.G. 1559*

Xenbuficin — *See* Xenbucin.

Xenipentone. $C_{17}H_{16}O$. 236.31. (*E*)-4-(4-Biphenylyl)-3-penten-2-one. *UNII-GP581VM303. CAS-55845-78-8.* INN.

Xenon Xe 127 (zee′ non). **USP.** A gas containing $100.0 \pm 15.0\%$ of the labeled amount of ^{127}Xe. *UNII-H95KBR1GDB. Diagnostic aid; gas, medicinal; radioactive agent.*

Xenon Xe 133 [*1971*] (zee′ non). **USP.** Xe. [Xenon (^{133}Xe) is INN; Xenon (^{133}Xe) Injection is JAN.] (1) Xenon, isotope of mass 133; (2) Xenon, isotope of mass 133. *UNII-X3P9A5HNYF. CAS-14932-42-4. Radioactive agent.* Xenon Xe 133 Gas Ampule (Medi-Physics†); Xenon Xe 133 Gas Vials (Medi-Physics†); Xeneisol (Mallinckrodt†); Xenon Xe 133-V.S.S. (Medi-Physics†)

Xenthiorate. $C_{22}H_{29}NOS$. 355.54. *S*-2-Diethylaminoethyl 2-(4-biphenyl)thiobutyrate. *UNII-0PM0Q96HVS. CAS-7009-79-2.* INN.

Xenygloxal. $C_{16}H_{10}O_4$. 266.25. 4,4′-Biphenyldiglyoxylaldehyde. *UNII-3C2T3HG40E. CAS-2673-23-6.* INN.

Xenyhexenic Acid. $C_{18}H_{18}O_2$. 266.33. 2-(4-Biphenylyl)-4-hexenoic acid. *UNII-4293LHY68W. CAS-964-82-9.* INN. ◇*CV 57533*

Xenysalate (INN, BAN) — *See* Biphenamine Hydrochloride.

Xenytropium Bromide. $C_{30}H_{34}BrNO_3$. 536.50. 8-(*p*-Phenylbenzyl)atropinium bromide. *CAS-511-55-7.* INN; MI. ◇*N-399*

Xibenolol. $C_{15}H_{25}NO_2$. 251.36. (±)-1-(*tert*-Butylamino)-3-(2,3-xylyloxy)-2-propanol. *UNII-0871JY946G. CAS-81584-06-7.* INN; MI.

Xibornol. $C_{18}H_{26}O$. 258.40. 6-Isobornyl-3,4-xylenol. *CAS-13741-18-9.* INN; DCF; MI; BAN.

Xidecaflur. $C_{22}H_{46}FNO_2$. 375.60. 2,2′-[(9Z)-9-Octadecenylimino]diethanol hydrofluoride. *UNII-OJK82QP37Q. CAS-207916-33-4.* INN.

Xilobam [*1978*] (zye′ loe bam). $C_{14}H_{19}N_3O$. 245.32. (1) Urea, *N*-(2,6-dimethylphenyl)-*N*′-(1-methyl-2-pyrrolidinylidene)-; (2) 1-(1-Methyl-2-pyrrolidinylidene)-3-(2,6-xylyl)urea. *CAS-50528-97-7.* INN. *Relaxant (muscle).* ◇*McN-3113*

Ximelagatran [*2002*] (zye″ mel a gat′ ran). C₂₄H₃₅N₅O₅. 473.57. (1) Glycine, *N*-[(1*R*)-1-cyclohexyl-2-[(2*S*)-2-[[[[4-[hydroxyamino)iminomethyl]phenyl]methyl]amino]carbonyl]-1-azetidinyl]-2-oxoethyl]-, ethyl ester; (2) Ethyl [[(1*R*)-1-cyclohexyl-2-[(2*S*)-2-[[4-(hydroxycarbamimidoyl)benzyl]carbamoyl]azetidin-1-yl-2-oxoethyl]amino]-acetate. *UNII-49HFB70472. CAS-192939-46-1.* INN. *Antithrombotic agent.* Exanta (proposed) (AstraZeneca) ✧*H 376/95*

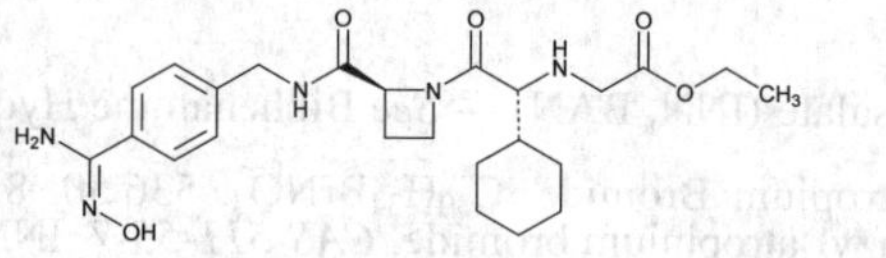

Ximoprofen. C₁₅H₁₉NO₃. 261.32. *p*-(3-Oxocyclohexyl)hydratropic acid oxime. *CAS-56187-89-4.* INN.

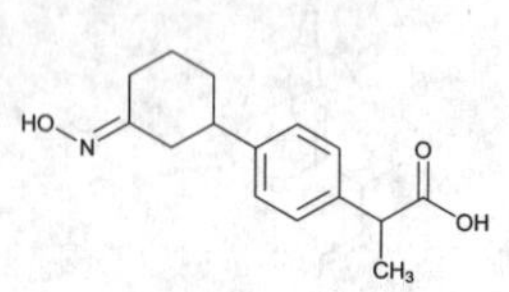

Xinidamine. C₁₇H₁₆N₂O₂. 280.32. 1-(2,4-Dimethylbenzyl)-1*H*-indazole-3-carboxylic acid. *UNII-8IVL8S1U34. CAS-50264-78-3.* INN.

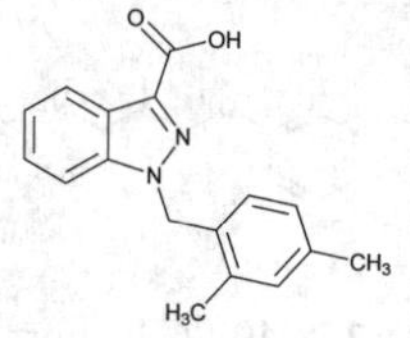

Xinomiline. C₅H₁₀N₂O. 114.15. 2-Amino-4,4-dimethyl-2-oxazoline. *UNII-3Q22EPG4O8. CAS-52832-91-4.* INN.

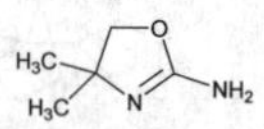

Xipamide [*1976*] (zip′ a mide). C₁₅H₁₅ClN₂O₄S. 354.81. (1) Benzamide, 5-(aminosulfonyl)-4-chloro-*N*-(2,6-dimethylphenyl)-2-hydroxy-; (2) 4-Chloro-5-sulfamoyl-2′,6′-salicyloxylidide. *CAS-14293-44-8.* INN; BAN. *Antihypertensive; diuretic.* ✧*MJF 10,938; Be-1293*

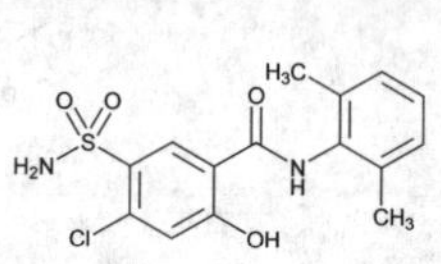

Xipranolol. C₂₃H₃₃NO₂. 355.51. 1-(Di-2,6-xylylmethoxy)-3-(isopropylamino)-2-propanol. *UNII-ZJI41P5WMH. CAS-19179-78-3.* INN. ✧*BS 7977 D [as dihydrochloride]*

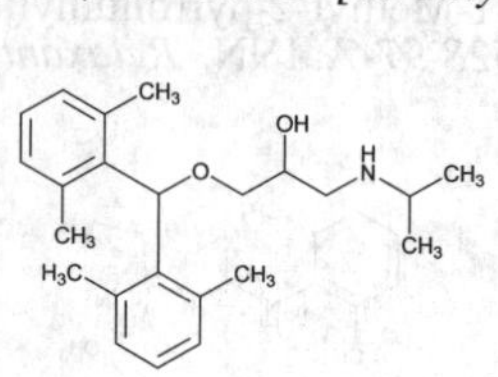

Xorphanol Mesylate [*1983*] (zor′ fa nol mes′ i late). C₂₃H₃₁NO.CH₄O₃S. 433.60. [Xorphanol is INN.] (1) Morphinan-3-ol, 17-(cyclobutylmethyl)-8-methyl-6-methylene-, (8*β*)-, methanesulfonate (salt); (2) 17-(Cyclobutylmethyl)-8*β*-methyl-6-methylenemorphinan-3-ol methanesulfonate (salt). *CAS-77287-90-2; CAS-77287-89-9* [xorphanol]. *Analgesic.* ✧*TR-5379M*

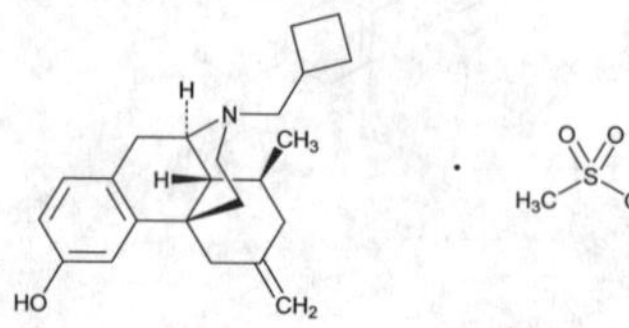

Xylamidine Tosylate [*1967*] (zye lam′ i deen tos′ i late). C₁₉H₂₄N₂O₂.C₇H₇SO₃H.½H₂O. 493.62. [Xylamidine Tosilate is INN; Xylamide Tosilate is BAN.] (1) Benzeneethanimidamide, *N*-[2-(3-methoxyphenoxy)propyl]-3-methyl-, mono(4-methylbenzenesulfonate); (2) *N*-[2-(*m*-Methoxyphenoxy)propyl]-2-*m*-tolylacetamidine mono-*p*-toluenesulfonate hemihydrate. *CAS-6443-40-9; CAS-6443-50-1* [xylamidine]. *Serotonin inhibitor.* [*Name previously used: Xylamide Tosylate.*]

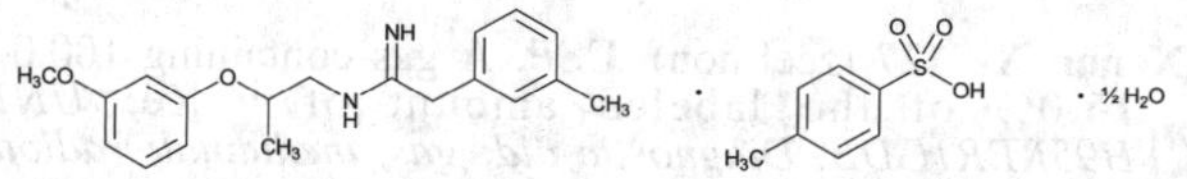

Xylazine (zye′ la zeen). USP. C₁₂H₁₆N₂S. 220.33. (1) 4*H*-1,3-Thiazin-2-amine, *N*-(2,6-dimethylphenyl)-5,6-dihydro-; (2) 5,6-Dihydro-2-(2,6-xylidino)-4*H*-1,3-thiazine. *UNII-2KFG9TP5V8. CAS-7361-61-7.* INN; BAN.

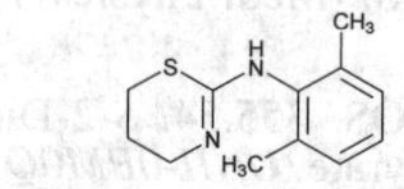

Xylazine Hydrochloride [*1972*] (zye′ la zeen hye″ droe klor′ ide). USP. C₁₂H₁₆N₂S.HCl. 256.79. (1) 4*H*-1,3-Thiazin-2-amine, *N*-(2,6-dimethylphenyl)-5,6-dihydro-, monohydrochloride; (2) 5,6-Dihydro-2-(2,6-xylidino)-4*H*-1,3-thiazine hydrochloride. *UNII-NGC3S0882S. CAS-23076-35-9. Analgesic; relaxant (muscle, veterinary).* Rompun (Bayer Animal Health) ✧*BAY Va 1470*

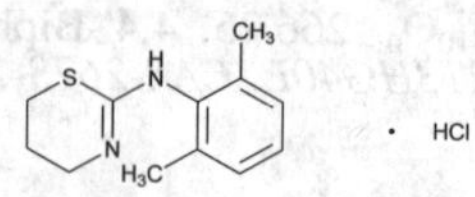

Xylitol (zye′ li tol). NF. C₅H₁₂O₅. 152.15. (1) Xylitol; (2) Xylitol. *UNII-VCQ006KQ1E. CAS-87-99-0.* BAN; JAN. *Pharmaceutic aid (vehicle, sweetened).*

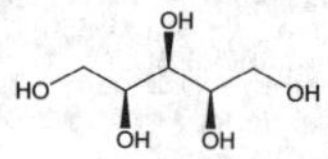

Xylocoumarol. $C_{17}H_{14}O_3$. 266.29. 4-Hydroxy-3-(3,5-xylyl)-coumarin. *UNII-J7I598ESCC. CAS-15301-97-0.* INN. ◇*B.S. 7173-D*

Xylofilcon A [*1986*] (zye″ loe fil′ kon). $(C_6H_9NO)_v$ $(C_5H_8O_2)_w(C_8H_{14}O_3)_x(C_{10}H_{16}O_2)_y(C_7H_{10}O_2)_z$. (1) 2-Pyrrolidinone, 1-ethenyl-, polymer with methyl 2-methyl-2-propenoate, 2-ethoxyethyl 2-methyl-2-propenoate, cyclohexyl 2-methyl-2-propenoate and 2-propenyl 2-methyl-2-propenoate; (2) 1-Vinyl-2-pyrrolidinone polymer with methyl methacrylate, 2-ethoxyethyl methacrylate, cyclohexyl methacrylate and allyl methacrylate. *CAS-84329-47-5. Contact lens material (hydrophilic).*

Xylometazoline Hydrochloride (zye″ loe me taz′ oh leen hye″ droe klor′ ide). **USP**. $C_{16}H_{24}N_2 \cdot HCl$. 280.84. [Xylometazoline is INN and BAN.] (1) 1*H*-Imidazole, 2-[[4-(1,1-dimethylethyl)-2,6-dimethylphenyl]methyl]-4,5-dihydro-, monohydrochloride; (2) 2-(4-*tert*-Butyl-2,6-dimethylbenzyl)-2-imidazoline monohydrochloride. *CAS-1218-35-5; CAS-526-36-3* [xylometazoline]. *Adrenergic (vasoconstrictor).* Neo-Synephrine II (Sterling Winthrop); Otrivin Hydrochloride (Ciba-Geigy†)

Xylose (zye′ lose). **USP**. $C_5H_{10}O_5$. 150.13. (1) D-Xylose; (2) D-Xylose. *UNII-A1TA934AKO. CAS-58-86-6* [acyclic form]; *CAS-7261-26-9* [D-Xylopyranose]; *CAS-6763-34-4* [α-D-Xylopyranose]; *CAS-2460-44-8* [β-D-Xylopyranose]. *Diagnostic aid (intestinal function determination).* Xylo-Pfan (Savage)

Xyloxemine. $C_{23}H_{33}NO_2$. 355.51. 2-[2-(Di-2,6-xylylmethoxy)ethoxy]-*N,N*-dimethylethylamine. *UNII-L95KV83PV9. CAS-1600-19-7.* INN. ◇*BS 6748*

^{169}Yb — *See* Pentetate Calcium Trisodium Yb 169.

^{169}Yb — *See* Ytterbium Yb 169 Pentetate.

Yeast, Dried. NF XIII; JAN; MI.

Yellow Fever Vaccine (yel′ oh fee′ ver vax′ een). **USP**. The attenuated strain that has been tested in monkeys for viscerotropism, immunogenicity, and neurotropism of living yellow fever virus selected for high antigenic activity and safety. *Immunizing agent (active).* YF-Vax (Bristol-Myers Squibb†)

Yellow Precipitate — *See* Mercuric Oxide, Yellow.

Yohimbic Acid. $C_{20}H_{24}N_2O_3$. 340.42. 17α-Hydroxyyohimban-16α-carboxylic acid. *UNII-35FAV1EVEG. CAS-522-87-2.* INN.

Yohimbine Hydrochloride (yoe him′ been hye″ droe klor′ ide). **USP**. $C_{21}H_{26}N_2O_3 \cdot HCl$. 390.90. 17α-Hydroxy-20-α-yohimban-16-β-carboxylic acid, methyl ester, hydrochloride. *UNII-NB2E1YP49F. CAS-65-19-0.* BAN.

Ytterbium Yb 169 Pentetate. $C_{14}H_{18}N_3Na_2O_{10}{}^{169}Yb$. (1) Ytterbate (2-)-$^{169}Yb$, [*N,N*-bis[2-[bis(carboxymethyl)amino]ethyl]glycinato(5-)]-, disodium; (2) Disodium [*N,N*-bis[2-[bis(carboxymethyl)amino]ethyl]glycinato(5-)]ytterbate(2-)-^{169}Yb. *CAS-81098-59-1.* USP XXII.

Yttrium Y 90 Epratuzumab [*2003*] (i′ tree um e″ pra tooz′ oo mab). (1) Immunoglobulin G1, anti-(human CD22 (antigen)) (human-mouse monoclonal hLL2 γ-chain), disulfide with human-mouse monoclonal hLL2 κ-chain, dimer, yttrium-90Y chelate; (2) Immunoglobulin G1 (human-mouse monoclonal hLL2 γ-chain anti-human antigen CD22), disulfide with human-mouse monoclonal hLL2 κ-chain, dimer, yttrium-90Y chelate. Molecular weight is approximately 150,000 daltons. *CAS-501423-23-0. Radioimmunotherapy (RAIT) for non-Hodgkin's B-cell lymphoma patients (monoclonal antibody).* LymphoCide (Immunomedics) ◇^{90}Y-*hLL2*

Yttrium Y 90 Epratuzumab Tetraxetan [*2004*] (i′ tree um e″ pra tooz′ oo mab te trax′ e tan). (1) Immunoglobulin G1, anti-(human CD22 (antigen)) (human-mouse monoclonal hLL2 γ-chain), disulfide with human-mouse monoclonal hLL2 κ-chain, dimer, 1,4,7,10-tetraazacyclododecane-1,4,7,10-tetraacetic acid conjugate, yttrium-90Y chelate; (2) Immunoglobulin G1 (human-mouse monoclonal hLL2 γ-chain anti-human antigen CD22), disulfide with human-

---

† Brand name formerly used, and/or firm no longer concerned with this product.

mouse monoclonal hLL2 κ-chain, dimer, 2,2',2'',2'''-(1,4,7,10-tetraazacyclododecane-1,4,7,10-tetryl)tetraacetic acid conjugate, yttrium-90Y. Molecular weight is approximately 150,000 daltons. *CAS-501423-25-2. Radioimmunotherapy (RAIT) for non-Hodgkin's B-cell lymphoma (monoclonal antibody).* ◇^{90}Y-DOTA-hLL2

Yttrium Y 90 Ibritumomab Tiuxetan (i' tree um eye'' bri toom' oh mab tye ux' e tan). **USP** [Injection]. The immunoconjugate resulting from a stable thiourea covalent bond between the monoclonal antibody ibritumomab and the linker-chelator tiuxetan [*N*-[2-bis(carboxymethyl)amino]-3-(*p*-isothiocyanatophenyl)propyl]-[*N*-[2-bis(carboxymethyl)amino]-2-(methyl)ethyl)glycine.

Yttrium Y 90 Labetuzumab [*2003*] (i' tree um la'' be tooz' oo mab). (1) Immunoglobulin G1, anti-(human carcinoembryonic antigen) (human-mouse monoclonal hMN-14 γ-chain), disulfide with human-mouse monoclonal hMN-14 κ-chain, dimer, yttrium-90Y chelate; (2) Immunoglobulin G1 (human-mouse monoclonal hMN-14 γ-chain anti-human carcinoembryonic antigen), disulfide with human-mouse monoclonal hMN-14 κ-chain, dimer, yttrium-90Y chelate. Molecular weight is approximately 150,000 daltons. *CAS-501423-27-4. Radioimmunotherapy (RAIT) of CEA-expressing tumors for use in the treatment of colorectal cancer (monoclonal antibody).* CEA-Cide (Immunomedics) ◇^{90}Y-hMN-14

Yttrium Y 90 Labetuzumab Tetraxetan [*2004*] (i' tree um la'' be tooz' oo mab te trax' e tan). (1) Immunoglobulin G1, anti-(human carcinoembryonic antigen) (human-mouse monoclonal hMN-14 γ-chain), disulfide with human-mouse monoclonal hMN-14 κ-chain, dimer, 1,4,7,10-tetraazacyclododecane-1,4,7,10-tetraacetic acid conjugate, yttrium-90Y chelate; (2) Immunoglobulin G1 (human-mouse monoclonal hMN-14 γ-chain anti-human carcinoembryonic antigen), disulfide with human-mouse monoclonal hMN-14 κ-chain, dimer, 2,2',2'',2'''-(1,4,7,10-tetraazacyclododecane-1,4,7,10-tetryl)tetraacetic acid conjugate, yttrium-90Y chelate. Molecular weight is approximately 150,000 daltons. *CAS-501423-30-9. Radioimmunotherapy (RAIT) for CEA-expressing tumors in colorectal, pancreatic, lung, breast, ovarian, and medullary thyroid cancer.* ◇^{90}Y-DOTA-hMN14

Yttrium Y 90 Tacatuzumab [*2004*] (i' tree um tak'' a tooz' oo mab). $C_{6470}H_{9971}N_{1712}O_{2007}S_{42}{}^{90}$Y. [Yttrium (^{90}Y) Tacatuzumab is INN.] Immunoglobulin G1, anti-(human α-fetoprotein) (human-mouse monoclonal hAFP-31 γ1-chain), disulfide with human-mouse monoclonal hAFP-31 κ-chain dimer, 1,4,7,10-tetraazacyclododecane-1,4,7,10-tetraacetic acid conjugate, yttrium-^{90}Y chelate. *CAS-476413-07-7. Tumor eradication.* AFP-Cide (Immunomedics) ◇*hAFP-31*

Yttrium Y 90 Tacatuzumab Tetraxetan [*2004*] (i' tree um tak'' a tooz' oo mab te trax' e tan). Immunoglobulin G1, anti-(human α-fetoprotein) (human-mouse monoclonal hAFP-31 γ1-chain), disulfide with human-mouse monoclonal hAFP-31 κ-chain dimer, 1,4,7,10-tetraazacyclododecane-1,4,7,10-tetraacetic acid conjugate, yttrium-^{90}Y chelate. *CAS-476413-07-7.* BAN. *Tumor eradication.* AFP-Cide (Immunomedics) ◇*hAFP-31*

Zabicipril. $C_{23}H_{32}N_2O_5$. 416.51. (3*S*)-2-[(2*S*)-*N*-[(1*S*)-1-Carboxy-3-phenylpropyl]alanyl]-2-azabicyclo[2.2.2]octane-3-carboxylic acid, 1-ethyl ester. *CAS-83059-56-7. INN.*

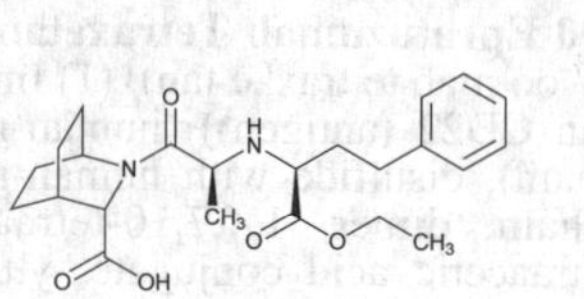

Zabiciprilat. $C_{21}H_{28}N_2O_5$. 388.46. (*S*)-2-[(*S*)-*N*-[(*S*)-1-Carboxy-3-phenylpropyl]alanyl]-2-azabicyclo[2.2.2]octane-3-carboxylic acid. *UNII-0A2D355316. CAS-90103-92-7.* INN.

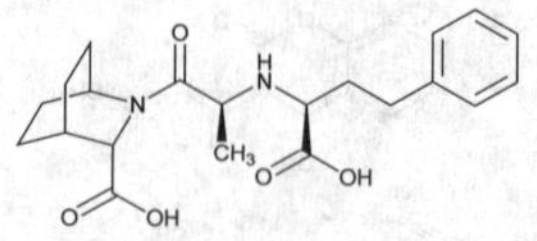

Zabofloxacin. $C_{19}H_{20}FN_5O_4$. 401.39. 1-Cyclopropyl-6-fluoro-7-[8-(methoxyimino)-2,6-diazaspiro[3.4]octan-6-yl]-4-oxo-1,4-dihydro-1,8-naphthyridine-3-carboxylic acid. *CAS-219680-11-2.* INN.

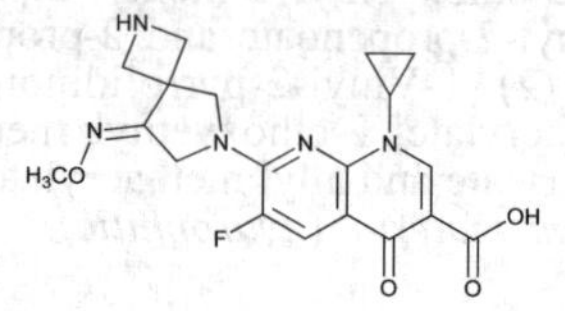

Zacopride Hydrochloride [*1986*] (za' koe pride hye'' droe klor' ide). $C_{15}H_{20}ClN_3O_2 \cdot HCl \cdot H_2O$. 364.27. [Zacopride is INN.] (1) Benzamide, 4-amino-*N*-1-azabicyclo[2.2.2]oct-3-yl-5-chloro-2-methoxy-, monohydrochloride, monohydrate; (2) 4-Amino-5-chloro-*N*-3-quinuclidinyl-*o*-anisamide monohydrochloride monohydrate. *CAS-99617-34-2; CAS-90182-92-6* [zacopride]. INN. *Anti-emetic; stimulant (peristaltic).* ◇*AHR-11190-B*

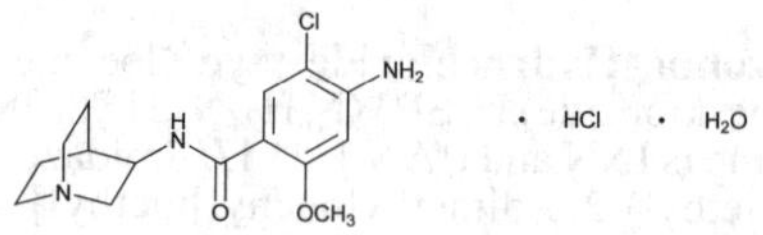

Zafirlukast [*1995*] (za'' fir loo' kast). $C_{31}H_{33}N_3O_6S$. 575.68. (1) Carbamic acid, [3-[[2-methoxy-4-[[[2-methylphenyl)sulfonyl]amino]carbonyl]phenyl]methyl]-1-methyl-1*H*-indol-5-yl]-, cyclopentyl ester; (2) Cyclopentyl 3-[2-methoxy-4-[(*o*-tolylsulfonyl)carbamoyl]benzyl]-1-methylindole-5-carbamate. *UNII-XZ629S5L50. CAS-107753-78-6.* INN; BAN. *Anti-asthmatic (leukotriene antagonist).* Accolate (AstraZeneca) ◇*ICI 204,219*

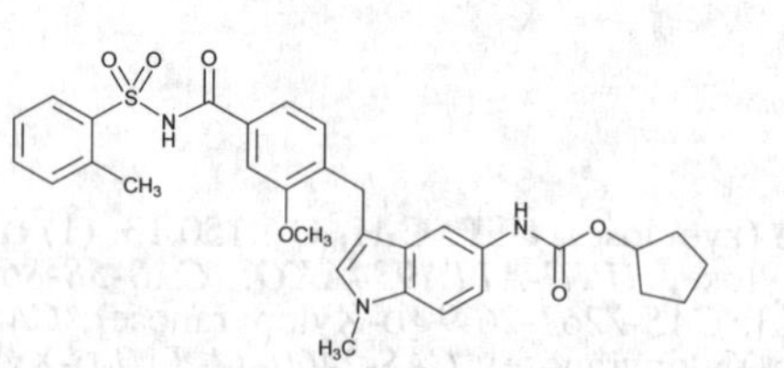

Zafuleptine. $C_{17}H_{26}FNO_2$. 295.39. (±)-7-[(*p*-Fluorobenzyl)amino]-8-methylnonanoic acid. *UNII-E697IIC25J. CAS-59209-97-1.* INN.

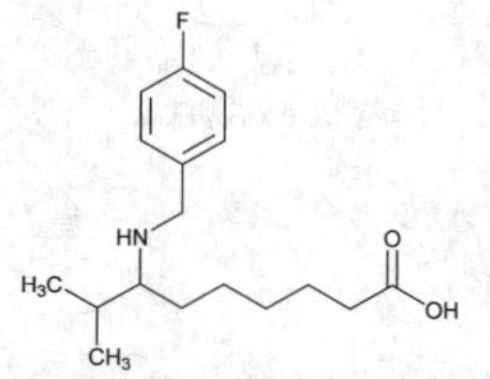

Zalcitabine [*1991*] (zal sye′ ta been). **USP.** $C_9H_{13}N_3O_3$. 211.22. (1) Cytidine, 2′,3′-dideoxy-; (2) 2′,3′-Dideoxycytidine. *UNII-6L3XT8CB3I.* *CAS-7481-89-2.* INN; BAN. *Antiviral.* Hivid (Roche) ◇*Ro 24-2027/000; NSC-606170*

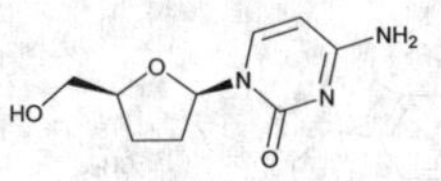

Zaldaride. $C_{26}H_{28}N_4O_2$. 428.53. (±)-1-[1-[(4-Methyl-4*H*,6*H*-pyrrolo[1,2-*α*][4,1]benzoxazepin-4-yl)methyl]-4-piperidyl]-2-benzimidazolinone. *UNII-GH66PET6S3.* *CAS-109826-26-8.* INN.

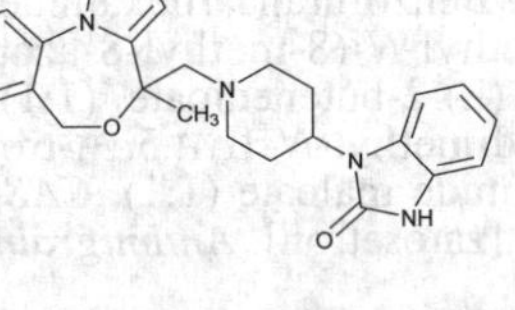

Zaleplon [*1994*] (zal′ e plon). $C_{17}H_{15}N_5O$. 305.33. (1) Acetamide, *N*-[3-(3-cyanopyrazolo[1,5-*α*]pyrimidin-7-yl)-phenyl]-*N*-ethyl-; (2) 3′-(3-Cyanopyrazolo[1,5-*α*]pyrimin-7-yl)-*N*-ethylacetanilide. *UNII-S62U433RMH.* *CAS-151319-34-5.* INN; BAN. *Sedative-hypnotic.* Sonata (King) ◇*CL 284,846; L846; LJC 10846; ZAL-846*

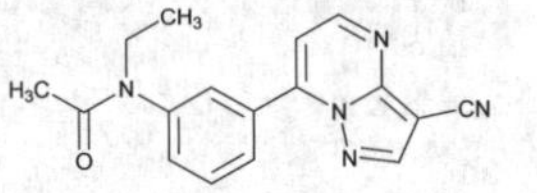

Zalospirone Hydrochloride [*1991*] (zal″ oh spye′ rone hye″ droe klor′ ide). $C_{24}H_{29}N_5O_2$·HCl. 455.98. [Zalospirone is INN.] (1) 4,7-Etheno-1*H*-cyclobut[*f*]isoindole-1,3(2*H*)-dione, 3a,4,4a,6a,7,7a-hexahydro-2-[4-[4-(2-pyrimidinyl)-1-piperazinyl]butyl]-, monohydrochloride, (3a*α*,4*β*,4a*α*,6a*α*,7*β*,7a*α*)-; (2) (1*R**,2*R**,5*S**,6*S**,7*S**,8*R**)-*N*-[4-[4-(2-Pyrimidinyl)-1-piperazinyl]butyl]tricyclo[4.2.2.0^{2,5}]deca-3,9-diene-7,8-dicarboximide monohydrochloride. *UNII-51EH2KC4M6.* *CAS-114374-97-9; CAS-114298-18-9* [zalospirone]. *Anti-anxiety agent.* ◇*WY-47846HCl*

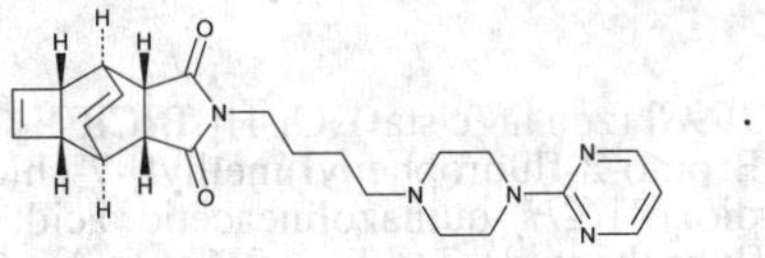

Zaltidine Hydrochloride [*1986*] (zal′ ti deen hye″ droe klor′ ide). $C_8H_{10}N_6S$·2HCl. 295.19. [Zaltidine is INN and BAN.] (1) Guanidine, [4-(2-methyl-1*H*-imidazol-5-yl)-2-thiazolyl]-, dihydrochloride; (2) [4-(2-Methylimidazol-5-yl)-2-thiazolyl]guanidine dihydrochloride. *CAS-90274-23-0; CAS-85604-00-8* [zaltidine]. *Antagonist (to histamine H_2receptors).* ◇*CP-57,361-01*

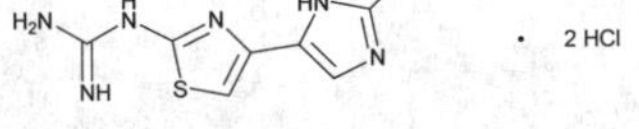

Zaltoprofen. $C_{17}H_{14}O_3S$. 298.36. (±)-10,11-Dihydro-*α*-methyl-10-oxodibenzo[*b*,*f*]thiepin-2-acetic acid. *UNII-H8635NG3PY.* *CAS-89482-00-8.* INN; JAN.

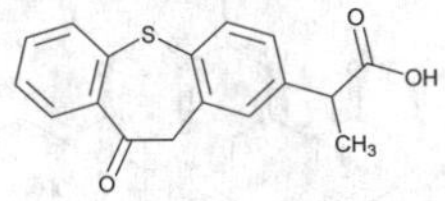

Zalutumumab. $C_{6512}H_{10074}N_{1734}O_{2032}S_{46}$. Immunoglobulin G1, anti-(human epidermal growth factor receptor)(human monoclonal 2F8 heavy chain), disulfide with human monoclonal 2F8 *κ*-chain, dimer. *CAS-667901-13-5.* INN.

Zamifenacin. $C_{27}H_{29}NO_3$. 415.52. (*R*)-3-(Diphenylmethoxy)-1-[3,4-(methylenedioxy)phenetyl]piperidene. *UNII-Y88Q418Y7M.* *CAS-127308-82-1.* INN. ◇*UK-76654-2 [as fumarate]*

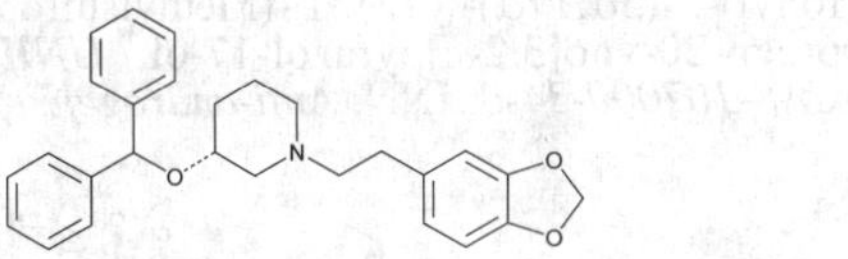

Zanamivir [*1997*] (zan am′ i vir). $C_{12}H_{20}N_4O_7$. 332.31. (1) D-*glycero*-D-*galacto*-Non-2-enonic acid, 5-(acetylamino)-4-[(aminoiminomethyl)amino]-2,6-anhydro-3,4,5-trideoxy-; (2) 5-Acetamido-2,6-anhydro-3,4,5-trideoxy-4-guanidino-D-*glycero*-D-*galacto*-non-2-enonic acid. *UNII-L6O3XI777I.* *CAS-139110-80-8.* INN; BAN. *Antiviral; inhibitor (influenza virus neuraminidase).* Relenza (GlaxoSmithKline) ◇*GR 121167X*

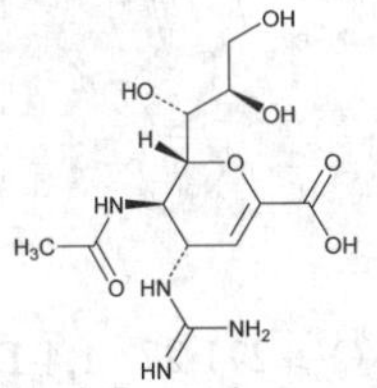

Zanapezil. $C_{25}H_{32}N_2O$. 376.53. 3-(1-Benzylpiperidin-4-yl)-1-(2,3,4,5-tetrahydro-1*H*-1-benzazepin-8-yl)propan-1-one. *UNII-0A0800O89N.* *CAS-142852-50-4.* INN.

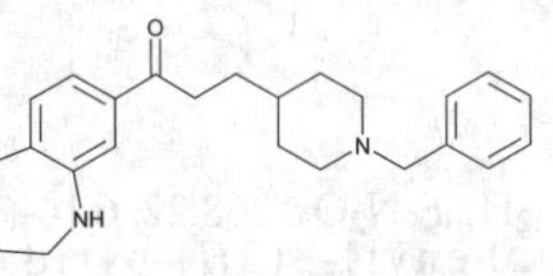

Zankiren Hydrochloride [*1993*] (zan kye′ ren hye″ droe klor′ ide). $C_{35}H_{55}N_5O_6S_2$·HCl. 742.43. [Zankiren is INN.] (1) 4-Thiazolepropanamide, *N*-[1-(cyclohexylmethyl)-2,3-dihydroxy-5-methylhexyl]-*α*-[[2-[[(4-methyl-1-piperazinyl)sulfonyl]methyl]-1-oxo-3-phenylpropyl]amino]-, monohydrochloride, [1*S*-[1*R**,[*R**(*R**)],2*S**,3*R**]]-; (2) (*S*)-*N*-(1*S*,2*R*,3*S*)-1-(Cyclohexylmethyl)-2,3-dihydroxy-5-methylhexyl]-*α*[(*α*S)-*α*-[[(4-methyl-1-piperazinyl)sulfo-

---

† Brand name formerly used, and/or firm no longer concerned with this product.

nyl]methyl]hydrocinnamamido]-4-thiazolepropionamide monohydrochloride. *CAS-138810-64-7; CAS-138742-43-5* [zankiren]. *Antihypertensive.* ◇*Abbott-72517*

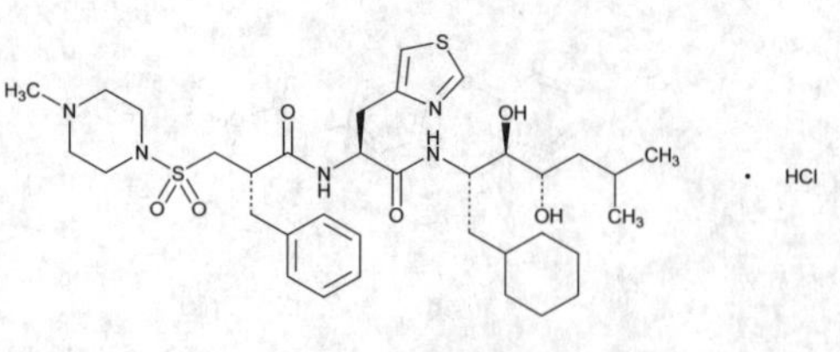

Zanolimumab [*2005*] (zan″ oh lim′ ue mab). Immunoglobulin, anti-(human CD4 antigen) (human monoclonal 6G5 heavy chain), disulfide with human monoclonal 6G5 light chain, dimer. Molecular weight is approximately 147,000 daltons. *CAS-652153-01-0.* INN. *Treatment of rheumatoid arthritis, psoriasis, cutaneous and peripheral T-cell lymphoma.* ◇*MDX-016; HuMax-CD4*

Zanoterone [*1992*] (zan oh′ ter one). $C_{23}H_{32}N_2O_3S$. 416.58. (1) 1′*H*-Pregn-20-yno[3,2-*c*]pyrazol-17-ol, 1′-(methylsulfonyl)-, (5α,17α)-; (2) 1′-(Methylsulfonyl)-1′*H*-5α,17α-pregn-20-yno[3,2-*c*]pyrazol-17-ol. *UNII-XQ5V1W49JG. CAS-107000-34-0.* INN. *Anti-androgen.* ◇*Win 49,596*

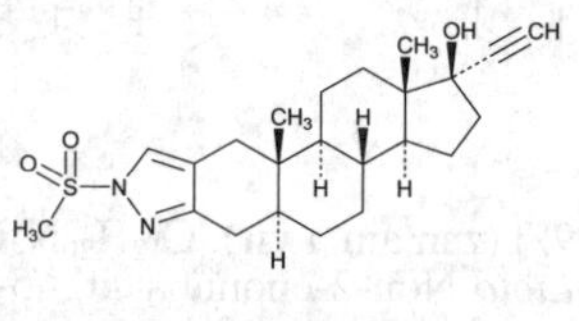

Zapizolam. $C_{15}H_9Cl_2N_5$. 330.17. 8-Chloro-6-(*o*-chlorophenyl)-4*H*-pyrido[2,3-*f*]-*s*-triazolo[4,3-*a*][1,4]diazepine. *UNII-MFF90009B9. CAS-64098-32-4.* INN.

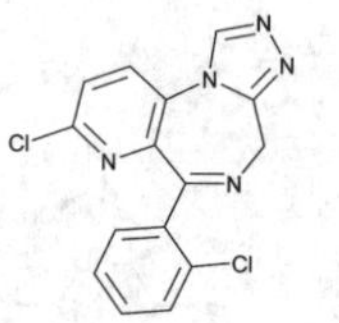

Zaprinast. $C_{13}H_{13}N_5O_2$. 271.27. 1,4-Dihydro-5-(2-propoxyphenyl)-1,2,3-triazolo[4,5-*d*]pyrimidin-7-one. *UNII-GXT25D5DS0. CAS-37762-06-4.* INN; BAN. ◇*M&B 22948*

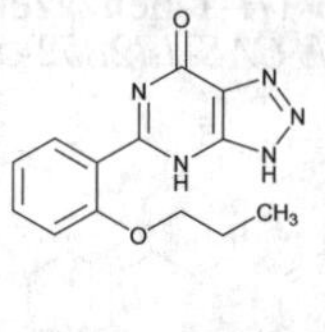

Zardaverine. $C_{12}H_{10}F_2N_2O_3$. 268.22. 6-[4-(Difluoromethoxy)-3-methoxyphenyl]-3(2*H*)-pyridazinone. *UNII-TQ358GWH6Y. CAS-101975-10-4.* INN.

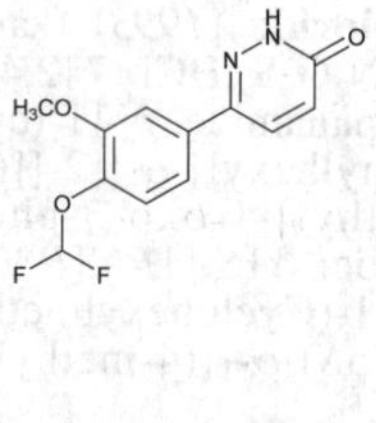

Zatebradine. $C_{26}H_{36}N_2O_5$. 456.57. 3-[3-[[(3,4-Dimethoxyphenethyl)methylamino]propyl]-1,3,4,5-tetrahydro-7,8-dimethoxy-2*H*-3-benzazepin-2-one. *UNII-TV27RY5876. CAS-85175-67-3.* INN.

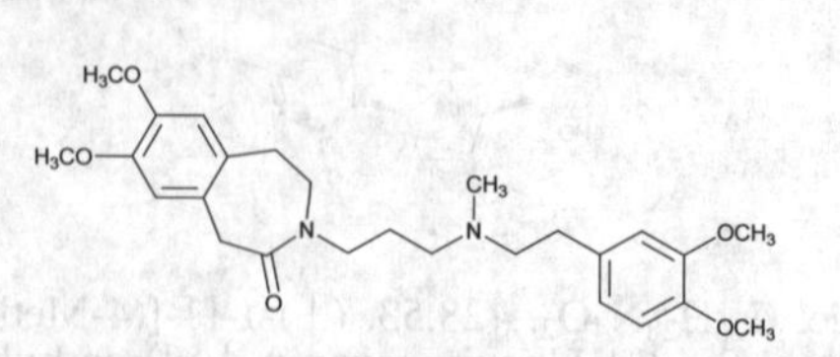

Zatosetron Maleate [*1990*] (za toe′ se tron mal′ ee ate). $C_{19}H_{25}ClN_2O_2 \cdot C_4H_4O_4$. 464.94. [Zatosetron is INN and BAN.] (1) 7-Benzofurancarboxamide, 5-chloro-2,3-dihydro-2,2-dimethyl-*N*-(8-methyl-8-azabicyclo[3.2.1]oct-3-yl)-, *endo*-, (*Z*)-2-butenedioate (1:1); (2) 5-Chloro-2,3-dihydro-2,2-dimethyl-*N*-1αH,5αH-tropan-3α-yl-7-benzofurancarboxamide maleate (1:1). *CAS-123482-23-5; CAS-123482-22-4* [zatosetron]. *Antimigraine.* ◇*LY277359 maleate*

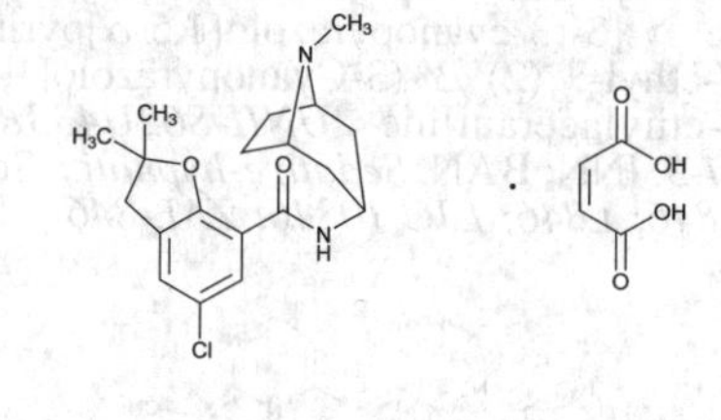

Zein (zee′ in). **NF**. A prolamine derived from corn (*Zea mays* Linné [Fam. Gramineae]). *Pharmaceutic aid (coating agent).*

Zelandopam. $C_{15}H_{15}NO_4$. 273.28. (-)-(*S*)-4-(3,4-Dihydroxyphenyl)-1,2,3,4-tetrahydro-7,8-isoquinolinediol. *UNII-IR6-XYD8SAX. CAS-139233-53-7.* INN.

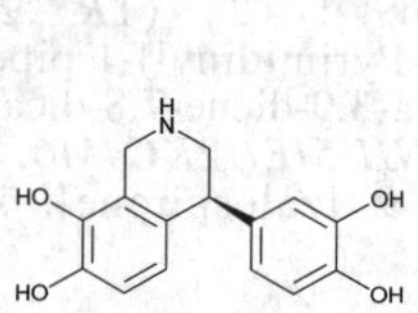

Zenarestat [*1998*] (zen ar′ e stat). $C_{17}H_{11}BrClFN_2O_4$. 441.64. (1) 3-[[4-Bromo-2-fluorophenyl)methyl]-7-chloro-3,4-dihydro-2,4-dioxo-1(2*H*)-quinazolineacetic acid; (2) 3-(4-Bromo-2-fluorobenzyl)-7-chloro-3,4-dihydro-2,4-dioxo-1(2*H*)-quinazolineacetic acid. *UNII-180C9PJ8JT. CAS-112733-06-9.* INN. *Treatment of diabetic neuropathy (aldose reductase inhibitor).* ◇*CI-1014; FK-366; FR-74366*

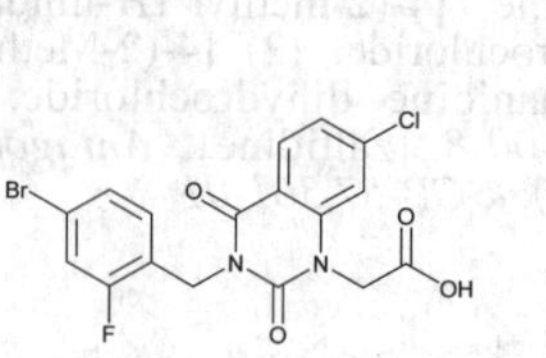

Zenazocine Mesylate [*1983*] (zen az′ oh seen mes′ i late). $C_{23}H_{35}NO_2 \cdot CH_4O_3S$. 453.64. (1) 3-Heptanone, 1-(1,2,3,4,5,6-hexahydro-8-hydroxy-3,6,11-trimethyl-2,6-methano-3-benzazocin-11-yl)-6-methyl-, (2α,6α,11*S**)-(±)-, methanesulfonate (salt); (2) (±)-1-[(2*R**,6*S**,11*S**)-1,2,3,4,5,6-Hexahydro-8-hydroxy-3,6,11-trimethyl-2,6-

methano-3-benzazocin-11-yl]-6-methyl-3-heptanone methanesulfonate (salt). *CAS-74559-85-6. Analgesic.* ◇*Win 42964-4*

Zeniplatin [*1990*] (zen″ i pla′ tin). $C_{11}H_{20}N_2O_6Pt$. 471.37. (1) Platinum, [2,2-bis(aminomethyl)-1,3-propanediol-*N,N′*][1,1-cyclobutanedicarboxylato(2-)]-, (*SP*-4-2)-; (2) *cis*-[2,2-Bis(aminomethyl)-1,3-propanediol](1,1-cyclobutanedicarboxylato)platinum. *CAS-111490-36-9. INN. Antineoplastic.* ◇*CL 286,558*

Zepastine. $C_{22}H_{26}N_2O_3S$. 398.52. 6,11-Dihydro-6-methyl-11-(1α*H*,5α*H*-tropan-3α-yloxy)dibenzo[*c,f*][1,2]thiazepine 5,5-dioxide. *UNII-27D37TX66Y. CAS-28810-23-3.* INN; DCF.

Zeranol [*1969*] (zer′ a nol). $C_{18}H_{26}O_5$. 322.40. (1) 1*H*-2-Benzoxacyclotetradecin-1-one, 3,4,5,6,7,8,9,10,11,12-decahydro-7,14,16-trihydroxy-3-methyl-, [3*S*-(3*R**,7*S**)]-; (2) (3*S*,7*X*)-3,4,5,6,7,8,9,10,11,12-Decahydro-7,14,16-trihydroxy-3-methyl-1*H*-2-benzoxacyclotetradecin-1-one; (3) (6*X*,10*S*)-6-(6,10-Dihydroxyundecyl)-β-resorcylic acid μ-lactone. *UNII-76LO2L2V39. CAS-26538-44-3.* INN; BAN. *Anabolic.* Ralabol (Pitman-Moore); Ralgro (Pitman-Moore) ◇*THFES (HM); P-1496; MK-188*

Zetidoline. $C_{16}H_{22}ClN_3O$. 307.82. 1-(*m*-Chlorophenyl)-3-[2-(3,3-dimethyl-1-azetidinyl)ethyl]-2-imidazolidinone. *UNII-3B5J9TG94X. CAS-51940-78-4.* INN; BAN.

Zibotentan [*2008*] (zye″ boe ten′ tan). $C_{19}H_{16}N_6O_4S$. 424.43. (1) 3-Pyridinesulfonamide, *N*-(3-methoxy-5-methyl-2-pyrazinyl)-2-[4-(1,3,4-oxadiazol-2-yl)phenyl]-; (2) *N*-(3-Methoxy-5-methylpyrazin-2-yl)-2-[4-(1,3,4-oxadiazol-2-yl)phenyl]pyridine-3-sulfonamide. *UNII-8054MM4902. CAS-186497-07-4.* INN. *Treatment of prostate cancer.* ◇*ZD4054*

Ziconotide [*1997*] (zye kon′ oh tide). $C_{102}H_{172}N_{36}O_{32}S_7$. 2639.13. (1) ω-Conotoxin M VIIA; (2) L-Cysteinyl-L-lysylglycyl-L-lysylglycyl-L-alanyl-L-lysyl-L-cysteinyl-L-seryl-L-arginyl-L-leucyl-L-methionyl-L-tyrosyl-L-α-aspartyl-L-cysteinyl-L-cysteinyl-L-threonylglycyl-L-seryl-L-cysteinyl-L-arginyl-L-serylglycyl-L-lysyl-L-cysteinamide cyclic (1→16),(8→20),(15→25)-tris(disulfide). *UNII-7I64C51O16. CAS-107452-89-1.* INN. *Treatment of and brain ischemia; analgesic.* Prialt (Elan) ◇*SNX-111*

CKGKGAKCSR LMYDCCTGSC RSGKC —NH₂

Zidapamide [*1983*] (zye dap′ a mide). $C_{16}H_{16}ClN_3O_3S$. 365.83. 4-Chloro-*N*-(1-methyl-2-isoindolinyl)-3-sulfamoylbenzamide. *CAS-75820-08-5.* INN.

Zidometacin [*1978*] (zye″ doe met′ a sin). $C_{19}H_{16}N_4O_4$. 364.35. (1) 1*H*-Indole-3-acetic acid, 1-(4-azidobenzoyl)-5-methoxy-2-methyl-; (2) 1-(*p*-Azidobenzoyl)-5-methoxy-2-methylindole-3-acetic acid. *UNII-446VQG66LC. CAS-62851-43-8.* INN. *Anti-inflammatory.*

Zidovudine [*1987*] (zye doe′ vue deen). **USP.** $C_{10}H_{13}N_5O_4$. 267.24. (1) Thymidine, 3′-azido-3′-deoxy-; (2) 3′-Azido-3′-deoxythymidine. *UNII-4B9XT59T7S. CAS-30516-87-1.* INN; BAN; JAN. *Antiviral.* Retrovir (GlaxoSmithKline) [*Name previously used: Azidothymidine.*] ◇*BW A509U; Compound S; AZT*

Zifrosilone [*1994*] (zye froe′ si lone). $C_{11}H_{13}F_3OSi$. 246.30. (1) Ethanone, 2,2,2-trifluoro-1-[3-(trimethylsilyl)phenyl]-; (2) 2,2,2-Trifluoro-3′-(trimethylsilyl)acetophenone. *CAS-132236-18-1.* INN. *Inhibitor (acetylcholinesterase).* ◇*MDL 73,745*

Zilantel [*1975*] (zil an′ tel). $C_{26}H_{38}N_2O_6P_2S_4$. 664.80. (1) Carbonimidodithioic acid, (diethoxyphosphinyl)-, 1,2-ethanediyl bis(phenylmethyl) ester; (2) Phosphonodithioimidocarbonic acid ethylene dibenzyl *P,P,P′,P′*-tetraethyl ester. *CAS-22012-72-2.* INN. *Anthelmintic.* ◇*Cl-64,976*

Zilascorb (^{2}H). 5,6-*O*-[(*RS*)-Benzylidene-α-*d*]-L-ascorbic acid. *CAS-122431-96-3.* INN.

Zileuton [*1990*] (zye loo′ ton). USP. $C_{11}H_{12}N_2O_2S$. 236.29. (1) Urea, *N*-(1-benzo[*b*]thien-2-ylethyl)-*N*-hydroxy-, (±)-; (2) (±)-1-(1-Benzo[*b*]thien-2-ylethyl)-1-hydroxyurea. *UNII-V1L22WVE2S. CAS-111406-87-2.* INN; BAN. *Inhibitor (5-lipoxygenase).* Zyflo (Sensus) ◇*Abbott-64077*

Zilpaterol. $C_{14}H_{19}N_3O_2$. 261.32. (±)-*trans*-4,5,6,7-Tetrahydro-7-hydroxy-6-(isopropylamino)imidazo[4,5,1-*jk*][1]benzazepin-2(1*H*)-one. *UNII-S384A1Y12J. CAS-117827-79-9.* INN.

Zimeldine Hydrochloride [*1977*] (zye mel′ deen hye″ droe klor′ ide). $C_{16}H_{17}BrN_2.2HCl.H_2O$. 408.16. [Zimeldine is INN and BAN.] (1) 2-Propen-1-amine, 3-(4-bromophenyl)-*N,N*-dimethyl-3-(3-pyridinyl)-, (*Z*)-, dihydrochloride monohydrate; (2) (*Z*)-3-[1-(*p*-Bromophenyl)-3-(dimethylamino)propenyl]pyridine dihydrochloride monohydrate. *CAS-61129-30-4; CAS-60525-15-7* [anhydrous]; *CAS-*

56775-88-3 [zimeldine]. *Antidepressant. [Name previously used: Zimelidine Hydrochloride]* ◇*H 102/09 Hydrochloride*

Zimelidine Hydrochloride (previously used name) — *See* Zimeldine Hydrochloride.

Zimidoben. $C_{12}H_{12}N_2O_2$. 216.24. 2-Imidazol-1-ylethyl benzoate *or* imidazole-1-ethanol benzoate (ester). *UNII-28810ORE8K. CAS-90697-56-6.* INN.

Zinc Acetate (zink as′ e tate). USP. $C_4H_6O_4Zn.2H_2O$. 219.50. (1) Acetic acid, zinc salt, dihydrate; (2) Zinc acetate dihydrate. *UNII-FM5526K07A. CAS-5970-45-6; CAS-557-34-6* [anhydrous]. Pharmaceutic necessity for Zinc-Eugenol Cement. Galzin (Teva)

Zinc Acetate, Basic. $C_{12}H_{18}O_{13}Zn_4$. 631.78. Hexakis(μ-acetato)-μ4-oxotetrazinc. *CAS-82279-57-0.* INN.

Zinc Carbonate [*1988*] (zink kar′ bo nate). USP. $3Zn(OH)_2.2ZnCO_3$. 548.96. (1) Bis[carbonato(2-)]hexahydroxypentazinc; (2)Bis[(carbonato)hexahydroxypentazinc; (3) Zinc subcarbonate. *UNII-EQR32Y7H0M. CAS-3486-35-9. Antiseptic (topical); astringent.*

Zinc Chloride (zink klor′ ide). USP. $ZnCl_2$. 136.29. (1) Zinc chloride; (2) Zinc chloride. *UNII-86Q357L16B. CAS-7646-85-7.* JAN. *Astringent; dentin desensitizer.*

Zinc Chloride Zn 65 [*1964*] (zink klor′ ide). $^{65}ZnCl_2$. (1) Zinc chloride ($^{65}ZnCl_2$); (2) Zinc chloride ($^{65}ZnCl_2$). *CAS-24359-56-6. Radioactive agent.*

Zinc Gelatin. *CAS-8047-36-7.* USP XXI.

Zinc Gluconate (zink gloo′ koe nate). USP. $C_{12}H_{22}O_{14}Zn$. 455.67. (1) Bis(D-gluconato-O^1,O^2) zinc; (2) Zinc D-gluconate (1:2). *CAS-4468-02-4. Supplement (trace mineral).*

Zinc Oleate. *UNII-7C247FL5FG. CAS-557-07-3.* NF III; MI.

Zinc Oxide (zink ox′ ide). **USP**. ZnO. 81.38. (1) Zinc oxide; (2) Zinc oxide. *UNII-SOI2LOH54Z. CAS-1314-13-2*. JAN. *Astringent; protectant (topical)*.

Zinc Peroxide, Medicinal. *CAS-1314-22-3*. USP XVII; MI.

Zinc Phenolsulfonate. [Phenolsulfonic Acid is JAN.] *CAS-127-82-2; CAS-98-67-9* [*p*-phenolsulfonic acid]. NF XI; MI.

Zinc Stearate (zink steer′ ate). **USP**. (1) Octadecanoic acid, zinc salt; (2) Zinc stearate. *CAS-557-05-1. Dusting powder; pharmaceutic aid (tablet and/or capsule lubricant)*.

Zinc Sulfate (zink sul′ fate). **USP**. $ZnSO_4.xH_2O$. 161.44 (anhydrous). (1) Sulfuric acid, zinc salt (1:1), hydrate; (2) Zinc sulfate (1:1) monohydrate; (3) Zinc sulfate (1:1) heptahydrate. *UNII-89DS0H96TB. CAS-7446-20-0* [heptahydrate]; *CAS-7733-02-0* [anhydrous]. JAN. *Astringent (ophthalmic)*.

Zinc Sulfocarbolate — *See* Zinc Phenolsulfonate.

Zinc Undecylenate (zink un de′ sil en ate). **USP**. $C_{22}H_{38}O_4Zn$. 431.91. (1) 10-Undecenoic acid, zinc (2+) salt; (2) Zinc 10-undecenoate. *UNII-388VZ25DUR; UNII-K3D86KJ24N* [undecylenic acid]. *CAS-557-08-4; CAS-112-38-9* [undecylenic acid]. JAN. *Antifungal*.

Zinc Valerate. USP IX; MI.

Zinc-Eugenol. USP XXI.

Zindotrine [*1986*] (zin′ doe treen). $C_{11}H_{15}N_5$. 217.27. (1) 1,2,4-Triazolo[4,3-*b*]pyridazine, 8-methyl-6-(1-piperidinyl)-; (2) 8-Methyl-6-piperidino-*s*-triazolo[4,3-*b*]pyridazine. *UNII-VQM3328PO0. CAS-56383-05-2*. INN. *Bronchodilator*. ◇MDL 257

Zindoxifene. $C_{21}H_{21}NO_4$. 351.40. 1-Ethyl-2-(*p*-hydroxyphenyl)-3-methylindol-5-ol diacetate (ester). *UNII-1IRS95M8DN. CAS-86111-26-4*. INN.

Zinoconazole Hydrochloride [*1983*] (zin″ oh kon′ a zole hye″ droe klor′ ide). $C_{15}H_{11}Cl_3N_4S.HCl$. 422.16. [Zinoconazole is INN.] (1) Ethanone, 1-(5-chloro-2-thienyl)-2-(1*H*-imidazol-1-yl)-, (2,6-dichlorophenyl)hydrazone, monohydrochloride, (*E*)-; (2) 5-Chloro-2-thienyl imidazol-1-ylmethyl ketone, (*E*)-(2,6-dichlorophenyl)hydrazone, monohydrochloride. *UNII-K8QJ749V4K. CAS-80168-44-1; CAS-84697-21-2* [zinoconazole]. *Antifungal*. ◇SC-38390

Zinostatin [*1978*] (zin″ oh stat′ in). [Zinostatin Stimalamer is INN and JAN.] Acidic, single-chain polypeptide, the molecular structure of which has not been fully elucidated. It is derived from *Streptomyces carzinostaticus* var. F-41. (1) Neocarzinostatin; (2) Neocarzinostatin. *CAS-9014-02-2; CAS-123760-07-6* [zinostatin stimalamer]. INN. *Antineoplastic. [Name previously used: Neocarzinostatin.]*

Zinterol Hydrochloride [*1977*] (zin′ ter ol hye″ droe klor′ ide). $C_{19}H_{26}N_2O_4S.HCl$. 414.95. [Zinterol is INN.] (1) Methanesulfonamide, *N*-[5-[2-[(1,1-dimethyl-2-phenylethyl)amino]-1-hydroxyethyl]-2-hydroxyphenyl]-, monohydrochloride; (2) 5′-[2-[(α,α-Dimethylphenethyl)amino]-1-hydroxyethyl]-2′-hydroxymethanesulfonanilide monohydrochloride. *CAS-38241-28-0; CAS-37000-20-7* [zinterol]. *Bronchodilator*. ◇MJ 9184-1

Zinviroxime [*1980*] (zin″ vir ox′ eem). $C_{17}H_{18}N_4O_3S$. 358.41. (1) 1*H*-Benzimidazol-2-amine, 6-[(hydroxyimino)phenylmethyl]-1-[(1-methylethyl)sulfonyl]-, (*Z*)-; (2) (*Z*)-2-Amino-6-benzoyl-1-(isopropylsulfonyl)benzimidazole oxime. *CAS-72301-78-1*. INN. *Antiviral*.

Zipeprol. $C_{23}H_{32}N_2O_3$. 384.51. α-(α-Methoxybenzyl)-4-(β-methoxyphenethyl)-1-piperazineethanol. *UNII-G5MUV8139H. CAS-34758-83-3*. INN; DCF; MI.

Ziprasidone Hydrochloride [*1994*] (zi pras′ i done hye″ droe klor′ ide). $C_{21}H_{21}ClN_4OS.HCl.H_2O$. 467.41. [Ziprasidone is INN and BAN.] (1) 2*H*-Indol-2-one, 5-[2-[4-(1,2-benzisothiazol-3-yl)-1-piperazinyl]ethyl]-6-chloro-1,3-dihydro-, monohydrochloride, monohydrate; (2) 5-[2-[4-(1,2-Benzisothiazol-3-yl)-1-piperazinyl]ethyl]-6-chloro-2-indolinone monohydrochloride, monohydrate. *UNII-216X081ORU;*

UNII-6UKA5VEJ6X [ziprasidone]. *CAS-138982-67-9; CAS-146939-27-7* [ziprasidone]. *Antipsychotic.* Geodon (Pfizer) ◇*CP-88,059-1*

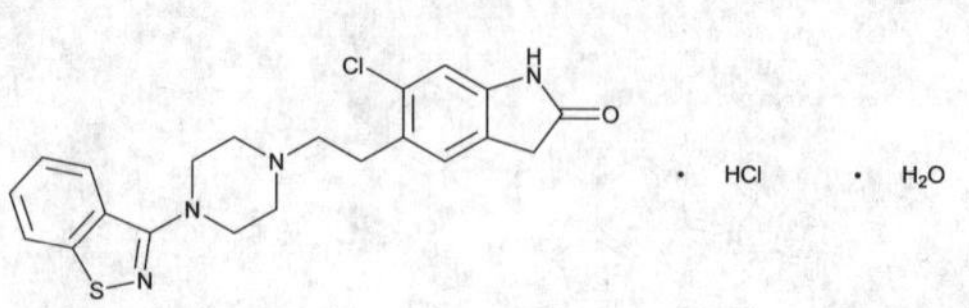

Ziprasidone Mesylate [*1999*] (zi pras′ i done mes′ i late). $C_{21}H_{21}ClN_4OS.CH_4O_3S.3H_2O$. 563.09. (1) 2*H*-Indol-2-one, 5-[2-[4-(1,2-benzisothiazol-3-yl)-1-piperazinyl]ethyl]-6-chloro-1,3-dihydro-, monomethanesulfonate, trihydrate; (2) 5-[2-[4-(1,2-Benzisothiazol-3-yl)-1-piperazinyl]ethyl]-6-chloro-2-indolinone monomethanesulfonate, trihydrate. *UNII-3X6SAX83JZ. CAS-199191-69-0. Antipsychotic (central D_2 and $5HT_2$ receptor antagonist).* Geodon (Pfizer) ◇*CP-88, 059-27*

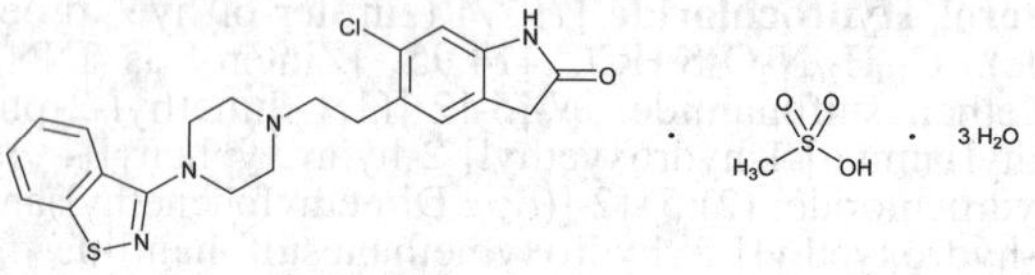

Ziralimumab. Immunoglobulin M, anti-(human antigen CD147) (human monoclonal ABX-RB2 μ-chain), disulfide with human monoclonal ABX-RB2 light chain, pentamer. INN.

^{65}Zn — *See* Zinc Chloride Zn 65.

Zocainone. $C_{22}H_{27}NO_3$. 353.45. (*E*)-3-[*o*-[2-(Diethylamino)ethoxy]phenoxy]-4-phenyl-3-buten-2-one. *UNII-W8U4S4XLWC. CAS-68876-74-4.* INN.

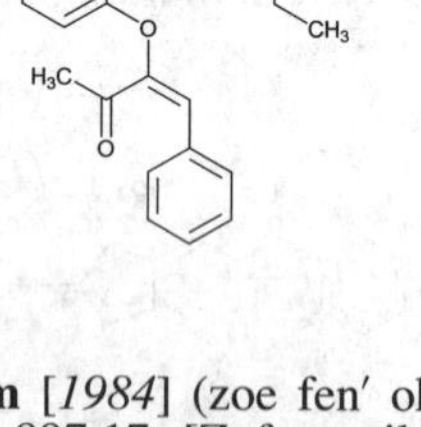

Zofenopril Calcium [*1984*] (zoe fen′ oh pril kal′ see um). $C_{44}H_{44}CaN_2O_8S_4$. 897.17. [Zofenopril is INN and BAN.] (1) L-Proline, 1-[3-(benzoylthio)-2-methyl-1-oxopropyl]-4-(phenylthio)-, calcium salt, [1(*R**),2α,4α]-; (2) (4*S*)-*N*-[(*S*)-3-Mercapto-2-methylpropionyl]-4-(phenylthio)-L-proline benzoate (ester), calcium salt. *CAS-81938-43-4; CAS-81872-10-8* [zofenopril]. *Enzyme inhibitor (angiotensin-converting).* Zoprace (Bristol-Myers Squibb†) ◇*SQ 26991*

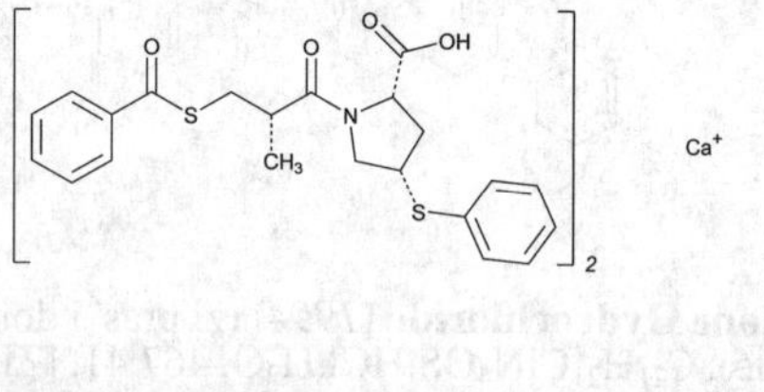

Zofenoprilat Arginine [*1990*] (zoe fen′ oh pril at). $C_{15}H_{19}NO_3S_2.C_6H_{14}N_4O_2$. 499.65. [Zofenoprilat is INN.] (1) L-Proline, 1-(3-mercapto-2-methyl-1-oxopropyl)-4-(phenylthio)-, [1(*R**),2α,4α]-, compd. with L-arginine (1:1); (2) (4*S*)-1-[(*S*)-3-Mercapto-2-methylpropionyl]-4-

(phenylthio)-L-proline, compound with L-arginine (1:1). *UNII-36F26ZSQ0D. CAS-81872-09-5; CAS-75176-37-3* [zofenoprilat]. *Antihypertensive.* ◇*SQ 26,703*

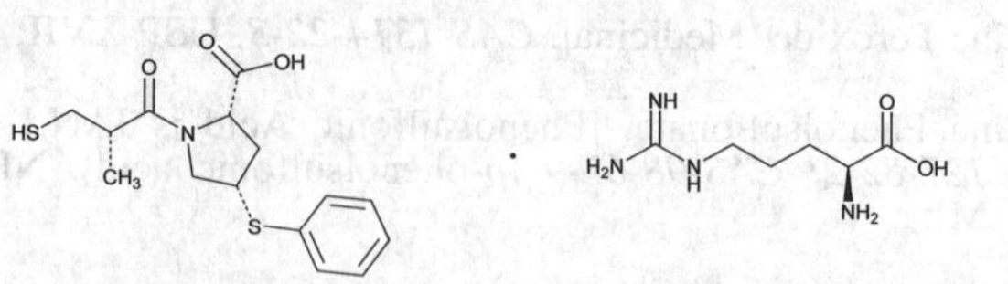

Zoficonazole. $C_{20}H_{19}Cl_3N_2O_2$. 425.74. 1-[2,4-Dichloro-β-[3-(*p*-chlorophenoxy)propoxy]phenethyl]imidazole. *UNII-FZA518V67A. CAS-71097-23-9.* INN.

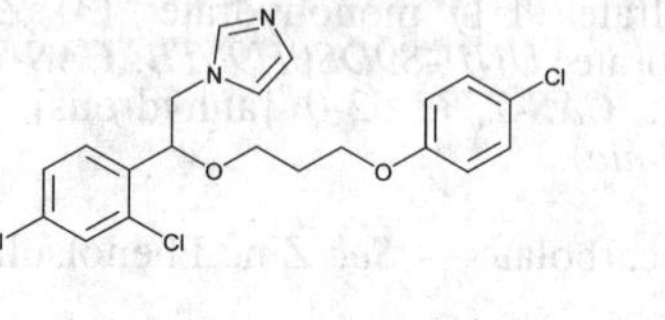

Zolamine Hydrochloride [*1967*] (zol′ a meen hye″ droe klor′ ide). $C_{15}H_{21}N_3OS.HCl$. 327.87. [Zolamine is INN.] (1) 1,2-Ethanediamine, *N*-[(4-methoxyphenyl)methyl]-*N*′,*N*′-dimethyl-*N*-2-thiazolyl-, monohydrochloride; (2) 2-[[2-(Dimethylamino)ethyl]-(*p*-methoxybenzyl)amino]thiazole monohydrochloride. *UNII-C2B9CF1640; UNII-NXB79TB0N2* [zolamine]. *CAS-1155-03-9; CAS-553-13-9* [zolamine]. *Antihistaminic; anesthetic (topical).* ◇*194-B; Wl 291*

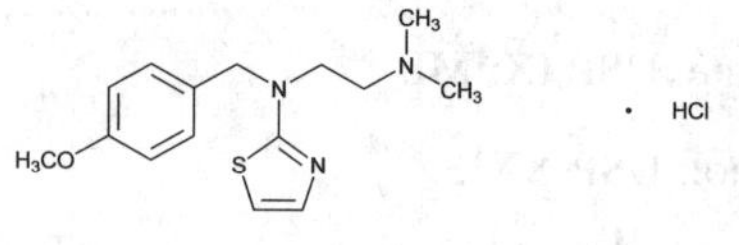

Zolasartan. $C_{24}H_{20}BrClN_6O_3$. 555.81. 1-[[3-Bromo-2-(*o*-1*H*-tetrazol-5-ylphenyl)-5-benzofuranyl]methyl]-2-butyl-4-chloroimidazole-5-carboxylic acid. *UNII-6NA6UHB9SW. CAS-145781-32-4.* INN; BAN. ◇*GR 117289C*

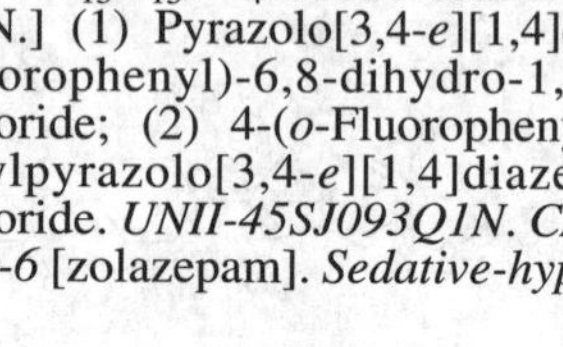

Zolazepam Hydrochloride [*1983*] (zoe laz′ e pam hye″ droe klor′ ide). **USP.** $C_{15}H_{15}FN_4O.HCl$. 322.77. [Zolazepam is INN and BAN.] (1) Pyrazolo[3,4-*e*][1,4]diazepin-7(1*H*)-one, 4-(2-fluorophenyl)-6,8-dihydro-1,3,8-trimethyl-, monohydrochloride; (2) 4-(*o*-Fluorophenyl)-6,8-dihydro-1,3,8-trimethylpyrazolo[3,4-*e*][1,4]diazepin-7(1*H*)-one monohydrochloride. *UNII-45SJ093Q1N. CAS-33754-49-3; CAS-31352-82-6* [zolazepam]. *Sedative-hypnotic.* ◇*CI-716*

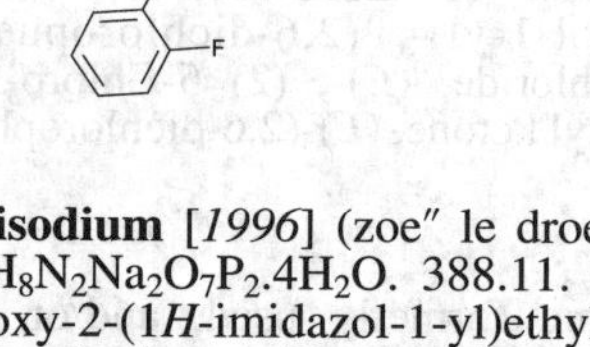

Zoledronate Disodium [*1996*] (zoe″ le droe′ nate dye soe′ dee um). $C_5H_8N_2Na_2O_7P_2.4H_2O$. 388.11. (1) Phosphonic acid, [1-hydroxy-2-(1*H*-imidazol-1-yl)ethylidene]bis-, disodium salt tetrahydrate; (2) Disodium dihydrogen (1-

hydroxy-2-imidazol-1-ylethylidene)diphosphonate, tetrahydrate. *UNII-7D7GS1SA24. CAS-165800-07-7. Bone resorption inhibitor; osteoporosis therapy adjunct. ✧CGP 42446A*

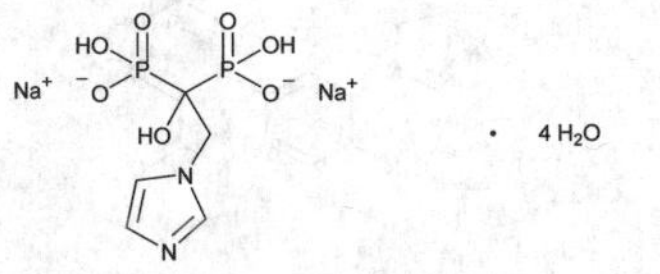

Zoledronate Trisodium [*1996*] (zoe″ le droe′ nate trye soe′ dee um). $(C_5H_7N_2Na_3O_7P_2)_5.2H_2O$. 1726.21. (1) Phosphonic acid, [1-hydroxy-2-(1*H*-imidazol-1-yl)ethylidene]bis-, trisodium salt hydrate (5:2); (2) Trisodium hydrogen (1-hydroxy-2-imidazol-1-ylethylidene)diphosphonate, hydrate (5:2). *CAS-165800-08-8. Bone resorption inhibitor; osteoporosis therapy adjunct. ✧CGP 42446B*

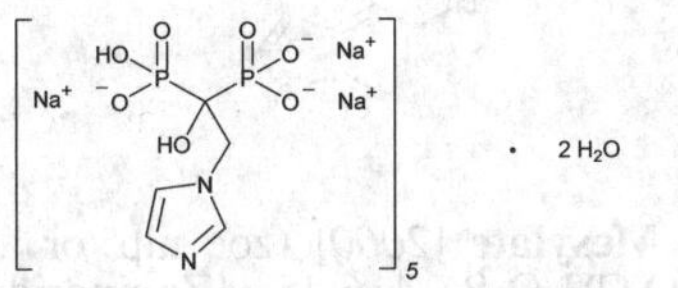

Zoledronic Acid [*1996*] (zoe″ le dron′ ik as′ id). $C_5H_{10}N_2O_7P_2.H_2O$. 290.10. (1) Phosphonic acid, [1-hydroxy-2-(1*H*-imidazol-1-yl)ethylidene]bis-, monohydrate; (2) (1-Hydroxy-2-imidazol-1-ylethylidene)diphosphonic acid, monohydrate. *UNII-6XC1PAD3KF. CAS-165800-06-6.* INN; BAN. *Osteoporosis therapy adjunct.* Reclast (Novartis) *✧CGP 42446*

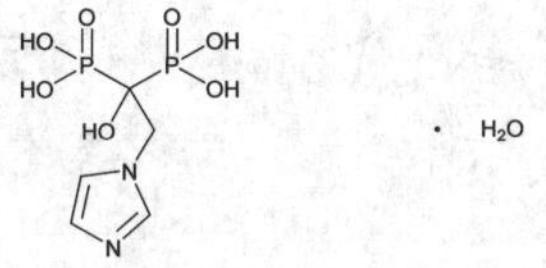

Zolenzepine. $C_{19}H_{24}N_6O_2$. 368.43. 4,9-Dihydro-1,3-dimethyl-4-[(4-methyl-1-piperazinyl)acetyl]pyrazolo[4,3-*b*][1,5]benzodiazepin-10(1*H*)-one. *UNII-O0XJ4L38Z3. CAS-78208-13-6.* INN.

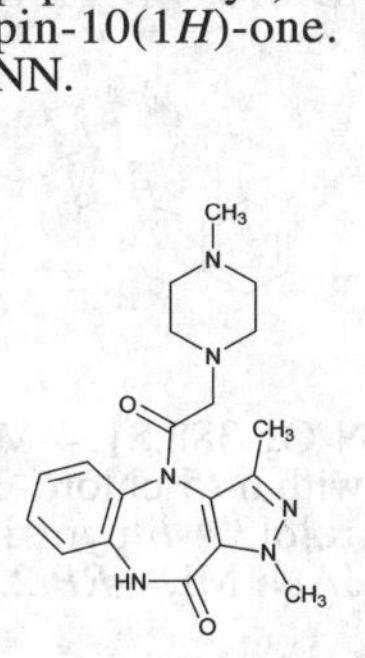

Zolertine Hydrochloride [*1966*] (zoe′ ler teen hye″ droe klor′ ide). $C_{13}H_{18}N_6.HCl$. 294.78. [Zolertine is INN.] (1) Piperazine, 1-phenyl-4-[2-(1*H*-tetrazol-5-yl)ethyl]-, monohydrochloride; (2) 1-Phenyl-4-[2-(1*H*-tetrazol-5-yl)ethyl]-piperazine monohydrochloride. *CAS-7241-94-3; CAS-4004-94-8* [zolertine]. *Anti-adrenergic; vasodilator. ✧MA 1277*

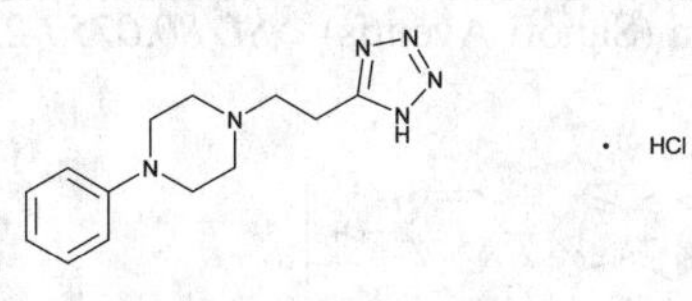

Zolimidine. $C_{14}H_{12}N_2O_2S$. 272.32. 2-[*p*-(Methylsulfonyl)phenyl]imidazol[1,2-*a*]pyridine. *UNII-YCF001N8QB. CAS-1222-57-7.* INN; MI.

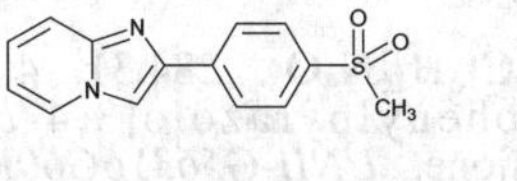

Zolimomab Aritox [*1993*] (zoe lim′ oh mab ar′ i tox). (1) Immunoglobulin G 1 (mouse monoclonal H65-RTA anti-human antigen CD 5 heavy chain), disulfide with mouse monoclonal H65-RTA light chain, dimer, disulfide with ricin (castor-oil plant A-chain protein moiety); (2) Immunoglobulin G 1 (mouse monoclonal H65-RTA anti-human antigen CD 5 heavy chain), disulfide with mouse monoclonal H65-RTA light chain, dimer, disulfide with ricin (castor-oil plant A-chain protein moiety). Molecular weight is approximately 210,000 daltons. *CAS-141483-72-9.* INN. *Monoclonal antibody (antithrombotic).* Orthozyme CD5 Plus (Xoma) *✧H65-RTA*

Zoliprofen. $C_{12}H_{11}NO_3S$. 249.29. (±)-*p*-(2-Thiazolyloxy)hydratropic acid. *UNII-J2GC047H27. CAS-56355-17-0.* INN.

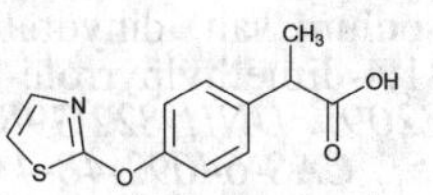

Zoliridine (DCF) — *See* Zolimidine.

Zolmitriptan [*1997*] (zole″ mi trip′ tan). $C_{16}H_{21}N_3O_2$. 287.36. (1) 2-Oxazolidinone, 4-[[3-[2-(dimethylamino)ethyl]-1*H*-indol-5-yl]methyl]-, (*S*)-; (2) (*S*)-4-[[3-[2-(Dimethylamino)ethyl]indol-5-yl]methyl]-2-oxazolidinone. *UNII-2FS66TH3YW. CAS-139264-17-8.* INN; BAN. *Antimigraine.* Zomig (AstraZeneca) *✧311C90*

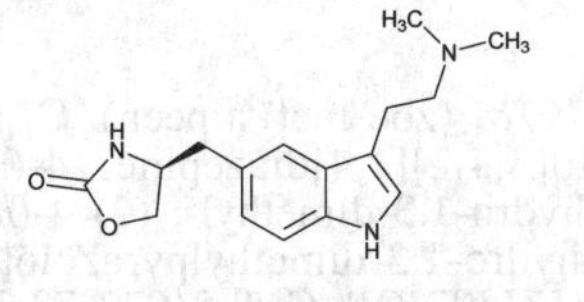

Zoloperone. $C_{22}H_{21}FN_3O_3$. 394.42. 4-(*p*-Fluorophenyl)-5-[2-[4-(*o*-methoxyphenyl)-1-piperazinyl]ethyl]-4-oxazolin-2-one. *UNII-3YU9TET43B. CAS-52867-74-0.* INN.

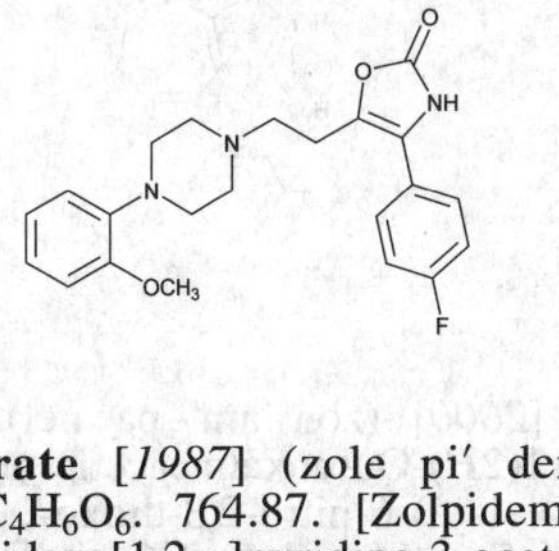

Zolpidem Tartrate [*1987*] (zole pi′ dem tar′ trate). $(C_{19}H_{21}N_3O)_2.C_4H_6O_6$. 764.87. [Zolpidem is INN and BAN.] (1) Imidazo[1,2-*a*]pyridine-3-acetamide, *N*,*N*,6-trimethyl-2-(4-methylphenyl)-, [*R*-(*R**,*R**)]-2,3-dihydrox-

† Brand name formerly used, and/or firm no longer concerned with this product.

ybutanedioate (2:1); (2) *N,N*,6-Trimethyl-2-*p*-tolylimidazo[1,2-*a*]pyridine-3-acetamide L-(+)-tartrate (2:1). *UNII-WY6W63843K; UNII-7K383OQI23* [zolpidem]. *CAS-99294-93-6; CAS-82626-48-0* [zolpidem]. *Sedative-hypnotic.* Ambien (Sanofi Aventis) ◇*SL 80.0750-23N*

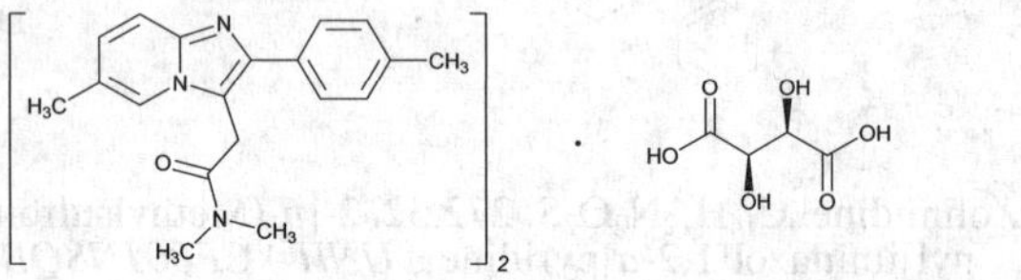

Zomebazam. $C_{15}H_{16}N_4O_2$. 284.31. 4,8-Dihydro-1,3,8-trimethyl-4-phenylpyrazolo[3,4-*b*][1,4]diazepine-5,7(1*H*,6*H*)dione. *UNII-G563Y6G60K. CAS-78466-70-3.* INN.

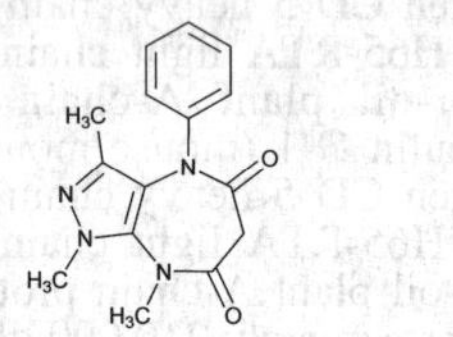

Zomepirac Sodium [*1978*] (zoe me′ pir ak soe′ dee um). $C_{15}H_{13}ClNNaO_3$.2H_2O. 349.74. [Zomepirac is INN and BAN.] (1) 1*H*-Pyrrole-2-acetic acid, 5-(4-chlorobenzoyl)-1,4-dimethyl-, sodium salt, dihydrate; (2) Sodium 5-(*p*-chlorobenzoyl)-1,4-dimethylpyrrole-2-acetate dihydrate. *UNII-Y0185WZ209; UNII-822G987U9J* [zomepirac]. *CAS-64092-49-5; CAS-64092-48-4* [anhydrous]; *CAS-33369-31-2* [zomepirac]. USP XXI. *Analgesic; antiinflammatory.* Zomax (Ortho-McNeil†) ◇*McN-2783-21-98*

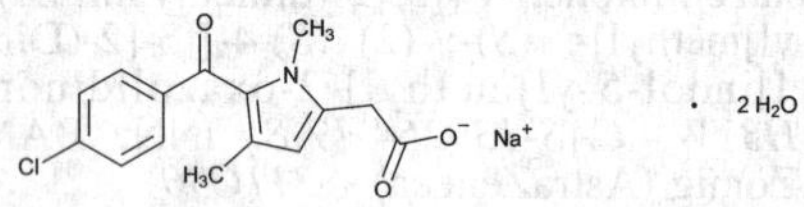

Zometapine [*1978*] (zoe met′ a peen). $C_{14}H_{15}ClN_4$. 274.75. (1) Pyrazolo[3,4-*e*][1,4]diazepine, 4-(3-chlorophenyl)-1,6,7,8-tetrahydro-1,3-dimethyl-; (2) 4-(*m*-Chlorophenyl)-1,6,7,8-tetrahydro-1,3-dimethylpyrazolo[3,4-*e*][1,4]diazepine. *UNII-9171J97IQP. CAS-51022-73-2. Antidepressant.* ◇*CI-781*

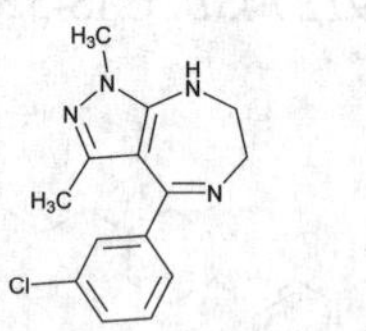

Zonampanel [*2000*] (zon am′ pa nel). $C_{13}H_9N_5O_6$.H_2O. 349.26. (1) 1(2*H*)-Quinoxalineacetic acid, 3,4-dihydro-7-(1*H*-imidazol-1-yl)-6-nitro-2,3-dioxo-, monohydrate; (2) 3,4-Dihydro-7-imidazol-1-yl-6-nitro-2,3-dioxo-1(2*H*)-quinoxalineacetic acid, monohydrate. *UNII-11G3FV7PG7.*

CAS-210245-80-0 [anhydrous]. INN. *Treatment of ischemic stroke (AMPA receptor antagonist offering neuroprotection).* (Yamanouchi) ◇*YM872*

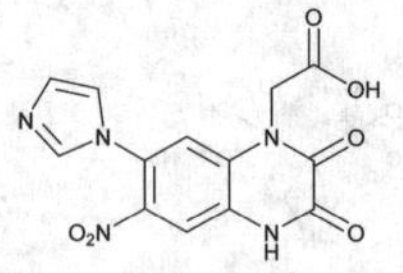

Zoniclezole Hydrochloride [*1992*] (zoe nik′ le zole hye″ droe klor′ ide). $C_{12}H_{10}ClN_3O$.HCl. 284.14. [Zoniclezole is INN.] (1) 1,2-Benzisoxazole, 5-chloro-3-[1-(1*H*-imidazol-1-yl)ethyl]-, monohydrochloride; (2) 5-Chloro-3-(1-imidazol-1-ylethyl)-1,2-benzisoxazole monohydrochloride. *CAS-121929-46-2; CAS-121929-20-2* [zoniclezole]. *Anticonvulsant.* ◇*CGS 18416A*

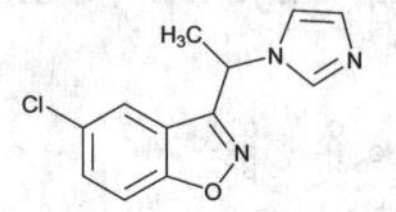

Zoniporide Mesylate [*2000*] (zoe nip′ or ide mes′ i late). $C_{17}H_{16}N_6O$.CH_4O_3S. 416.45. [Zoniporide is INN and BAN.] 1*H*-Pyrazole-4-carboxamide, *N*-(aminoiminomethyl)-5-cyclopropyl-1-(5-quinolinyl)-, monomethanesulfonate. *UNII-X4VP8104KI; UNII-8841R2UJPG* [zoniporide]. *CAS-249296-45-5* [anhydrous]; *CAS-241800-98-6* [zoniporide]. *Cardioprotective ((Na+-H+exchanger-1 NHE-1) inhibitor)).* (Pfizer) ◇*CP-597,396-27*

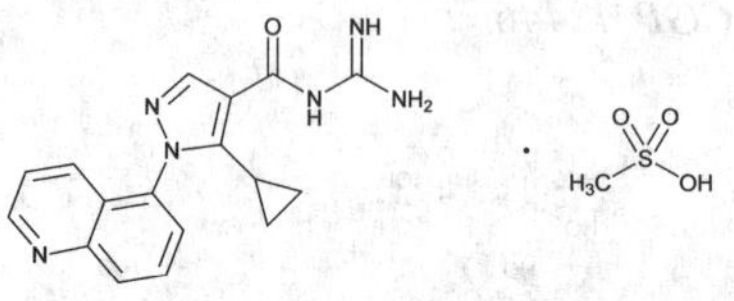

Zonisamide [*1985*] (zoe nis′ a mide). $C_8H_8N_2O_3S$. 212.23. 1,2-Benzisoxazole-3-methanesulfonamide. *UNII-459384H98V. CAS-68291-97-4.* INN; BAN; JAN. *Anticonvulsant.* Zonegran (Dainippon Pharmaceutical Co., Japan) ◇*CI-912; AD-810; PD-110843*

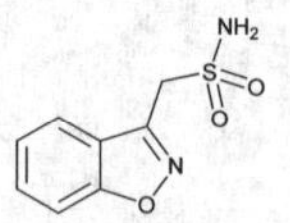

Zopiclone. $C_{17}H_{17}ClN_6O_3$. 388.81. 4-Methyl-1-piperazinecarboxylic acid ester with 6-(5-chloro-2-pyridyl)-6,7-dihydro-7-hydroxy-5*H*-pyrrolo[3,4-*b*]pyrazin-5-one. *CAS-43200-80-2.* INN; BAN; JAN; MI. ◇*RP 27267*

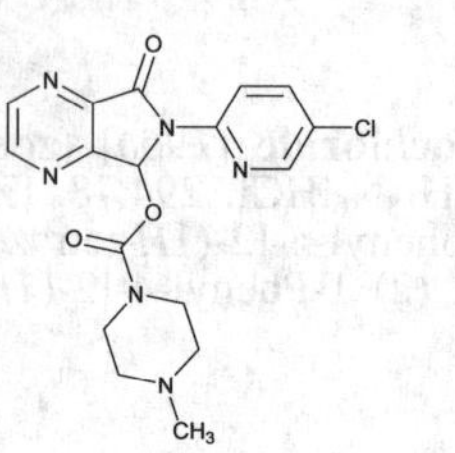

Zopolrestat [*1990*] (zoe pol′ re stat). $C_{19}H_{12}F_3N_3O_3S$. 419.38. (1) 1-Phthalazineacetic acid, 3,4-dihydro-4-oxo-3-[[5-(trifluoromethyl)-2-benzothiazolyl]methyl]-; (2) 3,4-Dihydro-4-oxo-3-[[5-(trifluoromethyl)-2-benzothiazolyl]methyl]-1-phthalazineacetic acid. *CAS-110703-94-1*. INN; BAN. *Antidiabetic; inhibitor (aldose reductase).* ◇*CP-73,850*

Zorbamycin [*1970*] (zor″ ba mye′ sin). Antibiotic derived from *Streptomyces bikiniensis* variant. (1) Zorbamycin; (2) Zorbamycin. *CAS-11056-20-5. Antibacterial.* ◇*U-30,604*

Zorubicin Hydrochloride [*1978*] (zoe roo′ bi sin hye″ droe klor′ ide). $C_{34}H_{35}N_3O_{10} \cdot HCl$. 682.12. [Zorubicin is INN.] (1) Benzoic acid [1-[4-[(3-amino-2,3,6-trideoxy-α-L-*lyxo*-hexopyranosyl)oxy]-1,2,3,4,6,11-hexahydro-2,5,12-trihydroxy-7-methoxy-6,11-dioxo-2-naphthacenyl]ethylidene]hydrazide, (2*S-cis*)-, monohydrochloride; (2) Benzoic acid hydrazide, 3-hydrazone with daunorubicin, monohydrochloride. *UNII-WXM8D9M6DE. CAS-36508-71-1; CAS-54083-22-6* [zorubicin]. *Antineoplastic.* ◇*RP 22,050 hydrochloride; NSC-164011*

Zosuquidar Trihydrochloride [*2002*] (zoe soo′ kwi dar trye hye″ droe klor′ ide). $C_{32}H_{31}F_2N_3O_2 \cdot 3HCl$. 636.99. [Zosuquidar is INN.] (1) 1-Piperazineethanol, 4-(1,1-difluoro-1,1a,6,10b-tetrahydrodibenzo[*a,e*]cyclopropa[*c*]cycloheptan-6-yl)-α-1[(5-quinolinyloxy)methyl]-, trihydrochloride, [6(*R*)-(1α,6α,10bα)]-; (2) (*R*)-4-[(1a*R*,6*R*,10b*S*)-1,2-Difluoro-1,1a,6,10b-tetrahydrodibenzo[*a,e*]cyclopropa[*c*]cycloheptan-6-yl]-α-[(5-quinoloyloxy)methyl]-1-piperazineethanol trihydrochloride. *UNII-813AGY3126; UNII-AB5K82X98Y* [zosuquidar]. *CAS-167465-36-3; CAS-167354-41-8* [zosuquidar]. *Treatment of multidrug resistance (modulator of P-gp resistance).* ◇*LY335979*

Zotarolimus [*2005*] (zoe″ tar oh′ li mus). $C_{52}H_{79}N_5O_{12}$. 966.21. (1) Rapamycin, 42-deoxy-42-(1*H*-tetrazol-1-yl)-, (42*S*)-; (2) (1*R*,9*S*,12*S*,15*R*,16*E*,18*R*,19*R*,21*R*,23-*S*,24*E*,26*E*,28*E*,30*S*,32*S*,35*R*)-1,18-Dihydroxy-19,30-dimethoxy-12-[(1*R*)-2-[(1*S*,3*R*,4*S*)-3-methoxy-4-(1*H*-tetrazol-1-yl)cyclohexyl]-1-methylethyl]-15,17,21,23,29,35-hexamethyl-11,36-dioxa-4-azatricyclo[30.3.1.0⁴,⁹]hexatriaconta-16,24,26,28-tetraene-2,3,10,14,20-pentone. *CAS-221877-54-9*. INN. *Drug component of phosphorycholine polymer coated drug-eluting stent currently under evaluation for the prevention of coronary restenosis following stent replacement.* ◇*ABT-578*

Zotepine. $C_{18}H_{18}ClNOS$. 331.86. 2-[(8-Chlorodibenzo[*b,f*]thiepin-10-yl)oxy]-*N,N*-dimethylethylamine. *UNII-U29O83JAZW. CAS-26615-21-4*. INN; BAN; JAN; MI.

Zoticasone. $C_{25}H_{30}F_2O_6S$. 496.56. *S*-[(3*R*)-2-Oxotetrahydrofuran-3-yl] 6α,9-difluoro-12β,17-dihydroxy-16α-methyl-3-oxoandrosta-1,4-diene-17β-carbothioate. *UNII-W1M09KX30C. CAS-192056-77-2*. INN; BAN. ◇*GR215864*

Zoxazolamine. $C_7H_5ClN_2O$. 168.58. 2-Amino-5-chlorobenzoxazole. *CAS-61-80-3*. NF XI; INN; BAN; MI.

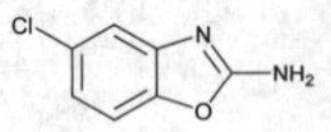

Zucapsaicin [*1994*] (zoo″ kap say′ sin). $C_{18}H_{27}NO_3$. 305.41. (1) 6-Nonenamide, *N*-[(4-hydroxy-3-methoxyphenyl)methyl]-8-methyl-, (*Z*)-; (2) (*Z*)-8-Methyl-*N*-vanillyl-6-nonenamide. *UNII-15OX67P384. CAS-25775-90-0*. INN. *Analgesic (topical)*.

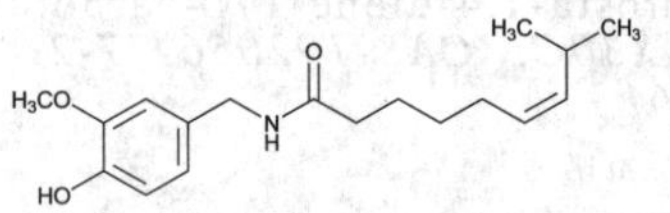

Zuclomifene (INN) — *See* Zuclomiphene.

Zuclomiphene [*1967*] (zoo kloe′ mi feen). $C_{26}H_{28}ClNO$. 405.96. [Zuclomifene is INN.] (1) Ethanamine, 2-[4-(2-chloro-1,2-diphenylethenyl)phenoxy]-*N,N*-diethyl-, (*Z*)-;

(2) (*Z*)-2-[*p*-(2-Chloro-1,2-diphenylvinyl)phenoxy]triethylamine. *UNII-3JU1DU3652. CAS-15690-55-8. [Name previously used: Transclomiphene.]* ◇*Isomer A; RMI 16,312*

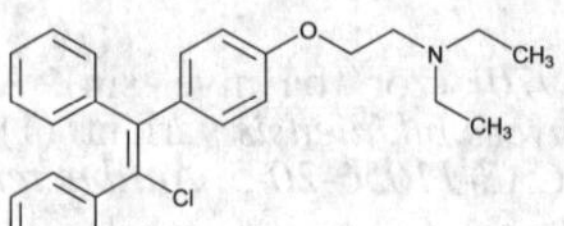

Zuclopenthixol. $C_{22}H_{25}ClN_2OS$. 400.96. (*Z*)-4-[3-(2-Chlorothioxanthen-9-ylidene)propyl]-1-piperazineethanol. *UNII-47ISU063SG. CAS-53772-83-1*. INN; BAN.

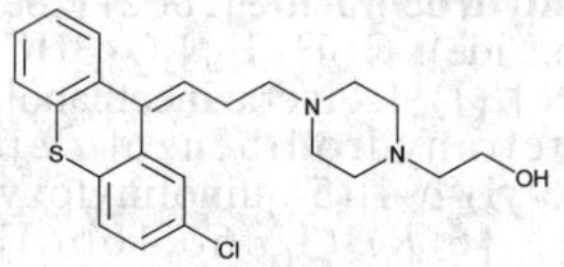

Zylofuramine. $C_{14}H_{21}NO$. 219.32. D-*threo*-α-Benzyl-*N*-ethyltetrahydrofurfurylamine. *CAS-3563-92-6*. INN.

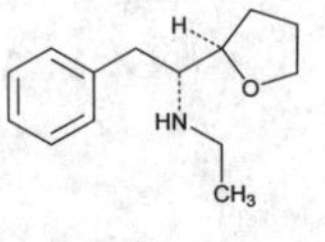

Appendix I
Brand Names for USAN and Other Nonpropriety Names

Abbokinase. Imarx brand of Urokinase.
Abegrin. MedImmune brand of Etaracizumab.
Abelcet. Enzon brand of Amphotericin B.
Abilify. Otsuka brand of Aripiprazole.
Abminthic. Pfizer† brand of Dithiazanine Iodide.
Abraxane. Abraxis brand of Paclitaxel.
Abreva. GlaxoSmithKline brand of Docosanol.
ABthrax. Human Genome Sciences brand of Raxibacumab.
Accelerase. Organon† brand of Pancrelipase.
Accolate. AstraZeneca brand of Zafirlukast.
Accuneb. Dey brand of Albuterol Sulfate.
Accupril. Pfizer brand of Quinapril Hydrochloride.
Accutane. Roche brand of Isotretinoin.
Ac-Di-Sol. FMC brand of Croscarmellose Sodium.
Aceon. Solvay Pharmaceuticals brand of Perindopril Erbumine.
Acephen. G & W brand of Acetaminophen.
Acetadote. Cumberland brand of Acetylcysteine.
Acetasol. Actavis brand of Acetic Acid, Glacial.
Achromycin. Lederle brand of Tetracycline Hydrochloride.
Acilac. Technilab brand of Lactulose.
Aciphex. Eisai Medical Research brand of Rabeprazole Sodium.
Aciquel. Ortho-McNeil† brand of Potassium Glucaldrate.
Aclovate. GlaxoSmithKline brand of Alclometasone Dipropionate.
Acne-Aid Cream. Stiefel† brand of Benzoyl Peroxide.
Acomplia. Sanofi-Synthelabo brand of Rimonabant.
Actase. Ortho Pharmaceutical† brand of Fibrinolysin, Human.
Acthar. Sanofi Aventis brand of Corticotropin.
Acthar Gel-Synthetic. Armour brand of Seractide Acetate.
Acthrel. Ferring Pharmaceuticals brand of Corticorelin Ovine Triflutate.
Actidil. GlaxoSmithKline brand of Triprolidine Hydrochloride.
Actigall. Watson brand of Ursodiol.
Actimmune. Genentech brand of Interferon Gamma-1b.
Actinex. University Of Arizonia Cancer Center brand of Masoprocol.
Actin-N. Sherwood brand of Nitrofurazone.
Actiq. Cephalon brand of Fentanyl Citrate.
Activase. Genentech brand of Alteplase.
Actonel. Procter & Gamble brand of Risedronate Sodium.
Actos. Takeda brand of Pioglitazone Hydrochloride.
Actron. Bayer brand of Ketoprofen.
Acular. Allergan brand of Ketorolac Tromethamine.
Acupan. 3M Pharmaceuticals brand of Nefopam Hydrochloride.
ACUVUE. Vistakon brand of Etafilcon A.
Acylanid. Novartis brand of Acetyldigitoxin.
Adagen. Enzon brand of Pegademase Bovine.
Adalat. Bayer brand of Nifedipine.
Adalin. Sterling Winthrop† brand of Carbromal.
Ademol. Bristol-Myers Squibb† brand of Flumethiazide.
Adenocard. Astellas brand of Adenosine.
Adenoscan. Astellas brand of Adenosine.
Adenyl. Wyeth-Ayerst brand of Adenosine Phosphate.
Adrenalin. King brand of Epinephrine.
Adriamycin. Bedford brand of Doxorubicin Hydrochloride.
Adriblastina. Farmitalia, Societa Farmaceutici Italia, Italy, brand of Doxorubicin.
Adrucil. Pfizer brand of Fluorouracil.

Advanced Pain Relief Callus Removers. Schering-Plough HealthCare brand of Salicylic Acid.
Advanced Pain Relief Corn Removers. Schering-Plough HealthCare brand of Salicylic Acid.
Advexin. Introgen Therapeutics brand of Contusugene Ladenovec.
Advil. Wyeth brand of Ibuprofen.
Aerbron. Angelini Francesco, Italy, brand of Proxazole.
Aerobid. Roche brand of Flunisolide.
Aerolone. Lilly brand of Isoproterenol Hydrochloride.
Aerospan. Forest brand of Flunisolide.
Aerosporin. GlaxoSmithKline brand of Polymyxin B Sulfate.
Affinitak. Isis brand of Aprinocarsen Sodium.
AFP-Cide. Immunomedics brand of Yttrium Y 90 Tacatuzumab.
AFP-Cide. Immunomedics brand of Yttrium Y 90 Tacatuzumab Tetraxetan.
Afrin 4 Hour Nasal Spray. Schering-Plough HealthCare brand of Phenylephrine Hydrochloride.
Afrinol. Schering-Plough brand of Pseudoephedrine Sulfate.
Aftate. Schering-Plough HealthCare brand of Tolnaftate.
Agenerase. GlaxoSmithKline brand of Amprenavir.
Aggrastat. Medicure brand of Tirofiban Hydrochloride.
Agribon [Veterinary]. Hoffmann-LaRoche brand of Sulfadimethoxine.
Agrylin. Shire brand of Anagrelide Hydrochloride.
A-hydrocort. Hospira brand of Hydrocortisone Sodium Succinate.
Aiviosin. ECO Animal Health brand of Tylvalosin Tartrate.
Aivlosin. ECO Animal Health brand of Tylvalosin.
Akbeta. Akorn brand of Levobunolol Hydrochloride.
Akineton. Knoll brand of Biperiden.
Akineton. Abbott brand of Biperiden Hydrochloride.
Akineton. Abbott brand of Biperiden Lactate.
Akpentolate. Akorn brand of Cyclopentolate Hydrochloride.
Akpro. Akorn brand of Dipivefrin Hydrochloride.
Akrinol. Schering brand of Acrisorcin.
Aktob. Akorn brand of Tobramycin.
Alamast. Sanofi Winthrop brand of Pemirolast Potassium.
Alavert. Wyeth brand of Loratadine.
Albalon. Allergan brand of Naphazoline Hydrochloride.
Albamycin. Pfizer brand of Novobiocin Sodium.
Albenza. GlaxoSmithKline brand of Albendazole.
Albon [Veterinary]. Hoffmann-LaRoche brand of Sulfadimethoxine.
Albuferon. Human Genome Sciences brand of Albinterferon Alfa-2b.
Albumotope I-125. Bristol-Myers Squibb† brand of Albumin, Iodinated I 125 Serum.
Albumotope I-131. Bristol-Myers Squibb† brand of Albumin, Iodinated I 131 Serum.
Albumotope-LS. Bristol-Myers Squibb† brand of Albumin, Aggregated Iodinated I 131 Serum.
Alcaine. Alcon brand of Proparacaine Hydrochloride.
Aldactone. Pfizer brand of Spironolactone.
Aldara. Graceway brand of Imiquimod.
Aldarsone. Abbott† brand of Phenarsone Sulfoxylate.
Aldomet. Merck brand of Methyldopa.
Aldomet. Merck brand of Methyldopate Hydrochloride.
Aleve. Bayer brand of Naproxen Sodium.
Alfenta. Akorn brand of Alfentanil Hydrochloride.

Alferon LDO. Interferon Sciences brand of Interferon Alfa-n3.

Alferon N Gel. Interferon Sciences brand of Interferon Alfa-n3.

Alferon N Injection. Interferon Sciences brand of Interferon Alfa-n3.

Alimta. Lilly brand of Pemetrexed Disodium.

Alinia. Romark brand of Nitazoxanide.

Alkeran. GlaxoSmithKline brand of Melphalan.

Alkergot. Sandoz brand of Ergoloid Mesylates.

Allegra. Sanofi Aventis brand of Fexofenadine Hydrochloride.

Alliance. CooperVision brand of Tetrafilcon A.

Alloferin. Hoffmann-LaRoche-International brand of Alcuronium Chloride.

Allovectin. Vical brand of Velimogene Aliplasmid.

Alminate. Bristol-Myers Squibb brand of Dihydroxyaluminum Aminoacetate.

Almora. Forest† brand of Magnesium Gluconate.

Alnovin. Hoechst-Roussel† brand of Fendosal.

Alomide. Alcon brand of Lodoxamide Tromethamine.

Alora. Watson brand of Estradiol.

Aloxi. Helsinn brand of Palonosetron Hydrochloride.

Alphacaine. Carlisle brand of Lidocaine.

Alphadrol. Pfizer brand of Fluprednisolone.

Alphagan. Allergan brand of Brimonidine Tartrate.

Alphanate. Alpha Therapeutic brand of Antihemophilic Factor.

AlphaNine. Alpha Therapeutic† brand of Factor IX Complex.

AlphaNine SD. Alpha Therapeutic brand of Factor IX Complex.

Alpharedisol. Merck brand of Hydroxocobalamin.

Alphatrex. Savage brand of Betamethasone Dipropionate.

Alredase. Wyeth-Ayerst brand of Tolrestat.

Alrex. Bausch & Lomb brand of Loteprednol Etabonate.

Altabax. GlaxoSmithKline brand of Retapamulin.

Altace. King brand of Ramipril.

ALternaGEL. Johnson & Johnson-Merck Consumer brand of Aluminum Hydroxide, Dried.

Altinil. Bristol-Myers Squibb† brand of Thiazesim Hydrochloride.

Altoprev. Teva brand of Lovastatin.

Alu-Cap. 3M Pharmaceuticals brand of Aluminum Hydroxide, Dried.

Alupent. Boehringer Ingelheim brand of Metaproterenol Sulfate.

Alurate. Hoffmann-LaRoche brand of Aprobarbital.

Alveograf. Sterling Winthrop brand of Durapatite.

Alvodine Ethanesulfonate. Sterling Winthrop† brand of Piminodine Esylate.

Alysine. Marion Merrell Dow† brand of Sodium Salicylate.

Amaryl. Sanofi Aventis brand of Glimepiride.

Ambenyl Cough Syrup. Parke-Davis† brand of Codeine Phosphate.

Amberlite IRP88 Resin. Rohm and Haas brand of Polacrilin Potassium.

Ambien. Sanofi Aventis brand of Zolpidem Tartrate.

Ambisome. Astellas brand of Amphotericin B.

Ambodryl. Pfizer brand of Bromodiphenhydramine Hydrochloride.

Amcill. Parke-Davis† brand of Ampicillin.

Amdray. Novartis brand of Valspodar.

Amenide. Sterling Winthrop brand of Quinfamide.

Amerge. GlaxoSmithKline brand of Naratriptan Hydrochloride.

Americaine. Fisons brand of Benzocaine.

Amerscan MDP. Nycomed Amersham† brand of Technetium Tc 99m Medronate Disodium.

Amethone Hydrochloride. Abbott† brand of Amolanone Hydrochloride.

Amicar. Xanodyne brand of Aminocaproic Acid.

Amidate. Hospira brand of Etomidate.

Amikin. Apothecon brand of Amikacin Sulfate.

Aminosol. Abbott brand of Protein Hydrolysate.

Amipaque. GE Healthcare brand of Metrizamide.

Amitiza. Takeda brand of Lubiprostone.

Amitril. Warner Chilcott brand of Amitriptyline Hydrochloride.

Ammivin. Marion Merrell Dow† brand of Khellin.

Amnesteem. Genpharm brand of Isotretinoin.

Amnestrogen. Bristol-Myers Squibb brand of Estrogens, Esterified.

Amoxil. GlaxoSmithKline brand of Amoxicillin.

Amphojel. Wyeth-Ayerst brand of Aluminum Hydroxide.

Amphotec. Three Rivers brand of Amphotericin B.

Amplimexon. Amplimed brand of Imexon.

Amprol [Veterinary]. Merial brand of Amprolium.

Amprovine [Veterinary]. Merial brand of Amprolium.

Amrix. Cephalon brand of Cyclobenzaprine Hydrochloride.

Amsidyl. Parke-Davis† brand of Amsacrine.

Amsof. Lombart brand of Deltafilcon B.

Amsof-Thin. Lombart brand of Deltafilcon B.

Amvaz. Dr. Reddy's brand of Amlodipine Maleate.

Amytal. Lilly brand of Amobarbital.

Amytal Sodium. Lilly brand of Amobarbital Sodium.

Anadrol. Alaven brand of Oxymetholone.

Anafranil. Tyco brand of Clomipramine Hydrochloride.

Anaspaz. Ascher brand of Hyoscyamine Sulfate.

Anatropin. Ortho Pharmaceutical† brand of Anagestone Acetate.

Ancef. GlaxoSmithKline brand of Cefazolin Sodium.

Ancobon. Valeant brand of Flucytosine.

Ancyte. Abbott† brand of Piposulfan.

Anderm. Wyeth-Ayerst† brand of Bufexamac.

Andriol. Diosynth B.V., Netherlands, brand of Testosterone Undecanoate.

Andriol. Organon brand of Testosterone Undecanoate.

Androderm. Watson brand of Testosterone.

Androgel. Unimed brand of Testosterone.

Android. Valeant brand of Fluoxymesterone.

Android. Valeant brand of Methyltestosterone.

AN-DTPA. CL Pharma AG, Austria, brand of Technetium Tc 99m Pentetate.

Anectine. Sandoz brand of Succinylcholine Chloride.

Angex. Janssen† brand of Lidoflazine.

Angiomax. The Medicines Company brand of Bivalirudin.

Anhydron. Lilly brand of Cyclothiazide.

AN-MAA. CL Pharma AG, Austria†, brand of Technetium Tc 99m Albumin Aggregated.

AN-MDP. CL Pharma AG, Austria, brand of Technetium Tc 99m Medronate.

Ansaid. Pfizer brand of Flurbiprofen.

Ansolysen. Wyeth brand of Pentolinium Tartrate.

Anspor. GlaxoSmithKline brand of Cephradine.

AN-Sulfur Colloid Kit. CL Pharma AG, Austria, brand of Technetium Tc 99m Sulfur Colloid.

Antabuse. Odyssey brand of Disulfiram.

Antara. Reliant brand of Fenofibrate.

Antepar. GlaxoSmithKline brand of Piperazine Citrate.

Anteron. Schering† brand of Gonadotropin, Serum.

Anthelcide EQ. SmithKline Beecham Animal Health brand of Oxibendazole.

Anthelvet. Ortho-McNeil† brand of Tetramisole Hydrochloride.

Anthra-Derm. Dermik brand of Anthralin.

Antidiar 200. Hoechst-Roussel† brand of Ethacridine Lactate.

Antidotum-Thallii-Heyl. Heyl, Germany, brand of Prussian Blue Insoluble.

Antilirium. Forest brand of Physostigmine Salicylate.

Antilon. Marion Merrell Dow† brand of Eterobarb.

Antiminth. Roerig brand of Pyrantel Pamoate.

Antisedan. Farmos Group Ltd., Finland, brand of Atipamezole.

Antivenin. Merck brand of Antivenin (Latrodectus mactans).

---

† Brand name formerly used, and/or firm no longer concerned with this product.

Antivert. Pfizer brand of Meclizine Hydrochloride.

Antizol. Jazz brand of Fomepizole.

Antrenyl. Novartis brand of Oxyphenonium Bromide.

Antril. Synergen brand of Anakinra.

Antrin. Pharmacyclics brand of Motexafin Lutetium.

Anturane. Novartis brand of Sulfinpyrazone.

Anzemet. Sanofi Aventis brand of Dolasetron Mesylate.

Aphthasol. Uluru brand of Amlexanox.

Apiquel. Ortho-McNeil† brand of Aminorex.

A.p.l. Ferring Pharmaceuticals brand of Gonadotropin, Chorionic.

Aplisol. Parke-Davis brand of Tuberculin.

Aplitest. Parke-Davis† brand of Tuberculin.

Apogen. King brand of Gentamicin Sulfate.

Apokyn. Vernalis brand of Apomorphine Hydrochloride.

Apresoline. Novartis brand of Hydralazine Hydrochloride.

Aptivus. Boehringer Ingelheim brand of Tipranavir.

Aqua Ivy, AP. Bayer† brand of Poison Ivy Extract, Alum Precipitated.

Aquacoat ECD. FMC brand of Ethylcellulose.

Aquamephyton. Merck brand of Phytonadione.

Aquasight. Lombart† brand of Deltafilcon B.

Aquasight-Thin. Lombart† brand of Deltafilcon B.

Aquasite. Ciba Vision, US Ophthalmics, brand of Dextran 70.

Aquasol A. AstraZeneca brand of Vitamin A.

Aquasol E. Astra brand of Vitamin E.

Aquatag. Solvay Pharmaceuticals brand of Benzthiazide.

AquaTar. Allergan Herbert brand of Coal Tar.

Aquatensen. Medpointe brand of Methyclothiazide.

Aquavan. Guilford brand of Fospropofol Disodium.

Aquex. Novartis† brand of Clopamide.

Aralen. Sanofi Aventis brand of Chloroquine Phosphate.

Aralen Hydrochloride. Sanofi Aventis brand of Chloroquine Hydrochloride.

Aramine. Merck brand of Metaraminol Bitartrate.

Arava. Sanofi Aventis brand of Leflunomide.

Arduan. Organon brand of Pipecuronium Bromide.

Aredia. Novartis brand of Pamidronate Disodium.

Arfonad. Roche brand of Trimethaphan Camsylate.

Aricept. Eisai Medical Research brand of Donepezil Hydrochloride.

Arimidex. AstraZeneca brand of Anastrozole.

Aristocort. Astellas brand of Triamcinolone.

Aristocort. Astellas brand of Triamcinolone Acetonide.

Aristocort. Astellas brand of Triamcinolone Diacetate.

Aristospan. Sandoz brand of Triamcinolone Hexacetonide.

Arixtra. GlaxoSmithKline brand of Fondaparinux Sodium.

Arkin. Otsuka America brand of Vesnarinone.

Arlacel 80. ICI Americas brand of Sorbitan Monooleate.

Arlacel 83. ICI Americas brand of Sorbitan Sesquioleate.

Arlacel 85. ICI Americas† brand of Sorbitan Trioleate.

Arlacel C. ICI Americas brand of Sorbitan Sesquioleate.

Arlamol E. ICI Americas brand of Polyoxypropylene 15 Stearyl Ether.

Arlatone UVB. ICI Americas† brand of Padimate O.

Arlef. Parke-Davis† brand of Flufenamic Acid.

Arlix. Hoechst-Roussel† brand of Piretanide.

Aromasin. Pfizer brand of Exemestane.

Arpocox. Merck brand of Arprinocid.

Arranon. GlaxoSmithKline brand of Nelarabine.

Arsumax. Knoll, Switzerland, brand of Artesunate.

Artane. Lederle brand of Trihexyphenidyl Hydrochloride.

Arthrex. Novartis brand of Proquazone.

Arthropan. Purdue Frederick brand of Choline Salicylate.

Artil. Hoechst-Roussel† brand of Isoxepac.

Aryplase. BioMarin brand of Galsulfase.

Asacol. Procter & Gamble brand of Mesalamine.

Asbron. Novartis brand of Theophylline Sodium Glycinate.

Ascorbicap. ICN† brand of Ascorbic Acid.

Ascorbin. Marion Merrell Dow† brand of Sodium Ascorbate.

Asendin. Lederle brand of Amoxapine.

Asmanex. Schering brand of Mometasone Furoate.

Astelin. Medpointe brand of Azelastine Hydrochloride.

Asterol [as dihydrochloride] [Veterinary]. Hoffmann-LaRoche† brand of Diamthazole.

Atabrine Hydrochloride. Sterling Winthrop brand of Quinacrine Hydrochloride.

Atacand. AstraZeneca brand of Candesartan Cilexetil.

Atarax. Pfizer brand of Hydroxyzine Hydrochloride.

Atgard. Boehringer Ingelheim Animal Health brand of Dichlorvos.

Athrombin. Purdue Frederick brand of Warfarin Sodium.

Athrombin-K. Purdue Frederick brand of Warfarin Potassium.

Ativan. Biovail brand of Lorazepam.

ATP. Medco Research brand of Adenosine Triphosphate Disodium.

Atpeg 300. ICI Americas† brand of Polyethylene Glycol.

Atpeg 4000. ICI Americas† brand of Polyethylene Glycol 4000.

Atridox. Tolmar brand of Doxycycline Hyclate.

Atromid. Wyeth brand of Clofibrate.

Atropen. Meridian brand of Atropine.

Atrovent. Boehringer Ingelheim brand of Ipratropium Bromide.

Atryn. GTC Biotherapeutics brand of Antithrombin Alfa.

Attenuvax. Merck brand of Measles Virus Vaccine Live.

Aurcoloid-198. Abbott† brand of Gold Au 198.

Aureomycin. Lederle brand of Chlortetracycline Hydrochloride.

Aureotope. Bristol-Myers Squibb† brand of Gold Au 198.

Aurexis. Avid Bioservices brand of Tefibazumab.

Auroscan-198. Abbott† brand of Gold Au 198.

Avage. Allergan brand of Tazarotene.

Avandia. GlaxoSmithKline brand of Rosiglitazone Maleate.

Avapro. Sanofi Aventis brand of Irbesartan.

Avatec [as sodium] [Veterinary]. Hoffmann-LaRoche brand of Lasalocid.

Avelox. Bayer brand of Moxifloxacin Hydrochloride.

Aventyl Hydrochloride. Ranbaxy brand of Nortriptyline Hydrochloride.

Avertin. Sterling Winthrop† brand of Tribromoethanol.

Avicel PH. FMC brand of Cellulose, Microcrystalline.

Avita. Mylan Bertek brand of Tretinoin.

Avodart. GlaxoSmithKline brand of Dutasteride.

Avomec [Veterinary]. Merial brand of Abamectin.

Award. Bausch & Lomb brand of Hilafilcon A.

Award. Bausch & Lomb brand of Hilafilcon B.

Axert. Ortho-McNeil brand of Almotriptan Malate.

Axid. Reliant brand of Nizatidine.

Axiquel. Ortho-McNeil† brand of Valnoctamide.

Axokine. Regeneron brand of Dapiclermin.

Aygestin. Duramed brand of Norethindrone Acetate.

Azactam. Bristol-Myers Squibb brand of Aztreonam.

Azasan. Aaipharma brand of Azathioprine.

Azasite. Inspire brand of Azithromycin.

Azelex. Allergan brand of Azelaic Acid.

Azilect. Teva brand of Rasagiline Mesylate.

Azlin. Bayer† brand of Azlocillin.

Azlin. Bayer brand of Azlocillin Sodium.

Azmacort. Abbott brand of Triamcinolone Acetonide.

Azolid. Sanofi Aventis brand of Phenylbutazone.

Azopt. Alcon brand of Brinzolamide.

Azulfidine. Pfizer brand of Sulfasalazine.

B & L 70. Bausch & Lomb brand of Lidofilcon A.

Baby Anbesol. Whitehall-Robins brand of Benzocaine.

Backache Caplets. Bristol-Myers Products brand of Magnesium Salicylate.

Bactocill. GlaxoSmithKline brand of Oxacillin Sodium.

Bactratycin. Wallace† brand of Tyrothricin.

Bactroban. GlaxoSmithKline brand of Mupirocin.

Bactroban. GlaxoSmithKline brand of Mupirocin Calcium.

Bal. Akorn brand of Dimercaprol.

Balneol. Solvay Pharmaceuticals brand of Mineral Oil.

Banamine [Veterinary]. Schering-Plough Animal Health brand of Flunixin Meglumine.

Bandol. Bristol-Myers Squibb† brand of Carbiphene Hydrochloride.

Banminth. Pfizer brand of Pyrantel Tartrate.

Banthine. Shire brand of Methantheline Bromide.

Baraclude. Bristol-Myers Squibb brand of Entecavir.

Baricon. Mallinckrodt† brand of Barium Sulfate.

Barocat. Mallinckrodt† brand of Barium Sulfate.

Barosperse. Mallinckrodt† brand of Barium Sulfate.

Barosperse II. Mallinckrodt† brand of Barium Sulfate.

Barotrast. Rhone-Poulenc Rorer† brand of Barium Sulfate.

Bar-test. Glenwood brand of Barium Sulfate.

Basaljel. Wyeth-Ayerst brand of Aluminum Carbonate, Basic.

Basen. Takeda brand of Voglibose.

Baycol. Bayer brand of Cerivastatin Sodium.

Bayer Select Backache. Sterling Health U.S.A. brand of Magnesium Salicylate.

BayGam. Bayer brand of Globulin, Immune.

BayHep B. Bayer brand of Hepatitis B Immune Globulin.

Baymix. Bayer Animal Health† brand of Coumaphos.

Baypress. Bayer brand of Nitrendipine.

BayRab. Bayer brand of Rabies Immune Globulin.

BayRho-D. Bayer brand of Rh₀ (D) Immune Globulin.

BayTet. Bayer brand of Tetanus Immune Globulin.

Baytril. Bayer Animal Health brand of Enrofloxacin.

Beclovent. GlaxoSmithKline brand of Beclomethasone Dipropionate.

Beconase. GlaxoSmithKline brand of Beclomethasone Dipropionate.

Becotin. Lilly brand of Vitamin B Complex.

Becozym. Hoffmann-LaRoche-International brand of Vitamin B Complex.

Beepen-vk. GlaxoSmithKline brand of Penicillin V Potassium.

Benadryl. McNeil brand of Diphenhydramine Hydrochloride.

Bendopa. Valeant brand of Levodopa.

BeneFix. Genetics Institute brand of Nonacog Alfa.

Benemid. Merck brand of Probenecid.

Benicar. Sankyo brand of Olmesartan Medoxomil.

Benoquin. Valeant brand of Monobenzone.

Benoral. Sterling Winthrop brand of Benorilate.

Benoxyl. Stiefel brand of Benzoyl Peroxide.

Bentyl. Axcan Scandipharm brand of Dicyclomine Hydrochloride.

Benylin DM. Parke-Davis brand of Dextromethorphan Hydrobromide.

BENZ 38. Benz Research and Development brand of Polymacon.

Benz 42. Benz Research and Development brand of Hefilcon A.

Benzac. Galderma brand of Benzoyl Peroxide.

Benzac W. Galderma brand of Benzoyl Peroxide.

Benzadrine. GlaxoSmithKline brand of Amphetamine Sulfate.

Benz-G 4X. Benz Research and Development brand of Hioxifilcon D.

Benz-G 5X. Benz Research and Development brand of Hioxifilcon A.

Benzocal. Marion Merrell Dow† brand of Polybenzarsol.

Bepadin. Medpointe brand of Bepridil Hydrochloride.

Berotec [as hydrobromide]. Boehringer Ingelheim brand of Fenoterol.

Berubigen. Pfizer brand of Cyanocobalamin.

Betaderm. Roaco brand of Betamethasone Valerate.

Betadine. Alcon brand of Povidone-Iodine.

Betagan. Allergan brand of Levobunolol Hydrochloride.

Betalin 12. Lilly brand of Cyanocobalamin.

Betalin Complex. Lilly brand of Vitamin B Complex.

Betalin Compound. Lilly brand of Vitamin B Complex.

Betalin S. Lilly brand of Thiamine Hydrochloride.

Betapace. Bayer brand of Sotalol Hydrochloride.

Betapar. Schering brand of Meprednisone.

Betapen-vk. Apothecon brand of Penicillin V Potassium.

Betaprone. Forest brand of Propiolactone.

Betaseron. Berlex brand of Interferon Beta-1b.

Betatrex. Savage brand of Betamethasone Valerate.

Beta-val. Teva brand of Betamethasone Valerate.

BetaVit. BASF brand of Beta Carotene.

Betaxon. Alcon brand of Levobetaxolol Hydrochloride.

Betimol. Sanofi Winthrop brand of Timolol.

Betoptic. Alcon brand of Betaxolol Hydrochloride.

Bextra. Interneuron brand of Pagoclone.

Bextra. Pfizer brand of Valdecoxib.

Biaxin. Abbott brand of Clarithromycin.

Bicillin. King brand of Penicillin G Benzathine.

Bicnu. Bristol-Myers Squibb brand of Carmustine.

Bilimiro. Bracco Industria Chimica S.p.A., Italy, brand of Iopronic Acid.

Bilimiron. Bracco Industria Chimica S.p.A., Italy, brand of Iopronic Acid.

Bilopaque. GE Healthcare brand of Tyropanoate Sodium.

Biltricide. Bayer brand of Praziquantel.

Bioclate. Centeon brand of Antihemophilic Factor.

Bioepiderm. Sterling Winthrop† brand of Biotin.

Biomydrin. Parke-Davis† brand of Phenylephrine Hydrochloride.

Bistrium Bromide. Bristol-Myers Squibb† brand of Hexamethonium Bromide.

Bitrex. Mac Farlan Smith, Scotland, brand of Denatonium Benzoate.

Black and White Bleaching Cream. Schering-Plough HealthCare† brand of Hydroquinone.

Blenoxane. Bristol-Myers Squibb brand of Bleomycin Sulfate.

Bleph. Allergan brand of Sulfacetamide Sodium.

Bloat Guard. SmithKline Beecham Animal Health brand of Poloxalene.

Blocadren. Merck brand of Timolol Maleate.

Blockain Hydrochloride. Sterling Winthrop† brand of Propoxycaine Hydrochloride.

Blutene. Abbott† brand of Tolonium Chloride.

BLyS. Human Genome Sciences brand of Ardenermin.

Bodyfolin. Merck Eprova AG brand of Levomefolate Calcium.

Bodyfolin. Merck Eprova AG brand of Levomefolic Acid.

Bonefos. Leiras Oy, Finland, brand of Clodronate Disodium.

Boniva. Roche brand of Ibandronate Sodium.

Bonomycin. Pfizer brand of Sancycline.

Bontril. Mallinckrodt brand of Phendimetrazine Tartrate.

Boston 7/30. Polymer Technology brand of Enflufocon A.

Botox. Allergan brand of Onaclostox.

Botox Cosmetic. Allergan brand of Onaclostox.

Bovatec [as sodium] [Veterinary]. Hoffmann-LaRoche brand of Lasalocid.

Bovitin [Veterinary]. Merial brand of Abamectin.

Bravavir. Bristol-Myers Squibb brand of Sorivudine.

Bravelle. Ferring Pharmaceuticals brand of Urofollitropin.

Breath-O. Toray, Japan, brand of Astifilcon A.

Brethaire. Novartis brand of Terbutaline Sulfate.

Brethine. Aaipharma brand of Terbutaline Sulfate.

Brevibloc. Baxter Healthcare brand of Esmolol Hydrochloride.

Brevital Sodium. King brand of Methohexital Sodium.

Brevoxyl. Stiefel brand of Benzoyl Peroxide.

Brij 30. ICI Americas brand of Laureth 4.

Brij 96. ICI Americas† brand of Polyoxyl 10 Oleyl Ether.

Brij 97. ICI Americas brand of Polyoxyl 10 Oleyl Ether.

---

† Brand name formerly used, and/or firm no longer concerned with this product.

Bristacycline. Bristol-Myers Squibb brand of Tetracycline Hydrochloride.

Bristamycin. Bristol-Myers Squibb brand of Erythromycin Stearate.

Bromural. Knoll† brand of Bromisovalum.

Bronitin. Wyeth brand of Epinephrine Bitartrate.

Bronkephrine. Sterling Winthrop brand of Ethylnorepinephrine Hydrochloride.

Bronkometer. Sanofi Aventis brand of Isoetharine Mesylate.

Bronkosol. Sanofi Aventis brand of Isoetharine Hydrochloride.

Bronsecur [as the base]. SmithKline Beecham† brand of Carbuterol Hydrochloride.

Brovana. Sepracor brand of Arformoterol Tartrate.

Bryrel. Sanofi Aventis brand of Piperazine Citrate.

Bucladin. Stuart brand of Buclizine Hydrochloride.

Bumex. Roche brand of Bumetanide.

Buphenyl. Medicis brand of Sodium Phenylbutyrate.

Buprenex. Reckitt Benckiser brand of Buprenorphine Hydrochloride.

Buro-Sol Concentrate. Doak brand of Aluminum Acetate.

Buspar. Bristol-Myers Squibb brand of Buspirone Hydrochloride.

Busulfex. PDL Biopharma brand of Busulfan.

Butalan. Lannett brand of Butabarbital Sodium.

Butaphyllamine. Marion Merrell Dow† brand of Ambuphylline.

Butazolidin. Novartis brand of Phenylbutazone.

Butesin. Abbott brand of Butamben.

Butisol Sodium. Medpointe brand of Butabarbital Sodium.

Butyn. Abbott† brand of Butacaine Sulfate.

Cafcit. Bristol-Myers Squibb brand of Caffeine Citrate.

Calan. Pfizer brand of Verapamil Hydrochloride.

Calcibind. Mission brand of Cellulose Sodium Phosphate.

Calcijex. Abbott brand of Calcitriol.

Calcimar. Rhone-Poulenc Rorer brand of Calcitonin.

Calciparine. Sanofi Aventis brand of Heparin Calcium.

Calcium Disodium Versenate. Graceway brand of Edetate Calcium Disodium.

Calderol. Organon brand of Calcifediol.

Calfspan Tablets [Veterinary]. Fort Dodge Animal Health brand of Sulfamethazine.

Calglucon. Novartis† brand of Calcium Gluconate.

Calpan. BASF brand of Calcium Pantothenate.

Calsed. Pharmion brand of Amrubicin Hydrochloride.

CalStar. FMC brand of Calcium Phosphate Dihydrate, Dibasic.

Cal-Sup. 3M Pharmaceuticals brand of Calcium Carbonate.

Camdan. Merck brand of Cambendazole.

Camoform Hydrochloride. Parke-Davis† brand of Bialamicol Hydrochloride.

Camoquin. Pfizer brand of Amodiaquine Hydrochloride.

Campath. Boehringer Ingelheim KG, Germany, brand of Alemtuzumab.

Campral. Forest brand of Acamprosate Calcium.

Camptosar. Pfizer brand of Irinotecan Hydrochloride.

Camvet [Veterinary]. Merial brand of Cambendazole.

Canasa. Axcan Scandipharm brand of Mesalamine.

Cancidas. Merck brand of Caspofungin Acetate.

Cantabiline. Lipha, S.A., France, brand of Hymecromone.

Cantil. Sanofi Aventis brand of Mepenzolate Bromide.

Cantor. Sanofi brand of Minaprine.

Canvaxin. Cancervax brand of Onamelatucel-L.

Capastat Sulfate. Lilly brand of Capreomycin Sulfate.

Capitrol. Westwood-Squibb brand of Chloroxine.

Capoten. Par brand of Captopril.

Carac. Sanofi Aventis brand of Fluorouracil.

Carafate. Axcan Scandipharm brand of Sucralfate.

Carbatrol. Shire brand of Carbamazepine.

Carbocaine. Hospira brand of Mepivacaine Hydrochloride.

Carbopol 910. Noveon brand of Carbomer 910.

Carbopol 934. Noveon brand of Carbomer 934.

Carbopol 934P. Noveon brand of Carbomer 934P.

Carbopol 940. Noveon brand of Carbomer 940.

Carbopol 941. Noveon brand of Carbomer 941.

Carbopol 971P. Noveon brand of Carbomer 941.

Carbopol 974P. Noveon brand of Carbomer 934P.

Carbopol 980. Noveon brand of Carbomer 940.

Carbopol 981. Noveon brand of Carbomer 941.

Carbopol 1342. Noveon brand of Carbomer 1342.

Carbowax Sentry. Union Carbide brand of Polyethylene Glycol.

Carbowax Sentry Methoxypolyethylene Glycol. Union Carbide brand of Polyethylene Glycol Monomethyl Ether.

Cardene. PDL Biopharma brand of Nicardipine Hydrochloride.

Cardiazol. Knoll† brand of Pentylenetetrazol.

Cardilate. Glaxo Wellcome† brand of Erythrityl Tetranitrate.

Cardiogen. Bristol-Myers Squibb† brand of Rubidium Chloride Rb 82.

Cardiografin. Bracco brand of Diatrizoate Meglumine.

Cardiolite. DuPont Merck brand of Technetium Tc 99m Sestamibi.

Cardiotec. Bracco Diagnostics brand of Technetium Tc 99m Teboroxime.

Cardiovasc. Recordati, Italy, brand of Lercanidipine Hydrochloride.

Cardizem. Biovail brand of Diltiazem Hydrochloride.

Cardrase. Pfizer brand of Ethoxzolamide.

Cardura. Pfizer brand of Doxazosin Mesylate.

Carmen. Recordati, Italy, brand of Lercanidipine Hydrochloride.

Carnitor. Sigma-Tau brand of Levocarnitine.

Caroid. Sterling Winthrop† brand of Papain.

Carraklenz Wound & Skin Cleanser. Carrington brand of Acemannan.

Carrisyn. Carrington brand of Acemannan.

Cartrol. Abbott brand of Carteolol Hydrochloride.

Casodex. AstraZeneca brand of Bicalutamide.

Cataflam. Novartis brand of Diclofenac Potassium.

Catapres. Boehringer Ingelheim brand of Clonidine.

Catapres. Boehringer Ingelheim brand of Clonidine Hydrochloride.

Catarase. Novartis brand of Chymotrypsin.

Catron Hydrochloride. Marion Merrell Dow† brand of Pheniprazine Hydrochloride.

Cattlyst [Veterinary]. Syntex brand of Laidlomycin Propionate Potassium.

Caverject. Pfizer brand of Alprostadil.

Cayston. Corus brand of Aztreonam Lysine.

CEA-CIDE. Immunomedics brand of Labetuzumab.

CEA-Cide. Immunomedics brand of Yttrium Y 90 Labetuzumab.

CEA-Scan. Immunomedics brand of Arcitumomab.

Cebione. Abbott† brand of Ascorbic Acid.

Ceclor. Lilly brand of Cefaclor.

Cecon. Abbott brand of Ascorbic Acid.

Cedax. Schering brand of Ceftibuten.

Cedilanid-D. Novartis brand of Deslanoside.

Ceenu. Bristol-Myers Squibb brand of Lomustine.

Ceepryn. Marion Merrell Dow† brand of Cetylpyridinium Chloride.

Cefadyl. Apothecon brand of Cephapirin Sodium.

Cefizox. Astellas brand of Ceftizoxime Sodium.

Cefmax. TAP brand of Cefmenoxime Hydrochloride.

Cefobid. Pfizer brand of Cefoperazone Sodium.

Cefomonil. TAP† brand of Cefsulodin Sodium.

Cefotan. Zeneca brand of Cefotetan.

Cefotan. AstraZeneca brand of Cefotetan Disodium.

Cefotaxime. Abraxis brand of Cefotaxime Sodium.

Cefrom. Hoechst-Roussel† brand of Cefpirome Sulfate.

Ceftin. GlaxoSmithKline brand of Cefuroxime Axetil.

Cefzil. Bristol-Myers Squibb brand of Cefprozil.

Celebrex. Pfizer brand of Celecoxib.

Celestone. Schering brand of Betamethasone.

Celestone. Schering brand of Betamethasone Sodium Phosphate.

Celexa. Forest brand of Citalopram Hydrobromide.

Cellcept. Roche brand of Mycophenolate Mofetil.

Cellcept. Roche brand of Mycophenolate Mofetil Hydrochloride.

Cellosize. Union Carbide brand of Hydroxyethyl Cellulose.

Celluvisc. Allergan brand of Carboxymethylcellulose Sodium.

Celontin. Pfizer brand of Methsuximide.

Celsis. Ortho-McNeil† brand of Cetiedil Citrate.

Cenolate. Abbott brand of Ascorbic Acid.

Centany. Johnson & Johnson brand of Mupirocin.

Centara. Centocor brand of Priliximab.

Centoxin. Centocor† brand of Nebacumab.

Centrac. Parke-Davis† brand of Profadol Hydrochloride.

Centrax. Pfizer brand of Prazepam.

Cepacol. Marion Merrell Dow† brand of Cetylpyridinium Chloride.

Ceradon. Takeda brand of Cefotiam Hydrochloride.

CerAxon. Interneuron brand of Citicoline Sodium.

Cerebyx. Pfizer brand of Fosphenytoin Sodium.

Ceredase. Genzyme brand of Alglucerase.

Ceresine. Cypros brand of Sodium Dichloroacetate.

Cerestat. Cambridge brand of Aptiganel Hydrochloride.

Ceretec. Nycomed Amersham brand of Technetium Tc 99m Exametazime.

Cerezyme. Genzyme brand of Imiglucerase.

Cerubidine. Bedford brand of Daunorubicin Hydrochloride.

Cervilaxin. Marion Merrell Dow† brand of Relaxin.

Cesamet. Valeant brand of Nabilone.

Cescan-131. Abbott† brand of Cesium Chloride Cs 131.

Cestex. SmithKline Beecham Animal Health brand of Epsiprantel.

Cetamide. Alcon brand of Sulfacetamide Sodium.

Cetane. Forest† brand of Ascorbic Acid.

Cetane-Caps TC. Forest† brand of Ascorbic Acid.

Cetrotide. Serono brand of Cetrorelix.

Cetrotide. Degussa A. G., Germany, brand of Cetrorelix Acetate.

Cevalin. Lilly brand of Ascorbic Acid.

Cevalin. Lilly brand of Sodium Ascorbate.

Cevex. Marion Merrell Dow† brand of Ascorbic Acid.

Chantix. Pfizer brand of Varenicline Tartrate.

Chemet. Ovation brand of Succimer.

Chemipen. Bristol-Myers Squibb† brand of Phenethicillin Potassium.

Chenix. Axcan Scandipharm brand of Chenodiol.

Children's Mylanta Upset Stomach Relief. Johnson & Johnson-Merck Consumer brand of Calcium Carbonate.

Chirocaine. Purdue brand of Levobupivacaine Hydrochloride.

Chloresium. Rystan brand of Chlorophyllin Copper Complex Sodium.

Chloretone. Parke-Davis brand of Chlorobutanol.

Chloromycetin. Pfizer brand of Chloramphenicol.

Chloromycetin. Pfizer brand of Chloramphenicol Sodium Succinate.

Chloromycetin Palmitate. Pfizer brand of Chloramphenicol Palmitate.

Chlor-Trimeton. Schering-Plough brand of Chlorpheniramine Maleate.

Chlorylen. Schering† brand of Trichloroethylene.

Cholac. Alra brand of Lactulose.

Cholebine (Japan). Mitsubishi Pharma brand of Colestilan Chloride.

Cholebrine. Mallinckrodt brand of Iocetamic Acid.

Choledyl. Warner Chilcott brand of Oxtriphylline.

Choletec. Bracco Diagnostics brand of Technetium Tc 99m Mebrofenin.

Cholografin. Bristol-Myers Squibb† brand of Iodipamide.

Cholografin Meglumine. Bracco brand of Iodipamide Meglumine.

Cholografin Sodium. Bracco brand of Iodipamide Sodium.

Cholovue. Bracco brand of Iodoxamate Meglumine.

Choloxin. Abbott brand of Dextrothyroxine Sodium.

Cholybar. Parke-Davis† brand of Cholestyramine Resin.

Chooz. Schering-Plough HealthCare brand of Calcium Carbonate.

Chromadax. Gloucester brand of Romidepsin.

Chromalbin. Bristol-Myers Squibb† brand of Albumin, Chromated Cr 51 Serum.

Chromitope Sodium. Bristol-Myers Squibb† brand of Sodium Chromate Cr 51.

Chromphosphotope. Bristol-Myers Squibb† brand of Chromic Phosphate P 32.

Chrysalin. OrthoLogic brand of Rusalatide Acetate.

Chymex. Savage brand of Bentiromide.

Chymodiactin. Abbott brand of Chymopapain.

Cialis. Lilly brand of Tadalafil.

Cibacalcin. Ciba-Geigy† brand of Calcitonin.

Cida-stat. Ecolab brand of Chlorhexidine Gluconate.

Ciloxan. Alcon brand of Ciprofloxacin Hydrochloride.

Cinobac. Lilly brand of Cinoxacin.

Cin-quin. Solvay Pharmaceuticals brand of Quinidine Sulfate.

Cipro. Bayer brand of Ciprofloxacin.

Cipro. Bayer brand of Ciprofloxacin Hydrochloride.

Circanol. 3M Pharmaceuticals brand of Ergoloid Mesylates.

Cisnoet. Berlex brand of Ditiocade Sodium.

Cisnoet. Berlex brand of Technetium Tc 99m Nitridocade.

CIS-PYRO. CL Pharma AG, Austria, brand of Technetium Tc 99m Pyrophosphate.

Citanest. AstraZeneca brand of Prilocaine Hydrochloride.

Citracal. Mission Pharmacal brand of Calcium Citrate.

Claforan. Sanofi Aventis brand of Cefotaxime Sodium.

Clamoxyl. Parke-Davis† brand of Clamoxyquin Hydrochloride.

Claravis. Barr brand of Isotretinoin.

Clarinex. Schering-Plough brand of Desloratadine.

Claritin. Schering-Plough brand of Loratadine.

CLD 2. Buckeye† brand of Croscarmellose Sodium.

Clear Away Wart Remover. Schering-Plough HealthCare brand of Salicylic Acid.

Clear By Design. SmithKline Beecham† brand of Benzoyl Peroxide.

Cleboril. Grupo Farmacéutico Almirall S.A., Spain, brand of Clebopride.

Clenicor. Symphar S.A., Switzerland, brand of Mifobate.

Cleocin. Pharmacia & Upjohn brand of Clindamycin.

Cleocin. Pfizer brand of Clindamycin Hydrochloride.

Cleocin. Pfizer brand of Clindamycin Palmitate Hydrochloride.

Cleocin. Pfizer brand of Clindamycin Phosphate.

Clevelox. The Medicines Company brand of Clevidipine Butyrate.

Climara. Bayer brand of Estradiol.

Clindagel. Galderma brand of Clindamycin Phosphate.

Clindesse. KV Pharmaceutical brand of Clindamycin Phosphate.

Clinium. Ortho-McNeil† brand of Lidoflazine.

Clinoril. Merck brand of Sulindac.

Clistin. McNeil brand of Carbinoxamine Maleate.

Clobex. Galderma brand of Clobetasol Propionate.

Cloderm. Coria brand of Clocortolone Pivalate.

Clolar. Genzyme brand of Clofarabine.

Clomid. Sanofi Aventis brand of Clomiphene Citrate.

Clopane Hydrochloride. Lilly† brand of Cyclopentamine Hydrochloride.

Cloradryn. Syntex brand of Cloprednol.

Cloretazine. Vion brand of Laromustine.

Clorpactin WCS-90. Guardian Laboratories brand of Oxychlorosene Sodium.

Cloxapen. GlaxoSmithKline brand of Cloxacillin Sodium.

Clozaril. Novartis brand of Clozapine.

---

† Brand name formerly used, and/or firm no longer concerned with this product.

Clysodrast. Rhone-Poulenc Rorer† brand of Bisacodyl Tannex.

Coactabs. Hoffmann-LaRoche† brand of Amdinocillin Pivoxil.

Coactin. Roche brand of Amdinocillin.

Coactinon. Mitsubishi Chemical Corporation, Japan, brand of Emivirine.

Coban [as sodium salt]. Lilly brand of Monensin.

Cobatope-57. Bristol-Myers Squibb† brand of Cobaltous Chloride Co 57.

Cobatope-60. Bristol-Myers Squibb† brand of Cobaltous Chloride Co 60.

Cobavite. Watson brand of Cyanocobalamin.

Cobefrin. Sterling Winthrop brand of Nordefrin Hydrochloride.

Coco-diazine. Lilly brand of Sulfadiazine.

Cogentin. Ovation brand of Benztropine Mesylate.

Cognex. Sciele brand of Tacrine Hydrochloride.

Colace. Roberts Pharmaceutical brand of Docusate Sodium.

Colazal. Salix brand of Balsalazide Disodium.

Colestid. Pfizer brand of Colestipol Hydrochloride.

Colloral. AutoImmune brand of Trinecol (pullus).

Cologel. Lilly brand of Methylcellulose.

Colrex Compound. Solvay Pharmaceuticals† brand of Codeine Phosphate.

Coly-mycin. King brand of Colistimethate Sodium.

Coly-mycin. King brand of Colistin Sulfate.

Combantrin. Pfizer brand of Pyrantel Pamoate.

Combidex. Advanced Magnetics brand of Ferumoxtran-10.

Combistrep. Pfizer brand of Streptoduocin.

Combotel. Bayer Animal Health† brand of Febantel.

Commit. GlaxoSmithKline brand of Nicotine Polacrilex.

Compazine. GlaxoSmithKline brand of Prochlorperazine.

Compazine. GlaxoSmithKline brand of Prochlorperazine Edisylate.

Compazine. GlaxoSmithKline brand of Prochlorperazine Maleate.

Complamin. 3M Pharmaceuticals† brand of Xanthinol Niacinate.

Compound W. Whitehall-Robins† brand of Salicylic Acid.

Comtan. Orion brand of Entacapone.

Conadil. 3M Pharmaceuticals† brand of Sulthiame.

Conceptrol. Ortho Pharmaceutical brand of Nonoxynol 9.

Concerta. ALZA brand of Methylphenidate Hydrochloride.

Condylox. Oclassen brand of Podofilox.

Conray. Mallinckrodt brand of Iothalamate Meglumine.

Conray. Mallinckrodt brand of Iothalamate Sodium.

Conray I 131. Mallinckrodt† brand of Iothalamate Sodium I 131.

Constilac. Alra brand of Lactulose.

Constulose. Actavis brand of Lactulose.

Contaflex GM3 49%. Contamac brand of Acofilcon B.

Contaflex GM3 58%. Contamac brand of Acofilcon A.

Contrapar. Wellcome, Great Britain, brand of Gloxazone.

Cooper Clear. CooperVision brand of Tetrafilcon A.

Cooper Thin. CooperVision brand of Polymacon.

Cooper Toric. CooperVision brand of Tetrafilcon A.

Copaxone. Teva brand of Glatiramer Acetate.

Copegus. Roche brand of Ribavirin.

Coramine. Ciba-Geigy† brand of Nikethamide.

Cordarone. Wyeth-Ayerst brand of Amiodarone.

Cordran. Oclassen brand of Flurandrenolide.

Corgard. King brand of Nadolol.

Corid [Veterinary]. Merial brand of Amprolium.

Corifeo. Recordati, Italy, brand of Lercanidipine Hydrochloride.

Corlopam. Hospira brand of Fenoldopam Mesylate.

Cormax. Healthpoint brand of Clobetasol Propionate.

Correctol Stool Softener Laxative. Schering-Plough HealthCare brand of Docusate Sodium.

Correctol Tablets, Caplets. Schering-Plough HealthCare brand of Bisacodyl.

Cortef. Pfizer brand of Hydrocortisone.

Cortef. Pfizer brand of Hydrocortisone Cypionate.

Cortef Acetate. Pfizer brand of Hydrocortisone Acetate.

Cortigel. Savage† brand of Corticotropin, Repository.

Cortone. Merck brand of Cortisone Acetate.

Cortril. Pfizer brand of Hydrocortisone.

Cortril. Pfizer brand of Hydrocortisone Acetate.

Cortrophin. Organon brand of Corticotropin.

Cortrophin Zinc ACTH. Organon† brand of Corticotropin Zinc Hydroxide.

Cortrosyn. Amphastar brand of Cosyntropin.

Corvaton. Hoechst-Roussel† brand of Molsidomine.

Corvert. Pfizer brand of Ibutilide Fumarate.

Cosmegen. Ovation brand of Dactinomycin.

Cotazym. Organon brand of Pancrelipase.

Cotazym-S. Organon brand of Pancrelipase.

Coumadin. Bristol-Myers Squibb brand of Warfarin Sodium.

Covera. Pfizer brand of Verapamil Hydrochloride.

Cozaar. Merck brand of Losartan Potassium.

Crasnitin. Bayer† brand of Asparaginase.

Cremophor EL. BASF brand of Polyoxyl 35 Castor Oil.

Cremophor ELP. BASF brand of Polyoxyl 35 Castor Oil.

Cremophor RH40. BASF brand of Polyoxyl 40 Hydrogenated Castor Oil.

Creon. Solvay Pharmaceuticals brand of Pancrelipase.

Crescent Bifocal. Bausch & Lomb† brand of Hefilcon A.

Crestor. AstraZeneca brand of Rosuvastatin Calcium.

Crinone. Columbia brand of Progesterone.

Criterion Ultra DW. Bausch & Lomb† brand of Polymacon.

Criterion Ultra FW. Bausch & Lomb† brand of Polymacon.

Criterion Ultra SP. Bausch & Lomb† brand of Polymacon.

Criterion Ultra Toric. Bausch & Lomb† brand of Hefilcon B.

Criterion XLT. Bausch & Lomb† brand of Polymacon.

Crixivan. Merck brand of Indinavir Sulfate.

Crolom. Bausch & Lomb brand of Cromolyn Sodium.

Crotan. Summers brand of Crotamiton.

Crystodigin. Lilly brand of Digitoxin.

Cubicin. Cubist brand of Daptomycin.

Cumopyran. Abbott† brand of Cyclocumarol.

Cumulase. Halozyme brand of Hyaluronidase (Human Recombinant).

Cuprimine. Merck brand of Penicillamine.

Curatrem [Veterinary]. Merial brand of Clorsulon.

Curosurf. Dey brand of Poractant Alfa.

Cutivate. Altana brand of Fluticasone Propionate.

Cyclaine. Merck brand of Hexylcaine Hydrochloride.

Cyclapen. Wyeth brand of Cyclacillin.

Cyclocort. Astellas brand of Amcinonide.

Cyclogyl. Alcon brand of Cyclopentolate Hydrochloride.

Cyclopar. Warner Chilcott brand of Tetracycline Hydrochloride.

Cyclospasmol. Wyeth-Ayerst brand of Cyclandelate.

Cyklokapron. Pfizer brand of Tranexamic Acid.

Cylert. Abbott brand of Pemoline.

Cymbalta. Lilly brand of Duloxetine Hydrochloride.

Cynt. Lilly brand of Moxonidine.

Cypentil. Abbott† brand of Piperidine Phosphate.

Cypromin. Schering† brand of Rolicyprine.

Cystadane. Rare brand of Betaine Hydrochloride.

Cystografin. Bracco brand of Diatrizoate Meglumine.

Cytadren. Novartis brand of Aminoglutethimide.

Cytellin. Lilly† brand of Sitosterols.

Cytolex. Abbott brand of Pexiganan Acetate.

Cytomel. King brand of Liothyronine Sodium.

Cytotec. Pfizer brand of Misoprostol.

Cytovene. Roche brand of Ganciclovir.

Cytoxan. Bristol-Myers Squibb brand of Cyclophosphamide.

Dacogen. MGI Pharma brand of Decitabine.

Dactil. Marion Merrell Dow† brand of Piperidolate Hydrochloride.

Dalgan. AstraZeneca brand of Dezocine.

Dalmane. Valeant brand of Flurazepam Hydrochloride.

Danocrine. Sanofi Aventis brand of Danazol.

Dantrium. Procter & Gamble brand of Dantrolene Sodium.

Daquin. 3M Pharmaceuticals† brand of Chlorazanil Hydrochloride.

Daranide. Merck brand of Dichlorphenamide.

Daraprim. GlaxoSmithKline brand of Pyrimethamine.

Darbid. GlaxoSmithKline brand of Isopropamide Iodide.

Darco. ICI Americas† brand of Carbon, Activated.

Daricon. Pfizer brand of Oxyphencyclimine Hydrochloride.

Darvon. Xanodyne brand of Propoxyphene Hydrochloride.

Darvon-N. Xanodyne brand of Propoxyphene Napsylate.

Daunoxome. Gilead Sciences brand of Daunorubicin Hydrochloride.

Daxid. Roerig brand of Xanthiol Hydrochloride.

1-Day ACUVUE. Vistakon brand of Etafilcon A.

Daypro. Pfizer brand of Oxaprozin.

Daytrana. Shire brand of Methylphenidate.

DBI. Ciba-Geigy† brand of Phenformin Hydrochloride.

D.C.P. Parke-Davis† brand of Calcium Phosphate Dihydrate, Dibasic.

Ddavp. Sanofi Aventis brand of Desmopressin Acetate.

Deaner. 3M Pharmaceuticals† brand of Deanol Acetamidobenzoate.

Deapril. Bristol-Myers Squibb brand of Ergoloid Mesylates.

Decabid. Lilly brand of Indecainide Hydrochloride.

Decadron. Merck brand of Dexamethasone.

Decadron. Merck brand of Dexamethasone Acetate.

Decadron. Merck brand of Dexamethasone Sodium Phosphate.

Decapryn. Sanofi Aventis brand of Doxylamine Succinate.

Decholin. Bayer† brand of Dehydrocholic Acid.

Decholin Sodium. Bayer† brand of Dehydrocholate Sodium.

Declinax. Hoffmann-LaRoche† brand of Debrisoquin Sulfate.

Declomycin. Stiefel brand of Demeclocycline Hydrochloride.

Definity. Bristol-Myers Squibb brand of Perflutren.

Deflamene. Farmitalia, Societa Farmaceutici Italia, Italy, brand of Formocortal.

Deladroxone. Bristol-Myers Squibb† brand of Algestone Acetophenide.

Delalutin. Bristol-Myers Squibb brand of Hydroxyprogesterone Caproate.

Delaprem. Savage† brand of Hexoprenaline Sulfate.

Delatestryl. Indevus brand of Testosterone Enanthate.

Delavan. Bayer† brand of Methylbenzethonium Chloride.

Delestrec. Bristol-Myers Squibb† brand of Estradiol Undecylate.

Delestrogen. King brand of Estradiol Valerate.

Delinal. Marion Merrell Dow† brand of Propenzolate Hydrochloride.

Delsym. Adams brand of Dextromethorphan Polistirex.

Delta-cortef. Pfizer brand of Prednisolone.

Delta-dome. Bayer brand of Prednisone.

Deltalin. Lilly brand of Ergocalciferol.

Deltasone. Pfizer brand of Prednisone.

Deltoin. Novartis† brand of Methetoin.

Demadex. Roche brand of Torsemide.

Demerol. Hospira brand of Meperidine Hydrochloride.

Demerol. Sanofi Aventis brand of Meperidine Hydrochloride.

Demser. Aton brand of Metyrosine.

Denagard. Boehringer Ingelheim Animal Health brand of Tiamulin.

Denavir. SmithKline Beecham brand of Penciclovir.

Denavir. Novartis brand of Penciclovir Sodium.

Dendrid. Alcon brand of Idoxuridine.

Depacon. Abbott brand of Valproate Sodium.

Depakene. Abbott brand of Valproic Acid.

Depakote. Abbott brand of Divalproex Sodium.

Depen. Medpointe brand of Penicillamine.

Depo. Pfizer brand of Estradiol Cypionate.

Depocyt. Skyepharma brand of Cytarabine.

Depo-medrol. Pfizer brand of Methylprednisolone Acetate.

Depo-testosterone. Pfizer brand of Testosterone Cypionate.

Derifil. Rystan brand of Chlorophyllin Copper Complex Sodium.

Dermabet. Taro brand of Betamethasone Valerate.

Derma-Smoothe/FS. Hill Dermac brand of Fluocinolone Acetonide.

Dermatop. Sanofi Aventis brand of Prednicarbate.

Desferal. Novartis brand of Deferoxamine Mesylate.

Desowen. Galderma brand of Desonide.

Desoxyn. Ovation brand of Methamphetamine Hydrochloride.

Desyrel. Apothecon brand of Trazodone Hydrochloride.

Detrol. Pfizer brand of Tolterodine Tartrate.

Devryl. SmithKline Beecham† brand of Clomacran Phosphate.

Dexacillin. Bristol-Myers Squibb† brand of Epicillin.

Dexampex. Teva brand of Dextroamphetamine Sulfate.

Dexawin. Sterling Winthrop† brand of Racephenicol.

Dexedrine. GlaxoSmithKline brand of Dextroamphetamine Sulfate.

Dexferrum. Luitpold brand of Iron Dextran.

Dexon. Davis & Geck brand of Polyglycolic Acid.

Dexone. Solvay Pharmaceuticals brand of Dexamethasone.

Dextromethorphan Hydrobromide OROS Tablets. Ciba-Geigy brand of Dextromethorphan Hydrobromide.

D.H.E. 45. Valeant brand of Dihydroergotamine Mesylate.

Diabeta. Sanofi Aventis brand of Glyburide.

Diabinese. Pfizer brand of Chlorpropamide.

Diagnex Blue. Bristol-Myers Squibb† brand of Azuresin.

Dial. Dial brand of Hexachlorophene.

Dialose. Johnson & Johnson-Merck Consumer brand of Docusate Sodium.

Dialume. Rhone-Poulenc Rorer† brand of Aluminum Hydroxide.

Diamox. Duramed brand of Acetazolamide.

Diamox. Duramed brand of Acetazolamide Sodium.

Diaparene. Sterling Winthrop brand of Methylbenzethonium Chloride.

Diapid. Novartis brand of Lypressin.

Diasone Sodium. Abbott brand of Sulfoxone Sodium.

Diastat. Valeant brand of Diazepam.

Dibenzyline. WellSpring brand of Phenoxybenzamine Hydrochloride.

Dibestil. Sterling Winthrop† brand of Diethylstilbestrol Dipropionate.

Dichlor-Mapharsen. Parke-Davis† brand of Dichlorophenarsine Hydrochloride.

Dickinson's Witch Hazel Formula. Dickinson brand of Witch Hazel.

Dicodid. Knoll† brand of Hydrocodone Bitartrate.

Didrex. Pfizer brand of Benzphetamine Hydrochloride.

Didronel. Procter & Gamble brand of Etidronate Disodium.

Differin. Galderma brand of Adapalene.

Diffusin. Ortho Pharmaceutical† brand of Hyaluronidase (Ovine).

Diflucan. Pfizer brand of Fluconazole.

Digifortis. Parke-Davis† brand of Digitalis.

Digiglusin. Lilly† brand of Digitalis.

Dilabil. Sterling Winthrop† brand of Dehydrocholic Acid.

Dilacor. Watson brand of Diltiazem Hydrochloride.

Dilantin. Pfizer brand of Phenytoin.

Dilantin. Parke-Davis brand of Phenytoin Sodium.

Dilatrate. Schwarz Pharma brand of Isosorbide Dinitrate.

Dilaudid. Abbott brand of Hydromorphone Hydrochloride.

Diloderm. Schering† brand of Dichlorisone Acetate.

Dimeray. Mallinckrodt† brand of Iocarmate Meglumine.

Dimetane. Wyeth brand of Brompheniramine Maleate.

Dimethylane. Marion Merrell Dow† brand of Promoxolane.

---

† Brand name formerly used, and/or firm no longer concerned with this product.

Dimorlin Tartrate. SmithKline Beecham† brand of Dextromoramide Tartrate.

Diodrast. Sterling Winthrop† brand of Iodopyracet.

Dionosil. GlaxoSmithKline brand of Propyliodone.

Diothane Hydrochloride. Marion Merrell Dow† brand of Diperodon Hydrochloride.

Diovan. Novartis brand of Valsartan.

Dioxatrine. Janssen Pharmaceutica, Belgium, brand of Benzetimide Hydrochloride.

Dioxyline. Laboratoires Franca Inc., Canada, brand of Benzoxiquine.

Di-Paralene. Abbott† brand of Chlorcyclizine Hydrochloride.

Dipentum. UCB brand of Olsalazine Sodium.

Diprivan. Abraxis brand of Propofol.

Diprofarn. Farmitalia, Societa Farmaceutici Italia, Italy, brand of Dipyrone.

Diprolene. Schering brand of Betamethasone Dipropionate.

Diprosone. Schering brand of Betamethasone Dipropionate.

Dirame. Bayer† brand of Propiram Fumarate.

Disalcid. 3M Pharmaceuticals brand of Salsalate.

Discase. Abbott brand of Chymopapain.

Dismutec. Sterling Winthrop brand of Pegorgotein.

Disomer. Schering brand of Dexbrompheniramine Maleate.

Dispermox. Ranbaxy brand of Amoxicillin.

Distrycin. Bristol-Myers Squibb† brand of Streptoduocin.

Ditropan. ALZA brand of Oxybutynin Chloride.

Diucardin. Wyeth brand of Hydroflumethiazide.

Diulo. Pfizer brand of Metolazone.

Diuril. Merck brand of Chlorothiazide.

Diuril. Ovation brand of Chlorothiazide Sodium.

DMSA Kidney Reagent. Medi-Physics brand of Technetium Tc 99m Succimer.

Dobutrex. Lilly brand of Dobutamine Hydrochloride.

Doca. Organon brand of Desoxycorticosterone Acetate.

Doctrin. Merck brand of Dexibuprofen Lysine.

Dogmatyl. Laboratoires Delagrange, France, brand of Sulpiride.

Dolinac. Wyeth-Ayerst brand of Felbinac.

Dolobid. Merck brand of Diflunisal.

Dolophine Hydrochloride. Xanodyne brand of Methadone Hydrochloride.

Domeboro. Bayer brand of Aluminum Acetate.

Domeform-HC. Bayer† brand of Clioquinol.

Dopacard. Fisons† brand of Dopexamine Hydrochloride.

Dopar. Shire brand of Levodopa.

Dopascan. Guilford brand of Iometopane I 123.

Dopram. Baxter Healthcare brand of Doxapram Hydrochloride.

Doral. Questcor brand of Quazepam.

Doratect [Veterinary]. Merial brand of Abamectin.

Dorbane. 3M Pharmaceuticals† brand of Danthron.

Doriden. Sanofi Aventis brand of Glutethimide.

Dormate. Medpointe brand of Mebutamate.

Dormison. Schering† brand of Meparfynol.

Doryx. Warner Chilcott brand of Doxycycline Hyclate.

Dostinex. Pfizer brand of Cabergoline.

Dovonex. Warner Chilcott brand of Calcipotriene.

Doxil. Ortho Biotech brand of Doxorubicin Hydrochloride.

Doxinate. Hoechst-Roussel† brand of Docusate Sodium.

Doxy. Abraxis brand of Doxycycline Hyclate.

D-Panthenol 50. BASF brand of Dexpanthenol.

Dr. Scholl's Athlete's Foot Spray. Schering-Plough HealthCare brand of Tolnaftate.

Dr. Scholl's Callus Removers. Schering-Plough HealthCare brand of Salicylic Acid.

Dr. Scholl's Corn Removers. Schering-Plough HealthCare brand of Salicylic Acid.

Dr. Scholl's Wart Remover Kit. Schering-Plough HealthCare brand of Salicylic Acid.

Dralzine. Teva brand of Hydralazine Hydrochloride.

Dramamine. Pfizer brand of Dimenhydrinate.

Drisdol. Sanofi Aventis brand of Ergocalciferol.

Dristan Inhaler. Whitehall-Robins† brand of Propylhexedrine.

DrithoCreme. Dermik brand of Anthralin.

Drithoscalp. Dermik brand of Anthralin.

Drixoral Cough. Schering-Plough HealthCare† brand of Dextromethorphan Hydrobromide.

Drolban. Lilly brand of Dromostanolone Propionate.

Dromos. Biosint S.p.A. brand of Levocarnitine Propionate Hydrochloride.

Droxia. Bristol-Myers Squibb brand of Hydroxyurea.

Droxone. Bristol-Myers Squibb† brand of Algestone Acetophenide.

Dry and Clear. Whitehall-Robins† brand of Benzoyl Peroxide.

D-S-S. Parke-Davis† brand of Docusate Sodium.

Dtic-Dome. Bayer brand of Dacarbazine.

Dulcolax. Boehringer Ingelheim brand of Bisacodyl.

Duofilm Wart Remover. Schering-Plough HealthCare brand of Salicylic Acid.

Duolip. L. Merckle, Germany, brand of Theofibrate.

Duolite AP143 Resin. Rohm and Haas brand of Cholestyramine Resin.

Duomectin [Veterinary]. Merial brand of Abamectin.

Duoplant. Stiefel† brand of Salicylic Acid.

Duotin [Veterinary]. Merial brand of Abamectin.

Durabolin. Organon brand of Nandrolone Decanoate.

Durabolin. Organon brand of Nandrolone Phenpropionate.

Duracillin. Lilly brand of Penicillin G Procaine.

Duraclon. Xanodyne brand of Clonidine Hydrochloride.

Duraflex. Ortho-McNeil† brand of Flumetramide.

Duragesic. ALZA brand of Fentanyl.

Duramorph. Baxter Healthcare brand of Morphine Sulfate.

Duranest [as hydrochloride]. Astra brand of Etidocaine.

Duraprep copolymer. 3M Specialty Materials brand of Iodine Povacrylex.

Duraquin. Warner Chilcott brand of Quinidine Gluconate.

DuraSoft 2. Wesley-Jessen brand of Phemfilcon A.

DuraSoft 3. Wesley-Jessen brand of Phemfilcon A.

Duricef. Warner Chilcott brand of Cefadroxil.

Duvoid. WellSpring brand of Bethanechol Chloride.

Dv. Sanofi Aventis brand of Dienestrol.

Dyclone. AstraZeneca brand of Dyclonine Hydrochloride.

Dymelor. Lilly brand of Acetohexamide.

Dynabac. Lilly brand of Dirithromycin.

Dynacin. Medicis brand of Minocycline Hydrochloride.

Dynacirc. Reliant brand of Isradipine.

Dyna-hex. Xttrium brand of Chlorhexidine Gluconate.

Dynamutilin. Bristol-Myers Squibb† brand of Tiamulin Fumarate.

Dynamyxin. Pfizer brand of Sulfomyxin.

Dynapen. Apothecon brand of Dicloxacillin Sodium.

Dynepo (pending). Aventis brand of Epoetin Delta.

Dynospheres M-035. Dyno Particles AS, Norway, brand of Ferristene.

Dyrenium. WellSpring brand of Triamterene.

Dytransin. Boots, England, brand of Ibufenac.

E5. Xoma brand of Edobacomab.

E-40. Lombart brand of Pentafilcon A.

E-50. Lombart brand of Pentafilcon A.

E-60. Lombart brand of Pentafilcon A.

"EASTMAN" 600. Eastman brand of Glyceryl Monostearate.

"EASTMAN" C-A-P. Eastman brand of Cellacefate.

"EASTMAN" Cellulose Acetate CA 398-10NF. Eastman brand of Cellulose Acetate.

"EASTMAN" HPMCP. Eastman brand of Hypromellose Phthalate.

"EASTMAN" Triacetin. Eastman brand of Triacetin.

"EASTMAN" Vitamin E TPGS. Eastman brand of Tocophersolan.

Ebesal. Hoechst-Roussel† brand of Allocupreide Sodium.

Edecrin. Aton brand of Ethacrynate Sodium.

Edecrin. Aton brand of Ethacrynic Acid.

Edex. Schwarz Pharma brand of Alprostadil.

Edronax. Pharmacia & Upjohn brand of Reboxetine Mesylate.

E.e.s. Abbott brand of Erythromycin Ethylsuccinate.

Effexor. Wyeth brand of Venlafaxine Hydrochloride.

Efudex. Valeant brand of Fluorouracil.

Ekomine. Hoechst-Roussel† brand of Methylatropine Nitrate.

Elavil. AstraZeneca brand of Amitriptyline Hydrochloride.

Eldepryl. Somerset brand of Selegiline Hydrochloride.

Eldisine. Lilly brand of Vindesine Sulfate.

Eldopaque Forte. ICN brand of Hydroquinone.

Eldoquin Forte. ICN brand of Hydroquinone.

Elestrim. Bradley brand of Estradiol.

Elidel. Novartis brand of Pimecrolimus.

Elimite. Allergan brand of Permethrin.

Elixophyllin. Forest brand of Theophylline.

Ellence. Pfizer brand of Epirubicin Hydrochloride.

Ellsyl. Marion Merrell Dow† brand of Metizoline Hydrochloride.

Elmiron. Ortho-McNeil brand of Pentosan Polysulfate Sodium.

Elocon. Schering brand of Mometasone Furoate.

Eloxatin. Sanofi Aventis brand of Oxaliplatin.

Elspar. Merck brand of Asparaginase.

Elvetil. Maggioni Farmaceutici S.p.A., Italy, brand of Stilonium Iodide.

Emadine. Alcon brand of Emedastine Difumarate.

Embeline. Healthpoint brand of Clobetasol Propionate.

Embutane. Hoechst-Roussel brand of Embutramide.

Emcyt. Pfizer brand of Estramustine Phosphate Sodium.

Emend. Merck brand of Aprepitant.

Emete-con. Roerig brand of Benzquinamide.

Emgel. Altana brand of Erythromycin.

Emko. Schering-Plough HealthCare brand of Nonoxynol 9.

Emsam. Somerset brand of Selegiline.

Emtriva. Gilead Sciences brand of Emtricitabine.

E-mycin. Abbott brand of Erythromycin.

E-mycin. Pfizer brand of Erythromycin Ethylsuccinate.

Enablex. Novartis brand of Darifenacin Hydrobromide.

Enbrel. Immunex brand of Etanercept.

Endecto. Merck brand of Abamectin.

Endep. Roche brand of Amitriptyline Hydrochloride.

Endobil. Bracco Industria Chimica S.p.A., Italy, brand of Iodoxamic Acid.

Endometrin. Ferring Pharmaceuticals brand of Progesterone.

Endometrion. Schering A.G., Germany, brand of Dienogest.

Endomirabil. Bracco Industria Chimica S.p.A., Italy, brand of Iodoxamic Acid.

Endrate. Hospira brand of Edetate Disodium.

Enduron. Abbott brand of Methyclothiazide.

Engerix-B. SmithKline Beecham brand of Hepatitis B Virus Vaccine Inactivated.

Enkaid. Bristol Labs† brand of Encainide Hydrochloride.

Enlon. Baxter Healthcare brand of Edrophonium Chloride.

Ensam. Somerset brand of Selegiline Hydrochloride.

Entodon. Sterling Winthrop† brand of Prolonium Iodide.

Entolase. Robins† brand of Pancrelipase.

Enulose. Actavis brand of Lactulose.

Envacar. Pfizer brand of Guanoxan Sulfate.

Enzactin. Whitehall-Robins† brand of Triacetin.

Enzec. Merck brand of Abamectin.

Enzek. Merck brand of Abamectin.

Enzodase. Bristol-Myers Squibb† brand of Hyaluronidase (Ovine).

Epi-C. Mallinckrodt† brand of Barium Sulfate.

Epi-Clear. Bristol-Myers Squibb† brand of Benzoyl Peroxide.

Epicon. Specialty UltraVision brand of Carbosilfocon A.

Epinal. Alcon brand of Epinephryl Borate.

Epipen. Meridian brand of Epinephrine.

Epi-Stat 57. Mallinckrodt† brand of Barium Sulfate.

Epi-Stat 61. Mallinckrodt† brand of Barium Sulfate.

Epitol. Teva brand of Carbamazepine.

Epivir. GlaxoSmithKline brand of Lamivudine.

Epogen. Amgen brand of Epoetin Alfa.

Epontol. Farbenfabriken Bayer A.G., Germany, brand of Propanidid.

Eppy/N. Pilkington Barnes Hind brand of Epinephryl Borate.

Eprinex [Veterinary]. Merial brand of Eprinomectin.

Eprolin. Lilly† brand of Vitamin E.

Equanil. Wyeth brand of Meprobamate.

Equetro. Shire brand of Carbamazepine.

Equigard. Boehringer Ingelheim Animal Health brand of Dichlorvos.

Equigel. Boehringer Ingelheim Animal Health† brand of Dichlorvos.

Equimate. Bayer Animal Health† brand of Fluprostenol Sodium.

Equioxx. Merial brand of Firocoxib.

Equipin. Mission brand of Homatropine Methylbromide.

Equipoise [Veterinary]. Fort Dodge Animal Health brand of Boldenone Undecylenate.

Equron [Veterinary]. Fort Dodge Animal Health brand of Hyaluronate Sodium.

Erasis. Orion Pharmaceutica, Finland, brand of Erythromycin Acistrate.

Eraxis. Pfizer brand of Anidulafungin.

Ergamisol. Janssen brand of Levamisole Hydrochloride.

Ergostat. Pfizer brand of Ergotamine Tartrate.

Ergotrate Maleate. Lilly brand of Ergonovine Maleate.

Eryc. Warner Chilcott brand of Erythromycin.

Eryderm. Abbott brand of Erythromycin.

Erygel. Merz brand of Erythromycin.

Erymax. Merz brand of Erythromycin.

Eryped. Abbott brand of Erythromycin Ethylsuccinate.

Erythrocin. Hospira brand of Erythromycin Lactobionate.

Erythrocin. Abbott brand of Erythromycin Stearate.

Escalol. ISP Van Dyk brand of Octinoxate.

Escalol. ISP Van Dyk brand of Octisalate.

Escalol 507. ISP Van Dyk brand of Padimate O.

Escorpal. Farbenfabriken Bayer A.G., Germany, brand of Phencarbamide.

Eserine Sulfate. Ciba Vision, US Ophthalmics, brand of Physostigmine Sulfate.

Esidrix. Novartis brand of Hydrochlorothiazide.

Eskabarb. SmithKline Beecham† brand of Phenobarbital.

Eskalith. JDS brand of Lithium Carbonate.

Esophotrast. Rhone-Poulenc Rorer† brand of Barium Sulfate.

Estergel. Merck brand of Isopropyl Myristate.

Estinyl. Schering brand of Ethinyl Estradiol.

Estrace. Warner Chilcott brand of Estradiol.

Estraderm. Novartis brand of Estradiol.

Estradurin. Wyeth brand of Polyestradiol Phosphate.

Estraguard. Solvay Pharmaceuticals brand of Dienestrol.

Estratab. Solvay Pharmaceuticals brand of Estrogens, Esterified.

Estring. Pfizer brand of Estradiol.

Estrogel. Ascend Therapeutics brand of Estradiol.

Estrovis. Pfizer brand of Quinestrol.

Estrumate. Bayer Animal Health brand of Cloprostenol Sodium.

Ethamide. Allergan brand of Ethoxzolamide.

Ethamolin. QOL brand of Ethanolamine Oleate.

Ethaquin. Ascher† brand of Ethaverine Hydrochloride.

Ethibond. Ethicon brand of Suture, Nonabsorbable Surgical.

Ethiflex. Ethicon† brand of Suture, Nonabsorbable Surgical.

Ethilon. Ethicon brand of Suture, Nonabsorbable Surgical.

Ethiodol. Savage brand of Ethiodized Oil.

---

† Brand name formerly used, and/or firm no longer concerned with this product.

Ethiodol-131. Abbott† brand of Ethiodized Oil I 131.

Ethmozine. Roberts Pharmaceutical brand of Moricizine.

Ethmozine. Shire brand of Moricizine Hydrochloride.

Ethnine Simplex. Purdue Frederick† brand of Pholcodine.

Ethocel. Dow Chemical brand of Ethylcellulose.

Ethrane. Baxter Healthcare brand of Enflurane.

Ethyol. MedImmune brand of Amifostine.

Etonin. Ortho-McNeil† brand of Etoperidone Hydrochloride.

Etopophos. Bristol-Myers Squibb brand of Etoposide Phosphate.

Etrenol. Sterling Winthrop brand of Hycanthone Mesylate.

Etrynit. Sterling Winthrop† brand of Propatyl Nitrate.

Eulexin. Schering brand of Flutamide.

Eumydrin. Sterling Winthrop† brand of Methylatropine Nitrate.

Eurax. Westwood-Squibb brand of Crotamiton.

Euresol. Knoll† brand of Resorcinol Monoacetate.

Eusolex. Rona Laboratories, Great Britain, brand of Enzacamene.

Eusolex. Rona Laboratories, Great Britain, brand of Homosalate.

Euthroid. Parke-Davis† brand of Liotrix.

Eutonyl. Abbott brand of Pargyline Hydrochloride.

Evac-Q-Tabs. Savage brand of Bisacodyl.

Evac-Q-Tabs. Savage† brand of Phenolphthalein.

Evipal. Sterling Winthrop† brand of Hexobarbital.

Evipal Sodium. Sterling Winthrop† brand of Hexobarbital Sodium.

Evista. Lilly brand of Raloxifene Hydrochloride.

Evoclin. Connetics brand of Clindamycin Phosphate.

Evoxac. Daiichi Pharmaceutical brand of Cevimeline Hydrochloride.

EVRA. R. W. Johnson brand of Norelgestromin.

Exanta (proposed). AstraZeneca brand of Ximelagatran.

Exelderm. Ranbaxy brand of Sulconazole Nitrate.

Exelon. Novartis brand of Rivastigmine.

Exjade. Novartis brand of Deferasirox.

Ex-Lax. Novartis brand of Phenolphthalein.

Exna. Robins brand of Benzthiazide.

Extraneal. Baxter Healthcare brand of Icodextrin.

E-z Scrub. Becton Dickinson Microbiology brand of Povidone-Iodine.

Factive. Oscient brand of Gemifloxacin Mesylate.

Factrel. Baxter Healthcare brand of Gonadorelin Hydrochloride.

Falmonox. Sterling Winthrop brand of Teclozan.

Famvir. Novartis brand of Famciclovir.

Fanasil. Hoffmann-LaRoche-International brand of Sulfadoxine.

Fanzil. Hoffmann-LaRoche† brand of Sulfadoxine.

Fareston. GTX brand of Toremifene Citrate.

Faslodex. AstraZeneca brand of Fulvestrant.

Fastin. GlaxoSmithKline brand of Phentermine Hydrochloride.

Favid. Favrille brand of Mitumprotimut-T.

Fazaclo. Azur brand of Clozapine.

Feen-a-Mint Gum. Schering-Plough HealthCare† brand of Phenolphthalein, Yellow.

Feen-a-Mint Tablets. Schering-Plough HealthCare brand of Bisacodyl.

Felbatol. Medpointe brand of Felbamate.

Feldene. Pfizer brand of Piroxicam.

Femara. Novartis brand of Letrozole.

Feminone. Pfizer brand of Ethinyl Estradiol.

Fempatch. Pfizer brand of Estradiol.

Femring. Warner Chilcott brand of Estradiol Acetate.

Femstat. Roche brand of Butoconazole Nitrate.

Femtrace. Warner Chilcott brand of Estradiol Acetate.

Fentora. Cephalon brand of Fentanyl Citrate.

Feosol. SmithKline Beecham brand of Ferrous Sulfate.

Feostat. Forest brand of Ferrous Fumarate.

Fergon. Sterling Health U.S.A. brand of Ferrous Gluconate.

Feridex. Advanced Magnetics brand of Ferumoxides.

Ferndex. Ferndale brand of Dextroamphetamine Sulfate.

Fero-Gradumet. Abbott† brand of Ferrous Sulfate.

Ferriseltz. Otsuka brand of Ferric Ammonium Citrate.

Ferrlecit. Watson brand of Sodium Ferric Gluconate Complex.

Ferro Drops. Parke-Davis† brand of Ferrous Lactate.

Ferrutope. Bristol-Myers Squibb† brand of Ferrous Citrate Fe 59.

Fertinex. Serono brand of Urofollitropin.

Fiblast. Scios Nova brand of Trafermin.

Fibocil. Lilly† brand of Aprindine Hydrochloride.

Fibriscint. Centocor† brand of Biciromab.

Fibrogen. Marion Merrell Dow† brand of Fibrinogen, Human.

Filaribits Plus. SmithKline Beecham Animal Health brand of Oxibendazole.

Finacea. Intendis brand of Azelaic Acid.

Finaplix. Roussel-UCLAF, France, brand of Trenbolone Acetate.

Firmagon. PolyPeptide brand of Degarelix Acetate.

Fisherman's Friend Lozenges. Bristol-Myers Products brand of Menthol.

Flagyl. Pfizer brand of Metronidazole.

Flagyl. Pfizer brand of Metronidazole Hydrochloride.

Flarex. Alcon brand of Fluorometholone Acetate.

Flavaxin. Sterling Winthrop† brand of Riboflavin.

Flavomycin. Hoechst-Roussel brand of Bambermycins.

Flaxedil. Davis & Geck brand of Gallamine Triethiodide.

Flectar. Maggioni Farmaceutici S.p.A., Italy, brand of Butixirate.

Flexeril. McNeil brand of Cyclobenzaprine Hydrochloride.

Flexfree. Wyeth-Ayerst brand of Felbinac.

Flolan. GlaxoSmithKline brand of Epoprostenol Sodium.

Flomax. Boehringer Ingelheim brand of Tamsulosin Hydrochloride.

Flonase. GlaxoSmithKline brand of Fluticasone Propionate.

Florone. Pfizer brand of Diflorasone Diacetate.

Floropryl. Merck brand of Isoflurophate.

Flovent. GlaxoSmithKline brand of Fluticasone Propionate.

Floxapen. Beecham Research Laboratories, England, brand of Floxacillin.

Floxin. Ortho-McNeil brand of Ofloxacin.

Flucort [Veterinary]. Syntex brand of Flumethasone.

Fludara. Bayer brand of Fludarabine Phosphate.

Fluderma. Farmitalia, Societa Farmaceutici Italia, Italy, brand of Formocortal.

Flumadine. Forest brand of Rimantadine Hydrochloride.

Fluocet. Alpharma brand of Fluocinolone Acetonide.

Fluogen. Parke-Davis† brand of Influenza Virus Vaccine.

Fluonid. Allergan brand of Fluocinolone Acetonide.

Fluorescite. Alcon brand of Fluorescein.

Fluorescite. Alcon brand of Fluorescein Sodium.

Fluorex 300. G.T. Laboratories brand of Flusilfocon C.

Fluorex 500. G.T. Laboratories brand of Flusilfocon B.

Fluorex 600. G.T. Laboratories brand of Flusilfocon E.

Fluorex 700. G.T. Laboratories brand of Flusilfocon A.

Fluorex 900. G.T. Laboratories brand of Flusilfocon D.

Fluorinse. Oral-B brand of Sodium Fluoride.

Fluoromar. Ohmeda brand of Fluroxene.

Fluoroperm 32. Paragon brand of Paflufocon C.

Fluoroperm 62. Paragon brand of Paflufocon B.

Fluoroperm 92. Paragon brand of Paflufocon A.

Fluoroperm 151. Paragon brand of Paflufocon D.

Fluoroplex. Allergan brand of Fluorouracil.

Fluothane. Wyeth brand of Halothane.

Fluotrex. Savage brand of Fluocinolone Acetonide.

Flurizan. Myriad brand of Tarenflurbil.

FluShield. Lederle brand of Influenza Virus Vaccine.

Fluxid. Schwarz Pharma brand of Famotidine.

Fluzone. Bristol-Myers Squibb† brand of Influenza Virus Vaccine.

Fml. Allergan brand of Fluorometholone.

Focalin. Novartis brand of Dexmethylphenidate Hydrochloride.

Fodosine. BioCryst brand of Forodesine.

Folicet. Mission brand of Folic Acid.

Follutein. Bristol-Myers Squibb brand of Gonadotropin, Chorionic.

Folvite. Wyeth brand of Folic Acid.

Foradil. Novartis brand of Formoterol Fumarate.

Forane. Baxter Healthcare brand of Isoflurane.

Forcaltonin. Unigene brand of Calcitonin.

Forhistal Maleate. Ciba-Geigy† brand of Dimethindene Maleate.

Forit. Sterling Winthrop brand of Oxypertine.

Formula 405. Doak brand of Pregnenolone Succinate.

Fortamet. Teva brand of Metformin Hydrochloride.

Fortaz. GlaxoSmithKline brand of Ceftazidime.

Fortical. Unigene brand of Calcitonin.

Fortizyme. Sterling Winthrop† brand of Alpha Amylase.

Fortovase. Roche brand of Saquinavir.

Fortral. Sterling Winthrop brand of Pentazocine.

Fosamax. Merck brand of Alendronate Sodium.

Foscavir. AstraZeneca brand of Foscarnet Sodium.

Fosrenol. Shire brand of Lanthanum Carbonate.

Fostex BPO Bar, Gel, and Wash. Bristol-Myers Products brand of Benzoyl Peroxide.

Fototar. ICN brand of Coal Tar.

Fragmin. Eisai Medical Research brand of Dalteparin Sodium.

Freezone. Whitehall-Robins† brand of Salicylic Acid.

FRE-FLEX. Optech brand of Focofilcon A.

Frenquel. Marion Merrell Dow† brand of Azacyclonol Hydrochloride.

Freon 11. DuPont Merck† brand of Trichloromonofluoromethane.

Fresh Look. Wesley-Jessen brand of Phemfilcon A.

Frova. Endo brand of Frovatriptan Succinate.

FS Shampoo. Galderma brand of Fluocinolone Acetonide.

Fuadin. Sterling Winthrop brand of Stibophen.

Fucidine. Bristol-Myers Squibb† brand of Fusidate Sodium.

Fulvicin Bolus [Veterinary]. Schering-Plough Animal Health† brand of Griseofulvin.

Fulvicin-P/G. Schering brand of Griseofulvin.

Fulvicin-U/F. Schering brand of Griseofulvin.

Fulvicin-U/F Powder and Tablets [Veterinary]. Schering-Plough Animal Health brand of Griseofulvin.

Fumidil. Abbott† brand of Fumagillin.

Funduscein. Novartis brand of Fluorescein Sodium.

Fungizone. Apothecon brand of Amphotericin B.

Furacin. Shire brand of Nitrofurazone.

Furadantin. Sciele brand of Nitrofurantoin.

Furanace. Dainippon Pharmaceutical Co., Japan, brand of Nifurpirinol.

Furmethide Iodide. SmithKline Beecham† brand of Furtrethonium Iodide.

Furoxone. Shire brand of Furazolidone.

Fuzeon. Roche brand of Enfuvirtide.

FW Toric. Bausch & Lomb† brand of Lidofilcon A.

Gabitril. Cephalon brand of Tiagabine Hydrochloride.

Gabren. Synthelabo Pharmacie, France, brand of Progabide.

Galida. AstraZeneca brand of Tesaglitazar.

Galzin. Teva brand of Zinc Acetate.

Gamimune N 5%. Bayer brand of Globulin, Immune.

Gamimune N 10%. Bayer brand of Globulin, Immune.

Gammagard. Hyland brand of Globulin, Immune.

Gammagee. Merck brand of Globulin, Immune.

Gammar. Centeon brand of Globulin, Immune.

Gammar-P I.V. Centeon brand of Globulin, Immune.

Gamophen. Arabrook brand of Hexachlorophene.

Gamulin. Marion Merrell Dow† brand of Globulin, Immune.

Gamulin Rh. Centeon brand of Rh₀ (D) Immune Globulin.

Ganite. Genta brand of Gallium Nitrate.

Gantanol. Roche brand of Sulfamethoxazole.

Gantrisin. Roche brand of Sulfisoxazole.

Gantrisin. Roche brand of Sulfisoxazole Acetyl.

Gantrisin. Roche brand of Sulfisoxazole Diolamine.

Garamycin. Schering brand of Gentamicin Sulfate.

Gardrin. Syntex brand of Enprostil.

Gastrocrom. Azur brand of Cromolyn Sodium.

Gastromark. Advanced Magnetics brand of Ferumoxsil.

Gas-X. Novartis brand of Simethicone.

Gem 91. Hybridon brand of Trecovirsen Sodium.

Gemonil. Abbott brand of Metharbital.

Gemzar. Lilly brand of Gemcitabine Hydrochloride.

Genasense. Genta brand of Oblimersen Sodium.

Generlac. Morton Grove brand of Lactulose.

Generx. Cardium Therapeutics brand of Alferminogene Tadenovec.

Genesa. Gensia brand of Arbutamine Hydrochloride.

Gengraf. Abbott brand of Cyclosporine.

Genoptic. Allergan brand of Gentamicin Sulfate.

Genotropin. Pfizer brand of Somatropin.

Gentak. Akorn brand of Gentamicin Sulfate.

GenTeal. Ciba Vision, US Ophthalmics, brand of Hypromellose.

Gentle Nature. Novartis brand of Sennosides.

Gentran 40. Baxter Healthcare brand of Dextran 40.

Gentran 75. Baxter Healthcare brand of Dextran 75.

Gen-xene. Alra brand of Clorazepate Dipotassium.

Geocillin. Pfizer brand of Carbenicillin Indanyl Sodium.

Geodon. Pfizer brand of Ziprasidone Hydrochloride.

Geodon. Pfizer brand of Ziprasidone Mesylate.

Geref. Serono brand of Sermorelin Acetate.

Gerimal. Watson brand of Ergoloid Mesylates.

Germa-medica. Huntington brand of Hexachlorophene.

Gitaligin. Schering† brand of Gitalin.

Glaucostat. Kingshill Pharmaceuticals, Inc., Switzerland, brand of Aceclidine.

Glaumeba. Marion Merrell Dow† brand of Glaucarubin.

Gleptosil. Fisons Pharmaceuticals Ltd., Great Britain, brand of Gleptoferron.

Gliadel. MGI Pharma brand of Carmustine.

Glionix. NovaRx brand of Ranagengliotucel-T.

Glofil-125. Abbott† brand of Iothalamate Sodium I 125.

Glofil-131. Abbott† brand of Iothalamate Sodium I 131.

Glucamide. Teva brand of Chlorpropamide.

Glucophage. Bristol-Myers Squibb brand of Metformin Hydrochloride.

Glucoscan. DuPont Merck brand of Technetium Tc 99m Gluceptate.

Glucose-40. Ciba Vision, US Ophthalmics, brand of Glucose, Liquid.

Glucotrol. Pfizer brand of Glipizide.

Glumal. Kyowa Hakko Kogyo Co., Ltd., Japan, brand of Aceglutamide Aluminum.

Glumetza. Depomed brand of Metformin Hydrochloride.

Glustat. Takeda brand of Voglibose.

Glutril. Hoffmann-LaRoche† brand of Glibornuride.

Glycolixir. Bristol-Myers Squibb† brand of Glycine.

Glynase. Pfizer brand of Glyburide.

Glysennid. Novartis† brand of Sennosides.

Glyset. Pfizer brand of Miglitol.

Gold Medalist Toric. Bausch & Lomb brand of Hefilcon C.

Gonal-F. Serono brand of Follitropin Alfa.

Goniosol. Ciba Vision, US Ophthalmics, brand of Hypromellose.

Gramoderm. Schering† brand of Gramicidin.

Grifulvin V. Ortho Pharmaceutical brand of Griseofulvin.

Grisactin. Wyeth-Ayerst brand of Griseofulvin.

Gris-PEG. Allergan Herbert brand of Griseofulvin.

Grolene. Pitman-Moore brand of Somfasepor.

GVAX Prostate. Cell Genesys brand of Galgenprostucel-L.

GVAX Prostate. Cell Genesys brand of Litgenprostucel-L.

Gvs. Savage brand of Gentian Violet.

---

† Brand name formerly used, and/or firm no longer concerned with this product.

Gynazole. KV Pharmaceutical brand of Butoconazole Nitrate.

Gyne-lotrimin. Schering-Plough brand of Clotrimazole.

Gynodiol. Duramed brand of Estradiol.

Gynol II. Ortho Pharmaceutical brand of Nonoxynol 9.

Gynorest. Solvay Pharmaceuticals brand of Dydrogesterone.

Haemate-P. Hoechst-Roussel brand of Antihemophilic Factor.

Halcion. Pfizer brand of Triazolam.

Haldol. Ortho-McNeil brand of Haloperidol.

Haldol. Ortho-McNeil brand of Haloperidol Decanoate.

Haldrone. Lilly brand of Paramethasone Acetate.

Halfan. GlaxoSmithKline brand of Halofantrine Hydrochloride.

Halog. Westwood-Squibb brand of Halcinonide.

Halotestin. Pfizer brand of Fluoxymesterone.

Halotex. Westwood-Squibb brand of Haloprogin.

Hansolar. Parke-Davis† brand of Acedapsone.

Harmonyl. Abbott brand of Deserpidine.

H-Big. Abbott† brand of Hepatitis B Immune Globulin.

H-B-Vax. Merck brand of Hepatitis B Virus Vaccine Inactivated.

Head & Shoulders Conditioner. Procter & Gamble brand of Pyrithione Zinc.

Heat Spray. Whitehall-Robins† brand of Methyl Nicotinate.

Hectorol. Genzyme brand of Doxercalciferol.

Hedulin. Sanofi Aventis brand of Phenindione.

Heliophan. Greeff brand of Homosalate.

Helixate. Centeon brand of Antihemophilic Factor.

Hemabate. Pfizer brand of Carboprost Tromethamine.

HemAssist. Baxter Healthcare brand of Hemoglobin Crosfumaril.

Hemofil M. Hyland brand of Antihemophilic Factor.

Hemokine. Novartis brand of Muplestim.

Hemolink. Hemosol, Canada, brand of Hemoglobin Raffimer.

Hemopure. Biopure brand of Hemoglobin Glutamer-250 (Bovine).

Hepatolite. DuPont Merck brand of Technetium Tc 99m Disofenin.

Hepato-Scan. Medi-Physics† brand of Lidofenin.

Hep-B-Gammagee. Merck brand of Hepatitis B Immune Globulin.

Hepicebrin [Tablets]. Lilly brand of Hexavitamin.

Hepsera. Gilead Sciences brand of Adefovir Dipivoxil.

Heptavax-B. Merck brand of Hepatitis B Virus Vaccine Inactivated.

Heptomer. Fisons Pharmaceuticals Ltd., Great Britain, brand of Gleptoferron.

Herperal. Farmitalia, Societa Farmaceutici Italia, Italy, brand of Stallimycin Hydrochloride.

Herplex. Allergan brand of Idoxuridine.

Hespan. DuPont Merck brand of Hetastarch.

Hetrazan. Lederle brand of Diethylcarbamazine Citrate.

Hexa-Betalin. Lilly brand of Pyridoxine Hydrochloride.

Hexadrol. Organon brand of Dexamethasone.

Hexadrol. Organon brand of Dexamethasone Sodium Phosphate.

Hexalen. MGI Pharma brand of Altretamine.

Hexamic Acid. Abbott brand of Cyclamic Acid.

Hexopal. Sterling Winthrop brand of Inositol Niacinate.

Hibiclens. Regent brand of Chlorhexidine Gluconate.

Hibistat. Regent brand of Chlorhexidine Gluconate.

Hippuran-125. Abbott† brand of Iodohippurate Sodium I 125.

Hippuran-131. Abbott† brand of Iodohippurate Sodium I 131.

Hippuran I 125. Mallinckrodt† brand of Iodohippurate Sodium I 125.

Hippuran I 131. Mallinckrodt brand of Iodohippurate Sodium I 131.

Hipputope. Bristol-Myers Squibb† brand of Iodohippurate Sodium I 131.

Hipputope I-125. Bristol-Myers Squibb† brand of Iodohippurate Sodium I 125.

Hiprex. Sanofi Aventis brand of Methenamine Hippurate.

Hismanal. Janssen brand of Astemizole.

Hispril. GlaxoSmithKline brand of Diphenylpyraline Hydrochloride.

Histalog. Lilly brand of Betazole Hydrochloride.

Hivid. Roche brand of Zalcitabine.

Hms. Allergan brand of Medrysone.

Holocaine Hydrochloride. Abbott† brand of Phenacaine Hydrochloride.

Homapin. Mission brand of Homatropine Methylbromide.

Homo-Tet. Savage† brand of Tetanus Immune Globulin.

H.P. Acthar Gel. Rhone-Poulenc Rorer brand of Corticotropin, Repository.

Humafac. Parke-Davis† brand of Antihemophilic Factor.

HumaSPECT. Intracel brand of Votumumab.

Humate-P. Centeon brand of Antihemophilic Factor.

Humatin. King brand of Paromomycin Sulfate.

Humatrope. Lilly brand of Somatropin.

Humegon. Organon brand of Menotropins.

Humorsol. Merck brand of Demecarium Bromide.

Humulin. Lilly brand of Insulin Human.

Hyazyme. Abbott† brand of Hyaluronidase (Ovine).

Hybri-CEAker. Hybritech brand of Indium In 111 Altumomab Pentetate.

Hybrid FS. Contamac brand of Hybufocon A.

Hycamtin. GlaxoSmithKline brand of Topotecan Hydrochloride.

Hydeltrasol. Merck brand of Prednisolone Sodium Phosphate.

Hydeltra-TBA. Merck brand of Prednisolone Tebutate.

Hydergine. Novartis brand of Ergoloid Mesylates.

Hydrasoft. CooperVision brand of Methafilcon B.

Hydrea. Bristol-Myers Squibb brand of Hydroxyurea.

Hydrocil Instant. Solvay Pharmaceuticals brand of Psyllium Husk.

Hydrocortone. Merck brand of Hydrocortisone.

Hydrocortone. Merck brand of Hydrocortisone Acetate.

Hydrocortone. Merck brand of Hydrocortisone Sodium Phosphate.

Hydrodiuril. Merck brand of Hydrochlorothiazide.

Hygroton. Sanofi Aventis brand of Chlorthalidone.

Hykinone. Abbott† brand of Menadione Sodium Bisulfite.

Hylenex. Halozyme brand of Hyaluronidase (Human Recombinant).

Hylorel. Pfizer brand of Guanadrel Sulfate.

Hy-Pam. Teva brand of Hydroxyzine Pamoate.

Hypaque. GE Healthcare brand of Diatrizoate Meglumine.

Hypaque. GE Healthcare brand of Diatrizoate Sodium.

Hyprotigen. B Braun brand of Protein Hydrolysate.

Hystrene 5016. Witco brand of Stearic Acid.

Hytakerol. Sterling Winthrop brand of Dihydrotachysterol.

Hytone. Dermik brand of Hydrocortisone.

Hytrin. Abbott brand of Terazosin Hydrochloride.

Iamin. ProCyte brand of Prezatide Copper Acetate.

Ibrin. Nycomed Amersham† brand of Fibrinogen I 125.

IC-Green. Akorn brand of Indocyanine Green.

Ichthymall. Mallinckrodt† brand of Ichthammol.

Idamycin. Bedford brand of Idarubicin Hydrochloride.

Idarac. Hoechst-Roussel† brand of Floctafenine.

Idro P₂. Maggioni Farmaceutici S.p.A., Italy, brand of Sulmarin.

Idro P₃. Maggioni Farmaceutici S.p.A., Italy, brand of Oxamarin Hydrochloride.

Idrolone. Maggioni Farmaceutici S.p.A., Italy, brand of Fenquizone.

Ifex. Bristol-Myers Squibb brand of Ifosfamide.

Igel 56. Igel Vision Care brand of Hefilcon C.

IHSA I-125. Mallinckrodt brand of Albumin, Iodinated I 125 Serum.

IHSA I-131. Mallinckrodt† brand of Albumin, Iodinated I 131 Serum.

Ilidar. Hoffmann-LaRoche† brand of Azapetine Phosphate.

Ilopan. Savage brand of Dexpanthenol.

Ilosone. Dista brand of Erythromycin Estolate.

Ilotycin. Dista brand of Erythromycin.

Ilotycin. Dista brand of Erythromycin Gluceptate.

Ilozyme. Savage brand of Pancrelipase.

Imagent. Alliance brand of Perflubron.

Imap. Ortho-McNeil† brand of Fluspirilene.

Imdur. Schering-Plough brand of Isosorbide Mononitrate.

Imitrex. GlaxoSmithKline brand of Sumatriptan.

Imitrex. GlaxoSmithKline brand of Sumatriptan Succinate.

Immu-G. Parke-Davis† brand of Globulin, Immune.

Immuglobin. Savage† brand of Globulin, Immune.

Immusine. ICN brand of Isatoribine.

Immu-Tetanus. Parke-Davis† brand of Tetanus Immune Globulin.

Imodium. McNeil brand of Loperamide Hydrochloride.

Implanon. Organon brand of Etonogestrel.

Imuran. Promethus brand of Azathioprine.

Imusay-125. Abbott† brand of Insulin I 125.

Imusay-131. Abbott† brand of Insulin I 131.

Inapsine. Akorn brand of Droperidol.

Inderal. Wyeth brand of Propranolol Hydrochloride.

INDICLOR. Nycomed Amersham brand of Indium In 111 Chloride.

Indigo Carmine. Becton Dickinson Microbiology† brand of Indigotindisulfonate Sodium.

Indium DTPA In 111. Medi-Physics brand of Indium In 111 Pentetate.

Indium Oxine. Nycomed Amersham brand of Indium In 111 Oxyquinoline.

Indium Oxine In 111. Medi-Physics brand of Indium In 111 Oxyquinoline.

Indocin. Merck brand of Indomethacin.

Indocin. Ovation brand of Indomethacin Sodium.

Indoklon. Ohmeda brand of Flurothyl.

Infants' Feverall. Actavis brand of Acetaminophen.

Infasurf. Ony brand of Calfactant.

Infed. Watson brand of Iron Dextran.

Inh. Novartis brand of Isoniazid.

Inhibace. Hoffmann-LaRoche brand of Cilazapril.

Injectapap. Ortho-McNeil brand of Acetaminophen.

Innofem. Novo Nordisk brand of Estradiol.

Innohep. Pharmion brand of Tinzaparin Sodium.

Innopran. Reliant brand of Propranolol Hydrochloride.

Inocor. Sterling Winthrop brand of Inamrinone.

Inomax. Ino brand of Nitric Oxide.

Inspra. Pfizer brand of Eplerenone.

Insta-Glucose. ICN brand of Glucose, Liquid.

Intal. King brand of Cromolyn Sodium.

Integrilin. Schering brand of Eptifibatide.

Intensain. Abbott† brand of Chromonar Hydrochloride.

Intercept. Ortho Pharmaceutical brand of Nonoxynol 9.

Intracaine Hydrochloride. Bristol-Myers Squibb† brand of Parethoxycaine Hydrochloride.

Intralipid. Fresenius brand of Soybean Oil.

Intron A. Schering brand of Interferon Alfa-2b.

Intron A HSA-free. Schering brand of Interferon Alfa-2b.

Intropin. Hospira brand of Dopamine Hydrochloride.

Invanz. Merck brand of Ertapenem Sodium.

Invega. Janssen brand of Paliperidone.

Inversine. Targacept brand of Mecamylamine Hydrochloride.

Invirase. Roche brand of Saquinavir Mesylate.

Iodosorb. Perstorp Carbotec, Sweden, brand of Cadexomer Iodine.

Iodotope I-125. Bristol-Myers Squibb† brand of Sodium Iodide I 125.

Iodotope I-131. Bristol-Myers Squibb† brand of Sodium Iodide I 131.

Iodotope Therapeutic. Bristol-Myers Squibb† brand of Sodium Iodide I 131.

Ionamin. Fisons brand of Phentermine.

Ionil. Galderma† brand of Salicylic Acid.

Ionil-Plus. Galderma† brand of Salicylic Acid.

Ionil-T. Galderma† brand of Coal Tar.

Ionil-T-Plus. Galderma† brand of Coal Tar.

Iopidine. Alcon brand of Apraclonidine Hydrochloride.

Ioquin. Abbott† brand of Iodoquinol.

Iosat. Anbex brand of Potassium Iodide.

Ipral Sodium. Bristol-Myers Squibb† brand of Probarbital Sodium.

Ipropran [Veterinary]. Hoffmann-LaRoche† brand of Ipronidazole.

Ipsatol. Key Pharmaceuticals† brand of Ipecac.

Iressa. AstraZeneca brand of Gefitinib.

Iriditope. Bristol-Myers Squibb† brand of Iridium Ir 192.

Ismelin. Novartis brand of Guanethidine Monosulfate.

Ismo. Dr. Reddy's brand of Isosorbide Mononitrate.

Ismotic. Alcon brand of Isosorbide.

Isocrin. Parke-Davis† brand of Oxyphenisatin Acetate.

Isofedrol. Boehringer Mannheim GmbH, Germany, brand of Ephedrine Sulfate.

Isolyte. McGaw brand of Potassium Phosphate, Dibasic.

Isoptin. Ranbaxy brand of Verapamil Hydrochloride.

Isopto Eserine. Alcon† brand of Physostigmine Salicylate.

Isopto Homatropine. Alcon brand of Homatropine Hydrobromide.

Isopto Hyoscine. Alcon brand of Scopolamine Hydrobromide.

Isopto Tears. Alcon brand of Hypromellose.

Isordil. Biovail brand of Isosorbide Dinitrate.

Isovue. Bracco brand of Iopamidol.

Istalol. Ista brand of Timolol Maleate.

Istizin. Sterling Winthrop† brand of Danthron.

Isuprel. Sanofi Aventis brand of Isoproterenol Hydrochloride.

Ivy Block. Stand Homeopath brand of Bentoquatam.

Jantoven. USl brand of Warfarin Sodium.

Januvia. Merck brand of Sitagliptin Phosphate.

Javlor. Middlebrook brand of Vinflunine Ditartrate.

Jefron. Marion Merrell Dow† brand of Polyferose.

Jodomiron. Bracco Industria Chimica S.p.A., Italy, brand of Iodamide.

Kabikinase. Pharmacia & Upjohn brand of Streptokinase.

Kadian. Alpharma brand of Morphine Sulfate.

Kafocin. Lilly brand of Cephaloglycin.

Kamoran. Lilly† brand of Actaplanin.

Kantrex. Apothecon brand of Kanamycin Sulfate.

Kaon. Savage† brand of Potassium Gluconate.

Kaon Cl. Savage brand of Potassium Chloride.

Kappadione. Lilly brand of Menadiol Sodium Diphosphate.

Karenitecin. BioNumerik brand of Cositecan.

Kayexalate. Sanofi Aventis brand of Sodium Polystyrene Sulfonate.

Kayquinone. Abbott brand of Menadione.

K-dur. Key brand of Potassium Chloride.

Keflet. Lilly brand of Cephalexin.

Keflex. Middlebrook brand of Cephalexin.

Keflin. Lilly brand of Cephalothin Sodium.

Kefloridin. Lilly† brand of Cephaloridine.

Keftab. Lilly brand of Cephalexin Hydrochloride.

Kefurox. Lilly brand of Cefuroxime Sodium.

Kefzol. Lilly brand of Cefazolin Sodium.

Kelfer. Laboratorio Mauricio Villela S. A., Brazil, brand of Ferriclate Calcium Sodium.

Kelfizina. Abbott† brand of Sulfalene.

Kemadrin. King brand of Procyclidine Hydrochloride.

Kemstro. Schwarz Pharma brand of Baclofen.

Kenacort. Bristol-Myers Squibb brand of Triamcinolone.

Kenacort. Bristol-Myers Squibb brand of Triamcinolone Diacetate.

Kenalog. Apothecon brand of Triamcinolone Acetonide.

Keppra. UCB brand of Levetiracetam.

Kerlone. Sanofi Aventis brand of Betaxolol Hydrochloride.

Kestine. Rhone-Poulenc Rorer brand of Ebastine.

Ketalar. King brand of Ketamine Hydrochloride.

Ketek. Sanofi Aventis brand of Telithromycin.

---

† Brand name formerly used, and/or firm no longer concerned with this product.

Ketozole. Taro brand of Ketoconazole.

Khelloyd. Hoechst-Roussel† brand of Khellin.

Kinevac. Bracco brand of Sincalide.

Klamar. Maggioni Farmaceutici S.p.A., Italy, brand of Guaiapate.

Klaron. Sanofi Aventis brand of Sulfacetamide Sodium.

Klebcil. King brand of Kanamycin Sulfate.

Klonopin. Roche brand of Clonazepam.

Klor-con. Upsher Smith brand of Potassium Chloride.

Klotogen. Abbott† brand of Menadione Sodium Bisulfite.

Klotrix. Apothecon brand of Potassium Chloride.

Koate-HP. Bayer brand of Antihemophilic Factor.

KOGENATE. Bayer brand of Antihemophilic Factor.

Kollicoat MAE 300. BASF brand of Methacrylic Acid Copolymer.

Kollidon 25, 30, 12PF, 17PF, 90F. BASF brand of Povidone.

Kollidon CL. BASF brand of Crospovidone.

Kollidon CLM. BASF brand of Crospovidone.

Konakion. Roche brand of Phytonadione.

Konyne 80. Bayer brand of Factor IX Complex.

Krypton Kr 81m Gas Generator. Medi-Physics brand of Krypton Kr 81m.

Ku-zyme HP. Schwarz Pharma brand of Pancrelipase.

Kwell. Reed & Carnrick brand of Lindane.

Kybernin. Hoechst-Roussel brand of Antithrombin III Human.

Kytril. Roche brand of Granisetron Hydrochloride.

Labrafil M1944CS. Gattefosse Etablissements, France, brand of Peglicol 5 Oleate.

Lacrisert. Aton brand of Hydroxypropyl Cellulose.

Lamictal. GlaxoSmithKline brand of Lamotrigine.

Lamisil. Novartis brand of Terbinafine.

Lamprene. Novartis brand of Clofazimine.

Lanoxin. GlaxoSmithKline brand of Digoxin.

Lantus. Hoechst Marion Roussel brand of Insulin Glargine.

Largon. Baxter Healthcare brand of Propiomazine Hydrochloride.

Lariam. Roche brand of Mefloquine Hydrochloride.

Larodopa. Roche brand of Levodopa.

Larotid. GlaxoSmithKline brand of Amoxicillin.

Lasan. Stiefel† brand of Anthralin.

Lasix. Sanofi Aventis brand of Furosemide.

Lavema. Sterling Winthrop† brand of Oxyphenisatin Acetate.

Laxilose. Technilab brand of Lactulose.

Leanstar. Pitman-Moore brand of Somfasepor.

Lectopam. Roche, Puerto Rico, brand of Bromazepam.

Legend. Bayer Animal Health brand of Hyaluronate Sodium.

Lendorm. Boehringer Ingelheim† brand of Brotizolam.

Lenetran. Marion Merrell Dow† brand of Mephenoxalone.

Lente. Novo Nordisk brand of Insulin Zinc.

Lente Iletin. Lilly brand of Insulin Zinc.

Lercadip. Recordati, Italy, brand of Lercanidipine Hydrochloride.

Lercan. Recordati, Italy, brand of Lercanidipine Hydrochloride.

Lercapin. Recordati, Italy, brand of Lercanidipine Hydrochloride.

Lercaton. Recordati, Italy, brand of Lercanidipine Hydrochloride.

Leritine. Merck brand of Anileridine Hydrochloride.

Lerkamen. Recordati, Italy, brand of Lercanidipine Hydrochloride.

Lerzam. Recordati, Italy, brand of Lercanidipine Hydrochloride.

Lescol. Novartis brand of Fluvastatin Sodium.

Letairis. Gilead Sciences brand of Ambrisentan.

Leukarrest. ICOS brand of Rovelizumab.

Leukeran. GlaxoSmithKline brand of Chlorambucil.

Leukine. Immunex brand of Sargramostim.

LeukoScan. Immunomedics brand of Sulesomab.

Leustatin. Ortho Biotech brand of Cladribine.

Leutech. Palatin brand of Technetium Tc 99m Fanolesomab.

Levaquin. Ortho-McNeil brand of Levofloxacin.

Levatol. Schwarz Pharma brand of Penbutolol Sulfate.

Levo-Dromoran. Valeant brand of Levorphanol Tartrate.

Levophed. Hospira brand of Norepinephrine Bitartrate.

Levoprome. Immunex brand of Levomepromazine.

Levoprome. Immunex brand of Methotrimeprazine.

Levo-t. Alara brand of Levothyroxine Sodium.

Levothroid. Lloyd brand of Levothyroxine Sodium.

Levoxyl. King brand of Levothyroxine Sodium.

Levsin. Schwarz Pharma brand of Hyoscyamine Sulfate.

Levsinex. Schwarz Pharma brand of Hyoscyamine Sulfate.

Levulan. Dusa brand of Aminolevulinic Acid Hydrochloride.

Lexapro. Forest brand of Escitalopram Oxalate.

Lexiva. GlaxoSmithKline brand of Fosamprenavir Calcium.

Liazal. Janssen brand of Liarozole Fumarate.

Librium. Valeant brand of Chlordiazepoxide Hydrochloride.

Lidanar. Novartis† brand of Mesoridazine.

Lidex. Medicis brand of Fluocinonide.

Lidoderm. Endo brand of Lidocaine.

Lidopen. Meridian brand of Lidocaine Hydrochloride.

Lincocin. Pfizer brand of Lincomycin Hydrochloride.

Linodil. Sterling Winthrop† brand of Inositol Niacinate.

Lioresal. Medtronic brand of Baclofen.

Liosol. Maggioni Farmaceutici S.p.A., Italy, brand of Xenbucin.

Lipitor. Pfizer brand of Atorvastatin Calcium.

Lipofen. Proethic brand of Fenofibrate.

Lipo-hepin. 3M Pharmaceuticals brand of Heparin Sodium.

Liposyn. Abbott brand of Safflower Oil.

Liposyn. Hospira brand of Soybean Oil.

Liquaemin Sodium. Organon brand of Heparin Sodium.

Liquamar. Organon brand of Phenprocoumon.

Liquamat. Galderma† brand of Sulfur, Precipitated.

Liquamycin [Veterinary]. Pfizer brand of Tetracycline.

Liquifilm Tears. Allergan brand of Polyvinyl Alcohol.

Lithobid. JDS brand of Lithium Carbonate.

Lithostat. Mission brand of Acetohydroxamic Acid.

Livostin. Novartis brand of Levocabastine Hydrochloride.

LL-38. Lombart brand of Polymacon.

Loceryl. Hoffmann-LaRoche brand of Amorolfine.

Locoid. Yamanouchi brand of Hydrocortisone Butyrate.

Locorten. Novartis brand of Flumethasone Pivalate.

Lodine. Wyeth brand of Etodolac.

Lodosyn. Bristol-Myers Squibb brand of Carbidopa.

Lofexidine. Rhone-Poulenc Rorer brand of Lofexidine Hydrochloride.

LoFrin. Abbott brand of Fenleuton.

Loniten. Pfizer brand of Minoxidil.

Lopid. Pfizer brand of Gemfibrozil.

Lopressor. Novartis brand of Metoprolol Fumarate.

Lopressor. Novartis brand of Metoprolol Tartrate.

Loprox. Medicis brand of Ciclopirox.

Loprox. Hoechst-Roussel brand of Ciclopirox Olamine.

Lora. Wallace† brand of Chlorhexadol.

Lorabid. King brand of Loracarbef.

Loranil. Sterling Winthrop† brand of Becanthone Hydrochloride.

Lorelco. Sanofi Aventis brand of Probucol.

Lorfan. Roche brand of Levallorphan Tartrate.

Loridine. Lilly† brand of Cephaloridine.

Lorothidol. Sterling Winthrop† brand of Bithionol.

Loroxide. Dermik brand of Benzoyl Peroxide.

Losec Sodium. Astra Pharmaceutical Production AB, Sweden, brand of Omeprazole Sodium.

Lotemax. Bausch & Lomb brand of Loteprednol Etabonate.

Lotensin. Novartis brand of Benazepril Hydrochloride.

Lotrimin. Schering brand of Butenafine Hydrochloride.

Lotrimin. Schering-Plough brand of Clotrimazole.

Lotronex. GlaxoSmithKline brand of Alosetron Hydrochloride.

Lotusate. Sanofi Aventis brand of Talbutal.

Lovaza. Reliant brand of Omega-3-acid Ethyl Esters.

Lovenox. Sanofi Aventis brand of Enoxaparin Sodium.

Loviscol. Wyeth-Ayerst brand of Carbocysteine.

Loxapine. Mylan brand of Loxapine Succinate.

Loxitane. Watson brand of Loxapine Succinate.

Loxitane Intramuscular [as hydrochloride]. Wyeth-Ayerst brand of Loxapine.

Loxitane-C Oral Suspension [as hydrochloride]. Wyeth-Ayerst brand of Loxapine.

Lozol. Sanofi Aventis brand of Indapamide.

Lucanix. NovaRx brand of Belagenpumatucel-L.

Lucaratin. BASF brand of Beta Carotene.

Ludiomil. Novartis brand of Maprotiline Hydrochloride.

Lufyllin. Medpointe brand of Dyphylline.

Lumigan. Allergan brand of Bimatoprost.

Luminal. Sterling Winthrop brand of Phenobarbital.

Luminal Sodium. Sterling Winthrop brand of Phenobarbital Sodium.

Lunesta. Sepracor brand of Eszopiclone.

Lupron. TAP brand of Leuprolide Acetate.

Lutrepulse. Ferring Pharmaceuticals brand of Gonadorelin Acetate.

Lutrin. Pharmacyclics brand of Motexafin Lutetium.

Lutrol E. BASF brand of Polyethylene Glycol.

Lutrol F. BASF brand of Poloxamer.

Luveris. Serono brand of Lutropin Alfa.

Luvox. Solvay Pharmaceuticals brand of Fluvoxamine Maleate.

Luxiq. Connetics brand of Betamethasone Valerate.

Lygranum. Bristol-Myers Squibb† brand of Lymphogranuloma Venereum Antigen.

Lymphazurin. US Surgical brand of Isosulfan Blue.

Lympho Scan. Immunomedics brand of Bectumomab.

Lymphocide. Immunomedics brand of Epratuzumab.

LymphoCide. Immunomedics brand of Yttrium Y 90 Epratuzumab.

LymphoStat-B. Human Genome Sciences brand of Belimumab.

Lynoral. Organon brand of Ethinyl Estradiol.

Lyrica. Pfizer brand of Pregabalin.

Lysodren. Bristol-Myers Squibb brand of Mitotane.

M50-50 Injection. Lemmon† brand of Diprenorphine.

M99 Injection. Lemmon† brand of Etorphine.

MAA I 131. Mallinckrodt† brand of Albumin, Aggregated Iodinated I 131 Serum.

Macmiror. Polichimica Sap, Italy, brand of Nifuratel.

Macrodantin. Procter & Gamble brand of Nitrofurantoin.

Macroscan-131. Abbott† brand of Albumin, Aggregated Iodinated I 131 Serum.

Macroscint. Johnson & Johnson brand of Immune Globulin Intravenous Pentetate.

Macrotec. Bracco Diagnostics brand of Technetium Tc 99m Albumin Aggregated.

Macstim. Genetics Institute brand of Cilmostim.

Macugen. Osi Eyetech brand of Pegaptanib Sodium.

Madribon. Hoffmann-LaRoche† brand of Sulfadimethoxine.

Magan. Savage brand of Magnesium Salicylate.

Magmilor. Polichimica Sap, Italy, brand of Nifuratel.

Magnacort. Pfizer brand of Hydrocortamate Hydrochloride.

Magnamycin. Pfizer brand of Carbomycin.

Magnevist. Bayer brand of Gadopentetate Dimeglumine.

Maliasin. Knoll† brand of Barbexaclone.

Mammol. Abbott brand of Bismuth Subnitrate.

Mandelamine. Parke-Davis brand of Methenamine Mandelate.

Mandol. Lilly brand of Cefamandole Nafate.

Mantomide. Sterling Winthrop† brand of Chlorbetamide.

Maolate. Pfizer brand of Chlorphenesin Carbamate.

Mapharsen. Parke-Davis† brand of Oxophenarsine Hydrochloride.

Marcaine. Hospira brand of Bupivacaine Hydrochloride.

Maretin. Bayer Animal Health† brand of Naftalofos.

Marezine. GlaxoSmithKline brand of Cyclizine Lactate.

Marine Colloids. FMC brand of Carrageenan.

Marinol. Unimed brand of Dronabinol.

Marogen. Chugai Pharmaceutical Co., Ltd., Japan, brand of Epoetin Beta.

Matromycin. Pfizer brand of Oleandomycin Phosphate.

Matulane. Sigma-Tau brand of Procarbazine Hydrochloride.

Mavik. Abbott brand of Trandolapril.

Maxair. Graceway brand of Pirbuterol Acetate.

Maxalt. Merck brand of Rizatriptan Benzoate.

Maxaquin. Pfizer brand of Lomefloxacin Hydrochloride.

Maxibolin. Organon brand of Ethylestrenol.

Maxicam. Parke-Davis† brand of Isoxicam.

Maxidex. Alcon brand of Dexamethasone.

Maxidex. Alcon brand of Dexamethasone Sodium Phosphate.

Maxipime. Squibb brand of Cefepime.

MaxiPost. Bristol-Myers Squibb brand of Flindokalner.

Maxivent. Roberts Pharmaceutical brand of Doxofylline.

Maxolon. King brand of Metoclopramide Hydrochloride.

Maxon. Davis & Geck brand of Polyglyconate.

Mazanor. Wyeth brand of Mazindol.

Md. Mallinckrodt brand of Diatrizoate Sodium.

MDP Kit. Medi-Physics brand of Technetium Tc 99m Medronate.

MDP-Bracco. Bracco Diagnostics brand of Technetium Tc 99m Medronate.

Mebaral. Sterling Winthrop brand of Mephobarbital.

Mebryl. SmithKline Beecham† brand of Embramine Hydrochloride.

Mecadox. Pfizer brand of Carbadox.

Meclan. Johnson & Johnson brand of Meclocycline Sulfosalicylate.

Meclomen. Pfizer brand of Meclofenamate Sodium.

Medalist. Bausch & Lomb brand of Polymacon.

Medalist Toric. Bausch & Lomb† brand of Lidofilcon A.

Medihaler-epi. 3M Pharmaceuticals brand of Epinephrine Bitartrate.

Medihaler-Tetracaine. 3M Pharmaceuticals† brand of Tetracaine.

Medrol. Pfizer brand of Methylprednisolone.

Mefoxin. Merck brand of Cefoxitin Sodium.

Megace. Bristol-Myers Squibb brand of Megestrol Acetate.

Megalone. Hoffmann-LaRoche brand of Fleroxacin.

Megazyme. SmithKline Beecham† brand of Asperkinase.

Megimide. Abbott† brand of Bemegride.

Meldane. Bayer Animal Health† brand of Coumaphos.

Mellaril. Novartis brand of Thioridazine.

Mellaril. Novartis brand of Thioridazine Hydrochloride.

Menest. King brand of Estrogens, Esterified.

Menostar. Bayer brand of Estradiol.

Menta-Bal. Marion Merrell Dow† brand of Mephobarbital.

Mentane. Hoechst-Roussel† brand of Velnacrine Maleate.

Mentax. Mylan Bertek brand of Butenafine Hydrochloride.

Mepron. GlaxoSmithKline brand of Atovaquone.

Meratran. Marion Merrell Dow† brand of Pipradrol Hydrochloride.

Mercloran. Parke-Davis† brand of Chlormerodrin.

Mercodinone. Marion Merrell Dow† brand of Hydrocodone Bitartrate.

Mercuhydrin. Marion Merrell Dow† brand of Meralluride.

Merdroxone Sodium. Sterling Winthrop† brand of Meragidone Sodium.

Meridia. Abbott brand of Sibutramine Hydrochloride.

Merital. Hoechst-Roussel† brand of Nomifensine Maleate.

Merprane. Bristol-Myers Squibb† brand of Merisoprol Hg 197.

Merrem. AstraZeneca brand of Meropenem.

Mersilene. Ethicon brand of Suture, Nonabsorbable Surgical.

Merthiolate. Lilly brand of Thimerosal.

Meruvax. Merck brand of Rubella Virus Vaccine Live.

Mervan. Continental Pharma, Belgium, brand of Alclofenac.

Mesantoin. Novartis brand of Mephenytoin.

Mesnex. Baxter Healthcare brand of Mesna.

---

† Brand name formerly used, and/or firm no longer concerned with this product.

Mestinon. Valeant brand of Pyridostigmine Bromide.

Metafolin. Merck Eprova AG brand of Levomefolate Calcium.

Metafolin. Merck Eprova AG brand of Levomefolic Acid.

Metahydrin. Sanofi Aventis brand of Trichlormethiazide.

Metandren. Novartis brand of Methyltestosterone.

Metastat. CollaGenex brand of Incyclinide.

Metastron. Nycomed Amersham brand of Strontium Chloride Sr 89.

Methadose. Mallinckrodt brand of Methadone Hydrochloride.

Metha-Meridiazine. Ortho-McNeil† brand of Trisulfapyrimidines.

Methergine. Novartis brand of Methylergonovine Maleate.

Methocel A. Dow Chemical brand of Methylcellulose.

Methocel E, F, J, K. Dow Chemical brand of Hypromellose.

Methostan. Schering† brand of Methandriol.

Methral. Pfizer brand of Fluperolone Acetate.

Methylin. Mallinckrodt brand of Methylphenidate Hydrochloride.

Meticortelone. Schering brand of Prednisolone Acetate.

Meticorten. Schering brand of Prednisone.

Meti-derm. Schering brand of Prednisolone.

Metopirone. Novartis brand of Metyrapone.

Metopirone Ditartrate. Ciba-Geigy† brand of Metyrapone Tartrate.

Metraspray. 3M Pharmaceuticals† brand of Tetracaine.

Metreton. Schering brand of Prednisolone Sodium Phosphate.

Metrodin. Serono brand of Urofollitropin.

Metrogel. Galderma brand of Metronidazole.

Metubine Iodide. Lilly brand of Metocurine Iodide.

Metvixia. PhotoCure, Norway, brand of Methyl Aminolevulinate Hydrochloride.

Metycaine Hydrochloride. Lilly† brand of Piperocaine Hydrochloride.

Mevacor. Merck brand of Lovastatin.

Mexate. Bristol-Myers Oncology† brand of Methotrexate.

Mezlin. Bayer brand of Mezlocillin Sodium.

Micardis. Boehringer Ingelheim brand of Telmisartan.

Micotil. Lilly brand of Tilmicosin.

MICRhoGAM. Ortho Diagnostic brand of Rh₀ (D) Immune Globulin.

Microderm. Johnson & Johnson brand of Chlorhexidine Gluconate.

Micro-k. KV Pharmaceutical brand of Potassium Chloride.

Microklenz. Carrington brand of Benzethonium Chloride.

Microlite. DuPont Merck brand of Technetium Tc 99m Albumin Colloid.

Microloid. Bristol-Myers Squibb† brand of Technetium Tc 99m Albumin Microaggregated.

Micronase. Pfizer brand of Glyburide.

Micronor. Ortho-McNeil brand of Norethindrone.

Midamor. Merck brand of Amiloride Hydrochloride.

Midicel. Parke-Davis† brand of Sulfamethoxypyridazine.

Midicel Acetyl. Parke-Davis† brand of Sulfamethoxypyridazine Acetyl.

Mifeprex. Danco brand of Mifepristone.

Migranal. Valeant brand of Dihydroergotamine Mesylate.

Migranal. Novartis brand of Endralazine Mesylate.

Milontin. Pfizer brand of Phensuximide.

Milophene. Milex brand of Clomiphene Citrate.

Miltown. Medpointe brand of Meprobamate.

Mini-Gamulin Rh. Centeon brand of Rh₀ (D) Immune Globulin.

Minipress. Pfizer brand of Prazosin Hydrochloride.

Minirin. Ferring Pharmaceuticals brand of Desmopressin Acetate.

Minitran. Graceway brand of Nitroglycerin.

Minocin. Triax brand of Minocycline Hydrochloride.

Mintezol. Merck brand of Thiabendazole.

Mint-O-Mag. Bristol-Myers Squibb† brand of Magnesia, [Milk of].

Minute-Gel. Oral-B brand of Sodium Fluoride.

Miochol. Novartis brand of Acetylcholine Chloride.

Miradon. Schering brand of Anisindione.

Mirapex. Boehringer Ingelheim brand of Pramipexole Dihydrochloride.

Mirena. Bayer brand of Levonorgestrel.

Mithracin. Pfizer brand of Plicamycin.

Mitrolan. Robins brand of Calcium Polycarbophil.

Mivacron. Abbott brand of Mivacurium Chloride.

Moban. Endo brand of Molindone Hydrochloride.

Mobic. Boehringer Ingelheim brand of Meloxicam.

Mobidin. Ascher brand of Magnesium Salicylate.

Mobisyl [as salicylate]. Ascher brand of Trolamine.

Moctanin. Exelixis brand of Monoctanoin.

Modane. Savage brand of Bisacodyl.

Modane. Savage† brand of Phenolphthalein.

Modane Bulk. Savage brand of Psyllium Husk.

Modane Soft. Savage brand of Docusate Sodium.

Moderil. Pfizer brand of Rescinnamine.

Modrastane. Bioenvision brand of Trilostane.

Modumate. Abbott† brand of Arginine Glutamate.

Mogadon. Hoffmann-LaRoche† brand of Nitrazepam.

Mol-Iron. Schering-Plough HealthCare† brand of Ferrous Sulfate.

Molofac. Bristol-Myers Squibb† brand of Docusate Sodium.

Momentum. Whitehall-Robins brand of Magnesium Salicylate.

Monacrin. Sterling Winthrop† brand of Aminacrine Hydrochloride.

Monistat. Johnson & Johnson brand of Miconazole.

Monistat. Johnson & Johnson brand of Miconazole Nitrate.

Monocid. GlaxoSmithKline brand of Cefonicid Sodium.

Monoclate-P. Centeon brand of Antihemophilic Factor.

Monodral Bromide. Sterling Winthrop brand of Penthienate Bromide.

Monoket. Schwarz Pharma brand of Isosorbide Mononitrate.

Mononine. Centeon brand of Factor IX Complex.

Monopril. Bristol-Myers Squibb brand of Fosinopril Sodium.

Monteban. Lilly brand of Narasin.

Monurol. Zambon brand of Fosfomycin Tromethamine.

Moroline. Schering-Plough HealthCare† brand of Petrolatum, White.

Motilium. Janssen brand of Domperidone.

Motilyn. Abbott† brand of Dexpanthenol.

Motrin. McNeil brand of Ibuprofen.

Moxam. Lilly brand of Moxalactam Disodium.

Ms Contin. Purdue Frederick brand of Morphine Sulfate.

Mucinex. Adams brand of Guaifenesin.

Mucofan. Wyeth-Ayerst brand of Carbocysteine.

Mucomyst. Apothecon brand of Acetylcysteine.

Mucosil. Dey brand of Acetylcysteine.

Multihance. Bracco brand of Gadobenate Dimeglumine.

Multocillin. Bayer† brand of Mezlocillin.

Mumpsvax. Merck brand of Mumps Virus Vaccine Live.

Murine Ear Drops. Ross brand of Carbamide Peroxide.

Muse. Vivus brand of Alprostadil.

Mustargen. Ovation brand of Mechlorethamine Hydrochloride.

Mutamycin. Bristol-Myers Squibb brand of Mitomycin.

Myambutol. Stat Trade brand of Ethambutol Hydrochloride.

My-B-Den. Bayer† brand of Adenosine Phosphate.

Mycamine. Astellas brand of Micafungin Sodium.

Mycelex. Bayer brand of Clotrimazole.

Mycifradin. Pfizer brand of Neomycin Sulfate.

Mycobutin. Pfizer brand of Rifabutin.

Mycograb. Novartis brand of Efungumab.

Mycospor. Bayer† brand of Bifonazole.

Mycostatin. Ranbaxy brand of Nystatin.

Mydfrin. Alcon brand of Phenylephrine Hydrochloride.

Mydriacyl. Alcon brand of Tropicamide.

Myfortic. Novartis brand of Mycophenolic Acid.

Myidyl. USl brand of Triprolidine Hydrochloride.

Mykrox. UCB brand of Metolazone.

Mylanta Fiber. Johnson & Johnson-Merck Consumer† brand of Psyllium Husk.

Mylanta Gas Relief. Johnson & Johnson-Merck Consumer brand of Simethicone.

Mylanta Soothing Lozenges. Johnson & Johnson-Merck Consumer brand of Calcium Carbonate.

Mylaramine. Morton Grove brand of Dexchlorpheniramine Maleate.

Mylaxen. Medpointe brand of Hexafluorenium Bromide.

Myleran. GlaxoSmithKline brand of Busulfan.

Mylicon Infant's Drops. Johnson & Johnson-Merck Consumer brand of Simethicone.

Mylotarg. Wyeth brand of Gemtuzumab Ozogamicin.

Myochrysine. Merck brand of Gold Sodium Thiomalate.

Myordil. Sterling Winthrop† brand of Amotriphene.

Myoscint. Centocor brand of Imciromab Pentetate.

Myotonachol. Glenwood brand of Bethanechol Chloride.

Myotrope. Wyeth-Ayerst brand of Pelrinone Hydrochloride.

Myotrophin. Cephalon-Chiron brand of Mecasermin.

Myoview. Nycomed Amersham brand of Technetium Tc 99m Tetrofosmin.

Myrj 52. ICI Americas brand of Polyoxyl 40 Stearate.

Myrj 53. ICI Americas brand of Polyoxyl 50 Stearate.

Mysoline. Valeant brand of Primidone.

Mytelase. Sanofi Aventis brand of Ambenonium Chloride.

Mytolon Chloride. Sterling Winthrop† brand of Benzoquinonium Chloride.

Mytozytrex. SuperGen brand of Mitomycin.

Myvacet. Eastman† brand of Mono- and Di-acetylated Monoglycerides.

Myverol. Eastman† brand of Mono- and Di-glycerides.

Nacton. Ortho-McNeil† brand of Poldine Methylsulfate.

Nafazair. Bausch & Lomb brand of Naphazoline Hydrochloride.

Naftin. Merz brand of Naftifine Hydrochloride.

Nalfon. Pedinol brand of Fenoprofen Calcium.

Nalline [Veterinary]. Merial brand of Nalorphine Hydrochloride.

Nallpen. GlaxoSmithKline brand of Nafcillin Sodium.

Namenda. Forest brand of Memantine Hydrochloride.

Napageln. Wyeth-Ayerst† brand of Felbinac.

Naphcon. Alcon brand of Naphazoline Hydrochloride.

Naprosyn. Roche brand of Naproxen.

Naqua. Schering brand of Trichlormethiazide.

Narapin. Astra brand of Ropivacaine Hydrochloride.

Narcan. Bristol-Myers Squibb brand of Naloxone Hydrochloride.

Nardil. Pfizer brand of Phenelzine Sulfate.

Nasacort. Sanofi Aventis brand of Triamcinolone Acetonide.

Nasalide. Teva brand of Flunisolide.

Nasarel. Teva brand of Flunisolide.

Nascobal. QOL brand of Cyanocobalamin.

Natabec. Parke-Davis† brand of Ferrous Sulfate.

Natacyn. Alcon brand of Natamycin.

Natopherol. Abbott† brand of Vitamin E.

Natrecor. Biochemie, Austria, brand of Nesiritide.

Natrecor. Biochemie, Austria, brand of Nesiritide Citrate.

Natritope Chloride. Bristol-Myers Squibb† brand of Sodium Chloride Na 22.

Naturetin. Apothecon brand of Bendroflumethiazide.

Naturvus. Milton Roy brand of Hefilcon B.

Navane. Pfizer brand of Thiothixene.

Navane. Pfizer brand of Thiothixene Hydrochloride.

Navelbine. Pierre brand of Vinorelbine Tartrate.

Nebcin. Lilly brand of Tobramycin Sulfate.

Nebupent [as isethionate]. Fujisawa brand of Pentamidine.

Nebupent. Abraxis brand of Pentamidine Isethionate.

Nefrosul. 3M Pharmaceuticals† brand of Sulfachlorpyridazine.

Negabot Plus Paste. Bayer Animal Health† brand of Febantel.

Neggram. Sanofi Aventis brand of Nalidixic Acid.

Nemazine. Parke-Davis† brand of Phenothiazine.

Nembutal. Ovation brand of Pentobarbital.

Nembutal Sodium. Ovation brand of Pentobarbital Sodium.

Neo Heliopan. H & R Florasynth brand of Amiloxate.

Neo Heliopan. Haarmann & Reimer, Germany, brand of Enzacamene.

Neo Heliopan. H & R Florasynth brand of Meradimate.

Neo Heliopan. H & R Florasynth brand of Octinoxate.

Neo Heliopan. Haarmann & Reimer, Germany, brand of Octisalate.

Neo Heliopan AP. Symrise GmbH brand of Bisdisulizole Disodium.

Neo-Calglucon. Novartis brand of Calcium Glubionate.

Neo-Cobefrin. Cook-Waite brand of Levonordefrin.

Neo-Cultol. Fisons† brand of Mineral Oil.

Neodrol. Pfizer brand of Stanolone.

Neodyne. Marion Merrell Dow† brand of Ethyl Dibunate.

Neoferon. Biogen brand of Interferon Beta-1a.

Neohydrin. Marion Merrell Dow† brand of Chlormerodrin.

Neohydrin-197. Abbott† brand of Chlormerodrin Hg 197.

Neohydrin-203. Abbott† brand of Chlormerodrin Hg 203.

Neo-Iopax. Schering† brand of Iodomethamate Sodium.

Neonal. Abbott† brand of Butethal.

Neopap. Polymedica brand of Acetaminophen.

Neoprofen. Ovation brand of Ibuprofen Lysine.

Neoquess. Forest† brand of Hyoscyamine Sulfate.

Neoral. Novartis brand of Cyclosporine.

Neoscan. Medi-Physics brand of Gallium Citrate Ga 67.

Neo-Synephrine. Sterling Health U.S.A. brand of Phenylephrine Hydrochloride.

Neo-Synephrine II. Sterling Winthrop brand of Xylometazoline Hydrochloride.

Neotrizine. Lilly† brand of Trisulfapyrimidines.

Neotrofin. NeoTherapeutics brand of Leteprinim Potassium.

Nephroflow. Medi-Physics† brand of Iodohippurate Sodium I 123.

Nesacaine. Abraxis brand of Chloroprocaine Hydrochloride.

Nethamine. Marion Merrell Dow† brand of Etafedrine Hydrochloride.

Netromycin. Schering brand of Netilmicin Sulfate.

Neumega. Genetics Institute brand of Oprelvekin.

Neupogen. Amgen brand of Filgrastim.

Neupro. Schwarz Pharma brand of Rotigotine.

Neurelan. Élan brand of Fampridine.

Neurolite. DuPont Merck brand of Technetium Tc 99m Bicisate.

Neurontin. Pfizer brand of Gabapentin.

Neutra Care. Oral-B brand of Sodium Fluoride.

Neutrapen. 3M Pharmaceuticals† brand of Penicillinase.

Neutrexin. MedImmune brand of Trimetrexate Glucuronate.

Neutrol TE. BASF brand of Edetol.

Neuvenge. Dendreon brand of Lapuleucel-T.

Nevanac. Alcon brand of Nepafenac.

Nexavar. Bayer HealthCare brand of Sorafenib.

Nexavar. Bayer brand of Sorafenib Tosylate.

Nexium. AstraZeneca brand of Esomeprazole Magnesium.

Nexium. AstraZeneca brand of Esomeprazole Sodium.

Niacor. Upsher Smith brand of Niacin.

Niaspan. Abbott brand of Niacin.

Niclocide. Bayer brand of Niclosamide.

Nicoderm. Sanofi Aventis brand of Nicotine.

Nicorette. GlaxoSmithKline brand of Nicotine Polacrilex.

Nicotrol. Pfizer brand of Nicotine.

Nigrin. Pfizer brand of Streptonigrin.

Nikethyl. Abbott† brand of Nikethamide.

Nilandron. Sanofi Aventis brand of Nilutamide.

Nimbex. Abbott brand of Cisatracurium Besylate.

Nimotop. Bayer brand of Nimodipine.

---

† Brand name formerly used, and/or firm no longer concerned with this product.

Nipent. Hospira brand of Pentostatin.

Niravam. Schwarz Pharma brand of Alprazolam.

Nisentil. Hoffmann-LaRoche† brand of Alphaprodine Hydrochloride.

Nisulfazole. Sterling Winthrop† brand of Para-Nitrosulfathiazole.

Nitranitol. Marion Merrell Dow† brand of Mannitol Hexanitrate.

Nitrazine Paper. Apothecon brand of Phenaphthazine.

Nitretamin. Bristol-Myers Squibb† brand of Trolnitrate Phosphate.

Nitro-bid. Sanofi Aventis brand of Nitroglycerin.

Nitro-dur. Key brand of Nitroglycerin.

Nitropress. Hospira brand of Sodium Nitroprusside.

Nitrostat. Pfizer brand of Nitroglycerin.

Nix. Insight brand of Permethrin.

Nizin. Broemmel† brand of Sulfanilate Zinc.

Nizoral. Janssen brand of Ketoconazole.

Nizoral. McNeil brand of Ketoconazole.

Nobrium. Hoffmann-LaRoche† brand of Medazepam Hydrochloride.

Nocertone. Labaz S.A., France, brand of Oxetorone Fumarate.

Noctec. Bristol-Myers Squibb† brand of Chloral Hydrate.

NoDoz Caplets and Chewable Tablets. Bristol-Myers Products brand of Caffeine.

Noludar. Roche brand of Methyprylon.

Nolvadex. AstraZeneca brand of Tamoxifen Citrate.

Norcalcin. Amgen brand of Tecalcet Hydrochloride.

Norcuron. Organon brand of Vecuronium Bromide.

Norcynt. Lilly brand of Moxonidine.

Norflex. 3M Pharmaceuticals brand of Orphenadrine Citrate.

Norisodrine. Abbott brand of Isoproterenol Hydrochloride.

Norisodrine. Abbott brand of Isoproterenol Sulfate.

Noritate. Sanofi Aventis brand of Metronidazole.

Norlutate. Pfizer brand of Norethindrone Acetate.

Norlutin. Pfizer brand of Norethindrone.

Normiflo. Pfizer brand of Ardeparin Sodium.

Normodyne. Schering brand of Labetalol Hydrochloride.

Noroxin. Merck brand of Norfloxacin.

Norpace. Pfizer brand of Disopyramide Phosphate.

Norplant. Population Council brand of Levonorgestrel.

Norpramin. Sanofi Aventis brand of Desipramine Hydrochloride.

Norvasc. Pfizer brand of Amlodipine Besylate.

Norvir. Abbott brand of Ritonavir.

Nostril. Boehringer Ingelheim† brand of Phenylephrine Hydrochloride.

Novafil. Davis & Geck brand of Polybutester.

Novaldin. Sterling Winthrop brand of Dipyrone.

Novantrone. Serono brand of Mitoxantrone Hydrochloride.

Noveon AA-1. Goodrich brand of Polycarbophil.

Noveon CA-1. Goodrich brand of Calcium Polycarbophil.

Noveon CA-2. Goodrich brand of Calcium Polycarbophil.

Novocain. Hospira brand of Procaine Hydrochloride.

Novolin. Novo Nordisk brand of Insulin Human.

Novrad. Lilly† brand of Levopropoxyphene Napsylate.

Noxafil. Schering brand of Posaconazole.

Nozinan. Aventis brand of Levomepromazine Hydrochloride.

Nozinan. Aventis brand of Levomepromazine Maleate.

NPH. Novo Nordisk brand of Insulin, Isophane.

NPH Iletin. Lilly brand of Insulin, Isophane.

Nubain. Endo brand of Nalbuphine Hydrochloride.

Nucynt. Lilly brand of Moxonidine.

Nuflor [Veterinary]. Schering-Plough Animal Health brand of Florfenicol.

Nujol. Schering-Plough HealthCare† brand of Mineral Oil.

Nulsa. Wallace† brand of Proglumide.

Numorphan. Endo brand of Oxymorphone Hydrochloride.

Nupercainal. Ciba-Geigy brand of Dibucaine.

Nupercaine. Novartis brand of Dibucaine Hydrochloride.

Nurolon. Ethicon brand of Suture, Nonabsorbable Surgical.

Nuromax. Abbott brand of Doxacurium Chloride.

Nutrestore. Nutritional Restart brand of Glutamine.

Nutrifolin. Merck Eprova AG brand of Levomefolate Calcium.

Nutrifolin. Merck Eprova AG brand of Levomefolic Acid.

Nutrilipid. B Braun brand of Soybean Oil.

Nutropin. Genentech brand of Somatropin.

Nuvion. Protein Design Labs brand of Visilizumab.

Nydrazid. Bristol-Myers Squibb brand of Isoniazid.

Occasions Multifocal. Bausch & Lomb brand of Polymacon.

Occasions Single Use. Bausch & Lomb brand of Polymacon.

Octin. Knoll† brand of Isometheptene Hydrochloride.

Octopirox. Hoechst AG, Germany, brand of Piroctone Olamine.

OctreoScan. Mallinckrodt brand of Indium In 111 Pentetreotide.

Ocuclear. Schering-Plough brand of Oxymetazoline Hydrochloride.

Ocufen. Allergan brand of Flurbiprofen Sodium.

Ocuflox. Allergan brand of Ofloxacin.

Ocupress. Novartis brand of Carteolol Hydrochloride.

Ocusert Pilo. Akorn brand of Pilocarpine.

Ocusulf. MIZA brand of Sulfacetamide Sodium.

Ogen. Pfizer brand of Estropipate.

Olaxin. SmithKline Beecham† brand of Clomacran Phosphate.

Oleotope. Bristol-Myers Squibb† brand of Oleic Acid I 131.

Oleotope Diagnostic. Bristol-Myers Squibb† brand of Oleic Acid I 131.

Oleotope I-125. Bristol-Myers Squibb† brand of Oleic Acid I 125.

Olux. Connetics brand of Clobetasol Propionate.

Omadine MDS. Olin brand of Bispyrithione Magsulfex.

Omnaris. Altana brand of Ciclesonide.

Omnicef. Abbott brand of Cefdinir.

Omniflox. Abbott† brand of Temafloxacin Hydrochloride.

Omnipaque. GE Healthcare brand of Iohexol.

Omnipen. Wyeth-Ayerst brand of Ampicillin.

Omnipen. Wyeth brand of Ampicillin Sodium.

Omnipred. Alcon brand of Prednisolone Acetate.

Omniscan. GE Healthcare brand of Gadodiamide.

Oncaspar. Enzon brand of Pegaspargase.

Onconase. Alfacell brand of Ranpirnase.

Oncophage. Antigenics brand of Vitespen.

OncoScint CR/OV. Cytogen brand of Indium In 111 Satumomab Pendetide.

Oncovin. Lilly brand of Vincristine Sulfate.

OP-2. Sterling Winthrop brand of Lotifocon B.

OP-6. Sterling Winthrop brand of Lotifocon C.

Opana. Endo brand of Oxymorphone Hydrochloride.

Ophthaine. Apothecon brand of Proparacaine Hydrochloride.

Ophthalgan. Wyeth-Ayerst brand of Glycerin.

Ophthetic. Allergan brand of Proparacaine Hydrochloride.

Optacryl 60. Paragon brand of Kolfocon A.

Optacryl Extra. Paragon brand of Kolfocon C.

Optacryl K. Paragon brand of Kolfocon B.

Optacryl Z. Paragon brand of Kolfocon D.

Opticrom. Allergan brand of Cromolyn Sodium.

Optiflex. Lilly brand of Somidobove.

Optikem 18. Optacryl brand of Kolfocon A.

Optikem 32. Optacryl brand of Kolfocon B.

Optim. Dow Chemical brand of Glycerin.

Optima 38. Bausch & Lomb brand of Polymacon.

Optima 38/SP. Bausch & Lomb brand of Polymacon.

Optima FW. Bausch & Lomb brand of Polymacon.

Optima Toric. Bausch & Lomb brand of Hefilcon B.

Optimark. Mallinckrodt brand of Gadoversetamide.

Optimil. Wallace† brand of Methaqualone Hydrochloride.

Optimine. Schering brand of Azatadine Maleate.

OptiPranolol. Bausch & Lomb Pharmaceuticals brand of Metipranolol.

Optiray. Mallinckrodt brand of Ioversol.

Optison. GE Healthcare brand of Albumin Human.

Optivar. Medpointe brand of Azelastine Hydrochloride.

Optrin. Pharmacyclics brand of Motexafin Lutetium.
Oraflex. Lilly† brand of Benoxaprofen.
Oragrafin Calcium. Bracco brand of Ipodate Calcium.
Oragrafin Sodium. Bracco brand of Ipodate Sodium.
Oralone. Taro brand of Triamcinolone Acetonide.
Ora-Lutin. Parke-Davis† brand of Ethisterone.
Oramorph. Xanodyne brand of Morphine Sulfate.
Orap. Teva brand of Pimozide.
Orapred. Medicis brand of Prednisolone Sodium Phosphate.
Orasone. Solvay Pharmaceuticals brand of Prednisone.
Oratel. Bayer Animal Health† brand of Febantel.
Ora-testryl. Bristol-Myers Squibb brand of Fluoxymesterone.
Oratrast. Rhone-Poulenc Rorer† brand of Barium Sulfate.
Oravue. Bristol-Myers Squibb† brand of Iopronic Acid.
Orbax. Schering-Plough Animal Health brand of Orbifloxacin.
Oretic. Abbott brand of Hydrochlorothiazide.
Oreton. Schering brand of Methyltestosterone.
Orfadin. Swedish Orphan brand of Nitisinone.
Organidin. Wallace brand of Glycerol, Iodinated.
Orgaran. Organon brand of Danaparoid Sodium.
Orimune. Lederle brand of Poliovirus Vaccine Live Oral.
Orinase. Pfizer brand of Tolbutamide.
Orinase Diagnostic. Pharmacia & Upjohn brand of Tolbutamide Sodium, Sterile.
Oriodide. Abbott† brand of Sodium Iodide I 131.
Orlaam. Roxane brand of Levomethadyl Acetate Hydrochloride.
Orlex. Procter & Gamble brand of Acetic Acid, Glacial.
Ornidyl. Sanofi Aventis brand of Eflornithine Hydrochloride.
ORTHO EVRA. R. W. Johnson brand of Norelgestromin.
Orthoclone OKT3. Ortho Pharmaceutical brand of Muromonab-CD3.
Ortho-est. Sun brand of Estropipate.
Orthozyme CD5 Plus. Xoma brand of Zolimomab Aritox.
Orudis. Wyeth brand of Ketoprofen.
Oruvail. Wyeth brand of Ketoprofen.
Orvaten. Upsher Smith brand of Midodrine Hydrochloride.
Osbil. Mallinckrodt† brand of Iobenzamic Acid.
Osmitrol. Baxter Healthcare brand of Mannitol.
Osmoglyn. Alcon brand of Glycerin.
Osmovist. Bayer brand of Iotrolan.
Ostamer. Marion Merrell Dow† brand of Polyurethane Foam.
Osteo D. Teva, Israel, brand of Secalciferol.
Osteolite. DuPont Merck brand of Technetium Tc 99m Medronate.
Otrivin Hydrochloride. Ciba-Geigy† brand of Xylometazoline Hydrochloride.
OvaRex. AltaRex brand of Oregovomab.
Ovide. Taro brand of Malathion.
Ovidrel. Serono brand of Choriogonadotropin Alfa.
Ovrette. Wyeth brand of Norgestrel.
Oxaine M. Wyeth-Ayerst† brand of Magnesium Hydroxide.
Oxandrin. Savient brand of Oxandrolone.
Oxilan. Guerbet brand of Ioxilan.
Oxistat. Altana brand of Oxiconazole Nitrate.
Oxivent. Boehringer Ingelheim brand of Oxitropium Bromide.
Oxsoralen. Valeant brand of Methoxsalen.
OxyContin. Purdue Frederick brand of Oxycodone.
Oxycontin. Purdue brand of Oxycodone Hydrochloride.
OxyCor. Bausch & Lomb brand of Balafilcon A.
Oxygent. Atofina brand of combination product; *See* Perflubrodec.
Oxyglobin Solution. Biopure brand of Hemoglobin Glutamer-200 (Bovine).
Oxylone. Pfizer brand of Fluorometholone.
Oxytrol. Watson brand of Oxybutynin.
Pacinox. Ortho-McNeil† brand of Capuride.

Pagitane. Lilly brand of Cycrimine Hydrochloride.
Palohex. Sterling Winthrop brand of Inositol Niacinate.
Palosein [Veterinary]. Oxis brand of Orgotein.
Paludrine. Zeneca brand of Chloroguanide Hydrochloride.
Pamelor. Tyco brand of Nortriptyline Hydrochloride.
Pamine. Bradley brand of Methscopolamine Bromide.
Panacur. Hoechst-Roussel brand of Fenbendazole.
Pancrease. Ortho-McNeil brand of Pancrelipase.
Pandel. Savage brand of Hydrocortisone Probutate.
Panheprin. Hospira brand of Heparin Sodium.
Panmycin. Pfizer brand of Tetracycline Hydrochloride.
Panolid. Novartis† brand of Ethybenztropine.
Panorex. Centocor brand of Edrecolomab.
PanOxyl. Stiefel brand of Benzoyl Peroxide.
Panretin. Eisai Medical Research brand of Alitretinoin.
Panteric. Parke-Davis† brand of Pancreatin.
Pantholin. Lilly† brand of Calcium Pantothenate.
Pantofenicol. Pluriquimica, Portugal, brand of Chloramphenicol Pantothenate Complex.
Pantopaque. Alcon brand of Iophendylate.
Panvac. Therion Biologics brand of Falimarev (CEA, MUC-1, fowlpox virus).
Panvac. Therion Biologics brand of Inalimarev (CEA, MUC-1, Vaccinia virus).
Paracaine. Optopics brand of Proparacaine Hydrochloride.
Paraderm. Wyeth-Ayerst brand of Bufexamac.
Paradione. Abbott brand of Paramethadione.
Paraflex. Ortho-McNeil brand of Chlorzoxazone.
Parafoil. Merck brand of Abamectin.
Parafon. Ortho-McNeil brand of Chlorzoxazone.
Paral. Forest brand of Paraldehyde.
Paraplatin. Bristol-Myers Squibb brand of Carboplatin.
Parasal. Panray brand of Aminosalicylic Acid.
Parasal Sodium. Panray brand of Aminosalicylate Sodium.
Parathar. Sanofi Aventis brand of Teriparatide Acetate.
Paredrine. Akorn brand of Hydroxyamphetamine Hydrobromide.
Parenzyme. Marion Merrell Dow† brand of Trypsin, Crystallized.
Parepectolin. Rhone-Poulenc Rorer† brand of Attapulgite, Activated.
Parest. Parke-Davis† brand of Methaqualone Hydrochloride.
Parfenac. Wyeth-Ayerst brand of Bufexamac.
Parlodel. Novartis brand of Bromocriptine Mesylate.
Parnate. GlaxoSmithKline brand of Tranylcypromine Sulfate.
Paroidin. Parke-Davis† brand of Parathyroid Hormone.
Parsidol. Pfizer brand of Ethopropazine Hydrochloride.
Parsol. Roche brand of Octinoxate.
Parsol 1789. Givaudan S.A., Switzerland, brand of Avobenzone.
Paser. Jacobus brand of Aminosalicylic Acid.
Patanol. Alcon brand of Olopatadine Hydrochloride.
Pathilon. Lederle brand of Tridihexethyl Chloride.
Pavabid. Hoechst Marion Roussel brand of Papaverine Hydrochloride.
Paveril Phosphate. Lilly† brand of Dioxyline Phosphate.
Pavulon. Organon brand of Pancuronium Bromide.
Paxil [as hydrochloride]. SmithKline Beecham brand of Paroxetine.
Paxil. GlaxoSmithKline brand of Paroxetine Hydrochloride.
Paxipam. Schering brand of Halazepam.
PBZ. Novartis brand of Tripelennamine Citrate.
PBZ. Novartis brand of Tripelennamine Hydrochloride.
PDS II. Ethicon brand of Polydioxanone.
Pedameth. Forest brand of Racemethionine.
PediaCare 1. McNeil Consumer brand of Dextromethorphan Hydrobromide.
Pediaflor. Ross brand of Sodium Fluoride.
Pediamycin. Ross brand of Erythromycin Ethylsuccinate.
Pediapred. UCB brand of Prednisolone Sodium Phosphate.
Peganone. Ovation brand of Ethotoin.

---

† Brand name formerly used, and/or firm no longer concerned with this product.

Pegasys. Hoffmann-LaRoche brand of Peginterferon Alfa-2a.

Pemulen TR-1. Noveon brand of Carbomer 1342.

Pemulen TR-2. Noveon brand of Carbomer 1342.

Penbritin. Wyeth brand of Ampicillin Sodium.

Penetrex. Sanofi Aventis brand of Enoxacin.

Pentacarinat [as isethionate]. Rhone-Poulenc Rorer brand of Pentamidine.

Pentam. Abraxis brand of Pentamidine Isethionate.

Pentam 300 [as isethionate]. Fujisawa brand of Pentamidine.

Pentasa. Shire brand of Mesalamine.

Pentaspan. DuPont Merck brand of Pentastarch.

Penthrane. Abbott brand of Methoxyflurane.

Pentids. Apothecon brand of Penicillin G Potassium.

Pentolair. Bausch & Lomb brand of Cyclopentolate Hydrochloride.

Pentothal. Abbott brand of Thiopental Sodium.

Pentoxil. Upsher Smith brand of Pentoxifylline.

Pentritol Tempules. Rhone-Poulenc Rorer† brand of Pentaerythritol Tetranitrate.

Pentyde. Immunetech brand of Pentigetide.

Pen-vee K. Wyeth brand of Penicillin V Potassium.

Pepcid. Merck brand of Famotidine.

Peptavlon. Wyeth brand of Pentagastrin.

Perceptin. Gliatech brand of Cipralisant Maleate.

Perchloracap. Mallinckrodt brand of Potassium Perchlorate.

Percorten. Novartis brand of Desoxycorticosterone Acetate.

Percorten. Novartis brand of Desoxycorticosterone Pivalate.

Perfan. Marion Merrell Dow brand of Enoximone.

Performist. Dey brand of Formoterol Fumarate.

Pergamid. Scios Nova brand of Perfosfamide.

Pergonal. Serono brand of Menotropins.

Periactin. Merck brand of Cyproheptadine Hydrochloride.

Peridex. 3M Pharmaceuticals brand of Chlorhexidine Gluconate.

Periochip. Dexcel brand of Chlorhexidine Gluconate.

Periogard. Colgate brand of Chlorhexidine Gluconate.

Periograf. Sterling Winthrop brand of Durapatite.

Periostat. CollaGenex brand of Doxycycline Hyclate.

Peritrate. Parke-Davis† brand of Pentaerythritol Tetranitrate.

Permaflex Naturals. CooperVision brand of Surfilcon A.

Permaflex UV Naturals 74. CooperVision brand of Vasurfilcon A.

Permalens. CooperVision brand of Perfilcon A.

Permapen. Pfizer brand of Penicillin G Benzathine.

Permax. Valeant brand of Pergolide Mesylate.

Permitil. Schering brand of Fluphenazine Hydrochloride.

Persa-Gel. Ortho Pharmaceutical brand of Benzoyl Peroxide.

Persantine. Boehringer Ingelheim brand of Dipyridamole.

Pertscan-99m. Abbott† brand of Sodium Pertechnetate Tc 99m.

Peson. Hoechst-Roussel† brand of Lyapolate Sodium.

Petrin. Parke-Davis† brand of Pentrinitrol.

Pexeva. JDS brand of Paroxetine Mesylate.

Pexid. Marion Merrell Dow† brand of Perhexiline Maleate.

Pfizerpen. Pfizer brand of Penicillin G Procaine.

Pfizerpen Vk. Pfizer brand of Penicillin V Potassium.

Phanodorn. Sterling Winthrop brand of Cyclobarbital.

Phanodorn Calcium. Sterling Winthrop† brand of Cyclobarbital Calcium.

Pharmaseal Scrub Care. Pharmaseal brand of Chlorhexidine Gluconate.

Phemerol Chloride. Parke-Davis brand of Benzethonium Chloride.

Phenergan. Wyeth brand of Promethazine Hydrochloride.

Phenmerzyl Nitrate. Marion Merrell Dow† brand of Phenylmercuric Nitrate.

Phenoxene. Marion Merrell Dow† brand of Chlorphenoxamine Hydrochloride.

Phenurone. Abbott brand of Phenacemide.

Pheny-Pas-Tebamin. Purdue Frederick brand of Phenyl Aminosalicylate.

Phillips Magnesia Tablets. Sterling Health U.S.A. brand of Magnesium Hydroxide.

Phillips Milk of Magnesia Liquid. Sterling Health U.S.A. brand of Magnesium Hydroxide.

Phisohex. Sanofi Aventis brand of Hexachlorophene.

Phoslo. Fresenius brand of Calcium Acetate.

Phosphaljel. Wyeth-Ayerst brand of Aluminum Phosphate.

Phosphocol P32. Mallinckrodt brand of Chromic Phosphate P 32.

Phospholine Iodide. Wyeth brand of Echothiophate Iodide.

Phosphotec. Bracco Diagnostics brand of Technetium Tc 99m Pyrophosphate.

Phosphotope. Bristol-Myers Squibb† brand of Sodium Phosphate P 32.

Photofrin. Axcan Scandipharm brand of Porfimer Sodium.

Pilagan. Allergan brand of Pilocarpine Nitrate.

Pilopine. Alcon brand of Pilocarpine Hydrochloride.

Pincets. Marion Merrell Dow† brand of Piperazine Phosphate.

Pindac. Leo brand of Pinacidil.

Pinsirup. Marion Merrell Dow† brand of Piperazine Phosphate.

Pipracil. Wyeth brand of Piperacillin Sodium.

Piptal. Marion Merrell Dow† brand of Pipenzolate Bromide.

Pirmavar. Parke-Davis brand of Pirmenol Hydrochloride.

Pitocin. King brand of Oxytocin.

Pitressin. Parke-Davis brand of Vasopressin.

Pitressin Tannate (Synthetic). Parke-Davis† brand of Argipressin Tannate.

Pitressin Tannate. King brand of Vasopressin Tannate.

Pituitrin [as injection]. Parke-Davis† brand of Pituitary, Posterior.

Pixykine. Immunex brand of Milodistim.

Placidyl. Abbott brand of Ethchlorvynol.

Plan B. Duramed brand of Levonorgestrel.

Plano T. Bausch & Lomb brand of Polymacon.

Plaquenil. Sanofi Aventis brand of Hydroxychloroquine Sulfate.

Plasdone. International Specialty Products brand of Povidone.

Plasma Plex. Centeon brand of Plasma Protein Fraction.

Plasmanate. Bayer brand of Plasma Protein Fraction.

Plasmatein. Alpha Therapeutic brand of Plasma Protein Fraction.

Platinol. Bristol-Myers Squibb brand of Cisplatin.

Plavix. Sanofi Aventis brand of Clopidogrel Bisulfate.

plegine. Wyeth brand of Phendimetrazine Tartrate.

Plenaxis. Praecis brand of Abarelix.

Plendil. AstraZeneca brand of Felodipine.

Pletal. Otsuka brand of Cilostazol.

Pluracare. BASF brand of Poloxamer.

Pluracol E. BASF brand of Polyethylene Glycol.

Pluronic. BASF brand of Poloxamer.

PLV-2. Novartis† brand of Felypressin.

Polaramine. Schering brand of Dexchlorpheniramine Maleate.

Polmiror. Polichimica Sap, Italy, brand of Nifuratel.

Polocaine. Abraxis brand of Mepivacaine Hydrochloride.

Polybrene. Abbott† brand of Hexadimethrine Bromide.

Polycillin. Apothecon† brand of Ampicillin.

Polycillin. Bristol-Myers Squibb brand of Ampicillin Sodium.

Polyglycol E 300, E 400, E 1450, E 8000. Dow Chemical brand of Polyethylene Glycol.

PolyHeme. Northfield brand of Hemoglobin Glutamer-256 (Human).

Polyplasdone. International Specialty Products brand of Crospovidone.

Polytaxin. Sterling Winthrop† brand of Hexavitamin.

Pondimin. Robins brand of Fenfluramine Hydrochloride.

Ponstel. Sciele brand of Mefenamic Acid.

Pontocaine. Sterling Winthrop brand of Tetracaine.

Pontocaine Hydrochloride. Sterling Winthrop brand of Tetracaine Hydrochloride.

Portyn. Parke-Davis† brand of Benzilonium Bromide.

Posicor. Hoffmann-LaRoche brand of Mibefradil Dihydrochloride.

Posilac. Monsanto brand of Sometribove.

Potaba. Glenwood brand of Aminobenzoate Potassium.

Povan. Pfizer brand of Pyrvinium Pamoate.

Pradaxa. Boehringer Ingelheim Pharma GmbH & Co. KG and Bidachem S.p.A. brand of Dabigatran.

Pradaxa. Boehringer Ingelheim Pharma GmbH & Co. KG and Bidachem S.p.A. brand of Dabigatran Etexilate.

Pradaxa. Boehringer Ingelheim Pharma GmbH & Co. KG and Bidachem S.p.A. brand of Dabigatran Etexilate Mesylate.

Prandin. Novo Nordisk brand of Repaglinide.

Pranone. Schering† brand of Ethisterone.

Prantal. Schering brand of Diphemanil Methylsulfate.

Pravachol. Bristol-Myers Squibb brand of Pravastatin Sodium.

Praxilene. Lipha, S.A., France, brand of Nafronyl Oxalate.

Precedex. Hospira brand of Dexmedetomidine.

Precef. Apothecon brand of Ceforanide.

Precose. Bayer brand of Acarbose.

Preference. CooperVision brand of Tetrafilcon A.

Preference Standard. CooperVision brand of Tetrafilcon A.

Preference Toric. CooperVision brand of Tetrafilcon A.

Pregnyl. Organon brand of Gonadotropin, Chorionic.

Prelay. Sankyo brand of Troglitazone.

Preludin. Boehringer Ingelheim brand of Phenmetrazine Hydrochloride.

Premarin. Wyeth brand of Estrogens, Conjugated.

Pre-op. Davis & Geck brand of Hexachlorophene.

Pre-Pen. Schwarz Pharma brand of Benzylpenicilloyl Polylysine.

Prequist Powder. Parke-Davis brand of Calcium Lactate.

Pre-Sate. Parke-Davis brand of Chlorphentermine Hydrochloride.

Prevacare. Johnson & Johnson brand of Chlorhexidine Gluconate.

Prevacid. TAP brand of Lansoprazole.

Prezios. Chugai Pharmaceutical Co., Ltd., Japan, brand of Maxacalcitol.

Prialt. Elan brand of Ziconotide.

Priftin. Sanofi Aventis brand of Rifapentine.

Prilosec. AstraZeneca brand of Omeprazole.

Prilosec. AstraZeneca brand of Omeprazole Magnesium.

Primacor. Sterling Winthrop brand of Milrinone.

Prinadol. SmithKline Beecham† brand of Phenazocine Hydrobromide.

Principen. Apothecon brand of Ampicillin.

Principen. Apothecon brand of Ampicillin Sodium.

Prinivil. Merck brand of Lisinopril.

Priodax. Schering† brand of Iodoalphionic Acid.

Priscoline. Novartis brand of Tolazoline Hydrochloride.

Proair. Teva brand of Albuterol Sulfate.

Pro-Air. Parke-Davis† brand of Procaterol Hydrochloride.

Proamatine. Shire brand of Midodrine Hydrochloride.

Pro-banthine. Shire brand of Propantheline Bromide.

Probkin. Parke-Davis brand of Piprozolin.

Procan. Pfizer brand of Procainamide Hydrochloride.

Procardia. Pfizer brand of Nifedipine.

Procholon. Bristol-Myers Squibb† brand of Dehydrocholic Acid.

Proclear. Biocompatibles brand of Omafilcon A.

Procrit. Ortho Biotech brand of Epoetin Alfa.

Prodorm. Parke-Davis† brand of Carbocloral.

Producil [Veterinary]. Merial brand of Efrotomycin.

Profenal. Alcon brand of Suprofen.

Proferdex. New River brand of Iron Dextran.

Profilate Heat-Treated. Alpha Therapeutic† brand of Antihemophilic Factor.

Profilate HP. Alpha Therapeutic† brand of Antihemophilic Factor.

Profilate OSD. Alpha Therapeutic brand of Antihemophilic Factor.

Profilate SD. Alpha Therapeutic† brand of Antihemophilic Factor.

Profilnine. Alpha Therapeutic† brand of Factor IX Complex.

Profilnine SD. Alpha Therapeutic brand of Factor IX Complex.

Proglycem. Baker Norton brand of Diazoxide.

Prograf. Astellas brand of Tacrolimus.

Prohance. Bracco brand of Gadoteridol.

Proketazine. Wyeth brand of Carphenazine Maleate.

Prolene. Ethicon brand of Suture, Nonabsorbable Surgical.

Prolergic. Schering† brand of Cycliramine Maleate.

Proleukin. Chiron brand of Aldesleukin.

Prolixin. Apothecon brand of Fluphenazine Enanthate.

Prolixin. Apothecon brand of Fluphenazine Hydrochloride.

Proloid. Pfizer brand of Thyroglobulin.

Proloprim. King brand of Trimethoprim.

Prolyse. Abbott brand of Nasaruplase Beta.

Promacetin. Parke-Davis† brand of Acetosulfone Sodium.

Prometa. Muro brand of Metaproterenol Sulfate.

Prometrium. Unimed brand of Progesterone.

Promizole. Parke-Davis† brand of Thiazosulfone.

Pronestyl. Apothecon brand of Procainamide Hydrochloride.

Propecia. Merck brand of Finasteride.

Propine. Allergan brand of Dipivefrin Hydrochloride.

Proplex T. Hyland brand of Factor IX Complex.

Propulsid. Janssen brand of Cisapride.

Proquin. Esprit brand of Ciprofloxacin Hydrochloride.

Proscar. Merck brand of Finasteride.

Prosom. Abbott brand of Estazolam.

Pro-Spot. Bayer Animal Health brand of Fenthion.

Prostaphlin. Apothecon brand of Oxacillin Sodium.

Prostigmine. ICN brand of Neostigmine Methylsulfate.

Prostin. Pfizer brand of Alprostadil.

Prostin E2. Pfizer brand of Dinoprostone.

Prostin F2 Alpha. Pfizer brand of Dinoprost Tromethamine.

Prosynap. Janssen brand of Lubeluzole.

Protalba. Marion Merrell Dow† brand of Protoveratrine A.

ProTec. Cell Therapeutics† brand of Lisofylline.

Protenate. Hyland brand of Plasma Protein Fraction.

Prothecan. Enzon brand of Pegamotecan.

Protonix. Wyeth brand of Pantoprazole Sodium.

Protopam Chloride. Wyeth brand of Pralidoxime Chloride.

Protopic. Astellas brand of Tacrolimus.

Protropin. Genentech brand of Somatrem.

Provenge. Dendreon brand of Sipuleucel-T.

Proventil. Schering brand of Albuterol.

Proventil. Schering brand of Albuterol Sulfate.

Provera. Pfizer brand of Medroxyprogesterone Acetate.

Provigil. Cephalon brand of Modafinil.

Provir. Shaman brand of Crofelemer.

Provocholine. Methapharm brand of Methacholine Chloride.

Prozac. Lilly brand of Fluoxetine Hydrochloride.

Prulet. Mission Pharmacal† brand of Phenolphthalein.

Pseudo. UCB brand of Pseudoephedrine Polistirex.

Psorcon. Sanofi Aventis brand of Diflorasone Diacetate.

Pulmicort. AstraZeneca brand of Budesonide.

Pulmolite. DuPont Merck brand of Technetium Tc 99m Albumin Aggregated.

Pulmozyme. Genentech brand of Dornase Alfa.

Puricase. Savient brand of Pegloticase.

Purinethol. Teva brand of Mercaptopurine.

PVS Basics. Paragon brand of Paflufocon E.

Pyridium. Warner Chilcott brand of Phenazopyridine Hydrochloride.

Pyrolite. DuPont Merck brand of Technetium Tc 99m (Pyro- and trimeta-) Phosphates.

Pyronil. Lilly† brand of Pyrrobutamine Phosphate.

Pyrophosphate Kit. Medi-Physics brand of Technetium Tc 99m Pyrophosphate.

Quadramet. Cytogen brand of Samarium Sm 153 Lexidronam Pentasodium.

Quadrol. BASF brand of Edetol.

---

† Brand name formerly used, and/or firm no longer concerned with this product.

Quantril. Roerig brand of Benzquinamide.
Quantum II. Polymer Technology brand of Hexafocon A.
Quarzan. Roche brand of Clidinium Bromide.
Quelicin. Hospira brand of Succinylcholine Chloride.
Questran. Bristol Labs brand of Cholestyramine Resin.
Questran Light. Bristol Labs brand of Cholestyramine Resin.
Quide. Dow Chemical brand of Piperacetazine.
Quinadome. Bayer† brand of Iodoquinol.
Quinaglute. Bayer brand of Quinidine Gluconate.
Quinidex. Wyeth brand of Quinidine Sulfate.
Quin-O-Creme. Marion Merrell Dow† brand of Clioquinol.
Quinolor. Bristol-Myers Squibb† brand of Halquinols.
Quinora. Schering brand of Quinidine Sulfate.
Quixin. Vistakon brand of Levofloxacin.
Rachromate. Abbott† brand of Sodium Chromate Cr 51.
Racobalamin-57. Abbott† brand of Cyanocobalamin Co 57.
Racobalamin-60. Abbott† brand of Cyanocobalamin Co 60.
Radinyl. Roberts Pharmaceutical brand of Etanidazole.
Radiocaps-131. Abbott† brand of Sodium Iodide I 131.
Radio-Cholografin. Bristol-Myers Squibb† brand of Iodipamide Sodium I 131.
Radiogardase-Cs. Heyl, Germany, brand of Prussian Blue Insoluble.
Ralabol. Pitman-Moore brand of Zeranol.
Ralgro. Pitman-Moore brand of Zeranol.
Rambazole. Barrier brand of Talarozole.
Ranestol. Parke-Davis† brand of Triclofenol Piperazine.
Ranexa. Sensus brand of Ranolazine.
Raniclor. Ranbaxy brand of Cefaclor.
Raoleic Acid-131. Abbott† brand of Oleic Acid I 131.
Raolein. Abbott† brand of Triolein I 131.
Rapamune. Wyeth brand of Sirolimus.
Raplon. Organon brand of Rapacuronium Bromide.
Raudixin. Apothecon brand of Rauwolfia Serpentina.
Rau-Sed. Bristol-Myers Squibb brand of Reserpine.
Rautensin. Novartis brand of Alseroxylon.
Rauwiloid. 3M Pharmaceuticals brand of Alseroxylon.
Ravocaine Hydrochloride. Cook-Waite brand of Propoxycaine Hydrochloride.
Raxar. Otsuka brand of Grepafloxacin Hydrochloride.
Razadyne. Ortho-McNeil brand of Galantamine Hydrobromide.
Rebetol. Schering-Plough brand of Ribavirin.
Recentin. AstraZeneca brand of Cediranib.
Recentin. AstraZeneca brand of Cediranib Maleate.
Reclast. Novartis brand of Zoledronic Acid.
Rectalad Enema. Wallace† brand of Docusate Potassium.
Redisol. Merck brand of Cyanocobalamin.
Reductol. Wyeth-Ayerst† brand of Acifran.
Redux. Interneuron brand of Dexfenfluramine Hydrochloride.
Refresh Plus, Cellufresh Formula. Allergan brand of Carboxymethylcellulose Sodium.
Regitine. Novartis brand of Phentolamine Mesylate.
Regitine Hydrochloride. Ciba-Geigy† brand of Phentolamine Hydrochloride.
Reglan. Schwarz Pharma brand of Metoclopramide Hydrochloride.
Regonol. Sandoz brand of Pyridostigmine Bromide.
Regranex. Johnson & Johnson brand of Becaplermin.
REGU-MATE. Roussel-UCLAF, France, brand of Altrenogest.
Rela. Schering brand of Carisoprodol.
Relafen. GlaxoSmithKline brand of Nabumetone.
Releasin. Parke-Davis† brand of Relaxin.
Relenza. GlaxoSmithKline brand of Zanamivir.
Relpax. Pfizer brand of Eletriptan Hydrobromide.
Remeflin. Wallace† brand of Dimefline Hydrochloride.
Remen. Parke-Davis† brand of Pramiracetam Hydrochloride.
Remeron. Organon brand of Mirtazapine.
Reminyl. Janssen Pharmaceutica, Belgium, brand of Galantamine.

Remodulin. United Therapeutics brand of Treprostinil.
Remsed. Bristol-Myers Squibb brand of Promethazine Hydrochloride.
Renagel. Genzyme brand of Sevelamer Hydrochloride.
Rencal. Bristol-Myers Squibb† brand of Phytate Sodium.
Renese. Pfizer brand of Polythiazide.
Reno. Bracco brand of Diatrizoate Meglumine.
Renoquid. Glenwood brand of Sulfacytine.
Renormax. Schering brand of Spirapril Hydrochloride.
Renova. Johnson & Johnson brand of Tretinoin.
Renovia. Recordati, Italy, brand of Lercanidipine Hydrochloride.
Renovue. Bracco brand of Iodamide Meglumine.
ReoPro. Lilly brand of Abciximab.
Replagal. Transkaryotic Therapies brand of Agalsidase Alfa.
Requip. GlaxoSmithKline brand of Ropinirole.
Requip. GlaxoSmithKline brand of Ropinirole Hydrochloride.
Rescriptor. Agouron brand of Delavirdine Mesylate.
Resectisol. B Braun brand of Mannitol.
Resinat. Marion Merrell Dow† brand of Polyamine-Methylene Resin.
Restasis. Allergan brand of Cyclosporine.
Restoril. Tyco brand of Temazepam.
Retin-A. Johnson & Johnson brand of Tretinoin.
Retisert. Bausch & Lomb brand of Fluocinolone Acetonide.
Retrovir. GlaxoSmithKline brand of Zidovudine.
Reverset. Incyte brand of Dexelvucitabine.
Rev-Eyes. Angelini brand of Dapiprazole Hydrochloride.
Revia. Duramed brand of Naltrexone Hydrochloride.
Revlimid. Celgene brand of Lenalidomide.
Reyataz. Bristol-Myers Squibb brand of Atazanavir Sulfate.
Rezifilm. Bristol-Myers Squibb† brand of Thiram.
Rezulin. Pfizer brand of Troglitazone.
R-gene 10. Pfizer brand of Arginine Hydrochloride.
Rheaform Boluses [Veterinary]. Fort Dodge Animal Health† brand of Clioquinol.
Rheumatrex. Wyeth-Ayerst brand of Methotrexate.
Rhinocort. AstraZeneca brand of Budesonide.
Rhodigel. Vanderbilt brand of Xanthan Gum.
RhoGAM. Ortho Diagnostic brand of Rh_o (D) Immune Globulin.
Rhus Tox Antigen. Lemmon† brand of Poison Ivy Extract, Alum Precipitated.
Ribasphere. Three Rivers brand of Ribavirin.
Ribomustine. Amcis AG, Switzerland, brand of Bendamustine Hydrochloride.
Ridaura. Promethus brand of Auranofin.
Rifadin. Sanofi Aventis brand of Rifampin.
Rilutek. Sanofi Aventis brand of Riluzole.
Rimactane. Actavis brand of Rifampin.
Rimadyl. Roche brand of Carprofen.
Rimso-50. Bioniche brand of Dimethyl Sulfoxide.
Rintal. Bayer Animal Health brand of Febantel.
Riomet. Ranbaxy brand of Metformin Hydrochloride.
Riopan. Whitehall-Robins brand of Magaldrate.
RISA-125. Abbott† brand of Albumin, Iodinated I 125 Serum.
RISA-131. Abbott† brand of Albumin, Iodinated I 131 Serum.
Risperdal. Janssen brand of Risperidone.
ritalin. Novartis brand of Methylphenidate Hydrochloride.
Rituxan. IDEC brand of Rituximab.
Rivanol. Hoechst-Roussel† brand of Ethacridine Lactate.
Rivizor. Janssen brand of Vorozole.
Robaxin. Schwarz Pharma brand of Methocarbamol.
Robengatope I-125. Bristol-Myers Squibb† brand of Rose Bengal Sodium I 125.
Robengatope I-131. Bristol-Myers Squibb† brand of Rose Bengal Sodium I 131.
Robinul. Sciele brand of Glycopyrrolate.
Rocaltrol. Roche brand of Calcitriol.
Roccal. Sterling Winthrop brand of Benzalkonium Chloride.

Rocephin. Roche brand of Ceftriaxone Sodium.

Roferon-A. Hoffmann-LaRoche brand of Interferon Alfa-2a.

Rogaine. Johnson & Johnson brand of Minoxidil.

Rohypnol. Roche, Puerto Rico†, brand of Flunitrazepam.

Rolaids. Parke-Davis brand of Dihydroxyaluminum Sodium Carbonate.

Romazicon. Roche brand of Flumazenil.

Romilar. Hoffmann-LaRoche-International brand of Dextromethorphan Hydrobromide.

Rompun. Bayer Animal Health brand of Xylazine Hydrochloride.

Rondomycin. Medpointe brand of Methacycline Hydrochloride.

Roniacol. Hoffmann-LaRoche† brand of Nicotinyl Alcohol.

Rovamycin. Rhone-Poulenc Rorer brand of Spiramycin.

Rowapraxin. Rowa Ltd., Ireland, brand of Pipoxolan Hydrochloride.

Rowasa. Alaven brand of Mesalamine.

Roxadyl. Sterling Winthrop brand of Rosoxacin.

Roxicodone. Roxane brand of Oxycodone Hydrochloride.

Rozerem. Takeda brand of Ramelteon.

Rubex. Bristol-Myers Squibb brand of Doxorubicin Hydrochloride.

Rubramin. Bristol-Myers Squibb brand of Cyanocobalamin.

Rubratope-57. Bristol-Myers Squibb† brand of Cyanocobalamin Co 57.

Rubratope-60. Bristol-Myers Squibb† brand of Cyanocobalamin Co 60.

r-UK. Abbott brand of Urokinase Alfa.

Rulide. Hoechst-Roussel† brand of Roxithromycin.

Rumensin [as sodium salt]. Lilly brand of Monensin.

RVPaba Lipstick. ICN† brand of Aminobenzoic Acid.

Rythmol. Reliant brand of Propafenone Hydrochloride.

Sabril. Hoechst Marion Roussel brand of Vigabatrin.

Saizen. Serono brand of Somatropin.

Salagen. MGI Pharma brand of Pilocarpine Hydrochloride.

Salicylic Acid Soap. Stiefel brand of Salicylic Acid.

Saligel. Stiefel† brand of Salicylic Acid.

Salisburystin. National Foundation for Cancer Research brand of Pentamustine.

Salizid. Parke-Davis† brand of Salinazid.

Salpix. Ortho-McNeil brand of Acetrizoate Sodium.

Saluron. Shire brand of Hydroflumethiazide.

Salyrgan. Sterling Winthrop† brand of Mersalyl.

Sanctura. Indevus brand of Trospium Chloride.

Sandimmune. Novartis brand of Cyclosporine.

Sandoglobulin. Novartis brand of Globulin, Immune.

Sandomigran. Novartis† brand of Pizotyline.

Sandopart. Novartis† brand of Demoxytocin.

Sandoptal. Novartis† brand of Butalbital.

Sandostatin. Novartis brand of Octreotide.

Sandostatin. Novartis brand of Octreotide Acetate.

Sandril. Lilly brand of Reserpine.

Sanorex. Novartis brand of Mazindol.

Sansert. Novartis brand of Methysergide Maleate.

Sarafem. Warner Chilcott brand of Fluoxetine Hydrochloride.

SaraFlox Injectable. Abbott brand of Sarafloxacin Hydrochloride.

SaraFlox WSP. Abbott brand of Sarafloxacin Hydrochloride.

Sarenin. Procter & Gamble brand of Saralasin Acetate.

Sarisol. Halsey brand of Butabarbital Sodium.

S.a.s. Solvay Pharmaceuticals brand of Sulfasalazine.

Sastid. Stiefel brand of Sulfur, Precipitated.

Sativex. GW Pharma Ltd brand of Nabiximols.

Scabene. Stiefel brand of Lindane.

Sclerosol. Bryan brand of Talc.

Seconal. Lilly† brand of Secobarbital.

Seconal Sodium. Ranbaxy brand of Secobarbital Sodium.

Secretin-Kabi. KabiVitrum, Sweden, brand of Secretin.

Sectral. Dr. Reddy's brand of Acebutolol Hydrochloride.

Sedamyl. 3M Pharmaceuticals† brand of Acecarbromal.

See3. Ciba Vision brand of Lotrafilcon A.

SeeQuence. Bausch & Lomb brand of Polymacon.

SeeQuence 2. Bausch & Lomb† brand of Polymacon.

Seffin. GlaxoSmithKline brand of Cephalothin Sodium.

Selacryn. SmithKline Beecham† brand of Ticrynafen.

Seldane. Merrell brand of Terfenadine.

Selecor. Rhone-Poulenc Rorer brand of Celiprolol Hydrochloride.

Selsun. Chattem brand of Selenium Sulfide.

Semap. Ortho-McNeil† brand of Penfluridol.

Semicid. Whitehall-Robins brand of Nonoxynol 9.

Semilente. Novo Nordisk† brand of Insulin Zinc, Prompt.

Semilente Iletin. Lilly brand of Insulin Zinc, Prompt.

Senokot. Purdue Frederick brand of Senna.

Sensipar. Amgen brand of Cinacalcet.

Sensipar. Amgen brand of Cinacalcet Hydrochloride.

Sensor. Abbott† brand of Fibrinogen I 125.

Sentry Dimethicone. Witco brand of Dimethicone.

Sentry Dimethicone Dispension. Witco brand of Dimethicone.

Sentry Polyox WSR. Union Carbide brand of Polyethylene Oxide.

Sentry Propylene Glycol. Union Carbide† brand of Propylene Glycol.

Sentry Simethicone. Witco brand of Simethicone.

Sentry Simethicone Emulsion. Witco brand of Simethicone.

Septanest. Cilag-Chemie, Switzerland, brand of Articaine Hydrochloride.

Septisol. Vestal brand of Hexachlorophene.

Septocaine. Cilag-Chemie, Switzerland, brand of Articaine Hydrochloride.

Serax. Alpharma brand of Oxazepam.

Serc. Unimed brand of Betahistine Hydrochloride.

Serenium. Bristol-Myers Squibb† brand of Ethoxazene Hydrochloride.

Serentil. Novartis brand of Mesoridazine Besylate.

Serevent. GlaxoSmithKline brand of Salmeterol Xinafoate.

SerLect. Abbott brand of Sertindole.

Sermion. Farmitalia, Societa Farmaceutici Italia, Italy, brand of Nicergoline.

Sernylan. Parke-Davis† brand of Phencyclidine Hydrochloride.

Seromycin. Lilly brand of Cycloserine.

Seroquel. AstraZeneca brand of Quetiapine Fumarate.

Serostim. Serono brand of Somatropin.

Serpasil. Novartis brand of Reserpine.

Serzone. Bristol-Myers Squibb brand of Nefazodone Hydrochloride.

Sethotope. Bristol-Myers Squibb† brand of Selenomethionine Se 75.

SGP 3. Permeable Technologies brand of Unifocon A.

Silsoft Aphakic. Bausch & Lomb brand of Elastofilcon A.

Silsoft Super Plus. Bausch & Lomb brand of Elastofilcon A.

Sil-Tech. Bausch & Lomb† brand of Elastofilcon A.

Silvadene. Hoechst Marion Roussel brand of Sulfadiazine, Silver.

Simdax. Orion Pharmaceutica, Finland, brand of Levosimendan.

Simulect. Novartis brand of Basiliximab.

Sinequan. Pfizer brand of Doxepin Hydrochloride.

Singulair. Merck brand of Montelukast Sodium.

Sirlene. Dow Chemical brand of Propylene Glycol.

Siseptin. Schering† brand of Sisomicin Sulfate.

SK-Bisacodyl. SmithKline Beecham† brand of Bisacodyl.

SK-Chloral Hydrate. SmithKline Beecham† brand of Chloral Hydrate.

Skelaxin. Jones brand of Metaxalone.

Skelaxin. King brand of Metaxalone.

Skelid. Sanofi Aventis brand of Tiludronate Disodium.

Skiodan Sodium. Sterling Winthrop† brand of Methiodal Sodium.

---

† Brand name formerly used, and/or firm no longer concerned with this product.

Slow-Fe. Ciba-Geigy† brand of Ferrous Sulfate.

Snow & Sun Sports Gel. Carrington brand of Acemannan.

Sodasorb. Grace brand of Soda Lime.

Sodium Omadine. Olin brand of Pyrithione Sodium.

Sodium Sulamyd. Schering brand of Sulfacetamide Sodium.

Soflens. Bausch & Lomb brand of Polymacon.

SofLens66. Bausch & Lomb brand of Alphafilcon A.

Sofspin. Bausch & Lomb brand of Polymacon.

Solacen. Wallace† brand of Tybamate.

Solaquin Forte. ICN brand of Hydroquinone.

Solaraze. Bioglan brand of Diclofenac Sodium.

Solatene. Hoffmann-LaRoche brand of Beta Carotene.

Solfoton. ECR† brand of Phenobarbital.

Solganal. Schering brand of Aurothioglucose.

Solodyn. Medicis brand of Minocycline Hydrochloride.

Soltamox. Rosemont brand of Tamoxifen Citrate.

Solu-cortef. Pfizer brand of Hydrocortisone Sodium Succinate.

Solu-medrol. Pfizer brand of Methylprednisolone Sodium Succinate.

Soma. Medpointe brand of Carisoprodol.

Somagard [as acetate]. Roberts Pharmaceutical brand of Deslorelin.

Somalgen. Laboratorio Bago, S.A., Argentina, brand of Talniflumate.

Somatokine. Avecia, UK, brand of Mecasermin Rinfabate.

Somavert. Pfizer brand of Pegvisomant.

Sombucaps. 3M Pharmaceuticals† brand of Hexobarbital.

Sombulex. 3M Pharmaceuticals† brand of Hexobarbital.

Somophyllin. Fisons brand of Aminophylline.

Sonacide. Wyeth-Ayerst brand of Glutaral.

Sonata. King brand of Zaleplon.

Sonazine. Sandoz brand of Chlorpromazine Hydrochloride.

Sonilyn. Carter-Wallace† brand of Sulfachlorpyridazine.

SonoVue (for the microbubble formulation). Ausimont brand of Sulfur Hexafluoride.

Sorbitrate. AstraZeneca brand of Isosorbide Dinitrate.

Sorboquel. Schering† brand of Calcium Polycarbophil.

Soriatane. Connetics brand of Acitretin.

Sorine. Upsher Smith brand of Sotalol Hydrochloride.

Sorlate. Abbott† brand of Polysorbate 80.

Sotradecol. Bioniche brand of Sodium Tetradecyl Sulfate.

Sotret. Ranbaxy brand of Isotretinoin.

Span 20. ICI Americas brand of Sorbitan Monolaurate.

Span 40. ICI Americas brand of Sorbitan Monopalmitate.

Span 60. ICI Americas brand of Sorbitan Monostearate.

Span 65. ICI Americas brand of Sorbitan Tristearate.

Span 80. ICI Americas brand of Sorbitan Monooleate.

Span 85. ICI Americas brand of Sorbitan Trioleate.

Sparine. Wyeth brand of Promazine Hydrochloride.

Spectazole. Johnson & Johnson brand of Econazole Nitrate.

Spectrobid. Pfizer brand of Bacampicillin Hydrochloride.

Spiriva. Boehringer Ingelheim KG, Germany, brand of Tiotropium Bromide.

Spiro-32. Unimed brand of Spirogermanium Hydrochloride.

Spiropitan. Janssen Pharmaceutica, Belgium, brand of Spiperone.

Spontin. Abbott† brand of Ristocetin.

Sporanox. Janssen brand of Itraconazole.

Spotton. Bayer Animal Health brand of Fenthion.

Sprycel. Bristol-Myers Squibb brand of Dasatinib.

St. Joseph Cough Syrup. Schering-Plough HealthCare† brand of Dextromethorphan Hydrobromide.

Stadol. Apothecon brand of Butorphanol Tartrate.

Stafac. SmithKline Beecham Animal Health brand of Virginiamycin.

Stanate. Torcan brand of Stannsoporfin.

Staphcillin. Apothecon brand of Methicillin Sodium.

Starfol Wax CG. Witco brand of Cetyl Esters Wax.

Starlix. Novartis brand of Nateglinide.

Stelazine. GlaxoSmithKline brand of Trifluoperazine Hydrochloride.

StemEx. Gamida Cell brand of Carlecortemcel-L.

StemEx. Teva, Israel, brand of Carlecortemcel-L.

Stenorol. Roussel-UCLAF, France, brand of Halofuginone Hydrobromide.

Sterane. Pfizer brand of Prednisolone.

Sterane. Pfizer brand of Prednisolone Acetate.

Sterisil. Parke-Davis† brand of Hexetidine.

Sterisol. Parke-Davis† brand of Hexedine.

Stilbestrol. Bristol-Myers Squibb brand of Diethylstilbestrol.

Stilbetin. Bristol-Myers Squibb brand of Diethylstilbestrol.

Stilphostrol. Bayer brand of Diethylstilbestrol Diphosphate.

Stimate. Behring brand of Desmopressin Acetate.

Stop. Oral-B brand of Stannous Fluoride.

Stovarsol. Abbott† brand of Acetarsone.

Stoxil. GlaxoSmithKline brand of Idoxuridine.

Strattera. Lilly brand of Atomoxetine Hydrochloride.

Streptase. Astra brand of Streptokinase.

Streptohydrazid. Pfizer brand of Streptonicozid.

Stresnil. Janssen Pharmaceutica, Belgium, brand of Azaperone.

Stri-Dex. Sterling Health U.S.A. brand of Salicylic Acid.

Stri-Dex Cleansing Bar. Sterling Health U.S.A. brand of Triclosan.

Stri-Dex Face Wash. Sterling Health U.S.A. brand of Triclosan.

Strifon. Ferndale brand of Chlorzoxazone.

Stromectol. Merck brand of Ivermectin.

Stronscan-85. Abbott† brand of Strontium Chloride Sr 85.

Strotope. Bristol-Myers Squibb† brand of Strontium Nitrate Sr 85.

Sublimaze. Akorn brand of Fentanyl Citrate.

Subose. Bristol-Myers Squibb† brand of Glyhexamide.

Subutex. Reckitt Benckiser brand of Buprenorphine Hydrochloride.

Sucaryl. Ross† brand of Saccharin Sodium.

Sucraid. QOL brand of Sacrosidase.

Sudafed. McNeil brand of Pseudoephedrine Hydrochloride.

Sufenta. Akorn brand of Sufentanil Citrate.

Suicalm. Janssen Pharmaceutica, Belgium, brand of Azaperone.

Sular. Sciele brand of Nisoldipine.

Sulfabid. Purdue Frederick brand of Sulfaphenazole.

Sulfacel. Optopics brand of Sulfacetamide Sodium.

Sulfamylon. Sterling Winthrop† brand of Mafenide.

Sulfamylon. UDL brand of Mafenide Acetate.

SulfaSURE SR Bolus [Veterinary]. Boehringer Ingelheim Animal Health brand of Sulfamethazine.

Sulfatryl. Wallace† brand of Trisulfapyrimidines.

Sulfonsol. Marion Merrell Dow† brand of Trisulfapyrimidines.

Sulfur Soap. Stiefel brand of Sulfur, Precipitated.

Sulka S Boluses [Veterinary]. Fort Dodge Animal Health brand of Sulfamethazine.

Sulla. Bayer brand of Sulfameter.

Sumycin. Par brand of Tetracycline Hydrochloride.

Sungard. Bayer† brand of Sulisobenzone.

Super Anahist. Parke-Davis brand of Thonzylamine Hydrochloride.

Superinone. Sterling Winthrop brand of Tyloxapol.

Supprelin. Roberts Pharmaceutical brand of Histrelin.

Suprane. Baxter Healthcare brand of Desflurane.

Suprax. Lupin brand of Cefixime.

Suprefact. Hoechst-Roussel† brand of Buserelin Acetate.

SUREVUE. Vistakon brand of Etafilcon A.

Surexin. Ortho-McNeil† brand of Pyrinoline.

Surfacaine. Lilly† brand of Cyclomethycaine Sulfate.

Surfak. Hoechst-Roussel† brand of Docusate Calcium.

Surgicel Absorbable Hemostat. Ethicon brand of Cellulose, Oxidized Regenerated.

Surgicel Fibrillar Absorbable Hemostat. Ethicon brand of Cellulose, Oxidized Regenerated.

Surgicel Nu-Knit Absorbable Hemostat. Ethicon brand of Cellulose, Oxidized Regenerated.

Surital. Parkdale brand of Thiamylal Sodium.

Surmax. Lilly brand of Avilamycin.

Surmontil. Wyeth-Ayerst brand of Trimipramine.

Surmontil. Odyssey brand of Trimipramine Maleate.

Survanta. Ross brand of Beractant.

Sustiva. Bristol-Myers Squibb brand of Efavirenz.

Sutent. Pfizer brand of Sunitinib Malate.

Sweeta. Bristol-Myers Squibb† brand of Saccharin.

Syllact. Carter-Wallace brand of Psyllium Husk.

Symadine. Solvay Pharmaceuticals brand of Amantadine Hydrochloride.

Symcor. Hoechst-Roussel† brand of Tiamenidine Hydrochloride.

Symcor Base TTS. Hoechst-Roussel† brand of Tiamenidine.

Symlin. Amylin brand of Pramlintide Acetate.

Symmetrel. Endo brand of Amantadine Hydrochloride.

Synacid [Veterinary]. Schering-Plough Animal Health brand of Hyaluronate Sodium.

Synalar. Medicis brand of Fluocinolone Acetonide.

Synanthic [Veterinary]. Syntex brand of Oxfendazole.

Synarel. Pfizer brand of Nafarelin Acetate.

Synchrocept [Veterinary]. Syntex brand of Prostalene.

Synchrocept B [Veterinary]. Syntex brand of Fenprostalene.

Syncillin. Bristol-Myers Squibb† brand of Phenethicillin Potassium.

Syncurine. GlaxoSmithKline brand of Decamethonium Bromide.

Synergeyes. Synergeyes brand of Paflufocon D-HEM-Iberfilcon A.

Syngestrotabs. Pfizer brand of Ethisterone.

Synkayvite. Roche brand of Menadiol Sodium Diphosphate.

Synsorb Pk. Synsorb brand of Galasomite.

Syntetrin. Bristol-Myers Squibb† brand of Rolitetracycline.

Synthroid. Abbott brand of Levothyroxine Sodium.

Syntocinon. Novartis brand of Oxytocin.

Syprine. Aton brand of Trientine Hydrochloride.

T-61. Hoechst-Roussel brand of Embutramide.

Tacaryl. Westwood-Squibb brand of Methdilazine.

Tacaryl. Westwood-Squibb brand of Methdilazine Hydrochloride.

Tace. Sanofi Aventis brand of Chlorotrianisene.

Tagamet. GlaxoSmithKline brand of Cimetidine.

Tagamet. GlaxoSmithKline brand of Cimetidine Hydrochloride.

Talamo. Marion Merrell Dow† brand of Amobarbital Sodium.

Talpheno. Marion Merrell Dow† brand of Phenobarbital.

Talsigel. Bristol-Myers Squibb† brand of Phthalylsulfacetamide.

Talwin. Sterling Winthrop brand of Pentazocine.

Talwin. Sanofi Aventis brand of Pentazocine Hydrochloride.

Talwin. Hospira brand of Pentazocine Lactate.

Tambocor. 3M Pharmaceuticals brand of Flecainide Acetate.

Tamiflu. Roche brand of Oseltamivir Phosphate.

TamoGel. Ascend Therapeutics brand of Afimoxifene.

Tandearil. Novartis brand of Oxyphenbutazone.

Tantum. Angelini Francesco, Italy, brand of Benzydamine Hydrochloride.

Tao. Pfizer brand of Troleandomycin.

Tapazole. King brand of Methimazole.

Taractan. Roche brand of Chlorprothixene.

Tarceva. Genentech brand of Erlotinib Hydrochloride.

Target. Wyeth-Ayerst brand of Felbinac.

Targocid. Hoechst Marion Roussel brand of Teicoplanin.

Targretin. Eisai Medical Research brand of Bexarotene.

TASK Tabs. Boehringer Ingelheim Animal Health brand of Dichlorvos.

Tasmaderm. Hoffmann-LaRoche† brand of Motretinide.

Tasmar. Valeant brand of Tolcapone.

Tavist. Novartis brand of Clemastine Fumarate.

Taxol. Bristol-Myers Squibb brand of Paclitaxel.

Taxotere. Sanofi Aventis brand of Docetaxel.

Tazicef. Hospira brand of Ceftazidime.

Tazidime. Lilly brand of Ceftazidime.

Tazorac. Allergan brand of Tazarotene.

Tc 99m DTPA Kit (chelate). Medi-Physics brand of Technetium Tc 99m Pentetate.

Tc 99m Generator. Medi-Physics brand of Sodium Pertechnetate Tc 99m.

TCC Soap. Monsanto† brand of Triclocarban.

Tearisol. Ciba Vision, US Ophthalmics, brand of Hypromellose.

Teceos. Hoechst-Roussel† brand of Butedronate Tetrasodium.

TechneColl. Mallinckrodt† brand of Technetium Tc 99m Sulfur Colloid.

Techneplex. Bracco Diagnostics brand of Technetium Tc 99m Pentetate.

TechneScan Gluceptate. Mallinckrodt brand of Technetium Tc 99m Gluceptate.

TechneScan HDP. Mallinckrodt brand of Technetium Tc 99m Oxidronate.

TechneScan HIDA. Mallinckrodt brand of Technetium Tc 99m Lidofenin.

TechneScan MAA. Mallinckrodt brand of Technetium Tc 99m Albumin Aggregated.

TechneScan MAG3. Mallinckrodt brand of Technetium Tc 99m Mertiatide.

TechneScan MDP. Mallinckrodt brand of Technetium Tc 99m Medronate.

TechneScan PYP. Mallinckrodt brand of Stannous Pyrophosphate.

TechneScan PYP Kit. Mallinckrodt brand of Technetium Tc 99m Pyrophosphate.

TechneScan Q-12. Mallinckrodt brand of Technetium Tc 99m Furifosmin.

TechneScan S.S.C. Mallinckrodt† brand of Stannous Sulfur Colloid.

TechneScan Sulfur Colloid. Mallinckrodt brand of Technetium Tc 99m Sulfur Colloid.

Technetium Tc 99m HSA. Medi-Physics brand of Technetium Tc 99m Albumin.

Technetium Tc 99m MAA. Medi-Physics brand of Technetium Tc 99m Albumin Aggregated.

Technetium Tc 99m TSC. Medi-Physics brand of Technetium Tc 99m Sulfur Colloid.

Teebacin. Consolidated Midland brand of Aminosalicylate Sodium.

Tegison. Roche brand of Etretinate.

Tegopen. Apothecon brand of Cloxacillin Sodium.

Tegretol. Novartis brand of Carbamazepine.

Telcyta. Telik brand of Canfosfamide Hydrochloride.

Teldrin. GlaxoSmithKline brand of Chlorpheniramine Maleate.

Telepaque. GE Healthcare brand of Iopanoic Acid.

Telintra. Telik brand of Ezatiostat Hydrochloride.

Telon. Novartis† brand of Benzpiperylon.

Telopar. Pfizer brand of Oxantel Pamoate.

Temaril. Allergan brand of Trimeprazine Tartrate.

Temodar. Schering brand of Temozolomide.

Temovate. Altana brand of Clobetasol Propionate.

Tempium. Hoffmann-LaRoche brand of Lazabemide Hydrochloride.

Tenex. Dr. Reddy's brand of Guanfacine Hydrochloride.

Tenormin. AstraZeneca brand of Atenolol.

Tenovil. Schering-Plough Research brand of Ilodecakin.

Tensilon. Valeant brand of Edrophonium Chloride.

Tenuate. Sanofi Aventis brand of Diethylpropion Hydrochloride.

Tepanil. 3M Pharmaceuticals brand of Diethylpropion Hydrochloride.

---

† Brand name formerly used, and/or firm no longer concerned with this product.

Tequin. Bristol-Myers Squibb brand of Gatifloxacin.

Terazol. Ortho-McNeil brand of Terconazole.

Terfonyl. Bristol-Myers Squibb† brand of Trisulfapyrimidines.

Teridax. Schering† brand of Iophenoxic Acid.

Teril. Taro brand of Carbamazepine.

Terramycin. Pfizer brand of Oxytetracycline.

Terramycin. Pfizer brand of Oxytetracycline Calcium.

Terramycin. Pfizer brand of Oxytetracycline Hydrochloride.

Teslac. Bristol-Myers Squibb brand of Testolactone.

Teslascan. GE Healthcare brand of Mangafodipir Trisodium.

Tessalon. Forest brand of Benzonatate.

Testim. Auxilium brand of Testosterone.

Testosterone. Pfizer brand of Testosterone Cypionate.

Testred. Valeant brand of Methyltestosterone.

Tesuloid. Bristol-Myers Squibb† brand of Technetium Tc 99m Sulfur Colloid.

Tetracyn. Pfizer brand of Tetracycline Hydrochloride.

Tetramet. Abbott† brand of Thyroxine I 125.

Tetrex. Bristol-Myers Squibb brand of Tetracycline Phosphate Complex.

Teveten. Abbott brand of Eprosartan Mesylate.

Thalamyd. Schering† brand of Phthalylsulfacetamide.

Thalitone. Monarch brand of Chlorthalidone.

Thalomid. Celgene brand of Thalidomide.

Tham. Hospira brand of Tromethamine.

The Alberta Lens SM2. Progressive Optical brand of Sulfocon B.

Theelin. Parkdale brand of Estrone.

Theelol. Parke-Davis† brand of Estriol.

Thenylene Hydrochloride. Abbott† brand of Methapyrilene Hydrochloride.

Theo-24. UCB brand of Theophylline.

Theocalcin. Knoll† brand of Theobromine Calcium Salicylate.

Theochron. Inwood brand of Theophylline.

Theocin. Sterling Winthrop† brand of Theophylline Sodium Acetate.

Theolair-sr. Graceway brand of Theophylline.

Thephorin. Hoffmann-LaRoche† brand of Phenindamine Tartrate.

Therabloat. SmithKline Beecham Animal Health brand of Poloxalene.

Theraclec. Altus brand of Liprotamase.

Therafectin. Greenwich brand of Amiprilose Hydrochloride.

Theralax. SmithKline Beecham† brand of Bisacodyl.

Therapeutic Mineral Ice. Bristol-Myers Products brand of Menthol.

Theriodide. Abbott† brand of Sodium Iodide I 131.

Thi-Di-Mer. Marion Merrell Dow† brand of Trisulfapyrimidines.

Thioban. Parke-Davis† brand of Thiocarbanidin.

Thiocymetin. Sterling Winthrop† brand of Thiamphenicol.

Thioplex. Immunex brand of Thiotepa.

Thiosulfil. Wyeth brand of Sulfamethizole.

Thonzide. Parke-Davis† brand of Thonzonium Bromide.

Thorazine. GlaxoSmithKline brand of Chlorpromazine.

Thorazine. GlaxoSmithKline brand of Chlorpromazine Hydrochloride.

THROMBATE III. Bayer brand of Antithrombin III Human.

Thrombostat. Parke-Davis brand of Thrombin.

Thypinone. Abbott brand of Protirelin.

Thyrel Trh. Ferring Pharmaceuticals brand of Protirelin.

Thyro-Block. Medpointe brand of Potassium Iodide.

Thyrogen. Genzyme brand of Thyrotropin Alfa.

Thyrolar. Forest brand of Liotrix.

Thyrosafe. R R Registrations brand of Potassium Iodide.

Thyroshield. Fleming brand of Potassium Iodide.

Thytropar. Sanofi Aventis brand of Thyrotropin.

Tiamate. Merck brand of Diltiazem Malate.

Tiazac. Biovail brand of Diltiazem Hydrochloride.

Ticar. GlaxoSmithKline brand of Ticarcillin Disodium.

Tice BCG. Organon brand of BCG Vaccine.

Ticlid. Roche brand of Ticlopidine Hydrochloride.

Tigan. King brand of Trimethobenzamide Hydrochloride.

Tigemen. Bristol-Myers Squibb† brand of Tigemonam Dicholine.

Tiguvon. Bayer Animal Health brand of Fenthion.

Tikosyn. Pfizer brand of Dofetilide.

Tilade. King brand of Nedocromil Sodium.

Timoptic. Merck brand of Timolol Maleate.

Tinactin. Schering-Plough HealthCare brand of Tolnaftate.

Tindal. Schering brand of Acetophenazine Maleate.

Tindamax. Mission brand of Tinidazole.

Tine Test. Lederle brand of Tuberculin.

Tine Test PPD. Lederle brand of Tuberculin.

Tinosorb M. Ciba Specialty Chemicals brand of Bisoctrizole.

Tinosorb S. Ciba Specialty Chemicals brand of Bemotrizinol.

Tiox [Veterinary]. Schering-Plough Animal Health† brand of Tioxidazole.

Tisercin. Egis brand of Levomepromazine Maleate.

Tiserton. Janssen brand of Ritanserin.

Tis-U-Sol. Baxter Healthcare brand of Pentalyte.

Tobi. Novartis brand of Tobramycin.

Tobrex. Alcon brand of Tobramycin.

Toclase. Pfizer brand of Carbetapentane Citrate.

Today Sponge. Whitehall-Robins† brand of Nonoxynol 9.

Tofranil. Tyco brand of Imipramine Hydrochloride.

Tolectin. Ortho-McNeil brand of Tolmetin Sodium.

Toleron. Mallinckrodt brand of Ferrous Fumarate.

Tolinase. Pfizer brand of Tolazamide.

Tolserol. Bristol-Myers Squibb† brand of Mephenesin.

Tomudex. Zeneca brand of Raltitrexed.

Toness. Angelini Francesco, Italy, brand of Proxazole Citrate.

Tonocard. AstraZeneca brand of Tocainide Hydrochloride.

Topamax. Ortho-McNeil brand of Topiramate.

Topicort. Taro brand of Desoximetasone.

Toprol. AstraZeneca brand of Metoprolol Succinate.

Toradol. Roche brand of Ketorolac Tromethamine.

Torecan. Novartis brand of Thiethylperazine Malate.

Torecan. Novartis brand of Thiethylperazine Maleate.

Tormosyl. Novartis† brand of Fluproquazone.

Tornalate. Sanofi Aventis brand of Bitolterol Mesylate.

Totacillin. GlaxoSmithKline brand of Ampicillin Sodium.

Tracervial-131. Abbott† brand of Sodium Iodide I 131.

Tracleer. Actelion brand of Bosentan.

Tracrium. Hospira brand of Atracurium Besylate.

Tradenal. Knoll† brand of Proscillaridin.

Tral. Abbott brand of Hexocyclium Methylsulfate.

Trancopal. Sanofi Aventis brand of Chlormezanone.

Trandate. Promethus brand of Labetalol Hydrochloride.

Transderm-Scop. Ciba-Geigy† brand of Scopolamine Hydrobromide.

Tranxene. Ovation brand of Clorazepate Dipotassium.

Trasicor. Novartis brand of Oxprenolol Hydrochloride.

Trasylol. Bayer brand of Aprotinin.

Travase. Abbott brand of Sutilains.

Travatan. Alcon brand of Travoprost.

Traxam. Wyeth-Ayerst brand of Felbinac.

Trecator. Wyeth brand of Ethionamide.

Trelstar. Watson brand of Triptorelin Pamoate.

Tremerase. Wyeth-Ayerst brand of Ciladopa Hydrochloride.

Tremin. Schering brand of Trihexyphenidyl Hydrochloride.

Trental. Sanofi Aventis brand of Pentoxifylline.

Trest. Novartis brand of Methixene Hydrochloride.

Triacet. Teva brand of Triamcinolone Acetonide.

Triazure. Parke-Davis† brand of Azaribine.

Triclos. Sanofi Aventis brand of Triclofos Sodium.

Tricor. Abbott brand of Fenofibrate.

Triderm. Del Ray brand of Triamcinolone Acetonide.

Tridione. Abbott brand of Trimethadione.

Triglide. Skyepharma brand of Fenofibrate.

Trilafon. Schering brand of Perphenazine.

Trileptal. Novartis brand of Oxcarbazepine.

Trimax. Sterling Winthrop brand of Magnesium Trisilicate.

Trimox. Apothecon brand of Amoxicillin.

Trimpex. Roche brand of Trimethoprim.

Trioleotope. Bristol-Myers Squibb† brand of Triolein I 131.

Triomet-125. Abbott† brand of Liothyronine I 125.

Triomet-131. Abbott† brand of Liothyronine I 131.

Triperidol. Ortho-McNeil† brand of Trifluperidol.

Trisenox. Cephalon brand of Arsenic Trioxide.

Trisoralen. Valeant brand of Trioxsalen.

Tritec. GlaxoSmithKline brand of Ranitidine Bismuth Citrate.

Tri-Thyrotope. Bristol-Myers Squibb† brand of Liothyronine I 131.

Tritin. Schering-Plough HealthCare† brand of Tolnaftate.

Tritiotope. Bristol-Myers Squibb† brand of Water, Tritiated.

Triton X-100. Union Carbide brand of Octoxynol 9.

Trizytek. Altus brand of Liprotamase.

Trobicin. Pfizer brand of Spectinomycin Hydrochloride.

Trocade. Hoffmann-LaRoche brand of Cipemastat.

Trofak. Synergen brand of Ersofermin.

Trolone. 3M Pharmaceuticals† brand of Sulthiame.

Tronolane. Ross brand of Pramoxine Hydrochloride.

Tronothane. Abbott brand of Pramoxine Hydrochloride.

Tropicacyl. Akorn brand of Tropicamide.

Trosinone. Abbott† brand of Ethisterone.

Trovan. Pfizer brand of Alatrofloxacin Mesylate.

Trovan. Pfizer brand of Trovafloxacin Mesylate.

Truozine. Abbott† brand of Trisulfapyrimidines.

Truphylline. G & W brand of Aminophylline.

Trusopt. Merck brand of Dorzolamide Hydrochloride.

Tuamine Sulfate. Lilly† brand of Tuaminoheptane Sulfate.

Tuasol 100. Marion Merrell Dow† brand of Tribromsalan.

Turgex. Xttrium brand of Hexachlorophene.

Tusscapine. Fisons† brand of Noscapine.

Tween 20. ICI Americas brand of Polysorbate 20.

Tween 40. ICI Americas brand of Polysorbate 40.

Tween 60. ICI Americas brand of Polysorbate 60.

Tween 65. ICI Americas brand of Polysorbate 65.

Tween 80. ICI Americas brand of Polysorbate 80.

Tween 85. ICI Americas brand of Polysorbate 85.

Twiston. Ortho-McNeil† brand of Rotoxamine Tartrate.

Twiston R-A. Ortho-McNeil† brand of Rotoxamine Tartrate.

Tydantil. Polichimica Sap, Italy, brand of Nifuratel.

Tygacil. Wyeth brand of Tigecycline.

Tykerb. GlaxoSmithKline brand of Lapatinib Ditosylate.

Tylan. Lilly brand of Tylosin.

Tylenol. McNeil brand of Acetaminophen.

Tymtran. Pfizer brand of Ceruletide Diethylamine.

Tyzeka. Idenix brand of Telbivudine.

Tyzine. Kenwood brand of Tetrahydrozoline Hydrochloride.

Ulcyn. Marion Merrell Dow† brand of Endobenzyline Bromide.

Ulo. 3M Pharmaceuticals brand of Chlophedianol Hydrochloride.

Ulpax. Hoffmann-LaRoche† brand of Ablukast Sodium.

Ultane. Abbott brand of Sevoflurane.

Ultiva. Abbott brand of Remifentanil Hydrochloride.

Ultra Tears. Alcon brand of Hypromellose.

Ultracaine. Hoechst AG, Germany, brand of Articaine Hydrochloride.

Ultracef. Bristol Labs† brand of Cefadroxil.

UltraCon. Specialty UltraVision brand of Carbosilfocon A.

Ultralente. Novo Nordisk† brand of Insulin Zinc, Extended.

Ultralente Iletin. Lilly brand of Insulin Zinc, Extended.

Ultram. Ortho-McNeil brand of Tramadol Hydrochloride.

UltraTag RBC. Mallinckrodt brand of Technetium Tc 99m Red Blood Cells.

Ultra-Technekow FM. Mallinckrodt brand of Sodium Pertechnetate Tc 99m.

Ultravist. Bayer brand of Iopromide.

Unilab Surgibone. Unilab brand of Surgibone.

Unipen. Wyeth brand of Nafcillin Sodium.

Uniphyl. Purdue Frederick brand of Theophylline.

Unisom. Pfizer brand of Doxylamine Succinate.

Unitensen. Medpointe brand of Cryptenamine Acetates.

Unithroid. Stevens J brand of Levothyroxine Sodium.

Unitop [Veterinary]. Hoffmann-LaRoche† brand of Cuprimyxin.

Univasc. Schwarz Pharma brand of Moexipril Hydrochloride.

Urbanyl. Hoechst-Roussel† brand of Clobazam.

Ureaphil. Hospira brand of Urea.

Urecholine. Odyssey brand of Bethanechol Chloride.

Urex. Vatring brand of Methenamine Hippurate.

Urispas. Ortho-McNeil brand of Flavoxate Hydrochloride.

Uritone. Parke-Davis† brand of Methenamine.

Urocit-K. Mission brand of Potassium Citrate.

Uromiro. Bracco Industria Chimica S.p.A., Italy, brand of Iodamide.

Uromiron. Bracco Industria Chimica S.p.A., Italy, brand of Iodamide.

Urotropin. Parke-Davis† brand of Methenamine.

Urovist Sodium. Berlex brand of Diatrizoate Sodium.

Uroxatral. Sanofi Aventis brand of Alfuzosin Hydrochloride.

Urso. Axcan Scandipharm brand of Ursodiol.

Utibid. Parke-Davis† brand of Oxolinic Acid.

Uticort. Pfizer brand of Betamethasone Benzoate.

Uvasorb HEB. 3V brand of Iscotrizinol.

Uvinul. BASF brand of Octisalate.

Uvinul M40. BASF brand of Oxybenzone.

Vagifem. Novo Nordisk brand of Estradiol.

Vagistat. Novartis brand of Tioconazole.

Valcor. Maggioni Farmaceutici S.p.A., Italy, brand of Droprenilamine.

Valcyte. Roche brand of Valganciclovir Hydrochloride.

Valisone. Schering brand of Betamethasone Valerate.

Valium. Roche brand of Diazepam.

Valmid. Dista brand of Ethinamate.

Valnac. Actavis brand of Betamethasone Valerate.

Valoron. Parke-Davis† brand of Tilidine Hydrochloride.

Valpin. Endo brand of Anisotropine Methylbromide.

Valstar. Indevus brand of Valrubicin.

Valtrex. GlaxoSmithKline brand of Valacyclovir Hydrochloride.

Vancenase. Schering brand of Beclomethasone Dipropionate.

Vanceril. Schering brand of Beclomethasone Dipropionate.

Vanclay. Vanderbilt brand of Kaolin.

Vancocin Hydrochloride. ViroPharma brand of Vancomycin Hydrochloride.

Vandazole. Teva brand of Metronidazole.

Vandid. 3M Pharmaceuticals† brand of Ethamivan.

Vaniqa. Skinmedica brand of Eflornithine Hydrochloride.

Vanobid. Sanofi Aventis brand of Candicidin.

Vanorm. Wyeth-Ayerst brand of Recainam Hydrochloride.

Vanos. Medicis brand of Fluocinonide.

Vanoxide. Dermik brand of Benzoyl Peroxide.

Vanseb-T. Allergan Herbert brand of Coal Tar.

Vansil. Pfizer brand of Oxamniquine.

Vantage. CooperVision brand of Tetrafilcon A.

Vantage Thin. CooperVision brand of Tetrafilcon A.

Vantin. Pfizer brand of Cefpodoxime Proxetil.

Vantol. Parke-Davis† brand of Bevantolol Hydrochloride.

Vaponefrin. Fisons† brand of Racepinephrine.

Vaprisol. Astellas brand of Conivaptan Hydrochloride.

Vascor. Johnson & Johnson brand of Bepridil Hydrochloride.

Vasocon. Novartis brand of Naphazoline Hydrochloride.

---

† Brand name formerly used, and/or firm no longer concerned with this product.

Vasodilan. Apothecon brand of Isoxsuprine Hydrochloride.
Vasodip. Recordati, Italy, brand of Lercanidipine Hydrochloride.
Vasotec. Biovail brand of Enalapril Maleate.
Vasotec. Biovail brand of Enalaprilat.
Vasoxyl. GlaxoSmithKline brand of Methoxamine Hydrochloride.
Vatensol. Pfizer brand of Guanoclor Sulfate.
V-Cillin. Lilly brand of Penicillin V.
V-cillin K. Lilly brand of Penicillin V Potassium.
Vectarion. Oril S.A., France, brand of Almitrine Mesylate.
Veegum. Vanderbilt brand of Magnesium Aluminum Silicate.
Veetids. Apothecon brand of Penicillin V Potassium.
Velban. Lilly brand of Vinblastine Sulfate.
Velcade. Millennium brand of Bortezomib.
Velosef. Apothecon brand of Cephradine.
Velosulin. Novo Nordisk brand of Insulin Human.
Venacil. Abbott† brand of Ancrod.
Venofer. American Regent brand of Iron Sucrose.
Venoglobulin-I. Alpha Therapeutic brand of Globulin, Immune.
Venoglobulin-S. Alpha Therapeutic brand of Globulin, Immune.
Ventaire. Sanofi Aventis brand of Protokylol Hydrochloride.
Ventavis. Actelion brand of Iloprost.
Ventolin. GlaxoSmithKline brand of Albuterol.
Ventolin. GlaxoSmithKline brand of Albuterol Sulfate.
Vepesid. Bristol-Myers Squibb brand of Etoposide.
Veramyst. GlaxoSmithKline brand of Fluticasone Furoate.
Vercyte. Abbott brand of Pipobroman.
Verecolene. Maggioni Farmaceutici S.p.A., Italy, brand of Fenci-butirol.
Veregen. Medigene brand of Sinecatechins.
Verelan. Elan brand of Verapamil Hydrochloride.
Veriloid. 3M Pharmaceuticals brand of Alkavervir.
Verluma. DuPont Merck brand of Technetium Tc 99m Nofetumo-mab Merpentan.
VersaLuma. DuPont Merck brand of Bisnafide Dimesylate.
Versapen. Bristol-Myers Squibb brand of Hetacillin.
Versapen-K. Bristol-Myers Squibb brand of Hetacillin Potassium.
Versed. Roche brand of Midazolam Hydrochloride.
Versene Acid. Dow Chemical brand of Edetic Acid.
Vertimil. Merck brand of Abamectin.
Vesanoid. Roche brand of Tretinoin.
Vesicare. Astellas brand of Solifenacin Succinate.
Vesprin. Apothecon brand of Triflupromazine.
Vesprin. Apothecon brand of Triflupromazine Hydrochloride.
Vetisulid [Veterinary]. Fort Dodge Animal Health brand of Sulfa-chlorpyridazine.
Vexol. Alcon brand of Rimexolone.
Vfend. Pfizer brand of Voriconazole.
Viadril. Pfizer brand of Hydroxydione Sodium Succinate.
Viadur. ALZA brand of Leuprolide Acetate.
Viagra. Pfizer brand of Sildenafil Citrate.
Vibramycin. Pfizer brand of Doxycycline.
Vibramycin. Pfizer brand of Doxycycline Calcium.
Vibramycin. Pfizer brand of Doxycycline Hyclate.
Vicks Formula 44. Procter & Gamble brand of Diphenhydramine Hydrochloride.
Vicryl. Ethicon brand of Polyglactin 910.
Vidaza. Pharmion brand of Azacitidine.
Videobil. Bracco Industria Chimica S.p.A., Italy, brand of Iopronic Acid.
Videocolangio. Bracco Industria Chimica S.p.A., Italy, brand of Io-doxamic Acid.
Videx. Bristol-Myers Squibb brand of Didanosine.
Vigamox. Alcon brand of Moxifloxacin Hydrochloride.
Vincrex. Bristol-Myers Squibb brand of Vincristine Sulfate.
Vinisil. Abbott† brand of Povidone.
Viocin Sulfate. Pfizer brand of Viomycin Sulfate.
Vioform. Ciba-Geigy† brand of Clioquinol.
Viokase. Robins brand of Pancrelipase.

Vioxx. Merck brand of Rofecoxib.
Viozan. AstraZeneca brand of Sibenadet Hydrochloride.
Vira-A. Parkdale brand of Vidarabine.
Viracept. Agouron brand of Nelfinavir Mesylate.
Viramidine. Valeant brand of Taribavirin Hydrochloride.
Viramune. Boehringer Ingelheim brand of Nevirapine.
Virazole. Valeant brand of Ribavirin.
Viread. Gilead Sciences brand of Tenofovir Disoproxil Fumarate.
Virend. Shaman brand of Crofelemer.
Viroptic. King brand of Trifluridine.
Visine. Pfizer brand of Oxymetazoline Hydrochloride.
Visipaque. GE Healthcare brand of Iodixanol.
Visken. Novartis brand of Pindolol.
Vistaril. Pfizer brand of Hydroxyzine Hydrochloride.
Vistaril. Pfizer brand of Hydroxyzine Pamoate.
Vistide. Gilead Sciences brand of Cidofovir.
Visudyne. QLT brand of Verteporfin.
Vitamin K1. Hospira brand of Phytonadione.
Vitrase. Biozyme Laboratories Ltd., UK, brand of Hyaluronidase (Ovine).
Vitrasert. Bausch & Lomb brand of Ganciclovir.
Vitravene. Novartis brand of Fomivirsen Sodium.
Vivactil. Odyssey brand of Protriptyline Hydrochloride.
Vivelle. Novartis brand of Estradiol.
Vivitrol. Alkermes brand of Naltrexone.
Vlemasque. Dermik† brand of Lime, Sulfurated.
Vlem-Dome. Bayer† brand of Lime, Sulfurated.
Volmax. Muro brand of Albuterol Sulfate.
Voltaren. Novartis brand of Diclofenac Sodium.
Voluven. Fresenius Kabi Deutschland GmbH brand of Hydro-xyethyl Starch 130/0.4.
Vonedrine. Marion Merrell Dow† brand of Phenpromethamine.
Vontil. SmithKline Beecham† brand of Thioproperazine Mesylate.
Vontrol. GlaxoSmithKline brand of Diphenidol Hydrochloride.
Vosol. Carter-Wallace brand of Acetic Acid.
VRX496. Virxsys brand of Lexgenleucel-T.
VS-7158. Witco brand of Cyclomethicone.
VS-7207. Witco brand of Cyclomethicone.
VS-7349. Witco brand of Cyclomethicone.
Vumon. Bristol-Myers Squibb brand of Teniposide.
Vyvanse. Shire brand of Lisdexamfetamine Dimesylate.
Weicon 60. Titmus Eurocon Kontaktlinsen GmbH & Co. KG, Ger-many, brand of Tefilcon A.
Welchol. Sankyo brand of Colesevelam Hydrochloride.
Wellbutrin. GlaxoSmithKline brand of Bupropion Hydrochloride.
Wellcovorin. GlaxoSmithKline brand of Leucovorin Calcium.
Wellferon. Glaxo Wellcome brand of Interferon Alfa-n1.
Wigrettes. Organon brand of Ergotamine Tartrate.
Winstrol. Ovation brand of Stanozolol.
Witcohol 66. Witco brand of Isostearyl Alcohol.
Witcohol 85. Witco brand of Oleyl Alcohol.
Witcohol 90. Witco brand of Oleyl Alcohol.
Wyamine Sulfate. Baxter Healthcare brand of Mephentermine Sul-fate.
Wyamycin. Wyeth brand of Erythromycin Ethylsuccinate.
Wydase. Wyeth-Ayerst brand of Hyaluronidase (Ovine).
Wytensin. Wyeth brand of Guanabenz Acetate.
Xalatan. Pfizer brand of Latanoprost.
Xanax. Pfizer brand of Alprazolam.
Xarelto. Bayer HealthCare brand of Sorafenib.
Xcytrin. Pharmacyclics brand of Motexafin Gadolinium.
Xeloda. Roche brand of Capecitabine.
Xeneisol. Mallinckrodt† brand of Xenon Xe 133.
Xenical. Roche brand of Orlistat.
Xenon Xe 133 Gas Ampule. Medi-Physics† brand of Xenon Xe 133.
Xenon Xe 133 Gas Vials. Medi-Physics† brand of Xenon Xe 133.
Xenon Xe 133-V.S.S. Medi-Physics† brand of Xenon Xe 133.

Xerecept. Hollister-Stier brand of Corticorelin Acetate.
Xibrom. Ista brand of Bromfenac Sodium.
Xifaxan. Salix brand of Rifaximin.
Xolair. Genentech brand of Omalizumab.
Xolegel. Barrier brand of Ketoconazole.
Xopenex. Sepracor brand of Levalbuterol Hydrochloride.
Xopenex. Sepracor brand of Levalbuterol Tartrate.
X-trozine. Shire Richwood brand of Phendimetrazine Tartrate.
Xylocaine. AstraZeneca brand of Lidocaine.
Xylocaine. Abraxis brand of Lidocaine Hydrochloride.
Xylo-Pfan. Savage brand of Xylose.
Xyotax. Amcis brand of Paclitaxel Poliglumex.
Xyrem. Jazz brand of Sodium Oxybate.
Xyzal. UCB brand of Levocetirizine Dihydrochloride.
YF-Vax. Bristol-Myers Squibb† brand of Yellow Fever Vaccine.
Yodoxin. Glenwood brand of Iodoquinol.
Yondelis. Pharma Mar brand of Trabectedin.
Yutopar. AstraZeneca brand of Ritodrine Hydrochloride.
Zactima. AstraZeneca brand of Vandetanib.
Zadaxin. SciClone brand of Thymalfasin.
Zaditor. Novartis brand of Ketotifen Fumarate.
Zagam. Mylan brand of Sparfloxacin.
Zanaflex. Acorda brand of Tizanidine Hydrochloride.
Zandip. Recordati, Italy, brand of Lercanidipine Hydrochloride.
Zanicor. Recordati, Italy, brand of Lercanidipine Hydrochloride.
Zanosar. Teva brand of Streptozocin.
Zantac. GlaxoSmithKline brand of Ranitidine Hydrochloride.
Zarontin. Pfizer brand of Ethosuximide.
Zaroxolyn. UCB brand of Metolazone.
Zavesca. Actelion brand of Miglustat.
Zaxopam. Quantum Pharmics brand of Oxazepam.
Zebeta. Duramed brand of Bisoprolol Fumarate.
Zectin. Merck brand of Abamectin.
Zefazone. Pfizer brand of Cefmetazole Sodium.
Zelapar. Valeant brand of Selegiline Hydrochloride.
Zelmac. Novartis brand of Tegaserod.
Zelnorm. Novartis brand of Tegaserod Maleate.
Zemiva. Molecular Insight brand of Iodofiltic Acid I 123.
Zemplar. Abbott brand of Paricalcitol.
Zemuron. Organon brand of Rocuronium Bromide.

Zenapax. Hoffmann-LaRoche brand of Daclizumab.
Zephiran Chloride. Sterling Winthrop brand of Benzalkonium Chloride.
Zerit. Bristol-Myers Squibb brand of Stavudine.
Zestril. AstraZeneca brand of Lisinopril.
Zetar. Dermik brand of Coal Tar.
Zetia. Merck/Schering-Plough brand of Ezetimibe.
Zettyn. Sterling Winthrop† brand of Cetalkonium Chloride.
Ziagen. GlaxoSmithKline brand of Abacavir Sulfate.
Zide. Solvay Pharmaceuticals brand of Hydrochlorothiazide.
Zinacef. GlaxoSmithKline brand of Cefuroxime Sodium.
Zinecard. Pharmacia & Upjohn brand of Dexrazoxane.
Zingo. Anesira brand of Lidocaine Hydrochloride.
Ziracin. Schering-Plough HealthCare brand of Evernimicin.
Zithromax. Pfizer brand of Azithromycin.
Zmax. Pfizer brand of Azithromycin.
Zocor. Merck brand of Simvastatin.
Zofran. GlaxoSmithKline brand of Ondansetron.
Zofran. GlaxoSmithKline brand of Ondansetron Hydrochloride.
Zoladex. Zeneca brand of Goserelin.
Zolinza. Merck brand of Vorinostat.
Zoloft. Pfizer brand of Sertraline Hydrochloride.
Zolyse. Alcon brand of Chymotrypsin.
Zomax. Ortho-McNeil† brand of Zomepirac Sodium.
Zomig. AstraZeneca brand of Zolmitriptan.
Zonalon. Bradley brand of Doxepin Hydrochloride.
Zonegran. Dainippon Pharmaceutical Co., Japan, brand of Zonisamide.
Zoprace. Bristol-Myers Squibb† brand of Zofenopril Calcium.
Zovirax. GlaxoSmithKline brand of Acyclovir.
Zovirax. GlaxoSmithKline brand of Acyclovir Sodium.
Zyban. GlaxoSmithKline brand of Bupropion Hydrochloride.
Zyflo. Sensus brand of Zileuton.
Zyloprim. Promethus brand of Allopurinol.
Zymar. Allergan brand of Gatifloxacin.
Zymase. Organon brand of Pancrelipase.
Zyprexa. Lilly brand of Olanzapine.
Zyrtec. Pfizer brand of Cetirizine Hydrochloride.
Zyvox. Pfizer brand of Linezolid.

---

† Brand name formerly used, and/or firm no longer concerned with this product.

Appendix II
USAN and USP and NF Names Listed by Category

The following list of names according to category of activity is compiled from the individual entries in the main list of the book. The compilation for this edition reflects an accommodation to several different pharmacologic and/or therapeutic classification schemes, with the result that some inconsistencies will be apparent. In the case of many new entries the sponsors of the USAN may not have complete information insofar as all of the categories of activity are concerned. Comments aimed toward the attainment of greater uniformity and usefulness in the pharmacologic classification system used herein will be welcomed, particularly if they are supported by authoritative information.

Abrasive

DENTAL
Pumice

Acaricide

VETERINARY
Nimidane

Acidifier
Ammonium Chloride (See also *Diuretic*)
Fumaric Acid
URINARY
Ascorbic Acid (See also *Vitamin (antiscorbutic)*)
Racemethionine

Adrenergic
Amidephrine Mesylate
Dopamine Hydrochloride
Ephedrine Sulfate
Epinephryl Borate
Esproquin Hydrochloride
Etafedrine Hydrochloride
Metaraminol Bitartrate
Prenalterol Hydrochloride
Tramazoline Hydrochloride
α₂-AGONIST
Apraclonidine Hydrochloride
α-BLOCKING
Dapiprazole Hydrochloride (See also *Antiglaucoma agent; Neuroleptic; Psychotropic*)
OPHTHALMIC
Adrenalone
Brimonidine Tartrate
Deterenol Hydrochloride
Dipivefrin
Epinephrine Bitartrate
Hydroxyamphetamine Hydrobromide
Oxidopamine
Phenylephrine Hydrochloride
VASOCONSTRICTOR
Epinephrine
Levonordefrin
Mephentermine Sulfate
Metizoline Hydrochloride
Naphazoline Hydrochloride
Norepinephrine Bitartrate
Octodrine (See also *Anesthetic (local)*)
Oxymetazoline Hydrochloride
Phenylpropanolamine Hydrochloride
Phenylpropanolamine Polistirex
Propylhexedrine
Pseudoephedrine Hydrochloride
Tetrahydrozoline Hydrochloride
Xylometazoline Hydrochloride

Adrenocortical steroid [See also **Glucocorticoid**]
Ciprocinonide
Dexamethasone Acetate
Flumoxonide
Hydrocortisone Hemisuccinate
Methylprednisolone Hemisuccinate
Procinonide
SALT-REGULATING
Desoxycorticosterone Acetate
Desoxycorticosterone Pivalate
Fludrocortisone Acetate
TOPICAL
Naflocort
Timobesone Acetate
Tipredane

Adrenocortical suppressant
Aminoglutethimide (See also *Antineoplastic*)
Trilostane

Adsorbant
Kaolin

Advanced colorectal cancer treatment
THYMIDYLATE SYNTHASE INHIBITOR
Raltitrexed

Aerosol propellant
Butane
Isobutane
Propane

Alcohol deterrent
Disulfiram

Aldosterone antagonist
Canrenoate Potassium
Canrenone
Dicirenone (See also *Hypotensive*)
Drospirenone
Eplerenone (See also *Antihypertensive*)
Mexrenoate Potassium
Prorenoate Potassium
Spironolactone (See also *Diuretic*)

Alkalizer
Potassium Citrate
Tromethamine
SYSTEMIC
Sodium Bicarbonate (See also *Replenisher (electrolyte)*)
Sodium Citrate
Tricitrates (See also *Alkalizer (urinary); Anti-urolithic (cystine calculi); Anti-urolithic (uric acid calculi); Buffer (neutralizing)*)
URINARY
Tricitrates (See also *Alkalizer (systemic); Anti-urolithic (cystine calculi); Anti-urolithic (uric acid calculi); Buffer (neutralizing)*)

Alzheimer's disease treatment

ADJUNCT
Cevimeline Hydrochloride
Donepezil Hydrochloride (See also *Dementia symptoms treatment adjunct; Cognition adjuvant; Inhibitor (acetylcholinesterase)*)
Sabcomeline Hydrochloride
CHOLINERGIC AGONIST
Tazomeline Citrate
Xanomeline
Xanomeline Tartrate
COGNITION ENHANCER
Besipirdine Hydrochloride
Icopezil Maleate (See also *Cognition adjuvant; Inhibitor (acetylcholinesterase)*)
Linopirdine
Sibopirdine (See also *Nootropic*)
MUSCARINIC M₁-AGONIST
Talsaclidine Fumarate

Amino acid
Alanine
Aspartic Acid
Cysteine Hydrochloride
Cystine
Histidine
Isoleucine
Leucine
Lysine
Lysine Acetate
Lysine Hydrochloride
Methionine
Phenylalanine
Proline
Serine

Threonine
Tryptophan
Tyrosine
Valine

Ammonia detoxicant
Arginine (See also *Diagnostic aid (pituitary function determination)*)
Arginine Glutamate
Arginine Hydrochloride

Amyotrophic lateral sclerosis treatment
Riluzole

Anabolic
Bolandiol Dipropionate
Bolasterone
Boldenone Undecylenate
Bolenol
Bolmantalate
Ethylestrenol
Methenolone Acetate
Methenolone Enanthate
Mibolerone (See also *Androgen*)
Nandrolone Cyclotate
Norbolethone
Pizotyline (See also *Antidepressant; Serotonin inhibitor (specific in migraine)*)
Quinbolone
Stenbolone Acetate
Zeranol

VETERINARY
Trenbolone Acetate

Analeptic
TREATMENT OF NARCOLEPSY AND HYPERSOMNIA
Modafinil

Analgesic
Acetaminophen (See also *Antipyretic*)
Aminobenzoate Potassium
Aminobenzoate Sodium
Anidoxime
Anilopam Hydrochloride
Anirolac (See also *Anti-inflammatory*)
Antipyrine
Aspirin (See also *Antipyretic; Antirheumatic*)
Benoxaprofen (See also *Anti-inflammatory*)
Benzydamine Hydrochloride (See also *Antipyretic; Anti-inflammatory*)
Bicifadine Hydrochloride
Bromadoline Maleate
Bromfenac Sodium
Buprenorphine Hydrochloride
Butacetin (See also *Antidepressant*)
Butixirate (See also *Antirheumatic*)
Butorphanol (See also *Antitussive*)
Butorphanol Tartrate (See also *Antitussive*)
Carbamazepine (See also *Anticonvulsant*)
Carbaspirin Calcium
Carbiphene Hydrochloride
Ciprefadol Succinate
Ciramadol
Ciramadol Hydrochloride

Clonixeril
Clonixin
Conorphone Hydrochloride
Cyclazocine
Dexibuprofen (See also *Anti-inflammatory*)
Dexoxadrol Hydrochloride (See also *Stimulant (central)*)
Dexpemedolac
Dezocine
Diflunisal (See also *Anti-inflammatory*)
Dihydrocodeine Bitartrate
Dimefadane
Dipyrone (See also *Antipyretic*)
Doxpicomine Hydrochloride
Drinidene
Enadoline Hydrochloride
Epirizole (See also *Anti-inflammatory*)
Ethoxazene Hydrochloride
Etofenamate (See also *Anti-inflammatory*)
Fenoprofen (See also *Anti-inflammatory*)
Fenoprofen Calcium (See also *Anti-inflammatory*)
Floctafenine
Flufenisal
Flunixin (See also *Anti-inflammatory*)
Flunixin Meglumine (See also *Anti-inflammatory*)
Flupirtine Maleate
Fluproquazone
Fluradoline Hydrochloride
Flurbiprofen (See also *Anti-inflammatory*)
Ibufenac (See also *Anti-inflammatory*)
Indoprofen (See also *Anti-inflammatory*)
Ketazocine
Ketorfanol
Ketorolac Tromethamine
Letimide Hydrochloride
Levonantradol Hydrochloride
Lofemizole Hydrochloride (See also *Anti-inflammatory; Antipyretic*)
Lorcinadol
Lornoxicam (See also *Anti-inflammatory*)
Magnesium Salicylate (See also *Antipyretic; Antirheumatic*)
Mefenamic Acid (See also *Anti-inflammatory*)
Menabitan Hydrochloride
Meptazinol Hydrochloride
Methopholine
Methotrimeprazine
Metkephamid Acetate
Mimbane Hydrochloride
Mirfentanil Hydrochloride
Molinazone
Moxazocine (See also *Antitussive*)
Nabitan Hydrochloride
Nalbuphine Hydrochloride (See also *Antagonist (to narcotics)*)
Nalmexone Hydrochloride (See also *Antagonist (to narcotics)*)
Namoxyrate
Nantradol Hydrochloride

Naproxen (See also *Anti-inflammatory; Antipyretic*)
Naproxen Sodium (See also *Anti-inflammatory; Antipyretic*)
Naproxol (See also *Anti-inflammatory; Antipyretic*)
Nefopam Hydrochloride
Nexeridine Hydrochloride
Noracymethadol Hydrochloride
Octazamide
Olvanil
Pemedolac
Pentazocine
Pentazocine Hydrochloride
Pentazocine Lactate
Phenyramidol Hydrochloride (See also *Relaxant (skeletal muscle)*)
Picenadol Hydrochloride
Pinadoline
Pirfenidone (See also *Anti-inflammatory; Antipyretic*)
Piroxicam Betadex (See also *Anti-inflammatory; Antirheumatic*)
Piroxicam Olamine (See also *Anti-inflammatory*)
Pravadoline Maleate
Prodilidine Hydrochloride
Profadol Hydrochloride
Propiram Fumarate
Propoxyphene Hydrochloride
Propoxyphene Napsylate
Proxazole (See also *Relaxant (smooth muscle); Anti-inflammatory*)
Proxazole Citrate (See also *Relaxant (smooth muscle); Anti-inflammatory*)
Proxorphan Tartrate (See also *Antitussive*)
Pyrroliphene Hydrochloride
Remifentanil Hydrochloride
Salcolex (See also *Anti-inflammatory; Antipyretic*)
Salethamide Maleate
Salicylamide
Salicylate Meglumine (See also *Antirheumatic*)
Salsalate (See also *Anti-inflammatory*)
Sodium Salicylate
Spiradoline Mesylate
Sufentanil
Talmetacin (See also *Anti-inflammatory; Antipyretic*)
Talniflumate (See also *Anti-inflammatory*)
Talosalate (See also *Anti-inflammatory*)
Tazadolene Succinate
Tebufelone (See also *Anti-inflammatory*)
Tetrydamine (See also *Anti-inflammatory*)
Tifurac Sodium
Tilidine Hydrochloride
Tiopinac (See also *Anti-inflammatory; Antipyretic*)
Tonazocine Mesylate
Tramadol Hydrochloride
Trefentanil Hydrochloride
Trolamine (See also *Pharmaceutic aid (alkalizing agent)*)

Veradoline Hydrochloride
Verilopam Hydrochloride
Volazocine
Xorphanol Mesylate
Xylazine Hydrochloride (See also *Relaxant (muscle, veterinary)*)
Zenazocine Mesylate
Zomepirac Sodium (See also *Anti-inflammatory*)

CYCLOOXYGENASE INHIBITOR
Dexibuprofen Lysine (See also *Anti-inflammatory*)

DENTAL
Eugenol

NARCOTIC
Alfentanil Hydrochloride
Anileridine
Anileridine Hydrochloride
Brifentanil Hydrochloride
Carfentanil Citrate
Codeine (See also *Antitussive*)
Codeine Phosphate (See also *Antitussive*)
Codeine Sulfate (See also *Antitussive*)
Fentanyl Citrate
Hydromorphone Hydrochloride
Levomethadyl Acetate
Levomethadyl Acetate Hydrochloride
Levorphanol Tartrate
Lofentanil Oxalate
Meperidine Hydrochloride
Methadone Hydrochloride
Methadyl Acetate
Morphine Sulfate
Ocfentanil Hydrochloride
Oxycodone
Oxycodone Hydrochloride
Oxycodone Terephthalate
Oxymorphone Hydrochloride
Pentamorphone
Sufentanil Citrate

SPECIFIC IN MIGRAINE
Ergotamine Tartrate
Oxetorone Fumarate

TOPICAL
Capsaicin (See also *Antineuralgic, specific pain syndromes, topical*)
Zucapsaicin

URINARY TRACT
Phenazopyridine Hydrochloride

VETERINARY
Detomidine Hydrochloride (See also *Sedative-hypnotic*)
Medetomidine Hydrochloride (See also *Sedative (veterinary)*)

Anaplasmodastat [See also **Antiprotozoal**]

VETERINARY
Gloxazone

Androgen
Fluoxymesterone
Mesterolone
Methyltestosterone
Mibolerone (See also *Anabolic*)
Nandrolone Decanoate
Nandrolone Phenpropionate

Nisterime Acetate
Oxandrolone
Oxymetholone
Silandrone
Stanozolol
Testosterone
Testosterone Cypionate
Testosterone Enanthate
Testosterone Ketolaurate
Testosterone Phenylacetate
Testosterone Propionate
Trestolone Acetate (See also *Antineoplastic*)

Anesthesia, adjunct to
Sodium Oxybate

Anesthesia
GENERAL
Veterinary
Embutramide

Anesthetic
Desflurane
Dexivacaine
Etoxadrol Hydrochloride
Ketamine Hydrochloride
Minaxolone
Phencyclidine Hydrochloride
Tiletamine Hydrochloride (See also *Anticonvulsant*)

INHALATION
Aliflurane
Cyclopropane
Enflurane
Ether
Fluroxene
Halothane
Isoflurane
Methoxyflurane
Nitrous Oxide
Norflurane
Roflurane
Sevoflurane
Teflurane

INJECTABLE
Midazolam Hydrochloride

INTRAVENOUS
Methohexital Sodium
Midazolam Maleate
Propanidid
Propofol
Thiamylal
Thiamylal Sodium
Thiopental Sodium (See also *Anticonvulsant*)

LOCAL
Bupivacaine Hydrochloride
Chloroprocaine Hydrochloride
Diamocaine Cyclamate
Dibucaine
Dibucaine Hydrochloride
Etidocaine
Levoxadrol Hydrochloride (See also *Relaxant (smooth muscle)*)
Lidocaine Hydrochloride
Mepivacaine Hydrochloride

Octodrine (See also *Adrenergic (vasoconstrictor)*)
Prilocaine
Prilocaine Hydrochloride
Procaine Hydrochloride
Propoxycaine Hydrochloride
Pyrrocaine
Risocaine
Rodocaine
Salicyl Alcohol
Tetracaine Hydrochloride

TOPICAL
Benoxinate Hydrochloride
Benzocaine
Biphenamine Hydrochloride (See also *Antibacterial; Antifungal*)
Butamben
Butamben Picrate
Cocaine
Cocaine Hydrochloride
Dyclonine Hydrochloride
Ethyl Chloride
Euprocin Hydrochloride
Isobutamben
Lidocaine
Oxethazaine
Pramoxine Hydrochloride
Tetracaine
Zolamine Hydrochloride (See also *Antihistaminic*)

Ophthalmic
Proparacaine Hydrochloride

Anhidrotic
Aluminum Chlorohydrate
Aluminum Chlorohydrex Polyethylene Glycol
Aluminum Chlorohydrex Propylene Glycol
Aluminum Dichlorohydrate
Aluminum Dichlorohydrex Polyethylene Glycol
Aluminum Dichlorohydrex Propylene Glycol
Aluminum Sesquichlorohydrate
Aluminum Sesquichlorohydrex Polyethylene Glycol
Aluminum Sesquichlorohydrex Propylene Glycol
Aluminum Zirconium Octachlorohydrate
Aluminum Zirconium Octachlorohydrex Gly
Aluminum Zirconium Pentachlorohydrate
Aluminum Zirconium Pentachlorohydrex Gly
Aluminum Zirconium Tetrachlorohydrate
Aluminum Zirconium Tetrachlorohydrex Gly
Aluminum Zirconium Trichlorohydrate
Aluminum Zirconium Trichlorohydrex Gly

Anorexic
Aminorex
Amphecloral
Chlorphentermine Hydrochloride

Clominorex
Clortermine Hydrochloride
Diethylpropion Hydrochloride
Fenfluramine Hydrochloride
Fenisorex
Fludorex (See also *Anti-emetic*)
Fluminorex
Levamfetamine Succinate
Mazindol
Mefenorex Hydrochloride
Phenmetrazine Hydrochloride
Phentermine
Sibutramine Hydrochloride (See also *Antidepressant*)

Antacid
Algeldrate
Almadrate Sulfate
Almagate
Aluminum Carbonate, Basic
Aluminum Hydroxide
Aluminum Hydroxide, Dried
Aluminum Phosphate
Bismuth Subsalicylate (See also *Antidiarrheal; Anti-ulcerative*)
Calcium Carbonate
Dihydroxyaluminum Aminoacetate
Dihydroxyaluminum Sodium Carbonate
Magaldrate
Magnesia, [Milk of] (See also *Laxative*)
Magnesium Carbonate
Magnesium Hydroxide (See also *Laxative*)
Magnesium Phosphate
Magnesium Trisilicate
Polyethadene
Potassium Glucaldrate
Silodrate

Antagonist
TO ALCOHOL AND NARCOTICS
Nadide
ANGIOTENSIN II RECEPTOR
Candesartan (See also *Antihypertensive*)
Candesartan Cilexetil (See also *Antihypertensive*)
Telmisartan (See also *Antihypertensive*)
α_2-RECEPTOR
Atipamezole
TO BENZODIAZEPINE
Flumazenil
BRADYKININ
Deltibant
Icatibant Acetate
TO CALCIUM
Tiapamil Hydrochloride
CALCIUM CHANNEL
Clentiazem Maleate
Isradipine
Nilvadipine
Teludipine Hydrochloride (See also *Antihypertensive*)
CHOLECYSTOKININ
Devazepide
ENDOTHELIN RECEPTOR
Bosentan

TO HISTAMINE H$_2$ AND H$_1$ RECEPTORS
Icotidine
TO HISTAMINE H$_2$ RECEPTORS
Cimetidine
Cimetidine Hydrochloride
Donetidine
Etintidine Hydrochloride
Famotidine
Metiamide
Oxmetidine Hydrochloride
Oxmetidine Mesylate
Ranitidine
Ranitidine Bismuth Citrate
Ranitidine Hydrochloride
Sufotidine
Tiotidine
Zaltidine Hydrochloride
Veterinary
Lupitidine Hydrochloride
LHRH
Abarelix (See also *Gonad-stimulating principle*)
Detirelix Acetate
TO NARCOTICS
Fenmetozole Hydrochloride (See also *Antidepressant*)
Nalbuphine Hydrochloride (See also *Analgesic*)
Nalmefene
Nalmexone Hydrochloride (See also *Analgesic*)
Naloxone Hydrochloride
Naltrexone
Oxilorphan
OPIOID
Quadazocine Mesylate
OXYTOCIN
Atosiban
THROMBOXANE A$_2$
Vapiprost Hydrochloride

Anterior pituitary activator
Epimestrol
FOR SWINE
Methallibure

Anterior pituitary suppressant
Danazol

Anthelmintic
Albendazole
Anthelmycin
Bromoxanide
Bunamidine Hydrochloride
Butonate
Cambendazole
Carbantel Lauryl Sulfate
Clioxanide
Closantel
Cyclobendazole
Dichlorvos
Diethylcarbamazine Citrate
Dribendazole
Dymanthine Hydrochloride
Etibendazole
Fenbendazole
Furodazole
Hexylresorcinol

Mebendazole
Morantel Tartrate
Niclosamide
Nitramisole Hydrochloride
Nitrodan
Oxantel Pamoate
Oxfendazole
Oxibendazole
Parbendazole
Piperamide Maleate
Piperazine
Piperazine Citrate
Piperazine Edetate Calcium
Proclonol (See also *Antifungal*)
Pyrantel Pamoate
Pyrantel Tartrate
Pyrvinium Pamoate
Rafoxanide
Stilbazium Iodide
Tetramisole Hydrochloride
Thiabendazole
Ticarbodine
Tioxidazole
Triclofenol Piperazine
Vincofos
Zilantel
VETERINARY
Butamisole Hydrochloride
Crufomate
Febantel
Fospirate
Imcarbofos
Lobendazole
Naftalofos
Netobimin
Nitroscanate
Phthalofyne
Praziquantel
Salantel
Thenium Closylate
Trichlorfon
Uredofos

Anti-acne
Adapalene
Azelaic Acid
Erythromycin Salnacedin
Inocoterone Acetate
Isotretinoin Anisatil

Anti-adrenergic
Bretylium Tosylate (See also *Cardiac depressant (anti-arrhythmic)*)
Dihydroergotamine Mesylate
Phentolamine Mesylate
Solypertine Tartrate
Zolertine Hydrochloride (See also *Vasodilator*)
α-RECEPTOR
Fenspiride Hydrochloride (See also *Bronchodilator*)
Labetalol Hydrochloride (See also *Anti-adrenergic (β-receptor)*)
Proroxan Hydrochloride
β-RECEPTOR
Acebutolol
Acebutolol Hydrochloride
Alprenolol Hydrochloride
Atenolol

Bunolol Hydrochloride
Carteolol Hydrochloride
Celiprolol Hydrochloride
Cetamolol Hydrochloride
Cicloprolol Hydrochloride
Dexpropranolol Hydrochloride (See also *Cardiac depressant (anti-arrhythmic)*)
Diacetolol Hydrochloride
Dilevalol Hydrochloride (See also *Antihypertensive*)
Esmolol Hydrochloride
Exaprolol Hydrochloride
Flestolol Sulfate
Labetalol Hydrochloride (See also *Antiadrenergic (α-receptor)*)
Levobetaxolol Hydrochloride
Levobunolol Hydrochloride
Metalol Hydrochloride
Metoprolol
Metoprolol Tartrate
Nadolol
Pamatolol Sulfate
Penbutolol Sulfate
Practolol
Propranolol Hydrochloride (See also *Cardiac depressant (anti-arrhythmic)*)
Sotalol Hydrochloride
Timolol
Timolol Maleate
Tiprenolol Hydrochloride
Tolamolol (See also *Vasodilator (coronary); Cardiac depressant (anti-arrhythmic)*)

Anti-allergic

Amlexanox
Astemizole (See also *Antihistaminic*)
Azelastine Hydrochloride (See also *Anti-asthmatic*)
Eclazolast (See also *Inhibitor (mediator release)*)
Emedastine Difumarate (See also *Antihistaminic, H₁-receptor; Asthma prophylactic*)
Lodoxamide Ethyl (See also *Anti-asthmatic*)
Lodoxamide Tromethamine (See also *Anti-asthmatic*)
Nivimedone Sodium
Olopatadine Hydrochloride
Oxatomide (See also *Anti-asthmatic*)
Pemirolast Potassium (See also *Inhibitor (mediator release)*)
Pentigetide
Pirquinozol
Poison Oak Extract
Proxicromil
Repirinast (See also *Anti-asthmatic*)
Tetrazolast Meglumine (See also *Anti-asthmatic*)
Thiazinamium Chloride
Tiacrilast
Tiacrilast Sodium
Tiprinast Meglumine
Tixanox
PROPHYLACTIC
Minocromil

Nedocromil
Nedocromil Calcium
Nedocromil Sodium
Probicromil Calcium

Anti-amebic [See also **Antiprotozoal**]

Berythromycin (See also *Antibacterial*)
Bialamicol Hydrochloride
Chloroquine (See also *Antimalarial*)
Chloroquine Hydrochloride (See also *Antimalarial*)
Chloroquine Phosphate (See also *Antimalarial; Suppressant (lupus erythematosus)*)
Clamoxyquin Hydrochloride
Clioquinol (See also *Anti-infective, topical*)
Emetine Hydrochloride
Iodoquinol
Paromomycin Sulfate
Quinfamide
Symetine Hydrochloride
Teclozan
Tetracycline (See also *Antibacterial; Antirickettsial*)
Tetracycline Hydrochloride (See also *Antibacterial; Antirickettsial*)

Anti-androgen

Benorterone
Cioteronel
Cyproterone Acetate
Delmadinone Acetate (See also *Progestin; Anti-estrogen*)
Topterone
Zanoterone

BENIGN PROSTATIC HYPERTROPHY
Oxendolone

Anti-anemic [See also **Hematinic**]

Epoetin Alfa (See also *Hematinic*)
Epoetin Beta (See also *Hematinic*)
Ferrous Sulfate, Dried
FOLATE DEFICIENCY
Leucovorin Calcium (See also *Antidote (to folic acid antagonists)*)

Anti-anginal

Amlodipine Besylate (See also *Antihypertensive*)
Amlodipine Maleate (See also *Antihypertensive*)
Betaxolol Hydrochloride (See also *Antihypertensive*)
Bevantolol Hydrochloride (See also *Antihypertensive; Cardiac depressant (anti-arrhythmic)*)
Butoprozine Hydrochloride (See also *Cardiac depressant (anti-arrhythmic)*)
Carvedilol (See also *Antihypertensive*)
Cinepazet Maleate
Metoprolol Succinate (See also *Antihypertensive*)
Molsidomine (See also *Vasodilator (coronary)*)
Monatepil Maleate (See also *Antihypertensive*)

Primidolol (See also *Antihypertensive; Cardiac depressant (anti-arrhythmic)*)
Ranolazine Hydrochloride
Tosifen
Verapamil Hydrochloride (See also *Cardiac depressant (anti-arrhythmic)*)

Anti-anxiety agent

Adatanserin Hydrochloride (See also *Antidepressant*)
Alpidem
Binospirone Mesylate
Bretazenil
Glemanserin
Ipsapirone Hydrochloride
Itasetron (See also *Antidepressant; Anti-emetic*)
Mirisetron Maleate
Ocinaplon
Ondansetron Hydrochloride (See also *Anti-emetic; Antischizophrenic*)
Pagoclone
Panadiplon
Pancopride (See also *Anti-emetic; Stimulant (peristaltic)*)
Pazinaclone
Serazapine Hydrochloride
Sunepitron Hydrochloride (See also *Antidepressant*)
Tandospirone Citrate
Zalospirone Hydrochloride

Anti-arthritic

Atiprimod Dihydrochloride (See also *Anti-inflammatory*)
Atiprimod Dimaleate (See also *Anti-inflammatory; Immunomodulator*)
Lodelaben (See also *Emphysema therapy adjunct*)

Anti-asthmatic

Atreleuton (See also *Inhibitor (5-lipoxygenase)*)
Azelastine Hydrochloride (See also *Anti-allergic*)
Bunaprolast
Cromitrile Sodium
Enofelast
Isamoxole
Ketotifen Fumarate
Levcromakalim (See also *Antihypertensive*)
Lodoxamide Ethyl (See also *Anti-allergic*)
Lodoxamide Tromethamine (See also *Anti-allergic*)
Oxarbazole
Oxatomide (See also *Anti-allergic*)
Piriprost
Piriprost Potassium
Pirolate
Quazolast (See also *Inhibitor (mediator release)*)
Quiflapon Sodium (See also *Suppressant (inflammatory bowel disease)*)
Repirinast (See also *Anti-allergic*)
Tetrazolast Meglumine (See also *Anti-allergic*)
Tiaramide Hydrochloride

Tibenelast Sodium (See also *Bronchodilator*)
Tranilast
Verofylline (See also *Bronchodilator*)

LEUKOTRIENE ANTAGONIST
Ablukast
Ablukast Sodium
Cinalukast
Montelukast Sodium
Ontazolast
Pobilukast Edamine
Ritolukast
Sulukast
Tomelukast
Verlukast
Zafirlukast

PROPHYLACTIC
Cromolyn Sodium

SELECTIVE PHOSPHODIESTERASE IV INHIBITOR
Filaminast

THROMBOXANE RECEPTOR ANTAGONIST
Seratrodast (See also *Anti-inflammatory* (*nonantihistaminic*))

TYPE IV PHOSPHODIESTERASE INHIBITOR
Arofylline (See also *Asthma prophylactic; Bronchodilator*)
Piclamilast

Anti-atherosclerotic
Mifobate
Pamaqueside (See also *Hypocholesterolemic*)
Timefurone

Antibacterial
Alamecin
Alatrofloxacin Mesylate
Alexidine
Amdinocillin
Amdinocillin Pivoxil
Amicycline
Amifloxacin
Amifloxacin Mesylate
Amikacin
Amikacin Sulfate
Amoxicillin
Amphomycin
Ampicillin
Ampicillin Sodium
Apalcillin Sodium
Apramycin
Aspartocin
Asperlin (See also *Antineoplastic*)
Astromicin Sulfate
Avilamycin
Avoparcin
Azithromycin
Azlocillin
Azlocillin Sodium
Bacampicillin Hydrochloride
Bacitracin
Bacitracin Methylene Disalicylate (See also *Food additive* (*veterinary*))
Bacitracin Zinc
Bambermycins
Berythromycin (See also *Anti-amebic*)
Betamicin Sulfate

Biapenem
Biniramycin
Biphenamine Hydrochloride (See also *Anesthetic* (*topical*)*; Antifungal*)
Bispyrithione Magsulfex (See also *Antidandruff; Antifungal*)
Butikacin
Butirosin Sulfate
Carbadox
Carbenicillin Disodium
Carbenicillin Indanyl Sodium
Carbenicillin Phenyl Sodium
Carbenicillin Potassium
Carumonam Sodium
Cefaclor
Cefadroxil
Cefamandole
Cefamandole Nafate
Cefamandole Sodium
Cefaparole
Cefatrizine
Cefazaflur Sodium
Cefbuperazone
Cefdinir
Cefepime
Cefepime Hydrochloride
Cefetecol
Cefixime
Cefmenoxime Hydrochloride
Cefmetazole
Cefmetazole Sodium
Cefonicid Monosodium
Cefonicid Sodium
Cefoperazone Sodium
Ceforanide
Cefotaxime Sodium
Cefotetan
Cefotetan Disodium
Cefotiam Hydrochloride
Cefoxitin
Cefoxitin Sodium
Cefpimizole
Cefpimizole Sodium
Cefpiramide
Cefpiramide Sodium
Cefpirome Sulfate
Cefpodoxime Proxetil
Cefprozil
Cefroxadine
Cefsulodin Sodium
Ceftazidime
Ceftibuten
Ceftizoxime Sodium
Ceftriaxone Sodium
Cefuroxime
Cefuroxime Axetil
Cefuroxime Pivoxetil
Cefuroxime Sodium
Cephacetrile Sodium
Cephalexin
Cephalexin Hydrochloride
Cephaloglycin
Cephaloridine
Cephalothin Sodium
Cephapirin Sodium
Cephradine
Cetocycline Hydrochloride
Cetophenicol

Chloramphenicol (See also *Antirickettsial*)
Chloramphenicol Palmitate (See also *Antirickettsial*)
Chloramphenicol Pantothenate Complex (See also *Antirickettsial*)
Chloramphenicol Sodium Succinate (See also *Antirickettsial*)
Chlorhexidine Phosphanilate
Chloroxylenol
Chlortetracycline Bisulfate (See also *Antiprotozoal*)
Chlortetracycline Hydrochloride (See also *Antiprotozoal*)
Cinoxacin
Ciprofloxacin
Ciprofloxacin Hydrochloride
Cirolemycin (See also *Antineoplastic*)
Clarithromycin
Clinafloxacin Hydrochloride
Clindamycin
Clindamycin Hydrochloride
Clindamycin Palmitate Hydrochloride
Clindamycin Phosphate
Cloxacillin Benzathine
Cloxacillin Sodium
Cloxyquin
Colistimethate Sodium
Colistin Sulfate
Coumermycin
Coumermycin Sodium
Cyclacillin
Dalfopristin
Daptomycin
Demeclocycline
Demeclocycline Hydrochloride
Demecycline
Denofungin (See also *Antifungal*)
Diaveridine
Dicloxacillin
Dicloxacillin Sodium
Dihydrostreptomycin Sulfate
Dipyrithione (See also *Antifungal*)
Dirithromycin
Doxycycline
Doxycycline Calcium (See also *Antiprotozoal*)
Doxycycline Fosfatex
Doxycycline Hyclate
Droxacin Sodium
Enoxacin
Eperezolid
Epicillin
Epitetracycline Hydrochloride
Erythromycin
Erythromycin Acistrate
Erythromycin Estolate
Erythromycin Ethylsuccinate
Erythromycin Gluceptate
Erythromycin Lactobionate
Erythromycin Propionate
Erythromycin Stearate
Fleroxacin
Floxacillin
Fludalanine
Flumequine
Fosfomycin
Fosfomycin Tromethamine

Fumoxicillin
Furazolium Chloride
Furazolium Tartrate
Fusidate Sodium
Fusidic Acid
Gatifloxacin
Gentamicin Sulfate
Gloximonam
Gramicidin
Grepafloxacin Hydrochloride
Haloprogin
Hetacillin
Hetacillin Potassium
Hexedine
Ibafloxacin
Imipenem
Isoconazole (See also *Antifungal*)
Josamycin
Kanamycin Sulfate
Kitasamycin
Levofloxacin
Levofuraltadone (See also *Antiprotozoal*)
Levopropylcillin Potassium
Lexithromycin
Lincomycin
Lincomycin Hydrochloride
Linezolid
Lomefloxacin
Lomefloxacin Hydrochloride
Lomefloxacin Mesylate
Loracarbef
Mafenide
Meclocycline
Meclocycline Sulfosalicylate
Megalomicin Potassium Phosphate
Mequidox
Meropenem
Methacycline
Methacycline Hydrochloride
Methicillin Sodium
Metioprim
Metronidazole Hydrochloride
Metronidazole Phosphate (See also *Antiprotozoal*)
Mezlocillin
Mezlocillin Sodium
Minocycline
Minocycline Hydrochloride
Mirincamycin Hydrochloride (See also *Antimalarial*)
Monensin (See also *Antiprotozoal; Antifungal*)
Monensin Sodium (See also *Antifungal; Antiprotozoal*)
Nafcillin Sodium
Nalidixate Sodium
Nalidixic Acid
Nebramycin
Neomycin Palmitate
Neomycin Sulfate
Neomycin Undecylenate (See also *Antifungal*)
Netilmicin Sulfate
Neutramycin
Nifuradene
Nifuraldezone

Nifuratel (See also *Antifungal; Antiprotozoal (Trichomonas)*)
Nifuratrone
Nifurdazil
Nifurimide
Nifurpirinol
Nifurquinazol
Nifurthiazole
Nitrocycline
Nitromide (See also *Coccidiostat (for poultry)*)
Norfloxacin
Novobiocin Sodium
Ofloxacin
Ormetoprim
Oxacillin Sodium
Oximonam
Oximonam Sodium
Oxolinic Acid
Oxytetracycline
Oxytetracycline Calcium
Oxytetracycline Hydrochloride (See also *Antirickettsial*)
Paldimycin
Paulomycin
Pefloxacin
Pefloxacin Mesylate
Penamecillin
Penicillin G Benzathine
Penicillin G Potassium
Penicillin G Procaine
Penicillin G Sodium
Penicillin V
Penicillin V Benzathine
Penicillin V Hydrabamine
Penicillin V Potassium
Pentizidone Sodium
Piperacillin
Piperacillin Sodium
Pirbenicillin Sodium
Piridicillin Sodium
Pirlimycin Hydrochloride
Pivampicillin Hydrochloride
Pivampicillin Pamoate
Pivampicillin Probenate
Polymyxin B Sulfate
Porfiromycin (See also *Antineoplastic*)
Propikacin
Pyrithione Zinc (See also *Antifungal; Antiseborrheic*)
Quindecamine Acetate
Quinupristin
Racephenicol
Ramoplanin
Ranimycin
Relomycin
Repromicin
Rifametane
Rifamexil
Rifamide
Rifampin
Rifapentine
Rifaximin
Rolitetracycline
Rolitetracycline Nitrate
Rosaramicin
Rosaramicin Butyrate
Rosaramicin Propionate

Rosaramicin Sodium Phosphate
Rosaramicin Stearate
Rosoxacin
Roxarsone
Roxithromycin
Sancycline
Sanfetrinem Cilexetil
Sanfetrinem Sodium
Sarmoxicillin
Sarpicillin
Scopafungin (See also *Antifungal*)
Sisomicin
Sisomicin Sulfate
Sparfloxacin
Spectinomycin Hydrochloride
Spiramycin
Stallimycin Hydrochloride
Steffimycin (See also *Antiviral*)
Streptonicozid
Sulfabenz (See also *Coccidiostat (for poultry)*)
Sulfabenzamide
Sulfacetamide
Sulfacetamide Sodium
Sulfacytine
Sulfadiazine
Sulfadiazine Sodium
Sulfadoxine
Sulfalene
Sulfamerazine
Sulfameter
Sulfamethazine
Sulfamethizole
Sulfamethoxazole
Sulfamonomethoxine
Sulfamoxole
Sulfanilate Zinc
Sulfanitran (See also *Coccidiostat (for poultry)*)
Sulfasalazine
Sulfasomizole
Sulfathiazole
Sulfazamet
Sulfisoxazole
Sulfisoxazole Acetyl
Sulfisoxazole Diolamine
Sulfomyxin
Sulopenem
Sultamicillin
Suncillin Sodium
Talampicillin Hydrochloride
Teicoplanin
Temocillin
Tetracycline (See also *Anti-amebic; Antirickettsial*)
Tetracycline Hydrochloride (See also *Anti-amebic; Antirickettsial*)
Tetracycline Phosphate Complex
Tetroxoprim
Thiamphenicol
Thiphencillin Potassium
Ticarcillin Cresyl Sodium
Ticarcillin Disodium
Ticarcillin Monosodium
Ticlatone (See also *Antifungal*)
Tiodonium Chloride
Tobramycin
Tobramycin Sulfate

Tosufloxacin
Trimethoprim
Trimethoprim Sulfate
Trisulfapyrimidines
Troleandomycin
Trospectomycin Sulfate
Trovafloxacin Mesylate
Tyrothricin
Vancomycin
Vancomycin Hydrochloride
Virginiamycin (See also *Food additive* (*veterinary*))
Zorbamycin

AMINOGLYCOSIDE
Isepamicin

ANTIMYCOBACTERIAL
Rifabutin
Rifalazil

LEPROSTATIC
Acedapsone (See also *Antimalarial*)
Acetosulfone Sodium
Clofazimine (See also *Antibacterial* (*tuberculostatic*))
Dapsone (See also *Suppressant* (*dermatitis herpetiformis*))

MICROBIAL DNA TOPOISOMERASE INHIBITOR
Temafloxacin Hydrochloride

OPHTHALMIC
Natamycin

SYSTEMIC
Cefazolin
Cefazolin Sodium

TOPICAL
Mupirocin
Mupirocin Calcium
Parachlorophenol

TUBERCULOSTATIC
Aminosalicylate Sodium
Aminosalicylic Acid
Benzoylpas Calcium
Capreomycin Sulfate
Clofazimine (See also *Antibacterial* (*leprostatic*))
Cycloserine
Ethambutol Hydrochloride
Ethionamide
Isoniazid
Phenyl Aminosalicylate
Pyrazinamide
Streptomycin Sulfate

URINARY
Methenamine
Methenamine Hippurate
Methenamine Mandelate
Nitrofurantoin

VETERINARY
Arsanilic Acid
Binfloxacin
Cefetamet
Cefquinome Sulfate
Ceftiofur Hydrochloride
Ceftiofur Sodium
Cinodine Hydrochloride
Cuprimyxin (See also *Antifungal*)
Danofloxacin Mesylate
Enrofloxacin

Florfenicol
Iprocinodine Hydrochloride
Nithiamide
Premafloxacin
Sedecamycin
Sulfachlorpyridazine
Thiostrepton
Tiamulin
Tiamulin Fumarate
Tilmicosin
Tilmicosin Phosphate

Antibacterial enzyme
Lysostaphin

Anticholelithic
DISSOLUTION OF GALLSTONES
Monoctanoin

Anticholelithogenic
Chenodiol
Ursodiol

Anticholinergic
Alverine Citrate
Anisotropine Methylbromide
Atropine
Atropine Oxide Hydrochloride
Benapryzine Hydrochloride
Benzetimide Hydrochloride
Benzilonium Bromide
Biperiden (See also *Antiparkinsonian*)
Biperiden Hydrochloride (See also *Antiparkinsonian*)
Biperiden Lactate (See also *Antiparkinsonian*)
Clidinium Bromide
Dexetimide
Dicyclomine Hydrochloride
Dihexyverine Hydrochloride
Domazoline Fumarate
Elantrine
Ethybenztropine
Glycopyrrolate
Heteronium Bromide
Homatropine Methylbromide
Hyoscyamine
Hyoscyamine Hydrobromide
Hyoscyamine Sulfate
Isopropamide Iodide
Mepenzolate Bromide
Methylatropine Nitrate
Metoquizine
Oxybutynin Chloride
Parapenzolate Bromide
Pentapiperium Methylsulfate
Phencarbamide
Poldine Methylsulfate
Proglumide
Propantheline Bromide
Propenzolate Hydrochloride
Tematropium Methylsulfate
Tofenacin Hydrochloride
Tolterodine
Toquizine
Triampyzine Sulfate
Trihexyphenidyl Hydrochloride (See also *Antiparkinsonian*)
GASTRIC
Elucaine

Tiquinamide Hydrochloride
OPHTHALMIC
Atropine Sulfate
Cyclopentolate Hydrochloride
Eucatropine Hydrochloride
Homatropine Hydrobromide
Scopolamine Hydrobromide
Tropicamide

Anticoagulant
Ancrod
Ardeparin Sodium
Argatroban
Bivalirudin (See also *Antithrombotic*)
Bromindione
Dalteparin Sodium (See also *Antithrombotic*)
Desirudin
Dicumarol
Heparin Calcium
Heparin Sodium
Lyapolate Sodium
Nafamostat Mesylate (See also *Antifibrinolytic*)
Phenprocoumon
Tinzaparin Sodium (See also *Antithrombotic*)
Warfarin Sodium

FOR PLASMA AND FOR BLOOD FOR FRACTIONATION
Anticoagulant Sodium Citrate
FOR STORAGE OF WHOLE BLOOD
Anticoagulant Citrate Dextrose
Anticoagulant Citrate Phosphate Dextrose
Anticoagulant Citrate Phosphate Dextrose Adenine
Anticoagulant Heparin

Anticoccidal
Maduramicin

Anticonvulsant
Albutoin
Ameltolide
Atolide
Buramate (See also *Antipsychotic*)
Carbamazepine (See also *Analgesic*)
Cinromide
Citenamide
Clonazepam
Cyheptamide
Dezinamide
Dimethadione
Divalproex Sodium
Eterobarb
Ethosuximide
Ethotoin
Flurazepam Hydrochloride (See also *Relaxant* (*muscle*); *Sedative-hypnotic*)
Fluzinamide
Fosphenytoin Sodium
Gabapentin
Ilepcimide
Lamotrigine
Magnesium Sulfate (See also *Laxative; Replenisher* (*electrolyte*))
Mephenytoin

Mephobarbital (See also *Sedative-hypnotic*)
Methetoin
Methsuximide
Milacemide Hydrochloride (See also *Antidepressant*)
Nabazenil
Nafimidone Hydrochloride
Nitrazepam (See also *Sedative-hypnotic*)
Phenacemide
Phenobarbital (See also *Sedative-hypnotic*)
Phenobarbital Sodium (See also *Sedative-hypnotic*)
Phensuximide
Phenytoin
Phenytoin Sodium
Pregabalin
Primidone
Progabide (See also *Relaxant (muscle)*)
Ralitoline
Ropizine
Sabeluzole (See also *Antihypoxic*)
Stiripentol
Sulthiame
Thiopental Sodium (See also *Anesthetic (intravenous)*)
Tiagabine Hydrochloride
Tiletamine Hydrochloride (See also *Anesthetic*)
Topiramate
Trimethadione
Valproate Sodium
Valproic Acid
Zoniclezole Hydrochloride
Zonisamide

NEUROPROTECTIVE
Remacemide Hydrochloride

TARDIVE DYSKINESIA
Vigabatrin

Antidandruff
Bispyrithione Magsulfex (See also *Antibacterial; Antifungal*)

Antidementia
PARTIAL MUSCARINIC AGONIST
Milameline Hydrochloride

Antidepressant
Adatanserin Hydrochloride (See also *Anti-anxiety agent*)
Adinazolam (See also *Sedative-hypnotic*)
Adinazolam Mesylate
Alaproclate
Aletamine Hydrochloride
Amedalin Hydrochloride
Amitriptyline Hydrochloride
Amoxapine
Aptazapine Maleate
Azaloxan Fumarate
Azepindole
Azipramine Hydrochloride
Beloxepin
Bipenamol Hydrochloride
Bupropion Hydrochloride
Butacetin (See also *Analgesic*)

Butriptyline Hydrochloride
Caroxazone
Cartazolate
Ciclazindol
Cidoxepin Hydrochloride
Cilobamine Mesylate
Clodazon Hydrochloride
Clomipramine Hydrochloride
Cotinine Fumarate
Cyclindole
Cypenamine Hydrochloride
Cyprolidol Hydrochloride
Cyproximide (See also *Antipsychotic*)
Daledalin Tosylate
Dapoxetine Hydrochloride
Dazadrol Maleate
Dazepinil Hydrochloride
Desipramine Hydrochloride
Dexamisole
Deximafen
Dibenzepin Hydrochloride
Dioxadrol Hydrochloride
Dothiepin Hydrochloride
Doxepin Hydrochloride
Duloxetine Hydrochloride
Eclanamine Maleate
Encyprate
Etoperidone Hydrochloride
Fantridone Hydrochloride
Fenmetozole Hydrochloride (See also *Antagonist (to narcotics)*)
Fenmetramide
Fezolamine Fumarate
Fluotracen Hydrochloride (See also *Antipsychotic*)
Fluoxetine
Fluoxetine Hydrochloride
Fluparoxan Hydrochloride
Gamfexine
Guanoxyfen Sulfate (See also *Antihypertensive*)
Imafen Hydrochloride
Imiloxan Hydrochloride
Imipramine Hydrochloride
Indeloxazine Hydrochloride
Intriptyline Hydrochloride
Iprindole
Isocarboxazid
Itasetron (See also *Anti-anxiety agent; Anti-emetic*)
Ketipramine Fumarate
Lofepramine Hydrochloride
Lortalamine
Maprotiline
Maprotiline Hydrochloride
Melitracen Hydrochloride
Milacemide Hydrochloride (See also *Anticonvulsant*)
Minaprine Hydrochloride
Mirtazapine
Moclobemide
Modaline Sulfate
Napactadine Hydrochloride
Napamezole Hydrochloride
Napitane Mesylate
Nefazodone Hydrochloride
Nisoxetine
Nitrafudam Hydrochloride

Nomifensine Maleate
Nortriptyline Hydrochloride
Octriptyline Phosphate
Opipramol Hydrochloride (See also *Antipsychotic*)
Oxaprotiline Hydrochloride
Oxypertine
Paroxetine
Phenelzine Sulfate
Pirandamine Hydrochloride
Pizotyline (See also *Anabolic; Serotonin inhibitor (specific in migraine)*)
Pramipexole (See also *Antiparkinsonian; Antischizophrenic; Dopamine agonist*)
Pramipexole Dihydrochloride (See also *Antiparkinsonian; Antischizophrenic; Dopamine agonist*)
Pridefine Hydrochloride
Prolintane Hydrochloride
Protriptyline Hydrochloride
Quipazine Maleate (See also *Oxytocic*)
Rolicyprine
Seproxetine Hydrochloride
Sertraline Hydrochloride
Sibutramine Hydrochloride (See also *Anorexic*)
Sulpiride
Sunepitron Hydrochloride (See also *Anti-anxiety agent*)
Suritozole
Tametraline Hydrochloride
Tampramine Fumarate
Tandamine Hydrochloride
Thiazesim Hydrochloride
Thozalinone
Trazodone Hydrochloride
Trebenzomine Hydrochloride
Trimipramine
Trimipramine Maleate
Venlafaxine Hydrochloride
Viloxazine Hydrochloride
Zimeldine Hydrochloride
Zometapine

Antidiabetic
Acetohexamide
Amlintide
Buformin
Butoxamine Hydrochloride (See also *Antihyperlipoproteinemic*)
Camiglibose
Chlorpropamide
Ciglitazone
Englitazone Sodium
Etoformin Hydrochloride
Gliamilide
Glibornuride
Glicetanile Sodium
Gliflumide
Glipizide
Glucagon
Glyburide
Glyhexamide
Glymidine Sodium
Glyoctamide
Glyparamide
Insulin
Insulin, Dalanated

Insulin Human
Insulin Human, Isophane
Insulin Human Zinc
Insulin Human Zinc, Extended
Insulin, Isophane
Insulin Lispro
Insulin, Neutral
Insulin Zinc
Insulin Zinc, Extended
Insulin Zinc, Prompt
Linogliride
Linogliride Fumarate
Metformin
Metformin Hydrochloride
Methyl Palmoxirate
Palmoxirate Sodium
Pioglitazone Hydrochloride
Pirogliride Tartrate
Pramlintide
Proinsulin Human
Rosiglitazone Maleate
Seglitide Acetate
Tolazamide
Tolbutamide
Tolpyrramide
Troglitazone
Zopolrestat (See also *Inhibitor (aldose reductase)*)

Antidiarrheal
Bismuth Subsalicylate (See also *Antacid; Anti-ulcerative*)
Rolgamidine

Antidiuretic
Argipressin Tannate
Desmopressin Acetate
Lypressin (See also *Vasoconstrictor*)

Antidote
ALCOHOL DEHYDROGENASE INHIBITOR
Fomepizole

TO ARSENIC AND GOLD AND MERCURY POISONING
Dimercaprol

TO CURARE PRINCIPLES
Edrophonium Chloride (See also *Diagnostic aid (myasthenia gravis)*)

TO CYANIDE POISONING
Methylene Blue (See also *Antimethemoglobinemic*)
Sodium Nitrite
Sodium Thiosulfate

TO FOLIC ACID ANTAGONISTS
Leucovorin Calcium (See also *Anti-anemic (folate deficiency)*)
Levoleucovorin Calcium

GENERAL PURPOSE
Charcoal, Activated (See also *Pharmaceutic aid (adsorbant)*)

TO HEPARIN
Protamine Sulfate

TO IRON POISONING
Deferoxamine Mesylate (See also *Chelating agent*)

TO PHOSPHORUS
Cupric Sulfate

Antidyskinetic
Cabergoline (See also *Antihyperprolactinemic; Dopamine agonist*)
Entacapone
Selegiline Hydrochloride (See also *Antiparkinsonian (in combination with levodopa/carbidopa)*)

IN GILLES DE LA TOURETTE'S DISEASE
Haloperidol (See also *Antipsychotic*)

Anti-eczematic
TOPICAL
Coal Tar

Anti-emetic
Alosetron Hydrochloride
Batanopride Hydrochloride
Bemesetron
Benzquinamide
Chlorpromazine (See also *Antipsychotic*)
Chlorpromazine Hydrochloride (See also *Antipsychotic*)
Clebopride
Cyclizine Hydrochloride
Dimenhydrinate
Diphenidol
Diphenidol Hydrochloride
Diphenidol Pamoate
Dolasetron Mesylate (See also *Antimigraine*)
Domperidone
Dronabinol
Fludorex (See also *Anorexic*)
Flumeridone
Galdansetron Hydrochloride
Granisetron
Granisetron Hydrochloride
Itasetron (See also *Anti-anxiety agent ; Antidepressant*)
Lurosetron Mesylate
Meclizine Hydrochloride
Metoclopramide Hydrochloride
Metopimazine
Ondansetron Hydrochloride (See also *Anti-anxiety agent ; Antischizophrenic*)
Palonosetron Hydrochloride (See also *Antinauseant*)
Pancopride (See also *Anti-anxiety agent ; Stimulant (peristaltic)*)
Prochlorperazine
Prochlorperazine Edisylate (See also *Antipsychotic*)
Prochlorperazine Maleate (See also *Antipsychotic*)
Promethazine Hydrochloride (See also *Antihistaminic*)
Thiethylperazine
Thiethylperazine Malate
Thiethylperazine Maleate
Trimethobenzamide Hydrochloride
Zacopride Hydrochloride (See also *Stimulant (peristaltic)*)

Anti-epileptic
Felbamate
Loreclezole

CONTROL OF ABNORMAL MOVEMENTS
Tolgabide

Anti-estrogen
Clometherone
Clomiphene Citrate
Delmadinone Acetate (See also *Progestin; Anti-androgen*)
Nafoxidine Hydrochloride
Nitromifene Citrate
Raloxifene Hydrochloride
Tamoxifen Citrate
Toremifene Citrate (See also *Antineoplastic*)
Trioxifene Mesylate

Antifibrinolytic
Nafamostat Mesylate (See also *Anticoagulant*)

Antiflatulent
Simethicone

Antifungal
Acrisorcin
Ambruticin
Amphotericin B
Azaconazole
Azaserine
Basifungin
Bifonazole
Biphenamine Hydrochloride (See also *Anesthetic (topical); Antibacterial*)
Bispyrithione Magsulfex (See also *Antibacterial; Antidandruff*)
Butenafine Hydrochloride
Butoconazole Nitrate
Calcium Undecylenate
Candicidin
Chlordantoin
Ciclopirox
Ciclopirox Olamine
Cilofungin
Cisconazole
Clotrimazole
Cuprimyxin (See also *Antibacterial (veterinary)*)
Denofungin (See also *Antibacterial*)
Dipyrithione (See also *Antibacterial*)
Doconazole
Econazole
Econazole Nitrate
Enilconazole
Ethonam Nitrate
Fenticonazole Nitrate
Filipin
Fluconazole
Flucytosine
Fungimycin
Griseofulvin
Hamycin
Isoconazole (See also *Antibacterial*)
Itraconazole
Kalafungin
Ketoconazole
Lomofungin
Lydimycin
Mepartricin (See also *Antiprotozoal*)
Metacresol (See also *Antiseptic (topical); Antifungal (veterinary)*)

Miconazole
Miconazole Nitrate
Monensin (See also *Antiprotozoal; Antibacterial*)
Monensin Sodium (See also *Antibacterial; Antiprotozoal*)
Naftifine Hydrochloride
Neomycin Undecylenate (See also *Antibacterial*)
Nifuratel (See also *Antibacterial; Antiprotozoal (Trichomonas)*)
Nifurmerone
Nitralamine Hydrochloride
Nystatin
Octanoic Acid
Omoconazole Nitrate
Orconazole Nitrate
Oxiconazole Nitrate
Oxifungin Hydrochloride
Parconazole Hydrochloride
Partricin (See also *Antiprotozoal*)
Potassium Iodide (See also *Expectorant; Supplement (iodine)*)
Proclonol (See also *Anthelmintic*)
Pyrithione Zinc (See also *Antibacterial; Antiseborrheic*)
Pyrrolnitrin
Rutamycin
Sanguinarium Chloride (See also *Anti-inflammatory; Antimicrobial*)
Saperconazole
Scopafungin (See also *Antibacterial*)
Selenium Sulfide (See also *Antiseborrheic*)
Sinefungin
Sulconazole Nitrate
Terbinafine
Terconazole
Thiram
Ticlatone (See also *Antibacterial*)
Tioconazole
Tolciclate
Tolindate
Tolnaftate
Triacetin
Triafungin
Undecylenic Acid
Viridofulvin
Zinc Undecylenate
Zinoconazole Hydrochloride

VETERINARY

Metacresol (See also *Antiseptic (topical); Antifungal*)

Antiglaucoma agent [See also **Adrenergic (ophthalmic) ; Cholinergic (ophthalmic)**]

Alprenoxime Hydrochloride
Brinzolamide
Colforsin
Dapiprazole Hydrochloride (See also *Adrenergic (α-blocking); Neuroleptic; Psychotropic*)
Dipivefrin Hydrochloride
Latanoprost
Naboctate Hydrochloride (See also *Antinauseant*)
Pilocarpine (See also *Cholinergic (ophthalmic)*)

Pirnabine

Antihemophilic
Antihemophilic Factor

Antihemorrhagic
Poliglusam

Antihistaminic
Acrivastine
Antazoline Phosphate
Astemizole (See also *Anti-allergic*)
Azatadine Maleate
Barmastine
Bromodiphenhydramine Hydrochloride
Brompheniramine Maleate
Carbinoxamine Maleate
Cetirizine Hydrochloride
Chlorpheniramine Maleate
Chlorpheniramine Polistirex
Cinnarizine
Clemastine
Clemastine Fumarate
Closiramine Aceturate
Cycliramine Maleate
Cyclizine
Cyproheptadine Hydrochloride (See also *Antipruritic*)
Dexbrompheniramine Maleate
Dexchlorpheniramine Maleate
Dimethindene Maleate
Diphenhydramine Citrate
Diphenhydramine Hydrochloride
Dorastine Hydrochloride
Doxylamine Succinate
Ebastine
Fexofenadine Hydrochloride
Levocabastine Hydrochloride
Loratadine
Mianserin Hydrochloride (See also *Serotonin inhibitor*)
Noberastine
Orphenadrine Citrate (See also *Relaxant (skeletal muscle)*)
Promethazine Hydrochloride (See also *Anti-emetic*)
Pyrabrom
Pyrilamine Maleate
Pyroxamine Maleate
Rocastine Hydrochloride
Rotoxamine
Tazifylline Hydrochloride
Temelastine
Terfenadine
Tripelennamine Citrate
Tripelennamine Hydrochloride
Triprolidine Hydrochloride
Zolamine Hydrochloride (See also *Anesthetic (topical)*)

Antihistaminic, H₁-receptor
Emedastine Difumarate (See also *Asthma prophylactic; Anti-allergic*)

Antihyperammonemic
Sodium Benzoate (See also *Pharmaceutic aid (antifungal agent)*)
Sodium Phenylacetate
Sodium Phenylbutyrate

Antihypercalcemic
Ibandronate Sodium (See also *Bone resorption inhibitor*)

Antihyperlipidemic
Cerivastatin Sodium (See also *Inhibitor (HMG-CoA reductase)*)
Cholestyramine Resin (See also *Ion-exchange resin (bile salts)*)
Clofibrate
Colesevelam Hydrochloride
Colestipol Hydrochloride
Crilvastatin
Dalvastatin
Dextrothyroxine Sodium
Eldacimibe
Fluvastatin Sodium (See also *Inhibitor (HMG-CoA reductase)*)
Gemfibrozil
Lecimibide
Lovastatin (See also *Inhibitor (HMG-CoA reductase)*)
Niacin (See also *Vitamin (enzyme cofactor)*)
Pravastatin Sodium
Probucol
Simvastatin
Tiqueside
Xenbucin

Antihyperlipoproteinemic
Acifran
Beloxamide
Bezafibrate
Boxidine
Butoxamine Hydrochloride (See also *Antidiabetic*)
Cetaben Sodium
Ciprofibrate
Gemcadiol
Halofenate (See also *Uricosuric*)
Lifibrate
Meglutol
Nafenopin
Pimetine Hydrochloride
Theofibrate
Tibric Acid
Treloxinate

Antihyperphosphatemic
Sevelamer Hydrochloride

Antihyperprolactinemic
Cabergoline (See also *Antidyskinetic; Dopamine agonist*)

Antihypertensive
Alipamide (See also *Diuretic*)
Althiazide
Amiquinsin Hydrochloride
Amlodipine Besylate (See also *Anti-anginal*)
Amlodipine Maleate (See also *Anti-anginal*)
Anaritide Acetate (See also *Diuretic*)
Atiprosin Maleate
Bemitradine (See also *Diuretic*)
Bendacalol Mesylate
Bendroflumethiazide (See also *Diuretic*)
Benzthiazide (See also *Diuretic*)

Betaxolol Hydrochloride (See also *Anti-anginal*)
Bethanidine Sulfate
Bevantolol Hydrochloride (See also *Anti-anginal; Cardiac depressant (anti-arrhythmic)*)
Bucindolol Hydrochloride
Bupicomide
Buthiazide (See also *Diuretic*)
Candesartan (See also *Antagonist (angiotensin II receptor)*)
Candesartan Cilexetil (See also *Antagonist (angiotensin II receptor)*)
Candoxatril
Candoxatrilat
Captopril (See also *Enzyme inhibitor (angiotensin-converting)*)
Carvedilol (See also *Anti-anginal*)
Ceronapril
Chlorothiazide Sodium (See also *Diuretic*)
Cicletanine
Cilazapril
Clonidine
Clonidine Hydrochloride
Clopamide (See also *Diuretic*)
Cyclopenthiazide
Cyclothiazide (See also *Diuretic*)
Darodipine (See also *Bronchodilator; Vasodilator*)
Debrisoquin Sulfate
Delapril Hydrochloride (See also *Enzyme inhibitor (angiotensin-converting)*)
Diapamide (See also *Diuretic*)
Diazoxide
Dilevalol Hydrochloride (See also *Anti-adrenergic (β-receptor)*)
Diltiazem Malate
Ditekiren
Doxazosin Mesylate
Ecadotril
Enalapril Maleate
Enalaprilat
Enalkiren
Endralazine Mesylate
Epithiazide (See also *Diuretic*)
Eplerenone (See also *Aldosterone antagonist*)
Eprosartan
Eprosartan Mesylate
Fenoldopam Mesylate (See also *Dopamine agonist*)
Flavodilol Maleate
Flordipine
Forasartan
Fosinopril Sodium (See also *Enzyme inhibitor (angiotensin-converting)*)
Fosinoprilat
Guanabenz
Guanabenz Acetate
Guanacline Sulfate
Guanadrel Sulfate
Guancydine
Guanethidine Monosulfate
Guanethidine Sulfate
Guanfacine Hydrochloride
Guanisoquin Sulfate

Guanoclor Sulfate
Guanoctine Hydrochloride
Guanoxabenz
Guanoxan Sulfate
Guanoxyfen Sulfate (See also *Antidepressant*)
Hydralazine Hydrochloride
Hydralazine Polistirex
Hydroflumethiazide (See also *Diuretic*)
Indacrinone (See also *Diuretic*)
Indapamide (See also *Diuretic*)
Indolapril Hydrochloride
Indoramin
Indoramin Hydrochloride
Indorenate Hydrochloride
Lacidipine
Leniquinsin
Levcromakalim (See also *Anti-asthmatic*)
Lisinopril
Lofexidine Hydrochloride
Losartan Potassium
Losulazine Hydrochloride
Mebutamate
Mecamylamine Hydrochloride
Medroxalol
Medroxalol Hydrochloride
Methalthiazide (See also *Diuretic*)
Methyclothiazide (See also *Diuretic*)
Methyldopa
Methyldopate Hydrochloride
Metolazone (See also *Diuretic*)
Metoprolol Fumarate
Metoprolol Succinate (See also *Anti-anginal*)
Metyrosine
Minoxidil (See also *Hair growth stimulant (topical)*)
Moexipril Hydrochloride (See also *Enzyme inhibitor (angiotensin-converting)*)
Monatepil Maleate (See also *Anti-anginal*)
Muzolimine (See also *Diuretic*)
Nitrendipine
Ofornine
Pargyline Hydrochloride
Pazoxide
Pelanserin Hydrochloride (See also *Vasodilator (serotonin S_2 and $α_1$ adrenergic receptor blocker)*)
Perindopril Erbumine
Phenoxybenzamine Hydrochloride
Pinacidil
Pivopril
Polythiazide (See also *Diuretic*)
Prazosin Hydrochloride
Primidolol (See also *Anti-anginal; Cardiac depressant (anti-arrhythmic)*)
Prizidilol Hydrochloride
Quinapril Hydrochloride (See also *Enzyme inhibitor (angiotensin-converting)*)
Quinaprilat (See also *Enzyme inhibitor (angiotensin-converting)*)
Quinazosin Hydrochloride
Quinelorane Hydrochloride (See also *Antiparkinsonian*)

Quinpirole Hydrochloride
Quinuclium Bromide
Ramipril (See also *Enzyme inhibitor (angiotensin-converting)*)
Rauwolfia Serpentina
Reserpine
Saprisartan Potassium
Saralasin Acetate
Sodium Nitroprusside
Sulfinalol Hydrochloride
Tasosartan
Telmisartan (See also *Antagonist (angiotensin II receptor)*)
Teludipine Hydrochloride (See also *Antagonist (calcium channel)*)
Temocapril Hydrochloride
Terazosin Hydrochloride
Terlakiren
Tiamenidine
Tiamenidine Hydrochloride
Ticrynafen (See also *Diuretic; Uricosuric*)
Tinabinol
Tiodazosin
Tipentosin Hydrochloride
Trichlormethiazide (See also *Diuretic*)
Trimazosin Hydrochloride
Trimethaphan Camsylate
Trimoxamine Hydrochloride
Tripamide (See also *Diuretic*)
Valsartan
Xipamide (See also *Diuretic*)
Zankiren Hydrochloride
Zofenoprilat Arginine

ANGIOTENSIN II RECEPTOR ANTAGONIST
Irbesartan

α-BLOCKER
Alfuzosin Hydrochloride

β-BLOCKER
Bisoprolol
Bisoprolol Fumarate
Nebivolol

Ophthalmic
Adaprolol Maleate
Metipranolol

CALCIUM CHANNEL BLOCKER
Belfosdil

VASODILATOR
Biclodil Hydrochloride
Flosequinan

Antihypotensive
Ciclafrine Hydrochloride
Midodrine Hydrochloride

Antihypoxic
Sabeluzole (See also *Anticonvulsant*)

Anti-infective
Lauryl Isoquinolinium Bromide
Moxalactam Disodium
Ornidazole
Pentisomicin

DNA GYRASE INHIBITOR
Difloxacin Hydrochloride
Sarafloxacin Hydrochloride

Anti-infective, topical
Alcohol (See also *Pharmaceutic aid (solvent)*)
Aminacrine Hydrochloride
Benzethonium Chloride (See also *Pharmaceutic aid (preservative)*)
Bithionolate Sodium
Bromchlorenone
Cetalkonium Chloride
Cetylpyridinium Chloride (See also *Pharmaceutic aid (preservative)*)
Chlorhexidine Hydrochloride
Clioquinol (See also *Anti-amebic*)
Domiphen Bromide
Fenticlor
Fludazonium Chloride
Fuchsin, Basic
Furazolidone (See also *Antiprotozoal (Trichomonas, topical)*)
Gentian Violet
Halquinols
Hexachlorophene (See also *Detergent*)
Hydrogen Peroxide
Ichthammol
Imidecyl Iodine
Iodine
Isopropyl Alcohol (See also *Pharmaceutic aid (solvent)*)
Mafenide Acetate
Meralein Sodium
Mercufenol Chloride
Mercury, Ammoniated
Methylbenzethonium Chloride
Nitrofurazone
Nitromersol
Octenidine Hydrochloride
Oxychlorosene
Oxychlorosene Sodium
Potassium Permanganate
Povidone-Iodine
Sepazonium Chloride
Silver Nitrate
Sulfadiazine, Silver
Symclosene
Thimerfonate Sodium
Thimerosal (See also *Pharmaceutic aid (preservative)*)
Troclosene Potassium
DENTAL
Carbamide Peroxide

Anti-inflammatory
Alclofenac
Algestone Acetonide
Alpha Amylase
Amcinafal
Amcinafide
Amfenac Sodium
Amiprilose Hydrochloride
Anirolac (See also *Analgesic*)
Apazone
Atiprimod Dihydrochloride (See also *Anti-arthritic*)
Atiprimod Dimaleate (See also *Anti-arthritic; Immunomodulator*)
Bendazac
Benoxaprofen (See also *Analgesic*)

Benzydamine Hydrochloride (See also *Analgesic; Antipyretic*)
Bromelains
Broperamole
Budesonide
Carprofen
Cicloprofen
Cintazone
Cliprofen
Clobetasol Propionate
Clobetasone Butyrate
Clopirac
Cloticasone Propionate
Cortodoxone
Deflazacort
Desonide
Desoximetasone
Dexibuprofen (See also *Analgesic*)
Dexibuprofen Lysine (See also *Analgesic (cyclooxygenase inhibitor)*)
Diclofenac Potassium
Diclofenac Sodium
Diflumidone Sodium
Diflunisal (See also *Analgesic*)
Difluprednate
Diftalone
Drocinonide
Enlimomab (See also *Monoclonal antibody*)
Enolicam Sodium (See also *Antirheumatic*)
Epirizole (See also *Analgesic*)
Etodolac
Etofenamate (See also *Analgesic*)
Felbinac
Fenamole
Fenbufen
Fenclofenac
Fenclorac
Fendosal
Fenoprofen (See also *Analgesic*)
Fenoprofen Calcium (See also *Analgesic*)
Fenpipalone
Fentiazac
Flazalone
Fluazacort
Flufenamic Acid
Flumizole
Flunisolide Acetate
Flunixin (See also *Analgesic*)
Flunixin Meglumine (See also *Analgesic*)
Fluocortin Butyl
Fluorometholone Acetate
Fluquazone
Flurbiprofen (See also *Analgesic*)
Fluretofen (See also *Antithrombotic*)
Fluticasone Propionate
Furaprofen
Furobufen
Ibufenac (See also *Analgesic*)
Ibuprofen
Ibuprofen Aluminum
Ilonidap
Indomethacin
Indomethacin Sodium
Indoprofen (See also *Analgesic*)

Indoxole (See also *Antipyretic*)
Intrazole
Isoflupredone Acetate
Isoxepac
Isoxicam
Ketoprofen
Lofemizole Hydrochloride (See also *Analgesic; Antipyretic*)
Lornoxicam (See also *Analgesic*)
Meclofenamate Sodium
Meclofenamic Acid
Mefenamic Acid (See also *Analgesic*)
Mesalamine
Meseclazone
Methylprednisolone Suleptanate
Morniflumate
Nabumetone
Naproxen (See also *Analgesic; Antipyretic*)
Naproxen Sodium (See also *Analgesic; Antipyretic*)
Naproxol (See also *Analgesic; Antipyretic*)
Nimazone
Orgotein (See also *Antirheumatic*)
Orpanoxin
Oxaprozin
Oxyphenbutazone (See also *Antirheumatic*)
Paranyline Hydrochloride
Phenbutazone Sodium Glycerate
Pirfenidone (See also *Analgesic; Antipyretic*)
Piroxicam
Piroxicam Betadex (See also *Analgesic; Antirheumatic*)
Piroxicam Cinnamate
Piroxicam Olamine (See also *Analgesic*)
Pirprofen
Prednazate
Prodolic Acid
Proquazone
Proxazole (See also *Relaxant (smooth muscle); Analgesic*)
Proxazole Citrate (See also *Relaxant (smooth muscle); Analgesic*)
Rimexolone
Romazarit (See also *Antirheumatic*)
Salcolex (See also *Analgesic; Antipyretic*)
Salsalate (See also *Analgesic*)
Sanguinarium Chloride (See also *Antifungal; Antimicrobial*)
Seclazone (See also *Uricosuric*)
Sermetacin
Sudoxicam
Sulindac
Suprofen
Talmetacin (See also *Analgesic; Antipyretic*)
Talniflumate (See also *Analgesic*)
Talosalate (See also *Analgesic*)
Tebufelone (See also *Analgesic*)
Tenoxicam
Tesicam
Tesimide
Tetrydamine (See also *Analgesic*)

Tiopinac (See also *Analgesic; Antipyretic*)
Tolmetin
Tolmetin Sodium
Triclonide
Triflumidate
Zidometacin
Zomepirac Sodium (See also *Analgesic*)

DERMATOLOGIC
Prifelone

GASTROINTESTINAL
Balsalazide Disodium
Olsalazine Sodium

INTERSTITIAL CYSTITIS
Pentosan Polysulfate Sodium

NONANTIHISTAMINIC
Seratrodast (See also *Anti-asthmatic (thromboxane receptor antagonist)*)

NONSTEROIDAL
Anakinra (See also *Suppressant (inflammatory bowel disease)*)
Meloxicam
Moxilubant Maleate (See also *Antirheumatic; Antipsoriatic*)

OSTEOARTHRITIS AND RHEUMATOID ARTHRITIS
Tenidap
Tenidap Sodium

STEROID
Dexamethasone Dipropionate

TOPICAL
Alclometasone Dipropionate
Anitrazafen
Cormethasone Acetate
Diflorasone Diacetate
Dimethyl Sulfoxide
Halcinonide
Halobetasol Propionate
Halopredone Acetate
Ibuprofen Piconol
Loteprednol Etabonate
Meclorisone Dibutyrate
Resocortol Butyrate
Salnacedin
Tixocortol Pivalate

Ophthalmic
Endrysone

VETERINARY
Flutiazin
Vedaprofen

Antikeratinizing agent
Doretinel
Linarotene
Pelretin

Antimalarial [See also **Antiprotozoal**]
Acedapsone (See also *Antibacterial (leprostatic)*)
Amodiaquine Hydrochloride
Amquinate
Arteflene
Chloroquine (See also *Anti-amebic*)
Chloroquine Hydrochloride (See also *Anti-amebic*)

Chloroquine Phosphate (See also *Anti-amebic; Suppressant (lupus erythematosus)*)
Cycloguanil Pamoate
Enpiroline Phosphate
Halofantrine Hydrochloride
Hydroxychloroquine Sulfate (See also *Suppressant (lupus erythematosus)*)
Mefloquine
Mefloquine Hydrochloride
Menoctone
Mirincamycin Hydrochloride (See also *Antibacterial*)
Primaquine Phosphate
Pyrimethamine
Quinine Sulfate
Tebuquine

Antimanic
Lithium Carbonate
Lithium Citrate
Lithium Hydroxide

Antimethemoglobinemic
Methylene Blue (See also *Antidote (to cyanide poisoning)*)

Antimicrobial
Aztreonam
Chlorhexidine Gluconate
Imidurea
Pirazmonam Sodium
Propionic Acid (See also *Pharmaceutic aid (acidifying agent)*)
Sanguinarium Chloride (See also *Antifungal; Anti-inflammatory*)
Tigemonam Dicholine

TOPICAL
Lycetamine
Nibroxane
Pyrithione Sodium

Antimigraine
Almotriptan
Alniditan Dihydrochloride
Avitriptan Fumarate
Dolasetron Mesylate (See also *Antiemetic*)
Naratriptan Hydrochloride
Rizatriptan Benzoate
Rizatriptan Sulfate
Sergolexole Maleate
Sumatriptan Succinate
Zatosetron Maleate
Zolmitriptan

Antimitotic
Podofilox

Antimycotic
Amorolfine

Antinauseant [See also **Anti-emetic**]
Buclizine Hydrochloride
Cyclizine Lactate
Naboctate Hydrochloride (See also *Antiglaucoma agent*)
Palonosetron Hydrochloride (See also *Anti-emetic*)

Antineoplastic
Acivicin
Aclarubicin
Acodazole Hydrochloride
Acronine
Adozelesin
Aldesleukin (See also *Biological response modifier; Immunostimulant*)
Altretamine
Ambomycin
Ametantrone Acetate
Aminoglutethimide (See also *Adrenocortical suppressant*)
Aminolevulinic Acid Hydrochloride
Amsacrine
Anastrozole
Anthramycin
Asparaginase
Asperlin (See also *Antibacterial*)
Azacitidine
Azetepa
Azotomycin
Batimastat
Benzodepa
Bicalutamide
Bisantrene Hydrochloride
Bisnafide Dimesylate
Bizelesin
Bleomycin Sulfate
Borocaptate Sodium B 10 (See also *Radioactive agent*)
Brequinar Sodium
Bropirimine (See also *Antiviral*)
Busulfan
Cactinomycin
Calusterone
Capecitabine
Caracemide
Carbetimer
Carboplatin
Carmustine
Carubicin Hydrochloride
Carzelesin
Chlorambucil
Cirolemycin (See also *Antibacterial*)
Cisplatin
Cladribine
Crisnatol Mesylate
Cyclophosphamide (See also *Immunosuppressant*)
Cytarabine (See also *Antiviral*)
Dacarbazine
Dactinomycin
Daunorubicin Hydrochloride
Decitabine
Denileukin Diftitox (See also *Biological response modifier*)
Dexormaplatin
Dezaguanine
Dezaguanine Mesylate
Diaziquone
Docetaxel
Doxorubicin
Doxorubicin Hydrochloride
Droloxifene
Droloxifene Citrate
Dromostanolone Propionate
Duazomycin

Edatrexate
Eflornithine Hydrochloride (See also *Antiprotozoal*)
Elsamitrucin
Enloplatin
Enpromate
Epipropidine
Epirubicin Hydrochloride
Esorubicin Hydrochloride
Estramustine
Estramustine Phosphate Sodium
Ethiodized Oil I 131 (See also *Radioactive agent*)
Etoposide
Etoposide Phosphate
Etoprine
Fadrozole Hydrochloride
Fazarabine
Fenretinide
Floxuridine (See also *Antiviral*)
Fludarabine Phosphate
Fluorouracil
Flurocitabine
Fosquidone
Fostriecin Sodium
Gemcitabine
Gemcitabine Hydrochloride
Gold Au 198 (See also *Diagnostic aid (liver imaging); Radioactive agent*)
Hydroxyurea
Idarubicin Hydrochloride
Idoxifene (See also *Hormone (replacement therapy, estrogen receptor antagonist); Osteoporosis treatment and prevention*)
Ifosfamide
Ilmofosine
Interferon Alfa-2a (See also *Biological response modifier*)
Interferon Alfa-2b (See also *Biological response modifier*)
Interferon Alfa-n1 (See also *Biological response modifier*)
Interferon Alfa-n3 (See also *Biological response modifier*)
Interferon Beta-1a (See also *Biological response modifier*)
Interferon Gamma-1b (See also *Biological response modifier; Immunoregulator*)
Iproplatin
Lanreotide Acetate
Letrozole
Leuprolide Acetate (See also *LHRH agonist*)
Liarozole Hydrochloride
Lometrexol Sodium
Lomustine
Losoxantrone Hydrochloride
Masoprocol
Maytansine
Mechlorethamine Hydrochloride
Megestrol Acetate
Melengestrol Acetate (See also *Progestin*)
Melphalan
Menogaril
Mercaptopurine

Methotrexate
Metoprine
Meturedepa
Mitindomide
Mitocarcin
Mitocromin
Mitogillin
Mitomalcin
Mitomycin
Mitosper
Mitotane
Mitoxantrone Hydrochloride
Mycophenolic Acid
Nelzarabine
Nilutamide
Nocodazole
Nogalamycin
Octreotide Pamoate
Ormaplatin
Oxisuran
Paclitaxel
Pegaspargase
Peldesine (See also *Antipsoriatic*)
Peliomycin
Pentamustine
Peplomycin Sulfate
Perfosfamide
Pipobroman
Piposulfan
Piroxantrone Hydrochloride
Plicamycin
Plomestane
Porfimer Sodium
Porfiromycin (See also *Antibacterial*)
Prednimustine
Procarbazine Hydrochloride
Puromycin (See also *Antiprotozoal (Trypanosoma)*)
Puromycin Hydrochloride (See also *Antiprotozoal (Trypanosoma)*)
Pyrazofurin
Riboprine
Rogletimide
Samarium Sm 153 Lexidronam Pentasodium (See also *Radioactive agent*)
Semustine
Simtrazene
Sodium Iodide I 131 (See also *Diagnostic aid (thyroid function determination); Radioactive agent*)
Sodium Phosphate P 32 (See also *Antipolycythemic; Diagnostic aid (neoplasm); Radioactive agent*)
Sparfosate Sodium
Sparsomycin
Spirogermanium Hydrochloride
Spiromustine
Spiroplatin
Streptonigrin
Streptozocin
Strontium Chloride Sr 89 (See also *Radioactive agent*)
Sulofenur
Suramin Hexasodium
Talisomycin
Tegafur
Teloxantrone Hydrochloride
Temoporfin

Teniposide
Teroxirone
Testolactone
Thiamiprine
Thioguanine
Thiotepa
Thymalfasin (See also *Hepatitis treatment; Infectious disease treatment; Vaccine enhancement*)
Tiazofurin
Tirapazamine
Toremifene Citrate (See also *Anti-estrogen*)
Trestolone Acetate (See also *Androgen*)
Triciribine Phosphate
Trimetrexate
Trimetrexate Glucuronate
Triptorelin
Uracil Mustard
Uredepa
Vapreotide
Verteporfin
Vinblastine Sulfate
Vincristine Sulfate
Vindesine
Vindesine Sulfate
Vinepidine Sulfate
Vinglycinate Sulfate
Vinleurosine Sulfate
Vinorelbine Tartrate
Vinrosidine Sulfate
Vinzolidine Sulfate
Vorozole
Zeniplatin
Zinostatin
Zorubicin Hydrochloride

ADJUNCT
Cedefingol (See also *Antipsoriatic*)
Elacridar Hydrochloride
Eniluracil
Erbulozole
Safingol (See also *Antipsoriatic*)
Safingol Hydrochloride (See also *Antipsoriatic*)
Tecogalan Sodium
Uracil

DNA TOPOISOMERASE I INHIBITOR
Irinotecan Hydrochloride
Lurtotecan Dihydrochloride
Topotecan Hydrochloride

DNA TOPOISOMERASE II INHIBITOR
Ledoxantrone Trihydrochloride
Sedoxantrone Trihydrochloride

HYPOXIC CELL RADIOSENSITIZER
Etanidazole

MATRIX METALLOPROTEINASE INHIBITOR
Marimastat

MICROTUBULE INHIBITOR
Mivobulin Isethionate
Rituximab (See also *Monoclonal antibody*)
Tubulozole Hydrochloride

SPECIFIC THYMIDYLATE SYNTHASE INHIBITOR
Metesind Glucuronate
Pemetrexed Disodium

Antineuralgic, specific pain syndromes, topical

Capsaicin (See also *Analgesic* (*topical*))

Antineutropenic

Daniplestim (See also *Hematopoietic stimulant*)

Filgrastim (See also *Hematopoietic stimulant*)

Lenograstim (See also *Hematopoietic stimulant*)

Milodistim (See also *Hematopoietic stimulant*)

Molgramostim (See also *Hematopoietic stimulant*)

Muplestim (See also *Hematopoietic stimulant*)

Regramostim (See also *Hematopoietic stimulant*)

Sargramostim (See also *Hematopoietic stimulant*)

Antiobsessional agent

Fluvoxamine Maleate

Antiparasitic

Abamectin

Clorsulon (See also *Fasciolicide*)

Ivermectin

VETERINARY

Doramectin

Eprinomectin

Moxidectin

Nemadectin

Antiparkinsonian

Benztropine Mesylate

Biperiden (See also *Anticholinergic*)

Biperiden Hydrochloride (See also *Anticholinergic*)

Biperiden Lactate (See also *Anticholinergic*)

Carmantadine

Ciladopa Hydrochloride (See also *Dopaminergic agent*)

Dopamantine

Ethopropazine Hydrochloride

Lazabemide

Levodopa

Lometraline Hydrochloride (See also *Antipsychotic*)

Mofegiline Hydrochloride

Naxagolide Hydrochloride (See also *Dopamine agonist*)

Pareptide Sulfate

Pramipexole (See also *Antidepressant; Antischizophrenic; Dopamine agonist*)

Pramipexole Dihydrochloride (See also *Antidepressant; Antischizophrenic; Dopamine agonist*)

Procyclidine Hydrochloride (See also *Relaxant* (*skeletal muscle*))

Quinelorane Hydrochloride (See also *Antihypertensive*)

Rasagiline Mesylate

Tolcapone

Trihexyphenidyl Hydrochloride (See also *Anticholinergic*)

D$_2$ RECEPTOR AGONIST

Ropinirole Hydrochloride

IN COMBINATION WITH LEVODOPA/CARBIDO-PA

Selegiline Hydrochloride (See also *Antidyskinetic*)

Antiperistaltic

Difenoximide Hydrochloride

Difenoxin

Diphenoxylate Hydrochloride

Fluperamide

Lidamidine Hydrochloride

Loperamide Hydrochloride

Malethamer

Nufenoxole

Paregoric

Antipneumocystic

Atovaquone

Antipolycythemic

Sodium Phosphate P 32 (See also *Antineoplastic; Diagnostic aid* (*neoplasm*); *Radioactive agent*)

Antiproliferative agent

Piritrexim Isethionate

Antiprostatic hypertrophy

Sitogluside

Antiprotozoal [See also Anaplasmodastat (veterinary); Anti-amebic; Antileishmanial; Antimalarial; Antischistosomal; Coccidiostat]

Amodiaquine

Azanidazole

Carnidazole

Chlortetracycline Bisulfate (See also *Antibacterial*)

Chlortetracycline Hydrochloride (See also *Antibacterial*)

Doxycycline Calcium (See also *Antibacterial*)

Eflornithine Hydrochloride (See also *Antineoplastic*)

Flubendazole

Flunidazole

Halofuginone Hydrobromide

Levofuraltadone (See also *Antibacterial*)

Mepartricin (See also *Antifungal*)

Metronidazole Phosphate (See also *Antibacterial*)

Monensin (See also *Antibacterial; Antifungal*)

Monensin Sodium (See also *Antibacterial; Antifungal*)

Partricin (See also *Antifungal*)

Ronidazole

Tinidazole

BABESIA

Imidocarb Hydrochloride

HISTOMONAS

Ipronidazole

Nitarsone

For poultry

Nifursemizone

Nifursol

TRICHOMONAS

Bamnidazole

Metronidazole

Misonidazole

Moxnidazole

Nifuratel (See also *Antibacterial; Antifungal*)

Sulnidazole

Topical

Furazolidone (See also *Anti-infective, topical*)

TRYPANOSOMA

Puromycin (See also *Antineoplastic*)

Puromycin Hydrochloride (See also *Antineoplastic*)

Antipruritic

Camphor

Cyproheptadine Hydrochloride (See also *Antihistaminic*)

Methdilazine

Methdilazine Hydrochloride

Trimeprazine Tartrate

TOPICAL

Ammonium Lactate

Colloidal Oatmeal

Menthol

Antipsoriatic

Acitretin

Anthralin

Azaribine

Calcipotriene

Cedefingol (See also *Antineoplastic* (*adjunct*))

Cycloheximide

Enazadrem Phosphate (See also *Inhibitor* (*5-lipoxygenase*))

Etretinate

Liarozole Fumarate

Lonapalene

Moxilubant Maleate (See also *Antirheumatic; Anti-inflammatory* (*nonsteroidal*))

Peldesine (See also *Antineoplastic*)

Safingol (See also *Antineoplastic* (*adjunct*))

Safingol Hydrochloride (See also *Antineoplastic* (*adjunct*))

Tepoxalin

Ticolubant

Antipsychotic

Acetophenazine Maleate

Alentemol Hydrobromide (See also *Dopamine agonist*)

Alpertine

Aripiprazole (See also *Antischizophrenic*)

Azaperone

Batelapine Maleate

Benperidol

Benzindopyrine Hydrochloride

Brofoxine

Bromperidol

Bromperidol Decanoate

Buramate (See also *Anticonvulsant*)

Butaclamol Hydrochloride

Butaperazine

Butaperazine Maleate
Carphenazine Maleate
Carvotroline Hydrochloride
Chlorpromazine (See also *Anti-emetic*)
Chlorpromazine Hydrochloride (See also *Anti-emetic*)
Chlorprothixene
Cinperene
Cintriamide
Clomacran Phosphate
Clopenthixol
Clopimozide
Clopipazan Mesylate
Cloroperone Hydrochloride
Clothiapine
Clothixamide Maleate
Clozapine
Cyclophenazine Hydrochloride
Cyproximide (See also *Antidepressant*)
Droperidol
Etazolate Hydrochloride
Fananserin
Fenimide
Flucindole
Flumezapine (See also *Neuroleptic*)
Fluotracen Hydrochloride (See also *Antidepressant*)
Fluphenazine Decanoate
Fluphenazine Enanthate
Fluphenazine Hydrochloride
Fluspiperone
Fluspirilene
Flutroline
Gevotroline Hydrochloride
Halopemide
Haloperidol (See also *Antidyskinetic (in Gilles de la Tourette's disease)*)
Haloperidol Decanoate
Iloperidone
Imidoline Hydrochloride
Lenperone
Lometraline Hydrochloride (See also *Antiparkinsonian*)
Mazapertine Succinate
Mesoridazine
Mesoridazine Besylate
Metiapine
Milenperone
Milipertine
Molindone Hydrochloride
Naranol Hydrochloride
Neflumozide Hydrochloride
Ocaperidone
Olanzapine
Opipramol Hydrochloride (See also *Antidepressant*)
Oxiperomide
Penfluridol
Pentiapine Maleate
Perphenazine
Pimozide
Pinoxepin Hydrochloride
Pipamperone
Piperacetazine
Pipotiazine Palmitate
Piquindone Hydrochloride
Prochlorperazine Edisylate (See also *Anti-emetic*)

Prochlorperazine Maleate (See also *Anti-emetic*)
Promazine Hydrochloride
Quetiapine Fumarate
Remoxipride
Remoxipride Hydrochloride
Rimcazole Hydrochloride
Seperidol Hydrochloride
Sertindole (See also *Neuroleptic*)
Setoperone
Spiperone
Thioridazine (See also *Sedative-hypnotic*)
Thioridazine Hydrochloride (See also *Sedative-hypnotic*)
Thiothixene
Thiothixene Hydrochloride
Tioperidone Hydrochloride
Tiospirone Hydrochloride
Trifluoperazine Hydrochloride (See also *Sedative-hypnotic*)
Trifluperidol
Triflupromazine
Triflupromazine Hydrochloride
Ziprasidone Hydrochloride

Antipyretic

Acetaminophen (See also *Analgesic*)
Aspirin (See also *Analgesic; Antirheumatic*)
Benzydamine Hydrochloride (See also *Analgesic; Anti-inflammatory*)
Dipyrone (See also *Analgesic*)
Indoxole (See also *Anti-inflammatory*)
Lofemizole Hydrochloride (See also *Anti-inflammatory; Analgesic*)
Magnesium Salicylate (See also *Analgesic; Antirheumatic*)
Naproxen (See also *Anti-inflammatory; Analgesic*)
Naproxen Sodium (See also *Anti-inflammatory; Analgesic*)
Naproxol (See also *Anti-inflammatory; Analgesic*)
Pirfenidone (See also *Analgesic; Anti-inflammatory*)
Salcolex (See also *Analgesic; Anti-inflammatory*)
Talmetacin (See also *Analgesic; Anti-inflammatory*)
Tiopinac (See also *Anti-inflammatory; Analgesic*)

Antirheumatic

Aspirin (See also *Analgesic; Antipyretic*)
Auranofin
Aurothioglucose
Bindarit
Butixirate (See also *Analgesic*)
Enolicam Sodium (See also *Anti-inflammatory*)
Gold Sodium Thiomalate
Lobenzarit Sodium
Magnesium Salicylate (See also *Analgesic; Antipyretic*)
Moxilubant Maleate (See also *Anti-inflammatory (nonsteroidal); Antipsoriatic*)

Orgotein (See also *Anti-inflammatory*)
Oxyphenbutazone (See also *Anti-inflammatory*)
Phenylbutazone
Pirazolac
Piroxicam Betadex (See also *Analgesic; Anti-inflammatory*)
Prinomide Tromethamine
Romazarit (See also *Anti-inflammatory*)
Salicylate Meglumine (See also *Analgesic*)
Seprilose

Antirickettsial

Chloramphenicol (See also *Antibacterial*)
Chloramphenicol Palmitate (See also *Antibacterial*)
Chloramphenicol Pantothenate Complex (See also *Antibacterial*)
Chloramphenicol Sodium Succinate (See also *Antibacterial*)
Oxytetracycline Hydrochloride (See also *Antibacterial*)
Tetracycline (See also *Anti-amebic; Antibacterial*)
Tetracycline Hydrochloride (See also *Anti-amebic; Antibacterial*)

Antischistosomal

Antimony Potassium Tartrate
Antimony Sodium Tartrate
Becanthone Hydrochloride
Hycanthone
Lucanthone Hydrochloride
Niridazole
Oxamniquine
Pararosaniline Pamoate
Teroxalene Hydrochloride

Antischizophrenic

Aripiprazole (See also *Antipsychotic*)
Ondansetron Hydrochloride (See also *Anti-anxiety agent ; Anti-emetic*)
Pramipexole (See also *Antidepressant; Antiparkinsonian; Dopamine agonist*)
Pramipexole Dihydrochloride (See also *Antidepressant; Antiparkinsonian; Dopamine agonist*)

Antiseborrheic

Chloroxine
Piroctone
Piroctone Olamine
Pyrithione Zinc (See also *Antibacterial; Antifungal*)
Resorcinol Monoacetate (See also *Keratolytic*)
Selenium Sulfide (See also *Antifungal*)

Antisecretory

Enprostil (See also *Anti-ulcerative*)
Nolinium Bromide (See also *Anti-ulcerative*)

GASTRIC
Arbaprostil
Deprostil
Fenoctimine Sulfate
Octreotide

Octreotide Acetate
Omeprazole Sodium
Rioprostil
Trimoprostil

Antisense antiviral used in the therapy of cytomegalovirus retinitis
Fomivirsen Sodium

Antiseptic
Cadexomer Iodine (See also *Anti-ulcerative*)
Chlorocresol (See also *Disinfectant*)
Disiquonium Chloride
Isomerol
Mecetronium Ethylsulfate
TOPICAL
Metacresol (See also *Antifungal; Antifungal (veterinary)*)
Zinc Carbonate (See also *Astringent*)

Antispasmodic
Stilonium Iodide
Tizanidine Hydrochloride

Antithrombotic
Anagrelide Hydrochloride
Bivalirudin (See also *Anticoagulant*)
Cilostazol (See also *Vasodilator; Inhibitor (platelet)*)
Dalteparin Sodium (See also *Anticoagulant*)
Danaparoid Sodium
Dazoxiben Hydrochloride
Efegatran Sulfate
Fluretofen (See also *Anti-inflammatory*)
Ifetroban
Ifetroban Sodium
Lamifiban
Lotrafiban Hydrochloride (See also *Platelet aggregation inhibitor*)
Napsagatran
Orbofiban Acetate (See also *Platelet aggregation inhibitor*)
Roxifiban Acetate (See also *Fibrinogen receptor antagonist*)
Sibrafiban (See also *Fibrinogen receptor antagonist; Platelet aggregation inhibitor*)
Tinzaparin Sodium (See also *Anticoagulant*)
Trifenagrel

Antitussive
Benzonatate
Butamirate Citrate
Butorphanol (See also *Analgesic*)
Butorphanol Tartrate (See also *Analgesic*)
Chlophedianol Hydrochloride
Codeine (See also *Analgesic (narcotic)*)
Codeine Phosphate (See also *Analgesic (narcotic)*)
Codeine Polistirex
Codeine Sulfate (See also *Analgesic (narcotic)*)
Codoxime
Dextromethorphan
Dextromethorphan Hydrobromide
Dextromethorphan Polistirex

Ethyl Dibunate
Guaiapate
Hydrocodone Bitartrate
Hydrocodone Polistirex
Levopropoxyphene Napsylate
Moxazocine (See also *Analgesic*)
Noscapine
Pemerid Nitrate
Pipazethate
Proxorphan Tartrate (See also *Analgesic*)
Suxemerid Sulfate

Anti-ulcerative
Aceglutamide Aluminum
Bismuth Subsalicylate (See also *Antidiarrheal; Antacid*)
Cadexomer Iodine (See also *Antiseptic*)
Enisoprost
Enprostil (See also *Antisecretory*)
Isotiquimide
Lansoprazole
Misoprostol
Nizatidine
Nolinium Bromide (See also *Antisecretory*)
Pantoprazole
Pirenzepine Hydrochloride
Rabeprazole Sodium (See also *Gastric acid pump inhibitor*)
Remiprostol
Roxatidine Acetate Hydrochloride
Sucrosofate Potassium
Tolimidone
GASTRIC
Pifarnine
GASTROINTESTINAL
Cetraxate Hydrochloride
Sucralfate
HISTAMINE H$_2$-RECEPTOR BLOCKER
Lavoltidine Succinate

Anti-urolithic
Cellulose Sodium Phosphate
CYSTINE CALCULI
Cysteamine
Cysteamine Hydrochloride
Tricitrates (See also *Alkalizer (systemic); Alkalizer (urinary); Anti-urolithic (uric acid calculi); Buffer (neutralizing)*)
URIC ACID CALCULI
Tricitrates (See also *Alkalizer (systemic); Alkalizer (urinary); Anti-urolithic (cystine calculi); Buffer (neutralizing)*)

Antiviral
Abacavir Succinate
Abacavir Sulfate
Acemannan (See also *Immunomodulator*)
Acyclovir
Acyclovir Sodium
Adefovir
Adefovir Dipivoxil
Afovirsen Sodium
Alovudine
Alvircept Sudotox

Amantadine Hydrochloride
Aranotin
Arildone
Atevirdine Mesylate
Avridine
Bropirimine (See also *Antineoplastic*)
Celgosivir Hydrochloride (See also *Inhibitor (α-glucosidase)*)
Cidofovir
Cipamfylline
Cytarabine (See also *Antineoplastic*)
Cytarabine Hydrochloride
Delavirdine Mesylate
Desciclovir
Didanosine
Disoxaril
Droxinavir Hydrochloride
Edoxudine
Enviradene
Enviroxime
Famciclovir
Famotine Hydrochloride
Felvizumab (See also *Monoclonal antibody (antiviral)*)
Fiacitabine
Fialuridine
Floxuridine (See also *Antineoplastic*)
Fosarilate
Foscarnet Sodium
Fosfonet Sodium
Ganciclovir
Ganciclovir Sodium
Indinavir
Indinavir Sulfate
Interferon Alfacon-1 (See also *Biological response modifier*)
Kethoxal
Lamivudine
Lobucavir
Lodenosine
Loviride
Memotine Hydrochloride
Methisazone
Nelfinavir Mesylate
Nevirapine
Palinavir
Penciclovir
Pirodavir
Pleconaril
Raluridine
Ribavirin
Rimantadine Hydrochloride
Ritonavir
Saquinavir Mesylate
Somantadine Hydrochloride
Sorivudine
Statolon
Stavudine
Steffimycin (See also *Antibacterial*)
Telinavir
Tilorone Hydrochloride
Trecovirsen Sodium
Valacyclovir Hydrochloride
Valganciclovir Hydrochloride
Vidarabine
Vidarabine Phosphate
Vidarabine Sodium Phosphate
Viroxime

Zalcitabine
Zanamivir (See also *Inhibitor (influenza virus neuraminidase)*)
Zidovudine
Zinviroxime

FOR POULTRY
Amidapsone

OPHTHALMIC
Idoxuridine
Trifluridine

Appetite stimulant
VETERINARY
Elfazepam

Appetite suppressant
SYSTEMIC
Dexfenfluramine Hydrochloride
Phendimetrazine Tartrate
Phentermine Hydrochloride

Asthma prophylactic
Arofylline (See also *Anti-asthmatic (type IV phosphodiesterase inhibitor); Bronchodilator*)
Emedastine Difumarate (See also *Antihistaminic, H_1-receptor; Anti-allergic*)
Levalbuterol Hydrochloride (See also *Bronchodilator*)
Levalbuterol Sulfate (See also *Bronchodilator*)

Astringent
Alcloxa (See also *Keratolytic*)
Aldioxa (See also *Keratolytic*)
Aluminum Acetate
Aluminum Subacetate
Calcium Hydroxide
Tannic Acid
Witch Hazel
Zinc Carbonate (See also *Antiseptic (topical)*)
Zinc Chloride (See also *Dentin desensitizer*)
Zinc Oxide (See also *Protectant (topical)*)

OPHTHALMIC
Zinc Sulfate

TOPICAL
Alum, Ammonium
Alum, Potassium
Aluminum Chloride
Aluminum Chlorohydrex

Barrier for the prevention of allergic contact dermatitis
Bentoquatam

Benign prostatic hyperplasia therapy agent
Tamsulosin Hydrochloride

Biological response modifier
Aldesleukin (See also *Antineoplastic; Immunostimulant*)
Denileukin Diftitox (See also *Antineoplastic*)
Interferon Alfa-2a (See also *Antineoplastic*)

Interferon Alfa-2b (See also *Antineoplastic*)
Interferon Alfacon-1 (See also *Antiviral*)
Interferon Alfa-n1 (See also *Antineoplastic*)
Interferon Alfa-n3 (See also *Antineoplastic*)
Interferon Beta-1a (See also *Antineoplastic*)
Interferon Gamma-1b (See also *Antineoplastic; Immunoregulator*)
Levamisole Hydrochloride
Roquinimex (See also *Immunomodulator*)

Blood flow adjuvant
Dextran 40 (See also *Plasma volume extender*)

Blood neutralizer
Blood Group Specific Substances A, B, and AB

Blood replenisher
Blood Cells, Red
Blood, Whole

Blood substitute
Perflubron

Blood volume supporter
Albumin Human
Plasma Protein Fraction

Bone resorption inhibitor
Alendronate Sodium
Etidronate Disodium
Ibandronate Sodium (See also *Antihypercalcemic*)
Pamidronate Disodium
Teriparatide (See also *Osteoporosis therapy adjunct*)
Zoledronate Disodium (See also *Osteoporosis therapy adjunct*)
Zoledronate Trisodium (See also *Osteoporosis therapy adjunct*)

Bronchodilator
Albuterol
Albuterol Sulfate
Arofylline (See also *Anti-asthmatic (type IV phosphodiesterase inhibitor); Asthma prophylactic*)
Azanator Maleate
Bamifylline Hydrochloride
Bitolterol Mesylate
Butaprost
Carbuterol Hydrochloride
Clorprenaline Hydrochloride
Colterol Mesylate
Darodipine (See also *Antihypertensive; Vasodilator*)
Doxaprost
Doxofylline
Dyphylline
Enprofylline
Ephedrine
Ephedrine Hydrochloride
Fenoterol

Fenspiride Hydrochloride (See also *Anti-adrenergic (α-receptor)*)
Formoterol Fumarate
Guaithylline (See also *Expectorant*)
Hexoprenaline Sulfate (See also *Tocolytic*)
Hoquizil Hydrochloride
Ipratropium Bromide
Isoetharine
Isoetharine Hydrochloride
Isoetharine Mesylate
Isoproterenol Hydrochloride
Isoproterenol Sulfate
Levalbuterol Hydrochloride (See also *Asthma prophylactic*)
Levalbuterol Sulfate (See also *Asthma prophylactic*)
Metaproterenol Polistirex
Metaproterenol Sulfate
Nisbuterol Mesylate
Oxtriphylline
Picumeterol Fumarate
Piquizil Hydrochloride
Pirbuterol Acetate
Pirbuterol Hydrochloride
Procaterol Hydrochloride
Quazodine (See also *Cardiotonic*)
Quinterenol Sulfate
Racepinephrine
Racepinephrine Hydrochloride
Reproterol Hydrochloride
Rimiterol Hydrobromide
Salmeterol
Salmeterol Xinafoate
Soterenol Hydrochloride
Sulfonterol Hydrochloride
Suloxifen Oxalate
Terbutaline Sulfate
Theophylline
Tibenelast Sodium (See also *Anti-asthmatic*)
Verofylline (See also *Anti-asthmatic*)
Xanoxate Sodium
Zindotrine
Zinterol Hydrochloride

ANTI-ALLERGIC
Fenprinast Hydrochloride

Buffer
NEUTRALIZING
Tricitrates (See also *Alkalizer (systemic); Alkalizer (urinary); Anti-urolithic (cystine calculi); Anti-urolithic (uric acid calculi)*)

Bulking agent for freeze drying
Creatinine

Carbon dioxide absorbant
Barium Hydroxide Lime
Soda Lime

Carbonic anhydrase inhibitor
Acetazolamide
Dichlorphenamide
Dorzolamide Hydrochloride
Methazolamide
Sezolamide Hydrochloride

Cardiac depressant
Acetylcholine Chloride (See also *Cholinergic; Miotic; Vasodilator (peripheral)*)
ANTI-ARRHYTHMIC
Acecainide Hydrochloride
Actisomide
Adenosine
Aprindine
Aprindine Hydrochloride
Artilide Fumarate
Azimilide Dihydrochloride
Bevantolol Hydrochloride (See also *Anti-anginal; Antihypertensive*)
Bidisomide
Bretylium Tosylate (See also *Anti-adrenergic*)
Bucainide Maleate
Bucromarone
Butoprozine Hydrochloride (See also *Anti-anginal*)
Capobenate Sodium
Capobenic Acid
Cifenline
Cifenline Succinate
Clofilium Phosphate
Dexpropranolol Hydrochloride (See also *Anti-adrenergic (β-receptor)*)
Dexsotalol Hydrochloride
Disobutamide
Disopyramide
Disopyramide Phosphate
Dofetilide
Drobuline
Edifolone Acetate
Emilium Tosylate
Encainide Hydrochloride
Flecainide Acetate
Ibutilide Fumarate
Indecainide Hydrochloride
Ipazilide Fumarate
Lorajmine Hydrochloride
Lorcainide Hydrochloride
Meobentine Sulfate
Mexiletine Hydrochloride
Modecainide
Moricizine
Oxiramide
Pirmenol Hydrochloride
Pirolazamide
Pranolium Chloride
Primidolol (See also *Antihypertensive; Anti-anginal*)
Procainamide Hydrochloride
Propafenone Hydrochloride
Propranolol Hydrochloride (See also *Anti-adrenergic (β-receptor)*)
Pyrinoline
Quindonium Bromide
Quinidine Gluconate
Quinidine Sulfate
Recainam Hydrochloride
Recainam Tosylate
Risotilide Hydrochloride
Ropitoin Hydrochloride
Sematilide Hydrochloride
Suricainide Maleate
Tocainide

Tocainide Hydrochloride
Tolamolol (See also *Vasodilator (coronary); Anti-adrenergic (β-receptor)*)
Transcainide
Verapamil Hydrochloride (See also *Anti-anginal*)
Ventricular
Amiodarone

Cardioprotectant
Dexrazoxane
Draflazine

Cardiotonic
Actodigin
Bemoradan
Butopamine
Carbazeran
Carsatrin Succinate
Deslanoside
Digitalis
Digitoxin
Digoxin
Dobutamine
Dobutamine Hydrochloride
Dobutamine Lactobionate
Dobutamine Tartrate
Enoximone
Imazodan Hydrochloride
Inamrinone
Indolidan
Isomazole Hydrochloride
Levdobutamine Lactobionate
Medorinone
Milrinone
Pelrinone Hydrochloride
Pimobendan
Piroximone
Prinoxodan
Proscillaridin
Quazinone
Quazodine (See also *Bronchodilator*)
Tazolol Hydrochloride
Toborinone
Vesnarinone
PHOSPHODIESTERASE INHIBITOR
Lixazinone Sulfate
POSITIVE INOTROPIC
Bemarinone Hydrochloride (See also *Cardiotonic (vasodilator)*)
VASODILATOR
Bemarinone Hydrochloride (See also *Cardiotonic (positive inotropic)*)

Cardiovascular agent
Dopexamine
Dopexamine Hydrochloride

Carminative
Capsicum (See also *Counterirritant (external); Stomachic*)
Capsicum Oleoresin (See also *Counterirritant (external); Stomachic*)

Caustic
Silver Nitrate, Toughened

Chelating agent
Deferoxamine Mesylate (See also *Antidote (to iron poisoning)*)

Edetate Sodium
Edetate Trisodium
Gluconolactone
Penicillamine
Trientine Hydrochloride
CALCIUM
Phytate Sodium
IRON
Deferoxamine
METAL
Edetate Calcium Disodium
Edetate Disodium (See also *Pharmaceutic aid (chelating agent)*)
PLUTONIUM
Pentetate Calcium Trisodium

Chemosterilant, avian
Azacosterol Hydrochloride

Choleretic
Dehydrocholic Acid
Fencibutirol
Hymecromone
Piprozolin
Sincalide
Tocamphyl

Cholinergic
Aceclidine
Acetylcholine Chloride (See also *Cardiac depressant; Miotic; Vasodilator (peripheral)*)
Bethanechol Chloride
Dexpanthenol
Methacholine Chloride
Neostigmine Bromide
Neostigmine Methylsulfate
Pyridostigmine Bromide
Quilostigmine
OPHTHALMIC
Carbachol
Demecarium Bromide
Echothiophate Iodide
Isoflurophate
Physostigmine
Physostigmine Salicylate
Physostigmine Sulfate
Pilocarpine (See also *Antiglaucoma agent*)
Pilocarpine Hydrochloride
Pilocarpine Nitrate

Cholinesterase reactivator
Obidoxime Chloride
Pralidoxime Chloride
Pralidoxime Iodide
Pralidoxime Mesylate

Chronic dermal ulcers treatment
PROMOTES THE PROLIFERATION OF MESENCHYMALLY-DERIVED CELLS
Becaplermin

Coccidiostat
Arprinocid
Narasin (See also *Growth stimulant (veterinary)*)
Semduramicin
Semduramicin Sodium

FOR PIGEONS
Clazuril

FOR POULTRY
Aklomide
Amprolium
Buquinolate
Clopidol
Cyproquinate
Decoquinate
Diclazuril
Dinsed
Lasalocid
Nequinate
Nitromide (See also *Antibacterial*)
Proquinolate
Robenidine Hydrochloride
Sulfabenz (See also *Antibacterial*)
Sulfanitran (See also *Antibacterial*)
Tiazuril

VETERINARY
Sulfaquinoxaline
Toltrazuril

Cognition adjuvant
Donepezil Hydrochloride (See also *Alzheimer's disease treatment* (adjunct); *Dementia symptoms treatment adjunct*; *Inhibitor* (acetylcholinesterase))
Ergoloid Mesylates
Icopezil Maleate (See also *Alzheimer's disease treatment* (cognition enhancer); *Inhibitor* (acetylcholinesterase))
Piracetam
Pramiracetam Hydrochloride
Pramiracetam Sulfate
Tacrine Hydrochloride (See also *Dementia symptoms treatment adjunct*)

Contact lens material
HYDROPHILIC
Abafilcon A
Alofilcon A
Alphafilcon A
Amfilcon A
Astifilcon A
Atlafilcon A
Balafilcon A
Bufilcon A
Crofilcon A
Cyclofilcon A
Deltafilcon A
Deltafilcon B
Dimefilcon A
Droxifilcon A
Elastofilcon A
Esterifilcon A
Etafilcon A
Focofilcon A
Govafilcon A
Hefilcon A
Hefilcon B
Hefilcon C
Hilafilcon A
Hioxifilcon A
Hydrofilcon A
Licryfilcon A
Licryfilcon B
Lidofilcon A

Lidofilcon B
Mafilcon A
Mesifilcon A
Methafilcon B
Mipafilcon A
Nelfilcon A
Netrafilcon A
Ocufilcon A
Ocufilcon B
Ocufilcon C
Ocufilcon D
Ocufilcon E
Ocufilcon F
Oxyfilcon A
Pentafilcon A
Perfilcon A
Phemfilcon A
Polymacon
Silafilcon A
Surfilcon A
Tetrafilcon A
Vifilcon A
Vifilcon B
Xylofilcon A

HYDROPHOBIC
Cabufocon A
Cabufocon B
Dimefocon A
Kolfocon A
Kolfocon B
Kolfocon C
Kolfocon D
Melafocon A
Nefocon A
Porofocon A
Porofocon B
Silafocon A
Tisilfocon A
Tolofocon A
Unifocon A
Vinafocon A

Counterirritant
EXTERNAL
Capsicum (See also *Carminative; Stomachic*)
Capsicum Oleoresin (See also *Carminative; Stomachic*)

Cystic fibrosis therapy adjunct
Dornase Alfa

Decongestant
Pseudoephedrine Sulfate

Dementia symptoms treatment adjunct
Donepezil Hydrochloride (See also *Alzheimer's disease treatment* (adjunct); *Cognition adjuvant; Inhibitor* (acetylcholinesterase))
Tacrine Hydrochloride (See also *Cognition adjuvant*)

Demulcent
Elm (See also *Pharmaceutic aid* (suspending agent))

Dental caries prophylactic
Dectaflur
Hetaflur

Ipexidine Mesylate
Olaflur
Sodium Fluoride
Sodium Monofluorophosphate
Stannous Fluoride

Dental plaque inhibitor
Octenidine Saccharin

Dental restoration agent
Gutta Percha

Dentin desensitizer
Zinc Chloride (See also *Astringent*)

Deodorant
Chlorophyllin Copper Complex

Depigmentor
Captamine Hydrochloride
Hydroquinone
Monobenzone

Depressant
GASTRIC ACID SECRETORY
Omeprazole

Detergent
Entsufon Sodium
Hexachlorophene (See also *Anti-infective, topical*)
Soap, Green
Sodium Ethasulfate
Thonzonium Bromide
Tyloxapol

Deterrent
SMOKING
Quinine Ascorbate

Detoxifying agent
Mesna

Diagnostic aid
Etifenin
Fludeoxyglucose F 18 (See also *Radioactive agent*)
Gadopentetate Dimeglumine
Gadoxanum
Gadozelite
Immune Globulin Intravenous Pentetate
Indium In 111 Oxyquinoline (See also *Radioactive agent*)
Indium In 111 Pentetreotide (See also *Radioactive agent*)
Iobenguane I 131 (See also *Radioactive agent*)
Iobenguane Sulfate I 131 (See also *Radioactive agent*)
Iodocetylic Acid I 123 (See also *Radioactive agent*)
Iofetamine Hydrochloride I 123 (See also *Radioactive agent*)
Iometopane I 123
Ioxilan
Mespiperone C 11 (See also *Radioactive agent*)
Pentetate Indium Disodium In 111 (See also *Radioactive agent*)
Pentetic Acid
Perflenapent
Perflisopent

Sermorelin Acetate (See also *Growth hormone-releasing hormone*)
Succimer
Tetrofosmin
Xenon Xe 127 (See also *Gas, medicinal; Radioactive agent*)

ADRENOCORTICAL INSUFFICIENCY
Corticorelin Ovine Triflutate (See also *Diagnostic aid (Cushing's syndrome); Hormone (corticotropin-releasing)*)
Corticotropin (See also *Hormone (adrenocorticotropic); Glucocorticoid*)
Corticotropin, Repository (See also *Hormone (adrenocorticotropic); Glucocorticoid*)
Corticotropin Zinc Hydroxide (See also *Hormone (adrenocorticotropic); Glucocorticoid*)

BLOOD

In vitro
Blood Grouping Serum, Anti-A
Blood Grouping Serum, Anti-B
Blood Grouping Serums Anti-D, Anti-C, Anti-E, Anti-c, Anti-e
Leukocyte Typing Serum

BLOOD VOLUME DETERMINATION
Albumin, Iodinated I 125 Serum (See also *Radioactive agent*)
Albumin, Iodinated I 131 Serum (See also *Diagnostic aid (intrathecal imaging); Radioactive agent*)
Carbon Monoxide C 11 (See also *Radioactive agent*)
Iodinated I 125 Albumin (See also *Radioactive agent*)
Iodinated I 131 Albumin (See also *Diagnostic aid (intrathecal imaging); Radioactive agent*)
Sodium Chromate Cr 51 (See also *Radioactive agent*)

BLOOD VOLUME AND CARDIAC OUTPUT DETERMINATION
Anazolene Sodium

BONE IMAGING
Butedronate Tetrasodium

BONE

Liver, and spleen imaging
Stannous Sulfur Colloid

BRAIN IMAGING
Fluorodopa F 18 (See also *Radioactive agent*)
Technetium Tc 99m Bicisate (See also *Radioactive agent*)
Technetium Tc 99m Siboroxime (See also *Radioactive agent*)

CARDIAC IMAGING
Ammonia N 13 (See also *Diagnostic aid (liver imaging); Radioactive agent*)

CARDIAC OUTPUT DETERMINATION
Indocyanine Green (See also *Diagnostic aid (hepatic function determination)*)

CARRIER AGENT
Disofenin

CORNEAL TRAUMA INDICATOR
Fluorescein

Fluorescein Sodium

CUSHING'S SYNDROME
Corticorelin Ovine Triflutate (See also *Diagnostic aid (adrenocortical insufficiency); Hormone (corticotropin-releasing)*)

CYSTOSCOPY
Indigotindisulfonate Sodium

DERMAL REACTIVITY INDICATOR
Coccidioidin
Diphtheria Toxin for Schick Test
Histoplasmin
Mumps Skin Test Antigen
Schick Test Control
Tuberculin

DIABETES
Tolbutamide Sodium, Sterile

GASTRIC SECRETION INDICATOR
Impromidine Hydrochloride
Pentagastrin

HEPATIC FUNCTION DETERMINATION
Arclofenin
Butilfenin
Indocyanine Green (See also *Diagnostic aid (cardiac output determination)*)
Iprofenin
Lidofenin
Rose Bengal Sodium I 131 (See also *Radioactive agent*)

HEPATOBILIARY FUNCTION DETERMINATION
Mebrofenin
Technetium Tc 99m Disofenin (See also *Radioactive agent*)

HYPOALBUMINEMIA
Tolpovidone I 131 (See also *Radioactive agent*)

HYPOCALCEMIA
Teriparatide Acetate

INTESTINAL FUNCTION DETERMINATION
Xylose

INTRATHECAL IMAGING
Albumin, Iodinated I 131 Serum (See also *Diagnostic aid (blood volume determination); Radioactive agent*)
Iodinated I 131 Albumin (See also *Diagnostic aid (blood volume determination); Radioactive agent*)

LIVER IMAGING
Ammonia N 13 (See also *Diagnostic aid (cardiac imaging); Radioactive agent*)
Gold Au 198 (See also *Antineoplastic; Radioactive agent*)

LUNG IMAGING
Albumin, Aggregated
Technetium Tc 99m Albumin Aggregated (See also *Radioactive agent*)

LYMPHANGIOGRAPHY
Isosulfan Blue

MYASTHENIA GRAVIS
Edrophonium Chloride (See also *Antidote (to curare principles)*)

NEOPLASM
Iomethin I 125 (See also *Radioactive agent*)

Iomethin I 131 (See also *Radioactive agent*)
Sodium Phosphate P 32 (See also *Antineoplastic; Antipolycythemic; Radioactive agent*)

OBSTETRICS
Quinaldine Blue

PANCREAS FUNCTION DETERMINATION
Bentiromide
Selenomethionine Se 75 (See also *Radioactive agent*)

PARAMAGNETIC
Ferristene
Ferucarbotran
Ferumoxides
Ferumoxsil
Ferumoxtran-10
Gadobenate Dimeglumine
Gadoteridol
Sprodiamide

Brain disorders; spine disorders
Gadodiamide
Gadoversetamide

PENICILLIN SENSITIVITY
Benzylpenicilloyl Polylysine

PERNICIOUS ANEMIA
Cyanocobalamin Co 57 (See also *Radioactive agent*)
Cyanocobalamin Co 60 (See also *Radioactive agent*)

PITUITARY FUNCTION DETERMINATION
Arginine (See also *Ammonia detoxicant*)
Metyrapone
Metyrapone Tartrate

RADIOACTIVE

Adrenomedullary disorders and neuroendocrine tumors
Iobenguane Sulfate I 123 (See also *Radioactive agent*)

Cardiac disease
Iocanlidic Acid I 123
Rubidium Chloride Rb 82 (See also *Radioactive agent*)
Technetium Tc 99m Furifosmin (See also *Radioactive agent*)

Vascular disorders
Technetium Tc 99m Apcitide
Water O 15 (See also *Radioactive agent*)

RADIONUCLIDE CISTERNOGRAPHY
Indium In 111 Pentetate (See also *Radioactive agent*)

RADIOPAQUE MEDIUM
Barium Sulfate
Diatrizoate Meglumine
Diatrizoate Sodium
Diatrizoic Acid
Ethiodized Oil
Gallium Citrate Ga 67 (See also *Radioactive agent*)
Iocarmate Meglumine
Iocarmic Acid
Iocetamic Acid
Iodamide
Iodamide Meglumine
Iodipamide Meglumine

Iodixanol
Iodoxamate Meglumine
Iodoxamic Acid
Ioglicic Acid
Ioglucol
Ioglucomide
Iogulamide
Iohexol
Iomeprol
Iopamidol
Iopanoic Acid
Iopentol
Iophendylate
Ioprocemic Acid
Iopromide
Iosefamic Acid
Ioseric Acid
Iosulamide Meglumine
Iosumetic Acid
Iotasul
Iotetric Acid
Iothalamate Meglumine
Iothalamate Sodium
Iothalamic Acid
Iotrolan
Iotroxic Acid
Ioversol
Ioxaglate Meglumine
Ioxaglate Sodium
Ioxaglic Acid
Ioxotrizoic Acid
Ipodate Calcium
Ipodate Sodium
Meglumine
Metrizamide
Metrizoate Sodium
Propyliodone
Thallous Chloride Tl 201 (See also *Radioactive agent*)

Bronchographic
Iopydol
Iopydone

Cardiac perfusion
Technetium Tc 99m Sestamibi (See also *Radioactive agent*)
Technetium Tc 99m Teboroxime (See also *Radioactive agent*)

Cholecystographic
Iobenzamic Acid
Ioglycamic Acid
Iopronic Acid
Tyropanoate Sodium

REGIONAL CEREBRAL PERFUSION IMAGING
Exametazime

RENAL FUNCTION DETERMINATION
Aminohippurate Sodium
Chlormerodrin Hg 197 (See also *Radioactive agent*)
Chlormerodrin Hg 203 (See also *Radioactive agent*)
Inulin
Iodohippurate Sodium I 123 (See also *Radioactive agent*)
Iodohippurate Sodium I 131 (See also *Radioactive agent*)
Mannitol (See also *Diuretic*)

Merisoprol Hg 197 (See also *Radioactive agent*)
Technetium Tc 99m Mertiatide (See also *Radioactive agent*)
Technetium Tc 99m Succimer (See also *Radioactive agent*)

SKELETAL IMAGING
Stannous Pyrophosphate
Technetium Tc 99m Medronate (See also *Radioactive agent*)
Technetium Tc 99m Oxidronate (See also *Radioactive agent*)

THYROID FUNCTION DETERMINATION
Sodium Iodide I 123 (See also *Radioactive agent*)
Sodium Iodide I 125 (See also *Radioactive agent*)
Sodium Iodide I 131 (See also *Antineoplastic; Radioactive agent*)

VASCULAR PATENCY
Fibrinogen I 125 (See also *Radioactive agent*)

Disinfectant
Bensalan
Benzoxiquine
Chlorocresol (See also *Antiseptic*)
Cloflucarban
Clorophene
Cresol
Dibromsalan
Fluorosalan
Formaldehyde
Fursalan
Glutaral
Halazone
Ictasol
Metabromsalan
Oxyquinoline
Phenolate Sodium
Propiolactone
Sodium Hypochlorite
Thiosalan
Tibrofan
Tribromsalan
Triclocarban
Triclosan

Diuretic
Alipamide (See also *Antihypertensive*)
Ambuphylline (See also *Relaxant (smooth muscle)*)
Ambuside
Amiloride Hydrochloride
Ammonium Chloride (See also *Acidifier*)
Anaritide Acetate (See also *Antihypertensive*)
Azolimine
Azosemide
Bemitradine (See also *Antihypertensive*)
Bendroflumethiazide (See also *Antihypertensive*)
Benzthiazide (See also *Antihypertensive*)
Brocrinat
Bumetanide
Buthiazide (See also *Antihypertensive*)
Chlorothiazide

Chlorothiazide Sodium (See also *Antihypertensive*)
Chlorthalidone
Clazolimine
Clopamide (See also *Antihypertensive*)
Clorexolone
Cyclothiazide (See also *Antihypertensive*)
Diapamide (See also *Antihypertensive*)
Epithiazide (See also *Antihypertensive*)
Ethacrynate Sodium
Ethacrynic Acid
Etozolin
Fenquizone
Furosemide
Hydrochlorothiazide
Hydroflumethiazide (See also *Antihypertensive*)
Indacrinone (See also *Antihypertensive*)
Indapamide (See also *Antihypertensive*)
Isosorbide
Mannitol (See also *Diagnostic aid (renal function determination)*)
Mefruside
Methalthiazide (See also *Antihypertensive*)
Methyclothiazide (See also *Antihypertensive*)
Metolazone (See also *Antihypertensive*)
Muzolimine (See also *Antihypertensive*)
Ozolinone
Piretanide
Polythiazide (See also *Antihypertensive*)
Spironolactone (See also *Aldosterone antagonist*)
Spiroxasone
Ticrynafen (See also *Uricosuric; Antihypertensive*)
Torsemide
Triamterene
Trichlormethiazide (See also *Antihypertensive*)
Triflocin
Tripamide (See also *Antihypertensive*)
Urea
Xipamide (See also *Antihypertensive*)

Dopamine agonist
Alentemol Hydrobromide (See also *Antipsychotic*)
Cabergoline (See also *Antidyskinetic; Antihyperprolactinemic*)
Fenoldopam Mesylate (See also *Antihypertensive*)
Naxagolide Hydrochloride (See also *Antiparkinsonian*)
Pergolide Mesylate
Pramipexole (See also *Antidepressant; Antiparkinsonian; Antischizophrenic*)
Pramipexole Dihydrochloride (See also *Antidepressant; Antiparkinsonian; Antischizophrenic*)

Dopaminergic agent
Ciladopa Hydrochloride (See also *Antiparkinsonian*)

PERIPHERAL
Ibopamine

Dusting powder
Starch (See also *Pharmaceutic aid*)
Starch, Topical
Talc (See also *Pharmaceutic aid (tablet and/or capsule lubricant)*)
Zinc Stearate (See also *Pharmaceutic aid (tablet and/or capsule lubricant)*)

Ectoparasiticide
Nifluridide
Permethrin
VETERINARY
Temefos

Electrolyte combination
Pentalyte
Salts, Rehydration

Emetic
Apomorphine Hydrochloride
Ipecac

Emphysema therapy adjunct
Lodelaben (See also *Anti-arthritic*)

Enzyme
DIGESTANT ADJUNCT
Cellulase
Pancreatin
Pancrelipase
PROTEOLYTIC
Chymopapain
Chymotrypsin
Papain
Sutilains
Trypsin, Crystallized

Enzyme inhibitor
Cilastatin Sodium
Sodium Amylosulfate
ALDOSE REDUCTASE
Alrestatin Sodium
Sorbinil
ANGIOTENSIN-CONVERTING
Benazepril Hydrochloride
Benazeprilat
Captopril (See also *Antihypertensive*)
Delapril Hydrochloride (See also *Antihypertensive*)
Fosinopril Sodium (See also *Antihypertensive*)
Libenzapril
Moexipril Hydrochloride (See also *Antihypertensive*)
Pentopril
Perindopril
Quinapril Hydrochloride (See also *Antihypertensive*)
Quinaprilat (See also *Antihypertensive*)
Ramipril (See also *Antihypertensive*)
Spirapril Hydrochloride
Spiraprilat
Teprotide
Zofenopril Calcium
GAUCHER'S DISEASE
Levcycloserine
GONADOTROPIN
Taleranol

Inhibitor
INFLUENZA VIRUS NEURAMINIDASE
Zanamivir (See also *Antiviral*)

Enzyme inhibitor
PEPSIN
Pepstatin
Polignate Sodium
PROLACTIN
Bromocriptine
Bromocriptine Mesylate
Lergotrile
Lergotrile Mesylate
PROTEINASE
Aprotinin
UREASE
Acetohydroxamic Acid
Benurestat
Flurofamide
Tolfamide

Enzyme replenisher
GLUCOCEREBROSIDASE
Alglucerase
Imiglucerase

Estrogen
Chlorotrianisene
Dienestrol
Diethylstilbestrol
Diethylstilbestrol Diphosphate
Equilin
Estradiol
Estradiol Cypionate
Estradiol Enanthate
Estradiol Undecylate
Estradiol Valerate
Estrazinol Hydrobromide
Estriol
Estrofurate
Estrogens, Conjugated
Estrogens, Esterified
Estrone
Estropipate
Ethinyl Estradiol
Fenestrel
Mestranol
Nylestriol
Quinestrol

Expectorant
Bromhexine Hydrochloride (See also *Mucolytic*)
Glycerol, Iodinated
Guaifenesin
Guaithylline (See also *Bronchodilator*)
Potassium Guaiacolsulfonate
Potassium Iodide (See also *Antifungal; Supplement (iodine)*)
Terpin Hydrate

Fasciolicide
Clorsulon (See also *Antiparasitic*)

Fibrinogen receptor antagonist
Roxifiban Acetate (See also *Antithrombotic*)
Sibrafiban (See also *Antithrombotic; Platelet aggregation inhibitor*)

Fibrinolytic
Anistreplase
Bisobrin Lactate
Brinolase

Fibroblast growth factor
Trafermin (See also *Stroke treatment*)

Food additive
Anoxomer (See also *Pharmaceutic aid (antioxidant)*)
Kasal
Polydextrose
VETERINARY
Amicloral
Bacitracin Methylene Disalicylate (See also *Antibacterial*)
Dicloralurea
Toliodium Chloride
Virginiamycin (See also *Antibacterial*)

Free oxygen radical scavenger
Pegorgotein

Galactopoietic agent
VETERINARY
Somagrebove
Somavubove

Gas, medicinal
Air, Medical
Oxygen
Oxygen 93 Percent
Xenon Xe 127 (See also *Diagnostic aid; Radioactive agent*)

Gases, diluent for
Helium

Gastric acid pump inhibitor
Rabeprazole Sodium (See also *Anti-ulcerative*)

Glomerulonephritis treatment
Sulotroban

Glucocorticoid
Amcinonide
Beclomethasone Dipropionate
Betamethasone
Betamethasone Acetate
Betamethasone Benzoate
Betamethasone Dipropionate
Betamethasone Sodium Phosphate
Betamethasone Valerate
Carbenoxolone Sodium
Clocortolone Acetate
Clocortolone Pivalate
Cloprednol
Corticotropin (See also *Hormone (adrenocorticotropic); Diagnostic aid (adrenocortical insufficiency)*)
Corticotropin, Repository (See also *Hormone (adrenocorticotropic); Diagnostic aid (adrenocortical insufficiency)*)
Corticotropin Zinc Hydroxide (See also *Hormone (adrenocorticotropic); Diagnostic aid (adrenocortical insufficiency)*)
Cortisone Acetate

Cortivazol
Descinolone Acetonide
Dexamethasone
Dexamethasone Sodium Phosphate
Diflucortolone
Diflucortolone Pivalate
Fluchloronide
Flumethasone
Flumethasone Pivalate
Flunisolide
Fluocinolone Acetonide
Fluocinonide
Fluocortolone
Fluocortolone Caproate
Fluorometholone
Fluperolone Acetate
Fluprednisolone
Fluprednisolone Valerate
Flurandrenolide
Formocortal
Hydrocortisone
Hydrocortisone Acetate
Hydrocortisone Butyrate
Hydrocortisone Probutate
Hydrocortisone Sodium Phosphate
Hydrocortisone Sodium Succinate
Hydrocortisone Valerate
Medrysone
Methylprednisolone
Methylprednisolone Acetate
Methylprednisolone Sodium Phosphate
Methylprednisolone Sodium Succinate
Nivazol
Paramethasone Acetate
Prednicarbate
Prednisolone
Prednisolone Acetate
Prednisolone Hemisuccinate
Prednisolone Sodium Phosphate
Prednisolone Sodium Succinate
Prednisolone Tebutate
Prednisone
Prednival
Ticabesone Propionate
Tralonide
Triamcinolone
Triamcinolone Acetonide
Triamcinolone Acetonide Sodium Phosphate
Triamcinolone Diacetate
Triamcinolone Hexacetonide

Gonad-stimulating principle
Abarelix (See also *Antagonist (LHRH)*)
Buserelin Acetate
Ganirelix Acetate
Gonadorelin Acetate
Gonadorelin Hydrochloride
Gonadotropin, Chorionic
Menotropins

Growth hormone releasing factor
Ibutamoren Mesylate
Pralmorelin Dihydrochloride

Growth hormone-releasing hormone
Rismorelin Porcine
Sermorelin Acetate (See also *Diagnostic aid*)

Growth stimulant
VETERINARY
Actaplanin
Alexomycin
Efrotomycin
Laidlomycin Propionate Potassium
Narasin (See also *Coccidiostat*)
Nosiheptide
Plauracin
Ractopamine Hydrochloride
Sometribove
Sometripor
Somfasepor
Sulbenox
Temodox

Hair growth stimulant
TOPICAL
Minoxidil (See also *Antihypertensive*)

Hematinic
Epoetin Alfa (See also *Anti-anemic*)
Epoetin Beta (See also *Anti-anemic*)
Ferric Fructose
Ferriclate Calcium Sodium
Ferrous Fumarate
Ferrous Gluconate
Ferrous Sulfate
Iron Dextran
Iron Sorbitex
Polyferose

VETERINARY
Gleptoferron

Hematopoietic
MACROPHAGE COLONY-STIMULATING FACTOR
Cilmostim

Hematopoietic inhibitor
Nagrestipen

Hematopoietic stimulant
Daniplestim (See also *Antineutropenic*)
Filgrastim (See also *Antineutropenic*)
Lenograstim (See also *Antineutropenic*)
Milodistim (See also *Antineutropenic*)
Molgramostim (See also *Antineutropenic*)
Muplestim (See also *Antineutropenic*)
Oprelvekin
Regramostim (See also *Antineutropenic*)
Sargramostim (See also *Antineutropenic*)

Hemostatic
Aminocaproic Acid
Ethamsylate
Factor IX Complex
Oxamarin Hydrochloride
Sulmarin
Tranexamic Acid

LOCAL
Cellulose, Oxidized
Cellulose, Oxidized Regenerated
Thrombin

Hepatitis treatment
Thymalfasin (See also *Antineoplastic; Infectious disease treatment; Vaccine enhancement*)

Hormone [See also **Adrenocortical steroid (salt-regulating); Androgen; Estrogen; Glucocorticoid; Gonad-stimulating principle; Prostaglandin; Thyroid hormone**]
Metogest
ADRENOCORTICOTROPIC
Corticotropin (See also *Glucocorticoid; Diagnostic aid (adrenocortical insufficiency)*)
Corticotropin, Repository (See also *Glucocorticoid; Diagnostic aid (adrenocortical insufficiency)*)
Corticotropin Zinc Hydroxide (See also *Glucocorticoid; Diagnostic aid (adrenocortical insufficiency)*)
Cosyntropin
Seractide Acetate
ANTIDIURETIC
Pituitary, Posterior
Vasopressin
CORTICOTROPIN-RELEASING
Corticorelin Ovine Triflutate (See also *Diagnostic aid (adrenocortical insufficiency); Diagnostic aid (Cushing's syndrome)*)
FOLLICLE-STIMULATING
Urofollitropin
GONADOTROPIN-RELEASING
Veterinary
Fertirelin Acetate
GROWTH
Somatrem
Somatropin
Porcine
Somalapor
Somenopor
Synthetic bovine
Somidobove
REPLACEMENT THERAPY
Estrogen receptor antagonist
Idoxifene (See also *Antineoplastic; Osteoporosis treatment and prevention*)

Hypocholesterolemic
Lifibrol
Pamaqueside (See also *Anti-atherosclerotic*)

Hypoglycemic
Glimepiride
ORAL
Darglitazone Sodium

Hypolipidemic
Azalanstat Dihydrochloride
Colestolone
Surfomer
Xenalipin

Hypotensive
Dicirenone (See also *Aldosterone antagonist*)

Viprostol (See also *Vasodilator*)

Immunizing agent

ACTIVE

BCG Vaccine
Cholera Vaccine
Diphtheria Toxoid
Diphtheria Toxoid Adsorbed
Hepatitis B Virus Vaccine Inactivated
Influenza Virus Vaccine
Measles Virus Vaccine Live
Meningococcal Polysaccharide Vaccine
  Group A
Meningococcal Polysaccharide Vaccine
  Group C
Mumps Virus Vaccine Live
Pertussis Vaccine
Pertussis Vaccine Adsorbed
Plague Vaccine
Poliovirus Vaccine Inactivated
Poliovirus Vaccine Live Oral
Rabies Vaccine
Rubella Virus Vaccine Live
Smallpox Vaccine
Tetanus Toxoid
Tetanus Toxoid Adsorbed
Typhoid Vaccine
Yellow Fever Vaccine

PASSIVE

Antirabies Serum
Antivenin (Latrodectus mactans)
Antivenin (Micrurus Fulvius)
Antivenin (Crotalidae) Polyvalent
Botulism Antitoxin
Diphtheria Antitoxin
Globulin, Immune
Hepatitis B Immune Globulin
Pertussis Immune Globulin
Rabies Immune Globulin
Rh$_o$ (D) Immune Globulin
Tetanus Antitoxin
Tetanus Immune Globulin
Vaccinia Immune Globulin
Varicella-Zoster Immune Globulin

Immunomodulator

Acemannan (See also *Antiviral*)
Atiprimod Dimaleate (See also *Anti-ar-
  thritic; Anti-inflammatory*)
Dimepranol Acedoben
Glatiramer Acetate
Imiquimod
Interferon Beta-1b
Lenercept
Lisofylline
Mycophenolate Mofetil
Prezatide Copper Acetate
Roquinimex (See also *Biological re-
  sponse modifier*)

Immunoregulator

Azarole
Fanetizole Mesylate
Frentizole
Interferon Gamma-1b (See also *Antine-
  oplastic; Biological response modifi-
  er*)
Oxamisole Hydrochloride
Ristianol Phosphate

Thymopentin
Tilomisole

Immunostimulant

Aldesleukin (See also *Antineoplastic;
  Biological response modifier*)
Loxoribine (See also *Vaccine adjuvant*)
Teceleukin

Immunosuppressant

Azathioprine
Azathioprine Sodium
Cedelizumab (See also *Monoclonal an-
  tibody*)
Cyclophosphamide (See also *Antineo-
  plastic*)
Cyclosporine
Daltroban
Gusperimus Trihydrochloride
Sirolimus
Tacrolimus

Impotence therapy

Sildenafil Citrate

Impotence therapy adjunct

Delequamine Hydrochloride

Infectious disease treatment

Thymalfasin (See also *Antineoplastic;
  Hepatitis treatment; Vaccine enhancement*)

Inhibitor

ADVANCED GLYCOSYLATION END-PRODUCT
FORMATION
Pimagedine Hydrochloride

α-GLUCOSIDASE
Acarbose
Celgosivir Hydrochloride (See also *An-
  tiviral*)
Miglitol

ALDOSE REDUCTASE
Minalrestat
Ponalrestat
Tolrestat
Zopolrestat (See also *Antidiabetic*)

ALPHA REDUCTASE
Epristeride
Finasteride

β-LACTAMASE
Clavulanate Potassium
Sulbactam Benzathine (See also *Syner-
  gist (penicillin/cephalosporin)*)
Sulbactam Pivoxil (See also *Synergist
  (penicillin/cephalosporin)*)
Sulbactam Sodium (See also *Synergist
  (penicillin/cephalosporin)*)
Tazobactam
Tazobactam Sodium

ACETYLCHOLINESTERASE
Donepezil Hydrochloride (See also *Alzheimer's disease treatment (adjunct);
  Dementia symptoms treatment adjunct; Cognition adjuvant*)
Icopezil Maleate (See also *Alzheimer's
  disease treatment (cognition enhancer); Cognition adjuvant*)
Zifrosilone

CHOLINESTERASE
Suronacrine Maleate
Velnacrine Maleate

COLLAGEN
Lufironil

DECARBOXYLASE
Benserazide
Carbidopa

HISTIDINE DECARBOXYLASE
Brocresine

HMG-COA REDUCTASE
Atorvastatin Calcium
Cerivastatin Sodium (See also *Antihy-
  perlipidemic*)
Fluvastatin Sodium (See also *Antihyper-
  lipidemic*)
Lovastatin (See also *Antihyperlipi-
  demic*)

LIPID PEROXIDATION
Tirilazad Mesylate

5-LIPOXYGENASE
Atreleuton (See also *Anti-asthmatic*)
Docebenone
Enazadrem Phosphate (See also *Anti-
  psoriatic*)
Zileuton

Veterinary
Fenleuton

MEDIATOR RELEASE
Eclazolast (See also *Anti-allergic*)
Pemirolast Potassium (See also *Anti-al-
  lergic*)
Quazolast (See also *Anti-asthmatic*)

PANCREATIC LIPASE
Orlistat

PLATELET
Cilostazol (See also *Vasodilator; Anti-
  thrombotic*)
Clopidogrel Bisulfate
Epoprostenol
Epoprostenol Sodium
Ticlopidine Hydrochloride

PROSTAGLANDIN SYNTHESIS
Flurbiprofen Sodium

THROMBOXANE SYNTHETASE
Dazmegrel
Furegrelate Sodium
Pirmagrel
Ridogrel

Insecticide

SYSTEMIC
Ronnel

VETERINARY
Cypothrin
Stirofos

Interceptive
Epostane

Ion-exchange resin

BILE SALTS
Cholestyramine Resin (See also *Antihyperlipidemic*)

POTASSIUM
Sodium Polystyrene Sulfonate

Ivy poisoning counteractant
Poison Ivy Extract, Alum Precipitated

Keratolytic
Alcloxa (See also *Astringent*)
Aldioxa (See also *Astringent*)
Benzoyl Peroxide
Dibenzothiophene
Etarotene
Isotretinoin
Motretinide
Picotrin Diolamine
Resorcinol
Resorcinol Monoacetate (See also *Anti-seborrheic*)
Salicylic Acid
Sumarotene
Tazarotene
Tretinoin
SYSTEMIC
Tetroquinone

Laxative
Bisacodyl
Bisacodyl Tannex
Bisoxatin Acetate
Calcium Polycarbophil
Casanthranol
Castor Oil
Lactulose
Magnesia, [Milk of] (See also *Antacid*)
Magnesium Citrate
Magnesium Hydroxide (See also *Antacid*)
Magnesium Sulfate (See also *Anticonvulsant; Replenisher (electrolyte)*)
Mineral Oil (See also *Pharmaceutic aid (solvent)*)
Oxyphenisatin Acetate
Phenolphthalein
Phenolphthalein, Yellow
Plantago Seed
Polycarbophil
Potassium Sodium Tartrate
Psyllium Husk
Senna
Sennosides
Sodium Phosphate, Dibasic

Leukopheresis adjunct
RED CELL SEDIMENTING AGENT
Pentastarch

LHRH agonist
Deslorelin
Goserelin
Histrelin
Leuprolide Acetate (See also *Antineoplastic*)
Lutrelin Acetate
Nafarelin Acetate

Liver disorder treatment
Malotilate

Lubricant and hydrophobing agent
Dimethicone (See also *Prosthetic aid (soft tissue)*)

Luteolysin
Fenprostalene

Memory adjuvant
Dimoxamine Hydrochloride
Ribaminol

Menopausal symptoms suppressant
Tibolone

Mental performance enhancer
Aniracetam

Miotic
Acetylcholine Chloride (See also *Cardiac depressant; Cholinergic; Vasodilator (peripheral)*)

Monoclonal antibody
Arcitumomab
Capromab Pendetide
Cedelizumab (See also *Immunosuppressant*)
Enlimomab (See also *Anti-inflammatory*)
Nerelimomab
Rituximab (See also *Antineoplastic (microtubule inhibitor)*)
Votumumab
ANTI-ENDOTOXIN
Edobacomab
Nebacumab
ANTIFIBRIN
Biciromab
ANTIMYOSIN
Imciromab Pentetate
ANTINEOPLASTIC ADJUVANT
Edrecolomab
ANTITHROMBOTIC
Abciximab
Zolimomab Aritox
ANTIVIRAL
Felvizumab (See also *Antiviral*)
Sevirumab
Tuvirumab
DIAGNOSTIC FOR THE DETECTION OF INFECTIOUS LESIONS
Sulesomab
DIAGNOSIS OF NON-HODGKIN'S LYMPHOMA AND DETECTION OF AIDS-RELATED LYMPHOMA
Bectumomab
IMMUNOSUPPRESSANT
Daclizumab
Muromonab-CD3
TREATMENT OF AUTOIMMUNE LYMPHOPROLIFERATIVE DISEASES AND IN ORGAN TRANSPLANTATION
Priliximab

Mood regulator
Fengabine

Mucolytic
Acetylcysteine
Bromhexine Hydrochloride (See also *Expectorant*)
Carbocysteine
Domiodol

Multiple sclerosis symptomatic treatment
Fampridine

Mydriatic
Berefrine

Myocardial infarction therapy
Reteplase (See also *Plasminogen activator*)

Myopathic
VETERINARY
Metrenperone

Nasal decongestant
Levmetamfetamine
Nemazoline Hydrochloride
Pseudoephedrine Polistirex

Neuroleptic
Dapiprazole Hydrochloride (See also *Adrenergic (α-blocking); Antiglaucoma agent; Psychotropic*)
Duoperone Fumarate
Flumezapine (See also *Antipsychotic*)
Risperidone
Sertindole (See also *Antipsychotic*)

Neuromuscular blocking agent
Atracurium Besylate
Cisatracurium Besylate
Doxacurium Chloride
Gallamine Triethiodide
Metocurine Iodide
Mivacurium Chloride
Pancuronium Bromide
Pipecuronium Bromide
Rapacuronium Bromide
Rocuronium Bromide
Succinylcholine Chloride
Tubocurarine Chloride
Vecuronium Bromide

Neuroprotective
Dizocilpine Maleate

NMDA antagonist
Licostinel
Selfotel

Non-hormonal sterol derivative
Pregnenolone Succinate

Nootropic
Sibopirdine (See also *Alzheimer's disease treatment (cognition enhancer)*)

Nutrient
Adenosine Phosphate
Fructose
Potassium Aspartate and Magnesium Aspartate

Nutritional supplement
Calcium Ascorbate

Osteoporosis therapy adjunct
Teriparatide (See also *Bone resorption inhibitor*)
Zoledronate Disodium (See also *Bone resorption inhibitor*)

Zoledronate Trisodium (See also *Bone resorption inhibitor*)

Zoledronic Acid

Osteoporosis treatment and prevention

Idoxifene (See also *Antineoplastic; Hormone (replacement therapy, estrogen receptor antagonist)*)

Tiludronate Disodium (See also *Paget's disease treatment*)

Oxytocic

Carboprost

Carboprost Methyl

Carboprost Tromethamine

Dinoprost (See also *Prostaglandin*)

Dinoprost Tromethamine (See also *Prostaglandin*)

Dinoprostone (See also *Prostaglandin*)

Ergonovine Maleate

Meteneprost (See also *Prostaglandin*)

Methylergonovine Maleate

Oxytocin

Quipazine Maleate (See also *Antidepressant*)

Sparteine Sulfate

Paget's disease treatment

Tiludronate Disodium (See also *Osteoporosis treatment and prevention*)

Pediculicide

Lindane (See also *Scabicide*)

Malathion

Pyrethrum Extract

Perfusion deficit disorders treatment

Hemoglobin Crosfumaril

Pharmaceutic aid

Ammonium Phosphate

Antimony Trisulfide Colloid

Betiatide

Caldiamide Sodium

Calteridol Calcium

Egtazic Acid

Gluceptate Sodium

Glucosamine

Medronate Disodium

Medronic Acid

Olive Oil

Phytate Persodium

Polacrilin

Polifeprosan 20

Silica, Dental-type

Sodium Polyphosphate

Sodium Pyrophosphate

Sodium Trimetaphosphate

Stannous Chloride

Starch (See also *Dusting powder*)

Tolu Balsam

Versetamide

ACIDIFYING AGENT

Acetic Acid

Acetic Acid, Glacial

Hydrochloric Acid

Malic Acid

Nitric Acid

Propionic Acid (See also *Antimicrobial*)

Sulfuric Acid

ADSORBANT

Charcoal, Activated (See also *Antidote (general purpose)*)

AEROSOL PROPELLANT

Dichlorodifluoromethane

Dichlorotetrafluoroethane

Trichloromonofluoromethane

AIR DISPLACEMENT

Nitrogen

ALCOHOL DENATURANT

Denatonium Benzoate (See also *Pharmaceutic aid (flavor)*)

Methyl Isobutyl Ketone

Sucrose Octaacetate

ALKALIZING AGENT

Diethanolamine

Edetol

Potassium Carbonate

Potassium Hydroxide

Sodium Borate

Sodium Carbonate

Sodium Hydroxide

Trolamine (See also *Analgesic*)

ANTIFUNGAL AGENT

Benzoic Acid

Butylparaben

Ethylparaben

Methylparaben

Propylparaben

Sodium Benzoate (See also *Antihyperammonemic*)

ANTIMICROBIAL AGENT

Benzyl Alcohol

Chlorobutanol

Phenylethyl Alcohol

Phenylmercuric Acetate

Phenylmercuric Nitrate

Potassium Sorbate

Sorbic Acid

ANTIMICROBIAL PRESERVATIVE

Methylparaben Sodium

Propylparaben Sodium

Sodium Dehydroacetate

ANTIOXIDANT

Anoxomer (See also *Food additive*)

Ascorbyl Palmitate

Butylated Hydroxyanisole

Butylated Hydroxytoluene

Hypophosphorous Acid

Potassium Metabisulfite

Propyl Gallate

Sodium Metabisulfite

Sulfur Dioxide

Tocopherols Excipient

BUFFERING AGENT

Calcium Acetate

Potassium Metaphosphate

Potassium Phosphate, Monobasic

Tartaric Acid

CHELATING AGENT

Edetate Dipotassium

Edetate Disodium (See also *Chelating agent (metal)*)

Edetic Acid

COATING AGENT

Ammonio Methacrylate Copolymer

Cellulose Acetate (See also *Polymer membrane, insoluble*)

Hypromellose Phthalate

Maltodextrin (See also *Pharmaceutic aid (tablet binder); Pharmaceutic aid (tablet and capsule diluent); Pharmaceutic aid (viscosity-increasing agent)*)

Polyvinyl Acetate Phthalate

Zein

COLOR

Caramel

Ferric Oxide

COMPLEXING AGENT

Gentisic Acid Ethanolamide

Oxyquinoline Sulfate

IN DIALYSIS SOLUTIONS

Sodium Acetate

DISPERSING AGENT

Poligeenan

DISPERSING AND SUSPENDING AGENT

Povidone

Silicon Dioxide

EMOLLIENT

Alkyl (C12-15) Benzoate (See also *Pharmaceutic aid (vehicle, oleaginous)*)

Isopropyl Myristate

Isostearyl Alcohol (See also *Pharmaceutic aid (solvent)*)

Oleyl Alcohol (See also *Pharmaceutic aid (emulsifying agent)*)

EMOLLIENT AND PERFUME

Almond Oil (See also *Pharmaceutic aid (vehicle, oleaginous)*)

EMULSIFYING AGENT

Carbomer 910 (See also *Pharmaceutic aid (suspending agent)*)

Carbomer 934 (See also *Pharmaceutic aid (suspending agent)*)

Carbomer 934P (See also *Pharmaceutic aid (suspending and/or viscosity agent); Pharmaceutic aid (thickening agent)*)

Carbomer 940 (See also *Pharmaceutic aid (suspending agent)*)

Carbomer 941 (See also *Pharmaceutic aid (suspending agent)*)

Carbomer 1342 (See also *Pharmaceutic aid (suspending agent)*)

Cetostearyl Alcohol

Cholesterol

Glyceryl Monostearate

Hydroxypropyl Cellulose (See also *Protectant (topical); Pharmaceutic aid (tablet coating agent)*)

Lanolin Alcohols

Lecithin

Mono- and Di-glycerides

Oleyl Alcohol (See also *Pharmaceutic aid (emollient)*)

Peglicol 5 Oleate

Pegoxol 7 Stearate

Polyoxyl 35 Castor Oil (See also *Pharmaceutic aid (surfactant)*)

Polyoxyl 40 Hydrogenated Castor Oil (See also *Pharmaceutic aid (surfactant)*)
Polyoxyl 50 Stearate (See also *Pharmaceutic aid (surfactant)*)
Propylene Glycol Monostearate
Wax, Emulsifying (See also *Pharmaceutic aid (stiffening agent)*)

EMULSIFYING AND STIFFENING AGENT
Cetyl Alcohol
Sodium Stearate

EMULSION ADJUNCT
Oleic Acid
Stearic Acid (See also *Pharmaceutic aid (tablet and/or capsule lubricant)*)
Stearyl Alcohol

ENCAPSULATING AGENT
Gelatin (See also *Pharmaceutic aid (suspending agent); Pharmaceutic aid (tablet binder); Pharmaceutic aid (tablet coating agent)*)

EXCIPIENT
Laurocapram
Polyethylene Glycol Monomethyl Ether

FILTERING MEDIUM
Siliceous Earth, Purified

FLAVOR
Anethole
Anise Oil
Benzaldehyde
Caraway
Caraway Oil
Cardamom
Cardamom Oil
Cherry Juice
Clove Oil
Denatonium Benzoate (See also *Pharmaceutic aid (alcohol denaturant)*)
Ethyl Vanillin
Fennel Oil
Lemon Oil
Methyl Salicylate
Monosodium Glutamate (See also *Pharmaceutic aid (perfume)*)
Orange Oil
Peppermint (See also *Pharmaceutic aid (perfume)*)
Peppermint Oil
Saccharin
Sorbitol (See also *Pharmaceutic aid (tablet excipient)*)
Sucrose (See also *Pharmaceutic aid (tablet excipient)*)
Sugar, Compressible (See also *Pharmaceutic aid (tablet excipient)*)
Sugar, Confectioner's (See also *Pharmaceutic aid (tablet excipient)*)
Vanilla
Vanillin

GELLING AGENT
Propylene Carbonate

HUMECTANT
Glycerin (See also *Pharmaceutic aid (solvent)*)
Hexylene Glycol (See also *Pharmaceutic aid (solvent)*)

Propylene Glycol (See also *Pharmaceutic aid (solvent); Pharmaceutic aid (suspending agent)*)

OINTMENT BASE
Petrolatum
Poloxamer (See also *Pharmaceutic aid (suppository base); Pharmaceutic aid (surfactant); Pharmaceutic aid (tablet binder and emulsifying agent); Pharmaceutic aid (tablet coating agent)*)
Polyethylene Glycol (See also *Pharmaceutic aid (suppository base); Pharmaceutic aid (solvent); Pharmaceutic aid (tablet excipient); Pharmaceutic aid (tablet and/or capsule lubricant)*)

Absorbent
Lanolin
Lanolin, Modified

Oleaginous
Petrolatum, White (See also *Protectant (topical)*)

PERFUME
Monosodium Glutamate (See also *Pharmaceutic aid (flavor)*)
Peppermint (See also *Pharmaceutic aid (flavor)*)
Rose Oil
Rose Water, Stronger

PLASTICIZER
Diacetylated Monoglycerides
Dibutyl Sebacate
Diethyl Phthalate
Mono- and Di-acetylated Monoglycerides
Octicizer
Triethyl Citrate

PRESERVATIVE
Benzalkonium Chloride
Benzethonium Chloride (See also *Anti-infective, topical*)
Cetylpyridinium Chloride (See also *Anti-infective, topical*)
Monothioglycerol
Phenol
Polixetonium Chloride
Potassium Benzoate
Sodium Formaldehyde Sulfoxylate
Sodium Propionate
Thimerosal (See also *Anti-infective, topical*)

SEQUESTERING AGENT
Betadex

SOLVENT
Acetone
Alcohol (See also *Anti-infective, topical*)
Amylene Hydrate
Butyl Alcohol
Corn Oil
Cottonseed Oil
Ethyl Acetate
Glycerin (See also *Pharmaceutic aid (humectant)*)
Hexylene Glycol (See also *Pharmaceutic aid (humectant)*)

Isopropyl Alcohol (See also *Anti-infective, topical*)
Isostearyl Alcohol (See also *Pharmaceutic aid (emollient)*)
Methyl Alcohol
Methylene Chloride
Mineral Oil (See also *Laxative*)
Peanut Oil
Phosphoric Acid
Polyethylene Glycol (See also *Pharmaceutic aid (ointment base); Pharmaceutic aid (suppository base); Pharmaceutic aid (tablet excipient); Pharmaceutic aid (tablet and/or capsule lubricant)*)
Polyoxypropylene 15 Stearyl Ether
Propylene Glycol (See also *Pharmaceutic aid (humectant); Pharmaceutic aid (suspending agent)*)
Propylene Glycol Diacetate
Sesame Oil (See also *Pharmaceutic aid (vehicle, oleaginous)*)

SOLVENT AND SOURCE OF AMMONIA
Ammonia Solution, Strong

SORBENT
Magnesium Oxide

SOURCE OF AMMONIA
Ammonium Carbonate

STABILIZER
Calcium Saccharate
Thymol

STIFFENING AGENT
Cetyl Esters Wax
Myristyl Alcohol
Paraffin
Paraffin, Synthetic
Wax, Emulsifying (See also *Pharmaceutic aid (emulsifying agent)*)
Wax, Microcrystalline (See also *Pharmaceutic aid (tablet coating agent)*)
Wax, White
Wax, Yellow

SUPPOSITORY BASE
Cocoa Butter
Fat, Hard
Poloxamer (See also *Pharmaceutic aid (ointment base); Pharmaceutic aid (surfactant); Pharmaceutic aid (tablet binder and emulsifying agent); Pharmaceutic aid (tablet coating agent)*)
Polyethylene Glycol (See also *Pharmaceutic aid (ointment base); Pharmaceutic aid (solvent); Pharmaceutic aid (tablet excipient); Pharmaceutic aid (tablet and/or capsule lubricant)*)

SURFACTANT
Docusate Sodium (See also *Stool softener*)
Lapyrium Chloride
Laureth 4
Laureth 9 (See also *Spermaticide*)
Monoethanolamine
Nonoxynol 4
Nonoxynol 10
Nonoxynol 15
Nonoxynol 30

Octoxynol 9
Poloxalene
Poloxamer (See also *Pharmaceutic aid (ointment base); Pharmaceutic aid (suppository base); Pharmaceutic aid (tablet binder and emulsifying agent); Pharmaceutic aid (tablet coating agent)*)
Polyoxyl 8 Stearate
Polyoxyl 10 Oleyl Ether
Polyoxyl 20 Cetostearyl Ether
Polyoxyl 35 Castor Oil (See also *Pharmaceutic aid (emulsifying agent)*)
Polyoxyl 40 Hydrogenated Castor Oil (See also *Pharmaceutic aid (emulsifying agent)*)
Polyoxyl 40 Stearate
Polyoxyl 50 Stearate (See also *Pharmaceutic aid (emulsifying agent)*)
Polysorbate 20
Polysorbate 40
Polysorbate 60
Polysorbate 65
Polysorbate 80
Polysorbate 85
Sodium Lauryl Sulfate
Sorbitan Monolaurate
Sorbitan Monooleate
Sorbitan Monopalmitate
Sorbitan Monostearate
Sorbitan Sesquioleate
Sorbitan Trioleate
Sorbitan Tristearate

SUSPENDING AGENT

Agar
Attapulgite, Activated
Bentonite
Carbomer 910 (See also *Pharmaceutic aid (emulsifying agent)*)
Carbomer 934 (See also *Pharmaceutic aid (emulsifying agent)*)
Carbomer 940 (See also *Pharmaceutic aid (emulsifying agent)*)
Carbomer 941 (See also *Pharmaceutic aid (emulsifying agent)*)
Carbomer 1342 (See also *Pharmaceutic aid (emulsifying agent)*)
Carboxymethylcellulose Sodium (See also *Pharmaceutic aid (tablet excipient); Pharmaceutic aid (viscosity-increasing agent)*)
Carboxymethylcellulose Sodium 12 (See also *Pharmaceutic aid (viscosity-increasing agent)*)
Carrageenan (See also *Pharmaceutic aid (viscosity-increasing agent)*)
Dextrin (See also *Pharmaceutic aid (viscosity-increasing agent); Pharmaceutic aid (tablet binder); Pharmaceutic aid (tablet and capsule diluent)*)
Elm (See also *Demulcent*)
Gelatin (See also *Pharmaceutic aid (encapsulating agent); Pharmaceutic aid (tablet binder); Pharmaceutic aid (tablet coating agent)*)

Hydroxyethyl Cellulose (See also *Pharmaceutic aid (viscosity-increasing agent)*)
Hypromellose (See also *Pharmaceutic aid (tablet excipient); Pharmaceutic aid (viscosity-increasing agent)*)
Magnesium Aluminum Silicate
Methylcellulose
Pectin (See also *Protectant*)
Pegoterate
Propylene Glycol (See also *Pharmaceutic aid (humectant); Pharmaceutic aid (solvent)*)
Propylene Glycol Alginate (See also *Pharmaceutic aid (viscosity-increasing agent)*)
Silicon Dioxide, Colloidal (See also *Pharmaceutic aid (tablet and capsule diluent); Pharmaceutic aid (thickening agent)*)
Sodium Alginate
Tragacanth
Xanthan Gum

SUSPENDING AND/OR VISCOSITY AGENT

Acacia
Carbomer 934P (See also *Pharmaceutic aid (emulsifying agent); Pharmaceutic aid (thickening agent)*)
Polyethylene Oxide (See also *Pharmaceutic aid (tablet binder)*)

TABLET BASE

Calcium Phosphate Dihydrate, Dibasic (See also *Replenisher (calcium)*)

TABLET BINDER

Dextrin (See also *Pharmaceutic aid (suspending agent); Pharmaceutic aid (viscosity-increasing agent); Pharmaceutic aid (tablet and capsule diluent)*)
Ethylcellulose
Gelatin (See also *Pharmaceutic aid (encapsulating agent); Pharmaceutic aid (suspending agent); Pharmaceutic aid (tablet coating agent)*)
Glucose, Liquid (See also *Pharmaceutic aid (tablet coating agent)*)
Guar Gum (See also *Pharmaceutic aid (tablet disintegrant)*)
Maltodextrin (See also *Pharmaceutic aid (coating agent); Pharmaceutic aid (tablet and capsule diluent); Pharmaceutic aid (viscosity-increasing agent)*)
Policapram
Polyethylene Oxide (See also *Pharmaceutic aid (suspending and/or viscosity agent)*)

TABLET BINDER AND DILUENT

Dextrates

TABLET BINDER AND EMULSIFYING AGENT

Alginic Acid
Poloxamer (See also *Pharmaceutic aid (ointment base); Pharmaceutic aid (suppository base); Pharmaceutic aid (surfactant); Pharmaceutic aid (tablet coating agent)*)

TABLET AND CAPSULE DILUENT

Calcium Sulfate
Cellulose, Microcrystalline
Dextrin (See also *Pharmaceutic aid (suspending agent); Pharmaceutic aid (viscosity-increasing agent); Pharmaceutic aid (tablet binder)*)
Lactose, Anhydrous
Lactose Monohydrate
Maltodextrin (See also *Pharmaceutic aid (coating agent); Pharmaceutic aid (tablet binder); Pharmaceutic aid (viscosity-increasing agent)*)
Silicon Dioxide, Colloidal (See also *Pharmaceutic aid (suspending agent); Pharmaceutic aid (thickening agent)*)

TABLET AND/OR CAPSULE LUBRICANT

Calcium Stearate
Glyceryl Behenate
Magnesium Stearate
Mineral Oil, Light (See also *Pharmaceutic aid (vehicle)*)
Polyethylene Glycol (See also *Pharmaceutic aid (ointment base); Pharmaceutic aid (suppository base); Pharmaceutic aid (solvent); Pharmaceutic aid (tablet excipient)*)
Sodium Stearyl Fumarate
Stearic Acid (See also *Pharmaceutic aid (emulsion adjunct)*)
Talc (See also *Dusting powder*)
Vegetable Oil, Hydrogenated
Zinc Stearate (See also *Dusting powder*)

TABLET COATING AGENT

Cellacefate
Gelatin (See also *Pharmaceutic aid (encapsulating agent); Pharmaceutic aid (suspending agent); Pharmaceutic aid (tablet binder)*)
Glaze, Pharmaceutical
Glucose, Liquid (See also *Pharmaceutic aid (tablet binder)*)
Hydroxypropyl Cellulose (See also *Protectant (topical); Pharmaceutic aid (emulsifying agent)*)
Methacrylic Acid Copolymer
Poloxamer (See also *Pharmaceutic aid (ointment base); Pharmaceutic aid (suppository base); Pharmaceutic aid (surfactant); Pharmaceutic aid (tablet binder and emulsifying agent)*)
Shellac
Wax, Carnauba
Wax, Microcrystalline (See also *Pharmaceutic aid (stiffening agent)*)

TABLET DISINTEGRANT

Carboxymethylcellulose Calcium
Croscarmellose Sodium
Guar Gum (See also *Pharmaceutic aid (tablet binder)*)
Polacrilin Potassium

TABLET EXCIPIENT

Calcium Silicate
Carboxymethylcellulose Sodium (See also *Pharmaceutic aid (suspending agent); Pharmaceutic aid (viscosity-increasing agent)*)

Crospovidone
Hypromellose (See also *Pharmaceutic aid (suspending agent); Pharmaceutic aid (viscosity-increasing agent)*)
Magnesium Silicate
Polipropene 25
Polyethylene Glycol (See also *Pharmaceutic aid (ointment base); Pharmaceutic aid (suppository base); Pharmaceutic aid (solvent); Pharmaceutic aid (tablet and/or capsule lubricant)*)
Sodium Starch Glycolate
Sorbitol (See also *Pharmaceutic aid (flavor)*)
Starch, Pregelatinized
Sucrose (See also *Pharmaceutic aid (flavor)*)
Sugar, Compressible (See also *Pharmaceutic aid (flavor)*)
Sugar, Confectioner's (See also *Pharmaceutic aid (flavor)*)

THICKENING AGENT
Carbomer 934P (See also *Pharmaceutic aid (emulsifying agent); Pharmaceutic aid (suspending and/or viscosity agent)*)
Glycol Distearate
Silicon Dioxide, Colloidal (See also *Pharmaceutic aid (suspending agent); Pharmaceutic aid (tablet and capsule diluent)*)

TONICITY AGENT
Sodium Chloride

VEHICLE
Ethyl Oleate
Mineral Oil, Light (See also *Pharmaceutic aid (tablet and/or capsule lubricant)*)

Oleaginous
Alkyl (C12-15) Benzoate (See also *Pharmaceutic aid (emollient)*)
Almond Oil (See also *Pharmaceutic aid (emollient and perfume)*)
Isopropyl Palmitate
Octyldodecanol
Safflower Oil
Sesame Oil (See also *Pharmaceutic aid (solvent)*)
Squalane

Solid carrier
Sugar Spheres

Sweetened
Xylitol

VISCOSITY-INCREASING AGENT
Carboxymethylcellulose Sodium (See also *Pharmaceutic aid (suspending agent); Pharmaceutic aid (tablet excipient)*)
Carboxymethylcellulose Sodium 12 (See also *Pharmaceutic aid (suspending agent)*)
Carrageenan (See also *Pharmaceutic aid (suspending agent)*)

Dextrin (See also *Pharmaceutic aid (suspending agent); Pharmaceutic aid (tablet binder); Pharmaceutic aid (tablet and capsule diluent)*)
Hydroxyethyl Cellulose (See also *Pharmaceutic aid (suspending agent)*)
Hypromellose (See also *Pharmaceutic aid (suspending agent); Pharmaceutic aid (tablet excipient)*)
Maltodextrin (See also *Pharmaceutic aid (coating agent); Pharmaceutic aid (tablet binder); Pharmaceutic aid (tablet and capsule diluent)*)
Polyvinyl Alcohol
Propylene Glycol Alginate (See also *Pharmaceutic aid (suspending agent)*)

WETTING AGENT
Cyclomethicone

WETTING AND/OR SOLUBILIZING AGENT
Nonoxynol 9 (See also *Spermaticide*)

Pharmaceutic necessity
Bismuth Subnitrate
Boric Acid
Juniper Tar
Lime
Podophyllum
Potassium Bicarbonate
Soybean Oil

Pigmentation agent
Methoxsalen
Trioxsalen

Plasma volume extender
Dextran 40 (See also *Blood flow adjuvant*)
Dextran 70
Dextran 75
Hetastarch

Plasminogen activator
Alteplase
Lanoteplase (See also *Thrombolytic*)
Reteplase (See also *Myocardial infarction therapy*)
Urokinase
Urokinase Alfa (See also *Thrombolytic*)

Platelet activating factor antagonist
Apafant
Lexipafant

Platelet aggregation inhibitor
Acadesine
Beraprost
Beraprost Sodium
Ciprostene Calcium
Itazigrel
Lifarizine
Lotrafiban Hydrochloride (See also *Antithrombotic*)
Orbofiban Acetate (See also *Antithrombotic*)
Oxagrelate
Sibrafiban (See also *Antithrombotic; Fibrinogen receptor antagonist*)

Polymer membrane, insoluble
Cellulose Acetate (See also *Pharmaceutic aid (coating agent)*)

Post-stroke and post-head trauma treatment
Citicoline Sodium

Potentiator
Pentostatin
CATECHOLAMINE
Talopram Hydrochloride

Prevention of post-recanalization reocclusion of coronary vessels
Xemilofiban Hydrochloride (See also *Treatment of unstable angina*)

Progestin
Algestone Acetophenide
Amadinone Acetate
Anagestone Acetate
Chlormadinone Acetate
Cingestol
Clogestone Acetate
Clomegestone Acetate
Delmadinone Acetate (See also *Anti-androgen; Anti-estrogen*)
Desogestrel
Dimethisterone
Dydrogesterone
Ethynerone
Ethynodiol Diacetate
Etonogestrel
Flurogestone Acetate
Gestaclone
Gestodene
Gestonorone Caproate
Gestrinone
Haloprogesterone
Hydroxyprogesterone Caproate
Levonorgestrel
Lynestrenol
Medrogestone
Medroxyprogesterone Acetate
Melengestrol Acetate (See also *Antineoplastic*)
Methynodiol Diacetate
Norethindrone
Norethindrone Acetate
Norethynodrel
Norgestimate
Norgestomet
Norgestrel
Oxogestone Phenpropionate
Progesterone
Quingestanol Acetate
Quingestrone
Tigestol
Trimegestone

VETERINARY
Altrenogest

Prostaglandin
Cloprostenol Sodium
Dinoprost (See also *Oxytocic*)
Dinoprost Tromethamine (See also *Oxytocic*)
Dinoprostone (See also *Oxytocic*)
Fluprostenol Sodium

Gemeprost
Meteneprost (See also *Oxytocic*)
Prostalene
Sulprostone
VETERINARY
Alfaprostol

Prostate growth inhibitor
Pentomone

Prosthetic aid
Durapatite
ARTERIAL
Artegraft
INTERNAL BONE SPLINT
Polyurethane Foam
Surgibone
SOFT TISSUE
Dimethicone (See also *Lubricant and hydrophobing agent*)
Dimethicone 350

Protectant
Pectin (See also *Pharmaceutic aid (suspending agent)*)
TOPICAL
Amifostine (See also *Radioprotector*)
Benzoin
Bismuth Subcarbonate
Calamine
Collodion
Hydroxypropyl Cellulose (See also *Pharmaceutic aid (emulsifying agent); Pharmaceutic aid (tablet coating agent)*)
Petrolatum, White (See also *Pharmaceutic aid (ointment base, oleaginous)*)
Titanium Dioxide
Zinc Oxide (See also *Astringent*)

Prothyrotropin
Protirelin

Psychotropic
Dapiprazole Hydrochloride (See also *Adrenergic (α-blocking); Antiglaucoma agent; Neuroleptic*)
Minaprine

Pulmonary surfactant
Beractant
Colfosceril Palmitate
Sinapultide

Radioactive agent
Albumin, Aggregated Iodinated I 131 Serum
Albumin, Chromated Cr 51 Serum
Albumin, Iodinated I 125 Serum (See also *Diagnostic aid (blood volume determination)*)
Albumin, Iodinated I 131 Serum (See also *Diagnostic aid (blood volume determination); Diagnostic aid (intrathecal imaging)*)
Ammonia N 13 (See also *Diagnostic aid (cardiac imaging); Diagnostic aid (liver imaging)*)

Borocaptate Sodium B 10 (See also *Antineoplastic*)
Calcium Chloride Ca 45
Calcium Chloride Ca 47
Carbon Monoxide C 11 (See also *Diagnostic aid (blood volume determination)*)
Cesium Chloride Cs 131
Chlormerodrin Hg 197 (See also *Diagnostic aid (renal function determination)*)
Chlormerodrin Hg 203 (See also *Diagnostic aid (renal function determination)*)
Chromic Chloride Cr 51
Chromic Phosphate Cr 51
Chromic Phosphate P 32
Cobaltous Chloride Co 57
Cobaltous Chloride Co 60
Cupric Acetate Cu 64
Cyanocobalamin Co 57 (See also *Diagnostic aid (pernicious anemia)*)
Cyanocobalamin Co 60 (See also *Diagnostic aid (pernicious anemia)*)
Deuterium Oxide
Diatrizoate Sodium I 125
Diatrizoate Sodium I 131
Diohippuric Acid I 125
Diohippuric Acid I 131
Diotyrosine I 125
Diotyrosine I 131
Ethiodized Oil I 131 (See also *Antineoplastic*)
Ferric Chloride Fe 59
Ferrous Citrate Fe 59
Ferrous Sulfate Fe 59
Fibrinogen I 125 (See also *Diagnostic aid (vascular patency)*)
Fludeoxyglucose F 18 (See also *Diagnostic aid*)
Fluorodopa F 18 (See also *Diagnostic aid (brain imaging)*)
Gallium Citrate Ga 67 (See also *Diagnostic aid (radiopaque medium)*)
Gold Au 198 (See also *Antineoplastic; Diagnostic aid (liver imaging)*)
Indium Chlorides In 113m
Indium In 111 Altumomab Pentetate (See also *Radiodiagnostic monoclonal antibody (anticarcinoembryonic antigen [CEA])*)
Indium In 111 Capromab Pendetide
Indium In 111 Chloride
Indium In 111 Oxyquinoline (See also *Diagnostic aid*)
Indium In 111 Pentetate (See also *Diagnostic aid (radionuclide cisternography)*)
Indium In 111 Pentetreotide (See also *Diagnostic aid*)
Indium In 111 Satumomab Pendetide (See also *Radiodiagnostic monoclonal antibody (ovarian and colorectal carcinoma)*)
Insulin I 125
Insulin I 131
Iobenguane I 123

Iobenguane I 131 (See also *Diagnostic aid*)
Iobenguane Sulfate I 123 (See also *Diagnostic aid (radioactive, adrenomedullary disorders and neuroendocrine tumors)*)
Iobenguane Sulfate I 131 (See also *Diagnostic aid*)
Iodinated I 125 Albumin (See also *Diagnostic aid (blood volume determination)*)
Iodinated I 131 Albumin (See also *Diagnostic aid (blood volume determination); Diagnostic aid (intrathecal imaging)*)
Iodinated I 131 Albumin Aggregated
Iodipamide Sodium I 131
Iodoantipyrine I 131
Iodocetylic Acid I 123 (See also *Diagnostic aid*)
Iodocholesterol I 131
Iodohippurate Sodium I 123 (See also *Diagnostic aid (renal function determination)*)
Iodohippurate Sodium I 125
Iodohippurate Sodium I 131 (See also *Diagnostic aid (renal function determination)*)
Iodopyracet I 125
Iodopyracet I 131
Iofetamine Hydrochloride I 123 (See also *Diagnostic aid*)
Iomethin I 125 (See also *Diagnostic aid (neoplasm)*)
Iomethin I 131 (See also *Diagnostic aid (neoplasm)*)
Iothalamate Sodium I 125
Iothalamate Sodium I 131
Iotyrosine I 131
Iridium Ir 192
Krypton Clathrate Kr 85
Krypton Kr 81m
Liothyronine I 125
Liothyronine I 131
Merisoprol Acetate Hg 197
Merisoprol Acetate Hg 203
Merisoprol Hg 197 (See also *Diagnostic aid (renal function determination)*)
Mespiperone C 11 (See also *Diagnostic aid*)
Methionine C 11
Oleic Acid I 125
Oleic Acid I 131
Pentetate Calcium Trisodium Yb 169
Pentetate Indium Disodium In 111 (See also *Diagnostic aid*)
Polymetaphosphate P 32
Potassium Chloride K 42
Povidone I 125
Povidone I 131
Raclopride C 11
Rose Bengal Sodium I 125
Rose Bengal Sodium I 131 (See also *Diagnostic aid (hepatic function determination)*)
Rubidium Chloride Rb 82 (See also *Diagnostic aid (radioactive, cardiac disease)*)

Rubidium Chloride Rb 86
Samarium Sm 153 Lexidronam Pentasodium (See also *Antineoplastic*)
Selenomethionine Se 75 (See also *Diagnostic aid (pancreas function determination)*)
Sodium Acetate C 11
Sodium Arsenate As 74
Sodium Chloride Na 22
Sodium Chromate Cr 51 (See also *Diagnostic aid (blood volume determination)*)
Sodium Fluoride F 18
Sodium Iodide I 123 (See also *Diagnostic aid (thyroid function determination)*)
Sodium Iodide I 125 (See also *Diagnostic aid (thyroid function determination)*)
Sodium Iodide I 131 (See also *Antineoplastic; Diagnostic aid (thyroid function determination)*)
Sodium Pertechnetate Tc 99m
Sodium Phosphate P 32 (See also *Antineoplastic; Antipolycythemic; Diagnostic aid (neoplasm)*)
Sodium Sulfate S 35
Strontium Chloride Sr 85
Strontium Chloride Sr 89 (See also *Antineoplastic*)
Strontium Nitrate Sr 85
Technetium Tc 99m Albumin
Technetium Tc 99m Albumin Aggregated (See also *Diagnostic aid (lung imaging)*)
Technetium Tc 99m Albumin Colloid
Technetium Tc 99m Albumin Microaggregated
Technetium Tc 99m Antimony Trisulfide Colloid
Technetium Tc 99m Arcitumomab
Technetium Tc 99m Bicisate (See also *Diagnostic aid (brain imaging)*)
Technetium Tc 99m Depreotide
Technetium Tc 99m Disofenin (See also *Diagnostic aid (hepatobiliary function determination)*)
Technetium Tc 99m Etidronate
Technetium Tc 99m Exametazime
Technetium Tc 99m Furifosmin (See also *Diagnostic aid (radioactive, cardiac disease)*)
Technetium Tc 99m Gluceptate
Technetium Tc 99m Lidofenin
Technetium Tc 99m Mebrofenin
Technetium Tc 99m Medronate (See also *Diagnostic aid (skeletal imaging)*)
Technetium Tc 99m Medronate Disodium
Technetium Tc 99m Mertiatide (See also *Diagnostic aid (renal function determination)*)
Technetium Tc 99m Oxidronate (See also *Diagnostic aid (skeletal imaging)*)
Technetium Tc 99m Pentetate

Technetium Tc 99m Pentetate Calcium Trisodium
Technetium Tc 99m (Pyro- and trimeta-) Phosphates
Technetium Tc 99m Pyrophosphate
Technetium Tc 99m Red Blood Cells
Technetium Tc 99m Sestamibi (See also *Diagnostic aid (radiopaque medium, cardiac perfusion)*)
Technetium Tc 99m Siboroxime (See also *Diagnostic aid (brain imaging)*)
Technetium Tc 99m Succimer (See also *Diagnostic aid (renal function determination)*)
Technetium Tc 99m Sulfur Colloid
Technetium Tc 99m Teboroxime (See also *Diagnostic aid (radiopaque medium, cardiac perfusion)*)
Technetium Tc 99m Tetrofosmin
Thallous Chloride Tl 201 (See also *Diagnostic aid (radiopaque medium)*)
Thyroxine I 125
Thyroxine I 131
Tolpovidone I 131 (See also *Diagnostic aid (hypoalbuminemia)*)
Triolein I 125
Triolein I 131
Water O 15 (See also *Diagnostic aid (radioactive, vascular disorders)*)
Water, Tritiated
Xenon Xe 127 (See also *Diagnostic aid; Gas, medicinal*)
Xenon Xe 133
Zinc Chloride Zn 65

Radiodiagnostic monoclonal antibody

ANTICARCINOEMBRYONIC ANTIGEN [CEA]
Indium In 111 Altumomab Pentetate (See also *Radioactive agent*)

OVARIAN AND COLORECTAL CARCINOMA
Indium In 111 Satumomab Pendetide (See also *Radioactive agent*)

Radionuclide carrier
Bibapcitide

Radioprotector
Amifostine (See also *Protectant (topical)*)

Regulator
CALCIUM
Calcifediol
Calcitonin
Calcitriol
Clodronic Acid
Dihydrotachysterol
Etidronic Acid
Gallium Nitrate
Oxidronic Acid
Piridronate Sodium
Potassium Phosphate, Dibasic
Risedronate Sodium
Secalciferol
Sodium Sulfate

Relaxant
MUSCLE
Baclofen

Benzoctamine Hydrochloride (See also *Sedative-hypnotic*)
Cinflumide
Cyclobenzaprine Hydrochloride
Flurazepam Hydrochloride (See also *Anticonvulsant; Sedative-hypnotic*)
Lorbamate
Nafomine Malate
Nelezaprine Maleate
Pipoxolan Hydrochloride
Progabide (See also *Anticonvulsant*)
Xilobam
Veterinary
Xylazine Hydrochloride (See also *Analgesic*)
SKELETAL MUSCLE
Alcuronium Chloride
Azumolene Sodium
Carisoprodol
Chlorphenesin Carbamate
Chlorzoxazone
Clodanolene
Dantrolene
Dantrolene Sodium
Fenyripol Hydrochloride
Fletazepam
Flumetramide
Hexafluorenium Bromide (See also *Synergist (succinylcholine)*)
Metaxalone
Methocarbamol
Orphenadrine Citrate (See also *Antihistaminic*)
Phenyramidol Hydrochloride (See also *Analgesic*)
Procyclidine Hydrochloride (See also *Antiparkinsonian*)
Rolodine
SMOOTH MUSCLE
Adiphenine Hydrochloride
Ambuphylline (See also *Diuretic*)
Aminophylline
Cinnamedrine
Fenalamide
Fetoxylate Hydrochloride
Flavoxate Hydrochloride
Isomylamine Hydrochloride
Levoxadrol Hydrochloride (See also *Anesthetic (local)*)
Mebeverine Hydrochloride
Mesuprine Hydrochloride (See also *Vasodilator*)
Methixene Hydrochloride
Papaverine Hydrochloride
Proxazole (See also *Analgesic; Anti-inflammatory*)
Proxazole Citrate (See also *Analgesic; Anti-inflammatory*)
Quinetolate
Ritodrine
Ritodrine Hydrochloride
Theophylline Sodium Glycinate
Thiphenamil Hydrochloride

Repartitioning agent
Cimaterol

Repellant, arthropod
Diethyltoluamide

Replacement therapy

ADENOSINE DEAMINASE DEFICIENCY
Pegademase Bovine

Replenisher

CALCIUM
Calcium Chloride
Calcium Glubionate
Calcium Gluceptate
Calcium Gluconate
Calcium Lactate
Calcium Levulinate
Calcium Phosphate Dihydrate, Dibasic
  (See also *Pharmaceutic aid* (*tablet
  base*))
Calcium Phosphate, Tribasic

CARNITINE
Levocarnitine

ELECTROLYTE
Magnesium Chloride
Magnesium Sulfate (See also *Anticon-
  vulsant; Laxative*)
Potassium Acetate
Potassium Chloride
Potassium Gluconate
Ringer's Injection (See also *Replenisher*
  (*fluid*))
Sodium Bicarbonate (See also *Alkalizer*
  (*systemic*))
Sodium Gluconate
Sodium Lactate
Trikates

FLUID
Ringer's Injection (See also *Replenisher*
  (*electrolyte*))

FLUID AND NUTRIENT
Dextrose
Protein Hydrolysate
Sugar, Invert

MAGNESIUM
Magnesium Gluconate

PLATELETS
Platelet Concentrate

Replenisher adjunct

ELECTROLYTE
Betaine Hydrochloride

Scabicide
Amitraz
Crotamiton
Lindane (See also *Pediculicide*)
Sulfur, Precipitated
Sulfur, Sublimed

Sclerosing agent
Ethanolamine Oleate
Morrhuate Sodium
Tribenoside

Sedative

PRE-ANESTHETIC
Propiomazine

VETERINARY
Acepromazine Maleate
Declenperone
Medetomidine Hydrochloride (See also
  Analgesic (*veterinary*))

Metoserpate Hydrochloride
Tameridone

Sedative-hypnotic
Adinazolam (See also *Antidepressant*)
Allobarbital
Alonimid
Alprazolam
Amobarbital Sodium
Bentazepam
Benzoctamine Hydrochloride (See also
  Relaxant (*muscle*))
Brotizolam
Butabarbital
Butabarbital Sodium
Butalbital
Capuride
Carbocloral
Chloral Betaine
Chloral Hydrate
Chlordiazepoxide Hydrochloride
Cloperidone Hydrochloride
Clorethate
Cyprazepam
Detomidine Hydrochloride (See also
  Analgesic (*veterinary*))
Dexclamol Hydrochloride
Diazepam
Dichloralphenazone
Estazolam
Ethchlorvynol
Etomidate
Fenobam
Flunitrazepam
Flurazepam Hydrochloride (See also
  Anticonvulsant; Relaxant (*muscle*))
Fosazepam
Glutethimide
Halazepam
Lormetazepam
Mecloqualone
Mephobarbital (See also *Anticonvul-
  sant*)
Meprobamate
Methaqualone
Midaflur
Nisobamate (See also *Tranquilizer*
  (*minor*))
Nitrazepam (See also *Anticonvulsant*)
Paraldehyde
Pentobarbital
Pentobarbital Sodium
Perlapine
Phenobarbital (See also *Anticonvulsant*)
Phenobarbital Sodium (See also *Anti-
  convulsant*)
Prazepam
Quazepam
Reclazepam
Roletamide
Secobarbital
Secobarbital Sodium
Suproclone
Thalidomide
Thioridazine (See also *Antipsychotic*)
Thioridazine Hydrochloride (See also
  Antipsychotic)
Tracazolate
Trepipam Maleate

Triazolam
Tricetamide
Triclofos Sodium
Trifluoperazine Hydrochloride (See also
  Antipsychotic)
Trimetozine
Uldazepam
Zaleplon
Zolazepam Hydrochloride
Zolpidem Tartrate

Selective adenosine A$_1$antagonist
Apaxifylline

Serotonin antagonist
Altanserin Tartrate
Amesergide
Ketanserin
Ritanserin

Serotonin inhibitor
Cinanserin Hydrochloride
Fenclonine
Fonazine Mesylate
Mianserin Hydrochloride (See also *An-
  tihistaminic*)
Xylamidine Tosylate

SPECIFIC IN MIGRAINE
Pizotyline (See also *Anabolic; Antidepressant*)

Serotonin receptor antagonist

SPECIFIC IN MIGRAINE
Tropanserin Hydrochloride

Smoking cessation adjunct
Nicotine
Nicotine Polacrilex

Spermaticide
Chlorindanol
Laureth 9 (See also *Pharmaceutic aid*
  (*surfactant*))
Laureth 10S
Nonoxynol 9 (See also *Pharmaceutic
  aid* (*wetting and/or solubilizing
  agent*))

Spreading agent
Hyaluronidase (Ovine)

Steroid

TOPICAL
Dexamethasone Acefurate
Mometasone Furoate

Stimulant

CARDIAC
Arbutamine Hydrochloride
Xamoterol
Xamoterol Fumarate

CENTRAL
Amfonelic Acid
Amphetamine Sulfate
Ampyzine Sulfate
Azabon
Caffeine
Dexoxadrol Hydrochloride (See also
  Analgesic)
Dextroamphetamine
Dextroamphetamine Sulfate

Difluanine Hydrochloride
Etryptamine Acetate
Fenethylline Hydrochloride
Flubanilate Hydrochloride
Flurothyl
Indriline Hydrochloride
Mefexamide
Methamphetamine Hydrochloride
Methylphenidate Hydrochloride
Pemoline
Pyrovalerone Hydrochloride

CENTRAL AND RESPIRATORY
Ethamivan

GASTRIC SECRETORY
Ceruletide
Ceruletide Diethylamine
Histamine Phosphate

PERISTALTIC
Cisapride
Dazopride Fumarate
Pancopride (See also *Anti-anxiety agent ; Anti-emetic*)
Zacopride Hydrochloride (See also *Anti-emetic*)

RESPIRATORY
Carbon Dioxide
Dimefline Hydrochloride
Doxapram Hydrochloride

Stomachic
Capsicum (See also *Carminative; Counterirritant (external)*)
Capsicum Oleoresin (See also *Carminative; Counterirritant (external)*)

Stool softener
Docusate Calcium
Docusate Potassium
Docusate Sodium (See also *Pharmaceutic aid (surfactant)*)

Stroke treatment
Lubeluzole
Trafermin (See also *Fibroblast growth factor*)

Stroke and traumatic brain injury treatment
NMDA ION CHANNEL BLOCKER
Aptiganel Hydrochloride

Sulfide, source of
Potash, Sulfurated

Sunscreen
Avobenzone
Ecamsule
Lisadimate
Roxadimate

Supplement
CALCIUM
Calcium Citrate
Calcium Lactobionate

IODINE
Potassium Iodide (See also *Antifungal; Expectorant*)
Sodium Iodide

TRACE MINERAL
Chromic Chloride

Copper Gluconate
Cupric Chloride
Manganese Chloride
Manganese Gluconate
Manganese Sulfate
Selenious Acid
Zinc Gluconate

Suppressant
DERMATITIS HERPETIFORMIS
Dapsone (See also *Antibacterial (leprostatic)*)
Sulfapyridine

GOUT
Amflutizole
Colchicine

INFLAMMATORY BOWEL DISEASE
Anakinra (See also *Anti-inflammatory (nonsteroidal)*)
Quiflapon Sodium (See also *Anti-asthmatic*)
Tazofelone

LUPUS ERYTHEMATOSUS
Chloroquine Phosphate (See also *Antimalarial; Anti-amebic*)
Hydroxychloroquine Sulfate (See also *Antimalarial*)

Surgical aid
Cotton, Purified
Rayon, Purified
Suture, Absorbable Surgical
Suture, Nonabsorbable Surgical
Tape, Adhesive

SURGICAL SUTURE COATING
Polybutilate

Absorbable
Poliglecaprone 90
Polyglactin 370

SURGICAL SUTURE MATERIAL
Polybutester
Polyglycolic Acid

Absorbable
Poliglecaprone 25
Polydioxanone
Polyglactin 910
Polyglyconate

TISSUE ADHESIVE
Bucrylate
Flucrylate
Mecrylate
Ocrylate

Surgical glove lubricant
Dusting Powder, Absorbable

Sweetener
Alitame
Aspartame
Maltitol
Melizame

NON-NUTRITIVE
Cyclamic Acid
Saccharin Calcium
Saccharin Sodium

Synergist
NON-SPECIFIC

Proadifen Hydrochloride
PENICILLIN/CEPHALOSPORIN
Sulbactam Benzathine (See also *Inhibitor (β-lactamase)*)
Sulbactam Pivoxil (See also *Inhibitor (β-lactamase)*)
Sulbactam Sodium (See also *Inhibitor (β-lactamase)*)

SUCCINYLCHOLINE
Hexafluorenium Bromide (See also *Relaxant (skeletal muscle)*)

Synovitis agent
VETERINARY
Hyaluronate Sodium

Thyroid hormone
Levothyroxine Sodium
Liothyronine Sodium
Liotrix
Thyroglobulin
Thyroid
Thyrotropin Alfa

Thyroid inhibitor
Methimazole
Propylthiouracil

Thrombolytic
Lanoteplase (See also *Plasminogen activator*)
Urokinase Alfa (See also *Plasminogen activator*)

Thyromimetic
Thyromedan Hydrochloride

Tocolytic
Hexoprenaline Sulfate (See also *Bronchodilator*)

Tranquilizer
Dexmedetomidine
Gepirone Hydrochloride
Pirenperone
Rolipram
Valnoctamide

MINOR
Bromazepam
Buspirone Hydrochloride
Chlordiazepoxide
Clazolam
Clobazam
Clorazepate Dipotassium
Clorazepate Monopotassium
Demoxepam
Enciprazine Hydrochloride
Hydroxyphenamate
Hydroxyzine Hydrochloride
Hydroxyzine Pamoate
Ketazolam
Lorazepam
Lorzafone
Loxapine
Loxapine Succinate
Medazepam Hydrochloride
Nabilone
Nisobamate (See also *Sedative-hypnotic*)
Oxazepam

Pentabamate
Ripazepam
Sulazepam
Taclamine Hydrochloride
Temazepam
Triflubazam
Tybamate

Treatment of unstable angina
Tirofiban Hydrochloride
Xemilofiban Hydrochloride (See also
*Prevention of post-recanalization re-
occlusion of coronary vessels*)

Ultraviolet screen
Actinoquinol Sodium
Aminobenzoic Acid
Beta Carotene
Bornelone
Bumetrizole
Cinoxate
Dioxybenzone
Drometrizole
Etocrylene
Homosalate
Octabenzone
Octocrylene
Octrizole
Oxybenzone
Padimate A
Padimate O
Sulisobenzone

Uricosuric
Benzbromarone
Halofenate (See also *Antihyperlipopro-
teinemic*)
Irtemazole
Probenecid
Seclazone (See also *Anti-inflammatory*)
Sulfinpyrazone
Ticrynafen (See also *Diuretic; Antihy-
pertensive*)

Vaccine adjuvant
Loxoribine (See also *Immunostimulant*)
Temurtide

Vaccine enhancement
Thymalfasin (See also *Antineoplastic;
Hepatitis treatment; Infectious dis-
ease treatment*)

Vasoconstrictor [See also **Adrenergic
(vasoconstrictor)**]
Angiotensin Amide
Felypressin
Lypressin (See also *Antidiuretic*)

SPECIFIC IN MIGRAINE
Methysergide
Methysergide Maleate

Vasodilator
Alprostadil
Amyl Nitrite
Bamethan Sulfate
Bepridil Hydrochloride
Betahistine Hydrochloride

Cilostazol (See also *Inhibitor (platelet);
Antithrombotic*)
Darodipine (See also *Antihypertensive;
Bronchodilator*)
Felodipine
Flunarizine Hydrochloride
Hexobendine
Iproxamine Hydrochloride
Isoxsuprine Hydrochloride
Mesuprine Hydrochloride (See also *Re-
laxant (smooth muscle)*)
Mibefradil Dihydrochloride
Nafronyl Oxalate
Nicardipine Hydrochloride
Nicergoline
Nimodipine
Oxfenicine
Pentaerythritol Tetranitrate
Pentoxifylline
Pindolol
Pirsidomine
Tipropidil Hydrochloride
Viprostol (See also *Hypotensive*)
Zolertine Hydrochloride (See also *Anti-
adrenergic*)

CALCIUM CHANNEL BLOCKER
Fostedil

CEREBRAL
Mefenidil
Mefenidil Fumarate

CORONARY
Azaclorzine Hydrochloride
Chromonar Hydrochloride
Clonitrate
Diltiazem Hydrochloride
Dipyridamole
Droprenilamine
Erythrityl Tetranitrate
Isosorbide Dinitrate
Isosorbide Mononitrate
Lidoflazine
Mioflazine Hydrochloride
Mixidine
Molsidomine (See also *Anti-anginal*)
Nicorandil
Nifedipine
Nisoldipine
Nitroglycerin
Oxprenolol Hydrochloride
Pentrinitrol
Perhexiline Maleate
Prenylamine
Propatyl Nitrate
Terodiline Hydrochloride
Tolamolol (See also *Cardiac depressant
(anti-arrhythmic); Anti-adrenergic (β
-receptor)*)
Verapamil

PERIPHERAL
Acetylcholine Chloride (See also *Cardi-
ac depressant; Cholinergic; Miotic*)
Buterizine
Cetiedil Citrate
Inositol Niacinate

Nicotinyl Alcohol
Suloctidil
Tolazoline Hydrochloride
Xanthinol Niacinate

SEROTONIN S$_2$ AND α$_1$ ADRENERGIC RECEP-
TOR BLOCKER
Pelanserin Hydrochloride (See also *An-
tihypertensive*)

Vasospastic therapy adjunct
Dextrorphan Hydrochloride

Vitamin
Adenine
Biotin
Panthenol
Riboflavin 5′-Phosphate Sodium

ANTIRACHITIC
Cholecalciferol
Ergocalciferol

ANTISCORBUTIC
Ascorbic Acid (See also *Acidifier (urin-
ary)*)
Sodium Ascorbate

ANTI-XEROPHTHALMIC
Vitamin A

ENZYME CO-FACTOR
Calcium Pantothenate
Calcium Pantothenate, Racemic
Niacin (See also *Antihyperlipidemic*)
Niacinamide
Pyridoxine Hydrochloride
Riboflavin
Thiamine Hydrochloride
Thiamine Mononitrate

HEMATOPOIETIC
Cyanocobalamin
Folic Acid
Hydroxocobalamin
Mecobalamin

PROTHROMBOGENIC
Menadiol Sodium Diphosphate
Menadione
Phytonadione

Vitamin E supplement
Tocophersolan
Vitamin E

Vitamins A and D, source of
Cod Liver Oil
Oleovitamin A and D

Vulnerary
TOPICAL
Allantoin

Wound healing agent
Ersofermin

Xanthine oxidase inhibitor
Allopurinol
Oxypurinol

Appendix III
Molecular Formulas

Molecular Formula	Non-proprietary Name
$_2(C_{16}H_{20}N_2O_2).C_4H_6O_6$	Ladostigil Tartrate
$[Ag(NH_3)_2]F$	Silver Diammine Fluoride
$AgNO_3$	Silver Nitrate
$AlCl_3.6H_2O$	Aluminum Chloride
$AlH_3O_3.xH_2O$	Algeldrate
$AlK(SO_4)_2.12H_2O$	Alum, Potassium
$AlNH_4(SO_4)_2.12H_2O$	Alum, Ammonium
$Al(OH)_3$	Aluminum Hydroxide
$Al(OH)_3$	Aluminum Hydroxide, Dried
$Al_y(OH)_{3y-z}Cl_z.H_2O$	Aluminum Chlorohydrate
$Al_y(OH)_{3y-z}Cl_z.nH_2O$	Aluminum Dichlorohydrate
$Al_y(OH)_{3y-z}Cl_z.nH_2O$	Aluminum Sesquichlorohydrate
$Al_y(OH)_{3y-z}Cl_z.nH_2O.mC_3H_8O_2$	Aluminum Chlorohydrex Propylene Glycol
$Al_y(OH)_{3y-z}Cl_z.nH_2O.mC_3H_8O_2$	Aluminum Dichlorohydrex Propylene Glycol
$Al_y(OH)_{3y-z}Cl_z.nH_2O.mC_3H_8O_2$	Aluminum Sesquichlorohydrex Propylene Glycol
$Al_y(OH)_{3y-z}Cl_z.nH_2O.m$ $H(OCH_2CH_2)_nOH$	Aluminum Chlorohydrex Polyethylene Glycol
$Al_y(OH)_{3y-z}Cl_z.nH_2O.m$ $H(OCH_2CH_2)_nOH$	Aluminum Dichlorohydrex Polyethylene Glycol
$Al_y(OH)_{3y-z}Cl_z.n\hat{H}_2O.m$ $H(OCH_2CH_2)_nOH$	Aluminum Sesquichlorohydrex Polyethylene Glycol
$Al_yZr(OH)_{3y+4-x}Cl_x.nH_2O$	Aluminum Zirconium Octachlorohydrate
$Al_yZr(OH)_{3y+4-x}Cl_x.nH_2O$	Aluminum Zirconium Pentachlorohydrate
$Al_yZr(OH)_{3y+4-x}Cl_x.nH_2O$	Aluminum Zirconium Tetrachlorohydrate
$Al_yZr(OH)_{3y+4-x}Cl_x.nH_2O$	Aluminum Zirconium Trichlorohydrate
$Al_2MgO_8Si_2.xH_2O$	Almasilate
$Al_2Mg_2O_{11}Si_3.xH_2O$	Silodrate
$Al_2Mg_4(OH)_{12}CO_3.3H_2O$	Vangatalcite
$Al_2(SO_4)_3.xH_2O$	Aluminum Sulfate
$Al_4H_6Mg_2O_{14}S.xH_2O$	Almadrate Sulfate
$Al_5Mg_{10}(OH)_{31}(SP_4)_2.xH_2O$	Magaldrate
$Al_6Bi_2O_{12}$	Bismuth Aluminate
$Al_7H_{17}O_{25}S_2.xH_2O$	Alusulf
$Al_8(OH)_{16}(C_{12}H_{14}O_{35}S_8)$ $[Al(OH)_3]_x[H_2O]_y$ in which $x = 8$ to 10, and $y = 22$ to 31	Sucralfate
$Al_{10}H_{26}Mg_5O_{39}S_2.nH_2O$	Almagodrate
As_2O_3	Arsenic Trioxide
$^{10}B_{12}H_{12}Na_2S$	Borocaptate Sodium B 10
$BaSO_4$	Barium Sulfate
$BiC_6H_5O_7$	Bismuth Citrate
$Bi_5O(OH)_9(NO_3)_4$	Bismuth Subnitrate
$CCaN_2$	Calcium Carbimide
CCl_2F_2	Dichlorodifluoromethane
CCl_3F	Trichloromonofluoromethane
CCl_4	Carbon Tetrachloride
$CHBr_3.C_6H_{12}N_4$	Brometenamine
$CHCl_3$	Chloroform
CHI_2NaO_3S	Dimethiodal Sodium
CHI_3	Iodoform
$CH_2AlNaO_5.nH_2O$	Carbaldrate
CH_2Cl_2	Methylene Chloride
$CH_2Cl_2Na_2O_6P_2.4H_2O$	Clodronate Disodium
CH_2INaO_3S	Methiodal Sodium
CH_2O	Formaldehyde
CH_3NaO_3S	Sodium Formaldehyde Sulfoxylate
$CH_3-(OCH_2CH_2)_n$ $OCH_2CH_2CH_2-$ $C_{781}H_{1288}N_{220}O_{220}S_7$	Pegacaristim
$CH_4Cl_2O_6P_2$	Clodronic Acid
CH_4N_2O	Urea
$^{13}CH_4N_2O$	Urea C 13
$^{14}CH_4N_2O$	Urea C 14
$CH_4N_2O_2$	Hydroxyurea
$CH_4Na_2O_6P_2$	Medronate Disodium
CH_4O	Methyl Alcohol
$CH_6N_2O_3$	Carbamide Peroxide
$CH_6N_4.HCl$	Pimagedine Hydrochloride
$CH_6O_6P_2$	Medronic Acid
$CH_6O_7P_2$	Oxidronic Acid
$CH_7AlMg_3O_{10}.2H_2O$	Almagate
$CH_{12}Fe_7Mg_4O_{15}.4H_2O$	Fermagate
$CH_{24}O_{11}$	Isomalt
CNa_3O_5P	Foscarnet Sodium
CO	Carbon Monoxide
^{11}CO	Carbon Monoxide C 11
CO_2	Carbon Dioxide
$C_2Cl_2F_4$	Dichlorotetrafluoroethane
C_2Cl_4	Tetrachloroethylene
$(C_2F_4)_n$	Polytef
$C_2HBrClF_3$	Halothane
C_2HBrF_4	Teflurane
$C_2HCl_2NaO_2$	Sodium Dichloroacetate
C_2HCl_3	Trichloroethylene
$C_2HCl_3O_2$	Trichloroacetic Acid
$C_2H_2F_4$	Norflurane
$(C_2H_2O_2)_n$	Polyglycolic Acid
$C_2H_3Cl_2NaO_4P$	Triclofos Sodium
$C_2H_3Cl_3O_2$	Chloral Hydrate
$C_2H_3KO_2$	Potassium Acetate
$C_2H_3NaO_2.3H_2O$	Sodium Acetate
$(C_2H_3NaO_3S)_n$ (n = approximately 25)	Lyapolate Sodium
$C_2H_3Na_2O_5P.H_2O$	Fosfonet Sodium
$C_2H_4Cl_2N_6$	Chloroazodin
$(C_2H_4O)_n$	Polyvinyl Alcohol
$(C_2H_4O)_n(C_2H_4O)_n$ $C_{302}H_{451}N_{85}O_{112}S_6$	Pegmusirudin
$(C_2H_4O)_nC_{16}H_{24}O$	Menfegol
$(C_2H_4O)_y(C_5H_8O_2)_z$	Atlafilcon A
$C_2H_4O_2$	Acetic Acid, Glacial
C_2H_5Cl	Ethyl Chloride
$C_2H_5NO_2$	Acetohydroxamic Acid

Molecular Formula	*Non-proprietary Name*
$C_2H_5NO_2$	Glycine
$C_2H_5NaO_3S_2$	Mesna
$C_2H_6AlNO_4.xH_2O$	Dihydroxyaluminum Aminoacetate
$C_2H_6N_2O_3$	Aminoethyl Nitrate
$C_2H_6N_2O_3.C_7H_8O_3S$	Itramin Tosylate
$C_2H_6Na_2O_7P_2$	Etidronate Disodium
C_2H_6O	Alcohol
C_2H_6OS	Dimethyl Sulfoxide
$(C_2H_6OSi)_a(C_{12}H_{10}OSi)_b$ $(C_3H_6OSi)_c(C_6H_5O_{3/2}Si)_d$ $(C_2H_7O_{1/2}Si)_e$	Silafilcon A
$(C_2H_6OSi)_n$	Cyclomethicone
$[[(C_2H_6OSi)_u]_3C_3H_7OSi]_v$ $(C_4H_6O_2)_w[C_8H_{10}O_3$ $(C_2H_4O)_n]_x(C_5H_9NO)_y$ $(C_5H_8O_2)_z$, $(n = 1, 2,$ or $3)$	Vinafocon A
$[[(C_2H_6OSi)_v]_3C_3H_7OSi]_w$ $(C_4H_6O_2)_x(C_6H_9NO)_y$ $(C_5H_8O_2)_z$	Oxyfilcon A
C_2H_7NO	Monoethanolamine
$C_2H_7NO_3S$	Taurine
C_2H_7NS	Cysteamine
$C_2H_7NS.HCl$	Cysteamine Hydrochloride
$C_2H_8N_2$	Ethylenediamine
$C_2H_8N_2O_3Pt$	Nedaplatin
$C_2H_8O_7P_2$	Etidronic Acid
$C_3Cl_2KN_3O_3$	Troclosene Potassium
$C_3Cl_3N_3O_3$	Symclosene
C_3F_8	Perflutren
C_3HF_7	Apaflurane
$C_3H_2ClF_5O$	Enflurane
$C_3H_2ClF_5O$	Isoflurane
$C_3H_2F_6O$	Desflurane
$C_3H_2N_4S$	Amitivir
$C_3H_4BrF_3O$	Roflurane
$C_3H_4Cl_2F_2O$	Methoxyflurane
$C_3H_4N_2S$	Aminothiazole
$C_3H_4O_2$	Propiolactone
$C_3H_5ClN_2O_6$	Clonitrate
$C_3H_5DFNO_2$	Fludalanine
$(C_3H_5GeO_{3.5})_n$	Propagermanium
$C_3H_5N_3O$	Cyacetacide
$C_3H_5N_3O_9$	Nitroglycerin
$C_3H_5NaO_2.xH_2O$	Sodium Propionate
$C_3H_5NaO_3$	Sodium Lactate
C_3H_6	Cyclopropane
$C_3H_6BrNO_3$	Debropol
$C_3H_6BrNO_4$	Bronopol
$C_3H_6N_2O_2$	Cycloserine
$C_3H_6N_2O_2$	Levcycloserine
$C_3H_6Na_2O_6S_2$	Eprodisate Disodium
C_3H_6O	Acetone
$C_3H_6O_2$	Propionic Acid
$C_3H_6O_3$	Dihydroxyacetone
$C_3H_6O_3$	Lactic Acid
$(C_3H_6)_n$	Polipropene 25
$C_3H_7NO_2$	Alanine
$C_3H_7NO_2$	Urethane
$C_3H_7NO_2S.HCl.H_2O$	Cysteine Hydrochloride
$C_3H_7NO_3$	Serine
$(C_3H_7N)_m(C_3H_5ClO)_n$ $(C_{12}H_{27}ClN_2)_o(C_{13}H_{27}N)_p.x$ HCl	Colesevelam Hydrochloride
$[(C_3H_7N)_m(C_3H_5ClO)_n].xCH_2O_3$	Sevelamer Carbonate
$(C_3H_7N)_m(C_3H_5ClO)_n.xHCl$	Sevelamer Hydrochloride

Molecular Formula	*Non-proprietary Name*
$C_3H_7N_3O_4$	Alanosine
$C_3H_7O_4P$	Fosfomycin
$C_3H_7O_4P.C_4H_{11}NO_3$	Fosfomycin Tromethamine
C_3H_8	Propane
$C_3H_8HgO_2$	Merisoprol Hg 197
$C_3H_8NO_6P$	Dexfosfoserine
$C_3H_8N_2OS$	Noxytiolin
$C_3H_8N_2O_2S$	Taurultam
C_3H_8O	Isopropyl Alcohol
$C_3H_8OS_2$	Dimercaprol
$C_3H_8O_2$	Propylene Glycol
$C_3H_8O_2S$	Monothioglycerol
$C_3H_8O_3$	Glycerin
$C_3H_8O_3$	Monoctanoin Component D
$C_3H_9NNa_2O_7P_2.5H_2O$	Pamidronate Disodium
$C_3H_9NO_3$	Ammonium Lactate
$C_3H_9NO_3S$	Tramiprosate
$C_3H_{11}NO_7P_2$	Pamidronic Acid
C_4F_{10}	Perflisobutane
C_4F_{10}	Perflubutane
C_4HI_4N	Iodol
$C_4H_2FeO_4$	Ferrous Fumarate
$C_4H_3AuNa_2O_4S+$ $C_4H_4AuNaO_4S$	Gold Sodium Thiomalate
$C_4H_3ClF_4O$	Aliflurane
$C_4H_3FN_2O_2$	Fluorouracil
$C_4H_3F_7O$	Sevoflurane
$C_4H_3IN_2OS$	Iodothiouracil
$C_4H_3N_3O_3S$	Forminitrazole
$C_4H_3N_3O_4$	Oteracil
$C_4H_4FN_3O$	Flucytosine
$C_4H_4F_6O$	Flurothyl
$C_4H_4KNaO_6.4H_2O$	Potassium Sodium Tartrate
$C_4H_4NO_4SK$	Acesulfame Potassium
$C_4H_4N_2O_2$	Uracil
$C_4H_4Na_2O_6.2H_2O$	Sodium Tartrate
$C_4H_4O_4$	Fumaric Acid
$C_4H_4O_4$	Maleic Acid
$(C_4H_4O_4)_m(C_4H_6O_3)_n$	Polyglyconate
$C_4H_5F_3O$	Fluroxene
$C_4H_5KO_6$	Potassium Bitartrate
$C_4H_5NO_4S$	Acesulfame
C_4H_5NS	Allyl Isothiocyanate
$C_4H_5N_3O$	Imexon
$C_4H_5N_4NaO_3S_2$	Acetazolamide Sodium
$C_4H_6CaO_4$	Calcium Acetate
$C_4H_6{}^{64}CuO_4$	Cupric Acetate Cu 64
$C_4H_6KNO_4.\frac{1}{2}H_2O$	Potassium Aspartate
$C_4H_6N_2$	Fomepizole
$(C_4H_6N_2.C_3H_5ClO)n$	Colestilan
$C_4H_6N_2S$	Methimazole
$C_4H_6N_4$	Praxadine
$C_4H_6N_4O.C_5H_4N_2O_4.2H_2O$	Orazamide
$C_4H_6N_4O_3$	Allantoin
$C_4H_6N_4O_3S_2$	Acetazolamide
$C_4H_6N_4O_{12}$	Erythrityl Tetranitrate
C_4H_6O	Vinyl Ether
$(C_4H_6O_2)_m(C_2H_5N)_n$	Polyethadene
$(C_4H_6O_2)_w(C_{10}H_{14}O_4)_x$ $(C_6H_{10}O_3)_y(C_6H_9NO)_z$	Vifilcon A
$(C_4H_6O_2)_w(C_{10}H_{14}O_4)_x$ $(C_6H_{10}O_3)_y(C_6H_9NO)_z$	Vifilcon B
$[(C_4H_6O_2)_x(C_{10}H_{10})_y](C_{10}H_{14}N_2)$	Nicotine Polacrilex
$C_4H_6O_3$	Propylene Carbonate
$(C_4H_6O_3)_n$	Polydioxanone
$C_4H_6O_4$	Succinic Acid

Molecular Formula	Non-proprietary Name
$C_4H_6O_4S_2$	Succimer
$C_4H_6O_4Zn.2H_2O$	Zinc Acetate
$C_4H_6O_5$	Malic Acid
$C_4H_6O_6$	Tartaric Acid
$C_4H_7AlN_4O_5$	Aldioxa
$C_4H_7AlO_5$	Aluminum Subacetate
$C_4H_7Cl_2O_4P$	Dichlorvos
$C_4H_7Cl_3N_2O_2$	Mecloralurea
$C_4H_7Cl_3O$	Chlorobutanol
$C_4H_7NO_2S$	Timonacic
$C_4H_7NO_4$	Aspartic Acid
$C_4H_7N_3O$	Creatinine
$C_4H_7NaO_2$	Sodium Butyrate
$C_4H_7NaO_3$	Sodium Oxybate
$C_4H_8Cl_3O_4P$	Metrifonate
$C_4H_8Cl_3O_4P$	Trichlorfon
$C_4H_8MgN_2O_4$	Magnesium Glycinate
$C_4H_8N_2O_3.H_2O$	Asparagine
$C_4H_8N_2S$	Allylthiourea
$C_4H_8N_3O_4P$	Fosfocreatinine
$C_4H_8Na_2O_6S_4$	Dimesna
$[(C_4H_8O)xH_2O]_m$ $(C_8H_6O_4)_n(C_4H_{10}O_2)_o$	Polybutester
$C_4H_8O_2$	Ethyl Acetate
$C_4H_9Al_2ClN_4O_7$	Alcloxa
$C_4H_9NO_2$	γ-Aminobutyric Acid
$C_4H_9NO_2S$	Mecysteine
$C_4H_9NO_3$	γ-Amino-β-hydroxybutyric acid
$C_4H_9NO_3$	Threonine
$C_4H_9Si-(C_2H_6OSi)_a$ $(C_{12}H_{10}OSi)_b$ $(C_3H_6OSi)_c-OSiC_4H_9$	Elastofilcon A
C_4H_{10}	Butane
C_4H_{10}	Isobutane
$C_4H_{10}NO_5P$	Fosmidomycin
$C_4H_{10}N_2$	Piperazine
$C_4H_{10}N_2.2C_6H_3Cl_3O$	Triclofenol Piperazine
$(C_4H_{10}N_2)_3.2C_6H_8O_7.xH_2O$	Piperazine Citrate
$C_4H_{10}N_2.H_3PO_4.H_2O$	Piperazine Phosphate
$C_4H_{10}O$	Butyl Alcohol
$C_4H_{10}O$	Ether
$C_4H_{10}O_2S$	Thiodiglycol
$C_4H_{10}O_4$	Erythritol
$C_4H_{11}Cl_2N_2O_2P$	Palifosfamide
$C_4H_{11}NO_2$	Diethanolamine
$C_4H_{11}NO_3$	Tromethamine
$C_4H_{11}NS.HCl$	Captamine Hydrochloride
$C_4H_{11}N_5$	Metformin
$C_4H_{11}N_5.HCl$	Metformin Hydrochloride
$C_4H_{12}NNaO_7P_2.3H_2O$	Alendronate Sodium
$C_4H_{12}N_3O_4P$	Creatinolfosfate
$C_4H_{13}NO_7P_2$	Alendronic Acid
C_5F_{12}	Perflenapent
C_5F_{12}	Perflisopent
$C_5H_3I_2NO$	Iopydone
$C_5H_4ClNO_2$	Gimeracil
$C_5H_4Cl_6O_3$	Clorethate
$C_5H_4FN_3O_2$	Favipiravir
C_5H_4NNaOS	Pyrithione Sodium
$C_5H_4N_2O_4$	Nifuroxime
$C_5H_4N_2O_4$	Orotic Acid
$C_5H_4N_4O$	Allopurinol
$C_5H_4N_4O_2$	Oxypurinol
$C_5H_4N_4S$	Tisopurine
$C_5H_4N_4S.H_2O$	Mercaptopurine

Molecular Formula	Non-proprietary Name
$C_5H_5NO_2$	Mecrylate
$C_5H_5N_3O$	Pyrazinamide
$C_5H_5N_3O_3S$	Nithiamide
$C_5H_5N_5$	Adenine
$C_5H_5N_5S.xH_2O$	Thioguanine
$C_5H_6Cl_6N_2O_3$	Dicloralurea
$C_5H_6N_2$	Fampridine
$C_5H_6N_2OS$	Methylthiouracil
$[C_5H_6Na_2O_{10}S_2]_n$ (n = 6 to 12)	Pentosan Polysulfate Sodium
$C_5H_6Na_4O_{10}P_2$	Butedronate Tetrasodium
$C_5H_7ClN_2O_3$	Acivicin
$C_5H_7NO_3$	Dimethadione
$C_5H_7NO_3$	Pidolic Acid
$C_5H_7NO_4S$	Tidiacic
$(C_5H_7N_2Na_3O_7P_2)_5.2H_2O$	Zoledronate Trisodium
$C_5H_7N_3$	Amifampridine
$C_5H_7N_3O_2$	Dimetridazole
$C_5H_7N_3O_4$	Azaserine
$C_5H_7N_5O$	Hydracarbazine
$C_5H_8BrNO_4$	Nibroxane
$C_5H_8Cl_3NO_3$	Carbocloral
$C_5H_8NNaO_4.H_2O$	Monosodium Glutamate
$C_5H_8N_2Na_2O_7P_2.4H_2O$	Zoledronate Disodium
$C_5H_8N_4O_3S_2$	Methazolamide
$C_5H_8N_4O_3S_2$	Propazolamide
$C_5H_8N_4O_{12}$	Pentaerythritol Tetranitrate
$C_5H_8O_2$	Glutaral
$[(C_5H_8O_2)_{n1}.(C_6H_9NO)_{n2}.$ $(C_{11}H_{20}O_2)_{n3}]_x.xINa.xI$	Iodine Povacrylex
$(C_5H_8O_2)_n(C_{10}H_{16}O_2)_m$ $(C_{19}H_{50}O_8Si_7)_x(C_{14}H_{22}O_6)_y$ $(C_6H_9NO)_z(C_{16}H_{14}F_{17}NO_4S)_g$ $(C_4H_6O_2)_q$	Sulfocon B
$(C_5H_8O_2)_v(C_4H_6O_2)_w$ $(C_{10}H_{14}O_4)_x(C_{16}H_{38}O_5Si_4)_y$ $(C_9H_{15}NO_2)_z$	Nefocon A
$(C_5H_8O_2)_x(C_5H_9NO)_y$ $(C_{10}H_{14}O_4)_z$	Netrafilcon A
$(C_5H_8O_2)_x(C_6H_9NO)_y$	Astifilcon A
$C_5H_8O_4S$	Danosteine
$C_5H_9Cl_2N_3O_2$	Carmustine
$C_5H_9IO_3$	Domiodol
$(C_5H_9NO)_u(C_6H_9NO)_v$ $(C_5H_8O_2)_w(C_8H_{14}O_3)_x$ $(C_{10}H_{14}O_4)_y(C_7H_{10}O_2)_z$	Mipafilcon A
$(C_5H_9NO)_w(C_{16}H_{38}O_5Si_4)_x$ $(C_{11}H_{14})_y(C_{10}H_{14}O_4)_z$	Abafilcon A
$C_5H_9NO_2$	Proline
$C_5H_9NO_2S$	Omonasteine
$C_5H_9NO_3.HCl$	Aminolevulinic Acid Hydrochloride
$C_5H_9NO_3S$	Acetylcysteine
$C_5H_9NO_3S$	Dextiopronin
$C_5H_9NO_3S$	Tiopronin
$C_5H_9NO_4$	Glutamic Acid
$(C_5H_9NO_4.C_3H_7NO_2$ $.C_6H_{14}N_2O_2.C_9H_{11}NO_3)_x.$ $xC_2H_4O_2$	Glatiramer Acetate
$C_5H_9NO_4S$	Carbocysteine
$C_5H_9N_3.2HCl$	Betazole Hydrochloride
$C_5H_9N_3.2HCl$	Histamine Dihydrochloride
$C_5H_9N_3.2H_3PO_4$	Histamine Phosphate
$C_5H_9N_3O_{10}$	Pentrinitrol
$C_5H_{10}ClN_3O_3$	Elmustine
$C_5H_{10}Cl_2O_2$	Loprodiol
$C_5H_{10}{}^{197}HgO_3$	Merisoprol Acetate Hg 197

Molecular Formula	*Non-proprietary Name*
$C_5H_{10}{}^{203}HgO_3$	Merisoprol Acetate Hg 203
$C_5H_{10}NNaOS_2.H_2O$	Ditiocade Sodium
$C_5H_{10}NNaS_2$	Ditiocarb Sodium
$C_5H_{10}N_2O$	Xinomiline
$C_5H_{10}N_2O_3$	Glutamine
$C_5H_{10}N_2O_7P_2.H_2O$	Zoledronic Acid
$C_5H_{10}O_3S$	Desmeninol
$C_5H_{10}O_5$	Xylose
$C_5H_{10}O_{10}P_2$	Butedronic Acid
$C_5H_{11}ClHgN_2O_2$	Chlormerodrin
$C_5H_{11}Cl^{197}HgN_2O_2$	Chlormerodrin Hg 197
$C_5H_{11}Cl^{203}HgN_2O_2$	Chlormerodrin Hg 203
$C_5H_{11}Cl_2N.HCl$	Mechlorethamine Hydrochloride
$C_5H_{11}N.H_3PO_4$	Piperidine Phosphate
$C_5H_{11}NO$	Isovaleramide
$C_5H_{11}NO_2$	Amyl Nitrite
$C_5H_{11}NO_2$	Valine
$C_5H_{11}NO_2.HCl$	Betaine Hydrochloride
$C_5H_{11}NO_2S$	Methionine
$C_5H_{11}NO_2S$	Penicillamine
$C_5H_{11}NO_2S$	Racemethionine
$C_5H_{11}NO_2Se$	Selenomethionine
$C_5H_{11}NO_2{}^{75}Se$	Selenomethionine Se 75
$C_5H_{12}N_2O_2$	Ornithine
$C_5H_{12}N_4O$	Tiformin
$C_5H_{12}N_8$	Mitoguazone
$C_5H_{12}O$	Amylene Hydrate
$C_5H_{12}O_5$	Xylitol
$C_5H_{13}ClN_2O_7$	Nitricholine Perchlorate
$C_5H_{13}NO.C_9H_9NO_3$	Dimepranol Acedoben
$C_5H_{13}N_2O_4P$	Alafosfalin
$C_5H_{14}ClNO$	Choline Chloride
$C_5H_{14}NO^+.C_{17}H_{14}ClO_4{}^-$	Choline Fenofibrate
$C_5H_{15}NO_7P_2$	Olpadronic Acid
$C_5H_{15}N_2O_3PS.3H_2O$	Amifostine
$C_5H_{16}N_2O_6P_2$	Lidadronic Acid
C_6F_{14}	Perflexane
$C_6HBiBr_4O_3$	Bibrocathol
$C_6H_4ClNO_4$	Nifurmerone
$C_6H_4N_2O_2$	Eniluracil
$C_6H_4O_6$	Tetroquinone
C_6H_5ClHgO	Mercufenol Chloride
C_6H_5ClO	Parachlorophenol
$C_6H_5{}^{67}GaO_7$	Gallium Citrate Ga 67
$C_6H_5K_3O_7.H_2O$	Potassium Citrate
$C_6H_5Li_3O_7.4H_2O$	Lithium Citrate
$C_6H_5NO_2$	Niacin
$C_6H_5NO_3$	Oxiniacic Acid
C_6H_5NaO	Phenolate Sodium
$C_6H_5NaO_4S.2H_2O$	Phenolsulphonate Sodium
$C_6H_5Na_3O_7$	Sodium Citrate
$C_6H_6AsCl_2NO.HCl$	Dichlorophenarsine Hydrochloride
$C_6H_6AsNO_2.HCl$	Oxophenarsine Hydrochloride
$C_6H_6AsNO_5$	Nitarsone
$C_6H_6AsNO_6$	Roxarsone
$C_6H_6Cl_2N_2O_4S_2$	Dichlorphenamide
$C_6H_6Cl_6$	Lindane
$C_6H_6N_2O$	Niacinamide
$C_6H_6N_2O_2$	Nicoxamat
$C_6H_6N_2O_3$	Acipimox
$C_6H_6N_4O$	Dezaguanine
$C_6H_6N_4O_3S$	Niridazole
$C_6H_6N_4O_4$	Nitrofurazone
$C_6H_6N_6O_2$	Temozolomide

Molecular Formula	*Non-proprietary Name*
$C_6H_6Na_{12}O_{24}P_6$	Phytate Persodium
C_6H_6O	Phenol
$C_6H_6O_2$	Hydroquinone
$C_6H_6O_2$	Resorcinol
$C_6H_6O_3$	Maltol
$C_6H_6O_3$	Phloroglucinol
$C_6H_6O_3$	Pyrogallol
$C_6H_6O_5S.C_4H_{11}N$	Ethamsylate
$C_6H_6O_8S_2$	Persilic Acid
$C_6H_7BHgO_3.C_6H_6HgO$	Phenylmercuric Borate
$C_6H_7ClN_2O_4S_2$	Clofenamide
$(C_6H_7F_3O_2)_t(C_{26}H_{58}O_9Si_6)_u$ $(C_5H_8O_2)_v(C_4H_6O_2)_w$ $(C_{13}H_{30}O_5Si_3)_x(C_{16}H_{38}O_5Si_4)_y$ $(C_{10}H_{14}O_4)_z$	Paflufocon A
$(C_6H_7F_3O_2)_s(C_{16}H_{38}O_5Si_4)_t$ $(C_{10}H_{20}O_5Si)_u(C_4H_6O_2)_y$ $(C_{26}H_{58}O_9Si_6)_w(C_{10}H_{14}O_4)_x$ $(C_6H_{10}O_3)_y(C_6H_9NO)_z$	Onsifocon A
$(C_6H_7F_3O_2)_t(C_{26}H_{58}O_8Si_6)_u$ $(C_5H_8O_2)_v(C_4H_6O_2)_w$ $(C_{13}H_{30}O_5Si_3)_x(C_{16}H_{38}O_5Si_4)_y$ $(C_{10}H_{14}O_4)_z$ (Component A: paflufocon D)	Paflufocon D-HEM-Iberfilcon A
$(C_6H_7F_3O_2)_u(C_{16}H_{38}O_5Si_4)_v$ $(C_{26}H_{58}O_9Si_6)_w(C_4H_6O_2)_x$ $(C_{10}H_{14}O_4)_y(C_6H_9NO)_z$	Hofocon A
$C_6H_7KO_2$	Potassium Sorbate
C_6H_7NO	Nicotinyl Alcohol
C_6H_7NO	Piconol
$C_6H_7NO_2$	Mepiroxol
$C_6H_7N_3O$	Isoniazid
$C_6H_7NaO_6$	Sodium Ascorbate
$C_6H_8AsNO_3$	Arsanilic Acid
$C_6H_8CaO_8.4H_2O$	Calcium Saccharate
C_6H_8ClNS	Clomethiazole
$C_6H_8ClN_7O.HCl.2H_2O$	Amiloride Hydrochloride
$C_6H_8NNa_2O_8P$	Sparfosate Sodium
$C_6H_8N_2$	Picolamine
$C_6H_8N_2O$	Cetohexazine
$C_6H_8N_2O_2$	Dimiracetam
$C_6H_8N_2O_2$	Gaboxadol
$C_6H_8N_2O_2S$	Sulfanilamide
$C_6H_8N_2O_8$	Isosorbide Dinitrate
$C_6H_8N_4O_4$	Ronidazole
$C_6H_8N_6$	Dametralast
$C_6H_8N_6O_{18}$	Mannitol Hexanitrate
$C_6H_8NaO_7Sb$	Sodium Antimonylgluconate
$C_6H_8O_2$	Sorbic Acid
$C_6H_8O_4$	Dimethyl Fumarate
$(C_6H_8O_4)_m(C_4H_4O_4)_n$	Polyglactin 370
$(C_6H_8O_4)_m(C_4H_4O_4)_n$	Polyglactin 910
$(C_6H_8O_6)_n$	Alginic Acid
$C_6H_8O_6$	Ascorbic Acid
$C_6H_8O_6$	Glucurolactone
$C_6H_8O_7$	Citric Acid, Anhydrous
$C_6H_8O_7.H_2O$	Citric Acid Monohydrate
$C_6H_9AlO_6$	Aluminum Acetate
$(C_6H_9NO)_n + (C_4H_6O_2)_m$	Copovidone
$(C_6H_9NO)_n$	Crospovidone
$(C_6H_9NO)_n$	Povidone
$(C_6H_9NO)_n\text{-}xI$	Povidone-Iodine
$(C_6H_9NO)_v(C_5H_8O_2)_w$ $(C_8H_{14}O_3)_x(C_{10}H_{16}O_2)_y$ $(C_7H_{10}O_2)_z$	Xylofilcon A

Molecular Formula	Non-proprietary Name
$(C_6H_9NO)_v(C_6H_{10}O_3)_w$ $(C_{16}H_{38}O_5Si_4)_x(C_7H_{10}O_2)_y$ $(C_4H_5O\text{-}(C_2H_4O)_a(C_2H_6OSi)_b$ $(C_2H_4O)_c\text{-}O_2C_4H_5)_z$	Mesifilcon A
$(C_6H_9NO)_w(C_5H_8O_2)_x$ $(C_7H_{10}O_2)_y(C_{10}H_{14}O_4)_z$	Lidofilcon A
$(C_6H_9NO)_w(C_5H_8O_2)_x$ $(C_{14}H_{22}O_6)_y(C_{12}H_{15}N_3O_3)_z$	Alofilcon A
$(C_6H_9NO)_x(C_5H_8O_2)_y$ $(C_7H_{10}O_2)_z$	Surfilcon A
$(C_6H_9NO)_x(C_{12}H_{14}O_2)_y$ $(C_9H_{14}O_3)_z$	Hydrofilcon A
$C_6H_9NO_2S$	Citiolone
$C_6H_9NO_3$	Trimethadione
$C_6H_9NO_6$	Isosorbide Mononitrate
$C_6H_9N_3.H_2SO_4$	Ampyzine Sulfate
$C_6H_9N_3O_2$	Histidine
$C_6H_9N_3O_2$	Medazomide
$C_6H_9N_3O_3$	Metronidazole
$C_6H_9N_3O_3.HCl$	Metronidazole Hydrochloride
$C_6H_9NaO_7.H_2O$	Sodium Glucuronate
$C_6H_9Na_9O_{24}P_6.$	Phytate Sodium
$C_6H_{10}CaO_6.xH_2O$	Calcium Lactate
$C_6H_{10}Cl_2N_2Pt$	Picoplatin
$(C_6H_{10}FeO_7)_nK_{n/2}$ $(n = 2$ to $100)$	Ferric Fructose
$C_6H_{10}N_2O_2$	Piracetam
$C_6H_{10}N_2O_3$	Oxiracetam
$C_6H_{10}N_2O_5$	Carglumic Acid
$C_6H_{10}N_3O_6P$	Metronidazole Phosphate
$C_6H_{10}N_4.$	Pentylenetetrazol
$C_6H_{10}N_4O_2$	Linsidomine
$C_6H_{10}N_6.$	Cyromazine
$C_6H_{10}N_6O$	Dacarbazine
$C_6H_{10}O$	Meparfynol
$C_6H_{10}O_2S_4$	Dixanthogen
$(C_6H_{10}O_2)_m(C_4H_4O_4)_n$	Poliglecaprone 25
$(C_6H_{10}O_2)_m(C_4H_4O_4)_n$	Poliglecaprone 90
$(C_6H_{10}O_3)_a(C_{17}H_{38}O_6Si_3)_b$ $(C_5H_9NO)_c(C_6H_9NO)_d$ $(C_{35}H_{92}O_{13}Si_{12})_e(C_{10}H_{14}O_4)_f$	Galyfilcon A
$(C_6H_{10}O_3)_n$	Polymacon
$(C_6H_{10}O_3)_u(C_{17}H_{38}O_6Si_3)_v$ $(C_5H_9NO)_w(C_6H_9NO)_x$ $(C_{35}H_{92}O_{13}Si_{12})_y(C_{16}H_{26}O_7)_z$	Senofilcon A
$(C_6H_{10}O_3)_v(C_4H_6O_2)_w$ $(C_8H_{14}O_2)_x(C_8H_{15}NO_2)_y$ $(C_{10}H_{14}O_4)_z$	Tefilcon A
$(C_6H_{10}O_3)_v(C_4H_6O_2)_w$ $(C_{18}H_{26}O_6)_x(C_8H_{14}O_2)_y$ $(C_{10}H_{16}O_2)_z$	Cyclofilcon A
$(C_6H_{10}O_3)_u(C_6H_9NO)_w$ $(C_{14}H_{24}O_3)_x(C_{10}H_{14}O_4)_y$ $(C_9H_{12}O_5)_z$	Alphafilcon A
$(C_6H_{10}O_3)_t(C_8H_{14}O_3)_w(C_4H_6O_2)_x$ $(C_4H_6O_2)_y(C_{10}H_{14}O_4)_z$	Govafilcon A
$(C_6H_{10}O_3)_t(C_9H_{15}NO_2)_w$ $(C_4H_6O_2)_x(C_5H_8O_2)_y$ $(C_{10}H_{14}O_4)_z$	Pentafilcon A
$(C_6H_{10}O_3)_v(C_9H_{16}O_2)_w(C_4H_6O_2)_x$ $(C_5H_8O_2)_y(C_{14}H_{12}O_3)_z$	Mafilcon A
$(C_6H_{10}O_3)_w(C_4H_6O_2)_x$ $(C_{10}H_{14}O_4)_y(C_8H_{14}O_4)_z$	Methafilcon B
$(C_6H_{10}O_3)_w(C_4H_6O_2)_x$ $(C_{18}H_{26}O_6)_y(C_8H_{14}O_2)_z$	Deltafilcon A
$(C_6H_{10}O_3)_w(C_4H_6O_2)_x$ $(C_{18}H_{26}O_6)_y(C_8H_{14}O_2)_z$	Deltafilcon B
$(C_6H_{10}O_3)_w(C_6H_9NO)_x$ $(C_7H_{10}O_2)_y(C_{10}H_{14}O_4)_z$	Hilafilcon A
$(C_6H_{10}O_3)_w(C_6H_9NO)_x$ $(C_7H_{10}O_2)_y(C_{10}H_{14}O_4)_z$	Hilafilcon B
$(C_6H_{10}O_3)_w(C_{10}H_{10})_x$ $(C_5H_8O_2)_y(C_6H_9NO)_z$	Tetrafilcon A
$(C_6H_{10}O_3)_x(C_4H_5NaO_2)_y$ $(C_{18}H_{26}O_6)_z$	Etafilcon A
$(C_6H_{10}O_3)_x(C_4H_6O_2)_y$	Focofilcon A
$(C_6H_{10}O_3)_x(C_4H_6O_2)_y(C_{10}H_{14}O_4)_z$	Amfilcon A
$(C_6H_{10}O_3)_x(C_4H_6O_2)_y(C_{10}H_{14}O_4)_z$	Ocufilcon A
$(C_6H_{10}O_3)_x(C_4H_6O_2)_y(C_{10}H_{14}O_4)_z$	Ocufilcon B
$(C_6H_{10}O_3)_x(C_4H_6O_2)_y(C_{10}H_{14}O_4)_z$	Ocufilcon C
$(C_6H_{10}O_3)_x(C_4H_6O_2)_y(C_{10}H_{14}O_4)_z$	Ocufilcon D
$(C_6H_{10}O_3)_x(C_4H_6O_2)_y(C_{10}H_{14}O_4)_z$	Ocufilcon E
$(C_6H_{10}O_3)_x(C_4H_6O_2)_y(C_{10}H_{14}O_4)_z$	Ocufilcon F
$(C_6H_{10}O_3)_x(C_4H_6O_2)_y(C_{16}H_{26}O_7)_z$	Genfilcon A
$(C_6H_{10}O_3)_x.(C_5H_8O_2)_y.(C_{14}H_{22}O_6)_z$	Dimefilcon A
$(C_6H_{10}O_3)_x(C_6H_9NO)_y(C_4H_6O_2)_z$	Perfilcon A
$(C_6H_{10}O_3)_x(C_6H_9NO)_y(C_{10}H_{14}O_4)_z$	Hefilcon A
$(C_6H_{10}O_3)_x(C_6H_9NO)_y(C_{10}H_{14}O_4)_z$	Hefilcon B
$(C_6H_{10}O_3)_x(C_6H_9NO)_y(C_{10}H_{14}O_4)_z$	Hefilcon C
$(C_6H_{10}O_3)_x(C_7H_{12}O_4)_y(C_{16}H_{26}O_7)_z$	Lenefilcon A
$(C_6H_{10}O_3)_x(C_8H_{14}O_3)_y.$	Phemfilcon A
$(C_6H_{10}O_3)_x(C_9H_{15}NO_2)_y$ $(C_{18}H_{26}O_6)_z.$	Bufilcon A
$(C_6H_{10}O_3)_x(C_{10}H_{14}O_4)_y$	Licryfilcon A
$(C_6H_{10}O_3)_x(C_{10}H_{14}O_4)_y$	Licryfilcon B
$(C_6H_{10}O_3)_x(C_{11}H_{22}NO_6P)_y$ $(C_{10}H_{14}O_4)_z$	Omafilcon A
$(C_6H_{10}O_3)_x(C_{14}H_{22}O_6)_y(C_6H_9NO)_z$	Droxifilcon A
$C_6H_{10}O_4$	Aceburic Acid
$C_6H_{10}O_4$	Adipic Acid
$C_6H_{10}O_4$	Isosorbide
$C_6H_{10}O_5$	Meglutol
$[C_6H_{10}O_5]_n$	Icodextrin
$C_6H_{10}O_6$	Gluconolactone
$C_6H_{11}AuO_5S$	Aurothioglucose
$C_6H_{11}BrN_2O_2$	Bromisovalum
$C_6H_{11}ClN_4O$	Giracodazole
$C_6H_{11}{}^{18}FO_5$	Fludeoxyglucose F 18
$C_6H_{11}IO_3$	Glycerol, Iodinated
$C_6H_{11}KO_7$	Potassium Gluconate
$(C_6H_{11}NO)_n$	Policapram
$C_6H_{11}NO_2$	Vigabatrin
$C_6H_{11}NO_3.HCl$	Methyl Aminolevulinate Hydrochloride
$C_6H_{11}NO_6$	Glucuronamide
$C_6H_{11}N_3O_4$	Caracemide
$C_6H_{11}N_3O_9$	Propatyl Nitrate
$C_6H_{11}NaO_7$	Sodium Gluconate
$C_6H_{11}Na_3O_{12}P_2.8H_2O.$	Fosfructose Trisodium
$C_6H_{11}O_5(C_6H_{10}O_5)_nOH.$	Inulin
$[C_6H_{11}O_7]_3Fe.3H_2O.$	Ferric Gluconate
$C_6H_{12}Br_2O_4$	Mitobronitol
$C_6H_{12}Br_2O_4$	Mitolactol
$(C_6H_{12}ClN)_n.C_{16}H_{36}Cl_2N_2O_6$	Polidronium Chloride
$C_6H_{12}Cl_3N$	Trichlormethine
$C_6H_{12}F_2N_2O_2.HCl.H_2O$	Eflornithine Hydrochloride
$C_6H_{12}NNaO_3S$	Sodium Cyclamate
$C_6H_{12}N_2Na_5O_{12}P_4{}^{153}Sm$	Samarium Sm 153 Lexidronam Pentasodium
$C_6H_{12}N_2O_4Pt$	Carboplatin
$C_6H_{12}N_2O_4S_2$	Cystine

Molecular Formula	Non-proprietary Name
$C_6H_{12}N_2O_{12}P_4{}^{153}Sm$	Samarium Sm 153 Lexidronam
$C_6H_{12}N_2S$	Mipimazole
$C_6H_{12}N_2S_4$	Thiram
$C_6H_{12}N_3PS$	Thiotepa
$C_6H_{12}N_4$	Methenamine
$C_6H_{12}N_4.C_8H_8O_3$	Methenamine Mandelate
$C_6H_{12}N_4.C_9H_9NO_3$	Methenamine Hippurate
$C_6H_{12}O$	Methyl Isobutyl Ketone
$C_6H_{12}O_3$	Paraldehyde
$C_6H_{12}O_4$	Kethoxal
$C_6H_{12}O_6$	Fructose
$C_6H_{12}O_6$	Galactose
$C_6H_{12}O_6$	Tagatose
$C_6H_{12}O_6.H_2O$	Dextrose
$C_6H_{13}NO_2$	Aminocaproic Acid
$C_6H_{13}NO_2$	Isoleucine
$C_6H_{13}NO_2$	Leucine
$(C_6H_{13}NO_2.C_6H_{11}NO_4)_n$	Leuciglumer
$C_6H_{13}NO_3$	Oxibetaine
$C_6H_{13}NO_3S$	Cyclamic Acid
$C_6H_{13}NO_3S$	Fudosteine
$C_6H_{13}NO_4.HCl$	Migalastat Hydrochloride
$C_6H_{13}NO_5$	Glucosamine
$C_6H_{13}NO_5.HCl$	Glucosamine Hydrochloride
$C_6H_{13}N_5$	Imeglimin
$C_6H_{13}N_5O$	Moroxydine
$C_6H_{14}ClNO_2S$	Methylmethionine Sulfonium Chloride
$C_6H_{14}ClN_3O_5S_2$	Laromustine
$C_6H_{14}Cl_4N_2Pt$	Dexormaplatin
$C_6H_{14}Cl_4N_2Pt$	Ormaplatin
$C_6H_{14}FO_3P$	Isoflurophate
$(C_6H_{14}NO_5)_2SO_4.2KCl$	Glucosamine Sulfate Potassium Chloride
$(C_6H_{14}NO_5)_2SO_4.2NaCl$	Glucosamine Sulfate Sodium Chloride
$C_6H_{14}N_2O_2$	Lysine
$C_6H_{14}N_2O_2$	Meldonium
$C_6H_{14}N_2O_2.C_2H_4O_2$	Lysine Acetate
$C_6H_{14}N_2O_2.C_{13}H_{18}O_2$	Ibuprofen Lysine
$C_6H_{14}N_2O_2.HCl$	Lysine Hydrochloride
$C_6H_{14}N_4O_2$	Arginine
$C_6H_{14}N_4O_2.C_5H_9NO_4$	Arginine Glutamate
$C_6H_{14}N_4O_2.HCl$	Arginine Hydrochloride
$C_6H_{14}O_2$	Hexylene Glycol
$C_6H_{14}O_3$	Diethylene Glycol Monoethyl Ether
$C_6H_{14}O_6$	Mannitol
$C_6H_{14}O_6$	Sorbitol
$C_6H_{14}O_6S_2$	Busulfan
$C_6H_{14}O_8S_2$	Treosulfan
$C_6H_{14}O_{12}P_2$	Fosfructose
$C_6H_{15}ClN_2O_2$	Carbachol
$C_6H_{15}NO_2$	Diisopropanolamine
$C_6H_{15}NO_3$	Trolamine
$C_6H_{15}N_5$	Buformin
$C_6H_{15}O_{15}P_3$	Atrinositol
$C_6H_{16}AlKO_{11}$	Potassium Glucaldrate
$C_6H_{17}NO_7P_2$	Neridronic Acid
$C_6H_{18}N_4.2HCl$	Trientine Hydrochloride
$C_6H_{18}N_4O_{17}P_2$	Trolnitrate Phosphate
$C_6H_{18}O_{24}P_6$	Phytic Acid
$C_6H_{20}Cl_2N_2O_2Pt$	Iproplatin
$C_7H_3BrClNO_2$	Bromchlorenone
$C_7H_3F_{12}N_3$	Midaflur
$C_7H_3IN_2O_3$	Nitroxinil
$C_7H_4ClNNa_2O_4S$	Monalazone Disodium
C_7H_4ClNOS	Ticlatone
$C_7H_4ClNO_2$	Chlorzoxazone
$C_7H_4NNaO_3S.2H_2O$	Saccharin Sodium
$C_7H_4O_3S$	Tioxolone
$C_7H_5BiO_4$	Bismuth Subsalicylate
$C_7H_5BiO_6$	Bismuth Subgallate
$C_7H_5ClN_2O$	Zoxazolamine
$C_7H_5ClN_2O_3$	Aklomide
$C_7H_5ClN_3NaO_4S_2$	Chlorothiazide Sodium
$C_7H_5Cl_2NO_4S$	Halazone
$C_7H_5HgNO_3$	Nitromersol
$C_7H_5KO_2$	Potassium Benzoate
$C_7H_5NO_3S$	Saccharin
$C_7H_5N_3O_5$	Nitromide
$C_7H_5NaO_2$	Sodium Benzoate
$C_7H_5NaO_3$	Sodium Salicylate
$C_7H_5NaO_4$	Sodium Gentisate
$C_7H_6ClN_3O_4S_2$	Chlorothiazide
$C_7H_6F_3NO_2$	Flucrylate
C_7H_6HgO	Isomerol
$C_7H_6KNO_2$	Aminobenzoate Potassium
$C_7H_6KNO_3$	Aminosalicylate Potassium
$C_7H_6NNaO_2$	Aminobenzoate Sodium
$C_7H_6NNaO_3.2H_2O$	Aminosalicylate Sodium
$C_7H_6N_4O_2$	Ciapilome
$C_7H_6N_4O_2$	Melizame
$C_7H_6N_4O_2$	Tirapazamine
$C_7H_6N_4O_5$	Nifuraldezone
$C_7H_6N_4S_2$	Citenazone
C_7H_6O	Benzaldehyde
$C_7H_6OCl_2(C_2H_4O)n$	Lemoxinol
$C_7H_6O_2$	Benzoic Acid
$C_7H_6O_3$	Salicylic Acid
$C_7H_7ClNNaO_2S$	Chloramine-T
$C_7H_7ClN_2O_3S$	Sulclamide
$C_7H_7ClN_6O_2$	Mitozolomide
$C_7H_7ClNa_2O_6P_2S$	Tiludronate Disodium
C_7H_7ClO	Chlorocresol
$C_7H_7Cl_2NO$	Clopidol
$C_7H_7Cl_3NO_4P$	Fospirate
$C_7H_7KO_5S.\frac{1}{2}H_2O$	Potassium Guaiacolsulfonate
$C_7H_7NO_2$	Aminobenzoic Acid
$C_7H_7NO_2$	Methyl Nicotinate
$C_7H_7NO_2$	Salicylamide
$C_7H_7NO_3$	Aminosalicylic Acid
$C_7H_7NO_3$	Mesalamine
$C_7H_7NO_4S$	Carzenide
$C_7H_7N_3O_4$	Nihydrazone
$C_7H_7N_5$	Fenamole
$C_7H_7O_6P$	Fosfosal
$C_7H_8AsNNa_2O_6S$	Phenarsone Sulfoxylate
$C_7H_8BrNO_2$	Brocresine
$C_7H_8ClN_3O_4S_2$	Hydrochlorothiazide
$(C_7H_8FeO_5)_n$	Ferropolimaler
$C_7H_8N_2O_5$	Nifuratrone
$C_7H_8N_4O_2.C_2H_7NO$	Theophylline Olamine
$C_7H_8N_4O_2.C_4H_{11}NO$	Ambuphylline
$C_7H_8N_4O_2.C_{10}H_{14}O_4$	Guaithylline
$C_7H_8N_4O_2.H_2O$	Theophylline
$C_7H_8N_4S$	Nicothiazone
C_7H_8O	Benzyl Alcohol
C_7H_8O	Cresol
C_7H_8O	Metacresol
$C_7H_8O_2$	Guaiacol
$C_7H_8O_2$	Mequinol

Molecular Formula	Non-proprietary Name
$C_7H_8O_2$	Salicyl Alcohol
$C_7H_8O_3$	Flamenol
$C_7H_9AsN_2O_4$	Carbarsone
$C_7H_9ClN_2O$	Pralidoxime Chloride
$C_7H_9ClN_2O_4S_2$	Disulfamide
C_7H_9ClO	Ethchlorvynol
$C_7H_9ClO_6P_2S$	Tiludronic Acid
$C_7H_9FN_3O_2P$	Flurofamide
$C_7H_9IN_2O$	Pralidoxime Iodide
$C_7H_9NO_2$	Deferiprone
$C_7H_9NO_2$	Metipirox
$C_7H_9NO_2$	Rolziracetam
$C_7H_9NO_2S$	Tizoprolic Acid
$C_7H_9NO_3$	Allomethadione
$C_7H_9NO_4S_2$	Taurosteine
$C_7H_9N_3O$	Phenicarbazide
$C_7H_9N_3O_2S_2$	Sulfathiourea
$C_7H_9N_3O_2S_2.C_7H_{10}N_2O_2S$	Sulfatolamide
$C_7H_9N_3O_3S$	Sulfacarbamide
$C_7H_9N_3O_4S$	Methaniazide
$C_7H_{10}ClNS$	Cloprothiazole
$C_7H_{10}ClN_3O_3$	Ornidazole
$C_7H_{10}NNaO_6P_2$	Piridronate Sodium
$C_7H_{10}NNaO_7P_2$	Risedronate Sodium
$C_7H_{10}N_2OS$	Olpimedone
$C_7H_{10}N_2OS$	Propylthiouracil
$C_7H_{10}N_2O_2S$	Carbimazole
$C_7H_{10}N_2O_2S$	Mafenide
$C_7H_{10}N_2O_2S.C_2H_4O_2$	Mafenide Acetate
$C_7H_{10}N_2O_5S_2$	Mesulfamide
$C_7H_{10}N_4O_2S$	Sulfaguanidine
$C_7H_{10}N_4O_4$	Bamnidazole
$C_7H_{10}N_4O_4$	Etanidazole
$C_7H_{10}N_4O_4S$	Dezaguanine Mesylate
$C_7H_{10}O_6S_3$	Ritiometan
$C_7H_{11}BrN_2O_2$	Bromacrylide
$C_7H_{11}Cl_3O_4$	Penthrichloral
$C_7H_{11}NO_2$	Ethosuximide
$C_7H_{11}NO_2$	Icofungipen
$C_7H_{11}NO_3$	Paramethadione
$C_7H_{11}NO_4$	Oxaceprol
$C_7H_{11}NO_4S$	Dacisteine
$C_7H_{11}NO_4S$	Telmesteine
$C_7H_{11}NO_6P_2$	Piridronic Acid
$C_7H_{11}NO_7P_2$	Risedronic Acid
$(C_7H_{11}N_2O.Cl)n$	Colestilan Chloride
$C_7H_{11}N_3$	Isaxonine
$C_7H_{11}N_3O_2$	Ipronidazole
$C_7H_{11}N_3O_3$	Secnidazole
$C_7H_{11}N_3O_3$	Ternidazole
$C_7H_{11}N_3O_4$	Misonidazole
$C_7H_{12}N_2O_2$	Ectylurea
$C_7H_{12}O_4$	Propylene Glycol Diacetate
$(C_7H_{12}O_4)_x.(C_6H_{10}O_3)_y.(C_{10}H_{14}O_4)_z$	Hioxifilcon D
$(C_7H_{12}O_4)_x(C_5H_8O_2)_y$	Crofilcon A
$(C_7H_{12}O_4)_x(C_6H_{10}O_3)_y(C_{10}H_{14}O_4)_z$	Hioxifilcon A
$C_7H_{13}BrN_2O_2$	Carbromal
$C_7H_{13}NO_3S_2$	Bucillamine
$C_7H_{13}NaO_8$	Gluceptate Sodium
$C_7H_{13}O_3P$	Fosmenic Acid
$C_7H_{14}BrNO$	Ibrotamide
$C_7H_{14}Cl_3NO_4$	Chloral Betaine
$C_7H_{14}NO_5P$	Selfotel
$C_7H_{14}N_2O_6S$	Glutaurine
$C_7H_{14}N_3O_3P$	Uredepa

Molecular Formula	Non-proprietary Name
$C_7H_{14}N_4$	Guancydine
$C_7H_{14}N_4S_2$	Methallibure
$C_7H_{15}ClN_4O_4S$	Tauromustine
$C_7H_{15}Cl_2N_2O_2P$	Ifosfamide
$C_7H_{15}Cl_2N_2O_2P.H_2O$	Cyclophosphamide
$C_7H_{15}Cl_2N_2O_4P$	Perfosfamide
$C_7H_{15}N$	Nanofin
$C_7H_{15}NO_2$	Emylcamate
$C_7H_{15}NO_3$	Carnitine
$C_7H_{15}NO_3$	Levocarnitine
$C_7H_{16}BrNO$	Meprochol
$C_7H_{16}ClNO_2$	Acetylcholine Chloride
$C_7H_{16}INO_2$	Oxapropanium Iodide
$C_7H_{16}N_2$	Cimemoxin
$C_7H_{16}N_2O.HCl$	Milacemide Hydrochloride
$C_7H_{16}N_4O_2.C_2H_4O_2$	Tilarginine Acetate
$C_7H_{16}N_4O_4S_2$	Taurolidine
$C_7H_{17}ClN_2O_2$	Bethanechol Chloride
$C_7H_{17}N$	Tuaminoheptane
$(C_7H_{17}N)_2.H_2SO_4$	Tuaminoheptane Sulfate
$C_7H_{17}NO_5$	Meglumine
$C_7H_{17}NO_5.C_7H_6O_3$	Salicylate Meglumine
$C_7H_{18}NO_2P$	Butafosfan
$C_7H_{23}F_3N_2O_2$	Flualamide
C_8BrF_{17}	Perflubron
$C_8H_3Cl_2N_3O_4$	Licostinel
$C_8H_3I_2NNa_2O_5$	Iodomethamate Sodium
$C_8H_4K_2O_{12}Sb_2.3H_2O$	Antimony Potassium Tartrate
$C_8H_4N_2S_2$	Bitoscanate
$C_8H_4Na_2O_{12}Sb_2$	Antimony Sodium Tartrate
$C_8H_5BrCl_6$	Bromociclen
$C_8H_5F_3N_2OS$	Riluzole
$C_8H_5NO_3$	Carsalam
$C_8H_5N_3O_3S_2$	Tenonitrozole
$C_8H_6Cl_3NO_2$	Triclacetamol
$C_8H_6F_3N_3O_4S_2$	Flumethiazide
$C_8H_6F_3O_6P$	Flufosal
$C_8H_6N_2O_2$	Fenadiazole
$C_8H_6N_2O_2$	Quindoxin
$C_8H_6N_2S_3$	Oltipraz
$C_8H_6N_4O_4S$	Nifurthiazole
$C_8H_6N_4O_5$	Nitrofurantoin
$C_8H_7ClN_2O_2S$	Diazoxide
$C_8H_7Cl_4N_3O_4S_2$	Teclothiazide
$C_8H_7IN_2OS$	Rimoprogin
$C_8H_7N_3O_5$	Dinitolmide
$C_8H_7N_3O_5$	Furazolidone
$C_8H_7NaO_2$	Sodium Phenylacetate
$C_8H_7NaO_3$	Methylparaben Sodium
$(C_8H_7NaO_3S)_n$	Tolevamer Sodium
$C_8H_7NaO_4$	Sodium Dehydroacetate
$(C_8H_7O_3S)_n.K_{(n-a)}Na_a$	Tolevamer Potassium Sodium
C_8H_8AuNOS	Aurothioglycanide
$C_8H_8BrCl_2O_3PS$	Bromofos
$C_8H_8BrNO_2$	Brosotamide
$C_8H_8CaNO_6P.3H_2O$	Pyridoxal Calcium Phosphate
$C_8H_8Cl_2IO_3PS$	Iodofenphos
$C_8H_8Cl_2N_4$	Guanabenz
$C_8H_8Cl_2N_4.C_2H_4O_2$	Guanabenz Acetate
$C_8H_8Cl_2N_4O$	Guanoxabenz
$C_8H_8Cl_2N_4O.HCl$	Biclodil Hydrochloride
$C_8H_8Cl_2O$	Dichloroxylenol
$C_8H_8Cl_3N_3O_4S_2$	Clorsulon
$C_8H_8Cl_3N_3O_4S_2$	Trichlormethiazide
$C_8H_8Cl_3O_3PS$	Ronnel
$C_8H_8F_3N_3O_4S_2$	Hydroflumethiazide

Molecular Formula	Non-proprietary Name
$C_8H_8HgO_2$	Phenylmercuric Acetate
$C_8H_8KNO_5$	Clavulanate Potassium
$C_8H_8N_2O_3S$	Zonisamide
$C_8H_8N_3Na_2O_6S^{99m}Tc$	Technetium Tc 99m Mertiatide
$C_8H_8N_4.HCl$	Hydralazine Hydrochloride
$C_8H_8N_4O_3S$	Thiofuradene
$C_8H_8N_4O_4$	Nifuradene
$C_8H_8O_3$	Hydroxytoluic Acid
$C_8H_8O_3$	Mandelic Acid
$C_8H_8O_3$	Methyl Salicylate
$C_8H_8O_3$	Methylparaben
$C_8H_8O_3$	Resorcinol Monoacetate
$C_8H_8O_3$	Vanillin
$C_8H_8O_4$	Dehydroacetic Acid
$C_8H_9AsBiNO_6$	Glycobiarsol
C_8H_9ClO	Chloroxylenol
$C_8H_9FN_2O_3$	Tegafur
$C_8H_9FO_2S$	Fluoresone
$C_8H_9HgNaO_3S_2$	Thimerfonate Sodium
$C_8H_9I_2NO_3$	Iopydol
$C_8H_9NO_2$	Acetaminophen
$C_8H_9NO_2$	Cresotamide
$C_8H_9NO_2$	Metacetamol
$C_8H_9NO_2S$	Oxisuran
$C_8H_9NO_3$	Oxfenicine
$C_8H_9NO_5$	Clavulanic Acid
$C_8H_9N_2NaO_3S.H_2O$	Sulfacetamide Sodium
$C_8H_9N_3O_4$	Nicorandil
$(C_8H_9O_4S)(C_8H_8O_4S)_n(C_7H_7O_4S)$	Policresulen
$C_8H_{10}AsNO_5$	Acetarsone
$C_8H_{10}AsN_2NaO_4.\frac{1}{2}H_2O$	Tryparsamide
$C_8H_{10}BrNO_3S$	Brobactam
$C_8H_{10}ClN_3O$	Lazabemide
$C_8H_{10}ClN_3O.HCl$	Lazabemide Hydrochloride
$C_8H_{10}ClN_3S$	Tiamenidine
$C_8H_{10}ClN_3S.HCl$	Tiamenidine Hydrochloride
$C_8H_{10}FN_3O_3S$	Emtricitabine
$(C_8H_{10}{}^{123}IN_3)_2.H_2SO_4$	Iobenguane I 123
$(C_8H_{10}{}^{131}IN_3)_2.H_2SO_4$	Iobenguane I 131
$(C_8H_{10}{}^{123}IN_3)_2.H_2SO_4$	Iobenguane Sulfate I 123
$(C_8H_{10}{}^{131}IN_3)_2.H_2SO_4$	Iobenguane Sulfate I 131
$C_8H_{10}NNaO_5S$	Sulbactam Sodium
$C_8H_{10}NO_6P.H_2O$	Pyridoxal Phosphate
$C_8H_{10}N_2OS$	Tenilsetam
$C_8H_{10}N_2O_3S$	Sulfacetamide
$C_8H_{10}N_2S$	Ethionamide
$C_8H_{10}N_4O_2$	Caffeine
$C_8H_{10}N_4O_2$	Enprofylline
$C_8H_{10}N_4O_4$	Nifursemizone
$C_8H_{10}N_4O_5$	Nidroxyzone
$C_8H_{10}N_5NaO_3$	Acyclovir Sodium
$C_8H_{10}N_6.H_2SO_4$	Dihydralazine Sulfate
$C_8H_{10}N_6S.2HCl$	Zaltidine Hydrochloride
$C_8H_{10}O$	Phenylethyl Alcohol
$C_8H_{10}O_2$	Phenoxyethanol
$C_8H_{11}Cl_2N_3O_2$	Uracil Mustard
$C_8H_{11}Cl_3O_6$	Chloralose
$(C_8H_{11}Cl_3O_6)_x(C_6H_{10}O_5)_y$	Amicloral
$C_8H_{11}NO$	Metyridine
$C_8H_{11}NOS.H_3PO_4$	Ristianol Phosphate
$C_8H_{11}NO_2$	Bucrylate
$C_8H_{11}NO_2$	Enbucrilate
$C_8H_{11}NO_2$	Norfenefrine
$C_8H_{11}NO_2$	Octopamine
$C_8H_{11}NO_2.HCl$	Dopamine Hydrochloride
$C_8H_{11}NO_3$	Oxidopamine

Molecular Formula	Non-proprietary Name
$C_8H_{11}NO_3.C_4H_6O_6.H_2O$	Norepinephrine Bitartrate
$C_8H_{11}NO_3.C_9H_{12}N_4O_6S$	Pyridofylline
$C_8H_{11}NO_3.HCl$	Pyridoxine Hydrochloride
$C_8H_{11}NO_3S.(Fe_2O_3)_{0.725}$	Ferristene
$C_8H_{11}NO_4$	Eglumetad
$C_8H_{11}NO_4S_2$	Erdosteine
$(C_8H_{11}NO_5S)_2.C_{16}H_{20}N_2$	Sulbactam Benzathine
$C_8H_{11}N_2NaO_3$	Barbital Sodium
$C_8H_{11}N_2NaO_3.\frac{1}{2}H_2O$	Pentizidone Sodium
$C_8H_{11}N_3O_2$	Caricotamide
$C_8H_{11}N_3O_3S$	Apricitabine
$C_8H_{11}N_3O_3S$	Lamivudine
$C_8H_{11}N_3O_4$	Troxacitabine
$C_8H_{11}N_5O_2$	Desciclovir
$C_8H_{11}N_5O_3$	Acyclovir
$C_8H_{11}N_5O_5S$	Satranidazole
$C_8H_{11}N_7S$	Ambazone
$C_8H_{12}CaN_2O_8.3H_2O$	Calcium L-Aspartate
$C_8H_{12}MgN_2O_8.4H_2O$	Magnesium Aspartate
$C_8H_{12}NO_5PS_2$	Cythioate
$C_8H_{12}N_2$	Mebanazine
$C_8H_{12}N_2.2HCl$	Betahistine Hydrochloride
$C_8H_{12}N_2.H_2SO_4$	Phenelzine Sulfate
$C_8H_{12}N_2O_3$	Barbital
$C_8H_{12}N_2O_4S$	Pralidoxime Mesylate
$C_8H_{12}N_2S$	Etrabamine
$C_8H_{12}N_3O_2P$	Tolfamide
$C_8H_{12}N_4O_3S$	Carnidazole
$C_8H_{12}N_4O_4$	Decitabine
$C_8H_{12}N_4O_5$	Azacitidine
$C_8H_{12}N_4O_5$	Fazarabine
$C_8H_{12}N_4O_5$	Ribavirin
$C_8H_{12}N_5O_4P$	Adefovir
$C_8H_{13}NO_2$	Bemegride
$C_8H_{13}NO_3$	Diethadione
$C_8H_{13}NO_3S_2$	Limazocic
$C_8H_{13}N_2O_5P.2H_2O$	Pyridoxamine Phosphate
$C_8H_{13}N_3O_4S$	Tinidazole
$C_8H_{13}N_3O_5S$	Mertiatide
$C_8H_{13}N_3O_6$	Doranidazole
$C_8H_{13}N_5O_4.HCl$	Taribavirin Hydrochloride
$C_8H_{14}Cl_3O_5P$	Butonate
$C_8H_{14}INO$	Furtrethonium Iodide
$C_8H_{14}N_2O.HCl$	Milameline Hydrochloride
$C_8H_{14}N_2O_2$	Etiracetam
$C_8H_{14}N_2O_2$	Levetiracetam
$C_8H_{14}N_2O_4Pt$	Oxaliplatin
$C_8H_{14}N_3O_6P.2H_2O$	Cidofovir
$C_8H_{14}N_5OPS$	Azetepa
$C_8H_{14}O_2S_2$	Lipoic Acid, Alpha
$C_8H_{14}O_2S_2$	Thioctic Acid
$(C_8H_{14}O_2)_x(C_7H_{12}O_2)_y(C_{10}H_{14}O_4)_z$	Esterifilcon A
$[[C_8H_{15}BrN_2O_2]_x[C_6H_{12}N_2O]_y]_n$	Azoximer Bromide
$C_8H_{15}Cl_3O_3$	Chlorhexadol
$C_8H_{15}NOS_2$	Thioctic Acid Amide
$C_8H_{15}NO_2$	Oxanamide
$C_8H_{15}NO_2$	Tranexamic Acid
$C_8H_{15}NO_2S$	Prenisteine
$C_8H_{15}NO_3$	Acetylleucine
$C_8H_{15}NO_3$	Acexamic Acid
$C_8H_{15}NO_3.HCl$	Tridolgosir Hydrochloride
$C_8H_{15}NO_3S$	Tizabrin
$C_8H_{15}N_2O_5P$	Midafotel
$C_8H_{15}N_3O_7$	Streptozocin
$C_8H_{15}N_5O$	Pildralazine
$C_8H_{15}N_5O_2$	Oxdralazine

Molecular Formula	Non-proprietary Name
$C_8H_{15}N_7O_2S_3$	Famotidine
$C_8H_{15}NaO_2$	Sodium Caprylate
$C_8H_{15}NaO_2$	Valproate Sodium
$C_8H_{16}ClN_3O_2$	Pentamustine
$C_8H_{16}N_2O_4$	Pentabamate
$C_8H_{16}N_6OS_2$	Gloxazone
$C_8H_{16}O_2$	Octanoic Acid
$C_8H_{16}O_2$	Valproic Acid
$C_8H_{17}Cl_2NO_2$	Diisopropylamine Dichloroacetate
$C_8H_{17}NO$	Valnoctamide
$C_8H_{17}NO$	Valpromide
$C_8H_{17}NO_2$	Pregabalin
$C_8H_{17}NO_5$	Miglitol
$(C_8H_{17}N_5.HCl)_n$	Polihexanide
$C_8H_{17}NaO_4S$	Sodium Ethasulfate
$C_8H_{18}BrNO_2$	Methacholine Bromide
$C_8H_{18}ClNO_2$	Carpronium Chloride
$C_8H_{18}ClNO_2$	Methacholine Chloride
$C_8H_{18}ClN_2O_5PS$	Sufosfamide
$C_8H_{18}N_2O_4PtS$	Spiroplatin
$C_8H_{18}O_3$	Terbuprol
$C_8H_{19}N$	Octodrine
$C_8H_{19}NO.HCl$	Heptaminol Hydrochloride
$C_8H_{19}NO_6P_2$	Incadronic Acid
$C_8H_{19}NO_6S_2$	Improsulfan
$C_8H_{19}N_5.HCl$	Etoformin Hydrochloride
$C_8H_{20}BrN$	Tetrylammonium Bromide
$C_8H_{20}NO_6P$	Choline Alfoscerate
$C_8H_{20}N_2$	Octamoxin
$C_8H_{20}N_4O_5S_2$	Argimesna
$C_8H_{20}O_7P_2$	Ethyl Pyrophosphate
$C_9F_{21}N$	Perfluamine
$C_9H_4Cl_3IO$	Haloprogin
$C_9H_5Br_2NO$	Broxyquinoline
C_9H_5ClINO	Clioquinol
$C_9H_5Cl_2NO$	Chloroxine
$C_9H_5Cl_3N_2O_2S$	Clotioxone
$C_9H_5I_2NO$	Iodoquinol
$C_9H_5I_3NNaO_3$	Acetrizoate Sodium
C_9H_6ClNO	Cloxyquin
$C_9H_6N_2O_3$	Nitroxoline
$C_9H_7Cl_2N_5$	Irsogladine
$C_9H_7Cl_2N_5$	Lamotrigine
$C_9H_7{}^{123}INNaO_3$	Iodohippurate Sodium I 123
$C_9H_7{}^{125}INNaO_3$	Iodohippurate Sodium I 125
$C_9H_7{}^{131}INNaO_3$	Iodohippurate Sodium I 131
$C_9H_7{}^{125}I_2NO_3$	Diohippuric Acid I 125
$C_9H_7{}^{131}I_2NO_3$	Diohippuric Acid I 131
C_9H_7NO	Oxyquinoline
$(C_9H_7NO)_2.H_2SO_4$	Oxyquinoline Sulfate
$C_9H_7N_3O_4S_2$	Para-Nitrosulfathiazole
$C_9H_7N_5O_3$	Acitazanolast
$C_9H_7N_5O_3$	Furalazine
$C_9H_7N_7O_2S$	Azathioprine
$C_9H_8CaN_3O_3$	Pyruvic Acid Calcium Isoniazid
$C_9H_8ClF_6NO_3S_2$	Begacestat
$C_9H_8ClNS_2$	Nimidane
$C_9H_8ClN_3O_3S$	Furazolium Chloride
$C_9H_8ClN_5.HCl$	Chlorazanil Hydrochloride
$C_9H_8ClN_5O$	Cloguanamil
$C_9H_8ClN_5S.HCl$	Tizanidine Hydrochloride
$C_9H_8Cl_2N_2O$	Clidafidine
$C_9H_8Cl_2N_6$	Nebidrazine
$C_9H_8N_2O$	Medorinone
$C_9H_8N_2O_2$	Pemoline

Molecular Formula	Non-proprietary Name
$C_9H_8N_2S_2$	Antienite
$C_9H_8N_4O_5$	Tretazicar
$C_9H_8N_4O_6$	Nifurtoinol
$C_9H_8N_8O_2S$	Thiamiprine
$C_9H_8O_4$	Aspirin
$C_9H_8O_4.C_6H_{14}N_2O_2$	Aspirin DL-Lysine
$C_9H_9BrFN_3$	Romifidine
$C_9H_9ClN_2O$	Clominorex
$C_9H_9ClN_2O_3$	Benurestat
C_9H_9ClO	Chlorindanol
$C_9H_9Cl_2NO_2$	Diloxanide
$C_9H_9Cl_2N_3$	Clonidine
$C_9H_9Cl_2N_3.HCl$	Clonidine Hydrochloride
$C_9H_9Cl_2N_3O.HCl$	Guanfacine Hydrochloride
$C_9H_9HgNaO_2S$	Thimerosal
$C_9H_9{}^{125}I_2NO_3$	Diotyrosine I 125
$C_9H_9{}^{131}I_2NO_3$	Diotyrosine I 131
$C_9H_9NO_2$	Noreximide
$C_9H_9NO_3$	Acedoben
$C_9H_9NO_3$	Salacetamide
$C_9H_9NO_6$	Hydroxypyridine Tartrate
$C_9H_9N_2NaO_3$	Aminohippurate Sodium
$C_9H_9N_3O_2S_2$	Sulfathiazole
$C_9H_9N_3O_2S_2$	Thiazosulfone
$C_9H_9N_3O_5$	Furmethoxadone
$C_9H_9N_3S$	Amiphenazole
$C_9H_9N_5$	Amanozine
$C_9H_{10}ClFN_2O_4$	Raluridine
$C_9H_{10}ClNO_2$	Fenclonine
$C_9H_{10}ClNO_3$	Carisbamate
$C_9H_{10}ClN_2O_5PS$	Azamethiphos
$C_9H_{10}ClN_3O_2S_2$	Tifenazoxide
$C_9H_{10}ClN_3S$	Timirdine
$C_9H_{10}Cl_2N_4$	Aganodine
$C_9H_{10}Cl_2N_4.HCl$	Apraclonidine Hydrochloride
$C_9H_{10}FIN_2O_5$	Fialuridine
$C_9H_{10}{}^{18}FNO_4$	Fluorodopa F 18
$C_9H_{10}FN_3O_3$	Dexelvucitabine
$C_9H_{10}FN_3O_3$	Elvucitabine
$C_9H_{10}FN_3O_4$	Flurocitabine
$C_9H_{10}{}^{131}INO_3$	Iotyrosine I 131
$C_9H_{10}N_2O$	Aminorex
$C_9H_{10}N_2O_2$	Phenacemide
$C_9H_{10}N_2O_2S$	Sulbenox
$C_9H_{10}N_2O_3$	Aminohippuric Acid
$C_9H_{10}N_2O_3$	Olmidine
$C_9H_{10}N_2O_3S_2$	Ethoxzolamide
$C_9H_{10}N_2S$	Etisazole
$C_9H_{10}N_4O_2S_2$	Sulfamethizole
$C_9H_{10}N_4O_3S_2$	Sulfametrole
$C_9H_{10}N_4O_4$	Nifurimide
$(C_9H_{10}N_4O_4)_2.C_4H_{10}N_2$	Acefylline Piperazine
$C_9H_{10}O_2$	Paroxypropione
$C_9H_{10}O_3$	Ethyl Vanillin
$C_9H_{10}O_3$	Ethylparaben
$C_9H_{10}O_4$	Flopropione
$C_9H_{11}BrN_2O_5$	Broxuridine
$C_9H_{11}ClN_2O.C_7H_{19}O_3S$	Tebanicline Tosylate
$C_9H_{11}ClN_2O_3S$	Diapamide
$C_9H_{11}Cl_2N_3O_4S_2$	Methyclothiazide
$C_9H_{11}FIN_3O_4$	Fiacitabine
$C_9H_{11}FN_2O_5$	Doxifluridine
$C_9H_{11}FN_2O_5$	Floxuridine
$C_9H_{11}F_2N_3O_4$	Gemcitabine
$C_9H_{11}F_2N_3O_4.HCl$	Gemcitabine Hydrochloride
$C_9H_{11}IN_2O_4$	Ropidoxuridine

Molecular Formula	Non-proprietary Name
$C_9H_{11}IN_2O_5$	Idoxuridine
$(C_9H_{11}N)_2.H_2SO_4$	Tranylcypromine Sulfate
$C_9H_{11}NO$	Cathinone
$C_9H_{11}NO_2$	Benzocaine
$C_9H_{11}NO_2$	Ethenzamide
$C_9H_{11}NO_2$	Parapropamol
$C_9H_{11}NO_2$	Phenylalanine
$C_9H_{11}NO_3$	Adrenalone
$C_9H_{11}NO_3$	Styramate
$C_9H_{11}NO_3$	Tyrosine
$C_9H_{11}NO_4$	Forfenimex
$C_9H_{11}NO_4$	Levodopa
$C_9H_{11}NO_5$	Droxidopa
$C_9H_{11}N_3O_4$	Ancitabine
$C_9H_{11}N_5O_4$	Navuridine
$C_9H_{12}BNO_4$	Epinephryl Borate
$C_9H_{12}ClN_3O_3S$	Alipamide
$C_9H_{12}ClN_3O_4S_2$	Ethiazide
$C_9H_{12}ClN_5O$	Moxonidine
$C_9H_{12}Cl_2N_4$	Guanclofine
$[C_9H_{12}Cl_2N_4O]_2.H_2SO_4$	Guanoclor Sulfate
$C_9H_{12}IN_3O_4$	Ibacitabine
$C_9H_{12}NO_5PS$	Fenitrothion
$C_9H_{12}N_2O_4S$	Pidotimod
$C_9H_{12}N_2O_5S$	Sulocarbilate
$C_9H_{12}N_2O_5S$	Tiazofurin
$C_9H_{12}N_2O_7P_2$	Minodronic Acid
$C_9H_{12}N_2S$	Protionamide
$C_9H_{12}N_3O_7P$	Cifostodine
$C_9H_{12}N_4O_3$	Etofylline
$(C_9H_{12}N_4O_3Zn)_n$	Polaprezinc
$C_9H_{12}N_5NaO_4$	Ganciclovir Sodium
$C_9H_{12}N_5Na_2O_3P.H_2O$	Benfosformin
$C_9H_{12}N_6$	Triethylenemelamine
$C_9H_{12}N_6O_3$	Amdoxovir
$C_9H_{12}O$	Phenylpropanol
$C_9H_{13}BrN_2O_2$	Pyridostigmine Bromide
$C_9H_{13}ClN_6O_2$	Nimustine
$C_9H_{13}N$	Dextroamphetamine
$C_9H_{13}N.C_4H_6O_4$	Levamfetamine Succinate
$(C_9H_{13}N)_2.H_2SO_4$	Amphetamine Sulfate
$(C_9H_{13}N)_2.H_2SO_4$	Dextroamphetamine Sulfate
$C_9H_{13}N.H_3PO_4$	Dextroamphetamine Phosphate
$C_9H_{13}NO$	Cathine
$C_9H_{13}NO$	Gepefrine
$C_9H_{13}NO.C_4H_6O_6$	Phenylpropanolamine Bitartrate
$C_9H_{13}NO.HBr$	Hydroxyamphetamine Hydrobromide
$C_9H_{13}NO.HCl$	Phenylpropanolamine Hydrochloride
$C_9H_{13}NO_2$	Ethinamate
$C_9H_{13}NO_2$	Oxedrine
$C_9H_{13}NO_2$	Pyrithyldione
$C_9H_{13}NO_2.C_4H_6O_6$	Metaraminol Bitartrate
$C_9H_{13}NO_2.C_4H_6O_6$	Phenylephrine Bitartrate
$C_9H_{13}NO_2.HCl$	Phenylephrine Hydrochloride
$C_9H_{13}NO_3$	Epinephrine
$C_9H_{13}NO_3$	Levonordefrin
$C_9H_{13}NO_3$	Racepinephrine
$C_9H_{13}NO_3.C_4H_6O_6$	Epinephrine Bitartrate
$C_9H_{13}NO_3.HCl$	Nordefrin Hydrochloride
$C_9H_{13}NO_3.HCl$	Racepinephrine Hydrochloride
$C_9H_{13}N_2NaO_3$	Probarbital Sodium
$C_9H_{13}N_2O_5P$	Perzinfotel
$C_9H_{13}N_3O$	Iproniazid
$C_9H_{13}N_3O_2$	Aminometradine

Molecular Formula	Non-proprietary Name
$C_9H_{13}N_3O_2$	Amisometradine
$C_9H_{13}N_3O_3$	Zalcitabine
$C_9H_{13}N_3O_4$	Torcitabine
$C_9H_{13}N_3O_5$	Cytarabine
$C_9H_{13}N_3O_5.HCl$	Cytarabine Hydrochloride
$C_9H_{13}N_3O_6$	Mizoribine
$C_9H_{13}N_3O_6$	Pyrazofurin
$C_9H_{13}N_5O_2$	Detiviciclovir
$C_9H_{13}N_5O_3$	Buciclovir
$C_9H_{13}N_5O_3$	Tiviciclovir
$C_9H_{13}N_5O_4$	Ganciclovir
$C_9H_{14}NO_2P$	Toldimfos
$C_9H_{14}NO_5P$	Fosopamine
$C_9H_{14}N_2$	Pheniprazine Hydrochloride
$C_9H_{14}N_2O$	Phenoxypropazine
$C_9H_{14}N_2O_3$	Metharbital
$C_9H_{14}N_2O_4S_2$	Cartasteine
$C_9H_{14}N_4O$	Azimexon
$C_9H_{14}N_4O_3$	Nimorazole
$C_9H_{14}N_4O_3S$	Sulnidazole
$C_9H_{14}N_4O_4$	Molsidomine
$C_9H_{14}N_4O_5$	Acadesine
$C_9H_{14}N_5O_4P.H_2O$	Tenofovir
$C_9H_{14}N_6O$	Oxonazine
$C_9H_{14}O_6$	Triacetin
$C_9H_{15}AlO_9$	Aluminum Lactate
$C_9H_{15}BrN_2O_2$	Broxaterol
$C_9H_{15}BrN_2O_3$	Acecarbromal
$C_9H_{15}NO_2$	Aceclidine
$C_9H_{15}NO_3S$	Captopril
$C_9H_{15}N_3$	Tetrydamine
$C_9H_{15}N_3.H_2SO_4$	Triampyzine Sulfate
$C_9H_{15}N_3O$	Azepexole
$C_9H_{15}N_5.C_4H_4O_4$	Alvameline Maleate
$C_9H_{15}N_5O$	Minoxidil
$C_9H_{15}N_5O_3.2HCl$	Sapropterin Dihydrochloride
$C_9H_{15}NaO_3$	Hexacyclonate Sodium
$C_9H_{15}O_3$	Cilexetil
$C_9H_{16}ClN_3O_2$	Lomustine
$C_9H_{16}N_2O_2S.HCl$	Tazolol Hydrochloride
$C_9H_{16}N_2O_3S$	Alonacic
$C_9H_{16}N_2O_4$	Bisorcic
$C_9H_{16}N_4O$	Darsidomine
$C_9H_{16}N_4O$	Rolgamidine
$C_9H_{16}N_4S_2$	Metiamide
$(C_9H_{16}O_2)_r(C_5H_8O_2)_s$ $(C_{11}H_6F_{12}O_4)_t(C_{16}H_{38}O_5Si_4)_u$ $(C_{13}H_{20}O_4)_v(C_{26}H_{58}O_9Si_6)_w$ $(C_4H_6O_2)_x(C_6H_9NO)_y$ $(C_{70}H_{188}O_{30}Si_{27})_z$	Enflufocon A
$(C_9H_{16}O_2)_r(C_5H_8O_2)_s$ $(C_{11}H_6F_{12}O_4)_t(C_{16}H_{38}O_5Si_4)_u$ $(C_{13}H_{20}O_4)_v(C_{26}H_{58}O_9Si_6)_w$ $(C_4H_6O_2)_x(C_6H_9NO)_y$ $(C_{70}H_{188}O_{30}Si_{27})_z$	Enflufocon B
$C_9H_{16}O_4$	Azelaic Acid
$C_9H_{17}NO$	Valdetamide
$C_9H_{17}NO_2$	Gabapentin
$C_9H_{17}NO_3$	Pivagabine
$C_9H_{18}Cl_3N_2O_2P$	Trofosfamide
$C_9H_{18}N_2O_2$	Capuride
$C_9H_{18}N_2O_3Pt$	Lobaplatin
$C_9H_{18}N_2O_4$	Meprobamate
$C_9H_{18}N_4.H_2SO_4.2H_2O$	Guanacline Sulfate
$C_9H_{18}N_6$	Altretamine
$C_9H_{19}BN_2O_3$	Talabostat

Molecular Formula	Non-proprietary Name
$C_9H_{19}BN_2O_3.CH_4O_3S$	Talabostat Mesylate
$C_9H_{19}ClN_3O_5P$	Fotemustine
$C_9H_{19}Cl_2N_2O_5PS_2$	Mafosfamide
$(C_9H_{19}N)_2.C_6H_{10}O_8$	Isometheptene Mucate
$C_9H_{19}N.HCl$	Cyclopentamine Hydrochloride
$C_9H_{19}N.HCl$	Isometheptene Hydrochloride
$C_9H_{19}NO_4$	Dexpanthenol
$C_9H_{19}NO_4$	Panthenol
$C_9H_{19}NO_7$	Choline Bitartrate
$C_9H_{20}Cl_3N_2O_3P$	Defosfamide
$C_9H_{20}N_4$	Guanazodine
$C_9H_{21}N_3.HCl$	Guanoctine Hydrochloride
$C_9H_{22}NNaO_7P_2.H_2O$	Ibandronate Sodium
$C_9H_{23}INO_3PS$	Echothiophate Iodide
$C_9H_{23}NO_7P_2$	Ibandronic Acid
$C_9H_{24}I_2N_2O$	Prolonium Iodide
$C_{10}BrF_{21}$	Perflubrodec
$C_{10}F_{18}$	Perflunafene
$C_{10}H_5Cl_3N_4S_3$	Subendazole
$C_{10}H_6Cl_2N_2O_2$	Pyrrolnitrin
$C_{10}H_6Cl_3N_3$	Loreclezole
$C_{10}H_6F_7N_3O_3$	Nifluridide
$C_{10}H_6N_4$	Strinoline
$C_{10}H_6N_8.C_7H_{17}NO_5.H_2O$	Tetrazolast Meglumine
$C_{10}H_6O_4$	Chromocarb
$C_{10}H_7Br_2NO$	Broquinaldol
$C_{10}H_7Cl_2IS$	Tiodonium Chloride
$C_{10}H_7Cl_2NO$	Chlorquinaldol
$C_{10}H_7Cl_2N_3O.HCl$	Anagrelide Hydrochloride
$C_{10}H_7F_3O_4$	Triflusal
$C_{10}H_7KN_6O$	Pemirolast Potassium
$C_{10}H_7N_3S$	Thiabendazole
$C_{10}H_7OS_2$	Anetholtrithion
$C_{10}H_8BrNO$	Tilbroquinol
$C_{10}H_8BrNO_2$	Brosuximide
$C_{10}H_8BrN_3O$	Bropirimine
$C_{10}H_8BrN_5OS$	Lomeguatrib
$C_{10}H_8ClNO_3$	Seclazone
$C_{10}H_8FN_5O_3$	Eflumast
$C_{10}H_8F_2N_4O$	Rufinamide
$C_{10}H_8HgNNaO_3S$	Otimerate Sodium
$C_{10}H_8MgN_2O_6S_3.3H_2O$	Bispyrithione Magsulfex
$C_{10}H_8N_2O_2S_2$	Dipyrithione
$C_{10}H_8N_2O_2S_2Zn$	Pyrithione Zinc
$C_{10}H_8N_4O_3$	Nifurprazine
$C_{10}H_8N_4O_3S_2$	Nitrodan
$C_{10}H_8N_4O_4$	Nitrefazole
$C_{10}H_8O_2$	Methylchromone
$C_{10}H_8O_3$	Hymecromone
$(C_{10}H_8O_4)_n$, in which $n = 20$ to 100	Pegoterate
$C_{10}H_8O_{10}S_2$	Sulmarin
$C_{10}H_9AgN_4O_2S$	Sulfadiazine, Silver
$C_{10}H_9ClN_2HCl$	Lofemizole Hydrochloride
$C_{10}H_9ClN_4O_2S$	Sulfachlorpyridazine
$C_{10}H_9ClN_4O_2S$	Sulfaclozine
$C_{10}H_9ClO_3$	Clorindanic Acid
$C_{10}H_9Cl_4O_4P$	Stirofos
$C_{10}H_9F_3N_2O$	Fluminorex
$C_{10}H_9I_3O_3$	Phenobutiodil
$C_{10}H_9NO$	Drinidene
$C_{10}H_9NO$	Tiliquinol
$C_{10}H_9NO_2$	Carfimate
$C_{10}H_9N_3O$	Inamrinone
$C_{10}H_9N_3S$	Tasuldine
$C_{10}H_9N_4NaO_2S$	Sulfadiazine Sodium

Molecular Formula	Non-proprietary Name
$C_{10}H_9N_7O$	Furterene
$C_{10}H_{10}BiNO_3$	Mebiquine
$C_{10}H_{10}BrNO_2$	Brofoxine
$C_{10}H_{10}ClNO_2$	Chlorthenoxazine
$C_{10}H_{10}ClN_3O$	Clazolimine
$C_{10}H_{10}Cl_2N_2O.HCl$	Fenmetozole Hydrochloride
$C_{10}H_{10}Cl_3NO_3$	Cloracetadol
$C_{10}H_{10}FNO_2.HCl.\frac{1}{2}H_2O$	Fluparoxan Hydrochloride
$C_{10}H_{10}FN_3S$	Suritozole
$C_{10}H_{10}N_2O$	Edaravone
$C_{10}H_{10}N_2OS$	Icodulinum
$C_{10}H_{10}N_2O_2$	Procodazole
$C_{10}H_{10}N_2O_2$	Caroxazone
$C_{10}H_{10}N_2O_3$	Imidazole Salicylate
$C_{10}H_{10}N_2O_3$	Mequidox
$C_{10}H_{10}N_2O_3$	Paraxazone
$C_{10}H_{10}N_2O_5$	Sinitrodil
$C_{10}H_{10}N_4OS$	Methisazone
$C_{10}H_{10}N_4O_2S$	Pirinidazole
$C_{10}H_{10}N_4O_2S$	Sulfadiazine
$C_{10}H_{10}N_4O_3$	Drazidox
$C_{10}H_{10}N_6O_2$	Azanidazole
$C_{10}H_{10}O_2$	Safrole
$C_{10}H_{10}O_8$	Aceglatone
$C_{10}H_{11}BrN_2O_3$	Brallobarbital
$C_{10}H_{11}ClFN_5O_3$	Clofarabine
$C_{10}H_{11}ClF_3N_3O_4S_3$	Epithiazide
$C_{10}H_{11}ClN_5O_6P$	Tocladesine
$C_{10}H_{11}ClO_3$	Clofibric Acid
$C_{10}H_{11}Cl_2N_3$	Sofinicline
$C_{10}H_{11}Cl_2N_3.C_6H_6O_3S$	Sofinicline Benzenesulfonate
$C_{10}H_{11}Cl_2N_3.HCl$	Nemazoline Hydrochloride
$C_{10}H_{11}F_3N_2O_5$	Trifluridine
$C_{10}H_{11}I_2NO_3$	Propyliodone
$C_{10}H_{11}NO_3$	Actarit
$C_{10}H_{11}NO_3$	Betamipron
$C_{10}H_{11}NO_3$	Diacetamate
$C_{10}H_{11}NO_4S$	Tenosiprol
$C_{10}H_{11}NO_4S_2$	Stepronin
$C_{10}H_{11}N_3O$	Azolimine
$C_{10}H_{11}N_3O$	Crotoniazide
$C_{10}H_{11}N_3O_2$	Lobendazole
$C_{10}H_{11}N_3O_2S_2$	Sulfasomizole
$C_{10}H_{11}N_3O_3S$	Sulfamethoxazole
$C_{10}H_{11}N_3O_5S$	Nifuratel
$C_{10}H_{11}N_4NaO_5S$	Carbazochrome Sodium Sulfonate
$C_{10}H_{11}N_4NaO_5S$	Tazobactam Sodium
$C_{10}H_{11}N_4O_7P$	Becampanel
$C_{10}H_{11}NaO_2$	Sodium Phenylbutyrate
$C_{10}H_{11}NaO_3$	Propylparaben Sodium
$[C_{10}H_{12}BrN_3]_2.H_2SO_4$	Guanisoquin Sulfate
$C_{10}H_{12}CaN_2Na_2O_8.xH_2O$	Edetate Calcium Disodium
$C_{10}H_{12}ClNO$	Beclamide
$C_{10}H_{12}ClNO_2$	Baclofen
$C_{10}H_{12}ClNO_4$	Chlorphenesin Carbamate
$C_{10}H_{12}ClN_3$	Tolonidine
$C_{10}H_{12}ClN_3O_3S$	Quinethazone
$C_{10}H_{12}ClN_3O_6S_2$	Carmetizide
$C_{10}H_{12}ClN_5O_3$	Cladribine
$C_{10}H_{12}Co_2N_2O_8$	Dicobalt Edetate
$C_{10}H_{12}FN_3$	Flutonidine
$C_{10}H_{12}FN_3O_4.H_2O$	Tezacitabine
$C_{10}H_{12}FN_5O_2$	Lodenosine
$C_{10}H_{12}FeN_2NaO_8$	Sodium Feredetate
$C_{10}H_{12}HgNNaO_5.C_7H_8N_4O_2$	Meragidone Sodium

Molecular Formula	Non-proprietary Name
$C_{10}H_{12}N_2.HCl$	Tolazoline Hydrochloride
$C_{10}H_{12}N_2Na_4O_8$	Edetate Sodium
$(C_{10}H_{12}N_2O)_2.C_4H_4O_4$	Cotinine Fumarate
$C_{10}H_{12}N_2O_2$	Nicopholine
$C_{10}H_{12}N_2O_3$	Allobarbital
$C_{10}H_{12}N_2O_4$	Stavudine
$C_{10}H_{12}N_2O_5S$	Sulfasuccinamide
$C_{10}H_{12}N_2O_6S$	Ritipenem
$C_{10}H_{12}N_4OS$	Amithiozone
$C_{10}H_{12}N_4O_2S_2$	Sulfaethidole
$C_{10}H_{12}N_4O_3$	Carbazochrome
$C_{10}H_{12}N_4O_3$	Didanosine
$C_{10}H_{12}N_4O_3.C_7H_5NaO_3$	Carbazochrome Salicylate
$C_{10}H_{12}N_4O_3S_2$	Sulfatrozole
$C_{10}H_{12}N_4O_4S$	Thioinosine
$C_{10}H_{12}N_4O_5$	Inosine
$C_{10}H_{12}N_4O_5$	Nifurdazil
$C_{10}H_{12}N_4O_5.C_{14}H_{22}N_2O_4$	Inosine Pranobex
$C_{10}H_{12}N_4O_5S$	Tazobactam
$C_{10}H_{12}N_4O_6S.H_2O$	Isatoribine
$C_{10}H_{12}N_5Na_2O_7P$	Vidarabine Sodium Phosphate
$C_{10}H_{12}O$	Anethole
$C_{10}H_{12}O_2$	Eugenol
$C_{10}H_{12}O_3$	Propylparaben
$(C_{10}H_{12}O_4)_v(C_7H_{12}O_4)_w$ $(C_6H_{10}O_3)_x(C_6H_9NO)_y$ $(C_5H_8O_2).yz$	Acofilcon A
$(C_{10}H_{12}O_4)_v (C_7H_{12}O_4)_w$ $(C_6H_{10}O_3)_x (C_6H_9NO)_y$ $(C_5H_8O_2).yz$	Acofilcon B
$C_{10}H_{12}O_5$	Asperlin
$C_{10}H_{12}O_5$	Propyl Gallate
$C_{10}H_{12}O_6S$	Sulprosal
$C_{10}H_{13}ClHgO$	Mercurobutol
$C_{10}H_{13}ClN_2O$	Lozilurea
$C_{10}H_{13}ClN_2O_2S.HCl$	Nitralamine Hydrochloride
$C_{10}H_{13}ClN_2O_3S$	Chlorpropamide
$C_{10}H_{13}ClN_2S$	Anpirtoline
$C_{10}H_{13}FN_2O_4$	Alovudine
$C_{10}H_{13}FN_2O_5$	Clevudine
$C_{10}H_{13}FN_5O_7P$	Fludarabine Phosphate
$C_{10}H_{13}NO$	Formetorex
$C_{10}H_{13}NO_2$	Homarylamine
$C_{10}H_{13}NO_2$	Phenacetin
$C_{10}H_{13}NO_2$	Phenprobamate
$C_{10}H_{13}NO_2$	Risocaine
$C_{10}H_{13}NO_2$	Tenamfetamine
$C_{10}H_{13}NO_3$	Buramate
$C_{10}H_{13}NO_3$	Fenacetinol
$C_{10}H_{13}NO_3$	Metyrosine
$C_{10}H_{13}NO_3$	Racemetirosine
$C_{10}H_{13}NO_4$	Lisadimate
$C_{10}H_{13}NO_4$	Melevodopa
$C_{10}H_{13}NO_4.1\frac{1}{2}H_2O$	Methyldopa
$C_{10}H_{13}NO_4S_2$	Meticrane
$C_{10}H_{13}NO_4S_2$	Tiprotimod
$C_{10}H_{13}NO_6.C_{10}H_{13}NO_6$	Piridoxilate
$C_{10}H_{13}N_2Na_3O_8$	Edetate Trisodium
$C_{10}H_{13}N_3.HCl$	Phenamazoline Hydrochloride
$(C_{10}H_{13}N_3)_2.H_2SO_4$	Debrisoquin Sulfate
$C_{10}H_{13}N_3O_2$	Guabenxan
$[C_{10}H_{13}N_3O_2]_2.H_2SO_4$	Guanoxan Sulfate
$C_{10}H_{13}N_3O_2S_2$	Subathizone
$C_{10}H_{13}N_3O_5S$	Nifurtimox
$C_{10}H_{13}N_5O_2.CH_4O_3S.H_2O$	Adrenochrome Monoaminoguanidine Mesilate
$C_{10}H_{13}N_5O_4$	Adenosine
$C_{10}H_{13}N_5O_4$	Zidovudine
$C_{10}H_{13}N_5O_4.H_2O$	Vidarabine
$C_{10}H_{14}CaO_6.2H_2O$	Calcium Levulinate
$C_{10}H_{14}ClN.HCl$	Chlorphentermine Hydrochloride
$C_{10}H_{14}ClN.HCl$	Clortermine Hydrochloride
$C_{10}H_{14}ClN_3OS$	Azintamide
$C_{10}H_{14}F_2N_2O_2$	Seletracetam
$C_{10}H_{14}K_2N_2O_8.2H_2O$	Edetate Dipotassium
$C_{10}H_{14}NO_5P$	*p*-Nitrophenyl-*O*-ethyl Ethylphosphonate
$C_{10}H_{14}N_2$	Nicotine
$C_{10}H_{14}N_2.2CH_4H_6O_6.2H_2O$	Nicotine Bitartrate
$(C_{10}H_{14}N_2)_2.C_6H_{10}O_8$	Rivanicline Galactarate
$C_{10}H_{14}N_2Na_2O_8.2H_2O$	Edetate Disodium
$C_{10}H_{14}N_2O$	Bupicomide
$C_{10}H_{14}N_2O$	Nikethamide
$C_{10}H_{14}N_2O_2$	Nerbacadol
$C_{10}H_{14}N_2O_3$	Aprobarbital
$C_{10}H_{14}N_2O_3S$	Lydimycin
$C_{10}H_{14}N_2O_4$	Proxibarbal
$C_{10}H_{14}N_2O_4$	Valofane
$C_{10}H_{14}N_2O_4.H_2O$	Carbidopa
$C_{10}H_{14}N_2O_4S_2$	Sulthiame
$C_{10}H_{14}N_2O_5$	Telbivudine
$C_{10}H_{14}N_4O_2$	Morinamide
$C_{10}H_{14}N_4O_3$	Protheobromine
$C_{10}H_{14}N_4O_3$	Proxyphylline
$C_{10}H_{14}N_4O_4$	Dyphylline
$C_{10}H_{14}N_5NaO_3$	Penciclovir Sodium
$C_{10}H_{14}N_5Na_2O_{13}P_3$	Adenosine Triphosphate Disodium
$C_{10}H_{14}N_5O_7P$	Adenosine Phosphate
$C_{10}H_{14}N_5O_7P$	Vidarabine Phosphate
$C_{10}H_{14}O$	Thymol
$C_{10}H_{14}O_2$	Idramantone
$(C_{10}H_{14}O_2)_u(C_{10}H_{10})_v$ $(C_{10}H_{14}O)_w(C_7H_8O_2)_x$ $(C_{16}H_{16}O_2)_y(C_7H_8O)_z$	Anoxomer
$C_{10}H_{14}O_3$	Mephenesin
$C_{10}H_{14}O_3S$	Tolmesoxide
$C_{10}H_{14}O_4$	Floverine
$C_{10}H_{14}O_4$	Guaifenesin
$C_{10}H_{15}N$	Levmetamfetamine
$C_{10}H_{15}N$	Ortetamine
$C_{10}H_{15}N$	Phenpromethamine
$C_{10}H_{15}N$	Phentermine
$C_{10}H_{15}N.HCl$	Methamphetamine Hydrochloride
$C_{10}H_{15}N.HCl$	Phentermine Hydrochloride
$C_{10}H_{15}NO$	Ephedrine
$C_{10}H_{15}NO$	Pholedrine
$C_{10}H_{15}NO.C_4H_4O_4$	Talsaclidine Fumarate
$C_{10}H_{15}NO.HCl$	Ephedrine Hydrochloride
$C_{10}H_{15}NO.HCl$	Pseudoephedrine Hydrochloride
$C_{10}H_{15}NO.HCl$	Racephedrine Hydrochloride
$(C_{10}H_{15}NO)_2.H_2SO_4$	Ephedrine Sulfate
$(C_{10}H_{15}NO)_2.H_2SO_4$	Pseudoephedrine Sulfate
$C_{10}H_{15}NO_2$	Ethypicone
$C_{10}H_{15}NO_2$	Etilefrine
$C_{10}H_{15}NO_2$	Hexapropymate
$C_{10}H_{15}NO_2$	Oxilofrine
$C_{10}H_{15}NO_3$	Dioxifedrine
$C_{10}H_{15}NO_3.HCl$	Ethylnorepinephrine Hydrochloride

Molecular Formula	Non-proprietary Name
$C_{10}H_{15}NO_4$	Kainic Acid
$C_{10}H_{15}N_2NaO_3$	Butabarbital Sodium
$C_{10}H_{15}N_3 \cdot \frac{1}{2}H_2SO_4$	Bethanidine Sulfate
$C_{10}H_{15}N_3 \cdot H_2SO_4$	Modaline Sulfate
$C_{10}H_{15}N_3O \cdot HCl$	Sabcomeline Hydrochloride
$(C_{10}H_{15}N_3O)_2 \cdot H_2SO_4$	Guanoxyfen Sulfate
$C_{10}H_{15}N_3O_5$	Benserazide
$C_{10}H_{15}N_3S$	Talipexole
$C_{10}H_{15}N_5$	Trapidil
$C_{10}H_{15}N_5 \cdot HCl$	Phenformin Hydrochloride
$C_{10}H_{15}N_5O_3$	Omaciclovir
$C_{10}H_{15}N_5O_3$	Penciclovir
$C_{10}H_{15}N_5O_4$	Nifurethazone
$C_{10}H_{16}$	*d*-Limonene
$C_{10}H_{16}Br_2N_2O_2$	Pipobroman
$C_{10}H_{16}ClNO$	Edrophonium Chloride
$C_{10}H_{16}N_2O$	Rilmenidine
$C_{10}H_{16}N_2OS$	Albutoin
$C_{10}H_{16}N_2O_2$	Fasoracetam
$C_{10}H_{16}N_2O_3$	Butabarbital
$C_{10}H_{16}N_2O_3$	Butethal
$C_{10}H_{16}N_2O_3S$	Biotin
$C_{10}H_{16}N_2O_3S \cdot CH_4O_3S$	Amidephrine Mesylate
$C_{10}H_{16}N_2O_4S_3 \cdot HCl$	Dorzolamide Hydrochloride
$C_{10}H_{16}N_2O_8$	Edetic Acid
$C_{10}H_{16}N_2S$	Manozodil
$C_{10}H_{16}N_4O_4$	Ipramidil
$C_{10}H_{16}N_6S$	Cimetidine
$C_{10}H_{16}N_6S \cdot HCl$	Cimetidine Hydrochloride
$C_{10}H_{16}N_8S_2$	Tiotidine
$C_{10}H_{16}O$	Camphor
$C_{10}H_{16}O_2$	Cicrotoic Acid
$(C_{10}H_{16}O_4)_n$	Polybutilate
$C_{10}H_{17}N \cdot HCl$	Amantadine Hydrochloride
$C_{10}H_{17}NOS \cdot HCl \cdot \frac{1}{2}H_2O$	Cevimeline Hydrochloride
$C_{10}H_{17}NO_2$	Methyprylon
$C_{10}H_{17}NO_4S_2$	Letosteine
$C_{10}H_{17}N_3$	Hexazole
$C_{10}H_{17}N_3O_6S$	Glutathione
$C_{10}H_{17}N_3S$	Pramipexole
$C_{10}H_{17}N_3S \cdot 2HCl \cdot H_2O$	Pramipexole Dihydrochloride
$C_{10}H_{17}N_9O_2S_3$	Tuvatidine
$C_{10}H_{18}ClN_3O_2$	Semustine
$C_{10}H_{18}ClN_3O_6$	Ecomustine
$C_{10}H_{18}ClN_3O_7$	Ranimustine
$C_{10}H_{18}Cl_2N_6O_4S_2$	Ditiomustine
$C_{10}H_{18}O$	Eucalyptol
$C_{10}H_{18}O_3$	Cyclobutoic Acid
$C_{10}H_{18}O_3$	Cyclobutyrol
$C_{10}H_{19}Cl_2NO_5$	Galamustine
$C_{10}H_{19}N$	Butynamine
$C_{10}H_{19}N$	Dropempine
$C_{10}H_{19}NO_2$	Procymate
$C_{10}H_{19}NO_5$	Hopantenic Acid
$C_{10}H_{19}N_2O_3Sb$	Ethylstibamine
$(C_{10}H_{19}N_3O_2)_2 \cdot H_2SO_4$	Guanadrel Sulfate
$C_{10}H_{19}O_6PS_2$	Malathion
$C_{10}H_{20}BN_3O_3$	Dutogliptin
$C_{10}H_{20}BN_3O_3 \cdot C_4H_6O_6$	Dutogliptin Tartrate
$C_{10}H_{20}CaN_2O_8S_2$	Acamprosate Calcium
$C_{10}H_{20}ClNO_4$	Levocarnitine Propionate Hydrochloride
$C_{10}H_{20}NO_4PS$	Propetamphos
$C_{10}H_{20}N_2O_2$	Valrocemide
$C_{10}H_{20}N_2O_4$	Mebutamate
$C_{10}H_{20}N_2S_3$	Sulfiram

Molecular Formula	Non-proprietary Name
$C_{10}H_{20}N_2S_4$	Disulfiram
$C_{10}H_{20}N_3O_2S_4{}^{99}Tc$	Technetium Tc 99m Nitridocade
$C_{10}H_{20}N_4$	Spirgetine
$C_{10}H_{20}O$	Cimepanol
$C_{10}H_{20}O$	Levomenthol
$C_{10}H_{20}O$	Menthol
$C_{10}H_{20}O$	Racementhol
$C_{10}H_{20}O_2 \cdot H_2O$	Terpin Hydrate
$C_{10}H_{20}O_3$	Promoxolane
$C_{10}H_{21}Cl_2N_2O_7P$	Glufosfamide
$C_{10}H_{21}N$	Levopropylhexedrine
$C_{10}H_{21}N$	Pempidine
$C_{10}H_{21}N$	Propylhexedrine
$C_{10}H_{21}NO_4$	Miglustat
$C_{10}H_{21}NO_7$	Voglibose
$C_{10}H_{21}N_3O \cdot C_6H_8O_7$	Diethylcarbamazine Citrate
$C_{10}H_{22}Cl_2N_2O_4$	Mannomustine
$C_{10}H_{22}Cl_2N_2O_4Pt$	Satraplatin
$C_{10}H_{22}N_4 \cdot H_2SO_4$	Guanethidine Monosulfate
$(C_{10}H_{22}N_4)_2 \cdot H_2SO_4$	Guanethidine Sulfate
$C_{10}H_{22}O_{14}S_4$	Mannosulfan
$C_{10}H_{23}N$	Diprobutine
$(C_{10}H_{24}Cl_2N_2O)_n$	Polixetonium Chloride
$C_{10}H_{24}N_2O_2 \cdot 2HCl$	Ethambutol Hydrochloride
$C_{10}H_{24}N_2O_8S_2$	Ritrosulfan
$C_{11}H_5BrCl_2NO_3S_2Na$	Tasisulam Sodium
$C_{11}H_6Br_3NOS$	Tibrofan
$C_{11}H_6ClN_3O_6 \cdot 2C_4H_{11}NO_3$	Lodoxamide Tromethamine
$C_{11}H_7Cl_2NO_2S$	Clantifen
$C_{11}H_7F_3N_2O_2S$	Amflutizole
$C_{11}H_7N_3O_2$	Dazoquinast
$C_{11}H_8ClNO_2$	Cyproximide
$C_{11}H_8ClNO_2S$	Fenclozic Acid
$C_{11}H_8F_3NO$	Flucarbril
$C_{11}H_8I_3N_2NaO_4$	Diatrizoate Sodium
$C_{11}H_8{}^{125}I_3N_2NaO_4$	Diatrizoate Sodium I 125
$C_{11}H_8{}^{131}I_3N_2NaO_4$	Diatrizoate Sodium I 131
$C_{11}H_8I_3N_2NaO_4$	Iothalamate Sodium
$C_{11}H_8{}^{125}I_3N_2NaO_4$	Iothalamate Sodium I 125
$C_{11}H_8{}^{131}I_3N_2NaO_4$	Iothalamate Sodium I 131
$C_{11}H_8NNaO_4 \cdot H_2O$	Nivimedone Sodium
$C_{11}H_8Na_2O_8S_2$	Menadiol Sodium Sulfate
$C_{11}H_8Na_4O_8P_2 \cdot 6H_2O$	Menadiol Sodium Diphosphate
$C_{11}H_8O_2$	Menadione
$C_{11}H_9BrO_4$	Bromebric Acid
$C_{11}H_9ClN_4O$	Nimazone
$C_{11}H_9ClO_2S$	Tianafac
$C_{11}H_9Cl_4NO_2$	Cloponone
$C_{11}H_9FN_2O_3$	Sorbinil
$C_{11}H_9I_3N_2O_4$	Diatrizoic Acid
$C_{11}H_9I_3N_2O_4$	Iothalamic Acid
$C_{11}H_9I_3N_2O_4 \cdot C_7H_{17}NO_5$	Diatrizoate Meglumine
$C_{11}H_9I_3N_2O_4 \cdot C_7H_{17}NO_5$	Iothalamate Meglumine
$C_{11}H_9I_3N_2O_5$	Ioxotrizoic Acid
$C_{11}H_9N_3O_2$	Naftazone
$C_{11}H_9N_3O_2$	Pirquinozol
$C_{11}H_9N_3O_3 \cdot HCl$	Nitrafudam Hydrochloride
$C_{11}H_9N_3O_4$	Nifurvidine
$C_{11}H_9NaO_5S \cdot 3H_2O$	Menadione Sodium Bisulfite
$C_{11}H_{10}BrN_5 \cdot C_4H_6O_6$	Brimonidine Tartrate
$C_{11}H_{10}ClNO_3$	Meseclazone
$C_{11}H_{10}ClN_3O$	Quazinone
$C_{11}H_{10}Cl_2N_4$	Metoprine
$C_{11}H_{10}CuN_2NaO_2S$	Allocupreide Sodium
$C_{11}H_{10}FNO_2S$	Flosequinan
$C_{11}H_{10}FN_3O_3$	Flunidazole

Molecular Formula	Non-proprietary Name
$C_{11}H_{10}F_3NO_2$	Flumetramide
$C_{11}H_{10}NNaO_4S$	Actinoquinol Sodium
$C_{11}H_{10}N_2O$	Amphenidone
$C_{11}H_{10}N_2O_2$	Tolimidone
$C_{11}H_{10}N_2S$	Antafenite
$C_{11}H_{10}N_4O_4$	Carbadox
$C_{11}H_{10}N_4O_6$	Nifurmazole
$C_{11}H_{10}N_6$	Bentemazole
$C_{11}H_{10}O_6$	Dipyrocetyl
$C_{11}H_{11}ClNNaO_4$	Salclobuzate Sodium
$C_{11}H_{11}ClN_4O_2$	Fenobam
$C_{11}H_{11}ClO_3$	Alclofenac
$C_{11}H_{11}Cl_2NO_3S$	Dichlormezanone
$C_{11}H_{11}Cl_2N_3O$	Muzolimine
$C_{11}H_{11}Cl_4NO_2$	Chlorbetamide
$C_{11}H_{11}F_3N_2O_2$	Dezinamide
$C_{11}H_{11}F_3N_2O_3$	Flutamide
$C_{11}H_{11}{}^{131}IN_2O$	Iodoantipyrine I 131
$C_{11}H_{11}I_3O_3$	Iophenoxic Acid
$C_{11}H_{11}NO_2$	Phensuximide
$C_{11}H_{11}NO_3S$	Nesosteine
$C_{11}H_{11}NO_4$	Pidobenzone
$C_{11}H_{11}NO_4S$	Deferitrin
$C_{11}H_{11}N_3O$	Metamfazone
$C_{11}H_{11}N_3O_2$	Mivazerol
$C_{11}H_{11}N_3O_2$	Piroximone
$C_{11}H_{11}N_3O_2S$	Sulfapyridine
$C_{11}H_{11}N_3O_2S.HCl$	Nitramisole Hydrochloride
$C_{11}H_{11}N_3S$	Tinazoline
$C_{11}H_{11}N_4NaO_2S$	Sulfamerazine Sodium [Injection]
$C_{11}H_{11}N_5.HCl$	Phenazopyridine Hydrochloride
$C_{11}H_{12}AsNO_5S_2$	Thiacetarsamide
$C_{11}H_{12}BrNO$	Cinromide
$C_{11}H_{12}ClNO_3S$	Chlormezanone
$C_{11}H_{12}ClNO_4$	Salclobuzic Acid
$C_{11}H_{12}Cl_2N_2O$	Dexlofexidine
$C_{11}H_{12}Cl_2N_2O$	Levlofexidine
$C_{11}H_{12}Cl_2N_2O.HCl$	Lofexidine Hydrochloride
$C_{11}H_{12}Cl_2N_2O_5$	Chloramphenicol
$(C_{11}H_{12}Cl_2N_2O_5)_4$	Chloramphenicol Pantothenate
$(C_{18}H_{32}CaN_2O_{10})$	Complex
$C_{11}H_{12}Cl_3N$	Amphecloral
$C_{11}H_{12}F_3NO$	Flumexadol
$C_{11}H_{12}I_3NO_2$	Iopanoic Acid
$C_{11}H_{12}NO_4PS_2$	Phosmet
$C_{11}H_{12}N_2O$	Antipyrine
$C_{11}H_{12}N_2O_2$	Ethotoin
$C_{11}H_{12}N_2O_2$	Fenozolone
$C_{11}H_{12}N_2O_2$	Idazoxan
$C_{11}H_{12}N_2O_2$	Ledazerol
$C_{11}H_{12}N_2O_2$	Metazamide
$C_{11}H_{12}N_2O_2$	Thozalinone
$C_{11}H_{12}N_2O_2$	Tryptophan
$C_{11}H_{12}N_2O_2.HCl.H_2O$	Amiquinsin Hydrochloride
$C_{11}H_{12}N_2O_2S$	Zileuton
$C_{11}H_{12}N_2O_2S_2$	Antazonite
$C_{11}H_{12}N_2O_3$	Nicoracetam
$C_{11}H_{12}N_2O_3$	Oxitriptan
$C_{11}H_{12}N_2O_3.HCl$	Bemarinone Hydrochloride
$C_{11}H_{12}N_2S$	Dexamisole
$C_{11}H_{12}N_2S.HCl$	Levamisole Hydrochloride
$C_{11}H_{12}N_2S.HCl$	Tetramisole Hydrochloride
$C_{11}H_{12}N_4O_2$	Molinazone
$C_{11}H_{12}N_4O_2$	Panidazole
$C_{11}H_{12}N_4O_2$	Todralazine
$C_{11}H_{12}N_4O_2S$	Sulfamerazine
$C_{11}H_{12}N_4O_2S$	Sulfaperin
$C_{11}H_{12}N_4O_3S$	Sulfalene
$C_{11}H_{12}N_4O_3S$	Sulfameter
$C_{11}H_{12}N_4O_3S$	Sulfamethoxypyridazine
$C_{11}H_{12}N_4O_3S$	Sulfamonomethoxine
$C_{11}H_{13}BrN_2O_5$	Brivudine
$C_{11}H_{13}BrN_2O_6$	Sorivudine
$C_{11}H_{13}ClF_3N_3O_4S_3$	Polythiazide
$C_{11}H_{13}Cl_3N_4O_4$	Triclofylline
$C_{11}H_{13}FN_4$	Isaglidole
$C_{11}H_{13}F_2N.HCl$	Mofegiline Hydrochloride
$C_{11}H_{13}F_3OSi$	Zifrosilone
$C_{11}H_{13}N.HCl$	Pargyline Hydrochloride
$C_{11}H_{13}NNa_2O_7S_2$	Disufenton Sodium
$C_{11}H_{13}NO_2$	Fenmetramide
$C_{11}H_{13}NO_2$	Idrocilamide
$C_{11}H_{13}NO_2S$	Tifemoxone
$C_{11}H_{13}NO_3$	Afalanine
$C_{11}H_{13}NO_3$	Thurfyl Nicotinate
$C_{11}H_{13}NO_3$	Toloxatone
$C_{11}H_{13}NO_3.HCl$	Hydrastinine Hydrochloride
$C_{11}H_{13}NO_4$	Mephenoxalone
$C_{11}H_{13}NO_4$	Moxadolen
$C_{11}H_{13}N_3$	Deximafen
$C_{11}H_{13}N_3.HCl$	Imafen Hydrochloride
$C_{11}H_{13}N_3O$	Ataquimast
$C_{11}H_{13}N_3O$	Ciamexon
$C_{11}H_{13}N_3O$	Feprosidnine
$C_{11}H_{13}N_3O$	Sumanirole
$C_{11}H_{13}N_3O_3S$	Sulfamoxole
$C_{11}H_{13}N_3O_3S$	Sulfatroxazole
$C_{11}H_{13}N_3O_3S$	Sulfisoxazole
$C_{11}H_{13}N_3O_3S.C_4H_{11}NO_2$	Sulfisoxazole Diolamine
$C_{11}H_{13}N_3O_5$	Propenidazole
$C_{11}H_{13}N_5$	Indanidine
$C_{11}H_{13}N_5O_2S$	Tivanidazole
$C_{11}H_{13}N_5O_5$	Azidamfenicol
$C_{11}H_{14}AsNO_3S_2$	Arsthinol
$C_{11}H_{14}ClN.HCl$	Lorcaserin Hydrochloride
$C_{11}H_{14}ClNO$	Fenaclon
$C_{11}H_{14}ClNO_2$	Buclosamide
$C_{11}H_{14}ClN_3O_3S$	Glyclopyramide
$C_{11}H_{14}ClN_3O_3S_2$	Tizolemide
$C_{11}H_{14}ClN_3O_4S_3$	Althiazide
$(C_{11}H_{14}ClN_5)_2.C_{23}H_{16}O_6$	Cycloguanil Pamoate
$C_{11}H_{14}F_3NO$	Fludorex
$C_{11}H_{14}N_2O$	Indantadol
$C_{11}H_{14}N_2O_2$	Pheneturide
$C_{11}H_{14}N_2O_3S$	Sulfadicramide
$C_{11}H_{14}N_2O_4$	Felbamate
$C_{11}H_{14}N_2S$	Isotiquimide
$C_{11}H_{14}N_2S.C_4H_6O_6$	Pyrantel Tartrate
$C_{11}H_{14}N_2S.C_{23}H_{16}O_6$	Pyrantel Pamoate
$C_{11}H_{14}N_2S.HCl$	Tiquinamide Hydrochloride
$C_{11}H_{14}N_2S_2$	Picartamide
$C_{11}H_{14}N_4O$	Idralfidine
$C_{11}H_{14}N_4O_2$	Epirizole
$C_{11}H_{14}N_4O_2S_2$	Glyprothiazol
$C_{11}H_{14}N_4O_2S_2$	Nestifylline
$C_{11}H_{14}N_4O_4$	Doxofylline
$C_{11}H_{14}N_4O_4$	Forodesine
$C_{11}H_{14}N_4O_4.HCl$	Forodesine Hydrochloride

Molecular Formula	Non-proprietary Name
$C_{11}H_{14}N_6$	Sardomozide
$C_{11}H_{14}O_3$	Butylparaben
$C_{11}H_{15}BrN_2O$	Bromamid
$C_{11}H_{15}ClN_2OS$	Fopirtoline
$C_{11}H_{15}ClN_2O_2$	Clormecaine
$C_{11}H_{15}ClN_2O_2$	Iproclozide
$C_{11}H_{15}ClO_2$	Metaglycodol
$C_{11}H_{15}ClO_2$	Phenaglycodol
$C_{11}H_{15}Cl_2N_5.HCl$	Chlorproguanil Hydrochloride
$C_{11}H_{15}N.HCl$	Aletamine Hydrochloride
$C_{11}H_{15}N.HCl$	Cypenamine Hydrochloride
$C_{11}H_{15}NO$	Metamfepramone
$C_{11}H_{15}NO.HCl$	Phenmetrazine Hydrochloride
$C_{11}H_{15}NO_2$	Butamben
$C_{11}H_{15}NO_2$	Exepanol
$C_{11}H_{15}NO_2$	Isobutamben
$C_{11}H_{15}NO_2$	Methoxyphedrine
$(C_{11}H_{15}NO_2)_2.C_6H_3N_3O_7$	Butamben Picrate
$C_{11}H_{15}NO_3$	Etosalamide
$C_{11}H_{15}NO_3$	Hydroxyphenamate
$C_{11}H_{15}NO_3$	Propoxur
$C_{11}H_{15}NO_3.HCl$	L-Tyrosine Ethylester Monohydrochloride
$C_{11}H_{15}NO_4$	Etilevodopa
$C_{11}H_{15}NO_4S$	Etebenecid
$C_{11}H_{15}NO_5$	Methocarbamol
$C_{11}H_{15}NO_5S$	Tosulur
$C_{11}H_{15}N_3O_4$	Pyricarbate
$C_{11}H_{15}N_3O_5$	Anaxirone
$C_{11}H_{15}N_3O_5S_2$	Rimeporide
$C_{11}H_{15}N_5$	Zindotrine
$C_{11}H_{15}N_5O_3$	Lobucavir
$C_{11}H_{15}N_5O_5$	Nelarabine
$C_{11}H_{15}N_5O_5$	Nelzarabine
$C_{11}H_{16}BrNO_2$	Brolamfetamine
$C_{11}H_{16}ClNO.HCl.H_2O$	Clorprenaline Hydrochloride
$C_{11}H_{16}ClN_3O_4S_2$	Buthiazide
$C_{11}H_{16}ClN_5.HCl$	Chloroguanide Hydrochloride
$C_{11}H_{16}ClO_2PS_3$	Carbofenotion
$C_{11}H_{16}FN_3O_3$	Carmofur
$C_{11}H_{16}I_2N_2O_5$	Iodopyracet
$C_{11}H_{16}{}^{125}I_2N_2O_5$	Iodopyracet I 125
$C_{11}H_{16}{}^{131}I_2N_2O_5$	Iodopyracet I 131
$C_{11}H_{16}N_2O$	Pozanicline
$C_{11}H_{16}N_2O$	Tocainide
$C_{11}H_{16}N_2O.C_4H_4O_6$	Pozanicline Tartrate
$C_{11}H_{16}N_2O.HCl$	Tocainide Hydrochloride
$C_{11}H_{16}N_2O_2$	Aloracetam
$C_{11}H_{16}N_2O_2$	Carbenzide
$C_{11}H_{16}N_2O_2$	Pilocarpine
$C_{11}H_{16}N_2O_2.HCl$	Pilocarpine Hydrochloride
$C_{11}H_{16}N_2O_2.HCl$	Safrazine Hydrochloride
$C_{11}H_{16}N_2O_2.HNO_3$	Pilocarpine Nitrate
$C_{11}H_{16}N_2O_3$	Butalbital
$C_{11}H_{16}N_2O_3$	Nifenalol
$C_{11}H_{16}N_2O_3$	Talbutal
$C_{11}H_{16}N_2O_3$	Vinbarbital
$C_{11}H_{16}N_2O_3$	Vinylbital
$C_{11}H_{16}N_2O_3S$	Caldaret
$C_{11}H_{16}N_2O_3S$	Ozolinone
$C_{11}H_{16}N_2O_5$	Edoxudine
$C_{11}H_{16}N_2O_5.HCl$	Talaglumetad Hydrochloride
$C_{11}H_{16}N_2O_8$	Isospaglumic Acid
$C_{11}H_{16}N_2O_8$	Spaglumic Acid

Molecular Formula	Non-proprietary Name
$C_{11}H_{16}N_4O.HCl$	Lidamidine Hydrochloride
$C_{11}H_{16}N_4O_2$	Isbufylline
$C_{11}H_{16}N_4O_4$	Dexrazoxane
$C_{11}H_{16}N_4O_4$	Pentostatin
$C_{11}H_{16}N_4O_4$	Razoxane
$C_{11}H_{16}N_4S$	Evandamine
$C_{11}H_{16}N_8O_8$	Imidurea
$C_{11}H_{16}O$	Fenipentol
$C_{11}H_{16}O_2$	Butylated Hydroxyanisole
$C_{11}H_{16}O_2$	Guaietolin
$C_{11}H_{16}O_4$	Mifobate
$C_{11}H_{17}ClO_7P_2$	Chlordantoin
$C_{11}H_{17}Cl_3N_2O_2S$	Dimetamfetamine
$C_{11}H_{17}N$	Etilamfetamine
$C_{11}H_{17}N$	Pentorex
$(C_{11}H_{17}N)_2.H_2SO_4$	Mephentermine Sulfate
$C_{11}H_{17}NO$	Methylephedrine
$C_{11}H_{17}NO.HCl$	Methoxyphenamine Hydrochloride
$C_{11}H_{17}NO.HCl$	Mexiletine Hydrochloride
$C_{11}H_{17}NO_2$	Metaterol
$C_{11}H_{17}NO_2.HCl$	Deterenol Hydrochloride
$C_{11}H_{17}NO_3$	Levisoprenaline
$C_{11}H_{17}NO_3.HCl$	Dioxethedrin Hydrochloride
$C_{11}H_{17}NO_3.HCl$	Isoproterenol Hydrochloride
$C_{11}H_{17}NO_3.HCl$	Methoxamine Hydrochloride
$(C_{11}H_{17}NO_3)_2.H_2SO_4$	Metaproterenol Sulfate
$(C_{11}H_{17}NO_3)_2.H_2SO_4.2H_2O$	Isoproterenol Sulfate
$C_{11}H_{17}NO_4$	Dimetofrine
$C_{11}H_{17}N_2NaO_2S$	Thiopental Sodium
$C_{11}H_{17}N_2NaO_3$	Amobarbital Sodium
$C_{11}H_{17}N_2NaO_3$	Pentobarbital Sodium
$(C_{11}H_{17}N_3O)_2.H_2SO_4$	Meobentine Sulfate
$C_{11}H_{17}N_3O_3$	Emorfazone
$C_{11}H_{17}N_3O_3S$	Carbutamide
$C_{11}H_{17}N_3O_5$	Carbubarb
$C_{11}H_{17}N_5O_2$	Dimethazan
$C_{11}H_{17}N_5O_3$	Cafaminol
$C_{11}H_{18}BrN_5O_3$	Pamabrom
$C_{11}H_{18}ClN_5S$	Mezilamine
$C_{11}H_{18}N_2O$	Prisotinol
$C_{11}H_{18}N_2OS$	Tamitinol
$C_{11}H_{18}N_2O_3$	Amobarbital
$C_{11}H_{18}N_2O_3$	Pentobarbital
$C_{11}H_{18}N_2O_3S.HCl$	Metalol Hydrochloride
$C_{11}H_{18}N_2O_4Pt$	Miboplatin
$C_{11}H_{18}N_2O_4S_3.HCl$	Sezolamide Hydrochloride
$C_{11}H_{18}N_2O_5$	Idrapril
$C_{11}H_{18}N_4O_3$	Imuracetam
$C_{11}H_{18}N_4O_3$	Pimonidazole
$C_{11}H_{19}NO_9$	Aceneuramic Acid
$C_{11}H_{20}FeNO_9$	Ferrocholinate
$C_{11}H_{20}N_2O_2$	Brivaracetam
$C_{11}H_{20}N_2O_4Pt$	Sebriplatin
$C_{11}H_{20}N_2O_6Pt$	Eptaplatin
$C_{11}H_{20}N_2O_6Pt$	Zeniplatin
$C_{11}H_{20}N_3O_3PS$	Pyrimitate
$C_{11}H_{20}O_2$	Undecylenic Acid
$C_{11}H_{21}Cl_2O_4P$	Vincofos
$C_{11}H_{21}N.HCl$	Mecamylamine Hydrochloride
$C_{11}H_{21}NO_3.HCl$	Hexaminolevulinate Hydrochloride
$C_{11}H_{22}N_2O_6$	Deanol Aceglumate
$C_{11}H_{22}N_3O_3P$	Meturedepa

Molecular Formula	Non-proprietary Name
$C_{11}H_{22}O_2$	Arundic Acid
$C_{11}H_{22}O_4$	Monoctanoin Component A
$C_{11}H_{23}N.CH_4O_3S$	Neramexane Mesylate
$C_{11}H_{23}NO$	Valdipromide
$C_{11}H_{23}N_7$	Meladrazine
$C_{11}H_{24}O_3$	Dibuprol
$C_{11}H_{25}N$	Iproheptine
$C_{11}H_{25}NO_8$	Choline Gluconate
$C_{11}H_{28}Br_2N_2$	Pentamethonium Bromide
$C_{11}H_{28}I_2N_2$	Pentamethonium Iodide
$C_{12}H_4Cl_2F_6N_4OS$	Fipronil
$C_{12}H_4Cl_4Na_2O_2S$	Bithionolate Sodium
$C_{12}H_4Na_5O_{16}S_4Sb.7H_2O$	Stibophen
$C_{12}H_6Cl_2N_2O_6$	Niclofolan
$C_{12}H_6Cl_4O_2S$	Bithionol
$C_{12}H_6Cl_4O_3S$	Bithionoloxide
$C_{12}H_6Cl_5I$	Feniodium Chloride
$C_{12}H_6N_2O_2$	Phanquone
$C_{12}H_6Na_6O_{12}S_6Sb_2$	Sodium Stibocaptate
$C_{12}H_7Br_4O_5P$	Bromofenofos
$C_{12}H_7ClN_2O_3$	Quazolast
$C_{12}H_7Cl_3O_2$	Triclosan
$C_{12}H_7N_5O_9$	Nifursol
$C_{12}H_8Cl_2N_2O_2$	Diclonixin
$C_{12}H_8Cl_2O_2$	Soneclosan
$C_{12}H_8Cl_2O_2S$	Fenticlor
$C_{12}H_8Cl_6O$	Dieldrin
$C_{12}H_8N_4O_6S$	Nifurzide
$C_{12}H_8O_4$	Methoxsalen
$C_{12}H_8O_4S$	Tenosal
$C_{12}H_8S$	Dibenzothiophene
$C_{12}H_9ClFN_5$	Arprinocid
$C_{12}H_9Cl_2NO_2S$	Eltenac
$C_{12}H_9Cl_3N_2O_2S$	Lotifazole
$C_{12}H_9F_3N_2O_2$	Leflunomide
$C_{12}H_9F_3N_2O_2$	Teriflunomide
$C_{12}H_9Li_6O_{12}S_3Sb$	Anthiolimine
$C_{12}H_9NO_6$	Miloxacin
$C_{12}H_9NS$	Phenothiazine
$C_{12}H_9N_2NaO_3S.H_2O$	Tiacrilast Sodium
$C_{12}H_9N_3O$	Milrinone
$C_{12}H_9N_3O_5$	Nifuroxazide
$C_{12}H_9N_3O_5S$	Nitazoxanide
$C_{12}H_9N_5O_3$	Ciadox
$C_{12}H_{10}BrNO_2S$	Brofezil
$C_{12}H_{10}CaO_{10}S_2$	Calcium Dobesilate
$C_{12}H_{10}Ca_3O_{14}.4H_2O$	Calcium Citrate
$C_{12}H_{10}ClN_3O.HCl$	Zoniclezole Hydrochloride
$C_{12}H_{10}Cl_2N_2O_2S$	Pazoxide
$C_{12}H_{10}FN_3O_4$	Fidarestat
$C_{12}H_{10}F_2N_2O_3$	Zardaverine
$C_{12}H_{10}F_3N_3O_4$	Nilutamide
$C_{12}H_{10}FeNa_4O_{14}$	Sodium Ferrous Citrate
$C_{12}H_{10}{}^{59}Fe_3O_{14}$	Ferrous Citrate Fe 59
$C_{12}H_{10}I_3N_2NaO_4$	Metrizoate Sodium
$C_{12}H_{10}Mg_3O_{14}$	Magnesium Citrate
$C_{12}H_{10}N_2O_3S$	Tiacrilast
$C_{12}H_{10}N_2O_4$	Nifurpirinol
$C_{12}H_{10}N_2O_5$	Cinoxacin
$C_{12}H_{10}N_2O_8S$	Ranelic Acid
$[(C_{12}H_{10})OSi]_a[C_2H_6OSi]_b$ $[C_3H_6OSi]_c[C_4H_9OSi]_d$	Dimefocon A
$C_{12}H_{10}O_3$	Spizofurone
$C_{12}H_{10}O_4$	Acifran
$C_{12}H_{10}O_6$	Metesculetol
$C_{12}H_{11}Br_3N_2O_5$	Broxitalamic Acid

Molecular Formula	Non-proprietary Name
$C_{12}H_{11}ClN_2O_5S$	Furosemide
$C_{12}H_{11}ClN_6O_2S_2$	Azosemide
$C_{12}H_{11}ClO_4$	Losigamone
$C_{12}H_{11}Cl_2N_3O_2$	Azaconazole
$C_{12}H_{11}I_3N_2O_4$	Iodamide
$C_{12}H_{11}I_3N_2O_4.C_7H_{17}NO_5$	Iodamide Meglumine
$C_{12}H_{11}I_3N_2O_5$	Ioxitalamic Acid
$C_{12}H_{11}NO$	Pirfenidone
$C_{12}H_{11}NO_2$	Carbaril
$C_{12}H_{11}NO_3S$	Zoliprofen
$C_{12}H_{11}NO_6$	Nitecapone
$C_{12}H_{11}N_2NaO_3$	Phenobarbital Sodium
$C_{12}H_{11}N_2NaO_3H_2O$	Nalidixate Sodium
$C_{12}H_{11}N_3$	Mefenidil
$C_{12}H_{11}N_3.C_4H_4O_4$	Mefenidil Fumarate
$C_{12}H_{11}N_3OS$	Dacopafant
$C_{12}H_{11}N_5O$	Peldesine
$C_{12}H_{11}N_5O.HCl$	Pelrinone Hydrochloride
$C_{12}H_{11}N_7$	Ampyrimine
$C_{12}H_{11}N_7$	Triamterene
$C_{12}H_{12}BrN_4NaO_2S.H_2O$	Sulfabromomethazine Sodium
$C_{12}H_{12}ClNO_4$	Eclazolast
$C_{12}H_{12}Cl_2N_4$	Etoprine
$C_{12}H_{12}FNO$	Cinflumide
$C_{12}H_{12}FN_3$	Sampirtine
$C_{12}H_{12}I_3N_2NaO_2$	Ipodate Sodium
$C_{12}H_{12}N_2O_2$	Cyclazodone
$C_{12}H_{12}N_2O_2$	Zimidoben
$C_{12}H_{12}N_2O_2S$	Dapsone
$C_{12}H_{12}N_2O_2S$	Enoximone
$C_{12}H_{12}N_2O_2S$	Sulfabenz
$C_{12}H_{12}N_2O_3$	Nalidixic Acid
$C_{12}H_{12}N_2O_3$	Phenobarbital
$C_{12}H_{12}N_2O_3.C_{10}H_{21}N$	Barbexaclone
$C_{12}H_{12}N_2O_3.HCl$	Dazoxiben Hydrochloride
$C_{12}H_{12}N_2O_4S$	Supidimide
$C_{12}H_{12}N_2O_5$	Temodox
$C_{12}H_{12}N_2O_6S_2Zn.4H_2O$	Sulfanilate Zinc
$C_{12}H_{12}N_4OS$	Motapizone
$C_{12}H_{12}N_4O_3$	Benznidazole
$C_{12}H_{12}N_4O_3$	Furafylline
$C_{12}H_{12}N_6Na_2O_{10}S_2$	Carumonam Sodium
$C_{12}H_{13}Br_2NO_3$	Fursalan
$C_{12}H_{13}ClN_4$	Pyrimethamine
$C_{12}H_{13}ClN_4O_2S$	Sulfaclomide
$C_{12}H_{13}ClN_4O_6S_2$	Sumetizide
$C_{12}H_{13}Cl_2N_3$	Alinidine
$C_{12}H_{13}Cl_2N_5$	Palatrigine
$C_{12}H_{13}F_3N_2O_2$	Fluzinamide
$C_{12}H_{13}I_3N_2O_3$	Iocetamic Acid
$C_{12}H_{13}I_3N_2O_3$	Iomeglamic Acid
$C_{12}H_{13}N.CH_4O_3S$	Rasagiline Mesylate
$C_{12}H_{13}NO.C_4H_6O_5$	Nafomine Malate
$C_{12}H_{13}NO_2$	Methsuximide
$C_{12}H_{13}NO_2S$	Phenylthilone
$C_{12}H_{13}NO_3$	Aniracetam
$C_{12}H_{13}NO_3S_2$	Beciparcil
$C_{12}H_{13}NO_3S_3$	Midesteine
$C_{12}H_{13}NO_5S$	Salnacedin
$C_{12}H_{13}N_3$	Gapicomine
$C_{12}H_{13}N_3O.HCl$	Fenyripol Hydrochloride
$C_{12}H_{13}N_3O_2$	Farampator
$C_{12}H_{13}N_3O_2$	Isocarboxazid
$C_{12}H_{13}N_3O_2$	Triaziquone
$C_{12}H_{13}N_3O_3S$	Fexinidazole
$C_{12}H_{13}N_3O_4$	Olaquindox

Molecular Formula	Non-proprietary Name
$C_{12}H_{13}N_4NaO_4S$	Sulfadimethoxine Sodium
$C_{12}H_{13}N_5O_4$	Carprazidil
$C_{12}H_{13}N_5O_5$	Nifurizone
$C_{12}H_{13}N_5O_9S_2.2(C_5H_{14}NO)$	Tigemonam Dicholine
$C_{12}H_{14}BiK_5O_{17}$	Bismuth Subcitrate Potassium
$C_{12}H_{14}CaO_{12}.2H_2O$	Calcium Ascorbate
$C_{12}H_{14}ClNO_4$	Diproxadol
$C_{12}H_{14}ClN_3O_2S_2$	Butadiazamide
$C_{12}H_{14}Cl_2FNO_4S$	Florfenicol
$C_{12}H_{14}Cl_2NO_3PS_2$	Benoxafos
$C_{12}H_{14}Cl_3O_4P$	Clorfenvinfos
$C_{12}H_{14}K_8O_{35}S_8.7H_2O$	Sucrosofate Potassium
$C_{12}H_{14}N_2$	Azepindole
$C_{12}H_{14}N_2$	Efetozole
$C_{12}H_{14}N_2.C_4H_4O_4$	Altinicline Maleate
$C_{12}H_{14}N_2.HCl$	Detomidine Hydrochloride
$C_{12}H_{14}N_2O$	Acetryptine
$C_{12}H_{14}N_2O_2$	Iminophenimide
$C_{12}H_{14}N_2O_2$	Mephenytoin
$C_{12}H_{14}N_2O_2$	Methetoin
$C_{12}H_{14}N_2O_2$	Primidone
$C_{12}H_{14}N_2O_2$	Quazodine
$C_{12}H_{14}N_2O_2$	Rogletimide
$C_{12}H_{14}N_2O_2S_2$	Bensuldazic Acid
$C_{12}H_{14}N_2O_3$	Deboxamet
$C_{12}H_{14}N_2O_3$	Diproqualone
$C_{12}H_{14}N_2O_3S$	Tioxidazole
$C_{12}H_{14}N_2O_3S.C_7H_{17}NO_5$	Tiprinast Meglumine
$C_{12}H_{14}N_2O_3S_3$	Mivotilate
$C_{12}H_{14}N_2O_4$	Ruvazone
$C_{12}H_{14}N_2O_6$	Netivudine
$C_{12}H_{14}N_3NaO_7.2H_2O$	Isoniazid Glucuronate Sodium
$C_{12}H_{14}N_4O_2S$	Sulfamethazine
$C_{12}H_{14}N_4O_2S$	Sulfisomidine
$C_{12}H_{14}N_4O_3S$	Sulfacytine
$C_{12}H_{14}N_4O_3S$	Sulfametomidine
$C_{12}H_{14}N_4O_4S$	Sulfadimethoxine
$C_{12}H_{14}N_4O_4S$	Sulfadoxine
$C_{12}H_{14}N_4O_4S$	Sulphamoprine
$C_{12}H_{14}N_5NaO_6S$	Oximonam Sodium
$C_{12}H_{14}O_2$	Fenabutene
$C_{12}H_{14}O_2S_2$	Ditophal
$C_{12}H_{14}O_3$	Furofenac
$C_{12}H_{14}O_4$	Diethyl Phthalate
$C_{12}H_{14}O_4$	Dimecrotic Acid
$C_{12}H_{14}O_5$	Cinametic Acid
$C_{12}H_{14}O_5$	Velaresol
$C_{12}H_{15}AsN_6OS_2$	Melarsoprol
$C_{12}H_{15}ClO_3$	Clofibrate
$C_{12}H_{15}Cl_2NO_5S$	Racephenicol
$C_{12}H_{15}Cl_2NO_5S$	Thiamphenicol
$C_{12}H_{15}Cl_2N_5O$	Clociguanil
$C_{12}H_{15}F_2NO_2$	Manifaxine
$C_{12}H_{15}HgNO_6$	Mercuderamide
$C_{12}H_{15}N.HCl$	Bicifadine Hydrochloride
$C_{12}H_{15}NO_3$	Metaxalone
$C_{12}H_{15}NO_3.HCl.H_2O$	Hydrocotarnine Hydrochloride
$C_{12}H_{15}NO_3S$	Vanitiolide
$C_{12}H_{15}NO_4$	Cintriamide
$C_{12}H_{15}NO_4$	Ethopabate
$C_{12}H_{15}NO_5S_3$	Sulopenem
$C_{12}H_{15}NO_6$	Benaxibine
$C_{12}H_{15}N_2O_3PS$	Phoxim
$C_{12}H_{15}N_3$	Indanazoline
$C_{12}H_{15}N_3O_2$	Pardoprunox
$C_{12}H_{15}N_3O_2.HCl$	Pardoprunox Hydrochloride

Molecular Formula	Non-proprietary Name
$C_{12}H_{15}N_3O_2S$	Albendazole
$C_{12}H_{15}N_3O_2S_2$	Glybuzole
$C_{12}H_{15}N_3O_3$	Oxibendazole
$C_{12}H_{15}N_3O_3S$	Albendazole Oxide
$C_{12}H_{15}N_3O_3S$	Glipalamide
$C_{12}H_{15}N_3O_5S$	Amezinium Metilsulfate
$C_{12}H_{15}N_3O_6$	Teroxirone
$C_{12}H_{15}N_5O_3.H_2O$	Entecavir
$C_{12}H_{15}N_5O_3S$	Sulfaguanole
$C_{12}H_{15}N_5O_6S$	Oximonam
$C_{12}H_{16}ClNO_3$	Meclofenoxate
$C_{12}H_{16}ClN_3O.C_{12}H_{26}O_4S$	Carbantel Lauryl Sulfate
$C_{12}H_{16}ClN_3O_3S.HCl$	Dabuzalgron Hydrochloride
$C_{12}H_{16}ClN_3O_4S_3$	Methalthiazide
$C_{12}H_{16}Cl_2N_4S$	Beclotiamine
$C_{12}H_{16}F_3N$	Levofenfluramine
$C_{12}H_{16}F_3N.HCl$	Dexfenfluramine Hydrochloride
$C_{12}H_{16}F_3N.HCl$	Fenfluramine Hydrochloride
$C_{12}H_{16}F_3NS$	Tiflorex
$[C_{12}H_{16}M_2O_{15}S_2]n$ (Nominal, the value of n is 30 to 60)	Poligeenan
$C_{12}H_{16}N_2$	Azaquinzole
$C_{12}H_{16}N_2$	Fenproporex
$C_{12}H_{16}N_2$	Ipidacrine
$C_{12}H_{16}N_2.C_2H_4O_2$	Etryptamine Acetate
$C_{12}H_{16}N_2O$	Nebracetam
$C_{12}H_{16}N_2OS_2$	Aprikalim
$C_{12}H_{16}N_2O_2$	Eltoprazine
$C_{12}H_{16}N_2O_2$	Phenylacetylglycine Dimethylamide
$C_{12}H_{16}N_2O_3$	Cyclobarbital
$C_{12}H_{16}N_2O_3$	Hexobarbital
$C_{12}H_{16}N_2O_3S$	Tolpyrramide
$C_{12}H_{16}N_2O_4S$	Tiapirinol
$C_{12}H_{16}N_2S$	Xylazine
$C_{12}H_{16}N_2S.C_4H_6O_6$	Morantel Tartrate
$C_{12}H_{16}N_2S.HCl$	Xylazine Hydrochloride
$C_{12}H_{16}N_2S_2$	Lucartamide
$C_{12}H_{16}N_3O_3P$	Benzodepa
$C_{12}H_{16}N_4O_2$	Taloximine
$C_{12}H_{16}N_4O_2S_2$	Glybuthiazol
$C_{12}H_{16}N_4O_3$	Iprazochrome
$C_{12}H_{16}N_6S.HCl$	Etintidine Hydrochloride
$C_{12}H_{16}O_2$	Ibufenac
$C_{12}H_{16}O_4$	Fepentolic Acid
$C_{12}H_{16}O_4S_2$	Malotilate
$C_{12}H_{16}O_6S$	Protiofate
$C_{12}H_{17}ClN_4OS.HCl$	Thiamine Hydrochloride
$C_{12}H_{17}ClO_2$	Fenpentadiol
$C_{12}H_{17}Cl_2NO$	Cericlamine
$C_{12}H_{17}NO$	Diethyltoluamide
$C_{12}H_{17}NO$	Indanorex
$C_{12}H_{17}NO.C_4H_6O_6$	Phendimetrazine Tartrate
$C_{12}H_{17}NO.HCl$	Trebenzomine Hydrochloride
$C_{12}H_{17}NOS.HCl$	Tiletamine Hydrochloride
$C_{12}H_{17}NO_2$	Butacetin
$C_{12}H_{17}NO_2$	Ciclopirox
$C_{12}H_{17}NO_2$	Pentalamide
$C_{12}H_{17}NO_2.C_2H_7NO$	Ciclopirox Olamine
$C_{12}H_{17}NO_3$	Bucetin
$C_{12}H_{17}NO_3$	Bufexamac
$C_{12}H_{17}NO_3$	Ethamivan
$C_{12}H_{17}NO_3$	Nicoboxil
$C_{12}H_{17}NO_3$	Norbudrine
$C_{12}H_{17}NO_3.HBr$	Rimiterol Hydrobromide

Molecular Formula	Non-proprietary Name
$C_{12}H_{17}NO_4.HCl$	Methyldopate Hydrochloride
$C_{12}H_{17}N_2NaO_2S$	Thiamylal Sodium
$C_{12}H_{17}N_2NaO_3$	Secobarbital Sodium
$C_{12}H_{17}N_2NaO_3S$	Tolbutamide Sodium, Sterile
$C_{12}H_{17}N_2O_4P$	Psilocybine
$C_{12}H_{17}N_3O$	Cimaterol
$C_{12}H_{17}N_3O_3S$	Cariporide
$C_{12}H_{17}N_3O_3S.CH_4O_3S$	Cariporide Mesylate
$C_{12}H_{17}N_3O_4S.H_2O$	Imipenem
$C_{12}H_{17}N_5$	Bumepidil
$C_{12}H_{17}N_5O_4$	Nifurpipone
$C_{12}H_{17}N_5O_4S$	Thiamine Mononitrate
$C_{12}H_{18}ClN.HCl$	Mefenorex Hydrochloride
$C_{12}H_{18}ClNO$	Etolorex
$C_{12}H_{18}ClNO$	Tulobuterol
$C_{12}H_{18}ClNO_2$	Meluadrine
$C_{12}H_{18}ClN_4O_4PS$	Monophosphothiamine
$C_{12}H_{18}Cl_2N_2O$	Clenbuterol
$C_{12}H_{18}FNO$	Flerobuterol
$C_{12}H_{18}{}^{123}IN.HCl$	Iofetamine Hydrochloride I 123
$C_{12}H_{18}N_2O$	Pivhydrazine
$C_{12}H_{18}N_2O_2$	Nicametate
$C_{12}H_{18}N_2O_2.HCl$	Doxpicomine Hydrochloride
$C_{12}H_{18}N_2O_2S$	Thiamylal
$C_{12}H_{18}N_2O_3$	Nealbarbital
$C_{12}H_{18}N_2O_3$	Secobarbital
$C_{12}H_{18}N_2O_3S$	Tolbutamide
$C_{12}H_{18}N_2O_4.HCl$	Midodrine Hydrochloride
$C_{12}H_{18}N_2O_5$	Epervudine
$C_{12}H_{18}N_2O_7$	Bicozamycin
$C_{12}H_{18}N_4O_2$	Verofylline
$C_{12}H_{18}N_4O_4$	Dupracetam
$C_{12}H_{18}O$	Amylmetacresol
$C_{12}H_{18}O$	Propofol
$C_{12}H_{18}O_2$	Hexylresorcinol
$C_{12}H_{18}O_2.C_{13}H_{10}N_2$	Acrisorcin
$C_{12}H_{18}O_6$	Ranimycin
$C_{12}H_{18}O_7$	Diprogulic Acid
$C_{12}H_{18}O_{13}Zn_4$	Zinc Acetate, Basic
$C_{12}H_{19}BrN_2O_2$	Neostigmine Bromide
$C_{12}H_{19}ClNO_3P$	Crufomate
$C_{12}H_{19}Cl_3O_8$	Sucralose
$C_{12}H_{19}NO.HCl$	Etafedrine Hydrochloride
$C_{12}H_{19}NO_2$	Fepradinol
$C_{12}H_{19}NO_2$	Ocrylate
$(C_{12}H_{19}NO_2)_2.H_2SO_4$	Bamethan Sulfate
$C_{12}H_{19}NO_3$	Metiprenaline
$C_{12}H_{19}NO_3.CH_4O_3S$	Colterol Mesylate
$C_{12}H_{19}NO_3.HCl$	Prenalterol Hydrochloride
$(C_{12}H_{19}NO_3)_2.H_2SO_4$	Terbutaline Sulfate
$C_{12}H_{19}NO_3S$	Lemidosul
$C_{12}H_{19}NO_4$	Choline Salicylate
$[C_{12}H_{19}NO_4]_2.MgSO_4.4H_2O$	Salcolex
$C_{12}H_{19}N_3O.HCl$	Procarbazine Hydrochloride
$C_{12}H_{19}N_8OP$	Pumitepa
$C_{12}H_{20}N_2$	Amiflamine
$C_{12}H_{20}N_2O$	Amiterol
$C_{12}H_{20}N_2O_2$	Isamoxole
$C_{12}H_{20}N_2O_2S$	Thiotetrabarbital
$C_{12}H_{20}N_2O_2S_2$	Methitural
$C_{12}H_{20}N_2O_3$	Tetrabarbital
$C_{12}H_{20}N_2O_3.C_2H_4O_2$	Pirbuterol Acetate
$C_{12}H_{20}N_2O_3.2HCl$	Pirbuterol Hydrochloride
$C_{12}H_{20}N_2O_3S.HCl$	Dexsotalol Hydrochloride
$C_{12}H_{20}N_2O_3S.HCl$	Sotalol Hydrochloride
$C_{12}H_{20}N_2O_4S.HCl$	Soterenol Hydrochloride

Molecular Formula	Non-proprietary Name
$C_{12}H_{20}N_4O_7$	Zanamivir
$C_{12}H_{20}N_4O_8P_2S$	Cocarboxylase
$C_{12}H_{20}O_2$	Bornyl Acetate
$C_{12}H_{20}O_7$	Triethyl Citrate
$C_{12}H_{21}N$	Memantine
$C_{12}H_{21}N.HCl$	Memantine Hydrochloride
$C_{12}H_{21}N.HCl$	Rimantadine Hydrochloride
$C_{12}H_{21}NO$	Pimeclone
$C_{12}H_{21}NO_5.HCl$	Celgosivir Hydrochloride
$C_{12}H_{21}NO_8S$	Topiramate
$C_{12}H_{21}N_2O_3PS$	Dimpylate
$C_{12}H_{21}N_2O_5S_2{}^{99m}Tc$	Technetium Tc 99m Bicisate
$C_{12}H_{21}N_3O_5S_3$	Brinzolamide
$C_{12}H_{21}N_3S$	Tebatizole
$C_{12}H_{21}N_5O_2S_2$	Nizatidine
$C_{12}H_{21}N_5O_3$	Cadralazine
$C_{12}H_{21}N_5O_3$	Oxtriphylline
$C_{12}H_{22}AsN_3O_6S$	Darinaparsin
$C_{12}H_{22}CaO_{14}$	Calcium Gluconate
$C_{12}H_{22}CuO_{14}$	Copper Gluconate
$C_{12}H_{22}FeO_{14}.2H_2O$	Ferrous Gluconate
$C_{12}H_{22}MgO_{14}.xH_2O$	Magnesium Gluconate
$C_{12}H_{22}MnO_{14}$	Manganese Gluconate
$C_{12}H_{22}N_2O$	Pexantel
$C_{12}H_{22}N_2O_2$	Crotetamide
$C_{12}H_{22}N_2O_4$	Lorbamate
$C_{12}H_{22}N_2O_8S_2$	Piposulfan
$C_{12}H_{22}O_3$	Ciclactate
$C_{12}H_{22}O_6$	Etoglucid
$C_{12}H_{22}O_{11}$	Lactulose
$C_{12}H_{22}O_{11}$	Maltose
$C_{12}H_{22}O_{11}$	Sucrose
$C_{12}H_{22}O_{14}Zn$	Zinc Gluconate
$C_{12}H_{23}N$	Dimecamine
$C_{12}H_{23}N$	Leptacline
$C_{12}H_{23}NO_3$	Icaridin
$C_{12}H_{23}N_3O$	Esaprazole
$C_{12}H_{24}FeN_2O_8$	Ferrotrenine
$C_{12}H_{24}N_2O_2$	Falintolol
$C_{12}H_{24}N_2O_4$	Carisoprodol
$C_{12}H_{24}O_{11}$	Lactitol
$C_{12}H_{24}O_{11}$	Maltitol
$C_{12}H_{25}NO_2$	Butoctamide
$C_{12}H_{26}I_2N_2O_2$	Trepirium Iodide
$C_{12}H_{26}O_6P_2S_4$	Dioxation
$C_{12}H_{27}O_3P$	Trifosmin
$C_{12}H_{30}Br_2N_2$	Hexamethonium Bromide
$C_{12}H_{30}I_2N_2$	Hexamethonium Iodide
$C_{12}H_{30}I_2N_2S$	Tiametonium Iodide
$C_{12}H_{44}CaFe_6Na_4O_{36}$	Ferriclate Calcium Sodium
$C_{12}H_{50}Cl_2N_{14}O_{12}Pt_3$	Triplatin Tetranitrate
$C_{12}H_{54}Al_{16}O_{75}S_8$	Lactalfate
$C_{13}H_6ClN_5O_2$	Traxanox
$C_{13}H_6Cl_5NO_3$	Oxyclozanide
$C_{13}H_6Cl_6O_2$	Hexachlorophene
$C_{13}H_6F_6NNaO_3S$	Batabulin Sodium
$C_{13}H_7F_6NO_3S$	Batabulin
$C_{13}H_8BrN_4NaO_3.2H_2O$	Azumolene Sodium
$C_{13}H_8Br_3NOS$	Thiosalan
$C_{13}H_8Br_3NO_2$	Tribromsalan
$C_{13}H_8ClN_3O$	Pifexole
$C_{13}H_8Cl_2N_2O_4$	Niclosamide
$C_{13}H_8Cl_2N_2O_6$	Nitroclofene
$C_{13}H_8Cl_2O_4S$	Ticrynafen
$C_{13}H_8F_2O_3$	Diflunisal
$C_{13}H_8N_2O_3$	Doqualast

Molecular Formula	Non-proprietary Name
$C_{13}H_8N_2O_3S$	Nitroscanate
$C_{13}H_9Br_2NO_2$	Dibromsalan
$C_{13}H_9Br_2NO_2$	Metabromsalan
$C_{13}H_9ClNO_2$	Clofenamic Acid
$C_{13}H_9Cl_2FN_2S$	Loflucarban
$C_{13}H_9Cl_3N_2O$	Triclocarban
$C_{13}H_9F_3N_2O_2$	Niflumic Acid
$C_{13}H_9F_3N_2O_2$	Triflocin
$C_{13}H_9NO$	Pyridarone
$C_{13}H_9NOSe$	Ebselen
$C_{13}H_9N_3O_2S$	Amoscanate
$C_{13}H_9N_5O_6.H_2O$	Zonampanel
$C_{13}H_{10}BrNO_3$	Resorantel
$C_{13}H_{10}ClN_3O_4S_2$	Lornoxicam
$C_{13}H_{10}Cl_2O_2$	Dichlorophen
$C_{13}H_{10}I_2O_3$	Furidarone
$C_{13}H_{10}N_2.HCl$	Aminacrine Hydrochloride
$C_{13}H_{10}N_2O_3S$	Ensulizole
$C_{13}H_{10}N_2O_4$	Thalidomide
$C_{13}H_{10}N_2O_5S$	Enoxamast
$C_{13}H_{10}N_4$	Triafungin
$C_{13}H_{10}N_4O_6.C_6H_8N_2O$	Nicarbazin
$C_{13}H_{10}O_3$	Giparmen
$C_{13}H_{10}O_7$	Exifone
$C_{13}H_{11}AsK_2N_6O_4S_2$	Melarsonyl Potassium
$C_{13}H_{11}ClN_2O_2$	Clonixin
$C_{13}H_{11}ClN_2O_2S$	Nuclomedone
$C_{13}H_{11}ClO$	Clorophene
$C_{13}H_{11}ClO_4$	Orpanoxin
$C_{13}H_{11}Cl_2NaO_4$	Ethacrynate Sodium
$C_{13}H_{11}F_6N_3O_5$	Topilutamide
$C_{13}H_{11}NO_2$	Balazipone
$C_{13}H_{11}NO_2$	Benzyl Nicotinate
$C_{13}H_{11}NO_3$	Osalmid
$C_{13}H_{11}NO_3$	Phenyl Aminosalicylate
$C_{13}H_{11}NO_5$	Oxolinic Acid
$C_{13}H_{11}N_3O$	Drometrizole
$C_{13}H_{11}N_3OS$	Timoprazole
$C_{13}H_{11}N_3O_2$	Salinazid
$C_{13}H_{11}N_3O_4$	Pomalidomide
$C_{13}H_{11}N_3O_4S_2$	Sudoxicam
$C_{13}H_{11}N_3O_4S_2$	Tenoxicam
$C_{13}H_{11}N_3O_5S$	Salazosulfamide
$C_{13}H_{11}N_3O_5S_2$	Maleylsulfathiazole
$C_{13}H_{12}ClNO_2S$	Ontianil
$C_{13}H_{12}Cl_2O_4$	Ethacrynic Acid
$C_{13}H_{12}F_2N_6O$	Fluconazole
$C_{13}H_{12}F_3N_6NaO_4S_3$	Cefazaflur Sodium
$C_{13}H_{12}I_3N_2NaO_4$	Diprotrizoate Sodium
$C_{13}H_{12}I_3N_3O_5$	Ioglicic Acid
$C_{13}H_{12}N_2O_2$	Ozagrel
$C_{13}H_{12}N_2O_2S$	Imitrodast
$C_{13}H_{12}N_2O_3S$	Sulfabenzamide
$C_{13}H_{12}N_2O_5S$	Nimesulide
$C_{13}H_{12}N_3NaO_6S$	Cephacetrile Sodium
$C_{13}H_{12}N_4O$	Quinezamide
$C_{13}H_{12}N_4O.HCl$	Imazodan Hydrochloride
$C_{13}H_{12}N_4O.HCl$	Oxifungin Hydrochloride
$C_{13}H_{12}N_4O_3$	Cinoquidox
$C_{13}H_{12}N_5NaO_5S_2$	Ceftizoxime Sodium
$C_{13}H_{12}N_8O_4S_3$	Ceftezole
$C_{13}H_{12}O_2$	Monobenzone
$C_{13}H_{12}O_2S$	Atliprofen
$C_{13}H_{12}O_7S_2$	Sultosilic Acid
$C_{13}H_{13}As_2N_2NaO_4S$	Neoarsphenamine
$C_{13}H_{13}BrN_4S$	Trovirdine

Molecular Formula	Non-proprietary Name
$C_{13}H_{13}ClN_2O_2S$	Ralitoline
$C_{13}H_{13}Cl_2N_3$	Proflavine Dihydrochloride
$C_{13}H_{13}F_2N_6O_4P$	Fosfluconazole
$C_{13}H_{13}N_3.C_4H_6O_6$	Varenicline Tartrate
$C_{13}H_{13}N_3O$	Dinaline
$C_{13}H_{13}N_3O$	Bemoradan
$C_{13}H_{13}N_3O_3$	Cyclobendazole
$C_{13}H_{13}N_3O_3$	Lenalidomide
$C_{13}H_{13}N_3O_3S$	Amidapsone
$C_{13}H_{13}N_3O_4$	Metronidazole Benzoate
$C_{13}H_{13}N_3O_5S_2.H_2O$	Succinylsulfathiazole
$C_{13}H_{13}N_3O_9S$	Furazolium Tartrate
$C_{13}H_{13}N_5O_2$	Zaprinast
$C_{13}H_{13}N_5O_4S$	Sulfachrysoidine
$C_{13}H_{13}NaO_4S$	Tibenelast Sodium
$C_{13}H_{14}ClNOS$	Alagebrium Chloride
$C_{13}H_{14}ClNO_2$	Pirprofen
$C_{13}H_{14}ClN_3O_2$	Imepition
$C_{13}H_{14}Cl_2O_3$	Ciprofibrate
$C_{13}H_{14}I_3NO_3$	Ioprocemic Acid
$C_{13}H_{14}N_2$	Lanicemine
$C_{13}H_{14}N_2.HCl.H_2O$	Tacrine Hydrochloride
$C_{13}H_{14}N_2O$	Fadolmidine
$C_{13}H_{14}N_2O$	Rofelodine
$C_{13}H_{14}N_2O.C_4H_4O_4$	Velnacrine Maleate
$C_{13}H_{14}N_2O.HCl$	Fadolmidine Hydrochloride
$C_{13}H_{14}N_2O.HCl$	Phenyramidol Hydrochloride
$C_{13}H_{14}N_2O_2$	Batoprazine
$C_{13}H_{14}N_2O_2$	Metomidate
$C_{13}H_{14}N_2O_2$	Naprodoxime
$C_{13}H_{14}N_2O_2$	Soretolide
$C_{13}H_{14}N_2O_2S$	Benzylsulfamide
$C_{13}H_{14}N_2O_3$	Mephobarbital
$C_{13}H_{14}N_2O_4$	Menadoxime
$C_{13}H_{14}N_2O_4$	Pidolacetamol
$C_{13}H_{14}N_2S.HCl$	Metizoline Hydrochloride
$C_{13}H_{14}N_3NaO_4S$	Glymidine Sodium
$C_{13}H_{14}N_4O_2$	Prinoxodan
$C_{13}H_{14}N_4O_4$	Pasiniazid
$C_{13}H_{14}N_6O_2$	Metazide
$C_{13}H_{14}O_4S$	Orazipone
$C_{13}H_{14}O_5S$	Esuprone
$C_{13}H_{14}O_6$	Baxitozine
$C_{13}H_{15}BrClNS$	Mitotenamine
$C_{13}H_{15}BrN_4O_2$	Brodimoprim
$C_{13}H_{15}Cl_2NO$	Clorgiline
$C_{13}H_{15}Cl_2NO_4$	Cetophenicol
$C_{13}H_{15}I_3N_2O_3$	Iosumetic Acid
$C_{13}H_{15}NO_2$	Fenimide
$C_{13}H_{15}NO_2$	Glutethimide
$C_{13}H_{15}NO_2$	Methastyridone
$C_{13}H_{15}NO_2$	Octazamide
$C_{13}H_{15}NO_2$	Securinine
$C_{13}H_{15}NO_3$	Mecarbinate
$C_{13}H_{15}NO_4S_2$	Rentiapril
$C_{13}H_{15}N_3.C_4H_4O_4$	Quipazine Maleate
$C_{13}H_{15}N_3O_4S$	Sulfisoxazole Acetyl
$C_{13}H_{15}N_3O_5S$	Asobamast
$C_{13}H_{15}N_5$	Epetirimod
$C_{13}H_{15}N_5.C_2H_6O_3S.H_2O$	Epetirimod Esylate
$C_{13}H_{15}N_5O_2$	Fasiplon
$C_{13}H_{15}N_5O_3$	Tazanolast
$C_{13}H_{15}N_5O_6$	Nifurfoline
$C_{13}H_{16}ClNO$	Esketamine
$C_{13}H_{16}ClNO.HCl$	Ketamine Hydrochloride
$C_{13}H_{16}ClN_3O_5S_2$	Ambuside

Molecular Formula	Non-proprietary Name
$C_{13}H_{16}Cl_{12}O_8$	Petrichloral
$C_{13}H_{16}HgNNaO_6$	Mersalyl
$C_{13}H_{16}N_2$	Demiditraz
$C_{13}H_{16}N_2$	Dexmedetomidine
$C_{13}H_{16}N_2.HCl$	Dexmedetomidine Hydrochloride
$C_{13}H_{16}N_2.HCl$	Medetomidine Hydrochloride
$C_{13}H_{16}N_2.HCl$	Tetrahydrozoline Hydrochloride
$C_{13}H_{16}N_2O$	Cirazoline
$C_{13}H_{16}N_2O$	Dexefaroxan
$C_{13}H_{16}N_2O$	Dianicline
$C_{13}H_{16}N_2O$	Efaroxan
$C_{13}H_{16}N_2O.C_{23}H_{16}O_6$	Oxantel Pamoate
$C_{13}H_{16}N_2O_2$	Aminoglutethimide
$C_{13}H_{16}N_2O_2$	Mofebutazone
$C_{13}H_{16}N_2O_2$	Pirmagrel
$C_{13}H_{16}N_2O_2S$	Thialbarbital
$C_{13}H_{16}N_2O_3$	Profexalone
$C_{13}H_{16}N_2O_3.HCl$	Indorenate Hydrochloride
$C_{13}H_{16}N_2O_4$	Domipizone
$C_{13}H_{16}N_2O_4S$	Taltrimide
$C_{13}H_{16}N_3NaO_4S.H_2O$	Dipyrone
$C_{13}H_{16}N_4$	Mifentidine
$C_{13}H_{16}N_4O_2$	Diaveridine
$C_{13}H_{16}N_4O_3S$	Cycotiamine
$C_{13}H_{16}N_4O_6$	Furaltadone
$C_{13}H_{16}N_4O_6$	Levofuraltadone
$C_{13}H_{16}O_3$	Cicloxilic Acid
$C_{13}H_{16}O_3$	Pibecarb
$C_{13}H_{17}Br_2NO_2$	Dembrexine
$C_{13}H_{17}ClN_2O_2$	Moclobemide
$C_{13}H_{17}N$	Selegiline
$C_{13}H_{17}N.HCl$	Selegiline Hydrochloride
$C_{13}H_{17}NO$	Crotamiton
$C_{13}H_{17}NO_2$	Alminoprofen
$C_{13}H_{17}NO_2$	Encyprate
$C_{13}H_{17}NO_3$	Romifenone
$C_{13}H_{17}NO_4$	Alibendol
$C_{13}H_{17}N_3.HCl$	Tramazoline Hydrochloride
$C_{13}H_{17}N_3O$	Aminopyrine
$C_{13}H_{17}N_3O.C_6H_{13}NO_3S$	Aminophenazone Cyclamate
$C_{13}H_{17}N_3O_2$	Parbendazole
$C_{13}H_{17}N_3O_3S_2$	Glysobuzole
$C_{13}H_{17}N_5O_2$	Aditeren
$C_{13}H_{17}N_5O_2$	Cipamfylline
$C_{13}H_{17}N_5O_2S$	Sulfasymazine
$C_{13}H_{17}N_5O_6$	Loxoribine
$C_{13}H_{17}N_5O_8S_2$	Aztreonam
$C_{13}H_{17}N_5O_8S_2.C_6H_{14}N_2O_2$	Aztreonam Lysine
$C_{13}H_{17}N_6O_7P$	Triciribine Phosphate
$C_{13}H_{18}Br_2N_2O$	Ambroxol
$C_{13}H_{18}ClF_3N_2O$	Mabuterol
$C_{13}H_{18}ClNO.HBr$	Bupropion Hydrobromide
$C_{13}H_{18}ClNO.HCl$	Bupropion Hydrochloride
$C_{13}H_{18}ClNO.HCl$	Lometraline Hydrochloride
$C_{13}H_{18}ClNO_2$	Alaproclate
$C_{13}H_{18}ClNO_2$	Cloforex
$C_{13}H_{18}ClNO_2.HCl$	Radafaxine Hydrochloride
$C_{13}H_{18}ClN_3O.HCl$	Imidoline Hydrochloride
$C_{13}H_{18}ClN_3O_3S$	Glypinamide
$C_{13}H_{18}ClN_3O_4S_2$	Cyclopenthiazide
$C_{13}H_{18}Cl_2N_2O_2$	Melphalan
$C_{13}H_{18}Cl_2N_2O_2$	Metamelfalan
$C_{13}H_{18}Cl_2N_2O_2$	Sarcolysin
$C_{13}H_{18}F_3N_3O_4S_2$	Penflutizide
$C_{13}H_{18}N_2$	Dicarbine

Molecular Formula	Non-proprietary Name
$C_{13}H_{18}N_2O.HCl$	Fenoxazoline Hydrochloride
$C_{13}H_{18}N_2O_3$	Heptabarbital
$C_{13}H_{18}N_2O_3$	Lacosamide
$C_{13}H_{18}N_2O_3S$	Tolpentamide
$C_{13}H_{18}N_2O_4S_2$	Almecillin
$C_{13}H_{18}N_4O_3$	Lomifylline
$C_{13}H_{18}N_4O_3$	Pentoxifylline
$C_{13}H_{18}N_6.HCl$	Zolertine Hydrochloride
$C_{13}H_{18}N_6O_5$	Moxnidazole
$C_{13}H_{18}O_2$	Dexibuprofen
$C_{13}H_{18}O_2$	Ibuprofen
$C_{13}H_{18}O_2.C_6H_{14}N_2O_2.H_2O$	Dexibuprofen Lysine
$C_{13}H_{19}ClN_2O$	Butanilicaine
$C_{13}H_{19}ClN_2O_2.HCl$	Chloroprocaine Hydrochloride
$C_{13}H_{19}ClN_2O_5S_2$	Mefruside
$C_{13}H_{19}Cl_2NO_2$	Cloranolol
$C_{13}H_{19}N$	Enefexine
$C_{13}H_{19}NO.HCl$	Diethylpropion Hydrochloride
$C_{13}H_{19}NO_2$	Butamoxane
$C_{13}H_{19}NO_2$	Exalamide
$C_{13}H_{19}NO_2$	Ibuproxam
$C_{13}H_{19}NO_2$	Ifoxetine
$C_{13}H_{19}NO_3$	Detanosal
$C_{13}H_{19}NO_3.HCl$	Viloxazine Hydrochloride
$C_{13}H_{19}NO_4S$	Probenecid
$C_{13}H_{19}N_3OS$	Dilopetine
$C_{13}H_{19}N_3OS.HCl.H_2O$	Rocastine Hydrochloride
$C_{13}H_{19}N_3O_2$	Amidantel
$C_{13}H_{19}N_3O_4$	Lufironil
$C_{13}H_{19}N_3O_5S_2$	Sparsomycin
$C_{13}H_{19}N_5.H_2O$	Pinacidil
$C_{13}H_{19}Na_2O_5P$	Fospropofol Disodium
$C_{13}H_{20}ClN_3O$	Declopramide
$C_{13}H_{20}ClN_3O_4S_2$	Mebutizide
$C_{13}H_{20}N_2O$	Prilocaine
$C_{13}H_{20}N_2O.HCl$	Prilocaine Hydrochloride
$C_{13}H_{20}N_2O_2$	Dropropizine
$C_{13}H_{20}N_2O_2$	Levodropropizine
$C_{13}H_{20}N_2O_2.C_4H_4O_4$	Salethamide Maleate
$C_{13}H_{20}N_2O_2.HCl$	Metabutethamine Hydrochloride
$C_{13}H_{20}N_2O_2.HCl$	Procaine Hydrochloride
$C_{13}H_{20}N_2O_3$	Hydroxyprocaine
$C_{13}H_{20}N_2O_3S$	Articaine
$C_{13}H_{20}N_2O_3S$	Dexetozoline
$C_{13}H_{20}N_2O_3S$	Etozolin
$C_{13}H_{20}N_2O_3S.HCl$	Articaine Hydrochloride
$C_{13}H_{20}N_4O_2$	Pentifylline
$C_{13}H_{20}N_4O_3$	Ciclosidomine
$C_{13}H_{20}N_4O_3$	Lisofylline
$C_{13}H_{20}N_6O_4.HCl$	Valacyclovir Hydrochloride
$C_{13}H_{20}O_3$	Febuprol
$C_{13}H_{21}AsN_8S_2$	Melarsomine
$C_{13}H_{21}NO_2$	Guaiactamine
$C_{13}H_{21}NO_2$	Tigloidine
$C_{13}H_{21}NO_2$	Toliprolol
$C_{13}H_{21}NO_2$	Tropigline
$C_{13}H_{21}NO_2.HCl$	Dimoxamine Hydrochloride
$C_{13}H_{21}NO_2S$	Ditolamide
$C_{13}H_{21}NO_2S.HCl$	Tiprenolol Hydrochloride
$C_{13}H_{21}NO_3$	Albuterol
$C_{13}H_{21}NO_3$	Isoetharine
$C_{13}H_{21}NO_3$	Levomoprolol
$C_{13}H_{21}NO_3$	Levosalbutamol
$C_{13}H_{21}NO_3$	Moprolol
$C_{13}H_{21}NO_3.CH_4O_3S$	Isoetharine Mesylate

Molecular Formula	Non-proprietary Name
$2(C_{13}H_{21}NO_3).C_4H_6O_6$	Levalbuterol Tartrate
$C_{13}H_{21}NO_3.HCl$	Isoetharine Hydrochloride
$C_{13}H_{21}NO_3.HCl$	Levalbuterol Hydrochloride
$(C_{13}H_{21}NO_3)_2.H_2SO_4$	Albuterol Sulfate
$C_{13}H_{21}NO_3.H_2SO_4$	Levalbuterol Sulfate
$C_{13}H_{21}NO_6$	Trolamine Salicylate
$C_{13}H_{21}N_2NaO_{11}S_2$	Glucosulfamide
$C_{13}H_{21}N_3.HCl$	Quinpirole Hydrochloride
$C_{13}H_{21}N_3O.HCl$	Procainamide Hydrochloride
$C_{13}H_{21}N_3O_3.HCl$	Carbuterol Hydrochloride
$C_{13}H_{21}N_3S_2$	Vedaclidine
$C_{13}H_{21}N_5O_2$	Etamiphyllin
$C_{13}H_{21}N_5O_2.H_2O$	Tezampanel
$C_{13}H_{21}N_5O_4.C_6H_5NO_2$	Xanthinol Niacinate
$C_{13}H_{21}N_5O_4.C_{10}H_{11}ClO_3$	Xantifibrate
$C_{13}H_{22}ClN_5S$	Iprozilamine
$C_{13}H_{22}N_2O_5Pt$	Enloplatin
$C_{13}H_{22}N_2O_6S$	Neostigmine Methylsulfate
$C_{13}H_{22}N_4O_3S$	Ranitidine
$C_{13}H_{22}N_4O_3S.C_6H_5BiO_7$	Ranitidine Bismuth Citrate
$C_{13}H_{22}N_4O_3S.HCl$	Ranitidine Hydrochloride
$C_{13}H_{24}N_2O_2$	Cropropamide
$C_{13}H_{24}N_2O_3$	Neboglamine
$C_{13}H_{24}N_3O_3PS$	Pirimiphos-ethyl
$C_{13}H_{24}N_4O_3S.C_4H_4O_4$	Timolol Maleate
$C_{13}H_{24}N_4O_3S.\frac{1}{2}H_2O$	Timolol
$C_{13}H_{25}B_5N_2O_{12}$	Procaine Borate
$C_{13}H_{25}NO_2$	Cyprodenate
$C_{13}H_{25}NO_9.1\frac{1}{2}H_2O$	Camiglibose
$C_{13}H_{25}N_2O_5$	Troxolamide
$C_{13}H_{26}N_2O_4$	Adelmidrol
$C_{13}H_{26}N_2O_4$	Nisobamate
$C_{13}H_{26}N_2O_4$	Tybamate
$C_{13}H_{26}O_4$	Monoctanoin Component B
$C_{13}H_{28}N_4O_2$	Exametazime
$C_{13}H_{29}N$	Octamylamine
$C_{13}H_{29}NO_2$	Decominol
$(C_{13}H_{30}Br_2N_2)n$	Hexadimethrine Bromide
$C_{13}H_{33}Br_2N_3$	Azamethonium Bromide
$C_{13}H_{38}N_2O_5S$	Fantofarone
$C_{14}{}^{11}CH_{20}Cl_2N_2O_3$	Raclopride C 11
$C_{14}H_6O_8$	Ellagic Acid
$C_{14}H_8Br_2F_3NO_2$	Fluorosalan
$C_{14}H_8CaN_2O_6S_2.3\frac{1}{2}H_2O$	Saccharin Calcium
$C_{14}H_8ClFN_2O_3S$	Ilonidap
$C_{14}H_8ClNNa_2O_4$	Lobenzarit Sodium
$C_{14}H_8ClN_2NaO_3S$	Tenidap Sodium
$C_{14}H_8F_3NO_2S$	Flutiazin
$C_{14}H_8NNaO_4$	Alrestatin Sodium
$C_{14}H_8N_2Na_2O_6$	Olsalazine Sodium
$C_{14}H_8N_2O_6$	Nifuroquine
$C_{14}H_8O_4$	Danthron
$C_{14}H_9ClF_3NO_2$	Efavirenz
$C_{14}H_9ClN_2O_3S$	Tenidap
$C_{14}H_9Cl_2F_3N_2O$	Cloflucarban
$C_{14}H_9Cl_2N_3O_2$	Lopirazepam
$C_{14}H_9Cl_2N_3O_3$	Clodanolene
$C_{14}H_9Cl_2N_3S_2$	Luliconazole
$C_{14}H_9Cl_3N_2OS$	Triclabendazole
$C_{14}H_9Cl_5$	Chlorophenothane
$C_{14}H_9F$	Fluretofen
$(C_{14}H_9F_3NO_2)_3Al$	Aluminum Flufenamate
$C_{14}H_9F_3O_2$	Xenalipin
$C_{14}H_9I_3O_4$	Tiratricol
$C_{14}H_9N_4NaO_5.3\frac{1}{2}H_2O$	Dantrolene Sodium
$C_{14}H_{10}BrN_3O$	Bromazepam
$C_{14}H_{10}Br_3NO_2$	Bensalan
$C_{14}H_{10}ClN_3S_2$	Lanoconazole
$C_{14}H_{10}Cl_2KNO_2$	Diclofenac Potassium
$C_{14}H_{10}Cl_2NNaO_2$	Diclofenac Sodium
$C_{14}H_{10}Cl_2NNaO_2.H_2O$	Meclofenamate Sodium
$C_{14}H_{10}Cl_2O_3$	Fenclofenac
$C_{14}H_{10}Cl_4$	Mitotane
$C_{14}H_{10}F_2NNaO_3S$	Diflumidone Sodium
$C_{14}H_{10}F_3NO_2$	Flufenamic Acid
$C_{14}H_{10}F_3NO_2$	Salfluverine
$C_{14}H_{10}F_3NO_5$	Nitisinone
$C_{14}H_{10}MgO_6.4H_2O$	Magnesium Salicylate
$C_{14}H_{10}N_4O$	Olprinone
$C_{14}H_{10}N_4O_5$	Dantrolene
$C_{14}H_{10}O_3$	Anthralin
$C_{14}H_{10}O_4$ (anhydrous)	Benzoyl Peroxide
$C_{14}H_{10}O_5$	Salsalate
$C_{14}H_{11}ClN_2O_4S$	Chlorthalidone
$C_{14}H_{11}ClO_3S$	Cliprofen
$C_{14}H_{11}Cl_2NO_2$	Meclofenamic Acid
$C_{14}H_{11}Cl_2NO_4$	Diloxanide Furoate
$C_{14}H_{11}F_3N_2O_2$	Flunixin
$C_{14}H_{11}F_3N_2O_2.C_7H_{17}NO_5$	Flunixin Meglumine
$C_{14}H_{11}NO_5$	Nebicapone
$C_{14}H_{11}NO_5$	Tolcapone
$C_{14}H_{11}N_3O_3S$	Nocodazole
$C_{14}H_{11}N_3O_4$	Stirimazole
$C_{14}H_{12}CaN_2O_6.3H_2O$	Aminosalicylate Calcium
$C_{14}H_{12}ClNO_2$	Cicletanine
$C_{14}H_{12}ClNO_2$	Tolfenamic Acid
$C_{14}H_{12}ClN_3O$	Bamaluzole
$C_{14}H_{12}ClN_3O_3S$	Fenquizone
$C_{14}H_{12}ClN_3O_4S_2$	Indisulam
$C_{14}H_{12}FNO_3$	Flumequine
$C_{14}H_{12}NNaO_4$	Droxacin Sodium
$C_{14}H_{12}N_2$	Bendazol
$C_{14}H_{12}N_2O_2$	Rolafagrel
$C_{14}H_{12}N_2O_2S$	Zolimidine
$C_{14}H_{12}N_2O_4$	Mitindomide
$C_{14}H_{12}N_2O_4S$	Tioxacin
$C_{14}H_{12}N_4$	Azarole
$C_{14}H_{12}N_4OS$	Nolatrexed
$C_{14}H_{12}N_4O_2S$	Sulfaquinoxaline
$C_{14}H_{12}N_6O$	Levosimendan
$C_{14}H_{12}N_6O$	Simendan
$C_{14}H_{12}N_6O_6$	Nitrovin
$C_{14}H_{12}OS$	Tibenzate
$C_{14}H_{12}O_2$	Benzyl Benzoate
$C_{14}H_{12}O_2$	Felbinac
$C_{14}H_{12}O_3$	Oxybenzone
$C_{14}H_{12}O_3$	Trioxsalen
$C_{14}H_{12}O_3S$	Suprofen
$C_{14}H_{12}O_3S$	Tiaprofenic Acid
$C_{14}H_{12}O_4$	Dioxybenzone
$C_{14}H_{12}O_5$	Evicromil
$C_{14}H_{12}O_5$	Khellin
$C_{14}H_{12}O_6S$	Sulisobenzone
$C_{14}H_{12}S_2$	Mesulfen
$C_{14}H_{13}AlCaN_2O_8.5H_2O$	Aluminoparaaminosalicylate Calcium
$C_{14}H_{13}ClFN_3O_4S_2$	Paraflutizide
$C_{14}H_{13}ClN_2$	Clonazoline
$C_{14}H_{13}ClN_2O$	Vincantril
$C_{14}H_{13}ClN_4O_2$	Arofylline
$C_{14}H_{13}ClO_3$	Lonaprofen
$C_{14}H_{13}NO$	Norletimol

Molecular Formula	Non-proprietary Name
$C_{14}H_{13}NO_2$	Diphenan
$C_{14}H_{13}NO_2$	Paxamate
$C_{14}H_{13}NO_3$	Alonimid
$C_{14}H_{13}NO_4$	Oxalinast
$C_{14}H_{13}N_2NaO_4S$	Acediasulfone Sodium
$C_{14}H_{13}N_3 \cdot HCl$	Fadrozole Hydrochloride
$C_{14}H_{13}N_3O_2S$	Sulmazole
$C_{14}H_{13}N_3O_2S \cdot HCl$	Isomazole Hydrochloride
$C_{14}H_{13}N_3O_3$	Ftivazide
$C_{14}H_{13}N_3O_4S_2$	Meloxicam
$C_{14}H_{13}N_3O_5S$	Isoxicam
$C_{14}H_{13}N_3O_5S$	Sulfanitran
$C_{14}H_{13}N_5$	Picodralazine
$C_{14}H_{13}N_5O_4S$	Nifuralide
$C_{14}H_{13}N_5O_5S_2$	Cefdinir
$C_{14}H_{13}N_8NaO_4S_3$	Cefazolin Sodium
$C_{14}H_{13}NaO_3$	Naproxen Sodium
$C_{14}H_{14}As_2N_2Na_2O_8S_2$	Sulfarsphenamine
$C_{14}H_{14}ClI$	Toliodium Chloride
$C_{14}H_{14}ClNO_2$	Clopirac
$C_{14}H_{14}ClNS \cdot HCl$	Ticlopidine Hydrochloride
$C_{14}H_{14}ClN_3O_2S$	Pirinixic Acid
$C_{14}H_{14}ClN_3O_4S_2$	Benzylhydrochlorothiazide
$C_{14}H_{14}ClN_3S$	Azuresin
$C_{14}H_{14}Cl_2N_2O$	Enilconazole
$C_{14}H_{14}Cl_3O_6P$	Haloxon
$C_{14}H_{14}I_3NO_4$	Propyl Docetrizoate
$C_{14}H_{14}N_2 \cdot HCl$	Naphazoline Hydrochloride
$C_{14}H_{14}N_2Na_2O_6S_3$	Sulfoxone Sodium
$C_{14}H_{14}N_2O$	Metyrapone
$C_{14}H_{14}N_2O \cdot 2C_4H_6O_6$	Metyrapone Tartrate
$C_{14}H_{14}N_2O_2$	Isonixin
$C_{14}H_{14}N_2O_2$	Metanixin
$C_{14}H_{14}N_2O_2$	Nixylic Acid
$C_{14}H_{14}N_2O_4S$	Tioxamast
$C_{14}H_{14}N_3NaO_5S_2$	Acetosulfone Sodium
$C_{14}H_{14}N_4$	Rolodine
$C_{14}H_{14}N_4O_2$	Razobazam
$C_{14}H_{14}N_4O_2S$	Cambendazole
$C_{14}H_{14}N_4O_4$	Terizidone
$C_{14}H_{14}N_4O_8S_2$	Dinsed
$C_{14}H_{14}N_8O_4S_3$	Cefazolin
$C_{14}H_{14}O_3$	Lexofenac
$C_{14}H_{14}O_3$	Naproxen
$C_{14}H_{14}O_4$	Phthalofyne
$C_{14}H_{14}O_6S$	Texacromil
$C_{14}H_{15}ClN_2O_3$	Itameline
$C_{14}H_{15}ClN_4$	Zometapine
$C_{14}H_{15}ClN_4O_2$	Aronixil
$C_{14}H_{15}ClO_2$	Clofurac
$C_{14}H_{15}Cl_2N$	Chlornaphazine
$C_{14}H_{15}FN_2$	Fipamezole
$C_{14}H_{15}FN_2O_2$	Flutomidate
$C_{14}H_{15}F_2N_3S \cdot HCl \cdot H_2O$	Nepicastat Hydrochloride
$C_{14}H_{15}F_3N_3O_6P$	Fanapanel
$C_{14}H_{15}NOS \cdot HCl$	Bipenamol Hydrochloride
$C_{14}H_{15}NO_2$	Acequinoline
$C_{14}H_{15}NO_4$	Oxazorone
$C_{14}H_{15}NO_5$	Folescutol
$C_{14}H_{15}NO_5S_2$	Linotroban
$C_{14}H_{15}NO_6S$	Isalsteine
$C_{14}H_{15}NO_6S$	Salmisteine
$C_{14}H_{15}N_2O_2P$	Fosenazide
$C_{14}H_{15}N_3O_2$	Indolidan
$C_{14}H_{15}N_3O_5$	Entacapone
$C_{14}H_{15}N_5O \cdot CH_4O_3S$	Endralazine Mesylate
$C_{14}H_{15}N_5O_2$	Taniplon
$C_{14}H_{15}N_5O_3$	Troquidazole
$C_{14}H_{15}N_5O_5S_2$	Cefetamet
$C_{14}H_{15}N_5O_6S_2$	Cefdaloxime
$C_{14}H_{15}N_7$	Diminazene
$C_{14}H_{16}BrNO_2$	Brofaromine
$C_{14}H_{16}ClNO$	Bexlosteride
$C_{14}H_{16}ClNO_4S$	Timofibrate
$C_{14}H_{16}ClN_3O_2$	Amipizone
$C_{14}H_{16}ClN_3O_4S_2$	Cyclothiazide
$C_{14}H_{16}ClO_5PS$	Coumaphos
$C_{14}H_{16}Cl_2N_4O_3$	Obidoxime Chloride
$C_{14}H_{16}Cl_2O_2$	Fenclorac
$C_{14}H_{16}Cl_6O_5$	Toloxychlorinol
$C_{14}H_{16}F_2N_2$	Flucindole
$C_{14}H_{16}N_2$	Atipamezole
$C_{14}H_{16}N_2 \cdot HCl$	Napactadine Hydrochloride
$C_{14}H_{16}N_2 \cdot HCl$	Napamezole Hydrochloride
$C_{14}H_{16}N_2O$	Coumazoline
$C_{14}H_{16}N_2O$	Prifuroline
$C_{14}H_{16}N_2O_2$	Etomidate
$C_{14}H_{16}N_2O_2$	Rolicyprine
$C_{14}H_{16}N_2O_2 \cdot HCl$	Imiloxan Hydrochloride
$C_{14}H_{16}N_2O_3$	Nadoxolol
$C_{14}H_{16}N_2O_3$	Phetharbital
$C_{14}H_{16}N_2O_4$	Oxagrelate
$C_{14}H_{16}N_2O_4$	Taglutimide
$C_{14}H_{16}N_4$	Budralazine
$C_{14}H_{16}N_4$	Imiquimod
$C_{14}H_{16}N_4$	Simtrazene
$C_{14}H_{16}N_4O \cdot HCl$	Ethoxazene Hydrochloride
$C_{14}H_{16}N_4O_3$	Piromidic Acid
$C_{14}H_{16}N_4O_3S$	Eniporide
$C_{14}H_{16}N_6O$	Siguazodan
$C_{14}H_{16}O_2$	Naproxol
$C_{14}H_{16}O_4S$	Esonarimod
$C_{14}H_{16}O_9$	Bergenin
$C_{14}H_{17}BrN_6O_2S_3$	Ebrotidine
$C_{14}H_{17}ClN_2O_3S$	Clorexolone
$C_{14}H_{17}ClN_4$	Lodinixil
$C_{14}H_{17}ClO_3$	Clomoxir
$C_{14}H_{17}Cl_2N_3O$	Piclonidine
$C_{14}H_{17}FN_2O_3$	Opaviraline
$C_{14}H_{17}NO_2$	Benzoclidine
$C_{14}H_{17}NO_2 \cdot HCl$	Indeloxazine Hydrochloride
$C_{14}H_{17}NO_4$	Mobecarb
$C_{14}H_{17}NO_5$	Fenamifuril
$C_{14}H_{17}NS_2$	Dimethylthiambutene
$C_{14}H_{17}N_2NaO_3$	Methohexital Sodium
$C_{14}H_{17}N_3O$	Frovatriptan
$C_{14}H_{17}N_3O \cdot C_4H_6O_4 \cdot H_2O$	Frovatriptan Succinate
$C_{14}H_{17}N_3O_2S$	Fasudil
$C_{14}H_{17}N_3O_5S$	Sulfacecole
$C_{14}H_{17}N_3O_9$	Azaribine
$C_{14}H_{17}N_5$	Sotirimod
$C_{14}H_{17}N_5O_3$	Pipemidic Acid
$C_{14}H_{18}As_2N_2O_6$	Difetarsone
$C_{14}H_{18}BrNO \cdot \tfrac{1}{2}H_2O$	Quinuclium Bromide
$C_{14}H_{18}CaN_3Na_3O_{10}$	Pentetate Calcium Trisodium
$C_{14}H_{18}ClN$	Picilorex
$C_{14}H_{18}ClNO_4S$	Tibric Acid
$C_{14}H_{18}ClN_3S \cdot C_6H_8O_7$	Chlorothen Citrate
$C_{14}H_{18}Cl_2N_2$	Clenpirin
$C_{14}H_{18}FNO_2 \cdot HCl$	Lubazodone Hydrochloride
$C_{14}H_{18}F_3NO$	Oxaflozane
$C_{14}H_{18}{}^{125}IN_3$	Iomethin I 125

Molecular Formula	Non-proprietary Name
$C_{14}H_{18}{}^{131}IN_3$	Iomethin I 131
$C_{14}H_{18}{}^{111}InN_3Na_2O_{10}$	Pentetate Indium Disodium In 111
$C_{14}H_{18}NNaO_5$	Sanfetrinem Sodium
$(C_{14}H_{18}NO_{17}S_2Na_3)_n$	Suleparoid Sodium
$C_{14}H_{18}N_2$	Cyclindole
$C_{14}H_{18}N_2$	Tefazoline
$C_{14}H_{18}N_2O$	Cilutazoline
$C_{14}H_{18}N_2O$	Ibudilast
$C_{14}H_{18}N_2O$	Propyphenazone
$C_{14}H_{18}N_2O_2$	Nefiracetam
$C_{14}H_{18}N_2O_2$	Parsalmide
$(C_{14}H_{18}N_2O_2)_2.H_2SO_4$	Quinterenol Sulfate
$C_{14}H_{18}N_2O_3$	Methohexital
$C_{14}H_{18}N_2O_3.HCl$	Letimide Hydrochloride
$C_{14}H_{18}N_2O_4$	Mofoxime
$C_{14}H_{18}N_2O_5$	Acitemate
$C_{14}H_{18}N_2O_5$	Aspartame
$C_{14}H_{18}N_2O_5$	Lidofenin
$C_{14}H_{18}N_2O_5S$	Tacapenem
$C_{14}H_{18}N_3NaO_{10}{}^{99m}Tc$	Technetium Tc 99m Pentetate
$C_{14}H_{18}N_3Na_2O_{10}{}^{169}Yb$	Ytterbium Yb 169 Pentetate
$C_{14}H_{18}N_4$	Bisfentidine
$C_{14}H_{18}N_4O_2$	Mexafylline
$C_{14}H_{18}N_4O_2$	Ormetoprim
$C_{14}H_{18}N_4O_2S$	Metioprim
$C_{14}H_{18}N_4O_3$	Trimethoprim
$(C_{14}H_{18}N_4O_3)_2.H_2SO_4$	Trimethoprim Sulfate
$C_{14}H_{18}N_4O_4S_2$	Thiophanate
$C_{14}H_{18}N_4O_9$	Caffeine Citrate
$C_{14}H_{18}N_6O.C_4H_6O_4$	Abacavir Succinate
$(C_{14}H_{18}N_6O)_2.H_2SO_4$	Abacavir Sulfate
$C_{14}H_{18}O_3$	Stiripentol
$C_{14}H_{18}O_4$	Cinoxate
$C_{14}H_{19}ClN_2O_2$	Eprobemide
$C_{14}H_{19}ClN_2O_3$	Cloximate
$C_{14}H_{19}ClN_4.HCl$	Amprolium
$C_{14}H_{19}ClN_4O_2$	Lintopride
$C_{14}H_{19}Cl_2NO_2$	Chlorambucil
$C_{14}H_{19}F_3N_2O_2.HCl$	Flubanilate Hydrochloride
$C_{14}H_{19}F_3N_4O$	Fluprazine
$C_{14}H_{19}IO$	Cicliomenol
$C_{14}H_{19}NO_2$	Levofacetoperane
$C_{14}H_{19}NO_2$	Methylphenidate
$C_{14}H_{19}NO_2$	Piperoxan
$C_{14}H_{19}NO_2.HCl$	Dexmethylphenidate Hydrochloride
$C_{14}H_{19}NO_2.HCl$	Methylphenidate Hydrochloride
$C_{14}H_{19}NO_4$	Daxalipram
$C_{14}H_{19}NO_4$	Filenadol
$C_{14}H_{19}NO_4S$	Tritiozine
$C_{14}H_{19}NO_5$	Trimetozine
$(C_{14}H_{19}NO_{14}SNa_2)_n$	Chondroitin Sulfate Sodium
$C_{14}H_{19}N_3O$	Oxolamine
$C_{14}H_{19}N_3O$	Ramifenazone
$C_{14}H_{19}N_3O$	Xilobam
$C_{14}H_{19}N_3O.2C_{12}H_{19}NO_3$	Quinetolate
$C_{14}H_{19}N_3O_2$	Zilpaterol
$C_{14}H_{19}N_3S$	Thenyldiamine
$(C_{14}H_{19}N_3S)_2.3C_4H_4O_4$	Methapyrilene Fumarate
$C_{14}H_{19}N_3S.HCl$	Methapyrilene Hydrochloride
$C_{14}H_{19}N_5O$	Mopidralazine
$C_{14}H_{19}N_5O_2.HCl$	Etazolate Hydrochloride
$C_{14}H_{19}N_5O_4$	Famciclovir
$C_{14}H_{19}N_5O_5$	Tecadenoson
$C_{14}H_{20}Br_2N_2.HCl$	Bromhexine Hydrochloride

Molecular Formula	Non-proprietary Name
$C_{14}H_{20}ClN_3O_2$	Bimoclomol
$C_{14}H_{20}ClN_3O_3$	Arimoclomol
$C_{14}H_{20}ClN_3O_3$	Ticalopride
$C_{14}H_{20}ClN_3O_3S$	Clopamide
$C_{14}H_{20}Cl_2N_2O_2$	Diclometide
$C_{14}H_{20}Cl_6N_2$	Chlorisondamine Chloride
$C_{14}H_{20}GdN_3O_{10}.2C_7H_{17}NO_5$	Gadopentetate Dimeglumine
$(C_{14}H_{20}NNaO_{11})_n$	Hyaluronate Sodium
$C_{14}H_{20}N_2$	Cipralisant
$C_{14}H_{20}N_2.C_4H_4O_4$	Cipralisant Maleate
$C_{14}H_{20}N_2O$	Aptocaine
$C_{14}H_{20}N_2O$	Pyrrocaine
$C_{14}H_{20}N_2O$	Tymazoline
$C_{14}H_{20}N_2O_2$	Bunitrolol
$C_{14}H_{20}N_2O_2$	Pindolol
$C_{14}H_{20}N_2O_2.C_4H_4O_4$	Domazoline Fumarate
$C_{14}H_{20}N_2O_2.HCl$	Piridocaine Hydrochloride
$C_{14}H_{20}N_2O_2S$	Azabon
$C_{14}H_{20}N_2O_3$	Propacetamol
$C_{14}H_{20}N_2O_3$	Vorinostat
$C_{14}H_{20}N_2O_3S$	Glycyclamide
$C_{14}H_{20}N_2O_3S_2$	Thiohexamide
$C_{14}H_{20}N_4O$	Imolamine
$C_{14}H_{20}N_4O$	Iroxanadine
$C_{14}H_{20}N_4O_7S_2$	Netobimin
$C_{14}H_{20}O$	Bornelone
$C_{14}H_{20}O$	Cyclomenol
$C_{14}H_{20}O_2$	Butibufen
$C_{14}H_{21}BO_2$	Tolboxane
$C_{14}H_{21}ClN_2O_2$	Clofexamide
$C_{14}H_{21}ClN_2O_2$	Clovoxamine
$C_{14}H_{21}ClN_2O_2.C_{19}H_{20}N_2O_2.2H_2O$	Clofezone
$C_{14}H_{21}N$	Eticyclidine
$C_{14}H_{21}NO$	Preclamol
$C_{14}H_{21}NO$	Zylofuramine
$C_{14}H_{21}NO.HCl$	Profadol Hydrochloride
$C_{14}H_{21}NOS.HCl$	Esproquin Hydrochloride
$C_{14}H_{21}NO_2$	Berefrine
$C_{14}H_{21}NO_2$	Carmantadine
$C_{14}H_{21}NO_2$	Padimate A
$C_{14}H_{21}NO_2.HCl$	Meprylcaine Hydrochloride
$C_{14}H_{21}NO_2.HCl$	Pentamoxane Hydrochloride
$C_{14}H_{21}NO_3$	Pivenfrine
$C_{14}H_{21}NO_3S$	Reparixin
$C_{14}H_{21}NO_4$	Ambenoxan
$C_{14}H_{21}NO_7S$	Sulbactam Pivoxil
$C_{14}H_{21}N_3O_2S$	Sumatriptan
$C_{14}H_{21}N_3O_2S.C_4H_6O_4$	Sumatriptan Succinate
$C_{14}H_{21}N_3O_3$	Oxamniquine
$C_{14}H_{21}N_3O_3S$	Metahexamide
$C_{14}H_{21}N_3O_3S$	Tolazamide
$C_{14}H_{21}N_3O_4S$	Sulmepride
$C_{14}H_{21}N_3O_6S$	Adicillin
$C_{14}H_{21}N_7$	Gapromidine
$C_{14}H_{22}BrN_3O_2$	Bromopride
$C_{14}H_{22}ClNO$	Clobutinol
$C_{14}H_{22}ClNO_2$	Bupranolol
$C_{14}H_{22}ClN_3O_2.HCl.H_2O$	Metoclopramide Hydrochloride
$C_{14}H_{22}ClN_3O_3S$	Lorapride
$C_{14}H_{22}N_2O$	Ispronicline
$C_{14}H_{22}N_2O$	Lidocaine
$C_{14}H_{22}N_2O$	Octacaine
$C_{14}H_{22}N_2O$	Quatacaine
$C_{14}H_{22}N_2O.HCl.H_2O$	Lidocaine Hydrochloride
$C_{14}H_{22}N_2O_2$	Propetamide

Molecular Formula	Non-proprietary Name
$C_{14}H_{22}N_2O_2$	Rivastigmine
$C_{14}H_{22}N_2O_2.HCl$	Naepaine Hydrochloride
$C_{14}H_{22}N_2O_3$	Atenolol
$C_{14}H_{22}N_2O_3$	Bucolome
$C_{14}H_{22}N_2O_3$	Esatenolol
$C_{14}H_{22}N_2O_3$	Practolol
$C_{14}H_{22}N_2O_3$	Trimetazidine
$C_{14}H_{22}N_2O_3S$	Piprozolin
$C_{14}H_{22}N_2O_7S$	Rimazolium Metilsulfate
$C_{14}H_{22}N_4.2HCl$	Quinelorane Hydrochloride
$C_{14}H_{22}N_4O_2$	Nosantine
$C_{14}H_{22}N_4O_3S$	Delfantrine
$C_{14}H_{22}N_4O_5.2HCl$	Valtorcitabine Dihydrochloride
$C_{14}H_{22}N_6O_5.HCl$	Valganciclovir Hydrochloride
$C_{14}H_{22}O_8$	Acetyltriethyl Citrate
$C_{14}H_{23}BrINO_3$	Fubrogonium Iodide
$C_{14}H_{23}Cl_2N_3O_2$	Spiromustine
$C_{14}H_{23}NO$	Tapentadol
$C_{14}H_{23}NO_2$	Piroctone
$C_{14}H_{23}NO_2.C_2H_7NO$	Piroctone Olamine
$C_{14}H_{23}NO_3$	Arnolol
$C_{14}H_{23}NO_3$	Crilvastatin
$C_{14}H_{23}NO_4S.HCl$	Sulfonterol Hydrochloride
$C_{14}H_{23}N_3OS$	Xanomeline
$C_{14}H_{23}N_3OS.C_4H_6O_6$	Xanomeline Tartrate
$C_{14}H_{23}N_3O_3S.HCl$	Sematilide Hydrochloride
$C_{14}H_{23}N_3O_{10}$	Pentetic Acid
$C_{14}H_{23}N_3S_2.C_6H_8O_7$	Tazomeline Citrate
$C_{14}H_{23}N_7S$	Sopromidine
$C_{14}H_{23}N_7S.3HCl$	Impromidine Hydrochloride
$C_{14}H_{24}CaN_4O_8$	Piperazine Edetate Calcium
$C_{14}H_{24}N_2O_7.2HCl.5H_2O$	Spectinomycin Hydrochloride
$C_{14}H_{24}N_2O_{10}$	Egtazic Acid
$C_{14}H_{25}N.HCl$	Somantadine Hydrochloride
$C_{14}H_{25}N_3O_4S.2\frac{1}{2}H_2O$	Alitame
$C_{14}H_{25}N_4NaO_{11}P_2$	Citicoline Sodium
$C_{14}H_{26}CaO_{16}$	Calcium Gluceptate
$[C_{14}H_{26}N_4O_3]_2.H_2SO_4$	Pareptide Sulfate
$C_{14}H_{26}O_2$	Loxanast
$C_{14}H_{26}O_3$	Menglytate
$C_{14}H_{26}O_4$	Valproate Pivoxil
$C_{14}H_{27}NO_6.HCl$	Amiprilose Hydrochloride
$C_{14}H_{27}N_3O_2.HCl$	Pramiracetam Hydrochloride
$C_{14}H_{27}N_3O_2.H_2SO_4$	Pramiracetam Sulfate
$C_{14}H_{28}N_9OP_3$	Fotretamine
$C_{14}H_{28}O_2$	Myristic Acid
$C_{14}H_{29}NaO_4S$	Sodium Tetradecyl Sulfate
$C_{14}H_{30}Br_2N_2O_4$	Suxamethonium Bromide
$C_{14}H_{30}Cl_2N_2O_4$	Succinylcholine Chloride
$C_{14}H_{30}I_2N_2O_2$	Dimecolonium Iodide
$C_{14}H_{30}N_4O_2$	Upenazime
$C_{14}H_{30}O$	Myristyl Alcohol
$C_{14}H_{30}O_2$	Gemcadiol
$C_{14}H_{30}O_2S_2$	Tiadenol
$C_{14}H_{32}N_2O_4$	Edetol
$C_{15}H_8F_2N_2O_2$	Imirestat
$C_{15}H_9BrFNO_4$	Brocrinat
$C_{15}H_9BrO_2$	Bromindione
$C_{15}H_9BrO_2$	Isobromindione
$C_{15}H_9ClO_2$	Clorindione
$C_{15}H_9Cl_2N_5$	Zapizolam
$C_{15}H_9FN_2O_3$	Ataluren
$C_{15}H_9FO_2$	Fluindione
$C_{15}H_9I_3O_5$	Acetiromate
$C_{15}H_{10}BrClN_4S$	Brotizolam
$C_{15}H_{10}Br_2ClNO_2S$	Brotianide

Molecular Formula	Non-proprietary Name
$C_{15}H_{10}ClI_2NO_3$	Clioxanide
$C_{15}H_{10}ClN_3O_3$	Clonazepam
$C_{15}H_{10}Cl_2N_2O$	Delorazepam
$C_{15}H_{10}Cl_2N_2O_2$	Lonidamine
$C_{15}H_{10}Cl_2N_2O_2$	Lorazepam
$C_{15}H_{10}Cl_3NO_6S$	Sulicrinat
$C_{15}H_{10}FNO_3$	Prinaberel
$C_{15}H_{10}F_7N_3O_2S_2$	Saviprazole
$C_{15}H_{10}I_4NNaO_4.xH_2O$	Dextrothyroxine Sodium
$C_{15}H_{10}I_4NNaO_4.xH_2O$	Levothyroxine Sodium
$C_{15}H_{10}NNaO_3.H_2O$	Furegrelate Sodium
$C_{15}H_{10}O_2$	Phenindione
$C_{15}H_{10}O_5S$	Tixanox
$C_{15}H_{11}BrCl_2N_2$	Nolinium Bromide
$C_{15}H_{11}BrNNaO_3.1\frac{1}{2}H_2O$	Bromfenac Sodium
$C_{15}H_{11}ClN_2O$	Mecloqualone
$C_{15}H_{11}ClN_2O$	Nordazepam
$C_{15}H_{11}ClN_2O_2$	Demoxepam
$C_{15}H_{11}ClN_2O_2$	Oxazepam
$C_{15}H_{11}ClO_2$	Cloridarol
$C_{15}H_{11}ClO_3$	Furcloprofen
$C_{15}H_{11}Cl_2F_5O_2$	Fenfluthrin
$C_{15}H_{11}Cl_2NO_4$	Clamidoxic Acid
$C_{15}H_{11}Cl_3N_4S.HCl$	Zinoconazole Hydrochloride
$C_{15}H_{11}FO_4$	Flufenisal
$C_{15}H_{11}F_3N_2O_2$	Manitimus
$C_{15}H_{11}I_3NNaO_4$	Liothyronine Sodium
$C_{15}H_{11}I_3O_4$	Thyropropic Acid
$C_{15}H_{11}{}^{125}I_4NO_4$	Thyroxine I 125
$C_{15}H_{11}{}^{131}I_4NO_4$	Thyroxine I 131
$C_{15}H_{11}NO_3$	Cridanimod
$C_{15}H_{11}N_2NaO_2$	Phenytoin Sodium
$C_{15}H_{11}N_3O$	Daniquidone
$C_{15}H_{11}N_3O_2.xH_2O$	Furodazole
$C_{15}H_{11}N_3O_3$	Nitrazepam
$C_{15}H_{11}N_9O$	Andolast
$C_{15}H_{12}ClNO_2$	Carprofen
$C_{15}H_{12}Cl_2N_2O_4$	Urefibrate
$C_{15}H_{12}FN_3O_5S$	Luxabendazole
$C_{15}H_{12}FNaO_2.2H_2O$	Flurbiprofen Sodium
$C_{15}H_{12}I_2O_3$	Iodoalphionic Acid
$C_{15}H_{12}I_3NO_4$	Detrothyronine
$C_{15}H_{12}{}^{125}I_3NO_4$	Liothyronine I 125
$C_{15}H_{12}{}^{131}I_3NO_4$	Liothyronine I 131
$C_{15}H_{12}I_3NO_4$	Rathyronine
$C_{15}H_{12}KN_5O_4$	Leteprinim Potassium
$C_{15}H_{12}NNaO_3.H_2O$	Amfenac Sodium
$C_{15}H_{12}N_2O$	Benhepazone
$C_{15}H_{12}N_2O$	Carbamazepine
$C_{15}H_{12}N_2O.HCl$	Nafimidone Hydrochloride
$C_{15}H_{12}N_2O_2$	Oxcarbazepine
$C_{15}H_{12}N_2O_2$	Phenytoin
$C_{15}H_{12}O_3$	Idronoxil
$C_{15}H_{12}O_5$	Tucaresol
$C_{15}H_{13}ClFNO_2$	Lumiracoxib
$C_{15}H_{13}ClNNaO_3.2H_2O$	Zomepirac Sodium
$C_{15}H_{13}ClN_2$	Chlormidazole
$C_{15}H_{13}ClN_2O$	Lofendazam
$C_{15}H_{13}Cl_2N_5.HCl$	Robenidine Hydrochloride
$C_{15}H_{13}FO_2$	Esflurbiprofen
$C_{15}H_{13}FO_2$	Fluprofen
$C_{15}H_{13}FO_2$	Flurbiprofen
$C_{15}H_{13}FO_2$	Tarenflurbil
$C_{15}H_{13}F_3N_2O_2$	Laflunimus
$C_{15}H_{13}NO_2S$	Metiazinic Acid
$C_{15}H_{13}NO_3$	Pranoprofen

Molecular Formula	Non-proprietary Name
$C_{15}H_{13}NO_3.C_4H_{11}NO_3$	Ketorolac Tromethamine
$C_{15}H_{13}NO_3S_2$	Epalrestat
$C_{15}H_{13}NO_4$	Acetaminosalol
$C_{15}H_{13}N_3O_2.C_4H_{11}NO_3$	Prinomide Tromethamine
$C_{15}H_{13}N_3O_2S$	Fenbendazole
$C_{15}H_{13}N_3O_2S$	Frentizole
$C_{15}H_{13}N_3O_3S$	Oxfendazole
$C_{15}H_{13}N_3O_4$	Aconiazide
$C_{15}H_{13}N_3O_4S$	Piroxicam
$C_{15}H_{13}N_3O_4S.C_2H_7NO$	Piroxicam Olamine
$(C_{15}H_{13}N_3O_4S)_2.(C_{42}H_{70}O_{35})_5$	Piroxicam Betadex
$C_{15}H_{13}N_5O_4$	Leteprinim
$C_{15}H_{14}ClNO_4S$	Aclantate
$C_{15}H_{14}ClN_3O.C_4H_4O_4$	Dazadrol Maleate
$C_{15}H_{14}ClN_3O_3$	Sarmazenil
$C_{15}H_{14}ClN_3O_4S.H_2O$	Cefaclor
$C_{15}H_{14}ClN_3O_4S_3$	Benzthiazide
$C_{15}H_{14}ClN_3O_6$	Acreozast
$C_{15}H_{14}ClN_3O_6$	Lodoxamide Ethyl
$C_{15}H_{14}FNO_3$	Ibafloxacin
$C_{15}H_{14}FN_3O_3$	Flumazenil
$C_{15}H_{14}F_3N_3O_3S$	Galosemide
$C_{15}H_{14}F_3N_3O_4S_2$	Bendroflumethiazide
$C_{15}H_{14}{}^{123}IN_3O_3$	Iomazenil (^{123}I)
$C_{15}H_{14}NNaO_3.2H_2O$	Tolmetin Sodium
$C_{15}H_{14}N_2Na_2O_6S_2$	Ticarcillin Disodium
$C_{15}H_{14}N_2O$	Doxenitoin
$C_{15}H_{14}N_2O$	Semaxanib
$C_{15}H_{14}N_2O_2$	Eslicarbazepine
$C_{15}H_{14}N_2O_2$	Licarbazepine
$C_{15}H_{14}N_2O_2$	Nepafenac
$C_{15}H_{14}N_2O_3$	Anilamate
$C_{15}H_{14}N_2O_4S$	Belinostat
$C_{15}H_{14}N_4O$	Fepitrizol
$C_{15}H_{14}N_4O$	Nevirapine
$C_{15}H_{14}N_4O$	Senazodan
$C_{15}H_{14}N_4O_2S$	Sulfaphenazole
$C_{15}H_{14}N_4O_6S_2$	Ceftibuten
$C_{15}H_{14}N_6O$	Meribendan
$C_{15}H_{14}N_8O_5S_4$	Cefmatilen
$C_{15}H_{14}O_3$	Fenoprofen
$C_{15}H_{14}O_3$	Mexenone
$C_{15}H_{14}O_4$	Furacrinic Acid
$C_{15}H_{14}O_4$	Menbutone
$C_{15}H_{14}O_5S$	Timefurone
$C_{15}H_{14}O_6$	Cianidanol
$C_{15}H_{14}O_7$	Leucocianidol
$C_{15}H_{15}BrN_2$	Nomelidine
$C_{15}H_{15}ClFNO$	Halonamine
$C_{15}H_{15}ClN_2O$	Nortetrazepam
$C_{15}H_{15}ClN_2O_4S$	Xipamide
$C_{15}H_{15}Cl_2N_2NaO_8$	Chloramphenicol Sodium Succinate
$C_{15}H_{15}Cl_2N_3O$	Endixaprine
$C_{15}H_{15}FN_4O.HCl$	Zolazepam Hydrochloride
$C_{15}H_{15}F_2NO$	Flunamine
$C_{15}H_{15}I_3NNaO_3$	Bunamiodyl Sodium
$C_{15}H_{15}I_3N_2O_6$	Ethyl Cartrizoate
$C_{15}H_{15}NO$	Oletimol
$C_{15}H_{15}NO_2$	Enfenamic Acid
$C_{15}H_{15}NO_2$	Mefenamic Acid
$C_{15}H_{15}NO_2$	Nafoxadol
$C_{15}H_{15}NO_2S$	Armodafinil
$C_{15}H_{15}NO_2S$	Modafinil
$C_{15}H_{15}NO_3$	Tolmetin
$C_{15}H_{15}NO_3S$	Adrafinil

Molecular Formula	Non-proprietary Name
$C_{15}H_{15}NO_4$	Zelandopam
$C_{15}H_{15}N_2NaO_6S_2.H_2O$	Ticarcillin Monosodium
$C_{15}H_{15}N_3O$	Nanterinone
$C_{15}H_{15}N_3O$	Premazepam
$C_{15}H_{15}N_3O.C_3H_6O_3.H_2O$	Ethacridine Lactate
$C_{15}H_{15}N_3O_2$	Tacedinaline
$C_{15}H_{15}N_3O_3$	Verazide
$C_{15}H_{15}N_7O_4S_3$	Cefivitril
$C_{15}H_{16}ClNO$	Setazindol
$C_{15}H_{16}ClNO_4$	Romazarit
$C_{15}H_{16}ClN_3O$	Lodaxaprine
$C_{15}H_{16}ClN_3O_3S$	Besulpamide
$C_{15}H_{16}ClN_3O_3S$	Glyparamide
$C_{15}H_{16}ClN_3O_4S_2$	Bemetizide
$C_{15}H_{16}ClN_3O_4S_3$	Hydrobentizide
$C_{15}H_{16}ClN_3S$	Tolonium Chloride
$C_{15}H_{16}Cl_3N_5$	Sipatrigine
$C_{15}H_{16}I_3NO_3$	Iolidonic Acid
$C_{15}H_{16}I_3NO_5$	Iobutoic Acid
$C_{15}H_{16}I_3N_3O_7$	Ioseric Acid
$C_{15}H_{16}N_2O$	Ameltolide
$C_{15}H_{16}N_2O$	Benmoxin
$C_{15}H_{16}N_2O$	Picobenzide
$C_{15}H_{16}N_2O_2$	Nafagrel
$C_{15}H_{16}N_2O_3$	Camonagrel
$C_{15}H_{16}N_2O_4$	Apaziquone
$C_{15}H_{16}N_2S$	Tienocarbine
$C_{15}H_{16}N_4O$	Ripazepam
$C_{15}H_{16}N_4O_2$	Nicaraven
$C_{15}H_{16}N_4O_2$	Zomebazam
$C_{15}H_{16}N_4O_3$	Melquinast
$C_{15}H_{16}N_6O$	Amicarbalide
$C_{15}H_{16}N_7NaO_5S_3$	Cefmetazole Sodium
$C_{15}H_{16}O_2$	Nabumetone
$C_{15}H_{16}O_6S$	Odiparcil
$C_{15}H_{16}O_8S_2$	Dicresulene
$C_{15}H_{17}BrN_2O_2$	Benzpyrinium Bromide
$C_{15}H_{17}ClFNO_4S$	Resatorvid
$C_{15}H_{17}ClN_2O_2$	Climbazole
$C_{15}H_{17}ClN_2O_2$	Lortalamine
$C_{15}H_{17}Cl_2NO_2$	Bemesetron
$C_{15}H_{17}FN_4O_2.C_4H_4O_4$	Flupirtine Maleate
$C_{15}H_{17}FN_4O_3$	Enoxacin
$C_{15}H_{17}FN_4O_3$	Esafloxacin
$C_{15}H_{17}I_3NNaO_3$	Tyropanoate Sodium
$C_{15}H_{17}N$	Dibemethine
$C_{15}H_{17}NO_2$	Agomelatine
$C_{15}H_{17}NO_3$	Ilepcimide
$C_{15}H_{17}NS_2$	Tipepidine
$C_{15}H_{17}N_3O$	Metralindole
$C_{15}H_{17}N_3O.HCl$	Cetoxime Hydrochloride
$C_{15}H_{17}N_3O_2S$	Pumosetrag
$C_{15}H_{17}N_3O_6S$	Betiatide
$C_{15}H_{17}N_5O$	Bemitradine
$C_{15}H_{17}N_5S.C_4H_4O_4$	Pentiapine Maleate
$C_{15}H_{17}N_7O_5S_3$	Cefmetazole
$C_{15}H_{17}NaO_3S$	Sodium Gualenate
$C_{15}H_{18}BrN_5O$	Broperamole
$C_{15}H_{18}Br_2N_4O_2$	Trimedoxime Bromide
$C_{15}H_{18}ClNO_3$	Enilospirone
$C_{15}H_{18}ClN_3O_2$	Famiraprinium Chloride
$C_{15}H_{18}ClN_3O_3S.HCl$	Tiaramide Hydrochloride
$C_{15}H_{18}Cl_2N_4O_3$	Ridazolol
$C_{15}H_{18}Cl_2N_2O_5$	Dichloralphenazone
$C_{15}H_{18}F_2N_6O_7S_2$	Flomoxef
$C_{15}H_{18}F_3NO$	Lanperisone

Molecular Formula	Non-proprietary Name
$C_{15}H_{18}F_3NO_5$	Befloxatone
$C_{15}H_{18}I_3NO_5$	Iolixanic Acid
$C_{15}H_{18}I_3NO_5$	Iopronic Acid
$C_{15}H_{18}N_2$	Pirlindole
$C_{15}H_{18}N_2O$	Isoprazone
$C_{15}H_{18}N_2O_2$	Propoxate
$C_{15}H_{18}N_2O_3$	Terbequinil
$C_{15}H_{18}N_4O_4S$	Biapenem
$C_{15}H_{18}N_4O_5$	Mitomycin
$C_{15}H_{18}N_6O_2$	Pimefylline
$C_{15}H_{18}N_8O_5.H_2O$	Regadenoson
$C_{15}H_{18}O_2$	Tetriprofen
$C_{15}H_{18}O_3$	Irofulven
$C_{15}H_{18}O_3$	Loxoprofen
$C_{15}H_{18}O_3$	Santonin
$C_{15}H_{18}O_3S$	Egualen
$C_{15}H_{18}O_5$	Raxofelast
$C_{15}H_{18}O_7.C_{15}H_{16}O_6$	Picrotoxin
$C_{15}H_{19}BrN_2O_5$	Mebrofenin
$C_{15}H_{19}Cl_2N_3O_4$	Maribavir
$C_{15}H_{19}FN_2O_2$	Fluzoperine
$C_{15}H_{19}F_3N_2S$	Ticarbodine
$C_{15}H_{19}NO$	Furfenorex
$C_{15}H_{19}NO$	Pronetalol
$C_{15}H_{19}NO_2$	Tasimelteon
$C_{15}H_{19}NO_3$	Ximoprofen
$C_{15}H_{19}NO_3S_2.C_6H_{14}N_4O_2$	Zofenoprilat Arginine
$C_{15}H_{19}NO_4S$	Bencisteine
$C_{15}H_{19}NO_4S_2$	Guaisteine
$C_{15}H_{19}NO_6$	Esculamine
$C_{15}H_{19}NS_2$	Ethylmethylthiambutene
$C_{15}H_{19}N_3OS.HCl$	Butamisole Hydrochloride
$C_{15}H_{19}N_3O_2S$	Dribendazole
$C_{15}H_{19}N_3O_4$	Abunidazole
$C_{15}H_{19}N_3O_4$	Tropabazate
$C_{15}H_{19}N_3O_5$	Carboquone
$C_{15}H_{19}N_5$	Naminidil
$C_{15}H_{19}N_5.C_7H_6O_2$	Rizatriptan Benzoate
$(C_{15}H_{19}N_5)_2.H_2SO_4.H_2O$	Rizatriptan Sulfate
$C_{15}H_{20}ClN_3O_2.HCl.H_2O$	Zacopride Hydrochloride
$C_{15}H_{20}ClN_5.HCl$	Spirotriazine Hydrochloride
$C_{15}H_{20}Cl_2N_2O$	Clibucaine
$C_{15}H_{20}FNO$	Primaperone
$C_{15}H_{20}NNaO_4$	Salcaprozate Sodium
$C_{15}H_{20}N_2$	Indalpine
$C_{15}H_{20}N_2.HCl$	Vabicaserin Hydrochloride
$C_{15}H_{20}N_2O$	Felipyrine
$C_{15}H_{20}N_2O_2.HCl$	Fenspiride Hydrochloride
$C_{15}H_{20}N_2O_2.HCl$	Oxamisole Hydrochloride
$C_{15}H_{20}N_2O_3$	Pifoxime
$C_{15}H_{20}N_2O_3S_2$	Talviraline
$C_{15}H_{20}N_2O_4$	Filaminast
$C_{15}H_{20}N_2O_4S$	Acetohexamide
$C_{15}H_{20}N_2O_4S$	Sumacetamol
$C_{15}H_{20}N_2O_5$	Iprofenin
$C_{15}H_{20}N_2S.HCl$	Methaphenilene Hydrochloride
$C_{15}H_{20}N_6O_4$	Azetirelin
$C_{15}H_{20}O_2$	Hexaprofen
$C_{15}H_{20}O_2$	Isoprofen
$C_{15}H_{20}O_3$	Amiloxate
$C_{15}H_{21}BrN_2O.C_4H_4O_4$	Bromadoline Maleate
$C_{15}H_{21}ClN_6$	Lesopitron
$C_{15}H_{21}Cl_2N_3O$	Acaprazine
$C_{15}H_{21}FN_6O$	Melogliptin
$C_{15}H_{21}F_3N_2O_2.C_4H_4O_4$	Fluvoxamine Maleate
$C_{15}H_{21}{}^{123}IN_2O_3$	Iolopride (^{123}I)
$C_{15}H_{21}N.HCl$	Fencamfamin Hydrochloride
$C_{15}H_{21}NO$	Eptazocine
$C_{15}H_{21}NO$	Metazocine
$C_{15}H_{21}NO$	Tofetridine
$C_{15}H_{21}NO_2$	Ciclonicate
$C_{15}H_{21}NO_2$	Indenolol
$C_{15}H_{21}NO_2$	Ketobemidone
$C_{15}H_{21}NO_2$	Tolpronine
$C_{15}H_{21}NO_2.HCl$	Ciclafrine Hydrochloride
$C_{15}H_{21}NO_2.HCl$	Isomolpan Hydrochloride
$C_{15}H_{21}NO_2.HCl$	Meperidine Hydrochloride
$C_{15}H_{21}NO_2.HCl$	Naxagolide Hydrochloride
$C_{15}H_{21}NO_2.HCl$	Prodilidine Hydrochloride
$C_{15}H_{21}NO_3$	Hydroxypethidine
$C_{15}H_{21}NO_3$	Metostilenol
$C_{15}H_{21}NO_4$	Afurolol
$C_{15}H_{21}NO_4$	Salcaprozic Acid
$C_{15}H_{21}N_3O$	Cizolirtine
$C_{15}H_{21}N_3O$	Etoprindole
$C_{15}H_{21}N_3O$	Quinocide
$C_{15}H_{21}N_3O.2H_3PO_4$	Primaquine Phosphate
$C_{15}H_{21}N_3OS.HCl$	Zolamine Hydrochloride
$C_{15}H_{21}N_3O_2$	Physostigmine
$C_{15}H_{21}N_3O_2.C_7H_6O_3$	Physostigmine Salicylate
$(C_{15}H_{21}N_3O_2)_2.H_2SO_4$	Physostigmine Sulfate
$C_{15}H_{21}N_3O_2S_3$	Arotinolol
$C_{15}H_{21}N_3O_3$	Eseridine
$C_{15}H_{21}N_3O_3S$	Gliclazide
$C_{15}H_{21}N_3O_4S$	Panipenem
$C_{15}H_{21}N_5O_2$	Aditoprim
$C_{15}H_{21}N_5O_4$	Riboprine
$C_{15}H_{22}FN_3O_4.H_2SO_4$	Flestolol Sulfate
$C_{15}H_{22}FN_3O_6$	Capecitabine
$C_{15}H_{22}N_2$	Etaminile
$C_{15}H_{22}N_2O$	Dexivacaine
$C_{15}H_{22}N_2O$	Levomilnacipran
$C_{15}H_{22}N_2O.HCl$	Mepivacaine Hydrochloride
$C_{15}H_{22}N_2O.HCl$	Milnacipran Hydrochloride
$C_{15}H_{22}N_2O.HCl.2H_2O$	Piquindone Hydrochloride
$C_{15}H_{22}N_2O_2$	Dabelotine
$C_{15}H_{22}N_2O_2$	Mepindolol
$C_{15}H_{22}N_2O_2$	Mixidine
$C_{15}H_{22}N_2O_2$	Penirolol
$C_{15}H_{22}N_2O_2.HCl$	Alprenoxime Hydrochloride
$C_{15}H_{22}N_2O_3$	Tolycaine
$C_{15}H_{22}N_2O_3S$	Heptolamide
$C_{15}H_{22}N_2O_4$	Troxipide
$C_{15}H_{22}N_2O_6$	Nipradilol
$C_{15}H_{22}N_4O_2$	Cartazolate
$C_{15}H_{22}N_4O_3$	Propentofylline
$C_{15}H_{22}N_6O_5S$	Ademetionine
$C_{15}H_{22}OS$	Tioctilate
$C_{15}H_{22}O_3$	Gemfibrozil
$C_{15}H_{22}O_3$	Octisalate
$C_{15}H_{22}O_5$	Artemisinin
$C_{15}H_{23}ClN_4O_2.C_4H_4O_4$	Dazopride Fumarate
$C_{15}H_{23}N.HCl$	Prolintane Hydrochloride
$C_{15}H_{23}NO$	Faxeladol
$C_{15}H_{23}NO.HCl$	Meptazinol Hydrochloride
$C_{15}H_{23}NO_2$	Ciramadol
$C_{15}H_{23}NO_2$	Mabuprofen
$C_{15}H_{23}NO_2$	Procinolol
$C_{15}H_{23}NO_2.HCl$	Alprenolol Hydrochloride
$C_{15}H_{23}NO_2.HCl$	Ciramadol Hydrochloride
$C_{15}H_{23}NO_2.HCl$	Isobucaine Hydrochloride
$C_{15}H_{23}NO_3$	Etilefrine Pivalate

Molecular Formula	Non-proprietary Name
$C_{15}H_{23}NO_3.HCl$	Ethomoxane Hydrochloride
$C_{15}H_{23}NO_3.HCl$	Oxprenolol Hydrochloride
$C_{15}H_{23}NO_3.HCl$	Parethoxycaine Hydrochloride
$C_{15}H_{23}NO_3.HCl$	Trimoxamine Hydrochloride
$C_{15}H_{23}NO_4$	Cycloheximide
$C_{15}H_{23}NO_4$	Roxadimate
$C_{15}H_{23}NS$	Tenocyclidine
$C_{15}H_{23}N_3$	Iquindamine
$C_{15}H_{23}N_3OS$	Diamthazole
$C_{15}H_{23}N_3O_2.HCl$	Acecainide Hydrochloride
$C_{15}H_{23}N_3O_3S$	Amdinocillin
$C_{15}H_{23}N_3O_4$	Safironil
$C_{15}H_{23}N_3O_4S$	Cyclacillin
$C_{15}H_{23}N_3O_4S$	Isosulpride
$C_{15}H_{23}N_3O_4S$	Levosulpiride
$C_{15}H_{23}N_3O_4S$	Sulpiride
$C_{15}H_{23}N_7O_5$	Sinefungin
$C_{15}H_{24}FNSi$	Silperisone
$C_{15}H_{24}N_2O$	Morforex
$C_{15}H_{24}N_2O$	Trimecaine
$C_{15}H_{24}N_2O_2$	Dimetholizine
$C_{15}H_{24}N_2O_2$	Tetracaine
$C_{15}H_{24}N_2O_2.HCl$	Tetracaine Hydrochloride
$C_{15}H_{24}N_2O_3$	Hydroxytetracaine
$C_{15}H_{24}N_2O_3$	Mefexamide
$C_{15}H_{24}N_2O_4S$	Tiapride
$C_{15}H_{24}N_4$	Nonapyrimine
$C_{15}H_{24}N_4O_2S_2$	Prosultiamine
$C_{15}H_{24}N_4O_6.2HCl$	Valopicitabine Dihydrochloride
$C_{15}H_{24}N_4O_6S_2$	Doripenem
$C_{15}H_{24}N_6O_4$	Valomaciclovir
$C_{15}H_{24}O$	Butylated Hydroxytoluene
$C_{15}H_{24}O(C_2H_4O)_n$	
(n = approximately 9)	Nonoxynol 9
$C_{15}H_{24}O_5$	Artenimol
$C_{15}H_{25}N$	Amfepentorex
$C_{15}H_{25}NO_2$	Edronocaine
$C_{15}H_{25}NO_2$	Xibenolol
$C_{15}H_{25}NO_3$	Metoprolol
$C_{15}H_{25}NO_3$	Piraxelate
$(C_{15}H_{25}NO_3)_2.C_4H_4O_4$	Metoprolol Fumarate
$(C_{15}H_{25}NO_3)_2.C_4H_6O_4$	Metoprolol Succinate
$(C_{15}H_{25}NO_3)_2.C_4H_6O_6$	Metoprolol Tartrate
$C_{15}H_{25}NO_3.HCl$	Butoxamine Hydrochloride
$C_{15}H_{25}N_3O$	Caproxamine
$C_{15}H_{25}N_3O.(CH_4O_3S)_2$	Lisdexamfetamine Dimesylate
$C_{15}H_{25}N_3O.HCl$	Recainam Hydrochloride
$C_{15}H_{25}N_5O_3$	Rociclovir
$C_{15}H_{26}N_2.H_2SO_4.5H_2O$	Sparteine Sulfate
$C_{15}H_{26}O$	Levomenol
$C_{15}H_{27}N_3O_4S_2.HCl$	Risotilide Hydrochloride
$C_{15}H_{28}N_4O_4.3H_2O$	Peramivir
$C_{15}H_{29}NO_4$	Dioxamate
$C_{15}H_{29}N_3O_5$	Marimastat
$C_{15}H_{30}O_3$	Trethocanoic Acid
$C_{15}H_{31}NO$	Octapinol
$C_{15}H_{31}NO_2$	Tradecamide
$C_{15}H_{32}N_2O.2HNO_3$	Pemerid Nitrate
$C_{15}H_{33}NO$	Laurixamine
$(C_{15}H_{37}NO_5Si_4)_w(C_6H_9NO)_x$	
$(C_{68}H_{184}O_{32}Si_{27})_y$	
$(C_6H_9NO_4)_z$	Balafilcon A
$C_{16}H_6Cl_3F_3N_6$	Fampronil
$C_{16}H_8N_2Na_2O_8S_2$	Indigotindisulfonate Sodium
$C_{16}H_8N_2O_5$	Pirenoxine
$C_{16}H_9F_3O_2$	Fluindarol

Molecular Formula	Non-proprietary Name
$C_{16}H_{10}ClF_3N_2O$	Fluquazone
$C_{16}H_{10}ClF_4NO_2$	Flindokalner
$C_{16}H_{10}ClKN_2O_3$	Clorazepate Monopotassium
$C_{16}H_{10}ClN_3$	Lotrifen
$C_{16}H_{10}KN_3O_5$	Potassium Nitrazepate
$C_{16}H_{10}O_4$	Xenygloxal
$C_{16}H_{11}ClK_2N_2O_4$	Clorazepate Dipotassium
$C_{16}H_{11}ClN_2O_3$	Tesicam
$C_{16}H_{11}ClN_4$	Estazolam
$C_{16}H_{11}F_4N_3O_2S$	Mavacoxib
$C_{16}H_{11}NO_2$	Benzoxiquine
$C_{16}H_{11}NO_2$	Cinchophen
$C_{16}H_{11}NO_3$	Oxycinchophen
$C_{16}H_{11}N_3O_5S$	Droxicam
$C_{16}H_{11}O_8P$	Foscolic Acid
$C_{16}H_{12}ClFN_2O$	Fludiazepam
$C_{16}H_{12}ClFN_2O_2$	Flutemazepam
$C_{16}H_{12}ClNO_3$	Benoxaprofen
$C_{16}H_{12}ClN_3O_3$	Meclonazepam
$C_{16}H_{12}Cl_2N_2O$	Cloroqualone
$C_{16}H_{12}Cl_2N_2O_2$	Lormetazepam
$C_{16}H_{12}Cl_2O_3$	Clofenoxyde
$C_{16}H_{12}Cl_2O_4$	Treloxinate
$C_{16}H_{12}FNO_3$	Flunoxaprofen
$C_{16}H_{12}FN_3O_3$	Flubendazole
$C_{16}H_{12}FN_3O_3$	Flunitrazepam
$C_{16}H_{12}N_2O_2$	Diftalone
$C_{16}H_{12}N_4O_5S_2$	Salazosulfathiazole
$C_{16}H_{12}O_3$	Anisindione
$C_{16}H_{12}O_3S$	Tiopinac
$C_{16}H_{12}O_4$	Furobufen
$C_{16}H_{12}O_4$	Isoxepac
$C_{16}H_{12}O_4$	Oxepinac
$C_{16}H_{12}O_6$	Kalafungin
$C_{16}H_{13}ClFN_3O_3S$	Cimicoxib
$C_{16}H_{13}ClN_2O$	Diazepam
$C_{16}H_{13}ClN_2O$	Mazindol
$C_{16}H_{13}ClN_2O_2$	Clobazam
$C_{16}H_{13}ClN_2O_2$	Temazepam
$C_{16}H_{13}ClN_2O_2$	Tolnidamine
$C_{16}H_{13}ClN_2O_4S$	Suclofenide
$C_{16}H_{13}ClN_2S$	Sulazepam
$C_{16}H_{13}ClN_6$	Vorozole
$C_{16}H_{13}Cl_2NO_4$	Aceclofenac
$C_{16}H_{13}Cl_2NO_4$	Quinfamide
$C_{16}H_{13}Cl_2N_3O$	Benclonidine
$C_{16}H_{13}Cl_3N_2OS$	Tioconazole
$C_{16}H_{13}FN_2O_3$	Irloxacin
$C_{16}H_{13}F_2NO_4S$	Flosulide
$C_{16}H_{13}F_3N_2O_3$	Colfenamate
$C_{16}H_{13}F_4NO_2$	Robenacoxib
$C_{16}H_{13}I_3N_2O_3$	Iobenzamic Acid
$C_{16}H_{13}NO$	Citenamide
$C_{16}H_{13}NO_2S$	Tazeprofen
$C_{16}H_{13}NO_4$	Papaveroline
$C_{16}H_{13}N_2Na_2O_6P$	Fosphenytoin Sodium
$C_{16}H_{13}N_3O_3$	Mebendazole
$C_{16}H_{13}N_3O_3$	Nimetazepam
$C_{16}H_{13}N_3O_4$	Nitraquazone
$C_{16}H_{13}N_3O_6$	Ipsalazide
$C_{16}H_{14}ClNO.HCl$	Famotine Hydrochloride
$C_{16}H_{14}ClN_3O$	Chlordiazepoxide
$C_{16}H_{14}ClN_3O.HCl$	Chlordiazepoxide Hydrochloride
$C_{16}H_{14}Cl_2O$	Proclonol
$C_{16}H_{14}Cl_2O_3$	Dulofibrate

Molecular Formula	*Non-proprietary Name*
$C_{16}H_{14}FN_3O$	Afloqualone
$C_{16}H_{14}F_2N_3NaO_4S.1.5H_2O$	Pantoprazole Sodium
$C_{16}H_{14}F_3NO_3S$	Tolrestat
$C_{16}H_{14}F_3N_3O_2S$	Dexlansoprazole
$C_{16}H_{14}F_3N_3O_2S$	Lansoprazole
$C_{16}H_{14}F_3N_3O_2S$	Levolansoprazole
$C_{16}H_{14}F_3N_5O$	Voriconazole
$C_{16}H_{14}N_2O$	Methaqualone
$C_{16}H_{14}N_2O.HCl$	Methaqualone Hydrochloride
$C_{16}H_{14}N_2O_2$	Doliracetam
$C_{16}H_{14}N_2O_2$	Miroprofen
$C_{16}H_{14}N_2O_3$	Bendazac
$C_{16}H_{14}N_2O_3S$	Valdecoxib
$C_{16}H_{14}N_2O_4$	Amlexanox
$C_{16}H_{14}N_2O_6S$	Phthalylsulfacetamide
$C_{16}H_{14}N_4O$	Adibendan
$C_{16}H_{14}OS_2$	Tenylidone
$C_{16}H_{14}O_2$	Cicloprofen
$C_{16}H_{14}O_3$	Dexketoprofen
$C_{16}H_{14}O_3$	Fenbufen
$C_{16}H_{14}O_3$	Ketoprofen
$(C_{16}H_{14}O_3)_x(C_2H_6OSi)_y$ $(C_5H_8O_2)_z$	Carbosilfocon A
$C_{16}H_{14}O_4$	Bakeprofen
$C_{16}H_{14}O_5$	Guacetisal
$C_{16}H_{14}O_5$	Guaimesal
$C_{16}H_{14}O_6$	Nanafrocin
$C_{16}H_{15}ClFN_3O_2$	Clanfenur
$C_{16}H_{15}ClN_2.HCl$	Medazepam Hydrochloride
$C_{16}H_{15}ClN_2OS$	Clotiazepam
$C_{16}H_{15}ClN_2O_3S$	Sulofenur
$C_{16}H_{15}ClN_2S$	Etasuline
$C_{16}H_{15}ClN_4O_2S$	Sulfaclorazole
$C_{16}H_{15}ClO_6$	Lonapalene
$C_{16}H_{15}Cl_2N$	Indatraline
$C_{16}H_{15}FN_2O_2S$	Atreleuton
$C_{16}H_{15}FN_2O_4$	Pazufloxacin
$C_{16}H_{15}FO$	Enofelast
$C_{16}H_{15}F_2N_3O_4S$	Pantoprazole
$C_{16}H_{15}F_3O$	Flumecinol
$C_{16}H_{15}F_6N_5O.H_3O_4P.H_2O$	Sitagliptin Phosphate
$C_{16}H_{15}N.C_4H_4O_4$	Dizocilpine Maleate
$C_{16}H_{15}NO$	Cyheptamide
$C_{16}H_{15}NO_2$	Tesimide
$C_{16}H_{15}NO_3$	Dilmefone
$C_{16}H_{15}NO_3$	Ftaxilide
$C_{16}H_{15}NO_4$	Anirolac
$C_{16}H_{15}NO_4$	Araprofen
$C_{16}H_{15}N_2NaO_6S_2$	Cephalothin Sodium
$C_{16}H_{15}N_3$	Epinastine
$C_{16}H_{15}N_3O$	Nicotredole
$C_{16}H_{15}N_3OS$	Tanaproget
$C_{16}H_{15}N_3O_4$	Mitonafide
$C_{16}H_{15}N_3O_5$	Opiniazide
$C_{16}H_{15}N_3O_5$	Pirolate
$C_{16}H_{15}N_3O_7S$	Sulfaloxic Acid
$C_{16}H_{15}N_4NaO_8S$	Cefuroxime Sodium
$C_{16}H_{15}N_5O_2$	Trizoxime
$C_{16}H_{15}N_5O_4S_3$	Cefetrizole
$C_{16}H_{15}N_5O_7S_2.3H_2O$	Cefixime
$C_{16}H_{15}N_7O_5S_4$	Cefuzonam
$C_{16}H_{16}ClHgN_2NaO_6$	Merbaphen
$C_{16}H_{16}ClNO_2$	Nicoclonate
$C_{16}H_{16}ClNO_2S.H_2SO_4$	Clopidogrel Bisulfate

Molecular Formula	*Non-proprietary Name*
$C_{16}H_{16}ClNO_3$	Clofeverine
$C_{16}H_{16}ClNO_3$	Nicofibrate
$C_{16}H_{16}ClNO_3.CH_4SO_3$	Fenoldopam Mesylate
$C_{16}H_{16}ClNO_4S$	Daltroban
$C_{16}H_{16}ClN_3O_3$	Indapamide
$C_{16}H_{16}ClN_3O_3S$	Metolazone
$C_{16}H_{16}ClN_3O_3S$	Zidapamide
$C_{16}H_{16}ClN_3O_4.H_2O$	Loracarbef
$C_{16}H_{16}ClN_3O_5S$	Cefedrolor
$C_{16}H_{16}ClN_5O.HCl.H_2O$	Fenprinast Hydrochloride
$C_{16}H_{16}FNO$	Fenisorex
$C_{16}H_{16}FN_3O_3S$	Ulifloxacin
$C_{16}H_{16}F_3NO.HCl$	Seproxetine Hydrochloride
$C_{16}H_{16}{}^2H_7NO$	Deutolperisone
$C_{16}H_{16}NO_6P$	Naftalofos
$C_{16}H_{16}N_2OS$	Dacemazine
$C_{16}H_{16}N_2O_2$	Nafazatrom
$C_{16}H_{16}N_2O_3S$	Febuxostat
$C_{16}H_{16}N_2O_4S$	Acedapsone
$C_{16}H_{16}N_2O_5S$	Succisulfone
$C_{16}H_{16}N_3NaO_7S_2$	Cefoxitin Sodium
$C_{16}H_{16}N_4O.2C_2H_6O_4S$	Hydroxystilbamidine Isethionate
$C_{16}H_{16}N_4O_2S$	Sulfazamet
$C_{16}H_{16}N_4O_5$	Nifurquinazol
$C_{16}H_{16}N_4O_8S$	Cefuroxime
$C_{16}H_{16}N_5NaO_7S_2$	Cefotaxime Sodium
$C_{16}H_{16}N_6Na_2O_{12}S_2Tc_2$	Technetium Tc 99m Tiatide
$C_{16}H_{16}O_2$	Naphthonone
$C_{16}H_{16}O_2$	Xenbucin
$C_{16}H_{16}O_2.C_4H_{11}NO$	Namoxyrate
$C_{16}H_{16}O_2.C_{12}H_{17}N$	Butixirate
$C_{16}H_{16}O_3$	Parvaquone
$C_{16}H_{16}O_6$	Meciadanol
$C_{16}H_{17}BrClN_3O_3.HBr$	Halofuginone Hydrobromide
$C_{16}H_{17}BrN_2.2HCl.H_2O$	Zimeldine Hydrochloride
$C_{16}H_{17}ClN_2O$	Tetrazepam
$C_{16}H_{17}ClN_2O_4$	Clonixeril
$C_{16}H_{17}FN_2S$	Tiflucarbine
$C_{16}H_{17}F_2N.HCl$	Delucemine Hydrochloride
$C_{16}H_{17}KN_2O_4S$	Penicillin G Potassium
$C_{16}H_{17}KN_2O_4S_2$	Thiphencillin Potassium
$C_{16}H_{17}KN_2O_5S$	Penicillin V Potassium
$C_{16}H_{17}NO_3$	Normorphine
$C_{16}H_{17}NO_5S$	Sulotroban
$C_{16}H_{17}N_2NaO_4S$	Penicillin G Sodium
$C_{16}H_{17}N_3$	Midaglizole
$C_{16}H_{17}N_3.HCl$	Besipirdine Hydrochloride
$C_{16}H_{17}N_3Na_2O_5$	Oglufanide Disodium
$C_{16}H_{17}N_3Na_2O_7S_2$	Suncillin Sodium
$C_{16}H_{17}N_3OS$	Bepiastine
$C_{16}H_{17}N_3OS_2$	Disuprazole
$C_{16}H_{17}N_3O_2$	Amonafide
$C_{16}H_{17}N_3O_2$	Dazmegrel
$C_{16}H_{17}N_3O_3$	Menitrazepam
$C_{16}H_{17}N_3O_3$	Niraxostat
$C_{16}H_{17}N_3O_4$	Anthramycin
$C_{16}H_{17}N_3O_4S.HCl.H_2O$	Cephalexin Hydrochloride
$C_{16}H_{17}N_3O_4S.H_2O$	Cephalexin
$C_{16}H_{17}N_3O_5S.H_2O$	Cefadroxil
$C_{16}H_{17}N_3O_7S_2$	Cefoxitin
$C_{16}H_{17}N_5O_4S$	Azidocillin
$C_{16}H_{17}N_5O_8S_2$	Ceftioxide
$C_{16}H_{17}N_9O_5S_2$	Cefteram

Molecular Formula	Non-proprietary Name
$(C_{16}H_{17}N_9O_5S_3)_2.HCl$	Cefmenoxime Hydrochloride
$C_{16}H_{18}ClN$	Clobenzorex
$C_{16}H_{18}ClN_3O_3$	Cebaracetam
$C_{16}H_{18}ClN_3S.3H_2O$	Methylene Blue
$C_{16}H_{18}Cl_2N_2O_2$	Valconazole
$C_{16}H_{18}FN_3O_2$	Retigabine
$C_{16}H_{18}FN_3O_3$	Norfloxacin
$C_{16}H_{18}N_2$	Metapramine
$C_{16}H_{18}N_2.C_4H_4O_4$	Nomifensine Maleate
$C_{16}H_{18}N_2O_2$	Butanixin
$C_{16}H_{18}N_2O_2$	Domoxin
$C_{16}H_{18}N_2O_2$	Pimetremide
$C_{16}H_{18}N_2O_2.HNO_3$	Ethonam Nitrate
$C_{16}H_{18}N_2O_3$	Cromakalim
$C_{16}H_{18}N_2O_3$	Levcromakalim
$C_{16}H_{18}N_2O_4S$	Benzylpenicillin
$C_{16}H_{18}N_2O_4S$	Sulfaproxyline
$C_{16}H_{18}N_2O_4S.C_{13}H_{20}N_2O_2.H_2O$	Penicillin G Procaine
$C_{16}H_{18}N_2O_4S.C_{15}H_{17}N$	Benethamine Penicillin
$(C_{16}H_{18}N_2O_4S)_2.C_{16}H_{18}N_2$	Phenyracillin
$(C_{16}H_{18}N_2O_4S)_2.C_{16}H_{20}N_2.4H_2O$	Penicillin G Benzathine
$C_{16}H_{18}N_2O_5S$	Penicillin V
$(C_{16}H_{18}N_2O_5S)_2.C_{16}H_{20}N_2$	Penicillin V Benzathine
$(C_{16}H_{18}N_2O_5S)_2.C_{42}H_{64}N_2$	Penicillin V Hydrabamine
$C_{16}H_{18}N_2O_7S_2$	Sulbenicillin
$C_{16}H_{18}N_2O_7S_2$	Temocillin
$C_{16}H_{18}N_2S$	Fenethazine
$C_{16}H_{18}N_3NaO_4S$	Ampicillin Sodium
$C_{16}H_{18}N_3NaO_5S$	Amoxicillin Sodium
$C_{16}H_{18}N_4O_2$	Nialamide
$C_{16}H_{18}N_4O_2$	Piribedil
$C_{16}H_{18}N_4O_3S$	Tenatoprazole
$C_{16}H_{18}O_2$	Nafcaproic Acid
$C_{16}H_{18}O_3$	Fenocinol
$C_{16}H_{18}O_3$	Pelubiprofen
$C_{16}H_{18}O_6S$	Iliparcil
$C_{16}H_{19}BrN_2.C_4H_4O_4$	Brompheniramine Maleate
$C_{16}H_{19}BrN_2.C_4H_4O_4$	Dexbrompheniramine Maleate
$C_{16}H_{19}ClN_2$	Tepirindole
$C_{16}H_{19}ClN_2.C_4H_4O_4$	Chlorpheniramine Maleate
$C_{16}H_{19}ClN_2.C_4H_4O_4$	Dexchlorpheniramine Maleate
$C_{16}H_{19}ClN_2O$	Rotoxamine
$C_{16}H_{19}ClN_2O.C_4H_4O_4$	Carbinoxamine Maleate
$C_{16}H_{19}ClN_4O_2S$	Pirinixil
$C_{16}H_{19}ClO_2$	Clidanac
$C_{16}H_{19}ClO_3$	Bucloxic Acid
$C_{16}H_{19}Cl_2NO$	Mitoclomine
$C_{16}H_{19}FN_2O_3S$	Tilmacoxib
$C_{16}H_{19}FN_4O_3$	Amifloxacin
$C_{16}H_{19}FN_4O_3.CH_4O_3S$	Amifloxacin Mesylate
$C_{16}H_{19}N$	Lefetamine
$C_{16}H_{19}NO$	Litoxetine
$C_{16}H_{19}NO_2$	Medifoxamine
$C_{16}H_{19}NO_2S$	Teniloxazine
$C_{16}H_{19}NO_3$	Prodolic Acid
$C_{16}H_{19}NO_4$	Roletamide
$C_{16}H_{19}N_3.C_4H_4O_4$	Aptazapine Maleate
$C_{16}H_{19}N_3O_3$	Prazitone
$C_{16}H_{19}N_3O_4S$	Ampicillin
$C_{16}H_{19}N_3O_4S$	Cephradine
$C_{16}H_{19}N_3O_5S$	Cefroxadine
$C_{16}H_{19}N_3O_5S.3H_2O$	Amoxicillin
$C_{16}H_{19}N_3S.HCl$	Isothipendyl Hydrochloride
$C_{16}H_{19}N_3S.HCl$	Prothipendyl Hydrochloride
$C_{16}H_{19}N_4O_5$	Golotimod
$C_{16}H_{19}N_5O$	Pipofezine

Molecular Formula	Non-proprietary Name
$C_{16}H_{19}N_5O_2$	Dimabefylline
$C_{16}H_{19}N_7O_5$	Orotirelin
$C_{16}H_{20}BrNO$	Quindonium Bromide
$C_{16}H_{20}ClNO_5S$	Serfibrate
$C_{16}H_{20}ClN_3$	Chloropyramine
$C_{16}H_{20}ClN_3O_3S$	Tripamide
$C_{16}H_{20}ClN_3S$	Tivirapine
$C_{16}H_{20}Cl_2N_2O$	Brasofensine
$C_{16}H_{20}Cl_2N_2O.C_4H_4O_4$	Brasofensine Maleate
$C_{16}H_{20}FN_3O_4$	Linezolid
$C_{16}H_{20}{}^{123}INO_2$	Iometopane I 123
$C_{16}H_{20}I_3N_3O_7$	Iotriside
$C_{16}H_{20}N_2.C_4H_4O_4$	Pheniramine Maleate
$C_{16}H_{20}N_2OS$	Voxergolide
$C_{16}H_{20}N_2O_2$	Perisoxal
$C_{16}H_{20}N_2O_2S$	Tipindole
$C_{16}H_{20}N_2O_3$	Morsuximide
$C_{16}H_{20}N_2O_4$	Diarbarone
$C_{16}H_{20}N_2O_4S_2$	Pyritinol
$C_{16}H_{20}N_2O_5$	Eterobarb
$C_{16}H_{20}N_4O_2$	Apazone
$C_{16}H_{20}N_4O_2$	Itasetron
$C_{16}H_{20}N_4O_3S$	Torsemide
$C_{16}H_{20}N_4O_5$	Porfiromycin
$C_{16}H_{20}N_4O_6$	Diaziquone
$C_{16}H_{20}N_6.C_4H_4O_4$	Batelapine Maleate
$C_{16}H_{20}O_2$	Fenestrel
$C_{16}H_{20}O_3$	Hexacyprone
$C_{16}H_{20}O_6P_2S_3$	Temefos
$C_{16}H_{21}ClN_4$	Enpiprazole
$C_{16}H_{21}ClN_4$	Mepiprazole
$C_{16}H_{21}Cl_2N_3O_2.HCl$	Bendamustine Hydrochloride
$C_{16}H_{21}IN_2O_5$	Galtifenin
$C_{16}H_{21}N.C_4H_6O_4$	Tazadolene Succinate
$C_{16}H_{21}NO$	Norlevorphanol
$C_{16}H_{21}NO_2$	Ramelteon
$C_{16}H_{21}NO_2.HCl$	Dexpropranolol Hydrochloride
$C_{16}H_{21}NO_2.HCl$	Propranolol Hydrochloride
$C_{16}H_{21}NO_3$	Rolipram
$C_{16}H_{21}NO_3.HBr$	Homatropine Hydrobromide
$C_{16}H_{21}NO_4$	Befunolol
$C_{16}H_{21}NO_4S$	Risarestat
$C_{16}H_{21}NO_5S$	Moguisteine
$C_{16}H_{21}NS_2$	Diethylthiambutene
$C_{16}H_{21}N_3$	Deriglidole
$C_{16}H_{21}N_3.C_6H_8O_7$	Tripelennamine Citrate
$C_{16}H_{21}N_3.HCl$	Tripelennamine Hydrochloride
$C_{16}H_{21}N_3O_2$	Zolmitriptan
$C_{16}H_{21}N_3O_3$	Bamaquimast
$C_{16}H_{21}N_3O_3S$	Ramixotidine
$C_{16}H_{21}N_3O_4S$	Epicillin
$C_{16}H_{21}N_5O_2$	Alizapride
$C_{16}H_{21}N_7O_7S_3$	Cefminox
$C_{16}H_{22}ClN$	Cloquinozine
$C_{16}H_{22}ClNO_4$	Clofibride
$C_{16}H_{22}ClN_3O$	Cletoquine
$C_{16}H_{22}ClN_3O$	Zetidoline
$C_{16}H_{22}ClN_3O_2$	Mezacopride
$C_{16}H_{22}ClN_3O_2$	Renzapride
$C_{16}H_{22}ClN_3O_4$	Plafibride
$C_{16}H_{22}Cl_2N_2O.C_4H_4O_4$	Eclanamine Maleate
$C_{16}H_{22}FNO$	Melperone
$C_{16}H_{22}NNaO_6$	Capobenate Sodium
$C_{16}H_{22}N_2O_2$	Isamoltan
$C_{16}H_{22}N_2O_3$	Ethyl Piperidinoacetylamino-benzoate

Molecular Formula	Non-proprietary Name
$C_{16}H_{22}N_2O_3.HCl$	Procaterol Hydrochloride
$C_{16}H_{22}N_2O_3S$	Glyhexamide
$C_{16}H_{22}N_2O_4$	Inproquone
$C_{16}H_{22}N_2O_5$	Butilfenin
$C_{16}H_{22}N_2O_5$	Etifenin
$C_{16}H_{22}N_3NaO_4S$	Dibupyrone
$C_{16}H_{22}N_4.C_4H_6O_6$	Pirogliride Tartrate
$C_{16}H_{22}N_4O$	Linogliride
$C_{16}H_{22}N_4O.C_4H_4O_4$	Linogliride Fumarate
$C_{16}H_{22}N_4O.HCl$	Thonzylamine Hydrochloride
$C_{16}H_{22}N_4O_3$	Apaxifylline
$C_{16}H_{22}N_4O_3$	Tomelukast
$C_{16}H_{22}N_4O_4$	Tetroxoprim
$C_{16}H_{22}N_4O_4S$	Acetiamine
$C_{16}H_{22}N_6O_4$	Protirelin
$C_{16}H_{22}N_6O_7$	Teopranitol
$C_{16}H_{22}O_2$	Geroquinol
$C_{16}H_{22}O_2$	Mexoprofen
$C_{16}H_{22}O_3$	Fencibutirol
$C_{16}H_{22}O_3$	Homosalate
$C_{16}H_{22}O_4$	Dibutyl Phthalate
$C_{16}H_{22}O_6$	Trepibutone
$C_{16}H_{23}BrN_2O_3$	Remoxipride
$C_{16}H_{23}BrN_2O_3.HCl.H_2O$	Remoxipride Hydrochloride
$C_{16}H_{23}ClN_2O_2$	Alloclamide
$C_{16}H_{23}N$	Rolicyclidine
$C_{16}H_{23}NO$	Anazocine
$C_{16}H_{23}NO$	Dezocine
$C_{16}H_{23}NO$	Inaperisone
$C_{16}H_{23}NO$	Tolperisone
$C_{16}H_{23}NO$	Tolquinzole
$C_{16}H_{23}NO.HCl$	Pyrovalerone Hydrochloride
$C_{16}H_{23}NO_2$	Betaprodine
$C_{16}H_{23}NO_2$	Bufuralol
$C_{16}H_{23}NO_2$	Idropranolol
$C_{16}H_{23}NO_2$	Metheptazine
$C_{16}H_{23}NO_2$	Properidine
$C_{16}H_{23}NO_2.C_6H_8O_7$	Ethoheptazine Citrate
$C_{16}H_{23}NO_2.HCl$	Alphaprodine Hydrochloride
$C_{16}H_{23}NO_2.HCl$	Etoxadrol Hydrochloride
$C_{16}H_{23}NO_2.HCl$	Hexylcaine Hydrochloride
$C_{16}H_{23}NO_2.HCl$	Piperocaine Hydrochloride
$C_{16}H_{23}NO_3$	Pargolol
$C_{16}H_{23}NO_3$	Pranosal
$C_{16}H_{23}NO_3$	Pribecaine
$C_{16}H_{23}NO_4$	Cinamolol
$C_{16}H_{23}NO_4$	Promolate
$C_{16}H_{23}NO_6$	Capobenic Acid
$C_{16}H_{23}NO_6$	Mofloverine
$C_{16}H_{23}N_3O_3S$	Glidazamide
$C_{16}H_{23}N_3O_4$	Gabexate
$C_{16}H_{23}N_5O$	Tegaserod
$C_{16}H_{23}N_5O.C_4H_4O_4$	Tegaserod Maleate
$C_{16}H_{23}N_7O_2$	Eptapirone
$C_{16}H_{24}N_2$	Isoaminile
$C_{16}H_{24}N_2.HCl$	Xylometazoline Hydrochloride
$C_{16}H_{24}N_2O$	Pincainide
$C_{16}H_{24}N_2O$	Ropinirole
$C_{16}H_{24}N_2O.HCl$	Oxymetazoline Hydrochloride
$C_{16}H_{24}N_2O.HCl$	Ropinirole Hydrochloride
$C_{16}H_{24}N_2O_2$	Droxicainide
$C_{16}H_{24}N_2O_2.HCl$	Molindone Hydrochloride
$C_{16}H_{24}N_2O_3.HCl$	Carteolol Hydrochloride
$C_{16}H_{24}N_2O_3S$	Glyoctamide
$C_{16}H_{24}N_2O_4$	Ubenimex
$C_{16}H_{24}N_2O_4.HCl$	Diacetolol Hydrochloride
$C_{16}H_{24}N_2O_5$	Tricetamide
$C_{16}H_{24}N_2O_6$	Pirisudanol
$C_{16}H_{24}N_4O_2$	Tracazolate
$C_{16}H_{24}N_4O_3$	Denbufylline
$C_{16}H_{24}N_{10}O_4$	Aminophylline
$C_{16}H_{24}O_5$	Exiproben
$C_{16}H_{25}GdN_4O_8$	Gadoteric Acid
$C_{16}H_{25}HgNNa_2O_6S$	Mercaptomerin Sodium
$C_{16}H_{25}NO$	Butidrine
$C_{16}H_{25}NO.HCl$	Picenadol Hydrochloride
$C_{16}H_{25}NO_2$	Butetamate
$C_{16}H_{25}NO_2$	Cyclexanone
$C_{16}H_{25}NO_2.C_4H_6O_4.H_2O$	Desvenlafaxine Succinate
$C_{16}H_{25}NO_2.HCl$	Tramadol Hydrochloride
$C_{16}H_{25}NO_2S$	Tertatolol
$C_{16}H_{25}NO_3$	Axomadol
$C_{16}H_{25}NO_3$	Moxisylyte
$C_{16}H_{25}NO_4$	Dioxadilol
$C_{16}H_{25}NO_4$	Floredil
$C_{16}H_{25}NO_4.HCl$	Esmolol Hydrochloride
$C_{16}H_{25}NS$	Gacyclidine
$C_{16}H_{25}N_2NaO_5S$	Cilastatin Sodium
$C_{16}H_{25}N_3O.C_4H_4O_4$	Propiram Fumarate
$C_{16}H_{25}N_3O_4S$	Prosulpride
$C_{16}H_{25}N_3O_5$	Xamoterol
$C_{16}H_{25}N_3O_5S$	Sulverapride
$C_{16}H_{25}N_5O_2$	Midaxifylline
$C_{16}H_{26}CaN_5NaO_8.xH_2O$	Caldiamide Sodium
$C_{16}H_{26}ClN_3O$	Clodacaine
$C_{16}H_{26}DyN_5O_8$	Sprodiamide
$C_{16}H_{26}GdN_5O_8$	Gadodiamide
$C_{16}H_{26}N_2.2HCl$	Pimetine Hydrochloride
$C_{16}H_{26}N_2O_3.HCl$	Proparacaine Hydrochloride
$C_{16}H_{26}N_2O_3.HCl$	Propoxycaine Hydrochloride
$C_{16}H_{26}N_2O_4.HCl$	Cetamolol Hydrochloride
$(C_{16}H_{26}N_2O_4)_2.H_2SO_4$	Pamatolol Sulfate
$C_{16}H_{26}N_4O_4$	Torbafylline
$C_{16}H_{26}O_5$	Artemether
$C_{16}H_{27}NO_3$	Amifloverine
$C_{16}H_{27}NO_4$	Guafecainol
$C_{16}H_{27}NO_4$	Valperinol
$C_{16}H_{27}NO_4S$	Pivopril
$C_{16}H_{27}NO_6$	Gabapentin Enacarbil
$C_{16}H_{28}CaO_5$	Gemcabene Calcium
$C_{16}H_{28}N_2O_2$	Epipropidine
$C_{16}H_{28}N_2O_2$	Tromantadine
$C_{16}H_{28}N_2O_4$	Oseltamivir
$C_{16}H_{28}N_2O_4.H_3PO_4$	Oseltamivir Phosphate
$C_{16}H_{28}N_4O_8$	Tetraxetan
$C_{16}H_{28}O_2$	Cioteronel
$C_{16}H_{29}BClN_6O_6{}^{99m}Tc$	Technetium Tc 99m Siboroxime
$C_{16}H_{30}O_6$	Seprilose
$C_{16}H_{31}{}^{123}IO_2$	Iodocetylic Acid I 123
$C_{16}H_{31}N_7O_6$	Thymotrinan
$(C_{16}H_{31}NaO_4)_n$	Divalproex Sodium
$C_{16}H_{32}O_2$	Palmitic Acid
$C_{16}H_{33}NO_2$	Delmopinol
$C_{16}H_{34}Cl_2N_2O_4$	Suxethonium Chloride
$C_{16}H_{34}I_2N_2O_2$	Dicolinium Iodide
$C_{16}H_{34}O$	Cetyl Alcohol
$C_{16}H_{35}N.HF$	Hetaflur
$C_{16}H_{38}Br_2N_2$	Decamethonium Bromide
$C_{16}H_{38}Cl_2N_2O$	Oxydipentonium Chloride
$(C_{16}H_{38}O_5Si_4)_u(C_{26}H_{58}O_9Si_6)_v$ $(C_5H_8O_2)_w(C_6H_7F_3O_2)_x$ $(C_4H_6O_2)_y(C_{10}H_{14}O_4)_z$	Lotifocon B

Molecular Formula	Non-proprietary Name
$(C_{16}H_{38}O_5Si_4)_u(C_{26}H_{58}O_9Si_6)_v$ $(C_5H_8O_2)_w(C_6H_7F_3O_2)_x$ $(C_4H_6O_2)_y(C_{10}H_{14}O_4)_z$	Lotifocon C
$(C_{16}H_{38}O_5Si_4)_v(C_5H_8O_2)_w$ $(C_8H_8F_6O_2)_x(C_4H_6O_2)_y$ $(C_{16}H_{26}O_7)_z$	Unifocon A
$(C_{16}H_{38}O_5Si_4)_v(C_6H_7F_3O_2)_w$ $(C_5H_8O_2)_x(C_4H_6O_2)_y$ $(C_{10}H_{14}O_4)_z$	Tolofocon A
$(C_{16}H_{38}O_5Si_4)_v(C_7H_6F_6O_2)_w$ $(C_4H_6O_2)_x(C_{13}H_{20}O_4)_y$ $(C_{70}H_{188}O_{30}Si_{27})_x$	Hexafocon A
$(C_{16}H_{38}O_5Si_4)_v(C_7H_6F_6O_2)_w$ $(C_6H_9NO)_x(C_4H_6O_2)_y$ $(C_{10}H_{14}O_4)_z$	Melafocon A
$(C_{16}H_{38}O_5Si_4)_w(C_5H_8O_2)_x$ $(C_4H_6O_2)_y(C_{10}H_{14}O_4)_z$	Kolfocon A
$(C_{16}H_{38}O_5Si_4)_w(C_6H_7F_3O_2)_x$ $(C_4H_6O_2)_y(C_{26}H_{58}O_9Si_6)_z$	Siflufocon A
$(C_{16}H_{38}O_6Si_4)_t(C_{26}H_{58}O_9Si_6)_u$ $(C_5H_8O_2)_v(C_6H_7F_3O_2)_w$ $(C_4H_6O_2)_x(C_9H_{15}NO_2)_y$ $(C_{14}H_{22}O_6)_z$	Flusilfocon A
$(C_{16}H_{38}O_6Si_4)_t(C_{26}H_{58}O_9Si_6)_u$ $(C_5H_8O_2)_v(C_6H_7F_3O_2)_w$ $(C_4H_6O_2)_x(C_9H_{15}NO_2)_y$ $(C_{14}H_{22}O_6)_z$	Flusilfocon B
$(C_{16}H_{38}O_6Si_4)_t(C_{26}H_{58}O_9Si_6)_u$ $(C_5H_8O_2)_v(C_6H_7F_3O_2)_w$ $(C_4H_6O_2)_x(C_9H_{15}NO_2)_y$ $(C_{14}H_{22}O_6)_z$	Flusilfocon C
$(C_{16}H_{38}O_6Si_4)_t(C_{26}H_{58}O_9Si_6)_u$ $(C_5H_8O_2)_v(C_6H_7F_3O_2)_w$ $(C_4H_6O_2)_x(C_9H_{15}NO_2)_y$ $(C_{14}H_{22}O_6)_z$	Flusilfocon D
$(C_{16}H_{38}O_6Si_4)_t(C_{26}H_{58}O_9Si_6)_u$ $(C_5H_8O_2)_v(C_6H_7F_3O_2)_w$ $(C_4H_6O_2)_x(C_9H_{15}NO_2)_y$ $(C_{14}H_{22}O_6)_z$	Flusilfocon E
$C_{17}H_8Cl_2F_8N_2O_3$	Lufenuron
$C_{17}H_9Cl_2FN_4O_2$	Letrazuril
$C_{17}H_9Cl_3N_4O_2$	Diclazuril
$C_{17}H_{10}CaO_8$	Probicromil Calcium
$C_{17}H_{10}Cl_2N_4O_2$	Clazuril
$C_{17}H_{10}F_6N_2O_2S$	Tiflamizole
$C_{17}H_{11}BrClFN_2O_4$	Zenarestat
$C_{17}H_{11}BrFN_3O_4$	Ranirestat
$C_{17}H_{11}Br_2NO_2$	Broxaldine
$C_{17}H_{11}ClF_4N_2S$	Quazepam
$C_{17}H_{11}ClN_2O_2S$	Tilomisole
$C_{17}H_{11}Cl_3NNaO_4S.H_2O$	Enolicam Sodium
$C_{17}H_{11}N_5$	Letrozole
$C_{17}H_{11}N_5O$	Ocinaplon
$C_{17}H_{12}BrFN_2O_3$	Ponalrestat
$C_{17}H_{12}Br_2O_3$	Benzbromarone
$C_{17}H_{12}ClFN_2O_2$	Pirazolac
$C_{17}H_{12}ClF_3N_2O$	Halazepam
$C_{17}H_{12}ClNO_2S$	Fentiazac
$C_{17}H_{12}ClN_5O$	Intrazole
$C_{17}H_{12}Cl_2N_2O_6S$	Lirimilast
$C_{17}H_{12}Cl_2N_4$	Triazolam
$C_{17}H_{12}Cl_3N_3O$	Alteconazole
$C_{17}H_{12}I_2O_3$	Benziodarone
$C_{17}H_{12}N_6O_3$	Quinotolast
$C_{17}H_{12}O_4$	Mitoflaxone
$C_{17}H_{12}O_6$	Talosalate

Molecular Formula	Non-proprietary Name
$C_{17}H_{13}ClF_4N_2$	Fletazepam
$C_{17}H_{13}ClN_2O_2$	Lonazolac
$C_{17}H_{13}ClN_4$	Alprazolam
$2C_{17}H_{13}ClN_4.3C_4H_4O_4$	Liarozole Fumarate
$C_{17}H_{13}ClN_4.HCl$	Liarozole Hydrochloride
$C_{17}H_{13}ClO_3$	Itanoxone
$C_{17}H_{13}F_3N_2O_2$	Triflubazam
$C_{17}H_{13}F_3N_2O_3S$	Ritolukast
$C_{17}H_{13}NO_3$	Napirimus
$C_{17}H_{13}N_3Na_2O_6.2H_2O$	Balsalazide Disodium
$C_{17}H_{13}N_3O_5S_2$	Phthalylsulfathiazole
$C_{17}H_{13}NaO_5$	Xanoxate Sodium
$C_{17}H_{14}BrFN_2O_2$	Haloxazolam
$C_{17}H_{14}ClFN_2O_3$	Doxefazepam
$C_{17}H_{14}ClN_3O_2S$	Tiazuril
$C_{17}H_{14}Cl_2F_2N_2O_3$	Roflumilast
$C_{17}H_{14}Cl_2N_2O_2$	Cloxazolam
$C_{17}H_{14}F_3NO_5S$	Triflumidate
$C_{17}H_{14}F_3N_3O_2S$	Celecoxib
$C_{17}H_{14}F_3N_3O_3S$	Deracoxib
$C_{17}H_{14}N_2O_2$	Bimakalim
$C_{17}H_{14}N_2O_2$	Oxapadol
$C_{17}H_{14}N_2O_3$	Adosopine
$C_{17}H_{14}N_2O_3$	Rosoxacin
$C_{17}H_{14}N_2O_6S$	Iguratimod
$C_{17}H_{14}N_2S_2$	Fezatione
$C_{17}H_{14}N_4O_5S_2$	Phthalylsulfamethizole
$C_{17}H_{14}O_3$	Benzarone
$C_{17}H_{14}O_3$	Furaprofen
$C_{17}H_{14}O_3$	Xylocoumarol
$C_{17}H_{14}O_3S$	Zaltoprofen
$C_{17}H_{14}O_4$	Oxindanac
$C_{17}H_{14}O_4$	Vadimezan
$C_{17}H_{14}O_4S$	Rofecoxib
$C_{17}H_{14}O_5$	Xanoxic Acid
$C_{17}H_{15}BrN_2$	Brolaconazole
$C_{17}H_{15}ClN_2O$	Ciclazindol
$C_{17}H_{15}ClN_2O_5S$	Alilusem
$C_{17}H_{15}ClN_4S$	Etizolam
$C_{17}H_{15}ClO_4$	Losmiprofen
$C_{17}H_{15}Cl_2N_3O_5S$	Sulazuril
$C_{17}H_{15}Cl_3N_2O_2$	Triclodazol
$C_{17}H_{15}FN_2O_3$	Fenleuton
$C_{17}H_{15}F_5O_2$	Pentafluranol
$C_{17}H_{15}NO_2$	Inicarone
$C_{17}H_{15}NO_3$	Dexindoprofen
$C_{17}H_{15}NO_3$	Indoprofen
$C_{17}H_{15}NO_5$	Benorilate
$C_{17}H_{15}NO_5$	Parcetasal
$C_{17}H_{15}N_3O_4$	Motrazepam
$C_{17}H_{15}N_5O$	Zaleplon
$C_{17}H_{15}N_7Na_2O_8S_4$	Cefotetan Disodium
$C_{17}H_{16}ClFN_2O_2$	Progabide
$C_{17}H_{16}ClNO.C_4H_4O_4$	Asenapine Maleate
$C_{17}H_{16}ClNO_4$	Meglitinide
$C_{17}H_{16}ClN_3O$	Amoxapine
$C_{17}H_{16}ClN_3O_2$	Carburazepam
$C_{17}H_{16}Cl_2N_2O$	Tuclazepam
$C_{17}H_{16}Cl_2N_2O_2$	Loviride
$C_{17}H_{16}Cl_2N_2O_3.HCl$	Parconazole Hydrochloride
$C_{17}H_{16}Cl_2N_2O_5$	Clefamide
$C_{17}H_{16}FNOS.HCl$	Fluradoline Hydrochloride
$C_{17}H_{16}F_6N_2O$	Mefloquine
$C_{17}H_{16}F_6N_2O.HCl$	Mefloquine Hydrochloride
$C_{17}H_{16}NO_2PS$	Quintiofos
$C_{17}H_{16}N_2Na_2O_6S$	Carbenicillin Disodium

Molecular Formula	Non-proprietary Name
$C_{17}H_{16}N_2O$	Etaqualone
$C_{17}H_{16}N_2O$	Nictindole
$C_{17}H_{16}N_2OS$	Bentazepam
$C_{17}H_{16}N_2O_2$	Xinidamine
$C_{17}H_{16}N_2O_3$	Emakalim
$C_{17}H_{16}N_2O_7S_2$	Sulosemide
$C_{17}H_{16}N_2S.CH_4O_3S$	Fanetizole Mesylate
$C_{17}H_{16}N_3NaO_6S_2$	Cephapirin Sodium
$C_{17}H_{16}N_4O_2$	Nifenazone
$C_{17}H_{16}N_4S_2$	Tenilapine
$C_{17}H_{16}N_6O.CH_4O_3S$	Zoniporide Mesylate
$C_{17}H_{16}O$	Xenipentone
$C_{17}H_{16}O_3$	Metbufen
$(C_{17}H_{16}O_6)_m(C_{10}H_{18}O_4)_n$	Polifeprosan 20
$C_{17}H_{17}ClFN_3O_3.HCl$	Clinafloxacin Hydrochloride
$C_{17}H_{17}ClN_2O$	Etifoxine
$C_{17}H_{17}ClN_6O_3$	Eszopiclone
$C_{17}H_{17}ClN_6O_3$	Zopiclone
$C_{17}H_{17}ClO_3$	Clobuzarit
$C_{17}H_{17}ClO_4$	Fenirofibrate
$C_{17}H_{17}ClO_6$	Griseofulvin
$C_{17}H_{17}Cl_2N.HCl$	Sertraline Hydrochloride
$C_{17}H_{17}Cl_2NO$	Diclofensine
$C_{17}H_{17}Cl_2NO$	Fengabine
$C_{17}H_{17}Cl_2NO_3$	Terofenamate
$C_{17}H_{17}FN_4O.CH_4O_3S$	Lurosetron Mesylate
$C_{17}H_{17}F_3N_6O_2$	Imanixil
$C_{17}H_{17}F_3O_2$	Terfluranol
$C_{17}H_{17}KN_2O_6S$	Carbenicillin Potassium
$C_{17}H_{17}NO_2$	Etazepine
$C_{17}H_{17}NO_2.HCl$	Memotine Hydrochloride
$C_{17}H_{17}NO_2.HCl.\tfrac{1}{2}H_2O$	Apomorphine Hydrochloride
$C_{17}H_{17}NO_3S$	Protizinic Acid
$C_{17}H_{17}NS$	Damotepine
$C_{17}H_{17}NS$	Tisoquone
$C_{17}H_{17}N_3O$	Ramosetron
$C_{17}H_{17}N_3O_2$	Divaplon
$C_{17}H_{17}N_3O_3S$	Picoprazole
$(C_{17}H_{17}N_3O_6S_2)_2.C_{16}H_{20}N_2$	Cephapirin Benzathine
$C_{17}H_{17}N_3O_8S$	Cefuracetime
$C_{17}H_{17}N_7O_8S_4$	Cefotetan
$C_{17}H_{18}Br_2N_4O_2$	Dibrompropamidine
$C_{17}H_{18}ClNO_4$	Pirifibrate
$C_{17}H_{18}ClNO_6$	Quincarbate
$C_{17}H_{18}ClN_3$	Lergotrile
$C_{17}H_{18}ClN_3.CH_4O_3S$	Lergotrile Mesylate
$C_{17}H_{18}ClN_3O$	Bumetrizole
$C_{17}H_{18}ClN_3O$	Clobenzepam
$C_{17}H_{18}ClN_3S$	Tilozepine
$C_{17}H_{18}Cl_2N_2O_5S$	Clometocillin
$C_{17}H_{18}FN_3$	Nerispirdine
$C_{17}H_{18}FN_3O_3$	Ciprofloxacin
$C_{17}H_{18}FN_3O_3.HCl.H_2O$	Ciprofloxacin Hydrochloride
$C_{17}H_{18}FN_3O_3S$	Rufloxacin
$C_{17}H_{18}FN_3S$	Timelotem
$C_{17}H_{18}F_2O_2$	Bifluranol
$C_{17}H_{18}F_3NO$	Fluoxetine
$C_{17}H_{18}F_3NO.HCl$	Fluoxetine Hydrochloride
$C_{17}H_{18}F_3N_3O_3$	Fleroxacin
$C_{17}H_{18}KN_3O_3S$	Esomeprazole Potassium
$C_{17}H_{18}N_2$	Amfetaminil
$C_{17}H_{18}N_2.HCl$	Dazepinil Hydrochloride
$C_{17}H_{18}N_2O_3$	Diphoxazide
$C_{17}H_{18}N_2O_3S$	Atibeprone
$C_{17}H_{18}N_2O_5S$	Piretanide
$C_{17}H_{18}N_2O_6$	Nifedipine

Molecular Formula	Non-proprietary Name
$C_{17}H_{18}N_2S_2$	Sulbentine
$C_{17}H_{18}N_3NaO_3S$	Omeprazole Sodium
$C_{17}H_{18}N_4O.HCl$	Alosetron Hydrochloride
$C_{17}H_{18}N_4O_3S$	Enviroxime
$C_{17}H_{18}N_4O_3S$	Viroxime
$C_{17}H_{18}N_4O_3S$	Viroxime Component A
$C_{17}H_{18}N_4O_3S$	Viroxime Component B
$C_{17}H_{18}N_4O_3S$	Zinviroxime
$C_{17}H_{18}N_5NaO_6S_2$	Cefovecin Sodium
$C_{17}H_{18}O_2S$	Namirotene
$C_{17}H_{18}O_4$	Procromil
$C_{17}H_{18}O_5$	Proxicromil
$C_{17}H_{19}ClN_2S$	Chlorpromazine
$C_{17}H_{19}ClN_2S.HCl$	Chlorpromazine Hydrochloride
$C_{17}H_{19}ClN_4$	Lorcinadol
$C_{17}H_{19}ClN_5O_4P.CH_4O_3S$	Pradefovir Mesylate
$C_{17}H_{19}FN_2O_2$	Ralfinamide
$C_{17}H_{19}FN_2O_2$	Safinamide
$C_{17}H_{19}FN_4O_4$	Marbofloxacin
$C_{17}H_{19}FN_4S$	Flumezapine
$C_{17}H_{19}F_2N_3O_3$	Lomefloxacin
$C_{17}H_{19}F_2N_3O_3.CH_4O_3S$	Lomefloxacin Mesylate
$C_{17}H_{19}F_2N_3O_3.HCl$	Lomefloxacin Hydrochloride
$C_{17}H_{19}KN_2O_5S$	Phenethicillin Potassium
$C_{17}H_{19}N$	Dimefadane
$C_{17}H_{19}N$	Etifelmine
$C_{17}H_{19}N.HCl$	Tametraline Hydrochloride
$C_{17}H_{19}NO.HCl$	Nefopam Hydrochloride
$C_{17}H_{19}NO_3$	Norcodeine
$C_{17}H_{19}NO_3$	Piperine
$C_{17}H_{19}NO_3.HCl$	Hydromorphone Hydrochloride
$(C_{17}H_{19}NO_3)_2.H_2SO_4.5H_2O$	Morphine Sulfate
$C_{17}H_{19}NO_4.HCl$	Amotosalen Hydrochloride
$C_{17}H_{19}NO_4.HCl$	Oxymorphone Hydrochloride
$C_{17}H_{19}NO_8S$	Faropenem Medoxomil
$C_{17}H_{19}N_2NaO_6S.H_2O$	Methicillin Sodium
$C_{17}H_{19}N_3$	Delergotrile
$C_{17}H_{19}N_3$	Esmirtazapine
$C_{17}H_{19}N_3$	Mirtazapine
$C_{17}H_{19}N_3.C_4H_4O_4$	Esmirtazapine Maleate
$C_{17}H_{19}N_3.HCl$	Antazoline Hydrochloride
$C_{17}H_{19}N_3.H_3PO_4$	Antazoline Phosphate
$C_{17}H_{19}N_3NaO_3S$	Esomeprazole Sodium
$C_{17}H_{19}N_3O$	Ofornine
$C_{17}H_{19}N_3O$	Piberaline
$C_{17}H_{19}N_3O.CH_4O_3S$	Phentolamine Mesylate
$C_{17}H_{19}N_3O.HCl$	Phentolamine Hydrochloride
$C_{17}H_{19}N_3O_2S$	Ufiprazole
$C_{17}H_{19}N_3O_3S$	Esomeprazole
$C_{17}H_{19}N_3O_3S$	Omeprazole
$C_{17}H_{19}N_3O_4S$	Metampicillin
$C_{17}H_{19}N_5$	Anastrozole
$C_{17}H_{19}N_5O$	Bazinaprine
$C_{17}H_{19}N_5O_2$	Pixantrone
$C_{17}H_{19}N_5O_2.C_2H_6O_4S$	Mivobulin Isethionate
$C_{17}H_{19}N_5O_2.C_2H_6O_4S$	Piritrexim Isethionate
$C_{17}H_{19}N_5O_6S_2$	Cefcapene
$C_{17}H_{19}NaO_6$	Mycophenolate Sodium
$C_{17}H_{20}BrNO.HCl$	Bromodiphenhydramine Hydrochloride
$C_{17}H_{20}ClNO$	Clemeprol
$C_{17}H_{20}ClNO.HCl$	Chlophedianol Hydrochloride
$C_{17}H_{20}ClN_3O_3$	Azasetron
$C_{17}H_{20}FN_3O_3$	Pefloxacin
$C_{17}H_{20}FN_3O_3.CH_4O_3S$	Pefloxacin Mesylate
$C_{17}H_{20}F_6N_2O_3.C_2H_4O_2$	Flecainide Acetate

Molecular Formula	Non-proprietary Name
$C_{17}H_{20}I_3N_3O_4$	Iomorinic Acid
$C_{17}H_{20}N_2O$	Vindeburnol
$C_{17}H_{20}N_2O.HCl$	Remacemide Hydrochloride
$C_{17}H_{20}N_2O_2$	Tropicamide
$C_{17}H_{20}N_2O_2$	Tropisetron
$C_{17}H_{20}N_2O_2S$	Etocarlide
$C_{17}H_{20}N_2O_2S$	Tinoridine
$C_{17}H_{20}N_2O_3S$	Tosifen
$C_{17}H_{20}N_2O_5S$	Bumetanide
$C_{17}H_{20}N_2S$	Tienopramine
$C_{17}H_{20}N_2S.C_7H_7ClN_4O_2$	Promethazine Teoclate
$C_{17}H_{20}N_2S.HCl$	Promazine Hydrochloride
$C_{17}H_{20}N_2S.HCl$	Promethazine Hydrochloride
$C_{17}H_{20}N_4NaO_9P.2H_2O$	Riboflavin 5′-Phosphate Sodium
$C_{17}H_{20}N_4O$	Propizepine
$C_{17}H_{20}N_4O.2HCl$	Vapitadine Dihydrochloride
$C_{17}H_{20}N_4O_2$	Propamidine
$C_{17}H_{20}N_4O_6$	Riboflavin
$C_{17}H_{20}N_4O_6S_2$	Cefsumide
$C_{17}H_{20}N_4S$	Olanzapine
$C_{17}H_{20}N_6$	Baquiloprim
$C_{17}H_{20}O_3$	Bunaprolast
$C_{17}H_{20}O_5S$	Firocoxib
$C_{17}H_{20}O_6$	Mycophenolic Acid
$C_{17}H_{21}Cl_2F_3N_5Na_4O_{12}P_3S_2$	Cangrelor Tetrasodium
$C_{17}H_{21}IO_2$	Phenyliodoundecynoate
$C_{17}H_{21}N$	Demelverine
$C_{17}H_{21}N.HCl$	Benzphetamine Hydrochloride
$C_{17}H_{21}NO$	Oxifentorex
$C_{17}H_{21}NO$	Phenyltoloxamine
$C_{17}H_{21}NO.C_6H_8O_7$	Diphenhydramine Citrate
$C_{17}H_{21}NO.C_6H_8O_7$	Phenyltoloxamine Citrate
$C_{17}H_{21}NO.C_7H_7ClN_4O_2$	Dimenhydrinate
$C_{17}H_{21}NO.HCl$	Atomoxetine Hydrochloride
$C_{17}H_{21}NO.HCl$	Diphenhydramine Hydrochloride
$C_{17}H_{21}NO.HCl$	Tofenacin Hydrochloride
$C_{17}H_{21}NO_2$	Desomorphine
$C_{17}H_{21}NO_2$	Nisoxetine
$C_{17}H_{21}NO_3$	Etodolac
$C_{17}H_{21}NO_3$	Galantamine
$C_{17}H_{21}NO_3$	Ritodrine
$C_{17}H_{21}NO_3.HBr$	Galantamine Hydrobromide
$C_{17}H_{21}NO_3.HCl$	Ritodrine Hydrochloride
$C_{17}H_{21}NO_4$	Cocaine
$C_{17}H_{21}NO_4$	Fenoterol
$C_{17}H_{21}NO_4$	Hydromorphinol
$C_{17}H_{21}NO_4.HBr.3H_2O$	Scopolamine Hydrobromide
$C_{17}H_{21}NO_4.HCl$	Cocaine Hydrochloride
$C_{17}H_{21}NO_5$	Proquinolate
$C_{17}H_{21}N_3O_2$	Nicogrelate
$C_{17}H_{21}N_3O_4$	Trimethamide
$C_{17}H_{21}N_5O$	Noberastine
$C_{17}H_{21}N_5O_5$	Theodrenaline
$C_{17}H_{22}BrNOS_2$	Timepidium Bromide
$C_{17}H_{22}I_3N_3O_8$	Iomeprol
$C_{17}H_{22}I_3N_3O_8$	Iopamidol
$C_{17}H_{22}N_2$	Bucricaine
$C_{17}H_{22}N_2$	Metrafazoline
$C_{17}H_{22}N_2O.C_4H_6O_4$	Doxylamine Succinate
$C_{17}H_{22}N_2OS$	Neticonazole
$C_{17}H_{22}N_2O_2$	Fenpipalone
$C_{17}H_{22}N_2O_3$	Catramilast
$C_{17}H_{22}N_2O_3$	Emivirine
$C_{17}H_{22}N_2O_6S_2$	Apratastat
$C_{17}H_{22}N_2S$	Thenalidine
$C_{17}H_{22}N_4O$	Minaprine
$C_{17}H_{22}N_4O.2HCl$	Minaprine Hydrochloride
$C_{17}H_{22}N_4O_2$	Moxiraprine
$C_{17}H_{22}N_4O_2$	Resiquimod
$C_{17}H_{22}N_4O_3$	Pirsidomine
$C_{17}H_{23}ClN_2O_2$	Bisaramil
$C_{17}H_{23}ClO_4$	Etomoxir
$C_{17}H_{23}Cl_2NO$	Tesofensine
$C_{17}H_{23}Cl_2NO.CH_4O_3S$	Cilobamine Mesylate
$C_{17}H_{23}FN_2O$	Azabuperone
$C_{17}H_{23}NO$	Racemorphan
$C_{17}H_{23}NO.C_4H_6O_6.2H_2O$	Levorphanol Tartrate
$C_{17}H_{23}NO.HCl$	Dextrorphan Hydrochloride
$C_{17}H_{23}NO.HCl$	Pirandamine Hydrochloride
$C_{17}H_{23}NO_2$	Dextilidine
$C_{17}H_{23}NO_2.HCl$	Tilidine Hydrochloride
$C_{17}H_{23}NO_2.HCl$	Tropanserin Hydrochloride
$C_{17}H_{23}NO_3$	Atropine
$C_{17}H_{23}NO_3$	Hyoscyamine
$C_{17}H_{23}NO_3$	Rotraxate
$C_{17}H_{23}NO_3.HBr$	Hyoscyamine Hydrobromide
$(C_{17}H_{23}NO_3)_2.H_2SO_4.H_2O$	Atropine Sulfate
$(C_{17}H_{23}NO_3)_2.H_2SO_4.2H_2O$	Hyoscyamine Sulfate
$C_{17}H_{23}NO_4$	Bucumolol
$C_{17}H_{23}NO_4.HCl$	Atropine Oxide Hydrochloride
$C_{17}H_{23}NO_4.HCl$	Cetraxate Hydrochloride
$C_{17}H_{23}N_3O$	Piperylone
$C_{17}H_{23}N_3O.C_4H_4O_4$	Pyrilamine Maleate
$C_{17}H_{23}N_3O_4$	Primidolol
$C_{17}H_{23}N_5O$	Indisetron
$C_{17}H_{23}N_5O_2.2HCl$	Quinazosin Hydrochloride
$C_{17}H_{23}N_5O_2.HCl$	Sunepitron Hydrochloride
$C_{17}H_{23}N_5O_4.C_2H_4O_2.\frac{1}{4}H_2O$	Orbofiban Acetate
$C_{17}H_{23}N_7O_5$	Taltirelin
$C_{17}H_{24}BrNO_3$	Homatropine Methylbromide
$C_{17}H_{24}ClN_3O.2HCl$	Clamoxyquin Hydrochloride
$C_{17}H_{24}ClN_3S$	Dazolicine
$C_{17}H_{24}F_3N_3O_3S$	Velneperit
$C_{17}H_{24}N_2O$	Pilsicainide
$C_{17}H_{24}N_2O.HCl$	Dimethisoquin Hydrochloride
$C_{17}H_{24}N_2O_2$	Phenglutarimide
$C_{17}H_{24}N_2O_3$	Carperidine
$C_{17}H_{24}N_2O_3$	Etacepride
$C_{17}H_{24}N_2O_3$	Tilisolol
$C_{17}H_{24}N_4$	Tolpiprazole
$C_{17}H_{24}N_4O_2S$	Disulergine
$C_{17}H_{24}N_4O_3$	Doreptide
$C_{17}H_{24}N_6O_4$	Selodenoson
$C_{17}H_{24}N_6O_4S$	Montirelin
$C_{17}H_{24}O_3$	Cyclandelate
$C_{17}H_{25}ClN_2O_3$	Eticlopride
$C_{17}H_{25}Cl_2F_3N_5O_{12}P_3S_2$	Cangrelor
$C_{17}H_{25}N.HCl$	Phencyclidine Hydrochloride
$C_{17}H_{25}NO$	Eperisone
$C_{17}H_{25}NO_2$	Alphameprodine
$C_{17}H_{25}NO_2$	Betameprodine
$C_{17}H_{25}NO_2$	Meradimate
$C_{17}H_{25}NO_2$	Metethoheptazine
$C_{17}H_{25}NO_2$	Proheptazine
$C_{17}H_{25}NO_2$	Propipocaine
$C_{17}H_{25}NO_2$	Trimeperidine
$C_{17}H_{25}NO_3$	Pecilocin
$C_{17}H_{25}NO_3.HCl$	Bunolol Hydrochloride
$C_{17}H_{25}NO_3.HCl$	Cyclopentolate Hydrochloride
$C_{17}H_{25}NO_3.HCl$	Eucatropine Hydrochloride
$C_{17}H_{25}NO_3.HCl$	Levobunolol Hydrochloride

Molecular Formula	Non-proprietary Name
$C_{17}H_{25}NO_4$	Buflomedil
$C_{17}H_{25}NO_4$	Ibopamine
$C_{17}H_{25}NO_4$	Trocimine
$C_{17}H_{25}NO_7$	Emiglitate
$C_{17}H_{25}N_3O$	Proxazole
$C_{17}H_{25}N_3O.C_6H_8O_7$	Proxazole Citrate
$C_{17}H_{25}N_3O_2$	Vildagliptin
$C_{17}H_{25}N_3O_2S$	Almotriptan
$C_{17}H_{25}N_3O_2S$	Naratriptan
$C_{17}H_{25}N_3O_2S.C_4H_6O_5$	Almotriptan Malate
$C_{17}H_{25}N_3O_2S.HCl$	Naratriptan Hydrochloride
$C_{17}H_{25}N_3O_4S$	Cipropride
$C_{17}H_{25}N_3O_5S$	Veralipride
$C_{17}H_{25}N_3O_5S.3H_2O$	Meropenem
$C_{17}H_{25}N_5O_2.2HCl.H_2O$	Prizidilol Hydrochloride
$C_{17}H_{25}N_7O_4$	Binodenoson
$C_{17}H_{26}ClN.HCl.H_2O$	Sibutramine Hydrochloride
$C_{17}H_{26}ClNO$	Tiprolisant
$C_{17}H_{26}ClN_3O_3.HCl$	Batanopride Hydrochloride
$C_{17}H_{26}FNO_2$	Zafuleptine
$C_{17}H_{26}FNO_3$	Butofilolol
$C_{17}H_{26}IN_3O$	Butopyrammonium Iodide
$C_{17}H_{26}N_2O$	Phenampromide
$C_{17}H_{26}N_2O.HCl.H_2O$	Ropivacaine Hydrochloride
$C_{17}H_{26}N_2O_2$	Paridocaine
$C_{17}H_{26}N_2O_3$	Dibusadol
$C_{17}H_{26}N_2O_3$	Soquinolol
$C_{17}H_{26}N_2O_4S$	Sultopride
$C_{17}H_{26}N_4O.2C_4H_4O_4$	Emedastine Difumarate
$C_{17}H_{26}N_4O.2HCl$	Alniditan Dihydrochloride
$C_{17}H_{26}N_4O_2$	Dalbraminol
$C_{17}H_{26}N_4O_3S_2$	Fursultiamine
$C_{17}H_{26}N_4O_4S$	Alpiropride
$C_{17}H_{26}N_4S_2$	Peratizole
$C_{17}H_{27}Cl_2N_5$	Olanexidine
$C_{17}H_{27}Cl_2N_5.HCl.\frac{1}{2}H_2O$	Olanexidine Hydrochloride
$C_{17}H_{27}N$	Gamfexine
$C_{17}H_{27}NO$	Amixetrine
$C_{17}H_{27}NO_2$	Padimate O
$C_{17}H_{27}NO_2.HCl$	Venlafaxine Hydrochloride
$C_{17}H_{27}NO_3$	Embutramide
$C_{17}H_{27}NO_3$	Nonivamide
$C_{17}H_{27}NO_3.HCl$	Pramoxine Hydrochloride
$C_{17}H_{27}NO_4$	Metipranolol
$C_{17}H_{27}NO_4$	Nadolol
$C_{17}H_{27}N_3O_3S$	Pitenodil
$C_{17}H_{27}N_3O_4S$	Amisulpride
$C_{17}H_{28}ClO_5P$	Fosarilate
$C_{17}H_{28}N_2O$	Etidocaine
$C_{17}H_{28}N_2O_2$	Ambucetamide
$C_{17}H_{28}N_2O_2$	Endomide
$C_{17}H_{28}N_2O_2$	Leucinocaine
$C_{17}H_{28}N_2O_2.HCl$	p-Butylaminobenzoyldiethylaminoethyl Hydrochloride
$C_{17}H_{28}N_2O_2.HCl$	Metabutoxycaine Hydrochloride
$C_{17}H_{28}N_2O_3$	Ambucaine
$C_{17}H_{28}N_2O_3.HCl$	Benoxinate Hydrochloride
$C_{17}H_{28}N_2O_5$	Perindoprilat
$C_{17}H_{28}N_4O.2C_4H_4O_4$	Piperamide Maleate
$C_{17}H_{28}N_4O_4$	Posatirelin
$C_{17}H_{28}O_5$	Artemotil
$C_{17}H_{29}GdN_4O_7$	Gadoteridol
$C_{17}H_{29}N$	Trimexiline
$C_{17}H_{29}N_3O_2$	Amoxecaine
$C_{17}H_{30}N_2O_5$	Aloxistatin

Molecular Formula	Non-proprietary Name
$C_{17}H_{30}N_2O_7.H_2SO_4.5H_2O$	Trospectomycin Sulfate
$C_{17}H_{30}N_4O_7P_2S_2$	Imcarbofos
$C_{17}H_{31}ClN_2O_5S.HCl.H_2O$	Pirlimycin Hydrochloride
$C_{17}H_{31}NO$	Myrtecaine
$C_{17}H_{31}NaO_3.2H_2O$	Palmoxirate Sodium
$C_{17}H_{32}BrNO_2$	Anisotropine Methylbromide
$C_{17}H_{34}N_4O_{10}$	Ribostamycin
$C_{17}H_{34}O_2$	Isopropyl Myristate
$(C_{17}H_{34}O_3Si_4)_u(C_7H_6F_6O_2)_v$ $(C_6H_9NO)_w(C_4H_6O_2)_x$ $(C_{10}H_{14}O_4)_y(C_{13}H_{14}O_2)_z$	Tisilfocon A
$C_{17}H_{35}IN_2O$	Opratonium Iodide
$C_{17}H_{35}N_5O_6.2H_2SO_4$	Astromicin Sulfate
$C_{17}H_{36}GeN_2.2HCl$	Spirogermanium Hydrochloride
$C_{17}H_{37}N_7O_3$	Tresperimus
$C_{17}H_{37}N_7O_3.3HCl$	Gusperimus Trihydrochloride
$C_{17}H_{38}BrN$	Tetradonium Bromide
$C_{18}Fe_7N_{18}$	Prussian Blue Insoluble
$C_{18}H_{10}I_6N_2O_7$	Ioglycamic Acid
$C_{18}H_{11}F_3N_2O_2S.H_2O$	Lidorestat
$C_{18}H_{12}ClF_3N_4O_4$	Delafloxacin
$C_{18}H_{12}ClF_3N_4O_4.C_7H_{17}NO_5$	Delafloxacin Meglumine
$C_{18}H_{12}ClN_3$	Climiqualine
$C_{18}H_{12}Cl_2N_2O$	Becliconazole
$C_{18}H_{12}Cl_2N_2O_3$	Gavestinel
$C_{18}H_{12}CuN_2O_{14}S_4.4C_4H_{11}N$	Cuproxoline
$C_{18}H_{12}N_3O_6Cr$	Chromium Picolinate
$C_{18}H_{13}ClFN_3.C_4H_4O_4$	Midazolam Maleate
$C_{18}H_{13}ClFN_3.HCl$	Midazolam Hydrochloride
$C_{18}H_{13}ClFN_3O_2$	Cinolazepam
$C_{18}H_{13}ClN_2O$	Pinazepam
$C_{18}H_{13}Cl_2NO_3S$	Tioxaprofen
$C_{18}H_{13}Cl_2N_3$	Climazolam
$C_{18}H_{13}Cl_2N_3O_2$	Reclazepam
$C_{18}H_{13}Cl_3N_2$	Aliconazole
$C_{18}H_{13}Cl_4N_3O.HNO_3$	Oxiconazole Nitrate
$C_{18}H_{13}NNa_2O_8S_2$	Sodium Picosulfate
$C_{18}H_{13}NNa_4O_8P_2$	Sodium Picofosfate
$C_{18}H_{13}NaO_4S.xH_2O$	Tifurac Sodium
$C_{18}H_{14}BrNO_4$	Intiquinatine
$C_{18}H_{14}ClFN_2O_3$	Ethyl Loflazepate
$C_{18}H_{14}ClN_3O_2S$	Denotivir
$C_{18}H_{14}Cl_2N_2$	Eberconazole
$C_{18}H_{14}Cl_2N_2O_3$	Ethyl Dirazepate
$C_{18}H_{14}Cl_2O_4$	Indacrinone
$C_{18}H_{14}Cl_4N_2O$	Isoconazole
$C_{18}H_{14}Cl_4N_2O$	Miconazole
$C_{18}H_{14}Cl_4N_2O.HNO_3$	Miconazole Nitrate
$C_{18}H_{14}F_3NO_2S$	Itazigrel
$C_{18}H_{14}F_3N_3O_4S$	Toltrazuril
$C_{18}H_{14}F_3N_3O_6S$	Ponazuril
$C_{18}H_{14}F_4N_2O_4S$	Bicalutamide
$C_{18}H_{14}N_4O_3$	Resequinil
$C_{18}H_{14}N_4O_5S$	Sulfasalazine
$C_{18}H_{14}O_6$	Cinfenoac
$C_{18}H_{15}ClN_2O$	Croconazole
$C_{18}H_{15}ClN_2O_2S$	Etoricoxib
$C_{18}H_{15}ClN_2O_3$	Benzotript
$C_{18}H_{15}ClN_2O_6S_2$	Sitaxentan
$C_{18}H_{15}ClO_4S$	Tibeglisene
$C_{18}H_{15}Cl_2N_3O$	Uldazepam
$C_{18}H_{15}Cl_2N_5O_5S_3$	Cefazedone
$C_{18}H_{15}Cl_3N_2O$	Econazole
$C_{18}H_{15}Cl_3N_2O.HNO_3$	Econazole Nitrate
$C_{18}H_{15}Cl_3N_2O.HNO_3$	Orconazole Nitrate
$C_{18}H_{15}Cl_3N_2S.HNO_3$	Sulconazole Nitrate

Molecular Formula	Non-proprietary Name
$C_{18}H_{15}FN_4O$	Finrozole
$C_{18}H_{15}F_3N_2O_2$	Flumizole
$C_{18}H_{15}NO_2$	Etocrylene
$C_{18}H_{15}NO_3$	Delmetacin
$C_{18}H_{15}NO_3$	Oxaprozin
$C_{18}H_{15}N_5O_6S$	Salazodine
$C_{18}H_{16}ClFN_2O_3$	Proflazepam
$C_{18}H_{16}Cl_2N_2O_2$	Mexazolam
$C_{18}H_{16}Cl_2O_4$	Ponfibrate
$C_{18}H_{16}FN_3O_4$	Etibendazole
$C_{18}H_{16}N_2O_3$	Amfonelic Acid
$C_{18}H_{16}N_2O_3$	Roquinimex
$C_{18}H_{16}N_2O_4$	Niometacin
$C_{18}H_{16}N_2O_6$	Bufrolin
$C_{18}H_{16}N_2O_6$	Minocromil
$C_{18}H_{16}N_4$	Irtemazole
$C_{18}H_{16}N_4O_6S$	Quinacillin
$C_{18}H_{16}N_6Na_2O_8S_3$	Cefonicid Sodium
$C_{18}H_{16}N_8Na_2O_7S_3.3\frac{1}{2}H_2O$	Ceftriaxone Sodium
$C_{18}H_{16}O_3$	Ipriflavone
$C_{18}H_{16}O_3$	Phenprocoumon
$C_{18}H_{16}O_4$	Bermoprofen
$C_{18}H_{16}O_4$	Butantrone
$C_{18}H_{17}Br_2NO_5$	Eprotirome
$C_{18}H_{17}ClN_2O$	Clazolam
$C_{18}H_{17}ClN_2O_2$	Girisopam
$C_{18}H_{17}ClN_2O_2$	Oxazolam
$C_{18}H_{17}ClN_2O_3$	Arfendazam
$C_{18}H_{17}ClO_2$	Lomevactone
$C_{18}H_{17}Cl_2N_3O_3.H_2O$	Lorzafone
$C_{18}H_{17}FN_2O$	Fluproquazone
$C_{18}H_{17}F_3N_2O_3$	Ridogrel
$C_{18}H_{17}F_3O_3S$	Pemaglitazar
$C_{18}H_{17}I_4NO_4$	Etiroxate
$C_{18}H_{17}NO_3$	Indobufen
$C_{18}H_{17}NO_3S_2$	Tazasubrate
$C_{18}H_{17}NO_5$	Tranilast
$C_{18}H_{17}N_3O_2$	Anitrazafen
$C_{18}H_{17}N_3O_2$	Pirodomast
$C_{18}H_{17}N_3O_4$	Pinafide
$C_{18}H_{17}N_5O_2$	Panadiplon
$C_{18}H_{17}N_6NaO_5S_2$	Cefamandole Sodium
$C_{18}H_{17}N_6NaO_8S_3$	Cefonicid Monosodium
$C_{18}H_{18}BrClN_2O$	Metaclazepam
$C_{18}H_{18}ClF_5N_6O.C_4H_4O_4.2H_2O$	Cevipabulin Fumarate
$C_{18}H_{18}ClF_5N_6O.C_4H_6O_4.2H_2O$	Cevipabulin Succinate
$C_{18}H_{18}ClNOS$	Zotepine
$C_{18}H_{18}ClNO_4$	Clanobutin
$C_{18}H_{18}ClNO_5$	Etofibrate
$C_{18}H_{18}ClNS$	Chlorprothixene
$C_{18}H_{18}ClN_2O_2P$	Fosazepam
$C_{18}H_{18}ClN_3O$	Loxapine
$C_{18}H_{18}ClN_3O.C_4H_6O_4$	Loxapine Succinate
$(C_{18}H_{18}ClN_3O)_w(C_6H_9NO)_x$ $(C_5H_8O_2)_y(C_7H_{10}O_2)_z$	Vasurfilcon A
$C_{18}H_{18}ClN_3O_2S_2$	Metibride
$C_{18}H_{18}ClN_3S$	Clothiapine
$C_{18}H_{18}Cl_2N_2O_2$	Tolgabide
$C_{18}H_{18}Cl_2N_2O_3$	Piclamilast
$C_{18}H_{18}FN_3.HCl$	Carvotroline Hydrochloride
$C_{18}H_{18}FN_7$	Adipiplon
$C_{18}H_{18}F_3NO_2$	Ufenamate
$C_{18}H_{18}F_3NO_4$	Etofenamate
$C_{18}H_{18}F_3N_3O_3$	Pleconaril
$C_{18}H_{18}N_2$	Cifenline
$C_{18}H_{18}N_2$	Fenharmane

Molecular Formula	Non-proprietary Name
$C_{18}H_{18}N_2.C_4H_6O_4$	Cifenline Succinate
$C_{18}H_{18}N_2O$	Demexiptiline
$C_{18}H_{18}N_2O$	Mariptiline
$C_{18}H_{18}N_2O$	Proquazone
$C_{18}H_{18}N_2O.C_4H_4O_4$	Azanator Maleate
$C_{18}H_{18}N_2O_3.C_4H_4O_4$	Aplindore Fumarate
$C_{18}H_{18}N_2O_6S$	Cefaloram
$C_{18}H_{18}N_4O_2$	Mesocarb
$C_{18}H_{18}N_6O_5S_2$	Cefamandole
$C_{18}H_{18}N_6O_5S_2$	Cefatrizine
$C_{18}H_{18}O_2$	Dienestrol
$C_{18}H_{18}O_2$	Xenyhexenic Acid
$C_{18}H_{18}O_4$	Metochalcone
$C_{18}H_{19}Br_2N_5O_2$	Brindoxime
$C_{18}H_{19}ClFN_7$	Falnidamol
$C_{18}H_{19}ClN_2.C_4H_4O_4$	Cycliramine Maleate
$C_{18}H_{19}ClN_2O_3$	Almoxatone
$C_{18}H_{19}ClN_2O_4$	Picafibrate
$C_{18}H_{19}ClN_4$	Clozapine
$C_{18}H_{19}Cl_2NO_4$	Felodipine
$C_{18}H_{19}F_2NO_5$	Riodipine
$C_{18}H_{19}F_2N_5S$	Ruzadolane
$C_{18}H_{19}F_3N_2S$	Triflupromazine
$C_{18}H_{19}F_3N_2S.HCl$	Triflupromazine Hydrochloride
$C_{18}H_{19}F_3N_6O_2$	Sabiporide
$C_{18}H_{19}N.HCl$	Benzoctamine Hydrochloride
$C_{18}H_{19}NOS$	Tolindate
$C_{18}H_{19}NOS.HCl$	Duloxetine Hydrochloride
$C_{18}H_{19}NO_2$	Isbogrel
$C_{18}H_{19}NO_3$	Glaziovine
$C_{18}H_{19}NS$	Prothixene
$C_{18}H_{19}N_3O$	Fabesetron
$C_{18}H_{19}N_3O$	Ondansetron
$C_{18}H_{19}N_3O.HCl$	Galdansetron Hydrochloride
$C_{18}H_{19}N_3O.HCl.2H_2O$	Ondansetron Hydrochloride
$C_{18}H_{19}N_3O_2$	Irampanel
$C_{18}H_{19}N_3O_2$	Nerisopam
$C_{18}H_{19}N_3O_2S$	Nepaprazole
$C_{18}H_{19}N_3O_3S.C_4H_4O_4$	Rosiglitazone Maleate
$C_{18}H_{19}N_3O_5S.H_2O$	Cefprozil
$C_{18}H_{19}N_3O_6S.2H_2O$	Cephaloglycin
$C_{18}H_{19}N_5O_3S.HCl$	Denibulin Hydrochloride
$C_{18}H_{19}N_5O_4S$	Voreloxin
$C_{18}H_{19}Na_2O_8P$	Fosbretabulin Disodium
$C_{18}H_{20}Br_2N_2O_2S$	Neltenexine
$C_{18}H_{20}ClNO.C_4H_4O_4$	Pyroxamine Maleate
$C_{18}H_{20}ClN_3O.HCl.H_2O$	Clodazon Hydrochloride
$C_{18}H_{20}ClN_3O_5S$	Glicondamide
$C_{18}H_{20}ClN_5O_5$	Sonedenoson
$C_{18}H_{20}FN_3O_4$	Ofloxacin
$C_{18}H_{20}FN_3O_4.\frac{1}{2}H_2O$	Levofloxacin
$C_{18}H_{20}FN_5O_4$	Gemifloxacin
$C_{18}H_{20}FN_5O_4.CH_4O_3S$	Gemifloxacin Mesylate
$C_{18}H_{20}NO_3PS$	Fostedil
$C_{18}H_{20}N_2$	Amezepine
$C_{18}H_{20}N_2$	Ciclopramine
$C_{18}H_{20}N_2.HCl$	Mianserin Hydrochloride
$C_{18}H_{20}N_2O.HCl.H_2O$	Fantridone Hydrochloride
$C_{18}H_{20}N_2O_2$	Vinconate
$C_{18}H_{20}N_2O_2S$	Liranaftate
$C_{18}H_{20}N_2O_6$	Nitrendipine
$C_{18}H_{20}N_2S$	Methdilazine
$C_{18}H_{20}N_2S.HCl$	Methdilazine Hydrochloride
$C_{18}H_{20}N_2S.HCl$	Pyrathiazine Hydrochloride
$C_{18}H_{20}N_3NaO_3S$	Rabeprazole Sodium
$C_{18}H_{20}N_4$	Lerisetron

Molecular Formula	*Non-proprietary Name*
$C_{18}H_{20}N_4O_2$	Nitracrine
$C_{18}H_{20}O_2$	Diethylstilbestrol
$C_{18}H_{20}O_2$	Equilin
$C_{18}H_{21}ClN_2.C_4H_4O_4$	Nelezaprine Maleate
$C_{18}H_{21}ClN_2.C_4H_7NO_3$	Closiramine Aceturate
$C_{18}H_{21}ClN_2.HCl$	Chlorcyclizine Hydrochloride
$C_{18}H_{21}ClN_2.H_3PO_4$	Clomacran Phosphate
$C_{18}H_{21}ClN_4$	Midamaline
$C_{18}H_{21}ClN_4O_9$	Bofumustine
$C_{18}H_{21}KN_2O_5S$	Levopropylcillin Potassium
$C_{18}H_{21}NO.HCl$	Azacyclonol Hydrochloride
$C_{18}H_{21}NO.HCl$	Pipradrol Hydrochloride
$C_{18}H_{21}NO_2$	Beloxamide
$C_{18}H_{21}NO_2$	Methyldesorphine
$C_{18}H_{21}NO_2.HCl$	Naranol Hydrochloride
$C_{18}H_{21}NO_3.C_4H_6O_6.2\frac{1}{2}H_2O$	Hydrocodone Bitartrate
$C_{18}H_{21}NO_3.HCl$	Metopon Hydrochloride
$C_{18}H_{21}NO_3.H_2O$	Codeine
$(C_{18}H_{21}NO_3)_2.H_2SO_4.3H_2O$	Codeine Sulfate
$C_{18}H_{21}NO_3.H_3PO_4.\frac{1}{2}H_2O$	Codeine Phosphate
$C_{18}H_{21}NO_4$	Oxycodone
$(C_{18}H_{21}NO_4)_2.C_8H_6O_4$	Oxycodone Terephthalate
$C_{18}H_{21}NO_4.HCl$	Oxycodone Hydrochloride
$C_{18}H_{21}NO_4.HCl$	Talibegron Hydrochloride
$C_{18}H_{21}NO_5$	Amikhelline
$C_{18}H_{21}NO_5.HCl$	Protokylol Hydrochloride
$C_{18}H_{21}NO_6$	Iprocrolol
$C_{18}H_{21}NO_6$	Naproxcinod
$C_{18}H_{21}N_3O$	Etofuradine
$C_{18}H_{21}N_3O.HCl$	Dibenzepin Hydrochloride
$C_{18}H_{21}N_3O.HCl$	Oxadimedine Hydrochloride
$C_{18}H_{21}N_3O_5S_2$	Prinomastat
$C_{18}H_{21}N_5O_2.C_7H_6O_2$	Alogliptin Benzoate
$C_{18}H_{21}N_5O_2S$	Amocarzine
$C_{18}H_{21}N_5O_3S$	Revospirone
$C_{18}H_{21}N_5O_4$	Metrifudil
$C_{18}H_{21}N_5S$	Tofimilast
$C_{18}H_{21}N_7O_4S$	Tiodazosin
$C_{18}H_{22}BrNO.HCl$	Embramine Hydrochloride
$C_{18}H_{22}BrNO_3S$	Heteronium Bromide
$C_{18}H_{22}ClNO.HCl$	Chlorphenoxamine Hydrochloride
$C_{18}H_{22}ClNO.HCl$	Phenoxybenzamine Hydrochloride
$C_{18}H_{22}ClNO.HCl$	Tecalcet Hydrochloride
$C_{18}H_{22}ClN_3O_2$	Carcainium Chloride
$C_{18}H_{22}Cl_2N_2O_3$	Diclofurime
$C_{18}H_{22}I_3N_3O_8$	Metrizamide
$C_{18}H_{22}N_2$	Cyclizine
$C_{18}H_{22}N_2$	Delfaprazine
$C_{18}H_{22}N_2$	Mezepine
$C_{18}H_{22}N_2$	Sifaprazine
$C_{18}H_{22}N_2.C_3H_6O_3$	Cyclizine Lactate
$C_{18}H_{22}N_2.HCl$	Cyclizine Hydrochloride
$C_{18}H_{22}N_2.HCl$	Desipramine Hydrochloride
$C_{18}H_{22}N_2O_2$	Carazolol
$C_{18}H_{22}N_2O_2.HCl.H_2O$	Phenacaine Hydrochloride
$C_{18}H_{22}N_2O_2S$	Oxomemazine
$C_{18}H_{22}N_2O_4S$	Besunide
$C_{18}H_{22}N_2O_5S$	Isopropicillin
$C_{18}H_{22}N_2O_5S$	Propicillin
$(C_{18}H_{22}N_2S)_2.C_4H_6O_6$	Trimeprazine Tartrate
$C_{18}H_{22}N_2S.HCl$	Diethazine Hydrochloride
$C_{18}H_{22}N_4Na_4O_{23}P_4$	Diquafosol Tetrasodium
$C_{18}H_{22}N_4O_4$	Tribendilol
$C_{18}H_{22}N_4O_4.HCl$	Xemilofiban Hydrochloride
$C_{18}H_{22}O$	Enzacamene
$C_{18}H_{22}O_2$	Estrone
$C_{18}H_{22}O_2$	Hexestrol
$C_{18}H_{22}O_2S$	Eprovafen
$C_{18}H_{22}O_3$	Methallenestril
$C_{18}H_{22}O_4$	Masoprocol
$C_{18}H_{22}O_4$	Terbucromil
$C_{18}H_{22}O_5S.C_4H_{10}N_2$	Estropipate
$C_{18}H_{22}O_8P_2$	Diethylstilbestrol Diphosphate
$(C_{18}H_{22})_m(O_4P)_n$ (Approximate)	Polyestradiol Phosphate
$C_{18}H_{23}ClN_2S$	Thiazinamium Chloride
$C_{18}H_{23}F^{123}INO_2$	Ioflupane (^{123}I)
$C_{18}H_{23}FN_2O_2$	Robalzotan
$C_{18}H_{23}FN_4O_5$	Eperezolid
$C_{18}H_{23}N$	Tolpropamine
$C_{18}H_{23}NO$	Bifemelane
$C_{18}H_{23}NO$	Dextrofemine
$C_{18}H_{23}NO$	Moxastine
$C_{18}H_{23}NO$	Racefemine
$C_{18}H_{23}NO.C_6H_8O_7$	Orphenadrine Citrate
$C_{18}H_{23}NO_2$	Butinazocine
$C_{18}H_{23}NO_2$	Ketazocine
$C_{18}H_{23}NO_2$	Medrylamine
$C_{18}H_{23}NO_3$	Butopamine
$C_{18}H_{23}NO_3$	Dobutamine
$C_{18}H_{23}NO_3$	Methyldihydromorphine
$C_{18}H_{23}NO_3$	Solpecainol
$C_{18}H_{23}NO_3.C_4H_6O_6$	Dihydrocodeine Bitartrate
$C_{18}H_{23}NO_3.C_4H_6O_6$	Dobutamine Tartrate
$C_{18}H_{23}NO_3.C_{12}H_{22}O_{12}$	Dobutamine Lactobionate
$C_{18}H_{23}NO_3.C_{12}H_{22}O_{12}$	Levdobutamine Lactobionate
$C_{18}H_{23}NO_3.HCl$	Dobutamine Hydrochloride
$C_{18}H_{23}NO_3.HCl$	Isoxsuprine Hydrochloride
$C_{18}H_{23}NO_3.HCl$	Ractopamine Hydrochloride
$C_{18}H_{23}NO_3S$	Ciglitazone
$C_{18}H_{23}NO_4$	Denopamine
$C_{18}H_{23}NO_4.HCl$	Arbutamine Hydrochloride
$C_{18}H_{23}NO_5$	Pentopril
$C_{18}H_{23}N_3O$	Acetergamine
$C_{18}H_{23}N_3O$	Atolide
$C_{18}H_{23}N_3O$	Vamicamide
$C_{18}H_{23}N_3O_2S$	Podilfen
$C_{18}H_{23}N_3O_3$	Buquiterine
$C_{18}H_{23}N_3O_6$	Imidaprilat
$C_{18}H_{23}N_5Na_4O_{21}P_4$	Denufosol Tetrasodium
$C_{18}H_{23}N_5O$	Binizolast
$C_{18}H_{23}N_5O_2.HCl$	Fenethylline Hydrochloride
$C_{18}H_{23}N_5O_3$	Cafedrine
$C_{18}H_{23}N_5O_5.HCl$	Reproterol Hydrochloride
$C_{18}H_{23}N_9O_4S_3.2HCl$	Cefotiam Hydrochloride
$C_{18}H_{23}NaO_3S$	Sodium Dibunate
$C_{18}H_{23}O_9N_3S$	Aspartame Acesulfame
$C_{18}H_{24}BrNO_3S$	Bretylium Tosylate
$C_{18}H_{24}BrNO_4$	Methscopolamine Bromide
$C_{18}H_{24}ClNO_2$	Clocanfamide
$C_{18}H_{24}ClNO_3$	Ericolol
$C_{18}H_{24}ClN_3O_2$	Pancopride
$C_{18}H_{24}FNO$	Nonaperone
$C_{18}H_{24}INO_2S$	Tiemonium Iodide
$C_{18}H_{24}I_3NO_8$	Iotrizoic Acid
$C_{18}H_{24}I_3N_3O_8$	Iopromide
$C_{18}H_{24}I_3N_3O_8$	Ioxilan
$C_{18}H_{24}I_3N_3O_9$	Ioglucol
$C_{18}H_{24}I_3N_3O_9$	Ioglunide
$C_{18}H_{24}I_3N_3O_9$	Ioversol
$C_{18}H_{24}N_2O$	Azaprocin

Molecular Formula	*Non-proprietary Name*
$C_{18}H_{24}N_2O$	Midazogrel
$C_{18}H_{24}N_2O$	Vintoperol
$C_{18}H_{24}N_2OS.C_2H_2O_4$	Suloxifen Oxalate
$C_{18}H_{24}N_2O_2S$	Darbufelone
$C_{18}H_{24}N_2O_2S.CH_4O_3S$	Darbufelone Mesylate
$C_{18}H_{24}N_2O_3$	Amquinate
$C_{18}H_{24}N_2O_3$	Atizoram
$C_{18}H_{24}N_2O_3$	Etanterol
$C_{18}H_{24}N_2O_4$	Ancarolol
$C_{18}H_{24}N_2O_5.2H_2O$	Enalaprilat
$C_{18}H_{24}N_2O_5S$	Amosulalol
$C_{18}H_{24}N_2O_6$	Cinepazic Acid
$C_{18}H_{24}N_4O$	Granisetron
$C_{18}H_{24}N_4O.HCl$	Granisetron Hydrochloride
$C_{18}H_{24}N_4O_3$	Naxifylline
$C_{18}H_{24}N_4O_4$	Carbazeran
$C_{18}H_{24}N_5O_8P$	Bucladesine
$C_{18}H_{24}N_6O$	Pexacerfont
$C_{18}H_{24}O_2$	Alfatradiol
$C_{18}H_{24}O_2$	Estradiol
$C_{18}H_{24}O_3$	Epiestriol
$C_{18}H_{24}O_3$	Estriol
$C_{18}H_{25}Br_2NO_3$	Oxabrexine
$C_{18}H_{25}ClN_2O$	Rodocaine
$C_{18}H_{25}ClO_2$	Norclostebol
$C_{18}H_{25}N$	Dimemorfan
$C_{18}H_{25}N$	Heptaverine
$C_{18}H_{25}N$	Volazocine
$C_{18}H_{25}NO$	Cyclazocine
$C_{18}H_{25}NO$	Dextromethorphan
$C_{18}H_{25}NO$	Levomethorphan
$C_{18}H_{25}NO$	Nepinalone
$C_{18}H_{25}NO$	Racemethorphan
$C_{18}H_{25}NO.HBr.H_2O$	Dextromethorphan Hydrobromide
$C_{18}H_{25}NO_2$	Allylprodine
$C_{18}H_{25}NO_2$	Moxazocine
$C_{18}H_{25}NO_3$	Atromepine
$C_{18}H_{25}N_3O.H_3O_4P$	Enazadrem Phosphate
$C_{18}H_{25}N_3O_3.C_4H_4O_4$	Azaloxan Fumarate
$C_{18}H_{25}N_3O_4$	Molracetam
$C_{18}H_{25}N_3O_5$	Carocainide
$C_{18}H_{25}N_3O_5$	Libenzapril
$C_{18}H_{25}N_5O_4$	Neldazosin
$C_{18}H_{25}N_5O_8S$	Gloximonam
$C_{18}H_{26}BrNOS_2$	Thihexinol Methylbromide
$C_{18}H_{26}BrNO_3$	Atropine Methylbromide
$C_{18}H_{26}ClNO_2$	Pranolium Chloride
$C_{18}H_{26}ClN_3$	Chloroquine
$C_{18}H_{26}ClN_3.(C_9H_6INO_4S)_2$	Cloquinate
$C_{18}H_{26}ClN_3.2HCl$	Chloroquine Hydrochloride
$C_{18}H_{26}ClN_3.2H_3PO_4$	Chloroquine Phosphate
$C_{18}H_{26}ClN_3O.H_2SO_4$	Hydroxychloroquine Sulfate
$C_{18}H_{26}ClN_3O_3$	Prucalopride
$C_{18}H_{26}N_2O$	Ipravacaine
$C_{18}H_{26}N_2O_3S.HCl$	Delequamine Hydrochloride
$C_{18}H_{26}N_2O_4$	Proglumide
$C_{18}H_{26}N_2O_4S$	Glibornuride
$C_{18}H_{26}N_2O_5$	Disofenin
$C_{18}H_{26}N_2O_6$	Methylatropine Nitrate
$C_{18}H_{26}N_2S.HCl$	Tandamine Hydrochloride
$C_{18}H_{26}N_4O_2S$	Mesulergine
$C_{18}H_{26}N_4O_3S$	Venritidine
$C_{18}H_{26}N_4O_5$	Denipride
$C_{18}H_{26}N_4O_6S$	Cetotiamine
$C_{18}H_{26}O$	Xibornol

Molecular Formula	*Non-proprietary Name*
$C_{18}H_{26}O_3$	Ibuverine
$C_{18}H_{26}O_3$	Inocoterone Acetate
$C_{18}H_{26}O_3$	Octinoxate
$C_{18}H_{26}O_5$	Taleranol
$C_{18}H_{26}O_5$	Zeranol
$(C_{18}H_{26}O_6)_w (C_{12}H_{16}O_3)_x$ $(C_7H_{12}O_3)_y (C_6H_{10}O_3)_z$ (Component B	Paflufocon D-HEM-Iberfilcon A
$C_{18}H_{27}IO_2S$	Hexasonium Iodide
$C_{18}H_{27}IO_3S$	Oxysonium Iodide
$C_{18}H_{27}NO_2$	Alifedrine
$C_{18}H_{27}NO_2$	Butaverine
$C_{18}H_{27}NO_2$	Pentapiperide
$C_{18}H_{27}NO_2.HCl$	Caramiphen Hydrochloride
$C_{18}H_{27}NO_2.HCl$	Dyclonine Hydrochloride
$C_{18}H_{27}NO_2S$	Tazofelone
$C_{18}H_{27}NO_3$	Capsaicin
$C_{18}H_{27}NO_3$	Droxypropine
$C_{18}H_{27}NO_3$	Minepentate
$C_{18}H_{27}NO_3$	Zucapsaicin
$C_{18}H_{27}NO_4$	Etoxeridine
$C_{18}H_{27}NO_5$	Propanidid
$C_{18}H_{27}NO_6$	Trixolane
$C_{18}H_{27}N_3O.H_3PO_4$	Pentaquine Phosphate
$C_{18}H_{27}N_3O_3$	Saxagliptin
$C_{18}H_{28}ClNO$	Clofenciclan
$C_{18}H_{28}N_2O$	Bumecaine
$C_{18}H_{28}N_2O$	Levobupivacaine
$C_{18}H_{28}N_2O.HCl$	Levobupivacaine Hydrochloride
$C_{18}H_{28}N_2O.HCl.H_2O$	Bupivacaine Hydrochloride
$C_{18}H_{28}N_2O_2$	Vadocaine
$C_{18}H_{28}N_2O_3S$	Almokalant
$C_{18}H_{28}N_2O_4$	Acebutolol
$C_{18}H_{28}N_2O_4.HCl$	Acebutolol Hydrochloride
$C_{18}H_{28}N_4O$	Butalamine
$C_{18}H_{28}N_6O$	Lamtidine
$C_{18}H_{28}O_4Si_4$	Quadrosilan
$C_{18}H_{29}NO_2$	Ketocaine
$C_{18}H_{29}NO_2$	Lotucaine
$C_{18}H_{29}NO_2.HCl$	Exaprolol Hydrochloride
$(C_{18}H_{29}NO_2)_2.H_2SO_4$	Penbutolol Sulfate
$C_{18}H_{29}NO_3.C_6H_8O_7$	Butamirate Citrate
$C_{18}H_{29}NO_3.HCl$	Betaxolol Hydrochloride
$C_{18}H_{29}NO_3.HCl$	Levobetaxolol Hydrochloride
$C_{18}H_{29}NO_4$	Bufetolol
$C_{18}H_{29}NO_4$	Guaiapate
$C_{18}H_{29}NO_4.HCl$	Cicloprolol Hydrochloride
$C_{18}H_{29}NO_4.HCl$	Iproxamine Hydrochloride
$C_{18}H_{29}N_3O_2$	Dalcotidine
$C_{18}H_{29}N_3O_5$	Bambuterol
$C_{18}H_{29}N_3O_5S$	Lenapenem
$C_{18}H_{30}BrNO_3S$	Penthienate Bromide
$(C_{18}H_{30}Ge_6O_{21})_n$	Repagermanium
$(C_{18}H_{30}N_2O_2)_2.H_2SO_4$	Butacaine Sulfate
$C_{18}H_{30}N_4O_{11}$	Almurtide
$C_{18}H_{30}O_2$	Gamolenic Acid
$C_{18}H_{31}GdN_4O_9$	Gadobutrol
$C_{18}H_{31}NO_2$	Ketocainol
$C_{18}H_{31}NO_4$	Bisoprolol
$(C_{18}H_{31}NO_4)_2.C_4H_4O_4$	Bisoprolol Fumarate
$C_{18}H_{31}N_3O_3$	Pafenolol
$C_{18}H_{31}N_3O_3S.C_4H_4O_4$	Suricainide Maleate
$C_{18}H_{32}Br_2Cl_2N_4O_2$	Dibrospidium Chloride
$C_{18}H_{32}CaN_2O_{10}$	Calcium Pantothenate
$C_{18}H_{32}CaN_2O_{10}$	Calcium Pantothenate, Racemic
$C_{18}H_{32}CaN_4O_9$	Calcobutrol

Molecular Formula	Non-proprietary Name
$C_{18}H_{32}CaO_{19}.H_2O$	Calcium Glubionate
$C_{18}H_{32}O_7$	Tributyl Citrate
$C_{18}H_{33}ClN_2O_5S$	Clindamycin
$C_{18}H_{33}ClN_2O_5S.HCl$	Clindamycin Hydrochloride
$C_{18}H_{34}ClN_2O_8PS$	Clindamycin Phosphate
$C_{18}H_{34}N_2O_6S$	Lincomycin
$C_{18}H_{34}N_2O_6S.HCl.H_2O$	Lincomycin Hydrochloride
$C_{18}H_{34}O_2$	Oleic Acid
$C_{18}H_{34}O_2.C_2H_7NO$	Ethanolamine Oleate
$C_{18}H_{34}O_3$	Methyl Palmoxirate
$C_{18}H_{34}O_3$	Rosaprostol
$C_{18}H_{34}O_4$	Dibutyl Sebacate
$C_{18}H_{34}O_6$	Sorbitan Monolaurate
$C_{18}H_{35}NO$	Laurocapram
$C_{18}H_{35}NO_2.HCl$	Isomylamine Hydrochloride
$C_{18}H_{36}Cl_4N_4O_2$	Prospidium Chloride
$C_{18}H_{36}N_4O_{11}.H_2SO_4$	Kanamycin Sulfate
$C_{18}H_{36}O$	Oleyl Alcohol
$C_{18}H_{37}N.HF$	Dectaflur
$C_{18}H_{37}NO_2$	Palmidrol
$C_{18}H_{37}N_5O_8$	Dibekacin
$C_{18}H_{37}N_5O_9$	Tobramycin
$(C_{18}H_{37}N_5O_9)_2.5H_2SO_4$	Tobramycin Sulfate
$C_{18}H_{37}N_5O_{10}$	Bekanamycin
$C_{18}H_{38}BrNO_2$	Laurcetium Bromide
$C_{18}H_{38}O$	Isostearyl Alcohol
$C_{18}H_{39}NO_2$	Safingol
$C_{18}H_{39}NO_2.HCl$	Safingol Hydrochloride
$C_{18}H_{39}N_3O_2$	Dodicin
$C_{18}H_{39}N_7O_3$	Anisperimus
$C_{18}H_{40}Br_2N_4O_4$	Hexcarbacholine Bromide
$C_{18}H_{40}O_4P_2$	Tetrofosmin
$C_{19}H_9HgI_2NaO_7S$	Meralein Sodium
$C_{19}H_{11}BrF_2N_2O_4$	Minalrestat
$C_{19}H_{11}Cl_2I_2NO_3$	Rafoxanide
$C_{19}H_{12}F_3N_3O_3S$	Zopolrestat
$C_{19}H_{12}F_6N_2O_7$	Flurantel
$C_{19}H_{12}O_6$	Dicumarol
$C_{19}H_{12}O_8$	Diacerein
$C_{19}H_{14}N_2OS_2$	Naftoxate
$C_{19}H_{14}N_4O_6$	Sivifene
$C_{19}H_{14}O_5S$	Phenolsulfonphthalein
$C_{19}H_{14}O_8$	Flavodic Acid
$C_{19}H_{15}CaNO_7$	Nedocromil Calcium
$C_{19}H_{15}ClNNaO_4.3H_2O$	Indomethacin Sodium
$C_{19}H_{15}ClN_2O_4$	Rebamipide
$C_{19}H_{15}Cl_3N_2O_2$	Democonazole
$C_{19}H_{15}F_3N_2OS$	Cisconazole
$C_{19}H_{15}F_3N_2O_3$	Tecovirimat
$C_{19}H_{15}F_3N_4O_3$	Tosufloxacin
$C_{19}H_{15}KO_4$	Warfarin Potassium
$C_{19}H_{15}NNa_2O_7$	Nedocromil Sodium
$C_{19}H_{15}NO_6$	Acenocoumarol
$C_{19}H_{15}NaO_4$	Warfarin Sodium
$C_{19}H_{16}ClFN_2O$	Flutoprazepam
$C_{19}H_{16}ClNO_4$	Clometacin
$C_{19}H_{16}ClNO_4$	Indomethacin
$C_{19}H_{16}ClNO_4$	Rilopirox
$C_{19}H_{16}Cl_2N_3NaO_5S.H_2O$	Dicloxacillin Sodium
$C_{19}H_{16}N_2O_2$	Lificiguat
$C_{19}H_{16}N_2O_4$	Benzobarbital
$C_{19}H_{16}N_4O_4$	Zidometacin
$C_{19}H_{16}N_5NaO_7S_3$	Ceftiofur Sodium
$C_{19}H_{16}N_6O_4S$	Zibotentan
$C_{19}H_{16}O_5$	Efloxate
$C_{19}H_{16}O_5$	Isocromil

Molecular Formula	Non-proprietary Name
$C_{19}H_{17}ClFN_3O_5S$	Floxacillin
$C_{19}H_{17}ClF_3NO_4$	Halofenate
$C_{19}H_{17}ClN_2NaO_3$	Laquinimod Sodium
$C_{19}H_{17}ClN_2O$	Prazepam
$C_{19}H_{17}ClN_2O_4$	Glafenine
$C_{19}H_{17}ClN_2O_4$	Oxametacin
$C_{19}H_{17}ClN_2O_6$	Arclofenin
$C_{19}H_{17}ClN_3NaO_5S.H_2O$	Cloxacillin Sodium
$C_{19}H_{17}Cl_2N_3O_5S$	Dicloxacillin
$C_{19}H_{17}Cl_3N_2S.HNO_3$	Butoconazole Nitrate
$C_{19}H_{17}NO$	Omigapil
$C_{19}H_{17}NOS$	Tolnaftate
$C_{19}H_{17}NO_2$	Neocinchophen
$C_{19}H_{17}NO_4S_2$	Naroparcil
$C_{19}H_{17}NO_5$	Mofezolac
$C_{19}H_{17}NO_7$	Incyclinide
$C_{19}H_{17}NO_7$	Nedocromil
$C_{19}H_{17}N_2NaO_4S$	Parecoxib Sodium
$C_{19}H_{17}N_3.HCl$	Fuchsin, Basic
$C_{19}H_{17}N_3O_4S_2$	Cephaloridine
$C_{19}H_{17}N_5O_2.2CH_4O_3S$	Nafamostat Mesylate
$C_{19}H_{17}N_5O_5S$	Salazosulfadimidine
$C_{19}H_{17}N_5O_7S_3.HCl$	Ceftiofur Hydrochloride
$C_{19}H_{17}N_6NaO_6S_2$	Cefamandole Nafate
$C_{19}H_{17}N_9O_5S_2$	Cefozopran
$C_{19}H_{18}BrClN_4O_2$	Parogrelil
$C_{19}H_{18}BrF_3N_2O_4$	Bromoxanide
$C_{19}H_{18}CaN_2O_9$	Carbaspirin Calcium
$C_{19}H_{18}ClFN_2O_3$	Flutazolam
$C_{19}H_{18}ClFN_2O_3S$	Elfazepam
$C_{19}H_{18}ClF_2N_3O_3.1\frac{1}{2}H_2O$	Sitafloxacin
$C_{19}H_{18}ClNO.CH_4O_3S$	Clopipazan Mesylate
$C_{19}H_{18}ClN_3O$	Cyprazepam
$C_{19}H_{18}ClN_3O_3$	Camazepam
$C_{19}H_{18}ClN_3O_4S$	Trazium Esilate
$C_{19}H_{18}ClN_3O_5S$	Rivaroxaban
$(C_{19}H_{18}ClN_3O_5S)_2.C_{16}H_{20}N_2$	Cloxacillin Benzathine
$C_{19}H_{18}ClN_5$	Adinazolam
$C_{19}H_{18}Cl_2N_2O_2$	Ciprazafone
$C_{19}H_{18}Cl_2N_4O_4S$	Prazocillin
$C_{19}H_{18}F_3NO_2$	Prefenamate
$C_{19}H_{18}F_6N_2O.H_3PO_4$	Enpiroline Phosphate
$C_{19}H_{18}F_6O_3$	Arteflene
$C_{19}H_{18}N_2O_2$	Ciproquazone
$C_{19}H_{18}N_2O_3$	Kebuzone
$C_{19}H_{18}N_2O_4$	Cimoxatone
$C_{19}H_{18}N_2O_4S$	Parecoxib
$C_{19}H_{18}N_2O_4S$	Tetomilast
$[(C_{19}H_{18}N_3)_2.C_{23}H_{14}O_6].2H_2O$	Pararosaniline Pamoate
$C_{19}H_{18}N_3NaO_5S.H_2O$	Oxacillin Sodium
$C_{19}H_{18}N_4O_2$	Pimobendan
$C_{19}H_{18}N_4O_2S$	Ilaprazole
$C_{19}H_{18}N_4O_5S_3$	Cefcanel
$C_{19}H_{18}N_6O_5S_3$	Cefditoren
$C_{19}H_{18}N_8Na_2O_5$	Aminopterin Sodium
$C_{19}H_{18}O_7$	Benfurodil Hemisuccinate
$C_{19}H_{19}BrClNO_2$	Berupipam
$C_{19}H_{19}ClN_2$	Desloratadine
$C_{19}H_{19}Cl_2N_3O_2$	Mipitroban
$C_{19}H_{19}Cl_2N_3O_3$	Elnadipine
$C_{19}H_{19}Cl_2N_3O_3$	Pinadoline
$C_{19}H_{19}F_2NO_2$	Flazalone
$C_{19}H_{19}N$	Setiptiline
$C_{19}H_{19}N.C_4H_6O_6$	Phenindamine Tartrate
$C_{19}H_{19}NO$	Maroxepin
$C_{19}H_{19}NOS.C_4H_4O_4$	Ketotifen Fumarate

Molecular Formula	Non-proprietary Name
$C_{19}H_{19}NO_6$	Etersalate
$C_{19}H_{19}NO_6S$	Indeglitazar
$C_{19}H_{19}NS$	Pimethixene
$C_{19}H_{19}N_2NaO_2.C_3H_8O_3$	Phenbutazone Sodium Glycerate
$C_{19}H_{19}N_3$	Perafensine
$C_{19}H_{19}N_3O_3$	Talampanel
$C_{19}H_{19}N_3O_6$	Nilvadipine
$C_{19}H_{19}N_5O_5S_3$	Cefaparole
$C_{19}H_{19}N_7O_6$	Folic Acid
$C_{19}H_{20}BrN_2O_4P$	Ibrolipim
$C_{19}H_{20}BrN_3O_3$	Bretazenil
$C_{19}H_{20}Br_2N_6O_4S$	Macitentan
$C_{19}H_{20}ClN$	Losindole
$C_{19}H_{20}ClNO$	Ecopipam
$C_{19}H_{20}ClNO.HCl$	Ecopipam Hydrochloride
$C_{19}H_{20}ClNO_2$	Odapipam
$C_{19}H_{20}ClNO_4$	Bezafibrate
$C_{19}H_{20}ClNO_5$	Ronifibrate
$C_{19}H_{20}ClN_3$	Clemizole
$C_{19}H_{20}ClN_3O$	Saripidem
$C_{19}H_{20}ClN_3O_4$	Siltenzepine
$C_{19}H_{20}ClN_3O_4S$	Piragliatin
$C_{19}H_{20}Cl_2N_2O_5$	Etofamide
$C_{19}H_{20}FNO_3$	Paroxetine
$C_{19}H_{20}FNO_3.CH_4O_4S$	Paroxetine Mesylate
$C_{19}H_{20}FNO_3.HCl$	Paroxetine Hydrochloride
$C_{19}H_{20}FN_3$	Fluperlapine
$C_{19}H_{20}FN_3.HCl$	Gevotroline Hydrochloride
$C_{19}H_{20}FN_3O_3.CH_4O_3S$	Danofloxacin Mesylate
$C_{19}H_{20}FN_5O_4$	Zabofloxacin
$C_{19}H_{20}F_2N_4O_4$	Pamapimod
$C_{19}H_{20}F_3NO$	Boxidine
$C_{19}H_{20}F_3NO_2$	Benfluorex
$C_{19}H_{20}F_3N_3O_3$	Morniflumate
$C_{19}H_{20}F_3N_3O_3$	Orbifloxacin
$C_{19}H_{20}F_3N_3O_4$	Cadrofloxacin
$C_{19}H_{20}F_6N_5O_5PS$	Alamifovir
$C_{19}H_{20}N_2$	Mebhydrolin
$C_{19}H_{20}N_2O$	Denzimol
$C_{19}H_{20}N_2O_2$	Phenylbutazone
$C_{19}H_{20}N_2O_3$	Amphotalide
$C_{19}H_{20}N_2O_3$	Bindarit
$C_{19}H_{20}N_2O_3$	Ditazole
$C_{19}H_{20}N_2O_3.CH_4O_3S.H_2O$	Dolasetron Mesylate
$C_{19}H_{20}N_2O_3.H_2O$	Oxyphenbutazone
$C_{19}H_{20}N_2O_3S$	Apricoxib
$C_{19}H_{20}N_2O_3S.HCl$	Pioglitazone Hydrochloride
$C_{19}H_{20}N_2O_7$	Aranidipine
$C_{19}H_{20}N_4O_2$	Nuvenzepine
$C_{19}H_{20}N_4O_2$	Rispenzepine
$C_{19}H_{20}N_4O_2S_2$	Elesclomol
$C_{19}H_{20}N_6O.2HCl$	Imidocarb Hydrochloride
$C_{19}H_{20}O_{10}$	Khelloside
$C_{19}H_{21}ClFN_3O_3.HCl$	Besifloxacin Hydrochloride
$C_{19}H_{21}ClN_2$	Elanzepine
$C_{19}H_{21}ClN_2OS$	Chloracyzine
$C_{19}H_{21}ClN_2OS$	Halethazole
$C_{19}H_{21}ClN_2O_3$	Oxazafone
$C_{19}H_{21}ClN_2S$	Clorotepine
$C_{19}H_{21}ClN_4O_5$	Acefylline Clofibrol
$C_{19}H_{21}ClN_4O_5$	Theofibrate
$C_{19}H_{21}FN_2O_2$	Eplivanserin
$C_{19}H_{21}FN_2O_4$	Levonadifloxacin
$C_{19}H_{21}FN_2O_4$	Nadifloxacin
$C_{19}H_{21}FN_4$	Tecastemizole

Molecular Formula	Non-proprietary Name
$C_{19}H_{21}FN_4O_3$	Ecenofloxacin
$C_{19}H_{21}F_3N_2S$	Trifluomeprazine
$C_{19}H_{21}F_3N_6O_2$	Opanixil
$C_{19}H_{21}N.HCl$	Indriline Hydrochloride
$C_{19}H_{21}N.HCl$	Nortriptyline Hydrochloride
$C_{19}H_{21}N.HCl$	Pridefine Hydrochloride
$C_{19}H_{21}N.HCl$	Protriptyline Hydrochloride
$C_{19}H_{21}NO.HCl$	Cidoxepin Hydrochloride
$C_{19}H_{21}NO.HCl$	Doxepin Hydrochloride
$C_{19}H_{21}NO_2$	Beloxepin
$C_{19}H_{21}NO_2$	Dimeprozan
$C_{19}H_{21}NO_2$	Oxitriptyline
$C_{19}H_{21}NO_3$	Spiroxepin
$C_{19}H_{21}NO_3.HCl$	Nalorphine Hydrochloride
$C_{19}H_{21}NO_4.HCl$	Naloxone Hydrochloride
$C_{19}H_{21}NO_5$	Osemozotan
$C_{19}H_{21}NO_5S$	Cinaproxen
$C_{19}H_{21}NO_6$	Oxodipine
$C_{19}H_{21}NS$	Pizotyline
$C_{19}H_{21}NS.HCl$	Dothiepin Hydrochloride
$C_{19}H_{21}N_3$	Perlapine
$C_{19}H_{21}N_3O$	Alcaftadine
$C_{19}H_{21}N_3O$	Talastine
$(C_{19}H_{21}N_3O)_2.C_4H_6O_6$	Zolpidem Tartrate
$C_{19}H_{21}N_3O_2S$	Enviradene
$C_{19}H_{21}N_3O_5$	Darodipine
$C_{19}H_{21}N_3O_5$	Isradipine
$C_{19}H_{21}N_3S$	Cyamemazine
$C_{19}H_{21}N_3S$	Metiapine
$C_{19}H_{21}N_5O_2.2HCl$	Pirenzepine Hydrochloride
$C_{19}H_{21}N_5O_3.2CH_4O_3S$	Oxmetidine Mesylate
$C_{19}H_{21}N_5O_3.2HCl$	Oxmetidine Hydrochloride
$C_{19}H_{21}N_5O_4.HCl$	Prazosin Hydrochloride
$C_{19}H_{22}BrNO_4S_2$	Tiotropium Bromide
$C_{19}H_{22}ClNO_2$	Chlordimorine
$C_{19}H_{22}ClNO_2.HCl$	Difencloxazine Hydrochloride
$C_{19}H_{22}ClN_3O_5S_2$	Clamikalant
$C_{19}H_{22}ClN_5O.HCl$	Trazodone Hydrochloride
$C_{19}H_{22}FN_3O$	Azaperone
$C_{19}H_{22}FN_3O_3$	Binfloxacin
$C_{19}H_{22}FN_3O_3$	Enrofloxacin
$C_{19}H_{22}FN_3O_3$	Vebufloxacin
$C_{19}H_{22}FN_3O_3.HCl$	Grepafloxacin Hydrochloride
$C_{19}H_{22}FN_3O_4.1½H_2O$	Gatifloxacin
$C_{19}H_{22}FN_3O_8$	Galocitabine
$C_{19}H_{22}F_2N_4O_3$	Sparfloxacin
$C_{19}H_{22}KN_3O_4S$	Hetacillin Potassium
$C_{19}H_{22}N_2$	Depramine
$C_{19}H_{22}N_2.HCl.H_2O$	Triprolidine Hydrochloride
$C_{19}H_{22}N_2O$	Noxiptiline
$C_{19}H_{22}N_2O$	Vinburnine
$C_{19}H_{22}N_2O.C_4H_4O_4$	Ketipramine Fumarate
$C_{19}H_{22}N_2O.HCl$	Amedalin Hydrochloride
$C_{19}H_{22}N_2OS$	Aceprometazine
$C_{19}H_{22}N_2OS.C_4H_4O_4$	Acepromazine Maleate
$C_{19}H_{22}N_2OS.HCl$	Thiazesim Hydrochloride
$C_{19}H_{22}N_2O_2$	Hydroxindasol
$C_{19}H_{22}N_2O_3$	Bumadizone
$C_{19}H_{22}N_2O_3S.HCl$	Dimethoxanate Hydrochloride
$C_{19}H_{22}N_2O_6S$	Penamecillin
$C_{19}H_{22}N_2S$	Dimelazine
$C_{19}H_{22}N_2S.C_2H_4O_2$	Mepazine Acetate
$C_{19}H_{22}N_4O$	Cianergoline
$C_{19}H_{22}N_4O_2$	Pumaprazole
$C_{19}H_{22}N_4O_2S$	Telenzepine
$C_{19}H_{22}N_4O_3$	Iclaprim

Molecular Formula	Non-proprietary Name
$C_{19}H_{22}N_4O_3.CH_4O_3S$	Iclaprim Mesylate
$C_{19}H_{22}N_8O_6S_2$	Cefoselis
$C_{19}H_{22}O_2$	Vedaprofen
$C_{19}H_{22}O_4$	Oxeglitazar
$C_{19}H_{23}ClN_2$	Homochlorcyclizine
$C_{19}H_{23}ClN_2.HCl$	Clomipramine Hydrochloride
$C_{19}H_{23}ClN_2O_2$	Traboxopine
$C_{19}H_{23}ClN_2S.HCl$	Chlorproethazine Hydrochloride
$C_{19}H_{23}FN_2O_3$	Roxoperone
$C_{19}H_{23}F_2N_3O_3$	Merafloxacin
$C_{19}H_{23}I_2NO_2$	Bufeniode
$C_{19}H_{23}NO$	Alimadol
$C_{19}H_{23}NO$	Cinnamedrine
$C_{19}H_{23}NO.C_7H_7ClN_4O_2$	Piprinhydrinate
$C_{19}H_{23}NO.HCl$	Diphenylpyraline Hydrochloride
$C_{19}H_{23}NO_2$	Elucaine
$C_{19}H_{23}NO_2$	Ibuprofen Piconol
$C_{19}H_{23}NO_2$	Minamestane
$C_{19}H_{23}NO_2.C_4H_4O_4$	Trepipam Maleate
$C_{19}H_{23}NO_2S$	Meprotixol
$C_{19}H_{23}NO_3$	Esreboxetine
$C_{19}H_{23}NO_3$	Oxyfedrine
$C_{19}H_{23}NO_3$	Reboxetine
$C_{19}H_{23}NO_3.CH_4O_3S.$	Reboxetine Mesylate
$C_{19}H_{23}NO_3.C_4H_6O_4$	Esreboxetine Succinate
$C_{19}H_{23}NO_3.HCl$	Biphenamine Hydrochloride
$C_{19}H_{23}NO_5$	Semorphone
$C_{19}H_{23}NO_5$	Tretoquinol
$C_{19}H_{23}NO_6$	Butocrolol
$C_{19}H_{23}N_3$	Amitraz
$C_{19}H_{23}N_3$	Binedaline
$C_{19}H_{23}N_3O.HCl$	Benzydamine Hydrochloride
$C_{19}H_{23}N_3OS$	Leminoprazole
$C_{19}H_{23}N_3O_2.C_4H_4O_4$	Ergonovine Maleate
$C_{19}H_{23}N_3O_3$	Coluracetam
$C_{19}H_{23}N_3O_3$	Espatropate
$C_{19}H_{23}N_3O_4S$	Hetacillin
$C_{19}H_{23}N_3O_5S$	Oxetacillin
$C_{19}H_{23}N_3S$	Dazidamine
$C_{19}H_{23}N_4O_6PS$	Benfotiamine
$C_{19}H_{23}N_5O_2$	Epiroprim
$C_{19}H_{23}N_5O_3$	Trimetrexate
$C_{19}H_{23}N_5O_3.C_6H_{10}O_7$	Trimetrexate Glucuronate
$C_{19}H_{23}N_5O_3S.HCl$	Ipsapirone Hydrochloride
$C_{19}H_{24}BrNS_2$	Tiquizium Bromide
$C_{19}H_{24}ClNO$	Mecloxamine
$C_{19}H_{24}INO_3$	Metocinium Iodide
$C_{19}H_{24}N_2$	Bamipine
$C_{19}H_{24}N_2$	Histapyrrodine
$C_{19}H_{24}N_2$	Monometacrine
$C_{19}H_{24}N_2$	Prazepine
$C_{19}H_{24}N_2.C_7H_8O_3S$	Daledalin Tosylate
$C_{19}H_{24}N_2.HCl$	Imipramine Hydrochloride
$C_{19}H_{24}N_2O$	Imipraminoxide
$C_{19}H_{24}N_2O$	Vincanol
$C_{19}H_{24}N_2O.HCl$	Palonosetron Hydrochloride
$C_{19}H_{24}N_2O.H_2SO_4$	Aminopentamide Sulfate
$C_{19}H_{24}N_2OS$	Levomepromazine
$C_{19}H_{24}N_2OS$	Methotrimeprazine
$C_{19}H_{24}N_2OS$	Phencarbamide
$C_{19}H_{24}N_2OS.C_4H_4O_4$	Levomepromazine Maleate
$C_{19}H_{24}N_2OS.HCl$	Levomepromazine Hydrochloride
$C_{19}H_{24}N_2O_2.CH_4O_3S$	Dicarfen

Molecular Formula	Non-proprietary Name
$C_{19}H_{24}N_2O_2$	Praziquantel
$C_{19}H_{24}N_2O_2$	Salverine
$C_{19}H_{24}N_2O_2.C_7H_7SO_3H.\frac{1}{2}H_2O$	Xylamidine Tosylate
$C_{19}H_{24}N_2O_3.HCl$	Dilevalol Hydrochloride
$C_{19}H_{24}N_2O_3.HCl$	Labetalol Hydrochloride
$C_{19}H_{24}N_2O_4$	Pipratecol
$C_{19}H_{24}N_2O_4$	Tolamolol
$(C_{19}H_{24}N_2O_4)_2.C_4H_4O_4$	Formoterol Fumarate
$C_{19}H_{24}N_2O_4.C_4H_6O_6$	Arformoterol Tartrate
$C_{19}H_{24}N_2O_4S$	Mesudipine
$C_{19}H_{24}N_2O_4S_2$	Omapatrilat
$C_{19}H_{24}N_2O_7S$	Furbucillin
$C_{19}H_{24}N_2S.HCl$	Ethopropazine Hydrochloride
$C_{19}H_{24}N_2S_2$	Levometiomeprazine
$C_{19}H_{24}N_2S_2.HCl$	Methiomeprazine Hydrochloride
$C_{19}H_{24}N_4O_2$	Pentamidine
$C_{19}H_{24}N_4O_3$	Pibutidine
$C_{19}H_{24}N_6O_2$	Zolenzepine
$C_{19}H_{24}N_6O_5S_2$	Cefepime
$C_{19}H_{24}O_2$	Almestrone
$C_{19}H_{24}O_2$	Metribolone
$C_{19}H_{24}O_2S$	Prifelone
$C_{19}H_{24}O_3$	Pirnabine
$C_{19}H_{24}O_3$	Testolactone
$C_{19}H_{25}BN_4O_4$	Bortezomib
$C_{19}H_{25}ClN_2O_2.C_4H_4O_4$	Zatosetron Maleate
$C_{19}H_{25}ClN_6O_5S_2.HCl.H_2O$	Cefepime Hydrochloride
$C_{19}H_{25}NO$	Drobuline
$C_{19}H_{25}NO$	Etoloxamine
$C_{19}H_{25}NO$	Hexapradol
$C_{19}H_{25}NO$	Tesmilifene
$C_{19}H_{25}NO.C_4H_6O_6$	Levallorphan Tartrate
$C_{19}H_{25}NO.HBr$	Alentemol Hydrobromide
$C_{19}H_{25}NO.HCl$	Tesmilifene Hydrochloride
$C_{19}H_{25}NOS$	Rotigotine
$C_{19}H_{25}NO_2$	Berlafenone
$C_{19}H_{25}NO_2$	Cliropamine
$C_{19}H_{25}NO_2$	Propinetidine
$(C_{19}H_{25}NO_2)_2.C_4H_6O_6$	Proxorphan Tartrate
$C_{19}H_{25}NO_2.HCl$	Nylidrin Hydrochloride
$C_{19}H_{25}NO_3$	Dopamantine
$C_{19}H_{25}NO_3$	Mitiglinide
$C_{19}H_{25}NO_3S$	Trethinium Tosilate
$C_{19}H_{25}NO_4$	Salmefamol
$C_{19}H_{25}NO_4$	Tetramethrin
$C_{19}H_{25}N_3$	Picoperine
$C_{19}H_{25}N_3O$	Milacainide
$C_{19}H_{25}N_3O$	Toprilidine
$C_{19}H_{25}N_3OS$	Thiambutosine
$C_{19}H_{25}N_3S$	Aminopromazine
$C_{19}H_{25}N_4O_6PS_2$	Uredofos
$C_{19}H_{25}N_5O_4.HCl.2H_2O$	Terazosin Hydrochloride
$C_{19}H_{26}BrNO$	Bibenzonium Bromide
$C_{19}H_{26}BrNO_3S$	Oxitefonium Bromide
$C_{19}H_{26}BrNO_4$	Oxitropium Bromide
$C_{19}H_{26}ClNO_6$	Arbaclofen Placarbil
$C_{19}H_{26}FeO$	Diciferron
$C_{19}H_{26}I_3N_3O_9$	Iohexol
$C_{19}H_{26}N_2O$	Naftypramide
$C_{19}H_{26}N_2O_3$	Benolizime
$C_{19}H_{26}N_2O_3$	Isoxaprolol
$C_{19}H_{26}N_2O_3$	Naminterol
$C_{19}H_{26}N_2O_4S$	Gemopatrilat
$C_{19}H_{26}N_2O_4S.HCl$	Zinterol Hydrochloride
$C_{19}H_{26}N_2O_4S_2$	Thiazinamium Metilsulfate

Molecular Formula	Non-proprietary Name
$C_{19}H_{26}N_2O_5S.HCl$	Mesuprine Hydrochloride
$C_{19}H_{26}N_2S.CH_4O_3S$	Pergolide Mesylate
$C_{19}H_{26}N_4O_4.HCl$	Piquizil Hydrochloride
$C_{19}H_{26}N_4O_5.HCl$	Hoquizil Hydrochloride
$C_{19}H_{26}N_6O$	Seliciclib
$C_{19}H_{26}NaO_9P$	Fostriecin Sodium
$C_{19}H_{26}O_2$	Androstenedione
$C_{19}H_{26}O_3$	Bioallethrin
$C_{19}H_{26}O_3$	Epimestrol
$C_{19}H_{26}O_3$	Formestane
$C_{19}H_{26}O_4.C_4H_{11}NO_2$	Tocamphyl
$C_{19}H_{27}ClO_2$	Clostebol
$C_{19}H_{27}FN_2O_3$	Carperone
$C_{19}H_{27}NO$	Pentazocine
$C_{19}H_{27}NO.C_3H_6O_3$	Pentazocine Lactate
$C_{19}H_{27}NO.C_4H_6O_4$	Ciprefadol Succinate
$C_{19}H_{27}NO.HCl$	Pentazocine Hydrochloride
$C_{19}H_{27}NO_2$	Mantabegron
$C_{19}H_{27}NO_3$	Nateglinide
$C_{19}H_{27}NO_3$	Tetrabenazine
$C_{19}H_{27}NO_4$	Cinoctramide
$C_{19}H_{27}NO_4$	Drotebanol
$C_{19}H_{27}NO_4$	Nolomirole
$C_{19}H_{27}NO_4S$	Emilium Tosylate
$C_{19}H_{27}NO_4S$	Revatropate
$C_{19}H_{27}NO_5S$	Mefenidramium Metilsulfate
$C_{19}H_{27}N_3O$	Ricasetron
$C_{19}H_{27}N_3O_4$	Semagacestat
$C_{19}H_{27}N_3O_4S$	Amantocillin
$C_{19}H_{27}N_3O_5$	Murocainide
$C_{19}H_{27}N_3O_5S_2$	Dofetilide
$C_{19}H_{27}N_5.HCl$	Dapiprazole Hydrochloride
$C_{19}H_{27}N_5O_3$	Bunazosin
$C_{19}H_{27}N_5O_4.HCl$	Alfuzosin Hydrochloride
$C_{19}H_{27}N_5O_5$	Nifekalant
$C_{19}H_{27}NaO_5S.2H_2O$	Sodium Prasterone Sulfate
$C_{19}H_{28}BrNO_3$	Glycopyrrolate
$C_{19}H_{28}BrNO_3$	Ritropirronium Bromide
$C_{19}H_{28}ClN_3O_5S.HCl$	Sulamserod Hydrochloride
$C_{19}H_{28}ClN_5O.HCl$	Etoperidone Hydrochloride
$C_{19}H_{28}N_2$	Iprindole
$C_{19}H_{28}N_2O_3$	Irolapride
$C_{19}H_{28}N_2O_4$	Carpindolol
$C_{19}H_{28}N_2O_4.HCl$	Roxatidine Acetate Hydrochloride
$C_{19}H_{28}N_4O_2S$	Etisulergine
$C_{19}H_{28}N_4O_5S_2$	Osutidine
$C_{19}H_{28}O_2$	Benorterone
$C_{19}H_{28}O_2$	Prasterone
$C_{19}H_{28}O_2$	Testosterone
$C_{19}H_{28}O_8$	Artesunate
$C_{19}H_{29}BClN_6O_6{}^{99m}Tc$	Technetium Tc 99m Teboroxime
$C_{19}H_{29}IO_2$	Iophendylate
$C_{19}H_{29}NO.HCl$	Cycrimine Hydrochloride
$C_{19}H_{29}NO.HCl$	Procyclidine Hydrochloride
$C_{19}H_{29}NO_2$	Bornaprolol
$C_{19}H_{29}NO_2.HCl$	Nexeridine Hydrochloride
$C_{19}H_{29}NO_3$	Butopiprine
$C_{19}H_{29}NO_3$	Nafetolol
$C_{19}H_{29}NO_4$	Perfomedil
$C_{19}H_{29}NO_5$	Burodiline
$C_{19}H_{29}NO_5$	Dipivefrin
$C_{19}H_{29}NO_5.HCl$	Dipivefrin Hydrochloride
$C_{19}H_{29}N_3O_2$	Amindocate
$C_{19}H_{29}N_3O_2$	Batebulast
$(C_{19}H_{29}N_5O_2)_2.C_4H_6O_4$	Lavoltidine Succinate
$C_{19}H_{29}N_5O_2.HCl$	Gepirone Hydrochloride
$C_{19}H_{30}N_2O_2$	Benrixate
$C_{19}H_{30}N_2O_2$	Camiverine
$C_{19}H_{30}N_2O_2$	Ebalzotan
$C_{19}H_{30}N_2O_2.HCl$	Bietamiverine Hydrochloride
$C_{19}H_{30}N_2O_3$	Fenalamide
$C_{19}H_{30}N_2O_5S$	Moveltipril
$C_{19}H_{30}N_2O_6S$	Tisocromide
$C_{19}H_{30}N_5O_{10}P.C_4H_4O_4$	Tenofovir Disoproxil Fumarate
$C_{19}H_{30}OS$	Epitiostanol
$C_{19}H_{30}O_2$	Androstenediol
$C_{19}H_{30}O_2$	Stanolone
$C_{19}H_{30}O_3$	Oxandrolone
$C_{19}H_{30}O_5$	Idebenone
$C_{19}H_{30}O_5$	Piperonyl Butoxide
$C_{19}H_{31}NO.C_4H_4O_4$	Bencyclane Fumarate
$C_{19}H_{31}NO_2$	Amafolone
$C_{19}H_{31}NO_4$	Decimemide
$C_{19}H_{31}NO_6S$	Artemisone
$C_{19}H_{31}N_7O_4$	Mopidamol
$C_{19}H_{32}BrNO_2$	Valethamate Bromide
$C_{19}H_{32}N_2$	Tedisamil
$2C_{19}H_{32}N_2.3C_4H_4O_4$	Tedisamil Sesquifumarate
$C_{19}H_{32}N_2O_2$	Camylofin
$C_{19}H_{32}N_2O_4.HCl$	Betoxycaine Hydrochloride
$C_{19}H_{32}N_2O_5$	Perindopril
$C_{19}H_{32}N_2O_5.C_4H_{11}N$	Perindopril Erbumine
$C_{19}H_{33}N$	Hexadiline
$C_{19}H_{33}NO_2.HCl$	Fingolimod Hydrochloride
$C_{19}H_{33}N_3O$	Pentisomide
$[C_{19}H_{34}N_2O_3S]_2.C_4H_4O_4$	Artilide Fumarate
$C_{19}H_{34}O_3$	Methoprene
$C_{19}H_{35}ClN_2O_5S.HCl$	Mirincamycin Hydrochloride
$C_{19}H_{35}N.C_4H_4O_4$	Perhexiline Maleate
$C_{19}H_{35}NO_2.HCl$	Dicyclomine Hydrochloride
$C_{19}H_{36}BrNO_2$	Sintropium Bromide
$C_{19}H_{36}N_2$	Bertosamil
$C_{19}H_{36}O_5$	Monoctanoin Component C
$C_{19}H_{37}N_5O_7$	Pentisomicin
$C_{19}H_{37}N_5O_7$	Sisomicin
$(C_{19}H_{37}N_5O_7)_2.5H_2SO_4$	Sisomicin Sulfate
$C_{19}H_{38}N_4O_{10}.xH_2SO_4$	Betamicin Sulfate
$C_{19}H_{38}O_2$	Isopropyl Palmitate
$C_{19}H_{39}NO_3$	Lopobutan
$C_{19}H_{40}I_2N_2$	Mebezonium Iodide
$C_{19}H_{40}N_2O_2$	Dapabutan
$C_{19}H_{41}NO_4$	Myralact
$C_{19}H_{42}BrN$	Cetrimonium Bromide
$C_{19}H_{42}N.C_6Cl_5O$	Trimethylcetylammonium Pentachlorophenate
$C_{19}H_{42}N_2O_8S_2$	Trimethidinium Methosulfate
$C_{20}H_2Cl_4{}^{125}I_4Na_2O_5$	Rose Bengal Sodium I 125
$C_{20}H_2Cl_4{}^{131}I_4Na_2O_5$	Rose Bengal Sodium I 131
$C_{20}H_6I_4Na_2O_5.H_2O$	Erythrosine Sodium
$C_{20}H_8Br_2HgNa_2O_6$	Merbromin
$C_{20}H_8Br_4Na_2O_{10}S_2$	Sulfobromophthalein Sodium
$C_{20}H_8I_4Na_2O_4$	Iodophthalein Sodium
$C_{20}H_{10}Cl_2F_5N_3O_3$	Fluazuron
$C_{20}H_{10}Na_2O_5$	Fluorescein Sodium
$C_{20}H_{11}Cl_2I_2NO_3$	Salantel
$C_{20}H_{12}{}^{131}I_6N_2Na_2O_6$	Iodipamide Sodium I 131
$C_{20}H_{12}N_4Na_2O_{12}S_4$	Bisdisulizole Disodium

Molecular Formula	*Non-proprietary Name*
$C_{20}H_{12}O_5$	Fluorescein
$C_{20}H_{13}ClF_3NO_3$	Floxacrine
$C_{20}H_{13}Cl_2F_2N_3O_5S$	Oglemilast
$C_{20}H_{13}F_6N_3O_2S$	Monepantel
$C_{20}H_{13}NO_2$	Mitoquidone
$C_{20}H_{14}ClNO_4$	Sanguinarium Chloride
$C_{20}H_{14}ClN_3O_3S$	Lintitript
$C_{20}H_{14}I_6N_2O_6$	Iodipamide
$C_{20}H_{14}I_6N_2O_6.2C_7H_{17}NO_5$	Iodipamide Meglumine
$C_{20}H_{14}N_5NaO_5$	Cromitrile Sodium
$C_{20}H_{14}O_3$	Florantyrone
$C_{20}H_{14}O_4$	Aloin
$C_{20}H_{14}O_4$	Phenolphthalein
$C_{20}H_{15}BrN_6O$	Etravirine
$C_{20}H_{15}ClN_4$	Vatalanib
$C_{20}H_{15}Cl_3N_2OS$	Arasertaconazole
$C_{20}H_{15}Cl_3N_2OS$	Sertaconazole
$C_{20}H_{15}F_2NO$	Senicapoc
$C_{20}H_{15}F_3N_4O_3.CH_4O_3S$	Trovafloxacin Mesylate
$C_{20}H_{15}N_3O_6$	Rubitecan
$C_{20}H_{16}ClF_2N_5O_2$	Albaconazole
$C_{20}H_{16}ClN_5O_3$	Telatinib
$C_{20}H_{16}F_3N_3O_3$	Cetefloxacin
$C_{20}H_{16}N_4O_2S$	Indiplon
$C_{20}H_{17}ClFN_3O_4$	Ethyl Carfluzepate
$C_{20}H_{17}ClN_2O_3$	Ketazolam
$C_{20}H_{17}Cl_3N_2O_2.HNO_3$	Omoconazole Nitrate
$C_{20}H_{17}FO_3S$	Sulindac
$C_{20}H_{17}FO_4S$	Exisulind
$C_{20}H_{17}F_2N_3O_3.HCl$	Sarafloxacin Hydrochloride
$C_{20}H_{17}F_3N_2O_4$	Floctafenine
$C_{20}H_{17}F_3N_2O_4$	Tasquinimod
$C_{20}H_{17}N_3O_4S$	Balaglitazone
$C_{20}H_{17}N_5O_9S_2.4H_2O$	Cefetecol
$C_{20}H_{18}BrClN_4S$	Ciclotizolam
$C_{20}H_{18}ClNO_4.xH_2O$	Berberine Chloride
$C_{20}H_{18}F_2N_4O_3$	Fandofloxacin
$C_{20}H_{18}F_3N_3O.C_7H_8O_3S$	Denagliptin Tosylate
$C_{20}H_{18}NNaO_3S$	Englitazone Sodium
$[C_{20}H_{18}NO_4]_2.SO_4.xH_2O$	Berberine Sulfate
$C_{20}H_{18}N_2O_3$	Cinnofuradione
$C_{20}H_{18}N_2O_7S_2$	Aranotin
$C_{20}H_{18}N_2S$	Citatepine
$C_{20}H_{18}N_4O_5S_2$	Cefalonium
$C_{20}H_{18}N_6Na_2O_9S$	Moxalactam Disodium
$C_{20}H_{18}N_8O_8S_3$	Ceftiolene
$C_{20}H_{19}ClFNO_4$	Tonabersat
$C_{20}H_{19}ClN_2O_3$	Pivoxazepam
$C_{20}H_{19}Cl_2NO_3$	Benzmalecene
$C_{20}H_{19}Cl_3N_2O_2$	Zoficonazole
$C_{20}H_{19}FN_4O_4$	Finafloxacin
$C_{20}H_{19}FN_8O_2$	Riociguat
$C_{20}H_{19}F_2NO_4$	Tidembersat
$C_{20}H_{19}F_3N_2O_4$	Sarakalim
$C_{20}H_{19}NO_3$	Acronine
$C_{20}H_{19}NO_3$	Oxazidione
$C_{20}H_{19}NO_4$	Satigrel
$C_{20}H_{19}NO_5$	Duometacin
$C_{20}H_{19}N_3.HCl$	Fuchsin, Basic
$C_{20}H_{19}N_3O.CH_4O_3S$	Obatoclax Mesylate
$C_{20}H_{19}N_3O_4S$	Rivoglitazone
$C_{20}H_{19}N_5$	Dapivirine
$C_{20}H_{19}N_5Na_2O_6$	Pemetrexed Disodium
$C_{20}H_{19}N_5O.HCl$	Acodazole Hydrochloride
$C_{20}H_{20}CaCl_2O_6$	Calcium Clofibrate
$C_{20}H_{20}ClNO$	Benzaprinoxide
$C_{20}H_{20}ClN_3O_3$	Tepoxalin
$C_{20}H_{20}ClN_5$	Amopyroquine
$C_{20}H_{20}ClN_5O_5S_2$	Suriclone
$C_{20}H_{20}Cl_2MgO_6$	Magnesium Clofibrate
$C_{20}H_{20}Cl_2N_4O_2S$	Capravirine
$C_{20}H_{20}FKN_6O_5$	Raltegravir Potassium
$C_{20}H_{20}FNO_3S.HCl$	Prasugrel Hydrochloride
$C_{20}H_{20}FNO_4$	Carabersat
$C_{20}H_{20}F_2N_4$	Liroldine
$C_{20}H_{20}N_2$	Milverine
$C_{20}H_{20}N_2O.C_4H_4O_4$	Suronacrine Maleate
$C_{20}H_{20}N_2O_2$	Befuraline
$C_{20}H_{20}N_2O_2$	Feprazone
$C_{20}H_{20}N_2O_2$	Odalprofen
$C_{20}H_{20}N_2O_3$	Denpidazone
$C_{20}H_{20}N_2O_3$	Elliptinium Acetate
$C_{20}H_{20}N_2O_4$	Leniquinsin
$C_{20}H_{20}N_4O_3.C_4H_4O_4$	Pafuramidine Maleate
$C_{20}H_{20}N_4O_4S$	Patamostat
$C_{20}H_{20}N_6O_7S_4$	Cefodizime
$C_{20}H_{21}AlCl_2O_7$	Aluminum Clofibrate
$C_{20}H_{21}BrFN_3OS$	Bederocin
$C_{20}H_{21}CaN_7O_6$	Folitixorin Calcium
$C_{20}H_{21}CaN_7O_7$	Leucovorin Calcium
$C_{20}H_{21}CaN_7O_7$	Levoleucovorin Calcium
$C_{20}H_{21}ClN_2O_2$	Dinazafone
$C_{20}H_{21}ClN_2O_4$	Fipexide
$C_{20}H_{21}ClO_4$	Fenofibrate
$C_{20}H_{21}Cl_2NO_4$	Biclofibrate
$C_{20}H_{21}Cl_2NO_4$	Lifibrate
$C_{20}H_{21}FN_2O$	Citalopram
$C_{20}H_{21}FN_2O$	Escitalopram
$C_{20}H_{21}FN_2O.C_2H_2O_4$	Escitalopram Oxalate
$C_{20}H_{21}FN_2O.HBr$	Citalopram Hydrobromide
$C_{20}H_{21}F_3N_2OS$	Fluacizine
$C_{20}H_{21}F_3N_2O_3$	Flucetorex
$C_{20}H_{21}F_3N_4O$	Flibanserin
$C_{20}H_{21}N.HCl$	Cyclobenzaprine Hydrochloride
$C_{20}H_{21}N.H_3PO_4$	Octriptyline Phosphate
$C_{20}H_{21}NO$	Butinoline
$C_{20}H_{21}NO$	Cotriptyline
$C_{20}H_{21}NO$	Danitracen
$C_{20}H_{21}NOS$	Tolciclate
$C_{20}H_{21}NOS_2$	Tinofedrine
$C_{20}H_{21}NO_2$	Moxaverine
$C_{20}H_{21}NO_3$	Mepixanox
$C_{20}H_{21}NO_3.HCl$	Dimefline Hydrochloride
$C_{20}H_{21}NO_4.HCl$	Papaverine Hydrochloride
$C_{20}H_{21}NO_5$	Repirinast
$C_{20}H_{21}N_2NaO_7S.4H_2O$	Sivelestat Sodium
$C_{20}H_{21}N_3.HCl$	Aptiganel Hydrochloride
$C_{20}H_{21}N_3O$	Cilansetron
$C_{20}H_{21}N_3O$	Imidafenacin
$C_{20}H_{21}N_3O.HCl.H_2O$	Cilansetron Hydrochloride
$C_{20}H_{21}N_3O_3$	Moquizone
$C_{20}H_{21}N_3O_4$	Fradafiban
$C_{20}H_{21}N_3O_7S$	Ampiroxicam
$C_{20}H_{21}N_7O_6S_2$	Ceforanide
$C_{20}H_{22}ClF_2N_3O$	Befiradol
$C_{20}H_{22}ClN.2H_3PO_4$	Pyrrobutamine Phosphate
$C_{20}H_{22}ClNO_4S$	Terutroban
$C_{20}H_{22}ClN_3.2HCl$	Dorastine Hydrochloride
$C_{20}H_{22}ClN_3O$	Amodiaquine
$C_{20}H_{22}ClN_3O.2HCl.2H_2O$	Amodiaquine Hydrochloride
$C_{20}H_{22}ClN_3O_4$	Peralopride
$C_{20}H_{22}ClN_5O_3S$	Adinazolam Mesylate

Molecular Formula	Non-proprietary Name
$C_{20}H_{22}Cl_2N_2O_4$	Dulozafone
$C_{20}H_{22}Cl_2N_2O_6$	Lemildipine
$C_{20}H_{22}FN_3O_6$	Norfloxacin Succinil
$C_{20}H_{22}NNaO_4$	Efaproxiral Sodium
$C_{20}H_{22}N_2$	Erizepine
$C_{20}H_{22}N_2.2C_4H_4O_4$	Azatadine Maleate
$C_{20}H_{22}N_2O_2$	Metoxepin
$C_{20}H_{22}N_2O_4$	Tilnoprofen Arbamel
$C_{20}H_{22}N_2O_7S$	Sivelestat
$C_{20}H_{22}N_2S$	Mequitazine
$C_{20}H_{22}N_4O$	Difenamizole
$C_{20}H_{22}N_4O_2$	Romergoline
$C_{20}H_{22}N_4O_4S$	Cefrotil
$C_{20}H_{22}N_4O_5$	Camostat
$C_{20}H_{22}N_4O_6S$	Febantel
$C_{20}H_{22}N_4O_6S_2$	Vanyldisulfamide
$C_{20}H_{22}N_4O_{10}S$	Cefuroxime Axetil
$C_{20}H_{22}N_5NaO_6S$	Azlocillin Sodium
$C_{20}H_{22}N_8O_5$	Methotrexate
$C_{20}H_{22}N_8O_6S_2$	Ceftobiprole
$C_{20}H_{22}O_2$	Norgestrienone
$C_{20}H_{22}O_3$	Avobenzone
$C_{20}H_{22}O_3$	Nafenopin
$C_{20}H_{23}BrClN_3O_2$	Broclepride
$C_{20}H_{23}BrN_2OS$	Propyromazine Bromide
$C_{20}H_{23}CaN_7O_6$	Levomefolate Calcium
$C_{20}H_{23}ClFNO$	Eliprodil
$C_{20}H_{23}ClN_2O_3$	Indopanolol
$C_{20}H_{23}ClN_4O_2$	Clonitazene
$C_{20}H_{23}ClO_2$	Ethynerone
$C_{20}H_{23}ClO_3$	Beclobrate
$C_{20}H_{23}Cl_2N_3O_2$	Peraclopone
$C_{20}H_{23}FN_4O_3$	Olamufloxacin
$C_{20}H_{23}HO_4$	Efaproxiral
$C_{20}H_{23}N$	Litracen
$C_{20}H_{23}N$	Maprotiline
$C_{20}H_{23}N.HCl$	Amitriptyline Hydrochloride
$C_{20}H_{23}N.HCl$	Maprotiline Hydrochloride
$C_{20}H_{23}NO$	Amitriptylinoxide
$C_{20}H_{23}NO$	Dexnafenodone
$C_{20}H_{23}NO$	Levoprotiline
$C_{20}H_{23}NO$	Nafenodone
$C_{20}H_{23}NO$	Quifenadine
$C_{20}H_{23}NO.HCl$	Oxaprotiline Hydrochloride
$C_{20}H_{23}NO_2$	Ciheptolane
$C_{20}H_{23}NO_2.HCl$	Amolanone Hydrochloride
$C_{20}H_{23}NO_2.HCl$	Dexoxadrol Hydrochloride
$C_{20}H_{23}NO_2.HCl$	Dioxadrol Hydrochloride
$C_{20}H_{23}NO_2.HCl$	Levoxadrol Hydrochloride
$C_{20}H_{23}NO_3$	Triclazate
$C_{20}H_{23}NO_4$	Naltrexone
$C_{20}H_{23}NO_4$	Thebacon
$C_{20}H_{23}NO_4.HCl$	Naltrexone Hydrochloride
$C_{20}H_{23}NO_5$	Cyproquinate
$C_{20}H_{23}NO_6.CH_4O_3S$	Bendacalol Mesylate
$C_{20}H_{23}NS.HCl.H_2O$	Methixene Hydrochloride
$C_{20}H_{23}N_3$	Cianopramine
$C_{20}H_{23}N_3.C_4H_4O_4$	Fezolamine Fumarate
$C_{20}H_{23}N_3OS$	Sopitazine
$C_{20}H_{23}N_3O_2$	Oxiperomide
$C_{20}H_{23}N_3O_4$	Epanolol
$C_{20}H_{23}N_5O$	Metrazifone
$C_{20}H_{23}N_5O_2$	Trazolopride
$C_{20}H_{23}N_5O_6S$	Azlocillin
$C_{20}H_{23}N_5S$	Timegadine
$C_{20}H_{24}BrNO_3$	Benzopyrronium Bromide

Molecular Formula	Non-proprietary Name
$C_{20}H_{24}ClNO$	Cloperastine
$C_{20}H_{24}ClNO_2$	Methopholine
$C_{20}H_{24}ClN_3O_2$	Clebopride
$C_{20}H_{24}ClN_3S$	Prochlorperazine
$C_{20}H_{24}ClN_3S.C_2H_6O_6S_2$	Prochlorperazine Edisylate
$C_{20}H_{24}ClN_3S.2C_4H_4O_4$	Prochlorperazine Maleate
$C_{20}H_{24}Cl_2N_{10}$	Picloxydine
$C_{20}H_{24}FN_3O_2$	Flupranone
$C_{20}H_{24}FN_3O_2$	Nardeterol
$C_{20}H_{24}FN_3O_4$	Balofloxacin
$C_{20}H_{24}FN_3O_4S$	Flubepride
$C_{20}H_{24}F_3N_3OS_2$	Flutizenol
$C_{20}H_{24}N_2$	Elantrine
$C_{20}H_{24}N_2$	Enprazepine
$C_{20}H_{24}N_2.C_4H_4O_4$	Dimethindene Maleate
$C_{20}H_{24}N_2O$	Ubisindine
$C_{20}H_{24}N_2O.HCl$	Indecainide Hydrochloride
$C_{20}H_{24}N_2OS$	Botiacrine
$C_{20}H_{24}N_2OS$	Propiomazine
$C_{20}H_{24}N_2OS.HCl$	Cinanserin Hydrochloride
$C_{20}H_{24}N_2OS.HCl$	Lucanthone Hydrochloride
$C_{20}H_{24}N_2OS.HCl$	Propiomazine Hydrochloride
$C_{20}H_{24}N_2O_2$	Quinidine
$C_{20}H_{24}N_2O_2$	Quinine
$C_{20}H_{24}N_2O_2$	Viquidil
$C_{20}H_{24}N_2O_2.2C_6H_8O_6$	Quinine Ascorbate
$C_{20}H_{24}N_2O_2.C_6H_{12}O_7$	Quinidine Gluconate
$(C_{20}H_{24}N_2O_2)_2.H_2SO_4.2H_2O$	Quinidine Sulfate
$(C_{20}H_{24}N_2O_2)_2.H_2SO_4.2H_2O$	Quinine Sulfate
$C_{20}H_{24}N_2O_2S$	Hycanthone
$C_{20}H_{24}N_2O_3$	Nofecainide
$C_{20}H_{24}N_2O_3$	Yohimbic Acid
$C_{20}H_{24}N_2O_5$	Codoxime
$C_{20}H_{24}N_2O_5$	Diamfenetide
$C_{20}H_{24}N_2O_5$	Medroxalol
$C_{20}H_{24}N_2O_5.HCl$	Medroxalol Hydrochloride
$C_{20}H_{24}N_2O_6$	Nisoldipine
$C_{20}H_{24}N_2S_2$	Metitepine
$C_{20}H_{24}N_4O_4$	Istradefylline
$C_{20}H_{24}N_6O_2$	Nortopixantrone
$C_{20}H_{24}O_2$	Ethinyl Estradiol
$C_{20}H_{24}O_2$	Exemestane
$C_{20}H_{24}O_3$	Trenbolone Acetate
$C_{20}H_{24}O_4$	Sobetirome
$C_{20}H_{24}O_5$	Terbufibrol
$C_{20}H_{24}O_7S$	Tesaglitazar
$C_{20}H_{25}BrN_4O$	Bromerguride
$C_{20}H_{25}ClN_2O$	Spiclamine
$C_{20}H_{25}ClN_2O_2$	Mefeclorazine
$C_{20}H_{25}ClN_2O_5.C_4H_4O_4$	Amlodipine Maleate
$C_{20}H_{25}ClN_2O_5.C_4H_6O_5$	Levamlodipine Malate
$C_{20}H_{25}ClN_2O_5.C_6H_6O_3S$	Amlodipine Besylate
$C_{20}H_{25}ClN_4OS$	Cloxypendyl
$C_{20}H_{25}ClO_4$	Osaterone
$C_{20}H_{25}Cl_3O_3$	Cloxestradiol
$C_{20}H_{25}FN_4O$	Niaprazine
$C_{20}H_{25}FN_8O_6S_2$	Cefluprenam
$C_{20}H_{25}N$	Prodipine
$C_{20}H_{25}N.HCl$	Fenpiprane Hydrochloride
$C_{20}H_{25}NO$	Difemetorex
$C_{20}H_{25}NO$	Glemanserin
$C_{20}H_{25}NO$	Normethadone
$C_{20}H_{25}NO$	Perastine
$C_{20}H_{25}NO$	Pridinol
$C_{20}H_{25}NO.HCl$	Talopram Hydrochloride
$C_{20}H_{25}NOS.HCl$	Thiphenamil Hydrochloride

Molecular Formula	Non-proprietary Name
$C_{20}H_{25}NO_2$	Dienogest
$C_{20}H_{25}NO_2$	Femoxetine
$C_{20}H_{25}NO_2$	Fomocaine
$C_{20}H_{25}NO_2$	Ketorfanol
$C_{20}H_{25}NO_2$	Propanocaine
$C_{20}H_{25}NO_2.HBr$	Estrazinol Hydrobromide
$C_{20}H_{25}NO_2.HCl$	Adiphenine Hydrochloride
$C_{20}H_{25}NO_2S_2.HCl$	Tiagabine Hydrochloride
$C_{20}H_{25}NO_3$	Benactyzine
$C_{20}H_{25}NO_3$	Dimenoxadol
$C_{20}H_{25}NO_3.CH_4O_3S.3H_2O$	Traxoprodil Mesylate
$C_{20}H_{25}NO_3.HCl$	Difemerine Hydrochloride
$C_{20}H_{25}NO_4$	Cilomilast
$C_{20}H_{25}NO_5$	Poskine
$C_{20}H_{25}NS$	Talsupram
$C_{20}H_{25}N_3O$	Lysergide
$C_{20}H_{25}N_3O$	Octrizole
$C_{20}H_{25}N_3O_2$	Propisergide
$C_{20}H_{25}N_3O_2.C_4H_4O_4$	Methylergonovine Maleate
$C_{20}H_{25}N_3O_3$	Imoxiterol
$C_{20}H_{25}N_3O_4$	Cinoxopazide
$C_{20}H_{25}N_3O_4$	Ecabapide
$C_{20}H_{25}N_3O_4$	Nemonoxacin
$C_{20}H_{25}N_3S.2C_{20}H_{14}O_4$	Perazine Fendizoate
$C_{20}H_{25}N_5O_3S$	Donetidine
$C_{20}H_{25}N_5O_6S$	Pelitrexol
$C_{20}H_{25}N_7O_6$	Levomefolic Acid
$C_{20}H_{26}Br_2N_2O$	Adamexine
$C_{20}H_{26}ClNO.HCl$	Clofenetamine Hydrochloride
$C_{20}H_{26}ClNO_3$	Adafenoxate
$C_{20}H_{26}ClNO_3$	Lachesine Chloride
$C_{20}H_{26}ClNO_5$	Cloricromen
$C_{20}H_{26}ClN_3O_2$	Piclopastine
$C_{20}H_{26}I_3N_3O_{12}$	Iogulamide
$C_{20}H_{26}N_2$	Dimetacrine
$C_{20}H_{26}N_2$	Trimipramine
$C_{20}H_{26}N_2.C_4H_4O_4$	Trimipramine Maleate
$C_{20}H_{26}N_2.HCl$	Mimbane Hydrochloride
$C_{20}H_{26}N_2O$	Ivoqualine
$C_{20}H_{26}N_2O$	Viqualine
$C_{20}H_{26}N_2O.2HCl$	Anilopam Hydrochloride
$C_{20}H_{26}N_2O_2$	Ajmaline
$C_{20}H_{26}N_2O_2$	Epsiprantel
$C_{20}H_{26}N_2O_2.2HCl$	Veradoline Hydrochloride
$C_{20}H_{26}N_2O_2.2HCl$	Verilopam Hydrochloride
$C_{20}H_{26}N_2O_3$	Cilostamide
$C_{20}H_{26}N_2O_3$	Disoxaril
$C_{20}H_{26}N_2O_4$	Itopride
$C_{20}H_{26}N_2O_4$	Ronactolol
$C_{20}H_{26}N_2O_4.CH_4O_3S$	Binospirone Mesylate
$C_{20}H_{26}N_2O_5S$	Alacepril
$C_{20}H_{26}N_2O_5S_2$	Spiraprilat
$C_{20}H_{26}N_2S.HCl$	Etymemazine Hydrochloride
$C_{20}H_{26}N_4O$	Lisuride
$C_{20}H_{26}N_4OS$	Oxypendyl
$C_{20}H_{26}N_4O_2$	Hexamidine
$C_{20}H_{26}N_4O_2$	Neraminol
$C_{20}H_{26}N_4O_5S$	Glisolamide
$C_{20}H_{26}N_4O_5S$	Niperotidine
$C_{20}H_{26}O_2$	Atamestane
$C_{20}H_{26}O_2$	Benzestrol
$C_{20}H_{26}O_2$	Methestrol
$C_{20}H_{26}O_2$	Norethindrone
$C_{20}H_{26}O_2$	Norethynodrel
$C_{20}H_{26}O_3$	Gestadienol
$C_{20}H_{27}BrN_2O_2S$	Dotefonium Bromide

Molecular Formula	Non-proprietary Name
$C_{20}H_{27}FN_2O_3$	Cicarperone
$C_{20}H_{27}N.C_6H_8O_7$	Alverine Citrate
$C_{20}H_{27}N.HCl$	Terodiline Hydrochloride
$C_{20}H_{27}NO$	Treptilamine
$C_{20}H_{27}NO_2$	Fenalcomine
$C_{20}H_{27}NO_2$	Oxilorphan
$C_{20}H_{27}NO_2$	Vetrabutine
$C_{20}H_{27}NO_3$	Trilostane
$C_{20}H_{27}NO_3Si_2$	Amsilarotene
$C_{20}H_{27}NO_4$	Prampine
$C_{20}H_{27}NO_4.HCl$	Bevantolol Hydrochloride
$C_{20}H_{27}NO_4S$	Domitroban
$C_{20}H_{27}NO_4S.HCl$	Sulfinalol Hydrochloride
$C_{20}H_{27}NO_5$	Buquinolate
$C_{20}H_{27}NO_5.HCl$	Chromonar Hydrochloride
$C_{20}H_{27}N_3O_5$	Cilazaprilat
$C_{20}H_{27}N_3O_5S$	Utibaprilat
$C_{20}H_{27}N_3O_6$	Febarbamate
$C_{20}H_{27}N_3O_6$	Imidapril
$C_{20}H_{27}N_5O_2$	Cilostazol
$C_{20}H_{27}N_5O_3.HCl$	Bamifylline Hydrochloride
$C_{20}H_{27}N_5O_5S$	Glisoxepide
$C_{20}H_{27}O_4P$	Octicizer
$C_{20}H_{28}BrN$	Emepronium Bromide
$C_{20}H_{28}Cl_4N_2O_4$	Teclozan
$C_{20}H_{28}FN_3O_3$	Carmegliptin
$C_{20}H_{28}FN_3O_3.2HCl$	Carmegliptin Dihydrochloride
$C_{20}H_{28}I_3N_3O_9$	Iobitridol
$C_{20}H_{28}I_3N_3O_9$	Iopentol
$C_{20}H_{28}I_3N_3O_{13}$	Ioglucomide
$C_{20}H_{28}N_2O$	Pytamine
$C_{20}H_{28}N_2O_3.HCl$	Oxyphencyclimine Hydrochloride
$C_{20}H_{28}N_2O_5.C_4H_4O_4$	Enalapril Maleate
$C_{20}H_{28}N_2O_5.HCl$	Remifentanil Hydrochloride
$C_{20}H_{28}N_2O_5S.HCl$	Tamsulosin Hydrochloride
$C_{20}H_{28}N_2O_6.C_4H_4O_4$	Cinepazet Maleate
$C_{20}H_{28}N_4O$	Terguride
$C_{20}H_{28}N_4O_2$	Rolofylline
$C_{20}H_{28}N_4O_4$	Ilomastat
$C_{20}H_{28}N_4O_6$	Sibrafiban
$C_{20}H_{28}N_4O_8S_2$	Stilbamidine Isethionate
$C_{20}H_{28}O$	Cingestol
$C_{20}H_{28}O$	Delanterone
$C_{20}H_{28}O$	Lynestrenol
$C_{20}H_{28}O$	Tigestol
$C_{20}H_{28}O_2$	Alitretinoin
$C_{20}H_{28}O_2$	Isotretinoin
$C_{20}H_{28}O_2$	Methandrostenolone
$C_{20}H_{28}O_2$	Nordinone
$C_{20}H_{28}O_2$	Norgesterone
$C_{20}H_{28}O_2$	Norvinisterone
$C_{20}H_{28}O_2$	Tebufelone
$C_{20}H_{28}O_2$	Tretinoin
$C_{20}H_{28}O_3$	Enestebol
$C_{20}H_{28}O_3S$	Ethyl Dibunate
$C_{20}H_{28}O_5S$	Ecabet
$C_{20}H_{28}O_6S$	Tiaprost
$C_{20}H_{29}ClO_4$	Arildone
$C_{20}H_{29}FN_6O_3.HCl$	Brifentanil Hydrochloride
$C_{20}H_{29}FO_3$	Fluoxymesterone
$C_{20}H_{29}NO$	Gemazocine
$C_{20}H_{29}NO$	Ibazocine
$C_{20}H_{29}NO_2$	Bremazocine
$C_{20}H_{29}NO_3$	Ipragratine
$C_{20}H_{29}NO_3.HCl$	Propenzolate Hydrochloride

Molecular Formula	Non-proprietary Name
$C_{20}H_{29}NO_4$	Fedrilate
$C_{20}H_{29}NO_6S$	Sultroponium
$C_{20}H_{29}N_3.C_4H_4O_4$	Atiprosin Maleate
$C_{20}H_{29}N_3O_2$	Dibucaine
$C_{20}H_{29}N_3O_2.HCl$	Dibucaine Hydrochloride
$C_{20}H_{29}N_3O_4S$	Tinisulpride
$C_{20}H_{29}N_3O_5S_3$	Fonazine Mesylate
$C_{20}H_{29}N_5O_3$	Buquineran
$C_{20}H_{29}N_5O_3$	Urapidil
$C_{20}H_{29}N_5O_4$	Dramedilol
$C_{20}H_{29}N_5O_6.HCl.H_2O$	Trimazosin Hydrochloride
$C_{20}H_{30}BrNO_2$	Cyclopyrronium Bromide
$C_{20}H_{30}BrNO_3$	Hexopyrronium Bromide
$C_{20}H_{30}BrNO_3.H_2O$	Ipratropium Bromide
$C_{20}H_{30}ClN_3O_4$	Dobupride
$C_{20}H_{30}N_2O_2$	Furazabol
$C_{20}H_{30}N_2O_2.2HCl$	Dipiproverine Hydrochloride
$C_{20}H_{30}N_2O_3$	Morpheridine
$C_{20}H_{30}N_2O_5$	Neotame
$C_{20}H_{30}O$	Retinol
$C_{20}H_{30}O_2$	Icosapent
$C_{20}H_{30}O_2$	Methyltestosterone
$C_{20}H_{30}O_2$	Metogest
$C_{20}H_{30}O_2$	Mibolerone
$C_{20}H_{30}O_2$	Norethandrolone
$C_{20}H_{30}O_2$	Oxendolone
$C_{20}H_{30}O_2$	Peretinoin
$C_{20}H_{30}O_3$	Oxymesterone
$C_{20}H_{31}NO$	Deramciclane
$C_{20}H_{31}NO.HCl$	Trihexyphenidyl Hydrochloride
$C_{20}H_{31}NO_2$	Drofenine
$C_{20}H_{31}NO_2.HCl$	Metcaraphen Hydrochloride
$C_{20}H_{31}NO_2S.C_6H_8O_7$	Cetiedil Citrate
$C_{20}H_{31}NO_3.C_6H_8O_7$	Carbetapentane Citrate
$C_{20}H_{31}NO_4.HCl$	Vernakalant Hydrochloride
$C_{20}H_{31}NO_5$	Ibuterol
$C_{20}H_{31}N_3O_6S$	Bacmecillinam
$C_{20}H_{31}N_5O_3S$	Sufotidine
$C_{20}H_{31}NaO_5$	Epoprostenol Sodium
$C_{20}H_{32}ClNO$	Tricyclamol Chloride
$C_{20}H_{32}F_2O_5$	Lubiprostone
$C_{20}H_{32}N_2O_4$	Furomine
$C_{20}H_{32}N_4O_5$	Solimastat
$C_{20}H_{32}N_5O_8P$	Adefovir Dipivoxil
$C_{20}H_{32}N_6O_{12}S_2$	Oxiglutatione
$C_{20}H_{32}O$	Bolenol
$C_{20}H_{32}O$	Ethylestrenol
$C_{20}H_{32}O_2$	Alkyl (C12-15) Benzoate
$C_{20}H_{32}O_2$	Mestanolone
$C_{20}H_{32}O_2$	Mesterolone
$C_{20}H_{32}O_2$	Methandriol
$C_{20}H_{32}O_3$	Icomucret
$C_{20}H_{32}O_5$	Dinoprostone
$C_{20}H_{32}O_5$	Epoprostenol
$C_{20}H_{33}NO_3$	Ganglefene
$C_{20}H_{33}NO_3$	Oxeladin
$C_{20}H_{33}NO_4S$	Tilsuprost
$C_{20}H_{33}NO_6S$	Pentapiperium Methylsulfate
$C_{20}H_{33}NO_7$	Candoxatrilat
$C_{20}H_{33}N_3O_3$	Talinolol
$C_{20}H_{33}N_3O_3S$	Quinagolide
$C_{20}H_{33}N_3O_4.HCl$	Celiprolol Hydrochloride
$C_{20}H_{33}N_5O_9$	Goralatide
$C_{20}H_{33}N_7O_3$	Stacofylline
$C_{20}H_{33}NaO_6S$	Entsufon Sodium
$C_{20}H_{34}AuO_9PS$	Auranofin

Molecular Formula	Non-proprietary Name
$C_{20}H_{34}GdN_5O_{10}$	Gadoversetamide
$C_{20}H_{34}N_2O_4$	Spiriprostil
$C_{20}H_{34}N_2O_5$	Orbutopril
$C_{20}H_{34}N_4O_{12}$	Temurtide
$C_{20}H_{34}O_2$	Plaunotol
$C_{20}H_{34}O_5$	Alprostadil
$C_{20}H_{34}O_5$	Dinoprost
$C_{20}H_{34}O_5.C_4H_{11}NO_3$	Dinoprost Tromethamine
$C_{20}H_{34}O_5.x(C_{36}H_{60}O_{30})$	Alprostadil Alfadex
$C_{20}H_{34}O_8$	Acetyltributyl Citrate
$C_{20}H_{35}NOS$	Suloctidil
$C_{20}H_{35}NO_2$	Dopropidil
$C_{20}H_{35}NO_2.HCl$	Dihexyverine Hydrochloride
$C_{20}H_{35}NO_2S.HCl$	Tipropidil Hydrochloride
$C_{20}H_{36}CaN_2O_{10}.\frac{1}{2}H_2O$	Calcium Hopantenate
$C_{20}H_{36}ClN$	Miripirium Chloride
$(C_{20}H_{36}N_2O_3S)_2.C_4H_4O_4$	Ibutilide Fumarate
$C_{20}H_{36}N_6O$	Lauroguadine
$C_{20}H_{36}O_2$	Ethyl Linoleate
$C_{20}H_{37}KO_7S$	Docusate Potassium
$C_{20}H_{37}NO_3$	Rociverine
$C_{20}H_{37}N_5O_{10}$	Versetamide
$C_{20}H_{37}NaO_7S$	Docusate Sodium
$C_{20}H_{38}BrNO_2$	Dipenine Bromide
$C_{20}H_{38}I_2O_2$	Iodetryl
$C_{20}H_{38}N_4O_4$	Dimorpholamine
$C_{20}H_{38}N_8S_2$	Bitipazone
$C_{20}H_{38}O_2$	Ethyl Oleate
$C_{20}H_{39}N_5O_7$	Etisomicin
$C_{20}H_{40}N_2O_{12}$	Hexamethonium Tartrate
$C_{20}H_{41}NO_3$	Cedefingol
$C_{20}H_{41}N_5O_7$	Micronomicin
$C_{20}H_{42}O$	Octyldodecanol
$C_{20}H_{42}O_5$	Laureth 4
$C_{20}H_{43}N.HCl$	Dymanthine Hydrochloride
$C_{21}H_{13}F_3N_2O_4$	Talniflumate
$C_{21}H_{15}N_3O_4$	Deferasirox
$C_{21}H_{16}ClF_3N_4O_3$	Sorafenib
$C_{21}H_{16}ClF_3N_4O_3.C_7H_8O_3S$	Sorafenib Tosylate
$C_{21}H_{16}FNO_3S$	Netoglitazone
$C_{21}H_{16}F_2N_2O_4$	Diflomotecan
$C_{21}H_{16}N_2.HCl$	Paranyline Hydrochloride
$C_{21}H_{16}N_2O_5S$	Susalimod
$C_{21}H_{16}N_4O_8S_2$	Nitrocefin
$C_{21}H_{16}O_7$	Coumetarol
$C_{21}H_{17}NO_9S_2$	Sulisatin
$C_{21}H_{18}ClNO_6$	Acemetacin
$C_{21}H_{18}ClN_3O_7S$	Cefoxazole
$C_{21}H_{18}F_3N_3O_3.HCl$	Temafloxacin Hydrochloride
$C_{21}H_{19}ClFNO_4S$	Laropiprant
$C_{21}H_{19}Cl_2N_3O_6S_3$	Ataciguat
$C_{21}H_{19}F_2N_3O_3.HCl$	Difloxacin Hydrochloride
$C_{21}H_{19}N.HCl$	Intriptyline Hydrochloride
$C_{21}H_{19}NO.HCl$	Cyprolidol Hydrochloride
$C_{21}H_{19}NO_4$	Cinmetacin
$C_{21}H_{19}NO_4$	Oxarbazole
$C_{21}H_{19}N_2NaO_5$	Varespladib Sodium
$C_{21}H_{19}N_3O_3S$	Amsacrine
$C_{21}H_{19}N_5O_2$	Sepimostat
$C_{21}H_{20}BrN_3$	Homidium Bromide
$C_{21}H_{20}ClNO_5.HCl$	Alvocidib
$C_{21}H_{20}ClNS$	Nuclotixene
$C_{21}H_{20}Cl_2FN_3O_2$	Lodiperone
$C_{21}H_{20}Cl_2N_6O_3$	Rilmazafone
$C_{21}H_{20}Cl_2O_3$	Permethrin
$C_{21}H_{20}FN_3O_4$	Radiprodil

Molecular Formula	Non-proprietary Name
$C_{21}H_{20}FN_3O_6S$	Prulifloxacin
$C_{21}H_{20}N_2O$	Tomoxiprole
$C_{21}H_{20}N_2O_5$	Varespladib
$C_{21}H_{20}N_4O_3$	Entinostat
$C_{21}H_{20}N_4O_3$	Picotamide
$C_{21}H_{20}N_6O$	Aminoquinuride
$C_{21}H_{21}ClFN_3O_2$	Alozafone
$C_{21}H_{21}ClN_2O_2$	Iclazepam
$C_{21}H_{21}ClN_2O_3$	Clodoxopone
$C_{21}H_{21}ClN_2O_8$	Demeclocycline
$C_{21}H_{21}ClN_2O_8.HCl$	Demeclocycline Hydrochloride
$C_{21}H_{21}ClN_4OS.CH_4O_3S.3H_2O$	Ziprasidone Mesylate
$C_{21}H_{21}ClN_4OS.HCl.H_2O$	Ziprasidone Hydrochloride
$C_{21}H_{21}ClN_4O_3$	Nizofenone
$C_{21}H_{21}ClO_3$	Clocoumarol
$C_{21}H_{21}Cl_3N_4O$	Rosonabant
$C_{21}H_{21}FN_2O_3$	Fludoxopone
$C_{21}H_{21}FN_2O_4S$	Ramatroban
$C_{21}H_{21}FN_4O_3$	Pradofloxacin
$C_{21}H_{21}FN_6O$	Dovitinib
$C_{21}H_{21}FN_6O.C_3H_6O_3.H_2O$	Dovitinib Lactate
$C_{21}H_{21}F_2N_3O_7$	Posizolid
$C_{21}H_{21}FeNa_6N_3O_{18}P_3$	Ferpifosate Sodium
$C_{21}H_{21}HgN_4NaO_8.H_2O$	Mercumatilin Sodium
$C_{21}H_{21}N.HCl$	Naftifine Hydrochloride
$C_{21}H_{21}N.HCl.1\frac{1}{2}H_2O$	Cyproheptadine Hydrochloride
$C_{21}H_{21}NO_2.C_4H_4O_4$	Oxetorone Fumarate
$C_{21}H_{21}NO_2S$	Tazarotene
$C_{21}H_{21}NO_4$	Zindoxifene
$C_{21}H_{21}NO_6$	Hydrastine
$C_{21}H_{21}N_2NaO_5S.H_2O$	Nafcillin Sodium
$C_{21}H_{21}N_3O_2$	Darenzepine
$C_{21}H_{21}N_3O_3$	Dizatrifone
$C_{21}H_{21}N_3O_3$	Ozenoxacin
$C_{21}H_{21}N_3O_6S$	Fumoxicillin
$C_{21}H_{21}N_3O_9$	Nitrocycline
$C_{21}H_{21}N_3S$	Tiomergine
$C_{21}H_{22}ClFN_4O_2$	Halopemide
$C_{21}H_{22}ClN_3O_3$	Axamozide
$C_{21}H_{22}F_3N_3OS$	Ftormetazine
$C_{21}H_{22}N_2O_2$	Bufezolac
$C_{21}H_{22}N_2O_2$	Strychnine
$C_{21}H_{22}N_2O_3$	Paquinimod
$C_{21}H_{22}N_2O_7$	Sancycline
$C_{21}H_{22}N_2O_8$	Demecycline
$C_{21}H_{22}N_4OS$	Abafungin
$C_{21}H_{22}N_4O_6S$	Raltitrexed
$C_{21}H_{23}BrFNO_2$	Bromperidol
$C_{21}H_{23}ClFNO_2$	Haloperidol
$C_{21}H_{23}ClFN_3O.2HCl$	Flurazepam Hydrochloride
$C_{21}H_{23}ClN_2O_4$	Rafabegron
$C_{21}H_{23}ClN_4O_2.HCl$	Cloperidone Hydrochloride
$C_{21}H_{23}Cl_2NO_6$	Clevidipine Butyrate
$C_{21}H_{23}Cl_2N_3O$	Alpidem
$C_{21}H_{23}FN_2O_3S$	Besonprodil
$C_{21}H_{23}F_3N_6O$	Vofopitant
$C_{21}H_{23}F_3N_6O.2HCl$	Vofopitant Dihydrochloride
$C_{21}H_{23}N.HCl$	Taclamine Hydrochloride
$C_{21}H_{23}NO.HCl$	Dapoxetine Hydrochloride
$C_{21}H_{23}NO_2$	Flavamine
$C_{21}H_{23}NO_3$	Pargeverine
$C_{21}H_{23}NO_3.HCl$	Olopatadine Hydrochloride
$C_{21}H_{23}NO_3.HCl$	Proroxan Hydrochloride
$C_{21}H_{23}NO_4.C_4H_4O_4$	Flavodilol Maleate
$C_{21}H_{23}NO_4S$	Dexecadotril
$C_{21}H_{23}NO_4S$	Ecadotril
$C_{21}H_{23}NO_4S$	Racecadotril
$C_{21}H_{23}NO_5S$	Rilmakalim
$C_{21}H_{23}NO_5S$	Sudexanox
$C_{21}H_{23}N_3OS$	Periciazine
$C_{21}H_{23}N_3O_2$	Panobinostat
$C_{21}H_{23}N_3O_7$	Amicycline
$C_{21}H_{23}N_3O_7S$	Lenampicillin
$C_{21}H_{23}N_5Na_2O_6$	Lometrexol Sodium
$C_{21}H_{23}N_5S$	Talarozole
$C_{21}H_{23}N_7O_2S.HCl$	Pazopanib Hydrochloride
$C_{21}H_{24}BrN_5O$	Temelastine
$C_{21}H_{24}ClNO$	Clobenztropine
$C_{21}H_{24}ClNO_2$	Quillifoline
$C_{21}H_{24}ClNO_4S_2$	Thenium Closylate
$C_{21}H_{24}ClNO_5$	Morclofone
$C_{21}H_{24}ClN_3OS$	Pipamazine
$C_{21}H_{24}ClN_3O_3$	Fominoben
$C_{21}H_{24}FN_3O_2S$	Setoperone
$C_{21}H_{24}FN_3O_4$	Moxifloxacin
$C_{21}H_{24}FN_3O_4.HCl$	Moxifloxacin Hydrochloride
$C_{21}H_{24}FN_5O_3$	Flufylline
$C_{21}H_{24}F_2N_2O_3$	Efletirizine
$C_{21}H_{24}F_2N_2O_3.2HCl$	Efletirizine Dihydrochloride
$C_{21}H_{24}F_3N.HCl$	Fluotracen Hydrochloride
$C_{21}H_{24}F_3N_3S.2HCl$	Trifluoperazine Hydrochloride
$C_{21}H_{24}I_3NO_4.HCl$	Thyromedan Hydrochloride
$C_{21}H_{24}N_2$	Quinupramine
$C_{21}H_{24}N_2$	Trazitiline
$C_{21}H_{24}N_2O$	Ciprafamide
$C_{21}H_{24}N_2O_2$	Apovincamine
$C_{21}H_{24}N_2O_3$	Hydroxindasate
$C_{21}H_{24}N_2O_4$	Carmoterol
$C_{21}H_{24}N_2O_4$	Cyclarbamate
$C_{21}H_{24}N_2O_4S$	Repinotan
$C_{21}H_{24}N_2O_5$	Toborinone
$C_{21}H_{24}N_2O_5S_2$	Temocaprilat
$C_{21}H_{24}N_2O_7$	Furnidipine
$C_{21}H_{24}N_4O$	Intoplicine
$C_{21}H_{24}N_4O_2.HCl$	Pelanserin Hydrochloride
$C_{21}H_{24}N_4O_2S$	Mirabegron
$C_{21}H_{24}N_4O_3S$	Vintiamol
$C_{21}H_{24}N_4O_7S$	Acefurtiamine
$C_{21}H_{24}NaN_5O_8S_2$	Mezlocillin Sodium
$C_{21}H_{24}O_2$	Gestrinone
$C_{21}H_{24}O_2$	Tosagestin
$C_{21}H_{24}O_7$	Visnadine
$C_{21}H_{25}BrN_2O_3$	Brovincamine
$C_{21}H_{25}ClFN_3O_3$	Mosapride
$C_{21}H_{25}ClN_2O_3$	Bepotastine
$C_{21}H_{25}ClN_2O_3$	Levocetirizine
$C_{21}H_{25}ClN_2O_3.2HCl$	Cetirizine Hydrochloride
$C_{21}H_{25}ClN_2O_3.2HCl$	Levocetirizine Dihydrochloride
$C_{21}H_{25}ClN_2O_4S$	Tianeptine
$C_{21}H_{25}ClO_2$	Trengestone
$C_{21}H_{25}ClO_5$	Cloprednol
$C_{21}H_{25}ClO_6.C_3H_8O_2.H_2O$	Dapagliflozin
$C_{21}H_{25}FN_2O_2$	Fluanisone
$C_{21}H_{25}FN_6$	Arpromidine
$C_{21}H_{25}IN_2S$	Mequitamium Iodide
$C_{21}H_{25}N$	Pyrophenindane
$C_{21}H_{25}N$	Terbinafine
$C_{21}H_{25}N.HCl$	Melitracen Hydrochloride
$C_{21}H_{25}NO$	Hepzidine
$C_{21}H_{25}NO.CH_4O_3S$	Benztropine Mesylate
$C_{21}H_{25}NO_2$	Cinnamaverine
$C_{21}H_{25}NO_2$	Myfadol

Molecular Formula	Non-proprietary Name
$C_{21}H_{25}NO_2.HCl$	Piperidolate Hydrochloride
$C_{21}H_{25}NO_3$	Nalmefene
$C_{21}H_{25}NO_3$	Piperilate
$C_{21}H_{25}NO_3S.HCl$	Tipentosin Hydrochloride
$C_{21}H_{25}NO_4.HCl$	Nalmexone Hydrochloride
$C_{21}H_{25}NO_5$	Demecolcine
$C_{21}H_{25}N_3O$	Ambasilide
$C_{21}H_{25}N_3O$	Ontazolast
$(C_{21}H_{25}N_3O_2S)_2.C_4H_4O_4$	Quetiapine Fumarate
$C_{21}H_{25}N_3O_2S_2$	Quisultazine
$C_{21}H_{25}N_3O_3$	Soraprazan
$C_{21}H_{25}N_3O_3$	Tiracizine
$C_{21}H_{25}N_3O_3S$	Pipazethate
$C_{21}H_{25}N_5O_2$	Icotidine
$C_{21}H_{25}N_5O_2$	Niprofazone
$C_{21}H_{25}N_5O_2.CH_4O_3S$	Atevirdine Mesylate
$C_{21}H_{25}N_5O_4.2HCl$	Piroxantrone Hydrochloride
$C_{21}H_{25}N_5O_4.2HCl.H_2O$	Teloxantrone Hydrochloride
$C_{21}H_{25}N_5O_8S_2$	Mezlocillin
$C_{21}H_{26}BrNO_3$	Mepenzolate Bromide
$C_{21}H_{26}BrNO_3$	Methantheline Bromide
$C_{21}H_{26}BrNO_3$	Parapenzolate Bromide
$C_{21}H_{26}BrNO_4$	Methylnaltrexone Bromide
$C_{21}H_{26}ClNO$	Clemastine
$C_{21}H_{26}ClNO.C_4H_4O_4$	Clemastine Fumarate
$C_{21}H_{26}ClN_3OS$	Perphenazine
$C_{21}H_{26}ClN_3O_2$	Nemonapride
$C_{21}H_{26}Cl_2N_2O_4$	Spiroglumide
$C_{21}H_{26}Cl_2O$	Clofoctol
$C_{21}H_{26}Cl_2O_2$	Biclotymol
$C_{21}H_{26}FN_3O_4$	Premafloxacin
$C_{21}H_{26}F_3N_5$	Lorpiprazole
$C_{21}H_{26}INO_3$	Etipirium Iodide
$C_{21}H_{26}N_2O$	Fenpipramide
$C_{21}H_{26}N_2O$	Tolnapersine
$C_{21}H_{26}N_2OS$	Oxyridazine
$C_{21}H_{26}N_2OS_2$	Mesoridazine
$C_{21}H_{26}N_2OS_2.C_6H_6O_3S$	Mesoridazine Besylate
$C_{21}H_{26}N_2O_2$	Epicainide
$C_{21}H_{26}N_2O_2S_2$	Sulforidazine
$C_{21}H_{26}N_2O_3$	Vincamine
$C_{21}H_{26}N_2O_3.HCl$	Yohimbine Hydrochloride
$C_{21}H_{26}N_2O_4.HCl$	Ciladopa Hydrochloride
$C_{21}H_{26}N_2O_6$	Ombrabulin
$C_{21}H_{26}N_2O_7$	Nimodipine
$C_{21}H_{26}N_2S_2$	Thioridazine
$C_{21}H_{26}N_2S_2.HCl$	Thioridazine Hydrochloride
$C_{21}H_{26}N_4O_2$	Linaprazan
$C_{21}H_{26}N_4O_5S$	Ersentilide
$C_{21}H_{26}N_6O_2$	Topixantrone
$C_{21}H_{26}N_8O_6S_2$	Cefclidin
$C_{21}H_{26}O_2$	Altrenogest
$C_{21}H_{26}O_2$	Cannabinol
$C_{21}H_{26}O_2$	Gestodene
$C_{21}H_{26}O_2$	Mestranol
$C_{21}H_{26}O_2$	Plomestane
$C_{21}H_{26}O_3$	Acitretin
$C_{21}H_{26}O_3$	Buparvaquone
$C_{21}H_{26}O_3$	Docebenone
$C_{21}H_{26}O_3$	Moxestrol
$C_{21}H_{26}O_3$	Octabenzone
$C_{21}H_{26}O_4$	Lifibrol
$C_{21}H_{26}O_5.H_2O$	Prednisone
$C_{21}H_{27}ClN_2O_2.C_{23}H_{16}O_6$	Hydroxyzine Pamoate
$C_{21}H_{27}ClN_2O_2.2HCl$	Hydroxyzine Hydrochloride
$C_{21}H_{27}ClO_3$	Cismadinone
$C_{21}H_{27}FN_2O_2$	Anisopirol
$C_{21}H_{27}FO_5$	Fluprednisolone
$C_{21}H_{27}FO_6$	Triamcinolone
$C_{21}H_{27}N$	Budipine
$C_{21}H_{27}N$	Pramiverine
$C_{21}H_{27}N$	Prozapine
$C_{21}H_{27}N.HCl$	Butriptyline Hydrochloride
$C_{21}H_{27}NO$	Benproperine
$C_{21}H_{27}NO$	Diphenidol
$C_{21}H_{27}NO$	Isomethadone
$C_{21}H_{27}NO$	Levomethadone
$(C_{21}H_{27}NO)_2.C_{23}H_{16}O_6$	Diphenidol Pamoate
$C_{21}H_{27}NO.HCl$	Diphenidol Hydrochloride
$C_{21}H_{27}NO.HCl$	Methadone Hydrochloride
$C_{21}H_{27}NOS$	Tibalosin
$C_{21}H_{27}NO_2$	Aprofene
$C_{21}H_{27}NO_2$	Dietifen
$C_{21}H_{27}NO_2$	Etafenone
$C_{21}H_{27}NO_2$	Ifenprodil
$C_{21}H_{27}NO_3.HCl$	Benapryzine Hydrochloride
$C_{21}H_{27}NO_3.HCl$	Diethylaminoethyl Diphenylhydroxypropionate Hydrochloride
$C_{21}H_{27}NO_3.HCl$	Propafenone Hydrochloride
$C_{21}H_{27}NO_3S_2$	Mazaticol
$C_{21}H_{27}NO_4.HCl$	Nalbuphine Hydrochloride
$C_{21}H_{27}NO_4S$	Diphemanil Methylsulfate
$C_{21}H_{27}NO_5$	Ritobegron
$C_{21}H_{27}N_3.2HCl$	Rimcazole Hydrochloride
$C_{21}H_{27}N_3O_2$	Methysergide
$C_{21}H_{27}N_3O_2.C_4H_4O_4$	Methysergide Maleate
$C_{21}H_{27}N_3O_3$	Anidoxime
$C_{21}H_{27}N_3O_3$	Bulaquine
$C_{21}H_{27}N_3O_3$	Nicainoprol
$C_{21}H_{27}N_3O_3$	Pirodavir
$C_{21}H_{27}N_3O_3S$	Sonepiprazole
$C_{21}H_{27}N_3O_3S.CH_4O_3S$	Sonepiprazole Mesylate
$C_{21}H_{27}N_3O_5$	Morocromen
$C_{21}H_{27}N_3O_5S$	Sarpicillin
$C_{21}H_{27}N_3O_6S$	Sarmoxicillin
$C_{21}H_{27}N_3O_7S.HCl$	Bacampicillin Hydrochloride
$C_{21}H_{27}N_5OS.3HCl$	Ledoxantrone Trihydrochloride
$C_{21}H_{27}N_5OS.3HCl$	Sedoxantrone Trihydrochloride
$C_{21}H_{27}N_5O_2S.3HCl$	Lupitidine Hydrochloride
$C_{21}H_{27}N_5O_4S$	Glipizide
$C_{21}H_{27}N_5O_7S$	Aspoxicillin
$C_{21}H_{27}N_5O_9S_2$	Cefpodoxime Proxetil
$C_{21}H_{27}N_7O_6$	Ketotrexate
$C_{21}H_{27}N_7O_{14}P_2$	Nadide
$C_{21}H_{27}Na_2O_8P$	Prednisolone Sodium Phosphate
$C_{21}H_{28}BrFO_2$	Haloprogesterone
$C_{21}H_{28}BrNO_3$	Methylbenactyzium Bromide
$C_{21}H_{28}BrNO_4$	Cimetropium Bromide
$C_{21}H_{28}FN_3O$	Enecadin
$C_{21}H_{28}N_2O$	Bifepramide
$C_{21}H_{28}N_2O$	Diampromide
$C_{21}H_{28}N_2O_2$	Decloxizine
$C_{21}H_{28}N_2O_5$	Ramiprilat
$C_{21}H_{28}N_2O_5$	Zabiciprilat
$C_{21}H_{28}N_2O_5.HCl$	Trimethobenzamide Hydrochloride
$C_{21}H_{28}N_2O_5S$	Tienoxolol
$C_{21}H_{28}N_2O_7$	Trigevolol
$C_{21}H_{28}N_4O_3.H_2SO_4.H_2O$	Lixazinone Sulfate
$C_{21}H_{28}N_4O_5$	Aderbasib
$C_{21}H_{28}O_2$	Demegestone

Molecular Formula	Non-proprietary Name
$C_{21}H_{28}O_2$	Dydrogesterone
$C_{21}H_{28}O_2$	Ethisterone
$C_{21}H_{28}O_2$	Levonorgestrel
$C_{21}H_{28}O_2$	Norgestrel
$C_{21}H_{28}O_2$	Tibolone
$C_{21}H_{28}O_3$	Segesterone
$C_{21}H_{28}O_4$	Deprodone
$C_{21}H_{28}O_4$	Formebolone
$C_{21}H_{28}O_5$	Aldosterone
$C_{21}H_{28}O_5$	Prednisolone
$C_{21}H_{28}O_5$	Roxibolone
$C_{21}H_{28}O_6$	Oxisopred
$C_{21}H_{29}ClO_3$	Hydromadinone
$C_{21}H_{29}ClO_6S$	Luprostil
$(C_{21}H_{29}Cl_2N_3O_2)_2.C_4H_4O_4$	Picumeterol Fumarate
$C_{21}H_{29}Cl_3O_3$	Cloxotestosterone
$C_{21}H_{29}FN_2O_2$	Fluciprazine
$C_{21}H_{29}FN_2O_3$	Fenaperone
$C_{21}H_{29}I_3N_4O_9$	Iosarcol
$C_{21}H_{29}N.HCl$	Diisopromine Hydrochloride
$C_{21}H_{29}NO$	Alphamethadol
$C_{21}H_{29}NO$	Betamethadol
$C_{21}H_{29}NO$	Biperiden
$C_{21}H_{29}NO$	Bufenadrine
$C_{21}H_{29}NO$	Dimepheptanol
$C_{21}H_{29}NO.C_3H_6O_3$	Biperiden Lactate
$C_{21}H_{29}NO.HCl$	Biperiden Hydrochloride
$C_{21}H_{29}NO_2$	Butorphanol
$C_{21}H_{29}NO_2$	Norelgestromin
$C_{21}H_{29}NO_2.C_4H_6O_6$	Butorphanol Tartrate
$C_{21}H_{29}NS_2.HCl$	Captodiame Hydrochloride
$C_{21}H_{29}N_3O$	Disopyramide
$C_{21}H_{29}N_3O.H_3PO_4$	Disopyramide Phosphate
$C_{21}H_{29}N_5O_2.C_6H_8O_7$	Tandospirone Citrate
$C_{21}H_{29}N_5O_6$	Gantofiban
$C_{21}H_{29}N_5O_6.C_2H_4O_2$	Roxifiban Acetate
$C_{21}H_{29}Na_2O_8P$	Hydrocortisone Sodium Phosphate
$C_{21}H_{30}BrNO_4$	Butylscopolamine Bromide
$C_{21}H_{30}Cl_2N_2O_5$	Dexloxiglumide
$C_{21}H_{30}Cl_2N_2O_5$	Loxiglumide
$C_{21}H_{30}FN_3O_2$	Pipamperone
$C_{21}H_{30}I_3N_3O_9$	Iosimide
$C_{21}H_{30}N_2O$	Bunaftine
$C_{21}H_{30}N_2O$	Hydroxystenozole
$C_{21}H_{30}N_2O$	Quinacainol
$C_{21}H_{30}N_2O_6$	Tosedostat
$C_{21}H_{30}N_2O_8S$	Docarpamine
$C_{21}H_{30}N_4O_3S$	Glibutimine
$C_{21}H_{30}N_4O_4$	Cinitapride
$C_{21}H_{30}N_4O_5S.HCl.3H_2O$	Acotiamide Hydrochloride
$C_{21}H_{30}O_2$ (A) THC	Nabiximols
$C_{21}H_{30}O_2$ (B) CBD	Nabiximols
$C_{21}H_{30}O_2$	Dronabinol
$C_{21}H_{30}O_2$	Progesterone
$C_{21}H_{30}O_3$	Trestolone Acetate
$C_{21}H_{30}O_4$	Cortodoxone
$C_{21}H_{30}O_5$	Hydrocortisone
$C_{21}H_{31}ClN_2O$	Viminol
$C_{21}H_{31}NO$	Cogazocine
$C_{21}H_{31}NO_2$	Bornaprine
$C_{21}H_{31}NO_2$	Fronepidil
$C_{21}H_{31}NO_3$	Spirendolol
$C_{21}H_{31}NO_4$	Furethidine
$C_{21}H_{31}NO_8S$	Tematropium Methylsulfate
$C_{21}H_{31}N_3O_5$	Cinpropazide

Molecular Formula	Non-proprietary Name
$C_{21}H_{31}N_3O_5.2H_2O$	Lisinopril
$C_{21}H_{31}N_5O.HCl$	Adatanserin Hydrochloride
$C_{21}H_{31}N_5O_2.HCl$	Buspirone Hydrochloride
$C_{21}H_{32}BrN$	Lauryl Isoquinolinium Bromide
$C_{21}H_{32}BrNO_3$	Oxypyrronium Bromide
$C_{21}H_{32}Cl_2N_4O$	Cariprazine
$C_{21}H_{32}N_2O$	Stanozolol
$C_{21}H_{32}N_2O_3$	Istaroxime
$C_{21}H_{32}N_2O_5S$	Camphotamide
$C_{21}H_{32}N_4O_5$	Pirepolol
$C_{21}H_{32}N_6O_3.HCl.H_2O$	Alfentanil Hydrochloride
$C_{21}H_{32}N_6O_3.H_2SO_4$	Efegatran Sulfate
$C_{21}H_{32}O$	Allylestrenol
$C_{21}H_{32}O_2$	Bolasterone
$C_{21}H_{32}O_2$	Calusterone
$C_{21}H_{32}O_2$	Cyclopregnol
$C_{21}H_{32}O_2$	Norbolethone
$C_{21}H_{32}O_3$	Alfaxalone
$C_{21}H_{32}O_3$	Oxymetholone
$C_{21}H_{32}O_3$	Renanolone
$C_{21}H_{32}O_4$	Alfadolone
$C_{21}H_{32}O_4$	Ataprost
$C_{21}H_{32}O_5$	Penprostene
$C_{21}H_{33}{}^{123}IO_2$	Iocanlidic Acid I 123
$C_{21}H_{33}NO$	Ramciclane
$C_{21}H_{33}N_2O_6P$	Ceronapril
$C_{21}H_{33}N_3O$	Sitamaquine
$C_{21}H_{33}N_3O_2$	Eptastigmine
$C_{21}H_{33}N_3O_3$	Terestigmine
$C_{21}H_{33}N_3O_5S$	Amdinocillin Pivoxil
$C_{21}H_{33}N_4O_6PS$	Managlinat Dialanetil
$C_{21}H_{34}BrNO_3$	Oxyphenonium Bromide
$C_{21}H_{34}ClN_3S_2$	Tropantiol
$C_{21}H_{34}F_2O_5$	Cobiprostone
$C_{21}H_{34}N_2O$	Sameridine
$C_{21}H_{34}O_2$	Eltanolone
$C_{21}H_{34}O_5$	Arbaprostil
$C_{21}H_{34}O_6$	Dimoxaprost
$C_{21}H_{34}O_6$	Eganoprost
$C_{21}H_{35}ClN_2O_3$	Lapyrium Chloride
$C_{21}H_{35}Cl_2MnN_5$	Imisopasem Manganese
$C_{21}H_{35}NO$	Amorolfine
$C_{21}H_{35}N_3.2C_4H_4O_4$	Bucainide Maleate
$C_{21}H_{36}ClNO$	Tridihexethyl Chloride
$C_{21}H_{36}INO$	Tridihexethyl Iodide
$C_{21}H_{36}N_2O_5S$	Hexocyclium Methylsulfate
$C_{21}H_{36}O_2$	Pregnandiol
$C_{21}H_{36}O_4$	Doxaprost
$C_{21}H_{36}O_5$	Carboprost
$C_{21}H_{36}O_5.C_4H_{11}NO_3$	Carboprost Tromethamine
$C_{21}H_{37}FN_2O_3S$	Trecetilide
$(C_{21}H_{37}FN_2O_3S)_2.C_4H_4O_4$	Trecetilide Fumarate
$C_{21}H_{38}ClN$	Benzododecinium Chloride
$C_{21}H_{38}ClN.H_2O$	Cetylpyridinium Chloride
$C_{21}H_{38}N_2.HCl$	Pirtenidine Hydrochloride
$C_{21}H_{38}N_6O_4$	Inogatran
$C_{21}H_{38}O_4$	Deprostil
$C_{21}H_{38}O_4$	Rioprostil
$C_{21}H_{39}ClNO_4P$	Clofilium Phosphate
$C_{21}H_{39}N_5O_{14}$	Bluensomycin
$(C_{21}H_{39}N_7O_{12})_2.3H_2SO_4$	Streptomycin Sulfate
$C_{21}H_{40}N_8O_5$	Icrocaptide
$C_{21}H_{40}N_8O_7$	Thymocartin
$(C_{21}H_{41}N_5O_7)_2.5H_2SO_4$	Netilmicin Sulfate
$C_{21}H_{41}N_5O_{11}$	Apramycin
$C_{21}H_{41}N_5O_{12}.2H_2SO_4.2H_2O$	Butirosin Sulfate

Molecular Formula	Non-proprietary Name
$(C_{21}H_{41}N_7O_{12})_2.3H_2SO_4$	Dihydrostreptomycin Sulfate
$C_{21}H_{43}N_5O_{12}$	Propikacin
$C_{21}H_{44}O_3$	Batilol
$C_{21}H_{45}N_3$	Hexetidine
$C_{21}H_{46}NO_4P$	Miltefosine
$C_{22}H_{14}Cl_2I_2N_2O_2$	Closantel
$C_{22}H_{16}ClN_3O_2$	Indibulin
$C_{22}H_{16}Cl_2O_4S$	Tioclomarol
$C_{22}H_{16}FN_7$	Etriciguat
$C_{22}H_{16}F_2N_2$	Flutrimazole
$C_{22}H_{16}N_4O_2S$	Rosabulin
$C_{22}H_{16}O_8$	Ethyl Biscoumacetate
$C_{22}H_{17}ClN_2$	Clotrimazole
$C_{22}H_{17}ClN_2$	Lombazole
$C_{22}H_{17}F_2N_5OS$	Isavuconazole
$C_{22}H_{17}F_2N_5OS$	Ravuconazole
$C_{22}H_{17}N_3O$	Piriqualone
$C_{22}H_{18}Cl_2FNO_3$	Cyfluthrin
$C_{22}H_{18}I_6N_2O_9$	Iotroxic Acid
$C_{22}H_{18}I_6N_2O_9.2C_7H_{17}NO_5$	Iotroxate Meglumine
$C_{22}H_{18}N_2$	Bifonazole
$C_{22}H_{18}N_4OS$	Axitinib
$C_{22}H_{18}N_6$	Rilpivirine
$C_{22}H_{18}O_3$	Anisacril
$C_{22}H_{19}Br$	Broparestrol
$C_{22}H_{19}Br_2NO_3$	Deltamethrin
$C_{22}H_{19}ClO_3$	Atovaquone
$C_{22}H_{19}Cl_2NO_3$	Alpha-Cypermethrin
$C_{22}H_{19}NO_2$	Indoxole
$C_{22}H_{19}NO_4$	Bisacodyl
$C_{22}H_{19}N_3O_4$	Tadalafil
$C_{22}H_{19}N_4NaO_8S_2$	Cefsulodin Sodium
$C_{22}H_{20}ClN_3$	Rilapine
$C_{22}H_{20}FN_3OS$	Tifluadom
$C_{22}H_{20}FN_3O_2$	Lufuradom
$C_{22}H_{20}N_2.HCl$	Benzindopyrine Hydrochloride
$C_{22}H_{20}N_2O_2$	Piketoprofen
$C_{22}H_{20}N_2O_5$	Reglitazar
$C_{22}H_{20}N_4O_5$	Talmetoprim
$C_{22}H_{20}N_6O_6$	Diniprofylline
$C_{22}H_{21}ClN_2O_6$	Sermetacin
$C_{22}H_{21}ClN_2O_8$	Meclocycline
$C_{22}H_{21}ClN_2O_8.C_7H_6O_6S$	Meclocycline Sulfosalicylate
$C_{22}H_{21}Cl_3N_4O$	Rimonabant
$C_{22}H_{21}FN_2O.HCl$	Sarizotan Hydrochloride
$C_{22}H_{21}FN_3O_3$	Zoloperone
$C_{22}H_{21}FN_4O$	Pruvanserin
$C_{22}H_{21}FN_4O.HCl$	Pruvanserin Hydrochloride
$C_{22}H_{21}NO_7.HCl$	Cetocycline Hydrochloride
$C_{22}H_{21}N_2NaO_6S_2$	Ticarcillin Cresyl Sodium
$C_{22}H_{21}N_3O_2$	Lusaperidone
$C_{22}H_{21}N_7O_6S_2$	Cefempidone
$C_{22}H_{21}N_8O_8PS_4.C_2H_4O_2.H_2O$	Ceftaroline Fosamil
$C_{22}H_{22}ClF_4NO_2.HCl$	Seperidol Hydrochloride
$C_{22}H_{22}ClKN_6O$	Losartan Potassium
$C_{22}H_{22}ClN_5O_2S$	Apafant
$C_{22}H_{22}ClN_5O_4S_2$	Suproclone
$C_{22}H_{22}FN_3O_2$	Belaperidone
$C_{22}H_{22}FN_3O_2$	Droperidol
$C_{22}H_{22}FN_3O_3$	Ketanserin
$C_{22}H_{22}F_3N$	Cinacalcet
$C_{22}H_{22}F_3N.HCl$	Cinacalcet Hydrochloride
$C_{22}H_{22}N_2O_2$	Cintazone
$C_{22}H_{22}N_2O_4$	Ambrisentan
$C_{22}H_{22}N_2O_5$	Varespladib Methyl
$C_{22}H_{22}N_2O_5S$	Fenbenicillin

Molecular Formula	Non-proprietary Name
$C_{22}H_{22}N_2O_6$	Darusentan
$C_{22}H_{22}N_2O_8$	Methacycline
$C_{22}H_{22}N_2O_8.HCl$	Methacycline Hydrochloride
$C_{22}H_{22}N_6O_5S_2.H_2SO_4$	Cefpirome Sulfate
$C_{22}H_{22}N_6O_7S_2.5H_2O$	Ceftazidime
$C_{22}H_{22}N_8.2HCl$	Bisantrene Hydrochloride
$C_{22}H_{22}N_{10}Na_2O_{12}S_2$	Pirazmonam Sodium
$C_{22}H_{22}O_5$	Cyclovalone
$C_{22}H_{22}O_8$	Podofilox
$C_{22}H_{23}ClFNO_2.HCl$	Cloroperone Hydrochloride
$C_{22}H_{23}ClFN_3O_2$	Milenperone
$C_{22}H_{23}ClFN_5O_2$	Flumeridone
$C_{22}H_{23}ClN_2O_2$	Loratadine
$C_{22}H_{23}ClN_2O_8.HCl$	Chlortetracycline Hydrochloride
$C_{22}H_{23}Cl_2N_3OS.C_6H_8O_7$	Elzasonan Citrate
$C_{22}H_{23}Cl_2N_3OS.HCl$	Elzasonan Hydrochloride
$C_{22}H_{23}FN_2O_5S$	Nesbuvir
$C_{22}H_{23}FN_4.HCl$	Revaprazan Hydrochloride
$C_{22}H_{23}FN_4O_2$	Rimacalib
$C_{22}H_{23}FN_4O_2.HCl$	Neflumozide Hydrochloride
$C_{22}H_{23}FN_6O_3$	Radezolid
$C_{22}H_{23}FN_6O_3.HCl$	Radezolid Hydrochloride
$C_{22}H_{23}F_2NO_2$	Lenperone
$C_{22}H_{23}F_4NO_2$	Trifluperidol
$C_{22}H_{23}NO_2$	Enpromate
$C_{22}H_{23}NO_3$	Dexpemedolac
$C_{22}H_{23}NO_3$	Pemedolac
$C_{22}H_{23}NO_4$	Nequinate
$C_{22}H_{23}NO_7$	Noscapine
$C_{22}H_{23}NS$	Tropatepine
$C_{22}H_{23}N_3O_2$	Isamfazone
$C_{22}H_{23}N_3O_2.HCl$	Serazapine Hydrochloride
$C_{22}H_{23}N_3O_4.HCl$	Erlotinib Hydrochloride
$C_{22}H_{23}N_5O$	Motesanib
$C_{22}H_{23}N_5O.2H_3O_4P$	Motesanib Diphosphate
$C_{22}H_{23}N_6Na_2O_8P$	Regrelor Disodium
$C_{22}H_{24}BrClN_4O_4$	Lodazecar
$C_{22}H_{24}BrFN_4O_2$	Vandetanib
$C_{22}H_{24}ClFN_4O_3$	Gefitinib
$C_{22}H_{24}ClNO_5$	Azaspirium Chloride
$C_{22}H_{24}ClN_3O.HCl$	Azelastine Hydrochloride
$C_{22}H_{24}ClN_3OS.2HCl$	Azaclorzine Hydrochloride
$C_{22}H_{24}ClN_3OS_2$	Spiclomazine
$C_{22}H_{24}ClN_3O_2S.2HCl$	Azalanstat Dihydrochloride
$C_{22}H_{24}ClN_5O$	Rabeximod
$C_{22}H_{24}ClN_5O_2$	Domperidone
$C_{22}H_{24}FN_3OS$	Timiperone
$C_{22}H_{24}FN_3O_2$	Benperidol
$C_{22}H_{24}FN_3O_2$	Declenperone
$C_{22}H_{24}FN_5O_4$	Brivanib Alaninate
$C_{22}H_{24}F_3N_3O_2S$	Ftorpropazine
$C_{22}H_{24}F_4N_2O$	Tefludazine
$C_{22}H_{24}N_2$	Pipequaline
$C_{22}H_{24}N_2O$	Tropirine
$C_{22}H_{24}N_2O_2$	Acrivastine
$C_{22}H_{24}N_2O_3$	Tribuzone
$C_{22}H_{24}N_2O_5$	Benazeprilat
$C_{22}H_{24}N_2O_7S$	Apremilast
$C_{22}H_{24}N_2O_8$	Tetracycline
$C_{22}H_{24}N_2O_8.HCl$	Epitetracycline Hydrochloride
$C_{22}H_{24}N_2O_8.HCl$	Tetracycline Hydrochloride
$(C_{22}H_{24}N_2O_8.HCl)_2.C_2H_6O.H_2O$	Doxycycline Hyclate
$C_{22}H_{24}N_2O_8.H_2O$	Doxycycline
$(C_{22}H_{24}N_2O_8)_3.NaPO_3.(HPO_3)_3$	Doxycycline Fosfatex

Molecular Formula	*Non-proprietary Name*
$C_{22}H_{24}N_2O_9$	Sornidipine
$C_{22}H_{24}N_2O_9.HCl$	Oxytetracycline Hydrochloride
$C_{22}H_{24}N_2O_9.2H_2O$	Oxytetracycline
$C_{22}H_{24}N_3NaO_7S$	Ertapenem Sodium
$C_{22}H_{24}N_4O_2.HCl$	Mirfentanil Hydrochloride
$C_{22}H_{25}ClN_2OS$	Clopenthixol
$C_{22}H_{25}ClN_2OS$	Zuclopenthixol
$C_{22}H_{25}ClN_2O_3$	Bifeprofen
$C_{22}H_{25}ClN_2O_4S.C_4H_4O_4$	Clentiazem Maleate
$C_{22}H_{25}Cl_2N_3O_2.2HCl$	Amustaline Dihydrochloride
$C_{22}H_{25}FN_4O_2$	Toceranib
$C_{22}H_{25}FN_4O_2.H_3O_4P$	Toceranib Phosphate
$C_{22}H_{25}F_2NO_4$	Dexnebivolol
$C_{22}H_{25}F_2NO_4$	Levonebivolol
$C_{22}H_{25}F_2NO_4$	Nebivolol
$C_{22}H_{25}F_2NO_4.HCl$	Nebivolol Hydrochloride
$C_{22}H_{25}F_2N_3O_2S$	Lubeluzole
$C_{22}H_{25}N$	Piroheptine
$C_{22}H_{25}NO_2.CH_4O_3S$	Napitane Mesylate
$C_{22}H_{25}NO_3$	Tamibarotene
$C_{22}H_{25}NO_3.HCl$	Pipoxolan Hydrochloride
$C_{22}H_{25}NO_4$	Dimoxyline
$C_{22}H_{25}NO_4$	Pitofenone
$C_{22}H_{25}NO_4S$	Adrogolide
$C_{22}H_{25}NO_4S.HCl$	Adrogolide Hydrochloride
$C_{22}H_{25}NO_6$	Colchicine
$C_{22}H_{25}N_3O$	Benzpiperylon
$C_{22}H_{25}N_3O$	Indoramin
$C_{22}H_{25}N_3O.HCl$	Indoramin Hydrochloride
$C_{22}H_{25}N_3O_2.HCl$	Bucindolol Hydrochloride
$C_{22}H_{25}N_3O_3$	Dacinostat
$C_{22}H_{25}N_3O_3$	Niravoline
$C_{22}H_{25}N_3O_3$	Spiroxatrine
$C_{22}H_{25}N_3O_3.C_4H_6O_6$	Solypertine Tartrate
$C_{22}H_{25}N_3O_4$	Abanoquil
$C_{22}H_{25}N_3O_4$	Vesnarinone
$C_{22}H_{25}N_3O_4S$	Moricizine
$C_{22}H_{25}N_3O_4S.HCl$	Moricizine Hydrochloride
$C_{22}H_{25}N_7O_5$	Edatrexate
$C_{22}H_{26}BrNO_3$	Clidinium Bromide
$C_{22}H_{26}ClNO_4$	Amibegron
$C_{22}H_{26}ClNO_4.HCl$	Amibegron Hydrochloride
$C_{22}H_{26}ClN_7O_2S.H_2O$	Dasatinib
$C_{22}H_{26}FNO_2$	Moperone
$C_{22}H_{26}FN_3O_2$	Spiramide
$C_{22}H_{26}FN_3O_2S$	Sabeluzole
$C_{22}H_{26}FN_3O_4$	Flesinoxan
$C_{22}H_{26}FN_5O_3$	Fluprofylline
$C_{22}H_{26}F_3N_3OS.2HCl$	Fluphenazine Hydrochloride
$C_{22}H_{26}N_2O_2$	Indocate
$C_{22}H_{26}N_2O_2$	Vinpocetine
$C_{22}H_{26}N_2O_2S$	Eletriptan
$C_{22}H_{26}N_2O_2S.HBr$	Eletriptan Hydrobromide
$C_{22}H_{26}N_2O_3S$	Zepastine
$C_{22}H_{26}N_2O_4$	Dextofisopam
$C_{22}H_{26}N_2O_4$	Levotofisopam
$C_{22}H_{26}N_2O_4$	Tofisoline
$C_{22}H_{26}N_2O_4$	Tofisopam
$C_{22}H_{26}N_2O_4S.C_4H_6O_5$	Diltiazem Malate
$C_{22}H_{26}N_2O_4S.HCl$	Diltiazem Hydrochloride
$C_{22}H_{26}N_6O_2$	Tameridone
$C_{22}H_{26}O_3$	Bioresmethrin
$C_{22}H_{26}O_4$	Seratrodast
$C_{22}H_{27}ClF_2O_3$	Halocortolone
$C_{22}H_{27}ClF_2O_5$	Halometasone
$C_{22}H_{27}ClN_2O.HCl$	Lorcainide Hydrochloride

Molecular Formula	*Non-proprietary Name*
$C_{22}H_{27}ClN_2O_3.HCl$	Lorajmine Hydrochloride
$C_{22}H_{27}ClN_4O_3$	Avizafone
$C_{22}H_{27}ClO_4$	Amadinone Acetate
$C_{22}H_{27}Cl_2N_3O_4$	Cloxacepride
$C_{22}H_{27}FN_2O_2.HCl$	Ocfentanil Hydrochloride
$2C_{22}H_{27}FN_3O_6S.Ca$	Rosuvastatin Calcium
$C_{22}H_{27}FN_4O_2.C_4H_6O_5$	Sunitinib Malate
$C_{22}H_{27}FO_5$	Fluprednidene
$C_{22}H_{27}MnN_4Na_3O_{14}P_2$	Mangafodipir Trisodium
$C_{22}H_{27}NO$	Ethybenztropine
$C_{22}H_{27}NO$	Sequifenadine
$C_{22}H_{27}NO.HBr$	Phenazocine Hydrobromide
$C_{22}H_{27}NO_2$	Amineptine
$C_{22}H_{27}NO_2$	Danazol
$C_{22}H_{27}NO_2$	Dexproxibutene
$C_{22}H_{27}NO_2$	Lobeline
$C_{22}H_{27}NO_2$	Pheneridine
$C_{22}H_{27}NO_2$	Pifenate
$C_{22}H_{27}NO_2$	Proxibutene
$C_{22}H_{27}NO_3$	Dioxaphetyl Butyrate
$C_{22}H_{27}NO_3$	Oxpheneridine
$C_{22}H_{27}NO_3$	Zocainone
$C_{22}H_{27}NO_4$	Isalmadol
$C_{22}H_{27}NO_6.CH_4O_3S$	Nisbuterol Mesylate
$C_{22}H_{27}N_3O_2$	Caroverine
$C_{22}H_{27}N_3O_2$	Omidoline
$C_{22}H_{27}N_3O_3$	Ganstigmine
$C_{22}H_{27}N_3O_3S_2$	Metopimazine
$C_{22}H_{27}N_3O_4.H_2O$	Diperodon
$C_{22}H_{27}N_3O_4S$	Metioxate
$C_{22}H_{27}N_3O_5S$	Glisentide
$C_{22}H_{27}N_5$	Pazelliptine
$C_{22}H_{27}N_5O$	Metoquizine
$C_{22}H_{27}N_5O_4.2HCl.\frac{1}{2}H_2O$	Losoxantrone Hydrochloride
$C_{22}H_{27}N_9O_4.HCl$	Stallimycin Hydrochloride
$C_{22}H_{28}BrN$	Prifinium Bromide
$C_{22}H_{28}BrNO_3$	Benzilonium Bromide
$C_{22}H_{28}BrNO_3$	Pipenzolate Bromide
$C_{22}H_{28}BrN_5O_5$	Dasantafil
$C_{22}H_{28}ClNO$	Setastine
$C_{22}H_{28}ClNaO_6$	Cloprostenol Sodium
$C_{22}H_{28}Cl_2N_2O_6$	Olradipine
$C_{22}H_{28}FNO_3$	Volinanserin
$C_{22}H_{28}FN_3O_3$	Mafoprazine
$C_{22}H_{28}FNa_2O_8P$	Betamethasone Sodium Phosphate
$C_{22}H_{28}FNa_2O_8P$	Dexamethasone Sodium Phosphate
$C_{22}H_{28}F_2O_4$	Diflucortolone
$C_{22}H_{28}F_2O_5$	Flumethasone
$C_{22}H_{28}GdN_3O_{11}.2C_7H_{17}NO_5$	Gadobenate Dimeglumine
$C_{22}H_{28}INO_2$	Diphenylpiperidinomethyl- dioxolan Iodide
$C_{22}H_{28}N_2$	Carbazocine
$C_{22}H_{28}N_2O$	Fentanyl
$C_{22}H_{28}N_2O.C_6H_8O_7$	Fentanyl Citrate
$C_{22}H_{28}N_2O_2$	Anileridine
$C_{22}H_{28}N_2O_2$	Brefonalol
$C_{22}H_{28}N_2O_2.2HCl$	Anileridine Hydrochloride
$C_{22}H_{28}N_2O_2.HCl$	Encainide Hydrochloride
$C_{22}H_{28}N_2O_2S$	Perimetazine
$C_{22}H_{28}N_2O_2S.HCl$	Becanthone Hydrochloride
$C_{22}H_{28}N_2O_3$	Modecainide
$C_{22}H_{28}N_2O_3$	Pentamorphone
$C_{22}H_{28}N_2O_5S$	Ilepatril
$C_{22}H_{28}N_2O_5S_2.HCl$	Sibenadet Hydrochloride

Molecular Formula	Non-proprietary Name
$C_{22}H_{28}N_4O_3$	Etonitazene
$C_{22}H_{28}N_4O_4.2C_2H_4O_2$	Ametantrone Acetate
$C_{22}H_{28}N_4O_6$	Banoxantrone
$C_{22}H_{28}N_4O_6.2HCl$	Mitoxantrone Hydrochloride
$C_{22}H_{28}N_6O_3S.CH_4O_3S$	Delavirdine Mesylate
$C_{22}H_{28}N_6O_8S_2$	Ceftizoxime Alapivoxil
$C_{22}H_{28}O_2$	Etonogestrel
$C_{22}H_{28}O_3$	Canrenone
$C_{22}H_{28}O_3$	Norethindrone Acetate
$C_{22}H_{28}O_5$	Isoprednidene
$C_{22}H_{28}O_5$	Meprednisone
$C_{22}H_{28}O_5$	Prednylidene
$C_{22}H_{29}BrN_2O$	Fenpiverinium Bromide
$C_{22}H_{29}FO_4$	Desoximetasone
$C_{22}H_{29}FO_4$	Doxibetasol
$C_{22}H_{29}FO_4$	Fluocortolone
$C_{22}H_{29}FO_4$	Fluorometholone
$C_{22}H_{29}FO_5$	Betamethasone
$C_{22}H_{29}FO_5$	Dexamethasone
$C_{22}H_{29}FO_5$	Flunoprost
$C_{22}H_{29}F_3N_2O_2$	Terciprazine
$C_{22}H_{29}F_3O_3$	Flumedroxone
$C_{22}H_{29}KO_4$	Canrenoate Potassium
$C_{22}H_{29}NOS$	Diprofene
$C_{22}H_{29}NOS$	Xenthiorate
$C_{22}H_{29}NO_2.C_{10}H_8O_3S.H_2O$	Levopropoxyphene Napsylate
$C_{22}H_{29}NO_2.C_{10}H_8O_3S.H_2O$	Propoxyphene Napsylate
$C_{22}H_{29}NO_2.C_{19}H_{20}N_2O_2$	Proxifezone
$C_{22}H_{29}NO_2.HCl$	Noracymethadol Hydrochloride
$C_{22}H_{29}NO_2.HCl$	Propoxyphene Hydrochloride
$C_{22}H_{29}NO_5$	Trimebutine
$C_{22}H_{29}NO_7S$	Poldine Methylsulfate
$C_{22}H_{29}N_3O_4$	Peradoxime
$C_{22}H_{29}N_3O_4S$	Lafutidine
$C_{22}H_{29}N_3O_6S.C_{13}H_{19}NO_4S$	Pivampicillin Probenate
$(C_{22}H_{29}N_3O_6S)_2.C_{23}H_{16}O_6$	Pivampicillin Pamoate
$C_{22}H_{29}N_3O_6S.HCl$	Pivampicillin Hydrochloride
$C_{22}H_{29}N_3S_2$	Thiethylperazine
$C_{22}H_{29}N_3S_2.2C_4H_4O_4$	Thiethylperazine Maleate
$C_{22}H_{29}N_3S_2.2C_4H_6O_5$	Thiethylperazine Malate
$C_{22}H_{29}N_7O_5$	Puromycin
$C_{22}H_{29}N_7O_5.2HCl$	Puromycin Hydrochloride
$C_{22}H_{29}N_9O_9S_2$	Cefbuperazone
$C_{22}H_{29}Na_2O_8P$	Methylprednisolone Sodium Phosphate
$C_{22}H_{29}O_8P.C_{13}H_{18}N_2O$	Prednazoline
$C_{22}H_{30}BrCl_2NO$	Halopenium Chloride
$C_{22}H_{30}BrNO$	Pirdonium Bromide
$C_{22}H_{30}ClN_3O_2$	Alepride
$C_{22}H_{30}Cl_2N_2O_2.CH_4O_3S$	Spiradoline Mesylate
$C_{22}H_{30}Cl_2N_{10}.2C_6H_8NO_3P$	Chlorhexidine Phosphanilate
$C_{22}H_{30}Cl_2N_{10}.2C_6H_{12}O_7$	Chlorhexidine Gluconate
$C_{22}H_{30}Cl_2N_{10}.2HCl$	Chlorhexidine Hydrochloride
$C_{22}H_{30}FNO_4$	Flusoxolol
$C_{22}H_{30}INO$	Stilonium Iodide
$C_{22}H_{30}MnN_4O_{14}P_2$	Mangafodipir
$C_{22}H_{30}N_2$	Aprindine
$C_{22}H_{30}N_2.HCl$	Aprindine Hydrochloride
$C_{22}H_{30}N_2O.HCl$	Pirmenol Hydrochloride
$C_{22}H_{30}N_2O_2$	Barucainide
$C_{22}H_{30}N_2O_2$	Eprozinol
$C_{22}H_{30}N_2O_2S$	Sufentanil
$C_{22}H_{30}N_2O_2S.C_6H_8O_7$	Sufentanil Citrate
$C_{22}H_{30}N_2O_3$	Davasaicin
$C_{22}H_{30}N_2O_5$	Trandolaprilat
$C_{22}H_{30}N_2O_5S_2.HCl$	Spirapril Hydrochloride

Molecular Formula	Non-proprietary Name
$C_{22}H_{30}N_2O_6$	Moxicoumone
$C_{22}H_{30}N_4O_2S_2.2CH_4O_3S$	Thioproperazine Mesylate
$C_{22}H_{30}N_6O_3S.C_4H_4O_4$	Avitriptan Fumarate
$C_{22}H_{30}N_6O_4S.C_6H_8O_7$	Sildenafil Citrate
$C_{22}H_{30}O$	Desogestrel
$C_{22}H_{30}O_2$	Promegestone
$C_{22}H_{30}O_2S$	Salirasib
$C_{22}H_{30}O_3$	Endrysone
$C_{22}H_{30}O_3$	Siccanin
$C_{22}H_{30}O_3$	Trimegestone
$C_{22}H_{30}O_4$	Terameprocol
$C_{22}H_{30}O_5$	Cicaprost
$C_{22}H_{30}O_5$	Methylprednisolone
$C_{22}H_{30}O_8$	Valtrate
$C_{22}H_{31}ClO_2$	Clometherone
$C_{22}H_{31}FO_2S_2$	Tipredane
$C_{22}H_{31}NO$	Tolterodine
$C_{22}H_{31}NO.C_4H_6O_6$	Tolterodine Tartrate
$C_{22}H_{31}NO_3$	Amicibone
$C_{22}H_{31}NO_3$	Epostane
$C_{22}H_{31}NO_3$	Oxybutynin
$C_{22}H_{31}NO_3.HCl$	Esoxybutynin Chloride
$C_{22}H_{31}NO_3.HCl$	Oxybutynin Chloride
$C_{22}H_{31}NO_4$	Fedotozine
$C_{22}H_{31}N_3O_2.HCl$	Piboserod Hydrochloride
$C_{22}H_{31}N_3O_3$	Taziprinone
$C_{22}H_{31}N_3O_4$	Adekalant
$C_{22}H_{31}N_3O_4S.HI$	Penethamate Hydriodide
$C_{22}H_{31}N_3O_5$	Cinepazide
$C_{22}H_{31}N_3O_5.H_2O$	Cilazapril
$C_{22}H_{31}N_3O_5S$	Utibapril
$C_{22}H_{31}N_3O_6S_2$	Tebipenem Pivoxil
$C_{22}H_{31}N_5O_4$	Melagatran
$C_{22}H_{32}BrNO_3$	Droclidinium Bromide
$C_{22}H_{32}Br_2N_4O_4$	Distigmine Bromide
$C_{22}H_{32}Cl_2N_2O_4$	Lorglumide
$C_{22}H_{32}N_2O_2$	Dopexamine
$C_{22}H_{32}N_2O_2.2HCl$	Dopexamine Hydrochloride
$C_{22}H_{32}N_2O_3$	Mociprazine
$C_{22}H_{32}N_2O_5$	Benzquinamide
$C_{22}H_{32}N_2O_6.H_2SO_4$	Hexoprenaline Sulfate
$C_{22}H_{32}N_4O$	Proterguride
$C_{22}H_{32}N_4O_4.H_2O$	Elarofiban
$C_{22}H_{32}N_4O_{14}P_2$	Fodipir
$C_{22}H_{32}O_2$	Doconexent
$C_{22}H_{32}O_2$	Promestriene
$C_{22}H_{32}O_3$	Medrysone
$C_{22}H_{32}O_3$	Methenolone Acetate
$C_{22}H_{32}O_3$	Stenbolone Acetate
$C_{22}H_{32}O_3$	Testosterone Propionate
$C_{22}H_{32}O_4$	Iloprost
$C_{22}H_{32}O_4$	Oxoprostol
$C_{22}H_{32}O_8$	Didrovaltrate
$C_{22}H_{33}ClN_2O$	Erocainide
$C_{22}H_{33}NO_3.H_2SO_4$	Cyclomethycaine Sulfate
$C_{22}H_{33}NO_5$	Nileprost
$C_{22}H_{33}N_3O_4S$	Recainam Tosylate
$C_{22}H_{34}BrNO$	Ciclonium Bromide
$C_{22}H_{34}ClN_3O_2$	Bidisomide
$C_{22}H_{34}GdN_5O_{10}$	Gadopenamide
$C_{22}H_{34}INO_2$	Oxapium Iodide
$C_{22}H_{34}N_2O$	Stirocainide
$C_{22}H_{34}N_2O_2$	Ipenoxazone
$C_{22}H_{34}N_2O_3$	Trapencaine
$C_{22}H_{34}N_2O_4.2HCl$	Oxamarin Hydrochloride
$C_{22}H_{34}N_4O_{10}$	Sobuzoxane

Molecular Formula	Non-proprietary Name
$C_{22}H_{34}O_2$ (EPA ethyl ester)	Omega-3-acid Ethyl Esters
$C_{22}H_{34}O_2$	Ethyl Icosapentate
$C_{22}H_{34}O_2$	Topterone
$C_{22}H_{34}O_5$	Pleuromulin
$C_{22}H_{34}O_7$	Colforsin
$C_{22}H_{35}[^{123}I]O_2$	Iodofiltic Acid I 123
$C_{22}H_{35}NO$	Pipoctanone
$C_{22}H_{35}NO_2$	Dexsecoverine
$C_{22}H_{35}NO_2$	Secoverine
$C_{22}H_{35}NO_4S$	Fenclexonium Metilsulfate
$C_{22}H_{35}NO_5$	Divabuterol
$C_{22}H_{35}NO_7$	Amoproxan
$C_{22}H_{35}N_3O_2$	Transcainide
$C_{22}H_{36}N_2O_3$	Fenetradil
$C_{22}H_{36}N_2O_4$	Arterolane
$C_{22}H_{36}N_2O_5S.HCl.H_2O$	Tirofiban Hydrochloride
$C_{22}H_{36}N_4O_5$	Cipemastat
$C_{22}H_{36}N_8O_{11}$	Pentigetide
$C_{22}H_{36}O_2$	Ganaxolone
$C_{22}H_{36}O_2Si$	Silandrone
$C_{22}H_{36}O_4$	Clinprost
$C_{22}H_{36}O_5$	Enisoprost
$C_{22}H_{36}O_5$	Limaprost
$C_{22}H_{36}O_5$	Prostalene
$C_{22}H_{37}ClO_4$	Nocloprost
$C_{22}H_{38}O_4Ca$	Calcium Undecylenate
$C_{22}H_{38}O_4Cu$	Copper Undecylenate
$C_{22}H_{38}O_4Zn$	Zinc Undecylenate
$C_{22}H_{38}O_5$	Carboprost Methyl
$C_{22}H_{38}O_5$	Misoprostol
$C_{22}H_{38}O_5$	Unoprostone
$C_{22}H_{38}O_7$	Ascorbyl Palmitate
$C_{22}H_{39}BrClNO$	Dodeclonium Bromide
$C_{22}H_{40}BrNO$	Domiphen Bromide
$(C_{22}H_{40}O_4)_n$	Surfomer
$C_{22}H_{42}N_4O_8S_2$	Pantethine
$C_{22}H_{42}O_6$ (Approximate)	Sorbitan Monopalmitate
$C_{22}H_{43}N_5O_{12}$	Isepamicin
$C_{22}H_{43}N_5O_{13}$	Amikacin
$C_{22}H_{43}N_5O_{13}.2H_2SO_4$	Amikacin Sulfate
$C_{22}H_{44}N_2.2C_4H_4O_4$	Atiprimod Dimaleate
$C_{22}H_{44}N_2.2HCl$	Atiprimod Dihydrochloride
$C_{22}H_{44}N_6O_{10}$	Arbekacin
$C_{22}H_{45}N_3$	Hexedine
$C_{22}H_{45}N_3O_3$	Teglicar
$C_{22}H_{45}N_5O_{12}$	Butikacin
$C_{22}H_{46}FNO_2$	Xidecaflur
$C_{22}H_{46}N_4O_3S_2V$	Naglivan
$C_{22}H_{46}O$	Docosanol
$C_{22}H_{47}N_3O$	Lycetamine
$C_{22}H_{49}NO_4S$	Mecetronium Ethylsulfate
$(C_{22}H_{56}O_8Si_7)_w(C_5H_8O_2)_x$ $(C_4H_6O_2)_y(C_{16}H_{26}O_7)_z$	Silafocon A
$C_{23}{}^{11}CH_{28}FN_3O_2$	Mespiperone C 11
$C_{23}H_{14}F_2NNaO_2$	Brequinar Sodium
$C_{23}H_{14}Na_2O_{11}$	Cromolyn Sodium
$C_{23}H_{15}N_3O$	Perampanel
$C_{23}H_{16}O_3$	Diphenadione
$C_{23}H_{16}O_6.C_{17}H_{20}N_4S.H_2O$	Olanzapine Pamoate
$C_{23}H_{18}F_2N_2O_2$	Fenflumizole
$C_{23}H_{18}N_2O_2$	Isofezolac
$C_{23}H_{18}N_2O_2$	Trifezolac
$C_{23}H_{18}N_4.H_2O$	Sibopirdine
$C_{23}H_{18}O_6$	Heliomycin
$C_{23}H_{19}ClF_3NO_3$	Cyhalothrin
$C_{23}H_{19}ClO_3S$	Tanomastat
$C_{23}H_{19}Cl_2NO_3S$	Ticolubant
$C_{23}H_{19}N_2NaO_4S$	Darglitazone Sodium
$C_{23}H_{20}Cl_2F_2N_2O_2S$	Drinabant
$C_{23}H_{20}Cl_2N_4O_2S$	Ibipinabant
$C_{23}H_{20}F_2N_2O_4.CH_4O_3S.H_2O$	Garenoxacin Mesylate
$C_{23}H_{20}N_2O_3S$	Sulfinpyrazone
$C_{23}H_{20}N_2O_5$	Bentiromide
$C_{23}H_{20}N_6O.2HBr$	Mocetinostat Dihydrobromide
$C_{23}H_{21}ClN_2O_4$	Gedocarnil
$C_{23}H_{21}ClN_6O_3$	Loprazolam
$C_{23}H_{21}ClO_3$	Chlorotrianisene
$C_{23}H_{21}F_4NO_3S_2$	Sodelglitazar
$C_{23}H_{21}F_7N_4O_3$	Aprepitant
$C_{23}H_{21}NO_4$	Xenazoic Acid
$C_{23}H_{21}N_2NaO_6S$	Carbenicillin Phenyl Sodium
$C_{23}H_{21}N_5O_5S$	Avosentan
$C_{23}H_{21}N_7O$	Tasosartan
$C_{23}H_{22}ClNO_2$	Licofelone
$C_{23}H_{22}ClN_3O_2$	Pagoclone
$C_{23}H_{22}ClN_5O_2S$	Bepafant
$C_{23}H_{22}ClN_5O_3$	Betrixaban
$C_{23}H_{22}FN_3O$	Elopiprazole
$C_{23}H_{22}F_3N_3O_2$	Florifenine
$C_{23}H_{22}F_7N_4O_6P.2C_7H_{17}NO_5$	Fosaprepitant Dimeglumine
$C_{23}H_{22}N_2O_4S$	Osmadizone
$C_{23}H_{22}N_8O$	Ripisartan
$C_{23}H_{23}BrCl_2N_4O$	Surinabant
$C_{23}H_{23}ClFNO_5$	Elvitegravir
$C_{23}H_{23}ClN_2O_3$	Mimopezil
$C_{23}H_{23}ClN_2O_3.HCl$	Solabegron Hydrochloride
$C_{23}H_{23}Cl_2N_3O_4S.HCl$	Tubulozole Hydrochloride
$C_{23}H_{23}IN_2S_2$	Dithiazanine Iodide
$C_{23}H_{23}NO_2.CH_4O_3S$	Crisnatol Mesylate
$C_{23}H_{23}NO_3$	Veliflapon
$C_{23}H_{23}N_3O_5.HCl$	Topotecan Hydrochloride
$C_{23}H_{23}N_5O_2$	Emapunil
$C_{23}H_{23}N_7O_5$	Pralatrexate
$C_{23}H_{24}ClFeN_3$	Ferroquine
$C_{23}H_{24}ClN_3O_2$	Piclozotan
$C_{23}H_{24}ClN_3O_5$	Ingliforib
$C_{23}H_{24}ClN_4NaO_4S$	Glicetanile Sodium
$C_{23}H_{24}FN_3O$	Cinuperone
$C_{23}H_{24}FN_3O_2$	Pirenperone
$C_{23}H_{24}FN_3O_2S$	Fananserin
$C_{23}H_{24}FN_3O_3$	Prideperone
$C_{23}H_{24}FN_6Na_2O_9P.6H_2O$	Fostamatinib Disodium
$C_{23}H_{24}F_3N_3OS$	Azaftozine
$C_{23}H_{24}F_7N_3O.CH_4O_3S$	Vestipitant Mesylate
$C_{23}H_{24}N_2O_4S$	Eprosartan
$C_{23}H_{24}N_2O_4S.CH_4O_3S$	Eprosartan Mesylate
$C_{23}H_{24}N_4.C_4H_4O_4$	Tampramine Fumarate
$C_{23}H_{24}N_4O_3S.C_6H_{10}O_7$	Metesind Glucuronate
$C_{23}H_{24}N_4O_6$	Merimepodib
$C_{23}H_{24}N_6O_5S_2.H_2SO_4$	Cefquinome Sulfate
$C_{23}H_{24}N_6O_7S_2$	Sulfamazone
$C_{23}H_{24}O_4$	Cyclofenil
$C_{23}H_{25}ClN_2O_9$	Clomocycline
$C_{23}H_{25}ClN_4O_4$	Capeserod
$C_{23}H_{25}ClN_6O_8S_3$	Cefmepidium Chloride
$C_{23}H_{25}F_2N_3O_2$	Fluspiperone
$C_{23}H_{25}F_3N_2OS$	Flupentixol
$C_{23}H_{25}N$	Fendiline
$C_{23}H_{25}NO$	Decitropine
$C_{23}H_{25}NO_6S$	Fasidotril
$C_{23}H_{25}N_3O_2.C_4H_4O_4$	Icopezil Maleate
$C_{23}H_{25}N_3O_6$	Lefradafiban

Molecular Formula	Non-proprietary Name
$C_{23}H_{25}N_5O_2$	Donitriptan
$C_{23}H_{25}N_5O_5.CH_4O_3S$	Doxazosin Mesylate
$C_{23}H_{26}BrNO_3$	Trantelinium Bromide
$C_{23}H_{26}ClN_7O_3$	Avanafil
$C_{23}H_{26}Cl_2O_6$	Simfibrate
$C_{23}H_{26}FN_3O_2$	Spiperone
$C_{23}H_{26}FN_6O_9P$	Fostamatinib
$C_{23}H_{26}F_3N_3S.2HCl$	Cyclophenazine Hydrochloride
$C_{23}H_{26}F_4N_2OS$	Teflutixol
$C_{23}H_{26}N_2O$	Roxindole
$C_{23}H_{26}N_2O_2$	Dexetimide
$C_{23}H_{26}N_2O_2.C_4H_6O_4$	Solifenacin Succinate
$C_{23}H_{26}N_2O_2.HCl$	Benzetimide Hydrochloride
$C_{23}H_{26}N_2O_3.C_4H_4O_4$	Pravadoline Maleate
$C_{23}H_{26}N_2O_5$	Quinaprilat
$C_{23}H_{26}N_2O_6$	Panamesine
$C_{23}H_{26}N_5NaO_7S$	Piperacillin Sodium
$C_{23}H_{26}N_6O_2$	Apilimod Mesylate
$C_{23}H_{26}O_3$	Phenothrin
$C_{23}H_{27}ClN_2O_2.2HCl$	Pinoxepin Hydrochloride
$C_{23}H_{27}ClO_2$	Gestaclone
$C_{23}H_{27}ClO_4$	Delmadinone Acetate
$C_{23}H_{27}ClO_6$	Chloroprednisone Acetate
$C_{23}H_{27}Cl_2N_3O_2$	Aripiprazole
$C_{23}H_{27}FN_4O_2$	Risperidone
$C_{23}H_{27}FN_4O_3$	Paliperidone
$C_{23}H_{27}F_3N_2O_2S$	Flupimazine
$C_{23}H_{27}N.HCl$	Butenafine Hydrochloride
$C_{23}H_{27}NO.C_6H_8O_7$	Deptropine Citrate
$C_{23}H_{27}NO_2$	Pituxate
$C_{23}H_{27}NO_3$	Etabenzarone
$C_{23}H_{27}NO_4$	Micinicate
$C_{23}H_{27}NO_5$	Diacetylnalorphine
$C_{23}H_{27}NO_5$	Octaverine
$C_{23}H_{27}NO_9$	Morphine Glucuronide
$C_{23}H_{27}N_3O$	Itrocainide
$C_{23}H_{27}N_3O$	Prenoxdiazine
$C_{23}H_{27}N_3O_2$	Morazone
$C_{23}H_{27}N_3O_2$	Parodilol
$C_{23}H_{27}N_3O_2$	Quilostigmine
$C_{23}H_{27}N_3O_3$	Benafentrine
$C_{23}H_{27}N_3O_4$	Benexate
$C_{23}H_{27}N_3O_4.HCl.C_{42}H_{70}O_{35}$	Benexate Hydrochloride Betadex
$C_{23}H_{27}N_3O_4S$	Tomeglovir
$C_{23}H_{27}N_3O_7$	Minocycline
$C_{23}H_{27}N_3O_7.HCl$	Minocycline Hydrochloride
$C_{23}H_{27}N_5O_2$	Terbogrel
$C_{23}H_{27}N_5O_7S.H_2O$	Piperacillin
$C_{23}H_{28}$	Temarotene
$C_{23}H_{28}ClN_3O$	Datelliptium Chloride
$C_{23}H_{28}ClN_3O_2S.2HCl$	Thiopropazate Hydrochloride
$C_{23}H_{28}ClN_3O_5S$	Glyburide
$C_{23}H_{28}ClN_5O_3.2HCl$	Azimilide Dihydrochloride
$C_{23}H_{28}Cl_2O_5$	Dichlorisone Acetate
$C_{23}H_{28}FN_5O_3$	Perbufylline
$C_{23}H_{28}F_2N_6O_4S$	Ticagrelor
$C_{23}H_{28}F_3N_3OS$	Homofenazine
$C_{23}H_{28}F_3NaO_6$	Fluprostenol Sodium
$C_{23}H_{28}GdN_3Na_2O_{11}$	Gadoxetate Disodium
$C_{23}H_{28}N_2$	Indopine
$C_{23}H_{28}N_2O$	Iferanserin
$C_{23}H_{28}N_2O$	Leiopyrrole
$C_{23}H_{28}N_2O_3$	Acoxatrine

Molecular Formula	Non-proprietary Name
$C_{23}H_{28}N_2O_3$	Bopindolol
$C_{23}H_{28}N_2O_3$	Mindodilol
$C_{23}H_{28}N_2O_3$	Tropapride
$C_{23}H_{28}N_2O_3S$	Cinalukast
$C_{23}H_{28}N_2O_4$	Pacrinolol
$C_{23}H_{28}N_2O_5S_2.HCl$	Temocapril Hydrochloride
$C_{23}H_{28}N_4O_4$	Nesapidil
$C_{23}H_{28}N_4O_4$	Peraquinsin
$C_{23}H_{28}N_4O_8S$	Vaneprim
$C_{23}H_{28}N_4O_{11}S$	Cefuroxime Pivoxetil
$C_{23}H_{28}N_6O_4$	Freselestat
$C_{23}H_{28}N_6O_6$	Mazokalim
$C_{23}H_{28}N_8$	Forasartan
$C_{23}H_{28}N_8OS$	Tozasertib
$C_{23}H_{28}N_8OS.xC_3H_6O_3$	Tozasertib Lactate
$C_{23}H_{28}O_2$	Pelretin
$C_{23}H_{28}O_6$	Enprostil
$C_{23}H_{28}O_7$	Besigomsin
$C_{23}H_{28}O_9$	Sergliflozin Etabonate
$C_{23}H_{29}ClFN_3O_4$	Cisapride
$C_{23}H_{29}ClN_2O_5S$	Sitalidone
$C_{23}H_{29}ClN_4O_3$	Ciltoprazine
$C_{23}H_{29}ClO_4$	Chlormadinone Acetate
$C_{23}H_{29}ClO_6$	Delprostenate
$C_{23}H_{29}FO_6$	Isoflupredone Acetate
$C_{23}H_{29}F_2N_3O$	Amperozide
$C_{23}H_{29}N$	Igmesine
$C_{23}H_{29}N.HCl$	Igmesine Hydrochloride
$C_{23}H_{29}NO$	Norpipanone
$C_{23}H_{29}NO_2$	Phenadoxone
$C_{23}H_{29}NO_2$	Pinolcaine
$C_{23}H_{29}NO_2.HCl$	Pyrroliphene Hydrochloride
$C_{23}H_{29}NO_3$	Benzethidine
$C_{23}H_{29}NO_3$	Fenbutrazate
$C_{23}H_{29}NO_3$	Phenoperidine
$C_{23}H_{29}NO_3$	Propiverine
$C_{23}H_{29}NO_3.HCl$	Conorphone Hydrochloride
$C_{23}H_{29}N_3O$	Necopidem
$C_{23}H_{29}N_3O$	Pirolazamide
$C_{23}H_{29}N_3O.2HCl$	Opipramol Hydrochloride
$C_{23}H_{29}N_3OS$	Apadoline
$C_{23}H_{29}N_3O_2$	Etomidoline
$C_{23}H_{29}N_3O_2$	Oxypertine
$C_{23}H_{29}N_3O_2S.2C_4H_4O_4$	Acetophenazine Maleate
$C_{23}H_{29}N_3O_2S_2$	Thiothixene
$C_{23}H_{29}N_3O_2S_2.2HCl.2H_2O$	Thiothixene Hydrochloride
$C_{23}H_{29}N_3O_3$	Eproxindine
$C_{23}H_{29}N_5O$	Toquizine
$C_{23}H_{30}BrNO_3$	Dimetipirium Bromide
$C_{23}H_{30}BrNO_3$	Propantheline Bromide
$C_{23}H_{30}BrN_3O_2$	Brazergoline
$C_{23}H_{30}ClNO$	Octastine
$C_{23}H_{30}ClN_3O.2HCl.2H_2O$	Quinacrine Hydrochloride
$C_{23}H_{30}Cl_2NNa_2O_6P$	Estramustine Phosphate Sodium
$C_{23}H_{30}FN_3$	Blonanserin
$C_{23}H_{30}GdN_3O_{11}$	Gadoxetic Acid
$C_{23}H_{30}N_2$	Emopamil
$C_{23}H_{30}N_2$	Levemopamil
$C_{23}H_{30}N_2O_2.C_2H_6O_3S$	Piminodine Esylate
$C_{23}H_{30}N_2O_2S$	Linarotene
$C_{23}H_{30}N_2O_3$	Vinpoline
$C_{23}H_{30}N_2O_4$	Pholcodine
$C_{23}H_{30}N_2O_5$	Fepromide
$C_{23}H_{30}N_4O_2S$	Perospirone

Molecular Formula	Non-proprietary Name
$C_{23}H_{30}N_4O_4S$	Lexipafant
$C_{23}H_{30}N_6O_4$	Teoprolol
$C_{23}H_{30}N_6O_6$	Apadenoson
$C_{23}H_{30}O_3$	Etretinate
$C_{23}H_{30}O_4$	Nomegestrol Acetate
$C_{23}H_{30}O_5$	Anecortave Acetate
$C_{23}H_{30}O_6$	Cortisone Acetate
$C_{23}H_{30}O_6$	Fenprostalene
$C_{23}H_{30}O_6$	Prednisolone Acetate
$C_{23}H_{31}CaN_3O_{11}$	Caloxetic Acid
$C_{23}H_{31}ClN_2O_3$	Etodroxizine
$C_{23}H_{31}Cl_2NO_3$	Estramustine
$C_{23}H_{31}Cl_3N_2OS$	Xanthiol Hydrochloride
$C_{23}H_{31}FO_4$	Dimesone
$C_{23}H_{31}FO_5$	Flurogestone Acetate
$C_{23}H_{31}FO_6$	Fludrocortisone Acetate
$C_{23}H_{31}IN_2O$	Buzepide Metiodide
$C_{23}H_{31}KO_4$	Prorenoate Potassium
$C_{23}H_{31}NO.CH_4O_3S$	Xorphanol Mesylate
$C_{23}H_{31}NO_2$	Alphacetylmethadol
$C_{23}H_{31}NO_2$	Betacetylmethadol
$C_{23}H_{31}NO_2$	Levomethadyl Acetate
$C_{23}H_{31}NO_2$	Methadyl Acetate
$C_{23}H_{31}NO_2$	Motretinide
$C_{23}H_{31}NO_2.HCl$	Levomethadyl Acetate Hydrochloride
$C_{23}H_{31}NO_2.HCl$	Proadifen Hydrochloride
$C_{23}H_{31}NO_3$	Diprafenone
$C_{23}H_{31}NO_3$	Norgestimate
$C_{23}H_{31}NO_7$	Mycophenolate Mofetil
$C_{23}H_{31}NO_7.HCl$	Mycophenolate Mofetil Hydrochloride
$C_{23}H_{31}NO_7S$	Bevonium Metilsulfate
$C_{23}H_{31}NO_7S$	Sulprostone
$C_{23}H_{31}N_3O_4S_2$	Batimastat
$C_{23}H_{31}N_5O_4S$	Glisamuride
$C_{23}H_{31}N_7O$	Dutacatib
$C_{23}H_{32}N_2O$	Moxaprindine
$C_{23}H_{32}N_2O_2S$	Tiocarlide
$C_{23}H_{32}N_2O_3$	Zipeprol
$C_{23}H_{32}N_2O_3S$	Zanoterone
$C_{23}H_{32}N_2O_5$	Ramipril
$C_{23}H_{32}N_2O_5$	Zabicipril
$C_{23}H_{32}N_2O_6.2HCl$	Enciprazine Hydrochloride
$C_{23}H_{32}N_4O_3S$	Nupafant
$C_{23}H_{32}N_4O_4.HCl$	Lotrafiban Hydrochloride
$C_{23}H_{32}N_4O_7S$	Libecillide
$C_{23}H_{32}N_6O_3S.2HCl$	Tazifylline Hydrochloride
$C_{23}H_{32}N_6O_4S$	Vardenafil
$C_{23}H_{32}N_6O_4S.2HCl$	Vardenafil Dihydrochloride
$C_{23}H_{32}O_2$	Medrogestone
$C_{23}H_{32}O_2.H_2O$	Dimethisterone
$C_{23}H_{32}O_3$	Estradiol Valerate
$C_{23}H_{32}O_3$	Quinestradol
$C_{23}H_{32}O_4$	Desoxycorticosterone Acetate
$C_{23}H_{32}O_4$	Norgestomet
$C_{23}H_{32}O_6$	Hydrocortisone Acetate
$C_{23}H_{33}FN_2O_2$	Propyperone
$C_{23}H_{33}IN_2O$	Isopropamide Iodide
$C_{23}H_{33}NO_2$	Azastene
$C_{23}H_{33}NO_2$	Nicanartine
$C_{23}H_{33}NO_2$	Xipranolol
$C_{23}H_{33}NO_2$	Xyloxemine
$C_{23}H_{33}NO_7S_2$	Suplatast Tosilate
$C_{23}H_{33}NO_8$	Sanfetrinem Cilexetil
$C_{23}H_{33}N_3O_6S$	Tameticillin

Molecular Formula	Non-proprietary Name
$C_{23}H_{33}N_5O_2$	Balicatib
$C_{23}H_{33}N_5O_5S$	Gliamilide
$C_{23}H_{34}IN_3O_3$	Beperidium Iodide
$C_{23}H_{34}NO_5P$	Fosinoprilat
$C_{23}H_{34}N_4O_5$	Inakalant
$C_{23}H_{34}N_6O$	Mapinastine
$C_{23}H_{34}O_2S$	Tinabinol
$C_{23}H_{34}O_4$	Rostafuroxin
$C_{23}H_{34}O_5$	Mevastatin
$C_{23}H_{34}O_5$	Treprostinil
$C_{23}H_{35}ClN_2O_2$	Pipramadol
$C_{23}H_{35}NO_2.CH_4O_3S$	Tonazocine Mesylate
$C_{23}H_{35}NO_2.CH_4O_3S$	Zenazocine Mesylate
$C_{23}H_{35}NO_2S$	Dalcetrapib
$C_{23}H_{35}N_3O$	Actisomide
$C_{23}H_{35}N_7O_6S$	Tomopenem
$C_{23}H_{35}NaO_7$	Pravastatin Sodium
$C_{23}H_{36}N_2O_2$	Finasteride
$C_{23}H_{36}N_4O_5S_3$	Octotiamine
$C_{23}H_{36}N_4O_{10}S_2$	Pentamidine Isethionate
$C_{23}H_{36}N_6O_5S.H_2O$	Argatroban
$C_{23}H_{36}O_2$	Becocalcidiol
$C_{23}H_{36}O_2$	Dimepregnen
$C_{23}H_{36}O_3$	Dromostanolone Propionate
$C_{23}H_{36}O_3$	Propetandrol
$C_{23}H_{36}O_5$	Viprostol
$C_{23}H_{38}ClN_3O$	Disobutamide
$C_{23}H_{38}NNaO_2$	Cetaben Sodium
$C_{23}H_{38}N_4O_3S$	Naluzotan
$C_{23}H_{38}N_4O_3S.HCl$	Naluzotan Hydrochloride
$C_{23}H_{38}O$	Teprenone
$C_{23}H_{38}O_2$	Rosterolone
$C_{23}H_{38}O_4$	Meteneprost
$C_{23}H_{38}O_4$	Trimoprostil
$C_{23}H_{38}O_5$	Gemeprost
$C_{23}H_{38}O_6$	Ornoprostil
$C_{23}H_{40}I_2N_2O_3$	Piprocurarium Iodide
$C_{23}H_{40}N_4O_{11}$	Murabutide
$C_{23}H_{40}O_5$ (Approximate)	Nonoxynol 4
$C_{23}H_{40}O_5$	Pimilprost
$C_{23}H_{40}O_6$	Mexiprostil
$C_{23}H_{41}ClN_2O$	Metalkonium Chloride
$C_{23}H_{41}N_5O_5S$	Rebimastat
$C_{23}H_{42}ClN$	Miristalkonium Chloride
$C_{23}H_{42}ClNO_2$	Benzoxonium Chloride
$C_{23}H_{42}N_2O_{12}$	Pentolinium Tartrate
$C_{23}H_{43}NO_4S$	Toloconium Metilsulfate
$C_{23}H_{45}N_5O_{14}.xH_2SO_4$	Paromomycin Sulfate
$C_{23}H_{46}N_2O_3$	Pendecamaine
$C_{23}H_{46}N_6O_{13}$	Framycetin
$C_{24}H_{16}F_3NO_4$	Tiplasinin
$C_{24}H_{19}ClN_4O_3$	Nicafenine
$C_{24}H_{19}NO_5$	Oxyphenisatin Acetate
$C_{24}H_{19}NO_6$	Bisoxatin Acetate
$C_{24}H_{19}N_2NaO_4S_2$	Edaglitazone Sodium
$C_{24}H_{19}N_3O_5S$	Piroxicam Cinnamate
$C_{24}H_{20}BrClN_6O_3$	Zolasartan
$C_{24}H_{20}Cl_2N_2OS.HNO_3$	Fenticonazole Nitrate
$C_{24}H_{20}Cl_2N_2O_3S$	Tolufazepam
$C_{24}H_{20}F_4N_8O_2.HCl$	Razaxaban Hydrochloride
$C_{24}H_{20}I_6N_4O_8$	Iocarmic Acid
$C_{24}H_{20}I_6N_4O_8.2C_7H_{17}NO_5$	Iocarmate Meglumine
$C_{24}H_{20}I_6N_5NaO_8$	Ioxaglate Sodium
$C_{24}H_{20}N_4O$	Scarlet Red
$C_{24}H_{20}N_6O_3$	Candesartan
$C_{24}H_{21}Br_3I_3N_5O_8$	Ioxabrolic Acid

Molecular Formula	Non-proprietary Name
$C_{24}H_{21}F_2NO_3$	Ezetimibe
$C_{24}H_{21}I_6N_5O_8$	Ioxaglic Acid
$C_{24}H_{21}I_6N_5O_8.C_7H_{17}NO_5$	Ioxaglate Meglumine
$C_{24}H_{21}N_5O_5S$	Nebentan
$C_{24}H_{22}ClFN_4O_4$	Eribaxaban
$C_{24}H_{22}FN_3O_4$	Exatecan
$C_{24}H_{22}FN_3O_4.CH_4O_3S.2H_2O$	Exatecan Mesylate
$C_{24}H_{22}F_3N$	Xaliproden
$C_{24}H_{22}I_6N_2O_9$	Iotranic Acid
$C_{24}H_{22}I_6N_2O_{10}$	Iotetric Acid
$C_{24}H_{23}ClFN_5O_2$	Pelitinib
$C_{24}H_{23}ClO_2$	Ospemifene
$C_{24}H_{23}FN_4O_3$	Olaparib
$C_{24}H_{23}NO_5S$	Aleglitazar
$C_{24}H_{23}N_3O_2$	Bifeprunox
$C_{24}H_{23}N_3O_2.CH_4O_3S$	Bifeprunox Mesylate
$C_{24}H_{23}N_3O_6S.HCl$	Talampicillin Hydrochloride
$C_{24}H_{24}CaI_6N_4O_4$	Ipodate Calcium
$C_{24}H_{24}ClNO_3$	Eniclobrate
$C_{24}H_{24}FN_3O_2$	Adoprazine
$C_{24}H_{24}FN_5O_2S$	Trelanserin
$C_{24}H_{24}N_2$	Acridorex
$C_{24}H_{24}N_2O_4$	Abecarnil
$C_{24}H_{24}N_2O_4$	Nicocodine
$C_{24}H_{24}N_2O_5$	Amtolmetin Guacil
$C_{24}H_{24}N_4O_4S$	Asulacrine
$C_{24}H_{24}N_4O_5S$	Lobeglitazone
$C_{24}H_{25}ClFN_5O_3.2HCl$	Canertinib Dihydrochloride
$C_{24}H_{25}FNNaO_4$	Fluvastatin Sodium
$C_{24}H_{25}FN_4O_2$	Ocaperidone
$C_{24}H_{25}FN_6O$	Mizolastine
$C_{24}H_{25}F_4NOS$	Piflutixol
$C_{24}H_{25}NO_4.HCl$	Flavoxate Hydrochloride
$C_{24}H_{25}NS$	Tixadil
$C_{24}H_{25}N_3O_2$	Panuramine
$C_{24}H_{25}N_6NaO_5S$	Pirbenicillin Sodium
$C_{24}H_{26}BrN_3O_3$	Nicergoline
$C_{24}H_{26}ClFN_4O$	Sertindole
$C_{24}H_{26}FN_3O$	Biriperone
$C_{24}H_{26}FN_3O_2$	Metrenperone
$C_{24}H_{26}FN_3O_3$	Butanserin
$C_{24}H_{26}N_2O$	Belarizine
$C_{24}H_{26}N_2OS_2$	Izonsteride
$C_{24}H_{26}N_2O_2$	Carmoxirole
$C_{24}H_{26}N_2O_4$	Carvedilol
$C_{24}H_{26}N_2O_4$	Nicodicodine
$C_{24}H_{26}N_2O_4.H_3O_4P.\frac{1}{2}H_2O$	Carvedilol Phosphate
$C_{24}H_{26}N_2O_6$	Suxibuzone
$C_{24}H_{26}N_4$	Ropizine
$C_{24}H_{26}N_6O_3$	Olmesartan
$C_{24}H_{26}O_4$	Estrofurate
$C_{24}H_{26}O_5$	Pentomone
$C_{24}H_{27}ClN_2O_3S$	Furomazine
$C_{24}H_{27}FN_2O_4$	Iloperidone
$C_{24}H_{27}FN_4O_2$	Lensiprazine
$C_{24}H_{27}N$	Prenylamine
$C_{24}H_{27}NO_2$	Cyheptropine
$C_{24}H_{27}NO_2$	Levophenacylmorphan
$C_{24}H_{27}NO_2$	Octocrylene
$C_{24}H_{27}NO_5S$	Troglitazone
$C_{24}H_{27}NO_6$	Mecinarone
$C_{24}H_{27}NS$	Tiopropamine
$C_{24}H_{27}N_3O_3$	Trequinsin
$C_{24}H_{27}N_3O_5S$	Erbulozole
$C_{24}H_{27}N_5O_5$	Carafiban
$C_{24}H_{27}NaO_9$	Omtriptolide Sodium

Molecular Formula	Non-proprietary Name
$C_{24}H_{28}Br_2N_2O_4$	Brovanexine
$C_{24}H_{28}ClFN_2O_2$	Amiperone
$C_{24}H_{28}ClNO_4$	Phenactropinium Chloride
$C_{24}H_{28}ClN_3OS.2C_4H_4O_4$	Clothixamide Maleate
$C_{24}H_{28}Cl_2F_2O_4$	Tralonide
$C_{24}H_{28}Cl_3FO_4$	Triclonide
$C_{24}H_{28}FN_3O$	Spirilene
$C_{24}H_{28}F_3N_3O_3$	Tafenoquine
$C_{24}H_{28}N_2O_2$	Meletimide
$C_{24}H_{28}N_2O_3$	Indacaterol
$C_{24}H_{28}N_2O_3$	Naftopidil
$C_{24}H_{28}N_2O_3.C_4H_4O_4$	Indacaterol Maleate
$C_{24}H_{28}N_2O_5.HCl$	Benazepril Hydrochloride
$C_{24}H_{28}N_4O_2$	Altapizone
$C_{24}H_{28}N_4O_5S$	Glisindamide
$C_{24}H_{28}N_4O_6$	Lamifiban
$C_{24}H_{28}N_4O_6.HCl$	Lamifiban Hydrochloride
$C_{24}H_{28}N_6O_5$	Spirofylline
$C_{24}H_{28}N_6O_{10}S$	Fomidacillin
$C_{24}H_{28}O_2$	Bexarotene
$C_{24}H_{28}O_3$	Spirorenone
$C_{24}H_{28}O_6Ti$	Budotitane
$C_{24}H_{29}BrFNO_3$	Flutropium Bromide
$C_{24}H_{29}BrN_2$	Darotropium Bromide
$C_{24}H_{29}ClO_4$	Cyproterone Acetate
$C_{24}H_{29}Cl_2FO_5$	Flucloronide
$C_{24}H_{29}FN_2O_2$	Aceperone
$C_{24}H_{29}FN_4O$	Irindalone
$C_{24}H_{29}FO_6$	Acrocinonide
$C_{24}H_{29}F_3O_6$	Cormethasone Acetate
$C_{24}H_{29}F_3O_6$	Froxiprost
$C_{24}H_{29}NO$	Phenomorphan
$C_{24}H_{29}NO.HCl$	Dexclamol Hydrochloride
$C_{24}H_{29}NO_3.HCl$	Donepezil Hydrochloride
$C_{24}H_{29}NO_4$	Pibaxizine
$C_{24}H_{29}NO_4.HCl$	Ethaverine Hydrochloride
$C_{24}H_{29}NO_4S$	Etolotifen
$C_{24}H_{29}NO_5S_2$	Sevitropium Mesilate
$C_{24}H_{29}N_3O_2$	Daporinad
$C_{24}H_{29}N_5O_2.HCl$	Zalospirone Hydrochloride
$C_{24}H_{29}N_5O_3$	Valsartan
$C_{24}H_{29}NaO_5$	Beraprost Sodium
$C_{24}H_{30}BrNO_4$	Tropenziline Bromide
$C_{24}H_{30}BrN_7O_3$	Pyrabrom
$C_{24}H_{30}ClFO_5$	Clocortolone Acetate
$C_{24}H_{30}ClN_7O_4S$	Edoxaban
$C_{24}H_{30}Cl_2O_6$	Etiprednol Dicloacetate
$C_{24}H_{30}FNa_2O_9P$	Triamcinolone Acetonide Sodium Phosphate
$C_{24}H_{30}F_2O_6$	Fluocinolone Acetonide
$C_{24}H_{30}N_2O_2$	Desmethylmoramide
$C_{24}H_{30}N_2O_2.HCl.H_2O$	Doxapram Hydrochloride
$C_{24}H_{30}N_2O_2S$	Piperacetazine
$C_{24}H_{30}N_2O_3.C_6H_8O_7$	Carfentanil Citrate
$C_{24}H_{30}N_2O_4$	Draquinolol
$C_{24}H_{30}N_2O_4S$	Siratiazem
$C_{24}H_{30}N_2O_8$	Mitopodozide
$C_{24}H_{30}N_4O.C_4H_4O_4$	Ipazilide Fumarate
$C_{24}H_{30}O_2$	Doretinel
$C_{24}H_{30}O_2S$	Sumarotene
$C_{24}H_{30}O_3$	Drospirenone
$C_{24}H_{30}O_5$	Beraprost
$C_{24}H_{30}O_5$	Taprostene
$C_{24}H_{30}O_6$	Eplerenone
$C_{24}H_{30}O_8$	Desaspidin
$C_{24}H_{31}ClO_4$	Clomegestone Acetate

Molecular Formula	Non-proprietary Name
$C_{24}H_{31}ClO_7$	Lanproston
$C_{24}H_{31}ClO_7$	Loteprednol Etabonate
$C_{24}H_{31}FO_3$	Dalvastatin
$C_{24}H_{31}FO_5$	Descinolone Acetonide
$C_{24}H_{31}FO_5$	Fluorometholone Acetate
$C_{24}H_{31}FO_5S$	Timobesone Acetate
$C_{24}H_{31}FO_6$	Betamethasone Acetate
$C_{24}H_{31}FO_6$	Fluperolone Acetate
$C_{24}H_{31}FO_6$	Paramethasone Acetate
$C_{24}H_{31}FO_6$	Triamcinolone Acetonide
$C_{24}H_{31}FO_6.H_2O$	Dexamethasone Acetate
$C_{24}H_{31}FO_6.\frac{1}{2}H_2O$	Flunisolide
$C_{24}H_{31}NO$	Abiraterone
$C_{24}H_{31}NO.HCl$	Dipipanone Hydrochloride
$C_{24}H_{31}NO_3$	Pipoxizine
$C_{24}H_{31}NO_3$	Terikalant
$C_{24}H_{31}NO_4$	Drotaverine
$C_{24}H_{31}NO_4$	Fenaftic Acid
$C_{24}H_{31}NO_6$	Sarpogrelate
$C_{24}H_{31}N_3O$	Famprofazone
$C_{24}H_{31}N_3O$	Homopipramol
$C_{24}H_{31}N_3OS$	Butaperazine
$C_{24}H_{31}N_3OS.2C_4H_4O_4$	Butaperazine Maleate
$C_{24}H_{31}N_3O_2.C_4H_4O_4$	Mirisetron Maleate
$C_{24}H_{31}N_3O_2S.2C_4H_4O_4$	Carphenazine Maleate
$C_{24}H_{31}N_3O_3$	Milipertine
$C_{24}H_{31}N_3O_3$	Selprazine
$C_{24}H_{31}N_5O_2$	Otenzepad
$C_{24}H_{32}ClFO_5$	Halcinonide
$C_{24}H_{32}N_2O_2$	Eprazinone
$C_{24}H_{32}N_2O_3.HCl$	Enadoline Hydrochloride
$C_{24}H_{32}N_2O_5$	Falipamil
$C_{24}H_{32}N_2O_5.HCl$	Metoserpate Hydrochloride
$2C_{24}H_{32}N_2O_5.H_2O_4S$	Bedoradrine Sulfate
$C_{24}H_{32}N_4O_2S.HCl$	Tiospirone Hydrochloride
$C_{24}H_{32}O_2$	Quinbolone
$C_{24}H_{32}O_3$	Menoctone
$C_{24}H_{32}O_4$	Bufogenin
$C_{24}H_{32}O_4$	Ethynodiol Diacetate
$C_{24}H_{32}O_4$	Megestrol Acetate
$C_{24}H_{32}O_4S$	Spironolactone
$C_{24}H_{32}O_6$	Desonide
$C_{24}H_{32}O_6$	Methylprednisolone Acetate
$C_{24}H_{32}O_7$	Etiproston
$C_{24}H_{32}O_{10}$	Acevaltrate
$C_{24}H_{33}FO_6$	Flurandrenolide
$C_{24}H_{33}KO_6.2H_2O$	Mexrenoate Potassium
$C_{24}H_{33}N$	Droprenilamine
$C_{24}H_{33}NO_3$	Denaverine
$C_{24}H_{33}NO_3.C_2H_2O_4$	Nafronyl Oxalate
$C_{24}H_{33}N_3O_4$	Ranolazine
$C_{24}H_{33}N_3O_4.2HCl$	Ranolazine Hydrochloride
$C_{24}H_{33}NaO_5$	Dehydrocholate Sodium
$C_{24}H_{34}N_2Na_2O_{18}S_3$	Glucosulfone
$C_{24}H_{34}N_2O.HCl.H_2O$	Bepridil Hydrochloride
$C_{24}H_{34}N_2O_2.2HCl$	Euprocin Hydrochloride
$C_{24}H_{34}N_2O_5$	Trandolapril
$C_{24}H_{34}N_2O_5.HCl$	Indolapril Hydrochloride
$C_{24}H_{34}N_4O_5S$	Glimepiride
$C_{24}H_{34}O_3$	Rimexolone
$C_{24}H_{34}O_3S$	Spiroxasone
$C_{24}H_{34}O_4$	Algestone Acetonide
$C_{24}H_{34}O_4$	Medroxyprogesterone Acetate
$C_{24}H_{34}O_4$	Proligestone
$C_{24}H_{34}O_4S_2$	Tiomesterone
$C_{24}H_{34}O_5$	Dehydrocholic Acid

Molecular Formula	Non-proprietary Name
$C_{24}H_{34}O_5$	Eptaloprost
$C_{24}H_{34}O_6S$	Rivenprost
$C_{24}H_{35}FO_6$	Drocinonide
$C_{24}H_{35}NO_3$	Temiverine
$C_{24}H_{35}NO_5$	Decoquinate
$C_{24}H_{35}N_5O_5$	Ximelagatran
$C_{24}H_{36}BrNO_2$	Ciclotropium Bromide
$C_{24}H_{36}ClN_3O_2$	Lirexapride
$C_{24}H_{36}N_4O_6S_2$	Romidepsin
$C_{24}H_{36}O_2$ (DHA ethyl ester)	Omega-3-acid Ethyl Esters
$C_{24}H_{36}O_3$	Anagestone Acetate
$C_{24}H_{36}O_3$	Nabilone
$C_{24}H_{36}O_4$	Bolandiol Dipropionate
$C_{24}H_{36}O_5$	Lovastatin
$C_{24}H_{36}O_7$	Ascorbyl Gamolenate
$C_{24}H_{37}ClN_2O_2$	Pipradimadol
$C_{24}H_{37}NO_4.C_2H_4O_2$	Edifolone Acetate
$C_{24}H_{38}N_2O_2$	Laurolinium Acetate
$C_{24}H_{38}N_2O_4$	Tomoglumide
$C_{24}H_{38}N_4O_2$	Moxipraquine
$C_{24}H_{38}N_4O_4S$	Azamulin
$C_{24}H_{38}O_3$	Canbisol
$C_{24}H_{38}O_5$	Alfaprostol
$C_{24}H_{39}N_3O_3$	Idaverine
$C_{24}H_{40}N_2.2HBr$	Conessine Hydrobromide
$C_{24}H_{40}N_2O_3$	Nexopamil
$C_{24}H_{40}N_8O_4$	Dipyridamole
$C_{24}H_{40}O_4$	Chenodiol
$C_{24}H_{40}O_4$	Ursodiol
$C_{24}H_{40}O_5$	Butaprost
$C_{24}H_{40}O_{10}S_2$	Ursulcholic Acid
$(C_{24}H_{40}O_{20})_n$	Betasizofiran
$(C_{24}H_{40}O_{20})_n$	Sizofiran
$C_{24}H_{42}CaO_{24}.2H_2O$	Calcium Lactobionate
$C_{24}H_{42}N_2$	Feclemine
$C_{24}H_{42}N_2O_3S$	Stearylsulfamide
$C_{24}H_{43}NO$	Clinolamide
$C_{24}H_{44}BCuF_4N_4O_4$	Copper Tetramibi Tetrafluoroborate
$C_{24}H_{44}N_2O_4.2H_2SO_4$	Suxemerid Sulfate
$C_{24}H_{44}N_4O_4S$	Sofigatran
$C_{24}H_{44}O_6$ (Approximate)	Sorbitan Monooleate
$C_{24}H_{46}O_6$ (Approximate)	Sorbitan Monostearate
$C_{24}H_{50}ClNO$	Cethexonium Chloride
$C_{25}H_{17}F_3KNO_5S$	Fandosentan Potassium
$C_{25}H_{18}ClN_5O_2S_2$	Capadenoson
$C_{25}H_{19}NO_2.C_4H_{11}NO_2$	Picotrin Diolamine
$C_{25}H_{19}NO_3$	Fendosal
$C_{25}H_{19}N_3O_2S$	Tulopafant
$C_{25}H_{20}N_4O_2$	Devazepide
$C_{25}H_{20}N_4O_5$	Azilsartan
$C_{25}H_{21}BrF_3KN_4O_4S$	Saprisartan Potassium
$C_{25}H_{21}ClN_2O_3S$	Pimetacin
$C_{25}H_{21}N_8O_2.C_5H_{14}NO$	Totrombopag Choline
$C_{25}H_{22}ClNO_3$	Fenvalerate
$C_{25}H_{22}N_2O_2$	Talnetant
$C_{25}H_{22}N_2O_2.HCl$	Talnetant Hydrochloride
$C_{25}H_{22}N_4O_4.2(C_2H_7NO)$	Eltrombopag Olamine
$C_{25}H_{22}N_4O_8$	Streptonigrin
$C_{25}H_{22}N_5NaO_6S$	Apalcillin Sodium
$C_{25}H_{22}N_6O_2.C_2H_4O_2$	Sotrastaurin Acetate
$C_{25}H_{22}O_{10}$	Silibinin
$C_{25}H_{22}O_{10}$	Silicristin
$C_{25}H_{22}O_{10}$	Silidianin
$C_{25}H_{23}ClN_2O_7$	Binifibrate
$C_{25}H_{23}ClN_4O_4$	Pazinaclone

Molecular Formula	Non-proprietary Name
$C_{25}H_{23}F_3N_4O_2$	Mubritinib
$C_{25}H_{23}N_5O_2S$	Bentamapimod
$C_{25}H_{23}N_8NaO_7S_2$	Cefpiramide Sodium
$C_{25}H_{23}N_9O_6S$	Clazosentan
$C_{25}H_{24}ClN_3O_3S$	Beminafil
$C_{25}H_{24}FNO_4$	Pitavastatin
$C_{25}H_{24}FNO_6$	Axitirome
$C_{25}H_{24}FN_5O_3$	Embusartan
$C_{25}H_{24}F_2N_2O_3$	Turofexorate Isopropyl
$C_{25}H_{24}F_2N_6O_5$	Fidexaban
$C_{25}H_{24}F_3NO_2$	Panomifene
$C_{25}H_{24}N_2O_4S$	Pamicogrel
$C_{25}H_{24}N_2O_6$	Pranidipine
$C_{25}H_{24}N_8O_7S_2$	Cefpiramide
$C_{25}H_{24}O_{12}$	Cynarine
$C_{25}H_{25}ClN_2$	Quinaldine Blue
$C_{25}H_{25}ClN_2O_4S$	Samixogrel
$C_{25}H_{25}Cl_2N_7O$	Otenabant
$C_{25}H_{25}Cl_2N_7O.HCl$	Otenabant Hydrochloride
$C_{25}H_{25}FN_2O_5$	Abaperidone
$C_{25}H_{25}NO_5$	Ragaglitazar
$C_{25}H_{25}NO_9$	Amrubicin
$C_{25}H_{25}NO_9.HCl$	Amrubicin Hydrochloride
$C_{25}H_{25}N_3O$	Trifenagrel
$C_{25}H_{25}N_3O_4S$	Sipoglitazar
$C_{25}H_{25}N_3O_5$	Gimatecan
$C_{25}H_{25}N_5O_4$	Apixaban
$C_{25}H_{25}N_7O_3$	Dabigatran
$C_{25}H_{26}F_2N_6OS.C_4H_6O_4$	Carsatrin Succinate
$C_{25}H_{26}F_2O_8$	Acefluranol
$C_{25}H_{26}F_6N_2O_2.HCl.H_2O$	Rolapitant Hydrochloride
$C_{25}H_{26}N_2O$	Savoxepin
$C_{25}H_{26}N_2O_2$	Medibazine
$C_{25}H_{26}N_4O_4$	Otamixaban
$C_{25}H_{26}N_6O$	Pratosartan
$C_{25}H_{26}N_6O_4S$	Taprizosin
$C_{25}H_{26}N_6O_8S$	Fuzlocillin
$C_{25}H_{26}N_9NaO_8S_2$	Cefoperazone Sodium
$C_{25}H_{26}O_6$	Naveglitazar
$C_{25}H_{27}ClN_2.2HCl.H_2O$	Meclizine Hydrochloride
$C_{25}H_{27}ClN_2O_8$	Glucametacin
$C_{25}H_{27}FN_4O_3$	Cediranib
$C_{25}H_{27}FN_4O_3.C_4H_4O_4$	Cediranib Maleate
$C_{25}H_{27}F_4N_3O_3S$	Odanacatib
$C_{25}H_{27}NO$	Cinfenine
$C_{25}H_{27}N_3O_4.HCl$	Belotecan Hydrochloride
$C_{25}H_{28}N_2O_2$	Cinperene
$C_{25}H_{28}N_2O_4Si$	Cositecan
$C_{25}H_{28}N_6O$	Irbesartan
$C_{25}H_{28}N_8O_2$	Linagliptin
$C_{25}H_{28}O_3$	Estradiol Benzoate
$C_{25}H_{28}O_3$	Etofenprox
$C_{25}H_{29}BrF_2O_7$	Halopredone Acetate
$C_{25}H_{29}ClN_2O_3$	Picumast
$C_{25}H_{29}FN_2O_2$	Mindoperone
$C_{25}H_{29}FN_2O_4S_2$	Viquidacin
$C_{25}H_{29}FN_4O_4S$	Gliflumide
$C_{25}H_{29}I_2NO_3$	Amiodarone
$C_{25}H_{29}NO_2$	Difeterol
$C_{25}H_{29}NO_2$	Prenoverine
$C_{25}H_{29}NO_4$	Tropodifene
$C_{25}H_{29}N_3O$	Nufenoxole
$C_{25}H_{29}N_3O_2$	Metergoline
$C_{25}H_{29}N_3O_3$	Adimolol
$C_{25}H_{29}N_3O_4.HCl$	Milveterol Hydrochloride
$C_{25}H_{29}N_5O_2$	Bisfenazone

Molecular Formula	Non-proprietary Name
$C_{25}H_{29}N_5O_7$	Visnafylline
$C_{25}H_{29}N_9O_3$	Preladenant
$C_{25}H_{30}ClNO_3$	Trospium Chloride
$C_{25}H_{30}ClN_3$	Gentian Violet
$C_{25}H_{30}ClN_5O_3$	Oberadilol
$C_{25}H_{30}FNO_6$	Fluazacort
$C_{25}H_{30}F_2O_6S$	Zoticasone
$C_{25}H_{30}N_2O_5$	Quinapril
$C_{25}H_{30}N_2O_5.HCl$	Quinapril Hydrochloride
$C_{25}H_{30}N_2O_7$	Moexiprilat
$C_{25}H_{30}N_4O_2$	Palosuran
$C_{25}H_{30}N_4O_5S$	Litomeglovir
$C_{25}H_{30}N_4O_9S_2$	Sultamicillin
$C_{25}H_{30}O_4S$	Mespirenone
$C_{25}H_{30}O_{10}$	Salprotoside
$C_{25}H_{31}ClF_2O_5$	Halobetasol Propionate
$C_{25}H_{31}ClF_2O_5S$	Cloticasone Propionate
$C_{25}H_{31}FN_6O_2.HCl$	Trefentanil Hydrochloride
$C_{25}H_{31}FO_8$	Triamcinolone Diacetate
$C_{25}H_{31}F_2NO_4.HCl$	Ronacaleret Hydrochloride
$C_{25}H_{31}F_3O_5S$	Fluticasone Propionate
$C_{25}H_{31}NO.HCl$	Butaclamol Hydrochloride
$C_{25}H_{31}NO_3$	Metindizate
$C_{25}H_{31}NO_4$	Fenperate
$C_{25}H_{31}NO_6$	Deflazacort
$C_{25}H_{31}N_2NaO_5$	Ifetroban Sodium
$C_{25}H_{31}N_3O_2$	Befiperide
$C_{25}H_{31}N_3O_4$	Alpertine
$C_{25}H_{31}N_5O_8$	Metescufylline
$C_{25}H_{31}N_7O_3$	Tanogitran
$C_{25}H_{31}NaO_8$	Prednisolone Sodium Succinate
$C_{25}H_{32}BrNOS$	Tipetropium Bromide
$C_{25}H_{32}ClFO_5$	Clobetasol Propionate
$C_{25}H_{32}ClN_5OS$	Imiclopazine
$C_{25}H_{32}ClN_5O_2.HCl$	Nefazodone Hydrochloride
$C_{25}H_{32}Cl_2O_6$	Clobenoside
$C_{25}H_{32}F_2O_5S$	Ticabesone Propionate
$C_{25}H_{32}F_3N_3O_4$	Silodosin
$C_{25}H_{32}N_2O$	Zanapezil
$C_{25}H_{32}N_2O_2$	Brinazarone
$C_{25}H_{32}N_2O_2$	Levomoramide
$C_{25}H_{32}N_2O_2$	Racemoramide
$C_{25}H_{32}N_2O_2.C_4H_6O_6$	Dextromoramide Tartrate
$C_{25}H_{32}N_2O_2S$	Sunagrel
$C_{25}H_{32}N_2O_3.C_2H_2O_4$	Lofentanil Oxalate
$C_{25}H_{32}N_2O_4.2H_2O$	Alvimopan
$C_{25}H_{32}N_2O_5$	Ifetroban
$C_{25}H_{32}N_2O_7$	Bometolol
$C_{25}H_{32}N_4O$	Retelliptine
$C_{25}H_{32}N_4O_2$	Pipebuzone
$C_{25}H_{32}N_4O_2S.HCl$	Tioperidone Hydrochloride
$C_{25}H_{32}O_2$	Quinestrol
$C_{25}H_{32}O_2S$	Etarotene
$C_{25}H_{32}O_3$	Nylestriol
$C_{25}H_{32}O_4$	Melengestrol Acetate
$C_{25}H_{32}O_4$	Naxaprostene
$C_{25}H_{32}O_8$	Prednisolone Hemisuccinate
$C_{25}H_{32}O_8.C_{21}H_{26}ClN_3OS$	Prednazate
$C_{25}H_{33}ClN_2O_2$	Lobuprofen
$C_{25}H_{33}ClO_5$	Clogestone Acetate
$C_{25}H_{33}NO_2$	Crobenetine
$C_{25}H_{33}NO_2$	Nonabine
$C_{25}H_{33}NO_4$	Etorphine
$C_{25}H_{33}NaO_8$	Hydrocortisone Sodium Succinate
$(C_{25}H_{34}FN_3O_2)_2.C_4H_6O_6$	Pimavanserin Tartrate

Molecular Formula	Non-proprietary Name
$C_{25}H_{34}F_2O_5$	Tafluprost
$C_{25}H_{34}F_2O_6$	Rofleponide
$C_{25}H_{34}N_2O_2$	Oxiramide
$C_{25}H_{34}N_2O_3.2HCl$	Tilorone Hydrochloride
$C_{25}H_{34}N_2O_4$	Fexicaine
$C_{25}H_{34}N_2O_8$	Niludipine
$C_{25}H_{34}N_3Na_2O_9PS$	Fosamprenavir Sodium
$C_{25}H_{34}O_4$	Methynodiol Diacetate
$C_{25}H_{34}O_6$	Budesonide
$C_{25}H_{34}O_6$	Dexbudesonide
$C_{25}H_{34}O_6$	Ingenol Mebutate
$C_{25}H_{34}O_8.H_2O$	Hydrocortisone Hemisuccinate
$C_{25}H_{35}NO_4$	Alprafenone
$C_{25}H_{35}NO_5.HCl$	Mebeverine Hydrochloride
$C_{25}H_{35}NO_8S$	Troxypyrrolium Tosilate
$C_{25}H_{35}N_3O$	Amesergide
$C_{25}H_{35}N_3O_6S$	Amprenavir
$C_{25}H_{35}N_5O_4$	Diisobutylaminobenzoyloxy-propyl Theophylline
$C_{25}H_{35}NaO_6$	Hydroxydione Sodium Succinate
$C_{25}H_{36}CaN_3O_9PS$	Fosamprenavir Calcium
$C_{25}H_{36}N_4O_3S$	Sulukast
$C_{25}H_{36}N_6O_4S$	Udenafil
$C_{25}H_{36}O_3$	Estradiol Enanthate
$C_{25}H_{36}O_5$	Pregnenolone Succinate
$C_{25}H_{36}O_5$	Remiprostol
$C_{25}H_{36}O_5S$	Butixocort
$C_{25}H_{36}O_6$	Hydrocortisone Butyrate
$C_{25}H_{37}KO_4$	Oxprenoate Potassium
$C_{25}H_{37}NO_2.CH_4O_3S$	Quadazocine Mesylate
$C_{25}H_{37}NO_3$	Episteride
$C_{25}H_{37}NO_4$	Bimatoprost
$C_{25}H_{37}NO_4$	Salmeterol
$C_{25}H_{37}NO_4.C_{11}H_8O_3$	Salmeterol Xinafoate
$C_{25}H_{37}NO_8S$	Troxonium Tosilate
$C_{25}H_{38}N_2O.HCl$	Bunamidine Hydrochloride
$C_{25}H_{38}O_2$	Penmesterol
$C_{25}H_{38}O_5$	Simvastatin
$C_{25}H_{39}NO_3$	Cetilistat
$C_{25}H_{39}N_3O_8$	Landiolol
$C_{25}H_{40}N_2O_3$	Pactimibe
$C_{25}H_{40}O_2S$	Mepitiostane
$C_{25}H_{41}ClO_3$	Lodelaben
$C_{25}H_{43}NO_3$	Minaxolone
$C_{25}H_{43}NO_{18}$	Acarbose
$C_{25}H_{43}N_{13}O_{10}$	Enviomycin
$C_{25}H_{44}ClN_3O_2$	Dofamium Chloride
$C_{25}H_{44}N_2O.2HCl$	Azacosterol Hydrochloride
$C_{25}H_{46}BrNO_2$	Amantanium Bromide
$C_{25}H_{46}ClN$	Cetalkonium Chloride
$C_{25}H_{48}N_6O_8$	Deferoxamine
$C_{25}H_{48}N_6O_8.CH_4O_3S$	Deferoxamine Mesylate
$C_{25}H_{48}N_6O_8.HCl$	Deferoxamine Hydrochloride
$C_{25}H_{52}NO_4P$	Perifosine
$C_{26}H_{16}N_3Na_3O_{10}S_3$	Anazolene Sodium
$C_{26}H_{18}CuN_4O_8$	Cuprimyxin
$C_{26}H_{19}FN_4O_2$	Pranazepide
$C_{26}H_{20}Cl_5FN_2O_2$	Fludazonium Chloride
$C_{26}H_{21}N_3O$	Linopirdine
$C_{26}H_{21}N_3O_4$	Lestaurtinib
$C_{26}H_{22}Cl_2N_2O_3$	Doconazole
$C_{26}H_{23}ClN_6OS_2$	Rocepafant
$C_{26}H_{23}ClN_6O_2S$	Setipafant
$C_{26}H_{23}Cl_5N_2O$	Sepazonium Chloride
$C_{26}H_{24}F_3N$	Paliroden

Molecular Formula	Non-proprietary Name
$C_{26}H_{25}ClN_2O_3$	Lirequinil
$C_{26}H_{25}ClN_2O_3$	Tolvaptan
$C_{26}H_{25}Cl_2N_3O$	Tebuquine
$C_{26}H_{25}FN_8O_4$	Plevitrexed
$C_{26}H_{25}F_3N_6O_5.CH_4O_3S$	Alatrofloxacin Mesylate
$C_{26}H_{25}F_9N_2O_4$	Torcetrapib
$C_{26}H_{25}IN_2S$	Bidimazium Iodide
$C_{26}H_{25}NO_3$	Ansoxetine
$C_{26}H_{25}N_2NaO_6S$	Carbenicillin Indanyl Sodium
$C_{26}H_{25}N_3O_3S$	Fenoverine
$C_{26}H_{25}N_8NaO_{11}S_2$	Ceftobiprole Medocaril
$C_{26}H_{26}ClN_3$	Rupatadine
$C_{26}H_{26}F_2N_2.2HCl$	Flunarizine Hydrochloride
$C_{26}H_{26}F_5KN_6O_3.C_2H_6O$	Telcagepant Potassium
$C_{26}H_{26}I_6N_2O_{10}$	Iodoxamic Acid
$C_{26}H_{26}I_6N_2O_{10}.2C_7H_{17}NO_5$	Iodoxamate Meglumine
$C_{26}H_{26}N_2.HCl$	Azipramine Hydrochloride
$C_{26}H_{26}N_4O_4S$	Bentiamine
$C_{26}H_{27}Br_2N_7$	Pyritidium Bromide
$C_{26}H_{27}ClN_2$	Clocinizine
$C_{26}H_{27}ClN_2O.HCl$	Lofepramine Hydrochloride
$C_{26}H_{27}ClN_2O_3S_2$	Verlukast
$C_{26}H_{27}ClO_3$	Fispemifene
$C_{26}H_{27}F_4N_3O_7$	Emricasan
$C_{26}H_{27}F_5N_6O_3$	Telcagepant
$C_{26}H_{27}NO_9.HCl$	Idarubicin Hydrochloride
$C_{26}H_{27}NO_{10}$	Medorubicin
$C_{26}H_{27}NO_{10}.HCl$	Carubicin Hydrochloride
$C_{26}H_{27}N_3O_4S$	Nictiazem
$C_{26}H_{27}N_5O_2$	Vilazodone
$C_{26}H_{28}ClNO$	Enclomiphene
$C_{26}H_{28}ClNO$	Zuclomiphene
$C_{26}H_{28}ClNO.C_6H_8O_7$	Clomiphene Citrate
$C_{26}H_{28}ClNO.C_6H_8O_7$	Toremifene Citrate
$C_{26}H_{28}ClNO_2$	Clomifenoxide
$C_{26}H_{28}ClN_3$	Pyrvinium Chloride
$C_{26}H_{28}ClN_3O_6S$	Fibracillin
$C_{26}H_{28}Cl_2N_4O_4$	Ketoconazole
$C_{26}H_{28}FN_3O_8S$	Altanserin Tartrate
$C_{26}H_{28}N_2$	Cinnarizine
$C_{26}H_{28}N_2.C_{10}H_{11}ClO_3$	Cinnarizine Clofibrate
$C_{26}H_{28}N_4O_2$	Zaldaride
$C_{26}H_{29}Cl_2N_5O_3$	Bosutinib
$C_{26}H_{29}FN_2O_2$	Cabastine
$C_{26}H_{29}FN_2O_2.HCl$	Levocabastine Hydrochloride
$C_{26}H_{29}F_2N_7.2CH_4O_3S$	Almitrine Mesylate
$C_{26}H_{29}NO.C_6H_8O_7$	Tamoxifen Citrate
$C_{26}H_{29}NO_2$	Afimoxifene
$C_{26}H_{29}NO_2$	Droloxifene
$C_{26}H_{29}NO_2.C_6H_8O_7$	Droloxifene Citrate
$C_{26}H_{29}NO_3$	Amotriphene
$C_{26}H_{29}NO_3$	Doxaminol
$C_{26}H_{29}NO_4$	Terflavoxate
$C_{26}H_{29}N_3O_6.HCl$	Nicardipine Hydrochloride
$C_{26}H_{29}N_5O_3$	Revizinone
$C_{26}H_{29}N_5O_7$	Pralnacasan
$C_{26}H_{30}BrNO_4S_2$	Aclidinium Bromide
$C_{26}H_{30}Cl_2F_3NO.HCl$	Halofantrine Hydrochloride
$C_{26}H_{30}FN_3O_6S$	Aseripide
$C_{26}H_{30}N_6O_3$	Danusertib
$C_{26}H_{30}Na_2O_9$	Estriol Sodium Succinate
$C_{26}H_{31}Cl_2N_3$	Aminoquinol
$C_{26}H_{31}Cl_2N_5O_3$	Terconazole
$C_{26}H_{31}FN_2O_4$	Lidanserin
$C_{26}H_{31}N_3O_2S$	Pretiadil
$C_{26}H_{31}N_5O_2$	Elbanizine

Molecular Formula	Non-proprietary Name
$C_{26}H_{31}N_5O_3$	Abitesartan
$C_{26}H_{32}ClFO_5$	Clobetasone Butyrate
$C_{26}H_{32}F_2O_7$	Diflorasone Diacetate
$C_{26}H_{32}F_2O_7$	Fluocinonide
$C_{26}H_{32}F_3N_3O_2S$	Oxaflumazine
$C_{26}H_{32}N_2O_5$	Ensaculin
$C_{26}H_{32}N_2O_5.HCl$	Delapril Hydrochloride
$C_{26}H_{32}N_2O_8$	Tritoqualine
$C_{26}H_{33}FNNaO_5$	Cerivastatin Sodium
$C_{26}H_{33}FO_7$	Flunisolide Acetate
$C_{26}H_{33}F_3N_2O_2$	Frabuprofen
$C_{26}H_{33}F_3N_2O_5$	Flordipine
$C_{26}H_{33}NO_2$	Fenretinide
$C_{26}H_{33}NO_4.HCl$	Cyprenorphine Hydrochloride
$C_{26}H_{33}NO_6$	Lacidipine
$C_{26}H_{33}NO_6$	Piprofurol
$C_{26}H_{33}N_3O_6$	Ecastolol
$C_{26}H_{33}N_5O_2$	Nilprazole
$C_{26}H_{33}NaO_8$	Methylprednisolone Sodium Succinate
$C_{26}H_{34}F_2O_7$	Flumoxonide
$C_{26}H_{34}F_3N_3O_3S$	Flosatidil
$C_{26}H_{34}KNO_4$	Piriprost Potassium
$C_{26}H_{34}N_6O_6S.H_2O$	Napsagatran
$C_{26}H_{34}O_4$	Posaraprost
$C_{26}H_{34}O_5S.C_2H_8N_2.H_2O$	Pobilukast Edamine
$C_{26}H_{34}O_7$	Fumagillin
$C_{26}H_{34}O_8$	Methylprednisolone Hemisuccinate
$C_{26}H_{35}AlO_5$	Ibuprofen Aluminum
$C_{26}H_{35}FO_5$	Fluocortin Butyl
$C_{26}H_{35}FO_6$	Amcinafal
$C_{26}H_{35}FO_6$	Amelometasone
$C_{26}H_{35}FO_6$	Fluprednisolone Valerate
$C_{26}H_{35}F_3O_6$	Travoprost
$C_{26}H_{35}NO_4$	Diprenorphine
$C_{26}H_{35}NO_4$	Diproteverine
$C_{26}H_{35}NO_4$	Piriprost
$C_{26}H_{35}N_3O_2.C_4H_6O_4$	Mazapertine Succinate
$C_{26}H_{35}N_3O_5.2HCl$	Dimethylaminoethyl Reserpilinate Dihydrochloride
$C_{26}H_{35}N_3O_7$ $(ML)+C_{45}H_{53}N_7O_{11}(D)$	Plauracin
$C_{26}H_{36}Cl_2N_2O_4$	Alestramustine
$C_{26}H_{36}N_2O_3$	Devapamil
$C_{26}H_{36}N_2O_3.C_4H_4O_4$	Sergolexole Maleate
$C_{26}H_{36}N_2O_4$	Amiglumide
$C_{26}H_{36}N_2O_4.2C_3H_6O_3$	Bisobrin Lactate
$C_{26}H_{36}N_2O_5$	Zatebradine
$C_{26}H_{36}O_3$	Estradiol Cypionate
$C_{26}H_{36}O_5$	Dicirenone
$C_{26}H_{36}O_5$	Domoprednate
$C_{26}H_{36}O_6$	Prednival
$C_{26}H_{36}O_7$	Hydrocortisone Aceponate
$C_{26}H_{37}NO_3.C_4H_4O_4$	Fesoterodine Fumarate
$C_{26}H_{37}NO_8S.HCl.H_2O$	Tiapamil Hydrochloride
$C_{26}H_{37}N_3O_4.C_4H_4O_4$	Moxilubant Maleate
$C_{26}H_{37}N_5O_2$	Cabergoline
$C_{26}H_{37}N_5O_5S$	Mirodenafil
$C_{26}H_{38}N_2O_4$	Alnespirone
$C_{26}H_{38}N_2O_4$	Mazipredone
$C_{26}H_{38}N_2O_6P_2S_4$	Zilantel
$C_{26}H_{38}N_2O_9$	Remogliflozin Etabonate
$C_{26}H_{38}O_2$	Quingestrone
$C_{26}H_{38}O_3$	Pentagestrone
$C_{26}H_{38}O_4$	Desoxycorticosterone Pivalate

Molecular Formula	Non-proprietary Name
$C_{26}H_{38}O_4$	Gestonorone Caproate
$C_{26}H_{38}O_4$	Oxabolone Cipionate
$C_{26}H_{38}O_5$	Edogestrone
$C_{26}H_{38}O_5$	Resocortol Butyrate
$C_{26}H_{38}O_5S$	Tixocortol Pivalate
$C_{26}H_{38}O_6$	Hydrocortisone Valerate
$C_{26}H_{39}NO_4.C_4H_4O_4$	Adaprolol Maleate
$C_{26}H_{40}Cl_4N_5O_{10}PS.HCl$	Canfosfamide Hydrochloride
$C_{26}H_{40}N_4O_9S$	Sampatrilat
$C_{26}H_{40}O_3$	Inecalcitol
$C_{26}H_{40}O_3$	Mesabolone
$C_{26}H_{40}O_3$	Testosterone Enanthate
$C_{26}H_{40}O_5$	Latanoprost
$C_{26}H_{41}Br_2NO_4$	Pinaverium Bromide
$C_{26}H_{41}NO$	Melinamide
$C_{26}H_{42}N_4O_5$	Sapacitabine
$C_{26}H_{42}O_4$	Maxacalcitol
$C_{26}H_{43}IN_2$	Stercuronium Iodide
$C_{26}H_{43}NO_3$	Olvanil
$C_{26}H_{44}O_4$	Obeticholic Acid
$C_{26}H_{44}O_9$	Mupirocin
$C_{26}H_{45}NO_7SSe$	Tauroselcholic Acid
$C_{26}H_{46}I_2N_2$	Candocuronium Iodide
$C_{26}H_{50}BrNO_2$	Penoctonium Bromide
$C_{26}H_{54}N_{10}O_2.2CH_4O_3S$	Ipexidine Mesylate
$C_{26}H_{56}NO_5PS$	Ilmofosine
$C_{26}H_{56}N_{10}$	Alexidine
$(C_{26}H_{58}O_9Si_6)_q(C_{16}H_{38}O_5Si_4)_r$ $(C_7H_{12}O_4)_s(C_7H_6F_6O_2)_t$ $(C_6H_{10}O_3)_u(C_6H_7F_3O_2)_v$ $(C_{14}H_{22}O_6)_w(C_7H_{10}O_2)_x$ $(C_5H_8O_2)_y(C_3H_4O_2)_z$	Hybufocon A
$C_{27}H_{18}{}^{111}InN_3O_3$	Indium In 111 Oxyquinoline
$C_{27}H_{20}ClNO_6$	Talmetacin
$C_{27}H_{20}N_4O$	Pyrinoline
$C_{27}H_{21}ClFN_3O_2$	Lixivaptan
$C_{27}H_{21}F_3N_2O_6S$	Cevoglitazar
$C_{27}H_{22}Cl_2N_4$	Clofazimine
$C_{27}H_{22}Cl_2N_4O$	Tipifarnib
$C_{27}H_{22}F_4N_4O_3S.HCl$	Losulazine Hydrochloride
$C_{27}H_{23}Cl_3N_2OS_2.(C_6H_3Cl_3O)_2$	Alazanine Triclofenate
$C_{27}H_{23}N_5O_4$	Pranlukast
$C_{27}H_{25}ClF_3N_3O_2$	Taranabant
$C_{27}H_{25}ClN_2O_4$	Feclobuzone
$C_{27}H_{25}F_2NO_4$	Omiloxetine
$C_{27}H_{25}F_2N_3OS$	Ritanserin
$C_{27}H_{25}F_3N_2O$	Flutroline
$C_{27}H_{25}F_3N_4O_3S$	Embeconazole
$C_{27}H_{26}FNO_3$	Glenvastatin
$C_{27}H_{26}N_4O_4S$	Inolitazone
$C_{27}H_{27}F_2NO_6$	Firategrast
$C_{27}H_{27}N_5O_9S_3$	Cefcanel Daloxate
$C_{27}H_{27}N_9O_6.H_3N$	Talotrexin Ammonium
$C_{27}H_{27}N_9O_6S$	Tezosentan
$C_{27}H_{28}N_2O_4$	Nitromifene
$C_{27}H_{28}N_2O_4.C_6H_8O_7$	Nitromifene Citrate
$C_{27}H_{28}N_2O_7$	Cilnidipine
$C_{27}H_{28}N_8O_9S_2$	Piroxicillin
$C_{27}H_{29}ClN_6O_5$	Elisartan
$C_{27}H_{29}F_3O_6S$	Fluticasone Furoate
$C_{27}H_{29}NO$	Trecadrine
$C_{27}H_{29}NO_3$	Zamifenacin
$C_{27}H_{29}NO_{10}$	Pirozadil
$C_{27}H_{29}NO_{10}.HCl$	Daunorubicin Hydrochloride
$C_{27}H_{29}NO_{10}.HCl$	Esorubicin Hydrochloride
$C_{27}H_{29}NO_{11}$	Doxorubicin

Molecular Formula	Non-proprietary Name
$C_{27}H_{29}NO_{11}.HCl$	Doxorubicin Hydrochloride
$C_{27}H_{29}NO_{11}.HCl$	Epirubicin Hydrochloride
$C_{27}H_{29}N_2O_2$	Mozavaptan
$C_{27}H_{29}N_3O_6$	Barnidipine
$C_{27}H_{29}N_5O$	Revenast
$C_{27}H_{29}N_5O_6S.H_2O$	Bosentan
$C_{27}H_{29}N_7O_2$	Barmastine
$C_{27}H_{30}ClFN_4O_3$	Talmapimod
$C_{27}H_{30}Cl_2O_6$	Mometasone Furoate
$C_{27}H_{30}F_2N_2O_3$	Lomerizine
$C_{27}H_{30}F_6N_2O_2$	Dutasteride
$C_{27}H_{30}N_2O_2$	Asimadoline
$C_{27}H_{30}N_2O_2$	Palovarotene
$C_{27}H_{30}N_2O_6S$	Tobicillin
$C_{27}H_{30}N_4O$	Oxatomide
$C_{27}H_{30}N_4O_4$	Saterinone
$C_{27}H_{30}O_6$	Sofalcone
$C_{27}H_{30}O_{16}.3H_2O$	Rutin
$C_{27}H_{31}Br_2ClN_4O_2$	Lonafarnib
$C_{27}H_{31}ClN_2O.2HCl$	Chlorbenzoxamine Hydrochloride
$C_{27}H_{31}ClN_2S$	Bentipimine
$C_{27}H_{31}ClO_{15}$	Keracyanin
$C_{27}H_{31}FN_2O_5$	Sagandipine
$C_{27}H_{31}F_6N_3O$	Figopitant
$C_{27}H_{31}NO_3$	Asocainol
$C_{27}H_{31}NO_4$	Estrapronicate
$C_{27}H_{31}N_2NaO_6S_2$	Isosulfan Blue
$C_{27}H_{31}N_5O_5$	Triletide
$C_{27}H_{31}N_7OS$	Fimasartan
$C_{27}H_{32}ClNO_2$	Triparanol
$C_{27}H_{32}ClN_5O_5$	Saracatinib
$C_{27}H_{32}N_2O_3$	Tamolarizine
$C_{27}H_{32}N_4O_6S$	Relacatib
$C_{27}H_{33}NO_{10}S$	Thiocolchicoside
$C_{27}H_{33}N_3O_6S$	Gliquidone
$C_{27}H_{33}N_3O_8$	Rolitetracycline
$C_{27}H_{33}N_3O_8.HNO_3.1\frac{1}{2}H_2O$	Rolitetracycline Nitrate
$C_{27}H_{33}N_9O_{15}P_2$	Flavin Adenin Dinucleotide
$C_{27}H_{34}F_2O_7$	Difluprednate
$C_{27}H_{34}F_2O_7$	Procinonide
$C_{27}H_{34}N_2Na_{16}O_{70}S_{16}$	Aprosulate Sodium
$C_{27}H_{34}N_2O_7.HCl$	Moexipril Hydrochloride
$C_{27}H_{34}N_4O$	Piritramide
$C_{27}H_{34}N_4O_5$	Retosiban
$C_{27}H_{34}N_4O_{10}$	Razinodil
$C_{27}H_{34}O_3$	Nandrolone Phenpropionate
$C_{27}H_{34}O_3$	Testosterone Phenylacetate
$C_{27}H_{35}ClN_2O_5$	Nisterime Acetate
$C_{27}H_{35}NO_4$	Alletorphine
$C_{27}H_{35}NO_4.HCl$	Levonantradol Hydrochloride
$C_{27}H_{35}NO_4.HCl$	Nantradol Hydrochloride
$C_{27}H_{35}NO_5$	Acetorphine
$C_{27}H_{35}NO_8$	Sedecamycin
$C_{27}H_{35}N_3O_6.HCl$	Ezatiostat Hydrochloride
$C_{27}H_{35}N_5O_7S$	Metenkefalin
$C_{27}H_{36}BN_3O_7$	Flovagatran
$C_{27}H_{36}ClFO_5$	Clocortolone Pivalate
$C_{27}H_{36}F_2O_5$	Diflucortolone Pivalate
$C_{27}H_{36}F_2O_6$	Flumethasone Pivalate
$C_{27}H_{36}N_2O_4$	Repaglinide
$C_{27}H_{36}N_2O_5$	Ivabradine
$C_{27}H_{36}N_2O_8$	Altoqualine
$C_{27}H_{36}N_4O_5S.CH_4O_3S$	Ibutamoren Mesylate
$C_{27}H_{36}O_3$	Orestrate
$C_{27}H_{36}O_3$	Quingestanol Acetate

Molecular Formula	Non-proprietary Name
$C_{27}H_{36}O_7$	Methylprednisolone Aceponate
$C_{27}H_{36}O_8$	Prednicarbate
$C_{27}H_{37}FO_6$	Betamethasone Valerate
$C_{27}H_{37}NO_6S$	Amoxydramine Camsilate
$C_{27}H_{37}N_3O_7S$	Darunavir
$C_{27}H_{38}F_6O_3$	Falecalcitriol
$C_{27}H_{38}N_2.H_2SO_4.\frac{1}{2}H_2O$	Fenoctimine Sulfate
$C_{27}H_{38}N_2O_4$	Dexverapamil
$C_{27}H_{38}N_2O_4$	Verapamil
$C_{27}H_{38}N_2O_4.HCl$	Verapamil Hydrochloride
$C_{27}H_{38}N_2O_8$	Prajmalium Bitartrate
$C_{27}H_{38}O_6$	Prednisolone Tebutate
$C_{27}H_{39}Cl_2N_3O$	Pentacynium Chloride
$C_{27}H_{39}NO_6$	Prednisolamate
$C_{27}H_{40}N_2O_2$	Pifarnine
$C_{27}H_{40}N_8O_7$	Cilengitide
$C_{27}H_{40}O_3$	Calcipotriene
$C_{27}H_{40}O_3$	Testosterone Cypionate
$C_{27}H_{40}O_4$	Hydroxyprogesterone Caproate
$C_{27}H_{41}NO_6.HCl$	Hydrocortamate Hydrochloride
$C_{27}H_{41}NO_6S$	Patupilone
$C_{27}H_{42}ClNO$	Octafonium Chloride
$C_{27}H_{42}ClNO_2$	Benzethonium Chloride
$C_{27}H_{42}Cl_2N_2O_6$	Chloramphenicol Palmitate
$C_{27}H_{42}N_2O_5S$	Ixabepilone
$C_{27}H_{42}O_3$	Methenolone Enanthate
$C_{27}H_{43}N_3O_4$	Taltobulin
$(C_{27}H_{44}N_{10}O_{12})_2.(H_2SO_4)_3$	Streptonicozid
$C_{27}H_{44}O$	Cholecalciferol
$C_{27}H_{44}O_2$	Alfacalcidol
$C_{27}H_{44}O_2$	Colestolone
$C_{27}H_{44}O_2$	Gefarnate
$C_{27}H_{44}O_2.H_2O$	Calcifediol
$C_{27}H_{44}O_3$	Calcitriol
$C_{27}H_{44}O_3$	Paricalcitol
$C_{27}H_{44}O_3$	Secalciferol
$C_{27}H_{44}O_3$	Tacalcitol
$C_{27}H_{45}^{131}IO$	Iodocholesterol I 131
$C_{27}H_{45}^{131}IO$	Norcholestenol Iodomethyl (^{131}I) [Injection]
$C_{27}H_{45}NO$	Olesoxime
$C_{27}H_{45}NO_4$	Stevaladil
$C_{27}H_{45}N_3O_3$	Turosteride
$C_{27}H_{45}N_3O_6$	Elacytarabine
$C_{27}H_{45}N_5O_5$	Boceprevir
$C_{27}H_{46}O$	Cholesterol
$C_{27}H_{48}O$	Epidihydrocholesterin
$C_{27}H_{49}N_5O_8$	Tabilautide
$C_{27}H_{50}O_6$	Tricaprilin
$C_{27}H_{50}O_7P_2$	Belfosdil
$C_{27}H_{58}NO_6P$	Edelfosine
$C_{27}H_{58}N_2O_3.2HF$	Olaflur
$C_{27}H_{60}ClNO_3Si$	Disiquonium Chloride
$C_{28}H_{19}FN_4O_8$	Emitefur
$C_{28}H_{20}CaN_2O_8.5H_2O$	Benzoylpas Calcium
$C_{28}H_{22}Cl_2FNO_3$	Flumethrin
$C_{28}H_{22}F_3N_7O$	Nilotinib
$C_{28}H_{22}NO_6P$	Fosquidone
$C_{28}H_{22}O_6$	Bencianol
$C_{28}H_{23}NO_3$	Cypothrin
$C_{28}H_{24}Br_2N_6$	Fazadinium Bromide
$C_{28}H_{24}N_4O_2$	Tarazepide
$C_{28}H_{24}O_6$	Furostilbestrol
$C_{28}H_{25}N_6NaO_{10}S_2$	Cefpimizole Sodium
$C_{28}H_{26}ClN_7$	Isometamidium Chloride
$C_{28}H_{26}F_4N_2OS.C_4H_4O_4$	Duoperone Fumarate

Molecular Formula	Non-proprietary Name
$C_{28}H_{26}N_2O_5$	Imiglitazar
$C_{28}H_{26}N_4O_2$	Tolpadol
$C_{28}H_{26}N_6O_{10}S_2$	Cefpimizole
$C_{28}H_{27}ClF_5NO$	Penfluridol
$C_{28}H_{27}Cl_2N_3O_7S$	Relcovaptan
$C_{28}H_{27}NO_3$	Aleplasinin
$C_{28}H_{27}NO_4S.HCl$	Raloxifene Hydrochloride
$C_{28}H_{28}ClF_2N_3O$	Clopimozide
$C_{28}H_{28}I_6N_4O_8$	Iosefamic Acid
$C_{28}H_{28}I_6N_4O_{10}S.C_7H_{17}NO_5$	Iosulamide Meglumine
$C_{28}H_{28}N_2O_2$	Difenoxin
$C_{28}H_{28}N_4O_3$	Ruboxistaurin
$C_{28}H_{28}N_6S_4$	Bisbendazole
$C_{28}H_{28}O_3$	Adapalene
$C_{28}H_{29}ClN_4S$	Israpafant
$C_{28}H_{29}F_2N_3O$	Pimozide
$C_{28}H_{29}F_5O_3$	Lonaprisan
$C_{28}H_{29}NO_4$	Bephenium Hydroxynaphthoate
$C_{28}H_{29}NO_4S$	Arzoxifene
$C_{28}H_{29}NO_4S.HCl$	Arzoxifene Hydrochloride
$C_{28}H_{29}N_5O_3.HCl$	Lecozotan Hydrochloride
$C_{28}H_{30}FN_3OS.C_4H_4O_4$	Monatepil Maleate
$C_{28}H_{30}F_2N_2O_2$	Trelnarizine
$C_{28}H_{30}INO$	Idoxifene
$C_{28}H_{30}N_2O_2$	Darifenacin
$C_{28}H_{30}N_2O_2.HBr$	Darifenacin Hydrobromide
$C_{28}H_{30}N_4O_2$	Fuprazole
$C_{28}H_{30}N_4O_6.2HCl$	Lurtotecan Dihydrochloride
$C_{28}H_{30}N_6OS$	Masitinib
$C_{28}H_{31}FN_2O$	Nivazol
$C_{28}H_{31}FN_4O$	Astemizole
$C_{28}H_{31}FN_4O_2$	Idenast
$C_{28}H_{31}FO_5$	Bervastatin
$C_{28}H_{31}F_2N_5O_2$	Icospiramide
$C_{28}H_{31}NO_2$	Lasofoxifene
$C_{28}H_{31}NO_2.C_4H_6O_6$	Lasofoxifene Tartrate
$C_{28}H_{31}NO_5$	Tobuterol
$C_{28}H_{31}NO_5.CH_4O_3S$	Bitolterol Mesylate
$C_{28}H_{31}NO_{10}$	Menogaril
$C_{28}H_{31}N_3O_4S$	Tolafentrine
$C_{28}H_{31}N_3O_6$	Benidipine
$C_{28}H_{31}N_3O_6$	Hepronicate
$C_{28}H_{31}N_5O_5S$	Rotamicillin
$C_{28}H_{32}F_2N_2O$	Vanoxerine
$C_{28}H_{32}IN_3S_2$	Tibezonium Iodide
$C_{28}H_{32}N_2O_5.HCl$	Nalfurafine Hydrochloride
$C_{28}H_{32}N_4O_5S.H_2O$	Edonentan
$C_{28}H_{32}O_6$	Mebenoside
$C_{28}H_{32}O_{15}$	Diosmin
$C_{28}H_{33}ClN_2.2HCl$	Buclizine Hydrochloride
$C_{28}H_{33}F_2N_3.3HCl$	Difluanine Hydrochloride
$C_{28}H_{33}NO_5$	Mepramidil
$C_{28}H_{33}NaO_8$	Ablukast Sodium
$C_{28}H_{34}F_2O_7$	Ciprocinonide
$C_{28}H_{34}N_2O_2$	Benderizine
$C_{28}H_{34}N_2O_2.HCl$	Carbiphene Hydrochloride
$C_{28}H_{34}N_2O_3.H_2O$	Denatonium Benzoate
$C_{28}H_{34}O_8$	Ablukast
$C_{28}H_{34}O_8S_2$	Ecamsule
$C_{28}H_{34}O_{15}$	Hesperidin
$C_{28}H_{35}ClN_4O$	Mosapramine
$C_{28}H_{35}FO_7$	Amcinonide
$C_{28}H_{35}NO_3$	Ulipristal
$C_{28}H_{35}NO_4$	Asoprisnil
$C_{28}H_{35}N_3O_7$	Virginiamycin Factor M_1
$C_{28}H_{35}N_5O_4.C_4H_6O_6$	Capromorelin Tartrate

Molecular Formula	Non-proprietary Name
$C_{28}H_{36}N_4O_2S.HCl$	Lurasidone Hydrochloride
$C_{28}H_{36}Na_2O_6S_3$ (Tentative)	Ictasol
$C_{28}H_{36}O_6$	Clinofibrate
$C_{28}H_{37}BrN_4O_3$	Ancriviroc
$C_{28}H_{37}ClN_4O$	Clocapramine
$C_{28}H_{37}ClO_7$	Alclometasone Dipropionate
$C_{28}H_{37}ClO_7$	Beclomethasone Dipropionate
$C_{28}H_{37}ClO_7$	Icometasone Enbutate
$C_{28}H_{37}FO_7$	Betamethasone Acibutate
$C_{28}H_{37}FO_7$	Betamethasone Dipropionate
$C_{28}H_{37}FO_7$	Dexamethasone Dipropionate
$C_{28}H_{37}NO_4$	Homprenorphine
$C_{28}H_{37}N_3O_3$	Bilastine
$C_{28}H_{37}N_3O_4$	Derquantel
$C_{28}H_{37}N_3O_7$	Volpristin
$C_{28}H_{38}BrNO_4$	Butropium Bromide
$C_{28}H_{38}FN_3O_6$	Flopristin
$C_{28}H_{38}F_3N_5O_2.C_4H_4O_4$	Vicriviroc Maleate
$C_{28}H_{38}N_2O_2.HCl$	Butoprozine Hydrochloride
$C_{28}H_{38}N_2O_4$	Febuverine
$C_{28}H_{38}N_2O_5$	Cilobradine
$C_{28}H_{38}N_2O_6$	Simetride
$C_{28}H_{38}N_2O_6.HCl$	Teludipine Hydrochloride
$C_{28}H_{38}N_4O.2HCl.H_2O$	Carpipramine Dihydrochloride
$C_{28}H_{38}N_4O_6$	Iganidipine
$C_{28}H_{38}O_3$	Nandrolone Cyclotate
$C_{28}H_{38}O_7$	Prednisolone Valerate Acetate
$C_{28}H_{38}O_{19}$	Sucrose Octaacetate
$C_{28}H_{39}FO_5$	Fluocortolone Caproate
$C_{28}H_{39}N_3O$	Alinastine
$C_{28}H_{39}N_7O_9$	Rotigaptide
$C_{28}H_{40}N_2O_2.2HCl$	Bialamicol Hydrochloride
$C_{28}H_{40}N_2O_5$	Gallopamil
$C_{28}H_{40}N_4O_5$	Umespirone
$C_{28}H_{40}N_4S$	Foropafant
$C_{28}H_{40}O_7$	Amebucort
$C_{28}H_{40}O_7$	Hydrocortisone Probutate
$C_{28}H_{41}ClN_2O.HCl$	Teroxalene Hydrochloride
$C_{28}H_{41}N_3O_3$	Oxethazaine
$C_{28}H_{41}N_3O_3$	Tiropramide
$C_{28}H_{42}Cl_4N_4O_2$	Ambenonium Chloride
$C_{28}H_{42}N_2O_5$	Fenoxedil
$C_{28}H_{42}N_4O_9$	Difebarbamate
$C_{28}H_{42}O_6$	Ambruticin
$C_{28}H_{44}ClNO_2.H_2O$	Methylbenzethonium Chloride
$C_{28}H_{44}O$	Ergocalciferol
$C_{28}H_{44}O_2$	Doxercalciferol
$C_{28}H_{44}O_3$	Nandrolone Decanoate
$C_{28}H_{46}CuN_{12}O_8.2C_2H_4O_2$	Prezatide Copper Acetate
$C_{28}H_{46}O$	Dihydrotachysterol
$C_{28}H_{47}NO_4S$	Tiamulin
$C_{28}H_{47}NO_4S.C_4H_4O_4$	Tiamulin Fumarate
$C_{28}H_{48}O_6$	Ecraprost
$C_{28}H_{54}N_8$	Plerixafor
$C_{28}H_{55}N_5O_2$	Impacarzine
$C_{28}H_{58}Br_2N_2O_6$	Prodeconium Bromide
$C_{28}H_{60}Al_{14}O_{71}S_7$	Dosmalfate
$C_{29}H_{24}N_4O_8$	Niceritrol
$C_{29}H_{25}N_3O_5$	Nicomorphine
$C_{29}H_{26}ClFN_4O_4S.2C_7H_8O_3S.$ H_2O	Lapatinib Ditosylate
$C_{29}H_{26}O_3$	Estradiol Acetate
$C_{29}H_{27}F_2N_3O$	Seganserin
$C_{29}H_{28}F_7NO_2$	Serlopitant
$C_{29}H_{28}N_2O_7$	Muraglitazar
$C_{29}H_{28}N_4O_{11}$	Edotecarin

Molecular Formula	Non-proprietary Name
$C_{29}H_{29}F_6N_3O_2$	Befetupitant
$C_{29}H_{29}IN_2S$	Pretamazium Iodide
$C_{29}H_{30}Cl_2F_2N_4O_2.2HCl.H_2O$	Mioflazine Hydrochloride
$C_{29}H_{30}FN_3O$	Flezelastine
$C_{29}H_{30}N_2O_3$	Octimibate
$C_{29}H_{30}N_6O_6$	Olmesartan Medoxomil
$C_{29}H_{30}O_8$	Enrasentan
$C_{29}H_{31}F_2N_3O$	Fluspirilene
$C_{29}H_{31}F_3N_2O_3$	Almorexant
$C_{29}H_{31}NO_2.HCl$	Nafoxidine Hydrochloride
$C_{29}H_{31}NO_4.HCl$	Acolbifene Hydrochloride
$C_{29}H_{31}NO_{11}S$	Ladirubicin
$C_{29}H_{31}N_7O$	Imatinib
$C_{29}H_{32}ClN_3O_4$	Elomotecan
$C_{29}H_{32}ClN_5O_2$	Pyronaridine
$C_{29}H_{32}N_2O_3$	Pipendoxifene
$C_{29}H_{32}N_2O_6S$	Levosemotiadil
$C_{29}H_{32}N_2O_6S$	Semotiadil
$C_{29}H_{32}N_4$	Lifarizine
$C_{29}H_{32}O_{13}$	Etoposide
$C_{29}H_{33}ClN_2O_2.HCl$	Loperamide Hydrochloride
$C_{29}H_{33}ClN_2O_3$	Loperamide Oxide
$C_{29}H_{33}FN_2O_6$	Elgodipine
$C_{29}H_{33}FO_4.H_2O$	Naflocort
$C_{29}H_{33}FO_6$	Amcinafide
$C_{29}H_{33}FO_6$	Betamethasone Benzoate
$C_{29}H_{33}FO_8$	Dexamethasone Acefurate
$C_{29}H_{33}NO_5$	Ecipramidil
$C_{29}H_{33}O_{16}P$	Etoposide Phosphate
$C_{29}H_{34}FN_3O_6$	Palonidipine
$C_{29}H_{34}N_2O_2$	Dotarizine
$C_{29}H_{34}O_6$	Tribenoside
$C_{29}H_{34}O_{17}$	Monoxerutin
$C_{29}H_{35}F_5$	Dexamethasone Beloxil
$C_{29}H_{35}NO_2$	Mifepristone
$C_{29}H_{35}NO_2$	Miproxifene
$C_{29}H_{35}N_3O_{10}$	Pecocycline
$C_{29}H_{36}N_2O_9$	Cinepaxadil
$C_{29}H_{36}N_6O_2$	Laprafylline
$C_{29}H_{36}O_4$	Algestone Acetophenide
$C_{29}H_{36}O_4$	Isotretinoin Anisatil
$C_{29}H_{37}ClFNO_7$	Cicortonide
$C_{29}H_{37}Cl_2NO_4$	Tefenperate
$C_{29}H_{37}NO_2$	Aglepristone
$C_{29}H_{37}NO_3$	Lilopristone
$C_{29}H_{37}NO_4$	Bucromarone
$C_{29}H_{37}N_3O_{13}$	Meglucycline
$C_{29}H_{38}ClFO_8$	Formocortal
$C_{29}H_{38}FN_3O_3.2HCl$	Mibefradil Dihydrochloride
$C_{29}H_{38}F_2O_9$	Itrocinonide
$C_{29}H_{38}F_3N_3O_2S$	Fluphenazine Enanthate
$C_{29}H_{38}N_2O_4$	Dehydroemetine
$C_{29}H_{38}N_2O_6.HCl$	Atrasentan Hydrochloride
$C_{29}H_{38}N_4O_9$	Pipacycline
$C_{29}H_{38}N_4O_{10}$	Lymecycline
$C_{29}H_{38}N_8O_8$	Guamecycline
$C_{29}H_{38}O_3$	Oxogestone Phenpropionate
$C_{29}H_{38}O_7$	Acrihellin
$C_{29}H_{38}O_7S$	Tipelukast
$C_{29}H_{39}Cl_2FN_4O_4S$	Ambamustine
$C_{29}H_{39}FO_7$	Betamethasone Butyrate Propionate
$C_{29}H_{39}NO_2$	Mofarotene
$C_{29}H_{39}NO_3$	Onapristone
$C_{29}H_{39}NO_9$	Omacetaxine Mepesuccinate
$C_{29}H_{39}N_3O_3$	Pumafentrine
$C_{29}H_{39}N_5O_8$	Tigecycline
$C_{29}H_{40}N_2O_3$	Lapisteride
$C_{29}H_{40}N_2O_4.2HCl$	Emetine Hydrochloride
$C_{29}H_{40}N_6O_6S.C_2H_4O_2$	Metkephamid Acetate
$C_{29}H_{40}O_3$	Bolmantalate
$C_{29}H_{41}F_2N_5O$	Maraviroc
$C_{29}H_{41}NO_4.HCl$	Buprenorphine Hydrochloride
$C_{29}H_{41}NO_7$	Candoxatril
$C_{29}H_{42}O_6$	Hydrocortisone Cypionate
$C_{29}H_{43}BrN_2O_4$	Otilonium Bromide
$C_{29}H_{43}FO_2$	Elocalcitol
$C_{29}H_{43}NO_2S$	Eflucimibe
$C_{29}H_{43}NO_4S$	Avasimibe
$C_{29}H_{43}N_3O_3$	Sevopramide
$C_{29}H_{44}ClNO_2$	Lauralkonium Chloride
$C_{29}H_{44}O_3$	Estradiol Undecylate
$C_{29}H_{44}O_6$	Ramnodigin
$C_{29}H_{44}O_9$	Actodigin
$C_{29}H_{44}O_{12}.8H_2O$	Ouabain
$C_{29}H_{45}NO_3$	Ecalcidene
$C_{29}H_{48}Br_2O_2$	Acebrochol
$C_{29}H_{48}O_4$	Lexacalcitol
$C_{29}H_{51}N_5O_4.HCl$	Droxinavir Hydrochloride
$C_{29}H_{52}N_6O_9$	Pimelautide
$C_{29}H_{53}NO_5$	Orlistat
$C_{29}H_{55}N_5O_{18}$	Lividomycin
$C_{30}H_{22}N_4O_4$	Adozelesin
$C_{30}H_{23}KN_4O_8$	Azilsartan Kamedoxomil
$C_{30}H_{23}N_3O_6$	Niceverine
$C_{30}H_{24}N_4O_8$	Azilsartan Medoxomil
$C_{30}H_{24}N_4O_{10}$	Nicofuranose
$C_{30}H_{25}F_{10}NO_3$	Anacetrapib
$C_{30}H_{26}CaO_6.2H_2O$	Fenoprofen Calcium
$C_{30}H_{26}F_6N_4O_2$	Antrafenine
$C_{30}H_{26}N_2O_{13}$	Oftasceine
$C_{30}H_{28}N_2Na_4O_{14}S_5$	Solasulfone
$C_{30}H_{29}ClN_6O_3$	Neratinib
$C_{30}H_{29}N_5O_4S$	Fiduxosin
$C_{30}H_{29}N_5O_4S.HCl$	Fiduxosin Hydrochloride
$C_{30}H_{30}N_2O_7$	Peliglitazar
$C_{30}H_{30}N_6O_3S$	Milfasartan
$C_{30}H_{31}FN_2O$	Siramesine
$C_{30}H_{31}F_3N_8O$	Bafetinib
$C_{30}H_{31}NO_3.CH_4O_3S$	Trioxifene Mesylate
$C_{30}H_{31}N_3O_3$	Dofequidar
$C_{30}H_{32}ClF_3N_2O_2$	Fluperamide
$C_{30}H_{32}ClN_3O_8$	Cronidipine
$C_{30}H_{32}ClN_3O_8S$	Nelivaptan
$C_{30}H_{32}ClN_7OS$	Balamapimod
$C_{30}H_{32}Cl_3NO$	Lumefantrine
$C_{30}H_{32}Cl_3N_3O_4.HCl$	Valategrast Hydrochloride
$C_{30}H_{32}FNO_{13}$	Galarubicin
$C_{30}H_{32}F_6N_4O$	Netupitant
$C_{30}H_{32}N_2O_2.HCl$	Diphenoxylate Hydrochloride
$C_{30}H_{32}N_2O_5$	Vinmegallate
$C_{30}H_{32}N_4O$	Cinprazole
$C_{30}H_{33}ClN_4O_2.CH_4O_3S$	Ispinesib Mesylate
$C_{30}H_{33}Cl_2F_2N_5O_2$	Draflazine
$C_{30}H_{33}N_3O_3.HCl$	Ropitoin Hydrochloride
$C_{30}H_{34}BrNO_3$	Xenytropium Bromide
$C_{30}H_{34}FN_5O_5$	Frakefamide
$C_{30}H_{34}N_2O_3.C_2H_4O_2$	Bazedoxifene Acetate
$C_{30}H_{35}BrN_{12}O_5$	Brostallicin
$C_{30}H_{35}FN_2O_3$	Mobenzoxamine
$C_{30}H_{35}F_2N_3O$	Lidoflazine
$C_{30}H_{35}F_7N_4O_2.CH_3SO_3H$	Casopitant Mesylate

Molecular Formula	Non-proprietary Name
$C_{30}H_{35}NO_3$	Levormeloxifene
$C_{30}H_{35}NO_3$	Ormeloxifene
$C_{30}H_{36}N_4O$	Tagorizine
$C_{30}H_{38}N_4.2C_2H_4O_2.2H_2O$	Quindecamine Acetate
$C_{30}H_{38}N_4O_{11}$	Apicycline
$C_{30}H_{39}NO_4.HCl$	Vapiprost Hydrochloride
$C_{30}H_{40}Cl_2N_4$	Dequalinium Chloride
$C_{30}H_{40}Cl_2O_6$	Meclorisone Dibutyrate
$C_{30}H_{41}FO_7$	Triamcinolone Hexacetonide
$C_{30}H_{41}NO_6S$	Sagopilone
$C_{30}H_{42}N_6O_5S$	Glicaramide
$C_{30}H_{42}O_8$	Proscillaridin
$C_{30}H_{44}N_2O_5$	Ivarimod
$C_{30}H_{44}N_2O_{10}$	Hexobendine
$C_{30}H_{44}O_3$	Boldenone Undecylenate
$C_{30}H_{44}O_4$	Terbuficin
$C_{30}H_{45}NNaO_7P$	Fosinopril Sodium
$C_{30}H_{46}N_2O_{14}S_2$	Aclatonium Napadisilate
$C_{30}H_{46}O_3$	Seocalcitol
$C_{30}H_{46}O_4$	Enoxolone
$C_{30}H_{47}NO_4S$	Retapamulin
$C_{30}H_{48}N_2O_2.2HCl$	Symetine Hydrochloride
$C_{30}H_{48}O_3$	Testosterone Undecanoate
$C_{30}H_{49}N_9O_9$	Thymopentin
$C_{30}H_{50}O_5$	Eldecalcitol
$C_{30}H_{53}NO_{11}$ (average)	Benzonatate
$C_{30}H_{53}N_3O_6$	Aliskiren
$(C_{30}H_{53}N_3O_6)_2.C_4H_4O_4$	Aliskiren Fumarate
$C_{30}H_{60}I_3N_3O_3$	Gallamine Triethiodide
$C_{30}H_{62}$	Squalane
$C_{30}H_{62}O_{10}$ (average)	Laureth 9
$C_{31}H_{27}BrO_3S$	Ertiprotafib
$C_{31}H_{28}N_4O_4$	Elinafide
$C_{31}H_{30}N_4O_2$	Pomisartan
$C_{31}H_{31}F_2NO_5$	Scopinast
$C_{31}H_{31}F_3N_2Na_2O_5S$	Tipranavir Disodium
$C_{31}H_{32}F_3N_3O_5S$	Masilukast
$C_{31}H_{32}N_2O_6$	Feloprentan
$C_{31}H_{32}N_4O_2$	Bezitramide
$C_{31}H_{33}F_3N_2O_5S$	Tipranavir
$C_{31}H_{33}N_3O_4$	Upidosin
$C_{31}H_{33}N_3O_6S$	Zafirlukast
$C_{31}H_{34}BrNO_4$	Fentonium Bromide
$C_{31}H_{35}Cl_2N_3O_2$	Saredutant
$C_{31}H_{35}F_7N_4O_2$	Orvepitant
$C_{31}H_{35}N_2NaO_{11}$	Novobiocin Sodium
$C_{31}H_{36}ClN_3O_5S$	Metofenazate
$C_{31}H_{36}IN_3$	Stilbazium Iodide
$C_{31}H_{36}I_6N_6O_{13}$	Iofratol
$C_{31}H_{36}I_6N_6O_{14}$	Iosimenol
$C_{31}H_{37}NO_7$	Nicocortonide
$C_{31}H_{37}N_5O_3$	Bamirastine
$C_{31}H_{37}N_5O_3$	Doramapimod
$C_{31}H_{38}F_2N_2O$	Flotrenizine
$C_{31}H_{38}N_2O$	Ezlopitant
$C_{31}H_{38}N_2O_6$	Daglutril
$C_{31}H_{38}N_4$	Buterizine
$C_{31}H_{39}FN_4O_7$	Rupintrivir
$C_{31}H_{39}NO_2$	Toripristone
$C_{31}H_{40}N_2O$	Trenizine
$C_{31}H_{40}N_2O_5$	Asoprisnil Ecamate
$C_{31}H_{40}N_6O_7S$	Ociltide
$C_{31}H_{40}O_2$	Menatetrenone
$C_{31}H_{41}BrFNO_3$	Bromperidol Decanoate
$C_{31}H_{41}ClFNO_3$	Haloperidol Decanoate
$C_{31}H_{41}Cl_2N_3O_5S_2$	Chlorphenoctium Amsonate

Molecular Formula	Non-proprietary Name
$C_{31}H_{41}N_5O_5.CH_4O_3S$ (dihydro-ergocornine mesylate)	Ergoloid Mesylates
$C_{31}H_{42}N_6O_3.HCl$	Anamorelin Hydrochloride
$C_{31}H_{42}N_6O_4$	Tandutinib
$C_{31}H_{43}N_3Na_{10}O_{49}S_8$	Fondaparinux Sodium
$C_{31}H_{43}N_3O_8$	Tanespimycin
$C_{31}H_{43}N_3O_8$	Terdecamycin
$C_{31}H_{44}N_2O_5S.HCl$	Dronedarone Hydrochloride
$C_{31}H_{44}N_2O_{10}$	Dilazep
$C_{31}H_{44}O_8$	Meproscillarin
$C_{31}H_{45}N_3O_8$	Retaspimycin
$C_{31}H_{45}N_3O_8.HCl$	Retaspimycin Hydrochloride
$C_{31}H_{46}O_2$	Phytonadione
$C_{31}H_{47}N_3O_9.H_2O$	Detajmium Bitartrate
$C_{31}H_{47}N_7O_{14}$	Pendetide
$C_{31}H_{47}NaO_4$	Fusidate Sodium
$C_{31}H_{48}N_4O_7S$	Terlakiren
$C_{31}H_{48}Na_2O_8P_2$	Phytonadiol Sodium Diphosphate
$C_{31}H_{48}O_2S_2$	Probucol
$C_{31}H_{48}O_4$	Testosterone Ketolaurate
$C_{31}H_{48}O_5$	Tisocalcitate
$C_{31}H_{48}O_6$	Fusidic Acid
$C_{31}H_{50}O_2$	Molfarnate
$C_{31}H_{51}NO_8$	Repromicin
$C_{31}H_{51}NO_9$	Rosaramicin
$C_{31}H_{51}NO_9.C_{18}H_{36}O_2$	Rosaramicin Stearate
$C_{31}H_{51}NO_9.NaH_2PO_4$	Rosaramicin Sodium Phosphate
$C_{31}H_{52}N_2O_5S$	Valnemulin
$C_{31}H_{55}N_3O_6$	Enocitabine
$C_{32}H_{16}N_8Zn$	Ciaftalan Zinc
$C_{32}H_{26}N_4O_2$	Conivaptan
$C_{32}H_{26}N_4O_2.HCl$	Conivaptan Hydrochloride
$C_{32}H_{28}N_6O_8.2CH_4O_3S$	Bisnafide Dimesylate
$C_{32}H_{29}F_5N_3NaO_5$	Elagolix Sodium
$C_{32}H_{29}N_5O_2.HCl$	Enzastaurin Hydrochloride
$C_{32}H_{30}F_5N_3O_5$	Elagolix
$C_{32}H_{31}ClN_4O_5$	Meclinertant
$C_{32}H_{31}F_2N_3O_2.3HCl$	Zosuquidar Trihydrochloride
$C_{32}H_{31}N_3O_4.HCl$	Difenoximide Hydrochloride
$C_{32}H_{31}N_5O$	Diaplasinin
$C_{32}H_{32}Cl_2O_{10}$	Salafibrate
$C_{32}H_{32}O_{13}S$	Teniposide
$C_{32}H_{34}N_4O_4S$	Diathymosulfone
$C_{32}H_{34}N_5NaO_{11}S_2$	Piridicillin Sodium
$C_{32}H_{36}BrClN_2O_2$	Rilozarone
$C_{32}H_{36}BrN_5O_8$	Pibrozelesin
$C_{32}H_{36}BrN_5O_8.HBr$	Pibrozelesin Hydrobromide
$C_{32}H_{36}N_2O_2$	Butoxylate
$C_{32}H_{37}ClN_2O_8$	Chloroserpidine
$C_{32}H_{37}NO_4$	Carebastine
$C_{32}H_{37}NO_{12}$	Pirarubicin
$C_{32}H_{37}NO_{13}$	Nemorubicin
$C_{32}H_{37}NO_{13}$	Sabarubicin
$C_{32}H_{37}N_3O_5$	Elziverine
$C_{32}H_{38}Cl_2N_{10}O_4$	Tallimustine
$C_{32}H_{38}N_2O_5$	Cortivazol
$C_{32}H_{38}N_2O_8$	Deserpidine
$C_{32}H_{38}N_2O_8$	Mefeserpine
$C_{32}H_{38}N_2O_{12}S_4$	Omocianine
$C_{32}H_{39}NO_2$	Ebastine
$C_{32}H_{39}NO_4.HCl$	Fexofenadine Hydrochloride
$C_{32}H_{40}BrN_5O_5$	Bromocriptine
$C_{32}H_{40}BrN_5O_5.CH_4SO_3$	Bromocriptine Mesylate
$C_{32}H_{40}N_2O.C_6H_8O_7.H_2O$	Maropitant Citrate
$C_{32}H_{40}N_2O_5S_2$	Trimethaphan Camsylate

Molecular Formula	*Non-proprietary Name*
$C_{32}H_{40}N_4O_3$	Tabimorelin
$C_{32}H_{41}NO_2$	Terfenadine
$C_{32}H_{43}N_5O_5$	Epicriptine
$C_{32}H_{43}N_5O_5.CH_4O_3S$ (dihydro-α-ergocryptine mesylate)	Ergoloid Mesylates
$C_{32}H_{43}N_5O_5.CH_4O_3S$ (dihydro-β-ergocryptin)	Ergoloid Mesylates
$C_{32}H_{44}O_7$	Ciclesonide
$C_{32}H_{45}N_3O_4S.CH_4O_3S$	Nelfinavir Mesylate
$C_{32}H_{45}N_5O_4$	Desocriptine
$C_{32}H_{46}N_8O_6S_2$	Bisbutytiamine
$C_{32}H_{46}N_8O_6S_2$	Sulbutiamine
$C_{32}H_{46}O_4$	Atocalcitol
$C_{32}H_{47}F_5O_3S$	Fulvestrant
$C_{32}H_{48}N_2$	Ronipamil
$C_{32}H_{48}N_2O_{10}$	Butobendine
$C_{32}H_{48}N_4O_8.HCl$	Alvespimycin Hydrochloride
$(C_{32}H_{48}O_{16})_n$	Porofocon A
$(C_{32}H_{48}O_{16})_n$	Porofocon B
$C_{32}H_{52}Br_2N_4O_4$	Demecarium Bromide
$C_{32}H_{53}BrN_2O_4$	Rocuronium Bromide
$C_{32}H_{55}BrN_4O$	Thonzonium Bromide
$C_{32}H_{55}N_9O_{10}$	Larazotide
$C_{32}H_{55}N_9O_{10}.C_2H_4O_2$	Larazotide Acetate
$C_{32}H_{58}N_6O_5.HCl$	Tasidotin Hydrochloride
$C_{32}H_{64}O_2$	Cetyl Palmitate
$C_{32}H_{66}O_{10}S$ (Approximate)	Laureth 10S
$C_{33}H_{24}Hg_2O_6S_2$	Hydrargaphen
$C_{33}H_{30}N_4O_2$	Telmisartan
$C_{33}H_{33}FO_6$	Etalocib
$C_{33}H_{34}Cl_2N_4O_7$	Becatecarin
$C_{33}H_{34}N_2O_5$	Amelubant
$C_{33}H_{34}N_4O_6$	Azelnidipine
$C_{33}H_{34}N_6O_6$	Candesartan Cilexetil
$C_{33}H_{35}FO_8$	Triamcinolone Furetonide
$C_{33}H_{35}NO_{13}$	Elsamitrucin
$(C_{33}H_{35}N_5O_5)_2.C_4H_6O_6$	Ergotamine Tartrate
$C_{33}H_{36}N_2O_{12}$	Cromoglicate Lisetil
$C_{33}H_{36}N_4O_3$	Mozenavir
$C_{33}H_{37}N_5O_5.CH_4O_3S$	Dihydroergotamine Mesylate
$C_{33}H_{38}N_2O_4$	Itriglumide
$C_{33}H_{38}N_2O_8$	Rescimetol
$C_{33}H_{38}N_4O_6.HCl.3H_2O$	Irinotecan Hydrochloride
$C_{33}H_{39}NO_{14}$	Detorubicin
$C_{33}H_{40}GdN_3Na_3O_{15}P$	Gadofosveset Trisodium
$C_{33}H_{40}N_2O_9$	Methoserpidine
$C_{33}H_{40}N_2O_9$	Reserpine
$C_{33}H_{40}N_2O_{12}$	Leurubicin
$C_{33}H_{40}N_6O_7$	Casokefamide
$C_{33}H_{41}ClN_2O_9$	Lapaquistat Acetate
$C_{33}H_{41}NO_{17}$	Ethoxazorutoside
$C_{33}H_{41}N_3O_{10}S_2$	Brecanavir
$C_{33}H_{42}O_{19}$	Troxerutin
$C_{33}H_{43}FN_{10}O_6.2C_2HF_3O_2$	Nemifitide Ditriflutate
$C_{33}H_{43}FO_7$	Dexamethasone Cipecilate
$C_{33}H_{43}N_3O_6.HCl$	Aplaviroc Hydrochloride
$C_{33}H_{43}N_5O_5$	Mergocriptine
$C_{33}H_{44}N_3O_{14}P$	Fosveset
$C_{33}H_{44}N_6O_5$	Telinavir
$C_{33}H_{45}NO_6S$	Tiprostanide
$C_{33}H_{45}N_3O_8S$	Satavaptan
$C_{33}H_{45}N_5O_3$	Lanepitant
$C_{33}H_{47}NO$	Moctamide
$C_{33}H_{47}NO_{13}$	Natamycin
$C_{33}H_{48}NNaO_{10}S$	Methylprednisolone Suleptanate
$C_{33}H_{50}N_4O_6S$	Remikiren
$C_{33}H_{50}O_4S_2$	Camobucol
$C_{33}H_{52}O_8$	Disogluside
$C_{33}H_{53}NO_3.HCl$	Naboctate Hydrochloride
$C_{33}H_{54}N_{12}O_{15}$	Nonathymulin
$C_{33}H_{54}O_5(C_2H_4O)_n$ (n = approximately 22)	Tocophersolan
$C_{33}H_{55}NO_8$	Disermolide
$C_{33}H_{58}Br_2N_2O_3$	Dacuronium Bromide
$C_{33}H_{58}N_6O_5$	Valomaciclovir Stearate
$C_{33}H_{58}N_{10}O_9$	Lagatide
$C_{33}H_{60}O_{6.5}$ (Approximate)	Sorbitan Sesquioleate
$C_{34}H_{24}N_6Na_4O_{14}S_4$	Evans Blue
$C_{34}H_{29}ClN_6O_3$	Modipafant
$C_{34}H_{30}N_2O_5$	Farglitazar
$C_{34}H_{32}N_4Na_2O_4$	Protoporphyrin Disodium
$C_{34}H_{32}N_4O_9$	Nicomol
$C_{34}H_{33}N_3O_5.HCl$	Elacridar Hydrochloride
$C_{34}H_{34}ClN_2NaO_3S$	Quiflapon Sodium
$C_{34}H_{35}NO_{11}.HCl$	Berubicin Hydrochloride
$C_{34}H_{35}N_3O_{10}.HCl$	Zorubicin Hydrochloride
$C_{34}H_{36}Cl_2N_4O_4Sn$	Stannsoporfin
$C_{34}H_{36}Cl_2N_6O_5S$	Anatibant
$C_{34}H_{36}F_3NO_{13}$	Valrubicin
$C_{34}H_{36}MgN_6O_6S_2$	Omeprazole Magnesium
$C_{34}H_{36}MgN_6O_6S_2.3H_2O$	Esomeprazole Magnesium
$C_{34}H_{37}N_5O_5$	Metergotamine
$C_{34}H_{38}N_2O_4$	Nafiverine
$C_{34}H_{38}N_3O_7P$	Efonidipine
$C_{34}H_{40}F_2N_4OS$	Lecimibide
$C_{34}H_{40}I_6N_4O_{12}$	Iozomic Acid
$C_{34}H_{41}N_3O_7$	Biricodar
$C_{34}H_{41}N_3O_7.2C_6H_8O_7$	Biricodar Dicitrate
$C_{34}H_{41}N_3O_{10}$	Cinecromen
$C_{34}H_{41}N_7O_5$	Dabigatran Etexilate
$C_{34}H_{41}N_7O_5.xCH_4O_3S$	Dabigatran Etexilate Mesylate
$C_{34}H_{46}ClN_3O_{10}$	Maytansine
$C_{34}H_{46}Cl_2N_2$	Hedaquinium Chloride
$C_{34}H_{47}NO_4$	Celivarone
$C_{34}H_{47}NO_{11}$	Aconitine
$C_{34}H_{48}Cl_2O_6S_2$	Tiafibrate
$C_{34}H_{48}Na_2O_7$	Carbenoxolone Sodium
$C_{34}H_{50}N_4O_9S$	Dalfopristin
$C_{34}H_{52}I_2N_2O_4$	Truxicurium Iodide
$C_{34}H_{52}N_2O_2$	Anipamil
$C_{34}H_{52}N_{18}O_2$	Semapimod
$C_{34}H_{52}O_6$	Deloxolone
$C_{34}H_{53}N_3O_3$	Dosergoside
$C_{34}H_{54}O_8$	Lasalocid
$C_{34}H_{54}O_{14}$	Neutramycin
$C_{34}H_{55}NO_{10}$	Rosaramicin Propionate
$C_{34}H_{57}BrN_2O_4$	Vecuronium Bromide
$C_{34}H_{58}Ca_3N_8O_{14}$	Calteridol Calcium
$C_{34}H_{62}FN_2O_{10}PS$	Fosfluridine Tidoxil
$C_{34}H_{63}ClN_2O_6S.HCl$	Clindamycin Palmitate Hydrochloride
$C_{34}H_{63}N_5O_9$	Pepstatin
$C_{34}H_{65}N_3O_5S.xC_3H_6O_3.yH_2O$	Squalamine Lactate
$C_{34}H_{68}N_2O_4Pt$	Miriplatin
$C_{34}H_{68}O_{10}$ (Approximate)	Polyoxyl 8 Stearate
$C_{35}H_{28}N_4O_{11}$	Nicofurate
$C_{35}H_{30}N_4O_4$	Midostaurin
$C_{35}H_{32}N_6O_4$	Dersalazine
$C_{35}H_{33}FN_6O_3$	Quarfloxin
$C_{35}H_{34}O_5$	Etamestrol
$C_{35}H_{35}ClF_2N_8O_5S$	Isavuconazonium Chloride
$C_{35}H_{35}ClNNaO_3S$	Montelukast Sodium

Molecular Formula	*Non-proprietary Name*
$C_{35}H_{37}N_3O_2$	Implitapide
$C_{35}H_{38}Cl_2N_8O_4$	Itraconazole
$C_{35}H_{38}F_2N_8O_4$	Saperconazole
$C_{35}H_{38}N_4O_6$	Manidipine 6300
$C_{35}H_{38}N_4O_6Pd$	Padoporfin
$C_{35}H_{39}F_2N_7O_4$	Pramiconazole
$C_{35}H_{40}N_2O_6$	Linetastine
$C_{35}H_{41}Cl_2N_3O_2$	Osanetant
$C_{35}H_{41}N_5O_5.CH_4O_3S$ (dihydro-ergocristine mesylate)	Ergoloid Mesylates
$C_{35}H_{42}FNO_8$	Triamcinolone Benetonide
$C_{35}H_{42}N_2O_9$	Rescinnamine
$C_{35}H_{42}N_2O_{11}$	Syrosingopine
$C_{35}H_{44}I_6N_6O_{15}$	Iodixanol
$C_{35}H_{44}I_6N_6O_{16}$	Iodecimol
$C_{35}H_{45}Cl_2NO_6$	Prednimustine
$C_{35}H_{46}N_6O_8S$	Amogastrin
$C_{35}H_{48}ClN_3O_{10}S$	Cantuzumab Mertansine
$C_{35}H_{48}N_{10}O_{15}$	Emideltide
$C_{35}H_{49}N_{11}O_9S_2$	Eptifibatide
$C_{35}H_{52}N_2O_3.HCl$	Nabitan Hydrochloride
$C_{35}H_{52}O_5S_2$	Succinobucol
$C_{35}H_{53}N_3O_9$	Lasinavir
$C_{35}H_{53}NaO_8$	Tetronasin Sodium
$C_{35}H_{54}O_4S_2$	Elsibucol
$C_{35}H_{54}O_8$	Tetronasin
$C_{35}H_{55}NO_3$	Nabazenil
$C_{35}H_{55}N_5O_6S_2.HCl$	Zankiren Hydrochloride
$C_{35}H_{56}N_6O_5$	Cemadotin
$C_{35}H_{56}N_6O_6$	Enalkiren
$C_{35}H_{57}NO_{10}$	Rosaramicin Butyrate
$C_{35}H_{58}O_{11}$	Filipin
$C_{35}H_{59}Al_3N_{10}O_{24}$	Aceglutamide Aluminum
$C_{35}H_{59}NaO_{11}$ (monensin B sodium)	Monensin Sodium
$C_{35}H_{60}Br_2N_2O_4$	Pancuronium Bromide
$C_{35}H_{60}O_6$	Sitogluside
$C_{35}H_{60}O_{11}$ (monensin B)	Monensin
$C_{35}H_{61}NO_{12}.H_3PO_4$	Oleandomycin Phosphate
$C_{35}H_{62}Br_2N_4O_4$	Pipecuronium Bromide
$C_{35}H_{64}FN_2O_8PS$	Fosalvudine Tidoxil
$C_{35}H_{64}N_5O_8PS$	Fozivudine Tidoxil
$C_{35}H_{72}BrN_3$	Pirralkonium Bromide
$C_{36}H_{28}N_6O_{10}$	Glunicate
$C_{36}H_{31}F_2N_5O_4S$	Sufugolix
$C_{36}H_{36}N_2O_3.HCl$	Fetoxylate Hydrochloride
$C_{36}H_{38}F_4N_4O_2S$	Darapladib
$C_{36}H_{39}NO_5$	Cinaciguat
$C_{36}H_{39}N_3O_6$	Dexniguldipine
$C_{36}H_{39}N_3O_6$	Niguldipine
$C_{36}H_{41}ClN_8O_4S$	Mitratapide
$C_{36}H_{41}N_3O_6.HCl$	Lercanidipine Hydrochloride
$C_{36}H_{42}Br_2N_2$	Hexafluorenium Bromide
$C_{36}H_{47}N_5O_4.H_2O$	Indinavir
$C_{36}H_{47}N_5O_4.H_2SO_4$	Indinavir Sulfate
$C_{36}H_{49}N_3NaO_{22}Sb_3$	Stibamine Glucoside
$C_{36}H_{50}Cl_2O_5$	Locicortolone Dicibate
$C_{36}H_{52}O_8$	Nemadectin
$C_{36}H_{53}N_7O_6$	Telaprevir
$C_{36}H_{54}N_6O_{14}$	Xamoterol Fumarate
$C_{36}H_{56}N_2O_4$	Dagapamil
$C_{36}H_{56}O_6.2C_7H_{17}NO_5$	Bevirimat Dimeglumine
$C_{36}H_{60}N_{10}O_{12}$	Davunetide
$C_{36}H_{60}O_{30}$	Alfadex
$C_{36}H_{61}NaO_{11}$ (monensin A sodium)	Monensin Sodium

Molecular Formula	*Non-proprietary Name*
$C_{36}H_{62}N_4.2(C_7H_5NO_3S)$	Octenidine Saccharin
$C_{36}H_{62}N_4.2HCl$	Octenidine Hydrochloride
$C_{36}H_{62}O_{11}$ (monensin A)	Monensin
$C_{36}H_{66}CaI_4O_4$	Diiodostearate Calcium
$C_{36}H_{66}N_6O_6^{99m}Tc$	Technetium Tc 99m Sestamibi
$C_{36}H_{68}O_2$	Oleyl Oleate
$C_{36}H_{74}Cl_2N_2$	Triclobisonium Chloride
$C_{37}H_{36}N_4O_3$	Laniquidar
$C_{37}H_{38}N_2O_6$	Cepharanthine
$C_{37}H_{39}NO_4$	Dapitant
$C_{37}H_{40}N_2O_8S$	Cortisuzol
$C_{37}H_{41}ClN_2O_6.HCl.5H_2O$	Tubocurarine Chloride
$C_{37}H_{42}Cl_2N_4O_2Sn$	Rostaporfin
$C_{37}H_{42}F_2N_8O_4$	Posaconazole
$C_{37}H_{42}N_6O_8S$	Tetragastrin
$C_{37}H_{43}N_5O_9PdS$	Padeliporfin
$C_{37}H_{47}NO_{12}$	Rifamycin
$C_{37}H_{48}I_6N_6O_{18}$	Iotrolan
$C_{37}H_{48}N_4O_4S$	Ibodutant
$C_{37}H_{48}N_4O_5$	Lopinavir
$C_{37}H_{48}N_6O_5S_2$	Ritonavir
$C_{37}H_{49}N_3O_5S$	Iprotiazem
$C_{37}H_{49}N_7O_9S$	Pentagastrin
$C_{37}H_{53}NO_8$	Moxidectin
$C_{37}H_{55}ClO_4$	Tocofenoxate
$C_{37}H_{55}N_5O_8S$	Ciprokiren
$C_{37}H_{56}N_2O_3.2HCl$	Menabitan Hydrochloride
$C_{37}H_{59}N_{13}O_{13}.xHCl$ (each component)	Cinodine Hydrochloride
$C_{37}H_{61}BrN_2O_4$	Rapacuronium Bromide
$C_{37}H_{61}NO_{13}$	Mirosamicin
$C_{37}H_{63}N_5O_7S_2$	Diamocaine Cyclamate
$C_{37}H_{63}NaO_{11}$ (monensin C sodium)	Monensin Sodium
$C_{37}H_{64}O_{11}$ (monensin C)	Monensin
$C_{37}H_{66}FNO_{13}$	Flurithromycin
$C_{37}H_{67}NO_{12}$	Berythromycin
$C_{37}H_{67}NO_{13}$	Erythromycin
$C_{37}H_{67}NO_{13}.C_7H_{14}O_8$	Erythromycin Gluceptate
$C_{37}H_{67}NO_{13}.C_{12}H_{13}NO_5S.2H_2O$	Erythromycin Salnacedin
$C_{37}H_{67}NO_{13}.C_{12}H_{22}O_{12}$	Erythromycin Lactobionate
$C_{37}H_{67}NO_{13}.C_{18}H_{36}O_2$	Erythromycin Stearate
$C_{37}H_{72}N_4O_5S$	Trodusquemine
$C_{38}H_{37}F_3O_8S$	Iralukast
$C_{38}H_{38}N_4O_6$	Tariquidar
$C_{38}H_{41}N_5Na_4O_9$	Talaporfin Sodium
$C_{38}H_{42}N_8O_6S_2$	Bisbentiamine
$C_{38}H_{47}Br_2N_9O_5$	Olcegepant
$C_{38}H_{49}N_3O_5$	Bemotrizinol
$C_{38}H_{49}N_9O_5$	Ipamorelin
$C_{38}H_{50}I_6N_6O_{14}S$	Iotasul
$C_{38}H_{50}N_6O_5$	Saquinavir
$C_{38}H_{50}N_6O_5.CH_4O_3S$	Saquinavir Mesylate
$C_{38}H_{51}NO_4$	Myrophine
$C_{38}H_{52}N_6O_2.CH_4O_3S.xH_2O$	Tirilazad Mesylate
$C_{38}H_{52}N_6O_7.H_2O_4S$	Atazanavir Sulfate
$C_{38}H_{55}Na_9O_{49}S_7$	Idraparinux Sodium
$C_{38}H_{56}I_2N_2O_4$	Truxipicurium Iodide
$C_{38}H_{56}O_7$	Cicloxolone
$C_{38}H_{58}O_{10} + C_{37}H_{56}O_{10}$	Dimadectin
$C_{38}H_{61}I_2N_3S_3$	Platonin
$C_{38}H_{63}NO_8S$	Roxolonium Metilsulfate
$C_{38}H_{66}Br_2N_2O_2$	Deditonium Bromide
$C_{38}H_{67}NO_{10}$	Alemcinal
$C_{38}H_{69}NO_{13}$	Clarithromycin
$C_{38}H_{70}N_2O_{13}$	Lexithromycin

Molecular Formula	Non-proprietary Name
$C_{38}H_{72}N_2O_{12}.xH_2O$	Azithromycin
$C_{38}H_{74}O_4$ (Predominant)	Glycol Distearate
$C_{39}H_{33}Cl_3N_2O_5S$	Ecopladib
$C_{39}H_{43}N_3O_{11}S$	Trabectedin
$C_{39}H_{43}N_5O_{12}S$	Penimocycline
$[C_{39}H_{46}N_6O_{14}[C_6H_{10}O_5]_x$ $[C_8H_{12}O_7]_y]_n$	Delimotecan
$C_{39}H_{49}NO_{16}$	Nogalamycin
$C_{39}H_{53}N_3O_9$	Bietaserpine
$C_{39}H_{57}FN_4O_4$	Paliperidone Palmitate
$C_{39}H_{58}N_2O_5$	Eldacimibe
$C_{39}H_{59}ClO_3$	Sitofibrate
$C_{39}H_{59}ClO_4$	Tocofibrate
$C_{39}H_{62}O_{14}$	Pamaqueside
$C_{39}H_{64}O_{13}$	Tiqueside
$C_{39}H_{67}N_5O_6$	Soblidotin
$C_{39}H_{68}N_2O_8$	Coleneuramide
$C_{39}H_{69}NO_{12}$	Idremcinal
$C_{39}H_{69}NO_{14}.C_{18}H_{35}O_2$	Erythromycin Acistrate
$C_{40}H_{30}Cl_2N_{10}O_6$	Nitroblue Tetrazolium Chloride
$C_{40}H_{33}F_3N_4O_3$	Dirlotapide
$C_{40}H_{35}Cl_3N_2O_4S$	Efipladib
$C_{40}H_{38}F_5N_3O_3S$	Rilapladib
$C_{40}H_{39}F_5N_4O_3$	Goxalapladib
$C_{40}H_{48}Cl_2N_2O_6$	Dimethyltubocurarinium Chloride
$C_{40}H_{48}I_2N_2O_6$	Metocurine Iodide
$C_{40}H_{50}N_6O_8S$	Ciluprevir
$C_{40}H_{56}$	Beta Carotene
$C_{40}H_{57}N_5O_7$	Carfilzomib
$C_{40}H_{58}O_4$	Gamma Oryzanol
$C_{40}H_{59}NO_{11}.CH_4O_3S$	Eribulin Mesylate
$C_{40}H_{63}N_3O_4S_2$	Pipotiazine Palmitate
$C_{40}H_{63}N_9O_8S$	Barusiban
$C_{40}H_{64}N_2O_2$	Bolazine
$C_{40}H_{65}KO_{13}$	Laidlomycin Propionate Potassium
$C_{40}H_{65}N_{13}O_{13}.xHCl$ (each component)	Iprocinodine Hydrochloride
$C_{40}H_{69}NO_{12}.\frac{1}{2}(C_4H_4O_4)$	Mitemcinal Fumarate
$C_{40}H_{71}NO_{14}$	Erythromycin Propionate
$C_{40}H_{71}NO_{14}.C_5H_9NO_3S$	Erythromycin Stinoprate
$C_{40}H_{71}NO_{14}.C_{12}H_{26}O_4S$	Erythromycin Estolate
$C_{40}H_{74}CaO_{14}S_2$	Docusate Calcium
$C_{40}H_{76}N_2O_{12}$	Gamithromycin
$C_{40}H_{80}NO_8P$	Colfosceril Palmitate
$C_{41}H_{36}ClF_3N_2O_4S$	Giripladib
$C_{41}H_{37}ClN_6O_5$	Carzelesin
$C_{41}H_{42}N_4O_6$	Vatanidipine
$C_{41}H_{42}N_4O_8$	Verteporfin
$C_{41}H_{47}Cl_2NO_6$	Atrimustine
$C_{41}H_{48}N_2O_9$	Pinokalant
$C_{41}H_{50}N_6O_2$	Bisoctrizole
$C_{41}H_{52}N_6O_5$	Palinavir
$C_{41}H_{56}O_5$	Cinoxolone
$C_{41}H_{57}NO_{10}S$	Fuladectin Component A_3
$C_{41}H_{63}GdN_4O_{14}$	Gadocoletic Acid
$C_{41}H_{63}NO_{14}$	Protoveratrine A
$C_{41}H_{64}O_8$	Prednisolone Steaglate
$C_{41}H_{64}O_{13}$	Digitoxin
$C_{41}H_{64}O_{14}$	Digoxin
$C_{41}H_{65}NO_{10}$ (factor A)	Spinosad
$C_{41}H_{67}NO_{15}$	Midecamycin
$C_{41}H_{67}NO_{15}$	Troleandomycin
$C_{41}H_{67}NO_{16}$	Maridomycin
$C_{41}H_{69}NO_{14}$	Diproleandomycin

Molecular Formula	Non-proprietary Name
$C_{41}H_{71}N_3O_8$	Tildipirosin
$C_{41}H_{76}N_2O_{15}$	Roxithromycin
$C_{41}H_{79}N_3O_{12}$ (components A & B)	Tulathromycin
$C_{42}H_{30}N_6O_{12}$	Inositol Niacinate
$C_{42}H_{32}N_6O_{12}$	Sorbinicate
$C_{42}H_{45}N_3O_7$	Pamaquine Naphthoate
$C_{42}H_{53}NO_{15}$	Aclarubicin
$C_{42}H_{54}Al_2Na_8O_{38}.2H_2O$	Sodium Glucaspaldrate
$C_{42}H_{55}N_3O_{11}S$	Rifamexil
$C_{42}H_{55}N_5O_8$	Barixibat
$C_{42}H_{59}NO_{10}S$	Fuladectin Component A_4
$C_{42}H_{59}N_3O_{10}$	Cethromycin
$C_{42}H_{60}K_2O_{16}$	Glycyrrhizinate Dipotassium
$C_{42}H_{62}O_{16}$	Glycyrrhizin
$C_{42}H_{64}N_{12}O_{12}S_2$	Aspartocin
$C_{42}H_{64}O_{15}$	Gitaloxin
$C_{42}H_{65}N_{11}O_{12}$	Cargutocin
$C_{42}H_{65}N_{13}O_{10}.xC_2H_4O_2.xH_2O$	Saralasin Acetate
$C_{42}H_{66}O_{14}$	Metildigoxin
$C_{42}H_{67}NO_{10}$ (factor D)	Spinosad
$C_{42}H_{68}N_2O_2$	Mebolazine
$C_{42}H_{69}NO_{15}$	Josamycin
$C_{42}H_{69}NO_{15}$	Rokitamycin
$C_{42}H_{70}O_{11}$	Salinomycin
$C_{42}H_{70}O_{35}$	Betadex
$C_{42}H_{70}O_{35}(C_3H_6O)_x$ where $x =\ _7$ MS, MS being Molar Substitution	Hydroxypropyl Betadex
$C_{42}H_{78}N_2O_{14}$	Dirithromycin
$C_{43}H_{36}Cl_2N_8O_5$	Bizelesin
$C_{43}H_{45}ClN_4O_6$	Timcodar
$C_{43}H_{45}ClN_4O_6.2CH_4O_3S$	Timcodar Dimesylate
$C_{43}H_{47}N_2NaO_6S_2$	Indocyanine Green
$C_{43}H_{49}N_7O_{10}$	Virginiamycin Factor S
$C_{43}H_{50}Cl_2N_2O_5S$	Nolpitantium Besilate
$C_{43}H_{51}N_3O_{11}$	Rifaximin
$C_{43}H_{53}NO_{14}.3H_2O$	Docetaxel
$C_{43}H_{55}N_5O_7$	Vindesine
$C_{43}H_{55}N_5O_7.H_2SO_4$	Vindesine Sulfate
$C_{43}H_{58}N_2O_{13}$	Rifamide
$C_{43}H_{58}N_4O_{12}$	Rifampin
$C_{43}H_{62}N_4O_{23}S_3$	Paldimycin B
$C_{43}H_{63}NO_{11}$	Selamectin
$C_{43}H_{65}N_5O_{10}$	Telithromycin
$C_{43}H_{65}N_{11}O_{12}S_2$	Demoxytocin
$C_{43}H_{66}N_{12}O_{12}S_2$	Oxytocin
$C_{43}H_{66}O_{14}$	Acetyldigitoxin
$C_{43}H_{67}N_9O_{13}$	Thymoctonan
$C_{43}H_{67}N_{11}O_{12}S_2$	Atosiban
$C_{43}H_{67}N_{15}O_{12}S_2$	Argiprestocin
$C_{43}H_{68}ClNO_{11}$	Pimecrolimus
$C_{43}H_{71}O_{11}$ (narasin B)	Narasin
$C_{43}H_{72}O_{11}$ (narasin A)	Narasin
$C_{43}H_{74}N_2O_{14}$	Spiramycin
$C_{43}H_{75}NO_{16}$	Erythromycin Ethylsuccinate
$C_{43}H_{78}N_6O_{13}$	Romurtide
$C_{43}H_{90}N_2O_2$	Avridine
$C_{44}H_{32}N_4O_4$	Temoporfin
$C_{44}H_{44}CaN_2O_8S_4$	Zofenopril Calcium
$C_{44}H_{46}CaN_4O_{18}$	Oxytetracycline Calcium
$C_{44}H_{48}N_4O_{10}$	Lemuteporfin
$C_{44}H_{50}Cl_2N_4O_2$	Alcuronium Chloride
$C_{44}H_{52}N_8O_{10}$	Efepristin
$C_{44}H_{55}NO_{16}$	Milataxel
$C_{44}H_{56}N_8O_7.C_2H_4O_2$	Seglitide Acetate

Molecular Formula	Non-proprietary Name
$C_{44}H_{57}NO_{17}$	Ortataxel
$C_{44}H_{59}N_7O_5$	Iscotrizinol
$C_{44}H_{60}N_4O_{12}$	Rifametane
$C_{44}H_{64}N_4O_4$	Bisdequalinium Diacetate
$C_{44}H_{64}N_4O_{23}S_3$	Paldimycin A
$C_{44}H_{69}NO_{12}.H_2O$	Tacrolimus
$C_{44}H_{70}CaO_8$	Ciprostene Calcium
$C_{44}H_{74}O_{11}$ (narasin D)	Narasin
$C_{44}H_{74}O_{11}$ (narasin I)	Narasin
$C_{44}H_{80}N_2O_{15}.2KH_2PO_4$	Megalomicin Potassium Phosphate
$C_{44}H_{84}ClN_2O_{10}P_2{}^{99m}Tc$	Technetium Tc 99m Furifosmin
$C_{45}H_{35}F_{10}O_{20}P$	Tafluposide
$C_{45}H_{49}N_7O_{11}S$	Afeletecan
$C_{45}H_{52}O_8$	Feneritrol
$C_{45}H_{53}NO_{14}$	Larotaxel
$C_{45}H_{54}F_2N_4O_8$	Vinflunine
$C_{45}H_{54}F_2N_4O_8.2C_4H_6O_6$	Vinflunine Ditartrate
$C_{45}H_{54}N_4O_8.2C_4H_6O_6$	Vinorelbine Tartrate
$C_{45}H_{55}N_9O_6.2HCl$	Pralmorelin Dihydrochloride
$C_{45}H_{56}N_6O_{14}S$	Penimepicycline
$C_{45}H_{57}NO_{14}$	Cabazitaxel
$C_{45}H_{58}N_{10}O_{13}$	Nepadutant
$C_{45}H_{63}N_{13}O_{12}S_2$	Ornipressin
$C_{45}H_{69}N_{11}O_{12}S$	Carbetocin
$C_{45}H_{75}NaO_{16}$	Semduramicin Sodium
$C_{45}H_{76}O_{16}$	Semduramicin
$C_{45}H_{84}O_{16}$ (Approximate)	Nonoxynol 15
$C_{46}H_{50}Cl_2N_6O_2$	Ditercalinium Chloride
$C_{46}H_{52}Na_2O_{16}$	Bimosiamose Disodium
$C_{46}H_{54}N_4O_{10}$	Vinformide
$C_{46}H_{54}N_8O_{12}S_2$	Derpanicate
$C_{46}H_{54}O_{16}$	Bimosiamose
$C_{46}H_{55}CoN_8O_{10}S$	Thiamine Cobalt Chlorophyllin Complex
$C_{46}H_{56}N_4O_9.H_2SO_4$	Vinepidine Sulfate
$C_{46}H_{56}N_4O_{10}.H_2SO_4$	Vincristine Sulfate
$C_{46}H_{57}NO_{15}S$	Simotaxel
$C_{46}H_{58}ClN_5O_8$	Proglumetacin
$C_{46}H_{58}N_4O_9.H_2SO_4$	Vinblastine Sulfate
$C_{46}H_{58}N_4O_9.xH_2SO_4$	Vinrosidine Sulfate
$C_{46}H_{60}FN_3O_{13}$	Tesetaxel
$C_{46}H_{61}NO_{11}$ (component A_3)	Latidectin
$C_{46}H_{62}N_4O_{11}$	Rifabutin
$C_{46}H_{64}O_{19}$	Gitoformate
$C_{46}H_{65}N_{13}O_{11}S_2$	Felypressin
$C_{46}H_{65}N_{13}O_{12}S_2$	Lypressin
$C_{46}H_{65}N_{13}O_{12}S_2$	Vasopressin
$C_{46}H_{65}N_{15}O_{12}S_2$	Vasopressin
$C_{46}H_{71}N_9O_{14}$	Ovemotide
$C_{46}H_{71}N_{11}O_{11}S$	Nacartocin
$C_{46}H_{73}ClN_4O_9$	Minopafant
$C_{46}H_{76}O_{14}$	Peliomycin
$C_{46}H_{77}NO_{17}$	Tylosin
$C_{46}H_{80}N_2O_{13}$	Tilmicosin
$C_{46}H_{80}N_2O_{13}.H_3O_4P$	Tilmicosin Phosphate
$C_{47}H_{51}NO_{14}$	Paclitaxel
$C_{47}H_{58}N_{12}O_6$	Examorelin
$C_{47}H_{62}N_{12}O_{11}S_2$	Lodenafil Carbonate
$C_{47}H_{63}NO_{11}$ (component A_4)	Latidectin
$C_{47}H_{64}N_4O_{12}$	Rifapentine
$C_{47}H_{70}O_{14}$	Abamectin Component B_{1b}
$C_{47}H_{72}O_{14}$ (Component H_2B_{1b})	Ivermectin
$C_{47}H_{72}O_{14}$	Ivermectin Component B_{1b}
$C_{47}H_{73}NO_{17}$	Amphotericin B
$C_{47}H_{74}N_{10}O_{14}S$	Disomotide
$C_{47}H_{74}O_{19}$	Deslanoside
$C_{47}H_{75}NO_{17}$	Nystatin
$C_{47}H_{83}NO_{17}$	Maduramicin
$C_{48}H_{58}ClN_5O_9.H_2SO_4$	Vinzolidine Sulfate
$C_{48}H_{63}N_5O_9.1\frac{1}{2}H_2SO_4$	Vinglycinate Sulfate
$C_{48}H_{64}N_2O_{17}$	Rodorubicin
$C_{48}H_{67}N_5O_{10}$	Motexafin
$C_{48}H_{67}N_{13}O_{11}$	Arfalasin
$C_{48}H_{68}N_{14}O_{14}S_2.3H_2O$	Desmopressin Acetate
$C_{48}H_{72}O_{14}$	Abamectin Component B_{1a}
$C_{48}H_{73}N_{11}O_{10}S$	Ebiratide
$C_{48}H_{74}N_{12}O_{22}$	Glaspimod
$C_{48}H_{74}O_{14}$ (Component H_2B_{1a})	Ivermectin
$C_{48}H_{74}O_{14}$	Ivermectin Component B_{1a}
$C_{48}H_{76}N_2O_4S$	Chaulmosulfone
$C_{49}H_{61}N_9O_{13}$	Desglugastrin
$C_{49}H_{62}N_{10}O_{16}S_3$	Sincalide
$C_{49}H_{66}N_{10}O_{10}S_2$	Octreotide
$C_{49}H_{66}N_{10}O_{10}S_2.C_{23}H_{16}O_6$	Octreotide Pamoate
$C_{49}H_{66}N_{10}O_{10}S_2.xC_2H_4O_2$	Octreotide Acetate
$C_{49}H_{70}N_{14}O_{11}$	Angiotensin Amide
$C_{49}H_{71}N_7O_{17}$	Cilofungin
$C_{49}H_{73}NO_{14}$	Eprinomectin Component B_{1b}
$C_{49}H_{75}N_{15}O_{12}S$	Labradimil
$C_{49}H_{76}O_3$	Tretinoin Tocoferil
$C_{49}H_{76}O_{20}$	Lanatoside C
$C_{50}H_{40}O_7$	Benzquercin
$C_{50}H_{44}N_6O_{13}\,[C_2H_4O]_n$	Pegamotecan
$C_{50}H_{60}Br_4N_6O_6S_2$	Cistinexine
$C_{50}H_{60}N_6O_{16}$	Etamocycline
$C_{50}H_{63}N_9O_{10}$	Linopristin
$C_{50}H_{68}N_{14}O_{10}$	Bremelanotide
$C_{50}H_{71}N_{13}O_{12}$	Angiotensin II
$C_{50}H_{74}O_{14}$	Doramectin
$C_{50}H_{75}NO_{14}$	Eprinomectin Component B_{1a}
$C_{50}H_{75}N_9O_8$	Ditekiren
$C_{50}H_{78}CaO_{12}$	Tenivastatin Calcium
$C_{51}H_{34}N_6Na_6O_{23}S_6$	Suramin Hexasodium
$C_{51}H_{43}N_{13}O_{12}S_6$	Nosiheptide
$C_{51}H_{57}NO_{18}$	Paclitaxel Ceribate
$C_{51}H_{63}N_3O_{11}S$	Fluorescein Lisicol
$C_{51}H_{64}N_4O_{13}$	Rifalazil
$C_{51}H_{69}N_5O_9$	Vinleucinol
$C_{51}H_{72}N_5O_{10}P$	Vinfosiltine
$C_{51}H_{73}N_{17}NaO_{20}S_5{}^{99m}Tc$	Technetium Tc 99m Apcitide
$C_{51}H_{74}O_{19}$	Pengitoxin
$C_{51}H_{79}NO_{13}$	Sirolimus
$C_{51}H_{98}O_6$	Tripalmitin
$(C_{52}H_{56}N_2O_{16})_n.(C_5H_7NO_3)_x$	Paclitaxel Poliglumex
$C_{52}H_{72}GdN_5O_{14}.xH_2O$ (where x is typically between $_0$ and $_2$)	Motexafin Gadolinium
$C_{52}H_{72}LuN_5O_{14}.xH_2O$ (where x is typically between $_0$ and $_2$)	Motexafin Lutetium
$C_{52}H_{74}Cl_2O_{18}$	Fidaxomicin
$C_{52}H_{74}N_{16}O_{15}S_2$	Terlipressin
$C_{52}H_{76}O_{24}$	Plicamycin
$C_{52}H_{79}N_5O_{12}$	Zotarolimus
$C_{52}H_{86}CaO_{18}.2H_2O$	Mupirocin Calcium
$C_{52}H_{88}N_{10}O_{15}$	Caspofungin
$C_{52}H_{88}N_{10}O_{15}.2C_2H_4O_2$	Caspofungin Acetate
$C_{52}H_{100}N_2O_{20}P_2$	Defoslimod
$C_{53}H_{67}N_9O_{10}S$	Quinupristin
$C_{53}H_{69}Cl_3N_2O_{14}$	Gantacurium Chloride
$C_{53}H_{76}N_{14}O_{12}$	Teprotide

Molecular Formula	Non-proprietary Name
$C_{53}H_{79}N_4Na_9O_{51}S_8$	Idrabiotaparinux Sodium
$C_{53}H_{83}NO_{14}$	Everolimus
$C_{53}H_{84}NO_{14}P$	Deforolimus
$C_{53}H_{87}NO_{19}$	Tylvalosin
$C_{53}H_{87}NO_{19}.xC_4H_6O_6$	Tylvalosin Tartrate
$C_{54}H_{69}N_{11}O_{10}S_2.x(C_2H_4O_2)$	Lanreotide Acetate
$C_{54}H_{80}N_2O_{16}S_2$	Laudexium Methylsulfate
$C_{54}H_{85}N_{13}O_{15}S$	Eledoisin
$C_{55}H_{57.6}N_5Na_{1.4}O_{20}$	Coumermycin Sodium
$C_{55}H_{59}N_5O_{20}$	Coumermycin
$C_{55}H_{75}N_{17}O_{13}.2HCl$	Gonadorelin Hydrochloride
$C_{55}H_{75}N_{17}O_{13}.xC_2H_4O_2.yH_2O$	Gonadorelin Acetate
$C_{55}H_{76}N_{16}O_{12}.C_2H_4O_2$	Fertirelin Acetate
$C_{55}H_{103}N_3O_{17}$	Primycin
$C_{56}H_{68}N_6O_9$	Vintriptol
$C_{56}H_{70}N_9NaO_{23}S$	Micafungin Sodium
$C_{56}H_{78}Cl_2N_2O_{16}$	Doxacurium Chloride
$C_{56}H_{87}NO_{16}$	Temsirolimus
$C_{57}H_{70}N_{12}O_9S_2$	Vapreotide
$C_{57}H_{82}O_{26}$	Chromomycin A_3
$C_{57}H_{87}N_7O_{15}$	Plitidepsin
$C_{57}H_{103}N_{16}Na_5O_{28}S_5$ (colistin B component)	Colistimethate Sodium
$C_{58}H_{66}N_{10}O_9$	Pasireotide
$C_{58}H_{73}N_7O_{17}$	Anidulafungin
$C_{58}H_{73}N_{13}O_{21}S_2$	Ceruletide
$C_{58}H_{73}N_{13}O_{21}S_2.xC_4H_{11}N$	Ceruletide Diethylamine
$C_{58}H_{80}Cl_2N_2O_{14}$	Mivacurium Chloride
$C_{58}H_{105}N_{16}Na_5O_{28}S_5$ (colistin A component)	Colistimethate Sodium
$C_{58}H_{114}O_{26}$ (Approximate)	Polysorbate 20
$C_{59}H_{74}N_{18}O_{14}$	Peforelin
$C_{59}H_{79}N_{15}O_{21}S_6$	Linaclotide
$C_{59}H_{79}N_{15}O_{21}S_6.C_2H_4O_2$	Linaclotide Acetate
$C_{59}H_{84}N_{16}O_{12}.(C_2H_4O_2)_n$ $n = 1$ or 2	Leuprolide Acetate
$C_{59}H_{84}N_{18}O_{14}$	Goserelin
$C_{59}H_{88}N_2O_{20}$	Efrotomycin
$C_{59}H_{89}N_{19}O_{13}S.xC_2H_4O_2$	Icatibant Acetate
$C_{59}H_{90}O_4$	Ubidecarenone
$C_{59}H_{103}N_3O_{18}$	Scopafungin
$C_{59}H_{105}N_{17}O_{11}.C_2H_4O_2$	Delmitide Acetate
$C_{59}H_{108}N_6NaO_{19}P.xH_2O$	Mifamurtide
$C_{60}H_{86}N_{16}O_{13}.C_2H_4O_2$	Buserelin Acetate
$C_{60}H_{90}N_6O_{14}$	Emodepside
$C_{60}H_{92}N_8O_{11}$	Basifungin
$C_{60}H_{92}N_{12}O_{10}$	Gramicidin S
$C_{60}H_{108}O_8$ (Approximate)	Sorbitan Trioleate
$C_{60}H_{114}O_8$ (Approximate)	Sorbitan Tristearate
$C_{61}H_{86}N_{10}O_{20}S_2$	Ilatreotide
$C_{61}H_{88}Cl_2O_{32}$ (Avilamycin A)	Avilamycin
$C_{61}H_{88}N_{18}O_{21}S_2.H_2SO_4$	Peplomycin Sulfate
$C_{61}H_{103}N_{16}Na_5O_{28}S_5$ (major component)	Sulfomyxin
$C_{62}H_{70}CaN_4O_{22}$	Novobiocin Calcium
$C_{62}H_{78}N_8O_{20}S_2$	Pantenicate
$C_{62}H_{86}N_{12}O_{16}$	Dactinomycin
$C_{62}H_{89}CoN_{13}O_{15}P$	Hydroxocobalamin
$C_{62}H_{111}N_{11}O_{12}$	Cyclosporine
$C_{62}H_{122}O_{26}$ (Approximate)	Polysorbate 40
$C_{63}H_{84}{}^{111}InN_{13}O_{19}S_2$	Indium In 111 Pentetreotide
$C_{63}H_{87}N_{13}O_{19}S_2$	Pentetreotide
$C_{63}H_{88}CoN_{14}O_{14}P$	Cyanocobalamin
$C_{63}H_{88}{}^{57}CoN_{14}O_{14}P$	Cyanocobalamin Co 57
$C_{63}H_{88}CoN_{14}O_{14}P$	Cyanocobalamin Co 58
$C_{63}H_{88}{}^{60}CoN_{14}O_{14}P$	Cyanocobalamin Co 60

Molecular Formula	Non-proprietary Name
$C_{63}H_{91}CoN_{13}O_{14}P$	Mecobalamin
$C_{63}H_{111}N_{11}O_{12}$	Valspodar
$C_{63}H_{111}N_{11}O_{12}$	Voclosporin
$C_{63}H_{113}N_{11}O_{12}$	Geclosporin
$C_{64}H_{82}N_{18}O_{13}$	Triptorelin
$C_{64}H_{82}N_{18}O_{13}.C_{23}H_{16}O_6$	Triptorelin Pamoate
$C_{64}H_{83}N_{17}O_{12}$	Deslorelin
$C_{64}H_{115}N_{11}O_{14}$	Oxeclosporin
$C_{64}H_{126}O_{26}$ (Approximate)	Polysorbate 60
$C_{65}H_{82}N_2O_{18}S_2$	Atracurium Besylate
$C_{65}H_{82}N_2O_{18}S_2$	Cisatracurium Besylate
$C_{65}H_{85}N_{17}O_{12}$	Avorelin
$C_{65}H_{85}N_{17}O_{12}.C_2H_4O_2$	Lutrelin Acetate
$C_{65}H_{92}N_{14}O_{18}S_2$	Edotreotide
$C_{65}H_{95}NO_{21}$ [empirical molecular formula]	Ganefromycin
$C_{65}H_{96}N_{16}O_{12}S_2$	Depreotide
$C_{66}H_{68}CaF_2N_4O_{10}$	Atorvastatin Calcium
$C_{66}H_{75}Cl_2N_9O_{24}$	Vancomycin
$C_{66}H_{75}Cl_2N_9O_{24}.HCl$	Vancomycin Hydrochloride
$C_{66}H_{83}N_{17}O_{13}.xC_2H_4O_2.yH_2O$	Nafarelin Acetate
$C_{66}H_{86}N_{18}O_{12}$	Histrelin
$C_{66}H_{122}N_2Na_4O_{19}P_2$	Eritoran Tetrasodium
$C_{68}H_{79}NO_{11}$	Cofisatin
$C_{68}H_{106}O_{12}$	Digalloyl Trioleate
$C_{68}H_{109}N_{17}O_{22}S_2$	Disitertide
$C_{68}H_{110}N_{22}O_{27}S_2$	Talisomycin
$C_{70}H_{92}ClN_{17}O_{14}$	Cetrorelix
$C_{70}H_{92}ClN_{17}O_{14}.xC_2H_4O_2$	Cetrorelix Acetate
$C_{70}H_{97}Cl_2NO_{38}$	Evernimicin
$C_{72-89}H_{68-99}Cl_2N_{8-9}O_{28-33}$	Teicoplanin
$C_{72}H_{68}Cl_2N_8O_{28}$	Teicoplanin A_{3-1}
$C_{72}H_{85}N_{19}O_{18}S_5$	Thiostrepton
$C_{72}H_{95}ClN_{14}O_{14}$	Abarelix
$C_{72}H_{96}ClN_{17}O_{14}$	Ozarelix
$C_{72}H_{100}CoN_{18}O_{17}P$	Cobamamide
$C_{72}H_{101}N_{17}O_{26}$	Daptomycin
$C_{72}H_{104}Na_8O_{48}S_8$	Sugammadex Sodium
$C_{72}H_{116}O_4$	Xantofyl Palmitate
$C_{73}H_{89}ClN_{10}O_{26}$ (Orienticine A)	Orientiparcin
$C_{73}H_{97}IN_6O_{25}S_3$	Ozogamicin
$C_{73}H_{129}N_3O_{30}$	Siagoside
$C_{74}H_{91}ClN_{10}O_{26}$ (Orienticine D)	Orientiparcin
$C_{74}H_{95}ClN_{16}O_{18}$	Ramorelix
$C_{74}H_{100}ClN_{15}O_{14}$	Teverelix
$C_{75}H_{70}N_6O_6$	Pyrvinium Pamoate
$C_{75}H_{106}N_{20}O_{19}S$	Tridecactide
$C_{75}H_{144}O_{31}$ (Approximate)	Nonoxynol 30
$C_{76}H_{104}N_{18}O_{19}S_2$	Somatostatin
$C_{76}H_{137}N_3O_{31}$	Mipragoside
$C_{78}H_{105}ClN_{18}O_{13}.2C_2H_4O_2$	Detirelix Acetate
$C_{78}H_{126}N_{30}O_{18}S_4.xHCl.yH_2O$	Iseganan Hydrochloride
$C_{80}H_{102}ClN_{23}O_{12}$	Prazarelix
$C_{80}H_{102}ClN_{23}O_{12}.C_2H_4O_2$	Prazarelix Acetate
$C_{80}H_{106}Cl_2N_{11}O_{27}P.HCl$	Telavancin Hydrochloride
$C_{80}H_{113}ClN_{18}O_{13}.2C_2H_4O_2$	Ganirelix Acetate
$C_{81}H_{82}Cl_4N_8O_{30}$ (aridicin A)	Ardacin
$C_{82}H_{84}Cl_4N_8O_{30}$ (aridicin B)	Ardacin
$C_{82}H_{103}ClN_{18}O_{16}$	Degarelix
$C_{82}H_{103}ClN_{18}O_{16}.xC_2H_4O_2.nH_2O$	Degarelix Acetate
$C_{82}H_{108}ClN_{17}O_{14}$	Iturelix
$C_{82}H_{119}N_{21}O_{34}S_3.C_2HF_3O_2$	Tigapotide Triflutate
$C_{83}H_{86}Cl_4N_8O_{30}$ (aridicin C)	Ardacin
$C_{83}H_{86}Cl_4N_8O_{30}$ (aridicin C_2)	Ardacin
$C_{85}H_{146}N_{26}O_{21}$	Tertomotide
$C_{86}H_{97}Cl_3N_{10}O_{26}$	Oritavancin

Molecular Formula	Non-proprietary Name
$C_{86}H_{97}Cl_3N_{10}O_{26}.2H_3PO_4$	Oritavancin Diphosphate
$C_{86}H_{135}N_{20}O_{19}{}^+$	Atilmotin
$C_{87}H_{143}N_{25}O_{20}$	Tiplimotide
$C_{88}H_{95}Cl_2N_9O_{33}$	Teicoplanin A_{2-1}
$C_{88}H_{97}Cl_2N_9O_{33}$	Teicoplanin A_{2-2}
$C_{88}H_{97}Cl_2N_9O_{33}$	Teicoplanin A_{2-3}
$C_{88}H_{100}Cl_2N_{10}O_{28}$	Dalbavancin
$C_{89}H_{99}Cl_2N_9O_{33}$	Teicoplanin A_{2-4}
$C_{89}H_{99}Cl_2N_9O_{33}$	Teicoplanin A_{2-5}
$C_{89}H_{125}N_{23}O_{25}S_3$	Lancovutide
$C_{90}H_{127}N_{27}O_{12}.5HCl$	Omiganan Pentahydrochloride
$C_{92}H_{141}N_{25}O_{26}$	Dirucotide
$C_{92}H_{141}N_{25}O_{26}.4C_2H_4O_2$	Dirucotide Acetate
$C_{93}H_{109}Cl_2N_{11}O_{32}$	Mideplanin
$(C_{97}H_{147}N_{29}O_{35}S)_3.(C_2H_4O_2)_2$	Rusalatide Acetate
$C_{98}H_{138}N_{24}O_{33}$	Bivalirudin
$C_{99}H_{155}N_{29}O_{21}S$	Alsactide
$C_{100}H_{156}N_{34}O_{22}S$	Giractide
$C_{100}H_{188}O_{28}$ (Approximate)	Polysorbate 85
$C_{100}H_{194}O_{28}$ (Approximate)	Polysorbate 65
$C_{101}H_{158}N_{30}O_{23}S$	Codactide
$C_{102}H_{172}N_{36}O_{32}S_7$	Ziconotide
$(C_{103}H_{217}N_3F_{36}O_{49}Si_{27})_a$ $(C_5H_9NO)_b(C_{16}H_{38}O_5Si_4)_c$ $(C_8H_8)_d$	Sifilcon A
$(C_{103}H_{217}N_3F_{36}O_{49}Si_{27})_x$ $(C_5H_9NO)_y(C_{16}H_{38}O_5Si_4)_z$	Lotrafilcon A
$(C_{103}H_{217}N_3F_{36}O_{49}Si_{27})_x$ $(C_5H_9NO)_y(C_{16}H_{38}O_5Si_4)_z$	Lotrafilcon B
$C_{107}H_{179}N_{35}O_{36}S_7$	Leconotide
$C_{111}H_{149}N_{27}O_{28}$	Edratide
$C_{112}H_{142}ClN_{21}O_{35}$	Ramoplanin A'_1
$C_{112}H_{162}N_{36}O_{43}S_{10}$	Bibapcitide
$C_{112}H_{175}N_{39}O_{35}S_3.xC_2H_4O_2$	Anaritide Acetate
$C_{113}H_{144}ClN_{21}O_{35}$	Ramoplanin A'_2
$C_{114}H_{146}ClN_{21}O_{35}$	Ramoplanin A'_3
$C_{118}H_{152}ClN_{21}O_{40}$	Ramoplanin A_1
$C_{119}H_{154}ClN_{21}O_{40}$	Ramoplanin A_2 (Main Component)
$C_{120}H_{156}ClN_{21}O_{40}$	Ramoplanin A_3
$C_{122}H_{172}N_{22}O_{40}$ (Nominal)	Colimecycline
$C_{122}H_{210}N_{32}O_{22}$	Pexiganan
$C_{122}H_{210}N_{32}O_{22}.xC_2H_4O_2$	Pexiganan Acetate
$C_{126}H_{238}N_{26}O_{22}$	Sinapultide
$C_{127}H_{203}N_{45}O_{39}S_3$	Carperitide
$C_{128}H_{194}N_{40}O_{28}S_2$	Deltibant
$C_{129}H_{215}N_{33}O_{55}$	Thymalfasin
$C_{130}H_{220}N_{44}O_{40}$ (human)	Secretin
$C_{130}H_{220}N_{44}O_{41}$ (porcine)	Secretin
$C_{131}H_{204}N_{40}O_{29}S$	Tricosactide
$C_{136}H_{210}N_{40}O_{31}S$	Cosyntropin
$C_{142}H_{222}N_{42}O_{31}$	Norleusactide
$C_{143}H_{244}N_{50}O_{42}S_4$	Nesiritide
$C_{143}H_{244}N_{50}O_{42}S_4.xC_6H_8O_7$	Nesiritide Citrate
$C_{145}H_{234}N_{52}O_{44}S_3$	Ularitide
$C_{145}H_{240}N_{44}O_{48}S_2$(salmon); $C_{151}H_{226}N_{40}O_{45}S_3$(human)	Calcitonin
$C_{147}H_{238}N_{44}O_{42}S$	Aviptadil
$C_{147}H_{243}N_{41}O_{46}$	Avicatonin
$C_{148}H_{244}N_{42}O_{47}$	Elcatonin
$C_{149}H_{246}N_{44}O_{42}S.xC_2H_4O_2.$ yH_2O	Sermorelin Acetate
$C_{150}H_{230}N_{44}O_{38}S$	Tosactide
$C_{152}H_{232}N_{40}O_{45}$	Taspoglutide
$C_{153}H_{225}N_{43}O_{49}S$	Glucagon
$C_{164}H_{252}N_{44}O_{55}S$	Teduglutide

Molecular Formula	Non-proprietary Name
$C_{165}H_{261}N_{51}O_{55}S_2$	Amlintide
$C_{171}H_{267}N_{51}O_{53}S_2$	Pramlintide
$C_{171}H_{267}N_{51}O_{53}S_2.xC_2H_4O_2.y$ H_2O (x and y are variable)	Pramlintide Acetate
$C_{172}H_{204}N_{62}Na_{17}O_{91}P_{17}S_{17}$	Oblimersen Sodium
$C_{172}H_{265}N_{43}O_{51}$	Liraglutide
$C_{175}H_{300}N_{56}O_{51}$	Semparatide
$C_{175}H_{300}N_{56}O_{51}.xC_2H_4O_2.yH_2O$	Semparatide Acetate
$C_{177}H_{225}N_{60}O_{94}P_{17}S_{17}$	Trabedersen
$C_{181}H_{291}N_{55}O_{51}S_2$	Teriparatide
$C_{181}H_{291}N_{55}O_{51}S_2.xH_2O.$ $yC_2H_4O_2$	Teriparatide Acetate
$C_{182}H_{310}N_{40}O_{35}$	Lusupultide
$C_{184}H_{282}N_{50}O_{60}S$	Exenatide
$C_{185}H_{288}N_{54}O_{55}S_2$	Obinepitide
$C_{187}H_{226}N_{62}Na_{19}O_{103}P_{19}S_{19}$	Cenersen Sodium
$C_{192}H_{225}N_{75}Na_{19}O_{98}P_{19}S_{19}$	Alicaforsen Sodium
$C_{192}H_{231}N_{57}Na_{19}O_{107}P_{19}S_{19}$	Afovirsen Sodium
$C_{196}H_{230}N_{68}Na_{19}O_{105}P_{19}S_{19}$	Aprinocarsen Sodium
$C_{204}H_{243}N_{63}Na_{20}O_{114}P_{20}S_{20}$	Fomivirsen Sodium
$C_{204}H_{301}N_{51}O_{64}$	Enfuvirtide
$C_{205}H_{339}N_{59}O_{63}S$ (ovine)	Corticorelin
$C_{205}H_{339}N_{59}O_{63}S.xC_2HF_3O_2.$	Corticorelin Ovine Triflutate
$C_{207}H_{308}N_{56}O_{58}S.(C_2H_4O_2)_x.$ xH_2O	Seractide Acetate
$C_{208}H_{344}N_{60}O_{63}S_2$ (human)	Corticorelin
$C_{208}H_{344}N_{60}O_{63}S_2$	Corticorelin Acetate
$C_{215}H_{347}N_{61}O_{65}S$	Lixisenatide
$C_{215}H_{358}N_{72}O_{66}S$	Somatorelin
$C_{218}H_{362}N_{72}O_{68}$	Dumorelin
$C_{221}H_{366}N_{72}O_{67}S$	Tesamorelin
$C_{221}H_{366}N_{72}O_{67}S.xC_2H_4O_2$	Tesamorelin Acetate
$C_{228}H_{313}Br_{12}GdN_{32}O_{116}$	Gadomelitol
$C_{230}H_{305}N_{67}Na_{19}O_{122}P_{19}S_{19}$	Mipomersen Sodium
$C_{231}H_{292}N_{78}Na_{20}O_{119}P_{20}S_{20}$	Custirsen Sodium
$C_{235}H_{341}N_{57}O_{67}$	Tifuvirtide
$C_{236}H_{303}N_{70}O_{133}P_{23}S_{23}$	Agatolimod
$C_{236}H_{303}N_{70}O_{133}P_{23}S_{23}Na_{23}$	Agatolimod Sodium
$C_{237}H_{286}N_{72}Na_{24}O_{131}P_{24}S_{24}$	Trecovirsen Sodium
$C_{245}H_{368}N_{64}O_{74}S_6$ (bovine)	Insulin Defalan
$C_{247}H_{372}N_{64}O_{75}S_6$ (porcine)	Insulin Defalan
$C_{254}H_{377}N_{65}O_{75}S_6$ (Insulin ox)	Insulin
$C_{256}H_{322}N_{95}O_{129}P_{25}S_{25}$	Litenimod
$C_{256}H_{361}N_{65}O_{73}S_6$	Insulin, Neutral [Injection] of Purified Porcine
$C_{256}H_{381}N_{65}O_{76}S_6$ (Insulin pig)	Insulin
$C_{256}H_{381}N_{65}O_{79}S_6$	Insulin Aspart
$C_{257}H_{375}N_{73}O_{83}S_7$	Murodermin
$C_{257}H_{383}N_{65}O_{77}S_6$	Insulin Human
$C_{257}H_{383}N_{65}O_{77}S_6$	Insulin Lispro
$C_{258}H_{384}N_{64}O_{78}S_6$	Insulin Glulisine
$C_{264}H_{350}K_{12}N_{48}O_{61}S_{12}$	Benpenolisin
$C_{267}H_{402}N_{64}O_{76}S_6$	Insulin Detemir
$C_{267}H_{404}N_{72}O_{78}S_6$	Insulin Glargine
$C_{269}H_{407}N_{73}O_{79}S_6$	Insulin Argine
$C_{270}H_{401}N_{73}O_{83}S_7$	Nepidermin
$C_{272}H_{318}N_{106}Na_{26}O_{138}P_{26}S_{26}$	Edifoligide Sodium
$C_{282}H_{412}N_{74}O_{75}S_6$	Depelestat
$C_{284}H_{432}N_{84}O_{79}S_7$	Aprotinin
$C_{287}H_{440}N_{80}O_{110}S_6$	Desirudin
$C_{287}H_{440}N_{80}O_{111}S_6$	Lepirudin
$C_{294}H_{342}F_{13}N_{107}Na_{28}O_{188}P_{28}$ $[C_2H_4O]_n$	Pegaptanib Sodium
$C_{305}H_{442}N_{88}O_{91}S_8$	Ecallantide
$C_{325}H_{557}N_{97}O_{95}S_6$	Garnocestim
$C_{331}H_{512}N_{94}O_{101}S_7$	Mecasermin

Molecular Formula	*Non-proprietary Name*
$C_{338}H_{516}N_{88}O_{108}S_4$	Nagrestipen
$C_{346}H_{585}N_{97}O_{102}S_5$	Iroplact
$C_{372}H_{600}N_{106}O_{106}S_4$	Emoctakin
$C_{379}H_{623}N_{127}O_{118}$	Rismorelin Porcine
$C_{380}H_{612}N_{112}O_{112}S_9$	Mirostipen
$C_{401}H_{463}N_{153}Na_{40}O_{290}P_{40}$	Bevasiranib Sodium
$C_{408}H_{674}N_{126}O_{126}S_2$	Parathyroid Hormone
$C_{410}H_{638}N_{114}O_{127}S_6$	Proinsulin Human
$C_{437}H_{682}N_{122}O_{134}S_{13}$ (α-subunit)	Follitropin Alfa
$C_{437}H_{682}N_{122}O_{134}S_{13}$ (α-subunit)	Follitropin Beta
$C_{437}H_{682}N_{122}O_{134}S_{13}$ (α-subunit)	Lutropin Alfa
$C_{437}H_{682}N_{122}O_{134}S_{13}$ (α-subunit)	Thyrotropin Alfa
$C_{437}H_{682}N_{122}O_{134}S_{13}$ (α-subunit); $C_{668}H_{1090}N_{196}O_{203}S_{13}$ (β-subunit)	Choriogonadotropin Alfa
$C_{502}H_{758}N_{154}O_{165}S_{16}$	Pegsunercept
$C_{520}H_{810}N_{142}O_{155}S_9$	Ranpirnase
$C_{538}H_{833}N_{145}O_{171}S_{13}$ (β-subunit)	Follitropin Alfa
$C_{538}H_{833}N_{145}O_{171}S_{13}$ (β-subunit)	Follitropin Beta
$C_{561}H_{887}N_{169}O_{136}S_4$	Rolipoltide
$C_{564}H_{909}N_{161}O_{166}S_5$	Daniplestim
$C_{577}H_{929}N_{165}O_{161}S_{14}$ (β-subunit)	Lutropin Alfa
$C_{585}H_{927}Gd_{24}N_{165}O_{213}$	Gadodenterate
$C_{587}H_{947}N_{177}S_{10}$	Abrineurin
$C_{602}H_{920}N_{152}O_{173}S_{14}$ (β-subunit)	Thyrotropin Alfa
$C_{637}H_{1003}N_{171}O_{187}S_8$ (protein moiety reduced)	Regramostim
$C_{639}H_{1002}N_{168}O_{196}S_8$ (protein moiety)	Sargramostim
$C_{639}H_{1007}N_{171}O_{196}S_8$ (protein moiety)	Molgramostim
$C_{651}H_{1054}N_{190}O_{200}S_8$	Pitrakinra
$C_{670}H_{1074}N_{186}O_{199}S_5$	Muplestim
$C_{676}H_{1087}N_{205}O_{203}S_8$	Denenicokin
$C_{679}H_{1083}N_{203}O_{224}S_4$	Ledismase
$C_{681}H_{1087}N_{203}O_{225}S_4$	Sudismase
$[C_{683}H_{1061}N_{197}O_{208}S_{10}]_2$	Eptotermin Alfa
$C_{685}H_{1071}N_{187}O_{194}S_3$ (αHb)	Hemoglobin Glutamer-256 (Human)
$C_{690}H_{1115}N_{177}O_{203}S_6$	Aldesleukin
$C_{693}H_{1118}N_{178}O_{203}S_7$	Celmoleukin
$C_{695}H_{1124}N_{180}O_{202}S_7$ (peptide)	Adargileukin Alfa
$C_{698}H_{1127}N_{179}O_{204}S_8$	Teceleukin
$C_{714}H_{1167}N_{191}O_{221}S_6$	Metreleptin
$C_{723}H_{1131}N_{209}O_{204}S_5$	Repifermin
$C_{724}H_{1119}N_{195}O_{201}S_3$ (βHb)	Hemoglobin Glutamer-256 (Human)
$C_{729}H_{1156}N_{204}O_{207}S_{10}$	Palifermin
$C_{734}H_{1166}N_{204}O_{216}S_5$	Interferon Gamma-1b
$C_{753}H_{1156}N_{228}O_{247}S_{25}$	Onercept
$C_{759}H_{1186}N_{208}O_{232}S_{10}$	Anakinra
$C_{761}H_{1206}N_{214}O_{225}S_6$	Interferon Gamma-1a
$C_{764}H_{1201}N_{217}O_{219}S_6$	Trafermin
$C_{767}H_{1204}N_{210}O_{229}S_2$	Sonermin
$C_{770}H_{1207}N_{193}O_{232}S_5$ (reduced protein)	Ardenermin
$C_{773}H_{1219}N_{201}O_{238}S_7$	Mobenakin
$C_{775}H_{1220}N_{220}O_{223}S_7$	Ersofermin
$C_{778}H_{1225}N_{215}O_{231}S_2$	Tasonermin
$C_{781}H_{1230}N_{216}O_{237}S_6$ (protein)	Tadekinig Alfa
$C_{800}H_{1300}N_{228}O_{24}S_5$	Darbepoetin Alfa
$C_{801}H_{1264}N_{212}O_{252}S_{10}$	Iboctadekin
$C_{809}H_{1301}N_{229}O_{240}S_5$ (amino acid sequence)	Epoetin Alfa
$C_{809}H_{1301}N_{229}O_{240}S_5$ (amino acid sequence)	Epoetin Beta
$C_{809}H_{1301}N_{229}O_{240}S_5$ (for non-glycosylated protein)	Epoetin Gamma
$C_{809}H_{1301}N_{229}O_{240}S_5$	Epoetin Delta
$C_{809}H_{1301}N_{229}O_{240}S_5$	Epoetin Epsilon
$C_{809}H_{1301}N_{229}O_{240}S_5$	Epoetin Kappa
$C_{809}H_{1301}N_{229}O_{240}S_5$	Epoetin Omega
$C_{809}H_{1301}N_{229}O_{240}S_5$	Epoetin Theta
$C_{809}H_{1301}N_{229}O_{240}S_5$	Epoetin Zeta
$C_{845}H_{1339}N_{223}O_{243}S_9$	Filgrastim
$C_{849}H_{1347}N_{223}O_{244}S_9 \cdot (C_2H_4O)_n$	Pegfilgrastim
$C_{850}H_{1344}N_{226}O_{245}S_8$ (for non-glycosylated protein)	Nartograstim
$C_{854}H_{1411}N_{253}O_{235}S_2$	Oprelvekin
$C_{858}H_{1259}N_{221}O_{289}S_{10}$	Votucalis
$C_{860}H_{1353}N_{227}O_{255}S_9$	Interferon Alfa-2a
$C_{860}H_{1353}N_{229}O_{255}S_9$	Interferon Alfa-2b
$C_{870}H_{1366}N_{236}O_{259}S_9$	Interferon Alfacon-1
$C_{871}H_{1329}N_{243}O_{260}S_4$	Dulanermin
$C_{903}H_{1399}N_{245}O_{252}S_5$	Interferon Beta-1b
$C_{908}H_{1406}N_{246}O_{252}S_7$ (protein moiety)	Interferon Beta-1a
$C_{917}H_{1483}N_{255}O_{288}S_9$	Atexakin Alfa
$C_{938}H_{1465}N_{257}O_{278}S_6$	Somfasepor
$C_{938}H_{1469}N_{255}O_{275}S_7$	Somenopor
$C_{945}H_{1482}N_{266}O_{278}S_3$	Dapiclermin
$C_{952}H_{1524}N_{266}O_{290}S_8$	Somatosalm
$C_{976}H_{1533}N_{265}O_{286}S_8$	Somavubove
$C_{977}H_{1527}N_{265}O_{287}S_7$	Somalapor
$C_{978}H_{1537}N_{265}O_{286}S_9$	Sometribove
$C_{979}H_{1527}N_{265}O_{287}S_8$	Sometripor
$C_{985}H_{1541}N_{285}O_{301}S_{12}$	Alfimeprase
$C_{987}H_{1550}N_{268}O_{291}S_9$	Somagrebove
$C_{990}H_{1528}N_{262}O_{300}S_7$	Somatropin
$C_{995}H_{1537}N_{263}O_{301}S_8$	Somatrem
$C_{1020}H_{1596}N_{274}O_{302}S_9$	Somidobove
$C_{1039}H_{1602}N_{274}O_{307}S_{27}$	Thyrotropin Alfa
$C_{1047}H_{1632}N_{306}O_{302}S_5$	Velafermin
$C_{1054}H_{1635}N_{293}O_{312}S_{16}$	Mirococept
$C_{1058}H_{1651}N_{277}O_{341}S_{14}$ (for non-glycosylated protein)	Mirimostim
$C_{1100}H_{1673}N_{271}O_{337}S_{10}$	Bifarcept
$C_{1128}H_{1702}N_{296}O_{336}S_{20}$	Avotermin
$C_{1132}H_{1716}N_{298}O_{330}S_{20}$	Cetermin
$C_{1170}H_{1764}N_{300}O_{387}S_{14}$	Eufauserase
$C_{1184}H_{1844}N_{330}O_{350}S_{22}$	Radotermin
$C_{1231}H_{1967}N_{371}O_{384}S_{20}$	Mecasermin Rinfabate
$C_{1244}H_{1947}N_{347}O_{418}S$ (protease)	Liprotamase
$C_{1251}H_{1956}N_{346}O_{374}S_5$ (A); $C_{1255}H_{1983}N_{363}O_{394}S_{15}$ (B)	Aviscumine
$C_{1290}H_{2210}N_{420}O_{394}S_{18}$	Liatermin
$C_{1317}H_{2043}N_{361}O_{395}S_9$ (monomer)	Romiplostim
$C_{1321}H_{1995}N_{339}O_{396}S_9$ (protein moiety)	Dornase Alfa
$C_{1336}H_{2116}N_{362}O_{410}S_{13}$	Milodistim
$C_{1400}H_{2167}N_{395}O_{422}S_{23}$	Tifacogin
$C_{1465}H_{2300}N_{402}O_{468}S_3$ (lipase)	Liprotamase
$C_{1511}H_{2342}N_{418}O_{436}S_{15}$	Thrombin Alfa
$C_{1523}H_{2383}N_{417}O_{462}S_7$ (monomer)	Rasburicase
$C_{1549}H_{2430}N_{408}O_{448}S_8$ (peptide monomer)	Pegloticase
$C_{1550}H_{2463}N_{425}O_{462}S_{12}$	Leridistim
$C_{1612}H_{2568}N_{500}O_{498}S_{44}$	Telbermin
$C_{1632}H_{1944}N_{610}Na_{156}O_{970}P_{156}S_4$	Abetimus Sodium
$C_{1632}H_{2100}N_{610}O_{970}P_{156}S_4$	Abetimus

Molecular Formula	Non-proprietary Name
$C_{1662}H_{2650}N_{422}O_{512}S_{18}$	Ancestim
$C_{1736}H_{2653}N_{499}O_{522}S_{22}$	Reteplase
$C_{1827}H_{2785}N_{493}O_{530}S_{11}$	Ismomultin Alfa
$C_{1950}H_{3157}N_{543}O_{599}S_{7}$ (monomer)	Glucarpidase
$(C_{1965}H_{3080}N_{479}O_{695}S_{16})$	Abatacept
$C_{1981}H_{3051}N_{561}O_{620}S_{27}$	Vatreptacog Alfa (activated)
$C_{1982}H_{3054}N_{560}O_{618}S_{28}$	Eptacog Alfa
$C_{1993}H_{3112}N_{562}O_{624}S_{34}$	Lenercept
$C_{2000}H_{3059}N_{559}O_{610}S_{31}$ (plus approximately 20% by weight Asn-linked carbohydrate)	Drotrecogin Alfa (activated)
$C_{2016}H_{3107}N_{545}O_{586}S_{14}$	Epafipase
$C_{2029}H_{3080}N_{544}O_{587}S_{27}$ (subunit protein moiety reduced)	Agalsidase Alfa
$C_{2029}H_{3080}N_{544}O_{587}S_{27}$ (subunit protein moiety reduced)	Agalsidase Beta
$C_{2031}H_{3121}N_{585}O_{601}S_{31}$ (amino acid sequence)	Nasaruplase Beta
$C_{2031}H_{3121}N_{585}O_{601}S_{31}$	Nasaruplase
$C_{2031}H_{3121}N_{585}O_{601}S_{31}$	Saruplase
$C_{2107}H_{3252}N_{562}O_{673}S_{12}$	Tadocizumab
$C_{2115}H_{3252}N_{556}O_{673}S_{16}$ (peptide)	Certolizumab Pegol
$C_{2146}H_{3346}N_{572}O_{686}S_{28}$	Lanimostim
$C_{2158}H_{3282}N_{562}O_{681}S_{12}$	Ranibizumab
$C_{2172}H_{3309}N_{627}O_{658}S_{34}$	Pamiteplase
$C_{2184}H_{3323}N_{633}O_{666}S_{29}$ (amino acid sequence)	Lanoteplase
$C_{2191}H_{3451}N_{583}O_{656}S_{18}$	Antithrombin Alfa
$C_{2198}H_{3424}N_{588}O_{704}S_{28}$ (protein moiety)	Cilmostim
$C_{2224}H_{3472}N_{618}O_{701}S_{36}$ (monomer)	Etanercept
$C_{2230}H_{3357}N_{633}O_{718}S_{50}$	Thrombomodulin Alfa
$C_{2234}H_{3512}N_{650}O_{682}S_{10}$	Cintredekin Besudotox
$C_{2327}H_{3553}N_{589}O_{667}S_{20}$	Hyaluronidase (Human Recombinant)
$C_{2342}H_{3521}N_{597}O_{742}S_{18}$ (amylase)	Liprotamase
$C_{2355}H_{3745}N_{613}O_{728}S_{17}$	Conestat Alfa
$C_{2367}H_{3577}N_{649}O_{772}S_{19}$	Blinatumomab
$C_{2529}H_{3843}N_{689}O_{716}S_{16}$	Galsulfase
$C_{2532}H_{3843}N_{671}O_{711}S_{16}$	Imiglucerase
$C_{2532}H_{3850}N_{672}O_{711}S_{16}$	Velaglucerase Alfa
$C_{2532}H_{3854}N_{672}O_{711}S_{16}$ (protein moiety)	Alglucerase
$C_{2558}H_{3872}N_{738}O_{781}S_{40}$	Tenecteplase
$C_{2560}H_{4036}N_{678}O_{799}S_{17}$	Denileukin Diftitox
$C_{2569}H_{3894}N_{746}O_{781}S_{40}$	Alteplase
$C_{2569}H_{3894}N_{746}O_{781}S_{40}$	Tisokinase
$C_{2569}H_{3896}N_{746}O_{783}S_{39}$	Monteplase
$C_{2580}H_{3948}N_{752}O_{784}S_{40}$ (non-glycosylated protein)	Silteplase
$C_{2600}H_{4040}N_{696}O_{774}S_{23}$ (peptide)	Hyaluronidase (Ovine)
$C_{2600}H_{4130}N_{748}O_{812}S_{10}$ (protein moiety)	Alvircept Sudotox
$C_{2689}H_{4057}N_{699}O_{792}S_{14}$ (reduced peptide sequence)	Idursulfase
$C_{2726}H_{4186}N_{710}O_{846}S_{20}$ (peptidic part)	Torapsel
$C_{2736}H_{4174}N_{914}O_{824}S_{46}$	Duteplase
$C_{2910}H_{4542}N_{814}O_{878}S_{24}$	Briobacept
$C_{2959}H_{4860}N_{810}O_{965}S_{16}$ (reduced peptide)	Verpasep Caltespen

Molecular Formula	Non-proprietary Name
$C_{3104}H_{4788}N_{856}O_{950}S_{44}$ (homodimer)	Atacicept
$C_{3232}H_{5032}N_{864}O_{979}S_{41}$	Albiglutide
$C_{3255}H_{5025}N_{855}O_{1050}S_{18}$	Naptumomab Estafenatox
$C_{3261}H_{5027}N_{855}O_{1034}S_{22}$	Senlizumab
$C_{3264}H_{5002}N_{840}O_{988}S_{20}$	Alefacept
$C_{3345}H_{5215}N_{963}O_{1015}S_{37}$ (protein)	Talactoferrin Alfa
$C_{3434}H_{5258}N_{894}O_{1041}S_{17}$	Bucelipase Alfa
$C_{3455}H_{5371}N_{921}O_{1060}S_{18}$	Citatuzumab Bogatox
$C_{3508}H_{5440}N_{922}O_{1096}S_{32}$	Belatacept
$C_{3567}H_{5645}N_{921}O_{1261}S_{12}P_{4}$	Laronidase
$C_{3708}H_{5735}N_{1013}O_{1111}S_{28}$	Catridecacog
$C_{3796}H_{5937}N_{1015}O_{1143}S_{50}$	Albinterferon Alfa-2b
$C_{3821}H_{5813}N_{1003}O_{1139}S_{35}$ + $C_{3547}H_{5400}N_{956}O_{1033}S_{35}$	Beroctocog Alfa
$C_{3875}H_{5917}N_{1107}O_{1190}S_{58}$	Troplasminogen Alfa
$C_{3953}H_{6020}N_{1040}O_{1158}S_{29}$ + $C_{3553}H_{5412}N_{956}O_{1028}S_{33}$	Moroctocog Alfa
$C_{3970}H_{6275}N_{1047}O_{1302}S_{21}$	Vitespen
$C_{4074}H_{6282}N_{1134}O_{1274}S_{68}$	Baminercept Alfa
$C_{4318}H_{6788}N_{1164}O_{1304}S_{32}$	Aflibercept
$C_{4758}H_{7262}N_{1274}O_{1369}S_{35}$	Alglucosidase Alfa
$C_{5992}H_{9317}N_{1641}O_{1834}S_{63}$	Transferrin Aldifitox
$C_{6320}H_{9794}N_{1702}O_{1998}S_{42}$	Raxibacumab
$C_{6330}H_{9748}N_{1672}O_{1998}S_{48}$	Stamulumab
$C_{6346}H_{9832}N_{1720}O_{2002}S_{42}$	Lexatumumab
$C_{6358}H_{9830}N_{1682}O_{1992}S_{38}$	Iratumumab
$C_{6374}H_{9864}N_{1692}O_{1996}S_{46}$	Ramucirumab
$C_{6388}H_{9856}N_{1712}O_{1998}S_{46}$	Mapatumumab
$C_{6392}H_{9908}N_{1732}O_{1996}S_{42}$	Etaracizumab
$C_{6394}H_{9888}N_{1696}O_{2012}S_{44}$ (protein moiety)	Daclizumab
$C_{6398}H_{9878}N_{1694}O_{2016}S_{48}$	Panitumumab
$C_{6400}H_{9908}N_{1716}O_{1998}S_{44}$	Foravirumab
$C_{6404}H_{9912}N_{1724}O_{2004}S_{50}$	Denosumab
$C_{6406}H_{9924}N_{1716}O_{2012}S_{46}$	Tigatuzumab
$C_{6414}H_{9934}N_{1718}O_{2010}S_{40}$	Urtoxazumab
$C_{6416}H_{9924}N_{1732}O_{1982}S_{44}$	Exbivirumab
$C_{6428}H_{9976}N_{1720}O_{2018}S_{42}$	Tocilizumab
$C_{6434}H_{9942}N_{1706}O_{2040}S_{52}$	Volociximab
$C_{6440}H_{9968}N_{1708}O_{2016}S_{42}$	Pritumumab
$C_{6446}H_{9946}N_{1702}O_{2042}S_{32}$	Bavituximab
$C_{6448}H_{9954}N_{1718}O_{2016}S_{42}$	Otelixizumab
$C_{6452}H_{9954}N_{1714}O_{2024}S_{46}$	Anrukinzumab
$C_{6452}H_{9958}N_{1722}O_{2010}S_{42}$	Canakinumab
$C_{6452}H_{9964}N_{1732}O_{1998}S_{42}$	Dacetuzumab
$C_{6458}H_{9918}N_{1706}O_{2026}S_{46}$	Veltuzumab
$C_{6462}H_{9938}N_{1738}O_{2022}S_{46}$	Teplizumab
$C_{6462}H_{9942}N_{1714}O_{2036}S_{46}$	Rafivirumab
$C_{6462}H_{9948}N_{1736}O_{2020}S_{54}$	Figitumumab
$C_{6462}H_{9996}N_{1728}O_{2028}S_{54}$	Pagibaximab
$C_{6464}H_{9942}N_{1706}O_{2026}S_{46}$	Tanezumab
$C_{6466}H_{10006}N_{1730}O_{2024}S_{40}$	Conatumumab
$C_{6466}H_{10018}N_{1734}O_{2026}S_{44}$ (peptide)	Bapineuzumab
$C_{6466}H_{9928}N_{1716}O_{2020}S_{42}$	Farletuzumab
$C_{6470}H_{9971}N_{1712}O_{2007}S_{42}{}^{90}Y$	Yttrium Y 90 Tacatuzumab
$C_{6472}H_{9972}N_{1732}O_{2004}S_{40}$	Ipilimumab
$C_{6476}H_{10014}N_{1706}O_{2008}S_{48}$	Motavizumab
$C_{6476}H_{9982}N_{1714}O_{2016}S_{42}$	Elotuzumab
$C_{6480}H_{10022}N_{1742}O_{2020}S_{44}$	Ofatumumab
$C_{6482}H_{10004}N_{1712}O_{2016}S_{46}$	Ustekinumab
$C_{6494}H_{9978}N_{1718}O_{2014}S_{46}$	Ocrelizumab
$C_{6496}H_{10072}N_{1740}O_{2024}S_{42}$	Gantenerumab
$C_{6500}H_{10052}N_{1724}O_{2036}S_{44}$	Cixutumumab
$C_{6500}H_{9974}N_{1726}O_{2026}S_{52}$	Tremelimumab

Molecular Formula	*Non-proprietary Name*
$C_{6512}H_{10060}N_{1712}O_{2020}S_{44}$	Afutuzumab
$C_{6512}H_{10074}N_{1734}O_{2032}S_{46}$	Zalutumumab
$C_{6518}H_{10020}N_{1728}O_{2036}S_{42}$	Talizumab
$C_{6518}H_{10002}N_{1738}O_{2036}S_{42}$	Inotuzumab Ozogamicin
$C_{6518}H_{10066}N_{1758}O_{2020}S_{40}$	Milatuzumab
$C_{6528}H_{10072}N_{1732}O_{2042}S_{42}$	Vedolizumab
$C_{6530}H_{10068}N_{1752}O_{2026}S_{44}$	Golimumab
$C_{6548}H_{10122}N_{1730}O_{2034}S_{44}$	Tefibazumab
$C_{6552}H_{10080}N_{1740}O_{2052}S_{46}$	Adecatumumab
$C_{6566}H_{10082}N_{1746}O_{2056}S_{40}$	Nimotuzumab
$C_{6598}H_{10232}N_{1788}O_{2060}S_{46}$	Libivirumab
$C_{6638}H_{10160}N_{1720}O_{2108}S_{44}$	Bevacizumab
$C_{6714}H_{10428}N_{1816}O_{2102}S_{52}$	Belimumab
$C_{6850}H_{10656}N_{1824}O_{2106}S_{50}$	Lumiliximab
$C_{7812}H_{12114}N_{2042}O_{2406}S_{60}$	Tucotuzumab Celmoleukin
$C_{9030}H_{13932}N_{2400}O_{2670}S_{74}$	Rilonacept
$CaBr_2$	Calcium Bromide
$CaCO_3$	Calcium Carbonate
$^{45}CaCl_2$	Calcium Chloride Ca 45
$^{47}CaCl_2$	Calcium Chloride Ca 47
$CaCl_2.2H_2O$	Calcium Chloride
$CaHPO_4.2H_2O$	Calcium Phosphate Dihydrate, Dibasic
CaO	Lime
$Ca(OH)_2$	Calcium Hydroxide
$CaSO_4$.	Calcium Sulfate
$Ca_5HO_{13}P_3$	Durapatite
$Ca_5(OH)(PO_4)_3$	Calcium Phosphate, Tribasic
$Cl^{82}Rb$	Rubidium Chloride Rb 82
$Cl_2H_6N_2Pt$	Cisplatin
$^{57}CoCl_2$	Cobaltous Chloride Co 57
$^{60}CoCl_2$	Cobaltous Chloride Co 60
$^{51}CrCl_3$	Chromic Chloride Cr 51
$CrCl_3.6H_2O$	Chromic Chloride
$^{51}CrPO_4$	Chromic Phosphate Cr 51
$Cr^{32}PO_4$	Chromic Phosphate P 32
Cr_2O_3	Dichromium Trioxide
$^{131}CsCl$	Cesium Chloride Cs 131
$CuCl_2.2H_2O$.	Cupric Chloride
$CuSO_4.5H_2O$	Cupric Sulfate
$Fe(C_5H_3O_4N_2)_2.7½H_2O$	Ferrous Orotate
$^{59}FeCl_3$	Ferric Chloride Fe 59
$(FeO)._1(Fe_2O_3)._{45}(C_6H_{10}O_5)._{41}$ (average formula)	Ferumoxtran-10
$(FeOOH)_m[HO-(C_6H_{10}O_5)_x-$ $C_7H_{13}O_7]_n$	Gleptoferron
$FeO_{1.49}$ (approximately); $C_{398}H_{646}O_{337}$ (coating)	Ferumoxytol
$^{59}FeSO_4$	Ferrous Sulfate Fe 59
$FeSO_4.7H_2O$	Ferrous Sulfate
$FeSO_4.xH_2O$	Ferrous Sulfate, Dried
$Fe^{III}_w([C_6H_{10}O_5]_aC_6H_{11}O_7)_x$ $(OH)_yO_z.nH_2O$	Ferric Carboxymaltose
$(Fe_2O_3)_m(FeO)_n$	Ferumoxides
$Fe_2(SO_4)_3.xH_2O$	Ferric Sulfate
$Fe_4(OH)_2(SO_4)_5$	Ferric Subsulfate
$GaN_3O_9.9H_2O$	Gallium Nitrate
HCl	Hydrochloric Acid
HNO_3	Nitric Acid
$H(OCH_2CH_2)_nOH$	Polyethylene Glycol
$HO(C_2H_4O)_a(C_3H_6O)_b$ $(C_2H_4O)_aH$	Poloxamer
$H_2^{15}O$	Water O 15
H_2O_2	Hydrogen Peroxide
H_2SO_4	Sulfuric Acid
H_2SeO_3	Selenious Acid

Molecular Formula	*Non-proprietary Name*
H_3BO_3	Boric Acid
$H_3^{13}N$	Ammonia N 13
H_3PO_2	Hypophosphorous Acid
H_3PO_4	Phosphoric Acid
He	Helium
$HgCl_2$	Mercuric Chloride
$Hg(NH_2)Cl$	Mercury, Ammoniated
I_2	Iodine
$[^{113m}In(H_2O)_6]Cl_3$, $[^{113m}In$ $(H_2O)_5Cl]Cl_2$, $[^{113m}In$ $(H_2O)_4Cl_2]Cl$, $^{113m}In(H_2O)_3Cl_3$ (Mixture)	Indium Chlorides In 113m
KBr	Potassium Bromide
KCl	Potassium Chloride
^{42}KCl	Potassium Chloride K 42
$KClO_4$.	Potassium Perchlorate
$KHCO_3$	Potassium Bicarbonate
KH_2PO_4 .	Potassium Phosphate, Monobasic
KI .	Potassium Iodide
$KMnO_4$.	Potassium Permanganate
KNO_3	Potassium Nitrate
KOH .	Potassium Hydroxide
KPO_3	Potassium Metaphosphate
K_2CO_3 .	Potassium Carbonate
K_2HPO_4 .	Potassium Phosphate, Dibasic
K_2SO_4	Potassium Sulfate
$K_2S_2O_5$	Potassium Metabisulfite
Kr 81m	Krypton Kr 81m
$La_2(CO_3)_3._xH_2O$	Lanthanum Carbonate
$LiOH.H_2O$	Lithium Hydroxide
Li_2CO_3	Lithium Carbonate
$MgCl_2.6H_2O$	Magnesium Chloride
MgO	Magnesium Oxide
$Mg(OH)_2$	Magnesia, [Milk of]
$Mg(OH)_2$	Magnesium Hydroxide
$2MgO.3SiO_2.xH_2O$	Magnesium Trisilicate
$MgSO_4.7H_2O$	Magnesium Sulfate
$Mg_3(PO_4)_2.5H_2O$	Magnesium Phosphate
$Mg_6Al_2(OH)_{16}CO_3.4H_2O$	Hydrotalcite
$MnCl_2.4H_2O$	Manganese Chloride
$MnSO_4.H_2O$	Manganese Sulfate
NH_3	Ammonia Solution, Strong
NH_4Cl	Ammonium Chloride
$(NH_4)_2HPO_4$	Ammonium Phosphate
$(NH_4)_6Mo_7O_{24}.4H_2O$	Ammonium Molybdate
$(NH_4)_2SO_4$	Ammonium Sulfate
NO	Nitric Oxide
N_2	Nitrogen
N_2O	Nitrous Oxide
$NaAl(OH)_2CO_3$	Dihydroxyaluminum Sodium Carbonate
$NaBO_3.H_2O$	Sodium Perborate Monohydrate
$NaBr$	Sodium Bromide
$NaCl$	Sodium Chloride
$^{22}NaCl$	Sodium Chloride Na 22
$NaClO$	Sodium Hypochlorite
NaF	Sodium Fluoride
$[NaFe_2O_3(C_6H_{11}O_7)$ $(C_{12}H_{22}O_{11})_5]_x$ (where x is approximately $_{200}$)	Sodium Ferric Gluconate Complex
$NaHCO_3$	Sodium Bicarbonate
$NaH_2PO_4.xH_2O$	Sodium Phosphate, Monobasic
NaI	Sodium Iodide
$Na^{125}I$	Sodium Iodide I 125
$Na^{131}I$	Sodium Iodide I 131

Molecular Formula	*Non-proprietary Name*
$NaNO_2$	Sodium Nitrite
$NaOH$	Sodium Hydroxide
$(NaPO_3)_n$	Sodium Polyphosphate
$Na^{99m}TcO_4$	Sodium Pertechnetate Tc 99m
$Na_2B_4O_7.10H_2O$	Sodium Borate
Na_2CO_3	Sodium Carbonate
$Na_2^{51}CrO_4$	Sodium Chromate Cr 51
$Na_2[Fe(CN)_5NO].2H_2O$	Sodium Nitroprusside
$Na_2HPO_4.xH_2O$	Sodium Phosphate, Dibasic
Na_2PFO_3	Sodium Monofluorophosphate
$Na_2S.9H_2O$	Sodium Sulfide
Na_2SO_3	Sodium Sulfite
$Na_2^{35}SO_4$	Sodium Sulfate S 35
$Na_2SO_4.10H_2O$	Sodium Sulfate
$Na_2S_2O_3.5H_2O$	Sodium Thiosulfate
$Na_2S_2O_5$	Sodium Metabisulfite
$Na_3Au(S_2O_3)_2.2H_2O$	Gold Sodium Thiosulfate
Na_3PO_4	Sodium Phosphate, Tribasic
$Na_3P_3O_9$	Sodium Trimetaphosphate
$Na_4P_2O_7$	Sodium Pyrophosphate
O_2	Oxygen
$^{86}RbCl$	Rubidium Chloride Rb 86
$^{81}RbOH$	Rubidium Hydroxide (^{81}Rb) [Injection]

Molecular Formula	*Non-proprietary Name*
S	Sulfur, Precipitated
S	Sulfur, Sublimed
SF_6	Sulfur Hexafluoride
SO_2	Sulfur Dioxide
Sb_2S_3	Antimony Trisulfide Colloid
SeS_2	Selenium Sulfide
SiO_2	Silicon Dioxide, Colloidal
$SiO_2.xH_2O$	Silicon Dioxide
$SnCl_2.2H_2O$	Stannous Chloride
SnF_2	Stannous Fluoride
$Sn_2P_2O_7$	Stannous Pyrophosphate
$^{85}SrCl_2$	Strontium Chloride Sr 85
$^{89}SrCl_2$	Strontium Chloride Sr 89
$^{85}Sr(NO_3)_2$	Strontium Nitrate Sr 85
TiO_2	Titanium Dioxide
$^{201}TlCl$	Thallous Chloride Tl 201
Xe	Xenon Xe 133
$ZnCl_2$	Zinc Chloride
$^{65}ZnCl_2$	Zinc Chloride Zn 65
ZnO	Zinc Oxide
$3Zn(OH)_2.2ZnCO_3$	Zinc Carbonate
$ZnSO_4.xH_2O$	Zinc Sulfate

Appendix IV
Code Designations for USAN and Other Non-proprietary Names

A-002. Code designation for Varespladib Methyl.

A 5MP. Code designation for Adenosine Phosphate.

A-007. Code designation for Sivifene.

A0026. Code designation for Faropenem Medoxomil.

A-41-304. Code designation for Desoximetasone.

A 46 745. Code designation for Gestrinone.

A-82. Code designation for Nitroxoline.

A110. Code designation for Pagibaximab.

A-118. Code designation for Sultroponium.

A-272. Code designation for Rutamycin.

A-1981-12. Code designation for Prodilidine Hydrochloride.

A-2205. Code designation for Profadol Hydrochloride.

A-2371. Code designation for Plicamycin.

A-2655. Code designation for Dioxamate.

A-3217. Code designation for Ocfentanil Hydrochloride.

A-3331. Code designation for Brifentanil Hydrochloride.

A-3508.HCl. Code designation for Mirfentanil Hydrochloride.

A-3665.HCl. Code designation for Trefentanil Hydrochloride.

A-4020 Linz. Code designation for Midodrine Hydrochloride.

A-4166. Code designation for Nateglinide.

A-4180. Code designation for Isometamidium Chloride.

A-4492. Code designation for Pentamorphone.

A-4696. Code designation for Actaplanin.

A-4828. Code designation for Trofosfamide.

A-5610. Code designation for Azelastine Hydrochloride.

A-7283. Code designation for Guanoctine Hydrochloride.

A-8103. Code designation for Pipobroman.

A 8999. Code designation for Aspartocin.

A-12253A. Code designation for Nebramycin.

A-16612. Code designation for Teroxalene Hydrochloride.

A-17624. Code designation for Ditolamide.

A-19120. Code designation for Pargyline Hydrochloride.

A-19757. Code designation for Encyprate.

A-20968. Code designation for Piposulfan.

A-27053. Code designation for Chromonar Hydrochloride.

A-32686. Code designation for Proscillaridin.

A 33547. Code designation for Remoxipride.

A 33547.HCl.H₂O. Code designation for Remoxipride Hydrochloride.

A-35957. Code designation for Altrenogest.

A-53986. Code designation for Fostedil.

A-60386X. Code designation for Beractant.

A-61589. Code designation for Docebenone.

A-65006. Code designation for Lansoprazole.

A-71100. Code designation for Voglibose.

A-73001. Code designation for Seratrodast.

A-75200 mesylate. Code designation for Napitane Mesylate.

A-77000. Code designation for Pazinaclone.

A-81229. Code designation for Alemcinal.

A-85761.0. Code designation for Atreleuton.

A-87089.0. Code designation for Pozanicline.

A-87089.74. Code designation for Pozanicline Tartrate.

A-93431.1. Code designation for Adrogolide Hydrochloride.

A-147627.1. Code designation for Atrasentan Hydrochloride.

A-154475.0. Code designation for Lestaurtinib.

A-157378.0. Code designation for Lopinavir.

A-165594. Code designation for Tebanicline Tosylate.

A-166594.47. Code designation for Tebanicline Tosylate.

A-174606.0. Code designation for Valomaciclovir Stearate.

A-182091.0. Code designation for Omaciclovir.

A-185980.1. Code designation for Fiduxosin Hydrochloride.

A-195773. Code designation for Cethromycin.

A-422894.0. Code designation for Sofinicline.

A-422894.112. Code designation for Sofinicline Benzenesulfonate.

A IX. Code designation for Demecycline.

A-A-1. Code designation for Dalbavancin.

AA-673. Code designation for Amlexanox.

AA-861. Code designation for Docebenone.

AA-2414. Code designation for Seratrodast.

AAB-001, humanized 3D-6 monoclonal antibody. Code designation for Bapineuzumab.

AAD 216. Code designation for Ardacin.

AAFC. Code designation for Flurocitabine.

AB08. Code designation for Doxycycline Fosfatex.

AB-100. Code designation for Uredepa.

AB-103. Code designation for Benzodepa.

AB-132. Code designation for Meturedepa.

AB-A 663. Code designation for Cimaterol.

Abbot-147627. Code designation for Atrasentan Hydrochloride.

Abbott-16900. Code designation for Teflurane.

Abbott-19957. Code designation for Lorbamate.

Abbott-22370. Code designation for Trimetozine.

Abbott-24091. Code designation for Berythromycin.

Abbott-34842. Code designation for Butamben Picrate.

Abbott-35616. Code designation for Clorazepate Dipotassium.

Abbott-36581. Code designation for Butamirate Citrate.

Abbott-38579. Code designation for Protirelin.

Abbott-38642. Code designation for Fosfonet Sodium.

Abbott-39083. Code designation for Clorazepate Monopotassium.

Abbott-40728. Code designation for Cetocycline Hydrochloride.

Abbott-41070. Code designation for Gonadorelin Acetate.

Abbott-43326. Code designation for Carteolol Hydrochloride.

Abbott-43818. Code designation for Leuprolide Acetate.

Abbott 44090. Code designation for Valproate Sodium.

Abbott-44747. Code designation for Astromicin Sulfate.

Abbott-45975. Code designation for Terazosin Hydrochloride.

Abbott-46811. Code designation for Cefsulodin Sodium.

Abbott-47631. Code designation for Estazolam.

Abbott-48999. Code designation for Cefotiam Hydrochloride.

Abbott-50192 (HCl). Code designation for Cefmenoxime Hydrochloride.

Abbott-50711. Code designation for Divalproex Sodium.

Abbott-56268. Code designation for Clarithromycin.

Abbott-56619. Code designation for Difloxacin Hydrochloride.

Abbott-56620. Code designation for Sarafloxacin Hydrochloride.

Abbott-57135 [sarafloxacin]. Code designation for Sarafloxacin Hydrochloride.

Abbott-61827. Code designation for Tosufloxacin.

Abbott-62254. Code designation for Temafloxacin Hydrochloride.

Abbott-64077. Code designation for Zileuton.

Abbott-64662. Code designation for Enalkiren.

Abbott-70569.1. Code designation for Tiagabine Hydrochloride.

Abbott-70569.HCl. Code designation for Tiagabine Hydrochloride.

Abbott-72517. Code designation for Zankiren Hydrochloride.

Abbott-73001. Code designation for Seratrodast.
Abbott-74187. Code designation for Nasaruplase Beta.
Abbott-76120. Code designation for Urokinase Alfa.
Abbott-76745. Code designation for Fenleuton.
Abbott-81229.0. Code designation for Alemcinal.
Abbott-84538. Code designation for Ritonavir.
Abbott-85761. Code designation for Atreleuton.
Abbott-195773. Code designation for Cethromycin.
ABC 12/3. Code designation for Doxofylline.
ABOB. Code designation for Moroxydine.
ABR-215062 sodium. Code designation for Laquinimod Sodium.
ABT-001. Code designation for Seratrodast.
ABT-089. Code designation for Pozanicline.
ABT-091. Code designation for Omaciclovir.
ABT-120. Code designation for Urokinase Alfa.
ABT-187. Code designation for Nasaruplase Beta.
ABT-229. Code designation for Alemcinal.
ABT-335. Code designation for Choline Fenofibrate.
ABT-378. Code designation for Lopinavir.
ABT-431. Code designation for Adrogolide Hydrochloride.
ABT-492. Code designation for Delafloxacin.
ABT-492. Code designation for Delafloxacin Meglumine.
ABT-569. Code designation for Tiagabine Hydrochloride.
ABT-578. Code designation for Zotarolimus.
ABT-594. Code designation for Tebanicline Tosylate.
ABT-606. Code designation for Valomaciclovir Stearate.
ABT-627. Code designation for Atrasentan Hydrochloride.
ABT-761. Code designation for Atreleuton.
ABT-773. Code designation for Cethromycin.
ABT-894. Code designation for Sofinicline.
ABT-980. Code designation for Fiduxosin Hydrochloride.
ABX-EGF. Code designation for Panitumumab.
AC001. Code designation for Amlintide.
AC0137. Code designation for Pramlintide.
AC0137. Code designation for Pramlintide Acetate.
AC-528. Code designation for Dioxation.
AC-601. Code designation for Buramate.
AC 1198. Code designation for Dimethadione.
AC 1370. Code designation for Cefpimizole.
AC002993. Code designation for Exenatide.
AC2993. Code designation for Exenatide.
AC 2993. Code designation for Exenatide.
AC-2993. Code designation for Exenatide.
AC2993A. Code designation for Exenatide.
AC 3810. Code designation for Bamifylline Hydrochloride.
AC4464. Code designation for Torsemide.
AC 263,780. Code designation for Cimaterol.
ACC-9089. Code designation for Flestolol Sulfate.
ACC-9653-010 (sodium salt). Code designation for Fosphenytoin Sodium.
ACEA 1021. Code designation for Licostinel.
ACH-126,443. Code designation for Elvucitabine.
ACP-103. Code designation for Pimavanserin Tartrate.
ACZ885. Code designation for Canakinumab.
Ad5CMV-p53. Code designation for Contusugene Ladenovec.
AD 32. Code designation for Valrubicin.
AD 106. Code designation for Cicrotoic Acid.
AD-810. Code designation for Zonisamide.
ADD-3878. Code designation for Ciglitazone.
ADD 243037. Code designation for Lacosamide.
ADL 8-2698. Code designation for Alvimopan.
ADR-033. Code designation for Tripamide.
ADR-529. Code designation for Dexrazoxane.
AE-9. Code designation for Feclobuzone.
AE-705W. Code designation for Neutramycin.
AEB071. Code designation for Sotrastaurin Acetate.
AF102B. Code designation for Cevimeline Hydrochloride.
AF0144. Code designation for Perflubrodec.

AF0150. Code designation for Perflexane.
AF-438 [as citrate]. Code designation for Oxolamine.
AF-634. Code designation for Proxazole Citrate.
AF-864. Code designation for Benzydamine Hydrochloride.
AF-1161. Code designation for Trazodone Hydrochloride.
AF 1934 [lysine]. Code designation for Bendazac.
AF 2139. Code designation for Dapiprazole Hydrochloride.
AF 2838. Code designation for Bindarit.
AG-3. Code designation for Chromonar Hydrochloride.
AG331. Code designation for Metesind Glucuronate.
AG1343. Code designation for Nelfinavir Mesylate.
AG-1749. Code designation for Lansoprazole.
AG2037. Code designation for Pelitrexol.
AG3340. Code designation for Prinomastat.
AG7088. Code designation for Rupintrivir.
AG-013736. Code designation for Axitinib.
AG 58107. Code designation for Ioxitalamic Acid.
AG-EE 623 ZW. Code designation for Repaglinide.
Agent M-01. Code designation for Sucrosofate Potassium.
AGI-1067. Code designation for Succinobucol.
AGI-1096. Code designation for Elsibucol.
AGIX-4207. Code designation for Camobucol.
AGN 20. Code designation for Metamfazone.
AGN 511 [as hydrochloride]. Code designation for Prazitone.
AGN 616. Code designation for Fantridone Hydrochloride.
AGN 190168. Code designation for Tazarotene.
AGN 190342-LF. Code designation for Brimonidine Tartrate.
AGN 192013. Code designation for Alitretinoin.
AGN 192024. Code designation for Bimatoprost.
AGR-1240. Code designation for Minaprine.
AH 3923. Code designation for Salmefamol.
AH 5158A. Code designation for Labetalol Hydrochloride.
AH 8165D. Code designation for Fazadinium Bromide.
AH 19065. Code designation for Ranitidine Hydrochloride.
AH 22216. Code designation for Lamtidine.
AH 23844 [lavoltidine]. Code designation for Lavoltidine Succinate.
AH 23844A. Code designation for Lavoltidine Succinate.
AH 25352X. Code designation for Sufotidine.
AHR-224. Code designation for Pyroxamine Maleate.
AHR-438. Code designation for Metaxalone.
AHR-504. Code designation for Glycopyrrolate.
AHR-619. Code designation for Doxapram Hydrochloride.
AHR-857. Code designation for Sulfameter.
AHR-1118. Code designation for Pridefine Hydrochloride.
AHR-1680. Code designation for Fenpipalone.
AHR-2277 [as hydrochloride]. Code designation for Lenperone.
AHR-2438B. Code designation for Polignate Sodium.
AHR-3000. Code designation for Butaperazine.
AHR-3002. Code designation for Fenfluramine Hydrochloride.
AHR-3015. Code designation for Cintazone.
AHR-3018. Code designation for Apazone.
AHR-3053. Code designation for Carbocysteine.
AHR-3070-C. Code designation for Metoclopramide Hydrochloride.
AHR-4698. Code designation for Isosorbide Mononitrate.
AHR-5531C. Code designation for Dazopride Fumarate.
AHR-5850D. Code designation for Amfenac Sodium.
AHR-6134. Code designation for Cloroperone Hydrochloride.
AHR 6646. Code designation for Duoperone Fumarate.
AHR-8559. Code designation for Fluzinamide.
AHR-9377. Code designation for Tampramine Fumarate.
AHR-9434. Code designation for Nepafenac.
AHR-10282B. Code designation for Bromfenac Sodium.
AHR-10718. Code designation for Suricainide Maleate.
AHR-11190-B. Code designation for Zacopride Hydrochloride.
AHR-11325-D. Code designation for Rocastine Hydrochloride.
AHR-11748. Code designation for Dezinamide.

AI-700. Code designation for Perflubutane.
AI-27,303. Code designation for Cetamolol Hydrochloride.
AICA. Code designation for Orazamide.
AIT-082. Code designation for Leteprinim Potassium.
AJ-2615. Code designation for Monatepil Maleate.
AL 20 [as hydrochloride]. Code designation for Clemizole.
AL-108. Code designation for Davunetide.
AL-208. Code designation for Davunetide.
Al-0361. Code designation for Hydroxyphenamate.
AL 0559. Code designation for Fenamole.
AL 842. Code designation for Deterenol Hydrochloride.
AL-1021. Code designation for Carperone.
AL1577A. Code designation for Levobetaxolol Hydrochloride.
AL02145. Code designation for Apraclonidine Hydrochloride.
AL02725. Code designation for Pyrithione Sodium.
AL-3432A. Code designation for Emedastine Difumarate.
AL-3789. Code designation for Anecortave Acetate.
AL-4862. Code designation for Brinzolamide.
AL-6221. Code designation for Travoprost.
AL-6515. Code designation for Nepafenac.
AL-12959. Code designation for Icomucret.
ALCA. Code designation for Alcloxa.
ALDA. Code designation for Aldioxa.
Allergan 211. Code designation for Idoxuridine.
ALO 1401-02. Code designation for Betaxolol Hydrochloride.
ALO 2184. Code designation for Resocortol Butyrate.
ALRT1057. Code designation for Alitretinoin.
AL-T30. Code designation for Vinafocon A.
AL-T150. Code designation for Oxyfilcon A.
ALT-711. Code designation for Alagebrium Chloride.
ALTU-135. Code designation for Liprotamase.
ALX1-11. Code designation for Parathyroid Hormone.
ALX 0600. Code designation for Teduglutide.
AM-684-Beta. Code designation for Relomycin.
AM-1155. Code designation for Gatifloxacin.
AMA 1080(2Na). Code designation for Carumonam Sodium.
AMD473. Code designation for Picoplatin.
AMD3100. Code designation for Plerixafor.
AMG073. Code designation for Cinacalcet.
AMG073 HCl. Code designation for Cinacalcet Hydrochloride.
AMG 162. Code designation for Denosumab.
AMG 655. Code designation for Conatumumab.
AMG 706. Code designation for Motesanib.
AMG 706. Code designation for Motesanib Diphosphate.
AMI-25. Code designation for Ferumoxides.
AMI-121. Code designation for Ferumoxsil.
AMN 107. Code designation for Nilotinib.
AMR-69. Code designation for Pirfenidone.
AN021. Code designation for Tizanidine Hydrochloride.
AN-051. Code designation for Dezinamide.
AN 1317. Code designation for Perimetazine.
AN 1324. Code designation for Glybuzole.
Anesthetic Compound No. 347. Code designation for Enflurane.
ANO-1020. Code designation for Tilarginine Acetate.
ANP 246. Code designation for Clofexamide.
ANP 3260. Code designation for Clofezone.
Antibiotic 241a. Code designation for Biniramycin.
Antibiotic A-5283. Code designation for Natamycin.
anti-CD11a. Code designation for Efalizumab.
anti-CD40L. Code designation for Toralizumab.
anti-CD154. Code designation for Toralizumab.
Antifoam A. Code designation for Simethicone.
Antifoam AF. Code designation for Simethicone.
anti-gp39. Code designation for Toralizumab.
anti-SSEA-1. Code designation for Technetium Tc 99m Fanoleso-
    mab.
ANX-510. Code designation for Folitixorin Calcium.
AO-128. Code designation for Voglibose.

AO-407. Code designation for Hydrofilcon A.
AOMA. Code designation for Surfomer.
AO-PLUTO. Code designation for Mesifilcon A.
AP 67. Code designation for Chlorthenoxazine.
AP23573. Code designation for Deforolimus.
APC8015. Code designation for Sipuleucel-T.
APC8024. Code designation for Lapuleucel-T.
APD356. Code designation for Lorcaserin Hydrochloride.
API-GP3. Code designation for Motexafin Gadolinium.
APM. Code designation for Aspartame.
Apo2L/TRAIL. Code designation for Dulanermin.
APSAC. Code designation for Anistreplase.
APT 070. Code designation for Mirococept.
AQ-110. Code designation for Tretoquinol.
AR-100. Code designation for Iclaprim.
AR-100.001. Code designation for Iclaprim Mesylate.
AR 12008. Code designation for Trapidil.
ara-A. Code designation for Vidarabine.
ara-AC. Code designation for Fazarabine.
AR-C68397AA. Code designation for Sibenadet Hydrochloride.
AR-C69931MX. Code designation for Cangrelor Tetrasodium.
AR-C69931XX. Code designation for Cangrelor.
AR-C126532XX. Code designation for Ticagrelor.
ARC I-K-1. Code designation for Methopholine.
ARDF 26. Code designation for Gliquidone.
AR-H039242XX. Code designation for Tesaglitazar.
AR-P900758XX. Code designation for Naproxcinod.
AS-013. Code designation for Ecraprost.
AS 101. Code designation for Arsanilic Acid.
AS-17665. Code designation for Nifurthiazole.
ASA 158/5 [as phosphate]. Code designation for Benproperine.
ASL-279. Code designation for Dopamine Hydrochloride.
ASL-601. Code designation for Acecainide Hydrochloride.
ASL-603. Code designation for Bretylium Tosylate.
ASL-607. Code designation for Pentastarch.
ASL-8052. Code designation for Esmolol Hydrochloride.
Asta 3746. Code designation for Ciclonium Bromide.
Astra 1512. Code designation for Prilocaine Hydrochloride.
Astra 1572. Code designation for Iron Sorbitex.
AT-101. Code designation for Isosorbide.
AT-125. Code designation for Acivicin.
AT 327. Code designation for Tipepidine.
AT-1001. Code designation for Larazotide Acetate.
AT-2266. Code designation for Enoxacin.
AT-2347. Code designation for Larazotide.
AT-4140. Code designation for Sparfloxacin.
ATC Code G03 GA Gonadotropins. Code designation for Chorio-
    gonadotropin Alfa.
ATC G03 GA Gonadotropins. Code designation for Lutropin Alfa.
ATI 01. Code designation for Sinapultide.
ATI 02. Code designation for Lucinactant.
ATL-962. Code designation for Cetilistat.
AVE0005. Code designation for Aflibercept.
AW 10. Code designation for Sitogluside.
AW 14′2333. Code designation for Perlapine.
AW-14′2446. Code designation for Clodazon Hydrochloride.
AW 105-843. Code designation for Naftifine Hydrochloride.
AY4166. Code designation for Nateglinide.
AY-5312. Code designation for Chlorhexidine Hydrochloride.
AY-5710. Code designation for Magaldrate.
AY-6108. Code designation for Ampicillin.
AY 6204 [as hydrochloride]. Code designation for Pronetalol.
AY-6608. Code designation for Pentagastrin.
AY-8682. Code designation for Cyheptamide.
AY-11,440. Code designation for Clogestone Acetate.
AY-11,483. Code designation for Estrofurate.
AY-15,613. Code designation for Citenamide.
AY-20,385. Code designation for Nequinate.

AY-20,694. Code designation for Dexpropranolol Hydrochloride.
AY-21,011. Code designation for Practolol.
AY-21,367. Code designation for Furobufen.
AY-21,554. Code designation for Talopram Hydrochloride.
AY-22,124. Code designation for Intriptyline Hydrochloride.
AY-22,214. Code designation for Taclamine Hydrochloride.
AY-22,241. Code designation for Actodigin.
AY-22,284A. Code designation for Alrestatin Sodium.
AY 22,469. Code designation for Deprostil.
AY-22989. Code designation for Sirolimus.
AY-23,028. Code designation for Butaclamol Hydrochloride.
AY-23,289. Code designation for Prodolic Acid.
AY-23,713. Code designation for Pirandamine Hydrochloride.
AY-23,946. Code designation for Tandamine Hydrochloride.
AY-24,031. Code designation for Gonadorelin Hydrochloride.
AY-24,169. Code designation for Dexclamol Hydrochloride.
AY-24,236. Code designation for Etodolac.
AY-24,269. Code designation for Proroxan Hydrochloride.
AY-24,559. Code designation for Doxaprost.
AY-24,856. Code designation for Pareptide Sulfate.
AY-25,329. Code designation for Azaclorzine Hydrochloride.
AY-25,712. Code designation for Acifran.
AY-27,110. Code designation for Ciladopa Hydrochloride.
AY-27,255. Code designation for Vinpocetine.
AY-27,773. Code designation for Tolrestat.
AY-28,228. Code designation for Atiprosin Maleate.
AY-28,768. Code designation for Pelrinone Hydrochloride.
AY-30,715. Code designation for Pemedolac.
AY-61122. Code designation for Methallibure.
AY-61123. Code designation for Clofibrate.
AY-62014. Code designation for Butriptyline Hydrochloride.
AY-62021. Code designation for Clopenthixol.
AY-62022. Code designation for Medrogestone.
AY 64043. Code designation for Propranolol Hydrochloride.
AZD2171. Code designation for Cediranib.
AZD2171 maleate. Code designation for Cediranib Maleate.
AZD2563. Code designation for Posizolid.
AZD3582. Code designation for Naproxcinod.
AZD6140. Code designation for Ticagrelor.
AZL O 211089. Code designation for Dimethyl Fumarate.
AZQ. Code designation for Diaziquone.
AZT. Code designation for Zidovudine.
B1 61.012. Code designation for Sargramostim.
B1Q 16. Code designation for Hedaquinium Chloride.
B28-Asp-Insulin. Code designation for Insulin Aspart.
B-360. Code designation for Paroxypropione.
B-436. Code designation for Prenylamine.
B992. Code designation for Stannsoporfin.
B1287. Code designation for Eritoran Tetrasodium.
B 1312 [as hydrochloride]. Code designation for Bupranolol.
B 1464. Code designation for Guanacline Sulfate.
B2036-PEG. Code designation for Pegvisomant.
B-2311. Code designation for Morinamide.
B-4130. Code designation for Iodamide.
B9302-107. Code designation for Roflumilast.
B9420-001. Code designation for Lusupultide.
B 10610. Code designation for Iodoxamic Acid.
B 11420. Code designation for Iopronic Acid.
B19036/7. Code designation for Gadobenate Dimeglumine.
B-35251. Code designation for Mitocromin.
BA 679 BR. Code designation for Tiotropium Bromide.
BA 4164-8. Code designation for Diflumidone Sodium.
BA 4197. Code designation for Flucrylate.
BA 4223. Code designation for Triflumidate.
BA 7602-06. Code designation for Talniflumate.
BA 7604-02. Code designation for Talosalate.
BA 7605-06. Code designation for Talmetacin.
Ba 13155 [as tartrate]. Code designation for Meladrazine.

Ba-20684. Code designation for Etonitazene.
Ba-29038. Code designation for Boldenone Undecylenate.
Ba-29837. Code designation for Deferoxamine Hydrochloride.
Ba-30803. Code designation for Benzoctamine Hydrochloride.
BA 32644. Code designation for Niridazole.
Ba-32968. Code designation for Delfantrine.
Ba-33112. Code designation for Deferoxamine Mesylate.
Ba-34,276 [as hydrochloride]. Code designation for Maprotiline.
Ba-34,647. Code designation for Baclofen.
BA 36278A. Code designation for Cephacetrile Sodium.
Ba-39,089. Code designation for Oxprenolol Hydrochloride.
Ba-40088. Code designation for Proxibutene.
Ba 41166/E. Code designation for Rifampin.
Ba-41795. Code designation for Codactide.
BAFF. Code designation for Ardenermin.
BAL5788. Code designation for Ceftobiprole Medocaril.
BAL5788-001. Code designation for Ceftobiprole Medocaril.
BAL9141-000. Code designation for Ceftobiprole.
BAQD 10. Code designation for Dequalinium Chloride.
BASF 43915. Code designation for Pelretin.
BASF 47011. Code designation for Doretinel.
BASF 52404. Code designation for Linarotene.
BAX 422Z. Code designation for Albutoin.
BAX 1400Z. Code designation for Dimethadione.
BAX 1515. Code designation for Sutilains.
BAX 1526. Code designation for Chymopapain.
BAX 2739Z. Code designation for Bamifylline Hydrochloride.
BAX-ACC-1638. Code designation for Atilmotin.
BAY 12-8039. Code designation for Moxifloxacin Hydrochloride.
BAY 12-9566. Code designation for Tanomastat.
BAY 43-9006. Code designation for Sorafenib.
BAY 54-9085. Code designation for Sorafenib Tosylate.
BAY 59-7939. Code designation for Rivaroxaban.
BAY 1500. Code designation for Mefruside.
BAY 1521. Code designation for Noxiptiline.
BAY 2353. Code designation for Niclosamide.
BAY 4059 Va. Code designation for Brotianide.
BAY 4503. Code designation for Propiram Fumarate.
BAY 5097. Code designation for Clotrimazole.
BAY 9002. Code designation for Naftalofos.
Bay a 1040. Code designation for Nifedipine.
BAY B 4231. Code designation for Glisoxepide.
Bay d 1107. Code designation for Etofenamate.
BAY d 8815 [hydrochloride]. Code designation for Amidantel.
Bay e 5009. Code designation for Nitrendipine.
BAY e 9736. Code designation for Nimodipine.
Bay g 2821. Code designation for Muzolimine.
Bay g 5421. Code designation for Acarbose.
Bay g 6575. Code designation for Nafazatrom.
BAY h 2049. Code designation for Daniquidone.
Bay h 4502. Code designation for Bifonazole.
Bay h 5757. Code designation for Febantel.
BAY i 3930. Code designation for Isomalt.
BAY i 7433. Code designation for Copovithane.
Bay k 5552. Code designation for Nisoldipine.
Bay m 1099. Code designation for Miglitol.
BAY o 1248. Code designation for Emiglitate.
Bay o 9867 monohydrate. Code designation for Ciprofloxacin
    Hydrochloride.
Bay q 3939. Code designation for Ciprofloxacin.
Bay q 4218. Code designation for Butaprost.
BAY q 7821. Code designation for Ipsapirone Hydrochloride.
BAY u 3405. Code designation for Ramatroban.
BAY V1 4718. Code designation for Etisomicin.
BAY V1 6045. Code designation for Flumethrin.
BAY Va 1470. Code designation for Xylazine Hydrochloride.
Bay VA 9387. Code designation for Etisazole.
BAY Va 9391. Code designation for Olaquindox.

BAY Vh 5757. Code designation for Febantel.
Bay Vi 9142. Code designation for Toltrazuril.
BAY Vk 4999. Code designation for Fuzlocillin.
Bay Vl 1704. Code designation for Cyfluthrin.
Bay Vn 6528. Code designation for Fenfluthrin.
Bay Vp 2674. Code designation for Enrofloxacin.
BAY w 6228. Code designation for Cerivastatin Sodium.
BAY w 6240. Code designation for Factor VIII (rDNA).
Bay w 6341. Code designation for Abafungin.
Bay x 1005. Code designation for Veliflapon.
BAY X 1351. Code designation for Nerelimomab.
BAY y 7432. Code designation for Ecadotril.
Bayer 1362. Code designation for Butaperazine.
Bayer 1420. Code designation for Propanidid.
Bayer 2502. Code designation for Nifurtimox.
Bayer 3231. Code designation for Triaziquone.
Bayer 5360. Code designation for Metronidazole.
Bayer 9015. Code designation for Niclofolan.
Bayer 9037. Code designation for Quintiofos.
Bayer 9053. Code designation for Phoxim.
Bayer 21199. Code designation for Coumaphos.
Bayer A 128. Code designation for Aprotinin.
Bayer L 1359. Code designation for Trichlorfon.
BAYNAC. Code designation for Fenfluthrin.
BB-94. Code designation for Batimastat.
BB-882. Code designation for Lexipafant.
BB-2516. Code designation for Marimastat.
BB-3644. Code designation for Solimastat.
BB-10010. Code designation for Nagrestipen.
BB-K8. Code designation for Amikacin Sulfate.
BBM-2478A. Code designation for Elsamitrucin.
BBR 2778. Code designation for Pixantrone.
BBR 3438. Code designation for Nortopixantrone.
BBR 3464. Code designation for Triplatin Tetranitrate.
BBR 3576 (dihydrochloride). Code designation for Topixantrone.
BC-105. Code designation for Pizotyline.
BCG65-E7. Code designation for Verpasep Caltespen.
BCH-4556. Code designation for Troxacitabine.
BCM. Code designation for Mannomustine.
BCNU. Code designation for Carmustine.
BCX-34. Code designation for Peldesine.
BCX-1777. Code designation for Forodesine.
BCX-1777. Code designation for Forodesine Hydrochloride.
BCX 2600. Code designation for Stiripentol.
BD 40A. Code designation for Formoterol Fumarate.
BDF5896. Code designation for Moxonidine.
BDH 1298. Code designation for Megestrol Acetate.
BDH 1921. Code designation for Melengestrol Acetate.
Be-100. Code designation for Ibuprofen Piconol.
BE 419. Code designation for Ioglycamic Acid.
Be-1293. Code designation for Xipamide.
BE5895. Code designation for Moxonidine.
BEC2. Code designation for Mitumomab.
BEMT. Code designation for Bemotrizinol.
BG 8301. Code designation for Teceleukin.
BG8967. Code designation for Bivalirudin.
BG9273. Code designation for Alefacept.
BG9588. Code designation for Ruplizumab.
BG9712. Code designation for Alefacept.
BG9719. Code designation for Naxifylline.
BG 9924. Code designation for Baminercept Alfa.
BI397. Code designation for Dalbavancin.
BIBR 277 SE. Code designation for Telmisartan.
BIBR 953 ZW. Code designation for Dabigatran.
BIBR 1048 BS RS1. Code designation for Dabigatran Etexilate.
BIBR 1048 MS. Code designation for Dabigatran Etexilate Mesylate.
BIBV 308 SE. Code designation for Terbogrel.

BIIP 20 XX. Code designation for Apaxifylline.
BI-L-239. Code designation for Enofelast.
BILA 2011 BS. Code designation for Palinavir.
BILN 2061 ZW. Code designation for Ciluprevir.
BIM-23014C. Code designation for Lanreotide Acetate.
BIMT 17. Code designation for Flibanserin.
BIMT 17 BS. Code designation for Flibanserin.
BIRG 0587. Code designation for Nevirapine.
BIRM-270. Code designation for Ontazolast.
BI-RR-0001. Code designation for Enlimomab.
BIRR004. Code designation for Tremacamra.
BL 191. Code designation for Pentoxifylline.
BL-3912A. Code designation for Dimoxamine Hydrochloride.
BL-4162a. Code designation for Anagrelide Hydrochloride.
BL-5111. Code designation for Tiodazosin.
BL-5572M. Code designation for Proxorphan Tartrate.
BL-5641A. Code designation for Etintidine Hydrochloride.
BL-P 804. Code designation for Hetacillin.
BL-P 1322. Code designation for Cephapirin Sodium.
BL-P 1462. Code designation for Suncillin Sodium.
BL-P1761. Code designation for Sarpicillin.
BL-P1780. Code designation for Sarmoxicillin.
BL-R 743. Code designation for Intrazole.
BL-S578. Code designation for Cefadroxil.
BL-S640. Code designation for Cefatrizine.
BL-S786. Code designation for Ceforanide.
BLyS. Code designation for Ardenermin.
BM01.004. Code designation for Metipranolol.
BM02.015. Code designation for Torsemide.
BM 06.019. Code designation for Epoetin Beta.
BM 06.022. Code designation for Reteplase.
BM 13.177. Code designation for Sulotroban.
BM 13.505. Code designation for Daltroban.
BM 14.190. Code designation for Carvedilol.
BM 15.075. Code designation for Bezafibrate.
BM 21.0955 · Na · H$_2$O. Code designation for Ibandronate Sodium.
BM 22.145. Code designation for Isosorbide Mononitrate.
BM 41.332. Code designation for Ciamexon.
BM 41.440. Code designation for Ilmofosine.
BM 51052. Code designation for Carazolol.
BMIPP. Code designation for Iodofiltic Acid I 123.
BMS068645. Code designation for Apadenoson.
BMS-180048. Code designation for Avitriptan Fumarate.
BMS-180048-02. Code designation for Avitriptan Fumarate.
BMS-180194. Code designation for Lobucavir.
BMS-180291. Code designation for Ifetroban.
BMS-180291-02. Code designation for Ifetroban Sodium.
BMS 180549. Code designation for Ferumoxtran-10.
BMS-181158. Code designation for Mequinol.
BMS-181173. Code designation for Gusperimus Trihydrochloride.
BMS-181176. Code designation for Becatecarin.
BMS-181339-01. Code designation for Paclitaxel.
BMS-182751. Code designation for Satraplatin.
BMS-186091. Code designation for Ammonium Lactate.
BMS-186295. Code designation for Irbesartan.
BMS-186716. Code designation for Omapatrilat.
BMS-186716-01. Code designation for Omapatrilat.
BMS-188667. Code designation for Abatacept.
BMS-189921. Code designation for Gemopatrilat.
BMS-200475-01. Code designation for Entecavir.
BMS-200980. Code designation for Lanoteplase.
BMS-204352. Code designation for Flindokalner.
BMS-204756-07. Code designation for Brasofensine Maleate.
BMS-205603-01. Code designation for Uracil.
BMS-206584-01. Code designation for Gatifloxacin.
BMS-207940-02. Code designation for Edonentan.
BMS-214778. Code designation for Tasimelteon.

BMS-217380-01. Code designation for Tesmilifene Hydrochloride.
BMS-224818. Code designation for Belatacept.
BMS-224819. Code designation for Teneliximab.
BMS-232632-05. Code designation for Atazanavir Sulfate.
BMS-234303-01. Code designation for Naminidil.
BMS 247550-01. Code designation for Ixabepilone.
BMS 275291-01. Code designation for Rebimastat.
BMS-284756-01. Code designation for Garenoxacin Mesylate.
BMS-298585. Code designation for Muraglitazar.
BMS-354825-03. Code designation for Dasatinib.
BMS-426707-1. Code designation for Peliglitazar.
BMS-477118-11. Code designation for Saxagliptin.
BMS-512148-05. Code designation for Dapagliflozin.
BMS-561389. Code designation for Razaxaban Hydrochloride.
BMS-562247-01. Code designation for Apixaban.
BMS-582664. Code designation for Brivanib Alaninate.
BMS-646256. Code designation for Ibipinabant.
BMS-710485. Code designation for Vinflunine Ditartrate.
BMY-05763-1-D. Code designation for Dexsotalol Hydrochloride.
BMY 13754. Code designation for Nefazodone Hydrochloride.
BMY 13805-1. Code designation for Gepirone Hydrochloride.
BMY 13859-1. Code designation for Tiospirone Hydrochloride.
BMY-21891. Code designation for Belfosdil.
BMY-25182. Code designation for Cefbuperazone.
BMY-25801-01. Code designation for Batanopride Hydrochloride.
BMY-26517. Code designation for Pemirolast Potassium.
BMY-27557. Code designation for Becatecarin.
BMY-27857. Code designation for Stavudine.
BMY-28090. Code designation for Elsamitrucin.
BMY-28100-03-800. Code designation for Cefprozil.
BMY-28142. Code designation for Cefepime.
BMY-28142 2HCl.H$_2$O. Code designation for Cefepime Hydrochloride.
BMY-30056. Code designation for Halobetasol Propionate.
BMY-30120. Code designation for Chlorhexidine Phosphanilate.
BMY-33419. Code designation for Tesmilifene Hydrochloride.
BMY-40327. Code designation for Modecainide.
BMY 40481. Code designation for Etoposide Phosphate.
BMY-40900. Code designation for Didanosine.
BMY-41606. Code designation for Vapreotide.
BMY-42215-1. Code designation for Gusperimus Trihydrochloride.
BMY-45594. Code designation for Satraplatin.
BN110 base. Code designation for Axomadol.
BN 200 (base). Code designation for Tapentadol.
(±)-BN-1270. Code designation for Cicletanine.
BNAG. Code designation for Donepezil Hydrochloride.
BNP-166. Code designation for Etiprednol Dicloacetate.
BNP1350. Code designation for Cositecan.
BOF-A2. Code designation for Emitefur.
BOL-303224-A. Code designation for Besifloxacin Hydrochloride.
BP 1.02. Code designation for Ecadotril.
BP-13. Code designation for Iosimenol.
BP 400. Code designation for Pimethixene.
BP-1184. Code designation for Guanoctine Hydrochloride.
BR-3-FC. Code designation for Briobacept.
BRI. Code designation for Sulfur Hexafluoride.
BRL-284. Code designation for Levopropylcillin Potassium.
BRL-804. Code designation for Hetacillin.
BRL-1241. Code designation for Methicillin Sodium.
BRL-1288. Code designation for Benapryzine Hydrochloride.
BRL-1341. Code designation for Ampicillin.
BRL-1621. Code designation for Cloxacillin Sodium.
BRL-1702. Code designation for Dicloxacillin.
BRL 2039. Code designation for Floxacillin.
BRL-2064. Code designation for Carbenicillin Disodium.

BRL 2288. Code designation for Ticarcillin Disodium.
BRL 2333. Code designation for Amoxicillin.
BRL-2333AB-B. Code designation for Amoxicillin Sodium.
BRL 2534. Code designation for Azidocillin.
BRL-3475. Code designation for Carbenicillin Phenyl Sodium.
BRL 4664. Code designation for Nonabine.
BRL 4910A. Code designation for Mupirocin.
BRL 4910F. Code designation for Mupirocin Calcium.
BRL 8988 Hydrochloride. Code designation for Talampicillin Hydrochloride.
BRL 12594. Code designation for Ticarcillin Cresyl Sodium.
BRL 13856. Code designation for Clopirac.
BRL 14151. Code designation for Clavulanic Acid.
BRL 14151K. Code designation for Clavulanate Potassium.
BRL 14777. Code designation for Nabumetone.
BRL 17421 [as sodium]. Code designation for Temocillin.
BRL 26921. Code designation for Anistreplase.
BRL 29060. Code designation for Paroxetine.
BRL 30892. Code designation for Denbufylline.
BRL 34915. Code designation for Cromakalim.
BRL-38227. Code designation for Levcromakalim.
BRL 38705. Code designation for Epsiprantel.
BRL-39123. Code designation for Penciclovir.
BRL-39123-D. Code designation for Penciclovir Sodium.
BRL 40015. Code designation for Diproteverine.
BRL-42810. Code designation for Famciclovir.
BRL 43694. Code designation for Granisetron.
BRL 43694A. Code designation for Granisetron Hydrochloride.
BRL-49653-C. Code designation for Rosiglitazone Maleate.
BRL 61063. Code designation for Cipamfylline.
BS 100-141. Code designation for Guanfacine Hydrochloride.
BS 749. Code designation for Metacetamol.
B.S. 6534. Code designation for Bufenadrine.
BS 6748. Code designation for Xyloxemine.
BS 6987. Code designation for Deptropine Citrate.
BS 7161 D [as hydrochloride]. Code designation for Pytamine.
B.S. 7173-D. Code designation for Xylocoumarol.
B.S. 7561 [as hydrochloride]. Code designation for Tixadil.
B.S. 7573-a. Code designation for Acridorex.
BS 7723 [as maleate]. Code designation for Tropirine.
BS 7977 D [as dihydrochloride]. Code designation for Xipranolol.
BSH. Code designation for Borocaptate Sodium B 10.
BSSG. Code designation for Sitogluside.
BT 621 [as hydrochloride]. Code designation for Todralazine.
BTPABA, PFT. Code designation for Bentiromide.
BTS 49 465. Code designation for Flosequinan.
BTS 7706. Code designation for Debropol.
BTS 13622. Code designation for Hexaprofen.
BTS 17345. Code designation for Fluprofen.
BTS 18,322. Code designation for Flurbiprofen.
BTS 24332. Code designation for Esflurbiprofen.
BTS 54524. Code designation for Sibutramine Hydrochloride.
BU-2231A. Code designation for Talisomycin.
BW 33A. Code designation for Atracurium Besylate.
BW 33-T-57. Code designation for Methisazone.
BW 49-210. Code designation for Diaveridine.
BW 56-72. Code designation for Trimethoprim.
BW 56-158. Code designation for Allopurinol.
BW-57-322. Code designation for Azathioprine.
BW 57-323. Code designation for Thiamiprine.
BW 58-271. Code designation for Rolodine.
BW-61-32. Code designation for Stilbazium Iodide.
BW 63-90. Code designation for Butacetin.
BW 64-9. Code designation for Butoxamine Hydrochloride.
BW 72U. Code designation for Trimethoprim Sulfate.
BW 207U. Code designation for Xenalipin.
BW 234U dihydrochloride. Code designation for Rimcazole Hydrochloride.

BW 248U sodium. Code designation for Acyclovir Sodium.
BW 301U isethionate. Code designation for Piritrexim Isethionate.
BW 323. Code designation for Bupropion Hydrochloride.
BW 325U. Code designation for Trifenagrel.
BW 356-C-61. Code designation for Gloxazone.
BW 430C. Code designation for Lamotrigine.
BW-467-C-60. Code designation for Bethanidine Sulfate.
BW-524W91. Code designation for Emtricitabine.
BW 532U. Code designation for Cinflumide.
BW 647U hydrochloride. Code designation for Bipenamol Hydrochloride.
BW 759U. Code designation for Ganciclovir.
BW 825C. Code designation for Acrivastine.
BW A256C. Code designation for Palatrigine.
BW A509U. Code designation for Zidovudine.
BW A515U. Code designation for Desciclovir.
BW A770U mesylate. Code designation for Crisnatol Mesylate.
BW A938U dichloride. Code designation for Doxacurium Chloride.
BW B109OU dichloride. Code designation for Mivacurium Chloride.
Bx 311. Code designation for Cinoxolone.
BX 341. Code designation for Bifluranol.
BX 363A [as disodium salt]. Code designation for Cicloxolone.
BX 591. Code designation for Acefluranol.
BX 650 A. Code designation for Ipsalazide.
BX661A. Code designation for Balsalazide Disodium.
BY217. Code designation for Roflumilast.
BY 1023. Code designation for Pantoprazole.
BYK20869. Code designation for Roflumilast.
BZ 55. Code designation for Carbutamide.
C-1. Code designation for Edrecolomab.
C-3. Code designation for Capobenate Sodium.
C-3. Code designation for Capobenic Acid.
C-4. Code designation for Imciromab Pentetate.
c7E3. Code designation for Abciximab.
C225. Code designation for Cetuximab.
C-238. Code designation for Pridinol.
C-434. Code designation for Trimedoxime Bromide.
C-1428. Code designation for Cyclarbamate.
C 1656. Code designation for Clometacin.
C-11925. Code designation for Phanquone.
C-12669. Code designation for Demecolcine.
C-49802B-Ba. Code designation for Oxaprotiline Hydrochloride.
CA4DP. Code designation for Fosbretabulin Disodium.
CA-7. Code designation for Brinolase.
Ca 1022. Code designation for Carbutamide.
CAB-2001. Code designation for Trafermin.
CAM-807. Code designation for Bialamicol Hydrochloride.
Cand5. Code designation for Bevasiranib Sodium.
CAS 276. Code designation for Molsidomine.
CAS 936. Code designation for Pirsidomine.
CB 11 [as hydrochloride]. Code designation for Phenadoxone.
CB-154. Code designation for Bromocriptine.
CB-154 mesylate. Code designation for Bromocriptine Mesylate.
CB 302. Code designation for Ferric Fructose.
CB 304. Code designation for Azaribine.
CB 309. Code designation for Fenabutene.
CB-311. Code designation for Somatropin.
CB 313. Code designation for Mitotane.
CB-337. Code designation for Meglutol.
CB 804. Code designation for Bucloxic Acid.
CB 1048. Code designation for Chlornaphazine.
CB 1664. Code designation for Aceprometazine.
CB 1678. Code designation for Propiomazine.
CB 2201. Code designation for Amfepentorex.
CB 3025. Code designation for Melphalan.
CB 3697. Code designation for Racefemine.

CB 4260. Code designation for Nortetrazepam.
CB 4261. Code designation for Tetrazepam.
CB 4857. Code designation for Menitrazepam.
CB 4985. Code designation for Acequinoline.
CB 7432. Code designation for Idoxifene.
CB 7598. Code designation for Abiraterone.
CB 7630 [as acetate]. Code designation for Abiraterone.
CB 10615. Code designation for Nifurmazole.
CB 11380. Code designation for Nifurizone.
CB 12592. Code designation for Subendazole.
CB-30038. Code designation for Minaprine.
CC-4047. Code designation for Pomalidomide.
CC-5013. Code designation for Lenalidomide.
CC-10004. Code designation for Apremilast.
CCA. Code designation for Lobenzarit Sodium.
CCD 1042. Code designation for Ganaxolone.
CCI-779. Code designation for Temsirolimus.
CCI 4725. Code designation for Clobetasol Propionate.
CCI 5537. Code designation for Clobetasone Butyrate.
C.C.I. 12923. Code designation for Minaxolone.
CCI 15641. Code designation for Cefuroxime Axetil.
CCI 18773. Code designation for Cloticasone Propionate.
CCI 18781. Code designation for Fluticasone Propionate.
CCI 23628. Code designation for Cefuroxime Pivoxetil.
CCNU. Code designation for Lomustine.
CCRG-81045. Code designation for Temozolomide.
CD 271. Code designation for Adapalene.
CDC-501. Code designation for Lenalidomide.
CDDD 1815. Code designation for Alprenoxime Hydrochloride.
CDDD 2803. Code designation for Adaprolol Maleate.
CDDD 3602. Code designation for Tematropium Methylsulfate.
CDDD 5604. Code designation for Loteprednol Etabonate.
CDP571. Code designation for Senlizumab.
CDP-771. Code designation for Gemtuzumab Ozogamicin.
CDP870. Code designation for Certolizumab Pegol.
CE-10. Code designation for Synthetic Conjugated Estrogens, B.
CEN 000029. Code designation for Priliximab.
CEP-151. Code designation for Mecasermin.
CEP-701. Code designation for Lestaurtinib.
CEP 1538. Code designation for Modafinil.
CEP-10953. Code designation for Armodafinil.
CEPH [as hydrochloride]. Code designation for Todralazine.
CERM 730. Code designation for Amoproxan.
CERM 1978. Code designation for Bepridil Hydrochloride.
CERM 10202. Code designation for Vedaprofen.
CG 201. Code designation for Bevonium Metilsulfate.
CG-315E. Code designation for Tramadol Hydrochloride.
CG1940. Code designation for Galgenprostucel-L.
CG5503 (base). Code designation for Tapentadol.
CG8711. Code designation for Litgenprostucel-L.
CG53135-05. Code designation for Velafermin.
CGA 18809. Code designation for Azamethiphos.
CGA-23654. Code designation for Nitroscanate.
CGA 72662. Code designation for Cyromazine.
CGP 2175C. Code designation for Metoprolol Fumarate.
CGP-2175E. Code designation for Metoprolol Tartrate.
CGP-7174/E. Code designation for Cefsulodin Sodium.
CGP 7760B. Code designation for Prenalterol Hydrochloride.
CGP 9000. Code designation for Cefroxadine.
CGP-14221/E. Code designation for Cefotiam Hydrochloride.
CGP-14,458. Code designation for Halobetasol Propionate.
CGP 21690E. Code designation for Oxiracetam.
CGP 23339AE. Code designation for Pamidronate Disodium.
CGP 25827A. Code designation for Formoterol Fumarate.
CGP 30694. Code designation for Edatrexate.
CGP 32349. Code designation for Formestane.
CGP 33101. Code designation for Rufinamide.
CGP 39393. Code designation for Desirudin.

CGP 41251. Code designation for Midostaurin.

CGP 42446. Code designation for Zoledronic Acid.

CGP 42446A. Code designation for Zoledronate Disodium.

CGP 42446B. Code designation for Zoledronate Trisodium.

CGP 45840B. Code designation for Diclofenac Potassium.

CGP 48933. Code designation for Valsartan.

CGS 5391B (anhydrous). Code designation for Enolicam Sodium.

CGS 7135A. Code designation for Azaloxan Fumarate.

CGS 7525A. Code designation for Aptazapine Maleate.

CGS 10078B. Code designation for Bendacalol Mesylate.

CGS 10746B. Code designation for Pentiapine Maleate.

CGS 10787D. Code designation for Prinomide Tromethamine.

CGS 13080. Code designation for Pirmagrel.

CGS 13429A. Code designation for Batelapine Maleate.

CGS 13945. Code designation for Pentopril.

CGS 14824A HCl. Code designation for Benazepril Hydrochloride.

CGS 14831. Code designation for Benazeprilat.

CGS 15040A. Code designation for Serazapine Hydrochloride.

CGS 15855A. Code designation for Isomolpan Hydrochloride.

CGS 16617. Code designation for Libenzapril.

CGS 16949A. Code designation for Fadrozole Hydrochloride.

CGS 18416A. Code designation for Zoniclezole Hydrochloride.

CGS 19755. Code designation for Selfotel.

CGS 20267. Code designation for Letrozole.

CGS 25019C. Code designation for Moxilubant Maleate.

CGS 26214. Code designation for Axitirome.

CGT003. Code designation for Edifoligide Sodium.

CGX-635. Code designation for Omacetaxine Mepesuccinate.

CH 3565. Code designation for Triclosan.

CH690001. Code designation for Tetronasin Sodium.

ChAglyCD3. Code designation for Otelixizumab.

CHIR-12.12. Code designation for Lucatumumab.

CHIR-258. Code designation for Dovitinib Lactate.

CHP. Code designation for Chlorhexidine Phosphanilate.

CHX-100. Code designation for Masoprocol.

CHX 3673. Code designation for Amlexanox.

CI-100. Code designation for Acetosulfone Sodium.

CI-107. Code designation for Argipressin Tannate.

CI-301. Code designation for Bialamicol Hydrochloride.

CI-336. Code designation for Carbocloral.

CI-366. Code designation for Ethosuximide.

CI-379. Code designation for Benzilonium Bromide.

CI-395. Code designation for Phencyclidine Hydrochloride.

CI 403A. Code designation for Pararosaniline Pamoate.

CI-406. Code designation for Oxymetholone.

CI-416. Code designation for Triclofenol Piperazine.

CI-419. Code designation for Fenimide.

CI 427. Code designation for Prodilidine Hydrochloride.

CI-433. Code designation for Clamoxyquin Hydrochloride.

CI 440. Code designation for Flufenamic Acid.

CI-456. Code designation for Diapamide.

CI-473. Code designation for Mefenamic Acid.

CI-501. Code designation for Cycloguanil Pamoate.

CI-515. Code designation for Guanoxyfen Sulfate.

CI-546. Code designation for Alipamide.

CI 556. Code designation for Acedapsone.

CI-572. Code designation for Profadol Hydrochloride.

CI-581. Code designation for Ketamine Hydrochloride.

CI-583. Code designation for Meclofenamic Acid.

CI-633. Code designation for Clioxanide.

CI-634. Code designation for Tiletamine Hydrochloride.

CI-636. Code designation for Sulfacytine.

CI-642. Code designation for Butirosin Sulfate.

CI 673. Code designation for Vidarabine.

CI-686.HCl. Code designation for Trebenzomine Hydrochloride.

CI-705. Code designation for Methaqualone.

CI-716. Code designation for Zolazepam Hydrochloride.

CI-718. Code designation for Bentazepam.

CI-719. Code designation for Gemfibrozil.

CI-720. Code designation for Gemcadiol.

CI-781. Code designation for Zometapine.

CI 787. Code designation for Tioperidone Hydrochloride.

CI-825. Code designation for Pentostatin.

CI-874. Code designation for Indeloxazine Hydrochloride.

CI-879. Code designation for Pramiracetam Hydrochloride.

CI-879 [sulfate]. Code designation for Pramiracetam Sulfate.

CI-880. Code designation for Amsacrine.

CI-881. Code designation for Ametantrone Acetate.

CI-882. Code designation for Sparfosate Sodium.

CI-888. Code designation for Procaterol Hydrochloride.

CI-897. Code designation for Tebuquine.

CI-898. Code designation for Trimetrexate.

CI-904. Code designation for Diaziquone.

CI-906. Code designation for Quinapril Hydrochloride.

CI-907. Code designation for Indolapril Hydrochloride.

CI-908. Code designation for Dezaguanine.

CI-908 mesylate. Code designation for Dezaguanine Mesylate.

CI-909. Code designation for Tiazofurin.

CI-911. Code designation for Rolziracetam.

CI-912. Code designation for Zonisamide.

CI-914. Code designation for Imazodan Hydrochloride.

CI-919. Code designation for Enoxacin.

CI-920. Code designation for Fostriecin Sodium.

CI-921. Code designation for Asulacrine.

CI 925. Code designation for Moexipril Hydrochloride.

CI-928. Code designation for Quinaprilat.

CI-942. Code designation for Piroxantrone Hydrochloride.

CI-945. Code designation for Gabapentin.

CI-946. Code designation for Ralitoline.

CI-958. Code designation for Ledoxantrone Trihydrochloride.

CI-958. Code designation for Sedoxantrone Trihydrochloride.

CI-960 HCl. Code designation for Clinafloxacin Hydrochloride.

CI-970. Code designation for Tacrine Hydrochloride.

CI-977. Code designation for Enadoline Hydrochloride.

CI-978. Code designation for Sparfloxacin.

CI-979. Code designation for Milameline Hydrochloride.

CI-980. Code designation for Mivobulin Isethionate.

CI-981. Code designation for Atorvastatin Calcium.

CI-982. Code designation for Fosphenytoin Sodium.

CI-983. Code designation for Cefdinir.

CI-991. Code designation for Troglitazone.

CI-994. Code designation for Tacedinaline.

CI-1003. Code designation for Suramin Hexasodium.

CI-1004. Code designation for Darbufelone Mesylate.

CI-1008. Code designation for Pregabalin.

CI-1011. Code designation for Avasimibe.

CI-1014. Code designation for Zenarestat.

CI-1019. Code designation for Igmesine Hydrochloride.

CI-1025. Code designation for Conivaptan Hydrochloride.

CI-1027. Code designation for Gemcabene Calcium.

CI-1033. Code designation for Canertinib Dihydrochloride.

CI-1034. Code designation for Fandosentan Potassium.

CI-1041. Code designation for Besonprodil.

CI-1042. Code designation for Lontucirev (Replicating Adenovirus).

CI-9148. Code designation for Cysteamine Hydrochloride.

CIBA 1906. Code designation for Thiambutosine.

CJ-11, 974. Code designation for Ezlopitant.

CJ 91B. Code designation for Olsalazine Sodium.

CJ-11,972. Code designation for Maropitant Citrate.

CK-0383. Code designation for Verofylline.

CK-0569 [as the base]. Code designation for Ipexidine Mesylate.

CK-1752A. Code designation for Sematilide Hydrochloride.

CK0238273. Code designation for Ispinesib Mesylate.

CKD-602. Code designation for Belotecan Hydrochloride.

CL09. Code designation for Icometasone Enbutate.

Cl 337. Code designation for Azaserine.

CL 369. Code designation for Ketamine Hydrochloride.

CL 399. Code designation for Tiletamine Hydrochloride.

Cl-583.Na salt. Code designation for Meclofenamate Sodium.

CL-639C. Code designation for Dioxadrol Hydrochloride.

Cl-661. Code designation for Oxiramide.

Cl-683. Code designation for Ripazepam.

Cl-775. Code designation for Bevantolol Hydrochloride.

Cl-808. Code designation for Vidarabine Phosphate.

Cl-808 sodium. Code designation for Vidarabine Sodium Phosphate.

Cl-845. Code designation for Pirmenol Hydrochloride.

CL-867. Code designation for Piridicillin Sodium.

Cl-871. Code designation for Piracetam.

CL-911C. Code designation for Dexoxadrol Hydrochloride.

CL-912C. Code designation for Levoxadrol Hydrochloride.

CL-1388R. Code designation for Guanadrel Sulfate.

CL-1848C. Code designation for Etoxadrol Hydrochloride.

CL 2422. Code designation for Guancydine.

CL 5,279. Code designation for Nithiamide.

CL 10304. Code designation for Aminocaproic Acid.

CL 12,625. Code designation for Natamycin.

CL 13,900. Code designation for Puromycin.

CL 14377. Code designation for Methotrexate.

CL 16,536. Code designation for Puromycin Hydrochloride.

CL 22415. Code designation for Demecycline.

CL 25477. Code designation for Azetepa.

CL 26193. Code designation for Simtrazene.

CL 27,071. Code designation for Descinolone Acetonide.

CL 34433. Code designation for Triamcinolone Hexacetonide.

CL 34699. Code designation for Amcinonide.

CL 36467. Code designation for Methotrimeprazine.

CL 39743. Code designation for Methotrimeprazine.

CL 39808. Code designation for Thozalinone.

CL 40881. Code designation for Ethambutol Hydrochloride.

CL 48156. Code designation for Imidoline Hydrochloride.

CL 53415. Code designation for Cyproximide.

CL 54131. Code designation for Piperamide Maleate.

CL 54998. Code designation for Brocresine.

CL 59112. Code designation for Roletamide.

CL 61965. Code designation for Triamcinolone Acetonide Sodium Phosphate.

CL 62,362. Code designation for Loxapine.

Cl-64,976. Code designation for Zilantel.

CL 65205. Code designation for Boxidine.

CL 65336. Code designation for Tranexamic Acid.

CL 65,562. Code designation for Triflocin.

CL 67,772. Code designation for Amoxapine.

CL 71563. Code designation for Loxapine Succinate.

CL 81,587. Code designation for Avoparcin.

CL 82,204. Code designation for Fenbufen.

CL 83,544. Code designation for Felbinac.

CL 84,633. Code designation for Nimidane.

CL 88,893. Code designation for Clazolimine.

CL 90,748. Code designation for Azolimine.

CL 98984. Code designation for Cinodine Hydrochloride.

CL 106359. Code designation for Triamcinolone Acetonide Sodium Phosphate.

CL 108,756. Code designation for Brocresine.

CL 112,302. Code designation for Buprenorphine Hydrochloride.

CL 115,347. Code designation for Viprostol.

CL 118,532. Code designation for Triptorelin.

CL 184,116. Code designation for Porfimer Sodium.

CL 184,824. Code designation for Alovudine.

CL 186,815. Code designation for Biapenem.

CL 203,821. Code designation for Cetaben Sodium.

CL 205925. Code designation for Iprocinodine Hydrochloride.

CL 206,214. Code designation for Butamisole Hydrochloride.

CL 206,576. Code designation for Sulbenox.

CL 206,797. Code designation for Cypothrin.

CL 216,942. Code designation for Bisantrene Hydrochloride.

CL 217,658. Code designation for Imcarbofos.

CL 220,075. Code designation for Bicifadine Hydrochloride.

CL 227,193. Code designation for Piperacillin Sodium.

CL 232,315. Code designation for Mitoxantrone Hydrochloride.

CL 273,547. Code designation for Ocinaplon.

CL 273,703. Code designation for Maduramicin.

CL 274,471. Code designation for Colestolone.

CL 284,635. Code designation for Cefixime.

CL 284,846. Code designation for Zaleplon.

CL 286,558. Code designation for Zeniplatin.

CL 287,088. Code designation for Nemadectin.

CL 287,110. Code designation for Enloplatin.

CL 287,389. Code designation for Nilvadipine.

CL 291,894. Code designation for Somagrebove.

CL 297,939. Code designation for Bisoprolol.

CL 297,939. Code designation for Bisoprolol Fumarate.

CL 298,741. Code designation for Tazobactam.

CL 301,423. Code designation for Moxidectin.

CL 307,579. Code designation for Tazobactam Sodium.

CL 307,782. Code designation for Levoleucovorin Calcium.

CL 318,952. Code designation for Verteporfin.

CLY-503. Code designation for Simfibrate.

CM 31-916. Code designation for Ceftiofur Sodium.

CMA-676. Code designation for Gemtuzumab Ozogamicin.

CMC-544. Code designation for Inotuzumab Ozogamicin.

CN-1883. Code designation for Acedapsone.

CN-5834-5931B. Code designation for Triclofenol Piperazine.

CN-10,395. Code designation for Ethosuximide.

CN-14,329-23A. Code designation for Cycloguanil Pamoate.

CN-15,573-23A. Code designation for Pararosaniline Pamoate.

CN-15,757. Code designation for Azaserine.

CN-16146. Code designation for Carbocloral.

CN-17,900-2B. Code designation for Clamoxyquin Hydrochloride.

CN-20,172-3. Code designation for Benzilonium Bromide.

CN-25,253-2. Code designation for Phencyclidine Hydrochloride.

CN-27,554. Code designation for Flufenamic Acid.

CN-34,799-5A. Code designation for Guanoxyfen Sulfate.

CN-35355. Code designation for Mefenamic Acid.

CN-36,337. Code designation for Diapamide.

CN-38,474. Code designation for Alipamide.

CN 38703. Code designation for Methaqualone.

CN-52,372-2. Code designation for Ketamine Hydrochloride.

CN-54521-2. Code designation for Tiletamine Hydrochloride.

CN 59,567. Code designation for Clioxanide.

CNS 1102. Code designation for Aptiganel Hydrochloride.

CNTO 148. Code designation for Golimumab.

CNTO 1275. Code designation for Ustekinumab.

CO 405. Code designation for Butidrine.

Co 200461. Code designation for Besonprodil.

Code 7227. Code designation for Ferumoxtran-10.

Code 7228. Code designation for Ferumoxytol.

CoFactor. Code designation for Folitixorin Calcium.

CO-I. Code designation for Nadide.

COL-3. Code designation for Incyclinide.

Compound 68-198. Code designation for Diamfenetide.

Compound 469. Code designation for Isoflurane.

Compound 497. Code designation for Dieldrin.

Compound 904. Code designation for Alexidine.

Compound 24266. Code designation for Pentetate Calcium Trisodium Yb 169.

Compound 42339. Code designation for Acronine.

Compound 49510. Code designation for Paricalcitol.

Compound 53616. Code designation for Frentizole.

Compound 56063. Code designation for Melizame.
Compound 57926. Code designation for Sinefungin.
Compound 79891. Code designation for Narasin.
Compound 81929. Code designation for Dobutamine.
Compound 83405. Code designation for Cefamandole.
Compound 83846. Code designation for Aprindine Hydrochloride.
Compound 85287. Code designation for Nibroxane.
Compound 89218. Code designation for Nisoxetine.
Compound 90459. Code designation for Benoxaprofen.
Compound 90606. Code designation for Isamoxole.
Compound 93819. Code designation for Fluretofen.
Compound 99170. Code designation for Aprindine.
Compound 99638. Code designation for Cefaclor.
Compound 109168. Code designation for Nifluridide.
Compound 112531. Code designation for Vindesine.
Compound 113878. Code designation for Ciprefadol Succinate.
Compound 113935. Code designation for Pentomone.
Compound 122587. Code designation for Drobuline.
Compound 133314. Code designation for Trioxifene Mesylate.
Compound LY 131126. Code designation for Butopamine.
Compound S. Code designation for Zidovudine.
Continuous Curve-CAB Contact Lens. Code designation for Porofocon B.
COP-1. Code designation for Glatiramer Acetate.
Copolymer-1. Code designation for Glatiramer Acetate.
Corus1020. Code designation for Aztreonam Lysine.
COX-189. Code designation for Lumiracoxib.
CP-15-639-2. Code designation for Carbenicillin Disodium.
CP-88, 059-27. Code designation for Ziprasidone Mesylate.
CP-0127. Code designation for Deltibant.
CP 172 AP. Code designation for Clopirac.
CP-556S. Code designation for Suloctidil.
CP 1044 J3. Code designation for Bufexamac.
CP 1552 S. Code designation for Milacemide Hydrochloride.
CP-10,188. Code designation for Fenclonine.
CP-10,303-8. Code designation for Quinterenol Sulfate.
CP-10,423-16. Code designation for Pyrantel Pamoate.
CP-10,423-18. Code designation for Pyrantel Tartrate.
CP-11,332-1. Code designation for Quinazosin Hydrochloride.
CP-12,009-18. Code designation for Morantel Tartrate.
CP-12,252-1. Code designation for Thiothixene Hydrochloride.
CP-12,299-1. Code designation for Prazosin Hydrochloride.
CP-12,521-1. Code designation for Piquizil Hydrochloride.
CP-12,574. Code designation for Tinidazole.
CP-13,608. Code designation for Tesicam.
CP-14,185-1. Code designation for Hoquizil Hydrochloride.
CP-14,368-1. Code designation for Lometraline Hydrochloride.
CP-14,445-16. Code designation for Oxantel Pamoate.
CP-15,464-2. Code designation for Carbenicillin Indanyl Sodium.
CP-15,467-61. Code designation for Lithium Carbonate.
CP-15,973. Code designation for Sudoxicam.
CP-16,171. Code designation for Piroxicam.
CP-16,171-85. Code designation for Piroxicam Olamine.
CP-16,533-1. Code designation for Verapamil.
CP-18,524. Code designation for Tibric Acid.
CP-19,106-1. Code designation for Trimazosin Hydrochloride.
CP-20,961. Code designation for Avridine.
CP-22,341. Code designation for Temodox.
CP-22,665. Code designation for Flumizole.
CP-24,314-1. Code designation for Pirbuterol Hydrochloride.
CP-24,314-14. Code designation for Pirbuterol Acetate.
CP-24,441-1. Code designation for Tametraline Hydrochloride.
CP-24,877. Code designation for Drinidene.
CP-25,673. Code designation for Tiazuril.
CP-26,154. Code designation for Tolimidone.
CP-27,634. Code designation for Gliamilide.
CP-28,720. Code designation for Glipizide.
CP-31,081. Code designation for Polydextrose.

CP-32,387. Code designation for Pirolate.
CP-33,994-2. Code designation for Pirbenicillin Sodium.
CP-34,089. Code designation for Sulprostone.
CP-36,584. Code designation for Flutroline.
CP-38,754. Code designation for Plauracin.
CP-44,001-1. Code designation for Nantradol Hydrochloride.
CP-45,634. Code designation for Sorbinil.
CP-45,899-2. Code designation for Sulbactam Sodium.
CP-45,899-99. Code designation for Sulbactam Benzathine.
CP-47,904. Code designation for Sulbactam Pivoxil.
CP-48,810-27. Code designation for Fanetizole Mesylate.
CP-48,867-9. Code designation for Ristianol Phosphate.
CP-49,952. Code designation for Sultamicillin.
CP-50,556-1. Code designation for Levonantradol Hydrochloride.
Cp-51,974-1. Code designation for Sertraline Hydrochloride.
CP-52,640-2. Code designation for Cefoperazone Sodium.
CP-54,802. Code designation for Alitame.
CP-57,361-01. Code designation for Zaltidine Hydrochloride.
CP-62,993. Code designation for Azithromycin.
CP-65703. Code designation for Ampiroxicam.
CP-66,248. Code designation for Tenidap.
CP-66,248-2. Code designation for Tenidap Sodium.
CP-70,429. Code designation for Sulopenem.
CP-70,490-09. Code designation for Enazadrem Phosphate.
CP-72,133. Code designation for Ilonidap.
CP-72,467-2. Code designation for Englitazone Sodium.
CP-73,049. Code designation for Binfloxacin.
CP-73,850. Code designation for Zopolrestat.
CP-76,136-27. Code designation for Danofloxacin Mesylate.
CP-80,794. Code designation for Terlakiren.
CP-86,325-2. Code designation for Darglitazone Sodium.
CP-88,059-1. Code designation for Ziprasidone Hydrochloride.
CP-88,818. Code designation for Tiqueside.
CP-93,393-1. Code designation for Sunepitron Hydrochloride.
CP-99,219-27. Code designation for Trovafloxacin Mesylate.
CP-101,606-27. Code designation for Traxoprodil Mesylate.
CP-116,517-27. Code designation for Alatrofloxacin Mesylate.
CP-118,954-11. Code designation for Icopezil Maleate.
CP-148,623. Code designation for Pamaqueside.
CP-325,366. Code designation for Tofimilast.
CP-336,156-CB. Code designation for Lasofoxifene Tartrate.
CP-358,774-01. Code designation for Erlotinib Hydrochloride.
CP-368,296. Code designation for Ingliforib.
CP-424,391-18. Code designation for Capromorelin Tartrate.
CP-448,187-01. Code designation for Elzasonan Hydrochloride.
CP-448,187-10. Code designation for Elzasonan Citrate.
CP-472,295. Code designation for Tulathromycin.
CP-526,555-18. Code designation for Varenicline Tartrate.
CP-529,414. Code designation for Torcetrapib.
CP-547,272. Code designation for Tulathromycin.
CP-597,396-27. Code designation for Zoniporide Mesylate.
CP-675,206. Code designation for Tremelimumab.
CP-742,033. Code designation for Dirlotapide.
CP-751,871. Code designation for Figitumumab.
CP-945,598. Code designation for Otenabant Hydrochloride.
CP-945,598. Code designation for Otenabant.
CPC-111. Code designation for Fosfructose Trisodium.
CPC-211. Code designation for Sodium Dichloroacetate.
Cpd. 5411. Code designation for Iopentol.
Cpd 109514. Code designation for Nabilone.
CR/662. Code designation for Tipepidine.
CRL 40476. Code designation for Modafinil.
CS-023. Code designation for Tomopenem.
CS-045. Code designation for Troglitazone.
CS-151. Code designation for Crofilcon A.
CS-514. Code designation for Pravastatin Sodium.
CS-622. Code designation for Temocapril Hydrochloride.
CS-706. Code designation for Apricoxib.

CS-807. Code designation for Cefpodoxime Proxetil.

CS-866. Code designation for Olmesartan Medoxomil.

CSAG-144. Code designation for Mebeverine Hydrochloride.

CT 1501R. Code designation for Lisofylline.

CT-2103. Code designation for Paclitaxel Poliglumex.

CT 53518. Code designation for Tandutinib.

CTR 6110. Code designation for Nitrodan.

CTX. Code designation for Lornoxicam.

CV-11974. Code designation for Candesartan.

CV 57533. Code designation for Xenyhexenic Acid.

CV 58903. Code designation for Xenazoic Acid.

CVT-124. Code designation for Naxifylline.

CVT-303. Code designation for Ranolazine.

CVT-510. Code designation for Tecadenoson.

CVT-3146. Code designation for Regadenoson.

CX691. Code designation for Farampator.

CX-3543. Code designation for Quarfloxin.

CY 39. Code designation for Psilocybine.

CY-116. Code designation for Aminocaproic Acid.

CY 153. Code designation for Acexamic Acid.

CY 216. Code designation for Nadroparin Calcium.

CYT-103^{111}In. Code designation for Indium In 111 Satumomab Pendetide.

CYT-356. Code designation for Capromab Pendetide.

CYT-424. Code designation for Samarium Sm 153 Lexidronam Pentasodium.

D2E7. Code designation for Adalimumab.

d4T. Code designation for Stavudine.

D 47. Code designation for Sulbentine.

D 00079. Code designation for Anoxomer.

D 237. Code designation for Cloforex.

D-254. Code designation for Pipazethate.

D-365. Code designation for Verapamil.

D-775. Code designation for Homofenazine.

D-1262. Code designation for Cloxypendyl.

D-1593. Code designation for Diapamide.

D-1721. Code designation for Alipamide.

D-1959.HCl. Code designation for Reproterol Hydrochloride.

D2083. Code designation for Desonide.

D2163. Code designation for Rebimastat.

D 4028. Code designation for Enprofylline.

D 7093. Code designation for Mesna.

D-9998. Code designation for Flupirtine Maleate.

D-18506. Code designation for Miltefosine.

D-20761. Code designation for Cetrorelix Acetate.

D-23129. Code designation for Retigabine.

D-24851. Code designation for Indibulin.

DA-398. Code designation for Epirizole.

DA 688. Code designation for Gefarnate.

DA-708. Code designation for Teflurane.

DA-808. Code designation for Nafcaproic Acid.

DA-893. Code designation for Roflurane.

DA-914. Code designation for Nafiverine.

DA-992. Code designation for Naftypramide.

DA 1773. Code designation for Sodium Picosulfate.

DA 2370. Code designation for Feprazone.

DAB$_{389}$IL2. Code designation for Denileukin Diftitox.

DAB-452. Code designation for Aplindore Fumarate.

DAC. Code designation for Decitabine.

DADDS. Code designation for Acedapsone.

(–)-DAPD. Code designation for Amdoxovir.

DAPD. Code designation for Amdoxovir.

D.A.T. Code designation for Acetiamine.

DATC. Code designation for Tiocarlide.

DAU6215CL. Code designation for Itasetron.

DB289. Code designation for Pafuramidine Maleate.

DBM. Code designation for Mitobronitol.

DBV. Code designation for Buformin.

DCA. Code designation for Sodium Dichloroacetate.

DCH 21 [as sodium salt]. Code designation for Exiproben.

DCLHb. Code designation for Hemoglobin Crosfumaril.

Cis-DDP. Code designation for Cisplatin.

DDVP. Code designation for Dichlorvos.

DETF. Code designation for Trichlorfon.

DF 118. Code designation for Dihydrocodeine Bitartrate.

DF 1681Y. Code designation for Reparixin.

DG-031. Code designation for Veliflapon.

DH-524. Code designation for Fenmetozole Hydrochloride.

DH-581. Code designation for Probucol.

DIC. Code designation for Dacarbazine.

Diethylhexyl butamido triazone (INCI). Code designation for Iscotrizinol.

DIM-SA. Code designation for Succimer.

DJN 608. Code designation for Nateglinide.

DK-7419. Code designation for Argatroban.

DL 152. Code designation for Bietaserpine.

DL-164. Code designation for Tiodonium Chloride.

DL-588. Code designation for Napactadine Hydrochloride.

DL-8280. Code designation for Ofloxacin.

dl HM-PAO. Code designation for Exametazime.

DMI. Code designation for Desipramine Hydrochloride.

DMO. Code designation for Dimethadione.

DMP 115. Code designation for Perflutren.

DMP 754. Code designation for Roxifiban Acetate.

DMP 840. Code designation for Bisnafide Dimesylate.

DMSA. Code designation for Succimer.

DMSC. Code designation for Doxycycline Fosfatex.

DMSO. Code designation for Dimethyl Sulfoxide.

DN-2327. Code designation for Pazinaclone.

DO6. Code designation for Lexipafant.

DOPS. Code designation for Droxidopa.

DOTA. Code designation for Tetraxetan.

DP178. Code designation for Enfuvirtide.

DPC-817. Code designation for Dexelvucitabine.

DPDP. Code designation for Fodipir.

DPE. Code designation for Dipivefrin.

DPN. Code designation for Nadide.

DPPE. Code designation for Tesmilifene Hydrochloride.

DR-3355. Code designation for Levofloxacin.

DS 103-282. Code designation for Tizanidine Hydrochloride.

DS-4152. Code designation for Tecogalan Sodium.

DSB*2NMG. Code designation for Bevirimat Dimeglumine.

DT-3. Code designation for Detrothyronine.

DT-327. Code designation for Clopamide.

DTI-0009. Code designation for Selodenoson.

DTIC. Code designation for Dacarbazine.

DTPA. Code designation for Pentetic Acid.

DTPA-SMS. Code designation for Pentetreotide.

D-Trp LHRH-PEA. Code designation for Deslorelin.

DU-6859a. Code designation for Sitafloxacin.

DU-21220. Code designation for Ritodrine.

DU-21445. Code designation for Tiprenolol Hydrochloride.

DU 22550 [as sulfate]. Code designation for Caproxamine.

DU23000. Code designation for Fluvoxamine Maleate.

DU-23187. Code designation for Quincarbate.

DU123265. Code designation for Cilansetron Hydrochloride.

DU 126891. Code designation for Pardoprunox.

DU 126891 hydrochloride. Code designation for Pardoprunox Hydrochloride.

DU127090. Code designation for Bifeprunox Mesylate.

DuP 128. Code designation for Lecimibide.

DuP 753. Code designation for Losartan Potassium.

Dup 785. Code designation for Brequinar Sodium.

DuP 921. Code designation for Sibopirdine.

DUP 937. Code designation for Teloxantrone Hydrochloride.

DUP 941. Code designation for Losoxantrone Hydrochloride.

DuP 996. Code designation for Linopirdine.
DV-1006. Code designation for Cetraxate Hydrochloride.
DW-61. Code designation for Flavoxate Hydrochloride.
DW-62. Code designation for Dimefline Hydrochloride.
DW 75. Code designation for Norleusactide.
DX-88. Code designation for Ecallantide.
DX-890. Code designation for Depelestat.
DX-8951f. Code designation for Exatecan Mesylate.
DyDTPA-BMA. Code designation for Sprodiamide.
E3A. Code designation for Estradiol Acetate.
E 39. Code designation for Inproquone.
E-52. Code designation for Pentafilcon A.
E-106-E [as cyclamate]. Code designation for Furfenorex.
E 141. Code designation for Ethamsylate.
E414. Code designation for Salcaprozate Sodium.
E-614. Code designation for Tripamide.
E-0659. Code designation for Azelastine Hydrochloride.
E-1000. Code designation for Amiloxate.
E2007. Code designation for Perampanel.
E2020. Code designation for Donepezil Hydrochloride.
E2080. Code designation for Rufinamide.
E-2663. Code designation for Bentiromide.
E-3810. Code designation for Rabeprazole Sodium.
E5564. Code designation for Eritoran Tetrasodium.
E7070. Code designation for Indisulam.
E7389. Code designation for Eribulin Mesylate.
E-7869. Code designation for Tarenflurbil.
E 9002. Code designation for Naftalofos.
EA-166. Code designation for Guanoxyfen Sulfate.
EAA-090. Code designation for Perzinfotel.
EACA. Code designation for Aminocaproic Acid.
EC 3.1.6.13. Code designation for Idursulfase.
EC 3.2.1.22. Code designation for Agalsidase Alfa.
EC 3.2.1.45. Code designation for Velaglucerase Alfa.
EDU. Code designation for Edoxudine.
EE$_3$ME. Code designation for Mestranol.
EF9. Code designation for Temoporfin.
EGTA. Code designation for Egtazic Acid.
EGYT 201. Code designation for Bencyclane Fumarate.
EHB 776. Code designation for Foscarnet Sodium.
EKB-569. Code designation for Pelitinib.
EL349. Code designation for Somidobove.
EL625. Code designation for Cenersen Sodium.
EL737. Code designation for Ractopamine Hydrochloride.
EL-857. Code designation for Apramycin.
EL870. Code designation for Tilmicosin.
EL-970. Code designation for Fampridine.
EL-974. Code designation for Ticarbodine.
ELD 950. Code designation for Eledoisin.
EM574. Code designation for Idremcinal.
EM906. Code designation for Faxeladol.
EM-1421. Code designation for Terameprocol.
EMBAY 8440. Code designation for Praziquantel.
EMD 15 700. Code designation for Nitrefazole.
EMD 33 512. Code designation for Bisoprolol.
EMD 9806. Code designation for Pramiverine.
EMD 19698 [as hydrogen maleate]. Code designation for Peratizole.
EMD 128130. Code designation for Sarizotan Hydrochloride.
EMD 273066. Code designation for Tucotuzumab Celmoleukin.
EMD 390920. Code designation for Pruvanserin.
EN-141. Code designation for Josamycin.
EN-313. Code designation for Moricizine.
EN-970. Code designation for Fluquazone.
EN-1010. Code designation for Pyrrocaine.
EN-1620A. Code designation for Nalmexone Hydrochloride.
EN-1639A. Code designation for Naltrexone Hydrochloride.
EN-1639A [as hydrochloride]. Code designation for Naltrexone.

EN-1661L. Code designation for Bisobrin Lactate.
EN-1733A. Code designation for Molindone Hydrochloride.
EN-2234A. Code designation for Nalbuphine Hydrochloride.
EN-15304. Code designation for Naloxone Hydrochloride.
EN 137774. Code designation for Ramatroban.
ENA-713. Code designation for Rivastigmine.
ENT-20852. Code designation for Butonate.
ENT-23969. Code designation for Carbaril.
ENT-25567. Code designation for Naftalofos.
ENT 29,106. Code designation for Nimidane.
EO9. Code designation for Apaziquone.
EPO. Code designation for Epoetin Alfa.
EPOCH. Code designation for Epoetin Beta.
ER-155055-90. Code designation for Perampanel.
ERB-041. Code designation for Prinaberel.
ERL 080. Code designation for Mycophenolate Sodium.
ES 304. Code designation for Nicofuranose.
estradiol-3-acetate. Code designation for Estradiol Acetate.
ET-394. Code designation for Tribromsalan.
ET-495. Code designation for Piribedil.
ET-743. Code designation for Trabectedin.
ETTN. Code designation for Propatyl Nitrate.
EU-1063. Code designation for Proquinolate.
EU-1085. Code designation for Leniquinsin.
EU-1093. Code designation for Buquinolate.
EU-1806. Code designation for Nafronyl Oxalate.
EU-2826. Code designation for Benurestat.
EU-2972. Code designation for Nolinium Bromide.
EU-3120. Code designation for Acodazole Hydrochloride.
EU-3325. Code designation for Triafungin.
EU-3421. Code designation for Oxifungin Hydrochloride.
EU-4093. Code designation for Azumolene Sodium.
EU-4200. Code designation for Piribedil.
EU-4534. Code designation for Flurofamide.
EU-4584. Code designation for Tolfamide.
EU-4891. Code designation for Diacetolol Hydrochloride.
EU-4906. Code designation for Sitogluside.
EU-5306. Code designation for Pefloxacin.
EUDR. Code designation for Edoxudine.
EV2-7. Code designation for Sevirumab.
EX 10-029-C. Code designation for Elantrine.
EX 10-781. Code designation for Metizoline Hydrochloride.
EX 12-095. Code designation for Eterobarb.
EX 4355. Code designation for Desipramine Hydrochloride.
EX 4810. Code designation for Ambuside.
Ex 4883. Code designation for Rolicyprine.
EXP-105-1. Code designation for Amantadine Hydrochloride.
EXP 126. Code designation for Rimantadine Hydrochloride.
EXP 338. Code designation for Midaflur.
EXP 999. Code designation for Metopimazine.
EYE001. Code designation for Pegaptanib Sodium.
EZ-246. Code designation for Pegamotecan.
F-368. Code designation for Dantrolene.
F-413. Code designation for Clodanolene.
F-440. Code designation for Dantrolene Sodium.
F-605 (as the sodium). Code designation for Clodanolene.
F-691. Code designation for Furodazole.
F-776. Code designation for Orpanoxin.
F-853. Code designation for Nitrafudam Hydrochloride.
F 1500. Code designation for Succisulfone.
F 1983. Code designation for Pyrovalerone Hydrochloride.
F 6066. Code designation for Cyclofenil.
F-12158. Code designation for Vinflunine Ditartrate.
F28249α. Code designation for Nemadectin.
Fa 402. Code designation for Fentonium Bromide.
FAT 70'884. Code designation for Bemotrizinol.
FAT 75'634. Code designation for Bisoctrizole.
FBA 1420. Code designation for Propanidid.

FBA 4059. Code designation for Brotianide.

FBB 4231. Code designation for Glisoxepide.

FBB 6896. Code designation for Clenpirin.

FC41-12 (Perflenapent/Perflisopent mixture). Code designation for Perflenapent.

FC41-12 (Perflenapent/Perflisopent mixture). Code designation for Perflisopent.

FC-1157a. Code designation for Toremifene Citrate.

Fc-1271. Code designation for Ospemifene.

FC-1271a. Code designation for Ospemifene.

FCE 20124. Code designation for Reboxetine Mesylate.

FCE 21336. Code designation for Cabergoline.

FCE24304. Code designation for Exemestane.

FCF 89. Code designation for Roquinimex.

F-ddA. Code designation for Lodenosine.

[18]FDG. Code designation for Fludeoxyglucose F 18.

FE200486 (as acetate salt). Code designation for Degarelix.

FE200486 (free base). Code designation for Degarelix Acetate.

FER-1443. Code designation for Ticlatone.

FG 5111. Code designation for Melperone.

FG-10571. Code designation for Panadiplon.

FI 5852. Code designation for Oxabolone Cipionate.

F.I. 6146. Code designation for Buzepide Metiodide.

FI 6337. Code designation for Metergoline.

FI 6339 [as the base]. Code designation for Daunorubicin Hydrochloride.

F.I. 6426. Code designation for Stallimycin Hydrochloride.

F.I. 6654. Code designation for Caroxazone.

F.I. 6820. Code designation for Brofoxine.

FK 027. Code designation for Cefixime.

FK228. Code designation for Romidepsin.

FK 235. Code designation for Nilvadipine.

FK-366. Code designation for Zenarestat.

FK463. Code designation for Micafungin Sodium.

FK 482. Code designation for Cefdinir.

FK 506. Code designation for Tacrolimus.

FK 749. Code designation for Ceftizoxime Sodium.

FKS-508. Code designation for Cevimeline Hydrochloride.

FLA 731. Code designation for Remoxipride.

FLA 731(−). Code designation for Remoxipride Hydrochloride.

FMdC. Code designation for Tezacitabine.

FP-GP1. Code designation for Motexafin Gadolinium.

FPL.670. Code designation for Cromolyn Sodium.

FPL 12924AA. Code designation for Remacemide Hydrochloride.

FPL 58668KC. Code designation for Probicromil Calcium.

FPL 59002. Code designation for Nedocromil.

FPL 59002KC. Code designation for Nedocromil Calcium.

FPL 59002KP. Code designation for Nedocromil Sodium.

FPL 59360. Code designation for Minocromil.

FPL 60278. Code designation for Dopexamine.

FPL 60278AR. Code designation for Dopexamine Hydrochloride.

FP-LP1. Code designation for Motexafin Lutetium.

FR 13749. Code designation for Ceftizoxime Sodium.

FR 17027. Code designation for Cefixime.

FR-74366. Code designation for Zenarestat.

FR900506. Code designation for Tacrolimus.

FR901228. Code designation for Romidepsin.

FS069. Code designation for Perflutren.

FSH. Code designation for Menotropins.

(−)-FTC. Code designation for Emtricitabine.

FTC-(−). Code designation for Emtricitabine.

FTS. Code designation for Salirasib.

FTY720. Code designation for Fingolimod Hydrochloride.

FU-02. Code designation for Fumoxicillin.

FUDR. Code designation for Floxuridine.

FUT-175. Code designation for Nafamostat Mesylate.

FWH 399. Code designation for Troxonium Tosilate.

FXR-450. Code designation for Turofexorate Isopropyl.

G-4. Code designation for Dichlorophen.

G-101, SCY-Er. Code designation for Erythromycin Salnacedin.

G-201,SCY. Code designation for Salnacedin.

G3139. Code designation for Oblimersen Sodium.

G-24480. Code designation for Dimpylate.

G-25178. Code designation for Prodeconium Bromide.

G-25766. Code designation for Clorindione.

G 26,872. Code designation for Phenbutazone Sodium Glycerate.

G 30320. Code designation for Clofazimine.

G-32883. Code designation for Carbamazepine.

G-33040. Code designation for Opipramol Hydrochloride.

G-33182. Code designation for Chlorthalidone.

G 34586. Code designation for Clomipramine Hydrochloride.

G-35020. Code designation for Desipramine Hydrochloride.

G 35259. Code designation for Ketipramine Fumarate.

G-704,650. Code designation for Alendronate Sodium.

GA101. Code designation for Afutuzumab.

gadolinium texaphyrin. Code designation for Motexafin Gadolinium.

GA-EPO. Code designation for Epoetin Delta.

GAP (Wyeth). Code designation for Rotigaptide.

GC-1. Code designation for Sobetirome.

GCR9905. Code designation for Faxeladol.

GD0039. Code designation for Tridolgosir Hydrochloride.

Gd texaphyrin. Code designation for Motexafin Gadolinium.

GdDTPA-BMA. Code designation for Gadodiamide.

Gd-Tex. Code designation for Motexafin Gadolinium.

GEA 654. Code designation for Alaproclate.

GER-11. Code designation for Pimagedine Hydrochloride.

GF 120918A. Code designation for Elacridar Hydrochloride.

GG-745. Code designation for Dutasteride.

GI 87084B. Code designation for Remifentanil Hydrochloride.

GI147211C. Code designation for Lurtotecan Dihydrochloride.

GI 198745. Code designation for Dutasteride.

GI262570X. Code designation for Farglitazar.

GM-611. Code designation for Mitemcinal Fumarate.

GMC 89-107. Code designation for Regramostim.

GM-CSF. Code designation for Regramostim.

GN1600. Code designation for Argatroban.

Go-560. Code designation for Febarbamate.

Go 919. Code designation for Piprozolin.

Go 1213. Code designation for Atolide.

Go 1733. Code designation for Suloxifen Oxalate.

Go 2782. Code designation for Iproxamine Hydrochloride.

Go 3026A. Code designation for Ciclafrine Hydrochloride.

GOE 3450. Code designation for Gabapentin.

GOE 5549. Code designation for Tacedinaline.

Goedecke 3282. Code designation for Ozolinone.

GP-1-110. Code designation for Acadesine.

GP-2-121-3. Code designation for Arbutamine Hydrochloride.

GP-121. Code designation for Phencyclidine Hydrochloride.

GP 31406. Code designation for Depramine.

GP 45840. Code designation for Diclofenac Sodium.

GP-47680. Code designation for Oxcarbazepine.

GP 51084. Code designation for Glibutimine.

GPA-878. Code designation for Metazamide.

GPI-200. Code designation for Iometopane I 123.

GR 2/234. Code designation for Alfaxalone.

GR 2/443 [as propionate]. Code designation for Doxibetasol.

GR 2/925. Code designation for Clobetasol Propionate.

GR 2/1214. Code designation for Clobetasone Butyrate.

GR 2/1574. Code designation for Alfadolone.

GR 412. Code designation for Dodeclonium Bromide.

GR 20263. Code designation for Ceftazidime.

GR 30921. Code designation for Mitoquidone.

GR 32191 [vapiprost]. Code designation for Vapiprost Hydrochloride.

GR 32191B. Code designation for Vapiprost Hydrochloride.

GR 33207. Code designation for Ovandrotone Albumin.

GR 33343 G. Code designation for Salmeterol Xinafoate.

GR 33343 X. Code designation for Salmeterol.

GR 38032F. Code designation for Ondansetron Hydrochloride.

GR 43175C. Code designation for Sumatriptan Succinate.

GR 43659X. Code designation for Lacidipine.

GR50360A. Code designation for Fluparoxan Hydrochloride.

GR 50692. Code designation for Cefempidone.

GR 53992B (GX 1296B). Code designation for Teludipine Hydrochloride.

GR 63178K. Code designation for Fosquidone.

GR 68755C. Code designation for Alosetron Hydrochloride.

GR 69153X. Code designation for Cefetecol.

GR 81225C. Code designation for Galdansetron Hydrochloride.

GR 81225X [as the base]. Code designation for Galdansetron Hydrochloride.

GR 85548A. Code designation for Naratriptan Hydrochloride.

GR 87442 N. Code designation for Lurosetron Mesylate.

GR92132X. Code designation for Troglitazone.

GR 109714X. Code designation for Lamivudine.

GR 114297A. Code designation for Picumeterol Fumarate.

GR 114297X [picumeterol]. Code designation for Picumeterol Fumarate.

GR 116526X. Code designation for Isotretinoin Anisatil.

GR 117289C. Code designation for Zolasartan.

GR 121167X. Code designation for Zanamivir.

GR 122311X. Code designation for Ranitidine Bismuth Citrate.

GR 138950C. Code designation for Saprisartan Potassium.

GR205171A. Code designation for Vofopitant Dihydrochloride.

GR215864. Code designation for Zoticasone.

GRT151 base. Code designation for Axomadol.

GRTA9906. Code designation for Faxeladol.

GRTA0009906. Code designation for Faxeladol.

GRT-TA300. Code designation for Faxeladol.

GS-95. Code designation for Thiethylperazine Maleate.

GS-0393. Code designation for Adefovir.

GS-0504. Code designation for Cidofovir.

GS-0840. Code designation for Adefovir Dipivoxil.

GS-1278. Code designation for Tenofovir.

GS-1339. Code designation for Dymanthine Hydrochloride.

GS 2147. Code designation for Sancycline.

GS-2876. Code designation for Methacycline.

GS-2989. Code designation for Meclocycline.

GS-3065. Code designation for Doxycycline.

GS-3159. Code designation for Carbenicillin Potassium.

GS-4331-05. Code designation for Tenofovir Disoproxil Fumarate.

GS-6244. Code designation for Carbadox.

GS-6742. Code designation for Sulfomyxin.

GS-7443. Code designation for Mequidox.

GS-9137. Code designation for Elvitegravir.

GSI-953. Code designation for Begacestat.

GSK159797C. Code designation for Milveterol Hydrochloride.

GSK221149A. Code designation for Retosiban.

GSK233705B. Code designation for Darotropium Bromide.

GSK716155. Code designation for Albiglutide.

GT16-026A. Code designation for Sevelamer Hydrochloride.

GT31-104HB. Code designation for Colesevelam Hydrochloride.

GT56-252. Code designation for Deferitrin.

GT160-246. Code designation for Tolevamer Sodium.

GT267-004. Code designation for Tolevamer Potassium Sodium.

GT335-012. Code designation for Sevelamer Carbonate.

GT-2331. Code designation for Cipralisant Maleate.

GV 104326B. Code designation for Sanfetrinem Sodium.

GV 118819X. Code designation for Sanfetrinem Cilexetil.

GV 150526X. Code designation for Gavestinel.

GW-1000. Code designation for Nabiximols.

GW64085X. Code designation for Brecanavir.

GW-80126. Code designation for Seprilose.

GW-280430A. Code designation for Gantacurium Chloride.

GW353162A. Code designation for Radafaxine Hydrochloride.

GW427353B. Code designation for Solabegron Hydrochloride.

GW 433908A. Code designation for Fosamprenavir Sodium.

GW 433908G. Code designation for Fosamprenavir Calcium.

GW572016F. Code designation for Lapatinib Ditosylate.

GW597588B. Code designation for Vestipitant Mesylate.

GW677954. Code designation for Sodelglitazar.

GW679769B. Code designation for Casopitant Mesylate.

GW685698X. Code designation for Fluticasone Furoate.

GW786034B. Code designation for Pazopanib Hydrochloride.

GW823093C. Code designation for Denagliptin Tosylate.

GW869682X. Code designation for Sergliflozin Etabonate.

GW873140A. Code designation for Aplaviroc Hydrochloride.

GW AH7673A. Code designation for Proguanil Hydrochloride.

GX15-070MS. Code designation for Obatoclax Mesylate.

^{2}H. Code designation for Deuterium Oxide.

H2G. Code designation for Omaciclovir.

h5G1.1. Code designation for Eculizumab.

h5G1.1 scFv. Code designation for Pexelizumab.

h5G1.1 scFv (CDR). Code designation for Pexelizumab.

h5G1.1VHC+h5G1.1VLC. Code designation for Eculizumab.

H 56/28. Code designation for Alprenolol Hydrochloride.

H65-RTA. Code designation for Zolimomab Aritox.

H 93/26 succinate. Code designation for Metoprolol Succinate.

H 102/09 Hydrochloride. Code designation for Zimeldine Hydrochloride.

H 104/08. Code designation for Pamatolol Sulfate.

H 133/22. Code designation for Prenalterol Hydrochloride.

H 154/82. Code designation for Felodipine.

H 168/68. Code designation for Omeprazole.

H 168/68 magnesium. Code designation for Omeprazole Magnesium.

H 168/68 sodium. Code designation for Omeprazole Sodium.

H199/18 magnesium trihydrate. Code designation for Esomeprazole Magnesium.

H199/18 sodium. Code designation for Esomeprazole Sodium.

H324/38. Code designation for Clevidipine Butyrate.

H 365. Code designation for Paroxypropione.

H 376/95. Code designation for Ximelagatran.

H 3774. Code designation for Alibendol.

H 4132. Code designation for Dotefonium Bromide.

H 4170. Code designation for Tolpiprazole.

H 4723. Code designation for Clobazam.

HA-1A. Code designation for Nebacumab.

hAFP-31. Code designation for Yttrium Y 90 Tacatuzumab.

hAFP-31. Code designation for Yttrium Y 90 Tacatuzumab Tetraxetan.

HB 115. Code designation for Nifurprazine.

HB 419. Code designation for Glyburide.

H.B.F. 386. Code designation for Cactinomycin.

HBOC-201. Code designation for Hemoglobin Glutamer-250 (Bovine).

HBOC-301. Code designation for Hemoglobin Glutamer-200 (Bovine).

HC 1528. Code designation for Decoquinate.

HC 20,511 fumarate. Code designation for Ketotifen Fumarate.

HCD-122. Code designation for Lucatumumab.

HCT 3012. Code designation for Naproxcinod.

HCV-796. Code designation for Nesbuvir.

HDPC. Code designation for Miltefosine.

HEOD. Code designation for Dieldrin.

Heparin Fragment Kabi 2165. Code designation for Dalteparin Sodium.

HEPP. Code designation for Pentigetide.

HES 130/0.4. Code designation for Hydroxyethyl Starch 130/0.4.

HF 241. Code designation for Bufeniode.

HF 1854. Code designation for Clozapine.

HF 1927. Code designation for Dibenzepin Hydrochloride.

HF-2159. Code designation for Clothiapine.

HFA-134-a. Code designation for Norflurane.

HFZ. Code designation for Homofenazine.

HGP-1. Code designation for Loteprednol Etabonate.

HGP-2. Code designation for Adaprolol Maleate.

HGP-5. Code designation for Alprenoxime Hydrochloride.

HGP-6. Code designation for Tematropium Methylsulfate.

HGS1018. Code designation for Lexatumumab.

HGS-ETR1. Code designation for Mapatumumab.

HGS-ETR2. Code designation for Lexatumumab.

HH105. Code designation for Butetamate.

HH 197. Code designation for Butamirate Citrate.

HIDA. Code designation for Lidofenin.

HKI-272. Code designation for Neratinib.

HL91. Code designation for Upenazime.

HL 267. Code designation for Dipenine Bromide.

HL 275. Code designation for Alvocidib.

HL 362. Code designation for Colforsin.

HL 523 [as hydrochloride]. Code designation for Tiformin.

HM-101. Code designation for Fispemifene.

HM-101a. Code designation for Fispemifene.

HMD. Code designation for Oxymetholone.

HMDP. Code designation for Oxidronic Acid.

HMG. Code designation for Menotropins.

hMN-14. Code designation for Labetuzumab.

HMR 1275. Code designation for Alvocidib.

HMR 1964. Code designation for Insulin Glulisine.

HMR3480. Code designation for Pralnacasan.

HMR3480/VX-740. Code designation for Pralnacasan.

HMR 3647. Code designation for Telithromycin.

HMR4396. Code designation for Epoetin Delta.

HOE 18 680. Code designation for Embutramide.

HOE 39-893d. Code designation for Penbutolol Sulfate.

HOE 42-440. Code designation for Tiamenidine Hydrochloride.

Hoe 045. Code designation for Articaine.

HOE 045. Code designation for Articaine Hydrochloride.

HOE 062 [Roxatidine]. Code designation for Roxatidine Acetate Hydrochloride.

HOE 71GT. Code designation for Insulin Glargine.

HOE 077. Code designation for Lufironil.

Hoe 105. Code designation for Citenazone.

HOE 118. Code designation for Piretanide.

HOE 140. Code designation for Icatibant Acetate.

HOE 216V. Code designation for Luxabendazole.

HOE 280. Code designation for Ofloxacin.

HOE 296. Code designation for Ciclopirox Olamine.

Hoe 296 V. Code designation for Resorantel.

HOE 296b. Code designation for Ciclopirox.

HOE 304. Code designation for Desoximetasone.

HOE 440. Code designation for Tiamenidine.

Hoe 473. Code designation for Aclantate.

HOE 490. Code designation for Glimepiride.

HOE 498. Code designation for Ramipril.

HOE 642. Code designation for Cariporide Mesylate.

HOE 760. Code designation for Roxatidine Acetate Hydrochloride.

HOE 766. Code designation for Buserelin Acetate.

HOE 777. Code designation for Prednicarbate.

Hoe 881V. Code designation for Fenbendazole.

HOE 893d. Code designation for Penbutolol Sulfate.

HOE 901. Code designation for Insulin Glargine.

HOE 984. Code designation for Nomifensine Maleate.

HOE 36801. Code designation for Etifoxine.

Hoechst 10495. Code designation for Norpipanone.

Hoechst 10582. Code designation for Normethadone.

Homoharringtonine. Code designation for Omacetaxine Mepesuccinate.

HP 029. Code designation for Velnacrine Maleate.

HP 128. Code designation for Suronacrine Maleate.

HP 290. Code designation for Quilostigmine.

HP 494. Code designation for Fluradoline Hydrochloride.

HP 522. Code designation for Brocrinat.

HP 549. Code designation for Isoxepac.

HP 749. Code designation for Besipirdine Hydrochloride.

HP 873. Code designation for Iloperidone.

HP 1598. Code designation for Guanoxyfen Sulfate.

HP 3522. Code designation for Brocrinat.

HPEK-1. Code designation for Tetroquinone.

hPTH 1-34 (acetate salt). Code designation for Teriparatide Acetate.

HR111V-sulfate. Code designation for Cefquinome Sulfate.

HR 221 [as sodium]. Code designation for Cefodizime.

HR 376. Code designation for Clobazam.

HR 756. Code designation for Cefotaxime Sodium.

HR 810 sulfate. Code designation for Cefpirome Sulfate.

HR 930. Code designation for Fosazepam.

HRP 543. Code designation for Dazepinil Hydrochloride.

HRP 913. Code designation for Neflumozide Hydrochloride.

HS-592. Code designation for Clemastine.

HSP90MAB. Code designation for Efungumab.

HSP 2986. Code designation for Pramiverine.

HspE7. Code designation for Verpasep Caltespen.

HSPPC-96. Code designation for Vitespen.

HT-11. Code designation for Cloperastine.

HTF 919. Code designation for Tegaserod.

HTF 919. Code designation for Tegaserod Maleate.

HTI-286. Code designation for Taltobulin.

HU1D10. Code designation for Apolizumab.

hu5c8. Code designation for Ruplizumab.

Hu23F2G. Code designation for Rovelizumab.

hu1124. Code designation for Efalizumab.

huC242-DM1. Code designation for Cantuzumab Mertansine.

HUF-2446. Code designation for Clodazon Hydrochloride.

HuLuc63. Code designation for Elotuzumab.

HuM291. Code designation for Visilizumab.

huMABCD20. Code designation for Afutuzumab.

HuMax-CD4. Code designation for Zanolimumab.

huS2C6. Code designation for Dacetuzumab.

HuZAF. Code designation for Fontolizumab.

HWA 285. Code designation for Propentofylline.

HWA-486. Code designation for Leflunomide.

HY-185. Code designation for Carbocloral.

HYO6A. Code designation for Hyaluronidase (Ovine).

I-653. Code designation for Desflurane.

I-2105. Code designation for Afovirsen Sodium.

[123]I labeled IMP. Code designation for Iofetamine Hydrochloride I 123.

IA-307. Code designation for Acetosulfone Sodium.

IB-367-03. Code designation for Iseganan Hydrochloride.

IBC. Code designation for Bucrylate.

IC351. Code designation for Tadalafil.

ICA-17043. Code designation for Senicapoc.

ICI 8173. Code designation for Quindoxin.

ICI 28257. Code designation for Clofibrate.

ICI 29661. Code designation for Pyrimitate.

ICI 32865. Code designation for Etoglucid.

ICI-33,828. Code designation for Methallibure.

ICI 35,868. Code designation for Propofol.

ICI 38174 [as hydrochloride]. Code designation for Pronetalol.

ICI 45520. Code designation for Propranolol Hydrochloride.

ICI 45763 [as hydrochloride]. Code designation for Toliprolol.

ICI 46,474. Code designation for Tamoxifen Citrate.

ICI 46683. Code designation for Oxyclozanide.

I.C.I. 47,319. Code designation for Dexpropranolol Hydrochloride.

ICI 48213. Code designation for Cyclofenil.

ICI 50,123. Code designation for Pentagastrin.

I.C.I. 50,172. Code designation for Practolol.

I.C.I. 54,450. Code designation for Fenclozic Acid.

ICI 54,594 [as sodium salt]. Code designation for Brofezil.

ICI 55,052. Code designation for Nequinate.

ICI 55,897. Code designation for Clobuzarit.

ICI 58,834. Code designation for Viloxazine Hydrochloride.

ICI 59118. Code designation for Razoxane.

ICI 66,082. Code designation for Atenolol.

ICI 80,008 [as sodium salt]. Code designation for Fluprostenol Sodium.

ICI 80,996. Code designation for Cloprostenol Sodium.

ICI 81,008. Code designation for Fluprostenol Sodium.

ICI 118,587. Code designation for Xamoterol Fumarate.

ICI 118,630. Code designation for Goserelin.

ICI 125,211. Code designation for Tiotidine.

ICI 128,436. Code designation for Ponalrestat.

ICI 136,753. Code designation for Tracazolate.

ICI 139603. Code designation for Tetronasin Sodium.

ICI 141,292. Code designation for Epanolol.

ICI 156,834. Code designation for Cefotetan.

ICI 176,334. Code designation for Bicalutamide.

ICI 182,780. Code designation for Fulvestrant.

ICI 194,660. Code designation for Meropenem.

ICI 204,219. Code designation for Zafirlukast.

ICI 204,636. Code designation for Quetiapine Fumarate.

ICI D1033. Code designation for Anastrozole.

ICID2079. Code designation for Talibegron Hydrochloride.

ICI-U.S. 457. Code designation for Octazamide.

ICJ 3393. Code designation for Iosimenol.

ICL670A. Code designation for Deferasirox.

ICN-542. Code designation for Ribaminol.

ICN-1256. Code designation for Tocladesine.

ICN-10146. Code designation for Isatoribine.

ICRF 159. Code designation for Razoxane.

ICRF-187. Code designation for Dexrazoxane.

IDD-676. Code designation for Lidorestat.

IDD-000676-01. Code designation for Lidorestat.

IDEC-102. Code designation for Rituximab.

IDEC-114. Code designation for Galiximab.

IDEC-129. Code designation for Ibritumomab Tiuxetan.

IDEC-152. Code designation for Gomiliximab.

IDEC-152. Code designation for Lumiliximab.

IDEC-C2B8. Code designation for Rituximab.

IDEC-Y2B8. Code designation for Ibritumomab Tiuxetan.

Id/KLH. Code designation for Mitumprotimut-T.

IDN 6556. Code designation for Emricasan.

IDU. Code designation for Idoxuridine.

IgE Pentapeptide. Code designation for Pentigetide.

IL-1 Trap. Code designation for Rilonacept.

IL13-PE38. Code designation for Cintredekin Besudotox.

IL-21. Code designation for Denenicokin.

IL 5902. Code designation for Spiramycin.

IL 6001. Code designation for Trimipramine.

IL-6302 mesylate. Code designation for Fonazine Mesylate.

IL-17803A. Code designation for Acebutolol Hydrochloride.

IL-19552. Code designation for Pipotiazine Palmitate.

IL 22811 HCl. Code designation for Meptazinol Hydrochloride.

ILX651. Code designation for Tasidotin Hydrochloride.

[123]I-M123. Code designation for Iofetamine Hydrochloride I 123.

IM862. Code designation for Oglufanide Disodium.

IMA-638. Code designation for Anrukinzumab.

IMC-1121B. Code designation for Ramucirumab.

IMC-A12. Code designation for Cixutumumab.

IMI-28. Code designation for Epirubicin Hydrochloride.

IMI 30. Code designation for Idarubicin Hydrochloride.

IMI 58. Code designation for Esorubicin Hydrochloride.

IMiD 3. Code designation for Pomalidomide.

IMMU-4. Code designation for Arcitumomab.

IMMU-106. Code designation for Veltuzumab.

IMMU-115. Code designation for Milatuzumab.

IMMU-hLL2. Code designation for Epratuzumab.

IMMU-LL2. Code designation for Bectumomab.

IMMU-MN3. Code designation for Sulesomab.

IN 29-5931B. Code designation for Triclofenol Piperazine.

IN 379. Code designation for Pimetine Hydrochloride.

IN 461. Code designation for Benzindopyrine Hydrochloride.

IN 511. Code designation for Phenyramidol Hydrochloride.

IN 836. Code designation for Fenyripol Hydrochloride.

IN 1060. Code designation for Cyprolidol Hydrochloride.

INA-X14. Code designation for Insulin Aspart.

INCB 007839. Code designation for Aderbasib.

INCB-8721. Code designation for Dexelvucitabine.

INF-1837. Code designation for Flufenamic Acid.

INF-3355. Code designation for Mefenamic Acid.

INF 4668. Code designation for Meclofenamic Acid.

INGN 201. Code designation for Contusugene Ladenovec.

INH-H2002. Code designation for Tefibazumab.

INN 00835. Code designation for Nemifitide Ditriflutate.

INS365. Code designation for Diquafosol Tetrasodium.

INS37217. Code designation for Denufosol Tetrasodium.

INS50589. Code designation for Regrelor Disodium.

Insulin X14. Code designation for Insulin Aspart.

INT-747. Code designation for Obeticholic Acid.

Interleukin-1 Trap. Code designation for Rilonacept.

IP 302 sodium. Code designation for Citicoline Sodium.

IP 456. Code designation for Pagoclone.

IP631. Code designation for Trospium Chloride.

IP-2105. Code designation for Afovirsen Sodium.

IPA. Code designation for Riboprine.

IPdR. Code designation for Ropidoxuridine.

IPI-504. Code designation for Retaspimycin.

IPI-504. Code designation for Retaspimycin Hydrochloride.

IPM. Code designation for Palifosfamide.

IPTD. Code designation for Glyprothiazol.

IS 5-MN. Code designation for Isosorbide Mononitrate.

I.S. 499. Code designation for Poldine Methylsulfate.

IS 2596. Code designation for Domoxin.

ISA247. Code designation for Voclosporin.

ISATX247. Code designation for Voclosporin.

ISIS-2105. Code designation for Afovirsen Sodium.

ISIS 2302. Code designation for Alicaforsen Sodium.

ISIS 2922. Code designation for Fomivirsen Sodium.

ISIS 5321. Code designation for Aprinocarsen Sodium.

ISIS 112989. Code designation for Custirsen Sodium.

ISIS 301012. Code designation for Mipomersen Sodium.

Isomer A. Code designation for Zuclomiphene.

Isomer B. Code designation for Enclomiphene.

J867. Code designation for Asoprisnil.

Janssen R 4929. Code designation for Benzetimide Hydrochloride.

JAV 852. Code designation for Benfosformin.

JB-8181. Code designation for Desipramine Hydrochloride.

JD-96. Code designation for Vinylbital.

JF-1. Code designation for Nalmefene.

JL 512. Code designation for Fenadiazole.

JL-1078. Code designation for Dihexyverine Hydrochloride.

JM-8. Code designation for Carboplatin.

JM-9. Code designation for Iproplatin.

JM-83. Code designation for Oxaliplatin.

JM-216. Code designation for Satraplatin.

JNJ-10234094. Code designation for Carisbamate.

JO-1784. Code designation for Igmesine Hydrochloride.

JTE-522. Code designation for Tilmacoxib.

JTK-303. Code designation for Elvitegravir.

JTP-19605. Code designation for Tilmacoxib.

K-17. Code designation for Thalidomide.
K-38. Code designation for Glycyclamide.
K85. Code designation for Omega-3-acid Ethyl Esters.
K-386. Code designation for Glycyclamide.
K-1900. Code designation for Nimorazole.
K 4024. Code designation for Glipizide.
K 4277. Code designation for Indoprofen.
K 9147. Code designation for Tolciclate.
K 11941. Code designation for Alfaprostol.
K 12148. Code designation for Lifibrol.
KABI 925. Code designation for Emylcamate.
Kabi 2234. Code designation for Tolterodine.
KAT 256 [as hydrochloride]. Code designation for Clobutinol.
KB 95. Code designation for Benzpiperylon.
KB-944. Code designation for Fostedil.
KC8857. Code designation for Tedisamil.
KC8857. Code designation for Tedisamil Sesquifumarate.
KC-9946. Code designation for Cilansetron.
KC-9946. Code designation for Cilansetron Hydrochloride.
KCA-757. Code designation for Tipelukast.
K-F 224. Code designation for Naftoxate.
KGF-2. Code designation for Repifermin.
KIN-493. Code designation for Oxcarbazepine.
Kita-ku Toyko. Code designation for Mitemcinal Fumarate.
KL₄-surfactant. Code designation for Lucinactant.
KL-255 [as hydrochloride]. Code designation for Bupranolol.
KM871. Code designation for Ecromeximab.
Ko 592 [as hydrochloride]. Code designation for Toliprolol.
Ko 1173 Cl. Code designation for Mexiletine Hydrochloride.
KO 1366. Code designation for Bunitrolol.
KOS-953. Code designation for Tanespimycin.
KOS-1022. Code designation for Alvespimycin Hydrochloride.
KP-363. Code designation for Butenafine Hydrochloride.
KRM-1648. Code designation for Rifalazil.
KRN-568. Code designation for Tecalcet Hydrochloride.
KS 33. Code designation for Oxyridazine.
KT5555. Code designation for Lestaurtinib.
KUR-1246. Code designation for Bedoradrine Sulfate.
KVX-478. Code designation for Amprenavir.
KW-110. Code designation for Aceglutamide Aluminum.
KW-2189. Code designation for Pibrozelesin Hydrobromide.
KW-2871. Code designation for Ecromeximab.
KW-3902. Code designation for Rolofylline.
KW4679; ALO4943A. Code designation for Olopatadine Hydrochloride.
KW-6002. Code designation for Istradefylline.
KWD 2019. Code designation for Terbutaline Sulfate.
L1. Code designation for Deferiprone.
L-8. Code designation for Lypressin.
L-67. Code designation for Prilocaine Hydrochloride.
L 75 1362B. Code designation for Colforsin.
L 86 8275. Code designation for Alvocidib.
L 542. Code designation for Mercurobutol.
L-554. Code designation for Tritoqualine.
L 566. Code designation for Dibemethine.
L-627. Code designation for Biapenem.
L-749. Code designation for Salacetamide.
L846. Code designation for Zaleplon.
L-1573. Code designation for Cysteamine.
L-1633. Code designation for Sodium Dibunate.
L-1718. Code designation for Osalmid.
L-1777. Code designation for Medazomide.
L 2197. Code designation for Benzarone.
L-2214. Code designation for Benzbromarone.
L 2329. Code designation for Benziodarone.
L 2642. Code designation for Etabenzarone.
L-3428. Code designation for Amiodarone.
L-4269. Code designation for Pyridarone.

L-5103 Lepetit. Code designation for Rifampin.
L-5418. Code designation for Diftalone.
L 5818 [as hydrochloride]. Code designation for Coumazoline.
L-6257. Code designation for Oxetorone Fumarate.
L-6400. Code designation for Fluazacort.
L 8027. Code designation for Nictindole.
L-9394. Code designation for Butoprozine Hydrochloride.
L-364,718. Code designation for Devazepide.
L-588357-0. Code designation for Metyrosine.
L-637,510. Code designation for Nelezaprine Maleate.
L-647,339. Code designation for Naxagolide Hydrochloride.
L-668,019. Code designation for Verlukast.
L-669,455. Code designation for Dexibuprofen Lysine.
L-700,462. Code designation for Tirofiban Hydrochloride.
L-735,524. Code designation for Indinavir Sulfate.
LA-012 [as hydrochloride]. Code designation for Quatacaine.
LA 391. Code designation for Sodium Picosulfate.
LA 1221 [as hydrochloride]. Code designation for Butalamine.
LA-6023. Code designation for Metformin.
LA-6023. Code designation for Metformin Hydrochloride.
LA III. Code designation for Diazepam.
LAAM. Code designation for Levomethadyl Acetate.
LAAM. Code designation for Levomethadyl Acetate Hydrochloride.
LAC-43. Code designation for Bupivacaine Hydrochloride.
LACI. Code designation for Tifacogin.
LAF237. Code designation for Vildagliptin.
LAS 3876. Code designation for Almagate.
LAS 9273. Code designation for Clebopride.
LAS 30451. Code designation for Pancopride.
LAS 31025. Code designation for Arofylline.
LAS 31416. Code designation for Almotriptan.
LAS 31416 D,L-malate acid. Code designation for Almotriptan Malate.
LAS 34273. Code designation for Aclidinium Bromide.
LAS 34273 micronized. Code designation for Aclidinium Bromide.
LAS W-090. Code designation for Ebastine.
LAS W-330. Code designation for Aclidinium Bromide.
LB-46. Code designation for Pindolol.
LB 125. Code designation for Cyprodenate.
LB-502. Code designation for Furosemide.
LB 20304a. Code designation for Gemifloxacin Mesylate.
LC 44. Code designation for Flupentixol.
LD 335. Code designation for Propyromazine Bromide.
LD 935. Code designation for Dipiproverine Hydrochloride.
LD 2351 [as hydrobromide]. Code designation for Butopiprine.
LD 2480. Code designation for Piprocurarium Iodide.
LD 2630. Code designation for Difencloxazine Hydrochloride.
LD 2988. Code designation for Folescutol.
LD 3055. Code designation for Oxypyrronium Bromide.
LD 3394. Code designation for Fenozolone.
LD 3612. Code designation for Paraflutizide.
LD 4644. Code designation for Pipebuzone.
L-DOPS. Code designation for Droxidopa.
LDP02. Code designation for Vedolizumab.
LDP-03. Code designation for Alemtuzumab.
LDP-341. Code designation for Bortezomib.
Leo 114. Code designation for Polyestradiol Phosphate.
levo-BC-2605. Code designation for Oxilorphan.
levo-BC-2627. Code designation for Butorphanol.
levo-BC-2627 tartrate. Code designation for Butorphanol Tartrate.
levo-BL-4566. Code designation for Moxazocine.
LF00. Code designation for Talactoferrin Alfa.
LF 08-0299. Code designation for Tresperimus.
LFA3TIP. Code designation for Alefacept.
L-FMAU. Code designation for Clevudine.
LG100057. Code designation for Alitretinoin.

LG100069. Code designation for Bexarotene.

LGD1057. Code designation for Alitretinoin.

LGD1069. Code designation for Bexarotene.

LJ 206. Code designation for Carbocysteine.

LJ C10,627. Code designation for Biapenem.

LJC 10,141. Code designation for Felbinac.

LJC 10846. Code designation for Zaleplon.

LJP 394. Code designation for Abetimus Sodium.

LL-705W. Code designation for Neutramycin.

LL 1530. Code designation for Nadoxolol.

LM-94. Code designation for Hymecromone.

LM 176. Code designation for Cobamamide.

LM 192. Code designation for Viquidil.

LM-427. Code designation for Rifabutin.

LM-1404. Code designation for Lortalamine.

LM 2717. Code designation for Clobazam.

LMCA. Code designation for Levomefolate Calcium.

LMD. Code designation for Dextran 40.

LMSR. Code designation for Levomefolic Acid.

L-MTP-PE. Code designation for Mifamurtide.

LMWD. Code designation for Dextran 40.

L.N. 107. Code designation for Broparestrol.

LRX-15. Code designation for Treprostinil.

LS-11. Code designation for Talaporfin Sodium.

LS-121. Code designation for Nafronyl Oxalate.

LS 519 Cl2. Code designation for Pirenzepine Hydrochloride.

LS 2616. Code designation for Roquinimex.

LSD. Code designation for Lysergide.

LSN2420586. Code designation for Pruvanserin Hydrochloride.

LSN2422347. Code designation for Pruvanserin.

Lu 02-030. Code designation for Gaboxadol.

LU3-010. Code designation for Talopram Hydrochloride.

Lu 10-171-B. Code designation for Citalopram Hydrobromide.

Lu 23-174. Code designation for Sertindole.

Lu 25-109-M. Code designation for Alvameline Maleate.

Lu 26-054-0. Code designation for Escitalopram Oxalate.

LU200134. Code designation for Adalimumab.

Lu texaphyrin. Code designation for Motexafin Lutetium.

lutetium texaphyrin. Code designation for Motexafin Lutetium.

Lu-Tex. Code designation for Motexafin Lutetium.

LVD. Code designation for Dextran 40.

LY 048 740. Code designation for Avilamycin.

LY9818. Code designation for Naveglitazar.

LY 12271-72. Code designation for Viroxime.

LY061188. Code designation for Cephalexin Hydrochloride.

LY097964. Code designation for Cefetamet.

LY099094. Code designation for Vindesine Sulfate.

LY104208. Code designation for Vinzolidine Sulfate.

LY 108380. Code designation for Doxpicomine Hydrochloride.

LY110140. Code designation for Fluoxetine Hydrochloride.

LY 119863. Code designation for Vinepidine Sulfate.

LY120363. Code designation for Flumezapine.

LY121019. Code designation for Cilofungin.

LY 122512. Code designation for Anitrazafen.

LY 122772. Code designation for Enviroxime.

LY 123508. Code designation for Lorzafone.

LY 127123. Code designation for Enviradene.

LY 127623. Code designation for Metkephamid Acetate.

LY 127809. Code designation for Pergolide Mesylate.

LY 127935. Code designation for Moxalactam Disodium.

LY 135837. Code designation for Indecainide Hydrochloride.

LY137998. Code designation for Somatropin.

LY 139037. Code designation for Nizatidine.

LY 139381. Code designation for Ceftazidime.

LY-139603. Code designation for Atomoxetine Hydrochloride.

LY 141894. Code designation for Amflutizole.

LY 146032. Code designation for Daptomycin.

LY 150378. Code designation for Clofilium Phosphate.

LY 150720. Code designation for Picenadol Hydrochloride.

LY156758. Code designation for Raloxifene Hydrochloride.

LY163502. Code designation for Quinelorane Hydrochloride.

LY163892 monohydrate. Code designation for Loracarbef.

LY167005. Code designation for Proinsulin Human.

LY170053. Code designation for Olanzapine.

LY170680. Code designation for Sulukast.

LY171555. Code designation for Quinpirole Hydrochloride.

LY171883. Code designation for Tomelukast.

LY 174008. Code designation for Dobutamine Tartrate.

LY 175326. Code designation for Isomazole Hydrochloride.

LY177370. Code designation for Tilmicosin.

LY177370 phosphate. Code designation for Tilmicosin Phosphate.

LY177837. Code designation for Somidobove.

LY186641. Code designation for Sulofenur.

LY 186655. Code designation for Tibenelast Sodium.

LY188011. Code designation for Gemcitabine.

LY188011 hydrochloride. Code designation for Gemcitabine Hydrochloride.

LY 195115. Code designation for Indolidan.

LY 201116. Code designation for Ameltolide.

LY203638. Code designation for Drotrecogin Alfa (activated).

LY206243 lactobionate. Code designation for Levdobutamine Lactobionate.

LY207506. Code designation for Dobutamine Lactobionate.

LY210448 HCl. Code designation for Dapoxetine Hydrochloride.

LY213829. Code designation for Tazofelone.

LY215229 hydrochloride. Code designation for Seproxetine Hydrochloride.

LY231514. Code designation for Pemetrexed Disodium.

LY-232105. Code designation for Spinosad.

LY 237216. Code designation for Dirithromycin.

LY237733. Code designation for Amesergide.

LY246708. Code designation for Xanomeline.

LY246708 tartrate. Code designation for Xanomeline Tartrate.

LY246736. Code designation for Alvimopan.

LY248686 HCl. Code designation for Duloxetine Hydrochloride.

LY253351. Code designation for Tamsulosin Hydrochloride.

LY264618 disodium. Code designation for Lometrexol Sodium.

LY275585. Code designation for Insulin Lispro.

LY277359 maleate. Code designation for Zatosetron Maleate.

LY281067. Code designation for Sergolexole Maleate.

LY287041. Code designation for Tazomeline Citrate.

LY293111. Code designation for Etalocib.

LY293404. Code designation for Rismorelin Porcine.

LY293558. Code designation for Tezampanel.

LY294468 sulfate. Code designation for Efegatran Sulfate.

LY295337. Code designation for Basifungin.

LY300502. Code designation for Bexlosteride.

LY303366. Code designation for Anidulafungin.

LY307640 sodium. Code designation for Rabeprazole Sodium.

LY315920-Na$^+$. Code designation for Varespladib Sodium.

LY317615. Code designation for Enzastaurin Hydrochloride.

LY320236. Code designation for Izonsteride.

LY326869. Code designation for Moxonidine.

LY333013. Code designation for Varespladib Methyl.

LY333328 diphosphate. Code designation for Oritavancin Diphosphate.

LY 333334. Code designation for Teriparatide.

LY335348. Code designation for Denileukin Diftitox.

LY335979. Code designation for Zosuquidar Trihydrochloride.

LY353381.HCl. Code designation for Arzoxifene Hydrochloride.

LY354740. Code designation for Eglumetad.

LY450139. Code designation for Semagacestat.

LY519818. Code designation for Naveglitazar.

LY544344 hydrochloride. Code designation for Talaglumetad Hydrochloride.

LY544349. Code designation for Sivelestat.

LY544349 Sodium Hydrate. Code designation for Sivelestat Sodium.

LY-570310. Code designation for Telaprevir.

LY-573636.Na. Code designation for Tasisulam Sodium.

LY640315. Code designation for Prasugrel Hydrochloride.

LY2148568. Code designation for Exenatide.

LY2420586. Code designation for Pruvanserin.

LY2422347 HCl. Code designation for Pruvanserin Hydrochloride.

LYO31537. Code designation for Ractopamine Hydrochloride.

M-14. Code designation for Rifamycin.

M. 99 [as hydrochloride]. Code designation for Etorphine.

M-141. Code designation for Spectinomycin Hydrochloride.

M200. Code designation for Volociximab.

M 285. Code designation for Cyprenorphine Hydrochloride.

M-811. Code designation for Salverine.

M-1028 (Meiji). Code designation for Haloprogin.

M. 5050. Code designation for Diprenorphine.

M 18575. Code designation for Dienogest.

M40403. Code designation for Imisopasem Manganese.

MA-540. Code designation for Quinuclium Bromide.

MA-593. Code designation for Salethamide Maleate.

MA 1277. Code designation for Zolertine Hydrochloride.

MA 1291. Code designation for Quipazine Maleate.

MA 1337. Code designation for Cloperidone Hydrochloride.

MA-1443. Code designation for Letimide Hydrochloride.

MAB35. Code designation for Indium In 111 Altumomab Pentetate.

MAb-B43.13. Code designation for Oregovomab.

m-AMSA. Code designation for Amsacrine.

MAS-1. Code designation for Polyglyconate.

Material A. Code designation for Pentetate Calcium Trisodium Yb 169.

MAY. Code designation for Nelarabine.

MAY. Code designation for Nelzarabine.

M&B 782 [as isethionate]. Code designation for Propamidine.

MB 800 [as isethionate]. Code designation for Pentamidine.

M&B 5062 A. Code designation for Amicarbalide.

M&B 9302. Code designation for Clorgiline.

M&B 15497. Code designation for Decoquinate.

M&B 16942A. Code designation for Diacetolol Hydrochloride.

M&B 17803A. Code designation for Acebutolol Hydrochloride.

M&B 22948. Code designation for Zaprinast.

M&B 33153. Code designation for Oxoprostol.

M&B 39831. Code designation for Temozolomide.

MB 46030. Code designation for Fipronil.

MBBT. Code designation for Bisoctrizole.

MBP8298. Code designation for Dirucotide.

MBR-4164-8. Code designation for Diflumidone Sodium.

MBR-4197. Code designation for Flucrylate.

MBR 4223. Code designation for Triflumidate.

MC 903. Code designation for Calcipotriene.

MCC-257. Code designation for Coleneuramide.

MCC 555. Code designation for Netoglitazone.

MCE. Code designation for Metergoline.

MCI-196. Code designation for Colestilan Chloride.

MCI-9038. Code designation for Argatroban.

McN-742. Code designation for Aminorex.

McN-1075. Code designation for Fenmetramide.

McN-1107. Code designation for Clominorex.

McN-1210. Code designation for Pyrinoline.

McN-1231. Code designation for Fluminorex.

McN-1546. Code designation for Flumetramide.

McN-1589. Code designation for Mixidine.

McN-2378. Code designation for Mefenidil.

McN-2378-46. Code designation for Mefenidil Fumarate.

McN-2453. Code designation for Azepindole.

McN-2559. Code designation for Tolmetin.

McN-2559-21-98. Code designation for Tolmetin Sodium.

McN-2783-21-98. Code designation for Zomepirac Sodium.

McN-3113. Code designation for Xilobam.

McN-3377-98. Code designation for Fenobam.

McN-3495. Code designation for Pirogliride Tartrate.

McN-3716. Code designation for Methyl Palmoxirate.

McN-3802 [anhydrous free acid]. Code designation for Palmoxirate Sodium.

McN-3802-21-98. Code designation for Palmoxirate Sodium.

McN 3935. Code designation for Linogliride.

McN-3935. Code designation for Linogliride Fumarate.

McN-4097-12-98. Code designation for Fenoctimine Sulfate.

McN-4853. Code designation for Topiramate.

McN-A-2673-11. Code designation for Etoperidone Hydrochloride.

McN-A-2833. Code designation for Perindopril.

McN-A-2833-109. Code designation for Perindopril Erbumine.

McN-JR-1625. Code designation for Haloperidol.

McN-JR-2498. Code designation for Trifluperidol.

McN-JR-4263-49. Code designation for Fentanyl Citrate.

McN-JR-4584. Code designation for Benperidol.

McN-JR-4749. Code designation for Droperidol.

McN-JR-4929-11. Code designation for Benzetimide Hydrochloride.

McN-JR-6218. Code designation for Fluspirilene.

McN-JR-6238. Code designation for Pimozide.

McN-JR-7242-11. Code designation for Difluanine Hydrochloride.

McN-JR-7904. Code designation for Lidoflazine.

McN-JR-8299-11. Code designation for Tetramisole Hydrochloride.

McN-JR-13,558-11. Code designation for Fetoxylate Hydrochloride.

McN-JR-15,403-11. Code designation for Difenoxin.

McN-JR-16,341. Code designation for Penfluridol.

McN-R-73-Z. Code designation for Rotoxamine.

McN-R-726-47. Code designation for Poldine Methylsulfate.

McN-R-1162-22. Code designation for Potassium Glucaldrate.

McN-R-1967. Code designation for Fenretinide.

McN-X-94. Code designation for Capuride.

McN-X-181. Code designation for Valnoctamide.

MD 141. Code designation for Ethamsylate.

MD-805. Code designation for Argatroban.

MD 2028. Code designation for Fluanisone.

MD 67350 [as maleate]. Code designation for Cinepazide.

MDL 257. Code designation for Zindotrine.

MDL 458. Code designation for Deflazacort.

MDL 473. Code designation for Rifapentine.

MDL 507. Code designation for Teicoplanin.

MDL 11,939. Code designation for Glemanserin.

MDL 14,042. Code designation for Lofexidine Hydrochloride.

MDL 16,455A. Code designation for Fexofenadine Hydrochloride.

MDL 17,043. Code designation for Enoximone.

MDL 18,962. Code designation for Plomestane.

MDL 19,205. Code designation for Piroximone.

MDL 19,744. Code designation for Tipentosin Hydrochloride.

MDL 26,024G0. Code designation for Tetrazolast Meglumine.

MDL 26,479. Code designation for Suritozole.

MDL 28,574A. Code designation for Celgosivir Hydrochloride.

MDL 62,198. Code designation for Ramoplanin.

MDL 62,769. Code designation for Rifamexil.

MDL 64,397. Code designation for Dalbavancin.

MDL 71,754. Code designation for Vigabatrin.

MDL 71,782 A. Code designation for Eflornithine Hydrochloride.

MDL 72,222. Code designation for Bemesetron.

MDL 72,422. Code designation for Tropanserin Hydrochloride.

MDL 72,974A. Code designation for Mofegiline Hydrochloride.

MDL 73,005EF. Code designation for Binospirone Mesylate.

MDL 73,147EF. Code designation for Dolasetron Mesylate.

MDL 73,745. Code designation for Zifrosilone.

MDL 73,945. Code designation for Camiglibose.

MDL 101,731. Code designation for Tezacitabine.

MDL 107,826A. Code designation for Alvocidib.

MDL-201129. Code designation for Beraprost Sodium.

MDL-201229. Code designation for Beraprost.

MDX-010. Code designation for Ipilimumab.

MDX-016. Code designation for Zanolimumab.

MDX-060. Code designation for Iratumumab.

MDX-CTLA-4. Code designation for Ipilimumab.

MEA. Code designation for Cysteamine.

MEDI-507. Code designation for Siplizumab.

MEDI-522. Code designation for Etaracizumab.

MEDI-524. Code designation for Motavizumab.

MEDI-538. Code designation for Blinatumomab.

MER-41. Code designation for Clomiphene Citrate.

meso-NDGA. Code designation for Masoprocol.

Methyl-CCNU. Code designation for Semustine.

MF 934. Code designation for Rufloxacin.

M.G. 143. Code designation for Sulmarin.

MG 559. Code designation for Metamfepramone.

M.G. 624. Code designation for Stilonium Iodide.

M.G. 652. Code designation for Oxamarin Hydrochloride.

M.G. 1559. Code designation for Xenbucin.

Mg 4833. Code designation for Fencibutirol.

M.G. 5454. Code designation for Guaiapate.

M.G. 5771. Code designation for Butixirate.

M.G. 8823. Code designation for Exaprolol Hydrochloride.

M.G. 8926 [as hydrochloride]. Code designation for Droprenilamine.

M.G. 13054. Code designation for Fenquizone.

M.G. 13608. Code designation for Domiodol.

MGA031. Code designation for Teplizumab.

MGI 114. Code designation for Irofulven.

MH-532. Code designation for Phenprobamate.

Mi-85. Code designation for Apazone.

MI-216. Code designation for Iothalamic Acid.

MIV 606. Code designation for Valomaciclovir Stearate.

MJ 505. Code designation for Phenyramidol Hydrochloride.

MJ 1986. Code designation for Indriline Hydrochloride.

MJ 1987. Code designation for Mesuprine Hydrochloride.

MJ 1988. Code designation for Quazodine.

MJ 1992. Code designation for Soterenol Hydrochloride.

MJ 1998. Code designation for Metalol Hydrochloride.

MJ 1999. Code designation for Sotalol Hydrochloride.

MJ 4309-1. Code designation for Oxybutynin Chloride.

MJ 9022-1. Code designation for Buspirone Hydrochloride.

MJ 9067-1. Code designation for Encainide Hydrochloride.

MJ 9184-1. Code designation for Zinterol Hydrochloride.

MJ 10061. Code designation for Benzbromarone.

MJ 12,175-170. Code designation for Tiprinast Meglumine.

MJ 12,880-1. Code designation for Tipropidil Hydrochloride.

MJ 13,105-1. Code designation for Bucindolol Hydrochloride.

MJ 13401-1-3. Code designation for Fenprinast Hydrochloride.

MJ 13,754-1. Code designation for Nefazodone Hydrochloride.

MJF 9325. Code designation for Ifosfamide.

MJF 10,938. Code designation for Xipamide.

MJF 11567-3. Code designation for Cefadroxil.

MJF-12264. Code designation for Tegafur.

MJF 12637. Code designation for Suloctidil.

MJR-35. Code designation for Dienogest.

MK 57. Code designation for Methyldesorphine.

MK-130 [as the base]. Code designation for Cyclobenzaprine
  Hydrochloride.

MK-188. Code designation for Zeranol.

MK-196. Code designation for Indacrinone.

MK-208. Code designation for Famotidine.

MK-217. Code designation for Alendronate Sodium.

MK-233. Code designation for Dexibuprofen Lysine.

MK-240. Code designation for Protriptyline Hydrochloride.

MK-250. Code designation for Emylcamate.

MK-329. Code designation for Devazepide.

MK-341. Code designation for Tranilast.

MK-351. Code designation for Methyldopa.

MK-360. Code designation for Thiabendazole.

MK-366. Code designation for Norfloxacin.

MK-383. Code designation for Tirofiban Hydrochloride.

MK-397. Code designation for Eprinomectin.

MK-401. Code designation for Clorsulon.

MK-417. Code designation for Sezolamide Hydrochloride.

MK-422. Code designation for Enalaprilat.

MK-0457. Code designation for Tozasertib Lactate.

MK-458. Code designation for Naxagolide Hydrochloride.

MK-0462. Code designation for Rizatriptan Benzoate.

MK-476. Code designation for Montelukast Sodium.

MK-507. Code designation for Dorzolamide Hydrochloride.

MK-0517. Code designation for Fosaprepitant Dimeglumine.

MK-0518. Code designation for Raltegravir Potassium.

MK-521. Code designation for Lisinopril.

MK-0524. Code designation for Laropiprant.

MK-591. Code designation for Quiflapon Sodium.

MK-595. Code designation for Ethacrynic Acid.

MK-621. Code designation for Efrotomycin.

MK-639. Code designation for Indinavir Sulfate.

MK-0663. Code designation for Etoricoxib.

MK-0677. Code designation for Ibutamoren Mesylate.

MK-678. Code designation for Seglitide Acetate.

MK-679. Code designation for Verlukast.

MK-0681. Code designation for Trientine Hydrochloride.

MK-733. Code designation for Simvastatin.

MK-781. Code designation for Metyrosine.

MK-0787. Code designation for Imipenem.

MK790. Code designation for Levomethadyl Acetate Hydrochloride.

MK-791. Code designation for Cilastatin Sodium.

MK-793. Code designation for Diltiazem Malate.

MK-801. Code designation for Dizocilpine Maleate.

MK-803. Code designation for Lovastatin.

MK-0826. Code designation for Ertapenem Sodium.

MK-0869. Code designation for Aprepitant.

MK-906. Code designation for Finasteride.

MK-0928. Code designation for Gaboxadol.

MK-0936. Code designation for Abamectin.

MK-0966. Code designation for Rofecoxib.

MK-0991. Code designation for Caspofungin Acetate.

MK-A462. Code designation for Rizatriptan Sulfate.

MKC-442. Code designation for Emivirine.

MKI-833. Code designation for Balamapimod.

ML-1024. Code designation for Theofibrate.

ML 1034. Code designation for Celucloral.

ML-1129. Code designation for Beraprost Sodium.

ML-1229. Code designation for Beraprost.

ML-1,709,460. Code designation for Gamithromycin.

ML-1,785,713. Code designation for Firocoxib.

MLN0002. Code designation for Vedolizumab.

MLN02. Code designation for Vedolizumab.

MM-416775. Code designation for Linaclotide Acetate.

MN-001. Code designation for Tipelukast.

MN-029. Code designation for Denibulin Hydrochloride.

MN-221. Code designation for Bedoradrine Sulfate.

MO-911. Code designation for Pargyline Hydrochloride.

MO-1255. Code designation for Encyprate.

MORAb-003. Code designation for Farletuzumab.

MOT-288. Code designation for Atilmotin.

MP-271. Code designation for Iosefamic Acid.

MP 302 (mixt. with Ioxaglate Sodium). Code designation for Ioxaglate Meglumine.

MP 328. Code designation for Ioversol.

MP-424. Code designation for Telaprevir.

MP-600. Code designation for Betiatide.

MP-620. Code designation for Iocetamic Acid.

MP-1051. Code designation for Silodrate.

MP-1177. Code designation for Gadoversetamide.

MP-1196. Code designation for Versetamide.

MP-1549. Code designation for Furomine.

MP-1554. Code designation for Technetium Tc 99m Furifosmin.

MP-1727. Code designation for Indium In 111 Pentetreotide.

MP 2032. Code designation for Iocarmic Acid.

MP 2032-Meglumine. Code designation for Iocarmate Meglumine.

MP-3047-04. Code designation for Iosimenol.

MP 4006. Code designation for Albumin, Aggregated.

MP 4018. Code designation for Stannous Pyrophosphate.

MP-6026. Code designation for Ioglucol.

MP 7010. Code designation for Stannous Sulfur Colloid.

MP-8000. Code designation for Ioglucomide.

MP-10013. Code designation for Iogulamide.

MPC-7869. Code designation for Tarenflurbil.

MPS-21. Code designation for Ovemotide.

MPS-22. Code designation for Disomotide.

MPV-253 AII. Code designation for Detomidine Hydrochloride.

MPV-785. Code designation for Medetomidine Hydrochloride.

MPV-1248. Code designation for Atipamezole.

MPV-1440. Code designation for Dexmedetomidine.

MPV-2426. Code designation for Fadolmidine Hydrochloride.

MR6S4. Code designation for Sevoflurane.

MRA. Code designation for Tocilizumab.

MRE0094. Code designation for Sonedenoson.

MRE0470. Code designation for Binodenoson.

MRL 38. Code designation for Hexadiline.

MRL-41. Code designation for Clomiphene Citrate.

MRP-10. Code designation for Pentetate Calcium Trisodium Yb 169.

MRX-115. Code designation for Perflutren.

MRZ 2663BR. Code designation for Methylnaltrexone Bromide.

MS 32520. Code designation for Gadofosveset Trisodium.

MS 325168A. Code designation for Fosveset.

MSI-78. Code designation for Pexiganan Acetate.

MSI-1256F. Code designation for Squalamine Lactate.

MSI-1436. Code designation for Trodusquemine.

MST-997. Code designation for Simotaxel.

MT-103. Code designation for Blinatumomab.

MTS 263. Code designation for Tropenziline Bromide.

MY-25 [as bitartrate]. Code designation for Metergotamine.

MY-33-7 [as hydrochloride]. Code designation for Lotucaine.

MY-5116. Code designation for Repirinast.

MYC123. Code designation for Efungumab.

MYC123A. Code designation for Efungumab.

MYC123B. Code designation for Efungumab.

MYC124. Code designation for Efungumab.

MYC 8003. Code designation for Mocimycin.

MYO-029. Code designation for Stamulumab.

MZ-144. Code designation for Rimazolium Metilsulfate.

N-3. Code designation for Methetoin.

N-137. Code designation for Carbetimer.

N-0252. Code designation for Laurocapram.

N-399. Code designation for Xenytropium Bromide.

N-553 [as hydrochloride]. Code designation for Tolperisone.

N-714. Code designation for Chlorprothixene.

N-746. Code designation for Clopenthixol.

N-7009. Code designation for Flupentixol.

N-7020. Code designation for Meprotixol.

N10146. Code designation for Isatoribine.

NA-66. Code designation for Pimeclone.

NA-119. Code designation for Bromamid.

NA 274. Code designation for Bromhexine Hydrochloride.

NAB 365. Code designation for Clenbuterol.

NAD. Code designation for Nadide.

NARI-10146. Code designation for Isatoribine.

NASH. Code designation for Borocaptate Sodium B 10.

NAT-327. Code designation for Trimoxamine Hydrochloride.

NAT-333. Code designation for Fenspiride Hydrochloride.

NB 68. Code designation for Dacuronium Bromide.

NBI-34060. Code designation for Indiplon.

NBI-56418. Code designation for Elagolix.

NBI-56418 Na. Code designation for Elagolix Sodium.

NC-123. Code designation for Mesoridazine.

NC 150. Code designation for Phenazopyridine Hydrochloride.

NC-503. Code designation for Eprodisate Disodium.

NC-758. Code designation for Tramiprosate.

NC 1264. Code designation for Thonzonium Bromide.

NC-1968. Code designation for Fungimycin.

NC-7197. Code designation for Esproquin Hydrochloride.

NC100697. Code designation for Tropantiol.

NCNU. Code designation for Pentamustine.

ND 50. Code designation for Octopamine.

NDC 0082-4155. Code designation for Daunorubicin Hydrochloride.

NDR 263. Code designation for Propenzolate Hydrochloride.

NDR 304. Code designation for Ethyl Dibunate.

NDR-5061A. Code designation for Aletamine Hydrochloride.

NDR-5523A. Code designation for Trimoxamine Hydrochloride.

NDR-5998A. Code designation for Fenspiride Hydrochloride.

NE-10064. Code designation for Azimilide Dihydrochloride.

NE 11740. Code designation for Tebufelone.

NE-19550. Code designation for Olvanil.

NE-58095. Code designation for Risedronate Sodium.

NE 97221. Code designation for Piridronate Sodium.

NESP. Code designation for Darbepoetin Alfa.

NEU 3002. Code designation for Corticorelin Acetate.

NF-71. Code designation for Nifurmerone.

NF-84. Code designation for Nifuraldezone.

NF-161. Code designation for Nifursemizone.

NF-246. Code designation for Nifuradene.

NF-602. Code designation for Levofuraltadone.

NF-902 [as hydrochloride]. Code designation for Levofuraltadone.

NF-963. Code designation for Furazolium Chloride.

NF-1010. Code designation for Nifurdazil.

NF-1088. Code designation for Nifurquinazol.

NF-1120. Code designation for Nifurimide.

NF-1425. Code designation for Furazolium Tartrate.

NFS1776. Code designation for Isovaleramide.

NG2-73. Code designation for Adipiplon.

NGX424. Code designation for Tezampanel.

NIB. Code designation for Nabitan Hydrochloride.

NIH 2933. Code designation for Dimepheptanol.

NIH 7574. Code designation for Benzethidine.

NIH 7607. Code designation for Etonitazene.

NIH 7667. Code designation for Noracymethadol Hydrochloride.

NIH 7672. Code designation for Methopholine.

NIH 8805. Code designation for Buprenorphine Hydrochloride.

NK 204. Code designation for Basifungin.

NK-631. Code designation for Peplomycin Sulfate.

NK 1006. Code designation for Bekanamycin.

NKK-105. Code designation for Malotilate.

NKT-01. Code designation for Gusperimus Trihydrochloride.

NM-147. Code designation for Valtorcitabine Dihydrochloride.

NM283. Code designation for Valopicitabine Dihydrochloride.

NN-304. Code designation for Insulin Detemir.

NN2211. Code designation for Liraglutide.

NNC-05-0328. Code designation for Tiagabine Hydrochloride.

NNC 90-1170. Code designation for Liraglutide.
NO-05-0328. Code designation for Tiagabine Hydrochloride.
NO-1886. Code designation for Ibrolipim.
NOET. Code designation for Ditiocade Sodium.
NOR-701. Code designation for Apaziquone.
NorMDP. Code designation for Almurtide.
NP. Code designation for Nifurpipone.
NPAP. Code designation for Prajmalium Bitartrate.
NPS 1506 · HCl. Code designation for Delucemine Hydrochloride.
NPS R-568. Code designation for Tecalcet Hydrochloride.
NPT 15392. Code designation for Nosantine.
NRP104. Code designation for Lisdexamfetamine Dimesylate.
NS-75A. Code designation for Cetrorelix Acetate.
NS 2214. Code designation for Brasofensine Maleate.
NSC 343499. Code designation for Asulacrine.
NSD 1055. Code designation for Brocresine.
NSP-989. Code designation for Tanaproget.
NU-445. Code designation for Sulfisoxazole Diolamine.
Nu-1779. Code designation for Betaprodine.
Nu-1932. Code designation for Betameprodine.
NU-2121. Code designation for Nicotinyl Alcohol.
NV-02B. Code designation for Telbivudine.
NV-02C. Code designation for Torcitabine.
NV-06. Code designation for Idronoxil.
NX 473. Code designation for Picoplatin.
NX1838. Code designation for Pegaptanib Sodium.
NXX-066. Code designation for Quilostigmine.
NXY-059. Code designation for Disufenton Sodium.
NY-198. Code designation for Lomefloxacin Hydrochloride.
OCT. Code designation for Maxacalcitol.
ODA 914. Code designation for Demoxytocin.
(–)-OddC. Code designation for Troxacitabine.
OGT 918. Code designation for Miglustat.
OGX-011. Code designation for Custirsen Sodium.
OHM-11638. Code designation for Atilmotin.
OHM-11771. Code designation for Nitric Oxide.
l-OHP. Code designation for Oxaliplatin.
OL(1)p53. Code designation for Cenersen Sodium.
OM-977. Code designation for Etaminile.
OMDS. Code designation for Dipyrithione.
OMS No 1825. Code designation for Azamethiphos.
ONO-1078. Code designation for Pranlukast.
ONO-5046. Code designation for Sivelestat.
ONO-5046.Na. Code designation for Sivelestat Sodium.
ONYX-015. Code designation for Lontucirev (Replicating Adeno-
   virus).
OP 21-23. Code designation for Parnaparin Sodium.
OP2000. Code designation for Deligoparin Sodium.
OPB-2045. Code designation for Olanexidine Hydrochloride.
OPC-21. Code designation for Cilostazol.
OPC-31. Code designation for Aripiprazole.
OPC-1085. Code designation for Carteolol Hydrochloride.
OPC-7251. Code designation for Nadifloxacin.
OPC-8212. Code designation for Vesnarinone.
OPC-13013. Code designation for Cilostazol.
OPC-14597. Code designation for Aripiprazole.
OPC-17116. Code designation for Grepafloxacin Hydrochloride.
OPC-18790. Code designation for Toborinone.
OPC-41061. Code designation for Tolvaptan.
OPF 009. Code designation for Ibrolipim.
OPT-80. Code designation for Fidaxomicin.
OR-611. Code designation for Entacapone.
(–)-OR-1259. Code designation for Levosimendan.
ORF-8063. Code designation for Triflubazam.
ORF 9326. Code designation for Nisterime Acetate.
ORF 10131. Code designation for Norgestimate.
ORF 11676. Code designation for Nalmefene.
ORF 15244. Code designation for Thymopentin.

ORF 15817. Code designation for Edoxudine.
ORF 15927. Code designation for Rioprostil.
ORF 16600. Code designation for Bemarinone Hydrochloride.
ORF 17070. Code designation for Histrelin.
ORF 18704. Code designation for Pelretin.
ORF 20257. Code designation for Doretinel.
ORF 20485. Code designation for Tepoxalin.
ORF 22164. Code designation for Atosiban.
ORF 22867. Code designation for Bemoradan.
Orf-32541. Code designation for Iturelix.
Org 538. Code designation for Testosterone Undecanoate.
Org 817. Code designation for Epimestrol.
ORG 2969. Code designation for Desogestrel.
ORG 3236. Code designation for Etonogestrel.
ORG 3770. Code designation for Mirtazapine.
Org 4428. Code designation for Beloxepin.
Org 5222. Code designation for Asenapine Maleate.
Org 6216. Code designation for Rimexolone.
ORG7417. Code designation for Resocortol Butyrate.
ORG 9426. Code designation for Rocuronium Bromide.
Org 9487. Code designation for Rapacuronium Bromide.
ORG 10172. Code designation for Danaparoid Sodium.
ORG 10486-0. Code designation for Nomegestrol Acetate.
Org 24448. Code designation for Farampator.
Org 25969. Code designation for Sugammadex Sodium.
Org 30659. Code designation for Tosagestin.
ORG 31540. Code designation for Fondaparinux Sodium.
Org 36286. Code designation for Corifollitropin Alfa.
Org 39141. Code designation for Ismomultin Alfa.
Org 50081. Code designation for Esmirtazapine Maleate.
Org GB 94. Code designation for Mianserin Hydrochloride.
Org NA 97. Code designation for Pancuronium Bromide.
ORG NC 45. Code designation for Vecuronium Bromide.
Org OD 14. Code designation for Tibolone.
OSI-774. Code designation for Erlotinib Hydrochloride.
P 7. Code designation for Lauroguadine.
P-12. Code designation for Oxacillin Sodium.
P-25. Code designation for Cloxacillin Sodium.
P-30 Protein. Code designation for Ranpirnase.
P-50. Code designation for Ampicillin.
P53. Code designation for Tetrofosmin.
P 071. Code designation for Cetirizine Hydrochloride.
P-71. Code designation for Lycetamine.
P 71-0129. Code designation for Fendosal.
P 76 2494A. Code designation for Fluradoline Hydrochloride.
P 76 2543. Code designation for Dazepinil Hydrochloride.
P 78 3522. Code designation for Brocrinat.
P79 3913. Code designation for Neflumozide Hydrochloride.
P83 6029A. Code designation for Velnacrine Maleate.
P-113. Code designation for Saralasin Acetate.
P-165. Code designation for Azaserine.
[99mTc]-P246. Code designation for Technetium Tc 99m Apcitide.
P-248. Code designation for Levopropylcillin Potassium.
P280. Code designation for Bibapcitide.
P-286. Code designation for Ioxaglic Acid.
P-301. Code designation for Hydroxyphenamate.
P-463. Code designation for Fenamole.
P-638. Code designation for Puromycin.
P829. Code designation for Depreotide.
P-1011. Code designation for Dicloxacillin Sodium.
P-1026. Code designation for Hexaminolevulinate Hydrochloride.
P-1202. Code designation for Methyl Aminolevulinate Hydro-
   chloride.
P-1306. Code designation for Glyparamide.
P-1496. Code designation for Zeranol.
P-1560. Code designation for Taleranol.
P-1742. Code designation for Fluperolone Acetate.
P-1779. Code designation for Althiazide.

P-1888. Code designation for Isosulfan Blue.

P-2105. Code designation for Epithiazide.

P-2525. Code designation for Polythiazide.

P-2530. Code designation for Methalthiazide.

P-2647. Code designation for Benzquinamide.

P-3232. Code designation for Somfasepor.

P-3693A. Code designation for Doxepin Hydrochloride.

P-3895. Code designation for Somfasepor.

P-3896. Code designation for Guanisoquin Sulfate.

P-4125. Code designation for Isosulfan Blue.

P-4385B. Code designation for Clothixamide Maleate.

P-4599. Code designation for Cidoxepin Hydrochloride.

P-4657 B. Code designation for Thiothixene.

P-5227. Code designation for Pinoxepin Hydrochloride.

P-5604. Code designation for Loteprednol Etabonate.

P-7138. Code designation for Nifurpirinol.

P 720549. Code designation for Isoxepac.

PA-144. Code designation for Plicamycin.

PA-457. Code designation for Bevirimat Dimeglumine.

PA-457 di-NMG. Code designation for Bevirimat Dimeglumine.

PA-457N. Code designation for Bevirimat Dimeglumine.

PA103001. Code designation for Bevirimat Dimeglumine.

PA103001-01. Code designation for Bevirimat Dimeglumine.

PA103001-04. Code designation for Bevirimat Dimeglumine.

PAA-701. Code designation for Bialamicol Hydrochloride.

PAA-3854. Code designation for Clamoxyquin Hydrochloride.

PAI-039. Code designation for Tiplasinin.

PAI-749. Code designation for Diaplasinin.

PAM-MR-807-23a. Code designation for Cycloguanil Pamoate.

PAM-MR-1165. Code designation for Acedapsone.

PAMN [as methonitrate]. Code designation for Prampine.

PAR-101. Code designation for Fidaxomicin.

PASIT. Code designation for Glyprothiazol.

PAT. Code designation for Fenamole.

PAZ-417. Code designation for Aleplasinin.

PB 89 [as hydrochloride]. Code designation for Fominoben.

p-BIDA. Code designation for Butilfenin.

PC-603. Code designation for Iproclozide.

PC1020 acetate. Code designation for Prezatide Copper Acetate.

PC-1421. Code designation for Piperacetazine.

PCI-0120. Code designation for Motexafin Gadolinium.

PCI-0123. Code designation for Motexafin Lutetium.

PCK3145. Code designation for Tigapotide Triflutate.

PD-93. Code designation for Piromidic Acid.

PD-0072953. Code designation for Gemcabene Calcium.

PD 81565. Code designation for Pentostatin.

PD 90,695-73. Code designation for Dezaguanine Mesylate.

PD 107779. Code designation for Enoxacin.

PD-110843. Code designation for Zonisamide.

PD 123654. Code designation for Tacedinaline.

PD 180988. Code designation for Fandosentan Potassium.

PD 180988-0016. Code designation for Fandosentan Potassium.

PD-183805. Code designation for Canertinib Dihydrochloride.

PD-0183805. Code designation for Canertinib Dihydrochloride.

PD 0196860. Code designation for Besonprodil.

PD 348,292. Code designation for Eribaxaban.

PDB. Code designation for Prifinium Bromide.

PDL063. Code designation for Elotuzumab.

PDL-063. Code designation for Elotuzumab.

PDLA. Code designation for Foscolic Acid.

PDX. Code designation for Pralatrexate.

PE1-1. Code designation for Tuvirumab.

PEG-SOD. Code designation for Pegorgotein.

Pentapeptide DSDPR. Code designation for Pentigetide.

PEP-005. Code designation for Ingenol Mebutate.

PF-26. Code designation for Mepramidil.

PF-00520904. Code designation for Derquantel.

PF-804950. Code designation for Edotecarin.

PF 03491390. Code designation for Emricasan.

PF-3512676. Code designation for Agatolimod.

PF-3512676. Code designation for Agatolimod Sodium.

PF-4383119. Code designation for Tanezumab.

PFA-186. Code designation for Salicylate Meglumine.

PG 430. Code designation for Febuverine.

PG490-88Na. Code designation for Omtriptolide Sodium.

PG-501. Code designation for Mazaticol.

$PGF_2\alpha$ THAM. Code designation for Dinoprost Tromethamine.

PH 218. Code designation for Edogestrone.

PH 5776. Code designation for Nitazoxanide.

PHA-290940AD. Code designation for Sunitinib Malate.

PHA-291639. Code designation for Toceranib.

PHA-291639E. Code designation for Toceranib Phosphate.

PHA-738144. Code designation for Certolizumab Pegol.

PHA 739,521. Code designation for Mavacoxib.

PHM-101. Code designation for Eufauserase.

PHX-1149. Code designation for Dutogliptin Tartrate.

PHX1149. Code designation for Dutogliptin.

PHXA41. Code designation for Latanoprost.

Pierrel-TQ 86. Code designation for Azipramine Hydrochloride.

PIXY321. Code designation for Milodistim.

PK 10169. Code designation for Enoxaparin Sodium.

PKC 412. Code designation for Midostaurin.

PLA-695. Code designation for Giripladib.

PLA-725. Code designation for Ecopladib.

PLA-902. Code designation for Efipladib.

PM 150. Code designation for Vedaprofen.

PM-671. Code designation for Ethosuximide.

PM 1807. Code designation for Fenimide.

PM-1952. Code designation for Fenacetinol.

PM-3944. Code designation for Flucetorex.

PM-185184. Code designation for Secnidazole.

PMD-387. Code designation for Crilvastatin.

PMPA. Code designation for Tenofovir.

PMPA Prodrug. Code designation for Tenofovir Disoproxil Fumarate.

PN 200-110. Code designation for Isradipine.

PNU-98528E. Code designation for Pramipexole Dihydrochloride.

PNU-101387G. Code designation for Sonepiprazole Mesylate.

PNU-140690E. Code designation for Tipranavir Disodium.

PNU-155950E. Code designation for Reboxetine Mesylate.

PNU-155971. Code designation for Exemestane.

PNU-165442G. Code designation for Esreboxetine Succinate.

PNU-180638E. Code designation for Almotriptan Malate.

PNU-200583E. Code designation for Tolterodine Tartrate.

POLI 67. Code designation for Tetrydamine.

POR 8. Code designation for Ornipressin.

POT.mes. Code designation for Paroxetine Mesylate.

PP-105. Code designation for Spinosad.

PP 563. Code designation for Cyhalothrin.

PPI-149. Code designation for Abarelix.

PPI-0903. Code designation for Ceftaroline Fosamil.

PPM-204. Code designation for Indeglitazar.

PR-171. Code designation for Carfilzomib.

PR-741-976A. Code designation for Somantadine Hydrochloride.

PR-0818-156A. Code designation for Verilopam Hydrochloride.

PR-870-714A. Code designation for Veradoline Hydrochloride.

PR-877-530L. Code designation for Flavodilol Maleate.

PR 879-317A. Code designation for Oxamisole Hydrochloride.

PR 934-423A. Code designation for Remacemide Hydrochloride.

PR-3847. Code designation for Teroxalene Hydrochloride.

PR070769. Code designation for Ocrelizumab.

PR-G 138-CL [as hydrochloride]. Code designation for Ciclosidomine.

Protease 1. Code designation for Brinolase.

PRT054021. Code designation for Betrixaban.

PRX-00023. Code designation for Naluzotan.

PS-341. Code designation for Bortezomib.
PS-1286. Code designation for Pararosaniline Pamoate.
PS 2383. Code designation for Trimetozine.
PT-9. Code designation for Betahistine Hydrochloride.
PT-100. Code designation for Talabostat.
PT-100. Code designation for Talabostat Mesylate.
PT-141. Code designation for Bremelanotide.
PT-523. Code designation for Talotrexin Ammonium.
PT523. Code designation for Talotrexin Ammonium.
PTC124. Code designation for Ataluren.
PTK787. Code designation for Vatalanib.
PTP-112. Code designation for Ertiprotafib.
PU-239. Code designation for Benzilonium Bromide.
PXD101. Code designation for Belinostat.
PY 108-068. Code designation for Darodipine.
PZ68. Code designation for Pentosan Polysulfate Sodium.
PZ 1511. Code designation for Carpipramine Dihydrochloride.
Q-12. Code designation for Technetium Tc 99m Furifosmin.
QAB149. Code designation for Indacaterol.
QAB149-AFA. Code designation for Indacaterol Maleate.
QB-1. Code designation for Cloquinozine.
QRX 101. Code designation for Becocalcidiol.
QRX-431. Code designation for Sobetirome.
QZ-2. Code designation for Methaqualone.
R 10.100. Code designation for Ethonam Nitrate.
R 48. Code designation for Chlornaphazine.
R 50 970. Code designation for Metrenperone.
R 51 163. Code designation for Tameridone.
R-52. Code designation for Mannosulfan.
R 62 818. Code designation for Lorcinadol.
R 64 766. Code designation for Risperidone.
R106-1. Code designation for Basifungin.
R-148. Code designation for Methaqualone.
R-411. Code designation for Valategrast Hydrochloride.
R 516. Code designation for Cinnarizine.
R-548. Code designation for Tricetamide.
R-568. Code designation for Tecalcet Hydrochloride.
R 610. Code designation for Racemoramide.
R 661. Code designation for Buzepide Metiodide.
R788 free acid. Code designation for Fostamatinib.
R788 sodium. Code designation for Fostamatinib Disodium.
R 798. Code designation for Rimiterol Hydrobromide.
R-803. Code designation for Furaprofen.
R 805. Code designation for Nimesulide.
R-830. Code designation for Prifelone.
R-830T. Code designation for Prifelone.
R-835. Code designation for Ibafloxacin.
R-837. Code designation for Imiquimod.
R-850. Code designation for Sotirimod.
R 1303. Code designation for Carbofenotion.
R 1406. Code designation for Phenoperidine.
R1439. Code designation for Aleglitazar.
R1450. Code designation for Gantenerumab.
R1503. Code designation for Pamapimod.
R-1558. Code designation for Tomopenem.
R 1575. Code designation for Cinnarizine.
R1579. Code designation for Carmegliptin.
R-1625. Code designation for Haloperidol.
R 1658. Code designation for Moperone.
R 1707. Code designation for Glafenine.
R 1881. Code designation for Metribolone.
R 1929. Code designation for Azaperone.
R 2028. Code designation for Fluanisone.
R 2113. Code designation for Desoximetasone.
R 2159. Code designation for Anisopirol.
R 2167. Code designation for Fluanisone.
R 2323. Code designation for Gestrinone.
R 2453. Code designation for Demegestone.

R-2498. Code designation for Trifluperidol.
R 2858. Code designation for Moxestrol.
R 2962. Code designation for Amiperone.
R 3248. Code designation for Aceperone.
R 3345. Code designation for Pipamperone.
R 3365. Code designation for Piritramide.
R3827. Code designation for Abarelix.
R 3959. Code designation for Clometacin.
R 4082. Code designation for Propyperone.
R-4263. Code designation for Fentanyl Citrate.
R 4318. Code designation for Floctafenine.
R 4444. Code designation for Duometacin.
R-4584. Code designation for Benperidol.
R 4714. Code designation for Oxiperomide.
R-4749. Code designation for Droperidol.
R 4845. Code designation for Bezitramide.
R 5046. Code designation for Cinperene.
R 5147. Code designation for Spiperone.
R 5188. Code designation for Spiroxatrine.
R 5385. Code designation for Acoxatrine.
R 5808. Code designation for Spiramide.
R 6109. Code designation for Spirilene.
R 6218. Code designation for Fluspirilene.
R 6238. Code designation for Pimozide.
R 6438. Code designation for Antazonite.
R 7242. Code designation for Difluanine Hydrochloride.
R 7464. Code designation for Propoxate.
R 7904. Code designation for Lidoflazine.
R 8025. Code designation for Antienite.
R 8141. Code designation for Antienite.
R-8193. Code designation for Antafenite.
R 8284. Code designation for Proclonol.
R 8299. Code designation for Tetramisole Hydrochloride.
R 9298. Code designation for Seperidol Hydrochloride.
R 10,948. Code designation for Diamocaine Cyclamate.
R 11,333. Code designation for Bromperidol.
R 12,563 [as hydrochloride]. Code designation for Dexamisole.
R 12,564. Code designation for Levamisole Hydrochloride.
R-13423. Code designation for Dicloxacillin.
R 13,558. Code designation for Fetoxylate Hydrochloride.
R-13,672. Code designation for Haloperidol Decanoate.
R 14,827. Code designation for Econazole Nitrate.
R 14,889. Code designation for Miconazole Nitrate.
R 14,950. Code designation for Flunarizine Hydrochloride.
R 15,403 [as hydrochloride]. Code designation for Difenoxin.
R-15,454 [as nitrate salt]. Code designation for Isoconazole.
R 15,556. Code designation for Orconazole Nitrate.
R 15,889. Code designation for Lorcainide Hydrochloride.
R 16,341. Code designation for Penfluridol.
R 16,470 [as hydrochloride]. Code designation for Dexetimide.
R 17,147. Code designation for Cyclobendazole.
R 17,635. Code designation for Mebendazole.
R 17,889. Code designation for Flubendazole.
R 17,934. Code designation for Nocodazole.
R 18,553. Code designation for Loperamide Hydrochloride.
R 18,910. Code designation for Fluperamide.
R 19,317. Code designation for Rodocaine.
R 22,700 [as hydrochloride]. Code designation for Rodocaine.
R 23,050. Code designation for Salantel.
R 23,633. Code designation for Fludazonium Chloride.
R 23,979. Code designation for Enilconazole.
R-25,061. Code designation for Suprofen.
R-25,160. Code designation for Cliprofen.
R 25,540. Code designation for Imafen Hydrochloride.
R 25,831 [as the free base]. Code designation for Carnidazole.
R 26,412. Code designation for Sulnidazole.
R 27,500. Code designation for Sepazonium Chloride.
R 28,096 [as hydrochloride]. Code designation for Carnidazole.

R-28,644. Code designation for Azaconazole.
R 28,930. Code designation for Fluspiperone.
R 29,764. Code designation for Clopimozide.
R 29,860. Code designation for Nitramisole Hydrochloride.
R 30,730. Code designation for Sufentanil.
R 31,520. Code designation for Closantel.
R 33,204. Code designation for Declenperone.
R 33,799. Code designation for Carfentanil Citrate.
R 33800. Code designation for Sufentanil Citrate.
R 33,812. Code designation for Domperidone.
R 34,000. Code designation for Doconazole.
R 34,009. Code designation for Milenperone.
R 34,301. Code designation for Halopemide.
R-34,803. Code designation for Etibendazole.
R 34,995. Code designation for Lofentanil Oxalate.
R 35,443. Code designation for Oxatomide.
R 38,198. Code designation for Buterizine.
R 39,209. Code designation for Alfentanil Hydrochloride.
R 39,500. Code designation for Parconazole Hydrochloride.
R 41,400. Code designation for Ketoconazole.
R-41,468. Code designation for Ketanserin.
R-42,470. Code designation for Terconazole.
R 43,512. Code designation for Astemizole.
R-43512. Code designation for Tecastemizole.
R-45,486. Code designation for Flumeridone.
R-46,541. Code designation for Bromperidol Decanoate.
R 46,846. Code designation for Tubulozole Hydrochloride.
R-47,465. Code designation for Pirenperone.
R 50,547. Code designation for Levocabastine Hydrochloride.
R 51,211. Code designation for Itraconazole.
R-51,469. Code designation for Mioflazine Hydrochloride.
R-51,619. Code designation for Cisapride.
R 52,245. Code designation for Setoperone.
R-53,200. Code designation for Altanserin Tartrate.
R 54,718. Code designation for Transcainide.
R 55104. Code designation for Erbulozole.
R 55,667. Code designation for Ritanserin.
R 57959. Code designation for Barmastine.
R58425. Code designation for Loperamide Oxide.
R 58735. Code designation for Sabeluzole.
R 60844. Code designation for Irtemazole.
R62,690. Code designation for Clazuril.
R64,433. Code designation for Diclazuril.
R 64947. Code designation for Noberastine.
R65,824. Code designation for Nebivolol.
R 66905. Code designation for Saperconazole.
R 67408. Code designation for Fenclofenac.
R067555. Code designation for Nebivolol Hydrochloride.
R 68070. Code designation for Ridogrel.
R 72063. Code designation for Loreclezole.
R 75231. Code designation for Draflazine.
R 75251. Code designation for Liarozole Hydrochloride.
R 77975. Code designation for Pirodavir.
R 79598. Code designation for Ocaperidone.
R 83842. Code designation for Vorozole.
R 85246. Code designation for Liarozole Fumarate.
R-87926. Code designation for Lubeluzole.
R-89439. Code designation for Loviride.
R 89674. Code designation for Alcaftadine.
R-91274. Code designation for Alniditan Dihydrochloride.
R103757. Code designation for Mitratapide.
R-106056. Code designation for Rivoglitazone.
R-109339. Code designation for Apricoxib.
R115500. Code designation for Catramilast.
R-115685. Code designation for Tomopenem.
R115777. Code designation for Tipifarnib.
R115866. Code designation for Talarozole.
R126638. Code designation for Pramiconazole.

R129160. Code designation for Vapitadine Dihydrochloride.
R935788 free acid. Code designation for Fostamatinib.
R935788 sodium. Code designation for Fostamatinib Disodium.
R04909832. Code designation for Gantenerumab.
RA-8. Code designation for Dipyridamole.
RA-C-384. Code designation for Iodocetylic Acid I 123.
RAD001. Code designation for Everolimus.
RB5 IgM. Code designation for Technetium Tc 99m Fanolesomab.
rBPI-$_{21}$. Code designation for Opebacan.
RC 61-91. Code designation for Ifenprodil.
RC-160. Code designation for Vapreotide.
RC-167. Code designation for Niceverine.
RC-172. Code designation for Aldioxa.
RC-173. Code designation for Alcloxa.
RC-1291 HCl. Code designation for Anamorelin Hydrochloride.
RC-27109. Code designation for Nifuroxazide.
RCH 314. Code designation for Benhepazone.
RCM 258. Code designation for Fepentolic Acid.
Rd 292. Code designation for Fenpentadiol.
RD 328. Code designation for Pasiniazid.
RD 406. Code designation for Cyprodenate.
RD 2801. Code designation for Pyritidium Bromide.
RD 9338 [as hydrochloride]. Code designation for Norbudrine.
RD 11654. Code designation for Ibufenac.
RD 17345. Code designation for Fluprofen.
rDSPA alpha 1. Code designation for Desmoteplase.
reboxetine. Code designation for Esreboxetine.
Rec 7/0267. Code designation for Dimefline Hydrochloride.
Rec 15 0122. Code designation for Nifurpipone.
Rec 15/1476. Code designation for Fenticonazole Nitrate.
Rec-15/2375. Code designation for Lercanidipine Hydrochloride.
REP 8839. Code designation for Bederocin.
REV 3659-(S). Code designation for Pivopril.
REV 6000A. Code designation for Delapril Hydrochloride.
RFS 2000. Code designation for Rubitecan.
RG 270. Code designation for Iomeglamic Acid.
RG 12561. Code designation for Dalvastatin.
RG 83606. Code designation for Diltiazem Hydrochloride.
rG-CSF. Code designation for Lenograstim.
RGH 1106. Code designation for Pipecuronium Bromide.
RGW-2938. Code designation for Prinoxodan.
RH-565. Code designation for Uredofos.
RH-32,565. Code designation for Uredofos.
RHC 2871. Code designation for Eclazolast.
RHC 2906. Code designation for Flordipine.
RHC 3659-(S). Code designation for Pivopril.
RHC 3988. Code designation for Quazolast.
rhGAA. Code designation for Alglucosidase Alfa.
rhGm-CSF. Code designation for Regramostim.
rhIGFBP-3. Code designation for Rinfabate.
rhIGF-I/rhIGFBP-3. Code designation for Mecasermin Rinfabate.
r-hTBP-1. Code designation for Onercept.
rhu GM-CSF. Code designation for Sargramostim.
rhu TNFR:Fc. Code designation for Etanercept.
rhuMab 2C4. Code designation for Pertuzumab.
rhuMAb CD18. Code designation for Erlizumab.
rhuMab-E25. Code designation for Omalizumab.
rHuPH20. Code designation for Hyaluronidase (Human Recombinant).
rhVEGF. Code designation for Telbermin.
RI-64. Code designation for Pifexole.
Rifamycin M-14. Code designation for Rifamide.
Riker 52G. Code designation for Aprotinin.
Riker 594. Code designation for Sulthiame.
Riker 595. Code designation for Butaperazine.
Riker 601. Code designation for Triaziquone.
rIL-21; recombinant human interleukin 21. Code designation for Denenicokin.

RIT 1140. Code designation for Apicycline.
RM 1601. Code designation for Fipronil.
r-metHuG-CSF. Code designation for Filgrastim.
r-metHuLeptin. Code designation for Metreleptin.
RMI 8090DJ. Code designation for Quindecamine Acetate.
RMI 9,384A. Code designation for Desipramine Hydrochloride.
RMI 9918. Code designation for Terfenadine.
RMI 10,482A. Code designation for Metizoline Hydrochloride.
RMI 16,238. Code designation for Eterobarb.
RMI 16,289. Code designation for Enclomiphene.
RMI 16,312. Code designation for Zuclomiphene.
RMI 80,029. Code designation for Elantrine.
RMI 81,182EF. Code designation for Cilobamine Mesylate.
RMI 81,968. Code designation for Medroxalol.
RMI 81,968 A. Code designation for Medroxalol Hydrochloride.
RMI 83,027. Code designation for Rolicyprine.
RMI 83,047. Code designation for Ambuside.
RMP-7. Code designation for Labradimil.
RN624. Code designation for Tanezumab.
RNH-5139. Code designation for Temocaprilat.
RNH-6270. Code designation for Olmesartan.
RO 1-5155. Code designation for Nicotinyl Alcohol.
Ro 01-6794/706; Ro 1-6794 (dextrorphan). Code designation for Dextrorphan Hydrochloride.
Ro 1-9334/19. Code designation for Dehydroemetine.
Ro 1-9569. Code designation for Tetrabenazine.
Ro 2-2985. Code designation for Lasalocid.
Ro 2-3773. Code designation for Clidinium Bromide.
Ro 2-9757. Code designation for Fluorouracil.
Ro 2-9915. Code designation for Flucytosine.
Ro 03-7355/000. Code designation for Avizafone.
Ro 03-8799. Code designation for Pimonidazole.
Ro 4-0403. Code designation for Chlorprothixene.
Ro 4-1544-6. Code designation for Sodium Stibocaptate.
Ro 4-1778/1. Code designation for Methopholine.
Ro 4-2130. Code designation for Sulfamethoxazole.
Ro 4-3780. Code designation for Isotretinoin.
RO 4-3816. Code designation for Alcuronium Chloride.
Ro 4-4393. Code designation for Sulfadoxine.
Ro 4-4602. Code designation for Benserazide.
Ro 4-5282. Code designation for Mefenorex Hydrochloride.
Ro 4-5360. Code designation for Nitrazepam.
Ro 4-6467/1. Code designation for Procarbazine Hydrochloride.
Ro 5-0690. Code designation for Chlordiazepoxide Hydrochloride.
Ro 5-2092. Code designation for Demoxepam.
Ro 5-2807. Code designation for Diazepam.
Ro 5-3059. Code designation for Nitrazepam.
RO 5-3307/1. Code designation for Debrisoquin Sulfate.
Ro 5-3350. Code designation for Bromazepam.
Ro 5-4023. Code designation for Clonazepam.
Ro 5-4200. Code designation for Flunitrazepam.
Ro 5-4556. Code designation for Medazepam Hydrochloride.
Ro 5-4645/010. Code designation for Coumermycin Sodium.
Ro 5-6901. Code designation for Flurazepam Hydrochloride.
Ro 5-9110/1. Code designation for Dorastine Hydrochloride.
Ro 5-9754. Code designation for Ormetoprim.
Ro 6-4563. Code designation for Glibornuride.
Ro 7-0207. Code designation for Ornidazole.
Ro 7-0582. Code designation for Misonidazole.
Ro 7-1554. Code designation for Ipronidazole.
Ro 7-4488/1. Code designation for Cuprimyxin.
Ro 09-1978/000. Code designation for Capecitabine.
Ro 10-1670/000. Code designation for Acitretin.
Ro 10-6338. Code designation for Bumetanide.
Ro 10-9070. Code designation for Amdinocillin.
Ro 10-9071. Code designation for Amdinocillin Pivoxil.
Ro 10-9359. Code designation for Etretinate.

Ro 11-1163/000. Code designation for Moclobemide.
Ro 11-1430. Code designation for Motretinide.
Ro 11-1781/023. Code designation for Tiapamil Hydrochloride.
Ro 12-0068/000. Code designation for Tenoxicam.
Ro 13-5057. Code designation for Aniracetam.
Ro 13-6438/006. Code designation for Quazinone.
Ro 13-8996. Code designation for Oxiconazole Nitrate.
Ro 13-9297. Code designation for Lornoxicam.
Ro 13-9904. Code designation for Ceftriaxone Sodium.
Ro 14-4767/000. Code designation for Amorolfine.
Ro 14-9706/000. Code designation for Sumarotene.
Ro 15-1570/000. Code designation for Etarotene.
Ro 15-1788/000. Code designation for Flumazenil.
Ro 16-6028/000. Code designation for Bretazenil.
Ro 17-2301/006. Code designation for Carumonam Sodium.
Ro 18-0647/002. Code designation for Orlistat.
Ro 19-6327/000. Code designation for Lazabemide.
Ro 19-6327/001. Code designation for Lazabemide Hydrochloride.
Ro 20-5720/000. Code designation for Carprofen.
Ro 21-0702. Code designation for Flurocitabine.
Ro 21-3981/001. Code designation for Midazolam Maleate.
Ro 21-3981/003. Code designation for Midazolam Hydrochloride.
Ro 21-5535. Code designation for Calcitriol.
Ro 21-5998. Code designation for Mefloquine.
Ro 21-5998/001. Code designation for Mefloquine Hydrochloride.
Ro 21-6937/000. Code designation for Trimoprostil.
Ro 21-8837/001. Code designation for Estramustine Phosphate Sodium.
Ro 22-1319/003. Code designation for Piquindone Hydrochloride.
Ro 22-2296/000. Code designation for Estramustine.
Ro 22-3747/000. Code designation for Tiacrilast.
Ro 22-3747/007. Code designation for Tiacrilast Sodium.
Ro 22-7796. Code designation for Cifenline.
Ro 22-7796/001. Code designation for Cifenline Succinate.
Ro 22-8181. Code designation for Interferon Alfa-2a.
Ro 22-9000. Code designation for Alfaprostol.
Ro 23-0731/000. Code designation for Sedecamycin.
Ro 23-3544/000. Code designation for Ablukast.
Ro 23-3544/001. Code designation for Ablukast Sodium.
Ro 23-6019. Code designation for Teceleukin.
Ro 23-6240/000. Code designation for Fleroxacin.
Ro 24-2027/000. Code designation for Zalcitabine.
Ro 24-5913. Code designation for Cinalukast.
Ro 24-7375. Code designation for Daclizumab.
Ro 24-7472/000. Code designation for Edodekin Alfa.
Ro 25-8310/000. Code designation for Peginterferon Alfa-2a.
Ro-25-8315/000. Code designation for Pegnartograstim.
Ro27-2441/002. Code designation for Valategrast Hydrochloride.
Ro 31-2848/006. Code designation for Cilazapril.
Ro 31-3113. Code designation for Cilazaprilat.
Ro 31-3948/000. Code designation for Romazarit.
Ro 31-8959/000. Code designation for Saquinavir.
Ro 31-8959/003. Code designation for Saquinavir Mesylate.
Ro 32-3555/000. Code designation for Cipemastat.
Ro 40-5967/001. Code designation for Mibefradil Dihydrochloride.
Ro 40-7592. Code designation for Tolcapone.
Ro 42-1611. Code designation for Arteflene.
Ro 44-9883/000. Code designation for Lamifiban.
Ro 44-9883/023. Code designation for Lamifiban Hydrochloride.
Ro 45-2081. Code designation for Lenercept.
Ro 46-6240/010. Code designation for Napsagatran.
Ro 47-0203/029. Code designation for Bosentan.
Ro 48-3657/001. Code designation for Sibrafiban.
Ro 63-9141. Code designation for Ceftobiprole.
Ro 64-0796/002. Code designation for Oseltamivir Phosphate.
Ro 65-5788. Code designation for Ceftobiprole Medocaril.

Ro 67-3189/000. Code designation for Netupitant.

Ro 67-5930. Code designation for Befetupitant.

Ro 70-0001/001. Code designation for Semparatide Acetate.

Ro 106-6271/297. Code designation for Semparatide Acetate.

Ro107-9070/194. Code designation for Valganciclovir Hydrochloride.

RO115-1240/190. Code designation for Dabuzalgron Hydrochloride.

Ro 48347. Code designation for Trengestone.

RO76477. Code designation for Paliperidone.

RO92670. Code designation for Paliperidone Palmitate.

Ro0272441/002. Code designation for Valategrast Hydrochloride.

RO 640796. Code designation for Oseltamivir.

RO0728804. Code designation for Aleglitazar.

RO2052349-602. Code designation for Edaglitazone Sodium.

RO3300074. Code designation for Palovarotene.

RO4389620-R1440. Code designation for Piragliatin.

Ro 4402257. Code designation for Pamapimod.

RO4607381. Code designation for Dalcetrapib.

RO4876904. Code designation for Carmegliptin.

RO4876904-001. Code designation for Carmegliptin Dihydrochloride.

RO4908463. Code designation for Tomopenem.

RO 5072759. Code designation for Afutuzumab.

R.P. 20 578. Code designation for Bamnidazole.

RP 2254. Code designation for Glyprothiazol.

RP 2259. Code designation for Glybuthiazol.

RP 2512 [as isethionate]. Code designation for Pentamidine.

RP 2921. Code designation for Aminothiazole.

RP 2987. Code designation for Diethazine Hydrochloride.

RP 3854. Code designation for Melarsoprol.

RP 4763 [as sodium salt]. Code designation for Difetarsone.

RP 5171. Code designation for Proadifen Hydrochloride.

RP 5337. Code designation for Spiramycin.

RP 6484. Code designation for Etymemazine Hydrochloride.

RP 6847. Code designation for Oxomemazine.

RP 6870. Code designation for Inproquone.

RP-7044. Code designation for Levomepromazine.

RP 7044. Code designation for Methotrimeprazine.

RP 7204. Code designation for Cyamemazine.

RP 7293. Code designation for Pristinamycin.

RP 7891. Code designation for Glybuzole.

RP 8595. Code designation for Dimetridazole.

RP 8823. Code designation for Metronidazole.

RP 8909. Code designation for Periciazine.

RP 9159. Code designation for Perimetazine.

RP 9671. Code designation for Nosiheptide.

RP 9778. Code designation for Protionamide.

RP 9921. Code designation for Aprotinin.

RP 9955. Code designation for Melarsonyl Potassium.

RP 12222. Code designation for Penmesterol.

RP 13057 [as the base]. Code designation for Daunorubicin Hydrochloride.

RP 13607. Code designation for Clotioxone.

RP 14539. Code designation for Secnidazole.

RP 16091. Code designation for Metiazinic Acid.

RP 19552. Code designation for Pipotiazine Palmitate.

R.P. 19,583. Code designation for Ketoprofen.

RP 22,050 hydrochloride. Code designation for Zorubicin Hydrochloride.

RP 22410. Code designation for Glisoxepide.

RP 27267. Code designation for Zopiclone.

RP 31264. Code designation for Suriclone.

RP 54274. Code designation for Riluzole.

RP 54476. Code designation for Dalfopristin.

RP 54563. Code designation for Enoxaparin Sodium.

RP-54780. Code designation for Oxaliplatin.

RP 56976. Code designation for Docetaxel.

RP 57669. Code designation for Quinupristin.

RP 60475. Code designation for Intoplicine.

RP 62203. Code designation for Fananserin.

RP 62955. Code designation for Pagoclone.

RP 64305. Code designation for Ebastine.

RP 73401. Code designation for Piclamilast.

rPAF-AH. Code designation for Epafipase.

RPR251526. Code designation for Ciclesonide.

RR No. 32705. Code designation for Rutamycin.

R&S 218-M. Code designation for Alletorphine.

RS-1301. Code designation for Delmadinone Acetate.

RS-1320. Code designation for Flunisolide Acetate.

RS-2208. Code designation for Amadinone Acetate.

RS-2252. Code designation for Flucloronide.

RS-2362. Code designation for Procinonide.

RS-2386. Code designation for Ciprocinonide.

RS-3268R. Code designation for Nandrolone Cyclotate.

RS-3540. Code designation for Naproxen.

RS-3650. Code designation for Naproxen Sodium.

RS-3694R. Code designation for Cormethasone Acetate.

RS-3999. Code designation for Flunisolide.

RS-4034. Code designation for Naproxol.

RS-4464. Code designation for Triclonide.

RS-4691. Code designation for Cloprednol.

R&S 5205-M. Code designation for Homprenorphine.

RS-6245. Code designation for Tazolol Hydrochloride.

RS-6818. Code designation for Xanoxate Sodium.

RS-7337. Code designation for Tixanox.

RS-8858. Code designation for Oxfendazole.

RS-9390. Code designation for Prostalene.

RS-10085-197. Code designation for Moexipril Hydrochloride.

RS-11988. Code designation for Laidlomycin Propionate Potassium.

RS-15385-197. Code designation for Delequamine Hydrochloride.

RS-21361. Code designation for Imiloxan Hydrochloride.

RS-21592. Code designation for Ganciclovir.

RS-21592 sodium. Code designation for Ganciclovir Sodium.

RS-21607-197. Code designation for Azalanstat Dihydrochloride.

RS-25259-197. Code designation for Palonosetron Hydrochloride.

RS-25560-197. Code designation for Nepicastat Hydrochloride.

RS-26306. Code designation for Ganirelix Acetate.

RS-35887. Code designation for Butoconazole Nitrate.

RS-35887-00-10-3. Code designation for Butoconazole Nitrate.

RS-35909-00-00-0. Code designation for Ticabesone Propionate.

RS-37326. Code designation for Anirolac.

RS-37449. Code designation for Temurtide.

RS-40584. Code designation for Flumoxonide.

RS-40974-00-00-0. Code designation for Tiopinac.

RS-43179. Code designation for Lonapalene.

RS-43285. Code designation for Ranolazine Hydrochloride.

RS-43285-003. Code designation for Ranolazine.

RS-44872. Code designation for Sulconazole Nitrate.

RS-44872-00-10-3. Code designation for Sulconazole Nitrate.

RS-49014. Code designation for Tazifylline Hydrochloride.

RS-61443. Code designation for Mycophenolate Mofetil.

RS-61443 [as mofetil]. Code designation for Mycophenolic Acid.

RS-61443-190. Code designation for Mycophenolate Mofetil Hydrochloride.

RS-66271-297. Code designation for Semparatide Acetate.

RS-68439. Code designation for Detirelix Acetate.

RS-69216. Code designation for Nicardipine Hydrochloride.

RS-69216-XX-07-0. Code designation for Nicardipine Hydrochloride.

RS-079070-194. Code designation for Valganciclovir Hydrochloride.

RS-82856. Code designation for Lixazinone Sulfate.

RS-82917-030. Code designation for Tifurac Sodium.

RS-84043. Code designation for Fenprostalene.

RS-84135. Code designation for Enprostil.

RS-85446-007. Code designation for Timobesone Acetate.

RS-87476-000. Code designation for Lifarizine.

RS-94991-298. Code designation for Nafarelin Acetate.

RS-100302-190. Code designation for Sulamserod Hydrochloride.

RSD1235. Code designation for Vernakalant Hydrochloride.

RSP58. Code designation for Delmitide Acetate.

RSR13. Code designation for Efaproxiral.

RSR13 sodium. Code designation for Efaproxiral Sodium.

RTA 744. Code designation for Berubicin Hydrochloride.

R-tofisopam. Code designation for Dextofisopam.

rt-PA. Code designation for Alteplase.

RU-0211. Code designation for Lubiprostone.

RU 486. Code designation for Mifepristone.

RU 882. Code designation for Inocoterone Acetate.

RU 965. Code designation for Roxithromycin.

RU-1697. Code designation for Trenbolone Acetate.

RU-2267. Code designation for Altrenogest.

RU 2323. Code designation for Gestrinone.

RU 15060. Code designation for Tiaprofenic Acid.

Ru 15750. Code designation for Floctafenine.

RU-19110. Code designation for Halofuginone Hydrobromide.

Ru 23908. Code designation for Nilutamide.

RU 24756. Code designation for Cefotaxime Sodium.

RU 27987. Code designation for Trimegestone.

RU 28965. Code designation for Roxithromycin.

RU35926. Code designation for Milameline Hydrochloride.

RU 38486. Code designation for Mifepristone.

RU 38882. Code designation for Inocoterone Acetate.

RU 44570. Code designation for Trandolapril.

RUF 331. Code designation for Rufinamide.

RWJ 10131. Code designation for Norgestimate.

RWJ-10553. Code designation for Norelgestromin.

RWJ 15817. Code designation for Edoxudine.

RWJ 15927. Code designation for Rioprostil.

RWJ 16600. Code designation for Bemarinone Hydrochloride.

RWJ-17021. Code designation for Topiramate.

RWJ 17070. Code designation for Histrelin.

RWJ 18704. Code designation for Pelretin.

RWJ 20257. Code designation for Doretinel.

RWJ 20485. Code designation for Tepoxalin.

RWJ 21757. Code designation for Loxoribine.

RWJ 22164. Code designation for Atosiban.

RWJ 24517. Code designation for Carsatrin Succinate.

RWJ 24834. Code designation for Linarotene.

RWJ-25213. Code designation for Levofloxacin.

RWJ 26251. Code designation for Cladribine.

RWJ 28299. Code designation for Immune Globulin Intravenous Pentetate.

RWJ 37796. Code designation for Mazapertine Succinate.

RWJ 47428. Code designation for Prazarelix Acetate.

RWJ 49004. Code designation for Cedelizumab.

RWJ-53308. Code designation for Elarofiban.

RWJ-57504. Code designation for Tilmacoxib.

RWJ 60235. Code designation for Becaplermin.

RWJ-241947. Code designation for Netoglitazone.

RWJ-270201. Code designation for Peramivir.

RWJ-333369. Code designation for Carisbamate.

RX-01_667. Code designation for Radezolid.

RX-01_667. Code designation for Radezolid Hydrochloride.

RX-103. Code designation for Radezolid.

RX-103. Code designation for Radezolid Hydrochloride.

RX-1741. Code designation for Radezolid.

RX-1741. Code designation for Radezolid Hydrochloride.

RX-3341. Code designation for Delafloxacin.

RX-3341. Code designation for Delafloxacin Meglumine.

RX 6029-M HCl. Code designation for Buprenorphine Hydrochloride.

Rx 67408. Code designation for Fenclofenac.

RX77989. Code designation for Pentamorphone.

R-(-)-YM-12617. Code designation for Tamsulosin Hydrochloride.

S 7. Code designation for Fenticlor.

S-041. Code designation for Gadodiamide.

S-043. Code designation for Sprodiamide.

S.049. Code designation for Ecadotril.

S-59. Code designation for Amotosalen Hydrochloride.

S-62. Code designation for Chlorphentermine Hydrochloride.

S 73 4118. Code designation for Piretanide.

S 77 0777. Code designation for Prednicarbate.

S 77 1221 B [as sodium]. Code designation for Cefodizime.

S-210. Code designation for Morsuximide.

S-222. Code designation for Ditazole.

S-303.2HCl. Code designation for Amustaline Dihydrochloride.

S 314. Code designation for Fusafungine.

S-940. Code designation for Naftalofos.

S-1153. Code designation for Capravirine.

S-1210. Code designation for Bietaserpine.

S-1320. Code designation for Budesonide.

S 1530. Code designation for Nimetazepam.

S-2367. Code designation for Velneperit.

S-2395. Code designation for Tertatolol.

S-2539F. Code designation for Phenothrin.

S-2620. Code designation for Almitrine Mesylate.

S-3013. Code designation for Varespladib Methyl.

S 4105. Code designation for Medibazine.

S-4522. Code designation for Rosuvastatin Calcium.

S-4661. Code designation for Doripenem.

S 5614 HCl. Code designation for Dexfenfluramine Hydrochloride.

S-9490. Code designation for Perindopril.

S-9490-3. Code designation for Perindopril Erbumine.

S-9780. Code designation for Perindoprilat.

S 10036. Code designation for Fotemustine.

S-16820. Code designation for Prifelone.

S-25930. Code designation for Ibafloxacin.

S26308. Code designation for Imiquimod.

S-30563. Code designation for Epetirimod.

S-30563-35-65. Code designation for Epetirimod Esylate.

S-30594. Code designation for Sotirimod.

SA-267. Code designation for Dipenine Bromide.

SANORG34006. Code designation for Idraparinux Sodium.

SB-075 acetate. Code designation for Cetrorelix Acetate.

SB 7505. Code designation for Ibopamine.

SB-202026-A. Code designation for Sabcomeline Hydrochloride.

SB-204269-EO. Code designation for Carabersat.

SB 205312. Code designation for Pranlukast.

SB-207266-A. Code designation for Piboserod Hydrochloride.

SB 207499. Code designation for Cilomilast.

SB-209247. Code designation for Ticolubant.

SB 209509-AX. Code designation for Frovatriptan Succinate.

SB 209763. Code designation for Felvizumab.

SB-214857-A. Code designation for Lotrafiban Hydrochloride.

SB-218842. Code designation for Tidembersat.

SB-220453. Code designation for Tonabersat.

SB-223030. Code designation for Idoxifene.

SB-223412-A. Code designation for Talnetant Hydrochloride.

SB-240563. Code designation for Mepolizumab.

SB-240683. Code designation for Pascolizumab.

SB-251353. Code designation for Garnocestim.

SB-265805-S. Code designation for Gemifloxacin Mesylate.

SB-275833. Code designation for Retapamulin.

SB-408075. Code designation for Cantuzumab Mertansine.

SB-462795. Code designation for Relacatib.

SB-480848. Code designation for Darapladib.

SB-485232. Code designation for Iboctadekin.

SB-497115-GR. Code designation for Eltrombopag Olamine.
SB-559448-AAA. Code designation for Totrombopag Choline.
SB-659032. Code designation for Rilapladib.
SB-683699. Code designation for Firategrast.
SB-715992-S. Code designation for Ispinesib Mesylate.
SB-751689-A. Code designation for Ronacaleret Hydrochloride.
SBI-0067. Code designation for Galasomite.
SBW-22. Code designation for Ketorfanol.
SC103. Code designation for Ascorbyl Gamolenate.
SC-0735. Code designation for Nitisinone.
SC 1749 [as sodium salt]. Code designation for Menbutone.
SC-4642. Code designation for Norethynodrel.
SC-7031. Code designation for Disopyramide.
SC-7294. Code designation for Propetandrol.
SC-7525. Code designation for Bolandiol Dipropionate.
SC-9376. Code designation for Canrenone.
SC-9880. Code designation for Flurogestone Acetate.
SC 10363. Code designation for Megestrol Acetate.
SC 11585. Code designation for Oxandrolone.
SC 11800. Code designation for Ethynodiol Diacetate.
SC-12350. Code designation for Nitralamine Hydrochloride.
SC-12937. Code designation for Azacosterol Hydrochloride.
SC-13504. Code designation for Ropizine.
SC-13957. Code designation for Disopyramide Phosphate.
SC-14207. Code designation for Metogest.
SC-14266. Code designation for Canrenoate Potassium.
SC-16148. Code designation for Silandrone.
SC-18862. Code designation for Aspartame.
SC-19198. Code designation for Methynodiol Diacetate.
SC-21009. Code designation for Norgestomet.
SC-23992. Code designation for Prorenoate Potassium.
SC-25469. Code designation for Pinadoline.
SC-26100. Code designation for Difenoximide Hydrochloride.
SC-26304. Code designation for Dicirenone.
SC-26438. Code designation for Pirolazamide.
SC-26714. Code designation for Mexrenoate Potassium.
SC-27123. Code designation for Octriptyline Phosphate.
SC-27166. Code designation for Nufenoxole.
SC-27761. Code designation for Pranolium Chloride.
SC-29333. Code designation for Misoprostol.
SC-31828. Code designation for Disobutamide.
SC-32642. Code designation for Metronidazole Hydrochloride.
SC-32840. Code designation for Oxagrelate.
SC-33643. Code designation for Bemitradine.
SC-33963. Code designation for Reclazepam.
SC-34301. Code designation for Enisoprost.
SC-35135. Code designation for Edifolone Acetate.
SC-36602. Code designation for Actisomide.
SC-37681. Code designation for Gemeprost.
SC-38390. Code designation for Zinoconazole Hydrochloride.
SC-39026. Code designation for Lodelaben.
SC-40230. Code designation for Bidisomide.
SC-47111. Code designation for Lomefloxacin Hydrochloride.
SC-47111A. Code designation for Lomefloxacin.
SC-47111B. Code designation for Lomefloxacin Mesylate.
SC-48834. Code designation for Remiprostol.
SC-52151. Code designation for Telinavir.
SC-52458. Code designation for Forasartan.
SC-54684A. Code designation for Xemilofiban Hydrochloride.
SC-55389A. Code designation for Droxinavir Hydrochloride.
SC-55494. Code designation for Daniplestim.
SC-57099B. Code designation for Orbofiban Acetate.
SC-58635. Code designation for Celecoxib.
SC-59046. Code designation for Deracoxib.
SC-59735. Code designation for Tifacogin.
SC-65872. Code designation for Valdecoxib.
SC-66110. Code designation for Eplerenone.
SC-69124. Code designation for Parecoxib.

SC-69124A. Code designation for Parecoxib Sodium.
SC-70935. Code designation for Leridistim.
SC-72325. Code designation for Imisopasem Manganese.
SCA-136. Code designation for Vabicaserin Hydrochloride.
SCE 963. Code designation for Cefotiam Hydrochloride.
SCE-1365 (Takeda) (base). Code designation for Cefmenoxime Hydrochloride.
Sch 1000-Br-monohydrate. Code designation for Ipratropium Bromide.
Sch 2544. Code designation for Cycliramine Maleate.
Sch 3444. Code designation for Parapenzolate Bromide.
Sch 4358. Code designation for Meprednisone.
Sch 4831. Code designation for Betamethasone.
Sch 4855. Code designation for Pseudoephedrine Sulfate.
Sch 6620. Code designation for Prednazate.
Sch 6673. Code designation for Acetophenazine Maleate.
Sch 6783. Code designation for Diazoxide.
Sch 7056. Code designation for Acrisorcin.
Sch 9384. Code designation for Oxymetazoline Hydrochloride.
Sch 9724. Code designation for Gentamicin Sulfate.
Sch 10144. Code designation for Tolnaftate.
Sch 10159. Code designation for Triclofos Sodium.
Sch 10304. Code designation for Clonixin.
Sch 10595. Code designation for Bupicomide.
Sch 10649. Code designation for Azatadine Maleate.
Sch 11460. Code designation for Betamethasone Dipropionate.
Sch 11572. Code designation for Meclorisone Dibutyrate.
Sch 11973. Code designation for Tosifen.
Sch 12041. Code designation for Halazepam.
Sch 12149. Code designation for Pazoxide.
Sch 12169. Code designation for Closiramine Aceturate.
Sch 12650. Code designation for Dazadrol Maleate.
Sch 12679. Code designation for Trepipam Maleate.
Sch 12707. Code designation for Clonixeril.
Sch 13166 D fumarate. Code designation for Domazoline Fumarate.
Sch 13430.2KH$_2$PO$_4$. Code designation for Megalomicin Potassium Phosphate.
Sch 13475 sulfate. Code designation for Sisomicin Sulfate.
Sch 13521. Code designation for Flutamide.
Sch 13949W Sulfate. Code designation for Albuterol Sulfate.
Sch 14342. Code designation for Betamicin Sulfate.
Sch 14714. Code designation for Flunixin.
Sch 14714 meglumine. Code designation for Flunixin Meglumine.
Sch 14947. Code designation for Rosaramicin.
Sch 14947 Stearate. Code designation for Rosaramicin Stearate.
Sch 14947.NaH$_2$PO$_4$. Code designation for Rosaramicin Sodium Phosphate.
Sch 15280. Code designation for Azanator Maleate.
Sch 15427. Code designation for Carmantadine.
Sch 15507. Code designation for Dopamantine.
Sch 15698. Code designation for Fletazepam.
Sch 15719W. Code designation for Labetalol Hydrochloride.
Sch 16134. Code designation for Quazepam.
Sch 16524. Code designation for Repromicin.
Sch 17894. Code designation for Rosaramicin Propionate.
Sch 18020W. Code designation for Beclomethasone Dipropionate.
Sch 18667. Code designation for Rosaramicin Butyrate.
Sch 19741. Code designation for Picotrin Diolamine.
Sch 19927. Code designation for Dilevalol Hydrochloride.
Sch 20569. Code designation for Netilmicin Sulfate.
Sch 21420. Code designation for Isepamicin.
Sch 21480. Code designation for Tioxidazole.
Sch 22219. Code designation for Alclometasone Dipropionate.
Sch 22591. Code designation for Pentisomicin.
Sch 25298. Code designation for Florfenicol.
SCH 27899. Code designation for Evernimicin.
Sch 28316Z. Code designation for Indenolol.

Sch 29851. Code designation for Loratadine.

Sch 30500. Code designation for Interferon Alfa-2b.

Sch 31353. Code designation for Dexamethasone Acefurate.

Sch 32088. Code designation for Mometasone Furoate.

Sch 32481. Code designation for Netobimin.

Sch 33844. Code designation for Spirapril Hydrochloride.

Sch 33861. Code designation for Spiraprilat.

SCH 34117. Code designation for Desloratadine.

Sch 35852. Code designation for Cisconazole.

SCH 39166. Code designation for Ecopipam Hydrochloride.

Sch 39300. Code designation for Molgramostim.

SCH 39400. Code designation for Binetrakin.

Sch 39720. Code designation for Ceftibuten.

SCH 40054 HCl. Code designation for Nemazoline Hydrochloride.

SCH 52000. Code designation for Ilodecakin.

SCH 52365. Code designation for Temozolomide.

SCH 55700. Code designation for Reslizumab.

SCH 56592. Code designation for Posaconazole.

SCH57068 · HCl. Code designation for Acolbifene Hydrochloride.

SCH58235. Code designation for Ezetimibe.

SCH 66336. Code designation for Lonafarnib.

SCH 209579. Code designation for Maxacalcitol.

SCH351125. Code designation for Ancriviroc.

SCH 417690. Code designation for Vicriviroc Maleate.

SCH 417849. Code designation for Talibegron Hydrochloride.

SCH 420814. Code designation for Preladenant.

SCH 446132. Code designation for Dasantafil.

SCH 503034. Code designation for Boceprevir.

SCH619734. Code designation for Rolapitant Hydrochloride.

Scha-306. Code designation for Cintazone.

SCIO 469. Code designation for Talmapimod.

SCL-70. Code designation for Alofilcon A.

SCTZ [as edisylate]. Code designation for Clomethiazole.

SCV-07. Code designation for Golotimod.

SD 25. Code designation for Dicarfen.

SD 149-01. Code designation for Feneritrol.

SD 270-07 [as succinate]. Code designation for Oxaprazine.

SD 270-31 [as disuccinate]. Code designation for Oxaflumazine.

SD 271-12. Code designation for Clobenzorex.

SD 286-03. Code designation for Cimemoxin.

SD 1223-01. Code designation for Trazitiline.

SD 1248-17 [as hydrochloride]. Code designation for Tropatepine.

SD 1750. Code designation for Dichlorvos.

SD 2102-18. Code designation for Acrocinonide.

SD 2124-01. Code designation for Procinolol.

SD 7859. Code designation for Clorfenvinfos.

SD 14112. Code designation for Sulclamide.

SD 15803. Code designation for Vincofos.

SD 17102. Code designation for Meticrane.

SD 27115 [as cyclamate]. Code designation for Furfenorex.

SDX-105. Code designation for Bendamustine Hydrochloride.

SDZ-212-713. Code designation for Rivastigmine.

SDZ 215-811. Code designation for Pentetreotide.

SDZ 215-811s. Code designation for Pentetreotide.

SDZ ASM 981. Code designation for Pimecrolimus.

SDZ DJN 608. Code designation for Nateglinide.

SDZ ILE 964. Code designation for Muplestim.

SDZ MSL 109. Code designation for Sevirumab.

SDZ OST 577. Code designation for Tuvirumab.

SDZ PSC 833. Code designation for Valspodar.

SDZ-CHI-621. Code designation for Basiliximab.

SDZ-ENA-713. Code designation for Rivastigmine.

SDZ-HTF-919. Code designation for Tegaserod.

SE 1702. Code designation for Gliclazide.

SeHCAT. Code designation for Tauroselcholic Acid.

SERM 3. Code designation for Arzoxifene Hydrochloride.

SF 86-327. Code designation for Terbinafine.

SF328. Code designation for Dirucotide.

SF328. Code designation for Dirucotide Acetate.

SF-R11. Code designation for Bovactant.

SG-75. Code designation for Nicorandil.

SGD 301-76. Code designation for Oxiconazole Nitrate.

SGN-40. Code designation for Dacetuzumab.

SGP 3. Code designation for Unifocon A.

SH 2.1139/H 248 AB. Code designation for Ioxotrizoic Acid.

SH 3.1168. Code designation for Gliflumide.

SH 100. Code designation for Oxapium Iodide.

SH 213 AB. Code designation for Iotroxic Acid.

SH 240. Code designation for Moxnidazole.

SH 263. Code designation for Droxacin Sodium.

SH 567. Code designation for Methenolone Acetate.

SH 582. Code designation for Gestonorone Caproate.

SH 601. Code designation for Methenolone Enanthate.

SH 714. Code designation for Cyproterone Acetate.

SH 717. Code designation for Glymidine Sodium.

SH 723. Code designation for Mesterolone.

SH 741. Code designation for Clomegestone Acetate.

SH 742. Code designation for Fluocortolone.

SH 770. Code designation for Fluocortolone Caproate.

SH 818. Code designation for Clocortolone Acetate.

SH 863. Code designation for Clocortolone Pivalate.

SH 926. Code designation for Iodamide.

SH 968. Code designation for Diflucortolone Pivalate.

SH 1040. Code designation for Gestaclone.

SH 1051. Code designation for Glicetanile Sodium.

SH B 331. Code designation for Gestodene.

SH E 199. Code designation for Etoformin Hydrochloride.

SH G 318 AB. Code designation for Sermetacin.

SH H 200 AB. Code designation for Ioglicic Acid.

SH H 239 AB. Code designation for Ioseric Acid.

SH K 203. Code designation for Fluocortin Butyl.

SH L 451 *A*. Code designation for Gadopentetate Dimeglumine.

SIB-1508Y. Code designation for Altinicline Maleate.

siga-246. Code designation for Tecovirimat.

SJ 1977. Code designation for Methixene Hydrochloride.

SK&F 51. Code designation for Octodrine.

SK&F 478. Code designation for Diphenidol.

SK&F 478-A. Code designation for Diphenidol Hydrochloride.

SK&F 478-J. Code designation for Diphenidol Pamoate.

SK&F 525-A. Code designation for Proadifen Hydrochloride.

SK&F 1340. Code designation for Dimefadane.

SK&F 1995. Code designation for Dicloralurea.

SK&F 2208. Code designation for Hetaflur.

SKF 2599. Code designation for Doxenitoin.

SK&F 3050. Code designation for Cortodoxone.

SK&F 5116. Code designation for Methotrimeprazine.

SK&F 6539. Code designation for Flurothyl.

SK&F 7690. Code designation for Benorterone.

SK&F 7988. Code designation for Virginiamycin.

SKF-8318. Code designation for Xenazoic Acid.

SK&F 8542. Code designation for Triamterene.

SKF 8898-A. Code designation for Moroxydine.

SKF 9976 [as citrate]. Code designation for Oxolamine.

SK&F 12866. Code designation for Clorethate.

SKF 13338. Code designation for Ampyrimine.

SK&F 13364-A. Code designation for Thyromedan Hydrochloride.

SK&F 14287. Code designation for Idoxuridine.

SK&F 14336. Code designation for Clomacran Phosphate.

SK&F 15601A. Code designation for Toliodium Chloride.

SKF 16046. Code designation for Anisacril.

SK&F 18,667. Code designation for Poloxalene.

SKF 20716. Code designation for Periciazine.

SK&F 24529. Code designation for Lobendazole.

SK&F 28175. Code designation for Fluotracen Hydrochloride.

SK&F 29044. Code designation for Parbendazole.
SK&F 30310. Code designation for Oxibendazole.
SKF 33134-A. Code designation for Amiodarone.
SK&F 38094. Code designation for Dectaflur.
SK&F 38095. Code designation for Olaflur.
SK&F 39162. Code designation for Auranofin.
SK&F 39186. Code designation for Amicloral.
SK&F 40383. Code designation for Carbuterol Hydrochloride.
SK&F 41558. Code designation for Cefazolin Sodium.
SK&F 53705-A. Code designation for Sulfonterol Hydrochloride.
SK&F 59962. Code designation for Cefazaflur Sodium.
SK&F 61636. Code designation for Bromoxanide.
SK&F 62698. Code designation for Ticrynafen.
SK&F 62979. Code designation for Albendazole.
SK&F 63797. Code designation for Dribendazole.
SK&F 69634. Code designation for Clopipazan Mesylate.
SK&F 70230-A. Code designation for Pipazethate.
SK&F 72517. Code designation for Elfazepam.
SK&F 82526-J. Code designation for Fenoldopam Mesylate.
SK&F 88373-Z. Code designation for Ceftizoxime Sodium.
SK&F 92058. Code designation for Metiamide.
SK&F 92657-A$_2$. Code designation for Prizidilol Hydrochloride.
SK&F 92676-A$_3$. Code designation for Impromidine Hydro-
  chloride.
SK&F 92994-A$_2$. Code designation for Oxmetidine Hydro-
  chloride.
SK&F 92994-J$_2$. Code designation for Oxmetidine Mesylate.
SK&F 93319. Code designation for Icotidine.
SK&F 93479. Code designation for Lupitidine Hydrochloride.
SK&F 93574. Code designation for Donetidine.
SK&F 93944. Code designation for Temelastine.
SK&F 94836. Code designation for Siguazodan.
SK&F 95587. Code designation for Sulotroban.
SK&F 96022. Code designation for Pantoprazole.
SK&F 96148. Code designation for Daltroban.
SK&F 100814. Code designation for Ardacin.
SK&F 101468. Code designation for Ropinirole.
SK&F 101468-A. Code designation for Ropinirole Hydrochloride.
SK&F 102,362. Code designation for Nilvadipine.
SK&F 104353-Q. Code designation for Pobilukast Edamine.
SK&F-105517-D. Code designation for Carvedilol Phosphate.
SK&F 105657. Code designation for Epristeride.
SK&F 106615-A2. Code designation for Atiprimod Dihydrochlor-
  ide.
SKF-106615-A2. Code designation for Atiprimod Dihydrochlor-
  ide.
SK&F 106615-I2. Code designation for Atiprimod Dimaleate.
SK&F 107647. Code designation for Glaspimod.
SK&F 108566. Code designation for Eprosartan.
SK&F 108566-J. Code designation for Eprosartan Mesylate.
SK&F D-39304. Code designation for Cephradine.
SK&F D-75073-Z. Code designation for Cefonicid Monosodium.
SK&F D-75073-Z$_2$. Code designation for Cefonicid Sodium.
SK&F S-104864-A. Code designation for Topotecan Hydro-
  chloride.
SKI-606. Code designation for Bosutinib.
SL 75 177-10. Code designation for Cicloprolol Hydrochloride.
SL 75.212-10. Code designation for Betaxolol Hydrochloride.
SL 76 002. Code designation for Progabide.
SL 77 499-10. Code designation for Alfuzosin Hydrochloride.
SL 79.229-00. Code designation for Fengabine.
SL 80.0342-00. Code designation for Alpidem.
SL 80.0750-23N. Code designation for Zolpidem Tartrate.
SL 81.0142-00. Code designation for Tolgabide.
SL 501. Code designation for Chlophedianol Hydrochloride.
SLV 308. Code designation for Pardoprunox.
SLV 308 hydrochloride. Code designation for Pardoprunox Hydro-
  chloride.

SLV-319. Code designation for Ibipinabant.
SM-50C. Code designation for Lubazodone Hydrochloride.
SM-1213 (free base). Code designation for Amiprilose Hydro-
  chloride.
SM-3997. Code designation for Tandospirone Citrate.
SM-5887. Code designation for Amrubicin Hydrochloride.
SM-7338. Code designation for Meropenem.
SM-13496. Code designation for Lurasidone Hydrochloride.
SMP 68-40. Code designation for Pyrabrom.
SMP-78 Acid S. Code designation for Ambruticin.
Sms2PA. Code designation for Strontium Chloride Sr 89.
SMS-201-995. Code designation for Octreotide.
SMS 201-995 ac. Code designation for Octreotide Acetate.
SMS 201-995 pa. Code designation for Octreotide Pamoate.
SMS pa. Code designation for Octreotide Pamoate.
SMT 487. Code designation for Edotreotide.
S.N. 44. Code designation for Insulin, Dalanated.
SN-166 [as the sodium salt]. Code designation for Glucosulfone.
SN-263. Code designation for Sodium Amylosulfate.
SN 654. Code designation for Mepartricin.
SNAC. Code designation for Salcaprozate Sodium.
SND919CL2Y. Code designation for Pramipexole Dihydrochlor-
  ide.
SND-5008. Code designation for Cevimeline Hydrochloride.
SNDX-275. Code designation for Entinostat.
SnET2. Code designation for Rostaporfin.
SNI-2011. Code designation for Cevimeline Hydrochloride.
SNK-508. Code designation for Cevimeline Hydrochloride.
SNR 1804. Code designation for Clamidoxic Acid.
SNS-595. Code designation for Voreloxin.
SNX-111. Code designation for Ziconotide.
SP54. Code designation for Pentosan Polysulfate Sodium.
SP63. Code designation for Otilonium Bromide.
SP-106. Code designation for Nabitan Hydrochloride.
SP-119. Code designation for Tinabinol.
SP-175. Code designation for Nabazenil.
SP-204. Code designation for Menabitan Hydrochloride.
SP-303. Code designation for Crofelemer.
SP-304. Code designation for Pirnabine.
SP-325. Code designation for Naboctate Hydrochloride.
SP924. Code designation for Lestaurtinib.
SPA-S-132. Code designation for Partricin.
SPA-S-160. Code designation for Mepartricin.
SPA-S-510. Code designation for Piroxicam Cinnamate.
SPA-S-565. Code designation for Rifametane.
SPC 297 D. Code designation for Azidocillin.
SPC-100270. Code designation for Safingol.
SPC-100271. Code designation for Safingol Hydrochloride.
SPC-101210. Code designation for Cedefingol.
SPI-77. Code designation for Mitopodozide.
SPI-8811. Code designation for Cobiprostone.
SPM 907. Code designation for Fesoterodine Fumarate.
SPM 925. Code designation for Moexipril Hydrochloride.
SPM 927. Code designation for Lacosamide.
SPM 962. Code designation for Rotigotine.
SPM 8272. Code designation for Fesoterodine Fumarate.
SPP100. Code designation for Aliskiren.
SPP100. Code designation for Aliskiren Fumarate.
SQ 1089. Code designation for Hydroxyurea.
SQ 1489. Code designation for Thiram.
SQ 2128. Code designation for Ethoxazene Hydrochloride.
SQ-6201. Code designation for Uracil.
SQ-7726. Code designation for Uracil.
SQ-8493. Code designation for Uracil.
SQ 9343. Code designation for Phytate Sodium.
SQ 9453. Code designation for Dimethyl Sulfoxide.
SQ 9538. Code designation for Testolactone.
SQ 9993. Code designation for Estradiol Undecylate.

SQ 10,269. Code designation for Carbiphene Hydrochloride.
SQ 10,496. Code designation for Thiazesim Hydrochloride.
SQ 10,643. Code designation for Cinanserin Hydrochloride.
SQ 11,302. Code designation for Epicillin.
SQ 11436. Code designation for Cephradine.
SQ 11725. Code designation for Nadolol.
SQ 13050. Code designation for Econazole Nitrate.
SQ 13,396. Code designation for Iopamidol.
SQ 13847. Code designation for Pirquinozol.
SQ 14055. Code designation for Tiamulin.
SQ 14,225. Code designation for Captopril.
SQ 15,101. Code designation for Algestone Acetophenide.
SQ 15,102. Code designation for Amcinafal.
SQ 15,112. Code designation for Amcinafide.
SQ 15,659. Code designation for Rolitetracycline.
SQ 15,860. Code designation for Glyhexamide.
SQ 15,874. Code designation for Pipazethate.
SQ 16,123. Code designation for Methicillin Sodium.
SQ 16,150. Code designation for Estradiol Enanthate.
SQ 16360. Code designation for Fusidate Sodium.
SQ 16374. Code designation for Methenolone Enanthate.
SQ 16,401. Code designation for Halquinols.
SQ 16,423. Code designation for Oxacillin Sodium.
SQ 16496. Code designation for Methenolone Acetate.
SQ 16,603. Code designation for Fusidic Acid.
SQ 18566. Code designation for Halcinonide.
SQ 19844. Code designation for Sincalide.
SQ 20009. Code designation for Etazolate Hydrochloride.
SQ 20824. Code designation for Cicloprofen.
SQ 20881. Code designation for Teprotide.
SQ 21982. Code designation for Iodoxamic Acid.
SQ 21983. Code designation for Iopronic Acid.
SQ 22022 [dihydrate]. Code designation for Cephradine.
SQ 22947. Code designation for Tiamulin Fumarate.
SQ 26490. Code designation for Naflocort.
SQ 26,703. Code designation for Zofenoprilat Arginine.
SQ 26776. Code designation for Aztreonam.
SQ 26962. Code designation for Mebrofenin.
SQ 26991. Code designation for Zofenopril Calcium.
SQ 27,239. Code designation for Tipredane.
SQ 27,519. Code designation for Fosinoprilat.
SQ 28555. Code designation for Fosinopril Sodium.
SQ 29,852. Code designation for Ceronapril.
SQ 30217. Code designation for Technetium Tc 99m Teboroxime.
SQ 30836. Code designation for Tigemonam Dicholine.
SQ-31,000. Code designation for Pravastatin Sodium.
SQ 32,097. Code designation for Technetium Tc 99m Siboroxime.
SQ 32,692. Code designation for Gadoteridol.
SQ 32,756. Code designation for Sorivudine.
SQ 33,248. Code designation for Calteridol Calcium.
SQ 34,514. Code designation for Lobucavir.
SQ34676. Code designation for Entecavir.
SQ 65396. Code designation for Cartazolate.
SQ 82291. Code designation for Oximonam.
SQ 82531. Code designation for Gloximonam.
SQ 82629. Code designation for Oximonam Sodium.
SQ 83360. Code designation for Pirazmonam Sodium.
SR-202. Code designation for Mifobate.
SR 720-22. Code designation for Metolazone.
SR 2508. Code designation for Etanidazole.
SR-7037. Code designation for Belfosdil.
SR 25990C. Code designation for Clopidogrel Bisulfate.
SR29142. Code designation for Rasburicase.
SR 33557. Code designation for Fantofarone.
SR33598B. Code designation for Dronedarone Hydrochloride.
SR 41319. Code designation for Tiludronic Acid.
SR 41319B. Code designation for Tiludronate Disodium.
SR 47436. Code designation for Irbesartan.

SR 57746. Code designation for Xaliproden.
SR58611. Code designation for Amibegron.
SR58611A. Code designation for Amibegron Hydrochloride.
SR 90107A. Code designation for Fondaparinux Sodium.
SR 96225. Code designation for Adenosine.
SR-96669. Code designation for Oxaliplatin.
SR141716. Code designation for Rimonabant.
SRA-333. Code designation for Lecozotan Hydrochloride.
SRG 95213. Code designation for Diazoxide.
SS734. Code designation for Besifloxacin Hydrochloride.
ST12. Code designation for Dexamethasone Dipropionate.
ST-155. Code designation for Clonidine Hydrochloride.
ST-155-BS. Code designation for Clonidine.
ST 261. Code designation for Levocarnitine Propionate Hydro-
  chloride.
ST 375. Code designation for Tolonidine.
St 567-BR [as hydrobromide]. Code designation for Alinidine.
ST 600. Code designation for Flutonidine.
ST-813. Code designation for Oxiconazole Nitrate.
St 1085 [as the base]. Code designation for Midodrine Hydro-
  chloride.
St 1411. Code designation for Dimepregnen.
ST1512/SO4. Code designation for Hexoprenaline Sulfate.
ST 9067. Code designation for Azintamide.
St. Peter 224. Code designation for Midodrine Hydrochloride.
STA-307. Code designation for Tiomesterone.
STA-4783. Code designation for Elesclomol.
STA-5312. Code designation for Rosabulin.
STA-5326 mesylate. Code designation for Apilimod Mesylate.
sTNF-RI. Code designation for Pegsunercept.
STS 557. Code designation for Dienogest.
SU101. Code designation for Leflunomide.
Su-4885. Code designation for Metyrapone Tartrate.
SU5416. Code designation for Semaxanib.
Su-5864. Code designation for Guanethidine Sulfate.
Su-6518. Code designation for Dimethindene Maleate.
Su-8341. Code designation for Cyclopenthiazide.
Su-9064. Code designation for Metoserpate Hydrochloride.
SU010398. Code designation for Sunitinib Malate.
Su-10568. Code designation for Clortermine Hydrochloride.
SU011248 L-malate salt. Code designation for Sunitinib Malate.
Su-13437. Code designation for Nafenopin.
Su-18137. Code designation for Cyproquinate.
Su 21524. Code designation for Pirprofen.
SUM 3170. Code designation for Loxapine.
SUN-0588 (Shiratori). Code designation for Sapropterin Dihy-
  drochloride.
SUN 4936. Code designation for Carperitide.
SUN 9216. Code designation for Lanoteplase.
SUR 2647. Code designation for Sumacetamol.
SYD-230. Code designation for Clioxanide.
Synthetic TRH. Code designation for Protirelin.
SYR-322. Code designation for Alogliptin Benzoate.
T2G1s. Code designation for Biciromab.
T20. Code designation for Enfuvirtide.
T67. Code designation for Batabulin.
T-1220. Code designation for Piperacillin Sodium.
T1401 (BioMarin). Code designation for Sapropterin Dihy-
  drochloride.
T-1551. Code designation for Cefoperazone Sodium.
T-1982. Code designation for Cefbuperazone.
T-2636. Code designation for Sedecamycin.
T-2636A. Code designation for Sedecamycin.
T-3811ME. Code designation for Garenoxacin Mesylate.
T138067. Code designation for Batabulin.
T138067-sodium. Code designation for Batabulin Sodium.
T-168390. Code designation for Dexlansoprazole.
TA-1790. Code designation for Avanafil.

TA-3090. Code designation for Clentiazem Maleate.

TA 5901. Code designation for Cefempidone.

TACI-Fc5. Code designation for Atacicept.

TAK-165. Code designation for Mubritinib.

TAK-375. Code designation for Ramelteon.

TAK-390. Code designation for Dexlansoprazole.

TAK 475. Code designation for Lapaquistat Acetate.

TAK-491. Code designation for Azilsartan Kamedoxomil.

TAK-491. Code designation for Azilsartan Medoxomil.

TAK-536. Code designation for Azilsartan.

TAK 599. Code designation for Ceftaroline Fosamil.

TALL-1. Code designation for Ardenermin.

TAP 031 (as the base). Code designation for Fertirelin Acetate.

TAP-144. Code designation for Leuprolide Acetate.

TAT-3. Code designation for Picoperine.

TATBA. Code designation for Triamcinolone Hexacetonide.

TBC1269z. Code designation for Bimosiamose Disodium.

Tc 99m anti-SSEA-1. Code designation for Technetium Tc 99m Fanolesomab.

Tc99m RB5 IgM. Code designation for Technetium Tc 99m Fanolesomab.

Tc99m RP-30A. Code designation for Technetium Tc 99m Sestamibi.

Tc99m-MP 4006. Code designation for Technetium Tc 99m Albumin Aggregated.

Tc 924 (DPD). Code designation for Butedronate Tetrasodium.

TC-01734. Code designation for Ispronicline.

TC-02403-12. Code designation for Rivanicline Galactarate.

TCC. Code designation for Triclocarban.

Tc-MAG$_3$. Code designation for Technetium Tc 99m Mertiatide.

^{99m}TcN-NOET. Code designation for Technetium Tc 99m Nitridocade.

TCV-116. Code designation for Candesartan Cilexetil.

Td-6424. Code designation for Telavancin Hydrochloride.

TE-031. Code designation for Clarithromycin.

TE 114. Code designation for Tiemonium Iodide.

TEAB. Code designation for Tetrylammonium Bromide.

Tenite Butyrate Formula 264 H4. Code designation for Cabufocon B.

TER199. Code designation for Ezatiostat Hydrochloride.

TER286. Code designation for Canfosfamide Hydrochloride.

TG01. Code designation for Apricoxib.

αTGI. Code designation for Teroxirone.

Th-152. Code designation for Metaproterenol Sulfate.

Th 322. Code designation for Metrifudil.

TH 1165a [as hydrobromide salt]. Code designation for Fenoterol.

TH-1321. Code designation for Protionamide.

TH-2151. Code designation for Hydracarbazine.

TH-2180. Code designation for Propanidid.

TH9507. Code designation for Tesamorelin.

TH9507. Code designation for Tesamorelin Acetate.

THANK. Code designation for Ardenermin.

THFES (HM). Code designation for Zeranol.

THQ. Code designation for Tetroquinone.

THR. Code designation for Troxerutin.

THR 221 [as sodium]. Code designation for Cefodizime.

TL7. Code designation for Ardenermin.

TL 057. Code designation for Batabulin.

TLK199. Code designation for Ezatiostat Hydrochloride.

TLK286. Code designation for Canfosfamide Hydrochloride.

TMB-4. Code designation for Trimedoxime Bromide.

TMC 114. Code designation for Darunavir.

TMC 125. Code designation for Etravirine.

TMI-005. Code designation for Apratastat.

TMX-67. Code designation for Febuxostat.

TNF MAb. Code designation for Nerelimomab.

TNFSBF13B. Code designation for Ardenermin.

TNFSF20. Code designation for Ardenermin.

TNK-tPA. Code designation for Tenecteplase.

TNO-6. Code designation for Spiroplatin.

TNX-355. Code designation for Ibalizumab.

TNX-901. Code designation for Talizumab.

(S)-tofisopam. Code designation for Levotofisopam.

TP-5. Code designation for Thymopentin.

TP-21. Code designation for Thioridazine.

TP 508. Code designation for Rusalatide Acetate.

TPGS. Code designation for Tocophersolan.

TPN-12. Code designation for Sulforidazine.

TPS-23. Code designation for Mesoridazine.

TR-495. Code designation for Methaqualone.

TR-2378. Code designation for Broperamole.

TR-2515. Code designation for Pelanserin Hydrochloride.

TR-2855. Code designation for Cromitrile Sodium.

TR-2985. Code designation for Ropitoin Hydrochloride.

TR-3369. Code designation for Indorenate Hydrochloride.

TR-4698. Code designation for Rioprostil.

TR-4979. Code designation for Butaprost.

TR-5109. Code designation for Conorphone Hydrochloride.

TR-5379M. Code designation for Xorphanol Mesylate.

TRAIL-R1 mAb. Code designation for Mapatumumab.

TRAIL-R2 mAb. Code designation for Conatumumab.

Trans AMCHA. Code designation for Tranexamic Acid.

TRAP-508. Code designation for Rusalatide Acetate.

TRK-100. Code designation for Beraprost Sodium.

TRK-820. Code designation for Nalfurafine Hydrochloride.

TRM-1. Code designation for Mapatumumab.

TRX4. Code designation for Otelixizumab.

TS 408. Code designation for Hydrocortisone Probutate.

TSAA-291. Code designation for Oxendolone.

TTFD. Code designation for Fursultiamine.

TTI-237. Code designation for Cevipabulin Fumarate.

TTI-237. Code designation for Cevipabulin Succinate.

TV-1203. Code designation for Etilevodopa.

TV-1901. Code designation for Valrocemide.

TV-3326. Code designation for Ladostigil Tartrate.

TV-4710. Code designation for Edratide.

TV-5600. Code designation for Laquinimod Sodium.

TVP-1012. Code designation for Rasagiline Mesylate.

TVX485. Code designation for Etofenamate.

TWSB. Code designation for Sodium Stibocaptate.

TX 066. Code designation for Nomegestrol Acetate.

U-935. Code designation for Amiquinsin Hydrochloride.

U-2032. Code designation for Kethoxal.

U-4527. Code designation for Cycloheximide.

U-5956. Code designation for Filipin.

U-6013. Code designation for Isoflupredone Acetate.

U-6987. Code designation for Carbutamide.

U-7743. Code designation for Mercufenol Chloride.

U-7750. Code designation for Streptovarycin.

U-7800. Code designation for Fluprednisolone.

U-8344. Code designation for Uracil Mustard.

U-8471. Code designation for Medrysone.

U-9889. Code designation for Streptozocin.

U-10,136. Code designation for Alprostadil.

U-10,149. Code designation for Lincomycin.

U-10,858. Code designation for Minoxidil.

U-10,974. Code designation for Flumethasone.

U-10,997. Code designation for Mibolerone.

U-11100A. Code designation for Nafoxidine Hydrochloride.

U-12,019E. Code designation for Methylprednisolone Sodium Phosphate.

U-12,062. Code designation for Dinoprostone.

U-12,241. Code designation for Cirolemycin.

U-12898. Code designation for Bluensomycin.

U-13,933. Code designation for Asperlin.

U-14,583. Code designation for Dinoprost.

U-14,583E. Code designation for Dinoprost Tromethamine.

U-14,743. Code designation for Porfiromycin.

U-15167. Code designation for Nogalamycin.

U-15,614. Code designation for Trestolone Acetate.

U-15,965. Code designation for Lydimycin.

U-17312E. Code designation for Etryptamine Acetate.

U-17,323. Code designation for Fluorometholone Acetate.

U-17835. Code designation for Tolazamide.

U-18,409AE. Code designation for Spectinomycin Hydrochloride.

U-18,496. Code designation for Azacitidine.

U-18,573. Code designation for Ibuprofen.

U-18,573G. Code designation for Ibuprofen Aluminum.

U-19183. Code designation for Sparsomycin.

U-19,646. Code designation for Chlorphenesin Carbamate.

U-19,718. Code designation for Kalafungin.

U-19763. Code designation for Bolasterone.

U-19,920. Code designation for Cytarabine.

U-19920A. Code designation for Cytarabine Hydrochloride.

U-20,661. Code designation for Steffimycin.

U-21,251. Code designation for Clindamycin.

U-22020. Code designation for Indoxole.

U-22,550. Code designation for Calusterone.

U-22,559A. Code designation for Dexoxadrol Hydrochloride.

U-24,729A. Code designation for Mirincamycin Hydrochloride.

U-24,792. Code designation for Lomofungin.

U-24,973A. Code designation for Melitracen Hydrochloride.

U-25,179 E. Code designation for Clindamycin Palmitate Hydrochloride.

U-25,873. Code designation for Ranimycin.

U-26,225A. Code designation for Tramadol Hydrochloride.

U-26,452. Code designation for Glyburide.

U-27,182. Code designation for Flurbiprofen.

U-28,009. Code designation for Denofungin.

U-28,288D. Code designation for Guanadrel Sulfate.

U-28,508. Code designation for Clindamycin Phosphate.

U-28,774. Code designation for Ketazolam.

U-29,479. Code designation for Scopafungin.

U-30,604. Code designation for Zorbamycin.

U-31,889. Code designation for Alprazolam.

U-31,920. Code designation for Uldazepam.

U-32,070E. Code designation for Calcifediol.

U-32,921. Code designation for Carboprost.

U-32,921E. Code designation for Carboprost Tromethamine.

U-33,030. Code designation for Triazolam.

U-34,865. Code designation for Diflorasone Diacetate.

U-36,059. Code designation for Amitraz.

U-36,384. Code designation for Carboprost Methyl.

U-41,123. Code designation for Adinazolam.

U-41,123F. Code designation for Adinazolam Mesylate.

U-42,126. Code designation for Acivicin.

U-42,585E. Code designation for Lodoxamide Tromethamine.

U-42,718. Code designation for Lodoxamide Ethyl.

U 42,842. Code designation for Arbaprostil.

U-43,120. Code designation for Paulomycin.

U-46,785. Code designation for Meteneprost.

U-47,931E. Code designation for Bromadoline Maleate.

U-48,753E. Code designation for Eclanamine Maleate.

U-52,047. Code designation for Menogaril.

U-53,059. Code designation for Itazigrel.

U-53,217. Code designation for Epoprostenol.

U-53,217A. Code designation for Epoprostenol Sodium.

U-53,996H. Code designation for Tazadolene Succinate.

U-54,461. Code designation for Bropirimine.

U-54,555. Code designation for Metronidazole Phosphate.

U-54,669F. Code designation for Losulazine Hydrochloride.

U-56,321. Code designation for Timefurone.

U-57,930E. Code designation for Pirlimycin Hydrochloride.

U-60,257. Code designation for Piriprost.

U-60,257B. Code designation for Piriprost Potassium.

U-61,431F. Code designation for Ciprostene Calcium.

U-62066E. Code designation for Spiradoline Mesylate.

U-63,196. Code designation for Cefpimizole.

U-63,196E. Code designation for Cefpimizole Sodium.

U-63287. Code designation for Ciglitazone.

U-63,366F. Code designation for Trospectomycin Sulfate.

U-63,557A. Code designation for Furegrelate Sodium.

U-64279A. Code designation for Ceftiofur Hydrochloride.

U-64279E. Code designation for Ceftiofur Sodium.

U-66858. Code designation for Bunaprolast.

U-67,590A. Code designation for Methylprednisolone.

U-67,590A. Code designation for Methylprednisolone Suleptanate.

U-68,553B. Code designation for Alentemol Hydrobromide.

U-69689E. Code designation for Fertirelin Acetate.

U-70138. Code designation for Paldimycin.

U-70226E. Code designation for Ibutilide Fumarate.

U-71038. Code designation for Ditekiren.

U-72107A. Code designation for Pioglitazone Hydrochloride.

U-72791. Code designation for Cefmetazole.

U-72791A. Code designation for Cefmetazole Sodium.

U-73,975. Code designation for Adozelesin.

U-74006F. Code designation for Tirilazad Mesylate.

U-75630. Code designation for Ibuprofen Piconol.

U-76252. Code designation for Cefpodoxime Proxetil.

U-77,233. Code designation for Ormaplatin.

U-77779. Code designation for Bizelesin.

U-78875. Code designation for Panadiplon.

U-78,938. Code designation for Dexormaplatin.

U-80244. Code designation for Carzelesin.

U-82127. Code designation for Alexomycin.

U-85,855. Code designation for Alvircept Sudotox.

U-87201E. Code designation for Atevirdine Mesylate.

U-88943E. Code designation for Artilide Fumarate.

U-90152S. Code designation for Delavirdine Mesylate.

U-95376. Code designation for Premafloxacin.

U-98079A. Code designation for Itasetron.

U-98528E; SUD919CL2Y. Code designation for Pramipexole.

U-100,592. Code designation for Eperezolid.

U-100,766. Code designation for Linezolid.

U-101,440E. Code designation for Irinotecan Hydrochloride.

U-108342E. Code designation for Trecetilide Fumarate.

UCB 1402. Code designation for Decloxizine.

UCB 1474. Code designation for Chlorbenzoxamine Hydrochloride.

UCB 1549. Code designation for Minepentate.

UCB 1967. Code designation for Dropropizine.

UCB 2073. Code designation for Etoxeridine.

UCB 3928. Code designation for Fedrilate.

UCB 4445. Code designation for Buclizine Hydrochloride.

ucb 22059. Code designation for Levetiracetam.

UCB 28556. Code designation for Levocetirizine Dihydrochloride.

ucb 28754. Code designation for Efletirizine Dihydrochloride.

ucb 34714. Code designation for Brivaracetam.

ucb 44212. Code designation for Seletracetam.

ucb L059. Code designation for Levetiracetam.

UDCG-115. Code designation for Pimobendan.

UH-AC 62XX. Code designation for Meloxicam.

UK-738. Code designation for Ethybenztropine.

UK-2054. Code designation for Famotine Hydrochloride.

UK-2371. Code designation for Memotine Hydrochloride.

UK-3540-1. Code designation for Amedalin Hydrochloride.

UK-3557-15. Code designation for Daledalin Tosylate.

UK-4271. Code designation for Oxamniquine.

UK-11,443. Code designation for Primidolol.

UK-14304-18. Code designation for Brimonidine Tartrate.

UK-18,892. Code designation for Butikacin.

UK-20,349. Code designation for Tioconazole.
UK-25,842. Code designation for Oxfenicine.
UK-31,214. Code designation for Propikacin.
UK-31,557. Code designation for Carbazeran.
UK-33,274-27. Code designation for Doxazosin Mesylate.
UK-37,248-01. Code designation for Dazoxiben Hydrochloride.
UK-38,485. Code designation for Dazmegrel.
UK-48,340-11. Code designation for Amlodipine Maleate.
UK-48,340-26. Code designation for Amlodipine Besylate.
UK-49,858. Code designation for Fluconazole.
UK-61260-27. Code designation for Nanterinone.
UK-61,689. Code designation for Semduramicin.
UK-61,689-2. Code designation for Semduramicin Sodium.
UK-67,994. Code designation for Doramectin.
UK-68,798. Code designation for Dofetilide.
UK-73,967. Code designation for Candoxatrilat.
UK-76654-2 [as fumarate]. Code designation for Zamifenacin.
UK-79,300. Code designation for Candoxatril.
UK-80067. Code designation for Modipafant.
UK-81,252. Code designation for Sampatrilat.
UK-88060. Code designation for Espatropate.
UK-88525. Code designation for Darifenacin.
UK-88525-04 (hydrobromide). Code designation for Darifenacin Hydrobromide.
UK-92,480-10. Code designation for Sildenafil Citrate.
UK-109,496. Code designation for Voriconazole.
UK-112,166. Code designation for Revatropate.
UK-112,166-04 [as hydrobromide]. Code designation for Revatropate.
UK-116,044. Code designation for Eletriptan.
UK-116,044-04. Code designation for Eletriptan Hydrobromide.
UK-116,044-04 [as hydrobromide]. Code designation for Eletriptan.
UK-124,114. Code designation for Selamectin.
UK-287,074-02. Code designation for Cefovecin Sodium.
UK-292,663. Code designation for Fosfluconazole.
UK-338,003. Code designation for Taprizosin.
UM 952. Code designation for Buprenorphine Hydrochloride.
UP 74. Code designation for Nixylic Acid.
UP 83. Code designation for Niflumic Acid.
UP 106. Code designation for Propizepine.
UP 107. Code designation for Bepiastine.
UP 164. Code designation for Morniflumate.
UR-4056. Code designation for Flutrimazole.
UR-9825. Code designation for Albaconazole.
USV 3659-(S). Code designation for Pivopril.
UT-15. Code designation for Treprostinil.
V-C 13. Code designation for Dichlofenthion.
VEC-162. Code designation for Tasimelteon.
VEGF Trap. Code designation for Aflibercept.
VER001. Code designation for Dalbavancin.
VI-21,497. Code designation for Merimepodib.
VIT-45. Code designation for Ferric Carboxymaltose.
VK-57. Code designation for Glyprothiazol.
VM-26. Code designation for Teniposide.
VML 251. Code designation for Frovatriptan Succinate.
VNP40101M. Code designation for Laromustine.
VP-16-213. Code designation for Etoposide.
VP 63843. Code designation for Pleconaril.
VRT-111950. Code designation for Telaprevir.
VRX496. Code designation for Lexgenleucel-T.
VUAB6453 (SPOFA). Code designation for Metipranolol.
VX-478. Code designation for Amprenavir.
VX-497. Code designation for Merimepodib.
VX-680. Code designation for Tozasertib Lactate.
VX-710-3. Code designation for Biricodar Dicitrate.
VX-740. Code designation for Pralnacasan.
VX-853-2. Code designation for Timcodar Dimesylate.

VX-950. Code designation for Telaprevir.
W 37. Code designation for Buformin.
W-554. Code designation for Felbamate.
W-583. Code designation for Mebutamate.
W 713. Code designation for Tybamate.
W-1015. Code designation for Nisobamate.
W-1372. Code designation for Beloxamide.
W 1655. Code designation for Phenazopyridine Hydrochloride.
W 1760A. Code designation for Namoxyrate.
W 1929. Code designation for Colistimethate Sodium.
W 2180. Code designation for Suxemerid Sulfate.
W 2197. Code designation for Pentrinitrol.
W 2291A. Code designation for Mimbane Hydrochloride.
W-2354. Code designation for Seclazone.
W 2394A. Code designation for Pemerid Nitrate.
W-2395. Code designation for Meseclazone.
W 2426. Code designation for Chlorphentermine Hydrochloride.
W 2900A. Code designation for Etozolin.
W-2946M. Code designation for Reproterol Hydrochloride.
W-2964M. Code designation for Flupirtine Maleate.
W 2965 A. Code designation for Acetryptine.
W-2979M. Code designation for Azelastine Hydrochloride.
W 3207B. Code designation for Modaline Sulfate.
W 3366A. Code designation for Quindonium Bromide.
W3395. Code designation for Algestone Acetonide.
W 3399. Code designation for Quingestrone.
W 3566. Code designation for Quinestrol.
W 3580B. Code designation for Ampyzine Sulfate.
W 3623. Code designation for Cyprazepam.
W 3676. Code designation for Sulazepam.
W 3699. Code designation for Piprozolin.
W 3746. Code designation for Cetophenicol.
W 3976B. Code designation for Triampyzine Sulfate.
W 4020. Code designation for Prazepam.
W 4425. Code designation for Almadrate Sulfate.
W 4454A. Code designation for Estrazinol Hydrobromide.
W 4540. Code designation for Quingestanol Acetate.
W 4565. Code designation for Oxolinic Acid.
W 4600. Code designation for Algeldrate.
W 4701. Code designation for Hexedine.
W 4744. Code designation for Mecloqualone.
W 4869. Code designation for Prednival.
W-5219. Code designation for Proglumide.
W 5494A. Code designation for Naranol Hydrochloride.
W 5733. Code designation for Atolide.
W 5759A. Code designation for Tilidine Hydrochloride.
W 5975. Code designation for Betamethasone Benzoate.
W 6309. Code designation for Difluprednate.
W 6412A. Code designation for Bunolol Hydrochloride.
W 6439A. Code designation for Suloxifen Oxalate.
W 6495. Code designation for Oxisuran.
W 7000A. Code designation for Levobunolol Hydrochloride.
W 7320. Code designation for Alclofenac.
W7783. Code designation for Ambruticin.
W 8495. Code designation for Isoxicam.
W 10168. Code designation for Vifilcon A.
W-19053 [as hydrochloride]. Code designation for Etidocaine.
W-36095. Code designation for Tocainide.
W 42782. Code designation for Iproxamine Hydrochloride.
W 43026A. Code designation for Ciclafrine Hydrochloride.
WA 184. Code designation for Sitogluside.
W-A 335. Code designation for Danitracen.
WAL 2014 FU. Code designation for Talsaclidine Fumarate.
WAY-140424. Code designation for Bazedoxifene Acetate.
WAY 164339. Code designation for Torapsel.
WAY-207294. Code designation for Inotuzumab Ozogamicin.
WAY-362450. Code designation for Turofexorate Isopropyl.
WAY-ACA-147. Code designation for Eldacimibe.

WAY-ANA-756. Code designation for Tasosartan.

WAY-ARI-509. Code designation for Minalrestat.

WAY-CMA-676. Code designation for Gemtuzumab Ozogamicin.

WAY-GAR-936. Code designation for Tigecycline.

WAY-GPA-748. Code designation for Pralmorelin Dihydrochloride.

WAY-PDA-641. Code designation for Filaminast.

WAY-PEM-420. Code designation for Dexpemedolac.

WAY-SEC-579. Code designation for Mirisetron Maleate.

WAY-VPA-985. Code designation for Lixivaptan.

WE352. Code designation for Triflubazam.

We 941. Code designation for Brotizolam.

We 973-BS. Code designation for Ciclotizolam.

WEB 2086 BS. Code designation for Apafant.

WG-253. Code designation for Rimiterol Hydrobromide.

WG 537 [as acetate]. Code designation for Flumedroxone.

WH 5668. Code designation for Propanidid.

WHR-539. Code designation for Fenclorac.

WHR-1051B. Code designation for Biclodil Hydrochloride.

WHR-1142A. Code designation for Lidamidine Hydrochloride.

WHR-2908A. Code designation for Lofepramine Hydrochloride.

WHR-5020. Code designation for Etofenamate.

Win 771. Code designation for Hydroxypethidine.

Win 1344. Code designation for Gamfexine.

Win 1783. Code designation for Isomethadone.

Win 3406. Code designation for Isoetharine.

Win 5063. Code designation for Racephenicol.

Win 5063-2. Code designation for Thiamphenicol.

Win 5563-3. Code designation for Colterol Mesylate.

Win 8851-2. Code designation for Tyropanoate Sodium.

Win 9154. Code designation for Inositol Niacinate.

Win 9317. Code designation for Propatyl Nitrate.

Win 11,318. Code designation for Bupivacaine Hydrochloride.

Win 11450. Code designation for Benorilate.

Win 11,464. Code designation for Fludorex.

Win 11,530. Code designation for Menoctone.

Win 11831. Code designation for Lorajmine Hydrochloride.

Win 13,146. Code designation for Teclozan.

Win 13820. Code designation for Becanthone Hydrochloride.

Win 14833. Code designation for Stanozolol.

Win 17625. Code designation for Azastene.

Win 17665. Code designation for Topterone.

Win 17,757. Code designation for Danazol.

Win 18,320. Code designation for Nalidixic Acid.

Win 18,320-3. Code designation for Nalidixate Sodium.

Win 18,413-2. Code designation for Solypertine Tartrate.

Win 18,501-2. Code designation for Oxypertine.

Win 18,935. Code designation for Milipertine.

Win 19356. Code designation for Clorindanic Acid.

Win 20,228. Code designation for Pentazocine.

Win 20,740. Code designation for Cyclazocine.

Win 21,904. Code designation for Alexidine.

WIN 22118. Code designation for Pegorgotein.

Win 23,200. Code designation for Volazocine.

Win 24,540. Code designation for Trilostane.

Win 24,933. Code designation for Hycanthone.

Win 25,347. Code designation for Nimazone.

Win 25,978. Code designation for Amfonelic Acid.

Win 27147-2. Code designation for Cyclindole.

Win 27,914. Code designation for Nivazol.

Win 29194-6. Code designation for Carbantel Lauryl Sulfate.

Win 31,665. Code designation for Alpertine.

Win 32,729. Code designation for Epostane.

Win 32,784. Code designation for Bitolterol Mesylate.

Win 34,276. Code designation for Ketazocine.

Win 34284. Code designation for Oxarbazole.

Win 34886. Code designation for Nisbuterol Mesylate.

Win 35150. Code designation for Flucindole.

Win 35,213. Code designation for Rosoxacin.

Win 35833. Code designation for Ciprofibrate.

Win 38020. Code designation for Arildone.

Win 38770. Code designation for Azarole.

Win 39103. Code designation for Metrizamide.

Win 39424. Code designation for Iohexol.

Win 40014. Code designation for Quinfamide.

Win 40350. Code designation for Durapatite.

Win 40680. Code designation for Inamrinone.

Win 40808-7. Code designation for Sulfinalol Hydrochloride.

Win 41464-2. Code designation for Octenidine Hydrochloride.

Win 41,464-6. Code designation for Octenidine Saccharin.

Win 41528-2. Code designation for Fezolamine Fumarate.

Win 42156-2. Code designation for Tonazocine Mesylate.

Win 42,202. Code designation for Fosarilate.

Win 42964-4. Code designation for Zenazocine Mesylate.

Win 44,441-3. Code designation for Quadazocine Mesylate.

Win 47,203-2. Code designation for Milrinone.

Win 48,049. Code designation for Ofornine.

Win 48,098-6. Code designation for Pravadoline Maleate.

Win 49,016. Code designation for Medorinone.

Win 49,375. Code designation for Amifloxacin.

Win 49,375-3. Code designation for Amifloxacin Mesylate.

Win 49,596. Code designation for Zanoterone.

Win 51,181-2. Code designation for Napamezole Hydrochloride.

Win 51,711. Code designation for Disoxaril.

WIN 52,172-2. Code designation for Pirtenidine Hydrochloride.

Win 54,177-4. Code designation for Ipazilide Fumarate.

WIN 59010. Code designation for Mangafodipir Trisodium.

WIN 59075. Code designation for Tirapazamine.

WIN 63843. Code designation for Pleconaril.

Win 90,000. Code designation for Cicletanine.

Wl 140. Code designation for Calcium Polycarbophil.

Wl 287. Code designation for Euprocin Hydrochloride.

Wl 291. Code designation for Zolamine Hydrochloride.

WP744. Code designation for Berubicin Hydrochloride.

WP-973. Code designation for Chlorhexidine Phosphanilate.

WQ-3034. Code designation for Delafloxacin.

WQ-3034. Code designation for Delafloxacin Meglumine.

WR-2721. Code designation for Amifostine.

WR 6026. Code designation for Sitamaquine.

WR 142,490. Code designation for Mefloquine.

WR-171669. Code designation for Halofantrine Hydrochloride.

WR 180,409. Code designation for Enpiroline Phosphate.

WR-228,258. Code designation for Tebuquine.

WR 238605. Code designation for Tafenoquine.

WV 569 [as hydrochloride]. Code designation for Norfenefrine.

WX 2412. Code designation for Fungimycin.

WX 14812. Code designation for Alofilcon A.

WX 14822. Code designation for Hydrofilcon A.

WY-460E. Code designation for Thiazinamium Chloride.

Wy-806. Code designation for Oxethazaine.

Wy-1359. Code designation for Propiomazine.

Wy-2039. Code designation for Etoxeridine.

Wy-2445. Code designation for Carphenazine Maleate.

Wy-2837. Code designation for Potassium Aspartate and Magnesium Aspartate.

Wy-2838. Code designation for Potassium Aspartate and Magnesium Aspartate.

Wy-3263. Code designation for Iprindole.

Wy-3277. Code designation for Nafcillin Sodium.

Wy-3467. Code designation for Diazepam.

Wy-3475. Code designation for Norbolethone.

Wy-3478. Code designation for Sodium Oxybate.

Wy-3498. Code designation for Oxazepam.

Wy-3707. Code designation for Norgestrel.

Wy-3917. Code designation for Temazepam.

Wy-4036. Code designation for Lorazepam.

WY-4082. Code designation for Lormetazepam.

Wy-4508. Code designation for Cyclacillin.

WY-5104. Code designation for Levonorgestrel.

Wy-8138. Code designation for Bisoxatin Acetate.

Wy-8678. Code designation for Guanabenz.

WY-8678 acetate. Code designation for Guanabenz Acetate.

WY-15,705. Code designation for Ciramadol.

WY-15,705 HCl. Code designation for Ciramadol Hydrochloride.

WY-16,225. Code designation for Dezocine.

WY-18,251. Code designation for Tilomisole.

WY-20,788. Code designation for Penamecillin.

WY-21,743. Code designation for Oxaprozin.

WY-21,894. Code designation for Fentiazac.

Wy 21901. Code designation for Indoramin.

WY-21,901 HCl. Code designation for Indoramin Hydrochloride.

WY 22811 HCl. Code designation for Meptazinol Hydrochloride.

WY-23,409. Code designation for Ciclazindol.

WY-24,081 HCl. Code designation for Tiquinamide Hydrochloride.

WY-24,377. Code designation for Isotiquimide.

WY-25,021. Code designation for Rolgamidine.

WY-40,972. Code designation for Lutrelin Acetate.

WY-42,362 HCl. Code designation for Recainam Hydrochloride.

WY-42,362 tosylate. Code designation for Recainam Tosylate.

WY-44,417 sodium. Code designation for Apalcillin Sodium.

WY-44,635. Code designation for Cefpiramide.

WY-44,635 sodium. Code designation for Cefpiramide Sodium.

WY-45,030. Code designation for Venlafaxine Hydrochloride.

Wy-45233. Code designation for Desvenlafaxine Succinate.

WY-47384. Code designation for Gevotroline Hydrochloride.

WY-47,663 acetate. Code designation for Anaritide Acetate.

WY-47791 HCl. Code designation for Carvotroline Hydrochloride.

WY-47846HCl. Code designation for Zalospirone Hydrochloride.

WY-48252. Code designation for Ritolukast.

Wy-48314. Code designation for Lexithromycin.

WY-48624. Code designation for Enciprazine Hydrochloride.

WY-48986. Code designation for Risotilide Hydrochloride.

WY-50324 HCl. Code designation for Adatanserin Hydrochloride.

WY-090217. Code designation for Sirolimus.

WY-90493 RD. Code designation for Ardeparin Sodium.

X-1497. Code designation for Methicillin Sodium.

XA41. Code designation for Latanoprost.

XDE-105. Code designation for Spinosad.

XI-921. Code designation for Iron Sucrose.

XL119. Code designation for Becatecarin.

XLG. Code designation for Polyglactin 910.

XM-72. Code designation for Polybutester.

XP03. Code designation for Levomepromazine.

XP13512. Code designation for Gabapentin Enacarbil.

XP19986. Code designation for Arbaclofen Placarbil.

XR9576. Code designation for Tariquidar.

XU 62-320. Code designation for Fluvastatin Sodium.

XZ-450. Code designation for Azithromycin.

Y 3642. Code designation for Tinoridine.

Y 4153 [as hydrochloride]. Code designation for Clocapramine.

Y 6124 [as hydrochloride]. Code designation for Bufetolol.

YC-93. Code designation for Nicardipine Hydrochloride.

^{90}Y-DOTA-hLL2. Code designation for Yttrium Y 90 Epratuzumab Tetraxetan.

^{90}Y-DOTA-hMN14. Code designation for Yttrium Y 90 Labetuzumab Tetraxetan.

YH1885. Code designation for Revaprazan Hydrochloride.

[90]Y-hLL2. Code designation for Yttrium Y 90 Epratuzumab.

[90]Y-hMN-14. Code designation for Yttrium Y 90 Labetuzumab.

YKP-509. Code designation for Carisbamate.

YM087. Code designation for Conivaptan Hydrochloride.

YM337. Code designation for Tadocizumab.

YM443. Code designation for Acotiamide Hydrochloride.

YM617. Code designation for Tamsulosin Hydrochloride.

YM872. Code designation for Zonampanel.

YM905. Code designation for Solifenacin Succinate.

YM992. Code designation for Lubazodone Hydrochloride.

YM-08316. Code designation for Formoterol Fumarate.

YM-09330. Code designation for Cefotetan Disodium.

YM-12617-1. Code designation for Tamsulosin Hydrochloride.

YM-35992. Code designation for Lubazodone Hydrochloride.

YM-67905. Code designation for Solifenacin Succinate.

YM67905. Code designation for Solifenacin Succinate.

YN-72. Code designation for Sorivudine.

YTR-830H. Code designation for Tazobactam.

YZ-817. Code designation for Dexelvucitabine.

Z 326. Code designation for Fentonium Bromide.

Z-338. Code designation for Acotiamide Hydrochloride.

Z 424. Code designation for Viminol.

Z 1282. Code designation for Fosfomycin Tromethamine.

Z-4828. Code designation for Trofosfamide.

Z4942. Code designation for Ifosfamide.

Z 6000. Code designation for Troxerutin.

ZAL-846. Code designation for Zaleplon.

ZCE025. Code designation for Indium In 111 Altumomab Pentetate.

ZD0473. Code designation for Picoplatin.

ZD1033. Code designation for Anastrozole.

ZD1694. Code designation for Raltitrexed.

ZD1839. Code designation for Gefitinib.

ZD2079. Code designation for Talibegron Hydrochloride.

ZD4054. Code designation for Zibotentan.

ZD4522 (calcium salt). Code designation for Rosuvastatin Calcium.

ZD5077. Code designation for Quetiapine Fumarate.

ZD6474. Code designation for Vandetanib.

ZD9238. Code designation for Fulvestrant.

ZD9331. Code designation for Plevitrexed.

ZIO-101. Code designation for Darinaparsin.

ZIO-201. Code designation for Palifosfamide.

ZIO-301. Code designation for Indibulin.

ZK 10 720. Code designation for Ioprocemic Acid.

ZK 39 482. Code designation for Iotrolan.

ZK 57 671. Code designation for Sulprostone.

ZK 62 711. Code designation for Rolipram.

ZK 71 630. Code designation for Iotetric Acid.

ZK 76 604. Code designation for Pirazolac.

ZK 79 112. Code designation for Iotasul.

ZK 30595. Code designation for Drospirenone.

ZK 35760. Code designation for Iopromide.

ZK 00036374. Code designation for Iloprost.

ZK 37659. Code designation for Dienogest.

ZK 62498. Code designation for Azelaic Acid.

ZK 00091106. Code designation for Clodronate Disodium.

ZK 132281. Code designation for Ferucarbotran.

ZK 139834. Code designation for Gadoxetate Disodium.

ZK 156942. Code designation for Tisocalcitate.

ZK 230211. Code designation for Lonaprisan.

ZK 807834. Code designation for Fidexaban.

ZM 204,636. Code designation for Quetiapine Fumarate.

(S)-Zopiclone. Code designation for Eszopiclone.

ZP-123 (Zealand). Code designation for Rotigaptide.

zTNF4. Code designation for Ardenermin.

ZYC101a. Code designation for Amolimogene Bepiplasmid.

14115700. Code designation for Aclidinium Bromide.

2-5410-3A. Code designation for Iodixanol.

2-HMHBG. Code designation for Omaciclovir.

2-PAM. Code designation for Pralidoxime Chloride.

2-PAM Chloride. Code designation for Pralidoxime Chloride.

3-01003. Code designation for Guanoxan Sulfate.

3-01029. Code designation for Guanoclor Sulfate.

3 MS. Code designation for Hydroxytoluic Acid.
4A65. Code designation for Imidocarb Hydrochloride.
4-C-32. Code designation for Ticlopidine Hydrochloride.
4-CNAB. Code designation for Salclobuzate Sodium.
4-HC. Code designation for Perfosfamide.
4-MP. Code designation for Fomepizole.
4-OHT. Code designation for Afimoxifene.
5-1 Ukima 5 Chome. Code designation for Mitemcinal Fumarate.
5-azacytosine arabinoside. Code designation for Fazarabine.
5-FU. Code designation for Fluorouracil.
5IUDR. Code designation for Idoxuridine.
8-Cl-cAMP. Code designation for Tocladesine.
10 80 07. Code designation for Omoconazole Nitrate.
12C. Code designation for Velaresol.
15AU81. Code designation for Treprostinil.
17-AAG. Code designation for Tanespimycin.
17-DMAG.HCl. Code designation for Alvespimycin Hydro-
    chloride.
22-708. Code designation for Endralazine Mesylate.
26P. Code designation for Aliflurane.
27-400. Code designation for Cyclosporine.
32-046. Code designation for Edetate Dipotassium.
36-801. Code designation for Etifoxine.
37 162 R.P. Code designation for Suproclone.
40 045. Code designation for Articaine.
40 045. Code designation for Articaine Hydrochloride.
41-123. Code designation for Clazolam.
41 982 RP. Code designation for Pefloxacin Mesylate.
42-348. Code designation for Lifibrate.
42-548. Code designation for Mazindol.
43-663. Code designation for Guanoxabenz.
43-715. Code designation for Proquazone.
46-790. Code designation for Fluproquazone.
46 R.P. Code designation for Benzylsulfamide.
47-210 [as sodium]. Code designation for Tetriprofen.
48-674. Code designation for Furacrinic Acid.
51W89. Code designation for Cisatracurium Besylate.
53-32C. Code designation for Ticlopidine Hydrochloride.
57C65. Code designation for Cloguanamil.
65-318. Code designation for Bidimazium Iodide.
66-269. Code designation for Pretamazium Iodide.
79 T61. Code designation for Lucanthone Hydrochloride.
88BV59H21-2V67-66. Code designation for Votumumab.
101M. Code designation for Laromustine.
115-8543 Japan. Code designation for Mitemcinal Fumarate.
125 I NM-113. Code designation for Iomethin I 125.
129Y83. Code designation for Colfosceril Palmitate.
131 I NM-113. Code designation for Iomethin I 131.
141W94. Code designation for Amprenavir.
177 J.D. Code designation for Aminocaproic Acid.
194-B. Code designation for Zolamine Hydrochloride.
205 E. Code designation for Calcium Dobesilate.
249-16. Code designation for Deditonium Bromide.
256U87 hydrochloride. Code designation for Valacyclovir Hydro-
    chloride.
311C90. Code designation for Zolmitriptan.
336U50. Code designation for Proguanil Hydrochloride.
349 C59. Code designation for Moxipraquine.
403. Code designation for Imisopasem Manganese.
506U. Code designation for Nelarabine.
506U. Code designation for Nelzarabine.
516 MD. Code designation for Cinnarizine.
524W91. Code designation for Emtricitabine.
566C. Code designation for Atovaquone.
566C80. Code designation for Atovaquone.
589C. Code designation for Tucaresol.
611 C 65. Code designation for Thenium Closylate.
619C89. Code designation for Sipatrigine.

640/1. Code designation for Cefuracetime.
640/359. Code designation for Cefuroxime.
673-082. Code designation for Nexeridine Hydrochloride.
711 SE. Code designation for Pipratecol.
776C85. Code designation for Eniluracil.
786-723. Code designation for Anilopam Hydrochloride.
851A. Code designation for Epetirimod.
851B. Code designation for Epetirimod Esylate.
882C87. Code designation for Netivudine.
935U83. Code designation for Raluridine.
1263W94. Code designation for Maribavir.
1314 TH. Code designation for Ethionamide.
1380U. Code designation for Baquiloprim.
1589 RB. Code designation for Pefloxacin.
1592U89. Code designation for Abacavir Succinate.
1592U89. Code designation for Abacavir Sulfate.
1709 CERM. Code designation for Niaprazine.
1875 CERM. Code designation for Fepromide.
2936. Code designation for Proscillaridin.
3123L. Code designation for Puromycin.
4091 C.B. Code designation for Benfurodil Hemisuccinate.
4306 CB. Code designation for Clorazepate Dipotassium.
4311 CB. Code designation for Clorazepate Monopotassium.
4909 RP. Code designation for Chlorproethazine Hydrochloride.
5048. Code designation for Dimethisterone.
5052. Code designation for Acetylcysteine.
5054. Code designation for Prodilidine Hydrochloride.
5058. Code designation for Oxybutynin Chloride.
5071. Code designation for Megestrol Acetate.
5107. Code designation for Chloral Betaine.
5190. Code designation for Amidephrine Mesylate.
5373. Code designation for Melengestrol Acetate.
6366A. Code designation for Imidaprilat.
7162 RP. Code designation for Trimipramine.
7432-S. Code designation for Ceftibuten.
8088 C.B. Code designation for Benfotiamine.
8102 CB. Code designation for Bamifylline Hydrochloride.
8599 R.P. mesylate. Code designation for Fonazine Mesylate.
10275-S. Code designation for Epitiostanol.
16726. Code designation for Symetine Hydrochloride.
16842. Code designation for Bitoscanate.
18894. Code designation for Nifungin.
20025. Code designation for Clorprenaline Hydrochloride.
21401-Ba. Code designation for Tribenoside.
21679-CH. Code designation for Malethamer.
24281. Code designation for Mitocarcin.
26383. Code designation for Thiphencillin Potassium.
27165. Code designation for Temefos.
28002. Code designation for Epipropidine.
29060-LE. Code designation for Vinblastine Sulfate.
29866. Code designation for Levopropoxyphene Napsylate.
30038CB. Code designation for Minaprine Hydrochloride.
30109. Code designation for Noracymethadol Hydrochloride.
30639. Code designation for Polyethadene.
31518. Code designation for Pyrroliphene Hydrochloride.
31595C. Code designation for Mitosper.
31814. Code designation for Heteronium Bromide.
32379. Code designation for Dromostanolone Propionate.
32645. Code designation for Vinleurosine Sulfate.
33006. Code designation for Acetohexamide.
33355. Code designation for Mestranol.
33379. Code designation for Flurandrenolide.
33876. Code designation for Anthelmycin.
34977. Code designation for Capreomycin Sulfate.
35483. Code designation for Cyclothiazide.
36781. Code designation for Vinrosidine Sulfate.
37231. Code designation for Vincristine Sulfate.
38000. Code designation for Clometherone.

38253. Code designation for Cephalothin Sodium.
38389. Code designation for Levopropylcillin Potassium.
38489. Code designation for Nortriptyline Hydrochloride.
38851. Code designation for Bolmantalate.
39435. Code designation for Cephaloglycin.
40045. Code designation for Trimetazidine.
40602. Code designation for Cephaloridine.
41071. Code designation for Cefalonium.
42406. Code designation for Metoquizine.
43853. Code designation for Clobenoside.
44089. Code designation for Valproic Acid.
44106. Code designation for Toquizine.
44328. Code designation for Dexproxibutene.
46083. Code designation for Cefazolin Sodium.
46236. Code designation for Dobutamine Hydrochloride.
47599. Code designation for Pyrazofurin.
47657. Code designation for Apramycin.
47663. Code designation for Tobramycin.
49040. Code designation for Vinglycinate Sulfate.
49825. Code designation for Nylestriol.

52230. Code designation for Pyrrolnitrin.
53183. Code designation for Aranotin.
53858. Code designation for Fenoprofen.
59156. Code designation for Enpromate.
60231/4. Code designation for Rufinamide.
60284. Code designation for Cyclophenazine Hydrochloride.
64716. Code designation for Cinoxacin.
66873. Code designation for Cephalexin.
67314. Code designation for Monensin.
68618. Code designation for Mycophenolic Acid.
69323. Code designation for Fenoprofen Calcium.
79907. Code designation for Lergotrile.
80066. Code designation for Bufilcon A.
83636. Code designation for Lergotrile Mesylate.
106223. Code designation for Cefamandole Nafate.
110264. Code designation for Cefaparole.
177501. Code designation for Clodronate Disodium.
1001277. Code designation for Bismuth Subcitrate Potassium.

Appendix V
UNII Codes for USAN and Other Nonproprietary Names

000F949089. Spirofylline

000TKM5BBQ. Ablukast

001L2FE0M3. Alvespimycin Hydrochloride [alvespimycin] (See also *612K359T69*)

0020414E5U. Minocycline Hydrochloride

0035H8M4YL. Heptaverine

003N66TS6T. Rasagiline Mesylate [rasagiline] (See also *LH8C2JI290*)

004T8726AU. Dexindoprofen

005MIM19QV. Quinezamide

005MKH0F6D. Proxifezone

005SYP50G5. Neostigmine Bromide (See also *3982TWQ96G*)

00DPD30SOY. Amsacrine

00EED65INL. Ancarolol

00FN6IH15D. Nortriptyline Hydrochloride (See also *BL03SY4LXB*)

00I7BI3BB7. Darsidomine

00IBG87IQW. Sermorelin Acetate (See also *89243S03TE*)

00JM91Q28F. Difemerine Hydrochloride

00L331RFEC. Batanopride Hydrochloride

00OT1QX5U4. Potassium Permanganate

00S0D0OEKR. Itasetron

00S42N58OM. Methapyrilene Hydrochloride

00T9G32ZVH. Closiramine Aceturate [closiramine]

00U7GX0NLM. Minaprine

00U7GX0NLM. Minaprine Hydrochloride [minaprine] (See also *82Y7NT6DFT*)

00V69U1QC7. Metioxate

012C11ZU6G. Terbinafine [terbinafine hydrochloride] (See also *G7RIW8S0XP*)

012LYD6KXM. Ambasilide

0163PVD2QZ. Hydroxystilbamidine Isethionate (See also *39J262E49W*)

01704YP3MO. Aminopyrine

0180PBK4FC. Nifuraldezone

018XNU6812. Alrestatin Sodium (See also *515DHK15LG*)

0199MV609F. Gadoteridol

01DZ4127G7. Belotecan Hydrochloride (See also *27Z82M2G1N*)

01J18G9G97. Aceglutamide Aluminum [aceglutamide] (See also *R7QTG0PMPX*)

01K63SUP8D. Fluoxetine

01L3E93T4C. Clometherone

01MI4Q9DI3. Pilocarpine

01MI4Q9DI3. Pilocarpine Nitrate [pilocarpine]

01Q9PC255D. Ammonium Chloride

01T23W89FR. Thiamylal

01YAE03M7J. Beta Carotene

021SEF3731. Albuterol Sulfate (See also *QF8SVZ843E*)

0223RD59PE. Remoxipride

022N12KJ0X. Oxibendazole

023C2WHX2V. Tromethamine

023D9E916L. Panamesine

023Z5BR09K. Ceftriaxone Sodium (See also *75J73V1629*)

0255AHR9GJ. Alminoprofen

025P9I542Y. Cyanocobalamin Co 57

02B8S6J90B. Mabuprofen

02DQX562CR. Mitoclomine

02F3473H9O. Magnesium Chloride (See also *59XN63C8VM*)

02L083W284. Ganciclovir Sodium (See also *P9G3CKZ4P5*)

02MNR4P2PM. Cianopramine

02N1TZF99F. Tolmetin Sodium

02NKI0ARRJ. Nupafant

02O55696WH. Carbinoxamine Maleate (See also *982A7M02H5*)

02OS7K758T. Metharbital

030PYR8953. Ropinirole

030Y90569U. Nebivolol

032WJR708Q. Botiacrine

033KF7V46H. Tinidazole

0343IGH41U. Tositumomab

0354RT7LG4. Buparvaquone

0374EZJ8CU. Clinofibrate

037S03TJ5M. Tinisulpride

0388G963HY. Hydrocortisone Sodium Phosphate

039G8U30HE. Fludazonium Chloride

039LU44I5M. Floxuridine

03CPZ5439O. Thihexinol Methylbromide

03DB58Y9DO. Betoxycaine Hydrochloride [betoxycaine] (See also *8II47759Z3*)

03F36JH21U. Etofamide

03F6B8N3QN. Cotarnine Chloride

03HN50ZAF0. Guanoxyfen Sulfate [guanoxyfen] (See also *47XBA61Y31*)

03J11K103C. Algeldrate

03J5ZE7KA5. Atropine Sulfate (See also *7C0697DR9I*)

03N9U5JAF6. Atipamezole

03NR868ICX. Amezinium Metilsulfate

03QB156W6I. Temocillin

03V657ZD3V. Methacholine Bromide [methacholine]

03V657ZD3V. Methacholine Chloride [methacholine] (See also *0W5ETF9M2K*)

04079A1RDZ. Cytarabine

04079A1RDZ. Cytarabine Hydrochloride [cytarabine] (See also *33K3DB6591*)

0414BW860U. Prifelone

04201GDN4R. Mometasone Furoate

042LAQ1IIS. Irinotecan Hydrochloride (See also *7673326042*)

043L86G83X. Edifolone Acetate (See also *4XE0U1P5FJ*)

045BU63E23. Ipronidazole

046O35D44R. Prilocaine

0475EA27Q3. Benzquinamide

0481JCC90T. Pibrozelesin Hydrobromide

048L81261F. Dexrazoxane

048UJ2MM65. Besulpamide

04B949KO6F. Denbufylline

04D148Z3VR. Aplaviroc Hydrochloride

04HCK0SD2O. Midazogrel

04JA59TNSJ. Phenylephrine Hydrochloride

04O7H69C4B. Sermetacin

04Q9AIZ7NO. Pemetrexed Disodium [pemetrexed] (See also *2PKU919BA9*)

04UZQ7O9SJ. Mosapramine

04WQU6T9QI. Levorphanol Tartrate (See also *27618J1N2X*)

04X6A188YW. Cypothrin

04XPW8C0FL. Aprotinin

04Y7590D77. Isoleucine

04Z20NMK31. Acedoben

04ZR38536J. Oxaliplatin
05186J17EP. Diclometide
0543W2JFRZ. Cariporide Mesylate
0578K3ELIO. Aceclidine
057SF9C1UZ. Bervastatin
057Y626693. Neomycin Sulfate (See also *I16QD7X297*)
05835HKX9S. Triampyzine Sulfate
059NUO2Z1L. Homidium Bromide
05G07285DK. Tasidotin Hydrochloride [tasidotin]
05KO5G76R2. Enfenamic Acid
05PB82Z52L. Repinotan
05RMF7YPWN. Hydrocortisone Butyrate
05TAA9I0Z8. Laidlomycin Propionate Potassium
05V02F2KDG. Rosiglitazone Maleate [rosiglitazone] (See also
   KX2339DP44)
05V5NVB5Y1. Flopropione
0600L2M6EZ. Phenampromide
060B6580LL. Iodoalphionic Acid
0619F35CGV. Tetracaine
063D2YI19E. Pumafentrine
065F7WPT0B. Forasartan
066975NG22. Dymanthine Hydrochloride [dymanthine] (See also
   JAD662Q3U7)
0678G6Q58A. Calusterone
068X84E056. Pramoxine Hydrochloride [pramoxine] (See also
   88AYB867L5)
06H9KWB6IB. Sitalidone
06KB629TKV. Tolnaftate
06LU7C9H1V. Liothyronine I 125 [liothyronine] (See also
   S1UAI9MKMG)
06LU7C9H1V. Liothyronine I 131 [liothyronine] (See also
   86AZ0G22V2)
06LU7C9H1V. Liothyronine Sodium [liothyronine] (See also
   GCA9VV7D2N)
06Q0V17SI9. Mitonafide
06XEA2VD56. Sorbitan Monooleate
06YTS68E0H. Delfaprazine
071P4J77HF. Clofexamide
0745KNO26J. Aspoxicillin
0757XV4DZR. Triclodazol
076WHW89TW. Follitropin Alfa
076WHW89TW. Follitropin Beta
0789652QUL. Mivotilate
078A24Q30O. Dyclonine Hydrochloride [dyclonine] (See also
   ZEC193879Q)
079X63S3DU. Cambendazole
07CJN646IN. Nofecainide
07H1561618. Ibrolipim
0813BZ6866. Clodronic Acid
08331R10RY. Mofegiline Hydrochloride
08379P260O. Tipelukast
08703R750L. Enoxamast
0871JY946G. Xibenolol
08760H16R0. Metyridine
088W05943X. Detiviciclovir
08AHL2YV5K. Panidazole
08AN7WA2G0. Triptorelin Pamoate
08GY9K1EUO. Rasburicase
08I79HTP27. Clopidogrel Bisulfate (See also *A74586SNO7*)
08IT6P8VHY. Cetraxate Hydrochloride
08J2K08A3Y. Stanolone
08K838NNTE. Aptocaine
08KL644731. Ethyl Biscoumacetate
08R5U8PYVO. Ipsapirone Hydrochloride (See also
   6J9B11MN0K)
08T7936572. Aminoquinuride
08V52GZ3H9. Tamibarotene
08X7F5UDJM. Dimethyl Phthalate

090519SAPF. Methantheline Bromide
090DE9CRP1. Timelotem
090O8Q78KU. Phenamazoline Hydrochloride (See also
   09L091X49E)
090XO8449J. Ciramadol Hydrochloride
0939APN2IR. Piclopastine
094ZI81Y45. Tamoxifen Citrate [tamoxifen] (See also
   7FRV7310N6)
098633Q42P. Cefluprenam
0990EG3K10. Telenzepine
09B57945V9. Propizepine
09HKW863J6. Diclofensine
09I93HJ3Y4. Tifemoxone
09L091X49E. Phenamazoline Hydrochloride [phenamazoline]
   (See also *090O8Q78KU*)
09Q5UV3747. Segesterone
09QF37C617. Examorelin
09TD6C5147. Biperiden Lactate (See also *0FRP6G56LD*)
09YNW8E5CT. Homopipramol
0A0800O89N. Zanapezil
0A09IUW5TP. Prucalopride
0A2D355316. Zabiciprilat
0A995E1KA6. Niprofazone
0ARR2L0V0A. Ponfibrate
0B50MLU3H1. Cefoselis
0B535E0BN0. Nedocromil
0B62S0B44U. Propyl Docetrizoate
0BI682BR2D. Cintazone
0BJK6B565B. Dofequidar
0BZK9FE5DE. Etisomicin
0C1SPQ0FSR. Epsiprantel
0C2796D6SB. Lofemizole Hydrochloride
0C39YBM73T. Oxisopred
0C50HW4FO1. Etravirine
0C78CV13XZ. Isobucaine Hydrochloride
0C94V6X681. Buclizine Hydrochloride [buclizine] (See also
   58FQD093NU)
0CD5FD6S2M. Fluocinolone Acetonide
0CDE7T54KW. Estrofurate
0CG6O25ZC4. Pecocycline
0CPP32S55X. Dimercaprol
0D2VUO6DCN. Cipropride
0D3Q044KCA. Galantamine
0D5204ZSIX. Pradefovir Mesylate (See also *GZE85Q9Q61*)
0D771IS0FH. Thiram
0DH9WUS03O. Terbequinil
0DHU5B8D6V. Citalopram
0DMO75HN8B. Carbantel Lauryl Sulfate
0DV09X6F21. Flumethasone Pivalate (See also *LR3CD8SX89*)
0E43V0BB57. Misoprostol
0E53J927NA. Magnesium Carbonate
0E6DA2DHBE. Sprodiamide [anhydrous]
0E8R4GDE2Q. Ritolukast
0EMF539HN0. Amedalin Hydrochloride
0EWG668W17. Phenazopyridine Hydrochloride (See also
   K2J09EMJ52)
0F1T12OCLX. Nicotredole
0F32U78V2Q. Chloroxylenol
0F5N573A2Y. Ether
0F65R8P09N. Goserelin
0FD207WKDU. Camostat
0FI451I3D5. Nafcaproic Acid
0FRP6G56LD. Biperiden
0FRP6G56LD. Biperiden Hydrochloride [biperiden] (See also
   K35N76CUHF)
0FRP6G56LD. Biperiden Lactate [biperiden] (See also
   09TD6C5147)
0FYM61NG4D. Histapyrrodine

0G389FZZ9M. Levocarnitine

0G3C18OH4D. Sulfoxone Sodium [sulfoxone] (See also *57OWB0Q221*)

0G3DE8943Y. Lanreotide Acetate [lanreotide] (See also *IEU56G3J9C*)

0G4X367WA3. Cromakalim

0G76K8X6C0. Methsuximide

0GEI24LG0J. Chenodiol

0GH9JX37C8. Butylscopolamine Bromide

0GSS0O37A8. Bemarinone Hydrochloride

0GXP746VXB. Cefotetan Disodium

0GZ72U84TN. Acedapsone

0H00N2AHSP. Dextrothyroxine Sodium (See also *4W9K63FION*)

0H73WJJ391. Topiramate

0HX1Z0A2MC. Carphenazine Maleate (See also *CLY16Y8Z7E*)

0HXY3M6S54. Octamoxin

0HZN7FV25R. Cyclobarbital Calcium

0I14K589E7. Etafenone

0I3V7S25AW. Myristic Acid

0I93JSA6L6. Tibenzate

0IMX38M2GG. Indomethacin Sodium

0J48LPH2TH. Hydrochlorothiazide

0J6174G60N. Saripidem

0J7USQ749M. Iodofiltic Acid I 123

0J8L4V3F81. Sulfaphenazole

0J9L7J6V8C. Nepafenac

0JJT8MQ49S. Flucetorex

0JS043FG0D. Doxibetasol

0K2I505OTV. Phentermine Hydrochloride (See also *C045TQL4WP*)

0K40CNM74K. Tioxacin

0K47UL67F2. Carvedilol

0K5C5T2QPG. Lansoprazole

0KJ20H1BLJ. Bibrocathol

0KJ2VE664U. Terconazole

0L0UGK6OOX. Derquantel

0L1S25NC1L. Cafaminol

0L55QF645F. Tolgabide

0L591QR10I. Azelastine Hydrochloride (See also *ZQI909440X*)

0L7AR6G18O. Isocromil

0LD7P9153C. Etofenprox

0LT9MW24NY. Calcium Lactophosphate

0M14O7T47Q. Lorpiprazole

0M1J60BWEX. Fencamfamin Hydrochloride

0M2W3TAG39. Amperozide (See also *8V2171U69N*)

0M3S43XK27. Benzphetamine Hydrochloride [benzphetamine] (See also *43DWT87QT7*)

0M52541M8X. Dorastine Hydrochloride

0M63DKI91K. Butethamine Hydrochloride

0M67U6Z98F. Droloxifene

0M8A98AD9H. Cyclobarbital

0M8OM373BS. Alafosfalin

0N2U15U85W. Azapetine Phosphate

0N4I6K95P2. Carbazeran

0N739K2A8A. Alamifovir

0N7609K889. Sulfadiazine

0N7609K889. Sulfadiazine, Silver [sulfadiazine]

0NB98NBX3D. Varespladib Methyl

0NJ98Y462X. Conivaptan

0NOY894QRB. Stepronin

0O501R1CSQ. Nafenodone

0O54ZQ14I9. Aminoglutethimide

0O653FA999. Azaloxan Fumarate [azaloxan] (See also *8605L38D80*)

0O6W0NP518. Clobenzepam

0O977R722D. Oxamniquine

0P1AN6K49Q. Flutizenol

0P1LKO80WN. Trovafloxacin Mesylate (See also *9F388J00UK*)

0P5B94FVD5. Bietaserpine

0P6C6ZOP5U. Roflumilast

0PG3PMK9YA. Tamolarizine

0PM0Q96HVS. Xenthiorate

0PV32JZB1J. Ampiroxicam

0Q1O6G98Q8. Parodilol

0Q3H898100. Oxonazine

0QAC3P785O. Inaperisone

0QGV8237I3. Lasinavir

0QJF08GDPE. Lorcaserin Hydrochloride

0QTW8Z7MCR. Rofecoxib

0R4888YXR5. Lefradafiban

0R8E9BWM4J. Tandospirone Citrate

0RE8K4LNJS. Isopropyl Myristate

0RH81L854J. Glutamine

0RO0SEU9AY. Melquinast

0S36458I44. Sanfetrinem Cilexetil [sanfetrinem]

0S3LDN5P7H. Etiroxate

0S9SLS3L93. Clofibride

0SUN4UF93Y. Picumeterol Fumarate (See also *86WEQ311WF*)

0SY050L61N. Chlormadinone Acetate

0T2EF4JQTU. Rimantadine Hydrochloride [rimantadine] (See also *JEI07OOS8Y*)

0T3Q181657. Ammonium Salicylate

0TTZ664R7Z. Phenoxybenzamine Hydrochloride [phenoxybenzamine] (See also *X1IEG24OHL*)

0U434950BU. Probicromil Calcium

0U575HR16Q. Denibulin Hydrochloride

0UT4JLE1CM. Aglepristone

0UX03A6JJC. Pentamethonium Bromide

0UYY5V4U2Q. Cafedrine

0V5436JAQW. Miglitol

0V7WAB3NV4. Clofurac

0V9VL751XU. Damotepine

0VCI53PK4A. Flupirtine Maleate (See also *MOH3ET196H*)

0VE05JYS2P. Cyclobenzaprine Hydrochloride (See also *69O5WQQ5TI*)

0VE4U49K15. Benoxinate Hydrochloride (See also *AXQ0-JYM303*)

0VN909S60Y. Dopexamine Hydrochloride

0VUA21238F. Lapatinib Ditosylate [lapatinib] (See also *G873GX646R*)

0W33021S30. Defosfamide

0W3C4GMZ2I. Metcaraphen Hydrochloride

0W5ETF9M2K. Methacholine Chloride (See also *03V657ZD3V*)

0WN4KYJ0C0. Biphenamine Hydrochloride

0WR771DJXV. Dobutamine Hydrochloride (See also *3S12J47372*)

0WVM2U8MFI. Dimetipirium Bromide

0WW6D218XJ. Pilocarpine Hydrochloride

0X2CW1QABJ. Fenoprofen Calcium (See also *RA33EAC7KY*)

0X60R85C0J. Chlorothen Citrate

0X748O646K. Ecopipam

0X97008FCC. Talopram Hydrochloride

0X9JDS6MF1. Platonin

0X9P7B60UD. Sulfaguanole

0X9PA28K43. Verteporfin

0XU0V77JVE. Amfetaminil

0Y25DT968Y. Draflazine

0Y299JY9V3. Carbromal

0Y2S3XUQ5H. Bumetanide

0Y84EU1HAA. Isoxaprolol

0YPR65R21J. Sodium Sulfate

0YZT43HS7D. Tetrahydrozoline Hydrochloride (See also *S9U025Y077*)

0Z4EEC962O. Succisulfone

0Z802HMY7H. Indoramin

0ZIP7YM8DI. Ascorbyl Gamolenate

0ZV4Q4L2FU. Acetyldigitoxin
1014KSJ86F. Erythromycin Ethylsuccinate
1018WH7F9I. Dexmedetomidine Hydrochloride
101V0R1N2E. Febuxostat
103G5E953K. Selodenoson
104NHK678E. Furbucillin
10661OD4VE. Proterguride
10BI795R7D. Hexestrol
10L39TRG1Z. Pentaerythritol Tetranitrate
10LGE70FSU. Ammonium Phosphate
10NHF3008V. Fidexaban
10T9CSU89I. Teriparatide
10TO0RP68C. Pranazepide
10X0709Y6I. Bisacodyl
10X0709Y6I. Bisacodyl Tannex [bisacodyl]
10X8X4P12Z. Naratriptan Hydrochloride (See also QX3KXL1ZA2)
10YM403FLS. Pirenzepine Hydrochloride (See also 3G0285N20N)
1133E05F6C. Fezolamine Fumarate [fezolamine] (See also I1GX0BGV7P)
1177I648L1. Alphameprodine
11DI31LWXF. Abafungin
11F6O06WN0. Brocresine
11G3FV7PG7. Zonampanel
11P9NUA12U. Nicarbazin
11S92G0TIW. Alfentanil Hydrochloride (See also 1N74HM2BS7)
11SV1951MR. Tamsulosin Hydrochloride (See also G3P28OM-L5I)
11YB79G1Y6. Atliprofen
11ZYL7QK34. Levotofisopam
1243654WZK. Menitrazepam
124I3FE35T. Telmesteine
124LSR3H2X. Delucemine Hydrochloride [delucemine] (See also P1I0CQY44Z)
124X2V25W4. Fosfosal
124XMA6YEI. Levocabastine Hydrochloride (See also H68BP06S81)
125267OAUF. Picumast
125OD7737X. Methocarbamol
127M91LHX5. Tradecamide
127X8DJ74M. Norpipanone
129FW80TG4. Mangafodipir Trisodium
12EA34U5B8. Neboglamine
12G01I6BBU. Retigabine
12H3K5QKN9. Potassium Gluconate
12I91IOS6Z. Acefylline Piperazine
12IMO9R11X. Benzoxonium Chloride
12L58GX4AS. Praxadine
12L83YI68T. Picafibrate
12L95QD6KV. Isomethadone
12LGO1XVPA. Hydroxyprocaine
12M44VTJ7B. Dalteparin Sodium
12R8659YM6. Tolycaine
12UHW9R67N. Isoflurophate
13097143QI. Lonazolac
134FM9ZZ6M. Pheniramine Maleate [pheniramine] (See also NYW905655B)
1351PE5UGS. Elotuzumab
1356SD6O2G. Talosalate
1364PS73AF. Acetone
136H45TB7B. Alclometasone Dipropionate [alclometasone] (See also S56PQL4N1V)
137KB7GYKB. Cefpiramide Sodium
137R1N49AD. Agomelatine
13AFD7670Q. Primidone
13H7H1ET2J. Butoxylate
13HX5F227D. Sulfaclorazole
13MIU3750H. Espatropate
13P4GX22ES. Lenperone
13RRH2218G. Rizatriptan Sulfate
13T4O6VMAM. Piroxicam
13X224L936. Piridoxilate
13Z9HTH115. Alosetron Hydrochloride [alosetron] (See also 2F5R1A46YW)
140QMO216E. Metronidazole
140QMO216E. Metronidazole Hydrochloride [metronidazole] (See also 76JC1633UF)
140T9JTG43. Butalamine
141A6AMN38. Cilastatin Sodium [cilastatin] (See also 5428WXZ74M)
14255EXE39. Ethylparaben
142M471B3J. Carbon Dioxide
143NQ3779B. Calcipotriene
144O8QL0L1. Diclofenac Potassium [diclofenac] (See also L4D5UA6CB4)
146D7G2I94. Rofelodine
146T0TU1JB. Penicillin V Potassium
14LS8QHX0U. Tiazuril
14NFL30YOH. Barucainide
14O50WS8JD. Octopamine
14PEC3LEVH. Pyrinoline
14U0D2SA4K. Fandosentan Potassium (See also 771E5ELJ7N)
14Y6444DRP. Diltiazem Malate
155R3B9K8H. Binospirone Mesylate
157NY06G9T. Pramiverine
1597304395. Etanterol
15C2VL427D. Aflibercept
15CC9BOH7Q. Soquinolol
15E9I74NZ8. Cyclomethycaine Sulfate [cyclomethycaine] (See also 7323N7T136)
15FIX9V2JP. Titanium Dioxide
15H5577CQD. Docetaxel
15JT14C3GI. Bekanamycin
15K99VDU5F. Beraprost Sodium (See also 35E3NJJ4O6)
15LTY5STY6. Omoconazole Nitrate (See also GQ8ADD54E1)
15OX67P384. Zucapsaicin
15QZ6NE84E. Indeloxazine Hydrochloride
15UQ94PT4P. Darbepoetin Alfa
15VZ5AL4JN. Mebeverine Hydrochloride
15XQ8043FN. Sulfaguanidine
1619C79FVJ. Pelubiprofen
1627CY4S8U. Dibuprol
162A01WTAJ. Anisopirol
1654W9611T. Tomopenem
16665T4A2X. Desoxycorticosterone Pivalate
1678OK0E08. Dexmethylphenidate Hydrochloride (See also M32RH9MFGP)
167NDD8MTE. Oxprenoate Potassium
16992A3UUS. Dametralast
1699G8679Z. Sodium Polystyrene Sulfonate
16C19Z7F4I. Fosenazide
16CHD79MIX. Iothalamate Sodium [iothalamic acid]
16CHD79MIX. Iothalamic Acid
16FL47B687. Iotrolan
170ZT3R958. Diphoxazide
17197F0KYM. Afimoxifene
172D4Q6LOW. Cloroqualone
172F2WN8DV. Oleyl Alcohol
173648DEO8. Bromacrylide
1754ZE4075. Metochalcone
176437APQH. Benzylhydrochlorothiazide
17682058OP. Cloperidone Hydrochloride
1768UW0XS1. Alpiropride
17B9PXO2SW. Tobuterol

1P441EE1PH. Ftormetazine
1P7H87IN75. Secobarbital
1P93TO196Z. Thiotetrabarbital
1P9D0Z171K. Butylated Hydroxytoluene
1P9E5C9137. Esproquin Hydrochloride (See also *3JYK9XFM9K*)
1P9L1B4UIC. Azipramine Hydrochloride [azipramine] (See also *U2508LW03T*)
1PA76KJ99Y. Cortisuzol
1PO9LWW5IN. Trazium Esilate
1PU994YJUH. Etosalamide
1Q1AWW2JET. Propisergide
1Q3CYC1YR6. Disulergine
1Q4C0XA9H4. Prizidilol Hydrochloride (See also *U6QG1RWA7B*)
1Q63WWP8G5. Carvotroline Hydrochloride [carvotroline]
1Q728MH9P9. Piridicillin Sodium (See also *6502ONO3L0*)
1Q73Q2JULR. Sodium Citrate
1Q8D39N37L. Amonafide
1QS9G4876X. Oxyclozanide
1QZ096EIEF. Endrysone
1R01BKB74A. Carpronium Chloride
1R0Y7O07NF. Dapabutan
1R754M4918. Lufenuron
1R7T67JP3G. Cimepanol
1RTH95874Z. Cioteronel
1RTM4PAL0V. Piperazine
1RTM4PAL0V. Piperazine Edetate Calcium [piperazine]
1RZ4ML637I. Doxaminol
1S169L7KAV. Nanterinone
1S3Z442A8N. Pirazmonam Sodium [pirazmonam] (See also *M89TPX4O2C*)
1S4CJB5ZGN. Estradiol Benzoate
1S50W1WU8T. Chaulmosulfone
1T0N3G9CRC. Trandolapril
1T1S98ONM1. Lorcainide Hydrochloride
1T3A50395T. Acriflavine
1T89100D5U. Sulconazole Nitrate (See also *5D9HAA5Q5S*)
1TBQ3A47P8. Fenalcomine
1TD8J48L61. Benzthiazide
1TR49121NP. Cypermethrin
1U4B477260. Tesmilifene Hydrochloride
1U511HHV4Z. Mexiletine Hydrochloride [mexiletine] (See also *606D60IS38*)
1U73ZZU4JK. Ectylurea
1UA8E65KDZ. Alitretinoin
1UA960P80H. Nicainoprol
1UD32YR59G. Tirapazamine
1UK146T40N. Chymopapain
1URW272384. Treptilamine
1UWS3T8EAB. Panuramine
1V339IMQ38. Dimepranol Acedoben
1V5135S169. Deximafen
1V7A1U282K. Prednisolone Tebutate
1V8X590XDP. Edotecarin
1VPU26JZZ4. Potassium Sorbate
1W306TDA6S. Rifabutin
1W5N8SZD9A. Glufosfamide
1W6L629B4K. Sulisobenzone
1W7R63X54A. Dibutoline Sulfate
1WAM1OQ30B. Amdinocillin Pivoxil
1WPQ720NCK. Trenizine
1X0094V6JV. Nafarelin Acetate [nafarelin] (See also *8ENZ0QJW4H*)
1X0MUE4C19. Clofenamic Acid
1X50HHA8FY. Valdetamide
1X9VK9O1SC. Fludarabine Phosphate (See also *P2K93U8740*)
1XA84ITL1H. Azastene
1XHL4Q8P7Y. Sulfiram

1XL6BJI034. Balsalazide Disodium (See also *P80AL8J7ZP*)
1XU086MM3H. Etibendazole
1Y17CTI5SR. Insulin Human
1Y58DO4MY1. Desipramine Hydrochloride (See also *TG537D343B*)
1Y6SNA8L5S. Edelfosine
1YF1KXP4QF. Nitraquazone
1YOQ7J9ACY. Cadrofloxacin
1YP2S94RVH. Brasofensine
1YTW0422YU. Salcaprozate Sodium
1Z0YFI05OO. Triflusal
1Z20MGK851. Leurubicin
1ZFB1FR98E. Etifelmine
1ZI8H16Z5I. Nixylic Acid
1ZK20VI6TY. Triamcinolone
200168S0CL. Ambroxol (See also *CC995ZMV90*)
202J683U97. Bromodiphenhydramine Hydrochloride (See also *T032BI7727*)
2046ZRO9VU. Physostigmine Salicylate (See also *9U1VM840SP*)
207LT9J9OC. Buspirone Hydrochloride (See also *TK65WKS8HL*)
207ZZ9QZ49. Methylphenidate
20O65J0B72. Sagandipine
20O93L6F9H. Oseltamivir
20P9NI883O. Aminopentamide Sulfate
21240MF57M. Sulfanilamide
2133JVQ6VE. Furalazine
2136B7T7KE. Sulazuril
2144G00Y7W. Cangrelor Tetrasodium
214IZI85K3. Trifluoperazine Hydrochloride [trifluoperazine] (See also *6P1Y2SNF5V*)
216X081ORU. Ziprasidone Hydrochloride (See also *6UKA5-VEJ6X*)
217727W28W. Sulfonethylmethane
21925K482H. Carisoprodol
21CP7826LC. Calcium Carbimide [cyanamide]
21FS93Y6OE. Antrafenine
21G64WZQ4I. Incyclinide
21G72T1950. Tolvaptan
21H450VP7K. Imcarbofos
21J54X4Z4Z. Betaprodine
21Q62BRI9U. Clocanfamide
220236ED28. Amodiaquine
220236ED28. Amodiaquine Hydrochloride [amodiaquine] (See also *K6PW2S574L*)
2208Y59985. Sufosfamide
2208ZLI77S. Eptazocine
221A91BQ2S. Etamiphyllin
2225PI3MOV. Thimerosal
224TL37A39. Pibaxizine
2260ZP67IT. Tipepidine
2285XW22DR. Cixutumumab
22966TX7J5. Epirubicin Hydrochloride (See also *3Z8479ZZ5X*)
229809935B. Methadone Hydrochloride (See also *UC6VBE7V1Z*)
229YMD7GRO. Naphthonone
22M9P70OQ9. Fenoterol
22QOO9B8KI. Eletriptan
22VKV8053U. Raltegravir Potassium [raltegravir] (See also *43Y000U234*)
22VUW43J2H. Butaperazine Maleate
22X328QOC4. Fulvestrant
22Z9Q44OIG. Fluindarol
2303MD51O1. Iocarmate Meglumine (See also *82PB24K6TZ; 6HG8UB2MUY*)
230447L0GL. Etiracetam
231HZQ66PD. Peraclopone
231RV72C8L. Doxefazepam
232HYX66HC. Capreomycin Sulfate [capreomycin] (See also *9H8D3J7V21*)

23310D4I19. Palonosetron Hydrochloride (See also *5D06587D6R*)

2331W47PSX. Horse Chestnut

234335M86K. Tozasertib

23473EC6BQ. Papaverine Hydrochloride (See also *DAA13NKG2Q*)

23521W1S24. Clavulanic Acid

238M5105OY. Naroparcil

238S75V9AV. Metopimazine

239IF5W61J. Bentiromide

23EDE20K1X. Lecozotan Hydrochloride (See also *48854OTZ5E*)

23OV73Q5G9. Acesulfame Potassium

23OW28RS7P. Quinupristin

23Q8M2HE6S. Meclocycline

23TF67G79M. Etofibrate

23X1185WBO. Iobenguane Sulfate I 123

23ZW4BG89C. Benzarone

241ATL177A. Soybean Oil

242Z0PM79Y. Propiomazine

242Z0PM79Y. Propiomazine Hydrochloride [propiomazine] (See also *70BO17YR03*)

2436VX1U9B. Ibutilide Fumarate [ibutilide] (See also *9L5X4M5L6I*)

243KJ527MC. Ciaftalan Zinc

244O1F90NA. Mizolastine

2456GO94TR. Diperodon

2456GO94TR. Diperodon Hydrochloride [diperodon] (See also *5YZ5R8I73Y*)

2494G1JF75. Lopinavir

2498Y783QT. Toremifene Citrate (See also *7NFE54O27T*)

24CU1YS91D. Danofloxacin Mesylate [danofloxacin] (See also *94F3SX3LEM*)

24F9PF7J3R. Toceranib Phosphate

24G45TQO8A. Revenast

24I7KUI7MK. Rose Bengal Sodium I 131

24MJ822NZ9. Pergolide Mesylate [pergolide] (See also *55B9HQY616*)

24MR6YLL3W. Difenamizole

24N16QE4S0. Pipoctanone

24PUW23GRX. Phthalylsulfacetamide

24S58UHU7N. Cefpimizole

24S58UHU7N. Cefpimizole Sodium [cefpimizole] (See also *X4628IMC52*)

24S79B9CX7. Arecoline Hydrobromide (See also *4ALN5933BH*)

24WE03BX2T. Levomenol

253GQW851Q. Vinorelbine Tartrate (See also *Q6C979R91Y*)

2579Z4P04J. Methyldopa Hydrochloride [methyldopate] (See also *7PX435DN5A*)

258J72S7TZ. Cefotaxime Sodium (See also *N2GI8B1GK7*)

25ATP958PA. Nealbarbital

25BB7EKE2E. Barium Sulfate

25CC4N0P8J. Nalfurafine Hydrochloride

25CJR2TJPW. Colterol Mesylate

25CO3X0R31. Seproxetine Hydrochloride [seproxetine] (See also *K4QYN23H2N*)

25E79B5CTM. Denileukin Diftitox

25G65PH99M. Impacarzine

25IH6R4SGF. Edetate Calcium Disodium (See also *9G34HU7RV0*)

25OIG0XCVX. Beperidium Iodide

25UR9N9041. Naftifine Hydrochloride (See also *4FB1TON47A*)

25W8454H16. Sulfamethizole

25X51I8RD4. Niacinamide

25Y9G9575K. Icotidine

25YF317R6S. Rescimetol

25YK75CYMX. Tridihexethyl Chloride

260080034N. Lacidipine

261MHO395H. Guaiactamine

262P8GS9L9. Tafenoquine

26337D5X88. Ceftizoxime Sodium (See also *C43C467DPE*)

263T0E9RR9. Dyphylline

26601THN1D. Bendazol

2679MF687A. Niacin

267GPF992J. Monalazone Disodium

2681D7P965. Phenelzine Sulfate (See also *O408N561GF*)

269K6498LD. Trimipramine Maleate

269M3QL74S. Dibrompropamidine

26G7YC77BU. Diampromide

26HUS7139V. Ocaperidone

26LUD4JO9K. Amitriptyline Hydrochloride (See also *1806D8D52K*)

26NAK24LS8. Hydralazine Hydrochloride [hydralazine] (See also *FD171B778Y*)

26PB1U68YF. Butedronic Acid

26POQ4GICP. Disulfamide

26R628272Q. Benactyzine [benactyzine hydrochloride] (See also *595EG71R3F*)

26RM326WVN. Cycloguanil Pamoate [cycloguanil]

26Y8H6WPAW. Vanitiolide

2728MV084C. Dextilidine

275L5M93QS. Barbital Sodium (See also *5WZ53ENE2P*)

27618J1N2X. Levorphanol Tartrate [levorphanol] (See also *04WQU6T9QI*)

276F2O42F5. Hydroxyprogesterone Caproate

277V92K32B. Serlopitant

2781UEP67S. Naftoxate

27D37TX66Y. Zepastine

27DXO59SAN. Tocainide

27J5OW8OGT. Metofenazate

27L0EP6IZK. Pirenoxine

27O3Q5ML57. Phenylephrine Bitartrate

27O7W4T232. Spironolactone

27P0WQO4ZB. Paxamate

27RL57FCYM. Amoproxan

27T1I13L6G. Amineptine

27T56C7KK0. Alglucerase

27X63J94GR. Nefazodone Hydrochloride (See also *59H4FCV1TF*)

27Y3KJK423. Aminophylline (See also *C229N9DX94*)

27Y876D139. Menatetrenone

27Z82M2G1N. Belotecan Hydrochloride [belotecan] (See also *01DZ4127G7*)

280111G160. Cefadroxil

280VGV0X4H. Declenperone

281Y036E0W. Aclantate

283383NO13. Racephenicol

286F595V8H. Tresperimus

2879S26V4P. Mitotenamine

287M0347EV. Dantrolene Sodium (See also *F64QU97QCR*)

2880D3468G. Levamisole Hydrochloride [levamisole] (See also *DL9055K809*)

28810ORE8K. Zimidoben

28A37T47QO. Phenyl Salicylate

28F9E0DJY6. Tannic Acid

28K6I5M16G. Palovarotene

28LQ20T5RC. Avasimibe

28N73Q6O7Y. Etisulergine

28O5C1J38A. Amfenac Sodium [amfenac]

28OQS360UJ. Debropol

28TV2P33KF. Ceftiolene

290YE8AR51. Trichloroethylene

2919279Q3W. Valdecoxib

291GX1YB65. Barbexaclone

292N180GYN. Melizame

292V8Q1MXQ. Vapiprost Hydrochloride (See also *H84XT1COAU*)

29610N9WR1. Picenadol Hydrochloride
2961Y60ATP. Proflavine Sulfate (See also *CY3RNB3K4T*)
2968PHW8QP. Citric Acid, Anhydrous [monohydrate] (See also *XF417D3PSL*)
29CS07FZII. Calcium Mandelate (See also *NH496X0UJX*)
29O079NTYT. Demeclocycline Hydrochloride (See also *5R5W9I-CI6O*)
29OE04A6C9. Thymotrinan
29OQ9EU4R1. Tiratricol
29PW75S82A. Carazolol
29UKX3A616. Sodium Iodide I 123
29VCO8ACHH. Sodium Iodide I 131
2A9QP32MD4. Melagatran
2ACZ6IPC6I. γ-Aminobutyric Acid
2AE8M83G3E. Rupatadine
2AHC415BQG. Valnemulin
2AV3RNM4HV. Tofisoline
2AY21R0U64. Erythromycin Gluceptate
2B2ZV6F5HG. Pipebuzone
2B3D399IVR. Litracen
2B562K7K56. Texacromil
2BMD2GNA4V. Lithium Carbonate
2BSS7XL60S. Azasetron [azasetron hydrochloride] (See also *77HC7URR9Z*)
2BTY8KH53L. Deferiprone
2BY2U8GO3M. Sarakalim
2C09NV773M. Pemirolast Potassium [pemirolast] (See also *497A17OUUE*)
2C21AN130I. Amifloxacin Mesylate (See also *5TU5227KYQ*)
2C29WCQ951. Piminodine Esylate
2C6NUM6878. Valrubicin
2CCC8CH216. Edonentan (See also *S5016F5ZH4*)
2CNI71214Y. Alanosine
2CSP4U82HK. Pazelliptine
2D4432ZP6M. Bidimazium Iodide
2D6A12Q12R. Temocaprilat
2DH4X8278M. Pravadoline Maleate
2DI9HA706A. Estrone
2DW6SEL94L. Metoquizine
2E18WX195X. Dabigatran Etexilate
2E2W0W5XIU. Eniluracil
2F5K551CB4. Tonazocine Mesylate
2F5R1A46YW. Alosetron Hydrochloride (See also *13Z9HTH115*)
2F5V2R6VX8. Cefcanel
2F70GCU00A. Diniprofylline
2F70KF5S0K. Mifentidine
2FS66TH3YW. Zolmitriptan
2FSU2FR80J. Etoperidone Hydrochloride (See also *KAI6M-VO39Z*)
2G222T03EY. Resequinil
2G25KE3954. Avitriptan Fumarate
2G86QN327L. Gelatin
2GHY1101MM. Flutoprazepam
2GT1D0TMX1. Moricizine (See also *71OK3Z1ESP*)
2GWV496552. Perifosine
2GZ0LIK7T4. Istradefylline
2H2HC19DYZ. Ethaverine Hydrochloride [ethaverine] (See also *6Z6T599E49*)
2H52Z9F2Q5. Pefloxacin
2H6ON8WA7L. Paraxazone
2HD55617I2. Semorphone
2HLC17MX9G. Agalsidase Alfa
2HX2OJH78L. Prothixene
2I4BC502BT. Salmeterol
2I8BD50I8B. Chloroxine
2I8RV6WL9A. Adaprolol Maleate (See also *XP991I1WL*)
2I8V5Q9A78. Resorantel
2IXX802851. Alatrofloxacin Mesylate

2IY97B405I. Tetrazolast Meglumine
2J1346C51H. Ladostigil Tartrate
2J6DQ1U5B5. Cilansetron
2JB27QJW3D. Prednisolone Valerate Acetate
2JEC1ITX7R. Indacaterol Maleate
2JH9LR1Y6S. Nitrocycline
2JMM46GA2V. Enefexine
2JQ3661CAD. Indopanolol
2K02669KWP. Ecabet
2K1V7GP655. Selegiline
2K3L8O9SOV. Chloropyramine
2K7I38CKN5. Tocainide Hydrochloride
2KFG9TP5V8. Xylazine
2KH13Z0S0Y. Eprosartan
2KL01R8ZV1. Diamthazole
2KN23X015H. Fludoxopone
2KNI5N06TI. Pyrazinamide
2KR89I4H1Y. Stearyl Alcohol
2KT2C544LR. Lubazodone Hydrochloride
2L2063955H. Cloridarol
2L6Q871829. Mipitroban
2L7I72RUHN. Butorphanol Tartrate (See also *QV897JC36D*)
2L8T9S52QM. Triprolidine Hydrochloride [triprolidine] (See also *YAN7R5L890*)
2LP301A921. Girisopam
2LXW0L6GWJ. Clomipramine Hydrochloride (See also *NUV44L116D*)
2M3055079H. Brivudine
2M36281008. Etodolac
2M3NG13839. Rolgamidine
2M3V3B8OEA. Depelestat
2MI60P494I. Ipazilide Fumarate
2MRO291B4U. Clobazam
2N2LI66RRO. Quinazosin Hydrochloride (See also *436XK6QFMR*)
2N4O9L084N. Nabilone
2N81MY12TE. Fosfomycin
2NL79NI1WS. Azalanstat Dihydrochloride [azalanstat] (See also *X30J960B4D*)
2NX48Z0A9G. Icodextrin
2O09BG0OWA. Farletuzumab
2OC4HKD3SF. Telbivudine
2OGQ81529L. Acetorphine
2OU4KS37EO. Cyclexanone
2OVL75B30W. Menadiol Sodium Diphosphate (See also *VQ093653DO*)
2P43Z53ESB. Tobicillin
2PKU919BA9. Pemetrexed Disodium (See also *04Q9AIZ7NO*)
2PO3M8FE7C. Ethypicone
2PP737Z523. Deanol Aceglumate
2Q9A409N0B. Clioxanide
2QW3FL6OPA. Metralindole
2R04ONI662. Eucalyptus Oil
2R4QO1868Y. Ridazolol
2R7O1ET613. Pranoprofen
2R880S54IS. Perimetazine
2RG1XQ1NYJ. Gonadorelin Acetate
2S068B75ZU. Fexofenadine Hydrochloride (See also *E6582LOH6V*)
2S3PL1B6UJ. Quetiapine Fumarate (See also *BGL0JSY5SI*)
2S713A4VP3. Podophyllum
2S9ZZM9Q9V. Bevacizumab
2SH16612I9. Aminorex
2SMM3M5ZMH. Delapril Hydrochloride (See also *W77UAL9THI*)
2STG09LA8F. Nitrodan
2T7T4YO42R. Triclofylline
2T7W4EA51W. Patamostat

2T8Q726O95. Lamivudine
2T90KE67L0. Ertapenem Sodium (See also *G32F6EID2H*)
2TB00A1Z7N. Cefpodoxime Proxetil (See also *7R4F94TVGY*)
2TP37O5J17. Isamoltan
2U1W68TROF. Maprotiline
2U7H1466GH. Methysergide Maleate
2U918O4BEV. Acrisorcin
2UB1JJT82D. Esorubicin Hydrochloride
2UG271VI0Z. Pheneridine
2URQ2N32W3. Calcium Lactate
2UTZ0QC864. Iscotrizinol
2UV6ZNQ92K. Perindoprilat
2UY4M2U3RA. Alendronate Sodium
2V16EO95H1. Palmitic Acid
2V6Z0JG2X0. Meladrazine
2VBY96ASWJ. Barnidipine
2VG7825GP4. Fenirofibrate
2VO6TC90PU. Butetamate
2VUW1087AD. Lirequinil
2W07HSP5PX. Furazabol
2W2V1U785A. Darotropium Bromide
2W4A77YPAN. Fluocinonide
2XCW01A0N5. Bismuth Potassium Tartrate
2XG66W44KF. Olopatadine Hydrochloride (See also *D27V6190PM*)
2XLN4Y044H. Regadenoson
2XRX3BD53M. Docebenone
2Y065P7MYR. Anitrazafen
2Y3Q6049LX. Fepentolic Acid
2Y7TIQ135H. Eriodictyon
2YF82QN5RY. Corticorelin Acetate
2YHB6175DO. Cyproheptadine Hydrochloride [cyproheptadine] (See also *NJ82J0F8QC*)
2Z07MYW1AZ. Anastrozole
2Z4E7E087J. Democonazole
2Z81WDX2ZH. Aditoprim
2Z86SYP11W. Ceftezole
2Z91X9052O. Diethylthiambutene
2Z9V171UEM. Flavodic Acid
2ZBF31C62F. Minepentate
2ZD004190S. Threonine
2ZL2BA06FU. Merimepodib
2ZM8CX04RZ. Insulin Glargine
2ZW8NEP6PQ. Itrocinonide
2ZYM2BH34M. Piriprost Potassium
304GTH6RNH. Etonogestrel
304NUG5GF4. Itraconazole
30555LM9SQ. Formetorex
305MB38V1C. Oxomemazine
30624AA6X2. Proadifen Hydrochloride
306ERL82IR. Fexinidazole
307YLU08D8. Guanisoquin Sulfate [guanisoquin] (See also *E4E8GE5LVJ*)
30868AY0IF. Fospropofol Disodium (See also *LZ257RZP7K*)
308EUN932K. Procymate
30905R8O7B. Methoxyflurane
309713XSKW. Cipralisant
30973N61ZF. Amisometradine
30CPC5LDEX. Sulfadimethoxine
30KYC7MIAI. Aspartic Acid
30KYC7MIAI. Potassium Aspartate and Magnesium Aspartate [aspartic acid]
30MUJ6YYUY. Montirelin
30OC46A3J9. Tripelennamine Citrate
30OGU6XH7S. Brotianide
30OMY4G3MK. Guanfacine Hydrochloride [guanfacine] (See also *PML56A160O*)
30Q7KI53AK. Epinephrine Bitartrate (See also *YKH834O4BH*)

30S4B46J8B. Sulfisoxazole Diolamine
310X6S84LW. Pyrvinium Pamoate
311154J4LN. Aprosulate Sodium
311WUU3BVY. Batebulast
313QE5199Z. Butynamine
3184855T90. Iotrizoic Acid
318F6L70J8. Granisetron Hydrochloride
318X4QY113. Gavestinel
319X2NFW0A. Colfosceril Palmitate
31C4KY9ESH. Nitric Oxide
31EPT7G9PL. Trimetozine
31IPX0ZD7R. Droprenilamine
31J5U3Q9ZN. Iothalamate Sodium I 125
31L760807H. Trimazosin Hydrochloride [trimazosin] (See also *827T79ILE7*)
31LA41942J. Picolamine
31PZ2VAU81. Carbamide Peroxide
31YX4A42L4. Fluquazone
32021T3D6N. Diphenidol Pamoate (See also *NQO8R319LY*)
320T6RNW1F. Mifepristone
320YC168LF. Halazepam
321US0I5R6. Quiflapon Sodium
322D5Y3Q0G. Nonapyrimine
322WXU4AU2. Ancriviroc
323A00CRO9. Amtolmetin Guacil
325OGW249P. Enoxacin
325PG708LF. Ciamexon
329I5805BP. Nanofin
32HRV3E3D5. Griseofulvin
32K9S228IK. Anpirtoline
32VY6L26ZW. Methixene Hydrochloride [methixene] (See also *84L8XK6N1G*)
32W4ZSE0X7. Clociguanil
33067B3N2M. Quinapril Hydrochloride (See also *RJ84Y44811*)
33361OE3AV. Diphenylpyraline Hydrochloride [diphenylpyraline] (See also *G9FU7F1E87*)
333M5986I5. Endralazine Mesylate
33482245B6. Dacuronium Bromide
334895S862. Doxycycline [doxycycline anhydrous] (See also *N12000U13O*)
336096P2WE. Racepinephrine Hydrochloride
336704VYVB. Dihexyverine Hydrochloride
337G83N988. Lasofoxifene
339NCG44TV. Phenol
33CM23913M. Carbamazepine
33H58I7GLQ. Erythromycin Lactobionate
33IAH5017S. Amitraz
33K3DB6591. Cytarabine Hydrochloride (See also *04079A1RDZ*)
33MG53C7XW. Vinflunine Ditartrate (See also *5BF646324K*)
33P8JV23L7. Tolboxane
33RU150WUN. Phenylpropanolamine Hydrochloride [phenylpropanolamine] (See also *8D5I63UE1Q*)
33S1GFG04E. Prinomide Tromethamine (See also *6NHC09L02I*)
33X04XA5AT. Lactic Acid
33XCH0HOCD. Propafenone Hydrochloride (See also *68IQX3-T69U*)
33Y9ANM545. Pazopanib Hydrochloride (See also *7RN5DR86CK*)
3405M6FD73. Periciazine
341YM32546. Menbutone
34237V843T. Isocarboxazid
342JR840KF. Cinchonine Sulfate
343BH0S0XR. Fluoresone
344S277G0Z. Allantoin
34711907NJ. Oxifungin Hydrochloride (See also *F14V3I66R3*)
347Q3OOJ13. Aceglatone
3483C2H13H. Hexamidine

34B0471E08. Bevonium Metilsulfate [bevonium] (See also *UW-C15E373Z*)

34E28BM822. Alnespirone

34E9Q468RT. Anilopam Hydrochloride [anilopam] (See also *JOT47SVI4K*)

34H206R8A5. Trecadrine

34K00NS0TZ. Tipropidil Hydrochloride

34S1S00GV3. Luxabendazole

34YTZ517S2. Bibenzonium Bromide [bibenzonium] (See also *4455J9277Q*)

34ZXW6ZV21. Bevantolol Hydrochloride

353613BU4U. Levallorphan Tartrate [levallorphan] (See also *U0VSF7HTN0*)

35421N8E8W. Glybuthiazol

356IB1O400. Flunixin

356IB1O400. Flunixin Meglumine [flunixin] (See also *8Y3JK0JW3U; 6HG8UB2MUY*)

357591W853. Diclonixin

3578QN1B5H. Lexofenac

3583H0GZAP. Loxoprofen

358S7VUE5N. Fluprostenol Sodium [fluprostenol] (See also *6H4ZY4O7NA*)

359HUE8FJC. Penciclovir

35C6UMO5SR. Tiospirone Hydrochloride [tiospirone] (See also *45Q1DF53NN*)

35E3NJJ4O6. Beraprost

35E3NJJ4O6. Beraprost Sodium [beraprost] (See also *15K99VDU5F*)

35FAV1EVEG. Yohimbic Acid

35LT29625A. Estramustine

35QK773Y96. Bepiastine

35S93Y190K. Procarbazine Hydrochloride [procarbazine] (See also *XH0NPH5ZX8*)

35VER614H0. Persilic Acid

35ZC5024YS. Iodol

3613ZY362L. Ecenofloxacin

362NW1LD6Z. Trimeprazine Tartrate (See also *76H78MJJ52*)

362O9ITL9D. Acetaminophen

362QBC4NL0. Piketoprofen

3642W81J7A. Cefsumide

36479UA8GL. Fenpiverinium Bromide

3666C56BBU. Begacestat

367589PJ2C. Mefenamic Acid

36780APV5N. Polythiazide

368GB5141J. Sodium Lauryl Sulfate

368IVD6M32. Nikethamide

36B82AMQ7N. Naloxone Hydrochloride [naloxone] (See also *F850569PQR*)

36DL76CZNI. Pifexole

36F26ZSQ0D. Zofenoprilat Arginine

36L0QUK8SY. Tienopramine

36M73UIK01. Ethyl Carfluzepate

36R61Y789T. Anaxirone

36S3EQV54C. Estazolam

36SG77D21B. Irloxacin

36W53O7109. Chlorocresol

36YG4ZMR69. Motrazepam

370694U45W. Thiocarbanidin

372MWC170E. Sifaprazine

37376U135T. Alilusem

3745QN167A. Piprofurol

374BH4KVRG. Aprikalim

374GJ0S41A. Melarsomine

375W3TA42N. Phenadoxone

37862HP2OM. Acepromazine Maleate

37CQ2C7X93. Canakinumab

37CW568NXL. Radezolid Hydrochloride

37JNS02E7V. Leuprolide Acetate

37Y9VR4W7A. Cefmetazole Sodium

382L14738L. Nonacog Alfa

382TLA8X28. Pribecaine

3858K104DQ. Cefquinome Sulfate

388K3TR36Z. Apramycin

388VZ25DUR. Zinc Undecylenate (See also *K3D86KJ24N*)

38EAO245ZX. Dutogliptin

38HR17LI0U. Trifosmin

38LVP0K73A. Sevoflurane

38M219L1OJ. Propoxyphene Napsylate

38PLP07BKC. Edratide

38QSU0IB5L. Esaprazole

38R2P4PIEI. Ericolol

38X7XS076H. Pralidoxime Chloride

39200FJ43J. Obatoclax Mesylate (See also *QN4128B52A*)

392TQL1E2Z. Glisentide

394E3P3B99. Arotinolol

39517A04PS. Episteride

395575MZO7. Pentostatin

3981541LXD. Diprogulic Acid

3982TWQ96G. Neostigmine Bromide [neostigmine] (See also *005SYP50G5*)

398E7Z7JB5. Dopexamine

398FD8EDAL. Pamicogrel

39IWK4M2UW. Carafiban

39J1LGJ30J. Tramadol Hydrochloride [tramadol] (See also *9N7R477WCK*)

39J262E49W. Hydroxystilbamidine Isethionate [hydroxystilbami-dine] (See also *0163PVD2QZ*)

39M9R3Q494. Butonate

39N9K8S2A4. Isosulfan Blue

39O1389K38. Sulfachrysoidine

39R4TAN1VT. Ferrous Sulfate

3A10ND4DWR. Tofenacin Hydrochloride (See also *C4A112M10H*)

3A189DH42V. Alemtuzumab

3A3N0634Q6. Rivoglitazone

3A3U0GI71G. Magnesium Oxide

3A58010674. Pegfilgrastim

3A64E3G5ZO. Bromocriptine

3A64E3G5ZO. Bromocriptine Mesylate [bromocriptine] (See also *FFP983J3OD*)

3A9RD92BS4. Maltol

3AA6IZ48YK. Benproperine

3ARD9VMM81. Levoxadrol Hydrochloride (See also *811X558HU0*)

3AVG9P140R. Binedaline

3AZF20DM1T. Indecainide Hydrochloride [indecainide] (See also *M76V0B96L5*)

3B03KPM27L. Casopitant Mesylate [casopitant] (See also *7VSV9BL497*)

3B46O2FH8I. Epirizole

3B5J9TG94X. Zetidoline

3B7O9ZC520. Prifinium Bromide

3B91HWA56M. Nalidixate Sodium [nalidixic acid] (See also *J17QL41ZAG*)

3B91HWA56M. Nalidixic Acid

3BR983K69O. Efonidipine [efonidipine hydrochloride] (See also *40ZTP2T37Q*)

3BT0VQG2GQ. Oxyphenisatin Acetate [oxyphenisatine]

3C2T3HG40E. Xenygloxal

3C9PSP36Z2. Hexamethonium Bromide [hexamethonium] (See also *8J77X3S603*)

3CD7R3856C. Diprotrizoate Sodium [diprotrizoic acid] (See also *3XJY028PJZ*)

3CF21QCB9J. Droxinavir Hydrochloride [droxinavir] (See also *7QZA627US7*)

3CIG2V70UB. Eflumast

3CO94WO6DJ. Eplivanserin
3D050LIQ3H. Dalcetrapib
3D49LE7HM2. Gluceptate Sodium
3D69H48U8Q. Potassium Nitrazepate
3D867NP06J. Pramipexole Dihydrochloride
3DE766VIG6. Baquiloprim
3DI2E1X18L. Cinnarizine
3DIZ9LF5Y9. Doxercalciferol
3DK1X2C37M. Eflucimibe
3DRR0X4728. Clazosentan
3DX3XEK1BN. Enrofloxacin
3DXB7KMD1F. Benafentrine
3E05NBH9V5. Ispronicline
3E3106052Y. Cinametic Acid
3E3V44J4Z9. Tranylcypromine Sulfate [tranylcypromine] (See
    also *7ZAT6ES870*)
3E44064G8N. Tenosiprol
3E74Y80MEY. Flavoxate Hydrochloride [flavoxate] (See also
    9C05J6089W)
3E93IV1U45. Sumanirole
3EVI8KD2BC. Valconazole
3F85I03NLO. Cicloxolone
3FDC82890Y. Monometacrine
3FTR44B32Q. Stannous Fluoride
3G0285N20N. Pirenzepine Hydrochloride [pirenzepine] (See also
    10YM403FLS)
3G05PH9FAS. Epervudine
3G6A5W338E. Caffeine
3G6A5W338E. Caffeine, Citrated [caffeine]
3GJC60U4Q8. Sitafloxacin [sitafloxacin anhydrous] (See also
    9TD681796G)
3GL26H7N6T. Lilopristone
3GQ9E911BI. Octodrine
3H0042311V. Dothiepin Hydrochloride (See also *W13O82Z7HL*)
3H04W2810V. Auranofin
3H48L0LPZQ. Ivabradine
3H4OD401LF. Carbazochrome Salicylate
3HA6AVV4EI. Trethinium Tosilate
3HP28R98LC. Tecalcet Hydrochloride (See also *8I16YLE4US*)
3HX21A3SQF. Ropidoxuridine
3HXR312Z9M. Obidoxime Chloride
3I12WH4EWF. Piromidic Acid
3I3H31VAS6. Timirdine
3I3T11UD2S. Paroxetine Hydrochloride
3I8Y076A0E. Thallous Chloride Tl 201
3IH6169RL0. Sodium Trimetaphosphate
3IN71E75Z5. Urethane
3IX8CWR24V. Siramesine
3J0KPB596Q. Tetrofosmin
3J50XA376E. Thymol
3J6WZA9PXS. Iodipamide Sodium
3J8Q1747Z2. Norgestrel
3J962UJT8H. Cefmetazole
3JB47N2Q2P. Natalizumab
3JGY52XJNA. Lutropin Alfa
3JI11Z5REF. Elgodipine
3JIJ299EWH. Fosfluconazole
3JU1DU3652. Zuclomiphene
3JYK9XFM9K. Esproquin Hydrochloride [esproquin] (See also
    1P9E5C9137)
3K01419ADP. Pyritidium Bromide
3K045XR58X. Oxtriphylline
3K0BN50QXD. Acefluranol
3K441526FO. Tetrabarbital
3K654P2M4J. Bufogenin
3K9958V90M. Alcohol
3KC089243P. Fenfluramine Hydrochloride
3KG76X4KJK. Biricodar

3KX376GY7L. Glutamic Acid
3KX376GY7L. Sodium Glutamate [glutamic acid]
3KXW0Y310I. Bezitramide
3L179F09D6. Sulfameter
3L1FU2EO79. Amoxydramine Camsilate
3L26N84757. Pirimiphos-ethyl
3L33UD42X4. Norgestomet
3L36P16U4R. Rabeprazole Sodium
3L5C5C8ZNG. Rosterolone
3L5TQ84570. Meclizine Hydrochloride [meclizine] (See also
    HDP7W44CIO)
3L83QP52XI. Efaproxiral Sodium
3LGR5S8101. Ioglicic Acid
3LNU79AO9S. Cinoxolone
3LPF0S0GVV. Ralfinamide
3LSZ7869T2. Parcetasal
3LY71185IQ. Ansoxetine
3M7OB98Y7H. Sildenafil Citrate [sildenafil] (See also
    BW9B0ZE037)
3M824XRO8N. Eptapirone
3M8608UQ61. Pravastatin Sodium (See also *KXO2KT9N0G*)
3MM99T8R5Q. Ioflupane (¹²³I)
3NM8B9838N. Tetrantoin
3NXW29V3WO. Hypromellose
3O2T2PJ89D. Donepezil Hydrochloride (See also *8SSC91326P*)
3O31P6T4G3. Levodropropizine
3O6AUX3I0J. Dexsecoverine
3OA32ZIB31. Bisfenazone
3OLH2HAK9F. Sulfatolamide
3OOH7Q4333. Cythioate
3OWL53L36A. Mannitol
3P4TQG94T1. Embutramide
3P5HNU5JTC. Acetophenazine Maleate
3PA0CDS0M5. Flumethiazide
3PFC574ITA. Gonadorelin Hydrochloride
3POA0Q644U. Histamine Dihydrochloride (See also
    820484N8I3)
3Q14SL1C0O. Flurantel
3Q22EPG4O8. Xinomiline
3Q2LQ1149L. Butafosfan
3Q6PPC19PO. Gadobenate Dimeglumine
3Q9L107XJB. Nelezaprine Maleate
3Q9Q0B929N. Dexchlorpheniramine Maleate [dexchlorphenira-
    mine] (See also *B10YD955QW*)
3QJA87N40S. Gadoxetic Acid
3QN8BYN5QF. Fingolimod Hydrochloride [fingolimod] (See also
    G926EC510T)
3QW5SNZ81H. Paranyline Hydrochloride (See also
    O2ILF29K8B)
3R77T835TA. Capobenic Acid
3R7NLP419C. Roxibolone
3RG8Q831DX. Tilozepine
3RLD929C4S. Etilefrine Pivalate
3RY07R55EE. Etryptamine Acetate (See also *GR181O3R32*)
3S12J47372. Dobutamine
3S12J47372. Dobutamine Hydrochloride [dobutamine] (See also
    0WR771DJXV)
3S182ET3UA. Tinzaparin Sodium
3S489RFX0J. Chlorbetamide
3S82268BKG. Talinolol
3SDG4RSP99. Iodecimol
3SHS7PS4PL. Chlordimorine
3ST302B24A. Losartan Potassium (See also *JMS50MPO89*)
3SZ9ZII529. Levofacetoperane
3T29053XGS. Profexalone
3T56HEP4NI. Cinoxopazide
3T93TS0430. Enofelast
3U02EL437C. Clindamycin

3U02EL437C. Clindamycin Hydrochloride [clindamycin] (See also *T20OQ1YN1W*)

3U02EL437C. Clindamycin Phosphate [clindamycin] (See also *EH6D7113I8*)

3U2FEE7NXX. Delergotrile

3U6IO1965U. Chlorpheniramine Maleate [chlorpheniramine] (See also *V1Q0O9OJ9Z*)

3U9A0FE9N5. Doxepin Hydrochloride (See also *5ASJ6HUZ7D*)

3UX6B304L3. Carbenicillin Potassium (See also *G42ZU72N5G*)

3UZ1CTQ989. Lamifiban Hydrochloride

3V0537Z59Q. Suclofenide

3V6I5962EM. Pivopril

3V721R4XYY. Phenyracillin

3V77J79MIF. Bisorcic

3VOW3G2JQC. Droxacin Sodium (See also *6XMB0871VB*)

3VPX99Q2D7. Iprotiazem

3VY58MWL7J. Pimetremide

3VZ2833V08. Fispemifene

3W0M245736. Betamipron

3W1JG795YI. Sunflower Oil

3W58ITX06Q. Vinylbital

3W7L15V40W. Revatropate

3W85193GZ4. Pifarnine

3WD5400T9N. Dichlorophenarsine Hydrochloride [dichlorophenarsine] (See also *571850CM3R*)

3X11EVM5SU. Loracarbef

3X6SAX83JZ. Ziprasidone Mesylate

3X7931PO74. Hydrocortisone Acetate

3XC8GUZ6CB. Sulfasalazine

3XJY028PJZ. Diprotrizoate Sodium (See also *3CD7R3856C*)

3XMK78S47O. Testosterone

3XQ12NYC0Q. Apalcillin Sodium

3Y1OT3J4NW. Rosoxacin

3YFV00531K. Lintitript

3YN0602W4W. Semagacestat

3YU9TET43B. Zoloperone

3YUZ4494BQ. Cefempidone

3YY13B9G25. Abitesartan

3Z3037LJTC. Licostinel

3Z6W3S36X5. Fomivirsen Sodium

3Z8479ZZ5X. Epirubicin Hydrochloride [epirubicin] (See also *22966TX7J5*)

3Z9Y7UWC1J. Apixaban

3ZLI4719J9. Cinmetacin

3ZZ5BJ9F2Q. Difenoxin

4006BCR8NJ. Burodiline

40257685LM. Azidamfenicol

403FO0NQG3. Benfluorex

403J23EMFA. Sodium Feredetate

4058H365ZB. Fiacitabine

406PGU9KGI. Etoprine

40755Z8956. Abaperidone

407JU2B9IS. Piperphenidol Hydrochloride

40AX66P76P. Atracurium Besylate

40D3SCR4GZ. Buprenorphine Hydrochloride [buprenorphine] (See also *56W8MW3EN1*)

40DK034DRC. Clentiazem Maleate [clentiazem]

40FH6D8CHK. Abacavir Succinate (See also *WR2TIP26VS*)

40JL785VD0. Cilansetron Hydrochloride

40P7XK9392. Flumazenil

40Q4C3O4V0. Ftivazide

40S1VHN69B. Bleomycin Sulfate [bleomycin] (See also *7DP3NTV15T*)

40SGR63TGL. Minodronic Acid

40SR2754GL. Ditophal

40X2P7DPGH. Ebselen

40Z22S8DO8. Ditercalinium Chloride

40ZTP2T37Q. Efonidipine (See also *3BR983K69O*)

411OG24QOU. Dinazafone

41391O1OAY2. Cyclandelate

413KH5ZJ73. Rosuvastatin Calcium [rosuvastatin] (See also *83MVU38M7Q*)

414P5USJ7F. Parethoxycaine Hydrochloride

4150VMF5EP. Capromorelin Tartrate

4155989DN5. Geroquinol

41622NK45V. Carburazepam

416P10SE9G. Fenfluthrin

41728CY7UX. Magnesium Salicylate

4182431BJH. Phenytoin Sodium

418546MT3A. Befunolol

418M5916WG. Chloral Hydrate

419A0R564U. Elopiprazole

41A1FCW148. Prethcamide

41KZS5432U. Aminobenzoate Potassium

41T4OAG59U. Aleglitazar

41VRH5220H. Paroxetine

41X3PWK4O2. Nateglinide

41X4FOR202. Troquidazole

41Z22TQD48. Cloracetadol

420HD787N9. Lazabemide

420IP921MB. Edetate Trisodium (See also *9G34HU7RV0*)

421105KRQE. Delavirdine Mesylate (See also *DOL5F9JD3E*)

421KAV3DHT. Edetate Dipotassium

42255P5X4D. Potassium Perchlorate

422L8173W8. Quinestradol

423D2T571U. Ethinyl Estradiol

423W026MA9. Amcinonide

42445HUU0O. Iclaprim

424DV0807X. Epalrestat

426QFE7XLK. Omeprazole Magnesium

426X066ELK. Forodesine

426X066ELK. Forodesine Hydrochloride [forodesine] (See also *6SN82Y9U73*)

427L2I2KIM. Senazodan

42932X67B5. Sodium Dichloroacetate

4293LHY68W. Xenyhexenic Acid

429ZT169UH. Acetazolamide Sodium

42B4PDY0AV. Adiphenine Hydrochloride

42BB1Y2586. Levomepromazine Hydrochloride

42C50P12AP. Chlophedianol Hydrochloride [chlophedianol] (See also *69QQ58998Y*)

42HK56048U. Tyrosine

42MB94QOSM. Emedastine Difumarate (See also *9J1H7Y9OJV*)

42O8UF5CJB. Fasoracetam

42R9MZG1DL. Cloxestradiol

42VPJ2980S. Proquazone

431LFF7I7J. Cephapirin Sodium

4326S15UIP. Linogliride Fumarate

432SI047GA. Eterobarb

433YPU24B8. Cetaben Sodium (See also *DTL5W0113X*)

4343OEZ18O. Allylprodine

43477QYX3D. Dexetimide

43502P7F0P. Methylprednisolone Acetate

436O5HM03C. Dihydroergotamine Mesylate [dihydroergotamine] (See also *81AXN7R2QT*)

436XK6QFMR. Quinazosin Hydrochloride [quinazosin] (See also *2N2LI66RRO*)

43A07PH183. Taurosteine

43DWT87QT7. Benzphetamine Hydrochloride (See also *0M3S43XK27*)

43K1W2T1M6. Interferon Alfa-2b

43S5D07K8G. Imafen Hydrochloride [imafen] (See also *W0X9P59ZQU*)

43SK4LAO7D. Racephedrine Hydrochloride

43VU4207NW. Chloramphenicol Palmitate

43XK6AW58D. Azamethonium Bromide [azamethonium] (See also *4K6NEI0MSR*)

43Y000U234. Raltegravir Potassium (See also *22VKV8053U*)

44413I5098G. Etebenecid

4419T9MX03. Iohexol

44277I316G. Timcodar Dimesylate

443O19GK1A. Guanabenz Acetate

4455J9277Q. Bibenzonium Bromide (See also *34YTZ517S2*)

445J9K442Z. Nesosteine

446254H55G. Croconazole

44665V00O8. Protriptyline Hydrochloride (See also *4NDU154T12*)

446VQG66LC. Zidometacin

448AZ21I6G. Fenoctimine Sulfate (See also *B45CF873F8*)

449NCX1P03. Etolorex

44EH625IUS. Laflunimus

44JHK6G39Q. Icomucret

44NWV6A237. Midaglizole

44P98H0A27. Cefrotil

44RAL3456C. Methamphetamine Hydrochloride [methamphetamine] (See also *997F43Z9CV*)

44YRR34555. Levetiracetam

45081SG6XT. Napirimus

451IFR0GXB. Scopolamine Hydrobromide (See also *DL48G20X8X*)

451W47IQ8X. Sodium Chloride

452VLY9402. Serine

4532264KW6. Nimetazepam

4550K0SC9B. Sodium Acetate

455E0S048W. Quinethazone

455Y914AKK. Tinabinol

45683D94EU. Azaconazole

456V4159SL. Teroxirone

458VC51857. Tegaserod

459384H98V. Zonisamide

45CO7XIN2K. Pralidoxime Mesylate

45I14D8O27. Choline Chloride

45P3261C7T. Sodium Carbonate

45PG892GO1. Evans Blue

45Q1DF53NN. Tiospirone Hydrochloride (See also *35C6UMO5SR*)

45S5605Q18. Cilostamide

45SJ093Q1N. Zolazepam Hydrochloride

45ZFO9E525. Dibekacin

463O18JU8V. Naepaine Hydrochloride

46475LV84I. Aptiganel Hydrochloride [aptiganel]

465N7P5U85. Nifuroxime

4661WA7OCU. Triclazate

46627O600J. Levodopa

467LU0UCUW. Sarizotan Hydrochloride [sarizotan] (See also *5P71E6YO9H*)

4685R51V7M. Esmirtazapine

468GE2241L. Propiverine

469GW8R486. Bromisovalum

469ULX0H4G. Nimorazole

46C1PX266N. Bufrolin

46HL4I09AH. Glafenine

46LG9K0Y24. Mobecarb

46QG38NC4U. Ethotoin

46V3V5EQAM. Etocarlide

46VZA7RX2B. Meclocycline Sulfosalicylate

46X4C9TILS. Dimoxyline

470XML6G45. Terbuficin

471LF4O004. Spiramide

4728AWF76J. Pituxate

4743XI19RY. Pareptide Sulfate [pareptide]

47602X79JF. Bifluranol

4784C8E03O. Triclabendazole

4791MN0PVE. Fubrogonium Iodide

4797W6I0T4. Carteolol Hydrochloride (See also *8NF31401XG*)

47E5O17Y3R. Phenylalanine

47ISU063SG. Zuclopenthixol

47JUM7D622. Fuprazole

47M74X9YT5. Cladribine

47RRR83SK7. Interferon Alfa-2a

47RU9546DX. Bephenium Hydroxynaphthoate

47UDJ8GA54. Oxetacillin

47XBA61Y31. Guanoxyfen Sulfate (See also *03HN50ZAF0*)

47Y56T6LEI. Rilmakalim

4805237NP5. Butoconazole Nitrate

4818HEA280. Perflubrodec

481GSD6F7Q. Danosteine

482M43SL0K. Oximonam

4839MB71E7. Nicofibrate

4846Q921YM. Calcium Sulfate [calcium sulfate dihydrate] (See also *WAT0DDB505*)

4858SN190E. Caramiphen Hydrochloride

4868V9LSKR. Furomazine

48854OTZ5E. Lecozotan Hydrochloride [lecozotan] (See also *23EDE20K1X*)

4888ME6C4E. Robenidine Hydrochloride [robenidine] (See also *8STT15Y392*)

48A5M73Z4Q. Atorvastatin Calcium (See also *A0JWA85V8F*)

48BX75B06D. Adatanserin Hydrochloride

48G1L28581. Dirucotide Acetate

48I5LU4ZWD. Meclofenamate Sodium [meclofenamic acid] (See also *94NJ818U2W*)

48I5LU4ZWD. Meclofenamic Acid

48IJA0E92C. Ifetroban Sodium

48N6U1781G. Sodium Phenylacetate

48P711MI2G. Dasantafil

48RW3M5575. Bisdequalinium Diacetate

48SPP0PA9Q. Cefotetan

48TCX9A1VT. Cystine

48TI67E57Q. Ecopladib

48U51W007F. Sulfamethazine

49030P3C8S. Benfosformin

490D9F069T. Lanthanum Carbonate

490DW6501Y. Alcuronium Chloride

4953C873N2. Nivimedone Sodium

4956DJR58O. Mecamylamine Hydrochloride (See also *6EE945-D3OK*)

495W7451VQ. Guaifenesin

4964P6T9RB. Aldosterone

4965G3J0F5. Sulfacetamide

4966RNG0BU. Tacrine Hydrochloride (See also *4VX7YNB537*)

49717AWG6K. Ribavirin

4975G9NM6T. Entacapone

497A17OUUE. Pemirolast Potassium (See also *2C09NV773M*)

499H4332KZ. Ipsalazide

499L7I0905. Benzquercin

49AB2PA48B. Talastine

49BR7256ZY. Quatacaine

49DCB7156W. Bipenamol Hydrochloride [bipenamol]

49DG2B481W. Sulfadimethoxine Sodium

49EEF6HRUS. Brequinar Sodium (See also *5XL19F49H6*)

49G3001BCK. Nafcillin Sodium (See also *4CNZ27M7RV*)

49HFB70472. Ximelagatran

49K58SMZ7U. Betahistine Hydrochloride

49NMI30XY2. Brosotamide

49S4O7ADLC. Lafutidine

49Y44QZL70. Thiopental Sodium (See also *JI8Z5M7NA3*)

49YNN75I8N. Buquiterine

4A3O49NGEZ. Oseltamivir Phosphate

4A3T9Z2TKX. Decominol

4A5352XI2A. Clobenzorex

4AF302ESOS. Ondansetron

4ALN5933BH. Arecoline Hydrobromide [arecoline] (See also *24S79B9CX7*)

4AO61I7SLB. Tomoglumide

4AOV43246G. Divaplon

4AW7F70MZO. Dimiracetam

4AZ2V8K4EK. Clefamide

4AZC6Y5A8G. Butofilolol

4B3SC438HI. Methylphenidate Hydrochloride

4B9XT59T7S. Zidovudine

4BA73M5E37. Ciprofloxacin Hydrochloride

4BMH7IZT98. Choline Fenofibrate

4BOC774388. Framycetin

4BXX0XNP9R. Azacyclonol Hydrochloride

4C5I4BQZ8F. Glymidine Sodium [glymidine]

4C9310B127. Eprovafen

4CNZ27M7RV. Nafcillin Sodium [nafcillin] (See also *49G3001BCK*)

4CZ1R38NDI. Pazufloxacin

4D4NC8MXLW. Dimecolonium Iodide

4D5D3422MW. Cefcapene

4D65PBX0VK. Dimenoxadol

4DN0TK4892. Belaperidone

4DN3AF1FU6. Noxytiolin

4DQ6T10R64. Revaprazan Hydrochloride (See also *5P184180P5*)

4E07GXB7AU. Desoximetasone

4E1MIA8QQL. Ceruletide Diethylamine

4E53T3611U. Bitolterol Mesylate (See also *9KY0QXD6LI*)

4E7858311F. Lanoconazole

4EAR229231. Bedoradrine Sulfate [bedoradrine] (See also *P875C0DV2V*)

4EVE5946BQ. Ketorolac Tromethamine (See also *YZI5105V0L*)

4F05V145YR. Tyropanoate Sodium [tyropanic acid] (See also *XRJ0P5FAYO*)

4F39T8N10K. Irindalone

4F44UQX9EV. Cethexonium Chloride

4F4L1E450W. Tixadil

4F4X42SYQ6. Rituximab

4F61F502T5. Dembrexine

4F86W47BR6. Raloxifene Hydrochloride (See also *YX9162EO3I*)

4F8YJZ690M. Iotranic Acid

4FA88HM3IX. Clortermine Hydrochloride [clortermine]

4FB1TON47A. Naftifine Hydrochloride [naftifine] (See also *25UR9N9041*)

4FBV0WY9OG. Domazoline Fumarate [domazoline] (See also *TQ4H2AG3JI*)

4FT78T86XV. Insulin Detemir

4G278XM8KC. Tolpentamide

4G4Z4676IS. Buciclovir

4G7DS2Q64Y. Progesterone

4G86N0SVV3. Lonaprofen

4GDQ854U53. Elvitegravir

4GY0AVT3L4. Tanespimycin

4H2LVB8X5O. Ioxotrizoic Acid

4H4JU6738Q. Clamidoxic Acid

4H75PAD8M3. Befloxatone

4H914M0CSP. Laquinimod Sodium (See also *908SY76S4G*)

4HZT2V9KX0. Dicloxacillin Sodium (See also *COF19H7WBK*)

4I5PG5VZ0V. Butopyronoxyl

4I8HAB65SZ. Nisoldipine

4I933V848G. Butanserin

4IHY34Y2NV. Iguratimod

4IU6VSV0EI. Chloramine-T

4J8I18ZP0A. Pelanserin Hydrochloride (See also *6SNR96E409*)

4J9726V5Y9. Lefetamine

4JB9426X1H. Pranosal

4JR41A10VP. Mizoribine

4JVD4X01MJ. Imidazole Salicylate

4K04IQ1OF4. Epoprostenol Sodium (See also *DCR9Z582X0*)

4K6NEI0MSR. Azamethonium Bromide (See also *43XK6AW58D*)

4K8KA8B61G. Repirinast

4KA5WHL8T2. Ecabapide

4KGX1STY2N. Rocepafant

4KV4X8IF6V. Dicyclomine Hydrochloride [dicyclomine] (See also *CQ903KQA31*)

4L066368AS. Fluvastatin Sodium [fluvastatin] (See also *PYF7O1FV7F*)

4L219Q1D16. Salazodine

4L6452S749. Inositol

4L6L92S51P. Dicolinium Iodide

4LJK511Z86. Gallium Citrate Ga 67

4M16098280. Balaglitazone

4MG6O8991R. Retapamulin

4MT4VIE29P. Atazanavir Sulfate (See also *QZU4H47A3S*)

4MYE3XA3GV. Berlafenone

4N3QA02VE5. Amoxecaine

4N7G8A6439. Satranidazole

4N8R018QB0. Ternidazole

4N8UJJ27IM. Perlapine

4NDU154T12. Protriptyline Hydrochloride [protriptyline] (See also *44665V00O8*)

4NH22NDW9H. Eflornithine Hydrochloride (See also *ZQN1G5V6SR*)

4NJ842U6BZ. Azimexon

4NM5039Y5X. Triclosan

4NN21HAX16. Tryparsamide

4NRT660KJQ. Sulfacetamide Sodium

4NW20GFQ7H. Iodohippurate Sodium I 123

4O4S742ANY. Escitalopram

4O5J85GJJB. Netilmicin Sulfate [netilmicin] (See also *S741ZJS97U*)

4OUL81K2RT. Carbenicillin Indanyl Sodium

4P3T9QF9NZ. Valganciclovir Hydrochloride (See also *GCU97FKN3R*)

4P63B997RT. Amphomycin

4PG8A6UTDX. Tiacrilast Sodium

4POG0RL69O. Benzbromarone

4Q13LY9Z8X. Methdilazine

4Q13LY9Z8X. Methdilazine Hydrochloride [methdilazine] (See also *T0GSO02UEZ*)

4Q1Q4V31K8. Medazomide

4Q52C550XK. Ibritumomab Tiuxetan

4Q81I59GXC. Mesalamine

4Q9N876YAJ. Butylphenamide

4QD397987E. Histidine

4QIH0N49E7. Pyrantel Tartrate [pyrantel]

4QWG6N8QKH. Hydroxychloroquine Sulfate [hydroxychloroquine] (See also *8Q2869CNVH*)

4QWV355536. Drofenine

4R1VB9P8V3. Stanozolol

4R5TV783X3. Cefetamet

4R73K9MRMX. Oxymesterone

4RII332OO R. Iodamide

4RII332OO R. Iodamide Meglumine [iodamide] (See also *6X283535A3; 6HG8UB2MUY*)

4RZ82L2GY5. Acetohydroxamic Acid

4S9081543Q. Ferpifosate Sodium

4S9CL2DY2H. Brimonidine Tartrate (See also *E6GNX3HHTE*)

4SDY4L68FP. Darenzepine

4SH0MFJ5HJ. Carbetapentane Citrate

4SYH0R661F. Pramiconazole

4T6H12BN9U. Petrolatum, White

4TI98Z838E. Estradiol

4U07F515LG. Eltrombopag Olamine (See also *S56D65XJ9G*)

4U1WVN6KUX. Phenaphthazine

4U5MP5IUD8. Niflumic Acid

4U7K4N52ZM. Oxytetracycline Hydrochloride (See also *X20I9EN955*)

4UQ3S81B25. Piboserod Hydrochloride [piboserod] (See also *61Z0VMM0AJ*)

4UWR086NOA. Alletorphine

4V3R166MB3. Carubicin Hydrochloride

4V44H1O8XI. Oxyphencyclimine Hydrochloride [oxyphencyclimine] (See also *GWO1432WOU*)

4V7M9137X9. Gabexate

4V7NMO33X6. Esculamine

4V9P667Y2G. Mocetinostat Dihydrobromide

4VD83UL6Y6. Kebuzone

4VFX2L7EM5. Mepivacaine Hydrochloride (See also *B6E06QE59J*)

4VX7YNB537. Tacrine Hydrochloride [tacrine] (See also *4966RNG0BU*)

4W0459ZA4V. Cefprozil

4W2P15D93M. Bepridil Hydrochloride

4W5HDS3936. Melengestrol Acetate

4W5IH7FLNY. Dibutyl Sebacate

4W9K63FION. Dextrothyroxine Sodium [dextrothyroxine] (See also *0H00N2AHSP*)

4WCI67NK8M. Thioridazine Hydrochloride

4WCY05C0SJ. Quipazine Maleate [quipazine] (See also *JY444CK9IG*)

4WQQ18VL49. Atilmotin

4X6E73CJ0Q. Spiperone

4X7Y0185J3. Bamnidazole

4XDY25L70B. Hydrocortisone Cypionate

4XE0U1P5FJ. Edifolone Acetate [edifolone] (See also *043L86G83X*)

4XKL2JJ08I. Alfaprostol

4XO7A09HQM. Fomocaine

4XRL9PL02Y. Pibutidine

4XS533X38C. Betameprodine

4XV7PTW3FZ. Dipiproverine Hydrochloride [dipiproverine] (See also *8UYY5B89ZU*)

4Y5P7MUD51. Octinoxate

4Y7UR6X2PO. Aranidipine

4YC2PY3AEU. Picloxydine

4YIR8202AX. Talbutal

4YK5Z54AT2. Denatonium Benzoate

4YSI0ZY4W9. Sulfaloxic Acid

4Z8R6ORS6L. Thalidomide

4Z8Y51M438. Procaine Borate [procaine]

4ZSF6GBG5S. Nisbuterol Mesylate

4ZXX17M1C4. Clopipazan Mesylate

5015H744JQ. Altanserin Tartrate [altanserin] (See also *9P204CHE8J*)

5018V4AEZ0. Bosutinib

501CFL162R. Hydroflumethiazide

501W00OOWA. Tarenflurbil

502FWN4Q32. Aliskiren

502H53WMM0. Quinuclium Bromide

504LR309YV. Sulnidazole

504R182ZX7. Apovincamine

504RN634MM. Ketotrexate

505434F98H. Capobenate Sodium

506T60A25R. Sorbitol

508ISH42Z9. Bolazine

509F88P9SZ. Permethrin

50D9XSG0VR. Mechlorethamine Hydrochloride [mechlorethamine] (See also *L0MR697HHI*)

50FH5AG9RW. Betamethasone Butyrate Propionate

50LQB69S1Z. Hydrocortisone Sodium Succinate

50LV9A548L. Lodoxamide Tromethamine (See also *SPU695OD73*)

50MD4SB4AP. Ciclopirox Olamine

50Q2Q042YR. Fosopamine

50SG953SK6. Mitomycin

50SZ4782J0. Atiprosin Maleate

50U0Z120RS. Nivazol

50VV3VW0TI. Atenolol

50Z1JVP72H. Antienite

51086HBW8G. Rizatriptan Benzoate [rizatriptan] (See also *WR978S7QHH*)

510M006KO6. Eltoprazine

511IU0826Z. Hexylcaine Hydrochloride [hexylcaine] (See also *V00NQ7SDYI*)

5123Q291S5. Pirdonium Bromide

51567MYG7V. Prodipine

515DHK15LG. Alrestatin Sodium [alrestatin] (See also *018XNU6812*)

519JDS089K. Broquinaldol

519MXN9YZR. Oxprenolol Hydrochloride [oxprenolol] (See also *F4XSI7SNIU*)

51AC49OLT7. Dichloroxylenol

51FOB87G3I. Ambenonium Chloride

51G6I8B902. Nilutamide

51HX72H34H. Aliconazole

51K3U6Q5ZN. Doreptide

51KFT71THG. Meseclazone

51V8U784H3. Isoetharine Hydrochloride (See also *YV0SN3276Q*)

520P4U8V2Z. Chlorproethazine Hydrochloride

5216EI628Q. Tacapenem

5253IGO5X3. Liranaftate

526U7A2651. Egtazic Acid

5286RBZ882. Pinazepam

5288I2K01S. Molfarnate

528XYJ8L1N. Etoposide Phosphate

52915ASM3D. Nestifylline

52936SIP7V. Phenyl Aminosalicylate

534I52PVWH. Decoquinate

5361814USE. Beclinazole

539M941Y9O. Neocinchophen

53A5V9FGN9. Paraflutizide

53C97244OY. Oxoprostol

53EY29W7EC. Miltefosine

53IEF47846. Acadesine

53J8I8O5EW. Hydroxydione Sodium Succinate

53PC6LO35W. Radezolid

53T7IN77LC. Fialuridine

53X71X3I1W. Carpipramine Dihydrochloride

5402501F0W. Pipamperone

541C7WS64R. Clorindione

541ZDL2E7U. Vanyldisulfamide

5428WXZ74M. Cilastatin Sodium (See also *141A6AMN38*)

543567RFQQ. Cycrimine Hydrochloride [cycrimine] (See also *9RB4L4K895*)

5437O7N5BH. Cinoxate

54473012UK. Sepazonium Chloride

544MD72T3H. Cloximate

544Y3D6MYH. Amoxicillin Sodium

5458S22S8I. Fenclorac

545MN0F125. Proflazepam

546994B3VA. Amiprilose Hydrochloride (See also *S0FG5X68QT*)

5491IVP21O. Dribendazole

54978VNA4T. Pirozadil

549TIC7B4R. Lorapride

54CA01C6JX. Diphenadione

54I81H0M9C. Amdoxovir

54N4UY1C7C. Protoporphyrin Disodium

54T0T0F4O2. Nifuroquine

5504169OQ8. Dofamium Chloride

551ME47I15. Dropempine

55408BLV3G. Fenamifuril
554Z48XN5E. Methimazole
555ERF3D9O. Nitrafudam Hydrochloride
556OP2G5M2. Mindoperone
55772LJ01V. Proligestone
5587267Z69. Domperidone
55B9HQY616. Pergolide Mesylate (See also *24MJ822NZ9*)
55C6RK944K. Decamethonium Bromide
55F75LJQ0V. Anamorelin Hydrochloride
55JG375S6M. Pregabalin
55P9TUL75S. Isoflupredone Acetate (See also *HYS0B45Z2S*)
55QM6Y09ZY. Bometolol
55TIT7J81D. Ozolinone
55X04QC32I. Sodium Hydroxide
56203T2K2X. Aluminum Clofibrate
562PDC2I9K. Hydrastine Hydrochloride
562RS6MC22. Cyanocobalamin Co 60
563KS2PQY5. Lacosamide
56588OP40D. Interferon Alfacon-1
5688UTC01R. Tretinoin
568ET80C3D. Calcium Pantothenate (See also *19F5HK2737*)
56B0591Y76. Sufotidine
56C9DTE69V. Flurithromycin
56G228IW9Q. Altoqualine
56LH93261Y. Methyldopa
56PE10F2EA. Salazosulfathiazole
56PPJ9MMPE. Cephradine [cephradine dihydrate] (See also
    F1BC02I72W)
56QH73D78K. Primidolol
56U7906FQW. Ganirelix Acetate
56W8MW3EN1. Buprenorphine Hydrochloride (See also
    40D3SCR4GZ)
56X54T817Q. Corticorelin Ovine Triflutate
571850CM3R. Dichlorophenarsine Hydrochloride (See also
    3WD5400T9N)
5726CF21KY. Peraquinsin
5743F6U086. Cinoquidox
5748P7L6IT. Cresotamide
576PU70Y8E. Terbutaline Sulfate (See also *N8ONU3L3PG*)
5776HBV7UD. Biriperone
578389D6D0. Clove Oil
578H0RMP25. Dirlotapide
57ANR1Z628. Betamethadol
57DQA39DO2. Bemegride
57F7CWY79K. Flualamide
57G776P4EJ. Morsuximide
57GNO57U7G. Finasteride
57O5S1QSAQ. Rolapitant Hydrochloride
57OWB0Q221. Sulfoxone Sodium (See also *0G3C18OH4D*)
57U5YI11WP. Chlorphenesin Carbamate
57WA9QZ5WH. Nimodipine
57WVB6I2W0. Atomoxetine Hydrochloride
57Y76R9ATQ. Naproxen
57Y76R9ATQ. Naproxen Sodium [naproxen] (See also
    9TN87S3A3C)
580655Z8RR. Mephentermine Sulfate (See also *TEZ91L71V4*)
5816OWJ81W. Valtorcitabine Dihydrochloride
5829E3D9I9. Fosmidomycin
582ILN204B. Clofenamide
58447S8P4L. Mafenide
58447S8P4L. Mafenide Hydrochloride [mafenide]
584A0O55XM. Clofeverine
584QS921R2. Cimemoxin
588N0603CT. Levisoprenaline
588X2YUY0A. Methylene Chloride
58FQD093NU. Buclizine Hydrochloride (See also *0C94V6X681*)
58H6RWO52I. Bacitracin

58H6RWO52I. Bacitracin Zinc [bacitracin] (See also
    89Y4M234ES)
58IFB293JI. Vorinostat
58NL35I27K. Benrixate
58SRQ4DV53. Fenclozic Acid
5909OF92EF. Fluzoperine
59375N1D0U. Acamprosate Calcium
5948VUI423. Elagolix Sodium
595CNE7RHB. Bolandiol Dipropionate
595EG71R3F. Benactyzine (See also *26R628272Q*)
595T4D0KQ3. Rilopirox
5965120SH1. Minoxidil
5968Y6H45M. Entecavir (See also *NNU2O4609D*)
5970HH9923. Mafosfamide
59762X5CLS. Tomelukast
5985O24GLM. Safrazine Hydrochloride
59AAO5F6HT. Fennel Oil
59H17J9F1B. Phencarbamide
59H4FCV1TF. Nefazodone Hydrochloride [nefazodone] (See also
    27X63J94GR)
59IG47SZ0E. Hydroxyamphetamine Hydrobromide (See also
    FQR280JW2N)
59JV96YTXV. Midodrine Hydrochloride (See also
    6YE7PBM15H)
59L7Y0530C. Toceranib
59NEE7PCAB. Lindane
59UA429E5G. Galsulfase
59X5ME2O06. Trifenagrel
59XE10C19C. Fusidate Sodium [fusidic acid] (See also
    J7P3696BCQ)
59XE10C19C. Fusidic Acid
59XN63C8VM. Magnesium Chloride [magnesium chloride anhy-
    drous] (See also *02F3473H9O*)
5A9SS67K16. Buzepide Metiodide
5AEP5YJ9MZ. Pafenolol
5AIJ4TGC6B. Sitamaquine
5APW73W3QZ. Moxalactam Disodium (See also *VUF6C936Z3*)
5AR83PR647. Razoxane
5ASJ6HUZ7D. Doxepin Hydrochloride [doxepin] (See also
    3U9A0FE9N5)
5B2546MB5Z. Elagolix
5B2658E0N2. Aminosalicylic Acid
5B266B85J1. Epithiazide
5B307S63B2. Beclomethasone Dipropionate (See also
    KGZ1SLC28Z)
5B3OM8452C. Pheniprazine Hydrochloride
5BF646324K. Vinflunine
5BF646324K. Vinflunine Ditartrate [vinflunine] (See also
    33MG53C7XW)
5BZF8S8IL5. Octacaine
5C0K1GQB2L. Domoxin
5C193VF4V3. Amindocate
5C5403N26O. Acacia
5C8KR48J61. Mepramidil
5C90PJN6E5. Ethoxazene Hydrochloride
5CA81DKM2L. Brindoxime
5CHW4JMR82. Propacetamol
5CKP8C2LLI. Cefamandole
5CKP8C2LLI. Cefamandole Nafate [cefamandole] (See also
    8HDO7941DO)
5COW40EV8M. Vesnarinone
5CYU0D0S8M. Flucindole
5D06587D6R. Palonosetron Hydrochloride [palonosetron] (See
    also *23310D4I19*)
5D1IB9AI6J. Dobutamine Tartrate
5D7022962A. Tofimilast
5D9HAA5Q5S. Sulconazole Nitrate [sulconazole] (See also
    1T89100D5U)

5DS173ODI4. Alemcinal
5DX9U76296. Vatalanib
5DXM29256P. Leptacline
5E4UI00UQJ. Siguazodan
5E7U48495E. Albiglutide
5E8K9I0O4U. Ciprofloxacin
5EOG8KQT0Y. Sulisatin
5EP74J9Q34. Imazodan Hydrochloride
5F8F2A90IA. Tipetropium Bromide
5FCH6YDY7Z. Eribaxaban
5FD1131I7S. Azithromycin [azithromycin dihydrate] (See also
    F94OW58Y8V; JTE4MNN1MD)
5FQG9774WD. Cefoperazone Sodium (See also *7U75I1278D*)
5G117T0TJZ. Khellin
5G2K7O5D8S. Flutazolam
5GF4B2I1DD. Acetrizoate Sodium
5GRO578KLP. Flurbiprofen
5H7I2IP58X. Boldenone Undecylenate [boldenone]
5H8F175RER. Mebutamate
5I159322PY. Chlorphenoxamine Hydrochloride
5I2Y40C5PX. Darbufelone Mesylate
5IAD0UV3FH. Pefloxacin Mesylate
5IE62321P4. Gramicidin
5IEH2KC4M6. Zalospirone Hydrochloride
5J49Q6B70F. Vincristine Sulfate [vincristine] (See also
    T5IRO3534A)
5J7C4JZ564. Plafibride
5J9CPU3RE0. Furazolidone
5JU4C2L5A0. Ferrous Lactate
5K0215OMQX. Dulofibrate
5K8EAX0G53. Tramiprosate
5K8WKN668K. Aminothiazole
5KN5Y9V01K. Levomepromazine Maleate
5KP3ZO1VLL. Bendacalol Mesylate (See also *BQ0I558X42*)
5KV86114PT. Monoethanolamine
5L0HB4V1EW. Carglumic Acid
5L16LKN964. Aniracetam
5L5GE3DV88. Triciribine Phosphate
5L7E7IY5EH. Dithiazanine Iodide [dithiazanine] (See also *8OE-*
    C3RA07X)
5LGN83G74V. Fluvoxamine Maleate (See also *O4L1XPO44W*)
5M64643B5U. Epicriptine
5M691HL4BO. Glatiramer Acetate
5M7Y6274ZE. Phenindione
5MB73H1ADH. Samixogrel
5ML58O200F. Ilepcimide
5MZ70CT96H. Bamaquimast
5N2K83R1L2. Fexicaine
5NC67NU76B. Mephobarbital
5NF5D4OPCI. Tetracaine Hydrochloride
5NPJ6BPX36. Propyliodone
5O564RN1QD. Creatinolfosfate
5O5U71P6VQ. Linsidomine
5O8R96XMH7. Vardenafil Dihydrochloride
5OFI9D9892. Dexecadotril
5OK523O4FU. Faropenem Medoxomil (See also *F52Y83BGH3*)
5OO7RKH9WL. Oxpheneridine
5OPO851W5L. Pargolol
5P184180P5. Revaprazan Hydrochloride [revaprazan] (See also
    4DQ6T10R64)
5P41KX11BT. Temodox
5P4DHS6ENR. Benzonatate
5P71E6YO9H. Sarizotan Hydrochloride (See also *467LU0U-*
    CUW)
5P7U986QGO. Feclemine
5P8VJ2I235. Arformoterol Tartrate (See also *F91H02EBWT*)
5PC250KSSH. Denufosol Tetrasodium [denufosol]
5PE5HV9NF0. Arteflene

5PE9FDE8GB. Clonazepam
5Q0Y96D5I8. Thiophanate
5Q36UVB8YA. Apadoline
5Q52X6ICJI. Bendroflumethiazide
5Q6TZN2HNM. Ecallantide
5QB0T2IUN0. Aluminum Hydroxide
5QH19BF6YG. Mefenidil Fumarate
5QTH9UHV0K. Dipivefrin Hydrochloride
5QZO15J2Z8. Famotidine
5R003655CR. Medrylamine
5R5W9ICI6O. Demeclocycline
5R5W9ICI6O. Demeclocycline Hydrochloride [demeclocycline]
    (See also *29O079NTYT*)
5R6712AY0K. Tetroxoprim
5R72CHP32S. Pardoprunox
5R78837D4A. Strontium Chloride Sr 89
5R97F5H93P. Estradiol Acetate
5RS1CY853F. Roxoperone
5RXY50Q01N. Oxabolone Cipionate
5S0W860XNR. Amprenavir
5S29HWU6QB. Cinnamon
5S6W795CQM. Naltrexone
5SEH9X1D1D. Ethosuximide
5SPW497X0Z. Levlofexidine
5SYZ8I05SH. Oxetorone Fumarate
5T619TQR3R. Tolterodine Tartrate
5T62Q3B36J. Sorafenib Tosylate
5T97333YZK. Ceftobiprole
5TAA004E22. Sargramostim
5TL50QU0W4. Peanut Oil
5TPM2EB426. Ertiprotafib
5TU5227KYQ. Amifloxacin
5TU5227KYQ. Amifloxacin Mesylate [amifloxacin] (See also
    2C21AN130I)
5U7IO9CV80. Azumolene Sodium [azumolene] (See also
    ISB31HSB8H)
5U85DBW7LO. Escitalopram Oxalate
5UBY8Y002G. Guanethidine Monosulfate (See also
    ZTI6C33Q2Q)
5UL276H6TF. Clemizole Penicillin
5UNK5C6QM5. Cetamolol Hydrochloride
5UTX5635HP. Oxyquinoline
5UTX5635HP. Oxyquinoline Sulfate [oxyquinoline] (See also
    61VUG75Y3P)
5UVC90J1LK. Diatrizoate Sodium [diatrizoic acid]
5UVC90J1LK. Diatrizoic Acid
5UX2SD1KE2. Cysteamine
5V141XK28X. Acemetacin
5V444H5WIC. Remifentanil Hydrochloride (See also
    P10582JYYK)
5V5IOJ8338. Pyridoxal Phosphate
5V71D8JOKK. Fazarabine
5V9KLZ54CY. Vinblastine Sulfate [vinblastine] (See also
    N00W22YO2B)
5VI1D4HYXC. Mindodilol
5VO597V509. Itameline
5VOM6GYJ0D. Valproate Sodium (See also *614OI1Z5WI*)
5VT6420TIG. Oteracil
5VV3MDU5IE. Idarubicin Hydrochloride (See also
    ZRP63D75JW)
5VZ26183XG. Sulocarbilate
5VZ7GZM43E. Nifekalant
5W494URQ81. Streptozocin
5W6YA9PKKH. Indinavir (See also *9MG78X43ZT*)
5W7SIA7YZW. Levonorgestrel
5W8JGG2651. Idursulfase
5WF7E9QC3F. Morantel Tartrate (See also *7NJ031HAX5*)
5WGM277OKR. Promolate

5WZ53ENE2P. Barbital

5WZ53ENE2P. Barbital Sodium [barbital] (See also *275L5M93QS*)

5X0D9H16IU. Eprodisate Disodium

5X4V82ZN30. Furaltadone

5X5HB3VZ3Z. Apricoxib

5X93W9OFZL. Drometrizole

5XE4NWM740. Mesoridazine

5XE7IWD0JX. Diprobutine

5XL19F49H6. Brequinar Sodium [brequinar] (See also *49EEF6H-RUS*)

5Y1CNW44Y5. Delmitide Acetate

5Y2EI94NBC. Oxymorphone Hydrochloride (See also *9VXA968E0C*)

5Y48085P9Q. Aprindine

5Y48085P9Q. Aprindine Hydrochloride [aprindine] (See also *PB5EKT7Q2V*)

5Y5F15120W. Protirelin

5Y9L3636O3. Mefloquine Hydrochloride

5YGV817KFT. Oxitriptyline

5YVB0POT2H. Chloroprocaine Hydrochloride [chloroprocaine] (See also *LT7Z1YW11H*)

5YZ5R8I73Y. Diperodon Hydrochloride (See also *2456GO94TR*)

5Z48ONN38P. Febarbamate

5Z492UNF9O. Propylene Glycol Diacetate

5Z5TRG74EY. Pivampicillin Pamoate

5Z6E9K79YV. Lithium Citrate

5Z7OO9FNFD. Difloxacin Hydrochloride [difloxacin] (See also *XJ0260HJ0O*)

5ZA2S6B08X. Cetyl Palmitate

5ZFR16F4QQ. Sepimostat

5ZZ84GCW8B. Formoterol Fumarate [formoterol] (See also *P3T5QA5J9N*)

600ZG213C3. Mivacurium Chloride

60158CV180. Nelarabine

60158CV180. Nelzarabine

601OJW5ILI. Cinprazole

601X8G3PCW. Dexnafenodone

60200PNZ7Q. Methohexital Sodium

606D60IS38. Mexiletine Hydrochloride (See also *1U511HHV4Z*)

60J29WG4Q6. Quisultazine

60V9STC53F. Ethylenediamine

60W3249T9M. Artesunate

610T1NWH34. Lucartamide

612K359T69. Alvespimycin Hydrochloride (See also *001L2FE0M3*)

614OI1Z5WI. Valproate Sodium [valproic acid] (See also *5VOM6-GYJ0D*)

614OI1Z5WI. Valproic Acid

6153CWM0CL. Warfarin Sodium

6158TKW0C5. Phenytoin

61AYL7492M. Peralopride

61D5V4OKTP. Demecarium Bromide

61H4T033E5. Orotic Acid

61JJC8N5ZK. Paromomycin Sulfate [paromomycin] (See also *845NU6GJPS*)

61K37E446T. Cefetrizole

61O17612T5. Iodothiouracil

61VUG75Y3P. Oxyquinoline Sulfate (See also *5UTX5635HP*)

61Z0VMM0AJ. Piboserod Hydrochloride (See also *4UQ3S81B25*)

6201E0JIF3. Flamenol

6208ZO6MLG. Revizinone

621BVT9M36. Fenbendazole

6239812J7L. Tosufloxacin [tosufloxacin monohydrate]

623OAC38YU. Dimemorfan

626DQ7N19L. Timiperone

6272R7515Q. Giparmen

62734PD6SM. Sultosilic Acid

62H10A1236. Ethynodiol Diacetate (See also *9E01C36A9S*)

62H4W26906. Bisnafide Dimesylate [bisnafide] (See also *J30IBO0LMA*)

62I3C8233L. Ipecac

62LN840SFZ. Mapinastine

62M960DHIL. Anisotropine Methylbromide

62NWQ924LH. Landiolol

62P526DC98. Desocriptine

62R1A43O49. Adekalant

62TEY51RR1. Bismuth Subsalicylate

62UXS86T64. Salinomycin

62V6QH821R. Argimesna

62VR67FK8E. Cistinexine

6308U1DL5F. Broxaldine

630F8M4Q1D. Etoformin Hydrochloride [etoformin] (See also *19HR3G3ESA*)

6315412YVF. Delafloxacin

631R1KON85. Teopranitol

632S1WU9Z2. Palinavir

632XD903SP. Gallic Acid

6337Z9RO7D. Cianergoline

6375T36951. Epostane

637C487Y09. Golotimod

638D8M316Y. Pirbenicillin Sodium (See also *8ARY01XRYU*)

63937KV33D. Erythromycin

63937KV33D. Erythromycin Estolate [erythromycin] (See also *XRJ2P631HP*)

63937KV33D. Erythromycin Propionate [erythromycin]

63CZ7GJN5I. Allopurinol

63FN7G03XY. Clorazepate Dipotassium (See also *D51WO0G0L4*)

63ISF1PDWX. Azanator Maleate (See also *699725286I*)

63KP7FXF2I. Piperazine Citrate

63M8RYN44N. Water O 15

63POE2M46Y. Elm

63T152J867. Becanthone Hydrochloride

63W7IE88K8. Iodoquinol

6413W06WR3. Choriogonadotropin Alfa

641EDA6X6L. Fenbenicillin

6429L0L52Y. Dipyrone

642I97LB5B. Crotetamide

644VL95AO6. Divalproex Sodium

646WTQ0G3E. Bietamiverine Hydrochloride

6490C9U457. Praziquantel

64ALC7F90C. Dipyridamole

64DXV166PH. Leucinocaine

64FS3BFH5W. Epoetin Alfa

64FS3BFH5W. Epoetin Beta

64FS3BFH5W. Epoetin Delta

64FS3BFH5W. Epoetin Epsilon

64FS3BFH5W. Epoetin Gamma

64FS3BFH5W. Epoetin Omega

64O047KTOA. Cetirizine Hydrochloride (See also *YO7261ME24*)

64O87U613H. Dagapamil

64OO8946ER. Mozenavir

64R4OHP8T0. Hyaluronidase (Ovine)

6502ONO3L0. Piridicillin Sodium [piridicillin] (See also *1Q728MH9P9*)

6513M33209. Andolast

6532B86WFG. Cefonicid Monosodium [cefonicid] (See also *QD9G66C5UF*)

653552FH1N. Pipamazine

653GN04T2G. Etersalate

654G2VCI4Q. Picotamide

655M5O3W0U. Telaprevir

659OIV373Y. Sibenadet Hydrochloride (See also *N32934RHGW*)

65LCB00B4Y. Cloxacillin Sodium

65M2UDR9AG. Etretinate
65NK71K78P. Avizafone
65Q28TV0ZY. Halopemide
65Q4QDG4KC. Rapacuronium Bromide
65UEH262IS. Safflower Oil
65VXC1MH0J. Fluocortolone
660932TPY6. Orbifloxacin
660YQ98I10. Potassium Chloride
66466QLM3S. Bamifylline Hydrochloride (See also
    ZTY15D026H)
66803GMO3G. Pincainide
668QM8QJFS. Tagorizine
668UF07O1P. Carzelesin
668Z8C33LU. Repaglinide
66974FR9Q1. Chloramphenicol
66ABP6C83F. Betazole Hydrochloride (See also 1C065P542O)
66JKK43S1Z. Bentazepam
66K342SF4G. Batelapine Maleate (See also P71TE299SG)
66VLQ6E6DL. Pratosartan
66WBM7N0NM. Trichlormethine
6702D36OG5. Paricalcitol
670P9AQR46. Aganodine
672T0ES47P. Romifenone
6734037O3L. Tesaglitazar
673LC5J4LQ. Pentamidine
677AYV0R9N. Lozilurea
677C126AET. Alvimopan
677Z1OCG11. Clantifen
67B255SI5F. Amotosalen Hydrochloride (See also
    K1LDZ0VBC0)
67JE11VN82. Elzasonan Citrate (See also 933PJL964R)
67M901L9NQ. Ammonium Lactate
67N58AU0IZ. Acrocinonide
67P356D8GH. Acebutolol
67P356D8GH. Acebutolol Hydrochloride [acebutolol] (See also
    B025Y34C54)
67U96J8P35. Meprednisone
67VB76HONO. Dexmedetomidine
67VKG5DY8W. Dibemethine
67WJC4Y2QY. Brolamfetamine
6804DJ8Z9U. Capecitabine
6822A07436. Ceftiofur Hydrochloride
6831EK981Y. Amprotropine Phosphate
684N1BF96B. Fenpiprane Hydrochloride (See also S2FVB1RL5X)
6856HDT30F. Cefdaloxime
685H843ULU. Carsalam
686WJT9102. Talotrexin Ammonium
6871619Q5X. Pantoprazole Sodium
68717P8FUZ. Hydrocortisone Valerate
6875L5852V. Phthalylsulfathiazole
68AYS9A614. Cediranib Maleate
68ENP3YGUF. Ciprefadol Succinate
68EP8R4PMV. Deriglidole
68IQX3T69U. Propafenone Hydrochloride [propafenone] (See
    also 33XCH0HOCD)
68JRS2HC1C. Homatropine Methylbromide
68P0556B0U. Cinolazepam
68QN45K12N. Krypton Kr 81m
68Y4CF58BV. Pyridoxine Hydrochloride (See also KV2JZ1BI6Z)
6908F93PY1. Lomefloxacin Mesylate
690G0D6V8H. Ketamine Hydrochloride [ketamine] (See also
    O18YUO0I83)
693SRA99OH. Pidolacetamol
695N30CINR. Methenamine Mandelate
6985IP0T80. Phendimetrazine Tartrate (See also AB2794W8KV)
6995V82D0B. Eplerenone
699725286I. Azanator Maleate [azanator] (See also
    63ISF1PDWX)

699Q1XT4EN. Tebuquine
69G8BD63PP. Bortezomib
69J8AO72Q3. Cinoctramide
69K7K19H4L. Cefaclor
69M5L7BXEK. Cloperastine
69MBN7JF59. Arildone
69MG3OZA0H. Adrogolide Hydrochloride
69O5WQQ5TI. Cyclobenzaprine Hydrochloride [cyclobenzapr-
    ine] (See also 0VE05JYS2P)
69PN84IO1A. Enalapril Maleate [enalapril] (See also
    9O25354EPJ)
69QQ58998Y. Chlophedianol Hydrochloride (See also
    42C50P12AP)
69VKY8P7EA. Dovitinib Lactate (See also I35H55G906)
69YP7Z48CW. Sulfaclozine
6A8BO41Z90. Bisbutytiamine
6A901E312A. Panitumumab
6AI06C00GW. Tizanidine Hydrochloride [tizanidine] (See also
    B53E3NMY5C)
6APJ3D1308. Acefurtiamine
6AQ1Y404U7. Cangrelor
6B5VVT93AR. Dichlorotetrafluoroethane
6BCE7KY501. Deditonium Bromide (See also B9JAY11T6C)
6BZN07BMW3. Torcitabine
6C1599T3OQ. Lofentanil Oxalate
6C816LUB1O. Idrocilamide
6CHG505391. Brolaconazole
6CTK2FB9QM. Hydracarbazine
6CW7F3G59X. Gabapentin
6D0JK5KM96. Cevoglitazar
6D1R3P86GX. Bitoscanate
6D7W9EAH22. Acodazole Hydrochloride
6DC9Q167V3. Propylene Glycol
6DF29U51Y7. Rociclovir
6DJ32STZ5W. Loreclezole
6DPV8NK46S. Amphetamine Sulfate (See also CK833KGX7E)
6DZB018428. Prazitone
6E0A168OB8. Desoxycorticosterone Acetate
6E17K3343P. Chloroquine Phosphate
6E6VJP68KR. Azimilide Dihydrochloride
6E89AM91SZ. Demegestone
6E8ZO8LRNM. Trazodone Hydrochloride (See also
    YBK48BXK30)
6EE945D3OK. Mecamylamine Hydrochloride [mecamylamine]
    (See also 4956DJR58O)
6EEL176LGY. Benaxibine
6EEL1GB72K. Clocapramine
6EH821150I. Abunidazole
6EIM3851UZ. Ethchlorvynol
6EJ6I44649. Ecipramidil
6EMF80C55F. Nolomirole
6ESF2Z39VZ. Brocrinat
6ET4K804XA. Benzmalecene
6EW8Q962A5. Salmeterol Xinafoate
6EYW73T7SG. Niometacin
6F39648E92. Galarubicin
6F5V775VPO. Phoxim
6FFV1V867C. Ufiprazole
6FG8041S5B. Omacetaxine Mepesuccinate
6FH145297U. Ametantrone Acetate
6FJ4B5B368. Homarylamine
6FY017I6S7. Talmetacin
6G3OCF528J. Setastine
6G4NNS4CW4. Disiquonium Chloride
6G973E04VI. Sodelglitazar
6GC8A4PAYH. Ethyl Icosapentate
6GDT77PQBW. Brifentanil Hydrochloride [brifentanil]

6GEY4W769K. Difenoximide Hydrochloride (See also *8UG1323C03*)

6GKB767I3M. Cogazocine

6GNT3Y5LMF. Levofloxacin

6GOW6DWN2A. Oxazepam

6GQP90I798. Adefovir

6GRI2J11N5. Clinprost

6GZW20TIOI. Belladonna Leaf

6H10WF5D0H. Trapencaine

6H13T09362. Fluperamide

6H35LF645A. Rivanicline Galactarate [rivanicline] (See also *VAS2V13A9H*)

6H4ZY4O7NA. Fluprostenol Sodium (See also *358S7VUE5N*)

6H6JXC52ME. Vincanol

6H925F8O5J. Tirofiban Hydrochloride (See also *GGX234SI5H*)

6HG8UB2MUY. Diatrizoate Meglumine [meglumine]

6HG8UB2MUY. Flunixin Meglumine [meglumine] (See also *8Y3JK0JW3U; 356IB1O400*)

6HG8UB2MUY. Iocarmate Meglumine [meglumine] (See also *2303MD51O1; 82PB24K6TZ*)

6HG8UB2MUY. Iodamide Meglumine [meglumine] (See also *6X283535A3; 4RII332O0R*)

6HG8UB2MUY. Iodipamide Meglumine [meglumine]

6HG8UB2MUY. Iodoxamate Meglumine [meglumine] (See also *CIX5G6J9R1; NS1Y283HW4*)

6HG8UB2MUY. Iosulamide Meglumine [meglumine]

6HG8UB2MUY. Iothalamate Meglumine [meglumine]

6HG8UB2MUY. Meglumine

6HG8UB2MUY. Salicylate Meglumine [meglumine]

6HJV9H13XS. Ferumoxsil

6HT8U7K3AM. Mequinol

6HWO3IJ4U9. Edronocaine

6I6JCF8EOE. Brobactam

6I97Z6S135. Bencyclane Fumarate [bencyclane] (See also *OZN2MG334O*)

6J4L7U7I9D. Sulbenox

6J92H2439Z. Fontolizumab

6J9B11MN0K. Ipsapirone Hydrochloride [ipsapirone] (See also *08R5U8PYVO*)

6J9BLA949Q. Testolactone

6JKA7MAH9C. Guaiacol

6K28Y098S7. Fenoxazoline Hydrochloride (See also *97JJW1W1R3*)

6K2W7T9V6Y. Choline Bitartrate

6K6FDA543A. Estrone Sodium Sulfate

6K7YS503HC. Docusate Calcium

6KI9M51JOG. Alitame

6KY687524K. Glimepiride

6L3991491R. Pyrithione Sodium

6L3XT8CB3I. Zalcitabine

6L8OF9XRDC. Fosaprepitant Dimeglumine [fosaprepitant] (See also *D35FM8T64X*)

6LL60J9E0O. Dimethindene Maleate

6LLN8EQ6TA. Drobuline

6LPU49W75V. Adamexine

6LUM696811. Sorbitan Tristearate

6LV4FOR43R. Butane

6M3C89ZY6R. Nicotine

6M452G7O1F. Ethyl Piperidinoacetylaminobenzoate

6M4IR9QY13. Fenaclon

6M7CVQ8PF8. Bucetin

6M8CV4TKXL. Thiohexamide

6M97XTV3HD. Olmesartan Medoxomil

6MB06022N0. Amadinone Acetate [amadinone]

6MCE3VTF0O. Tribromsalan

6MCT347Y2B. Lusupultide

6MDC25LQSR. Butoctamide

6MU6U599QZ. Regrelor Disodium

6MVF9U95DW. Letosteine

6N510JUL1Y. Oltipraz

6N5U4QFC3G. Ramiprilat

6NA6UHB9SW. Zolasartan

6NB119DLU7. Flosequinan

6NHC09L02I. Prinomide Tromethamine [prinomide] (See also *33S1GFG04E*)

6O0T5E048I. Pradofloxacin

6O2O36OL57. Linotroban

6O4754US88. Manidipine 6300

6O7C9P18WG. Ioseric Acid

6OEV9DX57Y. Cefoxitin

6OEV9DX57Y. Cefoxitin Sodium [cefoxitin] (See also *Q68050H03T*)

6OZP39ZG8H. Polysorbate 80

6P1Y2SNF5V. Trifluoperazine Hydrochloride (See also *214IZI85K3*)

6P52D0J76B. Bofumustine

6P92858988. Tricaprilin

6PL3DO2B30. Bithionoloxide

6PLQ3CP4P3. Etoposide

6PNS59HP4Y. Tiludronic Acid

6PU1E16C9W. Bronopol

6PZZ52D76Q. Eptastigmine

6Q0YU79408. Metamfazone

6Q18G1060S. Cerivastatin Sodium (See also *AM91H2KS67*)

6Q205EH1VU. Vancomycin

6Q99RDT97R. Pipobroman

6QK969R2IF. Phenolphthalein

6QO0F8648P. Loflucarban

6QR1645G9S. Pipramadol

6R8T1UDM3V. Palmidrol

6RC3ZT4HB0. Propiolactone

6RC5V8B7PO. Trihexyphenidyl Hydrochloride [trihexyphenidyl] (See also *AO61G82577*)

6RY56RB98P. Dabelotine

6RY6V6XM8T. Almitrine Mesylate (See also *9A1222NBG4*)

6RZ6XEZ3CR. Chlordiazepoxide

6RZ6XEZ3CR. Chlordiazepoxide Hydrochloride [chlordiazepoxide] (See also *MFM6K1XWDK*)

6S082C9NDT. Trimipramine

6SGF1AP698. Tazasubrate

6SK5U4T31I. Pentalamide

6SN82Y9U73. Forodesine Hydrochloride (See also *426X066ELK*)

6SNR96E409. Pelanserin Hydrochloride [pelanserin] (See also *4J8I18ZP0A*)

6SO6U10H04. Biotin

6SQ8M7ZSFV. Cemadotin

6T04V14CU9. Chlorproguanil Hydrochloride

6T84R30KC1. Tranexamic Acid

6T8C155666. Ipilimumab

6TK1G07BHZ. Posaconazole

6U5EA9RT2O. Levocetirizine

6U704SC0N2. Pyrimitate

6U85YRT588. Phenmetrazine Hydrochloride (See also *XA501VL3VR*)

6U9XA4JOD4. Furethidine

6UK191M53P. Elesclomol

6UKA5VEJ6X. Ziprasidone Hydrochloride [ziprasidone] (See also *216X081ORU*)

6V5034L121. Chlorotrianisene

6V9V2RYJ8N. Pseudoephedrine Hydrochloride (See also *7CUC9DDI9F*)

6VJE5G3D98. Cephalexin Hydrochloride

6W731X367Q. Selegiline Hydrochloride

6W9PS8B71J. Sorbitan Monolaurate

6WV4B8Q07H. Brofaromine

6WVL9C355G. Phensuximide

6WVM5HPV4T. Pirralkonium Bromide
6X1N18AU15. Mefenorex Hydrochloride
6X283535A3. Iodamide Meglumine (See also *4RII332OO0R; 6HG8UB2MUY*)
6X4F561V3W. Unoprostone
6X8764TW2J. Revospirone
6X97D2XT0O. Betaxolol Hydrochloride (See also *O0ZR1R6RZ2*)
6X9OC3H4II. Loperamide Hydrochloride [loperamide] (See also *77TI35393C*)
6XC1PAD3KF. Zoledronic Acid
6XK4G40F6W. Milacemide Hydrochloride
6XMB0871VB. Droxacin Sodium [droxacin] (See also *3VOW3G2JQC*)
6XN50U405Y. Tezampanel
6XSR933SRK. Ecadotril
6XXK617AU2. Fepromide
6Y24O4F92S. Bremelanotide
6Y42K4JRBJ. Fluprofylline
6Y556547YY. Moguisteine
6Y891C0JEV. Elarofiban
6YB4901Y90. Manganese Chloride [manganese chloride anhydrous]
6YE7PBM15H. Midodrine Hydrochloride [midodrine] (See also *59JV96YTXV*)
6YKS4Y3WQ7. Hydrocodone Bitartrate [hydrocodone] (See also *NO70W886KK*)
6YSS42VSEV. Fructose
6Z1Y2V4A7M. Econazole
6Z1Y2V4A7M. Econazole Nitrate [econazole] (See also *H438WYN10E*)
6Z5B6HVF6O. Latanoprost
6Z674O12T6. Rosabulin
6Z6T599E49. Ethaverine Hydrochloride (See also *2H2HC19DYZ*)
6Z9DV0V6TG. Ceftioxide
70097M6I30. Magnesium Stearate
702RHR475O. Fosbretabulin Disodium
704083NI0R. Clofoctol
70859437W3. Nardeterol
70968BVH2J. Donitriptan
70BO17YR03. Propiomazine Hydrochloride (See also *242Z0PM79Y*)
70C1507JU9. Phenacaine Hydrochloride
70J5AWG54Q. Azetirelin
70JE2N95KR. Tigecycline
70JKL15MUH. Citiolone
70QV580PA4. Propinetidine
70U2NQU0FP. Celgosivir Hydrochloride
71193OXG6S. Tallimustine
711S8Y0T33. Quinine Hydrochloride
712BAC33MZ. Iopromide
712MLZ30SB. Nitracrine
713BBL6840. Fluprazine
71IA9S35AJ. Semaxanib
71OK3Z1ESP. Moricizine [moricizine hydrochloride] (See also *2GT1D0TMX1*)
71OK3Z1ESP. Moricizine Hydrochloride
71OTZ9ZE0A. Imipenem
71P630M192. Thioproperazine Mesylate (See also *YJ050AQ56X*)
71Q1A3O279. Anileridine
71Q1A3O279. Anileridine Hydrochloride [anileridine] (See also *915Q054DLC*)
71WO621TJD. Vancomycin Hydrochloride
720J8565ZF. Lachesine Chloride
721809WQCP. Ruboxistaurin
721M9407IY. Propylthiouracil
722BFZ899Q. Ethylmethylthiambutene
723JX6CXY5. Menadione
723JX6CXY5. Menadione Sodium Bisulfite [menadione]

724377908B. Camphotamide
724L30Y2QR. Ursodiol
72531373MH. Clorindanic Acid
725P8AW50M. Cyclocumarol
726233N8L3. Cefmepidium Chloride
726I6TE06G. Pramlintide Acetate
72C4702BMV. Delfantrine
72FH6333M6. Hepzidine
72H8H6K34C. Darbufelone
72O4809PU1. Prazepine
72T37AL5JV. Dodicin
72W71I16EG. Sertaconazole
72YY86EA29. Cosyntropin
72ZJ154X86. Cyclacillin
73071MW2KM. Glyceryl Distearate
7318FJ13YJ. Thiothixene
731DCA35BT. Diethylstilbestrol
7323N7T136. Cyclomethycaine Sulfate (See also *15E9I74NZ8*)
73312P173G. Diphenoxylate Hydrochloride [diphenoxylate] (See also *W24OD7YW48*)
733BXR9780. Falintolol
7355X3ROTS. Dextromethorphan
7355X3ROTS. Dextromethorphan Hydrobromide [dextromethorphan] (See also *9D2RTI9KYH*)
7369R4J7S2. Ecomustine
736I6971TE. Cyclopentolate Hydrochloride (See also *I76F4SHP7J*)
737RR8Y409. Sivelestat Sodium
737T1YVX89. Metostilenol
73H7UDN6EC. Meldonium
73K4184T59. Digoxin
73NDV3S9Y7. Eucaine Hydrochloride
73OS0QIN3O. Medronic Acid
73P3618V2E. Octabenzone
73U81R979T. Biclofibrate
73W96524XT. Sulmarin
740T4C525W. Sulfisoxazole
7419T4YQQW. Mepixanox
742F5K270Q. Domitroban
742SXX0ICT. Tadalafil
746YWK1B07. Loxanast
74A4TNE8C3. Bromofos
74ATQ0K1LA. Tameridone
74B4VJV0WV. Cifostodine
74CQ4Q3N63. Cefteram
74FAA305EW. Ethyl Dirazepate
74GNV897RO. Bisantrene Hydrochloride
74KXF8I502. Aclarubicin
74L3DXN051. Tiacrilast
74RWP7W0J9. Betrixaban
74WY8560J7. Mefenidil
75046A1XTN. Alfuzosin Hydrochloride (See also *90347YTW5F*)
7506A6J57T. Besifloxacin Hydrochloride
7531I37BK3. Azaclorzine Hydrochloride (See also *7N4BHX8N3L*)
7531Q8398Y. Cinamolol
7539319JYI. Pomisartan
75473V2YZK. Bromopride
7560BB0BO3. Clorophene
756RDM536M. Flurazepam Hydrochloride (See also *IHP475989U*)
759N8462G8. Loprazolam
75C8DU40T0. Ciluprevir
75CL65GTYR. Benziodarone
75DLN707DO. Carebastine
75F375MT2N. Estramustine Phosphate Sodium
75J73V1629. Ceftriaxone Sodium [ceftriaxone] (See also *023Z5BR09K*)

75JR975T11. Ioxaglate Meglumine
75L57R6X36. Conivaptan Hydrochloride
75O9XHA4TU. Levobetaxolol Hydrochloride [levobetaxolol] (See also *8MR4W4O06J*)
75OCL1SPBQ. Gabapentin Enacarbil
75R0U2568I. Octreotide Acetate
75T64B71RP. Dexbrompheniramine Maleate [dexbromphenira-mine] (See also *BPA9UT29BS*)
75UI7QUZ5J. Sodium Aminobenzoate
7610629RVH. Prothipendyl Hydrochloride
7626GC95E5. Coriander Oil
762D3F7OY3. Morocromen
762OS3ZEJU. Benserazide
762RDY0Y2H. Clofarabine
765C9332T4. Guanadrel Sulfate [guanadrel] (See also *MT147RMO91*)
7662KG2R6K. Lubiprostone
76732QSQ30. Alvameline Maleate
7673326042. Irinotecan Hydrochloride [irinotecan] (See also *042LAQ1IIS*)
76755771U3. Hydroxyzine Hydrochloride
76845O8NMZ. Ethyl Acetate
7686S50JAH. Ingenol Mebutate
768T9DK07R. Bentipimine
76A0JE0FKJ. Adipic Acid
76H78MJJ52. Trimeprazine Tartrate [trimeprazine] (See also *362NW1LD6Z*)
76I7G6D29C. Morphine Hydrochloride [morphine]
76I7G6D29C. Morphine Sulfate [morphine] (See also *X3P646A2J0*)
76J0853EKA. Erdosteine
76JC1633UF. Metronidazole Hydrochloride (See also *140QMO216E*)
76K53XP4TO. Racecadotril
76LA80IG2G. Glucagon
76LO2L2V39. Zeranol
76S8CUH5MR. Nomifensine Maleate (See also *1LGS5JRP31*)
76W6J0943E. Flutamide
76YOO33643. Protionamide
771E5ELJ7N. Fandosentan Potassium [fandosentan] (See also *14U0D2SA4K*)
771H53976Q. Indinavir Sulfate
77243B845F. Oxazorone
7725983GSD. Butamoxane
772EN3BH6I. Dimethisoquin Hydrochloride [dimethisoquin] (See also *SMP2689462*)
7732P08TIR. Netupitant
776B62CQ27. Decitabine
776E09GMHQ. Cefivitril
776Q6XX45J. Ilaprazole
776XM7047L. Calcium Stearate
778XL6VBS8. Levoleucovorin Calcium
779291866J. Cyclarbamate
779619577M. Clobetasol Propionate (See also *ADN79D536H*)
77C3T28736. Depramine
77DUK856J7. Nonabine
77HC7URR9Z. Azasetron (See also *2BSS7XL60S*)
77K18757UK. Flezelastine
77K6Z421KU. Sorbitan Monopalmitate
77TI35393C. Loperamide Hydrochloride (See also *6X9OC3H4II*)
77W477J15H. Chlorothiazide
77W477J15H. Chlorothiazide Sodium [chlorothiazide] (See also *SN86FG7N2K*)
77WPB17ZK1. Topterone
77YW1RTU8V. Calcium Undecylenate
7812FUQ8VK. Cobaltous Chloride Co 60
7828VC80FJ. Diquafosol Tetrasodium [diquafosol] (See also *X8T9SBH9LL*)

783AHI015X. Chlorpheniramine Polistirex
7844H41L5Z. Tropantiol
785363R681. Pidotimod
7865D5D01M. Tretazicar
786Z46389E. Metformin Hydrochloride
787AQ35GHR. Befuraline
78D9U89TBG. Indocate
78E4J5IB5J. Mitotane
78G92X9EH7. Enpiprazole
78OY3Z0P7Z. Aminacrine Hydrochloride [aminacrine] (See also *OR5RM3Q5QL*)
78U6302ARL. Posatirelin
78VM28ZA2H. Binfloxacin
78W508SA0Q. Prideperone
78W62V43DY. Penbutolol Sulfate [penbutolol] (See also *US71433228*)
78XGN2K5RX. Erbulozole
78ZP3YR353. Bretylium Tosylate
7902N03BH0. Chlorindanol
795182TM5G. Paridocaine
79EDP2VHY8. Itrocainide
79QH89EV9M. Dutogliptin Tartrate
79QS8K2877. Alagebrium Chloride
79WCR09M2C. Nitricholine Perchlorate
7A2NOC3R88. Nizofenone
7A314HQM0I. Pentetate Calcium Trisodium [pentetic acid] (See also *G79YN26H5B*)
7A314HQM0I. Pentetic Acid
7A977PW795. Peradoxime
7AJ51I17KG. Ranitidine Bismuth Citrate
7AJO3BO7QN. Loratadine
7AK2FKB9AW. Bimosiamose Disodium
7AYY495RE0. Pumitepa
7B0ZZH8P2W. Pinacidil
7B1AVU9DJN. Methyl Nicotinate
7B5032XT6O. Carboprost
7B5032XT6O. Carboprost Tromethamine [carboprost] (See also *U4526F86FJ*)
7B58W7756G. Chlorisondamine Chloride
7B8PIR2954. Mephenesin
7BA3X03948. Berubicin Hydrochloride
7BA5G9Y06Q. Terfenadine
7BHQ856EJ5. Clioquinol
7BK02SCL3W. Betamethasone Sodium Phosphate
7BO8G1BYQU. Masoprocol
7BRF0Z81KG. Lomustine
7BVX6J0CGR. Feprazone
7C0697DR9I. Atropine
7C0697DR9I. Atropine Sulfate [atropine] (See also *03J5ZE7KA5*)
7C247FL5FG. Zinc Oleate
7C546U4DEN. Diflunisal
7C6TA32SD2. Clopimozide
7C782967RD. Ampicillin
7C8J54PVFI. Maprotiline Hydrochloride
7CLJ1MEZ8V. Razaxaban Hydrochloride
7CUC9DDI9F. Pseudoephedrine Hydrochloride [pseudo-ephedrine] (See also *6V9V2RYJ8N*)
7CZF3L922Y. Lypressin
7CZF3L922Y. Vasopressin [lysine form] (See also *Y4907O6MFD*)
7D0YB67S97. Abatacept
7D6EM3S13P. Lymecycline
7D7GS1SA24. Zoledronate Disodium
7D7RX5A8MO. Venlafaxine Hydrochloride (See also *GRZ5RCB1QG*)
7D96IR0PPM. Pegaspargase
7DP3NTV15T. Bleomycin Sulfate (See also *40S1VHN69B*)
7DR7H00HDT. Dromostanolone Propionate [dromostanolone] (See also *X20UZ57G4O*)

7DZO8EB0Z3. Amiloride Hydrochloride [amiloride] (See also *FZJ37245UC*)

7E136TJT00. Tivanidazole

7E1DV054LO. Estradiol Cypionate

7E3392891K. Cariporide

7E4PHP5N1D. Vecuronium Bromide

7E521JYJ4X. Linogliride

7E8Q32N75N. Piroxicam Cinnamate

7EE4K616KK. Difebarbamate

7ENI812SZS. Cipralisant Maleate

7ET381H9UA. Moxiraprine

7F228A0THI. Proxibutene

7F2X95XC2A. Naluzotan Hydrochloride

7F64A2K16Z. Fludiazepam

7FRV7310N6. Tamoxifen Citrate (See also *094ZI81Y45*)

7FXW6U30GY. Fosfomycin Tromethamine

7G29CRR596. Salacetamide

7G33012534. Sodium Oxybate

7G733H6RES. Prospidium Chloride

7GAQ2332NK. Pemoline

7GDN12Q42M. Dalbraminol

7GGP8DTV34. Trepirium Iodide

7GHI2O527Q. Sulclamide

7GR28W0FJI. Dacarbazine

7GR9I2683O. Mecasermin

7GVF119EM8. Mebezonium Iodide

7GWN8D7165. Tiprinast Meglumine

7H254VC0NT. Pralidoxime Iodide

7H634NXI03. Ciclonicate

7H6TM3CT4L. Oxandrolone

7HQ8UT1TPS. Piconol

7I22J7RY2A. Clovoxamine

7I64C51O16. Ziconotide

7I6MS3VHQE. Trazitiline

7IGS0KX75Q. Acoxatrine

7IO5LYA57N. Ropivacaine Hydrochloride [ropivacaine]

7J8897W37S. Dronabinol

7J9ZZ971AO. Pinokalant

7JEC65JCG2. Exalamide

7JEE2JF5OB. Tioctilate

7JHD84H15J. Astromicin Sulfate [astromicin] (See also *POY3S0T3BD*)

7JZ930H2M6. Picartamide

7K2B1728PB. Meprochol

7K383OQI23. Zolpidem Tartrate [zolpidem] (See also *WY6W63843K*)

7K50VT05OD. Naminidil

7K6U6T1360. Isofezolac

7KE5R66TSY. Pinoxepin Hydrochloride

7KKS9R192F. Gimatecan

7KNU786IT4. Valopicitabine Dihydrochloride (See also *I2T0B5G94M*)

7KYV510875. Pimecrolimus

7L38105Z6E. Setiptiline

7L3E358N9L. Dopamine Hydrochloride (See also *VTD58H1Z2X*)

7L93SJ2K9A. Carbiphene Hydrochloride

7L9H348XUO. Famotine Hydrochloride

7LG286J8GV. Carfentanil Citrate

7LJ087RS6F. Riluzole

7LKK855W8I. Letrozole

7LXU5N7ZO5. Furosemide

7M19191IKG. Teduglutide

7M1J3HN9VO. Disufenton Sodium

7M7YKX2N15. Topotecan Hydrochloride [topotecan] (See also *956S425ZCY*)

7MS1HEY2IZ. Taprostene

7N21461LKD. Aminosalicylate Potassium

7N3A092A5X. Heliomycin

7N4BHX8N3L. Azaclorzine Hydrochloride [azaclorzine] (See also *7531I37BK3*)

7N7IQB45VO. Erizepine

7NFE54O27T. Toremifene Citrate [toremifene] (See also *2498Y783QT*)

7NFK89B690. Medibazine

7NH28I651F. Isometamidium Chloride

7NJ031HAX5. Morantel Tartrate [morantel] (See also *5WF7E9QC3F*)

7NNO0D7S5M. Miconazole

7NNO0D7S5M. Miconazole Nitrate [miconazole] (See also *VW4H1CYW1K*)

7NZH2C1T6O. Vinbarbital

7NZH2C1T6O. Vinbarbital Sodium [Injection] [vinbarbital]

7OT95Q2G4E. Amipizone

7OW73204U1. Fumagillin

7P6B96QLKN. Teludipine Hydrochloride

7PV0B6ED98. Mebrofenin

7PX435DN5A. Methyldopate Hydrochloride (See also *2579Z4P04J*)

7PY8KH681I. Dizocilpine Maleate [dizocilpine]

7QCG0RP106. Rilapine

7QID3E7BG7. Dicumarol

7QZA627US7. Droxinavir Hydrochloride (See also *3CF21QCB9J*)

7R4F94TVGY. Cefpodoxime Proxetil [cefpodoxime] (See also *2TB00A1Z7N*)

7RDI07K19U. Mersalyl

7RE4N644YF. Benolizime

7RN5DR86CK. Pazopanib Hydrochloride [pazopanib] (See also *33Y9ANM545*)

7RNN0MXE38. Ecalcidene

7RS2Q8MCK8. Drotebanol

7S5I7G3JQL. Dexamethasone

7S73606O1A. Methyl Aminolevulinate Hydrochloride

7S79QT1T91. Dehydroemetine

7SEV7J4R1U. Talc

7SFC6U2VI5. Calcitonin [salmon] (See also *I0IO929019*)

7SGV5HQH8B. Acridorex

7SJF09406G. Verilopam Hydrochloride

7T1F30V5YH. Polysorbate 20

7T952LZM7T. Piperamide Maleate (See also *83B7UZO20C*)

7TJT8X832U. Tolfamide

7TQO7W3VT8. Bupivacaine Hydrochloride (See also *Y8335394RO*)

7TUY98X69L. Phenylacetylglycine Dimethylamide

7TXJ9MY5V9. Cronidipine

7U06D381UQ. Broparestrol

7U1EE4V452. Carbon Monoxide

7U248Z56LA. Linetastine

7U370BPS14. Dichlorvos

7U75I1278D. Cefoperazone Sodium [cefoperazone] (See also *5FQG9774WD*)

7U7O8Q48IO. Protokylol Hydrochloride (See also *8Y5Y4EEO2V*)

7U972CJ5AT. Iclaprim Mesylate

7UL287YTPJ. Amixetrine

7V31YC746X. Chloroform

7V49F22020. Salclobuzate Sodium

7VI3P2OT72. Dimelazine

7VLR55452Z. Fosphenytoin Sodium (See also *B4SF212641*)

7VSV9BL497. Casopitant Mesylate (See also *3B03KPM27L*)

7W2J09SCWX. Diflorasone Diacetate (See also *T2DHJ9645W*)

7W4TAI502Z. Perflisobutane

7WAL1X78KV. Angiotensin Amide

7WI4P02YN1. Ethopropazine Hydrochloride [ethopropazine] (See also *O00T1I1VRN*)

7WP69N3Y3Y. Tivirapine

7WU8BZ90TH. Candoxatrilat

7X6P5N8K2L. Farampator
7X768418RT. Aptazapine Maleate
7XIY785AZD. Insulin Glulisine
7XU7A7DROE. Amphotericin B
7XZB016MY5. Acebrochol
7Y0IV7N95Q. Balamapimod
7Y4N11PXO8. Troxerutin
7Y86X0D799. Cefazedone
7YA71JCD50. Treloxinate
7YB0YX4M89. Milacainide
7YO3254Y6B. Etazolate Hydrochloride (See also *I89Y79062L*)
7YQT311430. Caproxamine
7YRF8G0G0F. Amebucort
7Z32Z641H2. Pretamazium Iodide
7Z5X49W53P. Terlipressin
7Z6522T8N9. Testosterone Enanthate
7Z71845H3F. Ftaxilide
7Z7670589C. Fotretamine
7Z8O94ECSX. Alcaftadine
7Z9SP74BXF. Lobenzarit Sodium
7ZAT6ES870. Tranylcypromine Sulfate (See also *3E3V44J4Z9*)
7ZF18Q354W. Bumetrizole
7ZJ8PWY0XD. Amiphenazole
7ZNX9ET039. Oberadilol
7ZQK8VIO6V. Teloxantrone Hydrochloride (See also *96521WL61B*)
7ZRO0SC54Y. Ramosetron
7ZZN46QU1N. Flumeridone
80168379AG. Doxorubicin
80168379AG. Doxorubicin Hydrochloride [doxorubicin] (See also *82F2G7BL4E*)
8028PPX4PM. Disomotide
803BIX5JG5. Haloprogesterone
804826J2HU. Amoxicillin
8054MM4902. Zibotentan
806529YU1N. Acetarsone
8067S1388X. Protheobromine
807MP0MJ61. Vinconate
807N226MNL. Caroxazone
807PW4VQE3. Cefepime
80C9L8EP6V. Gepirone Hydrochloride (See also *JW5Y7B8Z18*)
80EHD8I43D. Aluminum Acetate
80K4H2RB8P. Indibulin
80M03YXJ7I. Valsartan
80O018LGCI. Spiroxepin
80O1E9JZLN. Lidanserin
80O63P88IS. Stallimycin Hydrochloride [stallimycin]
80Q9QWN15M. Quinagolide
80X61Y4X0B. Medorinone
80YS8O1MBS. Cisatracurium Besylate
810O95170J. Ditiomustine
811X558HU0. Levoxadrol Hydrochloride [levoxadrol] (See also *3ARD9VMM81*)
813AGY3126. Zosuquidar Trihydrochloride (See also *AB5K82-X98Y*)
813OG1OGVG. Tiliquinol
8163770L8P. Capeserod
817W3C6175. Timolol
818U2PZ2EH. Metaraminol Bitartrate [metaraminol] (See also *ZC4202M9P3*)
81AXN7R2QT. Dihydroergotamine Mesylate (See also *436O5HM03C*)
81BDR9Y8PS. Tazarotene
81BK194Z5M. Pyrantel Pamoate
81BMQ80QRL. Itopride
81F061RQS4. Carbazochrome
81G6I5V05I. Mebendazole
81HH79X39W. Cedefingol

81K9V7M3A3. Desogestrel
81QS09V3YW. Cefditoren
81U8A51CHK. Alestramustine
820484N8I3. Histamine Dihydrochloride [histamine] (See also *3POA0Q644U*)
8223RR9DWF. Prednisolone Sodium Succinate
82269ASB48. Varenicline Tartrate (See also *W6HS99O8ZO*)
822EC3XEJZ. Detorubicin
822G987U9J. Zomepirac Sodium [zomepirac] (See also *Y0185WZ209*)
826Y60901U. Betamethasone Dipropionate
827T79ILE7. Trimazosin Hydrochloride (See also *31L760807H*)
8286I9062N. Sulfasuccinamide
82CYO8A460. Butixirate
82F2G7BL4E. Doxorubicin Hydrochloride (See also *80168379AG*)
82J92E653W. Dioxethedrin Hydrochloride [dioxethedrin]
82KFT81F6W. Niclofolan
82PB24K6TZ. Iocarmate Meglumine [iocarmic acid] (See also *2303MD51O1; 6HG8UB2MUY*)
82PB24K6TZ. Iocarmic Acid
82V2M8K24R. Posizolid
82VFR53I78. Aripiprazole
82WI2L7Q6E. Dolasetron Mesylate [dolasetron] (See also *U3C8E5BWKR*)
82Y7NT6DFT. Minaprine Hydrochloride (See also *00U7GX0NLM*)
83619PEU5T. Pramipexole
838F01T721. Paliperidone
839184U8NM. Trimethamide
839F26EVAQ. Ipenoxazone
83B517YUVM. Milverine
83B7UZO20C. Piperamide Maleate [piperamide] (See also *7T952LZM7T*)
83CVD213TU. Cletoquine
83G67E21XI. Urokinase
83HN0GTJ6D. Cyclosporine
83L52U43TX. Iproxamine Hydrochloride (See also *URR853YL-ZA*)
83L91231V7. Pyridarone
83LCM6L2BY. Fomepizole
83MVU38M7Q. Rosuvastatin Calcium (See also *413KH5ZJ73*)
83NB50X92M. Quinacillin
8422DH508N. Cloxotestosterone
8427MP5VHD. Clobenoside
84319SGC3C. Amikacin
84319SGC3C. Amikacin Sulfate [amikacin] (See also *N6M33094FD*)
843CEN85DI. Apraclonidine Hydrochloride [apraclonidine] (See also *D2VW67N38H*)
845NU6GJPS. Paromomycin Sulfate (See also *61JJC8N5ZK*)
8483H94W1E. Tetradonium Bromide
849K45OH8R. Nifluridide
84C5PTP9X6. Iotroxic Acid
84CS1P306F. Sulfadiazine Sodium
84DZ9RW4WK. Acreozast
84F6U3J2R6. Gadodiamide
84L8XK6N1G. Methixene Hydrochloride (See also *32VY6L26ZW*)
84OPZ2Q0VB. Hexocyclium Methylsulfate
85061HTR8T. Clocortolone Acetate (See also *N8ZUB7XE0H*)
852A84Y8LS. Hexetidine
85474O1N9D. Cetalkonium Chloride
856DX0KJ84. Neramexane Mesylate [neramexane] (See also *9M85GXG84D*)
85713MT0EH. Arpromidine
858M12945S. Beclotiamine
858YGI5PIT. Bupranolol

85DV2PAF78. Nicanartine
85EW9V00UL. Elucaine
85H0HZU99M. Povidone-Iodine
85LCU5151G. Sulprosal
85P20FW39R. Timofibrate
85V47MCE4Z. Almoxatone
85W6I13D8M. Clemizole [hydrochloride] (See also *T97CB3796L*)
85X09V2GSO. Lasofoxifene Tartrate
8605L38D80. Azaloxan Fumarate (See also *0O653FA999*)
860MHI4WBA. Fepradinol
860MT00T7T. Cefuzonam
860O06CJWZ. Indorenate Hydrochloride
861J4K81C7. Etymemazine Hydrochloride [etymemazine] (See also *A7002E7T2Z*)
861R00J986. Cyclizine Lactate (See also *QRW9FCR9P2*)
862MFS0O74. Edaglitazone Sodium (See also *8GKF7V499B*)
864P0921DW. Bromfenac Sodium [bromfenac] (See also *8ECV571Y37*)
864V2Q084H. Amlodipine Besylate (See also *1J444QC288*)
8680B5Y37A. Pimefylline
8681H0C27P. Oleandomycin Phosphate (See also *P8ZQ646136*)
869PGR00AT. Ensaculin
86AZ0G22V2. Liothyronine I 131 (See also *06LU7C9H1V*)
86C4MRT55A. Pirinixic Acid
86DRW83R1H. Phentolamine Hydrochloride (See also *Z468598HBV*)
86EEZ49YVB. Fostamatinib Disodium
86KE25F200. Cyclobutoic Acid
86P6PQK0MU. Doxazosin Mesylate (See also *NW1291F1W8*)
86Q357L16B. Zinc Chloride
86Q50C824Z. Benanserin Hydrochloride
86TB3JLD8A. Furofenac
86TDZ5WP2B. Suxibuzone
86WEQ311WF. Picumeterol Fumarate [picumeterol] (See also *0SUN4UF93Y*)
870Q5BL2FN. Morazone
872109HX6B. Chloramphenicol Sodium Succinate
8738M34B4Y. Iosumetic Acid
8742T8ZQZA. Pamidronate Disodium
874HHB2V3S. Olpadronic Acid
876351L05K. Romifidine
876SH4764F. Glicondamide
877K0XW47A. Betamethasone Benzoate
8780F0K71U. Nifenazone
878CEJ4HGX. Pheneturide
879A12466H. Itriglumide
87C4V63NWI. Sulverapride
87CNY2EEBH. Calcium Bromide
87L38AY71R. Arofylline
87T4T8BO2E. Rotigotine
87TH1FJY1N. Cephacetrile Sodium
87V8H2Q8IH. Cliropamine
880XXO778K. Hydroxindasol
88174AK70T. Tinazoline
88181ACA0M. Norethynodrel
883G6DMT63. Isaxonine
883WKN7W8X. Cortisone Acetate (See also *V27W9254FZ*)
883YNL63WU. Eprazinone
8841R2UJPG. Zoniporide Mesylate [zoniporide] (See also *X4VP8104KI*)
88445508X3. Fenpipramide (See also *KJ2V75P034*)
88463U4SM5. Sulfadoxine
884KT10YB7. Ranitidine
886SAV9675. Cloprostenol Sodium
886U3H6UFF. Chloroquine
8871ZB4UGC. Pentabamate
887K2391VH. Dapagliflozin

887VHL8899. Glysobuzole
8883YP2R6D. Ivermectin
888Y08971B. Ceruletide
8890V3217X. Hydrastine
8892KM4U61. Imanixil
8896RX4S4J. Sumarotene
88AO1K4HJ3. Theophylline Sodium Acetate
88AYB867L5. Pramoxine Hydrochloride (See also *068X84E056*)
88C55N56UU. Secretin
88D34UY0QI. Dacemazine
88ETS2Q7LZ. Anidoxime
88M0X6627K. Fenclexonium Metilsulfate (See also *BV3N6F82WN*)
88XHZ13131. Ferrous Fumarate [fumaric acid] (See also *R5L488RY0Q*)
88XHZ13131. Fumaric Acid
89134SCM7M. Diloxanide
8915147A2B. Perazine Fendizoate [perazine]
891H89GFT4. Bufuralol
89243S03TE. Sermorelin Acetate [sermorelin] (See also *00IB-G87IQW*)
895X917GYE. Etilevodopa
89741L759Z. Osalmid
89846MU42L. Antafenite
898723IQHQ. Gleptoferron
89DS0H96TB. Zinc Sulfate
89Q735AA4A. Metrafazoline
89RAG7SB3B. Ronnel
89RBZ66NVC. Indisetron
89TPE33M27. Flurocitabine
89Y4M234ES. Bacitracin Zinc (See also *58H6RWO52I*)
8A5OIA91GT. Diproteverine
8A7F670F2Y. Sacrosidase
8A8NY1Z12E. Perfomedil
8A96H4311N. Hydroxytetracaine
8AQ60474G9. Guanethidine Sulfate (See also *ZTI6C33Q2Q*)
8ARY01XRYU. Pirbenicillin Sodium [pirbenicillin] (See also *638D8M316Y*)
8B1QWR724A. Reserpine
8B2807733D. Prednisolone Acetate
8B50X0IVEC. Semduramicin Sodium
8B830OJ2UX. Methoprene
8B9I31H724. Isopropamide Iodide [isopropamide] (See also *E0KNA372SZ*)
8BK5DLR67A. Cloxypendyl
8BT63DA42E. Indiplon
8C19ZXR2J2. Cyclopyrronium Bromide
8C3Z4148WZ. Alginic Acid
8CFL28PA3W. Morinamide
8CRQ2TH63M. Isopropyl Palmitate
8CY265YM5K. Pozanicline Tartrate
8D08K3S51E. Propylene Carbonate
8D4SNN7V92. Propyl Gallate
8D5I63UE1Q. Phenylpropanolamine Hydrochloride (See also *33RU150WUN*)
8DUH1N11BX. Tryptophan
8E92V52324. Phenoxypropazine
8ECV571Y37. Bromfenac Sodium (See also *864P0921DW*)
8ENZ0QJW4H. Nafarelin Acetate (See also *1X0094V6JV*)
8ET970D66K. Alimadol
8ETK1WAF6R. Thiethylperazine
8EUL29XUQT. Flurandrenolide
8F049NKY49. Calcium Polycarbophil
8F5X4B082E. Lixivaptan
8F63U28T2V. Imexon
8FVI4DU91L. Ethyl Cartrizoate
8G02RSW5CM. Oxametacin

8G167061QZ. Ethambutol Hydrochloride [ethambutol] (See also *QE4VW5FO07*)

8GKF7V499B. Edaglitazone Sodium [edaglitazone] (See also *862MFS0O74*)

8GM2J22278. Bacampicillin Hydrochloride [bacampicillin] (See also *PM034U953T*)

8GTS82S83M. Diphenhydramine Citrate [diphenhydramine]

8GZG754X6M. Gemtuzumab Ozogamicin

8HDO7941DO. Cefamandole Nafate (See also *5CKP8C2LLI*)

8HQJ711KH8. Clocinizine

8I16YLE4US. Tecalcet Hydrochloride [tecalcet] (See also *3HP28R98LC*)

8IF7HES548. Parconazole Hydrochloride (See also *8Z2Z19C8Z1*)

8II47759Z3. Betoxycaine Hydrochloride (See also *03DB58Y9DO*)

8IKK64FJVX. Chlormidazole

8IVL8S1U34. Xinidamine

8J11WBM781. Benzaprinoxide

8J763HFF5N. Clopidol

8J77X3S603. Hexamethonium Bromide (See also *3C9PSP36Z2*)

8J8O0MK4JG. Spirgetine

8J97CUZ4HX. Fenethazine

8JAK753213. Valdipromide

8JD13PH39Q. Quillifoline

8JSV4O30HQ. Menogaril

8KI671F2NS. Disogluside

8KK8CQ2K8G. Niclosamide

8L5014XET7. Terazosin Hydrochloride [terazosin] (See also *D32S14F082*)

8LXS95BSA9. Dihydrocodeine Bitartrate

8M09P36809. Piberaline

8M1YF8951V. Ceforanide

8M7Y72EP9K. Enpiroline Phosphate [enpiroline] (See also *QX39IR9V1D*)

8MB4MJ9R7L. Methoxamine Hydrochloride (See also *HUQ1K-C1YLI*)

8MDF5V39QO. Sodium Bicarbonate

8MF6L4447J. Flunoprost

8MKS280XJW. Imipraminoxide

8MR4W4O06J. Levobetaxolol Hydrochloride (See also *75O9XHA4TU*)

8N2L1NX8S3. Eprosartan Mesylate

8N3DW7272P. Cyclophosphamide

8N5BE1I42E. Amidapsone

8N86XTF9QD. Clinafloxacin Hydrochloride [clinafloxacin] (See also *G17M59V0FY*)

8NA5SWF92O. Lysergide

8NF31401XG. Carteolol Hydrochloride [carteolol] (See also *4797W6I0T4*)

8NJ5RWV39D. Cefazaflur Sodium

8NT43GG2HA. Allobarbital

8NT850T0YS. Bisoctrizole

8NVY8268MY. Mertiatide

8NZ41MIK1O. Enoxaparin Sodium

8O0C852CPO. Natamycin

8O4QYK6G4Y. Tisocalcitate

8OEC3RA07X. Dithiazanine Iodide (See also *5L7E7IY5EH*)

8OKQ9NS8MO. Aconiazide

8OMO7K4W74. Nuvenzepine

8OR09251MQ. Indacaterol

8P4W949T8K. Cefatrizine

8P6T83567P. Norbudrine

8P8TW6B25I. Ontazolast

8PDI6DY6GV. Lopirazepam

8PK70TXE1T. Carbarsone

8PUY50JWLU. Bentiamine

8PW272ITDS. Actinoquinol Sodium

8PW276HX8U. Dramedilol

8Q1PVL543G. Dipivefrin

8Q21Y09R21. Metabromsalan

8Q2869CNVH. Hydroxychloroquine Sulfate (See also *4QWG6N8QKH*)

8Q5153W1NW. Acetiromate

8R78F6L9VO. Sumatriptan

8R9E4766V4. Timepidium Bromide

8RSD11181G. Ciprazafone

8S09O559AQ. Pirlimycin Hydrochloride

8S4M0WS2UA. Isomylamine Hydrochloride

8S95DH25XC. Levomefolic Acid

8SKN0B0MIM. Benzoic Acid

8SSC91326P. Donepezil Hydrochloride [donepezil] (See also *3O2T2PJ89D*)

8STT15Y392. Robenidine Hydrochloride (See also *4888ME6C4E*)

8T3Q0X4G5G. Amogastrin

8T4L120N6M. Cyclobutyrol

8T66I31YNK. Aldioxa

8T96I3U713. Cadralazine

8TIF7T48FP. Piperazine Phosphate

8TUG8SF12T. Butaclamol Hydrochloride

8U0H6XI6EO. Clobetasone Butyrate

8U10GC2V6Y. Nicoracetam

8U27U3RIN4. Neridronic Acid

8UAL5421CL. Milfasartan

8UG1323C03. Difenoximide Hydrochloride [difenoximide] (See also *6GEY4W769K*)

8UYY5B89ZU. Dipiproverine Hydrochloride (See also *4XV7PTW3FZ*)

8V2171U69N. Amperozide [amperozide hydrochloride] (See also *0M2W3TAG39*)

8V32U4AOQU. Noscapine

8V6OK1I088. Meglitinide

8VLN5B44ZY. Oxymetazoline Hydrochloride [oxymetazoline] (See also *K89MJ0S5VY*)

8VY00AJ0RL. Dipipanone Hydrochloride (See also *X188638Y2V*)

8VZV102JFY. Fluconazole

8W1IQP3U10. Olmesartan

8W556014K9. Trimethaphan Camsylate

8W5C518302. Dapsone

8W8T17847W. Urea

8WNY0897ER. Sultroponium

8WTG4RSP9Y. Iprozilamine

8WWZ0E633P. Proxicromil

8X09WU898T. Marbofloxacin

8X1R260V33. Propicillin

8X50N88ZDP. Paramethasone Acetate (See also *VFC6ZX3584*)

8X7386QRLV. Gentamicin Sulfate (See also *T6Z9V48IKG*)

8XBV72641V. Nanafrocin

8XP74P4HO3. Tolpiprazole

8XU734C4NG. Isoxicam

8Y164V895Y. Carbachol

8Y3JK0JW3U. Flunixin Meglumine (See also *356IB1O400; 6HG8UB2MUY*)

8Y5377MMOO. Azaftozine

8Y5Y4EEO2V. Protokylol Hydrochloride [protokylol] (See also *7U7O8Q48IO*)

8Y7H79TF0I. Azaspirium Chloride

8YL4JT0L91. Dimorpholamine

8YX6HIZ0IP. Fenadiazole

8Z0ZXE70XL. Ketorfanol

8Z2Z19C8Z1. Parconazole Hydrochloride [parconazole] (See also *8IF7HES548*)

8Z96QXD6UM. Triethyl Citrate

8ZCA2I2L11. Ibopamine

8ZL07I20SB. Doxycycline Calcium

8ZYQ1474W7. Sodium Fluoride

900961Z8VR. Tubocurarine Chloride
9013DUQ28K. Anakinra
9014UFK50C. Edogestrone
9016E3VB47. Deserpidine
901AS54I69. Ramelteon
90347YTW5F. Alfuzosin Hydrochloride [alfuzosin] (See also *75046A1XTN*)
9042592173. Atromepine
9044SC542W. Duloxetine Hydrochloride (See also *O5TNM5N07U*)
904C84L01N. Glidazamide
905GLN509G. Betacetylmethadol
905Z5W3GKH. Thiotepa
906O0YJ6ZP. Monensin
9081Y98W2V. Triptorelin
90897H496X. Rotoxamine Tartrate (See also *VED9E376NC*)
908SY76S4G. Laquinimod Sodium [laquinimod] (See also *4H914M0CSP*)
90BEA145GY. Oxolamine
90ENL74SIG. Safinamide
90G868409O. Cephapirin Benzathine
90I02KLE8K. Dydrogesterone
90I96070LY. Betamethasone Acibutate
90X28IKH43. Vanoxerine
90Y4QC304K. Ketoprofen
9100L32L2N. Metformin
910906N64M. Serfibrate
910G0QIM2M. Domoprednate
910Q707V6F. Acecainide Hydrochloride [acecainide] (See also *B9K738KX14*)
911XR034RX. Doranidazole
913423W85V. Dizatrifone
914032762Y. Pentosan Polysulfate Sodium
915D88LM9O. Dimethylthiambutene
915Q054DLC. Anileridine Hydrochloride (See also *71QI A3O279*)
9164VT6ANB. Sodium Picofosfate
916GJF577D. Declopramide
9171J97IQP. Zometapine
918K9N56QZ. Lucanthone Hydrochloride
919C49XAYD. Decloxizine
91A0K1TY3Z. Halobetasol Propionate (See also *9P6159HM7T*)
91G29CI904. Ciltoprazine
91GW059KN7. Ethylene
91I69L5AY5. Enflurane
91MBZ8H3QO. Sodium Borate
91NGD0O6FZ. Penflutizide
91SZ6DGY86. Quinaldine Blue
91W6Z2N718. Cefotiam Hydrochloride [cefotiam] (See also *H7V12WDZ93*)
91XC93EU03. Phenformin Hydrochloride
91XW058U2C. Maleic Acid
91Y494NL0X. Butenafine Hydrochloride [butenafine] (See also *R8XA2029ZI*)
91ZE013933. Nequinate
91ZQW5JF1Z. Clidinium Bromide
9205LF98OL. Bencisteine
9242ECW6R0. Mycophenolate Mofetil
925FX3X776. Isoproterenol Sulfate
9266D9P3PQ. Bendamustine Hydrochloride [bendamustine] (See also *981Y8SX18M*)
927AH8112L. Nitrofurantoin (See also *E1QI2CQQ1I*)
927L42J563. Acyclovir Sodium
928Q33Q049. Retaspimycin Hydrochloride
9290ND070R. Gacyclidine
92D9H0A3WN. Setazindol
92KE01WH2P. Dazolicine
92M4C245D1. Dimetamfetamine

92S48G7U0W. Citatepine
931L4X5WMM. Impromidine Hydrochloride [impromidine] (See also *E57WP5Y41J*)
933N61G4SL. Cyprazepam
933PJL964R. Elzasonan Citrate [elzasonan] (See also *67JE11VN82*)
935E97BOY8. Folate Sodium [folic acid]
935E97BOY8. Folic Acid
936JST6JCN. Cetyl Alcohol
93AKI1U6QF. Spectinomycin Hydrochloride [spectinomycin] (See also *HWT06H303Z*)
93F1SP6QIN. Lithium Salicylate
93N13LB4Z2. Amrubicin
93VML10KA9. Enazadrem Phosphate (See also *GDV807GKAD*)
93X55PE38X. Fluorescein Sodium (See also *TPY09G7XIR*)
93X6A56W84. Eptaloprost
940ZL3AHKB. Sulfametomidine
942B99D5UK. Bacmecillinam
94301K998R. Clamikalant
9440R8149U. Azamethiphos
9451Z89515. Brinzolamide
947S0YZ36I. Reboxetine
94F21T5G3C. Spizofurone
94F3830Q73. Doxapram Hydrochloride [doxapram] (See also *P5RU6UOQ5Y*)
94F3SX3LEM. Danofloxacin Mesylate (See also *24CU1YS91D*)
94J1SMK20X. Droxypropine
94JPL25DUK. Fronepidil
94NJ818U2W. Meclofenamate Sodium (See also *48I5LU4ZWD*)
94Z39NID6C. Azatadine Maleate [azatadine] (See also *F3Q391WTX7*)
94ZLA3W45F. Arginine
94ZLA3W45F. Arginine Hydrochloride [arginine] (See also *F7LTH1E20Y*)
950O97NUPO. Preladenant
953357GACY. Pentolinium Tartrate
953A26OA1Y. Dornase Alfa
953AP1LBV8. Isothipendyl Hydrochloride
9566855ULN. Isobutamben
956S425ZCY. Topotecan Hydrochloride (See also *7M7YKX2N15*)
957E6438QA. Teniposide
957W618927. Ramixotidine
95818EH730. Amphotalide
95AK1A52I8. Tebipenem Pivoxil
95CO6N199Q. Amprolium
95H6S1X9CC. Timoprazole
95HR524N2M. Iron Dextran
95IK5KI84Z. Cycloserine
95IT3W8JZE. Silver Nitrate
95J02IOS74. Elanzepine
95K4LKB6QE. Detomidine Hydrochloride
95M8R751W8. Orlistat
95OOS7VE0Y. Oxybenzone
95PFX5932Y. Hetacillin Potassium (See also *TN4JSC48CV*)
95Q6WNP25P. Teniloxazine
95QB77JKPL. Doxylamine Succinate [doxylamine] (See also *V9BI9B5YI2*)
95QN29S1ID. Clemastine
95QN29S1ID. Clemastine Fumarate [clemastine] (See also *19259EGQ3D*)
95RFZ48151. Pentafluranol
95U4NV3X82. Cloroperone Hydrochloride
95URV01IDQ. Procaine Hydrochloride
964YS0OOG1. Foscarnet Sodium
96521WL61B. Teloxantrone Hydrochloride [teloxantrone] (See also *7ZQK8VIO6V*)
96600S6GLK. Mopidralazine
96789094BR. Spirendolol

9679TC07X4. Iodine
967RDI7Z6K. Ioxitalamic Acid
9684V5J83L. Sampirtine
969LVT6GJ2. Pirinixil
96D1L38S9Q. Etamocycline
96K6UQ3ZD4. Sucralose
96U2K78I3V. Spirapril Hydrochloride [spirapril] (See also *OCC25LM897*)
96Y4A9AODB. Pamaquine Naphthoate (See also *99QVL5KPSU*)
972FNV35ZM. Imuracetam
9738II2CCH. Tefazoline
9745E7HEBG. Furodazole
977A8K11XO. Dipenine Bromide
977BAL0NR7. Mepiprazole
97B5KCW80W. Bimosiamose
97C5T2UQ7J. Cholesterol
97I1C92E55. Cefixime
97JJW1W1R3. Fenoxazoline Hydrochloride [fenoxazoline] (See also *6K28Y098S7*)
97O6X78C53. Benperidol
97T5AZ1JIP. Cilnidipine
98138WON55. Chloroserpidine
981Y8SX18M. Bendamustine Hydrochloride (See also *9266D9P3PQ*)
9821373UA1. Doxpicomine Hydrochloride [doxpicomine]
982A7M02H5. Carbinoxamine Maleate [carbinoxamine] (See also *02O55696WH*)
982XCM1FOI. Tolbutamide
982XCM1FOI. Tolbutamide Sodium, Sterile [tolbutamide]
9842X06Q6M. Betamethasone
9844OS3B0J. Niludipine
984N9YTM4Y. Aceprometazine
988GU2F9PE. Suprofen
98C3QM4D0P. Lemidosul
98D603VP8V. Nelfinavir Mesylate (See also *HO3OGH5D7I*)
98F8Y85B6W. Chiniofon
98H1T17066. Pasireotide
98HS077RUP. Arnolol
98IMH7M386. Neostigmine Methylsulfate
98IW5HAV1N. Vedaclidine
98PDQ9OL4V. Nafagrel
98PI200987. Lidocaine
98QS4N58TW. Drotaverine
98SR74X50D. Tolufazepam
98WI44OHIQ. Ganaxolone
990TYB331R. Trichloromonofluoromethane
9927MT646M. Basiliximab
9959P4V12N. Teriparatide Acetate
995FT1W541. Idronoxil
9961SL881J. Chlorazanil Hydrochloride
9968S2UKFJ. Dalcotidine
9973I7EX5X. Bifeprofen
997F43Z9CV. Methamphetamine Hydrochloride (See also *44RAL3456C*)
99807U412Y. Amocarzine
9980ST005G. Litoxetine
99DK7FVK1H. Nevirapine
99LL28NYJ2. Propanocaine
99QVL5KPSU. Pamaquine Naphthoate [pamaquine] (See also *96Y4A9AODB*)
99T5TWO621. Chlormerodrin
99TA452185. Prenisteine
99W8X078CA. Alpha-Cypermethrin
99Y8VJ356G. Acitazanolast
99YI50276I. Rimazolium Metilsulfate
99YXE507IL. Tenofovir
9A1222NBG4. Almitrine Mesylate [almitrine] (See also *6RY6V6XM8T*)

9ABL5H8Y29. Pemerid Nitrate
9B1Z1V29C3. Desmethylmoramide
9BAN2XG1ZW. Tipranavir Disodium
9BRV734R3E. Iodohippurate Sodium I 131
9BW5T43J04. Thiodiglycol
9C05J6089W. Flavoxate Hydrochloride (See also *3E74Y80MEY*)
9C60Y73166. Plantago Seed
9C78O7JATH. Denzimol
9C8Z5F38D0. Isbufylline
9CAS0V66OI. Loxoribine
9CBM60191Z. Nithiamide
9CP4KB634M. Isovaleramide
9D2RTI9KYH. Dextromethorphan Hydrobromide (See also *7355X3ROTS*)
9D89762N7C. Guanclofine
9DES9QVH58. Pranidipine
9DLQ4CIU6V. Proline
9DRB973HUI. Dezaguanine
9DUJ3CMK8S. Nitromide
9E01C36A9S. Ethynodiol Diacetate [ethynodiol] (See also *62H10A1236*)
9E338QE28F. Meperidine Hydrochloride [meperidine] (See also *N8E7F7Q170*)
9E75N4A5HM. Triflupromazine Hydrochloride
9E75Q6SUUB. Pridinol
9E8EN393AL. Diisopromine Hydrochloride
9E96TNX6EZ. Fenharmane
9F388J00UK. Trovafloxacin Mesylate [trovafloxacin] (See also *0P1LKO80WN*)
9F5A05A29T. Valproate Pivoxil
9F90KA5Q8U. Triclofos Sodium
9FEN3M88VP. Xantifibrate
9FNZ7TFY4R. Bumepidil
9FPE56Z2TW. Nalorphine Hydrochloride
9FPE98DLZ5. Iganidipine
9G0LAW7ATQ. Levomepromazine
9G1OE216XY. Docosanol
9G34HU7RV0. Edetate Calcium Disodium [edetic acid] (See also *25IH6R4SGF*)
9G34HU7RV0. Edetate Disodium [edetic acid]
9G34HU7RV0. Edetate Sodium [edetic acid] (See also *MP1J8420LU*)
9G34HU7RV0. Edetate Trisodium [edetic acid] (See also *420IP921MB*)
9G34HU7RV0. Edetic Acid
9G3DCA3958. Lexacalcitol
9G64RSX1XD. Captopril
9G69D95443. Epiroprim
9GB927LAJW. Saxagliptin
9GC5JKP4BD. Milenperone
9GJ0N7ZAP0. Methacycline Hydrochloride (See also *IR235-I7C5P*)
9GXY5Z0873. Fenetradil
9H05937G3X. Fluprednisolone
9H440NF95E. Tamitinol
9H4570Q89D. Pleconaril
9H7VJE7A17. Fomidacillin
9H8D3J7V21. Capreomycin Sulfate (See also *232HYX66HC*)
9HLM53094I. Anidulafungin
9HPD98OUWN. Noberastine
9I4T8U1887. Nicoclonate
9I50C3I3OK. Fluorometholone Acetate (See also *SV0CSG527L*)
9I7LNY769Q. Meprobamate
9I7N9PR9J2. Captodiame Hydrochloride
9IFA5XM7R2. Betamethasone Valerate
9J1H7Y9OJV. Emedastine Difumarate [emedastine] (See also *42MB94QOSM*)
9J3ZB93FIE. Dicloralurea

9J68LNZ9ZL. Gloximonam
9J765S329G. Levothyroxine Sodium
9J8YA3ZT14. Ambutonium Bromide
9J92U4CVS0. Axomadol
9J97307Y1H. Florfenicol
9JDX055TW1. Dorzolamide Hydrochloride [dorzolamide] (See also *QZO5366EW7*)
9JFB58YK1E. Alverine Citrate
9JP0YSJ4IC. Suxemerid Sulfate
9JU12S4YFY. Fluoxymesterone
9KGC55KP6A. Epanolol
9KLU2E3573. Estrazinol Hydrobromide [estrazinol] (See also *P1NC244SOF*)
9KY0QXD6LI. Bitolterol Mesylate [bitolterol] (See also *4E53T3611U*)
9L0EXQ7125. Nitroxinil
9L2KA76MG5. Monobenzone
9L3Y3IJ2HI. Caldaret
9L5X4M5L6I. Ibutilide Fumarate (See also *2436VX1U9B*)
9L87N86R9A. Dipyrithione
9LHU78OQFD. Lovastatin
9LT1BRO48Q. Tolazamide
9LVF34296S. Hexazole
9M416Z9QNR. Ceftazidime
9M85GXG84D. Neramexane Mesylate (See also *856DX0KJ84*)
9MG4L920HS. Pretiadil
9MG78X43ZT. Indinavir [indinavir anhydrous] (See also *5W6YA9PKKH*)
9MM438AA0G. Bromoxanide
9MV14S8G3E. Pargyline Hydrochloride [pargyline] (See also *W70V6I2OMY*)
9N42CW7I54. Climbazole
9N7R477WCK. Tramadol Hydrochloride (See also *39J1LGJ30J*)
9NDF7JZ4M3. Rivaroxaban
9NGZ4GPE20. Binifibrate
9NQ109OW0G. Ciramadol
9NV2SR34P8. Betiatide
9NZ7H8YAHG. Aluminum Flufenamate
9O25354EPJ. Enalapril Maleate (See also *69PN84IO1A*)
9O52U70AP4. Piriqualone
9OGY4BOR8D. Mibolerone
9OQO0E343Z. Ammonia N 13
9P043590EX. Azabuperone
9P148IBA8M. Butantrone
9P1872D4OL. Exenatide
9P204CHE8J. Altanserin Tartrate (See also *5015H744JQ*)
9P5MH9F521. Epetirimod
9P6159HM7T. Halobetasol Propionate [halobetasol] (See also *91A0K1TY3Z*)
9PHQ9Y1OLM. Prednisolone
9Q79A81839. Enviradene
9QM8U7R83W. Hydrocortamate Hydrochloride (See also *Y3N00BK5WK*)
9RA9A22Z0W. Benurestat
9RB4L4K895. Cycrimine Hydrochloride (See also *543567RFQQ*)
9RMU91N5K2. Artemisinin
9S339BH15E. Glyparamide
9S44LIC7OJ. Norethindrone Acetate
9S7OD60EWP. Chlorprothixene
9SE2T8DW90. Tiamenidine Hydrochloride
9SUK9B7XVY. Mebhydrolin
9T08RAL174. Bucolome
9TD681796G. Sitafloxacin (See also *3GJC60U4Q8*)
9TF312056Y. Nicotinyl Alcohol
9TMU325RK3. Lanicemine
9TN87S3A3C. Naproxen Sodium (See also *57Y76R9ATQ*)
9TS4B3H261. Carbenicillin Disodium
9TUW81Y3CE. Parecoxib

9U1VM840SP. Physostigmine
9U1VM840SP. Physostigmine Salicylate [physostigmine] (See also *2046ZRO9VU*)
9U1VM840SP. Physostigmine Sulfate [physostigmine] (See also *G63V2J2N71*)
9U3GT3353T. Etonitazene
9U7D5QH5AE. Lactulose
9UUO2T61K7. Tiracizine
9UUW4V7G2H. Bunazosin
9VC7S3ZXXB. Lomefloxacin Hydrochloride
9VF16M7FWU. Aminosalicylate Calcium
9VXA968E0C. Oxymorphone Hydrochloride [oxymorphone] (See also *5Y2EI94NBC*)
9W0Z08C70V. Rodocaine
9WII5M0DU3. Dimefline Hydrochloride [dimefline] (See also *H0XB4R74ID*)
9WP59609J6. Chlorpromazine Hydrochloride (See also *U42B7VYA4P*)
9WQP0L619L. Biricodar Dicitrate
9WTD50I918. Butabarbital Sodium (See also *P0078O25A9*)
9X6F5H479X. Propikacin
9XE0V2SQYX. Promegestone
9XTM81VK2B. Sodium Caprylate
9Y0T619B3U. Bufenadrine
9Y54WZV1CJ. Anipamil
9Y8NXQ24VQ. Propranolol Hydrochloride [propranolol] (See also *F8A3652H1V*)
9YCX42I8IU. Sevelamer Carbonate
9YVR68W306. Enocitabine
9YX16459LE. Chloralformamide
9Z467FG2YK. Flurothyl
9Z4CJC3O5F. Isometheptene Hydrochloride (See also *Y7L24THH6T*)
9Z723VGH7J. Carmegliptin
9Z74BD3QPP. Lidorestat
9ZCS27634Y. Piperoxan
9ZOQ3TZI87. Sorafenib
9ZPC9768EH. Ipramidil
A01LX40298. Methapyrilene Fumarate [methapyrilene]
A034SE7857. Phytonadione
A051Q2099Q. Mirtazapine
A0BK6FM64M. Sumacetamol
A0CR5J8X17. Papaveroline
A0E0NMA80F. Diethylstilbestrol Diphosphate
A0JWA85V8F. Atorvastatin Calcium [atorvastatin] (See also *48A5M73Z4Q*)
A0Z3NAU9DP. Bicalutamide
A10SJL62JY. Ocrelizumab
A153L3JA99. Eltenac
A16F9MIN3Z. Dazoquinast
A1A1I8X02B. Diethylene Glycol Monoethyl Ether
A1L4914FMF. Ticlopidine Hydrochloride (See also *OM90-ZUW7M1*)
A1P35HS4XI. Darglitazone Sodium (See also *AVP9C03Z3K*)
A1TA934AKO. Xylose
A20F9XAI7W. Acrivastine
A221572SK5. Bromchlorenone
A2669OWX9N. Selamectin
A27512LR47. Benzestrol
A28G39IJ7K. Temarotene
A2BH18685W. Parvaquone
A2I8C7HI9T. Methylparaben
A2JGV5CNU4. Cyamemazine
A2P95OOCL0. Difeterol
A2Z7G2RGAH. Pimagedine Hydrochloride
A34YCH7N8A. Oxarbazole
A36BXO4PPX. Pentazocine Hydrochloride
A3N5ZCN45C. Bentonite

A3ULP0F556. Eculizumab

A3VLQ7024W. Dapiclermin

A4ER1Z8N9N. Grepafloxacin Hydrochloride (See also *L1M1U2HC31*)

A4JO90697G. Flotrenizine

A4P49JAZ9H. Ofloxacin

A4V5C6R9FB. Piroctone Olamine

A4VZ22K1WT. Coumarin

A4YJ7J11TG. Ioxilan

A53154FC4N. Terofenamate

A5Q7SNC216. Oxysonium Iodide

A5VAY2U3R8. Tedisamil

A60X6MBU6G. Becatecarin

A61RXM4375. Bexarotene

A6D97U294I. Sotalol Hydrochloride [sotalol] (See also *HEC37C70XX*)

A6IEZ5M406. Ranolazine

A6IEZ5M406. Ranolazine Hydrochloride [ranolazine] (See also *F71253DJUN*)

A6NT0I9X0K. Esafloxacin

A7002E7T2Z. Etymemazine Hydrochloride (See also *861J4K81C7*)

A73MM2Q32P. Triamcinolone Diacetate

A74586SNO7. Clopidogrel Bisulfate [clopidogrel] (See also *08I79HTP27*)

A75SB6QHEG. Ferric Hypophosphite

A76XI0HL37. Etizolam

A7D84513GV. Oxyphenbutazone [oxyphenbutazone anhydrous] (See also *H806S4B3NS*)

A7Q00A39MF. Dabuzalgron Hydrochloride (See also *LGX4GZ74WO*)

A7V27PHC7A. Quinine

A7V27PHC7A. Quinine Bisulfate [quinine]

A7V27PHC7A. Quinine Dihydrochloride [quinine]

A7V27PHC7A. Quinine Salicylate [quinine]

A7V27PHC7A. Quinine Tannate [quinine]

A886B5N5IM. Lisadimate

A8910SQJ1U. Solifenacin Succinate [solifenacin] (See also *KKA5DLD701*)

A89J34472U. Baxitozine

A8CO1VZK2Z. Alibendol

A8EU2FXY13. Topilutamide

A8M33244M6. Nitroxoline

A8Q8I19Q20. Pralatrexate

A937Z0MS6C. Midaxifylline

A948D8673W. Atevirdine Mesylate (See also *N24015WC6D*)

A960M0G5TP. Sarcolysin

A99MK953KZ. Inositol Niacinate

A9C8MNF7CA. Prinaberel

A9W1Q28TT2. Nerbacadol

AA0G3TW31W. Sultopride

AAK27WY74I. Irtemazole

AB2794W8KV. Phendimetrazine Tartrate [phendimetrazine] (See also *6985IP0T80*)

AB5K82X98Y. Zosuquidar Trihydrochloride [zosuquidar] (See also *813AGY3126*)

AB6MNQ6J6L. Succinic Acid

AB9DB0NX46. Dexpropranolol Hydrochloride

ABX8234H6M. Fenoxedil

ABY1GJ356X. Idenast

AC20PJ4101. Haloperidol Decanoate

AC79L7PV2G. Cloxacillin Benzathine (See also *O6X5QGC2VB*)

AC80WD7GPF. Ammonium Benzoate

ACZ6L64B41. Azintamide

ADC79EK5Q8. Ethylestrenol

ADD4H8T3K9. Piridronic Acid

ADN3S497AZ. Miglustat

ADN79D536H. Clobetasol Propionate [clobetasol] (See also *779619577M*)

ADN850L91I. Penthrichloral

ADS4I3E22M. Levalbuterol Tartrate

AE28F7PNPL. Methionine

AET4M101U3. Nilprazole

AF73293C2R. Acetylcholine Chloride

AFE2YW0IIZ. Sufentanil

AGG2FN16EV. Simvastatin

AI9376Y64P. Dexamethasone Sodium Phosphate

AI9WDT80FQ. Benzylsulfamide

AIQ630U6XO. Furtrethonium Iodide [furtrethonium] (See also *1D064NLD7G*)

AIU7053OWL. Haloprogin

AJ14S16J7N. Sulfonterol Hydrochloride (See also *Z540ZT2MI6*)

AJ6J4424XT. Furnidipine

AJS8S3P31H. Satavaptan

AJT2YN495R. Propatyl Nitrate

AK5Q5FZH2R. Pyritinol

AK7DRB7FMO. Levcycloserine

AL805O9OG9. Orphenadrine Citrate [orphenadrine] (See also *X0A40N8I4S*)

AL8499KM94. Ditolamide

AL8Z8K3P6S. Hexobarbital

AL8Z8K3P6S. Hexobarbital Sodium [hexobarbital] (See also *I788X867K7*)

AM2KZ47R0J. Delanterone

AM91H2KS67. Cerivastatin Sodium [cerivastatin] (See also *6Q18G1060S*)

AM94R510MS. Azathioprine Sodium

AMT77LS62O. Bithionol

AMT77LS62O. Bithionolate Sodium [bithionol]

AMW2MRV3OT. Dichlorisone Acetate [dichlorisone]

AMX8J6YS1H. Quindoxin

AN164J8Y0X. Trimethoprim

AO61G82577. Trihexyphenidyl Hydrochloride (See also *6RC5V8B7PO*)

AO9YF4MN30. Methicillin Sodium (See also *Q91FH1328A*)

AOX68RY4TV. Dinitolmide

AP3C1V2UPV. Sulfacecole

AP69E83Z79. Bifeprunox

APG9819VLM. Darifenacin

APG9819VLM. Darifenacin Hydrobromide [darifenacin] (See also *CR02EYQ8GV*)

APX8D32IX1. Mepenzolate Bromide

AR6Y753ARL. Piroheptine

ATD81G944M. Bumadizone

AV0X7V6CSE. Pilsicainide

AV4229D6CH. Domipizone

AV9U0660CW. Eribulin Mesylate

AVG0GBV8AP. Propiram Fumarate

AVP9C03Z3K. Darglitazone Sodium [darglitazone] (See also *A1P35HS4XI*)

AVX3D5A4LM. Thyrotropin Alfa

AWA682DH9Z. Pruvanserin Hydrochloride (See also *UL09X1-D9EM*)

AWC1VMS3HC. Buquineran

AX03A96739. Febuverine

AXA8K5U95M. Sulfaclomide

AXQ0JYM303. Benoxinate Hydrochloride [benoxinate] (See also *0VE4U49K15*)

AY28O44JGD. Pholedrine

AYI8EX34EU. Creatinine

AYN5T18K5R. Brovincamine

AZJ60Y1VSK. Flupimazine

B017BC5B1N. Meparfynol

B025Y34C54. Acebutolol Hydrochloride (See also *67P356D8GH*)

B07L15YAEV. Arbutamine Hydrochloride [arbutamine] (See also *K0NF2CPJ7F*)
B08O4ROE04. Pentacynium Chloride
B0E341RA20. Aklomide
B0F91K5U4N. Ibuprofen Piconol
B0P231ILBK. Ospemifene
B10YD955QW. Dexchlorpheniramine Maleate (See also *3Q9Q0B929N*)
B1E00KQ6NT. Talmapimod
B1H2FS2WPP. Bifepramide
B1H5V6OZSE. Iolidonic Acid
B1X701S0MV. Acifran
B255B0J51N. Tienocarbine
B28V86NGNK. Fonazine Mesylate
B2V233XGE7. Mestranol
B321AL142J. Molgramostim
B32804UAUQ. Azacosterol Hydrochloride
B3CRJ1EWJU. Thiothixene Hydrochloride
B453T1E8MP. Casokefamide
B45CF873F8. Fenoctimine Sulfate [fenoctimine] (See also *448AZ21I6G*)
B4J4M4939D. Carumonam Sodium
B4OB0JHI1X. Proparacaine Hydrochloride [proparacaine] (See also *U96OL57GOY*)
B4SF212641. Fosphenytoin Sodium [fosphenytoin] (See also *7VLR55452Z*)
B4XTR3PC33. Prampine
B51UC955KQ. Isaglidole
B53E3NMY5C. Tizanidine Hydrochloride (See also *6AI06C00GW*)
B54CW5KG52. Levomethadyl Acetate Hydrochloride
B57Z82EOGE. Alniditan Dihydrochloride [alniditan]
B5RKR9Y63Y. Febuprol
B5T2Z06Y9N. Glutaurine
B64NJG83K2. Hexafluorenium Bromide
B6831ORH7W. Salazosulfamide
B6C301298G. Efletirizine
B6CJY5K2ST. Adimolol
B6DRB5ZI7P. Metyrapone Tartrate (See also *ZS9KD92H6V*)
B6E06QE59J. Mepivacaine Hydrochloride [mepivacaine] (See also *4VFX2L7EM5*)
B72HH48FLU. Infliximab
B762XZ551X. Dioxybenzone
B76N6SBZ8R. Gemcitabine
B77K612SPZ. Bumecaine
B7IN85G1HY. Dinoprost
B8414665Y7. Pytamine
B8L03Q9MME. Ampyzine Sulfate
B8VQU4C05J. Adafenoxate
B8Z8J4400H. Sanguinarium Chloride
B908C4MV2R. Cefroxadine
B926Y9U4QN. Indacrinone
B9454PE93C. Cloricromen
B96UX1DDKS. Gemcabene Calcium [gemcabene] (See also *Z9AM8GST2F*)
B987T0L5FX. Benzetimide Hydrochloride [benzetimide] (See also *V6ERX20PHB*)
B9A98D632Z. Pipoxizine
B9JAY11T6C. Deditonium Bromide [deditonium] (See also *6BCE7KY501*)
B9K738KX14. Acecainide Hydrochloride (See also *910Q707V6F*)
BA484813BO. Salverine
BA5ALU2ZT9. Cefpirome Sulfate
BA9QH3P00T. Echothiophate Iodide
BB27ZR25WO. Cliprofen
BBL281NWFG. Cod Liver Oil
BBX060AN9V. Hydrogen Peroxide

BC621AC03L. Estrapronicate
BD07M97B2A. Alfaxalone
BD20Y3892A. Ioprocemic Acid
BD2A56I30W. Traxoprodil Mesylate
BD9T227F6M. Amikhelline
BDF1O1C72E. Nystatin
BDL7R8N38D. Guaiapate
BEW7469QZ0. Homatropine Hydrobromide
BF4C9Z1J53. Amantadine Hydrochloride [amantadine] (See also *M6Q1EO9TD0*)
BF6IGI53XH. Temelastine
BFE9UAV73M. Nifursemizone
BFG1TY61BG. Diacetamate
BG3F62OND5. Carboplatin
BGG1Y1ED0Y. Triclocarban
BGJ4Z7930W. Miproxifene
BGL0JSY5SI. Quetiapine Fumarate [quetiapine] (See also *2S3PL1B6UJ*)
BH210P244U. Medetomidine Hydrochloride
BH3B64OKL9. Fampridine
BH48F620JA. Fanetizole Mesylate [fanetizole] (See also *D3OG7B0G4M*)
BH6M93CIA0. Tiludronate Disodium
BHM1XXA2EZ. Desciclovir
BHV525JOBH. Doripenem
BI81Z4542G. Adrafinil
BIB7HG2V9E. Fasidotril
BIQ52YQ7VG. Araprofen
BIY8B0682Q. Salantel
BJ1N2V028P. Chlorphenoctium Amsonate
BJ4HF6IU1D. Pindolol
BJ507J4LKY. Tilorone Hydrochloride (See also *O6W7VEW6KS*)
BJ563H8V4W. Perastine
BK2633656Q. Dulozafone
BK349F52C9. Batimastat
BK76465IHM. Ranitidine Hydrochloride
BKE5Q1J60U. Imipramine Hydrochloride (See also *OGG85SX4E4*)
BKJ8M8G5HI. Imatinib
BKY8H56395. Fenbutrazate
BL03SY4LXB. Nortriptyline Hydrochloride [nortriptyline] (See also *00FN6IH15D*)
BL0L45OVKT. Fenthion
BL51M8CB8R. Relacatib
BLH9UKX9V1. Tesofensine
BLO7300903. Fenpentadiol
BM1HR7IP1L. Piragliatin
BN10X2TL6I. Cefoxazole
BN34FX42G3. Allyl Isothiocyanate
BO55Z3JL5K. Lamtidine
BO9LE4QFZF. Stavudine
BOD072YW0F. Lincomycin
BOD072YW0F. Lincomycin Hydrochloride [lincomycin] (See also *M6T05Z2B68*)
BOM1J10QQM. Dimetofrine
BP0YBT71AK. Endomide
BP76593251. Ronipamil
BPA9UT29BS. Dexbrompheniramine Maleate (See also *75T64B71RP*)
BPF36H1G6S. Cloxyquin
BQ0I558X42. Bendacalol Mesylate [bendacalol] (See also *5KP3ZO1VLL*)
BQ67CS3Q3E. Setoperone
BR2Z22465M. Mepiroxol
BR551134L6. Primaperone
BRL1C2459K. Amlexanox
BSC36V44TK. Subathizone
BT61K2O76Y. Nicopholine

BT9Y6D2DR0. Penirolol

BTS1Y6777M. Apadenoson

BV3N6F82WN. Fenclexonium Metilsulfate [fenclexonium] (See also *88M0X6627K*)

BVG9H4U2ZB. Divabuterol

BVM2UGN450. Dupracetam

BVS505O332. Chymotrypsin

BW7H1TJS22. Imidapril

BW9B0ZE037. Sildenafil Citrate (See also *3M7OB98Y7H*)

BWP53NPW3F. Gedocarnil

BX2MKR427K. Ciapilome

BXF83S0HEL. Alphacetylmethadol

BXO86P3XXW. Eltanolone

BXR49TP611. Isobutane

BXS8X8APGS. Ciclopramine

BY5RLE340B. Fosfonet Sodium

BYK4592A3Q. Ambazone

BYX6E7M5QE. Isonixin

BZ114NVM5P. Mitoxantrone Hydrochloride [mitoxantrone] (See also *U6USW86RD0*)

BZ1R15MTK7. Levomenthol

BZ5N591H97. Tetronasin

BZF2ZM0I5Z. Retaspimycin

C01407869B. Dimeprozan

C045TQL4WP. Phentermine

C045TQL4WP. Phentermine Hydrochloride [phentermine] (See also *0K2I505OTV*)

C04V6SGK8H. Faxeladol

C0HG40P7PY. Suloxifen Oxalate (See also *LD18TA6Q06*)

C0P8MP2SR5. Fenisorex

C11102TO53. Flunarizine Hydrochloride

C137DTR5RG. Theophylline

C137DTR5RG. Theophylline Olamine [theophylline]

C137DTR5RG. Theophylline Sodium Glycinate [theophylline]

C151H8M554. Sucrose

C1ENJ2TE6C. Oxycodone Hydrochloride (See also *CD35PMG570*)

C1LJO185Q9. Oxitriptan

C1PXF8V06N. Domiodol

C2087G0XX3. Furafylline

C229N9DX94. Aminophylline [aminophylline dihydrate] (See also *27Y3KJK423*)

C22G6EYP8B. Cephalothin Sodium (See also *R72LW146E6*)

C23W8PF2D4. Tilsuprost

C291HFX4DY. Norgestimate

C2B9CF1640. Zolamine Hydrochloride (See also *NXB79TB0N2*)

C2E1CI501T. Magnesium Trisilicate

C2QI4IOI2G. Medroxyprogesterone Acetate (See also *HSU1-C9YRES*)

C2R0GEU722. Lintopride

C3705I245K. Lifarizine

C38638H76Y. Ulifloxacin

C3QYZ005LS. Enolicam Sodium (See also *TEA6PI0H6H*)

C3XSG3DLPA. Clazolimine

C40N4EJY68. Glycyclamide

C43C467DPE. Ceftizoxime Sodium [ceftizoxime] (See also *26337D5X88*)

C460ZSU1OW. Eperezolid

C46317G8F0. Picobenzide

C49WS9N75L. Virginiamycin

C4A112M10H. Tofenacin Hydrochloride [tofenacin] (See also *3A10ND4DWR*)

C4A4TVM56F. Bencianol

C4A61P8A37. Motapizone

C4DT7VL6FU. Crotoniazide

C4DZ64560D. Troleandomycin

C4R42570ZO. Alaproclate

C4V95L5P6A. Bimethoxycaine Lactate

C4W7I532MX. Belarizine

C53598599T. Moxifloxacin Hydrochloride

C53SV0WO4V. Pivagabine

C5529G5JPQ. Ginger

C56709M5NH. Mazindol

C5KT601WPM. Quadrosilan

C5MKX7XOYA. Amustaline Dihydrochloride

C5W04GO61S. Tiopronin

C65T2BG75L. Cicarperone

C668Q9I33J. Oxiconazole Nitrate [oxiconazole] (See also *RQ8UL4C17S*)

C67IS11N0O. Amidantel

C69JI1BAU8. Amosulalol

C6BZ5263BJ. Apratastat

C6QE1Q1TKR. Procyclidine Hydrochloride [procyclidine] (See also *CQC932Z7YW*)

C6Y700V0M4. Inproquone

C6Z73MW6CR. Talsupram

C7B0AH4986. Fopirtoline

C7C2QDD75P. Gliquidone

C7D6T3H22J. Artemether

C7H9M9492J. Fumoxicillin

C7K8PK4Q0E. Stacofylline

C7Q3TBR3FP. Sequifenadine

C810JCZ56Q. Sodium Monofluorophosphate

C8A0P8G029. Aliskiren Fumarate

C8I4BVN78E. Glutethimide

C8MRZ07FDV. Oxytetracycline Calcium

C9734VZR4O. Brazergoline

C9LVQ0YUXG. Axitinib

C9Z9ICZ7YR. Tinoridine

CA49Y29RA9. Cyromazine

CB2TL9PS0T. Propoxyphene Hydrochloride

CBI6614BOL. Pipradimadol

CC9149U2QX. Sodium Ferric Gluconate Complex

CC995ZMV90. Ambroxol [ambroxol hydrochloride] (See also *200168S0CL*)

CD35PMG570. Oxycodone

CD35PMG570. Oxycodone Hydrochloride [oxycodone] (See also *C1ENJ2TE6C*)

CF48QOH154. Dioxifedrine

CFY01MZD5T. Cetefloxacin

CH1Y88E2AY. Aminoquinol

CH8C36F1MO. Stearylsulfamide

CHB1QD2QSS. Temazepam

CHG7QC509W. Cicletanine

CHH9H12AQ3. Tolazoline Hydrochloride [tolazoline] (See also *E669Z6S1JG*)

CHI530446X. Vanillin

CI0FAO63WC. Cefdinir

CI1S3XAK7O. Etodroxizine

CI71S98N1Z. Potassium Phosphate, Dibasic

CIF6334OLY. Tolcapone

CIK9F54ZHR. Docusate Potassium

CIW5S16655. Chlorophenothane

CIX5G6J9R1. Iodoxamate Meglumine (See also *NS1Y283HW4; 6HG8UB2MUY*)

CJ0O37KU29. Verapamil

CK0N3WH0SR. Perflutren

CK4M8AX1LN. Safironil

CK833KGX7E. Amphetamine Sulfate [amphetamine] (See also *6DPV8NK46S*)

CKM4S0R7LX. Ethynerone

CKS724B66O. Bepafant

CL2002R563. Pozanicline

CL2T97X0V0. Carbon Tetrachloride

CLO4JRD21F. Anatibant

CLY16Y8Z7E. Carphenazine Maleate [carphenazine] (See also *0HX1Z0A2MC*)
CLY7M0XD20. Migalastat Hydrochloride
CLY9MRR8FV. Orazamide
CM1N99QR1M. Metrizoate Sodium [metrizoic acid] (See also *O65Q227UIC*)
CM5J1V7AUT. Ebiratide
CMF6Z78SWL. Lobendazole
CN68E94R2X. Romazarit
CN8EF9N084. Tozasertib Lactate
CNG7995Y4B. Quinocide
CO51Q2EI5Z. Alphaprodine Hydrochloride
CO68M0Q897. Hydrocodone Polistirex
COF19H7WBK. Dicloxacillin
COF19H7WBK. Dicloxacillin Sodium [dicloxacillin] (See also *4HZT2V9KX0*)
COU3RRH769. Cabastine
CP1A26546Z. Tebanicline Tosylate
CQ27G2BZJM. Amlodipine Maleate
CQ903KQA31. Dicyclomine Hydrochloride (See also *4KV4X8IF6V*)
CQC932Z7YW. Procyclidine Hydrochloride (See also *C6QE1Q1TKR*)
CR02EYQ8GV. Darifenacin Hydrobromide (See also *APG9819VLM*)
CR6K9C2NHK. Methylparaben Sodium
CRS35BZ94Q. Desflurane
CT6BBQ5A68. Dinoprost Tromethamine
CTD060B1SS. Tretinoin Tocoferil
CU0X85F735. Ftorpropazine
CU3H37T766. Rilmazafone
CU8D464EDW. Somatrem
CU9463U2E2. Asenapine Maleate (See also *JKZ19V908O*)
CUI83R2732. Calcium Hypophosphite
CUT48I42ON. Methyprylon
CUZ39LUY82. Silodosin
CV07VSP2G8. Dazopride Fumarate [dazopride] (See also *J8ZC30U6CH*)
CV71VTP0VN. Ipidacrine
CVN9D598JL. Nantradol Hydrochloride
CW25IKJ202. Streptomycin Sulfate (See also *Y45QSO73OB*)
CWU66767HF. Bermoprofen
CX05Q7WO72. Broxitalamic Acid
CX3RPB4DVF. Flutomidate
CX9T97T0XH. Cinpropazide
CXJ7G6BYD7. Cyclindole
CY351D07GJ. Sulosemide
CY3RNB3K4T. Proflavine Dihydrochloride [proflavine]
CY3RNB3K4T. Proflavine Sulfate [proflavine] (See also *2961Y60ATP*)
CY5E0946P1. Broclepride
CYS9AKD70P. Isoflurane
CZ3T9T146K. Talnetant
CZ5312222S. Nicardipine Hydrochloride [nicardipine] (See also *K5BC5011K3*)
CZ5QG07777. Indopine [indopine hydrochloride] (See also *J57707EKBI*)
CZU6V3902K. Efloxate
D0514P112G. Anisperimus
D09L486R3J. Ciladopa Hydrochloride [ciladopa]
D0GX863OA5. Mupirocin
D0N7A2M3MU. Brallobarbital
D0NR12WK9J. Sulbentine
D0TAM1017B. Rentiapril
D0U312O2BE. Tenilapine
D0VK52NV5M. Asimadoline
D133ZRF50U. Tripalmitin
D1DE63830P. Nifenalol

D1FP3K444H. Diclofurime
D1Q7F6C2FP. Quazinone
D27V6190PM. Olopatadine Hydrochloride [olopatadine] (See also *2XG66W44KF*)
D28J6W18HY. Frovatriptan Succinate
D2JUE6GD5A. Erythromycin Ethylcarbonate
D2UFC189XF. Medrysone
D2UX06XLB5. Pomalidomide
D2VW67N38H. Apraclonidine Hydrochloride (See also *843CEN85DI*)
D32S14F082. Terazosin Hydrochloride (See also *8L5014XET7*)
D32TNF4T6G. Folescutol
D35FM8T64X. Fosaprepitant Dimeglumine (See also *6L8OF9XRDC*)
D3FM8FA78T. Pramlintide
D3OG7B0G4M. Fanetizole Mesylate (See also *BH48F620JA*)
D3R9B47JTE. Dimoxaprost
D3SQ406G9X. Articaine
D42O649ALL. Telcagepant
D42OWK5383. Acotiamide Hydrochloride [acotiamide] (See also *NMW7447A9A*)
D48MS3A6N9. Alvocidib
D4F329SL1O. Hexaminolevulinate Hydrochloride
D4SL77931L. Ritipenem
D51WO0G0L4. Clorazepate Dipotassium [clorazepic acid] (See also *63FN7G03XY*)
D51WO0G0L4. Clorazepate Monopotassium [clorazepic acid] (See also *MS63G8NQUI*)
D51WO0G0L4. Clorazepic Acid
D5340Y2I9G. Castor Oil
D57I4Z650L. Azetepa
D59N834676. Ezatiostat Hydrochloride
D59ZQ3VVMV. Lodaxaprine
D5H25D039V. Alprafenone
D61659OVD0. Fenticlor
D65DG142WK. Maltitol
D6FH7ALQ18. Etipirium Iodide
D6NBQ3H12U. Lenapenem
D6S4O4XD0H. Crotamiton
D6VHC87LLS. Chlorquinaldol
D762286A5N. Dotefonium Bromide
D7B8U8VA9J. Sulfamazone
D7CJB20DJO. Amicarbalide
D7ID553901. Clotioxone
D7UUO54C6N. Mafoprazine
D7ZD41RZI9. Ropinirole Hydrochloride
D83282DT06. Flucytosine
D86I0XLB13. Mitiglinide
D874R9PZ9T. Pactimibe
D87YGH4Z0Q. Omega-3-acid Ethyl Esters
D8K2JPN18B. Tolmetin
D8TST4O562. Pantoprazole
D8Z6E4IR2J. Renanolone
D933668QVX. Insulin Aspart
D959AE5USF. Clofazimine
D9693UHF82. Cefcanel Daloxate
D982V7VT3P. Echinacea Angustifolia
D9C330MD8B. Copovidone
D9FU86687U. Felipyrine
D9OM4SK49P. Cetylpyridinium Chloride
DA25635W9D. Etabenzarone
DA87705X9K. Erlotinib Hydrochloride (See also *J4T82NDH7E*)
DAA13NKG2Q. Papaverine Hydrochloride [papaverine] (See also *23473EC6BQ*)
DBE10Q8QF6. Mebiquine
DCR9Z582X0. Epoprostenol
DCR9Z582X0. Epoprostenol Sodium [epoprostenol] (See also *4K04IQ1OF4*)

DCV1328NH2. Tenidap Sodium
DE08037SAB. Magnesium Sulfate
DEE37CY4VO. Lomerizine
DES29595KX. Azolimine
DF7D3NY7EL. Noxiptiline
DG355XWQ4T. Diphenidol Hydrochloride (See also *NQO8R319LY*)
DGB1125380. Azepexole
DGN08QZ30G. Semotiadil
DH9E53K1Y8. Norflurane
DHT6E8M4KP. Pelitrexol
DI9132OQ3R. Seractide Acetate (See also *IGM44CEY2I*)
DIA2A74855. Isoproterenol Hydrochloride (See also *L628TT009W*)
DJ1N20F93D. Poskine
DJF293UV6K. Siltenzepine
DJH1LFU42E. Sulicrinat
DK0OIL461Z. Methaphenilene Hydrochloride
DK61ZER6T7. Mitindomide
DK95Z519WL. Pumaprazole
DKQ4T82YE6. Sulbactam Sodium
DL48G20X8X. Scopolamine Hydrobromide [scopolamine] (See also *451IFR0GXB*)
DL8Q24959P. Cefovecin Sodium
DL9055K809. Levamisole Hydrochloride (See also *2880D3468G*)
DM32B4GU70. Frakefamide
DO22K1PRDJ. Piribedil
DO2D32W0VC. Ancitabine
DO989GC5D1. Lestaurtinib
DOL5F9JD3E. Delavirdine Mesylate [delavirdine] (See also *421105KRQE*)
DOQ0J0TPF7. Metyrosine
DOS9ZOT21L. Denagliptin Tosylate [denagliptin] (See also *T47477CUF7*)
DOZ62MV6A5. Taltirelin
DQ0H2B8YKN. Fradafiban
DQ448MW7KS. Palivizumab
DQ61UZ670G. Etofuradine
DQ6KK6GV93. Piretanide
DQH6T6D8OY. Tiagabine Hydrochloride (See also *Z80I64HMNP*)
DR0QR50ALL. Spiroxatrine
DR5S136IVO. Avanafil
DS9UJN1I0X. Dapiprazole Hydrochloride
DT27W93DFF. Mesudipine
DT67WL708F. Delmopinol
DT7DT5E518. Enprofylline
DTI67O9503. Alglucosidase Alfa
DTL5W0113X. Cetaben Sodium [cetaben] (See also *433YPU24B8*)
DTN86H1ZWK. Napamezole Hydrochloride
DU65LYP662. Fantridone Hydrochloride
DUU9GVA746. Tribuzone
DV74WJ5PJB. Isoetharine Mesylate
DVO6SSG9S3. Brefonalol
DW310SVK6Q. Nicogrelate
DWG8UZD9HT. Acetomenaphthone
DWI62G0P59. Sivelestat
DWL616XF1K. Oxyfedrine
DWV1EFW947. Azlocillin Sodium
DX1U2629QE. Succimer
DX586KL1YX. Benzoylpas Calcium (See also *XEE879L727*)
DX60OV32AE. Sulmepride
DY38VHM5OD. Sodium Hypochlorite
DZY7AR1B0U. Epicainide
DZY9VU539P. Narasin
E0018IF0K4. Amelubant
E00MVC7O57. Balicatib

E0KNA372SZ. Isopropamide Iodide (See also *8B9I31H724*)
E1CR8487EN. Sodium Prasterone Sulfate
E1IO3ICJ9A. Tandutinib
E1L4ZW2F8O. Cathine
E1QI2CQQ1I. Nitrofurantoin [nitrofurantoin monohydrate] (See also *927AH8112L*)
E2287TKU04. Dexamethasone Acetate (See also *K7V8P532WP*)
E2EV7ZDD1M. Thiamiprine
E2M3325B1R. Fluacizine
E33L6C08A5. Pipratecol
E33TS05V6B. Aspirin Aluminum
E367I8C7FI. Brecanavir
E375EMI4HW. Brofezil
E377MF8EQ8. Trimethoprim Sulfate
E3AP71EM0O. Fanapanel
E3B2GI648A. Belatacept
E3M2R8Q947. Galdansetron Hydrochloride
E3N11DY0TA. Cartasteine
E3U7286V3W. Mitozolomide
E3U8347QWJ. Glycobiarsol
E3ZEH4F4CA. Etriciguat
E47C56IGOY. Acecarbromal
E4E8GE5LVJ. Guanisoquin Sulfate (See also *307YLU08D8*)
E4G31X93ZA. Atrasentan Hydrochloride (See also *V6D7VK2215*)
E4GA8884NN. Phosphoric Acid
E4RK86FAVR. Hepronicate
E51A927SNR. Triafungin
E521I6380L. Rilozarone
E524N2IXA3. Ornithine
E569WG6E60. Arzoxifene
E57WP5Y41J. Impromidine Hydrochloride (See also *931L4X5WMM*)
E5B7C16LFK. Tioclomarol
E5B8ND5IPE. Methohexital
E5GY4I6YCZ. Cinnamon Oil
E5XNT3RF5A. Tegaserod Maleate
E60VWA40D2. Mannomustine
E61Q31EK2F. Cyproterone Acetate [cyproterone]
E64XL9U38K. Chlorhexidine Hydrochloride
E6582LOH6V. Fexofenadine Hydrochloride [fexofenadine] (See also *2S068B75ZU*)
E65W20MU7A. Clorotepine
E669Z6S1JG. Tolazoline Hydrochloride (See also *CHH9H12AQ3*)
E66RIC936T. Toprilidine
E697IIC25J. Zafuleptine
E6GNX3HHTE. Brimonidine Tartrate [brimonidine] (See also *4S9CL2DY2H*)
E70CPL81IY. Relomycin
E70G3G5863. Bupropion Hydrobromide
E7199S1YWR. Lisinopril
E750O06Y6O. Hesperidin
E780TX33D2. Daniquidone
E7C6PMZ54M. Sulphamoprine
E7IDJ8DS1D. Alinidine
E7N3FX2T1J. Denpidazone
E7WED276I5. Mercaptopurine (See also *PKK6MUZ20G*)
E82B3Z65BN. Pirifibrate
E833KT807K. Ifetroban
E84FJ4KW3B. Duoperone Fumarate [duoperone] (See also *G7MM186D7U*)
E87N3L27KX. Adibendan
E8MZK2U45W. Ciclafrine Hydrochloride
E90NZP2L9U. Digitoxin
E9503DM633. Prozapine
E9584TMZ4M. Tiopropamine
E96467495S. Diflumidone Sodium [diflumidone]

E9730RXS4H. Donetidine
E9P274AJEW. Tibezonium Iodide
E9UO06K7CE. Bucindolol Hydrochloride [bucindolol]
EA590X615B. Alteconazole
EA6LD1M70M. Megestrol Acetate [megestrol] (See also *TJ2M0FR8ES*)
EAO03PE1TC. Sodium Nitroprusside
EB87433V6F. Parecoxib Sodium
ECA0E1PO91. Nexopamil
EDK3Z2X1IV. Nictindole
EE90ONI6FF. Potassium Citrate
EE92BBP03H. Diltiazem Hydrochloride [diltiazem] (See also *OLH94387TE*)
EEB95DS30P. Ecastolol
EEK88K197T. Tenosal
EEN99869SC. Alogliptin Benzoate (See also *JHC049LO86*)
EER9874LXT. Iodomethamate Sodium
EF0NX91490. Pentagastrin
EFW857872Q. Butamben
EG12MD1RMA. Moquizone
EG1ZDO6LRD. Clorsulon
EG3B69DFQ5. Tiflorex
EG6V6W7WDD. Mesulfen
EGV6V52K6N. Anaritide Acetate
EH28UP18IF. Isotretinoin
EH6D7113I8. Clindamycin Phosphate (See also *3U02EL437C*)
EH6H7VS52J. Glaucarubin
EHX04MU69R. Butopiprine
EJ9QI3Q1LT. Erocainide
EK22QV7701. Lidofenin
EK9LSW731R. Ethiazide
EKF7043SBU. Monoxerutin
EL461OY152. Forfenimex
ELK3V90G6C. Alefacept
EM8BM710ZC. Salicylamide
EMB5M4GMHP. Benzilonium Bromide
ENR1LLB0FP. Desmopressin Acetate [desmopressin] (See also *XB13HYU18U*)
ENV72C33QD. Thialbarbital
EOR26LQQ24. Ezetimibe
EOS1G6F668. Froxiprost
EOS72165S7. Fesoterodine Fumarate
EP3QG127N9. Vicriviroc Maleate (See also *TL515DW4QS*)
EPD1EH7F53. Propoxycaine Hydrochloride [propoxycaine] (See also *K490D39G46*)
EQ35YMS20Q. Fluindione
EQ8YV2D86Y. Taprizosin
EQR32Y7H0M. Zinc Carbonate
EQT531S367. Carvedilol Phosphate
ER09126G7A. Lornoxicam
ER0CTH01H9. Phenacetin
ERJ6X2MXV7. Sugammadex Sodium
ESH23ZBF8P. Dexproxibutene
ESJ56Q60GC. Ritodrine Hydrochloride
ET1UGF4A0B. Mexenone
ET36GPP4T7. Ioglycamic Acid
ET8IF4KS1T. Nedocromil Sodium
ETM878JC9K. Medazepam Hydrochloride (See also *P0J3387W3S*)
EUL532EI54. Closantel
EUT3557RT5. Arimoclomol
EVA0339N2N. Euprocin Hydrochloride
EWG253M961. Fluperlapine
EWP54G0J8F. Nitrocefin
EWQ57Q8I5X. Lactose Monohydrate
EX1ND80X1I. Isotiquimide
EX438O2MRT. Ferric Oxide, Yellow
EX637I77PC. Xantocillin

EYG5Y6355E. Trapidil
EYK815W3Z8. Nesbuvir
EYX738UZ5P. Demexiptiline
EZ15I5D6C1. Dextofisopam
EZ270U8Z9W. Amiquinsin Hydrochloride
EZ61NB05TG. Tabilautide
EZ948T2878. Tomoxiprole
EZN4D2O31B. Bemetizide
EZS5V8UN4Y. Spiroglumide
EZY3PL8Q0M. Batoprazine
F05Q2T2JA0. Docusate Sodium
F05RR5M463. Flerobuterol
F089I0511L. Indapamide
F0D4M5RASG. Bucainide Maleate [bucainide]
F0O89MB7QE. Propenidazole
F0P408N6V4. Lenalidomide
F0PVL84ZWR. Pimeclone
F0R68O7C4V. Asobamast
F0XDI6ZL63. Caspofungin
F0XVL451MO. Cinflumide
F0Z746KRKQ. Rubidium Chloride Rb 82
F14V3I66R3. Oxifungin Hydrochloride [oxifungin] (See also *34711907NJ*)
F1BC02I72W. Cephradine (See also *56PPJ9MMPE*)
F1DZD948G6. Nicafenine
F1T8QT9U8B. Digitalis
F1ZL87F3PM. Emakalim
F24ADO1E2D. Droxicam
F2613LO055. Bunitrolol
F2628ZD0FO. Arundic Acid
F2R8V82B84. Hyoscyamine Sulfate
F2S6Z4SB8T. Acaprazine
F2U67W4R4J. Iquindamine
F2VW3D43YT. Azelaic Acid
F37A9VKY5Q. Minocromil
F37S7G37O2. Esomeprazole Potassium
F38R0JR742. Lumefantrine
F39049Y068. Apomorphine Hydrochloride (See also *N21FAR7B4S*)
F39KSS6R80. Tidiacic
F3Q391WTX7. Azatadine Maleate (See also *94Z39NID6C*)
F41401512X. Nilotinib
F4216019LN. Albendazole
F446C597KA. Triamcinolone Acetonide
F49638UBDR. Oxilofrine
F4ER8Z6Q3U. Pivoxazepam
F4MW5166YH. Tritoqualine
F4X3L6068O. Ethopabate
F4XSI7SNIU. Oxprenolol Hydrochloride (See also *519MXN9YZR*)
F52Y83BGH3. Faropenem Medoxomil [faropenem] (See also *5OK523O4FU*)
F54EHJ34MV. Niceritrol
F551446KF3. Cyclopentamine Hydrochloride
F57Y390K2N. Nifurmerone
F5AK41IPQG. Sulfametrole
F5N0ALI65V. Beclamide
F5SXN2KNMR. Pixantrone
F5TD010360. Alprostadil
F5WR8N145C. Sodium Iodide
F5Z5EL4D26. Lonaprisan
F604ZKI910. Ipodate Calcium [ipodic acid]
F604ZKI910. Ipodate Sodium [ipodic acid]
F63SY70KV0. Butocrolol
F64QU97QCR. Dantrolene
F64QU97QCR. Dantrolene Sodium [dantrolene] (See also *287M0347EV*)
F69EA18270. Cefuracetime

F6G1K9WJU4. Anazolene Sodium
F6M52CDT0W. Varespladib Sodium
F6S91MHL3E. Alentemol Hydrobromide [alentemol] (See also *Y67FY3RWN1*)
F6Z53YN55N. Dimethiodal Sodium
F71253DJUN. Ranolazine Hydrochloride (See also *A6IEZ5M406*)
F738MWY53L. Abanoquil
F74MFL78A1. Cefonicid Sodium
F751MO69EV. Dexefaroxan
F76354LMGR. Propylene Glycol Monostearate
F777XEP0LL. Aceburic Acid
F7LTH1E20Y. Arginine Hydrochloride (See also *94ZLA3W45F*)
F83U6T74XR. Glisolamide
F84AE7X24P. Sarmazenil
F850569PQR. Naloxone Hydrochloride (See also *36B82AMQ7N*)
F8A3652H1V. Propranolol Hydrochloride (See also *9Y8NXQ24VQ*)
F8KLC2BD5Z. Dilazep
F8VB5M810T. Tetracycline
F8VB5M810T. Tetracycline Phosphate Complex [tetracycline]
F91H02EBWT. Arformoterol Tartrate [arformoterol] (See also *5P8VJ2I235*)
F925RR824R. Tecovirimat
F93C12LM0D. Furidarone
F93UJX4SWT. Ticarcillin Disodium [ticarcillin] (See also *G8TVV6DSYG*)
F94O7Q5JLM. Clodoxopone
F94OW58Y8V. Azithromycin (See also *5FD113117S; JTE4MNN1MD*)
F96TTB8728. Cidoxepin Hydrochloride [cidoxepin] (See also *XI27WMG8QK*)
F97OMS297F. Proxibarbal
F9NUX55P23. Azilsartan
FA0UYH6QUO. Flupentixol
FA1N0842KB. Salicyl Alcohol
FA2DM6879K. Vidarabine
FA2DM6879K. Vidarabine Phosphate [vidarabine]
FA2DM6879K. Vidarabine Sodium Phosphate [vidarabine]
FA36DV299Q. Dronedarone Hydrochloride (See also *JQZ1L091Y2*)
FA517NS3N7. Fluprednidene
FA675Q0E3E. Iocetamic Acid
FB0C1XZV4Y. Diethyltoluamide
FB2CIN6HMI. Intoplicine
FD171B778Y. Hydralazine Hydrochloride (See also *26NAK24LS8*)
FD6QP9BP8U. Fosquidone
FD72T13M0K. Proxazole
FD72T13M0K. Proxazole Citrate [proxazole]
FDP9A2F6YL. Alinastine
FE9794P71J. Iopanoic Acid
FEN504330V. Nadolol
FF28EJQ494. Promethazine Hydrochloride [promethazine] (See also *R61ZEH7III*)
FFL0D546HO. Carprofen
FFP983J3OD. Bromocriptine Mesylate (See also *3A64E3G5ZO*)
FFW2NGO18S. Afalanine
FGE8818GWA. Bromebric Acid
FGT82HNC7L. Exaprolol Hydrochloride (See also *Q4XX54I93R*)
FI96A8X663. Rilpivirine
FIP88CI9Y3. Protiofate
FKJ64U4XOB. Acequinoline
FL061Q6NMC. Iclazepam
FLQ7571NPM. Thiamphenicol
FM5526K07A. Zinc Acetate
FMS4X67Q96. Palonidipine
FMU62K1L3C. Fluphenazine Decanoate
FO21Z580M4. Saralasin Acetate (See also *H2AFV2HE66*)

FO2303MNI2. Dimethyl Fumarate
FO7JHA3G03. Fluroxene
FO8S2IW40N. Larazotide Acetate
FO90AO023F. Betamicin Sulfate
FO92091VP8. Tetrazepam
FP8Q8F72JH. Antazoline Hydrochloride
FQ3M2Y4BU3. Acetosulfone Sodium
FQI0PYJ799. Tiodazosin
FQR280JW2N. Hydroxyamphetamine Hydrobromide [hydroxyamphetamine] (See also *59IG47SZ0E*)
FRS4SO3K8D. Sodium Dibunate
FSF9L5AH4G. Clodazon Hydrochloride
FST467XS7D. Saccharin
FST467XS7D. Saccharin Calcium [saccharin]
FT8753F8R9. Cycotiamine
FTA7XXY4EZ. Perphenazine
FTK8U1GZNX. Thioguanine
FTX5V7543O. Amiperone
FU2BGC781U. Pildralazine
FV251T245M. Ubisindine
FV9J3JU8B1. Meropenem
FVF865388R. Desloratadine
FVL27C1DMG. Nomelidine
FVM336I71Y. Nipradilol
FVT2ESG270. Bisaramil
FVW7T75XP4. Mitratapide
FW0Z2U7O23. Dobupride
FWV8GJ56ZN. Tripelennamine Hydrochloride
FWY2578LP5. Pirazolac
FX3WJ41CMX. Perflexane
FX5AUU7Z8T. Perzinfotel
FX8Q9PI4VP. Disoxaril
FXC9231JVH. Calcitriol
FY2I4AJB16. Limazocic
FY38S0790W. Chromocarb
FYC8314117. Meluadrine
FYS6T7F842. Adalimumab
FYY3R43WGO. Minocycline
FZ2LZ7U304. Tiemonium Iodide
FZ7798X3IR. Camobucol
FZ7NYF5N8L. Iron Sucrose
FZ7ZH245CO. Tiprotimod
FZ989GH94E. Povidone
FZ99TBX0LI. Butanixin
FZA518V67A. Zoficonazole
FZJ37245UC. Amiloride Hydrochloride (See also *7DZO8EB0Z3*)
FZU1QI13O9. Aminopterin Sodium
G00490L21H. Efaroxan
G0313KNC7D. Amobarbital Sodium (See also *GWH6IJ239E*)
G04B77F772. Batabulin Sodium (See also *T4NP8G3K6Q*)
G07GZ97H65. Clotrimazole
G083B71P98. Pentetreotide
G0V6C994Q5. Oxacillin Sodium (See also *UH95VD7V76*)
G0WB531332. Etisazole
G162GK9U4W. Leflunomide
G17M59V0FY. Clinafloxacin Hydrochloride (See also *8N86XTF9QD*)
G1LN9045DK. Busulfan
G1M3398594. Celiprolol Hydrochloride
G1SCZ6N70K. Prefenamate
G1TGH6857X. Laurcetium Bromide
G1X2X9N95N. Ethybenztropine
G216926E9T. Butinoline
G25Z4785LV. Dioxadilol
G274R51QFV. Oximonam Sodium
G2753KSN40. Hexamethonium Iodide
G29272NCKL. Exametazime
G29272NCKL. Technetium Tc 99m Exametazime

G2B4VE5GH8. Aztreonam
G2M24F1I2A. Aseripide
G2S2V1ETBQ. Bemoradan
G2SH0XKK91. Retinol
G2V8248111. Spiclomazine
G31553PPJU. Furmethoxadone
G32F6EID2H. Ertapenem Sodium [ertapenem] (See also *2T90KE67L0*)
G359OL82VB. Halazone
G3E7RO42MB. Neldazosin
G3P28OML5I. Tamsulosin Hydrochloride [tamsulosin] (See also *11SV1951MR*)
G42ZU72N5G. Carbenicillin Potassium [carbenicillin] (See also *3UX6B304L3*)
G4449OF7S3. Benzopyrronium Bromide
G447S0T1VC. Valacyclovir Hydrochloride
G44PE6QB31. Minalrestat
G4A07F635U. Propetamphos
G4AG71204O. Bendazac
G4FQ3CKY5R. Asparaginase
G4G9J3Q65W. Difetarsone
G4N2F166MN. Necopidem
G4VS580P5E. Securinine
G510OWF4F4. Flubanilate Hydrochloride [flubanilate] (See also *GG0009389P*)
G563Y6G60K. Zomebazam
G56VK1HF36. Milnacipran Hydrochloride [milnacipran] (See also *RNZ43O5WW5*)
G59M7S0WS3. Nitroglycerin
G5C4M8847E. Incadronic Acid
G5MIG3753N. Broperamole
G5MUV8139H. Zipeprol
G6317AOI7K. Levobunolol Hydrochloride [levobunolol] (See also *O90S49LDHH*)
G63QQF2NOX. Avobenzone
G63V2J2N71. Physostigmine Sulfate (See also *9U1VM840SP*)
G69033J83V. Propyromazine Bromide
G6CS53NCVS. Methylprednisolone Suleptanate
G6G4YSZ601. Benzindopyrine Hydrochloride
G6N3J05W84. Ferumoxides
G6VI5P84SX. Tilmacoxib
G70B4ETF4S. Emtricitabine
G71TK93T5B. Doretinel
G751H98FY4. Dioxaphetyl Butyrate
G79YN26H5B. Pentetate Calcium Trisodium (See also *7A314HQM0I*)
G7M7YWO6CG. Nerispirdine
G7MM186D7U. Duoperone Fumarate (See also *E84FJ4KW3B*)
G7N11T8O78. Laropiprant
G7RIW8S0XP. Terbinafine (See also *012C11ZU6G*)
G7V6SLI20L. Arbekacin
G819A456D0. Abiraterone
G84189YY06. Benzoclidine
G84P716Z93. Ethonam Nitrate [ethonam] (See also *OT5Z8-RA5RQ*)
G87210HO7A. Locicortolone Dicibate
G873GX646R. Lapatinib Ditosylate (See also *0VUA21238F*)
G89JQ59I13. Prasugrel Hydrochloride
G8F3U654FU. Carbuterol Hydrochloride
G8RGG88B68. Peginterferon Alfa-2b
G8TVV6DSYG. Ticarcillin Disodium (See also *F93UJX4SWT*)
G8ZMP77RGJ. Terikalant
G905IN29U4. Beloxepin
G90E14A6I6. Clinolamide
G91KDP4M35. Sulfatrozole
G926EC510T. Fingolimod Hydrochloride (See also *3QN8BYN5QF*)
G9BH09J4JW. Phenoperidine

G9FU7F1E87. Diphenylpyraline Hydrochloride (See also *33361OE3AV*)
G9VC23W7W0. Orestrate
GAF9GJ18J5. Decimemide
GAK955D9Q5. Salfluverine
GAN16C9B8O. Glutathione
GB2433A4M3. Dapoxetine Hydrochloride [dapoxetine] (See also *U4OHT63MRI*)
GB901PL1KW. Visnafylline
GC4N5H35P2. Bromamid
GC87H8686G. Diproxadol
GCA9VV7D2N. Liothyronine Sodium (See also *06LU7C9H1V*)
GCU97FKN3R. Valganciclovir Hydrochloride [valganciclovir] (See also *4P3T9QF9NZ*)
GCW5E728OC. Panomifene
GDV807GKAD. Enazadrem Phosphate [enazadrem] (See also *93VML10KA9*)
GEB06NHM23. Metoprolol
GF00K3IIWE. Davunetide
GF6SPR73DW. Phentydrone
GFD7C86Q1W. *d*-Limonene
GFK50B8Y78. Racefemine
GFM415S5XL. Epinastine [epinastine hydrochloride] (See also *Q13WX941EF*)
GFO928U8MQ. Disopyramide
GFO928U8MQ. Disopyramide Phosphate [disopyramide] (See also *N6BOM1935W*)
GFX7QIS1II. Insulin Lispro
GG0009389P. Flubanilate Hydrochloride (See also *G510OWF4F4*)
GGX234SI5H. Tirofiban Hydrochloride [tirofiban] (See also *6H925F8O5J*)
GH09PRQ3FU. Bunaftine
GH500BOX75. Difencloxazine Hydrochloride (See also *M277CV2CL8*)
GH66PET6S3. Zaldaride
GH9IW85221. Rolitetracycline
GIE06H28OX. Retosiban
GJ20H50YF0. Metaproterenol Sulfate
GK3KFF4TIW. Flufosal
GKA5F0J75P. Cloprothiazole
GKH2KOV2RF. Ramifenazone
GLH0314RVC. Ticagrelor
GLI733V999. Balazipone
GLS2PGI8QG. Sevelamer Hydrochloride
GM8PQW6Q2J. Fosarilate
GMW67QNF9C. Leucine
GN5P7K3T8S. Phenbutazone Sodium Glycerate [phenylbutazone] (See also *RKC4AOX590*)
GN5P7K3T8S. Phenylbutazone
GN5XU2DXKV. Romiplostim
GN83C131XS. Ephedrine
GN8S7ZES0F. Methaniazide
GNG9ZD197L. Goxalapladib
GNN1DV99GX. Penicillamine
GNT396G9QT. Anagestone Acetate
GP568V9G19. Chlormezanone
GP581VM303. Xenipentone
GPN9HBH1HS. Alfimeprase
GQ8ADD54E1. Omoconazole Nitrate [omoconazole] (See also *15LTY5STY6*)
GQN5BVM24W. Pirolazamide
GR0L9S3J0F. Racepinephrine
GR181O3R32. Etryptamine Acetate [etryptamine] (See also *3RY07R55EE*)
GRE0P19C3Z. Benzoxiquine
GRX5L9Y3Z3. Dibrospidium Chloride
GRY6X9550R. Losmiprofen

GRZ5RCB1QG. Venlafaxine Hydrochloride [venlafaxine] (See also *7D7RX5A8MO*)

GS8D070P7W. Lufuradom

GS9EX7QNU6. Phenothiazine

GSL05Y1MN6. Codeine Phosphate

GSV7V79C63. Lotrafiban Hydrochloride

GTW8DB3OVN. Forminitrazole

GU9MLT8VE0. Intriptyline Hydrochloride [intriptyline] (See also *HK1HKT378E*)

GV0O7ES0R3. Enalaprilat

GV5ZHU20H9. Amantocillin

GVN71CAL3G. Alexidine

GVR41S4ZHJ. Flosulide

GVV4Z879SP. Sertindole

GW89575KF9. Squalane

GWH6IJ239E. Amobarbital

GWH6IJ239E. Amobarbital Sodium [amobarbital] (See also *G0313KNC7D*)

GWO1432WOU. Oxyphencyclimine Hydrochloride (See also *4V44H1O8XI*)

GX1Q848LV4. Bamaluzole

GXM4PER6WZ. Promestriene

GXT25D5DS0. Zaprinast

GYL649Z0HY. Cloxazolam

GYU56H6EBV. Cicliomenol

GZ1X96601Z. Tecadenoson

GZE85Q9Q61. Pradefovir Mesylate [pradefovir] (See also *0D5204ZSIX*)

GZM2484VQ4. Manozodil

H0982HF78B. Primaquine Phosphate (See also *MVR3634GX1*)

H0DE420U8G. Chlorzoxazone

H0G9379FGK. Calcium Carbonate

H0N246YG4Y. Icospiramide

H0XB4R74ID. Dimefline Hydrochloride (See also *9WII5M0DU3*)

H1187LU49Q. Trepibutone

H1250JIK0A. Clarithromycin

H16A5VCT9C. Testosterone Undecanoate

H191JFG8WA. Tromantadine

H19J064BA5. Bismuth Subnitrate

H1CGM4755H. Lesopitron

H1T03Z1G60. Dacopafant

H231GF11BV. Naphazoline Hydrochloride [naphazoline] (See also *MZ1131787D*)

H2AFV2HE66. Saralasin Acetate [saralasin] (See also *FO21Z580M4*)

H2BQI5Z8FT. Ditazole

H2V165956A. Fencibutirol

H3753190JS. Moexiprilat

H3H80F5CTY. Butoprozine Hydrochloride

H3SKB3662O. Sulfapyridine Sodium

H438WYN10E. Econazole Nitrate (See also *6Z1Y2V4A7M*)

H45187T098. Nandrolone Decanoate

H464ZO600O. Apaziquone

H48W1A97VB. Amiglumide

H4QBZ2LO84. Bethanechol Chloride

H50H3S3W74. Histrelin

H56CKB2FFV. Aranotin

H56TJ4554M. Dezaguanine Mesylate

H57G17P2FN. Brompheniramine Maleate [brompheniramine] (See also *IXA7C9ZN03*)

H5GU9YQL7L. Roxarsone

H5HKR8OEF3. Neraminol

H5L34MU3TQ. Artilide Fumarate [artilide]

H645GUL8KJ. Lisdexamfetamine Dimesylate [lisdexamfetamine] (See also *SJT761GEGS*)

H68BP06S81. Levocabastine Hydrochloride [levocabastine] (See also *124XMA6YEI*)

H68VTK0LL9. Cyclophenazine Hydrochloride

H6C0F5AD7D. Sudexanox

H743H7R6YE. Clodacaine

H77DL0Y630. Halofantrine Hydrochloride (See also *Q2OS4303HZ*)

H789N3FKE8. Baclofen

H7B263Z7AQ. Alloclamide

H7H9M0ICD7. Liroldine

H7SC0I332I. Glisoxepide

H7V12WDZ93. Cefotiam Hydrochloride (See also *91W6Z2N718*)

H806S4B3NS. Oxyphenbutazone (See also *A7D84513GV*)

H821664NPK. Perampanel

H82Q2D5WA7. Frovatriptan

H84XT1COAU. Vapiprost Hydrochloride [vapiprost] (See also *292V8Q1MXQ*)

H8635NG3PY. Zaltoprofen

H8A007M585. Tapentadol

H91334173C. Icodulinum

H92K6N217F. Epetirimod Esylate

H95KBR1GDB. Xenon Xe 127

H9JT455SZ7. Prosulpride

HA3R0MY016. Fenoldopam Mesylate (See also *INU8H2KAWG*)

HA82M3RAB2. Carmofur

HAY5MT18L3. Medronate Disodium

HB6PN45W4J. Idebenone

HBD503WORO. Ketotifen Fumarate (See also *X49220T18G*)

HC3NX54582. Trientine Hydrochloride (See also *SJ76Y07H5F*)

HD2D469W6U. Cephaloglycin [cephaloglycin anhydrous] (See also *NE7R11LA95*)

HDP7W44CIO. Meclizine Hydrochloride (See also *3L5TQ84570*)

HDU53A8A4S. Traxanox

HEC37C70XX. Sotalol Hydrochloride (See also *A6D97U294I*)

HF11NTT6MZ. Penoctonium Bromide

HFS3HB32J7. Etaqualone

HG18B9YRS7. Valine

HG22108KQK. Propyperone

HGB7P08R36. Isbogrel

HIE492ZZ3T. Phenoxyethanol

HII3IK0W0I. Sodium Iodide I 125

HJ57229JPX. Salafibrate

HJT0RXD7JK. Tobramycin Sulfate

HK1HKT378E. Intriptyline Hydrochloride (See also *GU9MLT8VE0*)

HL580335SI. Elinafide

HM4L00P85U. Acitemate

HM4YQM8WRC. Chlorobutanol

HM5641GA6F. Oprelvekin

HN0NCX453C. Famprofazone

HN3OFO5036. Cyclamic Acid

HO1A8B3YVV. Doramapimod

HO3OGH5D7I. Nelfinavir Mesylate [nelfinavir] (See also *98D603VP8V*)

HO6I89Z64J. Metesculetol

HOH9HJ2737. Pexantel

HOY74VZE0M. Gadoxetate Disodium

HP16WVP23Y. Butaprost

HP46XK89XB. Thiethylperazine Malate

HPE317O9TL. Pyrilamine Maleate [pyrilamine] (See also *R35D29L3ZA*)

HPI5A94GD9. Piroxicillin

HPN91K7FU3. Clofibrate

HQ43CN02U9. Ioxaglate Sodium

HQ7F53TO3L. Tioxamast

HSD1XP51CR. Simtrazene

HSU1C9YRES. Medroxyprogesterone Acetate [medroxyprogesterone] (See also *C2QI4IOI2G*)

HTV56CD308. Baminercept Alfa

HU9DX48N0T. Mycophenolic Acid

HUC352BGYM. Bucricaine

HUH663DN8F. Trimexiline
HUM6H389W0. Azlocillin
HUN219N434. Taleranol
HUQ1KC1YLI. Methoxamine Hydrochloride [methoxamine] (See also *8MB4MJ9R7L*)
HW3H7D91F6. Pegademase Bovine
HW5B6351RZ. Actarit
HW6NV07QEC. Ambrisentan
HW8W27HTXX. Iodixanol
HWR60H5GZB. Luprostiol
HWT06H303Z. Spectinomycin Hydrochloride (See also *93AKI1U6QF*)
HX1032V43M. Sodium Thiosulfate
HX58M2377W. Bromerguride
HY45T0EF6G. Tilnoprofen Arbamel
HYD2U48IAS. Bepotastine
HYS0B45Z2S. Isoflupredone Acetate [isoflupredone] (See also *55P9TUL75S*)
I04MF82GW9. Tosulur
I0IO929019. Calcitonin [human] (See also *7SFC6U2VI5*)
I0Q6O6740J. Ritodrine
I0VM4M70GC. Dabigatran
I16QD7X297. Neomycin Palmitate [neomycin]
I16QD7X297. Neomycin Sulfate [neomycin] (See also *057Y626693*)
I16QD7X297. Neomycin Undecylenate [neomycin]
I18M56OGME. Robalzotan
I18S89P20R. Degarelix Acetate
I1E9D14F36. Citalopram Hydrobromide
I1GX0BGV7P. Fezolamine Fumarate (See also *I133E05F6C*)
I1T8O1JTL6. Prochlorperazine Maleate
I20202Q8M8. Icofungipen
I29DRR8S3R. Rimiterol Hydrobromide
I2T0B5G94M. Valopicitabine Dihydrochloride [valopicitabine] (See also *7KNU786IT4*)
I2U18E6JKA. Esmirtazapine Maleate
I35H55G906. Dovitinib
I35H55G906. Dovitinib Lactate [dovitinib] (See also *69VKY8-P7EA*)
I36JP4Q9DF. Sarafloxacin Hydrochloride
I38846JP2L. Prodeconium Bromide
I3E2J32F37. Vetrabutine
I43T3ID6G2. Tesmilifene
I44VIC13P8. Cyprodenate
I4744080IR. Pentobarbital
I4744080IR. Pentobarbital Sodium [pentobarbital] (See also *NJJ0475N0S*)
I47IU4FOCO. Warfarin Potassium
I4I0Q76VHJ. Spirotriazine Hydrochloride
I4O62614HA. Gapromidine
I4O795Q03O. Tolonidine
I542T3H3T2. Metescufylline
I5MPG6F043. Susalimod
I5UTM533IP. Aronixil
I5ZZY3DC5G. Cloflucarban
I6406OC637. Fandofloxacin
I65MW4OFHZ. Rocuronium Bromide
I66ZZ0ZN0E. Troglitazone
I6B4B2U96P. Vildagliptin
I6CQM0F31V. Etidocaine
I6G9Y0J1OJ. Phenolsulfonphthalein
I6WP63U32H. Acenocoumarol
I7071G0W3C. Peratizole
I729P6N0P7. Parapropamol
I76F4SHP7J. Cyclopentolate Hydrochloride [cyclopentolate] (See also *736I6971TE*)
I788X867K7. Hexobarbital Sodium (See also *AL8Z8K3P6S*)
I7EKN1924Q. Meticrane

I7GT1U99Y9. Triamcinolone Hexacetonide
I898I67K6S. Chlorbenzoxamine Hydrochloride
I89Y79062L. Etazolate Hydrochloride [etazolate] (See also *7YO3254Y6B*)
I8AB3P944K. Ramciclane
I8MFJ1C0BY. Mosapride
I8X1O0607P. Cefepime Hydrochloride
I9L0DDD30I. Succinylcholine Chloride
I9NG89L275. Almokalant
I9Q51XHI1K. Delmetacin
I9W7N6B1KJ. Fluoxetine Hydrochloride
I9ZF7L6G2L. Nifedipine
IA16WBX317. Thiazinamium Metilsulfate
IA7306519N. Isosorbide Dinitrate
IAN371PP48. Ethinamate
IB1H345F24. Ambamustine
ICJ93X8X90. Canertinib Dihydrochloride
ID0YZQ2TCP. Trabectedin
ID1GU2627N. Fosamprenavir Calcium
IE65P4OE02. Cetiedil Citrate
IE9M6JG949. Metipirox
IEU56G3J9C. Lanreotide Acetate (See also *0G3DE8943Y*)
IFN18A4Y6B. Magnesium Glycinate
IFY5PE3ZRW. Norepinephrine Bitartrate (See also *X4W3ENH1CV*)
IG2442S013. Moxicoumone
IGA15S9H40. Manganese Sulfate [manganese sulfate anhydrous] (See also *W00LYS4T26*)
IGM44CEY2I. Seractide Acetate [seractide] (See also *DI9132OQ3R*)
IH245EI7CP. Tetronasin Sodium
IHK933KCIC. Pibrozelesin
IHP475989U. Flurazepam Hydrochloride [flurazepam] (See also *756RDM536M*)
IHS69L0Y4T. Cefazolin
II3F5A2G0F. Ataquimast
IJ21AK8IVJ. Eprozinol
IJ670B0H4A. Nebentan
IL298686U0. Diarbarone
IL870Q3Z8I. Cobiprostone
IM840F32VV. Mefeclorazine
IN1233R0JO. Trimecaine
INU8H2KAWG. Fenoldopam Mesylate [fenoldopam] (See also *HA3R0MY016*)
IO1C09Z674. Metoprolol Fumarate
IO7663S6D3. Dotarizine
IOW153004F. Lonafarnib
IP8QT76V17. Oxethazaine
IR235I7C5P. Methacycline
IR235I7C5P. Methacycline Hydrochloride [methacycline] (See also *9GJ0N7ZAP0*)
IR6XYD8SAX. Zelandopam
IR84JPZ1RK. Methylergonovine Maleate (See also *W53L6FE61V*)
IRH58115R1. Totrombopag Choline
IRZ1462XXF. Prazocillin
IS1UP79R56. Micafungin Sodium (See also *R10H71BSWG*)
IS7C3GTW01. Vintoperol
ISB31HSB8H. Azumolene Sodium (See also *5U7IO9CV80*)
ISQ9I6J12J. Linezolid
ITX08688JL. Quinidine
IU5QR144QX. Estrogens, Conjugated
IUH3AY74O3. Lapaquistat Acetate
IV021NXA9J. Prednisolone Sodium Phosphate
IV7T84QA4T. Technetium Tc 99m Apcitide
IW71N46B4Y. Ceftibuten
IWT50P9S79. Hyoscyamine Hydrobromide
IWW5FV6NK2. Hexachlorophene

IX0QAD6RD2. Afeletecan
IX6J1063HV. Indocyanine Green
IX8TM6153H. Losindole
IXA7C9ZN03. Brompheniramine Maleate (See also *H57G17P2FN*)
IY6234ODVR. Cefamandole Sodium
IY90U61Z3S. Argatroban (See also *OCY3U280Y3*)
IY9XDZ35W2. Dextrose
IZ1GXE233H. Flunamine
IZF55EH3CG. Telinavir
IZM1PNJ3JL. Abecarnil
J06Y7MXW4D. Deferoxamine
J06Y7MXW4D. Deferoxamine Hydrochloride [deferoxamine]
J06Y7MXW4D. Deferoxamine Mesylate [deferoxamine] (See also *V9TKO7EO6K*)
J0E2756Z7N. Irbesartan
J12U072QL0. Ibandronate Sodium
J13S2394HE. Quinidine Sulfate
J14M291SAO. Dioxadrol Hydrochloride
J17QL41ZAG. Nalidixate Sodium (See also *3B91HWA56M*)
J191YXB819. Dazidamine
J1A8830GE7. Calcobutrol
J1DOI7UV76. Phencyclidine Hydrochloride [phencyclidine] (See also *V1JZQ7GDTX*)
J1J54V24R4. Succinobucol
J1J87P409K. Isobromindione
J220T4J9Q2. Abacavir Sulfate
J23127WJYB. Clopirac
J280872D1O. Desonide
J28T4D661G. Bromociclen
J2C169J769. Eclanamine Maleate
J2D46N657D. Calomel
J2GC047H27. Zoliprofen
J2VZ07J96K. Polymyxin B Sulfate [polymyxin b] (See also *19371312D4*)
J30IBO0LMA. Bisnafide Dimesylate (See also *62H4W26906*)
J31IL9Z2EE. Oxatomide
J339Q7IM54. Benorterone
J39B52TV34. Albendazole Oxide
J3S205V4I2. Pipequaline
J3YYF867DV. Nimidane
J40338OKKT. Asocainol
J42298IESW. Prulifloxacin
J468V64WZ1. Cyclofenil
J4CLF34O60. Ticarbodine
J4LUG3IAAN. Etasuline
J4T82NDH7E. Erlotinib Hydrochloride [erlotinib] (See also *DA87705X9K*)
J4THI5N7O2. Bethanidine Sulfate
J4Z741D6O5. Gentian Violet
J4ZHN3HBTE. Lidoflazine
J50OIX95QV. Methenamine
J542BCR0IQ. Cycliramine Maleate
J57707EKBI. Indopine (See also *CZ5QG07777*)
J57CTF25XJ. Bropirimine
J57O328W4W. Flindokalner
J587DZQ8YB. Lauroguadine
J58862DTVD. Tariquidar
J60AR2IKIC. Clozapine
J613NI05SV. Apafant
J6292F8L3D. Haloperidol
J651EHI78N. Deprostil
J6793T658K. Pirbuterol Hydrochloride
J697UZ2A9J. Ipratropium Bromide
J6B56XB19T. Iopydone
J6D6912BXS. Taltobulin
J6UQP7JHOT. Fuzlocillin
J6W196LMV3. Droxicainide

J70472UD3D. Bazedoxifene Acetate (See also *Q16TT9C5BK*)
J778U505W5. Dextromoramide Tartrate
J7A92W69L7. Droxidopa
J7I598ESCC. Xylocoumarol
J7P3696BCQ. Fusidate Sodium (See also *59XE10C19C*)
J7RT0951E3. Alonacic
J81E81G364. Efaproxiral
J89LM8QVEE. Ritiometan
J8BDZ68989. Sumatriptan Succinate
J8IE53G2IV. Manifaxine
J8M468HBH4. Eticlopride
J8QB2W9908. Galosemide
J8U5694BCW. Flutemazepam
J8WA3K39B7. Melperone
J8ZC30U6CH. Dazopride Fumarate (See also *CV07VSP2G8*)
J998RDZ51I. Levobupivacaine
J998RDZ51I. Levobupivacaine Hydrochloride
J9QH779MEM. Sitaxentan
J9XW583M0N. Mimbane Hydrochloride [mimbane] (See also *O9NUI7UT2S*)
JA79OMG4QT. Pirmenol Hydrochloride
JAD662Q3U7. Dymanthine Hydrochloride (See also *066975NG22*)
JAJ86U8L6J. Azarole
JB937PER5C. Dimenhydrinate
JBP1N46HPN. Tiviciclovir
JC71GJ1F3L. Myrrh
JC82071PQS. Bufeniode
JCQ5G1KFHN. Imitrodast
JCX84Q7J1L. Celecoxib
JE42381TNV. Sulfamethoxazole
JE6H2O27P8. Efavirenz
JED5K35YGL. Iloprost
JEI07OOS8Y. Rimantadine Hydrochloride (See also *0T2EF4JQ-TU*)
JF3KQ40J31. Cyclobendazole
JF8V0828ZI. Quazepam
JFK78S0U9S. Talniflumate
JFN36L5S8K. Ampicillin Sodium
JFU09I87TR. Voriconazole
JGH8MYC891. Drotrecogin Alfa (activated)
JGS34J7L9I. Nebivolol Hydrochloride
JHC049LO86. Alogliptin Benzoate [alogliptin] (See also *EEN99869SC*)
JHU490RVYR. Propionic Acid
JI2B19CR0R. Thonzonium Bromide
JI688O846T. Bucromarone
JI8Z5M7NA3. Thiopental Sodium [thiopental] (See also *49Y44QZL70*)
JIL713Q00N. Cidofovir
JIO3275WGI. Tretoquinol
JJ768O327N. Dextroamphetamine Sulfate
JJH94R3PWB. Neratinib
JK517QTN4Q. Ciclotizolam
JKZ19V908O. Asenapine Maleate [asenapine] (See also *CU9463U2E2*)
JMS50MPO89. Losartan Potassium [losartan] (See also *3ST302B24A*)
JN9M0YN4VL. Furostilbestrol
JNJ23Q2COM. Lysine Hydrochloride
JOT47SVI4K. Anilopam Hydrochloride (See also *34E9Q468RT*)
JOV4UJY07O. Sulfamerazine Sodium [Injection] (See also *UR1-SAB295F*)
JP2EN8WORU. Nitarsone
JPW84AS66U. Ponazuril
JQ0A5VKV0Y. Iotetric Acid
JQ7ZT5MRA0. Efletirizine Dihydrochloride

JQT35NPK6C. Pioglitazone Hydrochloride (See also *X4OV71U42S*)

JQZ1L091Y2. Dronedarone Hydrochloride [dronedarone] (See also *FA36DV299Q*)

JR0N7XD5GZ. Quinestrol

JR13W81H44. Iopamidol

JRM708L703. Benazeprilat

JS492IR8Z6. Irolapride

JS86977WNV. Fluticasone Furoate

JSQ17GL1CN. Deanol Acetamidobenzoate

JSS1TEM917. Butibufen

JT4X6Z1HRR. Edatrexate

JTE4MNN1MD. Azithromycin [azithromycin monohydrate] (See also *F94OW58Y8V; 5FD1131I7S*)

JU9YAX04C7. Milrinone

JUT23379TN. Inamrinone

JV039JZZ3A. Betadex

JW3UZ4I1A8. Seclazone

JW5Y7B8Z18. Gepirone Hydrochloride [gepirone] (See also *80C9L8EP6V*)

JWF5YAW3QW. Valerian

JY0WD0UA60. Memantine Hydrochloride

JY444CK9IG. Quipazine Maleate (See also *4WCY05C0SJ*)

JY5N9F45AG. Dexoxadrol Hydrochloride [dexoxadrol] (See also *T0C1IR71L8*)

JZ963P0DIK. Pimavanserin Tartrate [pimavanserin] (See also *NA83F1SJSR*)

K0435HZQ57. Amantanium Bromide

K0744Q5ALP. Tribendilol

K08BK043YS. Vofopitant

K0KA807799. Carbocloral

K0NF2CPJ7F. Arbutamine Hydrochloride (See also *B07L15YAEV*)

K0T69WUD4Z. Frabuprofen

K0T77AAY7G. Urefibrate

K0U68Q2TXA. Corticotropin

K0YPY57FUQ. Isalsteine

K110K1B1VE. Diclazuril

K16AIQ8CTM. Pertuzumab

K16AME9I3V. Ataluren

K1LDZ0VBC0. Amotosalen Hydrochloride [amotosalen] (See also *67B255SI5F*)

K1M5RVL18S. Gaboxadol

K1U80DO9EB. Azaribine

K1YX059ML1. Apricitabine

K259Z4O1B3. Ciprokiren

K27005NP0A. Ixabepilone

K27F04K3A9. Pafuramidine Maleate

K29KWU39J0. Metioprim

K2A047674O. Parapenzolate Bromide

K2J09EMJ52. Phenazopyridine Hydrochloride [phenazopyridine] (See also *0EWG668W17*)

K2PM66M0VQ. Alifedrine

K2S5VMM2SG. Anazocine

K2VOT966ZI. Apazone

K3086GQJ9Z. Cefaloram

K356C79875. Strinoline

K35N76CUHF. Biperiden Hydrochloride (See also *0FRP6G56LD*)

K3B3L3Q0GV. Draquinolol

K3D86KJ24N. Undecylenic Acid

K3D86KJ24N. Zinc Undecylenate [undecylenic acid] (See also *388VZ25DUR*)

K3D9A0ICQ3. Ataticept

K3FRN4DDOY. Laniquidar

K3GDH6OH08. Didanosine

K3QML4J07E. Methisazone

K3UKR54YXW. Dexamethasone Dipropionate

K3V6HB0M57. Flutropium Bromide

K3Z4F929H6. Lysine

K40E7MO61Q. Norfloxacin Succinil

K41MYV7MPM. Ethacrynate Sodium (See also *M5DP350VZV*)

K43273G1CW. Guaimesal

K45001587E. Celivarone

K490D39G46. Propoxycaine Hydrochloride (See also *EP-D1EH7F53*)

K4MZ02M175. Dimethisterone

K4QYN23H2N. Seproxetine Hydrochloride (See also *25CO3X0R31*)

K59P7XNB8X. Dimetridazole

K5BC5011K3. Nicardipine Hydrochloride (See also *CZ5312222S*)

K5BN214699. Nitisinone

K5F4RU5VQJ. Imolamine

K65LB6598J. Phenyltoloxamine

K676NL63N7. Rolipram

K6A90IIZ19. Voreloxin

K6J75G277H. Lotrifen

K6PW2S574L. Amodiaquine Hydrochloride (See also *220236ED28*)

K6SU81C9V1. Oxdralazine

K72T3FS567. Adenosine

K76S41V71X. Acetylleucine

K7EB9E48ZE. Esuprone

K7Q1JQR04M. Dinoprostone

K7V8P532WP. Dexamethasone Acetate [dexamethasone acetate anhydrous] (See also *E2287TKU04*)

K80185F39X. Flumedroxone

K848JZ4886. Cysteine Hydrochloride [cysteine] (See also *ZT934N0X4W*)

K89MJ0S5VY. Oxymetazoline Hydrochloride (See also *8VLN5B44ZY*)

K8QJ749V4K. Zinoconazole Hydrochloride

K90ZOR23P1. Beciparcil

K94FTS1806. Flecainide Acetate [flecainide] (See also *M8U465Q1WQ*)

K97CJK0FXR. Pentorex

K9AY9IR2SD. Acipimox

K9CCS0RIBT. Ranelic Acid

K9P6MC7092. Oxybutynin

K9R83652CK. Carabersat

K9RLQ5L66X. Antazonite

K9V0CDQ56E. Cevimeline Hydrochloride [cevimeline] (See also *P81Q6V85NP*)

K9X45X0051. Anagrelide Hydrochloride [anagrelide] (See also *VNS4435G39*)

KA0B657LV3. Chlorthenoxazine

KAI6MVO39Z. Etoperidone Hydrochloride [etoperidone] (See also *2FSU2FR80J*)

KAM54NKT1Q. Clanfenur

KB1PCR9DMW. Chromic Chloride

KBO7409339. Metoserpate Hydrochloride (See also *X3G4L02XQU*)

KBZ4844CXN. Cefmenoxime Hydrochloride [cefmenoxime] (See also *NON736D32W*)

KC523G2996. Lanproston

KCC1V76AH8. Imidocarb Hydrochloride

KCJ747D3R4. Emylcamate

KD510K1IQW. Choline Salicylate

KDN276D83N. Iothalamate Sodium I 131

KDU8VH09O8. Xenazoic Acid

KE3U2023NP. Poractant Alfa

KE474IKG1W. Glyclopyramide

KE7J8A65P6. Glaziovine

KEN63D125F. Didrovaltrate

KF7Z0E0Q2B. Quinine Sulfate

KF7Z9K2T3W. Nandrolone Phenpropionate

KG60484QX9. Omeprazole

KGZ1SLC28Z. Beclomethasone Dipropionate [beclomethasone] (See also *5B307S63B2*)

KHS0AZ4JVK. Butalbital

KHV7ANE00E. Benderizine

KI24A9FF7S. Cloquinate

KI8H7H19WL. Telithromycin

KJ0091KAAH. Methylchromone

KJ2V75P034. Fenpipramide [fenpipramide hydrochloride] (See also *88445508X3*)

KK9WYJ6556. Dexetozoline

KKA5DLD701. Solifenacin Succinate (See also *A8910SQJ1U*)

KKV299446X. Daglutril

KL6248WNW4. Piperacetazine

KM2Z91756Z. Risedronic Acid

KN08449444. Adinazolam

KN08449444. Adinazolam Mesylate [adinazolam] (See also *NT8S62A727*)

KN82541NHV. Utibaprilat

KQJ4QI511C. Cotriptyline

KQT9O2462E. Tixanox

KR2L2A68XL. Normethadone

KRN50N3Y2T. Rotraxate

KU213XYO69. Fantofarone

KU8SPJ271W. Dexelvucitabine

KV03YZ6QLW. Omeprazole Sodium

KV2JZ1BI6Z. Pyridoxine Hydrochloride [pyridoxine] (See also *68Y4CF58BV*)

KV3495SGKS. Desaspidin

KV89R7ELF8. Bucloxic Acid

KVI301NA53. Pyridostigmine Bromide

KVL61ZF9UO. Neticonazole

KX2339DP44. Rosiglitazone Maleate (See also *05V02F2KDG*)

KX4D9BZA6X. Furegrelate Sodium [furegrelate]

KX7K68Z2UH. Enzastaurin Hydrochloride

KXC7811DBY. Acolbifene Hydrochloride

KXG0PR9DIH. Eganoprost

KXI2J76489. Iodoform

KXO2KT9N0G. Pravastatin Sodium [pravastatin] (See also *3M8608UQ61*)

KYT38QTB4K. Alpertine

KZ075BHY4P. Ciprostene Calcium [ciprostene]

KZ1O2SH88Z. Talabostat

L08SZ5Z5JC. Coumaphos

L0A22B22FT. Oxolinic Acid

L0FPV48Q5R. Trilostane

L0MR697HHI. Mechlorethamine Hydrochloride (See also *50D9XSG0VR*)

L0U38EHD86. Indanazoline

L11651398J. Calcium Gluceptate

L11K75P92J. Calcium Phosphate Dihydrate, Dibasic [calcium phosphate (1:1)] (See also *O7TSZ97GEP*)

L137U4A79K. Trimetrexate Glucuronate

L1E28E0J8F. Iralukast

L1F2Q2X956. Lisofylline

L1G37N4EBS. Mofloverine

L1M1U2HC31. Grepafloxacin Hydrochloride [grepafloxacin] (See also *A4ER1Z8N9N*)

L256JB984D. Ozagrel

L2B0WJF7ZY. Lactitol (See also *UH2K6W1Y64*)

L2C9GWQ43H. Esomeprazole Sodium

L2GWR3US1G. Supidimide

L2H26JSV0I. Enprazepine

L2JY6Z298S. Ersentilide

L2R75RQX26. Simfibrate

L2T84IQI2K. Nalbuphine Hydrochloride [nalbuphine] (See also *ZU4275277R*)

L31MM1385E. Halofuginone Hydrobromide [halofuginone]

L32B98BGJS. Feniodium Chloride

L35JN3I7SJ. Ramipril

L36H50F353. Podofilox

L36O5T016N. Rifaximin

L396QIB983. Tiplasinin

L39WTC366D. Procainamide Hydrochloride [procainamide] (See also *SI4064O0LX*)

L3H46UAC61. Methyclothiazide

L3J8QT828G. Racemoramide

L3JE09KZ2F. Saquinavir

L3M76J6S37. Dutacatib

L4618BD7KJ. Gatifloxacin

L4D5UA6CB4. Diclofenac Potassium (See also *144O8QL0L1*)

L4F80M873G. Aditeren

L4YEB44I46. Metoclopramide Hydrochloride [metoclopramide] (See also *W1792A2RVD*)

L51CBE03KF. Tabimorelin

L56P3532KI. Triclacetamol

L5U1X99Q9Z. Mexiprostil

L5U70J87J8. Besigomsin

L5W337AOUR. Aloxistatin

L5WVJ201KN. Duometacin

L628TT009W. Isoproterenol Hydrochloride [isoproterenol] (See also *DIA2A74855*)

L64N7M9BWR. Cetrimonium Bromide

L6867H5FR4. Entsufon Sodium

L6BR2WJD8V. Lomefloxacin

L6IE0KAZ8O. Lopobutan

L6JW2TJG99. Dibucaine

L6JW2TJG99. Dibucaine Hydrochloride [dibucaine] (See also *Z97702A5DG*)

L6O3XI777I. Zanamivir

L6UH7ZF8HC. Risperidone

L6V4Z7SX7S. Dimabefylline

L6X660925G. Enciprazine Hydrochloride [enciprazine]

L702S858Z6. Siccanin

L76T0ZCA8K. Oxymetholone

L7J6A1NE81. Benzoin

L84RBE4IDC. Bergenin

L8S50ZY490. Esreboxetine

L9026OPI2Z. Budipine

L94KSX715K. Avosentan

L95KV83PV9. Xyloxemine

L960UP2KRW. Hydromorphone Hydrochloride (See also *Q812464R06*)

L9806LPR7G. Nepinalone

L9F3D9RENQ. Oxybutynin Chloride

L9M34YK25C. Clometacin

L9P2881C3H. Plevitrexed

LAD1UQ73BE. Lorglumide

LAV5U5022Y. Methyl Salicylate

LB0T3NEB48. Isoprazone

LBU97HVE51. Etoprindole

LC5G1JUA39. Cetilistat

LC7FBL96A4. Remikiren

LCF9984C2K. Menadiol Sodium Sulfate

LCH760E9T7. Acitretin

LD18TA6Q06. Suloxifen Oxalate [suloxifen] (See also *C0HG40P7PY*)

LEC9GKY20K. Methylprednisolone Sodium Succinate

LER583670J. Loxapine

LER583670J. Loxapine Succinate [loxapine] (See also *X59SG0MRYU*)

LF1VBG4ZUK. Pexacerfont

LF2DT5DL6H. Benoxafos

LG64454O6I. Fenleuton

LGP81V5245. Idoxuridine

LGX4GZ74WO. Dabuzalgron Hydrochloride [dabuzalgron] (See also *A7Q00A39MF*)
LGX9OL562T. Indium In 111 Oxyquinoline
LH8C2JI290. Rasagiline Mesylate (See also *003N66TS6T*)
LHH887104B. Ifoxetine
LHX2B2R19F. Floredil
LI02075E1W. Flestolol Sulfate [flestolol] (See also *T5MWT8445U*)
LI81FMI713. Podilfen
LIJ2H8658W. Butriptyline Hydrochloride
LIU00Z1Z84. Hydrocortisone Hemisuccinate
LIX7OM008P. Taurultam
LJ1U13R8IK. Fenquizone
LJ25TI0CVT. Chlorothymol
LK279ER14X. Silicristin
LKG8494WBH. Benzyl Alcohol
LKO141R05V. Viomycin Sulfate (See also *YVU35998K5*)
LKX634SL5X. Oxeglitazar
LL0G25K7I2. Azilsartan Medoxomil
LL56J87F3X. Aleplasinin
LL60K9J05T. Cabergoline
LMK22VUH23. Cinoxacin
LND2P599LK. Elnadipine
LNV63FWR8M. Benapryzine Hydrochloride
LP80S8XS18. Ioxabrolic Acid
LQ54E5B4EW. Naluzotan
LQU92IU8LL. Propylhexedrine
LR3CD8SX89. Flumethasone
LR3CD8SX89. Flumethasone Pivalate [flumethasone] (See also *0DV09X6F21*)
LR57574HN8. Sodium Picosulfate
LR90117565. Cefuroxime Pivoxetil
LRX7AJ16DT. Cupric Sulfate
LS5O682BRO. Benzotript
LT12J5HVR8. Pipemidic Acid
LT7Z1YW11H. Chloroprocaine Hydrochloride (See also *5YVB0-POT2H*)
LT9004D9N0. Bemitradine
LU86E5P72A. Bornelone
LUO2Z7954T. Fluminorex
LVX8N1UT73. Sunitinib Malate (See also *V99T50803M*)
LVZ1VC61HB. Cephaloridine
LW0TIW155Z. Nabumetone
LW9S78L4M8. Eseridine
LWI5ZJ8WVL. Ferrocholinate
LWK91TU9AH. Piperonyl Butoxide
LWP0997QUF. Sumetizide
LX1OH63030. Isosorbide Mononitrate
LXD20TIK6Y. Stirocainide
LXK8EE245D. Ethoheptazine Citrate
LXN6S3999X. Maropitant Citrate
LXW024X05M. Erythromycin Stearate
LYH6F7I22E. Bromperidol
LYH6F7I22E. Bromperidol Decanoate [bromperidol]
LYJ16FZU9Q. Clorgiline
LZ257RZP7K. Fospropofol Disodium [fospropofol] (See also *30868AY0IF*)
LZ84VWN0U4. Razobazam
LZ9041E1BO. Scopinast
LZM2DSH251. Ronacaleret Hydrochloride
M03GIQ7Z6P. Sincalide
M04XWV43UF. Oxycodone Terephthalate
M084T66126. Dioxamate
M09BUF90C0. Elvucitabine
M09N8K7YJY. Pitofenone
M0TTH61XC5. Ibudilast
M0XW1UBI14. Testosterone Cypionate
M16PXG993G. Etidronate Disodium (See also *M2F465ROXU*)

M20215MUFR. Hydroxyzine Pamoate
M2108NUY0C. Tiflucarbine
M277CV2CL8. Difencloxazine Hydrochloride [difencloxazine] (See also *GH500BOX75*)
M2F465ROXU. Etidronate Disodium [etidronic acid] (See also *M16PXG993G*)
M2F465ROXU. Etidronic Acid
M2I27EKQ47. Climiqualine
M2X04R2E2Y. Carbadox
M329791L57. Methenamine Hippurate
M32RH9MFGP. Dexmethylphenidate Hydrochloride [dexmethylphenidate] (See also *1678OK0E08*)
M36927R46E. Amolanone Hydrochloride (See also *1ALL724WB1*)
M3EFS94984. Ormetoprim
M3EKF65MHG. Vaneprim
M3FU19R357. Glicetanile Sodium (See also *S39J3B52KS*)
M3MYK6R22U. Pivampicillin Probenate
M3PZW4O91B. Butopyrammonium Iodide
M41L2IN55T. Bismuth Subcarbonate
M41LMG25QB. Ataprost
M41W832TA3. Eletriptan Hydrobromide
M42D353K88. Propoxate
M44O63YPV9. Ethamivan
M45G7BJL52. Acediasulfone Sodium
M469UFX48N. Eniclobrate
M487QF2F4V. Amifostine
M4AW13H75T. Propylene Glycol Monolaurate
M4HBT852YO. Guanoclor Sulfate [guanoclor] (See also *Q1U97XK18R*)
M4I0D6VV5M. Calcium Chloride
M514041RF7. Emopamil
M572600E5P. Thiamine Hydrochloride (See also *X66NSO3N35*)
M575VKV19N. Iobenguane Sulfate I 131
M5DP350VZV. Ethacrynate Sodium [ethacrynic acid] (See also *K41MYV7MPM*)
M5DP350VZV. Ethacrynic Acid
M6142PTV7J. Devapamil
M61FM2VCSV. Amphenidone
M629807ATL. Imidurea
M652A5186T. Sulukast
M671F9NLEA. Canrenoate Potassium
M69H5TDQ1K. Perbufylline
M69O7IV78O. Teclothiazide
M6B59S6MEF. Arbaprostil
M6Q1EO9TD0. Amantadine Hydrochloride (See also *BF4C9Z1J53*)
M6T05Z2B68. Lincomycin Hydrochloride (See also *BOD072YW0F*)
M711N184JE. Paroxetine Mesylate
M76V0B96L5. Indecainide Hydrochloride (See also *3AZF20DM1T*)
M78TVM3G5Z. Doxacurium Chloride
M7G4B57ZCB. Ambucaine
M7R15X2683. Cinnamaverine
M801H13NRU. Azacitidine
M89TPX4O2C. Pirazmonam Sodium (See also *1S3Z442A8N*)
M8FR1KL85J. Flavodilol Maleate [flavodilol]
M8U465Q1WQ. Flecainide Acetate (See also *K94FTS1806*)
M911911U02. Potassium Acetate
M98T69Q7HP. Piperacillin Sodium
M99W4Q30OL. Delprostenate
M9C5T4Q638. Fepitrizol
M9JGK7U88V. Ethohexadiol
M9K14Z7S3L. Clocoumarol
MA3UYZ6K1H. Acesulfame
MAL9M0T5LV. Nitrofurantoin Sodium
MAT637500A. Tipifarnib

MBM1C4K26S. Pentifylline
MC09H30MFS. Caricotamide
MCG9O55T6K. Axamozide
MD0414799X. Hydroxyphenamate
MD6P741W8A. Maraviroc
MDY902UXSR. Esmolol Hydrochloride [esmolol] (See also V05260LC8D)
MEI78CAM16. Bisbentiamine
MF4NR5U03L. Trazolopride
MFF90009B9. Zapizolam
MFL71K7PU4. Buquinolate
MFM5450P3T. Ethylmorphine Hydrochloride
MFM6K1XWDK. Chlordiazepoxide Hydrochloride (See also 6RZ6XEZ3CR)
MGY2W95GWO. Echinacea pallida
MH4OU8RWCW. Remoxipride Hydrochloride
MH88D3N73W. Brosuximide
MHJ80W9LRB. Oxaprozin
MHM278SD3E. Montelukast Sodium [montelukast] (See also U1O3J18SFL)
MJ4PTD2VVW. Galantamine Hydrobromide
MJW015BAPH. Prilocaine Hydrochloride
MK73KA425L. Midamaline
MKO1PH93P2. Evicromil
ML4O3WYO2M. Nicametate
MN3L5RMN02. Clonidine
MN3L5RMN02. Clonidine Hydrochloride [clonidine] (See also W76I6XXF06)
MNX7R8C5VO. Carbidopa
MOA3SO592J. Pibecarb
MOH3ET196H. Flupirtine Maleate [flupirtine] (See also 0VCI53PK4A)
MOR84MUD8E. Chlorhexidine Gluconate (See also R4KO0-DY52L)
MP1J8420LU. Edetate Sodium (See also 9G34HU7RV0)
MP564IFE34. Indanidine
MPI4B0COZ7. Efetozole
MPM23GMO7Z. Doxofylline
MQG94M5EEO. Tesamorelin
MR28U787Z2. Nuclomedone
MR40VT1L8Z. Azosemide
MRG9KH7HF6. Gantofiban
MRK240IY2L. Azathioprine
MRU5XH3B48. Ergotamine Tartrate (See also PR834Q503T)
MS63G8NQUI. Clorazepate Monopotassium (See also D51WO0G0L4)
MT147RMO91. Guanadrel Sulfate (See also 765C9332T4)
MUN5LYG46H. Fentanyl Citrate (See also UF599785JZ)
MV4FO7V23V. Elantrine
MV715X4634. Plaunotol
MVC7EI41TU. Taziprinone
MVR3634GX1. Primaquine Phosphate [primaquine] (See also H0982HF78B)
MX0B07OP8M. Demelverine
MXF9G4I1V5. Sulfathiourea
MYS6082G8G. Ciclactate
MZ1131787D. Naphazoline Hydrochloride (See also H231GF11BV)
MZH0OM550M. Salirasib
N00W22YO2B. Vinblastine Sulfate (See also 5V9KLZ54CY)
N01ORX9D6S. Ibuprofen Lysine
N030400H8J. Clodronate Disodium
N04867Y76N. Bismuth Citrate
N0A3Z5XTC6. Tropicamide
N0F8P22L1P. Norfloxacin
N0TXR0XR5X. Linaclotide
N0U9G33XKT. Flupranone
N0V0Q7845W. Colfenamate

N12000U13O. Doxycycline (See also 334895S862)
N18A31MTB0. Almestrone
N1EXE5EHAN. Glucametacin
N1Q45E87DT. Thiabendazole
N1SN99T69T. Benazepril Hydrochloride (See also UDM7Q7QWP8)
N21FAR7B4S. Apomorphine Hydrochloride [apomorphine] (See also F39049Y068)
N24015WC6D. Atevirdine Mesylate [atevirdine] (See also A948D8673W)
N251Q608VU. Talibegron Hydrochloride
N274ZQ6PZJ. Fenoverine
N295J34A25. Drospirenone
N29QWW3BUO. Danazol
N2GI8B1GK7. Cefotaxime Sodium [cefotaxime] (See also 258J72S7TZ)
N2S0PKP5L5. Butidrine
N303OK87DT. Perospirone
N32934RHGW. Sibenadet Hydrochloride [sibenadet] (See also 659OIV373Y)
N33SZ2N85M. Lirexapride
N3D6TG58NI. Thioridazine
N3PA6559FT. Esomeprazole
N3RIB7X24K. Ioversol
N3RQ532IUT. Amiodarone
N40195UTPI. Protizinic Acid
N488540F94. Elacridar Hydrochloride [elacridar] (See also NX2BHH1A5B)
N5I18JI9D6. Pempidine
N5I6SR31GJ. Dimethoxanate Hydrochloride
N5MVC31W2N. Homochlorcyclizine
N673F6W2VH. Odanacatib
N6A93ZMN7U. Falipamil
N6BOM1935W. Disopyramide Phosphate (See also GFO928U8MQ)
N6M33094FD. Amikacin Sulfate (See also 84319SGC3C)
N70177JQTB. Doliracetam
N71M372MP4. Nimazone
N75R59YD0F. Becocalcidiol
N762921K75. Nitrogen
N78PI4C683. Versetamide
N7T6304257. Maleylsulfathiazole
N7U69T4SZR. Olanzapine
N7V53U4U4T. Delafloxacin Meglumine
N7Z035406B. Cilostazol
N804LDH51K. Fleroxacin
N824AOU5XV. Pegvisomant
N8516V0WOM. Buterizine
N863NB338G. Benzyl Benzoate
N8E7F7Q170. Meperidine Hydrochloride (See also 9E338QE28F)
N8F510M76F. Doqualast
N8ONU3L3PG. Terbutaline Sulfate [terbutaline] (See also 576PU70Y8E)
N8Y78OKP8D. Amafolone
N8ZUB7XE0H. Clocortolone Acetate [clocortolone] (See also 85061HTR8T)
N91BDP6H0X. Choline Dihydrogen Citrate [choline]
N986NI319S. Pralnacasan
N99027V28J. Ceftobiprole Medocaril
N9A0A0R9S8. Trimetazidine
N9EQE108I5. Conessine Hydrobromide
N9VWZ34G5E. Acetryptine
NA8320J834. Eptifibatide
NA83F1SJSR. Pimavanserin Tartrate (See also JZ963P0DIK)
NA91GV8GDJ. Lomifylline
NAT2FD82D7. Elmustine
NB2E1YP49F. Yohimbine Hydrochloride

NB2ZOX88RR. Clibucaine
NBB4EM8UXC. Benhepazone
NBY3IU407M. Leteprinim
NBZ3QY004S. Magnesium Hydroxide
NC11WKO35D. Bapineuzumab
NC32G269EF. Bensuldazic Acid [sodium bensuldazate] (See also *R8L0T98P0J*)
ND2M416302. Isopropyl Alcohol
NE25WV9C8S. Amiflamine
NE7R11LA95. Cephaloglycin (See also *HD2D469W6U*)
NE94J8CAMD. Cicaprost
NEZ417265P. Etoloxamine
NG99554ANW. Desvenlafaxine Succinate [desvenlafaxine] (See also *ZB22ENF0XR*)
NGC3S0882S. Xylazine Hydrochloride
NGU5H31YO9. Moxidectin
NH496X0UJX. Ammonium Mandelate [mandelic acid]
NH496X0UJX. Calcium Mandelate [mandelic acid] (See also *29CS07FZII*)
NH496X0UJX. Mandelic Acid
NH5000009I. Dehydrocholic Acid
NHI34IS56E. Ceftiofur Sodium
NHQ2X2AKZO. Molinazone
NHW07912O7. Chlorphentermine Hydrochloride [chlorphentermine] (See also *RL11HOJ7DM*)
NIG5418BXB. Estradiol Dipropionate
NIJ123W41V. Plicamycin
NJ82J0F8QC. Cyproheptadine Hydrochloride (See also *2YHB6175DO*)
NJJ0475N0S. Pentobarbital Sodium (See also *I4744080IR*)
NKF031O02G. Terflavoxate
NLD2X0VD2U. Ciheptolane
NLJ6390P1Z. Ephedrine Hydrochloride
NM87THP11P. Hexcarbacholine Bromide
NMH84OZK2B. Ondansetron Hydrochloride
NMW7447A9A. Acotiamide Hydrochloride (See also *D42OWK5383*)
NN00W8BQ8N. Conorphone Hydrochloride
NNB4I01PA7. Dimepheptanol
NNU2O4609D. Entecavir [entecavir anhydrous] (See also *5968Y6H45M*)
NO70W886KK. Hydrocodone Bitartrate (See also *6YKS4Y3WQ7*)
NOF9U9EYQ4. Adicillin
NON736D32W. Cefmenoxime Hydrochloride (See also *KBZ4844CXN*)
NPB7A7874U. Chlorcyclizine Hydrochloride
NQ74U9QR5D. Taltrimide
NQO8R319LY. Diphenidol
NQO8R319LY. Diphenidol Hydrochloride [diphenidol] (See also *DG355XWQ4T*)
NQO8R319LY. Diphenidol Pamoate [diphenidol] (See also *32021T3D6N*)
NQP2Y50Y6B. Sameridine
NQU9IPY4K9. Cediranib
NQX9KB6PCL. Somatropin
NR4B2SX17S. Chlortetracycline Calcium
NR7O1405Q9. Mesna
NRL66AVH63. Diaplasinin
NRU90S9ANF. Traboxopine
NS1Y283HW4. Iodoxamate Meglumine [iodoxamic acid] (See also *CIX5G6J9R1; 6HG8UB2MUY*)
NS1Y283HW4. Iodoxamic Acid
NS7PP85V4C. Cetohexazine
NSF067KU1M. Linaclotide Acetate
NSL1M7IFYP. Metazide
NT0758136A. Nitroclofene
NT0J0815S5. Chloroquine Hydrochloride
NT6K61736T. Sodium Phenylbutyrate

NT8S62A727. Adinazolam Mesylate (See also *KN08449444*)
NTI7T2IEIE. Bunamiodyl Sodium
NU8Y4C529J. Bazinaprine
NUV44L116D. Clomipramine Hydrochloride [clomipramine] (See also *2LXW0L6GWJ*)
NVW4Z03I9B. Bafetinib
NVZ4I0H58X. Sorbitan Monostearate
NW1291F1W8. Doxazosin Mesylate [doxazosin] (See also *86P6PQK0MU*)
NW2RTH6T2N. Fosinopril Sodium (See also *R43D2573WO*)
NWQ5N31VKK. Daptomycin
NX2BHH1A5B. Elacridar Hydrochloride (See also *N488540F94*)
NXB79TB0N2. Zolamine Hydrochloride [zolamine] (See also *C2B9CF1640*)
NY22HMQ4BX. Exemestane
NYM432G79C. Nosantine
NYW905655B. Pheniramine Maleate (See also *134FM9ZZ6M*)
NZ779Q5S0W. Sulazepam
NZP1W4BK07. Meletimide
NZW046NI85. Tioxidazole
O00T1I1VRN. Ethopropazine Hydrochloride (See also *7WI4-P02YN1*)
O00XM1O6TV. Cismadinone
O02SWY8981. Prostalene
O0417MPF6W. Difemetorex
O0J6XJN02I. Dutasteride
O0P4I5851I. Lurasidone Hydrochloride
O0U0E87X7F. Metocurine Iodide
O0X60K76I6. Acivicin
O0XJ4L38Z3. Zolenzepine
O0ZR1R6RZ2. Betaxolol Hydrochloride [betaxolol] (See also *6X97D2XT0O*)
O10DDW6JOO. Dihydroxyacetone
O12I24570R. Atiprimod Dihydrochloride
O14CWE893Z. Rilapladib
O14NF38MTL. Denaverine
O18YUO0I83. Ketamine Hydrochloride (See also *690G0D6V8H*)
O1GX33ON8R. Chlortetracycline Hydrochloride
O1R2462WA0. Clominorex
O1R9FJ93ED. Cefuroxime
O1R9FJ93ED. Cefuroxime Axetil [cefuroxime] (See also *Z49QDT0J8Z*)
O1ZB1046R1. Quinfamide
O26FZP769L. Lorazepam
O2GMZ0LF5W. Fluticasone Propionate
O2H0Q02M4P. Hetaflur [hexadecylamine] (See also *S58EH61Q1Y*)
O2ILF29K8B. Paranyline Hydrochloride [paranyline] (See also *3QW5SNZ81H*)
O316O1ZGEG. Pimilprost
O352864B8Z. Sodium Pyrophosphate
O3FX965V0I. Acetazolamide
O3J7H54KMD. Acetaminosalol
O3J8G9O825. Ritonavir
O3MCV749SW. Israpafant
O3PR2X907M. Benexate
O3S7RWT8R5. Benethamine Penicillin
O3TY87KJII. Cefedrolor
O408N561GF. Phenelzine Sulfate [phenelzine] (See also *2681D7P965*)
O40UQP6WCF. Sulfuric Acid
O414PZ4LPZ. Salicylic Acid
O494QX2F4D. Tazomeline Citrate
O49NOC9ROC. Triamcinolone Furetonide
O4L1XPO44W. Fluvoxamine Maleate [fluvoxamine] (See also *5LGN83G74V*)
O4Q7XM74N6. Tenilsetam
O52NM0A9YL. Buclosamide

O55EMK06L9. Carprazidil
O55N96CWOW. Dibusadol
O5CB12L4FN. Diazoxide
O5CSC6WH1T. Ibipinabant
O5TNM5N07U. Duloxetine Hydrochloride [duloxetine] (See also *9044SC542W*)
O609V24217. Sonepiprazole
O60O0JB93O. Acetergamine
O611591WAH. Moroxydine
O6550D6K3A. Hydrocortisone Probutate
O65Q227UIC. Metrizoate Sodium (See also *CM1N99QR1M*)
O68JXU1W09. Lergotrile
O6DDV91W1M. Bevirimat Dimeglumine
O6HVT48T15. Benzoquinonium Chloride
O6U9W3DMYT. Dimetholizine
O6W7VEW6KS. Tilorone Hydrochloride [tilorone] (See also *BJ507J4LKY*)
O6X5QGC2VB. Cloxacillin Benzathine [cloxacillin] (See also *AC79L7PV2G*)
O7M2E4264D. Rimexolone
O7T92N1Y8T. Elsibucol
O7TSZ97GEP. Calcium Phosphate Dihydrate, Dibasic (See also *L11K75P92J*)
O8G173034U. Flufylline
O8I1LL6A89. Eticyclidine
O8W0R05772. Clazuril
O90S49LDHH. Levobunolol Hydrochloride (See also *G6317AOI7K*)
O9643CJL3T. Pimelautide
O99X77ZQ8E. Diprofene
O9D004V63I. Picodralazine
O9J6ITY8UX. Morforex
O9KZB9HG1Y. Climazolam
O9M39HTM5W. Promazine Hydrochloride [promazine] (See also *U16EOR79U4*)
O9NUI7UT2S. Mimbane Hydrochloride (See also *J9XW583M0N*)
O9U0F09D5X. Droperidol
OA8TFX68PE. Lercanidipine Hydrochloride
OAY8ORS3CQ. Ethionamide
OBL58JN025. Octanoic Acid
OBN5I4B08W. Atolide
OBN7UDS42Y. Cephalexin
OC5IGJ7J6I. Temafloxacin Hydrochloride
OC71PP0F89. Exatecan
OCC25LM897. Spirapril Hydrochloride (See also *96U2K78I3V*)
OCS3IA7WA0. Thiphencillin Potassium (See also *Z4T2YRI005*)
OCW5XQQ13I. Oxyridazine
OCY3U280Y3. Argatroban [argatroban anhydrous] (See also *IY90U61Z3S*)
OE1C96974E. Alfadolone
OE6G20P68T. Bicifadine Hydrochloride
OED8FV75PY. Propyphenazone
OF4T2241HQ. Trifluomeprazine
OF5P57N2ZX. Alanine
OFG5EXG60L. Risedronate Sodium
OFM06SG1KO. Dichlorodifluoromethane
OG645J8RVW. Pirbuterol Acetate [pirbuterol] (See also *1EH73XKR9N*)
OG8HSX6N6H. Apaxifylline
OGG85SX4E4. Imipramine Hydrochloride [imipramine] (See also *BKE5Q1J60U*)
OGM0YHD1WF. Sibutramine Hydrochloride
OH2O403D1G. Mezlocillin
OI7443PDLB. Premazepam
OJ245FE5EU. Sodium Benzoate
OJF65U061Y. Metibride
OJK82QP37Q. Xidecaflur
OJY3SK9H5F. Firategrast

OKA45SU1Q4. Vadocaine
OKB1O47Q6F. Adosopine
OKG364O896. Estradiol Valerate
OKR68Y0E4T. Gemifloxacin
OKS0I0BBLP. Taniplon
OKX88EO7OI. Vedaprofen
OL961R6O2C. Felodipine
OLH94387TE. Diltiazem Hydrochloride (See also *EE92BBP03H*)
OM7J0XAL0S. Otenzepad
OM90ZUW7M1. Ticlopidine Hydrochloride [ticlopidine] (See also *A1L4914FMF*)
OMP2H17F9E. Oxfendazole
ONP3ME32DL. Temefos
ONU02D116S. Inocoterone Acetate
ONU5A67T2S. Eglumetad
OON1HFZ4BA. Cetrorelix
OP2V3XRV2Y. Prifuroline
OP401G7OJC. Etanercept
OP8B49OL1J. Gloxazone
OPC1BN901Y. Oxazidione
OPE7BD4AAA. Amfepentorex
OPL214POJ1. Adipiplon
OR0RPY2Y2V. Methoxypromazine Maleate
OR5RM3Q5QL. Aminacrine Hydrochloride (See also *78OY3Z0P7Z*)
ORE084U8IP. Glypinamide
OS1Z389K8S. Diethylcarbamazine Citrate (See also *V867Q8X3ZD*)
OSD78555ZM. Potassium Bromide
OSZ0E9DGOJ. Bretazenil
OT5Z8RA5RQ. Ethonam Nitrate (See also *G84P716Z93*)
OTT9J7900I. Tenofovir Disoproxil Fumarate
OU730881W5. Moperone
OW1N4G4R9W. Kanamycin Sulfate (See also *RUC37XUP2P*)
OWD9JI448N. Mitoquidone
OWY6DMB1YX. Metanixin
OXI6EF55FR. Garenoxacin Mesylate (See also *V72H9867WB*)
OYY3447OMC. Pamidronic Acid
OZN2MG334O. Bencyclane Fumarate (See also *6I97Z6S135*)
OZQ2XN817F. Prednisolone Steaglate
P0078O25A9. Butabarbital
P0078O25A9. Butabarbital Sodium [butabarbital] (See also *9WTD50I918*)
P06226385L. Penciclovir Sodium
P0GMS9N47Q. Emricasan
P0J3387W3S. Medazepam Hydrochloride [medazepam] (See also *ETM878JC9K*)
P0S37156TW. Tebatizole
P0T3ZRK3XV. Tianafac
P10582JYYK. Remifentanil Hydrochloride [remifentanil] (See also *5V444H5WIC*)
P110CQY44Z. Delucemine Hydrochloride (See also *124LSR3H2X*)
P13OO3FPZB. Ledazerol
P13TV5A758. Aplindore Fumarate
P14M0DWS2J. Cevipabulin Fumarate [cevipabulin] (See also *Q380BYV049*)
P188ANX8CK. Trastuzumab
P1ALI72U6C. Ramatroban
P1NC244SOF. Estrazinol Hydrobromide (See also *9KLU2E3573*)
P1QW714R7M. Imiquimod
P201BVY1MJ. Ethisterone
P21N4Z6JHO. Mezepine
P26FL0OO4P. Cinfenine
P2I071P32B. Lodinixil
P2I6R8W6UA. Dihydrostreptomycin Sulfate [dihydrostreptomy-cin] (See also *T7D48761UE*)

P2K93U8740. Fludarabine Phosphate [fludarabine] (See also *1X9VK9O1SC*)

P2Z71CIK5H. Betanaphthol

P2Z71CIK5H. Bismuth Betanaphthol [betanaphthol]

P32MG14U83. Piperilate

P37G7BTX8V. Arfendazam

P380M0454Z. Cefazolin Sodium

P3CTH044XJ. Probucol

P3P08Y1XJ4. Moxaverine

P3T5QA5J9N. Formoterol Fumarate (See also *5ZZ84GCW8B*)

P41PML4GHR. Nizatidine

P4BVX0D2MX. Clofenciclan

P4IE5B6D6U. Nitroscanate

P4QI4D1IUV. Bentemazole

P4SG24WI5Q. Colesevelam Hydrochloride

P5H9H0GK67. Nitralamine Hydrochloride

P5P95SB639. Palmoxirate Sodium (See also *R326X4TRBY*)

P5RU6UOQ5Y. Doxapram Hydrochloride (See also *94F3830Q73*)

P5T6BYS22Y. Licofelone

P6629XE33T. Dilevalol Hydrochloride [dilevalol]

P6708E7555. Selenomethionine Se 75

P67IM25ID8. Rilmenidine

P69N9N4Y9Y. Fluprofen

P6R62377KV. Tetracycline Hydrochloride

P6SB125NHA. Tilbroquinol

P6VXL377WL. Semduramicin

P6YC3EG204. Cyanocobalamin

P6YZ13C99Q. Calcifediol

P70VF8D9JJ. Besunide

P712T71Q3T. Monophosphothiamine

P71TE299SG. Batelapine Maleate [batelapine] (See also *66K342SF4G*)

P71U09G5BW. Cyclothiazide

P751RR158Y. Garnocestim

P771FDQ1WJ. Galamustine

P7725I9V3Z. Carisbamate

P78D9P90C0. Sulfachlorpyridazine

P7MDS492AC. Dicarfen

P7T269PR6S. Anacetrapib

P7U817352G. Oxiracetam

P7W01638W6. Norethandrolone

P7WI8UL647. Nesiritide

P80AL8J7ZP. Balsalazide Disodium [balsalazide] (See also *1XL6BJI034*)

P81Q6V85NP. Cevimeline Hydrochloride (See also *K9V0CDQ56E*)

P875C0DV2V. Bedoradrine Sulfate (See also *4EAR229231*)

P88XT4IS4D. Paclitaxel

P89DR4NY54. Octocog Alfa

P8S0GE5Q4I. Ciproquazone

P8T739L1FA. Pipofezine

P8W25X9B3K. Uredofos

P8Y54F701R. Timolol Maleate

P8ZQ646136. Oleandomycin Phosphate [oleandomycin] (See also *8681H0C27P*)

P936YA152N. Cefpiramide

P9BC99461E. Aluminum Monostearate

P9G3CKZ4P5. Ganciclovir

P9G3CKZ4P5. Ganciclovir Sodium [ganciclovir] (See also *02L083W284*)

P9HIK5V7WK. Guanoxabenz

P9J7O7YNSW. Avridine

P9VXV1408Y. Ceftaroline Fosamil

PA1123N395. Bilastine

PAI7J52V09. Phenacemide

PAP315WZIA. Estradiol Enanthate

PAU39W3CVB. Butacaine Sulfate

PB5EKT7Q2V. Aprindine Hydrochloride (See also *5Y48085P9Q*)

PD0931191Q. Fenflumizole

PD884XOZ9F. Clomoxir

PDC6A3C0OX. Glycerin

PDQ3ME68U3. Amibegron

PE8925K9EY. Alipamide

PEL7G6VRZ2. Homofenazine

PF3750D8AE. Oxepinac

PF3UC3747Y. Alozafone

PF4079THQO. Esonarimod

PF5DZW74VN. Calcium Hydroxide

PFM79PGI92. Clenpirin

PG20W5VQZS. Prochlorperazine Edisylate

PG53R0DWDQ. Alovudine

PGN54228S5. Puromycin Hydrochloride

PGQ9BY2MDE. Digalloyl Trioleate

PH2639TAB4. Nortopixantrone

PH41D05744. Benzethonium Chloride

PH7R4L7SNF. Fluprednisolone Valerate

PI150J9ZX1. Lazabemide Hydrochloride

PJ691WQY08. Ronactolol

PJP312605E. Almotriptan Malate

PK3852O88V. Prenoverine

PKI06M3IW0. Rivastigmine

PKK6MUZ20G. Mercaptopurine [mercaptopurine anhydrous] (See also *E7WED276I5*)

PL791XXJ7B. Aprofene

PM034U953T. Bacampicillin Hydrochloride (See also *8GM2J22278*)

PM28L0FHNP. Dexfenfluramine Hydrochloride

PML56A160O. Guanfacine Hydrochloride (See also *30OMY4G3MK*)

PN2ZH5LOQY. Erythrosine Sodium

PO572Z7917. Probenecid

POY3S0T3BD. Astromicin Sulfate (See also *7JHD84H15J*)

PP012U645Q. Voxergolide

PPM8SX5Q3V. Aminometradine

PQ3P6082I5. Pipacycline

PQ6CK8PD0R. Ascorbic Acid

PQ6CK8PD0R. Sodium Ascorbate [ascorbic acid]

PQK2N461KJ. Sulfabromomethazine Sodium [sulfabromomethazine]

PQS1L514CF. Ketobemidone

PQX0D8J21J. Cetuximab

PR3292R3H7. Atocalcitol

PR82C5R514. Arasertaconazole

PR834Q503T. Ergotamine Tartrate [ergotamine] (See also *MRU5XH3B48*)

PS51OZG63Z. Piroxantrone Hydrochloride

PSM3RT117Z. Triclonide

PU98C417NB. Ciprafamide

PUA774J9MP. Bufezolac

PV23P19YUG. Azelnidipine

PVH9FQC04V. Omtriptolide Sodium

PVI5M0M1GW. Filgrastim

PW08Y13465. Cefminox

PWL441R6EQ. Nortetrazepam

PWZ1720CBH. Bemotrizinol

PX44XO846X. Hyoscyamine

PYF7O1FV7F. Fluvastatin Sodium (See also *4L066368AS*)

PZ0O26OD9U. Caloxetic Acid

PZV3P03F1U. Atibeprone

Q022B63JPM. Balofloxacin

Q06WU8JY4F. Leteprinim Potassium

Q08SIO485D. Phenprocoumon

Q0CH43PGXS. Fasudil

Q0MQD1073Q. Chlorthalidone

Q0VL46026O. Fenabutene

Q0YKG9L6RF. Aprobarbital
Q1069WKM8G. Aliflurane
Q13WX941EF. Epinastine (See also *GFM415S5XL*)
Q16CT95N25. Bavituximab
Q16TT9C5BK. Bazedoxifene Acetate [bazedoxifene] (See also *J70472UD3D*)
Q1D0Q7R4D9. Perflubron
Q1M94GA18P. Iotyrosine I 131
Q1SUG5KBD6. Sodium Tetradecyl Sulfate
Q1U97XK18R. Guanoclor Sulfate (See also *M4HBT852YO*)
Q1UMG3UH45. Moexipril Hydrochloride
Q20Q21Q62J. Cisplatin
Q25MNP6OC1. Cebaracetam
Q2LN8K1MS7. Spiriprostil
Q2OS4303HZ. Halofantrine Hydrochloride [halofantrine] (See also *H77DL0Y630*)
Q2WXR1I0PK. Cromolyn Sodium (See also *Y0TK0FS77W*)
Q2XM6VR8DO. Ecraprost
Q30VCC064M. Prazepam
Q3254X40X2. Gallamine Triethiodide
Q326023R30. Bosentan
Q36R82SXRG. Lerisetron
Q380BYV049. Cevipabulin Fumarate (See also *P14M0DWS2J*)
Q3AP22Z9FJ. Carperone
Q3JEK5DO4K. Anethole
Q3JTX2Q7TU. Diazepam
Q3OKS62Q6X. Budesonide
Q3OKS62Q6X. Dexbudesonide
Q3U058H86V. Cloranolol
Q40Q9N063P. Acetic Acid
Q40Q9N063P. Acetic Acid, Glacial
Q40X8H422O. Hydroxocobalamin
Q41OR9510P. Melphalan
Q42OMW3AT8. Clavulanate Potassium
Q42T66VG0C. Benzylpenicillin
Q42T66VG0C. Penicillin Calcium [penicillin g]
Q42T66VG0C. Penicillin G Benzathine [penicillin g] (See also *RIT82F58GK*)
Q42T66VG0C. Penicillin G Hydrabamine [penicillin g]
Q42T66VG0C. Penicillin G Procaine [penicillin g]
Q461L7AK4R. Iobenguane I 131
Q46947FE7K. Peginterferon Alfa-2a
Q4K217VGA9. Calfactant
Q4MW9RM93A. Ralitoline
Q4R969U9FR. Edetol
Q4XX54I93R. Exaprolol Hydrochloride [exaprolol] (See also *FGT82HNC7L*)
Q5128GW9D4. Ropizine
Q56SEY8X9J. Salmefamol
Q58C92TUN0. Trichlormethiazide
Q5ELR5A7Y5. Ragaglitazar
Q60AU1LLNU. Oglufanide Disodium
Q6353VLJ8E. Befiperide
Q68050H03T. Cefoxitin Sodium (See also *6OEV9DX57Y*)
Q6C979R91Y. Vinorelbine Tartrate [vinorelbine] (See also *253GQW851Q*)
Q6U6J48BWY. Imiglucerase
Q6W1F7DJ2D. Rescinnamine
Q70OH404HR. Implitapide
Q71XPQ6R29. Guaiacol Carbonate
Q728680892. Cuprimyxin
Q76F3HAE5V. Oxypendyl
Q7FNA7HXLF. Mofoxime
Q812464R06. Hydromorphone Hydrochloride [hydromorphone] (See also *L960UP2KRW*)
Q830PW7520. Codeine
Q88T5P3444. Nemonapride
Q8BIH59O7H. Altretamine

Q8X02027X3. Gemfibrozil
Q90AGA787L. Sparfloxacin
Q91FH1328A. Methicillin Sodium [methicillin] (See also *AO9YF4MN30*)
Q94064N9NW. Debrisoquin Sulfate (See also *X31CDK040E*)
Q94YYU22B8. Diethylpropion Hydrochloride [diethylpropion] (See also *19V2PL39NG*)
Q9L0O73W7L. Coconut Oil
Q9S9NQ5YIY. Novobiocin Sodium
Q9XQ7N7ZRD. Dopropidil
QBL8IZH14X. Clocortolone Pivalate
QBX79NZC1D. Irsogladine
QCA39I2AP7. Lotucaine
QD8496WWYK. Libenzapril
QD9G66C5UF. Cefonicid Monosodium (See also *6532B86WFG*)
QE0G097358. Acronine
QE4VW5FO07. Ethambutol Hydrochloride (See also *8G167061QZ*)
QE6F49RPJ1. Sorbitan Trioleate
QF8SVZ843E. Albuterol
QF8SVZ843E. Albuterol Sulfate [albuterol] (See also *021SEF3731*)
QFP0P1DV7Z. Sitagliptin Phosphate [sitagliptin] (See also *TS63EW8X6F*)
QG05NRB077. Fenticonazole Nitrate [fenticonazole]
QG8198SR7M. Rimoprogin
QGC8W08I6I. Acetohexamide
QGH063955F. Fipronil
QGM18599H5. Butamisole Hydrochloride
QHO02LZ4H2. Chromic Phosphate P 32
QI0U3D4X3M. Sopitazine
QI846AL4NC. Dexivacaine
QIC03ANI02. Famciclovir
QIO667518T. Dilmefone
QJH0XA6AW9. Deboxamet
QK318GVY3Y. Cirazoline
QK4DYS664X. Flunisolide
QL5Z51GXKI. Flavamine
QM95LPV3CA. Mecetronium Ethylsulfate
QMS40680K6. Palifermin
QN4128B52A. Obatoclax Mesylate [obatoclax] (See also *39200FJ43J*)
QNG273A81O. Ticalopride
QNT09A162Y. Arsthinol
QO611KSM5P. Edrophonium Chloride
QOV2JZ647A. Netoglitazone
QP166M390Q. Ataciguat
QP1A5BD6K9. Menoctone
QR5PYD126V. Dexverapamil
QR6HQ1U73Z. Iodoantipyrine I 131
QRW683O56T. Amylocaine
QRW9FCR9P2. Cyclizine
QRW9FCR9P2. Cyclizine Hydrochloride [cyclizine] (See also *W0O1NHP4WE*)
QRW9FCR9P2. Cyclizine Lactate [cyclizine] (See also *861R00J986*)
QRY8KPT3QI. Nesapidil
QS9014Q792. Articaine Hydrochloride
QSB34YF0W9. Fluphenazine Enanthate
QT35T5T35Q. Sulfanitran
QTG126297Q. Diclofenac Sodium
QTO9JB4MDD. Sodium Tartrate
QTT17582CB. Hydrochloric Acid
QU6P2P8XLW. Simetride
QU72HVX338. Fabesetron
QU7E2XA9TG. Sodium Stearate
QUC7NX6WMB. Sertraline Hydrochloride [sertraline] (See also *UTI8907Y6X*)

QUF41MF56G. Tilisolol
QV3QF1EF2P. Toliodium Chloride
QV897JC36D. Butorphanol
QV897JC36D. Butorphanol Tartrate [butorphanol] (See also *2L7I72RUHN*)
QVF9Y6955W. Gadoteric Acid
QVZ3IAR3JS. Toltrazuril
QVZ4XA556B. Catramilast
QW7Y7ZR15U. Peramivir
QWB37T4WZZ. Histamine Phosphate
QWW7V29814. Pyridoxamine Phosphate
QX10HYY4QV. Sesame Oil
QX39IR9V1D. Enpiroline Phosphate (See also *8M7Y72EP9K*)
QX3KXL1ZA2. Naratriptan
QX3KXL1ZA2. Naratriptan Hydrochloride [naratriptan] (See also *10X8X4P12Z*)
QXS94885MZ. Bimatoprost
QY7HLH8V4L. Diproqualone
QZE8T5D680. Pazoxide
QZO5366EW7. Dorzolamide Hydrochloride (See also *9JDX055TW1*)
QZU4H47A3S. Atazanavir Sulfate [atazanavir] (See also *4MT4VIE29P*)
R01EZP92PU. Laurolinium Acetate
R0C9NIE5JJ. Chromonar Hydrochloride [chromonar]
R0OS2S9G4U. Sanfetrinem Sodium
R0TAY3X631. Norelgestromin
R10H71BSWG. Micafungin Sodium [micafungin] (See also *IS1UP79R56*)
R11SBP9F2B. Metocinium Iodide
R1308VH37P. Sobuzoxane
R133MWH7X1. Morniflumate
R1493W1CJ0. Properidine
R15UI3245N. Isoxsuprine Hydrochloride [isoxsuprine] (See also *V74TEQ36CO*)
R16CO5Y76E. Aspirin
R16SK8726X. Silperisone
R1SIA15KZ1. Sotrastaurin Acetate
R2GZD7LMYX. Irampanel
R2H3YN6E3L. Niaprazine
R326X4TRBY. Palmoxirate Sodium [palmoxiric acid] (See also *P5P95SB639*)
R337868TDW. Octenidine Saccharin
R3459K699K. Secnidazole
R35D29L3ZA. Pyrilamine Maleate (See also *HPE317O9TL*)
R3B1994K2E. Taribavirin Hydrochloride [taribavirin]
R3IOR5299G. Beminafil
R3TC4SEW5A. Clemeprol
R3TGX0K69Z. Etaminile
R3U09W4H4I. Xenbucin
R3UK8X3U3D. Modafinil
R40P36GDK6. Apaflurane
R40RXC296C. Topixantrone
R420KW629U. Mephenytoin
R43D2573WO. Fosinopril Sodium [fosinopril] (See also *NW2RTH6T2N*)
R46Y1C0ZR2. Dimecrotic Acid
R47KMF9589. Molracetam
R49EFA73Q7. Piroctone
R4AVR27MM8. Pralmorelin Dihydrochloride
R4CY19YS7C. Domiphen Bromide
R4K19W6S7Q. Mabuterol
R4KO0DY52L. Chlorhexidine Gluconate [chlorhexidine] (See also *MOR84MUD8E*)
R4KR9A9165. Amitivir
R4Z9X1N2ND. Dofetilide
R57ZHV85D4. Boric Acid
R5ELL4R7VD. Eclazolast

R5H8897N95. Labetalol Hydrochloride [labetalol] (See also *1GEV3BAW9J*)
R5L488RY0Q. Ferrous Fumarate (See also *88XHZ13131*)
R5O1XB5L3M. Iofetamine Hydrochloride I 123
R60L0SM5BC. Midazolam Maleate [midazolam]
R612XR8A9F. Vapitadine Dihydrochloride
R61ZEH7I1I. Promethazine Hydrochloride (See also *FF28EJQ494*)
R63VQ857OT. Amoxapine
R6875N380F. Quinidine Gluconate
R6889JIL5D. Feclobuzone
R6D2UI4FLS. Enclomiphene
R6D31YA2WK. Crisnatol Mesylate
R6DXU4WAY9. Esomeprazole Magnesium
R6G1M06TPO. Alepride
R6Q3791S76. Sodium Gluconate
R6ZMD4UH3D. Ispinesib Mesylate
R6ZTY81RE1. Pipecuronium Bromide
R71Y86M0WT. Chloroguanide Hydrochloride
R71Y86M0WT. Proguanil Hydrochloride
R72LW146E6. Cephalothin Sodium [cephalothin] (See also *C22G6EYP8B*)
R775Y233N3. Octrizole
R7GV3H6FQ4. Trimethadione
R7M676M8YV. Nicotine Bitartrate
R7P4D56J1Z. Piclonidine
R7QTG0PMPX. Aceglutamide Aluminum (See also *01J18G9G97*)
R802O5NILK. Piriprost
R81X549E70. Nordefrin Hydrochloride [nordefrin]
R85M2X0D68. Candesartan Cilexetil (See also *S8Q36MD2XX*)
R8869Q7R8I. Trifluperidol
R890C8J3N1. Carbaril
R8A7M9MY61. Cefuroxime Sodium
R8DWN01P1M. Bromadoline Maleate [bromadoline]
R8I97I2L24. Cinitapride
R8L0T98P0J. Bensuldazic Acid (See also *NC32G269EF*)
R8M46911LR. Flubendazole
R8XA2029ZI. Butenafine Hydrochloride (See also *91Y494NL0X*)
R8XDP7L3SL. Azidocillin
R92JB88O88. Ricasetron
R9400W927I. Ketoconazole
R953O2RHZ5. Pyrithione Zinc
R9IQ7GVL3E. Rofleponide
R9M4FJE48E. Dalfopristin
R9PHW59SFN. Naftopidil
R9QTB5E82N. Hexylresorcinol
R9Z042Z19E. Lithium Benzoate
RA33EAC7KY. Fenoprofen
RA33EAC7KY. Fenoprofen Calcium [fenoprofen] (See also *0X2CW1QABJ*)
RA6D4LW87K. Tioxaprofen
RAG2185DR1. Sibopirdine
RAP1D6110C. Leucocianidol
RB4XQ0T71U. Pivenfrine
RBZ1571X5H. Dasatinib
RE91AN4S8G. Luliconazole
REK4960K2U. Butylated Hydroxyanisole
RES9I0LGG5. Rolziracetam
RFO6IL3D3M. Methylnaltrexone Bromide
RFR2CH3QZK. Seletracetam
RFW2ET671P. Hydroxypropyl Cellulose
RG2371KXDE. Fosfocreatinine
RG277LF5B3. Sapropterin Dihydrochloride
RG38I2P540. Mupirocin Calcium
RG9G4Z82PY. Dinaline
RH5KI819JG. Carnidazole
RHH3W8F1CO. Metrizamide

RHW35E1G7E. Etoxeridine
RHW5BU180N. Novobiocin Calcium (See also *17EC19951N*)
RIT82F58GK. Penicillin G Benzathine (See also *Q42T66VG0C*)
RJ84Y44811. Quinapril
RJ84Y44811. Quinapril Hydrochloride [quinapril] (See also *33067B3N2M*)
RJ9V9V09VM. Altinicline Maleate [altinicline]
RJQ4G25ZRH. Methaqualone Hydrochloride
RK2972YZ2U. Tarazepide
RKC4AOX590. Phenbutazone Sodium Glycerate (See also *GN5P7K3T8S*)
RL11HOJ7DM. Chlorphentermine Hydrochloride (See also *NHW079127O*)
RL3HK1I66B. Symclosene
RLM74T3Z9D. Gadoversetamide
RM53R5R2BL. Elfazepam
RM5BP192F9. Aminophenazone Cyclamate
RML78EN3XE. Rimonabant
RMW9V5RW38. Trifluridine
RN145A0SVL. Arclofenin
RNZ43O5WW5. Milnacipran Hydrochloride (See also *G56VK1HF36*)
RO16TQF95Y. Triflupromazine
RP2J52327K. Butobendine
RP4A60D26L. Pentazocine
RPQ57D8S72. Docarpamine
RPR1R4C0P4. Leucovorin Calcium
RQ6L463N3B. Mecysteine
RQ6LP6Z0WY. Mafenide Acetate
RQ8UL4C17S. Oxiconazole Nitrate (See also *C668Q9I33J*)
RR5R8BAX26. Clormecaine
RR6866VL0O. Trandolaprilat
RRW32X4U1F. Dienestrol
RSH7NDI7MI. Befetupitant
RT3Y3QMF8N. Molindone Hydrochloride [molindone] (See also *1DWS68PNE6*)
RT6K0322Q7. Halopenium Chloride
RTN51LK7WL. Methscopolamine Bromide
RU10K34QRU. Vamicamide
RU19QYB9WZ. Giracodazole
RUC37XUP2P. Kanamycin Sulfate [kanamycin] (See also *OW1N4G4R9W*)
RUD5Y4SV0S. Trenbolone Acetate
RUK64CF26E. Thiethylperazine Maleate
RUM6K67ESG. Treprostinil
RV6J6604TK. Eucalyptol
RVJ0BV3H3Y. Mofezolac
RWM8CCW8GP. Octreotide
RYH2T97J77. Ranimustine
RZ5COP6XI5. Amezepine
RZD65TSM9U. Agalsidase Beta
S0177QHV2B. Budralazine
S01B3A38SK. Triflocin
S05RV1R3LZ. Tazeprofen
S07O44R1ZM. Capsaicin
S0FAJ1R9CD. Tioxolone
S0FG5X68QT. Amiprilose Hydrochloride [amiprilose] (See also *546994B3VA*)
S0GPJ58I2D. Iotriside
S0KXB0NKWN. Vincantril
S0QL3IT20J. Levamlodipine Malate
S0U059XF2E. Pinolcaine
S175C652YS. Symetine Hydrochloride (See also *UZ8WTY8051*)
S1IA7R2J48. Aminoethyl Nitrate
S1IC65Y242. Lorcinadol
S1UAI9MKMG. Liothyronine I 125 (See also *06LU7C9H1V*)
S1URO6678T. Leiopyrrole
S23189WW7E. Proheptazine

S2FVB1RL5X. Fenpiprane Hydrochloride [fenpiprane] (See also *684N1BF96B*)
S2QG84156O. Cupric Chloride
S312EY6ZT8. Fosinoprilat
S35880HLHZ. Brasofensine Maleate
S3709T25V6. Fadolmidine Hydrochloride
S384A1Y12J. Zilpaterol
S38B9W6AXW. Aminosalicylate Sodium
S39J3B52KS. Glicetanile Sodium [glicetanile] (See also *M3FU19R357*)
S39YD087F9. Elbanizine
S3IG39T94B. Amidephrine Mesylate
S3WF2KTK27. Linarotene
S48955N1AL. Letimide Hydrochloride [letimide]
S491HH391H. Prenoxdiazine
S4H62451TO. Iomeglamic Acid
S4TF6I2330. Sulbactam Benzathine [sulbactam]
S4YR4X39CA. Beloxamide
S4ZCE64Q3O. Tasuldine
S5016F5ZH4. Edonentan [edonentan anhydrous] (See also *2CCC8CH216*)
S547MDN7WX. Esoxybutynin Chloride
S56D65XJ9G. Eltrombopag Olamine [eltrombopag] (See also *4U07F515LG*)
S56PQL4N1V. Alclometasone Dipropionate (See also *136H45TB7B*)
S57Y5X1117. Tioconazole
S58EH61Q1Y. Hetaflur (See also *O2H0Q02M4P*)
S59502J185. Ciclesonide
S5969B6237. Mexazolam
S5D373PRDG. Camiverine
S5PUP23U26. Promethazine Teoclate
S5TJ79BX74. Tifurac Sodium
S62U433RMH. Zaleplon
S65743JHBS. Gefitinib
S69KXZ59AB. Aceperone
S6KDM312I5. Turofexorate Isopropyl
S6V5I726MH. Xanoxic Acid
S741ZJS97U. Netilmicin Sulfate (See also *4O5J85GJJB*)
S747T1ERAJ. Anisindione
S75C401OS1. Febantel
S76B51L5AM. Dextroamphetamine Phosphate (See also *TZ47U051FI*)
S77YM77P92. Floverine
S79265T71M. Lomeguatrib
S798V6YJRP. Edaravone
S7P608OW2O. Ciclosidomine
S7UT8VQG94. Florifenine
S7V92P67HO. Arsenic Trioxide
S866O45PIG. Beractant
S88072126Q. Diethazine Hydrochloride
S8K2JDR3NZ. Picilorex
S8P50T62B6. Asulacrine
S8Q36MD2XX. Candesartan
S8Q36MD2XX. Candesartan Cilexetil [candesartan] (See also *R85M2X0D68*)
S8S8451A4O. Teprenone
S90R21A2V2. Clonitazene
S915P5499N. Plerixafor
S9421HWB3Z. Oxyphenonium Bromide
S97YUG2A91. Efipladib
S9B9E35WUX. Anirolac
S9MFK45GY9. Acevaltrate
S9OX9692ZB. Galiximab
S9RZW428WX. Biclodil Hydrochloride
S9SDD93U5U. Aminopromazine
S9U025Y077. Tetrahydrozoline Hydrochloride [tetrahydrozoline] (See also *0YZT43HS7D*)

S9ZFX8403R. Sufentanil Citrate
SA9937IP23. Monoctanoin Component C
SAW16W26X6. Guabenxan
SB8ZUX40TY. Saccharin Sodium
SBC76K7XWC. Etazepine
SC80GNP08C. Candocuronium Iodide
SCK81AMR7R. Thrombin Alfa
SD507F5T2W. Danitracen
SD6QCT3TSU. Pentoxifylline
SE10G96M8W. Tazobactam
SE4TWR0K2C. Perflubutane
SE8X571K4C. Trelnarizine
SEF8X7MXO4. Chloroazodin
SF4NW7NH7C. Oxitropium Bromide
SG5IU7FD3R. Procodazole
SH1WY3R615. Nocodazole
SH55B0RQ9K. Oblimersen Sodium
SI4064O0LX. Procainamide Hydrochloride (See also
    L39WTC366D)
SI78RFJ7XI. Piprinhydrinate
SI86V6QNEG. Halcinonide
SID40G6U6D. Exiproben
SIG10953FN. Bamirastine
SIV03811UC. Kainic Acid
SIW4YR11ST. Carbubarb
SJ76Y07H5F. Trientine Hydrochloride [trientine] (See also
    HC3NX54582)
SJT761GEGS. Lisdexamfetamine Dimesylate (See also
    H645GUL8KJ)
SLF0D9077S. Oxytetracycline [oxytetracycline anhydrous] (See
    also *X20I9EN955*)
SLJ0HIL21J. Procinolol
SM0DJQ1HBT. Carcainium Chloride
SME6G1846X. Iodofenphos
SML2Y3J35T. Colchicine
SMP167WV5D. Cizolirtine
SMP2689462. Dimethisoquin Hydrochloride (See also *772EN3-
    BH6I*)
SN86FG7N2K. Chlorothiazide Sodium (See also *77W477J15H*)
SOA12P041N. Nitazoxanide
SOD6A38AGA. Levocetirizine Dihydrochloride
SOI2LOH54Z. Zinc Oxide
SP28AL52TM. Fenacetinol
SP86R356CC. Acetanilide
SPU695OD73. Lodoxamide Ethyl [lodoxamide]
SPU695OD73. Lodoxamide Tromethamine [lodoxamide] (See
    also *50LV9A548L*)
SPW36WUI5Z. Mofebutazone
SQ922M93PI. Clamoxyquin Hydrochloride
SQE6VB453K. Calcium Gluconate
SR60A3XG0F. Cinnamaldehyde
SS85U8K5ZN. Codeine Polistirex
SST9XCL51M. Gamma Oryzanol
ST0WR0R5X1. Cefetecol
STW31V60ZL. Pifenate
SU46BAM238. Ammonium Sulfate
SUC3551A8U. Quinotolast
SUG9176GRW. Practolol
SUO3KVS1O9. Aminohippurate Sodium
SV0CSG527L. Fluorometholone
SV0CSG527L. Fluorometholone Acetate [fluorometholone] (See
    also *9I50C3I3OK*)
SV6L22Y9QF. Amopyroquine
SVI38UY019. Estropipate
SW3OJS6TOD. Altapizone
SW9M9BB5K3. Phenobarbital Sodium
SX6K58TVWC. Glyburide
SY3J0147NB. Encainide Hydrochloride [encainide]

SYD411HZ3S. Radafaxine Hydrochloride
SYW4Z0B3KN. Nasaruplase Beta
SZ0F94M68J. Retelliptine
SZ83PVQ06I. Cilobamine Mesylate
T01B0RCE7T. Amelometasone
T0248823H1. Tazanolast
T032BI7727. Bromodiphenhydramine Hydrochloride [bromodi-
    phenhydramine] (See also *202J683U97*)
T034E4NS2Z. Sulfamethoxypyridazine
T034E4NS2Z. Sulfamethoxypyridazine Acetyl [sulfamethoxypyr-
    idazine]
T0785J3X40. Cefbuperazone
T0C1IR71L8. Dexoxadrol Hydrochloride (See also *JY5N9F45AG*)
T0GSO02UEZ. Methdilazine Hydrochloride (See also
    4Q13LY9Z8X)
T18F433X4S. Norethindrone
T1J0JOU64O. Dichlorophen
T1PE06G0VE. Camellia Oil
T1Y573BS7H. Apicycline
T20OQ1YN1W. Clindamycin Hydrochloride (See also
    3U02EL437C)
T2410KM04A. Heparin Sodium [heparin] (See also *ZZ45AB24-
    CA*)
T2DHJ9645W. Diflorasone Diacetate [diflorasone] (See also
    7W2J09SCWX)
T2GIP8IIG6. Furomine
T2OJ193WGR. Lometraline Hydrochloride
T30038QI8N. Nebracetam
T32BM3AM71. Proxorphan Tartrate
T38B9T1F30. Pyroxamine Maleate
T3C89M417N. Glutaral
T3CHA1B51H. Antipyrine
T3H6486135. Azaquinzole
T3RCY5OD7A. Epipropidine
T3Y0F5VOB8. Metazamide
T42P99266K. Methylene Blue
T4661K682A. Iopydol
T47477CUF7. Denagliptin Tosylate (See also *DOS9ZOT21L*)
T4C1IE36L0. Glisamuride
T4D9016A00. Lodazecar
T4G2I958J2. Mesoridazine Besylate
T4L2P3KH7K. Thiamylal Sodium
T4NP8G3K6Q. Batabulin
T4NP8G3K6Q. Batabulin Sodium [batabulin] (See also
    G04B77F772)
T4O2MP4507. Piroxicam Olamine
T51D685OXG. Dexamethasone Cipecilate
T5536Q4O60. Iodohippurate Sodium I 125
T58MSI464G. Acarbose
T5IBT2ZQS3. Denipride
T5IRO3534A. Vincristine Sulfate (See also *5J49Q6B70F*)
T5MWT8445U. Flestolol Sulfate (See also *LI02075E1W*)
T5RCK09KHV. Fipamezole
T6133SO781. Calcium Levulinate
T643E80J9K. Carocainide
T69Y9LDN44. Deferitrin
T6BL4ZC15G. Sulfalene
T6CRE6WE0W. Clorprenaline Hydrochloride
T6EKB9V2O2. Guacetisal
T6Q3060U91. Motesanib Diphosphate
T6Z9V48IKG. Gentamicin Sulfate [gentamicin] (See also
    8X7386QRLV)
T750UM24H8. Cefmatilen
T75W9911L6. Propane
T795873AJP. Sulfacytine
T7D4876IUE. Dihydrostreptomycin Sulfate (See also *P2I6R8-
    W6UA*)
T7ZM08F7FU. Bolasterone

T8593BT7B4. Lodiperone
T8KXA37068. Haloxon
T97CB3796L. Clemizole (See also *85W6I13D8M*)
T99M8X4T54. Dibupyrone
T9G78A1R21. Furaprofen
TA269SD04T. Benzaldehyde
TA9XO4D05J. Phthalofyne
TAY5ZBM0MO. Phthalylsulfamethizole
TB885DRP1J. Cyclomenol
TC0T0O9VYO. Raxofelast
TC2D6JAD40. Diphenhydramine Hydrochloride
TCN4MG2VXS. Dapivirine
TCU22W0APY. Etiproston
TDE8767O88. Levemopamil
TE7660XO1C. Glycine
TEA6PI0H6H. Enolicam Sodium [enolicam] (See also *C3QYZ005LS*)
TEZ91L71V4. Mephentermine Sulfate [mephentermine] (See also *580655Z8RR*)
TF9FPB4V3Y. Mefenidramium Metilsulfate
TG44VME01D. Fipexide
TG537D343B. Desipramine Hydrochloride [desipramine] (See also *1Y58DO4MY1*)
TH25PD4CCB. Metoprolol Succinate
THY6RIW44R. Etalocib
TI05AO53L7. Betamethasone Acetate
TJ2M0FR8ES. Megestrol Acetate (See also *EA6LD1M70M*)
TJ904HH8SN. Tetrachloroethylene
TK65WKS8HL. Buspirone Hydrochloride [buspirone] (See also *207LT9J9OC*)
TKL72421ZD. Famiraprinium Chloride
TKQ858A3VW. Iodipamide
TL2TJE8QTX. Aminobenzoic Acid
TL515DW4QS. Vicriviroc Maleate [vicriviroc] (See also *EP3QG127N9*)
TLE294X33A. Prussian Blue Insoluble
TLM2976OFR. Riboflavin
TM2TZD4G4A. Monoctanoin Component A
TML814419R. Mefloquine
TMZ3IBW2OW. Ebrotidine
TN4C52M5ZT. Moctamide
TN4JSC48CV. Hetacillin
TN4JSC48CV. Hetacillin Potassium [hetacillin] (See also *95PFX5932Y*)
TN9BEX005G. Bivalirudin
TO2JP2G53H. Lanperisone
TO4OC41XVI. Dichlormezanone
TOV02TDP9I. Nalmefene
TP71SPS85C. Lomevactone
TPC5Q8496G. Pipendoxifene
TPT3MH65LD. Clofezone
TPY09G7XIR. Fluorescein
TPY09G7XIR. Fluorescein Sodium [fluorescein] (See also *93X55PE38X*)
TQ358GWH6Y. Zardaverine
TQ4H2AG3JI. Domazoline Fumarate (See also *4FBV0WY9OG*)
TQD7Q784P1. Ebastine
TR0QT6QSUL. Remogliflozin Etabonate
TR3MLJ1UAI. Disulfiram
TR7Y641235. Coumazoline
TS63EW8X6F. Sitagliptin Phosphate (See also *QFP0P1DV7Z*)
TS6G201A6Q. Senicapoc
TSA7W27MF8. Pecilocin
TSQ6U39Q3G. Bulaquine
TT85QFR500. Calcium Clofibrate
TTD90R31WZ. Interferon Beta-1b
TTL6G7LIWZ. Lysine Acetate
TTN62ITH9I. Noscapine Hydrochloride

TU1X77K34Q. Arginine Glutamate
TU7HW0W0QT. Sodium Lactate
TUT9J99IMU. Bromoform
TV240CH11P. Demecycline
TV27RY5876. Zatebradine
TWN203TLYT. Tuvatidine
TX973XBY8N. Anthiolimine
TXG28R7G4Y. Upidosin
TXP4T9106S. Butaperazine
TY1X1WG26A. Furterene
TYG45UE07V. Pyrophenindane
TYR2U59WMA. Amitriptylinoxide
TZ47U051FI. Dextroamphetamine
TZ47U051FI. Dextroamphetamine Phosphate [dextroamphetamine] (See also *S76B51L5AM*)
TZ4OX61974. Tepoxalin
TZ7V40X7VX. Metolazone
TZ913SWN6M. Chloracyzine
TZX5469Z6I. Sodium Bisulfite
U0476M545B. Fludrocortisone Acetate [fludrocortisone] (See also *V47IF0PVH4*)
U09698V56W. Propipocaine
U0E93N6V2A. Cyanocobalamin Co 58
U0JZ726775. Desirudin
U0K8WHL37U. Dropropizine
U0RKZ75D0T. Aloracetam
U0VSF7HTN0. Levallorphan Tartrate (See also *353613BU4U*)
U129BBY8DB. Diphenan
U141W322WZ. Timcodar
U16EOR79U4. Promazine Hydrochloride (See also *O9M39HTM5W*)
U188XYD42P. Moxifloxacin
U1JK633AYI. Motesanib
U1K5BS2ABA. Loprodiol
U1O3J18SFL. Montelukast Sodium (See also *MHM278SD3E*)
U202363UOS. Fenofibrate
U2508LW03T. Azipramine Hydrochloride (See also *1P9L1B4UIC*)
U26EO4675Q. Caffeine Citrate
U29O83JAZW. Zotepine
U2Y5OFN795. Brivanib Alaninate
U301T88E1M. Atreleuton
U30C54N3MU. Netobimin
U3227B174V. Sulfasomizole
U347PV74IL. Gemcitabine Hydrochloride
U38E620NS6. Gestonorone Caproate
U38V3ZVV3V. Ferric Chloride
U3C8E5BWKR. Dolasetron Mesylate (See also *82WI2L7Q6E*)
U3H27498KS. Lamotrigine
U3P01618RT. Fluorouracil
U3RSY48JW5. Benzocaine
U40903X6V8. Pardoprunox Hydrochloride
U40Q9GE876. Quincarbate
U42703EIIO. Mepazine Acetate
U42B7VYA4P. Chlorpromazine
U42B7VYA4P. Chlorpromazine Hydrochloride [chlorpromazine] (See also *9WP59609J6*)
U4526F86FJ. Carboprost Tromethamine (See also *7B5032XT6O*)
U46E473275. Chlornaphazine
U4M5Y13FGM. Chromic Chloride Cr 51
U4OHT63MRI. Dapoxetine Hydrochloride (See also *GB2433A4M3*)
U4RY8MRX7C. Ethanolamine Oleate
U4TFJ7GB6T. Diamfenetide
U4THC4MHG7. Murocainide
U4VJ29L7BQ. Methoxsalen
U5026H7S5S. Suxethonium Chloride
U52APA00X7. Sabiporide

U5N7SU872W. Malathion
U5SYW473RQ. Telmisartan
U604E1NB3K. Reparixin
U64HJ4AK57. Etolotifen
U68WG3173Y. Carmustine
U6F3787206. Aminocaproic Acid
U6Q8Z01514. Adefovir Dipivoxil
U6QG1RWA7B. Prizidilol Hydrochloride [prizidilol hydrochloride anhydrous] (See also *1Q4C0XA9H4*)
U6USW86RD0. Mitoxantrone Hydrochloride (See also *BZ114NVM5P*)
U6X61U5ZEG. Ephedrine Sulfate
U700P169W2. Sulfamonomethoxine
U71XL721QK. Piperine
U863JGG2IA. Brivaracetam
U8687J667P. Hydroxindasate
U89MCO87LX. Halethazole
U8CJK0JH5M. Anthralin
U8QXS1WU8G. Ciglitazone
U8WVJ3501L. Bucumolol
U96OL57GOY. Proparacaine Hydrochloride (See also *B4OB0J-HI1X*)
U9LY9Y75X2. Pancuronium Bromide
U9R24EH050. Propetamide
U9YT4RM48N. Niceverine
UA6HM01WAK. Clidanac
UA8SE1325T. Gimeracil
UA8U0KJM72. Pamabrom
UAZ6V7728S. Cinacalcet
UAZ6V7728S. Cinacalcet Hydrochloride [cinacalcet] (See also *1K860WSG25*)
UC0DRK4OE0. Brinazarone
UC61HM8FX0. Pargeverine
UC6VBE7V1Z. Methadone Hydrochloride [methadone] (See also *229809935B*)
UCE6F4125H. Vardenafil
UD3030V43F. Poison Oak Extract
UD8PEV6JBD. Nicaraven
UD984I04LZ. Daunorubicin Hydrochloride (See also *ZS7284E0ZP*)
UDM7Q7QWP8. Benazepril Hydrochloride [benazepril] (See also *N1SN99T69T*)
UDX9AKS7GM. Arsanilic Acid
UEO8UW9V1Z. Etozolin
UF064M00AF. Diethyl Phthalate
UF599785JZ. Fentanyl
UF599785JZ. Fentanyl Citrate [fentanyl] (See also *MUN5-LYG46H*)
UFH8805FKA. St. John's Wort
UFN2Q54HS6. Setipafant
UH2K6W1Y64. Lactitol [lactitol monohydrate] (See also *L2B0WJF7ZY*)
UH95VD7V76. Oxacillin Sodium [oxacillin] (See also *G0V6C994Q5*)
UHB9Z3841A. Saquinavir Mesylate
UI1U1MYH09. Darapladib
UIF43N1HSV. Barmastine
UII7156WLU. Ingliforib
UJ1O5LVT0G. Razinodil
UK27RQ38IX. Diathymosulfone
UK4C618C8T. Broxyquinoline
UK5SR22C8Q. Glicaramide
UK6392GD5W. Oxycinchophen
UKC6GH80QR. Dicobalt Edetate
UKU5U19W9M. Flunoxaprofen
UL09X1D9EM. Pruvanserin
UL09X1D9EM. Pruvanserin Hydrochloride [pruvanserin] (See also *AWA682DH9Z*)

UL947A614K. Cicortonide
ULD9ZKE457. Palosuran
ULS5I8J03O. Olsalazine Sodium [olsalazine] (See also *Y7JEW0-XG7I*)
UM20QQM95Y. Ifosfamide
UMD07X179E. Certolizumab Pegol
UMD7G2653W. Ibandronic Acid
UMF554N5FG. Tacedinaline
UMH46V5U01. Dexamisole
UO003HH66V. Dietifen
UO1VQB3SPZ. Coumetarol
UOM2HMO524. Premafloxacin
UP7QBP99PN. Apremilast
UPN4ITI8T4. Trimetrexate
UPY9RD84AG. Fenocinol
UQG78PXR4W. Ketocainol
UQT9G45D1P. Halothane
UQW7UF9N91. Aclidinium Bromide
UR1SAB295F. Sulfamerazine
UR1SAB295F. Sulfamerazine Sodium [Injection] [sulfamerazine] (See also *JOV4UJY07O*)
UR59KN573L. Bisoprolol Fumarate
UR9VPI71PT. Fudosteine
URR853YLZA. Iproxamine Hydrochloride [iproxamine] (See also *83L52U43TX*)
URX5F7RDER. Eprobemide
US65H9WBNH. Tipindole
US71433228. Penbutolol Sulfate (See also *78W62V43DY*)
USE67B01YN. Gliflumide
USZ5MY269R. Beclobrate
UTI8907Y6X. Sertraline Hydrochloride (See also *QUC7NX6WMB*)
UU4X6T9FT5. Flubepride
UVG8VSP2SJ. Flumequine
UVL329170W. Cisapride
UWC15E373Z. Bevonium Metilsulfate (See also *34B0471E08*)
UX9Z118X9F. Propantheline Bromide
UXA545ABTT. Tazobactam Sodium
UXH81S8ZVB. Mycophenolate Mofetil Hydrochloride
UYE4T5I70X. Dexlansoprazole
UYN5I3I5YQ. Mipimazole
UZ5LMI200P. Florantyrone
UZ8WTY8051. Symetine Hydrochloride [symetine] (See also *S175C652YS*)
UZX80K71OE. Eszopiclone
V008L6478D. Levonordefrin
V00NQ7SDYI. Hexylcaine Hydrochloride (See also *5111U0826Z*)
V05260LC8D. Esmolol Hydrochloride (See also *MDY902UXSR*)
V09GC6329G. Floxacrine
V0N2VMB4FV. Keracyanin
V0Q53N427T. Fluspiperone
V0V73PEB8M. Cyhalothrin
V10579P3QZ. Amdinocillin
V10R70ML23. Heptabarbital
V13007Z41A. Lidocaine Hydrochloride
V17MYO89WO. Oxagrelate
V1J0B4P41O. Pirepolol
V1JK16Y2JP. Doxifluridine
V1JZQ7GDTX. Phencyclidine Hydrochloride (See also *J1DOI7UV76*)
V1L22WVE2S. Zileuton
V1Q0O9OJ9Z. Chlorpheniramine Maleate (See also *3U6IO1965U*)
V1V998DC17. Garlic
V1YC7T6LLI. Brodimoprim
V243ORA40X. Mezilamine
V27W9254FZ. Cortisone Acetate [cortisone] (See also *883WKN7W8X*)

V2P3K60DA2. Pentamidine Isethionate
V2W1791D7V. Xantofyl Palmitate
V35KBM8JGR. Aminolevulinic Acid Hydrochloride
V3888OEY5R. Verapamil Hydrochloride
V39YPH45FZ. Pirlindole
V3DMU7PVXF. Resiquimod
V477CK910J. Axitirome
V47IF0PVH4. Fludrocortisone Acetate (See also *U0476M545B*)
V4PW0S7ZP7. Panadiplon
V4WLW77V5Q. Oxaflozane
V51RRX51VH. Gepefrine
V51W472X6D. Cloponone
V52IY042L9. Furcloprofen
V55R69267Q. Etrabamine
V58CN2SY21. Tibenelast Sodium
V5F60UPD8P. Denopamine
V5QKF7Q20O. Datelliptium Chloride
V5VD430YW9. Aloe
V628N5FTX8. Fenaftic Acid
V63XWA605I. Armodafinil
V6D7VK2215. Atrasentan Hydrochloride [atrasentan] (See also *E4G31X93ZA*)
V6ERX20PHB. Benzetimide Hydrochloride (See also *B987T0L5FX*)
V6FL6O5GR7. Coluracetam
V6G94Z48FK. Triflumidate
V6OFU47K3W. Sulfinpyrazone
V6W7F1R86P. Fenaperone
V6X0RFU7AF. Tricetamide
V72H9867WB. Garenoxacin Mesylate [garenoxacin] (See also *OXI6EF55FR*)
V734AZP9BR. Mubritinib
V74TEQ36CO. Isoxsuprine Hydrochloride (See also *R15UI3245N*)
V797H4GG0Z. Aluminum Lactate
V7DXN0M42R. Clonixin
V7I71DQ432. Buflomedil
V7O1U41C9B. Eberconazole
V7O53S50SN. Lofendazam
V81J4OO2OT. Disuprazole
V82Q65924L. Crufomate
V8350F4A37. Phenylthilone
V83O1VOZ8L. Isoniazid
V8674RM5KM. Endixaprine
V867Q8X3ZD. Diethylcarbamazine Citrate [diethylcarbamazine] (See also *OS1Z389K8S*)
V8G4MOF2V9. Deferasirox
V8ZG4Y1B51. Talabostat Mesylate
V901LV1K7D. Prednicarbate
V91T9204HU. Lumiracoxib
V92884KHRI. Levonantradol Hydrochloride
V92SO9WP2I. Glycopyrrolate
V93U9DH62C. Emorfazone
V942ZCN81H. Metacetamol
V95R5KMY2B. Peppermint
V9783UEL0F. Flumexadol
V99T50803M. Sunitinib Malate [sunitinib] (See also *LVX8N1UT73*)
V9BI9B5YI2. Doxylamine Succinate (See also *95QB77JKPL*)
V9E5U5XF42. Flomoxef
V9EFU16ZIF. Methyltestosterone
V9HOC53L7L. Pivampicillin Hydrochloride
V9T15U399I. Dexamethasone Beloxil
V9TKO7EO6K. Deferoxamine Mesylate (See also *J06Y7MXW4D*)
V9YL6NEJ3G. Aderbasib
VA472258QN. Selprazine
VA5755GIJ8. Englitazone Sodium

VAS2V13A9H. Rivanicline Galactarate (See also *6H35LF645A*)
VB0PV6I7L6. Fluazuron
VB0R961HZT. Prednisone
VB4VCH77JV. Efegatran Sulfate (See also *VT0VK2474K*)
VB67O9FBGM. Pentamustine
VC7M3XD17L. Gadopenamide
VCQ006KQ1E. Xylitol
VD27I23138. Fosmenic Acid
VED9E376NC. Rotoxamine
VED9E376NC. Rotoxamine Tartrate [rotoxamine] (See also *90897H496X*)
VES82D23IB. Cericlamine
VF4N11KKKR. Ortetamine
VFC6ZX3584. Paramethasone Acetate [paramethasone] (See also *8X50N88ZDP*)
VFD629099M. Nitrefazole
VFU0OU98LO. Monoctanoin
VG2QF83CGL. Meloxicam
VGT0G37N5M. Tizoprolic Acid
VH2I1JN8Q1. Tazofelone
VHC779598X. Capravirine
VHX8K5SV4X. Dezocine
VI1001O2DI. Norclostebol
VIC0E207S4. Ditiocade Sodium
VIQ3X36S8C. Bialamicol Hydrochloride
VJB5FW9W9J. Ethyl Loflazepate
VJT6J7R4TR. Rifampin
VKH95UNQ6N. Prolonium Iodide
VL775ZTH4C. Penicillin G Potassium
VM4W7043SN. Miloxacin
VM88TV4OS5. Etamestrol
VMF4ELY9TZ. Thiacetarsamide
VMS3A207FA. Bakeprofen
VN04LI540Y. Phosmet
VN9A8JM7M7. Clindamycin Palmitate Hydrochloride
VNS4435G39. Anagrelide Hydrochloride (See also *K9X45X0051*)
VOU5V0B772. Ambuphylline
VOZ07VZP8G. Cromoglicate Lisetil
VP36V95O3T. Sodium Gentisate [gentisic acid]
VPR5FPH326. Antazoline Phosphate
VQ093653DO. Menadiol Sodium Diphosphate [menadiol] (See also *2OVL75B30W*)
VQM3328PO0. Zindotrine
VR021VC9TY. Doconazole
VR843X5GXG. Meprylcaine Hydrochloride
VRA0C6810N. Gallium Nitrate
VS041H42XC. Ergocalciferol
VSM36G5OTK. Fibracillin
VT0VK2474K. Efegatran Sulfate [efegatran] (See also *VB4VCH77JV*)
VTD58H1Z2X. Dopamine Hydrochloride [dopamine] (See also *7L3E358N9L*)
VTK01UQK3G. Sodium Sulfite
VUF6C936Z3. Moxalactam Disodium [moxalactam] (See also *5APW73W3QZ*)
VUW370O5QE. Caspofungin Acetate
VV0B5MP6VI. Oxydipentonium Chloride
VVJ6673MHY. Dichlorphenamide
VW4H1CYW1K. Miconazole Nitrate (See also *7NNO0D7S5M*)
VW6613KQ0H. Brometenamine
VWJ2QVH41J. Foropafant
VX29JB5XWV. Deracoxib
VXD0H11TQ7. Phenyliodoundecynoate
VXJ7Z24RN1. Dexlofexidine
VY62TIB872. Morclofone
VY6S496SVX. Trengestone
VYF3049W3N. Atrinositol
VZ8RRZ51VK. Tobramycin

VZI5B1W380. Oxcarbazepine

W00LYS4T26. Manganese Sulfate (See also *IGA15S9H40*)

W0194S5FOA. Fenproporex

W09SX84JTI. Amiterol

W0K2QLU43U. Ivoqualine

W0O1NHP4WE. Cyclizine Hydrochloride (See also *QRW9FCR9P2*)

W0X9P59ZQU. Imafen Hydrochloride (See also *43S5D07K8G*)

W11ET455ZI. Butinazocine

W12VDB26LB. Riodipine

W13O82Z7HL. Dothiepin Hydrochloride [dothiepin] (See also *3H0042311V*)

W14Z7581PA. Chlordantoin

W1792A2RVD. Metoclopramide Hydrochloride (See also *L4YEB44I46*)

W193003XW5. Drazidox

W1J43H2B3K. Hydroxypethidine

W1M09KX30C. Zoticasone

W1MKM70WQI. Muraglitazar

W1O4FV809G. Metrenperone

W24OD7YW48. Diphenoxylate Hydrochloride (See also *73312P173G*)

W2FH8O2BBE. Caraway

W2KGP0434Y. Binizolast

W2L3E1W827. Bamethan Sulfate (See also *Y08ZFJ9TFK*)

W2U467CIIL. Sinefungin

W2X096QY97. Trimethobenzamide Hydrochloride [trimethoben-zamide] (See also *WDQ5P1SX7Q*)

W2ZG23MGYI. Diphemanil Methylsulfate

W2ZU1RY8B0. Sinecatechins

W31X2H97FB. Torsemide

W33009B02O. Salazosulfadimidine

W36ZG6FT64. Sirolimus

W3D7B06505. Clobuzarit

W3G873MK03. Doxaprost

W4193719XR. Dehydrocholate Sodium

W41H6S09F4. Aloin

W456I35SKD. Monatepil Maleate

W486SJ5824. Abarelix

W4888I119H. Tartaric Acid

W4K0AE8XW9. Biclotymol

W4N6E1T46B. Dexamethasone Acefurate

W4P85FO7GS. Saterinone

W4VMH2E80M. Prinoxodan

W53L6FE61V. Methylergonovine Maleate [methylergonovine] (See also *IR84JPZ1RK*)

W5DCO14M05. Tecastemizole

W5E840UV9P. Sulfaperin

W5H7E45YT3. Banoxantrone

W5K3712F4H. Tiomesterone

W5P145L26T. Tefenperate

W5P1SSA8KD. Mivazerol

W5S57Y3A5L. Metoprolol Tartrate

W618Z2SMVL. Pirisudanol

W656S9I00W. Denotivir

W68DD2C7VG. Tolpyrramide

W6E275IURX. Losoxantrone Hydrochloride

W6HS99O8ZO. Varenicline Tartrate [varenicline] (See also *82269ASB48*)

W6Y945055S. Clanobutin

W70V6I2OMY. Pargyline Hydrochloride (See also *9MV14S8G3E*)

W733B0S9SD. Methazolamide

W76I6XXF06. Clonidine Hydrochloride (See also *MN3L5RMN02*)

VZ77UAL9THI. Delapril Hydrochloride [delapril] (See also *2SMM3M5ZMH*)

W7FHJ107MC. Cimicoxib

W7J490CUHM. Glipalamide

W7KQ46GJ8U. Uracil Mustard

W7TTW573JJ. Midazolam Hydrochloride

W7V2ZZ2FWB. Lasalocid

W86I18X716. Ronifibrate

W89H91R7VX. Arbaclofen Placarbil

W8F97XP38W. Carpindolol

W8M4X3Y7ZY. Fenitrothion

W8O17SJF3T. Memantine

W8OY9Y1132. Acetomeroctol

W8U4S4XLWC. Zocainone

W91CMS1V7Z. Belfosdil

W9769W09JF. Panipenem

W99LLM73R7. Rispenzepine

W9A18RJ49B. Quifenadine

W9BB98U6HP. Urofollitropin

W9CI6CR77M. Pyridofylline

W9F9H8GXWR. Tanaproget

W9O92HYT6I. Fiduxosin

W9WZN9A0GM. Benzoyl Peroxide

W9Y8L7GP4C. Cetrorelix Acetate

WA1RT89G9X. Ketocaine

WAS1IG4146. Xanoxate Sodium

WAT0DDB505. Calcium Sulfate (See also *4846Q921YM*)

WBL76FH528. Cilazaprilat

WBT5QH3KED. Sulfisoxazole Acetyl

WCC8Z95027. Elisartan

WDQ1526QJM. Levalbuterol Hydrochloride

WDQ5P1SX7Q. Trimethobenzamide Hydrochloride (See also *W2X096QY97*)

WEC6I2K1FC. Azilsartan Kamedoxomil

WEN3K83YKD. Todralazine

WF970ATW3T. Dacisteine

WFS7G78GYJ. Etomidoline

WFW942PR79. Rufinamide

WGD229O42W. Tenecteplase

WGL8B3MDAS. Imiclopazine

WH41D8433D. Ergonovine Maleate [ergonovine] (See also *YMH3D0ZJWV*)

WHE7A56U7K. Tolterodine

WI4X0X7BPJ. Hydrocortisone

WI93Z9138A. Testosterone Propionate

WIQ1H85SYP. Sodium Salicylate

WIU553VC0S. Pramiracetam Hydrochloride

WJ68R08KX9. Travoprost

WK1LBP1F3L. Ofornine

WK2XYI10QM. Ibuprofen

WK2XYI10QM. Ibuprofen Aluminum [ibuprofen] (See also *WK2XYI10QM*)

WK2XYI10QM. Ibuprofen Aluminum [ibuprofen] (See also *WK2XYI10QM*)

WKF2F316K6. Bunaprolast

WLK252Z51F. Sedecamycin

WLN5FGH1CY. Fadolmidine

WLT400RC9Q. Nafiverine

WM0HAQ4WNM. Tacrolimus

WMJ8TL7510. Benztropine Mesylate (See also *1NHL2J4X8K*)

WNW8115TM9. Sulfaquinoxaline

WO31V62797. Enilospirone

WP15DXU577. Colistin Sulfate (See also *Z67X93HJG1*)

WP8C6WF33S. Pendecamaine

WQ1WRV49R9. Afurolol

WQ29KQ9POT. Gluconolactone

WR2TIP26VS. Abacavir Succinate [abacavir] (See also *40FH6D8CHK*)

WR978S7QHH. Rizatriptan Benzoate (See also *51086HBW8G*)

WRO75M6RW2. Oxiperomide

WS1467RT9Z. Bufetolol

WS1IH75AJT. Dersalazine
WS821Z52LQ. Triamterene
WTM2C3IL2X. Chlorpropamide
WU6989IN6X. Perafensine
WUB68Y35M7. Rose Oil
WUF1DL156G. Terfluranol
WUI089UONU. Bisbendazole
WUU07Y30IA. Imidaprilat
WV4B56N49H. Ebalzotan
WVB6I50566. Dextrofemine
WWW0P95393. Gapicomine
WX877SQI1G. Mycophenolate Sodium
WXM8D9M6DE. Zorubicin Hydrochloride
WXR179L51S. Isosorbide
WY0R7196HP. Laurixamine
WY672D78VW. Acefylline Clofibrol
WY6W63843K. Zolpidem Tartrate (See also *7K383OQI23*)
WYQ7N0BPYC. Acetylcysteine
WZG3J2MCOL. Granisetron
X00B0D5O0E. Piperacillin
X04FQM7J4M. Sotirimod
X08N6BOT8Y. Dimepregnen
X0A40N8I4S. Orphenadrine Citrate (See also *AL805O9OG9*)
X0I74BAR02. Benzethidine
X0L78YB79M. Benzpyrinium Bromide
X0Q6N9USOZ. Fondaparinux Sodium
X0SMC42Q5O. Pyrathiazine Hydrochloride
X0Z7454B90. Prazosin Hydrochloride (See also *XM03YJ541D*)
X154DLC3EY. Amifloverine
X188638Y2V. Dipipanone Hydrochloride [dipipanone] (See also *8VY00AJ0RL*)
X1IEG24OHL. Phenoxybenzamine Hydrochloride (See also *0TTZ664R7Z*)
X1J18R4W8P. Alendronic Acid
X20I9EN955. Oxytetracycline (See also *SLF0D9077S*)
X20I9EN955. Oxytetracycline Hydrochloride [oxytetracycline] (See also *4U7K4N52ZM*)
X20UZ57G4O. Dromostanolone Propionate (See also *7DR7H00HDT*)
X235XX30GK. Tepirindole
X294K8K2PF. Dextiopronin
X2RN3Q8DNE. Galactose
X2T6O1TUNX. Lobuprofen
X2ZU9993TF. Litomeglovir
X30300EU7I. Talaglumetad Hydrochloride
X30J960B4D. Azalanstat Dihydrochloride (See also *2NL79NI1WS*)
X31CDK040E. Debrisoquin Sulfate [debrisoquin] (See also *Q94064N9NW*)
X38F62RR8L. Elzasonan Hydrochloride
X39AL81KEB. Metipranolol
X39TL7JDPF. Alacepril
X3D0O800AJ. Becampanel
X3FZE77O60. Fenipentol
X3G4L02XQU. Metoserpate Hydrochloride [metoserpate] (See also *KBO7409339*)
X3P646A2J0. Morphine Sulfate (See also *76I7G6D29C*)
X3P9A5HNYF. Xenon Xe 133
X3S33EX3KW. Ergoloid Mesylates
X43W7JDA8L. Amanozine
X44P41F7ZK. Nitroblue Tetrazolium Chloride
X4628IMC52. Cefpimizole Sodium (See also *24S58UHU7N*)
X49220T18G. Ketotifen Fumarate [ketotifen] (See also *HBD503WORO*)
X4HES1O11F. Acyclovir
X4OV71U42S. Pioglitazone Hydrochloride [pioglitazone] (See also *JQT35NPK6C*)
X4S9F8RL01. Gemifloxacin Mesylate

X4VP8104KI. Zoniporide Mesylate (See also *8841R2UJPG*)
X4W3ENH1CV. Norepinephrine Bitartrate [norepinephrine] (See also *IFY5PE3ZRW*)
X4W7ZR7023. Methylprednisolone
X4ZGP7K714. Sodium Formaldehyde Sulfoxylate
X50ZS5010Z. Quintiofos
X55XSL74YQ. Sisomicin
X55XSL74YQ. Sisomicin Sulfate [sisomicin]
X59SG0MRYU. Loxapine Succinate (See also *LER583670J*)
X5DWL380Z6. Pelitinib
X60881643X. Flurogestone Acetate
X66NSO3N35. Thiamine Hydrochloride [thiamine] (See also *M572600E5P*)
X66NSO3N35. Thiamine Mononitrate [thiamine]
X6Q56QN5QC. Hydroxyurea
X71N6E5IPO. Valofane
X72RBB02N8. Felbamate
X794618736. Ambruticin
X7D10K905G. Colestipol Hydrochloride
X7D2GSX1C1. Pidobenzone
X7S6Q4MHCB. Olanzapine Pamoate
X7WDT95N5C. Glipizide
X81L78B3RB. Spaglumic Acid
X83CZ0Y5TF. Furfenorex
X85G7936GV. Abciximab
X87G8IX72O. Emivirine
X88E147FCU. Salcaprozic Acid
X88TTO174Z. Racemetirosine
X8I39OJF4P. Fenprostalene
X8T9SBH9LL. Diquafosol Tetrasodium (See also *7828VC80FJ*)
X8W4CW0QHK. Talmetoprim
X8XI70B5Z6. Nitrofurazone
X91E9EME19. Cridanimod
X92J960C7P. Thiambutosine
X94OZJ468Y. Ethylnorepinephrine Hydrochloride
X9788XI79O. Galocitabine
X98U22RT62. Glenvastatin
X9N1XKR2OS. Carfimate
X9U622S114. Taranabant
XA501VL3VR. Phenmetrazine Hydrochloride [phenmetrazine] (See also *6U85YRT588*)
XB13HYU18U. Desmopressin Acetate (See also *ENR1LLB0FP*)
XBD99QNI42. Alphamethadol
XBP604F6UM. Secobarbital Sodium
XC0K09B7K4. Atrimustine
XC9FY2SGBG. Benmoxin
XCA050IPGB. Fasiplon
XD8BU85ZLK. Dodeclonium Bromide
XEE879L727. Benzoylpas Calcium [benzoylpas] (See also *DX586KL1YX*)
XF417D3PSL. Citric Acid, Anhydrous (See also *2968PHW8QP*)
XG4094G0OY. Maroxepin
XGL7GFB9YI. Artemotil
XH0NPH5ZX8. Procarbazine Hydrochloride (See also *35S93Y190K*)
XI27WMG8QK. Cidoxepin Hydrochloride (See also *F96TTB8728*)
XJ0260HJ0O. Difloxacin Hydrochloride (See also *5Z7OO9FNFD*)
XJ3W180C22. Trifezolac
XJ73B0K6KB. Caroverine
XJM390A33U. Rifapentine
XL025389JS. Methallenestril
XM03YJ541D. Prazosin Hydrochloride [prazosin] (See also *X0Z7454B90*)
XM930M133O. Camonagrel
XN95730F0N. Valategrast Hydrochloride
XNM7LT65NP. Aztreonam Lysine

XP343X1HJU. Protoveratrine A
XP9911I1WL. Adaprolol Maleate [adaprolol] (See also *2I8RV6WL9A*)
XPV71VQL72. Satigrel
XQ31741E9Q. Sobetirome
XQ5V1W49JG. Zanoterone
XQO13W6OCH. Esreboxetine Succinate
XRJ0P5FAYO. Tyropanoate Sodium (See also *4F05V145YR*)
XRJ2P631HP. Erythromycin Estolate (See also *63937KV33D*)
XRO4566Q4R. Interferon Beta-1a
XSD3N36UID. Camiglibose
XSG28FSA0W. Fosamprenavir Sodium
XTH861Q3CR. Bromofenofos
XTZ6AXU7KN. Clenbuterol
XUW8L8PW09. Isamfazone
XV74C1N1AE. Hydroquinone
XW0E5YS77G. Colistimethate Sodium
XWH5VH1L2F. Piperylone
XX112XZP0J. Tiotropium Bromide
XX2MN88N5D. Efalizumab
XXE1CET956. Indomethacin
XYS8INN1I6. Dequalinium Chloride
XZ3FK6LC67. Galtifenin
XZ629S5L50. Zafirlukast
XZA9HY6Z98. Methysergide
Y00SD533IW. Brovanexine
Y0185WZ209. Zomepirac Sodium (See also *822G987U9J*)
Y01JW64D01. Fenclofenac
Y08ZFJ9TFK. Bamethan Sulfate [bamethan] (See also *W2L3E1W827*)
Y09NU9DS9B. Detanosal
Y0EA50IJ3V. Dicarbine
Y0SNM34C6O. Dianicline
Y0TK0FS77W. Cromolyn Sodium [cromolyn] (See also *Q2WXR1I0PK*)
Y0WVV18VUI. Oxibetaine
Y11SP157PJ. Magnesium Clofibrate
Y134VQ304Y. Etafedrine Hydrochloride
Y19VNL22L0. Mesulfamide
Y1P25NQI7X. Piraxelate
Y24T9BT2Q2. Levmetamfetamine
Y3779XL39I. Iothiouracil Sodium
Y3834SIK5F. Porfimer Sodium
Y3FJ2C4H75. Sinitrodil
Y3I9520J7P. Ciclazindol
Y3N00BK5WK. Hydrocortamate Hydrochloride [hydrocortamate] (See also *9QM8U7R83W*)
Y41JS2NL6U. Bisoprolol
Y43GF64R34. Lepirudin
Y45QSO73OB. Streptomycin Sulfate [streptomycin] (See also *CW25IKJ202*)
Y4907O6MFD. Vasopressin [arginine form] (See also *7CZF3L922Y*)
Y4F9MIF6M1. Pirandamine Hydrochloride
Y4HRG433UU. Tedisamil Sesquifumarate
Y4S76JWI15. Methyl Alcohol
Y4Z8D13662. Benfurodil Hemisuccinate
Y521XM2900. Rufloxacin
Y5A751G47H. Benzododecinium Chloride
Y5G36EEA5Z. Diminazene
Y5GMK36KGY. Perindopril
Y5PAQ48WOO. Guaisteine
Y5V2N1KE8U. Sulfapyridine
Y67FY3RWN1. Alentemol Hydrobromide (See also *F6S91MHL3E*)
Y6BHZ28O92. Bamipine
Y6UY8OV51T. Trioxsalen
Y6V2W4S4WT. Firocoxib

Y7543E5K9T. Phentolamine Mesylate (See also *Z468598HBV*)
Y7FKS2XWQH. Sulfathiazole
Y7FKS2XWQH. Sulfathiazole Sodium [sulfathiazole]
Y7JEW0XG7I. Olsalazine Sodium (See also *ULS5I8J03O*)
Y7L24THH6T. Isometheptene Hydrochloride [isometheptene] (See also *9Z4CJC3O5F*)
Y80LB0Q7CB. Bunamidine Hydrochloride
Y8335394RO. Bupivacaine Hydrochloride [bupivacaine] (See also *7TQO7W3VT8*)
Y882YXF34X. Calcium Acetate
Y883P1Z2LT. Atovaquone
Y88Q418Y7M. Zamifenacin
Y98CK3J0OL. Diethylstilbestrol Dipropionate
Y995M7GM0G. Naveglitazar
Y9DL7QPE6B. Pseudoephedrine Sulfate
Y9FMC4513X. Pirenperone
Y9H1V576FH. Honey
Y9M3S784Z6. Ipamorelin
YAN7R5L890. Triprolidine Hydrochloride (See also *2L8T9S52QM*)
YAZ544QOFD. Carsatrin Succinate
YBK48BXK30. Trazodone Hydrochloride [trazodone] (See also *6E8ZO8LRNM*)
YBP650462L. Ambenoxan
YC3281G42A. Adrogolide
YC9ST449YJ. Ethyl Vanillin
YCF001N8QB. Zolimidine
YDA0W423G6. Probarbital Sodium
YDW24Y8IAB. Albaconazole
YEH1EZ96K6. Loteprednol Etabonate (See also *Z8CBU6KR16*)
YF1K15M17Y. Temozolomide
YFT7X7SR77. Mavacoxib
YFT8T83CF9. Filenadol
YGD81BG4SN. Nileprost
YGY317RK75. Deslanoside
YH9K692U9S. Clonazoline
YHP6YLT61T. Prochlorperazine
YI7VU623SF. Propofol
YI8LL014GF. Clometocillin
YIW503MI7V. Bismuth Subgallate
YIY0662KX9. Ritrosulfan
YJ050AQ56X. Thioproperazine Mesylate [thioproperazine] (See also *71P630M192*)
YJL42911RA. Reclazepam
YK3XA0K1O1. Picoperine
YKH834O4BH. Epinephrine
YKH834O4BH. Epinephrine Bitartrate [epinephrine] (See also *30Q7KI53AK*)
YL02E256HT. Pirinidazole
YL5FZ2Y5U1. Methotrexate
YMH3D0ZJWV. Ergonovine Maleate (See also *WH41D8433D*)
YN28Z5YZ73. Emideltide
YNJ78BD0AH. Benzobarbital
YNO268EI8T. Tenivastatin Calcium
YNU265SSR3. Atiprimod Dimaleate
YO1UK1S598. Isradipine
YO460OQ37K. Vandetanib
YO603Y8113. Darunavir
YO7261ME24. Cetirizine Hydrochloride [cetirizine] (See also *64O047KTOA*)
YOW8V9698H. Dimethyl Sulfoxide
YP0241BU76. Clomocycline
YP2Y0DRX4S. Azanidazole
YPP8YQZ13B. Bioresmethrin
YQE403BP4D. Phenobarbital
YQG0NJI5A7. Fengabine
YQH5093J7C. Parsalmide
YR5U3L9ZH1. Biapenem

YR841R53VW. Sulfaproxyline
YS08XHA860. Racementhol
YS5LY7JF4N. Penicillin G Sodium
YS7Z529O22. Tosagestin
YT3IDN1WR0. Subendazole
YU55MQ3IZY. Alprazolam
YUL4LO94HK. Resorcinol
YV0SN3276Q. Isoetharine
YV0SN3276Q. Isoetharine Hydrochloride [isoetharine] (See also *51V8U784H3*)
YV7QD1SJ9O. Bederocin
YVU35998K5. Viomycin Sulfate [viomycin] (See also *LKO141R05V*)
YX9162EO3I. Raloxifene Hydrochloride [raloxifene] (See also *4F86W47BR6*)
YY03Q39E6L. Oxiniacic Acid
YZI5105V0L. Ketorolac Tromethamine [ketorolac] (See also *4EVE5946BQ*)
Z06494074X. Cyclopregnol
Z0H242BBR1. Aspartame
Z0OMD60978. Tiametonium Iodide
Z0SPD4Z01X. Diethadione
Z1LH97KTRM. Alfadex
Z1R9N0A399. Tenoxicam
Z22628B598. Etomidate
Z243A6BHCS. Chloroprednisone Acetate
Z2MMV08KUQ. Formebolone
Z2Z439864Y. Ethyl Oleate
Z3614QOX8W. Pyrimethamine
Z380L7N00P. Deprodone
Z3D4AJ1R48. Dibenzothiophene
Z3H2D4MF7A. Nicoxamat
Z40X7EI2AF. Ioxaglic Acid
Z468598HBV. Phentolamine Hydrochloride [phentolamine] (See also *86DRW83R1H*)
Z468598HBV. Phentolamine Mesylate [phentolamine] (See also *Y7543E5K9T*)
Z49QDT0J8Z. Cefuroxime Axetil (See also *O1R9FJ93ED*)
Z4J6TAJ4FX. Cloxacepride
Z4OYQ8EJO8. Droclidinium Bromide
Z4T2YRI005. Thiphencillin Potassium [thiphencillin] (See also *OCS31A7WA0*)
Z4XE6IBF3V. Danthron
Z52H4811WX. Ethoxzolamide
Z540ZT2MI6. Sulfonterol Hydrochloride [sulfonterol] (See also *AJ14S16J7N*)
Z588009C7C. Robenacoxib
Z5B97MU9K4. Flurbiprofen Sodium
Z5M7SC6D5P. Tolnidamine
Z5R55CJ4CG. Mebanazine
Z615FRW64N. Paramethadione
Z61I075U2W. Penicillin V
Z61I075U2W. Penicillin V Benzathine [penicillin v]
Z61I075U2W. Penicillin V Hydrabamine [penicillin v]
Z6375YW9SF. Naltrexone Hydrochloride
Z67X93HJG1. Colistin Sulfate [colistin] (See also *WP15DXU577*)
Z69D9E381Q. Selenium Sulfide
Z6MXZ39302. Fenvalerate
Z6RX3C7B5V. Pimetacin
Z72930Q46K. Tetramethrin
Z7D4G976SH. Clostebol
Z80I64HMNP. Tiagabine Hydrochloride [tiagabine] (See also *DQH6T6D8OY*)
Z82YP691V7. Sornidipine
Z8CBU6KR16. Loteprednol Etabonate [loteprednol] (See also *YE-H1EZ96K6*)
Z8EZK2DSIT. Metoxepin
Z8IX2SC1OH. Propylparaben

Z8SRY7BR30. Ramnodigin
Z8T88FVW9V. Ocfentanil Hydrochloride
Z927X3UJ2W. Mecarbinate
Z94465H1Y7. Desmeninol
Z95Z9C2201. Pyrovalerone Hydrochloride
Z97702A5DG. Dibucaine Hydrochloride (See also *L6JW2TJG99*)
Z99269057A. Pentopril
Z99XUY03BK. Bisdisulizole Disodium
Z9AM8GST2F. Gemcabene Calcium (See also *B96UX1DDKS*)
Z9O08YRN8O. Tetrabenazine
ZAD9OKH9JC. Doconexent
ZB22ENF0XR. Desvenlafaxine Succinate (See also *NG99554ANW*)
ZB6F8MY53V. Etilefrine
ZBD6Y9UT6T. Fluciprazine
ZC4202M9P3. Metaraminol Bitartrate (See also *818U2PZ2EH*)
ZCC19F3X8K. Flutonidine
ZE3K6J8614. Trovirdine
ZE4IRB4DUC. Broxaterol
ZEC193879Q. Dyclonine Hydrochloride (See also *078A24Q30O*)
ZG2L2878MD. Evandamine
ZG7E5POY8O. Bupropion Hydrochloride
ZH3HEY032H. Hydroxytoluic Acid
ZH516LNZ10. Piracetam
ZHC772U9S3. Lombazole
ZIB93J9J6L. Pitenodil
ZIF514RVZR. Albumin Human
ZJC1Z4E09L. Iobutoic Acid
ZJI41P5WMH. Xipranolol
ZKV3GT35TR. Ruzadolane
ZL1R02VT79. Ranibizumab
ZL40NE83QQ. Cobaltous Chloride Co 57
ZL910H358R. Cilutazoline
ZN3R5560ZV. Larazotide
ZOU145W1XL. Fluphenazine Hydrochloride
ZP61X8C21F. Quinine Glycerophosphate
ZP7R667SGD. Butyl Chloride
ZPO6B92P5Y. Prisotinol
ZPY8VRF0GB. Cimaterol
ZQI909440X. Azelastine Hydrochloride [azelastine] (See also *0L591QR10I*)
ZQN1G5V6SR. Eflornithine Hydrochloride [eflornithine] (See also *4NH22NDW9H*)
ZR05N78276. Diflucortolone Pivalate
ZRP63D75JW. Idarubicin Hydrochloride [idarubicin] (See also *5VV3MDU5IE*)
ZS7284E0ZP. Daunorubicin Hydrochloride [daunorubicin] (See also *UD984I04LZ*)
ZS9KD92H6V. Metyrapone
ZS9KD92H6V. Metyrapone Tartrate [metyrapone] (See also *B6DRB5ZI7P*)
ZSJ254W6SF. Moxastine
ZT934N0X4W. Cysteine Hydrochloride (See also *K848JZ4886*)
ZTI6C33Q2Q. Guanethidine Monosulfate [guanethidine] (See also *5UBY8Y002G*)
ZTI6C33Q2Q. Guanethidine Sulfate [guanethidine] (See also *8AQ60474G9*)
ZTK4026YJ5. Iodopyracet
ZTY15D026H. Bamifylline Hydrochloride [bamifylline] (See also *66466QLM3S*)
ZU4275277R. Nalbuphine Hydrochloride (See also *L2T84IQI2K*)
ZWE0X0IG9D. Dalvastatin
ZY400R3BNT. Oxindanac
ZZ45AB24CA. Heparin Sodium (See also *T2410KM04A*)
ZZT404XD09. Tipranavir
ZZU2X307FG. Ioglucol

Appendix VI
CAS Registry Numbers and NSC Numbers

CAS REGISTRY NUMBERS

50-00-0. Formaldehyde

50-02-2. Dexamethasone

50-03-3. Hydrocortisone Acetate

50-04-4. Cortisone Acetate (See also *53-06-5*)

50-06-6. Phenobarbital

50-07-7. Mitomycin

50-09-9. Hexobarbital Sodium (See also *56-29-1*)

50-10-2. Oxyphenonium Bromide (See also *14214-84-7*)

50-11-3. Metharbital

50-12-4. Mephenytoin

50-13-5. Meperidine Hydrochloride (See also *57-42-1*)

50-14-6. Ergocalciferol

50-18-0. Cyclophosphamide [anhydrous] (See also *6055-19-2*)

50-19-1. Hydroxyphenamate

50-21-5. Lactic Acid

50-23-7. Hydrocortisone

50-24-8. Prednisolone [anhydrous] (See also *52438-85-4*)

50-27-1. Estriol (See also *514-68-1*)

50-28-2. Estradiol

50-29-3. Chlorophenothane

50-33-9. Phenbutazone Sodium Glycerate [phenylbutazone] (See also *34214-49-8; 28013-70-9*)

50-34-0. Propantheline Bromide (See also *298-50-0*)

50-35-1. Thalidomide

50-36-2. Cocaine

50-37-3. Lysergide

50-39-5. Protheobromine

50-41-9. Clomiphene Citrate (See also *911-45-5*)

50-42-0. Adiphenine Hydrochloride (See also *64-95-9*)

50-44-2. Mercaptopurine [anhydrous] (See also *6112-76-1*)

50-47-5. Desipramine Hydrochloride [desipramine] (See also *58-28-6*)

50-48-6. Amitriptyline Hydrochloride [amitriptyline] (See also *549-18-8*)

50-49-7. Imipramine Hydrochloride [imipramine] (See also *113-52-0*)

50-50-0. Estradiol Benzoate

50-52-2. Thioridazine

50-53-3. Chlorpromazine

50-54-4. Quinidine Sulfate [anhydrous] (See also *6591-63-5; 56-54-2*)

50-55-5. Reserpine

50-56-6. Oxytocin

50-57-7. Lypressin

50-58-8. Phendimetrazine Tartrate (See also *21102-82-9; 634-03-7*)

50-59-9. Cephaloridine

50-60-2. Phentolamine Hydrochloride [phentolamine] (See also *73-05-2*)

50-63-5. Chloroquine Phosphate (See also *54-05-7*)

50-65-7. Niclosamide

50-70-4. Sorbitol

50-76-0. Dactinomycin

50-78-2. Aspirin

50-81-7. Ascorbic Acid

50-91-9. Floxuridine

50-98-6. Ephedrine Hydrochloride [(–)-ephedrine hydrochloride] (See also *299-42-3*)

50-99-7. Dextrose [D-glucose, anhydrous] (See also *5996-10-1; 77029-61-9; 2280-44-6; 492-62-5; 492-61-5*)

51-03-6. Piperonyl Butoxide

51-05-8. Procaine Hydrochloride (See also *59-46-1*)

51-06-9. Procainamide Hydrochloride [procainamide] (See also *614-39-1*)

51-12-7. Nialamide

51-15-0. Pralidoxime Chloride

51-18-3. Triethylenemelamine

51-21-8. Fluorouracil

51-24-1. Tiratricol

51-26-3. Thyropropic Acid

51-30-9. Isoproterenol Hydrochloride (See also *7683-59-2*)

51-31-0. Levisoprenaline

51-34-3. Scopolamine Hydrobromide [scopolamine] (See also *6533-68-2; 114-49-8*)

51-40-1. Norepinephrine Bitartrate [anhydrous] (See also *69815-49-2; 5794-08-1; 51-41-2*)

51-41-2. Norepinephrine Bitartrate [norepinephrine] (See also *69815-49-2; 51-40-1; 5794-08-1*)

51-42-3. Epinephrine Bitartrate (See also *51-43-4*)

51-43-4. Epinephrine

51-45-6. Histamine Dihydrochloride [histamine]

51-48-9. Levothyroxine Sodium [L-thyroxine] (See also *25416-65-3; 55-03-8*)

51-49-0. Dextrothyroxine Sodium [dextrothyroxine] (See also *7054-08-2; 137-53-1*)

51-52-5. Propylthiouracil

51-55-8. Atropine

51-56-9. Homatropine Hydrobromide (See also *87-00-3*)

51-57-0. Methamphetamine Hydrochloride (See also *537-46-2*)

51-60-5. Neostigmine Methylsulfate (See also *59-99-4*)

51-61-6. Dopamine Hydrochloride [dopamine] (See also *62-31-7*)

51-63-8. Dextroamphetamine Sulfate (See also *51-64-9*)

51-64-9. Dextroamphetamine

51-68-3. Meclofenoxate

51-71-8. Phenelzine Sulfate [phenelzine] (See also *156-51-4*)

51-74-1. Histamine Phosphate

51-75-2. Mechlorethamine Hydrochloride [mechlorethamine] (See also *55-86-7*)

51-77-4. Gefarnate

51-79-6. Urethane

51-83-2. Carbachol

51-84-3. Acetylcholine Chloride [acetylcholine] (See also *60-31-1*)

51-98-9. Norethindrone Acetate

52-01-7. Spironolactone

52-21-1. Prednisolone Acetate

52-24-4. Thiotepa

52-26-6. Morphine Hydrochloride (See also *57-27-2*)

52-28-8. Codeine Phosphate [anhydrous] (See also *41444-62-6; 6059-47-8*)

52-31-3. Cyclobarbital

52-39-1. Aldosterone

52-43-7. Allobarbital

52-49-3. Trihexyphenidyl Hydrochloride (See also *144-11-6*)

52-51-7. Bronopol

52-53-9. Verapamil

52-62-0. Pentolinium Tartrate (See also *144-44-5*)

52-67-5. Penicillamine

52-68-6. Metrifonate

52-76-6. Lynestrenol

52-78-8. Norethandrolone

52-86-8. Haloperidol

52-88-0. Methylatropine Nitrate

52-89-1. Cysteine Hydrochloride [anhydrous] (See also *7048-04-6; 52-90-4*)

52-90-4. Cysteine Hydrochloride [cysteine] (See also *7048-04-6; 52-89-1*)

53-03-2. Prednisone

53-06-5. Cortisone Acetate [cortisone] (See also *50-04-4*)

53-10-1. Hydroxydione Sodium Succinate (See also *303-01-5*)

53-16-7. Estrone

53-18-9. Bietaserpine

53-19-0. Mitotane

53-21-4. Cocaine Hydrochloride (See also *50-36-2*)

53-31-6. Medibazine

53-33-8. Paramethasone Acetate [paramethasone] (See also *1597-82-6*)

53-34-9. Fluprednisolone

53-36-1. Methylprednisolone Acetate

53-39-4. Oxandrolone

53-43-0. Prasterone

53-46-3. Methantheline Bromide (See also *5818-17-7*)

53-60-1. Promazine Hydrochloride (See also *58-40-2*)

53-73-6. Angiotensin Amide

53-79-2. Puromycin

53-84-9. Nadide

53-86-1. Indomethacin

53-89-4. Benzpiperylon

54-03-5. Hexobendine

54-05-7. Chloroquine

54-11-5. Nicotine

54-21-7. Sodium Salicylate

54-30-8. Camylofin

54-31-9. Furosemide

54-32-0. Moxisylyte

54-35-3. Penicillin G Procaine [anhydrous] (See also *6130-64-9; 61-33-6*)

54-36-4. Metyrapone

54-42-2. Idoxuridine

54-47-7. Pyridoxal Calcium Phosphate

54-49-9. Metaraminol Bitartrate [metaraminol] (See also *33402-03-8; 17171-57-2*)

54-62-6. Aminopterin Sodium [aminopterin] (See also *58602-66-7*)

54-64-8. Thimerosal

54-71-7. Pilocarpine Hydrochloride (See also *92-13-7*)

54-80-8. Pronetalol

54-84-2. Cinanserin Hydrochloride (See also *1166-34-3*)

54-85-3. Isoniazid

54-87-5. Nitrofurantoin Sodium (See also *67-20-9*)

54-91-1. Pipobroman

54-92-2. Iproniazid (See also *305-33-9*)

54-95-5. Pentylenetetrazol

54-96-6. Amifampridine

55-03-8. Levothyroxine Sodium [anhydrous] (See also *25416-65-3; 51-48-9*)

55-06-1. Liothyronine Sodium (See also *6893-02-3*)

55-38-9. Fenthion

55-48-1. Atropine Sulfate [anhydrous] (See also *5908-99-6; 51-55-8*)

55-52-7. Pheniprazine Hydrochloride [pheniprazine] (See also *66-05-7*)

55-56-1. Chlorhexidine Gluconate [chlorhexidine] (See also *18472-51-0*)

55-63-0. Nitroglycerin

55-65-2. Guanethidine Monosulfate [guanethidine] (See also *645-43-2*)

55-68-5. Phenylmercuric Nitrate

55-73-2. Bethanidine Sulfate [bethanidine] (See also *114-85-2*)

55-86-7. Mechlorethamine Hydrochloride (See also *51-75-2*)

55-91-4. Isoflurophate

55-92-5. Methacholine Bromide [methacholine] (See also *333-31-3*)

55-94-7. Suxamethonium Bromide

55-97-0. Hexamethonium Bromide (See also *60-26-4*)

55-98-1. Busulfan

56-04-2. Methylthiouracil

56-12-2. γ-Aminobutyric Acid

56-23-5. Carbon Tetrachloride

56-28-0. Triclodazol

56-29-1. Hexobarbital

56-34-8. Tetraethylammonium Chloride

56-40-6. Dihydroxyaluminum Aminoacetate [aminoacetic acid] (See also *41354-48-7; 13682-92-3*)

56-41-7. Alanine [L]

56-45-1. Serine [L]

56-47-3. Desoxycorticosterone Acetate

56-53-1. Diethylstilbestrol

56-54-2. Quinidine

56-59-7. Felypressin

56-72-4. Coumaphos

56-75-7. Chloramphenicol

56-81-5. Glycerin

56-84-8. Aspartic Acid [L] (See also *6899-03-2*)

56-85-9. Glutamine

56-86-0. Glutamic Acid [L-glutamic acid] (See also *6899-05-4*)

56-87-1. Lysine [L]

56-89-3. Cystine [L]

56-94-0. Demecarium Bromide

56-97-3. Trimedoxime Bromide

57-06-7. Allyl Isothiocyanate

57-08-9. Acexamic Acid

57-09-0. Cetrimonium Bromide (See also *6899-10-1*)

57-10-3. Palmitic Acid

57-11-4. Stearic Acid

57-13-6. Urea

57-15-8. Chlorobutanol (See also *6001-64-5*)

57-22-7. Vincristine Sulfate [vincristine] (See also *2068-78-2*)

57-24-9. Strychnine

57-27-2. Morphine Hydrochloride [morphine] (See also *52-26-6*)

57-29-4. Nalorphine Hydrochloride (See also *62-67-9*)

57-30-7. Phenobarbital Sodium (See also *50-06-6*)

57-33-0. Pentobarbital Sodium (See also *76-74-4*)

57-37-4. Benactyzine [hydrochloride] (See also *302-40-9*)

57-41-0. Phenytoin

57-42-1. Meperidine Hydrochloride [meperidine] (See also *50-13-5*)

57-43-2. Amobarbital

57-44-3. Barbital

57-47-6. Physostigmine

57-48-7. Fructose

57-50-1. Sucrose

57-53-4. Meprobamate

57-55-6. Propylene Glycol

57-57-8. Propiolactone

57-62-5. Chlortetracycline Bisulfate [chlortetracycline] (See also *27823-62-7*)

57-63-6. Ethinyl Estradiol

57-64-7. Physostigmine Salicylate (See also *57-47-6*)

57-65-8. Thyromedan Hydrochloride (See also *15301-96-9*)

57-66-9. Probenecid

57-67-0. Sulfaguanidine

57-68-1. Sulfamethazine

57-83-0. Progesterone

57-85-2. Testosterone Propionate

57-88-5. Cholesterol

57-91-0. Alfatradiol

57-92-1. Streptomycin Sulfate [streptomycin] (See also *3810-74-0*)

57-94-3. Tubocurarine Chloride [anhydrous] (See also *6989-98-6; 41354-45-4; 57-95-4*)

57-95-4. Tubocurarine Chloride [tubocurarine] (See also *6989-98-6; 57-94-3; 41354-45-4*)

57-96-5. Sulfinpyrazone

58-00-4. Apomorphine Hydrochloride [apomorphine] (See also *41372-20-7; 314-19-2*)

58-05-9. Leucovorin Calcium [leucovorin] (See also *1492-18-8; 41927-89-3; 6035-45-6*)

58-08-2. Caffeine (See also *5743-12-4*)

58-14-0. Pyrimethamine

58-15-1. Aminopyrine

58-18-4. Methyltestosterone

58-19-5. Dromostanolone Propionate [dromostanolone] (See also *521-12-0*)

58-20-8. Testosterone Cypionate

58-22-0. Testosterone

58-25-3. Chlordiazepoxide

58-27-5. Menadione

58-28-6. Desipramine Hydrochloride (See also *50-47-5*)

58-32-2. Dipyridamole

58-33-3. Promethazine Hydrochloride (See also *60-87-7*)

58-34-4. Thiazinamium Metilsulfate (See also *2338-21-8*)

58-37-7. Aminopromazine

58-38-8. Prochlorperazine

58-39-9. Perphenazine

58-40-2. Promazine Hydrochloride [promazine] (See also *53-60-1*)

58-46-8. Tetrabenazine

58-54-8. Ethacrynate Sodium [ethacrynic acid] (See also *6500-81-8*)

58-55-9. Theophylline [anhydrous] (See also *5967-84-0*)

58-56-0. Pyridoxine Hydrochloride (See also *65-23-6*)

58-58-2. Puromycin Hydrochloride (See also *53-79-2*)

58-61-7. Adenosine

58-63-9. Inosine

58-71-9. Cephalothin Sodium (See also *153-61-7*)

58-73-1. Diphenhydramine Citrate [diphenhydramine] (See also *88637-37-0*)

58-74-2. Papaverine Hydrochloride [papaverine] (See also *61-25-6*)

58-85-5. Biotin

58-86-6. Xylose [acyclic form] (See also *7261-26-9; 6763-34-4; 2460-44-8*)

58-89-9. Lindane

58-93-5. Hydrochlorothiazide

58-94-6. Chlorothiazide

59-01-8. Kanamycin Sulfate [kanamycin] (See also *25389-94-0; 133-92-6*)

59-04-1. Paromomycin Sulfate [paromomycin, replaced] (See also *1263-89-4; 7542-37-2*)

59-05-2. Methotrexate

59-06-3. Ethopabate

59-14-3. Broxuridine

59-26-7. Nikethamide

59-30-3. Folate Sodium [folic acid] (See also *6484-89-5*)

59-32-5. Chloropyramine

59-33-6. Pyrilamine Maleate (See also *91-84-9*)

59-39-2. Piperoxan (See also *135-87-5*)

59-40-5. Sulfaquinoxaline

59-41-6. Bretylium Tosylate [bretylium] (See also *61-75-6*)

59-42-7. Phenylephrine Hydrochloride [phenylephrine] (See also *61-76-7*)

59-43-8. Thiamine Hydrochloride [thiamine] (See also *67-03-8*)

59-46-1. Procaine Borate [procaine] (See also *149-13-3*)

59-47-2. Mephenesin

59-50-7. Chlorocresol

59-51-8. Racemethionine

59-52-9. Dimercaprol

59-58-5. Prosultiamine

59-63-2. Isocarboxazid

59-66-5. Acetazolamide

59-67-6. Niacin

59-87-0. Nitrofurazone

59-92-7. Levodopa

59-96-1. Phenoxybenzamine Hydrochloride [phenoxybenzamine] (See also *63-92-3*)

59-97-2. Tolazoline Hydrochloride (See also *59-98-3*)

59-98-3. Tolazoline Hydrochloride [tolazoline] (See also *59-97-2*)

59-99-4. Neostigmine Bromide [neostigmine] (See also *114-80-7*)

60-00-4. Edetate Calcium Disodium [edetic acid] (See also *23411-34-9; 62-33-9*)

60-02-6. Guanethidine Sulfate (See also *55-65-2*)

60-12-8. Phenylethyl Alcohol

60-13-9. Amphetamine Sulfate (See also *300-62-9*)

60-18-4. Tyrosine [L]

60-23-1. Cysteamine

60-26-4. Hexamethonium Bromide [hexamethonium] (See also *55-97-0*)

60-27-5. Creatinine

60-29-7. Ether

60-30-0. Azamethonium Bromide [azamethonium] (See also *306-53-6*)

60-31-1. Acetylcholine Chloride (See also *51-84-3*)

60-32-2. Aminocaproic Acid

60-40-2. Mecamylamine Hydrochloride [mecamylamine] (See also *826-39-1*)

60-41-3. Strychnine Sulfate (See also *57-24-9*)

60-44-6. Penthienate Bromide (See also *22064-27-3*)

60-45-7. Fenimide

60-46-8. Aminopentamide Sulfate

60-49-1. Tridihexethyl Chloride [tridihexethyl] (See also *4310-35-4*)

60-54-8. Tetracycline (See also *6416-04-2*)

60-56-0. Methimazole

60-57-1. Dieldrin

60-79-7. Ergonovine Maleate [ergonovine] (See also *129-51-1*)

60-80-0. Antipyrine

60-87-7. Promethazine Hydrochloride [promethazine] (See also *58-33-3*)

60-89-9. Mepazine Acetate [mepazine] (See also *24360-97-2*)

60-91-3. Diethazine Hydrochloride [diethazine] (See also *341-70-8*)

60-93-5. Quinine Dihydrochloride (See also *130-95-0*)

60-99-1. Levomepromazine

61-00-7. Acepromazine Maleate [acepromazine] (See also *3598-37-6*)

61-01-8. Methoxypromazine Maleate [methoxypromazine] (See also *3403-42-7*)

61-12-1. Dibucaine Hydrochloride (See also *85-79-0*)

61-16-5. Methoxamine Hydrochloride (See also *390-28-3*)

61-19-8. Adenosine Phosphate

61-24-5. Cephalosporin C

61-25-6. Papaverine Hydrochloride (See also *58-74-2*)

61-32-5. Methicillin Sodium [methicillin] (See also *7246-14-2; 132-92-3*)

61-33-6. Benzylpenicillin

61-56-3. Sulthiame

61-57-4. Niridazole

61-68-7. Mefenamic Acid

61-72-3. Cloxacillin Benzathine [cloxacillin] (See also *23736-58-5*)

61-73-4. Methylene Blue [anhydrous] (See also *7220-79-3*)

61-74-5. Domoxin

61-75-6. Bretylium Tosylate (See also *59-41-6*)

61-76-7. Phenylephrine Hydrochloride (See also *59-42-7*)

61-78-9. Aminohippurate Sodium [aminohippuric acid] (See also *94-16-6*)

61-80-3. Zoxazolamine

61-90-5. Leucine [L]

62-31-7. Dopamine Hydrochloride (See also *51-61-6*)

62-33-9. Edetate Calcium Disodium [anhydrous] (See also *23411-34-9; 60-00-4*)

62-37-3. Chlormerodrin

62-38-4. Phenylmercuric Acetate

62-44-2. Phenacetin

62-46-4. Thioctic Acid

62-49-7. Choline Bitartrate [choline] (See also *87-67-2*)

62-51-1. Methacholine Chloride (See also *55-92-5*)

62-54-4. Calcium Acetate

62-67-9. Nalorphine Hydrochloride [nalorphine] (See also *57-29-4*)

62-68-0. Proadifen Hydrochloride (See also *302-33-0*)

62-73-7. Dichlorvos

62-90-8. Nandrolone Phenpropionate

62-97-5. Diphemanil Methylsulfate

63-05-8. Androstenedione

63-12-7. Benzquinamide

63-25-2. Carbaril

63-29-6. Glucurolactone

63-45-6. Primaquine Phosphate (See also *90-34-6*)

63-56-9. Thonzylamine Hydrochloride (See also *91-85-0*)

63-68-3. Methionine

63-74-1. Sulfanilamide

63-75-2. Arecoline Hydrobromide [arecoline] (See also *300-08-3*)

63-89-8. Colfosceril Palmitate

63-91-2. Phenylalanine

63-92-3. Phenoxybenzamine Hydrochloride (See also *59-96-1*)

63-98-9. Phenacemide

64-02-8. Edetate Sodium (See also *60-00-4*)

64-17-5. Alcohol

64-19-7. Acetic Acid

64-31-3. Morphine Sulfate [anhydrous] (See also *6211-15-0; 57-27-2*)

64-39-1. Trimeperidine

64-43-7. Amobarbital Sodium (See also *57-43-2*)

64-47-1. Physostigmine Sulfate (See also *57-47-6*)

64-55-1. Mebutamate

64-65-3. Bemegride

64-72-2. Chlortetracycline Hydrochloride

64-73-3. Demeclocycline Hydrochloride (See also *127-33-3*)

64-75-5. Tetracycline Hydrochloride (See also *60-54-8*)

64-77-7. Tolbutamide

64-86-8. Colchicine

64-95-9. Adiphenine Hydrochloride [adiphenine] (See also *50-42-0*)

65-19-0. Yohimbine Hydrochloride

65-23-6. Pyridoxine Hydrochloride [pyridoxine] (See also *58-56-0*)

65-28-1. Phentolamine Mesylate (See also *50-60-2*)

65-29-2. Gallamine Triethiodide (See also *153-76-4*)

65-31-6. Nicotine Bitartrate [anhydrous]

65-45-2. Salicylamide

65-49-6. Aminosalicylate Calcium [4-aminosalicylic acid] (See also *133-15-3; 6059-16-1*)

65-64-5. Mebanazine

65-85-0. Benzoic Acid

65-86-1. Orotic Acid

66-05-7. Pheniprazine Hydrochloride (See also *55-52-7*)

66-22-8. Uracil

66-32-0. Strychnine Nitrate (See also *57-24-9*)

66-75-1. Uracil Mustard

66-76-2. Dicumarol

66-79-5. Oxacillin Sodium [oxacillin] (See also *7240-38-2; 1173-88-2*)

66-81-9. Cycloheximide

66-84-2. Glucosamine Hydrochloride

67-03-8. Thiamine Hydrochloride (See also *59-43-8*)

67-20-9. Nitrofurantoin (See also *17140-81-7*)

67-28-7. Nihydrazone

67-42-5. Egtazic Acid

67-43-6. Pentetate Calcium Trisodium [pentetic acid] (See also *12111-24-9*)

67-45-8. Furazolidone

67-48-1. Choline Chloride (See also *62-49-7*)

67-56-1. Methyl Alcohol

67-63-0. Isopropyl Alcohol

67-64-1. Acetone

67-66-3. Chloroform

67-68-5. Dimethyl Sulfoxide

67-73-2. Fluocinolone Acetonide

67-78-7. Triamcinolone Diacetate

67-81-2. Penmesterol

67-92-5. Dicyclomine Hydrochloride (See also *77-19-0*)

67-95-8. Quingestrone

67-96-9. Dihydrotachysterol

67-97-0. Cholecalciferol

68-04-2. Sodium Citrate [anhydrous] (See also *6132-04-3*)

68-19-9. Cyanocobalamin

68-22-4. Norethindrone

68-23-5. Norethynodrel

68-26-8. Retinol

68-35-9. Sulfadiazine

68-41-7. Cycloserine

68-76-8. Triaziquone

68-88-2. Hydroxyzine Hydrochloride [hydroxyzine] (See also *2192-20-3*)

68-89-3. Dipyrone [anhydrous] (See also *5907-38-0*)

68-90-6. Benziodarone

68-91-7. Trimethaphan Camsylate

68-96-2. Hydroxyprogesterone Caproate [hydroxyprogesterone] (See also *630-56-8*)

69-05-6. Quinacrine Hydrochloride [anhydrous] (See also *6151-30-0; 83-89-6*)

69-09-0. Chlorpromazine Hydrochloride (See also *50-53-3*)

69-22-7. Caffeine Citrate

69-23-8. Fluphenazine Enanthate [fluphenazine] (See also *2746-81-8*)

69-25-0. Eledoisin

69-27-2. Chlorisondamine Chloride

69-43-2. Prenylamine [prenylamine lactate] (See also *390-64-7*)

69-44-3. Amodiaquine Hydrochloride [anhydrous] (See also *6398-98-7; 86-42-0*)

69-52-3. Ampicillin Sodium

69-53-4. Ampicillin (See also *7177-48-2*)

69-57-8. Penicillin G Sodium (See also *61-33-6*)

69-65-8. Mannitol

69-72-7. Salicylic Acid

69-74-9. Cytarabine Hydrochloride (See also *147-94-4*)

69-79-4. Maltose

69-81-8. Carbazochrome

70-00-8. Trifluridine

70-07-5. Mephenoxalone

70-10-0. Ticlatone

70-18-8. Glutathione

70-19-9. Thurfyl Nicotinate

70-26-8. Ornithine

70-30-4. Hexachlorophene

70-47-3. Asparagine [anhydrous] (See also *5794-13-8*)

70-49-5. Gold Sodium Thiomalate [thiomalic acid] (See also *12244-57-4*)

70-51-9. Deferoxamine

70-70-2. Paroxypropione

71-00-1. Histidine [L]

71-27-2. Succinylcholine Chloride (See also *6101-15-1*)

71-36-3. Butyl Alcohol

71-58-9. Medroxyprogesterone Acetate (See also *520-85-4*)

71-63-6. Digitoxin

71-67-0. Sulfobromophthalein Sodium (See also *297-83-6*)

71-68-1. Hydromorphone Hydrochloride (See also *466-99-9*)

71-73-8. Thiopental Sodium (See also *76-75-5*)

71-78-3. Pipradrol Hydrochloride (See also *467-60-7*)

71-81-8. Isopropamide Iodide (See also *7492-32-2*)

71-82-9. Levallorphan Tartrate (See also *152-02-3*)

71-91-0. Tetrylammonium Bromide

72-14-0. Sulfathiazole

72-17-3. Sodium Lactate

72-18-4. Valine [L]

72-19-5. Threonine [L]

72-33-3. Mestranol

72-44-6. Methaqualone

72-63-9. Methandrostenolone

72-69-5. Nortriptyline Hydrochloride [nortriptyline] (See also *894-71-3*)

72-80-0. Chlorquinaldol

73-05-2. Phentolamine Hydrochloride (See also *50-60-2*)

73-07-4. Prazepine

73-09-6. Etozolin

73-22-3. Tryptophan [L]

73-24-5. Adenine

73-32-5. Isoleucine

73-48-3. Bendroflumethiazide

73-49-4. Quinethazone

73-78-9. Lidocaine Hydrochloride [anhydrous] (See also *6108-05-0; 137-58-6*)

74-55-5. Ethambutol Hydrochloride [ethambutol] (See also *1070-11-7*)

74-79-3. Arginine

74-85-1. Ethylene

74-98-6. Propane

75-00-3. Ethyl Chloride

75-09-2. Methylene Chloride

75-19-4. Cyclopropane

75-25-2. Bromoform

75-28-5. Isobutane

75-47-8. Iodoform

75-60-5. Ferric Cacodylate [cacodylic acid] (See also *5968-84-3*)

75-69-4. Trichloromonofluoromethane

75-71-8. Dichlorodifluoromethane

75-80-9. Tribromoethanol

75-85-4. Amylene Hydrate

76-03-9. Trichloroacetic Acid

76-14-2. Dichlorotetrafluoroethane

76-19-7. Perflutren

76-20-0. Sulfonethylmethane

76-22-2. Camphor

76-23-3. Tetrabarbital

76-25-5. Triamcinolone Acetonide

76-29-9. Camphor, Monobromated

76-38-0. Methoxyflurane

76-41-5. Oxymorphone Hydrochloride [oxymorphone] (See also *357-07-3*)

76-42-6. Oxycodone

76-43-7. Fluoxymesterone

76-47-1. Hydrocortamate Hydrochloride [hydrocortamate] (See also *125-03-1*)

76-57-3. Codeine [anhydrous] (See also *6059-47-8*)

76-58-4. Ethylmorphine Hydrochloride [ethylmorphine] (See also *125-30-4*)

76-65-3. Amolanone Hydrochloride [amolanone] (See also *6009-67-2*)

76-73-3. Secobarbital

76-74-4. Pentobarbital

76-75-5. Thiopental Sodium [thiopental] (See also *71-73-8*)

76-76-6. Probarbital Sodium [probarbital] (See also *143-82-8*)

76-90-4. Mepenzolate Bromide (See also *25990-43-6*)

76-99-3. Methadone Hydrochloride [methadone] (See also *1095-90-5*)

77-01-0. Fenpipramide (See also *14007-53-5*)

77-02-1. Aprobarbital

77-04-3. Pyrithyldione

77-07-6. Levorphanol Tartrate [levorphanol] (See also *5985-38-6; 125-72-4; 6700-40-9*)

77-09-8. Phenolphthalein

77-10-1. Phencyclidine Hydrochloride [phencyclidine] (See also *956-90-1*)

77-12-3. Pentacynium Chloride

77-14-5. Proheptazine

77-15-6. Ethoheptazine Citrate [ethoheptazine] (See also *2085-42-9*)

77-19-0. Dicyclomine Hydrochloride [dicyclomine] (See also *67-92-5*)

77-20-3. Alphaprodine Hydrochloride [alphaprodine] (See also *561-78-4; 14405-05-1*)

77-21-4. Glutethimide

77-22-5. Caramiphen Hydrochloride [caramiphen] (See also *125-85-9*)

77-23-6. Carbetapentane Citrate [carbetapentane] (See also *23142-01-0*)

77-26-9. Butalbital

77-27-0. Thiamylal

77-28-1. Butethal

77-36-1. Chlorthalidone
77-37-2. Procyclidine Hydrochloride [procyclidine] (See also *1508-76-5*)
77-38-3. Chlorphenoxamine Hydrochloride [chlorphenoxamine] (See also *562-09-4*)
77-39-4. Cycrimine Hydrochloride [cycrimine] (See also *126-02-3*)
77-41-8. Methsuximide
77-46-3. Acedapsone
77-51-0. Isoaminile
77-65-6. Carbromal
77-66-7. Acecarbromal
77-67-8. Ethosuximide
77-75-8. Meparfynol
77-86-1. Tromethamine
77-89-4. Acetyltriethyl Citrate
77-90-7. Acetyltributyl Citrate
77-91-8. Choline Dihydrogen Citrate (See also *62-49-7*)
77-92-9. Citric Acid, Anhydrous (See also *5949-29-1*)
77-93-0. Triethyl Citrate
77-94-1. Tributyl Citrate
78-05-7. Octafonium Chloride
78-11-5. Pentaerythritol Tetranitrate
78-12-6. Petrichloral
78-28-4. Emylcamate
78-34-2. Dioxation
78-41-1. Triparanol
78-44-4. Carisoprodol
79-01-6. Trichloroethylene
79-09-4. Propionic Acid
79-17-4. Pimagedine Hydrochloride [pimagedine] (See also *1937-19-5*)
79-25-4. Sodium Formaldehyde Sulfoxylate [hydroxymethanesulfinic acid] (See also *6035-47-8; 149-44-0*)
79-55-0. Pempidine
79-57-2. Oxytetracycline [anhydrous] (See also *6153-64-6*)
79-61-8. Dichlorisone Acetate (See also *7008-26-6*)
79-64-1. Dimethisterone [anhydrous] (See also *41354-30-7*)
79-83-4. Calcium Pantothenate [pantothenic acid] (See also *137-08-6*)
79-90-3. Triclobisonium Chloride
79-93-6. Phenaglycodol
80-03-5. Acediasulfone Sodium [acediasulfone] (See also *127-60-6*)
80-08-0. Dapsone
80-13-7. Halazone
80-32-0. Sulfachlorpyridazine
80-34-2. Glyprothiazol
80-35-3. Sulfamethoxypyridazine
80-49-9. Homatropine Methylbromide (See also *87-00-3*)
80-50-2. Anisotropine Methylbromide
80-53-5. Terpin Hydrate [anhydrous] (See also *2451-01-6*)
80-74-0. Sulfisoxazole Acetyl
80-77-3. Chlormezanone
80-80-8. Acetosulfone Sodium [acetosulfone] (See also *128-12-1*)
80-92-2. Pregnandiol
81-07-2. Saccharin
81-13-0. Dexpanthenol

81-23-2. Dehydrocholate Sodium [dehydrocholic acid] (See also *145-41-5*)
81-81-2. Warfarin Potassium [warfarin] (See also *2610-86-8*)
82-02-0. Khellin
82-54-2. Cotarnine Chloride [cotarnine] (See also *10018-19-6*)
82-66-6. Diphenadione
82-88-2. Phenindamine Tartrate [phenindamine] (See also *569-59-5*)
82-92-8. Cyclizine
82-93-9. Chlorcyclizine Hydrochloride [chlorcyclizine] (See also *1620-21-9*)
82-95-1. Buclizine Hydrochloride [buclizine] (See also *129-74-8*)
82-98-4. Piperidolate Hydrochloride [piperidolate] (See also *129-77-1*)
82-99-5. Thiphenamil Hydrochloride [thiphenamil] (See also *548-68-5*)
83-12-5. Phenindione
83-40-9. Hydroxytoluic Acid
83-43-2. Methylprednisolone
83-67-0. Theobromine
83-73-8. Iodoquinol
83-75-0. Quinine Ethylcarbonate
83-86-3. Phytic Acid
83-88-5. Riboflavin
83-89-6. Quinacrine Hydrochloride [quinacrine] (See also *6151-30-0; 69-05-6*)
83-98-7. Orphenadrine Citrate [orphenadrine] (See also *4682-36-4*)
84-01-5. Chlorproethazine Hydrochloride [chlorproethazine] (See also *4611-02-3*)
84-02-6. Prochlorperazine Maleate (See also *58-38-8*)
84-04-8. Pipamazine
84-06-0. Thiopropazate Hydrochloride [thiopropazate]
84-08-2. Pyrathiazine Hydrochloride (See also *522-25-8*)
84-12-8. Phanquone
84-17-3. Dienestrol (See also *13029-44-2*)
84-22-0. Tetrahydrozoline Hydrochloride [tetrahydrozoline] (See also *522-48-5*)
84-36-6. Syrosingopine
84-55-9. Viquidil
84-66-2. Diethyl Phthalate
84-74-2. Dibutyl Phthalate
84-80-0. Phytonadione
84-96-8. Methylpromazine
84-97-9. Perazine Fendizoate [perazine] (See also *14516-56-4*)
84-98-0. Menadiol Sodium Diphosphate [menadiol bis(dihydrogen phosphate)] (See also *6700-42-1; 131-13-5; 481-85-6*)
85-16-5. Diprotrizoate Sodium [diprotrizoic acid] (See also *129-57-7*)
85-36-9. Acetrizoate Sodium [acetrizoic acid] (See also *129-63-5*)
85-73-4. Phthalylsulfathiazole
85-79-0. Dibucaine
85-83-6. Scarlet Red
85-90-5. Methylchromone
85-95-0. Benzestrol

86-12-4. Thenalidine
86-13-5. Benztropine Mesylate [benztropine] (See also *132-17-2*)
86-14-6. Diethylthiambutene
86-21-5. Pheniramine Maleate [pheniramine] (See also *132-20-7*)
86-22-6. Brompheniramine Maleate [brompheniramine] (See also *980-71-2*)
86-34-0. Phensuximide
86-35-1. Ethotoin
86-42-0. Amodiaquine
86-43-1. Propoxycaine Hydrochloride [propoxycaine] (See also *550-83-4*)
86-54-4. Hydralazine Hydrochloride [hydralazine] (See also *304-20-1*)
86-75-9. Benzoxiquine
86-78-2. Pentaquine Phosphate [pentaquine] (See also *5428-64-8*)
86-80-6. Dimethisoquin Hydrochloride [dimethisoquin] (See also *2773-92-4*)
87-00-3. Homatropine Hydrobromide [homatropine] (See also *51-56-9*)
87-08-1. Penicillin V
87-09-2. Almecillin
87-10-5. Tribromsalan
87-12-7. Dibromsalan
87-17-2. Salicylanilide
87-21-8. Piridocaine Hydrochloride [piridocaine]
87-27-4. Bismuth Subsalicylate [replaced] (See also *14882-18-9*)
87-33-2. Isosorbide Dinitrate
87-58-1. Iodol
87-66-1. Pyrogallol
87-67-2. Choline Bitartrate (See also *62-49-7*)
87-69-4. Tartaric Acid (See also *526-83-0*)
87-73-0. Calcium Saccharate [saccharic acid] (See also *5793-89-5*)
87-74-1. Gluceptate Sodium [D-*glycero*-D-*gulo*-heptonic acid] (See also *13007-85-7*)
87-76-3. Trimethylcetylammonium Pentachlorophenate
87-81-0. Tagatose
87-90-1. Symclosene
87-99-0. Xylitol
88-04-0. Chloroxylenol
88-46-0. Calcium Dobesilate [dobesilic acid] (See also *20123-80-2*)
89-25-8. Edaravone
89-57-6. Mesalamine
89-68-9. Chlorothymol
89-83-8. Thymol
90-01-7. Salicyl Alcohol
90-03-9. Mercufenol Chloride
90-05-1. Guaiacol
90-22-2. Valethamate Bromide
90-23-3. Piperphenidol Hydrochloride [piperphenidol] (See also *6091-56-1*)
90-33-5. Hymecromone
90-34-6. Primaquine Phosphate [primaquine] (See also *63-45-6*)
90-39-1. Sparteine Sulfate [sparteine] (See also *6160-12-9; 299-39-8*)
90-45-9. Aminacrine Hydrochloride [aminacrine] (See also *134-50-9*)

90-49-3. Pheneturide

90-54-0. Etafenone

90-64-2. Ammonium Mandelate [mandelic acid] (See also *530-31-4*)

90-69-7. Lobeline

90-80-2. Gluconolactone

90-81-3. Racephedrine Hydrochloride [racephedrine] (See also *134-71-4*)

90-82-4. Pseudoephedrine Hydrochloride [pseudoephedrine] (See also *345-78-8*)

90-84-6. Diethylpropion Hydrochloride [diethylpropion] (See also *134-80-5*)

90-86-8. Cinnamedrine

90-89-1. Diethylcarbamazine Citrate [diethylcarbamazine] (See also *1642-54-2*)

91-33-8. Benzthiazide

91-64-5. Coumarin

91-75-8. Antazoline Hydrochloride [antazoline] (See also *2508-72-7*)

91-79-2. Thenyldiamine (See also *958-93-0*)

91-80-5. Methapyrilene Fumarate [methapyrilene] (See also *33032-12-1*)

91-81-6. Tripelennamine Citrate [tripelennamine] (See also *6138-56-3*)

91-82-7. Pyrrobutamine Phosphate [pyrrobutamine] (See also *135-31-9*)

91-84-9. Pyrilamine Maleate [pyrilamine] (See also *59-33-6*)

91-85-0. Thonzylamine Hydrochloride [thonzylamine] (See also *63-56-9*)

92-12-6. Phenyltoloxamine (See also *1176-08-5*)

92-13-7. Pilocarpine

92-23-9. Leucinocaine

92-31-9. Tolonium Chloride

92-62-6. Proflavine Dihydrochloride [proflavine] (See also *531-73-7*)

92-84-2. Phenothiazine

92-97-7. Thiocarbanidin

93-14-1. Guaifenesin

93-23-2. Lauryl Isoquinolinium Bromide

93-30-1. Methoxyphenamine Hydrochloride [methoxyphenamine] (See also *5588-10-3*)

93-47-0. Verazide

93-54-9. Phenylpropanol

93-88-9. Phenpromethamine

94-07-5. Oxedrine

94-09-7. Benzocaine

94-10-0. Ethoxazene Hydrochloride [ethoxazene] (See also *2313-87-3*)

94-12-2. Risocaine

94-13-3. Propylparaben

94-14-4. Isobutamben

94-16-6. Aminohippurate Sodium (See also *61-78-9*)

94-19-9. Sulfaethidole

94-20-2. Chlorpropamide

94-23-5. Parethoxycaine Hydrochloride [parethoxycaine] (See also *136-46-9*)

94-24-6. Tetracaine

94-25-7. Butamben

94-26-8. Butylparaben

94-35-9. Styramate

94-36-0. Benzoyl Peroxide

94-44-0. Benzyl Nicotinate

94-62-2. Piperine

94-63-3. Pralidoxime Iodide

94-78-0. Phenazopyridine Hydrochloride [phenazopyridine] (See also *136-40-3*)

94-96-2. Ethohexadiol

95-04-5. Ectylurea

95-05-6. Sulfiram

95-25-0. Chlorzoxazone

95-27-2. Diamthazole (See also *136-96-9*)

95-48-7. Orthocresol

96-26-4. Dihydroxyacetone

96-27-5. Monothioglycerol

96-50-4. Aminothiazole

96-62-8. Dinsed

96-83-3. Iopanoic Acid

96-84-4. Iophenoxic Acid

96-88-8. Mepivacaine Hydrochloride [mepivacaine] (See also *1722-62-9*)

97-17-6. Dichlofenthion

97-18-7. Bithionol

97-23-4. Dichlorophen

97-24-5. Fenticlor

97-27-8. Chlorbetamide

97-44-9. Acetarsone

97-53-0. Eugenol

97-57-4. Tolpronine

97-59-6. Allantoin

97-77-8. Disulfiram

98-50-0. Arsanilic Acid

98-67-9. Zinc Phenolsulfonate [*p*-phenolsulfonic acid] (See also *127-82-2*)

98-72-6. Nitarsone

98-75-9. Propazolamide

98-79-3. Pidolic Acid

98-92-0. Niacinamide

98-96-4. Pyrazinamide

99-15-0. Acetylleucine

99-26-3. Bismuth Subgallate (See also *149-91-7*)

99-43-4. Benoxinate Hydrochloride [benoxinate] (See also *5987-82-6*)

99-45-6. Adrenalone

99-66-1. Valproate Sodium [valproic acid] (See also *1069-66-5*)

99-76-3. Methylparaben

100-33-4. Pentamidine

100-51-6. Benzyl Alcohol

100-52-7. Benzaldehyde

100-55-0. Nicotinyl Alcohol

100-56-1. Phenylmercuric Chloride

100-88-9. Cyclamic Acid

100-91-4. Eucatropine Hydrochloride [eucatropine] (See also *536-93-6*)

100-92-5. Mephentermine Sulfate [mephentermine] (See also *1212-72-2; 6190-60-9*)

100-95-8. Metalkonium Chloride

100-97-0. Methenamine

101-08-6. Diperodon [anhydrous] (See also *51552-99-9*)

101-20-2. Triclocarban

101-26-8. Pyridostigmine Bromide (See also *155-97-5*)

101-31-5. Hyoscyamine

101-40-6. Propylhexedrine

101-71-3. Diphenan

101-93-9. Phenacaine Hydrochloride [phenacaine] (See also *6153-19-1; 620-99-5*)

102-05-6. Dibemethine

102-29-4. Resorcinol Monoacetate

102-45-4. Cyclopentamine Hydrochloride [cyclopentamine, *N,α*-dimethylcyclopentaneethanamine] (See also *3459-06-1*)

102-60-3. Edetol

102-71-6. Trolamine

102-76-1. Triacetin

103-03-7. Phenicarbazide

103-16-2. Monobenzone

103-84-4. Acetanilide

103-86-6. Hydroxyamphetamine Hydrobromide [hydroxyamphetamine] (See also *306-21-8; 1518-86-1*)

103-90-2. Acetaminophen

104-06-3. Amithiozone

104-14-3. Octopamine

104-22-3. Benzylsulfamide

104-28-9. Cinoxate

104-29-0. Chlorphenesin Carbamate [chlorphenesin] (See also *886-74-8*)

104-31-4. Benzonatate

104-32-5. Propamidine

104-46-1. Anethole [synthetic] (See also *4180-23-8*)

104-55-2. Cinnamaldehyde

105-20-4. Betazole Hydrochloride [betazole] (See also *138-92-1*)

106-48-9. Parachlorophenol

106-97-8. Butane

107-15-3. Ethylenediamine

107-35-7. Taurine

107-41-5. Hexylene Glycol

107-43-7. Betaine Hydrochloride [betaine] (See also *590-46-5; 141-58-2*)

108-02-1. Captamine Hydrochloride [captamine] (See also *13242-44-9*)

108-10-1. Methyl Isobutyl Ketone

108-32-7. Propylene Carbonate

108-39-4. Metacresol

108-46-3. Resorcinol

108-73-6. Phloroglucinol

108-95-2. Phenol

109-00-2. Hydroxypyridine Tartrate [3-pyridinol] (See also *7008-17-5*)

109-43-3. Dibutyl Sebacate

109-57-9. Allylthiourea

109-69-3. Butyl Chloride

109-93-3. Vinyl Ether

109-95-5. Ethyl Nitrite [Spirit]

110-15-6. Succinic Acid

110-16-7. Maleic Acid

110-17-8. Ferrous Fumarate [fumaric acid] (See also *141-01-5*)

110-27-0. Isopropyl Myristate

110-44-1. Potassium Sorbate [sorbic acid] (See also *590-00-1; 24634-61-5; 22500-92-1*)

110-46-3. Amyl Nitrite (See also *8017-89-8*)

110-85-0. Piperazine

110-89-4. Piperidine Phosphate [piperidine] (See also *767-21-5*)

110-97-4. Diisopropanolamine

111-01-3. Squalane
111-30-8. Glutaral
111-42-2. Diethanolamine
111-48-8. Thiodiglycol
111-62-6. Ethyl Oleate
111-90-0. Diethylene Glycol Monoethyl Ether
112-24-3. Trientine Hydrochloride [trientine] (See also *38260-01-4*)
112-38-9. Undecylenic Acid
112-72-1. Myristyl Alcohol
112-80-1. Oleic Acid
112-92-5. Stearyl Alcohol
113-07-5. Doxapram Hydrochloride [anhydrous] (See also *7081-53-0; 309-29-5*)
113-15-5. Ergotamine Tartrate [ergotamine] (See also *379-79-3*)
113-18-8. Ethchlorvynol
113-22-4. Estriol Sodium Succinate
113-38-2. Estradiol Dipropionate
113-42-8. Methylergonovine Maleate [methylergonovine] (See also *57432-61-8; 7054-07-1*)
113-45-1. Methylphenidate
113-52-0. Imipramine Hydrochloride (See also *50-49-7*)
113-53-1. Dothiepin Hydrochloride [dothiepin] (See also *897-15-4*)
113-59-7. Chlorprothixene
113-73-5. Gramicidin S
113-78-0. Demoxytocin
113-79-1. Argipressin Tannate [argipressin]
113-80-4. Argiprestocin
113-92-8. Chlorpheniramine Maleate (See also *132-22-9*)
113-98-4. Penicillin G Potassium (See also *61-33-6*)
114-07-8. Erythromycin
114-26-1. Propoxur
114-43-2. Desaspidin
114-49-8. Scopolamine Hydrobromide [anhydrous] (See also *6533-68-2; 51-34-3*)
114-70-5. Sodium Phenylacetate
114-80-7. Neostigmine Bromide (See also *59-99-4*)
114-85-2. Bethanidine Sulfate (See also *55-73-2*)
114-86-3. Phenformin Hydrochloride [phenformin] (See also *834-28-6*)
114-90-9. Obidoxime Chloride
114-91-0. Metyridine
115-02-6. Azaserine
115-24-2. Sulfonmethane
115-33-3. Oxyphenisatin Acetate (See also *125-13-3*)
115-38-8. Mephobarbital
115-39-9. Bromophenol Blue
115-44-6. Talbutal
115-46-8. Azacyclonol Hydrochloride [azacyclonol] (See also *1798-50-1*)
115-51-5. Ambutonium Bromide (See also *14007-49-9*)
115-55-9. Phenylthilone
115-63-9. Hexocyclium Methylsulfate (See also *6004-98-4*)

115-67-3. Paramethadione
115-68-4. Sulfadicramide
115-79-7. Ambenonium Chloride (See also *52022-31-8; 7648-98-8*)
115-93-5. Cythioate
116-38-1. Edrophonium Chloride (See also *312-48-1*)
116-42-7. Sulfaproxyline
116-43-8. Succinylsulfathiazole
116-45-0. Sulfabromomethazine Sodium [sulfabromomethazine]
116-49-4. Glycobiarsol
116-52-9. Dicloralurea
117-10-2. Danthron
117-30-6. Dipiproverine Hydrochloride [dipiproverine] (See also *2404-18-4*)
117-37-3. Anisindione
117-89-5. Trifluoperazine Hydrochloride [trifluoperazine] (See also *440-17-5*)
117-96-4. Diatrizoate Meglumine [diatrizoic acid] (See also *131-49-7; 6284-40-8*)
118-08-1. Hydrastine
118-10-5. Cinchonine Sulfate [cinchonine] (See also *5949-16-6*)
118-23-0. Bromodiphenhydramine Hydrochloride [bromodiphenhydramine] (See also *1808-12-4*)
118-42-3. Hydroxychloroquine Sulfate [hydroxychloroquine] (See also *747-36-4*)
118-55-8. Phenyl Salicylate
118-56-9. Homosalate
118-57-0. Acetaminosalol
118-60-5. Octisalate
118-68-3. Etryptamine Acetate (See also *2235-90-7*)
118-71-8. Maltol
119-04-0. Framycetin
119-29-9. Ambucaine
119-36-8. Methyl Salicylate
119-41-5. Efloxate
119-48-2. Dimorpholamine
119-85-7. Vanyldisulfamide
119-93-7. Orthotolidine
119-96-0. Arsthinol
120-32-1. Clorophene
120-47-8. Ethylparaben
120-51-4. Benzyl Benzoate
120-91-2. Desmeninol
120-97-8. Dichlorphenamide
121-19-7. Roxarsone
121-25-5. Amprolium
121-32-4. Ethyl Vanillin
121-33-5. Vanillin
121-54-0. Benzethonium Chloride
121-55-1. Subathizone
121-57-3. Sulfanilate Zinc [sulfanilic acid] (See also *31884-76-1; 22484-64-6*)
121-59-5. Carbarsone
121-64-2. Sulocarbilate
121-75-5. Malathion
121-79-9. Propyl Gallate
121-81-3. Nitromide
122-06-5. Stilbamidine Isethionate [stilbamidine] (See also *140-59-0*)
122-09-8. Phentermine
122-11-2. Sulfadimethoxine

122-14-5. Fenitrothion
122-16-7. Sulfanitran
122-18-9. Cetalkonium Chloride
122-89-4. Mesulfamide
122-99-6. Phenoxyethanol
123-03-5. Cetylpyridinium Chloride [anhydrous] (See also *6004-24-6*)
123-31-9. Hydroquinone
123-47-7. Prolonium Iodide
123-56-8. Mercuric Succinimide [succinimide] (See also *584-43-0*)
123-63-7. Paraldehyde
123-76-2. Calcium Levulinate [levulinic acid] (See also *5743-49-7; 591-64-0*)
123-82-0. Tuaminoheptane
123-99-9. Azelaic Acid
124-04-9. Adipic Acid
124-07-2. Octanoic Acid
124-28-7. Dymanthine Hydrochloride [dymanthine] (See also *1613-17-8*)
124-29-8. Cetyl Alcohol (See also *36653-82-4*)
124-38-9. Carbon Dioxide
124-43-6. Carbamide Peroxide
124-65-2. Sodium Cacodylate (See also *75-60-5*)
124-72-1. Teflurane
124-87-8. Picrotoxin
124-88-9. Dimethiodal Sodium
124-90-3. Oxycodone Hydrochloride (See also *76-42-6*)
124-92-5. Metopon Hydrochloride (See also *143-52-2*)
124-94-7. Triamcinolone
125-02-0. Prednisolone Sodium Phosphate (See also *302-25-0*)
125-03-1. Hydrocortamate Hydrochloride (See also *76-47-1*)
125-04-2. Hydrocortisone Sodium Succinate (See also *2203-97-6*)
125-13-3. Oxyphenisatin Acetate [oxyphenisatine] (See also *115-33-3*)
125-28-0. Dihydrocodeine Bitartrate [dihydrocodeine] (See also *5965-13-9*)
125-29-1. Hydrocodone Bitartrate [hydrocodone] (See also *34195-34-1; 6190-38-1; 143-71-5*)
125-30-4. Ethylmorphine Hydrochloride (See also *76-58-4*)
125-33-7. Primidone
125-40-6. Butabarbital
125-42-8. Vinbarbital
125-45-1. Azetepa
125-51-9. Pipenzolate Bromide (See also *13473-38-6*)
125-52-0. Oxyphencyclimine Hydrochloride (See also *125-53-1*)
125-53-1. Oxyphencyclimine Hydrochloride [oxyphencyclimine] (See also *125-52-0*)
125-58-6. Levomethadone
125-60-0. Fenpiverinium Bromide
125-64-4. Methyprylon
125-65-5. Pleuromulin
125-69-9. Dextromethorphan Hydrobromide [anhydrous] (See also *6700-34-1; 125-71-3*)
125-70-2. Levomethorphan

125-71-3. Dextromethorphan

125-72-4. Levorphanol Tartrate [anhydrous] (See also *5985-38-6; 6700-40-9; 77-07-6*)

125-73-5. Dextrorphan Hydrochloride [dextrorphan] (See also *69376-27-8*)

125-84-8. Aminoglutethimide

125-85-9. Caramiphen Hydrochloride (See also *77-22-5*)

125-99-5. Tridihexethyl Iodide

126-02-3. Cycrimine Hydrochloride (See also *77-39-4*)

126-07-8. Griseofulvin

126-12-5. Anileridine Hydrochloride (See also *144-14-9*)

126-14-7. Sucrose Octaacetate

126-22-7. Butonate

126-27-2. Oxethazaine

126-31-8. Methiodal Sodium (See also *143-47-5*)

126-52-3. Ethinamate

126-92-1. Sodium Ethasulfate (See also *5254-16-0*)

126-93-2. Oxanamide

127-07-1. Hydroxyurea

127-08-2. Potassium Acetate

127-09-3. Sodium Acetate [anhydrous] (See also *6131-90-4*)

127-18-4. Tetrachloroethylene

127-31-1. Fludrocortisone Acetate [fludrocortisone] (See also *514-36-3*)

127-33-3. Demeclocycline (See also *13215-10-6*)

127-35-5. Phenazocine Hydrobromide [phenazocine] (See also *1239-04-9*)

127-48-0. Trimethadione

127-56-0. Sulfacetamide Sodium [anhydrous] (See also *6209-17-2; 144-80-9*)

127-57-1. Sulfapyridine Sodium (See also *144-83-2*)

127-58-2. Sulfamerazine Sodium [Injection] (See also *127-79-7*)

127-60-6. Acediasulfone Sodium (See also *80-03-5*)

127-65-1. Chloramine-T

127-69-5. Sulfisoxazole

127-71-9. Sulfabenzamide

127-77-5. Sulfabenz

127-79-7. Sulfamerazine

127-82-2. Zinc Phenolsulfonate (See also *98-67-9*)

128-09-6. Succinchlorimide

128-12-1. Acetosulfone Sodium (See also *80-80-8*)

128-13-2. Ursodiol

128-20-1. Eltanolone

128-37-0. Butylated Hydroxytoluene

128-44-9. Saccharin Sodium [anhydrous] (See also *6155-57-3; 81-07-2*)

128-46-1. Dihydrostreptomycin Sulfate [dihydrostreptomycin] (See also *5490-27-7*)

128-49-4. Docusate Calcium (See also *10041-19-7*)

128-62-1. Noscapine

129-03-3. Cyproheptadine Hydrochloride [cyproheptadine] (See also *41354-29-4; 969-33-5*)

129-06-6. Warfarin Sodium (See also *81-81-2*)

129-16-8. Merbromin

129-20-4. Oxyphenbutazone [anhydrous] (See also *7081-38-1*)

129-46-4. Suramin Hexasodium (See also *145-63-1*)

129-49-7. Methysergide Maleate (See also *361-37-5*)

129-51-1. Ergonovine Maleate (See also *60-79-7*)

129-57-7. Diprotrizoate Sodium (See also *85-16-5*)

129-63-5. Acetrizoate Sodium (See also *85-36-9*)

129-74-8. Buclizine Hydrochloride (See also *82-95-1*)

129-77-1. Piperidolate Hydrochloride (See also *82-98-4*)

129-83-9. Phenampromide

129-99-7. Meralluride [as sodium] (See also *8069-64-5*)

130-16-5. Cloxyquin

130-26-7. Clioquinol

130-37-0. Menadione Sodium Bisulfite [anhydrous] (See also *6147-37-1; 58-27-5*)

130-40-5. Riboflavin 5'-Phosphate Sodium [anhydrous]

130-61-0. Thioridazine Hydrochloride (See also *50-52-2*)

130-73-4. Methestrol

130-80-3. Diethylstilbestrol Dipropionate

130-81-4. Quindonium Bromide

130-83-6. Azapetine Phosphate

130-95-0. Quinine

131-01-1. Deserpidine

131-11-3. Dimethyl Phthalate

131-13-5. Menadiol Sodium Diphosphate [anhydrous] (See also *6700-42-1; 84-98-0; 481-85-6*)

131-48-6. Aceneuramic Acid

131-49-7. Diatrizoate Meglumine (See also *117-96-4; 6284-40-8*)

131-53-3. Dioxybenzone

131-57-7. Oxybenzone

131-67-9. Phthalofyne

131-69-1. Phthalylsulfacetamide

131-90-8. Butylphenamide

132-17-2. Benztropine Mesylate (See also *86-13-5*)

132-18-3. Diphenylpyraline Hydrochloride (See also *147-20-6*)

132-20-7. Pheniramine Maleate (See also *86-21-5*)

132-21-8. Dexbrompheniramine Maleate [dexbrompheniramine] (See also *2391-03-9*)

132-22-9. Chlorpheniramine Maleate [chlorpheniramine] (See also *113-92-8*)

132-35-4. Proxazole Citrate (See also *5696-09-3*)

132-60-5. Cinchophen

132-65-0. Dibenzothiophene

132-69-4. Benzydamine Hydrochloride (See also *642-72-8*)

132-89-8. Chlorthenoxazine

132-92-3. Methicillin Sodium [anhydrous] (See also *7246-14-2; 61-32-5*)

132-93-4. Phenethicillin Potassium (See also *147-55-7*)

132-98-9. Penicillin V Potassium (See also *87-08-1*)

133-09-5. Aminosalicylate Potassium [potassium 4-aminosalicylate] (See also *65-49-6*)

133-10-8. Aminosalicylate Sodium [anhydrous] (See also *6018-19-5; 65-49-6*)

133-11-9. Phenyl Aminosalicylate

133-15-3. Aminosalicylate Calcium [anhydrous] (See also *6059-16-1; 65-49-6*)

133-16-4. Chloroprocaine Hydrochloride [chloroprocaine] (See also *3858-89-7*)

133-53-9. Dichloroxylenol

133-58-4. Nitromersol

133-65-3. Solasulfone

133-67-5. Trichlormethiazide

133-92-6. Kanamycin Sulfate [replaced] (See also *25389-94-0; 59-01-8*)

134-03-2. Sodium Ascorbate (See also *50-81-7*)

134-09-8. Meradimate

134-31-6. Oxyquinoline Sulfate (See also *148-24-3*)

134-36-1. Erythromycin Propionate (See also *114-07-8*)

134-37-2. Amphenidone

134-49-6. Phenmetrazine Hydrochloride [phenmetrazine] (See also *1707-14-8*)

134-50-9. Aminacrine Hydrochloride (See also *90-45-9*)

134-53-2. Amprotropine Phosphate (See also *148-32-3*)

134-62-3. Diethyltoluamide

134-71-4. Racephedrine Hydrochloride (See also *90-81-3*)

134-72-5. Ephedrine Sulfate (See also *299-42-3*)

134-80-5. Diethylpropion Hydrochloride (See also *90-84-6*)

134-95-2. Calcium Mandelate (See also *90-64-2*)

135-07-9. Methyclothiazide

135-09-1. Hydroflumethiazide

135-19-3. Betanaphthol

135-23-9. Methapyrilene Hydrochloride (See also *91-80-5*)

135-31-9. Pyrrobutamine Phosphate (See also *91-82-7*)

135-43-3. Lauroguadine

135-58-0. Mesulfen

135-87-5. Piperoxan [hydrochloride] (See also *59-39-2*)

136-40-3. Phenazopyridine Hydrochloride (See also *94-78-0*)

136-44-7. Lisadimate

136-46-9. Parethoxycaine Hydrochloride (See also *94-23-5*)

136-47-0. Tetracaine Hydrochloride (See also *94-24-6*)

136-69-6. Protokylol Hydrochloride (See also *136-70-9*)

136-70-9. Protokylol Hydrochloride [protokylol] (See also *136-69-6*)

136-77-6. Hexylresorcinol

136-82-3. Piperocaine Hydrochloride [piperocaine] (See also *533-28-8*)

136-96-9. Diamthazole [dihydrochloride] (See also *95-27-2*)

137-05-3. Mecrylate

137-08-6. Calcium Pantothenate (See also *79-83-4*)

137-26-8. Thiram

137-40-6. Sodium Propionate [anhydrous] (See also *6700-17-0*)

137-53-1. Dextrothyroxine Sodium [anhydrous] (See also *7054-08-2; 51-49-0*)

137-58-6. Lidocaine

137-66-6. Ascorbyl Palmitate

137-76-8. Cetotiamine

137-86-0. Octotiamine

138-14-7. Deferoxamine Mesylate (See also *70-51-9*)

138-37-4. Mafenide Hydrochloride (See also *138-39-6*)

138-39-6. Mafenide

138-41-0. Carzenide

138-52-3. Salicin

138-56-7. Trimethobenzamide Hydrochloride [trimethobenzamide] (See also *554-92-7*)

138-84-1. Aminobenzoate Potassium (See also *150-13-0*)

138-86-3. *d*-Limonene [Limonene]

138-92-1. Betazole Hydrochloride (See also *105-20-4*)

139-02-6. Phenolate Sodium

139-05-9. Sodium Cyclamate

139-07-1. Benzododecinium Chloride (See also *10328-35-5*)

139-08-2. Miristalkonium Chloride

139-12-8. Aluminum Acetate

139-13-9. Bismuth Sodium Triglycollamate [triglycollamic acid] (See also *5798-43-6*)

139-33-3. Edetate Disodium [anhydrous] (See also *6381-92-6; 60-00-4*)

139-42-4. Cerium Oxalate

139-56-0. Salazosulfamide

139-62-8. Cyclomethycaine Sulfate [cyclomethycaine] (See also *50978-10-4; 537-61-1*)

139-88-8. Sodium Tetradecyl Sulfate (See also *4754-44-3*)

139-91-3. Furaltadone

139-93-5. Arsphenamine

140-40-9. Nithiamide

140-59-0. Stilbamidine Isethionate (See also *122-06-5*)

140-64-7. Pentamidine Isethionate

140-65-8. Pramoxine Hydrochloride [pramoxine] (See also *637-58-1*)

140-87-4. Cyacetacide

141-01-5. Ferrous Fumarate (See also *110-17-8*)

141-43-5. Monoethanolamine

141-58-2. Betaine Hydrochloride [replaced] (See also *590-46-5; 107-43-7*)

141-78-6. Ethyl Acetate

141-90-2. Thiouracil

141-94-6. Hexetidine

142-03-0. Aluminum Subacetate (See also *8000-61-1*)

142-47-2. Sodium Glutamate (See also *56-86-0*)

142-62-1. Sodium Caprylate [caproic acid] (See also *1984-06-1*)

142-91-6. Isopropyl Palmitate

143-27-1. Hetaflur [hexadecylamine] (See also *3151-59-5*)

143-28-2. Oleyl Alcohol

143-47-5. Methiodal Sodium [methiodal] (See also *126-31-8*)

143-52-2. Metopon Hydrochloride [metopon] (See also *124-92-5*)

143-57-7. Protoveratrine A

143-67-9. Vinblastine Sulfate (See also *865-21-4*)

143-71-5. Hydrocodone Bitartrate [anhydrous] (See also *34195-34-1; 6190-38-1; 125-29-1*)

143-74-8. Phenolsulfonphthalein

143-76-0. Cyclobarbital Calcium

143-81-7. Butabarbital Sodium (See also *125-40-6*)

143-82-8. Probarbital Sodium (See also *76-76-6*)

143-92-0. Tropenziline Bromide

144-02-5. Barbital Sodium (See also *57-44-3*)

144-11-6. Trihexyphenidyl Hydrochloride [trihexyphenidyl] (See also *52-49-3*)

144-12-7. Tiemonium Iodide (See also *6252-92-2*)

144-14-9. Anileridine

144-29-6. Piperazine Citrate [anhydrous] (See also *41372-10-5; 110-85-0*)

144-44-5. Pentolinium Tartrate [pentolinium] (See also *52-62-0*)

144-45-6. Spirgetine

144-55-8. Sodium Bicarbonate

144-74-1. Sulfathiazole Sodium (See also *72-14-0*)

144-75-2. Sulfoxone Sodium (See also *144-76-3*)

144-76-3. Sulfoxone Sodium [sulfoxone] (See also *144-75-2*)

144-80-9. Sulfacetamide

144-82-1. Sulfamethizole

144-83-2. Sulfapyridine

145-12-0. Oxymesterone

145-13-1. Pregnenolone Succinate [pregnenolone] (See also *4598-67-8*)

145-41-5. Dehydrocholate Sodium (See also *81-23-2*)

145-54-0. Propyromazine Bromide

145-63-1. Suramin Hexasodium [suramin] (See also *129-46-4*)

145-94-8. Chlorindanol

146-14-5. Flavin Adenin Dinucleotide

146-22-5. Nitrazepam

146-37-2. Laurolinium Acetate

146-40-7. Quinine Ascorbate

146-54-3. Triflupromazine

146-56-5. Fluphenazine Hydrochloride (See also *69-23-8*)

147-20-6. Diphenylpyraline Hydrochloride [diphenylpyraline] (See also *132-18-3*)

147-24-0. Diphenhydramine Hydrochloride

147-27-3. Dimoxyline

147-52-4. Nafcillin Sodium [nafcillin] (See also *7177-50-6; 985-16-0*)

147-55-7. Phenethicillin Potassium [phenethicillin] (See also *132-93-4*)

147-85-3. Proline [L]

147-94-4. Cytarabine

148-01-6. Dinitolmide

148-07-2. Benzmalecene

148-18-5. Ditiocarb Sodium

148-24-3. Oxyquinoline

148-32-3. Amprotropine Phosphate [amprotropine] (See also *134-53-2*)

148-56-1. Flumethiazide

148-64-1. Chlorothen Citrate (See also *148-65-2*)

148-65-2. Chlorothen Citrate [chlorothen] (See also *148-64-1*)

148-72-1. Pilocarpine Nitrate (See also *92-13-7*)

148-79-8. Thiabendazole

148-82-3. Melphalan

149-13-3. Procaine Borate (See also *59-46-1*)

149-15-5. Butacaine Sulfate (See also *149-16-6*)

149-16-6. Butacaine Sulfate [butacaine] (See also *149-15-5*)

149-17-7. Ftivazide

149-32-6. Erythritol

149-44-0. Sodium Formaldehyde Sulfoxylate [anhydrous] (See also *6035-47-8; 79-25-4*)

149-64-4. Butylscopolamine Bromide

149-91-7. Bismuth Subgallate [gallic acid] (See also *99-26-3*)

150-13-0. Aminobenzoate Potassium [*p*-aminobenzoic acid] (See also *138-84-1*)

150-38-9. Edetate Trisodium (See also *60-00-4*)

150-59-4. Alverine Citrate [alverine] (See also *5560-59-8*)

150-76-5. Mequinol

151-06-4. Chlorphentermine Hydrochloride (See also *461-78-9*)

151-21-3. Sodium Lauryl Sulfate (See also *151-41-7*)

151-41-7. Sodium Lauryl Sulfate [monododecyl hydrogen sulfate] (See also *151-21-3*)

151-67-7. Halothane

151-73-5. Betamethasone Sodium Phosphate (See also *360-63-4*)

152-02-3. Levallorphan Tartrate [levallorphan] (See also *71-82-9*)

152-11-4. Verapamil Hydrochloride

152-43-2. Quinestrol

152-47-6. Sulfalene

152-58-9. Cortodoxone

326-43-2. Phenyramidol Hydrochloride (See also *553-69-5*)

329-63-5. Racepinephrine Hydrochloride (See also *329-65-7*)

329-65-7. Racepinephrine

330-95-0. Nicarbazin

332-69-4. Bromamid

333-20-0. Potassium Thiocyanate

333-31-3. Methacholine Bromide (See also *55-92-5*)

333-36-8. Flurothyl

333-41-5. Dimpylate

337-47-3. Thiamylal Sodium

338-83-0. Perfluamine

338-95-4. Isoflupredone Acetate [isoflupredone] (See also *338-98-7*)

338-98-7. Isoflupredone Acetate (See also *338-95-4*)

339-43-5. Carbutamide

339-44-6. Glymidine Sodium [glymidine] (See also *3459-20-9*)

339-72-0. Levcycloserine

340-56-7. Methaqualone Hydrochloride (See also *72-44-6*)

340-57-8. Mecloqualone

341-00-4. Etifelmine

341-70-8. Diethazine Hydrochloride (See also *60-91-3*)

343-55-5. Dicloxacillin Sodium [anhydrous] (See also *13412-64-1; 3116-76-5*)

345-78-8. Pseudoephedrine Hydrochloride (See also *90-82-4*)

346-18-9. Polythiazide

350-12-9. Sulbentine

352-21-6. γ-Amino-β-hydroxybutyric acid

354-92-7. Perflisobutane

355-25-9. Perflubutane

355-42-0. Perflexane

356-12-7. Fluocinonide

357-07-3. Oxymorphone Hydrochloride (See also *76-41-5*)

357-08-4. Naloxone Hydrochloride (See also *51481-60-8; 465-65-6*)

357-56-2. Dextromoramide Tartrate [dextromoramide] (See also *2922-44-3*)

357-57-3. Brucine Sulfate [brucine] (See also *4845-99-2*)

357-66-4. Spirilene

357-67-5. Phetharbital

357-70-0. Galantamine

358-52-1. Hexapropymate

359-83-1. Pentazocine

360-63-4. Betamethasone Sodium Phosphate [betamethasone dihydrogen phosphate] (See also *151-73-5*)

360-70-3. Nandrolone Decanoate

361-37-5. Methysergide

362-29-8. Propiomazine

362-74-3. Bucladesine

363-13-3. Benhepazone

363-20-2. Tricetamide

363-24-6. Dinoprostone

364-62-5. Metoclopramide Hydrochloride [metoclopramide] (See also *54143-57-6; 7232-21-5*)

364-98-7. Diazoxide

365-26-4. Oxilofrine

366-70-1. Procarbazine Hydrochloride (See also *671-16-9*)

369-77-7. Cloflucarban

370-14-9. Pholedrine

372-66-7. Heptaminol Hydrochloride [heptaminol] (See also *543-15-7*)

378-44-9. Betamethasone

379-79-3. Ergotamine Tartrate (See also *113-15-5*)

382-67-2. Desoximetasone

382-82-1. Dicolinium Iodide

386-17-4. Iodophthalein Sodium [iodophthalein] (See also *632-73-5*)

388-51-2. Metofenazate

389-08-2. Nalidixate Sodium [nalidixic acid] (See also *15769-77-4; 3374-05-8*)

390-28-3. Methoxamine Hydrochloride [methoxamine] (See also *61-16-5*)

390-64-7. Prenylamine (See also *69-43-2*)

391-70-8. Troxonium Tosilate (See also *4386-76-9*)

395-28-8. Isoxsuprine Hydrochloride [isoxsuprine] (See also *579-56-6; 34331-89-0*)

396-01-0. Triamterene

404-82-0. Fenfluramine Hydrochloride (See also *458-24-2*)

404-86-4. Capsaicin

405-22-1. Nidroxyzone

406-90-6. Fluroxene

407-41-0. Dexfosfoserine

420-04-2. Calcium Carbimide [cyanamide] (See also *156-62-7*)

423-55-2. Perflubron

424-89-5. Clomegestone Acetate (See also *5367-84-0*)

426-13-1. Fluorometholone

427-00-9. Desomorphine

427-51-0. Cyproterone Acetate (See also *2098-66-0*)

428-07-9. Atromepine

428-37-5. Profadol Hydrochloride [profadol] (See also *2324-94-9*)

431-89-0. Apaflurane

432-60-0. Allylestrenol

434-03-7. Ethisterone

434-05-9. Methenolone Acetate (See also *153-00-4*)

434-07-1. Oxymetholone

434-43-5. Pentorex

435-97-2. Phenprocoumon

436-40-8. Inproquone

437-38-7. Fentanyl

437-74-1. Xanthinol Niacinate

438-41-5. Chlordiazepoxide Hydrochloride (See also *58-25-3*)

438-60-8. Protriptyline Hydrochloride [protriptyline] (See also *1225-55-4*)

438-67-5. Estrone Sodium Sulfate (See also *481-97-0*)

439-14-5. Diazepam

440-17-5. Trifluoperazine Hydrochloride (See also *117-89-5*)

440-58-4. Iodamide

441-61-2. Ethylmethylthiambutene

441-91-8. Benanserin Hydrochloride [benanserin] (See also *525-02-0*)

442-03-5. Anisopirol

442-16-0. Ethacridine Lactate [ethacridine] (See also *1837-57-6*)

442-52-4. Clemizole (See also *1163-36-6*)

443-48-1. Metronidazole (See also *13182-89-3*)

444-27-9. Timonacic

446-86-6. Azathioprine

447-41-6. Nylidrin Hydrochloride [nylidrin] (See also *849-55-8; 900-01-6*)

448-34-0. Azaprocin

451-71-8. Glyhexamide

451-77-4. Homarylamine (See also *533-10-8*)

452-35-7. Ethoxzolamide

455-83-4. Dichlorophenarsine Hydrochloride [dichlorophenarsine] (See also *536-29-8*)

456-59-7. Cyclandelate

457-60-3. Neoarsphenamine

457-87-4. Etilamfetamine

458-24-2. Fenfluramine Hydrochloride [fenfluramine] (See also *404-82-0*)

459-86-9. Mitoguazone

461-06-3. Carnitine

461-78-9. Chlorphentermine Hydrochloride [chlorphentermine] (See also *151-06-4*)

465-39-4. Bufogenin

465-53-2. Cyclopregnol

465-65-6. Naloxone Hydrochloride [naloxone] (See also *357-08-4; 51481-60-8*)

466-06-8. Proscillaridin

466-14-8. Ibrotamide

466-40-0. Isomethadone

466-90-0. Thebacon

466-97-7. Normorphine

466-99-9. Hydromorphone Hydrochloride [hydromorphone] (See also *71-68-1*)

467-15-2. Norcodeine

467-18-5. Myrophine

467-22-1. Carbiphene Hydrochloride (See also *15687-16-8*)

467-36-7. Thialbarbital

467-38-9. Thiotetrabarbital

467-43-6. Methitural

467-60-7. Pipradrol Hydrochloride [pipradrol] (See also *71-78-3*)

467-83-4. Dipipanone Hydrochloride [dipipanone] (See also *856-87-1*)

467-84-5. Phenadoxone

467-85-6. Normethadone

467-86-7. Dioxaphetyl Butyrate

467-90-3. Ethypicone

468-07-5. Phenomorphan

468-50-8. Betameprodine

468-51-9. Alphameprodine

468-56-4. Hydroxypethidine

468-59-7. Betaprodine

468-61-1. Oxeladin

469-21-6. Doxylamine Succinate [doxylamine] (See also *562-10-7*)

469-62-5. Propoxyphene Hydrochloride [propoxyphene] (See also *1639-60-7*)

469-78-3. Metheptazine

469-79-4. Ketobemidone
469-80-7. Pheneridine
469-81-8. Morpheridine
469-82-9. Etoxeridine
470-43-9. Promoxolane
470-82-6. Eucalyptol
470-90-6. Clorfenvinfos
471-34-1. Calcium Carbonate
471-53-4. Enoxolone
473-30-3. Thiazosulfone
473-32-5. Chaulmosulfone
473-41-6. Tolbutamide Sodium, Sterile (See also *64-77-7*)
473-42-7. Para-Nitrosulfathiazole
474-25-9. Chenodiol
474-58-8. Sitogluside
474-86-2. Equilin
476-66-4. Ellagic Acid
477-30-5. Demecolcine
477-32-7. Visnadine
477-80-5. Cinnofuradione
477-90-7. Bergenin
477-93-0. Dimethoxanate Hydrochloride [dimethoxanate] (See also *518-63-8*)
479-18-5. Dyphylline
479-50-5. Lucanthone Hydrochloride [lucanthone] (See also *548-57-2*)
479-68-5. Broparestrol
479-81-2. Bietamiverine Hydrochloride [bietamiverine]
479-92-5. Propyphenazone
480-17-1. Leucocianidol
480-22-8. Anthralin (See also *1143-38-0*)
480-30-8. Dichloralphenazone
480-49-9. Filipin
481-06-1. Santonin
481-49-2. Cepharanthine
481-85-6. Menadiol Sodium Diphosphate [menadiol] (See also *6700-42-1; 131-13-5; 84-98-0*)
481-97-0. Estrone Sodium Sulfate [estrone hydrogen sulfate] (See also *438-67-5*)
482-15-5. Isothipendyl Hydrochloride [isothipendyl] (See also *1225-60-1*)
482-44-0. Pentosalen
483-18-1. Emetine Hydrochloride [emetine] (See also *316-42-7*)
483-20-5. Indigotindisulfonate Sodium [5,5′-indigotindisulfonic acid] (See also *860-22-0*)
483-63-6. Crotamiton
484-23-1. Dihydralazine Sulfate [dihydralazine] (See also *7327-87-9*)
485-24-5. Phthalylsulfamethizole
485-34-7. Neocinchophen
485-41-6. Sulfachrysoidine
485-89-2. Oxycinchophen
486-12-4. Triprolidine Hydrochloride [triprolidine] (See also *6138-79-0; 550-70-9*)
486-16-8. Carbinoxamine Maleate [carbinoxamine] (See also *3505-38-2*)
486-17-9. Captodiame Hydrochloride [captodiame] (See also *904-04-1*)
486-47-5. Ethaverine Hydrochloride [ethaverine] (See also *985-13-7*)
486-56-6. Cotinine Fumarate [cotinine] (See also *5695-98-7*)

486-79-3. Dipyrocetyl
487-48-9. Salacetamide
487-53-6. Hydroxyprocaine
487-79-6. Kainic Acid
488-41-5. Mitobronitol
488-69-7. Fosfructose
490-55-1. Amiphenazole
490-79-9. Sodium Gentisate [gentisic acid] (See also *4955-90-2*)
490-98-2. Hydroxytetracaine
491-92-9. Pamaquine Naphthoate [pamaquine] (See also *635-05-2*)
492-18-2. Mersalyl
492-39-7. Cathine
492-61-5. Dextrose [β-D-glucopyranose, anhydrous] (See also *5996-10-1; 77029-61-9; 50-99-7; 2280-44-6; 492-62-5*)
492-62-5. Dextrose [α-D-glucopyranose, anhydrous] (See also *5996-10-1; 77029-61-9; 50-99-7; 2280-44-6; 492-61-5*)
492-85-3. Nicopholine
493-75-4. Bialamicol Hydrochloride [bialamicol] (See also *3624-96-2*)
493-76-5. Propanocaine
493-78-7. Methaphenilene Hydrochloride [methaphenilene] (See also *7084-07-3*)
493-80-1. Histapyrrodine
493-92-5. Prolintane Hydrochloride [prolintane] (See also *1211-28-5*)
494-03-1. Chlornaphazine
494-14-4. Chlordimorine
494-79-1. Melarsoprol
495-70-5. Meprylcaine Hydrochloride [meprylcaine] (See also *956-03-6*)
495-83-0. Tigloidine
495-84-1. Salinazid
495-99-8. Hydroxystilbamidine Isethionate [hydroxystilbamidine] (See also *533-22-2*)
496-00-4. Dibrompropamidine
496-38-8. Midamaline (See also *24360-03-0*)
496-67-3. Bromisovalum
497-19-8. Sodium Carbonate (See also *5968-11-6*)
497-75-6. Dioxethedrin Hydrochloride [dioxethedrin]
498-73-7. Mercurobutol
498-78-2. Stearylsulfamide
499-67-2. Proparacaine Hydrochloride [proparacaine] (See also *5875-06-9*)
500-08-3. Forminitrazole
500-34-5. Eucaine Hydrochloride [β-eucaine] (See also *555-28-2*)
500-42-5. Chlorazanil Hydrochloride [chlorazanil] (See also *2019-25-2*)
500-89-0. Thiambutosine
500-92-5. Chloroguanide Hydrochloride [chloroguanide] (See also *637-32-1*)
501-62-2. Phenamazoline Hydrochloride [phenamazoline] (See also *24359-77-1*)
501-68-8. Beclamide
502-55-6. Dixanthogen
502-59-0. Octamylamine

502-85-2. Sodium Oxybate (See also *591-81-1*)
502-98-7. Chloroazodin
503-01-5. Isometheptene Hydrochloride [isometheptene] (See also *6168-86-1*)
503-49-1. Meglutol
504-03-0. Nanofin
504-24-5. Fampridine
506-26-3. Gamolenic Acid
507-30-2. Choline Gluconate
508-99-6. Hydrocortisone Cypionate
509-56-8. Methyldihydromorphine
509-67-1. Pholcodine
509-74-0. Methadyl Acetate
509-78-4. Dimenoxadol
509-84-2. Metethoheptazine
509-86-4. Heptabarbital
510-53-2. Racemethorphan
510-74-7. Spiramide
510-90-7. Buthalital Sodium
511-12-6. Dihydroergotamine Mesylate [dihydroergotamine] (See also *6190-39-2*)
511-13-7. Chlophedianol Hydrochloride (See also *791-35-5*)
511-41-1. Diphoxazide
511-45-5. Pridinol
511-46-6. Clofenetamine Hydrochloride [clofenetamine] (See also *2019-16-1*)
511-55-7. Xenytropium Bromide
512-15-2. Cyclopentolate Hydrochloride [cyclopentolate] (See also *5870-29-1*)
512-16-3. Cyclobutyrol
512-48-1. Valdetamide
513-10-0. Echothiophate Iodide (See also *6736-03-4*)
514-36-3. Fludrocortisone Acetate (See also *127-31-1*)
514-50-1. Acebrochol
514-61-4. Normethandrone
514-65-8. Biperiden
514-68-1. Estriol [as succinate] (See also *50-27-1*)
514-73-8. Dithiazanine Iodide (See also *7187-55-5*)
515-49-1. Sulfathiourea
515-57-1. Maleylsulfathiazole
515-58-2. Salazosulfathiazole
515-64-0. Sulfisomidine
515-82-2. Chloralformamide
516-21-2. Cycloguanil Pamoate [cycloguanil] (See also *609-78-9*)
516-95-0. Epidihydrocholesterin
517-18-0. Methallenestril
518-20-7. Cyclocumarol
518-28-5. Podofilox
518-47-8. Fluorescein Sodium (See also *2321-07-5*)
518-61-6. Dacemazine
518-63-8. Dimethoxanate Hydrochloride (See also *477-93-0*)
519-26-6. Iodomethamate Sodium (See also *1951-53-7*)
519-30-2. Dimethazan
519-37-9. Etofylline
519-88-0. Ambucetamide
519-95-9. Florantyrone
520-20-7. Mepiperphenidol Bromide

520-26-3. Hesperidin

520-27-4. Diosmin

520-45-6. Dehydroacetic Acid [keto form] (See also *771-03-9*)

520-52-5. Psilocybine

520-85-4. Medroxyprogesterone Acetate [medroxyprogesterone] (See also *71-58-9*)

521-10-8. Methandriol

521-11-9. Mestanolone

521-12-0. Dromostanolone Propionate (See also *58-19-5*)

521-17-5. Androstenediol

521-18-6. Stanolone

521-35-7. Cannabinol

521-74-4. Broxyquinoline

521-78-8. Trimipramine Maleate (See also *739-71-9*)

522-00-9. Ethopropazine Hydrochloride [ethopropazine] (See also *1094-08-2*)

522-18-9. Chlorbenzoxamine Hydrochloride [chlorbenzoxamine] (See also *5576-62-5*)

522-24-7. Fenethazine

522-25-8. Pyrathiazine Hydrochloride (See also *84-08-2*)

522-40-7. Diethylstilbestrol Diphosphate

522-48-5. Tetrahydrozoline Hydrochloride (See also *84-22-0*)

522-51-0. Dequalinium Chloride (See also *6707-58-0*)

522-60-1. Ethylhydrocupreine Hydrochloride [ethylhydrocupreine] (See also *3413-58-9*)

522-87-2. Yohimbic Acid

523-54-6. Etymemazine Hydrochloride [etymemazine] (See also *3737-33-5*)

523-87-5. Dimenhydrinate

524-81-2. Mebhydrolin

524-83-4. Ethybenztropine

524-84-5. Dimethylthiambutene

524-99-2. Medrylamine

525-02-0. Benanserin Hydrochloride (See also *441-91-8*)

525-26-8. Cloperidone Hydrochloride (See also *4052-13-5*)

525-30-4. Mercuderamide

525-61-1. Quinocide

525-66-6. Propranolol Hydrochloride [propranolol] (See also *318-98-9*)

525-94-0. Adicillin

526-08-9. Sulfaphenazole

526-18-1. Osalmid

526-35-2. Allomethadione

526-36-3. Xylometazoline Hydrochloride [xylometazoline] (See also *1218-35-5*)

526-83-0. Tartaric Acid (See also *87-69-4*)

526-95-4. Calcium Gluconate [D-gluconic acid] (See also *299-28-5*)

527-07-1. Sodium Gluconate

527-09-3. Copper Gluconate

527-75-3. Berythromycin

528-94-9. Ammonium Salicylate

528-96-1. Benzoylpas Calcium [anhydrous] (See also *5631-00-5; 13898-58-3*)

529-96-4. Pyridoxamine Phosphate (anhydrous)

530-08-5. Isoetharine (See also *13725-16-1; 32095-14-0*)

530-10-9. Phenisonone Hydrobromide (See also *28227-96-5*)

530-31-4. Ammonium Mandelate (See also *90-64-2*)

530-43-8. Chloramphenicol Palmitate

530-54-1. Methoxyphedrine

530-78-9. Flufenamic Acid

531-72-6. Thiacetarsamide

531-73-7. Proflavine Dihydrochloride (See also *92-62-6*)

531-76-0. Sarcolysin

532-03-6. Methocarbamol

532-11-6. Anetholtrithion

532-32-1. Sodium Benzoate

532-34-3. Butopyronoxyl

532-40-1. Monophosphothiamine

532-43-4. Thiamine Mononitrate (See also *59-43-8*)

532-49-0. Dibutoline Sulfate

532-76-3. Hexylcaine Hydrochloride (See also *532-77-4*)

532-77-4. Hexylcaine Hydrochloride [hexylcaine] (See also *532-76-3*)

533-08-4. Tropigline

533-10-8. Homarylamine [hydrochloride] (See also *451-77-4*)

533-22-2. Hydroxystilbamidine Isethionate (See also *495-99-8*)

533-28-8. Piperocaine Hydrochloride (See also *136-82-3*)

533-45-9. Clomethiazole

534-84-9. Pimeclone

535-51-3. Phenarsone Sulfoxylate

535-65-9. Glybuthiazol

536-21-0. Norfenefrine

536-24-3. Ethylnorepinephrine Hydrochloride [ethylnorepinephrine] (See also *3198-07-0*)

536-29-8. Dichlorophenarsine Hydrochloride (See also *455-83-4*)

536-33-4. Ethionamide

536-43-6. Dyclonine Hydrochloride (See also *586-60-7*)

536-71-0. Diminazene

536-93-6. Eucatropine Hydrochloride (See also *100-91-4*)

537-12-2. Diperodon Hydrochloride (See also *101-08-6*)

537-17-7. Amanozine

537-21-3. Chlorproguanil Hydrochloride [chlorproguanil] (See also *15537-76-5*)

537-46-2. Methamphetamine Hydrochloride [methamphetamine] (See also *51-57-0*)

537-61-1. Cyclomethycaine Sulfate [hydrochloride] (See also *50978-10-4; 139-62-8*)

538-03-4. Oxophenarsine Hydrochloride (See also *306-12-7*)

538-23-8. Tricaprilin

538-71-6. Domiphen Bromide (See also *13900-14-6*)

539-54-8. Antimony Sodium Thioglycollate

539-68-4. Dihydroxyaluminum Sodium Carbonate [replaced] (See also *12011-77-7; 16482-55-6*)

540-10-3. Cetyl Palmitate

540-72-7. Thiocyanate Sodium

541-15-1. Levocarnitine

541-20-8. Pentamethonium Bromide (See also *2365-25-5*)

541-22-0. Decamethonium Bromide (See also *156-74-1*)

541-46-8. Isovaleramide

541-64-0. Furtrethonium Iodide (See also *7618-86-2*)

541-66-2. Oxapropanium Iodide (See also *5818-18-8*)

541-79-7. Carbocloral

543-15-7. Heptaminol Hydrochloride (See also *372-66-7*)

543-82-8. Octodrine

544-31-0. Palmidrol

544-35-4. Ethyl Linoleate

544-62-7. Batilol

544-63-8. Myristic Acid

545-59-5. Racemoramide

545-80-2. Poldine Methylsulfate (See also *596-50-9*)

545-90-4. Dimepheptanol

546-06-5. Conessine Hydrobromide [conessine] (See also *5913-82-6*)

546-32-7. Oxpheneridine

546-71-4. *p*-Nitrophenyl-*O*-ethyl Ethylphosphonate

546-88-3. Acetohydroxamic Acid

546-93-0. Magnesium Carbonate [anhydrous] (See also *23389-33-5; 39409-82-0*)

547-17-1. Xantofyl Palmitate

547-32-0. Sulfadiazine Sodium (See also *68-35-9*)

547-44-4. Sulfacarbamide

547-81-9. Epiestriol

548-00-5. Ethyl Biscoumacetate

548-57-2. Lucanthone Hydrochloride (See also *479-50-5*)

548-62-9. Gentian Violet

548-68-5. Thiphenamil Hydrochloride (See also *82-99-5*)

548-73-2. Droperidol

548-84-5. Pyrvinium Chloride

549-18-8. Amitriptyline Hydrochloride (See also *50-48-6*)

549-40-6. Furostilbestrol

549-56-4. Quinine Bisulfate (See also *130-95-0*)

549-68-8. Octaverine

550-01-6. Metabutoxycaine Hydrochloride (See also *3624-87-1*)

550-10-7. Hydrocotarnine Hydrochloride

550-28-7. Amisometradine

550-70-9. Triprolidine Hydrochloride [anhydrous] (See also *6138-79-0; 486-12-4*)

550-81-2. Amopyroquine

550-83-4. Propoxycaine Hydrochloride (See also *86-43-1*)

550-99-2. Naphazoline Hydrochloride (See also *835-31-4*)

551-11-1. Dinoprost

551-27-9. Propicillin

551-48-4. Guanoclor Sulfate (See also *5001-32-1*)

551-92-8. Dimetridazole

552-22-7. Thymol Iodide

552-25-0. Diampromide

552-79-4. Methylephedrine

552-92-1. Toloconium Metilsulfate

552-94-3. Salsalate

553-08-2. Thonzonium Bromide

553-13-9. Zolamine Hydrochloride [zolamine] (See also *1155-03-9*)

553-17-3. Guaiacol Carbonate

553-30-0. Proflavine Sulfate (See also *92-62-6*)

553-54-8. Lithium Benzoate

553-58-2. Metabutethamine Hydrochloride (See also *4439-25-2*)

553-65-1. Amoxecaine

553-68-4. Butethamine Hydrochloride (See also *2090-89-3*)

553-69-5. Phenyramidol Hydrochloride [phenyramidol] (See also *326-43-2*)

554-13-2. Lithium Carbonate

554-18-7. Glucosulfone

554-24-5. Phenobutiodil

554-57-4. Methazolamide

554-72-3. Tryparsamide

554-92-7. Trimethobenzamide Hydrochloride (See also *138-56-7*)

555-06-6. Sodium Aminobenzoate (See also *150-13-0*)

555-28-2. Eucaine Hydrochloride (See also *500-34-5*)

555-30-6. Methyldopa [anhydrous] (See also *41372-08-1*)

555-44-2. Tripalmitin

555-57-7. Pargyline Hydrochloride [pargyline] (See also *306-07-0*)

555-65-7. Brocresine

555-77-1. Trichlormethine

555-84-0. Nifuradene

555-90-8. Nicothiazone

556-08-1. Acedoben

556-12-7. Furalazine

557-04-0. Magnesium Stearate

557-05-1. Zinc Stearate

557-07-3. Zinc Oleate

557-08-4. Zinc Undecylenate (See also *112-38-9*)

557-34-6. Zinc Acetate [anhydrous] (See also *5970-45-6*)

561-27-3. Diacetylmorphine Hydrochloride [diacetylmorphine] (See also *1502-95-0*)

561-43-3. Oxypyrronium Bromide

561-48-8. Norpipanone

561-76-2. Properidine

561-77-3. Dihexyverine Hydrochloride [dihexyverine] (See also *5588-25-0*)

561-78-4. Alphaprodine Hydrochloride (See also *14405-05-1; 77-20-3*)

561-79-5. Metcaraphen Hydrochloride [metcaraphen] (See also *1950-31-8*)

561-83-1. Nealbarbital

561-86-4. Brallobarbital

562-09-4. Chlorphenoxamine Hydrochloride (See also *77-38-3*)

562-10-7. Doxylamine Succinate (See also *469-21-6*)

562-26-5. Phenoperidine

564-25-0. Doxycycline [anhydrous] (See also *17086-28-1*)

565-33-3. Metahexamide

565-99-1. Renanolone

566-48-3. Formestane

568-63-8. Erythrosine Sodium [anhydrous, open form] (See also *49746-10-3; 16423-68-0; 15905-32-5*)

569-57-3. Chlorotrianisene

569-59-5. Phenindamine Tartrate (See also *82-88-2*)

569-61-9. Pararosaniline Pamoate [pararosaniline] (See also *7232-51-1*)

569-65-3. Meclizine Hydrochloride [meclizine] (See also *31884-77-2; 1104-22-9*)

573-20-6. Acetomenaphthone

573-41-1. Theophylline Olamine (See also *58-55-9*)

573-58-0. Congo Red

574-25-4. Thioinosine

574-77-6. Papaveroline

574-79-8. Mercumatilin Sodium [replaced] (See also *60135-06-0; 43043-01-2*)

575-52-0. Penicillin O Chloroprocaine

575-74-6. Buclosamide

576-68-1. Mannomustine

577-11-7. Docusate Sodium (See also *10041-19-7*)

577-48-0. Butamben Picrate

577-91-3. Iodoalphionic Acid

578-89-2. Pimetremide

579-23-7. Cyclovalone

579-38-4. Diloxanide

579-56-6. Isoxsuprine Hydrochloride (See also *34331-89-0; 395-28-8*)

579-94-2. Menglytate

580-74-5. Xantocillin

581-88-4. Debrisoquin Sulfate (See also *1131-64-2*)

582-25-2. Potassium Benzoate

583-03-9. Fenipentol

584-08-7. Potassium Carbonate

584-18-9. Acetomeroctol

584-43-0. Mercuric Succinimide (See also *123-56-8*)

584-69-0. Ditophal

584-79-2. Bioallethrin

585-14-8. Poskine

585-86-4. Lactitol (See also *81025-03-8; 81025-04-9*)

585-88-6. Maltitol

586-06-1. Metaproterenol Polistirex [metaproterenol]

586-60-7. Dyclonine Hydrochloride [dyclonine] (See also *536-43-6*)

586-98-1. Piconol

587-23-5. Methenamine Mandelate (See also *100-97-0*)

587-46-2. Benzpyrinium Bromide

587-49-5. Salfluverine

587-61-1. Propyliodone

588-42-1. Trolnitrate Phosphate (See also *7077-34-1*)

590-00-1. Potassium Sorbate (See also *24634-61-5; 110-44-1; 22500-92-1*)

590-31-8. Meprochol

590-46-5. Betaine Hydrochloride (See also *141-58-2; 107-43-7*)

590-63-6. Bethanechol Chloride (See also *674-38-4*)

591-64-0. Calcium Levulinate [anhydrous] (See also *5743-49-7; 123-76-2*)

591-81-1. Sodium Oxybate [4-hydroxybutanoic acid] (See also *502-85-2*)

594-91-2. Perflisopent

595-33-5. Megestrol Acetate (See also *3562-63-8*)

595-77-7. Algestone Acetonide [algestone] (See also *4968-09-6*)

596-50-9. Poldine Methylsulfate [poldine] (See also *545-80-2*)

596-51-0. Glycopyrrolate

599-33-7. Prednylidene

599-54-2. Calcium Pantothenate, Racemic [DL-pantothenic acid] (See also *6381-63-1*)

599-79-1. Sulfasalazine

599-88-2. Sulfaperin

602-40-4. Cyheptropine

602-41-5. Thiocolchicoside

603-00-9. Proxyphylline

603-50-9. Bisacodyl

604-51-3. Deptropine Citrate [deptropine] (See also *2169-75-7*)

604-74-0. Bufenadrine

604-75-1. Oxazepam

606-04-2. Pamabrom

606-05-3. Pyrabrom

606-17-7. Iodipamide

606-90-6. Piprinhydrinate

609-78-9. Cycloguanil Pamoate (See also *516-21-2*)

611-53-0. Ibacitabine

611-75-6. Bromhexine Hydrochloride (See also *3572-43-8*)

614-39-1. Procainamide Hydrochloride (See also *51-06-9*)

614-42-6. Naepaine Hydrochloride (See also *2188-67-2*)

616-68-2. Trimecaine

616-91-1. Acetylcysteine

617-48-1. Malic Acid

618-82-6. Sulfarsphenamine

620-30-4. Racemetirosine

620-61-1. Hyoscyamine Sulfate [anhydrous] (See also *6835-16-1; 101-31-5*)

620-99-5. Phenacaine Hydrochloride [anhydrous] (See also *6153-19-1; 101-93-9*)

621-42-1. Metacetamol

621-72-7. Bendazol

624-49-7. Dimethyl Fumarate

627-83-8. Glycol Distearate

630-08-0. Carbon Monoxide

630-56-8. Hydroxyprogesterone Caproate (See also *68-96-2*)

630-60-4. Ouabain [anhydrous] (See also *11018-89-6*)

630-93-3. Phenytoin Sodium (See also *57-41-0*)

631-06-1. Dexoxadrol Hydrochloride (See also *4741-41-7*)

631-27-6. Glyclopyramide

632-00-8. Sulfasomizole

632-73-5. Iodophthalein Sodium (See also *386-17-4*)

632-99-5. Fuchsin, Basic

633-47-6. Cropropamide (See also *3544-46-5*)

633-65-8. Berberine Chloride (See also *2086-83-1*)

633-66-9. Berberine Sulfate

633-90-9. Cifostodine

634-03-7. Phendimetrazine Tartrate [phendimetrazine] (See also *50-58-8; 21102-82-9*)

634-08-2. Levofacetoperane

634-19-5. Phentydrone

635-05-2. Pamaquine Naphthoate (See also *491-92-9*)

635-41-6. Trimetozine

636-47-5. Stallimycin Hydrochloride [stallimycin] (See also *6576-51-8*)

636-54-4. Clopamide

637-07-0. Clofibrate

637-32-1. Chloroguanide Hydrochloride (See also *500-92-5*)

637-58-1. Pramoxine Hydrochloride (See also *140-65-8*)

638-94-8. Desonide

639-48-5. Nicomorphine

642-44-4. Aminometradine

642-72-8. Benzydamine Hydrochloride [benzydamine] (See also *132-69-4*)

642-78-4. Cloxacillin Sodium [anhydrous] (See also *7081-44-9*)

642-83-1. Aceglatone

643-22-1. Erythromycin Stearate (See also *114-07-8*)

644-26-8. Amylocaine

644-62-2. Meclofenamate Sodium [meclofenamic acid] (See also *6385-02-0*)

645-05-6. Altretamine

645-43-2. Guanethidine Monosulfate (See also *55-65-2*)

646-02-6. Aminoethyl Nitrate

651-06-9. Sulfameter

652-67-5. Isosorbide

653-03-2. Butaperazine

655-05-0. Thozalinone

655-35-6. Chromonar Hydrochloride (See also *804-10-4*)

657-24-9. Metformin

657-27-2. Lysine Hydrochloride (See also *56-87-1*)

659-40-5. Hexamidine [Hexamidine Isetionate] (See also *3811-75-4*)

660-27-5. Diisopropylamine Dichloroacetate

661-19-8. Docosanol

664-95-9. Glycyclamide

665-66-7. Amantadine Hydrochloride (See also *768-94-5*)

671-16-9. Procarbazine Hydrochloride [procarbazine] (See also *366-70-1*)

671-88-5. Disulfamide

671-95-4. Clofenamide

672-87-7. Metyrosine

673-31-4. Phenprobamate

674-38-4. Bethanechol Chloride [bethanechol] (See also *590-63-6*)

678-26-2. Perflenapent

679-90-3. Roflurane

692-13-7. Buformin

695-53-4. Dimethadione

702-54-5. Diethadione

709-55-7. Etilefrine

720-76-3. Fluminorex

721-19-7. Methastyridone

721-50-6. Prilocaine

723-42-2. Ditolamide

723-46-6. Sulfamethoxazole

728-88-1. Tolperisone

729-99-7. Sulfamoxole

730-07-4. Propetamide

732-11-6. Phosmet

735-52-4. Cetophenicol

735-64-8. Fenamifuril

737-31-5. Diatrizoate Sodium (See also *117-96-4*)

738-70-5. Trimethoprim

739-71-9. Trimipramine

742-20-1. Cyclopenthiazide

744-80-9. Benzobarbital

745-65-3. Alprostadil

747-30-8. Aminophenazone Cyclamate

747-36-4. Hydroxychloroquine Sulfate (See also *118-42-3*)

748-44-7. Acoxatrine

749-02-0. Spiperone

749-13-3. Trifluperidol

750-90-3. Quinine Salicylate (See also *130-95-0*)

751-84-8. Benethamine Penicillin

751-94-0. Fusidate Sodium (See also *6990-06-3*)

751-97-3. Rolitetracycline

767-21-5. Piperidine Phosphate (See also *110-89-4*)

768-94-5. Amantadine Hydrochloride [amantadine] (See also *665-66-7*)

771-03-9. Dehydroacetic Acid [enol form] (See also *520-45-6*)

773-76-2. Chloroxine

777-11-7. Haloprogin

786-19-6. Carbofenotion

787-93-9. Ameltolide

790-69-2. Loflucarban

791-35-5. Chlophedianol Hydrochloride [chlophedianol] (See also *511-13-7*)

796-29-2. Ketipramine Fumarate [ketipramine] (See also *17243-32-2*)

797-63-7. Levonorgestrel

800-22-6. Chloracyzine

801-52-5. Porfiromycin

804-10-4. Chromonar Hydrochloride [chromonar] (See also *655-35-6*)

804-30-8. Fursultiamine

804-36-4. Nitrovin

804-63-7. Quinine Sulfate [anhydrous] (See also *6119-70-6; 130-95-0*)

807-31-8. Aceperone

808-24-2. Nicodicodine

808-26-4. Sancycline

808-48-0. Desoxycorticosterone Pivalate

808-71-9. Penethamate Hydriodide

809-01-8. Edogestrone

811-97-2. Norflurane

813-93-4. Bismuth Citrate

814-80-2. Calcium Lactate [anhydrous] (See also *41372-22-9; 5743-47-5*)

822-16-2. Sodium Stearate

826-39-1. Mecamylamine Hydrochloride (See also *60-40-2*)

827-61-2. Aceclidine

829-74-3. Levonordefrin (See also *18829-78-2*)

830-89-7. Albutoin

834-28-6. Phenformin Hydrochloride (See also *114-86-3*)

835-31-4. Naphazoline Hydrochloride [naphazoline] (See also *550-99-2*)

841-73-6. Bucolome

844-26-8. Bithionoloxide

846-48-0. Boldenone Undecylenate [boldenone] (See also *13103-34-9*)

846-49-1. Lorazepam

846-50-4. Temazepam

847-20-1. Flubanilate Hydrochloride [flubanilate] (See also *967-48-6*)

847-25-6. Racephenicol

848-21-5. Norgestrienone

848-53-3. Homochlorcyclizine

848-75-9. Lormetazepam

849-55-8. Nylidrin Hydrochloride (See also *900-01-6; 447-41-6*)

850-52-2. Altrenogest

852-19-7. Sulfazamet

852-42-6. Guaiapate

853-34-9. Kebuzone

856-87-1. Dipipanone Hydrochloride (See also *467-83-4*)

859-07-4. Cefaloram

859-18-7. Lincomycin Hydrochloride [anhydrous] (See also *7179-49-9; 154-21-2*)

860-22-0. Indigotindisulfonate Sodium (See also *483-20-5*)

863-61-6. Menatetrenone

865-04-3. Methoserpidine

865-21-4. Vinblastine Sulfate [vinblastine] (See also *143-67-9*)

865-24-7. Vinglycinate Sulfate [vinglycinate] (See also *7281-31-4*)

866-84-2. Potassium Citrate [anhydrous] (See also *6100-05-6*)

868-14-4. Potassium Bitartrate

868-18-8. Sodium Tartrate

870-62-2. Hexamethonium Iodide

881-17-4. Iodohippurate Sodium I 131

882-09-7. Aluminum Clofibrate [clofibric acid] (See also *14613-01-5*)

886-08-8. Norletimol

886-74-8. Chlorphenesin Carbamate (See also *104-29-0*)

891-60-1. Declopramide

892-01-3. Hexacyprone

893-01-6. Tenylidone

894-71-3. Nortriptyline Hydrochloride (See also *72-69-5*)

896-71-9. Tigestol

897-15-4. Dothiepin Hydrochloride (See also *113-53-1*)

897-61-0. Penicillin O Potassium (See also *87-09-2*)

900-01-6. Nylidrin Hydrochloride [replaced] (See also *849-55-8; 447-41-6*)

900-77-6. Drocarbil

904-04-1. Captodiame Hydrochloride (See also *486-17-9*)

908-35-0. Metyrapone Tartrate (See also *54-36-4*)

909-39-7. Opipramol Hydrochloride (See also *315-72-0*)

910-86-1. Tiocarlide

911-45-5. Clomiphene Citrate [clomiphene] (See also *50-41-9*)

911-65-9. Etonitazene

912-60-7. Noscapine Hydrochloride (See also *128-62-1*)

914-00-1. Methacycline

915-30-0. Diphenoxylate Hydrochloride [diphenoxylate] (See also *3810-80-8*)

915-67-3. Amaranth

919-16-4. Lithium Citrate [anhydrous] (See also *6080-58-6*)

926-93-2. Methallibure

937-13-3. Oteracil

938-73-8. Ethenzamide

952-54-5. Morinamide

955-48-6. Metalol Hydrochloride (See also *7701-65-7*)

956-03-6. Meprylcaine Hydrochloride (See also *495-70-5*)

956-90-1. Phencyclidine Hydrochloride (See also *77-10-1*)

957-56-2. Fluindione

958-93-0. Thenyldiamine [hydrochloride] (See also *91-79-2*)

959-10-4. Xenbucin

959-14-8. Oxolamine

959-24-0. Sotalol Hydrochloride (See also *3930-20-9*)

960-05-4. Carbubarb

962-02-7. Nitrodan

963-39-3. Demoxepam

964-82-9. Xenyhexenic Acid

965-52-6. Nifuroxazide

965-90-2. Ethylestrenol

965-93-5. Metribolone

967-48-6. Flubanilate Hydrochloride (See also *847-20-1*)

968-63-8. Butinoline

968-81-0. Acetohexamide

968-93-4. Testolactone

969-33-5. Cyproheptadine Hydrochloride [anhydrous] (See also *41354-29-4; 129-03-3*)

972-02-1. Diphenidol

976-71-6. Canrenone

977-79-7. Medrogestone

979-32-8. Estradiol Valerate

980-71-2. Brompheniramine Maleate (See also *86-22-6*)

982-24-1. Clopenthixol

982-57-0. Chloramphenicol Sodium Succinate (See also *56-75-7*)

983-85-7. Penamecillin

985-13-7. Ethaverine Hydrochloride (See also *486-47-5*)

985-16-0. Nafcillin Sodium [anhydrous] (See also *7177-50-6; 147-52-4*)

987-02-0. Demecycline

987-24-6. Betamethasone Acetate

987-65-5. Adenosine Triphosphate Disodium

987-78-0. Citicoline Sodium [citicoline] (See also *33818-15-4; 1477-47-0*)

989-96-8. Triamcinolone Acetonide Sodium Phosphate [triamcinolone acetonide 21-(dihydrogen phosphate)] (See also *1997-15-5*)

990-73-8. Fentanyl Citrate·(See also *437-38-7*)

992-21-2. Lymecycline

1008-65-7. Fenadiazole

1018-34-4. Trepirium Iodide

1018-71-9. Pyrrolnitrin

1021-11-0. Guanoxyfen Sulfate (See also *13050-83-4*)

1027-87-8. Tolpentamide

1028-33-7. Pentifylline

1034-82-8. Heptolamide

1037-50-9. Sulfadimethoxine Sodium

1038-59-1. Glyoctamide

1042-42-8. Carcainium Chloride

1043-21-6. Pirenoxine

1046-17-9. Dibupyrone

1050-48-2. Benzilonium Bromide

1050-79-9. Moperone

1054-88-2. Spiroxatrine

1055-55-6. Bunamidine Hydrochloride (See also *3748-77-4*)

1063-55-4. Butaperazine Maleate

1066-17-7. Colistin Sulfate [colistin] (See also *1264-72-8*)

1069-55-2. Bucrylate

1069-66-5. Valproate Sodium (See also *99-66-1*)

1070-11-7. Ethambutol Hydrochloride (See also *74-55-5*)

1070-95-7. Guanoctine Hydrochloride (See also *3658-25-1*)

1077-28-7. Lipoic Acid, Alpha

1077-93-6. Ternidazole

1082-56-0. Tefazoline

1082-57-1. Tramazoline Hydrochloride [tramazoline] (See also *3715-90-0*)

1083-57-4. Bucetin

1084-65-7. Meticrane

1085-91-2. Nafcaproic Acid

1088-11-5. Nordazepam

1088-80-8. Metamelfalan

1088-92-2. Nifurtoinol

1092-46-2. Ketocaine

1093-58-9. Clostebol

1094-08-2. Ethopropazine Hydrochloride (See also *522-00-9*)

1095-90-5. Methadone Hydrochloride (See also *76-99-3*)

1096-72-6. Hepzidine

1098-60-8. Triflupromazine Hydrochloride (See also *146-54-3*)

1098-97-1. Pyritinol

1099-87-2. Sodium Prasterone Sulfate

1104-22-9. Meclizine Hydrochloride [anhydrous] (See also *31884-77-2; 569-65-3*)

1110-40-3. Cortivazol

1110-80-1. Pipacycline

1111-39-3. Acetyldigitoxin

1113-10-6. Guancydine

1115-70-4. Metformin Hydrochloride

1115-84-0. Methylmethionine Sulfonium Chloride

1119-34-2. Arginine Hydrochloride [L] (See also *74-79-3*)

1119-97-7. Tetradonium Bromide

1131-64-2. Debrisoquin Sulfate [debrisoquin] (See also *581-88-4*)

1134-47-0. Baclofen

1142-70-7. Butallylonal

1143-38-0. Anthralin (See also *480-22-8*)

1146-98-1. Bromindione

1146-99-2. Clorindione

1147-62-2. Pyrovalerone Hydrochloride (See also *3563-49-3*)

1150-20-5. Azabon

1151-11-7. Ipodate Calcium (See also *5587-89-3*)

1155-03-9. Zolamine Hydrochloride (See also *553-13-9*)

1156-05-4. Phenglutarimide

1156-19-0. Tolazamide

1157-87-5. Etoloxamine

1159-93-9. Clobenzepam

1161-88-2. Sulfatolamide

1163-36-6. Clemizole [hydrochloride] (See also *442-52-4*)

1164-38-1. Lachesine Chloride

1165-48-6. Dimefline Hydrochloride [dimefline] (See also *2740-04-7*)

1166-34-3. Cinanserin Hydrochloride [cinanserin] (See also *54-84-2*)

1169-79-5. Quinestradol

1172-18-5. Flurazepam Hydrochloride (See also *17617-23-1*)

1173-88-2. Oxacillin Sodium [anhydrous] (See also *7240-38-2; 66-79-5*)

1174-11-4. Xenazoic Acid

1176-08-5. Phenyltoloxamine [citrate] (See also *92-12-6*)

1177-87-3. Dexamethasone Acetate [anhydrous] (See also *55812-90-3*)

1178-28-5. Metoserpate Hydrochloride [metoserpate] (See also *1178-29-6*)

1178-29-6. Metoserpate Hydrochloride (See also *1178-28-5*)

1179-69-7. Thiethylperazine Maleate (See also *1420-55-9*)

1181-54-0. Clomocycline

1187-56-0. Selenomethionine Se 75

1188-38-1. Carglumic Acid

1191-80-6. Mercury Oleate

1195-16-0. Citiolone

1197-18-8. Tranexamic Acid

1197-21-3. Phentermine Hydrochloride (See also *122-09-8*)

1199-18-4. Oxidopamine

1209-98-9. Fencamfamin Hydrochloride [fencamfamin] (See also *2240-14-4*)

1211-28-5. Prolintane Hydrochloride (See also *493-92-5*)

1212-03-9. Metiprenaline

1212-72-2. Mephentermine Sulfate (See also *6190-60-9; 100-92-5*)

1212-83-5. Guanisoquin Sulfate (See also *154-73-4*)

1213-06-5. Etebenecid

1218-35-5. Xylometazoline Hydrochloride (See also *526-36-3*)

1219-35-8. Primaperone

1219-77-8. Bensuldazic Acid (See also *1950-15-8*)

1220-83-3. Sulfamonomethoxine

1221-56-3. Ipodate Sodium (See also *5587-89-3*)

1222-57-7. Zolimidine

1223-36-5. Clofexamide

1225-20-3. Iothalamate Sodium (See also *2276-90-6*)

1225-55-4. Protriptyline Hydrochloride (See also *438-60-8*)

1225-60-1. Isothipendyl Hydrochloride (See also *482-15-5*)

1225-65-6. Prothipendyl Hydrochloride (See also *303-69-5*)

1227-61-8. Mefexamide

1228-19-9. Glypinamide

1229-29-4. Doxepin Hydrochloride (See also *1668-19-5; 4698-39-9; 25127-31-5*)

1229-35-2. Methdilazine Hydrochloride (See also *1982-37-2*)

1231-93-2. Ethynodiol Diacetate [ethynodiol] (See also *297-76-7*)

1232-85-5. Elantrine

1233-53-0. Bunamiodyl Sodium [bunamiodyl] (See also *1923-76-8*)

1233-70-1. Diarbarone

1234-30-6. Etocarlide

1234-71-5. Namoxyrate

1235-15-0. Norbolethone

1235-82-1. Biperiden Hydrochloride (See also *514-65-8*)

1236-99-3. Levomepromazine Hydrochloride

1239-04-9. Phenazocine Hydrobromide (See also *127-35-5*)

1239-29-8. Furazabol

1239-45-8. Homidium Bromide

1240-15-9. Propiomazine Hydrochloride (See also *362-29-8*)

1241-94-7. Octicizer

1242-56-4. Stenbolone Acetate (See also *5197-58-0*)

1242-69-9. Decitropine

1243-33-0. Mefeclorazine

1247-42-3. Meprednisone

1249-84-9. Azacosterol Hydrochloride (See also *313-05-3*)

1252-69-3. Piperamide Maleate (See also *299-48-9*)

1253-28-7. Gestonorone Caproate

1254-35-9. Oxabolone Cipionate

1257-78-9. Prochlorperazine Edisylate (See also *58-38-8*)

1263-89-4. Paromomycin Sulfate (See also *7542-37-2; 59-04-1*)

1264-62-6. Erythromycin Ethylsuccinate (See also *114-07-8*)

1264-72-8. Colistin Sulfate (See also *1066-17-7*)

1300-94-3. Amylmetacresol

1301-42-4. Euprocin Hydrochloride [euprocin] (See also *18984-80-0*)

1301-70-8. Ferric Glycerophosphate (See also *27082-31-1*)

1302-78-9. Bentonite

1303-96-4. Sodium Borate (See also *1330-43-4*)

1304-85-4. Bismuth Subnitrate

1305-62-0. Calcium Hydroxide

1305-78-8. Lime

1306-06-5. Durapatite

1308-38-9. Dichromium Trioxide

1309-38-2. Ferumoxytol

1309-42-8. Magnesia, [Milk of]

1309-48-4. Magnesium Oxide

1310-45-8. Ferric Subsulfate (See also *8053-12-1*)

1310-58-3. Potassium Hydroxide

1310-65-2. Lithium Hydroxide [anhydrous] (See also *1310-66-3*)

1310-66-3. Lithium Hydroxide (See also *1310-65-2*)

1310-73-2. Sodium Hydroxide

1310-82-3. Rubidium Hydroxide (^{81}Rb) [Injection] [rubidium hydroxide]

1313-84-4. Sodium Sulfide

1314-13-2. Zinc Oxide

1314-22-3. Zinc Peroxide, Medicinal

1317-25-5. Alcloxa

1317-30-2. Potassium Glucaldrate [replaced] (See also *23835-15-6*)

1319-77-3. Cresol

1320-11-2. Iophendylate

1320-44-1. Methylbenzethonium Chloride (See also *25155-18-4*)

1322-14-1. Calcium Undecylenate

1323-39-3. Propylene Glycol Monostearate

1323-83-7. Glyceryl Distearate

1327-41-9. Aluminum Chlorohydrate [anhydrous] (See also *12042-91-0*)

1327-53-3. Arsenic Trioxide

1330-43-4. Sodium Borate [anhydrous] (See also *1303-96-4*)

1330-44-5. Algeldrate

1332-58-7. Kaolin

1332-96-3. Ferric Pyrophosphate, Soluble

1334-74-3. Sodium Glycerophosphate [anhydrous] (See also *55073-41-1; 27082-31-1*)

1336-20-5. Tetracycline Phosphate Complex (See also *60-54-8*)

1336-29-4. Bisacodyl Tannex (See also *603-50-9*)

1336-78-3. Imidecyl Iodine

1336-80-7. Ferrocholinate

1338-16-5. Iron Sorbitex

1338-39-2. Sorbitan Monolaurate

1338-41-6. Sorbitan Monostearate

1338-43-8. Sorbitan Monooleate

1338-54-1. Undecoylium Chloride-Iodine

1340-69-8. Bentoquatam

1344-34-9. Stibamine Glucoside

1345-04-6. Antimony Trisulfide Colloid

1362-89-6. Blastomycin

1391-36-2. Lancovutide

1391-41-9. Endomycin

1392-21-8. Kitasamycin (See also *37280-56-1*)

1393-25-5. Secretin (See also *108153-74-8; 17034-35-4*)

1393-48-2. Thiostrepton

1393-87-9. Fusafungine

1394-02-1. Hachimycin

1397-74-6. Acetyltannic Acid

1397-89-3. Amphotericin B

1398-11-4. Aspidosperma

1400-61-9. Nystatin

1401-55-4. Tannic Acid

1401-69-0. Tylosin

1402-81-9. Ambomycin

1402-82-0. Amphomycin

1402-84-2. Anthelmycin

1402-89-7. Aspartocin [replaced] (See also *4117-65-1*)

1403-17-4. Candicidin

1403-47-0. Duazomycin

1403-66-3. Gentamicin Sulfate [gentamicin] (See also *1405-41-0*)

1403-71-0. Hamycin

1403-99-2. Mitogillin

1404-04-2. Neomycin Palmitate [neomycin] (See also *1405-12-5*)

1404-08-6. Neutramycin

1404-15-5. Nogalamycin

1404-20-2. Peliomycin

1404-26-8. Polymyxin B Sulfate [polymyxin B] (See also *1405-20-5*)

1404-48-4. Relomycin

1404-55-3. Ristocetin

1404-59-7. Rutamycin

1404-64-4. Sparsomycin

1404-74-6. Streptovarycin

1404-87-1. Fungimycin

1404-88-2. Tyrothricin

1404-90-6. Vancomycin

1404-93-9. Vancomycin Hydrochloride (See also *1404-90-6*)

1404-95-1. Vinleurosine Sulfate (See also *23360-92-1*)

1405-00-1. Viridofulvin

1405-10-3. Neomycin Sulfate (See also *1404-04-2*)

1405-12-5. Neomycin Palmitate (See also *1404-04-2*)

1405-20-5. Polymyxin B Sulfate (See also *1404-26-8*)

1405-37-4. Capreomycin Sulfate (See also *11003-38-6*)

1405-41-0. Gentamicin Sulfate (See also *1403-66-3*)

1405-52-3. Sulfomyxin

1405-86-3. Glycyrrhizin

1405-87-4. Bacitracin

1405-89-6. Bacitracin Zinc (See also *1405-87-4*)

1405-97-6. Gramicidin

1406-04-8. Neomycin Undecylenate (See also *1404-04-2*)

1406-06-0. Penicillin Aluminum

1406-07-1. Penicillin Calcium (See also *61-33-6*)
1407-05-2. Methocidin
1407-83-6. Quinine Tannate (See also *130-95-0*)
1420-03-7. Propenzolate Hydrochloride (See also *4354-45-4*)
1420-53-7. Codeine Sulfate [anhydrous] (See also *6854-40-6; 6059-47-8*)
1420-55-9. Thiethylperazine
1421-14-3. Propanidid
1421-68-7. Amidephrine Mesylate (See also *3354-67-4; 37571-84-9*)
1424-00-6. Mesterolone
1424-27-7. Acetazolamide Sodium
1432-75-3. Nitralamine Hydrochloride (See also *71872-90-7*)
1456-52-6. Ioprocemic Acid
1461-15-0. Oftasceine
1463-28-1. Guanacline Sulfate [guanacline] (See also *23389-32-4; 1562-71-6*)
1464-42-2. Selenomethionine
1469-07-4. Damotepine
1470-35-5. Isobromindione
1476-53-5. Novobiocin Sodium
1477-19-6. Benzarone
1477-39-0. Noracymethadol Hydrochloride [noracymethadol] (See also *5633-25-0*)
1477-40-3. Levomethadyl Acetate [levomethadyl] (See also *34433-66-4*)
1477-47-0. Citicoline Sodium [citicoline, replaced] (See also *33818-15-4; 987-78-0*)
1480-19-9. Fluanisone
1490-04-6. Menthol
1491-41-4. Naftalofos
1491-59-4. Oxymetazoline Hydrochloride [oxymetazoline] (See also *2315-02-8*)
1491-81-2. Bolmantalate
1492-02-0. Glybuzole
1492-18-8. Leucovorin Calcium (See also *41927-89-3; 6035-45-6; 58-05-9*)
1501-84-4. Rimantadine Hydrochloride (See also *13392-28-4*)
1502-95-0. Diacetylmorphine Hydrochloride (See also *561-27-3*)
1505-95-9. Naftypramide
1508-45-8. Mitopodozide
1508-65-2. Oxybutynin Chloride
1508-75-4. Tropicamide
1508-76-5. Procyclidine Hydrochloride (See also *77-37-2*)
1518-86-1. Hydroxyamphetamine Hydrobromide [replaced] (See also *306-21-8; 103-86-6*)
1524-88-5. Flurandrenolide
1531-12-0. Norlevorphanol
1538-09-6. Penicillin G Benzathine [anhydrous] (See also *41372-02-5; 61-33-6*)
1539-39-5. Gapicomine
1553-34-0. Methixene Hydrochloride [anhydrous] (See also *7081-40-5; 4969-02-2*)
1553-60-2. Ibufenac

1562-71-6. Guanacline Sulfate [anhydrous] (See also *23389-32-4; 1463-28-1*)
1580-71-8. Amiperone
1580-83-2. Paraflutizide
1592-23-0. Calcium Stearate
1596-63-0. Quinacillin
1597-82-6. Paramethasone Acetate (See also *53-33-8*)
1600-19-7. Xyloxemine
1605-89-6. Bolasterone
1607-17-6. Pentrinitrol
1612-30-2. Menadiol Sodium Sulfate
1613-17-8. Dymanthine Hydrochloride (See also *124-28-7*)
1614-20-6. Nifurprazine
1617-90-9. Vincamine
1620-21-9. Chlorcyclizine Hydrochloride (See also *82-93-9*)
1622-61-3. Clonazepam
1622-62-4. Flunitrazepam
1639-60-7. Propoxyphene Hydrochloride (See also *469-62-5*)
1641-17-4. Mexenone
1642-54-2. Diethylcarbamazine Citrate (See also *90-89-1*)
1649-18-9. Azaperone
1661-29-6. Meturedepa
1665-48-1. Metaxalone
1668-19-5. Doxepin Hydrochloride [doxepin] (See also *1229-29-4; 4698-39-9; 25127-31-5*)
1673-06-9. Amphotalide
1675-66-7. Adelmidrol
1679-75-0. Cinnamaverine
1679-76-1. Drofenine
1684-40-8. Tacrine Hydrochloride (See also *321-64-2*)
1689-89-0. Nitroxinil
1693-37-4. Parapropamol
1695-77-8. Spectinomycin Hydrochloride [spectinomycin] (See also *22189-32-8; 21736-83-4*)
1696-79-3. Amiquinsin Hydrochloride [anhydrous] (See also *7125-70-4; 13425-92-8*)
1698-95-9. Proquinolate
1703-48-6. Dimabefylline
1707-14-8. Phenmetrazine Hydrochloride (See also *134-49-6*)
1707-15-9. Metazide
1715-33-9. Prednisolone Sodium Succinate (See also *2920-86-7*)
1715-40-8. Bromociclen
1716-12-7. Sodium Phenylbutyrate
1722-62-9. Mepivacaine Hydrochloride (See also *96-88-8*)
1729-61-9. Paranyline Hydrochloride [paranyline] (See also *5585-60-4*)
1740-22-3. Pyrinoline
1744-22-5. Riluzole
1748-43-2. Trethinium Tosilate
1759-09-7. Levometiomeprazine
1764-85-8. Epithiazide
1766-91-2. Penflutizide
1767-88-0. Desmethylmoramide
1776-83-6. Quintiofos
1786-81-8. Prilocaine Hydrochloride

1794-75-8. Laurcetium Bromide
1798-49-8. Difencloxazine Hydrochloride (See also *5617-26-5*)
1798-50-1. Azacyclonol Hydrochloride (See also *115-46-8*)
1808-12-4. Bromodiphenhydramine Hydrochloride (See also *118-23-0*)
1812-30-2. Bromazepam
1824-50-6. Benzylhydrochlorothiazide
1824-52-8. Bemetizide
1824-58-4. Ethiazide
1830-32-6. Azintamide
1837-57-6. Ethacridine Lactate (See also *442-16-0*)
1838-19-3. Dectaflur [9-octadecenylamine] (See also *36505-83-6*)
1841-19-6. Fluspirilene
1843-05-6. Octabenzone
1845-11-0. Nafoxidine Hydrochloride [nafoxidine] (See also *1847-63-8*)
1847-63-8. Nafoxidine Hydrochloride (See also *1845-11-0*)
1856-34-4. Clotioxone
1863-63-4. Ammonium Benzoate
1866-43-9. Rolodine
1867-66-9. Ketamine Hydrochloride (See also *6740-88-1*)
1879-77-2. Doxibetasol
1882-26-4. Pyricarbate
1884-24-8. Cynarine
1892-80-4. Fenethylline Hydrochloride (See also *3736-08-1*)
1893-33-0. Pipamperone
1897-89-8. Piriqualone
1900-13-6. Nifurvidine
1910-68-5. Methisazone
1923-76-8. Bunamiodyl Sodium (See also *1233-53-0*)
1926-48-3. Fenbenicillin
1926-49-4. Clometocillin
1937-19-5. Pimagedine Hydrochloride (See also *79-17-4*)
1947-37-1. Tetragastrin
1949-45-7. Metrizoate Sodium [metrizoic acid] (See also *7225-61-8*)
1950-15-8. Bensuldazic Acid [sodium bensuldazate] (See also *1219-77-8*)
1950-31-8. Metcaraphen Hydrochloride (See also *561-79-5*)
1950-39-6. Deferoxamine Hydrochloride (See also *70-51-9*)
1951-25-3. Amiodarone
1951-53-7. Iodomethamate Sodium [iodomethamate] (See also *519-26-6*)
1953-02-2. Tiopronin
1953-04-4. Galantamine Hydrobromide
1954-28-5. Etoglucid
1954-79-6. Mecloralurea
1961-77-9. Chlormadinone Acetate [chlormadinone] (See also *302-22-7*)
1972-08-3. Dronabinol
1977-10-2. Loxapine
1977-11-3. Perlapine
1980-45-6. Benzodepa
1980-49-0. Felipyrine
1982-37-2. Methdilazine
1984-06-1. Sodium Caprylate (See also *142-62-1*)

1984-15-2. Medronic Acid

1984-94-7. Sulfasymazine

1986-53-4. Bolandiol Dipropionate

1986-66-9. Sodium Stibocaptate [stibocaptate] (See also *3064-61-7*)

1997-15-5. Triamcinolone Acetonide Sodium Phosphate (See also *989-96-8*)

2001-81-2. Dipenine Bromide

2001-94-7. Edetate Dipotassium [anhydrous] (See also *25102-12-9; 58167-76-3*)

2002-29-1. Flumethasone Pivalate (See also *2135-17-3*)

2011-67-8. Nimetazepam

2013-58-3. Meclocycline

2016-36-6. Choline Salicylate

2016-63-9. Bamifylline Hydrochloride [bamifylline] (See also *20684-06-4*)

2016-88-8. Amiloride Hydrochloride [anhydrous] (See also *17440-83-4; 2609-46-3*)

2019-16-1. Clofenetamine Hydrochloride (See also *511-46-6*)

2019-25-2. Chlorazanil Hydrochloride (See also *500-42-5*)

2020-25-9. Phenyliodoundecynoate

2022-85-7. Flucytosine

2030-63-9. Clofazimine

2037-95-8. Carsalam

2042-50-4. Chlormerodrin Hg 203

2043-38-1. Buthiazide

2055-44-9. Perisoxal

2056-56-6. Cintazone

2058-46-0. Oxytetracycline Hydrochloride (See also *79-57-2*)

2058-52-8. Clothiapine

2062-78-4. Pimozide

2062-84-2. Benperidol

2066-89-9. Pasiniazid

2068-78-2. Vincristine Sulfate (See also *57-22-7*)

2078-54-8. Propofol

2079-78-9. Hexamethonium Tartrate

2085-42-9. Ethoheptazine Citrate (See also *77-15-6*)

2086-83-1. Berberine Chloride [berberine] (See also *633-65-8*)

2090-89-3. Butethamine Hydrochloride [butethamine] (See also *553-68-4*)

2098-66-0. Cyproterone Acetate [cyproterone] (See also *427-51-0*)

2104-96-3. Bromofos

2109-73-1. Butacetin

2119-75-7. Fluperolone Acetate (See also *3841-11-0*)

2127-01-7. Clorexolone

2135-14-0. Descinolone Acetonide

2135-17-3. Flumethasone

2139-47-1. Nifenazone

2152-34-3. Pemoline

2152-44-5. Betamethasone Valerate

2154-02-1. Methopholine

2156-27-6. Benproperine

2156-56-1. Sodium Dichloroacetate

2165-19-7. Guanoxan Sulfate [guanoxan] (See also *5714-04-5*)

2167-85-3. Pipazethate

2169-64-4. Azaribine

2169-75-7. Deptropine Citrate (See also *604-51-3*)

2174-16-5. Trolamine Salicylate

2174-64-3. Flamenol

2179-37-5. Bencyclane Fumarate [bencyclane] (See also *14286-84-1*)

2180-92-9. Bupivacaine Hydrochloride [bupivacaine] (See also *14252-80-3; 18010-40-7*)

2181-04-6. Canrenoate Potassium (See also *4138-96-9*)

2183-56-4. Hydromorphinol

2188-67-2. Naepaine Hydrochloride [naepaine] (See also *614-42-6*)

2192-20-3. Hydroxyzine Hydrochloride (See also *68-88-2*)

2193-87-5. Fluprednidene

2201-15-2. Eticyclidine

2201-39-0. Rolicyclidine

2203-97-6. Hydrocortisone Hemisuccinate [anhydrous] (See also *83784-20-7*)

2205-73-4. Tiomesterone

2207-50-3. Aminorex

2208-51-7. Pelanserin Hydrochloride [pelanserin] (See also *42877-18-9*)

2209-86-1. Loprodiol

2210-63-1. Mofebutazone

2210-64-2. Pyrrocaine Hydrochloride (See also *2210-77-7*)

2210-77-7. Pyrrocaine

2216-51-5. Levomenthol

2216-77-5. Dibuprol

2218-68-0. Chloral Betaine

2226-11-1. Bornelone

2235-90-7. Etryptamine Acetate [etryptamine] (See also *118-68-3*)

2240-14-4. Fencamfamin Hydrochloride (See also *1209-98-9*)

2240-21-3. Thiofuradene

2244-21-5. Troclosene Potassium (See also *2782-57-2*)

2259-96-3. Cyclothiazide

2260-08-4. Acetiromate

2261-94-1. Flucarbril

2272-11-9. Ethanolamine Oleate

2276-90-6. Iothalamate Meglumine [iothalamic acid] (See also *13087-53-1; 6284-40-8*)

2277-92-1. Oxyclozanide

2280-44-6. Dextrose [D-glucopyranose, anhydrous] (See also *5996-10-1; 77029-61-9; 50-99-7; 492-62-5; 492-61-5*)

2295-58-1. Flopropione

2313-87-3. Ethoxazene Hydrochloride (See also *94-10-0*)

2315-02-8. Oxymetazoline Hydrochloride (See also *1491-59-4*)

2315-08-4. Salazosulfadimidine

2320-86-7. Enestebol

2321-07-5. Fluorescein

2324-94-9. Profadol Hydrochloride (See also *428-37-5*)

2338-21-8. Thiazinamium Chloride [thiazinamium] (See also *4320-13-2*)

2338-37-6. Levopropoxyphene Napsylate [levopropoxyphene] (See also *55557-30-7; 5714-90-9; 5667-69-6*)

2347-80-0. Thioproperazine Mesylate (See also *316-81-4*)

2353-33-5. Decitabine

2363-58-8. Epitiostanol

2364-72-9. Cyprolidol Hydrochloride (See also *4904-00-1*)

2365-25-5. Pentamethonium Bromide [pentamethonium] (See also *541-20-8*)

2375-03-3. Methylprednisolone Sodium Succinate (See also *2921-57-5*)

2385-81-1. Furethidine

2387-59-9. Carbocysteine

2391-03-9. Dexbrompheniramine Maleate (See also *132-21-8*)

2392-39-4. Dexamethasone Sodium Phosphate (See also *312-93-6*)

2398-81-4. Oxiniacic Acid

2398-95-0. Foscolic Acid

2398-96-1. Tolnaftate

2401-56-1. Deditonium Bromide (See also *20462-53-7*)

2404-18-4. Dipiproverine Hydrochloride (See also *117-30-6*)

2409-26-9. Prazitone

2423-66-7. Quindoxin

2424-71-7. Metocinium Iodide

2430-27-5. Valpromide

2430-46-8. Tolboxane

2430-49-1. Vinylbital

2438-32-6. Dexchlorpheniramine Maleate (See also *25523-97-1*)

2438-72-4. Bufexamac

2440-22-4. Drometrizole

2441-88-5. Fenyripol Hydrochloride (See also *3607-24-7*)

2444-46-4. Nonivamide

2447-57-6. Sulfadoxine

2451-01-6. Terpin Hydrate (See also *80-53-5*)

2454-11-7. Formebolone

2455-84-7. Ambenoxan

2455-92-7. Sulclamide

2460-44-8. Xylose [β-D-Xylopyranose] (See also *58-86-6; 7261-26-9; 6763-34-4*)

2465-59-0. Oxypurinol

2485-62-3. Mecysteine (See also *18598-63-5*)

2487-63-0. Quinbolone

2490-97-3. Aceglutamide Aluminum [aceglutamide] (See also *12607-92-0*)

2507-91-7. Gloxazone

2508-72-7. Antazoline Hydrochloride (See also *91-75-8*)

2508-79-4. Methyldopate Hydrochloride (See also *5123-53-5; 2544-09-4*)

2521-01-9. Encyprate

2522-81-8. Pibecarb

2529-45-5. Flurogestone Acetate

2531-04-6. Piperylone

2537-29-3. Proxibarbal

2544-09-4. Methyldopate Hydrochloride [methyldopate] (See also *2508-79-4; 5123-53-5*)

2545-24-6. Niceverine

2545-39-3. Clamoxyquin Hydrochloride [clamoxyquin] (See also *4724-59-8*)

2551-62-4. Sulfur Hexafluoride

2557-49-5. Diflorasone Diacetate [diflorasone] (See also *33564-31-7*)

2576-92-3. Isoetharine Hydrochloride (See also *530-08-5*)

2577-72-2. Metabromsalan

2589-47-1. Prajmalium Bitartrate (See also *35080-11-6*)

2607-06-9. Diflucortolone

2608-24-4. Piposulfan

2609-46-3. Amiloride Hydrochloride [amiloride] (See also *17440-83-4; 2016-88-8*)

2610-86-8. Warfarin Potassium (See also *81-81-2*)

2612-33-1. Clonitrate

2618-25-9. Ioglycamic Acid

2618-26-0. Iodipamide Sodium (See also *606-17-7*)

2622-24-4. Prothixene

2622-26-6. Periciazine

2622-30-2. Carphenazine Maleate [carphenazine] (See also *2975-34-0*)

2622-37-9. Trifluomeprazine

2623-33-8. Diacetamate

2624-43-3. Cyclofenil

2624-44-4. Ethamsylate

2624-50-2. Trimethidinium Methosulfate [trimethidinium] (See also *14149-43-0*)

2627-69-2. Acadesine

2667-89-2. Bisbentiamine

2668-66-8. Medrysone

2673-23-6. Xenygloxal

2675-35-6. Sivifene

2709-56-0. Flupentixol

2740-04-7. Dimefline Hydrochloride (See also *1165-48-6*)

2740-52-5. Anagestone Acetate [anagestone] (See also *3137-73-3*)

2746-81-8. Fluphenazine Enanthate (See also *69-23-8*)

2748-74-5. Diacetylnalorphine

2748-88-1. Miripirium Chloride

2750-76-7. Rifamide

2751-09-9. Troleandomycin

2751-68-0. Acetophenazine Maleate [acetophenazine] (See also *5714-00-1*)

2753-45-9. Mebeverine Hydrochloride (See also *3625-06-7*)

2768-90-3. Quinaldine Blue

2773-92-4. Dimethisoquin Hydrochloride (See also *86-80-6*)

2779-55-7. Opiniazide

2782-57-2. Troclosene Potassium [troclosene] (See also *2244-21-5*)

2804-00-4. Roxoperone

2809-21-4. Etidronate Disodium [etidronic acid] (See also *7414-83-7*)

2825-60-7. Formocortal

2829-19-8. Rolicyprine

2856-74-8. Modaline Sulfate [modaline] (See also *2856-75-9*)

2856-75-9. Modaline Sulfate (See also *2856-74-8*)

2856-81-7. Azabuperone

2870-71-5. Atropine Methylbromide

2894-67-9. Delorazepam

2897-83-8. Alonimid

2898-11-5. Medazepam Hydrochloride (See also *2898-12-6*)

2898-12-6. Medazepam Hydrochloride [medazepam] (See also *2898-11-5*)

2898-13-7. Sulazepam

2901-75-9. Afalanine

2908-75-0. Esculamine

2917-94-4. Entsufon Sodium (See also *55837-16-6*)

2919-66-6. Melengestrol Acetate (See also *5633-18-1*)

2920-86-7. Prednisolone Hemisuccinate

2921-57-5. Methylprednisolone Hemisuccinate

2921-88-2. Chlorpyrifos

2921-92-8. Propatyl Nitrate

2922-20-5. Butoxamine Hydrochloride [butaxamine] (See also *5696-15-1*)

2922-44-3. Dextromoramide Tartrate (See also *357-56-2*)

2924-67-6. Fluoresone

2933-94-0. Toliprolol

2949-95-3. Tixadil

2955-38-6. Prazepam

2971-90-6. Clopidol

2975-34-0. Carphenazine Maleate (See also *2622-30-2*)

2988-32-1. Indriline Hydrochloride (See also *7395-90-6*)

2998-57-4. Estramustine

3000-39-3. Quingestanol Acetate (See also *10592-65-1*)

3006-10-8. Mecetronium Ethylsulfate

3011-89-0. Aklomide

3030-53-3. Clofenoxyde

3031-48-9. Acetergamine

3044-32-4. Clogestone Acetate (See also *20047-75-0*)

3055-99-0. Polidocanol

3056-17-5. Stavudine

3064-61-7. Sodium Stibocaptate (See also *1986-66-9*)

3074-35-9. Glidazamide

3092-17-9. Midodrine Hydrochloride (See also *42794-76-3*)

3093-35-4. Halcinonide

3094-09-5. Doxifluridine

3099-52-3. Nicametate

3102-00-9. Febuprol

3105-97-3. Hycanthone

3106-85-2. Isospaglumic Acid

3115-05-7. Iobenzamic Acid

3116-76-5. Dicloxacillin

3122-01-8. Thiazesim Hydrochloride (See also *5845-26-1*)

3124-93-4. Ethynerone

3130-96-9. Rathyronine

3137-73-3. Anagestone Acetate (See also *2740-52-5*)

3147-75-9. Octrizole

3151-59-5. Hetaflur (See also *143-27-1*)

3166-62-9. Methylbenactyzium Bromide

3168-01-2. Hydroxyhexamide

3176-03-2. Drotebanol

3184-59-6. Alipamide

3198-07-0. Ethylnorepinephrine Hydrochloride (See also *536-24-3*)

3200-06-4. Nafronyl Oxalate (See also *31329-57-4*)

3202-55-9. Benapryzine Hydrochloride (See also *22487-42-9*)

3207-50-9. Clinolamide

3215-70-1. Hexoprenaline Sulfate [hexoprenaline] (See also *32266-10-7*)

3239-44-9. Dexfenfluramine Hydrochloride [dexfenfluramine] (See also *3239-45-0*)

3239-45-0. Dexfenfluramine Hydrochloride (See also *3239-44-9*)

3240-20-8. Carbenzide

3253-60-9. Laudexium Methylsulfate

3254-89-5. Diphenidol Hydrochloride (See also *972-02-1*)

3254-93-1. Doxenitoin

3258-51-3. Valofane

3261-53-8. Gitaloxin

3270-71-1. Nifuraldezone

3277-59-6. Mimbane Hydrochloride [mimbane] (See also *5560-73-6*)

3286-46-2. Sulbutiamine

3313-26-6. Thiothixene [Z] (See also *5591-45-7*)

3329-14-4. Fenpiprane Hydrochloride (See also *3540-95-2*)

3342-61-8. Deanol Aceglumate

3344-16-9. Penicillin G Hydrabamine (See also *61-33-6*)

3344-18-1. Magnesium Citrate

3354-67-4. Amidephrine Mesylate [replaced] (See also *1421-68-7; 37571-84-9*)

3362-45-6. Noxiptiline

3363-58-4. Nifurfoline

3366-95-8. Secnidazole

3374-05-8. Nalidixate Sodium [anhydrous] (See also *15769-77-4; 389-08-2*)

3375-50-6. Mesna [2-mercaptoethanesulfonic acid] (See also *19767-45-4*)

3378-93-6. Clociguanil

3380-30-1. Soneclosan

3380-34-5. Triclosan

3383-96-8. Temefos

3385-03-3. Flunisolide [anhydrous] (See also *77326-96-6*)

3397-23-7. Ornipressin

3403-42-7. Methoxypromazine Maleate (See also *61-01-8*)

3413-58-9. Ethylhydrocupreine Hydrochloride (See also *522-60-1*)

3416-24-8. Glucosamine

3416-26-0. Lidoflazine

3424-98-4. Telbivudine

3425-97-6. Dimecolonium Iodide

3426-08-2. Prozapine

3428-05-5. Pyruvic Acid Calcium Isoniazid [anhydrous]

3432-99-3. Folitixorin Calcium [folitixorin] (See also *133978-75-3*)

3436-11-1. Delfantrine

3440-28-6. Betamipron

3447-95-8. Benfurodil Hemisuccinate

3459-06-1. Cyclopentamine Hydrochloride (See also *102-45-4*)

3459-20-9. Glymidine Sodium (See also *339-44-6*)
3459-96-9. Amicarbalide
3478-15-7. Etipirium Iodide
3485-14-1. Cyclacillin
3485-62-9. Clidinium Bromide
3486-35-9. Zinc Carbonate
3505-38-2. Carbinoxamine Maleate (See also *486-16-8*)
3506-31-8. Deterenol Hydrochloride [deterenol] (See also *23239-36-3*)
3511-16-8. Hetacillin
3521-62-8. Erythromycin Estolate (See also *114-07-8*)
3521-84-4. Iodipamide Meglumine (See also *606-17-7; 6284-40-8*)
3538-57-6. Haloprogesterone
3540-95-2. Fenpiprane Hydrochloride [fenpiprane] (See also *3329-14-4*)
3543-75-7. Bendamustine Hydrochloride (See also *16506-27-7*)
3544-35-2. Iproclozide
3544-46-5. Cropropamide [*E*] (See also *633-47-6*)
3545-67-3. Chloroquine Hydrochloride (See also *54-05-7*)
3546-03-0. Cyamemazine
3546-41-6. Pyrvinium Pamoate
3551-18-6. Acetryptine
3562-15-0. Isobucaine Hydrochloride (See also *14055-89-1*)
3562-55-8. Piprocurarium Iodide
3562-63-8. Megestrol Acetate [megestrol] (See also *595-33-5*)
3562-84-3. Benzbromarone
3562-99-0. Menbutone
3563-01-7. Aprofene
3563-14-2. Sulfasuccinamide
3563-49-3. Pyrovalerone Hydrochloride [pyrovalerone] (See also *1147-62-2*)
3563-58-4. Chlorhexadol
3563-92-6. Zylofuramine
3565-03-5. Pimetine Hydrochloride [pimetine] (See also *4991-68-8*)
3565-72-8. Embramine Hydrochloride [embramine] (See also *13977-28-1*)
3567-08-6. Glysobuzole
3567-38-2. Carfimate
3567-40-6. Dioxamate
3568-00-1. Mebutizide
3568-43-2. Sulfamethoxypyridazine Acetyl (See also *80-35-3*)
3569-26-4. Indopine (See also *24361-13-5*)
3569-58-2. Oxysonium Iodide
3569-59-3. Hexasonium Iodide
3569-77-5. Amidapsone
3570-07-8. Dimecamine
3570-10-3. Benorterone
3570-46-5. Ethomoxane Hydrochloride [ethomoxane] (See also *6038-78-4*)
3570-75-0. Nifurthiazole
3571-53-7. Estradiol Undecylate
3571-71-9. Metaterol
3571-88-8. Platonin
3572-43-8. Bromhexine Hydrochloride [bromhexine] (See also *611-75-6*)

3572-52-9. Biphenamine Hydrochloride [biphenamine] (See also *5560-62-3*)
3572-74-5. Moxastine
3572-80-3. Cyclazocine
3575-80-2. Melperone
3576-64-5. Clefamide
3577-01-3. Cephaloglycin [anhydrous] (See also *22202-75-1*)
3579-62-2. Denaverine
3583-64-0. Bumadizone
3590-16-7. Feclemine
3598-37-6. Acepromazine Maleate (See also *61-00-7*)
3599-32-4. Indocyanine Green
3601-19-2. Ropizine
3605-01-4. Piribedil
3607-18-9. Cidoxepin Hydrochloride [cidoxepin] (See also *25127-31-5*)
3607-24-7. Fenyripol Hydrochloride [fenyripol] (See also *2441-88-5*)
3611-72-1. Cloridarol
3612-98-4. Troxypyrrolium Tosilate
3614-30-0. Emepronium Bromide (See also *27892-33-7*)
3614-47-9. Hydracarbazine
3614-69-5. Dimethindene Maleate (See also *5636-83-9*)
3615-24-5. Ramifenazone
3615-74-5. Promolate
3616-05-5. Pyritidium Bromide [pyritidium] (See also *14222-46-9*)
3624-87-1. Metabutoxycaine Hydrochloride [metabutoxycaine] (See also *550-01-6*)
3624-96-2. Bialamicol Hydrochloride (See also *493-75-4*)
3625-06-7. Mebeverine Hydrochloride [mebeverine] (See also *2753-45-9*)
3625-07-8. Mebolazine
3626-67-3. Hexadiline
3632-91-5. Magnesium Gluconate [anhydrous] (See also *59625-89-7*)
3638-82-2. Propetandrol
3639-19-8. Difetarsone
3643-00-3. Oxogestone Phenpropionate [oxogestone] (See also *16915-80-3*)
3646-73-9. Galactose
3658-25-1. Guanoctine Hydrochloride [guanoctine] (See also *1070-95-7*)
3666-69-1. Dioxadrol Hydrochloride (See also *6495-46-1*)
3670-68-6. Propipocaine
3671-05-4. Fenocinol
3684-46-6. Broxaldine
3686-58-6. Tolycaine
3686-78-0. Dietifen
3687-18-1. Tramiprosate
3687-45-4. Oleyl Oleate
3688-66-2. Nicocodine
3688-85-5. Diapamide
3689-50-7. Oxomemazine
3689-76-7. Chlormidazole
3690-58-2. Fubrogonium Iodide
3690-61-7. Prodeconium Bromide
3691-78-9. Benzethidine
3692-44-2. Thiohexamide
3693-39-8. Flucloronide
3696-28-4. Dipyrithione

3697-42-5. Chlorhexidine Hydrochloride (See also *55-56-1*)
3703-76-2. Cloperastine
3703-79-5. Bamethan Sulfate [bamethan] (See also *5716-20-1*)
3704-09-4. Mibolerone
3715-90-0. Tramazoline Hydrochloride (See also *1082-57-1*)
3717-88-2. Flavoxate Hydrochloride (See also *15301-69-6*)
3731-52-0. Picolamine
3731-59-7. Moroxydine
3733-63-9. Decloxizine
3733-81-1. Defosfamide
3734-12-1. Hexopyrronium Bromide
3734-16-5. Prodilidine Hydrochloride (See also *3734-17-6*)
3734-17-6. Prodilidine Hydrochloride [prodilidine] (See also *3734-16-5*)
3734-33-6. Denatonium Benzoate [anhydrous] (See also *86398-53-0*)
3734-52-9. Metazocine
3735-45-3. Vetrabutine
3735-65-7. Butynamine
3735-84-0. Dimethylaminoethyl Reserpilinate Dihydrochloride
3735-85-1. Mefeserpine
3735-90-8. Phencarbamide
3736-08-1. Fenethylline Hydrochloride [fenethylline] (See also *1892-80-4*)
3736-12-7. Levopropylcillin Potassium [levopropylcillin] (See also *4803-44-5; 7245-75-2*)
3736-81-0. Diloxanide Furoate
3737-09-5. Disopyramide
3737-33-5. Etymemazine Hydrochloride (See also *523-54-6*)
3738-06-5. Phenylacetylglycine Dimethylamide
3748-77-4. Bunamidine Hydrochloride [bunamidine] (See also *1055-55-6*)
3754-19-6. Ambuside
3764-87-2. Trestolone Acetate [trestolone] (See also *6157-87-5*)
3771-19-5. Nafenopin
3772-76-7. Sulfametomidine
3776-93-0. Furfenorex
3778-73-2. Ifosfamide
3780-72-1. Morsuximide
3781-28-0. Propyperone
3784-89-2. Phenactropinium Chloride
3784-99-4. Stilbazium Iodide
3785-21-5. Butanilicaine
3785-44-2. Bisdequalinium Diacetate
3788-16-7. Cimemoxin
3791-63-7. Iodoantipyrine I 131
3795-88-8. Levofuraltadone
3801-06-7. Fluorometholone Acetate (See also *426-13-1*)
3810-35-3. Tenonitrozole
3810-74-0. Streptomycin Sulfate (See also *57-92-1*)
3810-80-8. Diphenoxylate Hydrochloride (See also *915-30-0*)
3811-25-4. Clorprenaline Hydrochloride [clorprenaline] (See also *5588-22-7; 6933-90-0*)
3811-53-8. Propinetidine

3811-56-1. Aminoquinuride

3811-75-4. Hexamidine (See also *659-40-5*)

3818-37-9. Phenoxypropazine

3818-50-6. Bephenium Hydroxynaphthoate (See also *7181-73-9*)

3818-62-0. Betoxycaine Hydrochloride [betoxycaine] (See also *5003-47-4*)

3818-88-0. Tricyclamol Chloride

3819-00-9. Piperacetazine

3820-67-5. Glafenine

3833-99-6. Homofenazine

3841-11-0. Fluperolone Acetate [fluperolone] (See also *2119-75-7*)

3845-22-5. Teroxalene Hydrochloride (See also *14728-33-7*)

3847-29-8. Erythromycin Lactobionate (See also *114-07-8*)

3851-30-7. Fenharmane

3858-89-7. Chloroprocaine Hydrochloride (See also *133-16-4*)

3861-73-2. Anazolene Sodium (See also *7488-76-8*)

3861-76-5. Clonitazene

3863-59-0. Hydrocortisone Sodium Phosphate [cortisol 21-(dihydrogen phosphate)] (See also *6000-74-4*)

3876-10-6. Clominorex

3896-11-5. Bumetrizole

3900-31-0. Fludiazepam

3902-71-4. Trioxsalen

3922-90-5. Oleandomycin Phosphate [oleandomycin] (See also *7060-74-4*)

3924-70-7. Amcinafal

3930-19-6. Streptonigrin

3930-20-9. Sotalol Hydrochloride [sotalol] (See also *959-24-0*)

3963-95-9. Methacycline Hydrochloride (See also *914-00-1*)

3964-81-6. Azatadine Maleate [azatadine] (See also *3978-86-7*)

3978-86-7. Azatadine Maleate (See also *3964-81-6*)

4004-94-8. Zolertine Hydrochloride [zolertine] (See also *7241-94-3*)

4008-48-4. Nitroxoline

4009-68-1. Adrenochrome Monoaminoguanidine Mesilate [Adrenochrome Guanylhydrazone Mesilate, anhydrous]

4015-18-3. Sulfaclomide

4015-32-1. Quazodine

4023-00-1. Praxadine

4042-30-2. Parvaquone

4044-65-9. Bitoscanate

4047-34-1. Trantelinium Bromide

4052-13-5. Cloperidone Hydrochloride [cloperidone] (See also *525-26-8*)

4065-45-6. Sulisobenzone

4070-80-8. Sodium Stearyl Fumarate

4075-88-1. Oxifentorex

4093-35-0. Bromopride

4117-65-1. Aspartocin (See also *1402-89-7*)

4138-96-9. Canrenoate Potassium [canrenoic acid] (See also *2181-04-6*)

4140-20-9. Estrapronicate

4148-16-7. Ritrosulfan

4171-13-5. Valnoctamide

4177-58-6. Clothixamide Maleate [clothixamide] (See also *4434-20-2*)

4180-23-8. Anethole (See also *104-46-1*)

4201-22-3. Tolonidine

4205-90-7. Clonidine

4205-91-8. Clonidine Hydrochloride (See also *4205-90-7*)

4210-97-3. Tiformin

4213-51-8. Bromacrylide

4214-72-6. Isaxonine

4245-41-4. Estradiol Acetate

4255-23-6. Aletamine Hydrochloride [aletamine] (See also *4255-24-7*)

4255-24-7. Aletamine Hydrochloride (See also *4255-23-6*)

4258-85-9. Clocortolone Acetate (See also *4828-27-7*)

4267-05-4. Teclothiazide

4267-81-6. Bolazine

4268-36-4. Tybamate

4291-63-8. Cladribine

4295-55-0. Clofenamic Acid

4295-63-0. Meprotixol

4298-15-1. Cletoquine

4299-60-9. Sulfisoxazole Diolamine (See also *127-69-5*)

4304-01-2. Truxicurium Iodide

4304-40-9. Thenium Closylate

4309-70-0. Novobiocin Calcium (See also *303-81-1*)

4310-35-4. Tridihexethyl Chloride (See also *60-49-1*)

4310-89-8. Hedaquinium Chloride

4317-14-0. Amitriptylinoxide

4320-13-2. Thiazinamium Chloride (See also *2338-21-8*)

4320-30-3. Arginine Glutamate

4330-99-8. Trimeprazine Tartrate (See also *41375-66-0; 84-96-8*)

4342-03-4. Dacarbazine

4350-09-8. Oxitriptan

4354-45-4. Propenzolate Hydrochloride [propenzolate] (See also *1420-03-7*)

4360-12-7. Ajmaline

4366-18-1. Coumetarol

4378-36-3. Fenbutrazate

4386-35-0. Meralein Sodium (See also *71872-91-8*)

4386-76-9. Troxonium Tosilate [troxonium] (See also *391-70-8*)

4388-82-3. Barbexaclone

4394-00-7. Niflumic Acid

4394-04-1. Metanixin

4394-05-2. Nixylic Acid

4397-91-5. Nicofurate

4406-22-8. Cyprenorphine Hydrochloride [cyprenorphine] (See also *16550-22-4*)

4408-78-0. Fosfonet Sodium [phosphonoacetic acid] (See also *54870-27-8; 36983-81-0*)

4418-26-2. Sodium Dehydroacetate

4419-39-0. Beclomethasone Dipropionate [beclomethasone] (See also *5534-09-8*)

4434-05-3. Coumermycin

4434-20-2. Clothixamide Maleate (See also *4177-58-6*)

4438-22-6. Atropine Oxide Hydrochloride [atropine oxide] (See also *4574-60-1*)

4439-25-2. Metabutethamine Hydrochloride [metabutethamine] (See also *553-58-2*)

4439-67-2. Amikhelline

4442-60-8. Butamoxane

4444-23-9. Persilic Acid

4448-96-8. Solypertine Tartrate [solypertine] (See also *5591-43-5*)

4468-02-4. Zinc Gluconate

4474-91-3. Angiotensin II

4498-32-2. Dibenzepin Hydrochloride [dibenzepin] (See also *315-80-0*)

4499-40-5. Oxtriphylline (See also *13930-27-3*)

4533-39-5. Nitracrine

4533-89-5. Flunisolide Acetate

4544-15-4. Piperilate [hydrochloride] (See also *4546-39-8*)

4546-39-8. Piperilate (See also *4544-15-4*)

4548-15-6. Flunidazole

4549-94-4. Dexsotalol Hydrochloride (See also *30236-32-9*)

4551-59-1. Fenalamide

4564-87-8. Carbomycin

4574-60-1. Atropine Oxide Hydrochloride (See also *4438-22-6*)

4575-34-2. Myfadol

4582-18-7. Endomide

4598-67-8. Pregnenolone Succinate (See also *145-13-1*)

4599-60-4. Penimepicycline

4611-02-3. Chlorproethazine Hydrochloride (See also *84-01-5*)

4618-18-2. Lactulose

4630-95-9. Prifinium Bromide (See also *10236-81-4*)

4662-17-3. Furidarone

4663-83-6. Buramate

4671-03-8. Hexazole

4682-36-4. Orphenadrine Citrate (See also *83-98-7*)

4684-87-1. Octamoxin

4696-76-8. Bekanamycin

4697-14-7. Ticarcillin Disodium (See also *34787-01-4*)

4697-36-3. Carbenicillin Disodium [carbenicillin] (See also *4800-94-6*)

4698-39-9. Doxepin Hydrochloride [(*E*)-isomer] (See also *1229-29-4; 1668-19-5; 25127-31-5*)

4724-59-8. Clamoxyquin Hydrochloride (See also *2545-39-3*)

4729-93-5. Pentamoxane Hydrochloride (See also *4730-07-8*)

4730-07-8. Pentamoxane Hydrochloride [pentamoxane] (See also *4729-93-5*)

4732-48-3. Meclorisone Dibutyrate [meclorisone] (See also *10549-91-4*)

4741-41-7. Dexoxadrol Hydrochloride [dexoxadrol] (See also *631-06-1*)

4754-44-3. Sodium Tetradecyl Sulfate [1-tetradecanol hydrogen sulfate] (See also *139-88-8*)

5581-52-2. Thiamiprine

5585-59-1. Nitrocycline

5585-60-4. Paranyline Hydrochloride (See also *1729-61-9*)

5585-62-6. Symetine Hydrochloride (See also *15599-45-8*)

5585-64-8. Amotriphene

5585-71-7. Benzindopyrine Hydrochloride

5585-73-9. Butriptyline Hydrochloride (See also *35941-65-2*)

5585-93-3. Oxypendyl

5586-87-8. Mefenorex Hydrochloride (See also *17243-57-1*)

5587-89-3. Ipodate Calcium [ipodic acid] (See also *1151-11-7*)

5587-93-9. Ampyrimine

5588-10-3. Methoxyphenamine Hydrochloride (See also *93-30-1*)

5588-16-9. Althiazide

5588-20-5. Chlordantoin

5588-21-6. Cintriamide

5588-22-7. Clorprenaline Hydrochloride (See also *6933-90-0; 3811-25-4*)

5588-23-8. Cypenamine Hydrochloride (See also *15301-54-9*)

5588-25-0. Dihexyverine Hydrochloride (See also *561-77-3*)

5588-29-4. Fenmetramide

5588-31-8. Imidoline Hydrochloride (See also *7303-78-8*)

5588-33-0. Mesoridazine

5588-38-5. Tolpyrramide

5591-22-0. Becanthone Hydrochloride (See also *15351-04-9*)

5591-27-5. Clometherone

5591-29-7. Etafedrine Hydrochloride (See also *7681-79-0*)

5591-33-3. Iosefamic Acid

5591-43-5. Solypertine Tartrate (See also *4448-96-8*)

5591-44-6. Pyrroliphene Hydrochloride (See also *15686-97-2*)

5591-45-7. Thiothixene (See also *3313-26-6*)

5591-47-9. Cyclomenol

5591-49-1. Anilamate

5593-20-4. Betamethasone Dipropionate

5598-52-7. Fospirate

5610-40-2. Securinine

5611-51-8. Triamcinolone Hexacetonide

5611-64-3. Methalthiazide

5617-26-5. Difencloxazine Hydrochloride [difencloxazine] (See also *1798-49-8*)

5626-25-5. Clodacaine

5626-34-6. Prednisolamate

5626-36-8. Nonapyrimine

5627-46-3. Clobenztropine

5630-53-5. Tibolone

5631-00-5. Benzoylpas Calcium (See also *528-96-1; 13898-58-3*)

5632-44-0. Tolpropamine

5632-52-0. Clofenciclan

5633-14-7. Benzetimide Hydrochloride (See also *119391-55-8*)

5633-16-9. Leiopyrrole

5633-18-1. Melengestrol Acetate [melengestrol] (See also *2919-66-6*)

5633-20-5. Oxybutynin

5633-25-0. Noracymethadol Hydrochloride (See also *1477-39-0*)

5634-34-4. Ambuphylline

5634-37-7. Clorethate

5634-38-8. Guaithylline

5634-39-9. Glycerol, Iodinated

5634-40-2. Levamfetamine Succinate (See also *156-34-3*)

5634-41-3. Parapenzolate Bromide

5634-42-4. Tocamphyl

5635-50-7. Hexestrol

5636-83-9. Dimethindene Maleate [dimethindene] (See also *3614-69-5*)

5636-92-0. Picloxydine

5638-76-6. Betahistine Hydrochloride [betahistine] (See also *5579-84-0*)

5657-61-4. Nicoxamat

5666-11-5. Levomoramide

5667-46-9. Dioxyline Phosphate

5667-69-6. Levopropoxyphene Napsylate [replaced] (See also *55557-30-7; 5714-90-9; 2338-37-6*)

5667-70-9. Pentabamate

5667-71-0. Streptonicozid

5668-06-4. Mecloxamine

5684-90-2. Penthrichloral

5695-98-7. Cotinine Fumarate (See also *486-56-6*)

5696-06-0. Methetoin

5696-09-3. Proxazole

5696-15-1. Butoxamine Hydrochloride (See also *2922-20-5*)

5696-17-3. Epipropidine

5697-56-3. Carbenoxolone Sodium [carbenoxolone] (See also *7421-40-1*)

5697-57-4. Hydroxystenozole

5704-03-0. Testosterone Phenylacetate

5711-40-0. Bromebric Acid

5714-00-1. Acetophenazine Maleate (See also *2751-68-0*)

5714-04-5. Guanoxan Sulfate (See also *2165-19-7*)

5714-05-6. Quindecamine Acetate (See also *19146-62-4; 19056-26-9*)

5714-08-9. Detrothyronine

5714-09-0. Ethyl Cartrizoate

5714-73-8. Methenamine Hippurate (See also *100-97-0*)

5714-75-0. Prednazate

5714-76-1. Quinetolate

5714-82-9. Triclofenol Piperazine

5714-90-9. Levopropoxyphene Napsylate [anhydrous] (See also *55557-30-7; 5667-69-6; 2338-37-6*)

5716-20-1. Bamethan Sulfate (See also *3703-79-5*)

5728-52-9. Felbinac

5741-22-0. Moprolol

5743-12-4. Caffeine [monohydrate] (See also *58-08-2*)

5743-27-1. Calcium Ascorbate [anhydrous] (See also *5743-28-2*)

5743-28-2. Calcium Ascorbate (See also *5743-27-1*)

5743-47-5. Calcium Lactate [pentahydrate] (See also *814-80-2; 41372-22-9*)

5743-49-7. Calcium Levulinate (See also *591-64-0; 123-76-2*)

5749-67-7. Carbaspirin Calcium

5779-54-4. Cyclarbamate

5779-59-9. Alazanine Triclofenate

5781-37-3. Cycliramine Maleate (See also *47128-12-1*)

5785-44-4. Calcium Citrate

5786-21-0. Clozapine

5786-68-5. Quipazine Maleate (See also *4774-24-7*)

5786-71-0. Fosfocreatinine

5789-72-0. Trimethamide

5793-04-4. Propisergide

5793-89-5. Calcium Saccharate (See also *87-73-0*)

5794-08-1. Norepinephrine Bitartrate [replaced] (See also *69815-49-2; 51-40-1; 51-41-2*)

5794-13-8. Asparagine (See also *70-47-3*)

5798-41-4. Bismuth Potassium Tartrate

5798-43-6. Bismuth Sodium Triglycollamate (See also *139-13-9*)

5800-19-1. Metiapine

5818-17-7. Methantheline Bromide [methantheline] (See also *53-46-3*)

5818-18-8. Oxapropanium Iodide [oxapropanium] (See also *541-66-2*)

5835-72-3. Diprofene

5845-26-1. Thiazesim Hydrochloride [thiazesim] (See also *3122-01-8*)

5854-93-3. Alanosine

5863-35-4. Nitromifene Citrate (See also *10448-84-7*)

5868-05-3. Niceritrol

5868-06-4. Fentonium Bromide

5870-29-1. Cyclopentolate Hydrochloride (See also *512-15-2*)

5874-95-3. Amicycline

5874-97-5. Metaproterenol Sulfate

5874-98-6. Testosterone Ketolaurate

5875-06-9. Proparacaine Hydrochloride (See also *499-67-2*)

5879-67-4. Oletimol

5892-10-4. Bismuth Subcarbonate

5897-19-8. Cyclizine Lactate (See also *82-92-8*)

5897-66-5. Aminophylline [dihydrate] (See also *317-34-0; 49746-06-7*)

5907-38-0. Dipyrone (See also *68-89-3*)

5908-99-6. Atropine Sulfate (See also *55-48-1; 51-55-8*)

5913-82-6. Conessine Hydrobromide (See also *546-06-5*)

5928-84-7. Penicillin V Benzathine (See also *63690-57-3; 87-08-1*)

5934-14-5. Succisulfone

5936-28-7. Hydrastine Hydrochloride (See also *118-08-1*)

5941-36-6. Estrazinol Hydrobromide [estrazinol] (See also *15179-97-2*)

5942-95-0. Carpipramine Dihydrochloride [carpipramine] (See also *7075-03-8*)

5949-16-6. Cinchonine Sulfate (See also *118-10-5*)

5949-29-1. Citric Acid, Anhydrous [monohydrate] (See also *77-92-9*)

5949-44-0. Testosterone Undecanoate

5964-24-9. Thimerfonate Sodium (See also *33305-56-5*)

5964-62-5. Diathymosulfone

5965-13-9. Dihydrocodeine Bitartrate (See also *125-28-0*)

5965-40-2. Allocupreide Sodium

5965-83-3. Sulfosalicylic Acid

5966-41-6. Diisopromine Hydrochloride [diisopromine] (See also *24358-65-4*)

5967-84-0. Theophylline (See also *58-55-9*)

5968-11-6. Sodium Carbonate [monohydrate] (See also *497-19-8*)

5968-84-3. Ferric Cacodylate (See also *75-60-5*)

5970-32-1. Mercuric Salicylate

5970-45-6. Zinc Acetate (See also *557-34-6*)

5972-85-0. Ammonium Valerate

5977-10-6. Fencibutirol

5980-31-4. Hexedine

5984-83-8. Fenabutene

5984-97-4. Iodothiouracil

5985-38-6. Levorphanol Tartrate (See also *125-72-4; 6700-40-9; 77-07-6*)

5987-82-6. Benoxinate Hydrochloride (See also *99-43-4*)

5988-22-7. Phytonadiol Sodium Diphosphate

5991-71-9. Clorazepate Monopotassium (See also *20432-69-3*)

5996-10-1. Dextrose [acyclic form] (See also *77029-61-9; 50-99-7; 2280-44-6; 492-62-5; 492-61-5*)

6000-74-4. Hydrocortisone Sodium Phosphate (See also *3863-59-0*)

6001-64-5. Chlorobutanol [hemihydrate] (See also *57-15-8*)

6004-24-6. Cetylpyridinium Chloride (See also *123-03-5*)

6004-98-4. Hexocyclium Methylsulfate [hexocyclium] (See also *115-63-9*)

6009-67-2. Amolanone Hydrochloride (See also *76-65-3*)

6011-12-7. Ambazone

6011-39-8. Clemizole Penicillin

6018-19-5. Aminosalicylate Sodium (See also *133-10-8; 65-49-6*)

6035-45-6. Leucovorin Calcium [pentahydrate] (See also *1492-18-8; 41927-89-3; 58-05-9*)

6035-47-8. Sodium Formaldehyde Sulfoxylate (See also *149-44-0; 79-25-4*)

6038-78-4. Ethomoxane Hydrochloride (See also *3570-46-5*)

6043-01-2. Domazoline Fumarate [domazoline] (See also *35100-41-5*)

6054-98-4. Olsalazine Sodium (See also *15722-48-2*)

6055-19-2. Cyclophosphamide (See also *50-18-0*)

6055-48-7. Toloxychlorinol

6059-16-1. Aminosalicylate Calcium [calcium 4-aminosalicylate] (See also *133-15-3; 65-49-6*)

6059-47-8. Codeine (See also *76-57-3*)

6064-83-1. Fosfosal

6080-58-6. Lithium Citrate (See also *919-16-4*)

6091-56-1. Piperphenidol Hydrochloride (See also *90-23-3*)

6092-18-8. Cycotiamine

6100-05-6. Potassium Citrate (See also *866-84-2*)

6100-16-9. Potassium Sodium Tartrate [replaced] (See also *6381-59-5; 304-59-6*)

6101-07-1. Strychnine Valerate (See also *57-24-9*)

6101-15-1. Succinylcholine Chloride [dihydrate] (See also *71-27-2*)

6108-05-0. Lidocaine Hydrochloride (See also *73-78-9; 137-58-6*)

6112-76-1. Mercaptopurine (See also *50-44-2*)

6119-47-7. Quinine Hydrochloride

6119-70-6. Quinine Sulfate (See also *804-63-7; 130-95-0*)

6130-64-9. Penicillin G Procaine (See also *54-35-3; 61-33-6*)

6131-90-4. Sodium Acetate (See also *127-09-3*)

6132-04-3. Sodium Citrate (See also *68-04-2*)

6138-56-3. Tripelennamine Citrate (See also *91-81-6*)

6138-79-0. Triprolidine Hydrochloride (See also *550-70-9; 486-12-4*)

6146-99-2. Menadoxime

6147-37-1. Menadione Sodium Bisulfite (See also *130-37-0; 58-27-5*)

6151-30-0. Quinacrine Hydrochloride (See also *69-05-6; 83-89-6*)

6153-19-1. Phenacaine Hydrochloride (See also *620-99-5; 101-93-9*)

6153-64-6. Oxytetracycline (See also *79-57-2*)

6155-57-3. Saccharin Sodium (See also *128-44-9; 81-07-2*)

6157-87-5. Trestolone Acetate (See also *3764-87-2*)

6160-12-9. Sparteine Sulfate (See also *299-39-8; 90-39-1*)

6168-76-9. Crotetamide

6168-86-1. Isometheptene Hydrochloride (See also *503-01-5*)

6170-69-0. Clamidoxic Acid

6184-06-1. Sorbinicate

6187-50-4. Tolquinzole

6190-38-1. Hydrocodone Bitartrate [replaced] (See also *34195-34-1; 143-71-5; 125-29-1*)

6190-39-2. Dihydroergotamine Mesylate (See also *511-12-6*)

6190-60-9. Mephentermine Sulfate [dihydrate] (See also *1212-72-2; 100-92-5*)

6192-97-8. Levopropylhexedrine

6196-08-3. Elanzepine

6197-30-4. Octocrylene

6202-23-9. Cyclobenzaprine Hydrochloride (See also *303-53-7*)

6209-17-2. Sulfacetamide Sodium (See also *127-56-0; 144-80-9*)

6211-15-0. Morphine Sulfate (See also *64-31-3; 57-27-2*)

6217-54-5. Doconexent

6223-35-4. Sodium Gualenate (See also *16915-32-5*)

6236-05-1. Nifuroxime

6252-92-2. Tiemonium Iodide [tiemonium] (See also *144-12-7*)

6272-74-8. Lapyrium Chloride

6281-26-1. Furmethoxadone

6284-40-8. Diatrizoate Meglumine [meglumine] (See also *131-49-7; 117-96-4*)

6303-21-5. Hypophosphorous Acid

6306-71-4. Lobendazole

6314-69-8. Oxadimedine Hydrochloride (See also *16485-05-5*)

6319-06-8. Noreximide

6340-87-0. Triclacetamol

6363-02-6. Nitramisole Hydrochloride [nitramisole] (See also *56689-44-2*)

6376-26-7. Salverine

6381-59-5. Potassium Sodium Tartrate (See also *304-59-6; 6100-16-9*)

6381-63-1. Calcium Pantothenate, Racemic (See also *599-54-2*)

6381-91-5. Saccharin Calcium (See also *6485-34-3; 81-07-2*)

6381-92-6. Edetate Disodium (See also *139-33-3; 60-00-4*)

6385-02-0. Meclofenamate Sodium (See also *644-62-2*)

6385-58-6. Bithionolate Sodium (See also *97-18-7*)

6398-98-7. Amodiaquine Hydrochloride (See also *69-44-3; 86-42-0*)

6411-75-2. Tuaminoheptane Sulfate (See also *123-82-0*)

6416-04-2. Tetracycline [trihydrate] (See also *60-54-8*)

6443-40-9. Xylamidine Tosylate (See also *6443-50-1*)

6443-50-1. Xylamidine Tosylate [xylamidine] (See also *6443-40-9*)

6452-71-7. Oxprenolol Hydrochloride [oxprenolol] (See also *6452-73-9*)

6452-73-9. Oxprenolol Hydrochloride (See also *6452-71-7*)

6469-36-9. Cloprothiazole

6484-89-5. Folate Sodium (See also *59-30-3*)

6485-34-3. Saccharin Calcium [anhydrous] (See also *6381-91-5; 81-07-2*)

6485-39-8. Manganese Gluconate (See also *84368-35-4*)

6489-97-0. Metampicillin

6493-05-6. Pentoxifylline

6495-46-1. Dioxadrol Hydrochloride [dioxadrol] (See also *3666-69-1*)

6500-81-8. Ethacrynate Sodium (See also *58-54-8*)

6503-95-3. Triampyzine Sulfate [triampyzine] (See also *7082-30-6*)

6506-37-2. Nimorazole

6533-00-2. Norgestrel

6533-68-2. Scopolamine Hydrobromide (See also *114-49-8; 51-34-3*)

6535-03-1. Stevaladil

6536-18-1. Morazone

6538-22-3. Dimeprozan

6539-57-7. Nordefrin Hydrochloride [nordefrin] (See also *155-60-2*)

6556-11-2. Inositol Niacinate

6576-51-8. Stallimycin Hydrochloride (See also *636-47-5*)

6577-41-9. Oxapium Iodide

6582-30-5. Lopobutan

6582-31-6. Dapabutan

6591-63-5. Quinidine Sulfate (See also *50-54-4; 56-54-2*)

6591-72-6. Penicillin V Hydrabamine (See also *87-08-1*)

6592-85-4. Hydrastinine Hydrochloride [hydrastinine] (See also *4884-68-8*)

6606-65-1. Enbucrilate

6620-60-6. Proglumide

6621-47-2. Perhexiline Maleate [perhexiline] (See also *6724-53-4*)

6673-35-4. Practolol

6673-97-8. Spiroxasone

6693-90-9. Prednazoline

6700-17-0. Sodium Propionate (See also *137-40-6*)

6700-34-1. Dextromethorphan Hydrobromide (See also *125-69-9; 125-71-3*)

6700-39-6. Isoproterenol Sulfate (See also *299-95-6; 7683-59-2*)

6700-40-9. Levorphanol Tartrate [replaced] (See also *5985-38-6; 125-72-4; 77-07-6*)

6700-42-1. Menadiol Sodium Diphosphate (See also *131-13-5; 84-98-0; 481-85-6*)

6700-54-5. Dextroamphetamine Phosphate [replaced] (See also *7528-00-9; 51-64-9*)

6701-17-3. Ocrylate

6707-58-0. Dequalinium Chloride [dequalinium] (See also *522-51-0*)

6723-40-6. Fluindarol

6724-53-4. Perhexiline Maleate (See also *6621-47-2*)

6736-03-4. Echothiophate Iodide [echothiophate] (See also *513-10-0*)

6740-88-1. Ketamine Hydrochloride [ketamine] (See also *1867-66-9*)

6763-34-4. Xylose [α-D-Xylopyranose] (See also *58-86-6; 7261-26-9; 2460-44-8*)

6795-60-4. Norvinisterone

6804-07-5. Carbadox

6818-37-7. Olaflur (See also *17671-49-1*)

6829-98-7. Imipraminoxide

6830-17-7. Oxamarin Hydrochloride [dihydrochloride] (See also *15301-80-1*)

6835-16-1. Hyoscyamine Sulfate (See also *620-61-1; 101-31-5*)

6843-97-6. Dodicin

6854-40-6. Codeine Sulfate (See also *1420-53-7; 6059-47-8*)

6893-02-3. Liothyronine I 125 [liothyronine] (See also *24359-14-6*)

6899-03-2. Aspartic Acid (See also *56-84-8*)

6899-05-4. Glutamic Acid (See also *56-86-0*)

6899-10-1. Cetrimonium Bromide [cetrimonium] (See also *57-09-0*)

6903-79-3. Creatinolfosfate

6915-57-7. Bibrocathol

6933-90-0. Clorprenaline Hydrochloride [anhydrous] (See also *5588-22-7; 3811-25-4*)

6961-46-2. Idrocilamide

6964-20-1. Tiadenol

6968-72-5. Mepiroxol

6981-18-6. Ormetoprim

6989-98-6. Tubocurarine Chloride (See also *57-94-3; 41354-45-4; 57-95-4*)

6990-06-3. Fusidate Sodium [fusidic acid] (See also *751-94-0*)

6998-60-3. Rifamycin

7001-56-1. Pentagestrone

7002-65-5. Oxibetaine

7004-98-0. Epimestrol

7007-76-3. Glucosulfamide

7007-81-0. Trethocanoic Acid

7007-88-7. Butadiazamide

7007-92-3. Cetohexazine

7007-96-7. Crotoniazide

7008-00-6. Dimetholizine

7008-02-8. Iodetryl

7008-13-1. Halopenium Chloride

7008-14-2. Hydroxindasate

7008-15-3. Hydroxindasol

7008-17-5. Hydroxypyridine Tartrate (See also *109-00-2*)

7008-18-6. Iminophenimide

7008-24-4. Chloroserpidine

7008-26-6. Dichlorisone Acetate [dichlorisone] (See also *79-61-8*)

7008-42-6. Acronine

7009-43-0. Methiomeprazine Hydrochloride [methiomeprazine]

7009-49-6. Hexacyclonate Sodium (See also *7491-42-1*)

7009-54-3. Pentapiperide

7009-65-6. Prampine

7009-68-9. Pyroxamine Maleate [pyroxamine] (See also *5560-75-8*)

7009-69-0. Pyrophenindane

7009-76-9. Triclazate

7009-79-2. Xenthiorate

7009-88-3. Phenyracillin

7009-91-8. Nitricholine Perchlorate

7013-41-4. Talopram Hydrochloride (See also *7182-51-6*)

7019-69-4. Thyroxine I 131

7035-04-3. Pyridarone

7036-58-0. Propoxate

7047-84-9. Aluminum Monostearate

7048-04-6. Cysteine Hydrochloride (See also *52-89-1; 52-90-4*)

7054-07-1. Methylergonovine Maleate [replaced] (See also *57432-61-8; 113-42-8*)

7054-08-2. Dextrothyroxine Sodium (See also *137-53-1; 51-49-0*)

7054-25-3. Quinidine Gluconate (See also *56-54-2*)

7059-24-7. Chromomycin A₃

7060-74-4. Oleandomycin Phosphate (See also *3922-90-5*)

7061-51-6. Polignate Sodium [sodium lignosulfonate] (See also *8061-51-6*)

7075-03-8. Carpipramine Dihydrochloride (See also *5942-95-0*)

7077-30-7. Butopyrammonium Iodide

7077-33-0. Febuverine

7077-34-1. Trolnitrate Phosphate [trolnitrate] (See also *588-42-1*)

7081-36-9. Tranylcypromine Sulfate [replaced] (See also *13492-01-8; 155-09-9*)

7081-38-1. Oxyphenbutazone (See also *129-20-4*)

7081-40-5. Methixene Hydrochloride (See also *1553-34-0; 4969-02-2*)

7081-44-9. Cloxacillin Sodium (See also *642-78-4*)

7081-52-9. Piminodine Esylate (See also *13495-09-5*)

7081-53-0. Doxapram Hydrochloride (See also *113-07-5; 309-29-5*)

7082-21-5. Terodiline Hydrochloride (See also *15793-40-5*)

7082-27-1. Trimoxamine Hydrochloride (See also *15686-23-4*)

7082-29-3. Ampyzine Sulfate (See also *5214-29-9*)

7082-30-6. Triampyzine Sulfate (See also *6503-95-3*)

7084-07-3. Methaphenilene Hydrochloride (See also *493-78-7*)

7085-44-1. Chlorothiazide Sodium (See also *58-94-6*)

7085-45-2. Biperiden Lactate (See also *514-65-8*)

7085-55-4. Troxerutin

7097-62-3. Meragidone Sodium

7101-51-1. Melevodopa

7104-38-3. Levomepromazine Maleate

7114-11-6. Naphthonone

7125-67-9. Metoquizine

7125-70-4. Amiquinsin Hydrochloride (See also *1696-79-3; 13425-92-8*)

7125-71-5. Toquizine

7125-73-7. Flumetramide

7125-76-0. Codoxime

7162-37-0. Paridocaine

7168-18-5. Chlorphenoctium Amsonate

7174-23-4. Oxydipentonium Chloride

7175-09-9. Tilbroquinol

7177-48-2. Ampicillin [trihydrate] (See also *69-53-4*)

7177-50-6. Nafcillin Sodium (See also *985-16-0; 147-52-4*)

7177-54-0. Penicillin O Sodium (See also *87-09-2*)

7179-49-9. Lincomycin Hydrochloride (See also *859-18-7; 154-21-2*)

7181-73-9. Bephenium Hydroxynaphthoate [bephenium] (See also *3818-50-6*)

7182-51-6. Talopram Hydrochloride [talopram] (See also *7013-41-4*)

7187-55-5. Dithiazanine Iodide [dithiazanine] (See also *514-73-8*)

7195-27-9. Mefruside

7199-29-3. Cyheptamide

7205-52-9. Phytate Sodium

7219-91-2. Thihexinol Methylbromide

7220-56-6. Flutiazin

7220-79-3. Methylene Blue (See also *61-73-4*)

7224-08-0. Imiclopazine

7225-61-8. Metrizoate Sodium (See also *1949-45-7*)

7230-65-1. Iodohippurate Sodium I 125

7232-21-5. Metoclopramide Hydrochloride [anhydrous] (See also *54143-57-6; 364-62-5*)

7232-51-1. Pararosaniline Pamoate (See also *569-61-9*)

7235-40-7. Beta Carotene

7237-81-2. Hepronicate

7240-38-2. Oxacillin Sodium (See also *1173-88-2; 66-79-5*)

7241-94-3. Zolertine Hydrochloride (See also *4004-94-8*)

7242-04-8. Pengitoxin

7245-75-2. Levopropylcillin Potassium [replaced] (See also *4803-44-5; 3736-12-7*)

7246-07-3. Actinoquinol Sodium (See also *15301-40-3*)

7246-14-2. Methicillin Sodium (See also *132-92-3; 61-32-5*)

7246-20-0. Triclofos Sodium (See also *306-52-5*)

7246-21-1. Tyropanoate Sodium (See also *27293-82-9*)

7247-57-6. Heteronium Bromide

7248-21-7. Iprazochrome

7261-26-9. Xylose [D-Xylopyranose] (See also *58-86-6; 6763-34-4; 2460-44-8*)

7261-97-4. Dantrolene

7262-00-2. Quinazosin Hydrochloride (See also *15793-38-1*)

7262-75-1. Lefetamine

7270-12-4. Cloquinate

7273-99-6. Gamfexine

7279-75-6. Isoetharine Mesylate (See also *530-08-5*)

7280-37-7. Estropipate (See also *481-97-0*)

7281-31-4. Vinglycinate Sulfate (See also *865-24-7*)

7296-30-2. Safrazine Hydrochloride (See also *33419-68-0*)

7297-25-8. Erythrityl Tetranitrate

7303-78-8. Imidoline Hydrochloride [imidoline] (See also *5588-31-8*)

7327-87-9. Dihydralazine Sulfate (See also *484-23-1*)

7332-27-6. Amcinafide

7361-61-7. Xylazine

7395-90-6. Indriline Hydrochloride [indriline] (See also *2988-32-1*)

7413-36-7. Nifenalol

7414-83-7. Etidronate Disodium (See also *2809-21-4*)

7416-34-4. Molindone Hydrochloride [molindone] (See also *15622-65-8*)

7421-40-1. Carbenoxolone Sodium (See also *5697-56-3*)

7424-00-2. Fenclonine

7432-25-9. Etaqualone

7433-10-5. Butidrine

7440-59-7. Helium

7446-09-5. Sulfur Dioxide

7446-20-0. Zinc Sulfate [heptahydrate] (See also *7733-02-0*)

7446-70-0. Aluminum Chloride [anhydrous] (See also *7784-13-6*)

7447-39-4. Cupric Chloride [anhydrous] (See also *10125-13-0*)

7447-40-7. Potassium Chloride

7455-39-2. Fonazine Mesylate (See also *7456-24-8*)

7456-24-8. Fonazine Mesylate [fonazine] (See also *7455-39-2*)

7460-12-0. Pseudoephedrine Sulfate (See also *90-82-4*)

7481-89-2. Zalcitabine

7483-09-2. Mesabolone

7487-88-9. Magnesium Sulfate [anhydrous] (See also *10034-99-8*)

7487-94-7. Mercuric Chloride

7488-56-4. Selenium Sulfide

7488-76-8. Anazolene Sodium [anazolene, acid] (See also *3861-73-2*)

7488-92-8. Ketocainol

7489-66-9. Tipindole

7491-09-0. Docusate Potassium (See also *10041-19-7*)

7491-42-1. Hexacyclonate Sodium [hexacyclonic acid] (See also *7009-49-6*)

7491-74-9. Piracetam

7492-29-7. Clazolam

7492-31-1. Isometheptene Mucate

7492-32-2. Isopropamide Iodide [isopropamide] (See also *71-81-8*)

7518-35-6. Mannosulfan

7527-91-5. Acrisorcin

7528-00-9. Dextroamphetamine Phosphate (See also *6700-54-5; 51-64-9*)

7528-13-4. Carperidine

7541-30-2. Mesuprine Hydrochloride [mesuprine] (See also *7660-71-1*)

7542-37-2. Paromomycin Sulfate [paromomycin] (See also *1263-89-4; 59-04-1*)

7546-28-3. Calcium Lactophosphate (See also *18365-82-7*)

7553-56-2. Iodine

7554-16-7. Benzoquinonium Chloride [benzoquinonium] (See also *311-09-1*)

7554-65-6. Fomepizole

7558-79-4. Sodium Phosphate, Dibasic [anhydrous] (See also *10140-65-5; 10039-32-4; 7782-85-6; 10028-24-7; 118830-14-1*)

7558-80-7. Sodium Phosphate, Monobasic [anhydrous] (See also *10049-21-5; 13472-35-0*)

7585-39-9. Betadex

7601-54-9. Sodium Phosphate, Tribasic [anhydrous] (See also *10101-89-0*)

7601-55-0. Metocurine Iodide

7617-74-5. Laurixamine

7618-86-2. Furtrethonium Iodide [furtrethonium] (See also *541-64-0*)

7631-86-9. Siliceous Earth, Purified

7631-90-5. Sodium Bisulfite

7632-00-0. Sodium Nitrite

7635-46-3. Sodium Phosphate P 32

7644-67-9. Azotomycin

7646-85-7. Zinc Chloride

7647-01-0. Hydrochloric Acid

7647-14-5. Sodium Chloride

7647-15-6. Sodium Bromide

7648-98-8. Ambenonium Chloride [ambenonium] (See also *115-79-7; 52022-31-8*)

7654-03-7. Benmoxin

7660-71-1. Mesuprine Hydrochloride (See also *7541-30-2*)

7664-38-2. Phosphoric Acid

7664-41-7. Ammonia Solution, Strong

7664-93-9. Sulfuric Acid

7681-11-0. Potassium Iodide

7681-14-3. Prednisolone Tebutate

7681-32-5. Rolitetracycline Nitrate [anhydrous] (See also *26657-13-6; 751-97-3*)

7681-49-4. Sodium Fluoride

7681-52-9. Sodium Hypochlorite

7681-53-0. Sodium Hypophosphite

7681-57-4. Sodium Metabisulfite

7681-76-7. Ronidazole

7681-78-9. Mebezonium Iodide

7681-79-0. Etafedrine Hydrochloride [etafedrine] (See also *5591-29-7*)

7681-80-3. Pentapiperium Methylsulfate (See also *26372-86-1*)

7681-82-5. Sodium Iodide

7681-93-8. Natamycin

7683-59-2. Isoproterenol Hydrochloride [isoproterenol] (See also *51-30-9*)

7685-23-6. Gitoformate

7690-08-6. Segesterone

7696-00-6. Mitotenamine

7696-12-0. Tetramethrin

7697-37-2. Nitric Acid

7698-97-7. Fenestrel

7700-17-6. Crotoxyfos

7701-65-7. Metalol Hydrochloride [metalol] (See also *955-48-6*)

7704-34-9. Sulfur, Precipitated

7706-67-4. Dimecrotic Acid

7712-50-7. Myrtecaine

7716-60-1. Etisazole

7720-78-7. Ferrous Sulfate [anhydrous] (See also *7782-63-0*)

7722-64-7. Potassium Permanganate

7722-84-1. Hydrogen Peroxide

7722-88-5. Sodium Pyrophosphate

7724-76-7. Rioprine

7727-37-9. Nitrogen

7727-43-7. Barium Sulfate

7727-73-3. Sodium Sulfate (See also *7757-82-6*)

7733-02-0. Zinc Sulfate [anhydrous] (See also *7446-20-0*)

7753-60-8. Anecortave Acetate

7757-79-1. Potassium Nitrate

7757-82-6. Sodium Sulfate [anhydrous] (See also *7727-73-3*)

7757-83-7. Sodium Sulfite

7757-87-1. Magnesium Phosphate [anhydrous] (See also *10233-87-1*)

7757-93-9. Calcium Phosphate Dihydrate, Dibasic [calcium phosphate (1:1)] (See also *7789-77-7*)

7758-02-3. Potassium Bromide

7758-11-4. Potassium Phosphate, Dibasic

7758-98-7. Cupric Sulfate [anhydrous] (See also *7758-99-8*)

7758-99-8. Cupric Sulfate (See also *7758-98-7*)

7761-45-7. Metoprine

7761-75-3. Furterene

7761-88-8. Silver Nitrate

7772-98-7. Sodium Thiosulfate [anhydrous] (See also *10102-17-7*)

7772-99-8. Stannous Chloride [anhydrous] (See also *10025-69-1*)

7773-01-5. Manganese Chloride [anhydrous] (See also *13446-34-9*)

7775-11-3. Sodium Chromate Cr 51

7778-18-9. Calcium Sulfate (See also *10101-41-4*)

7778-43-0. Sodium Arsenate, Exsiccated

7778-74-7. Potassium Perchlorate

7778-77-0. Potassium Phosphate, Monobasic

7778-80-5. Potassium Sulfate

7782-44-7. Oxygen

7782-63-0. Ferrous Sulfate (See also *7720-78-7*)

7782-85-6. Sodium Phosphate, Dibasic [heptahydrate] (See also *10140-65-5; 10039-32-4; 10028-24-7; 118830-14-1; 7558-79-4*)

7783-00-8. Selenious Acid

7783-20-2. Ammonium Sulfate

7783-28-0. Ammonium Phosphate

7783-33-7. Potassium Mercuric Iodide

7783-47-3. Stannous Fluoride

7783-83-7. Ferric Ammonium Sulfate

7783-84-8. Ferric Hypophosphite

7784-13-6. Aluminum Chloride (See also *7446-70-0*)

7784-24-9. Alum, Potassium (See also *10043-67-1*)

7784-25-0. Alum, Ammonium [anhydrous] (See also *7784-26-1*)

7784-26-1. Alum, Ammonium (See also *7784-25-0*)

7784-30-7. Aluminum Phosphate

7785-84-4. Sodium Trimetaphosphate

7785-87-7. Manganese Sulfate [anhydrous] (See also *10034-96-5; 6485-39-8; 84368-35-4*)

7786-30-3. Magnesium Chloride [anhydrous] (See also *7791-18-6*)

7789-20-0. Deuterium Oxide

7789-41-5. Calcium Bromide

7789-77-7. Calcium Phosphate Dihydrate, Dibasic (See also *7757-93-9*)

7789-79-9. Calcium Hypophosphite

7790-26-3. Sodium Iodide I 131

7790-53-6. Potassium Metaphosphate

7791-18-6. Magnesium Chloride (See also *7786-30-3*)

8000-10-0. Theophylline Sodium Glycinate (See also *58-55-9*)

8000-28-0. Lavender Oil

8000-34-8. Clove Oil

8000-42-8. Caraway [oil]

8000-48-4. Eucalyptus Oil

8000-61-1. Aluminum Subacetate (See also *142-03-0*)

8000-73-5. Ammonium Carbonate

8000-90-6. Potassium Aspartate and Magnesium Aspartate [replaced] (See also *14842-81-0; 56-84-8*)

8001-25-0. Olive Oil

8001-29-4. Cottonseed Oil

8001-31-8. Coconut Oil

8001-40-9. Iodized Oil

8001-54-5. Benzalkonium Chloride

8001-59-0. Creosote Carbonate

8001-79-4. Castor Oil

8001-95-4. Alseroxylon

8002-03-7. Peanut Oil

8002-31-1. Cocoa Butter

8002-74-2. Paraffin

8002-76-4. Papaveretum

8002-78-6. Persic Oil

8002-88-8. Theobromine Sodium Acetate (See also *83-67-0*)

8002-90-2. Chiniofon

8006-28-8. Soda Lime

8006-44-8. Candelilla Wax

8006-45-9. Chloriodized Oil

8006-90-4. Peppermint Oil

8007-00-9. Peruvian Balsam

8007-01-0. Rose Oil

8007-31-6. Silver Nitrate, Toughened

8007-43-0. Sorbitan Sesquioleate

8007-59-8. Sodium Hypochlorite [Solution, Diluted]

8007-69-0. Almond Oil

8007-70-3. Anise Oil

8007-80-5. Cinnamon Oil

8008-45-5. Nutmeg Oil

8008-53-5. Ethiodized Oil

8008-56-8. Lemon Oil

8008-74-0. Sesame Oil

8008-79-5. Spearmint Oil

8009-03-8. Petrolatum

8011-96-9. Calamine

8012-34-8. Mercurophylline

8012-89-3. Wax, Yellow

8012-95-1. Mineral Oil

8013-08-9. Eriodictyon

8013-10-3. Juniper Tar

8015-51-8. Prethcamide

8016-46-4. Pine Needle Oil

8016-70-4. Soybean Oil, Hydrogenated

8016-91-9. Trichinella Extract

8017-09-2. Tolu Balsam

8017-88-7. Phenylmercuric Borate

8017-89-8. Amyl Nitrite [mixture] (See also *110-46-3*)

8021-76-9. Sodium Psylliate [Injection]

8023-79-8. Palm Kernel Oil

8024-48-4. Casanthranol

8025-81-8. Spiramycin

8027-62-1. Raspberry Syrup

8028-66-8. Honey

8028-89-5. Caramel

8029-68-3. Ichthammol

8029-99-0. Paregoric

8030-26-0. Rose Water, Stronger

8030-62-4. Iso-alcoholic Elixir

8031-09-2. Morrhuate Sodium

8031-14-9. Oxychlorosene

8031-45-6. Hydroxystearin Sulfate

8039-60-9. Bismuth Betanaphthol (See also *135-19-3*)

8044-71-1. Cetrimide

8047-36-7. Zinc Gelatin

8047-67-4. Iron Sucrose

8048-31-5. Theobromine Sodium Salicylate (See also *83-67-0*)

8048-92-8. Decavitamin

8049-47-6. Pancreatin

8049-62-5. Insulin Human Zinc

8050-09-7. Rosin

8050-34-8. Azuresin

8050-35-9. Benzoin

8050-68-8. Starch Glycerite

8050-81-5. Simethicone

8052-16-2. Cactinomycin

8053-12-1. Ferric Subsulfate (See also *1310-45-8*)

8053-19-8. Styronate Resins

8058-76-2. Endobenzyline Bromide

8061-51-6. Polignate Sodium (See also *7061-51-6*)

8063-28-3. Ribaminol

8063-29-4. Insulin [Injection], Biphasic

8063-80-7. Polisaponin

8063-91-0. Mirincamycin Hydrochloride (See also *37217-18-8; 31101-25-4*)

8065-29-0. Liotrix

8066-49-7. Migrenin

8067-24-1. Ergoloid Mesylates (See also *11032-41-0*)

8067-69-4. Halquinols

8068-28-8. Colistimethate Sodium (See also *21362-08-3*)

8069-64-5. Meralluride (See also *129-99-7*)

9000-01-5. Acacia

9000-07-1. Carrageenan

9000-11-7. Carboxymethylcellulose Sodium [cellulose carboxymethyl ether] (See also *9004-32-4*)

9000-69-5. Pectin

9000-70-8. Gelatin

9000-90-2. Alpha Amylase

9000-92-4. Diastase

9000-99-1. Asperkinase

9001-00-7. Bromelains

9001-01-8. Kallidinogenase

9001-09-6. Chymopapain

9001-13-2. Hemocoagulase

9001-27-8. Beroctocog Alfa

9001-54-1. Hyaluronidase (Ovine) (See also *488712-31-8*)

9001-62-1. Rizolipase

9001-63-2. Lysozyme Chloride [lysozyme]

9001-73-4. Papain

9001-74-5. Penicillinase

9001-75-6. Saccharated Pepsin

9002-01-1. Streptokinase

9002-05-5. Thromboplastin

9002-60-2. Corticotropin

9002-61-3. Gonadotropin, Chorionic

9002-64-6. Parathyroid Hormone [parathyroid] (See also *68893-82-3; 345663-45-8*)

9002-68-0. Menotropins

9002-70-4. Gonadotropin, Serum

9002-71-5. Thyrotropin
9002-79-3. Intermedine
9002-84-0. Polytef
9002-89-5. Polyvinyl Alcohol
9002-90-8. Polyethylene Glycol [macrogol] (See also *25322-68-3*)
9002-92-0. Laureth 4
9002-93-1. Octoxynol 9
9003-01-4. Carbomer 910
9003-07-0. Polipropene 25
9003-11-6. Poloxalene
9003-23-0. Polyethadene
9003-27-4. Polyisobutylene
9003-39-8. Crospovidone
9003-68-3. Pegoterate
9003-97-8. Calcium Polycarbophil
9004-06-2. Elastase
9004-07-3. Chymotrypsin
9004-09-5. Fibrinolysin, Human
9004-12-0. Insulin, Dalanated
9004-14-2. Insulin, Neutral
9004-17-5. Insulin, Isophane
9004-32-4. Carboxymethylcellulose Sodium (See also *9000-11-7*)
9004-34-6. Cellulose, Microcrystalline
9004-35-7. Cellulose Acetate (See also *9035-69-2; 9012-09-3*)
9004-36-8. Cabufocon A
9004-38-0. Cellacefate
9004-51-7. Dextriferron
9004-53-9. Dextrin
9004-54-0. Dextran 40
9004-57-3. Ethylcellulose
9004-61-9. Hyaluronate Sodium [hyaluronic acid] (See also *9067-32-7*)
9004-62-0. Hydroxyethyl Cellulose
9004-64-2. Hydroxypropyl Cellulose
9004-65-3. Hydroxypropyl Methylcellulose 1828
9004-66-4. Iron Dextran
9004-67-5. Methylcellulose
9004-70-0. Pyroxylin
9004-74-4. Polyethylene Glycol Monomethyl Ether
9004-95-9. Cetomacrogol 1000
9004-96-0. Polyoxyl Oleate
9004-98-2. Polyoxyl 10 Oleyl Ether
9004-99-3. Polyoxyl 8 Stearate
9005-00-9. Polyoxyl Stearyl Ether
9005-25-8. Starch
9005-27-0. Hetastarch
9005-32-7. Alginic Acid
9005-36-1. Potassium Alginate
9005-38-3. Sodium Alginate (See also *9005-32-7*)
9005-49-6. Heparin Sodium [heparin] (See also *9041-08-1*)
9005-64-5. Polysorbate 20
9005-65-6. Polysorbate 80
9005-66-7. Polysorbate 40
9005-67-8. Polysorbate 60
9005-70-3. Polysorbate 85
9005-71-4. Polysorbate 65
9005-80-5. Inulin
9006-52-4. Albumin Tannate
9006-65-9. Dimethicone
9006-68-2. Polybenzarsol [replaced] (See also *54531-52-1*)

9007-12-9. Calcitonin (See also *47931-85-1; 21215-62-3*)
9007-43-6. Cytochrome C
9007-72-1. Ferric Carboxymaltose
9008-05-3. Histoplasmin
9008-11-1. Interferon
9009-29-4. Polyferose
9009-54-5. Polyurethane Foam
9009-65-8. Protamine Sulfate
9010-01-9. Sodium Amylosulfate
9010-34-8. Thyroglobulin
9010-53-1. Urogastrone
9011-01-2. Malethamer [replaced] (See also *67832-40-0; 29535-27-1[replaced]*)
9011-04-5. Hexadimethrine Bromide
9011-05-6. Polynoxylin
9011-93-2. Lysostaphin
9012-09-3. Cellulose Acetate [triacetate] (See also *9004-35-7; 9035-69-2*)
9012-54-8. Cellulase
9012-76-4. Poliglusam
9014-02-2. Zinostatin (See also *123760-07-6*)
9014-67-9. Aloxiprin
9014-89-5. Laureth 10S
9015-51-4. Silver Protein, Mild
9015-54-7. Protein Hydrolysate
9015-55-8. Lauromacrogol 400
9015-56-9. Polygeline
9015-62-7. Tolpovidone I 131
9015-68-3. Asparaginase
9015-73-0. Colextran
9016-01-7. Orgotein
9017-36-1. Polacrilin [replaced] (See also *50602-21-6*)
9026-00-0. Bucelipase Alfa
9031-11-2. Tilactase
9032-42-2. Hymetellose
9034-32-6. Psyllium Hemicellulose
9035-69-2. Cellulose Acetate [diacetate] (See also *9004-35-7; 9012-09-3*)
9039-53-6. Urokinase
9039-61-6. Batroxobin
9041-08-1. Ardeparin Sodium
9041-93-4. Bleomycin Sulfate (See also *11056-06-7*)
9042-14-2. Dextran Sulfate Sodium
9046-56-4. Ancrod
9048-49-1. Albumin, Iodinated I 125 Serum
9050-04-8. Carboxymethylcellulose Calcium
9050-67-3. Sizofiran
9050-75-3. Corticotropin Zinc Hydroxide
9067-32-7. Hyaluronate Sodium (See also *9004-61-9*)
9074-87-7. Glucarpidase
9087-70-1. Aprotinin (See also *12407-79-3; 11061-94-2*)
10001-13-5. Pexantel
10001-43-1. Pimefylline
10004-67-8. Amantocillin
10016-20-3. Alfadex
10018-19-6. Cotarnine Chloride (See also *82-54-2*)
10023-54-8. Aminoquinol
10024-97-2. Nitrous Oxide

10025-69-1. Stannous Chloride (See also *7772-99-8*)
10025-73-7. Chromic Chloride [anhydrous] (See also *10060-12-5*)
10025-77-1. Ferric Chloride
10025-82-8. Indium In 111 Chloride
10028-22-5. Ferric Sulfate [ferric tersulfate] (See also *142906-29-4*)
10028-24-7. Sodium Phosphate, Dibasic [dihydrate] (See also *10140-65-5; 10039-32-4; 7782-85-6; 118830-14-1; 7558-79-4*)
10034-96-5. Manganese Sulfate (See also *7785-87-7; 6485-39-8; 84368-35-4*)
10034-99-8. Magnesium Sulfate (See also *7487-88-9*)
10035-04-8. Calcium Chloride (See also *10043-52-4*)
10039-32-4. Sodium Phosphate, Dibasic [dodecahydrate] (See also *10140-65-5; 7782-85-6; 10028-24-7; 118830-14-1; 7558-79-4*)
10040-34-3. Sodium Picosulfate [picosulfuric acid] (See also *10040-45-6*)
10040-45-6. Sodium Picosulfate (See also *10040-34-3*)
10041-19-7. Docusate Calcium [1,4-bis(2-ethylhexyl)sulfosuccinate] (See also *128-49-4*)
10043-01-3. Aluminum Sulfate [anhydrous] (See also *17927-65-0*)
10043-35-3. Boric Acid
10043-49-9. Gold Au 198
10043-52-4. Calcium Chloride [anhydrous] (See also *10035-04-8*)
10043-67-1. Alum, Potassium [anhydrous] (See also *7784-24-9*)
10049-21-5. Sodium Phosphate, Monobasic [monohydrate] (See also *7558-80-7; 13472-35-0*)
10060-12-5. Chromic Chloride (See also *10025-73-7*)
10061-32-2. Levophenacylmorphan
10072-48-7. Acefurtiamine
10078-46-3. Roletamide
10085-81-1. Benzoctamine Hydrochloride (See also *17243-39-9*)
10087-89-5. Enpromate
10101-41-4. Calcium Sulfate [dihydrate] (See also *7778-18-9*)
10101-89-0. Sodium Phosphate, Tribasic [dodecahydrate] (See also *7601-54-9*)
10102-17-7. Sodium Thiosulfate (See also *7772-98-7*)
10102-43-9. Nitric Oxide
10112-91-1. Calomel
10116-22-0. Demegestone
10118-85-1. Lydimycin
10118-90-8. Minocycline
10124-48-8. Mercury, Ammoniated
10125-13-0. Cupric Chloride (See also *7447-39-4*)
10140-65-5. Sodium Phosphate, Dibasic (See also *10039-32-4; 7782-85-6; 10028-24-7; 118830-14-1; 7558-79-4*)
10161-33-8. Trenbolone Acetate [trenbolone] (See also *10161-34-9*)

10161-34-9. Trenbolone Acetate (See also *10161-33-8*)

10163-15-2. Sodium Monofluorophosphate

10189-94-3. Bepiastine

10202-40-1. Flutizenol

10206-21-0. Cephacetrile Sodium [cephacetrile] (See also *23239-41-0*)

10226-54-7. Lomifylline

10233-87-1. Magnesium Phosphate (See also *7757-87-1*)

10236-81-4. Prifinium Bromide [prifinium] (See also *4630-95-9*)

10238-21-8. Glyburide

10246-75-0. Hydroxyzine Pamoate (See also *68-88-2*)

10262-69-8. Maprotiline

10310-32-4. Tribenoside

10318-26-0. Mitolactol

10321-12-7. Propizepine

10322-73-3. Estrofurate

10328-35-5. Benzododecinium Chloride [benzododecinium] (See also *139-07-1*)

10329-60-9. Dioxifedrine

10331-57-4. Niclofolan

10347-81-6. Maprotiline Hydrochloride

10351-50-5. Leniquinsin

10355-14-3. Boxidine

10375-56-1. Chlormerodrin Hg 197

10379-11-0. Nortetrazepam

10379-14-3. Tetrazepam

10389-72-7. Clortermine Hydrochloride (See also *10389-73-8*)

10389-73-8. Clortermine Hydrochloride [clortermine] (See also *10389-72-7*)

10397-75-8. Iocarmate Meglumine [iocarmic acid] (See also *54605-45-7; 6284-40-8*)

10402-90-1. Eprazinone

10403-51-7. Mitindomide

10405-02-4. Trospium Chloride

10417-94-4. Icosapent

10418-03-8. Stanozolol

10423-37-7. Citenamide

10433-71-3. Tiametonium Iodide

10447-39-9. Quifenadine

10448-84-7. Nitromifene

10448-96-1. Almestrone

10456-04-9. Carbon Monoxide C 11

10457-66-6. Geroquinol

10457-90-6. Bromperidol

10457-91-7. Seperidol Hydrochloride [seperidol] (See also *17230-87-4*)

10488-36-5. Tofenacin Hydrochloride (See also *15301-93-6*)

10489-23-3. Tioctilate

10500-82-0. Famotine Hydrochloride (See also *18429-78-2*)

10539-19-2. Moxaverine

10540-29-1. Tamoxifen Citrate [tamoxifen] (See also *54965-24-1*)

10540-97-3. Memotine Hydrochloride (See also *18429-69-1*)

10549-91-4. Meclorisone Dibutyrate (See also *4732-48-3*)

10563-70-9. Melitracen Hydrochloride (See also *5118-29-6*)

10571-59-2. Nicoclonate

10572-34-6. Cicliomenol

10580-19-5. Phenolsulphonate Sodium

10592-65-1. Quingestanol Acetate [quingestanol] (See also *3000-39-3*)

10596-23-3. Clodronic Acid

11003-38-6. Capreomycin Sulfate [capreomycin] (See also *1405-37-4*)

11006-70-5. Olivomycin

11006-76-1. Mikamycin

11006-77-2. Statolon

11011-72-6. Bluensomycin

11014-70-3. Levorin

11015-37-5. Bambermycins

11018-89-6. Ouabain (See also *630-60-4*)

11029-70-2. Heliomycin

11032-41-0. Ergoloid Mesylates [dihydroergotoxine] (See also *8067-24-1*)

11033-34-4. Steffimycin

11041-12-6. Cholestyramine Resin

11042-64-1. Gamma Oryzanol

11043-98-4. Mitocromin

11043-99-5. Mitomalcin

11048-13-8. Nebramycin

11048-15-0. Kalafungin

11051-71-1. Avilamycin (See also *69787-79-7; 69787-80-0*)

11056-06-7. Bleomycin Sulfate [bleomycin] (See also *9041-93-4*)

11056-09-0. Ranimycin

11056-11-4. Biniramycin

11056-12-5. Cirolemycin

11056-13-6. Denofungin

11056-14-7. Mitocarcin

11056-15-8. Mitosper

11056-16-9. Nifungin

11056-18-1. Scopafungin

11056-20-5. Zorbamycin

11061-68-0. Insulin Human

11061-94-2. Aprotinin [ox pancreas basic reduced] (See also *9087-70-1; 12407-79-3*)

11070-73-8. Insulin [ox] (See also *12584-58-6*)

11071-15-1. Antimony Potassium Tartrate [anhydrous] (See also *28300-74-5*)

11091-62-6. Insulin Defalan [porcine] (See also *51798-72-2*)

11096-49-4. Partricin

11096-79-0. Alamecin

11097-68-0. Aluminum Sesquichlorohydrate

11115-82-5. Enramycin

11121-32-7. Mepartricin

11178-99-9. Neticonazole [replaced] (See also *130726-68-0; 130773-02-3*)

12002-30-1. Piperazine Edetate Calcium (See also *50322-15-1; 110-85-0; 60-00-4*)

12011-77-7. Dihydroxyaluminum Sodium Carbonate (See also *16482-55-6; 539-68-4*)

12040-73-2. Sucralox

12042-91-0. Aluminum Chlorohydrate [dihydrate] (See also *1327-41-9*)

12054-85-2. Ammonium Molybdate

12111-24-9. Pentetate Calcium Trisodium (See also *67-43-6*)

12125-02-9. Ammonium Chloride

12125-11-0. Almadrate Sulfate

12141-46-7. Aluminum Silicate, Natural

12167-74-7. Calcium Phosphate, Tribasic

12182-48-8. Glucalox

12192-57-3. Aurothioglucose

12211-28-8. Sutilains

12214-50-5. Sodium Glucaspaldrate

12244-57-4. Gold Sodium Thiomalate (See also *70-49-5*)

12262-77-0. Spirobarbital Sodium (See also *72035-36-0*)

12286-76-9. Ferric Fructose

12304-65-3. Hydrotalcite

12389-15-0. Ferrous Gluconate (See also *299-29-6; 526-95-4*)

12407-79-3. Aprotinin [ox pancreas basic] (See also *9087-70-1; 11061-94-2*)

12408-47-8. Silodrate

12542-33-5. Ictasol

12550-17-3. Sodium Antimonylgluconate

12569-38-9. Calcium Glubionate (See also *31959-85-0*)

12584-58-6. Insulin [pig] (See also *11070-73-8*)

12607-92-0. Aceglutamide Aluminum (See also *2490-97-3*)

12629-01-5. Somatropin

12650-69-0. Mupirocin

12678-07-8. Danaparoid Sodium [chondroitin, 6-(hydrogen sulfate), sodium salt] (See also *57459-72-0; 54328-33-5; 39455-18-0*)

12772-35-9. Butirosin Sulfate [butirosin] (See also *51022-98-1; 57549-48-1*)

13007-85-7. Gluceptate Sodium (See also *87-74-1*)

13007-93-7. Cuproxoline

13009-99-9. Mafenide Acetate

13010-47-4. Lomustine

13021-53-9. Terbuprol

13029-44-2. Dienestrol [*E,E*] (See also *84-17-3*)

13050-83-4. Guanoxyfen Sulfate [guanoxyfen] (See also *1021-11-0*)

13051-01-9. Carbazochrome Salicylate

13055-82-8. Reproterol Hydrochloride (See also *54063-54-6*)

13058-67-8. Lucimycin

13071-11-9. Dexpropranolol Hydrochloride (See also *5051-22-9*)

13074-00-5. Azastene

13085-08-0. Mazipredone

13087-53-1. Iothalamate Meglumine (See also *2276-90-6; 6284-40-8*)

13093-88-4. Perimetazine

13103-34-9. Boldenone Undecylenate (See also *846-48-0*)

13115-03-2. Cyanocobalamin Co 57 (See also *41559-38-0*)

13157-90-9. Benzquercin

13182-89-3. Metronidazole [benzoate] (See also *443-48-1*)

13189-98-5. Fudosteine

13215-10-6. Demeclocycline [sesquihydrate] (See also *127-33-3*)

13221-27-7. Tribuzone

13237-70-2. Fosmenic Acid

13242-44-9. Captamine Hydrochloride (See also *108-02-1*)

13246-02-1. Febarbamate

13254-33-6. Carpronium Chloride

13292-46-1. Rifampin

13311-84-7. Flutamide

13355-00-5. Melarsonyl Potassium (See also *37526-80-0*)

13364-32-4. Clobenzorex

13369-07-8. Sulfatrozole

13392-18-2. Fenoterol

13392-28-4. Rimantadine Hydrochloride [rimantadine] (See also *1501-84-4*)

13402-51-2. Tibenzate

13409-53-5. Podilfen

13410-86-1. Aconiazide

13411-16-0. Nifurpirinol

13412-64-1. Dicloxacillin Sodium (See also *343-55-5; 3116-76-5*)

13422-16-7. Triflocin

13422-51-0. Hydroxocobalamin

13422-53-2. Cyanocobalamin Co 60 [vitamin B₁₂-⁶⁰Co]

13422-55-4. Mecobalamin

13425-92-8. Amiquinsin Hydrochloride [amiquinsin] (See also *7125-70-4; 1696-79-3*)

13425-98-4. Improsulfan

13445-12-0. Iobutoic Acid

13445-63-1. Itramin Tosylate

13446-34-9. Manganese Chloride (See also *7773-01-5*)

13447-95-5. Methaniazide

13448-22-1. Clorotepine

13456-08-1. Bitipazone

13460-98-5. Theodrenaline

13461-01-3. Aceprometazine

13463-41-7. Pyrithione Zinc

13463-43-9. Ferrous Sulfate, Dried (See also *7720-78-7*)

13463-67-7. Titanium Dioxide

13471-78-8. Beclotiamine

13472-35-0. Sodium Phosphate, Monobasic [dihydrate] (See also *7558-80-7; 10049-21-5*)

13473-38-6. Pipenzolate Bromide [pipenzolate] (See also *125-51-9*)

13479-13-5. Pargeverine

13492-01-8. Tranylcypromine Sulfate (See also *7081-36-9; 155-09-9*)

13494-90-1. Gallium Nitrate [anhydrous] (See also *135886-70-3*)

13495-09-5. Piminodine Esylate [piminodine] (See also *7081-52-9*)

13523-86-9. Pindolol

13539-59-8. Apazone

13551-87-6. Misonidazole

13563-60-5. Norgesterone

13583-21-6. Norclostebol

13609-67-1. Hydrocortisone Butyrate

13614-98-7. Minocycline Hydrochloride (See also *10118-90-8*)

13642-52-9. Soterenol Hydrochloride [soterenol] (See also *14816-67-2*)

13647-35-3. Trilostane

13655-52-2. Alprenolol Hydrochloride [alprenolol] (See also *13707-88-5*)

13665-88-8. Mopidamol

13669-70-0. Nefopam Hydrochloride [nefopam] (See also *23327-57-3*)

13682-92-3. Dihydroxyaluminum Aminoacetate [anhydrous] (See also *41354-48-7; 56-40-6*)

13696-15-6. Benzopyrronium Bromide

13698-49-2. Delmadinone Acetate (See also *15262-77-8*)

13707-88-5. Alprenolol Hydrochloride (See also *13655-52-2*)

13710-19-5. Tolfenamic Acid

13717-04-9. Propiram Fumarate (See also *15686-91-6*)

13725-16-1. Isoetharine [replaced] (See also *530-08-5; 32095-14-0*)

13739-02-1. Diacerein

13741-18-9. Xibornol

13752-33-5. Panidazole

13755-38-9. Sodium Nitroprusside (See also *14402-89-2*)

13757-97-6. Quinterenol Sulfate [quinterenol] (See also *13758-23-1*)

13758-23-1. Quinterenol Sulfate (See also *13757-97-6*)

13799-03-6. Protizinic Acid

13838-08-9. Azidamfenicol

13838-16-9. Enflurane

13862-07-2. Difemetorex

13870-90-1. Cobamamide

13877-99-1. Minepentate

13885-31-9. Orestrate

13898-58-3. Benzoylpas Calcium [benzoylpas] (See also *5631-00-5; 528-96-1*)

13900-14-6. Domiphen Bromide [domiphen] (See also *538-71-6*)

13909-09-6. Semustine

13912-77-1. Octacaine

13912-80-6. Nicoboxil

13930-27-3. Oxtriphylline [replaced] (See also *4499-40-5*)

13930-34-2. Clormecaine

13931-64-1. Procymate

13946-02-6. Iproheptine

13956-29-1. Nabiximols [(A) CBD] (See also *1972-08-3*)

13957-36-3. Meladrazine

13957-38-5. Hydrobentizide

13958-40-2. Oxiramide

13967-73-2. Strontium Sr 85

13977-28-1. Embramine Hydrochloride (See also *3565-72-8*)

13977-33-8. Demelverine

13980-94-4. Metaglycodol

13993-65-2. Metiazinic Acid

13997-19-8. Nequinate

14007-49-9. Ambutonium Bromide [ambutonium] (See also *115-51-5*)

14007-53-5. Fenpipramide [hydrochloride] (See also *77-01-0*)

14007-64-8. Butetamate

14008-44-7. Metopimazine

14008-46-9. Pinoxepin Hydrochloride (See also *14008-66-3*)

14008-48-1. Bisoxatin Acetate (See also *17692-24-9*)

14008-60-7. Cresotamide

14008-66-3. Pinoxepin Hydrochloride [pinoxepin] (See also *14008-46-9*)

14008-71-0. Xanthiol Hydrochloride [xanthiol] (See also *17162-32-2*)

14009-24-6. Drotaverine

14028-44-5. Amoxapine

14038-43-8. Prussian Blue Insoluble

14055-89-1. Isobucaine Hydrochloride [isobucaine] (See also *3562-15-0*)

14058-90-3. Metazamide

14066-79-6. Chloroprednisone Acetate (See also *52080-57-6*)

14088-71-2. Proclonol

14089-84-0. Proxibutene

14107-37-0. Alfadolone

14144-06-0. Disogluside

14149-43-0. Trimethidinium Methosulfate (See also *2624-50-2*)

14166-26-8. Taglutimide

14176-10-4. Cetiedil Citrate [cetiedil] (See also *16286-69-4*)

14176-49-9. Tiletamine Hydrochloride [tiletamine] (See also *14176-50-2*)

14176-50-2. Tiletamine Hydrochloride (See also *14176-49-9*)

14214-84-7. Oxyphenonium Bromide [oxyphenonium] (See also *50-10-2*)

14222-46-9. Pyritidium Bromide (See also *3616-05-5*)

14222-60-7. Protionamide

14235-86-0. Hydrargaphen

14252-80-3. Bupivacaine Hydrochloride (See also *2180-92-9; 18010-40-7*)

14255-87-9. Parbendazole

14261-75-7. Cloforex

14262-80-7. Sodium Sulfate S 35

14286-84-1. Bencyclane Fumarate (See also *2179-37-5*)

14289-25-9. Diproleandomycin

14293-44-8. Xipamide

14320-04-8. Ciaftalan Zinc

14334-40-8. Pramiverine

14336-71-1. Calcium Chloride Ca 45

14357-78-9. Diprenorphine

14368-24-2. Trocimine

14376-16-0. Sulfaloxic Acid

14402-89-2. Sodium Nitroprusside [anhydrous] (See also *13755-38-9*)

14405-05-1. Alphaprodine Hydrochloride [stereononspecific] (See also *561-78-4; 77-20-3*)

14417-88-0. Melinamide

14437-41-3. Clioxanide

14461-91-7. Cyclazodone

14484-47-0. Deflazacort

14504-73-5. Tritoqualine

14516-56-4. Perazine Fendizoate [perazine maleate] (See also *84-97-9*)

14521-96-1. Etorphine

14538-56-8. Piperazine Phosphate [anhydrous] (See also *18534-18-4; 110-85-0*)

14543-09-0. Cobaltous Chloride Co 60

14556-46-8. Bupranolol

14561-42-3. Menoctone

14587-50-9. Difeterol

14611-51-9. Selegiline

14611-52-0. Selegiline Hydrochloride (See also *14611-51-9*)

14613-01-5. Aluminum Clofibrate (See also *882-09-7*)

14613-30-0. Magnesium Clofibrate

14636-12-5. Terlipressin

14639-25-9. Chromium Picolinate

14641-21-5. Aluminoparaaminosalicylate Calcium [anhydrous]

14663-23-1. Dantrolene Sodium [anhydrous] (See also *24868-20-0; 7261-97-4*)

14679-68-6. Diotyrosine I 131

14679-73-3. Todralazine

14694-69-0. Iridium Ir 192

14698-29-4. Oxolinic Acid

14728-33-7. Teroxalene Hydrochloride [teroxalene] (See also *3845-22-5*)

14745-50-7. Meletimide

14759-04-7. Oxyridazine

14759-06-9. Sulforidazine

14769-73-4. Levamisole Hydrochloride [levamisole] (See also *16595-80-5*)

14769-74-5. Dexamisole

14779-78-3. Padimate A

14783-68-7. Magnesium Glycinate

14785-50-3. Tiapirinol

14796-24-8. Cinperene

14796-28-2. Clodanolene

14807-96-6. Talc

14816-18-3. Phoxim

14816-67-2. Soterenol Hydrochloride (See also *13642-52-9*)

14817-09-5. Decimemide

14838-15-4. Phenylpropanolamine Hydrochloride [phenylpropanolamine] (See also *154-41-6*)

14842-81-0. Potassium Aspartate and Magnesium Aspartate (See also *8000-90-6; 56-84-8*)

14855-77-7. Diatrizoate Sodium I 131

14860-49-2. Clobutinol

14882-18-9. Bismuth Subsalicylate (See also *87-27-4*)

14885-29-1. Ipronidazole

14929-11-4. Simfibrate

14932-42-4. Xenon Xe 133

14976-57-9. Clemastine Fumarate (See also *15686-51-8*)

14984-34-0. Sodium Glucuronate

14987-04-3. Magnesium Trisilicate [anhydrous] (See also *39365-87-2*)

14992-59-7. Sodium Dibunate

15037-44-2. Ethonam Nitrate [ethonam] (See also *15037-55-5*)

15037-55-5. Ethonam Nitrate (See also *15037-44-2*)

15130-91-3. Sultroponium

15145-14-9. Ciclactate

15176-29-1. Edoxudine

15179-96-1. Nifurimide

15179-97-2. Estrazinol Hydrobromide (See also *5941-36-6*)

15180-00-4. Prednival

15180-02-6. Amfonelic Acid

15180-03-7. Alcuronium Chloride

15221-81-5. Fludorex

15228-71-4. Vinrosidine Sulfate [vinrosidine] (See also *18556-44-0*)

15250-13-2. Araprofen

15251-48-6. Oxytetracycline Calcium (See also *79-57-2*)

15256-58-3. Beloxamide

15262-77-8. Delmadinone Acetate [delmadinone] (See also *13698-49-2*)

15301-40-3. Actinoquinol Sodium [actinoquinol] (See also *7246-07-3*)

15301-45-8. Antafenite

15301-48-1. Bezitramide

15301-50-5. Cloponone

15301-52-7. Cyclexanone

15301-54-9. Cypenamine Hydrochloride [cypenamine] (See also *5588-23-8*)

15301-67-4. Feneritrol

15301-69-6. Flavoxate Hydrochloride [flavoxate] (See also *3717-88-2*)

15301-80-1. Oxamarin Hydrochloride [oxamarin] (See also *6830-17-7*)

15301-82-3. Pecocycline

15301-88-9. Pytamine

15301-89-0. Quillifoline

15301-93-6. Tofenacin Hydrochloride [tofenacin] (See also *10488-36-5*)

15301-96-9. Thyromedan Hydrochloride [thyromedan] (See also *57-65-8*)

15301-97-0. Xylocoumarol

15302-00-8. Acefylline Piperazine [replaced] (See also *18833-13-1*)

15302-05-3. Butoxylate

15302-10-0. Clibucaine

15302-12-2. Dimelazine

15302-15-5. Etosalamide

15302-16-6. Fenozolone

15302-18-8. Formetorex

15307-79-6. Diclofenac Sodium

15307-81-0. Diclofenac Potassium (See also *15307-86-5*)

15307-86-5. Diclofenac Potassium [diclofenac] (See also *15307-81-0*)

15311-77-0. Cloxypendyl

15318-45-3. Thiamphenicol

15339-50-1. Ferrotrenine

15350-99-9. Amoxydramine Camsilate

15351-04-9. Becanthone Hydrochloride [becanthone] (See also *5591-22-0*)

15351-05-0. Buzepide Metiodide

15351-09-4. Metamfepramone

15351-13-0. Nicofuranose

15356-70-4. Racementhol

15378-99-1. Anazocine

15387-10-7. Niprofazone

15387-18-5. Fezatione

15421-84-8. Trapidil

15468-10-7. Oxidronic Acid

15489-16-4. Stibophen (See also *23940-36-5; 16028-21-0*)

15500-66-0. Pancuronium Bromide

15518-76-0. Cyproximide

15518-82-8. Metescufylline

15518-84-0. Mobecarb

15518-87-3. Myralact

15534-05-1. Pipratecol

15534-92-6. Terbuficin

15537-76-5. Chlorproguanil Hydrochloride (See also *537-21-3*)

15574-49-9. Mecarbinate

15574-96-6. Pizotyline

15578-26-4. Stannous Pyrophosphate

15585-43-0. Rivanicline Galactarate [rivanicline] (See also *675132-86-2*)

15585-70-3. Bibenzonium Bromide (See also *59866-76-1*)

15585-71-4. Brometenamine

15585-86-1. Cyprodenate

15585-88-3. Dicarfen

15590-00-8. Etamocycline

15599-22-1. Cyclopyrronium Bromide

15599-26-5. Droxypropine

15599-27-6. Etaminile

15599-36-7. Halethazole

15599-37-8. Hexapradol

15599-39-0. Noxytiolin

15599-44-7. Spirotriazine Hydrochloride [spirotriazine]

15599-45-8. Symetine Hydrochloride [symetine] (See also *5585-62-6*)

15599-51-6. Apicycline

15599-52-7. Broquinaldol

15622-65-8. Molindone Hydrochloride (See also *7416-34-4*)

15639-50-6. Safingol

15663-27-1. Cisplatin

15676-16-1. Sulpiride

15678-91-8. Krypton Kr 81m

15686-23-4. Trimoxamine Hydrochloride [trimoxamine] (See also *7082-27-1*)

15686-27-8. Amfepentorex

15686-33-6. Biclotymol

15686-38-1. Carbazocine

15686-51-8. Clemastine

15686-60-9. Flavamine

15686-61-0. Fenproporex

15686-63-2. Etabenzarone

15686-68-7. Volazocine

15686-71-2. Cephalexin [anhydrous] (See also *23325-78-2*)

15686-72-3. Tibrofan

15686-74-5. Cyclophenazine Hydrochloride (See also *17692-26-1*)

15686-76-7. Bensalan

15686-77-8. Fursalan

15686-78-9. Thiosalan

15686-81-4. Norbudrine

15686-83-6. Pyrantel Pamoate [pyrantel] (See also *22204-24-6*)

15686-87-0. Pifenate

15686-91-6. Propiram Fumarate [propiram] (See also *13717-04-9*)

15686-97-2. Pyrroliphene Hydrochloride [pyrroliphene] (See also *5591-44-6*)

15686-98-3. Racefemine [replaced] (See also *22232-57-1*)

15687-05-5. Cloracetadol

15687-07-7. Cyprazepam

15687-08-8. Dextrofemine

15687-09-9. Difebarbamate

15687-13-5. Dodeclonium Bromide

15687-14-6. Embutramide

15687-16-8. Carbiphene Hydrochloride [carbiphene] (See also *467-22-1*)

15687-18-0. Fenpentadiol

15687-21-5. Flumedroxone

15687-22-6. Folescutol

15687-23-7. Guaiactamine

15687-27-1. Ibuprofen (See also *58560-75-1*)

15687-33-9. Metindizate

15687-37-3. Naftazone

15687-41-9. Oxyfedrine

15690-55-8. Zuclomiphene

15690-57-0. Enclomiphene

15690-63-8. Cesium Chloride Cs 131

15708-41-5. Sodium Feredetate

15722-48-2. Olsalazine Sodium [olsalazine] (See also *6054-98-4*)

15769-77-4. Nalidixate Sodium (See also *3374-05-8; 389-08-2*)

15790-02-0. Tropodifene

15793-38-1. Quinazosin Hydrochloride [quinazosin] (See also *7262-00-2*)

15793-40-5. Terodiline Hydrochloride [terodiline] (See also *7082-21-5*)

15825-70-4. Mannitol Hexanitrate

15826-37-6. Cromolyn Sodium (See also *16110-51-3*)

15845-96-2. Diflucortolone Pivalate

15845-98-4. Iothalamate Sodium I 131

15866-90-7. Incyclinide

15876-67-2. Distigmine Bromide

15879-93-3. Chloralose

15905-32-5. Erythrosine Sodium [erythrosine, phenolic] (See also *49746-10-3; 568-63-8; 16423-68-0*)

15922-78-8. Pyrithione Sodium

15949-72-1. Prazocillin

15992-13-9. Intrazole

15997-76-9. Nonaperone

16008-36-9. Methyldesorphine

16024-67-2. Iotrizoic Acid

16028-21-0. Stibophen [replaced] (See also *15489-16-4; 23940-36-5*)

16034-77-8. Iocetamic Acid

16037-91-5. Sodium Stibogluconate

16051-77-7. Isosorbide Mononitrate

16110-51-3. Cromolyn Sodium [cromolyn] (See also *15826-37-6*)

16112-96-2. Indanorex

16188-61-7. Talastine

16208-51-8. Dimesna

16231-75-7. Atolide

16259-34-0. Penimocycline

16284-59-6. Chromic Chloride Cr 51

16286-69-4. Cetiedil Citrate (See also *14176-10-4*)

16291-05-7. Nalmexone Hydrochloride [replaced] (See also *16676-27-0; 16676-26-9*)

16291-96-6. Charcoal, Activated

16320-04-0. Gestrinone (See also *40542-65-2*)

16378-21-5. Piroheptine

16401-80-2. Delmetacin

16413-89-1. Cobaltous Chloride Co 57

16423-68-0. Erythrosine Sodium [anhydrous, closed form] (See also *49746-10-3; 568-63-8; 15905-32-5*)

16426-83-8. Niometacin

16449-54-0. Aluminum Flufenamate

16469-74-2. Hydromadinone

16482-55-6. Dihydroxyaluminum Sodium Carbonate [coordination complex] (See also *12011-77-7; 539-68-4*)

16485-05-5. Oxadimedine Hydrochloride [oxadimedine] (See also *6314-69-8*)

16485-10-2. Panthenol

16488-48-5. *p*-Butylaminobenzoyldiethylaminoethyl Hydrochloride

16498-21-8. Oxaflumazine

16506-27-7. Bendamustine Hydrochloride [bendamustine] (See also *3543-75-7*)

16509-11-8. Otimerate Sodium

16543-10-5. Fosenazide

16545-11-2. Guamecycline

16549-56-7. Homprenorphine

16550-22-4. Cyprenorphine Hydrochloride (See also *4406-22-8*)

16562-98-4. Clantifen

16590-41-3. Naltrexone

16595-80-5. Levamisole Hydrochloride (See also *14769-73-4*)

16624-40-1. Iotyrosine I 131

16662-47-8. Gallopamil

16676-26-9. Nalmexone Hydrochloride [nalmexone] (See also *16676-27-0; 16291-05-7*)

16676-27-0. Nalmexone Hydrochloride (See also *16291-05-7; 16676-26-9*)

16676-29-2. Naltrexone Hydrochloride

16679-58-6. Desmopressin Acetate [desmopressin] (See also *62357-86-2; 62288-83-9*)

16731-55-8. Potassium Metabisulfite

16759-59-4. Benoxafos

16773-42-5. Ornidazole

16781-39-8. Etasuline

16816-67-4. Pantethine

16852-81-6. Benzoclidine

16870-37-4. Amogastrin

16915-32-5. Sodium Gualenate [gualenic acid] (See also *6223-35-4*)

16915-70-1. Nifursol

16915-71-2. Cingestol

16915-78-9. Bolenol

16915-79-0. Mequidox

16915-80-3. Oxogestone Phenpropionate (See also *3643-00-3*)

16925-51-2. Aurothioglycanide

16941-32-5. Glucagon

16960-16-0. Cosyntropin

16985-03-8. Nonabine

17021-26-0. Calusterone

17033-82-8. Iomethin I 125

17033-83-9. Iomethin I 131

17034-35-4. Secretin [porcine] (See also *108153-74-8; 1393-25-5*)

17035-90-4. Tilarginine Acetate [tilarginine] (See also *53308-83-1*)

17048-39-4. Digalloyl Trioleate

17086-28-1. Doxycycline (See also *564-25-0*)

17088-72-1. Penoctonium Bromide

17090-79-8. Monensin

17097-76-6. Calcium Hopantenate [anhydrous]

17112-21-9. Sodium Chloride Na 22

17127-48-9. Glaziovine

17140-78-2. Propoxyphene Napsylate [anhydrous] (See also *26570-10-5; 23239-43-2; 469-62-5*)

17140-81-7. Nitrofurantoin [monohydrate] (See also *67-20-9*)

17146-95-1. Pentazocine Lactate (See also *359-83-1*)

17162-32-2. Xanthiol Hydrochloride (See also *14008-71-0*)

17162-39-9. Phenylephrine Bitartrate

17171-57-2. Metaraminol Bitartrate [replaced] (See also *33402-03-8; 54-49-9*)

17176-17-9. Ademetionine

17194-00-2. Barium Hydroxide Lime

17196-88-2. Vincofos

17199-54-1. Alphamethadol

17199-55-2. Betamethadol

17199-58-5. Alphacetylmethadol

17199-59-6. Betacetylmethadol

17211-15-3. Phytate Persodium

17226-75-4. Khelloside

17230-85-2. Amquinate

17230-86-3. Carbenicillin Potassium (See also *4697-36-3*)

17230-87-4. Seperidol Hydrochloride (See also *10457-91-7*)

17230-88-5. Danazol

17230-89-6. Nimazone

17243-32-2. Ketipramine Fumarate (See also *796-29-2*)

17243-33-3. Fepentolic Acid

17243-38-8. Azidocillin

17243-39-9. Benzoctamine Hydrochloride [benzoctamine] (See also *10085-81-1*)

17243-49-1. Diclometide

17243-56-0. Visnafylline

17243-57-1. Mefenorex Hydrochloride [mefenorex] (See also *5586-87-8*)

17243-64-0. Piprozolin

17243-65-1. Pirralkonium Bromide

17243-68-4. Taloximine

17243-70-8. Triclofylline

17259-75-5. Oxdralazine

17279-39-9. Dimetamfetamine

17289-49-5. Tetrydamine

17316-67-5. Butafosfan

17321-77-6. Clomipramine Hydrochloride (See also *303-49-1*)

17332-61-5. Isoprednidene

17365-01-4. Etiroxate

17411-19-7. Dicarbine

17440-83-4. Amiloride Hydrochloride (See also *2016-88-8; 2609-46-3*)

17560-51-9. Metolazone

17575-22-3. Lanatoside C

17590-01-1. Amfetaminil

17598-65-1. Deslanoside

17605-73-1. Colterol Mesylate (See also *18866-78-9*)

17617-23-1. Flurazepam Hydrochloride [flurazepam] (See also *1172-18-5*)

17650-98-5. Ceruletide

17671-49-1. Olaflur [olaflur base] (See also *6818-37-7*)

17692-15-8. Furazolium Tartrate

17692-20-5. Cyclobutoic Acid

17692-22-7. Metizoline Hydrochloride [metizoline] (See also *5090-37-9*)

17692-23-8. Bentipimine

17692-24-9. Bisoxatin Acetate [bisoxatin] (See also *14008-48-1*)

17692-26-1. Cyclophenazine Hydrochloride [cyclophenazine] (See also *15686-74-5*)

17692-28-3. Clonazoline

17692-30-7. Diniprofylline

17692-31-8. Dropropizine

17692-34-1. Etodroxizine

17692-35-2. Etofuradine

17692-37-4. Fantridone Hydrochloride [fantridone] (See also *24390-12-3; 22461-13-8*)

17692-38-5. Fluprofen

17692-39-6. Fomocaine

17692-43-2. Picodralazine

17692-45-4. Quatacaine

17692-51-2. Metergoline

17692-54-5. Mitoclomine

17692-56-7. Moxicoumone

17692-62-5. Norleusactide

17692-63-6. Oxitefonium Bromide

17692-71-6. Vanitiolide

17692-74-9. Iothalamate Sodium I 125

17693-51-5. Promethazine Teoclate

17716-89-1. Pranosal

17737-65-4. Clonixin

17737-68-7. Diclonixin

17780-72-2. Clorgiline

17784-12-2. Sulfacytine

17854-59-0. Mepixanox

17902-23-7. Tegafur

17927-65-0. Aluminum Sulfate (See also *10043-01-3*)

17969-20-9. Fenclozic Acid

17969-45-8. Brofezil

18010-40-7. Bupivacaine Hydrochloride [anhydrous] (See also *14252-80-3; 2180-92-9*)

18016-80-3. Lisuride

18046-21-4. Fentiazac

18053-31-1. Fominoben

18109-80-3. Butamirate Citrate [butamirate] (See also *18109-81-4*)

18109-81-4. Butamirate Citrate (See also *18109-80-3*)

18118-80-4. Oxisopred

18174-58-8. Pipoxolan Hydrochloride (See also *23744-24-3*)

18181-70-9. Iodofenphos

18195-32-9. Cyanocobalamin Co 58

18296-44-1. Valtrate

18296-45-2. Didrovaltrate

18323-44-9. Clindamycin

18356-28-0. Rolziracetam

18365-82-7. Calcium Lactophosphate [lactophosphoric acid] (See also *7546-28-3*)

18378-89-7. Plicamycin

18429-69-1. Memotine Hydrochloride [memotine] (See also *10540-97-3*)

18429-78-2. Famotine Hydrochloride [famotine] (See also *10500-82-0*)

18464-39-6. Caroxazone

18467-77-1. Diprogulic Acid

18471-20-0. Ditazole

18472-51-0. Chlorhexidine Gluconate (See also *55-56-1*)

18481-23-7. Bisbutytiamine

18493-30-6. Metochalcone

18497-67-1. Ferric Chloride Fe 59

18507-89-6. Decoquinate

18534-18-4. Piperazine Phosphate (See also *14538-56-8; 110-85-0*)

18556-44-0. Vinrosidine Sulfate (See also *15228-71-4*)

18559-94-9. Albuterol

18588-57-3. Etoprine

18598-63-5. Mecysteine [hydrochloride] (See also *2485-62-3*)

18652-93-2. Methohexital

18656-21-8. Iodamide Meglumine (See also *440-58-4; 6284-40-8*)

18679-90-8. Hopantenic Acid

18683-91-5. Ambroxol (See also *23828-92-4*)

18694-40-1. Epirizole

18699-02-0. Actarit

18719-76-1. Keracyanin

18725-37-6. Dacisteine

18829-78-2. Levonordefrin [replaced] (See also *829-74-3*)

18833-13-1. Acefylline Piperazine (See also *15302-00-8*)

18840-47-6. Gepefrine

18841-58-2. Pipoctanone

18857-59-5. Nifurmazole

18866-78-9. Colterol Mesylate [colterol] (See also *17605-73-1*)

18883-66-4. Streptozocin

18910-65-1. Salmefamol

18917-89-0. Magnesium Salicylate [anhydrous] (See also *18917-95-8*)

18917-91-4. Aluminum Lactate

18917-95-8. Magnesium Salicylate (See also *18917-89-0*)

18965-97-4. Berlafenone

18966-32-0. Clocanfamide

18984-80-0. Euprocin Hydrochloride (See also *1301-42-4*)

19028-28-5. Toliodium Chloride

19056-26-9. Quindecamine Acetate [quindecamine] (See also *5714-05-6; 19146-62-4*)

19146-62-4. Quindecamine Acetate [anhydrous] (See also *5714-05-6; 19056-26-9*)

19171-19-8. Pomalidomide

19179-78-3. Xipranolol

19216-56-9. Prazosin Hydrochloride [prazosin] (See also *19237-84-4*)

19237-84-4. Prazosin Hydrochloride (See also *19216-56-9*)

19262-68-1. Dexmethylphenidate Hydrochloride (See also *40431-64-9*)

19281-29-9. Aptocaine

19291-69-1. Gestaclone

19356-17-3. Calcifediol [anhydrous] (See also *63283-36-3*)

19368-18-4. Ftaxilide

19379-90-9. Benzoxonium Chloride

19387-91-8. Tinidazole

19388-87-5. Taurolidine

19395-58-5. Moquizone

19410-02-7. Tropirine

19485-08-6. Cyproquinate

19486-61-4. Lauralkonium Chloride

19504-77-9. Pecilocin

19561-70-7. Nifuratrone

19562-30-2. Piromidic Acid

19705-61-4. Cicortonide

19767-45-4. Mesna (See also *3375-50-6*)

19794-93-5. Trazodone Hydrochloride [trazodone] (See also *25332-39-2*)

19825-63-9. Pirnabine (See also *68298-00-0*)

19863-06-0. Ioxotrizoic Acid

19877-89-5. Vincanol

19881-18-6. Nitroscanate

19885-51-9. Aranotin

19888-56-3. Fluazacort

19889-45-3. Guabenxan

19982-08-2. Memantine

19992-80-4. Butixirate

20047-75-0. Clogestone Acetate [clogestone] (See also *3044-32-4*)

20098-14-0. Idramantone

20123-80-2. Calcium Dobesilate (See also *88-46-0*)

20168-99-4. Cinmetacin

20170-20-1. Difenamizole

20187-55-7. Bendazac (See also *81919-14-4*)

20196-64-9. Liothyronine I 131 (See also *6893-02-3*)

20223-84-1. Mercaptomerin Sodium [mercaptomerin] (See also *21259-76-7*)

20228-27-7. Ruvazone

20229-30-5. Metitepine

20282-58-0. Tricosactide

20287-37-0. Fenquizone

20290-10-2. Morphine Glucuronide

20326-12-9. Mepiprazole

20326-13-0. Tolpiprazole

20380-58-9. Tilidine Hydrochloride [(±)-*trans*-tilidine] (See also *27107-79-5; 24357-97-9*)

20406-60-4. Mipimazole

20423-99-8. Deprodone

20432-69-3. Clorazepate Dipotassium [clorazepic acid] (See also *57109-90-7*)

20448-86-6. Bornaprine

20462-53-7. Deditonium Bromide [deditonium] (See also *2401-56-1*)

20537-88-6. Amifostine [anhydrous] (See also *112901-68-5*)

20559-55-1. Oxibendazole

20574-50-9. Morantel Tartrate [morantel] (See also *26155-31-7*)

20594-83-6. Nalbuphine Hydrochloride [nalbuphine] (See also *23277-43-2*)

20684-06-4. Bamifylline Hydrochloride (See also *2016-63-9*)

20788-07-2. Resorantel

20830-75-5. Digoxin

20830-81-3. Daunorubicin Hydrochloride [daunorubicin] (See also *23541-50-6*)

20977-50-8. Carperone

21031-72-1. Rubidium Chloride Rb 86

21059-46-1. Calcium L-Aspartate

21102-49-8. Volpristin

21102-82-9. Phendimetrazine Tartrate [replaced] (See also *50-58-8; 634-03-7*)

21132-59-2. Pazoxide

21187-98-4. Gliclazide

21208-26-4. Dimepregnen

21215-62-3. Calcitonin [human] (See also *47931-85-1; 9007-12-9*)

21216-78-4. Diphenylpiperidinomethyldioxolan Iodide

21221-18-1. Flazalone

21228-13-7. Dorastine Hydrochloride [dorastine] (See also *21228-28-4*)

21228-28-4. Dorastine Hydrochloride (See also *21228-13-7*)

21245-02-3. Padimate O

21256-18-8. Oxaprozin

21259-76-7. Mercaptomerin Sodium (See also *20223-84-1*)

21362-08-3. Colistimethate Sodium [replaced] (See also *8068-28-8*)

21362-69-6. Mepitiostane

21363-18-8. Viminol

21365-49-1. Tralonide

21370-21-8. Fenoxazoline Hydrochloride (See also *4846-91-7*)

21375-12-2. Moxestrol [replaced] (See also *34816-55-2*)

21411-53-0. Virginiamycin Factor M_1

21416-67-1. Razoxane [replaced] (See also *21416-87-5*)

21416-87-5. Razoxane (See also *21416-67-1*)

21434-91-3. Capobenate Sodium [capobenic acid] (See also *27276-25-1*)

21440-97-1. Brofoxine

21462-39-5. Clindamycin Hydrochloride (See also *58207-19-5; 18323-44-9*)

21466-07-9. Bromofenofos

21489-20-3. Talsupram

21498-08-8. Lofexidine Hydrochloride (See also *31036-80-3*)

21500-98-1. Tenocyclidine

21512-15-2. Citenazone

21535-47-7. Mianserin Hydrochloride (See also *24219-97-4*)

21560-58-7. Piquizil Hydrochloride [piquizil] (See also *23256-26-0*)

21560-59-8. Hoquizil Hydrochloride [hoquizil] (See also *23256-28-2*)

21590-91-0. Omidoline

21590-92-1. Etomidoline

21593-23-7. Cephapirin Sodium [cephapirin] (See also *24356-60-3*)

21626-89-1. Diftalone

21645-51-2. Aluminum Hydroxide

21649-57-0. Carbenicillin Phenyl Sodium (See also *27025-49-6*)

21662-79-3. Sulfacecole

21668-77-9. Eprodisate Disodium [eprodisate] (See also *36589-58-9*)

21679-14-1. Fludarabine Phosphate [fludarabine] (See also *75607-67-9*)

21686-10-2. Flupranone

21702-93-2. Cloguanamil

21715-46-8. Etifoxine

21721-92-6. Nitrefazole

21730-16-5. Metapramine

21736-83-4. Spectinomycin Hydrochloride [anhydrous] (See also *22189-32-8; 1695-77-8*)

21738-42-1. Oxamniquine

21755-66-8. Picoperine

21766-53-0. Iolidonic Acid

21791-39-9. Letimide Hydrochloride (See also *26513-90-6*)

21817-73-2. Bidimazium Iodide

21820-82-6. Fenpipalone

21829-22-1. Clonixeril

21829-25-4. Nifedipine

21888-98-2. Dexetimide

21908-53-2. Mercuric Oxide, Yellow

21919-05-1. Tretazicar

21925-88-2. Tesicam

22006-64-0. Tridecactide

22012-72-2. Zilantel

22013-23-6. Metoxepin

22033-87-0. Olesoxime

22059-60-5. Disopyramide Phosphate (See also *3737-09-5*)

22064-27-3. Penthienate Bromide [penthienate] (See also *60-44-6*)

22071-15-4. Ketoprofen

22089-22-1. Trofosfamide

22103-14-6. Bufeniode

22131-35-7. Butalamine

22131-79-9. Alclofenac

22136-26-1. Amedalin Hydrochloride [amedalin] (See also *22232-73-1*)

22136-27-2. Daledalin Tosylate [daledalin] (See also *23226-37-1; 30508-58-8*)

22150-28-3. Ipragratine

22151-68-4. Methohexital Sodium [replaced] (See also *309-36-4; 60634-69-7; 18652-93-2*)

22161-81-5. Dexketoprofen

22164-94-9. Suncillin Sodium [suncillin] (See also *23444-86-2*)

22189-31-7. Thiothixene Hydrochloride (See also *49746-09-0; 58513-59-0; 49746-04-5; 5591-45-7*)

22189-32-8. Spectinomycin Hydrochloride (See also *21736-83-4; 1695-77-8*)

22195-34-2. Guanadrel Sulfate (See also *40580-59-4*)

22199-08-2. Sulfadiazine, Silver (See also *68-35-9*)

22199-46-8. Clomacran Phosphate (See also *5310-55-4*)

22202-75-1. Cephaloglycin (See also *3577-01-3*)

22204-24-6. Pyrantel Pamoate (See also *15686-83-6*)

22204-29-1. Cetoxime Hydrochloride (See also *25394-78-9*)

22204-53-1. Naproxen

22204-91-7. Lifibrate

22232-54-8. Carbimazole

22232-57-1. Racefemine (See also *15686-98-3*)

22232-71-9. Mazindol

22232-73-1. Amedalin Hydrochloride (See also *22136-26-1*)

22248-79-9. Stirofos

22252-38-6. Methylprednisolone Sodium Phosphate [methylprednisolone 21-(dihydrogen phosphate)] (See also *5015-36-1*)

22254-24-6. Ipratropium Bromide [anhydrous] (See also *66985-17-9*)

22260-51-1. Bromocriptine Mesylate (See also *25614-03-3*)

22263-51-0. Nandrolone Cyclotate

22292-91-7. Naranol Hydrochloride [naranol] (See also *34256-91-2*)

22293-47-6. Feprosidnine

22298-29-9. Betamethasone Benzoate

22304-34-3. Amadinone Acetate (See also *30781-27-2*)

22316-47-8. Clobazam

22336-84-1. Metergotamine

22345-47-7. Tofisopam

22365-40-8. Triflubazam

22373-78-0. Monensin Sodium

22407-74-5. Bisobrin Lactate [bisobrin] (See also *24233-80-5*)

22443-11-4. Nepinalone

22457-89-2. Benfotiamine

22461-13-8. Fantridone Hydrochloride [anhydrous] (See also *24390-12-3; 17692-37-4*)

22484-64-6. Sulfanilate Zinc [anhydrous] (See also *31884-76-1; 121-57-3*)

22487-42-9. Benapryzine Hydrochloride [benapryzine] (See also *3202-55-9*)

22494-27-5. Flufenisal

22494-42-4. Diflunisal

22494-47-9. Clobuzarit

22500-92-1. Potassium Sorbate [(*E,E*)-sorbic acid] (See also *590-00-1; 24634-61-5; 110-44-1*)

22514-23-4. Fopirtoline

22521-79-5. Fenacetinol

22554-99-0. Sodium Fluoride F 18

22560-50-5. Clodronate Disodium [anhydrous]

22568-64-5. Diacetolol Hydrochloride [diacetolol] (See also *69796-04-9*)

22572-04-9. Codactide

22573-93-9. Alexidine (See also *22782-69-0*)

22609-73-0. Niludipine

22619-35-8. Tioclomarol

22632-06-0. Bupicomide

22661-76-3. Amoproxan

22662-39-1. Rafoxanide

22664-55-7. Metipranolol

22668-01-5. Etanidazole

22693-65-8. Olmidine

22730-86-5. Iolixanic Acid

22733-60-4. Siccanin

22736-85-2. Diflumidone Sodium [diflumidone] (See also *22737-01-5*)

22737-01-5. Diflumidone Sodium (See also *22736-85-2*)

22760-18-5. Proquazone

22782-69-0. Alexidine [replaced] (See also *22573-93-9*)

22790-84-7. Carbantel Lauryl Sulfate [carbantel] (See also *54644-15-4*)

22832-87-7. Miconazole Nitrate (See also *22916-47-8*)

22839-47-0. Aspartame (See also *53906-69-7*)

22855-57-8. Brosuximide

22881-35-2. Famprofazone

22888-70-6. Silibinin

22916-47-8. Miconazole

22933-72-8. Salazodine

22950-29-4. Dimetofrine

22994-85-0. Benznidazole

23023-91-8. Flucrylate

23031-25-6. Terbutaline Sulfate [terbutaline] (See also *23031-32-5*)

23031-32-5. Terbutaline Sulfate (See also *23031-25-6*)

23047-25-8. Lofepramine Hydrochloride [lofepramine] (See also *26786-32-3*)

23049-93-6. Enfenamic Acid

23067-13-2. Erythromycin Gluceptate (See also *114-07-8*)

23076-35-9. Xylazine Hydrochloride

23089-26-1. Levomenol

23092-17-3. Halazepam

23110-15-8. Fumagillin

23111-34-4. Feclobuzone

23142-01-0. Carbetapentane Citrate (See also *77-23-6*)

23152-29-6. Virginiamycin Factor S

23155-02-4. Fosfomycin

23163-42-0. Methynodiol Diacetate [methynodiol] (See also *23163-51-1*)

23163-51-1. Methynodiol Diacetate (See also *23163-42-0*)

23205-04-1. Iosulamide Meglumine [iosulamide] (See also *63534-64-5; 6284-40-8*)

23210-56-2. Ifenprodil

23214-92-8. Doxorubicin

23226-37-1. Daledalin Tosylate (See also *30508-58-8; 22136-27-2*)

23233-88-7. Brotianide

23239-36-3. Deterenol Hydrochloride (See also *3506-31-8*)

23239-37-4. Etoxadrol Hydrochloride (See also *28189-85-7*)

23239-41-0. Cephacetrile Sodium (See also *10206-21-0*)

23239-43-2. Propoxyphene Napsylate [replaced] (See also *26570-10-5; 17140-78-2; 469-62-5*)

23239-51-2. Ritodrine Hydrochloride

23239-78-3. Pridefine Hydrochloride (See also *5370-41-2*)

23247-36-1. Nafomine Malate (See also *46263-35-8*)

23249-97-0. Procodazole

23255-93-8. Hycanthone Mesylate (See also *3105-97-3*)

23256-09-9. Closiramine Aceturate (See also *47135-88-6*)

23256-23-7. Sulfatroxazole

23256-26-0. Piquizil Hydrochloride (See also *21560-58-7*)

23256-28-2. Hoquizil Hydrochloride (See also *21560-59-8*)

23256-30-6. Nifurtimox

23256-50-0. Guanabenz Acetate

23257-44-5. Fluprednisolone Valerate

23257-58-1. Levoxadrol Hydrochloride (See also *4792-18-1*)

23271-63-8. Amicibone

23271-74-1. Fedrilate

23277-43-2. Nalbuphine Hydrochloride (See also *20594-83-6*)

23277-50-1. Salicylate Meglumine (See also *6284-40-8*)

23288-49-5. Probucol

23288-60-0. Sodium Pertechnetate Tc 99m

23313-80-6. Epitetracycline Hydrochloride

23325-78-2. Cephalexin (See also *15686-71-2*)

23327-57-3. Nefopam Hydrochloride (See also *13669-70-0*)

23360-92-1. Vinleurosine Sulfate [vinleurosine] (See also *1404-95-1*)

23389-32-4. Guanacline Sulfate (See also *1562-71-6; 1463-28-1*)

23389-33-5. Magnesium Carbonate [normal, dihydrate] (See also *39409-82-0; 546-93-0*)

23411-34-9. Edetate Calcium Disodium (See also *62-33-9; 60-00-4*)

23413-80-1. Aspirin Aluminum

23444-86-2. Suncillin Sodium (See also *22164-94-9*)

23465-76-1. Caroverine

23469-05-8. Diamocaine Cyclamate (See also *27112-37-4*)

23476-83-7. Prospidium Chloride

23477-98-7. Sedecamycin

23486-22-8. Esproquin Hydrochloride (See also *37517-33-2*)

23492-69-5. Sopitazine

23505-41-1. Pirimiphos-ethyl

23541-50-6. Daunorubicin Hydrochloride (See also *20830-81-3*)

23564-06-9. Thiophanate

23573-66-2. Detanosal

23580-33-8. Furacrinic Acid

23593-75-1. Clotrimazole

23602-78-0. Benfluorex

23607-71-8. Fetoxylate Hydrochloride (See also *54063-45-5*)

23651-95-8. Droxidopa

23672-07-3. Levosulpiride

23674-86-4. Difluprednate

23694-81-7. Mepindolol

23696-28-8. Olaquindox

23707-33-7. Metrifudil

23712-05-2. Fenmetozole Hydrochloride (See also *41473-09-0*)

23736-58-5. Cloxacillin Benzathine (See also *61-72-3*)

23744-24-3. Pipoxolan Hydrochloride [pipoxolan] (See also *18174-58-8*)

23757-42-8. Midaflur

23758-80-7. Alletorphine

23779-99-9. Floctafenine

23790-08-1. Moxipraquine

23828-92-4. Ambroxol [hydrochloride] (See also *18683-91-5*)

23835-15-6. Potassium Glucaldrate (See also *1317-30-2*)

23869-24-1. Monoxerutin

23873-85-0. Proligestone

23887-41-4. Cinepazet Maleate [cinepazet] (See also *50679-07-7*)

23887-46-9. Cinepazide

23887-47-0. Cinpropazide

23891-60-3. Mepramidil

23910-07-8. Mebiquine

23915-73-3. Trebenzomine Hydrochloride [trebenzomine] (See also *23915-74-4*)

23915-74-4. Trebenzomine Hydrochloride (See also *23915-73-3*)

23930-19-0. Alfaxalone

23940-36-5. Stibophen [anhydrous] (See also *15489-16-4; 16028-21-0*)

23964-57-0. Articaine Hydrochloride

23964-58-1. Articaine

23980-14-5. Ethyl Dirazepate

24047-16-3. Caproxamine

24047-25-4. Guanoxabenz

24143-17-7. Oxazolam

24150-24-1. Terameprocol

24166-13-0. Cloxazolam

24219-97-4. Mianserin Hydrochloride [mianserin] (See also *21535-47-7*)

24233-80-5. Bisobrin Lactate (See also *22407-74-5*)

24237-54-5. Tinoridine

24243-89-8. Triflumidate

24243-97-8. Tymazoline

24279-91-2. Carboquone

24280-93-1. Mycophenolic Acid

24286-21-3. Water O 15

24305-27-9. Protirelin

24320-27-2. Halocortolone

24340-35-0. Piridoxilate

24353-45-5. Dibusadol

24353-88-6. Lorbamate (See also *30865-33-9*)

24356-60-3. Cephapirin Sodium (See also *21593-23-7*)

24356-66-9. Vidarabine (See also *5536-17-4*)

24356-94-3. Algestone Acetophenide

24357-97-9. Tilidine Hydrochloride [(+)-*trans-*] (See also *27107-79-5; 20380-58-9*)

24357-98-0. Isomylamine Hydrochloride (See also *28815-27-2*)

24358-29-0. Tibric Acid [nonstereospecific] (See also *37087-94-8*)

24358-65-4. Diisopromine Hydrochloride (See also *5966-41-6*)

24358-76-7. Nivazol

24358-84-7. Dexivacaine

24359-14-6. Liothyronine I 125 (See also *6893-02-3*)

24359-46-4. Strontium Chloride Sr 85

24359-50-0. Merisoprol Acetate Hg 203

24359-51-1. Merisoprol Acetate Hg 197

24359-56-6. Zinc Chloride Zn 65

24359-64-6. Sodium Iodide I 125

24359-77-1. Phenamazoline Hydrochloride (See also *501-62-2*)

24360-03-0. Midamaline [hydrochloride] (See also *496-38-8*)

24360-55-2. Milipertine

24360-58-5. Pentaphonate

24360-85-8. Iodipamide Sodium I 131

24360-97-2. Mepazine Acetate (See also *60-89-9*)

24361-13-5. Indopine [hydrochloride] (See also *3569-26-4*)

24381-55-3. Salethamide Maleate (See also *46803-81-0*)

24381-59-7. Strontium Nitrate Sr 85

24381-60-0. Chromic Phosphate P 32

24390-12-3. Fantridone Hydrochloride (See also *22461-13-8; 17692-37-4*)

24390-14-5. Doxycycline Hyclate (See also *564-25-0*)

24403-04-1. Debropol

24407-55-4. Bimethoxycaine Lactate

24428-71-5. Glicetanile Sodium (See also *24455-58-1*)

24455-58-1. Glicetanile Sodium [glicetanile] (See also *24428-71-5*)

24477-37-0. Glisolamide

24486-40-6. Thyroxine I 125

24526-64-5. Nomifensine Maleate [nomifensine] (See also *32795-47-4*)

24527-27-3. Spiclomazine

24584-09-6. Dexrazoxane

24622-72-8. Amixetrine

24632-47-1. Nifurpipone

24634-61-5. Potassium Sorbate [*E,E*] (See also *590-00-1; 110-44-1; 22500-92-1*)

24645-20-3. Hexaprofen

24671-26-9. Benrixate

24678-13-5. Lenperone

24701-51-7. Demexiptiline

24729-96-2. Clindamycin Phosphate (See also *18323-44-9*)

24815-24-5. Rescinnamine

24840-59-3. Pretamazium Iodide

24868-20-0. Dantrolene Sodium (See also *14663-23-1; 7261-97-4*)

24870-04-0. Giractide

24886-52-0. Pipofezine

24916-55-0. Rose Bengal Sodium I 131 [open form] (See also *50291-21-9*)

24936-97-8. Polybutilate

24967-93-9. Chondroitin Sulfate Sodium

25013-16-5. Butylated Hydroxyanisole

25038-54-4. Policapram

25046-79-1. Glisoxepide

25053-27-4. Lyapolate Sodium (See also *26101-52-0*)

25053-81-0. Licryfilcon A

25086-89-9. Copovidone

25092-07-3. Dimesone

25092-41-5. Norgestomet

25102-12-9. Edetate Dipotassium (See also *2001-94-7; 58167-76-3*)

25122-41-2. Clobetasol Propionate [clobetasol] (See also *25122-46-7*)

25122-46-7. Clobetasol Propionate (See also *25122-41-2*)

25122-57-0. Clobetasone Butyrate (See also *54063-32-0*)

25126-32-3. Sincalide

25127-31-5. Cidoxepin Hydrochloride (See also *3607-18-9*)

25129-81-1. Isoniazid Glucuronate Sodium [anhydrous]

25155-18-4. Methylbenzethonium Chloride [anhydrous] (See also *1320-44-1*)

25161-41-5. Acevaltrate

25214-48-6. Atlafilcon A

25229-42-9. Cicrotoic Acid

25231-21-4. Polyoxypropylene 15 Stearyl Ether

25269-04-9. Nisobamate

25287-60-9. Etofamide

25301-02-4. Tyloxapol

25314-87-8. Elucaine

25316-40-9. Doxorubicin Hydrochloride (See also *23214-92-8*)

25322-68-3. Polyethylene Glycol (See also *9002-90-8*)

25332-39-2. Trazodone Hydrochloride (See also *19794-93-5*)

25333-77-1. Acetorphine

25384-17-2. Allylprodine

25387-70-6. Dazadrol Maleate (See also *47029-84-5*)

25389-94-0. Kanamycin Sulfate (See also *133-92-6; 59-01-8*)

25392-50-1. Oxazorone

25394-78-9. Cetoxime Hydrochloride [cetoxime] (See also *22204-29-1*)

25416-65-3. Levothyroxine Sodium (See also *55-03-8; 51-48-9*)

25422-75-7. Antazonite

25451-15-4. Felbamate

25496-72-4. Glyceryl Monooleate

25507-04-4. Clindamycin Palmitate Hydrochloride (See also *36688-78-5*)

25509-07-3. Cloroqualone

25523-97-1. Dexchlorpheniramine Maleate [dexchlorpheniramine] (See also *2438-32-6*)

25526-93-6. Alovudine

25546-65-0. Ribostamycin

25573-43-7. Eseridine

25614-03-3. Bromocriptine

25655-01-0. Astifilcon A

25655-41-8. Povidone-Iodine

25681-89-4. Medronate Disodium

25683-71-0. Terizidone

25717-80-0. Molsidomine

25771-23-7. Duometacin

25775-90-0. Zucapsaicin

25803-14-9. Clometacin

25812-30-0. Gemfibrozil

25827-12-7. Suloxifen Oxalate [suloxifen] (See also *25827-13-8*)

25827-13-8. Suloxifen Oxalate (See also *25827-12-7*)

25827-76-3. Iomeglamic Acid

25859-76-1. Glibutimine

25875-50-7. Robenidine Hydrochloride (See also *25875-51-8*)

25875-51-8. Robenidine Hydrochloride [robenidine] (See also *25875-50-7*)

25905-77-5. Minaprine

25953-17-7. Minaprine Hydrochloride (See also *25905-77-5*)

25953-19-9. Cefazolin

25967-29-7. Flutoprazepam

25990-43-6. Mepenzolate Bromide [mepenzolate] (See also *76-90-4*)

25999-31-9. Lasalocid

26002-80-2. Phenothrin

26009-03-0. Polyglycolic Acid

26020-55-3. Oxetorone Fumarate [oxetorone] (See also *34522-46-8*)

26027-38-3. Nonoxynol 4

26058-50-4. Dotefonium Bromide

26070-23-5. Trazitiline

26070-78-0. Ubisindine

26095-59-0. Otilonium Bromide

26097-80-3. Cambendazole

26101-52-0. Lyapolate Sodium [ethenesulfonic acid homopolymer] (See also *25053-27-4*)

26130-02-9. Frentizole

26155-31-7. Morantel Tartrate (See also *20574-50-9*)

26159-34-2. Naproxen Sodium (See also *22204-53-1*)

26159-36-4. Naproxol

26171-23-3. Tolmetin

26225-59-2. Mecinarone

26242-33-1. Vintiamol

26266-57-9. Sorbitan Monopalmitate

26266-58-0. Sorbitan Trioleate

26281-69-6. Exiproben

26304-61-0. Azepindole

26305-03-3. Pepstatin (See also *39324-30-6*)

26308-28-1. Ripazepam

26309-95-5. Pivampicillin Hydrochloride (See also *33817-20-8*)

26328-53-0. Amoscanate

26350-39-0. Nifurizone

26363-46-2. Diphenidol Pamoate (See also *972-02-1*)

26372-86-1. Pentapiperium Methylsulfate [pentapiperium] (See also *7681-80-3*)

26481-51-6. Tiprenolol Hydrochloride [tiprenolol] (See also *39832-43-4*)

26513-79-1. Paraxazone

26513-90-6. Letimide Hydrochloride [letimide] (See also *21791-39-9*)

26538-44-3. Zeranol

26545-74-4. Glyceryl Monolinoleate

26552-51-2. Thiphencillin Potassium [thiphencillin] (See also *4803-45-6*)

26570-10-5. Propoxyphene Napsylate (See also *17140-78-2; 23239-43-2; 469-62-5*)

26605-69-6. Carbenicillin Indanyl Sodium (See also *35531-88-5*)

26615-21-4. Zotepine

26629-87-8. Oxaflozane

26631-90-3. Brobactam

26652-09-5. Ritodrine

26657-13-6. Rolitetracycline Nitrate (See also *7681-32-5; 751-97-3*)

26658-19-5. Sorbitan Tristearate

26658-42-4. Colestipol Hydrochloride [colestipol] (See also *37296-80-3*)

26675-46-7. Isoflurane

26717-47-5. Clofibride

26718-25-2. Halofenate

26750-81-2. Alibendol

26774-90-3. Epicillin

26780-50-7. Polyglactin 370

26786-32-3. Lofepramine Hydrochloride (See also *23047-25-8*)

26786-84-5. Lomofungin

26787-78-0. Amoxicillin [anhydrous] (See also *61336-70-7*)

26807-65-8. Indapamide

26833-87-4. Omacetaxine Mepesuccinate

26844-12-2. Indoramin

26849-57-0. Triclonide

26864-56-2. Penfluridol

26887-04-7. Iotranic Acid

26921-17-5. Timolol Maleate

26921-72-2. Melizame

26944-48-9. Glibornuride

26973-24-0. Ceftezole

26976-72-7. Aceburic Acid

27025-41-8. Oxiglutatione

27025-49-6. Carbenicillin Phenyl Sodium [carbenicillin phenyl] (See also *21649-57-0*)

27031-08-9. Sulfaguanole

27035-30-9. Oxametacin

27050-41-5. Clenpirin

27060-91-9. Flutazolam

27076-46-6. Alpertine

27082-31-1. Calcium Glycerophosphate [glycerophosphoric acid] (See also *27214-00-2*)

27107-79-5. Tilidine Hydrochloride [(±)-*trans*-] (See also *24357-97-9; 20380-58-9*)

27112-37-4. Diamocaine Cyclamate [diamocaine] (See also *23469-05-8*)

27112-40-9. Fenclexonium Metilsulfate [fenclexonium] (See also *30817-43-7*)

27115-86-2. Dacuronium Bromide

27164-46-1. Cefazolin Sodium

27199-40-2. Pifexole

27203-92-5. Tramadol Hydrochloride [tramadol] (See also *36282-47-0*)

27214-00-2. Calcium Glycerophosphate (See also *27082-31-1*)

27220-47-9. Econazole

27223-35-4. Ketazolam

27262-47-1. Levobupivacaine

27262-48-2. Levobupivacaine Hydrochloride

27276-25-1. Capobenate Sodium (See also *21434-91-3*)

27293-82-9. Tyropanoate Sodium [tyropanic acid] (See also *7246-21-1*)

27302-90-5. Oxisuran

27314-77-8. Drazidox

27314-97-2. Tirapazamine

27315-91-9. Pipebuzone

27318-86-1. Floverine

27325-36-6. Procinolol

27367-90-4. Niaprazine

27432-00-4. Mezepine

27450-21-1. Osmadizone

27466-27-9. Intriptyline Hydrochloride [intriptyline] (See also *27466-29-1*)

27466-29-1. Intriptyline Hydrochloride (See also *27466-27-9*)

27469-53-0. Almitrine Mesylate [almitrine] (See also *29608-49-9*)

27470-51-5. Suxibuzone

27503-81-7. Ensulizole

27511-99-5. Eterobarb

27523-40-6. Isoconazole

27574-24-9. Tropatepine

27581-02-8. Idropranolol

27589-33-9. Azosemide

27591-01-1. Bunolol Hydrochloride [bunolol] (See also *31969-05-8*)

27591-42-0. Oxazidione

27591-69-1. Tilorone Hydrochloride (See also *27591-97-5*)

27591-97-5. Tilorone Hydrochloride [tilorone] (See also *27591-69-1*)

27661-27-4. Benaxibine

27686-84-6. Masoprocol

27724-96-5. Cetraxate Hydrochloride (See also *34675-84-8*)

27736-80-7. Fenaftic Acid

27737-38-8. Mixidine (See also *42540-38-5*)

27762-78-3. Kethoxal

27823-62-7. Chlortetracycline Bisulfate (See also *57-62-5*)

27826-45-5. Libecillide

27833-64-3. Loxapine Succinate (See also *1977-10-2*)

27848-84-6. Nicergoline

27849-89-4. Chromium Cr 51 Edetate

27877-51-6. Tolindate

27885-92-3. Imidocarb Hydrochloride [imidocarb] (See also *5318-76-3*)

27890-59-1. Sulfaclozine

27892-33-7. Emepronium Bromide [emepronium] (See also *3614-30-0*)

27912-14-7. Levobunolol Hydrochloride (See also *47141-42-4*)

27959-26-8. Nicomol

28013-70-9. Phenbutazone Sodium Glycerate [replaced] (See also *34214-49-8; 50-33-9*)

28014-46-2. Polyestradiol Phosphate

28022-11-9. Megalomicin Potassium Phosphate [megalomicin] (See also *51481-68-6*)

28038-04-2. Salcolex (See also *54194-00-2*)

28038-50-8. Tolevamer Sodium (See also *28210-41-5*)

28069-65-0. Cuprimyxin

28125-87-3. Flutonidine

28168-10-7. Tetriprofen

28179-44-4. Ioxitalamic Acid

28189-85-7. Etoxadrol Hydrochloride [etoxadrol] (See also *23239-37-4*)

28210-41-5. Tolevamer Sodium [tolevamer] (See also *28038-50-8*)

28227-96-5. Phenisonone Hydrobromide [phenisonone] (See also *530-10-9*)

28240-18-8. Pinolcaine

28300-74-5. Antimony Potassium Tartrate (See also *11071-15-1*)

28319-77-9. Choline Alfoscerate

28395-03-1. Bumetanide

28434-01-7. Bioresmethrin

28523-86-6. Sevoflurane

28532-90-3. Furomazine

28546-58-9. Uldazepam

28598-08-5. Cinoctramine

28610-84-6. Rimazolium Metilsulfate (See also *35615-72-6*)

28657-80-9. Cinoxacin

28721-07-5. Oxcarbazepine

28757-48-4. Polihexanide [replaced] (See also *32289-58-0*)

28781-64-8. Menitrazepam

28782-42-5. Difenoxin

28797-61-7. Pirenzepine Hydrochloride [pirenzepine] (See also *29868-97-1*)

28810-23-3. Zepastine

28815-27-2. Isomylamine Hydrochloride [isomylamine] (See also *24357-98-0*)

28820-28-2. Naftoxate

28841-62-5. Atrinositol

28860-95-9. Carbidopa [anhydrous] (See also *38821-49-7*)

28911-01-5. Triazolam

28971-58-6. Acrocinonide

28981-97-7. Alprazolam

29025-14-7. Butropium Bromide

29039-00-7. Calcium Gluceptate

29050-11-1. Seclazone

29053-27-8. Meseclazone

29069-24-7. Prednimustine

29094-61-9. Glipizide

29098-15-5. Terofenamate

29110-47-2. Guanfacine Hydrochloride [guanfacine] (See also *29110-48-3*)

29110-48-3. Guanfacine Hydrochloride (See also *29110-47-2*)

29122-68-7. Atenolol

29125-56-2. Droclidinium Bromide

29144-42-1. Cetocycline Hydrochloride [cetocycline] (See also *56433-46-6; 53274-41-2*)

29176-29-2. Lofendazam

29177-84-2. Ethyl Loflazepate

29216-28-2. Mequitazine

29218-27-7. Toloxatone

29331-92-8. Licarbazepine

29334-07-4. Sulmarin

29335-92-0. Dextiopronin

29342-02-7. Metipirox

29342-05-0. Ciclopirox

29403-23-4. Phemfilcon A

29442-58-8. Motrazepam

29462-18-8. Bentazepam

29474-12-2. Cimepanol

29535-27-1[replaced]. Malethamer (See also *67832-40-0; 9011-01-2*)

29541-85-3. Oxitriptyline

29546-59-6. Ciclonium Bromide

29560-58-5. Moricizine [moricizine hydrochloride] (See also *31883-05-3*)

29608-49-9. Almitrine Mesylate (See also *27469-53-0*)

29619-86-1. Moctamide

29726-99-6. Tofisoline

29767-20-2. Teniposide

29782-68-1. Silidianin

29868-97-1. Pirenzepine Hydrochloride (See also *28797-61-7*)

29876-14-0. Nicotredole

29899-95-4. Clobenoside

29936-79-6. Mofoxime

29952-13-4. Peratizole

29975-16-4. Estazolam

29984-33-6. Vidarabine Phosphate (See also *5536-17-4*)

30033-10-4. Stercuronium Iodide

30034-03-8. Cefamandole Sodium

30097-06-4. Tidiacic

30103-44-7. Bumecaine

30223-48-4. Fluacizine

30236-32-9. Dexsotalol Hydrochloride [dexsotalol] (See also *4549-94-4*)

30271-85-3. Razinodil

30279-49-3. Suclofenide

30286-75-0. Oxitropium Bromide

30299-08-2. Clinofibrate

30387-51-0. Asperlin

30392-40-6. Bitolterol Mesylate [bitolterol] (See also *30392-41-7*)

30392-41-7. Bitolterol Mesylate (See also *30392-40-6*)

30418-38-3. Tretoquinol

30484-77-6. Flunarizine Hydrochloride (See also *52468-60-7*)

30508-58-8. Daledalin Tosylate [replaced] (See also *23226-37-1; 22136-27-2*)

30516-87-1. Zidovudine

30525-89-4. Paraformaldehyde

30529-16-9. Stirimazole

30531-86-3. Colfenamate

30533-89-2. Flurantel

30544-47-9. Etofenamate

30544-61-7. Clanobutin

30578-37-1. Amezinium Metilsulfate

30652-11-0. Deferiprone

30653-83-9. Parsalmide

30685-43-9. Metildigoxin

30709-69-4. Tizoprolic Acid

30716-01-9. Emilium Tosylate

30748-29-9. Feprazone

30751-05-4. Troxipide

30781-27-2. Amadinone Acetate [amadinone] (See also *22304-34-3*)

30817-43-7. Fenclexonium Metilsulfate (See also *27112-40-9*)

30840-27-8. Pretiadil

30851-76-4. Ethoxazorutoside

30865-33-9. Lorbamate [replaced] (See also *24353-88-6*)

30868-30-5. Pyrazofurin

30910-27-1. Treloxinate

30914-89-7. Flumexadol

30924-31-3. Cafaminol

30999-06-5. Tocophersolan

31002-79-6. Triamcinolone Benetonide

31036-80-3. Lofexidine Hydrochloride [lofexidine] (See also *21498-08-8*)

31101-25-4. Mirincamycin Hydrochloride [mirincamycin] (See also *8063-91-0; 37217-18-8*)

31112-62-6. Metrizamide

31127-82-9. Iodoxamate Meglumine [iodoxamic acid] (See also *51764-33-1; 6284-40-8*)

31218-83-4. Propetamphos

31221-85-9. Ibuverine

31224-92-7. Pifoxime

31232-26-5. Danitracen

31314-38-2. Prodipine

31329-57-4. Nafronyl Oxalate [nafronyl] (See also *3200-06-4*)

31342-36-6. Chloramphenicol Pantothenate Complex

31352-82-6. Zolazepam Hydrochloride [zolazepam] (See also *33754-49-3*)

31386-24-0. Amindocate

31386-25-1. Indocate

31428-61-2. Tiamenidine

31430-15-6. Flubendazole

31430-18-9. Nocodazole

31431-39-7. Mebendazole

31431-43-3. Cyclobendazole

31478-45-2. Bamnidazole

31512-74-0. Polixetonium Chloride

31566-31-1. Glyceryl Monostearate

31581-02-9. Cinoxolone

31598-07-9. Iozomic Acid

31621-87-1. Polydioxanone

31637-97-5. Etofibrate

31645-39-3. Palifosfamide

31677-93-7. Bupropion Hydrochloride (See also *34911-55-2*)

31690-09-2. Levomefolic Acid

31693-08-0. Focofilcon A

31698-14-3. Ancitabine

31721-17-2. Quinupramine

31729-24-5. Enpiprazole

31770-79-3. Meglucycline

31793-07-4. Pirprofen

31828-50-9. Cephradine [non-stoichiometric hydrate] (See also *38821-53-3; 58456-86-3*)

31828-71-4. Mexiletine Hydrochloride [mexiletine] (See also *5370-01-4*)

31842-01-0. Indoprofen

31842-61-2. Rimiterol Hydrobromide (See also *31931-97-2; 32953-89-2*)

31848-01-8. Morclofone

31868-18-5. Mexazolam

31879-05-7. Fenoprofen

31883-05-3. Moricizine (See also *29560-58-5*)

31884-76-1. Sulfanilate Zinc (See also *22484-64-6; 121-57-3*)

31884-77-2. Meclizine Hydrochloride (See also *1104-22-9; 569-65-3*)

31931-97-2. Rimiterol Hydrobromide [nonstereospecific] (See also *31842-61-2; 32953-89-2*)

31932-09-9. Ticarbodine

31959-85-0. Calcium Glubionate [anhydrous] (See also *12569-38-9*)

31959-88-3. Clodazon Hydrochloride (See also *4913-61-5; 4755-59-3*)

31969-05-8. Bunolol Hydrochloride (See also *27591-01-1*)

31980-29-7. Nicofibrate

32059-15-7. Guanazodine

32059-27-1. Sumetizide

32072-47-1. Squalamine Lactate (See also *148717-90-2*)

32095-14-0. Isoetharine [replaced] (See also *530-08-5; 13725-16-1*)

32195-33-8. Bisbendazole

32211-97-5. Cyclindole

32222-06-3. Calcitriol (See also *77326-95-5*)

32266-10-7. Hexoprenaline Sulfate (See also *3215-70-1*)

32289-58-0. Polihexanide (See also *28757-48-4*)

32295-18-4. Tosifen

32359-34-5. Medifoxamine

32385-11-8. Sisomicin

32421-46-8. Bunaftine

32447-90-8. Dextilidine

32462-30-9. Oxfenicine

32527-55-2. Tiaramide Hydrochloride [tiaramide] (See also *35941-71-0*)

32665-36-4. Eprozinol

32672-69-8. Mesoridazine Besylate (See also *5588-33-0*)

32710-91-1. Trifezolac

32780-64-6. Labetalol Hydrochloride (See also *36894-69-6*)

32795-44-1. Acecainide Hydrochloride [acecainide] (See also *34118-92-8*)

32795-47-4. Nomifensine Maleate (See also *24526-64-5*)

32797-92-5. Glisentide

32808-51-8. Bucloxic Acid

32828-81-2. Picotamide

32838-26-9. Butoctamide

32886-97-8. Amdinocillin Pivoxil

32887-01-7. Amdinocillin

32909-92-5. Sulfametrole

32953-89-2. Rimiterol Hydrobromide [rimiterol] (See also *31842-61-2; 31931-97-2*)

32954-43-1. Pendecamaine

32986-56-4. Tobramycin

32988-50-4. Viomycin Sulfate [viomycin] (See also *37883-00-4*)

33005-95-7. Tiaprofenic Acid

33025-33-1. Proroxan Hydrochloride (See also *33743-96-3*)

33032-12-1. Methapyrilene Fumarate (See also *91-80-5*)

33069-62-4. Paclitaxel

33089-61-1. Amitraz

33103-22-9. Enviomycin

33122-60-0. Nordinone

33124-50-4. Fluocortin Butyl [fluocortin] (See also *41767-29-7*)

33125-97-2. Etomidate

33144-79-5. Broperamole

33156-28-4. Ramnodigin

33159-27-2. Ecabet

33178-86-8. Alinidine

33204-76-1. Quadrosilan

33237-74-0. Aprindine Hydrochloride (See also *37640-71-4*)

33286-22-5. Diltiazem Hydrochloride (See also *42399-41-7*)

33305-56-5. Thimerfonate Sodium [thimerfonate] (See also *5964-24-9*)

33335-58-9. Dimethyltubocurarinium Chloride

33342-05-1. Gliquidone

33369-31-2. Zomepirac Sodium [zomepirac] (See also *64092-49-5; 64092-48-4*)

33371-53-8. Bevonium Metilsulfate [bevonium] (See also *5205-82-3*)

33386-08-2. Buspirone Hydrochloride (See also *36505-84-7*)

33396-37-1. Meproscillarin

33401-94-4. Pyrantel Tartrate (See also *15686-83-6*)
33402-03-8. Metaraminol Bitartrate (See also *17171-57-2; 54-49-9*)
33410-59-2. Amfilcon A
33414-30-1. Ftormetazine
33414-36-7. Ftorpropazine
33419-42-0. Etoposide
33419-68-0. Safrazine Hydrochloride [safrazine] (See also *7296-30-2*)
33453-23-5. Ciproquazone
33459-27-7. Xanoxate Sodium [xanoxic acid] (See also *41147-04-0*)
33515-09-2. Gonadorelin Acetate [gonadorelin] (See also *52699-48-6*)
33545-56-1. Ciclopramine
33564-30-6. Cefoxitin Sodium (See also *35607-66-0*)
33564-31-7. Diflorasone Diacetate (See also *2557-49-5*)
33588-20-4. Clidafidine
33605-67-3. Cargutocin
33605-94-6. Pirisudanol
33643-46-8. Esketamine
33665-90-6. Acesulfame
33671-46-4. Clotiazepam
33743-96-3. Proroxan Hydrochloride [proroxan] (See also *33025-33-1*)
33754-49-3. Zolazepam Hydrochloride (See also *31352-82-6*)
33765-68-3. Oxendolone
33774-52-6. Detajmium Bitartrate [anhydrous] (See also *53862-81-0*)
33779-37-2. Salprotoside
33813-84-2. Deprostil
33817-09-3. Levmetamfetamine
33817-20-8. Pivampicillin Hydrochloride [pivampicillin] (See also *26309-95-5*)
33818-15-4. Citicoline Sodium (See also *987-78-0; 1477-47-0*)
33876-97-0. Linsidomine
33889-69-9. Silicristin
33996-33-7. Oxaceprol
33996-58-6. Etiracetam
34024-41-4. Deboxamet
34031-32-8. Auranofin
34042-85-8. Sudoxicam
34061-33-1. Taclamine Hydrochloride [taclamine] (See also *34061-34-2*)
34061-34-2. Taclamine Hydrochloride (See also *34061-33-1*)
34089-81-1. Sodium Ferric Gluconate Complex
34097-16-0. Clocortolone Pivalate
34114-01-7. Pemerid Nitrate (See also *50432-78-5*)
34118-92-8. Acecainide Hydrochloride (See also *32795-44-1*)
34144-82-6. Suxemerid Sulfate (See also *47662-15-7*)
34148-01-1. Clidanac
34150-62-4. Ferriclate Calcium Sodium
34161-24-5. Fipexide
34183-22-7. Propafenone Hydrochloride (See also *54063-53-5*)
34184-77-5. Promegestone
34195-34-1. Hydrocodone Bitartrate (See also *6190-38-1; 143-71-5; 125-29-1*)

34214-49-8. Phenbutazone Sodium Glycerate (See also *28013-70-9; 50-33-9*)
34256-91-2. Naranol Hydrochloride (See also *22292-91-7*)
34262-84-5. Mesocarb
34273-10-4. Saralasin Acetate [saralasin] (See also *39698-78-7; 54194-01-3*)
34297-34-2. Anidoxime
34301-55-8. Isometamidium Chloride
34331-89-0. Isoxsuprine Hydrochloride (See also *579-56-6; 395-28-8*)
34368-04-2. Dobutamine
34381-68-5. Acebutolol Hydrochloride (See also *37517-30-9*)
34391-04-3. Levosalbutamol
34398-83-9. Amicloral
34427-79-7. Proxifezone
34433-66-4. Levomethadyl Acetate (See also *1477-40-3*)
34444-01-4. Cefamandole
34445-07-3. Silver Diammine Fluoride
34482-99-0. Fletazepam
34493-98-6. Dibekacin
34499-96-2. Temodox
34521-09-0. Antimony Sodium Tartrate
34522-46-8. Oxetorone Fumarate (See also *26020-55-3*)
34552-78-8. Lometraline Hydrochloride (See also *39951-65-0*)
34552-83-5. Loperamide Hydrochloride (See also *53179-11-6*)
34552-84-6. Isoxicam
34563-73-0. Feniodium Chloride
34580-13-7. Ketotifen Fumarate [ketotifen] (See also *34580-14-8*)
34580-14-8. Ketotifen Fumarate (See also *34580-13-7*)
34597-40-5. Fenoprofen Calcium [anhydrous] (See also *53746-45-5; 31879-05-7*)
34616-39-2. Fenalcomine
34633-34-6. Bifluranol
34642-77-8. Amoxicillin Sodium
34645-84-6. Fenclofenac
34661-75-1. Urapidil
34662-67-4. Cotriptyline
34675-84-8. Cetraxate Hydrochloride [cetraxate] (See also *27724-96-5*)
34703-49-6. Dropempine
34740-13-1. Profexalone
34753-46-3. Ciheptolane
34758-83-3. Zipeprol
34765-96-3. Alsactide
34779-28-7. Sulbenicillin
34784-64-0. Tertatolol
34787-01-4. Ticarcillin Disodium [ticarcillin] (See also *4697-14-7*)
34816-55-2. Moxestrol (See also *21375-12-2*)
34819-78-8. Ammonia N 13
34839-70-8. Metiamide
34866-46-1. Carbuterol Hydrochloride (See also *34866-47-2*)
34866-47-2. Carbuterol Hydrochloride [carbuterol] (See also *34866-46-1*)
34887-52-0. Fenisorex

34911-55-2. Bupropion Hydrochloride [amfebutamone] (See also *31677-93-7*)
34914-39-1. Ritiometan
34915-68-9. Bunitrolol
34919-98-7. Cetamolol Hydrochloride [cetamolol] (See also *77590-95-5*)
34959-30-3. Azaspirium Chloride
34966-41-1. Cartazolate
34976-39-1. Tioxacin
35035-05-3. Timepidium Bromide
35067-47-1. Droxacin Sodium [droxacin] (See also *57363-13-0*)
35080-11-6. Prajmalium Bitartrate [prajmalium] (See also *2589-47-1*)
35100-41-5. Domazoline Fumarate (See also *6043-01-2*)
35100-44-8. Endrysone
35115-60-7. Teprotide
35121-78-9. Epoprostenol
35135-01-4. Benafentrine
35135-67-2. Cormethasone Acetate (See also *35135-68-3*)
35135-68-3. Cormethasone Acetate [cormethasone] (See also *35135-67-2*)
35142-68-8. Homopipramol
35189-28-7. Norgestimate
35212-22-7. Ipriflavone
35265-50-0. Peraquinsin
35273-88-2. Gliflumide
35282-33-8. Benfosformin [anhydrous] (See also *52658-53-4*)
35285-69-9. Propylparaben Sodium
35301-24-7. Cedefingol
35319-70-1. Tiazuril
35322-07-7. Fosazepam
35398-15-3. Potassium Gluconate [monohydrate] (See also *299-27-4; 526-95-4*)
35423-09-7. Tesimide
35423-51-9. Tisocromide
35425-83-3. Quinuclium Bromide [anhydrous] (See also *64755-06-2*)
35449-36-6. Gemcadiol
35452-73-4. Ciprafamide
35457-80-8. Midecamycin
35515-77-6. Truxipicurium Iodide
35523-45-6. Fludalanine
35528-20-2. Vifilcon A
35531-88-5. Carbenicillin Indanyl Sodium [carbenicillin indanyl] (See also *26605-69-6*)
35554-44-0. Enilconazole
35575-96-3. Azamethiphos
35578-20-2. Oxarbazole
35604-67-2. Viloxazine Hydrochloride (See also *46817-91-8*)
35607-20-6. Avridine
35607-66-0. Cefoxitin
35615-72-6. Rimazolium Metilsulfate [rimazolium] (See also *28610-84-6*)
35619-65-9. Tritiozine
35620-67-8. Pirdonium Bromide
35700-21-1. Carboprost Methyl
35700-23-3. Carboprost
35703-32-3. Cinametic Acid
35710-57-7. Trizoxime

35711-34-3. Tolmetin Sodium [anhydrous] (See also *64490-92-2*)
35727-72-1. Ontianil
35764-73-9. Fluotracen Hydrochloride [fluotracen] (See also *57363-14-1*)
35775-82-7. Maridomycin
35795-16-5. Trimazosin Hydrochloride [trimazosin] (See also *53746-46-6; 35795-17-6*)
35795-17-6. Trimazosin Hydrochloride [anhydrous] (See also *53746-46-6; 35795-16-5*)
35834-26-5. Rosaramicin
35838-58-5. Etazolate Hydrochloride (See also *51022-77-6*)
35838-63-2. Clocoumarol
35843-07-3. Morocromen
35846-53-8. Maytansine
35891-93-1. Tocainide Hydrochloride
35898-87-4. Dilazep
35941-65-2. Butriptyline Hydrochloride [butriptyline] (See also *5585-73-9*)
35941-71-0. Tiaramide Hydrochloride [monohydrochloride] (See also *32527-55-2*)
36067-73-9. Azepexole
36093-47-7. Salantel
36104-80-0. Camazepam
36121-13-8. Burodiline
36141-82-9. Diamfenetide
36144-08-8. Mantabegron
36148-38-6. Besunide
36167-63-2. Halofantrine Hydrochloride (See also *69756-53-2; 66051-63-6*)
36175-05-0. Sodium Picofosfate
36199-78-7. Guafecainol
36282-47-0. Tramadol Hydrochloride (See also *27203-92-5*)
36291-32-4. Monoglyceride Citrate
36292-69-0. Ketazocine
36309-01-0. Dimemorfan
36322-90-4. Piroxicam
36330-85-5. Fenbufen
36364-49-5. Imidazole Salicylate
36425-29-3. Hefilcon A
36441-41-5. Lividomycin
36471-39-3. Nuclotixene
36499-65-7. Dicobalt Edetate
36504-64-0. Nictindole
36504-94-6. Butaclamol Hydrochloride (See also *51152-91-1*)
36505-82-5. Prodolic Acid
36505-83-6. Dectaflur [nonstereospecific] (See also *1838-19-3*)
36505-84-7. Buspirone Hydrochloride [buspirone] (See also *33386-08-2*)
36508-71-1. Zorubicin Hydrochloride (See also *54083-22-6*)
36518-02-2. Diproqualone
36531-26-7. Oxantel Pamoate [oxantel] (See also *68813-55-8*)
36589-58-9. Eprodisate Disodium (See also *21668-77-9*)
36590-19-9. Amocarzine
36616-52-1. Fenclorac
36637-18-0. Etidocaine
36637-22-6. Drocinonide

36653-82-4. Cetyl Alcohol (See also *124-29-8*)
36688-78-5. Clindamycin Palmitate Hydrochloride [clindamycin palmitate] (See also *25507-04-4*)
36703-88-5. Inosine Pranobex
36735-22-5. Quazepam
36740-73-5. Flumizole
36791-04-5. Ribavirin
36798-79-5. Budralazine
36861-47-9. Enzacamene
36889-15-3. Betamicin Sulfate [betamicin] (See also *43169-50-2*)
36894-69-6. Labetalol Hydrochloride [labetalol] (See also *32780-64-6*)
36920-48-6. Cefoxazole
36921-54-7. Xantifibrate (See also *882-09-7*)
36945-03-6. Lergotrile
36950-96-6. Cicloprofen
36980-34-4. Glicaramide
36983-69-4. Actodigin
36983-81-0. Fosfonet Sodium [anhydrous] (See also *54870-27-8; 4408-78-0*)
37000-20-7. Zinterol Hydrochloride [zinterol] (See also *38241-28-0*)
37017-46-2. Perfilcon A
37025-55-1. Carbetocin
37065-29-5. Miloxacin
37087-94-8. Tibric Acid (See also *24358-29-0*)
37091-65-9. Azlocillin Sodium
37091-66-0. Azlocillin
37106-97-1. Bentiromide
37115-32-5. Adinazolam
37132-72-2. Fotretamine
37148-27-9. Clenbuterol
37178-37-3. Etilevodopa
37209-31-7. Detralfate
37217-18-8. Mirincamycin Hydrochloride [replaced] (See also *8063-91-0; 31101-25-4*)
37280-56-1. Kitasamycin [tartrate] (See also *1392-21-8*)
37282-12-5. Polybutester
37286-92-3. Calcium Polystyrene Sulfonate
37294-43-2. Insulin I 131
37296-80-3. Colestipol Hydrochloride (See also *26658-42-4*)
37305-75-2. Actaplanin
37312-62-2. Serrapeptase
37321-09-8. Apramycin (See also *41194-16-5*)
37326-33-3. Hyalosidase
37332-99-3. Avoparcin
37340-82-2. Streptodornase
37350-58-6. Metoprolol (See also *54163-88-1*)
37398-31-5. Dilmefone
37415-62-6. Mycophenolate Sodium
37456-21-6. Terbucromil
37470-13-6. Flavodic Acid
37517-26-3. Pipotiazine Palmitate (See also *39860-99-6*)
37517-28-5. Amikacin
37517-30-9. Acebutolol

37517-33-2. Esproquin Hydrochloride [esproquin] (See also *23486-22-8*)
37526-80-0. Melarsonyl Potassium [melarsonyl] (See also *13355-00-5*)
37529-08-1. Mexoprofen
37554-40-8. Fluquazone
37561-27-6. Fenoverine
37571-84-9. Amidephrine Mesylate [amidephrine] (See also *1421-68-7; 3354-67-4*)
37577-24-5. Levofenfluramine
37598-94-0. Glipalamide
37612-13-8. Encainide Hydrochloride [encainide] (See also *66794-74-9*)
37640-71-4. Aprindine
37661-08-8. Bacampicillin Hydrochloride (See also *50972-17-3*)
37669-57-1. Arfendazam
37681-00-8. Coumazoline
37686-84-3. Terguride
37693-01-9. Clofoctol
37717-21-8. Flurocitabine
37723-78-7. Iopronic Acid
37750-83-7. Rimoprogin
37751-39-6. Ciclazindol
37753-10-9. Sufosfamide
37762-06-4. Zaprinast
37800-79-6. Difenoximide Hydrochloride (See also *47806-92-8*)
37855-80-4. Iprocrolol
37855-92-8. Azanator Maleate [azanator] (See also *39624-65-2*)
37863-70-0. Iosumetic Acid
37883-00-4. Viomycin Sulfate (See also *32988-50-4*)
37967-98-9. Tienopramine
38029-10-6. Pirbuterol Hydrochloride (See also *38677-81-5*)
38070-41-6. Tiodonium Chloride
38081-67-3. Carmantadine
38083-17-9. Climbazole
38101-59-6. Oglufanide Disodium [oglufanide] (See also *237068-57-4*)
38103-61-6. Tolamolol
38129-37-2. Bicozamycin
38184-50-8. Nitroblue Tetrazolium Chloride
38194-50-2. Sulindac
38234-21-8. Fertirelin Acetate [fertirelin] (See also *106756-71-2*)
38241-28-0. Zinterol Hydrochloride (See also *37000-20-7*)
38241-39-3. Tazolol Hydrochloride (See also *39832-48-9*)
38260-01-4. Trientine Hydrochloride (See also *112-24-3*)
38270-90-5. Strontium Chloride Sr 89
38274-54-3. Benurestat
38304-91-5. Minoxidil
38321-02-7. Dexverapamil
38349-38-1. Metrafazoline
38363-32-5. Penbutolol Sulfate (See also *38363-40-5*)
38363-40-5. Penbutolol Sulfate [penbutolol] (See also *38363-32-5*)
38373-83-0. Romifenone
38398-32-2. Ganaxolone
38452-29-8. Tolmesoxide

38562-01-5. Dinoprost Tromethamine
38609-97-1. Cridanimod
38647-79-9. Urefibrate
38668-01-8. Taurultam
38677-81-5. Pirbuterol Acetate [pirbuterol] (See also *65652-44-0*)
38677-85-9. Flunixin
38809-73-3. Surfilcon A
38821-49-7. Carbidopa (See also *28860-95-9*)
38821-52-2. Indoramin Hydrochloride
38821-53-3. Cephradine [anhydrous] (See also *58456-86-3; 31828-50-9*)
38821-80-6. Rodocaine
38873-55-1. Furobufen
38899-05-7. Glucosamine Sulfate Potassium Chloride
38916-34-6. Somatostatin
38955-22-5. Pinadoline
38957-41-4. Emorfazone
39022-39-4. Oxaprotiline Hydrochloride (See also *56433-44-4*)
39030-71-2. Pivampicillin Probenate [replaced] (See also *42190-91-0; 33817-20-8*)
39030-72-3. Pivampicillin Pamoate (See also *59549-62-1; 33817-20-8*)
39087-48-4. Calcium Clofibrate (See also *882-09-7*)
39099-98-4. Cinamolol
39123-11-0. Pituxate
39133-31-8. Trimebutine
39178-37-5. Inicarone
39186-49-7. Pirolazamide
39219-28-8. Promestriene
39224-48-1. Nitroclofene
39236-46-9. Imidurea
39294-79-6. Seractide Acetate [anhydrous] (See also *39295-97-1; 63304-56-3*)
39295-97-1. Seractide Acetate (See also *39294-79-6; 63304-56-3*)
39324-30-6. Pepstatin [nonspecific] (See also *26305-03-3*)
39365-87-2. Magnesium Trisilicate (See also *14987-04-3*)
39365-88-3. Potash, Sulfurated
39409-82-0. Magnesium Carbonate [basic] (See also *23389-33-5; 546-93-0*)
39455-18-0. Danaparoid Sodium [chondroitin, 4-(hydrogen sulfate), sodium salt] (See also *57459-72-0; 54328-33-5; 12678-07-8*)
39464-87-4. Betasizofiran
39492-01-8. Gabexate
39516-21-7. Tiopropamine
39537-99-0. Micinicate
39544-74-6. Benzotript
39552-01-7. Befunolol
39562-70-4. Nitrendipine
39563-28-5. Cloranolol
39567-20-9. Olpimedone
39577-19-0. Picumast
39624-65-2. Azanator Maleate (See also *37855-92-8*)
39624-66-3. Trepipam Maleate (See also *56030-50-3*)
39633-62-0. Aclantate

39640-15-8. Piberaline
39685-31-9. Cefuracetime
39698-78-7. Saralasin Acetate (See also *54194-01-3; 34273-10-4*)
39715-02-1. Endralazine Mesylate [endralazine] (See also *65322-72-7*)
39718-89-3. Alminoprofen
39731-05-0. Carpindolol
39754-64-8. Tifemoxone
39791-20-3. Nylestriol
39809-25-1. Penciclovir
39825-23-5. Bisorcic
39831-55-5. Amikacin Sulfate (See also *37517-28-5*)
39832-43-4. Tiprenolol Hydrochloride (See also *26481-51-6*)
39832-48-9. Tazolol Hydrochloride [tazolol] (See also *38241-39-3*)
39860-99-6. Pipotiazine Palmitate [pipotiazine] (See also *37517-26-3*)
39862-58-3. Strinoline
39878-70-1. Talampicillin Hydrochloride (See also *47747-56-8*)
39907-68-1. Dopamantine
39951-65-0. Lometraline Hydrochloride [lometraline] (See also *34552-78-8*)
39978-42-2. Nifurzide
40034-42-2. Rosoxacin
40054-69-1. Etizolam
40077-57-4. Aviptadil
40093-94-5. Torcitabine
40173-75-9. Tofetridine
40180-04-9. Ticrynafen
40198-53-6. Tioxaprofen
40256-99-3. Flucetorex
40372-00-7. Taribavirin Hydrochloride (See also *119567-79-2*)
40391-99-9. Pamidronic Acid
40431-64-9. Dexmethylphenidate Hydrochloride [dexmethylphenidate] (See also *19262-68-1*)
40507-23-1. Fluproquazone
40507-78-6. Indanazoline
40516-48-1. Tretinoin Tocoferil
40542-65-2. Gestrinone [replaced] (See also *16320-04-0*)
40580-59-4. Guanadrel Sulfate [guanadrel] (See also *22195-34-2*)
40594-09-0. Flucindole
40596-69-8. Methoprene
40665-92-7. Cloprostenol Sodium [cloprostenol] (See also *55028-72-3*)
40666-16-8. Fluprostenol Sodium [fluprostenol] (See also *55028-71-2*)
40680-87-3. Piprofurol
40691-50-7. Tixanox
40692-37-3. Tisoquone
40759-33-9. Nolinium Bromide
40762-15-0. Doxefazepam
40796-97-2. Bemesetron
40819-93-0. Lorajmine Hydrochloride (See also *47562-08-3*)
40828-44-2. Clazolimine
40828-45-3. Azolimine
40828-46-4. Suprofen
40912-73-0. Brosotamide
40966-79-8. Sarpicillin

41020-67-1. Mexrenoate Potassium [anhydrous] (See also *43169-54-6; 41020-68-2*)
41020-68-2. Mexrenoate Potassium [mexrenoic acid] (See also *43169-54-6; 41020-67-1*)
41020-79-5. Dicirenone
41078-02-8. Enprofylline
41094-88-6. Tracazolate
41100-52-1. Memantine Hydrochloride
41113-86-4. Bromoxanide
41147-04-0. Xanoxate Sodium (See also *33459-27-7*)
41152-17-4. Morforex
41183-64-6. Gallium Citrate Ga 67 (See also *52260-70-5*)
41194-16-5. Apramycin [replaced] (See also *37321-09-8*)
41294-56-8. Alfacalcidol
41340-25-4. Etodolac
41340-39-0. Impacarzine
41342-54-5. Carbaldrate
41354-29-4. Cyproheptadine Hydrochloride (See also *969-33-5; 129-03-3*)
41354-30-7. Dimethisterone (See also *79-64-1*)
41354-45-4. Tubocurarine Chloride [replaced] (See also *6989-98-6; 57-94-3; 57-95-4*)
41354-48-7. Dihydroxyaluminum Aminoacetate (See also *13682-92-3; 56-40-6*)
41372-02-5. Penicillin G Benzathine (See also *1538-09-6; 61-33-6*)
41372-08-1. Methyldopa (See also *555-30-6*)
41372-10-5. Piperazine Citrate (See also *144-29-6; 110-85-0*)
41372-20-7. Apomorphine Hydrochloride (See also *314-19-2; 58-00-4*)
41372-22-9. Calcium Lactate [hydrate] (See also *814-80-2; 5743-47-5*)
41375-66-0. Trimeprazine Tartrate [replaced] (See also *4330-99-8; 84-96-8*)
41385-14-2. Leuciglumer
41387-02-4. Lexofenac
41444-62-6. Codeine Phosphate (See also *52-28-8; 6059-47-8*)
41468-25-1. Pyridoxal Phosphate
41473-09-0. Fenmetozole Hydrochloride [fenmetozole] (See also *23712-05-2*)
41510-23-0. Biriperone
41559-38-0. Cyanocobalamin Co 57 (See also *13115-03-2*)
41570-61-0. Tulobuterol
41575-94-4. Carboplatin
41621-49-2. Ciclopirox Olamine
41653-21-8. Ethyl Piperidinoacetylaminobenzoate
41706-81-4. Poliglecaprone 25
41708-72-9. Tocainide
41717-30-0. Befuraline
41729-52-6. Dezaguanine
41767-29-7. Fluocortin Butyl (See also *33124-50-4*)
41791-49-5. Lonaprofen

41826-92-0. Trepibutone

41859-67-0. Bezafibrate

41906-86-9. Nitrocefin

41927-88-2. Sodium Iodide I 123

41927-89-3. Leucovorin Calcium [replaced] (See also *1492-18-8; 6035-45-6; 58-05-9*)

41941-56-4. Tocladesine

41952-52-7. Cefcanel

41964-07-2. Tolimidone

41992-22-7. Spirogermanium Hydrochloride (See also *41992-23-8*)

41992-23-8. Spirogermanium Hydrochloride [spirogermanium] (See also *41992-22-7*)

42024-98-6. Mazaticol

42050-23-7. Nafetolol

42061-52-9. Pumitepa

42110-58-7. Metioxate

42116-76-7. Carnidazole

42116-77-8. Deximafen (See also *60719-87-1*)

42190-91-0. Pivampicillin Probenate (See also *39030-71-2; 33817-20-8*)

42200-33-9. Nadolol

42220-21-3. Iodocholesterol I 131

42228-92-2. Acivicin

42239-60-1. Tilozepine

42281-59-4. Oxilorphan

42293-72-1. Bencisteine

42399-41-7. Diltiazem Hydrochloride [diltiazem] (See also *33286-22-5*)

42408-78-6. Pirandamine Hydrochloride (See also *42408-79-7*)

42408-79-7. Pirandamine Hydrochloride [pirandamine] (See also *42408-78-6*)

42408-80-0. Tandamine Hydrochloride [tandamine] (See also *58167-78-5*)

42408-82-2. Butorphanol

42422-68-4. Taleranol

42438-73-3. Denpidazone

42461-78-9. Sulfonterol Hydrochloride (See also *42461-79-0*)

42461-79-0. Sulfonterol Hydrochloride [sulfonterol] (See also *42461-78-9*)

42461-84-7. Flunixin Meglumine (See also *38677-85-9; 6284-40-8*)

42465-20-3. Acequinoline

42471-28-3. Nimustine

42540-38-5. Mixidine [replaced] (See also *27737-38-8*)

42540-40-9. Cefamandole Nafate (See also *34444-01-4*)

42583-55-1. Carmetizide

42597-57-9. Ronifibrate

42615-49-6. Amilomer

42615-60-1. Brinolase

42779-82-8. Clopirac

42792-26-7. Isosulpride

42794-76-3. Midodrine Hydrochloride [midodrine] (See also *3092-17-9*)

42835-25-6. Flumequine

42863-81-0. Lopirazepam

42864-78-8. Bevantolol Hydrochloride (See also *59170-23-9*)

42877-18-9. Pelanserin Hydrochloride (See also *2208-51-7*)

42879-47-0. Pranolium Chloride

42924-53-8. Nabumetone

42971-09-5. Vinpocetine

43033-72-3. Levomethadyl Acetate Hydrochloride

43043-01-2. Mercumatilin Sodium [mercumatilin] (See also *60135-06-0; 574-79-8*)

43169-50-2. Betamicin Sulfate (See also *36889-15-3*)

43169-54-6. Mexrenoate Potassium (See also *41020-67-1; 41020-68-2*)

43200-80-2. Zopiclone

43210-67-9. Fenbendazole

43229-80-7. Formoterol Fumarate (See also *73573-87-2*)

45086-03-1. Etoformin Hydrochloride [etoformin] (See also *53597-26-5*)

46263-35-8. Nafomine Malate [nafomine] (See also *23247-36-1*)

46464-11-3. Meobentine Sulfate [meobentine] (See also *58503-79-0*)

46803-81-0. Salethamide Maleate [salethamide] (See also *24381-55-3*)

46817-91-8. Viloxazine Hydrochloride [viloxazine] (See also *35604-67-2*)

47029-84-5. Dazadrol Maleate [dazadrol] (See also *25387-70-6*)

47082-97-3. Pargolol

47128-12-1. Cycliramine Maleate [cycliramine] (See also *5781-37-3*)

47135-88-6. Closiramine Aceturate [closiramine] (See also *23256-09-9*)

47141-42-4. Levobunolol Hydrochloride [levobunolol] (See also *27912-14-7*)

47166-67-6. Octriptyline Phosphate [octriptyline] (See also *51481-67-5*)

47206-15-5. Enprazepine

47254-05-7. Spiroxepin

47419-52-3. Dexproxibutene

47420-28-0. Trixolane

47487-22-9. Acridorex

47543-65-7. Prenoxdiazine

47562-08-3. Lorajmine Hydrochloride [lorajmine] (See also *40819-93-0*)

47662-15-7. Suxemerid Sulfate [suxemerid] (See also *34144-82-6*)

47682-41-7. Flupimazine

47739-98-0. Clocapramine

47747-56-8. Talampicillin Hydrochloride [talampicillin] (See also *39878-70-1*)

47806-92-8. Difenoximide Hydrochloride [difenoximide] (See also *37800-79-6*)

47917-41-9. Primycin

47931-80-6. Tosactide

47931-85-1. Calcitonin [salmon] (See also *21215-62-3; 9007-12-9*)

49561-92-4. Nivimedone Sodium [nivimedone] (See also *62077-09-2; 57441-90-4*)

49562-28-9. Fenofibrate

49564-56-9. Fazadinium Bromide

49637-08-3. Nabitan Hydrochloride (See also *66556-74-9*)

49697-38-3. Rimexolone

49745-00-8. Amidantel

49745-95-1. Dobutamine Hydrochloride (See also *34368-04-2*)

49746-00-1. Rotoxamine Tartrate (See also *5560-77-0*)

49746-04-5. Thiothixene Hydrochloride [anhydrous (*Z*)] (See also *22189-31-7; 49746-09-0; 58513-59-0; 5591-45-7*)

49746-06-7. Aminophylline [replaced] (See also *317-34-0; 5897-66-5*)

49746-09-0. Thiothixene Hydrochloride [*Z*] (See also *22189-31-7; 58513-59-0; 49746-04-5; 5591-45-7*)

49746-10-3. Erythrosine Sodium (See also *568-63-8; 16423-68-0; 15905-32-5*)

49755-67-1. Ioglicic Acid

49763-96-4. Stiripentol

49780-10-1. Azaclorzine Hydrochloride (See also *49864-70-2*)

49785-74-2. Supidimide

49847-97-4. Prorenoate Potassium

49864-70-2. Azaclorzine Hydrochloride [azaclorzine] (See also *49780-10-1*)

50264-69-2. Lonidamine

50264-78-3. Xinidamine

50270-32-1. Bufezolac

50270-33-2. Isofezolac

50291-21-9. Rose Bengal Sodium I 131 [closed form] (See also *24916-55-0*)

50293-90-8. Levalbuterol Hydrochloride

50322-15-1. Piperazine Edetate Calcium [dihydrate] (See also *12002-30-1; 110-85-0; 60-00-4*)

50335-55-2. Mezilamine

50366-32-0. Flunamine

50370-12-2. Cefadroxil [anhydrous] (See also *66592-87-8; 119922-85-9*)

50432-78-5. Pemerid Nitrate [pemerid] (See also *34114-01-7*)

50435-25-1. Nimidane

50450-03-8. Crofilcon A

50454-68-7. Tolnidamine

50465-39-9. Tocofibrate

50516-43-3. Nofecainide

50528-97-7. Xilobam

50583-06-7. Halonamine

50588-47-1. Amafolone

50602-21-6. Polacrilin (See also *9017-36-1*)

50629-82-8. Halometasone

50650-76-5. Piroctone

50673-97-7. Colestolone

50679-07-7. Cinepazet Maleate (See also *23887-41-4*)

50679-08-8. Terfenadine

50700-72-6. Vecuronium Bromide

50708-95-7. Tinabinol

50717-86-7. Sodium Ferrous Citrate

50801-44-0. Cortisuzol

50838-36-3. Tolciclate

50846-45-2. Bacmecillinam

50847-11-5. Ibudilast

50865-01-5. Protoporphyrin Disodium

50892-23-4. Pirinixic Acid

50906-05-3. Ephedrine [hemihydrate] (See also *299-42-3*)

50924-49-7. Mizoribine

50935-04-1. Carubicin Hydrochloride [carubicin] (See also *52794-97-5*)

50935-71-2. Mocimycin [trivial name] (See also *52212-85-8*)

50936-59-9. Idursulfase

50972-17-3. Bacampicillin Hydrochloride [bacampicillin] (See also *37661-08-8*)

50978-10-4. Cyclomethycaine Sulfate (See also *139-62-8; 537-61-1*)

50978-11-5. Diatrizoic Acid [dihydrate] (See also *117-96-4*)

51012-32-9. Tiapride

51022-69-6. Amcinonide

51022-70-9. Albuterol Sulfate (See also *18559-94-9*)

51022-71-0. Nabilone

51022-73-2. Zometapine

51022-74-3. Iotroxic Acid

51022-75-4. Cliprofen

51022-76-5. Sulnidazole

51022-77-6. Etazolate Hydrochloride [etazolate] (See also *35838-58-5*)

51022-98-1. Butirosin Sulfate (See also *57549-48-1; 12772-35-9*)

51025-85-5. Arbekacin

51037-30-0. Acipimox

51037-88-8. Tuclazepam

51047-24-6. Dimetipirium Bromide

51146-56-6. Dexibuprofen

51152-91-1. Butaclamol Hydrochloride [butaclamol] (See also *36504-94-6*)

51154-48-4. Fibracillin

51213-99-1. Clanfenur

51222-36-7. Ciclafrine Hydrochloride (See also *55694-98-9*)

51222-37-8. Iproxamine Hydrochloride (See also *52403-19-7*)

51234-28-7. Benoxaprofen

51264-14-3. Amsacrine

51274-83-0. Tiamenidine Hydrochloride

51287-57-1. Denotivir

51321-79-0. Sparfosate Sodium [sparfosic acid] (See also *66569-27-5*)

51322-75-9. Tizanidine Hydrochloride [tizanidine] (See also *64461-82-1*)

51333-22-3. Budesonide [11β,16α] (See also *51372-29-3; 51372-28-2*)

51354-31-5. Nisterime Acetate (See also *51354-32-6*)

51354-32-6. Nisterime Acetate [nisterime] (See also *51354-31-5*)

51372-28-2. Budesonide [(11β,16α[*S*])] (See also *51333-22-3; 51372-29-3*)

51372-29-3. Budesonide [(11β,16α[*R*])] (See also *51333-22-3; 51372-28-2*)

51395-42-7. Butedronic Acid

51411-04-2. Alrestatin Sodium [alrestatin] (See also *51876-97-2*)

51460-26-5. Carbazochrome Sodium Sulfonate

51473-23-5. Lergotrile Mesylate (See also *36945-03-6*)

51481-60-8. Naloxone Hydrochloride [dihydrate] (See also *357-08-4; 465-65-6*)

51481-61-9. Cimetidine

51481-62-0. Bucainide Maleate [bucainide] (See also *51481-63-1*)

51481-63-1. Bucainide Maleate (See also *51481-62-0*)

51481-64-2. Rosaramicin Propionate (See also *35834-26-5*)

51481-65-3. Mezlocillin

51481-67-5. Octriptyline Phosphate (See also *47166-67-6*)

51481-68-6. Megalomicin Potassium Phosphate (See also *28022-11-9*)

51493-19-7. Cinprazole

51497-09-7. Tenamfetamine

51527-19-6. Tianafac

51543-39-6. Esflurbiprofen

51543-40-9. Tarenflurbil

51547-64-9. Rosaramicin Stearate (See also *35834-26-5*)

51552-99-9. Diperodon (See also *101-08-6*)

51579-82-9. Amfenac Sodium [amfenac] (See also *61618-27-7*)

51598-60-8. Cimetropium Bromide

51627-14-6. Cefatrizine

51627-20-4. Cefaparole

51630-58-1. Fenvalerate

51762-05-1. Cefroxadine

51764-33-1. Iodoxamate Meglumine (See also *31127-82-9; 6284-40-8*)

51773-92-3. Mefloquine Hydrochloride

51781-06-7. Carteolol Hydrochloride [carteolol] (See also *51781-21-6*)

51781-21-6. Carteolol Hydrochloride (See also *51781-06-7*)

51798-72-2. Insulin Defalan [bovine] (See also *11091-62-6*)

51803-78-2. Nimesulide

51832-87-2. Picobenzide

51876-97-2. Alrestatin Sodium (See also *51411-04-2*)

51876-98-3. Gliamilide

51876-99-4. Ioseric Acid

51899-01-5. Ocrase

51934-76-0. Iomorinic Acid

51940-44-4. Pipemidic Acid

51940-78-4. Zetidoline

51952-41-1. Gonadorelin Hydrochloride (See also *33515-09-2*)

51953-95-8. Doxaprost

51987-65-6. Desglugastrin

52003-58-4. Ammonium Lactate

52014-67-2. Antithrombin III Human

52022-31-8. Ambenonium Chloride [tetrahydrate] (See also *115-79-7; 7648-98-8*)

52042-01-0. Elfazepam

52042-24-7. Diproxadol

52061-73-1. Valdipromide

52080-57-6. Chloroprednisone Acetate [chloroprednisone] (See also *14066-79-6*)

52093-21-7. Micronomicin

52094-70-9. Tetrantoin

52123-49-6. Cefazaflur Sodium (See also *58665-96-6*)

52128-35-5. Trimetrexate

52152-93-9. Cefsulodin Sodium (See also *62587-73-9*)

52157-83-2. Mindoperone

52157-91-2. Galosemide

52196-22-2. Ketotrexate

52205-73-9. Estramustine Phosphate Sodium

52212-02-9. Pipecuronium Bromide

52212-85-8. Mocimycin (See also *50935-71-2*)

52214-84-3. Ciprofibrate

52231-20-6. Cefrotil

52232-67-4. Teriparatide

52239-63-1. Thiethylperazine Malate (See also *1420-55-9*)

52247-86-6. Cicloxolone

52260-70-5. Gallium Citrate Ga 67 [replaced] (See also *41183-64-6*)

52279-58-0. Metogest

52279-59-1. Moxnidazole

52304-85-5. Lotucaine

52315-07-8. Cypermethrin

52340-25-7. Dexclamol Hydrochloride [dexclamol] (See also *52389-27-2*)

52365-63-6. Dipivefrin

52389-27-2. Dexclamol Hydrochloride (See also *52340-25-7*)

52391-89-6. Flutemazepam

52395-99-0. Belarizine

52403-19-7. Iproxamine Hydrochloride [iproxamine] (See also *51222-37-8*)

52406-01-6. Uredofos

52430-65-6. Glisamuride

52438-85-4. Prednisolone [sesquihydrate] (See also *50-24-8*)

52443-21-7. Glucametacin

52463-83-9. Pinazepam

52468-60-7. Flunarizine Hydrochloride [flunarazine] (See also *30484-77-6*)

52479-85-3. Exifone

52485-79-7. Buprenorphine Hydrochloride [buprenorphine] (See also *53152-21-9*)

52549-17-4. Pranoprofen

52618-67-4. Tioperidone Hydrochloride [tioperidone] (See also *52618-68-5*)

52618-68-5. Tioperidone Hydrochloride (See also *52618-67-4*)

52645-53-1. Permethrin

52658-53-4. Benfosformin (See also *35282-33-8*)

52663-86-2. Dimoxamine Hydrochloride (See also *52842-59-8*)

52699-48-6. Gonadorelin Acetate (See also *33515-09-2*)

52742-40-2. Alimadol

52757-95-6. Sevelamer Hydrochloride [sevelamer] (See also *182683-00-7*)

52758-02-8. Benzaprinoxide

52760-47-1. Tametraline Hydrochloride (See also *52795-02-5*)

52794-97-5. Carubicin Hydrochloride (See also *50935-04-1*)

52795-02-5. Tametraline Hydrochloride [tametraline] (See also *52760-47-1*)

52814-39-8. Metesculetol

52829-30-8. Proflazepam

52832-91-4. Xinomiline

52842-59-8. Dimoxamine Hydrochloride [dimoxamine] (See also *52663-86-2*)

52867-74-0. Zoloperone

52867-77-3. Fluzoperine

52906-84-0. Oxychlorosene Sodium (See also *8031-14-9*)

52918-63-5. Deltamethrin

52932-64-6. Cinodine Hydrochloride [antibiotic BM 123γ] (See also *68782-58-1*)

52934-83-5. Nanafrocin

52942-31-1. Etoperidone Hydrochloride [etoperidone] (See also *57775-22-1*)

52994-25-9. Glicondamide

53003-10-4. Salinomycin

53003-81-9. Ivarimod

53016-31-2. Norelgestromin

53026-85-0. Aluminum Chlorohydrex

53034-85-8. Ibuterol

53066-26-5. Lexithromycin

53076-26-9. Moxaprindine

53086-13-8. Dexindoprofen

53123-88-9. Sirolimus

53131-74-1. Ciapilome

53152-21-9. Buprenorphine Hydrochloride (See also *52485-79-7*)

53164-05-9. Acemetacin

53179-07-0. Nisoxetine

53179-09-2. Sisomicin Sulfate (See also *32385-11-8*)

53179-10-5. Fluperamide

53179-11-6. Loperamide Hydrochloride [loperamide] (See also *34552-83-5*)

53179-12-7. Clopimozide

53179-13-8. Pirfenidone

53230-10-7. Mefloquine

53251-94-8. Pinaverium Bromide (See also *59995-65-2*)

53267-01-9. Cifenline

53274-41-2. Cetocycline Hydrochloride [4α,4aβ,12aβ] (See also *56433-46-6; 29144-42-1*)

53308-83-1. Tilarginine Acetate (See also *17035-90-4*)

53341-49-4. Ponfibrate

53361-24-3. Imafen Hydrochloride (See also *59198-18-4*)

53370-90-4. Exalamide

53394-92-6. Drinidene

53400-67-2. Tiquinamide Hydrochloride [tiquinamide] (See also *53400-68-3*)

53400-68-3. Tiquinamide Hydrochloride (See also *53400-67-2*)

53403-97-7. Pyridofylline

53415-46-6. Fepitrizol

53421-38-3. Diethylaminoethyl Diphenylhydroxypropionate Hydrochloride

53449-58-4. Ciclonicate

53583-79-2. Sultopride

53597-26-5. Etoformin Hydrochloride (See also *45086-03-1*)

53597-27-6. Fendosal

53597-28-7. Fludazonium Chloride

53608-75-6. Pancrelipase

53608-96-1. Cloxotestosterone

53626-53-2. Tetrafilcon A

53643-48-4. Vindesine

53648-05-8. Ibuproxam

53648-55-8. Dezocine

53657-16-2. Dimepranol Acedoben [dimepranol] (See also *61990-51-0*)

53664-53-2. Lutropin Alfa [β-subunit] (See also *152923-57-4; 56832-30-5*)

53684-49-4. Bufetolol

53716-44-2. Rociverine

53716-45-3. Anilopam Hydrochloride (See also *53716-46-4*)

53716-46-4. Anilopam Hydrochloride [anilopam] (See also *53716-45-3*)

53716-47-5. Nexeridine Hydrochloride (See also *53716-48-6*)

53716-48-6. Nexeridine Hydrochloride [nexeridine] (See also *53716-47-5*)

53716-49-7. Carprofen

53716-50-0. Oxfendazole

53731-36-5. Floredil

53736-51-9. Cromitrile Sodium [cromitrile] (See also *53736-52-0*)

53736-52-0. Cromitrile Sodium (See also *53736-51-9*)

53746-45-5. Fenoprofen Calcium (See also *34597-40-5; 31879-05-7*)

53746-46-6. Trimazosin Hydrochloride (See also *35795-17-6; 35795-16-5*)

53772-83-1. Zuclopenthixol

53783-83-8. Tromantadine

53808-86-9. Ritropirronium Bromide

53808-87-0. Tetroxoprim

53808-88-1. Lonazolac

53813-83-5. Suriclone

53850-34-3. Thaumatin

53861-02-2. Oxetacillin

53862-80-9. Roxolonium Metilsulfate

53862-81-0. Detajmium Bitartrate (See also *33774-52-6*)

53882-12-5. Lodoxamide Ethyl [lodoxamide] (See also *53882-13-6*)

53882-13-6. Lodoxamide Ethyl (See also *53882-12-5*)

53885-35-1. Ticlopidine Hydrochloride (See also *55142-85-3*)

53902-12-8. Tranilast

53906-69-7. Aspartame [replaced] (See also *22839-47-0*)

53910-25-1. Pentostatin

53943-88-7. Letosteine

53966-34-0. Floxacrine

53973-98-1. Poligeenan

53983-00-9. Nibroxane

53993-67-2. Tiflorex

53994-73-3. Cefaclor [anhydrous] (See also *70356-03-5*)

54017-73-1. Murodermin

54022-49-0. Vinformide

54024-22-5. Desogestrel

54029-12-8. Albendazole Oxide

54048-10-1. Etonogestrel

54063-23-9. Cinepazic Acid

54063-24-0. Amifloverine

54063-25-1. Amiterol

54063-26-2. Azaftozine

54063-27-3. Biclofibrate

54063-28-4. Camiverine

54063-29-5. Cicarperone

54063-30-8. Ciltoprazine

54063-31-9. Cismadinone

54063-32-0. Clobetasone Butyrate [clobetasone] (See also *25122-57-0*)

54063-33-1. Cloxestradiol

54063-34-2. Cofisatin

54063-35-3. Dofamium Chloride

54063-36-4. Etolorex

54063-37-5. Etoprindole

54063-38-6. Fenaperone

54063-39-7. Fenetradil

54063-40-0. Fenoxedil

54063-41-1. Fepromide

54063-42-2. Ferric Citrate (^{59}Fe) [Injection]

54063-44-4. Ferropolimaler

54063-45-5. Fetoxylate Hydrochloride [fetoxylate] (See also *23607-71-8*)

54063-46-6. Fexicaine

54063-47-7. Gemazocine

54063-48-8. Heptaverine

54063-49-9. Metamfazone

54063-50-2. Mofloverine

54063-51-3. Nadoxolol

54063-52-4. Pitofenone

54063-53-5. Propafenone Hydrochloride [propafenone] (See also *34183-22-7*)

54063-54-6. Reproterol Hydrochloride [reproterol] (See also *13055-82-8*)

54063-55-7. Sulfaclorazole

54063-56-8. Suloctidil

54063-57-9. Suxethonium Chloride

54063-58-0. Toprilidine

54083-22-6. Zorubicin Hydrochloride [zorubicin] (See also *36508-71-1*)

54110-25-7. Pirozadil

54116-21-1. Netrafilcon A

54120-61-5. Prostalene

54141-87-6. Cinfenine

54143-54-3. Sepazonium Chloride

54143-55-4. Flecainide Acetate [flecainide] (See also *54143-56-5*)

54143-56-5. Flecainide Acetate (See also *54143-55-4*)

54143-57-6. Metoclopramide Hydrochloride (See also *7232-21-5; 364-62-5*)

54147-28-3. Tebatizole

54163-88-1. Metoprolol [replaced] (See also *37350-58-6*)

54182-58-0. Sucralfate

54182-59-1. Sulglicotide

54182-62-6. Polacrilin Potassium [replaced] (See also *65405-55-2; 50602-21-6*)

54182-63-7. Macrosalb (^{131}I)

54182-65-9. Azalomycin

54187-04-1. Rilmenidine

54188-38-4. Metralindole

54194-00-2. Salcolex [anhydrous] (See also *28038-04-2*)

54194-01-3. Saralasin Acetate [anhydrous] (See also *39698-78-7; 34273-10-4*)

54239-37-1. Cimaterol

54277-47-3. Macrosalb (^{99m}Tc)

54278-85-2. Candocuronium Iodide

54328-33-5. Danaparoid Sodium [dermatan, 4-(hydrogen sulfate), sodium salt] (See also *57459-72-0; 39455-18-0; 12678-07-8*)

54340-58-8. Meptazinol Hydrochloride [meptazinol] (See also *59263-76-2*)

54340-59-9. Quincarbate
54340-61-3. Brovanexine
54340-62-4. Bufuralol
54340-63-5. Clofeverine
54340-64-6. Fluciprazine
54340-65-7. Furbucillin
54340-66-8. Subendazole
54341-00-3. Dimefilcon A
54341-02-5. Piflutixol
54350-48-0. Etretinate
54376-91-9. Tipetropium Bromide
54400-59-8. Butamisole Hydrochloride [butamisole] (See also *54400-62-3*)
54400-62-3. Butamisole Hydrochloride (See also *54400-59-8*)
54419-31-7. Fenirofibrate
54451-24-0. Lanthanum Carbonate
54504-70-0. Theofibrate
54510-20-2. Iodocetylic Acid I 123
54527-84-3. Nicardipine Hydrochloride (See also *55985-32-5*)
54531-52-1. Polybenzarsol (See also *9006-68-2*)
54533-85-6. Nizofenone
54556-98-8. Propiverine [hydrochloride] (See also *60569-19-9*)
54573-75-0. Doxercalciferol
54592-27-7. Divabuterol
54605-45-7. Iocarmate Meglumine (See also *10397-75-8; 6284-40-8*)
54644-15-4. Carbantel Lauryl Sulfate (See also *22790-84-7*)
54657-96-4. Nifuralide
54657-98-6. Serfibrate
54663-47-7. Tibezonium Iodide
54739-18-3. Fluvoxamine Maleate [fluvoxamine] (See also *61718-82-9*)
54739-19-4. Clovoxamine
54785-02-3. Adamexine
54818-11-0. Cefsumide
54824-17-8. Mitonafide
54824-20-3. Pinafide
54845-95-3. Icomucret
54867-56-0. Bufrolin
54870-27-8. Fosfonet Sodium (See also *36983-81-0; 4408-78-0*)
54870-28-9. Meglitinide
54910-89-3. Fluoxetine
54935-03-4. Sulisatin
54965-21-8. Albendazole
54965-22-9. Fluspiperone
54965-24-1. Tamoxifen Citrate (See also *10540-29-1*)
55028-70-1. Arbaprostil
55028-71-2. Fluprostenol Sodium (See also *40666-16-8*)
55028-72-3. Cloprostenol Sodium (See also *40665-92-7*)
55073-41-1. Sodium Glycerophosphate (See also *1334-74-3; 27082-31-1*)
55077-30-0. Aclatonium Napadisilate
55079-83-9. Acitretin
55096-26-9. Nalmefene
55102-44-8. Bofumustine
55103-30-5. Rosaramicin Butyrate (See also *35834-26-5*)
55134-13-9. Narasin

55142-85-3. Ticlopidine Hydrochloride [ticlopidine] (See also *53885-35-1*)
55149-05-8. Pirolate
55150-67-9. Climiqualine
55162-26-0. Pirbenicillin Sodium (See also *55975-92-3*)
55165-22-5. Butocrolol
55172-29-7. Thallous Chloride Tl 201
55242-55-2. Propentofylline
55242-74-5. Oxifungin Hydrochloride (See also *64057-48-3*)
55242-77-8. Triafungin
55248-23-2. Nebidrazine
55268-74-1. Praziquantel
55268-75-2. Cefuroxime
55273-05-7. Impromidine Hydrochloride [impromidine] (See also *65573-02-6*)
55285-35-3. Butanixin
55285-45-5. Pirifibrate
55286-56-1. Doxaminol
55294-15-0. Muzolimine
55297-95-5. Tiamulin (See also *56142-71-3*)
55297-96-6. Tiamulin Fumarate (See also *55297-95-5*)
55299-10-0. Pivoxazepam
55299-11-1. Iquindamine
55300-29-3. Antrafenine
55313-67-2. Pipramadol
55432-15-0. Pirinidazole
55435-65-9. Acodazole Hydrochloride (See also *79152-85-5*)
55453-87-7. Isoxepac
55477-19-5. Iprozilamine
55482-89-8. Guacetisal
55485-20-6. Acaprazine
55530-41-1. Rotamicillin
55541-30-5. Dexamethasone Dipropionate
55557-30-7. Levopropoxyphene Napsylate (See also *5714-90-9; 5667-69-6; 2338-37-6*)
55560-96-8. Tixocortol Pivalate (See also *61951-99-3*)
55589-62-3. Acesulfame Potassium
55689-65-1. Oxepinac
55694-83-2. Pentizidone Sodium [pentizidone] (See also *59831-62-8*)
55694-98-9. Ciclafrine Hydrochloride [ciclafrine] (See also *51222-36-7*)
55695-56-2. Cloroperone Hydrochloride (See also *61764-61-2*)
55721-11-4. Secalciferol
55726-47-1. Enocitabine
55769-65-8. Butobendine
55779-06-1. Astromicin Sulfate [astromicin] (See also *72275-67-3; 66768-12-5*)
55779-18-5. Arprinocid
55812-90-3. Dexamethasone Acetate (See also *1177-87-3*)
55837-13-3. Piclopastine
55837-14-4. Butaverine
55837-15-5. Butopiprine
55837-16-6. Entsufon Sodium [entsufon] (See also *2917-94-4*)
55837-17-7. Brindoxime
55837-18-8. Butibufen

55837-19-9. Exaprolol Hydrochloride [exaprolol] (See also *59333-90-3*)
55837-20-2. Halofuginone Hydrobromide [halofuginone] (See also *64924-67-0*)
55837-21-3. Pipoxizine
55837-22-4. Pribecaine
55837-23-5. Teflutixol
55837-24-6. Bisfenazone
55837-25-7. Buflomedil
55837-26-8. Fenperate
55837-27-9. Piretanide
55837-28-0. Tiafibrate
55837-29-1. Tiropramide
55843-86-2. Miroprofen
55845-78-8. Xenipentone
55870-64-9. Pentisomicin
55872-82-7. Azarole
55902-02-8. Isamfazone
55902-93-7. Mebenoside
55902-94-8. Sitofibrate
55905-53-8. Clebopride
55926-23-3. Guanclofine
55937-99-0. Beclobrate
55975-92-3. Pirbenicillin Sodium [pirbenicillin] (See also *55162-26-0*)
55981-09-4. Nitazoxanide
55985-32-5. Nicardipine Hydrochloride [nicardipine] (See also *54527-84-3*)
55986-43-1. Cetaben Sodium [cetaben] (See also *64059-66-1*)
56030-50-3. Trepipam Maleate [trepipam] (See also *39624-66-3*)
56030-52-5. Bufilcon A
56030-54-7. Sufentanil
56038-13-2. Sucralose
56066-19-4. Aditeren
56066-63-8. Aditoprim
56079-80-2. Ropitoin Hydrochloride (See also *56079-81-3*)
56079-81-3. Ropitoin Hydrochloride [ropitoin] (See also *56079-80-2*)
56087-11-7. Dextranomer
56097-80-4. Valconazole
56119-96-1. Furodazole [anhydrous]
56124-62-0. Valrubicin
56142-71-3. Tiamulin [replaced] (See also *55297-95-5*)
56180-94-0. Acarbose
56187-47-4. Cefazedone
56187-89-4. Ximoprofen
56208-01-6. Pifarnine
56211-40-6. Torsemide
56211-43-9. Tameticillin
56219-57-9. Arildone
56227-39-5. Polidexide Sulfate [polidexide] (See also *63494-82-6*)
56238-63-2. Cefuroxime Sodium
56254-07-0. Iodohippurate Sodium I 123
56281-36-8. Motretinide
56283-74-0. Laidlomycin Propionate Potassium [laidlomycin] (See also *84799-02-0*)
56287-74-2. Afloqualone
56290-94-9. Medroxalol
56302-13-7. Satranidazole
56341-08-3. Mabuterol
56355-17-0. Zoliprofen
56377-79-8. Nosiheptide

56383-05-2. Zindotrine
56390-09-1. Epirubicin Hydrochloride (See also *56420-45-2*)
56391-55-0. Octazamide
56391-56-1. Netilmicin Sulfate [netilmicin] (See also *56391-57-2*)
56391-57-2. Netilmicin Sulfate (See also *56391-56-1*)
56392-17-7. Metoprolol Tartrate (See also *37350-58-6*)
56420-45-2. Epirubicin Hydrochloride [epirubicin] (See also *56390-09-1*)
56430-99-0. Flumecinol
56433-44-4. Oxaprotiline Hydrochloride [oxaprotiline] (See also *39022-39-4*)
56433-46-6. Cetocycline Hydrochloride (See also *53274-41-2; 29144-42-1*)
56463-68-4. Isoprazone
56481-43-7. Setazindol
56488-58-5. Tizolemide
56488-59-6. Terbufibrol
56488-60-9. Glutaurine
56488-61-0. Flubepride
56518-41-3. Brodimoprim
56551-60-1. Lidofilcon A
56562-79-9. Ioglunide
56585-33-2. Trimethoprim Sulfate (See also *738-70-5*)
56592-32-6. Efrotomycin
56605-16-4. Spiromustine
56611-65-5. Oxagrelate
56689-41-9. Aliflurane
56689-42-0. Repromicin
56689-43-1. Canbisol
56689-44-2. Nitramisole Hydrochloride (See also *6363-02-6*)
56689-45-3. Josamycin
56693-13-1. Mociprazine
56693-15-3. Terciprazine
56695-65-9. Rosaprostol
56717-18-1. Isotiquimide
56739-21-0. Nitraquazone
56741-95-8. Bropirimine
56767-76-1. Flurbiprofen Sodium
56775-88-3. Zimeldine Hydrochloride [zimeldine] (See also *61129-30-4; 60525-15-7*)
56784-39-5. Ozolinone
56796-20-4. Cefmetazole
56796-39-5. Cefmetazole Sodium
56824-20-5. Amiprilose Hydrochloride [amiprilose] (See also *60414-06-4*)
56832-30-5. Choriogonadotropin Alfa [α-subunit] (See also *177073-44-8; 56832-34-9*)
56832-34-9. Choriogonadotropin Alfa [β-subunit] (See also *177073-44-8; 56832-30-5*)
56897-09-7. Norcholestenol Iodomethyl (^{131}I) [Injection]
56917-29-4. Fluretofen
56959-18-3. Glusoferron
56969-22-3. Oxapadol
56980-93-9. Celiprolol Hydrochloride [celiprolol] (See also *57470-78-7*)
56983-13-2. Furofenac
56995-20-1. Flupirtine Maleate [flupirtine] (See also *75507-68-5*)

57009-15-1. Isocromil
57010-31-8. Tiapamil Hydrochloride [tiapamil] (See also *87434-83-1*)
57021-61-1. Isonixin
57041-67-5. Desflurane
57067-46-6. Isamoxole
57076-71-8. Denbufylline
57083-89-3. Peralopride
57109-90-7. Clorazepate Dipotassium (See also *20432-69-3*)
57132-53-3. Proglumetacin
57144-56-6. Isoprofen
57149-07-2. Naftopidil
57166-13-9. Napactadine Hydrochloride
57206-54-9. Efepristin
57227-17-5. Sevopramide
57237-97-5. Timoprazole
57248-88-1. Pamidronate Disodium [anhydrous] (See also *109552-15-0*)
57262-94-9. Setiptiline
57282-49-2. Lysine Acetate
57296-63-6. Indacrinone
57333-96-7. Tacalcitol
57363-13-0. Droxacin Sodium (See also *35067-47-1*)
57363-14-1. Fluotracen Hydrochloride (See also *35764-73-9*)
57381-26-7. Irsogladine
57432-61-8. Methylergonovine Maleate (See also *7054-07-1; 113-42-8*)
57435-86-6. Premazepam
57441-90-4. Nivimedone Sodium [anhydrous] (See also *62077-09-2; 49561-92-4*)
57459-72-0. Danaparoid Sodium [heparan, sulfate, sodium salt] (See also *54328-33-5; 39455-18-0; 12678-07-8*)
57460-41-0. Talinolol
57469-77-9. Ibuprofen Lysine
57470-78-7. Celiprolol Hydrochloride (See also *56980-93-9*)
57474-29-0. Nifuroquine
57475-17-9. Brovincamine
57479-88-6. Sulmepride
57524-89-7. Hydrocortisone Valerate
57526-81-5. Prenalterol Hydrochloride [prenalterol] (See also *61260-05-7*)
57529-83-6. Azipramine Hydrochloride (See also *58503-82-5*)
57548-79-5. Picafibrate
57549-48-1. Butirosin Sulfate [anhydrous] (See also *51022-98-1; 12772-35-9*)
57558-44-8. Secoverine
57574-09-1. Amineptine
57576-44-0. Aclarubicin
57645-05-3. Sermetacin
57647-79-7. Benclonidine
57648-21-2. Timiperone
57653-27-7. Droprenilamine
57653-28-8. Ibazocine
57653-29-9. Cogazocine
57666-60-1. Nitrafudam Hydrochloride (See also *64743-09-5*)
57680-55-4. Gleptoferron
57680-56-5. Sucrosofate Potassium [sucrosofate] (See also *76578-81-9*)
57694-27-6. Vinpoline

57695-04-2. Sitamaquine
57726-65-5. Nufenoxole
57734-69-7. Sequifenadine
57773-63-4. Triptorelin
57773-65-6. Deslorelin
57775-22-1. Etoperidone Hydrochloride (See also *52942-31-1*)
57775-26-5. Sultosilic Acid
57775-28-7. Prefenamate
57775-29-8. Carazolol
57781-14-3. Halopredone Acetate (See also *57781-15-4*)
57781-15-4. Halopredone Acetate [halopredone] (See also *57781-14-3*)
57801-81-7. Brotizolam
57808-63-6. Cicloxilic Acid
57808-64-7. Toldimfos
57808-65-8. Closantel
57808-66-9. Domperidone
57821-29-1. Sulodexide
57821-32-6. Menfegol
57847-69-5. Cefedrolor
57852-57-0. Idarubicin Hydrochloride (See also *58957-92-9*)
57916-70-8. Iclazepam
57925-64-1. Naprodoxime
57935-49-6. Tiomergine
57938-82-6. Adinazolam Mesylate (See also *37115-32-5*)
57982-77-1. Buserelin Acetate [buserelin] (See also *68630-75-1*)
57982-78-2. Budipine
57998-68-2. Diaziquone
58001-44-8. Clavulanic Acid
58012-63-8. Furcloprofen
58019-50-4. Menabitan Hydrochloride (See also *83784-21-8*)
58019-65-1. Nabazenil
58066-85-6. Miltefosine
58069-82-2. Urea C 13
58095-31-1. Sulbenox
58152-03-7. Isepamicin
58158-77-3. Amantanium Bromide
58166-83-9. Cafedrine
58167-74-1. Mafilcon A
58167-76-3. Edetate Dipotassium [monohydrate] (See also *25102-12-9; 2001-94-7*)
58167-78-5. Tandamine Hydrochloride (See also *42408-80-0*)
58182-63-1. Itanoxone
58186-27-9. Idebenone
58207-19-5. Clindamycin Hydrochloride [monohydrate] (See also *21462-39-5; 18323-44-9*)
58239-89-7. Moxazocine
58261-91-9. Mefenidil
58298-92-3. Colimecycline
58306-30-2. Febantel
58313-74-9. Treptilamine
58337-35-2. Elliptinium Acetate
58338-59-3. Dinaline
58409-59-9. Bucumolol
58416-00-5. Protiofate
58433-11-7. Tilomisole
58456-86-3. Cephradine [dihydrate] (See also *38821-53-3; 31828-50-9*)
58473-73-7. Drobuline

58473-74-8. Cinromide
58493-49-5. Olvanil
58497-00-0. Procinonide
58503-79-0. Meobentine Sulfate (See also *46464-11-3*)
58503-81-4. Droxifilcon A
58503-82-5. Azipramine Hydrochloride [azipramine] (See also *57529-83-6*)
58503-83-6. Penirolol
58513-59-0. Thiothixene Hydrochloride [anhydrous] (See also *22189-31-7; 49746-09-0; 49746-04-5; 5591-45-7*)
58524-83-7. Ciprocinonide
58546-54-6. Besigomsin
58551-69-2. Carboprost Tromethamine (See also *35700-23-3*)
58560-75-1. Ibuprofen [± mixture] (See also *15687-27-1*)
58569-55-4. Metenkefalin
58579-51-4. Anagrelide Hydrochloride (See also *68475-42-3*)
58581-89-8. Azelastine Hydrochloride [azelastine] (See also *79307-93-0*)
58602-66-7. Aminopterin Sodium (See also *54-62-6*)
58652-20-3. Nomegestrol Acetate (See also *58691-88-6*)
58662-84-3. Meclonazepam
58665-96-6. Cefazaflur Sodium [cefazaflur] (See also *52123-49-6*)
58691-88-6. Nomegestrol Acetate [nomegestrol] (See also *58652-20-3*)
58703-77-8. Sulprosal
58703-78-9. Cethexonium Chloride
58712-69-9. Traxanox
58754-46-4. Iferanserin
58757-61-2. Trimexiline
58761-87-8. Sudexanox
58765-21-2. Ciclotizolam
58769-17-8. Gestadienol
58786-99-5. Butorphanol Tartrate (See also *42408-82-2*)
58795-03-2. Apalcillin Sodium (See also *63469-19-2*)
58805-38-2. Probicromil Calcium [probicromil] (See also *71144-97-3*)
58832-68-1. Cloximate
58857-02-6. Ambruticin
58882-17-0. Roxadimate
58934-46-6. Lorcainide Hydrochloride (See also *59729-31-6*)
58944-73-3. Sinefungin
58957-92-9. Idarubicin Hydrochloride [idarubicin] (See also *57852-57-0*)
58970-76-6. Ubenimex
58985-93-6. Hydrofilcon A
58994-96-0. Ranimustine
59009-93-7. Carburazepam
59010-44-5. Prizidilol Hydrochloride [prizidilol] (See also *73398-12-6; 63642-19-3*)
59017-64-0. Ioxaglic Acid
59018-13-2. Ioxaglate Meglumine
59032-40-5. Disulergine
59040-30-1. Nafazatrom
59070-06-3. Ticarcillin Cresyl Sodium (See also *59070-07-4*)

59070-07-4. Ticarcillin Cresyl Sodium [ticarcillin cresyl] (See also *59070-06-3*)
59091-65-5. Delergotrile
59110-35-9. Pamatolol Sulfate [pamatolol] (See also *59954-01-7*)
59122-46-2. Misoprostol
59128-97-1. Haloxazolam
59160-29-1. Lidofenin
59170-23-9. Bevantolol Hydrochloride [bevantolol] (See also *42864-78-8*)
59179-95-2. Lorzafone [anhydrous] (See also *81603-65-8*)
59184-78-0. Buquineran
59198-18-4. Imafen Hydrochloride [imafen] (See also *53361-24-3*)
59209-97-1. Zafuleptine
59227-89-3. Laurocapram
59263-76-2. Meptazinol Hydrochloride (See also *54340-58-8*)
59277-89-3. Acyclovir
59333-67-4. Fluoxetine Hydrochloride
59333-90-3. Exaprolol Hydrochloride [monohydrochloride] (See also *55837-19-9*)
59338-93-1. Alizapride
59429-50-4. Tamitinol
59467-70-8. Midazolam Hydrochloride [midazolam] (See also *59467-96-8*)
59467-77-5. Climazolam
59467-94-6. Midazolam Maleate (See also *59467-70-8*)
59467-96-8. Midazolam Hydrochloride (See also *59467-70-8*)
59497-39-1. Naflocort [anhydrous] (See also *80738-47-2*)
59549-62-1. Pivampicillin Pamoate [replaced] (See also *39030-72-3; 33817-20-8*)
59619-81-7. Etiproston
59625-89-7. Magnesium Gluconate [dihydrate] (See also *3632-91-5*)
59643-91-3. Imexon
59653-73-5. Teroxirone
59703-84-3. Piperacillin Sodium
59708-52-0. Carfentanil Citrate [carfentanil] (See also *61380-27-6*)
59721-28-7. Camostat
59729-31-6. Lorcainide Hydrochloride [lorcainide] (See also *58934-46-6*)
59729-32-7. Citalopram Hydrobromide
59729-33-8. Citalopram
59729-37-2. Fexinidazole
59733-86-7. Butikacin
59752-23-7. Benderizine
59755-82-7. Enolicam Sodium [enolicam] (See also *73574-69-3; 59756-39-7*)
59756-39-7. Enolicam Sodium [anhydrous] (See also *73574-69-3; 59755-82-7*)
59767-12-3. Octastine
59776-90-8. Dupracetam
59794-18-2. Paulomycin
59798-30-0. Mezlocillin Sodium
59798-73-1. Enilospirone
59803-98-4. Brimonidine Tartrate [brimonidine] (See also *79570-19-7*)
59804-37-4. Tenoxicam

59828-07-8. Procaterol Hydrochloride (See also *72332-33-3; 60443-17-6*)
59831-62-8. Pentizidone Sodium (See also *55694-83-2*)
59831-63-9. Doconazole
59831-64-0. Milenperone
59831-65-1. Halopemide
59840-71-0. Pitenodil
59859-58-4. Femoxetine
59865-13-3. Cyclosporine
59866-76-1. Bibenzonium Bromide [bibenzonium] (See also *15585-70-3*)
59889-36-0. Ciprefadol Succinate [ciprefadol] (See also *60719-85-9*)
59917-39-4. Vindesine Sulfate (See also *53643-48-4*)
59937-28-9. Malotilate
59939-16-1. Cirazoline
59954-01-7. Pamatolol Sulfate (See also *59110-35-9*)
59973-80-7. Exisulind
59985-21-6. Diquafosol Tetrasodium [diquafosol] (See also *211427-08-6*)
59989-18-3. Eniluracil
59995-65-2. Pinaverium Bromide [pinaverium] (See also *53251-94-8*)
60019-19-4. Iotetric Acid
60019-20-7. Brazergoline
60023-92-9. Roxibolone
60070-14-6. Mariptiline
60084-10-8. Tiazofurin
60085-78-1. Clopipazan Mesylate [clopipazan] (See also *60086-22-8*)
60086-22-8. Clopipazan Mesylate (See also *60085-78-1*)
60104-29-2. Clofezone
60104-30-5. Orazamide
60135-06-0. Mercumatilin Sodium (See also *574-79-8; 43043-01-2*)
60135-22-0. Flumoxonide
60136-25-6. Epervudine
60142-96-3. Gabapentin
60148-52-9. Cypothrin
60166-93-0. Iopamidol
60173-73-1. Arfalasin
60175-95-3. Omonasteine
60200-06-8. Clorsulon
60207-31-0. Azaconazole
60209-20-3. Lycetamine
60239-18-1. Tetraxetan
60248-23-9. Fuprazole
60282-87-3. Gestodene
60324-59-6. Nomelidine
60325-46-4. Sulprostone
60400-86-4. Procromil
60400-92-2. Proxicromil
60414-06-4. Amiprilose Hydrochloride (See also *56824-20-5*)
60443-17-6. Procaterol Hydrochloride [replaced] (See also *59828-07-8; 72332-33-3*)
60525-15-7. Zimeldine Hydrochloride [anhydrous] (See also *61129-30-4; 56775-88-3*)
60560-33-0. Pinacidil [anhydrous] (See also *85371-64-8*)
60561-17-3. Sufentanil Citrate

60569-19-9. Propiverine (See also *54556-98-8*)

60575-32-8. Amezepine

60576-13-8. Piketoprofen

60607-34-3. Oxatomide

60607-35-4. Topterone

60607-68-3. Indenolol

60628-96-8. Bifonazole

60628-98-0. Lombazole

60634-69-7. Methohexital Sodium [±] (See also *309-36-4; 22151-68-4; 18652-93-2*)

60643-86-9. Vigabatrin

60653-25-0. Orpanoxin

60662-14-8. Pentetate Indium Disodium In 111

60662-16-0. Binedaline

60662-18-2. Eniclobrate

60662-19-3. Nilprazole

60668-24-8. Alafosfalin

60719-82-6. Alaproclate

60719-84-8. Inamrinone

60719-85-9. Ciprefadol Succinate (See also *59889-36-0*)

60719-87-1. Deximafen [replaced] (See also *42116-77-8*)

60731-46-6. Elcatonin

60734-87-4. Nisbuterol Mesylate [nisbuterol] (See also *60734-88-5*)

60734-88-5. Nisbuterol Mesylate (See also *60734-87-4*)

60746-64-7. Silafocon A

60762-57-4. Pirlindole

60763-49-7. Cinnarizine Clofibrate

60784-46-5. Elmustine

60802-40-6. Rosaramicin Sodium Phosphate (See also *35834-26-5*)

60812-35-3. Decominol

60837-57-2. Anoxomer

60840-55-3. Porofocon A

60925-61-3. Ceforanide

60940-34-3. Ebselen

60986-89-2. Clofurac

61036-62-2. Teicoplanin

61054-06-6. Ibuprofen Aluminum (See also *15687-27-1; 58560-75-1*)

61115-28-4. Alusulf

61129-30-4. Zimeldine Hydrochloride (See also *60525-15-7; 56775-88-3*)

61136-12-7. Almurtide

61177-45-5. Clavulanate Potassium

61197-73-7. Loprazolam

61220-69-7. Tiopinac

61260-05-7. Prenalterol Hydrochloride (See also *57526-81-5*)

61263-35-2. Meteneprost

61270-58-4. Cefonicid Monosodium [cefonicid] (See also *71420-79-6*)

61270-78-8. Cefonicid Sodium

61318-90-9. Sulconazole Nitrate [sulconazole] (See also *61318-91-0*)

61318-91-0. Sulconazole Nitrate (See also *61318-90-9*)

61325-80-2. Flumezapine

61336-70-7. Amoxicillin (See also *26787-78-0*)

61337-67-5. Mirtazapine [replaced] (See also *85650-52-8; 82601-27-2*)

61337-87-9. Esmirtazapine

61343-44-0. Tocofenoxate

61379-65-5. Rifapentine

61380-27-6. Carfentanil Citrate (See also *59708-52-0*)

61380-40-3. Lofentanil Oxalate [lofentanil] (See also *61380-41-4*)

61380-41-4. Lofentanil Oxalate (See also *61380-40-3*)

61400-59-7. Parconazole Hydrochloride [parconazole] (See also *62973-77-7*)

61413-54-5. Rolipram

61422-45-5. Carmofur

61444-62-0. Nifluridide

61463-79-4. Etafilcon A

61477-94-9. Pirmenol Hydrochloride (See also *68252-19-7*)

61477-95-0. Monalazone Disodium

61477-96-1. Piperacillin [anhydrous] (See also *66258-76-2*)

61477-97-2. Dazolicine

61484-38-6. Pareptide Sulfate [pareptide] (See also *61484-39-7*)

61484-39-7. Pareptide Sulfate (See also *61484-38-6*)

61545-06-0. Temocillin [temocillin sodium] (See also *66148-78-5*)

61557-12-8. Penprostene

61563-18-6. Soquinolol

61570-90-9. Tioxidazole

61618-27-7. Amfenac Sodium (See also *51579-82-9*)

61622-34-2. Cefotiam Hydrochloride [cefotiam] (See also *66309-69-1*)

61661-06-1. Levdobutamine Lactobionate [levdobutamine] (See also *129388-07-4*)

61718-82-9. Fluvoxamine Maleate (See also *54739-18-3*)

61764-61-2. Cloroperone Hydrochloride [cloroperone] (See also *55695-56-2*)

61822-36-4. Diprobutine

61825-94-3. Oxaliplatin

61849-14-7. Epoprostenol Sodium (See also *35121-78-9*)

61864-30-0. Benolizime

61869-07-6. Domiodol

61869-08-7. Paroxetine

61887-16-9. Dulofibrate

61914-43-0. Glucuronamide

61951-99-3. Tixocortol Pivalate [tixocortol] (See also *55560-96-8*)

61966-08-3. Triciribine Phosphate

61990-51-0. Dimepranol Acedoben (See also *53657-16-2*)

61990-92-9. Benpenolisin

62013-04-1. Dirithromycin

62030-88-0. Duoperone Fumarate [duoperone] (See also *62030-89-1*)

62030-89-1. Duoperone Fumarate (See also *62030-88-0*)

62052-97-5. Bumepidil

62077-09-2. Nivimedone Sodium (See also *57441-90-4; 49561-92-4*)

62087-72-3. Pentigetide

62087-96-1. Triletide

62107-94-2. Plauracin

62134-34-3. Butoprozine Hydrochloride (See also *62228-20-0*)

62220-58-0. Bipenamol Hydrochloride (See also *79467-22-4*)

62228-20-0. Butoprozine Hydrochloride [butoprozine] (See also *62134-34-3*)

62253-63-8. Nepidermin

62265-68-3. Quinfamide

62288-83-9. Desmopressin Acetate [anhydrous] (See also *62357-86-2; 16679-58-6*)

62304-98-7. Thymalfasin

62305-86-6. Orotirelin

62357-86-2. Desmopressin Acetate (See also *62288-83-9; 16679-58-6*)

62380-23-8. Cinecromen

62435-42-1. Perfosfamide

62473-79-4. Teniloxazine

62510-56-9. Picilorex

62524-99-6. Delprostenate

62559-74-4. Froxiprost

62568-57-4. Emideltide

62571-86-2. Captopril

62571-87-3. Minaxolone

62571-88-4. Evicromil

62587-73-9. Cefsulodin Sodium [cefsulodin] (See also *52152-93-9*)

62613-82-5. Oxiracetam

62625-18-7. Pirogliride Tartrate [pirogliride] (See also *62625-19-8*)

62625-19-8. Pirogliride Tartrate (See also *62625-18-7*)

62658-63-3. Bopindolol (See also *62658-64-4*)

62658-64-4. Bopindolol [malonate] (See also *62658-63-3*)

62658-88-2. Mesudipine

62666-20-0. Progabide

62732-44-9. Ipidacrine

62816-98-2. Ormaplatin

62851-43-8. Zidometacin

62882-99-9. Tinazoline

62893-19-0. Cefoperazone Sodium [cefoperazone] (See also *62893-20-3*)

62893-20-3. Cefoperazone Sodium (See also *62893-19-0*)

62894-89-7. Tiflamizole

62904-71-6. Doxpicomine Hydrochloride [doxpicomine] (See also *69494-04-8*)

62906-34-7. Deltafilcon A

62928-11-4. Iproplatin

62952-06-1. Aspirin DL-Lysine

62973-76-6. Azanidazole

62973-77-7. Parconazole Hydrochloride (See also *61400-59-7*)

62989-33-7. Sapropterin Dihydrochloride [sapropterin] (See also *69056-38-8*)

62992-61-4. Etersalate

63014-96-0. Delanterone

63074-08-8. Terazosin Hydrochloride [anhydrous] (See also *70024-40-7; 63590-64-7*)

63075-47-8. Fepradinol

63119-27-7. Anitrazafen

63132-38-7. Lidadronic Acid

63132-39-8. Olpadronic Acid

63204-23-9. Oxmetidine Hydrochloride (See also *72830-39-8*)

63245-28-3. Etifenin

63251-39-8. Sulfinalol Hydrochloride (See also *66264-77-5*)

63266-93-3. Eganoprost

63269-31-8. Ciramadol

63283-36-3. Calcifediol (See also *19356-17-3*)

63304-56-3. Seractide Acetate [seractide] (See also *39295-97-1; 39294-79-6*)

63323-46-6. Ciramadol Hydrochloride (See also *63269-31-8*)

63329-53-3. Lobenzarit Sodium [lobenzarit] (See also *64808-48-6*)

63358-49-6. Aspoxicillin

63388-37-4. Declenperone

63394-05-8. Plafibride

63409-12-1. Tylvalosin

63428-13-7. Tylvalosin Tartrate

63469-19-2. Apalcillin Sodium [apalcillin] (See also *58795-03-2*)

63472-04-8. Metbufen

63494-82-6. Polidexide Sulfate (See also *56227-39-5*)

63516-07-4. Flutropium Bromide

63521-85-7. Esorubicin Hydrochloride [esorubicin] (See also *63950-06-1*)

63527-52-6. Cefotaxime Sodium [cefotaxime] (See also *64485-93-4*)

63534-64-5. Iosulamide Meglumine (See also *23205-04-1; 6284-40-8*)

63540-28-3. Fenobam

63547-13-7. Adrafinil

63551-77-9. Sfericase

63585-09-1. Foscarnet Sodium

63590-64-7. Terazosin Hydrochloride [terazosin] (See also *70024-40-7; 63074-08-8*)

63610-08-2. Indobufen

63610-09-3. Lodoxamide Tromethamine (See also *53882-12-5*)

63612-50-0. Nilutamide

63619-84-1. Trioxifene Mesylate [trioxifene] (See also *68307-81-3*)

63638-91-5. Brofaromine

63642-19-3. Prizidilol Hydrochloride [anhydrous] (See also *73398-12-6; 59010-44-5*)

63659-12-1. Cicloprolol Hydrochloride [cicloprolol] (See also *63686-79-3*)

63659-18-7. Betaxolol Hydrochloride [betaxolol] (See also *63659-19-8*)

63659-19-8. Betaxolol Hydrochloride (See also *63659-18-7*)

63667-16-3. Dribendazole

63675-72-9. Nisoldipine

63686-79-3. Cicloprolol Hydrochloride (See also *63659-12-1*)

63690-57-3. Penicillin V Benzathine [tetrahydrate] (See also *5928-84-7; 87-08-1*)

63758-79-2. Indalpine

63824-12-4. Aliconazole

63834-83-3. Guaietolin

63927-95-7. Bentemazole

63941-73-1. Ioglucol

63941-74-2. Ioglucomide

63950-06-1. Esorubicin Hydrochloride (See also *63521-85-7*)

63958-90-7. Nonathymulin

63968-64-9. Artemisinin

63996-84-9. Tibalosin

64000-73-3. Pildralazine

64019-03-0. Doqualast

64019-93-8. Dipivefrin Hydrochloride

64024-15-3. Pentazocine Hydrochloride (See also *359-83-1*)

64039-88-9. Nicafenine

64057-48-3. Oxifungin Hydrochloride [oxifungin] (See also *55242-74-5*)

64059-66-1. Cetaben Sodium (See also *55986-43-1*)

64063-57-6. Picotrin Diolamine [picotrin] (See also *64063-83-8*)

64063-83-8. Picotrin Diolamine (See also *64063-57-6*)

64092-48-4. Zomepirac Sodium [anhydrous] (See also *64092-49-5; 33369-31-2*)

64092-49-5. Zomepirac Sodium (See also *64092-48-4; 33369-31-2*)

64098-32-4. Zapizolam

64099-44-1. Quisultazine

64118-86-1. Azimexon

64179-54-0. Timofibrate

64204-55-3. Esaprazole

64211-45-6. Oxiconazole Nitrate [oxiconazole] (See also *64211-46-7*)

64211-46-7. Oxiconazole Nitrate (See also *64211-45-6*)

64212-22-2. Nafimidone Hydrochloride [nafimidone] (See also *70891-37-1*)

64218-02-6. Plaunotol

64221-86-9. Imipenem [anhydrous] (See also *74431-23-5*)

64224-21-1. Oltipraz

64228-81-5. Atracurium Besylate

64241-34-5. Cadralazine

64294-94-6. Tropabazate

64294-95-7. Setastine

64314-52-9. Medorubicin

64318-79-2. Gemeprost

64336-55-6. Oxycodone Terephthalate

64379-93-7. Cinflumide

64396-09-4. Terfluranol

64420-40-2. Etibendazole

64440-87-5. Cideferron

64461-82-1. Tizanidine Hydrochloride (See also *51322-75-9*)

64485-93-4. Cefotaxime Sodium (See also *63527-52-6*)

64490-92-2. Tolmetin Sodium (See also *35711-34-3*)

64496-66-8. Salafibrate

64506-49-6. Sofalcone

64519-82-0. Isomalt [dihydrate]

64521-35-3. Ferrous Citrate Fe 59

64544-07-6. Cefuroxime Axetil (See also *55268-75-2*)

64552-16-5. Ecipramidil

64552-17-6. Butofilolol

64557-97-7. Cinoquidox

64603-91-4. Gaboxadol

64638-07-9. Brolamfetamine

64743-08-4. Diclofurime

64743-09-5. Nitrafudam Hydrochloride [nitrafudam] (See also *57666-60-1*)

64748-79-4. Azumolene Sodium [azumolene] (See also *91524-18-4*)

64755-06-2. Quinuclium Bromide (See also *35425-83-3*)

64779-98-2. Irolapride

64795-23-9. Etisulergine

64795-35-3. Mesulergine

64808-48-6. Lobenzarit Sodium (See also *63329-53-3*)

64840-90-0. Eperisone

64860-67-9. Valperinol

64872-76-0. Butoconazole Nitrate [butoconazole] (See also *64872-77-1*)

64872-77-1. Butoconazole Nitrate (See also *64872-76-0*)

64881-21-6. Caricotamide

64924-67-0. Halofuginone Hydrobromide (See also *55837-20-2*)

64952-97-2. Moxalactam Disodium [moxalactam] (See also *64953-12-4*)

64953-12-4. Moxalactam Disodium (See also *64952-97-2*)

65002-17-7. Bucillamine

65008-93-7. Bometolol

65009-35-0. Lidamidine Hydrochloride (See also *66871-56-5*)

65043-22-3. Indeloxazine Hydrochloride

65052-63-3. Cefetamet

65057-90-1. Talisomycin

65085-01-0. Cefmenoxime Hydrochloride [cefmenoxime] (See also *75738-58-8*)

65089-17-0. Pirinixil

65141-46-0. Nicorandil

65184-10-3. Teoprolol

65195-55-3. Abamectin [Component B$_{1a}$] (See also *65195-56-4*)

65195-56-4. Abamectin [Component B$_{1b}$] (See also *65195-55-3*)

65222-35-7. Pazelliptine

65236-29-5. Prenoverine

65271-80-9. Mitoxantrone Hydrochloride [mitoxantrone] (See also *70476-82-3*)

65277-42-1. Ketoconazole

65285-58-7. Vincantril

65307-12-2. Cefetrizole

65322-72-7. Endralazine Mesylate [monomethanesulfonate] (See also *39715-02-1*)

65329-79-5. Mobenzoxamine

65350-86-9. Meciadanol

65389-08-4. Indium In 111 Oxyquinoline

65400-85-3. Ethyl Carfluzepate

65405-55-2. Polacrilin Potassium (See also *54182-62-6; 50602-21-6*)

65415-41-0. Nicocortonide

65415-42-1. Oxabrexine

65429-87-0. Spirendolol

65454-61-7. Technetium Tc 99m Pentetate

65472-88-0. Naftifine Hydrochloride [naftifine] (See also *65473-14-5*)

65473-14-5. Naftifine Hydrochloride (See also *65472-88-0*)

65509-24-2. Maroxepin

65509-66-2. Citatepine

65511-41-3. Nantradol Hydrochloride [nantradol] (See also *65511-42-4*)

65511-42-4. Nantradol Hydrochloride (See also *65511-41-3*)
65517-27-3. Metaclazepam
65569-29-1. Cloxacepride
65571-68-8. Lofemizole Hydrochloride [lofemizole] (See also *70169-80-1*)
65573-02-6. Impromidine Hydrochloride (See also *55273-05-7*)
65576-45-6. Asenapine Maleate [asenapine] (See also *85650-56-2*)
65606-61-3. Diciferron
65617-86-9. Avizafone
65634-39-1. Pentafluranol
65646-68-6. Fenretinide
65652-44-0. Pirbuterol Acetate (See also *38677-81-5*)
65655-59-6. Pacrinolol
65708-37-4. Flufosal
65717-97-7. Disofenin
65761-24-2. Sulfamazone
65776-67-2. Afurolol
65807-02-5. Goserelin
65847-85-0. Morniflumate
65884-46-0. Ciadox
65886-71-7. Fazarabine
65896-14-2. Romifidine [hydrochloride] (See also *65896-16-4*)
65896-16-4. Romifidine (See also *65896-14-2*)
65899-72-1. Alozafone
65899-73-2. Tioconazole
65928-58-7. Dienogest
65950-99-4. Pirquinozol
66051-63-6. Halofantrine Hydrochloride [[±]-halofantrine] (See also *36167-63-2; 69756-53-2*)
66085-59-4. Nimodipine
66093-35-4. Talmetoprim
66104-22-1. Pergolide Mesylate [pergolide] (See also *66104-23-2*)
66104-23-2. Pergolide Mesylate (See also *66104-22-1*)
66108-95-0. Iohexol
66112-59-2. Temurtide
66148-78-5. Temocillin (See also *61545-06-0*)
66172-75-6. Verofylline
66195-31-1. Ibopamine
66203-00-7. Carocainide
66203-94-9. Murocainide
66208-11-5. Ifoxetine
66211-92-5. Detorubicin
66215-27-8. Cyromazine
66258-76-2. Piperacillin (See also *61477-96-1*)
66264-77-5. Sulfinalol Hydrochloride [sulfinalol] (See also *63251-39-8*)
66292-52-2. Butilfenin
66292-53-3. Iprofenin
66304-03-8. Epicainide
66309-69-1. Cefotiam Hydrochloride (See also *61622-34-2*)
66327-51-3. Fuzlocillin
66357-35-5. Ranitidine
66357-59-3. Ranitidine Hydrochloride
66364-73-6. Enpiroline Phosphate [enpiroline] (See also *66364-74-7*)

66364-74-7. Enpiroline Phosphate (See also *66364-73-6*)
66376-36-1. Alendronic Acid
66451-06-7. Bornaprolol
66474-36-0. Cefivitril
66504-75-4. Bicifadine Hydrochloride (See also *71195-57-8*)
66508-53-0. Fosmidomycin
66516-09-4. Mertiatide
66529-17-7. Midaglizole
66532-85-2. Propacetamol
66535-86-2. Lotrifen
66556-74-9. Nabitan Hydrochloride [nabitan] (See also *49637-08-3*)
66564-14-5. Cinitapride
66564-15-6. Aleptide
66564-16-7. Ciclosidomine
66569-27-5. Sparfosate Sodium [disodium salt] (See also *51321-79-0*)
66575-29-9. Colforsin
66592-87-8. Cefadroxil (See also *50370-12-2; 119922-85-9*)
66608-04-6. Rolgamidine
66608-32-0. Imcarbofos
66635-85-6. Anirolac
66644-81-3. Veralipride
66711-21-5. Apraclonidine Hydrochloride [apraclonidine] (See also *73218-79-8*)
66722-44-9. Bisoprolol
66734-12-1. Butopamine
66734-13-2. Alclometasone Dipropionate (See also *67452-97-5*)
66759-48-6. Desocriptine
66768-12-5. Astromicin Sulfate [xH_2SO_4] (See also *72275-67-3; 55779-06-1*)
66778-37-8. Orconazole Nitrate [orconazole] (See also *66778-38-9*)
66778-38-9. Orconazole Nitrate (See also *66778-37-8*)
66788-41-8. Tinofedrine
66794-74-9. Encainide Hydrochloride (See also *37612-13-8*)
66813-51-2. Alexitol Sodium
66827-12-1. Almagate (See also *72526-11-5*)
66834-24-0. Cianopramine
66852-54-8. Halobetasol Propionate (See also *98651-66-2*)
66866-63-5. Lutrelin Acetate [lutrelin] (See also *83784-18-3*)
66871-56-5. Lidamidine Hydrochloride [lidamidine] (See also *65009-35-0*)
66877-67-6. Domoprednate
66887-96-5. Propikacin
66898-60-0. Talosalate
66898-62-2. Talniflumate
66934-18-7. Flunoxaprofen
66960-34-7. Metkephamid Acetate [metkephamid] (See also *66960-35-8*)
66960-35-8. Metkephamid Acetate (See also *66960-34-7*)
66969-81-1. Tiodazosin
66981-73-5. Tianeptine
66984-59-6. Cinfenoac
66985-17-9. Ipratropium Bromide (See also *22254-24-6*)

67037-37-0. Eflornithine Hydrochloride [eflornithine] (See also *96020-91-6*)
67040-53-3. Tiprostanide
67101-27-3. Alofilcon A
67102-87-8. Pentomone
67110-79-6. Luprostiol
67121-76-0. Fluperlapine
67165-56-4. Diclofensine
67182-81-4. Bispyrithione Magsulfex
67199-66-0. Daniquidone
67227-55-8. Primidolol
67227-56-9. Fenoldopam Mesylate [fenoldopam] (See also *67227-57-0*)
67227-57-0. Fenoldopam Mesylate (See also *67227-56-9*)
67244-90-0. Phenylpropanolamine Bitartrate
67254-81-3. Peradoxime
67268-43-3. Giparmen
67330-25-0. Ufenamate
67337-44-4. Sarmoxicillin
67346-49-0. Arformoterol Tartrate [arformoterol] (See also *200815-49-2*)
67375-30-8. Alpha-Cypermethrin
67392-87-4. Drospirenone
67394-31-4. Verilopam Hydrochloride (See also *68318-20-7*)
67422-14-4. Proinsulin Human
67452-97-5. Alclometasone Dipropionate [alclometasone] (See also *66734-13-2*)
67469-69-6. Vanoxerine
67489-39-8. Talmetacin
67527-59-7. Iprocinodine Hydrochloride [*N*-(1-methylethyl)antibiotic BM 123γ] (See also *68782-59-2*)
67542-41-0. Imuracetam
67577-23-5. Pivenfrine
67579-24-2. Bromadoline Maleate [bromadoline] (See also *81447-81-6*)
67696-82-6. Acrihellin
67699-41-6. Vinzolidine Sulfate
67700-30-5. Furaprofen
67765-04-2. Enefexine
67793-71-9. Draquinolol
67832-40-0. Malethamer (See also *29535-27-1[replaced]; 9011-01-2*)
67915-31-5. Terconazole
67992-58-9. Ioxaglate Sodium
68020-77-9. Carprazidil
68045-74-9. Copovithane
68085-85-8. Cyhalothrin
68134-81-6. Gacyclidine
68170-69-4. Vinepidine Sulfate [vinepidine] (See also *83200-11-7*)
68170-97-8. Palmoxirate Sodium [palmoxiric acid] (See also *79069-97-9*)
68206-94-0. Cloricromen
68238-36-8. Isosulfan Blue
68247-85-8. Peplomycin Sulfate [peplomycin] (See also *70384-29-1*)
68252-19-7. Pirmenol Hydrochloride [pirmenol] (See also *61477-94-9*)
68284-69-5. Disobutamide
68289-14-5. Metrazifone
68291-97-4. Zonisamide
68298-00-0. Pirnabine [(±)-pirnabine] (See also *19825-63-9*)

68302-57-8. Amlexanox

68307-81-3. Trioxifene Mesylate (See also *63619-84-1*)

68318-20-7. Verilopam Hydrochloride [verilopam] (See also *67394-31-4*)

68359-37-5. Cyfluthrin

68367-52-2. Sorbinil

68373-14-8. Sulbactam Benzathine [sulbactam] (See also *83031-43-0*)

68377-92-4. Arotinolol

68379-03-3. Clofilium Phosphate

68392-35-8. Afimoxifene

68401-81-0. Ceftizoxime Sodium [ceftizoxime] (See also *68401-82-1*)

68401-82-1. Ceftizoxime Sodium (See also *68401-81-0*)

68411-27-8. Alkyl (C12-15) Benzoate

68424-04-4. Polydextrose

68444-58-6. Cellulose Sodium Phosphate

68475-40-1. Cipropride

68475-42-3. Anagrelide Hydrochloride [anagrelide] (See also *58579-51-4*)

68497-62-1. Pramiracetam Hydrochloride [pramiracetam] (See also *75733-50-5*)

68548-99-2. Oxindanac

68550-75-4. Cilostamide

68556-59-2. Prosulpride

68562-41-4. Mecasermin

68567-30-6. Solpecainol

68576-86-3. Enciprazine Hydrochloride [enciprazine] (See also *68576-88-5*)

68576-88-5. Enciprazine Hydrochloride (See also *68576-86-3*)

68616-83-1. Pentamorphone

68630-75-1. Buserelin Acetate (See also *57982-77-1*)

68635-50-7. Deloxolone

68677-06-5. Lorapride

68693-11-8. Modafinil

68693-30-1. Somantadine Hydrochloride (See also *79594-24-4*)

68741-18-4. Buterizine

68767-14-6. Loxoprofen

68782-58-1. Cinodine Hydrochloride (See also *52932-64-6*)

68782-59-2. Iprocinodine Hydrochloride (See also *67527-59-7*)

68786-66-3. Triclabendazole

68788-56-7. Etacepride

68797-29-5. Pipradimadol

68797-31-9. Econazole Nitrate (See also *27220-47-9*)

68813-55-8. Oxantel Pamoate (See also *36531-26-7*)

68844-77-9. Astemizole

68859-20-1. Insulin Argine

68876-74-4. Zocainone

68890-66-4. Piroctone Olamine (See also *50650-76-5*)

68893-82-3. Parathyroid Hormone [human] (See also *345663-45-8; 9002-64-6*)

68902-57-8. Metioprim

68959-20-6. Disiquonium Chloride

69004-03-1. Toltrazuril

69004-04-2. Ponazuril

69014-14-8. Tiotidine

69017-89-6. Ipexidine Mesylate [ipexidine] (See also *69017-90-9*)

69017-90-9. Ipexidine Mesylate (See also *69017-89-6*)

69047-39-8. Binifibrate

69049-06-5. Alfentanil Hydrochloride [anhydrous] (See also *70879-28-6; 71195-58-9*)

69049-73-6. Nedocromil

69049-74-7. Nedocromil Sodium

69056-38-8. Sapropterin Dihydrochloride (See also *62989-33-7*)

69118-25-8. Cinepaxadil

69123-90-6. Fiacitabine

69123-98-4. Fialuridine

69175-77-5. Losindole

69198-10-3. Metronidazole Hydrochloride (See also *443-48-1*)

69207-52-9. Methyl Palmoxirate

69217-67-0. Sumacetamol

69304-47-8. Brivudine

69365-65-7. Fenoctimine Sulfate [fenoctimine] (See also *69365-66-8; 69365-67-9*)

69365-66-8. Fenoctimine Sulfate (See also *69365-67-9; 69365-65-7*)

69365-67-9. Fenoctimine Sulfate [anhydrous] (See also *69365-66-8; 69365-65-7*)

69372-19-6. Pemirolast Potassium [pemirolast] (See also *100299-08-9*)

69373-95-1. Diproteverine

69376-27-8. Dextrorphan Hydrochloride (See also *125-73-5*)

69381-94-8. Fenprostalene

69387-87-7. Tinisulpride

69388-79-0. Sulbactam Pivoxil

69388-84-7. Sulbactam Sodium (See also *68373-14-8*)

69402-03-5. Piridicillin Sodium (See also *69414-41-1*)

69408-81-7. Amonafide

69414-41-1. Piridicillin Sodium [piridicillin] (See also *69402-03-5*)

69425-13-4. Prifelone

69429-84-1. Cilobamine Mesylate [cilobamine] (See also *69429-85-2*)

69429-85-2. Cilobamine Mesylate (See also *69429-84-1*)

69430-24-6. Cyclomethicone

69479-26-1. Pirepolol

69494-04-8. Doxpicomine Hydrochloride (See also *62904-71-6*)

69539-53-3. Etintidine Hydrochloride [etintidine] (See also *71807-56-2*)

69542-93-4. Pivagabine

69558-55-0. Thymopentin

69624-60-8. Nelezaprine Maleate [nelezaprine] (See also *107407-62-5*)

69635-63-8. Amipizone

69648-38-0. Butaprost

69648-40-4. Oxoprostol

69655-05-6. Didanosine

69657-51-8. Acyclovir Sodium

69712-56-7. Cefotetan

69739-16-8. Cefodizime (See also *86329-79-5*)

69756-53-2. Halofantrine Hydrochloride [halofantrine] (See also *36167-63-2; 66051-63-6*)

69787-79-7. Avilamycin [avilamycin A] (See also *11051-71-1; 69787-80-0*)

69787-80-0. Avilamycin [avilamycin C] (See also *11051-71-1; 69787-79-7*)

69796-04-9. Diacetolol Hydrochloride (See also *22568-64-5*)

69815-38-9. Proxorphan Tartrate [proxorphan] (See also *69815-39-0*)

69815-39-0. Proxorphan Tartrate (See also *69815-38-9*)

69815-49-2. Norepinephrine Bitartrate (See also *51-40-1; 5794-08-1; 51-41-2*)

69819-86-9. Darinaparsin

69900-72-7. Trimoprostil

69907-17-1. Indopanolol

69915-62-4. Loxanast

69956-77-0. Pelubiprofen

69975-86-6. Doxofylline

70009-66-4. Oxalinast

70018-51-8. Quazinone

70024-40-7. Terazosin Hydrochloride (See also *63074-08-8; 63590-64-7*)

70059-30-2. Cimetidine Hydrochloride

70132-50-2. Pimonidazole

70145-52-7. Cyclofilcon A

70161-09-0. Democonazole

70161-10-3. Medroxalol Hydrochloride (See also *56290-94-9*)

70161-11-4. Ivermectin [component B_{1a}] (See also *70288-86-7; 70209-81-3*)

70169-80-1. Lofemizole Hydrochloride (See also *65571-68-8*)

70181-03-2. Dazopride Fumarate [dazopride] (See also *81957-25-7*)

70209-81-3. Ivermectin [component B_{1b}] (See also *70288-86-7; 70161-11-4*)

70222-86-5. Levonantradol Hydrochloride (See also *71048-87-8*)

70260-53-6. Mindodilol

70288-86-7. Ivermectin (See also *70161-11-4; 70209-81-3*)

70312-00-4. Tolnapersine

70356-03-5. Cefaclor (See also *53994-73-3*)

70356-09-1. Avobenzone

70369-47-0. Bucindolol Hydrochloride (See also *71119-11-4*)

70374-39-9. Lornoxicam

70384-29-1. Peplomycin Sulfate [sulfate salt, 1:1] (See also *68247-85-8*)

70384-91-7. Lortalamine

70458-92-3. Pefloxacin

70458-95-6. Pefloxacin Mesylate

70458-96-7. Norfloxacin

70476-82-3. Mitoxantrone Hydrochloride (See also *65271-80-9*)

70529-35-0. Itazigrel

70541-17-2. Oxazafone

70590-58-8. Etrabamine

70639-48-4. Etisomicin

70641-51-9. Edelfosine

70667-26-4. Ornoprostil

70696-66-1. Napirimus

70704-03-9. Vinconate

70711-40-9. Ametantrone Acetate

70724-25-3. Carbazeran

70774-25-3. Leurubicin

70775-75-6. Octenidine Hydrochloride (See also *71251-02-0*)

70788-27-1. Acefylline Clofibrol

70788-28-2. Flurofamide

70788-29-3. Tolfamide

70797-11-4. Cefpiramide

70801-02-4. Flutroline

70833-07-7. Prifuroline

70865-14-4. Conorphone Hydrochloride (See also *72060-05-0*)

70879-28-6. Alfentanil Hydrochloride (See also *69049-06-5; 71195-58-9*)

70891-37-1. Nafimidone Hydrochloride (See also *64212-22-2*)

70895-39-5. Tipropidil Hydrochloride (See also *70895-45-3*)

70895-45-3. Tipropidil Hydrochloride [tipropidil] (See also *70895-39-5*)

70976-76-0. Bifepramide

70977-46-7. Eflumast

71002-09-0. Pirazolac

71002-10-3. Vidarabine Sodium Phosphate (See also *29984-33-6; 5536-17-4*)

71010-45-2. Glisindamide

71010-52-1. Gellan Gum

71027-13-9. Eclanamine Maleate [eclanamine] (See also *71027-14-0*)

71027-14-0. Eclanamine Maleate (See also *71027-13-9*)

71031-15-7. Cathinone

71048-87-8. Levonantradol Hydrochloride [levonantradol] (See also *70222-86-5*)

71048-88-9. Ceftioxide

71079-19-1. Timegadine

71097-23-9. Zoficonazole

71097-83-1. Nileprost

71109-09-6. Vedaprofen

71116-82-0. Tiaprost

71119-10-3. Lotifazole

71119-11-4. Bucindolol Hydrochloride [bucindolol] (See also *70369-47-0*)

71119-12-5. Dinazafone

71125-38-7. Meloxicam

71138-71-1. Octapinol

71138-97-1. Hypromellose Acetate Succinate

71144-97-3. Probicromil Calcium [Ca salt (1:1)] (See also *58805-38-2*)

71195-56-7. Broclepride

71195-57-8. Bicifadine Hydrochloride [bicifadine] (See also *66504-75-4*)

71195-58-9. Alfentanil Hydrochloride [alfentanil] (See also *70879-28-6; 69049-06-5*)

71205-22-6. Almasilate

71247-25-1. Ceruletide Diethylamine [x salt]

71251-02-0. Octenidine Hydrochloride [octenidine] (See also *70775-75-6*)

71251-04-2. Surfomer

71276-43-2. Quadazocine Mesylate [quadazocine] (See also *71276-44-3*)

71276-44-3. Quadazocine Mesylate (See also *71276-43-2*)

71316-84-2. Fluradoline Hydrochloride [fluradoline] (See also *77590-97-7*)

71320-77-9. Moclobemide

71351-79-6. Icotidine

71420-79-6. Cefonicid Monosodium (See also *61270-58-4*)

71439-68-4. Bisantrene Hydrochloride (See also *78186-34-2*)

71461-18-2. Tonazocine Mesylate [tonazocine] (See also *73789-00-1*)

71475-35-9. Lozilurea

71486-22-1. Vinorelbine Tartrate [vinorelbine] (See also *125317-39-7*)

71576-40-4. Aptazapine Maleate [aptazapine] (See also *71576-41-5*)

71576-41-5. Aptazapine Maleate (See also *71576-40-4*)

71617-10-2. Amiloxate

71628-96-1. Menogaril

71653-63-9. Riodipine

71675-85-9. Amisulpride

71680-63-2. Dametralast

71731-58-3. Tiquizium Bromide

71767-13-0. Iotasul

71771-90-9. Denopamine

71807-56-2. Etintidine Hydrochloride (See also *69539-53-3*)

71827-56-0. Clemeprol

71872-90-7. Nitralamine Hydrochloride [nitralamine] (See also *1432-75-3*)

71872-91-8. Meralein Sodium [meralein] (See also *4386-35-0*)

71923-29-0. Fludoxopone

71923-34-7. Clodoxopone

71963-77-4. Artemether

71990-00-6. Bremazocine

72005-58-4. Vadocaine

72035-36-0. Spirobarbital Sodium [spirobarbital] (See also *12262-77-0*)

72060-05-0. Conorphone Hydrochloride [conorphone] (See also *70865-14-4*)

72064-79-0. Prednisolone Valerate Acetate

72131-33-0. Sulotroban

72238-02-9. Retelliptine

72275-67-3. Astromicin Sulfate (See also *66768-12-5; 55779-06-1*)

72301-78-1. Viroxime [zinviroxime] (See also *72301-79-2*)

72301-79-2. Enviroxime

72318-55-9. Indorenate Hydrochloride

72324-18-6. Stepronin

72332-33-3. Procaterol Hydrochloride [procaterol] (See also *59828-07-8; 60443-17-6*)

72420-38-3. Acifran

72432-03-2. Miglitol

72432-10-1. Aniracetam

72444-62-3. Perafensine

72444-63-4. Lodiperone

72467-44-8. Piclonidine

72479-26-6. Fenticonazole Nitrate [fenticonazole] (See also *73151-29-8*)

72481-99-3. Brocrinat

72492-12-7. Spizofurone

72496-41-4. Pirarubicin

72509-76-3. Felodipine (See also *86189-69-7*)

72522-13-5. Eptazocine

72526-11-5. Almagate [anhydrous] (See also *66827-12-1*)

72526-12-6. Isomerol [a] (See also *72526-13-7*)

72526-13-7. Isomerol [b] (See also *72526-12-6*)

72558-82-8. Ceftazidime [anhydrous] (See also *78439-06-2*)

72559-06-9. Rifabutin

72573-82-1. Gadoteric Acid

72590-77-3. Hydrocortisone Probutate

72599-27-0. Miglustat

72619-34-2. Bermoprofen

72702-95-5. Ponalrestat

72714-74-0. Viqualine

72714-75-1. Ivoqualine

72716-75-7. Lupitidine Hydrochloride (See also *83903-06-4*)

72732-56-0. Piritrexim Isethionate [piritrexim] (See also *79483-69-5*)

72741-87-8. Tridolgosir Hydrochloride [tridolgosir] (See also *214462-68-7*)

72803-02-2. Darodipine

72808-81-2. Tepirindole

72822-12-9. Dapiprazole Hydrochloride [dapiprazole] (See also *72822-13-0*)

72822-13-0. Dapiprazole Hydrochloride (See also *72822-12-9*)

72822-56-1. Azaloxan Fumarate [azaloxan] (See also *86116-60-1*)

72830-39-8. Oxmetidine Hydrochloride [oxmetidine] (See also *63204-23-9*)

72869-16-0. Pramiracetam Sulfate (See also *68497-62-1*)

72895-88-6. Eltenac

72956-09-3. Carvedilol

72973-11-6. Forfenimex

73080-51-0. Repirinast

73090-70-7. Epiroprim

73105-03-0. Pentamustine

73121-56-9. Enprostil

73151-29-8. Fenticonazole Nitrate (See also *72479-26-6*)

73205-13-7. Ticabesone Propionate (See also *74131-77-4*)

73218-79-8. Apraclonidine Hydrochloride (See also *66711-21-5*)

73232-52-7. Methylnaltrexone Bromide

73278-54-3. Lamtidine

73310-10-8. Ethyl Icosapentate

73334-05-1. Metronidazole Phosphate

73334-07-3. Iopromide

73384-59-5. Ceftriaxone Sodium [ceftriaxone] (See also *104376-79-6*)

73384-60-8. Sulmazole

73398-12-6. Prizidilol Hydrochloride (See also *63642-19-3; 59010-44-5*)

73445-46-2. Fenflumizole

73514-87-1. Fosarilate

73573-42-9. Rescimetol

73573-87-2. Formoterol Fumarate [formoterol] (See also *43229-80-7*)

73573-88-3. Mevastatin

73574-69-3. Enolicam Sodium [monohydrate] (See also *59756-39-7; 59755-82-7*)
73590-58-6. Omeprazole
73590-85-9. Ufiprazole
73647-73-1. Viprostol
73681-12-6. Indecainide Hydrochloride (See also *74517-78-5*)
73684-69-2. Mirosamicin
73725-85-6. Lidanserin
73747-20-3. Sulverapride
73747-21-4. Naboctate Hydrochloride
73764-72-4. Etamestrol
73771-04-7. Prednicarbate
73789-00-1. Tonazocine Mesylate (See also *71461-18-2*)
73803-48-2. Tripamide
73815-11-9. Cimoxatone
73816-42-9. Meclocycline Sulfosalicylate (See also *2013-58-3*)
73865-18-6. Nardeterol
73873-87-7[replaced]. Iloprost (See also *78919-13-8*)
73931-96-1. Denzimol
73963-72-1. Cilostazol
74011-58-8. Enoxacin
74014-51-0. Rokitamycin
74050-20-7. Hydrocortisone Aceponate
74050-97-8. Haloperidol Decanoate
74050-98-9. Ketanserin
74103-06-3. Ketorolac Tromethamine [ketorolac] (See also *74103-07-4*)
74103-07-4. Ketorolac Tromethamine (See also *74103-06-3*)
74129-03-6. Tebuquine
74131-77-4. Ticabesone Propionate [ticabesone] (See also *73205-13-7*)
74168-08-4. Losmiprofen
74176-31-1. Alfaprostol
74191-85-8. Doxazosin Mesylate [doxazosin] (See also *77883-43-3*)
74220-07-8. Spirorenone
74226-22-5. Dazoxiben Hydrochloride (See also *78218-09-4*)
74252-25-8. Indomethacin Sodium
74258-86-9. Alacepril
74356-00-6. Cefotetan Disodium
74381-53-6. Leuprolide Acetate
74431-23-5. Imipenem (See also *64221-86-9*)
74436-00-3. Geclosporin
74512-12-2. Omoconazole Nitrate [omoconazole] (See also *83621-06-1*)
74513-62-5. Trimegestone
74517-42-3. Ditercalinium Chloride
74517-78-5. Indecainide Hydrochloride [indecainide] (See also *73681-12-6*)
74531-88-7. Tioxamast
74559-85-6. Zenazocine Mesylate
74604-76-5. Enoxamast
74627-35-3. Cianergoline
74639-40-0. Docarpamine
74682-62-5. Ticarcillin Monosodium [anhydrous]
74685-16-8. Picenadol Hydrochloride (See also *79201-85-7*)
74709-54-9. Vindeburnol

74738-24-2. Recainam Hydrochloride [recainam] (See also *74752-07-1*)
74752-07-1. Recainam Hydrochloride (See also *74738-24-2*)
74752-08-2. Recainam Tosylate
74764-40-2. Bepridil Hydrochloride
74772-77-3. Ciglitazone
74790-08-2. Spiroplatin
74817-61-1. Murabutide
74847-35-1. Pyronaridine
74849-93-7. Cefpiramide Sodium
74855-17-7. Iocanlidic Acid I 123
74863-84-6. Argatroban [anhydrous] (See also *141396-28-3*)
74899-71-1. Interferon Beta
74899-72-2. Interferon Alfa
74978-16-8. Magaldrate
75018-71-2. Tauroselcholic Acid
75067-66-2. Bromperidol Decanoate (See also *10457-90-6*)
75078-91-0. Temarotene
75139-05-8. Tetronasin Sodium
75139-06-9. Tetronasin
75172-81-5. Migalastat Hydrochloride (See also *108147-54-2*)
75176-37-3. Zofenoprilat Arginine [zofenoprilat] (See also *81872-09-5*)
75184-94-0. Fenprinast Hydrochloride [fenprinast] (See also *77482-47-4*)
75219-46-4. Atrimustine
75330-75-5. Lovastatin
75345-27-6. Polidronium Chloride
75358-37-1. Linogliride
75437-14-8. Milverine
75438-57-2. Moxonidine
75444-64-3. Flumeridone
75444-65-4. Pirenperone
75458-65-0. Tienocarbine
75464-11-8. Butantrone
75481-73-1. Cefminox
75507-68-5. Flupirtine Maleate (See also *56995-20-1*)
75522-73-5. Dazidamine
75529-73-6. Amperozide [hydrochloride] (See also *75558-90-6*)
75530-68-6. Nilvadipine
75558-90-6. Amperozide (See also *75529-73-6*)
75564-40-8. Biclodil Hydrochloride (See also *85125-49-1*)
75567-37-2. Ingenol Mebutate
75607-67-9. Fludarabine Phosphate (See also *21679-14-1*)
75616-02-3. Dulozafone
75616-03-4. Ciprazafone
75626-99-2. Tobuterol
75659-07-3. Dilevalol Hydrochloride [dilevalol] (See also *75659-08-4*)
75659-08-4. Dilevalol Hydrochloride (See also *75659-07-3*)
75689-93-9. Imanixil
75695-93-1. Isradipine
75696-02-5. Cinolazepam
75706-12-6. Leflunomide
75733-50-5. Pramiracetam Hydrochloride (See also *68497-62-1*)
75734-93-9. Polyglyconate

75738-58-8. Cefmenoxime Hydrochloride (See also *65085-01-0*)
75747-14-7. Tanespimycin
75748-50-4. Ancarolol
75751-89-2. Iogulamide
75755-07-6. Piridronic Acid
75820-08-5. Zidapamide
75841-82-6. Mopidralazine
75847-73-3. Enalapril Maleate [enalapril] (See also *76095-16-4*)
75859-03-9. Rimcazole Hydrochloride (See also *75859-04-0*)
75859-04-0. Rimcazole Hydrochloride [rimcazole] (See also *75859-03-9*)
75867-00-4. Fenfluthrin
75887-54-6. Artemotil
75889-62-2. Fostedil
75949-60-9. Isoxaprolol
75949-61-0. Pafenolol
75963-52-9. Nuclomedone
75970-99-9. Tecastemizole
75985-31-8. Ciamexon
75991-49-0. Dazepinil Hydrochloride (See also *75991-50-3*)
75991-50-3. Dazepinil Hydrochloride [dazepinil] (See also *75991-49-0*)
75992-53-9. Moxadolen
76002-75-0. Dazoquinast
76053-16-2. Reclazepam
76095-16-4. Enalapril Maleate (See also *75847-73-3*)
76144-81-5. Meldonium
76145-76-1. Tomoxiprole
76168-82-6. Ramoplanin
76252-06-7. Nicainoprol
76263-13-3. Fluzinamide
76301-19-4. Timefurone
76330-71-7. Altanserin Tartrate [altanserin] (See also *79449-96-0*)
76352-13-1. Tropapride
76420-72-9. Enalaprilat [anhydrous] (See also *84680-54-6*)
76448-31-2. Propenidazole
76448-47-0. Veradoline Hydrochloride (See also *79201-80-2*)
76470-66-1. Loracarbef [anhydrous] (See also *121961-22-6*)
76496-68-9. Levoprotiline
76497-13-7. Sultamicillin
76530-44-4. Azamulin
76536-74-8. Buquiterine
76541-72-5. Mifobate
76543-88-9. Interferon Alfa-2a
76547-98-3. Lisinopril [anhydrous] (See also *83915-83-7*)
76568-02-0. Flosequinan
76578-81-9. Sucrosofate Potassium (See also *57680-56-5*)
76584-70-8. Divalproex Sodium
76596-57-1. Broxaterol
76600-30-1. Nosantine
76610-84-9. Cefbuperazone
76631-46-4. Detomidine Hydrochloride [detomidine] (See also *90038-01-0*)
76639-94-6. Florfenicol
76675-97-3. Resocortol Butyrate [resocortol] (See also *76738-96-0*)
76676-34-1. Oxprenoate Potassium

76696-97-4. Rofelodine
76712-82-8. Histrelin
76716-60-4. Fluprazine
76732-75-7. Picartamide
76738-96-0. Resocortol Butyrate (See also *76675-97-3*)
76743-10-7. Lucartamide
76812-98-1. Trigevolol
76824-35-6. Famotidine
76894-77-4. Dazmegrel
76932-56-4. Nafarelin Acetate [nafarelin] (See also *86220-42-0*)
76953-65-6. Dramedilol
76956-02-0. Lavoltidine Succinate [lavoltidine] (See also *86160-82-9*)
76963-41-2. Nizatidine
76990-56-2. Milacemide Hydrochloride [milacemide] (See also *76990-85-7*)
76990-85-7. Milacemide Hydrochloride (See also *76990-56-2*)
77005-28-8. Texacromil
77016-85-4. Plomestane
77029-61-9. Dextrose [D-glucopyranose monohydrate] (See also *5996-10-1; 50-99-7; 2280-44-6; 492-62-5; 492-61-5*)
77086-21-6. Dizocilpine Maleate [dizocilpine] (See also *77086-22-7*)
77086-22-7. Dizocilpine Maleate (See also *77086-21-6*)
77146-42-0. Chlorhexidine Phosphanilate
77164-20-6. Levomoprolol
77175-51-0. Croconazole
77181-69-2. Sorivudine
77191-36-7. Nefiracetam
77197-48-9. Quinezamide
77257-42-2. Stilonium Iodide
77287-05-9. Rioprostil
77287-89-9. Xorphanol Mesylate [xorphanol] (See also *77287-90-2*)
77287-90-2. Xorphanol Mesylate (See also *77287-89-9*)
77326-95-5. Calcitriol [monohydrate] (See also *32222-06-3*)
77326-96-6. Flunisolide (See also *3385-03-3*)
77337-73-6. Acamprosate Calcium (See also *77337-76-9*)
77337-76-9. Acamprosate Calcium [acamprosate] (See also *77337-73-6*)
77342-26-8. Tefenperate
77360-52-2. Ceftiolene
77372-61-3. Valproate Pivoxil
77400-65-8. Asocainol
77416-65-0. Exepanol
77472-98-1. Pipequaline
77482-47-4. Fenprinast Hydrochloride (See also *75184-94-0*)
77495-92-2. Pirlimycin Hydrochloride [monohydrate]
77502-27-3. Tolpadol
77518-07-1. Amiflamine
77519-25-6. Dexetozoline
77528-67-7. Manozodil
77590-92-2. Suproclone
77590-95-5. Cetamolol Hydrochloride (See also *34919-98-7*)
77590-96-6. Flordipine

77590-97-7. Fluradoline Hydrochloride (See also *71316-84-2*)
77599-17-8. Panomifene
77639-66-8. Prinomide Tromethamine [prinomide] (See also *109636-76-2*)
77650-95-4. Proterguride
77658-97-0. Anaxirone
77671-31-9. Enoximone
77679-27-7. Iobenguane I 131
77695-52-4. Ecastolol
77727-10-7. Nacartocin
77858-21-0. Velaresol
77862-92-1. Falipamil
77883-43-3. Doxazosin Mesylate (See also *74191-85-8*)
77989-60-7. Metibride
78088-46-7. Tabilautide
78090-11-6. Picoprazole
78092-66-7. Ristianol Phosphate
78110-38-0. Aztreonam
78113-36-7. Romurtide
78168-92-0. Filenadol
78186-33-1. Fumoxicillin
78186-34-2. Bisantrene Hydrochloride [bisantrene] (See also *71439-68-4*)
78208-13-6. Zolenzepine
78218-09-4. Dazoxiben Hydrochloride [dazoxiben] (See also *74226-22-5*)
78246-49-8. Paroxetine Hydrochloride
78247-49-1. Potassium Guaiacolsulfonate
78266-06-5. Mebrofenin
78273-80-0. Roxatidine Acetate Hydrochloride [roxatidine] (See also *93793-83-0; 78628-28-1*)
78281-72-8. Nepafenac
78299-53-3. Tiacrilast
78370-13-5. Emopamil
78371-66-1. Bucromarone
78372-26-6. Tefilcon A
78372-27-7. Stirocainide
78410-57-8. Ociltide
78415-72-2. Milrinone
78421-12-2. Droxicainide
78439-06-2. Ceftazidime (See also *72558-82-8*)
78459-19-5. Adimolol
78466-70-3. Zomebazam
78466-98-5. Razobazam
78467-68-2. Locicortolone Dicibate
78480-14-5. Dicresulene
78512-63-7. Pimelautide
78541-97-6. Piquindone Hydrochloride [piquindone] (See also *83784-19-4*)
78613-35-1. Amorolfine (See also *78613-38-4*)
78613-38-4. Amorolfine [hydrochloride] (See also *78613-35-1*)
78628-28-1. Roxatidine Acetate Hydrochloride [roxatidine acetate] (See also *93793-83-0; 78273-80-0*)
78628-80-5. Terbinafine [hydrochloride] (See also *91161-71-6*)
78649-41-9. Iomeprol
78664-73-0. Posatirelin
78718-52-2. Benexate
78755-81-4. Flumazenil
78756-61-3. Alifedrine
78771-13-8. Sarmazenil

78782-47-5. Linogliride Fumarate
78919-13-8. Iloprost (See also *73873-87-7[replaced]*)
78964-85-9. Fosfomycin Tromethamine
78967-07-4. Mofezolac
78994-23-7. Levormeloxifene
78994-24-8. Ormeloxifene
78997-40-7. Prisotinol
79069-94-6. Fanetizole Mesylate [fanetizole] (See also *79069-95-7*)
79069-95-7. Fanetizole Mesylate (See also *79069-94-6*)
79069-97-9. Palmoxirate Sodium (See also *68170-97-8*)
79071-15-1. Tazasubrate
79094-20-5. Daltroban
79130-64-6. Ansoxetine
79152-85-5. Acodazole Hydrochloride [acodazole] (See also *55435-65-9*)
79201-80-2. Veradoline Hydrochloride [veradoline] (See also *76448-47-0*)
79201-85-7. Picenadol Hydrochloride [picenadol] (See also *74685-16-8*)
79211-10-2. Iosimide
79211-34-0. Iotriside
79243-67-7. Rosterolone
79253-92-2. Taziprinone
79262-46-7. Savoxepin
79282-39-6. Rilozarone
79286-77-4. Esafloxacin
79307-93-0. Azelastine Hydrochloride (See also *58581-89-8*)
79313-75-0. Sopromidine
79350-37-1. Cefixime
79360-43-3. Nocloprost
79404-91-4. Cilofungin
79416-27-6. Methyl Aminolevulinate Hydrochloride
79449-96-0. Altanserin Tartrate (See also *76330-71-7*)
79449-98-2. Cabastine
79449-99-3. Icospiramide
79455-30-4. Nicaraven
79467-19-9. Sintropium Bromide
79467-22-4. Bipenamol Hydrochloride [bipenamol] (See also *62220-58-0*)
79467-23-5. Mioflazine Hydrochloride [mioflazine] (See also *79467-24-6*)
79467-24-6. Mioflazine Hydrochloride (See also *79467-23-5*)
79483-69-5. Piritrexim Isethionate (See also *72732-56-0*)
79516-68-0. Levocabastine Hydrochloride [levocabastine] (See also *79547-78-7*)
79517-01-4. Octreotide Acetate
79547-78-7. Levocabastine Hydrochloride (See also *79516-68-0*)
79559-97-0. Sertraline Hydrochloride (See also *79617-96-2*)
79570-19-7. Brimonidine Tartrate (See also *59803-98-4*)
79578-14-6. Timobesone Acetate (See also *87116-72-1*)
79594-24-4. Somantadine Hydrochloride [somantadine] (See also *68693-30-1*)
79617-96-2. Sertraline Hydrochloride [sertraline] (See also *79559-97-0*)

79619-31-1. Flavodilol Maleate [flavodilol] (See also *79619-32-2*)

79619-32-2. Flavodilol Maleate (See also *79619-31-1*)

79644-90-9. Vebufloxacin

79645-27-5. Tobramycin Sulfate

79660-72-3. Fleroxacin

79672-88-1. Piriprost

79700-61-1. Dopropidil

79700-63-3. Fronepidil

79712-53-1. Tazifylline Hydrochloride (See also *79712-55-3*)

79712-55-3. Tazifylline Hydrochloride [tazifylline] (See also *79712-53-1*)

79714-31-1. Risarestat

79770-24-4. Iotrolan

79778-41-9. Neridronic Acid

79781-95-6. Rilapine

79784-22-8. Barucainide

79794-75-5. Loratadine

79798-39-3. Ketorfanol

79855-88-2. Trequinsin

79874-76-3. Delmopinol

79902-63-9. Simvastatin

79944-58-4. Idazoxan

79992-71-5. Pimetacin

80012-43-7. Epinastine (See also *80012-44-8*)

80012-44-8. Epinastine [hydrochloride] (See also *80012-43-7*)

80018-06-0. Fengabine

80109-27-9. Ciladopa Hydrochloride [ciladopa] (See also *83529-09-3*)

80125-14-0. Remoxipride

80168-44-1. Zinoconazole Hydrochloride (See also *84697-21-2*)

80195-36-4. Cefdaloxime

80210-62-4. Cefpodoxime Proxetil [cefpodoxime] (See also *87239-81-4*)

80214-83-1. Roxithromycin

80225-28-1. Tilsuprost

80263-73-6. Eclazolast

80288-49-9. Furafylline

80294-25-3. Mexafylline

80295-38-1. Conestat Alfa

80343-63-1. Sufotidine

80349-58-2. Panuramine

80370-57-6. Ceftiofur Hydrochloride [ceftiofur] (See also *103980-44-5*)

80387-96-8. Difemerine Hydrochloride [difemerine]

80410-36-2. Fezolamine Fumarate [fezolamine] (See also *80410-37-3*)

80410-37-3. Fezolamine Fumarate (See also *80410-36-2*)

80428-29-1. Mafoprazine

80433-71-2. Levoleucovorin Calcium

80471-63-2. Epostane

80474-14-2. Fluticasone Propionate (See also *90566-53-3*)

80486-69-7. Cloticasone Propionate (See also *87556-66-9*)

80529-93-7. Gadopentetate Dimeglumine [gadopentetic acid] (See also *86050-77-3*)

80573-03-1. Ipsalazide

80573-04-2. Balsalazide Disodium [balsalazide] (See also *150399-21-6*)

80576-83-6. Edatrexate

80595-73-9. Acefluranol

80614-21-7. Nicogrelate

80614-27-3. Midazogrel

80621-81-4. Rifaximin

80680-05-3. Tivanidazole

80680-06-4. Tefludazine

80738-47-2. Naflocort (See also *59497-39-1*)

80743-08-4. Dioxadilol

80755-51-7. Bunazosin

80763-86-6. Glunicate

80809-81-0. Docebenone

80828-32-6. Indolapril Hydrochloride (See also *80876-01-3*)

80830-42-8. Rentiapril

80841-47-0. Asulacrine

80844-07-1. Etofenprox

80863-62-3. Alitame [anhydrous] (See also *99016-42-9*)

80876-01-3. Indolapril Hydrochloride [indolapril] (See also *80828-32-6*)

80879-63-6. Emiglitate

80880-90-6. Telenzepine

80883-55-2. Enviradene

80937-31-1. Flosulide

81025-03-8. Lactitol [dihydrate] (See also *585-86-4; 81025-04-9*)

81025-04-9. Lactitol [monohydrate] (See also *585-86-4; 81025-03-8*)

81026-63-3. Enisoprost

81028-91-3. Fosfructose Trisodium

81043-56-3. Metrenperone

81045-33-2. Iodecimol

81045-50-3. Pivopril

81093-37-0. Pravastatin Sodium [pravastatin] (See also *81131-70-6*)

81098-59-1. Ytterbium Yb 169 Pentetate

81098-60-4. Cisapride

81103-11-9. Clarithromycin

81110-73-8. Racecadotril

81129-83-1. Cilastatin Sodium (See also *82009-34-5*)

81131-70-6. Pravastatin Sodium (See also *81093-37-0*)

81161-17-3. Esmolol Hydrochloride (See also *103598-03-4*)

81167-16-0. Imiloxan Hydrochloride [imiloxan] (See also *86710-23-8*)

81267-65-4. Idronoxil

81377-02-8. Seglitide Acetate [seglitide] (See also *99248-33-6*)

81382-52-7. Pentiapine Maleate

81403-68-1. Alfuzosin Hydrochloride (See also *81403-80-7*)

81403-80-7. Alfuzosin Hydrochloride [alfuzosin] (See also *81403-68-1*)

81409-90-7. Cabergoline

81424-67-1. Caracemide

81428-04-8. Taltrimide

81435-67-8. Losulazine Hydrochloride

81447-78-1. Levlofexidine

81447-79-2. Dexlofexidine

81447-80-5. Diprafenone

81447-81-6. Bromadoline Maleate (See also *67579-24-2*)

81478-25-3. Lomevactone

81485-25-8. Peretinoin

81486-22-8. Nipradilol

81496-81-3. Artenimol

81523-49-1. Vaneprim

81525-10-2. Nafamostat Mesylate [nafamostat] (See also *82956-11-4*)

81528-80-5. Dalbraminol

81571-28-0. Vinleucinol

81584-06-7. Xibenolol

81600-06-8. Vintriptol

81603-65-8. Lorzafone (See also *59179-95-2*)

81656-30-6. Tifluadom

81669-57-0. Anistreplase

81674-79-5. Guaimesal

81703-42-6. Bendacalol Mesylate [bendacalol] (See also *81737-62-4*)

81703-55-1. Ciprostene Calcium (See also *81845-44-5*)

81732-65-2. Bambuterol

81737-62-4. Bendacalol Mesylate (See also *81703-42-6*)

81792-35-0. Teopranitol

81801-12-9. Xamoterol

81840-15-5. Vesnarinone

81845-44-5. Ciprostene Calcium [ciprostene] (See also *81703-55-1*)

81846-19-7. Treprostinil

81872-09-5. Zofenoprilat Arginine (See also *75176-37-3*)

81872-10-8. Zofenopril Calcium [zofenopril] (See also *81938-43-4*)

81907-78-0. Batebulast

81919-14-4. Bendazac [lysine] (See also *20187-55-7*)

81926-94-5. Omega-3-acid Ethyl Esters [DHA ethyl ester] (See also *86227-47-6*)

81938-43-4. Zofenopril Calcium (See also *81872-10-8*)

81957-25-7. Dazopride Fumarate (See also *70181-03-2*)

81968-16-3. Mergocriptine

81982-32-3. Alpiropride

81988-87-6. Ramoplanin A_1

81988-88-7. Ramoplanin A_2 (Main Component)

81988-89-8. Ramoplanin A_3

81998-90-5. Tolevamer Potassium Sodium (See also *1011713-07-7*)

82009-34-5. Cilastatin Sodium [cilastatin] (See also *81129-83-1*)

82030-87-3. Somatrem

82034-46-6. Loteprednol Etabonate (See also *129260-79-3*)

82059-50-5. Dextofisopam

82059-51-6. Levotofisopam

82101-10-8. Flerobuterol

82114-19-0. Amflutizole

82117-51-9. Cinuperone

82140-22-5. Etolotifen

82159-09-9. Epalrestat

82168-26-1. Adafenoxate

82186-77-4. Lumefantrine

82190-91-8. Flufylline

82190-92-9. Flotrenizine

82190-93-0. Trenizine

82209-39-0. Piraxelate

82219-78-1. Cefuzonam

82227-39-2. Pibaxizine
82230-03-3. Carbetimer
82230-53-3. Girisopam
82239-52-9. Moxiraprine
82248-59-7. Atomoxetine Hydrochloride (See also *83015-26-3*)
82279-57-0. Zinc Acetate, Basic
82356-44-3. Hioxifilcon A
82410-32-0. Ganciclovir
82413-20-5. Droloxifene
82419-36-1. Ofloxacin
82509-56-6. Piroxicillin
82522-70-1. Modecainide
82547-58-8. Cefteram
82571-53-7. Ozagrel
82571-55-9. Pentafilcon A
82586-52-5. Moexipril Hydrochloride (See also *103775-10-6*)
82586-55-8. Quinapril Hydrochloride (See also *85441-61-8*)
82599-22-2. Ditiomustine
82601-27-2. Mirtazapine [replaced] (See also *85650-52-8; 61337-67-5*)
82626-01-5. Alpidem
82626-48-0. Zolpidem Tartrate [zolpidem] (See also *99294-93-6*)
82640-04-8. Raloxifene Hydrochloride (See also *84449-90-1*)
82650-83-7. Tenilapine
82664-20-8. Flurithromycin
82666-62-4. Sulosemide
82747-56-6. Cicletanine [cicletanine hydrochloride] (See also *89943-82-8*)
82752-99-6. Nefazodone Hydrochloride (See also *83366-66-9*)
82821-47-4. Mabuprofen
82834-16-0. Perindopril
82857-82-7. Ilepcimide
82924-03-6. Pentopril
82952-64-5. Trimetrexate Glucuronate
82956-11-4. Nafamostat Mesylate (See also *81525-10-2*)
82964-04-3. Tolrestat
82989-25-1. Tazanolast
83015-26-3. Atomoxetine Hydrochloride [tomoxetine] (See also *82248-59-7*)
83031-43-0. Sulbactam Benzathine (See also *68373-14-8*)
83038-87-3. Doxycycline Fosfatex
83059-56-7. Zabicipril
83150-76-9. Octreotide
83153-38-2. Mefenidil Fumarate (See also *58261-91-9*)
83153-39-3. Tiprinast Meglumine [tiprinast] (See also *83198-90-7*)
83166-17-0. Tampramine Fumarate [tampramine] (See also *83166-18-1*)
83166-18-1. Tampramine Fumarate (See also *83166-17-0*)
83184-43-4. Mifentidine
83198-90-7. Tiprinast Meglumine (See also *83153-39-3*)
83200-08-2. Eproxindine
83200-09-3. Dembrexine
83200-10-6. Anipamil
83200-11-7. Vinepidine Sulfate (See also *68170-69-4*)
83275-56-3. Tiracizine

83366-66-9. Nefazodone Hydrochloride [nefazodone] (See also *82752-99-6*)
83395-21-5. Ridazolol
83435-66-9. Delapril Hydrochloride [delapril] (See also *83435-67-0*)
83435-67-0. Delapril Hydrochloride (See also *83435-66-9*)
83455-48-5. Bromerguride
83461-56-7. Mifamurtide (See also *838853-48-8*)
83471-41-4. Pincainide
83480-29-9. Voglibose
83482-77-3. Vinmegallate
83529-08-2. Tubulozole Hydrochloride (See also *84697-22-3*)
83529-09-3. Ciladopa Hydrochloride (See also *80109-27-9*)
83573-53-9. Tizabrin
83602-05-5. Spiraprilat
83621-06-1. Omoconazole Nitrate (See also *74512-12-2*)
83622-85-9. Trifosmin
83625-35-8. Amebucort
83646-86-0. Inocoterone Acetate (See also *83646-97-3*)
83646-97-3. Inocoterone Acetate [inocoterone] (See also *83646-86-0*)
83647-97-6. Spirapril Hydrochloride [spirapril] (See also *94841-17-5*)
83656-38-6. Ipramidil
83689-23-0. Molfarnate
83784-18-3. Lutrelin Acetate (See also *66866-63-5*)
83784-19-4. Piquindone Hydrochloride (See also *78541-97-6*)
83784-20-7. Hydrocortisone Hemisuccinate (See also *2203-97-6*)
83784-21-8. Menabitan Hydrochloride [menabitan] (See also *58019-50-4*)
83799-24-0. Fexofenadine Hydrochloride [fexofenadine] (See also *153439-40-8; 138452-21-8*)
83805-11-2. Falecalcitriol
83863-79-0. Florifenine
83880-70-0. Dexamethasone Acefurate
83881-51-0. Cetirizine Hydrochloride [cetirizine] (See also *83881-52-1*)
83881-52-1. Cetirizine Hydrochloride (See also *83881-51-0*)
83903-06-4. Lupitidine Hydrochloride [lupitidine] (See also *72716-75-7*)
83905-01-5. Azithromycin [anhydrous] (See also *121479-24-4; 117772-70-0*)
83915-83-7. Lisinopril (See also *76547-98-3*)
83919-23-7. Mometasone Furoate
83928-66-9. Gepirone Hydrochloride (See also *83928-76-1*)
83928-76-1. Gepirone Hydrochloride [gepirone] (See also *83928-66-9*)
83930-13-6. Somatorelin
83991-25-7. Ambasilide
83997-19-7. Ataprost
84057-84-1. Lamotrigine
84057-95-4. Ropivacaine Hydrochloride [ropivacaine] (See also *132112-35-7*)
84057-96-5. Flusoxolol
84071-15-8. Ramixotidine

84088-42-6. Roquinimex
84145-89-1. Almoxatone
84145-90-4. Nafoxadol
84203-09-8. Trifenagrel
84225-95-6. Raclopride C 11 [raclopride] (See also *97849-54-2*)
84226-12-0. Eticlopride
84233-61-4. Nesosteine
84243-58-3. Imazodan Hydrochloride [imazodan] (See also *89198-09-4*)
84252-03-9. Erythromycin Stinoprate
84290-27-7. Tucaresol
84329-47-5. Xylofilcon A
84368-35-4. Manganese Gluconate [replaced] (See also *6485-39-8*)
84371-65-3. Mifepristone
84379-13-5. Bretazenil
84386-11-8. Baxitozine
84392-17-6. Xenalipin
84408-37-7. Desciclovir
84449-90-1. Raloxifene Hydrochloride [raloxifene] (See also *82640-04-8*)
84455-52-7. Oxmetidine Mesylate
84472-85-5. Navuridine
84485-00-7. Sibutramine Hydrochloride [anhydrous] (See also *125494-59-9; 106650-56-0*)
84490-12-0. Piroximone
84558-93-0. Netivudine
84611-23-4. Erdosteine
84625-59-2. Dotarizine
84625-61-6. Itraconazole
84680-54-6. Enalaprilat (See also *76420-72-9*)
84681-71-0. Rapeseed Oil, Fully Hydrogenated
84697-21-2. Zinoconazole Hydrochloride [zinoconazole] (See also *80168-44-1*)
84697-22-3. Tubulozole Hydrochloride [free base] (See also *83529-08-2*)
84720-88-7. Antithrombin Alfa
84799-02-0. Laidlomycin Propionate Potassium (See also *56283-74-0*)
84845-57-8. Ritipenem
84845-75-0. Niperotidine
84878-61-5. Maduramicin
84880-03-5. Cefpimizole
84901-45-1. Doliracetam
84937-45-1. Gusperimus Trihydrochloride [hydrochloride] (See also *85468-01-5; 104317-84-2*)
84957-29-9. Cefpirome Sulfate [cefpirome] (See also *98753-19-6*)
84957-30-2. Cefquinome Sulfate [cefquinome] (See also *118443-89-3*)
84962-75-4. Flutomidate
85053-46-9. Suricainide Maleate [suricainide] (See also *85053-47-0*)
85053-47-0. Suricainide Maleate (See also *85053-46-9*)
85056-47-9. Piroxicam Olamine
85068-76-4. Iofetamine Hydrochloride I 123
85076-06-8. Axamozide
85118-42-9. Lufuradom
85118-43-0. Fluprofylline
85118-44-1. Minocromil

85125-49-1. Biclodil Hydrochloride [biclodil] (See also *75564-40-8*)
85136-71-6. Tilisolol
85166-20-7. Ciclotropium Bromide
85175-67-3. Zatebradine
85181-38-0. Tropanserin Hydrochloride (See also *85181-40-4*)
85181-40-4. Tropanserin Hydrochloride [tropanserin] (See also *85181-38-0*)
85197-77-9. Tipredane
85247-76-3. Dagapamil
85247-77-4. Ronipamil
85287-61-2. Cefpimizole Sodium (See also *84880-03-5*)
85320-67-8. Ericolol
85320-68-9. Amosulalol
85371-64-8. Pinacidil (See also *60560-33-0*)
85392-79-6. Indanidine
85418-85-5. Sunagrel
85441-60-7. Quinaprilat
85441-61-8. Quinapril
85443-48-7. Bencianol
85465-82-3. Thymotrinan
85466-18-8. Thymocartin
85468-01-5. Gusperimus Trihydrochloride (See also *104317-84-2; 84937-45-1*)
85505-64-2. Vapiprost Hydrochloride [vapiprost] (See also *87248-13-3*)
85604-00-8. Zaltidine Hydrochloride [zaltidine] (See also *90274-23-0*)
85622-93-1. Temozolomide
85622-95-3. Mitozolomide
85650-52-8. Mirtazapine (See also *61337-67-5; 82601-27-2*)
85650-56-2. Asenapine Maleate (See also *65576-45-6*)
85666-24-6. Furegrelate Sodium [furegrelate] (See also *87463-91-0*)
85673-87-6. Revenast
85691-74-3. Pirmagrel
85702-89-2. Tazeprofen
85721-33-1. Ciprofloxacin
85750-38-5. Erocainide
85750-39-6. Etilefrine Pivalate
85754-59-2. Ambamustine
85760-74-3. Quinpirole Hydrochloride [quinpirole] (See also *85798-08-9*)
85798-08-9. Quinpirole Hydrochloride (See also *85760-74-3*)
85856-54-8. Moveltipril
85897-35-4. Sacrosidase
85966-89-8. Preclamol
85969-07-9. Budotitane
85977-49-7. Tauromustine
86015-38-5. Neflumozide Hydrochloride (See also *86636-93-3*)
86024-64-8. Quinacainol
86042-50-4. Cistinexine
86048-40-0. Quazolast
86050-77-3. Gadopentetate Dimeglumine (See also *80529-93-7*)
86111-26-4. Zindoxifene
86116-60-1. Azaloxan Fumarate (See also *72822-56-1*)
86140-10-5. Neraminol
86160-82-9. Lavoltidine Succinate (See also *76956-02-0*)

86168-78-7. Sermorelin Acetate [sermorelin] (See also *114466-38-5*)
86181-42-2. Temelastine
86189-69-7. Felodipine (See also *72509-76-3*)
86197-47-9. Dopexamine
86216-41-3. Broxitalamic Acid
86220-42-0. Nafarelin Acetate (See also *76932-56-4*)
86227-47-6. Omega-3-acid Ethyl Esters [EPA ethyl ester] (See also *81926-94-5*)
86273-18-9. Lenampicillin
86273-92-9. Tolufazepam
86304-28-1. Buciclovir
86315-52-8. Isomazole Hydrochloride [isomazole] (See also *87359-33-9*)
86329-79-5. Cefodizime [as sodium] (See also *69739-16-8*)
86347-14-0. Medetomidine Hydrochloride [medetomidine] (See also *86347-15-1*)
86347-15-1. Medetomidine Hydrochloride (See also *86347-14-0*)
86348-98-3. Flunoprost
86365-92-6. Trazolopride
86386-73-4. Fluconazole
86393-32-0. Ciprofloxacin Hydrochloride
86393-37-5. Amifloxacin
86398-53-0. Denatonium Benzoate (See also *3734-33-6*)
86401-95-8. Methylprednisolone Aceponate
86433-40-1. Terflavoxate
86434-57-3. Beperidium Iodide
86484-91-5. Dopexamine Hydrochloride
86487-64-1. Setoperone
86541-74-4. Benazepril Hydrochloride (See also *86541-75-5*)
86541-75-5. Benazepril Hydrochloride [benazepril] (See also *86541-74-4*)
86541-78-8. Benazeprilat
86627-15-8. Aronixil
86627-50-1. Lodinixil
86636-93-3. Neflumozide Hydrochloride [neflumozide] (See also *86015-38-5*)
86641-76-1. Dibrospidium Chloride
86662-54-6. Binizolast
86696-86-8. Tenilsetam
86696-87-9. Aganodine
86696-88-0. Frabuprofen
86710-23-8. Imiloxan Hydrochloride (See also *81167-16-0*)
86767-75-1. Octenidine Saccharin
86780-90-7. Aranidipine
86784-80-7. Corticorelin Acetate
86811-09-8. Litoxetine
86811-58-7. Fluazuron
86832-68-0. Carumonam Sodium (See also *87638-04-8*)
86880-51-5. Epanolol
86914-11-6. Tolgabide
86939-10-8. Indatraline
87034-87-5. Bamaluzole
87051-13-6. Tosulur
87051-43-2. Ritanserin
87051-46-5. Butanserin

87056-78-8. Quinagolide (See also *94424-50-7*)
87071-16-7. Arclofenin
87116-72-1. Timobesone Acetate [timobesone] (See also *79578-14-6*)
87129-71-3. Arnolol
87151-85-7. Spiradoline Mesylate [spiradoline] (See also *87173-97-5*)
87173-97-5. Spiradoline Mesylate (See also *87151-85-7*)
87178-42-5. Dosergoside
87233-61-2. Emedastine Difumarate [emedastine] (See also *87233-62-3*)
87233-62-3. Emedastine Difumarate (See also *87233-61-2*)
87234-24-0. Piroxicam Cinnamate
87239-81-4. Cefpodoxime Proxetil (See also *80210-62-4*)
87248-13-3. Vapiprost Hydrochloride (See also *85505-64-2*)
87269-59-8. Naxaprostene
87269-97-4. Ramiprilat
87333-19-5. Ramipril
87344-06-7. Amtolmetin Guacil
87359-33-9. Isomazole Hydrochloride (See also *86315-52-8*)
87434-82-0. Dezaguanine Mesylate
87434-83-1. Tiapamil Hydrochloride (See also *57010-31-8*)
87463-91-0. Furegrelate Sodium (See also *85666-24-6*)
87495-31-6. Disoxaril
87495-33-8. Napamezole Hydrochloride (See also *91524-14-0*)
87549-36-8. Parcetasal
87556-66-9. Cloticasone Propionate [cloticasone] (See also *80486-69-7*)
87573-01-1. Salnacedin
87611-28-7. Melquinast
87626-55-9. Mitoflaxone
87638-04-8. Carumonam Sodium [carumonam] (See also *86832-68-0*)
87646-83-1. Lodazecar
87679-37-6. Trandolapril
87679-71-8. Trandolaprilat
87691-91-6. Tiospirone Hydrochloride [tiospirone] (See also *87691-92-7*)
87691-92-7. Tiospirone Hydrochloride (See also *87691-91-6*)
87719-32-2. Etarotene
87721-62-8. Flestolol Sulfate [flestolol] (See also *88844-73-9*)
87726-17-8. Panipenem
87729-89-3. Seganserin
87760-53-0. Tandospirone Citrate [tandospirone] (See also *112457-95-1*)
87771-40-2. Ioversol
87784-12-1. Ofornine
87806-31-3. Porfimer Sodium
87810-56-8. Fostriecin Sodium [fostriecin] (See also *87860-39-7*)
87848-99-5. Acrivastine
87860-39-7. Fostriecin Sodium (See also *87810-56-8*)
87901-11-9. Coumermycin Sodium
87936-75-2. Tazadolene Succinate [tazadolene] (See also *87936-82-1*)

87936-82-1. Tazadolene Succinate (See also *87936-75-2*)
87940-60-1. Eprobemide
87952-98-5. Mespirenone
88036-80-0. Amifloxacin Mesylate (See also *86393-37-5*)
88040-23-7. Cefepime
88041-40-1. Lemidosul
88053-05-8. Cinoxopazide
88058-88-2. Naxagolide Hydrochloride [naxagolide] (See also *99705-65-4*)
88069-67-4. Pilsicainide
88107-10-2. Tomelukast
88124-26-9. Adosopine
88124-27-0. Etazepine
88133-11-3. Bemitradine
88150-42-9. Amlodipine Besylate [amlodipine] (See also *111470-99-6*)
88150-47-4. Amlodipine Maleate
88199-75-1. Sevitropium Mesilate
88255-01-0. Netobimin
88296-61-1. Medorinone
88296-62-2. Transcainide
88303-60-0. Losoxantrone Hydrochloride [losoxantrone] (See also *132937-89-4*)
88321-09-9. Aloxistatin
88426-32-8. Ursulcholic Acid
88426-33-9. Buparvaquone
88430-50-6. Beraprost
88431-47-4. Clomoxir
88475-69-8. Beraprost Sodium (See also *88430-50-6*)
88495-63-0. Artesunate [replaced] (See also *182824-33-5*)
88578-07-8. Imoxiterol
88579-39-9. Tasuldine
88637-37-0. Diphenhydramine Citrate (See also *58-73-1*)
88660-47-3. Epicriptine
88669-04-9. Trospectomycin Sulfate [trospectomycin] (See also *88851-61-0*)
88678-31-3. Liranaftate
88721-77-1. Renzapride
88768-40-5. Cilazapril [anhydrous] (See also *92077-78-6*)
88844-73-9. Flestolol Sulfate (See also *87721-62-8*)
88851-61-0. Trospectomycin Sulfate (See also *88669-04-9*)
88851-62-1. Piriprost Potassium
88852-12-4. Limaprost
88859-04-5. Mafosfamide
88889-14-9. Fosinopril Sodium (See also *98048-97-6*)
88931-51-5. Clinprost
88939-40-6. Semorphone
88980-20-5. Mexiprostil
89163-44-0. Cinaproxen
89194-77-4. Bisaramil
89197-32-0. Efaroxan
89198-09-4. Imazodan Hydrochloride (See also *84243-58-3*)
89213-87-6. Carperitide
89232-84-8. Pelrinone Hydrochloride (See also *94386-65-9*)
89303-63-9. Atiprosin Maleate [atiprosin] (See also *89303-64-0*)

89303-64-0. Atiprosin Maleate (See also *89303-63-9*)
89315-55-9. Ilmofosine
89365-50-4. Salmeterol
89371-37-9. Imidapril (See also *89396-94-1*)
89371-44-8. Imidaprilat
89383-13-1. Somidobove
89391-50-4. Imirestat
89396-94-1. Imidapril [hydrochloride] (See also *89371-37-9*)
89419-40-9. Mosapramine
89482-00-8. Zaltoprofen
89558-90-7. Genfilcon A
89565-68-4. Tropisetron
89613-77-4. Mezacopride
89622-90-2. Brinazarone
89651-00-3. Voxergolide
89662-30-6. Detirelix Acetate [detirelix] (See also *102583-46-0*)
89667-40-3. Isbogrel
89672-11-7. Cioteronel
89767-59-9. Salmisteine
89778-26-7. Toremifene Citrate [toremifene] (See also *89778-27-8*)
89778-27-8. Toremifene Citrate (See also *89778-26-7*)
89781-55-5. Rolafagrel
89785-84-2. Tazobactam Sodium
89786-04-9. Tazobactam
89796-99-6. Aceclofenac
89797-00-2. Iopentol
89838-96-0. Octimibate
89875-86-5. Tiflucarbine
89943-82-8. Cicletanine (See also *82747-56-6*)
89957-37-9. Gantenerumab
89987-06-4. Tiludronic Acid
90038-01-0. Detomidine Hydrochloride (See also *76631-46-4*)
90055-97-3. Tienoxolol
90060-42-7. Nolomirole
90101-16-9. Droxicam
90103-92-7. Zabiciprilat
90104-48-6. Doreptide
90139-06-3. Cilazaprilat
90162-60-0. Isbufylline
90182-92-6. Zacopride Hydrochloride [zacopride] (See also *99617-34-2*)
90207-12-8. Sulicrinat
90237-04-0. Dexsecoverine
90243-66-6. Montirelin
90243-97-3. Spiclamine
90243-98-4. Dimoxaprost
90274-22-9. Darenzepine
90274-23-0. Zaltidine Hydrochloride (See also *85604-00-8*)
90274-24-1. Ractopamine Hydrochloride (See also *97825-25-7*)
90293-01-9. Bifemelane
90326-85-5. Nesapidil
90350-40-6. Methylprednisolone Suleptanate
90357-06-5. Bicalutamide
90402-40-7. Abanoquil
90409-78-2. Polifeprosan 20
90509-02-7. Luxabendazole

90566-53-3. Fluticasone Propionate [fluticasone] (See also *80474-14-2*)
90581-63-8. Falintolol
90693-76-8. Eptaloprost
90697-56-6. Zimidoben
90697-57-7. Motapizone
90729-41-2. Oxodipine
90729-42-3. Carebastine
90729-43-4. Ebastine
90730-93-1. Xamoterol Fumarate
90733-40-7. Edifolone Acetate [edifolone] (See also *90733-42-9*)
90733-42-9. Edifolone Acetate (See also *90733-40-7*)
90749-32-9. Laprafylline
90779-69-4. Atosiban
90808-12-1. Divaplon
90828-99-2. Itrocainide
90845-56-0. Trecadrine
90849-08-4. Oximonam Sodium
90850-05-8. Gloximonam
90895-85-5. Ronactolol
90898-90-1. Oximonam
90961-53-8. Tedisamil
90992-25-9. Besulpamide
91017-58-2. Abunidazole
91032-26-7. Teicoplanin A$_{2-2}$
91032-34-7. Teicoplanin A$_{2-1}$
91032-36-9. Teicoplanin A$_{2-3}$
91032-37-0. Teicoplanin A$_{2-4}$
91032-38-1. Teicoplanin A$_{2-5}$
91077-32-6. Dezinamide
91161-71-6. Terbinafine (See also *78628-80-5*)
91257-14-6. Tuvatidine
91296-86-5. Difloxacin Hydrochloride (See also *98106-17-3*)
91296-87-6. Sarafloxacin Hydrochloride (See also *98105-99-8*)
91374-20-8. Ropinirole Hydrochloride (See also *91374-21-9*)
91374-21-9. Ropinirole
91406-11-0. Esuprone
91421-42-0. Rubitecan
91431-42-4. Lonapalene
91441-23-5. Piroxantrone Hydrochloride [piroxantrone] (See also *105118-12-5*)
91441-48-4. Teloxantrone Hydrochloride [teloxantrone] (See also *132937-88-3*)
91524-13-9. Nefocon A
91524-14-0. Napamezole Hydrochloride [napamezole] (See also *87495-33-8*)
91524-15-1. Irloxacin
91524-16-2. Timolol
91524-18-4. Azumolene Sodium (See also *64748-79-4*)
91587-01-8. Pelretin
91618-36-9. Ibafloxacin
91714-94-2. Bromfenac Sodium [bromfenac] (See also *120638-55-3*)
91753-07-0. Mitoquidone
91832-40-5. Cefdinir
91833-77-1. Rocastine Hydrochloride [rocastine] (See also *99617-35-3*)
91935-26-1. Toripristone
92071-51-7. Rotraxate

92077-78-6. Cilazapril (See also *88768-40-5*)

92118-27-9. Fotemustine

92134-98-0. Fosphenytoin Sodium (See also *93390-81-9*)

92210-43-0. Bemarinone Hydrochloride [bemarinone] (See also *101626-69-1*)

92257-40-4. Dizatrifone

92262-58-3. Valrocemide

92268-40-1. Perfomedil

92302-55-1. Devapamil

92339-11-2. Iodixanol

92569-65-8. Aprikalim

92589-98-5. Ipsapirone Hydrochloride (See also *95847-70-4*)

92615-20-8. Nafenodone

92623-83-1. Pravadoline Maleate [pravadoline] (See also *92623-84-2*)

92623-84-2. Pravadoline Maleate (See also *92623-83-1*)

92623-85-3. Milnacipran Hydrochloride [milnacipran] (See also *101152-94-7*)

92629-87-3. Dexnafenodone

92665-29-7. Cefprozil [anhydrous] (See also *121123-17-9*)

92761-26-7. Ecamsule

92812-82-3. Fluorodopa F 18

92981-78-7. Tesmilifene Hydrochloride

93047-39-3. Etanterol

93047-40-6. Naminterol

93064-63-2. Venritidine

93105-81-8. Lodelaben [replaced] (See also *111149-90-7*)

93106-60-6. Enrofloxacin

93181-81-8. Lodaxaprine

93181-85-2. Endixaprine

93221-48-8. Levobetaxolol Hydrochloride [levobetaxolol] (See also *116209-55-3*)

93265-81-7. Ropidoxuridine

93277-96-4. Altapizone

93379-54-5. Esatenolol

93384-43-1. Onaclostox

93390-81-9. Fosphenytoin Sodium [fosphenytoin] (See also *92134-98-0*)

93413-62-8. Desvenlafaxine Succinate [desvenlafaxine] (See also *386750-22-7*)

93413-69-5. Venlafaxine Hydrochloride [venlafaxine] (See also *99300-78-4*)

93479-96-0. Alteconazole

93479-97-1. Glimepiride

93616-27-4. Teicoplanin A$_{3-1}$

93664-94-9. Nemonapride

93738-40-0. Ralitoline

93793-83-0. Roxatidine Acetate Hydrochloride (See also *78273-80-0; 78628-28-1*)

93821-75-1. Butinazocine

93957-54-1. Fluvastatin Sodium [fluvastatin] (See also *93957-55-2*)

93957-55-2. Fluvastatin Sodium (See also *93957-54-1*)

94011-82-2. Bazinaprine

94035-02-6. Hydroxypropyl Betadex

94055-76-2. Suplatast Tosilate

94088-85-4. Doxycycline Calcium

94149-41-4. Midesteine

94153-50-1. Mespiperone C 11

94168-98-6. Rifametane

94192-59-3. Lixazinone Sulfate [lixazinone] (See also *101626-67-9*)

94218-72-1. Celmoleukin

94218-75-4. Teceleukin [reduced protein moiety] (See also *136279-32-8*)

94386-65-9. Pelrinone Hydrochloride [pelrinone] (See also *89232-84-8*)

94424-50-7. Quinagolide [hydrochloride] (See also *87056-78-8*)

94470-67-4. Cromakalim

94497-51-5. Tamibarotene

94535-50-9. Levcromakalim

94746-78-8. Molracetam

94749-08-3. Salmeterol Xinafoate

94820-09-4. Cadexomer Iodine

94841-17-5. Spirapril Hydrochloride (See also *83647-97-6*)

94948-59-1. Tasonermin

95058-70-1. Nictiazem

95058-81-4. Gemcitabine

95104-27-1. Tetrazolast Meglumine [tetrazolast] (See also *133008-33-0; 121762-69-4*)

95105-77-4. Sornidipine

95153-31-4. Perindoprilat

95232-68-1. Tenosal

95233-18-4. Atovaquone

95268-62-5. Upenazime

95355-10-5. Domipizone

95374-52-0. Prideperone

95382-33-5. Omeprazole Magnesium

95399-71-6. Fosinoprilat

95510-70-6. Omeprazole Sodium

95520-81-3. Elziverine

95522-45-5. Colestilan

95588-08-2. Tipentosin Hydrochloride [tipentosin] (See also *95588-10-6*)

95588-10-6. Tipentosin Hydrochloride (See also *95588-08-2*)

95634-82-5. Batelapine Maleate [batelapine] (See also *120360-10-3*)

95635-55-5. Ranolazine

95635-56-6. Ranolazine Hydrochloride (See also *95635-55-5*)

95668-38-5. Idralfidine

95722-07-9. Cicaprost

95729-65-0. Azetirelin

95734-82-0. Nedaplatin

95847-70-4. Ipsapirone Hydrochloride [ipsapirone] (See also *92589-98-5*)

95847-87-3. Revospirone

95896-08-5. Anaritide Acetate [anaritide] (See also *104595-79-1*)

96020-91-6. Eflornithine Hydrochloride (See also *67037-37-0*)

96036-03-2. Meropenem [anhydrous] (See also *119478-56-7*)

96055-45-7. Nicotine Polacrilex

96125-53-0. Clentiazem Maleate [clentiazem] (See also *96128-92-6*)

96128-89-1. Erythromycin Acistrate

96128-90-4. Lobuprofen

96128-92-6. Clentiazem Maleate (See also *96125-53-0*)

96153-56-9. Bisfentidine

96164-19-1. Peraclopone

96187-53-0. Brequinar Sodium [brequinar] (See also *96201-88-6*)

96191-65-0. Ioxabrolic Acid

96201-88-6. Brequinar Sodium (See also *96187-53-0*)

96258-13-8. Tribendilol

96301-34-7. Atamestane

96306-34-2. Timelotem

96346-61-1. Onapristone

96353-48-9. Somagrebove

96389-68-3. Crisnatol Mesylate [crisnatol] (See also *96389-69-4*)

96389-69-4. Crisnatol Mesylate (See also *96389-68-3*)

96392-96-0. Dexormaplatin

96427-12-2. Lactalfate

96449-05-7. Rispenzepine

96478-43-2. Irindalone

96487-37-5. Nuvenzepine

96497-67-5. Rodorubicin

96513-83-6. Pentisomide

96515-73-0. Palonidipine

96565-55-8. Ablukast Sodium

96566-25-5. Ablukast

96604-21-6. Ocinaplon

96609-16-4. Lifibrol

96645-87-3. Erizepine

96684-40-1. Piroxicam Betadex

96743-96-3. Ramciclane

96829-58-2. Orlistat

96847-55-1. Levomilnacipran

96914-39-5. Actisomide

96922-80-4. Pantenicate

96946-42-8. Cisatracurium Besylate

97048-13-0. Urofollitropin

97068-30-9. Elsamitrucin

97110-59-3. Trazium Esilate

97240-79-4. Topiramate

97275-40-6. Cefcanel Daloxate

97322-87-7. Troglitazone

97466-90-5. Quinelorane Hydrochloride [quinelorane] (See also *97548-97-5*)

97468-37-6. Cephapirin Benzathine

97483-17-5. Tifurac Sodium [tifurac] (See also *102488-97-1*)

97519-39-6. Ceftibuten

97546-74-2. Troxolamide

97548-97-5. Quinelorane Hydrochloride (See also *97466-90-5*)

97642-74-5. Clomifenoxide

97682-44-5. Irinotecan Hydrochloride [irinotecan] (See also *136572-09-3*)

97702-82-4. Iosarcol

97747-88-1. Lilopristone

97752-20-0. Droloxifene Citrate

97772-98-0. Butedronate Tetrasodium

97825-25-7. Ractopamine Hydrochloride [ractopamine] (See also *90274-24-1*)

97845-62-0. Penciclovir Sodium

97849-54-2. Raclopride C 11 (See also *84225-95-6*)

97901-21-8. Nafagrel

97964-54-0. Tomoglumide

97964-56-2. Lorglumide

98048-07-8. Fomidacillin

98048-97-6. Fosinopril Sodium [fosinopril] (See also *88889-14-9*)

98059-18-8. Interferon Gamma-1a

98059-61-1. Interferon Gamma-1b
98079-51-7. Lomefloxacin
98079-52-8. Lomefloxacin Hydrochloride
98105-99-8. Sarafloxacin Hydrochloride [sarafloxacin] (See also *91296-87-6*)
98106-17-3. Difloxacin Hydrochloride [difloxacin] (See also *91296-86-5*)
98116-53-1. Sulukast
98123-83-2. Epsiprantel
98204-48-9. Spirofylline
98206-10-1. Flesinoxan
98224-03-4. Eltoprazine
98319-26-7. Finasteride
98323-83-2. Carmoxirole
98326-32-0. Senazodan
98330-05-3. Anpirtoline
98374-54-0. Siltenzepine
98383-18-7. Ecomustine
98410-36-7. Palatrigine
98418-47-4. Metoprolol Succinate
98530-76-8. Drotrecogin Alfa (activated)
98631-95-9. Sobuzoxane
98651-66-2. Halobetasol Propionate [halobetasol] (See also *66852-54-8*)
98753-19-6. Cefpirome Sulfate (See also *84957-29-9*)
98769-81-4. Reboxetine
98769-84-7. Reboxetine Mesylate
98774-23-3. Tesmilifene
98815-38-4. Casokefamide
98819-76-2. Esreboxetine
98833-92-2. Stacofylline
99011-02-6. Imiquimod
99016-42-9. Alitame (See also *80863-62-3*)
99107-52-5. Bunaprolast
99149-95-8. Saruplase
99156-66-8. Barmastine
99210-65-8. Interferon Alfa-2b
99248-32-5. Donetidine
99248-33-6. Seglitide Acetate (See also *81377-02-8*)
99258-55-6. Oxamisole Hydrochloride (See also *99258-56-7*)
99258-56-7. Oxamisole Hydrochloride [oxamisole] (See also *99258-55-6*)
99283-10-0. Molgramostim
99287-30-6. Egualen
99291-25-5. Levodropropizine
99294-93-6. Zolpidem Tartrate (See also *82626-48-0*)
99294-94-7. Teriparatide Acetate
99300-78-4. Venlafaxine Hydrochloride (See also *93413-69-5*)
99323-21-4. Inaperisone
99453-84-6. Neltenexine
99464-64-9. Ampiroxicam
99499-40-8. Disuprazole
99500-54-6. Efetozole
99518-29-3. Derpanicate
99522-79-9. Pranidipine
99592-32-2. Sertaconazole
99593-25-6. Rilmazafone
99614-02-5. Ondansetron (See also *108303-49-1; 116002-70-1*)
99617-34-2. Zacopride Hydrochloride (See also *90182-92-6*)

99617-35-3. Rocastine Hydrochloride (See also *91833-77-1*)
99665-00-6. Flomoxef
99705-65-4. Naxagolide Hydrochloride (See also *88058-88-2*)
99755-59-6. Rotigotine
99759-19-0. Tiqueside
99803-72-2. Nerbacadol
99821-44-0. Nasaruplase
99821-47-3. Urokinase Alfa
100035-75-4. Evandamine
100158-38-1. Otenzepad
100188-33-8. Piridronate Sodium
100227-05-2. Pirtenidine Hydrochloride (See also *103923-27-9*)
100299-08-9. Pemirolast Potassium (See also *69372-19-6*)
100324-81-0. Lisofylline
100345-64-0. Siagoside
100417-09-2. Timirdine
100427-26-7. Lercanidipine Hydrochloride [lercanidipine] (See also *132866-11-6*)
100510-33-6. Adibendan
100551-63-1. Exametazime [replaced] (See also *105613-48-7*)
100587-52-8. Norfloxacin Succinil
100643-71-8. Desloratadine
100643-96-7. Indolidan
100678-32-8. Cifenline Succinate
100680-33-9. Cefuroxime Pivoxetil
100927-13-7. Idaverine
100927-14-8. Befiperide
100981-43-9. Ebrotidine
101001-34-7. Pamicogrel
101152-94-7. Milnacipran Hydrochloride (See also *92623-85-3*)
101193-40-2. Quinotolast
101197-99-3. Acitemate
101238-51-1. Levemopamil
101246-68-8. Eptastigmine
101312-92-9. Valnemulin
101335-99-3. Eprovafen
101343-69-5. Ocfentanil Hydrochloride [ocfentanil] (See also *112964-97-3*)
101345-71-5. Brifentanil Hydrochloride [brifentanil] (See also *117268-95-8*)
101363-10-4. Rufloxacin
101396-42-3. Mequitamium Iodide
101411-70-5. Paldimycin A
101411-71-6. Paldimycin B
101418-00-2. Policresulen
101477-55-8. Lomerizine
101479-70-3. Adaprolol Maleate [adaprolol] (See also *121009-31-2*)
101506-83-6. Namirotene
101526-62-9. Sematilide Hydrochloride (See also *101526-83-4*)
101526-83-4. Sematilide Hydrochloride [sematilide] (See also *101526-62-9*)
101530-10-3. Lanoconazole
101626-66-8. Dobutamine Tartrate
101626-67-9. Lixazinone Sulfate (See also *94192-59-3*)
101626-68-0. Nedocromil Calcium
101626-69-1. Bemarinone Hydrochloride (See also *92210-43-0*)
101626-70-4. Talipexole

101827-46-7. Butenafine Hydrochloride (See also *101828-21-1*)
101828-21-1. Butenafine Hydrochloride [butenafine] (See also *101827-46-7*)
101831-36-1. Clazuril
101831-37-2. Diclazuril
101973-77-7. Esonarimod
101975-10-4. Zardaverine
102130-84-7. Nemadectin
102144-78-5. Tameridone
102280-35-3. Baquiloprim
102426-96-0. Paldimycin
102488-97-1. Tifurac Sodium (See also *97483-17-5*)
102507-71-1. Tigemonam Dicholine [tigemonam] (See also *102916-21-2*)
102583-46-0. Detirelix Acetate (See also *89662-30-6*)
102625-70-7. Pantoprazole
102669-89-6. Saterinone
102670-46-2. Batanopride Hydrochloride [batanopride] (See also *102670-59-7*)
102670-59-7. Batanopride Hydrochloride (See also *102670-46-2*)
102676-47-1. Fadrozole Hydrochloride [fadrozole] (See also *102676-96-0*)
102676-96-0. Fadrozole Hydrochloride (See also *102676-47-1*)
102733-72-2. Sometripor
102744-97-8. Sometribove
102767-28-2. Levetiracetam
102771-12-0. Nerisopam
102786-61-8. Eptacog Alfa
102791-47-9. Nanterinone (See also *102791-74-2*)
102791-74-2. Nanterinone [mesylate] (See also *102791-47-9*)
102908-59-8. Binospirone Mesylate [binospirone] (See also *124756-23-6*)
102916-21-2. Tigemonam Dicholine (See also *102507-71-1*)
103024-93-7. Tiviciclovir
103055-07-8. Lufenuron
103060-53-3. Daptomycin
103129-82-4. Levamlodipine Malate [levamlodipine] (See also *736178-83-9*)
103177-37-3. Pranlukast
103181-72-2. Guaisteine
103186-19-2. Seratrodast (See also *112665-43-7*)
103222-11-3. Vapreotide
103238-56-8. Parodilol
103238-57-9. Cefempidone
103255-66-9. Pazinaclone
103300-74-9. Taltirelin
103336-05-6. Ditekiren
103337-74-2. Letrazuril
103420-77-5. Devazepide
103451-84-9. Avicatonin
103466-73-5. Icometasone Enbutate
103475-41-8. Tepoxalin
103486-79-9. Belfosdil
103577-45-3. Lansoprazole
103597-45-1. Bisoctrizole
103598-03-4. Esmolol Hydrochloride [esmolol] (See also *81161-17-3*)
103624-59-5. Traboxopine
103628-46-2. Sumatriptan

103628-48-4. Sumatriptan Succinate (See also *103628-46-2*)

103639-04-9. Ondansetron Hydrochloride

103725-47-9. Betiatide

103745-39-7. Fasudil

103766-25-2. Gimeracil

103775-10-6. Moexipril Hydrochloride [moexipril] (See also *82586-52-5*)

103775-14-0. Moexiprilat

103775-75-3. Miboplatin

103810-45-3. Bidisomide

103831-41-0. Borocaptate Sodium B 10

103844-77-5. Necopidem

103844-86-6. Saripidem

103878-83-7. Lazabemide Hydrochloride

103878-84-8. Lazabemide

103878-96-2. Fosopamine

103890-78-4. Lacidipine

103909-75-7. Maxacalcitol

103922-33-4. Pibutidine

103923-27-9. Pirtenidine Hydrochloride [pirtenidine] (See also *100227-05-2*)

103926-64-3. Sepimostat

103946-15-2. Elnadipine

103980-44-5. Ceftiofur Hydrochloride (See also *80370-57-6*)

103980-45-6. Metostilenol

103997-59-7. Selprazine

104010-37-9. Ceftiofur Sodium

104051-20-9. Brefonalol

104054-27-5. Atipamezole

104121-92-8. Eldecalcitol

104138-64-9. Agalsidase Alfa

104145-95-1. Cefditoren (See also *117467-28-4*)

104153-37-9. Rilopirox

104206-65-7. Nitisinone

104227-87-4. Famciclovir

104317-84-2. Gusperimus Trihydrochloride [gusperimus] (See also *85468-01-5; 84937-45-1*)

104340-86-5. Leminoprazole

104344-23-2. Bisoprolol Fumarate

104348-91-6. Technetium Tc 99m Tiatide [anion]

104376-79-6. Ceftriaxone Sodium (See also *73384-59-5*)

104383-17-7. Sabeluzole

104393-00-2. Pirazmonam Sodium (See also *108319-07-9*)

104454-71-9. Ipenoxazone

104456-79-3. Cisconazole

104485-01-0. Trapencaine

104486-81-9. Mupirocin Calcium [anhydrous] (See also *115074-43-6*)

104561-36-6. Doretinel

104564-71-8. Dobutamine Lactobionate

104595-79-1. Anaritide Acetate (See also *95896-08-5*)

104632-26-0. Pramipexole

104675-29-8. Velnacrine Maleate [velnacrine] (See also *118909-22-1*)

104675-35-6. Suronacrine Maleate [suronacrine] (See also *113108-86-4*)

104713-75-9. Barnidipine

104716-22-5. Technetium Tc 99m Teboroxime

104719-71-3. Lorcinadol

104746-04-5. Eslicarbazepine

104775-36-2. Ecabapide

104777-03-9. Asobamast

104868-24-8. Mipafilcon A

104902-08-1. Cilutazoline

104987-11-3. Tacrolimus [anhydrous] (See also *109581-93-3*)

105051-87-4. Minamestane

105102-18-9. Tibenelast Sodium

105102-20-3. Liroldine

105102-21-4. Torbafylline

105118-12-5. Piroxantrone Hydrochloride (See also *91441-23-5*)

105118-13-6. Iprotiazem

105118-14-7. Datelliptium Chloride

105149-04-0. Osaterone

105182-45-4. Fluparoxan Hydrochloride [fluparoxan] (See also *111793-41-0*)

105219-56-5. Apafant

105239-91-6. Cefclidin

105250-86-0. Ebiratide

105292-70-4. Alonacic

105431-72-9. Linopirdine

105462-24-6. Risedronic Acid

105523-37-3. Tiprotimod

105567-83-7. Berefrine

105581-52-0. Tolofocon A

105613-48-7. Exametazime (See also *100551-63-1*)

105618-02-8. Galamustine

105674-77-9. Lanproston

105685-11-8. Batoprazine

105687-93-2. Sumarotene

105784-61-0. Temafloxacin Hydrochloride (See also *108319-06-8*)

105806-65-3. Efegatran Sulfate [efegatran] (See also *126721-07-1*)

105816-04-4. Nateglinide

105851-17-0. Fludeoxyglucose F 18

105857-23-6. Alteplase

105879-42-3. Cephalexin Hydrochloride

105920-77-2. Camonagrel

105953-59-1. Dumorelin

105956-97-6. Clinafloxacin Hydrochloride [clinafloxacin] (See also *105956-99-8*)

105956-99-8. Clinafloxacin Hydrochloride (See also *105956-97-6*)

105979-17-7. Benidipine

106033-96-9. Itrocinonide

106073-01-2. Taniplon

106083-71-0. Radafaxine Hydrochloride (See also *192374-14-4*)

106100-65-6. Fasiplon

106133-20-4. Tamsulosin Hydrochloride [tamsulosin] (See also *106463-17-6*)

106266-06-2. Risperidone

106282-98-8. Somalapor

106308-44-5. Rufinamide

106344-20-1. Stannsoporfin

106372-55-8. Aspartame Acesulfame

106392-12-5. Poloxamer [block copolymer] (See also *9003-11-6*)

106400-81-1. Lometrexol Sodium [lometrexol] (See also *120408-07-3*)

106417-28-1. Technetium Tc 99m Siboroxime

106463-17-6. Tamsulosin Hydrochloride (See also *106133-20-4*)

106498-99-1. Vintoperol

106516-24-9. Sertindole

106560-14-9. Faropenem Medoxomil [faropenem] (See also *141702-36-5*)

106635-80-7. Tafenoquine

106650-56-0. Sibutramine Hydrochloride [sibutramine] (See also *125494-59-9; 84485-00-7*)

106669-71-0. Arpromidine

106685-40-9. Adapalene

106686-40-2. Gapromidine

106707-51-1. Dobupride

106719-74-8. Galtifenin

106730-54-5. Olprinone

106756-71-2. Fertirelin Acetate (See also *38234-21-8*)

106819-53-8. Doxacurium Chloride

106854-46-0. Argimesna

106861-44-3. Mivacurium Chloride

106900-12-3. Loperamide Oxide

106941-25-7. Adefovir

106972-33-2. Denipride

107000-34-0. Zanoterone

107007-99-8. Granisetron Hydrochloride

107023-41-6. Pobilukast Edamine [pobilukast] (See also *137232-03-2*)

107052-56-2. Romergoline

107078-89-7. Melafocon A

107097-79-0. Tosufloxacin [monohydrate] (See also *108138-46-1*)

107097-80-3. Loxiglumide

107133-36-8. Perindopril Erbumine

107233-08-9. Cevimeline Hydrochloride [cevimeline] (See also *153504-70-2*)

107266-06-8. Gevotroline Hydrochloride [gevotroline] (See also *112243-58-0*)

107266-08-0. Carvotroline Hydrochloride [carvotroline] (See also *136777-43-0*)

107320-86-5. Isomolpan Hydrochloride [isomolpan] (See also *121096-86-4*)

107361-33-1. Enazadrem Phosphate [enazadrem] (See also *132956-22-0*)

107407-62-5. Nelezaprine Maleate (See also *69624-60-8*)

107429-63-0. Lintopride

107452-79-9. Cefmepidium Chloride

107452-89-1. Ziconotide

107489-37-2. Thymoctonan

107667-60-7. Polaprezinc

107703-78-6. Glemanserin (See also *132553-86-7*)

107724-20-9. Eplerenone

107736-98-1. Umespirone

107753-78-6. Zafirlukast

107793-72-6. Ioxilan

107868-30-4. Exemestane

107910-75-8. Ganciclovir Sodium (See also *82410-32-0*)

108001-60-1. Troquidazole

108050-54-0. Tilmicosin

108138-46-1. Tosufloxacin [anhydrous (±)] (See also *107097-79-0*)

108147-54-2. Migalastat Hydrochloride [migalastat] (See also *75172-81-5*)

108153-74-8. Secretin [human] (See also *17034-35-4; 1393-25-5*)

108210-73-7. Bifeprofen

108258-89-5. Sulazuril

108303-49-1. Ondansetron [replaced] (See also *99614-02-5; 116002-70-1*)

108310-20-9. Pirodomast

108319-06-8. Temafloxacin Hydrochloride [temafloxacin] (See also *105784-61-0*)

108319-07-9. Pirazmonam Sodium [pirazmonam] (See also *104393-00-2*)

108391-88-4. Orbutopril

108436-80-2. Rociclovir

108437-28-1. Binfloxacin

108605-62-5. Teriflunomide

108612-45-9. Mizolastine

108674-86-8. Sergolexole Maleate [sergolexole] (See also *108674-87-9*)

108674-87-9. Sergolexole Maleate (See also *108674-86-8*)

108674-88-0. Idenast

108687-08-7. Teludipine Hydrochloride [teludipine] (See also *108700-03-4*)

108700-03-4. Teludipine Hydrochloride (See also *108687-08-7*)

108736-35-2. Lanreotide Acetate [lanreotide] (See also *127984-74-1*)

108778-82-1. Beractant

108785-69-9. Lorpiprazole

108852-90-0. Nemorubicin

108894-39-9. Sitalidone

108894-40-2. Brolaconazole

108894-41-3. Famiraprinium Chloride

108912-17-0. Atliprofen

108945-35-3. Taprostene

109214-55-3. Libenzapril

109229-57-4. Englitazone Sodium (See also *109229-58-5*)

109229-58-5. Englitazone Sodium [englitazone] (See also *109229-57-4*)

109525-44-2. Cliropamine

109543-76-2. Romazarit

109545-84-8. Evernimicin

109550-08-5. Paflufocon A

109552-15-0. Pamidronate Disodium (See also *57248-88-1*)

109581-73-9. Technetium Tc 99m Sestamibi

109581-93-3. Tacrolimus (See also *104987-11-3*)

109623-97-4. Gedocarnil

109636-76-2. Prinomide Tromethamine (See also *77639-66-8*)

109683-61-6. Utibapril

109683-79-6. Utibaprilat

109713-79-3. Neldazosin

109791-32-4. Ascorbyl Gamolenate

109826-26-8. Zaldaride

109889-09-0. Granisetron

110013-21-3. Merafloxacin

110042-95-0. Acemannan

110072-15-6. Tosagestin

110078-46-1. Plerixafor

110101-66-1. Tirilazad Mesylate [tirilazad] (See also *149042-61-5*)

110140-89-1. Ridogrel

110143-10-7. Lodenosine

110172-45-7. Sebriplatin

110221-44-8. Temocapril Hydrochloride (See also *111902-57-9*)

110221-53-9. Temocaprilat

110230-98-3. Talaporfin Sodium [talaporfin] (See also *220201-34-3*)

110267-81-7. Amrubicin

110294-55-8. Sudismase

110299-05-3. Selodenoson

110311-27-8. Sulofenur

110311-30-3. Amrubicin Hydrochloride

110314-48-2. Adozelesin

110347-85-8. Selfotel

110390-84-6. Perbufylline

110480-13-2. Idremcinal

110588-56-2. Noberastine

110588-57-3. Saperconazole

110605-64-6. Isaglidole

110623-33-1. Suritozole

110629-41-9. Elbanizine

110638-68-1. Calcium Lactobionate

110690-43-2. Emitefur

110703-94-1. Zopolrestat

110816-79-0. Cromoglicate Lisetil

110845-89-1. Remiprostol

110871-86-8. Sparfloxacin

110883-46-0. Giracodazole

110909-60-9. Follitropin Alfa [β-subunit] (See also *146479-72-3; 56832-30-5*)

110942-02-4. Aldesleukin

110958-19-5. Fasoracetam

111011-63-3. Efonidipine (See also *111011-76-8*)

111011-76-8. Efonidipine [hydrochloride] (See also *111011-63-3*)

111025-46-8. Pioglitazone Hydrochloride [pioglitazone] (See also *112529-15-4*)

111073-18-8. Nemazoline Hydrochloride (See also *130759-56-7*)

111073-20-2. Orientiparcin [Orienticine A] (See also *159445-62-2; 112848-46-1*)

111149-90-7. Lodelaben (See also *93105-81-8*)

111212-85-2. Ersofermin

111223-26-8. Ceronapril

111358-88-4. Lestaurtinib

111393-84-1. Amitivir

111406-87-2. Zileuton

111470-99-6. Amlodipine Besylate (See also *88150-42-9*)

111490-36-9. Zeniplatin

111523-41-2. Enloplatin

111686-79-4. Remacemide Hydrochloride (See also *128298-28-2*)

111753-73-2. Satigrel

111786-07-3. Prinoxodan

111793-41-0. Fluparoxan Hydrochloride (See also *105182-45-4*)

111841-85-1. Abecarnil

111868-63-4. Tiacrilast Sodium

111902-57-9. Temocapril Hydrochloride [temocapril] (See also *110221-44-8*)

111911-87-6. Rebamipide

111974-60-8. Ritolukast

111974-69-7. Quetiapine Fumarate [quetiapine] (See also *111974-72-2*)

111974-72-2. Quetiapine Fumarate (See also *111974-69-7*)

112017-99-9. Ibuprofen Piconol

112018-00-5. Tebufelone

112018-01-6. Bemoradan

112108-01-7. Ecopipam

112111-43-0. Armodafinil

112192-04-8. Roxindole

112243-58-0. Gevotroline Hydrochloride (See also *107266-06-8*)

112362-50-2. Dalfopristin

112398-08-0. Danofloxacin Mesylate [danofloxacin] (See also *119478-55-6*)

112457-95-1. Tandospirone Citrate (See also *87760-53-0*)

112522-64-2. Tacedinaline

112529-15-4. Pioglitazone Hydrochloride (See also *111025-46-8*)

112568-12-4. Iturelix

112573-72-5. Dexecadotril

112573-73-6. Ecadotril

112665-43-7. Seratrodast (See also *103186-19-2*)

112721-39-8. Pifonakin

112733-06-9. Zenarestat

112809-51-5. Letrozole

112848-46-1. Orientiparcin [Orienticine D] (See also *159445-62-2; 111073-20-2*)

112856-44-7. Losigamone

112885-41-3. Mosapride

112887-68-0. Raltitrexed

112891-97-1. Alentemol Hydrobromide [alentemol] (See also *112892-81-6*)

112892-81-6. Alentemol Hydrobromide (See also *112891-97-1*)

112893-26-2. Becliconazole

112901-68-5. Amifostine (See also *20537-88-6*)

112922-55-1. Cericlamine

112964-97-3. Ocfentanil Hydrochloride (See also *101343-69-5*)

112965-21-6. Calcipotriene

112966-96-8. Domitroban

112984-60-8. Ulifloxacin

113079-82-6. Terbequinil

113082-98-7. Enalkiren

113102-19-5. Rifamexil

113108-86-4. Suronacrine Maleate (See also *104675-35-6*)

113165-32-5. Niguldipine

113167-61-6. Terdecamycin

113359-04-9. Cefozopran

113378-31-7. Semduramicin

113378-32-8. Kolfocon A

113403-10-4. Dexibuprofen Lysine [anhydrous] (See also *141505-32-0*)

113427-24-0. Epoetin Alfa

113457-05-9. Ledoxantrone Trihydrochloride [ledoxantrone] (See also *119221-49-7*)

113507-06-5. Moxidectin

113593-34-3. Flosatidil

113617-63-3. Orbifloxacin

113662-23-0. Gadobenate Dimeglumine [gadobenic acid] (See also *127000-20-8*)

113665-84-2. Clopidogrel Bisulfate [clopidogrel] (See also *120202-66-6*)

113712-98-4. Tenatoprazole

113716-48-6. Iolopride (^{123}I)

113759-50-5. Cronidipine

113775-47-6. Dexmedetomidine

113806-05-6. Olopatadine Hydrochloride [olopatadine] (See also *140462-76-6*)

113852-37-2. Cidofovir [anhydrous] (See also *149394-66-1*)

113857-87-7. Talotrexin Ammonium [talotrexin] (See also *648420-92-2*)

113932-41-5. Tematropium Methylsulfate

113957-09-8. Cebaracetam

114030-44-3. Dexpemedolac

114084-78-5. Ibandronic Acid

114298-18-9. Zalospirone Hydrochloride [zalospirone] (See also *114374-97-9*)

114374-97-9. Zalospirone Hydrochloride (See also *114298-18-9*)

114394-67-1. Lomefloxacin Mesylate

114432-13-2. Fantofarone

114451-30-8. Ganefromycin [component β] (See also *114451-31-9*)

114451-31-9. Ganefromycin [component α] (See also *114451-30-8*)

114466-38-5. Sermorelin Acetate (See also *86168-78-7*)

114485-92-6. Pidolacetamol

114517-02-1. Fosquidone

114560-48-4. Apaziquone

114568-26-2. Patamostat

114607-46-4. Acitazanolast

114686-12-3. Imitrodast

114716-16-4. Pemedolac

114776-28-2. Bepafant

114798-26-4. Losartan Potassium [losartan] (See also *124750-99-8*)

114856-44-9. Oberadilol

114870-03-0. Fondaparinux Sodium

114899-77-3. Trabectedin

114977-28-5. Docetaxel [anhydrous] (See also *148408-66-6*)

115007-34-6. Mycophenolate Mofetil

115074-43-6. Mupirocin Calcium (See also *104486-81-9*)

115103-54-3. Tiagabine Hydrochloride [tiagabine] (See also *145821-59-6*)

115256-11-6. Dofetilide

115288-27-2. Methafilcon B

115308-98-0. Tallimustine

115313-22-9. Serazapine Hydrochloride [serazapine] (See also *117581-05-2*)

115344-47-3. Siguazodan

115436-72-1. Risedronate Sodium

115436-73-2. Ipazilide Fumarate [ipazilide] (See also *115436-74-3*)

115436-74-3. Ipazilide Fumarate (See also *115436-73-2*)

115464-77-2. Elopiprazole

115550-35-1. Marbofloxacin

115574-30-6. Irtemazole

115575-11-6. Liarozole Fumarate [liarozole] (See also *145858-52-2; 145858-51-1*)

115762-17-9. Ruzadolane

115911-28-9. Sampirtine

115956-12-2. Dolasetron Mesylate [dolasetron] (See also *115956-13-3*)

115956-13-3. Dolasetron Mesylate (See also *115956-12-2*)

115972-78-6. Olradipine

116001-96-8. Pentosan Polysulfate Sodium [replaced] (See also *140207-93-8*)

116002-70-1. Ondansetron [replaced] (See also *99614-02-5; 108303-49-1*)

116041-13-5. Nebracetam

116057-75-1. Idoxifene

116094-23-6. Insulin Aspart

116209-55-3. Levobetaxolol Hydrochloride (See also *93221-48-8*)

116287-14-0. Lanperisone

116289-53-3. Tulopafant

116308-55-5. Vatanidipine

116313-94-1. Nitecapone

116476-13-2. Semotiadil

116476-16-5. Levosemotiadil

116539-59-4. Duloxetine Hydrochloride [duloxetine] (See also *136434-34-9*)

116644-53-2. Mibefradil Dihydrochloride [mibefradil] (See also *116666-63-8*)

116649-85-5. Ramatroban

116666-63-8. Mibefradil Dihydrochloride (See also *116644-53-2*)

116680-01-4. Mycophenolate Mofetil Hydrochloride

116684-92-5. Galdansetron Hydrochloride [galdansetron] (See also *156712-35-5*)

116763-36-1. Nestifylline

116795-97-2. Ledazerol

116818-99-6. Isalsteine

116853-25-9. Cefluprenam

116861-00-8. Isamoltan

116907-13-2. Risotilide Hydrochloride (See also *120688-08-6*)

117086-68-7. Ricasetron

117091-64-2. Etoposide Phosphate

117268-95-8. Brifentanil Hydrochloride (See also *101345-71-5*)

117276-75-2. Lanimostim

117279-73-9. Israpafant

117305-33-6. Telimomab Aritox

117414-74-1. Midafotel

117467-28-4. Cefditoren [pivoxil] (See also *104145-95-1*)

117523-47-4. Mirfentanil Hydrochloride [mirfentanil] (See also *119413-53-5*)

117545-11-6. Bimakalim

117570-53-3. Vadimezan

117581-05-2. Serazapine Hydrochloride (See also *115313-22-9*)

117591-79-4. Remoxipride Hydrochloride

117704-25-3. Doramectin

117742-13-9. Ardacin

117772-70-0. Azithromycin [dihydrate] (See also *83905-01-5; 121479-24-4*)

117819-25-7. Bakeprofen

117827-79-9. Zilpaterol

117827-80-2. Gadopenamide

117827-81-3. Delfaprazine

117857-45-1. Loreclezole

117976-89-3. Rabeprazole Sodium [rabeprazole] (See also *117976-90-6*)

117976-90-6. Rabeprazole Sodium (See also *117976-89-3*)

118248-91-2. Fodipir

118288-08-7. Lafutidine

118292-40-3. Tazarotene

118390-30-0. Interferon Alfacon-1

118420-47-6. Tagorizine

118428-36-7. Pimobendan

118443-89-3. Cefquinome Sulfate (See also *84957-30-2*)

118457-14-0. Nebivolol

118457-15-1. Dexnebivolol

118457-16-2. Levonebivolol

118812-69-4. Ularitide

118830-14-1. Sodium Phosphate, Dibasic [monohydrate] (See also *10140-65-5; 10039-32-4; 7782-85-6; 10028-24-7; 7558-79-4*)

118909-22-1. Velnacrine Maleate (See also *104675-29-8*)

118976-38-8. Dabelotine

119006-77-8. Flutrimazole

119068-77-8. Semduramicin Sodium

119141-88-7. Esomeprazole

119169-78-7. Epristeride

119175-48-3. Fermagate

119221-49-7. Ledoxantrone Trihydrochloride (See also *113457-05-9*)

119229-65-1. Nerispirdine

119257-34-0. Besipirdine Hydrochloride [besipirdine] (See also *130953-69-4*)

119271-78-2. Sezolamide Hydrochloride (See also *123308-22-5*)

119302-91-9. Rocuronium Bromide

119322-27-9. Meribendan

119356-77-3. Dapoxetine Hydrochloride [dapoxetine] (See also *129938-20-1*)

119363-62-1. Amiglumide

119386-96-8. Mofegiline Hydrochloride [free base] (See also *120635-25-8*)

119391-55-8. Benzetimide Hydrochloride [benzetimide] (See also *5633-14-7*)

119413-53-5. Mirfentanil Hydrochloride (See also *117523-47-4*)

119413-54-6. Topotecan Hydrochloride (See also *123948-87-8*)

119413-55-7. Elgodipine

119431-25-3. Eliprodil

119478-55-6. Danofloxacin Mesylate (See also *112398-08-0*)

119478-56-7. Meropenem (See also *96036-03-2*)

119514-66-8. Lifarizine

119515-38-7. Icaridin

119567-79-2. Taribavirin Hydrochloride [taribavirin] (See also *40372-00-7*)

119610-26-3. Aloracetam

119618-22-3. Esoxybutynin Chloride [esoxybutynin] (See also *230949-16-3*)

119625-78-4. Terlakiren

119637-66-0. Metoprolol Fumarate

119637-67-1. Moguisteine

119644-22-3. Raluridine

119673-08-4. Becatecarin

119683-68-0. Ferumoxides

119687-33-1. Iganidipine

119693-74-2. Somenopor

119719-11-8. Ilatreotide

119784-94-0. Tenidap Sodium

119793-66-7. Levocarnitine Propionate Hydrochloride

119813-10-4. Carzelesin
119817-90-2. Dexloxiglumide
119905-05-4. Delequamine Hydrochloride [delequamine] (See also *119942-75-5*)
119914-60-2. Grepafloxacin Hydrochloride [grepafloxacin] (See also *161967-81-3*)
119922-85-9. Cefadroxil [hemihydrate] (See also *66592-87-8; 50370-12-2*)
119942-75-5. Delequamine Hydrochloride (See also *119905-05-4*)
120014-06-4. Donepezil Hydrochloride [donepezil] (See also *142057-77-0*)
120054-86-6. Dexniguldipine
120066-54-8. Gadoteridol
120068-37-3. Fipronil
120081-14-3. Goralatide
120092-68-4. Manidipine 6300
120138-50-3. Quinupristin
120202-66-6. Clopidogrel Bisulfate (See also *113665-84-2*)
120210-48-2. Tenidap
120241-31-8. Alvameline Maleate [alvameline] (See also *219581-36-9*)
120279-96-1. Dorzolamide Hydrochloride [dorzolamide] (See also *130693-82-2*)
120287-85-6. Cetrorelix
120313-91-9. Thrombomodulin Alfa
120360-10-3. Batelapine Maleate (See also *95634-82-5*)
120373-36-6. Unoprostone
120408-07-3. Lometrexol Sodium (See also *106400-81-1*)
120410-24-4. Biapenem
120443-16-5. Verlukast
120444-71-5. Deramciclane
120511-73-1. Anastrozole
120551-59-9. Crilvastatin
120608-46-0. Duteplase
120635-25-8. Mofegiline Hydrochloride (See also *119386-96-8*)
120635-74-7. Cilansetron
120638-55-3. Bromfenac Sodium (See also *91714-94-2*)
120656-74-8. Trefentanil Hydrochloride [trefentanil] (See also *120656-93-1*)
120656-93-1. Trefentanil Hydrochloride (See also *120656-74-8*)
120685-11-2. Midostaurin
120688-08-6. Risotilide Hydrochloride [risotilide] (See also *116907-13-2*)
120770-34-5. Draflazine
120788-07-0. Sulopenem
120815-74-9. Butixocort
120819-70-7. Naroparcil
120824-08-0. Linotroban
120958-90-9. Dalcotidine
120993-53-5. Desirudin
121009-30-1. Alprenoxime Hydrochloride
121009-31-2. Adaprolol Maleate (See also *101479-70-3*)
121009-77-6. Tenivastatin Calcium [tenivastatin] (See also *151006-18-7*)
121029-11-6. Altoqualine
121032-29-9. Nelarabine

121096-86-4. Isomolpan Hydrochloride (See also *107320-86-5*)
121104-96-9. Celgosivir Hydrochloride [celgosivir] (See also *141117-12-6*)
121123-17-9. Cefprozil (See also *92665-29-7*)
121181-53-1. Filgrastim
121243-20-7. Pancopride [nonstereospecific] (See also *121650-80-4*)
121249-14-7. Corticorelin Ovine Triflutate
121268-17-5. Alendronate Sodium
121277-96-1. Terikalant
121281-41-2. Technetium Tc 99m Bicisate
121288-39-9. Loxoribine
121479-24-4. Azithromycin [monohydrate] (See also *83905-01-5; 117772-70-0*)
121524-08-1. Amibegron
121524-09-2. Amibegron Hydrochloride
121547-04-4. Mirimostim
121584-18-7. Valspodar
121588-75-8. Amesergide
121617-11-6. Saviprazole
121650-80-4. Pancopride [±] (See also *121243-20-7*)
121679-13-8. Naratriptan
121750-57-0. Itameline
121762-69-4. Tetrazolast Meglumine [anhydrous] (See also *133008-33-0; 95104-27-1*)
121808-62-6. Pidotimod
121840-95-7. Rogletimide
121915-83-1. Calteridol Calcium (See also *132722-73-7*)
121929-20-2. Zoniclezole Hydrochloride [zoniclezole] (See also *121929-46-2*)
121929-46-2. Zoniclezole Hydrochloride (See also *121929-20-2*)
121961-22-6. Loracarbef (See also *76470-66-1*)
122111-03-9. Gemcitabine Hydrochloride
122173-74-4. Mideplanin
122254-45-9. Glenvastatin
122312-54-3. Epoetin Beta
122312-55-4. Dosmalfate
122320-73-4. Rosiglitazone Maleate [rosiglitazone] (See also *155141-29-0*)
122332-18-7. Mivobulin Isethionate [mivobulin] (See also *126268-81-3*)
122341-38-2. Temoporfin
122384-88-7. Amlintide
122431-96-3. Zilascorb (^{2}H)
122575-28-4. Naglivan
122647-31-8. Ibutilide Fumarate [ibutilide] (See also *122647-32-9*)
122647-32-9. Ibutilide Fumarate (See also *122647-31-8*)
122760-91-2. Caldiamide Sodium (See also *128326-81-8*)
122830-14-2. Deriglidole
122841-10-5. Cefoselis
122852-42-0. Alosetron Hydrochloride [alosetron] (See also *122852-69-1*)
122852-69-1. Alosetron Hydrochloride (See also *122852-42-0*)
122898-67-3. Itopride
122946-42-3. Spiriprostil
122946-43-4. Telmesteine

122956-68-7. Modipafant [racemate] (See also *122957-06-6*)
122957-06-6. Modipafant (See also *122956-68-7*)
122970-40-5. Isatoribine [anhydrous] (See also *198832-38-1*)
123013-22-9. Amelometasone
123018-47-3. Atiprimod Dihydrochloride [atiprimod] (See also *130065-61-1*)
123040-69-7. Azasetron (See also *141922-90-9*)
123072-45-7. Aprosulate Sodium
123120-99-0. Ecogramostim
123122-54-3. Candoxatrilat
123122-55-4. Candoxatril
123171-59-5. Cefepime Hydrochloride
123205-52-7. Trelnarizine
123212-08-8. Somatosalm
123258-84-4. Itasetron
123286-00-0. Vinfosiltine
123308-22-5. Sezolamide Hydrochloride [sezolamide] (See also *119271-78-2*)
123318-82-1. Clofarabine
123407-36-3. Arteflene
123441-03-2. Rivastigmine
123447-62-1. Prulifloxacin
123482-22-4. Zatosetron Maleate [zatosetron] (See also *123482-23-5*)
123482-23-5. Zatosetron Maleate (See also *123482-22-4*)
123524-52-7. Azelnidipine
123548-56-1. Acreozast
123618-00-8. Fedotozine
123663-49-0. Iguratimod
123748-56-1. Iodofiltic Acid I 123
123760-07-6. Zinostatin [zinostatin stimalamer] (See also *9014-02-2*)
123774-72-1. Sargramostim
123948-87-8. Topotecan Hydrochloride [topotecan] (See also *119413-54-6*)
123955-10-2. Almokalant
123997-26-2. Eprinomectin (See also *133305-88-1; 133305-89-2*)
124012-42-6. Galocitabine
124066-33-7. Taurosteine
124083-20-1. Etomoxir
124146-64-1. Mobenakin
124265-89-0. Omaciclovir
124316-02-5. Alprafenone
124351-85-5. Incadronic Acid
124378-77-4. Enadoline Hydrochloride [enadoline] (See also *124439-07-2*)
124423-84-3. Panadiplon
124436-59-5. Pirodavir
124439-07-2. Enadoline Hydrochloride (See also *124378-77-4*)
124478-60-0. Aglepristone
124508-66-3. Triptorelin Pamoate
124584-08-3. Nesiritide
124750-99-8. Losartan Potassium (See also *114798-26-4*)
124756-23-6. Binospirone Mesylate (See also *102908-59-8*)
124784-31-2. Erbulozole
124832-26-4. Valacyclovir Hydrochloride [valacyclovir] (See also *124832-27-5*)

124832-27-5. Valacyclovir Hydrochloride (See also *124832-26-4*)
124858-35-1. Nadifloxacin
124884-28-2. Ramoplanin A′₁
124884-29-3. Ramoplanin A′₂
124884-30-6. Ramoplanin A′₃
124904-93-4. Ganirelix Acetate [ganirelix] (See also *129311-55-3*)
124937-51-5. Tolterodine
124937-52-6. Tolterodine Tartrate
125224-05-7. Technetium Tc 99m Mertiatide
125251-66-3. Arbutamine Hydrochloride (See also *128470-16-6*)
125279-79-0. Ersentilide
125317-39-7. Vinorelbine Tartrate (See also *71486-22-1*)
125363-87-3. Carsatrin Succinate [carsatrin] (See also *132199-13-4*)
125372-33-0. Dacopafant
125472-02-8. Mivazerol
125494-59-9. Sibutramine Hydrochloride [monohydrate] (See also *84485-00-7; 106650-56-0*)
125533-88-2. Mofarotene
125602-71-3. Bepotastine
125729-29-5. Lemildipine
125926-17-2. Sarpogrelate
125961-82-2. Tipelukast
125973-56-0. Amsilarotene
125974-72-3. Intoplicine
126100-97-8. Dimiracetam
126222-34-2. Remikiren
126268-81-3. Mivobulin Isethionate (See also *122332-18-7*)
126294-30-2. Sagandipine
126544-47-6. Ciclesonide (See also *141845-82-1*)
126721-07-1. Efegatran Sulfate (See also *105806-65-3*)
126752-39-4. Somavubove
126825-36-3. Bertosamil
126871-95-2. Unifocon A
126924-38-7. Seproxetine Hydrochloride [seproxetine] (See also *127685-30-7*)
127000-20-8. Gadobenate Dimeglumine (See also *113662-23-0*)
127035-60-3. Enofelast
127045-41-4. Pazufloxacin
127182-67-6. Cefetecol
127254-12-0. Sitafloxacin [anhydrous] (See also *163253-35-8*)
127266-56-2. Adatanserin Hydrochloride [adatanserin] (See also *144966-96-1*)
127294-70-6. Balofloxacin
127304-28-3. Linarotene
127308-82-1. Zamifenacin
127373-66-4. Sivelestat
127396-36-5. Iomazenil (¹²³I)
127420-24-0. Idrapril
127471-94-7. Isotretinoin Anisatil
127502-06-1. Tetrofosmin
127625-29-0. Fananserin
127657-42-5. Minodronic Acid
127685-30-7. Seproxetine Hydrochloride (See also *126924-38-7*)
127757-91-9. Regramostim
127757-92-0. Maslimomab

127759-89-1. Lobucavir
127779-20-8. Saquinavir
127785-64-2. Basifungin
127932-90-5. Ramorelix
127943-53-7. Disermolide
127984-74-1. Lanreotide Acetate (See also *108736-35-2*)
128075-79-6. Lufironil
128196-01-0. Escitalopram
128229-52-7. Tamolarizine
128232-14-4. Raxofelast
128253-31-6. Veliflapon
128270-60-0. Bivalirudin
128298-28-2. Remacemide Hydrochloride [remacemide] (See also *111686-79-4*)
128312-51-6. Cinalukast
128326-80-7. Nicoracetam
128326-81-8. Caldiamide Sodium [caldiamide] (See also *122760-91-2*)
128326-82-9. Eberconazole
128345-62-0. Ranitidine Bismuth Citrate
128420-61-1. Minopafant
128470-15-5. Melarsomine
128470-16-6. Arbutamine Hydrochloride [arbutamine] (See also *125251-66-3*)
128470-17-7. Sprodiamide [anhydrous]
128486-54-4. Lurosetron Mesylate [lurosetron] (See also *143486-90-2*)
128517-07-7. Romidepsin
128607-22-7. Ospemifene
128620-82-6. Limazocic
129009-83-2. Versetamide
129029-23-8. Ocaperidone
129069-19-8. Poractant Alfa
129260-79-3. Loteprednol Etabonate [loteprednol] (See also *82034-46-6*)
129300-27-2. Fabesetron
129311-55-3. Ganirelix Acetate (See also *124904-93-4*)
129336-81-8. Tenosiprol
129388-07-4. Levdobutamine Lactobionate (See also *61661-06-1*)
129453-61-8. Fulvestrant
129497-78-5. Verteporfin
129566-95-6. Somfasepor
129580-63-8. Satraplatin
129612-87-9. Miproxifene
129618-40-2. Nevirapine
129639-79-8. Abafungin
129655-21-6. Bizelesin
129688-50-2. Minalrestat
129716-58-1. Dofequidar
129722-12-9. Aripiprazole
129729-66-4. Emakalim
129731-10-8. Vorozole
129731-11-9. Tibeglisene
129791-92-0. Rifalazil
129805-33-0. Eptotermin Alfa
129938-20-1. Dapoxetine Hydrochloride (See also *119356-77-3*)
129981-36-8. Sampatrilat
130018-77-8. Levocetirizine
130018-87-0. Levocetirizine Dihydrochloride
130065-61-1. Atiprimod Dihydrochloride (See also *123018-47-3*)
130112-42-4. Mivotilate

130120-54-6. Lenograstim [component 2] (See also *135968-09-1; 130120-55-7*)
130120-55-7. Lenograstim [component 1] (See also *135968-09-1; 130120-54-6*)
130120-57-9. Prezatide Copper Acetate
130152-35-1. Igmesine Hydrochloride
130167-69-0. Pegaspargase
130209-82-4. Latanoprost
130306-02-4. Tezacitabine [anhydrous] (See also *171176-43-5*)
130308-48-4. Icatibant Acetate [icatibant] (See also *138614-30-9*)
130370-60-4. Batimastat
130403-08-6. Soretolide
130455-76-4. Epoetin Gamma
130493-03-7. Bimoclomol
130579-75-8. Eplivanserin
130610-93-4. Niravoline
130636-43-0. Nifekalant
130641-36-0. Picumeterol Fumarate [picumeterol] (See also *130641-37-1*)
130641-37-1. Picumeterol Fumarate (See also *130641-36-0*)
130641-38-2. Bindarit
130693-82-2. Dorzolamide Hydrochloride (See also *120279-96-1*)
130726-68-0. Neticonazole (See also *11178-99-9; 130773-02-3*)
130759-56-7. Nemazoline Hydrochloride [nemazoline] (See also *111073-18-8*)
130773-02-3. Neticonazole [hydrochloride] (See also *130726-68-0; 11178-99-9*)
130782-54-6. Beciparcil
130800-90-7. Sipatrigine
130804-35-2. Lecimibide
130929-57-6. Entacapone
130953-69-4. Besipirdine Hydrochloride (See also *119257-34-0*)
131069-91-5. Gadoversetamide
131081-40-8. Silteplase
131094-16-1. Trafermin
131129-98-1. Mipragoside
131179-95-8. Efaproxiral
131410-48-5. Gadodiamide [anhydrous]
131517-13-0. Govafilcon A
131577-81-6. Lenefilcon A
131608-78-1. Technetium Tc 99m Nitridocade
131635-06-8. Sifaprazine
131740-09-5. Alvocidib (See also *146426-40-6*)
131741-08-7. Simendan
131796-63-9. Odapipam
131865-88-8. Sonedenoson
131875-08-6. Lexacalcitol
131918-61-1. Paricalcitol
131929-60-7. Spinosad [factor A] (See also *131929-63-0*)
131929-63-0. Spinosad [factor D] (See also *131929-60-7*)
131986-45-3. Xanomeline
131987-54-7. Tazomeline Citrate [tazomeline] (See also *175615-45-9*)
132014-21-2. Rilmakalim
132017-01-7. Bervastatin
132019-54-6. Monatepil Maleate [monatepil] (See also *132046-06-1*)

132036-88-5. Ramosetron

132046-06-1. Monatepil Maleate (See also *132019-54-6*)

132100-55-1. Dalvastatin

132112-35-7. Ropivacaine Hydrochloride (See also *84057-95-4*)

132199-13-4. Carsatrin Succinate (See also *125363-87-3*)

132203-70-4. Cilnidipine

132210-43-6. Cipamfylline

132236-18-1. Zifrosilone

132245-57-9. Dexamethasone Cipecilate

132373-81-0. Vamicamide

132418-35-0. Setipafant

132418-36-1. Rocepafant

132438-21-2. Camiglibose

132449-46-8. Lesopitron

132486-03-4. Rubidium Chloride Rb 82

132539-06-1. Olanzapine

132539-07-2. Remifentanil Hydrochloride (See also *132875-61-7*)

132553-86-7. Glemanserin [(±)] (See also *107703-78-6*)

132640-22-3. Andolast

132682-98-5. Glufosfamide

132722-73-7. Calteridol Calcium [calteridol] (See also *121915-83-1*)

132722-74-8. Pirsidomine

132787-19-0. Tradecamide

132810-10-7. Blonanserin

132829-83-5. Espatropate

132866-11-6. Lercanidipine Hydrochloride (See also *100427-26-7*)

132875-61-7. Remifentanil Hydrochloride [remifentanil] (See also *132539-07-2*)

132937-88-3. Teloxantrone Hydrochloride (See also *91441-48-4*)

132937-89-4. Losoxantrone Hydrochloride (See also *88303-60-0*)

132956-22-0. Enazadrem Phosphate (See also *107361-33-1*)

132978-98-4. Tisilfocon A

133008-33-0. Tetrazolast Meglumine (See also *121762-69-4; 95104-27-1*)

133040-01-4. Eprosartan

133099-04-4. Darifenacin

133099-07-7. Darifenacin Hydrobromide (See also *133099-04-4*)

133107-64-9. Insulin Lispro

133208-93-2. Ibrolipim

133242-30-5. Landiolol

133267-19-3. Artilide Fumarate [artilide] (See also *133267-20-6*)

133267-20-6. Artilide Fumarate (See also *133267-19-3*)

133276-80-9. Samixogrel

133305-88-1. Eprinomectin [component B₁ₐ] (See also *123997-26-2; 133305-89-2*)

133305-89-2. Eprinomectin [component B₁ᵦ] (See also *123997-26-2; 133305-88-1*)

133432-71-0. Peldesine

133454-47-4. Iloperidone

133652-38-7. Reteplase

133692-55-4. Seprilose

133718-29-3. Revizinone

133737-32-3. Pagoclone

133804-44-1. Caldaret

133865-88-0. Ralfinamide

133865-89-1. Safinamide

133978-75-3. Folitixorin Calcium (See also *3432-99-3*)

134088-74-7. Nartograstim

134143-28-5. Glaspimod

134183-95-2. Fampronil

134208-17-6. Mazapertine Succinate [mazapertine] (See also *134208-18-7*)

134208-18-7. Mazapertine Succinate (See also *134208-17-6*)

134234-12-1. Traxoprodil Mesylate [traxoprodil] (See also *189894-57-3*)

134308-13-7. Tolcapone

134377-69-8. Safironil

134379-77-4. Dexelvucitabine

134404-52-7. Seocalcitol

134457-28-6. Prazarelix

134485-10-2. Prazarelix Acetate

134523-00-5. Atorvastatin Calcium [atorvastatin] (See also *134523-03-8*)

134523-03-8. Atorvastatin Calcium (See also *134523-00-5*)

134564-82-2. Befloxatone

134633-29-7. Tecogalan Sodium

134678-17-4. Lamivudine

134774-45-1. Rasburicase

134865-33-1. Meluadrine

135003-30-4. Apadoline

135038-57-2. Fasidotril

135062-02-1. Repaglinide

135202-79-8. Ilonidap

135306-39-7. Manifaxine

135306-78-4. Caloxetic Acid

135326-11-3. Gadoxetic Acid

135326-22-6. Gadoxetate Disodium

135354-02-8. Xaliproden

135381-77-0. Flezelastine

135459-90-4. Ranelic Acid

135463-81-9. Coluracetam

135467-16-2. Octreotide Pamoate

135548-15-1. Oxeclosporin

135558-11-1. Lobaplatin

135637-46-6. Atizoram

135729-56-5. Palonosetron Hydrochloride [palonosetron] (See also *135729-62-3*)

135729-62-3. Palonosetron Hydrochloride (See also *135729-56-5*)

135779-82-7. Bamaquimast

135821-54-4. Ceftizoxime Alapivoxil

135886-70-3. Gallium Nitrate (See also *13494-90-1*)

135889-00-8. Cefcapene

135905-89-4. Mirisetron Maleate [mirisetron] (See also *148611-75-0*)

135928-30-2. Beloxepin

135968-09-1. Lenograstim (See also *130120-55-7; 130120-54-6*)

136033-49-3. Nexopamil

136087-85-9. Fidarestat

136122-46-8. Mipitroban

136145-07-8. Arofylline

136199-02-5. Rolofylline

136236-51-6. Rasagiline Mesylate [rasagiline] (See also *161735-79-1*)

136279-32-8. Teceleukin (See also *94218-75-4*)

136310-93-5. Tiotropium Bromide (See also *139404-48-1*)

136381-85-6. Lintitript

136433-51-7. Tazofelone

136434-34-9. Duloxetine Hydrochloride (See also *116539-59-4*)

136468-36-5. Foropafant

136470-65-0. Banoxantrone

136470-78-5. Abacavir Succinate [abacavir] (See also *168146-84-7*)

136564-68-6. Masilukast

136572-09-3. Irinotecan Hydrochloride (See also *97682-44-5*)

136653-69-5. Nasaruplase Beta

136668-42-3. Quiflapon Sodium [quiflapon] (See also *147030-01-1*)

136777-43-0. Carvotroline Hydrochloride (See also *107266-08-0*)

136790-76-6. Lubiprostone

136794-86-0. Iometopane I 123

136816-75-6. Atevirdine Mesylate [atevirdine] (See also *138540-32-6*)

136817-59-9. Delavirdine Mesylate [delavirdine] (See also *147221-93-0*)

136892-64-3. Ecraprost

136949-58-1. Iobitridol

137071-32-0. Pimecrolimus

137099-09-3. Turosteride

137109-71-8. Balazipone

137109-78-5. Orazipone

137159-92-3. Aptiganel Hydrochloride [aptiganel] (See also *137160-11-3*)

137160-11-3. Aptiganel Hydrochloride (See also *137159-92-3*)

137214-72-3. Iliparcil

137215-12-4. Odiparcil

137219-37-5. Plitidepsin

137232-03-2. Pobilukast Edamine (See also *107023-41-6*)

137234-62-9. Voriconazole

137275-81-1. Osemozotan

137281-23-3. Pemetrexed Disodium [pemetrexed] (See also *150399-23-8*)

137330-13-3. Tilmicosin Phosphate

137332-54-8. Tivirapine

137460-88-9. Odalprofen

137463-76-4. Milodistim

137487-62-8. Alvircept Sudotox

137500-42-6. Darsidomine

137795-35-8. Spiroglumide

137862-53-4. Valsartan

137882-98-5. Abitesartan

137975-06-5. Mozavaptan

138068-37-8. Lepirudin

138071-82-6. Gadobutrol

138112-76-2. Agomelatine

138117-50-7. Leteprinim

138199-71-0. Levofloxacin

138298-79-0. Alnespirone

138330-98-0. Afovirsen Sodium (See also *151356-08-0*)

138384-68-6. Metesind Glucuronate [metesind] (See also *157182-23-5*)

138402-11-6. Irbesartan

138452-21-8. Fexofenadine Hydrochloride [replaced] (See also *153439-40-8; 83799-24-0*)

138506-45-3. Pidobenzone

138511-81-6. Icodulinum

138530-94-6. Dexlansoprazole

138530-95-7. Levolansoprazole

138531-07-4. Sinapultide

138540-32-6. Atevirdine Mesylate (See also *136816-75-6*)

138614-30-9. Icatibant Acetate (See also *130308-48-4*)

138660-96-5. Sevirumab

138660-97-6. Tuvirumab

138660-99-8. Imciromab Pentetate (See also *138661-00-4*)

138661-00-4. Imciromab Pentetate [indium In 111 imciromab pentetate] (See also *138660-99-8*)

138661-01-5. Nebacumab

138661-02-6. Pentetreotide

138661-03-7. Furnidipine

138708-32-4. Ferpifosate Sodium

138729-47-2. Eszopiclone

138742-43-5. Zankiren Hydrochloride [zankiren] (See also *138810-64-7*)

138778-28-6. Siratiazem

138783-13-8. Biciromab (See also *138783-14-9*)

138783-14-9. Biciromab [technetium Tc 99m biciromab] (See also *138783-13-8*)

138810-64-7. Zankiren Hydrochloride (See also *138742-43-5*)

138890-62-7. Brinzolamide

138926-19-9. Ibandronate Sodium

138955-26-7. Indium In 111 Satumomab Pendetide [satumomab pendetide monoclonal-linker/chelator] (See also *138955-27-8; 144058-40-2*)

138955-27-8. Indium In 111 Satumomab Pendetide (See also *138955-26-7; 144058-40-2*)

138982-67-9. Ziprasidone Hydrochloride (See also *146939-27-7*)

139039-69-3. Indium In 111 Altumomab Pentetate [altumomab pentetate monoclonal conjugate] (See also *139039-70-6*)

139039-70-6. Indium In 111 Altumomab Pentetate (See also *139039-69-3*)

139076-62-3. Octocog Alfa

139096-04-1. Indium In 111 Pentetreotide

139110-80-8. Zanamivir

139133-26-9. Lexipafant

139133-27-0. Nupafant

139145-27-0. Parogrelil

139225-22-2. Panamesine

139226-28-1. Darbufelone

139233-53-7. Zelandopam

139264-17-8. Zolmitriptan

139290-65-6. Volinanserin

139308-65-9. Tolafentrine

139314-01-5. Quilostigmine

139340-56-0. Darbufelone Mesylate

139402-18-9. Alestramustine

139403-31-9. Pimilprost

139404-48-1. Tiotropium Bromide [hydrate] (See also *136310-93-5*)

139481-59-7. Candesartan

139755-79-6. Safingol Hydrochloride

139755-80-9. Iobenguane I 123

139755-83-2. Sildenafil Citrate [sildenafil] (See also *171599-83-0*)

139781-09-2. Sibopirdine

139886-04-7. Milameline Hydrochloride (See also *139886-32-1*)

139886-32-1. Milameline Hydrochloride [milameline] (See also *139886-04-7*)

140128-74-1. Cefmatilen

140207-93-8. Pentosan Polysulfate Sodium (See also *116001-96-8*)

140462-76-6. Olopatadine Hydrochloride (See also *113806-05-6*)

140616-46-2. Fluorescein Lisicol

140637-86-1. Galarubicin

140661-97-8. Deltibant

140678-14-4. Mangafodipir Trisodium

140695-21-2. Osutidine

140703-49-7. Avorelin

140703-51-1. Examorelin

140850-73-3. Igmesine

140898-91-5. Hexaminolevulinate Hydrochloride

140944-31-6. Silperisone

140945-32-0. Mapinastine

141117-12-6. Celgosivir Hydrochloride (See also *121104-96-9*)

141184-34-1. Filaminast

141195-77-9. Cefovecin Sodium (See also *234096-34-5*)

141200-24-0. Darglitazone Sodium [darglitazone] (See also *141683-98-9*)

141374-81-4. Tarazepide

141388-76-3. Besifloxacin Hydrochloride [besifloxacin] (See also *405165-61-9*)

141396-28-3. Argatroban (See also *74863-84-6*)

141410-98-2. Edobacomab

141483-72-9. Zolimomab Aritox

141505-32-0. Dexibuprofen Lysine (See also *113403-10-4*)

141505-33-1. Levosimendan

141549-75-9. Indisetron

141575-50-0. Vedaclidine

141579-54-6. Fenleuton

141611-76-9. Sanfetrinem Sodium

141625-93-6. Dronedarone Hydrochloride (See also *141626-36-0*)

141626-36-0. Dronedarone Hydrochloride [dronedarone] (See also *141625-93-6*)

141646-08-4. Sanfetrinem Cilexetil (See also *156769-21-0*)

141660-63-1. Iofratol

141683-98-9. Darglitazone Sodium (See also *141200-24-0*)

141702-36-5. Faropenem Medoxomil (See also *106560-14-9*)

141725-10-2. Milacainide

141725-88-4. Cetefloxacin

141732-76-5. Exenatide (See also *141758-74-9*)

141758-74-9. Exenatide (See also *141732-76-5*)

141790-23-0. Fozivudine Tidoxil

141845-82-1. Ciclesonide (See also *126544-47-6*)

141922-90-9. Azasetron [hydrochloride] (See also *123040-69-7*)

141977-79-9. Miriplatin

141993-70-6. Eldacimibe

142001-63-6. Saredutant

142057-77-0. Donepezil Hydrochloride (See also *120014-06-4*)

142139-60-4. Lapisteride

142155-43-9. Cizolirtine

142217-69-4. Entecavir [anhydrous] (See also *209216-23-9*)

142261-03-8. Hemoglobin Crosfumaril

142298-00-8. Emoctakin

142340-99-6. Adefovir Dipivoxil

142373-60-2. Tirofiban Hydrochloride [anhydrous] (See also *150915-40-5; 144494-65-5*)

142481-95-6. Technetium Tc 99m Furifosmin

142852-50-4. Zanapezil

142864-19-5. Enlimomab

142880-36-2. Ilomastat

142906-29-4. Ferric Sulfate [hydrate] (See also *10028-22-5*)

142996-66-5. Furomine

143003-46-7. Alglucerase

143090-92-0. Anakinra

143201-11-0. Cerivastatin Sodium (See also *145599-86-6*)

143224-34-4. Telinavir

143248-63-9. Sinitrodil

143249-88-1. Dexefaroxan

143257-97-0. Sameridine

143257-98-1. Lerisetron

143322-58-1. Eletriptan

143343-83-3. Toborinone

143383-65-7. Premafloxacin

143388-64-1. Naratriptan Hydrochloride (See also *121679-13-8*)

143393-27-5. Azalanstat Dihydrochloride [azalanstat] (See also *143484-82-6*)

143443-90-7. Ifetroban

143484-82-6. Azalanstat Dihydrochloride (See also *143393-27-5*)

143486-90-2. Lurosetron Mesylate (See also *128486-54-4*)

143491-57-0. Emtricitabine

143631-61-2. Atexakin Alfa

143631-62-3. Ciprokiren

143653-53-6. Abciximab

143664-11-3. Elacridar Hydrochloride [elacridar] (See also *143851-98-3*)

143831-71-4. Dornase Alfa

143851-98-3. Elacridar Hydrochloride (See also *143664-11-3*)

143943-73-1. Lirequinil

144031-34-5. Lotifocon B

144034-80-0. Rizatriptan Benzoate [rizatriptan] (See also *145202-66-0*)

144035-83-6. Piclamilast

144056-32-6. Omafilcon A

144058-40-2. Indium In 111 Satumomab Pendetide [satumomab] (See also *138955-27-8; 138955-26-7*)

144060-53-7. Febuxostat

144143-96-4. Eprosartan Mesylate

144245-52-3. Fomivirsen Sodium [fomivirsen] (See also *160369-77-7*)

144348-08-3. Binodenoson

144412-49-7. Lamifiban

144459-70-1. Rofleponide

144494-65-5. Tirofiban Hydrochloride [tirofiban] (See also *150915-40-5; 142373-60-2*)

144506-11-6. Alilusem

144510-96-3. Pixantrone

144598-75-4. Paliperidone

144604-00-2. Diltiazem Malate

144665-07-6. Lubeluzole

144689-24-7. Olmesartan

144689-63-4. Olmesartan Medoxomil

144701-48-4. Telmisartan

144702-17-0. Pomisartan

144743-92-0. Teverelix

144849-63-8. Bisnafide Dimesylate [bisnafide] (See also *145124-30-7*)

144875-48-9. Resiquimod

144912-63-0. Perzinfotel

144916-42-7. Sonermin

144966-96-1. Adatanserin Hydrochloride (See also *127266-56-2*)

144980-29-0. Repinotan

145040-37-5. Candesartan Cilexetil (See also *139481-59-7*)

145108-58-3. Dexmedetomidine Hydrochloride

145124-30-7. Bisnafide Dimesylate (See also *144849-63-8*)

145137-38-8. Desmoteplase

145155-23-3. Interferon Beta-1b

145158-71-0. Tegaserod

145202-66-0. Rizatriptan Benzoate (See also *144034-80-0*)

145216-43-9. Forasartan

145258-61-3. Interferon Beta-1a

145375-43-5. Mitiglinide

145414-12-6. Lirexapride

145435-72-9. Gamithromycin

145464-27-3. Immune Globulin Intravenous Pentetate

145464-28-4. Capromab Pendetide (See also *151763-64-3*)

145497-36-5. Alphafilcon A

145508-78-7. Icopezil Maleate [icopezil] (See also *145815-98-1*)

145514-04-1. Amdoxovir

145574-90-9. Scopinast

145599-86-6. Cerivastatin Sodium [cerivastatin] (See also *143201-11-0*)

145672-81-7. Cetrorelix Acetate

145733-36-4. Tasosartan

145739-56-6. Tetomilast

145781-32-4. Zolasartan

145815-98-1. Icopezil Maleate (See also *145508-78-7*)

145821-59-6. Tiagabine Hydrochloride (See also *115103-54-3*)

145832-33-3. Detumomab

145858-50-0. Liarozole Hydrochloride

145858-51-1. Liarozole Fumarate [deleted] (See also *145858-52-2; 115575-11-6*)

145858-52-2. Liarozole Fumarate (See also *115575-11-6; 145858-51-1*)

145918-75-8. Troxacitabine

145941-26-0. Oprelvekin

146362-70-1. Meclinertant

146376-58-1. Talibegron Hydrochloride [talibegron] (See also *178600-17-4*)

146426-40-6. Alvocidib (See also *131740-09-5*)

146464-95-1. Pralatrexate

146479-72-3. Follitropin Alfa (See also *56832-30-5; 110909-60-9*)

146510-36-3. Olanexidine

146613-90-3. Saprisartan Potassium (See also *146623-69-0*)

146623-69-0. Saprisartan Potassium [saprisartan] (See also *146613-90-3*)

146665-77-2. Eptaplatin

146706-68-5. Rismorelin Porcine

146939-27-7. Ziprasidone Hydrochloride [ziprasidone] (See also *138982-67-9*)

146978-48-5. Moxilubant Maleate [moxilubant] (See also *147398-01-4*)

147025-53-4. Talsaclidine Fumarate [talsaclidine] (See also *147025-54-5*)

147025-54-5. Talsaclidine Fumarate (See also *147025-53-4*)

147030-01-1. Quiflapon Sodium (See also *136668-42-3*)

147059-72-1. Trovafloxacin Mesylate [trovafloxacin] (See also *147059-75-4*)

147059-75-4. Trovafloxacin Mesylate (See also *147059-72-1*)

147076-36-6. Laflunimus

147084-10-4. Alcaftadine

147098-20-2. Rosuvastatin Calcium (See also *287714-41-4*)

147116-64-1. Ezlopitant

147116-67-4. Maropitant Citrate [maropitant] (See also *359875-09-5*)

147127-20-6. Tenofovir

147149-76-6. Nolatrexed

147191-91-1. Priliximab

147221-93-0. Delavirdine Mesylate (See also *136817-59-9*)

147245-92-9. Glatiramer Acetate

147254-64-6. Ranirestat

147362-57-0. Loviride

147398-01-4. Moxilubant Maleate (See also *146978-48-5*)

147403-03-0. Azilsartan

147432-77-7. Ontazolast

147497-64-1. Davasaicin

147511-69-1. Pitavastatin

147536-97-0. Bosentan [anhydrous] (See also *157212-55-0*)

147568-66-9. Carmoterol

147650-57-5. Terestigmine

147664-63-9. Pexiganan

147817-50-3. Siramesine

147859-97-0. Peforelin

148016-81-3. Doripenem

148031-34-9. Eptifibatide

148152-63-0. Napitane Mesylate [napitane] (See also *149189-73-1*)

148189-70-2. Votumumab

148363-16-0. Epoetin Omega

148396-36-5. Fradafiban

148408-65-5. Sunepitron Hydrochloride

148408-66-6. Docetaxel (See also *114977-28-5*)

148430-28-8. Sarakalim

148465-45-6. Crofelemer

148504-51-2. Ripisartan

148553-50-9. Pregabalin

148563-16-0. Levalbuterol Sulfate

148564-47-0. Milfasartan

148611-75-0. Mirisetron Maleate (See also *135905-89-4*)

148637-05-2. Cilmostim

148641-02-5. Muplestim

148717-54-8. Tecalcet Hydrochloride [tecalcet] (See also *177172-49-5*)

148717-90-2. Squalamine Lactate [squalamine] (See also *32072-47-1*)

148778-32-9. Pibrozelesin Hydrobromide

148883-56-1. Tifacogin

148905-78-6. Bexlosteride

148998-94-1. Trecovirsen Sodium [trecovirsen] (See also *170274-79-0*)

149042-61-5. Tirilazad Mesylate (See also *110101-66-1*)

149079-51-6. Cartasteine

149189-73-1. Napitane Mesylate (See also *148152-63-0*)

149210-33-3. Iobenguane Sulfate I 131

149394-66-1. Cidofovir (See also *113852-37-2*)

149394-67-2. Ledismase

149400-88-4. Sardomozide

149488-17-5. Trovirdine

149494-37-1. Ebalzotan

149503-79-7. Lefradafiban

149556-49-0. Susalimod

149606-27-9. Soblidotin

149647-78-9. Vorinostat

149682-77-9. Talabostat

149759-26-2. Pinokalant

149820-74-6. Xemilofiban Hydrochloride [xemilofiban] (See also *156586-91-3*)

149824-15-7. Ilodecakin

149838-23-3. Doranidazole

149845-06-7. Saquinavir Mesylate

149845-07-8. Tiludronate Disodium

149882-10-0. Lurtotecan Dihydrochloride [lurtotecan] (See also *155773-58-3*)

149888-94-8. Azimilide Dihydrochloride (See also *149908-53-2*)

149908-23-6. Erythromycin Salnacedin

149908-53-2. Azimilide Dihydrochloride [azimilide] (See also *149888-94-8*)

149920-56-9. Idraparinux Sodium

149926-91-0. Revatropate

149950-60-7. Emivirine

149951-16-6. Lenapenem

149979-74-8. Terbogrel

150080-09-4. Talabostat Mesylate

150322-43-3. Prasugrel Hydrochloride [prasugrel] (See also *389574-19-0*)

150332-35-7. Pamaqueside

150337-94-3. Ecalcidene

150375-75-0. Relcovaptan

150378-17-9. Indinavir [anhydrous] (See also *180683-37-8*)

150399-21-6. Balsalazide Disodium (See also *80573-04-2*)

150399-23-8. Pemetrexed Disodium (See also *137281-23-3*)

150408-73-4. Pranazepide

150443-71-3. Nicanartine

150490-84-9. Follitropin Beta [replaced] (See also *146479-72-3; 56832-30-5; 110909-60-9*)

150490-85-0. Berupipam

150501-62-5. Tedisamil Sesquifumarate

150586-58-6. Fipamezole

150587-07-8. Dexamethasone Beloxil

150631-27-9. Nacolomab Tafenatox

150683-30-0. Tolvaptan

150702-32-2. Fuladectin Component A_4

150702-33-3. Fuladectin Component A_3

150756-35-7. Efletirizine

150785-53-8. Alemcinal

150812-12-7. Retigabine

150915-40-5. Tirofiban Hydrochloride (See also *142373-60-2; 144494-65-5*)

150915-41-6. Perospirone

151006-18-7. Tenivastatin Calcium [anhydrous] (See also *121009-77-6*)

151096-09-2. Moxifloxacin

151126-32-8. Pramlintide

151140-96-4. Avitriptan Fumarate [avitriptan] (See also *171171-42-9*)

151159-23-8. Midaxifylline

151287-22-8. Tobicillin

151319-34-5. Zaleplon

151356-08-0. Afovirsen Sodium [afovirsen] (See also *138330-98-0*)

151533-22-1. Levomefolate Calcium

151581-23-6. Apaxifylline

151581-24-7. Iralukast

151763-64-3. Capromab Pendetide [capromab] (See also *145464-28-4*)

151767-02-1. Montelukast Sodium (See also *158966-92-8*)

151823-14-2. Sapacitabine

151878-23-8. Calcobutrol

151879-73-1. Aprinocarsen Sodium [for base substance]

151912-11-7. Amediplase

151912-42-4. Pamiteplase

152044-54-7. Patupilone

152074-97-0. Dirucotide

152317-89-0. Alniditan Dihydrochloride [alniditan] (See also *155428-00-5*)

152459-95-5. Imatinib

152520-56-4. Nebivolol Hydrochloride

152657-84-6. Nalfurafine Hydrochloride [nalfurafine] (See also *152658-17-8*)

152658-17-8. Nalfurafine Hydrochloride (See also *152657-84-6*)

152735-23-4. Upidosin

152811-62-6. Piboserod Hydrochloride [piboserod] (See also *178273-87-5*)

152854-19-8. Xanomeline Tartrate

152923-56-3. Daclizumab

152923-57-4. Lutropin Alfa (See also *56832-30-5; 53664-53-2*)

152939-42-9. Opanixil

152981-31-2. Inolimomab

153062-94-3. Pumosetrag

153101-26-9. Regavirumab

153168-05-9. Pleconaril

153205-46-0. Asimadoline

153242-02-5. Aseripide

153259-65-5. Cilomilast

153322-05-5. Lanicemine

153420-96-3. Atibeprone

153436-22-7. Gavestinel

153438-49-4. Dapitant

153439-40-8. Fexofenadine Hydrochloride (See also *138452-21-8; 83799-24-0*)

153504-70-2. Cevimeline Hydrochloride (See also *107233-08-9*)

153504-81-5. Licostinel

153507-46-1. Bibapcitide

153537-73-6. Plevitrexed

153559-49-0. Bexarotene

153804-05-8. Pratosartan

153808-85-6. Cadrofloxacin

153832-38-3. Ertapenem Sodium (See also *153832-46-3*)

153832-46-3. Ertapenem Sodium [ertapenem] (See also *153832-38-3*)

154039-60-8. Marimastat

154082-13-0. Omocianine

154189-24-9. Sibenadet Hydrochloride (See also *154189-40-0*)

154189-40-0. Sibenadet Hydrochloride [sibenadet] (See also *154189-24-9*)

154229-19-3. Abiraterone

154248-96-1. Iroplact

154248-97-2. Imiglucerase

154323-57-6. Almotriptan

154355-76-7. Atreleuton

154357-42-3. Levonadifloxacin

154361-48-5. Arcitumomab (See also *154361-49-6*)

154361-49-6. Arcitumomab [technetium Tc 99m arcitumomab] (See also *154361-48-5*)

154361-50-9. Capecitabine

154413-61-3. Ticolubant

154427-83-5. Samarium Sm 153 Lexidronam

154541-72-7. Alinastine

154598-52-4. Efavirenz

154612-39-2. Palinavir

154652-83-2. Tezampanel [anhydrous] (See also *317819-68-4*)

154702-15-5. Iscotrizinol

154725-65-2. Epoetin Epsilon

154738-42-8. Mitemcinal Fumarate [mitemcinal] (See also *154802-96-7*)

154802-96-7. Mitemcinal Fumarate (See also *154738-42-8*)

154889-68-6. Pibrozelesin

154906-40-8. Semparatide

155030-63-0. Emodepside

155141-29-0. Rosiglitazone Maleate (See also *122320-73-4*)

155206-00-1. Bimatoprost

155213-67-5. Ritonavir

155270-99-8. Istradefylline

155319-91-8. Mangafodipir

155415-08-0. Inogatran

155418-06-7. Nolpitantium Besilate

155428-00-5. Alniditan Dihydrochloride (See also *152317-89-0*)

155576-45-7. Tremacamra

155662-50-3. Droxinavir Hydrochloride (See also *159910-86-8*)

155773-56-1. Ferristene

155773-57-2. Pegorgotein

155773-58-3. Lurtotecan Dihydrochloride (See also *149882-10-0*)

155773-59-4. Ensaculin

155798-07-5. Ioflupane (^{123}I)

155974-00-8. Ivabradine

156001-18-2. Embusartan

156053-89-3. Alvimopan [anhydrous] (See also *170098-38-1*)

156090-17-4. Nortopixantrone

156090-18-5. Topixantrone

156131-91-8. Dimadectin

156137-99-4. Rapacuronium Bromide

156165-55-8. Enflufocon B

156227-98-4. Afelimomab

156294-36-9. Larotaxel

156436-89-4. Motexafin Gadolinium

156436-90-7. Motexafin Lutetium

156586-89-9. Edrecolomab

156586-90-2. Cedelizumab

156586-91-3. Xemilofiban Hydrochloride (See also *149820-74-6*)

156601-79-5. Nepaprazole

156616-23-8. Monteplase

156679-34-4. Lenercept

156712-35-5. Galdansetron Hydrochloride (See also *116684-92-5*)

156715-37-6. Ifetroban Sodium

156722-18-8. Rostafuroxin

156740-57-7. Axitirome

156769-21-0. Sanfetrinem Cilexetil [sanfetrinem] (See also *141646-08-4*)

156862-51-0. Belaperidone

156897-06-2. Licofelone

156965-06-9. Tisocalcitate

157182-23-5. Metesind Glucuronate (See also *138384-68-6*)

157182-32-6. Alatrofloxacin Mesylate [alatrofloxacin] (See also *157605-25-9*)

157212-55-0. Bosentan (See also *147536-97-0*)

157238-32-9. Cetermin

157283-68-6. Travoprost

157476-76-1. Technetium (^{99m}Tc) Pintumomab

157476-77-2. Lagatide

157605-25-9. Alatrofloxacin Mesylate (See also *157182-32-6*)

157716-52-4. Perifosine

157810-81-6. Indinavir Sulfate

158318-63-9. Bectumomab

158364-59-1. Pumaprazole

158382-37-7. Canfosfamide Hydrochloride [canfosfamide] (See also *439943-59-6*)

158440-71-2. Irofulven

158483-22-8. Balafilcon A

158682-68-9. Elisartan

158747-02-5. Frovatriptan

158751-64-5. Clamikalant

158827-34-0. Pralmorelin Dihydrochloride (See also *158861-67-7*)

158861-67-7. Pralmorelin Dihydrochloride [pralmorelin] (See also *158827-34-0*)
158876-82-5. Rupatadine
158930-17-7. Frovatriptan Succinate
158966-92-8. Montelukast Sodium [montelukast] (See also *151767-02-1*)
159073-29-7. Nelfilcon A
159075-60-2. Emfilermin
159098-79-0. Tilnoprofen Arbamel
159138-80-4. Cariporide
159138-81-5. Cariporide Mesylate (See also *159138-80-4*)
159351-69-6. Everolimus
159445-62-2. Orientiparcin (See also *111073-20-2; 112848-46-1*)
159445-63-3. Nateplase
159445-64-4. Odulimomab
159519-65-0. Enfuvirtide
159634-47-6. Ibutamoren Mesylate [ibutamoren] (See also *159752-10-0*)
159668-20-9. Napsagatran
159752-10-0. Ibutamoren Mesylate (See also *159634-47-6*)
159768-75-9. Labradimil
159776-67-7. Rizatriptan Sulfate (See also *144034-80-0*)
159776-68-8. Linetastine
159776-69-9. Cemadotin
159776-70-2. Melagatran
159811-51-5. Ulipristal
159910-86-8. Droxinavir Hydrochloride [droxinavir] (See also *155662-50-3*)
159912-53-5. Sabcomeline Hydrochloride [sabcomeline] (See also *159912-58-0*)
159912-58-0. Sabcomeline Hydrochloride (See also *159912-53-5*)
159989-64-7. Nelfinavir Mesylate [nelfinavir] (See also *159989-65-8*)
159989-65-8. Nelfinavir Mesylate (See also *159989-64-7*)
159997-94-1. Biricodar
160135-92-2. Gemopatrilat
160146-17-8. Finrozole
160337-95-1. Insulin Glargine
160369-77-7. Fomivirsen Sodium (See also *144245-52-3*)
160369-78-8. Samarium Sm 153 Lexidronam Pentasodium (See also *154427-83-5*)
160492-56-8. Osanetant
160677-67-8. Tresperimus
160707-69-7. Apricitabine
160970-54-7. Silodosin
161172-51-6. Etalocib
161178-07-0. Lubazodone Hydrochloride [lubazodone] (See also *161178-10-5*)
161178-10-5. Lubazodone Hydrochloride (See also *161178-07-0*)
161262-29-9. Amotosalen Hydrochloride (See also *161262-29-9*)
161417-03-4. Pozanicline
161600-01-7. Netoglitazone
161605-73-8. Fanapanel
161715-24-8. Tebipenem Pivoxil
161735-79-1. Rasagiline Mesylate (See also *136236-51-6*)

161753-30-6. Daniplestim
161796-78-7. Esomeprazole Sodium
161796-84-5. Esomeprazole Potassium
161814-49-9. Amprenavir
161832-65-1. Talampanel
161967-81-3. Grepafloxacin Hydrochloride (See also *119914-60-2*)
161982-62-3. Depreotide
162011-90-7. Rofecoxib
162301-05-5. Ecenofloxacin
162359-55-9. Fingolimod Hydrochloride [fingolimod] (See also *162359-56-0*)
162359-56-0. Fingolimod Hydrochloride (See also *162359-55-9*)
162394-19-6. Palifermin
162401-32-3. Roflumilast
162520-00-5. Salirasib
162635-04-3. Temsirolimus
162652-95-1. Vinflunine
162706-37-8. Elinafide
162774-06-3. Nerelimomab
162808-62-0. Caspofungin
163000-63-3. Neboglamine
163133-43-5. Naproxcinod
163217-09-2. Inecalcitol
163222-33-1. Ezetimibe
163250-90-6. Orbofiban Acetate [orbofiban] (See also *165800-05-5*)
163252-36-6. Clevudine
163253-35-8. Sitafloxacin (See also *127254-12-0*)
163521-12-8. Vilazodone
163545-26-4. Ancestim
163706-06-7. Cangrelor
163706-36-3. Cangrelor Tetrasodium
163796-60-9. Bifarcept
164150-99-6. Fandofloxacin
164178-54-5. Mazokalim
164579-32-2. Pantoprazole Sodium
164656-23-9. Dutasteride
165101-50-8. Alexomycin
165101-51-9. Becaplermin
165108-07-6. Selamectin
165253-33-8. Abafilcon A
165450-17-9. Neotame
165538-40-9. Terutroban
165668-41-7. Indisulam
165800-03-3. Linezolid
165800-04-4. Eperezolid
165800-05-5. Orbofiban Acetate (See also *163250-90-6*)
165800-06-6. Zoledronic Acid
165800-07-7. Zoledronate Disodium
165800-08-8. Zoledronate Trisodium
165942-79-0. Technetium Tc 99m Nofetumomab Merpentan
166089-32-3. Lintuzumab
166089-33-4. Nagrestipen
166181-63-1. Ipravacaine
166374-49-8. Naxifylline
166432-28-6. Clevidipine Butyrate [clevidipine] (See also *167221-71-8*)
166518-60-1. Avasimibe
166591-11-3. Adrogolide Hydrochloride
166663-25-8. Anidulafungin
167221-71-8. Clevidipine Butyrate (See also *166432-28-6*)
167256-08-8. Enrasentan

167305-00-2. Omapatrilat
167354-41-8. Zosuquidar Trihydrochloride [zosuquidar] (See also *167465-36-3*)
167362-48-3. Abetimus
167465-36-3. Zosuquidar Trihydrochloride (See also *167354-41-8*)
167747-19-5. Sulesomab
167747-20-8. Felvizumab
167816-91-3. Faralimomab
167887-97-0. Olamufloxacin
167933-07-5. Flibanserin
168021-79-2. Disufenton Sodium
168079-32-1. Lixivaptan
168146-84-7. Abacavir Succinate (See also *136470-78-5*)
168266-51-1. Vofopitant Dihydrochloride
168266-90-8. Vofopitant
168273-06-1. Rimonabant
168626-94-6. Conivaptan Hydrochloride
168682-53-9. Ezatiostat Hydrochloride [ezatiostat] (See also *286942-97-0*)
169147-32-4. Abetimus Sodium
169148-63-4. Insulin Detemir
169312-27-0. Talviraline
169543-49-1. Icrocaptide
169590-40-3. Flusilfocon E
169590-41-4. Deracoxib
169590-42-5. Celecoxib
169758-66-1. Robalzotan
169802-84-0. Enlimomab Pegol
169939-94-0. Ruboxistaurin
170098-38-1. Alvimopan (See also *156053-89-3*)
170105-16-5. Imidafenacin
170274-79-0. Trecovirsen Sodium (See also *148998-94-1*)
170277-31-3. Infliximab
170364-57-5. Enzastaurin Hydrochloride [enzastaurin] (See also *359017-79-1*)
170368-04-4. Anisperimus
170566-84-4. Lanepitant
170569-88-7. Mavacoxib
170632-47-0. Lificiguat
170729-80-3. Aprepitant
170787-99-2. Efaproxiral Sodium
170851-70-4. Ipamorelin
170858-33-0. Sonepiprazole
170858-34-1. Sonepiprazole Mesylate
170861-63-9. Reglitazar
170902-47-3. Roxifiban Acetate [roxifiban] (See also *176022-59-6*)
170912-52-4. Donitriptan
171047-47-5. Ladirubicin
171049-14-2. Lotrafiban Hydrochloride [lotrafiban] (See also *179599-82-7*)
171092-39-0. Defoslimod
171099-57-3. Oritavancin
171171-42-9. Avitriptan Fumarate (See also *151140-96-4*)
171176-43-5. Tezacitabine (See also *130306-02-4*)
171228-49-2. Posaconazole
171335-80-1. Exatecan
171500-79-1. Dalbavancin
171596-29-5. Tadalafil
171599-83-0. Sildenafil Citrate (See also *139755-83-2*)

171655-91-7. Brasofensine

171714-84-4. Darusentan

171752-56-0. Adrogolide

171870-23-8. Lanoteplase

172152-36-2. Ilaprazole

172673-20-0. Fosaprepitant Dimeglumine [fosaprepitant] (See also *265121-04-8*)

172732-68-2. Varespladib

172733-08-3. Varespladib Methyl

172733-42-5. Varespladib Sodium (See also *172732-68-2*)

172740-14-6. Posaraprost

172820-23-4. Pexiganan Acetate

172903-00-3. Triplatin Tetranitrate

172927-65-0. Sibrafiban

173146-27-5. Denileukin Diftitox

173240-15-9. Nemifitide Ditriflutate [nemifitide] (See also *204992-09-6*)

173324-94-2. Temiverine

173334-57-1. Aliskiren

173334-58-2. Aliskiren Fumarate

173424-77-6. Laromustine

173830-14-3. Brasofensine Maleate

173838-31-8. Telithromycin (See also *191114-48-4*)

173937-91-2. Atrasentan Hydrochloride [atrasentan] (See also *195733-43-8*)

173997-05-2. Nepicastat Hydrochloride [nepicastat] (See also *177645-08-8*)

174022-42-5. Bevirimat Dimeglumine [bevirimat] (See also *823821-85-8*)

174254-13-8. Biricodar Dicitrate

174391-92-5. Mozenavir

174402-32-5. Edotecarin

174484-41-4. Tipranavir

174636-32-9. Talnetant

174638-15-4. Fosfluridine Tidoxil

174722-30-6. Keliximab

174722-31-7. Rituximab

175013-73-7. Tidembersat

175013-84-0. Tonabersat

175385-62-3. Lasinavir

175414-77-4. Voreloxin

175481-36-4. Lacosamide

175591-23-8. Tapentadol

175615-45-9. Tazomeline Citrate (See also *131987-54-7*)

175865-59-5. Valganciclovir Hydrochloride (See also *175865-60-8*)

175865-60-8. Valganciclovir Hydrochloride [valganciclovir] (See also *175865-59-5*)

176022-59-6. Roxifiban Acetate (See also *170902-47-3*)

176161-24-3. Maribavir

176199-48-7. Eglumetad [anhydrous] (See also *209216-09-1*)

176644-21-6. Eniporide

176894-09-0. Omiloxetine

176975-26-1. Izonsteride

177036-94-1. Ambrisentan

177072-49-0. Gadoxanum

177073-44-8. Choriogonadotropin Alfa (See also *56832-30-5; 56832-34-9*)

177172-49-5. Tecalcet Hydrochloride (See also *148717-54-8*)

177469-96-4. Implitapide

177563-40-5. Carafiban

177645-08-8. Nepicastat Hydrochloride (See also *173997-05-2*)

177834-92-3. Eletriptan Hydrobromide

177975-08-5. Sarizotan Hydrochloride [sarizotan, replaced] (See also *195068-07-6; 351862-32-3*)

178040-94-3. Opaviraline

178273-87-5. Piboserod Hydrochloride (See also *152811-62-6*)

178307-42-1. Revaprazan Hydrochloride (See also *199463-33-7*)

178535-92-7. Abrineurin (See also *178535-93-8*)

178535-93-8. Abrineurin [monomer] (See also *178535-92-7*)

178600-17-4. Talibegron Hydrochloride (See also *146376-58-1*)

178823-49-9. Tiplimotide

178959-14-3. Technetium Tc 99m Apcitide

178979-85-6. Capravirine

179033-51-3. Timcodar

179045-86-4. Basiliximab

179067-42-6. Tafluposide

179120-92-4. Altinicline Maleate [altinicline] (See also *192231-16-6*)

179324-69-7. Bortezomib

179386-43-7. Sumanirole

179463-17-3. Caspofungin Acetate

179472-53-8. Evans Blue [replaced] (See also *314-13-6*)

179474-81-8. Prucalopride

179545-77-8. Tanomastat

179599-82-7. Lotrafiban Hydrochloride (See also *171049-14-2*)

179602-65-4. Mitratapide

179756-85-5. Eptapirone

180200-66-2. Gatifloxacin

180200-68-4. Tilmacoxib

180288-69-1. Trastuzumab

180384-56-9. Clazosentan

180384-57-0. Tezosentan

180683-37-8. Indinavir (See also *150378-17-9*)

180694-97-7. Mimopezil

180898-37-7. Bisdisulizole Disodium

180916-16-9. Lasofoxifene

180918-68-7. Trecetilide

181054-95-5. Nonacog Alfa

181183-52-8. Almotriptan Malate

181296-84-4. Omigapil

181477-43-0. Disomotide

181477-91-8. Ovemotide

181630-15-9. Picoplatin

181695-72-7. Valdecoxib

181785-84-2. Elvucitabine

181816-48-8. Ombrabulin

181872-90-2. Iosimenol

182133-25-1. Arzoxifene

182133-27-3. Arzoxifene Hydrochloride

182167-02-8. Acolbifene Hydrochloride [acolbifene] (See also *252555-01-4*)

182212-66-4. Avotermin

182316-31-0. Ataquimast

182415-09-4. Piclozotan

182683-00-7. Sevelamer Hydrochloride (See also *52757-95-6*)

182760-06-1. Ravuconazole

182815-43-6. Colesevelam Hydrochloride [colesevelam] (See also *182815-44-7*)

182815-44-7. Colesevelam Hydrochloride (See also *182815-43-6*)

182821-27-8. Daglutril

182824-33-5. Artesunate (See also *88495-63-0*)

183063-72-1. Atiprimod Dimaleate

183133-96-2. Cabazitaxel

183293-82-5. Gemcabene Calcium [gemcabene] (See also *209789-08-2*)

183305-24-0. Fidexaban

183313-30-6. Timcodar Dimesylate

183319-69-9. Erlotinib Hydrochloride (See also *183321-74-6*)

183321-74-6. Erlotinib Hydrochloride [erlotinib] (See also *183319-69-9*)

183325-78-2. Calfactant

183547-57-1. Gantofiban

183552-38-7. Abarelix

183659-72-5. Catramilast

183747-35-5. Nepadutant

183849-43-6. Abaperidone

183990-46-7. Salcaprozic Acid

184036-34-8. Sitaxentan

184159-40-8. Sulamserod Hydrochloride (See also *219757-90-1*)

184475-35-2. Gefitinib

184653-84-7. Carabersat

185055-67-8. Ferroquine

185106-16-5. Acotiamide Hydrochloride [acotiamide] (See also *773092-05-0*)

185229-68-9. Alicaforsen Sodium [alicaforsen] (See also *331257-52-4*)

185243-69-0. Etanercept

185428-18-6. Rivoglitazone

185517-21-9. Arundic Acid

185913-78-4. Satavaptan

185954-27-2. Tofimilast

185954-98-7. Eritoran Tetrasodium (See also *185955-34-4*)

185955-34-4. Eritoran Tetrasodium [eritoran] (See also *185954-98-7*)

186018-45-1. Metreleptin

186040-50-6. Paclitaxel Ceribate

186139-09-3. Trodusquemine

186348-23-2. Ortataxel

186392-65-4. Ingliforib

186495-49-8. Delucemine Hydrochloride [delucemine] (See also *186495-99-8*)

186495-99-8. Delucemine Hydrochloride (See also *186495-49-8*)

186497-07-4. Zibotentan

186638-10-8. Pegmusirudin

186692-46-6. Seliciclib

186826-86-8. Moxifloxacin Hydrochloride

186953-56-0. Pafuramidine Maleate [pafuramidine] (See also *837369-26-3*)

187139-68-0. Pegacaristim

187164-19-8. Luliconazole

187219-99-4. Axomadol

187269-40-5. Bimosiamose

187269-60-9. Bimosiamose Disodium

187348-17-0. Edodekin Alfa

187393-00-6. Bemotrizinol

187523-35-9. Flindokalner
187602-11-5. Sofigatran
187852-63-7. Delimotecan [for Na salt]
187865-22-1. Derquantel
187870-78-6. Rimeporide
187949-02-6. Albaconazole
188039-54-5. Palivizumab
188062-50-2. Abacavir Sulfate
188063-80-1. Hilafilcon A
188106-30-1. Semparatide Acetate
188116-07-6. Imepition
188181-42-2. Elacytarabine
188196-22-7. Frakefamide
188396-77-2. Paliroden
188630-14-0. Liatermin
188696-80-2. Becampanel
188913-58-8. Dersalazine
188968-51-6. Cilengitide
189003-92-7. Trelanserin
189032-40-4. Nesiritide Citrate
189047-99-2. Ferumoxtran-10
189059-71-0. Lapaquistat Acetate [lapa-
    quistat] (See also *189060-13-7*)
189060-13-7. Lapaquistat Acetate (See
    also *189059-71-0*)
189188-57-6. Tegaserod Maleate
189198-30-9. Pactimibe
189261-10-7. Natalizumab
189279-58-1. Delafloxacin
189353-31-9. Fadolmidine
189353-32-0. Fadolmidine Hydrochloride
189385-65-7. Hexafocon A
189681-70-7. Aplindore Fumarate [aplin-
    dore] (See also *189681-71-8*)
189681-71-8. Aplindore Fumarate (See
    also *189681-70-7*)
189691-06-3. Bremelanotide
189752-49-6. Motexafin
189894-57-3. Traxoprodil Mesylate (See
    also *134234-12-1*)
189940-24-7. Daxalipram
189950-11-6. Tropantiol
189954-96-9. Firocoxib
190133-94-9. Ecopipam Hydrochloride
190258-12-9. Edronocaine
190648-49-8. Cipemastat
190791-29-8. Lasofoxifene Tartrate
190977-41-4. Oblimersen Sodium
191114-48-4. Telithromycin (See also
    173838-31-8)
191150-83-1. Tipranavir Disodium
191217-81-9. Pramipexole Dihydrochlor-
    ide
191349-60-7. Trecetilide Fumarate
191588-94-0. Tenecteplase
191732-72-6. Lenalidomide
192056-77-2. Zoticasone
192185-72-1. Tipifarnib
192230-36-7. Hemoglobin Glutamer-250
    (Bovine)
192230-37-8. Hemoglobin Glutamer-200
    (Bovine)
192231-16-6. Altinicline Maleate (See
    also *179120-92-4*)
192314-93-5. Iclaprim
192329-42-3. Prinomastat
192374-14-4. Radafaxine Hydrochloride
    [radafaxine] (See also *106083-71-0*)

192391-48-3. Tositumomab
192441-08-0. Lomeguatrib
192564-13-9. Leteprinim Potassium
192564-14-0. Oritavancin Diphosphate
192658-64-3. Tasidotin Hydrochloride [ta-
    sidotin] (See also *623174-20-9*)
192725-17-0. Lopinavir
192755-52-5. Pralnacasan
192939-46-1. Ximelagatran
193079-69-5. Tabimorelin
193153-04-7. Otamixaban
193273-66-4. Capromorelin Tartrate [ca-
    promorelin] (See also *193273-69-7*)
193273-69-7. Capromorelin Tartrate (See
    also *193273-66-4*)
193275-84-2. Lonafarnib
193681-12-8. Alamifovir
193700-51-5. Leridistim
193811-33-5. Tacapenem
193901-90-5. Gadofosveset Trisodium
    [anhydrous] (See also *211570-55-7*)
193901-91-6. Fosveset
194085-75-1. Carisbamate
194100-83-9. Thyrotropin Alfa
194413-58-6. Semaxanib
194468-36-5. Vinflunine Ditartrate (See
    also *162652-95-1*)
194785-19-8. Bedoradrine Sulfate [bed-
    oradrine] (See also *194785-31-4*)
194785-31-4. Bedoradrine Sulfate (See
    also *194785-19-8*)
194798-83-9. Fosfluconazole
194804-75-6. Garenoxacin Mesylate [gar-
    enoxacin] (See also *223652-90-2*)
195068-07-6. Sarizotan Hydrochloride
    (See also *351862-32-3; 177975-08-5*)
195156-77-5. Valomaciclovir Stearate
195157-34-7. Valomaciclovir
195158-85-1. Vepalimomab
195189-17-4. Minretumomab
195532-12-8. Pradofloxacin
195533-53-0. Batabulin
195533-98-3. Batabulin Sodium (See also
    195533-53-0)
195733-43-8. Atrasentan Hydrochloride
    (See also *173937-91-2*)
195875-84-4. Tesofensine
195883-06-8. Omtriptolide Sodium [om-
    triptolide] (See also *195883-09-1*)
195883-09-1. Omtriptolide Sodium (See
    also *195883-06-8*)
195962-23-3. Corifollitropin Alfa
196078-29-2. Mepolizumab
196078-30-5. Pramlintide Acetate
196488-72-9. Ranpirnase
196597-26-9. Ramelteon
196612-93-8. Falnidamol
196618-13-0. Oseltamivir
196808-45-4. Farglitazar
197099-66-4. Rovelizumab
197462-97-8. Hemoglobin Raffimer
197502-82-2. Parecoxib Sodium
197509-46-9. Laniquidar
197720-53-9. Exatecan Mesylate
197904-84-0. Apricoxib
198022-65-0. Icofungipen
198153-51-4. Peginterferon Alfa-2a

198283-73-7. Tebanicline Tosylate [teba-
    nicline] (See also *198283-74-8*)
198283-74-8. Tebanicline Tosylate (See
    also *198283-73-7*)
198470-84-7. Parecoxib
198480-55-6. Pipendoxifene
198481-32-2. Bazedoxifene Acetate [ba-
    zedoxifene] (See also *198481-33-3*)
198481-33-3. Bazedoxifene Acetate (See
    also *198481-32-2*)
198821-22-6. Merimepodib
198832-38-1. Isatoribine (See also
    122970-40-5)
198904-31-3. Atazanavir Sulfate [atazana-
    vir] (See also *229975-97-7*)
198958-88-2. Elarofiban [anhydrous] (See
    also *221005-96-5*)
199113-98-9. Balaglitazone
199191-69-0. Ziprasidone Mesylate
199331-40-3. Etiprednol Dicloacetate
199396-76-4. Asoprisnil
199463-33-7. Revaprazan Hydrochloride
    [revaprazan] (See also *178307-42-1*)
199685-57-9. Onercept
199739-10-1. Paliperidone Palmitate
199798-84-0. Elocalcitol
200074-80-2. Lusupultide
200815-49-2. Arformoterol Tartrate (See
    also *67346-49-0*)
201034-75-5. Daporinad
201410-53-9. Talarozole
201530-41-8. Deferasirox
201605-51-8. Itriglumide
201677-61-4. Sivelestat Sodium
202057-76-9. Manitimus
202138-50-9. Tenofovir Disoproxil Fuma-
    rate
202189-78-4. Bilastine
202340-45-2. Eflucimibe
202409-33-4. Etoricoxib
202590-69-0. Ticalopride
202833-07-6. Morolimumab
202833-08-7. Atorolimumab
202844-10-8. Indantadol
203170-33-3. Lotrafilcon A
203258-60-0. Brostallicin
203737-93-3. Istaroxime
203787-91-1. Salcaprozate Sodium
203923-89-1. Cositecan
204200-47-5. Coleneuramide
204205-90-3. Indibulin
204248-78-2. Omiganan Pentahydrochlor-
    ide [omiganan] (See also *269062-93-
    3*)
204255-11-8. Oseltamivir Phosphate
204267-33-4. Feloprentan
204318-14-9. Edotreotide
204512-90-3. Tecadenoson
204519-64-2. Gemifloxacin
204519-65-3. Gemifloxacin Mesylate
204519-66-4. Talnetant Hydrochloride
204565-76-4. Pegnartograstim
204656-20-2. Liraglutide
204658-47-9. Torapsel
204697-65-4. Olcegepant
204992-09-6. Nemifitide Ditriflutate (See
    also *173240-15-9*)
205110-48-1. Cethromycin

205887-54-3. Telbermin
205923-56-4. Cetuximab
205923-57-5. Epratuzumab
206181-63-7. Ibritumomab Tiuxetan
206254-79-7. Opebacan
206260-33-5. Irampanel
206361-99-1. Darunavir
206873-63-4. Tariquidar
206884-98-2. Niraxostat
207137-56-2. Binetrakin
207623-20-9. Agatolimod
207748-29-6. Insulin Glulisine
207916-33-4. Xidecaflur
207993-12-2. Pumafentrine
208110-64-9. Befiradol
208265-92-3. Pegfilgrastim
208538-73-2. Micafungin Sodium (See also *235114-32-6*)
208576-22-1. Epafipase
208848-19-5. Freselestat
208992-74-9. Fiduxosin Hydrochloride
208993-54-8. Fiduxosin
209216-09-1. Eglumetad (See also *176199-48-7*)
209216-23-9. Entecavir (See also *142217-69-4*)
209342-40-5. Finafloxacin
209394-27-4. Ladostigil Tartrate [ladostigil] (See also *209394-46-7*)
209394-46-7. Ladostigil Tartrate (See also *209394-27-4*)
209467-52-7. Ceftobiprole
209733-45-9. Anatibant
209783-80-2. Entinostat
209789-08-2. Gemcabene Calcium (See also *183293-82-5*)
209799-67-7. Forodesine
209810-58-2. Darbepoetin Alfa
209859-87-0. Cilansetron Hydrochloride (See also *120635-74-7*)
209860-87-7. Tafluprost
210101-16-9. Conivaptan
210245-80-0. Zonampanel [anhydrous]
210419-36-6. Opratonium Iodide
210538-44-6. Taprizosin
210584-54-6. Amustaline Dihydrochloride
210589-09-6. Laronidase
210891-04-6. Edonentan [anhydrous] (See also *264609-13-4*)
211100-13-9. Sabarubicin
211110-63-3. Sobetirome
211254-73-8. Lonaprisan
211323-03-4. Erlizumab
211427-08-6. Diquafosol Tetrasodium (See also *59985-21-6*)
211439-12-2. Davunetide
211448-85-0. Denufosol Tetrasodium [denufosol] (See also *318250-11-2*)
211513-37-0. Dalcetrapib
211570-55-7. Gadofosveset Trisodium (See also *193901-90-5*)
211735-76-1. Farampator
211914-51-1. Dabigatran
211915-06-9. Dabigatran Etexilate
212115-71-4. Trinecol (pullus)
212141-54-3. Vatalanib
213027-19-1. Cipralisant

213327-37-8. Oregovomab
213411-83-7. Edaglitazone Sodium [edaglitazone] (See also *369631-81-2*)
213819-48-8. Belotecan Hydrochloride (See also *256411-32-2*)
213998-46-0. Gantacurium Chloride
214462-68-7. Tridolgosir Hydrochloride (See also *72741-87-8*)
214548-46-6. Lusaperidone
214559-60-1. Bivatuzumab
214745-43-4. Efalizumab
214766-78-6. Degarelix
215174-50-8. Rimacalib
215529-47-8. Bamirastine
215604-75-4. Afeletecan
215647-85-1. Peginterferon Alfa-2b
215808-49-4. Lemuteporfin
216167-82-7. Succinobucol
216167-92-9. Camobucol
216167-95-2. Elsibucol
216503-57-0. Alemtuzumab
216503-58-1. Mitumomab
216669-97-5. Sibrotuzumab
216974-75-3. Bevacizumab
217087-09-7. Esomeprazole Magnesium
217500-96-4. Tulathromycin (component A) (See also *280755-12-6*)
217797-14-3. Paroxetine Mesylate
218282-71-4. Olanexidine Hydrochloride
218298-21-6. Razaxaban Hydrochloride [razaxaban] (See also *405940-76-3*)
218791-21-0. Imisopasem Manganese
218949-48-5. Tesamorelin
219311-43-0. Dabuzalgron Hydrochloride (See also *219311-44-1*)
219311-44-1. Dabuzalgron Hydrochloride [dabuzalgron] (See also *219311-43-0*)
219527-63-6. Repifermin
219581-36-9. Alvameline Maleate (See also *120241-31-8*)
219649-07-7. Labetuzumab
219680-11-2. Zabofloxacin
219685-50-4. Eculizumab
219685-93-5. Pexelizumab
219716-33-3. Visilizumab
219757-90-1. Sulamserod Hydrochloride [sulamserod] (See also *184159-40-8*)
219810-59-0. Neramexane Mesylate [neramexane] (See also *457068-92-7*)
219846-31-8. Resequinil
219861-08-2. Escitalopram Oxalate
219923-85-0. Pramiconazole
219989-84-1. Ixabepilone
220201-34-3. Talaporfin Sodium (See also *110230-98-3*)
220322-05-4. Elzasonan Hydrochloride
220578-59-6. Gemtuzumab Ozogamicin
220620-09-7. Tigecycline
220641-11-2. Naminidil
220651-94-5. Ruplizumab
220712-29-8. Tadekinig Alfa
220847-86-9. Valategrast Hydrochloride [valategrast] (See also *828271-96-1*)
220984-26-9. Detiviciclovir
220991-20-8. Lumiracoxib
220991-32-2. Robenacoxib
220997-97-7. Diflomotecan

220998-10-7. Elomotecan
221005-96-5. Elarofiban (See also *198958-88-2*)
221019-25-6. Crobenetine
221241-63-0. Fandosentan Potassium [fandosentan] (See also *221246-12-4*)
221246-12-4. Fandosentan Potassium (See also *221241-63-0*)
221373-18-8. Olanzapine Pamoate
221877-54-9. Zotarolimus
222030-63-9. Fosbretabulin Disodium
222400-20-6. Tomopenem
222535-22-0. Alefacept
222551-17-9. Adoprazine
222716-86-1. Pegaptanib Sodium
222732-94-7. Asoprisnil Ecamate
222834-30-2. Ragaglitazar
223132-37-4. Inolitazone
223420-20-0. Cipralisant Maleate
223537-30-2. Rupintrivir
223577-45-5. Aviscumine
223652-90-2. Garenoxacin Mesylate (See also *194804-75-6*)
223661-25-4. Bulaquine
223673-61-8. Mirabegron
224452-66-8. Retapamulin
224785-90-4. Vardenafil
224789-15-5. Vardenafil Dihydrochloride
225239-31-6. Technetium Tc 99m Fanolesomab
225367-66-8. Efletirizine Dihydrochloride
226072-63-5. Solimastat
226256-56-0. Cinacalcet
226700-79-4. Fosamprenavir Sodium [fosamprenavir] (See also *226700-80-7*)
226700-80-7. Fosamprenavir Sodium (See also *226700-79-4*)
226700-81-8. Fosamprenavir Calcium
226954-04-7. Emapunil
227318-71-0. Epetirimod
227318-75-4. Sotirimod
227622-74-4. Gadomelitol
227940-00-3. Adekalant
228266-40-8. Taltobulin
229305-39-9. Golotimod
229614-55-5. Peramivir (monohydrate)
229975-97-7. Atazanavir Sulfate (See also *198904-31-3*)
230949-16-3. Esoxybutynin Chloride (See also *119618-22-3*)
231277-92-2. Lapatinib Ditosylate [lapatinib] (See also *388082-78-8*)
233254-24-5. Tomeglovir
234096-34-5. Cefovecin Sodium [cefovecin] (See also *141195-77-9*)
235114-32-6. Micafungin Sodium [micafungin] (See also *208538-73-2*)
235428-87-2. Taplitumomab Paptox
237068-57-4. Oglufanide Disodium (See also *38101-59-6*)
238750-77-1. Tosedostat
239101-33-8. Deferitrin
241473-69-8. Reslizumab
241479-67-4. Isavuconazole
241800-98-6. Zoniporide Mesylate [zoniporide] (See also *249296-45-5*)
242138-07-4. Omalizumab
242148-62-5. Hofocon A

242478-37-1. Solifenacin Succinate [solifenacin] (See also *242478-38-2*)
242478-38-2. Solifenacin Succinate (See also *242478-37-1*)
243835-65-6. Lamifiban Hydrochloride
243984-11-4. Resatorvid
244015-05-2. Iseganan Hydrochloride (See also *257277-05-7*)
244081-42-3. Rafabegron
244096-20-6. Gavilimomab
244130-01-6. Mirostipen
244767-67-7. Dapivirine
245116-90-9. Lidorestat [anhydrous]
245765-41-7. Ozenoxacin
246527-99-1. Mureletecan
246539-15-1. Dibotermin Alfa
246861-96-1. Garnocestim
247046-52-2. Dilopetine
247207-64-3. Leconotide
247257-48-3. Fimasartan
248281-84-7. Laquinimod Sodium [laquinimod] (See also *248282-07-7*)
248282-01-1. Paquinimod
248282-07-7. Laquinimod Sodium (See also *248281-84-7*)
248919-64-4. Linaprazan
249296-44-4. Varenicline Tartrate [varenicline] (See also *375815-87-5*)
249296-45-5. Zoniporide Mesylate [anhydrous] (See also *241800-98-6*)
250242-54-7. Lemalesomab
250386-15-3. Apadenoson
250601-04-8. Imiglitazar
250694-07-6. Teglicar
250710-65-7. Adargileukin Alfa
251303-04-5. Ertiprotafib
251562-00-2. Tifuvirtide
251565-85-2. Tesaglitazar
252188-71-9. Ceftobiprole Medocaril (See also *376653-43-9*)
252260-06-3. Posizolid
252555-01-4. Acolbifene Hydrochloride (See also *182167-02-8*)
252662-47-8. Toralizumab
252870-53-4. Ispronicline
252920-94-8. Solabegron Hydrochloride [solabegron] (See also *451470-34-1*)
253128-41-5. Eribulin Mesylate [eribulin] (See also *441045-17-6*)
253450-09-8. Besonprodil
254750-02-2. Emricasan
254877-67-3. Ataciguat
254964-60-8. Tasquinimod
255730-18-8. Artemisone
255734-04-4. Ritobegron
256382-08-8. Rivenprost
256411-32-2. Belotecan Hydrochloride [belotecan] (See also *213819-48-8*)
257277-05-7. Iseganan Hydrochloride [iseganan] (See also *244015-05-2*)
257933-82-7. Pelitinib
258516-87-9. Fospropofol Disodium (See also *258516-89-1*)
258516-89-1. Fospropofol Disodium [fospropofol] (See also *258516-87-9*)
258818-34-7. Larazotide
259074-76-5. Alfimeprase
259188-38-0. Rebimastat

259525-01-4. Enecadin
259793-96-9. Favipiravir
260980-89-0. Topilutamide
261356-80-3. Epoetin Delta
261944-46-1. Soraprazan
262352-17-0. Torcetrapib
263351-82-2. Paclitaxel Poliglumex
263547-71-3. Epitumomab Cituxetan
263562-28-3. Barixibat
264609-13-4. Edonentan (See also *210891-04-6*)
265114-23-6. Cimicoxib
265121-04-8. Fosaprepitant Dimeglumine (See also *172673-20-0*)
266359-83-5. Reparixin
267227-08-7. Apolizumab
267243-28-7. Canertinib Dihydrochloride [canertinib] (See also *289499-45-2*)
267639-76-9. Romiplostim
268203-93-6. Udenafil
269055-15-4. Etravirine
269062-93-3. Omiganan Pentahydrochloride (See also *204248-78-2*)
269079-62-1. Isalmadol
269718-83-4. Pardoprunox Hydrochloride
269718-84-5. Pardoprunox
272105-42-7. Disitertide
272780-74-2. Metelimumab
274679-00-4. Padoporfin
274693-27-5. Ticagrelor
274901-16-5. Vildagliptin
274925-86-9. Nebicapone
275371-94-3. Taspoglutide
276690-58-5. Iroxanadine
279215-43-9. Tifenazoxide
279253-83-7. Vapitadine Dihydrochloride (See also *793655-64-8*)
280585-34-4. Oxeglitazar
280755-12-6. Tulathromycin (component B) (See also *217500-96-4*)
280776-87-6. Gadocoletic Acid
280782-97-0. Managlinat Dialanetil
282526-98-1. Cetilistat
284019-34-7. Denibulin Hydrochloride [denibulin] (See also *779356-64-8*)
284041-10-7. Rostaporfin
284461-73-0. Sorafenib
284490-13-7. Forodesine Hydrochloride (See also *209799-67-7*)
285571-64-4. Barusiban
285983-48-4. Doramapimod
285985-06-0. Lerdelimumab
286930-03-8. Fesoterodine Fumarate
286942-97-0. Ezatiostat Hydrochloride (See also *168682-53-9*)
287096-87-1. Delmitide Acetate [delmitide] (See also *501019-16-5*)
287405-51-0. Apratastat
287714-30-1. Teduglutide
287714-41-4. Rosuvastatin Calcium [rosuvastatin] (See also *147098-20-2*)
288104-79-0. Surinabant
288383-20-0. Cediranib
288392-69-8. Siplizumab
289499-45-2. Canertinib Dihydrochloride (See also *267243-28-7*)
289656-45-7. Senicapoc
289893-25-0. Arimoclomol

290296-68-3. Befetupitant
290297-26-6. Netupitant
290815-26-8. Avosentan
292618-32-7. Gimatecan
292634-27-6. Dianicline
292819-64-8. Ecromeximab
293736-67-1. Berubicin Hydrochloride (See also *677017-23-1*)
295350-45-7. Ozarelix
295371-00-5. Verpasep Caltespen
296251-72-4. Velimogene Aliplasmid
299423-37-3. Teneliximab
300832-84-2. Ciluprevir
302904-82-1. Atocalcitol
304853-42-7. Tanaproget
305391-49-5. Ardenermin
305841-29-6. Sagopilone
306296-47-9. Vicriviroc Maleate [vicriviroc] (See also *599179-03-0*)
308240-58-6. Talactoferrin Alfa
308831-61-0. Sufugolix
309913-83-5. Talmapimod
311330-20-8. Onsifocon A
312753-06-3. Indacaterol
313348-27-5. Regadenoson [anhydrous] (See also *875148-45-1*)
313682-08-5. Brecanavir
317819-68-4. Tezampanel (See also *154652-83-2*)
318250-11-2. Denufosol Tetrasodium (See also *211448-85-0*)
318498-76-9. Flopristin
319460-85-0. Axitinib
320345-99-1. Aclidinium Bromide
320367-13-3. Lixisenatide
321915-31-5. Litomeglovir
324758-66-9. Sabiporide
325715-02-4. Indiplon
325965-23-9. Linopristin
326859-36-3. Fontolizumab
327026-93-7. Lensiprazine
328538-04-1. Edifoligide Sodium [for the base substance]
328898-40-4. Tildipirosin
329306-27-6. Lirimilast
329744-44-7. Embeconazole
329773-35-5. Cinaciguat
330784-47-9. Avanafil
330942-05-7. Betrixaban
330988-75-5. Pegsunercept
331243-22-2. Pascolizumab
331257-52-4. Alicaforsen Sodium (See also *185229-68-9*)
331731-18-1. Adalimumab
331741-94-7. Muraglitazar [free acid]
331744-64-0. Peliglitazar
332012-40-5. Telatinib
332348-12-6. Abatacept
333754-36-2. Tesetaxel
333963-42-1. Cobiprostone
334476-46-9. Vestipitant Mesylate [vestipitant] (See also *334476-64-1*)
334476-64-1. Vestipitant Mesylate (See also *334476-46-9*)
335619-18-6. Inakalant
336113-53-2. Ispinesib Mesylate [ispinesib] (See also *514820-03-2*)
336128-48-4. Senlizumab

336801-86-6. Vapaliximab

337376-15-5. Icodextrin

338990-84-4. Isavuconazonium Chloride

338992-00-0. Vandetanib [replaced] (See also *443913-73-3*)

339086-80-5. Tadocizumab

339177-26-3. Panitumumab

339186-68-4. Matuzumab

339986-90-2. Tucotuzumab Celmoleukin

341028-37-3. Alagebrium Chloride

341031-54-7. Sunitinib Malate (See also *557795-19-4*)

341524-89-8. Fispemifene

342026-92-0. Sipoglitazar

342577-38-2. Velneperit

343306-71-8. Sugammadex Sodium [sugammadex] (See also *343306-79-6*)

343306-79-6. Sugammadex Sodium (See also *343306-71-8*)

345663-45-8. Parathyroid Hormone [human recombinant] (See also *68893-82-3; 9002-64-6*)

346735-24-8. Amelubant

347396-82-1. Ranibizumab

348119-84-6. Obinepitide

350992-10-8. Bifeprunox

350992-13-1. Bifeprunox Mesylate

351862-32-3. Sarizotan Hydrochloride [sarizotan] (See also *195068-07-6; 177975-08-5*)

352458-37-8. Delafloxacin Meglumine

352513-83-8. Semapimod

354813-19-7. Balicatib

355129-15-6. Eprotirome

355151-12-1. Rotigaptide

356057-34-6. Darapladib

356068-94-5. Toceranib

356547-88-1. Belimumab

357336-20-0. Brivaracetam

357336-74-4. Seletracetam

357613-77-5. Galiximab

357613-86-6. Gomiliximab

358970-97-5. Drinabant

359017-79-1. Enzastaurin Hydrochloride (See also *170364-57-5*)

359689-54-6. Valtorcitabine Dihydrochloride (See also *380886-95-3*)

359875-09-5. Maropitant Citrate (See also *147116-67-4*)

361343-19-3. Elzasonan Citrate [elzasonan] (See also *361343-20-6*)

361343-20-6. Elzasonan Citrate (See also *361343-19-3*)

361442-04-8. Saxagliptin [anhydrous] (See also *945667-22-1*)

362505-84-8. Relacatib

362665-56-3. Tiprolisant

364782-34-3. Cinacalcet Hydrochloride (See also *226256-56-0*)

366017-09-6. Mubritinib

366789-02-8. Rivaroxaban

367514-87-2. Lurasidone Hydrochloride [lurasidone] (See also *367514-88-3*)

367514-88-3. Lurasidone Hydrochloride (See also *367514-87-2*)

369631-81-2. Edaglitazone Sodium (See also *213411-83-7*)

370893-06-4. Ancriviroc

371918-44-4. Latidectin [component A.i4] (See also *371918-51-3*)

371918-51-3. Latidectin [component A_3] (See also *371918-44-4*)

372075-36-0. Cintredekin Besudotox

372075-37-1. Sontuzumab

372151-71-8. Telavancin Hydrochloride [telavancin] (See also *560130-42-9*)

375348-49-5. Bertilimumab

375815-87-5. Varenicline Tartrate (See also *249296-44-4*)

375823-41-9. Tocilizumab

376348-65-1. Maraviroc

376592-42-6. Totrombopag Choline [totrombopag] (See also *851606-62-7*)

376653-43-9. Ceftobiprole Medocaril (See also *252188-71-9*)

377727-87-2. Preladenant

378746-64-6. Nemonoxacin

379231-04-6. Saracatinib

380610-22-0. Talizumab

380610-27-5. Pertuzumab

380843-75-4. Bosutinib

380886-95-3. Valtorcitabine Dihydrochloride [valtorcitabine] (See also *359689-54-6*)

380917-97-5. Perampanel

381683-92-7. Ecopladib

381683-94-9. Efipladib

386750-22-7. Desvenlafaxine Succinate (See also *93413-62-8*)

387825-03-8. Salclobuzic Acid

387825-07-2. Salclobuzate Sodium

387867-13-2. Tandutinib

388082-78-8. Lapatinib Ditosylate (See also *231277-92-2*)

389574-19-0. Prasugrel Hydrochloride (See also *150322-43-3*)

393101-41-2. Milataxel

393105-53-8. Tiplasinin

394730-60-0. Boceprevir

395639-53-9. Aselizumab

396091-73-9. Pasireotide

397864-44-7. Fluticasone Furoate

398507-55-6. Lodenafil Carbonate

400010-39-1. Cantuzumab Mertansine

400046-53-9. Ozogamicin

401925-43-7. Celivarone

402567-16-2. Firategrast

402595-29-3. Etriciguat

402710-25-2. Canakinumab [variable heavy γ1 chain] (See also *402710-27-4*)

402710-27-4. Canakinumab [variable light κ chain] (See also *402710-25-2*)

402957-28-2. Telaprevir

403483-39-6. Hybufocon A

403483-42-1. Acofilcon A

403604-85-3. Nebentan

404950-80-7. Panobinostat

404951-53-7. Dacinostat

405159-59-3. Idrabiotaparinux Sodium

405165-61-9. Besifloxacin Hydrochloride (See also *141388-76-3*)

405169-16-6. Dovitinib

405341-12-0. Rinfabate

405940-76-3. Razaxaban Hydrochloride (See also *218298-21-6*)

408504-26-7. Sergliflozin Etabonate

410528-02-8. Palovarotene

412950-08-4. Rilapladib

412950-27-7. Goxalapladib

414864-00-9. Belinostat

414910-27-3. Casopitant Mesylate [casopitant] (See also *414910-30-8*)

414910-30-8. Casopitant Mesylate (See also *414910-27-3*)

420794-05-0. Alglucosidase Alfa

425386-60-3. Semagacestat

425637-18-9. Sotrastaurin Acetate [sotrastaurin] (See also *908351-31-5*)

428863-50-7. Certolizumab Pegol

433265-65-7. Faxeladol

433282-68-9. Lecozotan Hydrochloride (See also *434283-16-6*)

433922-67-9. Edratide

434283-16-6. Lecozotan Hydrochloride [lecozotan] (See also *433282-68-9*)

437981-77-6. Lontucirev (Replicating Adenovirus)

439687-69-1. Nelivaptan

439943-59-6. Canfosfamide Hydrochloride (See also *158382-37-7*)

441045-17-6. Eribulin Mesylate (See also *253128-41-5*)

441765-97-5. Talaglumetad Hydrochloride (See also *441765-98-6*)

441765-98-6. Talaglumetad Hydrochloride [talaglumetad] (See also *441765-97-5*)

441798-33-0. Macitentan

442201-24-3. Remogliflozin Etabonate

443144-26-1. Pruvanserin

443144-27-2. Pruvanserin Hydrochloride (See also *443144-26-1*)

443913-73-3. Vandetanib (See also *338992-00-0*)

444069-80-1. Dapiclermin

444190-52-7. Ditiocade Sodium

444731-52-6. Pazopanib Hydrochloride [pazopanib] (See also *635702-64-6*)

445041-75-8. Intiquinatine

446022-33-9. Pelitrexol

446264-97-7. Galyfilcon A

447406-78-2. Sodelglitazar

449811-01-2. Pamapimod

451470-34-1. Solabegron Hydrochloride (See also *252920-94-8*)

453562-69-1. Motesanib

457068-92-7. Neramexane Mesylate (See also *219810-59-0*)

457075-21-7. Ganstigmine

457913-93-8. Ismomultin Alfa

459789-99-2. Obeticholic Acid

459856-18-9. Pexacerfont

460738-38-9. Ecallantide

461023-63-2. Aplaviroc Hydrochloride (See also *461443-59-4*)

461443-59-4. Aplaviroc Hydrochloride [aplaviroc] (See also *461023-63-2*)

464213-10-3. Ibipinabant

465540-87-8. Taneptacogin Alfa

467214-20-6. Alvespimycin Hydrochloride [alvespimycin] (See also *467214-21-7*)

467214-21-7. Alvespimycin Hydrochloride (See also *467214-20-6*)

468715-71-1. Elsilimomab
472960-22-8. Albinterferon Alfa-2b
473289-62-2. Ilepatril
473553-86-5. Alferminogene Tadenovec
474641-19-5. Deutolperisone
474793-41-4. Iclaprim Mesylate (See also *192314-93-5*)
475207-59-1. Sorafenib Tosylate
475479-34-6. Aleglitazar
476181-74-5. Golimumab
476413-07-7. Yttrium Y 90 Tacatuzumab
476436-68-7. Naveglitazar
477202-00-9. Ipilimumab
478166-15-3. Mecasermin Rinfabate
478296-72-9. Gabapentin Enacarbil
478799-92-7. Senofilcon A
479198-61-3. Iboctadekin
480449-70-5. Edoxaban
481629-87-2. Aleplasinin
481631-45-2. Diaplasinin
481658-94-0. Dirlotapide
483369-58-0. Denagliptin Tosylate [denagliptin] (See also *811432-66-3*)
486460-32-6. Sitagliptin Phosphate [sitagliptin] (See also *654671-77-9*)
488712-31-8. Hyaluronidase (Ovine) (See also *9001-54-1*)
488832-69-5. Elesclomol
492448-75-6. Vitespen
496050-39-6. Pemaglitazar
496054-87-6. Radiprodil
496775-61-2. Eltrombopag Olamine [eltrombopag] (See also *496775-62-3*)
496775-62-3. Eltrombopag Olamine (See also *496775-61-2*)
497221-38-2. Rusalatide Acetate [rusalatide] (See also *875455-82-6*)
499212-74-7. Pritumumab
500287-72-9. Rilpivirine
501000-36-8. Dutacatib
501019-16-5. Delmitide Acetate (See also *287096-87-1*)
501081-76-1. Rilonacept
501423-23-0. Yttrium Y 90 Epratuzumab
501423-25-2. Yttrium Y 90 Epratuzumab Tetraxetan
501423-27-4. Yttrium Y 90 Labetuzumab
501423-30-9. Yttrium Y 90 Labetuzumab Tetraxetan
501948-05-6. Rosabulin
502422-74-4. Figopitant
502496-16-4. Urtoxazumab
503605-66-1. Adecatumumab
503612-47-3. Apixaban
506433-25-6. Depelestat
507453-82-9. Mirococept
509077-98-9. Catumaxomab
509077-99-0. Ertumaxomab
514820-03-2. Ispinesib Mesylate (See also *336113-53-2*)
515814-01-4. Voclosporin
518048-05-0. Raltegravir Potassium [raltegravir] (See also *871038-72-1*)
519055-62-0. Tasisulam Sodium [tasisulam] (See also *519055-63-1*)
519055-63-1. Tasisulam Sodium (See also *519055-62-0*)
521079-87-8. Tefibazumab

522664-63-7. Ibodutant
524067-21-8. Becocalcidiol
524684-52-4. Prinaberel
533927-56-9. Atilmotin
536748-46-6. Eribaxaban
537694-98-7. Besilesomab
540769-28-6. Palosuran
541547-35-7. Agatolimod Sodium
541550-19-0. Apilimod Mesylate [apilimod] (See also *870087-36-8*)
544417-40-5. Capadenoson
544697-52-1. Gadodenterate
552292-08-7. Rolapitant Hydrochloride [rolapitant] (See also *914462-92-3*)
552858-79-4. Galsulfase
557795-19-4. Sunitinib Malate [sunitinib] (See also *341031-54-7*)
558480-40-3. Volociximab
560130-42-9. Telavancin Hydrochloride (See also *372151-71-8*)
565451-13-0. Raxibacumab
566906-50-1. Beminafil
569351-91-3. Dasantafil
569658-79-3. Libivirumab
569658-80-6. Exbivirumab
571170-77-9. Laropiprant
572924-54-0. Deforolimus
575458-75-2. Radotermin
579475-18-6. Orvepitant
581079-18-7. Pegamotecan
583057-48-1. Arasertaconazole
592557-41-0. Tenatumomab [heavy chain] (See also *592557-43-2*)
592557-43-2. Tenatumomab [light chain] (See also *592557-41-0*)
593282-20-3. Dabigatran Etexilate Mesylate
595566-61-3. Pagibaximab
599179-03-0. Vicriviroc Maleate (See also *306296-47-9*)
600735-73-7. Contusugene Ladenovec
603139-19-1. Odanacatib
604802-70-2. Epoetin Zeta
606138-08-3. Catridecacog
607723-33-1. Lobeglitazone
608137-32-2. Lisdexamfetamine Dimesylate [lisdexamfetamine] (See also *608137-33-3*)
608137-33-3. Lisdexamfetamine Dimesylate (See also *608137-32-2*)
608141-41-9. Apremilast
609799-22-6. Tasimelteon
610309-89-2. Carvedilol Phosphate
615258-40-7. Denosumab
616202-92-7. Lorcaserin Hydrochloride [lorcaserin] (See also *846589-98-8*)
620948-34-7. Vabicaserin Hydrochloride (See also *620948-93-8*)
620948-93-8. Vabicaserin Hydrochloride [vabicaserin] (See also *620948-34-7*)
623174-20-9. Tasidotin Hydrochloride (See also *192658-64-3*)
625095-60-5. Pradefovir Mesylate [pradefovir] (See also *625095-61-6*)
625095-61-6. Pradefovir Mesylate (See also *625095-60-5*)
625114-41-2. Piragliatin
625115-55-1. Riociguat

627861-07-8. Beperminogene Perplasmid
629167-92-6. Mipomersen Sodium (See also *1000120-98-8*)
629664-81-9. Turofexorate Isopropyl
635702-64-6. Pazopanib Hydrochloride (See also *444731-52-6*)
635715-01-4. Inotuzumab Ozogamicin
635724-55-9. Esreboxetine Succinate
637328-69-9. Tanogitran
637334-45-3. Ocrelizumab
639089-54-6. Tozasertib
640281-90-9. Valopicitabine Dihydrochloride [valopicitabine] (See also *640725-71-9*)
640725-71-9. Valopicitabine Dihydrochloride (See also *640281-90-9*)
640735-09-7. Iratumumab
641571-10-0. Nilotinib
643094-49-9. Fasobegron
648420-92-2. Talotrexin Ammonium (See also *113857-87-7*)
648895-38-9. Bapineuzumab
648904-28-3. Bavituximab
649735-63-7. Brivanib Alaninate
652153-01-0. Zanolimumab
652990-07-3. Milveterol Hydrochloride [milveterol] (See also *804518-03-4*)
654671-77-9. Sitagliptin Phosphate (See also *486460-32-6*)
658052-09-6. Mapatumumab
661464-94-4. Levalbuterol Tartrate
664338-39-0. Arterolane
667901-13-5. Zalutumumab
668270-12-0. Linagliptin
675132-86-2. Rivanicline Galactarate (See also *15585-43-0*)
676251-22-2. Regrelor Disodium (See also *787548-03-2*)
676258-98-3. Naptumomab Estafenatox
677010-34-3. Motavizumab
677017-23-1. Berubicin Hydrochloride [berubicin] (See also *293736-67-1*)
679404-95-6. Hemoglobin Glutamer-256 (Human)
679809-58-6. Enoxaparin Sodium
679818-59-8. Ofatumumab
680188-33-4. Ibalizumab
680993-85-5. Esmirtazapine Maleate
685563-13-7. Inalimarev (CEA, MUC-1, Vaccinia virus)
685563-14-8. Falimarev (CEA, MUC-1, fowlpox virus)
685922-56-9. Custirsen Sodium (See also *903916-27-8*)
686344-29-6. Otenabant
686347-12-6. Otenabant Hydrochloride
691852-58-1. Nesbuvir
697761-98-1. Elvitegravir
697766-75-9. Velafermin
698387-09-6. Neratinib
698389-00-3. Rolipoltide
701977-09-5. Taranabant
702686-96-2. Ronacaleret Hydrochloride (See also *753449-67-1*)
705287-60-1. Stamulumab
706779-91-1. Pimavanserin Tartrate [pimavanserin] (See also *706782-28-7*)

706782-28-7. Pimavanserin Tartrate (See also *706779-91-1*)

706808-37-9. Belatacept

716840-32-3. Denenicokin

721946-42-5. Transferrin Aldifitox

728917-18-8. Veltuzumab

736178-83-9. Levamlodipine Malate (See also *103129-82-4*)

740873-06-7. Naluzotan

740873-82-9. Naluzotan Hydrochloride

745013-59-6. Tremelimumab

748810-28-8. Vernakalant Hydrochloride (See also *794466-70-9*)

753449-67-1. Ronacaleret Hydrochloride [ronacaleret] (See also *702686-96-2*)

753498-25-8. Indacaterol Maleate

757942-43-1. Bederocin

757971-58-7. Hyaluronidase (Human Recombinant)

759457-82-4. Padeliporfin

760937-92-6. Teneligliptin

762260-74-2. Efungumab

762263-14-9. Epoetin Theta

763113-22-0. Olaparib

763903-67-9. Fosalvudine Tidoxil

769169-27-9. Begacestat

769901-96-4. Capeserod

773092-05-0. Acotiamide Hydrochloride (See also *185106-16-5*)

775304-57-9. Ataluren

775351-65-0. Imeglimin

778576-62-8. Oglemilast

779356-64-8. Denibulin Hydrochloride (See also *284019-34-7*)

781649-09-0. Telcagepant

781666-30-6. Dirucotide Acetate

782500-75-8. Albiglutide

787548-03-2. Regrelor Disodium [regrelor] (See also *676251-22-2*)

790299-79-5. Masitinib

791635-59-1. Simotaxel

791828-58-5. Aderbasib

792921-10-9. Abagovomab

793655-64-8. Vapitadine Dihydrochloride [vapitadine] (See also *279253-83-7*)

794466-70-9. Vernakalant Hydrochloride [vernakalant] (See also *748810-28-8*)

799279-80-4. Sofinicline

803712-67-6. Obatoclax Mesylate [obatoclax] (See also *803712-79-0*)

803712-79-0. Obatoclax Mesylate (See also *803712-67-6*)

804518-03-4. Milveterol Hydrochloride (See also *652990-07-3*)

811420-59-4. Sinecatechins

811432-66-3. Denagliptin Tosylate (See also *483369-58-0*)

813452-14-1. Carmegliptin Dihydrochloride

813452-18-5. Carmegliptin

815610-63-0. Ustekinumab

820957-38-8. Retosiban

823821-85-8. Bevirimat Dimeglumine (See also *174022-42-5*)

827318-97-8. Danusertib

827611-49-4. Aztreonam Lysine

828271-96-1. Valategrast Hydrochloride (See also *220847-86-9*)

828933-51-3. Nimotuzumab

832720-36-2. Elagolix Sodium

834153-87-6. Elagolix

835619-41-5. Indeglitazar

837369-26-3. Pafuramidine Maleate (See also *186953-56-0*)

838853-48-8. Mifamurtide (See also *83461-56-7*)

839673-52-8. Cevoglitazar

839712-12-8. Cariprazine

840486-93-3. Adipiplon

845264-92-8. Atacicept

845273-93-0. Sevelamer Carbonate

845736-10-9. Iodine Povacrylex

845816-02-6. Lexatumumab

846589-98-8. Lorcaserin Hydrochloride (See also *616202-92-7*)

847353-30-4. Arbaclofen Placarbil

847923-13-1. Paflufocon D-HEM-Iberfilcon A (iberfilcon A) (See also *109550-08-5*)

848084-83-3. Tigapotide Triflutate [tigapotide] (See also *848084-84-4*)

848084-84-4. Tigapotide Triflutate (See also *848084-83-3*)

848344-36-5. Bentamapimod

849550-05-6. Cevipabulin Fumarate [cevipabulin] (See also *849550-69-2*)

849550-69-2. Cevipabulin Fumarate (See also *849550-05-6*)

849758-52-7. Bevasiranib Sodium (See also *959961-96-7*)

850607-58-8. Darotropium Bromide

850649-61-5. Alogliptin Benzoate [alogliptin] (See also *850649-62-6*)

850649-62-6. Alogliptin Benzoate (See also *850649-61-5*)

851199-59-2. Linaclotide

851199-60-5. Linaclotide Acetate (See also *851199-59-2*)

851606-62-7. Totrombopag Choline (See also *376592-42-6*)

852313-25-8. Litenimod

852329-66-9. Dutogliptin

852954-81-5. Cevipabulin Succinate

853426-35-4. Blinatumomab

856676-23-8. Choline Fenofibrate

857036-77-2. Cediranib Maleate

857402-23-4. Retaspimycin

857402-63-2. Retaspimycin Hydrochloride

857876-30-3. Motesanib Diphosphate

860642-69-9. Serlopitant

861151-12-4. Rosonabant

861998-00-7. Anamorelin Hydrochloride

862111-32-8. Aflibercept

862189-95-5. Mirodenafil

863029-99-6. Balamapimod

863031-21-4. Azilsartan Medoxomil

863031-24-7. Azilsartan Kamedoxomil

863127-77-9. Dasatinib

865200-20-0. Giripladib

865311-47-3. Quarfloxin

866021-48-9. Ceftaroline Fosamil

867153-61-5. Dulanermin

867217-46-7. Sifilcon A

868540-17-4. Carfilzomib

868771-57-7. Melogliptin

869572-92-9. Tecovirimat

869858-13-9. Thrombin Alfa

869881-54-9. Briobacept

869884-77-5. Radezolid Hydrochloride

869884-78-6. Radezolid

870087-36-8. Apilimod Mesylate (See also *541550-19-0*)

870524-46-2. Amolimogene Bepiplasmid

871038-72-1. Raltegravir Potassium (See also *518048-05-0*)

871224-64-5. Almorexant

871576-03-3. Flovagatran

872178-65-9. Rabeximod

872525-61-6. Votucalis

872847-66-0. Cenersen Sodium

873857-62-6. Fidaxomicin

874819-74-6. Toceranib Phosphate

875148-45-1. Regadenoson (See also *313348-27-5*)

875446-37-0. Anacetrapib

875455-82-6. Rusalatide Acetate (See also *497221-38-2*)

876170-44-4. Sofinicline Benzenesulfonate

876387-05-2. Teplizumab

879555-13-2. Epoetin Kappa

880149-29-1. Bismuth Subcitrate Potassium

880266-57-9. Tanezumab

880486-59-9. Dacetuzumab

881191-44-2. Otelixizumab

881851-50-9. Larazotide Acetate (See also *258818-34-7*)

884502-91-4. Liprotamase

884604-91-5. Velaglucerase Alfa

885051-90-1. Pegloticase

887148-69-8. Monepantel

887650-05-7. Bafetinib

890402-81-0. Dutogliptin Tartrate

892497-01-7. Azoximer Bromide

892553-42-3. Etaracizumab

896444-34-1. Epetirimod Esylate

896723-44-7. Farletuzumab

896731-82-1. Conatumumab

897936-89-9. Vatreptacog Alfa (activated)

898830-54-1. Sitimagene Ceradenovec

899796-83-9. Milatuzumab

899827-04-4. Tozasertib Lactate

901119-35-5. Fostamatinib

901758-09-6. Tesamorelin Acetate

903512-50-5. Lucatumumab

903916-27-8. Custirsen Sodium [custirsen] (See also *685922-56-9*)

904302-98-3. Viquidacin

905818-69-1. Bupropion Hydrobromide

908351-31-5. Sotrastaurin Acetate (See also *425637-18-9*)

909110-25-4. Baminercept Alfa

910649-32-0. Anrukinzumab

914295-16-2. Fostamatinib Disodium

914462-92-3. Rolapitant Hydrochloride (See also *552292-08-7*)

915019-08-8. Tertomotide

915296-00-3. Elotuzumab

915769-50-5. Dovitinib Lactate (See also *405169-16-6*)

918127-53-4. Tigatuzumab

925681-61-4. Trabedersen

929881-05-0. Alipogene Tiparvovec
931101-84-7. Troplasminogen Alfa
934216-54-3. Alacizumab Pegol
934246-14-7. Degarelix Acetate
943453-46-1. Figitumumab
943609-66-3. Vedolizumab
944263-65-4. Demiditraz
944537-89-7. Mocetinostat Dihydrobromide

944548-37-2. Rafivirumab
944548-38-3. Foravirumab
945228-49-9. Citatuzumab Bogatox
945405-37-8. Pozanicline Tartrate
945667-22-1. Saxagliptin (See also *361442-04-8*)
947687-12-9. Cixutumumab
947687-13-0. Ramucirumab
949142-50-1. Afutuzumab

953077-35-5. Telcagepant Potassium
959961-96-7. Bevasiranib Sodium [bevasiranib] (See also *849758-52-7*)
960404-48-2. Dapagliflozin
1000120-98-8. Mipomersen Sodium [mipomersen] (See also *629167-92-6*)
1011713-07-7. Tolevamer Potassium Sodium (See also *81998-90-5*)

NSC NUMBERS

675. Benzoyl Peroxide
739. Aminopterin Sodium [as the base]
740. Methotrexate
742. Azaserine
746. Urethane
750. Busulfan
752. Thioguanine
755. Mercaptopurine
762. Mechlorethamine Hydrochloride
763. Dimethyl Sulfoxide
1390. Allopurinol
1771. Thiram
1879. Phenazopyridine Hydrochloride
2101. Roxarsone
2619. Sulfabenz
2834. Paroxypropione
3053. Dactinomycin
3055. Puromycin Hydrochloride
3088. Chlorambucil
3096. Demecolcine
3184. Nifuraldezone
3364. Filipin
3590. Leucovorin Calcium
3951. Benzoxiquine
4112. Fenticlor
5085. Nitarsone
5109. Dinsed
5366. Noscapine
5547. Dymanthine Hydrochloride
5648. Thonzonium Bromide
6091. Dapsone
6365. Tromethamine
6386. Bialamicol Hydrochloride
6396. Thiotepa
6470. Nifuradene
6738. Dichlorvos
7214. Ethoxazene Hydrochloride
7571. Aminacrine Hydrochloride
7760. Pralidoxime Iodide
7778. Oxybenzone
8806. Melphalan [as hydrochloride]
9120. Prednisolone
9166. Testosterone Propionate
9324. Allobarbital
9564. Norethindrone
9565. Ethisterone
9566. Estradiol Benzoate
9698. Mannomustine [as hydrochloride]
9701. Methyltestosterone
9704. Progesterone
9706. Triethylenemelamine
9894. Hexestrol

9895. Estradiol
10023. Prednisone
10039. Normethandrone
10108. Chlorotrianisene
10483. Hydrocortisone
10973. Ethinyl Estradiol
12165. Fluoxymesterone
12198. Dromostanolone Propionate
13875. Altretamine
14279. Pyrabrom
14574. Lucanthone Hydrochloride
15200. Gallium Nitrate
15432. Norethynodrel
15796. Becanthone Hydrochloride
16895. Lithium Carbonate
17261. Inproquone
17590. Estradiol Valerate
17591. Testosterone Enanthate
17592. Hydroxyprogesterone Caproate
17777. Phenyramidol Hydrochloride
17789. Benzindopyrine Hydrochloride
18268. Cactinomycin
18317. Cortodoxone
19043. Oxycodone
19477. Hexafluorenium Bromide
19893. Fluorouracil
19987. Methylprednisolone
20246. Clamoxyquin Hydrochloride
20264. Adenosine Phosphate
20272. Nadide
20293. Estradiol [as the alpha form]
20526. Tribromsalan
20527. Dibromsalan
21626. Propiolactone
23162. Nandrolone Phenpropionate
23516. Risocaine
23759. Testolactone
24559. Plicamycin
24970. Bromchlorenone
25141. Buclizine Hydrochloride
25154. Pipobroman
25159. Pemoline
25413. Fenamole
25614. Phthalofyne
26154. Aminocaproic Acid
26271. Cyclophosphamide
26386. Medroxyprogesterone Acetate
26492. Thyroid
26980. Mitomycin
27178. Capuride
27640. Floxuridine
28120. Amidapsone

29215. Triaziquone
29863. Guanethidine Sulfate
30152. Dimethadione
30223. Buramate
32065. Hydroxyurea
32363. Valnoctamide
32942. Cetalkonium Chloride
33077. Carbocloral
33659. Lapyrium Chloride
34249. Pentetate Calcium Trisodium
34462. Uracil Mustard
34632. Mafenide
34652. Mephenytoin
35770. Clomiphene Citrate
37095. Uredepa
37096. Benzodepa
37725. Lynestrenol
38721. Mitotane
38887. Thiamiprine
39084. Azathioprine
39415. Domiphen Bromide
39470. Betamethasone
39661. Idoxuridine
39690. Proadifen Hydrochloride
40144. Phenyl Aminosalicylate
40725. Isosorbide
40902. Phencyclidine Hydrochloride
42044. Lobendazole
42722. Methandrostenolone
43183. Fenyripol Hydrochloride
43193. Stanozolol
43798. Pargyline Hydrochloride
44827. Descinolone Acetonide
45383. Streptonigrin
45388. Dacarbazine
45463. Captamine Hydrochloride
46077. Demoxepam
47439. Fluprednisolone
47774. Piposulfan
49171. Salsalate
49506. Inositol Niacinate
49842. Vinblastine Sulfate
50364. Metronidazole
51001. Carbomycin
51097. Duazomycin
51325. Meturedepa
51812. Sancycline [as hydrochloride]
52644. Pyrrocaine
53397. Ambomycin
54702. Flumethasone
55926. Spiramycin
55975. Epimestrol

56308. Epipropidine
56410. Porfiromycin
56654. Azotomycin
56769. Dioxybenzone
56808. Quinaldine Blue
58775. Nitrazepam
59687. Oxyphenisatin Acetate
59729. Sparsomycin
59989. Clorophene
60584. Sulisobenzone
60719. Nitromide
61815. Diatrizoate Sodium
62939. Trimetozine
63278. Medrysone
63878. Cytarabine Hydrochloride
63963. Etryptamine Acetate
64013. Ethosuximide
64087. Clopenthixol
64198. Diazoxide
64375. Benzquinamide
64393. Spiramycin [as hydrochloride]
64540. Pyroxamine Maleate
64826. Azetepa
64967. Methenolone Enanthate
65411. Flurogestone Acetate
66233. Bolasterone
66847. Thalidomide
66952. Aminorex
67068. Oxandrolone
67239. Azaribine
67574. Vincristine Sulfate
68982. Guanabenz
69200. Chlorthalidone
69529. Mitogillin
69536. Methallibure
69811. Methisazone
69948. Trestolone Acetate
70600. Acetophenazine Maleate
70731. Lincomycin Hydrochloride
70735. Nafoxidine Hydrochloride
70762. Tolazamide
70845. Nogalamycin
70933. Cycliramine Maleate
70968. Melengestrol Acetate
71047. Trioxsalen
71423. Megestrol Acetate
71755. Carphenazine Maleate
71901. Statolon
72005. Triclocarban
72274. Mitopodozide
73205. Dipyrone
73713. Dextroamphetamine
74226. Methenolone Acetate
75054. Mesterolone
76098. Chlorphentermine Hydrochloride
76239. Oxypurinol
76455. Peliomycin
77120. Sulfanitran
77213. Procarbazine Hydrochloride
77370. Fenclonine
77471. Mitocromin
77518. Diazepam
77625. Triamterene
77747. Triclofenol Piperazine
77830. Cycloguanil Pamoate
78194. Methixene Hydrochloride
78502. Meclocycline
78559. Flurazepam Hydrochloride

78714. Clothixamide Maleate
78987. Isomylamine Hydrochloride
79037. Lomustine
79389. Clofibrate
80998. Cortivazol
81430. Cyproterone Acetate
82116. Gloxazone
82151. Daunorubicin Hydrochloride
82174. Nalidixic Acid
82261. Gentamicin Sulfate
82699. Flufenamic Acid
83653. Amantadine Hydrochloride
83799. Simtrazene
84054. Gestonorone Caproate
84223. Sodium Oxybate
84973. Cyprolidol Hydrochloride
85791. Ethacrynic Acid
85998. Streptozocin
88536. Calusterone
89277. Modaline Sulfate
91523. Propranolol Hydrochloride
92336. Dydrogesterone
92338. Chlormadinone Acetate
92339. Fluocinolone Acetonide
93158. Asperlin
94219. Candicidin
95072. Ormetoprim
95147. Silandrone
95441. Semustine
100071. Haloprogin
100638. Amfonelic Acid
101791. Fluocinonide
102629. Flazalone
102816. Azacitidine
102824. Apazone
102825. Cintazone
103336. Menoctone
105546. Riboprine
106563. Bethanidine Sulfate
106564. Butacetin
106565. Butoxamine Hydrochloride
106566. Erythrityl Tetranitrate
106568. Trimethoprim
106569. Thenium Closylate
106570. Rolodine
106571. Bunamidine Hydrochloride
106572. Tolpyrramide
106959. Carbiphene Hydrochloride
106960. Glyhexamide
106962. Ipodate Sodium
106995. Lomofungin
107041. Scopafungin
107079. Chymopapain
107412. Coumermycin
107429. Cyclazocine
107430. Pentazocine
107431. Metrizoate Sodium
107433. Teclozan
107434. Tyropanoate Sodium
107528. Acetosulfone Sodium
107529. Pararosaniline Pamoate
107654. Pyrrolnitrin
107677. Dimethindene Maleate
107678. Angiotensin Amide
107679. Cyclopenthiazide
107680. Flumethasone Pivalate
108034. Hydroxyphenamate
108160. Doxepin Hydrochloride

108161. Polythiazide
108163. Guanoclor Sulfate
108164. Epithiazide
108165. Thiothixene
108166. Troleandomycin
109212. Ipronidazole
109229. Asparaginase
109724. Ifosfamide
110364. Oxolinic Acid
110430. Chromonar Hydrochloride
110431. Methyclothiazide
110432. Methoxyflurane
110433. Sulfalene
111071. Carbenicillin Disodium
111180. Acetylcysteine
112682. Enpromate
112931. Tetroquinone
113233. Mitomalcin
113926. Rifampin
114649. Flavoxate Hydrochloride
114650. Dimefline Hydrochloride
114901. Desipramine Hydrochloride
115748. Chlordiazepoxide Hydrochloride
115944. Enflurane
117032. Mitosper
119875. Cisplatin
122758. Tretinoin
123018. Medrogestone
123127. Doxorubicin Hydrochloride
125717. Cinanserin Hydrochloride
125973. Paclitaxel
127716. Decitabine
129185. Mycophenolic Acid
129224. Adiphenine Hydrochloride
130044. Thiethylperazine Maleate
133099. Rifamide
134434. Hycanthone
134454. Dronabinol
136947. Niridazole
137443. Kalafungin
139593. Sulfasomizole
141046. Clofazimine
142005. Mecloqualone
143969. Tilorone Hydrochloride
148958. Tegafur
153858. Maytansine
157658. Denatonium Benzoate
158565. Chlorindanol
164011. Zorubicin Hydrochloride
169780. Dexrazoxane
172112. Spiromustine
181815. Perfosfamide
182986. Diaziquone
192965. Spirogermanium Hydrochloride
208734. Aclarubicin
218321. Pentostatin
241240. Carboplatin
245467. Vindesine Sulfate
246131. Valrubicin
249992. Amsacrine
253272. Caracemide
256927. Iproplatin
261726. Dezaguanine
262168. Diatrizoic Acid
266046. Oxaliplatin
269148. Menogaril
280594. Triciribine Phosphate
281272. Fazarabine

284356. Mitindomide
286193. Tiazofurin
296934. Teroxirone
296961. Amifostine
301467. Etanidazole
305884. Acodazole Hydrochloride
311056. Spiroplatin
312887. Fludarabine Phosphate
355644. Teloxantrone Hydrochloride
356894. Gusperimus Trihydrochloride
357885. Losoxantrone Hydrochloride
362856. Temozolomide
368390. Brequinar Sodium
403169. Acronine

405124. Symclosene
406087. Ethamivan
406239. Sorbitan Monooleate
408735. Diaveridine
409962. Carmustine
515776. Dipyridamole
524411. Methetoin
525334. Nifurthiazole
526046. Nicotinyl Alcohol
526062. Dexoxadrol Hydrochloride
526063. Levoxadrol Hydrochloride
526280. Metabromsalan
527579. Meprednisone
527604. Deferoxamine

527986. Levofuraltadone
528004. Vinleurosine Sulfate
528880. Pimetine Hydrochloride
528986. Ampicillin
606170. Zalcitabine
613792. Lodenosine
614491. Tocladesine
649890. Alvocidib
655649. Becatecarin
659772. Alitretinoin
712783. Talotrexin Ammonium

Appendix VII
Guiding Principles for Coining United States Adopted Names for Drugs

By definition, nonproprietary names are not subject to proprietary trademark rights but are entirely in the public domain. This distinguishes them from the trademarked names that have been registered for private use. A United States Adopted Name (USAN) is a nonproprietary name selected by the USAN Council according to principles developed to assure safety, consistency, and logic in the choice of names. These principles take into account practical considerations, such as the existence of trademarks and the fact that the intended uses of substances for which names are being selected may change. These guidelines are and must be sufficiently flexible to be revised if this is considered to be desirable and/or necessary.

General Rules

1. A nonproprietary name should be useful primarily to health practitioners, especially physicians, pharmacists, nurses, educators, dentists, and veterinarians.
   a. The primary criterion for judging usefulness is suitability, including safety for use in the routine processes of prescribing, ordering, dispensing, and administering drugs throughout the United States.
   b. The second criterion is suitability for use in educational programs for students in medically oriented professions and for use in scientific and lay publications.
   c. The third criterion is suitability for use internationally for drug identification, for the exchange of information and translation into different languages.
2. Attributes that contribute to usefulness are simplicity (brevity and ease of pronunciation), euphony, and ready recognition and recall.
   a. The name for the active moiety of a drug should be a single word, preferably with no more than four syllables.
   b. The name for the active moiety may be modified by a single term, preferably with no more than four syllables, to show a chemical modification, such as salt or ester formation (e.g., cortisone acetate from cortisone, cefamandole sodium from cefamandole, erythromycin acistrate from erythromycin).
   c. Only under compelling circumstances is a name with more than one modifying term acceptable (e.g., pharmaceuticals containing radioactive isotopes, the different classes of interferons).
   d. Acronyms, initials, and condensed words may be acceptable in otherwise appropriate terminology.
3. A name should reflect characteristics and relationships that will be of practical value to the users.
   a. A common, simple word element (a "stem") should be incorporated in the names of all members of a group of related drugs when pertinent, common characteristics can be identified (e.g., similarity of pharmacological action). When pharmacological similarity is found in drugs of distinctly different chemical nature, stems should differ (e.g., the antipsychotics, promazine and haloperidol; the nonsteroidal anti-inflammatory agents [NSAID], ibuprofen, etodolac, and isoxicam).

b. Distinctive terminology should be used for specific drugs or groups (e.g., insulin I 131, dextran 40, interferon alfa-2a and interferon alfa-n1; licryfilcon A and licryfilcon B; epoetin alfa and epoetin beta).
4. A name should be free from conflict with other nonproprietary names and with established trademarks and should be neither confusing nor chemically misleading.
   a. Prefixes that imply "better," "newer," or "more effective," or evoke the name of the manufacturer, dosage form, duration of action or rate of drug release should not be used.
   b. Prefixes that refer to an anatomical connotation or medical condition are not acceptable.
   c. Prefixes that indicate a chemical element or compound (Ca, Ni, and Stannous) are not acceptable.
5. Preference should be given to names of established usage provided they conform to these guiding principles and are determined to be free from conflict with existing nonproprietary names and trademarks.
6. Identical negotiations submitted by two or more manufacturers will be conducted in accordance with the Council's practice of maintaining confidentiality. The applicants involved will not be notified of the multiple sources of the submission. However, the name selected by the USAN Council will need to be accepted by each manufacturer involved in the negotiation process.
7. A request for a USAN should be made after the drug manufacturer or sponsor has submitted an Investigational New Drug (IND) application to the Food and Drug Administration (FDA) to obtain permission to initiate studies on humans.
8. Deferred Negotiations:
   a. The USAN Council Secretariat will defer an ongoing negotiation for six (6) months plus one additional three-month extension upon receipt of a written request from the manufacturer. If the USAN Council has selected a name candidate and recommended this name to the manufacturer, the maximum deferral is one six-month period.
   b. The negotiation will be canceled after the maximum nine-month deferral has lapsed.
   c. If the negotiation is to be reopened at a later time, it will receive a new USAN file number and will be treated as a new application. The manufacturer will be expected to submit a new USAN negotiation form, update the background information, and submit the appropriate user's fee.

Specific Rules

1. Because of the international exchange of drug information, specific guidelines have been formulated to ensure appropriate translation of nonproprietary names into other languages. The following rules of preferred spelling should be used when coining USAN designations:
   a. the letter "f" should be used instead of "ph"
   b. the letter "t" should be used instead of "th"

c. the letter "e" should be used instead of "ae" or "oe"
d. the letter "i" should be used instead of "y"
e. the letter "h" should be avoided
f. the letter "k" should be avoided.
g. the letter "j" should be avoided.
h. the letter "w" should be avoided.
i. "ar", "rac", "lev", "dex", or "es" are reserved for stereochemical configurations

2. Additionally, these letter combinations are restricted until further notice. Please avoid the following prefixes:
   a. the beginning letter combination of "me"
   b. the beginning letter combination of "str"
   c. chemical connotations such as "ben", "bu", "cat", "cel", "fen", "flu", "piro"
   d. chemical symbols unless present in the compound, "al", "ba", "ca", "li", "ni"

   In order to facilitate the development of names that will be accepted on an international level please note:

   A. The following letter combinations pose pronunciation problems in several languages:
      -ch-
      -rs-
      -xn
   B. The letter sequence "-m" and "-n" followed by consonants may be regarded as difficult.
      (1) "-m" before a consonant other than "p", "n", or "b"
      (2) -nb-, and -np- should be avoided
   C. The letter sequence "-vr" should be avoided.
   D. In addition, it should be kept in mind that there is, in some languages, no distinction between:
      "b" and "v" or "p"
      "l" and "r"
      "z" and "g"

3. Isolated letters, numbers, or hyphenations are restricted to those groups of substances for which such usage fulfills a clearly demonstrable purpose (e.g., interferon alfa-2b, paflufocon A, technetium Tc 99m siboroxime).

4. Group relationships in a name preferably should be indicated by use of syllables or stems; conversely, use of the stem for other than the appropriate group should be avoided. When multiple stems are available, the stem conveying the most information should be used.

5. Esters, salts, chelates, and complexes ordinarily require a two-word name to indicate the inactive as well as the active portion.

6. The preferred order for the name of an inorganic salt is cation-anion (e.g., sodium bromide). The same order is preferred for well-known salts of simple organic acids (e.g., sodium lactate, magnesium citrate, potassium acetate). However, for more complex organic compounds, the pharmacologically active portion should be identified first (e.g., oxacillin sodium, ibuprofen piconol, dexibuprofen lysine).

7. A name for a salt or ester generally should be derived from the name of the pharmacologically active moiety or corresponding acid (e.g., sodium acetate or ethyl acetate, derived from acetic acid). When a nonacid suffix is used, as in the penicillin series, a salt should be named without modification of the parent acid name (e.g., oxacillin sodium, derived from oxacillin). Names for different salts or esters of the same active moiety should differ only in the name of the inactive portion; exceptions are permissible when the salt and ester forms possess pharmacologic activity.

8. A name for the salt form of the pharmacologically active moiety is specific to the number of molecules used to react with the active moiety (e.g., balsalazide <u>di</u>sodium, gusperimus <u>tri</u>hydrochloride). If only one molecule is used to react with the active moiety, the designation for the salt name is used without reference to the mono-prefix (e.g., besipirdine hydrochloride, afovirsen hydrochloride). [This rule was formulated and approved in January 1993; different requirements were applied prior to this date.]

9. A name for a quaternary ammonium substance should designate the cation and anion separately (e.g., octonium bromide, not octonine methylbromide). The name assigned to the cation must contain the *-ium* suffix stem.

10. A name for a complex of two or more components should list the name of the principal active ingredient followed by a coined designation for the second component ending with an *-ex* suffix to indicate "complex" (e.g., bisacodyl tann<u>ex</u>, doxycycline fosfat<u>ex</u>). Complexes formed from sulfonated diethenylbenzene-ethenylbenzene copolymers and an active ingredient should list the name of the principal active ingredient followed by "polistirex" (e.g., chlorpheniramine <u>poli-stirex</u>, codeine <u>polistirex</u>).

11. A name for a drug containing a radioactive atom should list, in the order given: (1) the name of the drug containing the radioactive atom, (2) the element symbol, (3) the isotope number, and (4) the name of the carrier agent, if any (e.g., rose bengal sodium I 131, cyanocobalamin Co 60, potassium bromide Br 82, technetium Tc 99m butilfenin, technetium Tc 99m medronate, indium In 111 oxyquinoline, indium In 111 satumomab pendetide).

12. A name for a substance generally should not indicate the state of hydration, the morphology, or the mode of preparation. Reference to the water of hydration is retained in the chemical information (chemical names, formulas, weight) but is excluded from the nonproprietary name. The degree of hydration becomes a part of the chemical entity identified by the USAN.

13. Under the terms of the Orphan Drug Act of 1983, the development and marketing of drug products that are of limited commercial application but that are potentially useful in relatively rare disease conditions are encouraged. The selection of a name for an orphan drug may be based on special considerations. Therefore, when the name for an orphan drug appears to follow a more chemically oriented terminology style than is customary for drug nomenclature generally, this is not to be regarded as a basis or a precedent for a future selection of a USAN.

14. A name coined for a new chemical entity routinely does not specify the stereoisomeric form of the molecule in the nonproprietary name. If the stereochemical configuration has been determined, this information is presented in the chemical name(s) and is reflected in the structural formula. A USAN can, therefore, identify the racemic mixture (e.g., carnitine, ibuprofen, tetramisole), the levo isomer (e.g., remoxipride, quadazocine), or the dextro form (e.g., butopamine). Subsequently, if a name is needed for a different enantiomer or for the racemic form, the following prefixes should be added to the existing name:
   a. For the racemate, the rac-/race- prefix is used (e.g., race-methionine, racepinephrine, ractopamine).
   b. For the levo rotatory form, the "(S)" isomer, the lev-/levo- prefix is used (e.g., levocarnitine, levamisole, lev-cromakalim, levdobutamine).
   c. For the levo rotatory form but for the "(R)" isomer, ["R(-)"-isomer], the "ar-" prefix is added to the base name.
   d. For the dextro rotatory form, the "(R)" isomer, the dex-/dextro- prefix is used (e.g., dexamisole, dexibuprofen, dextroamphetamine, dexverapamil, dexrazoxane, dexfosfoserine, dexniguldipine).
   e. For the dextro rotatory form but for the "(S)" isomer ["S(+)"-isomer], the "es-" prefix is added to the base name.

15. Official names have been selected for a number of radicals and adducts used to form salts or esters of the pharmacologically active moiety. In a majority of cases, these names represent contractions of the chemical name assigned to the radical or adduct. In four specific cases, the official name identifies a multicomponent adduct:

- *acistrate* identifies the 2′-acetate (ester) **and** octadecanoate (salt) (e.g., erythromycin acistrate).
- *probutate* identifies the double ester—1-oxobutoxy **and** 1-oxopropoxy (e.g., hydrocortisone probutate).
- *estolate* identifies the double salt—propanoate **and** dodecyl sulfate (e.g., erythromycin estolate).
- *hyclate* identifies the monohydrochloride salt, hemiethanolate, hemihydrate combination (e.g., doxyclin hyclate).
- For the complete list of official names for radicals, see the end of this Appendix.

Nomenclature for Biological Products

The USAN Council has been involved in coining names for various biological products: the insulins, interferons, interleukins, growth hormones, colony-stimulating factors, cytokines, and monoclonal antibodies. With increasing development of highly purified biological extracts and recombinant materials, the Council expects to have an increasingly greater role in assigning names and developing nomenclature rules for these agents.

Listed below are specific guidelines created by the USAN Council, in conjunction with the Food and Drug Administration (FDA), the US FDA Center for Biologics Evaluation and Research (CBER), and the World Health Organization (WHO) International Nonproprietary Names (INN) Committee.

Interferons

The following multitiered style for creating nonproprietary names for interferons was adopted by the USAN Council:

(1) The word interferon is the first element in the name. Interferon is defined as the class name for a family of species-specific proteins (or glycoproteins) that are produced according to information encoded by species of interferon genes and exert complex antineoplastic, antiviral, and immunomodulating effects. The three main forms of interferon used in therapy are interferon alfa (formerly leukocyte or lymphoblastoid interferon), interferon beta (formerly fibroblast interferon), and interferon gamma (formerly immune interferon).

(2) The appropriate Greek letter (spelled out) is the second word of the name:

alfa, beta, gamma.

(3) An appropriate Arabic numeral and letter are appended to the Greek letter by a hyphen (no space) to delineate subcategories. The numbers conform to the recommendation of the Interferon Nomenclature Committee. The lowercase letter is assigned by the drug nomenclature agencies to differentiate one manufacturer's interferon from another's. Examples of pure interferon substances are:

interferon alfa-2a
interferon alfa-2b
interferon beta-1a
interferon beta-1b
interferon gamma-1a

(4) For mixtures of naturally occurring interferons, the lower case letter "n" precedes the number. Examples of names of mixtures of interferons obtained from a natural source, whether the exact percentage of a mixture is known or not, are:

interferon alfa-n1
interferon alfa-n2

Interleukins

The suffix *-kin* is used in naming interleukin-type substances except for interleukin 3 (IL-3) which was classified as a pleiotropic colony-stimulating factor and assigned the "plestim" stem (e.g., daniplestim). The "kin" nomenclature series was divided into subgroups with an adjuvant stem representing the numerical class of the interleukin followed by the kin suffix. The subgroups are:

-nakin	interleukin 1 derivatives
-onakin	interleukin 1α derivatives
-benakin	interleukin 1β derivatives
-leukin	interleukin 2 derivatives
-trakin	interleukin 4 derivatives
-penkin	interleukin 5 derivatives
-exakin	interleukin 6 derivatives
-eptakin	interleukin 7 derivatives
-octakin	interleukin 8 derivatives
-nonakin	interleukin 9 derivatives
-decakin	interleukin 10 derivatives
-elvekin	interleukin 11 derivatives
-dodekin	interleukin 12 derivatives

Somatotropins

The following guidelines have been developed for somatotropin analogs:

(1) The *som-* prefix is used for growth hormone derivatives, e.g.,
somatropin for human growth hormone
somatrem for methionyl human growth hormone

(2) The *som-* prefix and the *-bove* suffix are required for bovine somatotropin derivatives, e.g.,
somidobove
sometribove
somagrebove

(3) The *som-* prefix and the *-por* suffix are required for porcine somatotropin derivatives, e.g.,
somalapor
somenopor
sometripor
somfasepor

Colony-Stimulating Factors

The following guidelines have been developed for recombinant colony-stimulating factors:

(1) The suffix *-grastim* is used for granulocyte colony-stimulating factors (G-CSF), e.g.,
lenograstim
filgrastim

(2) The suffix *-gramostim* is used for granulocyte macrophage colony-stimulating factors (GM-CSF), e.g.,
molgramostim
regramostim
sargramostim

(3) The suffix *-mostim* is used for macrophage colony-stimulating factors (M-CSF), e.g.,
mirimostim

(4) The suffix *-plestim* is used for interleukin 3 (IL-3) factors classified as pleiotropic colony-stimulating factors, e.g.,
muplestim
daniplestim

(5) The suffix *-distim* is used for conjugates of two different types of colony-stimulating factors, e.g.,
milodistim

(6) The suffix *-cestim* is used for stem cell stimulating factors, e.g., ancestim.

Erythropoietins

The word *epoetin* is used for recombinant human erythropoietin, followed by the appropriate Greek letter (spelled out). "Epoetin" describes erythropoietin preparations that have an amino acid sequence identical to the endogenous cytokine; the words alfa, beta, gamma, etc. are added to designate preparations that differ in the composition and the nature of the carbohydrate moieties. Erythropoietins assigned a USAN are:

epoetin alfa
epoetin beta
epoetin gamma

Monoclonal Antibodies

The following guidelines have been developed for monoclonal antibodies:

(1) The suffix -*mab* is used for monoclonal antibodies and fragments.

(2) Identification of the animal source of the product is an important safety factor based on the number of products that may cause source-specific antibodies to develop in patients. The following letters were approved as product source identifiers:

u = human   e = hamster
o = mouse   i = primate
a = rat   xi = chimera
zu = humanized

These identifiers are used as infixes preceding the -*mab* suffix stem, e.g.,

-umab (human)
-omab (mouse)
-ximab (chimera)
-zumab (humanized)

(3) The general disease state subclass must be incorporated into the name by use of a code syllable. The following disease state subclasses were approved based on products currently before the Council. Additional subclasses will be added as necessary.

Disease or Target Class:
Viral   -vir-
Bacterial   -bac-
Immune   -lim-
Infectious Lesions   -les-
Tumors
colon   -col-
melanoma   -mel-
mammary   -mar-
testis   -got-
ovary   -gov-
prostate   -pr(o)-
miscellaneous   -tum-

(4) In order to create a unique name, a distinct, compatible syllable should be selected as the starting prefix.

(5) Sequence of stems. The order for combining the key elements is as follows: Infix representing the target disease state, the source of the product, the monoclonal root -*mab* used as a suffix (e.g., bi*ciromab*, sa*tumomab*, ne*bacumab*, se*virumab*, tu*virumab*). When combining a target or disease infix stem with the source stem for chimeric monoclonal antibody, the last consonant of the target/disease syllable is dropped, e.g.:

target	source	-mab stem	USAN
-cir-	-xi	-mab	abciximab
-lim-	-zu	-mab	daclizumab

These modifications were deemed necessary to facilitate pronunciation of the resultant designation.

(6) If the product is radiolabeled or conjugated to another chemical such as a toxin, identification of this conjugate is accomplished by use of a separate, second word or other acceptable chemical designation. For monoclonals conjugated to a toxin, the "-*tox*" stem must be included as part of the name selected for the toxin (e.g., zolimomab *aritox*, the designation *aritox* was selected to identify ricin A-chain). For radiolabeled products, the word order is: name of the isotope, element symbol, isotope number, and name of the monoclonal antibody: e.g., *technetium Tc 99m biciromab indium In 111 altumomab pentetate*.

(7) A separate, distinct name must be assigned to any linker/chelator used to conjugate the monoclonal antibody to a toxin, isotope, or for pegylated monoclonal antibodies, e.g.,

telimomab aritox
indium In 111 satumomab pendetide
enlimomab pegol

For the USAN Council to initiate the selection of a nonproprietary name for a monoclonal antibody or fragment, the nomenclature application must provide the following relevant information:

(1) The immunoglobulin class and subclass and the type of associated light chain.

(2) Identity of the fragment of the immunoglobulin used (if applicable).

(3) Species source from which the coding region for the immunoglobulin originated and specific, complete origin of all parts of chimeric, humanized, or semisynthetic immunoglobulins.

(4) The antigen specificity of the immunoglobulin, including its source.

(5) The clone designation (specify if vector or vector-cell combination).

(6) For conjugated monoclonal antibodies, the identity of any linkers, chelators, toxins, and/or isotopes present in the product.

(7) Identity of other modifications to the antibody, e.g., reduction of disulfide bonds, glycosylation or deglycosylation, amino acid modification, or substitution.

List of Stems Used by the USAN Council

This list represents common stems for which chemical and/or pharmacologic parameters have been established. These stems and their definitions have been approved by the USAN Council and are recommended for use in coining new nonproprietary names for drugs that belong to an established series of related agents. The list is not exhaustive in that it does not include all stems used by the Council and other national or international nomenclature groups. It is the nature of the nomenclature process that new, potential stems are constantly being created and that definitions of older stems may need to be modified as new information becomes available. (Updated July 2008)

Stem	Definition	Examples
-abine	(see -arabine, -citabine)	
-ac	anti-inflammatory agents (acetic acid derivatives)	bromfen*ac*, dexpemedol*ac*
-acetam	(see -racetam)	
-actide	synthetic corticotropins	ser*actide*
-adol or -adol-	analgesics (mixed opiate receptor agonists/antagonists)	taz*adol*ene, spir*adol*ene, levonantr*adol*
-adox	antibacterials (quinoline dioxide derivatives)	carb*adox*
-afenone	antiarrhythmics (propafenone derivatives)	alpr*afenone*, dipr*afenone*x
-afil	PDE5 inhibitors	tadal*afil*
-aj-	antiarrhythmics (ajmaline derivatives)	lor*aj*mine
-aldrate	antacid aluminum salts	mag*aldrate*
-algron	alpha$_1$ and alpha$_2$-adrenoreceptor agonists	dabuz*algron*
-alol	combined alpha and beta blockers	labet*alol*, medrox*alol*
-amivir	(see -vir)	
-ampa	ionotropic non-NMDA glutamate receptors (AMPA and/or KA receptors)	
-ampanel	antagonists	bec*ampanel*
-ampator	modulators	for*ampator*
-andr-	androgens	n*andr*olone
-anib	angiogenesis inhibitors	semax*anib*
-anserin	serotonin 5-HT$_2$ receptor antagonists	alt*anserin*, trop*anserin*, adat*anserin*
-antel	anthelmintics (undefined group)	carb*antel*
-antrone	antineoplastics; anthraquinone derivatives	pix*antrone*
-apsel	P-selectin antagonists	tor*apsel*
-arabine	antineoplastics (arabinofuranosyl derivatives)	faz*arabine*, flud*arabine*
aril-, -aril, -aril-	antiviral (arildone derivatives)	plecon*aril*, *aril*done, fos*aril*ate
-arit	antirheumatics (lobenzarit type)	lobenz*arit*, clobuz*arit*
-arol	anticoagulants (dicumarol type)	dicum*arol*
-arone	antiarrhythmics	amiod*arone*, droned*arone*
-arot-	arotinoids	et*arot*ene, sum*arot*ene, taz*arot*ene
-arotene	arotinoid derivatives	bex*arotene*, lin*arotene*, taz*arotene*
arte-	antimalarials (artemisin derivatives)	*arte*flene
-ase	enzymes	algluce*rase*, dor*nase* alfa
subgroup:		
-dismase	superoxide dismutase activity (exception: orgotein)	su*dismase*
-teplase	tissue-type plasminogen activators	al*teplase*, du*teplase*, sil*teplase*
-uplase	urokinase-type plasminogen activators	sar*uplase*, nasar*uplase*

Stem	Definition	Examples
-ast	antiasthmatics/antiallergics (not acting primarily as antihistamines; leukotriene biosynthesis inhibitors)	
subgroup:		
-lukast	leukotriene receptor antagonists	cina*lukast*, pobi*lukast*
-milast	type IV phosphodiesterase inhibitors	picla*milast*
-trodast	thromboxane A$_2$ receptor antagonists	sera*trodast*
-zolast	benzoxazole derivatives	ecla*zolast*, onta*zolast*
-tegr-	integrin antagonists	vala*tegr*ast
-(a)tadine	tricyclic histaminic-H$_1$ receptor antagonists, loratadine derivatives	deslor*atadine*, rup*atadine*, soman*tadine*
-astine	antihistaminics (histamine H$_1$ receptor antagonists)	eb*astine*
-atadine	tricyclic antiasthmatics	olop*atadine*, lor*atadine*
-axine	antianxiety, antidepressant inhibitor of norepinephrine and dopamine re-uptake	
-(f)axine		rad*faxine*
-azenil	benzodiazepine receptor agonists/antagonists	bret*azenil*, flum*azenil*
-azepam	antianxiety agents (diazepam type)	lor*azepam*
-azepide	cholecystokinin receptor antagonists	dev*azepide*
-azocine	narcotic antagonists/agonists (6,7-benzomorphan derivatives)	quad*azocine*, ket*azocine*
-azoline	antihistamines/local vasoconstrictors (antazoline type)	ant*azoline*
-azosin	antihypertensives (prazosin type)	dox*azosin*
-bactam	beta-lactamase inhibitors	sul*bactam*
-bamate	tranquilizers/antiepileptics (propanediol and pentanediol groups)	mepro*bamate*, fel*bamate*
-barb or -barb-	barbituric acid derivatives	pheno*barb*ital, seco*barb*ital, etero*barb*
-begron	beta 3 adrenoreceptor agonist	tali*begron*
-bendazole	anthelmintics (tibendazole type)	cam*bendazole*
-berel	beta estrogen receptor agonist	prina*berel*
-bersat	anticonvulsants; antimigraine (benzoylamino-benzpyran derivatives)	cara*bersat*, tidem*bersat*
bol- or -bol-	anabolic steroids	*bol*andiol, mi*bol*erone
-bufen	non-steroidal anti-inflammatory agents, fenbufen derivatives	indo*bufen*
-bulin	antineoplastics (mitotic inhibitors; tubulin binders)	mivo*bulin*
-butan	antiseptics (dapabutan type)	dapa*butan*, lopo*butan*
-butazone	anti-inflammatory analgesics (phenylbutazone type)	mofe*butazone*

Stem	Definition	Examples
-caine	local anesthetics	dibucaine
calci- or -calci-	vitamin D analogues	calcipotriene tacalcitol
-camra	antivirals (intracellular adhesion molecules, icam-1 derivatives)	tremacamra
-camsule	camphorsulfonic acid derivatives used as UVA sunscreens	ecamsule
-capoc	agonists of the Gardos channel, or the calcium activated potassium channel of intermediate conductance	senicapoc
-carbef	antibiotics (carbacephem derivatives)	loracarbef
-casan	caspase (interleukin $-1b$) converting enzyme inhibitors	pralnacasan
-caserin	serotonin receptor agonists, primarily 5-HT$_2$	lorcaserin vabicaserin
-castat	(see -stat)	
-catib	cathespin inhibitors	balicatib
-cavir	(see -vir)	
cef-	cephalosporins	cefazolin
-cept	receptor molecules, native or modified (a preceding infix should designate the target) subgroups:	alvircept
-co-	complement receptors	micrococept
-facept	lymphocyte function-associated with antigen 3 (LFA) receptor	alefacept
-farcept	interferon receptors	pifarcept
-lefacept	lymphocyte function-associated antigen 3	alefacept
-nercept	tumor necrosis factor receptors	lenercept
-tacept	cytotoxic T lymphocyte-associated antigen 4 (CTLA-4)	belatacept
-vircept	antiviral receptors	alvircept
-cet	receptors (small molecule) subgroup:	
-calcet	calcium	tecalcet
-cetrapib	cholesterol ester transfer protein inhibitors	torcetrapib
-cic	hepatoprotectives (timonacic type)	limazocic
-ciclib	cyclin dependent kinase inhibitors	seliciclib
-ciclovir	(see -vir)	
-cidib	cyclin dependent kinase inhibitor	alvocidib
-cidin	natural antibiotics (undefined group)	gramicidin
-ciguat	guanaline cyclase activator	ataciguat atriciguat
-cillin	penicillins	ampicillin
-citabine	nucleoside antiviral or antineoplastic agents, cytarabine or azarabine derivatives	gemcitabine fiacitabine zalcitabine
-clidine	muscarinic agonists (various indications)	vedaclidine talsaclidine
-clomol	heat-shock protein inducers (bimoclomal type)	elescomol

Stem	Definition	Examples
-clone	hypnotics/tranquilizers (zopiclone type)	pagoclone
-cog	blood coagulation factors subgroups:	
-eptacog	blood coagulation factor VII	eptacog alfa (activated)
-nonacog	blood coagulation factor IX	nonacog alfa
-octocog	blood coagulation factor VIII	moroctocog alfa octocog alfa
-cogin	blood coagulation cascade inhibitor	tifacogin
-conazole	systemic antifungals (miconazole type)	fluconazole oxiconazole
-cort-	cortisone derivatives	hydrocortisone
-coxib	cyclooxygenase-2 inhibitors	celecoxib parecoxib valdecoxib
-cridar	(see -dar)	
-crinat	diuretics (ethacrynic acid derivatives)	brocrinat
-crine	acridine derivatives	amsacrine quinacrine
-cromil	antiallergics (cromoglicic acid derivatives)	nedocromil
-curium	neuromuscular blocking agents (quaternary) (also ammonium compounds)	atracurium
-curonium		alcuronium pipecuronium
-cycline	antibiotics (tetracycline derivatives)	minocycline
-dan	positive inotropic agents (pimobendan type)	prinoxodan indolidan
-dapsone	antimycobacterials (diaminodiphenylsulfone derivatives)	acedapsone
-dar	multidrug resistance inhibitors subgroups:	
-cridar	acridine carboxamide derivatives	elacridar
-icodar	pipecolic acid derivatives	biricodar
-quidar	qunioline derivatives	lamiquidar zozuquidar
-spodar	ciclosporin D derivatives	valspodar
-denoson	adenosine A receptor agonists	tecadenoson binodenoson
-depsin	depsipeptide derivatives	romidepsin
-dermin	(see -ermin)	
dil-, -dil- or -dil	vasodilators (undefined group)	fostedil
-dipine	phenylpyridine vasodilators (nifedipine type)	darodipine felodipine
-dismase	(see -ase)	
-distim	(see -stim)	
-ditan	antimigraine (5-HT$_1$ receptor agonists)	alniditan
-dopa	dopamine receptor agonists	levodopa
-dore	dopamine D$_2$D$_3$ receptor modulators	aplindore fumarate
-dotin	synthetic analogs of the dolastatin series	tasidotin HCl
-dralazine	antihypertensives (hydrazine-phthalazines)	hydralazine endralazine

Stem	Definition	Examples
-dronate	calcium metabolism regulators	etidronate, tiludronate
-dutant	(see -tant)	
-ectedin	ecteinascodin derivatives	monectedin
-ectin	antiparasitics (ivermectin type)	doramectin, moxidectin
-elestat	(see -stat)	
-elvakin	(see -kin)	
-emcinal	erythromycin derivatives lacking antibiotic activity	mitemcinal
-entan	endothelin receptor antagonists	bosentan
-eptacog	(see -cog)	
-eptakin	(see -kin)	
-erg-	ergot alkaloid derivatives	pergolide
-eridine	analgesics (meperidine type)	anileridine
-ermin	growth factors subgroups:	
-bermin	vascular endothelial growth factors	telbermin
-dermin	epidermal growth factors	murodermin
-fermin	fibroblast growth factors	ersofermin
-nermin	tumor necrosis factors	sonermin, tasonermin
-plermin	platelet derived growth factors	becaplermin
-sermin	insulin-like growth factors	mecasermin
-termin	transforming growth factors	cetermin
-otermin	bone morphogenetic proteins	dibotermin alfa
estr- or -estr-	estrogens	estrone fenestrel
-estrant	estrogen antagonists	fulvestrant
-etanide	diuretics (piretanide type)	bumetanide
-exakin	(see -kin)	
-ezolid	oxazolidinone antibacterials	eperezolid, linezolid
-farnib	farnesyl transferase inhibitor	tipifarnib
-fenamate	"fenamic acid" ester or salt derivatives	etofenamate
-fenamic acid	anti-inflammatory agents (anthranilic acid derivatives)	flufenamic acid
-fenin	diagnostic aids [(phenylcarbamoyl)methyl iminodiacetic acid derivatives]	arclofenin
-fenine	analgesics (fenamic acid subgroup)	floctafenine
-fentanil	narcotic analgesics (fentanyl derivatives)	alfentanil, mirfentanil, brifentanil
-fentrine	phosphodiesterase inhibitor	pumafentrine
-fermin	(see -ermin)	
-fetamin(e)	amfetamine derivatives	levmetamfetamine
-fiban	fibrinogen receptor antagonists (glycoprotein IIb/ IIIa receptor antagonist)	lamifiban, tirofiban
-fibatide	(see -tide)	
-fibrate	antihyperlipidemics (clofibrate type)	bezafibrate
-filcon	hydrophilic contact lens materials	alphafilcon A, xylofilcon A, mipafilcon A
-fingol	sphingosine derivatives	cedefingol, safingol
-flapon	5-lipoxygenase-activating protein (FLAP) inhibitors	quiflapon

Stem	Definition	Examples
-flurane	general inhalation anesthetics (halogenated alkane derivatives)	enflurane
-fo-	phosphoro-derivatives	adefovir
-focon	hydrophobic contact lens materials	trifocon A, pasifocon B, satafocon A
-formin	hypoglycemics (phenformin type)	buformin
-fosfamide	isophosphoramide mustard derivatives	palifosfamide
-fradil	calcium channel blockers acting as vasodilators	mibefradil
-fulven	antineoplastic, acylfulven derivatives	viridofulven
-fungin	antifungal antibiotics (undefined group)	kalafungin
-fylline	theophylline derivatives	enprofylline, bamifylline, cipamfylline
-gab-	gabamimetics	fengabine
gado-	gadolinium derivatives (principally for diagnostic use)	gadodiamide, gadoteridol, gadobenate
-gapil	neuronal apoptosis inhibitors; GAPDH	omigapil
-ganan	antimicrobial, bactericidal permeability increasing polypeptide	iseganan, pexiganan
-gatran	thrombin inhibitors (argatroban type)	efegatran
-gest-	progestins	megestrol
-giline	MAO inhibitors, type B	selegiline
-gillin	antibiotics (*Aspergillus* strains)	mitogillin
gli-	antihypoglycemics	gliflumide
-gliflozin	phlorozin derivatives, phenolic glycosides	sergliflozin
-glinide	antidiabetic, SGLT2 inhibitors, not phlorozin derivatives	repaglinide, mitiglinide
-gliptin	dipeptidyl aminopeptidase-IV inhibitors	vildagliptin
-glitazar	PPAR agonists (not thiazolidene derivatives)	farglitazar
-glitazone	PPST agonists (thiazolidene derivatives)	ciglitazone, rosiglitazone
-glumide	CCK antagonists, antiulcer, anxiolytic agent	amiglumide, itriglumide
-golix	GnRH receptor antagonists (nonpeptide)	rupugolixo
-gosivir	(see -vir)	
-gramostim	(see -stim)	
-grastim	(see -stim)	
-grel- or -grel	platelet aggregation inhibitors (undefined group)	itazigrel, dimetagrel, furegrelate
guan-	antihypertensives (guanidine derivatives)	guanoctine
-ibat	ileal bile acid transport inhibitor	barixibat
-icam	anti-inflammatory agents (isoxicam type)	enolicam, tenoxicam
-icodar	(see -dar)	

Stem	Definition	Examples
-ifen(e)	antiestrogens of the clomifene and tamoxifen groups	nitrom*ifene* ralox*ifene* drolox*ifene*
-ilide	class III antiarrhythmic agents	ibut*ilide* risot*ilide* dofet*ilide*
-imepodib	inosine monophosphate dehydrogenase inhibitors	mer*imepodib*
-imex	immunostimulants	forfen*imex* roquin*imex* uben*imex*
-imibe-	antihyperlipidaemics, acyl CoA: cholesterol acyltransferase (ACAT) inhibitors	eldac*imibe* avas*imibe* pact*imibe*
-imod	immunomodulators	ivar*imod* pidot*imod*
	subgroup:	
-mapimod	mitogen-activated protein (MAP) kinase inhibitors	dorm*apimod*
-imus	immunosuppressives	tacrol*imus* napir*imus* gusper*imus*
	subgroup:	
-rolimus	immunosuppressant, rapamycin derivatives	sirol*imus*
io-	iodine-containing contrast media	*io*damide
-irudin	anticoagulants (hirudin type)	des*irudin*
-isant	histamine H3 receptor antagonists	cipral*isant*
-isomide	antiarrhythmics (disopyramide derivatives)	bid*isomide*
-ium (also -onium)	quaternary ammonium derivatives	clidin*ium* disiqu*onium* polixet*onium*
-ixafor	CXCR4 antagonists	pler*ixafor*
-kacin	antibiotics obtained from *Streptomyces kanamyceticus* (related to kanamycin)	ami*kacin*
-kalant	potassium channel antagonists	almo*kalant* teri*kalant*
-kalim	potassium channel agonists	croma*kalim* apri*kalim*
-kalner	opener of large conductance calcium-activated (maxi-k) K+ channels	flindo*kalner*
-kef-	enkephalin agonists (various indications)	met*keph*amidc caso*kef*amide
-kin	interleukin type substances	
	subgroups:	
-decakin	interleukin-10 analogues and derivatives	ilo*decakin*
-dodekin	interleukin-12 analogues and derivatives	e*dodekin* alfa
-elvekin	interleukin-11 analogues and derivatives	opr*elvekin*
-enicokin	interleukin-21 analogues and derivatives	den*enicokin*
-eptakin	interleukin-7 analogues and derivatives	
-exakin	interleukin-6 analogues and derivatives	at*exakin* alfa
-leukin	interleukin-2 analogues and derivatives	tec*eleukin* aldes*leukin*

Stem	Definition	Examples
-nakin	interleukin-1 analogues and derivatives	
	subgroups:	
-onakin	interleukin 1-α analogues and derivatives	pit*onakin*
-benakin	interleukin 1-β analogues and derivatives	mo*benakin*
-nonakin	interleukin-9 analogues and derivatives	
-octakin	interleukin-8 analogues and derivatives	em*octakin*
-penkin	interleukin-5 analogues and derivatives	
-trakin	interleukin-4 analogues and derivatives	bine*trakin*
-kinra	interleukin receptor antagonists	
	subgroups:	
-nakinra	interleukin 1 (IL-1) receptor antagonists	a*nakinra*
-kiren	renin inhibitors	dite*kiren* terla*kiren* zan*kiren*
-lazad	lipid peroxidation inhibitors	tiri*lazad*
-leptin	leptin derivatives	metre*leptin*
-leukin	(see -kin)	
-lipim	lipoprotein lipase activators	ibro*lipim*
-locib	antineoplastics that inhibit the formation of 5-LO, LTB$_4$, LTC$_4$, and thromboxane B$_2$ (TxB$_2$); and Activate PPARγ nuclear receptors	eta*locib*
-locib	antineoplastics that inhibit the formation of 5-LO, LTB$_4$, LTC$_4$, and trhomboxane B$_2$ (TxB$_2$); and Activate PPARγ nuclear receptors	eta*locib*
-lubant	leukotriene receptor antagonists (treatment of inflammatory skin disorders)	tico*lubant*
-lukast	(see -ast)	
-luren	inducers of ribosomal readthrough of nonsense mutation in mRNA stop codons	ata*luren*
-lutamide	antiandrogens	bica*lutamide* *flutamide*
-lutril	neutral endopeptidase inhibitors possessing additional endothelin converting enzyme inhibitory activity	dag*lutril*
-mab	monoclonal antibodies	imciro*mab* abcixi*mab* capro*mab* daclixi*mab* detumo*mab* enlimo*mab*
	subgroup:	
-axo-	rat-murine hybrid antibodies	
-les-	infix for inflammatory/infectious lesions	
-neu(r)-	nervous system	bapin*euzumab*
-os-	bone	den*osumab*
-toxa-	toxin as a target	ur*toxazumab*
-mantadine or -mantine	antivirals/antiparkinsonians (adamantane derivatives)	ri*mantadine* dopa*mantine*
-mastat	(see -stat)	

Stem	Definition	Examples
-meline	cholinergic agonists (arecoline derivatives used in treatment of Alzheimer's disease)	xano*meline*
-melteon	selective melatonin receptor agonist	ra*melteon*
-mer	polymers	cadex*omer* carbeti*mer*
-mesine	sigma receptor ligands	ig*mesine* pana*mesine*
-mestane	antineoplastics (aromatase inhibitors)	plo*mestane*
-metacin	anti-inflammatory agents (indomethacin type)	zido*metacin*
-micin	antibiotics (*Micromonospora* strains)	madura*micin* genta*micin*
-monam	monobactam antibiotics	gloxi*monam* oxi*monam* tige*monam*
-morelin	(see -relin)	
-moren	non-peptidic growth hormone secretagogues	ibuta*moren*
-mostim	(see -stim)	
-motine	antivirals (quinoline derivatives)	fa*motine*
-moxin	monoamine oxidase inhibitors (hydrazine derivatives)	ben*moxin* do*moxin*
-mulin	antibacterials, pleuromulin derivatives	retapa*mulin*
-multin	mucosal tolerance inductors	ismo*multin*
-mustine	antineoplastics (chloroethylamine derivatives)	car*mustine*
-mycin	antibiotics (*Streptomyces* strains)	linco*mycin*
nab- or -nab-	cannabinol derivatives	*nab*azenil dro*nab*inol
-nakalant	mixed sodium/potassium channel blockers	ver*nakalant*
-nakin	(see -kin)	
nal-	narcotic agonists/antagonists (normorphine type)	*nal*mefene
-navir	(see vir-)	
-nercept	(see -cept)	
-nermin	(see -ermin)	
-nertant	neurotensin receptor antagonists	remi*nertant*
-nesib	kinesin inhibitors	isp*inesib*
-netant	(see -tant)	
-neurin	neurotensin receptor antagonists; neurotropins	abri*neurin*
-nicline	nicotinic acetylcholine receptor partial agonists/agonists	alti*nicline*
-nidap	nonsteroidal anti-inflammatory agents (tenidap type)	ilo*nidap* te*nidap*
-nidazole	antiprotozoal substances (metronidazole type)	ti*nidazole*
nifur-	5-nitrofuran derivatives	*nifur*atel *nifur*atrone
-nil	benzodiazepine receptor antagonists/agonists subgroup:	
-punil	mitochondrial benzodiazepine receptor (MBR) selective, partial, or inverse agonists (purine derivatives)	ema*punil*
-quinil	benzodiazepine receptor agonists, also partial or inverse (quinoline derivatives)	lire*quinil*
-nixin	anti-inflammatory agents (anilinonicotinic acid derivatives)	clo*nixin*
-nonacog	(see -cog)	
-nonakin	(see -kin)	
-octacog	(see -cog)	
-octakin	(see -kin)	
-olol	beta-blockers (propranolol type)	tim*olol* aten*olol*
-olone	steroids (*not* prednisolone derivatives)	minax*olone*
-onide	topical steroids (acetal derivatives)	amcin*onide*
-opilone	epothilone	fil*opilone*
-orex	anorexians	flud*orex*
-orphan	narcotic antagonists/agonists (morphinan derivatives)	dextro meth*orphan* dextr*orphan*
-osuran	urotensin receptor antagonists	pal*osuran*
-otilate	hepatoprotectants, di-isopropyl-1,3-dithiol-malonate derivatives	miv*otilate*
-oxacin	antibacterials (quinolone derivatives)	diflo*xacin* ciproflo*xacin*
-oxan	alpha-adrenoceptor antagonists (benzodioxane derivatives)	imil*oxan*
-oxanide	antiparasitics (salicylanilide derivatives)	brom*oxanide*
-oxef	antibiotics (oxacefalosporanic acid derivatives)	flom*oxef*
-oxetine	antidepressants (fluoxetine type)	dap*oxetine* sepr*oxetine*
-oxin	fluoroquinolone derivatives, nonantibacterial indications (e.g. antineoplastic antibiotics)	vorel*oxin*
-pafant	platelet-activating factor antagonists	apa*fant* daco*pafant* tulo*pafant* lexi*pafant*
-pamide	diuretics (sulfamoylbenzoic acid derivatives)	ali*pamide*
-pamil	coronary vasodilators (verapamil type)	tia*pamil*
-pamine	dopaminergics (butopamine type)	foso*pamine* ibo*pamine*
-panel	AMPA receptor antagonists	fana*panel* irum*panel* talam*panel*
-parcil	antithrombotics	beci*parcil* ili*parcil*
-parcin	glycopeptide antibiotics	avo*parcin*
-parib	poly-ADP-ribose polymerase inhibitors	ola*parib*
-parin	heparin derivatives and low molecular weight (or depolymerized) heparins	he*parin* tinza*parin* dalte*parin*
-parinux	antithrombotic indirect selective synthetic factor Xa inhibitors	fonda*parinux*

Stem	Definition	Examples
-paroid	antithrombotics (heparinoid type)	dana*paroid* sul*paroid*
-peg	PEGylated compounds	*peg*caristim *peg*nartograstim *peg*visomant
-penem	antibacterial antibiotics (carbapenem derivatives)	imi*penem*
-penkin	(see -kin)	
perflu-	blood substitutes and/or diagnostics (perfluorochemicals)	*perflu*bron *perflu*nafene
-peridol	antipsychotics (haloperidol type)	halo*peridol*
-peridone	antipsychotics (risperidone type)	ris*peridone* ilo*peridone* oca*peridone*
-perit	neuropeptide Y receptor modulators	velne*perit*
-neperit	neuropeptide Y5	
-perone	antianxiety agents/neuroleptics (4'-fluoro-4-piperidinobutyrophenone derivatives)	duo*perone*
-pezil	acetylcholinesterase inhibitors used in the treatment of Alzheimer's disease	ico*pezil* done*pezil*
-pidem	hypnotics/sedatives (zolpidem type)	zol*pidem* al*pidem*
-pirdine	cognition enhancers	lino*pirdine* besi*pirdine* sibo*pirdine*
-pirox	antimycotics (pyridone derivatives)	ciclo*pirox*
-pitant	(see -tant)	
-plact	platelet factor 4 analogs and derivatives	iro*plact*
-pladib	phospholipase A2 inhibitors	eco*pladib*
-planin	antibacterials (*Actinoplanes* strains)	mide*planin* ramo*planin* teico*planin*
-platin	antineoplastics (platinum derivatives)	cis*platin*
-plasinin	inhibitors of plasminogen activator inhibitors—type 1	ti*plasinin*
-plermin	(see -ermin)	
-plestim	(see -stim)	
-plon	non-benzodiazepine anxiolytics, sedatives, hypnotics	ocina*plon* zale*plon*
-poetin	erythropoietins	*epoetin* alfa *epoetin* beta
-porfin	benzoporphyrin derivatives	verte*porfin* temo*porfin*
-pramine	antidepressants (imipramine type)	lofe*pramine*
-prazan	acid pump inhibitors, not dependent on acid activation	omida*prazan*
-prazole	antiulcer agents (benzimidazole derivatives) subgroup:	ome*prazole* disu*prazole*
-maprazole	acid pump inhibitors	pu*maprazole*
pred-, -pred- or -pred	prednisone and prednisolone derivatives	*pred*nicarbate clo*pred*nol oxiso*pred*
-pressin	vasoconstrictors (vasopressin derivatives)	desmo*pressin*

Stem	Definition	Examples
-pride	sulpiride derivatives	remoxi*pride* zaco*pride*
-pril	antihypertensives (ACE inhibitors)	enala*pril* temoca*pril* spira*pril*
-prilat	antihypertensives (ACE inhibitors) (diacid analogs of the -pril entity)	enala*prilat* spira*prilat*
-prim	antibacterials (trimethoprim type)	ormeto*prim*
-prinim	nootropic agents, purine derivatives	lete*prinim*
-prisnil	selective progesterone receptor modulators (SPRM)	aso*prisnil*
-pristin	antibacterials, pristinamycin derivatives	quinu*pristin* efe*pristin*
-pristone	progesterone receptor antagonists	mife*pristone*
-profen	anti-inflammatory/analgesic agents (ibuprofen type)	flurbi*profen*
-proget	nonsteroidal ligand for the progesterone receptor	tana*proget*
-prost- or -prost	prostaglandin derivatives	rio*prost*il dino*prost*
-protafib	protein tyrosine phosphatase 1B inhibitors	erti*protafib*
-pultide	(see -tide)	
-queside	cholesterol sequestrants (glycosides)	pama*queside*
-racetam	nootropes (piracetam type)	pi*racetam*
-racil	uracil type antineoplastics	enilu*racil* gemer*acil* oter*acil*
-rafenib	Raf kinase inhibitors	sor*afenib*
-relin	prehormones or hormone-release stimulating peptides subgroups:	nafa*relin*
-morelin	growth hormone-release stimulating peptides	du*morelin*
-tirelin	thyrotropin releasing hormone analogues	pro*tirelin*
-relix	hormone-release inhibiting peptides	deti*relix*
-renone	aldosterone antagonists (spironolactone type)	can*renone*
-restat	(see -stat)	
-retin- or -retin	retinol derivatives	etr*etinate* pel*retin*
-rev	therapeutic virus	
-tucirev	tumoricidal	lon*tucirev*
-ribine	ribofuranil derivatives (pyrazofurin type)	loxo*ribine*
rifa-	antibiotics (rifamycin derivatives)	*rifa*pentine *rifa*mpin
-rinone	cardiotonics (amrinone type)	mil*rinone*
-rozole	aromatase inhibitors (imidazole/triazole derivatives)	let*rozole* fad*rozole* tala*rozole* vo*rozole*
-rsen	antisense oligonucleotides	alicafo*rsen*
-rubicin	antineoplastic antibiotics (daunorubicin type)	eso*rubicin* ida*rubicin*
sal-, -sal- or -sal	anti-inflammatory agents (salicylic acid derivatives)	me*sal*amine difluni*sal* bal*sal*azide

Stem	Definition	Examples
-sartan	angiotensin II receptor antagonists	los*artan* epro*sartan*
-semide	diuretics (furosemide type)	azo*semide*
-sermin	(see -ermin)	
-serod	serotonin receptor antagonists and partial agonists	pibo*serod*
-serpine	*Rauwolfia* alkaloid derivatives	re*serpine*
-setron	serotonin 5-HT₃ antagonists	ondan*setron* grani*setron* luro*setron*
-siban	oxytocin antagonists	baru*siban*
-sidomine	antianginals (sydnone derivatives)	pir*sidomine* mol*sidomine* lin*sidomine*
som-	growth hormone derivatives	*som*atrem *som*atropin
som- -bove	bovine somatotropin derivatives	*som*etri*bove*
som- -por	porcine somatotropin derivatives	*som*etri*por* *som* agre*por*
-sonan	5-HT₁ᵦ receptor antagonists	elza*sonan*
-spirone	anxiolytics (buspirone type)	zalo*spirone* tio*spirone*
-spodar	(see -dar)	
-sporin	immunosuppressants (cyclosporine type)	gecle*sporin* oxeclo*sporin*
-stat or -stat-	enzyme inhibitors subgroups:	
-castat	dopamine β-hydrolase (DBH) inhibitors	nepi*castat*
-elestat	elastase inhibitors	sive*lestat*
-inostat	inhibitors of histone deacetylase	daci*nostat*
-listat	gastrointestinal lipase inhibitors)	ceti*listat*
-mastat	antineoplastics (matrix metalloproteinase inhibitors)	bati*mastat*
-(a)mostat	proteolytic enzyme inhibitors	nafa*mostat*
-restat- or -restat	aldose-reductase inhibitors	ponal*restat* tol*restat*
-vastatin	antihyperlipidemics (HMG-CoA inhibitors) (other series members)	ator*vastatin* lo*vastatin* pra*vastatin*
	urease inhibitor	ben*urestat*
	renal dehydropeptidase inhibitor	cila*statin*
	pepsin inhibitor	pep*statin*
-ster-	steroids (androgens, anabolics)	testo*sterone*
-steride	testosterone reductase inhibitors	epri*steride* fena*steride*
-stigmine	cholinesterase inhibitors (physostigmine type)	quilo*stigmine* teser*stigmine*
-stim	colony-stimulating factors subgroups:	
-distim	conjugates of two different types of colony-stimulating factors	milo*distim*
-gramo- stim	granulocyte macrophage colony-stimulating factors (GM-CSF)	mol*gramostim* re*gramostim* sar*gramostim* eco*gramostim*
-grastim	granulocyte colony-stimulating factors (G-CSF)	fil*grastim* leno*grastim*
-mostim	macrophage colony-stimulating factors (M-CSF)	miri*mostim*
-plestim	interleukin-3 derivatives; pleiotropic colony-stimulating factors	dani*plestim*
-stinel	(*N*-methyl-ᴅ-asparate) NMDA receptor antagonists (glycine recognition site)	lico*stinel*
-sulam	antineoplastics, apoptosis inducing sulfonamide	indi*sulam*
sulfa-	antimicrobials (sulfonamides derivatives)	*sulfa*salazine
-sulfan	antineoplastics, alkylating agents (methanesulfonate derivatives) subgroups:	bu*sulfan*
-lind	pro-apoptotic cGMP phosphodiesterase inhibitors	racta*lind*
-sulind	sulfone metabolite	exi*sulind* dracta*lind*
-tant	tachykinin (neurokinin) receptor antagonists subgroups:	
-dutant	NK₂ receptor antagonists	sare*dutant*
-netant	NK₃ receptor antagonists	osa*netant*
-pitant	NK₁ receptor antagonists	da*pitant* zina*pitant* lane*pitant*
-tapide	microsomal triglyceride transfer protein (MTP) inhibitors	impli*tapide*
-taxel	antineoplastics, taxane derivatives	pacli*taxel*
-tecan	antineoplastics (camptothecine derivatives)	topo*tecan* irino*tecan*
-tecarin	antineoplastics (rebeccamycin derivatives)	beca*tecarin*
-tepa	antineoplastics (thiotepa derivatives)	aze*tepa*
-teplase	(see -ase)	
-termin	(see -ermin)	
-terol	bronchodilators (phenethylamine derivatives)	albu*terol*
-tesind	thymidilate synthetase inhibitors (benzindole derivatives)	me*tesind*
-texafin	texaphryn derivatives	mo*texafin*
-thiazide	diuretics (thiazide derivatives)	chloro*thiazide*
-tiapine	antipsychotics (dibenzothiazepine derivatives)	qui*tiapine*
-tiazem	calcium channel blockers (diltiazem type)	dil*tiazem* clen*tiazem* ipro*tiazem*
-tibant	antiasthmatics (bradykinin antagonists)	ica*tibant*
-tide	peptides and glycopeptides subgroups:	octreo*tide*
-fibatide	platelet aggregation inhibitors (glycoprotein IIb/IIIa receptor antagonists)	epti*fibatide*
-murtide	peptides with muranic acid present	mifa*murtide*

Stem	Definition	Examples
-pultide	peptides used as pulmonary surfactants	sina*pultide*
-zotide	zonulin antagonists	lara*zotide*
-tidine	H_2-receptor antagonists (cimetidine type)	lupi*tidine* done*tidine* rani*tidine*
-tinib	tyrosine kinase inhibitors	caner*tinib* ima*tinib* mubri*tinib*
-tirelin	(see -relin)	
-tirome	antihyperlidaemic, thyromimetic derivatives	anti*tirome* axi*tirome* sobe*tirome*
-tocin	oxytocin derivatives	oxy*tocin*
-toclax	antineoplastic, BLC-2 inhibitor	oba*toclax*
-toin	antiepileptics (hydantoin derivatives)	albu*toin*
-toran	TLR4 receptor antagonists	eri*toran*
-tox(a)-	toxins	ur*toxa*zumab
-traposin	aP2 inhibitors	sel*traposin*
-trexate	antimetabolites (folic acid derivatives)	metho*trexate*
-trexed	antineoplastic thymidylate synthetase inhibitors	peme*trexed* rali*trexed* nola*trexed*
-tricin	antibiotics (polyene derivatives)	mepar*tricin*
-tril or -trilat	endopeptidase inhibitors	candoxa*tril* candoxa*trilat*
-triptan	antimigraine agents (5-HT_1 receptor agonists)	nara*triptan* oxi*triptan* suma*triptan*
-triptyline	antidepressants (dibenzo[*a,d*]cycloheptane derivatives)	ami*triptyline*
-troban	antithrombotics (thromboxane A_2 receptor antagonists)	dal*troban* sulo*troban*
-trodast	(see -ast)	
-troline	antipsychotics (dopamine D_2 antagonists)	carvo*troline* gevo*troline*
-trombopag	thrombopoetin agonists	el*trombopag*
trop- or -trop-	atropine derivatives	benz*trop*ine
-uclin	mucosal tolerance inhibitors	
-uplase	(see -ase)	
-uracil	uracil derivatives used as thyroid antagonists and as antineoplastics	fluoro*uracil*
-(ur)amidine	pentamidine derivatives/analogues	pa*furamidine*
-uridine	antivirals; antineoplastics (uridine derivatives)	idox*uridine*
-vaptan	vasopressin receptor antagonists	coni*vaptan* relco*vaptan*
-vastatin	(see -stat)	
-verine	spasmolytic agents (papaverine type)	mebe*verine*

Stem	Definition	Examples
vin- or -vin-	vinca alkaloids	*vin*epidine apo*vin*camine
vir-, -vir- or -vir	antiviral substances (undefined group)	ganciclo*vir* en*vir*adine *vir*oxime al*vir*cept dela*vir*dine
	subgroups:	
-amivir	neuraminidase inhibitors	zan*amivir*
-cavir	carbocyclic nucleosides	lobu*cavir*
-ciclovir or -cyclovir	antivirals (acyclovir type)	des*ciclovir* fam*ciclovir* pen*ciclovir*
-gosivir	glucosidase inhibitor	cel*gosivir*
-navir	HIV protease inhibitors (saquinavir type)	droxi*navir* indi*navir* rito*navir*
-virdine	antivirals (non-nucleoside reverse transcriptase inhibitors; pyridine derivatives)	ate*virdine* dela*virdine*
-virenz	antivirals (non-nucleoside reverse transcriptase inhibitors; benzoxazinone derivatives)	efa*virenz*
-virsen	antivirals (antisense)	afo*virsen* fomi*virsen* treco*virsen*
-vircept	(see -cept)	
-virdine	(see vir)	
-virenz	(see vir)	
-virimat	antiviral, disrupts viral maturation	be*virimat*
-viroc	CCR5 antagonists	mara*viroc*
-criviroc	CCR5 antagonists, immunomodulators	an*criviroc*
-vudine	antineoplastics; antivirals (zidovudine group) (exception: edoxudine)	sta*vudine* lami*vudine* alo*vudine*
-xaban	antithrombotic: blood coagulation factor X^A inhibitors	tami*xaban*
-xanox	antiallergic respiratory tract drugs (xanoxic acid derivatives)	ti*xanox*
-(x)antrone	antineoplastics, mitoxantrone derivatives aza-anthracenedione class of antitumor agents	pix*antrone*
-zolamide	carbonic anhydrase inhibitors	brin*zolamide* dor*zolamide* se*zolamide*
-zolast	(see -ast)	
-zomib	proteozome inhibitors	borte*zomib*
-zotan	5-HT_{1A} receptor agonists/antagonists acting primarily as neuroprotectors	robal*zotan* sari*zotan* ibal*zotan* leco*zotan*

Organic Moieties, Counterions, and Solvent Molecules Used in Coining Two-Word Names

Note: names for carboxylic acid or sulfonate anions would also be applied to the parent acids or their esters.

Name Used	Chemical Name and/or Formula
acefurate	acetate ester and furan-2-carboxylate ester
acetate	acetate
acetonide	isopropylidenedioxy, or acetonide
aceturate	*N*-acetylglycinate
acistrate	acetate ester and stearate salt
acoxil	(acetyloxy)methyl
anisatil	2-(4-methoxyphenyl)-2-oxoethyl
arbamel	2-(dimethylamino)-2-oxoethyl
argine	$30^B\alpha$-L-arginine-$30^B\beta$-L-arginine —Arg—Arg
aspart	38^B-L-aspartic acid —Asp—
axetil	(*RS*)-1-(acetyloxy)ethyl
beloxil	benzyloxy
benzoate	benzoate
besylate INN: besilate	benzenesulfonate

Name Used	Chemical Name and/or Formula
betadex	β-cyclodextrin
bromide	Br^-
buciclate	*trans*-4-butylcyclohexanecarboxylate
butyrate INN: butirate	butyrate
calcium	Ca^{2+}
camsylate INN: camsilate	(1*S*)-(+)-(7,7-dimethyl-2-oxobicyclo[2.2.1]heptan-1-yl)methanesulfonate or (1*S*)-(+)-10-camphorsulfonate
caproate	hexanoate
chloride	Cl^-
cilexetil	(*RS*)-1-[[(cyclohexyloxy)carbonyl]oxy]ethyl
citrate	2-hydroxypropane-1,2,3-tricarboxylate
closylate INN: closilate	4-chlorobenzene-1-sulfonate
crosfumaril	(2*E*)-but-2-enedioyl
cyclotate INN: ciclotate	4-methylbicyclo[2.2.2]oct-2-ene-1-carboxylate

Name Used	Chemical Name and/or Formula
cypionate INN: cipionate	cyclopentane propionate 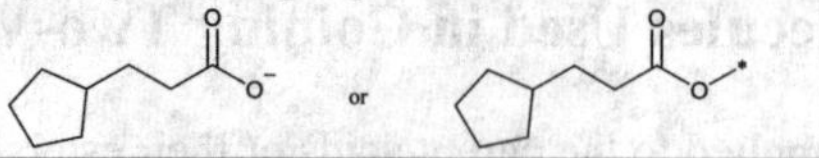
dapropate INN: daropate	*N,N*-dimethyl-β-alaninate or 3-(dimethylamino)propanoate 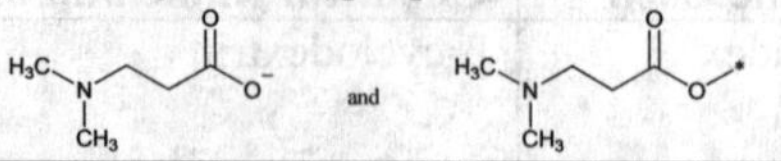
detemir	tetradecanoyl 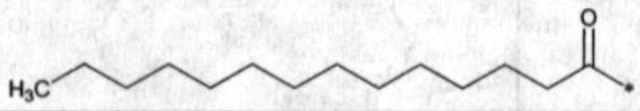
diftitox	*N*-L-methionyl-387-L-histidine-388-L-alanine-1-388-toxin (*Corynebacterium diptheriae* strain C7) (388→2')-protein
diolamine	2,2'-azanediyldiethanol or diethanolamine 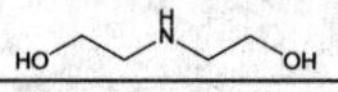
edamine	ethane-1,2-diamine or ethylenediamine 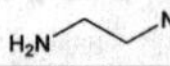
edetate (formerly edathamil)	ethylenediaminetetraacetate, and all anions derived from edetic acid (EDTA) 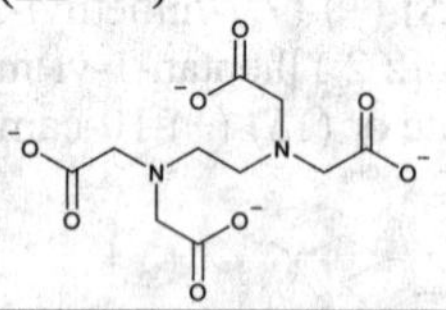
edisylate	1,2-ethanedisulfonate 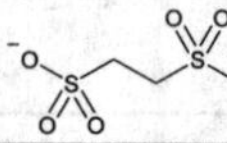
enanthate INN: enantate	heptanoate 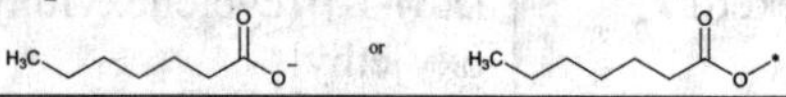
epolamine	2-(pyrrolidin-1-yl)ethanol 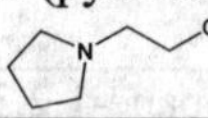
erbumine	*tert*-butylamine 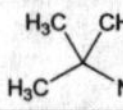
estolate	propionate ester and dodecyl sulfate salt 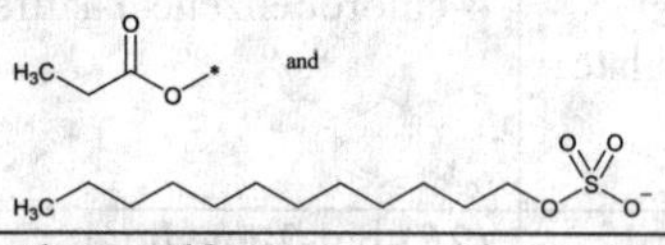
esylate INN: esilate	ethanesulfonate 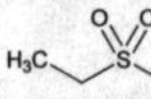
etabonate	ethyl carbonate 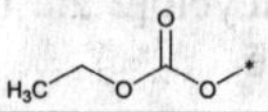
ethylsulfate INN: etilsulfate	ethyl sulfate 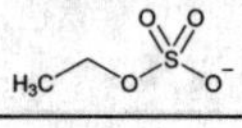

Name Used	Chemical Name and/or Formula
fostedate	tetradecyl hydrogen phosphate 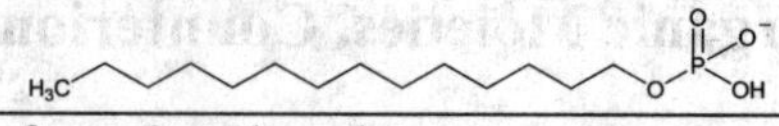
furoate	furan-2-carboxylate 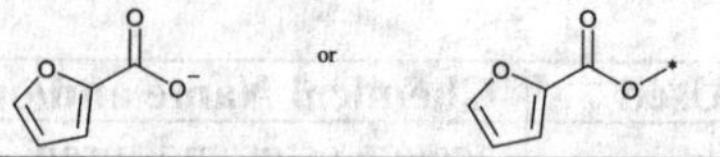
glargine	21^A-glycine-30^{B}α-L-arginine-30^{B}β-L-arginine —Gly— and —Arg—Arg
gluceptate	D-*glycero*-D-*gulo*-heptanoate 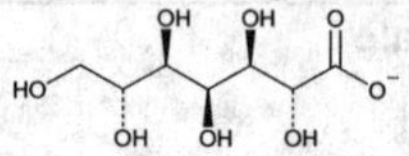
gluconate	(2*R*,3*S*,4*R*,5*R*)-2,3,4,5,6-pentahydroxyhexanoate 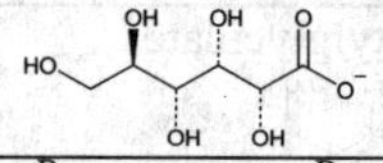
glulisine	3^B-L-lysine,29 ^{B}-L-glutamic acid —Lys— and —Glu—
hemisuccinate	3-carboxypropanoate 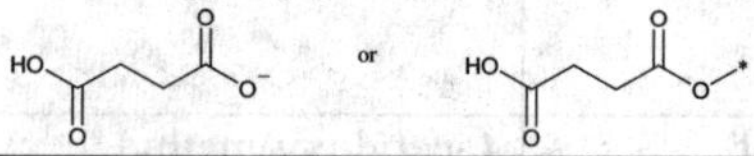
hexacetonide	3,3-dimethylbutyrate ester and acetonide 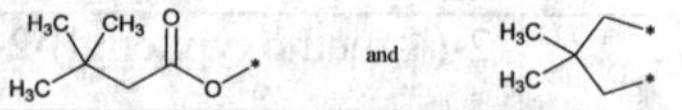
hybenzate INN: hibenzate	2-(4-hydroxylbenzoyl)benzoate 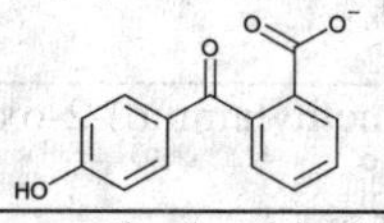
hyclate	monohydrochloride, hemiethanolate, and hemihydrate HCl · ½ C$_2$H$_5$OH · ½ H$_2$O
hydrochloride	hydrochloric acid HCl
hydroxide	OH$^-$
iodide	I$^-$
isethionate INN: isetionate	2-hydroxyethane-1-sulfonate 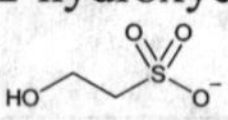
isoproxil	isopropoxycarbonyloxymethyl 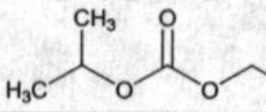
lactate	2-hydroxypropanoate 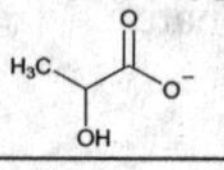

Name Used	Chemical Name and/or Formula
laurate	dodecanoate 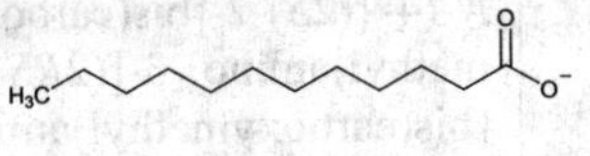 or 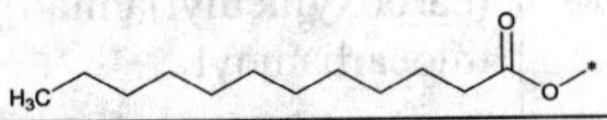
lispro	28^{B}-L-lysine-29^{B}-L-proline —Lys—Pro
medoxomil	(5-methyl-2-oxo-1,3-dioxol-4-yl)methyl 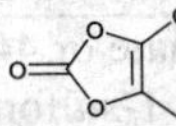
meglumine	*N*-methylglucamine 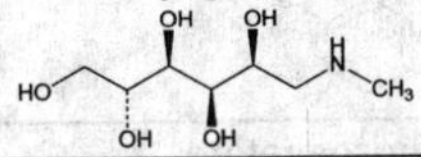
merpentan	4,5-bis(2-mercaptoacetamido)valeric acid and anions derived from this acid 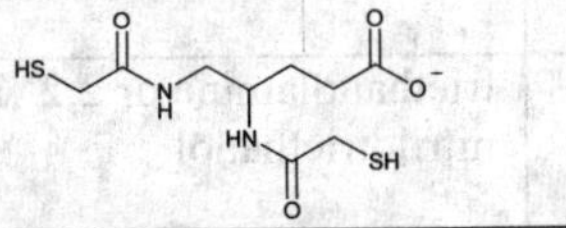
mertansine	tetrakis{(4*RS*)-4[(3-{[(1*S*)-2-{[(1*S*,2*R*,3*S*,5*S*,6*S*,16*E*,18*E*,20*R*,21*S*)-11-chloro-21-hydroxy-12,20-dimethoxy-2,5,9,16-tetramethyl-8,23-dioxo-4,24-dioxa-9,22-diazatetracyclo[19.3.1.110,14.03,5]-hexacosa-10,12,14(26),16,18-pentaen-6-yl]oxy}1-methyl-2-oxoethyl]methylamino}-3-oxopropyl)disulfanyl]pentanoyl} 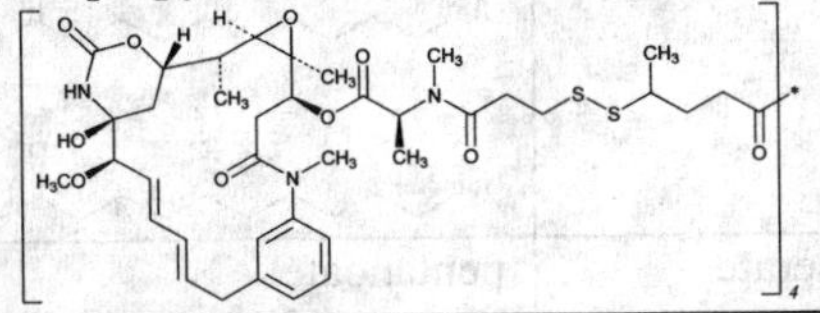
mesylate INN: mesilate	methanesulfonate 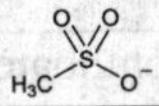
mofetil	2-(4-morpholin-4-yl)ethyl 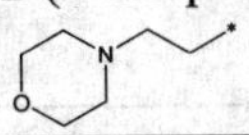
napsylate INN: napsilate	2-naphthalenesulfonate 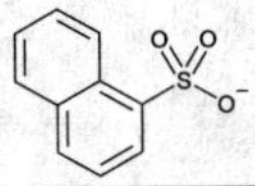
nicotinate	pyridine-3-carboxylate 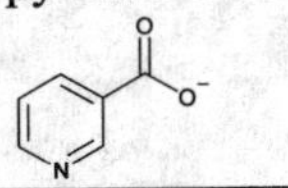 or 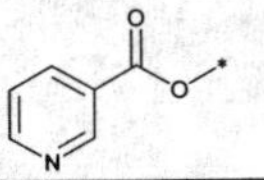
nitrate	nitric acid or nitrate salt HNO_3 or NO_3^-
olamine	ethanolamine or 2-aminoethanol 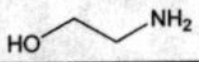
oleate	(9*Z*)-octadec-9-enoate 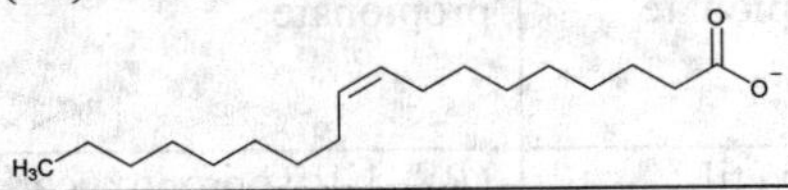
palmitate	hexadecanoate 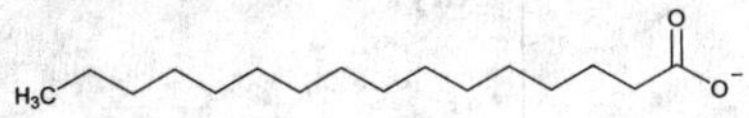 or 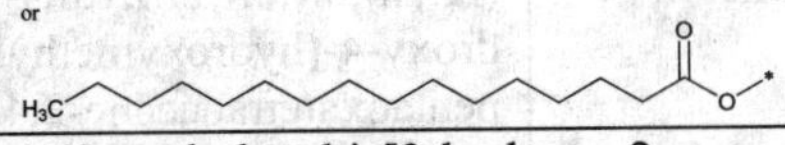
pamoate INN: embonate	4,4'-methylenebis[3-hydroxy-2-naphthoate] 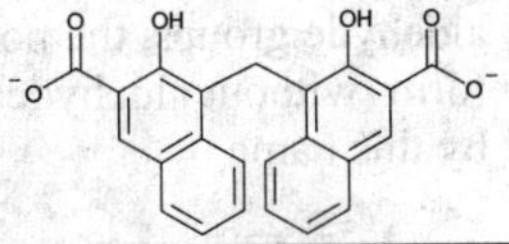
pegol	α-(2-carboxyethyl)-ω-methoxypoly(oxyethane-1,2-diyl) 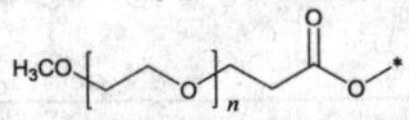
pendetide	N^6-[*N*-[2-[[2-[bis(carboxymethyl)-amino]ethyl] (carboxymethyl)amino]-ethyl]-*N*-(carboxymethyl)glycyl]-N^2-(*N*-glycyl-L-tyrosyl)-L-lysine 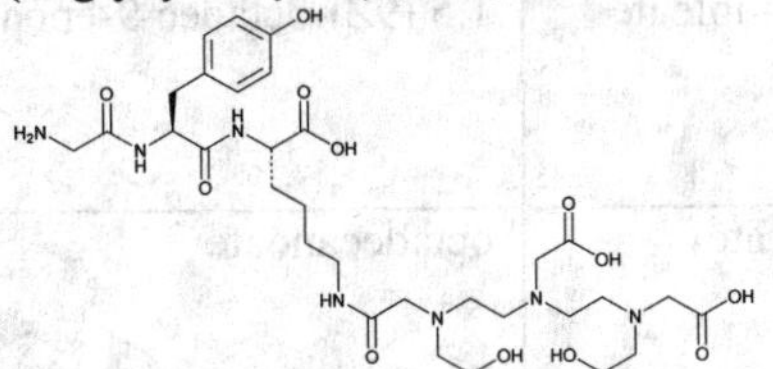
perchlorate	perchloric acid or perchlorate salt $HClO_4$, ClO_4^-
peroxide	H_2O_2
phenpropionate	3-phenylpropionate 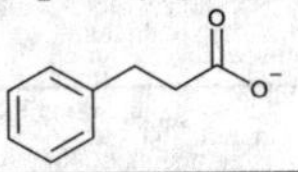 or 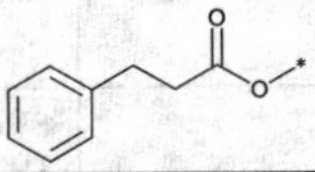
phosphate	phosphoric acid and salts derived from phosphoric acid H_3PO_4, $H_2PO_4^-$, HPO_4^{2-} or PO_4^{3-}
pivalate	pivalate or trimethylacetate 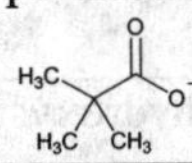 or 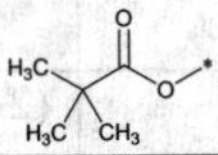
pivoxetil	1-[(2-methoxy-2-methylpropionyl)-oxy]ethyl 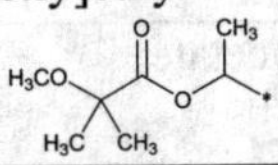
potassium	K^+
probutate INN: buteprate	propionate ester and butyrate ester 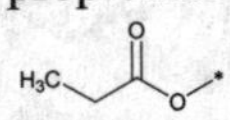 and 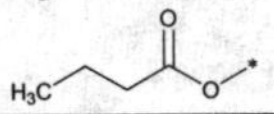

Name Used	Chemical Name and/or Formula
propionate	propionate 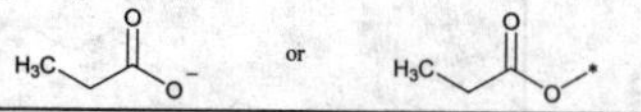
proxetil	(*RS*)-1-[(isopropoxycarbonyl)oxy]-ethyl 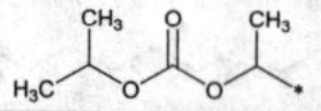
raffimer	(2*R*,4*S*,6*R*,8*R*,11*S*,13*R*)-1,14-dihydroxy-4-(hydroxymethyl)-3,5,7,10,12-pentaoxatetradecane-2,4,6,8,11,13-hexacarbaldehyde, a cross-linking agent (i.e., hemoglobin raffimer) that polymerizes with reaction at the aldehyde groups, the polymerized form (without aldehydes) is also called by this name 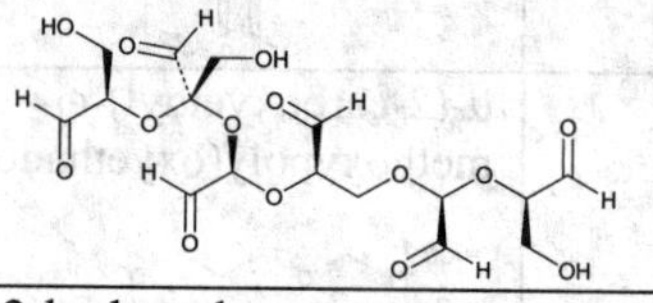
salicylate	2-hydroxybenzoate 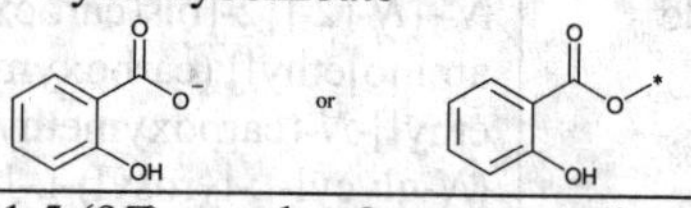
sesquioleate	1.5 (9*Z*)-octadec-9-enoate sodium 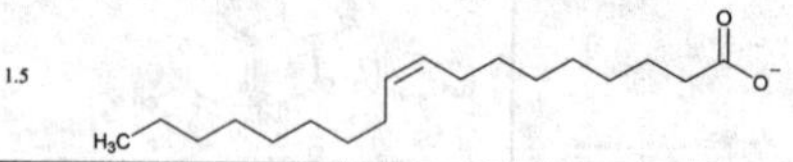
stearate	octadecanoate 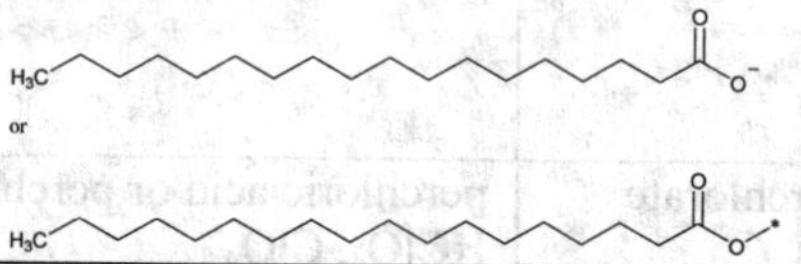
succinate	succinate 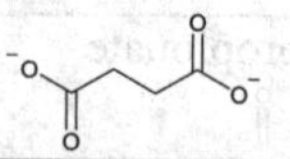
sulfate	sulfate SO_4^{2-}
suleptanate	sodium 7-methyl[(2-sulfoethyl)carbamoyl]heptanoyl 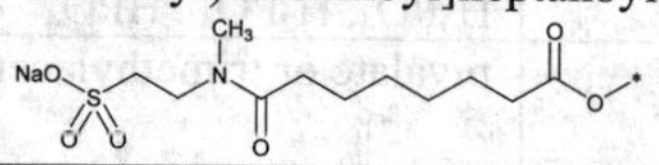
tartrate	(2*R*,3*R*)-2,3-dihydroxysuccinate 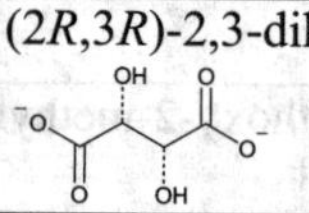
tebutate	*tert*-butylacetate 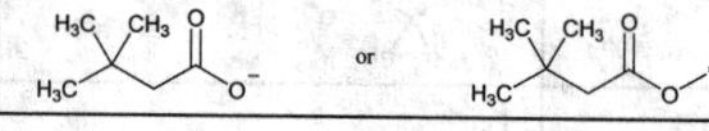

Name Used	Chemical Name and/or Formula
tiuxetan	*N*-(4-{(2*S*)-2-[bis(carboxymethyl)amino]-3-[(2*RS*)-{2-[bis(carboxymethyl)amino]propyl}-(carboxymethyl)amino]propyl}phenyl)thiocarbamoyl 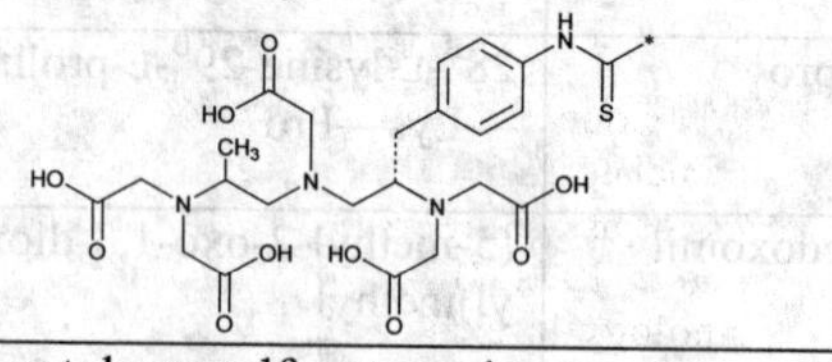
tosylate INN: tosilate	*p*-toluenesulfonate or 4-methylbenzene-1-sulfonate 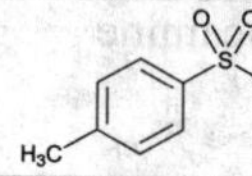
triflutate	trifluoroacetate 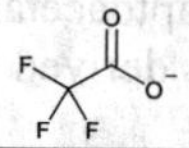
trolamine	triethanolamine or 2,2',2''-nitrilotriethanol 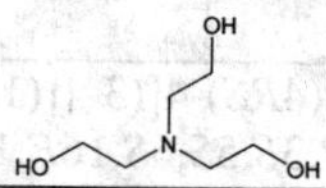
undecylate	undecanoate 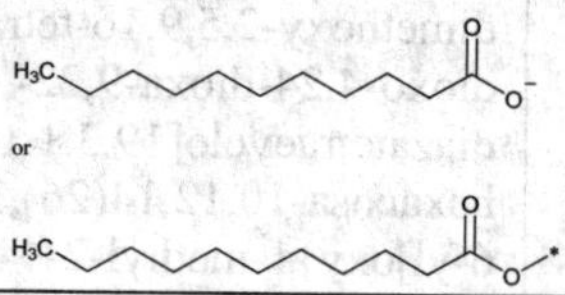
undecylenate	undec-10-enoate 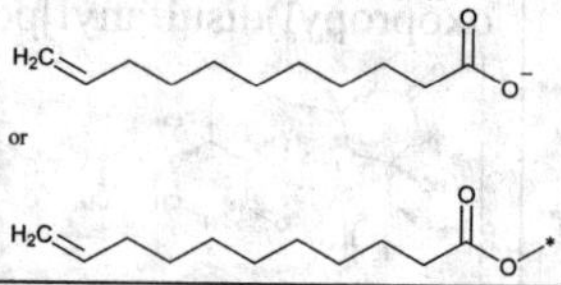
valerate	pentanoate 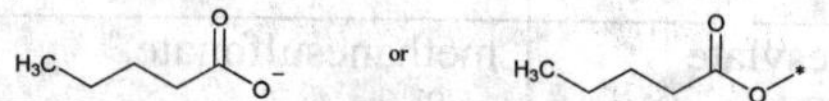
xinafoate	1-hydroxy-2-naphthoate 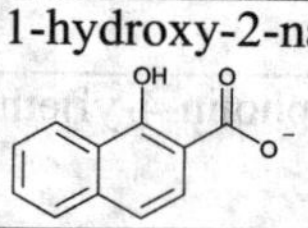

Appendix VIII

Guiding Principles for Coining United States Adopted Names for Contact Lens Materials

The USAN Council began its involvement in the area of polymer nomenclature in 1971 and formulated the first nomenclature rules for assigning nonproprietary names to contact lens materials in 1972. Based on available information on polymer technology in existence at that time as well as information from the U.S. Food and Drug Administration (FDA), lens polymers were divided into the *filcon* (hydrophilic) and the *focon* (hydrophobic) series.

The following nomenclature rules, approved by the USAN Council in 1994, represent several expansions and revisions of the initial guidelines.

General Rules

1. For nomenclature purposes, contact lens materials are divided into hydrophilic and hydrophobic groups, depending on their water content. The hydrophilic lens materials with water content equal to or more than 10 percent (10%) by weight at ambient temperature ($23 \pm 2°$ C) are assigned "-filcon" names; "-focon" names are assigned to hydrophobic lens materials with water content less than 10 percent (10%).

2. In addition to water content, nomenclature for contact lens materials depends primarily on the polymeric composition, i.e., the repeating monomer units comprising the lens material. These repeating units include linear monomers, and crosslinking entrapped color additives or ultraviolet absorbers are excluded in establishing the polymeric composition of the contact lens material for nomenclature purposes.

3. The first member of a series is assigned a unique nonproprietary name containing the proper *-filcon* or *-focon* suffix stem. A separate capital letter "A" is added after each parent designation. Subsequent designations for polymers consisting of identical monomers receive the same parent name but a different appended letter (B, C, D, etc.). These letters are needed to differentiate between polymers of identical monomeric units but with different ratios of units that have different physiochemical properties, as determined by water content, oxygen permeability [Dk] value, specific gravity, refractive index, surface charge, wetting angle, elasticity, and toughness of the lens.

4. A contact lens material having the same repeating monomeric units as a named substance but made by a different manufacturing process (e.g., lathe-cut versus cast-molded) is not required to obtain a new USAN if the lens material has the same water content and oxygen permeability as the initially named polymer.

5. The addition of a surface treatment to an existing lens material that has been assigned a USAN does not require a new USAN.

   a. A new USAN will not be assigned to contact lens materials containing chemically bound or physically entrapped color additives. The USAN Council defers to FDA labeling rules to identify color additives used to make tinted lenses.

   b. A new USAN will not be assigned to contact lens materials containing either chemically bound or physically entrapped ultraviolet absorbers. The USAN Council defers to FDA labeling rules to identify UV absorber used to make these lenses.

   ô

6. A revision of the guiding principles regarding the publication timeframe of USAN for contact lens materials was approved by the USAN Council at their February 10, 2003, meeting. Therefore, information on USAN for contact lens materials will not be published until after the manufacturer files a Premarket Approval Application (PMA) with the FDA Center for Devices and Radiological Health (CDRH) and this notice appears in the database.

7. Contact lens materials are not assigned nonproprietary names by the World Health Organization (WHO) International Nonproprietary Names (INN) Committee. Names for contact lens polymers have USAN status only.

USAN Assigned to Hydrophilic Contact Lens Materials

USAN	Year Approved	Manufacturer	Trademark
abafilcon A	1995	Pilkington Barnes Hind	
acofilcon A	2002	Contamac, Ltd.	Contaflex GM3 58%
acofilcon B	2002	Contamac, Ltd.	
acquafilcon A	2002	Vistakon, Division of Johnson & Johnson Vision Products	
alofilcon A	1979	Parke-Davis	
alphafilcon A	1993	Bausch & Lomb, Inc.	
amfilcon A (reclassified to ocufilcon series)	1985	Applied Optics	
astifilcon A	1985	Toray Industries, Inc. (Japan)	Breath-O
atlafilcon A	1989	Ciba Vision	Excellens
balafilcon A	1994	Bausch & Lomb	
bisfilcon A	1996	Vistakon	
bufilcon A	1977	Soft Lenses	Hydrocurve II; Sportmate
		Pilkington Barnes-Hind	Softmate Custom-Eyes
		CTL, Inc.	Custom Eyes-45L; Softmate I
comfilcon A	2005	CooperVision	
crofilcon A	1974	Pilkington Barnes-Hind	CSI; Orion; Azteh; CSI Colors
cyclofilcon A	1979	Burton, Parsons	
darfilcon A	1984	Pilkington Barnes-Hind	
deltafilcon A	1978	Alcon	
		Aquarius	Aqua-Soft
		Lombart Lens Ltd.	Amsoft
		Medicornea	Softflow
		Custom Contact Lenses	Custo-Flex
		Custom Contact Lenses	Tri Pol 43
		Advanced Soft Optics	Softics
		Metrosoft	Metrosoft
		Contact Lens Corp. of America	Softnet
deltafilcon B	1985	Lombart Lens Ltd.	Amsof; Amsof-Thin; Aquasight; Aquasight-Thin
dimefilcon A	1975		Geflex
droxifilcon A	1977	Accugel Labs	Accugel
elastofilcon A	1980	Bausch & Lomb	B & L Silsoft
epsifilcon A	1997	CooperVision, Inc.	
esterifilcon A	1982		
etafilcon A	1977	Vistakon	Acuvue; Hydromarc; Vistamark; Euvilens
		Bausch & Lomb	B & L 58
focofilcon A	1985	Optech	Fre-Flex
galyfilcon A	2002	Vistakon, Division of Johnson & Johnson Vision Products	
genfilcon A	1996	Vistakon	
govafilcon A	1991	Menicon (Japan)	
hefilcon A	1974	Soft Lenses, Inc.	Hydrocurve
		Bausch & Lomb	Naturvue
		Benz Research	Benz 42
		Flexlens	Flexlens
		University Optical Prod.	Alges
		Unilens Corp.	Unilens
		Western Contact Lens	Technicon-45 Soft
hefilcon B	1979	Bausch & Lomb	Miracon
		Softside	Softside
hefilcon C	1989	Bausch & Lomb	Bausch & Lomb Toric
hilafilcon A	1997	Bausch & Lomb	Award
hilafilcon B	1999	Bausch & Lomb	Award
hioxifilcon A	1995	Benz Research	Benz 55G
hioxifilcon B	1995	Benz Research	Benz-G45
hioxifilcon C	2003	Benz Research	Benz-G® 10X
hydrofilcon A	1979	Parke-Davis	
lenefilcon A	1998	Vistakon	
licryfilcon A	1981		
licryfilcon B	1981		

USAN	Year Approved	Manufacturer	Trademark
lidofilcon A	1977	Bausch & Lomb	B & L 70; FW Toric
		N & N Contact Lens	N & N 70
		Vision Tech, Inc.	VT 70
		Cooper Vision	CV 70
		CTL, Inc.	Custom Eyes-70L
		Lombart Lenses, Ltd.	Genesis-4; LL-70
		Product Dev. Consortium	IC-70
		Allergan Optical	Hydron X-70; M-70; Omniflex Sofblue
lidofilcon B	1977	Bausch & Lomb	CW 79
		N & N Contact Lens	N & N PW
		CTL, Inc.	Custom Eyes-79L
		Vision Tech, Inc.	Sauflon PW: VT-79; Genesis-79
		Kontur Kontact Lenses	Kontur Soft
		Coast Contact Lens, Inc.	Hydrosoft Colors; Hydrosoft XW; Hydrosoft; Hydrosoft EZC
lotrafilcon A	1996	CIBA Vision	
lotrafilcon B	2000	CIBA Vision	
mafilcon A	1977	N & N Contact Lens	N & N Menicon
mesifilcon A	1980		
methafilcon B	1990	CoastVision	Hydrosoft
mipafilcon A	1993	Menicon Co., Ltd (Japan)	
nelfilcon A	1996	CIBA Vision	
netrafilcon A	1990	Pilkington Barnes-Hind	Signature
ocufilcon A	1977	N & N Contact Lens	Tresoft
ocufilcon B	1978	Ocu-Ease Optical	Ocu-Flex 53; VT-53; Am Flex II
		Unilens Corp.	Unilens 53
		GBF Contact Lenses, Inc.	GBF Sherex; GBF Torex
ocufilcon C	1981	N & N Contact Lens	Soft Touch
		Optical Plastic Research	O.P.R.-55
		United Contact Lens	UCL-55
ocufilcon D	1989	Allergan Optical	Hydron
ocufilcon E	1990	Ocu-Ease Optical	Ocu-Flex 65
ofilcon A	1984	Wesley-Jessen	Dursoft 4
omafilcon A	1995	Biocompatibles International, Inc.	Proclear
oxyfilcon A	1981		
pentafilcon A	1983	Lombart Lens Ltd.	E-40; E-50; E-60
perfilcon A	1978	CooperVision	Permalens
pevafilcon A	1984	3 M	
phemfilcon A	1977	Wesley-Jessen	Durasoft; Durasoft 2; Durasoft 2 Colors; Durasoft 2 Lite Tint
polymacon	1971	Bausch & Lomb	Softlens; Sofspin; Softlens Optima 38; Natureltint; Sofscreen; SeeQuence; PA-1; Bi-Tech; Custom Eyes-38
		Allergan Optical	Hydron; Omega; NuView; SoftView; Acclaim; Zero 4; Zero 6
		Ocular Sciences/American Hydron	Zero 4; Zero 4F; Sofblue/Softint; Edge III; Proactive; Ultraflex; Smart Choice; Echelon Bifocal; Custom Toric; CQ4
		Capital Contact Lenses	PCD
		GBF Contacts Lenses	ABA-11; V/X
		CooperVision	Cooper 38; Mystique; CopperThin
		Salvatori Ophthalmics	Soft-Form II
		Metro Optics	Metrosoft II; Metrotint; Metrolite
		Pilkington Barnes-Hind	Custom Eyes-38; CTL-M; CTL-Lite; Natural Touch
		Ideal Optics	Ideal Soft PS; PS-45
		Vision-Ease Contact Lens	VE Soft
		Product Dev. Corp.	PDC
		Epcon Labs	Epcon Soft
		Lombart Lens Ltd.	LL-38
		Westcon Contact Lens	Horizon 38; Westhin Toric
		Contact Lens Corp. of America	Softact II; Fulfocus
		Fashion	Cellusoft

USAN	Year Approved	Manufacturer	Trademark
senofilcon A	2003	Vistakon, Division of Johnson & Johnson Vision Care, Inc.	
silafilcon A	1978	Bausch & Lomb	Silicon
siloxyfilcon A	1994	Permeable Technologies	LifeStyle MultiSoft
surfilcon A	1985	CooperVision	Permaflex Naturals 74
tefilcon A	1981	Ciba Vision	CibaThin; CibaSoft; ToriSoft; Softint; Bisoft; Opaque
		Vision Tech	VT-38
tetrafilcon A	1976	Ciba Vision	Aosoft
		CooperVision	Permathin; CV Classic; Permaflex Thin 43
		UCO Optical	Aquaflex
		CTL, Inc.	Customer Eyes-42L; CTL-M Tinted
		Wesley-Jessen	Aquaflex LiteTint; Aquaflex
trifilcon A	1982	Bausch & Lomb	
vifilcon A	1974	Ciba Vision	Softcon; Spectrum; NewVue; Softcolors; Focus Vistint
vifilcon B	1987		
xylofilcon A	1986	Igel Optics	Igel 67
		Salvatori Ophthalmics	PDC Sof-Form 67
		Advanced Optical	Softics
		Contact Lens Corp. of America	Softact II; Fulfocus
		Pilkington Barnes-Hind	Custom Eyes S ET-3; Custom Eyes S ET-4

USAN Assigned to Hydrophobic Contact Lens Materials

USAN	Year Approved	Manufacturer	Trademark
amefocon A	1983	Bausch & Lomb	B & L RGP
amsilfocon A	1989	Bentec Engineering, Inc.	Trans-Aire; Bis 56
aquilafocon A	2004	CibaVision	
arfocon A	1984	Wesley-Jessen	Airlens
cabufocon A	1976	Danker Labs	Meso
cabufocon B	1979		
carbosilfocon A	1997	Specialty UltraVision	UltraConEpiCon
crilfocon A	1996	G.T. Laboratories	Sil-O-Flex IV
crilfocon B	1996	G.T. Laboratories	Sil-O-Flex II
dimefocon A	1979	Danker Labs	Sila Rx
		Pilkington Barnes-Hind	Dansel
enflufocon A	1994	Polymer Technology Corp.	Boston® 7/30
enflofocon B	1997	Polymer Technology	
erifocon A	1987	Paragon Vision Sciences	
flurofocon A	1983	Ocular Sciences/American Hydron	Advent
flusilfocon A	1989	G.T. Labs	Fluorex 700
flusilfocon B	1989	G.T. Labs	Fluorex 500
flusilfocon C	1989	G.T. Labs	Fluorex 300
flusilfocon D	1989	G.T. Labs	Fluorex 800
flusilfocon E	1996	G.T. Labs	Fluorex 600
hexafocon A	1997	Wilmington Partners L.P. Polymer Technology Div.	Quantum II
itabisfluorofocon A	1997	Wilmington Partners L.P. Polymer Technology Div.	Boston RXD
itafluorofocon A	1997	Wilmington Partners L.P. Polymer Technology Div.	Boston Equalens
itafocon A	1983	Wilmington Partners L.P. Polymer Technology Div.	Boston II
		Bausch & Lomb	B & L GP 26
		UCO Optics	Aquaflex HGP
itafocon B	1985	Wilmington Partners L.P. Polymer Technology Div.	Boston IV
kolfocon A	1989	Paragon Vision Sciences	Optacryl 60
		Innovative Optics, Inc.	I.O.-18
		Vista Optics, Ltd.	Vista Optics; Optacryl 18

USAN	Year Approved	Manufacturer	Trademark
kolfocon B	1989	Paragon Vision Sciences	Optacryl K; Uvasorb-K
		Innovative Optics, Inc.	I.O.-32
		Vista Optics, Ltd.	Vista Optics; Optacryl 32
kolfocon C	1989	Paragon Vision Sciences	Optacryl Extra
kolfocon D	1989	Paragon Vision Sciences	Optacryl Z
lotifocon A	1992	Stellar Contact Lens, Inc.	OP-3
lotifocon B	1994	Stellar Contact Lens, Inc.	OP-2
lotifocon C	1994	Stellar Contact Lens, Inc.	OP-6
melafocon A	1988	Menicon (Japan)	Menicon SF-P
migafocon A	2002	Paragon Vision Sciences	
nefocon A	1985	Oculus Contact Lens Co.	Ocusil
nefocon B	1987	Neefe Optical Supply	Opti-Perm
nefocon C	1987	Eagle Plastics Intl.	Trans Aire
onsifocon A	2001	The Lagado Corporation	
oprifocon A	1997	Polymer Technology	Boston Equalens II
oxyflufocon A	1989	Ideal Optics, Inc.	O → Perm F60
paflufocon A	1987	Paragon Vision Sciences	Fluoroperm 92
paflufocon B	1987	Paragon Vision Sciences	Fluoroperm 60
paflufocon C	1987	Paragon Vision Sciences	Fluoroperm 30
paflufocon D	1990	Paragon Vision Sciences	Fluoroperm 151
paflufocon E	1998	Paragon Vision Sciences	PVS Basics
paflufocon F	2001	Paragon Vision Sciences	
pasifocon A	1985	Paragon Vision Sciences	Paraperm O_2
		Con-Cise Contact Lens Co.	Oxyflow 39
pasifocon B	1985	Paragon Vision Sciences	Paraperm II
pasifocon C	1985	Paragon Vision Sciences	Paraperm EW
pasifocon D	1985	Paragon Vision Sciences	Paraperm III
pasifocon E	1985	Paragon Vision Sciences	Paraperm IV
pemufocon A	1994	Innovision, Inc.	AccuCon
porofocon A	1977	Rynco Scientific Corp.	RX-56
porofocon B	1977	Soft Lenses	Cabcurve
roflufocon A	2004	Contamac Ltd.	Contaperm
roflufocon B	2004	Contamac Ltd.	Contaperm
roflufocon C	2004	Contamac Ltd.	Contaperm
roflufocon D	2004	Contamac Ltd.	Contaperm
roflufocon E	2004	Contamac Ltd.	Contaperm
rosilfocon A	1990	Ocutec Corp.	Novalens
satafocon A	1994	Polymer Technology Corp.	Boston VII
siflufocon A	1987	Bausch & Lomb	
silafocon A	1978	Pilkington Barnes-Hind	Polycon II; Polycon HDK; Diffrax
sterafocon A	1995	Optical Polymer Research	O → PERM30
sulfocon A	1990	Progressive Optical Research (Canada)	The Alberta Lens "S"
sulfocon B	2001	Progressive Optical Research, Ltd.	The Alberta Lens™ SM2
telafocon A	1984	Permeable Technologies	SGP Lens
tisilfocon A	1991	Menicon (Japan)	
tolofocon A	1986	Toyo (Japan)	
trifocon A	1986	Permeable Technologies	PCL II Lens
unifocon A	1990	Permeable Technologies	SGP 3
vinafocon A	1983		
wilofocon A	1995	Futuristic Drug Designs	Flosi

Appendix IX
USAN Submission Forms

The application forms on the next pages may be photocopied and submitted as part of a new negotiation. An editable version of the USAN application form is available as a MS-Word document at the USAN Program website, www.ama-assn.org/go/usan.

An official USAN application must be used for the purpose of applying for a USAN, and forwarded to the American Medical Association/United States Adopted Names (USAN) Council at the address below.

American Medical Association
Attn: USAN Program
515 North State Street
Chicago, IL 60610

Send a check payable to the American Medical Association/USAN for the appropriate amount and send to the following address:

American Medical Association
Attn: Remittance
515 North State Street
Chicago, IL 60610

Please make sure to reference that the payment is for a USAN application. Electronic credit card payments cannot be accepted at this time; however, electronic fund transfers are possible. Please call 312-464-4906 for details.

Form A
USAN Application for Single Entity Drug and Salt Form
UNITED STATES ADOPTED NAMES COUNCIL
AMERICAN MEDICAL ASSOCIATION
515 N. STATE ST.
CHICAGO, IL 60610
312-464-4046

**REQUEST FOR A UNITED STATES
ADOPTED NAME (USAN) FOR A SINGLE
ENTITY DRUG AND USAN MODIFIED**

(for USAN staff use only)

File No. (Single Entity):   Acknowledged:
File No. (Modified):   WHO No.:
INN Status:

SUGGESTED NAME(S) IN ORDER OF PREFERENCE FOR SINGLE ENTITY:
(Please attach verification of the absence of conflicts with existing chemical names,
insecticides, other nonproprietary names or trademarks)

1.
2.
3.

DESIGNATION FOR SALT FORM (e.g. hydrochloride, sodium, etc.)

CHEMICAL NAME(S) OR DESCRIPTION FOR SINGLE ENTITY:
(Chemical Abstracts Service Index Name must be supplied)

CHEMICAL NAME(S) OR DESCRIPTION FOR SALT FORM:
(Chemical Abstracts Service Index Name must be supplied)

STRUCTURAL FORMULA FOR SINGLE ENTITY:
(Provide stereochemistry)

STRUCTURAL FORMULA FOR SALT FORM:
(Provide stereochemistry)

MOLECULAR FORMULA FOR SINGLE ENTITY:

MOLECULAR FORMULA FOR SALT FORM:

MOLECULAR WEIGHT FOR SINGLE ENTITY:

MOLECULAR WEIGHT FOR SALT FORM:

CHEMICAL ABSTRACTS SERVICE (CAS) REGISTRY NUMBER FOR SINGLE ENTITY:
(CAS Registry number must be supplied)

CHEMICAL ABSTRACTS SERVICE (CAS) REGISTRY NUMBER FOR SALT FORM:

(CAS Registry number must be supplied)

CODE DESIGNATION(S) FOR SINGLE ENTITY:

CODE DESIGNATION(S) FOR SALT FORM:

TRADEMARK(S):

TRIVIAL NAME(S):

MANUFACTURER(S):

PRINCIPAL THERAPEUTIC USE(S):

PHARMACOLOGIC ACTION:

1. **The process of selecting a USAN should be initiated during that period of investigation when the compound is undergoing clinical studies.**

Please indicate the date clinical trials began:

IND Application Number(s):

2. **The undersigned confirms that the CAS registry numbers and Index names are correct. Permission is granted to USAN to utilize this information in USAN-generated publications.**

3. **Permission is granted for the USAN Council Secretariat to secure the International Union of Pure and Applied Chemistry (IUPAC) chemical names for the compounds submitted.**

4. **Permission is granted for the USAN Council Secretariat to submit the negotiated nonproprietary name to the World Health Organization (WHO) Nomenclature Committee for consideration. A fee of $6,000.00 assessed by the WHO is payable by check to the WHO; payment will be made when the name is forwarded to WHO for consideration. If the name is already an International Nonproprietary Name (INN), permission is granted to forward it to WHO as a matter of information.**

5. **This submission is made with the understanding that insofar as is known, none of the suggested names are trademarked or the subject of pending registration. It is further understood that the adopted USAN will remain free and unrestricted nonproprietary names that will not be trademarked.**

6. **This submission is made with the understanding that names submitted to the USAN Council for this compound will be posted on the USAN Web site as "names under consideration."**

7. **The undersigned understands and acknowledges that because "names under consideration" as well as adoption statements are published on the USAN Web site, there is a possibility that unaffiliated third parties might register a name as an Internet domain without the prior knowledge of the USAN Progam. The undersigned waives all liability of USAN if this is to occur.**

8. **When naming biologics please take note of the following reminders:**

    a. **The complete amino acid sequence is required for proteins, peptides or antibodies, or the nucleotide sequence for oligonucleotides, in a MS Word document.**
    b. **For a glycoprotein/glycopeptide, the glycosylation pattern including the sites of glycosylation, type of sugars, etc.**
    c. **Please supply CDR-IMGT and FR-IMGT; the origin of each chain; sites of disulfide-bridges; Ig-subclass; name/structure of the antigen against which the monoclonal antibody is directed.**

       d.   **Include expression system and comparison with the native sequence.**

9. **Please enclose $15,000 as the appropriate fee-for-service for names for a single entity drug and salt form.**

10. **Make check payable to American Medical Association/USAN. Please call 312-464-4046 to request information on an electronic fund transfer.   If check is not enclosed or is to be sent separately, please send to the following address:**

American Medical Association
Attn: Remittance
515 N. State St.
Chicago, IL 60610

Please make sure to note that payment is for a USAN application and include code designations or other relevant reference information.

Submitted by:

Applicant: (Name of firm, sponsor or legal representative)

Address:

Telephone:

Fax:

Name of Contact Person:

Title:

Email Address:

Signature:

Date:

Form B
USAN Application for Single Entity Drug
UNITED STATES ADOPTED NAMES COUNCIL
AMERICAN MEDICAL ASSOCIATION
515 N. STATE ST.
CHICAGO, IL 60610
312-464-4046

**REQUEST FOR A UNITED STATES
ADOPTED NAME (USAN) FOR A SINGLE
ENTITY DRUG**

(for USAN staff use only)

File No. (Single Entity):   Acknowledged:
INN Status: WHO No.:

SUGGESTED NAME(S) IN ORDER OF PREFERENCE:
(Please attach verification of the absence of conflicts with existing chemical names,
insecticides, other nonproprietary names or trademarks)

1.

2.

3.

CHEMICAL NAME(S) OR DESCRIPTION:
(Chemical Abstracts Service Index Name must be supplied)

STRUCTURAL FORMULA:
(Provide stereochemistry)

MOLECULAR FORMULA:

MOLECULAR WEIGHT:

CHEMICAL ABSTRACTS SERVICE (CAS) REGISTRY NUMBER:
(CAS Registry number must be supplied)

CODE DESIGNATION(S):

TRADEMARK(S):

TRIVIAL NAME(S):

MANUFACTURER(S):

PRINCIPAL THERAPEUTIC USE(S):

PHARMACOLOGIC ACTION:

1. The process of selecting a USAN should be initiated during that period of
    investigation when the compound is undergoing clinical studies.

    Please indicate the date clinical trials began:

    IND Application Number(s):

2. The undersigned confirms that the CAS registry numbers and Index names
    are correct. Permission is granted to USAN to utilize this information in
    USAN-generated publications.

3. Permission is granted for the USAN Council Secretariat to secure the
    International Union of Pure and Applied Chemistry (IUPAC) chemical
    names for the compounds submitted.

4. Permission is granted for the USAN Council Secretariat to submit the
    negotiated nonproprietary name to the World Health Organization (WHO)
    Nomenclature Committee for consideration. A fee of $6,000.00 assessed
    by the WHO is payable by check to the WHO; payment will be made when
    the name is forwarded to WHO for consideration. If the name is already an
    International Nonproprietary Name (INN), permission is granted to forward
    it to WHO as a matter of information.

5. This submission is made with the understanding that insofar as is known,
    none of the suggested names are trademarked or the subject of pending
    registration. It is further understood that the adopted USAN will remain
    a free and unrestricted nonproprietary name that will not be trademarked.

6. This submission is made with the understanding that names submitted
    to the USAN Council for this compound will be posted on the USAN Web
    site as "names under consideration."

7. The undersigned understands and acknowledges that because "names under
    consideration" as well as adoption statements are published on the USAN Web
    site, there is a possibility that unaffiliated third parties might register a name as
    an Internet domain without the prior knowledge of the USAN Progam. The
    undersigned waives all liability of USAN if this is to occur.

8. When naming biologics please take note of the following reminders:

    a. The complete amino acid sequence is required for proteins, peptides
        or antibodies, or the nucleotide sequence for oligonucleotides, in a
        MS Word document.
    b. For a glycoprotein/glycopeptide, the glycosylation pattern including
        the sites of glycosylation, type of sugars, etc.
    c. Please supply CDR-IMGT and FR-IMGT; the origin of each chain;
        sites of disulfide-bridges; Ig-subclass; name/structure of the antigen
        against which the monoclonal antibody is directed.

    d.   Include expression system and comparison with the native sequence.

9. Please enclose $10,000 as the appropriate fee-for-service.

10. Make check payable to American Medical Association/USAN. Please call 312-464-4046 to request information on an electronic fund transfer.   If check is not enclosed or is to be sent separately, please send to the following address:

American Medical Association
Attn: Remittance
515 N. State St.
Chicago, IL 60610

Please make sure to note that payment is for a USAN application and include code designations or other relevant reference information.

Submitted by:

Applicant: (Name of firm, sponsor or legal representative)

Address:

Telephone:

Fax:

Name of Contact Person:

Title:

Email Address:

Signature:

Date:

Form C
USAN Modified Application
UNITED STATES ADOPTED NAMES COUNCIL
AMERICAN MEDICAL ASSOCIATION
515 N. STATE ST.
CHICAGO, IL 60610
312-464-4046

**REQUEST FOR A UNITED STATES
ADOPTED NAME (USAN) FOR A USAN
MODIFIED**

(for USAN staff use only)

File No: Acknowledged:
INN Status: INN No. for the base:

Use this form to request a USAN for a salt of a substance that already received a USAN.
Please attach a copy of the adoption statement for the substance that has received a
USAN, from which the substance to be named is derived (if available).

SUGGESTED NAME:
(Documentation of a trademark/linguistics search is not required, if the name is derived
from an existing USAN.)

1.

CHEMICAL NAME(S) OR DESCRIPTION:
(Chemical Abstracts Service Index name)

STRUCTURAL FORMULA:
(Provide stereochemistry, if known)

MOLECULAR FORMULA:

MOLECULAR WEIGHT:

CHEMICAL ABSTRACTS SERVICE (CAS) Registry Number:
(A separate CAS Registry Number is required for each new form of a substance)

CODE DESIGNATIONS:
(List any changes or additions to the code designations since the first USAN was adopted)

TRADEMARK(S):
(Include any trade names obtained since first USAN was adopted)

TRIVIAL NAME:
(Include any changes or additions since the first USAN was adopted)

NAME AND ADDRESS OF MANUFACTURER:

PRINCIPAL THERAPEUTIC USE(S):

1. **The process of selecting a USAN should be initiated during that period of investigation when the compound is undergoing clinical studies.**

   Please indicate the date clinical trials began:

   IND Application Number(s):

2. **The undersigned confirms that the CAS registry numbers and Index names are correct. Permission is granted to USAN to utilize this information in USAN-generated publications.**

3. Permission is granted for the USAN Council Secretariat to secure the
    International Union of Pure and Applied Chemistry (IUPAC) chemical
    names for the compounds submitted.

4. Permission is granted for the USAN Council Secretariat to forward the name
    to WHO as a matter of information.

5. This submission is made with the understanding that insofar as is known,
    none of the suggested names are trademarked or the subject of pending
    registration. It is further understood that the adopted USAN will remain
    a free and unrestricted nonproprietary name that will not be trademarked.

6. This submission is made with the understanding that names submitted
    to the USAN Council for this compound will be posted on the USAN Web
    site as "names under consideration."

7. The undersigned understands and acknowledges that because "names under
    consideration" as well as adoption statements are published on the USAN Web
    site, there is a possibility that unaffiliated third parties might register a name as
    an Internet domain without the prior knowledge of the USAN Progam. The
    undersigned waives all liability of USAN if this is to occur.

8. When naming biologics please take note of the following reminders:

    a. The complete amino acid sequence is required for proteins, peptides
        or antibodies, or the nucleotide sequence for oligonucleotides, in a
        MS Word document.
    b. For a glycoprotein/glycopeptide, the glycosylation pattern including
        the sites of glycosylation, type of sugars, etc.
    c. Please supply CDR-IMGT and FR-IMGT; the origin of each chain;
        sites of disulfide-bridges; Ig-subclass; name/structure of the antigen
        against which the monoclonal antibody is directed.
    d. Include expression system and comparison with the native
        sequence.

9. Please enclose $5,000 as the appropriate fee-for-service.

10. Make check payable to American Medical Association/USAN. Please call 312-464-
    4046 to request information on an electronic fund transfer. If check is not
    enclosed or is to be sent separately, please send to the following address:

American Medical Association
Attn: Remittance
515 N. State St.
Chicago, IL 60610

*Please make sure to note that payment is for a USAN application and
include code designations or other relevant reference information.*

Submitted by:

Applicant: (Name of firm, sponsor or legal representative)

Address:

Telephone:

Fax:

Name of Contact Person:

Title:

Email Address:

Signature:

Date:

Form D
USAN Revised Application
UNITED STATES ADOPTED NAMES COUNCIL
AMERICAN MEDICAL ASSOCIATION
515 N. STATE ST.
CHICAGO, IL 60610
312-464-4046

**REQUEST FOR A UNITED STATES
ADOPTED NAME (USAN) FOR A USAN
REVISED**

(for USAN staff use only)

File No: Acknowledged:
INN Status: WHO No.:

Use this form to request revisions to a published adoption statement. Please attach a copy of the adoption statement, if available. Please take note of the following when submitting this application:

1. For requests to change the molecular formula, molecular weight or structural formula, attach documentation of new chemical information for this compound.

2. For requests to change the CAS Registry Number, attach documentation that CAS has changed it.

3. For requests to change manufacturer or other supporting information, please provide documentation detailing these changes.

NAME FOR WHICH YOU ARE REQUESTING A REVISION:

REASON FOR REVISION:

Please describe revisions to any of the following.

CHEMICAL NAMES:

STRUCTURAL FORMULA:

MOLECULAR FORMULA:

MOLECULAR WEIGHT:

CAS REGISTRY NUMBER:

CODE DESIGNATIONS:

TRADEMARK:

MANUFACTURER:

INDICATIONS/THERAPEUTIC CLAIM:

1. The process of selecting a USAN should be initiated during that period of investigation when the compound is undergoing clinical studies.

   Please indicate the date clinical trials began:

   IND Application Number(s):

2. The undersigned confirms that the CAS registry numbers and Index names are correct. Permission is granted to USAN to utilize this information in USAN-generated publications.

3. Permission is granted for the USAN Council Secretariat to secure the
    International Union of Pure and Applied Chemistry (IUPAC) chemical
    names for the compounds submitted.

4. Permission is granted for the USAN Council Secretariat to forward
    the USAN Revised to WHO as a matter of information.

5. This submission is made with the understanding that insofar as is known,
    none of the suggested names are trademarked or the subject of pending
    registration. It is further understood that the adopted USAN will remain
    a free and unrestricted nonproprietary name that will not be trademarked.

6. The undersigned understands and acknowledges that because "names under
    consideration" as well as adoption statements are published on the USAN Web
    site, there is a possibility that unaffiliated third parties might register a name as
    an Internet domain without the prior knowledge of the USAN Progam. The
    undersigned waives all liability of USAN if this is to occur.

7. When revising biologics please take note of the following reminders:

    a.   The complete amino acid sequence is required for proteins, peptides
         or antibodies, or the nucleotide sequence for oligonucleotides, in a
         MS Word document.
    b.   For a glycoprotein/glycopeptide, the glycosylation pattern including
         the sites of glycosylation, type of sugars, etc.
    c.   Please supply CDR-IMGT and FR-IMGT; the origin of each chain;
         sites of disulfide-bridges; Ig-subclass; name/structure of the antigen
         against which the monoclonal antibody is directed.
    d.   Include expression system and comparison with the native
         sequence.

8. Please enclose $2,500 as the appropriate fee-for-service.

9. Make check payable to American Medical Association/USAN. Please call 312-464-
    4046 to request information on an electronic fund transfer.   If check is
    not enclosed or is to be sent separately, please send to the following address:

American Medical Association
Attn: Remittance
515 N. State St.
Chicago, IL 60610

*Please make sure to note that payment is for a USAN application and
include code designations or other relevant reference information.*

Submitted by:

Applicant: (Name of firm, sponsor or legal representative)

Address:

Telephone:

Fax:

Name of Contact Person:

Title:

Email Address:

Signature:

Date:

Form E
USAN Application for Contact Lens Material
UNITED STATES ADOPTED NAMES COUNCIL
AMERICAN MEDICAL ASSOCIATION
515 N. STATE ST.
CHICAGO, IL 60610
312-464-4046

**REQUEST FOR A UNITED STATES
ADOPTED NAME (USAN) FOR CONTACT
LENS MATERIAL**

(for USAN staff use only)

File No: Acknowledged:

SUGGESTED NAME(S) IN ORDER OF PREFERENCE:
Please attach verification of the absence of conflicts with existing chemical names,
insecticides, other nonproprietary names or trademarks

1.	
2.	
3.	

CHEMICAL NAME(S):
Chemical Abstracts Service Index Names for the polymer and each monomer must be
supplied. If this is a submission for a hybrid lens material, please supply information for
both the soft skirt and hard center.

STRUCTURAL FORMULAS:
Structural formulas and stereochemistry, if known, must be supplied for each monomer. If
this is a submission for a hybrid lens material, please supply information for both the soft
skirt and hard center.

MOLECULAR FORMULA:

List the formula for each monomer, and for the whole polymer. If this is a submission for a hybrid lens material, please supply information for both the soft skirt and hard center.

CHEMICAL ABSTRACTS SERVICE (CAS) Registry Number:

Separate CAS Registry Numbers must be supplied for the entire polymer and for each monomer. If this is a submission for a hybrid lens material, please supply information for both the soft skirt and hard center.

PURITY OF 2-hydroxyethyl methacrylate (if applicable):

WATER CONTENT at ambient temperature (23 ± 2°C):

[mean value ± standard deviation __________; number of measurements__________]

OXYGEN PERMEABILITY AT 35°C:

[mean value ± standard deviation __________; number of measurements__________]

METHOD USED TO DETERMINE OXYGEN PERMEABILITY:

TRADEMARK(S):

MANUFACTURER(S):

1. **The process of selecting a USAN should be initiated during that period of investigation when the compound is undergoing clinical studies.**

   Please indicate the date clinical trials began:

2. The undersigned confirms that the CAS registry numbers and Index names are correct. Permission is granted to USAN to utilize this information in USAN-generated publications.

3. Permission is granted for the USAN Council Secretariat to secure the International Union of Pure and Applied Chemistry (IUPAC) chemical names for the compounds submitted.

4. This submission is made with the understanding that insofar as is known, none of the suggested names are trademarked or the subject of pending registration. It is further understood that the adopted USAN will remain a free and unrestricted nonproprietary name that will not be trademarked.

5. This submission is made with the understanding that accepted names for contact lens materials will be posted on the USAN Web site.

6. The undersigned understands and acknowledges that because names as well as adoption statements are published on the USAN Web site, there is a possibility that unaffiliated third parties might register a name as an Internet domain without the prior knowledge of the USAN Progam. The undersigned waives all liability of USAN if this is to occur.

7. The appropriate fee-for-service is enclosed. Check one:

Name for a new contact lens material	$10,000.00
USAN modified (name for a contact lens material for which an adopted USAN already exists)	$5,000.00
USAN revised (revision of support information used to define a USAN or USAN modified, resulting in a revised adoption and/or revised publication)	$2,500.00

8. Make check payable to American Medical Association/USAN. Please call 312-464-4046 to request information on an electronic fund transfer. If check is not enclosed or is to be sent separately, please send to the following address:

American Medical Association
Attn: Remittance
515 N. State St.
Chicago, IL 60610

Please make sure to note that payment is for a USAN application and include code designations or other relevant reference information.

Submitted by:

Applicant: (Name of firm, sponsor or legal representative)

Address:

Telephone:

Fax:

Name of Contact Person:

Title:

Email Address:

Signature:

Date:

HISTORICAL NOTE

The organization responsible for the periodic revision and publication of the United States Pharmacopeia came into existence in January 1820, and was incorporated in 1900 under the name, The United States Pharmacopeial Convention. In keeping with the growth of the medical and pharmaceutical professions and over a century and a half of medical progress, the Convention has continued to draw upon the organizations that are broadly representative of the teaching and practice of these and allied professions in providing a base of authority for the Pharmacopeia.

From the outset and over the years since 1820, those physicians and pharmacists who have devoted countless hours to creating and maintaining the Pharmacopeia have been deeply concerned with the names by which drugs are commonly known. Indeed, encouraging the use of standard names for drugs has been almost as important a function of the Pharmacopeia as that of providing high standards of quality for them.

The acquisition by the USP Convention of the National Formulary, on January 2, 1975, consolidated the responsibility for the names in the USP and NF, the legally recognized compendia of standards for drugs. The standards-setting process, however, is such that the USP Council of Experts ordinarily has not entered the picture until after the drug names, both those for nonproprietary use and those protected by trademarks, have been selected and put into use.

The foundations of the United States Adopted Names (USAN) Council were established in June 1961, when the American Medical Association and the United States Pharmacopeial Convention formed the AMA-USP Nomenclature Committee. The American Pharmaceutical Association became the third sponsor in 1964. At that time, the name of the committee was changed to the United States Adopted Names Council, and "United States Adopted Name" or "USAN" was designated as the term to describe any nonproprietary name formally adopted by the council. In 1967, the U.S. Food and Drug Administration began its participation in the USAN Council through appointment of a liaison representative to the council. The FDA later strengthened this relationship by publishing in the Federal Register regulations which state in part that "Interested persons, in the absence of the designation by the Food and Drug Administration of an official name, may rely on as the established name for any drug the current compendial name or the USAN. . . ."